MANN'S SURGERY OF THE FOOT AND ANKLE

Volume 1

MANN'S SURGERY OF THE FOOT AND ANKLE

NINTH EDITION

Michael J. Coughlin, MD

Director, Saint Alphonsus Foot and Ankle Clinic, Boise, Idaho
Clinical Professor, Department of Orthopaedic Surgery
University of California, San Francisco, San Francisco, California
Past-president, American Orthopedic, Foot and Ankle Society
Past-president, International Federation of Foot and Ankle Societies

Charles L. Saltzman, MD

Chairman, Department of Orthopaedics
Louis S. Peery MD Endowed Presidential Professor, University of Utah
University Orthopaedic Center, Salt Lake City, Utah
Past-president, American Orthopaedic Foot and Ankle Society
Vice President, International Federation of Foot and Ankle Societies

Robert B. Anderson, MD

Chief, Foot and Ankle Service
Vice-chair, Department of Orthopaedic Surgery, Carolinas Medical Center
OrthoCarolina Foot and Ankle Institute, Charlotte, North Carolina
Past-president, American Orthopaedic Foot and Ankle Society

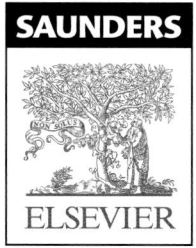

SAUNDERS

ELSEVIER

5/14
mAtt.
#405.00

ELSEVIER
SAUNDERS

1600 John F. Kennedy Blvd.
Ste 1800
Philadelphia, PA 19103-2899

MANN'S SURGERY OF THE FOOT AND ANKLE

ISBN: 978-0-323-07242-7
Volume 1 Part Number: 9996074684
Volume 2 Part Number: 9996074749

Notices

Knowledge and best practice in this field are constantly changing. As new research and experience broaden our understanding, changes in research methods, professional practices, or medical treatment may become necessary.

Practitioners and researchers must always rely on their own experience and knowledge in evaluating and using any information, methods, compounds, or experiments described herein. In using such information or methods they should be mindful of their own safety and the safety of others, including parties for whom they have a professional responsibility.

With respect to any drug or pharmaceutical products identified, readers are advised to check the most current information provided (i) on procedures featured or (ii) by the manufacturer of each product to be administered, to verify the recommended dose or formula, the method and duration of administration, and contraindications. It is the responsibility of practitioners, relying on their own experience and knowledge of their patients, to make diagnoses, to determine dosages and the best treatment for each individual patient, and to take all appropriate safety precautions.

To the fullest extent of the law, neither the Publisher nor the authors, contributors, or editors assume any liability for any injury and/or damage to persons or property as a matter of products liability, negligence or otherwise, or from any use or operation of any methods, products, instructions, or ideas contained in the material herein.

Library of Congress Cataloging-in-Publication Data
Mann's surgery of the foot and ankle / [edited by] Michael J. Coughlin, Charles Saltzman, Robert B. Anderson.—Ninth edition.
      p. ; cm.
    Surgery of the foot and ankle
    Preceded by Surgery of the foot and ankle / edited by Michael J. Coughlin, Roger A. Mann, Charles L. Salzmann. 8th ed. c2007.
    Includes bibliographical references and index.
    ISBN 978-0-323-07242-7 (set : hardcover : alk. paper)
    I. Coughlin, Michael J., editor of compilation.   II. Saltzman, Charles L., editor of compilation.   III. Anderson, Robert B. (Robert Bentley), 1957- editor of compilation.   IV. Title: Surgery of the foot and ankle.
    [DNLM: 1. Ankle—surgery. 2. Foot—surgery. 3. Ankle Injuries—surgery. 4. Foot Diseases—surgery. WE 880]
    RD563
    617.5′85059—dc23
                                                                                    2013017557

Executive Content Strategist: Dolores Meloni
Content Development Manager: Lucia Gunzel
Publishing Services Manager: Anne Altepeter
Project Manager: Cindy Thoms
Design Direction: Louis Forgione

Printed in China

Last digit is the print number: 9 8 7 6 5 4 3 2 1

ELSEVIER | Book Aid International | Working together to grow libraries in developing countries

www.elsevier.com • www.bookaid.org

To our parents—

Martha and Jim,
Abraham and Ruth,
and Dottie and Dick,

for the opportunities they presented to us;

to our wives—

Kirsten, Ingrid, and Jean,

for their support and encouragement;

and to our children—

Erin and Elizabeth;
Hanna and Erik;
and Ryan, Tyler, and Michael,

*for the happiness, enthusiasm,
and joy that they bring
to our families*

Contributors

Richard G. Alvarez, MD
Professor and Chair
Department of Orthopaedic Surgery
Director of Foot and Ankle
University of Tennessee College of Medicine
Chattanooga, Tennessee
Chapter 11: Toenail Abnormalities

John G. Anderson, MD
Associate Professor
Department of Orthopaedic Surgery
Michigan State University College of Human Medicine
Chairman, Spectrum Health Hospitals
Department of Orthopaedic Surgery
Co-Director, Grand Rapids Orthopaedic Foot and Ankle
Fellowship
Co-Director, Grand Rapids Orthopaedic Residency Program
Grand Rapids, Michigan
Chapter 37: Ankle Fractures

Robert B. Anderson, MD
Chief, Foot and Ankle Service
Vice-chair, Department of Orthopaedic Surgery
Carolinas Medical Center
OrthoCarolina Foot and Ankle Institute
Charlotte, North Carolina
Chapter 2: Principles of the Physical Examination
of the Foot and Ankle
Chapter 6: Hallux Valgus
Chapter 31: Stress Fractures of the Foot and Ankle
Chapter 40: Fractures of the Midfoot and Forefoot

Rahul Banerjee, MD
Assistant Professor
Department of Orthopaedic Surgery
University of Texas Southwestern Medical Center
Dallas, Texas
Chapter 39: Fractures and Fracture-Dislocations
of the Talus

Alexej Barg, MD
Attending Surgeon
Orthopaedic Department
University Hospital of Basel
Basel, Switzerland;
Research Fellow
Harold K. Dunn Orthopaedic Research Laboratory
University Orthopaedic Center
University of Utah
Salt Lake City, Utah
Chapter 22: Ankle Replacement

Judith F. Baumhauer, MD, MPH
Professor and Associate Chair of Academic Affairs
Department of Orthopaedic Surgery
Foot and Ankle Division
University of Rochester
Rochester, New York
Chapter 13: Plantar Heel Pain

Timothy C. Beals, MD
Associate Professor
Director of Foot and Ankle Fellowship
Department of Orthopaedics
University of Utah
Salt Lake City, Utah
Rosenberg Cooley Metcalf Clinic
Park City, Utah
Chapter 34: Congenital and Acquired Neurologic
Disorders

Douglas Beaman, MD
Summit Orthopaedics, LLP
Portland, Oregon
Chapter 23: Ring External Fixation in the
Foot and Ankle

James H. Beaty, MD
Professor of Orthopaedics
Department of Orthopaedic Surgery
University of Tennessee-Campbell Clinic
Memphis, Tennessee
Chapter 33: Congenital Foot Deformities

Alireza Behboudi, DO
Orthopaedics
East Texas Medical Center
Tyler, Texas
Chapter 37: Ankle Fractures

Gary M. Berke, MS, CP
Adjunct Clinical Assistant Professor
Department of Orthopaedic Surgery
Stanford University
Palo Alto, California
Private Practitioner
Gary M. Berke Prosthetics/Orthotics
Redwood City, California
Chapter 29: Lower Limb Prosthetics

Mark J. Berkowitz, MD
Associate Staff Orthopaedic Surgeon
Orthopaedic and Rheumatologic Institute
Cleveland Clinic Foundation
Cleveland, Ohio
Chapter 35: Dislocations of the Foot

Brad D. Blankenhorn, MD
Assistant Professor
Department of Orthopaedic Surgery
University of New Mexico
Albuquerque, New Mexico
Chapter 21: Ankle Arthritis

Donald R. Bohay, MD, FACS
Professor
Department of Orthopaedic Surgery
Michigan State University College of Human Medicine
Director, Grand Rapids Orthopaedic Foot and Ankle
Fellowship Program
Grand Rapids, Michigan
Chapter 37: Ankle Fractures

James W. Brodsky, MD
Clinical Professor of Orthopaedic Surgery
University of Texas Southwestern Medical School
Director, Foot and Ankle Surgery Fellowship Program
Baylor University Medical Center
Professor of Orthopaedic Surgery
Texas A&M University, College of Medicine
Dallas, Texas
Chapter 27: Diabetes
Chapter 28: Amputations of the Foot and Ankle

George T. Calvert, MD
Assistant Professor
Division of Orthopaedic Surgery
City of Hope National Medical Center
Duarte, California
Chapter 18: Soft Tissue and Bone Tumors

Loretta B. Chou, MD
Professor and Chief of Foot and Ankle Surgery
Department of Orthopaedic Surgery
Stanford University
Stanford, California
Chapter 4: Conservative Treatment of the Foot

Thomas O. Clanton, MD
Director, Foot and Ankle Sports Medicine
The Steadman Clinic
Vail, Colorado
Chapter 30: Athletic Injuries to the Soft Tissue of the Foot and Ankle

J. Chris Coetzee, MD
Orthopedic Foot and Ankle Surgeon
Twin Cities Orthopedics
Minneapolis, Minnesota
Chapter 20: Treatment of Hindfoot and Midfoot Arthritis

Bruce E. Cohen, MD
Assistant Residency Program Director
Department of Orthopaedic Surgery
Carolinas Medical Center;
Fellowship Director, OrthoCarolina Foot and Ankle Institute
Charlotte, North Carolina
Chapter 31: Stress Fractures of the Foot and Ankle

Michael J. Coughlin, MD
Director, Saint Alphonsus Foot and Ankle Clinic
Boise, Idaho
Clinical Professor, Department of Orthopaedic Surgery
University of California, San Francisco
San Francisco, California
Chapter 6: Hallux Valgus
Chapter 7: Lesser Toe Deformities
Chapter 9: Bunionettes
Chapter 10: Sesamoids and Accessory Bones of the Foot
Chapter 11: Toenail Abnormalities
Chapter 19: Arthritis of the Foot and Ankle
Chapter 24: Disorders of Tendons

Jennifer J. Davis, MD
Associate Professor
Department of Anesthesiology
University of Utah
Salt Lake City, Utah
Chapter 5: Anesthesia

W. Hodges Davis, MD
OrthoCarolina Foot and Ankle Institute
Charlotte, North Carolina
Chapter 2: Principles of the Physical Examination of the Foot and Ankle

Laura K. Dawson, MD
Orthopaedic Foot and Ankle Fellow
Department of Orthopaedics and Rehabilitation
University of Rochester
Rochester, New York
Chapter 13: Plantar Heel Pain

Jonathan T. Deland, MD
Chief, Foot and Ankle Service
Hospital for Special Surgery
New York, New York
Chapter 25: Pes Planus

Brian D. Dierckman, MD
Attending Surgeon
American Health Network Bone and Spine
Carmel, Indiana
Chapter 32: Arthroscopy of the Foot and Ankle

Benedict F. DiGiovanni, MD
Professor
Department of Orthopaedics and Rehabilitation
Director, Musculoskeletal Curriculum
University of Rochester
Rochester, New York
Chapter 13: Plantar Heel Pain

Matthew B. Dobbs, MD
Department of Orthopaedic Surgery
Barnes-Jewish Hospital at Washington University
School of Medicine
Saint Louis Shriners Hospital
Saint Louis, Missouri
Chapter 33: Congenital Foot Deformities

Jesse F. Doty, MD
Clinical Instructor
Department of Orthopaedic Surgery
University of Tennessee College of Medicine
Chattanooga, Tennessee
Chapter 11: Toenail Abnormalities

J. Kent Ellington, MD
OrthoCarolina Foot and Ankle Institute
Charlotte, North Carolina
Chapter 40: Fractures of the Midfoot and Forefoot

Richard D. Ferkel, MD
Assistant Clinical Professor of Orthopedic Surgery
UCLA Center for the Health Sciences
Director of Sports Medicine Fellowship
Southern California Orthopedic Institute
Van Nuys, California
Chapter 32: Arthroscopy of the Foot and Ankle

Richard E. Gellman, MD
Summit Orthopaedics, LLP
Portland, Oregon
Chapter 23: Ring External Fixation in the Foot and Ankle

J. Speight Grimes Jr., MD
Assistant Professor
Department of Orthopaedics
Texas Tech Health Sciences Center
Lubbock, Texas
Chapter 15: Infections of the Foot

Gregory P. Guyton, MD
Attending Orthopaedic Surgeon
Department of Orthopaedic Surgery
Medstar Union Memorial Hospital
Baltimore, Maryland
Chapter 26: Pes Cavus

Steven L. Haddad, MD
Senior Attending
Illinois Bone and Joint Institute, LLC
Glenview, Illinois
Chapter 25: Pes Planus

Andrew Haskell, MD
Department of Orthopaedics
Palo Alto Medical Clinic
Palo Alto, California
Assistant Clinical Professor
Department of Orthopaedic Surgery
University of California, San Francisco
San Francisco, California
Chapter 1: Biomechanics of the Foot and Ankle

Catherine L. Hayter, MBBS, FRANZCR
Radiologist
Castlereagh Sports Imaging
St Leonards, New South Wales, Australia
Chapter 3: Imaging of the Foot and Ankle

Christopher B. Hirose, MD
Private Practice of Orthopaedic Foot and Ankle Surgery
Coughlin Clinic
Saint Alphonsus Regional Medical Center
Boise, Idaho
Chapter 19: Arthritis of the Foot and Ankle

Kenneth J. Hunt, MD
Assistant Professor
Department of Orthopaedic Surgery
Stanford University
Palo Alto, California
Chapter 34: Congenital and Acquired Neurologic Disorders

Todd A. Irwin, MD
Assistant Professor
Department of Orthopaedic Surgery
University of Michigan
Ann Arbor, Michigan
Chapter 2: Principles of the Physical Examination
of the Foot and Ankle

J. Benjamin Jackson III, MD
Chief Resident
Carolinas Medical Center
OrthoCarolina Foot and Ankle Institute
Charlotte, North Carolina
Chapter 40: Fractures of the Midfoot and Forefoot

Jeffrey E. Johnson, MD
Professor
Department of Orthopaedic Surgery
Chief, Foot and Ankle Service
Barnes-Jewish Hospital at Washington University
School of Medicine
Saint Louis, Missouri
Chapter 27: Diabetes

Ari J. Kaz, MD
Orthopaedic Surgeon
Illinois Bone and Joint Institute, LLC
Assistant Professor of Clinical Orthopaedics
Department of Orthopaedic Surgery
University of Illinois–Chicago
Chicago, Illinois
Chapter 8: Keratotic Disorders of the Plantar Skin

Travis J. Kemp, MD
Coughlin Foot and Ankle Clinic
Saint Alphonsus Regional Medical Center
Boise, Idaho
Chapter 23: Ring External Fixation in the Foot and Ankle

John P. Ketz, MD
Assistant Professor
Department of Orthopaedics
University of Rochester
Rochester, New York
Chapter 36: Pilon Fractures

Sandra E. Klein, MD
Assistant Professor
Department of Orthopaedic Surgery
Barnes-Jewish Hospital at Washington University
School of Medicine
Saint Louis, Missouri
Chapter 27: Diabetes

Stephen J. Kovach, MD
Assistant Professor
Department of Surgery—Plastic Surgery
University of Pennsylvania Health System
Philadelphia, Pennsylvania
Chapter 17: Soft Tissue Reconstruction for the
Foot and Ankle

Fabian G. Krause, MD
Assistant Professor
Department of Orthopaedic Surgery
Inselspital, University of Berne
Berne, Switzerland
Chapter 26: Pes Cavus

Douglas W. Kress, MD
Division of Pediatric Dermatology
Children's Hospital of Pittsburgh
Wexford, Pennsylvania
Chapter 16: Dermatology of the Foot and
Lower Extremity

L. Scott Levin, MD, FACS
Paul B. Magnuson Professor of Bone and Joint Surgery
Chairman
Professor of Orthopaedic Surgery
Department of Orthopaedic Surgery
Professor of Surgery, Division of Plastic Surgery
Department of Surgery
University of Pennsylvania Health System
Philadelphia, Pennsylvania
Chapter 17: Soft Tissue Reconstruction for the Foot
and Ankle

James M. Linklater, MBBS, FRANZCR
Castlereagh Sports Imaging
St Leonards, New South Wales, Australia
Chapter 3: Imaging of the Foot and Ankle

Roger A. Mann, MD
Private Practice Orthopaedic Surgery
Oakland, California
Director, Foot Fellowship Program
Associate Clinical Professor of Orthopaedic Surgery
University of California School of Medicine
San Francisco, California
Chapter 1: Biomechanics of the Foot and Ankle
Chapter 8: Keratotic Disorders of the Plantar Skin

Florian Nickisch, MD
Assistant Professor
Department of Orthopaedics
University of Utah
Salt Lake City, Utah
Chapter 39: Fractures and Fracture-Dislocations
of the Talus

David I. Pedowitz, MS, MD
Assistant Professor
Department of Orthopedic Surgery
Thomas Jefferson University
Rothman Institute
Philadelphia, Pennsylvania
Chapter 14: Soft Tissue Disorders of the Foot

Walter J. Pedowitz, MD
Clinical Professor
Department of Othopaedic Surgery
Columbia University
New York, New York
Union County Orthopaedic Group
Linden, New Jersey
Chapter 14: Soft Tissue Disorders of the Foot

Phinit Phisitkul, MD
Clinical Assistant Professor
Department of Orthopaedics and Rehabilitation
University of Iowa
Iowa City, Iowa
Chapter 32: Arthroscopy of the Foot and Ankle

Stefan Rammelt, MD, PhD
Professor of Surgery
Department of Trauma and Reconstructive Surgery
University Hospital Carl Gustav Carus
Technische Universität Dresden
Dresden, Germany
Chapter 38: Fractures of the Calcaneus

R. Lor Randall, MD, FACS
The L.B. & Olive S. Young Endowed Chair for Cancer Research
Director, Sarcoma Services and Chief, SARC Lab
Professor of Orthopaedics
Huntsman Cancer Institute and Primary Children's Medical Center
University of Utah
Salt Lake City, Utah
Chapter 18: Soft Tissue and Bone Tumors

John W. Read, MBBS, FRANZCR, DDU
Radiologist
Castlereagh Sports Imaging
St Leonards, New South Wales, Australia
Chapter 3: Imaging of the Foot and Ankle

Mark A. Reed, MD
Private Practice of Orthopedic Surgery
Orthopaedic Specialists of Seattle
Seattle, Washington
Chapter 12: Disorders of the Nerves

Charles L. Saltzman, MD
Chairman, Department of Orthopaedics
Louis S. Peery MD Endowed Presidential Professor
University of Utah
University Orthopaedic Center
Salt Lake City, Utah
Chapter 21: Ankle Arthritis
Chapter 22: Ankle Replacement
Chapter 28: Amputations of the Foot and Ankle

Roy W. Sanders, MD
Chief, Department of Orthopaedic Surgery
Tampa General Hospital
Director, Orthopaedic Trauma Services
Florida Orthopaedic Institute
Tampa, Florida
Chapter 35: Dislocations of the Foot
Chapter 36: Pilon Fractures
Chapter 37: Ankle Fractures
Chapter 38: Fractures of the Calcaneus

Lew C. Schon, MD
Attending Orthopaedic Surgeon
Department of Orthopaedic Surgery
Chief, Foot and Ankle Fellowship and Orthobiologic Laboratory
MedStar Union Memorial Hospital
Assistant Professor Orthopaedics
Johns Hopkins School of Medicine
Assistant Professor
Biomedical Engineering, Johns Hopkins University
Baltimore, Maryland
Associate Professor of Orthopaedics
Georgetown School of Medicine
Washington, DC
Chapter 12: Disorders of the Nerves
Chapter 24: Disorders of Tendons

Faustin R. Stevens, MD
Private Practice of Foot and Ankle Surgery
Tri-City Orthopaedics
Kennewick, Washington
Chapter 19: Arthritis of the Foot and Ankle

Jeffrey Swenson, MD
Professor of Anesthesiology
University of Utah
Salt Lake City, Utah
Chapter 5: Anesthesia

Norman E. Waldrop, III, MD
Director, Foot and Ankle Orthopaedic Surgery
Andrews Sports Medicine
American Sports Medicine Institute
Birmingham, Alabama
Chapter 30: Athletic Injuries to the Soft Tissues of the Foot and Ankle

Art Walling, MD
Foot and Ankle Surgery
Musculoskeletal Oncology
Florida Orthopaedic Institute
Tampa, Florida
Chapter 37: Ankle Fractures

Keith L. Wapner, MD, FACS
Clinical Professor of Orthopaedic Surgery
Director, Foot and Ankle Division
Director, Foot and Ankle Fellowship Program
University of Pennsylvania
Adjunct Professor of Orthopedic Surgery
Drexel College of Medicine
Philadelphia, Pennsylvania
Chapter 4: Conservative Treatment of the Foot

Preface

In 1959, Henri L. DuVries, MD, published the first edition of *Surgery of the Foot*. This text summarized his 30-year personal experience in diagnosing and treating disorders, deformities, and injuries of the foot and ankle. His book became a classic, but it was also significant because it was written by a physician who originally had obtained his training as a podiatrist and then subsequently became a doctor of medicine.

In 1965, Dr. DuVries expanded the book to include several other contributors, taking a form that is a model even for the current textbook. Included in this second edition were Verne T. Inman, MD, chairman of the Department of Orthopaedic Surgery at the University of California, San Francisco, and Roger A. Mann, MD, a senior resident in orthopaedic surgery. Eight years later, in 1973, Dr. Inman succeeded Dr. DuVries as the editor of the third edition of *Surgery of the Foot*. Again, with this text, an expanded objective included discussion of the ankle joint as well as an in-depth analysis of the biomechanics of the foot and ankle. Five years later, in 1978, Dr. Mann became the editor of the fourth edition. Dr. Mann, having been a resident under Dr. Inman and having served a fellowship under Dr. DuVries, was presented with a unique opportunity to blend the special interests of these two unique clinicians—Dr. Inman's basic biomechanical research and Dr. DuVries' wealth of clinical knowledge. In 1986, Dr. Mann edited a revised fifth edition.

In 1978, as Dr. Mann's first foot and ankle fellow, I had the opportunity to be exposed to both his philosophy of patient care and the creativity with which he addressed the evaluation and treatment of his patients. His meticulous surgical technique and comprehensive postoperative program were coupled with an introspective method of assessing the results of specific procedures to delineate the preferred treatment regimen. Dr. Mann's 45 years in private practice, stimulated by more than 75 foot and ankle fellows, have complemented my interaction with him. In 1999, I initiated my own fellowship program and have learned a great deal from the 15 fellows who I have trained. I also have frequently reviewed the surgical procedures used in my everyday practice, with the common goal of defining the strengths of individual procedures as well as their weaknesses. From the 34 years that I have been in private practice in Boise, Idaho, I have come to believe that the principles initially espoused by Drs. Inman and DuVries and expanded on by Dr. Mann have given me a unique perspective.

In 1993, Dr. Mann and I collaborated on the sixth edition, which was expanded to a comprehensive two-volume text. In 1999, this was revised by us as the seventh edition and, in 2005, it was published as a colorized eighth edition, in which we were joined by, Dr. Charles L. Saltzman, as a co-editor.

This is a living text and has continued to evolve from the initial work of Henri L. DuVries. Much of our orthopaedic careers have been devoted to working with this text; Dr. Mann has contributed to or edited all but one of the first eight editions, and I have contributed to or edited half of the editions. However, change and growth are important! As of this edition, Dr. Mann has become an editor emeritus but has continued to give us his input and valued advice. To recognize and honor his invaluable contributions to the textbook, we have named this ninth edition *Mann's Surgery of the Foot and Ankle*. Most important, Robert B. Anderson, MD, a past fellow of John Gould, MD, joins Dr. Saltzman and me as an editor of this text. Dr. Anderson brings a wealth of clinical knowledge and a sports medicine background to this association. Just as Dr. DuVries complemented his text by adding Dr. Inman, and Dr. Inman introduced Dr. Mann, we feel strongly that Dr. Anderson's addition will make this a stronger and more well-rounded work. The ninth edition is also enhanced by the work of many of our excellent fellows and colleagues from around the world who have made substantial sacrifices to contribute to this textbook. In this edition, 25 authors continue to contribute, but 42 new authors have been added. These contributing authors are at the forefront of their specific area of foot and ankle surgery. Each contributing author has covered a specific topic in a comprehensive fashion, which we believe will leave the reader with a clear, concise appreciation of the subject. Although this book is not meant to be encyclopedic in nature, our goal has always been to provide the reader with a method of evaluating and treating a particular problem. More than 40% of the ninth edition has been completely rewritten by both new and returning contributors, and the remaining chapters have been updated.

In 1990, Dr. Mann and I published the *Video Textbook of Foot and Ankle Surgery,* the second volume of which appeared in 1995. This enabled foot and ankle surgeons to view a surgical procedure while simultaneously reading about the operative technique. Encouraged by the success of this endeavor, the eighth edition of *Surgery of the Foot and Ankle* incorporated, for the first time, 60 edited videos on two DVDs. This unique addition has now become an industry standard. To enhance the current edition, we have retained 45 classic videos narrated by Dr. Mann and added 75 new videos contributed by us as well as many other colleagues. Furthermore, advances in Internet and online learning have enhanced the electronic version of the ninth edition textbook and video compilation to allow viewing on smartphone and tablet devices before performing surgical procedures, affecting both learning and improving patient care.

This new edition has been divided into 10 sections that have been subdivided into chapters. Specific surgical techniques within the chapters are described and illustrated in detail to afford the reader an understanding of the indications for each procedure and insight into the performance of the technique. Although many different treatment regimens are presented, our goal is to recommend a specific treatment plan for each pathologic entity. Furthermore, some topics are presented in more than one section, enabling the reader to appreciate the varying points of view presented by individual contributors. It is our goal to provide the reader with an accurate assessment of both the attributes and the deficiencies of specific orthopaedic foot and ankle procedures, new and old. In this edition, we present our most up-to-date thinking regarding the diagnosis, treatment, and specific surgical care of foot and ankle problems.

In **Part I,** *General Considerations,* the biomechanics, examination, and conservative treatment of foot and ankle problems are addressed. In large part, the initial principles advocated by Dr. DuVries, Dr. Inman, and Dr. Mann, as presented in their early editions, are included in this portion of the text but have been updated. Anesthetic techniques have been completely rewritten and have been updated to include popliteal blocks and indwelling catheters. Discussions of imaging methods, an integral part of the evaluation process for foot and ankle disorders, have also been completely rewritten and include in-depth coverage of magnetic resonance imaging and computed tomography.

In **Part II,** *Forefoot,* an extensive analysis of deformities of the great toe, along with complications associated with individual hallux valgus procedures, has been completely revised to make the reader aware of primary surgical techniques as well as salvage techniques used for postsurgical complications. Inclusion of newer, popular surgical techniques has been added. The chapter on lesser toes has been completely rewritten and updated because of the vast number of advances made in the area of

plantar plate tears and treatment of this complex problem. The chapters on sesamoids, keratotic disorders, and toenail abnormalities have all been updated as well.

Part III, *Nerve Disorders,* **and Part IV,** *Miscellaneous,* have been completely updated to cover both acquired and static neurologic disorders; the material about heel pain has been rewritten and updated by new authors.

Part V, *Soft Tissue Disorders of the Foot and Ankle,* includes revised chapters on infection, dermatology, and soft tissue reconstruction and a completely new chapter on tumors of the foot and ankle.

Part VI, *Arthritis, Postural Disorders, and Tendon Disorders,* has been completely revamped, updating our current knowledge and treatment of systemic inflammatory arthritis, traumatic arthritis, and osteoarthritis. The chapter on total ankle arthroplasty presents substantial changes because of the dramatic developments that have occurred over the past decade in ankle joint replacement. Revisions of the chapters on pes planus and pes cavus are included. The chapter on arthrodesis of the foot has been replaced by one on arthritis of the hindfoot and midfoot, containing both assessment and surgical treatment of conditions in this region. The chapter on tendon abnormalities has been extensively rewritten to reflect significant technical advances in this area.

A separate section, **Part VII,** *Diabetes,* contains three completely updated chapters on diabetes, amputations, and prostheses of the foot and ankle.

Part VIII, *Sports Medicine,* includes a comprehensive chapter on athletic soft tissue injuries as well as specific chapters regarding stress fractures and arthroscopy; all three chapters have been revised and updated to familiarize the reader with this exciting and evolving area of orthopaedic technology.

Pediatrics is covered in **Part IX** with two chapters: a general pediatric chapter and a separate chapter on congenital and acquired neurologic disorders, where new authors have added significant new information.

Finally, **Part X,** *Trauma,* includes six chapters. These chapters, which have been updated and revised, include discussion of fractures of the distal tibia; ankle; dislocations of the foot and ankle; and calcaneus talus, midfoot, and forefoot fractures, which are covered in a comprehensive fashion.

As Roger Mann stated in the preface of the fifth edition, "As medicine continues to progress, the information of this textbook will again need to be upgraded. The principles presented, however, are basic in their approach and will not change significantly over the years." We believe that the ninth edition of *Mann's Surgery of the Foot and Ankle* will strongly enhance this dynamic and exciting field of orthopaedics and will complement the learning experience of the resident and fellow-in-training as well as the practicing surgeon.

Michael J. Coughlin, MD

Acknowledgments

We acknowledge those who have assisted us in the preparation of this text:

Video productions: Boise, Idaho
Travis J. Kemp, MD—surgical videography, video editing, and video production; Saint Alphonsus Hospital day surgery employees for their assistance in surgical videography; Eileen Brown, LPN, for assistance in surgical procedures and videography

Artwork: Boise, Idaho
Barbara Kirk of Graphic Source—color artwork

Clinical and literary assistance: Boise, Idaho
Margaret C. Collins, RN, ONC—patient follow-up photography and patient verification; Sandra Hight—librarian, the Kissler Medical Family Library

Executive and administrative support: Saint Alphonsus Health Care Systems, Boise, Idaho
Sally Jeffcoat, President and CEO of Saint Alphonsus Health Systems; David F. Kirk, MHA, Director of Operations, Saint Alphonsus Medical Group; Annie T. Sutton, MBA, Clinic Manager, Coughlin Foot and Ankle Clinic at Saint Alphonsus Hospital

Secretarial and technical support: Salt Lake City, Utah
Rebecca Nielson

We acknowledge the previous editions of this text and the editors of each edition:

SURGERY OF THE FOOT
1st Edition, 1959, editor: Henri L. DuVries, MD
2nd Edition, 1965, editor: Henri L. DuVries, MD
3rd Edition, 1973, editor: Verne T. Inman, MD
4th Edition, 1978, editor: Roger A. Mann, MD
5th Edition, 1986, editor: Roger A. Mann, MD

SURGERY OF THE FOOT AND ANKLE
6th Edition, 1993, editors: Roger A. Mann, MD, and Michael J. Coughlin, MD

7th Edition, 1999, editors: Michael J. Coughlin, MD, and Roger A. Mann, MD
8th Edition, 2007, editors: Michael J. Coughlin, MD; Roger A. Mann, MD; and Charles L. Saltzman, MD

MANN'S SURGERY OF THE FOOT AND ANKLE
9th Edition, 2014, editors: Michael J. Coughlin, MD; Charles L. Saltzman, MD; and Robert B. Anderson, MD

Michael J. Coughlin, MD
Charles L. Saltzman, MD
Robert B. Anderson, MD

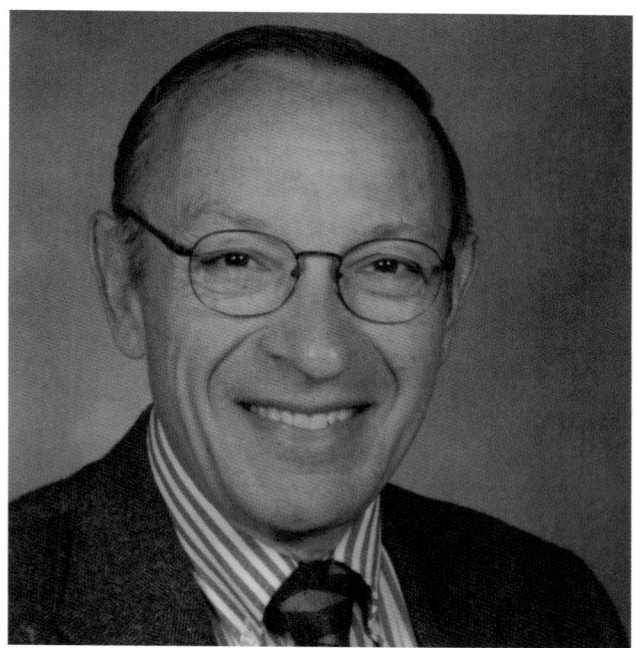

We are proud to dedicate the ninth edition of *Surgery of the Foot and Ankle* to Roger A. Mann, MD, and have changed the official name to *Mann's Surgery of the Foot and Ankle*. Dr. Mann served as a mentor and teacher at a time when there were few foot and ankle fellowships or fellows. He guided the *American Orthopaedic Foot and Ankle Society* in its early years and promoted education of residents and surgeons in active practice through programs at the *American Academy of Orthopedic Surgeons* and the *American Orthopaedic Foot and Ankle Society* meetings. Prolific in his studies and publications, he has introduced more than 75 fellows to his methods of investigation and surgery, thus truly changing surgery in America during his time. He took the rather small primer entitled *Surgery of the Foot* and changed it to a two-volume color textbook—*Surgery of the Foot and Ankle*, with a video supplement—that has become the definitive textbook for foot and ankle surgery in the world.

His vision and action are proof that one man can truly make a difference, and he has done that.

Contents

Volume 2

List of Video Clips

Video Editing by Travis J. Kemp, MD
Most voiceovers by Michael J. Coughlin, MD, and Roger A. Mann, MD

PART I

GENERAL CONSIDERATIONS

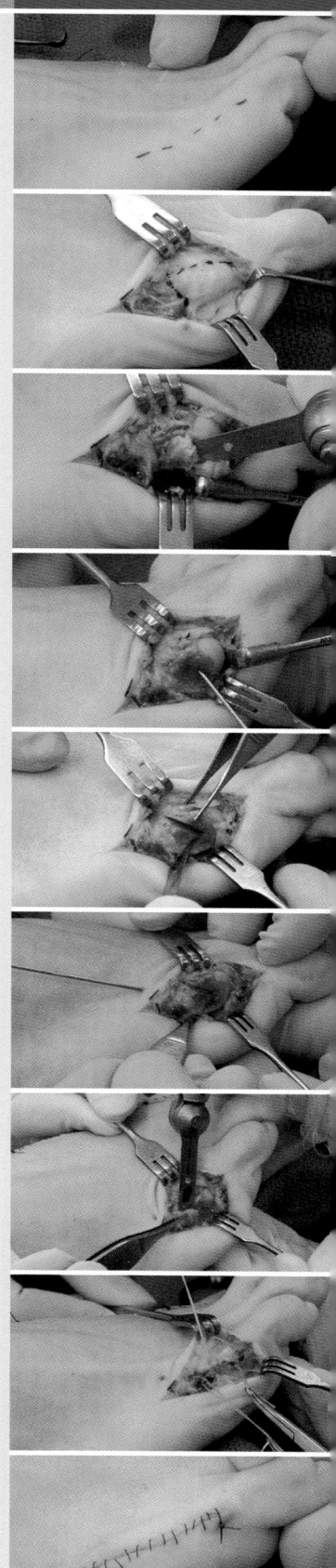

Chapter 1

Biomechanics of the Foot and Ankle

Andrew Haskell, Roger A. Mann

The human foot is an intricate mechanism that functions interdependently with other components of the locomotor system. Failure of the functioning of a single part, whether by disease, external forces, or surgical manipulation, will alter the functions of the remaining parts. To further complicate things, wide variations occur in the normal component parts of the foot and ankle, and these variations affect the degree of contribution of each part to the function of the entire foot. Depending on the contributions of an individual component, the loss or functional modification of that component by surgical intervention may result in minor or major alterations in the function of adjacent components. This variation helps to explain why the same procedure performed on the foot of one person produces a satisfactory result, whereas in another person the result is unsatisfactory.

Yet the surgeon is called on constantly to change the anatomic and structural components of the foot. When so doing, awareness of the consequences of these changes is fundamental to achieving desired results. Put another way, an understanding of interrelationships between foot and ankle components and how they interact with the greater locomotor system is critical to achieving predictable outcomes when altering these components surgically.

Understanding the biomechanics of the foot and ankle also contributes to sound surgical decision making and adds to the success of postoperative treatment. Appreciating the mechanical behavior of the foot allows the physician to differentiate foot disabilities that may be successfully treated by nonsurgical procedures rather than approached surgically. Furthermore, some operative procedures that fail to completely achieve the desired result can be improved by minor alterations in the behavior of adjacent components through shoe modification or the use of orthotic inserts or braces.

With increased attention being given to athletics, the physician must have a basic knowledge of the mechanics that occur during running. Many of the same basic mechanisms that will be described for the biomechanics of the foot and ankle are not significantly altered during running. The same stabilization mechanism within the foot occurs during running as during walking. The major differences observed during running are that the gait cycle is altered considerably, the amount of force generated (as measured by force plate data) is markedly increased, the range of motion of the joints of the lower extremities is increased, and the phasic activity of the muscles of the lower extremities is altered. Differences between walking and running will be highlighted in the following sections.

Starting this textbook with a chapter focused on foot and ankle biomechanics is meant to provide a foundation for the reader upon which the remaining chapters are built. It has been assumed that the orthopaedic surgeon possesses an accurate knowledge of the anatomy of the foot and ankle. If this knowledge is lacking, textbooks of anatomy are available that depict in detail the precise anatomic structures constituting this part of the human body.[46,49] In this chapter, the gait cycle is reviewed, kinematic and kinetic aspects of gait are explored, and specific anatomic interrelationships of the foot and ankle are emphasized. Throughout this discussion, mechanics that differentiate running from walking are described. Finally, clinical examples are explored, and methods for functional evaluation of the foot are presented as practical demonstrations of the concepts within.

GAIT CYCLE

Walking Cycle

Human gait is a rhythmic, cyclic forward progression involving motion of all body segments. A single cycle is often defined as the motion between the heel strike of one step and the heel strike of the same foot on the subsequent step. Gait parameters, such as stride length, velocity, and cadence, are easy to measure based on this definition.

A single cycle can be divided further. The walking cycle for one limb is broken into a stance phase and a swing phase. The stance phase typically constitutes 62% of the cycle and the swing phase 38%. The stance phase is further divided into a period of double limb support (from 0% to 12%), in which both feet are on the ground, followed by a period of single limb support (from 12% to 50%) and a second period of double limb support (from 50% to 62%), after which the swing phase begins (Fig. 1-1).

The opposite leg also goes through a predictable sequence during a gait cycle. The position and activities of this contralateral leg can be seen at predictable times. For instance, contralateral toe-off is typically at 12% of the gait cycle, occurring after the ipsilateral foot has reached a foot-flat position. Ipsilateral heel rise begins at

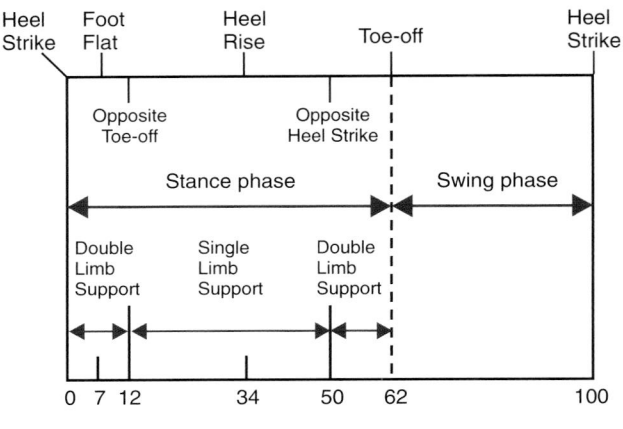

Figure 1-1 Phases of the walking cycle. Stance phase constitutes approximately 62%, and swing phase 38% of cycle. During stance phase of walking, there are two periods of double limb support and one period of single limb support. Stance phase is further divided into three intervals: from heel strike to foot flat at approximately 7% of the gait cycle, foot flat to heel rise at approximately 34% of the gait cycle, and heel rise to toe-off at approximately 62% of the gait cycle.

34% as the contralateral leg swings through and passes the stance foot. Finally, contralateral heel strike occurs at 50% of the gait cycle.

In a patient with spasticity, the initial heel strike may be toe contact, and foot flat may not occur by 7% of the cycle. Heel rise may be premature if spasticity or an equinus contracture is present or delayed in the case of weakness of the gastrocnemius–soleus muscle group. Weakness of anterior compartment leg musculature resulting in a footdrop may lead to accentuated hip and knee flexion during swing-through and alteration in attaining a foot-flat position.

The walking cycle being one of continuous motion is difficult to appreciate in its entirety because so many events occur simultaneously. To help appreciate the different activities and functions of the components of the foot and ankle during gait, the stance phase can be divided into three intervals: the first interval, extending from initial heel strike to the foot laying flat on the floor; the second interval, occurring during the period of foot flat as the body passes over the foot; and the third interval, extending from the beginning of ankle joint plantar flexion as the heel rises from the floor to when the toes lift from the floor.

First Interval

The first interval occurs during approximately the first 15% of the walking cycle and is defined from the moment of initial heel strike to when the foot becomes flat on the floor. Typically, the opposite heel has lifted from the floor, but weight remains on the forefoot. During the first interval, the foot helps to absorb and dissipate the forces generated by the foot striking the ground.

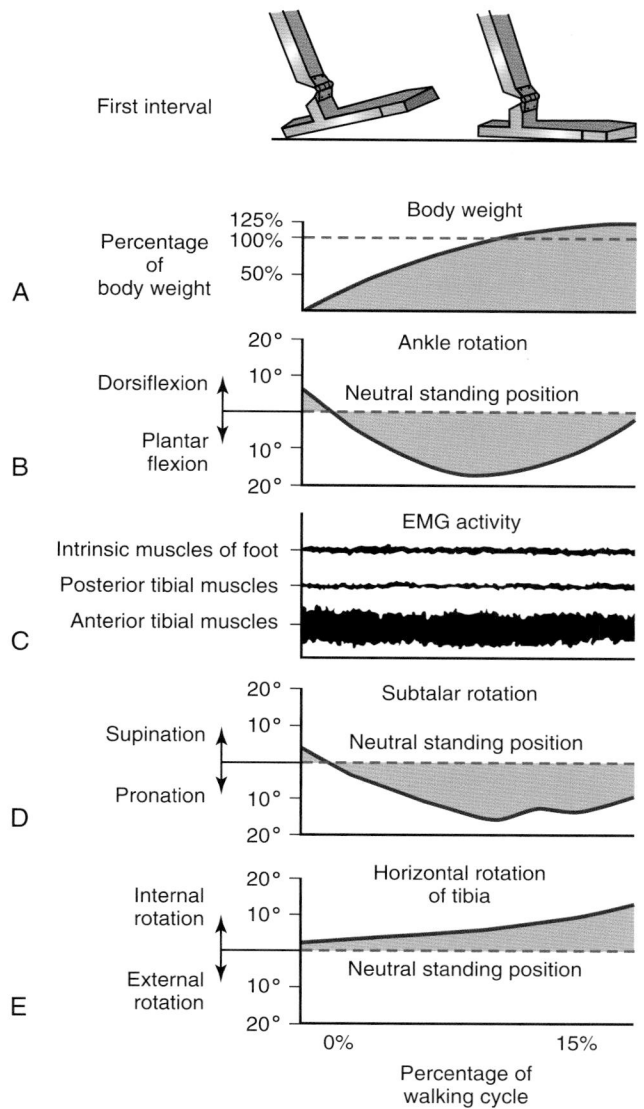

Figure 1-2 Composite of events of first interval of walking, or period that extends from heel strike to foot flat. *EMG,* electromyograph.

The ankle joint undergoes rapid plantar flexion from heel strike until foot flat is achieved. At approximately 7% of the walking cycle, dorsiflexion begins (Fig. 1-2B).

As the foot is loaded with the weight of the body during the first interval, the calcaneus rapidly everts and the longitudinal arch flattens. This flattening of the arch originates in the subtalar joint and reaches a maximum during this interval (Fig. 1-2D). The hindfoot is often mildly supinated at initial ground contact associated with ankle dorsiflexion during swing-through. The hindfoot moving from supination to pronation during the first interval is a passive mechanism, and the amount of motion appears to depend entirely on the configuration of the articulating surfaces, their capsular attachments, and ligamentous support. No significant muscle function appears to play a role in restricting this motion at initial ground contact.

The subtalar joint links rotation of the hindfoot to rotation of the leg. During the first interval, eversion of the calcaneus is translated by the subtalar joint into inward rotation that is transmitted proximally across the ankle joint into the lower extremity (Fig. 1-2E). Distally, this hindfoot eversion unlocks the transverse tarsal joint (Fig. 1-2D), allowing the midfoot joints to become supple. This allows the flattening of the longitudinal arch that contributes to energy dissipation during this phase.

At heel strike, the center of gravity of the body is decelerated by ground contact, then immediately accelerated upward to carry it over the extending lower extremity. The heel's impact and body's center of gravity shift accounts for a vertical floor reaction that exceeds body weight by 15% to 25% (Fig. 1-2A).

Eccentric contraction of the anterior compartment leg muscles slows the rapid ankle plantar flexion during this phase from heel strike until a foot-flat position is reached. The posterior calf muscles all are electrically quiet, as are the intrinsic muscles in the sole of the foot (Fig. 1-2C). There is no muscular response in those muscles usually considered important in supporting the longitudinal arch of the foot. Weakness of the anterior compartment muscles leads to a loss of this deceleration and a characteristic slap foot gait.

Second Interval

The second interval extends from 15% to 40% of the walking cycle. During this interval, the body's center of gravity passes from behind to in front of the weight-bearing leg. It reaches a maximum height as it passes over the leg at about 35% of the cycle, after which it commences to fall. During this interval, the foot transitions from a flexible, energy-absorbing structure to a more rigid one, capable of bearing the body's weight.

The ankle joint undergoes progressive dorsiflexion during the second interval, reaching its peak at 40% of the walking cycle. This is when the force across the ankle joint has reached a maximum of 4.5 times body weight. Heel rise begins at 34% of the cycle as the contralateral leg passes by the stance foot and precedes the onset of plantar flexion, which begins at 40% (Fig. 1-3B).

During the second interval, the subtalar joint progressively inverts. This starts at about 30% of the cycle in a normal foot and at about 15% of the cycle in a flatfoot (Fig. 1-3D). Multiple factors contribute to this inversion, but precisely which plays the greatest role is unclear. Above the subtalar joint, the swinging contralateral limb externally rotates the stance limb. This external rotation torque is translated by the subtalar joint into hindfoot inversion. The oblique nature of the ankle joint axis, the oblique setting of the metatarsal break, and the function of the plantar aponeurosis also contribute to hindfoot inversion. Inversion of the subtalar joint is passed distally into the midfoot, increasing the stability of the transverse

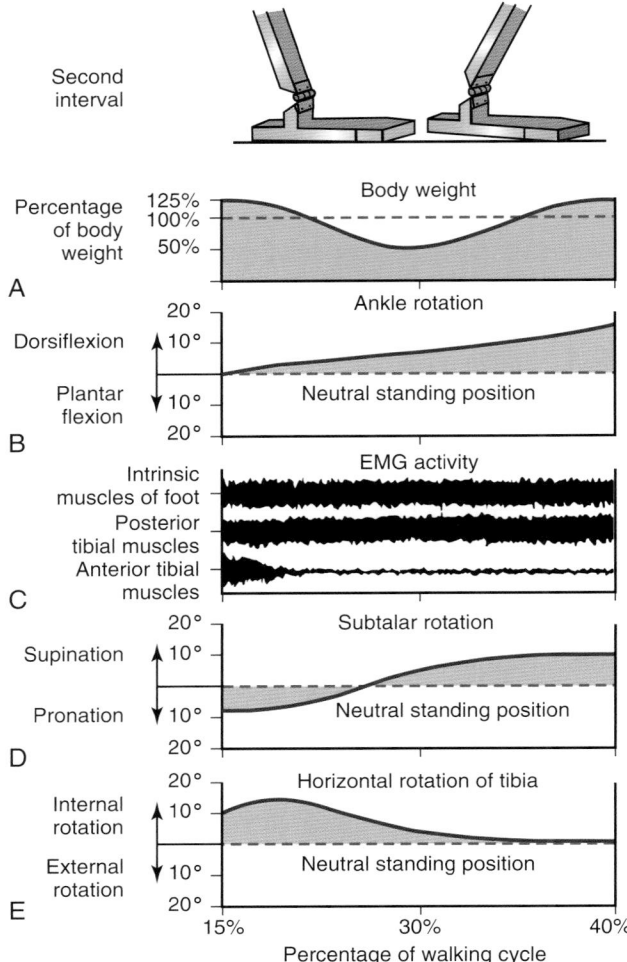

Figure 1-3 Composite of events of second interval of walking, or period of foot flat. *EMG*, electromyograph.

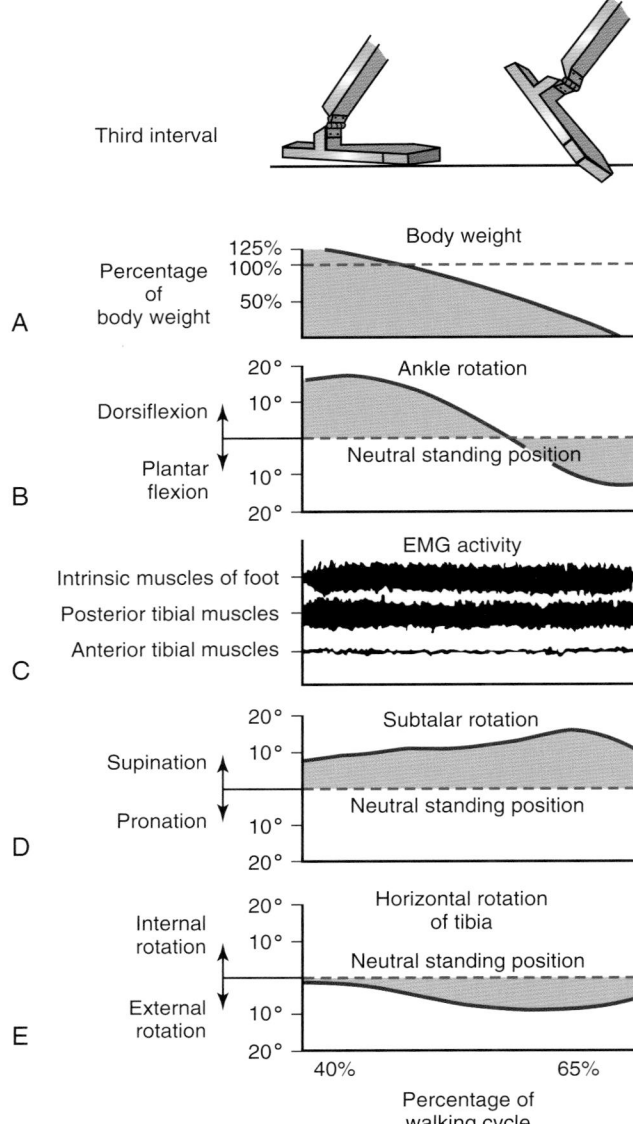

Figure 1-4 Composite of all events of third interval of walking, or period extending from foot flat to toe-off. *EMG*, electromyograph.

tarsal articulation and transforming the flexible midfoot into a rigid structure.

During this interval, full body weight is not borne on the foot, smoothing the transition to single limb support. Force plate recordings show that the load on the foot may be as low as 70% to 80% of actual body weight (Fig. 1-3A).

During the second interval, important functional changes occur in both the foot and leg, which are the result of muscular action. The posterior and lateral compartment leg muscles (triceps surae, peroneals, tibialis posterior, long toe flexors) and intrinsic muscles in the sole of the foot demonstrate electrical activity (Fig. 1-3C). Intrinsic muscle activity of the normal foot begins at 30% of the cycle, whereas in flatfoot, activity begins at 15% of the cycle. The posterior calf musculature slows the forward movement of the tibia over the fixed foot, which permits the contralateral limb to increase its step length. Weakness of the posterior compartment muscles may lead to premature contralateral heel strike and shortened stride length.

Third Interval

The third interval constitutes the last of the stance phase and extends from 40% to 62% of the walking cycle.

The ankle joint demonstrates rapid plantar flexion during this interval as the foot essentially extends the stance, effective length. The subtalar joint continues to invert during this interval, reaching its maximum at toe-off (Fig. 1-4D). This completes the conversion of the forefoot from the flexible structure observed in the first interval at the time of weight acceptance to a rigid structure at the end of the third interval in preparation for toe-off. The inversion is a continuation of the processes that began in the second interval. These include external rotation of limb above the foot passing across the ankle and subtalar joints as well as mechanisms in the foot such as the obliquity of the ankle joint, the function of the plantar aponeurosis, and obliquity of the metatarsal break. Distally, the transverse tarsal joint is converted from a flexible structure into a rigid one by the progressive inversion of the calcaneus. The talonavicular joint also is stabilized during this period by the pressure placed across the joint by both body weight and the intrinsic force created by the plantar aponeurosis.

At the beginning of the third interval, force plate recordings demonstrate an increase in the percentage of body weight borne by the foot resulting from the center of gravity falling. The load on the foot exceeds body weight by approximately 20%. Later in the interval, the vertical floor reaction force falls to zero as the body's weight is transferred to the opposite foot (Fig. 1-4A).

Ankle plantar flexion during the third interval is caused primarily by the concentric contraction of the posterior calf musculature, in particular the triceps surae (Fig. 1-4B). The plantar flexion leads to relative elongation of the extremity. Although full plantar flexion at the ankle joint occurs during this interval, electrical activity is observed only until 50% of the cycle, after which there is no longer electrical activity in the extrinsic muscles (Fig. 1-4C). The remainder of ankle joint plantar flexion occurs because of the transfer of weight from the stance leg to the contralateral limb. The intrinsic muscles of the foot are active until toe-off. Although the intrinsic muscles help to stabilize the longitudinal arch, the main stabilizer is the plantar aponeurosis, which is functioning maximally during this period as the toes are brought into dorsiflexion and the plantar aponeurosis is wrapped around the metatarsal heads, forcing them into plantar flexion and elevating the longitudinal arch. The anterior compartment muscles become active in the last 5% of this interval, probably to initiate dorsiflexion of the ankle joint immediately after toe-off.

Running Cycle

The changes that occur in the gait cycle during running relative to walking are illustrated in Figure 1-5. During walking, one foot is always in contact with the ground; as the speed of gait increases, a transition occurs wherein a float phase is incorporated, during which time both feet are off the ground. Rather than a period of double limb support as occurs during walking, there is a period of no limb support. As the speed of gait continues to increase, the time the foot spends on the ground, both in real time and in percentage of cycle, decreases considerably. The speed at which one transitions from walking to running is greater than the speed at which one transitions back from running to walking.

KINEMATICS OF HUMAN LOCOMOTION

Humans use a unique and characteristic orthograde bipedal mode of locomotion. But walking is more than

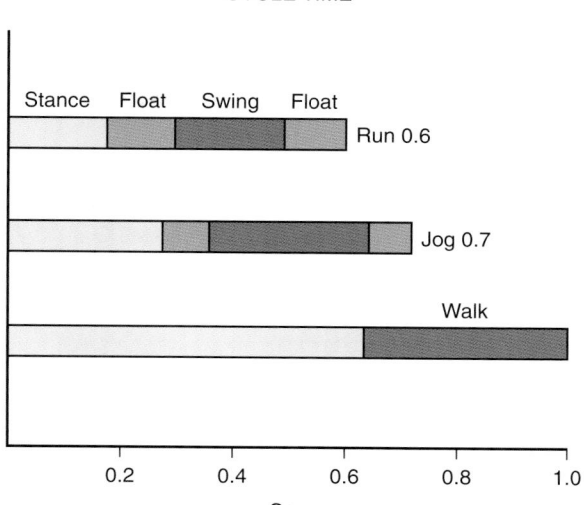

Figure 1-5 Variations in gait cycle for running, jogging, and walking. Note that as the speed of gait increases, stance phase decreases. In this illustration, subject is walking at 3.75 miles per hour, jogging at about 1 mile per 9 minutes, and running about 1 mile per 5 minutes.

merely placing one foot in front the other. During walking, all major segments of the body are in motion. Displacements of the body segments occur in a well-preserved fashion and can be accurately described. Kinematics is the study of the motion of these body segments.

Human locomotion is a learned process; it does not develop as the result of an inborn reflex.[59] The first few steps of an infant holding onto his or her parent's hand exemplify the learning process necessary to achieve orthograde progression. The result of this learning process is the integration of the neuromusculoskeletal mechanisms, with their gross similarities and individual variations, into an adequately functioning system of locomotion. Once a person has learned to walk, the mechanisms of ambulation are adaptable and work whether the person is an amputee learning to use a prosthesis, a long-distance runner, or a high-heeled shoe wearer.

A smoothly performing locomotor system results from the harmonious integration of many components. Because human locomotion involves all major segments of the body, certain suprapedal movements demand specific functions from the foot, and the manner in which the foot functions or fails to function may be reflected in patterns of movement in the other segments of the body. Similarly, alterations in movements above, such as a stiff knee or hip from arthritis or knee hyperextension from postpolio quadriceps weakness, may be reflected below by changes in the behavior of the foot.

Although bipedal locomotion imposes gross similarities in the manner in which all of us walk, each of us exhibits minor individual differences that allow us to be recognized by a friend or acquaintance, even from a distance. The causes of these individual characteristics of

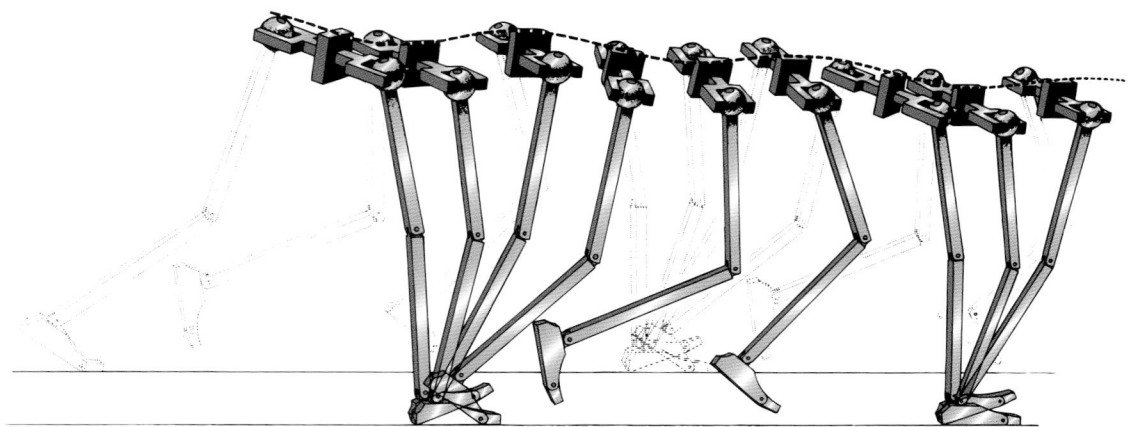

Figure 1-6 Displacement of center of gravity of body in smooth sinusoidal path. (From Saunders JB, Inman VT, Eberhart HD: The major determinants in normal and pathological gait. *J Bone Joint Surg Am* 35A:543-558, 1953.)

locomotion are many. Each of us differs somewhat in the length and distribution of mass of the various segments of the body, segments that must be moved by muscles of varying fiber length. Furthermore, individual differences occur in the position of axes of movement of the joints, with concomitant variations in effective lever arms. These and many more such factors combine to establish in each of us a final idiosyncratic manner of locomotion.

Just as no two people walk exactly alike, gait kinematics will not always be identical even within the same individual. The contribution of a single component varies under different circumstances. Type of shoe, amount of fatigue, weight of load carried, and other such variables can cause diminished functioning of some components, with compensatory increased functioning of others. An enormous number of variations in the behavior of individual components are possible; however, the diversely functioning components, when integrated, are complementary and will produce smooth forward progression.

Average values of single anthropometric observations of gait kinematic parameters are alone of little value. The surgeon should be alert to the anthropometric variations that occur within the population, but it is more important to understand the functional interrelationships among the various components. This is particularly true in the case of the foot, where anatomic variations are extensive. If average values are the only bases of comparison, it becomes difficult to explain why some feet function adequately and asymptomatically, although their measurements deviate from the average, whereas others function symptomatically, even though their measurements approximate the average. Therefore, in this chapter, emphasis is placed on functional interrelationships and not on lists of kinematic measurements.

Vertical Body Displacements

The rhythmic upward and downward displacement of the body during walking is familiar to everyone, and is particularly noticeable when someone is out of step in a parade. These displacements in the vertical plane are a necessary concomitant of bipedal locomotion. When the legs are separated, as during transmission of the body weight from one leg to the other (double weight bearing), the distance between the trunk and the floor must be less than when it passes over a relatively extended leg, as during midstance.

Smoothing and minimizing vertical oscillations of the body's center of gravity minimizes energy expenditure. Physics principles tell us that much more energy is needed to lift the body against gravity and slow its descent (vertical displacement) than to move perpendicular to gravity's pull (fore–aft or lateral displacement). Because the nature of bipedal locomotion demands such vertical oscillations of the body, they should occur in a smooth manner. The center of gravity of the body does displace in a smooth sinusoidal path; the amplitude of displacement is approximately 4 to 5 cm (Fig. 1-6).[65,66] The body's center of gravity reaches its maximum elevation immediately after passage over the weight-bearing leg and then begins to fall. This fall is stopped at the termination of the swing phase of the opposite leg as the heel strikes the ground.

Much of the coordination of motion between the different segments of the lower limbs results in minimizing the vertical displacement of the body's center of gravity. Although movements of the pelvis and hip modify the amplitude of the sinusoidal pathway, the knee, ankle, and foot are particularly involved in converting what would be a series of intersecting arcs into a smooth, sinusoidal curve.[66] This conversion requires both simultaneous and precise sequential motions in the knee, ankle, and foot.

In a well-functioning system, the body's falling center of gravity is smoothly decelerated, because relative shortening of the leg occurs at the time of impact against a gradually increasing resistance. The knee flexes against a graded contraction of the quadriceps muscle; the ankle plantar flexes against the resisting anterior tibial muscle. After the foot-flat position is reached, further shortening is achieved by pronation of the foot to a degree permitted by the ligamentous structures within.

So, to reemphasize, hindfoot pronation constitutes an important additional factor to that of knee flexion and ankle plantar flexion needed to smoothly decelerate and finally to stop the downward path of the body. If one were forced to walk stiff-kneed or without a mobile foot and ankle, the downward deceleration of the center of gravity at heel strike would be instantaneous. The body would be subjected to a severe jarring force, and the locomotor system would lose kinetic energy.

After reaching its nadir, the center of gravity moves upward to propel it over the stance leg. The leg functionally elongates by transitory extension of the knee, further plantar flexion of the ankle as the heel elevates, and supination of the foot. Elevation of the heel is the major component contributing to upward acceleration of the center of gravity at this time.

Lateral Body Displacements

When a person is walking, the body does not remain precisely in the plane of progression but oscillates slightly from side to side to keep the center of gravity approximately over the weight-bearing foot. Watching someone walk from behind highlights this subtle side-to-side shift of their center of gravity toward the stance limb. When walking side by side with a companion, if one gets out of step with the other, their bodies may bump from this side-to-side sway.

The body is shifted slightly over the weight-bearing leg, with each step creating a sinusoidal lateral displacement of the center of gravity of approximately 4 to 5 cm with each complete stride. This lateral displacement can be increased by walking with the feet more widely separated and decreased by keeping the feet close to the plan of progression (Fig. 1-7). Normally, the slight valgus of the tibiofemoral angle (physiologic genu valgum) permits the tibia to remain essentially vertical and the feet close together while the femurs diverge to articulate with the pelvis, minimizing the lateral displacement.

Horizontal Limb Rotation

In addition to vertical and lateral displacements of the body, a series of axial rotatory movements occur that can be measured in the horizontal (transverse) plane. Rotations of the pelvis and the shoulder girdle are easy to see

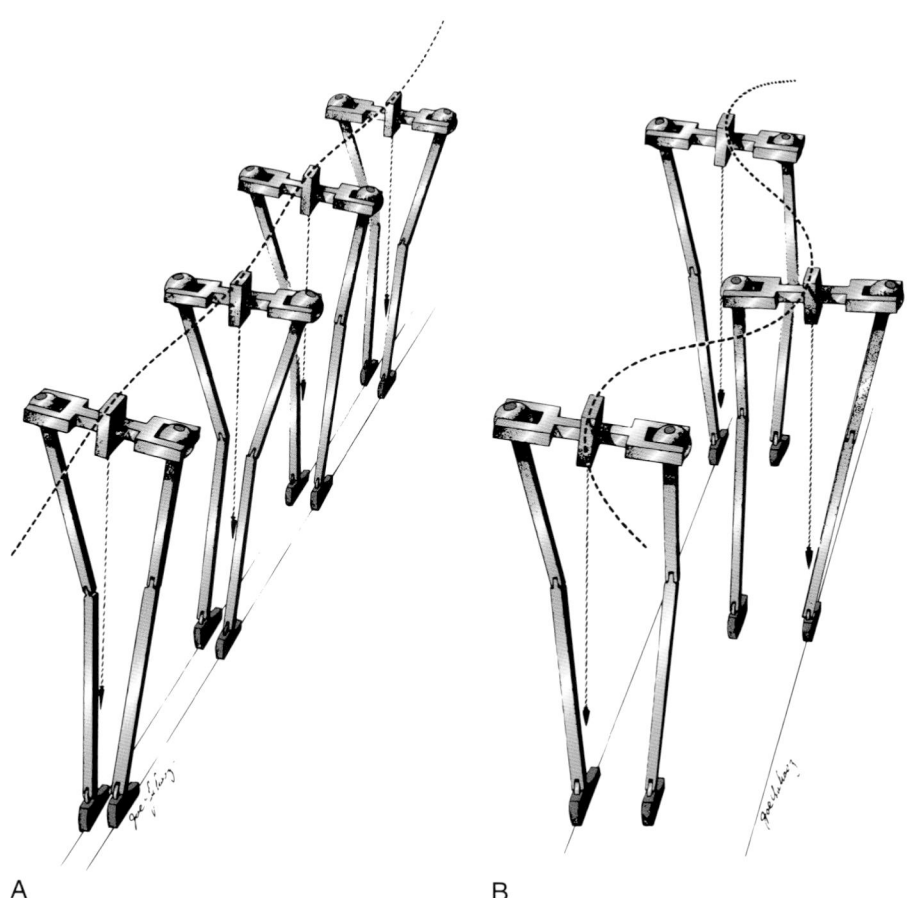

A   B

Figure 1-7 **A,** Slight lateral displacement of body occurring during walking with feet close together. **B,** Increased lateral displacement of body occurring during walking with feet wide apart. (From Saunders JB, Inman VT, Eberhart HD: The major determinants in normal and pathological gait. *J Bone Joint Surg Am* 35A:543-558, 1953.)

when watching someone walk. Similar horizontal rotations occur in the femoral and tibial segments of the extremities. The tibias rotate about their long axes, internally during swing phase and into the first interval of stance phase and externally during the latter phases of stance. The degree of these rotations is subject to marked individual variations. In a series of 12 male subjects, the recorded average horizontal rotation of the tibia was 19 degrees during a gait cycle but varied between 13 and 25 degrees.[48]

At heel strike, progressive inward rotation occurs in the lower extremity, which consists of the pelvis, femur, and tibia, and this inward rotation reaches a maximum at the time of foot flat. The internal rotation at heel strike is initiated by the collapse of the subtalar joint into valgus, and its magnitude is determined by the flexibility of the foot and its ligamentous support. After contralateral toe-off, at about 12% of the cycle, progressive outward rotation occurs, which reaches a maximum at the time of toe-off, when inward rotation resumes (Fig. 1-8). Once the foot is on the ground, progressive external rotation is probably initiated by the contralateral swinging limb, which rotates the pelvis forward, imparting a certain degree of external rotation to the stance limb. This external rotation subsequently is passed from the pelvis distally to the femur and tibia, across the ankle joint, and is translated by the subtalar joint into inversion, which reaches its maximum at toe-off. The external rotation is enhanced by the external rotation of the ankle joint axis, the oblique metatarsal break, and the plantar aponeurosis after heel rise begins.

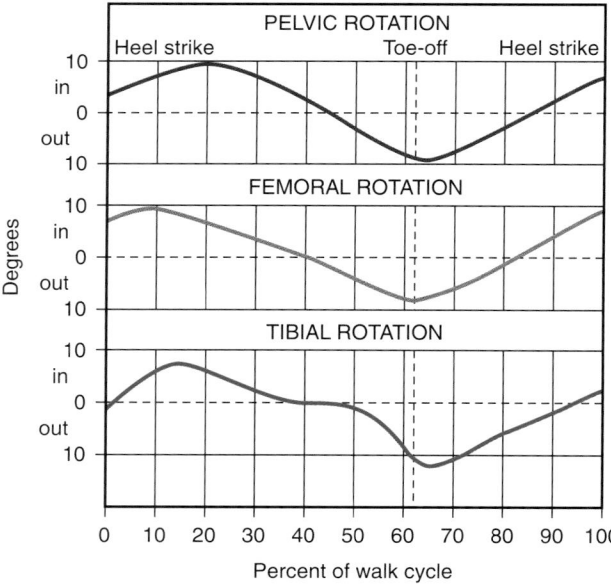

Figure 1-8 Transverse rotation occurring in the lower extremity during walking. Internal rotation occurs until approximately 15% of cycle, at which time progressive external rotation occurs until toe-off, when internal rotation begins again.

KINETICS OF HUMAN LOCOMOTION

To begin a review of gait kinetics, one must recognize that the ambulating human is both a physical machine and a biologic organism subject to physical laws and beholden to muscular action. Gait kinematics and lower-extremity anatomic interrelationships strive to achieve a system that takes us from one spot to another with the least expenditure of energy.[60] Said another way, human locomotion is a blending of physical and biologic forces that combine to achieve maximum efficiency at minimum cost. Kinetics is the study of these energy expenditures.

All characteristics of muscular behavior are exploited in locomotion. Muscle groups may accelerate or decelerate body segments at different points in the gait cycle. They may contract concentrically (as they shorten) or eccentrically (as they lengthen). Part of energy conservation during the gait cycle involves having muscles work near their peak efficiency, which tends to be at or longer than their resting length.[14,17,65] When motion in the skeletal segments is decelerated or when external forces work on the body, activated muscles become efficient. Activated muscles, in fact, are approximately six times as efficient when resisting elongation (eccentric contraction) as when shortening to perform external work.[1,5,6] In addition, noncontractile elements in muscles and specific connective tissue structures assist muscular action by providing an elastic component that stores and later releases kinetic energy.

Assessment of the forces and torques imparted by the ground on the lower extremity has illuminated the biomechanical processes at work during gait. Investigation of the pressures experienced by the various regions of the plantar foot has provided insight into the pathogenesis and treatment of many foot and ankle disorders. A number of tools have evolved to study gait kinetics. These are described in detail in the next section, followed by an analysis of kinetics during gait.

Measuring Whole Body Kinetics and Plantar Pressure

Studying the foot's interaction with the ground has a long history, ranging from examining footprints in soil to real-time mapping of plantar pressure under natural conditions. Plantar pressure and ground reaction force measurements are well established in the research realm and have been instrumental in refining our understanding of foot and ankle biomechanics. In conjunction with other technology, including high-speed cameras, video motion-sensing equipment, electrogoniometers, and electromyograph (EMG) devices, the study of the ground–foot interaction has aided the understanding of gait kinetics and kinematics.

Despite improvements in available measurement methods, however, practical collection of clinically novel information remains difficult. The wide variability of normal measures makes clinical comparisons difficult.

The large number of measurement systems and equally large number of data analysis techniques make it difficult to generalize results.

Although confirmation of areas of excess pressure and monitoring the effects of treatment may prove useful, there is little specificity between plantar pressure patterns and clinical syndromes.

Types of Studies

A variety of measurement techniques have been used to study the interaction of the foot with the ground. Indirect techniques rely on correlating other measurable gait parameters to plantar characteristics and offer the advantage of not relying on expensive and often bulky equipment. For example, an estimation of ground reaction force can be made based on a simple-to-measure temporal variable, foot–ground contact time.[13]

Direct measurement techniques rely on physical properties or electronic transducers to translate the interaction between the foot and the ground into a measurable quantity. Multiple direct measurement systems are available that use a variety of strategies to record plantar pressure or ground reaction force. Unfortunately, results obtained with different systems under similar conditions are not always similar, and even qualitative comparisons may not be appropriate.[38] Spatial resolution and sample rate affect the ability of a system to record true peak plantar pressures and to isolate particular areas under the foot.

The earliest direct measurement methods relied on physical properties of a material to capture the interaction of the foot with the ground. Casts of the foot in clay, plaster, or soil were used with the assumption that areas of deeper penetration represented areas of highest pressure.[10,21] Rubber mats incorporating longitudinal ridges,[54] pyramidal projections,[21] or a multilevel grid (such as the Harris-Beath mat),[67,78] use the elastic property of rubber which, when stood or walked on, distorts in proportion to the pressure applied (Fig. 1-9). Although fast, inexpensive, and portable, these methods have low measurement resolution and lack temporal discrimination.[67]

Optically based systems rely on visualizing the plantar aspect of the foot during stance or gait. The simplest allows observation or photographic recording of the plantar foot through a clear platform (Fig. 1-10). This provides an accurate, dynamic, qualitative representation of foot morphology. Addition of a physical transduction device between the foot and glass plate allows quantification of regionalized plantar pressures and adds the temporal component missed using a physical transduction system alone.[21] The pedobarograph places a thin plastic sheet over the clear plate.[4] The sheet is illuminated at the edges, and pressure on the plastic distorts the light in

Figure 1-9 Pressure distribution on plantar aspect of foot as demonstrated by use of barograph. As dots get larger and denser, pressure distribution is greater. (From Elftman H: A cinematic study of the distribution of pressure in the human foot. *Anat Rec* 59:481-491, 1934.)

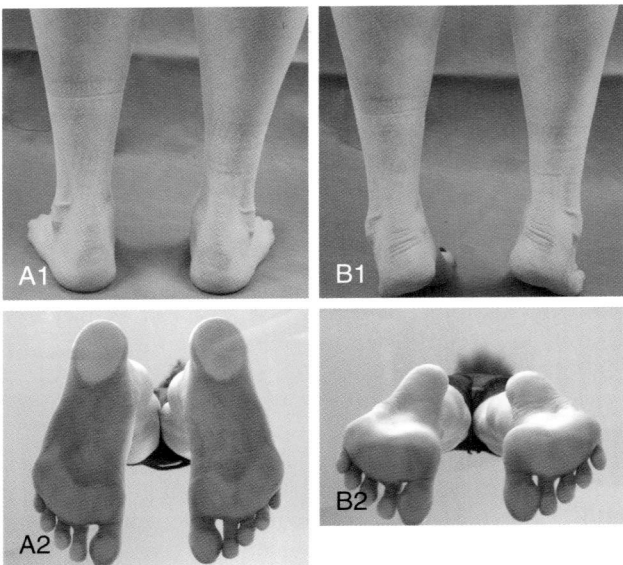

Figure 1-10 Feet and legs of person standing on barograph. **A,** Weight bearing with muscles relaxed. **B,** Rising on toes.

proportion to the pressure applied. The images can be recorded and calibrated to provide a spatial resolution and temporal responsiveness not found with the Harris-Beath mat. However, slow responsiveness at high forces may bias results.[36]

A force plate measures the ground reaction force, that is, the force exerted by the ground on the foot, in three degrees of freedom (vertical force, forward shear, side shear), and allows calculation of the torques around the foot and ankle (axial torque, sagittal torque, coronal torque). Force transducers are configured in orthogonal planes at the corners of a section of floor. The resulting data provide a representation of the average forces experienced by the foot over the gait cycle (Fig. 1-11). One advantage of this type of system is that shear forces and torques can be measured in addition to vertical force. The limitations include the lack of ability to map specific regions of plantar pressure. This limitation can be circumvented with the addition of an optical diffraction system, as described above, or with a series of smaller force plates placed in tandem.[71]

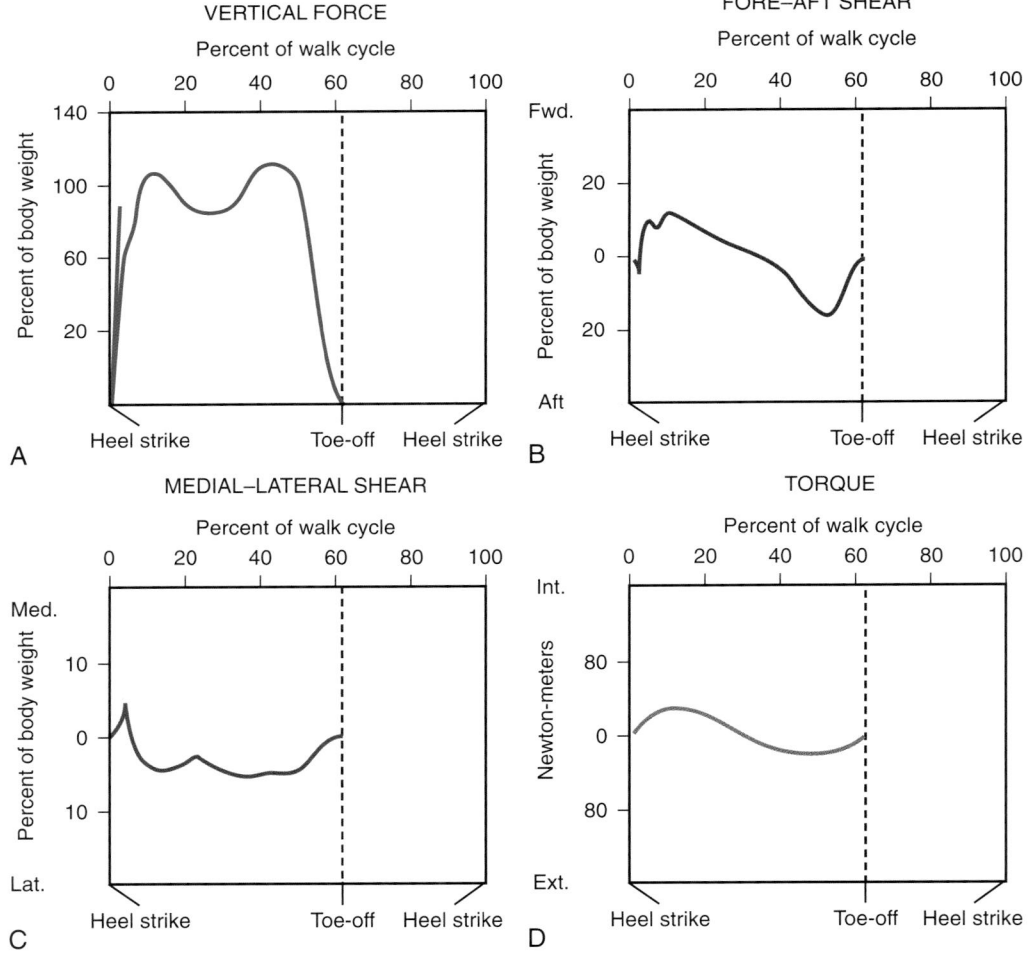

Figure 1-11 Ground reaction to walking. **A,** Vertical force. **B,** Fore–aft shear. **C,** Medial–lateral shear. **D,** Torque. *Ext.,* External; *Fwd.,* forward; *Int.,* internal; *Lat.,* lateral; *Med.,* medial.

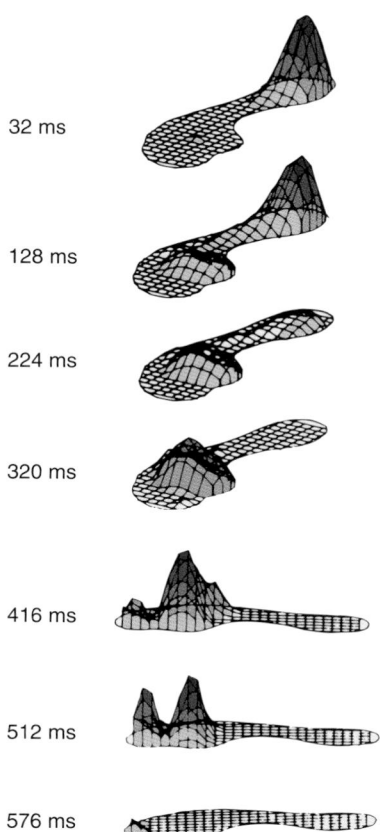

32 ms

128 ms

224 ms

320 ms

416 ms

512 ms

576 ms

Figure 1-12 Pressure distribution under bare foot during walking. Height of display above ground is proportional to pressure. (From Clarke TE: *The pressure distribution under the foot during barefoot walking* [doctoral dissertation], University Park, Pa, 1980, Pennsylvania State University.)

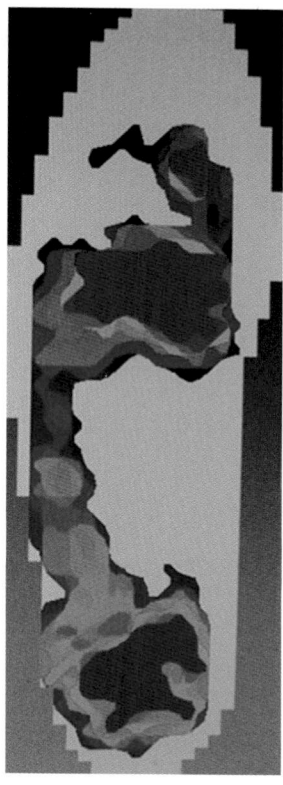

Figure 1-13 Peak plantar pressure map using an in-shoe thin-film pressure transducer. *Red* represents areas of relatively high pressure, and *violet*, areas of low pressure. (Courtesy Ken Hunt, MD.)

The ability to place pressure transducers on discrete parts of the foot has become possible, as their size has shrunk. They can be placed on strategic points of the foot, or an array can be created to map the pressures exerted by the foot during stance or gait. These data provide a spatial and temporal map of plantar pressure over the gait cycle[54,62] (Fig. 1-12). Many of these systems use a floor mat or platform built into the floor with a grid of pressure-sensitive transducers. An alternative is to place a thin film containing a pressure transduction array into a shoe (Fig. 1-13). In this way, the plantar pressures experienced by the foot can be measured in a wider variety of settings and under multiple impacts as well as account for the effect of shoe wear.[42,77] For example, feet experience 10% to 50% higher plantar pressures in a flat, flexible shoe compared with a soft shoe with a firm rubber sole.[63] The floor mat and in-shoe methods correlate well when the shoe used has a firm sole or when barefoot.[7]

A number of system-specific and analysis-dependent factors affect the results of pressure transducer array measurements, including pressure transducer density, responsiveness, linearity, resolution, and range of the transducers. Methods of analyzing the data also differ, including reporting results as force versus pressure, peak values versus sum of values over time, and strategies of regionalizing the foot's plantar surface. Increasing pressure transducer density provides better spatial representation of plantar pressure, whereas systems with relatively lower transducer density may underestimate measurements, such as peak pressure, because the true peak may be missed. Some transducers may have a nonlinear response at the extremes of their measurable range or have a low-level cutoff. The maximum sample rate affects contact time measurements, and low sample rates may underestimate peak pressure measurements because the true peak pressure may be missed.

Data Representations

Output from the different measurement systems reflects the nature of their measurement mechanisms. The Harris mat reports pedal pressure but does not vary with time. The force plate reports a true ground reaction force but in not spatially discriminative. The optical systems and the transduction arrays each report pedal pressure that varies with time. The data measured by these systems is subject to sensor density, resolution, and sample rate limitations discussed above. To simplify the information and allow comparisons between subjects or after treatments, a variety of derivative parameters have been

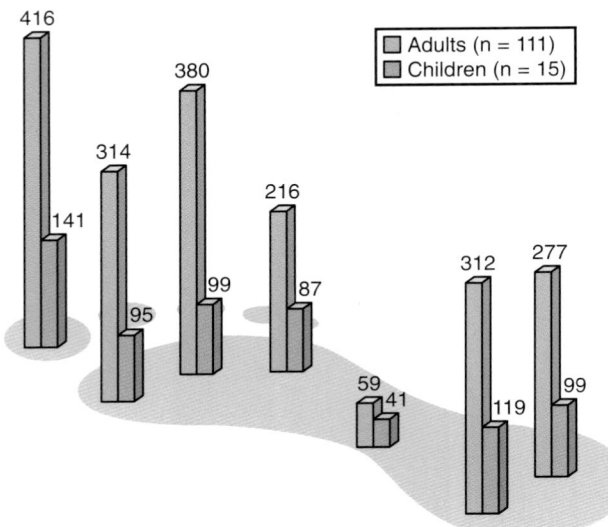

Figure 1-14 Peak pressure values under selected foot regions demonstrate impact in heel region, minimal weight bearing in midfoot, buildup of pressure beneath metatarsal heads, and transfer of weight to great toe region. (From Hennig EM, Rosenbaum D: Pressure distribution patterns under the feet of children in comparison with adults. *Foot Ankle* 11:306-311, 1991.)

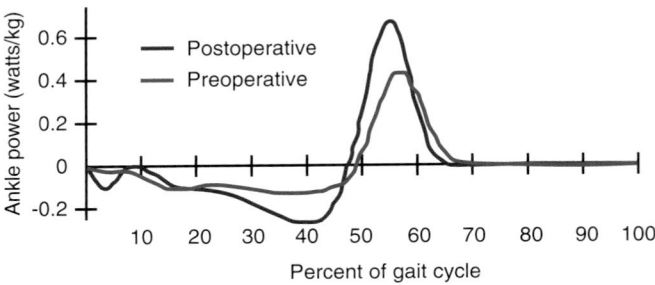

Figure 1-15 Joint power generated (positive) or absorbed (negative) during the gait cycle before and after total ankle replacement. (Modified from Brodsky JW, Polo FE, Coleman SC, Bruck N: Changes in gait following the Scandinavian Total Ankle Replacement. *J Bone Joint Surg Am* 93:1890-1896, 2011.)

defined based on these raw data. Not all systems or measurement methods are able to derive all of these measurements.

The ground reaction force is a vector quantity varying temporally and spatially over the gait cycle that represents the average reciprocal force exerted by the floor in response to the foot. It has a magnitude and direction, and the starting point may be projected onto a representation of the plantar foot at the point of average maximum vertical force (Fig. 1-14). The ground reaction force can be deconstructed into vertical force, anterior–posterior shear, and medial–lateral shear. The vertical ground reaction force represents the force of the ground pushing upward on the foot, and can be calculated from systems that measure plantar pressure for the whole foot or for defined regions of the foot.[76] Typically, it has two peaks; the first peak occurs as the body weight is transferred from dual- to single-leg stance and the second as the body weight moves forward over the metatarsal heads. Studies of ground reaction forces may focus on the magnitude of one or the other vertical peak or the timing of the peaks and valleys. Torque (moment) and power around a joint also can be calculated from the ground reaction force, joint geometry, timing parameters, and kinematics.

Another frequently reported measurement is the maximum pressure recorded, or peak pressure. It is usually reported over a spatially subdivided map of the plantar foot. Peak pressure for areas such as the heel, individual or grouped metatarsal heads, and toes are common. Alternatively, peak pressure can be reported as a temporally varying measure by displaying its location

and magnitude on a diagram of the foot. Peak force can be calculated from peak pressure because the size of the pressure transducers is known. Calculated joint moments represent the torque applied by muscles to counteract the measured ground reaction force, and joint power is calculated from the joint moment and angular velocity (Fig. 1-15).

Timing measurements can also be made. The time intervals from heel strike to metatarsal strike, toe strike, heel-off, metatarsal-off, and toe-off can be calculated. The pressure · time integral, or impulse, for the whole foot or defined regions can be calculated. This may be standardized for each region as a percentage of the total impulse for a given foot. The impulse may characterize plantar loading better than peak pressure by taking both pressure and time into consideration.

Finally, the pattern of plantar loading can be categorized based on the pressure measurements. Patients may tend to load the medial ray, the medial and central rays, the central rays, or the central and lateral rays.[35] Put another way, there is an inverse relationship between peak pressure under the first metatarsal head and toe relative to the lesser metatarsal heads.[25] As walking speed increases, a medialization of forefoot pressure occurs such that peak pressure under the first metatarsal head increases and that under the lesser metatarsal heads decreases.[64]

Measurement Variability

Many sources of variability affect the results of these measurements. Separating important clinical or research findings from differences based on testing apparatus, measurement methodology, patient demographic factors, or analysis methodology requires an understanding of how these factors affect the measured results. Differences between the different testing apparatus have been described above. Other sources of variability can be divided into methodology, analysis, and patient-specific factors.

Walking speed affects the magnitude of plantar pressures during gait. Velocity is linearly related to peak vertical and fore–aft ground reaction forces,[3,57] and inversely related to the pressure · time integral.[81] As velocity increases, peak pressures on the heel, medial metatarsal heads, and the first toe increase while peak pressure in the fifth metatarsal head decreases.[35,64] This medialization may be related to increased magnitude and velocity of hindfoot eversion and medial shear force at heel strike. Timing measurements also change with increasing speed. The normalized time to peak pressure is decreased on the heel but unchanged in the midfoot and forefoot, suggesting the rollover process is mainly accelerated by reducing the time from heel strike to foot flat.[64] To minimize variability introduced because of walking speed, subjects may walk at a fixed rate or at their natural pace.[81]

Deviations from a normal gait pattern can occur if the subject has to take a long or short stride in an effort to place the foot on the appropriate measurement area of floor-based systems. To minimize this effect, the measurement platform is placed flush with the floor and hidden from the subject with a thin, uniform floor covering. The traditional midgait method uses a short lead-up walk before the foot strikes the measurement platform. A three-step or two-step lead-up is as reproducible, but a one-step lead-up is not adequate.[15,56]

Variability of the measurements is also dependent on the type of gait. For example, plantar pressures measured when standing differ from pressures measured during gait.[10] Variations in walking patterns, such as a shuffling-type gait, alter the peak forces on the foot.[82] Gait pattern alteration can be seen in certain conditions, such as after ankle fracture fixation or with concurrent knee pathology.[3,8]

Drift and calibration of the measurement systems affect the variability of measurements. Plantar pressure measurement systems need to be calibrated to allow comparisons between systems. Transducer output varies between different transducers, with temperature, when an in-shoe system is removed and reinserted, and with the number of trials performed. Pressure can vary by as much as 20% with repeated measurements on the same insert.[63] There may be an offset that drifts with time.[56] The measurements may be adequate for relative ranking purposes but need repeated calibration with a fixed system if accurate values are needed.

Variability is also introduced in the methods by which the acquired data are analyzed. For example, peak pressure can be reported for the whole surface of the foot during a gait cycle, but the clinical utility of this is limited because different regions of the foot experience different plantar pressures during the gait cycle. Subdividing the regions of the plantar foot and recording peak pressures in each of these areas over the gait cycle provides more meaningful data. The heel is often represented as a single region but may be subdivided into medial, central, and lateral.[64] Midfoot peak pressures may be useful in pathologic conditions, such as rocker-bottom deformity, and can classify foot morphology into planus, normal, and cavus categories.[64] The base of the fifth metatarsal can be included as part of the midfoot or can be identified as a separate pressure zone. Improvements in sensor technology have allowed measurement of individual metatarsal heads and toe forefoot pressures.[25,37] Definition of these regions (masks) is still a manual process and is repeated for each trial. Having a single person define the regions may decrease variability.[37]

Subject-specific characteristics also introduce variability. Children's feet have a dramatically different loading pattern and lower peak pressure because of high relative foot area[27] (see Fig. 1-14). Differences in joint mobility and forefoot pressure based on a subject's ethnicity have been shown in neuropathic diabetics.[73] The patient's dominant side may experience greater static and dynamic vertical force,[42] although others have found no side dominance.[29] Foot morphology also affects plantar pressure; cavus feet have different midfoot loading characteristics and rate and degree of hindfoot eversion than flatfeet.[64] During running, fatigued subjects tend to have decreased step time, decreased peak and integral force and pressure under heel, and medialization of forces.[77] After a hindfoot fusion, greater contact force at heel strike has been observed.[45,69] This could be due to the inability of the calcaneus to move into a valgus position after heel strike.[2]

The effect of body weight on plantar pressure is less direct than might be expected. Although some have correlated maximum vertical force during gait and body weight,[42] many other studies found little correlation.[26,27,39] In children, the correlation of body weight to peak plantar pressures is clear and plays a greater role in determining peak pressure than in adults.[27,35] The area of peak pressure most highly correlated with body weight in children is the fourth metatarsal head,[35] and in adults may be the fourth metatarsal head or the midfoot.[27,35]

Individuals load the foot with different spatial patterns as well. After heel strike, the forefoot may be loaded more medially or laterally across the metatarsal heads and may load the metatarsals and toes simultaneously or in turn. A variety of classification systems have been proposed to group these types of loading, and biomechanical theories have been proposed to explain the different loading patterns.[35,37,76] Finally, there is an inherent variability in an individual's gait from step to step that ranges from less than 1% for vertical ground reaction force to much higher for timing-dependent variables and values calculated as a product of measures.[29] Measured values may vary by more than 10% under identical testing conditions. Averaging data from as few as three trials improves the reliability of the measurement.[39]

Kinetics of Walking

Force plates measure the force felt by the floor produced by displacement of the body's center of gravity. By Newton's law of equal and opposite forces, this is the same force experienced by the foot and represents the effect of gravitational forces on the whole body while walking.[19] The principle of the force plate is seen when one stands on a bathroom scale and flexes and extends the knees to raise and lower the body. The indicator on the dial moves abruptly as vertical floor reaction is registered.

Whole Body Kinetics

The only forces that can produce motion in the human body are those created by gravity, by muscular activity, and, in a few instances, by the elasticity of specific connective tissue structures. A force plate instantaneously records the forces imposed by the body through the foot onto the floor. These measurements include vertical floor reactions, fore and aft shears, medial and lateral shears, and horizontal torques. During the stance phase of walking, the floor reactions in all four categories are continuously changing. Figure 1-11 demonstrates the force plate data obtained during normal walking. The slower an individual walks, the less the center of gravity moves, and the resultant forces are less. Conversely, the faster the gait, the greater the movement of the center of gravity, and hence a larger force is experienced. When shoes are donned, these forces are transmitted through the interface between the sole of the shoe and the walking surface. This can attenuate rapid spikes, such as the heel striking the ground, and distribute the force over a larger area of the foot, diminishing peak plantar pressures.

The vertical element of ground reaction force is the largest of the component vectors and represents the force required to oppose the pull of gravity. It demonstrates an initial spike and rapid decline as the heel contacts the ground. Shoe material can alter the magnitude of the spike: a softer heel will result in a smaller initial spike, and a harder heel in a larger spike. The vertical ground reaction force curve then has two peaks during the stance phase. The first whole body vertical force peak is 10% to 15% greater than body weight and is caused by the upward acceleration of the body's center of gravity. This is followed by a dip to approximately 20% less than body weight as the center of gravity reaches the top of its trajectory and begins to fall. A second peak of 10% to 15% greater than body weight results from resisting the falling of the center of gravity as the body moves over the stance leg. After this, the force rapidly declines to zero at toe-off as weight transfers to the opposite limb (see Fig. 1-11A). We see from the lack of a vertical ground reaction peak at the end of stance phase that the toes do not push off but rather are lifted from the floor as the weight transfers to the other side.

Forward shear occurs at initial heel strike representing the braking of the body as it resists forward momentum. After the center of gravity has passed in front of the weight-bearing foot, an aft shear occurs. The aft shear reaches a maximum as the opposite limb strikes the ground at 50% of the walking cycle. The aft shear approaches zero at the time of toe off, once again showing the lack of push off during normal walking gait. The magnitude of the fore–aft shear, however, is only about 10% to 15% of body weight (see Fig. 1-11B).

Medial shear is the force exerted toward the midline at the time of heel strike, after which there is a persistent lateral shear until opposite heel strike at 50% of the cycle. A medial shear is not seen in persons with an above-knee amputation in whom a lateral shear mode is always present because of lack of abductor control of the prosthesis. The magnitude of the medial–lateral shear is about 5% of body weight (see Fig. 1-11C).

Lower extremity rotation during the stance phase causes a torque of the foot against the ground. After heel strike, there is an internal torque that reaches maximum at the time of foot flat, after which there is a progressive external torque that reaches a maximum just before toe-off. This torque corresponds to the inward and outward rotation of the lower extremity (see Fig. 1-11D). The majority of this rotation occurs with the foot firmly placed on the floor. The rotations, therefore, generate an internal torque of 7 to 8 newton-meters, which is of considerable magnitude.[19] The ankle and subtalar joints facilitate the transmission of rotatory forces between the foot and lower limb.

The movement of the ground reaction force vector along the bottom of a normal foot follows a consistent pattern[41] (Fig. 1-16). After heel strike, it moves rapidly forward until it reaches the metatarsal area, where it dwells for about half of the stance phase, then passes distally to the great toe. In a patient with a rheumatoid arthritis–related hallux valgus deformity and significant metatarsalgia, the center of pressure remains in the posterior aspect of the foot, avoiding the painful metatarsal area, then rapidly passes over the metatarsal heads along the middle of the foot (Fig. 1-17).[24] In patients with amputation of the great toe, the center of pressure passes in a more lateral direction (Fig. 1-18).[51]

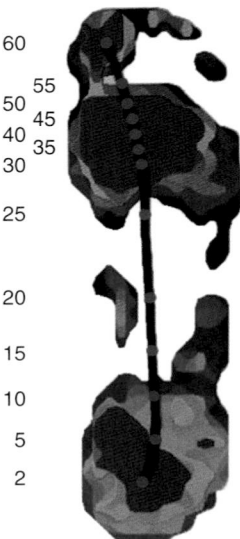

Figure 1-16 Peak plantar pressure map with superimposed path of instantaneous center of ground reaction force *(black line)*. The *red dots* and corresponding labels represent the location of the ground reaction force at a given percentage of the gait cycle.

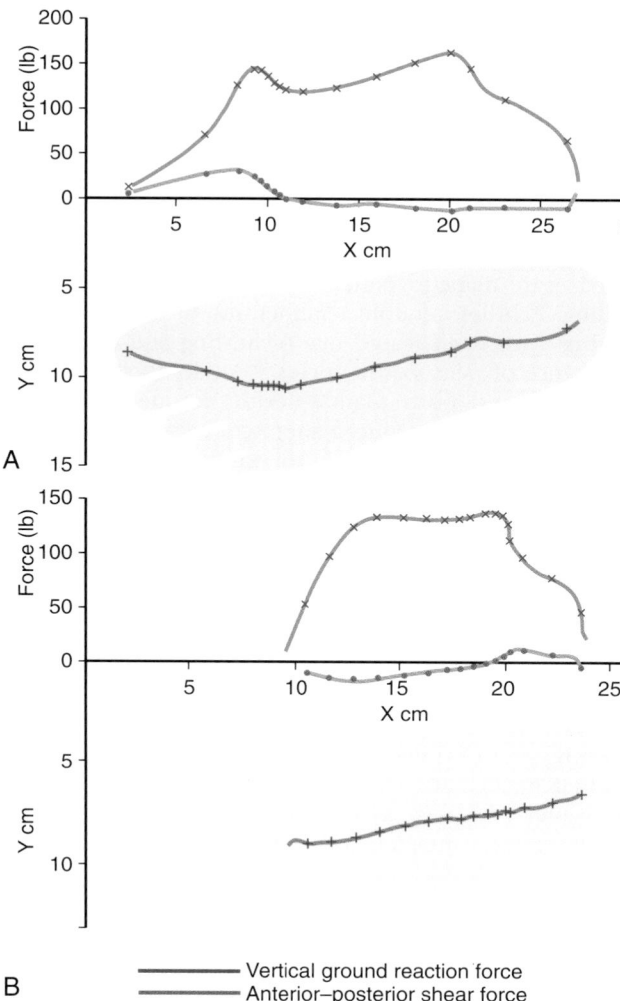

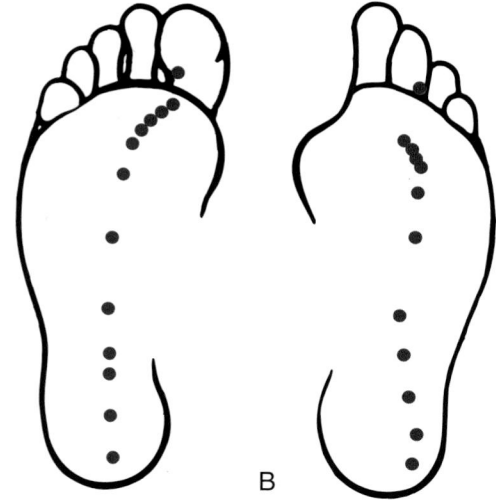

Figure 1-18 Movement of center of pressure after amputation of great toe. **A,** Normal progression of center of pressure. **B,** Abnormal movement of center of pressure after amputation of great toe. Note that pressure tends to dwell more laterally in the metatarsal area, then passes out toward the third toe rather than the great toe. (From Mann RA, Poppen NK, O'Konski M: Amputation of the great toe. a clinical and biomechanical study. *Clin Orthop* 226:192-205, 1988.)

———— Vertical ground reaction force
———— Anterior–posterior shear force

Figure 1-17 Progression of center of pressure in normal and abnormal foot, beginning at the right and progressing to the left. *Blue line* is the vertical component of ground reaction force, and *tan line* is anterior–posterior shear component of ground reaction force. Marks along the path represent ⅟₂₅-second intervals. **A,** Note progression of center of pressure from heel toward toes during normal walking cycle. The center of pressure moves rapidly from the heel, dwells in metatarsal head region, then passes rapidly to the great toe at toe-off. **B,** Progression of center of pressure in a patient with rheumatoid arthritis with severe hallux valgus deformity and significant metatarsalgia. Note that the center of pressure remains toward the heel, then rapidly progress across the metatarsal head area with little or no pressure borne by the great toe. Patients with rheumatoid arthritis or significant metatarsalgia keep their weight in the posterior aspect of foot to avoid pressure over the painful portion of foot, which may lead to a shuffling gait. (From Grundy M, Tosh PA, McLeish RD, Smidt L: An investigation of the centres of pressure under the foot while walking. *J Bone Joint Surg Br* 57:98-103, 1975.)

Plantar Pressure Kinetics

Research on plantar pressure during gait has proved useful in a number of clinically relevant areas, including forefoot pressure involving a number of clinical syndromes. Increased forefoot pressures may lead to metatarsalgia or neuropathic ulceration and is mitigated by simple insole modifications. Diabetic and neuropathic foot ulceration correlate with areas of increased vertical and shear forces.[58] The weight-bearing pattern in these patients tends to shift from the medial to the lateral border of the forefoot, and the load taken by the toes is reduced.[18] The rheumatoid foot demonstrates similar findings.[2] A soft pad placed proximal to the metatarsal heads decreases metatarsal head pressure from 12 to 60%.[34] Placement of a ½-inch lateral heel wedge decreased pressure under the third through fifth metatarsal heads by 24% and increased pressure under first and second metatarsal heads by 21%.[63] A ½-inch medial heel wedge decreased the pressure under the first and second metatarsal heads by 28% and under the first toe by 31%.

Patients with hallux valgus may develop transfer metatarsalgia as plantar pressure increases under the lesser metatarsal heads and decreases under the first toe in relation to the size of the deformity.[11,40] Those patients with hallux valgus and lesser toe metatarsalgia have greater peak pressure and peak pressure · time integral under the second through fifth metatarsal heads than those without metatarsalgia.[74] Measurement of plantar pressure may be predictive because no patients with less than 20 N · cm⁻²

peak pressure had metatarsalgia, and all patients with more than 70 N · cm⁻² peak pressure had metatarsalgia. Hallux valgus correction with proximal first metatarsal osteotomy and distal soft tissue procedure decreases peak pressure under the second and third metatarsal heads.[80] After a distal chevron osteotomy for mild-to-moderate hallux valgus, the degree of plantar displacement of the distal first metatarsal osteotomy correlates with increased pressure under the first metatarsal head and to a decrease in clinical metatarsalgia.[75] Procedures that destabilize the first metatarsophalangeal joint, such as Keller resection arthroplasty and silicone (Silastic) implant arthroplasty, increase pressure on the lesser metatarsal heads (Fig. 1-19).[20,28,40,70]

The Achilles tendon and plantar fascia also influence plantar pressure and gait biomechanics.[33] The Achilles tendon contributes to heel rise, leading to a reduction in the vertical displacement of the center of gravity and minimizing energy expenditure.[47] During the stance phase, energy is stored in the gastrocnemius–soleus complex as the ankle dorsiflexes, and the tendon is elastically stretched and is returned after heel rise as the ankle plantar flexes. This elastic recoil facilitates shortening of the gastrocnemius–soleus complex at rates well above those possible by maximal muscle contraction and allows the muscles to act at a rate and length of maximum efficiency over the gait cycle.[31,32] Gastrocnemius–soleus work increases with step length, effectively lengthening the limb by plantar flexing the ankle.[32] A chronically elongated or ruptured tendon leads to a paradoxically rigid ankle by recruiting other ankle stabilizers.[12] The time to initial peak vertical force is shortened, highlighting a loss of shock absorption, but the second peak vertical force, representing metatarsal head pressure, is not diminished.[72] In diabetic patients with plantar ulceration, adding Achilles tendon lengthening to total contact casting leads to increased rate of healing and decreased recurrence of neuropathic ulcers.[55] Ankle dorsiflexion is increased, and both plantar-flexion torque and peak plantar pressure are reduced after Achilles tendon lengthening initially, but plantar-flexor torque and peak pressure return by 7 months even though accentuated dorsiflexion remains.[55] This suggests that the decrease in peak plantar pressure may be related to a weakening of ankle plantar flexors rather than to an increase in ankle dorsiflexion.

Kinetics of Running

The forces involved during running are considerable, reaching 2.5 to 3 times body weight (Fig. 1-20). The larger forces generated are related to increased displacement of the center of gravity as the speed of gait increases. At initial ground contact, increasing the range of motion at the ankle, knee, and hip joints helps absorb these larger forces. As the speed of gait further increases, the degree of motion in these joints also increases to help absorb the added impact. Muscles are active over a greater percentage of the gait cycle during running. The gastrocnemius–soleus contribution to forward propulsion is minimal during normal walking but plays a larger role as walking speed increases.[23]

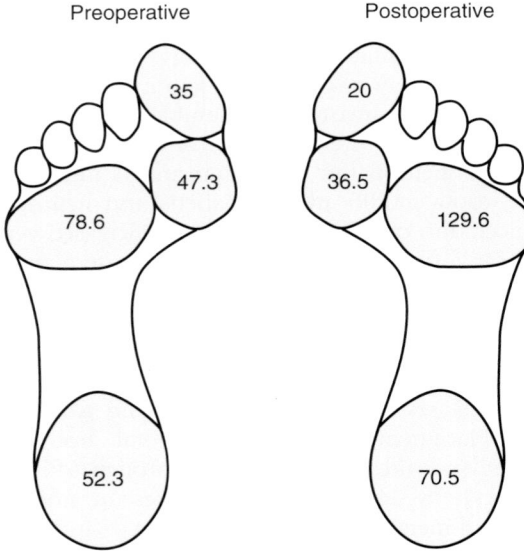

Preoperative   Postoperative

Figure 1-19 Peak forces (in newtons) measured in four areas of foot before and after silicone arthroplasty of first metatarsophalangeal joint. Preoperatively, there is significant weight bearing by first metatarsal and great toe relative to lateral metatarsals. Postoperatively, there is decreased weight bearing by first metatarsal and great toe and increased weight bearing beneath lesser metatarsal head region. This demonstrates effect of loss of windlass mechanism, by which pressure is transferred to great toe, which, in turn, depresses first metatarsal head. (From Beverly MC, Horan FT, Hutton WC: Load cell analysis following silastic arthroplasty of the hallux. *Int Orthop* 9:101-104, 1985.)

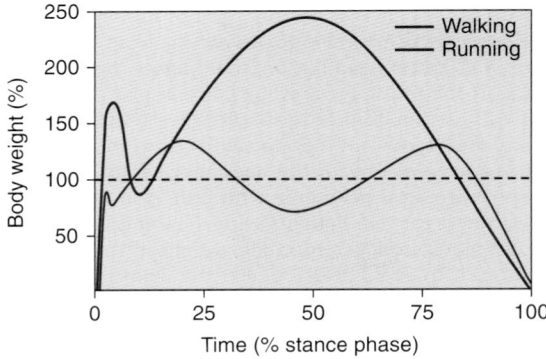

Figure 1-20 Comparison of vertical ground reaction for walking *(blue line)* and jogging *(red line)*. The horizontal axis is scaled as a percentage of total time in stance phase for walking (0.6 sec) and running (0.24 sec). The vertical axis is shown as a percentage of body weight. (From DeLee JC, Drez D, Miller MD, editors: *DeLee & Drez's orthopaedic sports medicine*, 3rd ed, New York, 2009, Elsevier.)

BIOMECHANICS OF THE COMPONENT OF THE LOCOMOTOR SYSTEM

The human foot too often is viewed as a semirigid base whose principal function is to provide a stable support for the superincumbent body. Instead, it has evolved as a dynamic mechanism functioning as an integral part of the locomotor system. From the moment of heel strike to the instant of toe-off, floor reactions, joint motions, and muscular activity are changing constantly. Floor reactions and pedal pressure measurements demonstrate the forces transmitted through the foot, continuous geometric measurements record joint motion, and electromyographic studies show the phasic activity of the intrinsic and extrinsic muscles during gait. To make it easier to understand the various events that occur during a step, a discussion of the biomechanics of the various articulations and muscles that control their function is presented. The discussion divides the gait cycle into two separate themes. The first discusses mechanisms by which the foot and ankle contribute to energy absorption during the early phases of stance, followed by a section discussing mechanisms by which the foot converts from a supple to a rigid platform allowing heel rise and toe-off. Swing phase is discussed, and finally, distinctions between walking and running gait are highlighted.

Heel Strike to Foot Flat: Supple for Impact Absorption

Ankle Joint

At heel strike, the ankle is initially dorsiflexed from swing-through and rapidly plantar flexes, reaching a maximum of 10 degrees at 7% of the cycle once foot flat has occurred

(see Fig 1-2). After heel strike, the anterior compartment leg muscles function as a group to slow the rapid ankle plantar flexion rotation. This activity continues until plantar flexion is complete. During this time, the muscle undergoes an eccentric (lengthening) contraction that helps absorb the energy of heel strike and transfer of weight from the opposite leg. Clinically, if the anterior tibial muscle group is not functioning, a foot slap is noted after heel strike, resulting from lack of control of initial ankle plantar flexion.

The direction of the ankle axis in the transverse plane of the leg dictates the vertical plane in which the foot will flex and extend. In the clinical literature, this plane of ankle motion in relation to the sagittal plane of the leg is referred to as the degree of tibial torsion. Rotation of the ankle axis in the horizontal plane can affect only the amount of toeing-out or toeing-in of the foot. Although it is common knowledge that the ankle axis is directed laterally as projected on the transverse plane of the leg, it is not widely appreciated that the ankle axis is also directed laterally and downward, as seen in the coronal plane. Inman, in anthropometric studies, found that, in the coronal plane, the axis of the ankle may deviate 88 to 100 degrees from the vertical axis of the leg (Fig. 1-21A).[43] The axis of the ankle passes just distal to the tip of each malleolus, allowing the examiner to obtain a reasonably accurate estimate of the position of the empiric axis by placing the tips of the index fingers at the most distal bony tips of the malleoli (Figs. 1-21B and 1-22).

Because the ankle joint axis is obliquely oriented, an apparent rotation of the foot relative to the horizontal plane of the leg occurs with movements of the ankle. With the foot free and the leg fixed, the oblique ankle joint axis causes the foot to deviate outward on dorsiflexion and

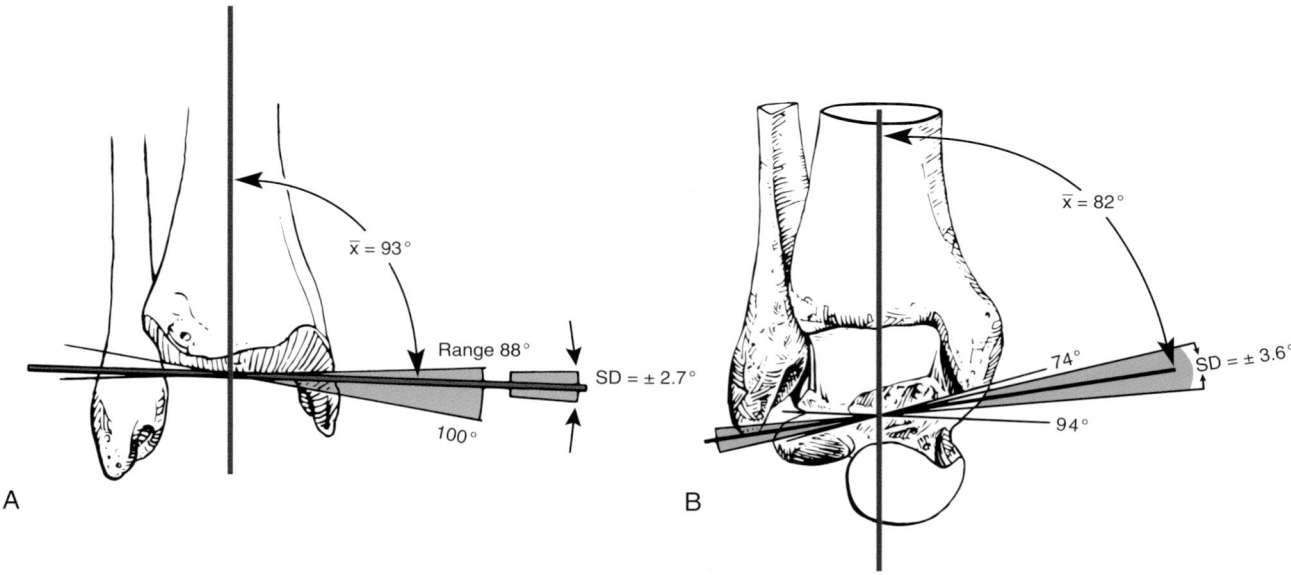

Figure 1-21 **A,** Variations in angle between midline of tibia and plafond of mortise. **B,** Variations in angle between midline of tibia and empiric axis of ankle. *SD,* Standard deviation; x̄, arithmetic mean. (From Inman VT: *The joints of the ankle,* Baltimore, 1976, Williams & Wilkins.)

inward on plantar flexion, as seen by the projection of the foot onto the transverse plane (Fig. 1-23). The amount of this rotation will vary with the obliquity of the ankle axis and the amount of dorsiflexion and plantar flexion. Conversely, with the foot fixed to the floor, the oblique ankle axis causes the tibia to rotate internally with dorsiflexion and externally with plantar flexion.

Rotations of the leg and movements of the foot caused by an oblique ankle axis, when observed independently, are qualitatively and temporarily in agreement. However, when the magnitudes of the various displacements are studied, it becomes clear that rotation of the leg attributable to ankle axis obliquity is much smaller than the degree of horizontal rotation of the leg that actually occurs. In normal locomotion, ankle motion ranges from 20 to 36 degrees, with an average of 24 degrees.[9,65] The obliquity of the ankle axis ranges from 88 to 100 degrees,

with an average of 93 degrees from the vertical.[43] Even in the most oblique axis and movement of the ankle through the maximum range of 36 degrees, only 11 degrees of rotation of the leg around a vertical axis will occur.

Subtalar Joint

The subtalar joint works in cooperation with the ankle to account for the additional leg rotation not explained by the obliquity of the ankle joint axis. The subtalar joint is a sliding single-axis joint that acts like a mitered hinge connecting the talus and the calcaneus. The axis of the subtalar joint passes from medial to lateral at an angle of approximately 16 degrees and from the horizontal plane approximately 42 degrees[17,53] (Fig. 1-24). Individual variations are extensive and impart variability to the behavior of this joint during locomotion. Furthermore, the subtalar joint appears to be a determinative joint of the foot,

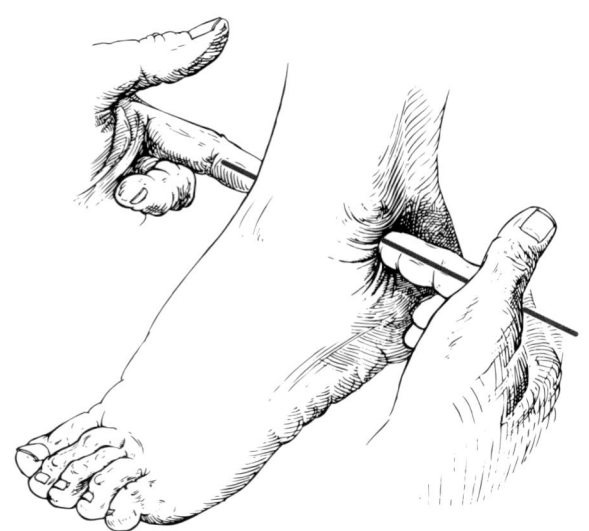

Figure 1-22 Estimation of obliquity of empirical ankle axis by palpating tips of malleoli.

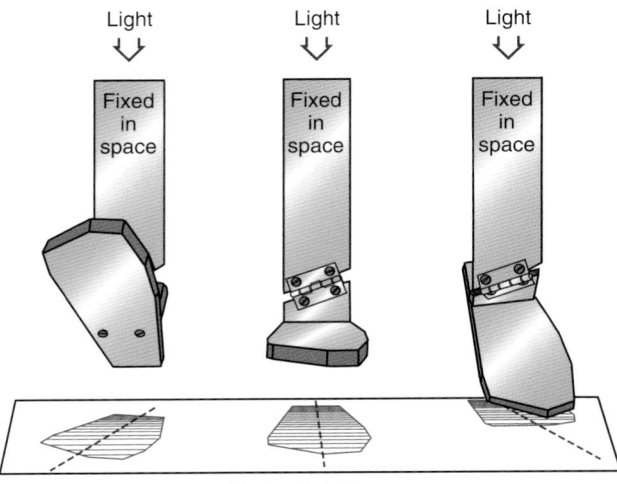

Figure 1-23 Effect of obliquely placed ankle axis on rotation of foot in horizontal plane during plantar flexion and dorsiflexion, with foot free. Displacement is reflected in shadows of foot.

Figure 1-24 Variations in subtalar joint axes. **A,** In transverse plane, subtalar axis deviates approximately 23 degrees medial to long axis of foot, with range of 4 to 47 degrees. **B,** In horizontal plane, axis approximates 41 degrees, with range of 21 to 69 degrees. $\bar{x}$, arithmetic mean. (Modified from Isman RE, Inman VT: Anthropometric studies of the human foot and ankle. *Bull Prosthet Res* 10:97, 1969.)

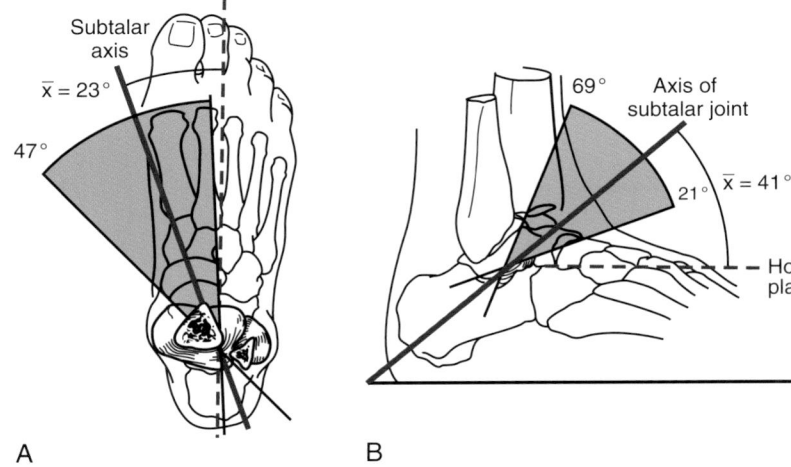

A   B

influencing the performance of the more distal articulations and modifying the forces imposed on the skeletal and soft tissues.

Based on its inclined axis, the subtalar joint functions essentially like a hinge connecting the talus and the calcaneus. The functional relationships that result from such a mechanical arrangement are illustrated in Figure 1-25A, which shows two boards jointed by a hinge. The vertical board represents the tibia and the horizontal board the foot. If the axis of the hinge is at 45 degrees, a simple torque converter has been created. Rotation of the vertical member causes equal rotation of the horizontal member. Changing the angle of the hinge alters this one-to-one relationship such that a more horizontally placed hinge causes a greater rotation of the horizontal member for each degree of rotation of the vertical member; the reverse holds true if the hinge is placed more vertically.

The model can be refined further (Fig. 1-25B) by dividing the horizontal "foot" segment into a short proximal and a long distal segment, with a pivot between the two segments. This pivot represents the transverse tarsal joint complex, which consists of the talonavicular and calcaneocuboid joints. The longer distal segment remains fixed to the floor in this model, and rotation at the transverse tarsal joint complex accommodates hindfoot inversion and eversion during stance phase. Thus the distal segment remains stationary, and only the short segment adjacent to the hinge rotates. The specific mechanics of this joint complex are discussed in the following section.

The interrelated rotation described by these models helps to demonstrate motion of the subtalar joint during walking.[79] At the time of heel strike, the subtalar joint is slightly inverted and rapidly everts, reaching a maximum at foot flat, after which progressive inversion occurs until the time of toe-off. In the normal foot, approximately 6 degrees of rotation occurs. Although quantification of subtalar joint motion remains elusive because of the

complexity of the movement, subsequent studies have confirmed qualitatively the direction of movement, namely, eversion after heel strike until foot flat, then inversion until toe-off (Fig. 1-26). Eversion of the hindfoot at heel strike occurs passively, dictated by the lateral

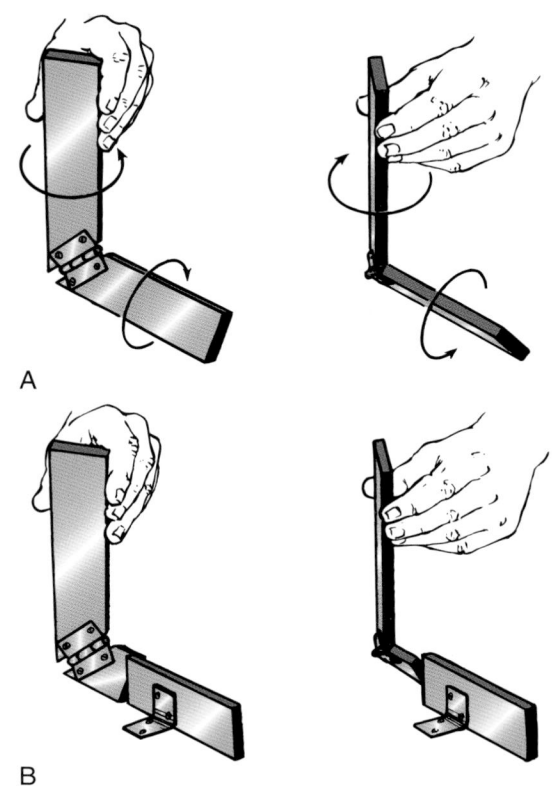

Figure 1-25 Simple mechanism demonstrating functional relationships. **A,** Action of mitered hinge. **B,** Addition of pivot between two segments of mechanism.

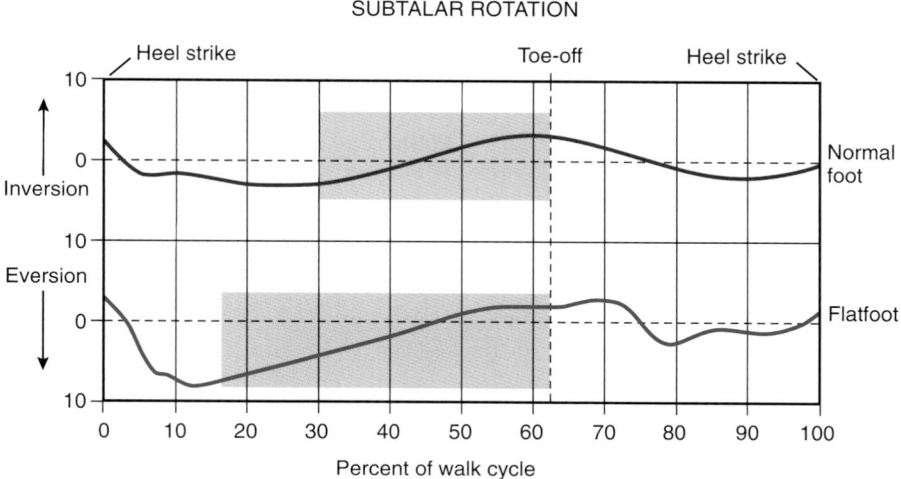

Figure 1-26 Subtalar joint motion in normal foot and flatfoot. Shaded areas indicate period of activity of intrinsic muscles in normal foot and flatfoot.

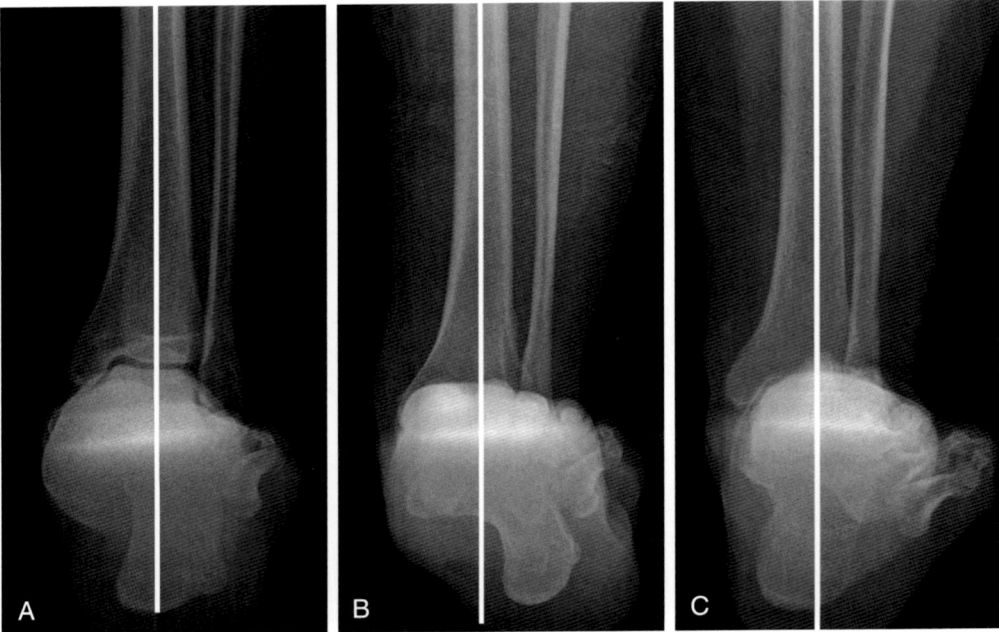

Figure 1-27 Hindfoot alignment radiographs demonstrating placement of the calcaneus relative to the weight-bearing axis of the tibia. **A,** A hindfoot with physiologic valgus shows the weight-bearing axis of the lower extremity passing through the medial aspect of the calcaneus. **B,** A flatfoot with calcaneus valgus shows the weight-bearing axis passing medial to the calcaneus. **C,** A cavus foot with calcaneus varus shows the weight-bearing axis passing through the lateral aspect of the calcaneus.

placement of the subtalar axis relative to the weight-bearing axis through the tibia (Fig. 1-27). Energy is passively absorbed by the stretch of the surrounding ligaments that control subtalar eversion.

At heel strike, there is also progressive inward rotation in the lower extremity, reaching a maximum at the time of foot flat. The internal rotation at heel strike is initiated by the collapse of the subtalar joint into eversion through the obliquity of the subtalar joint axis. The flexibility of the foot and its surrounding ligamentous support determine the magnitude of this rotation. The recording of torques imposed on a force plate substantiates these rotations. Magnitudes vary but range from 7 to 8 newton-meters.[19] Because the foot does not typically rotate on the floor, this torque is absorbed by the joint complexes and surrounding ligaments, further contributing to energy absorption during this part of stance phase.

Of interest, in persons with flatfeet, the axis of the subtalar joint is more horizontal than in persons with "normal" feet; therefore the same amount of rotation of the leg imposes greater supinatory and pronatory effects on the foot. Furthermore, people with asymptomatic flatfeet usually show a greater range of subtalar motion than do persons with more neutrally aligned hindfeet. In the neutral foot, approximately 6 degrees of rotation occurs, and in flatfoot, about 12 degrees (see Fig. 1-26). The reverse holds true for people with pes cavus, in whom the generalized rigidity of the foot, more vertical subtalar axis, and limited motion in the subtalar joint often are observed.

Transverse Tarsal Joint Complex

The calcaneocuboid and talonavicular articulations together often are considered to make up the transverse tarsal joint complex. Each possesses some independent motion and has been subjected to intensive study.[22] However, from a functional standpoint, they perform together.

Elftman[22] demonstrated that the axes of these two joints are parallel when the calcaneus is in an everted position and are nonparallel when the calcaneus is in an inverted position. The importance of this is that, when the axes are parallel, there is flexibility within the transverse tarsal joint, whereas when the axes are nonparallel, there is rigidity at the transverse tarsal joint (Fig. 1-28). Imagine a door where the hinges all line up and will open and close easily, whereas if the hinges of a door diverge, the door will be stuck in one position.

The transverse tarsal joint transmits the motion that occurs in the hindfoot distally into the forefoot, which is fixed to the ground. To approach the true anatomic situation of the human foot even more closely, the wooden foot model described above is modified to split the distal portion of the horizontal member into two structures (Fig. 1-29A and B). The medial one represents the three medial rays of the foot that articulate through the navicular and cuneiform bones to the talus; the lateral one represents the two lateral rays that articulate through the cuboid to the calcaneus. In Figure 1-29C and D, the entire mechanism has been placed into the leg and foot to demonstrate the mechanical linkages resulting in specific

EVERSION   INVERSION

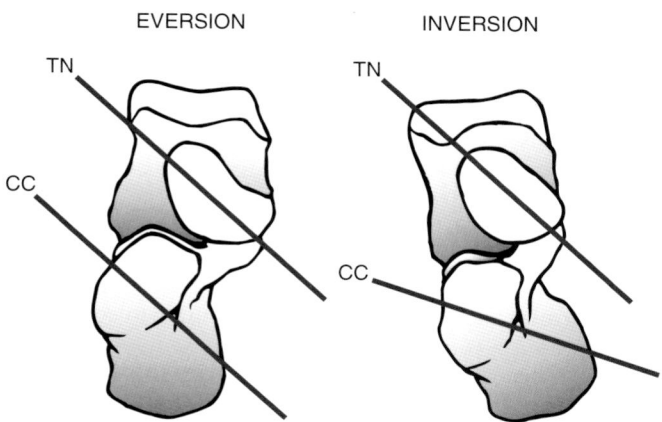

Figure 1-28 Function of transverse tarsal joint, (as described by Elftman H: The transverse tarsal joint and its control, Clin Orthop Relat Res 16:41-46, 1960.) demonstrates that when the calcaneus is in eversion, the resultant axes of talonavicular *(TN)* and calcaneocuboid *(CC)* joints are parallel. When the subtalar joint is in an inverted position, the axes are nonparallel, giving increased stability to the midfoot.

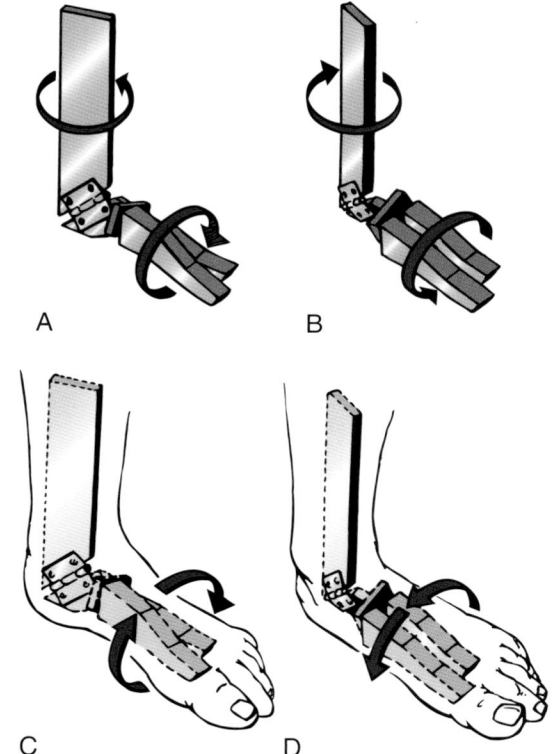

A   B

C   D

Figure 1-29 Distal portion of horizontal member replaced by two structures. **A** and **B**, Mechanical analog of principal components of foot. **C** and **D**, Mechanical components inserted into foot and leg.

movements in the leg and foot. External rotation of the leg causes inversion of the heel, elevation of the medial side of the foot, and depression of the lateral side. Internal rotation of the leg produces the opposite effect on the foot.

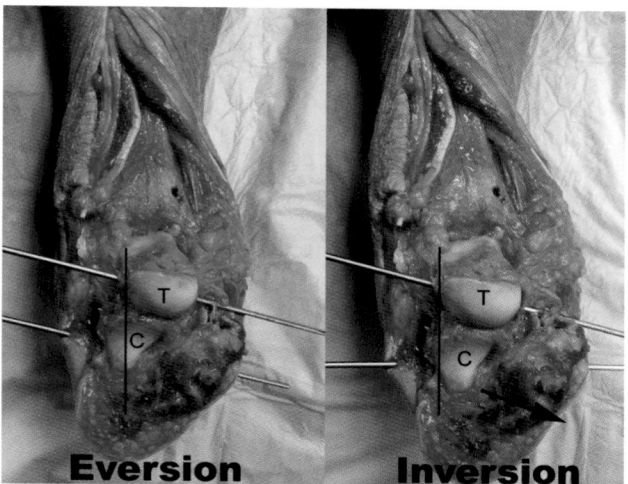

Eversion   Inversion

Figure 1-30 Anatomic specimen with the foot removed at the transverse tarsal joint complex, demonstrating the relationship between talus and calcaneus during hindfoot motion. The talar head *(T)* and calcaneal side of the calcaneocuboid joint *(C)* are shown. The *vertical line* highlights motion of the calcaneus relative to the talus. K-wires mark the axes of the respective joints. When the calcaneus is in the everted position, the talonavicular and calcaneocuboid joint axes are parallel, and the transverse tarsal joint complex is mobile. When the calcaneus is in an inverted position, following the direction of the arrow, the talonavicular and calcaneocuboid joint axes diverge, and the transverse tarsal joint complex is locked.

At the time of heel strike, as the calcaneus moves into eversion, the joints of the transverse tarsal joint complex become parallel, and the midfoot becomes flexible. Although quantification of motion in this joint has not been achieved, Figure 1-30 visually demonstrates the degree of motion that occurs in the transverse tarsal joint when the hindfoot is everted, contrasted to when it is inverted. The suppleness of the midfoot and stretch of surrounding ligaments further contributes to energy absorption during the period from heel strike to foot flat. From a clinical standpoint, the importance of this joint is observed if a subtalar arthrodesis is placed into too much inversion, resulting in stiffness of the midfoot region and causing excessive weight on the lateral border of the foot and a tendency to vault over the rigid midfoot.

Foot Flat to Toe-Off: Progression to a Rigid Platform

All of the essential mechanisms discussed in this section are pictorially summarized in Figure 1-10. The two lower photographs, taken with the subject standing on a barograph, reveal the distribution of pressure between the foot and the weight-bearing surface. (A barograph records reflected light through a transparent plastic platform; the intensity of the light is roughly proportionate to the pressure the foot imposes on the plate.) In Figure 1-10A, the subject was asked to stand with muscles relaxed. Note that the leg is moderately rotated internally and the heel is slightly everted (in valgus position). The body weight is placed on the heel, the outer side of the foot, and the metatarsal heads. In Figure 1-10B, the subject was asked to rise on his toes. Note that the leg is now externally rotated, the heel is inverted (in varus position), and the longitudinal arch is elevated. The weight is concentrated on the metatarsal heads and is shared equally by the metatarsal heads and the toes. Contraction of the intrinsic and extrinsic muscles contributes to stability of the foot and ankle as the body weight is transferred to the forefoot and the heel is raised. Dorsiflexion of the toes tightens the plantar aponeurosis and assists in inversion of the heel. The supinatory twist activates the "locking" mechanism in the transverse tarsal articulation and talonavicular joint, thus converting a flexible foot into a rigid lever. The following sections describe these changes in detail.

Ankle Joint

With the foot fixed on the ground during midstance, the body passing over the foot produces dorsiflexion of the ankle (see Fig. 1-3). The ankle undergoes progressive dorsiflexion until approximately 40% of the gait cycle, at which time plantar flexion once again begins, reaching a maximum at the time of toe-off (see Fig 1-4). The oblique ankle axis initially imposes an internal rotation on the leg, the degree of which depends on the amount of dorsiflexion and the obliquity of the ankle axis (Fig. 1-31).[48] During midstance, as the ankle dorsiflexes, a resulting internal rotational torque to the leg occurs. As the heel rises in preparation for lift-off, the ankle is plantar flexed.

This, in turn, reverses the horizontal rotation, causing the leg to rotate externally.

The posterior calf muscles basically function as a group, although the tibialis posterior and peroneus longus muscles usually begin functioning by about 10% of the stance phase, whereas the other posterior calf muscles tend to become functional at about 20% of the stance phase. As the ankle joint undergoes progressive dorsiflexion from foot flat until heel rise at 40% of the cycle, these muscles contract eccentrically. After heel rise, as ankle plantar flexion begins, they continue to contract, but now via a concentric contraction. It is interesting to note, however, that by 50% of the cycle, the electrical activity in these muscles ceases, and the remainder of the plantar flexion of the ankle joint is a passive event. High-speed motion pictures have demonstrated that during steady-state walking, at the time of toe-off, the foot is lifted from the ground, and the toes do not actively push off.

The function of the posterior calf group during stance phase is to control the forward movement of the tibia on the fixed foot.[68,72] Control of the forward movement of the stance leg tibia is critical to normal gait because it permits the contralateral leg to take a longer step, increasing stride length and improving walking efficiency. In pathologic states in which the calf muscle is weak, the stride length shortens, and dorsiflexion occurs at the ankle joint after heel strike because it is a position of stability. Paradoxically, the ankle is held more rigidly by secondary stabilizers to make up for the inability to control ankle dorsiflexion.[12]

Forces across the ankle joint reach a peak at approximately 40% of the cycle, which is when the transition from dorsiflexion to plantar flexion occurs (Fig. 1-32). The force across the ankle joint reaches approximately 4.5

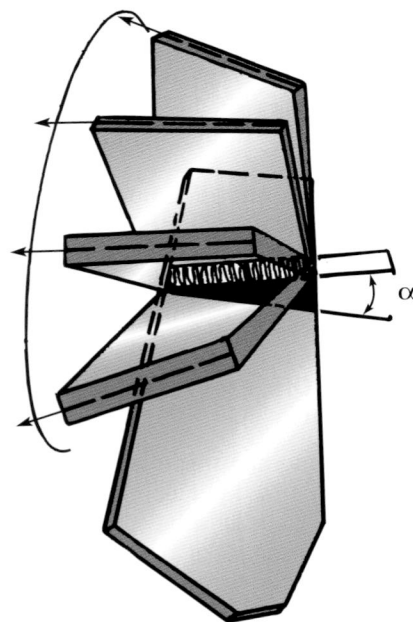

Figure 1-31 Foot fixed to floor. Plantar flexion and dorsiflexion of ankle produce horizontal rotation of leg because of obliquity of ankle axis.

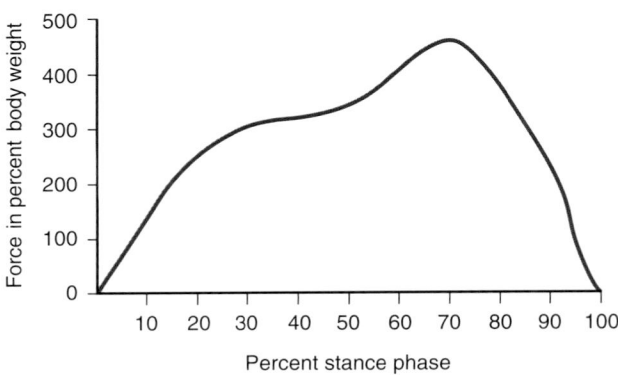

Figure 1-32 Compressive forces across ankle joint during stance phase of walking. Note that for normal subjects, force across ankle joint is approximately 4.5 times body weight at 60% to 70% of stance phase. This corresponds to 40% of walking cycle when ankle plantar flexion is beginning. (From Stauffer RN, Chao EY, Brewster RC: Force and motion analysis of the normal, diseased, and prosthetic ankle joint. *Clin Orthop* 127:189-196, 1977.)

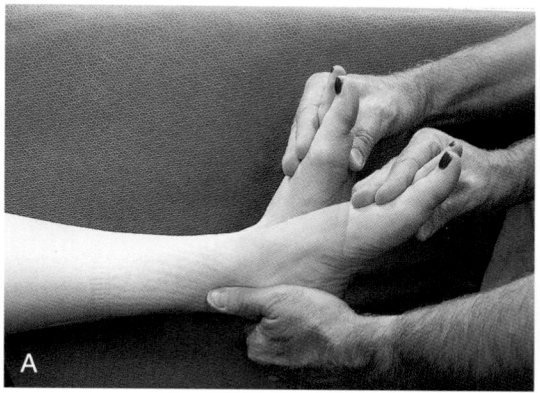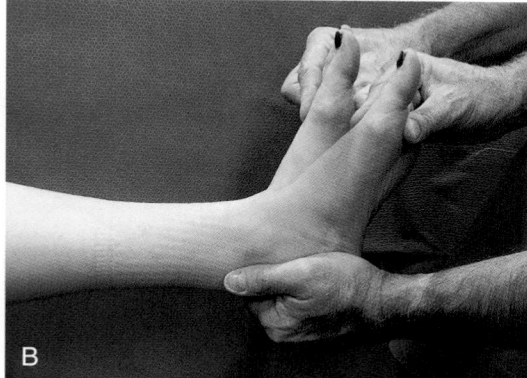

Figure 1-33 Rearrangement of skeletal components of foot. **A,** Supination of forefoot and eversion of heel permitting maximal motion in all components of foot. **B,** Pronation of forefoot and inversion of heel resulting in locking of all components of foot and producing rigid structure.

times body weight. This much force confined to a small surface area probably is one reason the components of total ankle joints may loosen and why malreduced ankle fractures rapidly progress to arthritis.

Subtalar Joint

After the hindfoot reaches maximal eversion during the initial phase of stance, it progressively inverts from the foot-flat phase through toe-off for a total arc of 6 degrees in a normal foot (see Fig. 1-26). Both passive and active mechanisms lead to this progressive inversion of the hindfoot. Hindfoot inversion stabilizes the midfoot during the later stages of stance phase by producing a rigid transverse tarsal articulation.

Muscle activity in the deep posterior compartment contributes to hindfoot inversion (see Fig. 1-3). As the posterior tibial muscle–tendon complex contracts, the hindfoot is pulled into inversion. Activity of the intrinsic muscles of the foot also contributes to midfoot stability and correlates fairly closely with the degree of subtalar joint rotation. In the normal foot, the intrinsic muscles become active at about 30% of the walking cycle, whereas in flatfoot, they become active during the first 15% of the walking cycle (see Fig. 1-26).[50]

Passive mechanisms contributing to hindfoot inversion and midfoot stabilization include the plantar aponeurosis and metatarsophalangeal break, which will be described below. Linkage of leg rotation to hindfoot motion also contributes to hindfoot inversion during the later stages of stance. The pelvis, thigh, and leg rotate externally during the last two thirds of stance. This external rotation is converted to hindfoot inversion through the oblique axis subtalar joint.[19]

Transverse Tarsal Articulation

The importance of the transverse tarsal articulation lies not in its axes of motion while non–weight bearing but in how it functions during the stance phase when the foot is required to support the body's weight. The amount of motion achievable by the transverse tarsal articulation with the forefoot fixed depends on the position of the heel. This phenomenon can be seen when examining the foot. If the examiner holds the hindfoot in an everted position, it seems the midfoot becomes "unlocked" and that maximum motion is possible in the transverse tarsal articulation. However, if the hindfoot is inverted and held firmly in one hand, the transverse tarsal articulation appears to become "locked." The previously elicited motions all become suppressed, and the midfoot becomes rigid (Fig. 1-33). The phenomenon is explained by convergence and divergence of the transverse tarsal joint axes (see Fig. 1-30).

The same relationship between hindfoot position and midfoot suppleness holds during the stance phase of gait. At the time of heel strike, as the calcaneus moves into eversion, there is flexibility in the transverse tarsal joint, and at the time of toe-off, the calcaneus is in an inverted position, resulting in stability of the transverse tarsal joint and hence the longitudinal arch of the foot. This relationship contributes to longitudinal arch stability as the heel rises from the floor, allowing the foot to act as an extension of the leg and improving stride length.

Plantar Aponeurosis

The plantar aponeurosis is a band of fibrous tissue arising from the tubercle of the calcaneus and passing distally to insert into the base of the proximal phalanx. As the plantar aponeurosis passes the plantar aspect of the metatarsophalangeal joints, it combines with the joint capsule to form the plantar plate. The function of the plantar aponeurosis has been likened to a windlass mechanism (Fig. 1-34).[30]

The plantar aponeurosis is the most significant stabilizer of the longitudinal arch between heel rise and toe-off. As the body moves over the fixed foot and the heel begins to rise, the proximal phalanges dorsiflex, pulling the plantar aponeurosis over the metatarsal heads. This tightens the plantar fascia, resulting in a depression of the

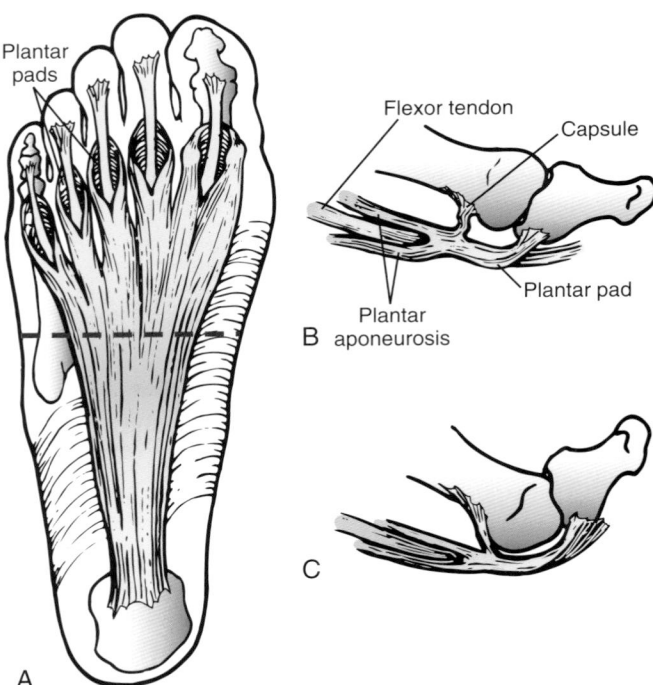

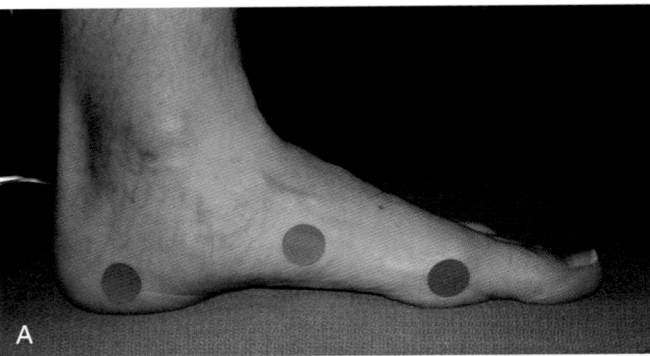

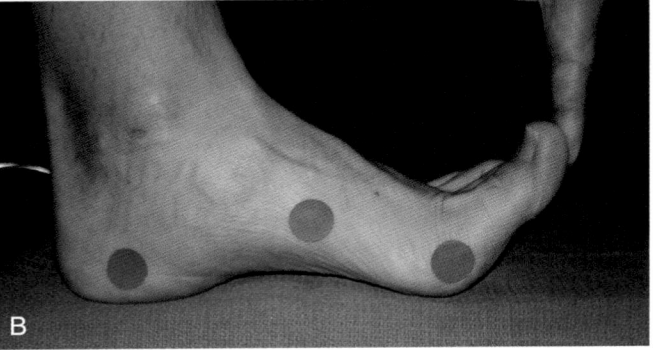

Figure 1-34 Plantar aponeurosis. **A,** Division of plantar aponeurosis around flexor tendons. **B,** Components of plantar pad and its insertion into base of proximal phalanx. **C,** Extension of toes draws plantar pad over metatarsal head, pushing it into plantar flexion.

metatarsal heads and an elevation of the longitudinal arch (Fig. 1-35). This mechanism is passive in that no muscle function per se brings about this stabilization.

The plantar aponeurosis is most functional on the medial side of the foot and becomes less functional as one moves laterally toward the fifth metatarsophalangeal articulation. Based on its medial attachment to the calcaneus, plantar fascia tightening also contributes to hindfoot inversion, tibial external rotation, and transverse tarsal joint stabilization.[16] These changes stabilize the midfoot and allow the foot to act as a rigid lever during the toe-off phase of gait.

The mechanics of the windlass mechanism can be demonstrated clinically by having an individual stand and forcing the great toe into dorsiflexion. As this occurs, one observes elevation of the longitudinal arch by the depression of the first metatarsal by the proximal phalanx, and, at the same time, inversion of the calcaneus. Careful observation of the tibia demonstrates that it externally rotates in response to this calcaneal inversion.

Metatarsophalangeal Break

The metatarsophalangeal break refers to the axis formed by the unequal forward extension of the metatarsals. The head of the second metatarsal is the most distal head; that of the fifth metatarsal is the most proximal. Although the first metatarsal usually is shorter than the second (because the first metatarsal head is slightly elevated and is

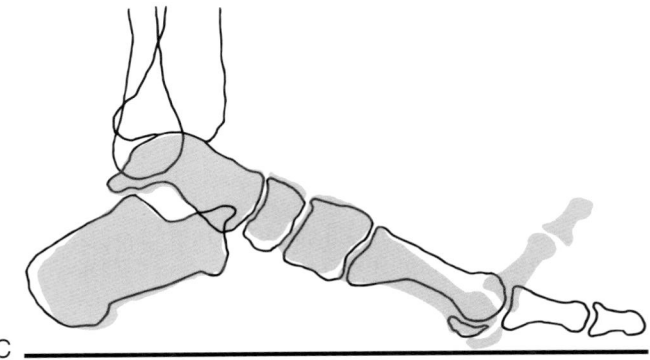

Figure 1-35 Dynamic function of plantar aponeurosis. **A,** Foot at rest. **B,** Dorsiflexion of metatarsophalangeal joints, which activates windlass mechanisms, brings about elevation of longitudinal arch, plantar flexion of metatarsal heads, and inversion of heel. **C,** Superimposed tracing of lateral radiographs of the foot at rest *(outline)* and with first ray dorsiflexion *(gray figure)*. Notice that dorsiflexion of the first toe tightens the plantar aponeurosis, which results in depression of the metatarsal heads, elevation and shortening of the longitudinal arch, inversion of the calcaneus, and elevation of the calcaneal pitch. (From DeLee JC, Drez D, Miller MD, editors: *DeLee & Drez's orthopaedic sports medicine,* 3rd ed, New York, 2009, Elsevier.)

supported by the two sesamoid bones), it often functionally approximates the length of the second.

When the heel is elevated during standing or at the time of toe lift-off, all the metatarsal heads normally share the weight of the body. To achieve this fair division, the foot must supinate slightly and deviate laterally. After

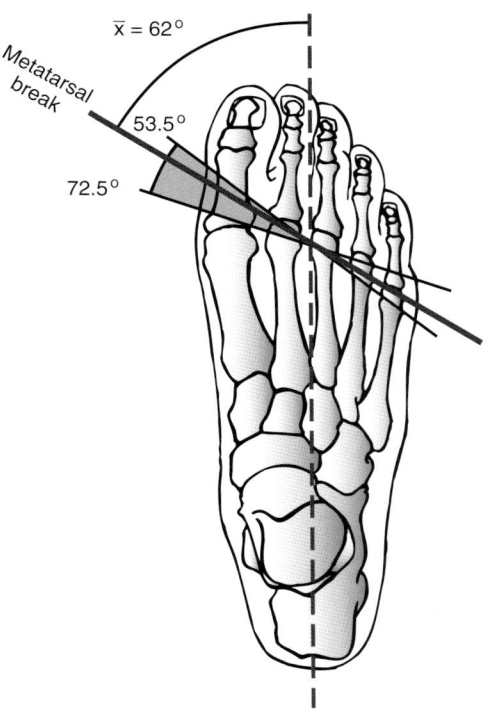

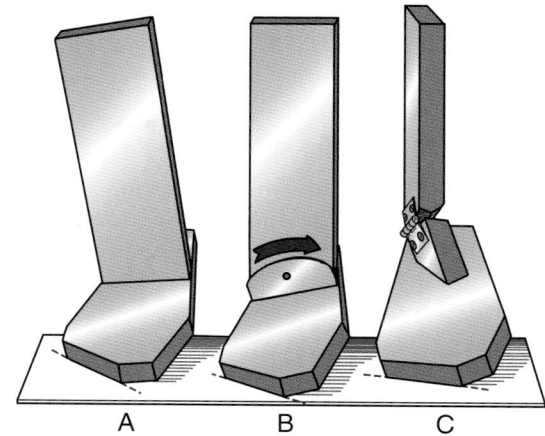

Figure 1-37 Supination and lateral deviation of foot during raising of heel caused by oblique metatarsophalangeal break. **A,** Wooden mechanism without articulation. If no articulation is present, leg deviates laterally. **B,** Wooden mechanism with articulation. Leg remains vertical; hence some type of articulation must exist between foot and leg. **C,** Articulation similar to that of subtalar joint. In addition to its other complex functions, subtalar joint also functions to permit leg to remain vertical.

Figure 1-36 Variations in metatarsal break in relation to longitudinal axis of foot. (From Isman RE, Inman VT: Anthropometric studies of the human foot and ankle. *Bull Prosthet Res* 10:97, 1969.)

wearing a new pair of shoes for a while, one notices the appearance of an oblique crease in the area overlying the metatarsophalangeal articulation (Fig. 1-36). This oblique crease demonstrates the metatarsophalangeal break. The angle between the metatarsophalangeal break and the long axis of the foot may vary from 50 to 70 degrees.[44] The more oblique the metatarsophalangeal break, the more the foot must supinate and deviate laterally after heel rise.

If the leg and foot acted as a single rigid member without ankle, subtalar, or transverse tarsal articulations, the metatarsophalangeal break would cause lateral inclination and external rotation of the leg (Fig. 1-37A). However, the subtalar joint accommodates this supination and permits the leg to remain in a vertical plane during walking (Fig. 1-37B and C).

Talonavicular Joint

The talonavicular joint morphology adds additional stability to the longitudinal arch when force is applied across it during the last half of the stance phase. The joint surface has different curvature of radius in the anteroposterior and lateral projections (Fig. 1-38). When force is applied across a joint of this shape, stability is enhanced. This occurs at toe-off, when the plantar aponeurosis has stabilized the longitudinal arch and most of the body weight is being borne by the forefoot and medial longitudinal arch.

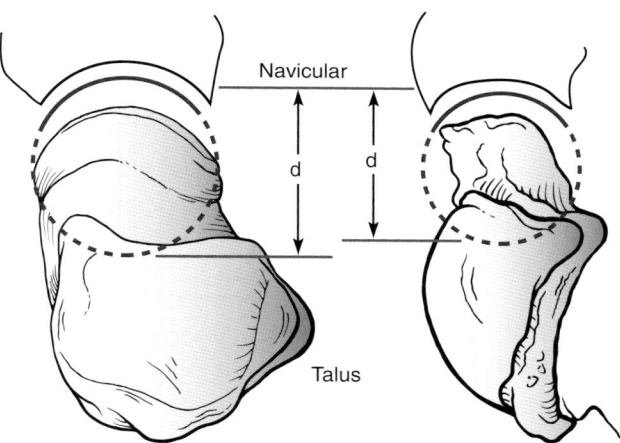

Figure 1-38 Talonavicular joint. *Left,* Anterior view. *Right,* Lateral view. Relationship of head of talus to navicular bone shows differing diameters of head of talus. (From Mann RA: Intractable Plantar Keratoses. In Nicholas JA, Hershman EB, editors: *The lower extremity and spine in sports medicine,* ed 2, St Louis, 1995, Mosby.)

Swing Phase

During swing phase, dorsiflexion occurs at the ankle joint. Beginning at about 55% of the cycle and throughout swing phase, the anterior compartment muscles contract concentrically to dorsiflex the ankle. The medial insertion of the tibialis anterior tendon pulls the hindfoot into slight inversion during swing phase such that the calcaneus is slightly inverted at initial heel strike. This is why most people will wear down the outer edge of the heel in their shoes asymmetrically. Anterior compartment musculature weakness results in a footdrop gait, characterized by accentuated hip flexion or circumduction of the hip during swing phase to avoid the toes of the dropped foot hitting the floor during swing-through.

Component Mechanics of Running

During running, the stance phase is diminished from approximately 0.6 second while walking to 0.2 second while sprinting (Fig. 1-39). During this brief period of stance phase, the forces involved in the vertical plane are increased to 2.5 to 3 times body weight. The range of

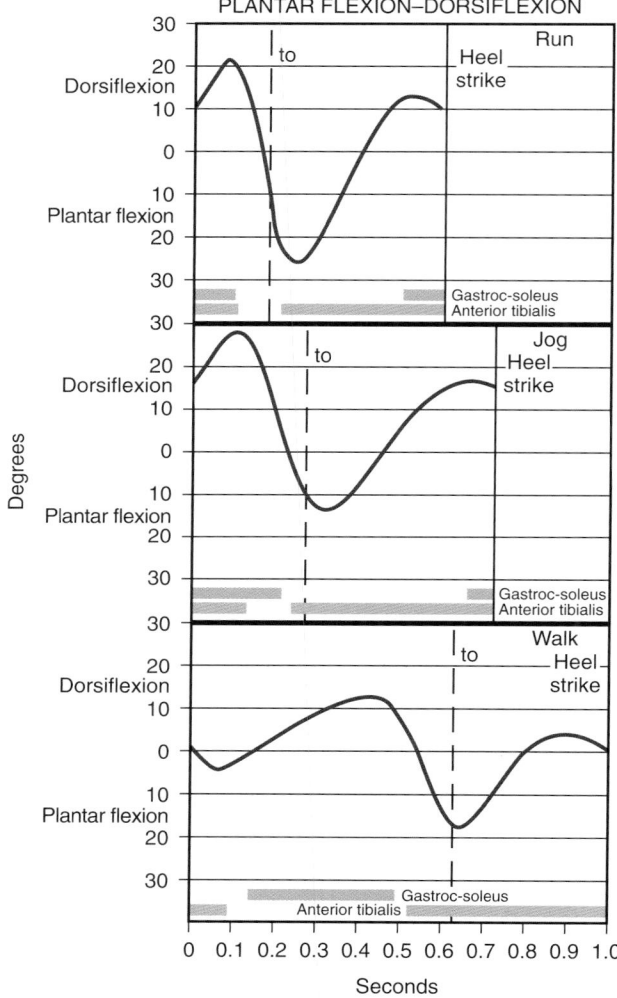

Figure 1-39 Ankle joint dorsiflexion–plantar flexion during running, jogging, and walking. Note that time of walking cycle decreases from 1 second for walking to approximately 0.6 second for running. Stance-phase time decreases significantly, as well. Muscle function is characterized by gastrocnemius–soleus muscle group and anterior tibial muscle. Note that gastrocnemius–soleus muscle group becomes active in late swing phase for jogging and running, compared with stance-phase muscle for walking. (From Mann RA: Intractable Plantar Keratoses. In Nicholas JA, Hershmann EB, editors: *The lower extremity and spine in sports medicine*, ed 2, St Louis, 1995, Mosby.)

motion of the joints is increased approximately 50%, and the muscles in the lower extremity must control these motions over a short time when measured in real time but over a considerable period when expressed as percentage of the gait cycle. It is probably because of the increased forces and muscle action required over a shorter period of time, and the repetitive nature of sport, that overuse injuries occur during running.

Considerable alterations occur around the ankle joint when comparing jogging or running with walking. The gait cycle time progressively decreases from 1 second to 0.6 second. The ankle's total arc of motion increases from 30 degrees during walking to 45 degrees during running. This motion occurs during 0.6 second for walking and 0.2 second for running. The direction of motion also changes: during walking, plantar flexion occurs at heel strike, whereas during jogging and running, there is progressive dorsiflexion. Rapid plantar flexion occurs at toe-off during all speeds of gait.

Along with this increase in the range of motion and in the forces generated during running, the muscle function in the lower extremity also is altered. In real time, the phasic activity of most muscles decreases; however, when considered as a percentage of the gait cycle, the period of activity of these muscles increases considerably. Generally speaking, at initial ground contact, the majority of the muscles about the hip, knee, and ankle joints are active, and their period of activity, which begins during the late float phase, increases as the speed of gait increases. This is probably related to the rapid motion required by these joints in preparation for the impact of ground contact. During walking, there is adequate time for most of the preparation for ground contact to be carried out rather passively, but with the markedly increased range and speed of motion of these joints during running, muscle function plays a more active role. As the speed of gait increases, the muscle function in the posterior calf group changes significantly. During walking, the posterior calf group functions in stance phase, and during jogging and running, it performs in late swing phase; its activity is ongoing from the time of initial ground contact through most of the stance phase. The muscle group controls the ankle dorsiflexion that occurs after initial ground contact, the forward movement of the tibia, and brings about plantar flexion of the ankle joint. Similar changes in both the magnitude of motion and muscle function occur about the hip and knee joints as well. During running and changing direction, as well as acceleration and deceleration, the toes play an active role in push-off, whereas push-off is minimal during steady-state walking.

SURGICAL IMPLICATIONS OF BIOMECHANICS OF THE FOOT AND ANKLE

The purpose of this section is to correlate the biomechanical principles discussed thus far with some of the surgical procedures carried out about the foot and ankle. The decisions made by the orthopaedic surgeon when planning and undertaking a surgical procedure depend on a thorough understanding of biomechanical principles.

Biomechanical Considerations in Ankle Arthrodesis

Because the subtalar and ankle joints work together during gait, it is important that certain anatomic facts be kept in mind when carrying out an ankle arthrodesis. An arthrodesis of the ankle joint places increased stress on the subtalar joint below and the knee joint above. The degree of internal or external tibial torsion, genu varum or genu valgum, proximal muscle weakness, and configuration of the longitudinal arch should be considered.

When an ankle arthrodesis is carried out, the degree of transverse rotation placed in the ankle mortise must be carefully considered so that increased stress is not caused within the foot. If the ankle is placed into excessive internal rotation, the patient experiences difficulty when the center of gravity passes over the foot. The position of internal rotation places increased stress on the subtalar and midtarsal joint region, which may become painful as a result of increased stress. Knee pain, and possibly hip pain, also may develop secondarily as a result of attempts to externally rotate the lower limb to help compensate for the abnormal position of the foot. If the ankle is placed into too much external rotation, the patient tends to roll over the medial border of the foot. This position permits the patient to easily roll over the foot, but in turn, it places increased stress on the medial side of the first metatarsophalangeal joint, which can lead to a hallux valgus deformity. It may also cause increased stress along the medial side of the knee joint.

The degree of varus or valgus tilt of the ankle joint must be carefully considered and should be related to the degree of subtalar joint motion and the overall alignment of the knee and tibia. If the subtalar joint is stiff and unable to compensate for any malalignment, it is imperative to place the ankle joint into sufficient valgus position to obtain a plantigrade foot. If the ankle joint is placed into varus position, the patient will walk on the lateral border of the foot. This not only causes the patient discomfort because of localized weight bearing in a relatively small area, but the persistent varus position of the subtalar joint keeps the transverse tarsal joint in a semirigid state, resulting in a rather immobile forefoot that is difficult for the body to pass over during the stance phase.

The degree of dorsiflexion and plantar flexion of the ankle joint must also be carefully considered when carrying out an ankle arthrodesis. If there is a short lower extremity or an unstable knee joint as a result of weakness or loss of quadriceps function, the ankle joint should be placed into plantar flexion (10 to 15 degrees) to help give stability to the knee joint. If the pathologic process involves only the ankle joint, a neutral position is considered the position of choice. If the ankle joint is placed into excessive plantar flexion, the involved limb is lengthened, which, in turn, causes a back-knee thrust on the knee joint, uneven gait pattern, and stress across the midfoot. If the ankle is placed into too much dorsiflexion, the impact of ground contact is concentrated in one small area of the heel, which may result in chronic pain. After an ankle arthrodesis, patients usually develop increased motion in the sagittal plane, which helps to compensate for loss of ankle motion. In our study of 81 ankle fusions, the sagittal arc of motion of the talar first metatarsal averaged 24 degrees (9 to 43 degrees), at the talonavicular joint 14 ± 5 degrees, and at the talocalcaneal joint 8 ± 6 degrees (Fig. 1-40).[52]

Hindfoot Alignment

Rotation occurs in the transverse plane during normal walking. This transverse rotation increases as we proceed from the pelvis to the ankle. Internal rotation occurs at initial ground contact, followed by external rotation until toe-off, when internal rotation begins again (see Fig. 1-8). This transverse rotation passes across the ankle joint and is translated by the subtalar joint to the calcaneus and foot. The loss of subtalar joint motion may result from trauma, arthritis, surgery, or congenital abnormality. This loss of rotation causes increased stress to be placed on the

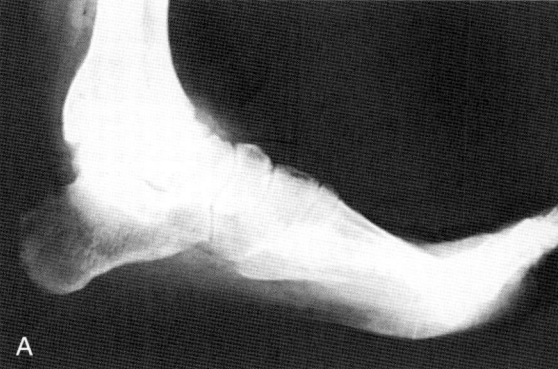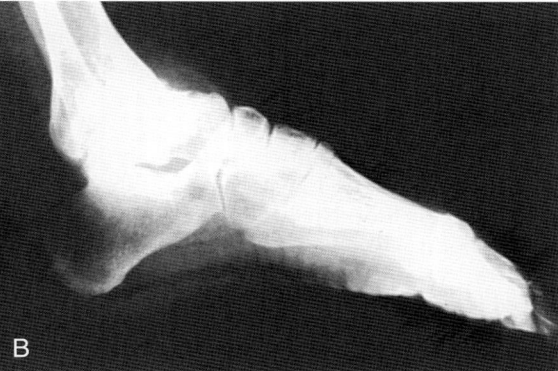

Figure 1-40 Increased motion in transverse tarsal and subtalar joints to compensate for ankle arthrodesis. **A,** Dorsiflexion. **B,** Plantar flexion.

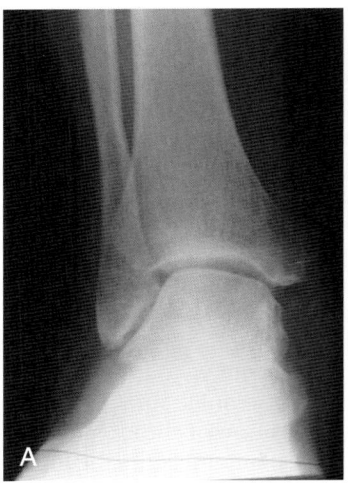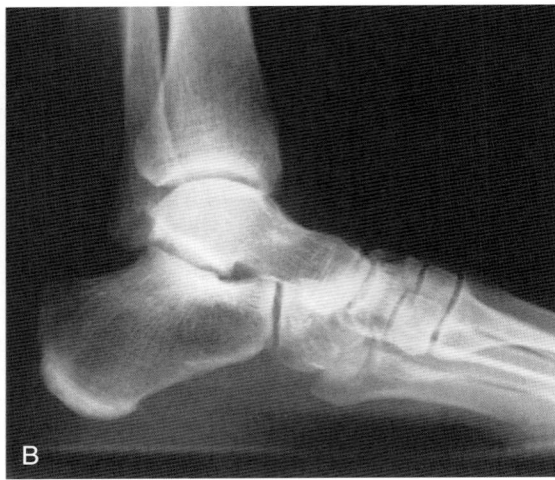

Figure 1-41 Etiology of a ball-and-socket ankle joint in adults. **A,** As a result of a congenital abnormality of the subtalar joint that eliminated subtalar motion, the ankle joint absorbed transverse rotation that normally occurs in subtalar joint. **B,** A congenital talonavicular fusion, which results in loss of subtalar joint motion, causes the ankle to absorb transverse rotation, resulting in a ball-and-socket ankle joint.

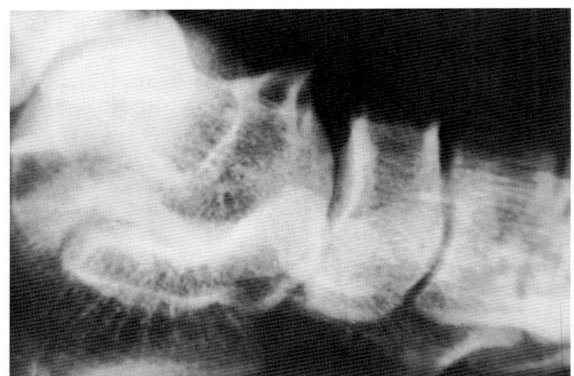

Figure 1-42 Talar beaking after increased stress as result of subtalar coalition.

joint above (ankle) and below (transverse tarsal) the immobile joint. These changes brought on by lack of subtalar joint function may lead to chronic pain. The increased stress may cause secondary changes to occur in some individuals, which may take the form of a ball-and-socket ankle joint (Fig. 1-41). At other times, beaking may occur in the talonavicular joint in a patient with a subtalar coalition (Fig. 1-42).

When a subtalar joint is fused, the transverse rotation that occurs in the lower extremity is partially absorbed in the ankle joint because it no longer can pass through the subtalar joint into the foot. The varus or valgus alignment of the subtalar joint will affect the position of the forefoot, so accurate alignment is essential. If the subtalar joint is placed into too much varus, the forefoot is rotated into supination, and the weight-bearing line of the extremity then passes laterally to the calcaneus and fifth metatarsal. This results in increased stress on the lateral collateral ligament structure and abnormal weight bearing along the lateral aspect of the foot. This position also holds the forefoot in a semirigid position, so the patient must either vault over it or place the foot in external rotation to roll over the medial aspect.

The position of choice is a valgus tilt of about 5 degrees in the subtalar joint because this permits satisfactory stability of the ankle joint, and the weight-bearing line of the body will pass medial to the calcaneus; therefore no stress will be placed on the lateral collateral ligament structure. This position results in slight pronation of the forefoot, which permits even distribution of weight on the plantar aspect of the foot. The slight valgus position also allows the forefoot to remain flexible so that the body can more easily pass over it.

Midfoot Alignment

When surgical stabilization of the talonavicular or transverse tarsal joint is carried out, motion in the subtalar joint is largely eliminated. For motion to occur in the subtalar joint, rotation of the navicular over the head of the talus must occur. If it cannot, there is essentially no subtalar joint motion. An isolated fusion of the calcaneocuboid joint results in about a 30% loss of subtalar joint motion. Motion of the subtalar joint directly affects the stability of the foot through its control of the transverse tarsal joint. When the subtalar joint is in valgus position, the transverse tarsal joint is unlocked and the forefoot is flexible. Conversely, when the subtalar joint is inverted, the transverse tarsal joint is locked and the forefoot is fairly rigid. Because of the role the transverse tarsal joint plays in controlling the forefoot, it is essential that the foot be placed in a plantigrade position when the joints are stabilized. If the foot is placed into too much supination, the medial border of the foot is elevated, and undue stress is placed on the lateral aspect of the foot. It also creates a rigid forefoot. The position of choice is neutral rotation or slight pronation, which ensures a flexible plantigrade foot.

When a triple arthrodesis is carried out, the position of choice is 5 degrees of valgus for the subtalar joint and neutral rotation of the transverse tarsal joint. It should be emphasized, however, that it is better to err on the side of too much valgus and pronation to keep the weight-bearing line medial to the calcaneus because that produces a more flexible plantigrade foot. When carrying out a pantalar arthrodesis, the same basic principles apply.

Surgical stabilization of the intertarsal and medial three tarsometatarsal joints can be carried out with minimum loss of function or increased stress on the other joints in the foot. The intertarsal joints, which are distal to the transverse tarsal joint and proximal to the metatarsophalangeal joints, have little or no motion between them. The lateral two tarsometatarsal joints are more flexible, and surgically, strategies that maintain flexibility are favored to fusion.

Forefoot Principles

Removal of the base of the proximal phalanx of the great toe causes instability of the medial longitudinal arch as a result of disruption of the plantar aponeurosis and the windlass mechanism. This leads to decreased weight bearing of the first metatarsal head, which results in weight being transferred to the lesser metatarsal heads. Surgical techniques that remove the proximal phalanx base but preserve the plantar plate may lessen this effect. If the base of the proximal phalanx of one of the lesser toes is removed, a similar problem of instability occurs, but to a much lesser degree, particularly moving laterally across the foot. Conversely, resection of the metatarsal head, except in severe disease states such as rheumatoid arthritis or diabetes, results in a similar problem because the windlass mechanism is destroyed as a result of the relative shortening of the ray. This also causes increased stress and callus formation beneath the adjacent metatarsal head, which is subjected to increased weight bearing.

When carrying out an arthrodesis of the first metatarsophalangeal joint for such conditions as hallux rigidus, recurrent hallux valgus, or degenerative arthritis, the alignment of the arthrodesis site is critical. The metatarsophalangeal joint should be placed into approximately 10 to 15 degrees of valgus and 15 to 25 degrees of dorsiflexion in relation to the first metatarsal shaft. The degree of dorsiflexion depends to a certain extent on the heel height of the shoe that the patient desires to wear. An arthrodesis of the first metatarsophalangeal joint has a minimum effect on gait. The arthrodesis places increased stress on the interphalangeal joint of the hallux. This increased stress may result in degenerative changes over time, but these rarely become symptomatic. From a theoretic standpoint, increased stress is placed on the first metatarsocuneiform joint after arthrodesis of the metatarsophalangeal joint, but it is unusual to see any form of degenerative change.

An isolated arthrodesis of the interphalangeal joint of the great toe does not seem to have any significant effect on the biomechanics of gait, nor does an arthrodesis of the proximal and distal interphalangeal joints of the lesser toes.

Resection of a single sesamoid bone because of a pathologic condition, such as a fracture, avascular necrosis, or intractable plantar keratosis, may be done with relative impunity. If, however, one sesamoid already has been removed, the second sesamoid probably should not be removed because of risk of a cock-up deformity of the metatarsophalangeal joint. This occurs because the intrinsic muscle insertion into the proximal phalanx of the great toe encompasses the sesamoids, and when the sesamoid is removed, this insertion is impaired to a varying degree. If adequate intrinsic function is not present, flexion of the proximal phalanx cannot be brought about, and a cock-up deformity results.

Tendon Transfers

When evaluating muscle weakness or loss about the foot and ankle, the diagram in Figure 1-43 can be useful. It demonstrates the motion that occurs around each joint axis and the location of the muscles in relation to the axes. By considering the muscles in relation to the axes, it is possible to carefully note which muscles are functioning and thereby determine which muscles might be transferred to rebalance the foot and ankle. Generally speaking, if inadequate strength is present to balance the foot adequately, it is important to establish adequate plantar flexion function over that of dorsiflexion; an equinus gait is not as disabling as a calcaneal-type gait. Also keep in mind that it is much more difficult to retrain a muscle that has been a stance-phase muscle to become a swing-phase muscle than to retrain a swing-phase muscle to become a stance-phase muscle. Therefore, if possible, an in-phase muscle transfer will produce a more satisfactory result because no phase conversion is necessary.

Ligaments of the Ankle Joint

The configuration and alignment of the ligamentous structures of the ankle are such that they permit free movement of the ankle and subtalar joints to occur simultaneously. Because the configuration of the trochlear surface of the talus is curved to produce a cone-shaped articulation whose apex is directed medially, the single fan-shaped deltoid ligament is adequate to provide stability to the medial side of the ankle joint (Fig. 1-44). On the lateral aspect of the ankle joint, however, where there is a larger area to be covered by a ligamentous structure, the ligament is divided into three bands: the anterior and posterior talofibular ligaments and the calcaneofibular ligament. The relationship of these ligaments to each other and to the axes of the subtalar and ankle joints must

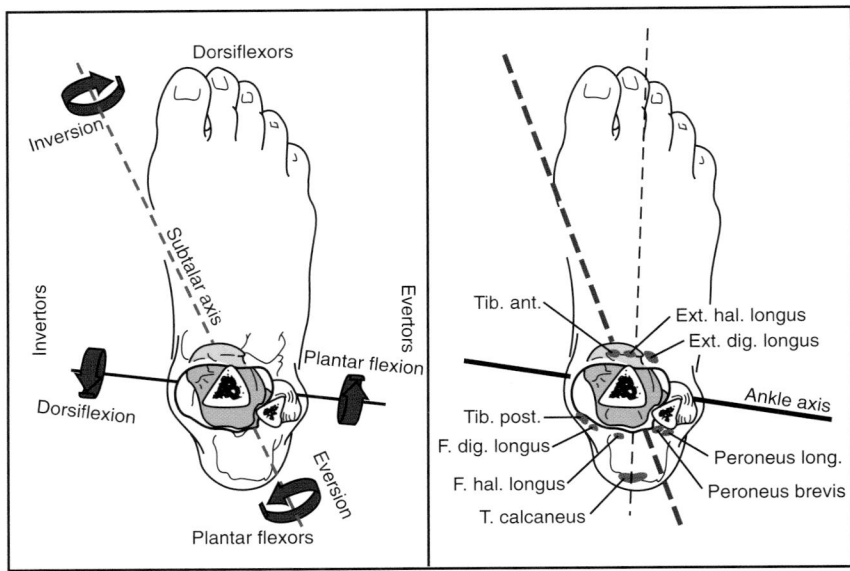

Figure 1-43 *Left,* Diagram demonstrates rotation that occurs about subtalar and ankle axes. *Right,* Diagram demonstrates relationship of various muscles about subtalar and ankle axes. (From Haskell A, Mann RA. Chapter 23: Biomechanics of the Foot. In American Academy of Orthopaedic Surgeons: *Atlas of Orthoses and Assistive Devices,* ed 4, Philadelphia, 2008, Mosby.)

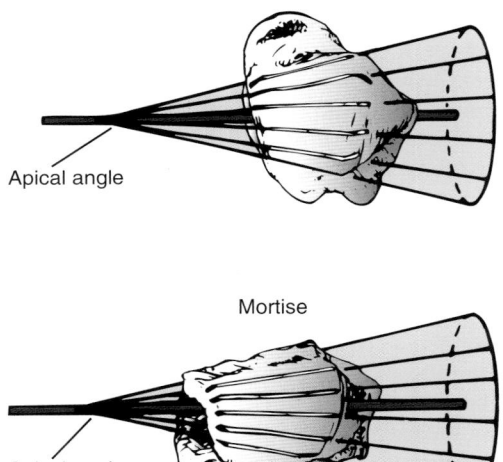

Figure 1-44 Curvature of trochlear surface of talus creates cone whose apex is based medially. From this configuration, one can observe that the deltoid ligament is well suited to function along the medial side of ankle joint, whereas laterally, where more rotation occurs, three separate ligaments are necessary. (From Inman VT: *The joints of the ankle,* Baltimore, 1976, Williams & Wilkins.)

always be considered carefully when these joints are examined or ligamentous surgery is contemplated.

Figure 1-45 demonstrates the anterior talofibular and calcaneofibular ligaments in relation to the subtalar joint axis. The calcaneofibular ligament is parallel to the subtalar joint axis in the sagittal plane. As the ankle joint is dorsiflexed and plantar flexed, this relationship between the calcaneofibular ligament and the subtalar joint axis

does not change. Furthermore, the calcaneofibular ligament crosses both the ankle and the subtalar joint. This ligament is constructed to permit motion to occur in both of these joints simultaneously. It is important to appreciate that, when the ankle joint is in neutral position, the calcaneofibular ligament is angulated posteriorly, but as the ankle joint is brought into more dorsiflexion, the calcaneofibular ligament is brought into line with the fibula, thereby becoming a true collateral ligament. Conversely, as the ankle joint is brought into plantar flexion, the calcaneofibular ligament becomes horizontal to the ground. In this position, it provides little or no stability for resisting inversion stress. The anterior talofibular ligament, on the other hand, is brought into line with the fibula when the ankle joint is plantar flexed, thereby acting as a collateral ligament. When the ankle joint is brought up into dorsiflexion, the anterior talofibular ligament becomes sufficiently horizontal so that it does not function as a collateral ligament. It can thus be appreciated that, depending on the position of the ankle joint, either the calcaneofibular or the anterior talofibular ligament will be a true collateral ligament with regard to providing stability to the lateral side of the ankle joint.

The relationship between these two ligaments has been quantified and is presented in Figure 1-46. This demonstrates the relationship of the angle produced by the calcaneofibular and the anterior talofibular ligaments to one another. The average angle in the sagittal plane is approximately 105 degrees, although there is considerable variation, from 70 to 140 degrees. This is important because, from a clinical standpoint, it partially explains why some persons have lax collateral ligaments. If we assume that when the ankle is in full dorsiflexion the calcaneofibular ligament provides most of the stability

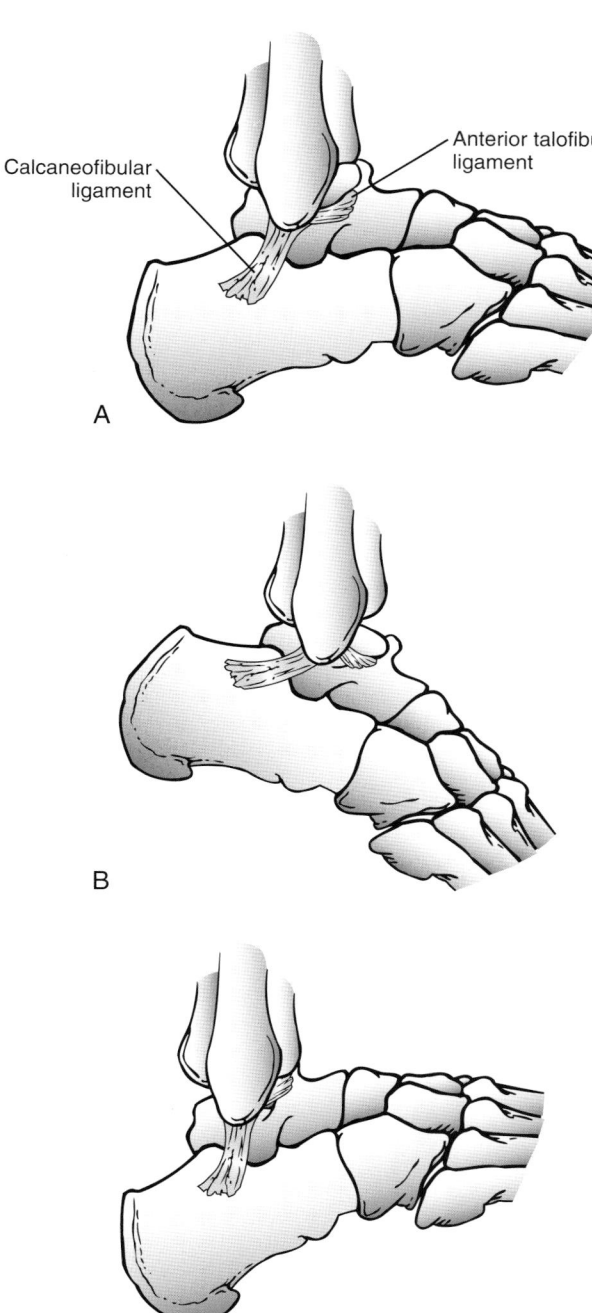

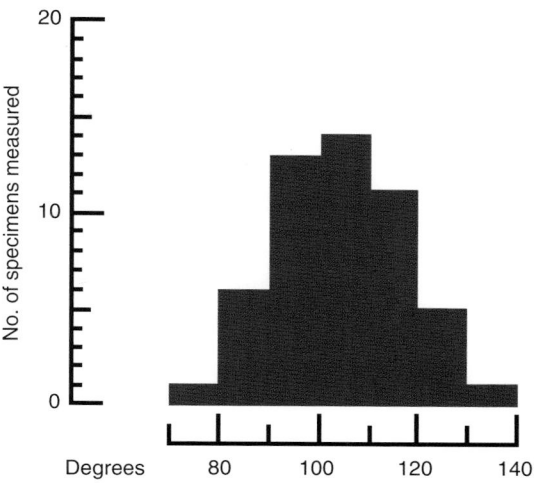

Figure 1-46 Average angle between calcaneofibular and talofibular ligaments in sagittal plane. Although the average angle is 105 degrees, there is considerable variation, from 70 to 140 degrees. (From Inman VT: *The joints of the ankle*, Baltimore, 1976, Williams & Wilkins.)

Figure 1-45 Calcaneal fibular ligament and anterior talofibular ligament. **A,** In neutral position of ankle joint, both anterior talofibular and calcaneofibular ligaments provide support to joint. **B,** In plantar flexion, anterior talofibular ligament is in line with fibula and provides most of support to lateral aspect of ankle joint. **C,** In dorsiflexion, calcaneofibular ligament is in line with the fibula and provides support to the lateral aspect of ankle joint. (From Inman VT: *The joints of the ankle*, Baltimore, 1976, Williams & Wilkins.)

and that in full plantar flexion the anterior talofibular ligament provides stability, then as we pass from dorsiflexion to plantar flexion and back there will be a certain period in which neither ligament is functioning as a true collateral ligament. If we assume there is an average angle of approximately 105 degrees between these ligaments, then generally speaking, an area in which an insufficient lateral collateral ligament is present is unusual; however, if we have angulation of 130 to 140 degrees between these two ligaments, there is a significant interval while the ankle is passing from dorsiflexion to plantar flexion and back in which neither ligament is functioning as a collateral ligament. This may explain why some persons are susceptible to chronic ankle sprains. Some patients who are thought to have ligamentous laxity may, in reality, possess this anatomic configuration of lateral collateral ligaments.

The other factor that needs to be considered is the relationship of the calcaneofibular ligament to subtalar joint motion. The primary stabilizers of the subtalar joint are the interosseus talocalcaneal ligaments that reside within the sinus tarsi, not the calcaneofibular ligament.[61] Because motion in the subtalar joint occurs about an axis that deviates from dorsal-medial to plantar-lateral (see Fig. 1-24), and the calcaneal attachment of the calcaneofibular ligament lies on the subtalar joint axis, motion of the subtalar joint around this axis occurs with minimal change in calcaneofibular length. Instead, as the subtalar joint moves, the calcaneofibular ligament moves along a path approximating the surface of a cone whose apex is the intersection of the ligament and the subtalar joint axis.[43] This relationship of the calcaneofibular ligament to the ankle and subtalar joint axes is critical when contemplating ligamentous reconstruction because any ligament reconstruction that fails to take this normal

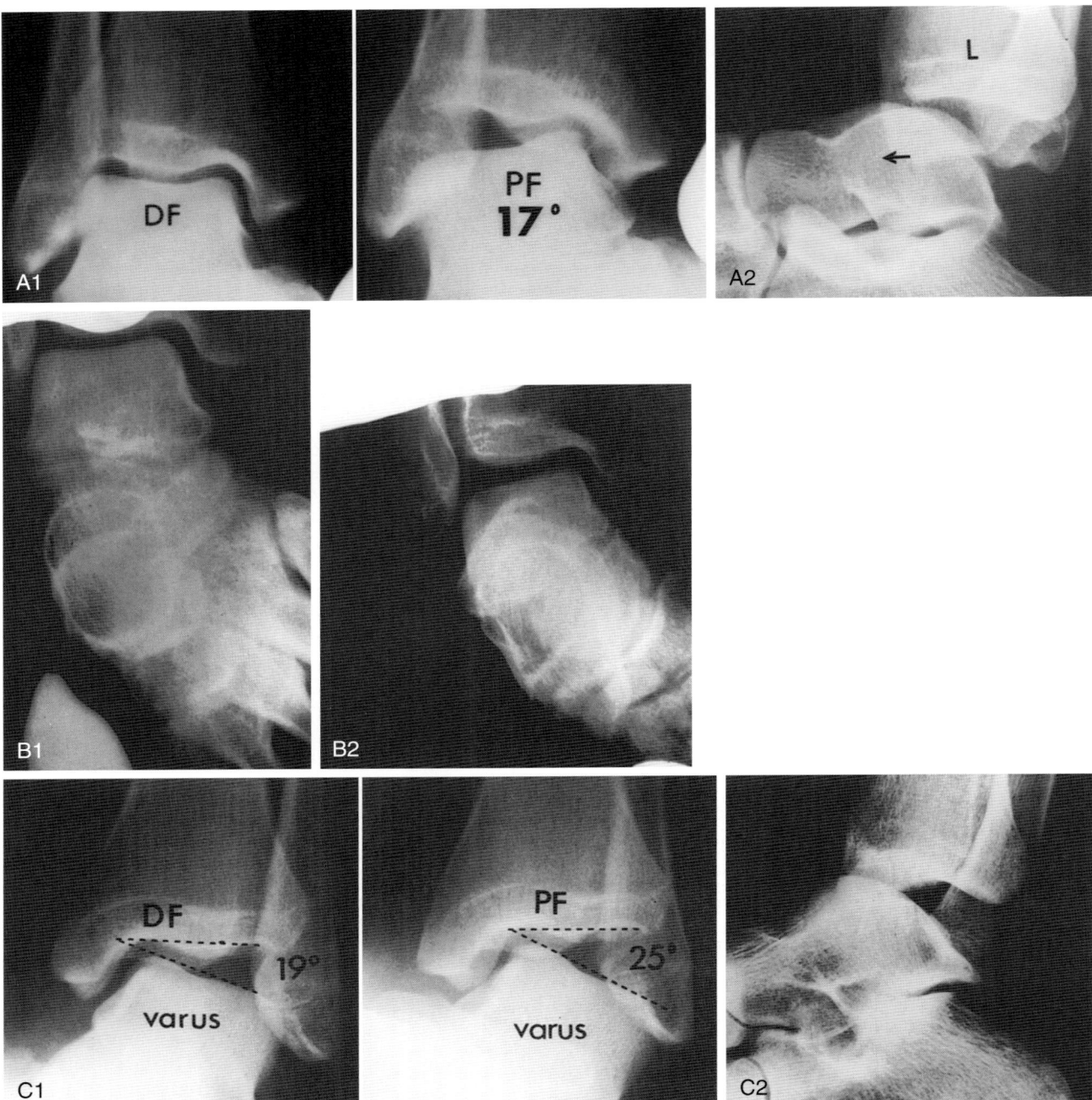

Figure 1-47 **A,** Stress radiographs of ankle in dorsiflexion *(DF)* demonstrate no instability in calcaneofibular ligament. Same ankle stressed in plantar flexion *(PF)* demonstrates loss of stability caused by disruption of anterior talofibular ligament. Note anterior subluxation present when this ligament *(L)* is torn (anterior drawer sign). **B,** Stress radiograph of ankle in plantar flexion demonstrates no ligamentous instability. Same ankle stressed in dorsiflexion demonstrates laxity of calcaneofibular ligament. **C,** Stress radiograph of ankle joint in dorsiflexion, plantar flexion, and anteriorly all demonstrate evidence of ligamentous disruption. This indicates complete tear of lateral collateral ligament structure.

anatomic configuration into consideration results in a situation in which motion in one or both of these joints is restricted.

From a clinical standpoint, when one is evaluating the stability of the lateral collateral ligament structure, the ankle joint should be tested in dorsiflexion to demonstrate the competency of the calcaneofibular ligament and in plantar flexion to test the competency of the anterior talofibular ligament. If both ligaments are completely disrupted, there will be no stability in either position. Furthermore, to test for stability of the anterior talofibular ligament, the anterior drawer sign should be elicited, with the ankle joint in neutral position, when the anterior talofibular ligament is in a position to resist anterior displacement of the talus from the ankle mortise (Fig. 1-47).

REFERENCES

1. Abbott BC, Bigland B, Ritchie JM: The physiological cost of negative work. *J Physiol* 117:380–390, 1952.
2. Alexander IJ, Chao EY, Johnson KA: The assessment of dynamic foot-to-ground contact forces and plantar pressure distribution: a review of the evolution of current techniques and clinical applications. *Foot Ankle* 11:152–167, 1990.
3. Andriacchi TP, Ogle JA, Galante JO: Walking speed as a basis for normal and abnormal gait measurements. *J Biomech* 10:261–268, 1977.
4. Arcan M, Brull MA: A fundamental characteristic of the human body and foot, the foot-ground pressure pattern. *J Biomech* 9:453–457, 1976.
5. Asmussen E: Positive and negative muscular work. *Acta Physiol Scand* 28:364–382, 1953.
6. Banister E, Brown S: The relative energy requirements of physical activity. In Falls H, editor: *Exercise physiology*, New York, 1968, Academic Press.
7. Barnett S, Cunningham JL, West S: A comparison of vertical force and temporal parameters produced by an in-shoe pressure measuring system and a force platform. *Clin Biomech (Bristol, Avon)* 15:781–785, 2000.
8. Becker HP, Rosenbaum D, Kriese T, et al: Gait asymmetry following successful surgical treatment of ankle fractures in young adults. *Clin Orthop* 311:262–269, 1995.
9. Berry FJ: Angle variation patterns of normal hip, knee and ankle in different operations. *Univ Calif Prosthet Devices Res Proj Rep* Ser 11, February 1952.
10. Betts RP, Franks CI, Duckworth T, et al: Static and dynamic foot-pressure measurements in clinical orthopaedics. *Med Biol Eng Comput* 18:674–684, 1980.
11. Blomgren M, Turan I, Agadir M: Gait analysis in hallux valgus. *J Foot Surg* 30:70–71, 1991.
12. Boyden EM, Kitaoka HB, Cahalan TD, et al: Late versus early repair of Achilles tendon rupture. Clinical and biomechanical evaluation. *Clin Orthop* 317:150–158, 1995.
13. Breit GA, Whalen RT: Prediction of human gait parameters from temporal measures of foot-ground contact. *Med Sci Sports Exerc* 29:540–547, 1997.
14. Bresler B, Berry F: Energy and power in the leg during normal level walking. *Univ Calif Prosthet Devices Res Proj Rep* Ser 11, May 1951.
15. Bryant A, Singer K, Tinley P: Comparison of the reliability of plantar pressure measurements using the two-step and midgait methods of data collection. *Foot Ankle Int* 20:646–650, 1999.
16. Carlson RE, Fleming LL, Hutton WC: The biomechanical relationship between the tendoachilles, plantar fascia and metatarsophalangeal joint dorsiflexion angle. *Foot Ankle Int* 21:18–25, 2000.
17. Close J, Inman V: The action of the subtalar joint. *Univ Calif Prosthet Devices Res Proj Rep* Ser 11, May 1953.
18. Ctercteko GC, Dhanendran M, Hutton WC, et al: Vertical forces acting on the feet of diabetic patients with neuropathic ulceration. *Br J Surg* 68:608–614, 1981.
19. Cunningham D: Components of floor reaction during walking. *Univ Calif Prosthet Devices Res Proj Rep* Ser 11, November 1950.
20. Duckworth T, Betts RP, Franks CI, et al: The measurement of pressures under the foot. *Foot Ankle* 3:130–141, 1982.
21. Elftman H: A cinematic study of the distribution of pressure in the human foot. *Anat Rec* 59:481–491, 1934.
22. Elftman H: The transverse tarsal joint and its control. *Clin Orthop Relat Res* 16:41–46, 1960.
23. Fujita M, Matsusaka N, Norimatsu T, et al: The role of the ankle plantar flexors in level walking. In Winter DA, editor: *Biomechanics IX-A*, Champaign, Ill, 1985, Human Kinetics Publishers, pp 484–488.
24. Grundy M, Tosh PA, McLeish RD, et al: An investigation of the centres of pressure under the foot while walking. *J Bone Joint Surg Br* 57:98–103, 1975.
25. Hayafune N, Hayafune Y, Jacob AC: Pressure and force distribution characteristics under the normal foot during push-off phase in gait. *Foot* 9:88–92, 1999.
26. Hennig EM, Rosenbaum D: Pressure distribution patterns under the feet of children in comparison with adults. *Foot Ankle* 11:306–311, 1991.
27. Hennig EM, Staats A, Rosenbaum D: Plantar pressure distribution patterns of young school children in comparison to adults. *Foot Ankle Int* 15:35–40, 1994.
28. Henry AP, Waugh W, Wood H: The use of footprints in assessing the results of operations for hallux valgus. A comparison of Keller's operation and arthrodesis. *J Bone Joint Surg Br* 57:478–481, 1975.
29. Herzog W, Nigg BM, Read LJ, et al: Asymmetries in ground reaction force patterns in normal human gait. *Med Sci Sports Exerc* 21:110–114, 1989.
30. Hicks JH: The mechanics of the foot. II. The plantar aponeurosis and the arch. *J Anat* 88:25–30, 1954.
31. Hof AL: In vivo measurement of the series elasticity release curve of human triceps surae muscle. *J Biomech* 31:793–800, 1998.
32. Hof AL, Geelen BA, Van den Berg J: Calf muscle moment, work and efficiency in level walking; role of series elasticity. *J Biomech* 16:523–537, 1983.
33. Hof AL, Van Zandwijk JP, Bobbert MF: Mechanics of human triceps surae muscle in walking, running and jumping. *Acta Physiol Scand* 174:17–30, 2002.
34. Holmes GB Jr, Timmerman L: A quantitative assessment of the effect of metatarsal pads on plantar pressures. *Foot Ankle* 11:141–145, 1990.
35. Hughes J, Clark P, Jagoe JR, et al: The pattern of pressure distribution under the weightbearing forefoot. *Foot* 1:117–124, 1991.
36. Hughes J, Clark P, Klenerman L: The importance of the toes in walking. *J Bone Joint Surg Br* 72:245–251, 1990.
37. Hughes J, Clark P, Linge K, et al: A comparison of two studies of the pressure distribution under the feet of normal subjects using different equipment. *Foot Ankle* 14:514–519, 1993.
38. Hughes J, Kriss S, Klenerman L: A clinician's view of foot pressure: a comparison of three different methods of measurement. *Foot Ankle* 7:277–284, 1987.
39. Hughes J, Pratt L, Linge K, et al: Reliability of pressure measurements: the EMED F system. *Clin Biomech* 6:14–18, 1991.
40. Hutton WC, Dhanendran M: The mechanics of normal and hallux valgus feet—a quantitative study. *Clin Orthop* 157:7–13, 1981.
41. Hutton WC, Stott JRR, Stokes JAF: The mechanics of the foot. In Klenerman L, editor: *The foot and its allied disorders*, Oxford, 1982, Blackwell Scientific Publications, p 42.
42. Imamura M, Imamura ST, Salomao O, et al: Pedobarometric evaluation of the normal adult male foot. *Foot Ankle Int* 23:804–810, 2002.
43. Inman V: *The joints of the ankle*, Baltimore, 1976, Williams & Wilkins.
44. Isman R, Inman V: Anthropometric studies of the human foot and ankle. *Bull Prosthet Res* 10-11:97, 1969.
45. Katoh Y, Chao EY, Laughman RK, et al: Biomechanical analysis of foot function during gait and clinical applications. *Clin Orthop Relat Res* 177:23–33, 1983.

46. Kelikian AS, Sarrafian SK: *Anatomy of the foot and ankle,* ed 3, Philadelphia, 2011, JB Lippincott.
47. Kerrigan DC, Della Croce U, Marciello M, et al: A refined view of the determinants of gait: significance of heel rise. *Arch Phys Med Rehabil* 81:1077–1080, 2000.
48. Levens A, Inman V, Blosser J: Transverse rotation of the segments of the lower extremity in locomotion. *J Bone Joint Surg Am* 30A:859–872, 1948.
49. Logan BM, Hutchings RT: *McMinn's color atlas of foot and ankle anatomy,* ed 4, St Louis, 2012, Elsevier.
50. Mann R, Inman VT: Phasic activity of intrinsic muscles of the foot. *J Bone Joint Surg Am* 46:469–481, 1964.
51. Mann RA, Poppen NK, O'Konski M: Amputation of the great toe. A clinical and biomechanical study. *Clin Orthop Relat Res* 226:192–205, 1988.
52. Mann RA, Rongstad KM: Arthrodesis of the ankle: a critical analysis. *Foot Ankle Int* 19:3–9, 1998.
53. Manter J: Movements of the subtalar and transverse tarsal joints. *Anat Rec* 80:397–410, 1941.
54. Morton DJ: Structural factors in static disorders of the foot. *Am J Surg* 9:315–328, 1930.
55. Mueller MJ, Sinacore DR, Hastings MK, et al: Effect of Achilles tendon lengthening on neuropathic plantar ulcers. A randomized clinical trial. *J Bone Joint Surg Am* 85-A:1436–1445, 2003.
56. Mueller MJ, Strube MJ: Generalizability of in-shoe peak pressure measures using the F-scan system. *Clin Biomech (Bristol, Avon)* 11:159–164, 1996.
57. Nilsson J, Thorstensson A: Ground reaction forces at different speeds of human walking and running. *Acta Physiol Scand* 136:217–227, 1989.
58. Pollard JP, Le Quesne LP, Tappin JW: Forces under the foot. *J Biomed Eng* 5:37–40, 1983.
59. Popova T: Quoted in Issledovaniia po biodinamike lokomotsii. In Bernstein N, editor: *Biodinamika khod'by normal'nogo vzroslogo muzhchiny,* Moscow, 1935, Idat Vsesoiuz Instit Eksper Med.
60. Ralston HJ: Energy-speed relation and optimal speed during level walking. *Int Z Angew Physiol* 17:277–283, 1958.
61. Ringleb SI, Dhakal A, Anderson CD, et al: Effects of lateral ligament sectioning on the stability of the ankle and subtalar joint. *J Orthop Res* 29:1459–1464, 2011.
62. Rodgers MM, Cavanagh PR: Pressure distribution in Morton's foot structure. *Med Sci Sports Exerc* 21:23–28, 1989.
63. Rose NE, Feiwell LA, Cracchiolo A 3rd: A method for measuring foot pressures using a high resolution, computerized insole sensor: the effect of heel wedges on plantar pressure distribution and center of force. *Foot Ankle* 13:263–270, 1992.
64. Rosenbaum D, Hautmann S, Gold M, et al: Effects of walking speed on plantar pressure patterns and hindfoot angular motion. *Gait Posture* 2:191–197, 1994.
65. Ryker NJ: Glass walkway studies of normal subjects during normal walking. *Univ Calif Prosthet Devices Res Proj Rep* Ser 11, January 1952.
66. Saunders JB, Inman VT, Eberhart HD: The major determinants in normal and pathological gait. *J Bone Joint Surg Am* 35-A:543–558, 1953.
67. Silvino N, Evanski PM, Waugh TR: The Harris and Beath foot-printing mat: diagnostic validity and clinical use. *Clin Orthop* 151:265–269, 1980.
68. Simon SR, Mann RA, Hagy JL, et al: Role of the posterior calf muscles in normal gait. *J Bone Joint Surg Am* 60:465–472, 1978.
69. Stein H, Simkin A, Joseph K: The foot-ground pressure distribution following triple arthrodesis. *Arch Orthop Trauma Surg* 98:263–269, 1981.
70. Stokes IA, Hutton WC, Stott JR, et al: Forces under the hallux valgus foot before and after surgery. *Clin Orthop Relat Res* 142:64–72, 1979.
71. Stott JR, Hutton WC, Stokes IA: Forces under the foot. *J Bone Joint Surg Br* 55:335–344, 1973.
72. Sutherland DH, Cooper L, Daniel D: The role of the ankle plantar flexors in normal walking. *J Bone Joint Surg Am* 62:354–363, 1980.
73. Veves A, Sarnow MR, Giurini JM, et al: Differences in joint mobility and foot pressures between black and white diabetic patients. *Diabet Med* 12:585–589, 1995.
74. Waldecker U: Metatarsalgia in hallux valgus deformity: a pedographic analysis. *J Foot Ankle Surg* 41:300–308, 2002.
75. Wanivenhaus A, Brettschneider W: Influence of metatarsal head displacement on metatarsal pressure distribution after hallux valgus surgery. *Foot Ankle* 14:85–89, 1993.
76. Wearing SC, Urry SR, Smeathers JE: Ground reaction forces at discrete sites of the foot derived from pressure plate measurements. *Foot Ankle Int* 22:653–661, 2001.
77. Willson JD, Kernozek TW: Plantar loading and cadence alterations with fatigue. *Med Sci Sports Exerc* 31:1828–1833, 1999.
78. Winson IG, Rawlinson J, Broughton NS: Treatment of metatarsalgia by sliding distal metatarsal osteotomy. *Foot Ankle* 9:2–6, 1988.
79. Wright DG, Desai SM, Henderson WH: Action of the subtalar and ankle-joint complex during the stance phase of walking. *J Bone Joint Surg Am* 46:361–382, 1964.
80. Yamamoto H, Muneta T, Asahina S, et al: Forefoot pressures during walking in feet affected with hallux valgus. *Clin Orthop* 323:247–253, 1996.
81. Zhu H, Wertsch JJ, Harris GF, et al: Walking cadence effect on plantar pressures. *Arch Phys Med Rehabil* 76:1000–1005, 1995.
82. Zhu HS, Wertsch JJ, Harris GF, et al: Foot pressure distribution during walking and shuffling. *Arch Phys Med Rehabil* 72:390–397, 1991.

Chapter 2

Principles of the Physical Examination of the Foot and Ankle

Todd A. Irwin, Robert B. Anderson, W. Hodges Davis

You may not see it, but it sees you.
Jack Hughston, MD, discussing the physical examination

The foot, ankle, and leg are parts of the body that are readily accessible to careful physical examination. In the vast majority of cases, a definitive diagnosis can be reached by obtaining a careful history, conducting a proper physical examination, and using the indicated ancillary diagnostic procedures. Effective examination of the lower extremity can be dependent on the patient's age and receptiveness to examination.

In this chapter, the focus is on examination of the mature foot and ankle. The reader will receive a framework for a systematic approach to the normal examination. This will give a background for understanding the pathology described in subsequent chapters. In addition, a detailed description of the topographic anatomy of the foot and ankle is provided. It is with this knowledge that the practitioner can best evaluate the abnormalities in this easily palpable body part. It must be stressed that one sees only what one is looking for, or, in the words of a wise Southern gentleman physician "you may not see it [foot pathology], but it sees you." Keep your eyes wide open.

OVERVIEW

To prevent overlooking pertinent findings, the examiner should follow a rigorous routine. The particular routine adopted will vary depending on personal preference and arrangement of office facilities. The suggestion is to consciously formulate this routine and school oneself to deviate rarely from it. This will best ensure nothing is missed. However, no matter what procedure is used, the examiner must consider the foot and ankle from three different points of view.

First, the foot and ankle should be seen systemically or as part of the greater body. In the detailed examination, the effects of systemic problems cannot be underestimated. The foot examination can reveal the presence of systemic disease as well as give evidence of circulatory, neuropathic, metabolic, and cutaneous abnormalities. The examiner should not be so focused on the foot as to miss a much more illustrative and often treatable global disease.

Second, the foot and ankle should be considered an important component of the locomotor system. They play reciprocal roles with the suprapedal segments, and abnormal function of any part of the locomotor apparatus is reflected in adaptive changes in the normal parts. Therefore it is helpful for the examiner to observe the patient walking over an appreciable distance.

Third, the human foot and ankle should be viewed as relatively recent evolutionary acquisitions; thus they are subject to considerable individual anatomic and functional variation. It is regrettable that in most of the anatomic and orthopaedic literature, only average values for the positions of axes of the major articulations and for ranges of motion about these axes are given (see Chapter 1). It so happens that an average person is difficult to find, particularly among patients seeking help in our offices. The examiner should be aware of these variations and should also be cognizant of their functional implications. In most patients, the luxury of a "normal" contralateral extremity allows the examiner the most definitive pertinent comparison. Only with such knowledge and insight can the examiner determine the proper therapeutic course and realistically evaluate the chances of success or failure of that choice.

SEQUENCE OF EXAMINATION

When examining the foot and ankle, the examiner should follow as closely as possible the procedural sequence taught in courses in introductory physical diagnosis. After taking an adequate history, the examiner first inspects, then palpates, and finally (in an orthopaedic examination) manipulates. This sequence must be modified and repeated several times as the patient performs tasks in various positions and under various stresses.

The following outline for the examination of the foot and ankle has proved useful. In subsequent sections, the authors detail specific portions of the particular examination that should be stressed.

It is helpful for the patients to be in shorts, skirts, or loose-fitting trousers to allow easy observation of the legs and knees. In general, all socks or hose are removed. The examination area should allow gait and stance observation from front and rear.

The usual sequence of examination begins with the examiner first observing the patient walking because this often can be done even before taking the history. Second is the standing examination, which is done from front and rear, and must include visualization of the knee and its alignment. Third, the bulk of the examination is done with the patient sitting on a table slightly above the examiner. This allows for easy inspection, palpation, and manipulation of both extremities. Examination with the patient prone or supine is optional and is done as the first three portions of the examination dictate. The amount of time spent on each portion of this examination sequence depends on the patient's presentation.

TOPOGRAPHIC ANATOMY

The importance of topographic anatomy to the examination of the foot and ankle cannot be overstated. The

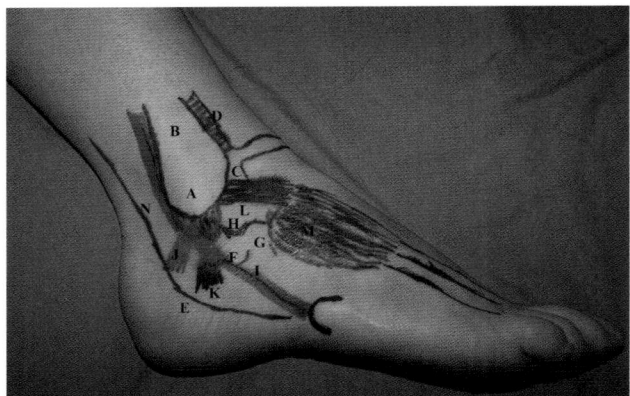

Figure 2-1 Lateral ankle and hindfoot topography, anterior lateral view. *A*, Distal fibula; *B*, fibular shaft; *C*, lateral gutter of the ankle; *D*, distal syndesmosis; *E*, lateral wall of the calcaneus; *F*, the peroneal tubercle; *G*, sinus tarsi; *H*, lateral talar process; *I*, peroneal tendons; *J*, insertion point of the superior peroneal retinaculum; *K*, calcaneofibular ligament; *L*, anterior talofibular ligament; *M*, extensor digitorum brevis muscle; *N*, sural nerve.

experienced examiner can palpate the vast majority of the pathologic structures and use radiographic tests for confirmation only. The authors divide this discussion into anatomic regions, with the palpable bones, joints, nerves and vascular structures, and ligaments and tendons highlighted.

Ankle and Hindfoot

Lateral Ankle

The examination of the osteology of the lateral ankle begins with the easily palpable tip of the fibula (Fig. 2-1). From the tip, the distal fibula *(A)* and the shaft *(B)* can be felt in its entirety by running the examiner's fingers proximally. The lateral gutter of the ankle joint *(C)* can be found by running the thumb medially over the anterior and medial edge of the fibula. The lateral shoulder of the talus can be felt at the joint line by dorsiflexing and plantar flexing the ankle. The distal syndesmosis *(D)* is felt by following the medial edge of the fibula superior to the joint line. The lateral wall of the calcaneus *(E)* can be palpated with little difficulty inferior and posterior to the tip of the fibula. If this lateral wall is palpated distal and inferior to the tip of the fibula, the peroneal tubercle *(F)* can be felt as the calcaneal neck nears the calcaneocuboid joint. The sinus tarsi *(G)* (the space in front of the posterior facet of the subtalar joint) is a palpable soft spot approximately 1 cm distal and 1 cm inferior to the tip of the fibula. The anterior portion of the posterior facet of the subtalar joint can be located with deep thumb palpation into the sinus tarsi. The lateral talar process *(H)* is palpated on the posterior wall of the sinus tarsi. The anterior process of the calcaneus is the anterior wall of the sinus tarsi.

The palpable tendons, muscles, and ligaments in the lateral ankle and hindfoot can best be referenced from the tip of the fibula. Superior and posterior to the tip of the fibula are the peroneal tendons *(I)*. The peroneus brevis is deep to the peroneus longus. The tendons can be felt in the groove, and the anterior edge of the fibular groove is sharp and is the insertion point of the superior peroneal retinaculum *(J)*. Inferior and extending posterior and inferior is the calcaneofibular ligament *(K)*. It passes deep to the peroneal tendons as the tendons clear the fibula. From the tip of the fibula, if the examiner runs a finger 1 to 1.5 cm along the anterior edge, the anterior talofibular ligament *(L)* can be felt. In the uninjured patient, it can be felt as a soft tissue thickening that can be rolled against the anterior lateral talar shoulder.

If the examiner continues to run a finger superior on the anterior fibula up to the junction with the distal tibiofibular connection, the most inferior fibers of the syndesmotic ligament *(D)* can be felt (anterior distal tibiofibular ligament). The remainder of the anterior syndesmotic ligament can be felt by palpating directly superior to the tibia and fibula junction. To truly assess this portion of the syndesmosis requires deep palpation. The extensor digitorum brevis muscle *(M)* can be located by palpating the sinus tarsi *(G)* because this muscle covers this space. The peroneal tendons can be felt on the lateral calcaneal wall, extending from the distal end of the fibular groove, which runs inferior then distal. The brevis is dorsal as the tendons turn distal. The peroneus brevis is also dorsal at the peroneal tubercle, and the peroneus longus is plantar. In this area, the tendons can be felt in their separate sheaths created by the inferior peroneal retinaculum and the tubercle.

The nervous topography in this region is fairly straightforward. The sural nerve can be felt in the fatty soft spot directly posterior to the peroneal tendons running in the fibular groove (Fig. 2-2). In a thin patient, this nerve can be rolled under a finger, just posterior to the course of the peroneal tendons as the tendons enter the lateral midfoot. The superficial peroneal nerve can first be palpated as a number of branches just superior to the distal ankle

syndesmosis. Again, it is best seen and palpated by rolling the branch under a finger as the ankle is plantar flexed.

Medial Ankle

The topography of the medial ankle and hindfoot (Fig. 2-3) is as accessible as the lateral. The reference point here is the tip of the medial malleolus *(A)*, which also allows a reference for medial ankle osteology. The tip of the malleolus is the most distal bony prominence palpated on the medial tibia. From this point, the anterior medial tibiotalar joint line *(B)* can be located by sliding a thumb 2 cm superior and then lateral until the thumb feels a soft spot. This is the medial gutter, the articular space between the medial malleolus and the medial talar body. Following the gutter proximally allows palpation of the anterior distal tibial plafond. This can be followed laterally across the joint. Following the malleolus posteriorly and proximally allows palpation of the entire posterior medial edge of the malleolus and tibia.

From the tip of the medial malleolus, with the ankle at neutral, a line drawn distal and slightly plantar will run through the navicular bone *(C)*. The navicular is best felt with the hindfoot slightly supinated. With the hindfoot pronated and the midfoot abducted, the talar head *(D)* can be felt on the medial foot just proximal to the navicular. The medial talonavicular joint can be delineated by adducting and abducting the transverse tarsal joint. If the line between the navicular and the medial malleolus is divided in half and drops plantarward 1 to 1.5 cm, the sustentaculum tali *(E)*—a medial ossicle of the calcaneus—can be palpated.

The palpable tendons and ligaments of the medial hindfoot can also be referenced from the tip of the medial malleolus. The superficial deltoid ligament *(F)* fans out from the malleolus but can best be palpated anterior and distal to it. The anterior fascicles of the deltoid can be felt by following the anterior edge of the malleolus only

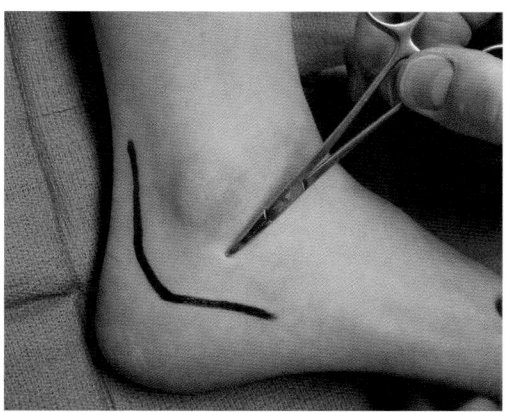

Figure 2-2 Sural nerve, surface anatomy.

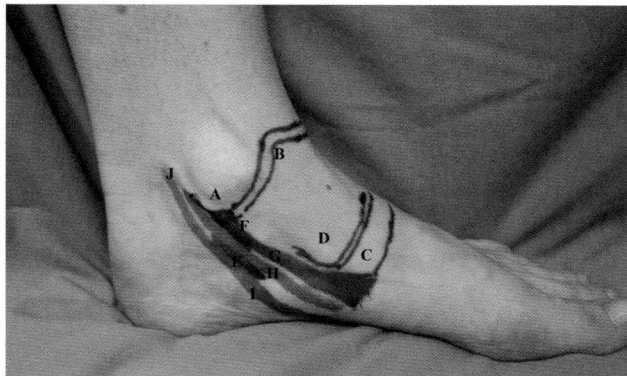

Figure 2-3 Medial ankle and hindfoot topography, direct medial view. *A,* Tip of the medial malleolus; *B,* anterior medial tibiotalar joint line; *C,* navicular bone; *D,* the talar head; *E,* sustentaculum tali; *F,* superficial deltoid ligament; *G,* posterior tibial tendon; *H,* flexor digitorum longus; *I,* flexor hallucis longus; *J,* pulse of the posterior tibial artery.

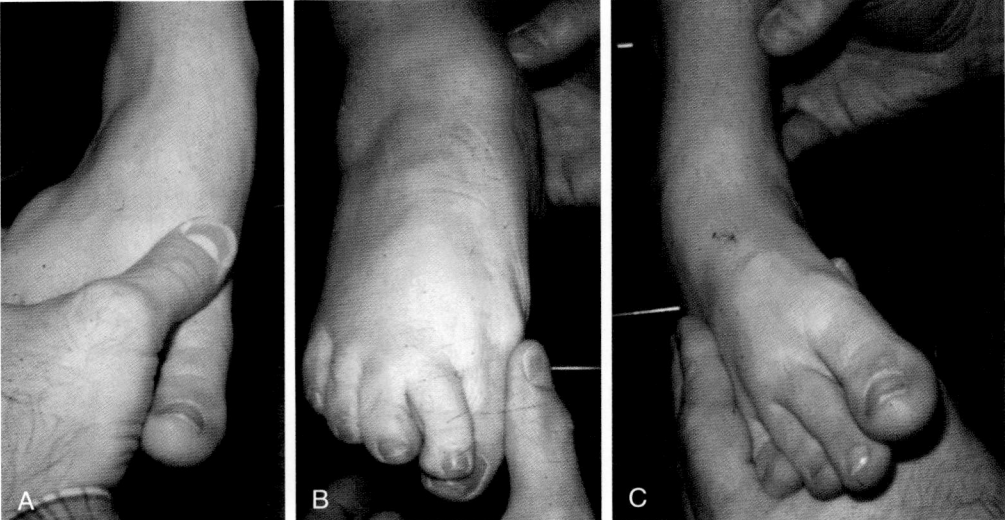

Figure 2-4 Examination of the posterior tibial tendon. **A,** The foot is plantar flexed and abducted to neutralize the pull of the anterior tibial tendon. **B,** The posterior tibial tendon is palpated. **C,** The patient attempts to adduct the foot, and the strength of the posterior tibial tendon is assessed.

1 cm. If the examiner feels the medial gutter, the origin of the superficial deltoid has been passed. The most anterior fascicles of the superficial deltoid (anterior tibionavicular and anterior tibioligamentous) can be palpated because they originate from the anterior ridge of the malleolus. The portion of the superficial deltoid originating from the tip of the malleolus can be located as it courses deep to the tendons of the medial ankle. The individual fasicles of the deep deltoid ligament cannot be isolated by palpation. The more posterior aspects of the superficial deltoid cannot be palpated directly.

The posterior tibial tendon *(G)* can be appreciated along its entire course. It begins at the musculotendinous junction, 5 to 7 cm from the tip of the medial malleolus, just off the posterior bony margin of the distal tibia, and travels distally, almost adherent to the posterior aspect of the medial malleolus. The tendon curves around the medial malleolus and then extends distally to the plantar medial insertion on the navicular.

The flexor digitorum longus (FDL) *(H)* is easily palpated posterior and medial to the posterior tibialis tendon at a level 1 to 2 cm from the tip of the malleolus. It can be felt again in the midfoot as it crosses deep to the flexor hallucis longus (FHL) tendon. The FHL tendon *(I)* is best palpated in the ankle slightly posterior and deep to the posterior tibial artery and nerve at the level 1 to 2 cm proximal to the medial malleolus. The FHL also can be felt as it passes plantar to the sustentaculum tali. The superomedial aspect of the spring ligament (superomedial calcaneonavicular ligament) is palpated plantar and deep to the posterior tibial tendon, just proximal to the tendon's insertion on the plantar-medial navicular (Fig. 2-4).

It is import to locate the neurovascular structures of the medial ankle. The pulse of the posterior tibial artery

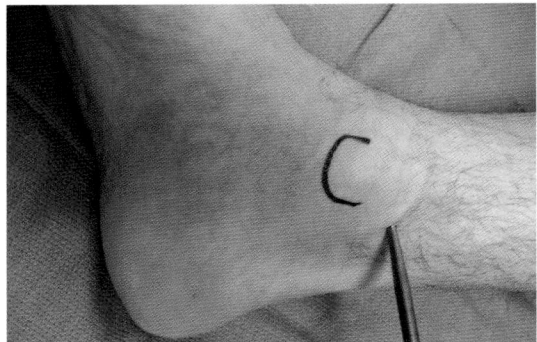

Figure 2-5 The posterior tibial artery pulse is best felt 2 cm from the malleolar tip.

(see *J* in Fig. 2-3) can be felt 1 to 2 cm posterior and medial to the medial edge of the medial malleolus. The pulse is strongest approximately 2 cm posterior to the malleolar tip (Fig. 2-5). The posterior tibial nerve runs with the artery in the tarsal tunnel. The nerve bifurcates into the medial and lateral plantar nerves at the level of the tip of the malleolus. The medial branch courses distally and plantarly and can be palpated as it runs under the abductor hallucis muscle at the level of the medial gutter of the ankle joint (Fig. 2-6). The lateral plantar nerve travels straight inferior from the tarsal tunnel and can be palpated as it runs deep to the abductor hallucis. The saphenous nerve can sometimes be palpated on the medial malleolus by rolling it gently under the fingers.

Posterior Ankle

The Achilles tendon (Fig. 2-7A) defines the posterior ankle and hindfoot. This large tendon can best be examined with the patient prone. The tendon transects the

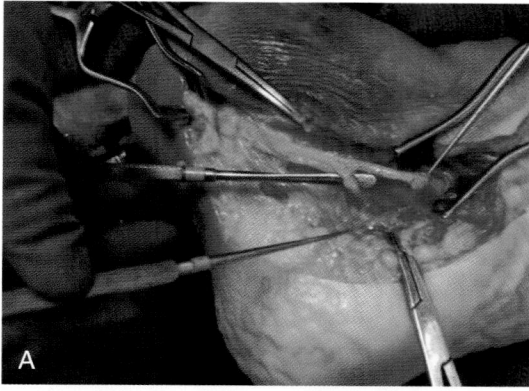

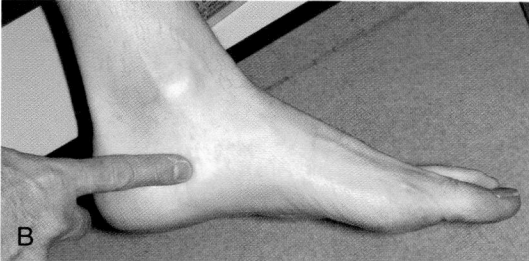

Figure 2-6 **A,** Anatomic specimen demonstrating the posterior tibial nerve. **B,** The posterior tibial nerve may be palpated just inferior to the medial malleolus.

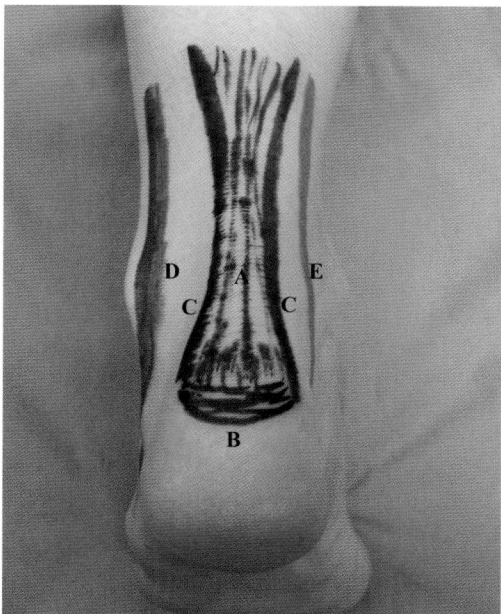

Figure 2-7 Posterior ankle and hindfoot. *A,* Achilles tendon; *B,* the Achilles insertional ridge of the calcaneus; *C,* retrocalcaneal space; *D,* the peroneal tendons; *E,* flexor hallucis longus tendon.

posterior ankle and can be easily palpated because of the tendon's subcutaneous course. The tendon inserts into the calcaneus broadly, and the Achilles insertional ridge of the calcaneus *(B)* is palpated at the distal insertion of the tendon. The posterior calcaneus is palpated medially,

laterally, and posteriorly. The retrocalcaneal space *(C),* which is deep to the Achilles at its insertion, can be easily pinched by pressure from either medial or lateral. The space or its bursa (or both) is an area that is easily delineated from the Achilles proper. The posterior lateral ankle is another access point for the peroneal tendons *(D)* as they pass posterior to the fibula and can be an easier way to feel both tendons in the fibular groove. The same can be said for the FHL tendon *(E),* which is a posteromedial ankle tendon at this point (Fig. 2-8).

Anterior Ankle

The anterior ankle (Fig. 2-9) is defined by the readily palpable anterior tibialis tendon *(A).* The tendon is found by asking the patient to actively dorsiflex the ankle. The anterior tibialis, first felt at or near the midanterior ankle just proximal to the malleoli, is the largest tendon structure that passes more medially as it travels distally. Its insertion on the plantar medial cuneiform and plantar first metatarsal is defined with the same dorsiflexion maneuver (Fig. 2-10).

On either side of the anterior tibialis tendon, the anterior ankle joint *(B)* can be felt by deep palpation. The distinction between the tibia and the talus is more easily felt with gentle dorsiflexion and plantar flexion of the ankle joint. The transition from anterior tibia to anterior fibula is quite superficial and can help guide the estimation of the location of the less superficial midanterior tibia and talus. The branches of the superficial peroneal nerve *(C)* are palpated by gently rolling the fingers over the superficial portions of the anterior ankle (Fig. 2-11). All of these branches are found lateral to the anterior tibialis. The pulse of the dorsalis pedis artery is usually felt not at the ankle but in the dorsal midfoot.

The remaining tendons of the anterior ankle (see Fig. 2-9) are all found lateral to the anterior tibialis. From medial to lateral, these easily palpable tendons are the extensor hallucis longus (EHL) *(D),* the extensor digitorum longus (EDL) *(E),* and the peroneus tertius *(F)* (found in most people). The examination of these tendons can be made easier by active dorsiflexion or passive plantar flexion of the toes and ankle. Medial to the anterior tibialis, no tendons are normally present.

Plantar Hindfoot

Examination of the plantar-lateral aspect of the hindfoot is all about defining the anatomy of the lateral calcaneal area (Fig. 2-12). If the examiner begins at the posterior-most aspect of the calcaneus and runs a finger distal to it, the lateral edge of the calcaneus can be felt as separate from the lateral aspect of the plantar fat pad (Fig. 2-13). The fat pad begins to be prominent as the skin texture changes from thin to thick as the weight-bearing surface of the heel becomes apparent. On the plantar surface (see Fig. 2-12), the lateral band of the plantar fascia and the abductor digiti minimi *(A)* are most often indistinguishable as a pinchable band originating from the palpable lateral calcaneus and extending distal to the fifth

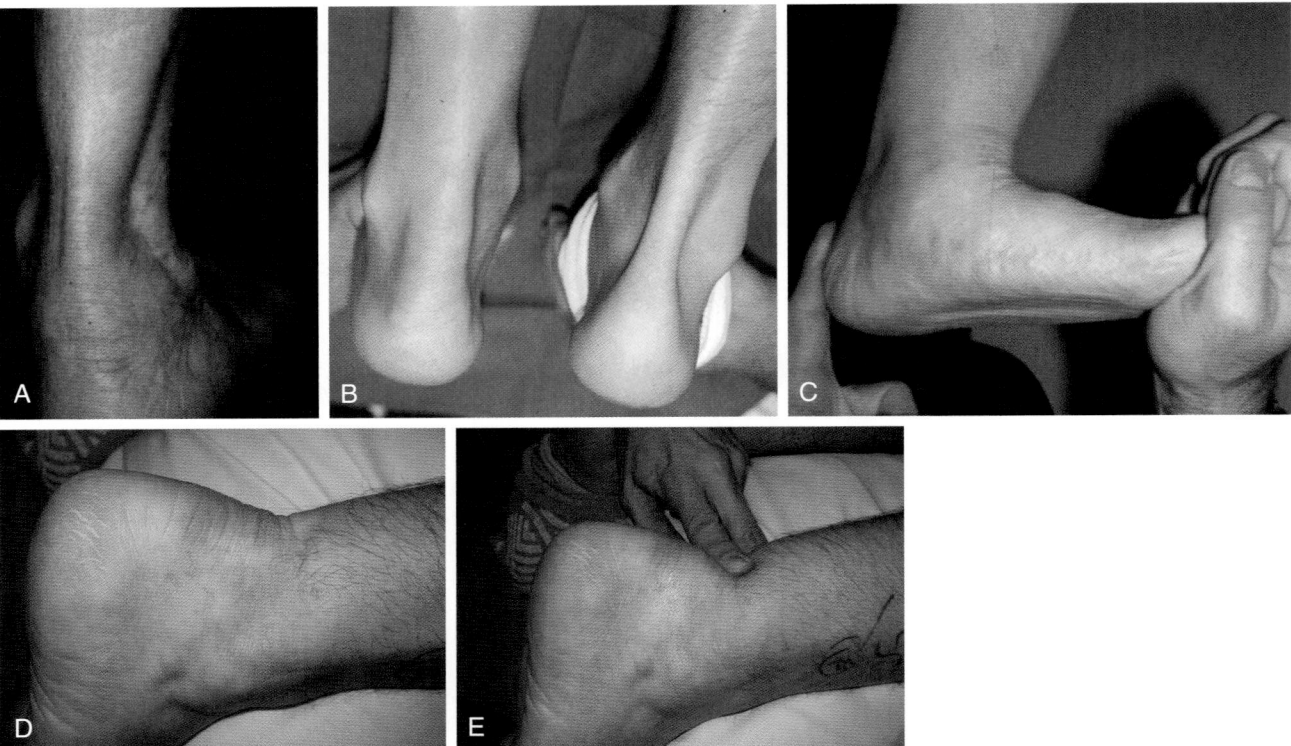

Figure 2-8 Achilles tendon. **A,** The normal tendon is examined from behind. **B,** Tendinosis is seen in the Achilles tendon on the left. **C,** Excursion of the ankle joint is noted. A defect in the Achilles tendon after a rupture is observed **(D)** and palpated **(E)** on examination.

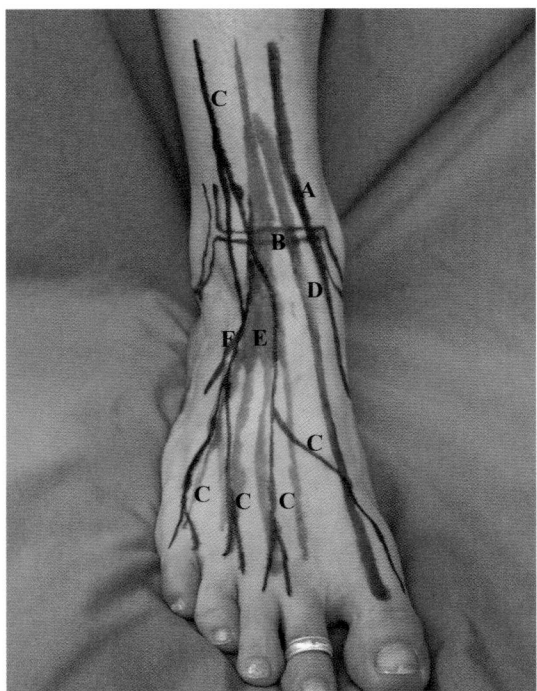

Figure 2-9 Anterior ankle. *A,* Anterior tibialis tendon; *B,* anterior ankle joint; *C,* branches of the superficial peroneal nerve; *D,* extensor hallucis longus; *E,* extensor digitorum longus; *F,* peroneus tertius.

metatarsal head. The sural nerve can be felt as a cord just plantar to the peroneal tendons as they run along the calcaneal wall.

The plantar-medial hindfoot is best located from the posterior calcaneus by running a finger along the plantar-medial border of the bone. Soon, the bone becomes less subcuticular as the soft tissues of the arch are more prominent. The abductor hallucis muscle *(B)* can be palpated as it originates from the plantar-medial calcaneus and extends distally to insert on the plantar-medial first metatarsophalangeal (MTP) joint. The medial cord of the plantar fascia *(C)* is palpated just plantar and lateral to the abductor hallucis. It is felt most readily by passively dorsiflexing the toes.

The origin of the medial cord of the plantar fascia is best felt by passively dorsiflexing the toes and then running a thumb posterior until it is felt on the proximal plantar calcaneus. Deep palpation is required, as the examiner feels posteriorly, because the thick plantar fat pad *(D)* covers this area by covering the posterior-plantar calcaneus. The heel pad is thinner as the plantar hindfoot transitions to the non–weight-bearing arch. There are no palpable neural or vascular structures in the plantar hindfoot, but the medial and lateral plantar nerves are just deep to the abductor hallucis muscle as they cross into the plantar hindfoot. Deep palpation can elicit tenderness in the respective distributions of these nerves.

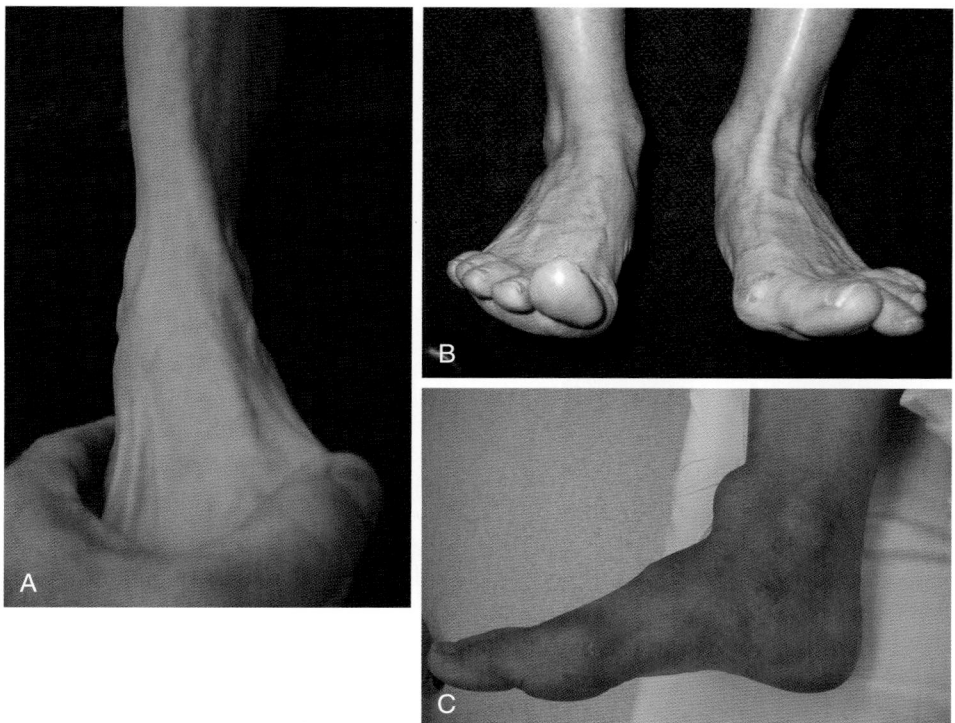

Figure 2-10 **A,** Normal anterior tibial tendon. **B,** Rupture of anterior tibial tendon noted on *left* (right foot). **C,** Rupture and contraction leaves a mass on the anterior ankle. (**B** and **C,** Courtesy L. Schoen, MD.)

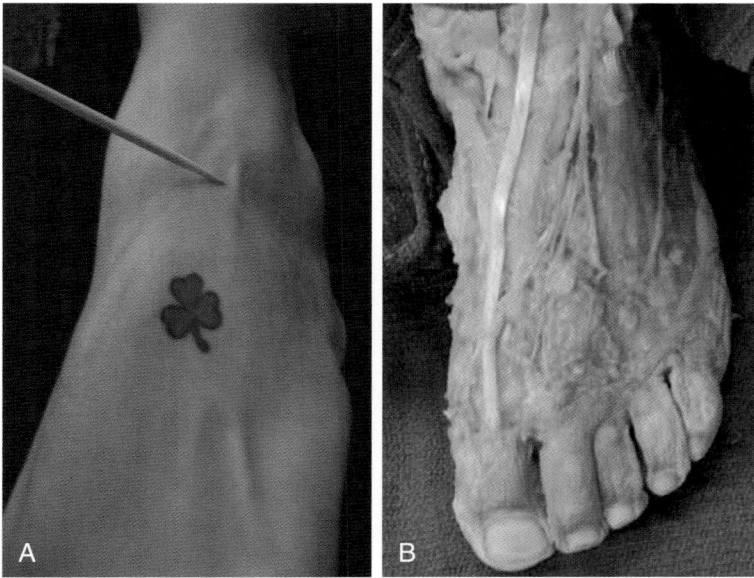

Figure 2-11 Superficial peroneal nerves. **A,** Superficial anatomy. **B,** Anatomic dissection demonstrating superficial peroneal nerve branches.

Midfoot

The structures of the dorsal midfoot, in most cases, can be appreciated with a careful examination (Fig. 2-14A and B). The bones of the midfoot can all be palpated most readily on the dorsum. The osteology of the dorsal midfoot is best felt by starting proximal at the talonavicular joint *(A)*. The detail of the bony edges can be defined by the palpable joints. The talonavicular joint can be felt as the most mobile joint on the medial side. By moving the foot into abduction and supination, the mobility of

43

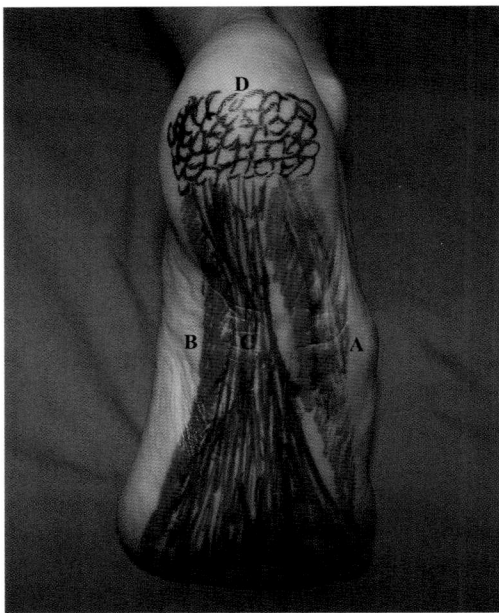

Figure 2-12 Plantar hindfoot. *A,* Lateral band of the plantar fascia and the abductor digiti minimi; *B,* abductor hallucis muscle; *C,* medial cord of the plantar fascia; *D,* plantar fat pad.

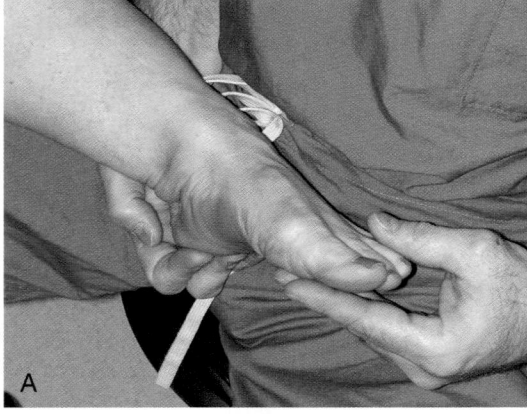

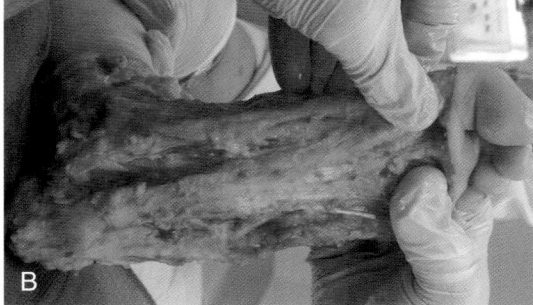

Figure 2-13 Plantar fascia. **A,** Clinical examination of plantar fascia. **B,** Anatomic dissection demonstrating the plantar fascia.

the joint can be felt. Whereas some motion is present in the more distal joints, in the normal foot, the talonavicular joint is most mobile.

Once the talonavicular joint is found medially, the dorsal joint can be felt by running a finger along the navicular. Palpating distally while staying dorsal, the examiner will feel a subtle ridge or thickening at the navicular cuneiform joint and the first tarsometatarsal joint *(B)*. The edges of the joints can be followed to define the bony architecture of the corresponding bones. The bases of the lesser tarsometatarsal joints are best isolated by following the lesser metatarsal shafts from distal to proximal. The second base is proximal to the first base, inset between the first and the third *(C)*.

The lateral aspect of the midfoot is more mobile than the medial and is best referenced from the prominent base of the fifth metatarsal *(D)*. This is the most lateral bony area on the lateral midfoot. It is both prominent and mobile. The calcaneocuboid joint *(E)* is isolated by holding the hindfoot stable and then dorsiflexing and plantar flexing the midfoot. The calcaneocuboid joint is the mobile segment just proximal to the base of the fifth metatarsal as the examiner feels along the lateral calcaneal wall. The anterior process of the calcaneus *(F)* is found by running a finger dorsally on the calcaneocuboid joint. The most dorsal palpable bony structure on this line is the anterior process of the calcaneus. The fourth and fifth tarsometatarsal joint can be located by the same dorsiflexion and plantar flexion used for the calcaneocuboid joint, but the fifth joint is at the base of the fifth metatarsal, and the fourth joint is slightly medial and dorsal to the fifth metatarsal.

The midfoot represents the insertion area of many of the ankle tendons. The medial midfoot is the insertion area for the posterior tibialis, the anterior tibialis, and the peroneus longus tendons. The insertion of the posterior tibialis *(G)* is best felt at the navicular. When a patient actively supinates and inverts the foot, the tendon can be isolated proximally at the medial malleolus and followed to its insertion. The same can be done for the anterior tibialis *(H)* as it inserts on the plantar-medial aspect of the cuneiform and plantar proximal first metatarsal.

The insertion of the peroneus longus cannot be palpated specifically except in very thin patients, but its insertion on the plantar base of the first metatarsal is an area that can be mobile with peroneus longus activity. Asking the patient to actively plantar flex the first metatarsal can isolate the peroneus longus tendon (see Fig. 2-14C and D).

The medial midfoot is an area where the examiner can palpate extrinsic tendons that insert distal in the forefoot. Directly plantar to the medial cuneiform (Fig. 2-15), the point where the FHL and FDL cross (see Fig. 2-14), the master knot of Henry *(I)* can be located by deep palpation. This is made easier by active plantar flexion of the five toes. The medial cord of the plantar fascia covers the knot, but the moving tendons can be felt deep and medial to the medial cord of the static fascia. The EHL and EDL

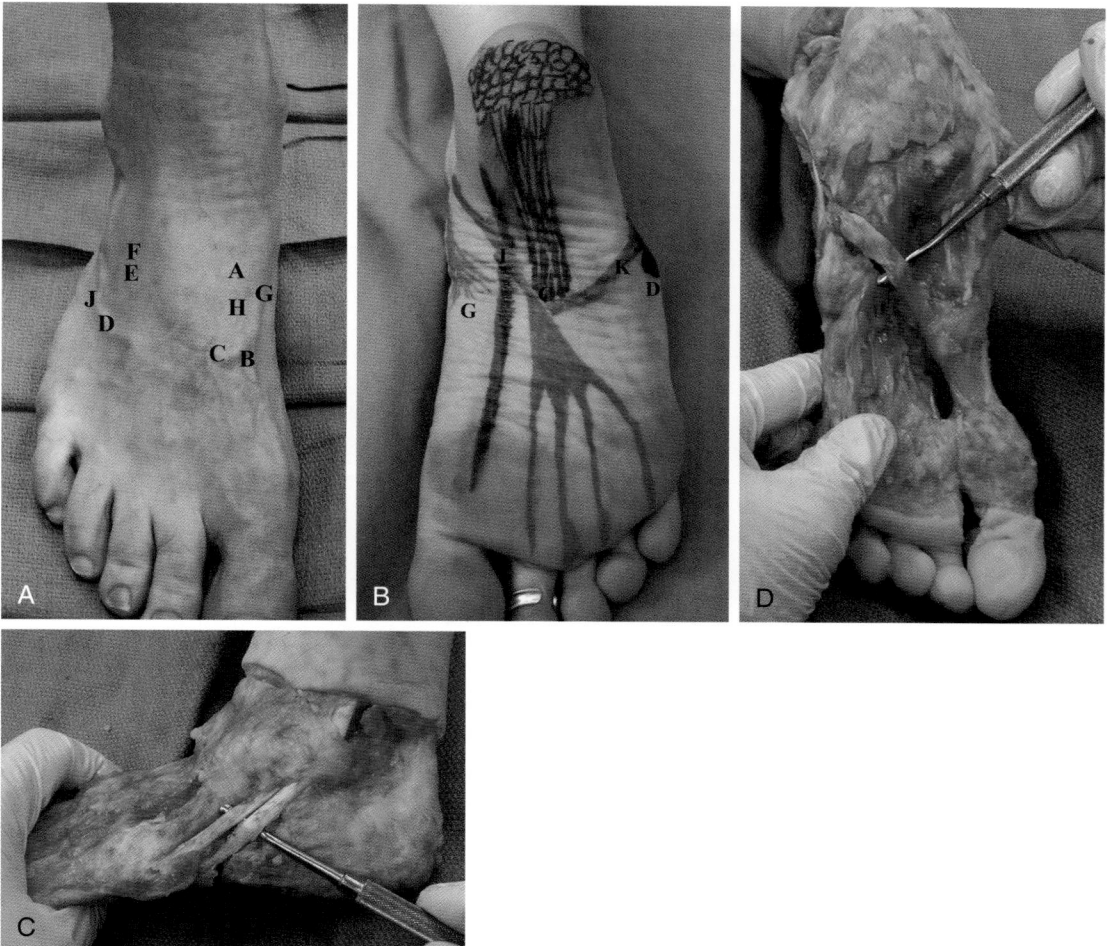

Figure 2-14 Midfoot. **A,** Dorsal view. *A,* Talonavicular joint; *B,* first tarsometatarsal joint; *C,* second metatarsal base; *D,* base of the fifth metatarsal; *E,* calcaneocuboid joint; *F,* anterior process of the calcaneus; *G,* insertion of the posterior tibialis; *H,* insertion of the anterior tibialis; *J,* peroneus brevis insertion. **B,** Plantar view. *D,* base of the fifth metatarsal; *G,* insertion of the posterior tibialis; *I,* master knot of Henry; *J,* peroneus brevis insertion; *K,* cuboid tunnel. **C,** Anatomic specimen demonstrating peroneus longus and brevis. **D,** Plantar view of peroneus longus insertion.

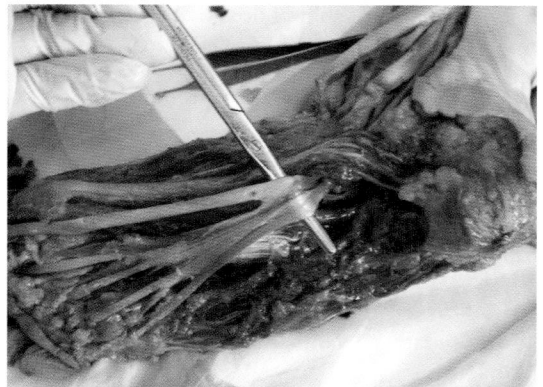

Figure 2-15 Anatomic specimen demonstrating the knot of Henry.

cross the dorsal medial midfoot and also are best palpated after active dorsiflexion of the toes.

On the lateral side, the peroneus brevis insertion *(J)* on the base of the fifth metatarsal is best appreciated with active eversion. The peroneus longus can be palpated as it exits the inferior peroneal retinaculum plantar to the peroneus brevis. As the peroneus longus crosses superficial to the calcaneocuboid joint, it is felt as it dives plantar to head into the cuboid tunnel *(K)* and then across the bottom of the foot to the base of the first metatarsal. The cuboid tunnel and the peroneus longus in it can be palpated by deep pressure at the plantar-lateral cuboid.

The plantar fascia (PF) can be appreciated on the plantar foot with passive dorsiflexion of the toes (the Windlass mechanism). At the midfoot, the PF is wider than and not as thick as it is in the hindfoot. At this point, the examiner also can see the PF inserting to the five toes. The intrinsic foot muscles can be palpated as a group, but,

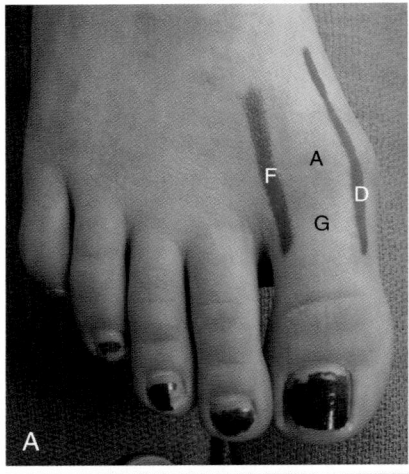
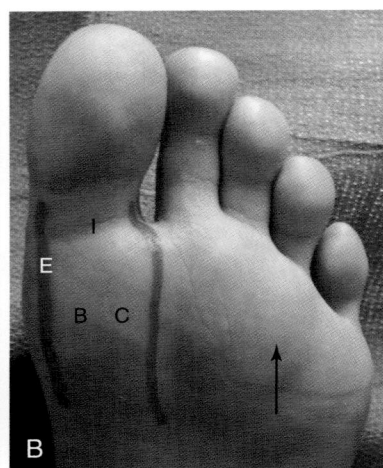
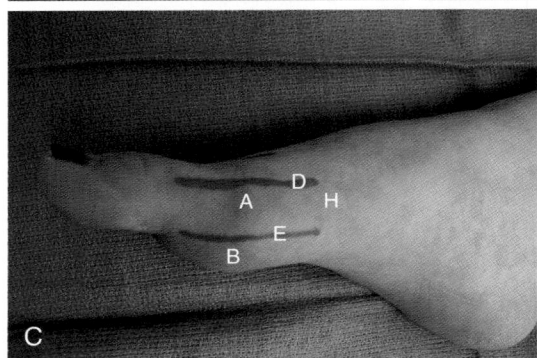

Figure 2-16 Hallux complex. **A,** Dorsal view. *A,* Head of the first metatarsal; *D,* dorsal medial hallucal nerve; *F,* dorsal lateral hallucal nerve; *G,* extensor hallucis longus. **B,** Plantar view. *B,* Tibial (medial) sesamoid; *C,* fibular (lateral) sesamoid; *E,* plantar medial hallucal nerve; *I,* flexor hallucis longus. **C,** Medial view. *A,* Head of the first metatarsal; *B,* tibial (medial) sesamoid; *D,* dorsal medial hallucal nerve; *E,* plantar medial hallucal nerve; *H,* abductor hallucis tendon.

other than the abductor hallucis (medial) and abductor digiti minimi (lateral), the specific muscles cannot be isolated.

Forefoot

Hallux Complex

The forefoot examination often begins with the hallux and its surrounding complex (Fig. 2-16). The first metatarsal can be palpated along its entire course. Beginning with the base of the proximal metatarsal, the first metatarsal can be followed distally to the head of the metatarsal *(A)*. At the first metatarsal's distal plantar extent, the tibial (medial) *(B)* and fibular (lateral) sesamoids *(C)* can be appreciated. They can best be felt by passive dorsiflexion of the hallux MTP joint and deep palpation of the fat pad plantar to the joint. The proximal phalanx is very superficial and can be felt almost circumferentially. The hallux interphalangeal joint and the distal phalanx of the hallux can also be palpated circumferentially.

The sensory nerves of the hallux are very superficial and can be palpated in a thin patient. The clinically significant nerves are the dorsal hallucal nerve and the plantar medial hallucal nerve. The dorsal hallucal nerve *(D)* is felt as a rounded cord on the dorsomedial edge of the medial eminence of the first metatarsal. The plantar-medial hallucal nerve *(E)* is found on the plantar-medial

first metatarsal, just medial and dorsal to the tibial sesamoid bone and the dorsal lateral hallucal nerve *(F)* on the lateral aspect of the hallux. The dorsalis pedis artery pulse is appreciated proximal to the bases of the first and second metatarsals as the artery goes to the plantar foot.

The tendons of the hallux are palpated circumferentially. Dorsally, the EHL *(G)* (larger) and EHB (smaller and lateral) can best be seen with active dorsiflexion of the hallux (Fig. 2-17). The abductor hallucis tendon (see Fig. 2-16) *(H)* is appreciated dorsal to the tibial sesamoid at the joint line of the hallux MTP joint. The FHL *(I)* is appreciated between the sesamoids plantarly. It can be found lying on the proximal phalanx by rolling a finger across the plantar proximal phalanx all the way to the FHL insertion on the plantar base of the distal phalanx. The flexor hallucis brevis cannot be felt directly, but its location can be estimated by allowing a finger to slide proximally and distally on the sesamoids.

Lesser Metatarsals and Toes

The lesser metatarsals and the corresponding toes can be discussed as a group (Fig. 2-18A and B). As in the hallux, the bony anatomy is quite superficial. The metatarsal shafts can be palpated their entire length dorsally. The shafts are best located at the midmetatarsal and can be palpated distally or proximally as indicated. The plantar metatarsals cannot be directly palpated until the distal

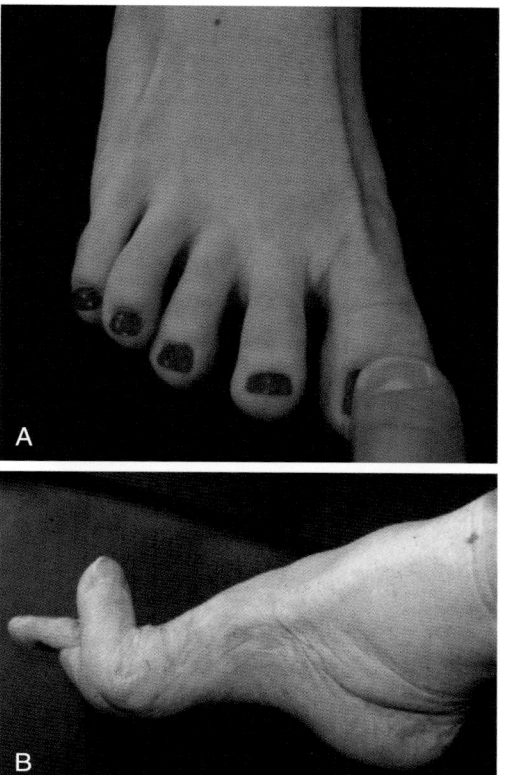

Figure 2-17 **A,** Normal appearance of the extensor hallucis longus (EHL). **B,** After a cerebrovascular accident, an overactive EHL causes excess dorsiflexion of the hallux.

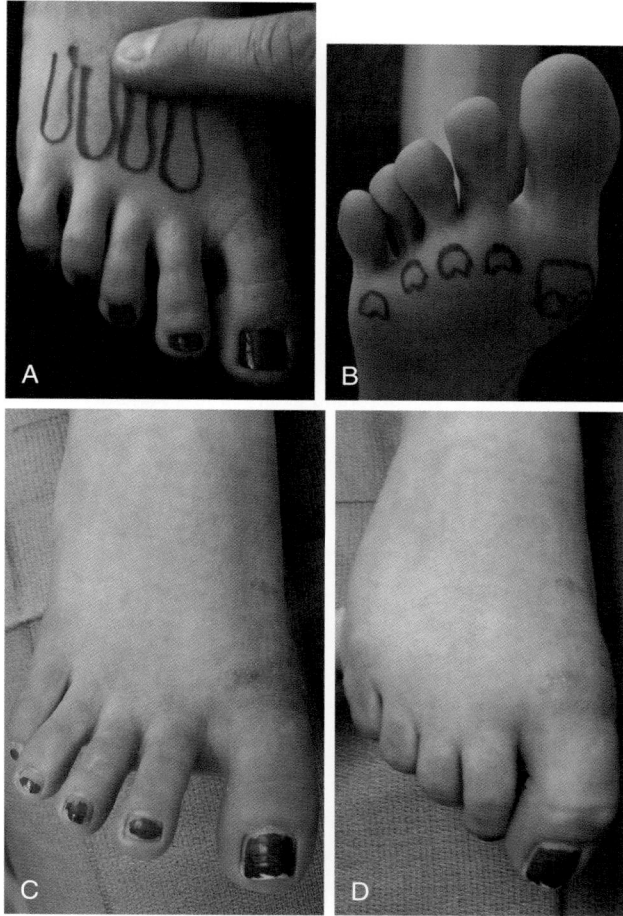

Figure 2-18 Forefoot. Dorsal **(A)** and plantar **(B)** views of the lesser metatarsals and toes. **C,** Extension of lesser toes. **D,** Flexion of lesser toes.

end or head. The metatarsal heads are always felt, but the detail is variable depending on the thickness of the plantar fat pad. The dorsal toe bones are easier to palpate than the plantar bones. Regardless, the MTP joints can be appreciated by passive plantar and dorsiflexion of the toes. The proximal interphalangeal (PIP) and distal interphalangeal (DIP) joints can be appreciated by passive or active plantar flexion of the joints (Fig. 2-18C and D). As the toes get smaller, the joints become less active and more passive. The fifth toe has little active control.

The tendons of the lesser toes move as a unit and are best examined together. The EDL can be seen best with active dorsiflexion of the toes. The EDB can usually be seen with the same maneuver in the second and third toes, but it is less accessible in the fourth. The FDL can be best palpated plantar at the base of the toes with a finger sweep in the transverse direction. Active flexion of the toes can help with this. The plantar plate of the MTP joint is in the space between the plantar metatarsal head and the base of the proximal phalanges.

EXAMINATION IN SEQUENCE

As mentioned earlier, the systematic sequence of the foot and ankle examination allows the examiner to be thorough and complete. Observation is the key first

component to the physical examination. The standing examination is performed, followed by a thorough seated examination. Supine and prone examinations are helpful for specific situations. Finally, if necessary, observation of the patient's gait and evaluation of footwear can add important information.

Standing Examination

The standing examination can provide the examiner with a tremendous amount of information. Asymmetry is best addressed on standing examination by using a direct visual comparison with the opposite extremity.

First, the patient is asked to stand facing the examiner, either on the floor or on a raised stool, with feet shoulder width apart (Fig. 2-19). This allows visualization of the anterior pelvis, the patellae, and the tibial tubercle. Using these anatomic landmarks, the rotation of the foot in relation to the tibia, hip, and pelvis can be established. To estimate pelvic tilt from the front, the examiner places an index finger on either the anterior superior iliac spines or the iliac crests. An anatomic or functional shortening

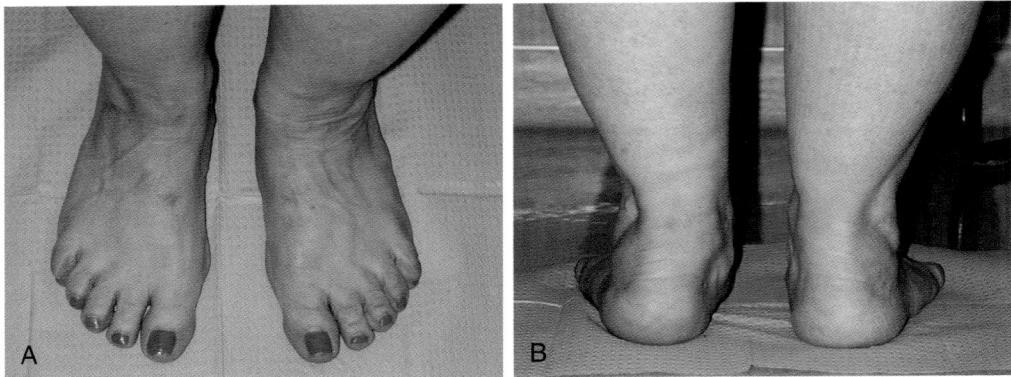

Figure 2-19 Standing examination. **A,** Patient facing the examiner. **B,** Patient facing away from the examiner.

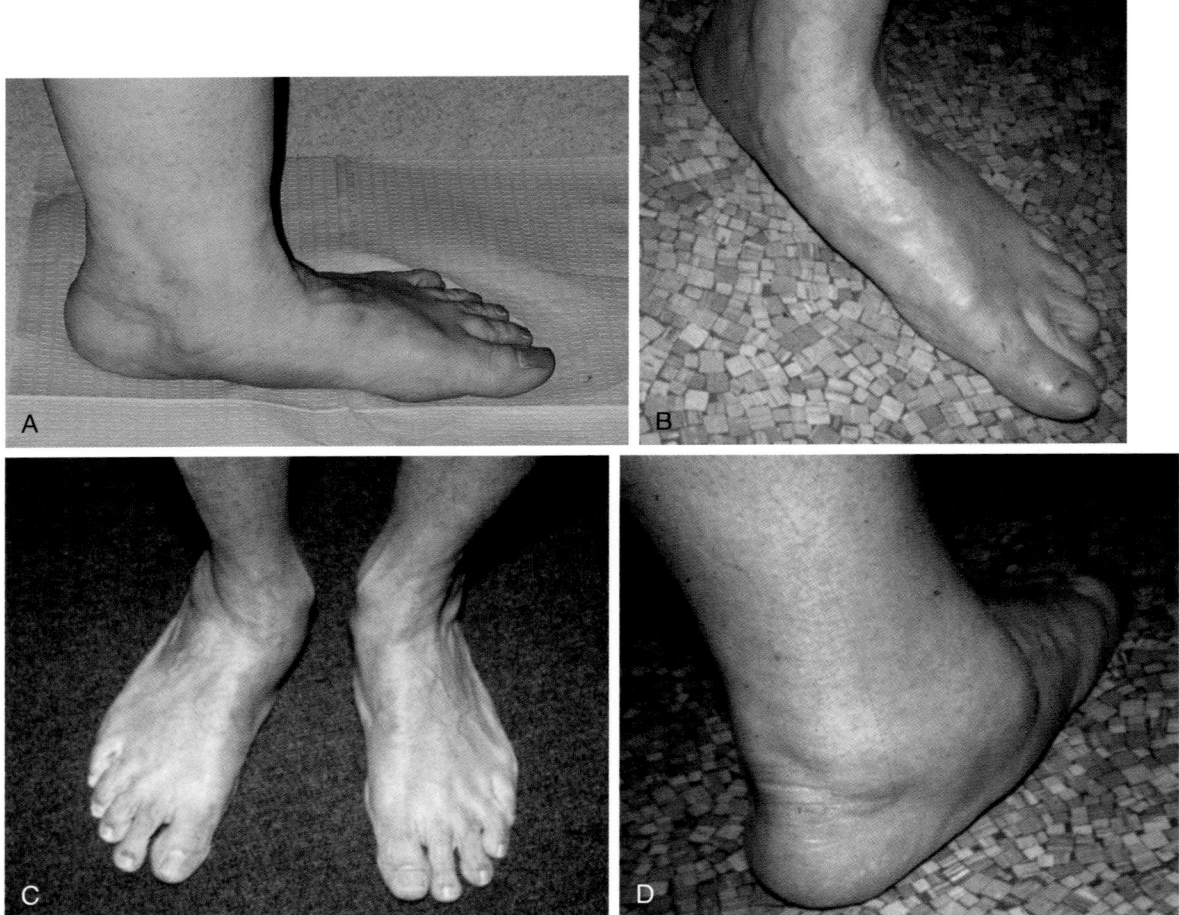

Figure 2-20 Examples of pes planus. **A,** Severe pes planus. **B to D,** Varying degrees of pes planus.

of one leg can be seen readily if the shortening is greater than ¼ inch. Inspection of the popliteal creases reveals whether major shortening is in the thigh or in the lower leg. Gross abnormalities of the lower extremity, including circumference difference of the thighs and calves and excessive deviation in skeletal alignment in all planes (varus, valgus, flexion, extension, and rotation), are best appreciated during the standing examination.

Once overall leg alignment is established, inspection of the foot and ankle begins with the medial longitudinal arch. The presence of pes planus or pes cavus can be determined. There are least two general categories of pes planus for the purposes of the physical examination. In one category, the longitudinal arch is depressed, with a relatively normal valgus hindfoot position and straight midfoot and forefoot (Fig. 2-20A and B). In addition, the

Achilles tendon remains relatively in line with the hindfoot. In the second category, the foot appears to have fallen inward, like the tilting of a half-hemisphere (Fig. 2-20C and D). The heel is in excessive valgus, the outer border of the foot shows angulation at the midfoot, and the forefoot is abducted, creating a more complex deformity. In contrast to the first category, the Achilles tendon deviates laterally when the patient bears weight on the relaxed foot. The pathologic implications of these two types of flatfoot are different.

The pes cavus or high arch foot also has two main types, although the two are often combined. In the first, the heel is in neutral to slight valgus, but the forefoot flexibility allows good ground accommodation through forefoot pronation or a plantar-flexed first ray (Fig. 2-21A). In the second, the heel is fixed in varus and the midfoot and forefoot have compensated by forefoot adduction, which results in lateral column overload (Fig. 2-21B). The presence of heel varus during the front-facing examination is indicated by the ability to visualize the medial border of the heel. Again, the pathologic process associated with the two types is different. The Coleman block test is an excellent way to determine whether the cavus foot position is being driven by the forefoot or the hindfoot (see Chapter 6). Both flatfoot and cavus foot consist of a spectrum of deformities that involve both bony and soft tissue components, the majority of which are normal physiologic variations. However, a consistent definition of "normal," when speaking of flatfoot and cavus foot, is unclear.

Finally, the front-facing standing examination gives a good view of the toes and how they contact the ground. The valgus or varus position of the hallux is highlighted with weight bearing. The pronation of the hallux in relation to the rest of the foot is seen best in this posture. The lesser toes can also be appreciated in this way. Crossover deformities, cock-up deformities, joint contractures, floating toes, and dynamic location of callus (terminal or dorsal) are most efficiently examined with the patient standing on a stool. The examiner also should note whether the toes touch the ground (Figs. 2-22A and B).

At this point, the patient should be observed while facing away from the seated examiner (see Fig. 2-19B). Again, the feet should be shoulder width apart to ascertain the true hindfoot alignment. The pelvis, femur, thigh, knee, tibia, and calf symmetry is reexamined from this view. In particular, the relationship of the heel axis to the ankle joint and the rest of the foot are appreciated. Excessive heel valgus or varus should be noted. The lateral metatarsal and toes are seen normally from this view, although the ability to visualize more toes on one side compared with the other may indicate a pathologic flatfoot deformity. Asymmetry in this examination goes a long way in illustrating the cause and solution in hindfoot, midfoot, and ankle disorder.

While the patient is facing away from the examiner, it is helpful to have the patient elevate to balance on the toes. If the foot is functioning normally, the heel promptly inverts, the longitudinal arch rises, and the leg rotates externally (Fig. 2-23). Failure of these movements to occur can indicate a weak foot or a specific pathologic process. The patient should also be asked to single-limb toe raise on each foot (Fig. 2-24). This can demonstrate early weakness, especially when the patient is asked to do it multiple times, or marked weakness if the patient is unable to single-limb toe raise at all. In patients who are able to perform the task, it is importation to ask if it elicits pain and where the pain occurs. Do not place too much stock in the single-limb toe raise in elderly patients, because many elderly patients are unable to accomplish this maneuver even when all joints and tendons are normal.

Inversion of the heel is achieved through proper performance of the subtalar and transverse tarsal articulations and the tendons that act across these joints. Failure of the heel to invert or eliciting pain during the maneuver should immediately focus the examiner's attention on possible malfunction of these structures. Some conditions that can limit activity in these joints are muscle weakness, dysfunction of the tibialis posterior, arthritic changes in the hindfoot, and such skeletal abnormalities as vertical talus and tarsal coalition.

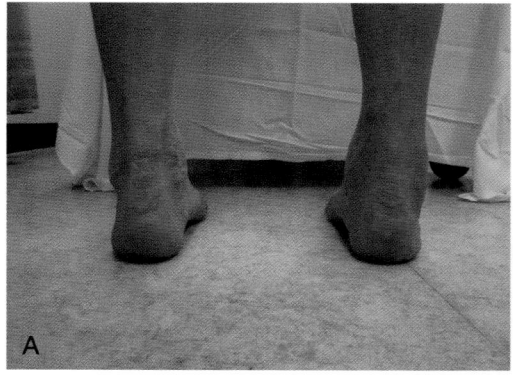 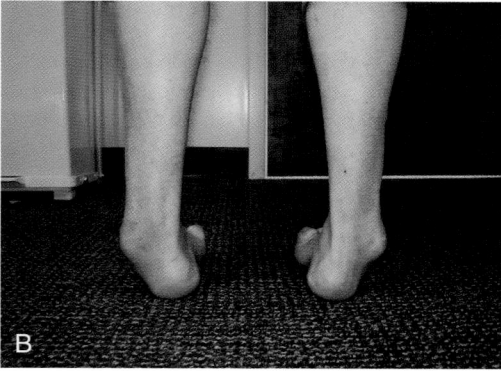

Figure 2-21 A, View of the lower extremity from behind, highlighting cavus foot with neutral hindfoot alignment. **B,** Cavovarus foot posture with lateral column overload.

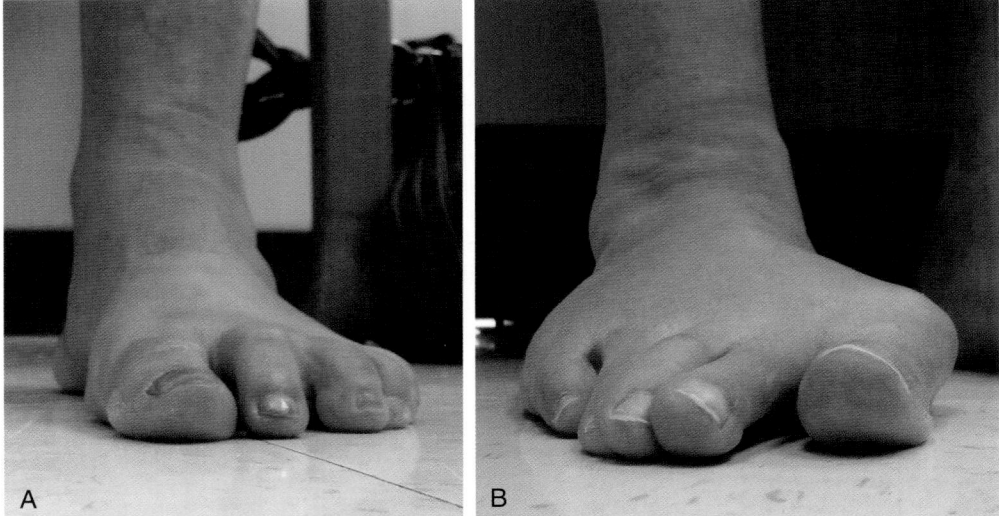

Figure 2-22 **A,** The neutral or unpronated hallux, which is considered normal. **B,** Significant pronation (malrotation) of the hallux in association with valgus malalignment.

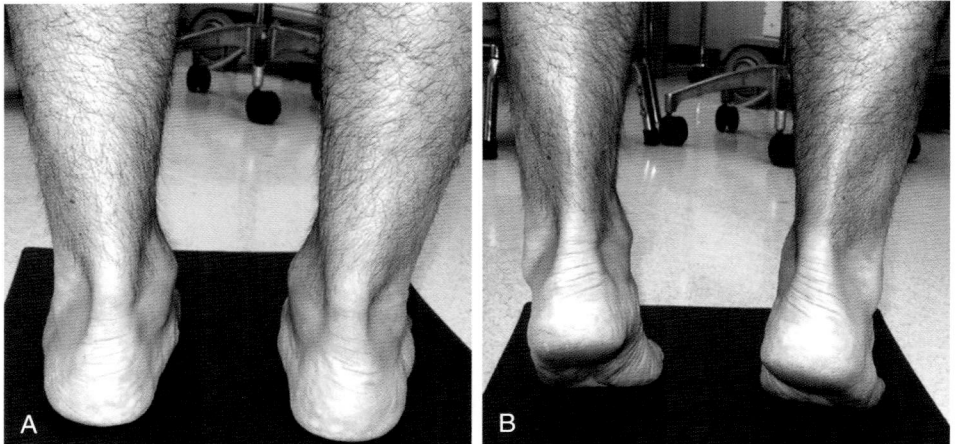

Figure 2-23 Dynamic arch creation. **A,** Flatfoot at stance. **B,** Arch creation at toe-off.

Sitting Examination

The patient is asked to sit on the edge of the table with the legs dangling over the edge (Fig. 2-25). The examiner should sit lower on a stool. This allows for easy inspection, palpation, and manipulation of both extremities. It is at this point that the lessons learned in the topographic anatomy section are best used.

General Visual Overview

Any visible abnormalities should be noted at this time. Varicosities, areas of telangiectasia, erythema, and ecchymosis, and generalized edema should be noted. The skin is examined for local areas of swelling, and the structures in these areas are palpated. The skin over joints normally is cooler than the skin over muscular areas of the extremity. The examiner should observe the various muscle groups, looking for atrophy in the anterior, lateral, and posterior calf region, as well as the medial side of the foot.

The distribution of hair on the foot should be carefully noted. Loss of distal foot or toe hair can suggest a systemic disorder, such as peripheral vascular disease or lupus.

The skin on the plantar aspect of the foot and about the toes is inspected carefully for callus formation, which often indicates abnormal pressure on the foot. All scars, wounds, and ulcerations should be noted, surgical or otherwise, because this can give the examiner insight into the history of that particular foot.

General Skeletal Overview

Gross skeletal deformities are readily discernible and can hardly be overlooked even by the most inexperienced examiner. Deviation in the hallux MTP joints, lesser toe

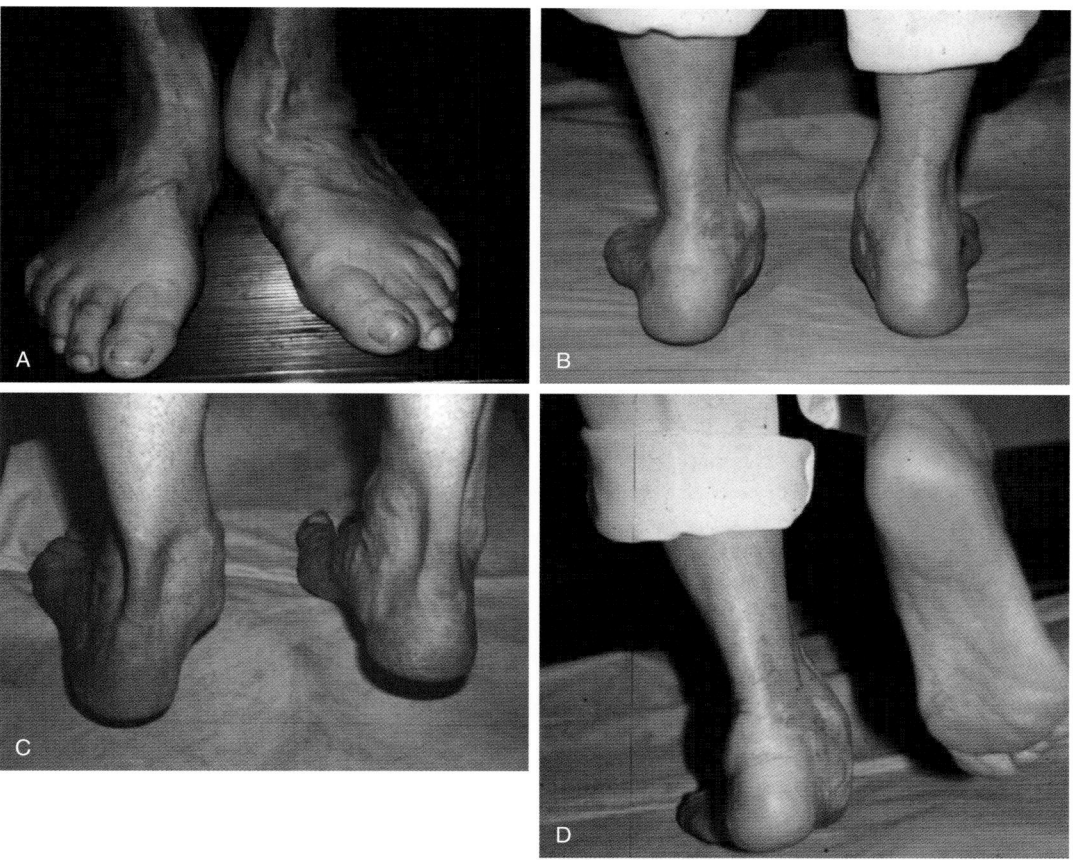

Figure 2-24 Single-limb toe-raise examination. **A,** Anterior view. **B,** Posterior view before examination (patient's left foot has a ruptured posterior tibial tendon). **C,** Patient is able to stand on tip toe on the right foot without difficulty. **D,** On the left foot, the arch sags; the patient is not able to perform a repetitive toe raise.

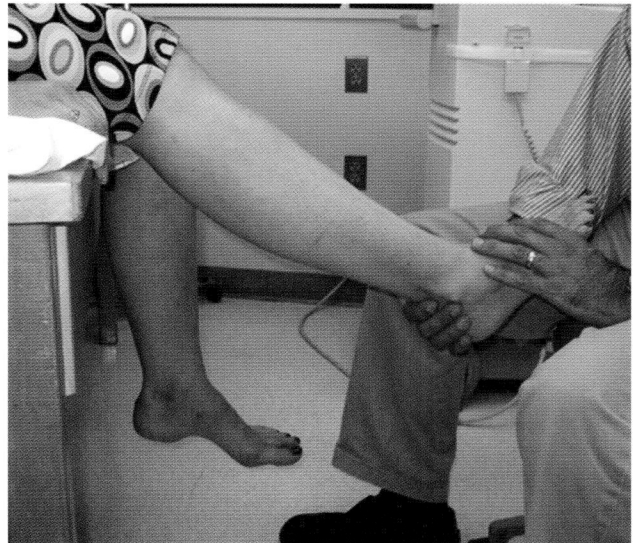

Figure 2-25 Sitting examination. Note the position of the examiner.

deformities, and asymmetric midfoot deformity can be observed grossly at this point. The bony prominences about the foot are carefully noted. A prominence over the region of the tarsometatarsal joints may be the first sign of arthrosis of these joints, and a prominence over the fifth metatarsal head can indicate a bunionette deformity. Difficulties in making a diagnosis are more likely to arise in patients whose feet, on casual inspection, appear relatively normal.

Neurovascular Examination

Evaluating the neurovascular status should be performed after inspection as it can offer clues to systemic or focal issues present. The posterior tibial and dorsalis pedis pulses should be palpated and their strength noted. When the pulses are difficult to palpate, testing capillary refill time by compressing the distal nail bed and measuring time to reperfusion is a helpful way to gauge overall perfusion. Normal capillary refill time is considered to be less than 2 seconds. Weak or absent pulses may indicate problems such as peripheral vascular disease, systemic autoimmune disorders, or diabetes, which are important considerations, especially in surgical candidates.

The detailed peripheral nerve evaluation is best directed by the history. When the patient complains of a burning type of pain, often accompanied by a feeling of numbness, a careful sensory examination should be conducted because this is most often nerve pain. Such complaints often indicate peripheral nerve disorders and may be early symptoms of a generalized neuritis or neuropathy. Systemic disorders, such as diabetes and sensory axonal neuropathy, are commonly first suspected after a careful foot examination. Simple office tools, such as the Semmes-Weinstein monofilament test (Fig. 2-26), can be used to assess the degree of sensory deficit in the patient. The examiner should check not only for deficits in cutaneous sensation and reflexes but also for diminished positional and vibratory sensation.

There are several areas in the foot in which the peripheral nerve may be locally entrapped and irritated. The most common site is the tibial nerve as it passes through the tarsal tunnel, which is located behind the medial malleolus. Percussion along the course of the nerve as it passes through the tunnel to elicit tingling can indicate compression or irritation of the nerve. The deep peroneal nerve can be entrapped beneath the extensor retinaculum of the dorsum of the foot and ankle; this is known as *anterior tarsal tunnel syndrome*. When the diagnosis is suspected, the examiner should carefully percuss over the inferior extensor retinaculum and along the course of the deep peroneal nerve to look for evidence of tingling, which indicates irritability of the nerve. Besides being compressed at the level of the extensor retinaculum, the irritation of the nerve may occur as it passes over a dorsal exostosis at the talonavicular joint or more distally at the tarsometatarsal articulation.

Burning pain that radiates to the web space between the third and fourth toes should raise suspicion of interdigital neuroma. Firm palpation in the plantar web space usually reproduces the neuritic symptoms. Palpation of the plantar metatarsal heads should be performed at the same time because metatarsalgia is another common cause of plantar foot pain, in particular when the complaints are centered around the first and second web space. Mediolateral compression of the foot, particularly when examining the third web space, can result in a click and pain radiating toward the toes. Finally, direct palpation in the distal aspect of the web space while dorsiflexing the toes is a sensitive test for interdigital neuroma, because this maneuver pulls the interdigital nerve against the offending intermetatarsal ligament.

On rare occasions, a tight band of transverse crural fascia entraps the superficial peroneal nerves. This is detected by carefully percussing along the inferior margin of the crural fascia when examining a patient who complains of discomfort over the dorsum of the foot. Nerve entrapment also can occur around a surgical scar or in an area that has been crushed, and these areas should be carefully noted. The sural nerve is particularly at risk for surgical scar entrapment or injury after lateral hindfoot procedures, such as the extensile lateral approach for calcaneus fractures.

Range of Motion of the Joints

While the patient remains on the table, the joints of the foot and ankle should be assessed for motion. The passive and active range of motion of all major articulations of the foot should be checked for limitation of motion, painful movement, and crepitus. These findings can occur separately or in any combination or sequence.

ANKLE JOINT

The ankle joint should be moved through its full range of motion (Fig. 2-27). Normal ankle range of motion is approximately 10 to 15 degrees of dorsiflexion to 45 to 50 degrees of plantar flexion. Although the ankle is essentially a single-axis joint, its axis travels along a line that is reasonably estimated by placing the tips of the index fingers just below the most distal projections of the two malleoli (Fig. 2-28). Therefore the axis travels posteriorly and inferiorly from a medial to lateral direction. In

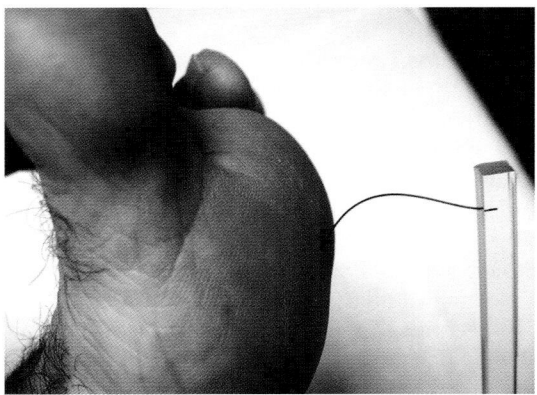

Figure 2-26 Semmes-Weinstein monofilament.

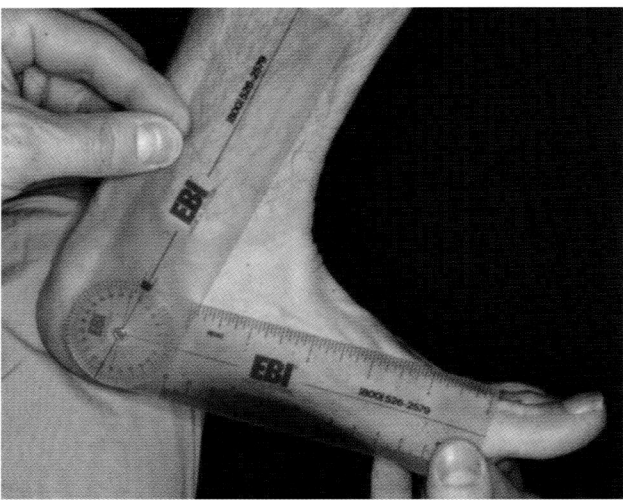

Figure 2-27 Ankle range of motion documented on the lateral aspect with a goniometer.

addition, based on the conical nature of the talus, with the radius of curvature being longer laterally than medially, rotation of the ankle joint results in medial deviation of the foot in plantar flexion and lateral deviation of the foot in dorsiflexion. Because an oblique axis of the ankle assists in absorbing the horizontal rotation of the leg, its range of motion on gross examination is related to the range of motion in the subtalar joint.

The ankle joint should also be checked for instability in the sagittal, coronal, and rotational planes. The anterior drawer examination and the inversion stress test examine the stability of the lateral ankle ligaments (in particular the anterior talofibular ligament [ATFL] and calcaneofibular ligament [CFL], respectively) (Fig. 2-29A and B). Adding an external rotation moment to the anterior drawer examination can check the stability of the deltoid ligament, although this can be a very subtle finding. Normally, there is no lateral shift of the talus in the mortise even when the foot is in full plantar flexion. Any lateral or medial displacement of the talus within the

mortise that is seen on examination indicates an abnormality of the mortise. The stability of the syndesmosis is checked by both the calf compression test and the external rotation test (Fig. 2-30A and B). Actual laxity is often difficult to appreciate, although, if either of these tests creates pain along the syndesmosis, an injury to these ligaments should be suspected. When checking stability, it is extremely important and helpful to use the opposite extremity for comparison.

SUBTALAR JOINT

The amount of motion in the subtalar joint varies. Isman and Inman[1] found a minimum of 20 degrees and a maximum of 60 degrees of motion in a series of feet in cadaver specimens. Motion in the subtalar joint is intimately involved with motion in the talonavicular joint and calcaneocuboid joint. If one of these joints is stiff or arthritic, it can significantly affect the motion seen in the other joints. A gross method of determining the degree of subtalar motion is to apply rotatory force on the calcaneus in the coronal plane while permitting the rest of the foot to move passively. When this is combined with a rotatory force applied to the forefoot, the foot proceeds through large displacements in motion through the talonavicular and calcaneocuboid joints that are additive to subtalar motion. This method allows gross analysis of the flexibility or rigidity of the hindfoot, which can be important in certain clinical situations, such as adult-acquired flatfoot (see Chapter 25).

The most accurate, but not practical, method of determining the degree of subtalar motion is to place the patient prone and flex the knee to approximately 135 degrees. The axis of the subtalar joint now lies close to the horizontal plane. The examiner then passively inverts and everts the heel while measuring the extent of motion with a gravity goniometer or level (Fig. 2-31). This method is used primarily for research purposes.

A more practical method of determining the degree of subtalar motion is accomplished while the patient is sitting on the examining table. The calcaneus is placed in

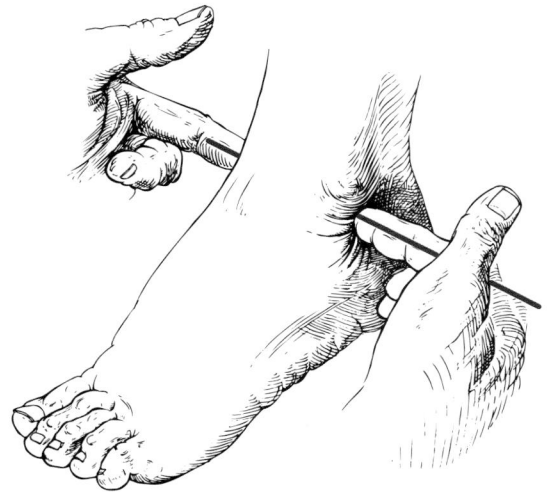

Figure 2-28 Estimating the location of the ankle axis.

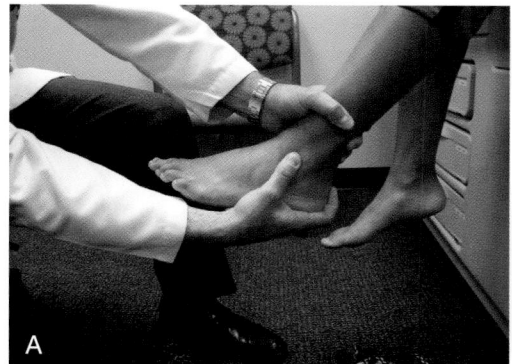
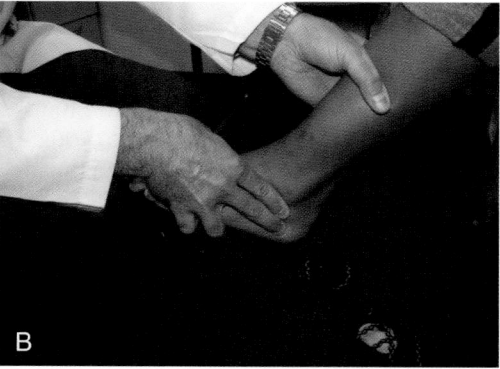

Figure 2-29 **A,** The anterior drawer examination. The foot is pulled anteriorly, with the ankle in slight plantar flexion and counterpressure applied to the anterior tibia. **B,** Inversion or talar tilt stress test. The heel is inverted while maintaining the ankle in a neutral dorsiflexed position. A finger placed on the lateral talar process during inversion will assist in determining that the instability is arising from the ankle and not subtalar joint.

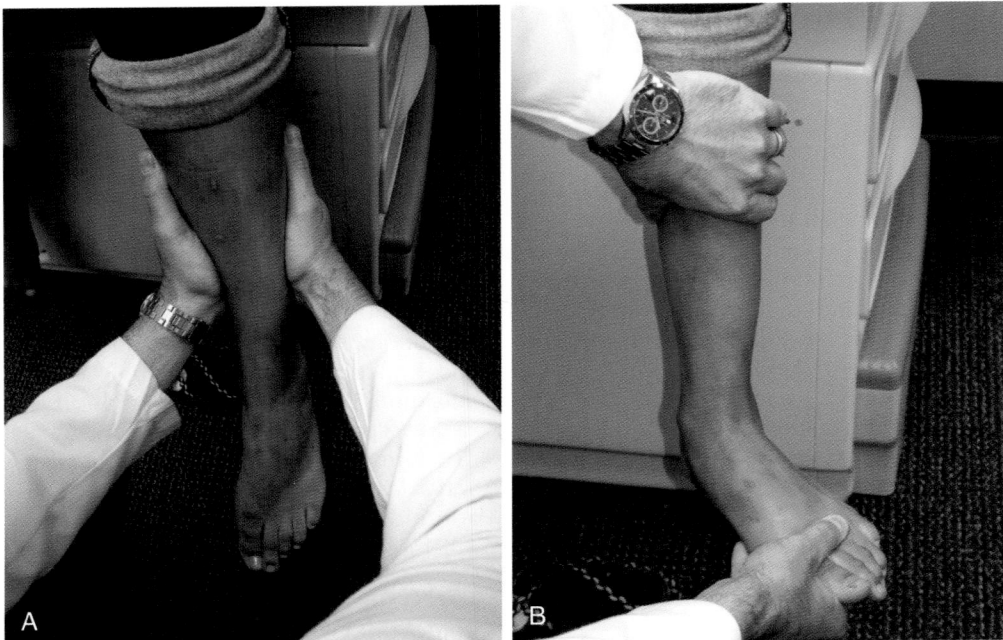

Figure 2-30 **A,** The calf compression or "squeeze" test. Pain elicited with this maneuver is suggestive of a syndesmotic injury. **B,** External rotation stress test may identify a syndesmotic injury with production of pain or instability. With the knee flexed, rotate the foot externally while maintaining the leg in a fixed position.

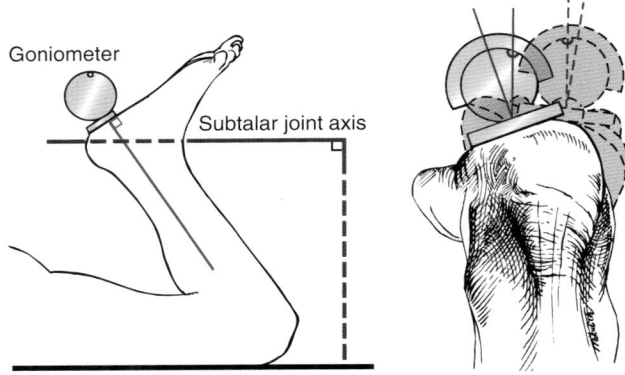

Figure 2-31 Spheric goniometer attached to the calcaneus to measure the degree of subtalar motion.

line with the long axis of the tibia. With the calcaneus held in one hand and the forefoot (including the transverse tarsal joint) in the other, the subtalar joint is brought into inversion and eversion. It is helpful to place a fingertip on the lateral process of the talus to determine if any of the inversion is occurring through the ankle joint. While carrying out this motion, it is important to note not only the total range of motion but also the amount of inversion and eversion. There usually is twice as much inversion as eversion. Occasionally, in a patient with flatfoot, although there is full total range of motion, the plane of motion is such that little or no inversion occurs. It also is important to observe any asymmetry of subtalar motion in a percentage fashion. This is often the most

reproducible measurement for this joint. Lack of subtalar motion should alert the examiner to the possibility of arthrosis of the subtalar joint, peroneal spastic flatfoot, or an anatomic abnormality such as tarsal coalition.

TRANSVERSE TARSAL JOINT

The motion of the transverse tarsal joint (talonavicular and calcaneocubiod joints) is observed by holding the calcaneus in line with the long axis of the tibia (the subtalar neutral position) and the forefoot parallel to the floor. Adduction and abduction of this joint can be isolated (Fig. 2-32). Although these measurements are somewhat variable, a general rule is that there is twice as much adduction as abduction at the transverse tarsal joint. As with the subtalar joint, it is imperative that the total range of motion is noted as well as the degree of adduction and abduction. In some pathologic states, such as posterior tibial tendon dysfunction or arthrosis of the midtarsal joints, the foot is maintained in a chronically abducted position, and a neutral position cannot be achieved. This fixed abduction should be noted to highlight the joints with the primary disorder.

TARSOMETATARSAL JOINTS

The first metatarsocuneiform joint has variable range of motion in both the sagittal and coronal plane. To test this motion in the sagittal plane, the four lesser metatarsal heads should be held in one hand while the first metatarsal head should be translated dorsally and plantarly. This test determines first-ray mobility, which is important in hallux valgus pathology. Hypermobility of this joint is

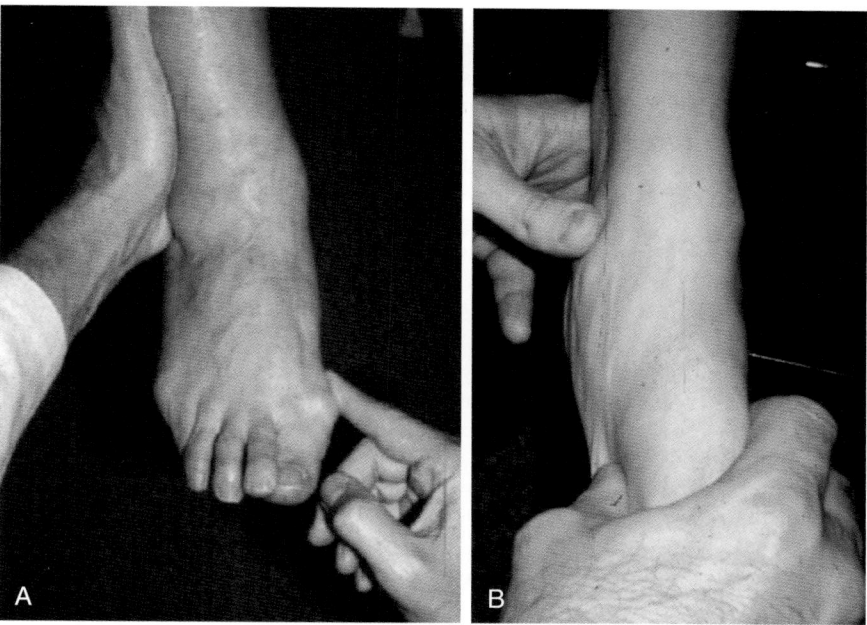

Figure 2-32 Evaluation of the transverse tarsal joint. The hindfoot is stabilized and the forefoot is abducted **(A)** and adducted **(B)**.

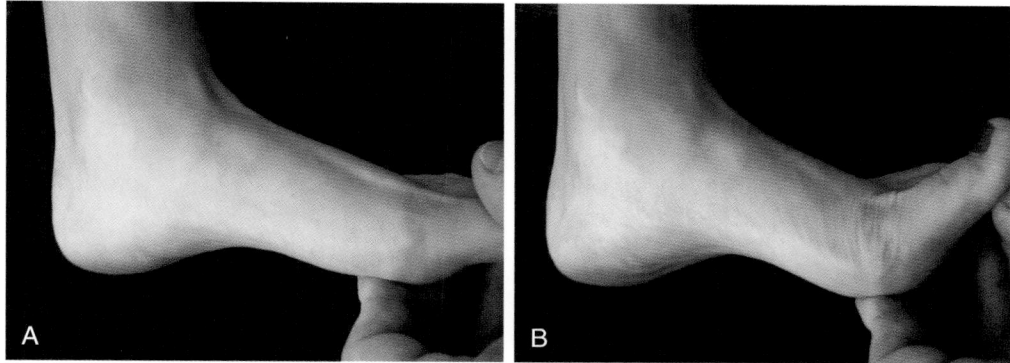

Figure 2-33 Range of motion of the first metatarsophalangeal joint. **A,** Normal resting position. **B,** Passive dorsiflexion.

not well defined and is examiner dependent, although getting a sense of the normal range of mobility comes with experience. The second and third metatarsocuneiform joints have minimal motion in the normal setting. The fourth and fifth tarsometatarsal joints are extremely flexible in the sagittal plane and can also be isolated by holding the medial three metatarsal heads while translating the fourth and fifth dorsally and plantarly. Axial rotation of the forefoot while holding the subtalar neutral position can elicit midfoot pain in the setting of tarsometatarsal arthrosis.

METATARSOPHALANGEAL JOINTS

Motion at the MTP joints is measured by placing the ankle at a right angle and having the patient actively dorsiflex and plantar flex the MTP joints and the interphalangeal joints. Then passive motion can be

determined at the same time. Again, there is a great deal of individual variability, with dorsiflexion ranging from 45 to 90 degrees and plantar flexion from 10 to 40 degrees, depending on the mobility of the individual joints. Dorsal translation of the lesser MTP joints can be tested by holding the metatarsal head in one hand and the base of the proximal phalanx in the other hand and directing a dorsal force with the thumb. This examination tests the integrity of the plantar plate and is especially important in the second and third MTP joint. The critical factor is, again, to compare the sides for asymmetry. The motion of the interphalangeal joints is likewise observed (Fig. 2-33).

Relationship of Forefoot to Hindfoot

After the range of motion of the foot has been determined, the relationship of the hindfoot to the forefoot should be ascertained. This relationship is important because it can be the underlying cause of the patient's clinical problem. Determination of this relationship is best carried out with the patient sitting on the examining table with the knees flexed at 90 degrees.

The hindfoot is grasped and placed into its neutral position (the calcaneus in line with the long axis of the leg or the Achilles). When examining the right foot, the heel is grasped with the examiner's right hand, and the area of the fifth metatarsal head is grasped with the left hand. The examiner's right thumb is placed over the talonavicular joint, and this joint is manipulated until the examiner feels that the head of the talus is covered by the navicular. This movement is brought about by the examiner's left hand moving the forefoot in relation to the hindfoot. Once the neutral hindfoot position has been achieved, the relationship of the forefoot, as projected by a plane parallel to the metatarsals, is related to a plane perpendicular to the long axis of the calcaneus.

Based on this measurement, the forefoot will be in one of three positions in relation to the hindfoot:

- *Neutral*: The plane of the metatarsals and the plane of the calcaneus are perpendicular to each other.
- *Forefoot varus*: The lateral aspect of the foot is more plantar flexed than the medial aspect, placing the forefoot in a supinated position (Fig. 2-34).
- *Forefoot valgus*: The medial border of the foot is more plantar flexed in relation to the lateral border of the foot, placing the foot in a pronated position.

This measurement should be carried out two or three times to be sure an error is not made (Fig. 2-35).

The importance of this measurement is that by relating the position of the forefoot to the hindfoot, various types of clinical problems can be identified. In the normal foot, the forefoot and hindfoot planes are almost perpendicular to each other, although a moderate degree of variability in the measurement is of no clinical significance. The relation of the forefoot to the hindfoot may be supple or rigid. This determination is important when considering

surgery to create a plantigrade foot. A fixed varus or valgus forefoot deformity does not permit the foot to become plantigrade once the hindfoot is placed into neutral position, and thus the extent of the fusion mass needs to include the transverse tarsal joint in order to realign the forefoot. Conversely, when the forefoot is supple or neutral, realignment of the hindfoot alone permits the forefoot to be plantigrade.

Direct Palpation

The importance of direct palpation cannot be emphasized enough in the examination of the foot and ankle. The ready access to the bony, tendinous, and ligamentous

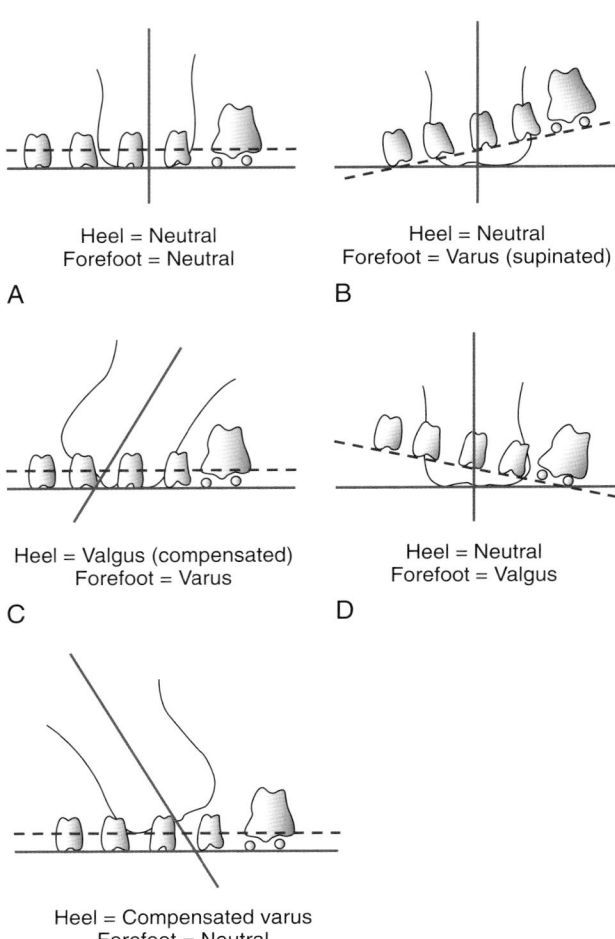

Heel = Neutral
Forefoot = Neutral

A

Heel = Neutral
Forefoot = Varus (supinated)

B

Heel = Valgus (compensated)
Forefoot = Varus

C

Heel = Neutral
Forefoot = Valgus

D

Heel = Compensated varus
Forefoot = Neutral

E

Figure 2-35 Relationship of hindfoot to forefoot. **A,** Normal alignment; forefoot perpendicular to calcaneus. **B,** Forefoot varus (uncompensated); lateral aspect of the forefoot is plantar flexed in relation to the medial aspect. **C,** Forefoot varus (compensated); with the forefoot flat on the floor, the heel assumes a valgus position, which can result in impingement of the calcaneus against the fibula. **D,** Forefoot valgus (uncompensated); the medial aspect of the forefoot is plantar flexed in relation to the lateral aspect. **E,** Forefoot valgus (compensated); with the forefoot flat on the floor, the heel assumes a varus position.

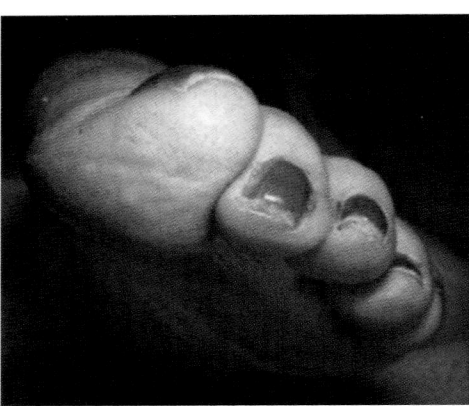

Figure 2-34 Forefoot varus.

structures, in combination with a focused history, is essential to finally determining the exact structure that is pathologic. The distance between the tender area in two medial tendons, FHL and posterior tibialis, is only a few millimeters but makes a world of difference in treatment and prognosis. Careful study of the topographic anatomy (see earlier) allows a mastery of this portion of the seated examination. The systematic palpation must be done carefully and directly. The tools used most often are the tip of the examiner's dominant index finger or, for deeper structures, the tip of the thumb. It is not unusual to arrive at a diagnosis after a careful history and a single palpation with a question: *Does it hurt here?*

One important structure to palpate is the plantar aponeurosis or plantar fascia, which should be palpated along its entire surface. Dorsiflexion of the toes makes the fascia more prominent and facilitates palpation (Fig. 2-36). In the case of a suspected plantar fascial rupture, palpating the proximal portion of both plantar fascias while dorsiflexing the toes will demonstrate a fullness and loss of discrete medial fascial border on the affected side.

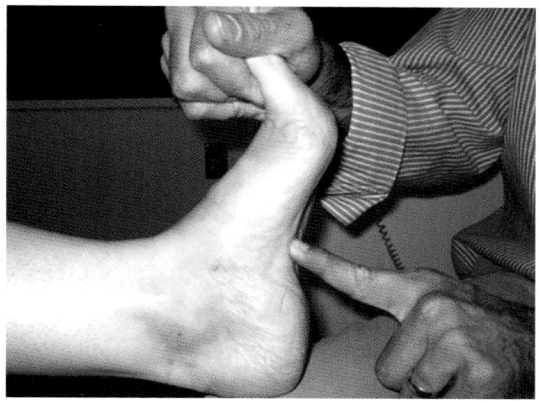

Figure 2-36 Palpation of the plantar aponeurosis facilitated by dorsiflexion of the toes.

Muscle Function

Muscle function about the foot and ankle should be carefully tested. Most of the testing is done while the patient is seated. It is important to observe the strength of each muscle, particularly in a patient who has demonstrated some evidence of muscle weakness. It is also helpful to palpate each tendon to be sure that compensation by another muscle is not masking loss of function. It is imperative that the examiner considers all the information gleaned during each component of the physical examination. For example, a patient who is unable to actively dorsiflex his or her ankle may have a ruptured tibialis anterior tendon, a peroneal nerve palsy, or a significant Achilles contracture. The adept examiner will be able to combine the findings, correlate with the history, and arrive at a presumptive diagnosis. Sometimes, specific muscle groups lead to confusion.

The function of the tibialis posterior is important to assess because it is the principal invertor of the foot. However, the tibialis anterior acts as a secondary invertor as well. To isolate tibialis posterior function from tibialis anterior function, it is important to keep the foot plantar flexed while having the patient actively invert the foot against resistance and palpating the tibialis posterior tendon. In addition, the foot should be placed into an everted position, and then the patient is asked to invert against some resistance. In some patients, this can be done easiest with the patient's legs crossed (Fig. 2-37). Another helpful technique is to ask the patient to point each foot down and in toward the other foot. Asymmetry in the amount of foot inversion is an indication of posterior tibial tendon pathology.

The extrinsic muscles of the lateral foot can lead to similar difficulties. The peroneus brevis muscle functions mainly to evert the foot, and the peroneus longus functions mainly to plantar flex the medial column of the foot. To get a sense of peroneal strength, the patient should be asked to externally rotate the foot against resistance both from an externally rotated and internally rotated position. The eversion function of the peroneus

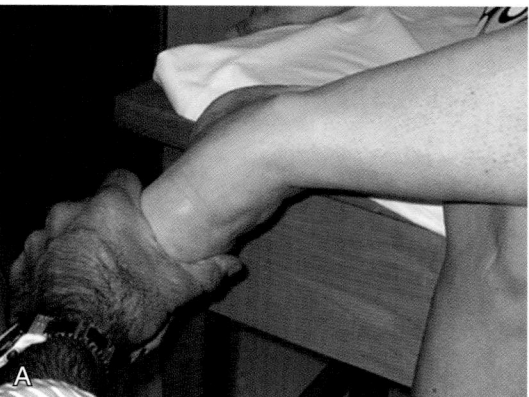 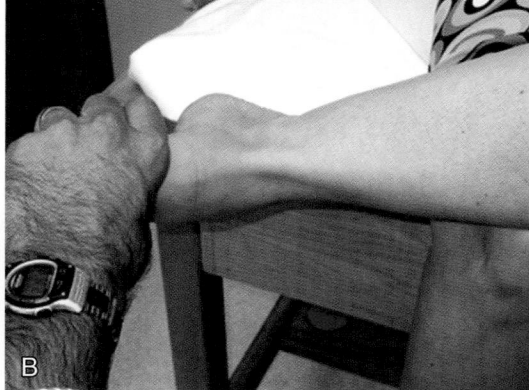

Figure 2-37 Isolation of posterior tibialis muscle function. **A,** The muscle is tested with the patient's foot dependent to gravity with the legs crossed. **B,** The strength is tested from full eversion to full inversion.

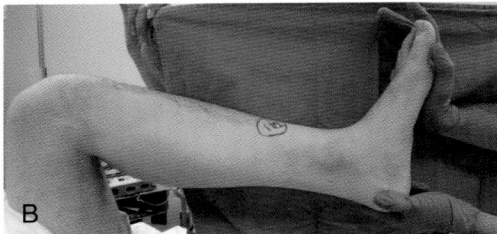

Figure 2-38 Demonstration of the Silverskiold test for determining origin of an Achilles contracture. Dorsiflex the ankle with subtalar neutral and knee extended **(A)**, and then flex the knee **(B).** If ankle dorsiflexion improves with knee flexion, as in this case, then the gastrocnemius portion of the gastrocnemius–soleus complex is considered to be the primary origin.

brevis is tested by simply asking the patient to evert against the resistance. The eversion function of the peroneus longus is quite weak. To isolate the peroneus longus, the patient should be asked to plantar flex the medial side of the foot while the examiner resists beneath the first metatarsal head. This is also an opportune time to examine the stability of the peroneal tendons in the retrofibular groove. The patient is asked to dorsiflex and evert the foot against resistance while the examiner gently palpates the lateral ridge of the distal fibula. An insufficient superior peroneal retinaculum will lead to subluxation of the tendons over the fibular ridge. Circumduction of the foot can also help assess for tendon stability, as well as elicit tendon snapping or intrasheath subluxation.[2]

Not only should the strength of each muscle group be tested, but it is also important to determine whether a contracture is present. In the hindfoot, the most common contracture is the calf muscle complex. To check the gastrocnemius–soleus complex for contracture, with the knee flexed, the hindfoot is first placed into neutral position, and the navicular is centered over the head of the talus. With the foot in neutral position, passive dorsiflexion of the ankle to approximately 10 to 15 degrees should be possible. If not, there is an element of contracture of the muscle group. The knee is then fully extended and the same maneuver carried out. If dorsiflexion past neutral cannot be achieved, then the gastrocnemius portion of the gastrocnemius–soleus complex is contracted. If the subtalar joint is permitted to pass into valgus while the examiner is attempting to measure dorsiflexion at the ankle joint, the presence of a contracture can easily be masked (Fig. 2-38A and B).

Specific Examination Components for Individual Consideration

Supine Examination

The supine examination is mentioned for completeness. The most common use of the supine examination is for a detailed inspection of the plantar foot. In particular, in an obese patient, body habitus prevents adequate inspection of the bottom of the foot while sitting. Rotational and length discrepancies of the lower extremity can also

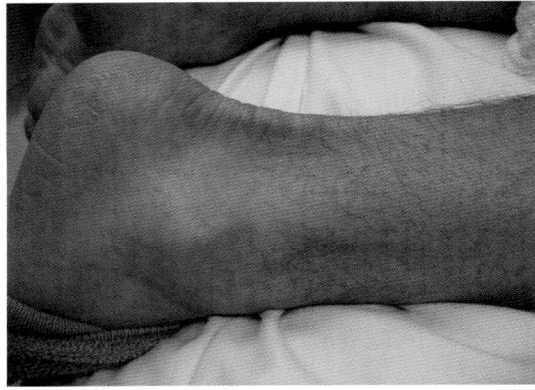

Figure 2-39 Prone examination.

be confirmed or further evaluated during the supine examination.

Prone Examination

The prone examination is a specialty examination that can make certain areas of the foot and ankle more readily accessible (Fig. 2-39). In particular, the posterior calcaneus, Achilles tendon, and calf are best examined prone. The tendon can be palpated along its entirety under direct vision. This allows access to defects and masses. Resting tension of the Achilles is best evaluated prone by asking the patients to flex both knees and visualizing the position of the foot from the end of the bed. Normal resting tension of the Achilles should result in about 10 to 15 degrees of plantar flexion; an asymmetric drop of one foot indicates insufficiency or tear of the Achilles. A Thompson test should also be performed in this position, which consists of squeezing the gastrocnemius–soleus muscle mass and visualizing whether the foot plantar flexes. Lack of plantar flexion in this test indicates discontinuity of the Achilles tendon, most commonly a rupture. The skin over the tendon can also be manipulated in this position to differentiate between a number of Achilles pathologies. The posterior calcaneus can best be viewed and palpated from this approach, in particular at the insertional ridge where the Achilles attaches.

Gait

Evaluation of a patient's gait is an important component of the physical examination in certain clinical scenarios. Because many diagnoses and treatment plans can be made without observing gait, it is helpful to reserve this component of the examination toward the end, when it is clinically relevant. It is important to observe the patient walking at various speeds and with shoes on and off. The hands should be empty and arms hanging freely at the sides. The following observations should be made:

1. *Detect obvious abnormalities of locomotion.* This is best observed, for examination purposes, by trying to examine each leg through a number of strides individually. This allows the examiner to separate out sidedness on loss of stride length and gait phase of a limp.

2. *Perceive asymmetric behavior of the two sides of the body.* This asymmetry can be in torso rotation, upper extremity swing, or lower extremity unilateral gait disturbances. As a rule, the shoulders rotate 180 degrees out of phase with the pelvis; this is a passive response to pelvic rotation. If there are no abnormalities in the spine or upper extremities, rotation of the shoulders is reflected in equal and symmetric arm swing. If the arm swing is asymmetric, horizontal rotation of the pelvis also is asymmetric. Because such asymmetric pelvic rotation can be the result of abnormality in any of the components of the lower extremity, it is mandatory that the practitioner take extra care in examining not only the foot and ankle but also the knees and hips.

3. *Observe the position of the patella and tibial tubercle in standing and walking.* They are indicators of the degree of horizontal rotation of the leg in the axial plane and can guide the examiner to look more proximal for the primary pathologic process.

4. *Observe the degree of toeing in or out* (Fig. 2-40). The phase of gait when this deformity occurs is the key to understanding the cause. At toe-off, the leg has achieved its maximal external rotation, and the foot toes out slightly. During swing phase, the entire leg and foot rotate internally. The average amount of rotation is about 15 degrees, but this varies greatly from person to person. It may be almost imperceptible (3 degrees) or considerable (30 degrees).[3] At the time of heel strike, the long axis of the foot has approached, to a varying degree, the plane of progression. The degree of parallelism between the long axis of the foot and the plane of progression at this point is subject to considerable individual variation. However, the transition from heel strike to foot flat, which occurs rapidly, should be carefully observed. Some persons show an increase in toe-in during the very short period of plantar flexion of the ankle, indicating a greater degree of obliquity of the ankle axis (see Chapter 1).

5. *Observe the longitudinal arch during the first half of stance phase walking* (see Fig. 2-23). Look for dynamic pronation or supination at the stance phase to assess midstance stability. Normally, the foot pronates as it is loaded with the body weight during the first half of stance phase. The amount of pronation is subject to extreme individual variation. The important factor, however, is whether the foot remains pronated during the period of heel rise and lift-off. In the normally functioning foot, as the heel rises, there is almost instantaneous inversion of the heel. If the heel fails to invert at this time, the examiner should check the strength of the intrinsic and extrinsic muscles of the foot and the range of motion in the articulations of the hindfoot and midfoot.

6. *Note the amount of heel inversion and supination of the foot during lift-off* and the presence or absence of rotatory slippage of the forefoot on the floor. Except on

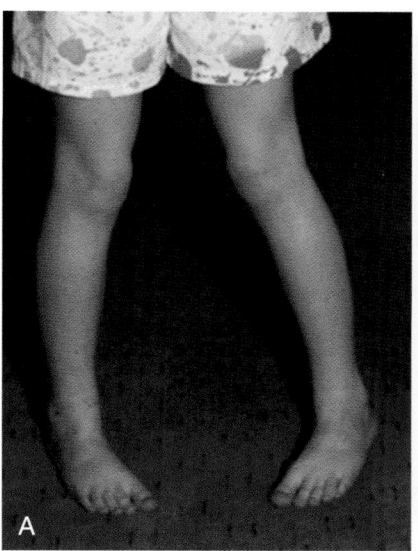
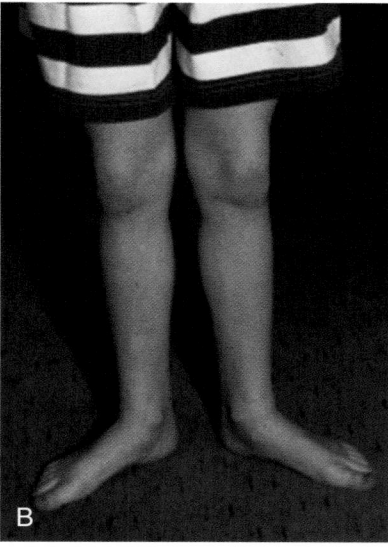

Figure 2-40 Examination of patella and tibial tubercle position. **A,** Intoeing in a child. **B,** External rotation of lower extremities.

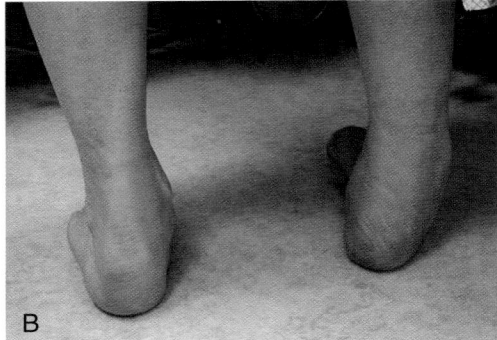

Figure 2-41 Position of heel in stance phase. **A,** Excess heel valgus *(right foot).* **B,** Excess heel varus *(right foot).*

slippery surfaces, the shoe does not visibly rotate externally or slip on the floor at the time of lift-off. Failure of the ankle and subtalar joints to permit adequate external rotation of the leg during this phase of walking can result in direct transmission of the rotatory forces to the interface between the sole of the shoe and the walking surface, with resultant rotatory slippage of the shoe on the floor. On noting slippage, the examiner should look for possible muscle imbalance and should check the obliquity of the ankle axis and the range of motion in the subtalar joint (Fig. 2-41).

7. *Observe the position of the foot in relation to the floor at the time of heel strike.* Normally, the heel strikes the ground first, followed by rapid plantar flexion. If this sequence does not occur, further investigation is indicated. In pathologic conditions, the patient might contact the ground with the foot flat or possibly on the toes. The time of heel rise also should be carefully noted; it occurs normally at 34% of the walking cycle just after the swinging leg has passed the stance foot. Early heel rise can indicate tightness of the gastrocnemius–soleus muscle complex. A delay in heel rise can indicate weakness in the same muscle group.

If the implications of the preceding statements are not readily apparent, it is suggested that the reader review Chapter 1.

Shoe Examination

Because the type of shoe and the heel height affect the way a person walks, they must be noted in the history and in the examination sequence. When wearing high heels, for example, women show less ankle-joint motion than when wearing flat heels, and in tennis shoes they show little difference from men in gait.

It is most convenient for the examiner to inspect the shoes during the history taking, although the information

gleaned from this inspection should be correlated with the gait analysis. The examination should include

1. *Path of wear from heel to toe:* Early lateral hindshoe and midshoe wear indicates a supination deformity. Loss of the medial sole and counter indicates a pronation deformity.
2. *Presence of supportive devices or corrections in the shoes:* Arch supports, heel pads, heel wedges, leather manipulation to accommodate deformity, or forefoot pads indicate previous difficulties.
3. *Obliquity of the angle of the crease in the toe of the shoe:* The angle varies from person to person; the greater the obliquity of the crease in the shoe to its long axis, the greater the amount of subtalar motion required to distribute the body weight evenly over the metatarsal heads.
4. *Impression the forefoot has made on the insole of the shoe:* This can often give important information about the patient's force distribution on the plantar foot.
5. *Presence or absence of circular wear on the sole of the shoe:* Such wear indicates rotatory slippage of the foot on the floor during lift-off, from lack of subtalar motion.
6. *The shape of the shoe compared with the shape of the foot:* This gives the examiner clues as to the proper sizing of the patient's shoes. The shape of the shoe (e.g., narrow pointed shoe or broad toe box), and the overall shape of the foot when the patient is weight bearing should be carefully observed.

REFERENCES
1. Isman RE, Inman VT: Anthropometric studies of the human foot and ankle, *Bull Prosthet Res* 10–11:97–129, 1969.
2. Raikin SM, Elias I, Nazarian LN: Intrasheath subluxation of the peroneal tendons, *J Bone Joint Surg Am* 90:992–999, 2008.
3. Levens AS, Inman VT, Blosser JA: Transverse rotation of the segments of the lower extremity in locomotion, *J Bone Joint Surg Am* 30:859–872, 1948.

Chapter 3

Imaging of the Foot and Ankle

James M. Linklater, John W. Read, Catherine L. Hayter

Imaging is an essential component in the diagnostic workup of many conditions of the foot and ankle. This chapter reviews the basic principles of imaging, with the aim of providing a solid foundation for routine clinical practice. In the limited space available, the authors' approach will be clinically pragmatic and focused on general concepts, rather than individual conditions.

ROLE OF IMAGING

For the foot and ankle surgeon, imaging is often central to diagnosis, management, and treatment planning. It offers a noninvasive window into the nature of anatomic derangements about which surgical decisions must be made. Imaging can assist with accurate early diagnosis, assessment of lesion grade and extent, assessment of treatment response, objective documentation of pathology in medicolegal settings, exclusion of sinister or systemic processes, and preoperative planning. With the advent of minimally invasive surgical techniques, the need to assess lesion suitability for arthroscopic treatment has further increased the importance of imaging. Various percutaneous needle interventions are also now possible using various imaging modalities for accurate guidance.

Effective Use of Imaging

Although valuable as a diagnostic tool, imaging should only be requested if the result will be used to guide management and is most effective when used to confirm or exclude a specific clinical hypothesis or to narrow a clinical differential. In this setting, the test has a specific purpose, and the result has direct clinical meaning. The importance of a thorough clinical assessment therefore cannot be overemphasized, because it is only on the basis of specific questions that arise from the history and physical examination that the most appropriate imaging test(s) can be chosen. A valid clinical role for imaging can include the detection or exclusion of sinister or systemic disease when clinical "red flags" are present (Table 3-1).

It is important that the request form should, apart from describing the general symptomatic context (e.g., forefoot pain), further state the actual question(s) to be answered (e.g., "stress fracture second metatarsal?"). This allows the supervising radiologist to both optimize the imaging protocol and provide a clinically relevant report.

Incidental imaging findings are common and can include normal variants, age-related degenerative changes, old posttraumatic changes and old surgical changes. Such findings can be problematic, particularly when imaging is used in place of a proper physical examination.

Choice of Test

Any imaging workup should generally commence with plain radiographs. This low-cost approach carries an acceptable low radiation dose and provides basic diagnostic information that cannot be readily obtained by any other means (e.g., bone alignment in the weight-bearing foot). When combined with a careful clinical assessment,

plain films alone are often sufficient for both diagnosis and management. When negative, they are still useful in ruling out common differential considerations and demonstrating features that sophisticated tests alone, such as magnetic resonance imaging (MRI) and ultrasound, may otherwise entirely miss or misinterpret (e.g., soft tissue calcifications, foreign bodies, bone spurs and loose bodies, accessory centers of ossification, deformities and malalignments, old injuries, anatomic predispositions, bone tumor characterization). Particularly in the current era of MRI, the fundamental and enduring importance of plain radiographs should never be forgotten.

When further imaging is required, the choice of exactly which test to order can sometimes be challenging because a wide range of imaging tests and variations in imaging technology are available. In general, the specialist foot and ankle surgeon who is expected to resolve a difficult clinical problem should select the locally available test that is most reliable for the diagnosis under consideration. This may vary in any given locale for reasons such as equipment availability and radiologist expertise. Other factors that may influence the choice of imaging test can include (1) patient concerns, such as cost, convenience, discomfort; (2) safety risks, including patient age, radiation dose, and contrast sensitivity; and (3) costs to third parties, such as sporting clubs, insurers, or the taxpayer.

Radiation Safety

Plain radiographs, computed tomography (CT) scans and isotope bone scans all expose patients to ionizing radiation that carries a risk of both cancer induction and genetic damage. This risk is well established at high doses (e.g., Hiroshima victims) but remains uncertain at low doses, such as those used in medical imaging. Because all populations are exposed to the natural background radiation of cosmic rays (Table 3-2) and also have an incidence of cancers arising from causes other than radiation, it is statistically difficult to evaluate the cancer risk associated with medical radiations at doses of 100 mSv or less.[25] A cautious "linear no-threshold model" has therefore been adopted that assumes that even the smallest radiation dose carries a level of risk and that this risk increases linearly with cumulative lifetime exposure. It is also well recognized that, depending on age, children can be up to 10 times more sensitive to ionizing radiation than adults, and an actual effect equivalent to one excess case of leukemia and one excess case of brain tumor per 10,000

Table 3-1 Clinical Red Fags

Age > 50 years
Constitutional symptoms
Atypical symptoms
Risk factors (e.g., diabetes, immune deficiency)
Nonmechanical pain (e.g., night pain at rest)
Complex past history
Previous malignancy
Family history of arthritis
Other clues (e.g., progressive neurologic deficit, urinary
  symptoms)
Poor response to therapy

Table 3-2 Typical Effective Radiation Dose[3,42,44]

Average U.S. background radiation/yr	3.0 mSv
Single trans-Atlantic flight	0.04 mSv
Radiograph: chest (PA)	0.02 mSv
Radiograph: foot (single exposure)	0.001 mSv
Computed tomography: ankle	0.07 mSv
Isotope (Tc-99m–MDP) bone scan	6.3 mSv

MDP, methylene diphosphonate; *PA,* posteroanterior.

head CT scans has recently been shown for the first time in children younger than 10 years who underwent multiple CT head scans with a cumulative dose of 50 to 60 mGy.[57]

These risks should be kept in perspective. The radiation dose associated with a basic three-view foot radiograph is at least 10 times lower than the exposure associated with a single trans-Atlantic air flight (Table 3-2), and it is generally accepted that medical imaging tests are justified if there is a reasonable likelihood they will provide a health benefit or inform patient management.[6] Nevertheless, medical exposures should always be kept "As Low As Reasonably Achievable" (ALARA principle), and alternative tests, such as ultrasound and MRI, which avoid ionizing radiations altogether are preferable to CT or isotope studies whenever they offer equivalent or superior diagnostic efficacy, particularly in children and especially for follow-up imaging. In clinical practice, radiologists normally exercise caution and specify imaging protocols that minimize the ionizing radiation dose. The surgeon should also feel comfortable that the doses involved in foot and ankle imaging are mostly extremely low (see Table 3-2). Last, the American Association of Physicists in Medicine has recently issued a reassuring policy statement that asserts that "the risks of medical imaging at effective doses below 50 mSv for single procedures or 100 mSv for multiple procedures over short time periods are too low to be detectable and may be nonexistent."[1]

RADIOGRAPHS

An effective radiographic examination provides fine anatomic detail and comprises appropriate views that have been correctly positioned. Poor radiographic technique may contribute to diagnostic error by invalidating established radiographic signs, measurements, and alignment criteria. Whenever the relevant anatomy of clinical interest has not been clearly demonstrated, the examination is technically inadequate and should be repeated.[2]

Film interpretation requires knowledge of (1) normal bone development in the pediatric patient[65] (Fig. 3-1) and (2) normal anatomic variants at all ages. Secondary centers of ossification and sesamoids of the foot can both be mistaken for fractures[65] (Fig. 3-2). A full discussion of normal variants is beyond the scope of this chapter, but appropriate references should be consulted when in doubt.[30,66]

The *routine ankle series* consists of an anteroposterior (AP) view, mortise view, and lateral view (Fig. 3-3). The *routine foot series* consists of an AP view (Fig. 3-4), oblique view (Fig. 3-5) and a lateral view (Fig. 3-6). The optimal assessment of alignment and joint space at the foot and ankle *requires weight-bearing views whenever possible* (Figs. 3-7 to 3-10). The diagnostic impact of weight-bearing views can be substantial (Fig. 3-11). Depending upon clinical context, a limited number of *additional views* may be warranted.

1. *Ankle impingement:* Lateral dorsiflexion or plantarflexion views (Fig. 3-12); "lazy" lateral view (Fig. 3-13)
2. *Talocalcaneal coalition:* Harris-Beath view (Fig. 3-14), oblique views (Fig. 3-15), Brodén views (Fig. 3-16)
3. *Trauma:* AP view of proximal fibula if Maisonneuve fracture suspected (Fig. 3-17); reverse oblique view of ankle if medial malleolus fracture suspected (Fig. 3-18)

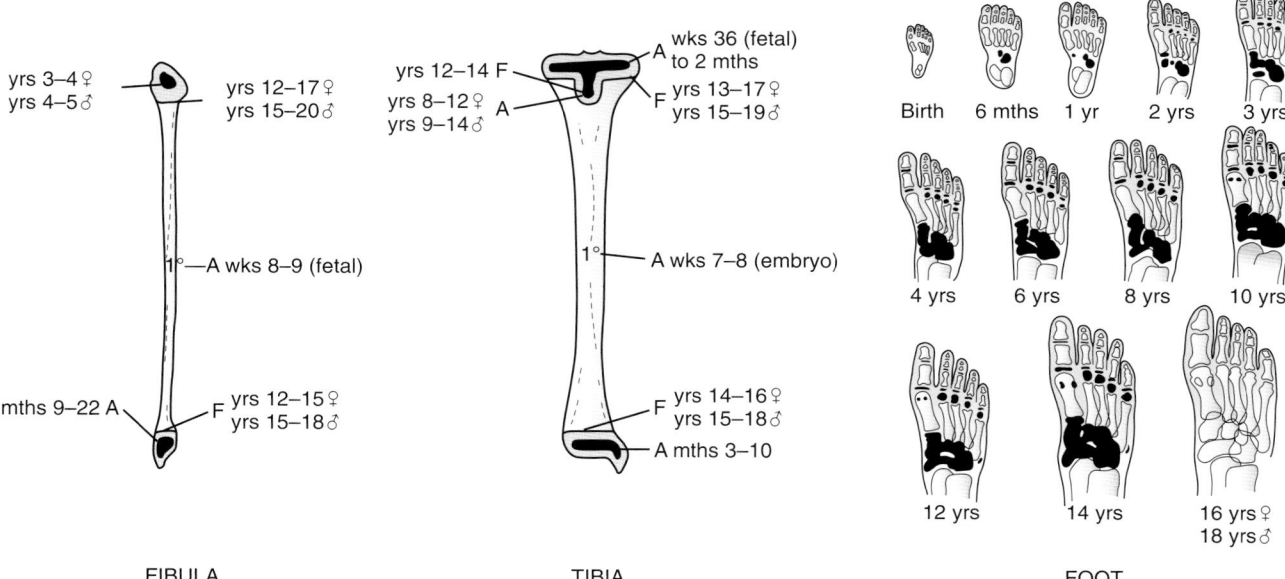

Figure 3-1 Stages of normal osseous development of the foot and ankle. *1°*, primary center of ossification: stippled areas and regions shaded black indicate secondary centers of ossification; *A*, age at first appearance; *F*, age at fusion. (From Scheuer L, Black S: *Developmental juvenile osteology*, Oxford, England, 2000, Elsevier Academic Press.)

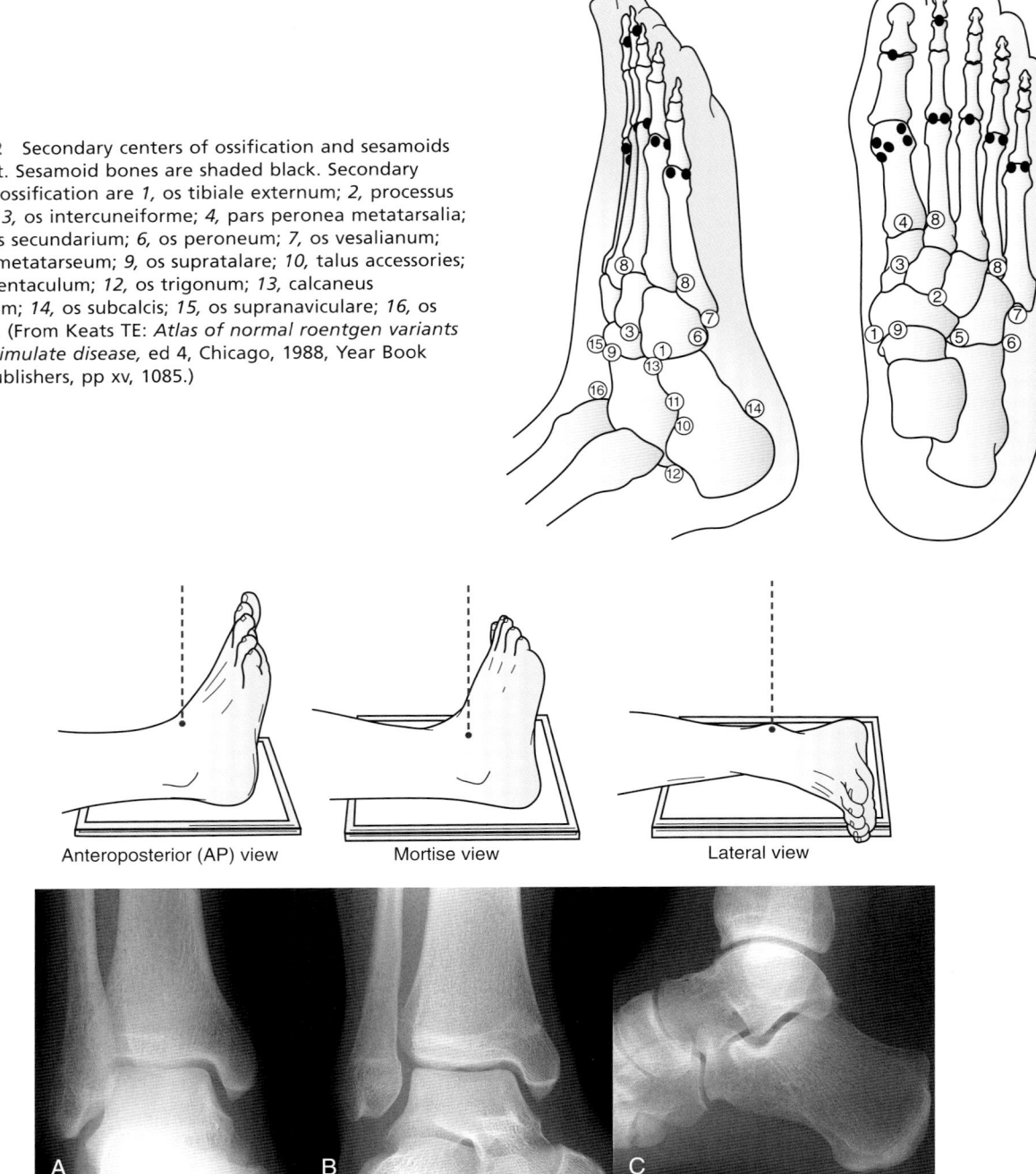

Figure 3-2 Secondary centers of ossification and sesamoids of the foot. Sesamoid bones are shaded black. Secondary centers of ossification are *1,* os tibiale externum; *2,* processus uncinatus; *3,* os intercuneiforme; *4,* pars peronea metatarsalia; *5,* cuboides secundarium; *6,* os peroneum; *7,* os vesalianum; *8,* os intermetatarseum; *9,* os supratalare; *10,* talus accessories; *11,* os sustentaculum; *12,* os trigonum; *13,* calcaneus secundarium; *14,* os subcalcis; *15,* os supranaviculare; *16,* os talotibiale. (From Keats TE: *Atlas of normal roentgen variants that may simulate disease,* ed 4, Chicago, 1988, Year Book Medical Publishers, pp xv, 1085.)

Anteroposterior (AP) view   Mortise view   Lateral view

A   B   C

Figure 3-3 Non–weight-bearing views of the ankle. **A,** The anteroposterior (AP) view is obtained with the toes pointing directly upward and a vertical primary beam centered on the ankle joint. In this position, the talus is slightly externally rotated, the lateral gutter of ankle joint is partially obscured by the lateral malleolus, and the anterior tubercle of the tibia overlaps the distal fibula. **B,** The mortise view is obtained by internally rotating the foot 15 to 20 degrees to bring the talus into its true AP position and the malleoli equidistant from the cassette. In this position, the entire profile of the talar dome is well seen, and both the medial and lateral clear spaces of ankle joint are well displayed and may be compared. The primary beam must be centered on the joint space, and the foot should be dorsiflexed to avoid the tip of the lateral malleolus being overlapped by the calcaneus. **C,** The lateral view requires a straight tube centered on the ankle joint and superimposition of the medial and lateral malleoli, but it is often poorly taken. An ankle joint effusion can be readily appreciated as water density distending the anterior joint recess on a correctly positioned and exposed lateral view. Note the fractured base of fifth metatarsal in the example shown here. (From Anderson IF, Read JW: *Atlas of imaging in sports medicine,* ed 2, Sydney, 2008, McGraw-Hill and Jones CP, Younger ASE: Imaging of the foot and ankle. In Coughlin MJ, Mann RA, Saltzman CL, editors: *Surgery of the foot and ankle,* ed 8, Philadelphia, 2007, Mosby Elsevier.)

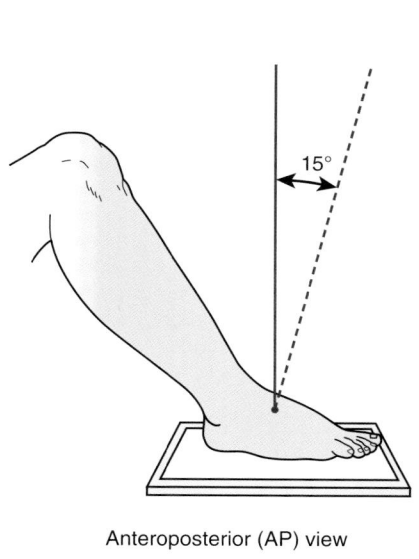

Anteroposterior (AP) view

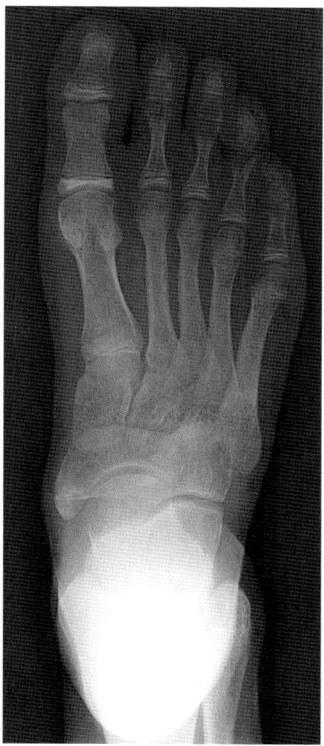

Figure 3-4 Non–weight-bearing anteroposterior (AP) view of the foot. The AP view is obtained with the primary beam centered on the base of third metatarsal and angled 15 degrees cephalad. Note the prominent os tibiale externum in the example shown here with the related synchondrosis showing overlying soft tissue swelling of active stress reaction. (Diagram from Jones CP, Younger ASE: Imaging of the foot and ankle. In Coughlin MJ, Mann RA, Saltzman CL, editors: *Surgery of the foot and ankle*, ed 8, Philadelphia, 2007, Mosby Elsevier.)

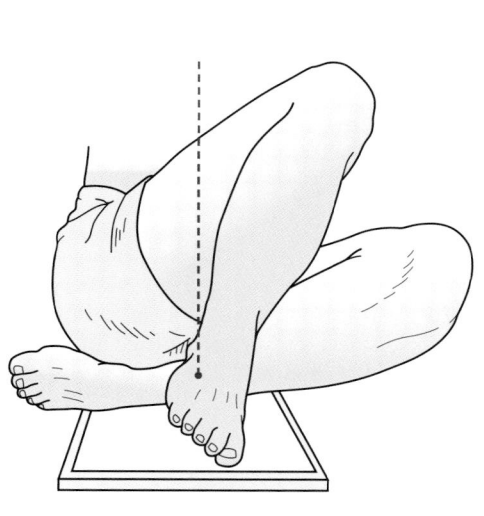

Oblique view

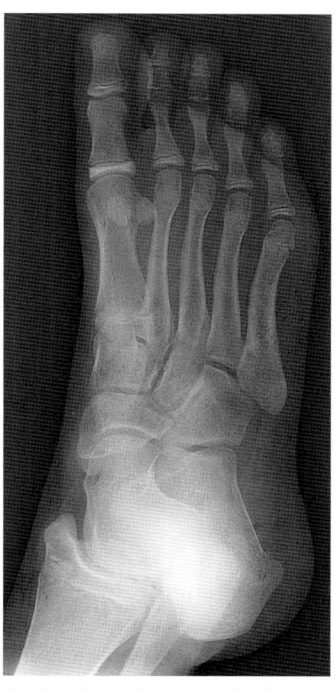

Figure 3-5 Non–weight-bearing oblique view of the foot. This view is obtained by elevating the lateral border of foot 30 degrees and directing the primary beam at the base of fifth metatarsal. It is used to assess the toes, metatarsals, and tarsal bones anterior to the ankle joint. The oblique view is particularly helpful in assessing calcaneonavicular coalitions and the lateral tarsometatarsal articulations. Note prominent os tibiale externum in the example shown here. (Diagram from Jones CP, Younger ASE: Imaging of the foot and ankle. In Coughlin MJ, Mann RA, Saltzman CL, editors: *Surgery of the foot and ankle*, ed 8, Philadelphia, 2007, Mosby Elsevier.)

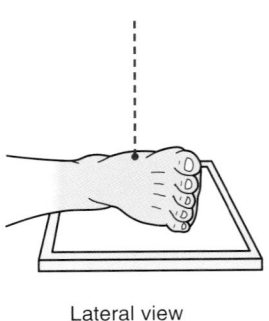

Lateral view

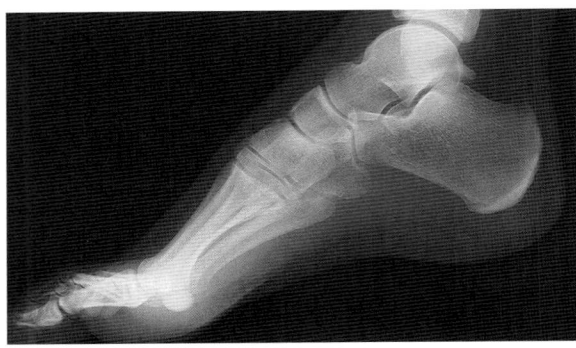

Figure 3-6 Non–weight-bearing lateral view of foot. This view provides a critical overview of foot anatomy and is also used to assess the plantar soft tissues in clinical settings such as foreign body and plantar fasciitis. Lateral radiographs are obtained with the primary beam directed perpendicular to a point just above the base of fifth metatarsal. Note that non–weight-bearing lateral views are inferred when the tibia is *not* vertical to the talus. (From Anderson IF, Read JW: *Atlas of imaging in sports medicine,* ed 2, Sydney, 2008, McGraw-Hill and Jones CP, Younger ASE: Imaging of the foot and ankle. In Coughlin MJ, Mann RA, Saltzman CL, editors: *Surgery of the foot and ankle,* ed 8, Philadelphia, 2007, Mosby Elsevier.)

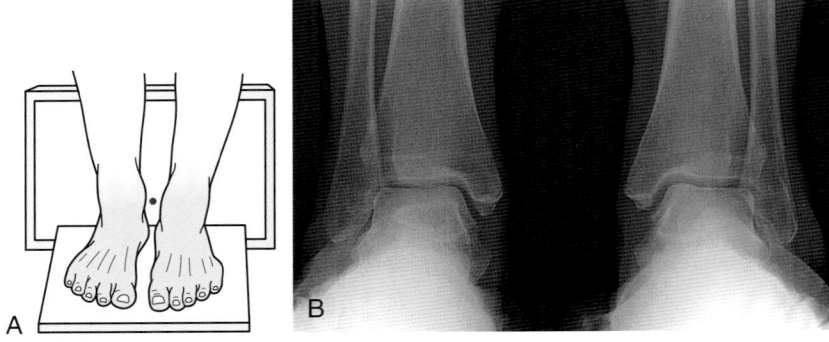

Figure 3-7 Weight-bearing anteroposterior view of ankles. **A,** The patient is positioned on a 5-cm block, with the film cassette behind the heels and a horizontal beam centered between the ankle joints at joint level. **B,** Radiograph illustrates essentially symmetric joints with slight tilt of talar articular surface. The angle of the talar articular surface can normally be a few degrees off horizontal in either a medial or lateral direction. (Diagram from Jones CP, Younger ASE: Imaging of the foot and ankle. In Coughlin MJ, Mann RA, Saltzman CL, editors: *Surgery of the foot and ankle,* ed 8, Philadelphia, 2007, Mosby Elsevier.)

4. *Ankle instability:* Stress views of ankle joint (Figs. 3-19 and 3-20); stress view of distal tibiofibular syndesmosis (Fig. 3-21)
5. *Heel:* Lateral and axial views of calcaneus (Fig. 3-22)
6. *Navicular:* Navicular view (Fig. 3-23)
7. *Talus:* Talar neck view (Fig. 3-24).
8. *Tarsometatarsal joints or base of second metatarsal:* Plantar-dorsal projection of midfoot (Fig. 3-25)
9. *Toes:* Lateral and lateral-oblique phalangeal views (Fig. 3-26)
10. *Sesamoids:* Axial, medial-oblique, lateromedial, and stress views of sesamoids (Figs. 3-27 to 3-30).

Common radiographic measurements used to assess foot deformities are shown in Figures 3-31 to 3-37. However, the significance of any apparent radiographic abnormality should always be weighed in the overall clinical context because radiographic measurements are subject to a wide range of normal variation and are also susceptible to error through poor radiographic technique.

ULTRASOUND

Basic Science

Ultrasound (US) uses the SONAR (SOund NAvigation and Ranging) principle to build up cross-sectional images of soft tissue anatomy. Sound waves above the pitch of human hearing (typically in the 5- to 18-MHz range for musculoskeletal imaging) are generated by a handheld transducer applied to the skin. These propagate through the tissues and are reflected by various acoustic tissue interfaces as returning echoes of differing intensity and

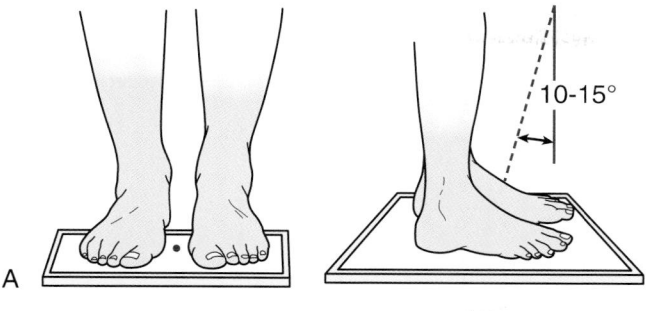

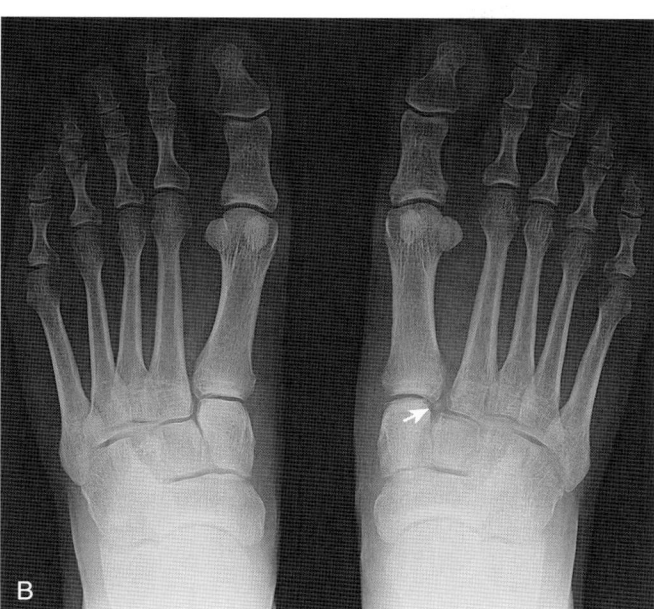

Figure 3-8 Weight-bearing anteroposterior (AP) view of feet. Weight-bearing views of the feet provide functional information and are recommended for all evaluations unless clinically contraindicated. There are significant measurement differences between weight-bearing and non–weight-bearing views when assessing alignment abnormalities. Lisfranc diastasis injuries are often missed if no weight-bearing view has been obtained. **A,** Diagrams show patient positioning for simultaneous AP views with the primary beam centered between the feet at the first metatarsophalangeal joint and with a 10- to 15-degree cephalad tube tilt. **B,** Weight-bearing AP radiograph shows a Lisfranc fracture-dislocation on the right, with widened proximal 1–2 metastarsal interspace, malalignment at the second tarsometatarsal joint (TMTJ2), and a small avulsion fracture fragment *(arrow).* (Diagrams from Jones CP, Younger ASE: Imaging of the foot and ankle. In Coughlin MJ, Mann RA, Saltzman CL, editors: *Surgery of the foot and ankle,* ed 8, Philadelphia, 2007, Mosby Elsevier. Radiographs from Anderson IF, Read JW: *Atlas of imaging in sports medicine,* ed 2, Sydney, 2008, McGraw-Hill.)

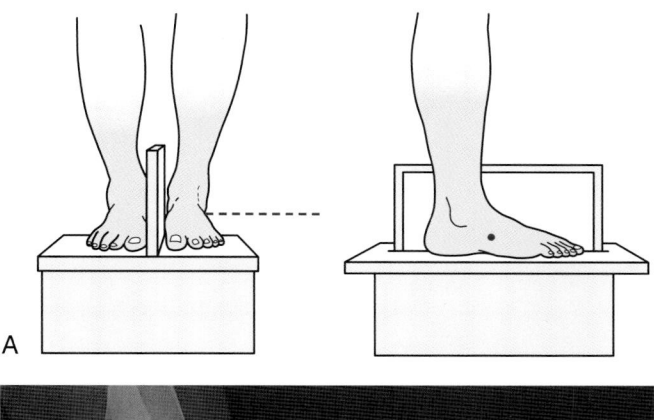

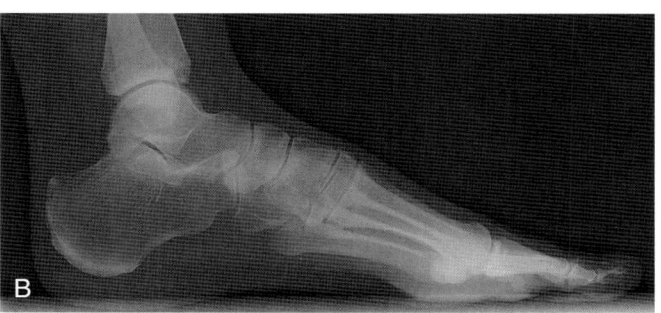

Figure 3-9 Weight-bearing lateral view of foot. Lateral weight-bearing views must be taken individually. **A,** Diagrams show patient positioning. **B,** Normal weight-bearing lateral radiograph. (Diagram from Jones CP, Younger ASE: Imaging of the foot and ankle. In Coughlin MJ, Mann RA, Saltzman CL, editors: *Surgery of the foot and ankle,* ed 8, Philadelphia, 2007, Mosby Elsevier.)

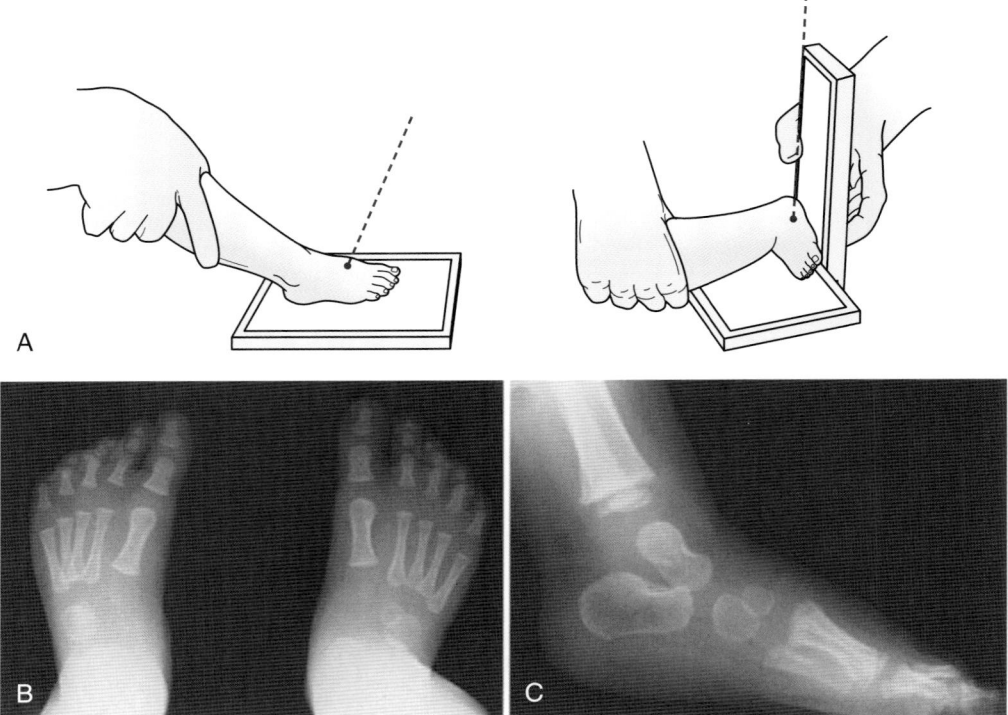

Figure 3-10 Infant weight-bearing views of foot. Special techniques are required to obtain adequate foot views in young children and infants. These involve active immobilization and compression by a gloved assistant or a static immobilization system. Radiographs of the contralateral foot may be helpful for comparison. **A,** Positioning for anteroposterior (AP) and lateral views with immobilization technique. **B,** AP radiograph. **C,** Lateral radiograph. (From Jones CP, Younger ASE: Imaging of the foot and ankle. In Coughlin MJ, Mann RA, Saltzman CL, editors: *Surgery of the foot and ankle,* ed 8, Philadelphia, 2007, Mosby Elsevier.)

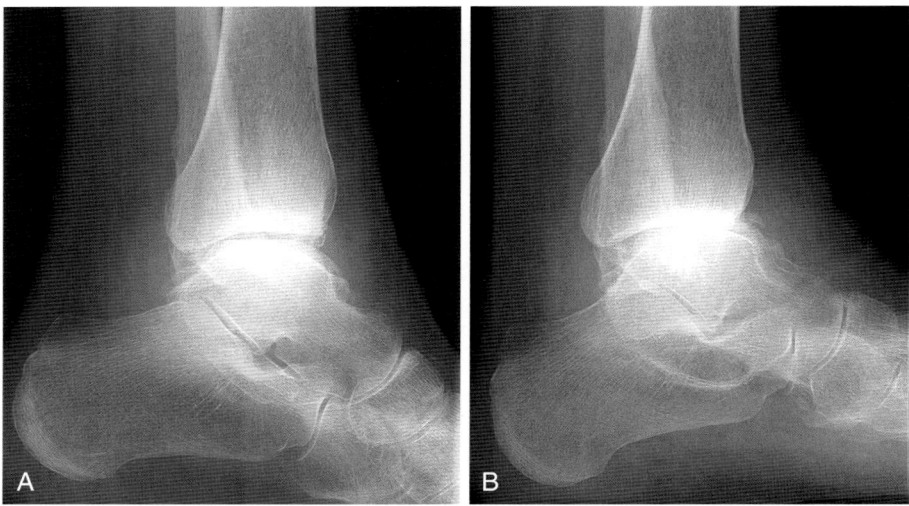

Figure 3-11 Effect of weight bearing. Non–weight-bearing **(A)** and weight-bearing **(B)** lateral views of the ankle show the value of functional loading. Marked joint space narrowing is revealed on the weight-bearing view in this example of ankle arthrosis. (From Anderson IF, Read JW: *Atlas of imaging in sports medicine,* ed 2, Sydney, 2008, McGraw-Hill.)

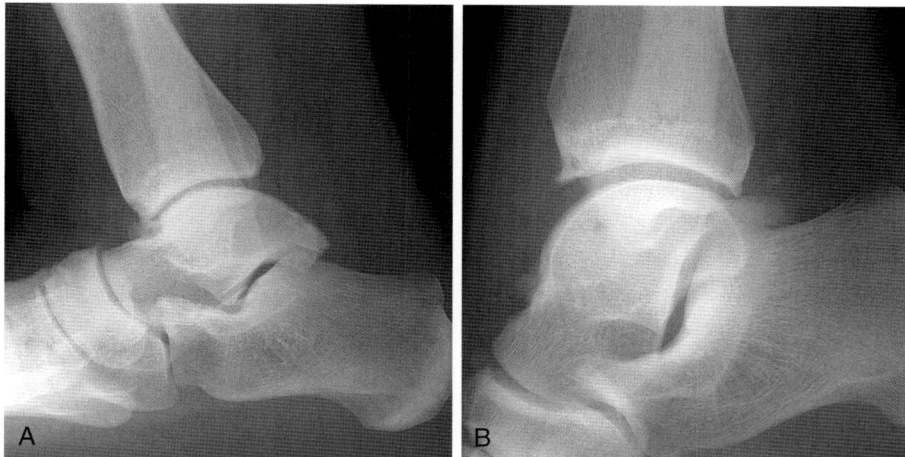

Figure 3-12 Ankle impingement views. These views are used to assess any bony contribution to ankle impingement. The *anterior impingement* or *"lunge" view* **(A)** is a weight-bearing lateral view obtained in maximum ankle dorsiflexion, with the example shown here demonstrating direct bony abutment between an anterior tibial bone spur and new bone formation at the dorsal neck of talus. The *posterior impingement view* **(B)** is a weight-bearing lateral view obtained in extreme plantar flexion, with the example shown here demonstrating direct bony abutment between a posterior tibial bone spur and a prominent posterior process of talus. This case also shows loose ossific bodies posteriorly, and osteophyte at the anterior margin of ankle joint that would predispose to concomitant anterior impingement symptoms. (From Anderson IF, Read JW: *Atlas of imaging in sports medicine,* ed 2, Sydney, 2008, McGraw-Hill.)

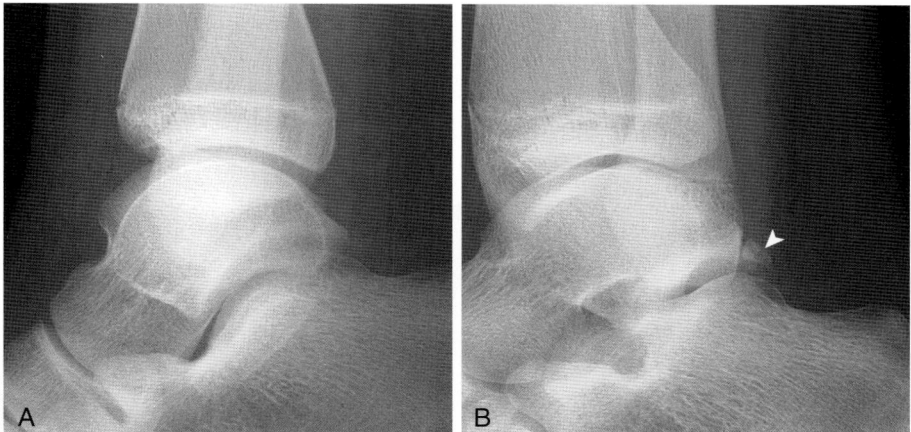

Figure 3-13 Lazy lateral view of ankle. This view profiles the lateral tubercle of the posterior process of talus (posterolateral process talus) and is used to identify a small os trigonum that may be contributing to posterior ankle impingement yet remains invisible on the standard lateral view of ankle. It is obtained as a lateral projection with the foot in 10 to 15 degrees of external rotation to profile the lateral rather than medial tubercle (posterolateral process). In the example shown here, the true lateral view of ankle **(A)** appears normal, but the lazy lateral view **(B)** reveals an os trigonum *(arrowhead)*. (From Anderson IF, Read JW: *Atlas of imaging in sports medicine,* ed 2, Sydney, 2008, McGraw-Hill.)

time-of-flight that are then assembled line by line to form a "gray-scale" image. The whole process occurs rapidly enough to allow real-time imaging.

Use of Ultrasound

The advantages of US include low cost, patient comfort, an absence of hazardous ionizing radiation, the clinically interactive nature of the test (Fig. 3-38), the ability to assess tissue dynamics such as tendon glide and stability (Fig. 3-39), the ability of Doppler techniques to detect soft tissue hyperemia and neovascularity (Fig. 3-40), and the ability to guide diagnostic and/or therapeutic injections accurately (Fig. 3-41). The clinical aspect of directly probing the visualized anatomy with an US transducer allows the operator to accurately correlate any site(s) of

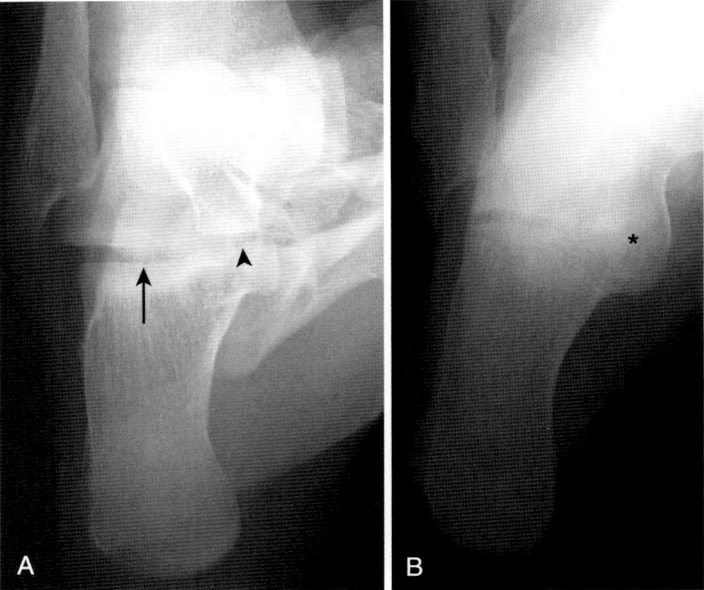

Figure 3-14 Harris-Beath view. This view profiles the posterior and middle subtalar joints. The patient is seated on the x-ray table with the leg extended and heel resting on the film cassette. The ankle is then placed in dorsiflexion and held in this position by the patient using a strap to apply traction to the forefoot. The x-ray tube is angled 45 degrees cephalad, with the primary beam entering the sole of the foot at the level of the base of fifth metatarsal. Slight internal rotation of the foot will improve the view by bringing the sustentaculum tali into profile. **A,** A normal hindfoot is shown with the *arrow* indicating the posterior subtalar joint and *arrowhead* indicating the middle subtalar joint. **B,** Osseous coalition of the middle subtalar joint *(asterisk).* (From Anderson IF, Read JW: *Atlas of imaging in sports medicine,* ed 2, Sydney, 2008, McGraw-Hill.)

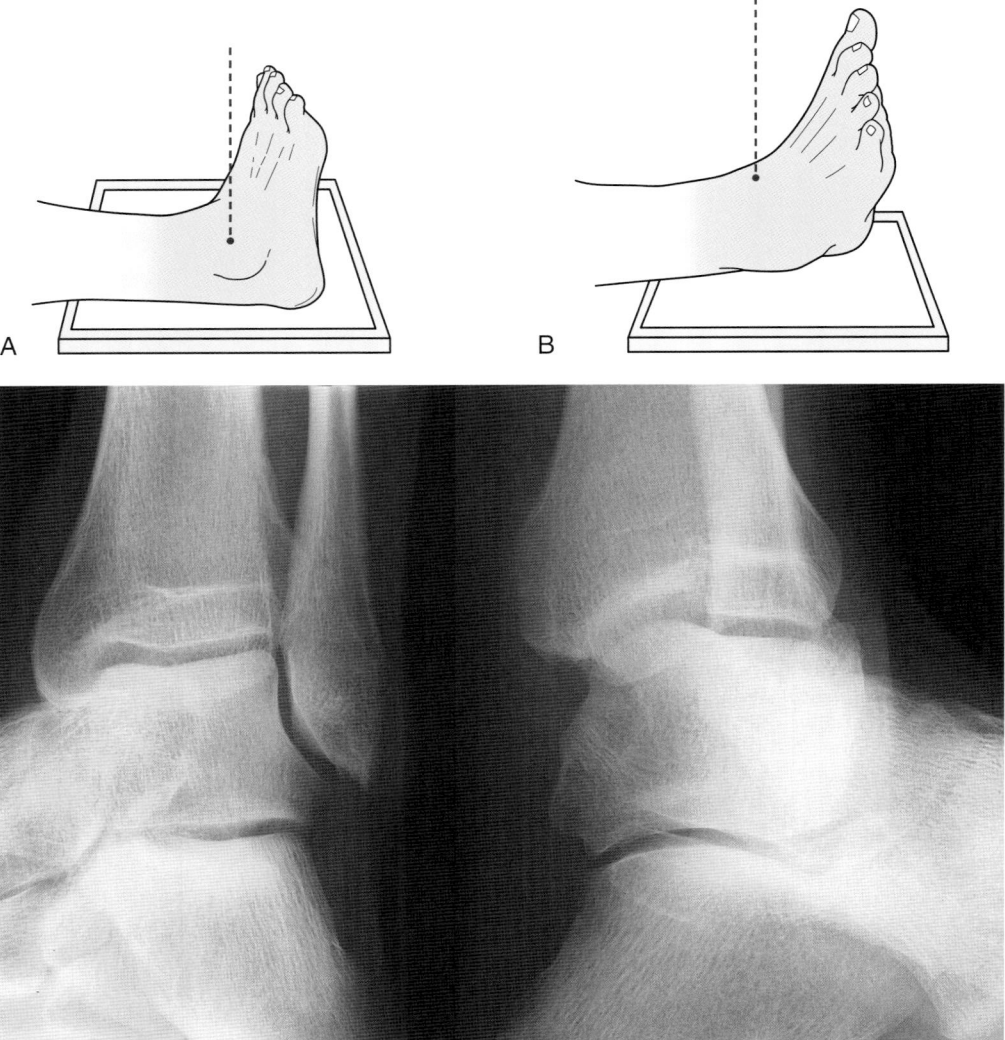

Figure 3-15 Oblique views of subtalar joint. **A,** Internal oblique view is similar to mortise view but with more plantar flexion and 45 degrees of internal rotation. **B,** External oblique view is obtained with a straight tube and 45 degrees of external rotation. (Diagram from Jones CP, Younger ASE: Imaging of the foot and ankle. In Coughlin MJ, Mann RA, Saltzman CL, editors: *Surgery of the foot and ankle,* ed 8, Philadelphia, 2007, Mosby Elsevier. Radiograph from Anderson IF, Read JW: *Atlas of imaging in sports medicine,* ed 2, Sydney, 2008, McGraw-Hill.)

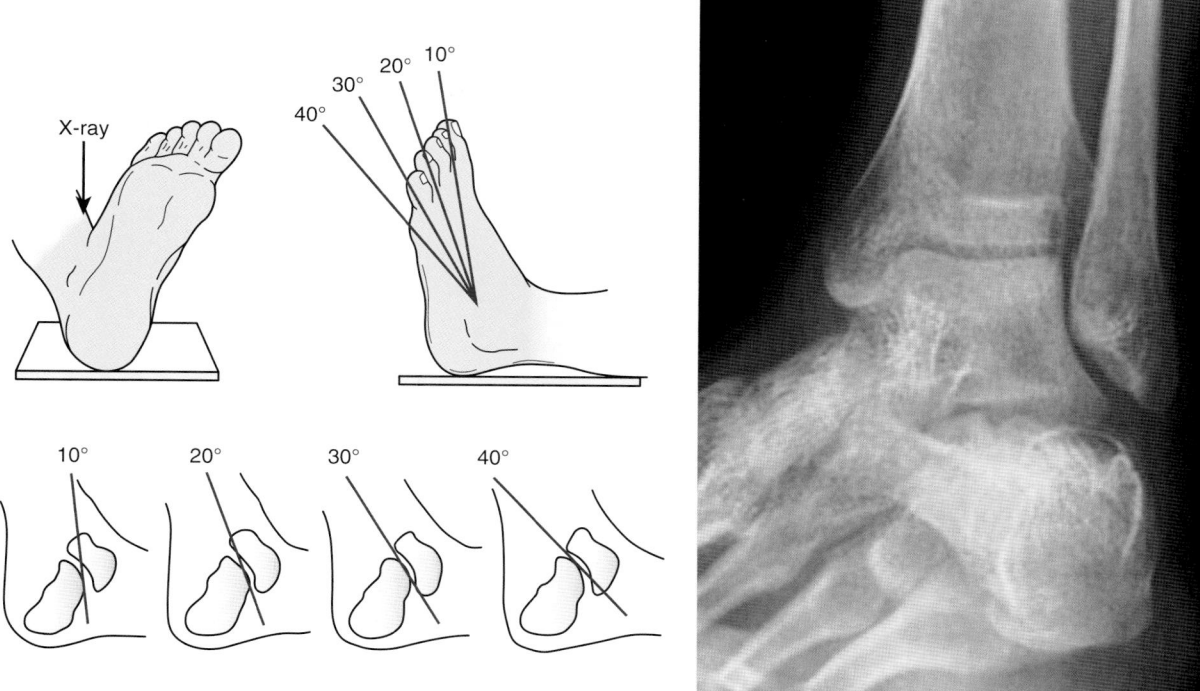

Figure 3-16 Brodén view. This technique profiles the posterior subtalar facet for the evaluation of subtalar coalitions and intraarticular fractures of the calcaneus. Brodén views are obtained with the ankle in neutral dorsiflexion, the leg internally rotated 30 degrees, and the x-ray beam centered over the lateral malleolus, with cephalad tube tilt varying between 10 and 40 degrees to tangent-differing segments of the curved posterior subtalar facet. The radiograph shown here demonstrates an intraarticular fracture of the calcaneus. (Diagrams from Jones CP, Younger ASE: Imaging of the foot and ankle. In Coughlin MJ, Mann RA, Saltzman CL, editors: *Surgery of the foot and ankle,* ed 8, Philadelphia, 2007, Mosby Elsevier, and Burdeaux BD Jr: The medial approach for calcaneal fractures. *Clin Orthop Rel Res* 290:96–107, 1993. Radiograph from Lee KB, Park CH, Seon JK, Kim MS: Arthroscopic subtalar arthrodesis using a posterior 2-portal approach in the prone position. *Arthroscopy* 26:230–238, 2010.)

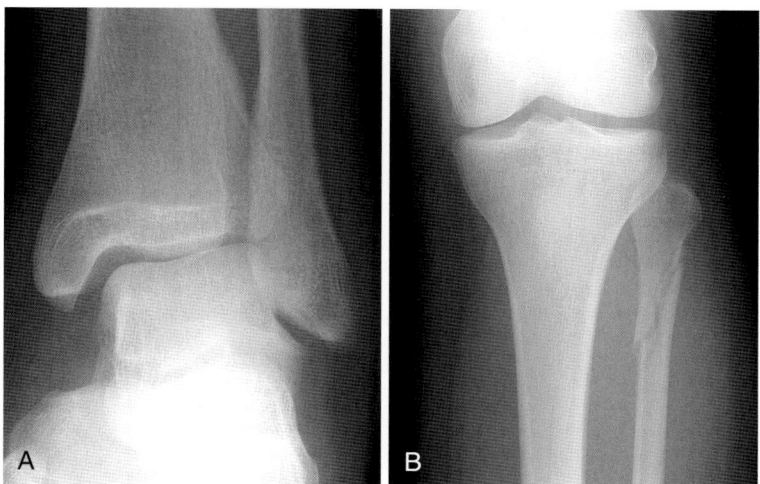

Figure 3-17 Anteroposterior (AP) view of proximal fibula. Maisonneuve fractures can easily be overlooked if the symptoms and signs at the ankle level dominate. An AP view of fibula should therefore be obtained whenever standard ankle views raise suspicion on the basis of either lateral talar displacement or tibiofibular widening without distal fibular fracture, or if there is a seemingly isolated fracture of posterior malleolus. In the example shown here, the AP view of the ankle **(A)** shows widening of the medial ankle gutter and tibiofibular syndesmosis in keeping with tibiofibular diastasis injury. An AP view of fibula **(B)** subsequently confirmed a Maisonneuve fracture. Radiograph B from Anderson IF, Read JW: *Atlas of imaging in sports medicine,* ed 2, Sydney, 2008, McGraw-Hill.)

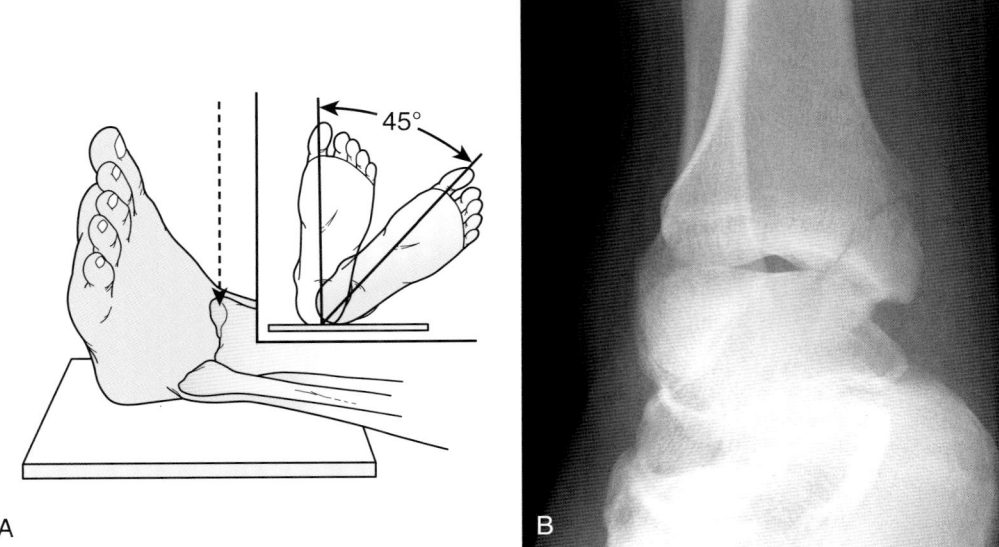

Figure 3-18 Reverse oblique view of ankle. This view is used to assess fractures of the medial malleolus. **A,** A straight beam is centered on the joint space with the ankle positioned in 45-degree external rotation. **B,** A reverse oblique view shows a fracture of medial malleolus. (Radiograph from Anderson IF, Read JW: *Atlas of imaging in sports medicine,* ed 2, Sydney, 2008, McGraw-Hill.)

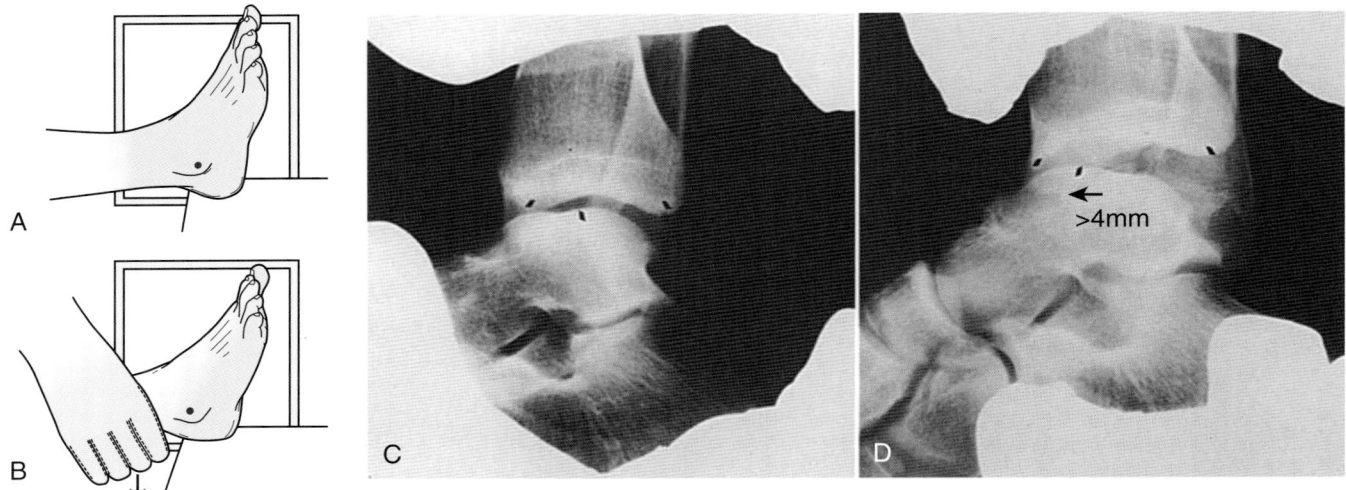

Figure 3-19 Anterior drawer stress view of ankle. This technique detects anterior talofibular ligament insufficiency. Cross-table lateral views of the ankle both at rest **(A)** and with vertical stress applied **(B)** are taken with the heel elevated on a support. A positive examination shows greater than 4 mm anterior displacement *(arrow)* of the talus when vertical stress is applied, illustrated in images **C** and **D.** (From Jones CP, Younger ASE: Imaging of the foot and ankle. In Coughlin MJ, Mann RA, Saltzman CL, editors: *Surgery of the foot and ankle,* ed 8, Philadelphia, 2007, Mosby Elsevier.)

pain and/or tenderness with the imaging appearance. This has been described as "sonopalpation" and can be very helpful in confirming a symptomatic structure or clinically relevant finding. Similarly, the demonstration of locally increased tissue vascularity using Doppler techniques serves to increase the likelihood of a gray-scale finding being relevant to symptoms.[62]

The limitations of US include an inability to see through bone/gas/metal, image quality degraded by obesity and marked subcutaneous edema, reduced resolution and sensitivity at tissue depths greater than 3 cm, the local availability of a reliable and well-trained operator, the "keyhole" nature of images that may be difficult for the surgeon to orient and understand, and image

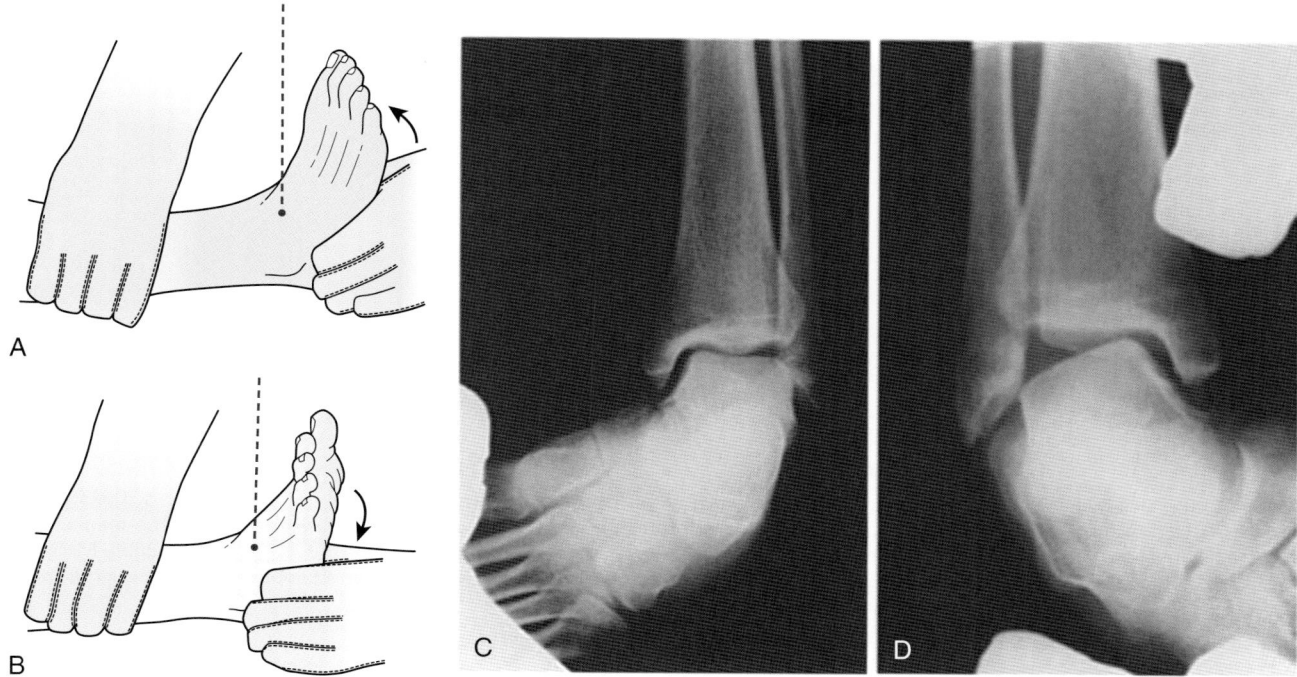

Figure 3-20 **Varus and valgus stress views of the ankle.** Positioning for varus **(A)** and valgus **(B)** stress views of the ankle is illustrated. Varus stress in ankle plantar flexion tests for anterior talofibular and calcaneofibular ligament insufficiency. Valgus stress tests for deltoid ligament insufficiency. The use of stress radiography remains controversial because reliability may be compromised by the large range of normal variation in joint laxity. In the acute trauma setting, local analgesia probably increases accuracy. An abnormal varus or valgus stress examination is regarded as demonstrating either (a) talar tilt greater than or equal to 10 degrees more than the normal side, or (b) greater than or equal to 3 mm discrepancy in lateral ankle joint opening distance between the injured and normal side, as measured from the most lateral aspect of the talar dome to the adjacent tibial articular surface. In the example here, an abnormal varus stress radiograph **(D)** is shown relative to the normal side **(C)**. (From Jones CP, Younger ASE: Imaging of the foot and ankle. In Coughlin MJ, Mann RA, Saltzman CL, editors: *Surgery of the foot and ankle,* ed 8, Philadelphia, 2007, Mosby Elsevier.)

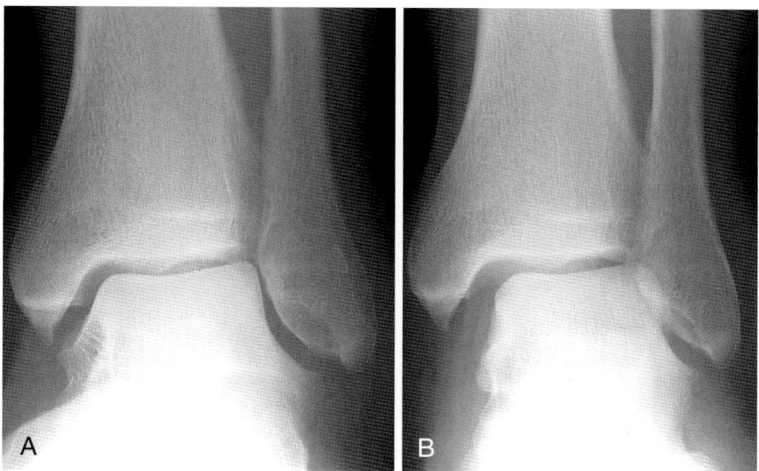

Figure 3-21 Stress view of distal tibiofibular syndesmosis. This view can be helpful when distal tibiofibular disastasis is suspected but the initial radiographs are negative. An anteroposterior view is obtained with maximum external rotation stress applied to the foot against a firmly held tibia. An abnormal syndesmosis will widen with applied stress. In the example shown here, the medial clear space of ankle joint and distal tibiofibular syndesmosis are both questionably widened on the nonstressed view **(A)** but clearly open on the stress view **(B).** This indicates injury of both the syndesmosis and deltoid ligament. (From Anderson IF, Read JW: *Atlas of imaging in sports medicine,* ed 2, Sydney, 2008, McGraw-Hill.)

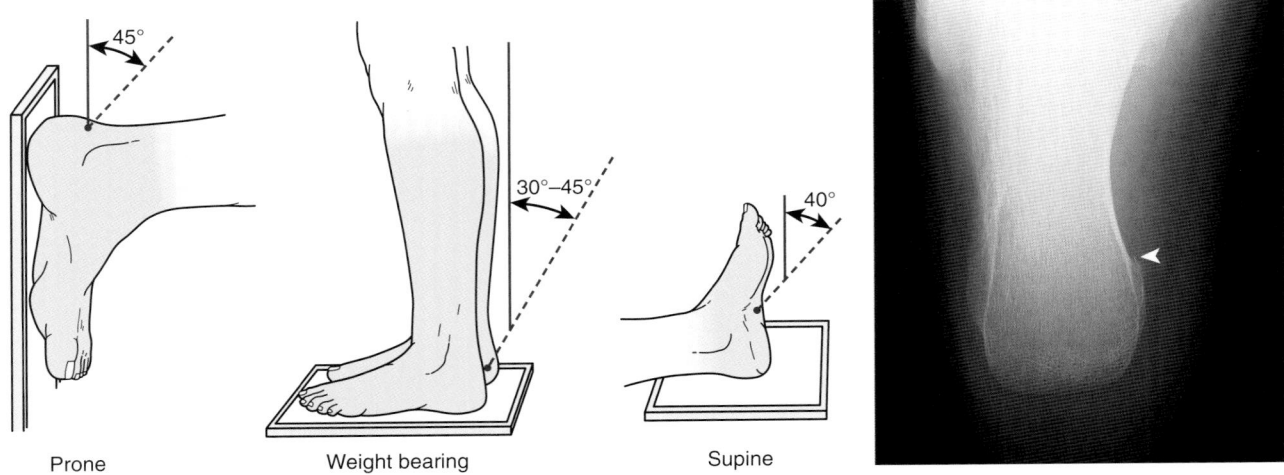

Figure 3-22 Axial view of calcaneus. Diagrams show various methods of obtaining an axial view of the calcaneus. The supine or prone positions may be used in trauma. The actual radiograph shown here demonstrates a subtle fracture of the medial calcaneal tuberosity *(arrowhead)*. (From Anderson IF, Read JW: *Atlas of imaging in sports medicine,* ed 2, Sydney, 2008, McGraw-Hill; Jones CP, Younger ASE: Imaging of the foot and ankle. In Coughlin MJ Mann RA, Saltzman CL, editors: *Surgery of the foot and ankle,* ed 8, Philadelphia, 2007, Mosby Elsevier.)

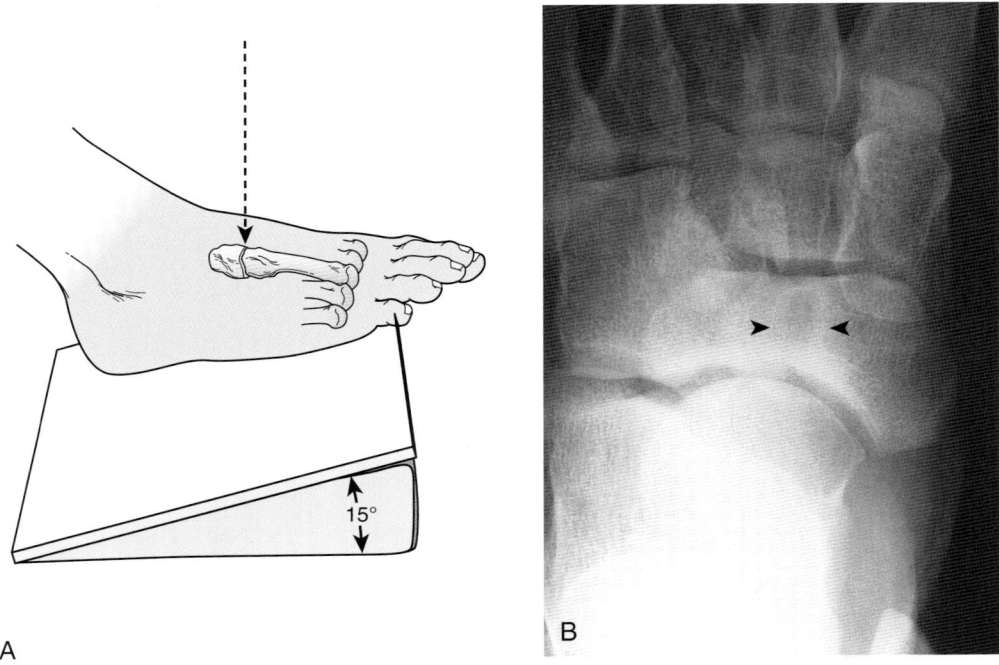

Figure 3-23 Navicular view. This view facilitates the detection of subtle navicular stress fractures. **A,** The forefoot is elevated on a 15-degree wedge to optimally profile the proximal and distal articular surfaces of the navicular. Detail resolution is improved by coning to the region of interest. **B,** This example shows a chronic complete stress fracture disrupting the middle third of the navicular *(arrowheads)*. (From Anderson IF, Read JW: *Atlas of imaging in sports medicine,* ed 2, Sydney, 2008, McGraw-Hill.)

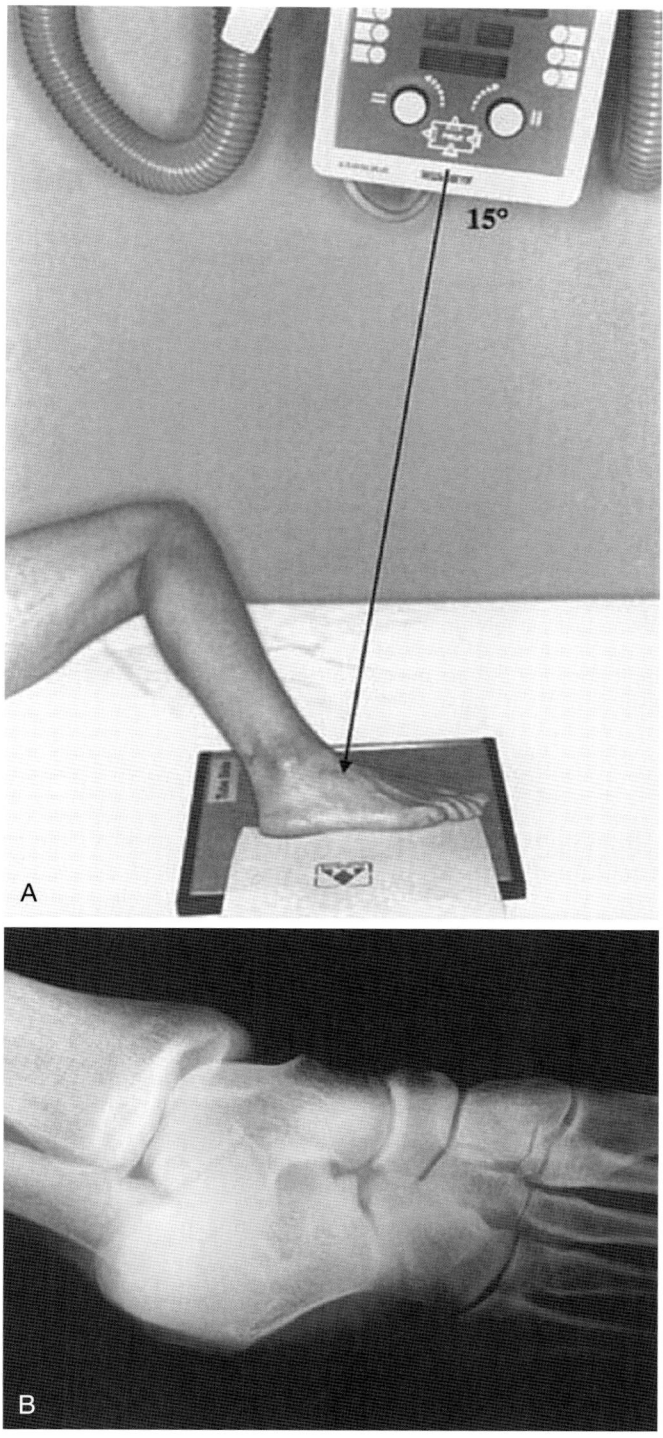

Figure 3-24 Talar neck view. This view is used to evaluate fractures. **A,** The ankle is placed in maximum equinus with the foot pronated 15 degrees, the x-ray beam angled 15 degrees cephalad and centered on the talar neck. **B,** The talar neck is viewed in the frontal plane. (From Myerson M, editor: *Foot and ankle disorders,* Philadelphia, 1999, WB Saunders.)

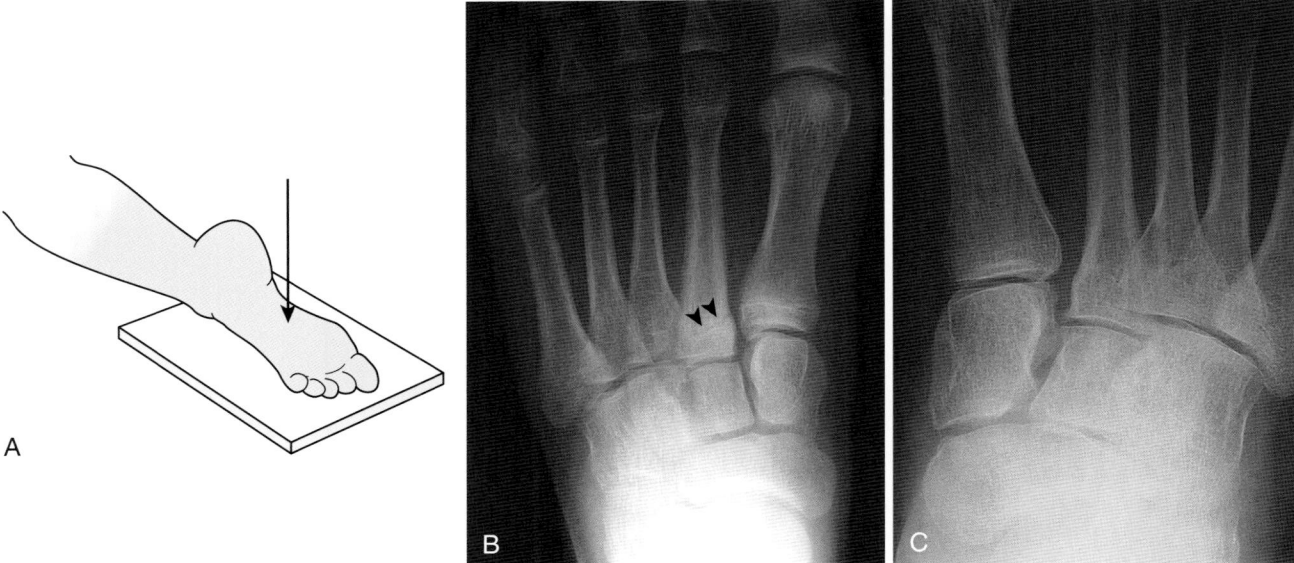

Figure 3-25 Planto-dorsal view of midfoot. This view optimally profiles the tarsometatarsal joint spaces and is extremely valuable when evaluating for tarsometatarsal joint injury or stress fractures at the base of second metatarsal. **A,** The patient is placed in prone position with the dorsal surface of foot flat against the film cassette and a straight tube centered on the base of second metatarsal. **B,** An example showing a stress fracture of second metatarsal *(arrowheads).* **C,** An example showing a sagittal diastasis injury involving the 1–2 intermetatarsal, medial intercuneiform, and naviculomedial cuneiform joints.

artifacts that can limit visualization of some tendon segments or be a diagnostic pitfall for the inexperienced (Fig. 3-42).

US is well suited to the assessment of many superficial tendons and ligaments (Figs. 3-43 and 3-44), foreign bodies, ganglion cysts (Fig. 3-45), and other superficial masses (Fig. 3-46; see Fig. 3-38). In addition, because metal does not distort the sonographic image, US is a good alternative to MRI for the assessment of soft tissue structures adjacent to orthopedic hardware (Fig. 3-47).

NUCLEAR MEDICINE

The major role of nuclear medicine imaging around the ankle is to identify bone injuries and other processes that are occult on plain radiographs or CT scanning. In this regard, nuclear imaging offers an alternative to MRI. Radiographically occult fractures are common around the ankle because of complex anatomy and curved surfaces. Nuclear medicine bone scans are also valuable for demonstrating marrow changes that may be associated with bone contusion, overuse injury, reflex sympathetic dystrophy, tumors, or pain of unknown origin.

Basic Science

Nuclear medicine imaging is based on the injection, into a patient, of radiopharmaceutical agents, which emit radiation that can then be detected and used to form a

diagnostic image. A large number of radiopharmaceutical agents have been developed to address a variety of medical conditions. Nuclear medicine imaging therefore has the advantage of providing both anatomic and physiologic information.[26]

After administration of the radiopharmaceutical agent, a gamma camera is used to record the pattern of radiopharmaceutical distribution in the patient. The radioactivity emitted passes through a lead collimator and interacts with scintillator crystals in the camera. A resultant reaction gives off photons of light, which are coupled to photomultiplier tubes. These, in turn, release an amplified number of electrons, proportional to the intensity of the incident light. The electrons produce an image, which can be recorded on film or by a computer for further processing. The collimator is a major factor determining image resolution, and the type of collimator used can be adjusted depending on imaging needs. For example, pinhole collimators have high spatial resolution and are useful for imaging small body parts (such as the ankle), although they suffer from lower sensitivity.

The radiopharmaceutical agents most commonly used for evaluation of the musculoskeletal system include technetium-99m (Tc-99m) diphosphonates (bone scan), gallium-67 (Ga-67) citrate (gallium scan), and indium-111 (In-111)– or Tc-99m–labeled leukocytes (white blood cell/leukocyte scan). The specific agent used will depend on the clinical question to be answered.

Text continued on p. 82

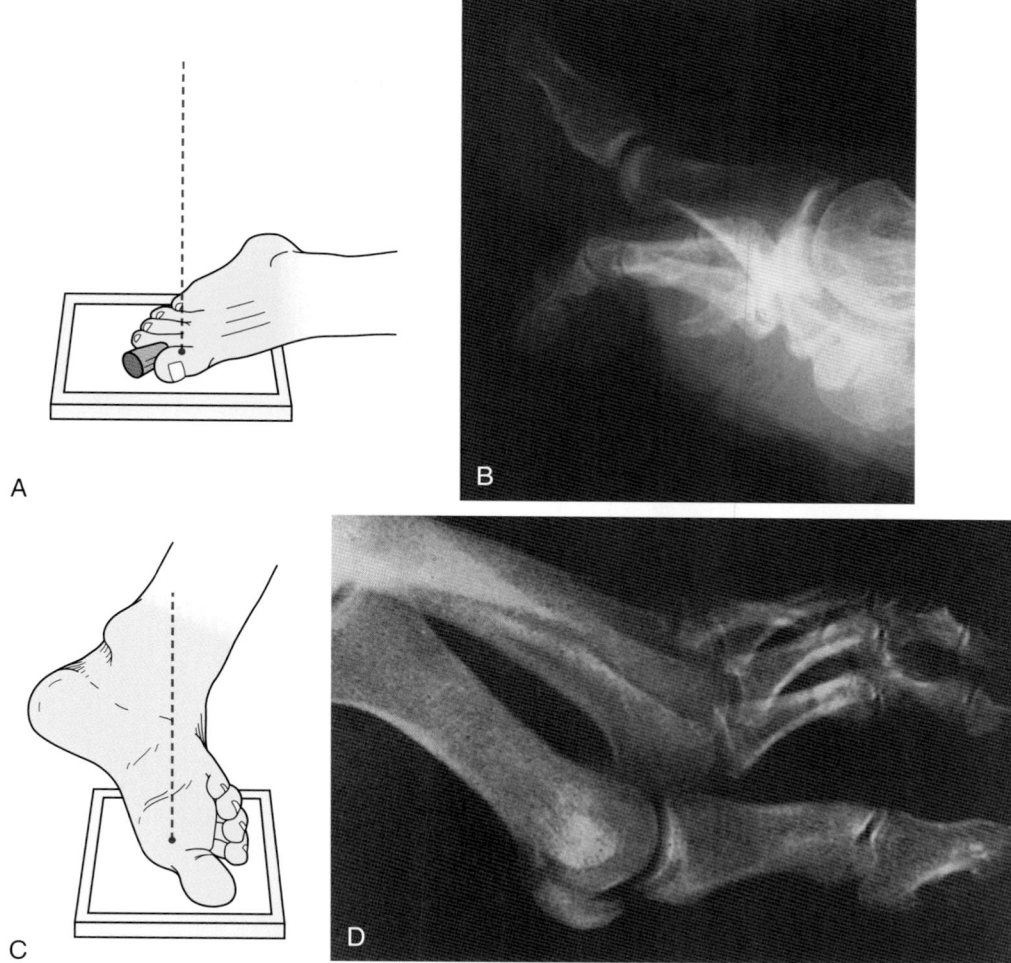

Figure 3-26 Additional phalangeal views. When detailed evaluation of the phalanges is required, the standard views of the foot may be supplemented with lateral and/or lateral-oblique views of the toes. **A,** For a *lateral phalangeal view,* the foot is laterally positioned with the uninvolved toes flexed and, if possible, the involved toe extended by padding. **B,** An illustrative lateral radiograph of the great toe shows a fracture. **C,** For a *lateral-oblique phalangeal view,* the plantar surface of the foot is obliquely oriented as shown in the diagram, with the primary beam centered on the first metatarsophalangeal joint. **D,** A lateral-oblique radiograph illustrates improved visualization of phalanges, particularly the great toe. (Drawings and images from Jones CP, Younger ASE: Imaging of the foot and ankle. In Coughlin MJ, Mann RA, Saltzman CL, editors: *Surgery of the foot and ankle,* ed 8, Philadelphia, 2007, Mosby Elsevier; source, in turn, borrowed image **D** from Clarke KC: *Positioning in radiography,* ed 9, London, 1973, Ilford.)

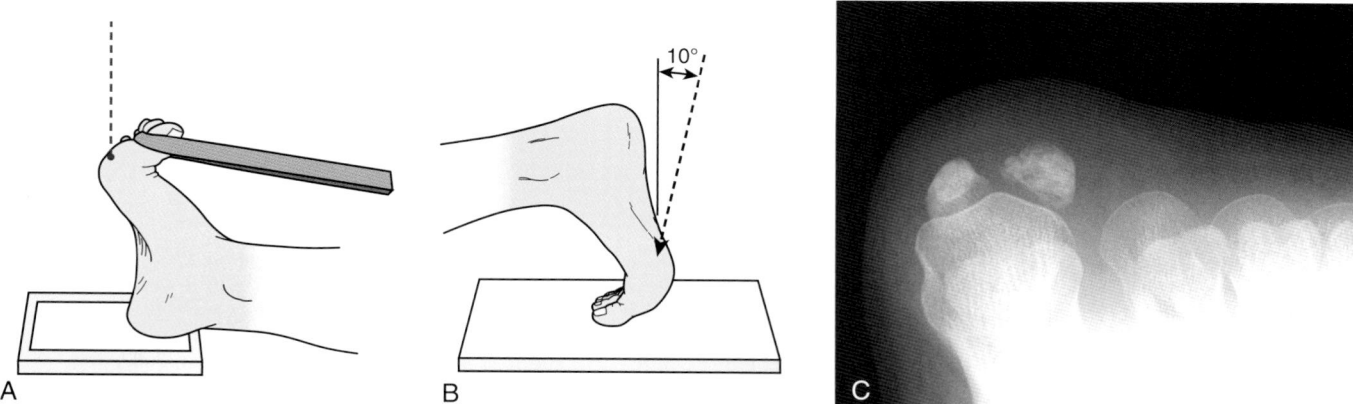

Figure 3-27 Axial sesamoid view. The axial (or "skyline") sesamoid view profiles the sesamoid bones, metatarsosesamoid articulations, and median articular ridge of the first metatarsal. **A,** Supine patient positioning using a straight beam, with the toes dorsiflexed and the plantar surface of the foot at a 75-degree angle to the cassette. **B,** Preferred prone patient positioning with 10-degree cephalad tube angulation and the toes held in dorsiflexion by pressure against the cassette. **C,** Radiograph shows a case of chronic lateral sesamoid bone stress with sclerosis, cystic change, and probable fracture. (Diagram from Jones CP, Younger ASE: Imaging of the foot and ankle. In Coughlin MJ, Mann RA, Saltzman CL, editors: *Surgery of the foot and ankle,* ed 8, Philadelphia, 2007, Mosby Elsevier. Radiograph from Anderson IF, Read JW: *Atlas of imaging in sports medicine,* ed 2, Sydney, 2008, McGraw-Hill.)

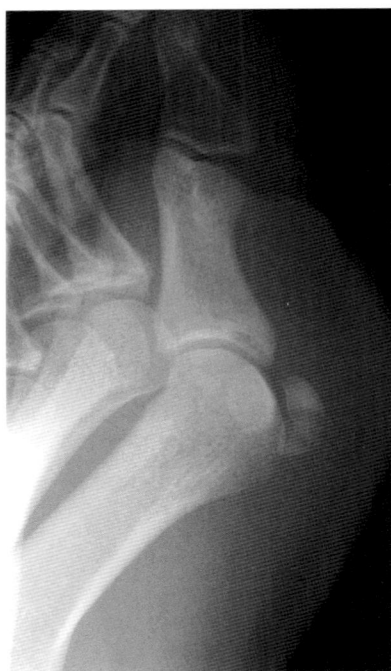

Figure 3-28 Medial oblique sesamoid view. The medial sesamoid may be further assessed in oblique projection by raising the medial side of the foot and centering on the first metatarsal head. The example here shows a fracture of the medial sesamoid with cystic change at the fracture margins. (From Anderson IF, Read JW: *Atlas of imaging in sports medicine,* ed 2, Sydney, 2008, McGraw-Hill.)

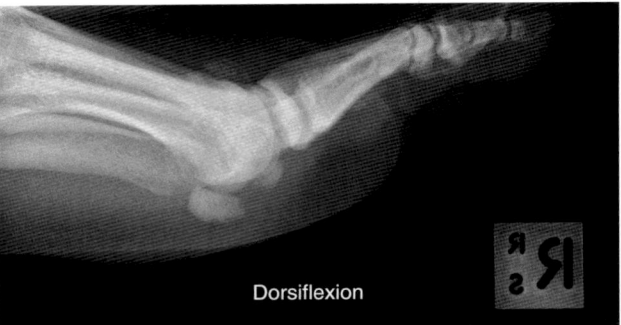

Dorsiflexion

Figure 3-30 Sesamoid stress view. A lateral radiograph with the first metatarsophalangeal joint (MTPJ1) in dorsiflexion demonstrates disruption of the synchondrosis of the medial sesamoid, which was not clearly evident on standard radiographs of the foot.

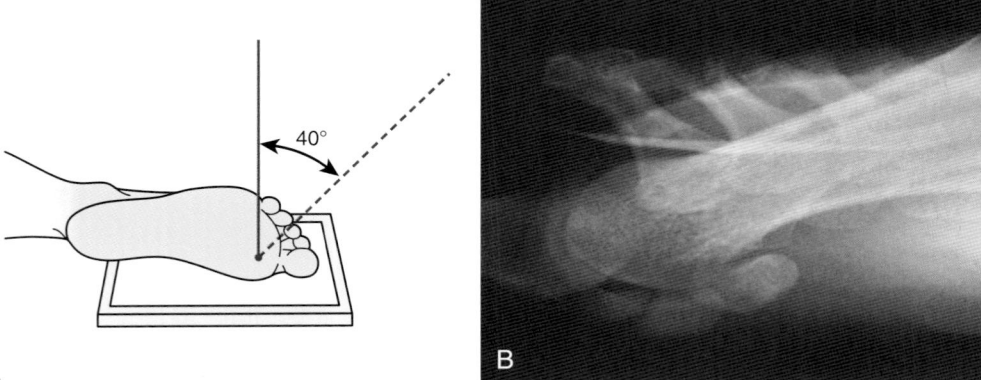

A

B

Figure 3-29 Lateromedial sesamoid view. This oblique projection can provide good anatomic detail of the medial and lateral sesamoids with minimized bony overlap. **A,** The patient is positioned with the medial side of the foot against the cassette to give a lateral projection of the first metatarsophalangeal joint and the x-ray beam angled 40 degrees toward the heel. **B,** Radiograph illustrates separation of sesamoids and improved anatomic detail. (From Jones CP, Younger ASE: Imaging of the foot and ankle. In Coughlin MJ, Mann RA, Saltzman CL, editors: *Surgery of the foot and ankle,* ed 8, Philadelphia, 2007, Mosby Elsevier.)

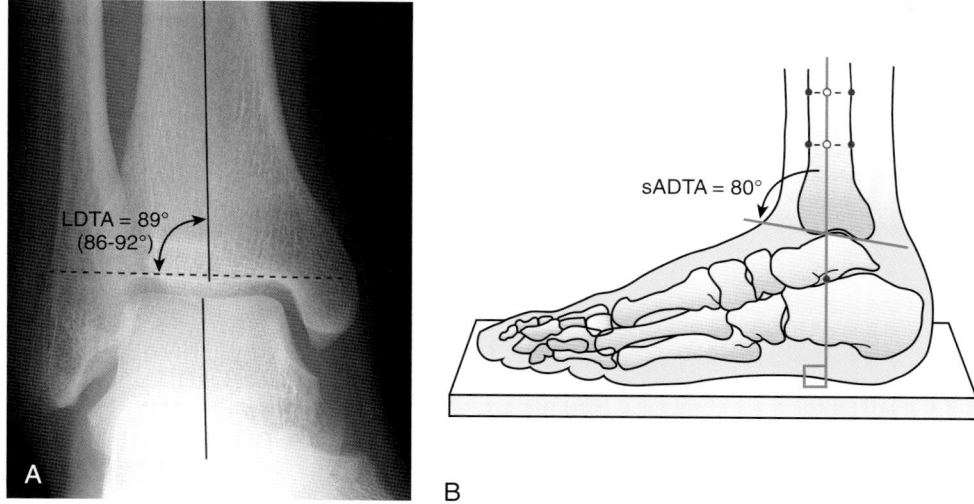

Figure 3-31 Talotibial angles. **A,** On the anteroposterior projection of ankle, the average lateral distal tibial angle *(LDTA)* between the central diaphyseal axis of tibia and the talar dome is 89 degrees, and the axis of the tibia lies slightly medial to the center of talus. **B,** On the lateral weight-bearing view of ankle, the central axis of the tibia normally passes through the lateral process of talus, and the anterior-to-posterior distal tibial angle *(sADTA)* measures 80 degrees. (**A,** Modified from Paley D: *Principles of deformity correction,* New York, 2002, Springer-Verlag. Diagram from Jones CP, Younger ASE: Imaging of the foot and ankle. In Coughlin MJ, Mann RA, Saltzman CL, editors: *Surgery of the foot and ankle,* ed 8, Philadelphia, 2007, Mosby Elsevier; source, in turn, redrawn from Paley D: *Principles of deformity correction,* New York, 2002, Springer-Verlag.)

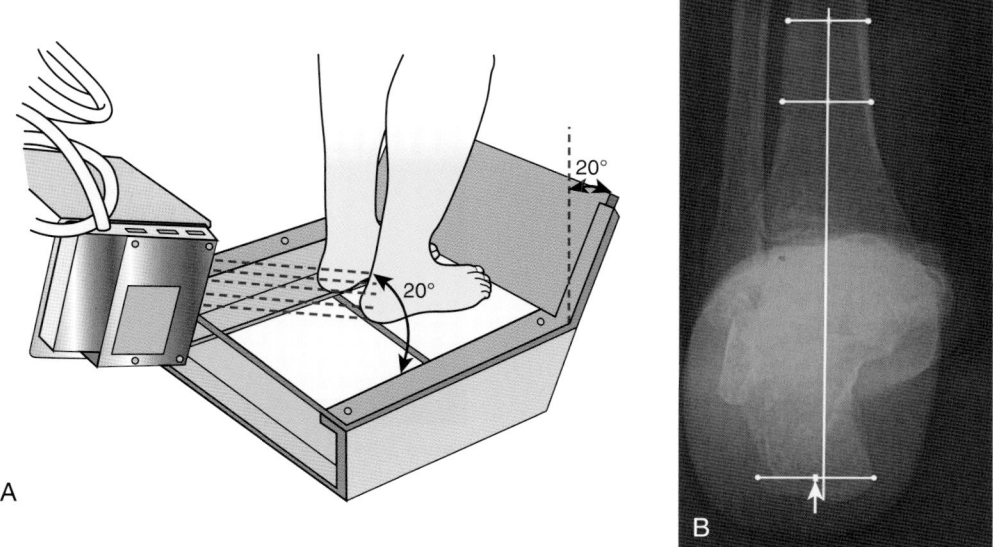

Figure 3-32 Hindfoot alignment view. **A,** The hindfoot alignment view is obtained with the patient standing on an elevated platform with the x-ray beam posterior to the heel, angled 20 degrees caudal from the horizontal. The cassette is placed in front of the patient, perpendicular to the beam, angled 20 degrees off the vertical. It is critical that the long axis of second metatarsal is oriented rectangular to the film cassette because rotation of the foot will alter the measurement of hindfoot alignment angle. **B,** The midline of the calcaneal tuberosity *(arrow)* normally lies slightly lateral to the middiaphyseal axis of the tibia, giving a normal hindfoot angle of 0 to 5 degrees valgus. (Drawing A modified from Jones CP, Younger ASE: Imaging of the foot and ankle. In Coughlin MJ, Mann RA, Saltzman CL, editors: *Surgery of the foot and ankle,* ed 8, Philadelphia, 2007, Mosby Elsevier; Image B modified from Buck FM, Hoffmann A, Mamisch-Saupe N, Espinosa N, et al: Hindfoot alignment measurements: rotation-stability of measurement techniques on hindfoot alignment view and long axial view radiographs, *AJR Am J Roentgenol* 197:578–582, 2011.)

Figure 3-33 Lateral weight-bearing foot measurements. Commonly used measurements and their normal values are illustrated. The talar–first metatarsal angle (Meary angle) assesses the longitudinal arch of the medial column of foot and is measured between *(A)* the long axis of talus drawn from the midheight of talar body through the middiameter of talonavicular joint, and *(B)* the long axis of the first metatarsal is obtained by finding the diaphyseal centers at both proximal and distal shaft levels. The fifth metatarsal base height is a measure of the longitudinal arch of the lateral column of foot. (From Meary R: On the measurement of the angle between the talus and the first metatarsal, *Rev Chir Orthop* 53:389, 1967.)

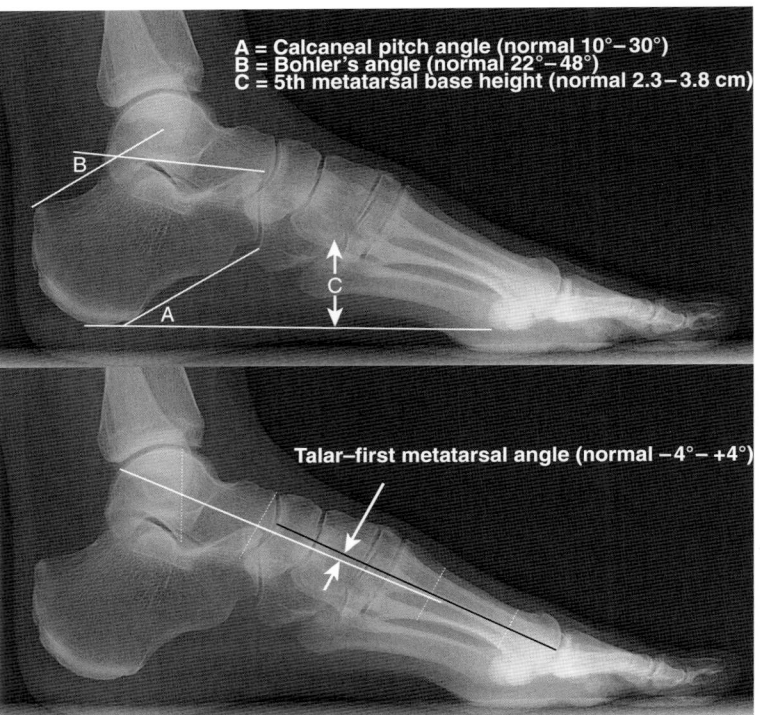

A = Calcaneal pitch angle (normal 10°–30°)
B = Bohler's angle (normal 22°–48°)
C = 5th metatarsal base height (normal 2.3–3.8 cm)

Talar–first metatarsal angle (normal −4°– +4°)

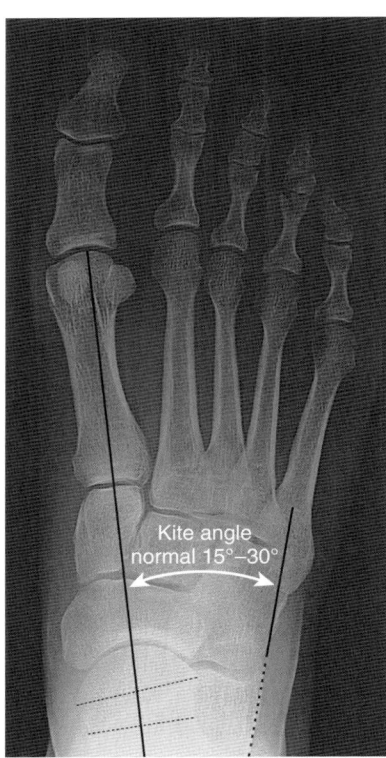

Kite angle
normal 15°–30°

Figure 3-34 Anteroposterior (AP) talocalcaneal angle. The AP talocalcaneal angle (Kite angle) is formed between the long axis of the talus and a line drawn along the lateral surface of the calcaneus, but it can be difficult to measure because of poor penetration of the hindfoot on many weight-bearing AP projections. In the adult foot, angles greater than 30 degrees indicate hindfoot valgus, and angles less than 15 degrees indicate hindfoot varus. Note that the long axis of talus normally extends along the first metatarsal, and the central long axis of calcaneus normally extends along the fourth metatarsal.

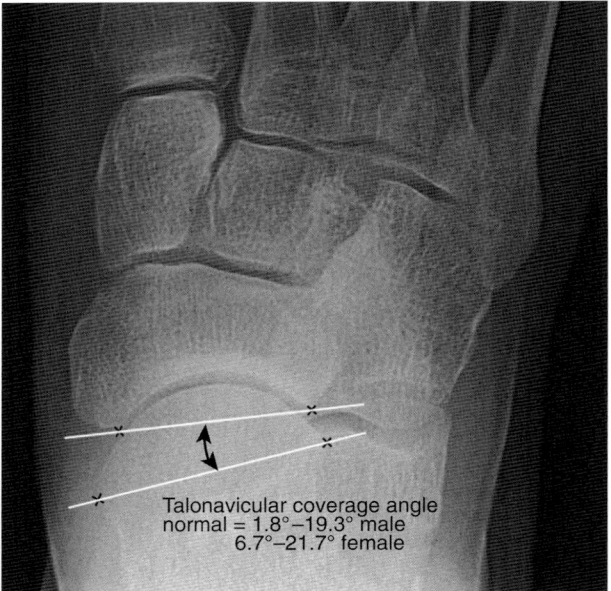

Talonavicular coverage angle
normal = 1.8°–19.3° male
6.7°–21.7° female

Figure 3-35 Talonavicular coverage angle. An anteroposterior (AP) weight-bearing view is used to assess "coverage" of the talar head by the navicular. With pes planus, there is *lateral* peritalar subluxation of the navicular and abduction of the forefoot. With pes cavus, there is *medial* peritalar subluxation of the navicular and supination of the forefoot. The talonavicular coverage angle is measured between lines drawn across the respective articular corners of talus and navicular. The normal values shown here have been taken from a recent study by Murley et al. (From Murley GS, Menz HB, Landorf KB: A protocol for classifying normal- and flat-arched foot posture for research studies using clinical and radiographic measurements, *J Foot Ankle Res* 2:22, 2009.)

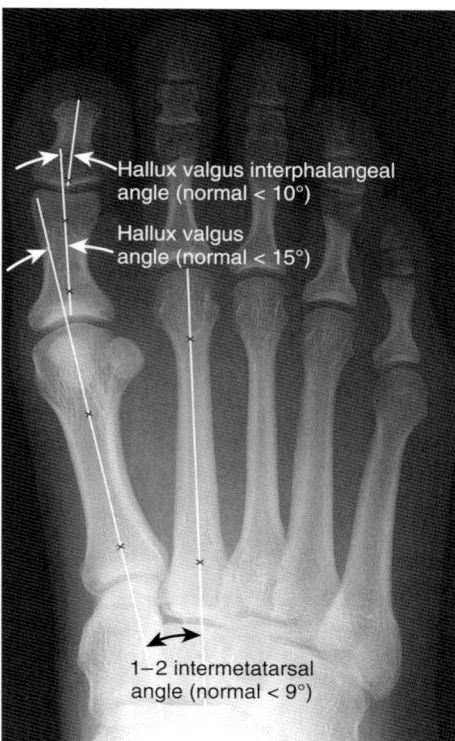

Figure 3-36 Hallux valgus assessment. An anteroposterior weight-bearing view is required to assess great toe malalignment when planning a surgical correction of hallux valgus deformity. The long axes of the metatarsals and phalanges are determined by finding the diaphyseal midpoints at metadiaphyseal level ("x" calipers). Normal hallux alignment values are shown.

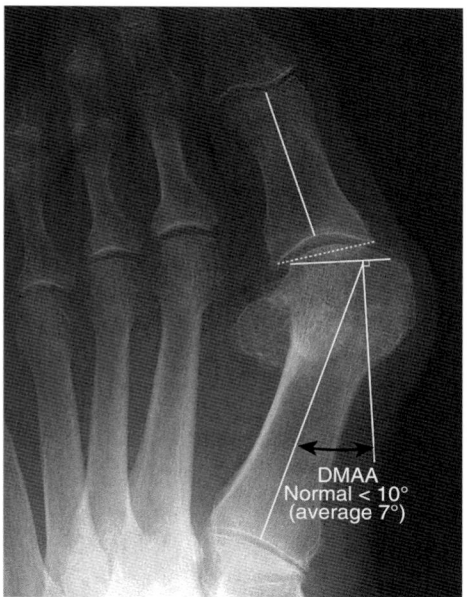

Figure 3-37 Distal metatarsal articular angle *(DMAA)* assessment. Although radiographic assessment of the DMAA is limited by poor interobserver reliability, this measurement is relevant when a distal medial closing-wedge osteotomy is being considered for the surgical treatment of hallux valgus deformity. The DMAA is the lateral slope of the articular surface of first metatarsal head relative to the long axis of first ray, normally measuring less than 10 degrees. The significance of an increased DMAA is determined by joint congruity. A congruent joint exists when lines drawn across the articular corners of both the proximal phalanx *(dotted line)* and first metatarsal head *(DMAA line)* are parallel. Hallux valgus is usually associated with an incongruent or subluxed joint that will benefit from surgical correction to restore alignment (as in the example shown here). However, some cases of hallux valgus with increased DMAA retain normal joint congruence. In these instances, a conventional surgical correction may result in a stiff joint or recurrent deformity, and an extraarticular approach to osteotomy is instead required to avoid causing an incongruent joint.

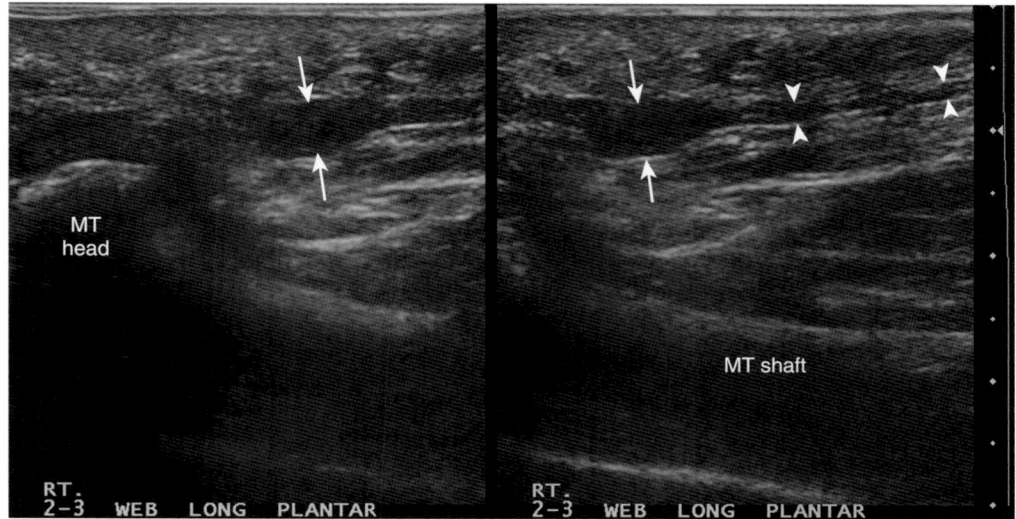

Figure 3-38 Value of sonopalpation. Long-axis ultrasound images obtained over the plantar aspect of the 2–3 metatarsal *(MT)* interspace in a patient with recurrent metatarsalgia after a Morton neurectomy showed a bulbous hypoechoic swelling of "stump" neuroma *(arrows)*, in continuity with the common plantar digital nerve *(arrowheads)*. Palpation directly over this point reproduced the clinical complaint and confirmed the relevance of the imaging observation.

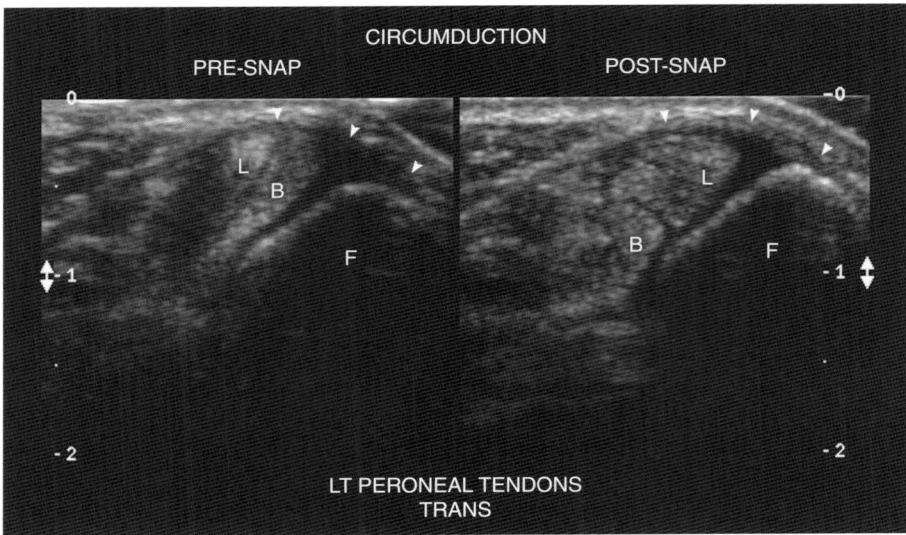

Figure 3-39 Value of dynamic ultrasound. Preclick and postclick cine-loop frames from a real-time ultrasound examination obtained during active ankle circumduction in a patient with painful retrofibular clicking demonstrate *intrasheath subluxation* of the peroneus brevis tendon. Transverse images showed the click to correspond with sudden displacement of the peroneus brevis *(B)* tendon from beneath peroneus longus *(L)* tendon, although both remained within the retromalleolar space *(F)*. Note the intact overlying superior peroneal retinaculum *(arrowheads)* and also the predisposing convexity of the peroneal groove. (From Anderson IF, Read JW: *Atlas of imaging in sports medicine,* ed 2, Sydney, 2008, McGraw-Hill.)

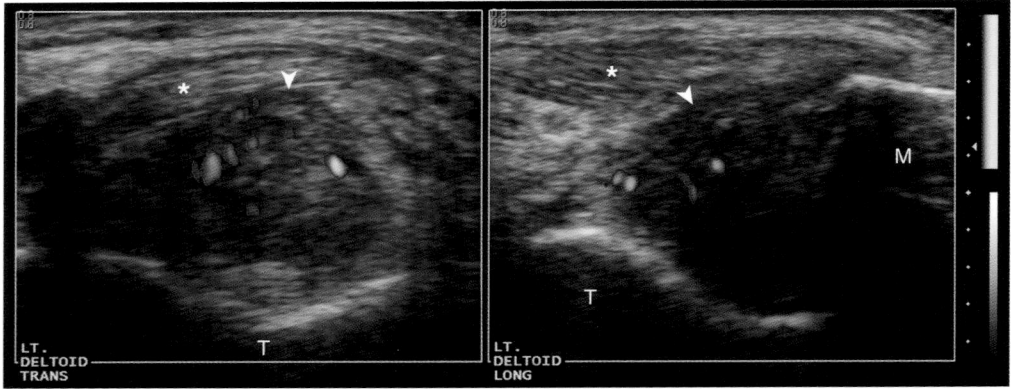

Figure 3-40 Value of Doppler ultrasound. A case of chronic medial ankle pain and tenderness persisting more than 10 months after ankle inversion injury was thought clinically to be due to tibialis posterior tendonopathy. However, transverse and long-axis power Doppler ultrasound images instead showed features of deltoid desmitis with a thickened hypoechoic deltoid ligament demonstrating convex bulge of the outer surface *(arrowheads)* and accompanying interstitial hyperemia *(colored pixels)*. Note overlying normal tibialis posterior tendon *(asterisk)*. M, medial malleolus; T, talus. (From Anderson IF, Read JW: *Atlas of imaging in sports medicine,* ed 2, Sydney, 2008, McGraw-Hill.)

Technetium-99m–Methylene Diphosphonate Bone Scanning

Technetium-99m (Tc-99m)–methylene diphosphonate (MDP) bone scanning provides a map of osteoblastic activity and is one of the staples of nuclear medicine scanning. Vigorous osteoblastic activity occurs in the growth plates of the juvenile skeleton, healing fractures, and pathologic conditions stimulating skeletal blood flow and bone repair. Bone scanning takes advantage of the fact that there is normally a continuous balance between bone breakdown and new bone formation in the skeleton. Focal increased or decreased uptake of the Tc-99m–MDP can be recognized as abnormal and highlight sites of pathology. Although bone scanning is sensitive, it is not specific because increased metabolic activity is a final common pathway for many diseases that alter osteoblast activity.

Tc-99m–MDP is administered intravenously and is delivered to the skeletal system based on vascular distribution. Within minutes, osteoblasts begin to assemble

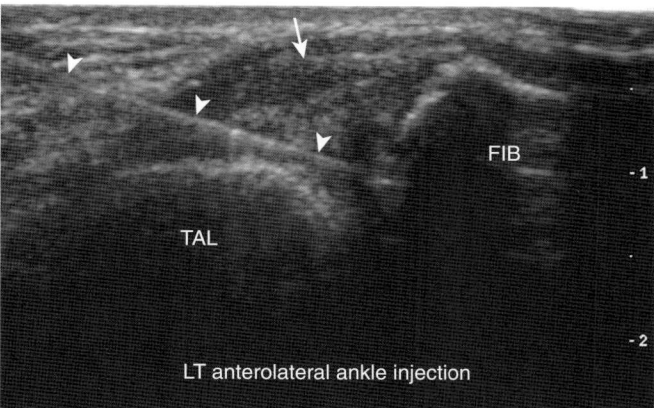

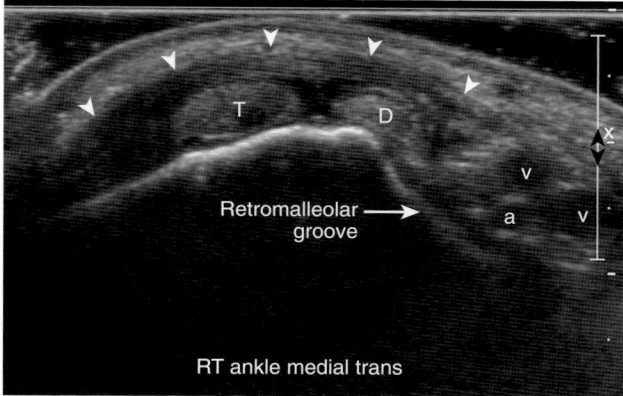

Figure 3-41 Accurate needle guidance. By directing a needle within the imaging plane of the ultrasound transducer, an advancing needle tip can be visualized in real time and accurately guided into specific anatomic spaces. In a case of anterolateral ankle impingement because of hypertrophic posttraumatic scarring of the anterior talofibular ligament *(arrow)*, a needle *(arrowheads)* was directed into the anterolateral recess of ankle joint at the deep margin of the pathologically thickened ligament for the purpose of corticosteroid injection. *FIB,* fibula; *LT,* left; *TAL,* talus.

Figure 3-43 Tibialis posterior tendon dislocation. Transverse ultrasound image over the medial malleolus shows avulsion of the flexor retinaculum *(arrowheads)* and anteromedial dislocation of both the tibialis posterior *(T)* and flexor digitorum longus *(D)* tendons. Posterior tibial artery *(a)* and veins *(v)* are indicated. *RT,* right; *trans,* transverse.

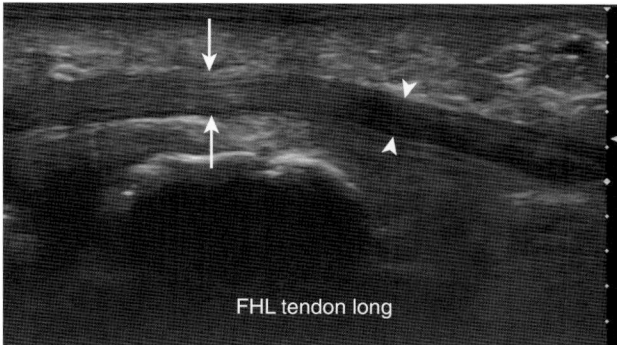

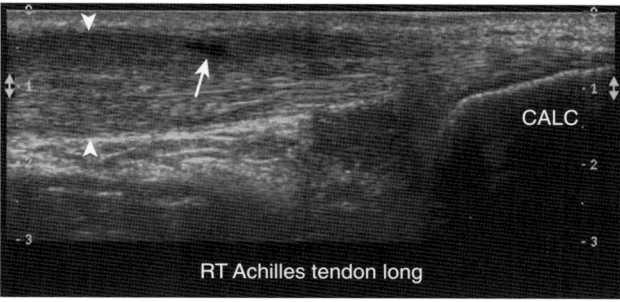

Figure 3-44 Achilles tendon partial-thickness tear. Long-axis ultrasound image shows chronic noninsertional Achilles tendonosis (fusiform hypoechoic thickening indicated by *arrowheads*) with small transverse anechoic defect in fiber continuity because of complicating partial-thickness tear *(arrow)*. *CALC,* calcaneus, *RT,* right.

Figure 3-42 Anisotropy. Ultrasound image artifacts can be a diagnostic pitfall for the inexperienced. One of the most important of these is the result of tissue reflectivity varying according to the angle of beam incidence (anisotropy). Structures with highly organized and regular fiber orientation, such as tendons and ligaments, are affected by anisotropy, as shown in this example of normal flexor hallucis longus *(FHL)* tendon, where the segment that is perpendicular to the insonating beam is accurately represented with echogenic fibers *(arrows)*, but the segment that is oblique to the beam appeared falsely hypoechoic *(arrowheads)*.

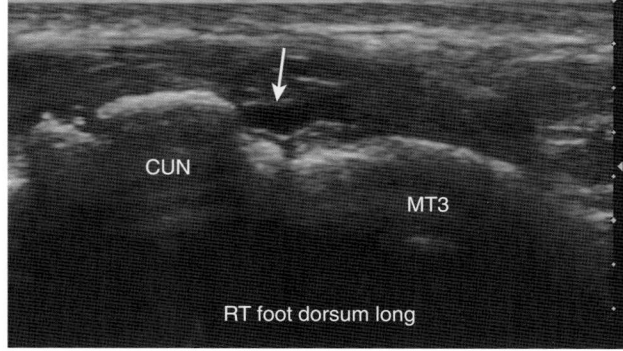

the labeled diphosphonates into the hydration shell of hyroxyapatite crystals as they are formed and modified. Three-phase and four-phase bone scans are used to determine the vascular nature of the lesion and to separate soft tissue injury or infection from focal osseous disease. Phase 1 ("blood flow") is a dynamically acquired arterial phase. Phase 2 ("blood pool") is a set of static images, representing the blood pool and soft tissue phase. Phase 3 ("delayed") is acquired 3 to 4 hours later and represents delayed skeletal uptake. Phase 4 can be acquired the

Figure 3-45 Midfoot ganglion. Although no mass was clinically palpable, the site of pain indicated by the patient corresponded with a small, rounded, anechoic space-occupying lesion located directly over the tarsometatarsal joint line with no perceptible wall thickness *(arrow)*. These features are consistent with a tarsometatarsal joint ganglion. *CUN,* lateral cuneiform; *MT3,* third metatarsal; *RT,* right.

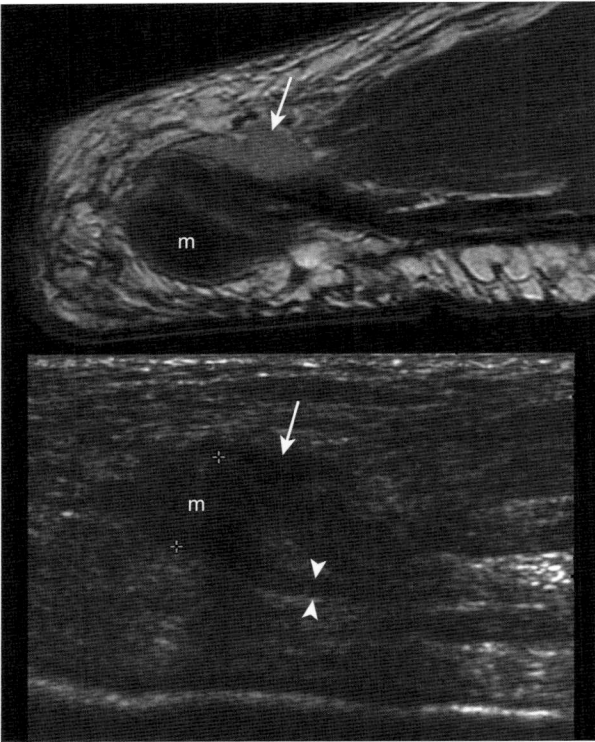

Figure 3-46 Morton neuroma. Long-axis proton-density–weighted magnetic resonance image and corresponding long-axis ultrasound image have been obtained over the distal metatarsal interspace at metatarsophalangeal joint level and show the typical position and appearance of a Morton neuroma. The neuroma *(m)* is appreciated on ultrasound as an ovoid hypoechoic thickening that shows smoothly tapering continuity with the more proximal segment of common plantar digital nerve *(arrowheads)*. Fluid is seen within the adjacent intermetatarsal bursa *(arrows)*.

following morning if better skeletal detail is required, usually when the patient has poor renal function (e.g., diabetic foot infection).

Single-Photon Emission Computed Tomography

Single photon emission computed tomography (SPECT) is an imaging alternative to routine planar scanning, providing images with improved contrast and spatial resolution. A series of planar images are obtained by means of a gamma camera, which travels in an arc around the patient. Information from these acquisitions is postprocessed to produce axial images, which can be reformatted in sagittal and coronal planes.

SPECT is a new diagnostic tool that combines a multihead gamma camera and CT scanner mounted together with a common imaging table. This allows the morphologic information of CT to be fused with the biologic information of bone scanning, allowing precise localization of pathology.[8,27] SPECT has been shown to be useful in evaluating midfoot arthritis, where the number and configuration of joints are complex,[55] and assessing the precise location of pathology in patients presenting with obscure foot and ankle pain.[76] SPECT may be useful in the management of osteochondral lesions of the talus by demonstrating the degree of activity of the lesion and the precise location of the active segment in multiple lesions.[33,43]

Gallium Scanning and White Cell Scanning

Gallium-67 is an agent that accumulates in infections, areas of inflammation, and in some tumors.[56] It is also a weak bone scanning agent. After administration of Ga-67, imaging is performed at 24, 48, and 72 hours. Whole-body imaging is usually performed, but scanning can be

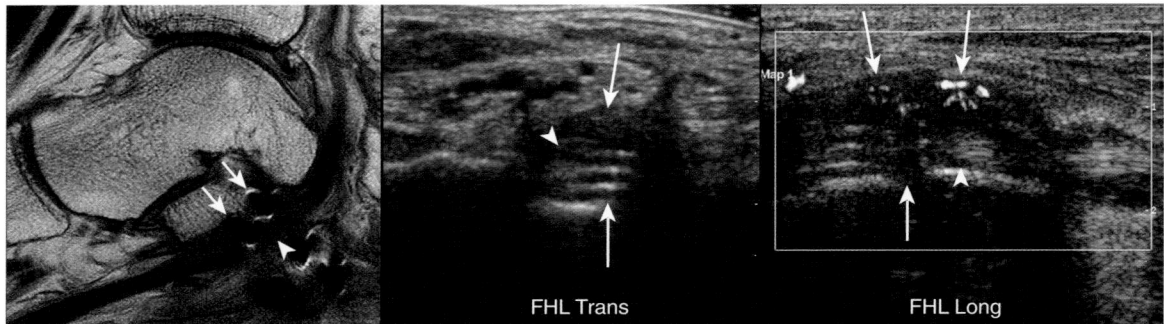

Figure 3-47 Imaging adjacent to metal. Ultrasound is useful in assessing the soft tissues adjacent to metallic surgical hardware (when magnetic resonance imaging may be nondiagnostic). This is illustrated in a case of flexor hallucis longus *(FHL)* tendinosis and peritendonitis secondary to impingement by surgical screws after internal fixation of a calcaneal fracture. The FHL tendon at the level of sustentaculum tali is shown on a sagittal proton-density–weighted magnetic resonance image *(left)*, a transverse gray-scale ultrasound image *(middle)*, and a long-axis power Doppler ultrasound image *(right)*. Surgical screws *(short arrows)* directly impinge upon a distorted segment of FHL tendon *(arrowheads)*. A markedly thickened and hyperemic peritendon *(long arrows)* is best appreciated on ultrasound.

limited to the area of interest. Ga-67 is limited by its poor photon yield per disintegration; therefore it is a suboptimal imaging agent. Ga-67 scanning has been replaced by leukocyte scanning for evaluation of osteomyelitis in most regions of the skeleton, but it remains the procedure of choice for diagnosing spinal osteomyelitis.

Leukocyte scanning is an alternative technique used to detection of infection or inflammation. Radionuclides available for leukocyte scanning include In-111 and Tc-99m. Whole blood is drawn from the patient and is centrifuged to extract the leukocytes. The leukocytes are then incubated with the radionuclide and reinjected into the patient.[38] Imaging is performed at 4 hours and at 24 hours. Because the majority of leukocytes labeled are neutrophils, the procedure is most useful for identifying neutrophil-mediated inflammatory processes, such as bacterial infections.

Use of Nuclear Scanning

Nuclear medicine scanning is increasingly being replaced by MRI in the field of musculoskeletal imaging. Bone scanning, however, remains the primary means of evaluating the entire skeleton for a potentially polyostotic process, such as metastatic disease, bone dysplasias, or diffuse arthritis. Evaluation of foot and ankle pain of unknown cause also is another common indication for bone scanning. Bone scanning can detect bone stress, occult fractures, osteochondral injuries, osteoid osteomas, and arthritis (Figs. 3-48 to 3-50).[26] Radionuclide uptake in occult fractures occurs within 72 hours of

injury, even in patients with osteoporosis.[41] Bone scanning will be positive in patients with midfoot sprain and normal radiographs[54]; however, uptake on bone scan is nonspecific and can also occur with chronic instability or osteoarthritis.

Reflex sympathetic dystrophy, or complex regional pain syndrome, can also be diagnosed with bone scans.[12] Because of the inappropriately increased vascular

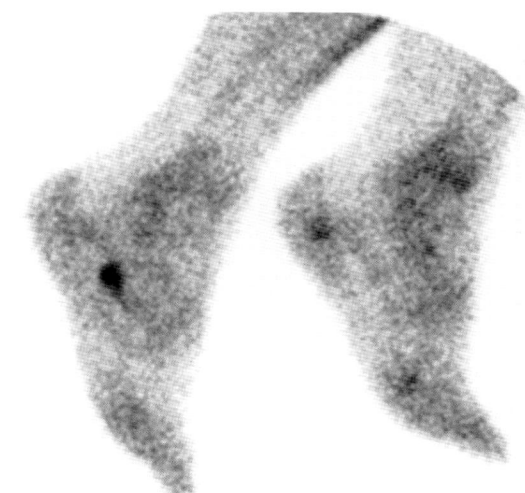

Figure 3-48 Painful os peroneum syndrome. Delayed-phase bone scan image demonstrating increased radiotracer uptake in an os peroneum that was tender to palpation, consistent with painful os peroneum syndrome (POPS).

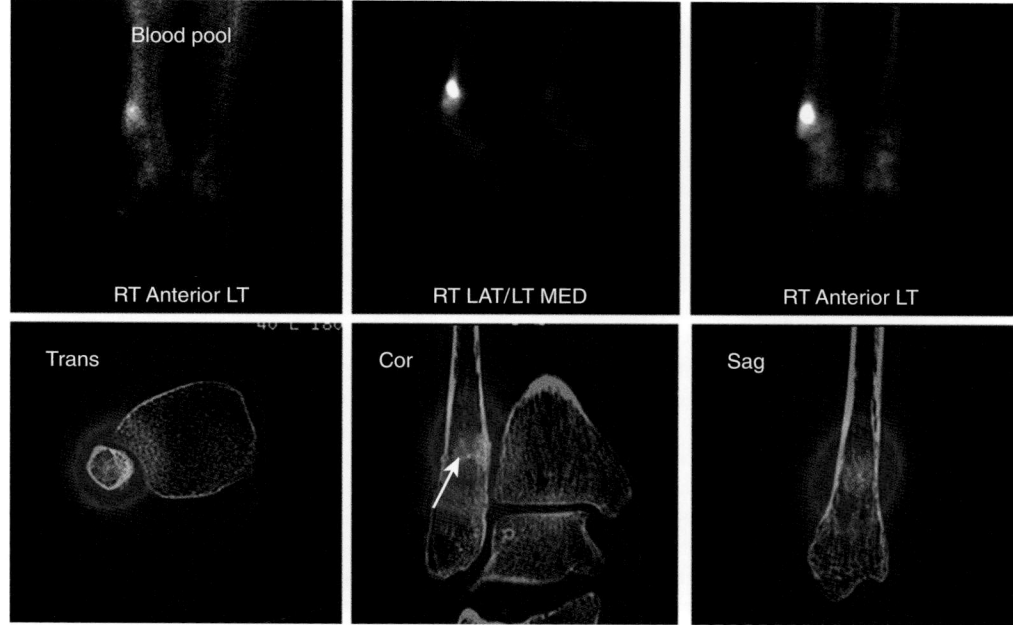

Figure 3-49 Fibular stress fracture. A single-photon emission computed tomography (SPECT) study demonstrates a stress fracture of the distal fibula that was not evident on plain radiographs. Blood pool image *(top left)* and delayed planar images *(top middle and right)* demonstrate increased radiotracer uptake at the distal fibula. *Cor,* coronal; *LAT,* lateral; *LT,* left; *MED,* medial; *RT,* right; *Sag,* sagittal; *Trans,* transverse. (Image courtesy Dr. Hans Van Der Wall.)

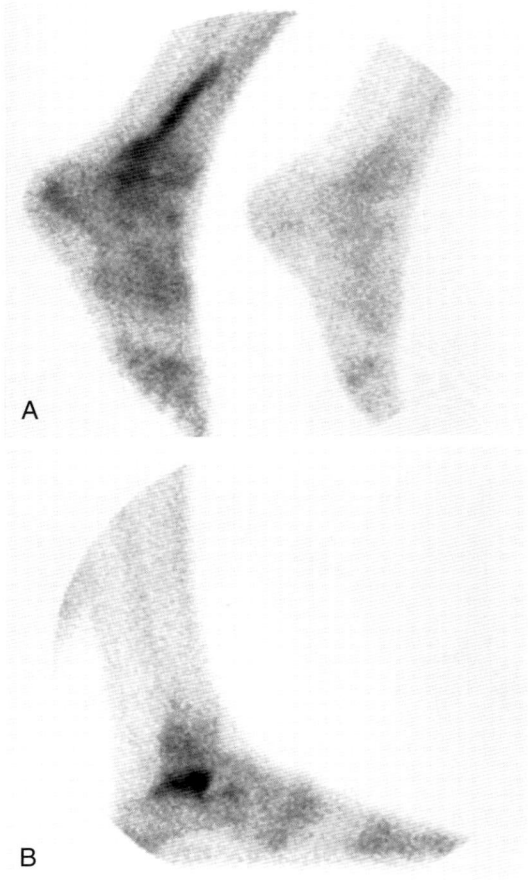

Figure 3-50 Depiction of occult fractures. Bone scanning demonstrates a vertical fracture of the distal fibula **(A)** and a fracture of the body of the talus, adjacent to the subtalar joint **(B)**. Neither fracture was evident on the prior radiographs.

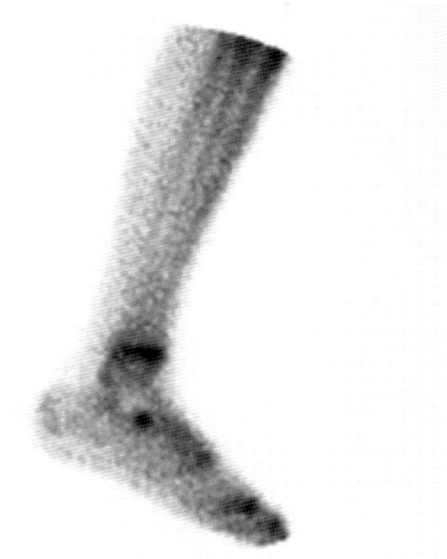

Figure 3-51 Physiologic technetium-99m–methylene diphosphonate uptake in an athlete. Multiple sites of increased isotope uptake are present in the foot and ankle of this young athlete.

response, one extremity will demonstrate diffuse increased tracer uptake on blood flow, blood pool, and delayed-phase scans.

In the highly trained athlete, areas of increased isotope uptake in the foot and ankle are incredibly common and may therefore be considered almost "normal." This is particularly so in the adolescent athlete.[10] Consequently, the clinical history and presentation must be carefully considered before interpreting the significance of an area of increased isotope uptake (Fig. 3-51).

Infection is another indication for radionuclide scanning. In-111–labeled leukocyte scanning, combined with bone scanning, is the most common method used to diagnose osteomyelitis. Nuclear medicine scanning is particularly useful in imaging for occult infection because whole body images can be obtained. When infection is clearly localized to a particular area, MRI is more accurate in assessing the extent of osseous and soft tissue involvement and detecting complications such as bone abscess and soft tissue collections.[46,77]

COMPUTED TOMOGRAPHY

Computed tomography provides excellent bony anatomic detail and is particularly useful in evaluation of the complex anatomy of the foot and ankle. Multidetector CT (MDCT) technology produces high-resolution thin-slice images that can be obtained in any plane, aiding in the visualization of fractures and assisting preoperative planning. CT is also useful to define loose bodies and avulsed fragments and to assess the tibiofibular syndesmosis for disruption.

Basic Science

A CT scanner consists of a scanning gantry, an x-ray generator, a computerized data processing system, and a movable patient table. A narrow, collimated beam of x-rays is generated on one side of the patient. After passing through the patient, the attenuated x-ray beam is detected by a fixed ring of detectors within the scanning gantry. Attenuation or absorption of the x-ray beam reflects the density of the imaged tissue. The x-ray tube rotates 360 degrees around the patient, and these measurements of x-ray transmission are repeated many times from different directions. A computer is used to mathematically reconstruct a cross-sectional image of the body from measurements of x-ray transmission through thin slices of patient tissue.

The computer analyzes the average attenuation in a three-dimensional (3D) volume, or voxel, of tissue. The number is converted into a gray-scale value and is displayed on the screen as a pixel. CT pixel numbers are proportional to the difference between average x-ray attenuation of the tissues within the voxel and that of water. The Hounsfield unit (HU) scale is used, whereby water is assigned a value of 0 HU. Hounsfield units are therefore not absolute values but are relative values that vary from one CT system to another. In general, bone is +400 to + 1000 HU, soft tissue is +40 to +80 HU, fat is −60 to −100 HU, and air is −1000 HU. The range and center of gray-scale value can be manipulated by altering the window width and window level, respectively. Narrow window widths and low window levels result in "soft tissue windows." Wider window widths and higher window levels result in "bone windows."

The computer algorithm chosen for image reconstruction and the thickness of the scanned slice determines the voxel dimensions. In general, imaging the foot and ankle requires high-resolution scanning, with a slice thickness of 0.5 to 1 mm. Scanning is performed in the axial plane; images may be reformatted in sagittal, coronal, or oblique planes or as three-dimensional reconstructions.

CT scanners have evolved from conventional scanners, which obtained a single slice at each indexed table interval with a short pause between images, to *helical* or *spiral* CT scanners. Multidetector helical CT (MDCT) is the current technology used by most scanners. It uses the principles of helical CT, whereby the patient table is moved at a constant speed through the CT gantry while the x-ray tube rotates continuously around the patient, but the instrument incorporates multiple rows of detector rings. This allows the acquisition of multiple slices per tube rotation, therefore increasing the area of the patient that can be scanned in a given time by the x-ray beam. Available systems have moved from 2 slices to 320 slices,

which covers 40 mm of patient length for each rotation of the x-ray tube. The advantage of MDCT includes faster imaging times and the ability to obtain thin (0.625 mm) slices, allowing the creation of isotropic voxels that can be reconstructed into any imaging plane without loss of resolution.

The limitations of CT scanning include radiation dose (see Table 3-2), cost, and the limited ability of CT to assess soft tissues. Dual source CT (DSCT) is a new technology, originally developed for cardiac imaging, which can decrease radiation dose by more than half. A DSCT scanner is equipped with two x-ray tubes and two corresponding detectors that are oriented in the gantry at an angular offset of 90 degrees. This allows an increase in temporal resolution, increase in speed of acquisition, and decrease in radiation dose to the patient. By using x-ray beams at two different energy levels, DSCT can also allow the differentiation of different materials, based on their energy attenuation profiles. In the foot and ankle, this has been shown to be useful in distinguishing monosodium urate crystals from calcium hydroxyapatite crystals in the prospective diagnosis of gout.[22] DSCT can also facilitate a reduction in artifact in the setting of in situ metal hardware.

Use of Computed Tomography Scanning

CT scanning provides high-resolution images of bony anatomy, which can be reconstructed in any plane. This is useful in the imaging of complex fractures of the foot and ankle, which may be radiographically occult or difficult to evaluate on plain radiographs. CT scanning is particularly helpful in the assessment of traumatic injuries to the midfoot (Fig. 3-52).[24] CT of calcaneal fractures

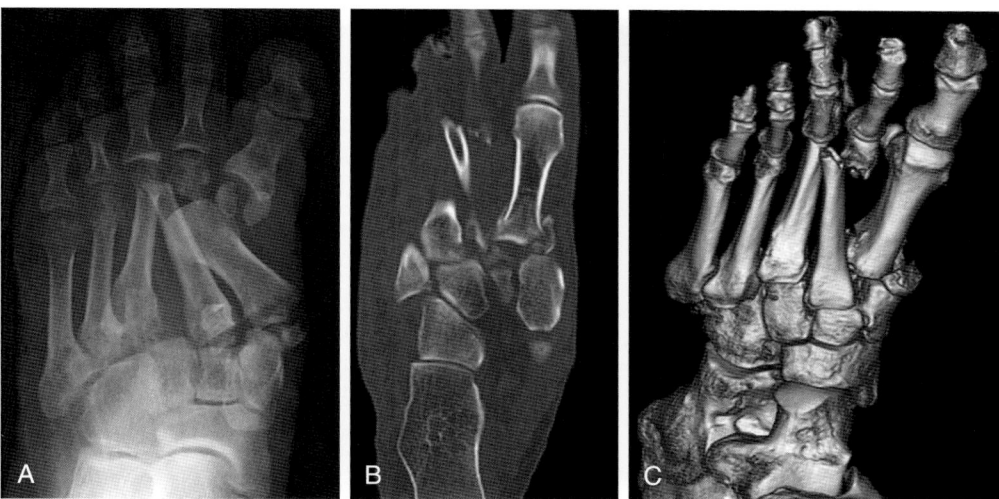

Figure 3-52 Assessment of midfoot fractures using three-dimensional (3D) multidetector computed tomography (MDCT). Radiographs **(A)** demonstrate fracture-dislocations of the tarsometatarsal joints, fracture of the neck of the second metatarsal, and dislocations of the third and first metatarsophalangeal joints. Axial CT **(B)** is difficult to interpret, but 3D MDCT **(C)** helps in preoperative assessment of the complex injury and allows better understanding of the deformities. (From Anderson IF, Read JW: *Atlas of imaging in sports medicine,* ed 2, Sydney, 2008, McGraw-Hill.)

can identify involvement of the posterior subtalar joint, sustentaculum tali, and calcaneocuboid joint (Fig. 3-53).[18] Impingement by fracture fragments on adjacent soft tissue structures, such as the peroneal tendons, can also be identified.[20,64] CT provides useful information in the evaluation of triplane, Tillaux, pilon, and trimalleolar fractures, aiding preoperative planning (Fig. 3-54).[45] Three-dimensional reconstructions are particularly helpful for preoperative planning in these complex injuries.

CT scanning can be useful in the assessment of tarsal coalitions (Fig. 3-55), neoplasms (Fig. 3-56), foreign bodies, osteochondral injuries, and subtalar joint arthritis. In the postoperative patient, CT scanning can evaluate for osseous fusion at a site of arthrodesis or at sites of internal fixation of fractures or osteotomies (Fig. 3-57). If a patient is unable to undergo MRI (e.g., because of a cardiac pacemaker), CT arthrography offers an alternative imaging modality to assess osteochondral injuries of the ankle joint.

MAGNETIC RESONANCE IMAGING

MRI is an increasingly valuable tool in foot and ankle imaging because of its superior soft tissue contrast and ability to assess articular cartilage and detect subtle bone marrow edema and occult fractures. MRI is particularly useful in the detection and characterization of ligament injuries, bone contusion, chondral and osteochondral lesions, and impingement syndromes.

Basic Science

MRI is a technique that produces tomographic images by means of magnetic fields and radio waves. Although CT evaluates only a single tissue parameter—attenuation of the x-ray beam—MRI can analyze multiple tissue characteristics, including proton (hydrogen) density, T1 and T2 relaxation times of tissue, and blood flow. Although a detailed description of MRI physics is beyond the scope of this chapter, it is helpful to have a basic understanding

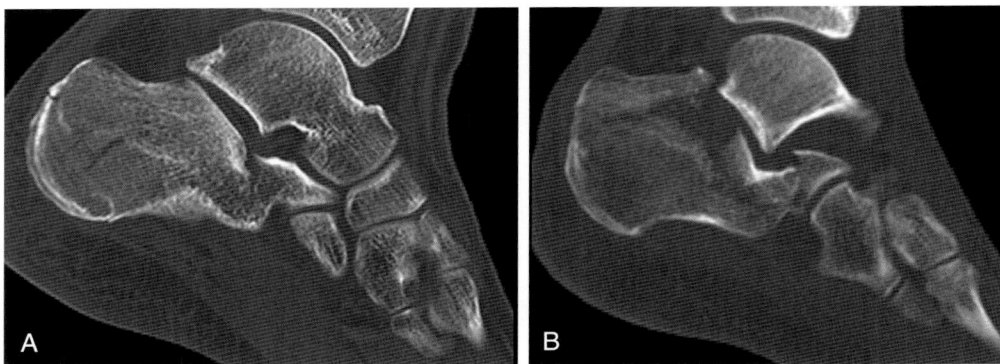

Figure 3-53 Assessment of calcaneal fractures using multidetector computed tomography (MDCT). The morphology of comminuted calcaneal fractures and involvement of the subtalar joints is well displayed by MDCT images through the medial **(A)** and lateral **(B)** aspects of the posterior subtalar joint. (From Anderson IF, Read JW: *Atlas of imaging in sports medicine*, ed 2, Sydney, 2008, McGraw-Hill.)

Figure 3-54 Multidetector computed tomography of ankle fractures. Coronal CT **(A)** demonstrates an oblique fracture through the distal tibia, involving the growth plate and distal tibial eipiphysis. Three-dimensional reconstruction **(B)** clearly shows the injury to be a triplane fracture. (From Anderson IF, Read JW: *Atlas of imaging in sports medicine*, ed 2, Sydney, 2008, McGraw-Hill.)

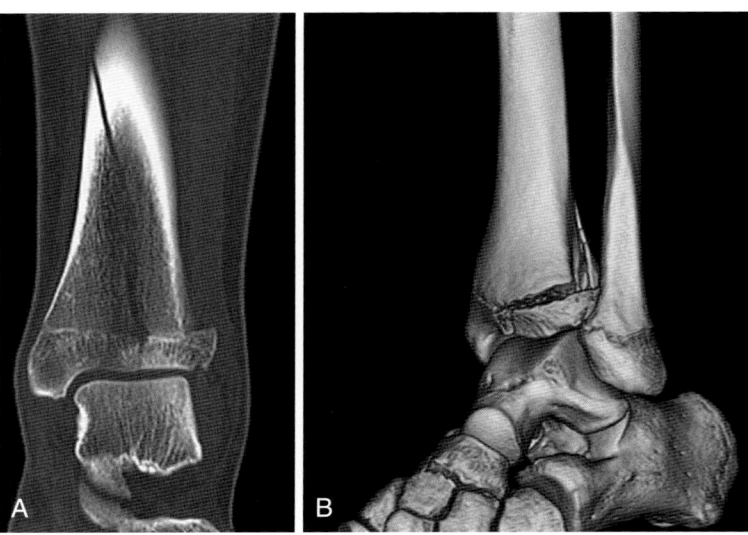

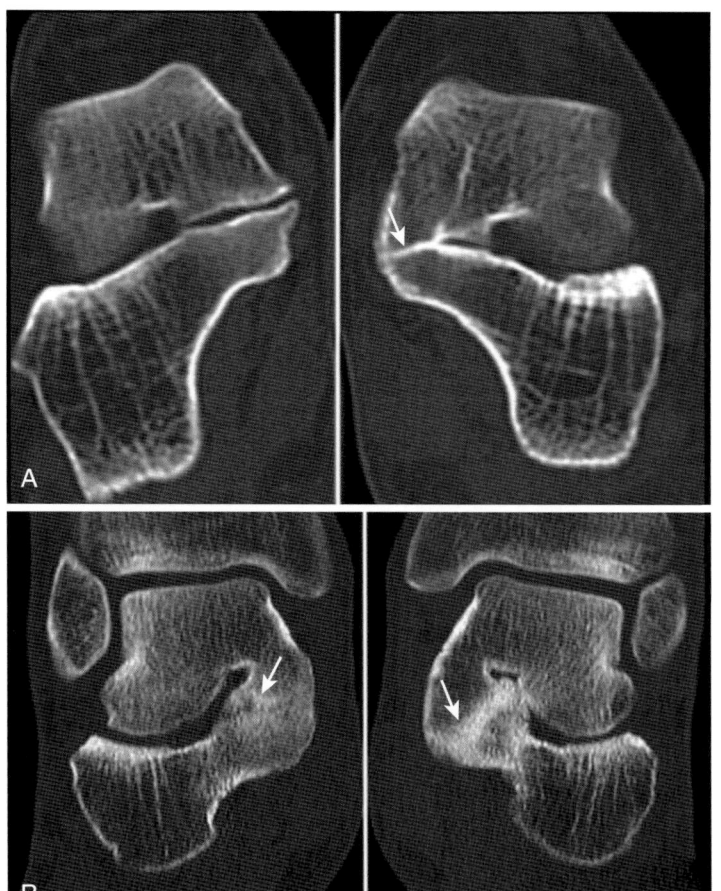

Figure 3-55 Computed tomography (CT) assessment of coalition. **A,** CT demonstrates narrowing and irregularity of the left middle subtalar joint *(white arrow)* resulting from a cartilaginous coalition. **B,** In another patient, there are bilateral osseous coalitions of the middle subtalar joints *(arrows)*. (From Anderson IF, Read JW: *Atlas of imaging in sports medicine,* ed 2, Sydney, 2008, McGraw-Hill.)

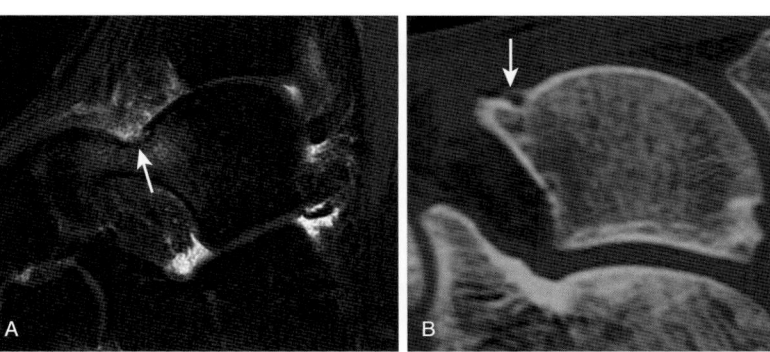

Figure 3-56 Computed tomography (CT) for assessment of tumors. A 26-year-old ballerina presented with persistent pain and symptoms of anterior ankle impingement. On magnetic resonance imaging **(A),** there is questionable shallow cortical erosion of the dorsal talar neck *(arrow)* with subcortical bone marrow edema and adjacent soft tissue edema. On CT **(B),** there is an intracortical nidus *(arrow),* consistent with an osteoid osteoma. (From Anderson IF, Read JW: *Atlas of imaging in sports medicine,* ed 2, Sydney, 2008, McGraw-Hill.)

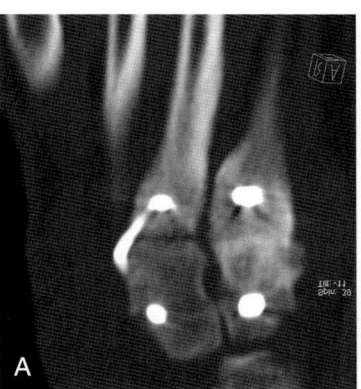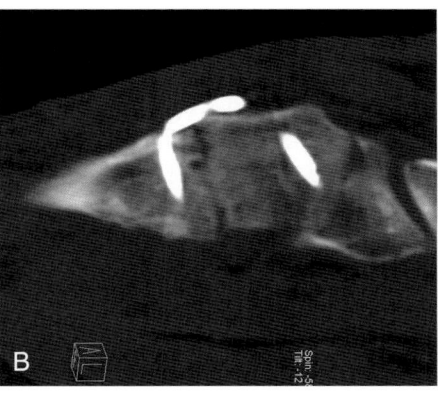

Figure 3-57 Computed tomography (CT) for assessment of arthrodesis. Dual-energy CT demonstrating solid first tarsometatarsal joint arthrodesis **(A)** and nonunion of an attempted second tarsometatarsal joint arthrodesis **(A and B).**

of the method, terminology, and image characteristics involved. The following discussion has been adapted from Anderson and Read.[2]

Routine MRI utilizes the magnetic properties of unpaired hydrogen protons, and the chemical and magnetic environments in which they are found, to produce images of biologic tissues. The spin of the positively charged hydrogen proton makes it behave like a tiny bar magnet. When placed in a strong external magnetic field, these protons align themselves with the external magnetic field. Electromagnetic energy is then pulsed at the natural or "resonant" frequency of the proton (a radiofrequency, or RF, pulse), temporarily exciting the protons to a higher energy state. When this external RF pulse is switched off, the protons "relax" back into alignment with the external magnetic field (a lower energy state). This emits a corresponding amount of RF energy that can be detected and used to form an image.

After the RF pulse is turned off, the protons return to their prior orientation in the field and gradually return to a random precession. This emits a radiowave signal, known as a T1 and T2. The signal characteristics and subsequent image formation depend on the ratio of the T1 and T2 information plus proton density (PD). Each tissue's composition has a unique T1 and T2 character.

The rate and nature of hydrogen proton relaxation are determined by the local chemical, structural, and magnetic environments in which these protons are found (e.g., lipids, free water, proteins). Different tissues therefore exhibit significant differences in their resonant behavior, which is the source of the superb image contrast provided by MRI. Most tissues can be differentiated by differences in their characteristic T1 and T2 relaxation times. T1 (spin-lattice [longitudinal] relaxation time) is a measure of a protons ability to exchange energy with its surrounding chemical matrix and represents a measure of how quickly a tissue can become magnetized. T2 (spin-spin [transverse] relaxation time) conveys how quickly a given tissue loses its magnetization.

External RF energy is introduced in a series of pulses (known as a pulse sequence), the timing of which determines which type of proton relaxation is emphasized in the resultant image, that is, whether an image is T1 weighted or T2 weighted. The two most important pulse parameters are time to repetition (TR) and time to echo (TE). TR is the amount of time between consecutive groups of RF pulses, and TE is the time between the initial RF pulse and subsequent signal detection. Using a short TR (≤500 msec) and short TE (≤20 msec) will produce a T1-weighted image, while using a long TR (≥2000 msec) and long TE (≥70 msec) will produce a T2-weighted image. Using a long TR (≥2000 msec) and intermediate TE (25-30 msec) will minimize the effects of T1 and T2 weighting and will instead produce an image reflecting hydrogen density: a proton-density–weighted image.

The coils or antennae that detect and measure the RF signal returning from the patient are critical determinants of image quality. These receiver coils were initially incorporated into the wall of the magnet (body coils). The role of MRI in characterizing the musculoskeletal system did not expand until the introduction of specialized extremity coils (surface coils) in the late 1980s. Surface coils are positioned close to the structures of interest, thereby improving signal-to-noise ratio and allowing the acquisition of high-resolution images. More recently, there have been even further improvements in image quality by combining multiple coils into a phased-array configuration.

Magnetic resonance scanners can be classified as low field, midfield, and high field, depending on the strength of the external magnet, which is measured in tesla (T) units. The most common magnetic resonance scanners in current use are midfield 1.5 T and high-field 3 T scanners. Ultrahigh-field 7 T scanners are currently being used in research applications.[29] High-field scanners offer improved resolution for small body parts and decreased imaging times.

Magnetic Resonance Imaging Clinical Sequences

The early years of clinical MRI were dominated by conventional spin-echo pulse sequences. These were prolonged acquisitions that were susceptible to patient movement, usually taking between 10 and 15 minutes each. The development of faster techniques has allowed high-resolution sequences to be performed in reasonable time frames of 2 and 5 minutes each. Fast spin-echo (FSE) sequences have now become the general workhorse of musculoskeletal imaging. These sequences are usually used in combination with supplementary sequences, such as short tau inversion recovery (STIR) or gradient-recalled echo (GRE). FSE techniques have also incorporated strategies to suppress the bright signal emanating from fat, which can obscure the high signal of pathology (fat suppression).

T1-Weighted Fast Spin-Echo Sequences

T1-weighted FSE sequences utilize short imaging parameters (TR ≤ 500 msec, TE ≤ 20 msec at 1.5 T) and reflect the T1 characteristics of tissue within the image. Fat, proteinaceous fluid, subacute hemorrhage, and gadolinium contrast will appear high signal (bright). Fluid (i.e., water) will appear low signal (dark). T1-weighted images have a high signal-to-noise ratio and therefore have the advantage of providing good anatomic detail. However, T1-weighted images result in poor delineation between the intermediate signal intensity cartilage and the low signal intensity joint fluid. T1-weighted images are insensitive to edema (fluid), and fat will appear high signal, which can mask adjacent pathology. The "magic angle" phenomenon (discussed below) is most conspicuous on T1 images. These factors can all cloud the delineation of anatomy or pathology and therefore limit the clinical value of T1-weighted images in musculoskeletal imaging. T1-weighted sequences, however, remain useful for the demonstration of fractures and tumor tissue characterization.

T2-Weighted Fast Spin-Echo Sequences

T2-weighted FSE sequences utilize long imaging parameters (TR ≥ 2000 msec, TE ≥ 70 msec at 1.5 T) and reflect the T2 characteristics of tissue within the image. T2 images emphasize fluid and edema, which will appear high signal. On T2-weighted FSE sequences, fat is moderately high signal intensity, and muscle appears as intermediate signal. Tendons and ligaments appear low signal. The magic angle phenomenon is minimized because of the long TE; therefore T2-weighted sequences can be helpful whenever the magic angle phenomenon may confound image interpretation. T2-weighted sequences are often combined with fat-suppression techniques to highlight edema and are useful in assessing tissue characteristics of tumors.

Proton-Density–Weighted Fast Spin-Echo Sequences

Proton-density–weighted FSE sequences utilize intermediate imaging parameters (TR ≥ 2000 msec, TE = 25-40 msec at 1.5 T) and reflect the concentration of hydrogen protons, rather than the T1 or T2 characteristics of tissue within the image. PD-weighted sequences have become the general workhorse of musculoskeletal MRI because they provide high contrast resolution and high spatial resolution images with relatively high signal-to-noise ratio (i.e., good anatomic resolution), allowing for reasonably fast scan times.

PD-weighted FSE sequences are particularly useful for assessment of articular cartilage. At 1.5 T, optimal image contrast between articular cartilage and joint fluid is obtained using TE values of 25 to 35 msec. This produces good contrast between the intermediate signal intensity articular cartilage, the low signal intensity fibrocartilage and subchondral bone and the high signal intensity synovial fluid. On PD-weighted FSE images, articular cartilage demonstrates a normal gray-scale stratification, which corresponds to the cartilage zonal anatomy. Partial thickness chondral lesions and chondral flaps are also well depicted with thin slice PD-weighted FSE sequences. The disadvantage of PD-weighted images is that the magic angle artifact remains moderately conspicuous and should not be misinterpreted as pathology.

Short Tau Inversion Recovery or "Fat-Sat" Sequences

The application of fat suppression to FSE images overcomes the problem of high signal fat obscuring edema and increases the contrast differences between cartilage, fluid, and synovium. The two most common imaging techniques used to achieve fat suppression in musculoskeletal imaging are frequency-selective fat-suppression techniques and STIR sequences. These produce images with low signal intensity fat and bone marrow but high signal intensity fluid and tissue edema.

Frequency-selective fat-saturation ("fat-sat") techniques achieve fat suppression by applying an initial RF pulse that sets the magnetization of fat to zero ("nulling") before the imaging pulses. This results in images with good spatial resolution and faster acquisition times when compared with STIR images. The images are, however, highly sensitive to magnetic field inhomogeneity and are therefore vulnerable to uneven fat suppression when imaging off-center in the magnet or when imaging curved body parts, such as the foot and ankle. They are also ineffective in the setting of metal. In these settings, inversion recovery techniques provide more robust fat suppression.

STIR images achieve fat suppression by acquiring signal at a particular time in an inversion recovery pulse sequence (inversion time or TI ≈ 140 msec at 1.5 T), when the signal from fat is almost nulled, while maintaining water and soft tissue signal. STIR sequences provide robust fat suppression, even in the presence of metal, but carry a penalty of longer acquisition times and, consequently, reduced spatial resolution.

Gradient-Recalled Echo Sequences

GRE sequences are another distinct technique that utilizes an additional parameter known as "flip angle." At large flip angles (45-90 degrees), the sequences give T1-weighted images, and at low flip angles (5-20 degrees), they give a unique type of image described as having "T2-star" (T2*) weighting. GRE sequences provide high signal-to-noise ratio (i.e., high spatial resolution images) and can also be obtained as volumetric (3D) acquisitions, allowing reconstructions in any imaging plane. Fat-suppressed T1 gradient-recalled echo sequences are more sensitive than conventional proton-density or fat-suppressed T2 sequences in demonstrating Achilles tendinosis. The disadvantages of GRE sequences include relatively long scan times and marked accentuation of magnetic susceptibility artifacts in the setting of metal (for example, residual micorometallic debris after surgery) or gas.

Tissues with an increased concentration of paramagnetic compounds, such as methemoglobin, melanin, iron, and manganese have a "blooming" effect on GRE images, making the affected areas appear larger than on corresponding FSE sequences. In practice, this property of GRE sequences can be exploited when imaging hemosiderin (e.g., pigmented villonodular synovitis (PVNS), hemachromatosis), calcification, or loose bodies.

Magnetic Resonance Arthrogaphy

Routine MRI of the foot and ankle is usually performed using a nonarthrographic technique. MR arthrography has, however, been suggested to be helpful in the evaluation of osteochondral lesions and ankle soft tissue impingement.[31,63] Under ultrasound or fluoroscopic guidance, dilute gadolinium is injected into the joint before MRI. The injected contrast separates the articular capsule from other structures and, because of the T1 shortening effect of gadolinium, outlines intraarticular structures on T1-weighted images.[69] Although MR arthrography is still used in some centers, with the advent of high-resolution imaging and high-field (3 T) scanners, the authors consider the indications for MR arthrography in the foot and ankle to be extremely limited.

New Magnetic Resonance Imaging Technique: Biochemical Imaging

The integrity of articular cartilage and cartilage repair has traditionally been assessed using conventional PD-weighted FSE techniques or fat-suppressed 3D GRE images. Quantitative MR imaging techniques that allow a more sophisticated assessment of cartilage degeneration and cartilage repair are now being developed. These techniques detect changes in the ultrastructure of cartilage and provide an assessment of cartilage biochemistry. They therefore have the potential to detect changes in cartilage biochemistry that may precede discernible cartilage thinning found with traditional MR techniques. Quantitative MR imaging techniques are classified into those that detect alterations in collagen fiber orientation (T2 mapping) and those that detect alterations in the proteolgycan content (delayed gadolinium-enhanced magnetic resonance imaging of cartilage [dGEMRIC], T1 rho mapping).

T2 Mapping

T2 mapping is performed by acquiring several images at different echo times at the same slice location. The T2 calculation is performed on a pixel-by-pixel basis, by fitting the signal intensity from each echo image and the corresponding echo time, to an exponential decay equation. The T2 map of articular cartilage reflects the collagen fiber orientation and the mobile water content[47] and is displayed using a color-coded map. Prolongation of T2 relaxation times is associated with osteoarthritis and breakdown in cartilage structure.[48] Quantitative T2 measurements demonstrate excellent interobserver and intraobserver reliability,[21,49] thereby offering a tool for reproducible assessment of cartilage status over time.

Delayed Gadolinium-Enhanced Magnetic Resonance Imaging of Cartilage

dGEMRIC exploits the fixed charge property of articular cartilage through the use of an injection of (negatively charged) gadolinium contrast. The fixed charge density in cartilage is largely the result of the concentration and distribution of the negatively charged glycosaminoglycan chains within the proteolgycan macromolecules. Gadolinium is administered intravenously; the patient performs 10 minutes of exercise; and, after a 90-minute delay, T1-weighted maps are obtained, usually through the use of a specialized inversion recovery pulse sequence.[4] The gadolinium penetrates the articular cartilage; the amount of penetration is inversely proportional

to the glycosaminoglycan content. The gadolinium acts to shorten T1 relaxation times, allowing for the generation of T1 maps. In areas with depleted glycosaminoglycan content, there will be an increased distribution of gadolinium and therefore a higher T1 signal, which is reflected by a diminished "relative glycosaminoglycan index."

T1 Rho (ρ) Mapping

T1 rho (ρ) is a technique used to assess the low-frequency interactions between hydrogen in macromolecules and free water.[74] Similar to T2 mapping, T1 rho is calculated on a pixel-by-pixel basis by fitting the signal intensity from each spin-lock image and the corresponding spin-lock length to an exponential decay equation. T1 rho has been shown to reflect proteolgycan content in articular cartilage. Subjects with osteoarthritis have longer T1 rho values than asymptomatic controls, and T1 rho may be even more sensitive to early cartilage degeneration than T2 mapping alone.[34] Although clinically feasible at 1.5 T, T1 rho is largely applied at 3 T and is a promising technique to detect changes in proteolgycan content in early cartilage degeneration.

Contraindications to Magnetic Resonance Imaging

Contraindications to MRI include cardiac pacemakers (except in limited circumstances), ferromagnetic foreign bodies (particularly those near vital structures, such as intraocular foreign bodies), and certain metallic and electronic implants, including ferromagnetic cerebral aneurysm clips. MRI units screen patients for the presence of these implants with extensive prescan questionnaires and interviews.

Pitfalls and Artifacts in Magnetic Resonance Imaging

Magic Angle Phenomenon

The signal intensity of ordered tissues, such as cartilage and tendons, depends on the orientation of the collagen fibers relative to the external magnetic field, which in a conventional MR scanner, runs parallel to the long axis of the patient's body. When highly structured tissues are imaged at 55 degrees to the external magnetic field, using a short TE (i.e., T1, PD, and GRE sequences), there is a normal prolongation of T2 values, a phenomenon known as the magic angle effect.[16] The magic angle phenomenon is observed within tendons, articular cartilage, or menisci and results in a spurious high signal, which can mimic pathology. A common example in foot and ankle imaging is seen in the peroneal tendons at the submalleolar level when the ankle is scanned in neutral flexion. T2-weighted sequences can be helpful whenever magic angle phenomenon may cloud image interpretation because true pathology is usually brighter on T2 than on T1- or PD-weighted images.

Bone Marrow "Edema"

A marrow edema-like signal is defined as focal areas of T2 hyperintensity and T1 hypointensity. This is a nonspecific finding that can be due to a number of causes, including hematopoietic marrow, infection, trauma, and tumor. The bone marrow edema pattern is relatively common in foot and ankle MRI and may not always indicate true pathology.

Foci of high T2 signal can be seen in the tarsal bones of asymptomatic patients, particularly those younger than 15 years. These foci are thought to be due to perivascular foci of red marrow, physiologic stress, or increased bone turnover resulting from weight-bearing or normal skeletal growth.[32,68] High T2 signal, rounded foci are often also seen in the anterior calcaneus at the angle of Gissane and should not be misinterpreted as pathologic.[78] These foci are thought to represent nutrient channels or intraosseous ganglion cysts. A similar appearance may be seen in the dorsal talar neck and along the plantar surface of the sinus tarsi, which are also though to relate to vascular channels.[23] Finally, a bone marrow edema pattern has been described in the foot and ankle within the first 12 weeks after immobilization. This pattern was not found to correlate with pain or the clinical syndrome of reflex symphathetic dystrophy and tended to resolve by 18 weeks postimmoblization.[14] Presumably this relates to disuse osteopenia.

Use of Magnetic Resonance Imaging

Indications for MRI include the assessment of acute or chronic trauma, instability, impingement, osteochondral pathology, occult fractures or stress reactions, osteonecrosis, soft tissue and osseous tumors, nerve entrapment syndromes, arthropathies, tendon pathology, and infection.

These conditions and the role of MRI are discussed in more detail in the following section of this chapter.

IMAGING OF FOOT AND ANKLE PATHOLOGY

Imaging Ligament Injury

Ligaments in the foot and ankle are in general uniformly hypointense (dark) on commonly utilized MR imaging sequences. Although some ligaments may be visualized completely on a single MR image, it is not uncommon for the ligaments to lie in a plane that is slightly oblique to the MR image plane such that ligament assessment requires review of multiple contiguous images. If the ligament is superficially situated and amenable to ultrasound assessment, it usually demonstrates a mildly fibrillar sonographic architecture, provided the ultrasound beam is perpendicular to the ligament fibers. CT lacks sufficient contrast resolution to provide direct assessment of ligament injury.

The spectrum of acute ligament injury demonstrable on imaging ranges from minor strain injury to complete tear. On MRI, minor strain injury manifests as subtle intraligament signal hyperintensity, often with mild ligament thickening and periligamentous edema. On ultrasound, ligamentous strain injury manifests as hypoechoic ligament thickening, often with associated reactive hyperemia on color Doppler assessment. Acute complete ligament tears usually demonstrate clear-cut ligament fiber discontinuity on MRI and ultrasound, with fluid evident at the point of tear (Figs. 3-58 to 3-60). In the subacute stage of ligament injury, the injured ligament usually appears thickened and edematous, and the point of ligament fiber discontinuity will often be obscured by early scar response (Fig. 3-61). The potential for scar

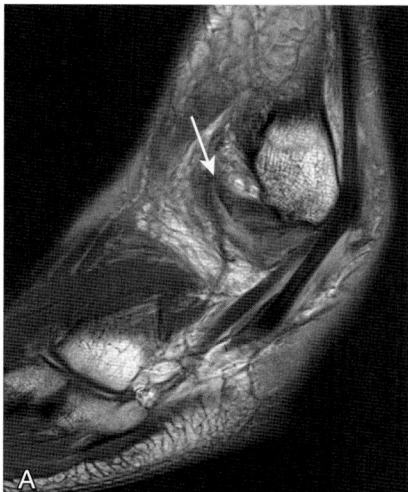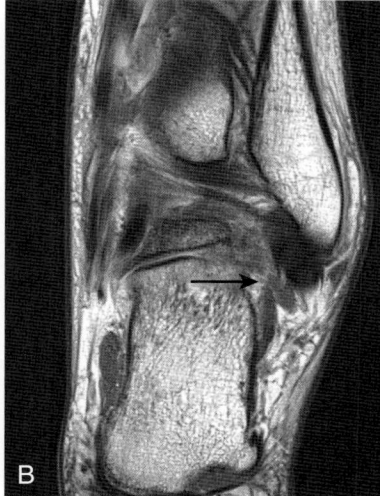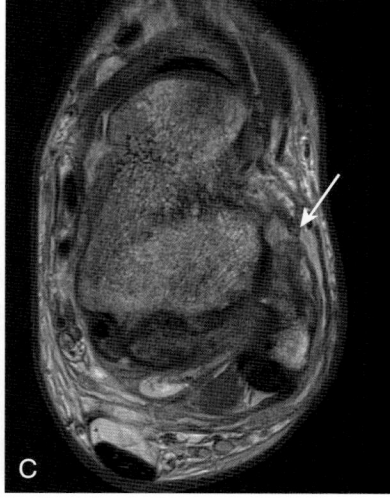

Figure 3-58 Acute lateral ligament tear. Sagittal **(A)**, coronal **(B)**, and axial **(C)** proton-density fast spin-echo magnetic resonance images demonstrate an acute complete tear of the distal anterior talofibular ligament (*arrow* in **A** and **C**) and an avulsion of the calcaneofibular ligament from the fibula (*arrow* in **B**).

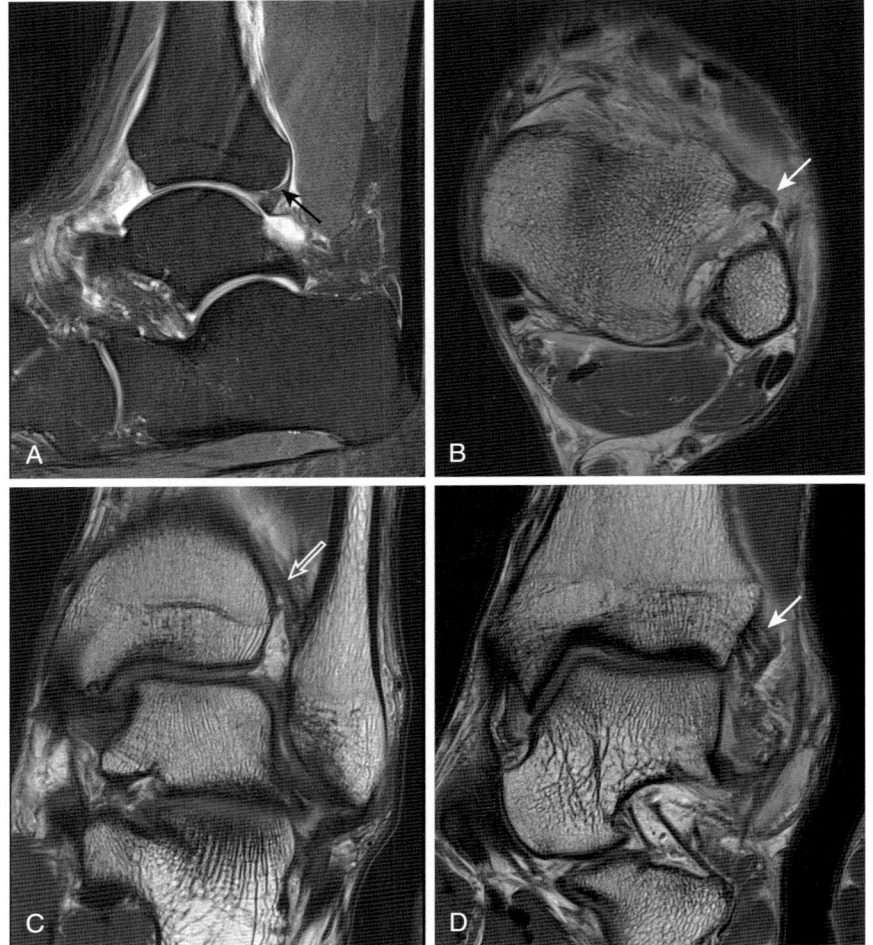

Figure 3-59 Triligamentous syndesmotic ligament complex injury. Sagittal proton-density (PD) fat-saturated **(A)**, axial PD **(B)**, and coronal PD fast spin-echo (**C** and **D**) magnetic resonance images demonstrate a complete tear of the anterior-inferior talofibular ligament (AITFL) from the fibula (*white arrow* in images **B** and **D**), moderate-grade partial tear of the inferior interossous ligament (*open arrow* in **C**), and high-grade partial tear of the posterior-inferior talofibular ligament (PITFL) from the tibia (*black arrow* in images **A** and **B**).

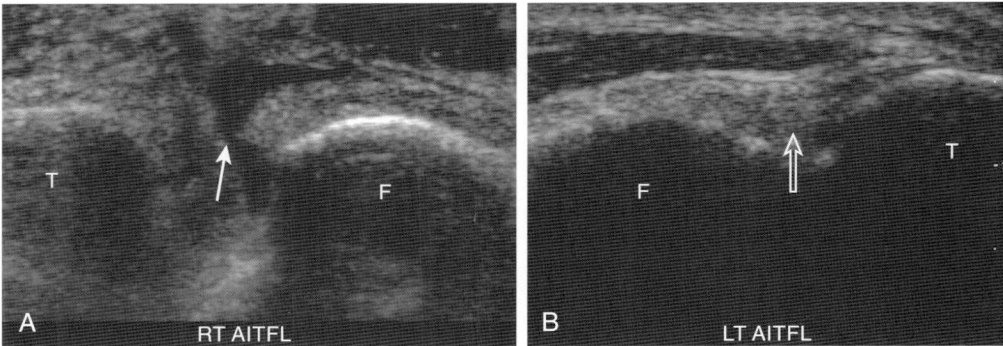

Figure 3-60 Ultrasound of syndesmotic injury. On the symptomatic right side **(A)**, there is an acute complete midsubtance tear of the anterior-inferior talofibular ligament *(AITFL)* with a transversely oriented hypoechoic defect and fiber discontinuity *(arrow)*. This contrasts with the normal left side **(B)**, where the AITFL *(open arrow)* is intact. *F,* fibula; *T,* tibia.

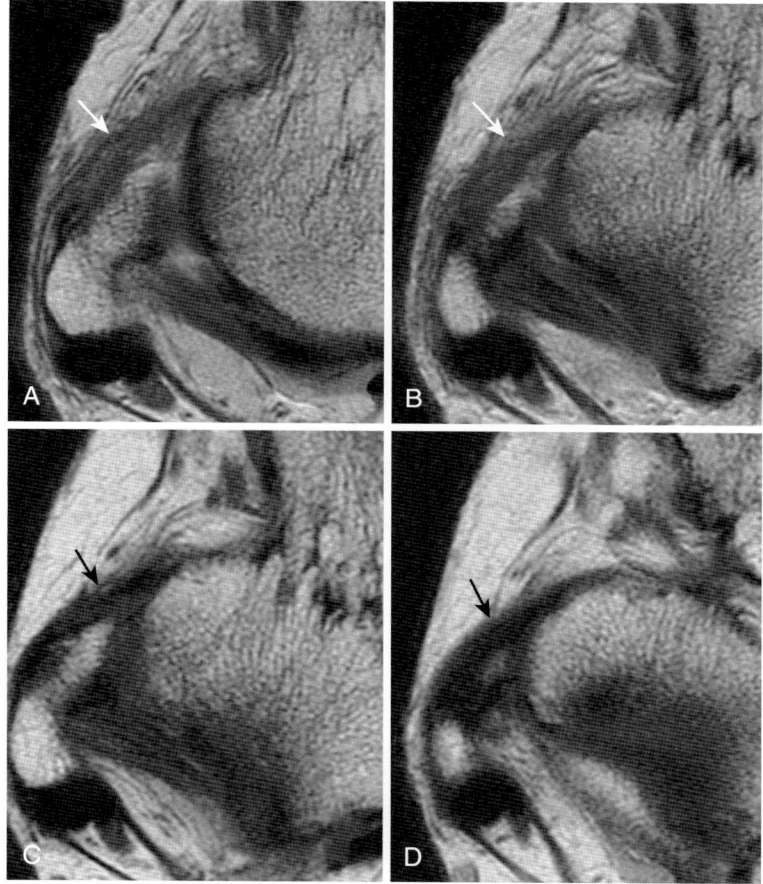

Figure 3-61 Ligament remodeling on magnetic resonance imaging. Axial proton-density (**A** and **B**) images 6 weeks postinversion injury demonstrate early remodeling of the anterior talofibular ligament, which remains hyperintense and thickened *(white arrow)*. At 20 weeks postinjury (**C** and **D**), there is mature scar remodeling of the ligament *(black arrow)*, which now appears uniformly hypointense and only marginally thickened.

remodeling of injured ligaments in the foot and ankle is substantial, particularly the anterior talofibular ligament (ATFL) and calcaneofibular ligament (CFL), such that a previously injured ligament may appear near normal on imaging once it has undergone mature scar remodeling, a process that may continue to evolve over 12 to 18 months. Although imaging is helpful in assessing ligament injury and scar healing, it does not provide direct assessment of ligament laxity.

Ankle and Transverse Tarsal Joint Ligament Complex Injury

Because most acute ankle sprains settle without significant complication, the role of imaging in the acute trauma setting is mainly to exclude ancillary pathology that might require early intervention. To this end, the Ottawa Ankle Rules can be used to decide whether a plain radiograph is initially warranted.[70] These guidelines state that an examiner is unlikely to miss a clinically significant fracture if there is no bony tenderness and the patient is able to bear weight for at least four steps. Failing this, or

if symptoms/signs persist more than 4 weeks after injury, a plain radiograph examination should be performed. Although plain radiography will detect gross diastasis of the distal tibiofibular joint, a significant proportion of syndesmotic injuries will remain occult to plain radiographic assessment.

Although more sophisticated imaging tests are *generally not* indicated in the assessment of acute ankle injuries in the general population, early MRI of the sprained ankle in the elite or professional athlete is now commonly performed to distinguish between injury to the lateral ankle ligament complex (Fig. 3-62), syndesmotic ligament complex,[15] and transverse tarsal joint complex (Fig. 3-63), and to clarify extent of injury and prognosis. A targeted ultrasound examination is a valid alternative to MRI for the differentiation of lateral ankle ligament injury from syndesmosis injury (see Fig. 3-60).

The scar healing potential of injuries to the lateral ankle ligament complex, syndesmotic and transverse tarsal joint complex, with appropriate treatment, is very good. At 6 to 12 weeks postinjury, complete ATFL tears

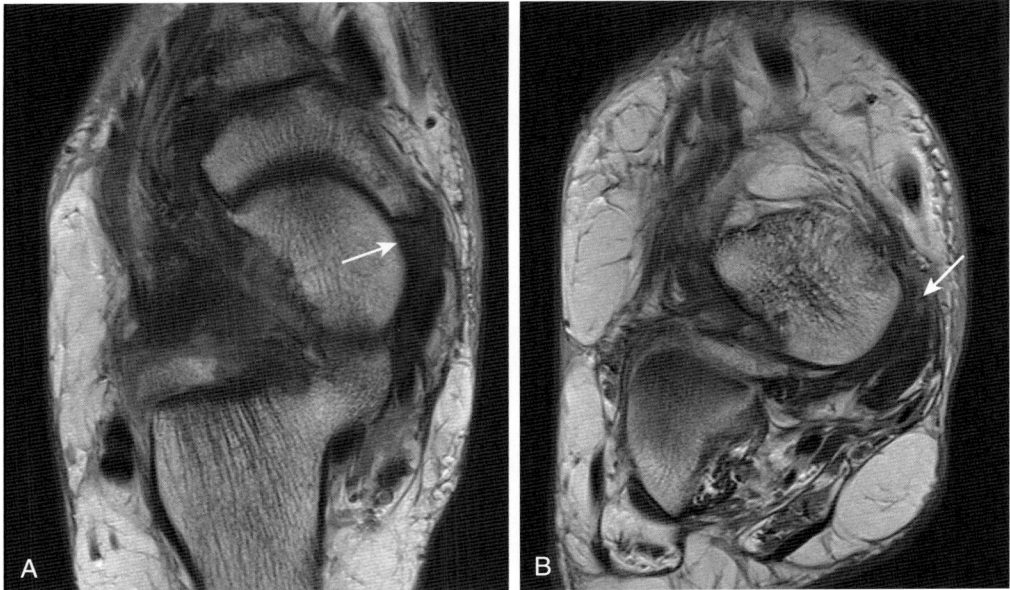

Figure 3-62 Partial-tear superomedial fibers of the spring ligament. Axial **(A)** and coronal **(B)** proton-density imaging of a moderate-grade partial tear of the superomedial fibers of the spring ligament.

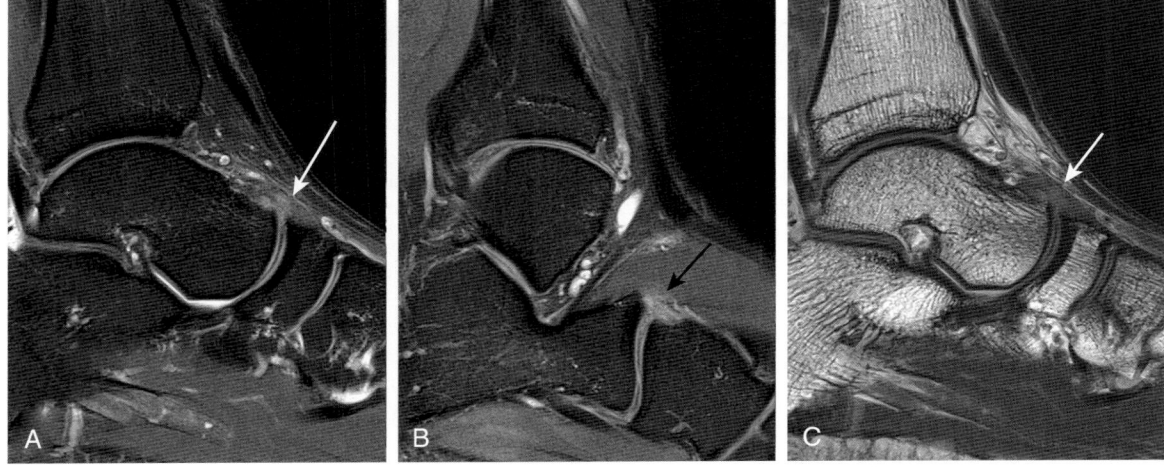

Figure 3-63 Transverse tarsal joint sprain. Sagittal proton-density (PD) fat-saturated **(A and B)** and PD fast spin-echo **(C)** magnetic resonance images demonstrate a subacute sprain of the dorsal talonavicular joint capsule, with thickened edematous immaturely scarred dorsal capsule (*white arrows* in **A** and **C**) and subacute sprain of the lateral limb of the bifurcate ligament and dorsal capsule of the calcaneocuboid joint (*black arrow* in **B**).

commonly show ill-defined bridging scar tissue of intermediate signal on MRI and no evidence of residual laxity on physical examination.[11] Eventually, most injured ligaments remodel with mature scar and appear as well-defined structures of homogeneously low signal (see Fig. 3-61).

Isolated spring ligament tears are an uncommon but important cause of posttraumatic planovalgus deformity that is readily demonstrated on MRI (see Fig. 3-62) and may be suspected on ultrasound.

Midfoot Ligamentous Injury

Significantly displaced midfoot injuries are generally imaged with radiographs and CT. There is some variation in the approach to the imaging assessment and management of subtle Lisfranc ligament complex injuries in which there is no or minimal displacement on weight-bearing radiographs. Some surgeons find stress radiography under anesthesia useful in determining whether to internally fix the midfoot.[60] Others advocate the use of MRI in determining the extent of capsuloligamentous

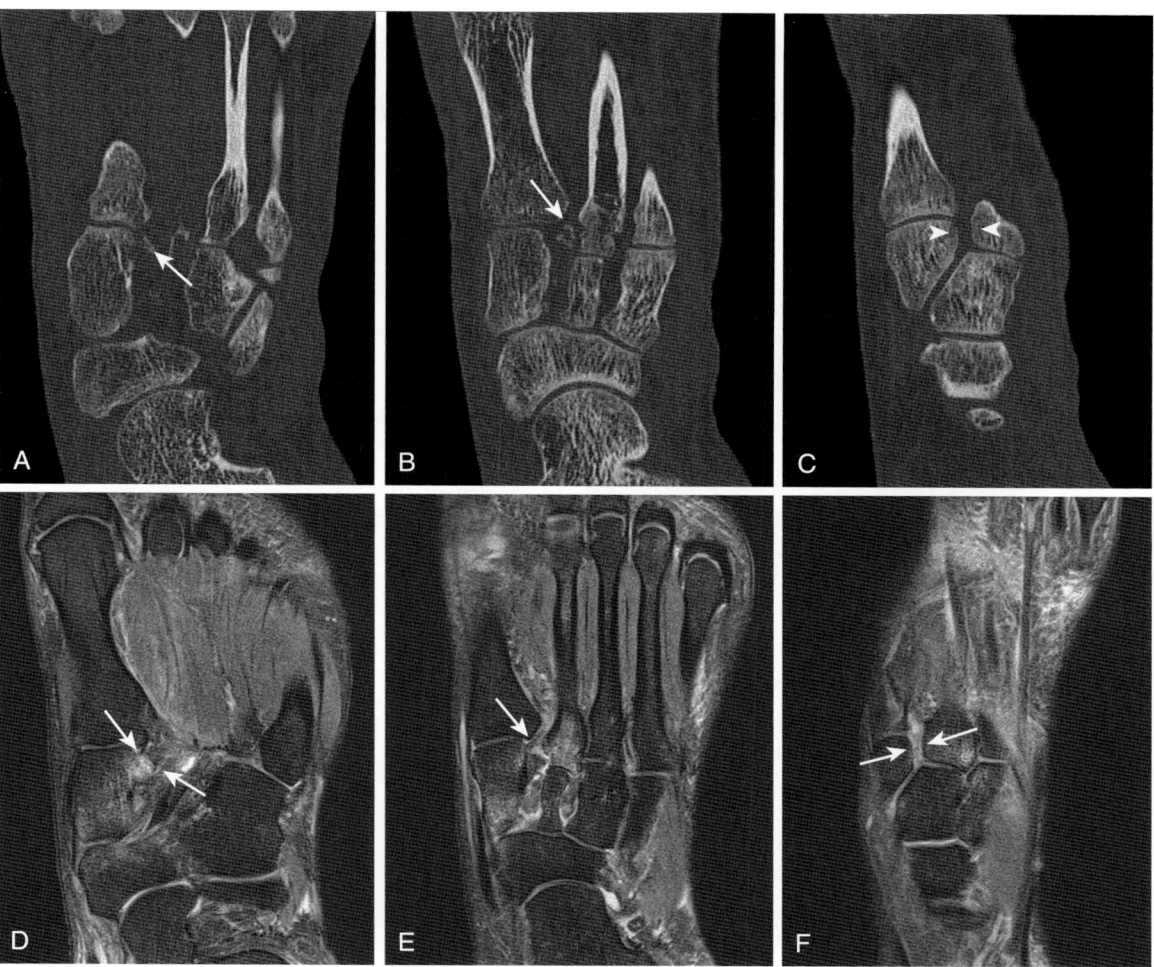

Figure 3-64 Acute Lisfranc ligament complex disruption on computed tomography (CT) and magnetic resonance imaging (MRI). Long-axis CT images demonstrate flake avulsion fracture fragment *(arrow,* **A***)* related to medial cuneiform avulsion of the plantar oblique C1–M3 ligament flake avulsion fracture fragment *(arrow,* **B***)* related to metatarsal avulsion of the interosseous Lisfranc ligament and CT widening of the C1–M2 interval dorsally *(arrowheads,* **C***)*. Corresponding MR images demonstrate the C1–M3 ligament stump *(arrows,* **D***)*, the interosseous Lisfranc ligament stump *(arrow,* **E***)*, and the widening of the C1–M2 interval *(arrows,* **F***)*. The flake avulsion fragments are difficult to appreciate on MRI.

injury and using this to determine whether to proceed to examination under anesthesia[58] (Fig. 3-64). Some surgeons use the increased sensitivity of CT in detecting subtle displacement and cortical flake avulsion fragments not evident on plain radiographs[59] (see Fig. 3-64).

Forefoot Ligament Injury

Injuries to the first metatarsophalangeal (MTP) joint capsuloligamentous complex are relatively common and may involve the collateral ligaments and plantar or dorsal capsule. In the setting of plantar plate (sesamophalangeal ligament) disruption, the diagnosis may be inferred by demonstrating proximal sesamoid migration on weight-bearing radiographs (Fig. 3-65). MRI provides direct assessment of the capsuloligamentous disruption (see Fig. 3-65).[37]

Degeneration and tear of the lateral plantar plate of the second MTP joint is a common cause of metatarsalgia. Although the presence of a lateral plantar plate tear can be inferred by the presence of varus drift of the second toe on clinical assessment or weight-bearing radiographs, ultrasound and MRI can readily demonstrate the nature of the plantar plate pathology, allowing differentiation between attritional attenuation-elongation and frank tear, aiding preoperative assessment (Fig. 3-66).[37]

Imaging Chondral and Osteochondral Lesions

Isolated chondral lesions in the ankle and foot generally remain occult to plain radiographic assessment. If there is an associated acute traumatic fracture of the subchondral plate and cancellous subchondral bone, the fracture

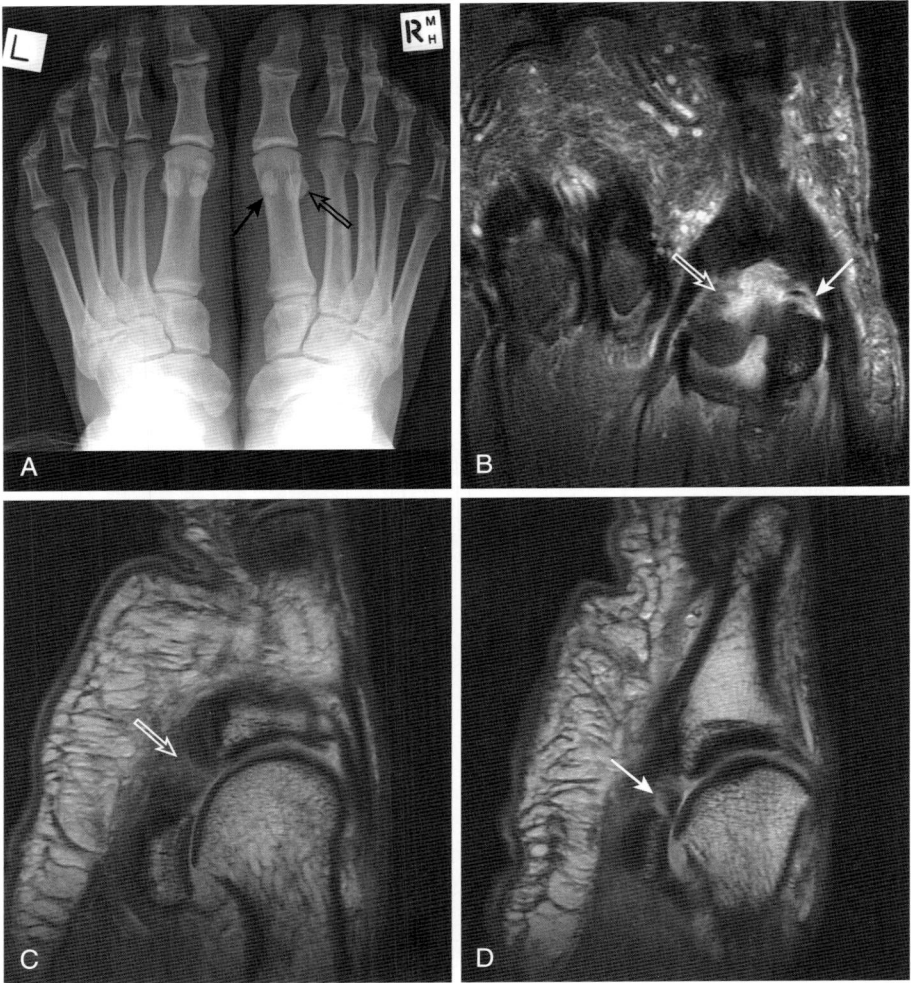

Figure 3-65 Turf toe. Weight-bearing radiograph **(A)** demonstrates retraction of the medial sesamoid *(black arrow)* and lateral sesamoid *(open black arrow)* of the right first metatarsophalangeal joint. Long-axis fat-saturated proton-density (PD) **(B)** and sagittal PD **(C** and **D)** magnetic resonance images demonstrate avulsion of the medial plantar plate off the medial sesamoid. with an associated flake fracture fragment *(white arrow)*. There is avulsion of the lateral plantar plate off the base of the proximal phalanx *(open white arrow)*.

line may be demonstrable on plain radiographs (Fig. 3-67). With chronicity, central osteophyte formation, subchondral cystic change, or sclerosis may develop locally at the site of the chondral lesion. There may also be osteophyte formation at the joint margins. CT is more sensitive in demonstrating and characterizing undisplaced fracture, subchondral cystic change, sclerosis, and central osteophyte formation. However, it does not provide direct assessment of articular cartilage and will not demonstrate subchondral bone marrow edema. High-resolution MRI provides direct assessment of articular cartilage and will demonstrate bone marrow edema that anecdotally correlates with activity of the osteochondral lesion. In addition to demonstrating chondral pathology in the ankle, high-resolution MRI has the ability to demonstrate chondral pathology in the subtalar joint, midfoot, and forefoot (Figs. 3-68 and 3-69).

Imaging Articular Cartilage Repair

Talar dome chondral injuries may spontaneously heal or repair may be surgically assisted using either arthroscopic techniques (e.g., debridement, curettage, and drilling) or chondral or osteochondral grafts. Spontaneous repair and marrow stimulation techniques both attempt to fill a chondral or osteochondral defect with reparative fibrocartilage, which lacks the resilience and durability of normal hyaline cartilage. The bony component of an osteochondral defect will often fail to spontaneously fill with new bone. Autologous osteochondral grafting (e.g., mosaicplasty) and autologous chondrocyte implantation (ACI) are alternative surgical techniques that attempt to deliver a more physiologic, stable, and durable reconstruction of the joint surface. MRI provides the best assessment of progress after these surgical procedures (Figs. 3-70 and

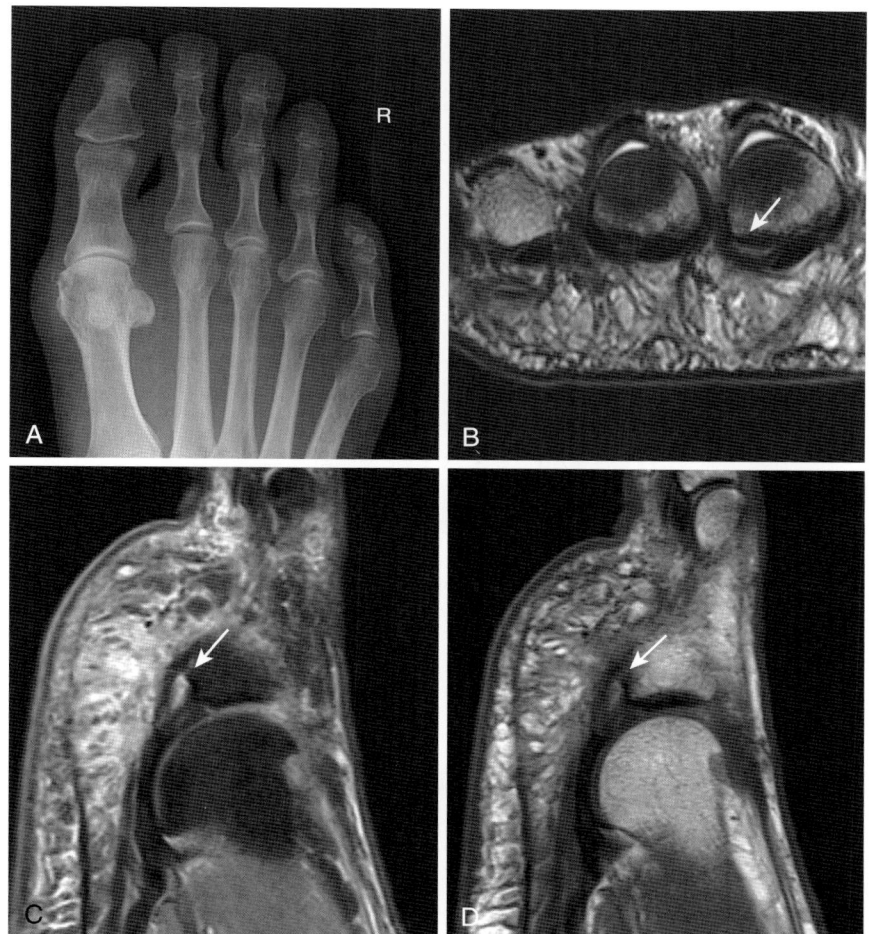

Figure 3-66 Tear of the lateral plantar plate second metatarsophalangeal (MTP) joint. On the radiograph **(A)**, there is slight varus drift of the second toe and a relatively short first metatarsal, with resultant second metatarsal head protrusion, predisposing to overload of the second ray. Short-axis PD **(B)**, sagittal proton-density (PD) fat-saturated **(C)**, and sagittal PD **(D)** magnetic resonance images demonstrate degeneration and high-grade partial-thickness tear of the lateral plantar plate of the second MTP joint *(arrows)*.

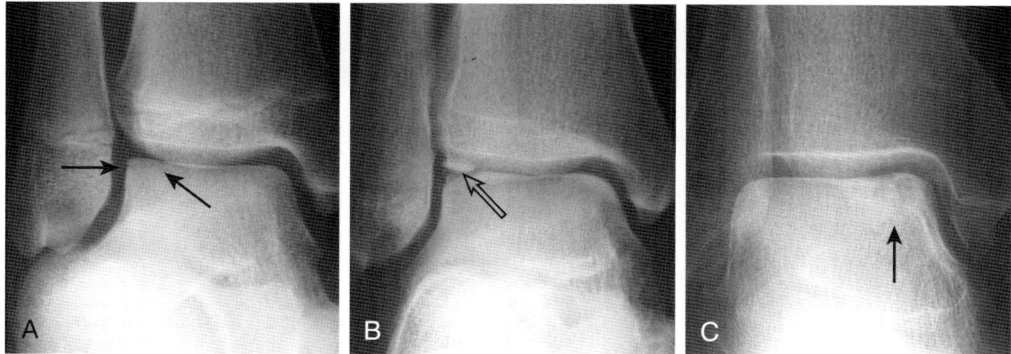

Figure 3-67 Talar dome osteochondral lesion. Plain radiographs demonstrate undisplaced *arrows*, **(A)** and a displaced *double arrow*, **(B)** osteochondral fractures of the lateral talar dome and a chronic medial talar dome osteochondral lesion with subchondral cystic change and sclerosis *(arrow, C)*. (From Anderson IF, Read JW: *Atlas of imaging in sports medicine*, ed 2, Sydney, 2008, McGraw-Hill.)

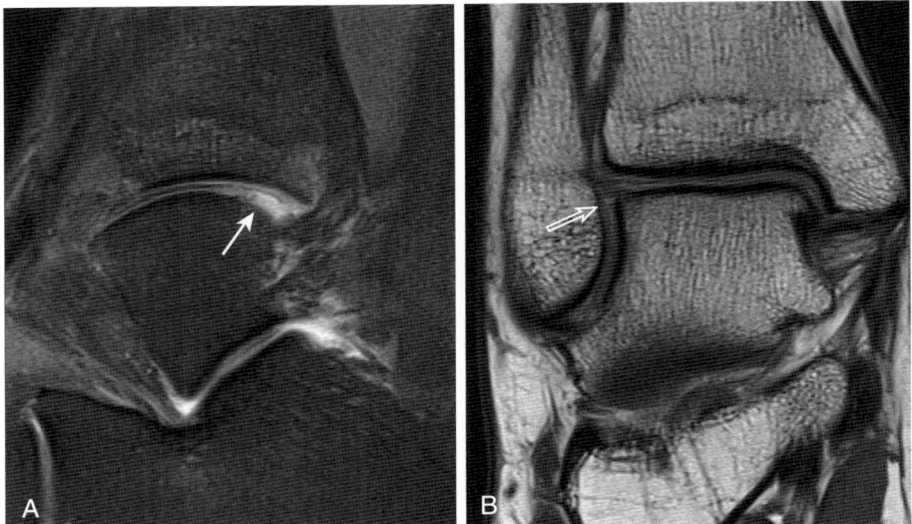

Figure 3-68 Talar dome chondral flap. Sagittal proton-density (PD) fat-saturated **(A)** and coronal PD **(B)** magnetic resonance images demonstrate an arthroscopically confirmed in situ full-thickness chondral flap at the lateral talar dome, with breach of the chondral surface at the superior margin of the lateral gutter articular facet *(open arrow)* and basal delamination at the weight-bearing aspect. There is minor subchondral sclerosis without an adjacent bone marrow pattern.

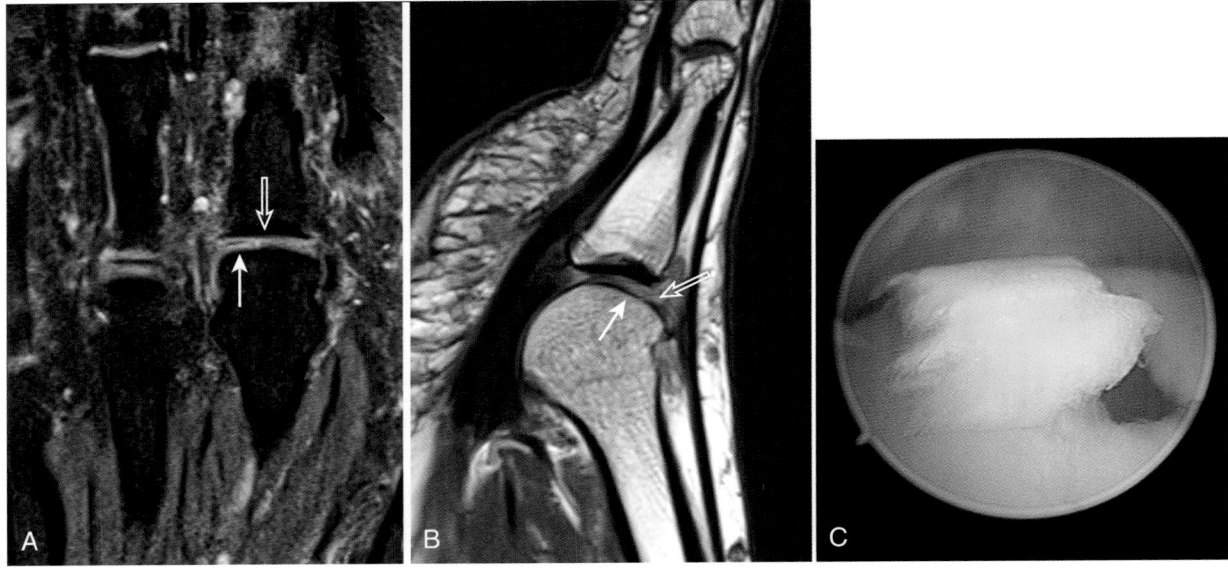

Figure 3-69 Chondral flap second metatatarsal head. Long-axis fat-saturated proton-density (PD) **(A)** and sagittal PD **(B)** magnetic resonance images demonstrate an in situ full-thickness chondral flap at the mid-to-dorsal aspect of the second metatarsal head *(white arrows),* with breach of the chondral surface at the dorsal and medial margins *(open arrows).* There is no subchondral bone marrow edema. **C,** Arthroscopic image in the same patient demonstrates the chondral flap.

3-71), although the signal characteristics of a graft do not allow reparative fibrocartilage to be reliably differentiated from hyaline-like articular cartilage.[72] Quantitative MR techniques, such as dGEMRIC, T1 rho, and T2 mapping, show some promise in this regard.[72]

Imaging Impingement Syndromes

Impingement is a clinical syndrome of end-range joint pain and/or motion restriction resulting from the direct mechanical abutment of bone and/or soft tissues. Impingement syndromes at the ankle may occur after

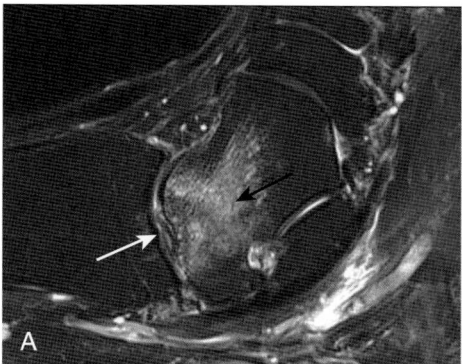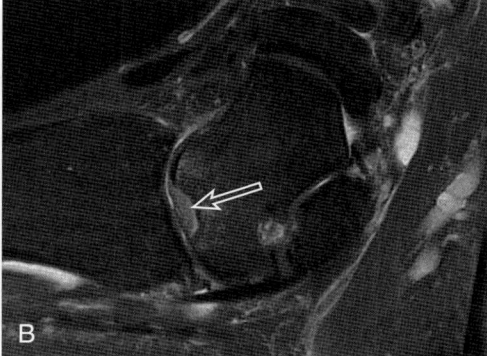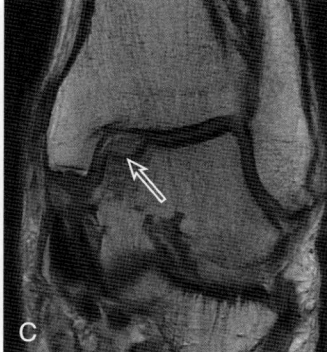

Figure 3-70 **A,** Sagittal fat-suppressed proton-density (PD) magnetic resonance (MR) image demonstrating a chronic medial talar dome osteochondral lesion with in situ unstable osteochondral fragment *(white arrow)* and cystic change and extensive bone marrow edema at the margins of the potential osteochondral crater *(black arrow).* **B,** Postarthroscopic excision of the osteochondral fragment, deroofing of the cystic change, and osteoplasty. On sagittal fat-suppressed PD MR sequencing, there is 100% fill of the crater, with reparative fibrocartilage that demonstrates a smooth surface. There has been substantial reduction in the extent of bone marrow edema. No residual cystic change is evident. On sagittal fat-suppressed PD **(B)** and coronal PD **(C)** sequencing, signal hyperintensity at the basal layer of the reparative fibrocartilage indicates immature basal integration *(open arrows).*

either acute macrotrauma or repetitive microtrauma. Various underlying pathologies and anatomic variations may predispose to impingement. Modern imaging modalities can usefully demonstrate these changes and assist with patient management.[36] Implicit in the definition of impingement as a clinical syndrome is that the diagnosis remains "clinical" because imaging changes alone do not reliably predict symptoms or clinical relevance.

Impingement syndromes in the ankle may be classified according to location and by the type of underlying pathology—soft tissue or bony. Posttraumatic synovitis, intraarticular fibrous bands–scar tissue, capsular scarring, or developmental and acquired bony spurs or prominences are the most common causes of ankle impingement. Sites of impingement at the ankle include anterolateral, anterior, anteromedial, posteromedial, and posterior.[36]

Bony impingment lesions at the ankle may be confirmed on plain radiographs, often supplemented by specific views, for instance, oblique radiographs of the foot for anteromedial impingement spurs and a lazy lateral view to show an os trigonum. MRI may demonstrate bone marrow edema at the site of an active impingement lesion and adjacent synovitis, capsular thickening, and pericapsular edema (Fig. 3-72 to 3-74).[36] Soft tissue impingement lesions around the ankle are usually best demonstrated on MRI. MR arthrography and the use of intravenous contrast have been advocated as means of increasing the sensitivity of MRI for detecting impingement lesions. In routine clinical practice, a high-resolution nonarthrographic approach is usually adequate. Ultrasound can be helpful in the diagnosis of soft tissue impingement lesions and can be used to guide corticosteroid injections.

Imaging Tendon Pathology

Tendons connect muscles and bones, transmitting forces generated by muscle contraction on to bone, allowing movement of joints. The basic constituents of tendon are collagen bundles, tenocytes, and ground substance, which is rich in proteoglycans. Collagen bundles provide tensile strength, while ground substance provides structural support for the collagen fibers and regulates the maturation of collagen. Tenocytes synthesize ground substance and collagen. Tendinosis is characterized by degeneration of tendon cells and collagen fibers and an increase in noncollagenous matrix. Intratendon inflammation is not a feature of tendinosis. However, peritendon inflammation is commonly seen in association with tendinosis or in isolation, being described as a tenosynovitis, if there is a tendon sheath, or paratenonitis, if there is a paratenon, such as in the Achilles tendon.

Tendinosis

Tendinosis may be demonstrated on ultrasound or MRI. On ultrasound, tendinosis manifests as a hypoechoic echotextural change, with alteration of the normal fibrillar architecture of the tendon (Fig. 3-75). If the ultrasound beam is not perpendicular to the tendon, then it may appear artifactually hypoechoic because of anisotropy, which, if unrecognized, can lead to a false-positive diagnosis of tendinosis. Ultrasound has the advantage of providing assessment of tendon and peritendon blood flow by using color Doppler. Tendon and peritendon hyperemia is commonly seen in tendinosis and peritendinitis and may be a marker of activity of the pathology (Fig. 3-76).

On MRI, tendinosis usually first manifests on fat-suppressed T1 GRE sequencing as a subtle increase in

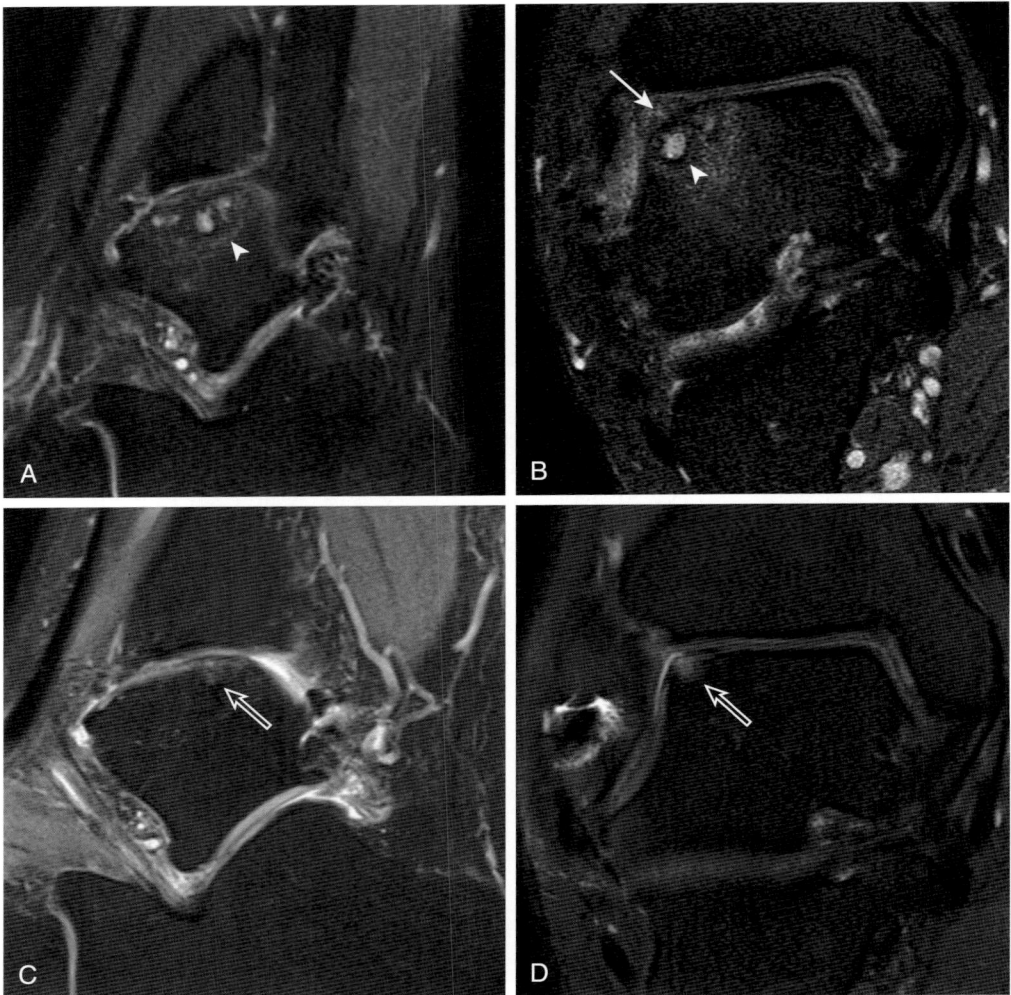

Figure 3-71 Autologous chondrocyte implantation (ACI) of a lateral talar dome osteochondral lesion. Despite multiple prior arthroscopic debridements, the lateral talar dome lesion remained symptomatic. Pre-ACI sagittal **(A)** and coronal **(B)** fat-suppressed proton-density (PD) magnetic resonance (MR) images demonstrate multilocular subchondral cystic change and surrounding bone marrow edema *(arrowhead)* and incomplete basal delamination of reparative fibrocartilage anteriorly *(white arrow)*. One year post-ACI, sagittal **(C)** and coronal **(D)** fat-suppressed PD MR images demonstrate there has been resolution of the subchondral cystic change and bone marrow edema, 100% fill of the graft with smooth graft surface, and evidence of mature basal and peripheral integration *(double arrows)*.

signal intensity (Fig. 3-77). If the tendon fibers are at 55 degrees to the longitudinal axis of the magnetic field in the MR unit, then the magic angle phenomenon can result in tendon signal hyperintensity in normal tendons, mimicking tendinosis. This is commonly seen in the peroneal tendons at the submalleolar level and may be seen in the posterior tibial tendon at the submalleolar level. The magic angle phenomenon is largely absent on a heavily T2-weighted sequence. Peritendon inflammation may be seen on ultrasound as a thickened peritendon space, tendon sheath effusion, and tenosynovial thickening with associated hyperemia on color Doppler. An inert-appearing tendon sheath effusion is not diagnostic of a peritendonitis. On MRI, thickening of

the peritendon space and tenosynovial thickening may be more subtle when compared with ultrasound. There may edema in the fat plane adjacent to the tendon sheath/paratenon. Use of intravenous contrast may help distinguish an inert tendon sheath effusion from a tenosynovitis.

Insertional Achilles tendinosis differs from noninsertional tendinosis seen in the Achilles tendon and other tendons. Impingement may play a role in the pathogenesis of insertional Achilles tendinosis resulting from bony overgrowth of the posterosuperior process of the calcaneus, usually with an associated retrocalcaneal bursitis. However, a subgroup of insertional Achiless tendinosis does not involve impingement and is often

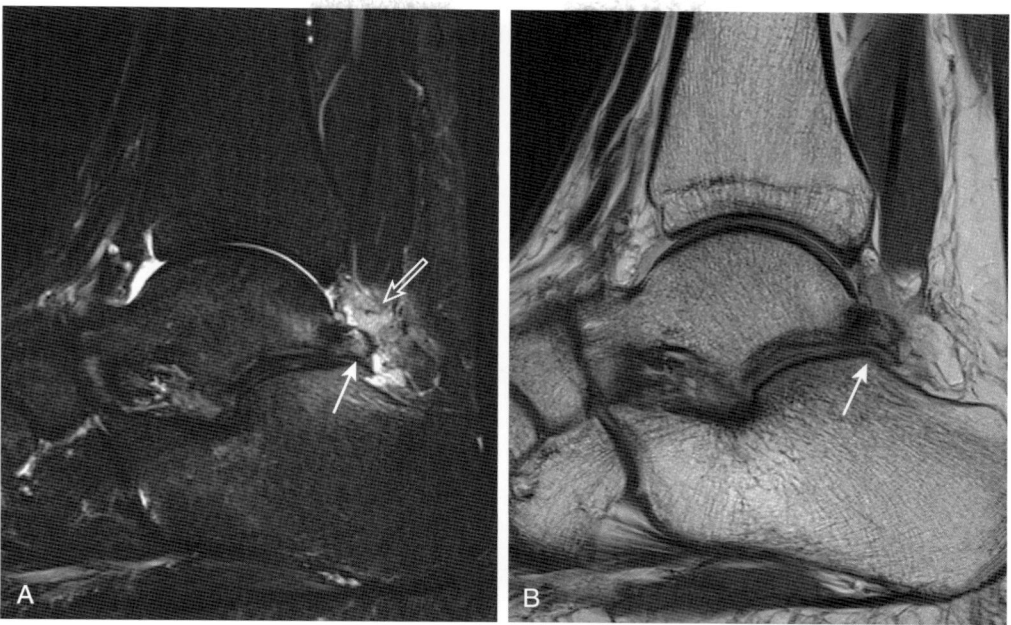

Figure 3-72 Posterior ankle impingement. Sagittal proton-density (PD) fat-saturated **(A)** and PD **(B)** magnetic resonance images demonstrate a moderate-sized os trigonum *(white arrow)* with a bone marrow edema pattern across the synchondrosis *(white arrows)*, synovitis in the posterior recess of the ankle and subtalar joint, and adjacent pericapsular edema *(open arrow)*. The findings are suggestive of active posterior impingement.

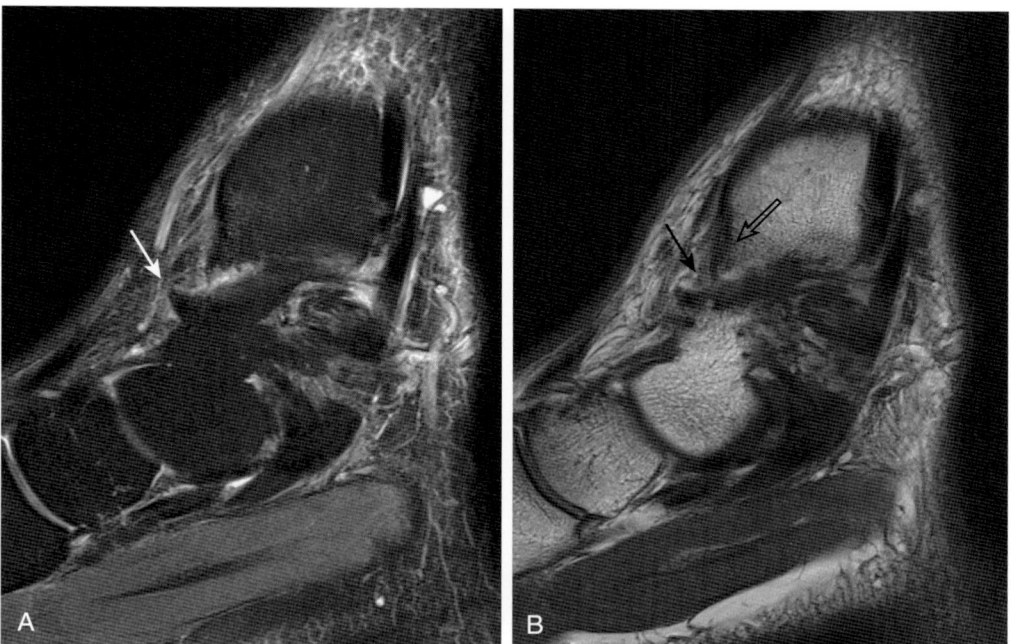

Figure 3-73 Anteromedial ankle impingement. Sagittal proton-density (PD) fat-saturated **(A)** and sagittal PD **(B)** magnetic resonance images demonstrate a prominent dorsomedial talar neck spur *(black arrow)* and moderate anteromedial plafond spur *(open black arrow)*, respectively. There is capsulosynovial thickening in the anteromedial gutter, with adjacent pericapsular edema *(white arrow)*. The findings would predispose to anteromedial impingement symptoms.

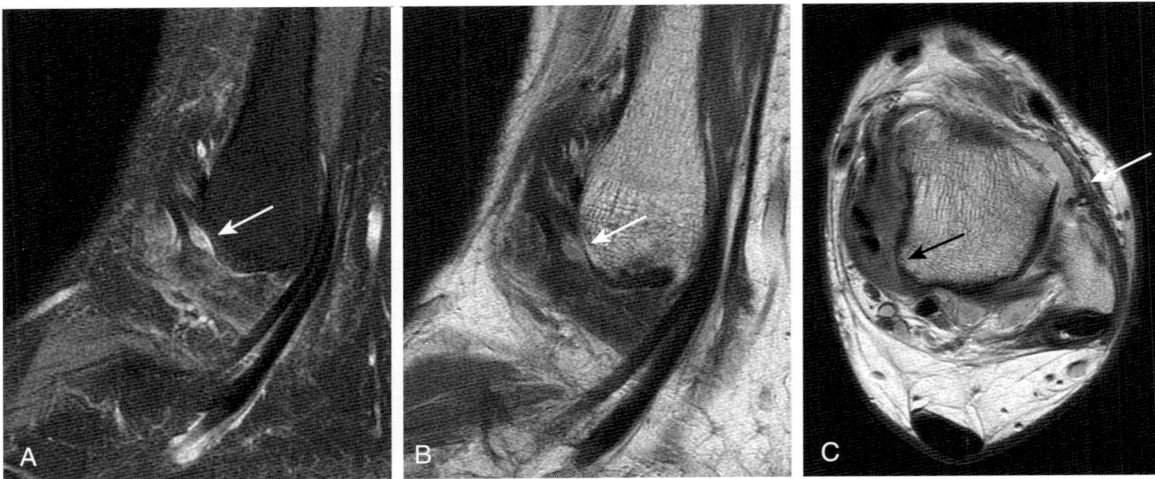

Figure 3-74 Anterolateral impingement and meniscoid lesion and posteromedial impingement (POMI) lesion. Sagittal proton-density (PD) fat-saturated **(A)**, sagittal PD **(B)**, and axial PD **(C)** magnetic resonance images in a patient 3 months postinversion injury, with ongoing pain. There is a dense traumatic synovitis in the anterolateral gutter, with an immature meniscoid lesion *(white arrow)*. There is hypertrophic scarring of the deep fibers of the deltoid ligament, with protrusion into the medial gutter posteriorly *(black arrow)*, predisposing to POMI.

Figure 3-75 Acute tibialis anterior tendinosis and peritendinitis. Longitudinal ultrasound images from a cyclist who presented with acute right anterior lower leg pain. On the symptomatic right side, there is subcutaneous edema *(open arrow)*, thickening of the tibialis anterior tendon, mild decrease in echogenicity *(arrow pointing superiorly)*, and thickening of the peritendon space *(oblique arrow pointing inferiorly)*, when compared with the asymptomatic left side.

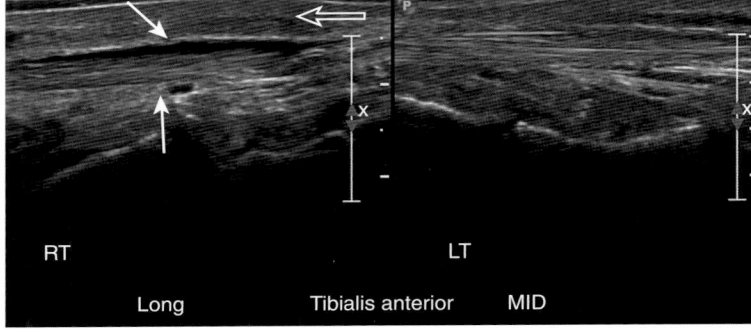

Figure 3-76 Stenosing peroneus longus tenosynovitis. **A,** Transverse ultrasound image of the peroneal tendons at the level of a prominent peroneal tubercle demonstrating thickening of the inferior peroneal retinaculum toward the insertion on the peroneal tubercle *(white arrow)*, manifesting as a hypoechoic thickened septum between the peroneus longus and brevis tendons, with adjacent thickening of the peroneus longus tendon and peritendon space. **B,** Longitudinal power Doppler image demonstrates moderate hyperemia within the thickened peritendon space *(open arrow)*, indicating a peritendinitis. *TNS,* tendons.

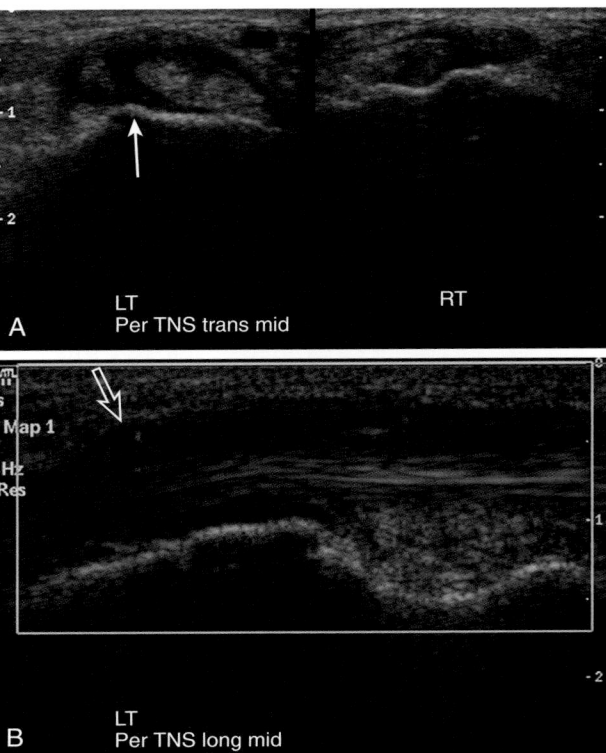

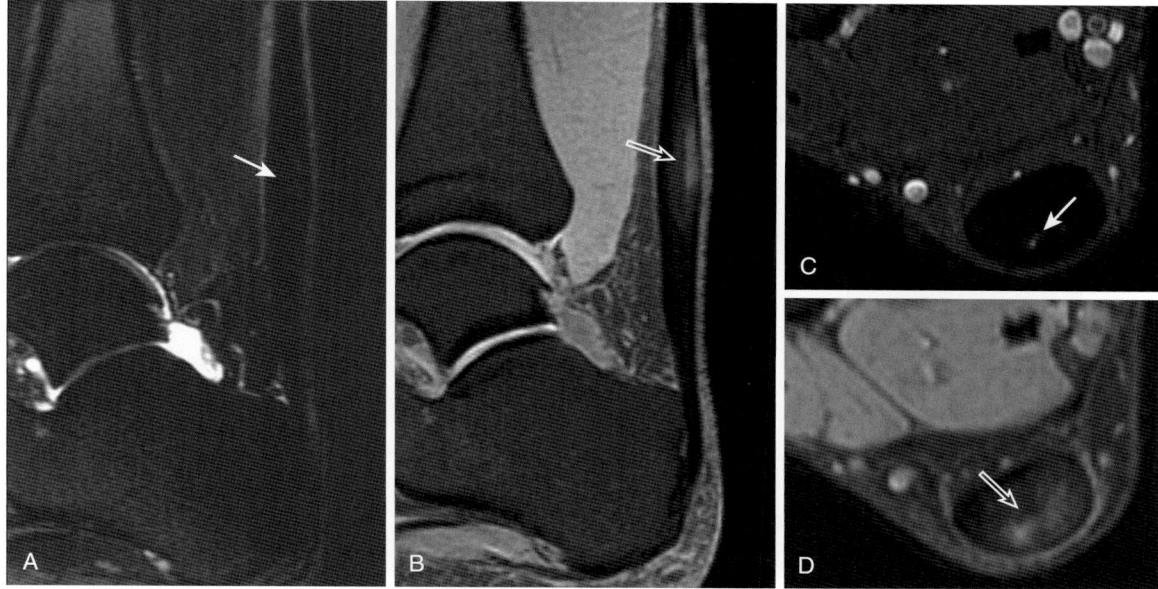

Figure 3-77 Active Achilles tendinosis. Sagittal **(A)** and axial **(C)** fat-suppressed T2 magnetic resonance (MR) images demonstrate fusiform thickening of the midfibers of the Achilles tendon, with an instrasubtance longitudinal fissure *(arrows)* and moderately active surrounding tendinosis, only appreciable on sagittal **(B)** and axial **(D)** fat-suppressed T1 gradient-recalled echo MR images as an area of ill-defined signal hyperintensity *(open arrow)*.

characterized by dystrophic intratendon ossification and enthesial bony spurring (Fig. 3-78).

Stenosing Tenosynovitis

A stenosing tenosynovitis may involve the peroneal tendons, typically at the level of the peroneal tubercle. The imaging findings in this setting are often very subtle and are not totally specific, consisting of thickening of the inferior peroneal retinaculum, usually with prominence of the peroneal tubercle. A stenosing tenosynovitis may also affect the flexor hallucis longus tendon at the level of the fibroosseous tunnel.

Tendon Tears

Acute tendon tears in the foot and ankle may range from complete tears, most commonly seen in the mid-Achilles tendon, to small intrasubstance transversely oriented tears. Although, clinically, most acute complete tendon tears are obvious to the foot and ankle surgeon and do not necessarily require imaging, the patient will often have already undergone imaging of the injured tendon before their index presentation to the foot and ankle surgeon. Not uncommonly, ultrasound examinations of a complete tear of the Achilles tendon may be misinterpreted by the inexperienced sonologist as indicating a partial tear. In this setting, MRI may be required to document the complete tear. Imaging can also provide information on the quality of the tendon edge, the distance between the two tendon edges, and the degree, if any, of muscle atrophy (Figs. 3-79 and 3-80).

Attritional longitudinal tears are commonly seen in the peroneus brevis tendon and posterior tibial tendon and may also be seen in the peroneus longus tendon, Achilles tendon, and distal fibers of the tibialis anterior tendon (Fig. 3-81). When using ultrasound and MRI, it sometimes can be a struggle to characterize peroneal tendon split tears at the retromalleolar sulcus level, that is, caused by close apposition of the peroneus longus and brevis tendons to the lateral malleolus as the tendons curve around the malleolus.

Imaging Inflammatory Arthropathies

The role of imaging in the evaluation of the patient with an inflammatory arthropathy in the foot and ankle may range from initial diagnosis (Fig. 3-82), evaluating extent of disease, assessing for active inflammation, and differentiating active inflammation from a secondary degenerative arthropathy or a complication of treatment such as avascular necrosis.

Occasionally, imaging may play a role in the diagnosis of psoriatic arthritis in a patient presenting with a dactylitis, helping rule out infection and other differential diagnoses (Fig. 3-83). Occasionally, a patient's index presentation of an inflammatory arthropathy may consist of a rheumatoid nodule in the foot and ankle or an MTP joint synovitis or intermetatarsal bursitis.

Initial imaging assessment of the patient with a suspected inflammatory arthropathy should commence with plain radiography, which in the early stages will be

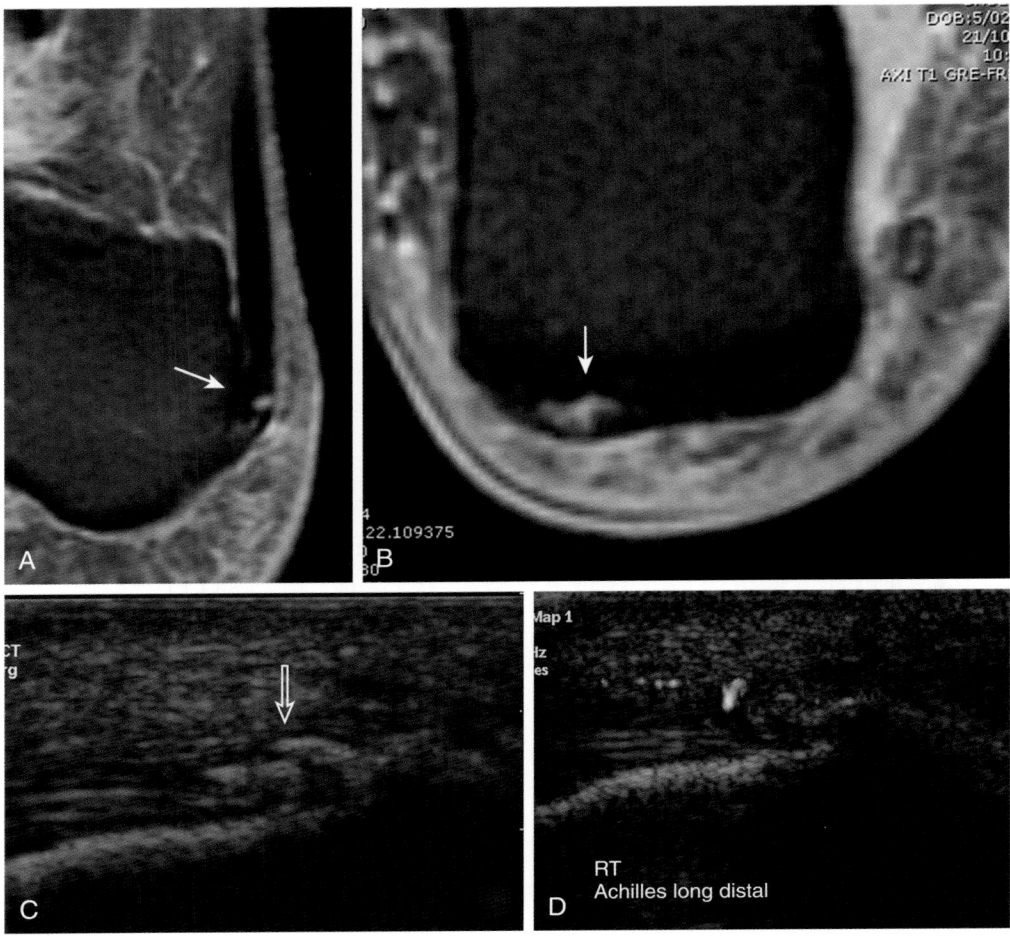

Figure 3-78 Insertional Achilles tendinosis with dystrophic tendon calcification-ossification. Sagittal **(A)** and axial **(B)** fat-suppressed T1 gradient-recalled echo magnetic resonance images demonstrating focal insertional Achilles tendon thickening and signal hyperintensity toward the superficial margin *(arrow)*, with overlying low-grade adventitial bursopathy, and small bony spur at the superficial margin. No intratendon calcification-ossification is evident. **C,** Longitudinal ultrasound image of the corresponding area demonstrates echogenic foci consistent with dystrophic calcification-ossification *(open arrow)*. **D,** On power Doppler, there is corresponding tendon and peritendon hyperemia.

negative. MRI and ultrasound are more sensitive in detecting and characterizing the extent of an inflammatory arthropathy. Use of intravenous contrast may provide further insight into the extent and severity of an inflammatory arthropathy and may help differentiate between an inert joint effusion and an active synovitis. Intravenous contrast administration can be combined with an MR angiographic sequence, providing further information on the degree of hyperemia associated with an inflammatory arthropathy. MR angiography can also be helpful in assessing a peripheral vasculitis. Ultrasound, with the use of color Doppler, provides a noninvasive assessment for hyperemic synovitis and can also assess periarticular erosions.

In the setting of an advanced inflammatory arthropathy with secondary degenerative change, plain radiography often provides sufficient imaging assessment, sometimes supplemented with CT or MRI. Some

seronegative inflammatory arthropathies may present with an isolated enthesitis, which can be a more challenging diagnosis. MRI may demonstrate enthesial bone marrow edema and contrast enhancement, although, in more advanced cases, bony erosion and proliferative bony reaction may be evident (Fig. 3-84). These latter changes may be evident on plain radiographs. Nuclear medicine bone scan provides a nonspecific but reasonably sensitive means of assessing for an inflammatory arthropathy.

Gout, when presenting in typical fashion in the first MTP joint, rarely needs cross-sectional imaging. In acute gout in the early stages of the disease, plain radiographs will often only demonstrate soft tissue swelling. With chronicity, punched out periarticular erosions may be seen. Less commonly, gout may present with involvement of other sites, including tendons around the foot and ankle and the joints of the hindfoot. In such cases, there

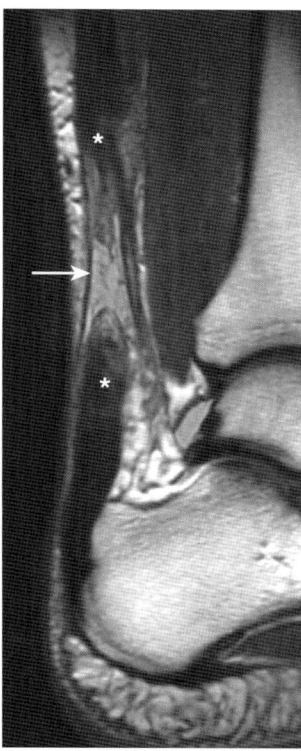

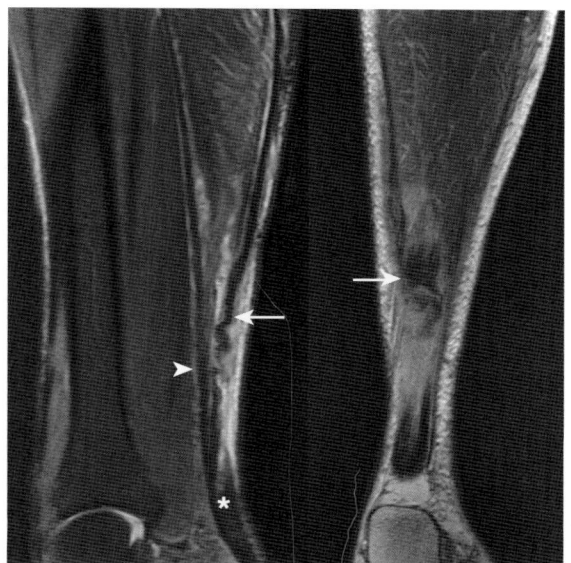

Figure 3-79 Complete midsegment Achilles tendon rupture. A sagittal proton-density–weighted magnetic resonance image shows a complete tear appreciated as a gap in tendon continuity produced by retraction of the proximal stump and filled largely by fat *(arrow)*. There are changes of underlying tendonosis at the separated proximal and distal tendon stumps *(asterisks)*.

Figure 3-80 Complex partial tear of triceps surae complex in a 51-year-old recreational soccer player with acute-onset calf pain. Coronal proton-density (PD) *(right)* and fat-suppressed sagittal PD *(left)* magnetic resonance images show a mildly retracted tear of the medial head gastrocnemius tendon component of the triceps surae complex *(arrows)*, a largely intact soleal component *(arrowhead)*, and background changes of proximal Achilles tendonosis *(asterisk)*. The patient was successfully managed conservatively.

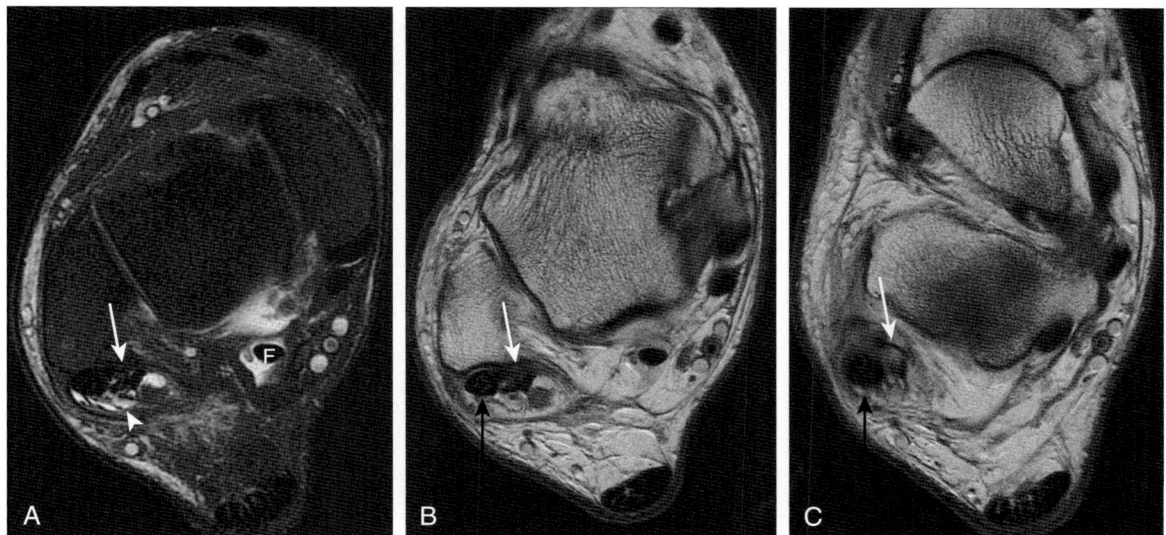

Figure 3-81 Longitudinal split-tear peroneus brevis tendon and peroneal peritendonitis. Axial fat-suppressed axial T2-weighted **(A)** and axial proton-density–weighted **(B and C)** magnetic resonance images show the peroneus brevis tendon *(white arrows)* separated into two halves by a line of high signal. The adjacent peroneus longus tendon *(black arrows)* is thickened and demonstrates intrasubstance tendonosis signal. The peroneal tendon sheath is distended by effusion *(white arrowhead)* and shows contained stranding indicative of synovitis. There is fluid within the flexor hallucis longus tendon sheath *(F)*.

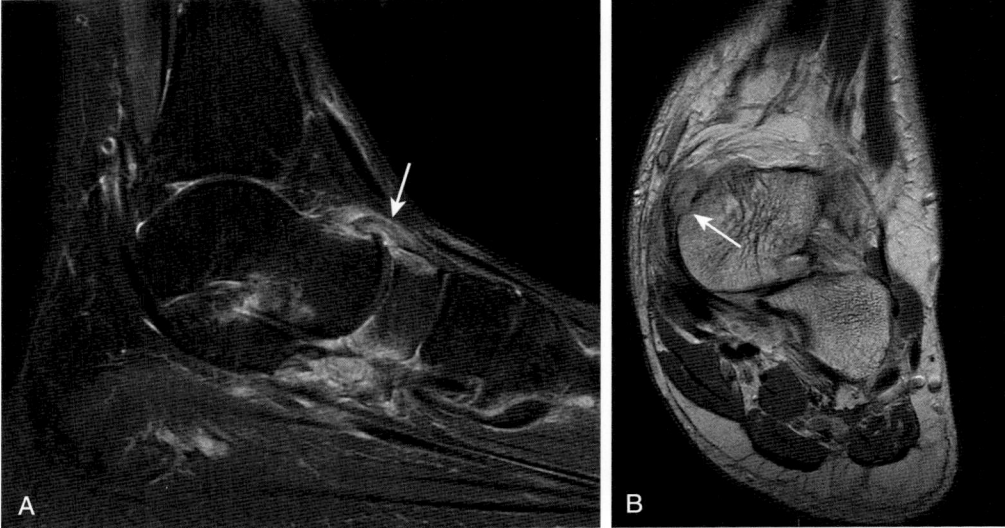

Figure 3-82 Inflammatory synovitis with periarticular erosion. **A,** Sagittal fat-suppressed proton-density (PD) magnetic resonance (MR) image demonstrating talonavicular middle subtalar joint synovitis, with thickened edematous dorsal capsule *(white arrow)* and periarticular bone marrow edema at the capsular insertions. **B,** Coronal PD MR image demonstrating a periarticular erosion at the dorsomedial aspect of the talar head *(white arrow),* with moderate adjacent synovial thickening.

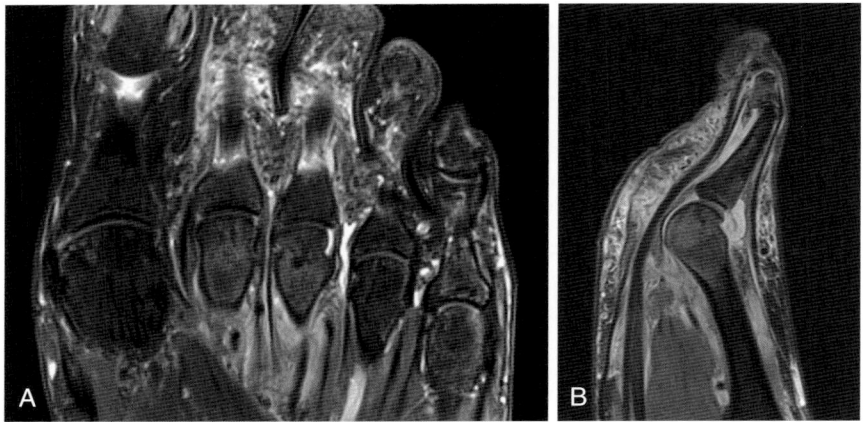

Figure 3-83 Psoriatic arthropathy related dactylitis mimics infection. Long-axis **(A)** and sagittal fat-suppressed proton-density **(B)** magnetic resonance images demonstrate a dactylitis involving the second and third toes, with subcutaneous edema, metatarsophalangeal and interphalangeal joint effusions, and flexor tendon sheath effusions.

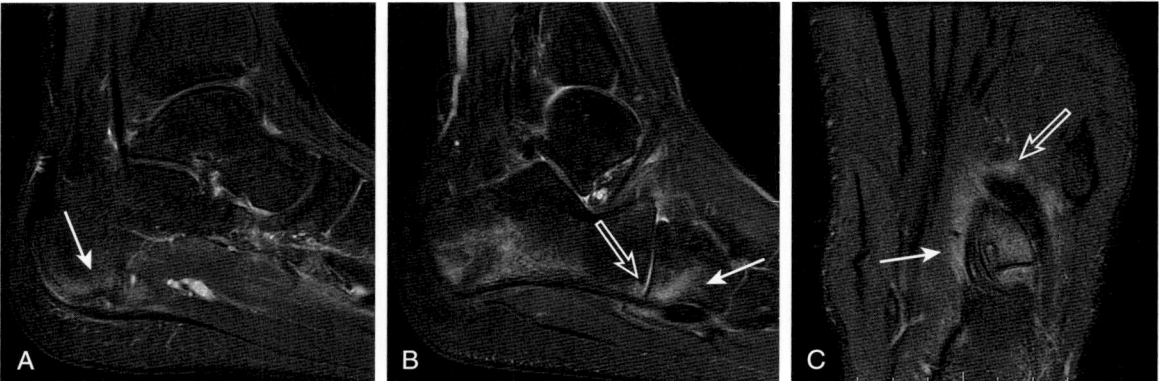

Figure 3-84 Seronegative inflammatory arthropathy presenting with enthesitis, synovitis, and tenosynovitis. **A,** Sagittal fat-suppressed proton-density (PD) magnetic resonance (MR) image demonstrating extensive bone marrow edema at the calcaneal origin of the plantar fascia, with mild adjacent fascial signal hyperintensity *(white arrow),* compatible with an enthesitis. **B,** Sagittal fat-suppressed PD MR image demonstrating bone marrow edema at the margins of the cuboid tunnel for the peroneus longus tendon *(white arrow)* and a small calcaneocuboid joint effusion and mild synovitis *(open arrow).* **C,** Axial fat-suppressed PD MR image demonstrating a thickened edematous long plantar ligament *(white arrow)* with periligamentous soft tissue edema and enthesial bone marrow edema at the cuboid insertion. Note also the changes of peroneus longus peritendinitis at cuboid tunnel level *(open arrow).*

may be a role for cross-sectional imaging in establishing a diagnosis and assessing disease severity. The recent development of dual energy CT allows differentiation of gout crystals from calcium hydroxyapatite.

Imaging Nerve Pathology in the Foot and Ankle

Advances in MRI and ultrasound technology now allow direct high-resolution visualization of peripheral nerves in the foot and ankle. The most frequent application of this technology is in the assessment of Morton neuroma. High-resolution techniques can accurately assess for neural thickening, infiltration of the perineural fat plane, and intermetatarsal bursopathy (Figs. 3-85 to 3-87). Some studies have cast doubt on the accuracy of imaging in assessing for Morton neuroma. This in part reflects that some Morton neuromas may be asymptomatic and that some patients may have a painful common plantar digital nerve without a Morton neuroma being present. Of note, however, both ultrasound and MRI of the central forefoot can be technically demanding and have a significant learning curve.

Imaging plays a role in assessing the patient with suspected tarsal tunnel syndrome by way of identifying compressive neural lesions, such as ganglia or accessory flexor muscles, and identifying focal neural pathology, such as benign peripheral nerve sheath tumor, posttraumatic neuroma, and perineural fibrosis (Figs. 3-88 to 3-90). Both ultrasound and MRI are efficacious in this regard, with the exception that perineural fibrosis may be more conspicuous on MRI and that ultrasound assessment of

the distal tarsal tunnel is technically more demanding than MRI. Both ultrasound and MRI can be helpful in the assessment of superficial peroneal nerve and sural nerve pathology (see Fig. 3-89)

In addition to providing direct assessment of peripheral nerves in the foot and ankle, MRI, and to a lesser extent, ultrasound can demonstrate a denervation effect in the intrinsic muscles of the foot in the distribution of

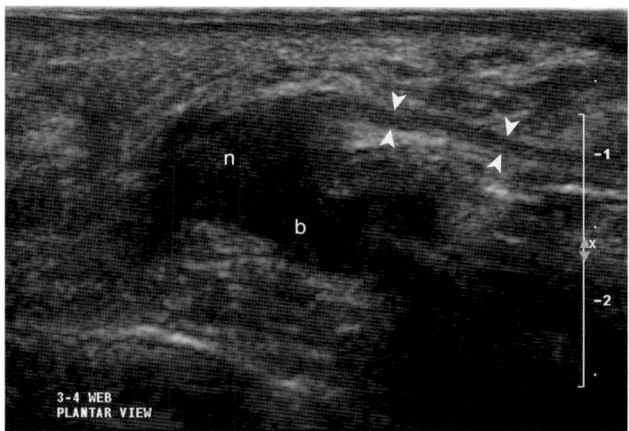

Figure 3-85 Ultrasound of Morton neuroma. A long-axis view has been obtained over the plantar aspect of the 3–4 web space at metatarsophalangeal joint level. An ovoid hypoechoic thickening *(n)* of the common digital nerve consistent with a Morton neuroma is demonstrated. *Arrowheads* indicate the normal segment of common digital nerve proximal to the neuroma. Fluid is seen within the adjacent intermetatarsal bursa *(b)*.

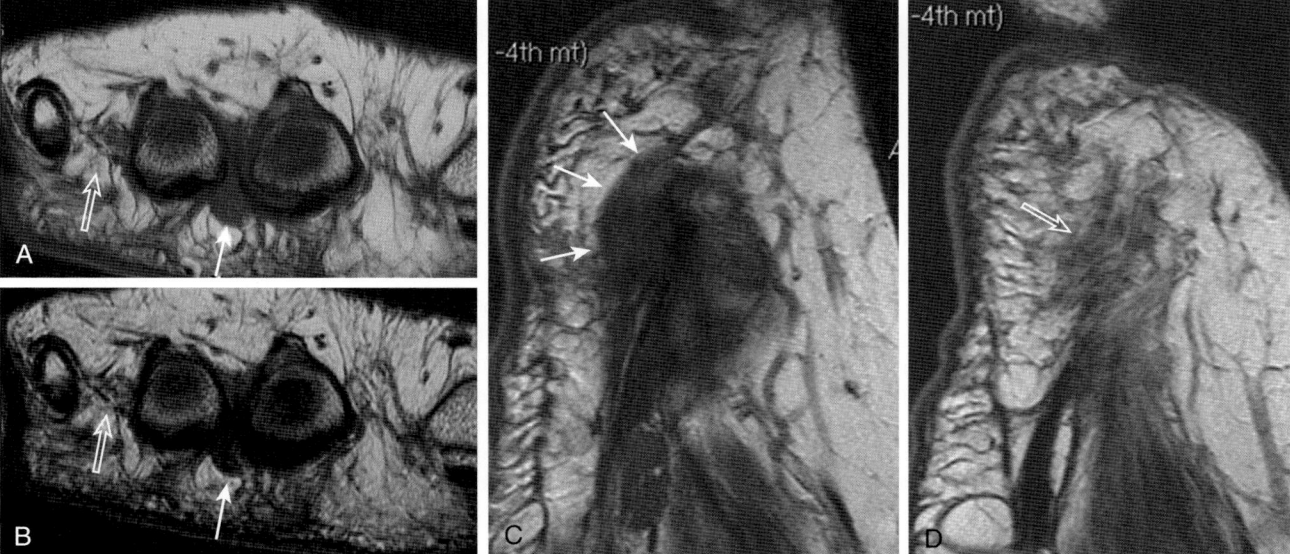

Figure 3-86 Magnetic resonance (MR) imaging of Morton neuroma. Coronal (short axis) T1 **(A)** and T2 **(B)** MR images demonstrating a moderate-sized 2–3 web-space Morton neuroma *(white arrows)*. Note the normal neurovascular bundle in the 3–4 web space *(open arrow)*. **C,** In sagittal cross section, the fusiform morphology of the Morton neuroma is readily appreciated *(white arrows)*. **D,** In contrast, note the normal neurovascular bundle in sagittal cross section *(open arrow)*.

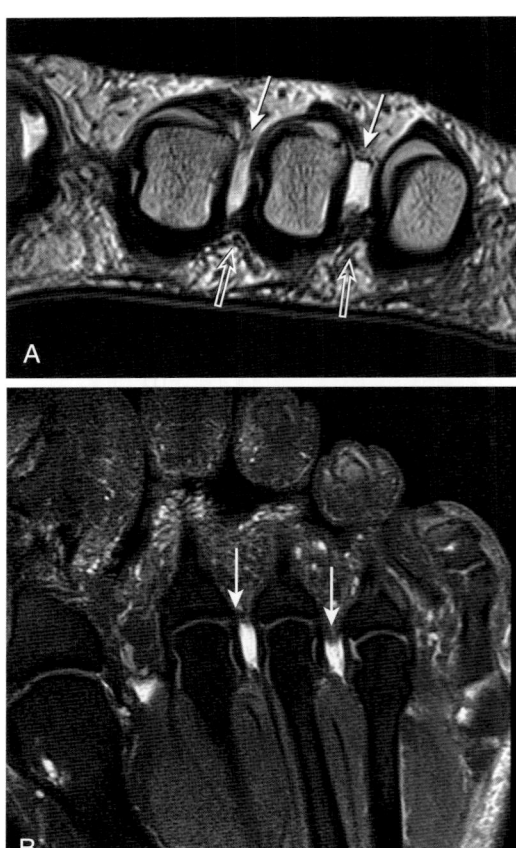

Figure 3-87 Magnetic resonance (MR) imaging of intermetatarsal effusion. **A,** Coronal T2-weighted MR image demonstrating 2–3 and 3–4 intermetatarsal effusions *(white arrows),* seen as confluent high (fluid) signal at the mid-to-dorsal aspect of the web spaces. Note the normal neurovascular bundles at the plantar aspects of the web spaces *(open arrows).* **B,** Long-axis fat-suppressed proton-density MR image again demonstrates the intermetatarsal bursal effusions *(white arrows),* rendered more conspicuous by the use of fat suppression.

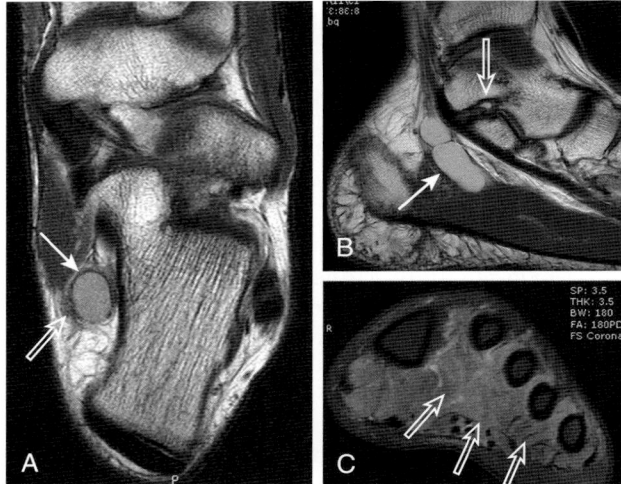

Figure 3-88 Tarsal tunnel ganglion with lateral plantar nerve (LPN) denervation effect. **A,** Axial proton-density (PD) magnetic resonance (MR) image demonstrating a tarsal tunnel ganglion cyst *(white arrow)* displacing and compressing the LPN *(open arrow).* **B,** Sagittal PD MR image demonstrating the tarsal tunnel ganglion cyst *(white arrow)* arising from a fibrous extraarticular talocalcaneal coalition *(open arrow).* **C,** Short-axis MR image through the forefoot demonstrating subacute denervation effect in the interossei and adductor hallucis muscles *(open arrows).* Note normal signal intensity of the two heads of flexor hallucis brevis and abductor hallucis.

the affected nerve, providing a secondary sign of peripheral nerve pathology (see Fig. 3-88). In the case of denervation effect involving the abductor digiti minimi muscle, imaging often fails to demonstrate the site of the nerve abnormality.

In the postoperative setting, MRI and ultrasound are both well suited to demonstrating posttraumatic neuroma formation. Ultrasound because of its unlimited multiplanar capability is often better able to demonstrate neural abnormalities in longitudinal cross section when compared with MRI. Ultrasound is also superior to MRI in demonstrating surgical sutures traversing a nerve.

Imaging Tumors in the Foot and Ankle

Approximately 7% of bone and soft tissue tumors occur in the foot and ankle, and most are benign or nonneoplastic soft tissue tumors. Benign soft tissue tumors include lipoma, angioleiomyoma, vascular malformation, schwannoma, and superficial acral fibromyxoma. Nonneoplastic soft tissue lesions occurring in the foot and ankle include giant cell tumor of tendon sheath, pigmented villonodular synovitis, fibroma of tendon sheath, plantar fibroma, Morton neuroma, reactive pseudotumor (reactive periostitis, bizarre parosteal osteochondromatous proliferation [BPOP]) subungual exostosis, and turret exostosis, ganglia, and adventitial bursae. Bone tumors are also more commonly benign than malignant. Common benign bone tumors include enchondroma, periosteal chondroma, osteochondroma, chondromyxoid fibroma, chondroblastoma, osteoid osteoma, osteoblastoma, and nonneoplastic lesions, such as aneurysmal bone cyst and simple bone cyst.

Notwithstanding that they are uncommon, sarcomas do occur in the foot and ankle, and, as a consequence, all masses in the foot and ankle require detailed and rigorous imaging assessment. In general, benign soft tissue tumors are superficial in location and less than 5 cm in size. Soft tissue sarcomas are more commonly located in the deeper tissue layers and are often relatively large at presentation. Synovial sarcoma is the commonest sarcoma in the foot and ankle and is usually seen in young adults (Fig. 3-91). It deserves special mention because of the relatively high frequency of delay in diagnosis resulting from misinterpretation on imaging as a ganglion or plantar fibroma.

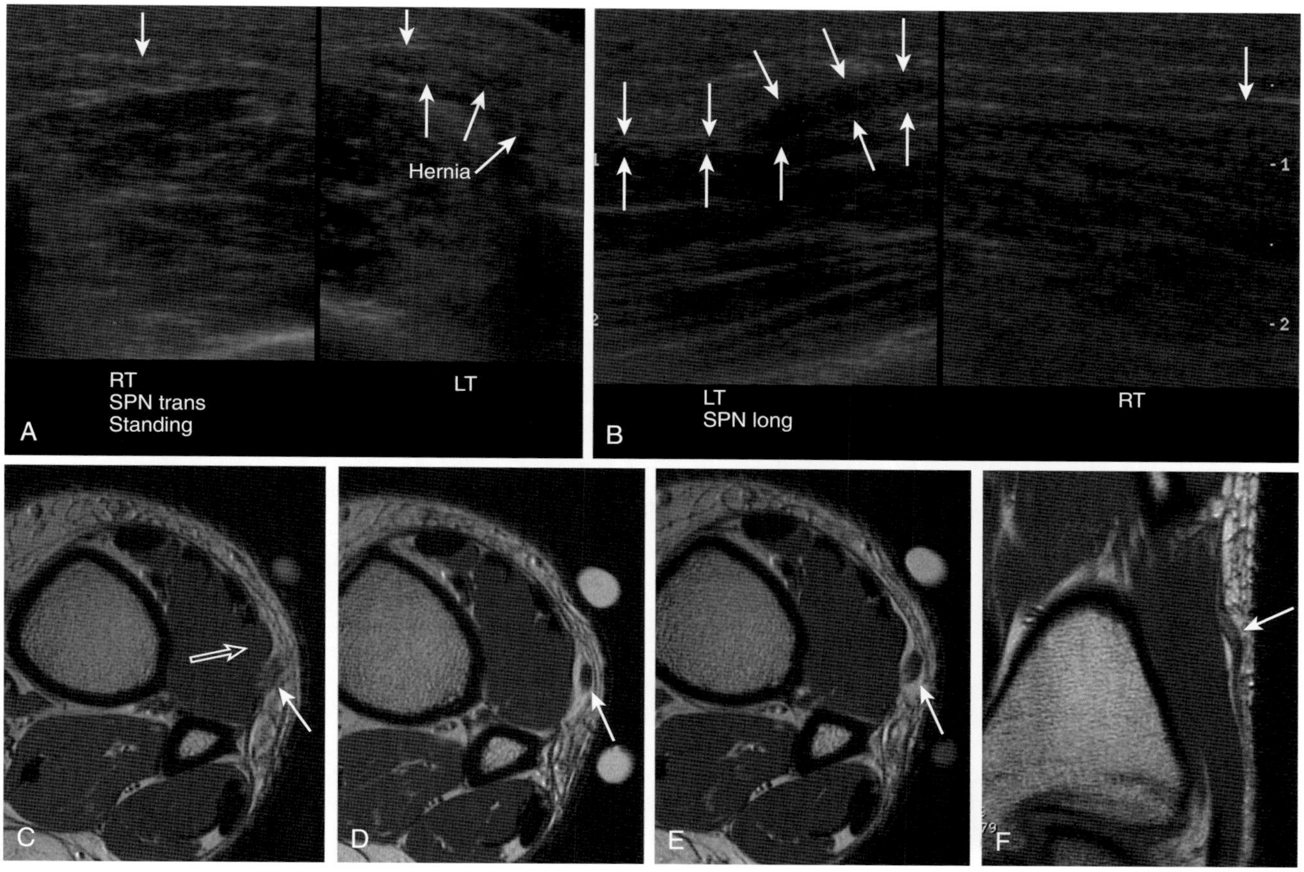

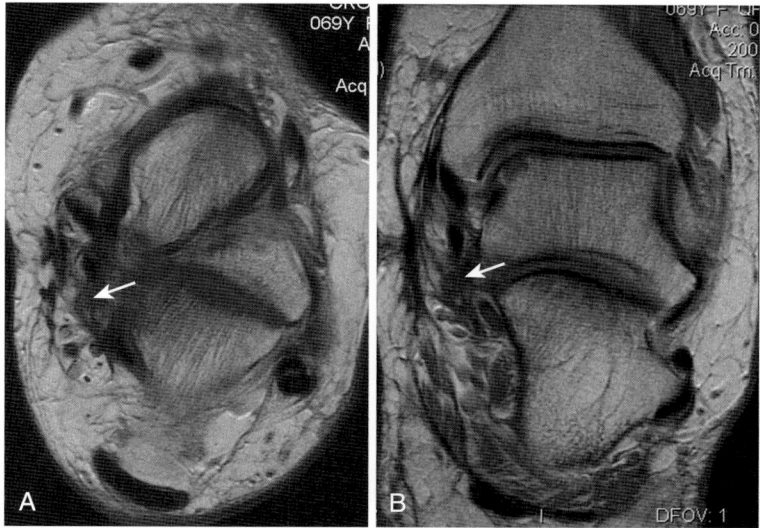

Figure 3-89 Posttraumatic neuroma superficial peroneal nerve *(SPN)* and adjacent muscle hernia. **A,** Transverse ultrasound image performed with the patient standing demonstrates thickening of the left SPN in the lower leg and bulging in contour of the investing fascia of the anterior compartment consistent with a muscle hernia. Note normal right SPN and investing fascia. **B,** Long-axis ultrasound image demonstrating transition in caliber of the SPN as it emerges from the deep fascia *(arrows).* **C, D** and **E,** Descending transverse proton-density (PD) magnetic resonance images demonstrate the muscle hernia *(open arrow)* and thickening of the SPN *(white arrows).* **F,** Long-axis PD MR image demonstrates thickening of the SPN as it emerges from the deep fascia *(white arrow).*

Figure 3-90 Perineural scar after prior tarsal tunnel release. **A,** Axial proton-density (PD) magnetic resonance image demonstrating perineural scar encasement of the medial plantar nerve and neural thickening and edema *(white arrow),* with similar findings on a coronal PD image **(B).**

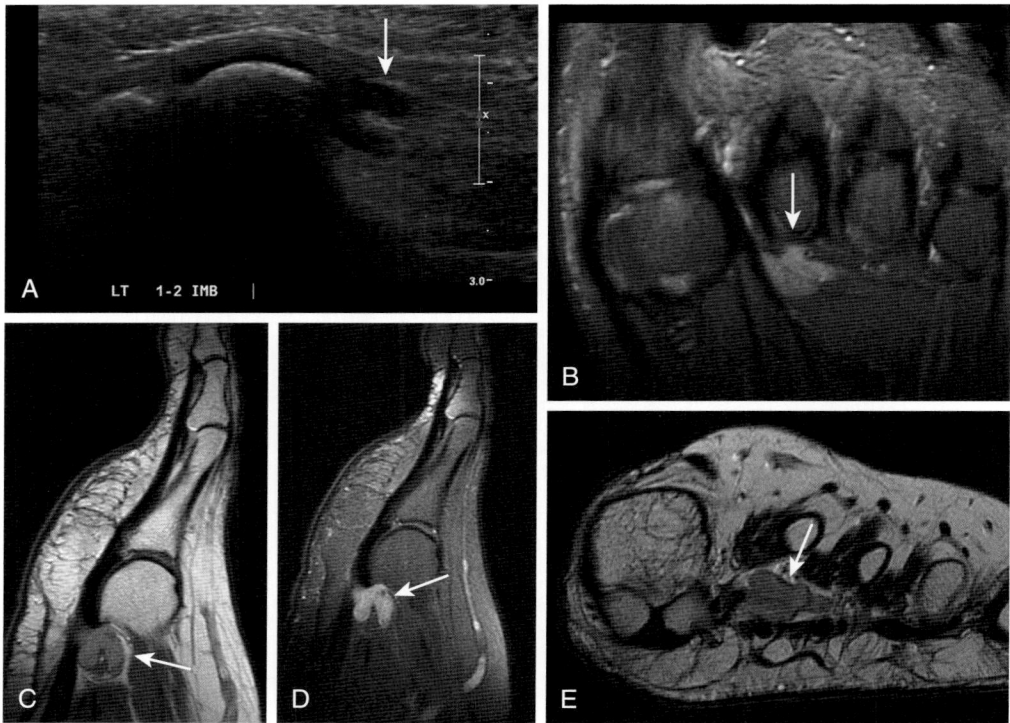

Figure 3-91 Synovial sarcoma. **A,** Sagittal ultrasound image demonstrates a nonspecific bilobular hypoechoic lesion in the region of the 1–2 intermetatarsal bursa *(white arrow).* **B,** Long-axis fat-suppressed proton-density (PD), **C,** sagittal PD, and **D,** fat-suppressed PD and **E,** short-axis T2 magnetic resonance images demonstrate a solid T2 hyperintense lesion, which, on excision biopsy, was a synovial sarcoma *(white arrows).*

Malignant bone tumors in the foot and ankle, when they occur, are most commonly chondrosarcomas, osteogenic sarcoma, or Ewing tumors (Fig. 3-92).

Radiographs and MRI are the main initial imaging investigations in the workup of a tumor in the foot and ankle. In suspected malignant tumors, positron emission tomography (PET) and chest CT are indicated to assess for metastatic disease. A radiograph is helpful in demonstrating calcifications in soft tissue tumors and in characterizing the matrix of bone tumors. A radiograph is also useful in demonstrating periosteal reaction, bone destruction and expansion, and pressure erosion. Ultrasound can be helpful in the diagnosis of Morton neuroma and ganglia. It is critical to adhere to strict sonographic criteria for a diagnosis of a ganglion to avoid misdiagnosis of solid tumors as ganglia. MRI is superior to ultrasound with respect to providing an overview of the region of interest and in its ability to characterize the tumor and its extent. Intravenous contrast administration is generally indicated when characterizing a tumor, providing further insight into lesion vascularity and extent.

If there is uncertainty regarding a potential diagnosis of a bone or soft tissue tumor in the foot and ankle, or if the lesion is thought to be malignant, then a diagnostic biopsy should be performed, preferably at a center where there is a multidisciplinary team that includes a radiologist, oncologic surgeon, and a pathologist. A core biopsy may be performed percutaneously under imaging guidance by a radiologist, or an open surgical biopsy may be performed. In general, fine needle biopsy, as opposed to core biopsy, does not provide sufficient material for accurate diagnosis.

Imaging Infections in the Foot and Ankle

Although diagnostic imaging can demonstrate imaging features compatible with infection, the diagnosis of infection must take into account the clinical picture, the results of serum markers of inflammation, and appropriate aspirates or biopsy of suspected infected tissue. The commonest clinical scenarios of infection in the foot and ankle are hematogenous spread of osteomyelitis in the skeletally immature, the infected diabetic foot, and postoperative infection.

Imaging assessment of suspected infection should commence with plain radiographs. In the setting of osteomyelitis, plain radiographic findings may range from being normal to demonstrating localized osteolysis, periosteal reaction, and possibly a sequestrum. CT scanning may demonstrate subtle areas of osteolysis, periosteal reaction, and sequestrum formation that are not readily appreciated with plain radiography. Ultrasound can be helpful in confirming the presence of a soft tissue collection, joint or tendon sheath effusion, and can provide

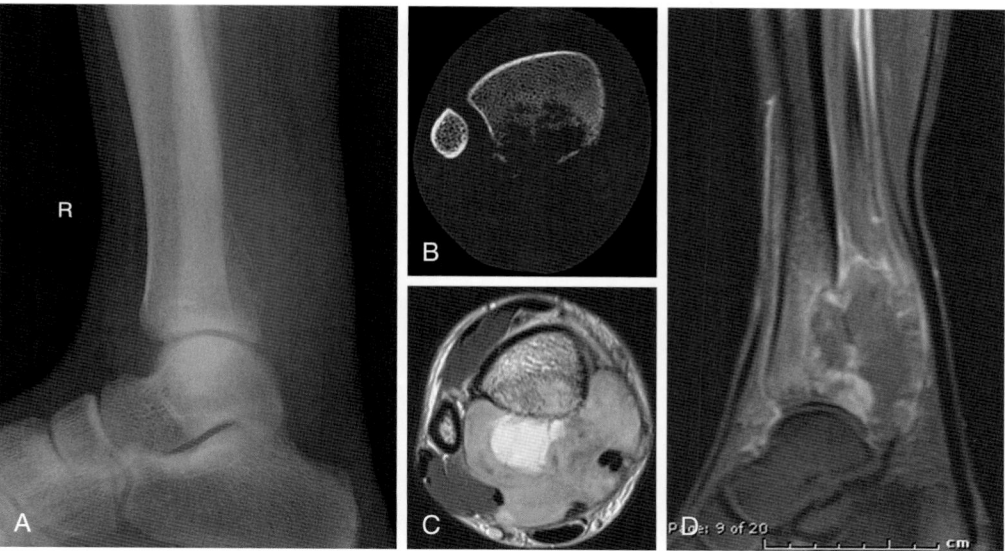

Figure 3-92 Ewing sarcoma in distal tibia. **A,** Lateral radiograph of the ankle demonstrates a lytic lesion in the distal tibia posteriorly, with adjacent soft tissue mass. **B,** Computed tomography scan demonstrates aggressive pattern of permeative osteolysis. Axial proton-density **(C)** and postintravenous contrast sagittal fat-suppressed T1 **(D)** magnetic resonance images demonstrate the extensive associated soft tissue mass.

guidance for aspiration and microbiologic assessment. Contrast-enhanced MRI, with its greater contrast resolution, is the modality of choice for the evaluation of most suspected soft tissue and osseous infections in the foot and ankle (Fig. 3-93). The typical MR finding in infection consists of edema, manifesting as high signal on fat-suppressed PD or T2 sequencing and low signal on T1 sequencing, with a corresponding thick rind of contrast enhancement. For osseous infections, bone scans (high sensitivity, low specificity), radiolabeled leukocyte scans (higher specificity than bone scan), and F-18–fluorodeoxyglucose positron emission tomography (^{18}F-FDG PET) (high sensitivity, intermediate specificity) can be used to detect and localize sites of infection in the ankle and foot. Note that in the diabetic foot false-negative nuclear medicine scans may occur because of ischemia and resultant insufficient accumulation of radiotracer in the focus of osteomyelitis.

Miscellaneous Conditions in the Foot and Ankle

Complex Regional Pain Syndrome

Complex regional pain syndrome (CRPS) is a complex and poorly understood condition of severe pain that follows trauma or surgery and exhibits features such as local vasomotor disturbances, trophic changes (e.g., hair loss, thin skin, increased sweating, a sensation of cold), and restricted or painful movement.[67] CRPS can easily be overlooked, and mild forms of this condition often go unrecognized, but physical examination is the mainstay of diagnosis. Plain radiographs are usually normal in early-stage CRPS (0-3 months) and show only nonspecific osteopenia in 60% of cases (Fig. 3-94) during the later stages (3-12 months)[75] but must be performed to rule out associated disorders. Joint effusions may be variably associated with the early stages of CRPS. Power Doppler US *may* show soft tissue hyperemia in the affected lower limb.[52] MRI (Fig. 3-95) is unreliable and does *not* have an established role in the diagnosis of CRPS.[75] *Isotope bone scan* remains the only sensitive, specific, and generally accepted diagnostic imaging modality in the lower extremity.[39]

Arthrofibrosis

Arthrofibrosis is an exaggerated fibrosis of joint capsule after trauma or surgery that results in joint stiffness, pain, and impingement symptoms.[35] Any joint may be affected, but the knee, elbow, shoulder, wrist, hand, and ankle are most frequent. Relative postsurgical or posttraumatic immobility is a known risk factor[15] and rationale for postoperative range of motion exercises. The likelihood of arthrofibrosis is also related to the severity of the initiating injury, with an increased incidence when multiple ligaments have been injured or multiple procedures have been performed.[53] Fibrosis and associated capsular contracture can result in abnormal joint surface contact pressures and predispose to osteoarthrosis. Although the diagnosis is usually clinical, MRI can be helpful in atypical or unsuspected cases, or if concomitant pathology exists that may confuse the clinical picture. The MRI findings in cases of established ankle arthrofibrosis are those of a thickened joint capsule (usually >3 mm) with low signal intensity (Fig. 3-96).

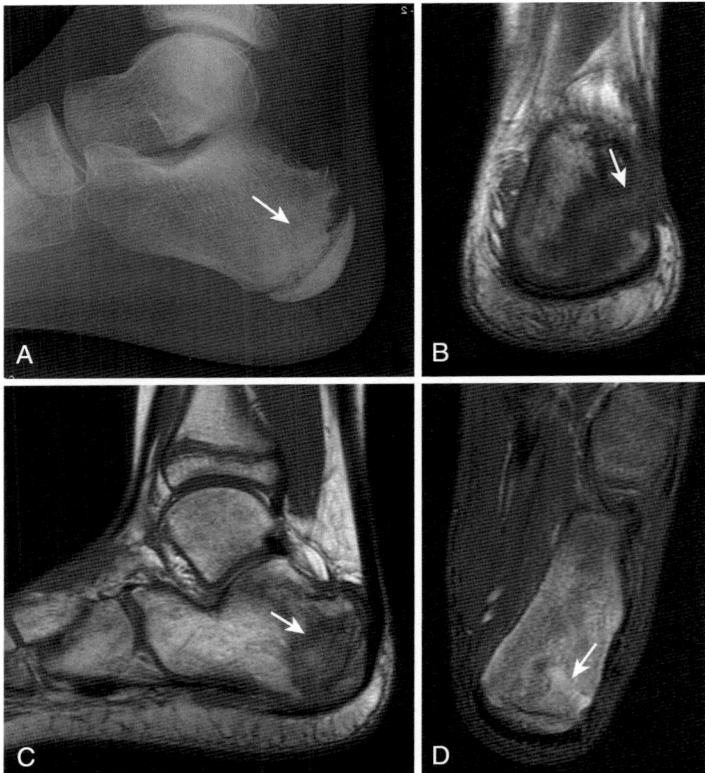

Figure 3-93 Chronic osteomyelitis calcaneus with cloaca. Lateral radiograph **(A)** of the heel demonstrates ill-defined sclerosis *(white arrow)* in the calcaneus adjacent to the calcaneal apophysis. Coronal proton-density (PD) **(B)**, sagittal PD **(C)**, and axial fat-suppressed T2 sequencing **(D)** demonstrates a lytic lesion in the posterior tubercle of the calcaneus adjacent to the apophysis, with a cloaca at the lateral border *(white arrows)* and infiltration of the overlying subcutaneous fat.

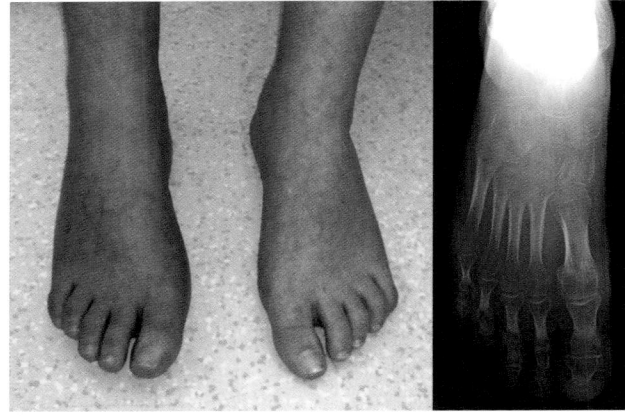

Figure 3-94 Clinical photograph *(left)* of cutaneous vasomotor disturbance and radiograph *(right)* of nonspecific osteopenia in complex regional pain syndrome.

Posttraumatic Fat Necrosis

Posttraumatic fat necrosis is a painful condition involving subcutaneous fat that follows direct contusion, crush, or shear injury and is characterized by organizing hemorrhage, fat necrosis, and fibrosis.[73] There is often a delay of weeks before a tender palpable lump is appreciated, and a majority of patients do not recall any inciting injury. In the early stages, there may be a visible ecchymosis and corresponding high signal on MRI. This resolves and, in the later stages, MRI may show only low signal and a loss of subcutaneous fat volume. On ultrasound, there is a thickened, tender, and indurated subcutaneous fat space containing poorly-marginated areas of increased echogenicity with variable hyperemia. Of importance, imaging does not show any discrete mass apart from an occasional oil cyst (Fig. 3-97). Fat necrosis may occur at any age, is more common in women, and is most frequent at sites prone to direct trauma (e.g., breast, thigh, shin). The tender lump may take months to subside. Fat necrosis can cause skin contour deformity resulting from fibrosis, oil cysts, and radiographic calcifications.

Foreign Bodies

Foreign body localization and removal can be challenging. Appropriate imaging is often a key to surgical success. Plain radiographs should *always* be obtained, with any additional advanced imaging choices based on those results and the character of the injury. Ultrasound can generally be used to identify, mark the overlying skin, provide a depth to target, and assess the pertinent anatomic relationships of radiolucent foreign bodies.

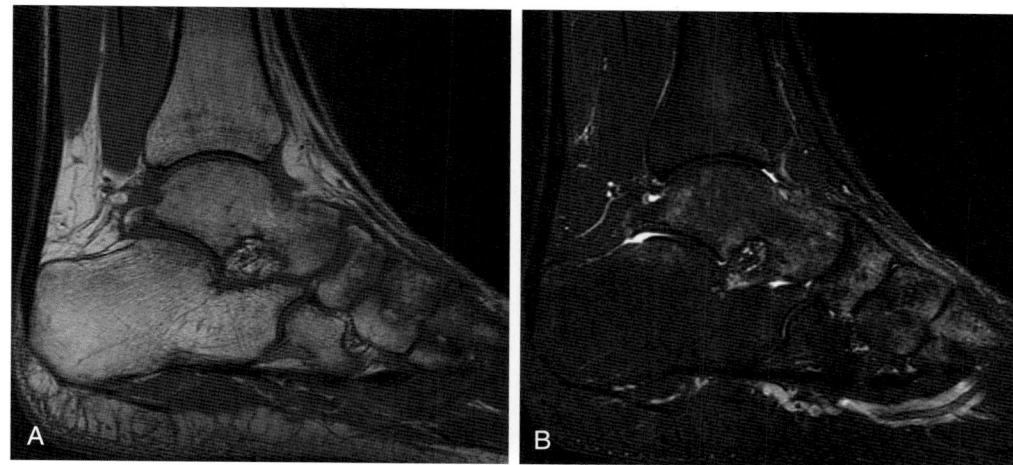

Figure 3-95 Magnetic resonance imaging appearance in a case of warm-phase reflex sympathetic dystrophy (RSD). Sagittal T1 **(A)** and sagittal STIR **(B)** images show a coarse blotchy pattern of diffuse marrow edema involving multiple bones. There is also an area of soft tissue edema over the dorsum of midfoot. (From Anderson IF, Read JW: *Atlas of imaging in sports medicine,* ed 2, Sydney, 2008, McGraw-Hill.)

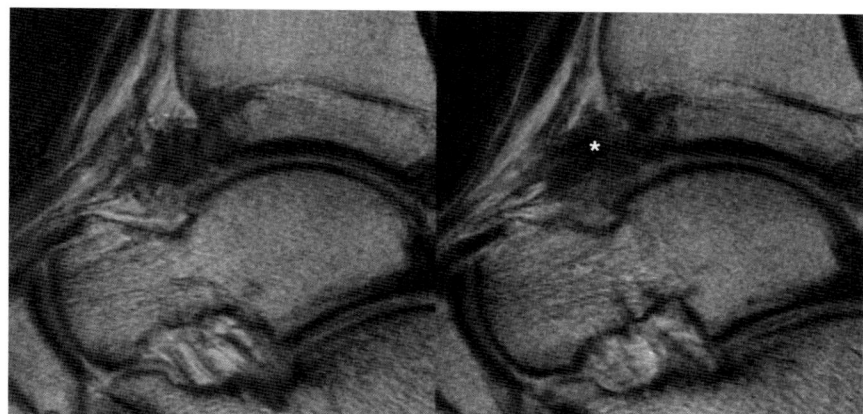

Figure 3-96 Arthrofibrosis. Sagittal proton-density–weighted magnetic resonance images show focal thickening of the anterior ankle capsule *(asterisk)* consistent with arthrofibrotic change after arthroscopy. (From Anderson IF, Read JW: *Atlas of imaging in sports medicine,* ed 2, Sydney, 2008, McGraw-Hill.)

Preoperative hookwire localization under CT guidance has also been described.[5]

Avascular Necrosis of Bone in the Foot and Ankle

Avascular necrosis (AVN) is an uncommon pathology in the foot and ankle, usually seen in the talus as a complication of a talar neck fracture but also described in virtually all bones in the foot and ankle. Imaging diagnosis of established AVN relies on the demonstration of demarcated sclerosis resulting from laying down of new bone over necrotic trabeculae, with revascularization and resorption at the edge of the osteonecrotic segment, accounting for the demarcated margins (Fig. 3-98). The reparative interface between necrotic tissue and viable granulation tissue may be seen as the "double-line sign" on MRI, a low signal intensity rim in which the inner aspect becomes high signal on T2-weighted images. Although this sign is characteristic of AVN of the femoral head, it is less frequently seen in the ankle and foot.[7] Early diagnosis of avascular necrosis can be difficult. In the talus, the absence of subchondral osteopenia in the talar dome at 4 to 8 weeks posttalar neck fracture (Hawkin sign) has been reported to have an association with avascular necrosis of the talus; however, it lacks specificity.[61] Bone marrow edema on MRI is also a nonspecific imaging finding, particularly in the setting of recent fracture.[7,51] Dynamic contrast-enhanced (DCE) MRI has been used to attempt to characterize the perfusion status in the setting of suspected early avascular necrosis.[51] At this stage, there are no validated criteria for DCE MRI diagnosis of avascular necrosis, and there has been no demonstrated superiority of DCE MRI over conventional MRI in the diagnosis

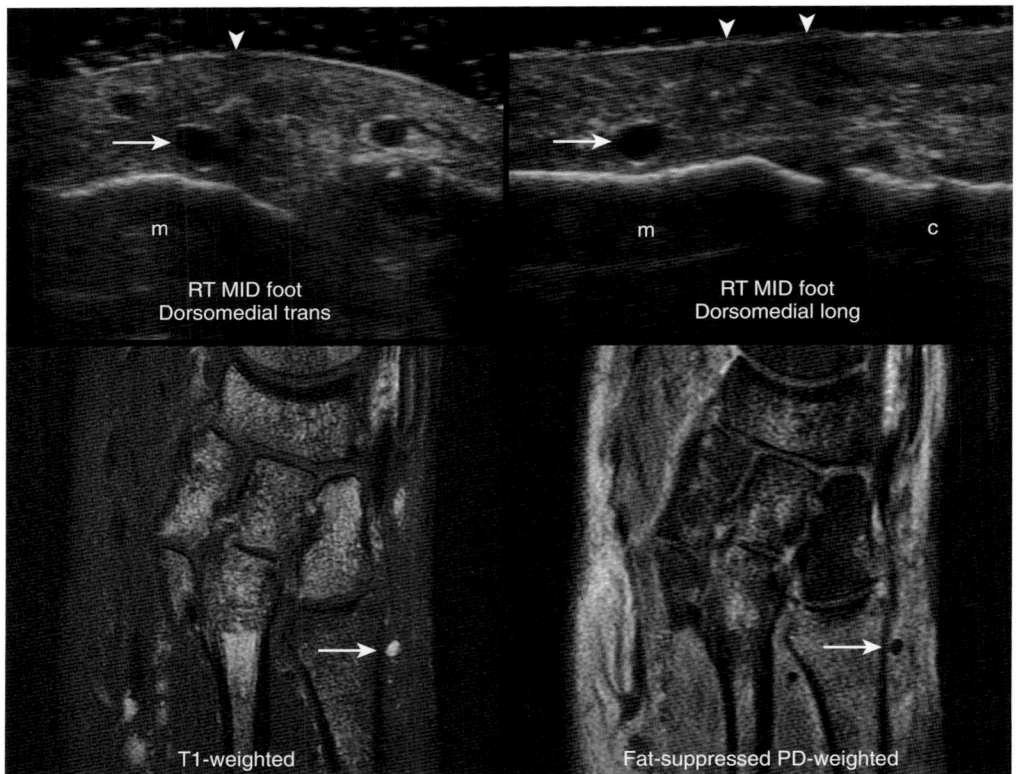

Figure 3-97 Fat necrosis. This example of fat necrosis was imaged 3 weeks after crush injury of the foot. Ultrasound *(top)* shows thickened echogenic subcutaneous space and small oil cyst *(arrows)*. *Arrowheads* indicate a cutaneous laceration that had been sutured. Magnetic resonance image *(bottom)* confirms the oily nature of the cyst seen on ultrasound because the lesion shows high T1 signal that completely suppresses with fat saturation *(arrows)*. Also note extensive marrow edema resulting from bone bruising.

of AVN.[13,71] In the early stage of avascular necrosis, relatively increased enhancement may be seen because of venous stasis, with reduced time to peak enhancement,[9] which is paradoxic to the expected decreased perfusion in an avascular necrotic segment and creates difficulties in the interpretation of such studies.

INTERVENTIONAL RADIOLOGY IN THE FOOT AND ANKLE

Imaging guidance can facilitate accurate delivery of an injectate in the foot and ankle. Corticosteroid formulations are most commonly injected. There is increasing use of platelet-rich plasma (PRP) injections for the treatment of tendinopathy and plantar fasciosis. Other newer injection therapies include the use of cultured autologous tenocytes for treatment of tendinopathy and adipocyte-derived stem cells for the treatment of osteoarthritis. Other interventional procedures that may be done under imaging guidance include RF ablation of nerves or neural lesions such as a Morton neuroma.

The choice of imaging modality for image guidance will vary with local expertise and availability. There has been a substantial increase in the proportion of

ultrasound-guided procedures over the last 10 years. These include ganglion aspiration, Morton neuroma injection, joint injection, tendon sheath injection, Achilles paratenon brisement, plantar fascia injection (with steroid or PRP), and dry needling. One limitation of ultrasound-guided joint injection is that there is only limited ability to demonstrate on static images the distribution of the injectate. Fluoroscopic-guided joint injections have the advantage of showing the distribution of contrast within the joint after injection. Computed tomography has a limited role in imaging-guided procedures in the foot and ankle. Its principal role lies in guiding radiofrequency ablation of osteoid osteoma.

Minimally invasive imaging-guided percutaneous intervention has grown enormously in recent years. Although clinical guidance is adequate for some injections, others may benefit from a more precise and controlled procedure under direct imaging control. The radiologist is uniquely placed to perform these more demanding interventions by using a variety of imaging tools (e.g., fluoroscopy, CT, ultrasound). Such procedures may include joint injections (Fig. 3-99), tendon sheath injections, bursal injections, platelet-rich plasma injections, perineural injections (Fig. 3-100),[40] aspirations of

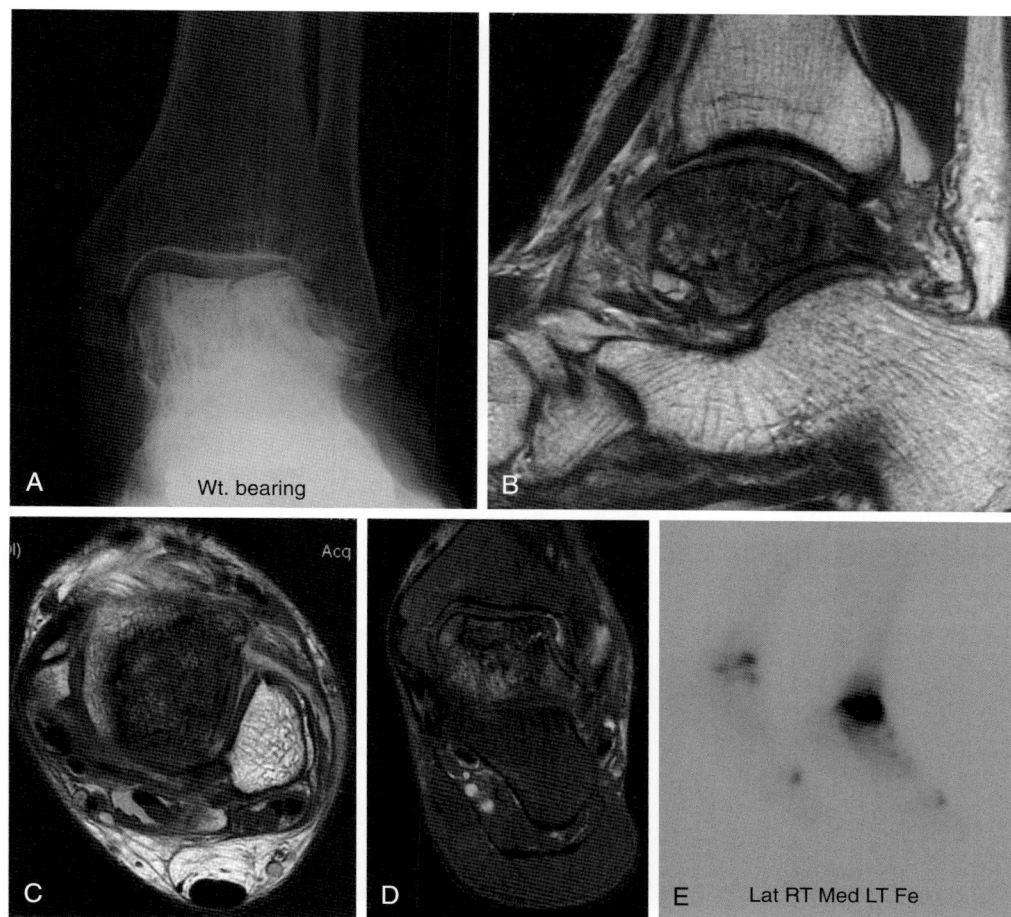

Figure 3-98 Spontaneous avascular necrosis of the talar dome in a 50-year-old male with a remote background history of ankle trauma. **A,** Anteroposterior radiograph demonstrates sclerosis, fragmentation, and partial collapse of the talar dome, and old posttraumatic changes at the medial and lateral malleoli. **B** and **C,** Sagittal and axial proton-density magnetic resonance (MR) images demonstrate geographically marginated, mildly heterogeneous, low signal consistent with sclerosis. A linear high-signal fracture line is also evident. Note the sparing of the medial portion of the talar dome. **D,** Coronal fat-suppressed MR image demonstrates edema-like signal in a mildly heterogeneous distribution within the osteonecrotic segment. **E,** Corresponding increased radiotracer uptake is evident on bone scan. *Fe,* feet; *Lat,* lateral; *LT,* left; *Med,* medial; *RT,* right; *Wt.,* weight.

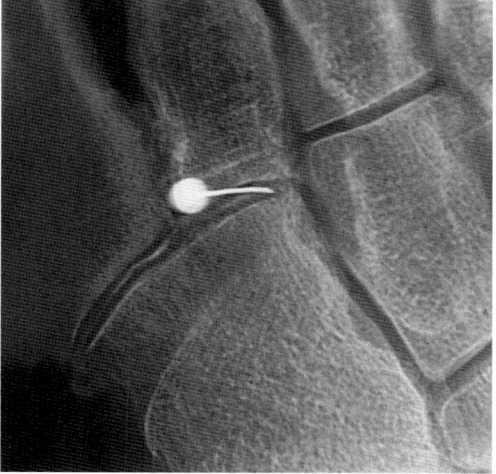

Figure 3-99 Fluoroscopic guidance has allowed accurate needle placement within the fourth tarsometatarsal joint, further confirmed with the injection of a small amount of radiopaque contrast material. Procedures of this type can document unequivocally the site injected, providing the surgeon with a high level of confidence and sometimes detecting unexpected communications with other joints, tendon sleeves or periarticular cysts. (From Anderson IF, Read JW: *Atlas of imaging in sports medicine,* ed 2, Sydney, 2008, McGraw-Hill.)

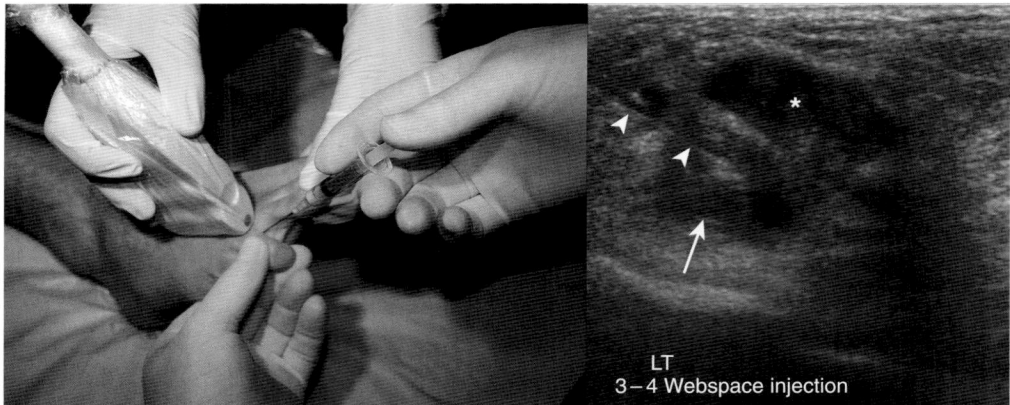

Figure 3-100 An ultrasound-guided technique of corticosteroid injection for a Morton neuroma is illustrated. The transducer is placed over the dorsum of the foot and oriented in the long axis of the relevant web space. The needle is then advanced from a distal interdigital approach to allow direct visualization *(arrowheads)* as the tip is placed within the zone of neural/perineural thickening *(arrow)*, and corticosteroid is then instilled. Note some spillage of injectate into the adjacent intermetatarsal bursa *(asterisk)*.

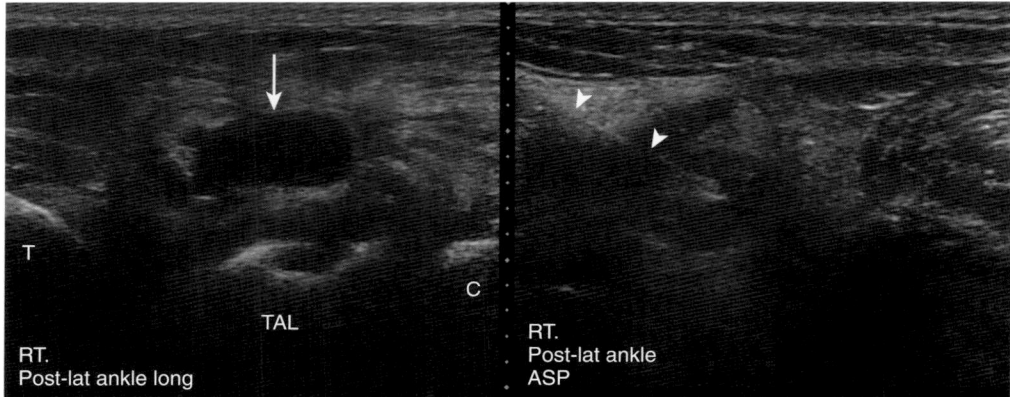

Figure 3-101 A posterior ankle ganglion is shown on the preaspiration image *(arrow)*. After needle placement *(arrowheads)* and aspiration, the cyst was completely emptied. *C,* calcaneus; *lat,* lateral; *RT,* right; *T,* tibia; *TAL,* talus.

ganglion cysts (Fig. 3-101) and other fluid collections, alcohol[17,28,50] or radiofrequency[19] ablations of Morton neuromas.

REFERENCES

1. AAPM position statement on radiation risks from medical imaging procedures. December 13, 2011. Policy Number PP 25-A. [database on the Internet]. American Association of Physicists in Medicine. Available at http://www.aapm.org/org/policies/details.asp?id=318andtype=PPandcurrent=true. Accessed August 12, 2012.
2. Anderson IF, Read JW: *Atlas of imaging in sports medicine,* ed 2, Sydney, 2008, McGraw-Hill.
3. Bagshaw M: Cosmic radiation in commercial aviation, 2009. Available at http://www.iaasm.org/documents/Cosmic_Radiation.pdf. Accessed July 21, 2012.
4. Bashir A, Gray ML, Burstein D: Gd-DTPA2- as a measure of cartilage degeneration, *Magn Reson Med* 36:665–673, 1996.
5. Bissonnette RT, Connell DG, Fitzpatrick DG: Preoperative localization of low-density foreign bodies under CT guidance, *Can Assoc Radiol J* 39:286–287, 1988.
6. Brady Z, Cain TM, Johnston PN: Justifying referrals for paediatric CT, *Med J Aust* 197:95–98, 2012.
7. Buchan CA, Pearce DH, Lau J, White LM: Imaging of postoperative avascular necrosis of the ankle and foot, *Semin Musculoskelet Radiol* 16:192–204, 2012.
8. Bunyaviroch T, Aggarwa A, Oates ME: Optimized scintigraphic evaluation of infection and inflammation: role of single-photon emission computed tomography/computed tomography fusion imaging, *Semin Nucl Med* 36:295–311, 2006.
9. Chan WP, Liu YJ, Huang GS, et al: Relationship of idiopathic osteonecrosis of the femoral head to perfusion changes in the proximal femur by dynamic contrast-enhanced MRI, *Am J Roentgenol* 196:637–643, 2011.
10. Cooper R, Allwright S, Anderson J: *Atlas of nuclear imaging in sports medicine,* Sydney, 2003, McGraw-Hill.
11. De Simoni C, Wetz HH, Zanetti M, et al: Clinical examination and magnetic resonance imaging in the assessment of ankle sprains treated with an orthosis, *Foot Ankle Int* 17:177–182, 1996.
12. Demangeat JL, Constantinesco A, Brunot B, et al: Three-phase bone scanning in reflex sympathetic dystrophy of the hand, *J Nucl Med* 29:26–32, 1988.

13. Donati OF, Zanetti M, Nagy L, et al: Is dynamic gadolinium enhancement needed in MR imaging for the preoperative assessment of scaphoidal viability in patients with scaphoid nonunion? *Radiology* 260:808–816, 2011.

14. Elias I, Zoga AC, Schweitzer ME, et al: A specific bone marrow edema around the foot and ankle following trauma and immobilization therapy: pattern description and potential clinical relevance, *Foot Ankle Int* 28:463–471, 2007.

15. Enneking WF, Horowitz M: The intra-articular effects of immobilization on the human knee, *J Bone Joint Surg Am* 54:973–985, 1972.

16. Erickson SJ, Prost RW, Timins ME: The "magic angle" effect: background physics and clinical relevance, *Radiology* 188:23–25, 1993.

17. Fanucci E, Masala S, Fabiano S, et al: Treatment of intermetatarsal Morton's neuroma with alcohol injection under US guide: 10-month follow-up, *Eur Radiol* 14:514–518, 2004.

18. Forrester DM, Kerr R: Trauma to the foot, *Radiol Clin North Am* 28:422–433, 1990.

19. Genon MP, Chin TY, Bedi HS, Blackney MC: Radio-frequency ablation for the treatment of Morton's neuroma, *ANZ J Surg* 80:583–585, 2010.

20. Giachino AA, Uhthoff HK: Intra-articular fractures of the calcaneus, *J Bone Joint Surg Am* 71:794–797, 1989.

21. Glaser C, Mendlik T, Dinges J et al: Global and regional reproducibility of T2 relaxation time measurements in human patellar cartilage, *Magn Reson Med* 56:527–534, 2006.

22. Glazenbrook KN, Guimaraes L, Murthy NS, et al: Identification of intraarticular and periarticular uric acid crystals with dual-energy CT: initial evaluation, *Radiology* 261:516–524, 2011.

23. Gyftopoulos S, Bencardino JT: Normal variants and pitfalls in MRI imaging of the ankle and foot, *Magn Res Clin North Am* 18:691–705, 2010.

24. Hapamaki V, Kiuru M, Koskinen S: Lisfranc fracture-dislocation in patients with multiple trauma: diagnosis with multidetector computed tomography, *Foot Ankle Int* 25:614–619, 2004.

25. Health risks from exposure to low levels of ionizing radiation: BEIR VII Phase 2, Washington, DC, 2006, National Academies Press. Available at http://www.nap.edu/openbook.php?record_id=11340. Accessed August 12, 2012.

26. Holder LE: Clinical radionuclide bone imaging, *Radiology* 176:607–614, 1990.

27. Horger M, Bares R: The role of single-photon emission computed tomography/computed tomography in benign and malignant bone disease, *Semin Nucl Med* 36:286–294, 2006.

28. Hughes RJ, Ali K, Jones H, et al: Treatment of Morton's neuroma with alcohol injection under sonographic guidance: follow-up of 101 cases, *AJR Am J Roentgenol* 188:1535–1539, 2007.

29. Juras V, Welsch G, Bar P, et al: Comparison of 3T and 7T MRI clinical sequences for ankle imaging, *Eur J Radiol* 81:1846–1850, 2012.

30. Keats TE, Anderson MW: *Atlas of normal roentgen variants that may simulate disease*, ed 8, Philadelphia, 2007, Mosby Elsevier, pp xxii, 1321.

31. Kramer J, Stiglbauer R, Engel A, et al: MR contrast arthrography (MRA) in osteochondritis dissecans, *J Comput Assist Tomogr* 16:254–260, 1992.

32. Laor T, Jaramillo D: MR insights into skeletal maturation: what is normal? *Radiology* 250:28–38, 2009.

33. Leumann A, Valderrabano V, Plaass C, et al: A novel imaging method for osteochondral lesions of the talus—comparison of SPECT-CT with MRI, *Am J Sports Med* 39:1095–1101, 2011.

34. Li X, Han ET, Ma CB, et al: In vivo 3T spiral imaging based multi-slice T(1rho) mapping of knee articular cartilage in osteoarthritis, *Magn Reson Med* 54:929–936, 2005.

35. Lindenfeld TN, Wojtys EM, Husain A: Surgical treatment of arthrofibrosis of the knee, *Instr Course Lect* 49:211–221, 2000.

36. Linklater J: MR imaging of ankle impingement lesions [review], *Magn Reson Imaging Clin N Am* 17:775–800, vii-viii, 2009.

37. Linklater JM: Imaging of sports injuries in the foot, *AJR Am J Roentgenol* 199:500–508, 2012.

38. Love C, Palestro CL: Radionclude imaging of infection, *J Nucl Med Technol* 32:47–57, 2004.

39. Mackinnon SE, Holder LE: The use of three-phase radionuclide bone scanning in the diagnosis of reflex sympathetic dystrophy, *J Hand Surg Am* 9:556–563, 1984.

40. Markovic M, Crichton K, Read JW, et al: Effectiveness of ultrasound-guided corticosteroid injection in the treatment of Morton's neuroma, *Foot Ankle Int* 29:483–487, 2008.

41. Matin P: The appearance of bone scans following fractures, including immediate and long-term studies, *J Nucl Med* 20:1227–1231, 1979.

42. National Council on Radiation Protection and Measurements: *Ionizing radiation exposure of the population of the United States. Report No. 93*, Bethesda, Md, 1987, NCRP Publishers.

43. Meftah M, Katchis SD, Scharf SC, et al: SPECT/CT in the management of osteochondral lesions of the talus, *Foot Ankle Int* 32:233–238, 2011.

44. Mettler FA Jr, Huda W, Yoshizumi TT, Mahesh M: Effective doses in radiology and diagnostic nuclear medicine: a catalog, *Radiology* 248:254–263, 2008.

45. Mitchell MJ, Ho C, Howard BA, et al: Diagnostic imaging of trauma to the ankle and foot; IV: fractures of the calcaneus, *J Foot Surg* 28:479–484, 1989.

46. Morrison WB, Schweitzer ME, Wapner KL, et al: Osteomyelitis in feet of diabetics: clinical accuracy, surgical utility and cost-effectiveness of MR imaging, *Radiology* 196:557–564, 1995.

47. Mosher TJ, Dardzinski BL: Cartilage MRI T2 relaxation time mapping: overview and applications, *Semin Musculoskelet Radiol* 8:355–368, 2004.

48. Mosher TJ, Dardzinski BL, Smith MB: Human articular cartilage: influence of aging and early symptomatic degeneration on the spatial variation of T2—preliminary findings at 3T, *Radiology* 214:259–266, 2000.

49. Mosher TJ, Zhang Z, Reddy R, et al: Knee articular cartilage damage in osteoarthritis; analysis of MRI image biomarker reproducibility in ACRIN-PA 4001 multicenter trial, *Radiology* 258:832–842, 2011.

50. Musson RE, Sawhney JS, Lamb L, et al: Ultrasound guided alcohol ablation of Morton's neuroma, *Foot Ankle Int* 33:196–201, 2012.

51. Myerson M, Christensen JC, Steck JK, Schuberth JM: Avascular necrosis of the foot and ankle, *Foot Ankle Spec* 5:128–136, 2012.

52. Nazarian LN, Schweitzer ME, Mandel S, et al: Increased soft-tissue blood flow in patients with reflex sympathetic dystrophy of the lower extremity revealed by power Doppler sonography, *AJR Am J Roentgenol* 171:1245–1250, 1998.

53. Noyes FR, Barber-Westin SD: Reconstruction of the anterior and posterior cruciate ligaments after knee dislocation. Use of early protected postoperative motion to decrease arthrofibrosis, *Am J Sports Med* 25:769–778, 1997.

54. Nunley JA, Vertullo CJ: Classification, investigation and management of midfoot sprains: Lisfranc injuries in the athlete, *Am J Sports Med* 30:871–878, 2002.

55. Pagenstert GI, Barg A, Leumann AG, et al: SPECT-CT in degenerative joint disease of the foot and ankle, *J Bone Joint Surg Br* 91:1191–1196, 2009.

56. Palestro CJ: The current role of gallium imaging in infection, *Semin Nucl Med* 24:128–141, 1994.

57. Pearce MS, Salotti JA, Little MP, et al: Radiation exposure from CT scans in childhood and subsequent risk of leukaemia and brain tumours: a retrospective cohort study, *Lancet* 380:499–505, 2012. doi:10.1016/S0140-6736(12)60815-0.

58. Potter HG, Deland JT, Gusmer PB, et al: Magnetic resonance imaging of the Lisfranc ligament of the foot, *Foot Ankle Int* 19:438–446, 1998.

59. Preidler KW, Peicha G, Lajtai G, et al: Conventional radiography, CT, and MR imaging in patients with hyperflexion injuries of the foot: diagnostic accuracy in the detection of bony and ligamentous changes, *AJR Am J Roentgenol* 173:1673–1677, 1999.

60. Raikin SM, Elias I, Dheer S, et al: Prediction of midfoot instability in the subtle Lisfranc injury, *J Bone Joint Surg Am* 91:892–899, 2009.

61. Rammelt S, Zwipp H: Talar neck and body fractures, *Injury* 40:120–135, 2009.

62. Reiter M, Ulreich N, Dirisamer A, et al: Colour and power Doppler sonography in symptomatic Achilles tendon disease, *Int J Sports Med* 25:301–305, 2004.

63. Robinson P, White LM, Salonen D, Ogilivie-Harris D: Anteromedial impingment of the ankle: using MR arthrography to assess the anteromedial recess, *AJR Am J Roentgenol* 178:601–604, 2002.

64. Rosenberg ZS, Feldman F, Singson RD, Price G: Peroneal tendon injury associated with calcaneal fractures: CT findings, *AJR Am J Roengenol* 149:125–129, 1987.

65. Scheuer LB, Black S: *Developmental juvenile osteology*, Oxford, England, 2000, Elsevier Academic Press.

66. Schmidt H, Köhler A, Zimmer EA, et al: *Borderlands of normal and early pathologic findings in skeletal radiography*, ed 4, New York, 1993, Thieme Medical Publishers.

67. Schutzer SF, Gossling HR: The treatment of reflex sympathetic dystrophy syndrome, *J Bone Joint Surg Am* 66:625–629, 1984.

68. Shabshin N, Schweitzer ME, Morrison WB, et al: High-signal T2 changes of the bone marrow of the foot and ankle in children: red marrow or traumatic changes? *Pediatr Radiol* 36:670–676, 2006.

69. Steinbach LS, Palmer WE, Schweitzer ME: Special focus session. MR arthrography, *Radiographics* 22:1223–1246, 2002.

70. Stiell IG, McKnight RD, Greenberg GH, et al: Implementation of the Ottawa ankle rules, *JAMA* 271:827–832, 1994.

71. Takao M, Sugano N, Nishii T, et al: Different magnetic resonance imaging features in two types of nontraumatic rabbit osteonecrosis models, *Magn Reson Imaging* 27:233–239, 2009.

72. Trattnig S, Welsch G, Domayer S, Apprich S: MR imaging of postoperative talar dome lesions, *Semin Musculoskelet Radiol* 16:177–184, 2012. [Epub Jul 31, 2012].

73. Tsai TS, Evans HA, Donnelly LF, et al: Fat necrosis after trauma: a benign cause of palpable lumps in children, *AJR Am J Roentgenol* 169:1623–1626, 1997.

74. Wheaton AJ, Dodge GR, Borthakur A, et al: Detection of changes in articular cartilage proteoglycan by T(1rho) magnetic resonance imaging, *J Orthop Res* 23:102–108, 2005.

75. Wheeless CR 3rd: Reflex sympathetic dystrophy imaging [database on the Internet]. *Wheeless' textbook of orthopaedics.* Available at http://www.wheelessonline.com/ortho/rsd_role_of_bone_scans. Accessed July 12, 2012.

76. Williams T, Cullen N, Goldberg A, Singh D: SPECT-CT imaging of obscure foot and ankle pain, *Foot Ankle Surg* 18:30–33, 2012.

77. Yuj WT, Corosn JD, Baraniewski HM, et al: Osteomyelitis of the foot in diabetic patients: evaluation with plain film, 99 m Tc-MDP bone scintigraphy and MR imaging, *AJR Am J Roentgenol* 152:795–800, 1989.

78. Zubler V, Mengiardi B, Pfirmann CW, et al: Bone marrow changes on STIR MR images of asymptomatic feet and ankles, *Eur Radiol* 17:3066–3072, 2007.

Chapter 4

Conservative Treatment of the Foot

Loretta B. Chou, Keith L. Wapner

GENERAL CONSIDERATIONS

Conservative treatment of foot and ankle disorders is important and often successful. Nonoperative regimens are relatively inexpensive and can be easily accomplished. The treating physician and surgeon should have thorough knowledge and understanding of the interaction of the foot and the shoe or device applied. Also, the biomechanics of normal foot function and the effect of the disease entity being treated should be analyzed. The anatomy of the normal shoe, the function of each component, and the effect of modifying each of these components must be appreciated.[4,5,7,23,24] Furthermore, the practitioner should be familiar with over-the-counter devices as well as with prescribed inserts and orthoses. The desired results of these devices on the foot and ankle should be fully recognized.[8,15]

The majority of adult forefoot deformities are acquired and the result of ill-fitting footwear. The most common of these deformities are hallux valgus, hammer toes, hard corns, interdigital neuromas, and plantar keratoses.

The foremost component of conservative treatment begins with patient education about the effects of ill-fitting shoes and high heels. Forefoot loading is increased by the foot sliding forward into the toe box.[22] Female patients may not comply with this initial treatment because ill-fitting shoes continue to be inherent in high fashion. It is often necessary to remind patients that, for daily dress, there is no other part of the body they would consider putting in a container whose shape is so drastically different from that body part. A useful tool is comparing an outline of the patient's foot to his or her current footwear; this is usually effective in conveying this point (Fig. 4-1). Unless the patient is willing to accept that a change in footwear is indicated, both conservative and operative intervention may be futile.

A proper-fitting shoe should accommodate the variations in the person's foot.[16] A set of consumer guidelines has been developed by the National Shoe Retailers Association, the Pedorthic Footwear Association, and the American Orthopaedic Foot and Ankle Society (Table 4-1). It is imperative to measure the shoe with the foot in a standing position because the width of the foot can increase up to two sizes and length by one-half size from the sitting to standing position. In addition, the foot should be measured late in the day because the foot expands in volume as much as 4% by the end of the day. Shoes should be fitted with the normally worn socks. There should be a full finger breadth between the tip of the shoe and the end of the longest toe, with the toes fully extended.

Recently, walking- and running-type athletic shoes have made proper-fitting shoes more socially acceptable. Currently, women have more choices in the appropriate and acceptable type of footwear in many workplace environments. Acceptance of proper fit over trends in style may adequately relieve a patient's symptoms.

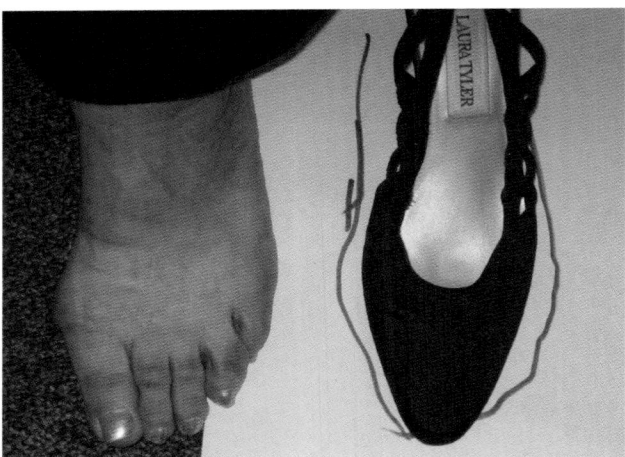

Figure 4-1 Comparing the outline of a foot to a woman's dress shoe demonstrates the disparity in shape.

Table 4-1	10 Points of Proper Shoe Fit

1. Sizes vary among shoe brands and styles. Do not select shoes by the size marked inside the shoe. Judge the shoe by how it fits on your foot.
2. Select a shoe that conforms as nearly as possible to the shape of your foot.
3. Have your feet measured regularly. The size of your feet changes as you grow older.
4. Have both feet measured. For most persons, one foot is larger than the other. Fit to the larger foot.
5. Fit at the end of the day when the feet are largest.
6. Stand during the fitting process and check that there is adequate space ($\frac{3}{8}$ to $\frac{1}{2}$ inch) for your longest toe at the end of each shoe.
7. Make sure the ball of your foot fits snugly into the widest part of the shoe.
8. Do not purchase shoes that feel too tight, expecting them to stretch.
9. Your heel should fit comfortably in the shoe with a minimum amount of slippage.
10. Walk in the shoe to make sure it fits and feels right.

National Shoe Retailers Association, the Pedorthic Footwear Association, and the American Orthopedic Foot and Ankle Society: *10 Points of Proper Shoe Fit.* Columbia, Md, National Shoe Retailers Association, 1995.

Modification of footwear or use of orthoses can be used to treat deformities of the foot. Disease can compromise motor function, joint function, skin integrity, sensation, and proprioception. Once the effects have been assessed, the appropriate modifications should be prescribed to attempt to restore normal function or protect the affected limb from further breakdown.

FOOT ORTHOSES

Foot orthoses are devices that can be placed in a shoe to help accommodate deformities or to decrease abnormal pressure or stress at a specific site on the foot or ankle.

Orthoses function by applying a force on the body in a controlled manner to achieve a desired result, that is, transfer of pressure or restriction of motion. These devices range from simple shoe insoles to ankle–foot orthoses (AFOs). The popularity of shoe inserts for runners has led to many anecdotal claims about the efficacy of their use. However, there are few controlled studies to confirm these claims.

It should be remembered that although orthoses may correct foot position and accommodate deformity, there is no evidence that an orthosis can correct or prevent the development of a hallux valgus or other structural deformities. Also, these devices may not prevent knee, hip, or back arthritis. The goals of foot orthoses include providing shock absorption, cushioning tender areas of the foot, relieving high plantar pressure areas by redistributing weight-bearing pressures covering the entire plantar surface, supporting and protecting healed fracture using the total-contact concept, controlling and supporting flexible deformities, limiting motion of joints, and accommodating fixed deformities with soft moldable materials.[17]

It is not always necessary to use a custom orthosis. For the accommodation of many forefoot- and heel-related problems, over-the-counter inserts may be effective in relieving symptoms, and at a lower cost. The abuse and overprescribing of custom inserts has led most medical insurance companies to deny payment for these inserts. Familiarity with the over-the-counter devices allows the treating physician to direct the patient on how to use these devices efficaciously and may be useful for initial treatment.

Over-the-Counter Inserts

With the advances in materials used in shoe manufacturing, it is often possible to accomplish many of the goals of orthosis without the expense of custom-molded inlays. Several companies offer padded insoles for shock absorption and heel cushioning (Fig. 4-2). Spenco, Viscopeds, Dr. Scholl's, and other companies provide padded insoles and inlays that can provide relief for metatarsalgia and fat-pad atrophy. The addition of metatarsal supports, such as the Hapad longitudinal metatarsal pad on a cushioned inlay or in a shoe with a soft sole, can effectively relieve metatarsalgia or neuroma symptoms. Various heel inserts, such as Visco heels or Tuli heel cups, are often helpful in treating plantar heel pain. These devices are readily available through medical supply catalogs and are often found in pharmacies and athletic shoe stores. Patients should be educated on their proper placement and use.

Once the patient has been evaluated and the desired correction chosen, the proper footwear should be selected. In some instances, this may be all that is needed. If additional correction is needed, off-the-shelf items should be considered. The cost to the patient is considerable for custom orthoses, and more insurance companies now refuse payment for any orthosis that does not cross the

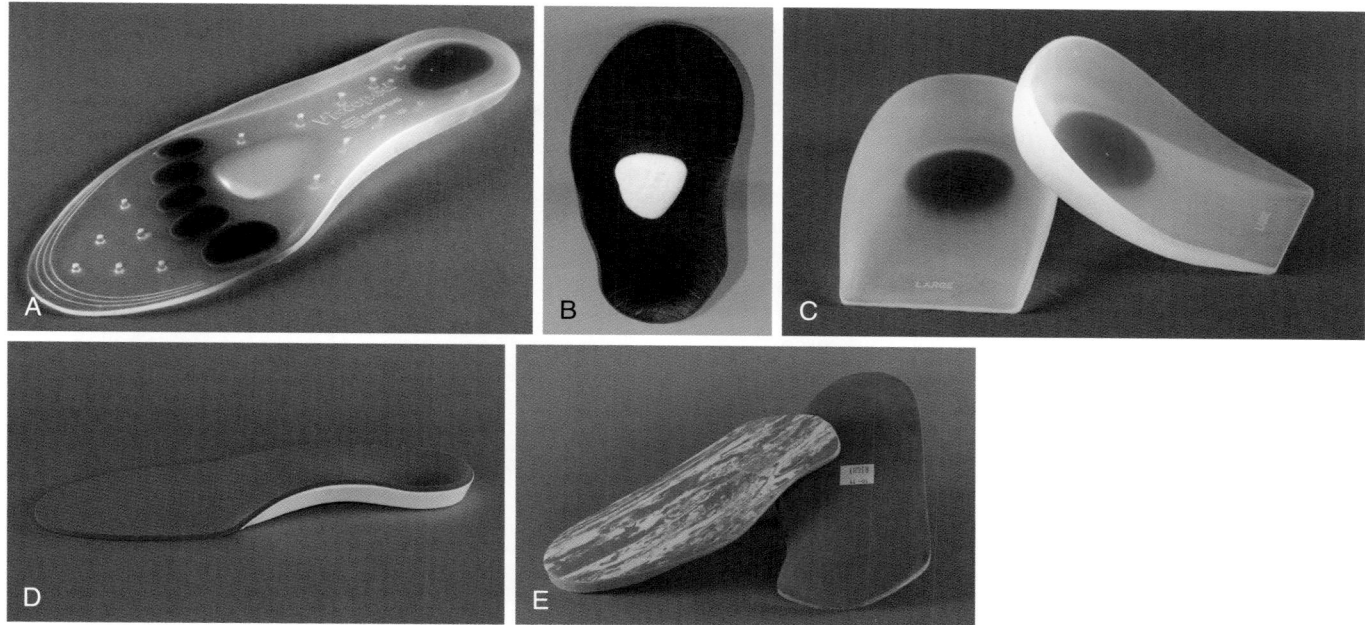

Figure 4-2 Over-the-counter inserts. **A,** Viscoped. **B,** Combination liner and Hapad metatarsal pad. **C,** Visco heel cushion. **D,** Full-length insole. **E,** Three-quarter–length insole.

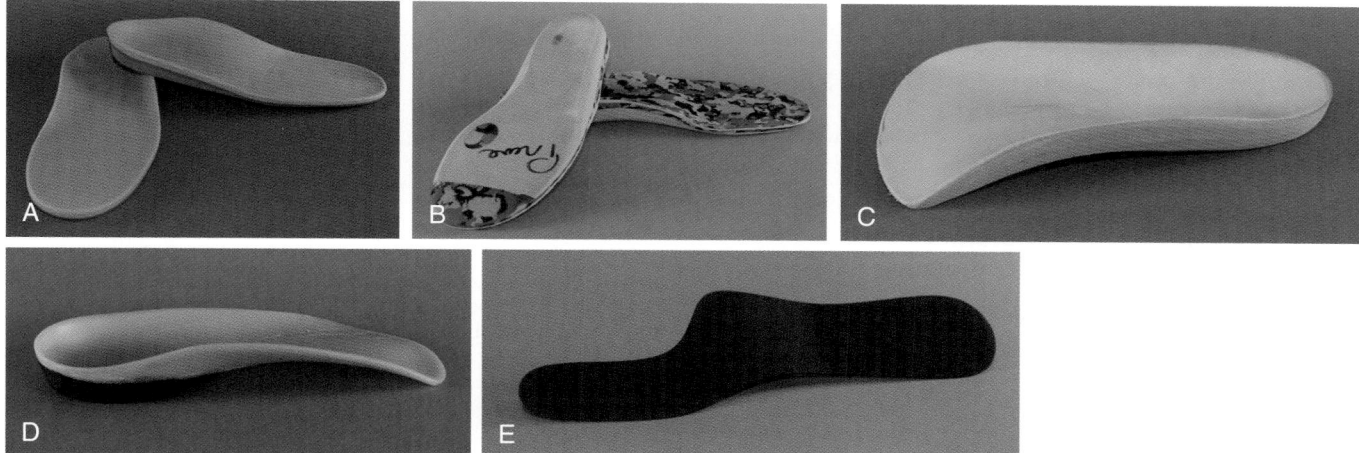

Figure 4-3 Common types of custom orthoses. **A,** Plastazote insole, a soft material ideal for patients with rheumatoid arthritis or diabetes mellitus. **B,** Full-length orthosis with relief for the first metatarsal head, such as for sesamoiditis. **C,** Three-quarter–length foot orthosis indicated for hindfoot disorders. **D,** Rigid foot orthosis. **E,** Morton carbon fiber plate used for turf toe or hallux rigidus.

ankle joint. If adequate correction cannot be accomplished, custom orthoses can be prescribed.

Custom Foot Orthoses

If the patient has a deformity or disorder that is not amenable to treatment with an over-the-counter device, a custom orthoses may be appropriate. There are three general types of custom inserts: soft, semirigid, and rigid (Fig. 4-3).

Soft orthoses are made with materials that may include polyurethane foam, polyvinyl chloride foam, ethylene vinyl acetate, and latex foam. These materials are used when the effect is cushioning, impact absorption, and reducing shear forces of friction. This is particularly important for use in the insensate foot. Also, soft inserts are beneficial for use with fixed deformities, especially those with bony prominences. Soft materials can be used with semirigid material underneath to gain better mechanical properties. These inserts are generally thicker than the rigid orthoses and may require the use of an extra-depth shoe, depending on the pathology.

Semirigid orthoses are the most commonly prescribed inserts. Unlike rigid orthoses, they offer shock absorption and some flexibility while still providing tensile strength and durability. They are used to support and stabilize flexible deformities and relieve pressure by weight transfer. Combinations of materials are often used; the inserts are generally thicker than rigid inserts and might require the patient to wear a deeper shoe. The materials used include leather, polyethylene compounds, closed or open cellular rubber compounds, cork, felt, and viscoelastic polymers.

Rigid orthoses are used to decrease or control motion, such as in the treatment of arthritis of the midfoot or forefoot. The device stiffens the shoe and functions similar to a steel shank within the shoe. Of note, patients with plantar prominences or significant fat-pad atrophy might find these too uncomfortable to wear. A rigid orthosis is often prescribed to block pronation but may be no more effective than a semirigid device and may be more difficult to tolerate. Furthermore, rigid orthoses offer no shock-absorbing properties and should be avoided in patients with impaired sensation. The materials used are thermoplastics or carbon fiber.

Custom orthoses are generally made from a foam impression of the feet of patients, in which the foot is pressed into the foam box evenly. The use of plantar pressure data obtained from new technology with the EMED-D pressure platform (Novel, Munich, Germany) with four sensors/cm^2 yields superior off-loading capacity of insoles.[20]

University of California Biomechanics Laboratory (UCBL) Foot Orthoses

Another type of foot orthosis is the UCBL insert, which controls flexible postural deformities by controlling the hindfoot.[15] The orthosis should be molded with the heel in neutral position. To work successfully, the orthosis must be able to grasp the heel and prevent it from moving into valgus. By keeping the calcaneus in neutral position, the orthosis stiffens the transverse tarsal joints, and pronation and forefoot abduction can be diminished. It may be necessary to add medial posting to the heel and forefoot to keep the heel out of valgus. As medial posting is added, it may be necessary to lower the medial trim line to avoid impingement on the medial malleolus.

With fxed deformities, such as arthritis of the midfoot, a UCBL insert can decrease motion and reduce pain. The foot is molded in situ, and the polypropylene should have a relief over the area of bony prominence. The orthosis can be lined with a material for pressure absorption, such as polyurethane foam (PPT) in the relief, and then the entire orthosis can be covered with a material such as polyethylene foam (Plastazote) for comfort (Fig. 4-4).

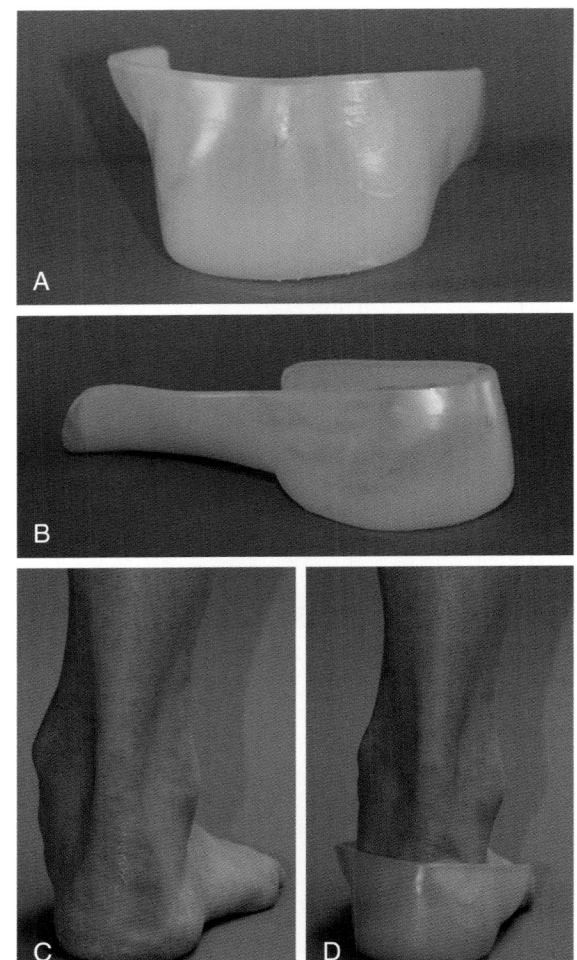

Figure 4-4 University of California Biomechanics Laboratory (UCBL) insert. **A,** Posterior view. **B,** Medial view. **C,** Posterior view of a patient with posterior tibial tendon dysfunction demonstrating hindfoot valgus, pes planus, and forefoot abduction. **D,** UCBL insert controlling foot deformity.

ANKLE–FOOT ORTHOSES

The most common type of orthosis that has proved useful in treating foot and ankle problems is the ankle–foot orthosis (AFO), made of either molded polypropylene or double-upright construction.

AFOs can be made from double uprights attached to the shoe or molded polypropylene, either as a posterior shell or incorporated into a leather lacer (Arizona brace) (Fig. 4-5). The molded AFO is more potent in most instances. The AFO can be made with a fixed or hinged ankle. The orthosis is manufactured from a positive cast of the lower limb. Modifications can be made through reliefs over bony prominences to accommodate fit, and these can be lined with material to provide comfort and protect the foot and deformity. These modifications of the orthosis allow better control of deformities and expand the use of these orthoses to rigid as well as flexible deformities.

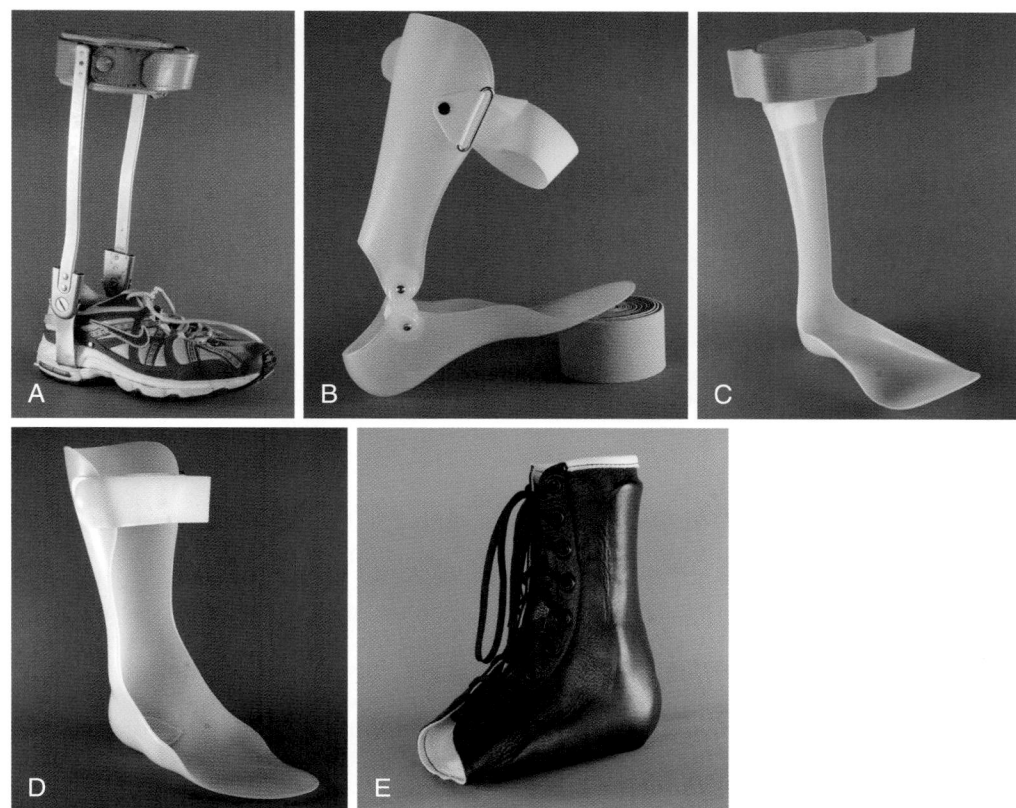

Figure 4-5 Ankle–foot orthoses (AFOs). **A,** Double upright AFO for solid control of the ankle. **B,** Dorsi-assist AFO used for patients with footdrop or foot instability. **C,** Posterior leaf spring AFO, prefabricated for stable foot and ankle and supports dropfoot. **D,** Solid ankle AFO prescribed for ankle arthritis pain and control of the foot and ankle. **E,** Arizona-style AFO.

The molded AFO can provide stability to one or several joints of the foot and ankle complex. The trim lines can be modified, depending on the rigidity desired. To diminish ankle motion, the trim lines should extend anteriorly to the midline of the malleoli, but the foot plate can end proximal or just distal to the metatarsal heads. If intending to control subtalar or transverse tarsal motion, the trim lines can be cut behind the malleoli to allow some ankle motion. If intending to control midfoot arthritis, it may be necessary to use a full foot plate to prevent pain during normal gait.

The Arizona brace AFO can be constructed with either lace or hook-and-loop (Velcro) closures. It provides stability to the hindfoot through three-point fixation similar to a short-leg cast. It has the advantage of being lower than a standard molded AFO and might have better patient acceptance.

APPLIANCES

Various appliances have been developed for the treatment of forefoot deformities. Pads and cushions can be effective in relieving pain but will not correct deformities. Padding is effective only if the shoe is the correct shape and material. Pads take up additional space within the shoe and can increase pressure if the toe box is too small.

A toe crest can be effective in relieving pressure on the tips of the toes from hammer toe and mallet toe deformities. Corn and callus pads can also relieve pressure but are more effective if the overlying callus and corn tissue is removed and the shoe is stretched over the offending prominence or a wider toe box is used. Foam or gel (Silipos) sleeves can also effectively relieve pressure (Fig. 4-6). Toe separators can be used, but lamb's wool can be equally effective between the toes and has the advantage of better absorption of moisture than the separators have.

TREATMENT OF SPECIFIC DISORDERS

Arthritis

The use of orthoses can be beneficial in the conservative therapy of arthritis of the foot and ankle by decreasing the pressure and motion across the affected joint. Orthoses should be custom molded and padded appropriately over any bony deformity. The patient must understand that an orthosis does not cure the problem but can offer a good means of controlling symptoms if he or she wishes to avoid an operation.

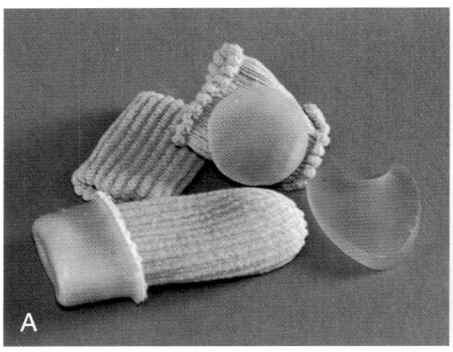 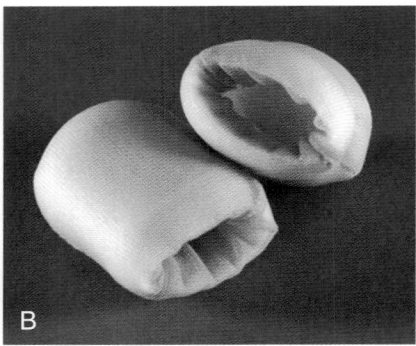 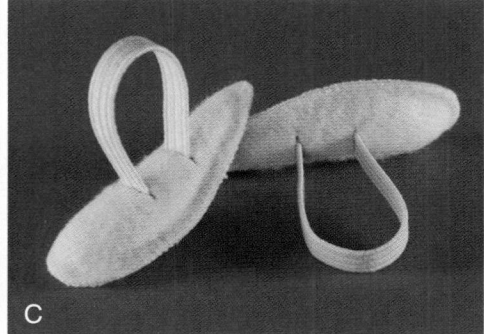

Figure 4-6 Appliances used for forefoot deformities. **A,** Silipos digital cap to relieve pressure on tip of toe; digital pads for hard corns and hammer toes; toe separators for soft corns and hallux valgus. **B,** Toe cushion digital pads. **C,** Toe crests to elevate tips of toes for hammer and mallet toe deformities.

Ankle arthritis is treated with a molded AFO with a fixed ankle or Arizona brace. In patients with normal ankles and arthritis restricted to the subtalar joint, a molded AFO with a hinged ankle or a UCBL with high trim lines can be prescribed. A solid ankle cushion heel (SACH) and rocker-bottom sole on the shoe can increase the beneficial results of the orthosis and afford the patient a more normal gait pattern. Also, if a full foot plate is used, a rocker-bottom sole should be considered. In patients with a normal ankle joint, a hinged ankle orthosis may be used to allow ankle motion.

Midfoot arthritis can be very painful and limit weight-bearing activities. In general, arthritis in this area can be treated successfully with an orthotic device. This is achieved by stabilizing affected joints and still allowing function.[21] The use of the UCBL or a carbon fiber plate may be indicated. More severe cases may be treated with an AFO and accommodative arch support. Patients often need to change the lacing pattern on their shoes to avoid pressure over dorsal spurs. A rocker-bottom sole may provide additional relief of pain and improved function.

Tendon Disorders

Chronic tendon tears can lead to significant pain and deformity if left untreated. Although surgical reconstruction has proved successful, some patients are not candidates for surgery because of concomitant medical conditions, whereas others do not wish to undergo surgical intervention. For chronic dysfunction of the Achilles, peroneal, and anterior and posterior tibial tendons, a custom-molded AFO[1,7] or Arizona brace[2] is capable of controlling symptoms. A custom articulated AFO may be one of the most potent ways to produce the greatest improvement in a flexible flatfoot deformity caused by posterior tibial tendon dysfunction (stage II). It allows some correction of the deformity and yet allows ankle motion.[1] If necessary, these orthoses can be combined with a good-quality running shoe, rocker-bottom heel, or SACH to yield a better gait pattern.

Patients should understand that the purpose of the orthosis is to control the position of the foot and hopefully prevent progression of any deformity. If significant tendon damage is present, the orthosis will not be curative, and the patient can decide between using a permanent orthosis or having reconstructive surgery.

In instances of tendinitis or early tendinosis, prolonged use of a molded AFO for ambulation can allow for healing.[26] Bracing is continued until the swelling and tenderness have resolved, and then progressive mobilization and physical therapy are prescribed. If the objective changes have not resolved within 6 months, bracing has proved not curative, and the patient has the option of continuing with bracing as the elected form of treatment or choosing surgical correction. If healing occurs, then a patient may progress to less restrictive devices before returning to full activity without appropriate support. This may involve the use of a flexible foot orthosis.

In patients with complete tendon rupture, orthoses can be used for producing pain relief and providing improved function. With chronic tendon tears or dysfunction, there can be a fixed deformity of the foot and ankle complex. For the orthosis to give the desired result, the mold must incorporate reliefs and padding over areas of deformities. An outflare heel may be needed to support the orthosis in the shoe and provide an adequate base of support in advanced deformities.

For posterior tibial tendon dysfunction (PTTD), stage I may be treated with a cast or a removeable walking boot. Once acute symptoms subside, the patient can use a foot orthosis. Stage II deformity requires a more significant support, such as an over-the-counter ankle–stirrup brace, a UCBL orthosis, or an AFO.[1,2,18] For a fixed deformity, or stage III deformity, an Arizona brace or AFO may be necessary to decrease pain, increase support, and improve function.

Heel Pain

Orthoses are frequently used to treat chronic heel pain syndrome.[3,9] Because of the difficulty in diagnosing a specific cause of heel pain, recommendations for the type of inserts vary, from the use of a rigid orthosis to soft, pliable inserts.[19] Some studies cast doubt on inserts being effective in the treatment of heel pain, but this might reflect the overprescription of these devices without the proper indications.[12,13]

In patients with atrophy of the heel fat pad, soft inserts and a well-padded shoe would be indicated. For chronic plantar fasciitis, soft inserts may be fruitful for shock absorption if overuse is a causative factor. Over-the-counter devices and appropriate shoes can be as effective as custom devices at significantly less cost. This treatment should be combined with other treatment modalities.

Night splints for the treatment of chronic plantar fasciitis maintain foot position and have been shown to be a useful treatment.[27] Although the original studies were performed using a custom-molded AFO with full foot plates, over-the-counter alternatives are now readily available and appear to be equally successful. The prefabricated foot orthosis has been found to increase the midfoot contact area, resulting in greater redistribution of force, thus reducing pressure under the heel.[3] Recent finite element analysis of the heel model quantified the effects of insole conformity, insole thickness, and insole material on pressure relief.[14] It appears that a conforming profile insert is the most important design for reducing heel-pad plantar pressure during walking. In addition, although thicker insoles give secondary pressure relief, conforming insoles should be made from stiffer material to avoid bottoming out. Flat insoles are less potent in reducing pressure.

LESSER TOE DISORDERS

Lesser toe deformities may be caused by ill-fitting footwear, such as high heels and narrow–toe box shoes. Other etiologies include those of traumatic, arthritic, idiopathic, or neuromuscular origin. Initial treatment consists of proper footwear, that is, a deeper and wider toe box. Stretching the shoe over the deformity or use of over-the-counter insoles with metatarsal pads or bars is effective. Severe or fixed deformities may need more significant treatment, such as rocker-bottom shoes, accommodative shoes, and a custom orthosis.

Calluses and Corns

Callus and corn formation occurs in response to excessive pressure over a bony prominence. This may be the consequence of a loss of the normal fat pad without deformity, secondary to pressure developing in response to deformity, or improper footwear that causes pressure on a bony prominence. Adequate management of these problems requires patient education and acceptance of appropriate shoes. Removal of the overlying hyperkeratotic tissue by paring the lesion produces significant relief of symptoms (Fig. 4-7).[28] To prevent recurrence of the

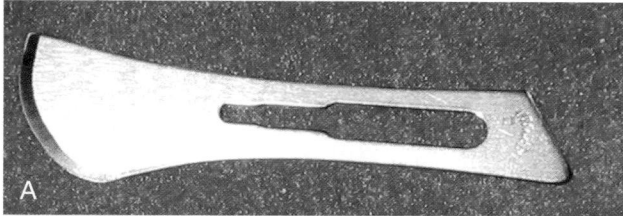
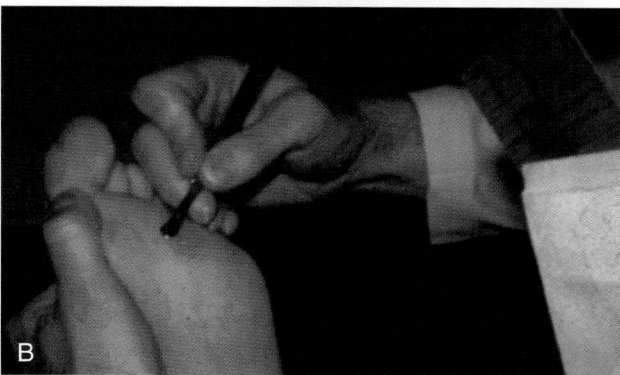

Figure 4-7 **A,** Number 17 blade for paring callus has no sharp points but rounded edges. **B,** Paring callus.

lesion, the shoe must be modified to keep pressure off the affected area.

With plantar callosities, recurrence can be prevented by an appropriately sized metatarsal pad placed proximal to the metatarsal heads. The pad can be placed directly in the shoe or integrated in a custom foot orthosis. Patients prefer the later because it can be transferred from shoe to shoe. For dorsal corns, after the removal of the hyperkeratotic tissue, toe sleeves or toe crests may be effective (see Fig. 4-6). Stretching the toe box above the affected toe also helps relieve pressure and decreases the rate and incidence of corn formation.

The commonly found corn over the dorsal and lateral aspects of the fifth toe without deformity is seen in patients wearing pointed dress shoes. Paring is initially effective; however, the lesion recurs if the footwear is not modified. If the patient is unwilling to change his or her footwear, the shoe should be prestretched with a shoemaker's wand over the affected toe to help decrease the pressure. In this instance, surgery is rarely successful if the patient is unwilling to change his or her shoe style. The success of shoe modifications when accepted by the patient makes surgery rarely indicated.

Hammer toe deformities can be treated, in part, with a metatarsal pad to relieve plantar pain. In addition, taping can add stability to the metatarsophalangeal joint with a hammer toe deformity. A strip of ¼-inch tape can be looped over the base of the toe to mimic the force of the intrinsic muscles and plantar plate (Fig. 4-8). This loop should be applied in the morning and removed at the end of the day. It can help patients with crossover toe deformities and subluxating hammer toe deformities. Another method is to use an over-the-counter toe sling or toe sleeve (see Fig. 4-6).

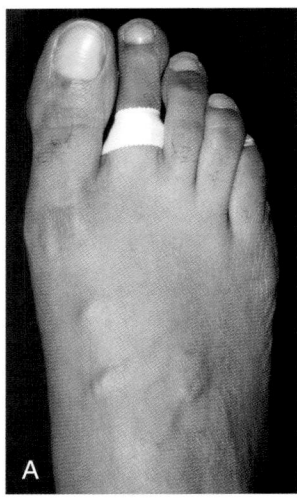
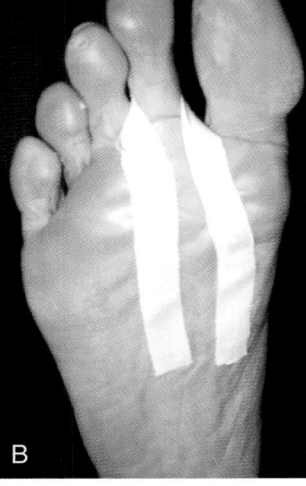

Figure 4-8 Toe taped for instability of the metatarsophalangeal joint. **A,** Dorsal view. **B,** Plantar view.

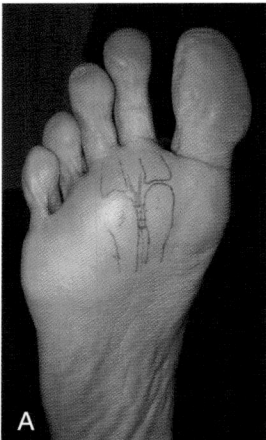
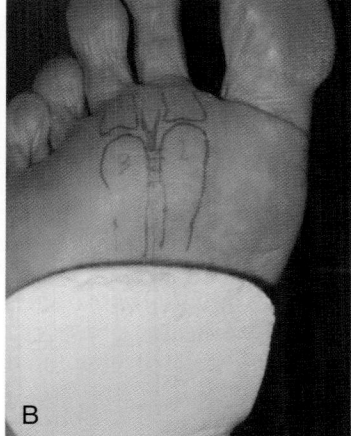

Figure 4-9 **A,** Diagram of location of Morton neuroma at the level of the transverse metatarsal ligament. **B,** Pad placement to relieve pressure proximal to the neuroma.

Neuromas

Interdigital neuromas, or Morton neuromas, can often be successfully treated with a wider shoe and appropriately placed and sized metatarsal pad (Fig. 4-9). The effect is to prevent squeezing the metatarsal heads together, as with a narrow–toe box shoe, and providing a pad to spread the metatarsals and alleviate pressure on the affected neuroma. When using these pads, the patient should be instructed to break in these devices gradually. In most cases, patients start with a small size and may increase the size of the pad if their symptoms have not been relieved once they are wearing the pad all day. Or, a custom-molded orthosis may be help decrease symptoms. If a custom orthosis is prescribed, rigid material at the distal end of the orthosis should be avoided because it may aggravate symptoms.

Bunionettes

Bunionettes can often be treated successfully by pre-stretching the shoe to avoid pressure over the bony prominence. A rounded or squared toe box can help prevent progression of the deformity.

FIRST METATARSOPHALANGEAL JOINT

Hallux Valgus Deformities

Hallux valgus deformities cannot be prevented or corrected by orthotic devices, and such devices should not be prescribed for that purpose.[10] In patients with excessive pronation, an orthotic device to reduce pronation may be helpful and can relieve valgus stress on the great toe. Nonoperative treatment of hallux valgus revolves around the choice of proper footwear to accommodate the present deformity and prevent increased valgus pressure on the great toe to reduce progression.[10] The choice of shoes is determined by the severity of the deformity. Pre-stretching of the shoe above the first metatarsophalangeal joint can be useful to relieve pressure.

In moderate-to-severe deformities, an extra-wide shoe may be required. The shoe can be pre-stretched over the bunion, and a soft leather upper should be used.

Hallux Rigidus

Hallux rigidus is an arthritic condition, and nonoperative management involves accommodating the dorsal exostosis in a roomy comfortable shoe.[25] A computational modeling approach with a three-dimensional finite element model of the first ray showed increased hallux pressures as much as 223% with restriction of metatarsophalangeal joint dorsiflexion, as with hallux rigidus.[6] The increase in pressure can be reduced using flat insoles. Therefore initial treatment consists of wearing a stiff-soled shoe. A carbon fiber plate or custom orthosis with a Morton extension can be effective in decreasing symptoms (see Fig. 4-3F). Alternatively, a shoe with a steel shank and rocker bottom can be used. Symptoms from a prominent dorsal eminence may be treated with stretching of the toe box or use of an extra-depth shoe.

Sesamoid Disorders

The sesamoids can be afflicted by inflammation, injury, or fracture. Inflammation of the sesamoids is known as sesamoiditis, and the pain is localized to the medial or lateral sesamoid. Treatment consists of casting to decrease the severe acute pain. Then a metatarsal pad placed just proximal to the sesamoids can be used. Some patients benefit from a custom orthosis with a metatarsal pad for relief at the sesamoid (see Fig. 4-3C). Adjustments may be needed for recovery, which is generally expected.

SHOE ANATOMY

The shoe protects the foot from the external environment. It is also used to decrease pressure with weight bearing, and in cases of disease or deformities, shoes are helpful in decreasing shear forces, while supporting and accommodating the foot.

The basic shoe types used are the traditional Oxford-type shoe, which allows for 0.25- to 0.375-inch depth.[17] The extra depth will allow for deformities and can accept an insert (Fig. 4-10). The shoe can be modified to improve propulsion, improve ambulation and motion, increase stability and proprioception, and to off-load areas of high pressure. These are accomplished by using flares, extended shanks, rocker soles, and relasting.

The basic anatomy of the shoe includes standard parts of the upper, outsole, heel, insole, shank, ball, forepart, toe box, and vamp (Fig. 4-11). First, the upper is the top portion of the shoe, while the outsole and heel form the bottom of the shoe. The outsole and heel has contact with the ground. On the inside of the shoe is the insole, which contacts the plantar aspect of the foot.

The shank extends from the heel breast (the front of the heel) to the ball of the shoe. The ball is the area under the metatarsal heads. The forepart extends from the ball to the tip, or end of the shoe. The toe box describes the height of the shoe at this level. The vamp, part of the upper, extends from the tip back over the ball and instep to the quarters, which join in the back of the shoe at the back seam. The Balmoral, or Bal last, shoe has the quarters meeting at the front of the throat of the shoe, with the vamp extending as the tongue beneath them. The Blucher last has the quarters loose at the inner edge and is made to be laced over the vamp and tongue.

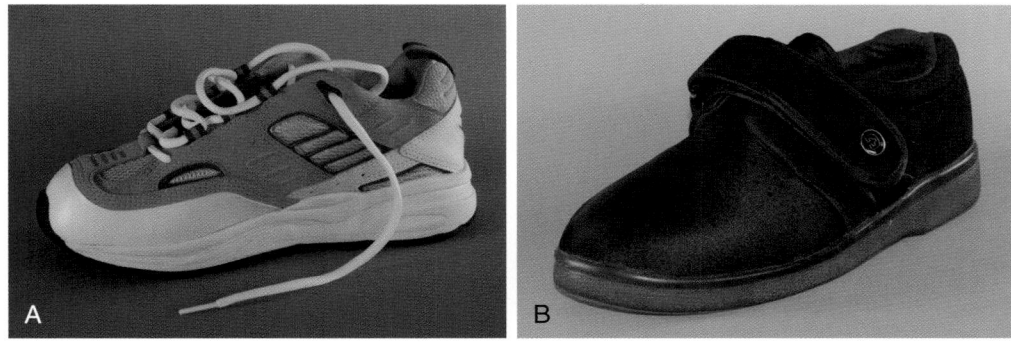

Figure 4-10 **A,** Extra-depth shoe to accommodate forefoot deformity or for use with an orthosis. **B,** Extra-depth shoe with soft material for diabetes mellitus patients.

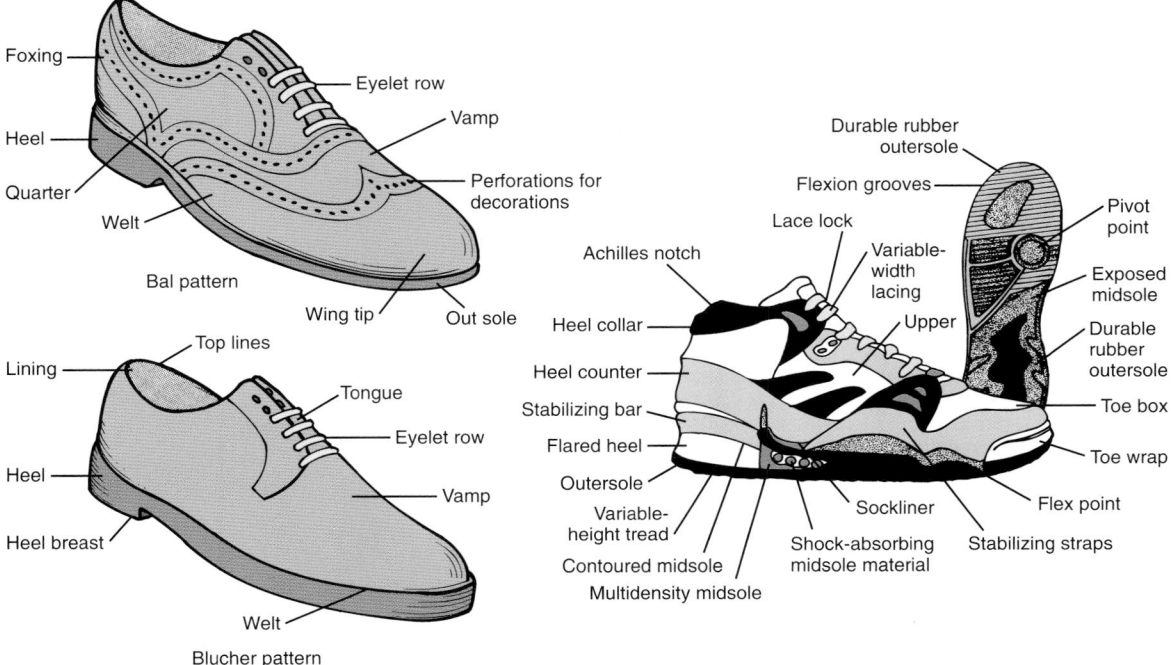

Figure 4-11 Structural components of the shoe.

The last is the three-dimensional form that the upper of the shoe is made from (Fig. 4-12). Historically, all lasts were made by hand with no distinction between the left and right foot until about 1820. In the 1850s, the ability to duplicate shoe lasts, mold the leather uppers, and attach them to the soles by machine allowed the shoemaker to progress from making 1 pair of shoes per day to more than 600 per day. Over the next century and a half, the technology of manufacturing has rapidly progressed, just as the materials available have.[15]

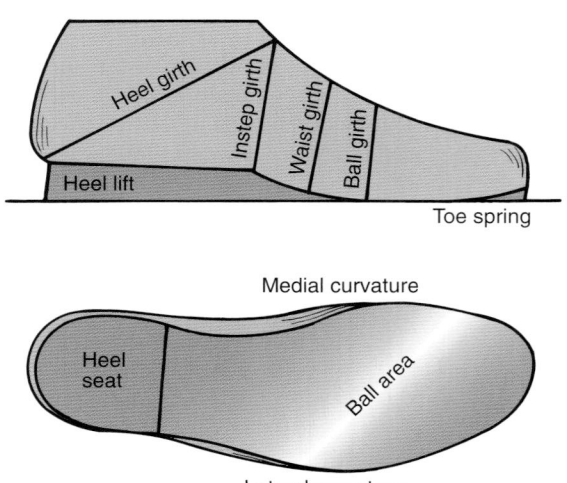

Figure 4-12 Diagram of the last, the form on which the shoe is made. (Modified from Frey C: Shoe wear and pedorthic devices. In Lutter LD, Mizel MS, Pfeffer GB, editors: *Orthopedic knowledge update: foot and ankle,* Rosemont, Ill, 1994, American Academy of Orthopaedic Surgeons.)

Lasting also describes the bottoming method that is used to attach the upper to the sole. Many techniques have been used, and one shoe can be lasted with more than one method, called *combination lasting. Slip lasting* involves sewing the upper pieces together moccasin style and gluing this to the midsole, giving a flexible construction. With *board lasting,* the upper is glued to a firm board, providing a stiff shoe; this method is often used in athletic shoes to decrease pronation. A combination last can provide stability from a board-lasted heel and flexibility from a slip-lasted forefoot (Fig. 4-13).

Types of Uppers

Many different materials are available for constructing the upper of the shoe. Traditionally, leather has been used because of its durability, moldability, and breathability. Athletic shoes are made from soft nylon, mesh nylon, and canvas reinforced at the counter, toe box, or vamp with leather, rubber, or plastics for added stability. This combination allows the shoe to be lighter but still stable. The nylon mesh shoe may be useful in accommodating deformities of the lesser toes.

Leather uppers can be stretched to accommodate forefoot deformities, but the extent of shoe deformation is limited. The toe box should have the height and width to properly fit the foot. If friction against the skin is a concern, as in a neuropathic foot, a heat-moldable foam (Thermold) upper may be used.

Several patterns of lace stays are available, and each has its own advantage (Fig. 4-14). The Blucher pattern, with no seam across the instep, has the advantage of allowing easier entry into the shoe. The Bal pattern can provide

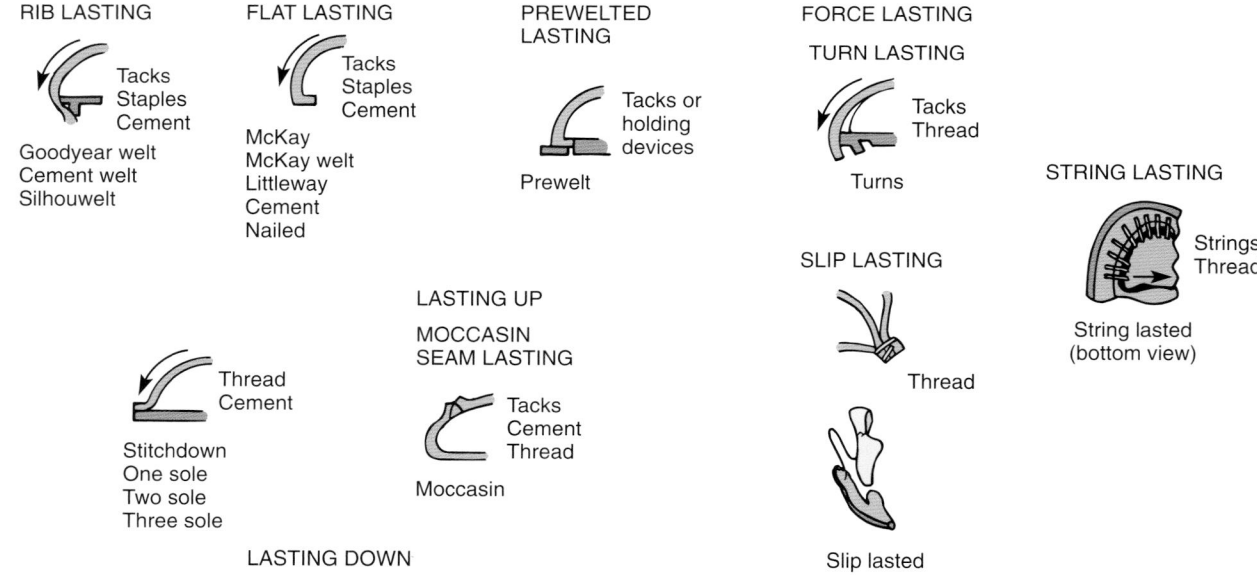

Figure 4-13 Lasting techniques used to attach the upper to the sole. (Modified from Gould N: Footwear: shoes and shoe modifications. In Jahss MH, editor: *Disorders of the foot and ankle: medical and surgical management,* ed 2, vol 3, Philadelphia, 1991, WB Saunders, p 2885.)

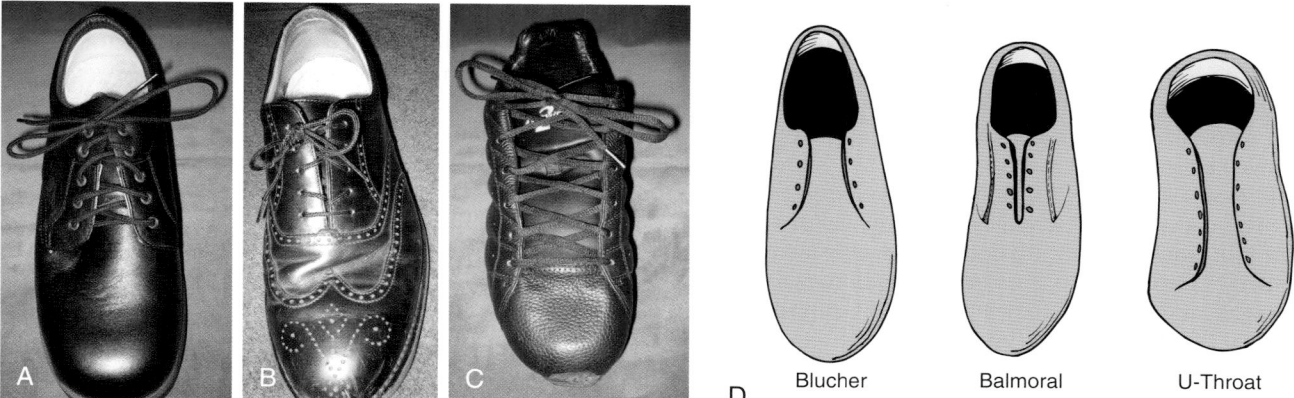

Figure 4-14   Lace stay patterns. **A,** Blucher pattern, with no seam across the instep, has the advantage of allowing easy entry into the shoe. **B,** Balmoral pattern may provide more stability, but the entry is limited and might not accept an orthotic device. **C,** The U-throat or lace-toe pattern allows the shoe to open even wider and may be useful in accepting an orthosis or allowing entry into the shoe after hindfoot fusion. **D,** Diagram of patterns of lace stays.

Blucher   Balmoral   U-Throat

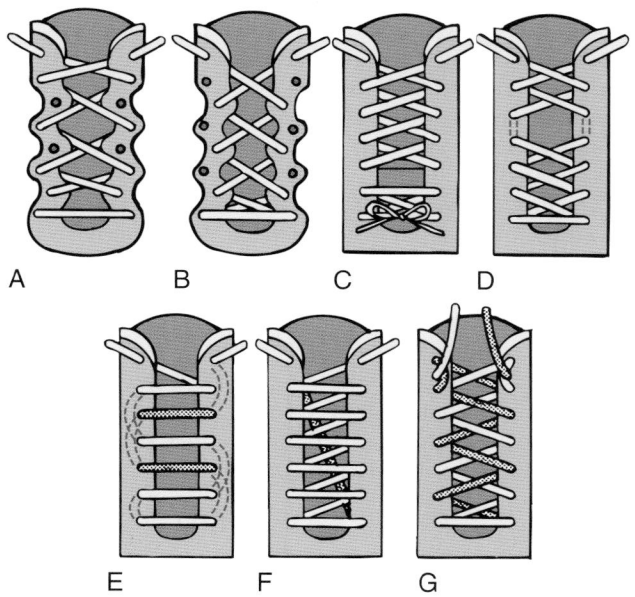

Figure 4-15   Patterns of lacing. **A,** Variable for wide fit. **B,** Variable for narrow fit. **C,** Independent, using two laces. **D,** Crisscross to avoid bony prominences. **E,** High arch pattern to avoid lacing crossing top of foot. **F,** Pull-up pattern to allow relief of pressure on toes. **G,** Crisscross loop pattern to avoid heel blisters. (Modified from Frey C: Shoe wear and pedorthic devices. In Lutter LD, Mizel MS, Pfeffer GB, editors: *Orthopedic knowledge update: foot and ankle,* Rosemont, Ill, 1994, American Academy of Orthopaedic Surgeons, p 78.)

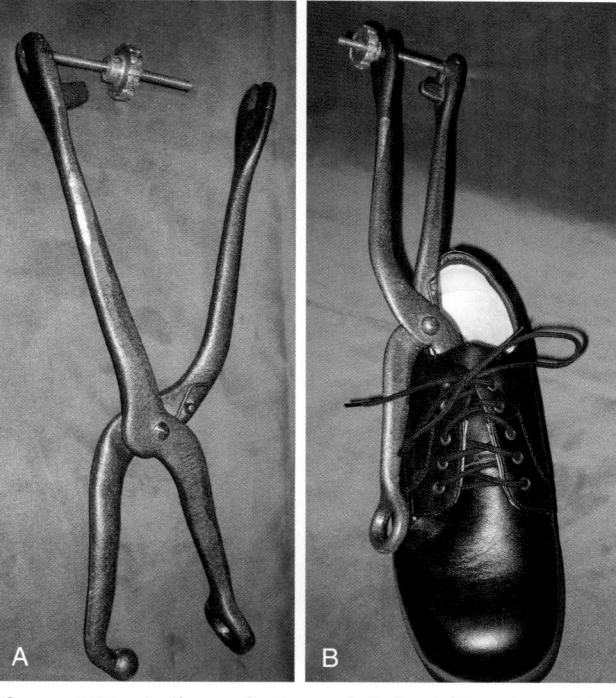

Figure 4-16   **A,** Shoemaker's wand. **B,** Stretching shoe with the wand.

more stability, but the entry is limited and might not accept an orthotic device. The U-throat and lace-toe patterns allow the shoe to open even wider and may be useful in accepting an orthosis or allowing entry into the shoe after hindfoot fusion.

Many lacing patterns can secure a better fit of the shoe (Fig. 4-15). Athletic shoes often have multiple eyelets to allow different lacing techniques. By changing the lacing to avoid crossing the dorsum of the foot, pressure can be relieved over bony prominences or a high-arched foot. Wide or narrow feet can be secured by different lacing patterns.

Once the proper material, shape, and lacing pattern of the shoe have been determined, it may still be necessary to stretch the upper to avoid pressure over bony deformities. With the patient standing and bearing full weight on the affected foot, the area of impingement can be identified and marked. A shoemaker's wand can stretch the shoe at this area (Fig. 4-16).

Types of Lasts

Shoe manufacturers have many different lasts, and there is great variation in the fit of shoes that are labeled with the same size. A shoe manufacturer might have 30 to 60 active last styles with 80 to 90 sizes for as many as 5000 different lasts.[15] Thus it is difficult to define a normal last.

The concept of a *corrective last* is not accurate because the last cannot correct a deformity. Lasts come in several general categories (Fig. 4-17). A conventional last is made in right- and left-foot shapes. A straight last has a straight medial border from heel to toe, without curving at the

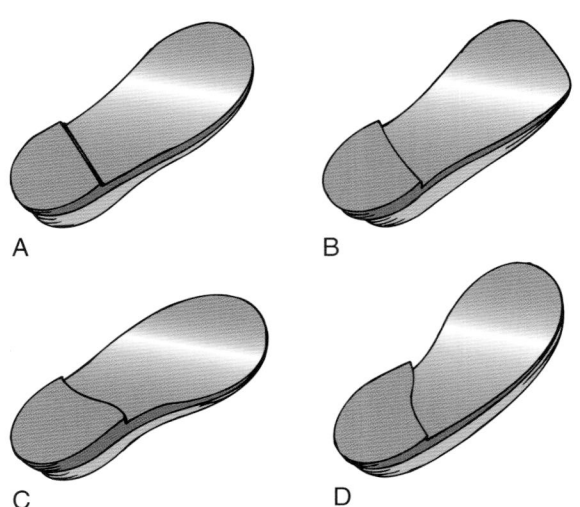

Figure 4-17 Lasts. **A,** Conventional. **B,** Straight. **C,** Outflare. **D,** Inflare. (Modified from Gould N: Footwear: Shoes and shoe modifications. In Jahss MH, editor: *Disorders of the foot and ankle: medical and surgical management,* ed 2, vol 3, Philadelphia, 1991, WB Saunders, p 2903.)

toe box. Women's dress shoes can simulate a straight last on the medial side and have the point of the toe box at the end of the great toe. The outflare last, or reverse last, flares to the lateral side of the shoe and is often used after treatment for metatarsus adductus. The inflare last curves medially and is used in athletic shoes, with a 7-degree curve to allow greater mobility of the foot.[11]

Types of Soles

Traditionally, soles of shoes were constructed of leather. In dress shoes, this material is still commonly used. Soles in athletic, work, and recreational shoes are generally made from rubber compounds. Microcellular blown rubber compounds and polyurethane are used for midsole and wedges. Black carbon rubber and styrene-butadiene are very hard-wearing compounds used for outsoles. Ethyl vinyl acetate is also commonly used in running shoes for its flexibility and impact-absorbing properties. Manufacturers often combine the blown rubber for impact resistance covered by black carbon rubber for wear on the outsole. The superior impact absorption of these rubber and synthetic materials can be used to decrease pressure and loading of the foot and ankle. As a result, many manufacturers now offer dress shoes with soles made of these materials.

Traction between the shoe and the floor can be influenced by the material of the sole and the pattern on the outsole. Various patterns have been developed for different sports. The pattern and amount of friction can also influence how well a patient with balance or proprioceptive loss can tolerate a shoe. Too much friction can cause a patient to stumble, whereas loss of friction with a slick surface can be equally dangerous.

The outsole of the shoe can be modified (Fig. 4-18). A medial wedge can be used to decrease forefoot eversion,

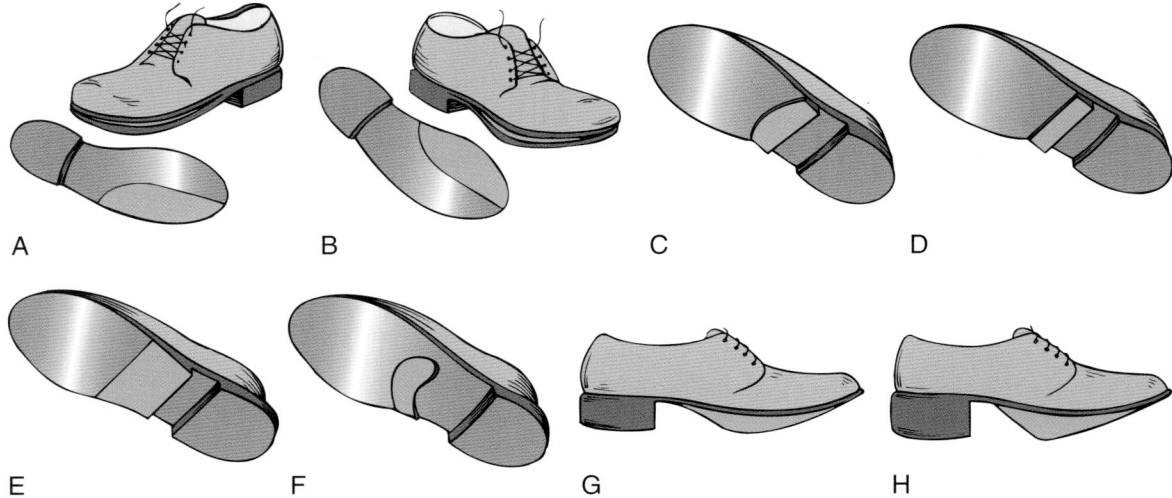

Figure 4-18 Outsole modifications. **A,** Lateral sole wedge. **B,** Medial sole wedge. **C,** Mayo metatarsal bar. **D,** Flush's metatarsal bar. **E,** Denver heel. **F,** Hauser bar. **G,** Rocker sole. **H,** Extended rocker sole. (Modified from Gould N: Footwear: shoes and shoe modifications. In Jahss MH, editor: *Disorders of the foot and ankle: medical and surgical management,* ed 2, vol 3, Philadelphia, 1991, WB Saunders, p 2907.)

and a lateral wedge can be used to decrease forefoot inversion in a flexible foot.

Various metatarsal bars have been described for treating metatarsalgia. The principle is to have the bar placed proximal to the metatarsal heads to adequately relieve pressure under the area of greatest loading.

Rocker soles are often useful in unloading the forefoot and decreasing the need for metatarsophalangeal joint dorsiflexion. Rocker soles allow a better gait pattern when used with rigid bracing of the foot and ankle (Fig. 4-19). There are five basic types of rocker soles.[17,23] The mild rocker sole is the most popular type and results in notable improvement in mild metatarsal pressure and gait by increasing forward propulsion. The other types

include heel-to-toe, toe-only, severe angle, negative heel, and double-rocker soles.

Types of Heels

The materials used for the heel are similar to those used for the sole. The decision about the material used should stem from the demands placed on the foot. Many modifications of the heel have been described (Fig. 4-20). The Thomas and Stone heels were used to help prevent pronation. Medial and lateral heel wedges help block heel eversion and inversion, respectively. These wedges should be used with a rigid heel counter to effectively grip the heel and produce the desired effect. External heel wedges have

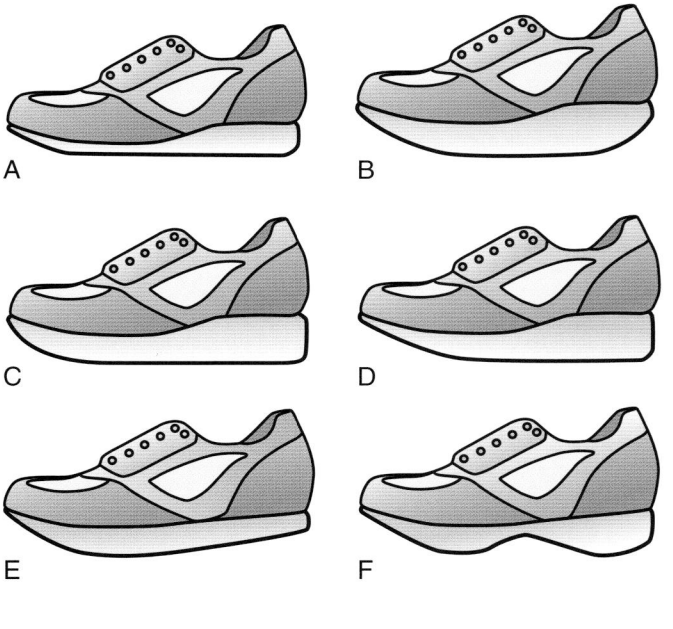

Figure 4-19 Variations of rocker soles. **A,** Mild rocker sole is the most common type used to relieve metatarsal pressure and assist in gait. **B,** Heel-to-toe sole used for increased propulsion at toe-off, decreased pressure on heel strike, and reduced need for ankle motion, such as for patients with ankle or subtalar fusion. **C,** Toe-only rocker sole is used for patients with forefoot problems, because it increases weight bearing proximal to the metatarsal heads. **D,** Severe angle is prescribed for extreme relief of metatarsal head or toe tip ulcerations. **E,** Negative heel accommodates a foot fixed in dorsiflexion or relieves forefoot pressures. **F,** Double sole is helpful for patients with midfoot pathology, such as Charcot foot. (Redrawn from Janisse DJ, Janisse E: Shoe modification and the use of orthoses in the treatment of foot and ankle pathology. *J Am Acad Orthop Surg* 16:152-158, 2008.)

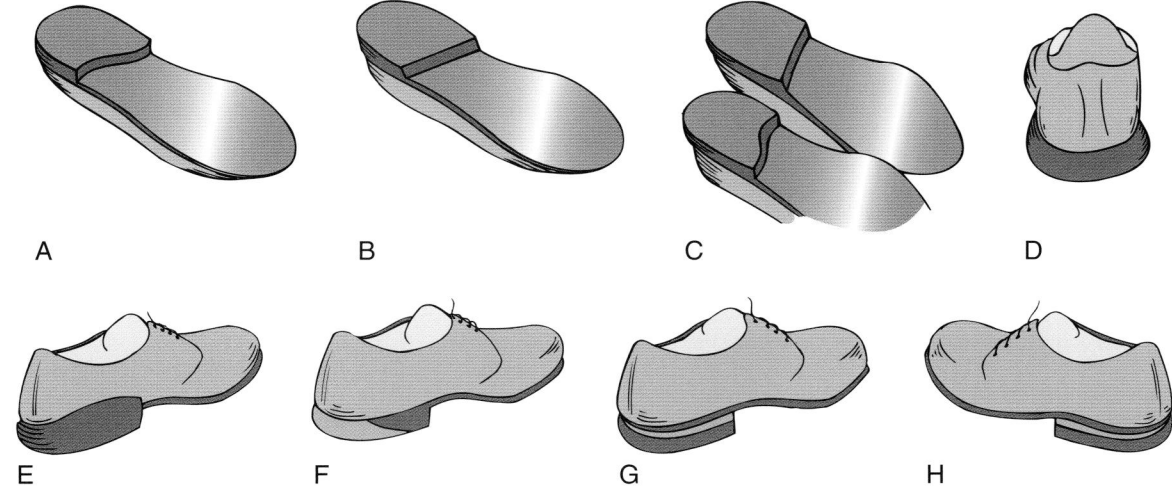

Figure 4-20 Heel modifications. **A,** Thomas heel. **B,** Stone heel. **C,** Reverse Thomas and Stone heel. **D,** Flare heel. **E,** Offset heel. **F,** Plantar flexion heel. **G,** Medial wedge heel. **H,** Lateral wedge heel. (Modified from Gould N: Footwear: shoes and shoe modifications. In Jahss MH, editor: *Disorders of the foot and ankle: medical and surgical management,* ed 2, vol 3, Philadelphia, 1991, WB Saunders, p 2906.)

an advantage over inserts by not raising the heel out of the counter, which allows for a better grasp of the heel.

Flared and offset heels allow for a broader base of support in walking. These heels decrease the amount of subtalar motion in patients with arthritis. A lateral flare can help prevent ankle sprains in patients with chronic instability. The offset heel is often useful with bracing in patients with advanced hindfoot deformities.

The SACH, or plantar flexion heel, is also useful with bracing when ankle motion is lost (see Fig. 4-20G and H). It uses a wedge of soft compressible material within the heel. It may be combined with a rocker sole to compensate for decreased ankle dorsiflexion and plantar flexion. The degree of rocker-bottom effect is controlled by the height of the heel, thickness of the wedge, and position of the rocker bottom.

Heel lifts are used to compensate for leg-length discrepancy. These may be all external or combined with an internal device on the shoe. These are often useful as a temporary device when the opposite extremity is placed in a prefabricated walking cast. These walking casts usually have a built-in rocker bottom and are higher than the patient's normal shoe. Patients who have difficulty with this temporary leg-length discrepancy can be helped by application of a lift to the opposite shoe to compensate. A heel lift may also be used when a SACH and rocker bottom have been applied to the opposite shoe.

When the outsole and heel of the shoe for postural abnormalities are modified, the shank of the shoe should afford some flexibility to allow the foot to respond to the correction applied. When arthritic conditions of the midfoot and forefoot are treated, the shank should be stiffened to decrease the motion of the foot.

The advances in shoe manufacturing and materials have led to a new popularity of running and walking shoes. In general, these shoes allow better fit of the forefoot and greater cushioning of the foot and ankle. The popularity of these shoes helps in the treatment of many foot and ankle problems without the need to prescribe the traditional orthopaedic Oxford. Patient acceptance of this type of footwear affords greater compliance with treatment.

REFERENCES

1. Alvarez RG, Marini A, Schmitt C, Saltzman CL: Stage I and II posterior tibial tendon dysfunction treated by a structured nonoperative management protocol: an orthosis and exercise program, *Foot Ankle Int* 27:2–8, 2006.
2. Augustin JF, Lin SS, Berberian WA, Johnson JE: Nonoperative treatment of adult acquired flat foot with the Arizona brace, *Foot Ankle Clin* 8:491–502, 2003.
3. Bonanno DR, Landorf KB, Menz HB: Pressure-relieving properties of various shoe inserts in older people with plantar heel pain, *Gait Posture* 33:385–389, 2011.
4. Bordelon RL: Correction of hypermobile flatfoot in children by molded inserts, *Foot Ankle Int* 1:143–150, 1980.
5. Bordelon RL: Hypermobile flatfoot in children. Comprehension, evaluation, and treatment, *Clin Orthop Relat Res* 181:7–14, 1983.
6. Budhabhatti SP, Erdemir A, Petre M, et al: Finite element modeling of the first ray of the foot: a tool for the design of interventions, *J Biomech Eng* 129:750–756, 2007.
7. Cavanagh PR, Ulbrecht JS, Zanine W, et al: A method for investigation of the effects of outsole modifications in therapeutic footwear, *Foot Ankle Int* 17:706–708, 1996.
8. Chao W, Wapner KL, Lee TH, et al: Nonoperative treatment of posterior tibial tendon dysfunction, *Foot Ankle Int* 17:736–741, 1996.
9. Drake M, Bittenbender C, Boyles RE: The short-term effects of treating plantar fasciitis with a temporary custom foot orthosis and stretching, *J Orthop Sports Phys Ther* 41:221–231, 2011.
10. Easley ME, Trnka HJ: Current concepts review: hallux valgus part 1: pathomechanics, clinical assessment, and nonoperative management, *Foot Ankle Int* 28:654–659, 2007.
11. Frey C: Shoe wear and pedorthic devices. In Lutter LD, Mizel MS, Pfeffer GB, editors: *Orthopaedic knowledge update: foot and ankle*, Rosemont, Ill, 1994, American Academy of Orthopaedic Surgeons.
12. Gill LH: Plantar fasciitis: diagnosis and conservative management, *J Am Acad Orthop Surg* 5:109–117, 1997.
13. Gill LH, Kiebzak GM: Outcome of nonsurgical treatment for plantar fasciitis, *Foot Ankle Int* 17:527–532, 1996.
14. Goske S, Erdemir A, Petre M, et al: Reduction of plantar heel pressures: insole design using finite element analysis, *J Biomech* 39:2363–2370, 2006.
15. Gould N: Footwear: Shoes and shoe modifications. In Jahss MH, editor: *Disorders of the foot and ankle: medical and surgical management*, ed 2, vol 3. Philadelphia, 1991, WB Saunders, pp 73–88.
16. Janisse DJ: The art and science of fitting shoes, *Foot Ankle Int* 13:257–262, 1992.
17. Janisse DJ, Janisse E: Shoe modification and the use of orthoses in the treatment of foot and ankle pathology, *J Am Acad Orthop Surg* 16:152–158, 2008.
18. Krause F, Bosshard A, Lehmann O, Weber M: Shell brace for stage II posterior tibial tendon insufficiency, *Foot Ankle Int* 29:1095–1100, 2008.
19. Mizel MS, Marymount JV, Trepman E: Treatment of plantar fasciitis with a night splint and shoe modification consisting of a steel shank and anterior rocker bottom, *Foot Ankle Int* 17:732–735, 1996.
20. Owings TM, Woerner JL, Frampton JD, et al: Custom therapeutic insoles based on both foot shape and plantar pressure measurement provide enhanced pressure relief, *Diabetes Care* 31:839–844, 2008.
21. Patel A, Rao S, Nawoczenski D, et al: Midfoot arthritis, *J Am Acad Orthop Surg* 18:417–425, 2010.
22. Perera AM, Mason L, Stephens MM: The pathogenesis of hallux valgus, *J Bone Joint Surg Am* 93:1650–1661, 2011.
23. Perry JE, Ulbrecht JS, Derr JA, et al: The use of running shoes to reduce plantar pressures in patients who have diabetes, *J Bone Joint Surg Am* 77:1819–1826, 1995.
24. Rozema A, Ulbrecht MB, Pammer SE, et al: In-shoe plantar pressures during activities of daily living: implications for therapeutic footwear design, *Foot Ankle Int* 17:352–359, 1996.
25. Shurnas PS: Hallux rigidus: etiology, biomechanics, and nonoperative treatment, *Foot Ankle Clin* 14:1–8, 2009.
26. Solan M, Davies M: Management of insertional tendinopathy of the Achilles tendon, *Foot Ankle Clin* 12:597–615, 2007.
27. Wapner KL, Sharkey PF: The use of night splints for treatment of recalcitrant plantar fasciitis, *Foot Ankle Int* 12:135–137, 1991.
28. Young MJ, Cavanagh PR, Thomas G, et al: The effect of callus removal on dynamic foot pressures in diabetic patients, *Diabet Med* 9:55–57, 1992.

Anesthesia

Jeffrey Swenson, Jennifer J. Davis

OVERVIEW

This chapter contains a review of the pharmacologic and procedural therapies available for pain control after foot and ankle surgery. The focus is on new techniques and pharmacologic agents. Recent progress in acute pain management is a product of changing patient demographics as well as advances in technology.

For several years, opioids have been used as a primary therapy to provide postoperative analgesia. However, as the population ages and has a higher rate of obesity, the side effects of opioids become more concerning. Opioid-induced respiratory depression is a life-threatening risk that increases with age and obesity. Nausea, vomiting, constipation, and pruritus are major sources of patient dissatisfaction that must be overcome as more procedures are performed in an ambulatory setting. Finally, many more patients are now treated with opioids for chronic pain conditions. For patients consuming opioids chronically, efficacy in the acute pain setting is markedly reduced. All of these factors contribute to a growing interest in finding effective methods to reduce opioid requirements by using "nonopioid" alternatives for pain control.

A CHANGING ROLE FOR OPIOIDS

The American Society of Anesthesiologists and the American College of Chest Physicians have both published guidelines for the perioperative management of patients with known or suspected obstructive sleep apnea (OSA).[2,45] These guidelines highlight the association of opioids with adverse respiratory events during the postoperative period. They also stress the importance of screening patients preoperatively for signs or symptoms of OSA because up to 70% of patients who suffer from this disorder have not been diagnosed at the time of surgery.[37] A common theme in all guidelines for perioperative management of OSA is the need to reduce or eliminate opioid analgesics during the postoperative period.

The rate of opioid prescription in the United States has changed dramatically in response to increased pressure placed on physicians to treat pain. The Centers for Disease Control and Prevention report that the distribution of prescription opioids through the pharmaceutical supply chain increased more than 600% between 1997 and 2007.[73] Since 2003, opioid analgesics have been the cause of more deaths from overdose than cocaine and heroin combined.[73] This increase in opioid abuse and accidental deaths has also been a catalyst for efforts to decrease the role of opioids as the primary analgesics after surgery.

MULTIMODAL ANALGESIA

Multimodal analgesia is the practice of combining more than one type of analgesic to optimize pain control while minimizing the adverse effects of individual agents.[70,90,109]

Table 5-1 Drug Categories That Can Be Used Concurrently in Multimodal Analgesia

Drug Category	Mechanism of Action	Dosing	Special Considerations
Gabapentinoids			
Pregabalin	Voltage-dependent calcium channels at central/peripheral nerves	75-100 mg bid	Reduces opioid use and opioid side effects
			May reduce chronic pain at surgery site
NSAIDs			NSAIDs (nonspecific):
Ibuprofen (oral)	Inhibition of cyclooxygenase (nonspecific)	400-800 mg tid	Potential renal toxicity
			Platelet inhibition
Ketorolac (IV)		15-30 mg qid	Cardiovascular risk
			Gastric mucosa effects
			Potent analgesic
			Higher gastric mucosa
			Toxicity compared with other
Celecoxib	COX-2 specific	200 mg bid	NSAIDs:
			Reduced platelet effect
			Reduced gastric toxicity
			Cardiovascular risk
			Potential renal toxicity
Acetaminophen	CNS inhibition of cyclooxygenase, modulation of central serotonin		Well tolerated
			Caution with hepatic disease
Acetaminophen (IV) (paracetamol)		Up to 1 g qid	Reliable plasma levels in the perioperative period
Acetaminophen (oral)		Up to 1 g qid	May not produce therapeutic levels in perioperative period
Combined Mu Agonist/ Norepinephrine-Serotonin Reuptake Inhibitors	Mu agonist/inhibition of norepinephrine-serotonin reuptake		Caution with other serotonin reuptake inhibitors such as antidepressants
Tramadol	Inhibits both serotonin and norepinephrine reuptake	50-100 mg qid	Lower risk of tolerance, dependence
Tapentadol	Norepinephrine reuptake inhibition only	50-75 mg qid	Lower risk of tolerance, dependence, nausea, constipation

bid, Two times per day; *COX-2,* cyclooxygenase-2; *CNS,* central nervous system; *IV,* intravenous; *NSAIDs,* nonsteroidal antiiflammatory drugs; *qid,* four times per day; *tid,* three times per day.

It is a promising way to decrease or eliminate the role of opioids in postoperative pain control. A number of pharmacologic agents can be used concurrently to provide analgesia, including nonsteroidal antiinflammatory drugs (NSAIDs), acetaminophen, gabapentinoids, mu agonists, and serotonin/norepinephrine reuptake inhibitors (Table 5-1). Peripheral nerve blocks also provide a major component in reducing opioid requirements.[48] The increased availability of high-resolution ultrasound has greatly facilitated the use of peripheral nerve blocks as a component of multimodal analgesia.

COMPONENTS OF MULTIMODAL ANALGESIA

Nonsteroidal Antiinflammatory Drugs

Nonsteroidal antiinflammatory drugs belong to broad class of medications used to treat pain and inflammation. The mechanism of action for these agents is to block the production of prostaglandins. This effect is achieved by the inhibition of cyclooxygenase. At least two isoenzymes

(COX-1, COX-2) have been identified for cyclooxygenase. The COX-1 isoenzyme has been called a "housekeeping" enzyme responsible for maintaining physiologic functions of the gastrointestinal tract, platelets, and kidneys. The COX-2 isoenzyme is involved primarily in production of prostaglandins that intensify the inflammatory response.[15]

Nonspecific NSAIDs are effective for relieving pain and inflammation but are also associated with platelet dysfunction, gastrointestinal toxicity, renal toxicity, cardiovascular risk, and the potential for impaired bone and connective tissue healing. The introduction of COX-2–specific NSAIDs (referred to as coxibs) has been an attempt to reduce or eliminate two of these unwanted effects, namely, gastrointestinal and platelet effects.[43,88] At present, celecoxib is the only COX-2–specific NSAID available for use in the United States. Other coxibs, such as rofecoxib and valdecoxib, have been removed amid concerns that they are associated with increased cardiovascular risk. Clinicians should be mindful that all NSAIDs (COX-2–specific and nonspecific NSAIDs) must be used with caution in patients at increased risk of cardiovascular disease.[63,85]

Gastrointestinal side effects of NSAIDs are more common in older patients, those with a prior history of peptic ulcer disease, and those receiving aspirin.[91] The improved gastrointestinal tolerance with celecoxib and other COX-2–specific NSAIDs is expected because these drugs were developed in part to reduce gastrointestinal side effects. When using nonspecific COX inhibitors, however, the incidence of gastrointestinal side effects can also be significantly reduced with proton pump inhibitors.[52,57]

Although all NSAIDs can be associated with cardiovascular risk, the COX-2–specific drugs have been the subject of most recent reports of edema, ventricular dysfunction, and cardiac ischemia. The cardiovascular risk associated with these drugs is thought to be partly the result of a relative imbalance of prostacyclin and thromboxane.[49] At present, only one COX-2 inhibitor (celecoxib) remains approved for use in the United States by the Food and Drug Administration (FDA). The early clinical evidence suggesting cardiovascular risk related to NSAIDs was largely associated with prolonged use; however, recent studies suggest that increased cardiovascular risk occurs almost immediately after initiation of therapy.[85]

Bone and soft tissue healing are additional concerns with the use of all NSAIDs. Reviews of in vitro and animal studies document changes in bone and soft tissue healing associated with NSAID use.[16,78] Although clinical data do not consistently show outcome differences in patients treated with NSAIDs,[51] there is enough evidence to justify careful consideration before their use. A reasonable approach for the use of NSAIDs in the perioperative period is to limit or avoid their use in patient populations or procedures that typically have high rates of failure or nonunion.[6,75]

A common question that arises with the use of celecoxib is whether it can be used safely in patients who have a history of allergy to sulfonamide antibiotics. Meta-analyses suggest there is a greater incidence of allergic reactions, in general, among patients with sulfonamide hypersensitivity; however, there is not an increased risk specific to celecoxib.[72,92]

Acetaminophen and Paracetamol

Acetaminophen and its parenteral form, paracetamol, are commonly used in conjunction with opioids for postoperative analgesia. The mechanisms of action for these drugs is not well defined but has been linked to cyclooxygenase inhibition in the central nervous system (CNS) as well as central modulation of the serotonin system.[13,44] Both agents are well tolerated, with relatively few side effects.

Paracetamol, the intravenous formulation of acetaminophen, was approved for use in the United States in 2011. A unique application for paracetamol is for patients who cannot take oral acetaminophen. There seems to be little difference in analgesic efficacy between oral and parenteral forms of acetaminophen if therapeutic levels are achieved. However, at least two studies comparing plasma levels in surgical patients after preoperative dosing of oral acetaminophen or parenteral paracetamol show therapeutic plasma levels are reliably achieved only when intravenous paracetamol is used.[17,99] In fact, less than 50% of subjects receiving oral doses achieved therapeutic plasma concentrations.[17]

Combining Paracetamol (Acetaminophen) and Nonsteroidal Antiinflammatory Drugs

An important aspect of multimodal analgesia that can be easily overlooked is the simple practice of combining acetaminophen (or paracetamol) with an NSAID. This approach has been evaluated in the setting of paracetamol alone versus the combination as well as NSAIDs alone versus the combination. In both situations, there were significant reductions in both pain scores and opioid requirements.[55,68] An especially appealing aspect of this practice is that many of the studies showing improved pain control involved ibuprofen and acetaminophen, which are inexpensive and easily accessible by patients.

Pregabalin and Gabapentin

Pregabalin and gabapentin are unique drugs that are structurally related to gamma-aminobutyric acid. They act by binding to voltage-dependent calcium channels in the central and peripheral nervous system and thereby alter the release of excitatory neurotransmitters.[40] These actions produce anticonvulsant, antihyperalgesic, and anxiolytic effects.[110]

Although both drugs are used for pain control, pregabalin has some unique characteristics that make it well suited for postoperative analgesia. Compared with gabapentin, pregabalin has faster onset, more predictable plasma concentrations, and fewer side effects.[40] Pregabalin has been studied in a number of perioperative settings and found to reduce opioid requirements as well as opioid-related side effects.[4,14,35,97] The most commonly reported side effects of pregabalin are dizziness and somnolence.

Clinical effect is achieved rapidly after oral administration of pregabalin. There is early onset of analgesia, and peak plasma concentrations are reached within 1 hour.[10] Pregabalin has been studied in a range of doses as an adjunct for postoperative pain control. Although a typical starting dose is 75 mg bid, effective doses for reducing perioperative opioid requirements ranged up to 150 mg bid.[58,110]

A unique finding in patients treated with pregabalin in the perioperative period is a lower incidence of chronic pain associated with surgery. For example, patients treated with pregabalin after total knee arthroplasty had a significantly lower incidence of chronic neuropathic pain

---

at 6 months compared with controls.[20] Likewise, functional outcomes and pain scores at 3 months after lumbar diskectomy were improved in patients treated perioperatively with pregabalin.[19]

Opioid Agonists

Opioids produce analgesia through agonist activity at mu receptors in the central nervous system. However, in addition to analgesia, all opioids are associated with abuse potential, respiratory depression, nausea, constipation, and pruritus. Despite these unwanted side effects, opioids still are the primary analgesics prescribed by most clinicians.

Anecdotal differences with respect to nausea, pruritus, and analgesic efficacy are a common reason for "opioid swapping" in clinical practice. However, the continued publication of reviews on the management of opioid-related side effects suggests that no particular opioid has emerged as "clearly superior" with respect to side-effect profile.[8,93] Opioids such as oxycodone, hydrocodone, and hydromorphone may differ with respect to potency and dosing interval; however, they are surprisingly similar in terms of analgesic efficacy and side-effect profile when compared in equipotent doses.

The most successful measures for reducing opioid-related side effects have resulted from reducing their dose requirements through multimodal analgesia.[61]

Combined Opioid Agonist–Monoamine Reuptake Inhibitors

Tramadol and tapentadol are analgesics that act through a dual mechanism of opioid receptor activity and mono-amine reuptake inhibition.[67] In the case of tramadol, reuptake of both serotonin and norepinephrine are inhibited.[32] For tapentadol, only norepinephrine levels are affected.[38]

A notable difference between tramadol and tapentadol and equipotent doses of traditional opioids is their potential for respiratory depression. These drugs do not rely on mu agonist activity as their sole mechanism for analgesia. As such, there is some evidence to suggest they may associated with less respiratory depression than conventional opioids at doses providing comparable levels of analgesia.[53,76,77,87] Respiratory depression is always a concern when treating postoperative pain, and certain patient populations are especially at risk. Thus tramadol and tapentadol, while still associated with respiratory depression, may be preferable for patients at risk for obstructive sleep apnea or with other specific risk factors for respiratory depression.

A unique characteristic of tapentadol is its low incidence of gastrointestinal side effects. Compared with other commonly prescribed opioids, tapentadol causes significantly less nausea, vomiting, and constipation.[47,67] Thus, in patients in whom these symptoms are problematic, tapentadol may be especially advantageous. This decrease in nausea and other gastrointestinal side effects has not been observed to the same degree for tramadol.

Serotonin and norepinephrine reuptake inhibition have been shown to produce analgesia even in the absence of mu receptor activity. Duloxetine, a selective serotonin and norepinephrine reuptake inhibitor, has been reported to significantly reduce opioid requirements by more than 30% after knee arthroplasty.[50]

In light of their effect on monoamine reuptake inhibition, caution should be used before prescribing tramadol or tapentadol in combination with other drugs that might increase CNS serotonin or norepinephrine concentrations. Serotonin syndrome is a potentially life-threatening condition that may develop in patients treated with drugs whose mechanism of action involves increased CNS serotonin and norepinephrine levels.[67] This syndrome is also known to be associated with the use of this class of drugs in patients treated with opioid analgesics.

PATIENTS WHO REQUIRE SPECIAL CONSIDERATION

Obstructive Sleep Apnea

Obstructive sleep apnea is a breathing disorder that is often not diagnosed until surgery. In a recent review, it was reported that more than 70% of patients with OSA were not diagnosed until their preoperative evaluation.[2] Unfortunately, OSA may first be detected in the perioperative period as a result of a respiratory or cardiac complication. After surgery, OSA may manifest as hypoxemia, cardiac ischemia, delirium, and arrhythmias. Because of its association with obesity and increased age, the prevalence of OSA has increased steadily in recent years.

The American College of Chest Physicians and the American Society of Anesthesiologists (ASA) have outlined treatment guidelines for screening and perioperative management of OSA patients.[2,45] Their recommendations include specific aspects of the preoperative, intraoperative, and postoperative care.

In the preoperative evaluation, it is important to conduct a directed history and physical examination in all patients because many with OSA are undiagnosed at the time of surgery. Specific questionnaires have been developed to screen for OSA. These include the STOP-BANG and ASA questionnaires that stratify patients as low or high risk for OSA. The STOP-BANG scoring system uses a mnemonic to present an eight-point evaluation validated by Chung et al.[27] Specifically, the questionnaire identifies loud snoring (S), daytime tiredness (T), observed apnea during sleep (O), and treatment for high blood pressure (P). The other characteristics associated with OSA are body mass index (BMI) greater than 35 kg/m^2 (B), age greater than 50 years (A), neck circumference greater than 40 cm (N), and male gender (G). Patients with three or more of these eight criteria are considered high risk for OSA.

The intraoperative management of patients with OSA is focused on avoiding anesthetics that have a prolonged effect on recovery of spontaneous ventilation. Thus it seems reasonable to favor regional over general anesthesia and to use short-acting anesthetics whenever possible. However, despite the logic of these strategies, there are no prospective trials showing improved outcomes with any specific anesthetic technique.[28] There is consensus, however, about the practice of minimizing the use of opioids in the perioperative period. Patients with OSA have an increased sensitivity to respiratory depression caused by opioid analgesics compared with controls without OSA.[18,103]

An important question with respect to postoperative management of OSA patients is whether they should be candidates for ambulatory surgery. There is little prospective information on outcome for OSA patients having outpatient surgery. The ASA has suggested that management of OSA patients should be based on three factors. These factors include the severity of their OSA symptoms, the scale of surgery/anesthesia performed, and the anticipated need for postoperative opioid analgesics. Only patients who have minimally invasive procedures requiring little or no postoperative opioids are considered for ambulatory surgery. Table 5-2 contains a summary of the preoperative, intraoperative, and postoperative considerations in patients at risk for OSA.

Chronic Opioid-Consuming Patients

In recent years, there has been a significant increase in the number of patients treated chronically with opioids. These patients present a unique challenge in the perioperative period for several reasons. First, tolerance can develop very rapidly after initiating therapy with opioid analgesics.[25,46,100] There is considerable evidence to suggest that chronic opioid use may even cause a hyperalgesic state in some patients.[60] Thus, during the postoperative period, chronic opioid-consuming patients may report higher pain scores despite having higher levels of sedation when compared with opioid-naïve controls.[79] In fact, the incidence of severe sedation postoperatively in opioid-tolerant patients is more than twice that of opioid-naïve controls. It has been suggested that lethal overdoses of opioid in chronic users may be due to a narrowing of the ratio between analgesic and lethal plasma concentrations.[104]

As with OSA patients, nonopioid analgesics and peripheral nerve blocks should be utilized wherever possible to provide improved pain control. Use caution when trying to achieve a specific "pain score." As previously stated, chronic opioid-consuming patients typically report higher pain scores at rest and with movement despite having higher levels of sedation.[79] Thus an objective measure of opioid effect, such as respiratory rate, is appropriate for maintaining safety.

When dosing opioids in the postoperative period, it should be noted that opioid-tolerant patients may require

Table 5-2 Perioperative Management of Patients with Obstructive Sleep Apnea

Preoperative Management
Screen all patients for signs/symptoms of obstructive sleep apnea (OSA) with a validated protocol such as STOP-BANG.[27]
S—Loud Snoring
T—Daytime Fatique, Tiredness
O—Observed Apnea during Sleep
P—High Blood Pressure

B—Body Mass Index (BMI) > 35 kg/m^2
A—Age > 50 years
N—Neck Circumference > 40 cm
G—Male Gender
Patients with a documented history of OSA or with three or more positive findings on STOP-BANG screening should be identified as high risk for OSA and informed of the likely need for hospital admission after surgery.
Patients with a known history of OSA who are already treated with continuous positive airway pressure (CPAP) should bring their device from home.

Intraoperative Management
Where reasonable, regional anesthesia or peripheral nerve block for anesthesia and postoperative analgesia should be provided.
Use short-acting anesthetics and minimize the use of opioids.

Postoperative Management
Ambulatory surgery may be appropriate for the following patients:
Those who have had only regional or local anesthesia
Those who require minimal or no postoperative opioid analgesics
For Hospitalized Patients
Consider nonopioid analgesia and peripheral nerve blocks wherever possible.
Maintain patient in semiupright position to avoid airway obstruction (avoid supine position).
Continue the use of CPAP for patients already on this therapy at home.
Monitor with continuous pulse-oximetry.

See references 2, 27, 28, and 45.

significantly greater doses than opioid-naïve patients.[31,71] Patients should have their preoperative opioid doses restarted as soon as it is practical. Additional analgesia should be provided ideally with nerve blocks and nonopioid analgesics. Additional opioids should be available "prn" but not as long-acting, scheduled doses. Practical considerations for the postoperative management of opioid tolerant patients are found in Table 5-3.

Because of the increased potential for opioid-related respiratory depression, inpatient monitoring and supplemental oxygen should be considered for opioid-tolerant patients having surgery associated with significant postoperative pain. Consideration should also be given to scheduling these patients earlier in the day to allow adequate time in the perioperative anesthetic care unit (PACU) to safely determine appropriate postoperative care and disposition (inpatient or ambulatory).

Table 5-3 Practical Considerations for Chronic Opioid-Consuming Patients

1. Instruct the patient and family that safety is the primary goal. For that reason, respiratory rate and level of consciousness will be used to regulate opioid administration rather than by pain score alone.
2. Preoperative opioid doses should restarted as soon as is practical. Additional opioids to treat acute pain should be prescribed as immediate-release only and scheduled on a "prn" basis.
3. Schedule these patients early in the day to allow adequate time in the perioperative anesthetic care unit and in the patient's room (if hospitalized) to observe the planned analgesic regimen and adjust as needed during normal working hours.
4. Utilize all additional elements of multimodal analgesics where appropriate, including nonsteroidal antiiflammatory drugs, pregabalin, acetaminophen (paracetamol), peripheral nerve blocks, and mixed mu agonist/monoamine reuptake inhibitors (tramadol/tapentadol).
5. Patients requiring large doses of opioids should be cared for in a monitored setting with continuous pulse oximetry and supplemental oxygen.

REGIONAL ANESTHESIA

Recent advances in technology have had a significant impact on regional anesthesia. The introduction of portable, high-resolution ultrasound (US) is largely responsible for a resurgence of interest in peripheral nerve blocks. Ultrasound use has increased dramatically as a result of the combined effects of decreased equipment cost and remarkable improvement in image quality. In addition, imaging platforms are now extremely portable, with many devices being as small as hand-held computers.

Significant advances have also been made in the use of continuous peripheral nerve blocks. As more complex procedures are performed on an outpatient basis, there is an increased need to provide safe and effective analgesia without relying solely on opioid analgesics. Continuous peripheral nerve blocks can facilitate pain management in a number of patients for whom opioids are unsuitable.

Ultrasound-Guided Peripheral Nerve Blocks

For many years, electrical nerve stimulation (NS) was the "gold standard" technique for performing nerve blocks. Despite an absence of data showing a consistent relationship between the stimulating needle current and the distance to the nerve,[12,81,82,98] NS remained popular due to the lack of any alternative method to guide needle placement.

A troubling aspect of NS-guided blocks is the frequency with which they result in unintentional needle trauma and intraneural injection.[82] In a recent study of sciatic nerve (SN) blocks performed using NS guidance, 94% of patients experienced unintended nerve penetration and intraneural injection.[83] This high rate of intraneural injection reflects the inability to consistently produce motor response from the stimulating needle even when it is positioned on or within the target nerve.[82,98]

There is considerable disparity in the rate of neurologic complications reported for patients having NS-guided blocks. For example, in the previously mentioned study, where the authors described a 94% rate of intraneural injection, there were no reported neuropathies.[83] By contrast, in a larger series of NS-guided SN catheters placed for foot and ankle surgery, 41% of patients reported postoperative neuropathic symptoms. Of these patients, 11% required extra hospital visits specifically for treatment of neurologic symptoms.[41] Thus, although the actual incidence of nerve injury associated with NS block may vary, laboratory and clinical data confirm that needle trauma and intraneural injection are not only uncomfortable for the patient[36] but injurious to the nerve as well.[29,39,80,86,106]

The introduction of high-resolution US has been an important development in regional anesthesia. Although initially viewed by some as a novelty or merely a supplement to NS techniques,[11] US is now established as the preferred method for performing nerve blocks. Indeed, when compared with NS techniques, blocks performed using US have higher success rates, less procedure-related pain, fewer vascular punctures, fewer needle passes, lower local anesthetic requirements, and shorter performance times.[1,42,59,62,64,74] Perhaps even more compelling, when NS is used in an attempt to supplement US guidance, nerve blocks take longer to perform and require more needle passes.[34,89]

Continuous Peripheral Nerve Block (Video Clips 7)

After orthopedic surgery, severe pain may persist for 2 to 3 days. Although single-injection nerve blocks (SINB) can provide analgesia for up to 24 hours, blocks of this duration require large volumes of concentrated local anesthetics and are associated with dense motor and sensory effect. By contrast, continuous peripheral nerve block (CPNB) can be used to provide prolonged analgesia by using low volumes of dilute local anesthetic. Thus flexibility with respect to duration and block density can be achieved while avoiding the need for large and potentially toxic doses of local anesthetic.

The ability to provide prolonged analgesia without dense motor and sensory effect is appealing because many patients report decreased satisfaction when the extremity is "too numb" or "immobile." Limb neglect caused by dense motor and sensory block may also result in positioning injury and falls.[84,94,107] Emerging data for dilute local anesthetic infusions suggest that lower concentrations are associated with improved motor function without compromise in pain scores or patient satisfaction. After shoulder surgery, low concentration interscalene blocks (0.125% vs. 0.25% bupivacaine) provided comparable analgesia and patient satisfaction but with improved diaphragm function and higher oxygen saturation.[96]

Continuous nerve block can facilitate outpatient management for procedures that historically have required hospital admission for pain control. In one series, patients were successfully treated as outpatients after open treatment of calcaneus fracture.[54] This resulted in a cost savings of more than $4000 per patient. Thus CPNB may not only provide excellent analgesia, but may also result in reduced health care costs.

The benefits of CPNB are increasingly apparent as more complex procedures are performed on an outpatient basis. It should be noted, however, that there is considerable variability between institutions regarding placement and management of continuous peripheral catheters. Some common trends, however, include a dominant influence of ultrasound to guide catheter placement and recognition that patients can manage and remove their catheters at home with minimal supervision.

Equipment costs are important in all aspects of patient care. With this in mind, it should be noted that a wide variety of infusion pumps are available for continuous peripheral nerve blocks. Although some very costly pumps are programmable and feature variable infusion rates with bolus capability,[56] excellent results can be obtained using less expensive fixed-rate elastomeric pumps.[94,105] In comparisons between simple, fixed-rate elastomeric pumps and pumps featuring variable-rate and bolus capability, fixed-rate elastomeric pumps were associated with higher patient satisfaction and fewer technical problems.[23] Thus many institutions experienced in the use of CPNB have adopted the use of simple elastomeric pumps for both economic and patient satisfaction reasons.

Nerve Blocks above the Knee

Sciatic Nerve Block at the Level of the Popliteal Fossa (Video Clips 6)

Sciatic nerve block at the level of the popliteal fossa is widely used because the nerve is easily visualized with US at this level. Moreover, a single injection can block all the nerves of the foot and ankle, with the exception of the saphenous nerve. The sciatic nerve, popliteal artery, and popliteal vein are easy to visualize within the popliteal fossa by using US guidance. As seen in Figure 5-1, the popliteal fossa is bordered medially by the semimembranosus/semitendinosus muscles and laterally by the biceps femoris muscle. This nerve can be located by imaging superficial and lateral to the popliteal artery and vein, which are useful landmarks when imaging with ultrasound. Division of the sciatic nerve into the tibial and peroneal nerves occurs approximately 5 to 7 cm superior to the popliteal crease.[101]

Many early techniques for sciatic nerve block are based on the belief that the nerve is closely enveloped within the popliteal space by an impermeable connective tissue sheath.[102] This would require the injecting needle to

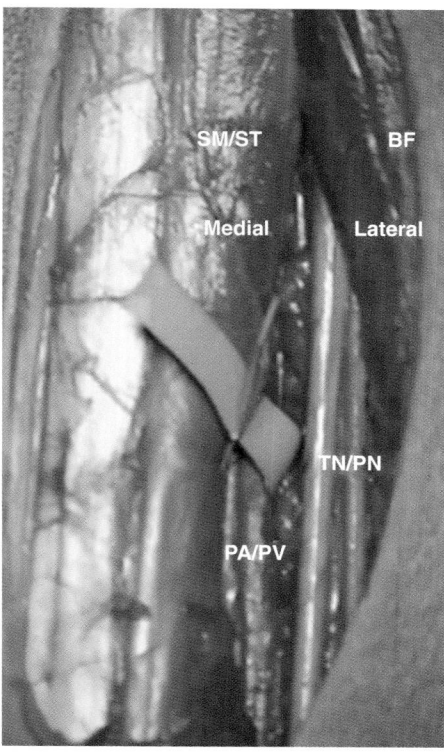

Figure 5-1 The tibial (TN) and peroneal nerves (PN) are displayed within the popliteal fossa distal to the division of the sciatic nerve. The popliteal artery (PA) and popliteal vein (PV) are medial to the nerves and are marked with a vessel loop. The biceps femoris (BF) muscle forms the lateral border of the popliteal fossa. Its medial border is formed by a confluence of the semimembranosus/semitendinosis (SM/ST) muscles.

penetrate this sheath to achieve successful nerve block. However, in Figure 5-2, the distribution pattern of methylene blue dye injected 0.5 cm medial to the sciatic nerve is demonstrated. It is clear from this image that methylene blue dye spreads from the medial to lateral border of the space as well as for a considerable distance proximal to the injection point. This extensive distribution of injectate suggests that successful sciatic nerve block at the level of the popliteal fossa can be performed without contact or immediate proximity between the injecting needle and the sciatic nerve. Clinical and laboratory outcomes confirm the efficacy of this technique.[54,94] Excellent analgesia is achieved while injecting a safe distance from the nerve.

In Figure 5-3, an ultrasound image of the sciatic nerve within the popliteal fossa is demonstrated. In this view, the biceps femoris muscle is visible at the lateral border of the space, while the semimembranosus/semitendinosus muscles are seen medially. The popliteal artery and vein are hypoechoic (black) structures seen deep and medial to the nerve. Figure 5-4 demonstrates the ultrasound appearance of local anesthetic injected 0.5 cm medial to the sciatic nerve. An extensive black (hypoechoic) area of local anesthetic surrounds the nerve.

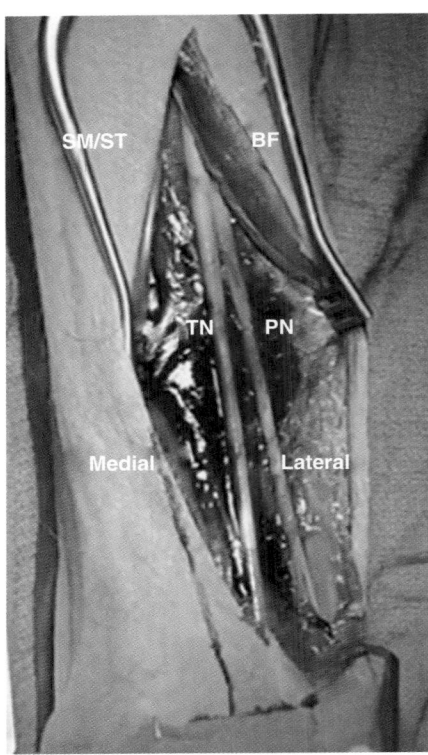

Figure 5-2 The distribution of methylene blue dye throughout the popliteal space from a single injection point within the popliteal space demonstrates how successful sciatic nerve block does not require immediate proximity to the nerve. The sciatic nerve *(SN)* is shown proximal to its division into the tibial *(TN)* and peroneal nerves *(PN)*. The biceps femoris *(BF)* muscle as well as the semimembranosus/semitendinosus *(SM/ST)* muscles are also labeled as borders of the popliteal fossa.

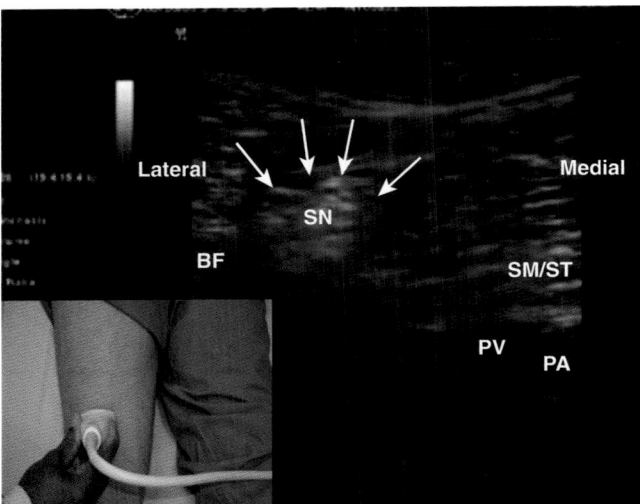

Figure 5-3 Axial ultrasound image of the popliteal space approximately 5 cm superior to the popliteal crease. The popliteal artery *(PA)* and vein *(PV)* are visible medial and deep to the sciatic nerve *(SN)*. The borders of the popliteal space are formed by the biceps femoris muscle (BF) laterally and the semimembranosus/semitendinosis muscles *(SM/ST)* medially. The *white arrows* highlight the superficial border of the SN.

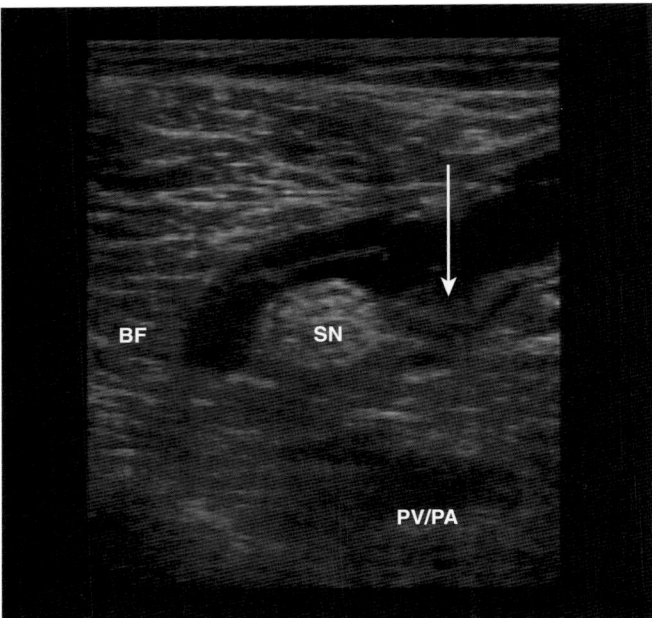

Figure 5-4 Axial image of the popliteal space approximately 5 cm superior to the popliteal crease during ultrasound-guided injection. The *white arrow* represents the position of the needle approximately 1 cm medial to the superficial surface of the sciatic nerve *(SN)*. The hypoechoic (black) area superficial and lateral to the nerve is local anesthetic. The popliteal artery *(PA)* and vein *(PV)* are visible medial and deep to the SN.

The Saphenous Nerve above the Knee

The saphenous nerve is a pure sensory branch of the femoral nerve. At the level of the superior pole of the patella, it exits the adductor canal in a tissue plane between the vastus medialis and sartorius muscles (Fig. 5-5). Figure 5-6 demonstrates the tissue plane between the vastus medialis and the sartorius that is readily visible with ultrasound. Although the saphenous nerve itself is rarely visible within this tissue plane, it can be reliably blocked by injection of local anesthetic into this compartment. In Figure 5-7, the fascial plane between the vastus medialis and the sartorius muscles has been distended with local anesthetic. This will effectively block the saphenous nerve.

Nerve Blocks below the Knee

Historically, nerve blocks below the knee have been limited to the ankle, where surface landmarks can be used to identify injection sites. With US guidance, nerves can be visualized and blocked for a considerable distance proximal to the ankle if necessary. This greatly increases the versatility of block placement in cases where traditional landmarks for injection at the ankle might be affected by edema, erythema, or skin breakdown. Another advantage of US is the ability to inject local anesthetic without needle trauma to nerves or blood vessels. Thus

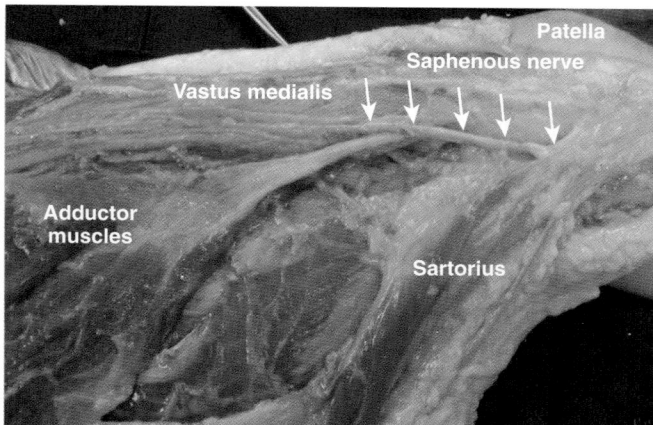

Figure 5-5 This image shows the medial aspect of the thigh immediately superior to the patella. The sartorius muscle has been transected and reflected medially to expose the saphenous nerve. The saphenous nerve passes superficial to the tendinous insertion of the adductor muscles to a fascial plane between the vastus medialis and the sartorius muscle.

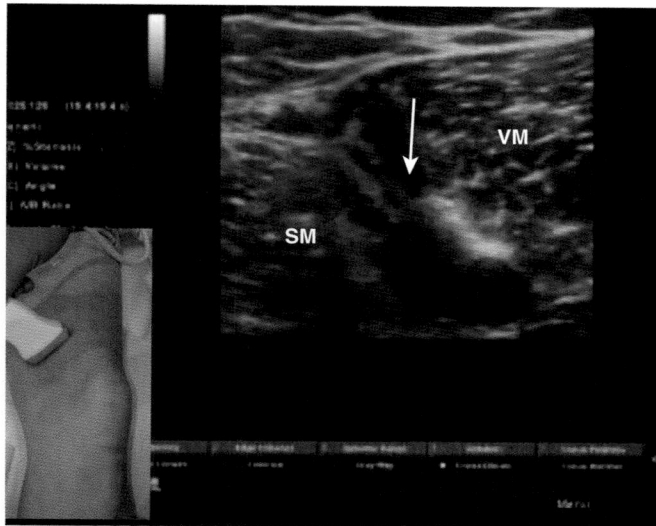

Figure 5-7 Axial ultrasound view of the medial aspect of the thigh immediately after injection of 15 mL of local anesthetic into the fascial plane between the sartorius *(SM)* and the vastus medialis *(VM)* muscles. The saphenous nerve itself is not usually visible at this level but can be reliably blocked by injection within this fascial plane.

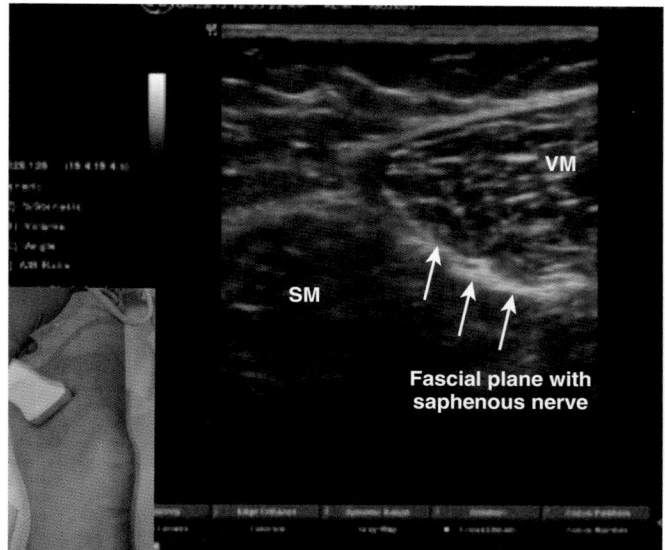

Figure 5-6 Ultrasound image showing an axial view of the medial aspect of the thigh at the level of the superior pole of the patella. The fascial plane between the sartorius *(SM)* and the vastus medialis *(VM)* contains the saphenous nerve. The saphenous nerve itself is not usually visible in this plane.

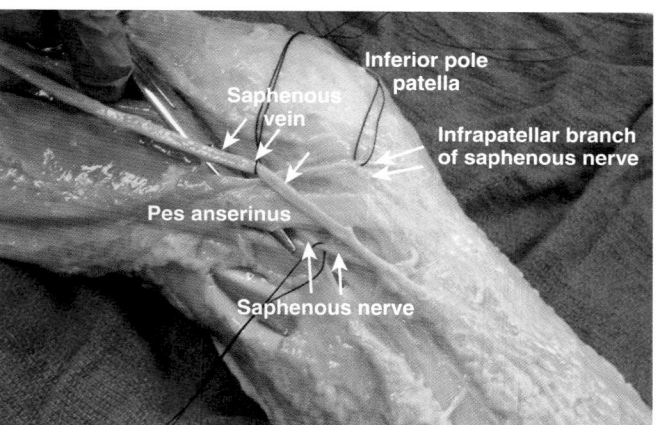

Figure 5-8 The relationship of the saphenous vein, saphenous nerve, and the pes anserinus. Inferior to the pes anserinus, the saphenous vein and nerve are in close proximity to one other within the subcutaneous tissue. Proximally, the nerve passes deep to the pes anserinus, while the vein remains in the subcutaneous tissue. When using the saphenous vein as a landmark for saphenous nerve block, injection should be immediately inferior to the pes anserinus.

ultrasound provides an added degree of versatility because nerves of the foot and ankle can be visualized along most of their length and blocked where most appropriate.

The Saphenous Nerve

The saphenous nerve can be blocked below the knee at the level of the tibial plateau. Figure 5-8 shows the saphenous nerve as it emerges from beneath the pes anserinus. After emerging from deep to the pes anserinus, the saphenous nerve travels in the subcutaneous tissue with the saphenous vein see (see Fig. 5-8) on the medial aspect of the tibia. A common mistake in blocking the saphenous nerve at this level is to inject only in an anterior direction across the medial tibial plateau. Although this will effectively block the infrapatellar branch of the saphenous nerve, the more distal portion should be

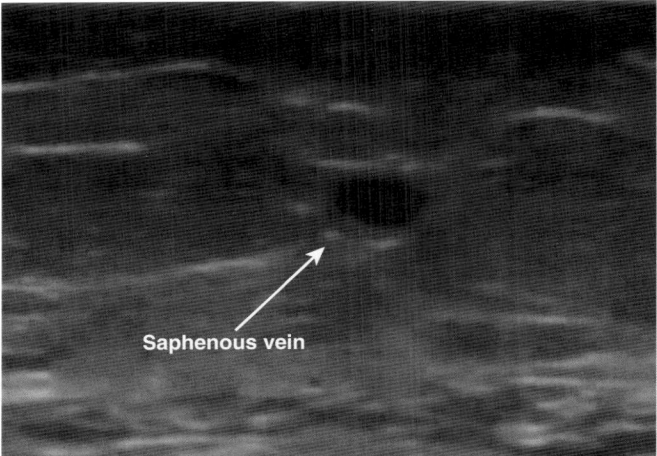

Figure 5-9 Ultrasound image of the medial aspect of the leg shows the appearance of the saphenous vein *(SV)* immediately inferior to the pes anserinus. Note the saphenous nerve is not visible in this image, and injection is performed using the vein as a marker for the position of the saphenous nerve. This image must be obtained using extremely light pressure with the ultrasound transducer, to avoid compression of the saphenous vein.

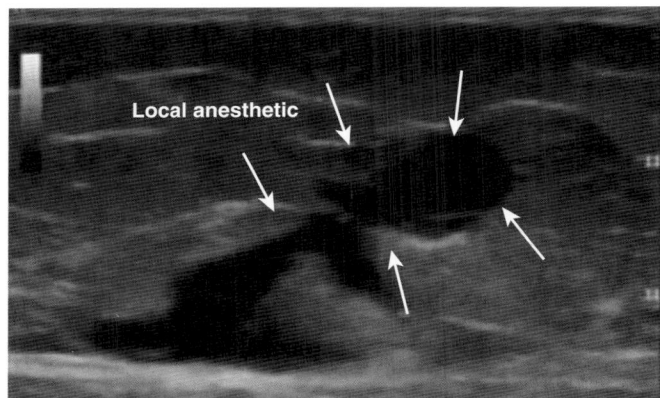

Figure 5-10 Axial view of local anesthetic (hypoechoic) after infiltration around the saphenous vein. Injection is performed using the saphenous vein inferior to the pes anserinus as a landmark.

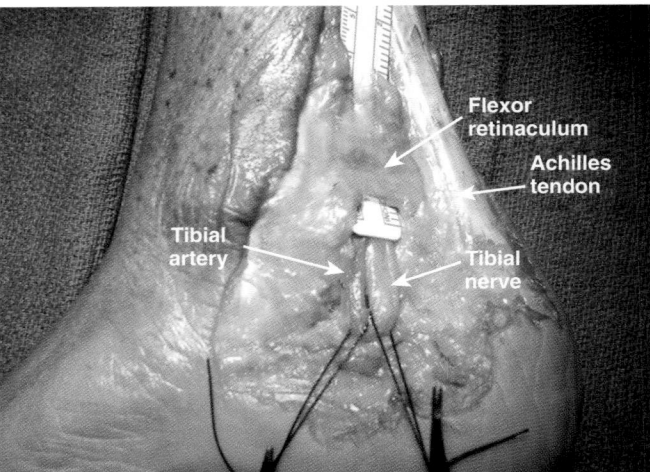

Figure 5-11 A dissection of the medial aspect of the right ankle shows the flexor retinaculum, which has been cut away inferiorly. The tibial nerve is seen posterior to the tibial artery.

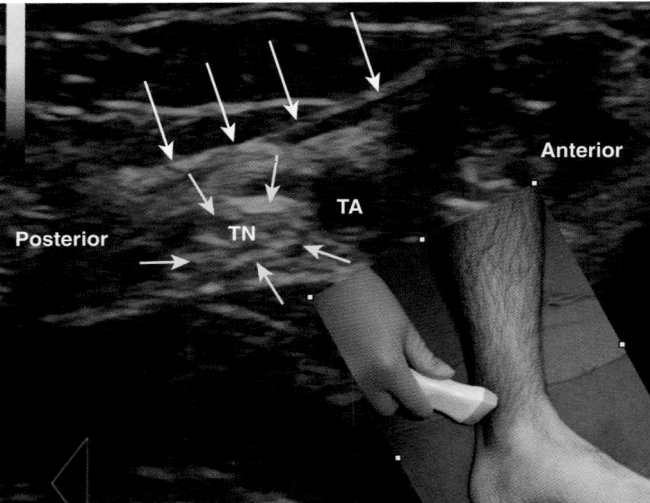

Figure 5-12 Ultrasound image of the medial aspect of the left ankle immediately superior to the malleolus. The image shows the relationship between the tibial artery *(TA)* and the tibial nerve *(TN)* (whose borders are defined by *yellow arrows*). Note that both structures are deep to the flexor retinaculum that is outlined by *white arrows*.

blocked by infiltration around the saphenous vein as shown in Figures 5-9 and 5-10. Note in these US images that the saphenous nerve is not visible and that successful block is achieved by injecting in proximity to the saphenous vein.

The Tibial Nerve (Video Clip 5)

The tibial nerve is readily visualized with US at the level of the medial malleolus. Here, it is located deep to the flexor retinaculum and posterior to the tibial artery (Fig. 5-11). Using ultrasound, the injecting needle can be advanced either anterior or posterior to the nerve and

deep to the flexor retinaculum (Fig. 5-12). The proximal course of the tibial nerve can be followed as it runs with the tibial artery in a plane between the flexor digitorum longus anteriorly and the flexor hallucis longus posteriorly. Figure 5-13 shows the ultrasound appearance of the tibial nerve at the level of the midtibia. It is readily visualized adjacent to the tibial artery in a tissue plane between the flexor digitorum longus and the flexor hallucis longus. Injection can be made in the tissue plane between the flexor digitorum longus and the flexor hallucis longus.

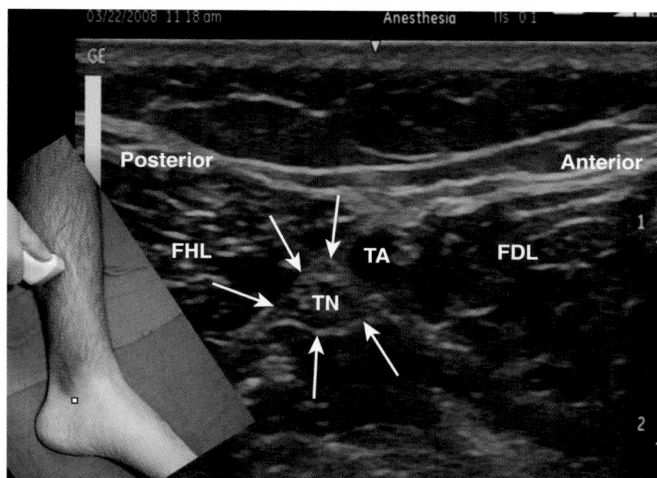

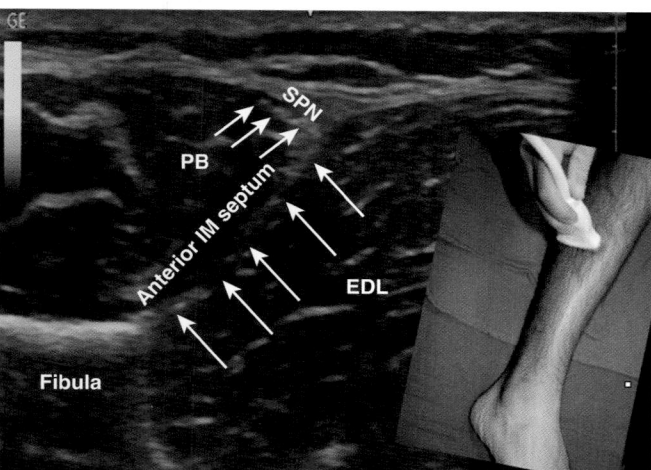

Figure 5-13 The medial aspect of the left leg is at the level of the midtibia. The tibial nerve *(TN)* and tibial artery *(TA)* continue in close proximity to one another. They are bordered anteriorly by the flexor digitorum longus *(FDL)* and posteriorly by the flexor hallucis longus *(FHL)*.

Figure 5-15 Ultrasound image of the lateral aspect of the right leg at the level of the midfibula. The superficial peroneal nerve *(SPN)* at this level is deep to the investing fascia of the leg and lies on the superficial surface of the peroneus brevis muscle *(PB)*. The anterior intermuscular septum is a useful landmark because the nerve lies immediately posterior to this septum. The extensor digitorum longus muscle *(EDL)* borders the anterior surface of the intermuscular septum.

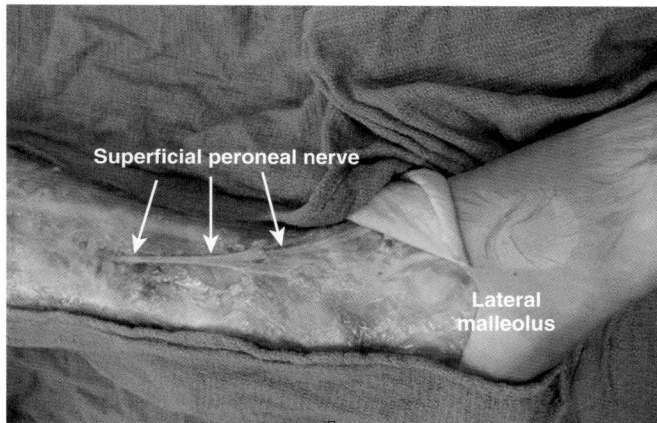

Figure 5-14 In this dissection of the right lower leg, the superficial peroneal nerve is seen as it pierces the investing fascia near the anterior intermuscular septum. As it passes distally to the ankle, it divides extensively over the dorsum of the foot.

The Deep Peroneal Nerve

The deep peroneal nerve can be visualized at the superior level of the malleoli, where it lies on the anterior surface of the tibia immediately lateral to the anterior tibial artery. At this level, both the artery and the nerve pass between the tendons of the extensor hallucis longus and the extensor digitorum longus (Fig. 5-16). When using ultrasound, the pulsatile anterior tibial artery is easily visualized and is a useful point of reference for the deep peroneal nerve at the level of the ankle (Fig. 5-17). If more a proximal block is required, the artery and nerve can be followed proximally, where they lie on the anterior surface of the interosseous membrane (Fig. 5-18). At this level, the nerve is rarely visible but can be successfully blocked by injecting in a plane between the interosseous membrane and the anterior tibial artery.

The Sural Nerve

At the level of the lateral malleolus, the sural nerve can be identified, using ultrasound, by its proximity to the small saphenous vein. The vein and nerve are adjacent to one another in the subcutaneous tissue between the Achilles tendon posteriorly and the tendons of the peroneus longus and brevis anteriorly (Fig. 5-19). The nerve and vein can be traced proximally to a position midline between the medial and lateral heads of the gastrocnemius muscle. At this level, the nerve pierces the investing fascia of the leg (Fig. 5-20). In Figure 5-21, the small saphenous vein and the sural nerve are visible in the midline between the medial and lateral heads of the gastrocnemius muscle. Here the nerve is still in the

The Superficial Peroneal Nerve

The superficial peroneal nerve branches extensively as it passes in the subcutaneous tissue from the lower leg to the ankle (Fig. 5-14). It is typically not visible with ultrasound at this level but can be blocked at the ankle with a subcutaneous injection between the medial and lateral malleoli. At the level of the midfibula, the nerve pierces the investing fascia of the leg. Using ultrasound at this level, the nerve can be visualized immediately deep to the investing fascia of the leg on the surface of the peroneus brevis muscle and lateral to the anterior intermuscular septum (Fig. 5-15).

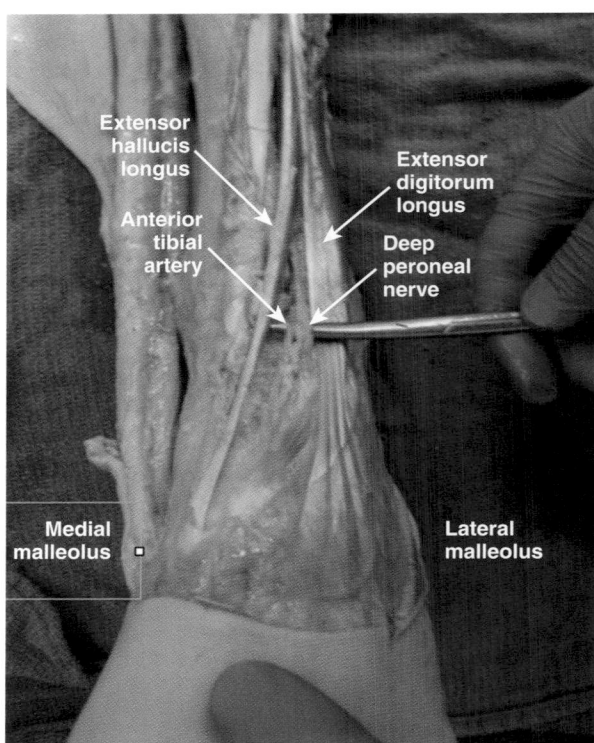

Figure 5-16 In this dissection of the ankle, the extensor retinaculum has been removed to reveal the deep peroneal nerve in a position lateral to the anterior tibial artery. These two structures are between the extensor hallucis longus and extensor digitorum longus tendons.

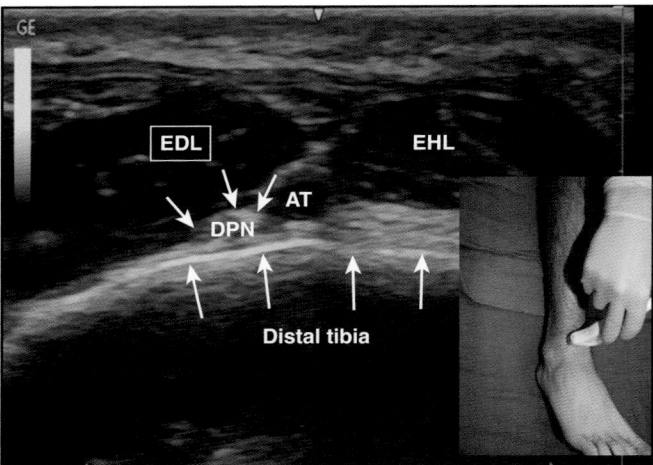

Figure 5-17 Ultrasound image immediately superior to the malleoli shows the anterior tibial artery *(AT)* medial to the deep peroneal nerve *(DPN)*. Both structures are on the anterior surface of the tibia. The extensor digitorum longus *(EDL)* and extensor hallucis longus *(EHL)* muscles are superficial to the nerve and artery.

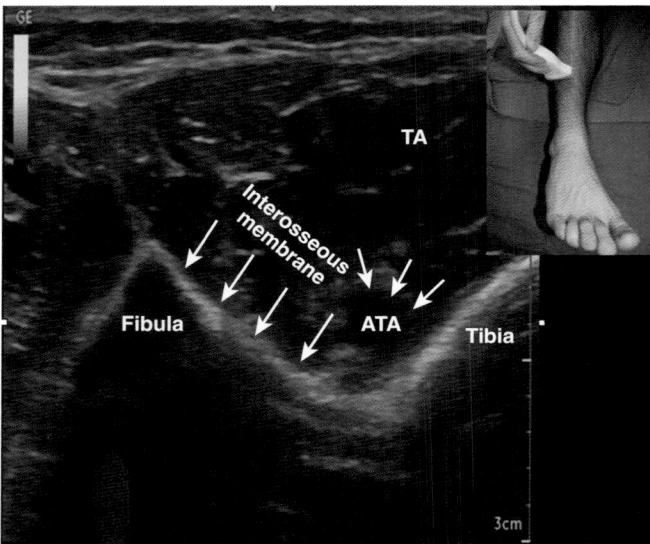

Figure 5-18 The deep peroneal nerve is not usually visible above the ankle when using ultrasound. However, because this nerve travels in close proximity to the anterior tibial artery *(ATA)*, this vessel can be used as a marker for successful injection. Injection between the interosseous membrane and the ATA will result in successful block at this level. The tibialis anterior muscle *(TA)* is seen in this view anterior to the artery and nerve.

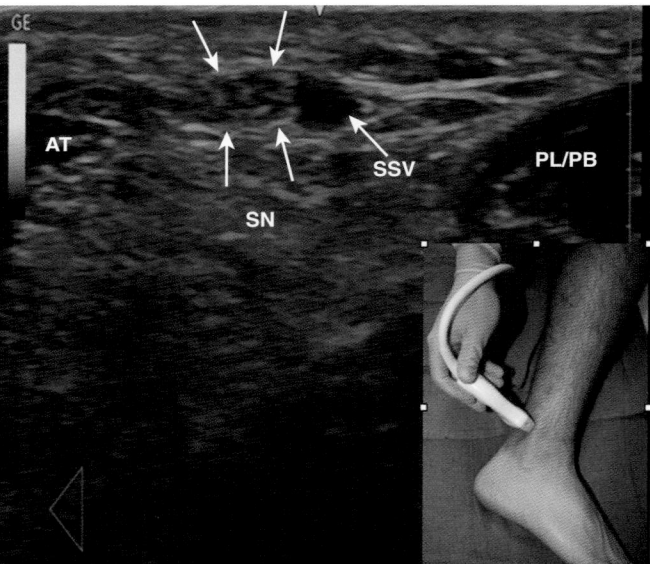

Figure 5-19 Ultrasound image at the level of the lateral malleolus, the sural nerve (SN) is seen adjacent to the small saphenous vein *(SSV)*. Both the vein and the nerve are in the subcutaneous tissue between the Achilles tendon *(AT)* posteriorly and the tendons of the peroneus longus and peroneus brevis *(PL/PB)* anteriorly. The small saphenous vein *(SSV)* is a useful landmark that is consistently adjacent to the sural nerve *(SN)* at this level.

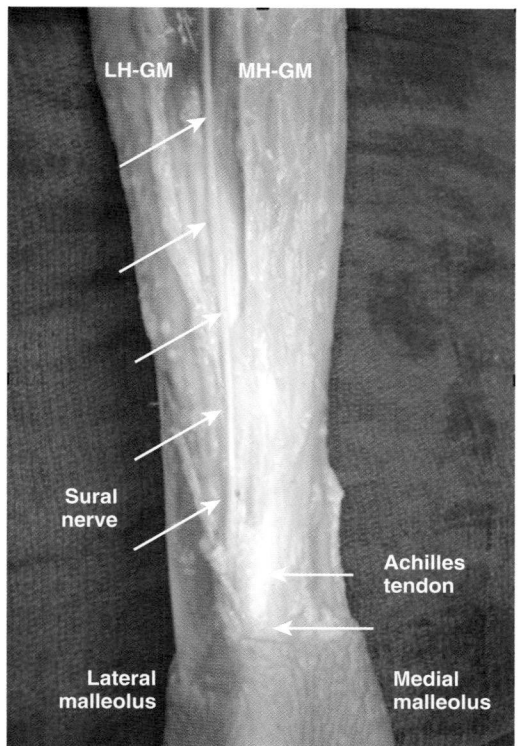

Figure 5-20 In this image of the posterior aspect of the lower leg, the proximal sural nerve is visible in the midline between the medial *(MH-GM)* and lateral *(LH-GM)* heads of the gastrocnemius muscle. The distal position of the nerve is between the Achilles tendon and the lateral malleolus.

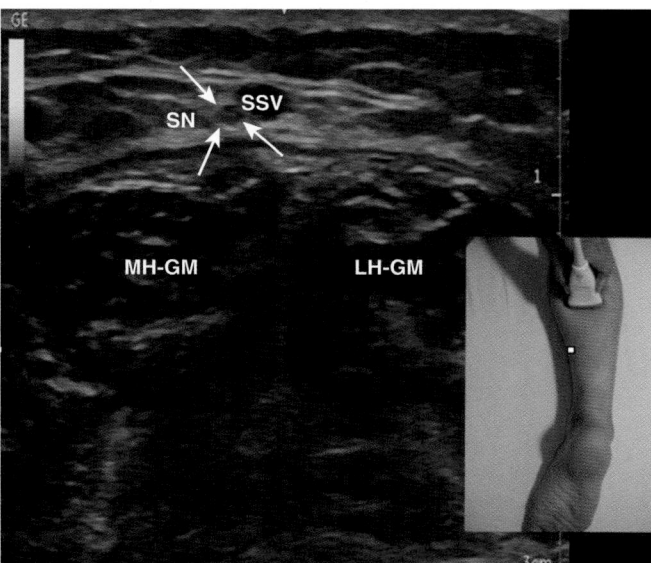

Figure 5-21 Ultrasound image of the posterior aspect of the lower leg shows the small saphenous vein *(SSV)* and the sural nerve *(SN)* in a position midline between the medial *(MH-GM)* and lateral *(LH-GM)* heads of the gastrocnemius muscle.

subcutaneous tissue and has not pierced the investing fascia of the leg.

NERVE BLOCK COMPLICATIONS

Peripheral nerve blocks provide excellent pain relief after surgery, but are not considered an indispensible component of perioperative care. Because all medical procedures are associated with the risk of injury, it is appropriate to reserve nerve blocks for patients in whom there is a clear benefit. The obvious goal for regional anesthesia is to reduce the risk of nerve blocks to a level that is favorable for all patients experiencing moderate-to-severe postoperative pain.

Complications occurring during the performance of nerve blocks include intravascular injection of local anesthetic, nerve injury, and vascular injury. However, injury may also result from the loss of motor and sensory function in the affected extremity. For example, patients are vulnerable to compression injuries and falls during any period of dense motor and sensory block.[84,94,107] Thus it is important to take appropriate safety measures both during nerve block placement and for the duration of its effect.

Intravascular Injection of Local Anesthetic

Accidental intravascular injection of local anesthetic can manifest as symptoms and signs ranging from perioral numbness and agitation to grand mal seizures and cardiovascular collapse. A local anesthetic dose that is completely safe for injection into tissue can be toxic if injected intravascularly. Thus it is important to recognize that published guidelines for "allowable doses" of local anesthetic do not apply to rapid intravascular administration.[33]

The use of ultrasound has introduced new methods for detecting intravascular injection. First, blood vessels can be visualized during the procedure, and needle position can be adjusted accordingly. Next, injection of even small volumes of local anesthetic (0.5-1.0 mL) within a blood vessel causes turbulence that can be seen on the ultrasound image as "hyperechoic contrast," alerting the operator to intravascular injection. Finally, during normal injection, there should be obvious displacement of tissue by the injectate that is visibly hypoechoic (black). Examples of the hypoechoic appearance of injectate are seen in Figures 5-4 and 5-10. If tissue displacement is not apparent during injection, the procedure is halted until intravascular injection can be ruled out.

Studies comparing ultrasound guided nerve blocks with nerve stimulator techniques demonstrate that fewer vascular punctures as well as fewer seizures caused by intravascular injection occur when using ultrasound guidance.[1,69] Thus ultrasound has already had a significant impact on one of the most serious complications of regional anesthesia.

Nerve Injury

The reported incidence of injury after peripheral nerve block in the lower extremity varies greatly. This is due to several factors, including what defines "nerve injury." Transient sensory changes, lasting days or weeks after nerve block, have been reported in up to 41% of patients treated with peripheral nerve block performed using nerve stimulator guidance.[41] By contrast, prolonged neurologic deficits are reported to be as low as 0.05% in other large series.[3]

The cause of perioperative nerve injury is often difficult to identify. Some recognized factors related to nerve block include needle trauma, intraneural injection, and toxicity of injectate.[5,65] Equally important, however, are injuries related to trauma or compression of the extremity during a period of dense motor and sensory block. Thus the postoperative care of patients with long-acting nerve blocks should include precautions with respect to limb positioning, padding of the extremity, and assessing perfusion.

Several studies show superiority of ultrasound over nerve stimulation when comparing success rate, patient acceptance, efficiency, and local anesthetic requirements.[1,59,74] However, there is little evidence confirming a decreased incidence of nerve injury for blocks placed using ultrasound compared with nerve stimulation. The apparent lack of improvement with respect to nerve injury when blocks are placed with ultrasound may reflect reluctance on the part of anesthesiologists to modify existing block techniques. Before the availability of ultrasound, nerve stimulation was used to position the injecting needle in contact with or in immediate proximity to the nerve. With the transition away from nerve stimulation, many practitioners have simply converted ultrasound into the visual equivalent of a nerve stimulator. In other words, ultrasound rather than nerve stimulation is used to position the needle in immediate proximity or contact with the nerve. The result of this practice has been a continued high rate of nerve penetration and intraneural injection that is the subject of considerable discussion and investigation.[9,26,95]

Because needle trauma and intraneural injection are known to be associated with nerve injury,[29,39,80,86,106] it would seem wise to use every possible tool to avoid these risk factors. In fact, existing anatomic studies demonstrate that most nerves such as the brachial plexus, femoral nerve, and the sciatic nerve are all contained within distinct fascial compartments.[7,30,108] Moreover, these nerves can be successfully blocked by injection into these fascial compartments and without immediate proximity to the nerve. Ultrasound is particularly suited for these techniques because it can be used to position the needle in the correct fascial compartment for successful block without proximity to the nerve. Thus two of the known causes of nerve injury—needle trauma and intraneural injection—can be avoided. Recent clinical data confirm success rates approaching 100% for blocks performed using ultrasound to guide fascial compartment injection without proximity to the nerve.[94]

Infection

Although infection can occur with any type of nerve block, this complication is most commonly associated with continuous indwelling catheters. The majority of studies reporting infection associated with indwelling catheters are from hospitalized patients. In these reports, the infection rate ranges from 0% to 3.2%.[24,66] For outpatients, the reported rates are less than 1%.[21,94] Guidelines for sterile precautions during catheter placement are largely extrapolations from data pertaining to central venous access techniques. In addition to sterile precautions for catheter placement, it is important to follow all pharmacy standards and sterile precautions during the preparation and filling of infusion pumps used with continuous catheter techniques. At least one report of deep cellulitis has been attributed to an infusion pump that was not filled under sterile conditions.[22]

Although tunneling of peripheral nerve catheters has been recommended to reduce bacterial colonization, this has not been proven to reduce infection. Specific risk factors identified with catheter infection include duration of catheter use longer than 48 hours, lack of antibiotic prophylaxis, and position in the axillary or inguinal region.[21]

SUMMARY

The postoperative management of surgical patients has undergone important developments in recent years. These developments are the result of changing patient demographics as well as technologic advances in medical devices and pharmaceuticals.

An aging and more obese population has increased the risk of perioperative respiratory events in patients with diagnosed and undiagnosed obstructive sleep apnea. The increasing use and abuse of opioids in the overall population changes the safety and efficacy of this widely prescribed class of drugs. Lastly, economic pressures to perform more complex procedures on an ambulatory basis have steadily increased.

Fortunately, the tools to provide safe and effective patient care in the face of these challenges are developing as well. Of necessity, the greatest paradigm shift will be away from a reliance on opioids as the dominant analgesic for postoperative pain control.

REFERENCES

1. Abrahams MS, Aziz MF, Fu RF, Horn JL: Ultrasound guidance compared with electrical neurostimulation for peripheral nerve block: a systematic review and meta-analysis of randomized controlled trials, Br J Anaesth 102:408–417, 2009.
2. Adesanya AO, Lee W, Greilich NB, Joshi GP: Perioperative management of obstructive sleep apnea, Chest 138:1489–1498, 2010.

3. Auroy Y, Benhamou D, Bargues L, et al: Major complications of regional anesthesia in France: the SOS Regional Anesthesia Hotline Service, *Anesthesiology* 97:1274–1280, 2002.

4. Balaban F, Yagar S, Ozgok A, et al: A randomized, placebo-controlled study of pregabalin for postoperative pain intensity after laparoscopic cholecystectomy, *J Clin Anesth* 24:175–178, 2012.

5. Barrington MJ, Snyder GL: Neurologic complications of regional anesthesia, *Curr Opin Anaesthesiol* 24:554–560, 2011.

6. Beck A, Salem K, Krischak G, et al: Nonsteroidal anti-inflammatory drugs (NSAIDs) in the perioperative phase in traumatology and orthopedics effects on bone healing, *Oper Orthop Traumatol* 17:569–578, 2005.

7. Beck GP: Anterior approach to sciatic nerve block, *Anesthesiology* 24:222–224, 1963.

8. Benyamin R, Trescot AM, Datta S, et al: Opioid complications and side effects, *Pain Physician* 11(Suppl 2):S105–S120, 2008.

9. Bigeleisen PE, Chelly J: An unsubstantiated condemnation of intraneural injection, *Reg Anesth Pain Med* 36:95, 2011; author reply 95–97, 98–99.

10. Bockbrader HN, Radulovic LL, Posvar EL, et al: Clinical pharmacokinetics of pregabalin in healthy volunteers, *J Clin Pharmacol* 50:941–950, 2010.

11. Boezaart AP: Perineural infusion of local anesthetics, *Anesthesiology* 104:872–880, 2006.

12. Bollini CA, Urmey WF, Vascello L, Cacheiro F: Relationship between evoked motor response and sensory paresthesia in interscalene brachial plexus block, *Reg Anesth Pain Med* 28:384–388, 2003.

13. Bonnefont J, Courade JP, Alloui A, Eschalier A: [Antinociceptive mechanism of action of paracetamol], *Drugs* 63(Spec No 2):1–4, 2003.

14. Bornemann-Cimenti H, Lederer AJ, Wejbora M, et al: Preoperative pregabalin administration significantly reduces postoperative opioid consumption and mechanical hyperalgesia after transperitoneal nephrectomy, *Br J Anaesth* 108:845–849, 2012.

15. Botting RM: Inhibitors of cyclooxygenases: mechanisms, selectivity and uses, *J Physiol Pharmacol* 57(Suppl 5):113–124, 2006.

16. Boursinos LA, Karachalios T, Poultsides L, Malizos KN: Do steroids, conventional non-steroidal anti-inflammatory drugs and selective Cox-2 inhibitors adversely affect fracture healing? *J Musculoskel Neuronal Interact* 9:44–52, 2009.

17. Brett CN, Barnett SG, Pearson J: Postoperative plasma paracetamol levels following oral or intravenous paracetamol administration: a double-blind randomised controlled trial, *Anaesth Intensive Care* 40:166–171, 2012.

18. Brown KA, Laferriere A, Lakheeram I, Moss IR: Recurrent hypoxemia in children is associated with increased analgesic sensitivity to opiates, *Anesthesiol* 105:665–669, 2006.

19. Burke SM, Shorten GD: Perioperative pregabalin improves pain and functional outcomes 3 months after lumbar discectomy, *Anesth Analg* 110:1180–1185, 2010.

20. Buvanendran A, Kroin JS, Della Valle CJ, et al: Perioperative oral pregabalin reduces chronic pain after total knee arthroplasty: a prospective, controlled trial, *Anesth Analg* 110:199–207, 2010.

21. Capdevila X, Bringuier S, Borgeat A: Infectious risk of continuous peripheral nerve blocks, *Anesthesiology* 110:182–188, 2009.

22. Capdevila X, Jaber S, Pesonen P, et al: Acute neck cellulitis and mediastinitis complicating a continuous interscalene block, *Anesth Analg* 107:1419–1421, 2008.

23. Capdevila X, Macaire P, Aknin P, et al: Patient-controlled perineural analgesia after ambulatory orthopedic surgery: a comparison of electronic versus elastomeric pumps, *Anesth Analg* 96:414–417, 2003.

24. Capdevila X, Pirat P, Bringuier S, et al: Continuous peripheral nerve blocks in hospital wards after orthopedic surgery: a multicenter prospective analysis of the quality of postoperative analgesia and complications in 1,416 patients, *Anesthesiology* 103:1035–1045, 2005.

25. Chia YY, Liu K, Wang JJ, et al: Intraoperative high-dose fentanyl induces postoperative fentanyl tolerance, *Can J Anaesth* 46:872–877, 1999.

26. Choquet O, Morau D, Biboulet P, Capdevila X: Where should the tip of the needle be located in ultrasound-guided peripheral nerve blocks? *Curr Opin Anaesthesiol* 25:596–602, 2012.

27. Chung F, Yegneswaran B, Liao P, et al: STOP questionnaire: a tool to screen patients for obstructive sleep apnea, *Anesthesiology* 108:812–821, 2008.

28. Chung SA, Yuan H, Chung F: A systemic review of obstructive sleep apnea and its implications for anesthesiologists, *Anesth Analg* 107:1543–1563, 2008.

29. Cohen JM, Gray AT: Functional deficits after intraneural injection during interscalene block, *Reg Anesthesia Pain Med* 35:397–399, 2010.

30. Dalens B, Vanneuville G, Tanguy A: Comparison of the fascia iliaca compartment block with the 3-in-1 block in children, *Anesth Analg* 69:705–713, 1989.

31. Davis JJ, Johnson KB, Egan TD, et al: Preoperative fentanyl infusion with pharmacokinetic simulation for anesthetic and perioperative management of an opioid-tolerant patient, *Anesth Analg* 97:1661–1662, 2003.

32. Dayer P, Desmeules J, Collart L: [Pharmacology of tramadol], *Drugs* 53(Suppl 2):18–24, 1997.

33. Dillane D, Finucane BT: Local anesthetic systemic toxicity, *Can J Anaesth* 57:368–380, 2010.

34. Dingemans E, Williams SR, Arcand G, et al: Neurostimulation in ultrasound-guided infraclavicular block: a prospective randomized trial, *Anesth Analg* 104:1275–1280, 2007.

35. Durkin B, Page C, Glass P: Pregabalin for the treatment of postsurgical pain, *Expert Opin Pharmacother* 11:2751–2758, 2010.

36. Fanelli G, Casati A, Garancini P, Torri G: Nerve stimulator and multiple injection technique for upper and lower limb blockade: failure rate, patient acceptance, and neurologic complications. Study Group on Regional Anesthesia, *Anesth Analg* 88:847–852, 1999.

37. Finkel KJ, Searleman AC, Tymkew H, et al: Prevalence of undiagnosed obstructive sleep apnea among adult surgical patients in an academic medical center, *Sleep Med* 10:753–758, 2009.

38. Frampton JE. Tapentadol immediate release: a review of its use in the treatment of moderate to severe acute pain, *Drugs* 70:1719–1743, 2010.

39. Fredrickson MJ: Case report: neurological deficit associated with intraneural needle placement without injection, *Can J Anaesth* 56:935–938, 2009.

40. Gajraj NM: Pregabalin: its pharmacology and use in pain management, *Anesth Analg* 105:1805–1815, 2007.

41. Gartke K, Portner O, Taljaard M: Neuropathic symptoms following continuous popliteal block after foot and ankle surgery, *Foot Ankle Int* 33:267–274, 2012.

42. Gelfand HJ, Ouanes JP, Lesley MR, et al: Analgesic efficacy of ultrasound-guided regional anesthesia: a meta-analysis, *J Clinl Anesth* 23:90–96, 2011.

43. Graff J, Skarke C, Klinkhardt U, et al: Effects of selective COX-2 inhibition on prostanoids and platelet physiology in young healthy volunteers, *J Thromb Haemost* 5:2376–2385, 2007.

44. Graham GG, Scott KF: Mechanism of action of paracetamol, *Am J Ther* 12:46–55, 2005.

45. Gross JB, Bachenberg KL, Benumof JL, et al: Practice guidelines for the perioperative management of patients with obstructive

sleep apnea: a report by the American Society of Anesthesiologists Task Force on Perioperative Management of patients with obstructive sleep apnea, *Anesthesiology* 104:1081–1093, 2006; quiz 117–118.

46. Guignard B, Bossard AE, Coste C, et al: Acute opioid tolerance: intraoperative remifentanil increases postoperative pain and morphine requirement, *Anesthesiology* 93:409–417, 2000.

47. Hartrick C, Van Hove I, Stegmann JU, et al: Efficacy and tolerability of tapentadol immediate release and oxycodone HCl immediate release in patients awaiting primary joint replacement surgery for end-stage joint disease: a 10-day, phase III, randomized, double-blind, active- and placebo-controlled study, *Clin Ther* 31:260–271, 2009.

48. Hebl JR, Dilger JA, Byer DE, et al: A pre-emptive multimodal pathway featuring peripheral nerve block improves perioperative outcomes after major orthopedic surgery, *Reg Anesth Pain Med* 33:510–517, 2008.

49. Hinz B, Renner B, Brune K: Drug insight: cyclo-oxygenase-2 inhibitors—a critical appraisal, *Nat Clin Pract Rheumatol* 3:552–560, 2007.

50. Ho KY, Tay W, Yeo MC, et al: Duloxetine reduces morphine requirements after knee replacement surgery, *Br J Anaesth* 105:371–376, 2010.

51. Hofmann AA, Bloebaum RD, Koller KE, Lahav A: Does celecoxib have an adverse effect on bone remodeling and ingrowth in humans? *Clin Orthop Rel Res* 452:200–204, 2006.

52. Hooper L, Brown TJ, Elliott R, et al: The effectiveness of five strategies for the prevention of gastrointestinal toxicity induced by non-steroidal anti-inflammatory drugs: systematic review, *BMJ* 329:948, 2004.

53. Houmes RJ, Voets MA, Verkaaik A, et al: Efficacy and safety of tramadol versus morphine for moderate and severe postoperative pain with special regard to respiratory depression, *Anesth Analg* 74:510–514, 1992.

54. Hunt KJ, Higgins TF, Carlston CV, et al: Continuous peripheral nerve blockade as postoperative analgesia for open treatment of calcaneal fractures, *J Orthop Trauma* 24:148–155, 2010.

55. Hyllested M, Jones S, Pedersen JL, Kehlet H: Comparative effect of paracetamol, NSAIDs or their combination in postoperative pain management: a qualitative review, *Br J Anaesth* 88:199–214, 2002.

56. Ilfeld BM, Enneking FK: Continuous peripheral nerve blocks at home: a review, *Anesth Analg* 100:1822–1833, 2005.

57. Jacobsen RB, Phillips BB: Reducing clinically significant gastrointestinal toxicity associated with nonsteroidal antiinflammatory drugs, *Anns Pharmacother* 38:1469–1481, 2004.

58. Kim JC, Choi YS, Kim KN, et al: Effective dose of peri-operative oral pregabalin as an adjunct to multimodal analgesic regimen in lumbar spinal fusion surgery, *Spine* 36:428–433, 2011.

59. Koscielniak-Nielsen ZJ: Ultrasound-guided peripheral nerve blocks: what are the benefits? *Acta Anaesthesiol Scand* 52:727–737, 2008.

60. Lee M, Silverman SM, Hansen H, et al: A comprehensive review of opioid-induced hyperalgesia, *Pain Physician* 14:145–161, 2011.

61. Maheshwari AV, Blum YC, Shekhar L, et al: Multimodal pain management after total hip and knee arthroplasty at the Ranawat Orthopaedic Center, *Clin Orthop Rel Res* 467:1418–1423, 2009.

62. Mariano ER, Loland VJ, Sandhu NS, et al: Comparative efficacy of ultrasound-guided and stimulating popliteal-sciatic perineural catheters for postoperative analgesia, *Can J Anaesth* 57:919–926, 2010.

63. McGettigan P, Henry D: Cardiovascular risk with non-steroidal anti-inflammatory drugs: systematic review of population-based controlled observational studies, *PLoS Med* 8:e1001098, 2011.

64. McNaught A, Shastri U, Carmichael N, et al: Ultrasound reduces the minimum effective local anaesthetic volume compared with peripheral nerve stimulation for interscalene block, *Br J Anaesth* 106:124–130, 2011.

65. Neal JM, Bernards CM, Hadzic A, et al: ASRA Practice Advisory on Neurologic Complications in Regional Anesthesia and Pain Medicine, *Reg Anesth Pain Med* 33:404–415, 2008.

66. Neuburger M, Buttner J, Blumenthal S, et al: Inflammation and infection complications of 2285 perineural catheters: a prospective study, *Acta Anaesthesiol Scand* 51:108–114, 2007.

67. Nossaman VE, Ramadhyani U, Kadowitz PJ, Nossaman BD: Advances in perioperative pain management: use of medications with dual analgesic mechanisms, tramadol and tapentadol, *Anesthesiol Clin* 28:647–666, 2010.

68. Ong CK, Seymour RA, Lirk P, Merry AF: Combining paracetamol (acetaminophen) with nonsteroidal antiinflammatory drugs: a qualitative systematic review of analgesic efficacy for acute postoperative pain, *Anesth Analg* 110:1170–1179, 2010.

69. Orebaugh SL, Williams BA, Vallejo M, Kentor ML: Adverse outcomes associated with stimulator-based peripheral nerve blocks with versus without ultrasound visualization, *Reg Anesth Pain Med* 34:251–255, 2009.

70. Parvizi J, Miller AG, Gandhi K: Multimodal pain management after total joint arthroplasty, *J Bone Joint Surg Am* 93:1075–1084, 2011.

71. Patanwala AE, Jarzyna DL, Miller MD, Erstad BL: Comparison of opioid requirements and analgesic response in opioid-tolerant versus opioid-naive patients after total knee arthroplasty, *Pharmacotherapy* 28:1453–1460, 2008.

72. Patterson R, Bello AE, Lefkowith J: Immunologic tolerability profile of celecoxib, *Clin Therap* 21:2065–2079, 1999.

73. Centers for Disease Control and Prevention (CDC): CDC grand rounds: prescription drug overdoses—a U.S. epidemic, *MMWR Morb Mortal Wkly Rep* 61:10–13, 2012.

74. Perlas A, Brull R, Chan VW, et al: Ultrasound guidance improves the success of sciatic nerve block at the popliteal fossa, *Reg Anesth Pain Med* 33:259–265, 2008.

75. Pountos I, Georgouli T, Calori GM, Giannoudis PV: Do nonsteroidal anti-inflammatory drugs affect bone healing? A critical analysis, *Scientific World Journal* 2012:606404, 2012.

76. Prommer EE: Tramadol: does it have a role in cancer pain management? *J Opioid Manag* 1:131–138, 2005.

77. Radbruch L, Grond S, Lehmann KA: A risk-benefit assessment of tramadol in the management of pain, *Drug Safety* 15:8–29, 1996.

78. Randelli P, Randelli F, Cabitza P, Vaienti L: The effects of COX-2 anti-inflammatory drugs on soft tissue healing: a review of the literature, *J Biol Regul Homeostatic Agents* 24:107–114, 2010.

79. Rapp SE, Ready LB, Nessly ML: Acute pain management in patients with prior opioid consumption: a case-controlled retrospective review, *Pain* 61:195–201, 1995.

80. Rice AS, McMahon SB: Peripheral nerve injury caused by injection needles used in regional anaesthesia: influence of bevel configuration, studied in a rat model, *Br J Anaesth* 69:433–438, 1992.

81. Rigaud M, Filip P, Lirk P, et al: Guidance of block needle insertion by electrical nerve stimulation: a pilot study of the resulting distribution of injected solution in dogs, *Anesthesiology* 2008;109:473–478.

82. Robards C, Hadzic A, Somasundaram L, et al: Intraneural injection with low-current stimulation during popliteal sciatic nerve block, *Anesth Analg* 109:673–677, 2009.

83. Sala-Blanch X, Lopez AM, Pomes J, et al: No clinical or electrophysiologic evidence of nerve injury after intraneural injection during sciatic popliteal block, *Anesthesiology* 115:589–595, 2011.

84. Saporito A, Sturini E, Petri J, et al: Case report: unusual complication during outpatient continuous regional popliteal analgesia, *Can J Anaesth* 59:958–962, 2012.

85. Schjerning Olsen AM, Fosbol EL, Lindhardsen J, et al: Duration of treatment with nonsteroidal anti-inflammatory drugs and impact on risk of death and recurrent myocardial infarction in patients with prior myocardial infarction: a nationwide cohort study, *Circulation* 123:2226–2235, 2011.

86. Selander D, Dhuner KG, Lundborg G: Peripheral nerve injury due to injection needles used for regional anesthesia. An experimental study of the acute effects of needle point trauma, *Acta Anaesthesiol Scand* 21:182–188, 1977.

87. Shipton EA: Tramadol—present and future, *Anaesth Intensive Care* 28:363–374, 2000.

88. Silverstein FE, Faich G, Goldstein JL, et al: Gastrointestinal toxicity with celecoxib vs nonsteroidal anti-inflammatory drugs for osteoarthritis and rheumatoid arthritis: the CLASS study: a randomized controlled trial. Celecoxib Long-term Arthritis Safety Study, *JAMA* 284:1247–1255, 2000.

89. Sites BD, Beach ML, Chinn CD, et al: A comparison of sensory and motor loss after a femoral nerve block conducted with ultrasound versus ultrasound and nerve stimulation, *Reg Anesth Pain Med* 34:508–513, 2009.

90. Skinner HB: Multimodal acute pain management, *Am J Orthop* 33(Suppl 5):5–9, 2004.

91. Sostres C, Gargallo CJ, Arroyo MT, Lanas A: Adverse effects of non-steroidal anti-inflammatory drugs (NSAIDs, aspirin and coxibs) on upper gastrointestinal tract, *Best Pract Res Clin Gastroenterol* 24:121–132, 2010.

92. Strom BL, Schinnar R, Apter AJ, et al: Absence of cross-reactivity between sulfonamide antibiotics and sulfonamide nonantibiotics, *N Engl J Med* 349:1628–1635, 2003.

93. Swegle JM, Logemann C: Management of common opioid-induced adverse effects, *Am Fam Physician* 74:1347–1354, 2006.

94. Swenson JD, Bay N, Loose E, et al: Outpatient management of continuous peripheral nerve catheters placed using ultrasound guidance: an experience in 620 patients, *Anesth Analg* 103:1436–1443, 2006.

95. Swenson JD, Davis JJ: No clinical or electrophysiologic evidence proving intraneural injection is safe, *Anesthesiology* 116:1152, 2012; author reply 1153–1154.

96. Thackeray EM, Swenson JD, Gertsch MC, et al: Diaphragm function after interscalene brachila plexus block: a double-blind, randomized comparison of 0.25% and 0.125% bupivacaine, *J Shoulder Elbow Surg* 2012. [Epub ahead of print.]

97. Tiippana EM, Hamunen K, Kontinen VK, Kalso E: Do surgical patients benefit from perioperative gabapentin/pregabalin? A systematic review of efficacy and safety, *Anesth Analg* 104:1545–1556, 2007.

98. Urmey WF, Stanton J: Inability to consistently elicit a motor response following sensory paresthesia during interscalene block administration, *Anesthesiology* 96:552–554, 2002.

99. van der Westhuizen J, Kuo PY, Reed PW, Holder K: Randomised controlled trial comparing oral and intravenous paracetamol (acetaminophen) plasma levels when given as preoperative analgesia, *Anaesth Intensive Care* 39:242–246, 2011.

100. Vinik HR, Kissin I: Rapid development of tolerance to analgesia during remifentanil infusion in humans, *Anesth Analg* 86:1307–1311, 1998.

101. Vloka JD, Hadzic A, April E, Thys DM: The division of the sciatic nerve in the popliteal fossa: anatomical implications for popliteal nerve blockade, *Anesth Analg* 92:215–217, 2001.

102. Vloka JD, Hadzic A, Lesser JB, et al: A common epineural sheath for the nerves in the popliteal fossa and its possible implications for sciatic nerve block, *Anesth Analg* 84:387–390, 1997.

103. Waters KA, McBrien F, Stewart P, et al: Effects of OSA, inhalational anesthesia, and fentanyl on the airway and ventilation of children, *J Appl Physiol* 92:1987–1994, 2002.

104. White JM, Irvine RJ: Mechanisms of fatal opioid overdose, *Addiction* 94:961–972, 1999.

105. White PF, Issioui T, Skrivanek GD, et al: The use of a continuous popliteal sciatic nerve block after surgery involving the foot and ankle: does it improve the quality of recovery? *Anesth Analg* 97:1303–1309, 2003.

106. Whitlock EL, Brenner MJ, Fox IK, et al: Ropivacaine-induced peripheral nerve injection injury in the rodent model, *Anesth Analg* 111:214–220, 2010.

107. Williams BA, Kentor ML, Bottegal MT: The incidence of falls at home in patients with perineural femoral catheters: a retrospective summary of a randomized clinical trial, *Anesth Analg* 104:1002, 2007.

108. Winnie AP: Interscalene brachial plexus block, *Anesth Analg* 49:455–466, 1970.

109. Young A, Buvanendran A: Recent advances in multimodal analgesia, *Anesthesiol Clin* 30:91–100, 2012.

110. Zhang J, Ho KY, Wang Y: Efficacy of pregabalin in acute postoperative pain: a meta-analysis, *Br J Anaesth* 106:454–462, 2011.

FOREFOOT

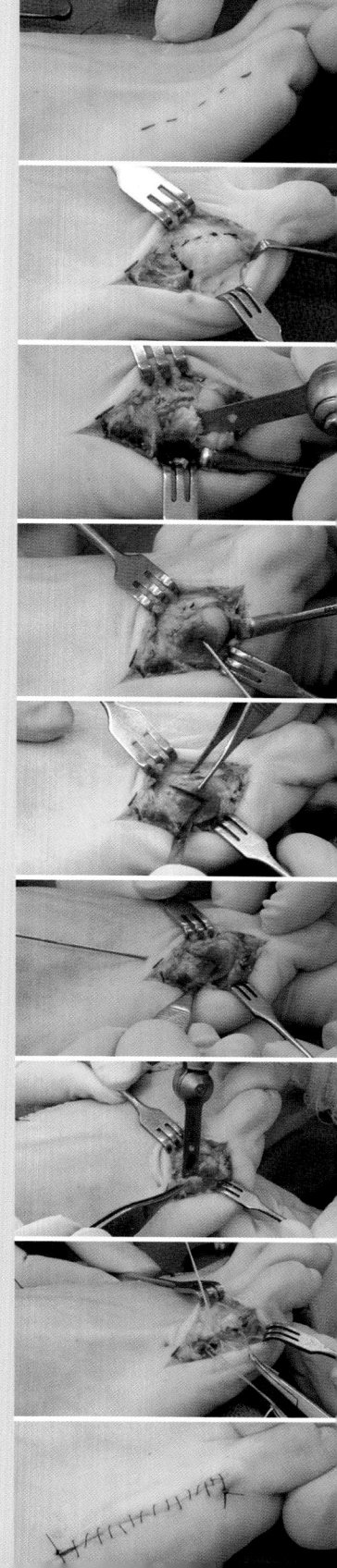

Chapter 6

Hallux Valgus

Michael J. Coughlin, Robert B. Anderson

OVERVIEW

The term *bunion* is derived from the Latin word *bunio*, meaning turnip, which has led to some confusing misapplications regarding disorders of the first metatarsophalangeal (MTP) joint. The word *bunion* has been used to denote any enlargement or deformity of the MTP joint, including such diverse diagnoses as an enlarged bursa, overlying ganglion, gouty arthropathy, and hallux valgus, as well as proliferative osseous changes that can develop secondary to MTP joint arthrosis (Fig. 6-1).

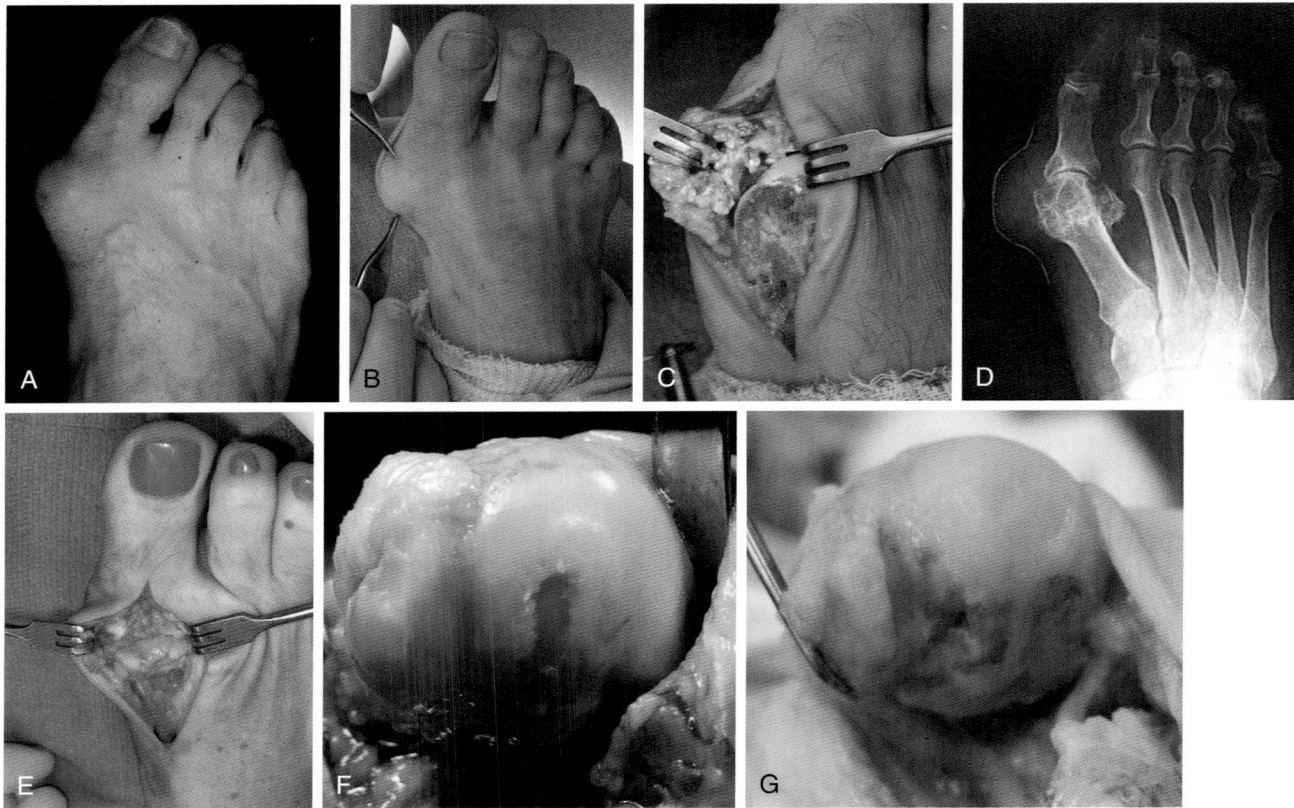

Figure 6-1 **A,** Appearance of hallux valgus deformity. **B,** Gouty arthropathy with a similar appearance. **C,** Intraoperative appearance with gouty tophi causing medial enlargement. **D,** Ganglion over the medial eminence causing enlargement. **E,** Enlargement due to hallux rigidus. **F** and **G,** As the cristae is worn, full-thickness cartilaginous erosions occur on the plantar aspect of the first metatarsal head. These are largely not observed, unless exposed during the dissection. They can be a source of postoperative diminished motion and intraarticular pain.

The term *hallux valgus* was introduced by Carl Hueter[230] to define a static subluxation of the first MTP joint characterized by lateral deviation of the great toe and medial deviation of the first metatarsal. It is now recognized, particularly in juvenile patients, that a hallux valgus deformity can originate because of lateral deviation of the articular surface of the metatarsal head without subluxation of the first MTP joint.[97-99]

A hallux valgus deformity can also be associated with abnormal foot mechanics, such as a contracted Achilles tendon; severe pes planus; generalized neuromuscular disease, such as cerebral palsy or a cerebrovascular accident (CVA, stroke); or an acquired deformity of the hindfoot secondary to rupture of the posterior tibial tendon. It can likewise be associated with various inflammatory arthritic conditions, such as rheumatoid arthritis (Fig. 6-2).

ANATOMY

The specialized articulation of the first MTP joint of the great toe differs from that of the lesser toes in that it has a sesamoid mechanism. The head of the first metatarsal is round and covered by cartilage and articulates with the

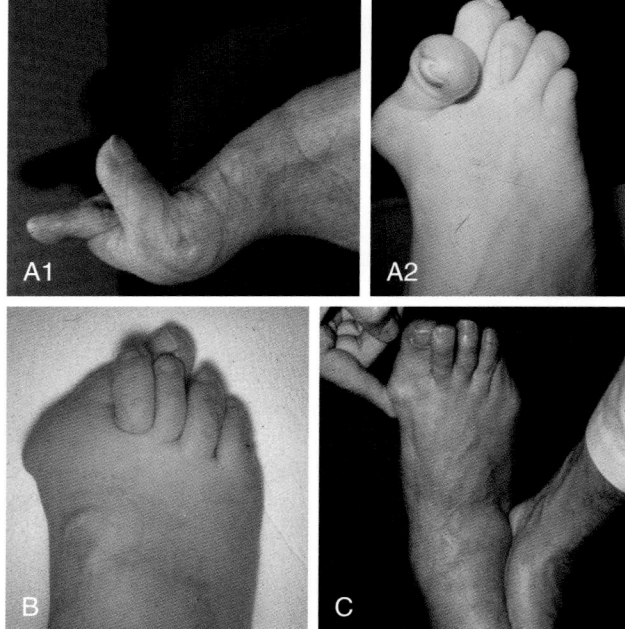

Figure 6-2 Hallux valgus deformity after a cerebral vascular accident (**A1** and **A2**), rheumatoid arthritis (**B**), and ruptured posterior tibial tendon (**C**).

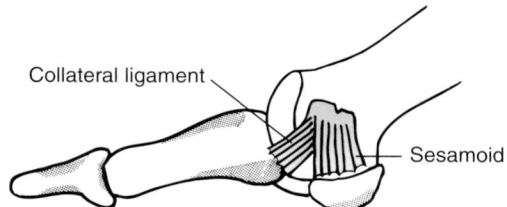

Figure 6-3 Collateral ligament structure around the first metatarsal head.

somewhat smaller, concave elliptic base of the proximal phalanx. A fan-shaped ligamentous band originates from the medial and lateral metatarsal epicondyles and constitutes the collateral ligaments of the MTP joint (Fig. 6-3). These ligaments interdigitate with ligaments of the sesamoids. The strong collateral ligaments run distally and plantarward to the base of the proximal phalanx, whereas the sesamoid ligaments fan out plantarward to the margins of the sesamoid and the plantar plate. The two tendons of the flexor hallucis brevis, the abductor and adductor hallucis, the plantar aponeurosis, and the joint capsule condense on the plantar aspect of the MTP joint to form the plantar plate (Fig. 6-4A).

Located on the plantar surface of the metatarsal head are two longitudinal cartilage-covered grooves separated by a rounded ridge (the crista). A sesamoid bone is contained in each tendon of the flexor hallucis brevis and articulates by means of cartilage-covered convex facets on its superior surface, with the corresponding longitudinal grooves on the inferior surface of the first metatarsal head. Distally, the two sesamoids are attached by the fibrous plantar plate (sesamoid-phalangeal ligament) to the base of the proximal phalanx; thus the sesamoid complex is attached to the base of the proximal phalanx rather than the metatarsal head. The sesamoids are connected by the intersesamoidal ligament, and this recess conforms to the crista on the plantar surface of the metatarsal head (Fig. 6-4B).

The tendons and muscles that move the great toe are arranged around the MTP joint in four groups. The dorsal group is composed of the long and short extensor tendons, which pass dorsally, with the extensor hallucis longus anchored, medially and laterally by the hood ligament (Fig. 6-5). The extensor hallucis brevis inserts beneath the hood ligament into the dorsal aspect of the base of the proximal phalanx. The plantar group contains the long and short flexor tendons, which pass across the plantar surface, with the tendon of the flexor hallucis longus coursing through a centrally located tendon sheath on the plantar aspect of the sesamoid complex. This tendon is firmly anchored by this tunnel within the sesamoid complex. The last two groups are composed of the tendons of the abductor and adductor hallucis, which pass medially and laterally, respectively, but closer to the plantar surface than the dorsal surface. Thus the dorsomedial and dorsolateral aspects of the joint capsule are covered only

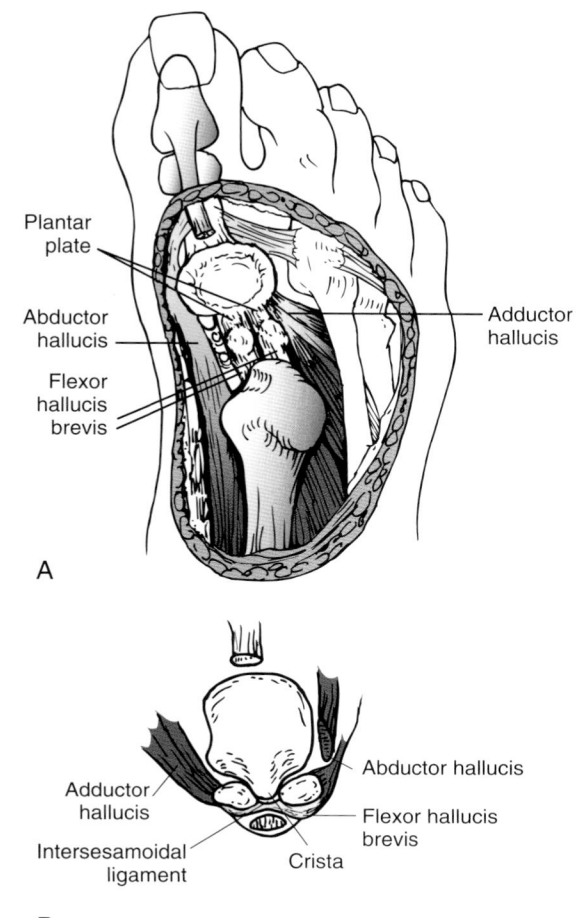

A

B

Figure 6-4 **A,** Dorsal view of first metatarsophalangeal (MTP) joint with the toe in plantar flexion. **B,** Cross section through the MTP joint demonstrating the relationship of the sesamoids and tendons to the first metatarsal head.

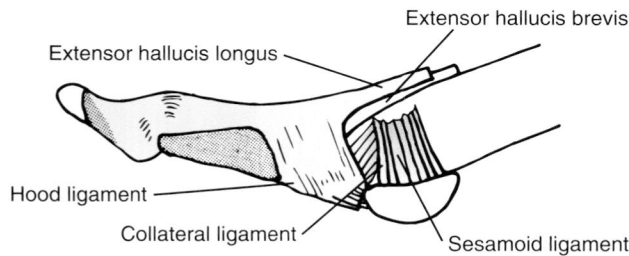

Figure 6-5 Collateral ligament structure and extensor mechanism around the first metatarsophalangeal joint.

by the hood ligaments, which maintain alignment of the extensor hallucis longus tendon.

The adductor hallucis, arising from the lesser metatarsal shafts, is made up of two segments, the transverse and the oblique heads, which insert on the plantar lateral aspect of the base of the proximal phalanx and also blend with the plantar plate and the sesamoid complex. The adductor hallucis balances the abductor forces of the abductor hallucis (Fig. 6-6). Acting in a line parallel to this bone and using the head of the first metatarsal as a fulcrum, the abductor hallucis pushes the first metatarsal toward the second metatarsal.

The base of the first metatarsal has a mildly sinusoidal articular surface that articulates with the distal articular surface of the first cuneiform. The joint has a slight medial plantar inclination. The medial lateral dimension is approximately half the length of the dorsoplantar dimension. The joint is stabilized by capsular ligaments and is bordered laterally by the proximal aspect of the second metatarsal, which extends more cephalad and offers a stabilizing lateral buttress to the first metatarsocuneiform (MTC) articulation. ElSaid et al,[146] in a cadaveric evaluation of 239 specimens, observed a facet to be present in 25% of cases; however, these were not specimens with hallux valgus. Coughlin and Jones[101] observed the radiographic presence of a facet between the proximal first and second metatarsals in 7% of 122 cases review with a bunion deformity (Fig. 6-7). The orientation of the MTC joint may determine the amount of metatarsus primus varus, and the shape of the articulation may affect metatarsal mobility. A medial inclination of up to 8 degrees at the MTC joint is normal. Increased obliquity at this joint can increase the degree of metatarsus primus varus. The axis of motion of the MTC joint is aligned to permit motion in a dorsal-medial to plantar-lateral plane.

The tarsometatarsal articulation is quite stable in the central portion because of interlocking of the central metatarsals and cuneiforms (Fig. 6-8). This is not necessarily the case for the first and fifth metatarsals, where stability is determined not only by the inherent stability of the tarsometatarsal articulation but also by the surrounding capsular structures. Therefore, when ligamentous laxity is present, the first metatarsal may deviate medially and the fifth metatarsal laterally in the development of a splay foot deformity (Fig. 6-9).

PATHOANATOMY

Because no muscle inserts on the metatarsal head, it is vulnerable to extrinsic forces, in particular, constricting

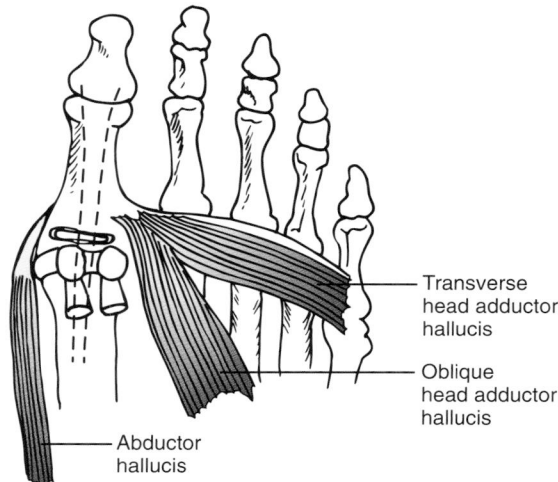

Figure 6-6 Normal anatomic configuration of the first metatarsophalangeal joint demonstrating the stabilizing effect of the abductor and adductor hallucis muscles.

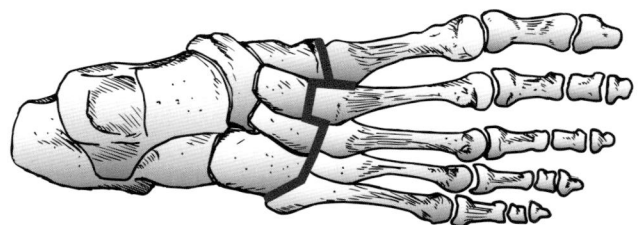

Figure 6-8 Stability of the tarsometatarsal articulation is maintained by interlocking of the central metatarsals.

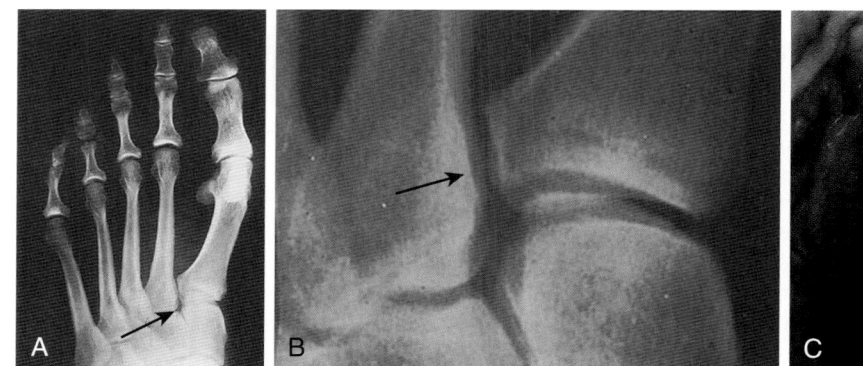
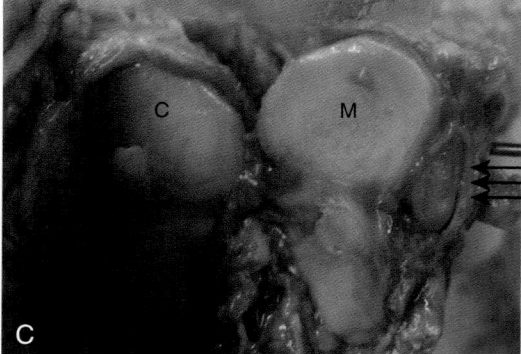

Figure 6-7 **A,** Anteroposterior radiograph demonstrating the irreducibility of the 1–2 intermetatarsal (IM) angle because of IM facet. **B,** Close-up demonstrating facet between proximal first and second metatarsal. **C,** Anatomic specimen showing close-up of the first metatarsal proximal facet (M) *(on right)* and cuneiform articular surface (C) on left. The first metatarsal has been folded back, exposing the cuneiform and metatarsal articular surfaces and the corresponding facets. The accessory facet is noted with three arrows. (Courtesy Faustin R. Stevens, MD.)

footwear. Once the metatarsal becomes destabilized and begins to subluxate medially, the tendons about the MTP joint drift laterally. The muscles that previously acted to stabilize the joint become deforming forces because their pull is lateral to the longitudinal axis of the first ray. The plantar aponeurosis and the windlass mechanism contribute significantly to stabilization of the first ray[450,460]; with progression of a hallux valgus deformity, their stabilizing influence is diminished (Fig. 6-10).[102,190] As the hallux valgus deformity progresses, the soft tissues on the lateral aspect of the first MTP joint become contracted, and those on the medial aspect become attenuated. The metatarsal head is pushed in a medial direction by the lateral deviation of the proximal phalanx, thereby progressively exposing the sesamoids, which are anchored in place by the transverse metatarsal ligament and the adductor hallucis muscle. As the metatarsal head continues to deviate medially off the sesamoids, the crista, which normally acts to stabilize the sesamoids, is gradually eroded (see Fig. 6-1F and G).[35,449,496] These lesions are rarely seen on the plantar surface of the first metatarsal unless an effort is made intraoperatively to inspect this area. Bock et al[35] reported on a large series of patients treat for hallux valgus, and found that 57% had significant plantar erosive lesions. Roukis et al,[449] reporting on 166 feet that underwent bunion surgery, noted that almost every joint had some element of articular cartilage erosion on the plantar metatarsal head. In more severe deformities, this erosion becomes more pronounced and extensive.[35,449] As the sesamoid sling slides beneath the first metatarsal head, the hallux gradually pronates. As this dynamic joint

deformity occurs, the medial eminence often becomes more prominent (Fig. 6-11).

The hallux and the first MTP joint play a significant role in the transfer of weight-bearing forces during locomotion. The plantar aponeurosis also plays a key role in this process by plantar flexing the first metatarsal as weight is transferred to the hallux. As the hallux is dorsiflexed at the first MTP joint, the first metatarsal is depressed, which results in increased weight bearing beneath the first metatarsal head and stabilization of the medial longitudinal arch (Fig. 6-12). Certain pathologic conditions, either acquired or iatrogenic, diminish the ability of the first MTP joint and hallux to function as weight-bearing structures. This results in transfer of weight to the lateral aspect of the forefoot, which often leads to the development of a transfer lesion beneath the second or third metatarsal head. As less weight is borne by the first ray, transfer metatarsalgia and lesser toe deformities may develop. Coughlin and Jones[100] reported a 48% incidence of second MTP joint symptoms in a prospective study of adult patients undergoing repair of moderate and severe hallux valgus deformity.

PATHOPHYSIOLOGY

The dynamics of the hallux valgus deformity can best be understood by first examining the articulation where the deformity occurs, that is, the MTP and MTC joints. The most stable MTP articulation has a flat articular surface, and conversely, the most unstable has a rounded head (Fig. 6-13).[88,139,155,336] Coughlin and Jones[101] noted this in 71% of patients in a large series of cases of hallux valgus

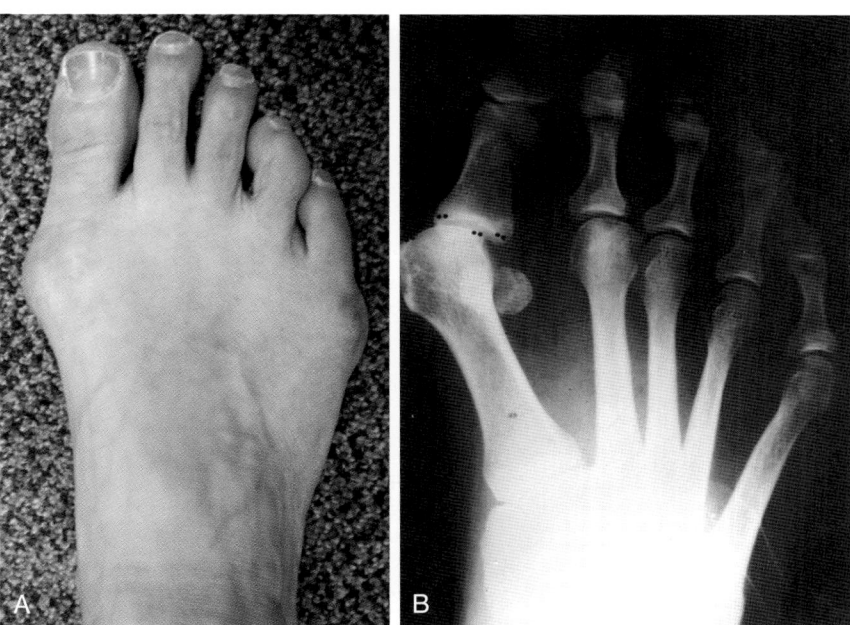

Figure 6-9 Splayed foot deformity. **A,** Clinical appearance. **B,** Radiograph.

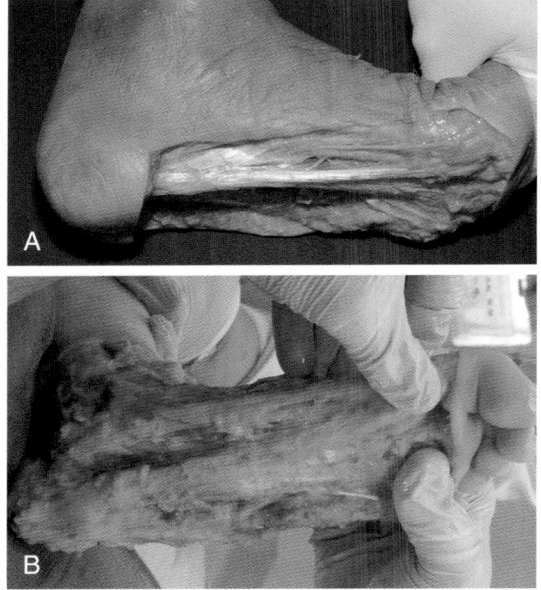

Figure 6-10 **A,** Medial view of the plantar aponeurosis. **B,** From beneath, the insertion into the hallux stabilizes the first ray.

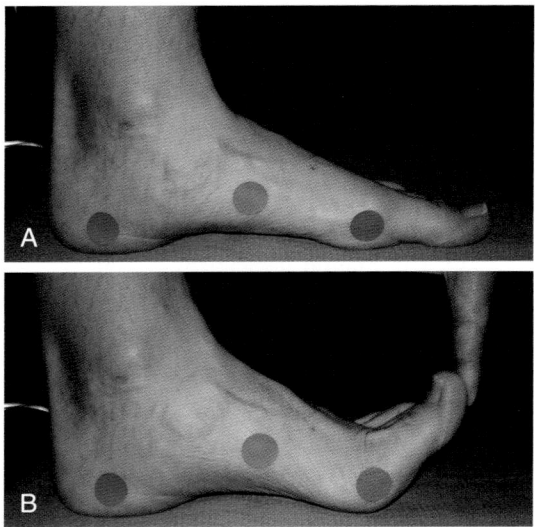

Figure 6-12 Dynamic function of the plantar aponeurosis. **A,** Foot at rest. **B,** Dorsiflexion of the metatarsophalangeal joints, which activates windlass mechanisms and brings about elevation of the longitudinal arch, plantar flexion of the metatarsal heads, and inversion of the heel.

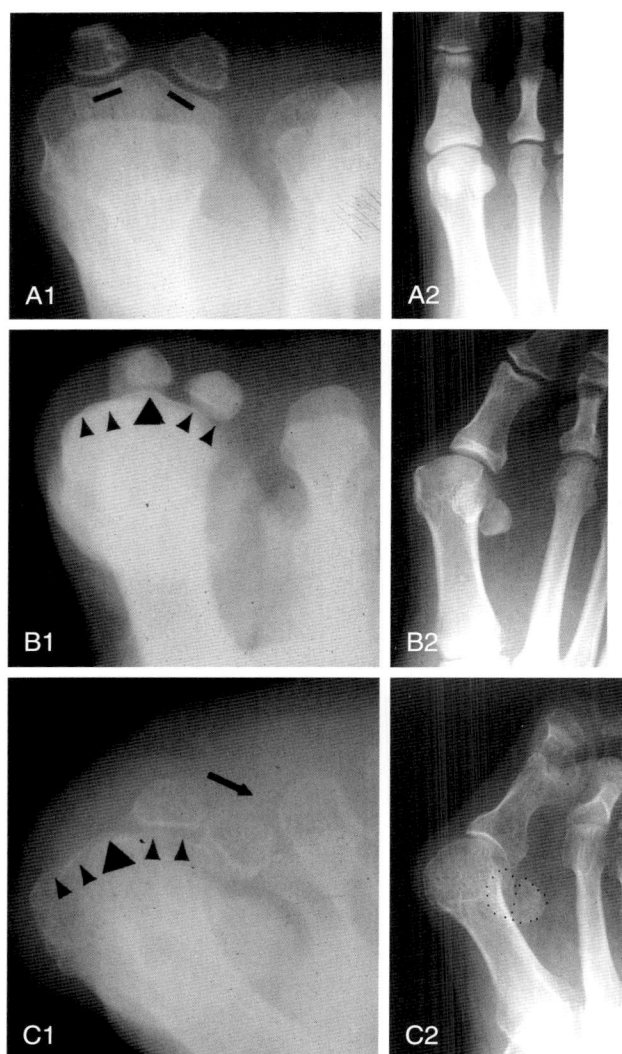

Figure 6-11 Sesamoid **(A1)** and anteroposterior (AP) **(A2)** views of a normal foot. Sesamoid **(B1)** view and AP **(B2)** views of moderate deformity. Sesamoid **(C1)** and AP **(C2)** views of severe deformity.

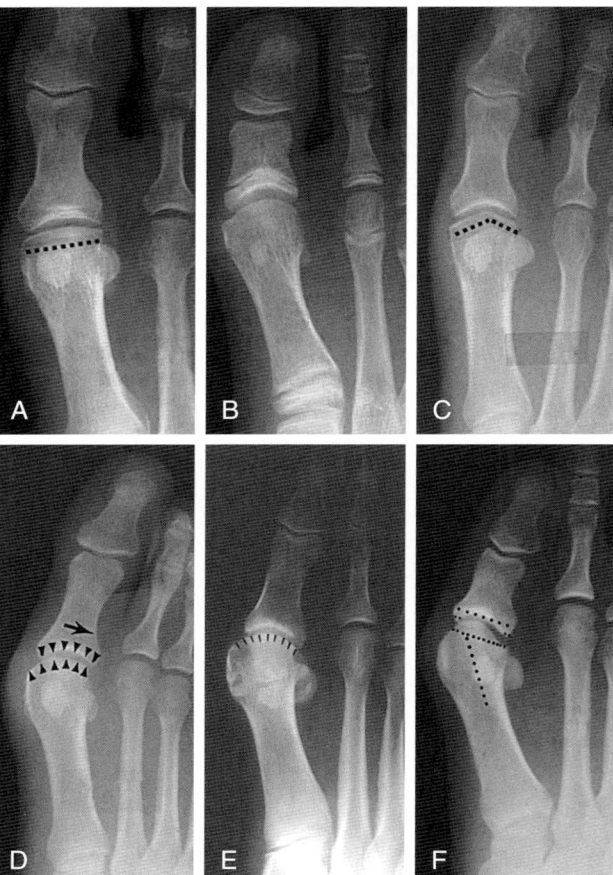

Figure 6-13 Anteroposterior radiographs demonstrating varying shapes of the metatarsophalangeal (MTP) articular surface. **A,** Flat MTP joint surface. Chevron-shaped surface in a juvenile **(B)** and in an adult **(C)** without subluxation. **D** and **E,** A rounded articular surface is more prone to subluxation of the MTP joint **(D,** mild subluxation (arrow denotes lateral subluxation of proximal phalanx); **E,** moderate subluxation). **F,** Congruent MTP joint with hallux valgus.

they examined. Okuda et al[394] also observed an increased incidence of a rounded first metatarsal head associated with hallux valgus. A congruent MTP joint likewise is more stable than an incongruent or subluxated joint. A congruent joint tends to remain stable, whereas once a joint has begun to subluxate, the deformity tends to progress with the passing of time (Fig. 6-14).

A patient with more than 10 to 15 degrees of lateral deviation of the distal metatarsal articular surface may have a significant hallux valgus deformity that is symptomatic because of the presence of a prominent medial eminence, even though the joint is congruent and tends to be stable.

In some circumstances, alignment of the first MTP joint is normal but a valgus deformity is present because of a deformity within the proximal phalanx, and a hallux valgus interphalangeus (HVI) deformity results (Fig. 6-15).

No muscle inserts into the first metatarsal head, and as a result its position is influenced by the position of the proximal phalanx. Because medial and lateral movement of the first metatarsal is to a great extent controlled by the position of the proximal phalanx, a certain degree of mobility at the MTC joint must exist for this to occur. A horizontal orientation tends to resist an increase in the intermetatarsal (IM) angle, whereas an oblique orientation is a less stable articulation.

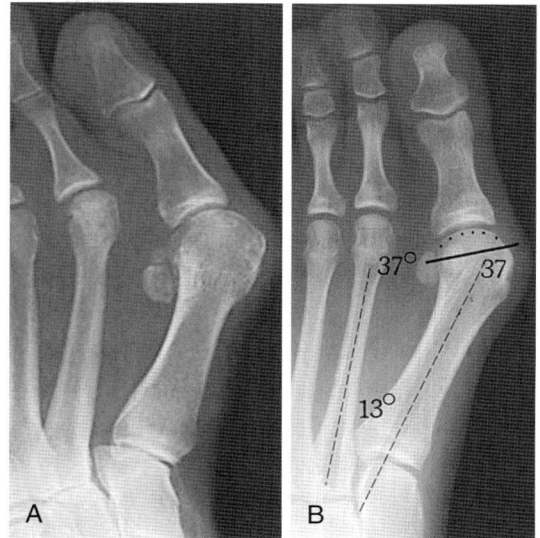

Figure 6-14 **A,** Subluxated metatarsophalangeal (MTP) joint with a hallux valgus deformity. **B,** Moderate metatarsus adductus with a congruent MTP joint (distal metatarsal articular angle, 37 degrees; hallux valgus angle, 37 degrees).

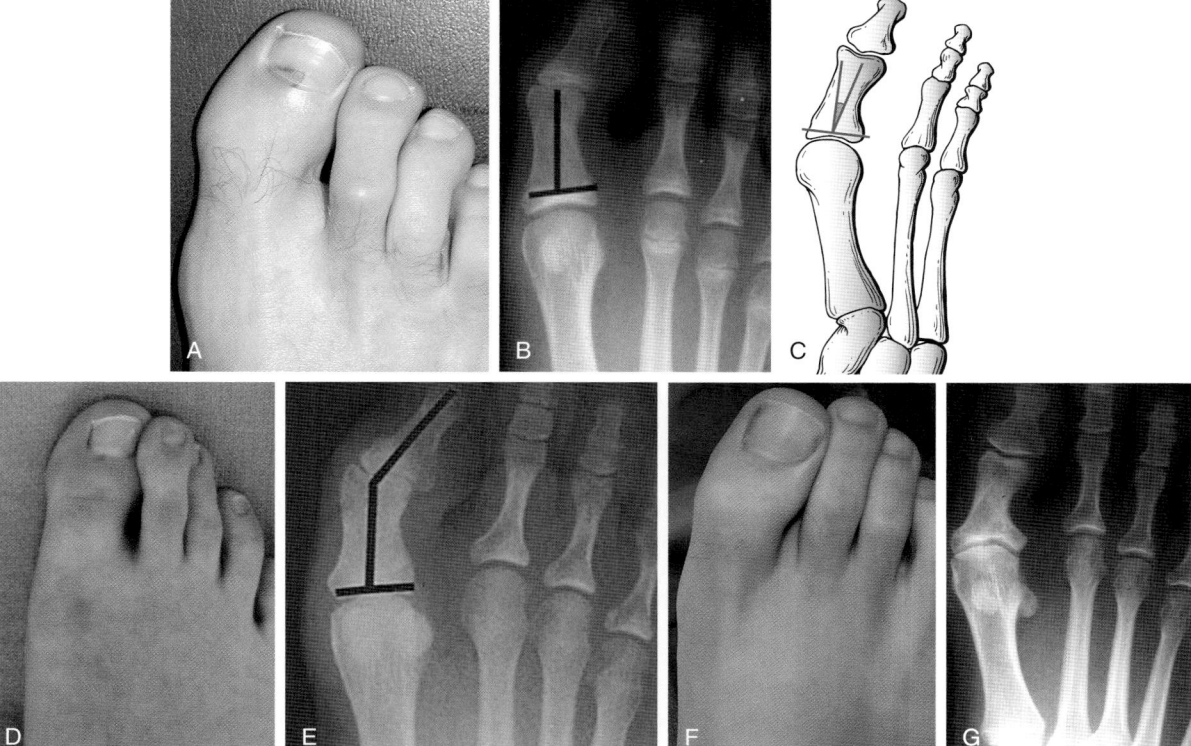

Figure 6-15 Hallux valgus interphalangeus. **A,** Clinical photo. **B,** Radiographic appearance. **C,** Schematic diagram of the abnormality. **D,** Clinical appearance of the distal interphalangeus. **E,** Radiographic appearance. **F,** Clinical appearance. **G,** Radiographic appearance of the interphalangeus that developed after an epiphyseal injury in adolescence.

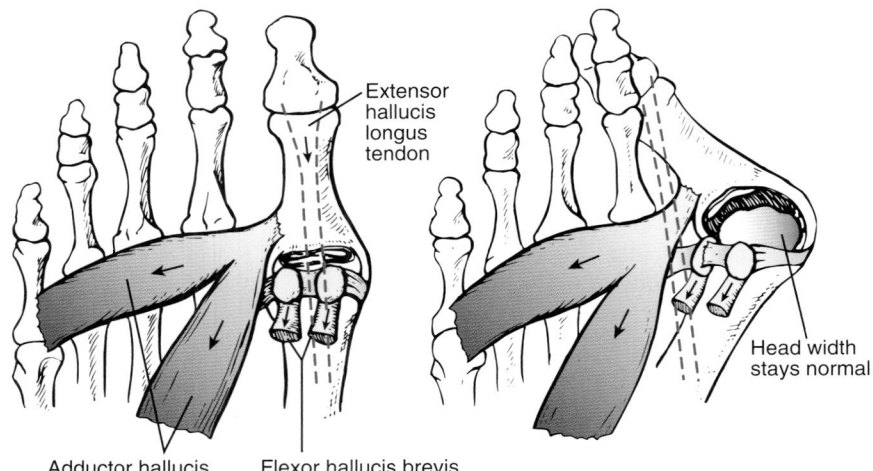

Extensor hallucis longus tendon

Head width stays normal

Adductor hallucis   Flexor hallucis brevis

Figure 6-16 Pathophysiology of hallux valgus deformity. Normally, the metatarsal head is stabilized within the sleeve of ligaments and tendons, which provide stability to the joint. As the proximal phalanx deviates laterally, it places pressure on the metatarsal head, which deviates medially. This results in attenuation of the medial joint capsule and contracture of the lateral joint capsule.

The pathophysiology of a hallux valgus deformity varies, depending on the nature of the deformity. With a congruent hallux valgus deformity, the basic deformity consists of the prominent medial eminence (the bunion), which results in pressure against the shoe and thus a painful bursa or cutaneous nerve over the prominence. The MTP joint itself is stable, and the deformity does not usually progress in adults.

With an incongruent or subluxated hallux valgus deformity, there is usually a progressive deformity. As the proximal phalanx moves laterally on the metatarsal head, it exerts pressure against the metatarsal head, which pushes it medially and results in an increased IM angle. As this process occurs, there is progressive attenuation of the medial joint capsule, as well as a progressive contracture of the lateral joint capsule (Figs. 6-16 and 6-17).

While this deformity is occurring, the sesamoid sling, which is anchored laterally by the insertion of the adductor hallucis muscle and the transverse metatarsal ligament, remains in place as the metatarsal head moves medially and thereby creates pressure on the medial joint capsule. The weakest portion of the medial joint capsule lies just above the abductor hallucis tendon, and with chronic pressure, this portion of the capsule gives way; as a result, the abductor hallucis muscle gradually slides beneath the medially deviating metatarsal head. As this process slowly progresses, atrophy of the crista occurs beneath the first metatarsal head, which normally helps stabilize the sesamoids (Fig. 6-18).

Once the abductor hallucis slides beneath the first metatarsal head, two events occur. First, the intrinsic muscles no longer act to stabilize the MTP joint but actually help enhance the deformity. Second, as the abductor hallucis rotates beneath the metatarsal head, because it is connected to the proximal phalanx, it will spin the proximal phalanx around on its long axis and give rise to

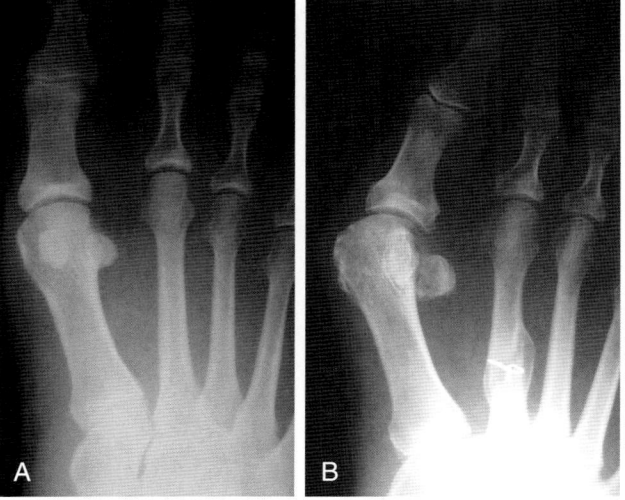

Figure 6-17 Progression of both hallux valgus and a 1–2 intermetatarsal angular deformity over a 5-year period. **A,** Initial radiograph. **B,** Twenty years later, a simultaneous increase in both angular deformities has occurred.

varying degrees of pronation (Fig. 6-19). It has been well established that as the hallux valgus deformity progresses, so does the degree of pronation.[336,344]

Because of this abnormal rotation, calluses may develop along the medial aspect of the interphalangeal (IP) joint. Ultimately, as the MTP joint becomes less stable, the hallux carries less weight, body weight is transferred laterally in the forefoot, and callus may develop beneath the second, third, or both metatarsal heads. Increased pressure may lead to capsulitis, instability, or deviation of the second MTP joint as well.

With severe hallux valgus deformities, the extensor hallucis longus tendon is displaced laterally as the medial

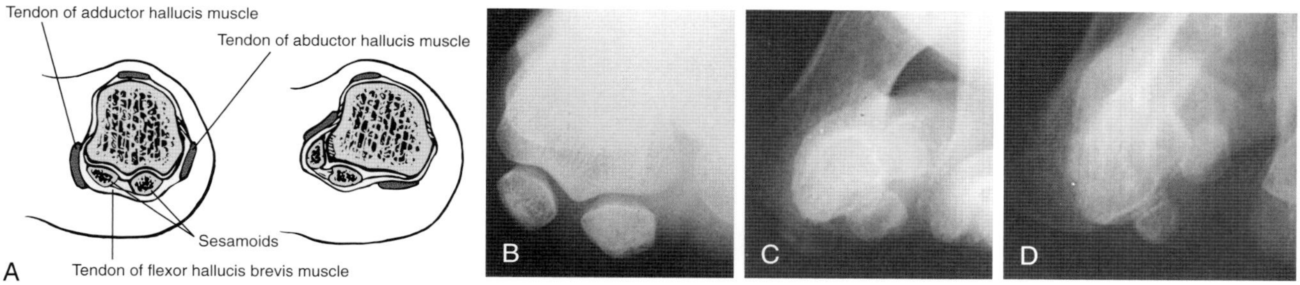

Figure 6-18 Relationship of the sesamoids to the metatarsal head. **A,** Diagram demonstrating the sesamoids stabilized by the crista, followed by atrophy of the crista as the metatarsal head deviates medially off the sesamoids. **B,** Normal relationship of the sesamoids to the crista. **C,** Moderate hallux valgus deformity. **D,** Severe hallux valgus deformity.

hood ligament and capsule become stretched. As a result, when the extensor hallucis contracts, it not only extends the toe but also tends to adduct it, thus further aggravating the deformity. The abductor hallucis tendon, by migrating plantarward, loses its remaining abduction power. The flexor hallucis longus tendon, which retains its relationship to the sesamoids, moves laterally and also becomes a dynamic deforming force.

In rare circumstances, if the progressive deformity of the MTP joint continues unabated, dislocation of the MTP joint may occur over time, with the fibular and tibial sesamoids becoming dislocated into the first IM space (Fig. 6-20).

Normally, a small eminence is present on the medial aspect of the first metatarsal head. The size of the medial eminence varies, and sometimes most of the enlargement is on the dorsomedial aspect of the head and is thus not apparent on anteroposterior (AP) radiographs. Volkman[540] and Truslow[527] both suggested that new bone formation occurred with bunion formation, whereas Lane[293] and Haines and McDougall[200] suggested that merely a segment of the first metatrsal head had become exposed with lateral deviation of the hallux. Thordarson and Krewer[515] and Coughlin and Jones[101] have both demonstrated that the size of the medial eminence was similar in subjects with and without bunions, and the authors concluded that bony proliferation was not a component of bunion formation. The overall width of the distal metatarsal head does not enlarge with progression of a hallux valgus deformity. Thordarson and Krewer reported an average width of the medial eminence of 4.4 mm, whereas Coughlin and Jones[101] reported the mean width to be 4.6 mm in subjects with bunions (Fig. 6-21). The medial eminence develops with lateral migration of the proximal phalanx, but it is not characterized by new bone formation or hypertrophy of the medial first metatarsal head.

As the hallux valgus deformity develops, progressive medial deviation of the metatarsal head occurs and becomes symptomatic because of pressure against the shoe. Individuals who wear a broad, soft shoe or sandal are not usually bothered by the enlarged medial eminence, in contrast to persons who wear dress or high-heeled shoes. At times, an inflamed or thickened bursa

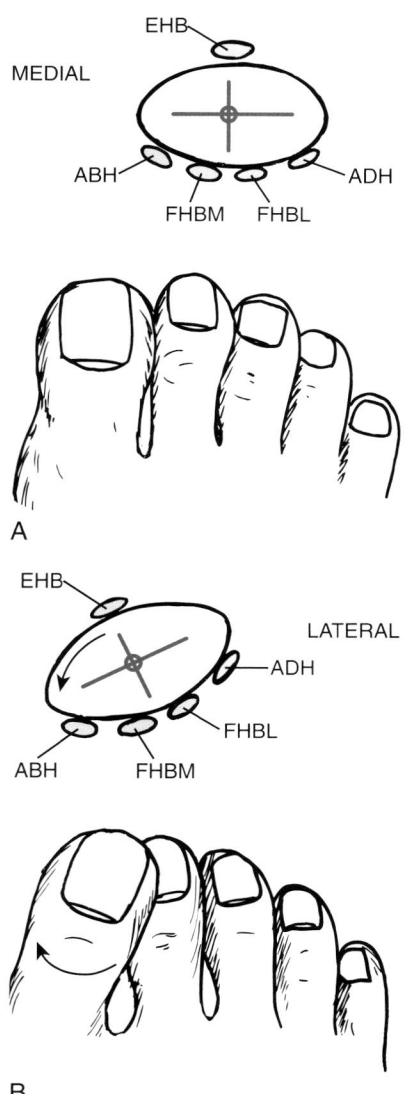

Figure 6-19 Schematic representation of tendons around the first metatarsal head. **A,** Normal articulation in a balanced state. **B,** Relationship of the tendons in hallux valgus deformity. *ABH,* abductor hallucis; *ADH,* adductor hallucis; *EHB,* extensor hallucis brevis; *FHBL,* flexor hallucis brevis lateral head; *FHBM,* flexor hallucis brevis medial head.

163

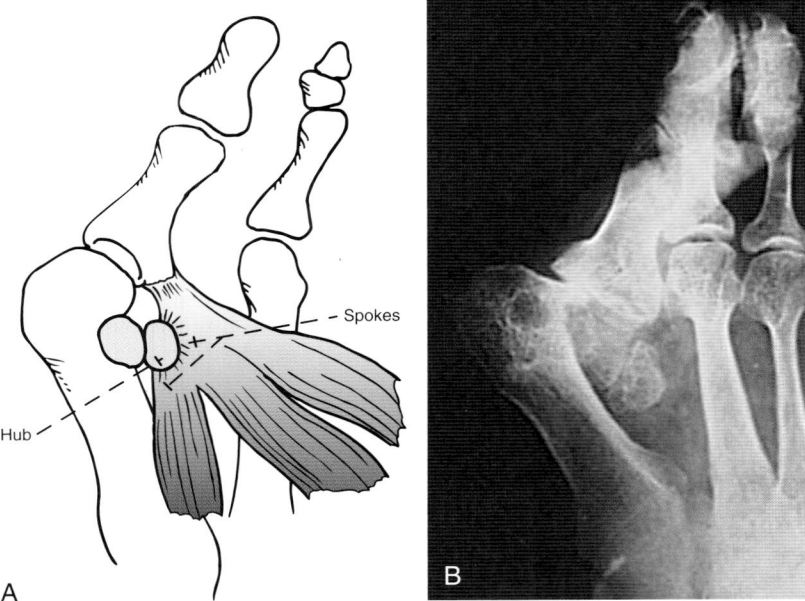

Figure 6-20 **A,** Diagram of severe hallux valgus. **B,** Severe end-stage hallux valgus deformity with dislocation of metatarsophalangeal joint and sesamoid mechanism into first web space.

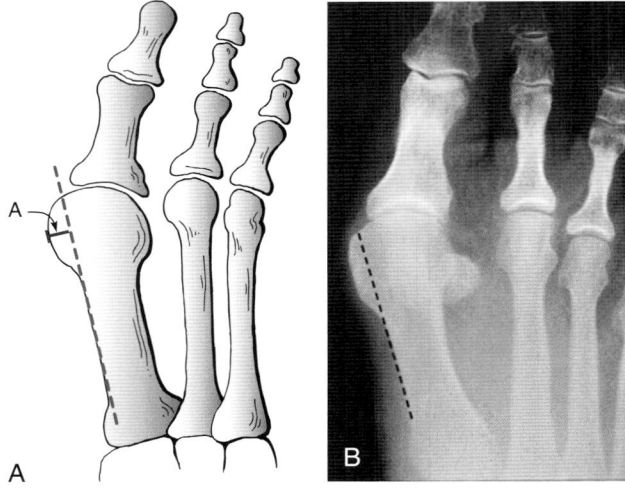

Figure 6-21 Technique of measuring the medial eminence. **A,** A longitudinal line is drawn along the medial diaphyseal shaft of the first metatarsal. A perpendicular line *(A)* is then drawn at the widest extent on the medial eminence and measured. **B,** Radiograph.

may aggravate the problem. On rare occasions and usually in older patients, the skin over the medial eminence can break down and result in a draining sinus. On other occasions, a ganglion arising from the medial side of the joint can erode the joint capsule and make the eventual hallux valgus repair technically much more difficult (see Fig. 6-1D).

The splayed appearance of the forefoot in more severe cases of hallux valgus (see Fig. 6-9) occurs primarily because the first metatarsal head is no longer contained within the sesamoid sling and is displaced in a medially deviated position. The middle metatarsals do not splay because of the stable articulation at their tarsometatarsal joints. On occasion, the fifth metatarsal lacks stability and drifts laterally, thereby completing the appearance of a splayed foot.

As the hallux drifts laterally, the lesser toes, particularly the second toe, are under increasing pressure. In response to this pressure, the second MTP joint may remain stable, and the great toe may drift beneath the second toe or occasionally on top of it. At other times, progressive subluxation or complete dislocation of the second MTP joint occurs. On occasion, no subluxation affects the second MTP joint; rather, all the lesser toes are pushed into lateral deviation or a "wind-swept" appearance resulting from extrinsic pressure from the hallux.

DEMOGRAPHICS

Age of Onset

Piggott[414] reported on a series of adult patients evaluated for hallux valgus deformities. Fifty-seven percent of the patients interviewed recalled an onset of the deformity during their adolescent years, whereas only 5% recalled development of the bunion deformity after 20 years of age. In a long-term review of patients with hallux valgus deformities, Hardy and Clapham[208] reported that 46% of bunion deformities occurred before the age of 20. Although Scranton[471] stated that a hallux valgus deformity rarely develops before 10 years of age, Coughlin[95] reported on a series of juvenile patients with bunions in whom the average age at onset was 12 years; 40% of these patients noted that the onset of their deformity occurred at the age of 10 years or younger. Thus development probably occurs much earlier than has previously been appreciated.*

In contrast, Coughlin[91] reported onset by decade in a group of men and noted that 21 of 34 (62%) patients dated the development of their bunion to the third to fifth decade of life. Only 7 of 34 (20%) recalled onset in the adolescent years. Later, Coughlin and Jones[101] stated that 65% of adults reported the onset of their deformity in the third through fifth decades and only 4% in the first decade. Although the onset of hallux valgus indeed peaked during the third decade, the incidence of occurrence was almost equal throughout the second through fifth decades. There was not relationship between the severity of the deformity and the decade of onset.

At what age a patient recognizes a hallux valgus deformity is obviously dependent on understanding the deformity, the symptoms, magnitude of the deformity, family history, and keenness of a patient's observation skills. Many deformities can begin in the adolescent years but progress in magnitude in later decades when they become more symptomatic. The date when surgery was performed should not be confused with the age at onset. Coughlin and Jones[101] noted that although patients recalled the onset of their bunion deformity at a mean age of 31 years, the average age at which surgery was performed was 50 years. Increasing age was not associated with increasing magnitude of angular deformity. In a retrospective study, Coughlin and Thompson[112] reviewed more than 800 cases and reported the mean age at surgery to be 60 years. Of importance is the fact that late development after skeletal maturity occurs in a foot that at one point most likely had a normal structure, whereas an early onset in the juvenile years occurs before maturation in a foot that most likely "never had a normal structure." Coughlin[95] observed, in a series of patients with juvenile hallux valgus, that early onset of hallux valgus (before 10 years of age) was associated with a much higher distal metatarsal articular angle (DMAA), a finding that would probably alter the choice of operative technique in these patients.

Gender

Although several studies have provided statistical data showing some predilection in the female population for the development of hallux valgus, this may be merely a reflection of a specific person's choice of footwear. Wilkins,[552] in a study of schoolchildren's feet, reported a female preponderance of 2:1. Hewitt et al[221] and Marwil and Brantingham,[350] in investigating male and female military recruits, found a predilection of approximately 3:1 in the female population. Creer[114] and Hardy and Clapham,[207] in reporting statistics from their surgical practices, found this ratio to be approximately 15:1 in

---

*References 10, 58, 170, 195, 364, 471, and 472.

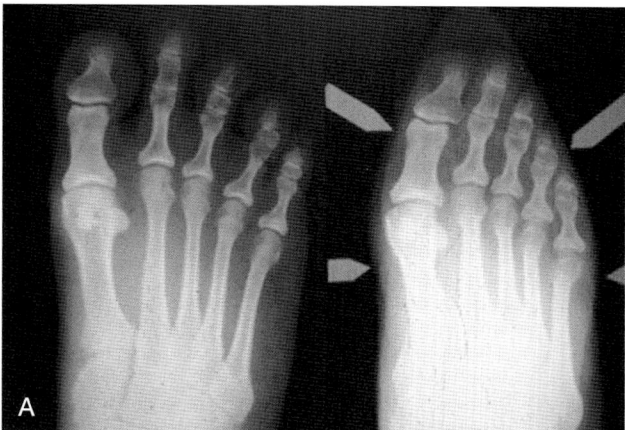

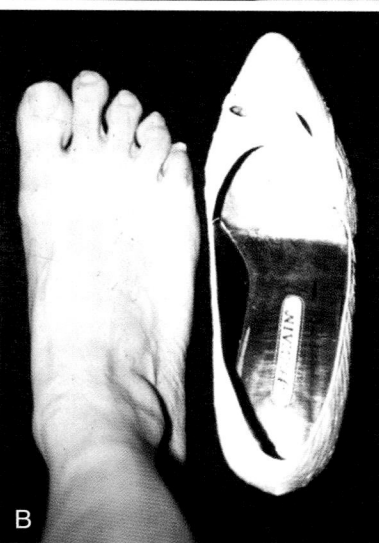

Figure 6-22 **A,** Normal foot on the *left,* foot in a fashionable shoe on the *right.* **B,** Photograph of the foot and shoe.

adult patients. The reported incidence of females in the juvenile population undergoing surgical correction for hallux valgus deformities varies from 84% to 100%.* Several studies on adult patients report females make up 90% or more of the patient population.† Coughlin and Jones[101] found that the proportion of females in their report on moderate and severe hallux valgus deformities was 92% ($P < .01$). Certainly, shoes worn by women are generally less physiologic than those worn by men, and shoes of any type can lead to hallux valgus in susceptible persons; however, it is also likely that heredity plays a substantial role in the development of bunion deformities (Fig. 6-22). On the contrary, Akinbo et al,[3] in a study of young Nigerians, reported close to equal female (56%) and male (44%) involvement in an adolescent population. Pique-Vidal et al[419] observed that gender did not

---

*References 73, 217, 370, 513, 514, and 526.
†References 34, 38, 73, 74, 112, 207, 255, 312, 318, 336, 352, 370, and 414.

effect the severity of the angular deformity. Pique-Vidal[419] did not note an association between gender and severity of deformity in his series of 350 subjects.

Bilaterality

The authors previously believed that hallux valgus deformities commonly occurred as unilateral deformities.[339] This notion was based on reports of the results of surgical procedures in which a majority of patients underwent unilateral surgery.* However, this information does not truly document the incidence of bilaterality. Patients may have bilateral deformities yet have surgery performed on only one side. They may undergo bilateral surgery yet have only the index surgery performed during the period of study. Even though many reports cite unilateral occurrence, the author's prospective evaluation of moderate and severe hallux valgus deformities demonstrated that although 84% of patients had bilateral hallux valgus deformities, only 18% had both feet corrected during the study period.[101] The remaining surgery occurred either before or after the reported study. There was no association between bilateral deformities and handedness, family history, or the magnitude of the preoperative deformity. There was a strong correlation between bilateralism and a family history of bunions ($P < .01$). Symptoms and varying magnitudes of deformity may lead a person to desire unilateral correction despite having bilateral hallux valgus deformities. The authors believe that the majority of patients have bilateral hallux valgus deformities of differing magnitude.

Handedness

Ninety percent of the population is right handed,[550] but how this translates to foot dominance is unknown.[549] Coughlin and Jones[101] reported that 91% of patients who underwent bunion surgery were right handed and were unable to find a correlation between handedness and foot side involved, age of onset, or severity of the hallux valgus deformity. Although most series report the number of right and left feet involved, it is unknown whether handedness makes a difference in development of the deformity.

Frequency of Occurrence

Myerson[384] has suggested that hallux valgus deformities develop in 2% to 4% of the population. Although no published study has reported the frequency of development or the rate of surgical correction of hallux valgus deformities in the United States, Coughlin and Thompson[112,513] estimated that more than 200,000 hallux valgus corrections are performed in the United States each year. This figure is probably an underestimate of both the incidence of the deformity and the frequency of surgical correction.

---

*References 73, 140, 344, 348, 454, and 535.

ETIOLOGY

Extrinsic Causes

Footwear

Hallux valgus occurs almost exclusively in persons who wear shoes but does occasionally occur in unshod people (Fig. 6-23). The notion of footwear being the principal

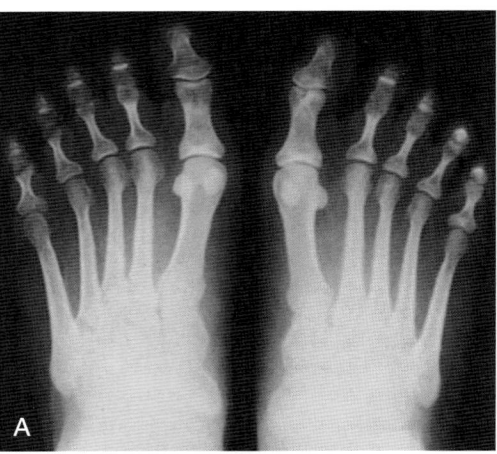
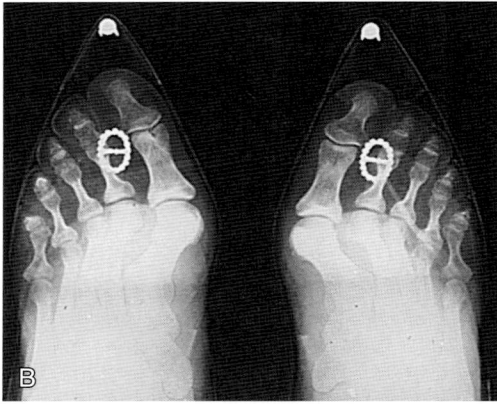
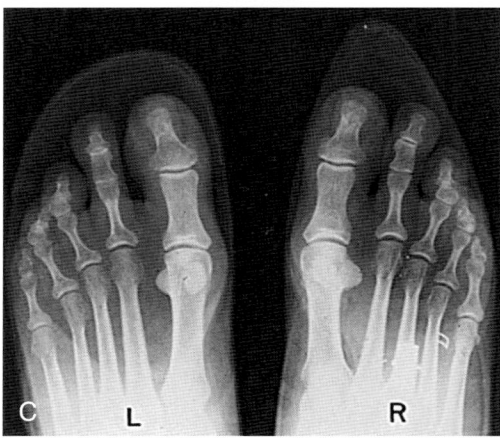

Figure 6-23 **A,** Normal feet of young woman during weight bearing. **B,** Feet in shoes during weight bearing. Note the developing hallux valgus. **C,** Effects of different types of shoes. The left shoe permits freedom of forefoot function; the right shoe restricts function of the four lesser toes.

contributor to the development of hallux valgus was substantiated by a study of Sim-Fook and Hodgson[487] in which 33% of shod persons had some degree of hallux valgus as compared with 2% of unshod persons. Owoeye et al[3,398] reported a very low incidence of hallux valgus in Nigerian youth in a typically unshod population. Hallux valgus deformities were also extremely rare in the Japanese because of the nature of their traditional footwear, the tabi sandal (Fig. 6-24). When the manufacture of fashionable leather shoes greatly exceeded the manufacture of traditional sandals in the 1970s, the incidence of hallux valgus deformity increased substantially.[259] Conversely, physicians in France referred to the development of hallux valgus deformities as early as the 18th century. Before that time, the common footwear was a Greco-Roman style, flat-soled sandal. Studies by Maclennan[322] in New Guinea, Wells[547] in South Africa, Barnicot and Hardy[21] in West Africa, Engle and Morton[148] in the Belgian Congo, and James[239] in the Solomon Islands found some element of metatarsus primus varus and an occasional asymptomatic hallux valgus deformity in the indigenous populations (Fig. 6-25). Cho et al[67] has reported in a study from a rural Korean community, that female subject

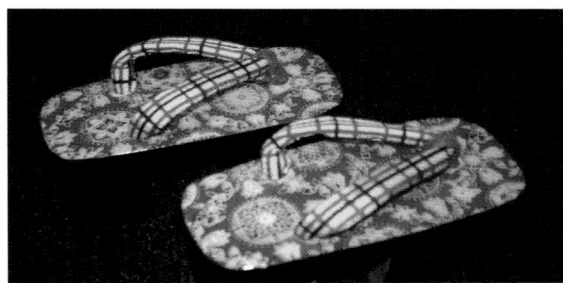

Figure 6-24 Traditional Japanese sandal.

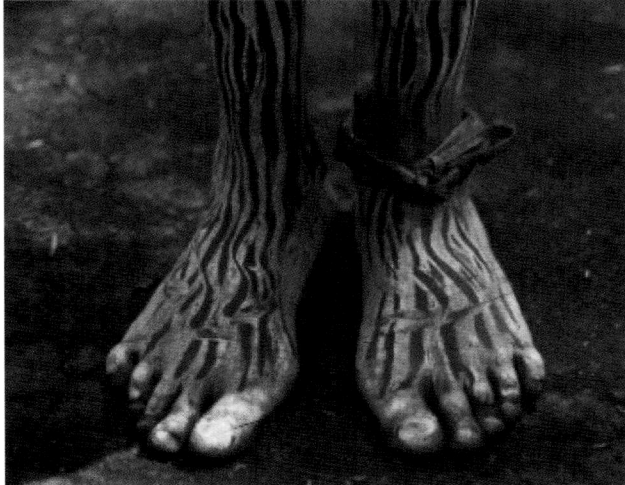

Figure 6-25 Kenyan tribesman with an asymptomatic hallux valgus deformity. (Courtesy J.J. Coughlin, MD.)

in the fourth through seventh decades had a higher incidence of deformity.

One can conclude from these studies that an asymptomatic hallux valgus deformity in an unshod person may be attributed to hereditary causes. In shoe-wearing populations, however, a symptomatic and painful bunion would be expected to develop more commonly.[113,221] A wide or splayed forefoot forced into a constricting shoe might thus lead to symptoms over the medial eminence.

Although shoes appear to be an essential extrinsic factor in the development of hallux valgus, the deformity does not develop in many people who wear fashionable footwear. Therefore some intrinsic predisposing factors must make some feet more vulnerable to the effect of footwear and likewise predispose some unshod feet to the development of hallux valgus. Although high-fashion footwear has been implicated in the progression of hallux valgus deformities in adults,* Hardy and Clapham[207] and others[95,249] have suggested that in most cases a juvenile hallux valgus deformity does not appear to be influenced by a history of constricting footwear. Poorly fitting shoes play a small role in juvenile hallux valgus. In a prospective study of adults with hallux valgus, Coughlin and Jones[101] reported that only 34% of patients undergoing surgical correction implicated constricting footwear as a cause of their deformity. In an earlier report, Coughlin[91] found that 60% of men with hallux valgus who had undergone surgical correction implicated ill-fitting shoes as a cause of their deformity.

Occupation
Cathcart[62] and Creer[114] have implicated occupation as a cause of hallux valgus. Again, objective evidence in the small percentage of patients who claim that their occupation contributed to their hallux valgus deformity is lacking. Coughlin and Jones[101] reported that patients considered occupation an infrequent cause of their deformity, with 17% implicating their job as a cause of their hallux valgus deformity. However, there was not a correlation between the magnitude of the angular deformity and those who attributed their deformity to either occupation or constricting shoewear.

Trauma
Trauma to the forefoot may be a cause of acute deformity or chronic deviation to the MTP joint. Rupture of the medial joint capsule has been recognized as a cause leading to development of a bunion deformity.[151] Johal et al[241] reported a bunion deformity that followed a tibial shaft fracture with entrapment and injury to the medial plantar nerve. Bohay et al[37] reported seven cases in which a Lisfranc joint injury led to first MTC joint instability and later bunion deformity. Surgical correction with a standard bunion correction in several of these cases led to realignment of the first ray.

---

*References 5, 105, 164, 361, 471, and 487.

Intrinsic Causes

Heredity

The notion that a hallux valgus deformity is inherited has indeed been suggested by many authors.* A positive family history of hallux valgus in 58% to 88% has been reported in five different series of adult patients.[73,184,207,370,427] Coughlin and Jones[101] stated that 86 of 103 adult patients (84%) reported a family history (parents, grandparents) of hallux valgus deformities.

In 1956, Johnston[248] reported an in-depth genetic history on subjects with hallux valgus. Based on a single-family case report, he proposed that this trait was auto-somal dominant with incomplete penetrance. Juvenile hallux valgus deformities have been characterized by their familial tendency. Coughlin[95] reported a family history in 72% of patients in his retrospective study on juveniles and noted that a bunion was identified in 94% of 31 mothers of children with a family history of hallux valgus deformity. Of the 31 patients with a positive family history for the deformity, four females noted an unbroken four-generation history of hallux valgus transmission from maternal great-grandmother to maternal grandmother to mother to patient (Fig. 6-26). Eleven females reported a three-generation history of transmission from maternal grandmother to mother to patient, and 11 patients noted a two-generation history of mother-to-patient transmission. Of three males with hallux valgus in this same series, two reported their mothers to have had a bunion and one reported a three-generation history of maternal transmission to the patient. Thus 29 of 31 patients (94%) with a family history showed a pattern consistent with maternal transmission. The preoperative hallux valgus deformity in these patients was reported to be 5 degrees greater in those with a family history, although the average postoperative hallux valgus correction was similar in patients with and without a family history.

Pique-Vidal et al,[419] in a report of 350 patients with hallux valgus, constructed a three-generation pedigree. The gender ratio was male:female 1:15; juveniles comprised only 5% of the series. Ninety percent of the subjects had at least one other relative with a bunion; 70% of the subjects had at least three relatives with bunion involvement. The authors also observed that severity of the deformity was not affected by gender or the magnitude of deformity in other relatives.

Both Bonney and Macnab[38] and Coughlin[95] observed an earlier onset of deformity in patients with a family history of hallux valgus. The high rate of maternal transmission noted in previous reports[95,207] makes it difficult to avoid a conclusion that there is a genetic predisposition for hallux valgus deformities in the female population. However, the chapter authors believe that although this trait can be associated with X-linked dominant transmission or polygenic transmission, it more commonly is

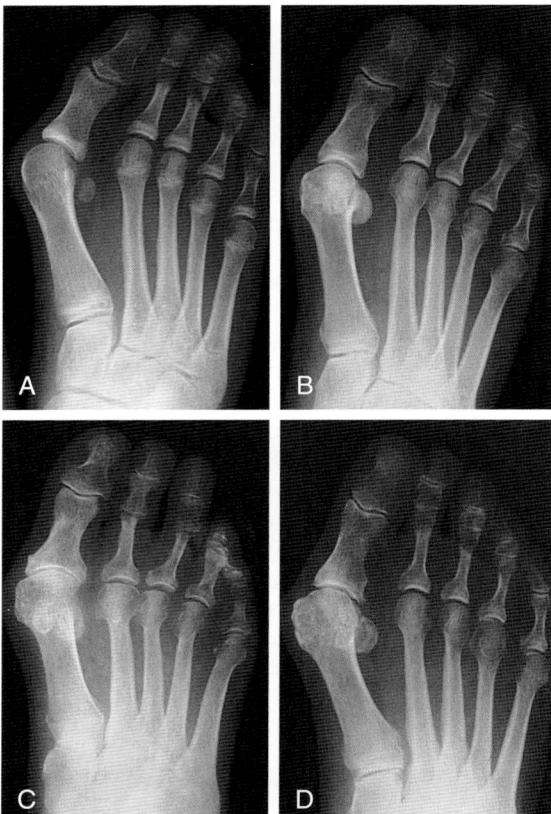

Figure 6-26 A family history of juvenile hallux valgus is common. **A,** Hallux valgus in a 16-year-old girl. **B,** Hallux valgus of long-standing duration in her 33-year-old mother. **C,** Hallux valgus in her 60-year-old grandmother. **D,** Hallux valgus in her 85-year-old great-grandmother, present since her youth.

an autosomal dominant transmission with incomplete penetrance.[95,419]

Pes Planus

The association of pes planus with the development of a hallux valgus deformity is controversial. A low incidence of advanced pes planus in adults with hallux valgus led Mann and Coughlin to conclude that the occurrence of hallux valgus with pes planus is uncommon in patients without neuromuscular disorders.[336] The incidence of pes planus in the general population was defined in a review of normal adult military recruits by Harris and Beath.[210] They reported a 20% incidence of pes planus. Half of these cases represented an asymptomatic "simple depression of the longitudinal arch." In general, pes planus may be no more common in those with hallux valgus than in the general population.* Pouliart et al[427] did not observe any relationship between the degree of pes planus and the severity of hallux valgus. Kilmartin and Wallace[272] found that the incidence of pes planus in the normal

---

*References 38, 58, 95, 101, 110, 138, 145, 170, 184, 197, 201, 318, 419, 472, and 514.

*References 95, 101, 110, 272, 336, 459, and 526.

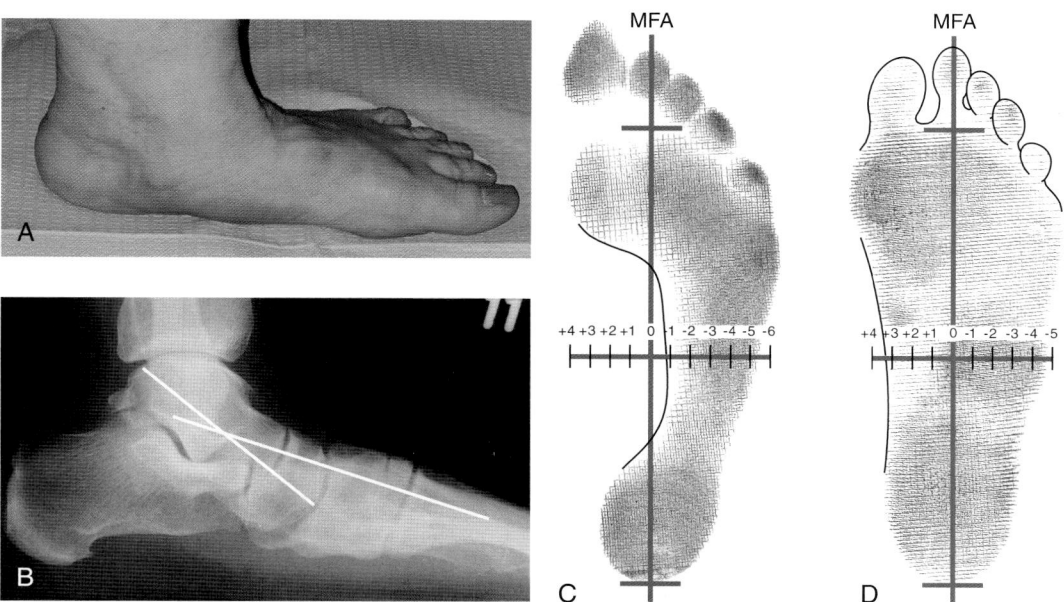

Figure 6-27 **A,** Pes planus deformity. **B,** Lateral talometatarsal angle demonstrating pes planus. Harris mat imprint **(C)** demonstrating a normal arch and a pes planus deformity **(D)** (*MFA,* midline foot axis, a line drawn from the middle of the second toe imprint to the center of the heel imprint. An imprint medial to the MFA represents a low-arched foot or pes planus). **(C** and **D,** Used with permission from Grebing B, Coughlin M: Evaluation of Morton's theory of second metatarsal hypertrophy. *J Bone Joint Surg Am* 86:1375-1386, 2004.)

population and in those with a hallux valgus deformity was essentially the same. They concluded that pes planus in juveniles had no significant association either with the magnitude of the preoperative hallux valgus deformity or with the postoperative success or failure rate of a surgical repair. This finding was confirmed by Coughlin[95] and Trott,[526] and McCluney and Tinley,[359] who all noted no increased incidence of pes planus in juvenile patients. Studies by Canale et al,[58] Coughlin[95] and Kilmartin and Wallace[272] have reported no correlation between pes planus and the success rate of surgical repair of a hallux valgus deformity. Coughlin and Jones[100,101] reported a 15% incidence of moderate and severe pes planus in their surgical series of 122 feet with hallux valgus.

Arch height has been quantified by both Harris mat imprints and radiographic measurements (Fig. 6-27).[103,110] Coughlin and Kaz[103] reported good correlation between Harris mat imprints and physical examination and angular measurements, such as the lateral talometatarsal angle, lateral talocalcaneal angle, calcaneal pitch, and the AP taolnavicular angle. Grebing and Coughlin[192] used Harris mat imprints to assess arch height and demonstrated that a low arch was significantly more common in an adult group with hallux valgus than in a control group. They reported an 11% incidence of pes planus in a normal control group and a 24% incidence in a group with hallux valgus but also found no correlation between the hallux valgus angle and pes planus or between pes planus and first-ray mobility. Saragas and Becker[459] did not find an increased incidence of pes planus when they examined

the calcaneal pitch angle and found no association between the degree of pes planus and the severity of hallux valgus deformity. King and Toolan[275] observed an association between the hallux valgus angle and both the Meary line (lateral talometatarsal angle) and the AP talo-navicular coverage angle in those with pes planus.

Other authors have suggested that a hallux valgus deformity tends to develop in a pronated foot.* Hohmann[225] was the most definitive and asserted that hallux valgus was always associated with pes planus and that pes planus is always a causative factor in hallux valgus. In attempting to resolve this contradiction, the chapter authors believe that a patient with a pes planus deformity in whom hallux valgus develops will have more rapid progression of the deformity. However, hallux valgus does not develop in most patients with pes planus.

Models and radiographs can demonstrate the role of pronation in the pathophysiology of hallux valgus in a normal foot (Figs. 6-28 to 6-31). Although an excellent demonstration of the effect of pronation on the foot and hallux. They do not enable determination of what initiates a hallux valgus deformity. In Figure 6-28, a pendulum has been attached to the nail of the great toe. As the foot is pronated, rotation of the first ray around its longitudinal axis is clearly seen. In Figure 6-29, a skeletal model has been photographed. With longitudinal rotation of the

---

*References 9, 28, 73, 89, 90, 113, 138, 150, 165, 205, 223, 230, 235, 254, 255, 353, 354, 385, 444, 462, 466, 486, 503, and 534.

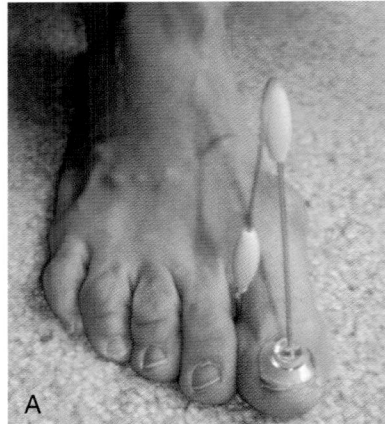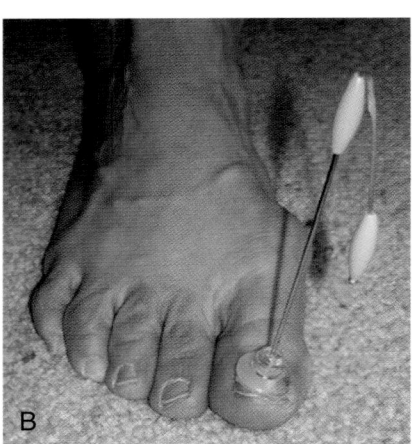

Figure 6-28 Longitudinal rotation of the first ray. **A,** Supination. **B,** Pronation. A pendulum is attached to the toenail of the great toe.

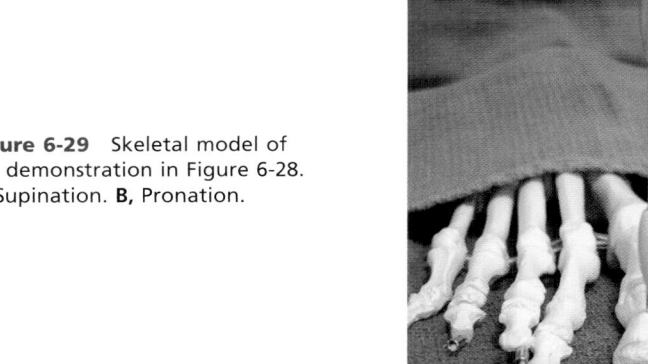

Figure 6-29 Skeletal model of the demonstration in Figure 6-28. **A,** Supination. **B,** Pronation.

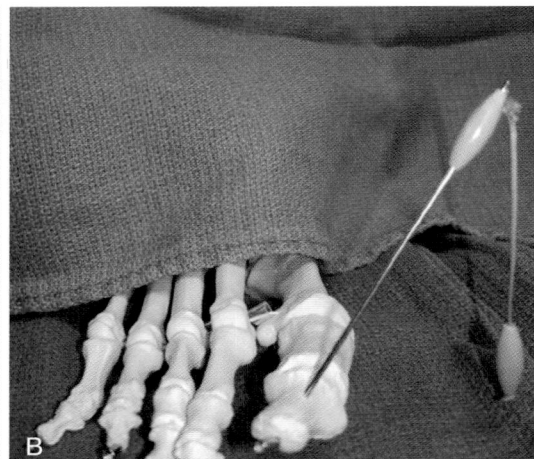

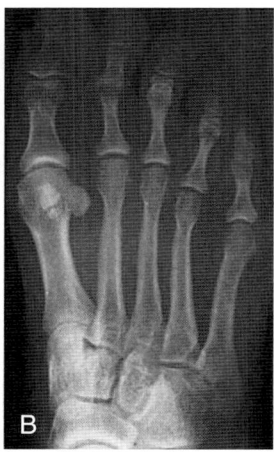

Figure 6-30 Foot during weight bearing. **A,** Supination. **B,** Pronation. Note the apparent lateral displacement of the sesamoids.

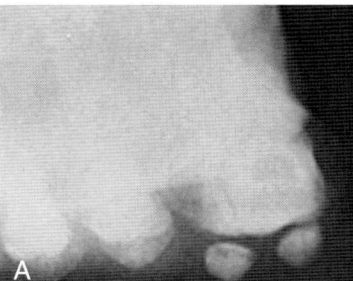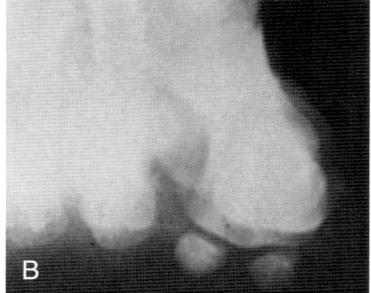

Figure 6-31 Tangential views of the sesamoids during weight bearing. **A,** Supination. **B,** Pronation. The degree of longitudinal rotation of the metatarsal is clearly demonstrated by the position of the sesamoids, which still retain a normal relationship to their facets beneath the metatarsal head.

first metatarsal head, the fibular sesamoid becomes visible on the lateral side of the first metatarsal head. Figure 6-30 shows a dorsoplantar weight-bearing radiograph; with the pronated position of the sesamoids, they appear to have been displaced laterally. The fibular sesamoid is now visible in the interval between the first and second metatarsals, as would be anticipated from the skeletal model in Figure 6-31. Tangential or sesamoid views of the foot show that this appearance is caused solely by longitudinal rotation of the first metatarsal, not by actual lateral displacement; the sesamoids remain in a normal relationship with their facets located on the plantar surface of the metatarsal head (see Fig. 6-31).

Pronation of the foot imposes a longitudinal rotation of the first ray (metatarsal and phalanges) that places the axis of the MTP joint in an oblique plane relative to the floor. In this position, the foot appears to be less able to withstand the deforming pressures exerted on it by either shoes or weight bearing.[255] No data are available on the relationship between the degree of pes planus and the degree of hallux valgus in the small percentage of unshod persons in whom the condition develops. Furthermore, authors who have noted a relationship between pes planus and hallux valgus in shod people have presented no quantitative data.*

To discount pronation entirely, however, is not appropriate because in some cases it can play a substantial role in the development and progression of specific hallux valgus deformities. Pronation of the foot does alter the axis of the first ray.[258] With weight bearing, the first MTP joint assumes an oblique orientation with the ground. In some pronated feet, especially in patients with ligamentous laxity, pressure exerted on the medial capsule of the first MTP joint can lead to progression of a hallux valgus deformity because the soft tissue supporting structures are unable to withstand these deforming forces. In such pathologic situations, a physician should be aware of possible progression of deformity, as well as postoperative recurrence. The use of prefabricated or custom orthoses in these patients may be beneficial. Persons with a mild hallux valgus deformity may experience rapid progression of the deformity if instability of the hindfoot secondary to rupture of the posterior tibial tendon, hindfoot valgus secondary to rheumatoid arthritis, or instability of the first MTC joint develops. Therefore pronation of the foot can be a factor predisposing to hallux valgus in certain conditions because the medial capsular structures offer limited resistance to the strong deforming forces.

Hypermobility of the Metatarsocuneiform Joint

The concept of hypermobility of the first ray was introduced by Morton in 1928.[376,377] Later, Lapidus[294-296] suggested an association between increased mobility of the first MTC joint and hallux valgus. Many reports dealing with correction of hallux valgus implicate first-ray hypermobility as a cause yet offer no proof regarding the

---

*References 28, 73, 138, 205, 225, 235, 246, and 466.

magnitude of preoperative or postoperative mobility.* The notion of this theory has been advanced by Hansen, Sangeorzan, and others.[73,205,456]

Others have disputed the significance of first-ray mobility as a cause of hallux valgus.† In reports on series involving the treatment of hallux valgus, Dreeben and Mann[136] and others[99,110] have found no evidence of first-ray hypermobility after surgical correction of a hallux valgus deformity. Wanivenhaus and Pretterklieber[544] reported a 7% incidence of MTC joint instability. Coughlin and Jones[100] reported that 23 of 122 patients (10%) with moderate or severe halllux valgus preoperatively were observed to have increased first-ray mobility.

Clinical assessment of sagittal plane mobility of the first ray was described by Morton,[376,377] who suggested that with the ankle in neutral position, the examiner stabilize the lateral aspect of the forefoot with one hand and then grasp the first ray with the other hand (Fig. 6-32). The first ray was translated in a dorsal plantar direction until a soft end point was reached. First-ray hypermobility was defined as excess motion on this examination. The biomechanical axis of the first MTC joint is obliquely placed, which permits motion of the metatarsal head to occur in a dorsomedial to plantar-lateral direction (Fig. 6-33). This oblique motion of the joint can indeed be qualitatively observed on physical examination, but attempting to quantify it clinically has been difficult. Although Morton claimed that first-ray hypermobility led to a multitude of foot problems,[376,377] he concluded that there was no reliable method by which he could quantify the magnitude of first-ray hypermobility.[377] Efforts to quantify MTC mobility have proved difficult,[162,386,456] and surprisingly, no report of the results of first MTC joint arthrodesis has provided data on the preoperative and postoperative magnitude of first-ray mobility.[386,456] Attempts to quantify first-ray mobility have measured motion in either degrees[152,236,544] or millimeters of either dorsal displacement or total excursion[176-181] (Fig. 6-34). Efforts to accurately measure first-ray mobility have evolved to the use of external calipers in recent years. Klaue, Hansen, and Masquelet[279] described a noninvasive caliper consisting of a modified ankle–foot orthosis and an external micrometer to quantify first-ray mobility. The authors found measurable, repeatable values for both normal and hypermobile first rays and concluded that hypermobility was often associated with the development of hallux valgus. They reported that normal adult patients had approximately 5 mm of flexibility at the MTC joint, and patients with hallux valgus had 9 mm or more of mobility. Although the applied force is not standardized when using this device, both the examination and the position of the foot and ankle are actually quite similar to the manual examination as originally described by Morton.[377,539] Jones et al[252] have substantiated that the

---

*References 14, 28, 73, 88, 204, 205, 219, 279, 305, 383, 385, 386, 456, and 466.
†References 110, 111, 136, 190, 208, 448, and 492.

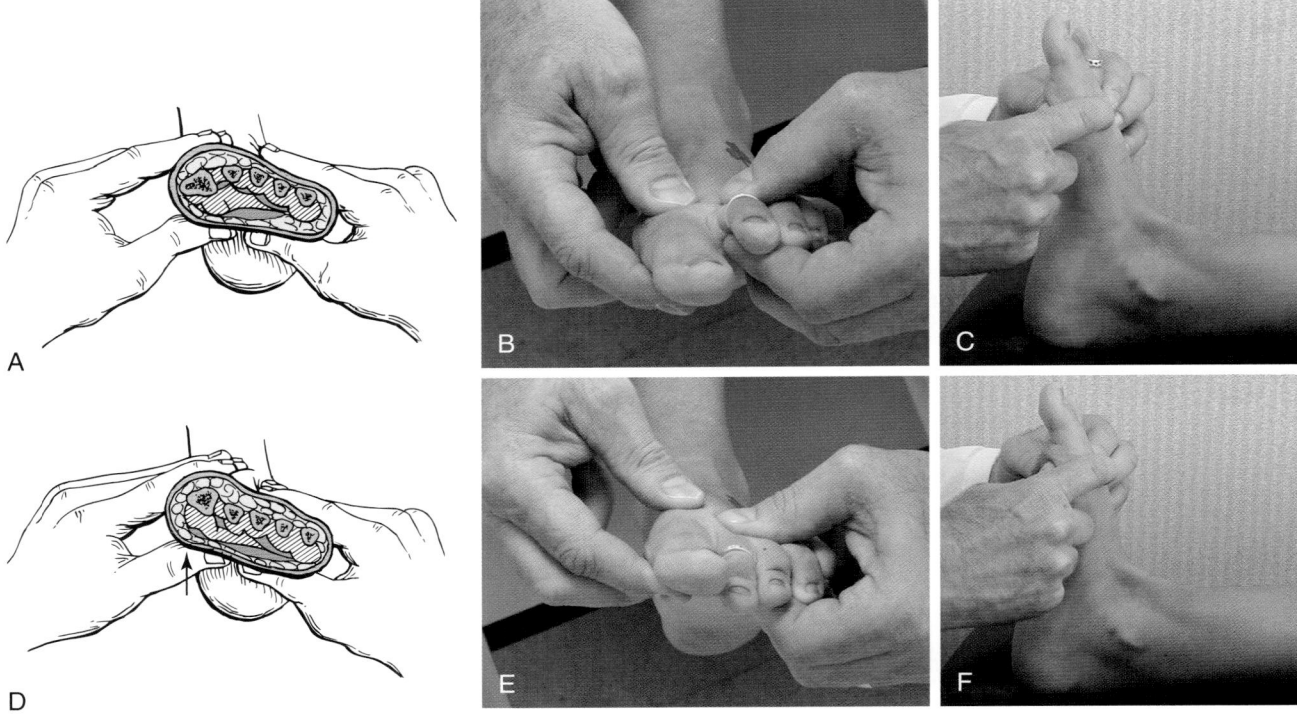

Figure 6-32 Examination for metatarsophalangeal (MTC) instability of the first ray. **A** and **B,** The lesser metatarsals are grasped between the index finger and the thumb of one hand, and the first metatarsal is grasped with the other hand. With the ankle in neutral position, the first metatarsal head is moved in the dorsoplantar direction. With a stable MTC joint, the distal ray does not become excessively elevated. **C** and **D,** With hypermobility, the first metatarsal head can be pushed in a dorsal direction above the sagittal plate axis of the lesser metatarsal heads. **E** and **F,** The ankle must be maintained in neutral position, or "false hypermobility" may be diagnosed.

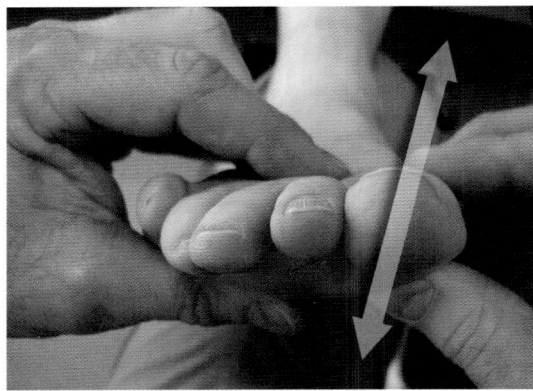

Figure 6-33 The mechanical axis of the first metatarsocuneiform joint is from plantar lateral to dorsomedial.

Klaue device is reliable and gives reproducible measurements of first-ray excursion.[252] Glasoe et al[179,180] demonstrated comparability of both the Klaue device and the Glasoe device for external measurement of first-ray mobility.

Other reports have also demonstrated that external calipers are reliable in quantifying first-ray motion.[84,176-178,181]

Klaue et al[279] and others[176,192] used external calipers to measure first-ray mobility and reported greater mobility in patients with hallux valgus deformities than in control subjects. However, both Glasoe et al[177] and Cornwall et al[84] reported that the manual testing technique, as described by Hansen[204] and others,* was quite unreliable and not reproducible when compared with mechanical testing techniques. Using the Klaue device to assess postoperative first-ray mobility after treatment with various hallux valgus surgical techniques, Coughlin et al[99] reported that the measured mobility was 4 mm after MTP arthrodesis and 5 mm after distal soft tissue reconstruction with proximal first metatarsal osteotomy.[110] In both series, no first-ray hypermobility was observed after correction of the bunion. However, in neither of these studies were measurements made before correction of the hallux valgus (because this measurement device had not been available).

Sarrafian[460] observed that the position of the ankle secondarily affects tension on the plantar aponeurosis (Fig. 6-35). Rush et al[450] suggested that first-ray motion could affect tension on the plantar aponeurosis and windlass mechanism, thus secondarily diminishing first-ray mobility.

---

*References 28, 73, 144, 204, 383, 385, 386, 456, and 262.

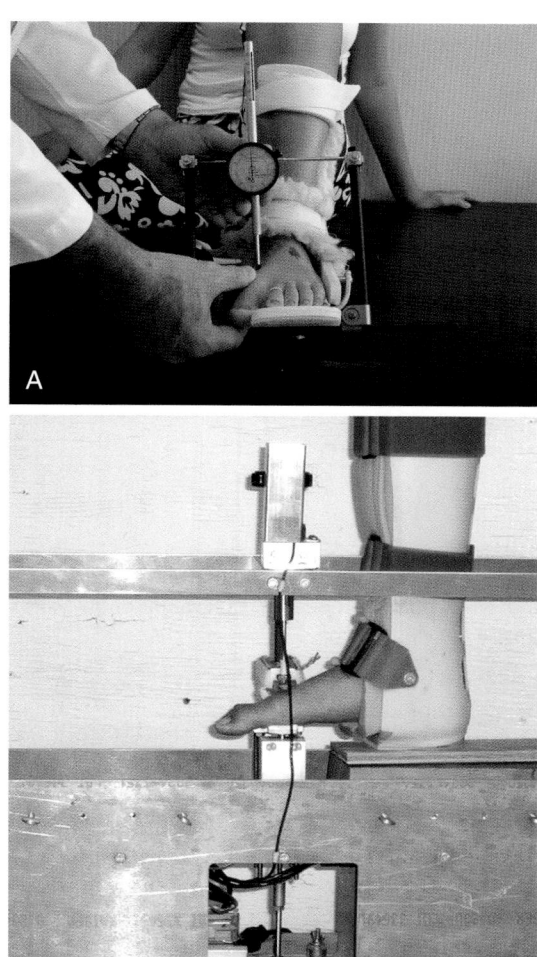

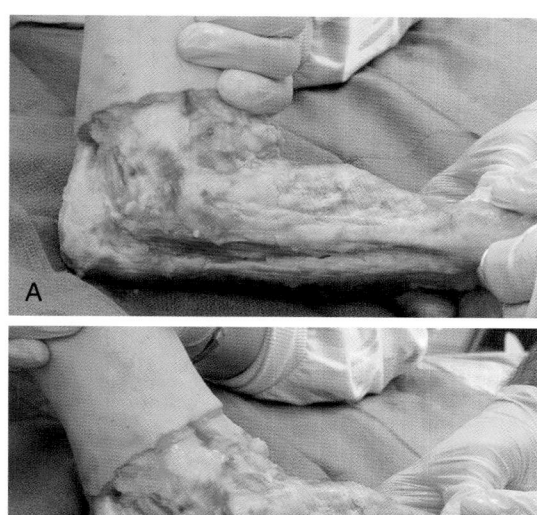

Figure 6-35 Plantar aponeurosis in neutral position **(A)** and plantar flexion of the ankle **(B).** Lax aponeurosis may play a significant role in first-ray hypermobility when the examination is conducted with the ankle in plantar flexion.

Figure 6-34 Two examples of external devices used to quantify first-ray hypermobility. **A,** Klaue device. **B,** Glasoe device. (Courtesy Ward Glasoe.)

It was Grebing and Coughlin[190] who defined the position of manual examination by investigating a group of patients with a modified Klaue device that enabled them to dorsiflex and plantar flex the ankle while measuring first-ray mobility (Fig. 6-36). A control group (mean mobility, 5 mm), a group with moderate and severe hallux valgus (mean mobility, 7.0 mm), a group that had previously undergone first MTP arthrodesis (mean mobility, 4.4 mm), and a group that had previously undergone plantar fasciectomy (mean mobility, 7.4 mm) were studied. When the ankle was placed in 5 degrees of dorsiflexion, first-ray mobility was significantly diminished in all four groups. When the ankle was placed in 30 degrees of plantar flexion, there was significantly increased mobility in the first three groups; however, the group that previously underwent plantar fasciectomy did not experience an increase in first-ray mobility. Of interest is that in the hallux valgus group, when examined in neutral position, 21% were considered hypermobile, but when they

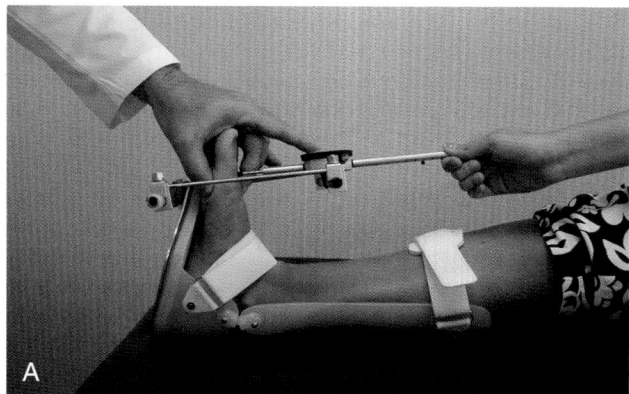

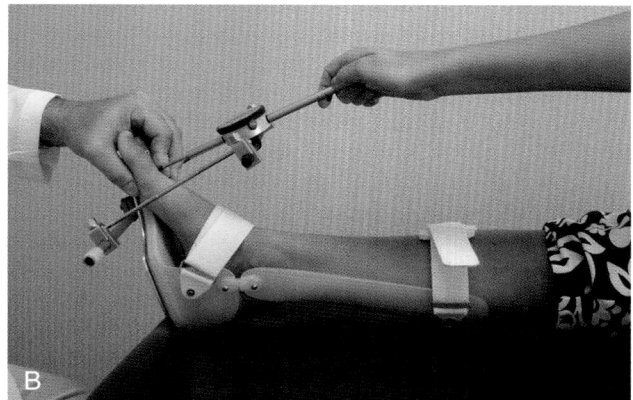

Figure 6-36 Modified Klaue device in dorsiflexion **(A)** and plantar flexion **(B)** demonstrating a substantial difference in first-ray mobility.

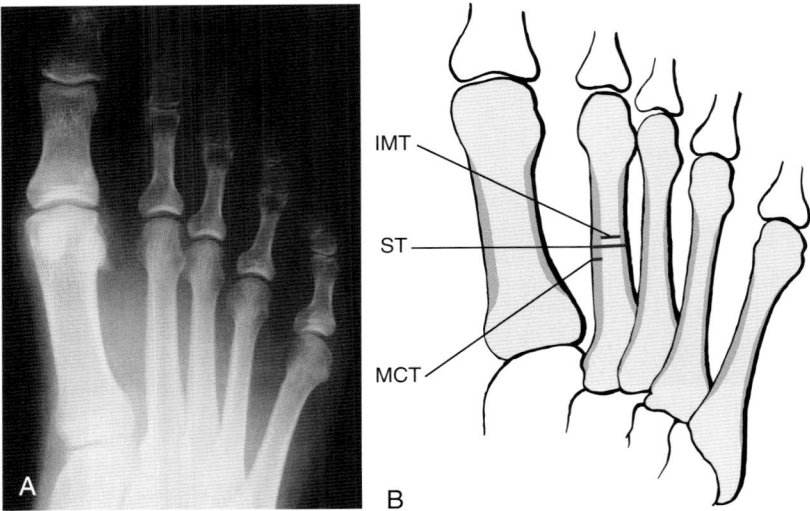

Figure 6-37 **A,** Anteroposterior radiograph of an asymptomatic foot with medial cortical hypertrophy. **B,** Measurements of medial cortical thickness *(MCT)*, intramedullary thickness *(IMT)*, and shaft thickness *(ST)* demonstrate no correlation with hypermobility of the first ray and hallux valgus. (**B,** Used with permission from Grebing B, Coughlin M: Evaluation of Morton's theory of second metatarsal hypertrophy. *J Bone Joint Surg Am* 86:1375-1386, 2004.)

were examined in plantar flexion, 92% were considered hypermobile. Thus the position of the ankle substantially influences the perceived first-ray mobility. When the ankle is plantar flexed 30 degrees, the amount of first-ray mobility is increased almost twofold.

Coughlin et al,[102] in a cadaver study of specimens with hallux valgus, reported that first-ray mobility as measured with the Klaue device was 11 mm preoperatively. After distal soft tissue repair and proximal osteotomy to correct the deformity, mean first-ray mobility was 5 mm. In a follow-up prospective study in which a similar operative repair was performed on 122 feet with moderate and severe hallux valgus deformities, Coughlin and Jones[100,101] reported first-ray mobility to have a preoperative mean of 7.3 mm that was reduced to a mean of 4.5 mm after surgical correction. Thus, with the ability to actually quantify first-ray mobility, the authors concluded that first-ray mobility is an effect of the hallux valgus deformity rather than a cause in most cases. The fact that it is reduced to a normal level after distal surgical realignment or proximal first metatarsal osteotomy that spares the MTC joint[101,102,110] makes a strong case for increased first-ray mobility being a secondary rather than a primary cause. First-ray stability is probably a function of first-ray alignment and the effectiveness of the intrinsic and extrinsic muscles and the plantar aponeurosis and not an intrinsic characteristic of the first MTC joint. Coughlin and Jones[101] reported no correlation between first-ray mobility and the magnitude of the hallux valgus angular deformities.

Although Morton[377] claimed that first-ray hypermobility was characterized by increased mobility on manual clinical examination, he concluded that the most notable structural feature of first-ray hypermobility was hypertrophy of the second metatarsal diaphysis as demonstrated

on an AP radiograph (1928). Prieskorn et al[429] attempted to relate mobility of the first MTC joint to thickening of the second metatarsal shaft and found no correlation. Grebing and Coughlin[192] analyzed second metatarsal shaft width and medial cortical hypertrophy (in a series of 172 patients, with 25,000 data points) and found no association with hallux valgus, first-ray mobility, or first metatarsal length. They concluded that using second metatarsal cortical hypertrophy or shaft width was an inappropriate indication for first MTC joint arthrodesis in the treatment of a hallux valgus deformity (Fig. 6-37). Opsomer et al,[396] in a later study of second-ray medial cortical thickness after hallux valgus correction, reported osseous diminution of the cortical thickness in as little as 11 months after surgery. In their series of 13 patients in which differences were measured in hundreths of millimeters, their claim that redistribution of weight-bearing patterns led to cortical thinning is questionable. The significance of the preoperative measurement, as well as the postoperative changes will require a much more rigorous process with a larger study, and longer-term follow-up.

Coughlin and Jones[101] and Cooper et al[81] have reported no correlation between measured first-ray mobility and any radiographic angular measurements defining pes planus (Meary's line, calcaneal pitch, AP talonavicular coverage, lateral talocalcaneal angle). Myerson[384] and King and Toolan[275] suggested that a radiographic gap on the plantar aspect of the first MTC joint is associated with both hallux valgus and first MTC joint instability. The incidence of this finding is unknown. Coughlin and Jones,[100] in a prospective study of moderate and severe hallux valgus deformities, reported a 23% incidence of plantar gapping. Of those 122 cases, the average first-ray mobility as measured by the Klaue device was 7.2 mm. The mean hallux valgus angle for these cases was 30

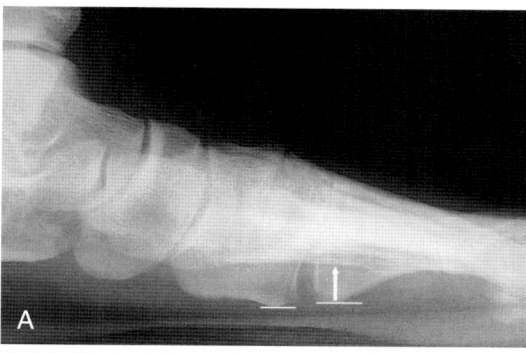

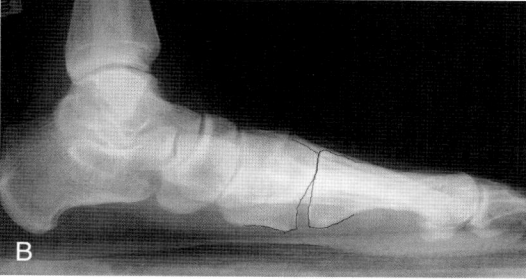

Figure 6-38 A, The first metatarsal lift is the difference in the perpendicular distance between the inferior border of the base of the first metatarsal and the inferior border of the first cuneiform. **B,** The first metatarsal–medial cuneiform angle is demonstrated on the lateral radiograph. (Courtesy Chris Coetzee, MD.)

degrees. With respect to the preoperative presence of plantar MTC joint gapping, there was no significant difference in first-ray mobility between those with and without gapping. Of interest, one third of those joints with a gap resolved after distal realignment of the bunion deformity. It is likely that the plantar gapping as seen on the lateral radiograph is indicative of sagittal plane instability, just as metatarsus primus varus is indicative of axial plane instability.

King and Toolan,[275] in a small series (25 cases), described the first metatarsal medial cuneiform angle (MMCA) as a possibly being a reliable measure of dorsiflexion or plantar wedging of the first MTC joint (Fig. 6-38). All patients in King and Toolan's series were considered to have first-ray instability when assessed by manual examination, although the magnitude of mobility was not quantified or reported. They described increased dorsiflexion through the first MTC joint (hallux valgus patients, 2 degrees; controls, 0.2 degree) and concluded that this demonstrated an association between the clinical and radiographic findings of first-ray hypermobility and hallux valgus. In the Coughlin study,[100] in which a much larger cohort was examined, no evidence was found to support King and Toolan's notion[275] that an increase in first metatarsal-cuneiform angle was associated with increased first-ray mobility.

If increased sagittal motion of the first ray is a primary factor that predisposes to the onset of a hallux valgus deformity, one would not expect a substantial reduction in first-ray mobility after a surgical realignment distal to the first MTC joint. Postcorrection measurements of first-ray mobility (using Klaue device measurements) after a distal realignment procedure (both in vivo and in vitro) demonstrate consistent and regular reduction of first-ray mobility.[91,99,100,102,274] Sarrafian[460] has suggested that the plantar aponeurosis plays a key role in first-ray stability. The chapter authors believe that realignment of the first ray restores normal anatomic relationships (intrinsic and extrinsic muscles, plantar aponeurosis) and that this, in turn, leads to a diminution in first-ray mobility. Thus the stability of the first ray, in most cases, is a function of the alignment of the first ray and is not an intrinsic characteristic of the first MTC joint.

Ligamentous Laxity

Carl et al[59] observed mild generalized ligamentous laxity in a small series of patients with hallux valgus. Clark et al,[73] in a report on juveniles, noted that 69% of patients in their series had generalized laxity on physical examination. Others[88,336,385] have mentioned ligamentous laxity as an etiologic factor.

Beighton and Bird[29] defined ligamentous laxity with a 9-point scale in which 2 points were awarded for hyperextension of both elbows beyond 10 degrees (1 point for only one elbow), 2 points for hyperextension of both knees beyond 10 degrees (1 point for only one knee), 2 points for extension of the little finger beyond 90 degrees (1 point for each hand), 2 points for extension of the thumb flat with the wrist (1 point for each hand), and 1 point for the ability to place the hands flat on the ground with the knees extended. A total of 9 points can be accumulated on the examination. A score greater than 6 points indicated generalized ligamentous laxity or hypermobility. Beighton noted that most individuals (94% of males and 80% of females) score 2 or fewer points (Fig. 6-39). Although studies[88,336,385] have correlated hyperflexibility of the thumb with hypermobility of the first ray, no study has documented the preoperative and postoperative laxity of patients with Beighton and Bird's method. In one retrospective study[99] of a group of patients with moderate and severe hallux valgus deformities treated by first MTP arthrodesis (mean hallux valgus angle, 42 degrees), 17 of 19 patients demonstrated no evidence of any laxity on the 9-point examination (0 points). Although postoperative recurrence may be a concern in treating patients with ligamentous laxity, the incidence is most likely quite low. Grimes and Coughlin[196] evaluated a series of subjects treated with first MTP joint arthrodesis for previously failed hallux valgus surgery. They closely evaluated this series of 29 patients (33 feet) with the Beighton examination and found only 5 of 29 (14%) had confirmed ligamentous laxity. Of interest, only two patients had first-ray hypermobility as confirmed on the Klaue apparatus. Nonetheless, attention should be addressed to ligamentous laxity in any evaluation before correction of hallux valgus. Although the finding of ligamentous laxity is probably uncommon in the typical adult patient with hallux valgus, patients with Ehlers-Danlos or Marfan syndrome may be better treated conservatively because they may have an increased risk of postoperative recurrence.

Achilles Contracture

Morton[377] defined normal ankle dorsiflexion as requiring 15 degrees. Mann and Coughlin[336] and others[28,88,89,205]

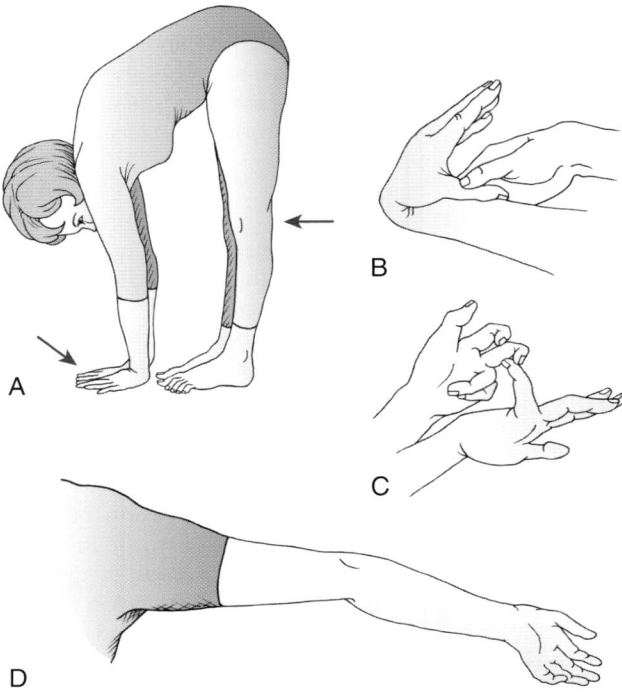

Figure 6-39 Beighton criteria for ligamentous laxity. The 9-point scoring system awards points for hyper-laxity: able to touch palms of hands on the floor with knees extended = 1 point for each side **(A)**, able to touch thumb to radial forearm = 1 point for each side **(B)**, able to touch index finger to extensor surface of forearm = 1 point for each side **(C)**, and elbow hyperextension = 1 point for each side **(D)**. Values over 5 points are considered to indicate ligamentous laxity in the patient.

have suggested that on occasion, a contracted Achilles tendon is associated with the development of hallux valgus. In contrast, Coughlin and Shurnas[110] noted an absence of heel cord tightness in their series and found no correlation between ankle dorsiflexion and hallux valgus (Fig. 6-40).

DiGiovanni et al,[134] when using 10 degrees or less of ankle dorsiflexion as a guideline, noted that 44% demonstrated "restricted dorsiflexion." When using 5 degrees or less of ankle dorsiflexion as a guideline for surgical intervention, they observed that 8 of 34 normal subjects (24%) had restricted dorsiflexion and recommended surgical lengthening of the Achilles complex.

Grebing and Coughlin[192] studied the incidence of ankle range of motion in normal subjects and patients with hallux valgus. In the control group, the mean ankle dorsiflexion was 9 degrees, and in the hallux valgus group it averaged 11 degrees. They reported that 19% of normal patients they studied had ankle dorsiflexion of 5 degrees or less. In a similarly sized group of patients with hallux valgus, 21% demonstrated ankle dorsiflexion of 5 degrees or less. Grebing and Coughlin noted that 81% of controls and 67% of those with hallux valgus had 10 degrees or less of ankle dorsiflexion. No correlation was found between ankle dorsiflexion and the magnitude of hallux valgus. In the report by Coughlin and Jones,[101] no correlation was demonstrated between ankle dorsiflexion and the hallux valgus angle.

Gastrocnemius lengthening has been recommended for patients with a limitation of 5 degrees or more.[204] However, none of the patients in the series reported by Grebing and Coughlin[192] were symptomatic, and no Achilles tendon lengthening were performed in the course of their treatment. An Achilles tendon contracture secondary to any cause can produce a gait pattern in which the person slightly externally rotates the foot or tends to roll off the medial border of the foot. This repetitive stress against the hallux has been postulated to lead to a hallux valgus deformity. This can be observed in patients with

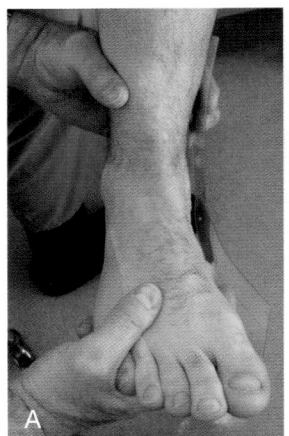
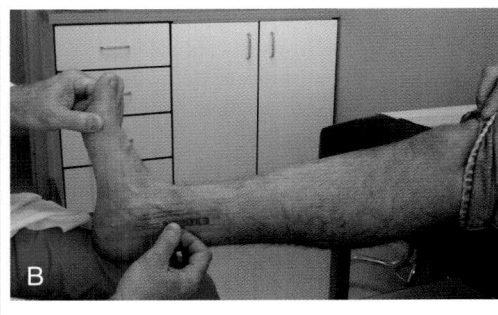
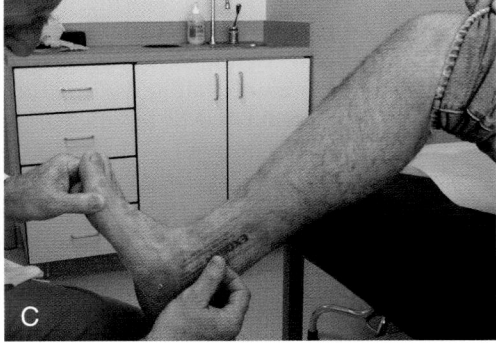

Figure 6-40 Ankle range of motion is quantified with the hindfoot in neutral position **(A)** and the knee both extended **(B)** and flexed **(C)**.

neuromuscular disorders (e.g., cerebral palsy, poliomyelitis) or patients who have had a CVA.

Although DiGiovanni et al[134] suggested that gastrocnemius lengthening be performed in patients undergoing foot surgery with dorsiflexion of less than 5 degrees, the fact that 81% of subjects demonstrated less than 10 degrees of ankle dorsiflexion suggests that this finding may not be abnormal. Furthermore, Coughlin and Jones[101] reported an incidence of 12% to 54% in patients with moderate and severe hallux valgus who had either less than 5 degrees (14 feet, 12%) or less than 10 degrees (66 feet, 54%) of ankle dorsiflexion. Of the 122 feet in the series, in no case was an Achilles tendon lengthening or gastrocnemius slide procedure performed in conjunction with the bunion correction. There was no correlation between the success of surgery and the tightness of the gastrocnemius–soleus complex. Although on occasion a gastrocnemius–soleus contracture may accompany a hallux valgus deformity, the chapter authors believe this to be uncommon, and lengthening is recommended in the uncommon patients with substantial restriction in ankle dorsiflexion.

Miscellaneous Factors
Obesity or an increased body mass index (BMI) has been shown to present an increased risk factor for tendonitis, plantar fasciitis, and degenerative arthritis of the lower extremity, but has not been associated with an increased risk of hallux valgus.[160]

Amputation of the second toe often results in a hallux valgus deformity, probably from loss of the support afforded by the second toe (Fig. 6-41). Mild hallux valgus may be seen after resection of the second metatarsal head.

Syndacylization of the first and second toes has been reported to occur with a hallux valgus deformity.[432]

Cystic degeneration of the medial capsule of the first MTP joint can occur. The resulting ganglion formation may sufficiently attenuate the capsule to permit the development of a hallux valgus deformity (see Fig. 6-1D).

Hallux valgus has been reported to occur with the development of a space occupying mass in the first IM space (Fig. 6-42).[566]

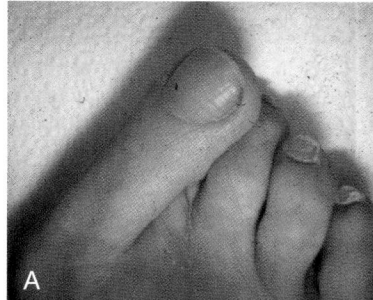
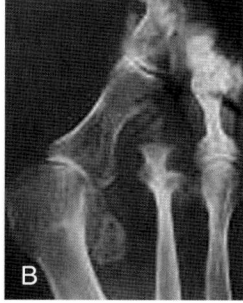

Figure 6-41 **A,** Clinical appearance. **B,** Radiograph of severe hallux valgus after amputation of the second toe.

ANATOMIC AND RADIOGRAPHIC CONSIDERATIONS

Angular Measurements

Radiographs of the foot should always be taken with the patient in the weight-bearing position. The basic studies should include AP, lateral, and oblique views. The AP radiographs are obtained with a tube-to-film distance of 1 m and the x-ray tube centered on the tarsometatarsal joint and angled 15 degrees toward the ankle joint, relative to the plantar aspect of the foot.[106]

Hallux Valgus Angle
On an AP weight-bearing radiograph, axes are drawn on the first metatarsal and proximal phalanx so that they bisect metaphyseal reference points in the proximal and distal metaphyseal regions that are equidistant from the medial and lateral cortices of the proximal phalanx and the first metatarsal. The angle created by the intersection of these axes forms the hallux valgus angle. A normal angle is less than 15 degrees,[207] mild deformity is less than 20 degrees, moderate deformity is 20 to 40 degrees, and severe deformity is greater than 40 degrees[88] (Fig. 6-43).

1–2 Intermetatarsal Angle
On an AP weight-bearing radiograph, reference points are placed in the proximal and distal metaphyseal regions equidistant from the medial and lateral cortices of the first and second metatarsals.[106] The angle created by the intersection of these axes forms the 1–2 intermetatarsal angle. Normal is less than 9 degrees,[207] mild deformity is 11 degrees or less, moderate deformity is greater than 11 and less than 16 degrees, and severe deformity is greater than 16 degrees[88] (Fig. 6-44).

Hallux Interphalangeal Angle
On an AP weight-bearing radiograph, reference points are placed in the proximal and distal metaphyseal regions equidistant from the medial and lateral cortices of the proximal phalanx to create an axis of the proximal phalanx.[108] Reference points are placed at the center of the base of the distal phalanx and at the tip of the distal phalanx, and a second axis is drawn. The intersection of these two axes forms the hallux IP angle (Fig. 6-45).

Distal Metatarsal Articular Angle
On an AP weight-bearing radiograph, the DMAA defines the relationship of the distal first metatarsal articular surface to the longitudinal axis of the first metatarsal.[98] Points are placed at the most medial and lateral extent on the distal first metatarsal articular surface. A line connecting these points defines the lateral slope of the articular surface. Another line is drawn perpendicular to this articular line. The angle subtended by this perpendicular line and the longitudinal diaphyseal axis of the first metatarsal defines the DMAA. Normal is regarded as 6 degrees or less of lateral deviation (Fig. 6-46).[438]

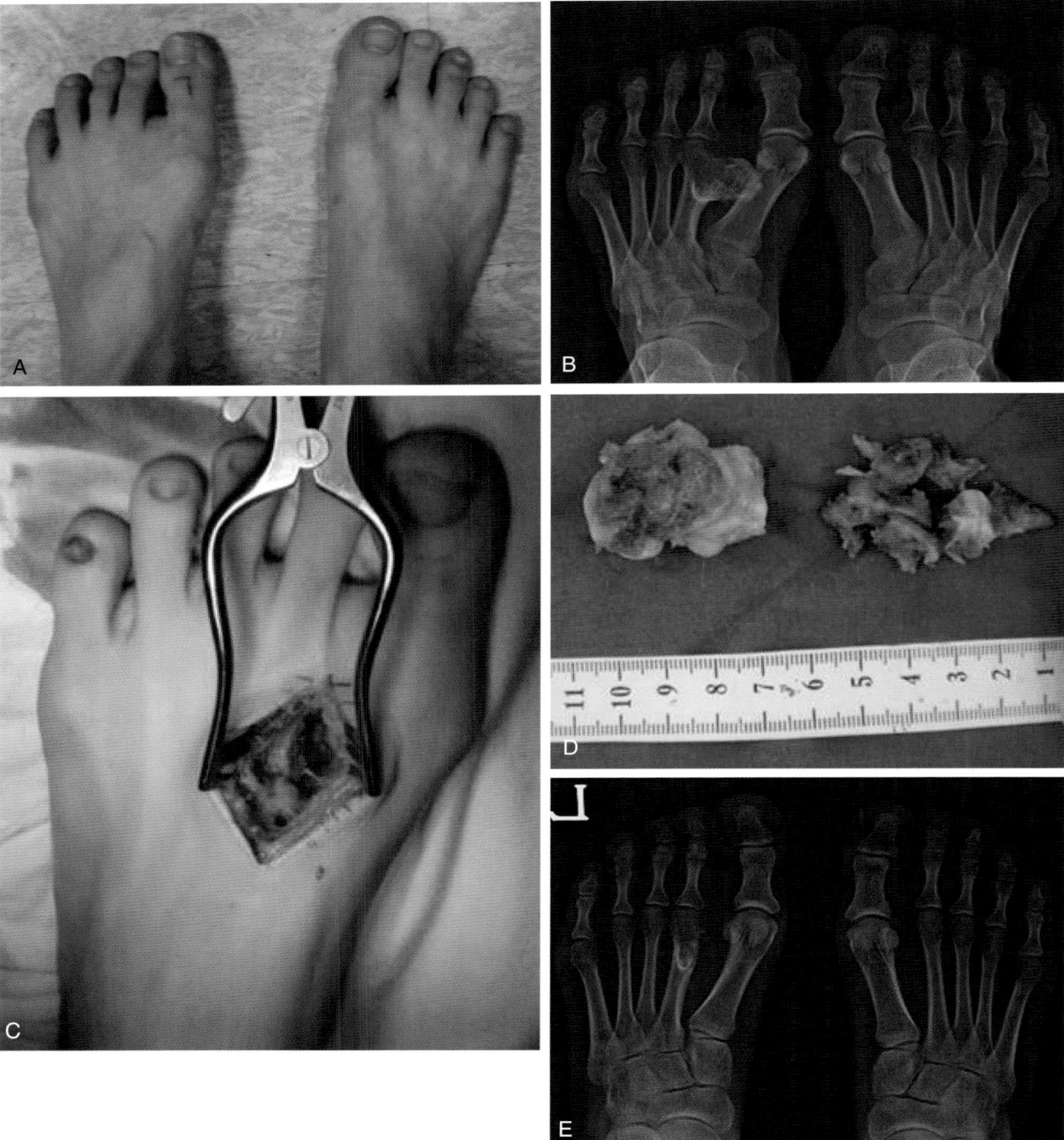

Figure 6-42 **A,** Clinical photograph demonstrating hallux valgus deformity on left. **B,** Anteroposterior radiograph showing large osseous lesion on second metatarsal creating widening of the 1–2 intermetatarsal (IM) angle. **C,** Intraoperative photograph showing bony lesions. **D,** Resected specimen. **E,** After removal of the mass, a marked reduction in the IM angle has occurred. (Courtesy Young Koo Lee, MD. Used with permission. From Young KW, Lee KT, Kwak JJ, et al: Mass-induced unilateral hallux valgus. *Orthopedics* 33:927, 2010.)

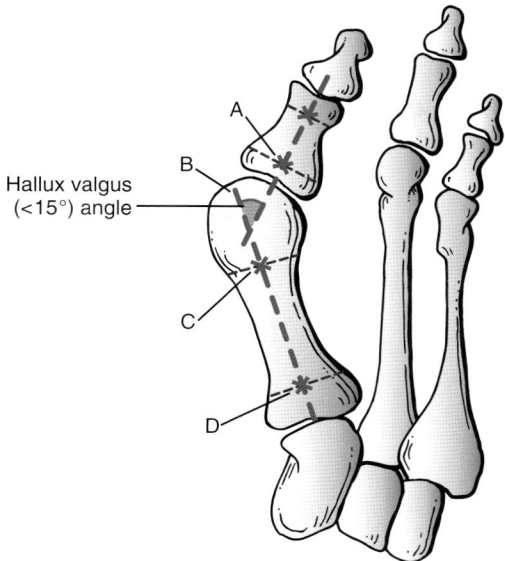

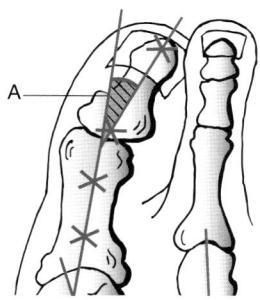

Figure 6-45 Hallux valgus interphalangeal (HVIP) angle. Middiaphyseal reference points are drawn on the proximal phalanx, and on the distal phalanx, a reference point is placed at the distal tip of the phalanx and at the midpoint of the articular surface of the distal phalanx. A line is drawn to connect the reference points for the axes of each phalanx. The intersection of the axis of the distal phalanx with the longitudinal axis of the proximal phalanx forms the HVIP axis.

Figure 6-43 Hallux valgus angle. Marks are placed in the middiaphyseal region of the proximal phalanx and the first metatarsal at an equal distance from the medial and lateral cortices. The longitudinal axis of the proximal phalanx is determined by an axis drawn though points *A* and *B,* and the longitudinal axis of the first metatarsal is determined by a line drawn through points *C* and *D.* The hallux valgus angle is formed by the intersection of the diaphyseal axes of the first metatarsal *(line CD)* and the proximal phalanx *(line AB).*

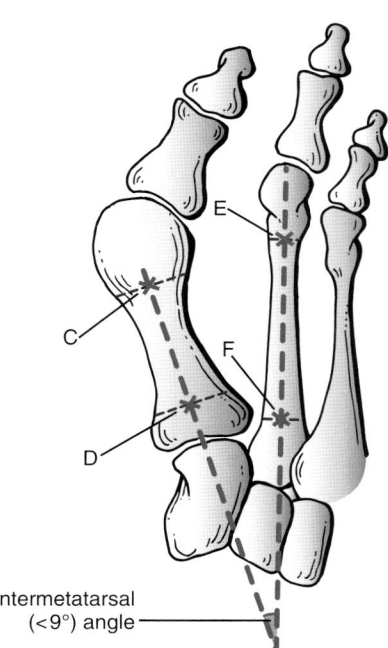

Figure 6-44 1–2 Intermetatarsal (IM) angle. Middiaphyseal reference points are placed equidistant from the medial and lateral cortices of the first and second metatarsals in both the proximal and distal middiaphyseal region. The longitudinal axis is drawn for both the first metatarsal *(line CD)* and the second metatarsal *(line EF).* The 1–2 IM angle is formed by the intersection of these two axes *(line CD* and *line EF).*

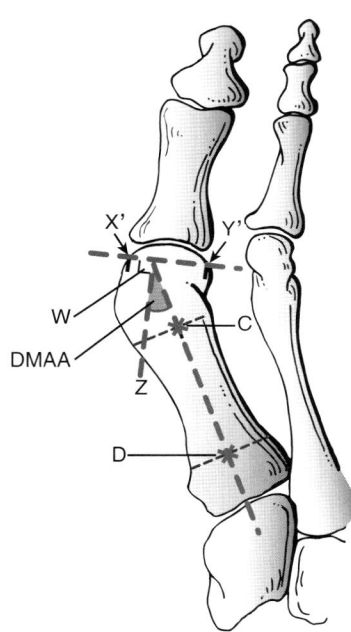

Figure 6-46 Distal metatarsal articular angle (DMAA). The DMAA defines the relationship of the articular surface of the distal first metatarsal with the longitudinal axis of the first metatarsal. Points are placed on the most medial and lateral extent of the distal metatarsal articular surface *(X′, Y′).* A line drawn to connect these two points defines the "slope laterally of the articular surface." Another line through points *(W, Z)* is drawn perpendicular to the first line *X′-Y′.* A third line through points *(C, D)* defines the longitudinal axis of the first metatarsal. The angle subtended by the perpendicular line *(W, Z)* and the longitudinal axis of the first metatarsal *(C, D)* defines the DMAA.

Metatarsophalangeal Joint Congruency

On an AP weight-bearing radiograph, the congruency of the MTP joint is determined by inspecting the relationship of the articular surfaces of the base of the proximal phalanx and the first metatarsal head. Individual reference points are placed at the most medial and lateral extents of the phalangeal articular surface and the distal metatarsal articular surface.[98] With a subluxated (noncongruent) hallux valgus deformity, the corresponding points on the proximal phalanx migrate laterally in relation to the corresponding points on the metatarsal head. With a nonsubluxated (congruent) hallux valgus deformity, concentric apposition of these points on the corresponding metatarsal and phalangeal joint articular surfaces occurs. No lateral shift of the proximal phalanx takes place with a congruent hallux valgus deformity (Figs. 6-47 to 6-49).[91]

Medial Eminence

One of the key components of a hallux valgus deformity is the size of the medial eminence. It is frequently this prominence that is the focus of pain and footwear intolerance by patients.[101] The size of the medial eminence is measured by drawing a line along the medial diaphyseal border of the first metatarsal. A perpendicular line is then drawn at the widest extent of the medial eminence and measured in millimeters (see Fig. 6-21).[515]

Both Haines and McDougall[200] and Lane[293] suggested that the medial eminence was not a new growth but merely a portion of the metatarsal that had become exposed with lateral deviation of the proximal phalanx.

The size of the articular surface diminishes as the sagittal sulcus migrates lateralward. The sagittal sulcus forms a border between the medial eminence and the remaining articular surface. Volkman[540] and Truslow[527] suggested that there was actually new bone formation with development of a bunion. Thordarson and Krewer[515] reviewed a

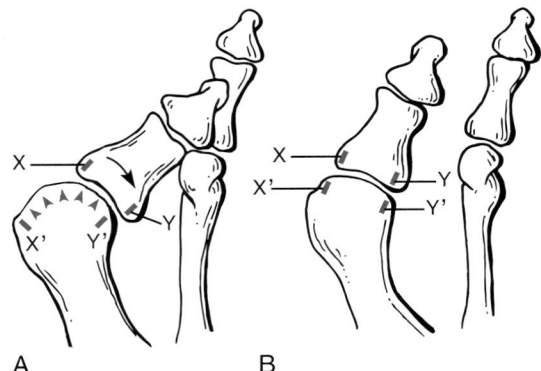

Figure 6-47 ■ Congruency versus subluxation. **A,** Hallux valgus deformity with subluxation (noncongruent joint) is characterized by lateral deviation of the articular surface of the proximal phalanx in relation to the articular surface of the distal first metatarsal. **B,** Hallux valgus deformity with a nonsubluxated (congruent) metatarsophalangeal joint is caused most often by lateral inclination of the distal metatarsal articular surface. Points *X* and *Y* determine the medial and lateral extent of the articular surface of the proximal phalanx; points *X'* and *Y'* determine the medial and lateral extent of the metatarsal articular surface. Note the lateral slope of the distal metatarsal articular surface.

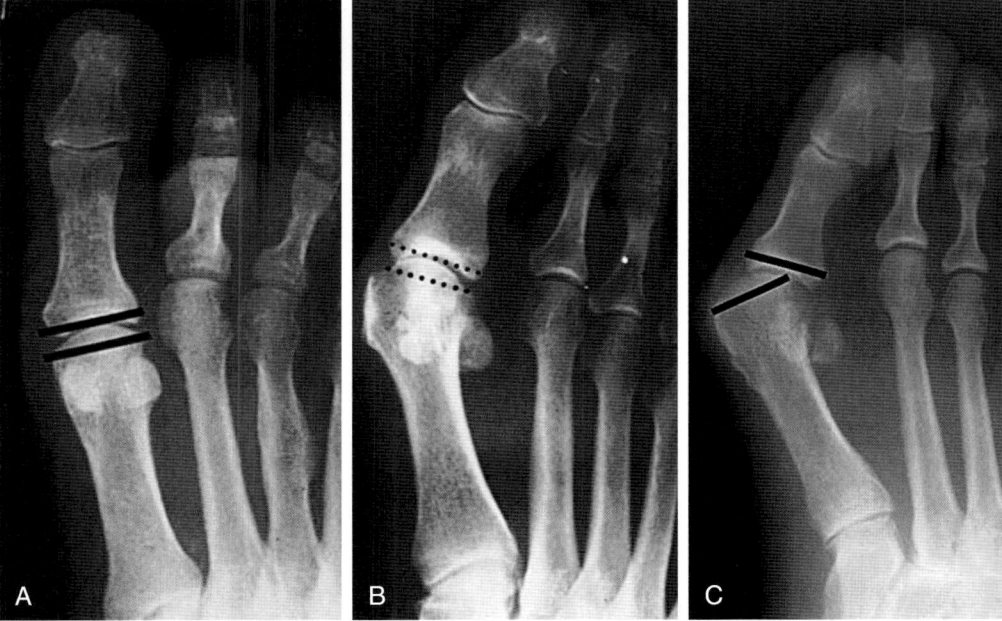

Figure 6-48 ■ Relationship of the proximal phalanx to the metatarsal head. **A,** A congruent joint is one in which the articular surfaces are parallel. In this case, the distal metatarsal articular angle (DMAA) is normal. **B,** Congruent joint with DMAA increased to 27 degrees. **C,** With an incongruent or subluxated metatarsophalangeal joint, joint surfaces are no longer parallel, thus creating an unstable situation.

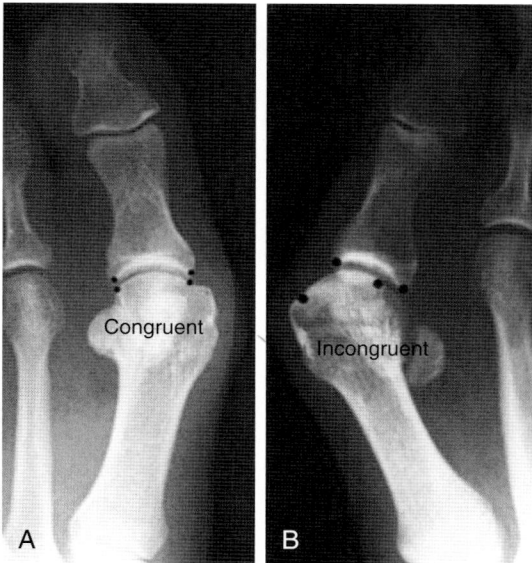

Figure 6-49 Examples of congruent **(A)** and incongruent **(B)** (subluxated) metatarsophalangeal joints. When a congruent joint is present, the proximal phalanx cannot be moved on the metatarsal head without creating an incongruent situation. An incongruent or subluxated joint can be corrected by rotating the proximal phalanx on the metatarsal head.

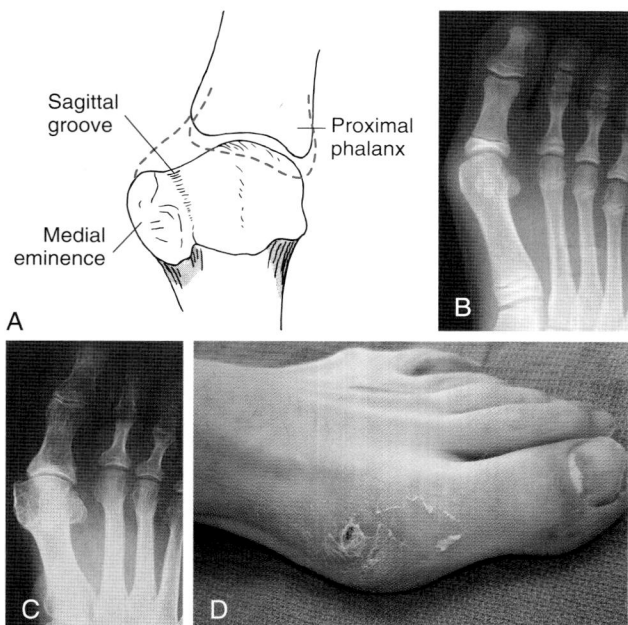

Figure 6-50 **A,** Diagramatic representation of the medial eminence and sagittal groove. **B,** Juvenile hallux valgus deformity with no significant medial eminence and no degenerative changes. Note the open epiphysis. **C,** Moderate hallux valgus deformity with a large medial eminence. **D,** Ulceration may develop over the medial eminence secondary to chronic pressure against the medial eminence and overlying bursa.

series of feet and reported that the size of the medial eminence is similar in patients who undergo bunion surgery and those without a hallux valgus deformity (Fig. 6-50). They concluded that bone proliferation did not occur with bunion formation. Thordarson and Krewer[515] reported that the mean thickness of the measured medial eminence was 4.4 mm in those with hallux valgus and 4.1 mm in those with normal feet. The mean difference was 0.2 mm. Coughlin and Jones[101] also concluded that the medial eminence does not reflect new bone formation. Resection of the medial eminence is a standard component of most hallux valgus repairs. Reducing a prominent medial eminence does aid in narrowing the forefoot; however, it is important to stress that the sagittal sulcus is not a reliable landmark for gauging resection of the medial eminence and may lead to excessive resection and subsequent hallux varus if a disproportionate amount of bone is removed.

Metatarsus Primus Varus

The simultaneous occurrence of hallux valgus and metatarsus varus has been noted frequently in the literature (Fig. 6-51). Hardy and Clapham[207,208] and others[101,110,192] have reported a correlation between the degree of hallux valgus and the size of the IM angle. Of all the variables considered in their study, Hardy and Clapham[207] noted that the highest correlation was between metatarsus primus varus and hallux valgus ($P = .71$). The question of cause and effect between medial deviation of the first

metatarsal and valgus of the great toe continues to be debated, but the findings indicate a combined deformity to a greater or lesser extent in most patients. Truslow[527] proposed the term *metatarsus primus varus* to describe a congenital anomaly that, if present, "inevitably resulted in hallux valgus" when the person was forced to wear shoes. Others have also supported his notion that the primary deformity is an increased 1–2 IM angle.*

Studies by Hardy and Clapham[207] and Craigmile,[113] in contrast, indicate that metatarsus primus varus is secondary to the hallux valgus deformity. Others have supported this notion that lateral migration of the hallux leads to medial deviation of the first metatarsal.[208,254,336,352,357] A close relationship exists between the degree of metatarsus primus varus and hallux valgus, which must be considered in any corrective surgery. Metatarsus primus varus may predispose a foot at risk, and poor footwear may enhance the development of a hallux valgus deformity.

The current authors believe that metatarsus primus varus is more frequently associated with the juvenile form of hallux valgus than the adult form and is probably a strong predisposing factor. In adults, metatarsus primus varus is probably more often a secondary change. Metatarsus primus varus can be associated with an adducted forefoot as well. Based on our analysis of available

---

*References 38, 73, 150, 280, 295, 370, and 493.

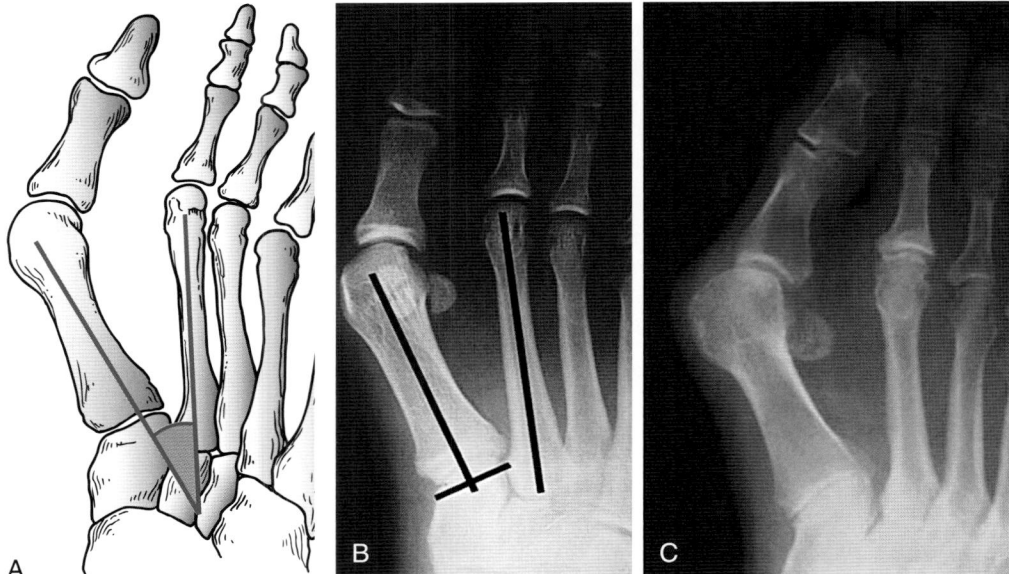

Figure 6-51 A, Diagramatic representation of metatarsus primus varus in a juvenile patient. **B,** Radiograph of an 18-year-old woman. **C,** Radiograph of a 55-year-old woman with metatarsus primus varus.

information, the authors are unable to conclude which is the primary deformity and can assert only the correlation between the two.

Hallux Valgus Interphalangeus

The relationship between the proximal and the distal phalanx of the hallux demonstrates that a line drawn perpendicular to the articular surface of the base of the proximal phalanx will usually not deviate laterally more than 10 degrees. When this line deviates more than 10 degrees laterally as it passes through the proximal phalanx, it gives rise to a hallux valgus interphalangeus deformity (see Fig. 6-15A-C). On occasion, the distal articular surface of the proximal phalanx deviates in a lateral direction, which creates a more severe HVI deformity (see Fig. 6-15D and E). An epiphyseal injury can lead to deformity as well (see Fig. 6-15F and G). At times, an HVI deformity coexists with a hallux valgus deformity and must be considered when correction of hallux valgus is carried out or the correction is incomplete. Park et al[404] has suggested that the interphalangeus angle may be artificially reduced because of pronation of the hallux associated with increasing deformity. They reported an average HVI angle of 13 degrees, and advocated an Akin osteotomy for those with a great HVI angle.

Sorto et al[499] suggested that there is an inverse relationship between the hallux valgus angle and the hallux valgus interphalangeal (HVIP) angle. They concluded that an increased hallux valgus angle indicates MTP joint instability, whereas a decreased angle indicates joint stability. Sorto et al[498] reported that in a normal foot the HVIP angle averages 13 degrees. They concluded that an increase in the HVIP angle is dependent on transverse

plane stability at the MTP joint. An increase in the HVIP angle is associated with a low hallux valgus angle and increased transverse plane stability. Conversely, decreased stability (hallux valgus) is associated with a high hallux valgus angle and a low HVIP angle.

Barnett[20] reported that a normal value for the HVIP angle was 10 degrees or less. Bryant et al[52] reported that the average HVIP angle was 5 degrees for those with hallux valgus and 15 degrees for those with hallux rigidus. Coughlin and Shurnas[108] reported that the average HVIP angle was 18 degrees in those with hallux rigidus. They hypothesized that as the MTP joint becomes more resistant to a transverse plane deformity, the hallux becomes predisposed to an increase in the HVIP angle. In a report by Coughlin and Jones,[101] the average HVIP angle in this group with hallux valgus was 6.7 degrees. There were only 13 of 122 subjects with an HVI angle greater than 10 degees. The current authors suggest that in those with hallux valgus there is less resistance to transverse plane deformity, thus explaining the decreased HVIP angle.

First Metatarsal Length

The length of the first metatarsal in comparison to the second metatarsal, with regard to a possible association with hallux valgus, is controversial. Based on minimal supporting data, both a short[28,211,377,537] and a long* first metatarsal have been implicated as essential factors in the development of hallux valgus deformities. The method of metatarsal measurement appears to influence the measured frequency of a long or short first metatarsal.

---

*References 52, 200, 208, 329, 353, 354, 359, 380, 489, and 509.

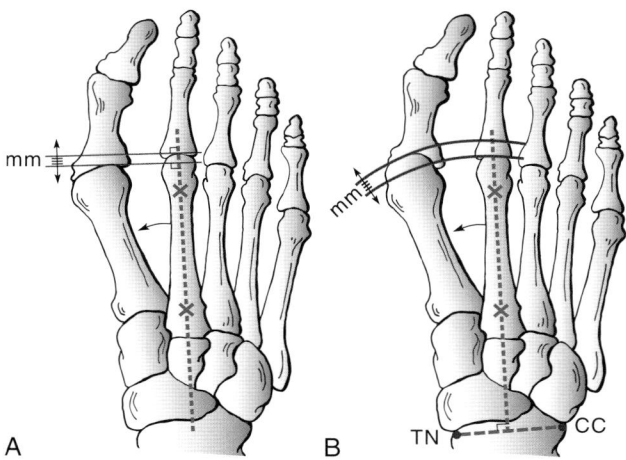

Figure 6-52 Method of measurement of first metatarsal length. **A,** Morton's method[377] using transverse lines. **B,** Hardy and Clapham's method[207] using arcs is not influenced by varying angular deformities.

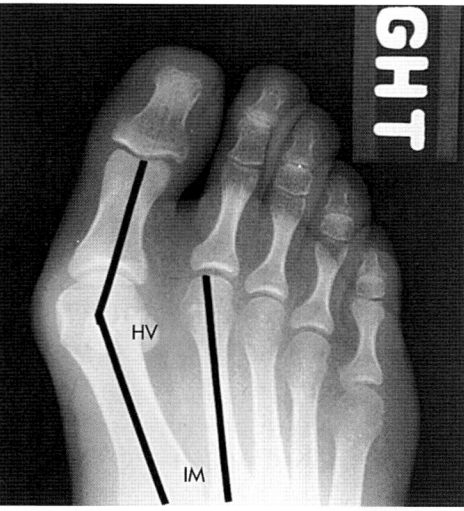

Figure 6-53 Note the long first metatarsal despite an increased hallux valgus *(HV)* and intermetatarsal *(IM)* angle.

Morton[377] suggested drawing a transverse line between the distal extent of the first and second metatarsals to compare their relative lengths (Fig. 6-52A). Hardy and Clapham[207] thought that this method was influenced by angular deformities (hallux valgus, metatarsus primus varus, metatarsus adductus) (Fig. 6-52B). Using the arc method, Harris and Beath[211] reported 32% with short first metatarsals, 37% with equal lengths of the first and second metatarsals, and 31% with long first metatarsals in the general population. In his evaluation of juvenile patients with hallux valgus, Coughlin[95] reported short first metatarsals in 28%, first and second metatarsals of equal length in 42%, and long first metatarsals in 30%—data closely concurring with that previously reported by Harris and Beath.[211]

Munuera et al[380] reported that in comparing males and females with hallux valgus both genders had a first ray that was longer (mean, 3.6 mm) than normal. Males characteristically had a longer hallux and first metatarsal, although females only had a long first metatarsal.

Mancuso et al[329] reported that 77% of patients with a hallux valgus deformity had a first metatarsal length equal to or longer than the second metatarsal. Mancuso et al[329] and Grebing and Coughlin[192] recognized that Morton's method of measurement had inherent problems (Fig. 6-53). As the 1–2 IM angle increases, there is apparent shortening of the first metatarsal. Grebing and Coughlin[192] compared the two methods of measurement in a control group and in a group with hallux valgus. In the control group, 30% of the first metatarsals were short with the arc method and 53% were short with Morton's method of measurement. In the group with hallux valgus, only 5% had a short first metatarsal with the arc method, whereas 63% were short when Morton's method was used. The normal group compared closely with results previously reported by Hardy and Clapham.[208] The

chapter authors believe that the notion of first metatarsal shortness, as suggested by Morton,[377] is largely an artifact based solely on his novel measurement technique. In fact, when the arc method of measurement is used, rarely is a short first metatarsal associated with a hallux valgus deformity.[192] The relationship between metatarsal length and the development of hallux valgus seems to be incidental, with decreased first metatarsal length playing essentially no role and increased length being of questionable significance.[95,211,336,459] Slight shortening of the first metatarsal typically occurs after many surgical procedures involving first metatarsal osteotomies. This may be an acceptable development because of the incidence of long first metatarsals in patients with hallux valgus.[504]

Metatarsophalangeal Joint Shape

The shape of the head of the first metatarsal varies considerably from a round dome-shaped structure to a flat articular surface. The orientation and shape of the metatarsal and phalangeal articular surfaces have an important effect on the intrinsic stability of the first MTP joint. These respective articular surfaces may resist or predispose the hallux to deformity. The association of a curved metatarsal articular surface with hallux valgus has been proposed by several authors,[46,95,339,384,394] the variability of specific joint shapes in the general population is thought to be substantial. Okuda et al,[394] in a comparison of a control group and a group with hallux valgus, found a 78% incidence of a rounded metatarsal head in a cohort (76 feet) with a bunion and 2% in the control group (60 feet) (Fig. 6-54). Schweitzer et al[469] reported no difference in the shape of the MTP joint when they compared patients with hallux valgus or hallux rigidus. DuVries[139] and others[88,336,339] have suggested that a curved surface is less stable and more prone to progressive hallux valgus deformity.

Patients with hallux valgus have been shown to have a high incidence of rounded metatarsal heads, varying in frequency from 71% to 91%.[100,155,329]

A flat or chevron-shaped MTP articulation (see Fig. 6-13A-C) is stable, tends to resist increased progressive valgus deformation, and is associated with hallux rigidus.[108] Coughlin and Shurnas[108] found that only 29 of 110 (26%) MTP joints in a group of patients with hallux rigidus had an oval or curved articular joint surface (see Fig. 6-13D and E). Coughlin and Jones[101] reported that a curved articulation was present in 71% of those with a moderate or severe hallux valgus deformity. The current authors believe that a flattened or chevron-shaped articulation is more stable and tends to resist subluxation and that a curved joint shape is less resistant to transverse plane deformity and predisposes to a hallux valgus deformity.

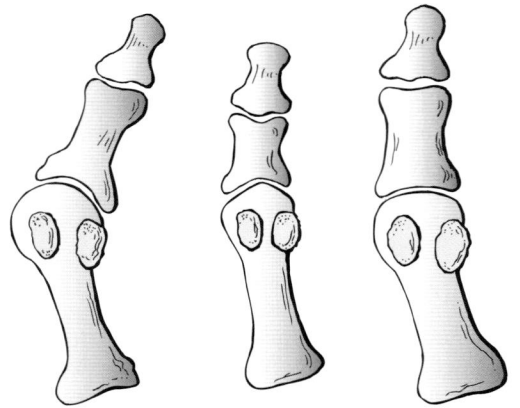

Figure 6-54 Diagram demonstrating curved, chevron, and flat metatarsophalangeal articulations.

Joint Congruity

Congruity is the term used to describe the relationship of the metatarsal and phalangeal articular surfaces. A congruent hallux valgus deformity occurs when the corresponding articular surfaces of the metatarsal and phalanx are concentrically aligned[88,95,414] (see Fig. 6-13A-C and F). When the proximal phalanx has migrated laterally off the metatarsal articular surface, the deformity is deemed a noncongruous or subluxated articulation (Fig. 6-55; see Fig. 6-13D and E). Piggott[414] suggested that mild subluxation of the first MTP joint can progress to significant subluxation and leave the medial metatarsal articular surface uncovered (see Figs. 6-17, 6-41B, and 6-48C). Congruency of the first MTP joint was initially described by Piggott,[414] who noted that a congruous joint was typically stable, and hallux valgus did not appear to increase with time (Fig. 6-56). Thus the valgus orientation of the hallux can be caused by either joint subluxation or sloping of the metatarsal articular surface or the phalangeal articular surface in relation to the diaphyseal axis of their respective bones. With a congruent hallux valgus deformity, the magnitude of hallux valgus is determined by the magnitude of the DMAA. Piggott,[414] in an analysis of 215 adult feet with hallux valgus, determined that 9% had a congruent joint (see Fig. 6-49A). Significant hallux valgus can occur with a congruent joint. In a patient with a symptomatic hallux valgus deformity and a congruent MTP joint, who requires surgical intervention, intraarticular MTP joint realignment may create an incongruent joint.[12,70,92,216,217] This sloping of the joint articular surface may predispose the patient to a recurrent hallux valgus deformity[48,88,97,339] or the development of postoperative degenerative joint disease (Fig. 6-57).[5,70,92,216,217]

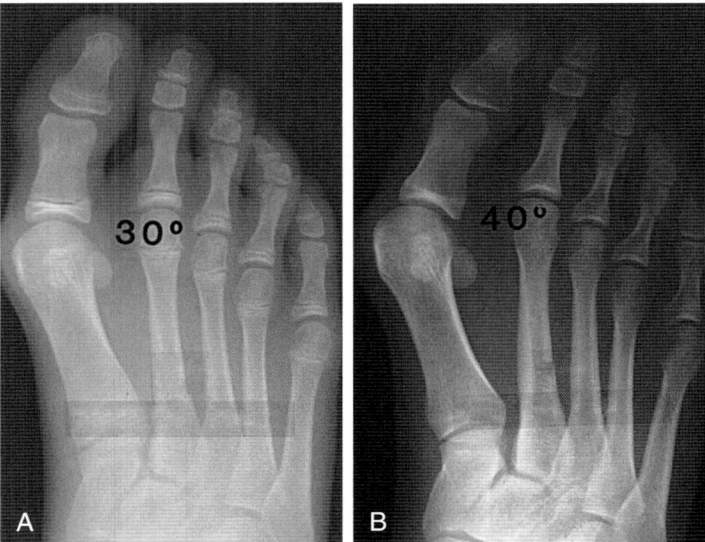

Figure 6-55 **A,** Moderate hallux valgus deformity in 10-year-old girl. **B,** At 19 years of age, before surgical correction, the deformity has increased, and the patient became much more symptomatic.

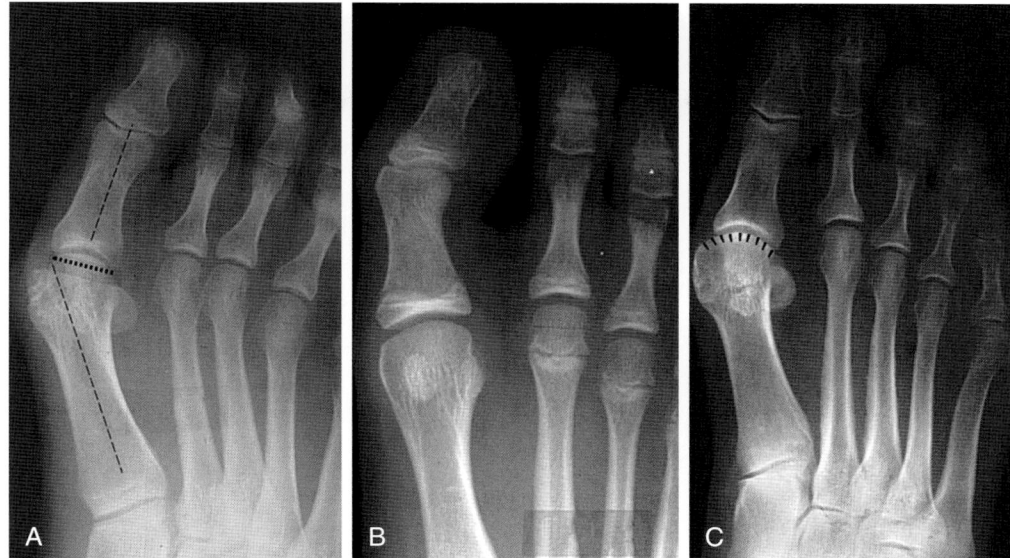

Figure 6-56 **A,** Radiograph demonstrating moderate hallux valgus deformity without subluxation of the first metatarsophalangeal (MTP) joint. The hallux valgus angle is caused primarily by 25 degrees of lateral angulation of the distal metatarsal articular angle. A sagittal sulcus has developed medial to the articular surface. There is a prominent medial eminence. The *dotted line* demonstrates the lateral slope of the distal metatarsal articular surface. **B,** Hallux valgus interphalangeus deformity. **C,** Subluxated MTP joint with a hallux valgus deformity caused primarily by subluxation of the first MTP joint.

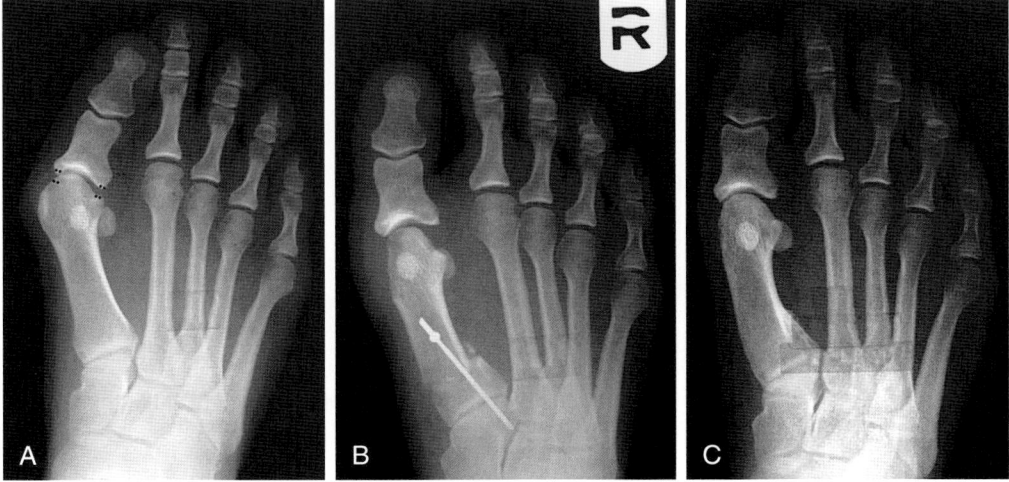

Figure 6-57 **A,** Preoperative radiograph demonstrating a hallux valgus deformity with a congruent metatarsophalangeal (MTP) joint. **B,** Radiograph after first metatarsal osteotomy and distal soft tissue repair. Note the lack of congruency at the MTP joint. **C,** Thirteen years later, a radiograph demonstrates incongruent MTP joint with narrowing of the medial joint space. The patient complained of greatly restricted MTP motion.

Chi et al[65] reported great difficulty in consistently and accurately assessing joint congruity, whereas Pique-Vidal et al[418] reported a much higher accuracy. Others have reported varing degrees of accuracy in quantifying the DMAA. Coughlin and Freund[98] found variable accuracy in their much larger study, with differing accuracy by some reviewers, and also found some radiographs more difficult to assess. Radiographs of skeletally immature feet are much more difficult to assess regarding congruency.

Although some feet are difficult to assess, others are clearly congruent, and it is these particular feet that warrant careful and specific surgical treatment (Fig. 6-58).

In a study dealing just with juveniles with hallux valgus, Coughlin[95] demonstrated that 47% were noted to have a congruent joint with a laterally sloping DMAA (Fig. 6-59). For those with a subluxated first MTP joint, the average DMAA was 8 degrees. For congruent joints, the average lateral slope or DMAA was 15 degrees. The

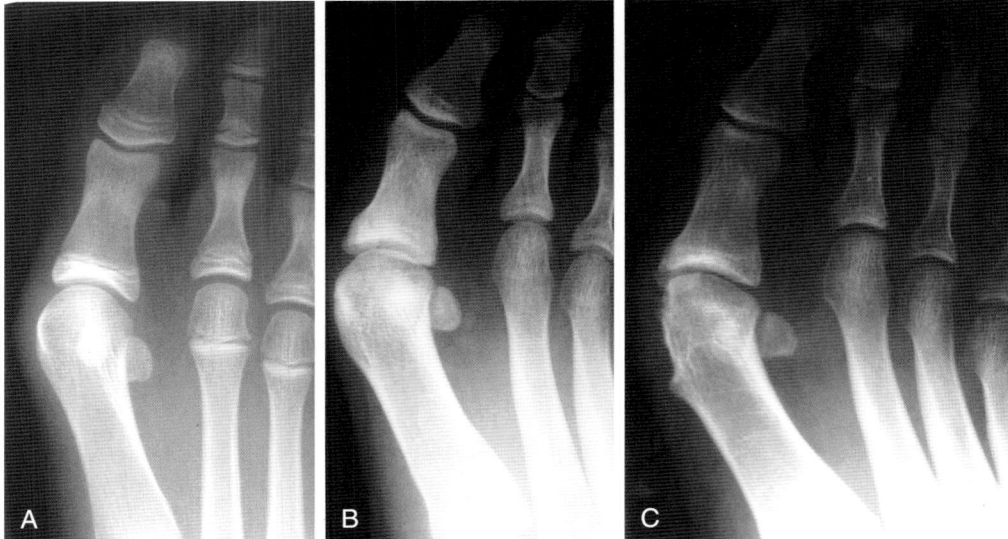

Figure 6-58 **A,** Juvenile hallux valgus deformity with a metatarsophalangeal (MTP) joint in which congruency is difficult to assess. **B,** Skeletally mature individual with a similar MTP joint that is difficult to assess. **C,** It is only with the unsuccessful surgical procedure that the congruent joint becomes more apparent.

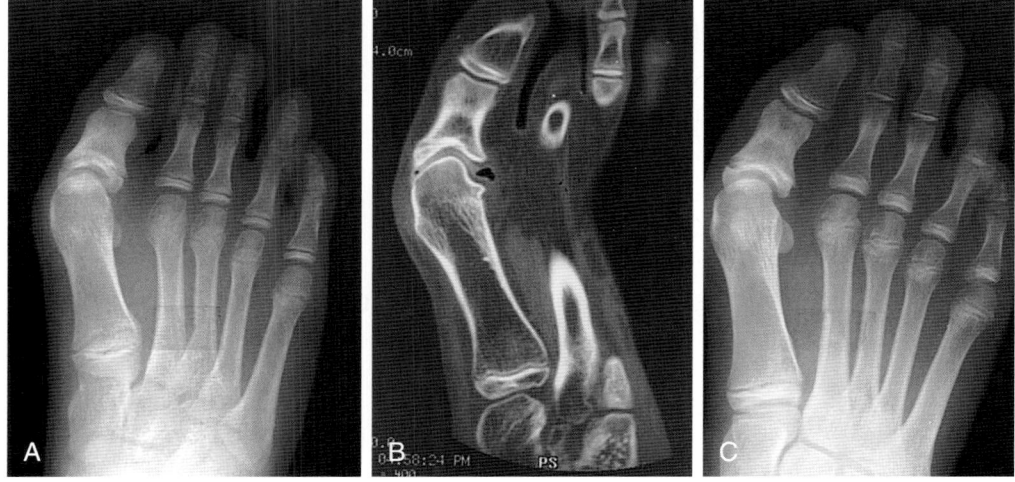

Figure 6-59 **A,** Anteroposterior radiograph demonstrating a congruent metatarsophalangeal (MTP) joint with hallux valgus in a 10-year-old skeletally immature girl. **B,** Air contrast CT scan demonstrating congruent articular surfaces. **C,** Congruent MTP joint in a skeletally mature female.

DMAA was noted to be significantly higher in patients with a positive family history, in those with early-onset of hallux valgus (younger than 10 years), and in those with a long first metatarsal. The DMAA was not affected by the presence of metatarsus adductus. An increased DMAA is the defining characteristic of many juvenile hallux valgus deformities.

Coughlin[91] reported that a congruent joint was present in 37% of males with hallux valgus; the measured DMAA was twice as high (21 degrees) in congruent joints than in subluxated joints. When the postoperative hallux valgus angle was compared in the two groups, in those with a congruent joint, the preoperative DMAA and postoperative hallux valgus angle closely correlated.

Distal Metatarsal Articular Angle and Proximal Articular Set Angle

On an AP radiograph, the DMAA (or proximal articular set angle) defines the relationship of the articular surface of the distal first metatarsal to the axis of the first metatarsal (see Fig. 6-46). The radiograph may demonstrate that the articular surfaces of the distal first metatarsal and the proximal phalanx are not oriented at right angles to the long axis of the metatarsal and phalanx (see Figs. 6-48B and 6-49A). Slight valgus alignment allows lateral inclination of the great toe, and thus a hallux valgus angle of 15 degrees or less is considered normal.[207,228]

To measure the DMAA, a point is placed on the most medial extent of the metatarsal articular surface and a second point on the most lateral extent of the metatarsal articular surface. A line is then drawn connecting these two points. The angle subtended by the longitudinal axis of the first metatarsal and a line drawn perpendicular to the distal metatarsal articular surface defines the magnitude of the DMAA. The reported normal value of the DMAA in adults varies in the literature (6.3-18 degrees).[6,95,194,438,502] Lateral sloping of the articular surface of the distal first metatarsal or the base of the proximal phalanx may be the cause of a static valgus orientation of the great toe (see Fig. 6-56A). As the DMAA increases, the magnitude of the hallux valgus angle increases.

Piggott[414] stated that over time, this congruent orientation can lead to pain but that it is unusual for a deformity of this type to progress to a more severe abnormality. Measurement of this angle is extremely important when evaluating a patient with a hallux valgus deformity because it will in part determine what type of operative procedure should be performed. Richardson et al[438] demonstrated in adults that the DMAA can be reliably quantified on an AP radiograph, although others have had difficulty in measuring the DMAA.[418,417,442] Robinson et al[442] has observed variation in the measurement of the DMAA with both rotation and inclination of the first ray. Pontious et al[423] observed that it is much more difficult to measure the DMAA in a young person before bone maturation. Coughlin[95] observed that in juvenile patients younger than 10 years with hallux valgus, the DMAA averaged 15 degrees, and in those older than 10 years, it averaged 9 degrees. In a series of juvenile hallux valgus deformities treated with a soft tissue realignment of the first MTP joint, lack of recognition of the DMAA resulted in suboptimal correction of the deformity.[412] Coughlin and Jones,[101] after eliminating all congruous hallux valgus deformities from their study, analyzed the remaining deformities, which were all deemed noncongruous or subluxated, and they measured the magnitude of the DMAA in these cases. The mean DMAA for these subluxated joints was 10.6 degrees. Coughlin[95] noted that the DMAA averaged 16 degrees in those with a long first metatarsal and 6.0 degrees in those with a short first metatarsal ($P = .002$). Of interest is that Breslauer and Cohen[48] observed that an increased DMAA greater than 15 degrees was associated with erosion of the plantar metatarsal articular surface.

The proximal phalangeal articular angle (PPAA, or the distal articular set angle) defines the orientation of the proximal phalangeal articular surface in relation to the long axis of the proximal phalanx (see Fig. 6-15). Although slight valgus inclination is often present in the proximal phalanx, it rarely exceeds 5 degrees. When this angle exceeds 5 degrees, an HVI deformity occurs. Hallux valgus interphalangeus as a separate entity occurs infrequently (3%).[95]

A static hallux valgus abnormality can develop as a result of an abnormally large DMAA or PPAA or a combination of both. Hallux valgus deformities caused by angulation of the articular surfaces are considered a static structural abnormality; although symptoms may develop, these deformities are unlikely to progress over time.[105,414] Coughlin and Shurnas[110] confirmed earlier findings that the preoperative DMAA measurement correlated with the magnitude of postoperative hallux valgus correction in men with hallux valgus deformities. The DMAA has not been linked with the magnitude of preoperative hallux valgus, or with 1–2 internmatetarsal or HVI angles.[101]

First Metatarsocuneiform Joint

The first MTC joint is a key factor in the development of both an enlarged 1–2 IM angle and an increased hallux valgus angle. The shape of the MTC joint has a variable medial deviation. The orientation and flexibility of the MTC joint play an important role in development of the deformity at the MTP joint. On an AP radiograph, the angle formed by the intersection of the longitudinal axes of the first and second metatarsals defines the 1–2 IM angle.[13,60,138,428] Metatarsus primus varus or a 1–2 IM angle of 9 degrees or greater is considered abnormal[207] (see Fig. 6-44). The proximal articular surface of the first metatarsal articulates with the distal articular surface of the first cuneiform. This elliptic concave joint surface is oriented in the transverse (coronal) plane.[200,460] Normally, it is deviated medially, but in some cases, it may have a marked degree of medial inclination, which is thought to result in joint instability. Both Ewald[150] and Berntsen[32] observed that when the first MTC joint was obliquely oriented, the first metatarsal was inclined medially and a hallux valgus deformity was much more prevalent. The MTC joint is difficult to visualize on plain radiographs. It is questionable whether a horizontal orientation, oblique orientation, or curved MTC articulation correlates with an increased 1–2 IM angle (Fig. 6-60). Simon[489] and Brage et al[45] have questioned the "apparent orientation" of this joint and suggested that some of the apparent radiographic findings were indeed artifacts. After anatomic dissection of the MTC joint, Haines and McDougall[200] and Truslow[527] concluded that a hallux valgus deformity is often associated with an oblique orientation of the first MTC joint. Haines and McDougall[200] hypothesized that an abnormality in the first metatarsal base leads to a metatarsus primus varus deformity. First MTC joint orientation is the major factor associated with an increased magnitude of the 1–2 IM angle. Mitchell et al[370] concluded that an increased 1–2 IM angle is the result of an abnormal first MTC joint articulation. The chapter authors have observed the complex nature of this facet in dissections. The distal first cuneiform articular surface is typically convex dorsally (Fig. 6-61) and flat or concave plantarward. There is a medial inclination of this joint that is variable. Depending upon the angle of the radiographic beam, the joint may appear rounded or flat or oblique. Further investigation of this joint is important in

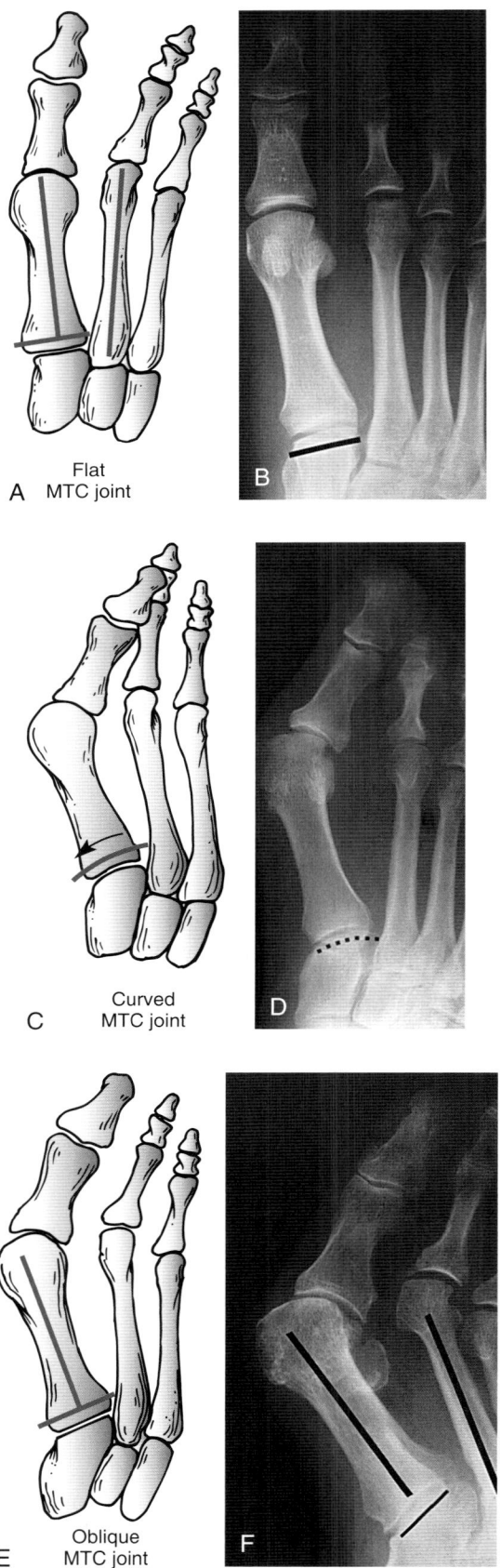

Flat
A MTC joint

B

Curved
C MTC joint

D

Oblique
E MTC joint

F

Figure 6-60 **A** and **B,** Flat metatarsocuneiform (MTC) joint. **C** and **D,** Curved MTC joint. **E,** Oblique MTC joint. **F,** Oblique MTC joint with severe metatarsus adductus and hallux valgus.

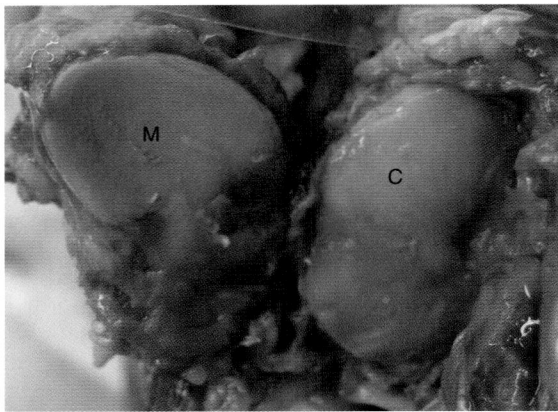

Figure 6-61 Dissection of the first metatarsocuneiform joint. Base of the first metatarsal is on the *left (M),* the articular surface of the distal cuneiform is on the *right (C).* Note the convex dorsal surface of the first cuneiform and concave or flattened inferior surface of the first cuneiform.

defining what is obviously a key joint in the development of hallux valgus deformities.

Inman[235] and Piggott[414] suggested that with subluxation of the MTP joint a simultaneous concomitant increase occurs in the 1–2 IM angle (Fig. 6-62). DuVries[139] stated that in juveniles, the increased 1–2 IM angle was responsible for the development of hallux valgus, whereas in adults, the increased 1–2 IM angle was a secondary change after first MTP joint subluxation. The belief that in juveniles an increased 1–2 IM angle is a primary deformity and the hallux valgus deformity is a secondary or acquired deformity is not new.*

When a hallux valgus deformity occurs with a concomitant increase in the 1–2 IM angle, inherent flexibility at the first MTC joint may be present. In this situation, adequate correction of a hallux valgus deformity can be achieved by performing a distal soft tissue realignment without metatarsal osteotomy.[105,336] Antrobus[10] hypothesized that after a distal soft tissue repair (without a first metatarsal osteotomy) to correct a hallux valgus deformity, if the 1–2 IM angle corrected to a normal range, the metatarsus primus varus deformity was secondary to the distal hallux valgus deformity. The inherent flexibility of the first MTC joint plays an integral role in the success of any hallux valgus surgical correction. MTC joint flexibility, however, can often be assessed only intraoperatively. Most distal first metatarsal osteotomies, MTP joint arthroplasties, and soft tissue realignments achieve correction of the 1–2 IM angle by realignment of the MTP joint.

*References 38, 60, 70, 138, 249, and 556.

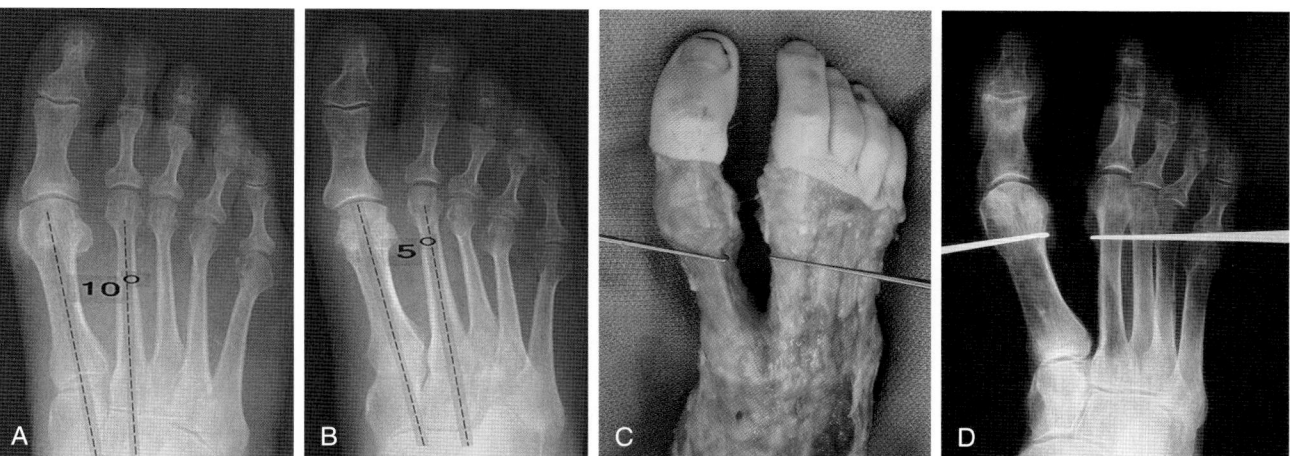

Figure 6-62 **A,** Mild to low-moderate hallux valgus deformity. **B,** Falling distal soft tissue repair. The hallux valgus deformity is corrected, but the 1–2 intermetatarsal angle is reduced because of distal soft tissue realignment. **C,** Anatomic specimen. **D,** Radiographic examination demonstrating the magnitude of MTC joint mobility.

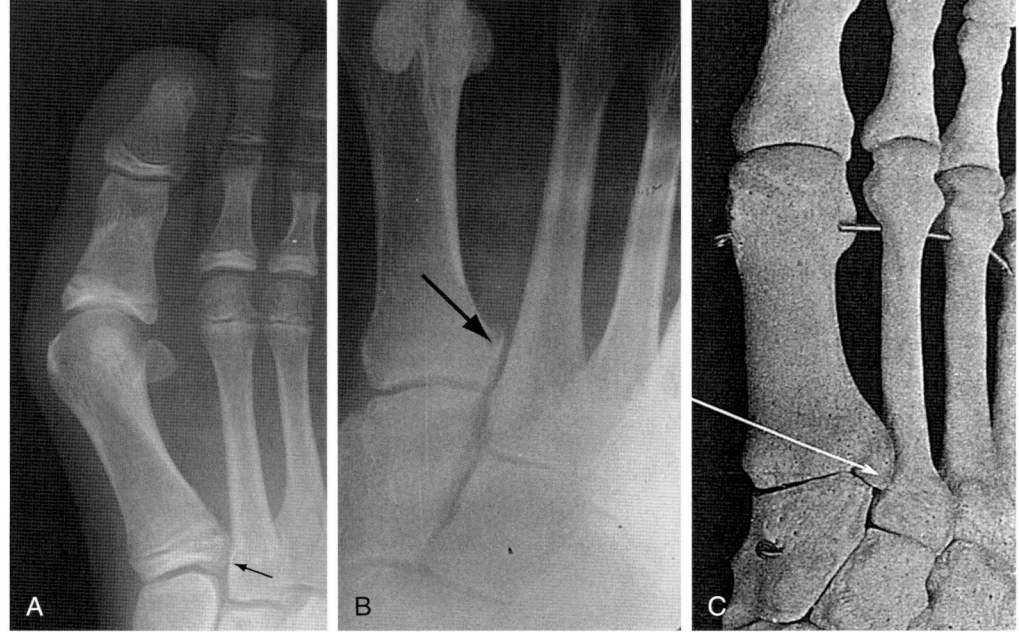

Figure 6-63 An intermetatarsal (IM) facet (*arrows* in all three images denote intermetatarsal facet) may limit correction of the 1–2 IM angle if a first metatarsal osteotomy is not performed. **A,** Intermetatarsal facet associated with a juvenile hallux valgus deformity. **B,** Facet in an adult patient. **C,** Anatomic dissection demonstrating an IM facet. (**C,** From Dwight T: *Variations of the bones of the hands and feet: a clinical atlas,* Philadelphia, 1907, JB Lippincott.)

Mann and Coughlin[336] reported an average decrease in the 1–2 IM angle of 5.2 degrees after a modified McBride procedure in adults (without a first metatarsal osteotomy). Hawkins et al[214] reported an average 5.2-degree decrease in the 1–2 IM angle after the Mitchell procedure. One can infer from these studies that sufficient flexibility often exists at the MTC articulation and allows a reduction in the 1–2 IM angle after either a distal first metatarsal osteotomy or distal soft tissue realignment. This is an important issue because flexibility of the MTC joint can influence both the development of hallux valgus and the appropriate type of surgical repair used to achieve a successful outcome.

Intermetatarsal Facet / Os Intermetatarseum

An intermetatarsal facet located between the proximal lateral base of the first metatarsal and the proximal medial base of the second metatarsal (Fig. 6-63) may create a rigid MTC articulation that is resistant to surgical

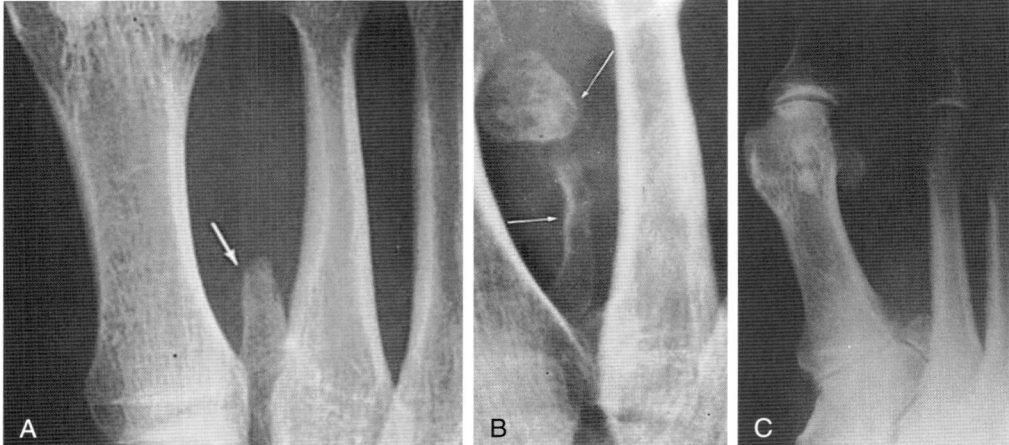

Figure 6-64 Os intermetatarseum. **A,** Os intermetatarseum with an increase in the 1–2 intermetatarsal (IM) angle *(arrow)*. A first metatarsal osteotomy will be necessary to correct the IM angle. **B,** Two examples of the variable appearance of an os intermetatarseum *(arrows)*. **C,** Hallux valgus deformity with an os intermetatarseum. This deformity will require a proximal osteotomy to achieve correction of the deformity. (**B,** From Keats TE: *Atlas of normal roentgen variants that simulate disease,* 4th ed, St Louis, 1987, CV Mosby.)

reduction after a distal osteotomy or distal soft tissue procedure.[294,296,335,543] Likewise, the presence of an os intermetatarseum (Fig. 6-64) may create a rigid MTC articulation that resists correction of the 1–2 IM angle.[335,527] The presence of an IM facet or os intermetatarseum[336,339] in the proximal interval between the first and second metatarsals has been suggested to be incompatible with successful distal soft tissue repair because it is an impediment to diminution of the 1–2 intermetatarsal angle. On the contrary,[234] Ellington et al[144] have suggested that the presence of an os intermatarseum is associated with first-ray hypermobility although they present no evidence to substantiate this claim (see Fig. 6-7C). Coughlin and Jones[101] demonstrated that the incidence of os intermetatarseum was 7% and that of an IM facet was 7%.

Metatarsus Adductus

On an AP radiograph, the longitudinal axis of the lesser tarsus is used to measure the magnitude of metatarsus adductus.[147,297] A line is drawn on the lateral aspect of the foot between two points marking the most lateral extent of the calcaneocuboid joint and the most lateral extent of the fifth metatarsocuboid joint (Fig. 6-65). A second line is drawn along the medial lesser tarsus between two other points: the most medial extent of the talonavicular joint and the most medial extent of the first MTC joint. At the midpoint of these separate lines, a connecting line is drawn that bisects the lesser tarsus. Then a line is drawn perpendicular to the lesser tarsus bisection line. The angle that this line forms with the longitudinal axis of the second metatarsal determines the relationship of the forefoot to the lesser tarsus and thus the magnitude of metatarsus adductus. A normal value is 0 to 15 degrees, mild metatarsus adductus is 16 to 19 degrees, moderate

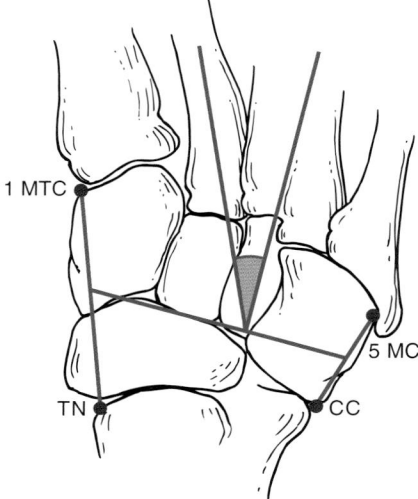

Figure 6-65 The magnitude of metatarsus adductus is determined by creating a longitudinal axis of the lesser tarsus and measuring its relationship to the longitudinal axis of the second metatarsal. A normal value is 0 to 15 degrees, mild metatarsus adductus is 16 to 19 degrees, moderate metatarsus adductus is 20 to 25 degrees, and severe metatarsus adductus is greater than 25 degrees. *CC,* most lateral extent of the calcaneocuboid joint; *5 MC,* most lateral extent of the fifth metatarsal cuboid joint; *TN,* most medial extent of the talonavicular joint; *1 MTC,* most medial extent of the first metatarsocuneiform joint. A line connecting the midpoint of these two lines (*1 MTC–TN* and *5 MC–CC*) defines the axis of the lesser tarsus. The intersection of a line perpendicular to this axis forms an angle with the longitudinal axis of the second metatarsal and defines the magnitude of metatarsus adductus.

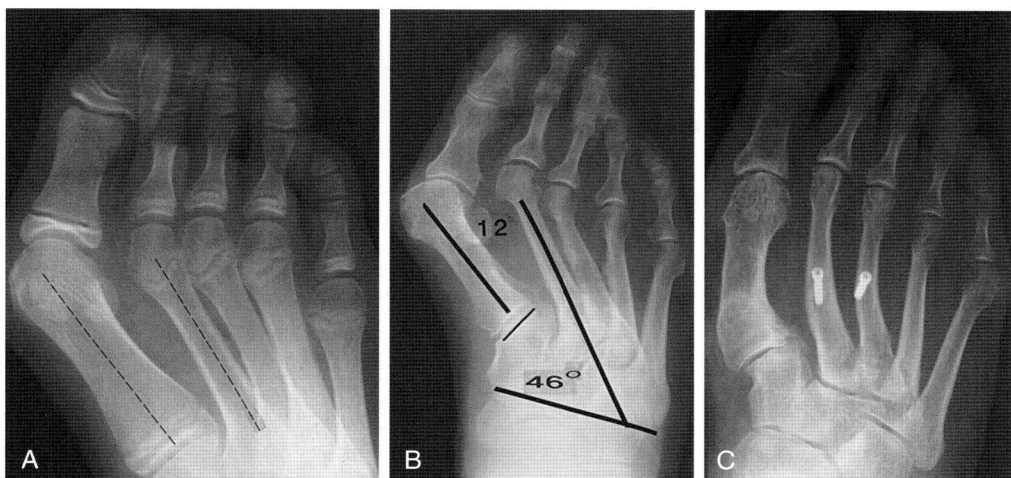

Figure 6-66 A, Juvenile hallux valgus with severe metatarsus adductus. Although the 1–2 intermetatarsal (IM) angle measures 2 degrees and parallelism exists between the first and second metatarsals, the 1–2 IM angle would be approximately 35 degrees with a normal forefoot. **B,** Metatarsus adductus combined with metatarsus primus varus and a subluxated metatarsophalangeal joint. The metatarsus adductus angle measures 46 degrees, and the 1–2 IM angle measures 12 degrees. With normal forefoot alignment, however, metatarsus primus varus might exceed 40 degrees. **C,** Correction of hallux valgus and osteotomies of the second and third metatarsals for metatarsus adductus. (Courtesy R. Okuda, MD.)

metatarsus adductus is 20 to 25 degrees, and severe metatarsus adductus is greater than 25 degrees.[18,95,147,297] In the presence of metatarsus adductus, a hallux valgus deformity is characterized by an abnormally low 1–2 IM angle resulting from medial deviation of both the first and second metatarsals.[259]

The incidence of metatarsus adductus in the general population is 1 in 1000.[564] Griffiths and Palladino[194] found no relationship between hallux valgus and the metatarsus adductus angle with regard to gender. Ferrari and Malone-Lee[156] found that all women in their series with an abnormal metatarsus adductus angle had an increase in the hallux valgus angle. Men with metatarsus adductus, on the other hand, had a normal hallux valgus angle. Coughlin and Shurnas[110] and others[52,101,269] have found no association with hallux valgus in men (Fig. 6-66), and Coughlin and Jones[101] also reported that there was no a correlation between preoperative hallux valgus and metatarsus adductus in a series that was largely female.

Whereas Staheli[500] and others[359] have suggested that there was no association of metatarsus adductus and juvenile hallux valgus, others have observed an increased incidence of hallux valgus and metatarsus adductus, mainly in the juvenile population.* Coughlin[95] reported a 22% incidence of metatarsus adductus in his series of patients with juvenile hallux valgus, and Banks et al[18] reported a linear correlation between an increasing hallux valgus angle and an increased incidence of metatarsus adductus. Mahan and Jacko[326] reported an increased recurrence rate after hallux valgus repair when metatarsus adductus was

---

*References 18, 95, 186, 194, 197, 201, 270, 297, 326, 423, and 526.

present, but Coughlin[95] was unable to substantiate this finding.

Metatarsus adductus associated with a hallux valgus deformity is a difficult condition to treat because there is little room to realign the first metatarsal laterally. Coughlin[95] reported no significant increase in the metatarsus adductus angle in patients with a positive family history of juvenile hallux valgus. Martinelli et al[349] have advocated a multiple metatarsal osteotomies in combination with a hallux valgus repair as a means to correct the forefoot deformity.

Blood Supply to the First Metatarsal Head

The blood supply to the first metatarsal passes through a nutrient artery traversing the lateral cortex of the midshaft of the metatarsal in a distal direction. The vessel divides within the medullary canal and sends branches both distally and proximally. Whereas the blood supply through the nutrient artery demonstrates little variation, the blood supply to the metatarsal head and to the base of the metatarsal does demonstrate variability (Fig. 6-67). According to Shereff et al,[478] the primary sources of circulation to the metatarsal head emanate from the first dorsal metatarsal artery, the first plantar metatarsal artery, and the superficial branch of the medial plantar artery. The majority of this blood supply penetrates the capsule in the general area along the dorsal and lateral aspects of the joint. Figure 6-68 shows the geographic distribution of the intraosseous blood supply to the metatarsal head. Proximally, the blood supply is centered around the area of the old epiphyseal plate region and seems to demonstrate a more uniform pattern. The surgical significance is that after medial capsulorrhaphy and distal metatarsal

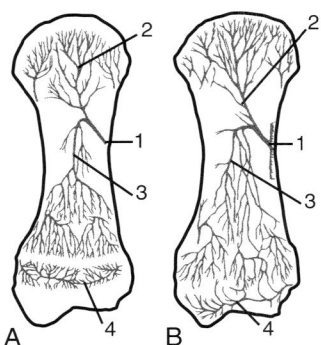 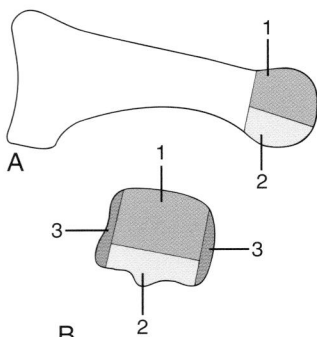

Figure 6-67 Blood supply to first metatarsal bone in an adolescent aged 12 to 13 years **(A)** and in an adult **(B).** The nutrient artery *(1)* divides into a short distal branch *(2)* and a long proximal branch *(3).* The distal branch anastomoses with the distal metaphyseal and capital vessels. The proximal branch is longer and is directed proximally toward epiphysis, which in turn is supplied by arterial branches entering from its mediolateral side. *4,* Epiphyseal vessels. (From Sarrafian SK: *Anatomy of the foot and ankle,* Philadelphia, 1983, JB Lippincott.)

Figure 6-68 Geographic distribution of the intraosseous blood supply to the metatarsal head. **A,** Lateral view. **B,** Axial view. Note the dorsal metaphyseal vessels *(1),* which supply the dorsal two thirds of the head; plantar metaphyseal vessels *(2),* which supply the plantar third of the head; and capital arteries *(3),* which supply the medial and lateral fourth of the head. (From Shereff MJ, Yang QM, Kummer FJ: Extraosseous and intraosseous arterial supply to the first metatarsal and metatarsophalangeal joints. *Foot Ankle* 8:81-93, 1987.)

Figure 6-69 Epiphyses at the base of the proximal phalanx and first metatarsal present in a juvenile with hallux valgus must be protected at the time of surgery. **A,** Diagram. **B,** Radiograph.

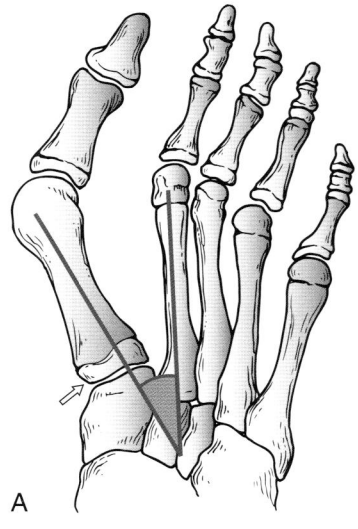 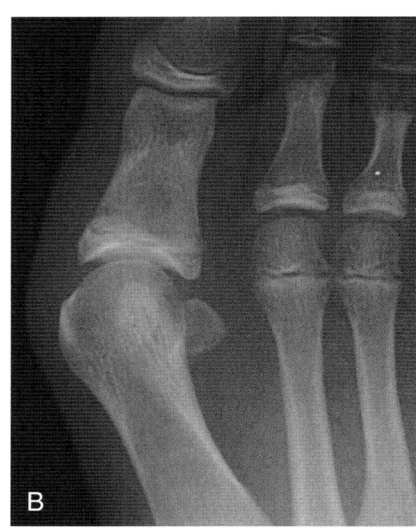

osteotomy, the vascular supply to the metatarsal head depends on the remaining metaphyseal vessels. Wide soft tissue dissection may imperil the circulation of the capital fragment and lead to avascular necrosis (AVN).

Open Epiphysis

A juvenile hallux valgus deformity may be further complicated by the presence of an open epiphysis at the base of the proximal phalanx and first metatarsal (Fig. 6-69). Postoperative recurrence of a hallux valgus deformity attributable to further epiphyseal growth has been speculated as a cause of recurrence and has led to the recommendation that surgical intervention be postponed until skeletal maturity has been achieved.* Helal[216] and Bonney

and Macnab[35] have cautioned against early surgery because of the poor prognosis, but Goldner and Gaines[186] stated that "early surgery" may allow for remodeling of the articular cartilage. These authors and others[95,170,171,488] have noted no contraindications to early surgery. Coughlin[95] observed that patients who underwent surgical correction with an open epiphysis had greater correction of the hallux valgus angle.

The high recurrence rate in patients with an open epiphysis may be explained not only by a more severe deformity in those who undergo early surgery but also by a corresponding increased DMAA in younger patients with severe deformity. Coughlin[95] noted that in patients

---

*References 38, 70, 105, 201, 361, 364, 472, and 488.

with an onset of hallux valgus before the age of 10, the average hallux valgus deformity was 32 degrees; in patients 10 years or older, the average preoperative deformity was 25 degrees. Significantly greater correction was achieved in patients with early-onset of deformity. The average hallux valgus correction in the younger group was 24 degrees, and the average correction in the older group was 15 degrees ($P = .0001$).

The average DMAA of patients who underwent correction of hallux valgus in the presence of an open epiphysis was 21 degrees, whereas the average DMAA of those who underwent correction after the epiphysis was closed was 10 degrees. Greater deformity may have been a factor influencing early correction of a hallux valgus deformity with an open epiphysis. The magnitude of the DMAA in these patients was two times greater than in those with a closed epiphysis. Luba and Rosman[319] hypothesize that medial inclination of the first metatarsal epiphysis causes tension forces to develop on the lateral aspect of the epiphysis and compression forces to develop on the medial aspect of the epiphysis, thereby leading to increased growth of the lateral epiphysis with subsequent increased medial inclination of the first metatarsal. They further hypothesized that the surgical correction achieved by a first metatarsal osteotomy distal to an open first metatarsal epiphysis may decrease with time because of lateral epiphyseal overgrowth. However, no evidence supports the premise that "epiphyseal overgrowth" of the proximal first metatarsal is the cause of recurrent hallux valgus in juvenile patients. A large DMAA in juvenile hallux valgus deformities treated by intraarticular correction (i.e., a distal soft tissue procedure) is associated with a high recurrence rate.[95] An increased DMAA may have led to the previous conclusion that surgery in the presence of an open epiphysis is contraindicated. Rather, in the presence of a large DMAA (often associated with severe deformity at a younger age), intraarticular correction is contraindicated.

A partial lateral first metatarsal epiphyseal arrest procedure in the early adolescent years may theoretically achieve gradual diminution of the 1–2 IM angle. Ellis[145] and others[119,159,292,474,479] have proposed partial lateral epiphyseal arrest to achieve a gradual decrease in metatarsus primus varus.[145] Ellis, in reporting on 20 cases of partial epiphyseal arrest, noted a high failure rate; others[156,479] report only anecdotal short-term experience with this technique. Davids et al[119] reported on a 4-year follow-up on 11 feet treated with lateral epiphyseodesis. Although they concluded that no foot clinically worsened, and that they achieved a significant correction in 6 of 11 feet, the average angular correction was mediocre at best (hallux valgus angle correction of 3.5 degrees, 1–2 IM angle correction of 2 degrees). The efficacy of this technique remains hypothetical and is not recommended.

The possibility of an epiphyseal injury at the base of either the first metatarsal or the proximal phalanx after an osteotomy must be considered when surgery is to be performed on a growing child, and this is probably the

major reason for delaying surgical intervention. Anderson et al[8] analyzed the rate of growth in the female foot and determined that full foot growth is usually achieved by 14 years of age. At 12 years of age, an average of less than 1 cm of total longitudinal foot growth remains. Less than 50% of this growth occurs at the proximal first metatarsal epiphysis, and thus a relatively small amount of growth occurs in the first ray after 12 years of age.[8] In adolescent boys, completion of growth tends to occur at an average age of 16 years. By age 12, however, boys still have almost 3 cm of total longitudinal foot growth remaining. Again, with an estimated 50% of the remaining longitudinal foot growth occurring at the first metatarsal epiphysis, approximately 1.5 cm of metatarsal growth remains.

The presence of an open epiphysis is not a contraindication to either surgical correction or an osteotomy in either the proximal phalanx or the proximal first metatarsal. At surgery it is important to determine the exact location of the phalangeal or metatarsal epiphysis to avoid causing an iatrogenic epiphyseal injury (Fig. 6-70). Reconstruction of a short 1st metatarsal may be a complex and difficult salvage.[232] Correction of hallux valgus in a juvenile patient frequently requires an osteotomy to achieve complete correction. When either a phalangeal or a metatarsal osteotomy is planned in a patient 10 years or younger, it is important to ascertain the amount of growth that can be expected postoperatively, not only in the foot but also in the first metatarsal. If an iatrogenic epiphyseal injury does occur, one can then hypothesize its effect on ultimate phalangeal or metatarsal longitudinal growth. In an older juvenile patient, iatrogenic epiphyseal arrest or partial epiphyseal plate closure after surgery will have little effect on first-ray length at this age. Surgery in a younger child is not contraindicated and may allow adaptation or remodeling of the MTP articular surfaces postoperatively.[186]

JUVENILE HALLUX VALGUS

To qualify as a juvenile hallux valgus deformity, the onset of the deformity must occur in the preteen or teenage years. Despite development during this period, however, a patient may choose to seek medical treatment later in life. Coughlin and Mann[105] and others[88,97] have observed that in adults, certain hallux valgus deformities are much more difficult to correct surgically than others. These same patients appear to have a much higher risk of postoperative recurrence of deformity (Fig. 6-71). The authors hypothesized that these bunions occur in adults because of specific anatomic characteristics that developed during the juvenile and adolescent years.

Juvenile and adult hallux valgus deformities can be differentiated by several characteristics. Degenerative arthritis of the first MTP joint is rarely associated with a juvenile hallux valgus deformity but is more often associated with an adult bunion (Fig. 6-72).* Likewise, whereas

*References 105, 201, 364, 423, 471, and 475.

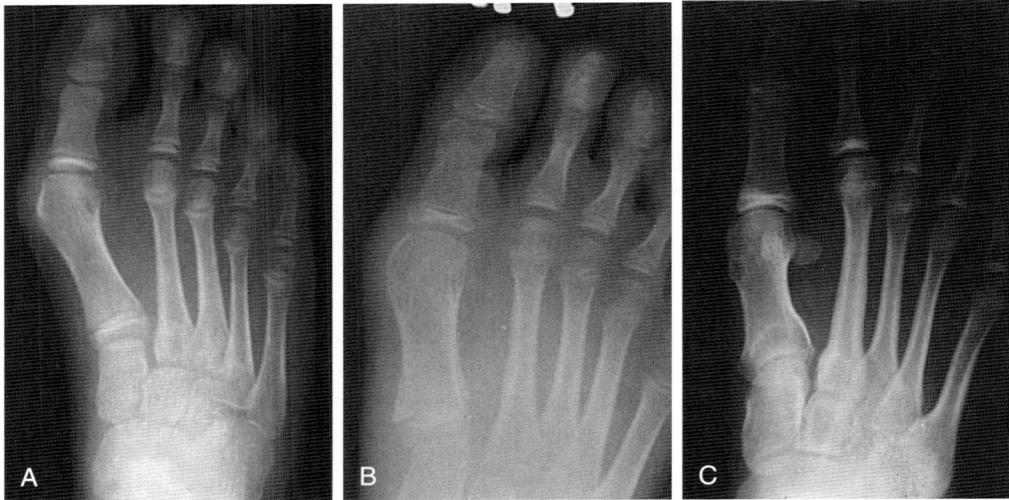

Figure 6-70 **A,** Radiograph before a proximal first metatarsal osteotomy with an open epiphysis. **B,** After proximal first metatarsal osteotomy, injury to the proximal first metatarsal epiphysis has occurred. **C,** A radiograph later demonstrates a shortened first metatarsal after an epiphyseal injury.

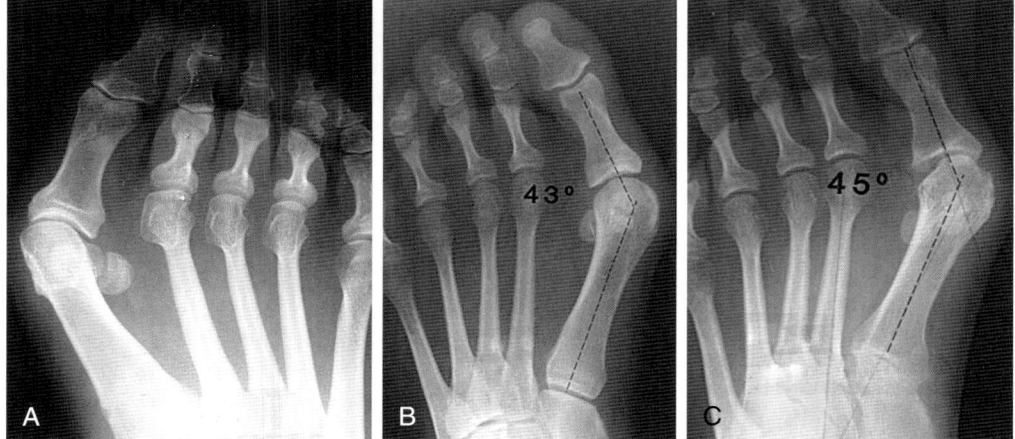

Figure 6-71 **A,** Postoperative recurrence in a patient with metatarsus adductus and a congruent metatarsophalangeal joint who underwent surgery in the teenage years. Hallux valgus deformity may develop in the adolescent years but can be surgically treated years later. Many juvenile deformities have pathologic elements that are extremely difficult to treat. **B** and **C,** Preoperative and postoperative radiographs, respectively, in a juvenile who had rapid recurrence 8 weeks after surgical repair.

bursal thickening over the medial eminence is typically found in older patients, it is rarely present in a juvenile with hallux valgus.* The epiphyseal growth plates at the base of the first metatarsal and proximal phalanges are frequently open in early adolescence.[105,364] In juveniles and adolescents with hallux valgus, the prominence of the medial eminence is of lesser magnitude[105,197,423,488] and the magnitude of the 1–2 IM angle is often increased,[105] but the hallux valgus angle is typically of lesser magnitude.[105,197,201,364] Pronation of the hallux is much less common in juvenile patients.[197,423,475] Hypermobility of the first MTC articulation may be associated with a juvenile bunion.[73] However, a very rigid MTC joint

articulation may also occur and make surgical repair resistant to correction without a metatarsal osteotomy.

CLASSIFICATION

The main purpose of a classification of hallux valgus deformities is to facilitate the decision-making process on how to treat the deformity. No one classification is perfect, and the numbers used to define a mild, moderate, or severe deformity are not "etched in stone." Classification should be used only as a general guide. With experience, the clinician will be able to appreciate which procedures can be "pushed" past these limits and which yield a satisfactory result when used for midrange conditions in the classification. As with any surgery, the finesse needed to

---

*References 138, 195, 361, 364, 471, and 472.

carry out a good bunion procedure can be gained only through clinical experience.

With a mild bunion deformity, the hallux valgus angle is less than 20 degrees, and part of the deformity may result from an HVIdeformity. The MTP joint is often congruent, and the IM angle is usually 11 degrees or less

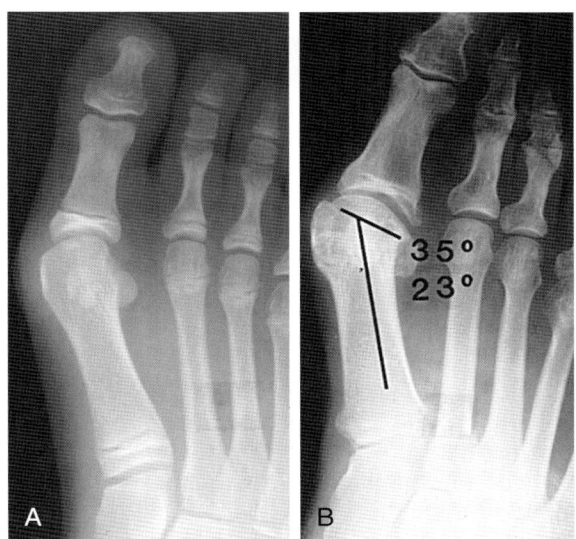

Figure 6-72 **A,** Juvenile hallux valgus deformity with no significant medial eminence and no degenerative changes. Note the open epiphysis. **B,** Hallux valgus deformity in an adult. Note the sagittal sulcus, degenerative changes at the first metatarsophalangeal joint, enlarged medial eminence, substantial subluxation of the sesamoids, and increased distal metatarsal articular angle (23 degrees).

(Fig. 6-73A). These patients typically complain of a painful medial eminence that frequently has a sharp ridge along the dorsomedial aspect. Radiographs generally demonstrate that the sesamoids are maintained in anatomic position. On occasion, however, about 50% subluxation of the fibular sesamoid may be present.

A moderate hallux valgus deformity usually demonstrates subluxation of the MTP joint, unless the DMAA is abnormal. The hallux valgus angular deformity is 20 to 40 degrees, and the great toe may exert some pressure against the second toe. The hallux is typically pronated. The IM angle varies from 11 to 16 degrees. The fibular sesamoid is usually displaced 75% to 100%.

A severe hallux valgus deformity has greater than 40 degrees of lateral deviation of the hallux, and this often results in an underriding or overriding deformity of the second toe. The hallux is moderately or severely pronated. Because of the functional loss of the first MTP joint with a severe deformity, a painful transfer lesion may develop beneath the second metatarsal head. Radiographic examination demonstrates significant subluxation of the MTP joint and usually 100% lateral subluxation of the fibular sesamoid. The IM angle is generally greater than 16 to 18 degrees (Fig. 6-73B).

PATIENT EVALUATION

History and Physical Examination

Evaluation of hallux valgus begins with a careful history of the patient's condition. This should include the chief complaint, which in the authors' series of bunions is pain over the medial eminence in 70% to 75% of patients.[101,344]

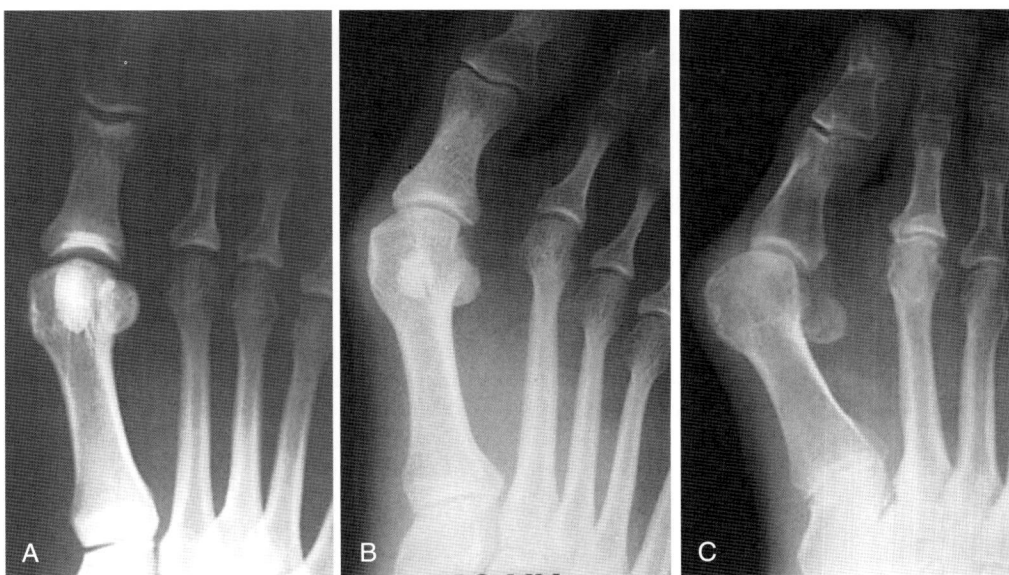

Figure 6-73 **A,** Radiograph of mild hallux valgus deformity, which has up to 20 degrees of angulation at the metatarsophalangeal joint. **B,** Radiograph of moderate hallux valgus deformity, which has between 20 and 40 degrees of angulation at the metatarsophalangeal joint. **C,** Radiographs of severe hallux valgus deformity demonstrate displacement of the metatarsal head off the sesamoids.

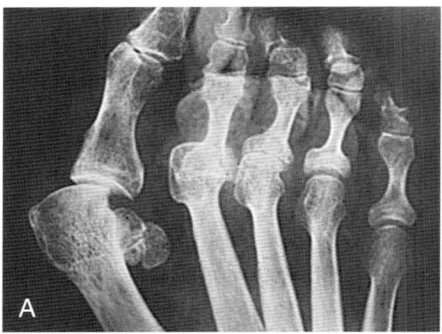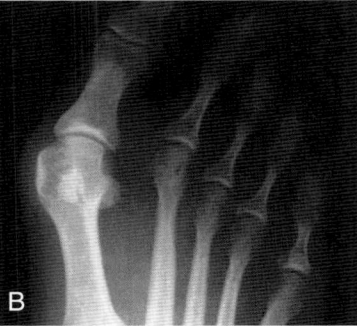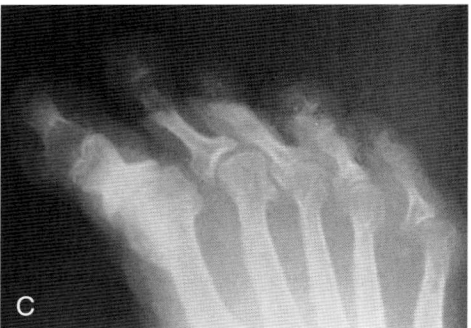

Figure 6-74 Deformities of lesser metatarsophalangeal (MTP) joints resulting from deviation of hallux. **A,** Dislocation of the second MTP joint and subluxation of the third MTP joint associated with hallux valgus deformity. **B,** Lateral deviation of all lesser MTP joints associated with hallux valgus deformity. **C,** Medial deviation of all lesser MTP joints associated with hallux varus deformity.

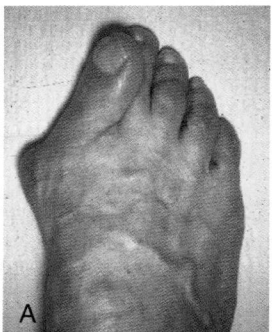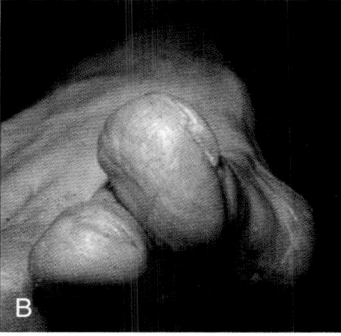

Figure 6-75 **A** and **B,** Pronation of the hallux is common with more severe deformities. This may lead to an ingrown toenail along the medial border of the great toe.[282]

A symptomatic intractable plantar keratosis beneath the second metatarsal head was present in about 40% of patients in the earlier study.[344] Symptomatic metatarsalgia was present in 48% of patients in a later study.[101] Other associated problems include instability of the lesser MTP joints, interdigital neuromas, lesser toe deformities, corns, and calluses (Fig. 6-74). Information should be obtained regarding the patient's level of activity, occupation, athletic inclinations, preference for specific types of footwear, and reasons for choosing surgery. The patient's medical history should be obtained as well.

The physical examination is carried out by observing the patient's gait and then carefully observing the foot with the patient both standing and sitting. The magnitude of the deformity of the hallux and lesser toes is noted and the longitudinal arch and hindfoot position observed. The magnitude of pronation of the hallux is assessed (Fig. 6-75). Typically, with more severe deformities, the magnitude of pronation increases.[110,336]

With the patient sitting, range of motion of the ankle, subtalar, transverse tarsal, and MTP joints is examined. Ankle range of motion is carefully assessed while the knee is both flexed and extended, with attention directed to gastrocnemius–soleus muscle tightness (restricted ankle dorsiflexion) (see Fig. 6-40). Care is taken to ensure that the foot is held in a neutral position (with the talonavicular joint reduced to eliminate transverse tarsal or subtalar motion)[39,192,210] with respect to the forefoot and hindfoot during assessment of the gastrocnemius–soleus. Ankle joint motion is measured by placing a goniometer on the lateral aspect of the foot and ankle and using the fibula and plantar lateral border of the foot as landmarks for each limb of the goniometer. A right angle is considered a neutral position.

The posture of the forefoot is assessed (e.g., forefoot varus, valgus, neutral). The first MTP joint is carefully palpated for evidence of synovitis and crepitus, as well as for specific areas of pain.

Active and passive range of MTP joint motion is assessed with the patient sitting and measured with a goniometer by using the plantar aspect of the foot and the medial axis of the proximal phalanx as points of reference.[495] A neutral position is recorded as 0 degrees, and dorsiflexion and plantar flexion are measured from this point. Joseph[256] reported that the average passive range of motion of the first MTP joint in adults older than 45 years was 87 degrees (67 degrees of dorsiflexion and 20 degrees of plantar flexion).

Palpation over the dorsomedial cutaneous nerve often demonstrates irritability if there is a large medial eminence. Attention should also be directed to the plantarmedial hallucial nerve, which courses over the dorsal border of the medial sesamoid.[413] While gently dorsiflexing and plantar flexing the first MTP joint, an attempt is made to manually reduce the deformity to determine how much correction can be achieved. At times, particularly with a long-standing hallux valgus deformity, a reduction in dorsiflexion occurs as the great toe is brought out of lateral deviation. This suggests that the distal metatarsal articular surface may be laterally deviated or that the articular cartilage has deteriorated to such an extent that dorsiflexion may be reduced after surgical realignment.

The mobility of the first MTC joint is also evaluated. This examination is performed with the patient sitting, the knee flexed, and the ankle positioned at a 90-degree angle or in neutral position.[190] The forefoot is stabilized

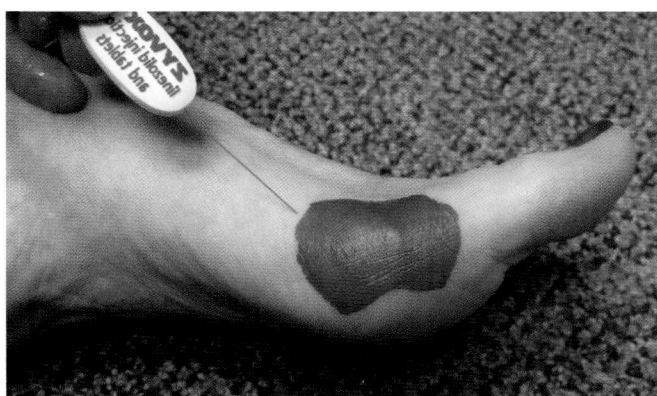

Figure 6-76 Sensory deficit over the medial eminence with progression of a bunion deformity. The diminished sensory area is marked in red. Sensation is checked with a Symes-Weinstein filament.

with one hand, and the first metatarsal is grasped between the thumb and index finger of the opposite hand. The first metatarsal is then moved from a dorsomedial to a plantar-lateral direction and compared with the opposite side (see Figs. 6-32 and 6-33). In our experience, pathologic hypermobility exists in approximately 10% to 15% of patients with a hallux valgus deformity; however, mobility may be substantially treated and reduced with realignment merely of the first MTP joint.[91,99-101,110] The plantar aspect of the foot is then examined for the presence of an intractable plantar keratosis, which most frequently is located beneath the second metatarsal head. On occasion, one can form beneath the tibial sesamoid because of its centralized position beneath the metatarsal head. The IM spaces are carefully palpated for evidence of neuritic symptoms. The lesser toes are then examined for evidence of lesser MTP joint instability, hammer toes, mallet toes, or interdigital corns.

Vascular evaluation includes palpation of the dorsalis pedis and posterior tibial pulses, observation of capillary filling of the toes, and assessment of the skin and hair pattern. If there is any question regarding the circulatory status of the foot, a Doppler evaluation is obtained.

The neurologic examination focuses on sensation, vibratory sense, and strength of the intrinsic and extrinsic muscles. Often, a sensory deficit may develop with reduced sensation over the medial eminence and medial hallux (Fig. 6-76). This is likely due to either traction on or pressure from the bunion on the dorsal medial sensory nerve to the hallux. Careful attention to this nerve during the surgical dissection is important; the sensory deficit often diminishes during the postoperative period.

CONSERVATIVE TREATMENT

Conservative care in most patients with a bunion deformity is adequate to relieve symptoms.[141] A symptomatic mild hallux valgus deformity should be periodically examined and radiographs obtained to evaluate any

progression in the magnitude of the deformity. A custom or prefabricated orthotic device may assist in the treatment of a flexible flatfoot deformity or in a patient with ligamentous laxity and hallux valgus associated with pes planus (Fig. 6-77A).* Groiso[197] recommended the use of bunion night splints and exercises and noted a 50% improvement in hallux valgus deformities in a 7-year study of juvenile patients. Others have tried physical therapy and night splints,[137] and even injections of botulinum toxin[431], but there are no long-term studies that conclusively demonstate successful long-term correction of a deformity.

The physician should encourage the use of roomy footwear to reduce pressure over the medial eminence. A soft leather shoe with a wide toe box and, preferably, a soft sole may give significant relief of symptoms. A pedorthist can modify shoes by stretching and relieving pressure points over the bunion. On occasion, custom-made footwear may help patients with severe hallux valgus deformities who are reluctant to undergo surgical correction. The use of bunion pads, night splints, bunion posts, and other commercial appliances may also help in relieving symptoms (Fig. 6-77B-D). Modification of footwear is probably the most important factor in achieving symptomatic relief of pain in a patient with a bunion deformity. It is difficult to achieve compliance in any patient with regard to wearing roomy footwear. Constricting footwear increases symptoms in patients with a hallux valgus deformity. Shoes with a low heel, an adequate toe box, and a soft upper tend to diminish symptoms.

The use of prefabricated or custom orthotics is controversial in the treatment of a patient with hallux valgus. It has not been demonstrated that orthotic devices prevent progression of the deformity. An orthotic device may be uncomfortable for a patient because it occupies space within the shoe. It may place increased pressure against the medial eminence and result in increased symptoms rather than relief of pressure on the first metatarsal head. Durman[138] and others[170,195,326,361,472] recommend their use postoperatively, but Canale et al[58] and others[95,268] have not used them. Kilmartin et al,[268] curiously, found that the hallux valgus angle increased more in patients who used orthotics and concluded that orthoses did not prevent progression of a hallux valgus deformity.

If conservative care has not led to a diminution of symptoms or the deformity has progressed, surgical correction can be considered.† Rapid progression of a hallux valgus deformity is unusual, and frequently, a hallux valgus deformity can be observed over a lengthy period (see Fig. 6-17). Although cosmesis is mentioned as a possible indication for surgery,[60,319,471,488,556] pain and discomfort should be the major considerations for surgical correction. It may be difficult on occasion to distinguish between a patient's concern for cosmesis and actual discomfort.[559]

---

*References 70, 95, 105, 170, 186, 414, 471, 472, and 488.
†References 135, 337, 355, 356, 358, and 367.

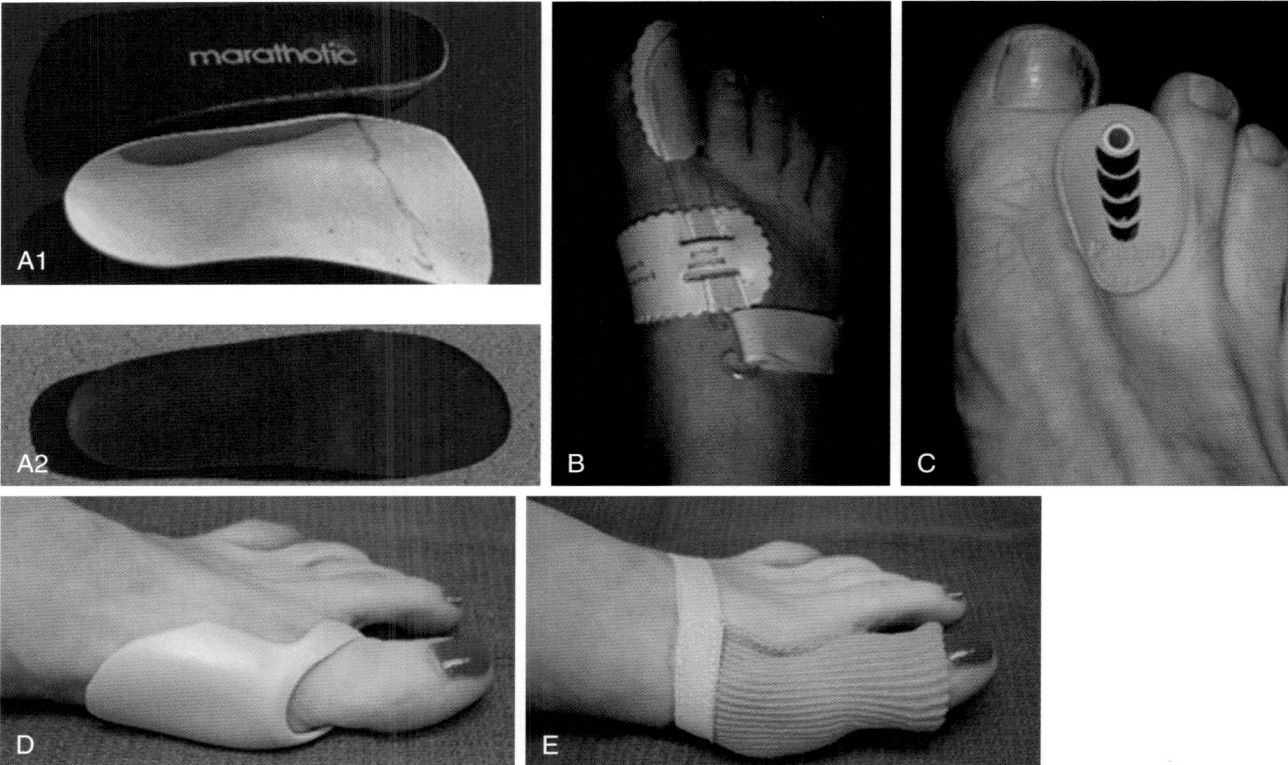

Figure 6-77 Conservative measures for the treatment of hallux valgus. **A1** and **A2,** Orthotics. **B,** Night splint. **C,** Bunion post. **D** and **E,** Bunion pad.

Nonsurgical care should also be considered in patients with hyperelasticity, ligamentous laxity, or neuromuscular disorders because of the high recurrence rate. Surgery is not urgent. When contemplating surgery, careful decision making may decrease the incidence of postsurgical recurrence of a hallux valgus deformity. Radovic and Shah[431] have reported the use of botulinum toxin A to temporarily diminish the strength of the adductor hallucis and secondarily the angular deformity of the hallux and first metatarsal in a nonsurgical candidate with small corrections noted in the hallux valgus and intermetatarsal angles. Whether this modality will have a place in future therapy remains to be seen.

Considerations with Surgical Intervention

Anesthesia and Pain Control

The vast majority of forefoot surgery is done in an outpatient setting. Peripheral nerve blocks may be used either for the surgery or as a method of postoperative pain management. Discussion of the technique and methods of anesthesia are contained in Chapter 5. However, the recovery process may be modified by use of analgesics, antiinflammatory medications, local injections, and/or continuous infusion of anesthetic agent to maintain a nerve block during the immediate postoperative period.

Adequate anesthesia is necessary when using a tourniquet. A more peripheral location allows a more distal

nerve block. A lower ankle level tourniquet does allow a distal nerve block as opposed to a thigh or upper calf pneumatic tourniquet. Grebing and Coughlin[191] showed an ankle Esmark tourniquet to be safe and reliable in achieving tourniquet pressures in a safe range that allowed forefoot surgery with a bloodless field.

Mattila et al[351] administered one dose of oral dexamethazone both preoperatively and postoperatively in association with bunion surgery and noted reduced nausea and pain levels in the immediate postoperative period. Brattwall et al[47] in a study of postoperative bunion patients reported that oral administration of a cyclooxygenase (COX)-2 inhibitor for a week after surgery achieved much better pain relief than sustained release tramadol in a controlled study. They also reported on computed tomography (CT) scan follow-up on these patients and noted no sign of impaired bone healing at 12 weeks after surgery. Daniels et al[117] reported the use of low-dose immediate-release oral diclofenac (used for 4 days after bunionectomies), and noted, compared to a placebo, that there was shorter time to pain reduction, reduced use of opoids, and superior pain relief.

White et al[551] reported the use of a continuous infusion of 0.25% bupivacaine for 72 hours after foot and ankle surgery. They noted significant reduction in postoperative pain and the use of opiod analgesics, and a substantial improvement in patient satisfaction levels after surgery. Gallardo et al[166] reported on the use of continuous popliteal block with bupivicaine after total ankle replacement and noted lower requirement of opiates, good pain control, and a higher level of postoperative satisfaction. Kim et al,[273] in the evaluation of 30 patients who underwent bunion surgery, compared a placebo group to those with a subcutaneous injection of a mixture of ketorolac, epinephreine, morphine, and ropivicaine. Those with the multidrug injection had substantial pain relief for 1.5 days after surgery.

Foot and ankle surgery can be particularly painful in the immediate postoperative period, and the use of oral and parenteral medication can mitigate pain to a significant degree. The use of a peripheral nerve block at surgery, infiltration of the region where surgery has been performed with a mixture of analgesics and antiinflammatory medications, and the continuous infusion of anesthetic agents[551] to achieve a longer-acting nerve block all hold promise in reducing postoperative discomfort and improving patient satisfaction.

Miscellaneous Factors

Healing of soft tissue and osseous structures may be effected by cigarette smoking. Krannitz et al[285] reported that the healing time of a distal first metatarsal osteotomy was delayed in primary smokers. It took 1.73 times longer to achieve bony consolidation in smokers. Time to healing in nonsmokers averaged 69 days, and took 120 days in smokers. Of interest, in those who were exposed to second hand smoke, the average time to bony healing was 78 days. Patients with a smoking history or a history of someone who smokes in their presence should be alerted to the increased risk of delay healing.

The issue of bilateral versus unilateral surgery is a controversial topic in hallux valgus surgery. The age of a patient, his or her dexterity, the particular procedure being preformed, and the quality of assistance for each patient plays a role is the decision-making process. Coughlin and Jones[100] reported virtually all of 122 cases were done separately as unilateral procedures. Fridman et al,[161,302] have noted no substantial difference in complications, angular correction, or clinical outcomes with unilateral or bilateral bunion surgeries.

Postoperative physical therapy is likewise a decision that is best individualized by the treating physician for each patient. Jones et al,[251] in a cadaveric study, reported a mean loss of MTP motion of 23 degrees after a distal soft tissue realignment with proximal first metatarsal osteotomy. Most of the loss of motion occurred with dorsiflexion of 22 degrees, with minimal reduction of MTP joint plantar flexion. Thus attention must be directed early to the patient who has difficulty with regaining MTP joint motion. Schuh et al[467] reported a significant increase in postoperative range of motion, especially MTP joint dorsiflexion, after a 4- to 6-week course of physical therapy. Improved weight bearing, gait, and range of motion were noted in this group of 30 patients.

Attention to lesser toe deformities associated with a hallux valgus deformity may identify the presence of lesser toe malalignment,[100,101] necessitating realignment of one or more lesser toes.[132]

SURGICAL TREATMENT

Decision Making

The decision-making process in hallux valgus surgery must begin with the understanding that not all hallux valgus deformities are equal. In the past, one repair was attempted for all types of hallux valgus deformity. Many different factors must be considered when evaluating a deformity. If a single procedure is used to correct all these various deformities, the possibility of success in most patients will be less than satisfactory.

The following issues should be considered in the decision-making process for hallux valgus surgery:

- The patient's chief complaint, occupation, and athletic interests
- Physical findings
- Radiographic evaluation, which should include the magnitude of the hallux valgus, intermetatarsal, and interphalangeal angles; the magnitude of the DMAA; the presence of a congruent or incongruent joint; the extent of MTP and MTC joint arthrosis; and the degree of pronation of the hallux
- The patient's age
- Neurovascular status of the foot
- The patient's expectations

Most of these issues can be quantified, but a patient's expectations of the procedure cannot. People who undergo bunion surgery often do not fully appreciate what outcome to expect. Many patients are unhappy after bunion surgery, mainly because they did not realize that they may not be able to return to their previous level of activity. They were not made fully aware of the potential postsurgical complications, or they fail to remember preoperative discussions.[482] Shurnas and Coughlin[482] reported that, after preoperative discussion of risks and complications, recall of individual risks averaged 10% or less. Nonetheless, an attempt must be made to educate the patient about the benefits as well as the risks of surgery. A patient must fully understand that some residual stiffness, pain, or deformity may occur after surgery. Some patients have bunion surgery only because they believe that they will then be able to wear a more fashionable shoe and are subsequently disappointed when this goal cannot be achieved. In reviewing more than 300 bunion cases,[101,336,344] the authors have observed that a third of patients could wear the shoes that they wanted before surgery and that two thirds could after surgery. Unfortunately, this still leaves a third of patients unable to wear their shoe of choice, and this should be explained to the patient preoperatively.

Another group of patients who pose a specific problem are those in professional sports or dance, who rely on

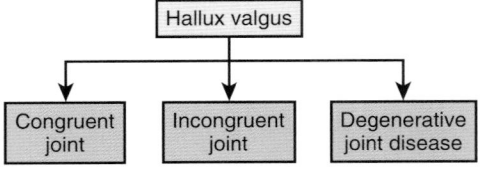

Figure 6-78 The initial algorithm for decision making divides hallux valgus deformities into those with a congruent joint, those with an incongruent joint, and joints with degenerative arthritis.

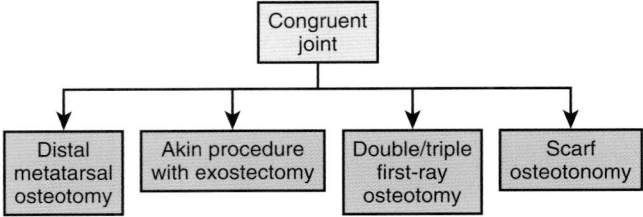

Figure 6-79 If a patient has a congruent joint, these procedures will result in satisfactory correction.

their feet for their livelihood. Until it is no longer possible to perform in their chosen field, bunion surgery should probably be deferred.[90] If patients can eventually resume their previous level of activity after surgery, they will be much more satisfied with the outcome.[90]

With more than 100 surgical procedures described in the literature to correct a hallux valgus deformity, no procedure is adequate to correct all bunion deformities. The authors have developed an algorithm that gives the clinician a logical scheme with which to approach a patient with a hallux valgus deformity. The deformity is placed into one of three main groups according to the radiographic appearance: a congruent joint, an incongruent (subluxated) joint, or a joint with arthrosis (Fig. 6-78). Using these three basic groups, the algorithm correlates the radiographic appearance of the joint with procedures that provide optimal correction of the hallux valgus deformity. No algorithm is all-inclusive, nor can it include all operative procedures, but this algorithm helps organize the surgical considerations and uses proven surgical techniques that have been shown to withstand the test of time.

In using the algorithm, the clinician first must decide whether the hallux valgus deformity is accompanied by a congruent or incongruent (subluxated) MTP joint. A congruent MTP joint has no subluxation of the proximal phalanx on the metatarsal head. Therefore the proximal phalanx, in theory, cannot be rotated back on the metatarsal head, or an incongruent situation might result. A surgical technique must respect a congruent joint when present, and no attempt should be made to alter joint congruency. Most patients with a congruent MTP joint will complain of pain over the medial eminence, although exceptions do exist when significant lateral deviation of the articular surface (increased DMAA) occurs and creates a hallux valgus deformity (see Figs. 6-57 to 6-59). For a mild hallux valgus deformity with a congruous MTP joint, an extraarticular repair (distal metatarsal osteotomy) is preferable because a distal soft tissue realignment may change a congruous joint into an incongruous joint. In patients with a congruent joint, the following procedures will produce a satisfactory result (Fig. 6-79):

- Distal metatarsal osteotomy (Fig. 6-80A-C)
- An Akin procedure with excision of the medial eminence (see Fig. 6-80D and E)

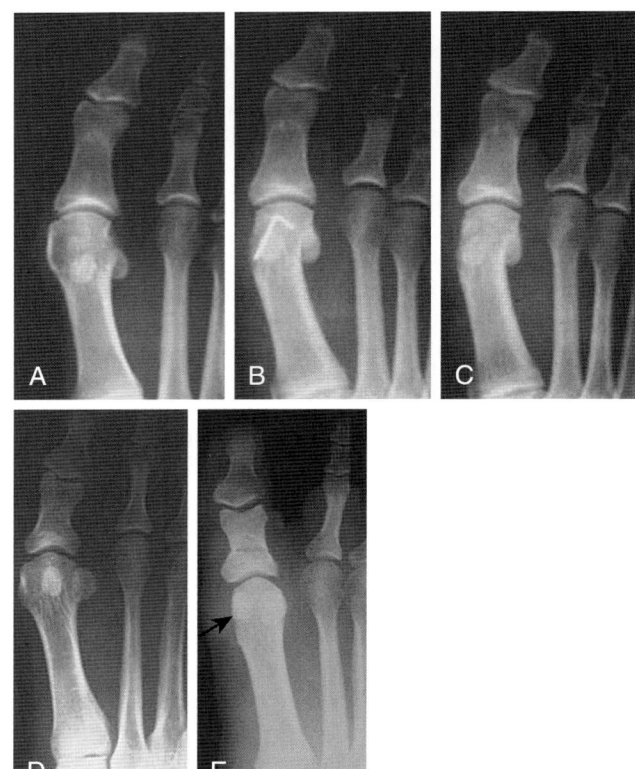

Figure 6-80 Preoperative **(A)** and postoperative **(B and C)** radiographs after correction of hallux valgus with a congruent joint. A chevron procedure was performed. Preoperative **(D)** and postoperative **(E)** radiographs after correction of hallux valgus. An Akin procedure with excision of the medial eminence was performed *(arrow)*.

- Double/triple first-ray osteotomy (Fig 6-81)
- Scarf osteotomy

An incongruent hallux valgus deformity (i.e., the proximal phalanx is subluxated laterally on the metatarsal head) requires a procedure that can move the proximal phalanx back onto the metatarsal head to reestablish a congruent joint. The key component of all these procedures is the use of a distal soft tissue repair and realignment. Although the components of these procedures may vary, the philosophy of a soft tissue realignment remains the same. Because the magnitude of a hallux valgus

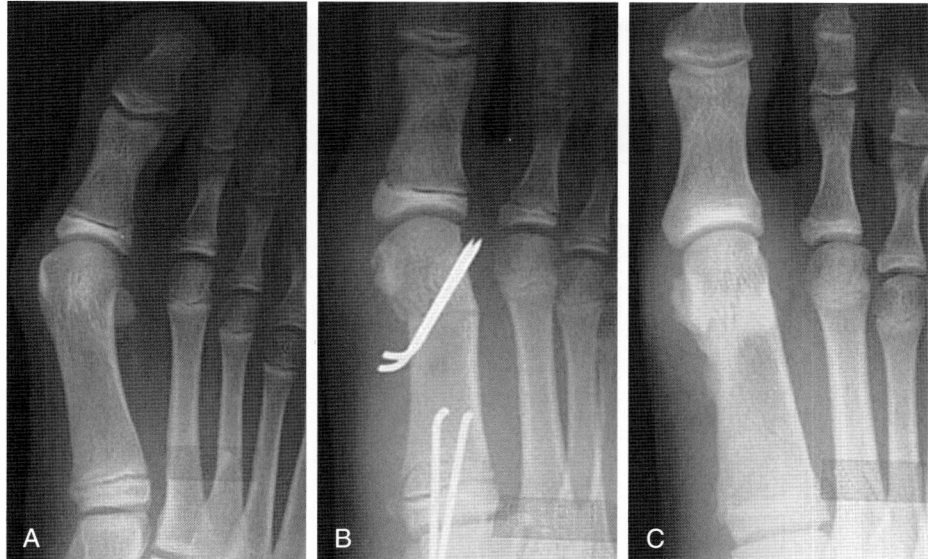

Figure 6-81 **A,** Anteroposterior radiograph of a 14-year-old girl demonstrating progression of deformity. **B,** After distal first metatarsal closing wedge osteotomy and proximal first metatarsal osteotomy, alignment is improved. **C,** A 2-year follow-up radiograph shows acceptable alignment.

deformity varies, the procedure of choice depends on the severity of the deformity. The authors have divided severity into three groups: mild, moderate, and severe. These groups will obviously overlap, but the procedures described for each degree of deformity will probably produce the best overall results (Fig. 6-82).

With a *mild deformity,* the hallux valgus angle is *less than 20 degrees,* and the IM angle is *less than 11 degrees.* The following procedures are used:

■ Distal metatarsal osteotomy (i.e., chevron, Bosch) (see Fig. 6-80)
■ Distal soft tissue procedure with or without proximal metatarsal osteotomy (Figs. 6-83 and 6-84)
■ Midshaft osteotomy (scarf) (Fig. 6-85)

With a *moderate deformity,* the hallux valgus angle is *less than 40 degrees,* and the IM angle is *greater than 13 degrees.* The following procedures are recommended:

■ Distal soft tissue procedure with a proximal metatarsal osteotomy (see Fig. 6-84)
■ Midshaft scarf osteotomy (see Fig. 6-85)
■ Distal metatarsal osteotomy (see Fig. 6-80)

The chevron procedure is not included for treatment of moderate hallux valgus deformity because consistently reliable correction of the deformity in the upper ranges of the moderate group will often not occur. In the lower range of the moderate group, a chevron procedure may result in satisfactory correction.

With a *severe deformity,* the hallux valgus angle is *greater than 40 degrees,* and the IM angle is *greater than 20 degrees.* The following procedures are recommended:

■ Distal soft tissue procedure with proximal metatarsal osteotomy (see Fig. 6-84)
■ Scarf osteotomy (see Fig. 6-85)
■ A Lapidus procedure (Fig. 6-86)
■ Arthrodesis of the first MTP joint (Fig. 6-87)

A distal osteotomy is not recommended for a severe deformity because of its inability to consistently correct the deformity when the hallux valgus angle exceeds 40 degrees and the IM angle exceeds 20 degrees. Severe deformities with or without associated first-ray hypermobility, or those with degeneration of the first MTC joint, can be treated with a distal soft tissue procedure and first MTC joint arthrodesis (the Lapidus procedure) (see Fig. 6-86).

Significant arthrosis of the MTP joint negates the possibility of carrying out most realignment procedures because stiffness and pain of the MTP joint will usually result. Thus the authors recommend performing an arthrodesis. This procedure produces a stable, painless joint that will not deteriorate over time. The use of an MTP joint prosthesis in patients with hallux valgus do not stand up to the test of time and frequently require revision or removal.

Surgical Procedures

Hallux valgus repair requires careful consideration of the surgical goals. The obvious objective is to correct the deformity anatomically so that a long-term satisfactory result is achieved. Thus the ideal hallux valgus repair anatomically realigns the MTP joint without disrupting the biomechanics or normal weight-bearing function of the first MTP joint complex. Procedures that lead to excessive metatarsal shortening or dorsal displacement of the

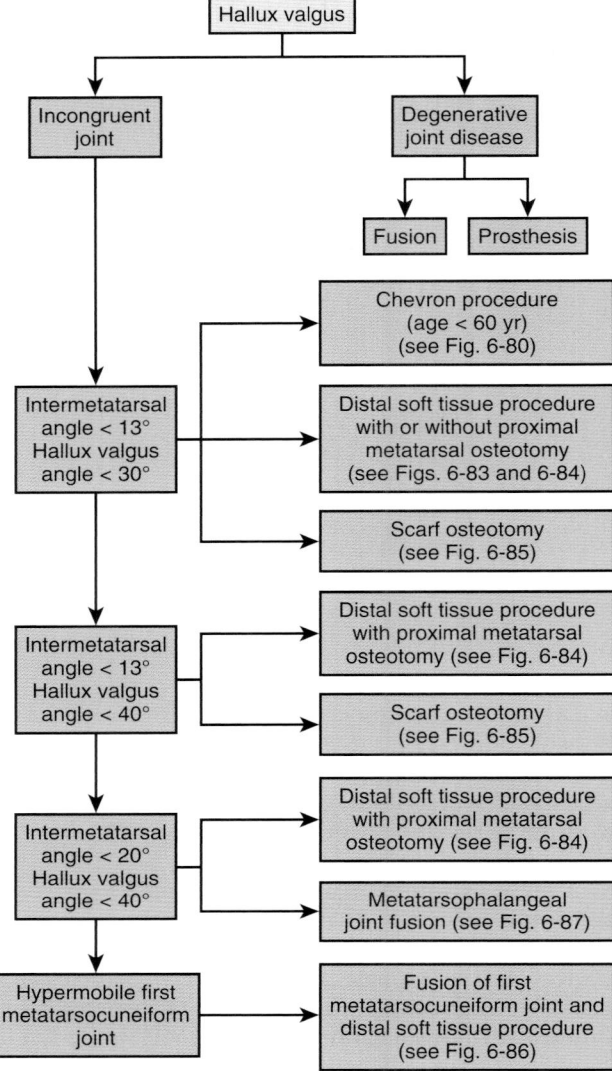

Figure 6-82 Algorithm for a patient with an incongruent joint. The procedure is based on the severity of deformity. For degenerative joint disease, the authos recommend fusion and rarely a prosthesis.

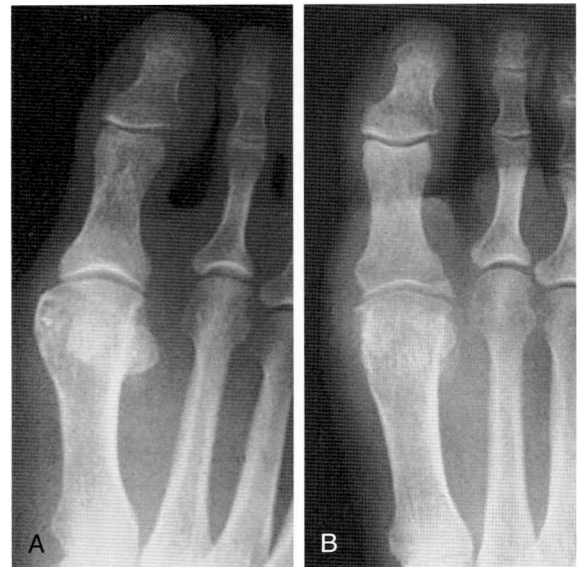

Figure 6-83 Preoperative (A) and postoperative (B) radiographs of a hallux valgus deformity with an incongruent joint that was corrected with a distal soft tissue procedure.

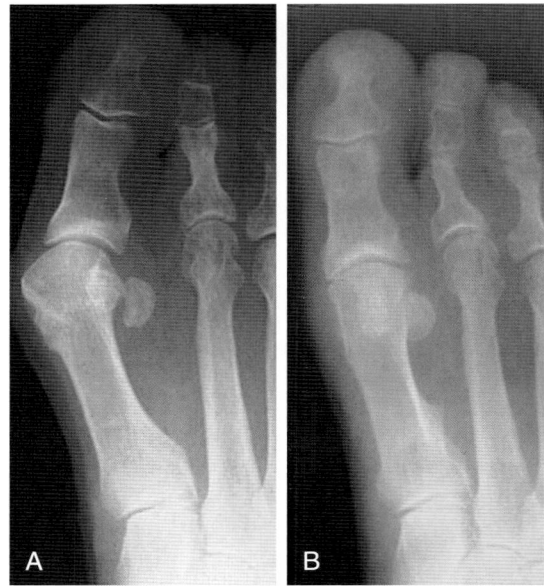

Figure 6-84 Preoperative (A) and postoperative (B) radiographs of a hallux valgus deformity with an incongruent joint that was corrected with a distal soft tissue procedure and proximal metatarsal osteotomy.

metatarsal head, that are associated with an excessive risk of AVN, or that use foreign materials that incite a local reaction or fail within the perioperative period should be avoided.

Most surgical procedures described here have been carefully reviewed in the authors' own patient series and in some cases have been modified to enable achieving the best possible result.

The following procedures are described in detail:

■ Distal soft tissue procedure
■ Akin procedure
■ Distal chevron osteotomy procedure
  ■ Alternative transverse distal osteotomy (e.g., Mitchell/Bosch)

■ Distal soft tissue procedure with proximal metatarsal osteotomy (various types are presented)
■ Scarf osteotomy
■ Multiple first-ray osteotomies
■ Lapidus procedure
■ Keller procedure
■ MTP arthrodesis

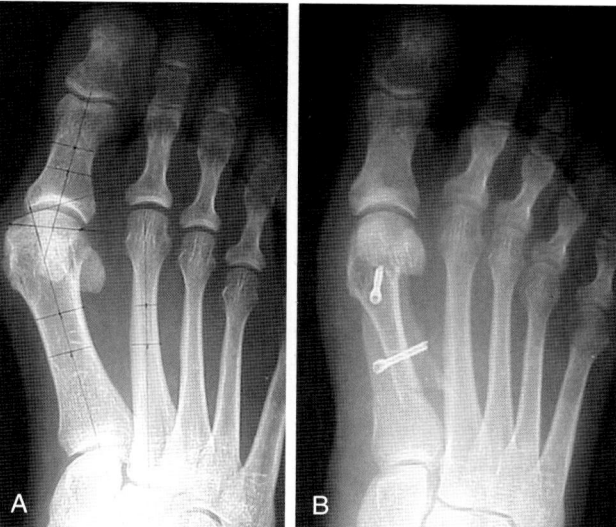

Figure 6-85 **A,** Preoperative radiograph. **B,** After a scarf osteotomy.

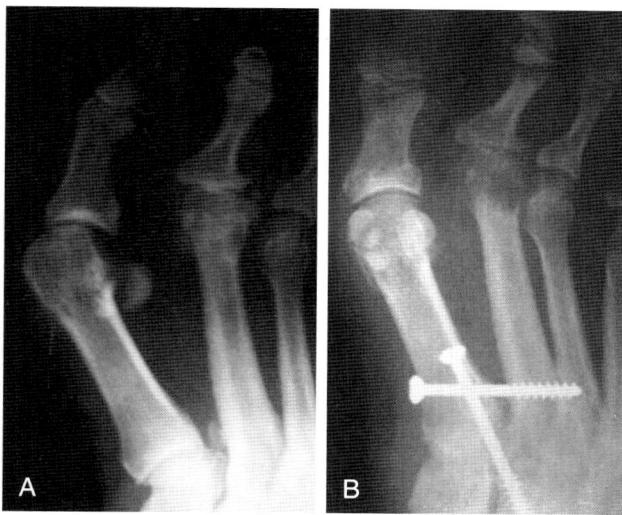

Figure 6-86 Preoperative **(A)** and postoperative **(B)** radiographs of a severe hallux valgus deformity with an incongruent metatarsophalangeal joint and an unstable metatarsocuneiform (MTC) joint that was corrected with a distal soft tissue procedure and first MTC arthrodesis.

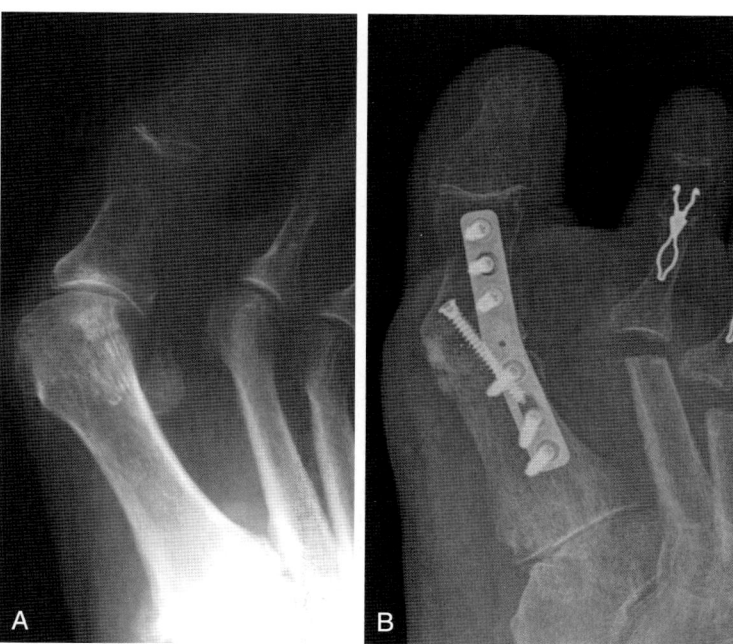

Figure 6-87 Preoperative **(A)** and postoperative **(B)** radiographs of a severe hallux valgus deformity with incongruent joint corrected by arthrodesis of metatarsophalangeal joint. Note the dramatic reduction in the 1–2 intermetatarsal angle.

DISTAL SOFT TISSUE PROCEDURE

Distal soft tissue realignment as correction for a hallux valgus deformity has been advocated in several reports.[260,373,397,567] It was Silver,[486] however, who popularized the technique of medial capsulorrhaphy, medial exostectomy, and lateral capsular and adductor release. Later, McBride[355,356,358] modified this technique by removal of the lateral sesamoid and transfer of the conjoined adductor tendon to the lateral first metatarsal head. DuVries[139] and others[334-336,338,343] modified this procedure so extensively that the eponym "McBride" is no longer appropriate. Mann and Coughlin[336] and later Mann and Pfeffinger,[343] after reviewing the results of this procedure in adults, recommended that the fibular sesamoid be preserved because of the high rate of hallux varus after sesamoid excision.

The basis of this procedure is that the contracted lateral joint structures (i.e., the adductor hallucis, lateral joint capsule, transverse metatarsal ligament) are released, thereby permitting the proximal phalanx to be realigned on the metatarsal head (Video Clip 55). The problematic medial eminence is exposed via a capsulotomy of the first MTP joint, of which there are a number of variations. The attenuated medial capsule is plicated after the medial eminence has been excised. The limiting factor with this technique is the magnitude of metatarsal primus varus present. Because this is only a soft tissue realignment, if there is a fixed malalignment with a 1–2 IM angle of more than 10 degrees, long-lasting correction is unlikely. Therefore the first MTC joint must have sufficient mobility to permit correction of the IM angle from its preoperative position into a normal range postoperatively, or the hallux valgus deformity will recur.

Indications

A distal soft tissue procedure is indicated in a patient with an incongruent (or subluxated) joint, a hallux valgus deformity of less than 30 degrees, and an IM angle of less than 11 degrees. If the indications for the procedure are pushed beyond this magnitude of deformity, sufficient mobility must exist at the MTC joint to allow reduction of the IM angle. If the IM angle does not reduce, the hallux valgus deformity often recurs, so a proximal metatarsal osteotomy is added to the distal soft tissue procedure to provide complete correction. This procedure is applicable to all age groups, from juvenile through octogenarian. An MTC arthrodesis can also be used in association with a distal soft tissue realignment.

Contraindications

The main contraindication to a distal soft tissue procedure is a deformity that exceeds the procedure's capability to gain adequate correction. If the hallux valgus angle is greater than 30 degrees and the IM angle is greater than 11 degrees, this procedure will usually not result in a durable or predictable correction. In many cases, early recurrence often develops because the fixed IM angle has not been adequately corrected. Another contraindication is the presence of a congruent joint with significant lateral deviation of the distal metatarsal articular surface (a DMAA greater than 15 degrees) (see Figs. 6-49, 6-57, and 6-58). In these circumstances, a distal soft tissue procedure is contraindicated because it cannot correct the deformity and will transform a congruent into an incongruent joint. Other contraindications include advanced arthrosis of the MTP joint, spasticity of any type (e.g., cerebral palsy, CVA, head injury), and ligamentous laxity.

Technique

The surgical technique consists of three steps: release of the first web space, preparation of the medial aspect of the MTP joint with excision of the medial eminence, and subsequent reconstruction of the MTP joint. In addition, some authors have described augmenting the procedure with intermetatarsal fixation to help support the soft tissue reconstruction.[352,560]

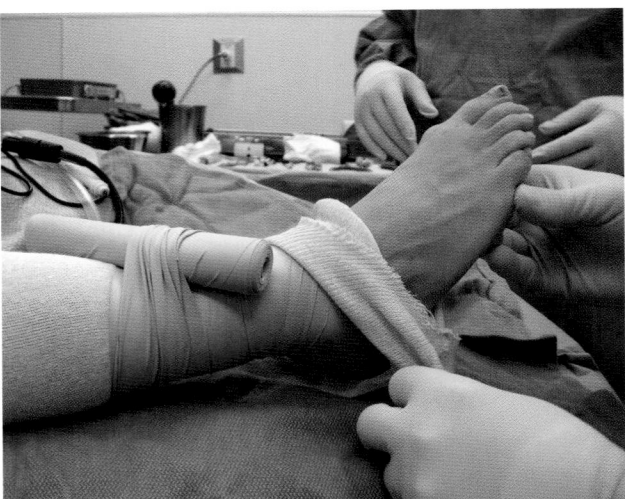

Figure 6-88 An Esmark bandage is often used to exsanguinate the extremity and then is used as a tourniquet above the level of the malleoli.

Release of the First Web Space

1. A peripheral nerve block is typically used for anesthesia, and a tourniquet is applied in the supramalleolar region (Fig. 6-88). A 2-cm dorsal longitudinal incision is centered in the first intermetatarsal web space (Figs. 6-89A and 6-90A). The incision is deepened in the midline through the subcutaneous tissue and fat until the adventitious bursa is identified between the two heads. The dissection is made in the midline to protect the superficial branches of the deep peroneal nerve, which pass on either side of the web space.

2. A Weitlaner retractor or lamina spreader is inserted between the first and second metatarsal heads to facilitate exposure of the web space (see Fig. 6-89B). The adductor hallucis tendon is identified along the dorsal aspect of the fibular sesamoid and the lateral aspect of the metatarsal head. The scalpel blade is inserted into this interval with the blade lying between the metatarsal head dorsally and the fibular sesamoid plantarward. The blade is directed distally until it strikes the base of the proximal phalanx; the knife is turned laterally against the adductor tendon, and the tendon is released from the base of the proximal phalanx. The knife is then brought proximally in the same plane between the metatarsal head and sesamoid to cut the remainder of the capsule between the sesamoid and metatarsal (see Fig. 6-90B and C).

3. The distal end of the adductor tendon that was released from the base of the proximal phalanx is dissected from the lateral aspect of the fibular sesamoid until the junction of the flexor hallucis brevis and adductor hallucis muscle fibers is reached. The fibular sesamoid is inspected by pushing it plantarward with a Freer elevator. It is important to preserve the lateral head of the flexor hallucis brevis tendon so as to reduce the risk of postoperative hallux varus. For the same reason, the

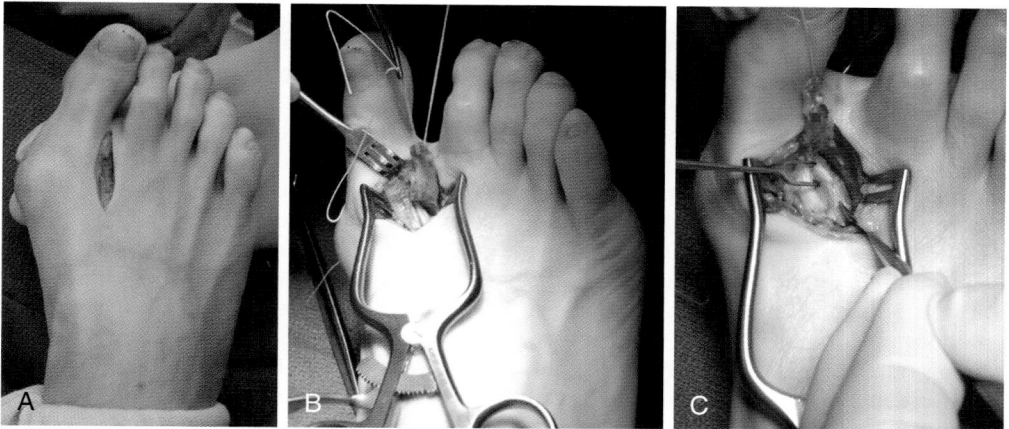

Figure 6-89 **A,** The initial skin incision is made in the web space between the first and second metatarsals. **B,** A Weitlaner retractor is used to expose the conjoined adductor tendon, which is released. **C,** The lateral sesamoid is freed up but not routinely excised.

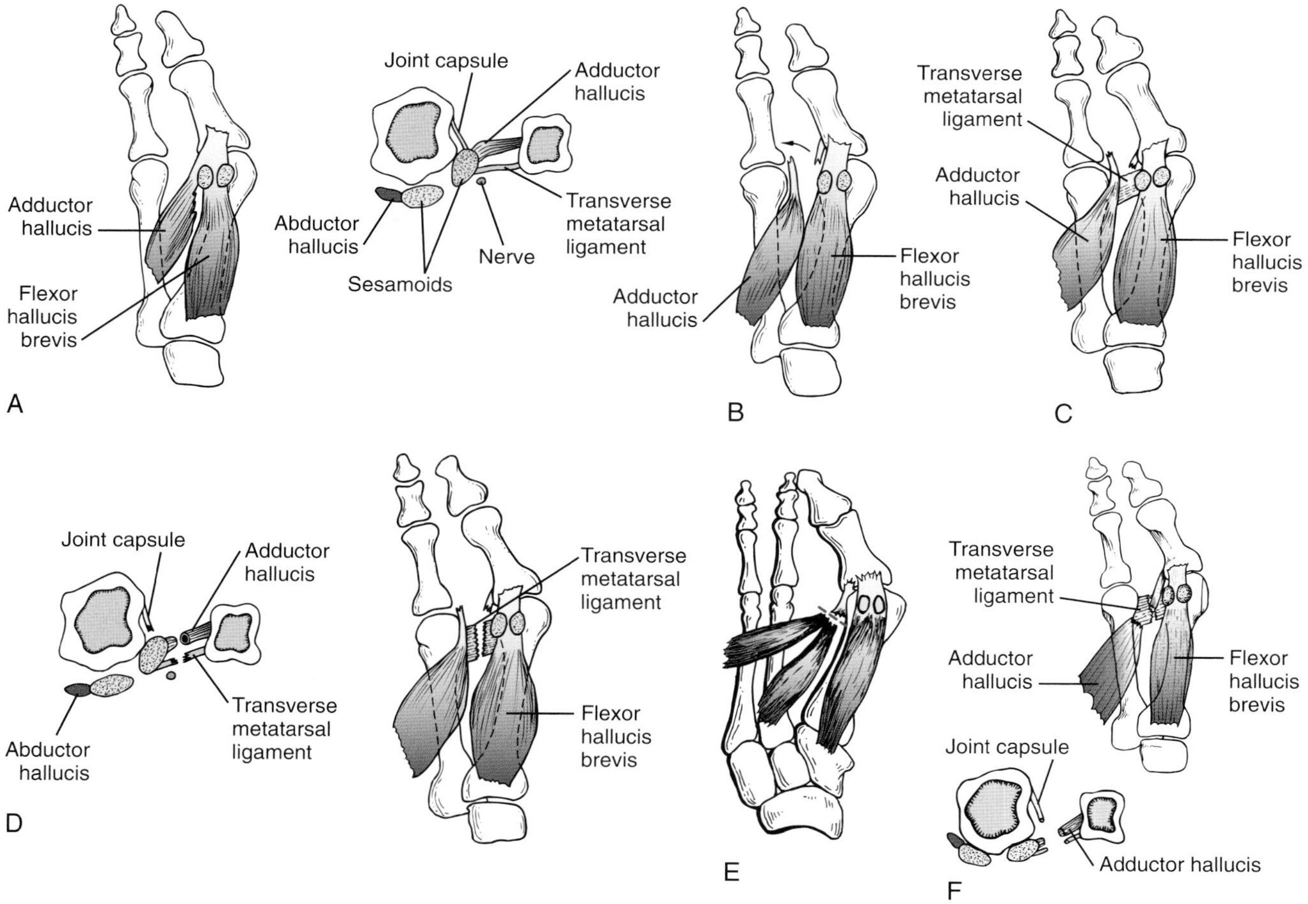

Figure 6-90 Technique for carrying out a distal soft tissue procedure. **A,** The adductor tendon inserts into the lateral aspect of the fibular sesamoid and into the base of the proximal phalanx. The *inset* demonstrates contracted tissue in cross section. **B,** The adductor tendon is released from its insertion into the lateral aspect of the fibular sesamoid and the base of the proximal phalanx. **C,** The transverse metatarsal ligament is noted to pass from the second metatarsal into the fibular sesamoid. **D,** The transverse metatarsal ligament has been transected. The *inset* demonstrates that at this point, contracted lateral structures (i.e., the lateral joint capsule, adductor hallucis, transverse metatarsal ligament) have been released. **E** and **F,** Alternative lateral release involving retention of a distal 2-cm stump of adductor tendon for the lateral capsular repair.

fibular sesamoid is rarely excised unless significant degenerative changes are seen at the sesamoid-metatarsal articulation.

Alternative Technique[93]: The distal adductor tendon insertion is left attached to the base of the proximal phalanx (2 cm in length) (see Figs. 6-90E and 6-89B and C). The tendon is released at the level of the musculotendinous junction to allow the proximal adductor hallucis tendon to retract. The distal stump of the tendon is later sutured to the lateral aspect of the metatarsal capsule. This maneuver may help to lessen the risk for hallux varus.

4. The self-retaining retractor is placed deeper into the wound, and the first and second metatarsals are spread apart to place tension on the transverse metatarsal ligament, which passes from the second metatarsal into the fibular sesamoid. The ligament is transected cautiously to prevent injury to the underlying common digital nerve and vessels in the first web space (see Fig. 6-90D). Once the ligament is released, an elevator is passed along the plantar aspect of the fibular sesamoid to ensure that the sesamoids can be relocated beneath the metatarsal head. In the rare case where the fibular sesamoid has been excised, the tendon of the flexor hallucis longus is inspected to ensure that it was not inadvertently transected.

5. The lateral capsule is perforated with several puncture wounds, and the toe is angulated medially to disrupt the remaining lateral capsule. (The purpose of this tearing technique is to leave some lateral capsular tissue present so that with healing it will stabilize the lateral MTP joint and minimize the risk of development of a postoperative hallux varus deformity.) Alternatively, a distally based capsular flap can be developed by detaching the lateral capsule from the lateral first metatarsal head. The stump of conjoined tendon that has been preserved is later sutured into the lateral metatarsal capsule and soft tissue for reinforcement of the lateral capsule to minimize varus inclination. If a distally based cuff of lateral capsule has been developed, it is later sutured into the proximal capsular tissue. If the lateral capsule has been released at the level of the MTP joint, three interrupted 2-0 absorbable sutures are used to approximate the first and second MTP joint capsules. These sutures are later tied at the conclusion of the procedure.

This completes release of the lateral contracture of the MTP joint, and attention is directed to its medial aspect (see Fig. 6-90F).

Preparation of the Medial Aspect of the Metatarsophalangeal Joint

1. The medial incision is made in the midline and begins distally at the midportion of the proximal phalanx and continues proximally 1 cm beyond the medial eminence (Fig. 6-91A). The incision is deepened through the subcutaneous tissue to the joint capsule, and dissection is carried out along the capsular plane. It is important to create a full-thickness flap to prevent any

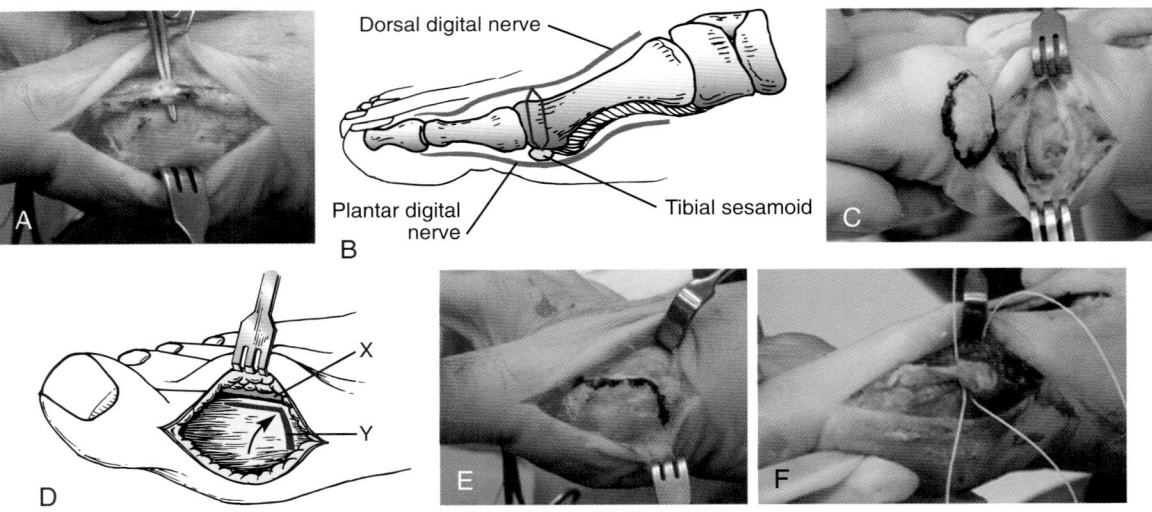

Figure 6-91 A, The medial incision is made in midline, beginning at the midportion of the proximal phalanx and continuing proximally 1 cm beyond the medial eminence. A clamp is used to elevate the dorsomedial cutaneous nerve, which must be protected. **B,** Diagram demonstrating the medial capsular incision, which begins 2 to 3 mm proximal to the base of the proximal phalanx. A second incision is made 3 to 8 mm more proximal to remove a flap of tissue. The size of the flap is determined by the severity of the deformity. **C,** Two parallel cuts in the medial capsule are shown. A wedge of tissue measuring approximately 6 mm has been removed. Note how the capsular cut is directed in a V configuration down through the abductor hallucis tendon, with the apex at the tibial sesamoid. Dorsally, the apex of the V is about 1 cm medial to the extensor tendon. **D** and **E,** An L-shaped capsulotomy releases the dorsal and proximal metatarsophalangeal joint capsule. **F,** A drill hole is made in the metaphysis to secure the dorsal proximal capsule.

possible skin slough. By reflecting the flaps dorsally and plantarward, the dorsal and plantar medial cutaneous nerves can be identified and retracted.

2. The dorsal and plantar flaps are retracted to expose the joint capsule. As mentioned above, there are multiple capsulotomies described. One technique is a vertical capsular incision placed approximately 2 to 3 mm proximal to the base of the proximal phalanx. A second parallel incision is then made in the capsule, 4 to 8 mm more proximal, depending on the severity of the deformity (Fig. 6-91B and C). The capsular incisions are connected dorsally by an inverted-V incision approximately 5 to 10 mm medial to the extensor hallucis longus tendon. The capsular flap is now exposed plantarward, where a V-shaped incision is made through the abductor hallucis tendon. When making this incision through the abductor tendon, the surgeon must keep the knife blade inside the joint to prevent any damage to the plantar-medial cutaneous nerve, which passes just plantar to the sesamoid. If the surgeon attempts to make this incision from outside the capsule in, the plantar-medial cutaneous nerve might be cut by the blade's tip. By working from the inside out, however, the sesamoid prevents the knife from passing too far plantarward, thereby protecting the plantar medial cutaneous nerve. (If by chance this nerve is transected, it should be freed up proximally and buried beneath the abductor hallucis muscle to prevent a neuroma from forming along the plantar medial aspect of the foot.) The medial eminence is exposed by creating a flap of capsule that is based proximally and plantarward. This is done by making an incision along the dorsomedial aspect of the capsule and carefully dissecting it from the medial eminence until it is exposed in its entirety. With a severe deformity, the dorsal portion of the joint capsule is often flimsy and could tear. This is not a cause for concern, however, because the plantar half of the capsule is the most important in the capsular repair.

Alternative Capsular Incision[93]: An L- or V-shaped, distally based capsular flap is developed to release the capsular attachments on the dorsal and proximal aspects (Fig. 6-91D and E). If the capsular tissue is of poor quality, as can occur in situations of severe attenuation, a drill hole is made on the dorsomedial aspect of the metaphysis of the first metatarsal. At the time of capsular repair, the proximal capsule is secured with interrupted absorbable suture through this drill hole (Fig. 6-91F). Several interrupted 2-0 absorbable sutures are then used to repair the proximal as well as the dorsal capsular incision.

3. The MTP joint is inspected and the condition of the articular cartilage noted.

4. The sagittal sulcus is identified and the medial eminence removed, starting approximately 1 to 2 mm medial to the sagittal sulcus in a line parallel with the medial diaphyseal cortex of the first metatarsal (Fig. 6-92). Care is taken to not remove an excessive amount of medial eminence to avoid narrowing the metatarsal head and creating medial instability that may lead to a hallux varus deformity. Scalloping and excessive resection can be avoided by beginning the bone cut along the dorsal aspect of the first metatarsal. Before removing the medial eminence, the radiographs should be inspected; a line is projected along the medial aspect of the metatarsal distally through the medial eminence (see Fig. 6-92D and E). This line provides a general idea about how much medial eminence should be excised. The osteotomized edges are smoothed with a rongeur, especially in the area of the dorsomedial corner of the metatarsal head, an area that often has a sharp prominence. This completes the preparation of the medial capsular structures.

Reconstruction of the Metatarsophalangeal Joint

1. After release of the soft tissue structures around the first metatarsal head, the mobility of the first MTC joint is assessed by pushing the first metatarsal head lateralward (Fig. 6-93A). If the first metatarsal head is easily translated lateralward with little resistance or tendency to spread, one can assume that the IM angle will probably reduce with only a soft tissue procedure. If, however, the first metatarsal head tends to "spring back" medially as though resisting realignment, a distal soft tissue procedure alone will probably be inadequate, and a proximal metatarsal osteotomy should be performed as well. The authors tend to perform an osteotomy in approximately 95% of cases. If the first and second metatarsals tend to spring open, there will probably be residual widening of the IM space and early recurrence of the deformity (Fig. 6-93B and C). As a general rule, if there is any question about whether to perform an osteotomy, it should probably be performed, as the authors do in the vast majority of cases. The osteotomy technique is described later.

2. If an osteotomy is not necessary, the soft tissues on the lateral aspect of the MTP joint are repaired by identifying the adductor tendon in the plantar web space and placing two sutures between it and the remaining lateral capsular cuff of the first metatarsal head. These sutures secure the transferred adductor tendon along the lateral aspect of the first MTP joint. The authors believe that the adductor tendon helps re-form the capsular tissue on the lateral aspect of the MTP joint (Fig. 6-94).

3. The hallux is placed in correct alignment during repair of the medial joint capsule. This position consists of neither varus nor valgus. The base of the phalanx is aligned with the long axis of the first metatarsal. Any pronation is corrected by slightly supinating the hallux as the sutures are placed. The derotation of the phalanx ensures that the sesamoids, which are connected to the base of the proximal phalanx, are realigned beneath the first metatarsal head. The edge of the tibial sesamoid should be clearly visible in the base of the medial wound with the toe in a corrected position. (If such is

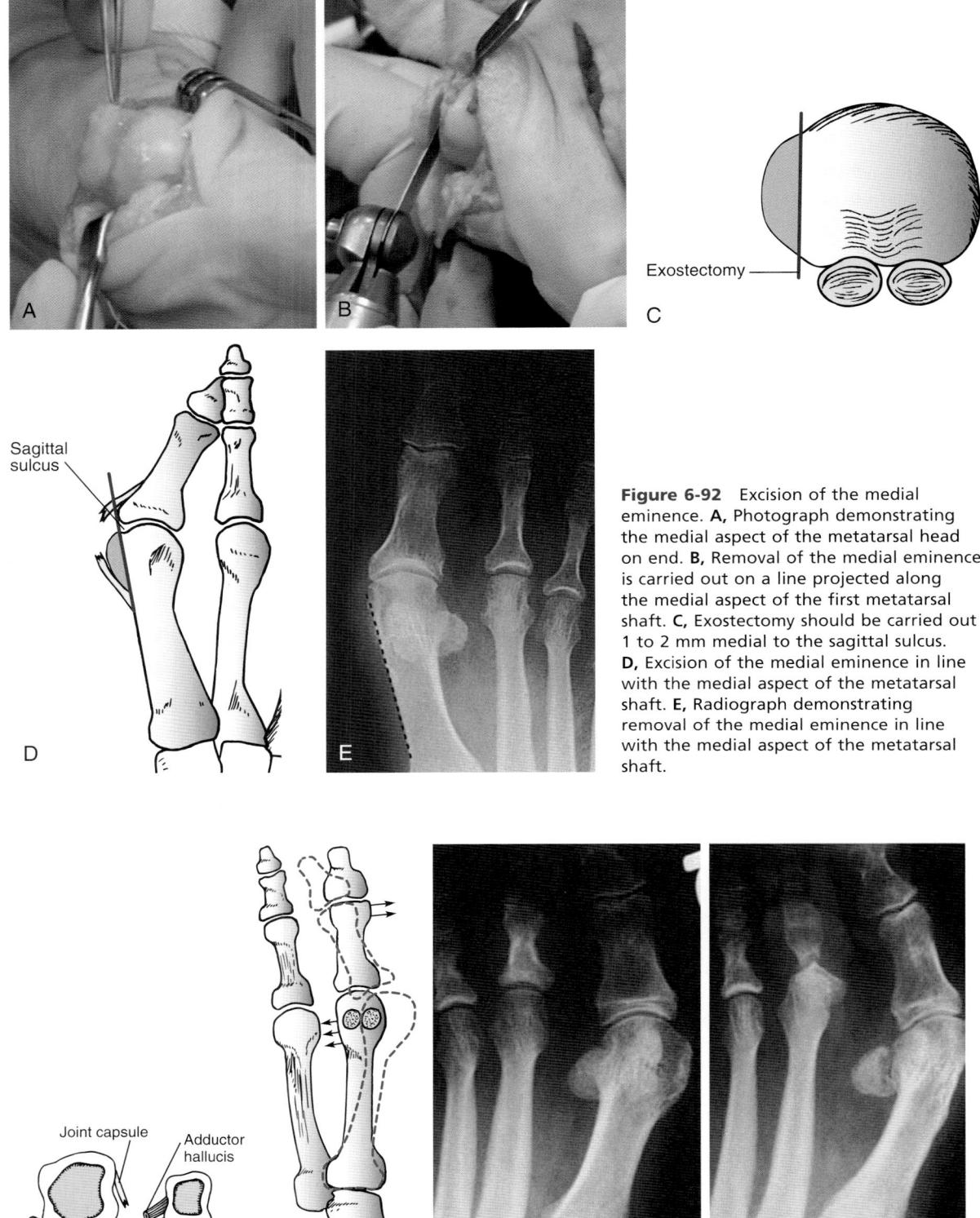

Figure 6-92 Excision of the medial eminence. **A,** Photograph demonstrating the medial aspect of the metatarsal head on end. **B,** Removal of the medial eminence is carried out on a line projected along the medial aspect of the first metatarsal shaft. **C,** Exostectomy should be carried out 1 to 2 mm medial to the sagittal sulcus. **D,** Excision of the medial eminence in line with the medial aspect of the metatarsal shaft. **E,** Radiograph demonstrating removal of the medial eminence in line with the medial aspect of the metatarsal shaft.

Figure 6-93 **A,** To determine whether an osteotomy is necessary after soft tissue releases have been carried out, the first metatarsal head is pushed laterally. If the metatarsal head tends to spring back medially, an osteotomy should be considered. The authors perform an osteotomy about 95% of the time. Preoperative **(B)** and postoperative **(C)** radiographs demonstrate a recurrent hallux valgus deformity caused by lack of correction of the intermetatarsal angle.

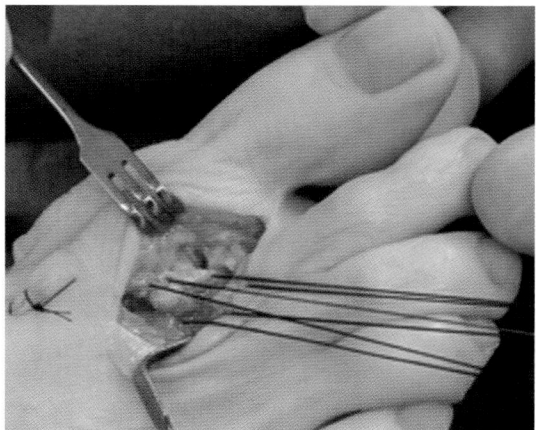

Figure 6-94 Two or three sutures are used to reef the capsule of the first and second metatarsophalangeal joints, with incorporation of the adductor tendon within the sutures.

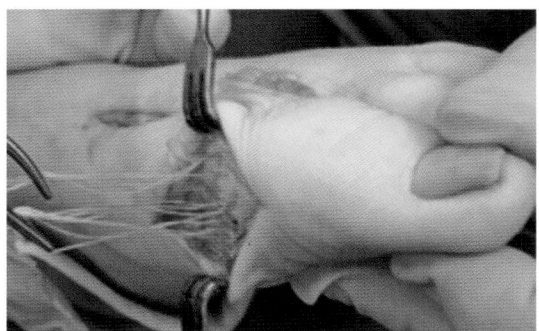

Figure 6-95 Plication of the medial joint capsule is carried out while the great toe is held in line with the first metatarsal, 2 to 3 degrees of varus, and rotated to place the sesamoids beneath the metatarsal head. The medial capsular flap then is approximated, and if redundant capsule still exists, more capsular tissue can be removed.

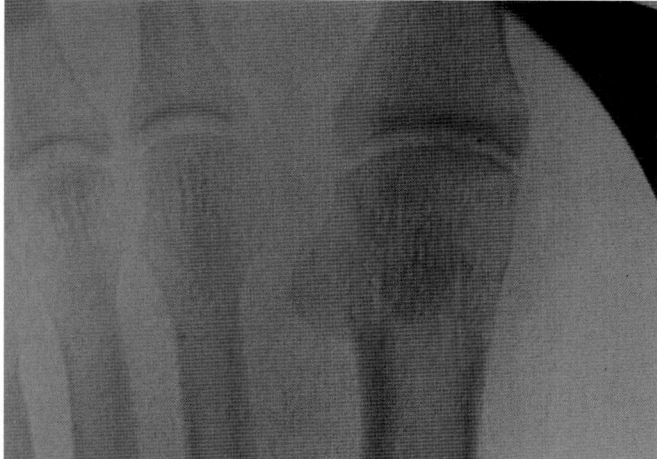

Figure 6-96 Intaoperative fluoroscopic image of the foot with simulated weight bearing. Proper joint alignment is confirmed, and the image can be repeated after the dressing has been applied to avoid overcorrection.

not the case, release of any remaining lateral joint contracture is necessary so that the sesamoid sling can be rotated beneath the metatarsal head (Fig. 6-95).

4. The medial capsule is repaired with four or five interrupted sutures. The most important part of the capsular repair is the plantar half, which includes the abductor hallucis tendon and the thickest portion of the joint capsule. Repair of the abductor hallucis tendon is very important.[391] Before placing the sutures, the two edges of the capsule are brought into apposition to ensure that sufficient capsular tissue has been removed. If there appears to be redundant capsule remaining, it is excised to allow the two capsular edges to be opposed with the capsular closure. On completion of the medial capsular repair, the hallux should be satisfactorily aligned. A slight degree of residual varus can usually be corrected with the postoperative dressings. If, however, the amount of correction is inadequate, that is, if there is residual valgus, the capsular sutures should be removed, more medial capsule

resected, and the structures reapproximated. Obtaining an intraoperative fluoroscopic image is helpful in ensuring that proper alignment is achieved (Fig. 6-96).
5. The sutures in the first web space are tied.
6. The skin is approximated with fine interrupted suture, and a sterile compression dressing is applied for 12 to 24 hours.

Intermetatarsal (Interosseous) Fixation

1. Cerclage sutures, screws, and suture-button devices have been advocated to assist with intermetatarsal correction.
2. The approach used for intermetatarsal fixation, and stabilization is dependent upon the device selected. Sutures cerclaging the first and second metatarsals in the distal third have been described, although others have advocated more proximal fixation with 3- to 4-mm screws.[352,560] There have also been numerous reports describing suture-button placement at multiple levels on the metatarsals.[261,265,422,548]
3. Basic to the techniques described is the use of fluoroscopic imaging to assist with the manual reduction of the IM 1–2 angle and placement of the fixation device.
4. Once the intermetatarsal fixation is secured, a medial capsulorrhapy of the hallux metatarsophalangeal joint is completed (Fig. 6-97).

Postoperative Care

Each surgeon will adopt a postoperative program for timing of patient visits, dressing techniques and radiographic follow-up that best suits their practice and the patient's needs. The compression dressing is removed in the office within the first 1 to 2 weeks after the procedure, and a new dressing consisting of 2-inch Kling gauze and ½-inch adhesive tape is applied to hold the toe in anatomic alignment. The postoperative dressings are

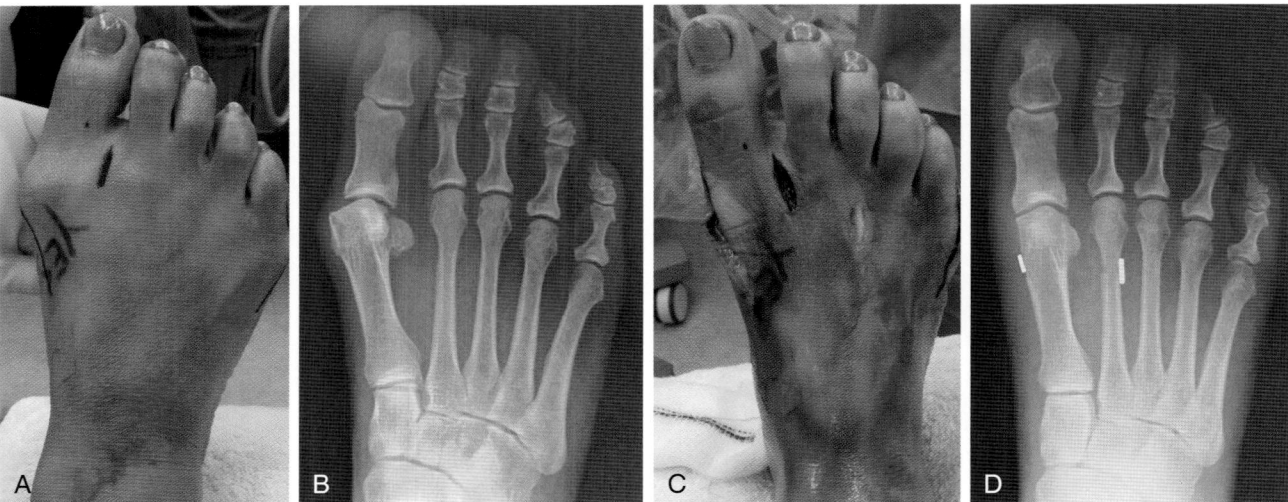

Figure 6-97 Preoperative appearance **(A)** of a bunion deformity in an adult woman with accompanying anteroposterior (AP) **(B)** standing radiograph. Deformity was managed with resection of the medial eminence, formal first web-space release, and placement of an interosseous fixation device between the first and second metatarsals, via a 1.1-mm drill hole. Postoperative appearance **(C)** and standing AP radiograph at 13 weeks postoperatively **(D)**.

critical in obtaining satisfactory alignment after a hallux valgus repair. During the first 3 to 4 weeks after surgery, the dressings can influence the position of the toe. The purpose of the dressing is to bind the metatarsal heads tightly together, after which a spica-like dressing is placed around the hallux, either holding it in a neutral position or adjusting it into slight varus or valgus, depending on the desired correction. To ensure that the sesamoids remain reduced beneath the metatarsal head, the gauze around the hallux of the right foot (when dressing the foot from the bottom of the bed) is wrapped in a counterclockwise direction and that of the left foot in a clockwise direction (Fig. 6-98). This ensures that the correct rotational torque is placed on the hallux to maintain acceptable alignment of the sesamoids. After surgery, the patient is permitted to ambulate as tolerated in a stiff-soled postoperative shoe. Initially, the patient ambulates on the heel and lateral aspect of the foot. It usually takes 2 to 4 weeks before the typical patient applies any significant pressure along the medial aspect of the foot.

The postoperative dressings are changed weekly for the first 4 weeks, and if the position of the hallux is satisfactory, they are changed every 10 to 14 days for the second 4 weeks. The authors do not believe that cast immobilization is necessary after this procedure. With the foot covered by a cast, the first MTP joint cannot be adequately observed, and thus fine adjustments to the alignment cannot be performed.

At the first postoperative visit, an AP radiograph is obtained, with as much weight bearing as possible. This identifies the alignment of the first MTP joint, and the toe is dressed into neutral, varus, or valgus alignment with the subsequent dressings. During the postoperative period, even with dressings in place, the patient is encouraged to perform active and passive range-of-motion

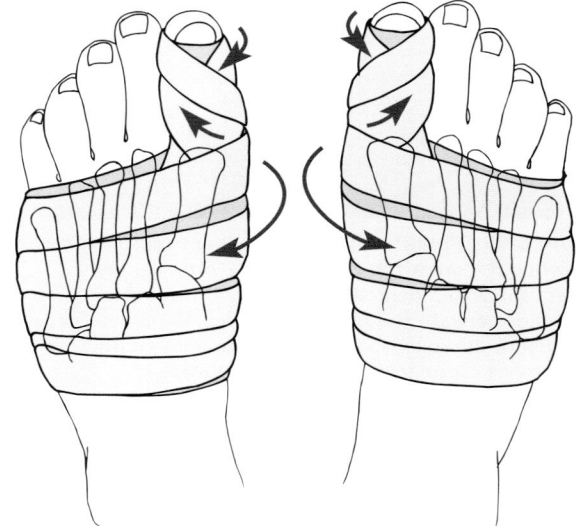

Figure 6-98 Postoperative dressings after correction of hallux valgus. Note that the metatarsal heads are firmly bound together with Kling bandage and that the great toe is rotated to keep the sesamoids realigned beneath the metatarsal head. This necessitates dressing the right toe in a counterclockwise direction and the left toe in a clockwise direction when one is standing at the foot of the bed.

exercises to reestablish dorsiflexion and plantar flexion (Fig. 6-99).

After 6 to 8 weeks of immobilization, the dressing is discontinued and a foam toe separator may be instituted for day hours (Fig. 6-100). As the swelling and thickening about the first MTP joint subsides, the patient can progress from a sandal or broad-toed shoe eventually to fashionable footwear. The patient is encouraged to wear wide, soft shoes rather than narrow, high-heeled

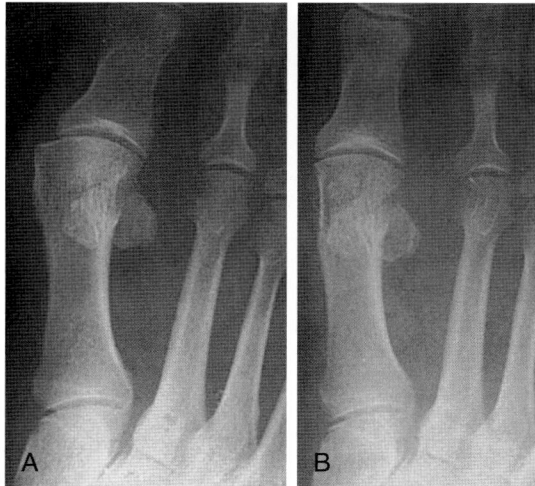

Figure 6-99 Results after correction of hallux valgus deformity with a distal soft tissue procedure.

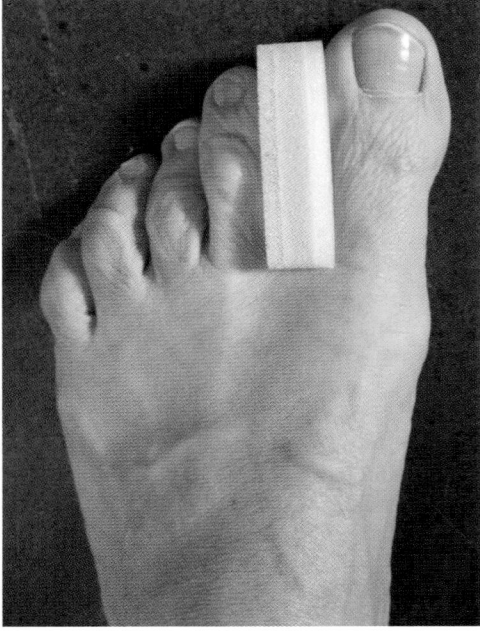

Figure 6-100 An inexpensive foam toe separator may be used after dressings are removed in an effort to protect the hallux from extrinsic pressures.

shoes. The time required for the swelling to adequately subside varies greatly from patient to patient and may exceed 3 months. If the toe is noted to drift into a slight valgus position after removal of the dressings, a night bunion splint may be indicated (see Fig. 6-77B).

Results

Although Silver[486] advocated resection of the medial eminence and release of the lateral soft tissues, he did not report his results with this procedure. In a review of simple bunionectomies with or without lateral capsulotomy in 33 adult patients, Kitaoka et al[277] reported a

Table 6-1	Summary of 72 Feet before and after a Distal Soft Tissue Procedure	
Angle	**Preoperative**	**Postoperative**
Average hallux valgus	32.4°	15.9°
Average first/second intermetatarsal	14.3°	8.8°

From reference 343.

5-degree increase in the hallux valgus angle postoperatively and a 2-degree increase in the 1–2 IM angle at long-term follow-up. A failure rate of 24% was reported. Bonney and Macnab[38] reported generally poor results after simple exostectomy, with 37% of patients requiring additional treatment. Meyer et al[367] and others[245,336,343] have reported a high rate of success in the treatment of mild and moderate hallux valgus deformities in adults with a distal soft tissue realignment. Mann and Coughlin[336] reported an average 15-degree correction of the hallux valgus angle and an average 5.2-degree correction of the 1–2 IM angle. However, with a severe hallux valgus deformity, distal soft tissue realignment alone achieves only a 50% correction of the deformity. Thus the indications for distal soft tissue reconstruction alone are limited to a mild deformity (hallux valgus angle < 30 degrees and IM angle < 11 degrees). To the current authors' knowledge, there have been no prospective studies evaluating the effectiveness of intermetarsal (interosseous) fixation.

A high failure rate of the McBride procedure in juvenile patients that varies from 43% to 75% has been reported in the literature.[38,95,216,217,472] This technique in juveniles confirms the wider experience in the literature that this procedure has limited ability to correct a hallux valgus deformity with an increased DMAA. For a subluxated MTP joint with a moderate or severe hallux valgus deformity (hallux valgus angle requiring > 20 degrees correction or an IM angle > 15 degrees), a proximal metatarsal osteotomy has been recommended in conjunction with a distal soft tissue realignment.*

In a subsequent review of 72 feet in 47 patients undergoing distal soft tissue realignment, Mann and Pfeffinger[343] reported postoperative satisfaction in 92% of patients. The main reason for satisfaction was pain relief, decreased deformity, and diminution in bunion size. Unrestricted footwear was possible in 20% of patients preoperatively and 53% postoperatively. This still left 47% of patients unable to wear the shoes of their choice. The overall level of activity increased in 66% of patients and was unchanged in 34%.

Table 6-1 presents the preoperative and postoperative hallux valgus and IM angles for the entire group, and Table 6-2 lists the results by severity of the deformity. These results once again confirm that a satisfactory outcome can be obtained in the treatment of mild and

---

*References 69, 82, 101, 122, 136, 140, 142, 153, 167, 168, 186, 233, 303, 306, 344, 387, 392, 409, 416, 443, 457, 481, 508, 516, and 535.

Table 6-2 Summary of Results of Distal Soft Tissue Procedures by Severity of Deformity

Varus	Mild (<20°)	Moderate (21°–40°)	Severe (>40°)	Patients with Postoperative Hallux
Number of feet	4	57	11	6
Mean age (yr)	51	55	57	56
Mean Hallux Valgus Angle				
Preoperative	18°	31°	46°	37°
Postoperative	11°	15°	19°	−7.5°
Mean First/Second Intermetatarsal Angle				
Preoperative	10.7°	14°	17°	17°
Postoperative	8.5°	8.6°	10°	5°

From Reference 343.

Table 6-3 Postoperative Correction before and after Distal Soft Tissue Procedures

	Preoperative Intermetatarsal Angle	
Hallux Valgus Angle	≤15°	>15°
Preoperative	28	38
Postoperative	11	18
Correction	17	20

From Reference 343.

moderate hallux valgus deformities. However, with a severe deformity, a distal soft tissue procedure alone will not usually result in a satisfactory outcome. Table 6-3 compares the results in patients with an IM angle of less than 15 degrees and greater than 15 degrees and demonstrates that with severe deformity, a distal soft tissue procedure alone is routinely incapable of achieving satisfactory realignment. In the entire series, only 41% of feet had a residual hallux valgus angle of less than 16 degrees. This figure emphasizes that the reliability of this procedure, particularly for a more advanced deformity, is not good, and the procedure is indicated mainly for mild and low-end moderate deformities.

Complications

Recurrence of Deformity. Recurrence may be related to one or more of the following factors:

■ Inadequate postoperative dressings
■ Insufficient plication of the medial joint capsule
■ Inadequate release of the lateral joint contracture, which may include the capsule, adductor hallucis tendon, or transverse metatarsal ligament
■ Insufficient medial capsular tissues secondary to degenerative changes or cyst formation
■ Failure to recognize and treat metatarsus primus varus
■ Failure to recognize a congruent joint

Arthrofibrosis. Slight loss of motion occurred after surgery.[343] Range-of-motion measurements demonstrated 67 degrees of dorsiflexion and 8 degrees of plantar flexion, compared with 75 and 16 degrees, respectively, in the uninvolved foot. Arthrofibrosis may be caused by the following:

■ Postoperative infection
■ Unrecognized arthrosis of the MTP joint
■ Unrecognized causes
■ Realignment of a congruent joint

Peripheral Nerve Entrapment. On occasion, the dorsal or plantar cutaneous nerve to the great toe becomes injured or entrapped, which can cause pain if a large neuroma develops. Use of the incisions as described in this section reduces this complication to a minimum.

Hallux Varus. The major complication encountered in the series of Mann et al[344] was an 8% incidence of hallux varus deformity, which averaged 7.5 degrees (Fig. 6-101). The position of the proximal phalanx influenced the IM angle; the IM angle was corrected 12 degrees in feet with hallux varus versus 5 degrees in those without overcorrection. In all cases of hallux varus, the tibial sesamoid subluxated medially; however, in only half the feet with medial sesamoid subluxation did a hallux varus deformity develop. Preoperatively, the feet in which a hallux varus deformity developed were characterized by more severe deformities. Mann and Coughlin[339] recommended that release of the lateral MTP joint capsule be performed without a lateral sesamoidectomy. After this modification, a reduced rate of hallux varus was reported.[335,337] Use of the stump of conjoined adductor tendon and cuff of the lateral MTP capsule to reinforce the lateral capsule at the time of surgical correction may also help minimize the incidence of postoperative hallux varus.[93]

See page 300 at the end of this chapter for a discussion of hallux varus.

Intermetatarsal (Interosseous) Fixation. There have been several reports of second metatarsal stress fractures with the use of cerclage suture techniques and with suture-button fixation devices.[261,265,323,422] This has lead to modifications of the technique, not only downsizing the device but also placing it in a more proximal location in the second metatarsal. The technique is avoided in those patients with osteopenia.

AKIN PROCEDURE

An Akin procedure[2] achieves correction of a hallux valgus deformity by means of a medial capsulorrhaphy, resection of the medial eminence, and medial closing-wedge

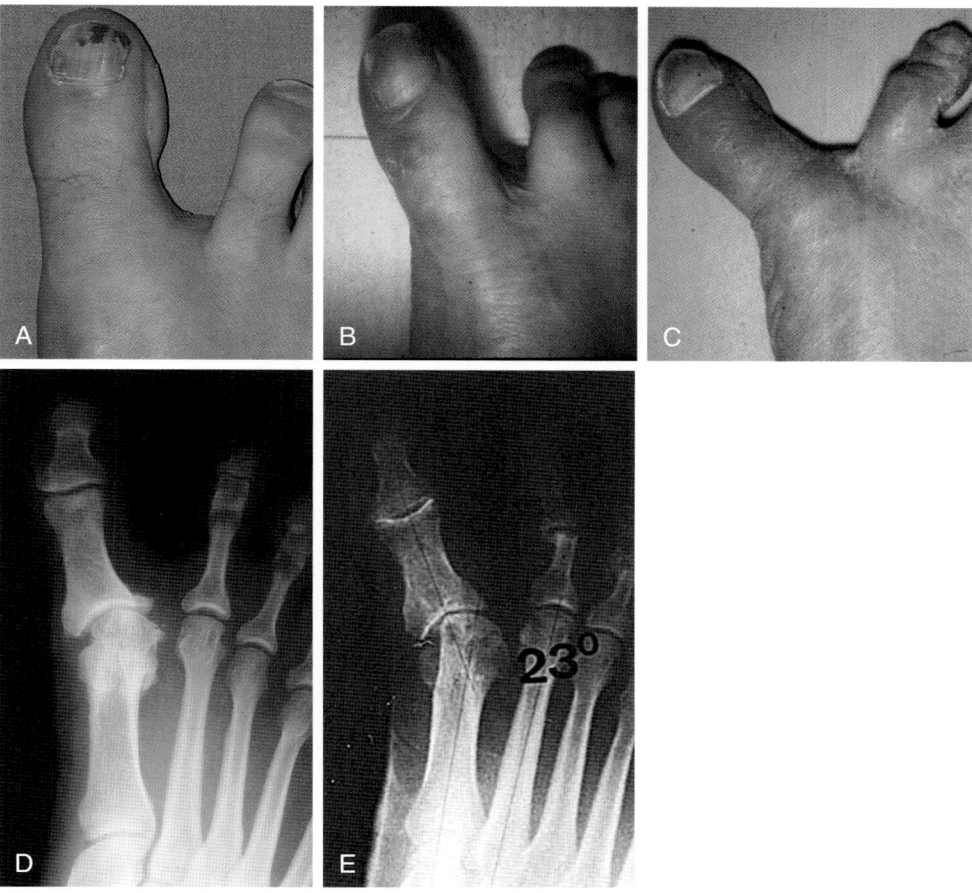

Figure 6-101 Hallux varus deformity after a distal soft tissue procedure with excision of the fibular sesamoid. **A,** Mild. **B,** Moderate. **C,** Severe deformity with medial deviation of the lesser toes. **D** and **E,** Postoperative radiographs demonstrating moderately severe hallux varus deformity with subluxation of the medial sesamoid.

phalangeal osteotomy (Video Clips 52 and 53).[11,404,476,520,538] This procedure can produce a satisfactory result in the treatment of specific types of deformities but is not indicated in the presence of MTP joint subluxation.

Indications

The primary indication for this procedure is a hallux valgus interphalangeus (HVI) deformity (Fig. 6-102).[420] In the presence of a congruous MTP joint with a significant hallux valgus deformity and an increased IM angle, extraarticular repair can be achieved by a combination of proximal phalangeal osteotomy and first metatarsal osteotomy (Fig. 6-103).[80,371,404,520] The use of an extraarticular repair may prevent disturbance of a congruent MTP articulation.[97,186] It is also useful to achieve derotation of a pronated hallux,[404,447,468] and shortening in patients with a long proximal phalanx.[224,447]

After an initial surgical procedure complicated by recurrent deformity, if any residual lateral deviation of the hallux results in pressure against the second toe, a phalangeal osteotomy can angulate the hallux medially away from the adjacent second toe. The procedure can also be used in conjunction with almost any bunion

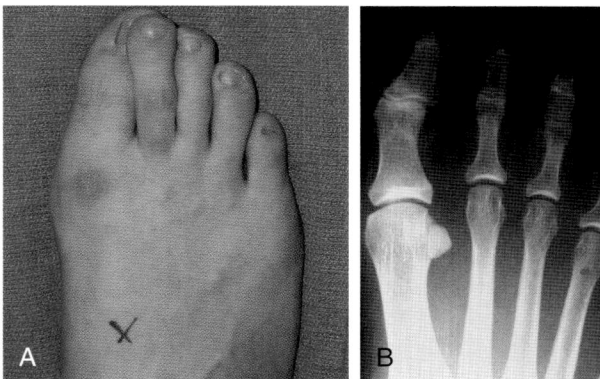

Figure 6-102 Hallux valgus interphalangeus: clinical **(A)** and radiographic **(B)** appearance.

correction in which some valgus of the hallux is still present.[80,101,371,404,520] A phalangeal osteotomy can be combined with a more proximal first-ray osteotomy (Fig. 6-104).[101,404,520] On occasion, a phalangeal osteotomy can be used without a medial eminence resection and medial capsular reefing if only an osteotomy is indicated to realign the great toe.

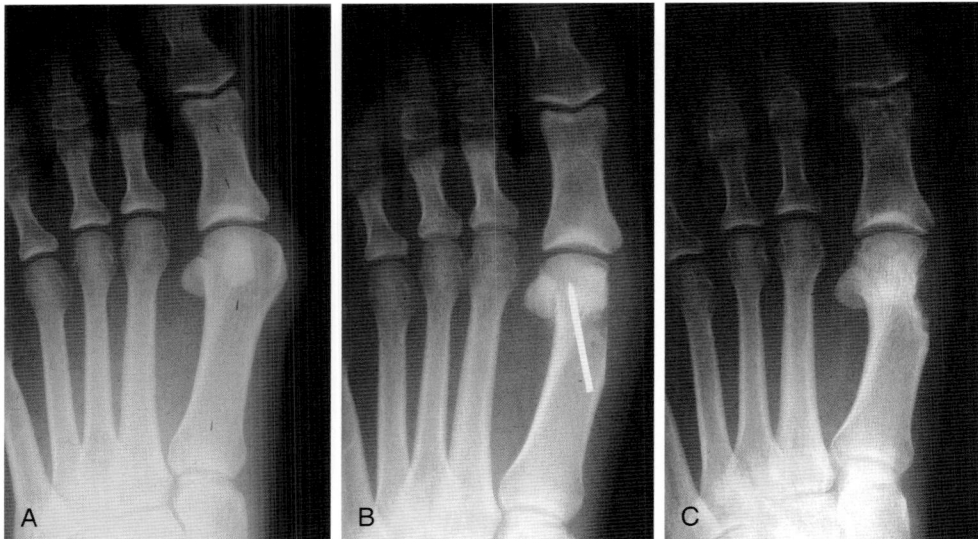

Figure 6-103 Moderate hallux valgus deformity. **A,** Preoperative radiographic appearance. **B,** Radiograph after a chevron osteotomy with correction of the hallux valgus angle. **C,** Twelve-year follow-up after the procedure.

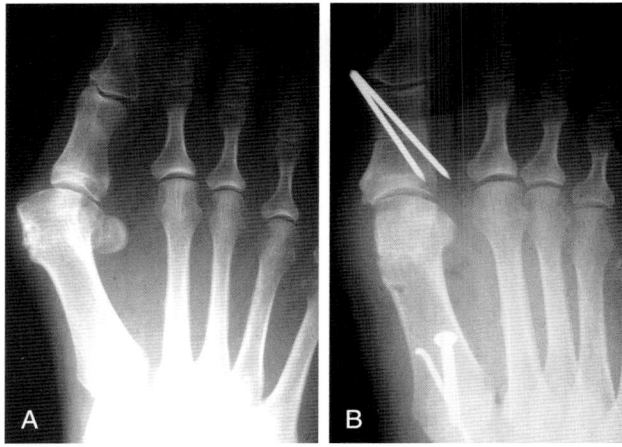

Figure 6-104 A, Preoperative radiograph. **B,** After a Mann-Akin procedure.

Contraindications

The Akin procedure is contraindicated as a primary procedure to correct a hallux valgus deformity if there is any subluxation of the MTP joint. An Akin procedure does not decrease the 1–2 IM angle; therefore, with a significant metatarsus primus varus deformity, an Akin procedure alone is insufficient to correct the deformity. This procedure can actually lead to destabilization of the MTP joint if used as a primary procedure to correct a hallux valgus deformity characterized by a subluxated MTP joint.[420]

Technique

The surgical technique for the Akin procedure is divided into exposure, performance of the osteotomy, and reconstruction of the joint capsule and osteotomy.

Surgical Exposure

1. A medial longitudinal skin incision is centered over the medial eminence, just proximal to the IP joint and extended 1 cm proximal to the medial eminence. Dorsal and plantar full-thickness skin flaps are created, with care taken to protect the dorsomedial and plantar medial cutaneous nerves.
2. An L-shaped, distally based capsular flap is created. With this L-shaped flap, the dorsal and proximal MTP joint capsular attachments are released while the distal and plantar capsular attachments remain intact. The capsule is carefully dissected off the medial eminence (see Fig. 6-91D).
3. Through this same exposure, subperiosteal dissection is used to expose the phalangeal metaphyseal region, with care taken to protect the distally based capsular flap. The soft tissue is not stripped past the dorsomedial and plantar medial surfaces of the proximal phalanx.

    Alternative to Step 2: A vertical capsulotomy is made with a No. 11 blade, starting 2 to 3 mm proximal to the base of the proximal phalanx. A second cut is made parallel to the first, with no more than 2 to 4 mm of capsular tissue removed. The amount of capsular excision depends on the size of the medial eminence (see Fig. 6-91B).

Technique of Resection of the Medial Eminence and Phalangeal Osteotomy

1. With an oscillating saw, the medial eminence is resected in line with the first metatarsal medial cortex. The osteotomy is begun slightly medial to the sagittal sulcus and extended proximally along the medial border of the first metatarsal. The remaining edges,

particularly on the dorsomedial aspect of the metatarsal head, are smoothed with a rongeur.

2. A small, medially based wedge of bone is resected in the metaphyseal, diaphyseal-metaphyseal, or diaphyseal region. The location of the osteotomy depends on the site of maximal deformity, which in the proximal phalanx may be central, proximal, or distal (Figs. 6-105A and B and 6-106).[447] (A mini–image intensifier can be used to check the location of the phalangeal osteotomy site in reference to the location of the MTP joint, IP joint, and, in a juvenile patient, open epiphysis.)

3. The lateral cortex of the phalanx is left intact (minimally), and the osteotomy site is closed. Routinely, a 2- to 3-mm–wide resection is performed with the apex at the lateral base; however, depending on the magnitude of the deformity, the closing-wedge osteotomy may be smaller or larger (see Fig. 6-105C and D). In addition, the surgeon must keep in mind that the phalangeal surface of the MTP joint is concave. When performing the initial osteotomy, there is a risk of penetrating the joint with the saw blade. A second cut is made slightly distal to the first, and usually 3 to 4 mm of bone is removed at the medial aspect of the

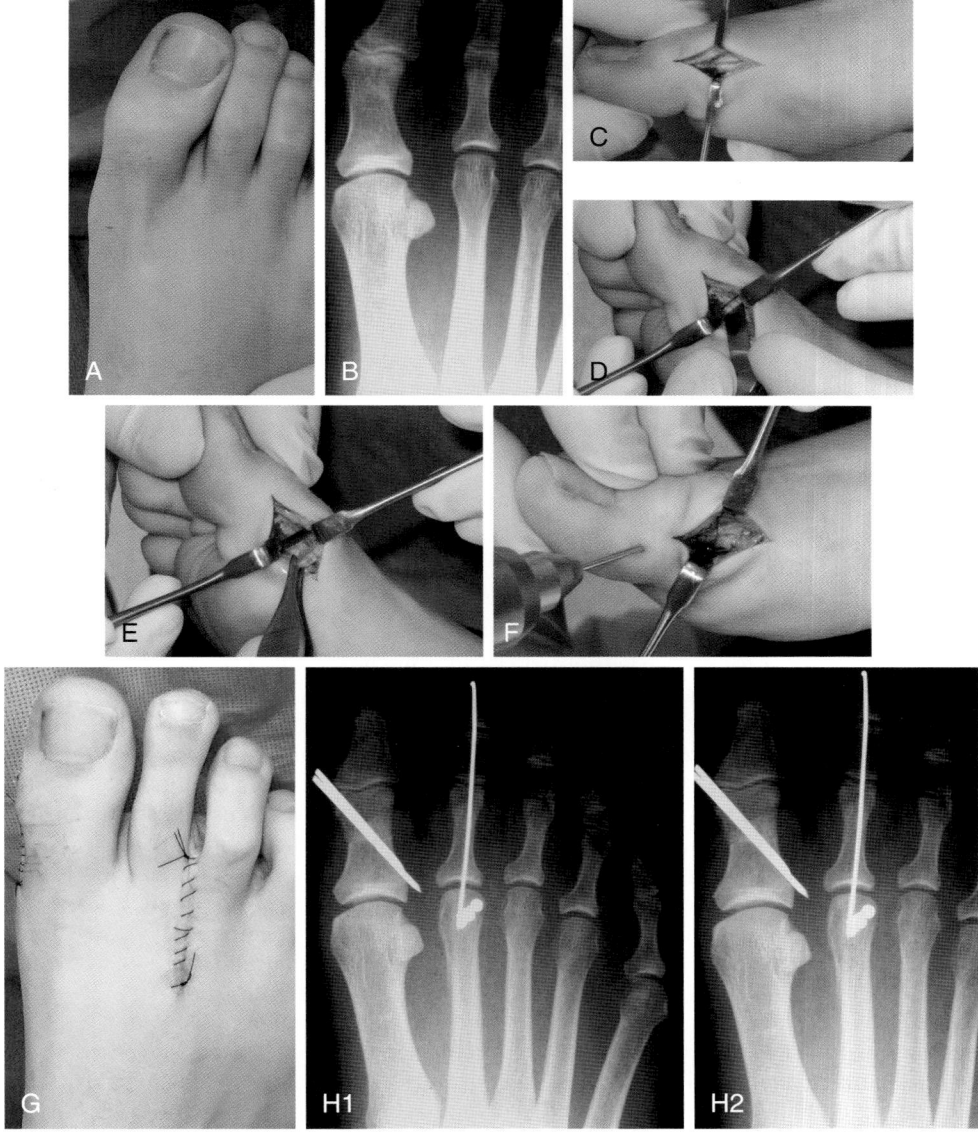

Figure 6-105 Technique of Akin phalangeal osteotomy. Preoperative clinical **(A)** and radiographic **(B)** appearance. **C,** Operative incision for just phalangeal osteotomy. **D,** Two parallel cuts are made for the medially based closing-wedge osteotomy. **E,** The wedge is removed. **F,** The osteotomy is closed and fixed with two Kirschner wires. Postoperative clinical **(G)** and radiographic **(H1 and H2)** appearance after osteotomy. (An interdigital neuroma and Weil osteotomy was performed as well.)

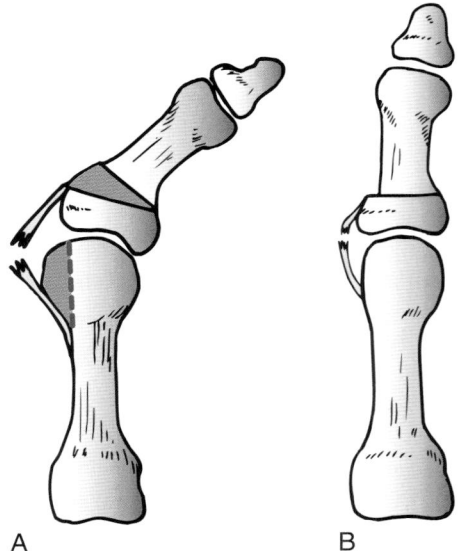

Figure 6-106 **A,** Proposed phalangeal osteotomy. **B,** After the osteotomy.

osteotomy site. One should attempt to maintain a periosteal hinge laterally. If pronation of the hallux is present, the hallux can be derotated at the osteotomy site before placement of fixation to correct any remaining deformity (see Fig. 6-105E).

Reconstruction of the Joint Capsule and Osteotomy

1. The medial joint capsule is repaired because, after this step, one can predict how much correction must be gained from the phalangeal osteotomy. The MTP capsule is repaired with interrupted absorbable suture. If insufficient capsule is present on the dorsal proximal aspect of the MTP joint, a small hole can be drilled in the metaphysis to anchor the capsular flap.

2. After capsular repair, the osteotomy site is approximated medially to assess alignment of the hallux. If the alignment is inadequate, more bone can be resected. The osteotomy site is stabilized with one or two 0.062-inch Kirschner wires (K-wires) (see Fig. 6-105F-H). The pin or pins are placed obliquely from a distal medial location. Care is taken to avoid penetration of the IP and MTP joints. Intraoperative fluoroscopy or intraoperative radiography can be used to visualize the final position of the K-wire. The pins are cut flush with the level of the skin to aid in later removal.

3. An alternative method of fixation of the osteotomy site can be achieved by using a staple, heavy suture, or wire placed through two pairs of medial drill holes, one on the dorsomedial aspect and one on the plantar medial aspect of the osteotomy site. This suture is passed through the drill holes and tied to stabilize the osteotomy (Fig. 6-107A). A compression staple[520] can also be used (Fig. 6-107B); multiple K-wires (Fig. 6-107C),

compression pin (Fig. 6-107D), or screws (Fig. 6-107E) may be used to stabilize the osteotomy site.

4. The skin is approximated with interrupted sutures and a compression dressing applied.

Postoperative Care

A gauze-and-tape toe spica compression dressing is applied after surgery (Fig. 6-108). The patient is permitted to ambulate in a postoperative shoe with weight borne on the outer aspect of the foot. The dressing is changed 1 to 2 days after surgery and then on a weekly basis. The toe is held in a neutral or slight varus position during this healing phase to allow the capsular tissues and osteotomy site to heal adequately. Rarely is casting necessary after a phalangeal osteotomy. The dressing is maintained until the osteotomy site has healed, which typically takes 6 to 8 weeks. If K-wires were used for internal fixation, they are removed 3 to 6 weeks after surgery. Motion of the IP and MTP joints is initiated at this time.

Results

The best indication for the use of an isolated Akin phalangeal osteotomy is hallux valgus interphalangeus (Fig. 6-109). There are no studies that report the results of isolated Akin osteotomies for interphalangeal deformities alone. When used to correct a mild residual deformity after a previous hallux valgus correction, a phalangeal osteotomy can produce a satisfactory result, provided that the MTP joint is congruent and the residual valgus is caused by lateral sloping of the distal phalangeal articular surface (Fig. 6-110). The use of internal fixation is helpful in maintaining the operative correction and should achieve rigid stabilization of the osteotomy; malunion and nonunion are uncommon (Fig. 6-111).[473] The Akin procedure achieves little correction of the 1–2 IM angle.[185,420] In reporting on a series of 22 adult patients, Plattner and Van Manen[420] initially observed an average 13-degree correction of the hallux valgus angle; however, at long-term follow-up, this correction diminished to only 6 degrees of correction. Seelenfreund et al[473] and Goldberg et al[185] reported high recurrence rates (16%-21%) and a high rate of postoperative dissatisfaction and concluded that isolated phalangeal osteotomy as treatment of a hallux valgus deformity does not have a sound biomechanical basis and is contraindicated as an isolated procedure (Figs. 6-112 and 6-113). Toth et al[520] reported on 22 consecutive Akin osteotomies and noted an average correction of 9 degrees at the osteotomy site. All were done in combination with a first metatarsal osteotomy. No delayed or nonunions were noted. The average shortening of the phalanx was 2 mm.

Shannak et al,[476] who suggested the Akin procedure can reliably achieve approximately 10 degrees of angular correction, recommended locating the osteotomy 5 mm distal to the apex of the proximal phalangeal MTP articular surface.

Although Akin[2] and Colloff and Weitz[80] advocated lateral MTP capsular release, the chapter authors believe

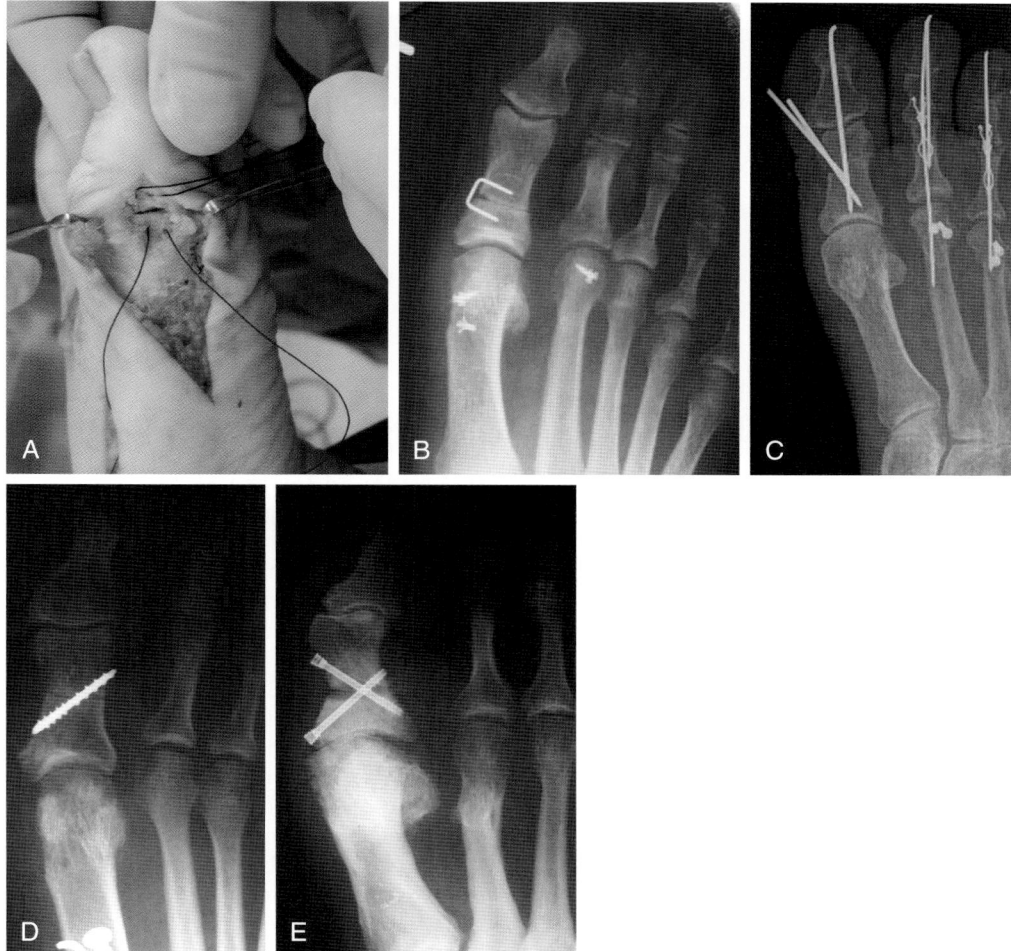

Figure 6-107 Alternative means of osteotomy fixation. **A,** Osteotomy site. Heavy suture material has been placed through drill holes on either side, after which the osteotomy site is closed and the sutures tied to secure the osteotomy in place. **B,** Small compression staple. **C,** Akin osteotomy fixed with multiple Kirschner wires. **D,** Fixation with compression pin. **E,** Fixation with cross-compression screws.

that, in general, a wide capsular release should be avoided because it has the potential for devascularizing the proximal phalangeal fragment or the epiphysis in a younger patient. Extensive soft tissue stripping of the proximal phalanx should be avoided because it may lead to vascular compromise of the proximal fragment. Intraarticular extension of the osteotomy with subsequent arthritis occurs infrequently.[447]

Complications

Overcorrection can develop because of an excessively large medial-wedge resection.[476,538] Shannak et al[476] advised a wedge resection of approximately 3 mm, although they cautioned that males (with typically increased width of the proximal phalanx) required a larger wedge than females. Vilas et al[538] reported performing a medial exostectomy of the IP joint after overcorrection with an Akin ostetomy.

The main complication of the Akin procedure is recurrence or progression of a deformity when the procedure was used to treat a deformity characterized by an incongruent or subluxated MTP joint (see Fig. 6-112). On occasion, when a phalangeal osteotomy is used to treat a hallux valgus deformity characterized by a congruent joint, the MTP joint may sublux postoperatively. Significant loss of IP joint plantar flexion of the great toe may occur, especially if the osteotomy is carried out distal to the midportion of the phalanx. If care is not taken, the tendon of the flexor or extensor hallucis longus could be inadvertently severed, particularly when the osteotomy is performed in the distal portion of the phalanx. AVN of the proximal phalanx may occur after excessive soft tissue stripping or excessive retraction of the soft tissues (Fig. 6-114). Other reported complications with this procedure include a poor cosmetic appearance and a high rate of subjective dissatisfaction postoperatively.[42,185,473]

DISTAL METATARSAL OSTEOTOMY (CHEVRON PROCEDURE)

The technique for a distal chevron osteotomy was initially described by Austin and Leventen[12,13] and Corless.[83] With a chevron osteotomy, resection of the medial eminence,

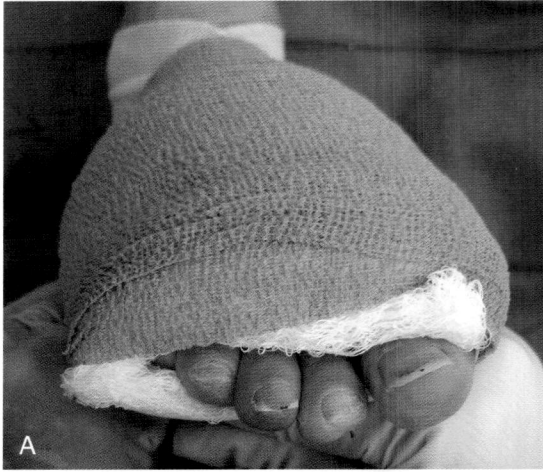

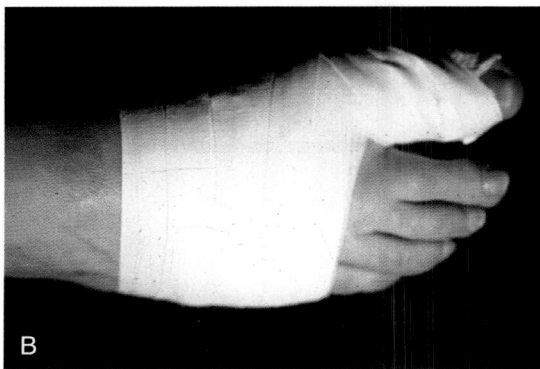

Figure 6-108 **A,** Immediate postoperative dressing. **B,** Dressing used for the remainder of treatment.

distal metatarsal osteotomy, and medial capsulorrhaphy are used to realign the hallux, thereby producing some narrowing of the forefoot (Video Clip 54). Since its initial description, several modifications in the technical part of the procedure have been made, including the angle of the osteotomy and the use of various alternative methods of internal fixation. An Akin procedure has been added by some[371] to augment the angular correction. There have been numerous modifications made in an attempt to use this technique for more moderate bunion deformities*

Indications

In general, a chevron osteotomy is indicated for mild and low-moderate hallux valgus deformities (hallux valgus angle < 30 degrees or 1–2 IM angle < 13 degrees) with subluxation of the first MTP joint.[92,222,365,415] When used in patients with a greater deformity, particularly the IM angle, the procedure's capability of achieving correction diminishes. The limits of the osteotomy rest in the width of the metatarsal neck available for displacement. A chevron osteotomy provides an extraarticular correction and can also be for the treatment of a hallux valgus deformity with a congruous first MTP joint if the DMAA is 15 degrees or less. For the occasional patient with a DMAA greater than 15 degrees or in the presence of a congruent or minimally subluxated hallux valgus deformity, the end result can be enhanced by removal of a small wedge of bone from the medial aspect of the chevron cut to enable the articular surface to be rotated more perpendicular to the long axis of the metatarsal (Fig. 6-115) (Video Clip 62).[71] Modifications have been described for this scenario as well, allowing reproducible biplanar correction to diminish an increased DMMA.[85,128,408,517,518] Likewise, moving the apex of the

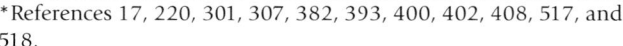

*References 17, 220, 301, 307, 382, 393, 400, 402, 408, 517, and 518.

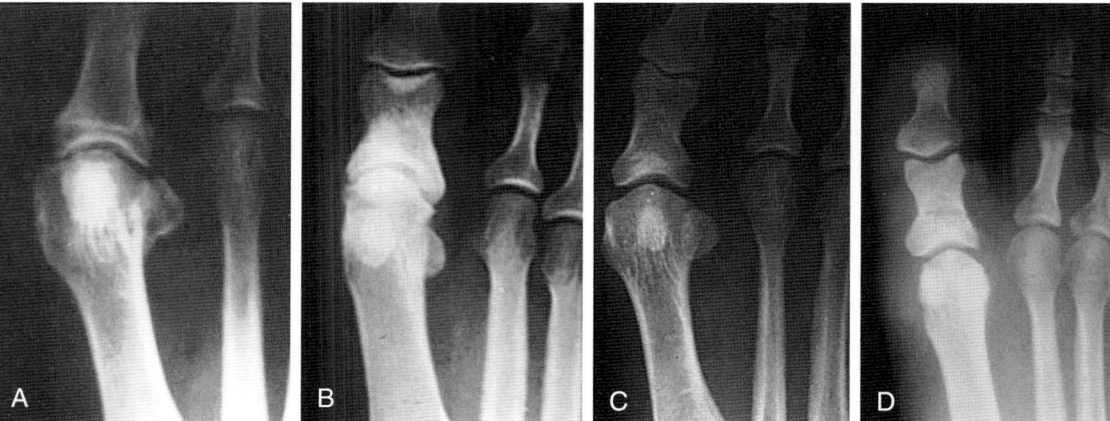

Figure 6-109 **A,** Preoperative radiograph demonstrating an irregularly shaped metatarsal head. This metatarsal head will not permit correction by medial displacement because an incongruent articular surface will result. **B,** Postoperative radiograph demonstrating satisfactory alignment after an Akin procedure, with removal of the medial eminence without affecting the articular surface. Preoperative **(C)** and postoperative **(D)** radiographs of hallux valgus demonstrate correction with the Akin procedure and excision of the medial eminence.

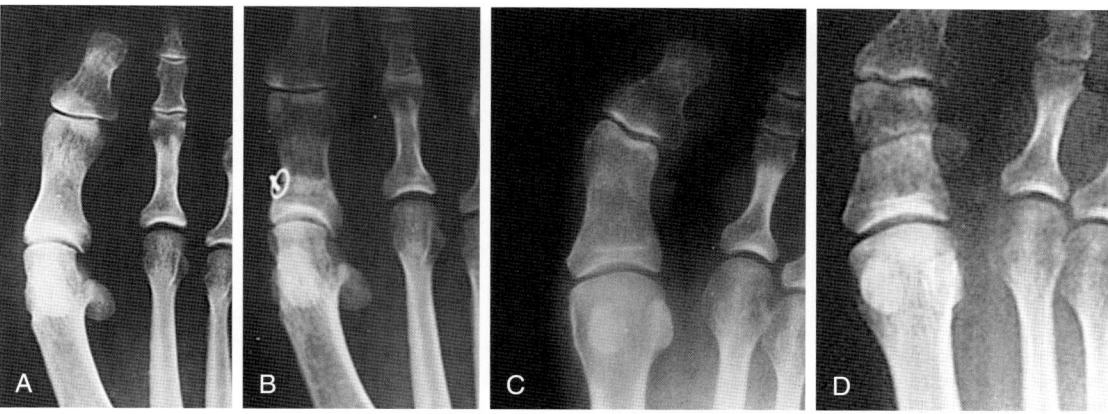

Figure 6-110 A, Preoperative radiograph of mild recurrence of hallux valgus deformity. **B,** Correction of recurrence with the Akin procedure. Preoperative **(C)** and postoperative **(D)** radiographs demonstrate correction of hallux valgus interphalangeus with the Akin procedure. Note that the osteotomy site is near the apex of the deformity, whereas in a routine Akin procedure, it is carried out in the proximal portion of the phalanx.

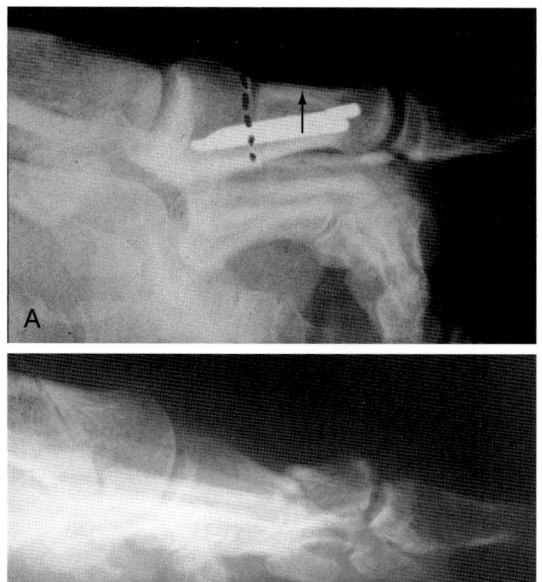

Figure 6-111 A, Rigid internal fixation holds the osteotomy. **B,** Dorsiflexion malunion resulting from early weight bearing.

osteotomy slightly proximal tends to increase the angular correction that can be achieved. A chevron osteotomy does not correct hallux pronation and only partially corrects sesamoid subluxation. The indications for a chevron osteotomy, when combined with a phalangeal osteotomy,[371] include a hallux valgus deformity with a congruous first MTP joint (DMAA < 20 degrees), as well as mild or moderate pronation of the hallux. Whereas Hattrup and Johnson[213] initially suggested that postoperative patient satisfaction seemed to decrease somewhat in patients older than 60 years, Trnka[523,524,525] reported high levels of satisfaction in even older age groups.

Contraindications

The main contraindication to a traditional chevron osteotomy is a moderate-to-severe deformity, with the hallux valgus angle exceeding 35 degrees, the IM angle exceeding 15 degrees, and a congruous first MTP joint with a DMAA greater than 15 degrees. Moderate or severe pronation of the hallux is difficult to correct with the chevron procedure. Advanced age is only a relative contraindication, but it may be associated with decreased MTP joint motion. In patients with moderate or advanced joint arthrosis, stiffness usually develops after a chevron procedure, and thus an alternative procedure should be considered.

Medial Approach and Exposure of the Metatarsal Head

1. A longitudinal incision is centered over the medial eminence beginning at the midportion of the proximal phalanx and extending 1 cm proximal to the medial eminence (Fig. 6-116A). The dissection is carried down to the joint capsule, and full-thickness dorsal and plantar skin flaps are created. As the dorsal flap is created, caution is exercised to avoid damage to the dorsomedial cutaneous nerve. As the plantar flap is created, the surgeon must avoid the plantar medial cutaneous nerve.
2. An L- or V-shaped, distally based capsular flap is developed as previously described for a distal soft tissue procedure (Fig. 6-116B and C), with detachment of the dorsal and proximal capsular attachments.[309]

    Alternative Technique: A vertical capsular incision is made approximately 2 to 3 mm proximal and parallel to the base of the proximal phalanx. A second capsular incision is made 2 to 4 mm more proximal but parallel to the first cut. The two capsular incisions are joined dorsally by an inverted-V cut (see Fig. 6-91B and C). The capsular flap is then grasped with forceps and dissected plantarward, and a second V cut is made through

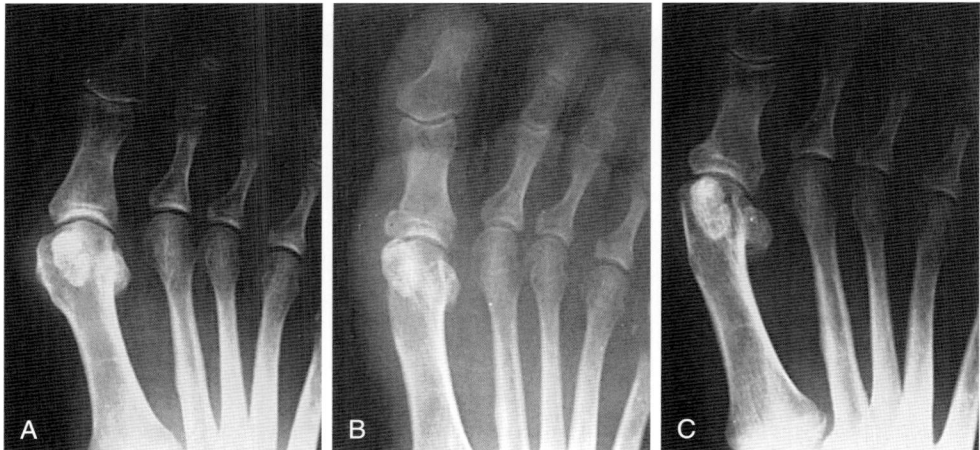

Figure 6-112 **A,** Preoperative radiograph demonstrating moderate hallux valgus deformity in a 25-year-old woman. **B,** After an Akin osteotomy and resection of the medial eminence, the 1–2 intermetatarsal angle has not been corrected. **C,** At final follow-up, the radiograph demonstrates recurrence of the deformity with subluxation of the metatarsophalangeal joint.

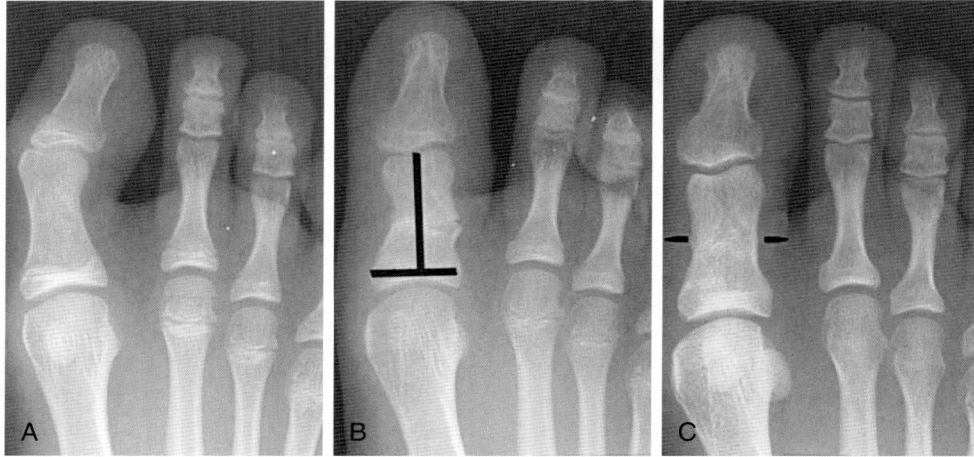

Figure 6-113 **A,** Preoperative radiograph demonstrating a hallux valgus interphalangeus deformity. **B,** Radiograph after an Akin phalangeal osteotomy. **C,** Seven years later, a radiograph demonstrates acceptable long-term alignment. (Note: medial capsulorrhaphy and medial eminence resection were not performed.)

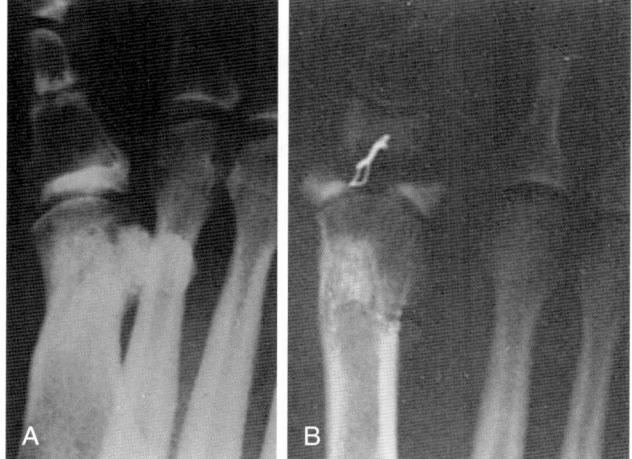

Figure 6-114 Complications after the Akin procedure. **A,** Delayed union or nonunion of the osteotomy site. **B,** Avascular necrosis.

the abductor hallucis tendon. With this inferior cut, the knife blade must remain inside the joint and come to rest against the tibial sesamoid at the apex of the plantar cut, to prevent damage to the plantar medial cutaneous nerve. (Rarely is more than 4 mm of capsule removed.) An incision is made along the dorsomedial aspect of the metatarsal head to create a capsular flap, which when retracted exposes the medial eminence. Soft tissue reflection should be limited to a degree necessary for exposure of the medial prominence and sulcus. Care should also be taken to avoid excessive soft tissue stripping with Hohmann retractors.

Technique of Osteotomy

1. The medial eminence is resected with an oscillating saw (or osteotome) in a line parallel with the medial border of the foot (Fig. 6-116D). The plane of the osteotomy through the medial eminence is not parallel to the metatarsal shaft but rather slightly oblique,

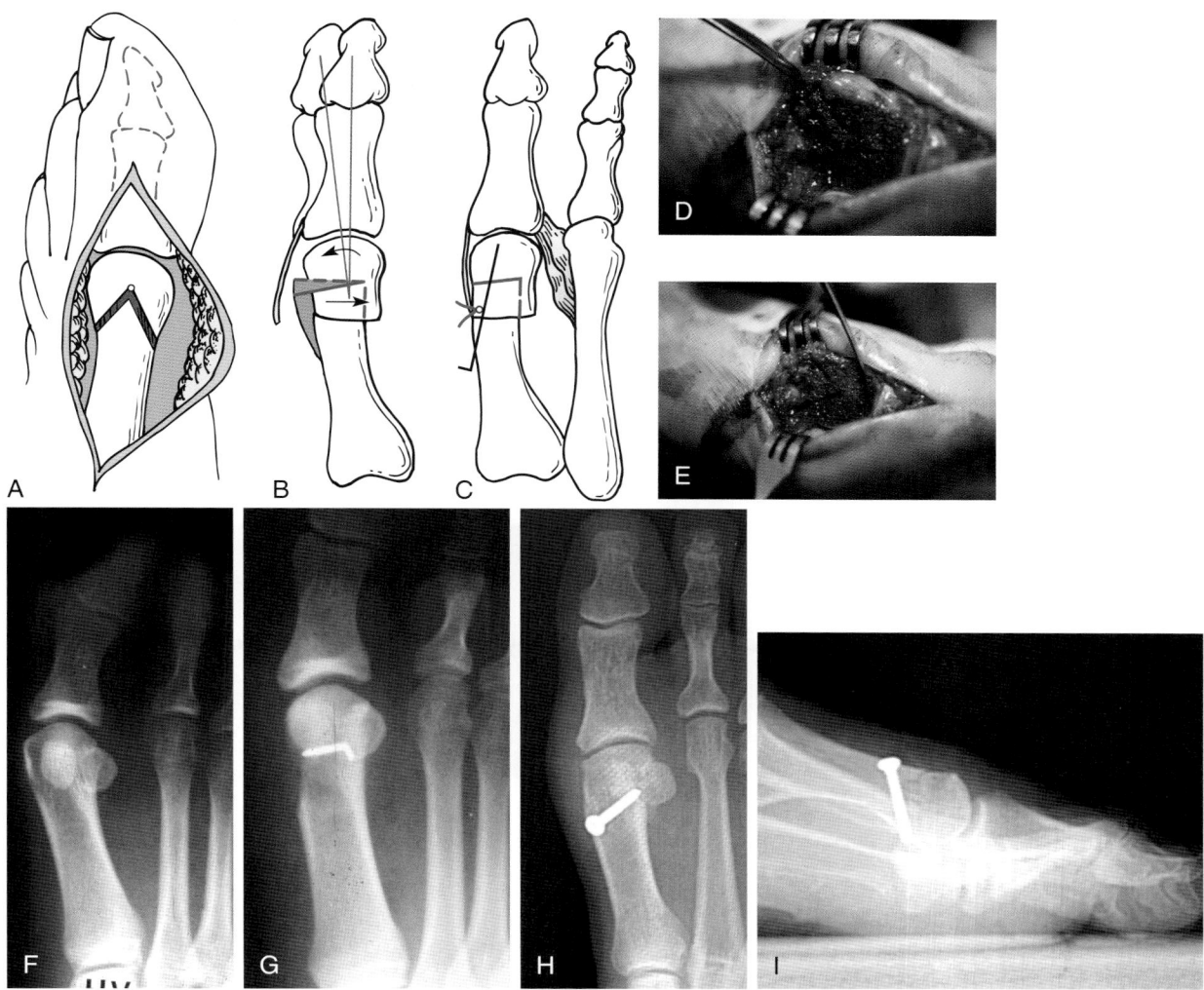

Figure 6-115 Biplanar chevron osteotomy. With an increased distal metatarsal articular angle, a biplanar chevron osteotomy is performed. A transverse chevron osteotomy is placed in a similar location. **A,** However, more bone is removed from the dorsomedial and plantar medial limb of the osteotomy to allow realignment (**B** and **C**) of a congruent metatarsophalangeal joint articulation with lateral translation of the capital fragment. **D,** Closing-wedge osteotomy. **E,** Closure of the osteotomy site. **F,** Preoperative radiograph. **G,** Postoperative radiograph after a biplanar chevron osteotomy. **H** and **I,** With screw fixation.

which creates a broad base of the capital fragment that adds stability to the osteotomy site as it is displaced laterally. The cut begins at the lateral edge of the sagittal sulcus and is carried proximally (Fig. 6-117A). Any osteophytes, including the medial ridge of the sagittal sulcus, are removed with a rongeur.

2. Although the authors do not routinely release the adductor tendon and lateral capsular structures, others have successfully performed a release in conjunction with a chevron osteotomy.[193,281,410,421,523] Some surgeons reach through the joint and release the lateral capsule,[307,505] whereas others choose an open exposure with a separate intermetatarsal dissection.* Excessive soft tissue stripping is avoided because it may endanger circulation to the metatarsal head. Most of the

*References 19, 63, 193, 410, 464, 523, and 524.

blood supply emanates from the dorsal and plantar aspects of the metatarsal head.[410] The authors believe, however, that if the deformity is so severe as to require a formal lateral release, rather than stretching the indications for a chevron osteotomy, another procedure might be preferable because the risk for vascular compromise would be eliminated.

3. The distal chevron osteotomy is carried out in the metaphyseal region because this area provides a large surface area for bone contact that is quite stable and aids in rapid healing (Fig. 6-117B). A 2-mm drill hole is useful to mark the apex of the osteotomy on the metatarsal head. The drill hole is placed at the center of an imaginary circle in which the radius is the distal articular surface (see Fig. 6-116E). The hole is made in a lateral direction, parallel to the bottom of the foot and articular surface. A horizontal osteotomy is

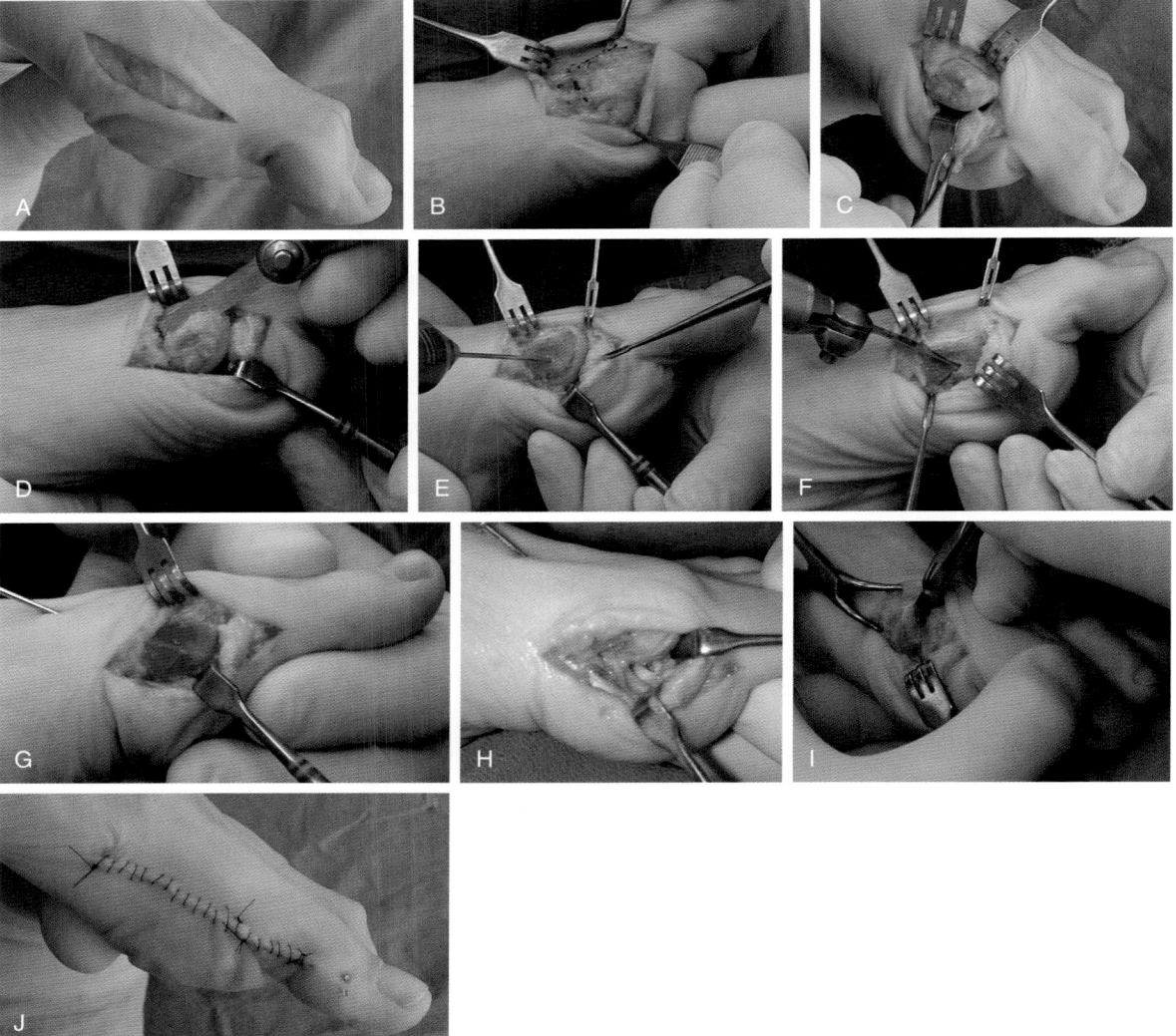

Figure 6-116 Technique for the chevron procedure. **A,** The skin incision is centered over the medial aspect of the metatarsophalangeal joint, starting at the midportion of the proximal phalanx and carried proximally about 6 cm. **B,** An L-shaped capsular flap is used to expose the medial eminence and is retracted **(C). D,** The medial eminence is resected. **E,** A hole is drilled in the center of the metatarsal head to mark the apex of the osteotomy. **F,** The chevron osteotomy is performed at a 60-degree angle. **G,** The osteotomy is fixed with a dorsoplantar pin. **H,** Care is taken to avoid excess plantar placement of the pin. **I,** The medial flare is resected. **J,** Skin closure.

created with an oscillating saw blade that has a fine in-line tooth configuration so as to avoid excessive bone resection. The angle of the chevron cut diverges at approximately a 60-degree angle; the base is oriented proximally (see Fig. 6-116F). The plantar cut must exit proximal to the sesamoids, which places it just proximal to the synovial fold, thereby making it extraarticular. As the osteotomy is performed, the surgeon can feel the saw blade meet and penetrate the lateral cortex; care must be taken to not overpenetrate the cortex and enter the lateral soft tissues, which may damage the blood supply to the metatarsal head (Fig. 6-117E).[71] It is critical that the osteotomy arms do not venture proximally, because this would create

further shortening and the risk of transfer metatarsalgia. Badwey et al[15] reported that the capital fragment can be displaced laterally up to 6 mm in males and 5 mm in females, which constitutes displacement of approximately 30% of the metatarsal's width. To displace the osteotomy, it is sometimes useful to hold the proximal portion of the metatarsal with a small towel clip while pushing the metatarsal head laterally (Fig. 6-117C).

4. *Alternative Technique:* The authors have also used a vertical distal osteotomy with a longitudinal plantar cut as an alternative to a chevron osteotomy. This enables placement of a dorsoplantar screw and is also more adaptable for a biplanar osteotomy (Fig. 6-118).

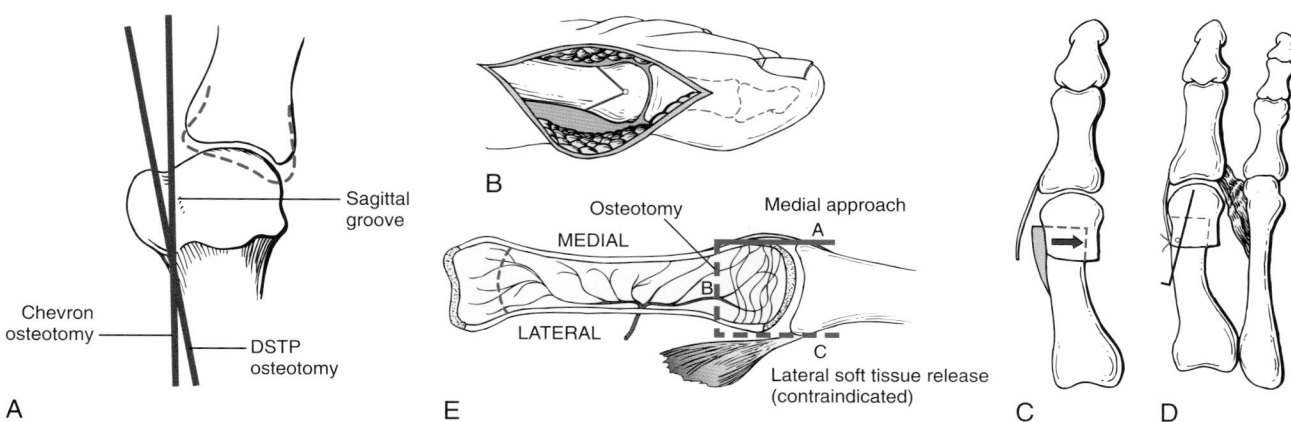

Figure 6-117 A, With a chevron osteotomy, resection of the medial eminence proceeds in line with the medial border of the foot. (With a distal soft tissue repair, the resection is in line with the medial border of the first metatarsal.) **B,** A drill hole is placed equidistant from the dorsal, distal, and plantar metatarsal articular surface. This point marks the apex of the osteotomy, with the chevron osteotomy oriented in a mediolateral plane. **C,** The capital fragment is translated laterally *(arrow).* **D,** The osteotomy is stabilized with a Kirschner wire, and the capsule is anchored by suture through the metaphyseal drill hole. **E,** Dorsal view of the first metatarsal demonstrating the vascular supply to the first metatarsal head. Distal metatarsal osteotomy *(B)* combined with extensive lateral soft tissue release *(C)* and medial capsulorrhaphy *(A)* may compromise the vascularity of the capital fragment. *DSTP,* distal soft tissue procedure.

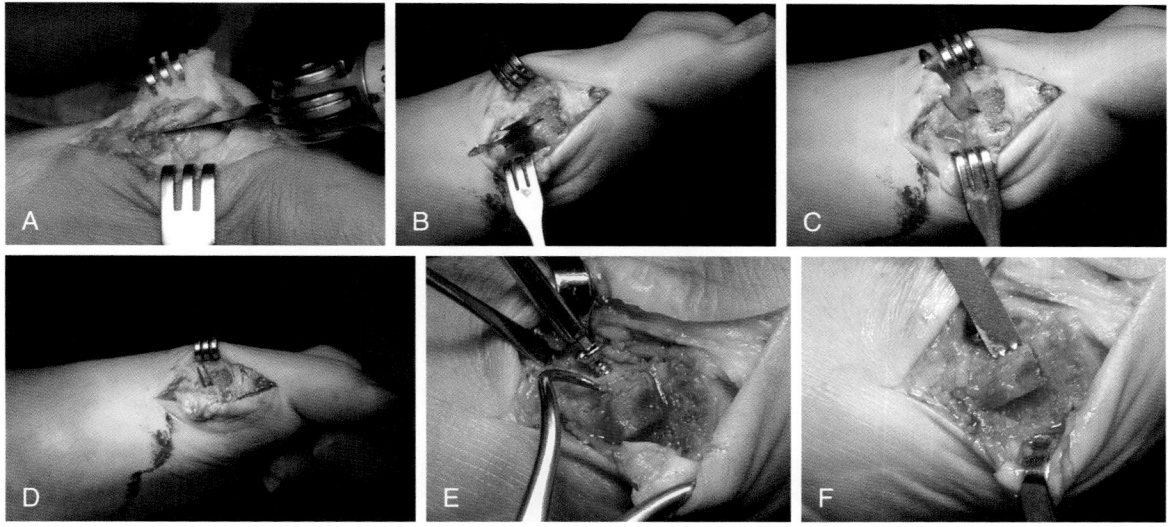

Figure 6-118 A, Through a medial approach, the eminence is resected. **B,** A longitudinal osteotomy is made parallel to the plantar surface of the foot, exiting above the sesamoid articulation. **C,** A vertical cut is made proximal to the articular surface. **D,** If biplanar correction is necessary, a single medial-based wedge is removed. **E,** A compression screw is placed. **F,** The medial flare is shaved with a saw.

Reconstruction of the Joint

1. Once the osteotomy is displaced and the proximal phalanx centered on the articular surface of the metatarsal head, if a significant degree of valgus still remains, a uniplanar or biplanar chevron osteotomy is added to produce a medial closing-wedge effect[128] (Figs. 6-119 and 6-120). Two to 3 mm of bone can be removed from the medial aspect of the metatarsal cut to produce this medial closing osteotomy and realignment of the

articular surface. Rarely is it necessary to remove more than this amount of bone. After the initial chevron osteotomy, the surgeon retracts the capital fragment distally by grasping the osteotomized surface with a small, two-pronged bone hook. An oscillating saw is then used to resect a small, medially based wedge of bone from the medial superior (and medial inferior surfaces if biplanar), with the resection beveled toward the lateral aspect of the metatarsal metaphysis. When

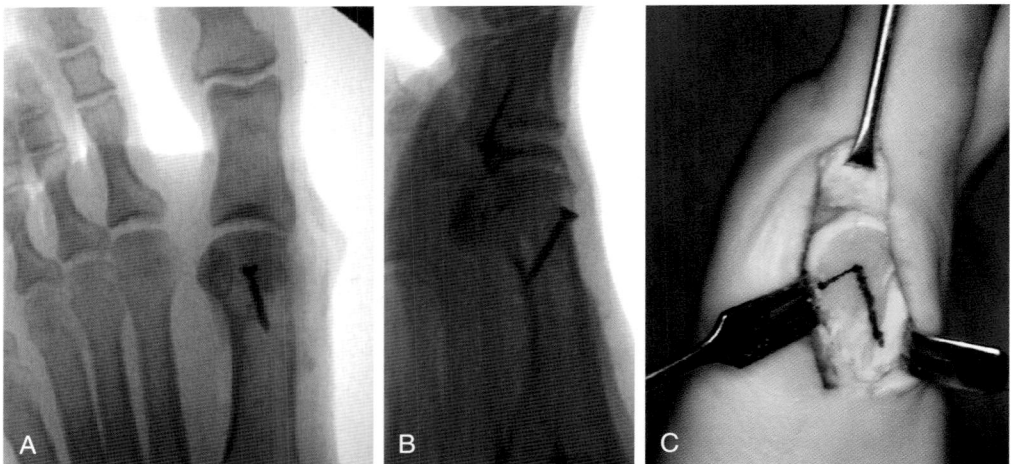

Figure 6-119 Intraoperative fluoroscopic anteroposterior **(A)** and lateral **(B)** radiographs illustrating internal fixation of a distal metatarsal osteotomy with 3-mm bicortical screw. Note the modified osteotomy, in this case a longer dorsal arm **(C)**, to allow for screw fixation.

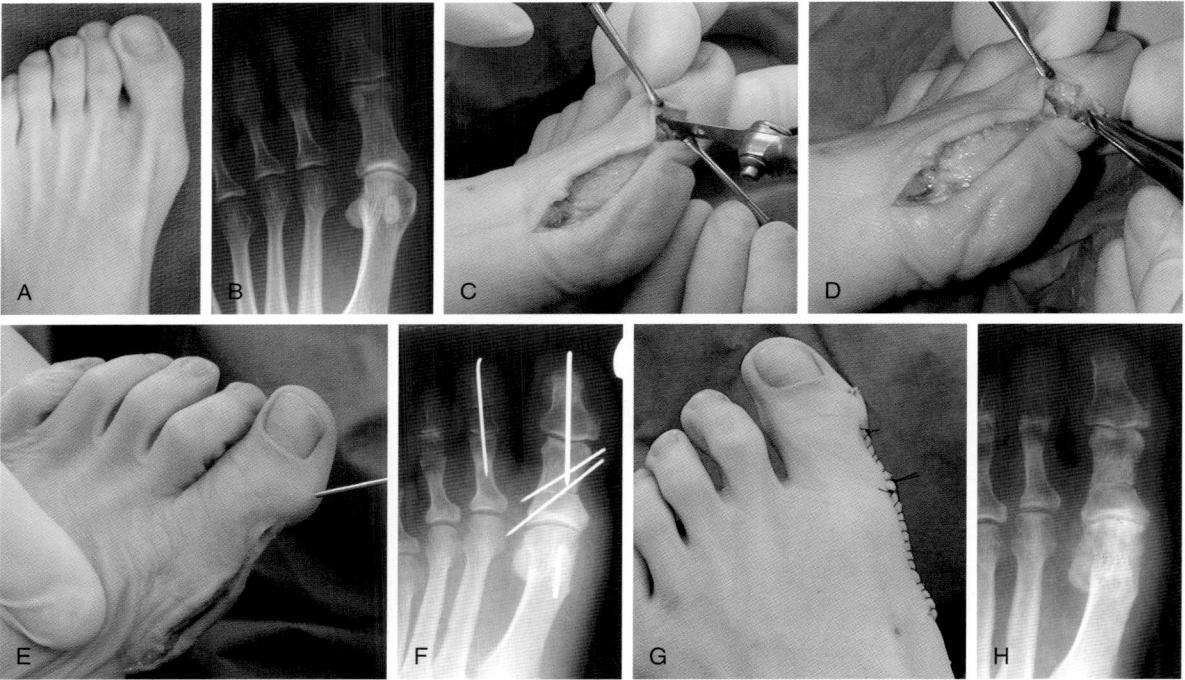

Figure 6-120 Combined chevron-Akin procedure. Preoperative clinical **(A)** and radiographic **(B)** appearance. **C** and **D,** Phalangeal osteotomy. **E,** Kirschner wire fixation. **F,** Internal fixation. **G,** Postoperative clinical appearance. **H,** Final radiographic appearance.

the osteotomy site is closed, the capital fragment is angulated in a more medial direction than with a routine chevron osteotomy.

2. With either technique (standard or biplanar), the capital fragment is then impacted on the proximal fragment and fixed with a 0.062-inch K-wire, or 2.5- to 3.0-mm screw, directed from a dorsal to plantar direction (see Figs. 6-116G and 6-118E). The use of a screw will typically require a longer osteotomy arm (either dorsal or plantar) to allow perpendicular and bicortical fixation (see Fig. 6-119A-C). Care is taken to avoid penetrating the MTP joint with the fixation device (see Fig. 6-116H).

3. The prominent metaphyseal flare created by displacement at the osteotomy site is beveled with an oscillating saw (see Fig. 6-116I).

4. The medial capsular flap is repaired with interrupted absorbable sutures, with the toe held in neutral to

slight varus position. If correction is incomplete because of inadequate excision of capsular tissue, more capsule should be removed. Intraoperative fluoroscopic imaging is helpful in confirming desired joint alignment. When there is insufficient dorsomedial capsule with which to repair the capsular flap, a dorsal metaphyseal drill hole can be used to anchor the capsular repair (see Fig. 6-91F). The skin is closed in routine fashion (see Fig. 6-116J).

5. Inadequate correction of valgus results from one of three anatomic problems: More capsular tissue may need to be removed from the medial joint capsule, the DMAA may be increased and should be corrected by the addition of a medial closing osteotomy at the chevron site, or an HVI deformity may be present and requires correction via a phalangeal osteotomy (see Fig. 6-120).

6. Before placing a compression dressing, the foot is inspected to ensure that there is no excessive skin tension over the pin site, if used. If present, a small incision should be made in the skin to release this tension.

Postoperative Care

The gauze-and-tape compression dressing applied at surgery is removed 1 to 2 weeks later, after which the foot is covered in a firm toe-spica dressing consisting of 2-inch Kling gauze and $\frac{1}{2}$-inch adhesive tape, similar to that used after a distal soft tissue procedure (see Fig. 6-108). If any pronation is present, the dressing must be wrapped in such a way that the toe is held in correct alignment to eliminate or minimize the pronation. The dressing is changed weekly. Sutures are removed 2 to 3 weeks after surgery. The patient is allowed to ambulate in a postoperative shoe with weight borne on the heel and outer aspect of the foot. At initial follow-up, a radiograph is obtained to assess alignment of the first ray, and subsequent dressings are used to correct any residual varus or valgus deformity. The dressing is changed at 10-day intervals over an 8-week period after surgery, assuming that the alignment is satisfactory. If used, the K-wire is removed 4 weeks after surgery in an office setting, and dressings can be discontinued 6 weeks after the procedure. Patients are started on a program of active and passive range-of-motion exercises, as pain permits; they are permitted to ambulate in a soft shoe 6 to 8 weeks after surgery.

Results

After a chevron osteotomy the satisfaction rate is relatively high, with the reported average correction of the hallux valgus angle being 12 to 15 degrees[*] and the average correction of the 1–2 IM angle varying from 4 to 5 degrees[†] (see Fig. 6-103). Reported postoperative narrowing of the forefoot varies from 3 to 6 mm after a chevron osteotomy. Zimmer et al[569] published a report on the

effectiveness of the chevron procedure in juvenile patients and reported a 20% recurrence rate. Extrapolating from these results, the limits of the procedure for a consistently reproducible outcome are a hallux valgus angle of less than 30 degrees and an IM angle of less than 12 to 13 degrees. Expansion of the indications for this procedure to more severe deformities appears to increase the risk of patient dissatisfaction and complications. Reporting on 50 adults who underwent distal metatarsal osteotomy for hallux valgus, Meier and Kenzora[365] noted a 74% satisfaction rate when the 1–2 IM angle was greater than 12 degrees and a 94% satisfaction rate when the 1–2 IM angle was 12 degrees or less. In general, Harper[209] noted that 1 degree of correction is obtained for every 1 mm of lateral translation of the capital fragment. Greater correction has been achieved by Trnka et al[524] and Stienstra et al,[505] who reported 18 degrees of correction of the hallux valgus angle. In both studies, a lateral release was performed. Stienstra et al[505] reported that they translated the capital fragment almost 10 mm laterally. No cases of delayed union, nonunion, or AVN developed. Trnka et al[524] performed a retrospective study on 100 feet treated with a chevron osteotomy and translation of the capital fragment 3 to 6 mm, and they achieved 87% good or excellent results. They also released the lateral capsule, the adductor tendon, and the transverse intermetatarsal ligament. In a follow-up study,[523] there was no deterioration of the results or subjective satisfaction at 5-year follow-up.

In a series of 17 patients and 23 feet, Mann and Donatto[340] carefully analyzed the degree of correction of the hallux valgus angle, IM angle, and the fibular sesamoid position to carefully define the true correction after a chevron procedure. They measured the hallux valgus and IM angles by drawing lines that bisected the shafts of the first and second metatarsals and then compared the results with those from the center-of-head method, which measures the angle formed by a line drawn from the center of the first metatarsal head and middle of the metatarsal base and a line bisecting the second metatarsal shaft.[106] In the method in which both metatarsals were bisected, the preoperative and postoperative IM angle was 11 degrees. In the center-of-head method, the IM angle was 9 degrees preoperatively and 7 degrees postoperatively. When the hallux valgus angle was measured with one line through the longitudinal axis of the first metatarsal and the other through the proximal phalanx, as opposed to one line through the center of the first metatarsal head, the results demonstrated a correction of 5 degrees for the former and 8 degrees for the latter. Basically, this demonstrates that the degree of correction possible with the chevron procedure is quite small, which must be considered when selecting patients for this procedure. The position of the fibular sesamoid was essentially unchanged.

The chevron osteotomy has limited capability to correct a hallux valgus deformity with an increased DMAA.[95] Because of the limited correction achieved with a chevron osteotomy, it must be reserved for mild and

---

[*]References 129, 213, 220, 222, 245, 310, 410, 421, 461, and 523.
[†]References 213, 220, 222, 245, 309, 310, and 421.

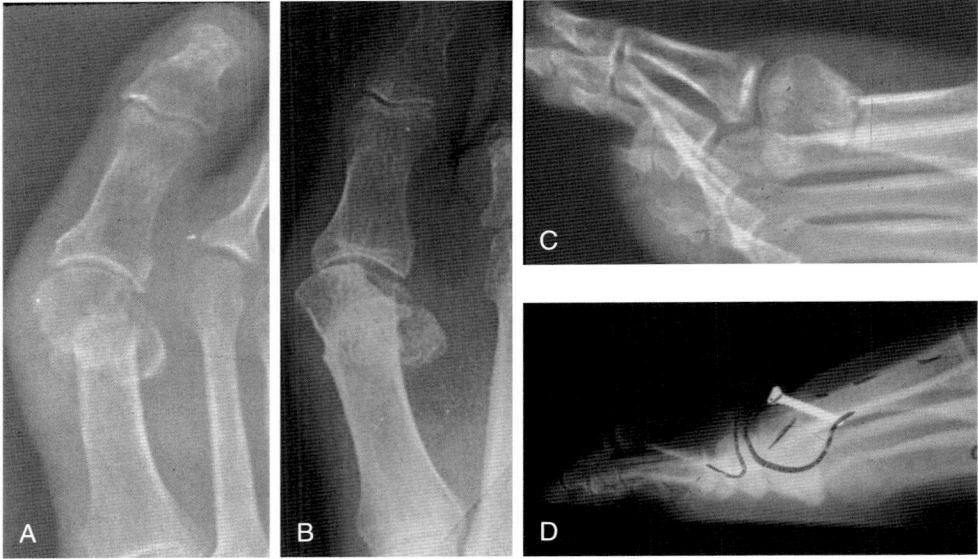

Figure 6-121 Malunion can occur in any plane. Medial **(A)**, lateral **(B)**, and dorsal **(C)** displacement because of lack of internal fixation. **D,** Plantar displacement with internal fixation.

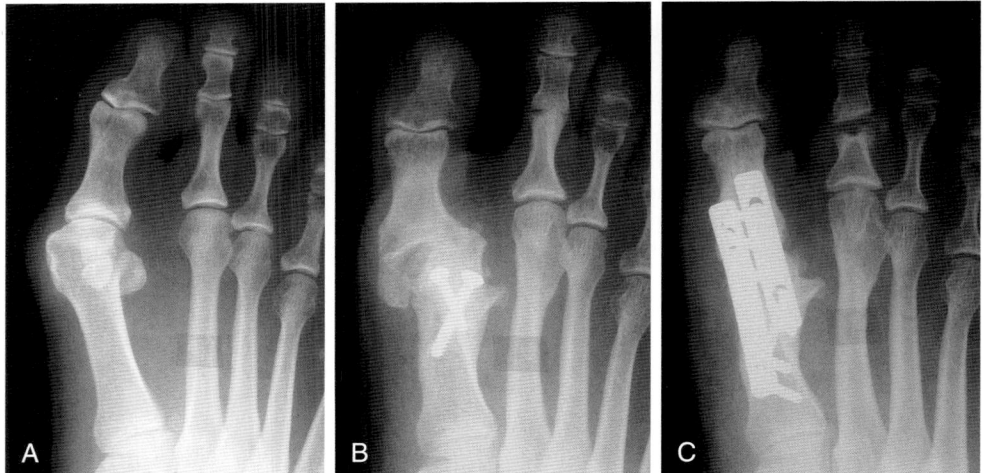

Figure 6-122 Malunion because of poor alignment of the osteotomy. **A,** Preoperative. **B,** Poor postoperative malalignment. **C,** Salvage with metatarsophalangeal joint arthrodesis.

moderate hallux valgus deformities. Chou et al[71] reported on 14 patients who had undergone a biplanar chevron osteotomy for mild and moderate hallux valgus deformities in which an average 7-degree correction of the DMAA was achieved.

Postoperative displacement of the osteotomy site varied from 1.8% of 225 cases reported by Hattrup and Johnson[213] to 12% reported by Johnson et al[244] and can lead to overcorrection or undercorrection (Fig. 6-121).[222] The incidence of postoperative displacement of the capital fragment medially or laterally or deviation dorsally or plantarward can be minimized by the use of some form of internal fixation rather than relying on impaction of

the osteotomy site as was initially recommended,[13,245,524] especially in those for whom greater displacement of the osteotomy is desired (Fig. 6-122).

Most surgeons have transitioned from wire fixation to a variety of screws to decrease the inherent risks of loosening, skin irritation, and infection. Early reports on internal fixation with absorbable implants demonstrated evidence of a foreign body reaction.[406] Recent reports using poly-L-lactic acid[19,54,129,222,375,406] demonstrated less common side effects of osteolysis or granuloma formation. Gill et al[173] reported a 10% incidence of pin-tract osteolysis when using polydioxanone (PDS) bioabsorbable pins to internally fix a chevron osteotomy.

Complications

Complications after the chevron procedure are similar to those noted with other osteotomy procedures: pain, recurrence of the hallux valgus deformity, transfer metatarsalgia secondary to shortening, MTP joint arthrofibrosis, nonunion, and postoperative neuritic symptoms secondary to entrapment of a cutaneous nerve. The most frequent complications reported with the chevron osteotomy are recurrence and undercorrection of a hallux valgus deformity, which vary in frequency from 10% to 20% (Fig. 6-123).[12,222,310]

Recurrence of hallux valgus deformity occurs in about 10% of cases.[6,164] The 10% recurrence rate can probably be significantly lessened if the indications for the procedure are not overextended. In the series reported by Hirvensalo et al,[222] the deformity recurred when the preoperative hallux valgus averaged 37 degrees, and the IM angle averaged 13 degrees. Hattrup and Johnson[213] noted recurrence of the deformity in 18 of 225 procedures; they reported that the average preoperative hallux valgus angle of 37 degrees was corrected to an average of 31 degrees postoperatively. Other authors have not documented the severity of the preoperative hallux valgus deformity when discussing recurrence. If there are no intraarticular symptoms or advanced degeneration, recurrent hallux valgus can be managed with an Akin osteotomy (Fig. 6-124A and B).

Mean shortening of the first metatarsal averaged 2 to 2.5 mm in two series[222,340] and was as high as 6 mm in 28 cases reported by Pring et al.[430] Shortening can develop as a result of excessive bone loss[12,222,365] or be due to bone necrosis or resection at the osteotomy site. Klosok et al[281] reported the development of postoperative transfer lesions in 12% and postoperative metatarsalgia in 43% of patients after a chevron osteotomy (Fig. 6-125).

Although cutaneous nerve injury can occur with this procedure, the use of a medial midline surgical approach substantially reduces the incidence of nerve entrapment when compared with performance of the osteotomy through a dorsal or dorsomedial incision.

Excessive soft tissue stripping and and overpenetration of the lateral cortex at the level of the osteotomy should be avoided to minimize the risk for nonunion (Fig. 6-126A and B). The location of the two limbs of the osteotomy, particularly the plantar limb, is critical. The plantar limb should be extraarticular, if possible, both to avoid injury to the sesamoids and to minimize the development of MTP joint adhesions between the sesamoids and the metatarsal head, which can lead to resultant loss of MTP joint motion. Trnka et al[523] noted that passive range

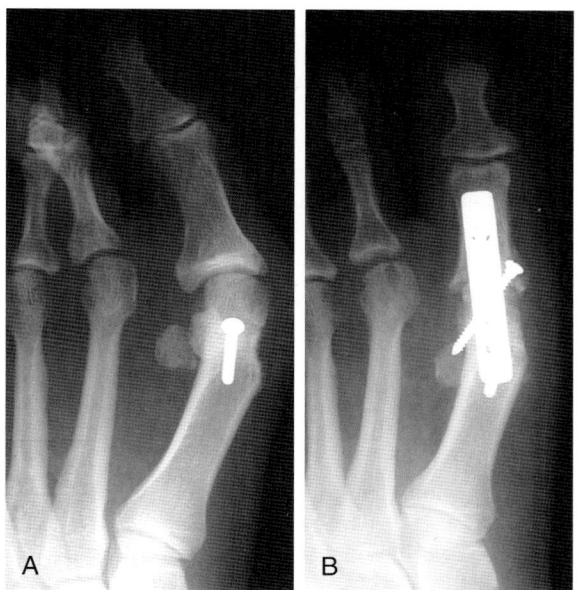

Figure 6-123 **A,** Recurrence after the chevron procedure. **B,** Salvage with metatarsophalangeal joint arthrodesis.

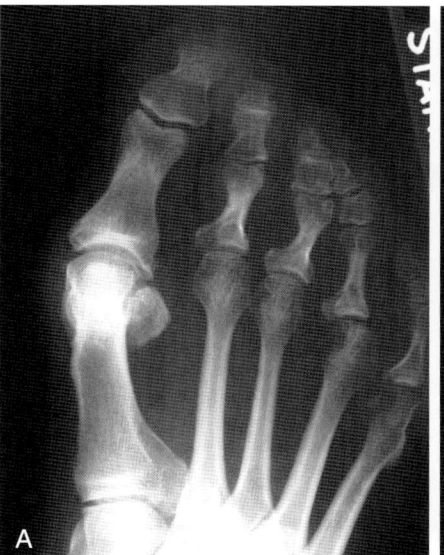 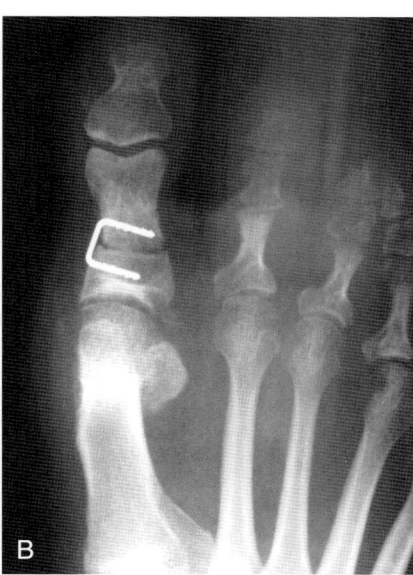

Figure 6-124 **A,** Preoperative anteroposterior standing radiograph in a patient with recurrent hallux valgus after a distal metatarsal osteotomy. **B,** Postoperative radiograph 7 weeks after correction, using a medial closing-wedge osteotomy of the proximal phalanx.

of motion was 72 degrees preoperatively and 61 and 62 degrees at the 1-year and 2-year follow-up after a chevron osteotomy. A patient should be counseled that decreased MTP range of motion may occur after the procedure (Fig. 6-127).

Hallux varus may develop because of lateral displacement of the capital fragment, medial subluxation of the tibial sesamoid, excessive excision of the medial eminence resulting in inappropriate narrowing of the metatarsal head, and AVN of the medial aspect of the capital fragment. Although these complications are uncommon, awareness of them may help in their prevention (Fig. 6-128).

The most serious complication after a chevron osteotomy is AVN (Fig. 6-129). The incidence of AVN varies from 4% to 20%.[193,227,244,410] In an early report, Meier and Kenzora[365] noted AVN in 20% of patients after a chevron osteotomy, and this figure increased to 40% when combined with an adductor tenotomy. Shereff et al[478] cautioned that lateral release increases the risk of AVN (Fig. 6-130). No AVN, however, was observed in a series of chevron procedures reported by Hattrup and Johnson.[213] Green et al[193] identified no evidence of first metatarsal AVN after release of the conjoined adductor tendon, sesamoidal ligament, and fibular sesamoid ligament through an intermetatarsal incision. Although excessive capsular dissection has been implicated in the development of AVN, careful surgical technique and preservation of the distal vascular structures can help avoid AVN. Peterson et al[410] reported a case of AVN after lateral release. They suggested that a carefully performed chevron procedure preserves the dorsal and plantar blood supply and did not believe that a lateral capsular release above the sesamoids or an adductor tendon release interrupted the vascular supply. Trnka et al[524] performed a lateral release through a separate incision; after dissecting out and releasing the tarsometatarsal ligament and the lateral capsule, they reported no evidence of AVN at final follow-up. Trnka et al[523] then reviewed the combined series of Pochatko, Trnka, and Peterson[410,421,524,525] of 224 chevron procedures and found that only four cases of AVN developed (2%), and in three of these cases, excessive stripping was documented. Most recently, Pontenza's series[426] noted only one case of asymptomatic AVN and concluded that a lateral release was safe in those patients with mild-to-moderate hallux valgus.

AVN is a potential problem that may not be preventable in certain cases because of peculiarities in the blood supply to the capital fragment,[328] but this does not necessarily preclude a successful end result.[477] When performing a chevron procedure, however, excessive soft tissue stripping should be minimized. Excess lateral penetration of the saw blade should also be avoided because it can damage the lateral capsular circulation to the metatarsal head (Fig. 6-131). Malal recommended a longer plantar osteotomy arm to avoid the plantar-lateral corner of the metatarsal neck, where blood supply enters the metatarsal

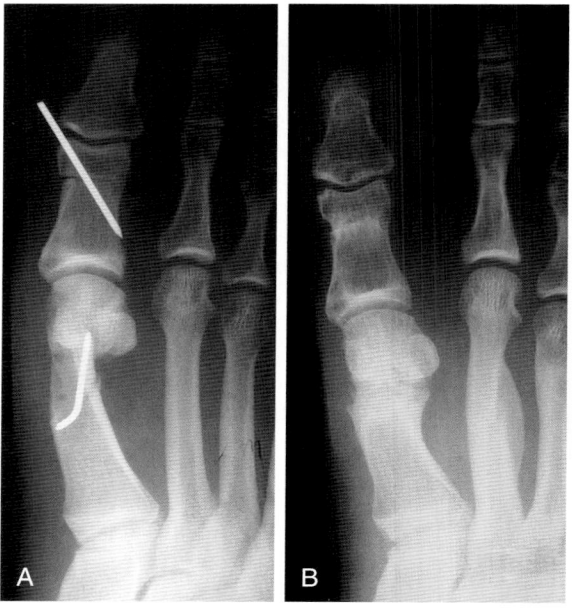

Figure 6-125 **A,** After a combined chevron-Akin procedure. **B,** Stress fracture of the second metatarsal 4 months after surgery.

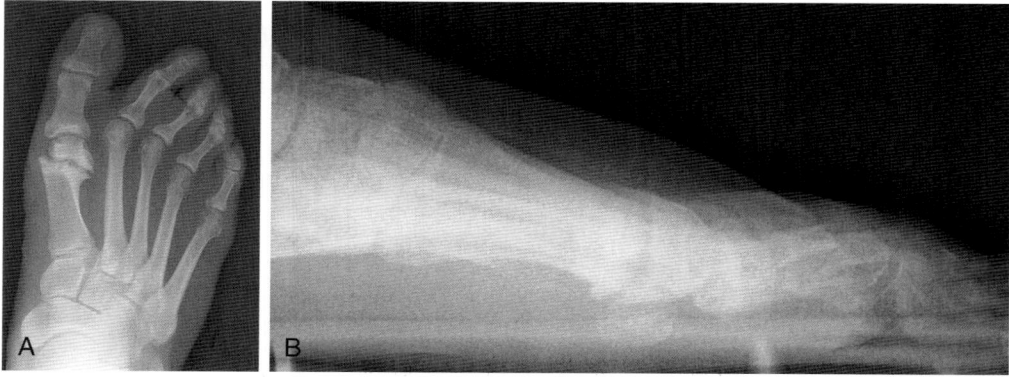

Figure 6-126 Anteroposterior **(A)** and lateral **(B)** radiographs depicting a nonunion of a distal chevron osteotomy.

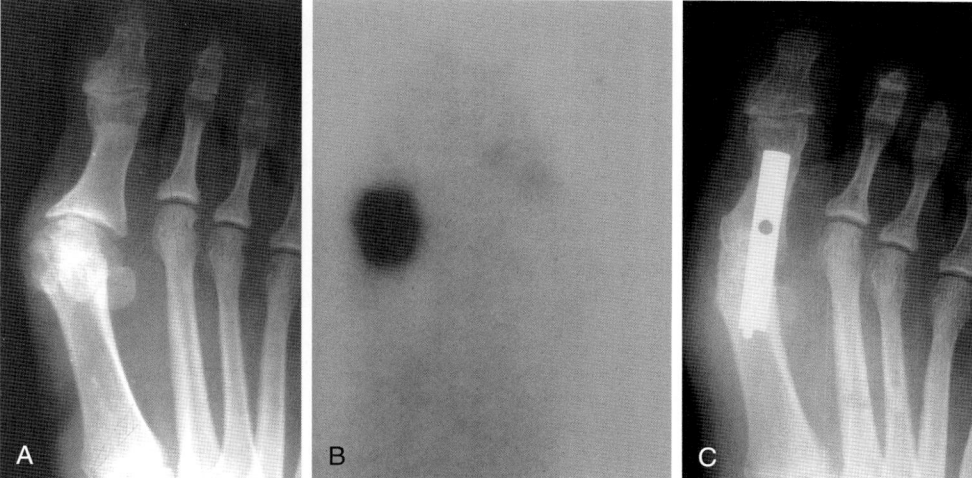

Figure 6-127 Patient with severe restriction of metatarsophalangeal (MTP) joint motion. **A,** Degenerative arthritis versus avascular necrosis 2 years after a chevron procedure. **B,** Increased uptake on bone scan at the MTP joint. **C,** Salvage with MTP joint arthrodesis.

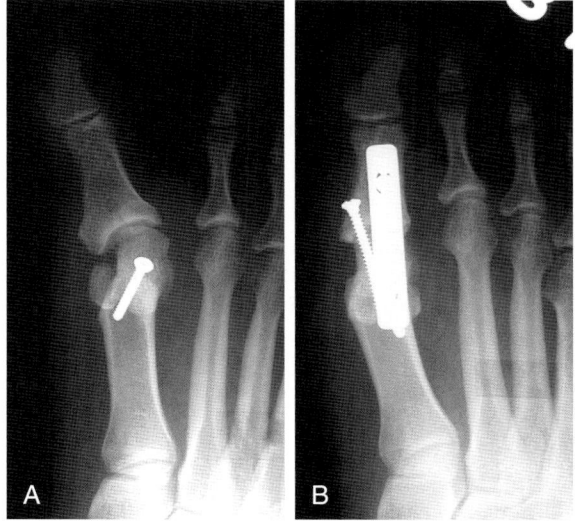

Figure 6-128 **A,** Hallux varus after a chevron procedure. **B,** Salvage with metatarsophalangeal arthrodesis. (Same patient as shown in Fig. 6-123 after recurrence on the contralateral side.)

head—a finding contrary to the work of Shereff.[478] Release of the lateral structures may enable greater correction but, if done extensively, can increase the risk of AVN.[238,309,365,555] Thomas et al[511] performed lateral soft tissue release and, frequently, fibular sesamoidectomy through a plantar incision. In a review of 80 of their chevron procedures, the radiographic changes suggested vascular compromise in 76% (61 of 80) of the feet, but at follow-up, none had progressed to AVN. Wilkinson et al[554] postoperatively evaluated 20 patients with magnetic resonance imaging after chevron osteotomy. Fifty percent had evidence of AVN, mostly in the dorsal metatarsal head, although none of the patients were symptomatic. The authors also

performed McBride procedures as controls, and none showed evidence of decreased vascularity to the metatarsal head.

The question of whether to release the lateral capsular structures when performing a chevron procedure depends on the perceived risk of AVN. Based on the literature,* careful, meticulous release of contracted lateral structures at the level of the joint is probably safe because it is distal to the blood supply to the metatarsal head. However, in the presence of a more severe deformity, it may be a better alternative to choose another procedure that does not have any risk of development of AVN. More extensive dissection along the lateral aspect of the metatarsal head, such as with excision of the fibular sesamoid, should be avoided because this dissection carries a higher risk of disturbing the blood supply along the lateral aspect of the metatarsal head.

DISTAL METATARSAL OSTEOTOMY (MITCHELL, BOSCH TYPES)

Correction of a hallux valgus deformity by means of a distal first metatarsal osteotomy was first described by Reverdin[436] in 1881 and later by both Peabody[407] and Hohmann.[225] However, it was Mitchell[214,370] who described and popularized the technique of a biplanar metaphyseal osteotomy, which achieves lateral and plantar displacement of the capital fragment, as well as shortening of the first metatarsal. Wilson[558] and others[188,374,463,530] described an oblique metaphyseal osteotomy, Bosch[42,43] and Kramer,[283] a transverse osteotomy, and Magnan,[26,330,331] a percutaneous osteotomy. The Mitchell procedure, as described by Hawkins et al,[214] is a double step-cut osteotomy through the neck of the first metatarsal. Several modifications have been made to this procedure through the years, including changes in the design of

---

*References 12, 281, 328, 410, 421, 511, and 524.

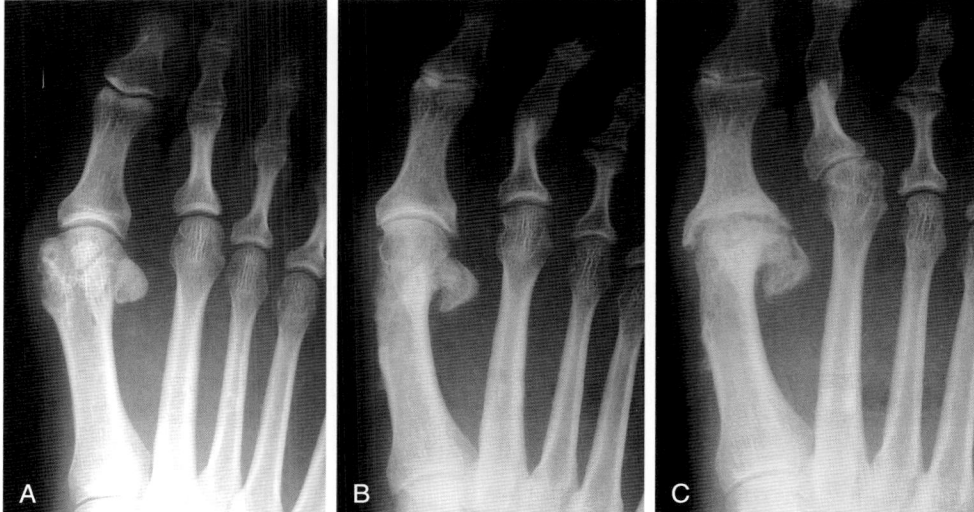

Figure 6-129 Avascular necrosis of the metatarsal head after distal osteotomy. **A,** Preoperative radiograph. **B,** After surgery. **C,** Five years after surgery, complete chondrolysis and avascular necrosis have developed.

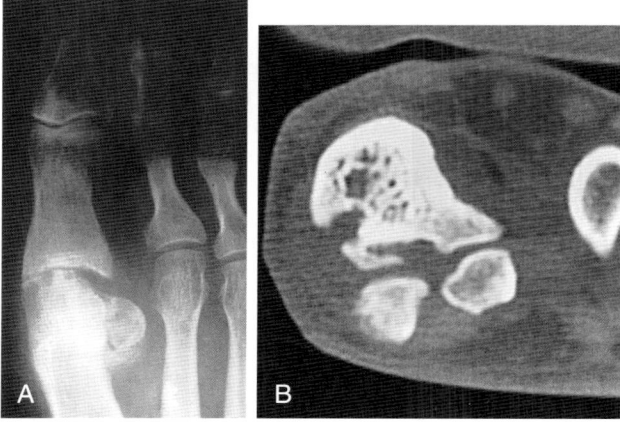

Figure 6-130 **A,** Avascular necrosis after a chevron procedure. **B,** Computed tomography scan demonstrating marked cystic degeneration.

the medial capsulorrhaphy,[49,369,374,463] the osteotomy technique,[*] the method of internal fixation,[†] and postoperative care.[49,374,507] The changes described make the eponym Mitchell somewhat inadequate to describe the procedure as now performed in many series. Nonetheless, Mitchell's important principles remain—that shortening should be kept to a minimum, plantar flexion of the capital fragment should consistently be achieved, and rotation of the capital fragment to realign the distal articular metatarsal surface is occasionally indicated.

The Bosch osteotomy is much like the Mitchell in principle. However, it has received considerable attention

_____

*References 42, 43, 49, 284, 330, 331, 374, 425, 463, 530, 558, 561, and 562.
†References 49, 127, 158, 290, 342, 366, 372, 374, 425, 463, 507, 561, and 562.

of late as one[324] amenable to minimally invasive techniques.[26,330,331] Minimal incision surgery has also been applied to the chevron and other distal first metatarsal osteotomies. Arthroscopic-assisted surgeries have also been described.[321,484]

Indications
Distal metatarsal osteotomies (whether oblique or transverse) are indicated for a moderate or moderately severe hallux valgus deformity with a subluxed MTP joint. If the DMAA is not substantial (<15 degrees), this osteotomy is still indicated. The upper limit is 35 to 40 degrees for hallux valgus angular deformity and 15 degrees for the 1–2 IM angle. As a general rule, satisfactory results seem to diminish significantly with more severe deformities and in patients older than 60 years.[158] The location of the osteotomy in the proximal region of the distal metaphysis enables it to achieve slightly more correction than a chevron osteotomy does.

Contraindications
The procedure should not be used to treat patients with mild hallux valgus deformity, a short first metatarsal, lateral metatarsalgia, a DMAA greater than 20 degrees, or more-than-mild MTP joint arthrosis.

Technique
The surgical technique for a distal metatarsal osteotomy is divided into the surgical approach, technique of the metatarsal osteotomy, and reconstruction of the osteotomy and MTP joint.

Surgical Approach
1. A longitudinal skin incision is made over the dorsomedial aspect of the first MTP joint. The incision begins distally at the midportion of the proximal

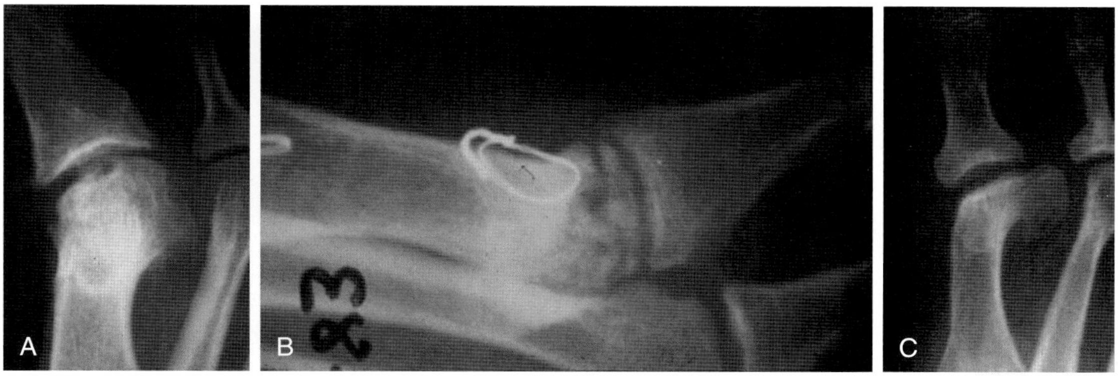

Figure 6-131 Avascular necrosis leading to varus deformity **(A)** and subchondral lysis **(B). C,** Collapse and dissolution of the metatarsal head.

phalanx and is carried proximally 6 cm over the meta-tarsal shaft. Care is taken to protect the dorsomedial and plantar medial cutaneous nerves of the hallux.

2. A distally based capsular flap[49] or a V/Y-shaped capsu-lar flap[370] is developed over the medial aspect of the MTP joint to expose the medial eminence.

3. Subperiosteal dissection is carried out along the dor-somedial aspect of the distal metatarsal. Extensive dis-section is avoided, especially in the area of the dorsal lateral capsular area. The adductor tendon and lateral capsular attachments are not released to avoid disrupt-ing the blood supply to the metatarsal head.[365]

4. The medial eminence is exposed and excised in line with the medial aspect of the metatarsal shaft, starting about 1 mm medial to the sagittal sulcus.

Technique of First Metatarsal Osteotomy

1. A double osteotomy is performed in the distal first metatarsal metaphyses. The initial cut of the double osteotomy is an incomplete cut that is commenced 2 cm proximal to the distal metatarsal articular surface (Fig. 6-132A). The depth of this cut depends on the amount of correction desired. The wider the lateral shelf, the less correction obtained. Typically, a lateral bridge of bone measuring 4 to 5 mm is left. The plantar aspect of the metatarsal is inspected as the osteotomy is performed to ensure that the cut is proximal to the sesamoids.

2. Although in the classic description of the procedure by Mitchell et al[370] holes are drilled above and below the osteotomy for placement of cerclage suture, more rigid internal fixation is preferable. Either a $\frac{5}{64}$-inch Stein-mann pin or two K-wires are commonly used to fix the shaft and the capital fragment.[18,158,290]

3. The second parallel osteotomy is cut completely through the metatarsal approximately 2 mm proximal and parallel to the initial cut in a medial-to-lateral direction. The magnitude of the deformity determines the amount of shortening desired, the thickness of the resection, and the width of the lateral shelf that is left. This cut is angled so that 2 mm more of bone is

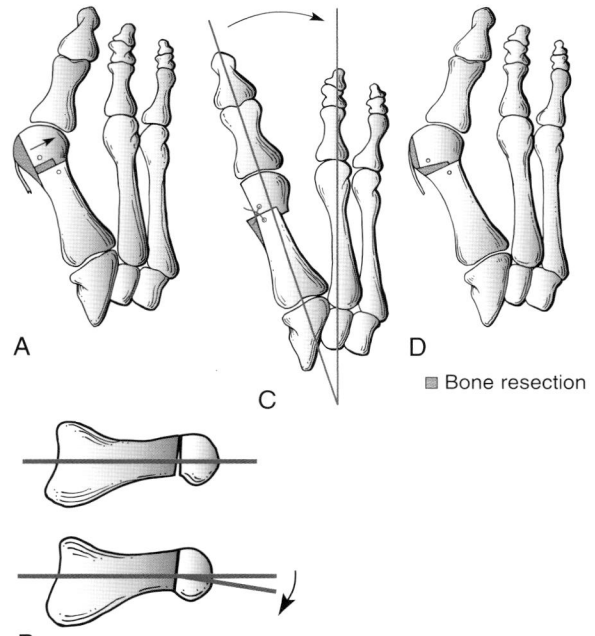

Figure 6-132 A, The proposed osteotomy for moderate hallux valgus deformity necessitates bone resection and shortening. The width of lateral shelf determines the amount of displacement of the capital fragment. The wider the shelf, the greater the lateral displacement. **B,** Slightly more bone is resected on the plantar aspect of the osteotomy site to decrease the prevalence of postoperative transfer lesions. **C,** After displacement and shortening, the capital fragment is translated laterally. The medial metaphyseal flare is removed. **D,** With an increased distal metatarsal articular angle, biplanar resection allows realignment of congruent metatarsophalangeal joint articulation.

removed on the plantar aspect, thereby tilting the oste-otomy site plantarward (Fig. 6-132C). The width of the lateral spike on the distal fragment depends on the magnitude of the IM angle. With a severe deformity, the spike may constitute approximately one third of

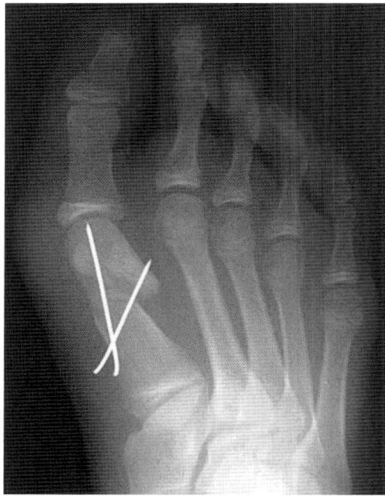

Figure 6-133 Internal fixation with two Kirschner wires.

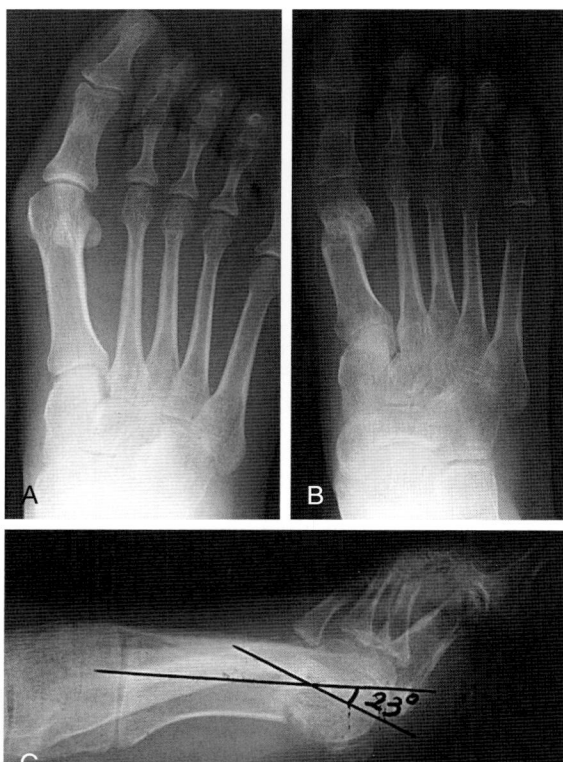

Figure 6-134 **A,** Preoperative radiograph demonstrating a moderate hallux valgus deformity. **B,** Radiograph after a Mitchell osteotomy. **C,** Lateral radiograph demonstrating plantar flexion of the capital fragment. (Courtesy Kent Wu, MD.)

the metatarsal shaft, whereas with a more moderate deformity, it consists of only about one sixth of the metatarsal's width. The degree of plantar tilting depends on the length of the first metatarsal and whether a plantar lesion is present under the second metatarsal.

Reconstruction of the Osteotomy and Metatarsophalangeal Joint

1. The osteotomy site is displaced laterally 4 to 5 mm until the lateral shelf locks over the edge of the proximal fragment, and the position is carefully checked to ensure that slight plantar flexion is present. Blum[34] reported that rather than removing more bone off the metatarsal's plantar aspect, the capital fragment was displaced plantarward 2 to 4 mm to compensate for this shortening (Fig. 6-132B). If the distal metatarsal articular surface is sloped laterally (increased DMAA), more bone can be removed from the medial aspect of the metatarsal, and the capital fragment is then rotated to align the articular surface more perpendicular to the metatarsal shaft (Fig. 6-132D).
2. The osteotomy site is stabilized with K-wires,[158,222,228,290,507] screws,[561,562] staples,[49] or an oblique $\frac{5}{64}$-inch Steinmann pin (Fig. 6-133).
3. The remaining medial metaphyseal flare created by the lateral displacement of the capital fragment is then resected with a power saw (Fig. 6-134).
4. The MTP joint is brought into a neutral or slight varus position, and the medial capsular tissues are plicated with interrupted sutures.
5. The skin is closed with interrupted sutures and a firm compression dressing is applied.

Technique of Bosch (Percutaneous Osteotomy)

Magnan et al[330,331] advocate a transverse osteotomy in the proximal metaphyseal region in which the metatarsal

head is translated medialward without resection of the medial eminence. It is fixed with a longitudinal Steinmann pin (Fig. 6-135).

Postoperative Care

A gauze-and-tape compressing dressing is applied after completion of the surgical procedure. One to 2 weeks after surgery, the compression dressing is removed, and the patient placed in a firm spica-like dressing consisting of 2-inch Kling gauze and $\frac{1}{2}$-inch adhesive tape dressing. Some authors will fashion a slipper cast to immobilize the hallux and forefoot. Most authors prefer that the patient remain non–weight bearing for 4 weeks after surgery because the osteotomy site is not as stable as some of the other osteotomies previously described. One to 3 weeks after surgery, the sutures are removed and a radiograph obtained with as much weight bearing as tolerated to assess alignment of the MTP joint. The dressing changes are then based on this radiograph. If pins are used, they are generally removed 4 to 6 weeks after surgery, and the patient is then permitted to ambulate in either a postoperative shoe or a removable cast boot until the osteotomy site has healed, which typically occurs at approximately 6 to 8 weeks after surgery.

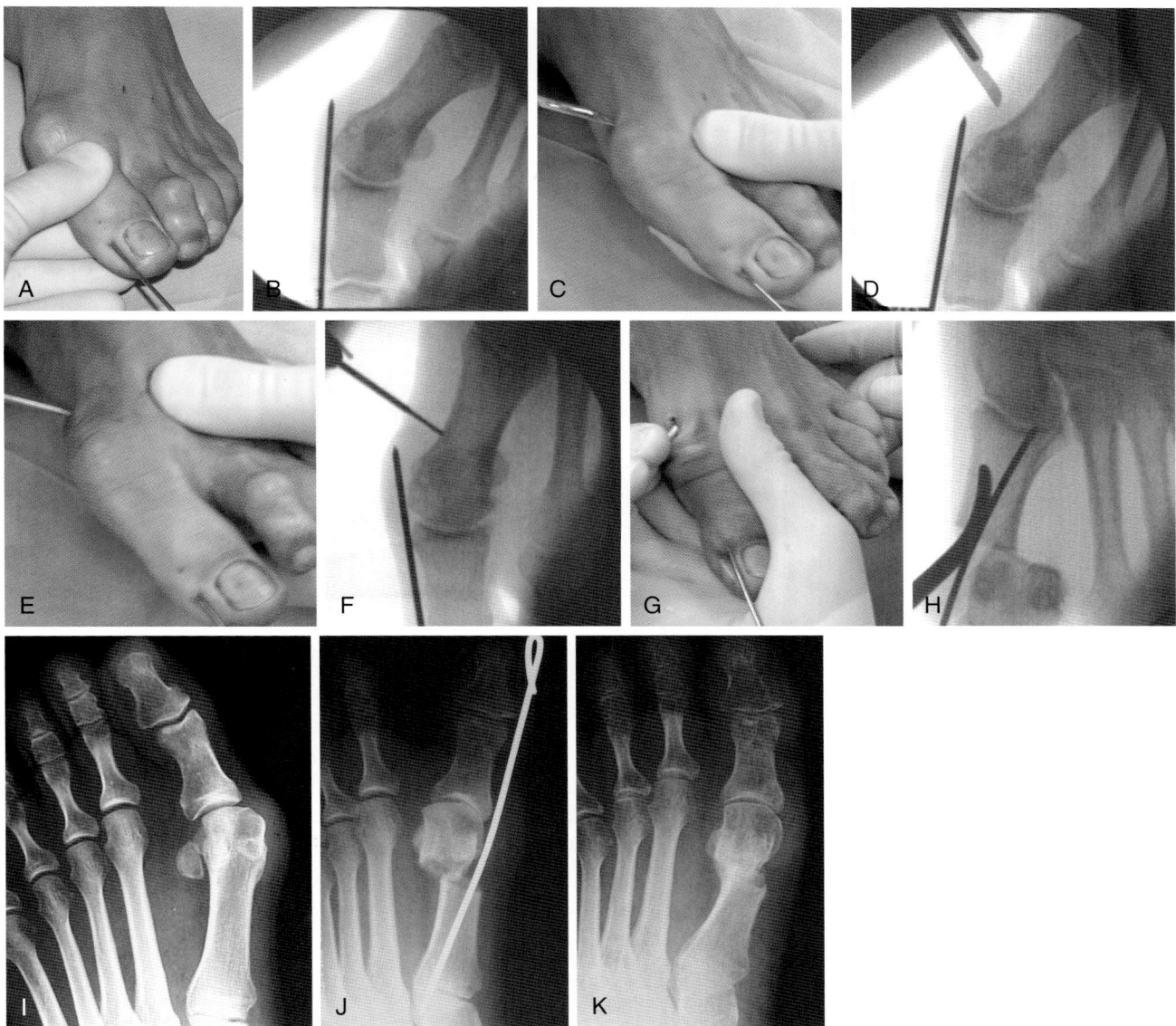

Figure 6-135 Percutaneous osteotomy: introduction of a Kirschner wire at the tip of the toe. **A,** Operative photograph. **B,** Fluoroscopic view. **C,** Small incision. **D,** Fluoroscopic view. **E,** Osteotomy of the metaphysis. **F,** Fluoroscopic view. **G,** Reduction of the intermetatarsal angle. **H,** Fixation placed in the intramedullary canal. **I,** Preoperative radiograph. **J,** Intraoperative radiograph. **K,** Four months after surgery. (Courtesy B. Magnan, MD.)

Results

The Mitchell procedure is of historical interest, and prior reports noted high patient satisfaction and satisfactory correction of the hallux valgus and intermetatarsal angular deformities. The overall experience with both the Mitchell osteotomy and the modified Mitchell-type distal metatarsal osteotomies is that satisfactory correction is achieved in 82% to 97% of cases.* In two of the largest series, Blum[34] reported that 185 of 204 patients (91%) and Hawkins et al[214] reported that 182 of 188 patients (97%) were satisfied with the procedure. The average reported correction of the hallux valgus angle varies from 10 to 25 degrees,* and the average correction of the 1–2 IM angle varies from 5 to 10 degrees.† Shortening of the first metatarsal is a key component in achieving correction of the hallux valgus deformity (Fig. 6-136J); however, it places the patient at risk for postoperative metatarsalgia.[214,393] Excessive shortening is the most common cause of lesser MTP joint pain and callus formation after a distal first metatarsal osteotomy for correction of hallux valgus.‡ Merkel et al[366] reported an average first metatarsal shortening of 7 mm. In patients who had more than 10 mm

---

*References 34, 49, 60, 158, 184, 276, 371, 561, and 562.

*References 34, 49, 158, 184, 276, 290, 561, and 562.
†References 34, 49, 158, 184, 214, 276, 561, and 562.
‡References 60, 158, 184, 214, 276, 370, 463, and 558.

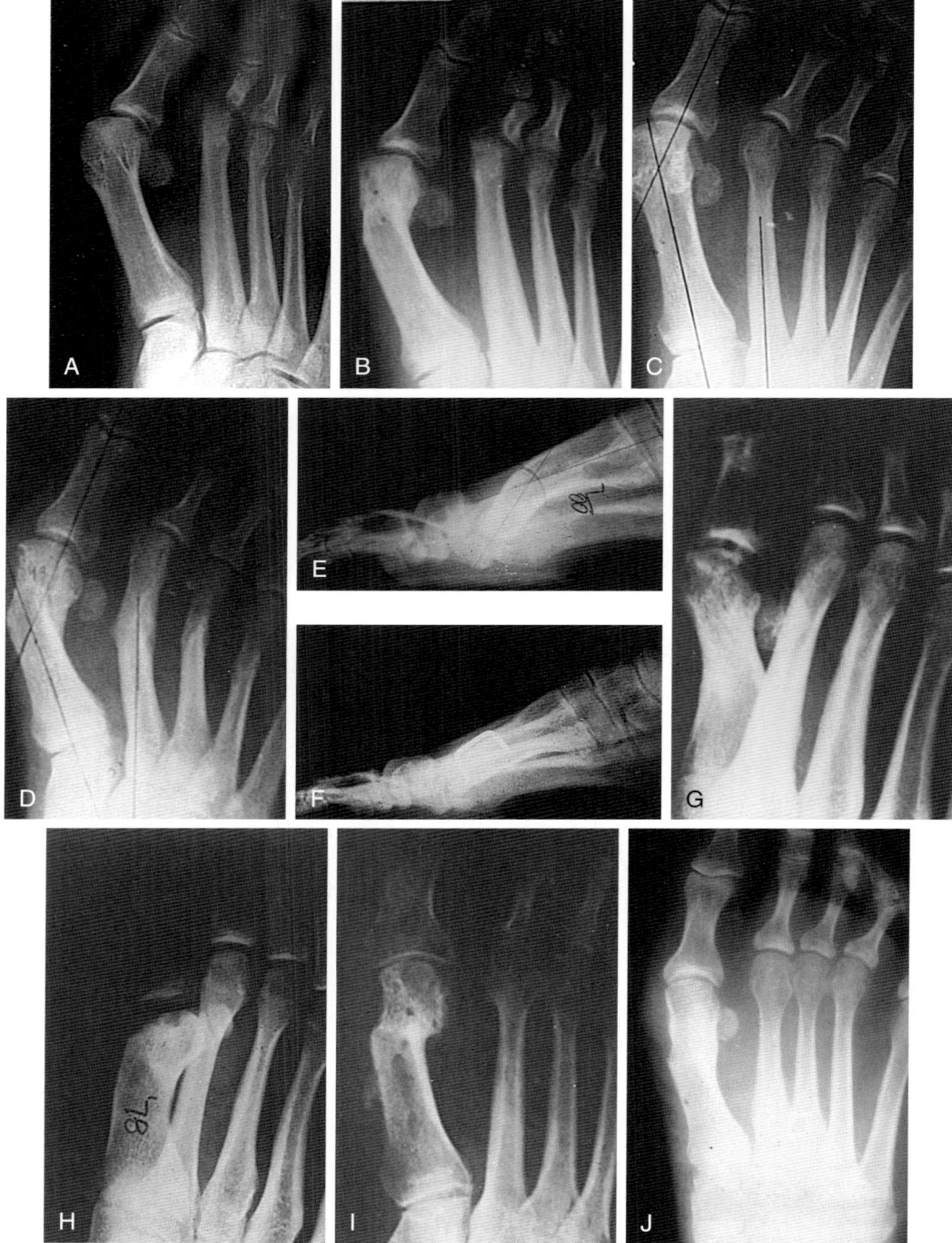

Figure 6-136 Complications after the Mitchell procedure. **A,** Preoperative radiograph. **B,** Postoperative radiograph showing incomplete correction because the deformity is too severe to be corrected by the Mitchell procedure. **C,** Preoperative radiograph. **D,** Postoperative radiograph showing lateral deviation of the capital fragment. **E,** Radiograph demonstrating plantar flexion of the capital fragment. **F,** Realignment after a dorsal closing wedge metatarsal osteotomy. **G,** Dorsiflexion of the distal fragment. **H,** Plantar flexion of the distal fragment. **I,** Avascular changes in the metatarsal head. **J,** Shortening of the first ray.

of shortening, a higher rate of dissatisfaction and a higher incidence of metatarsalgia were reported. Rates of postoperative metatarsalgia have been reported to vary from 10% to 40%,[214,276,290,561] with a 31% incidence reported by Hawkins et al[214] in the largest series. Plantar angulation[34,184,214,370] or plantar displacement[366,561,562] of the capital fragment has been advocated to diminish the ill effects of first metatarsal shortening. Dorsal angulation at the osteotomy site is associated with patient dissatisfaction because it tends to compound the effects of first metatarsal shortening.[49,366,561,562] Dumon's recent paper highlights the long-term success of the procedure, aided by internal fixation.[131]

As mentioned above, the Bosch technique applies a minimally invasive approach for accomplishing the distal metatarsal osteotomy. Several authors have found good results by using this method, with shorter operating time, improved rates of healing and fewer complications.[26,330,331] A more recent report highlights a number of potential complications with the technique, including osteonecrosis, nonunion, malunion, and recurrence.[257] In addition, Huang noted an unacceptable recurrence of radiographic hallux valgus and recommended that the procedure be avoided in those patients with moderate-to-severe deformity.[229]

Complications

Recurrence and undercorrection of hallux valgus deformity have also been recognized as complications after distal metatarsal osteotomy (Fig. 6-137). These complications have been reported to occur in approximately 10% of cases.* Use of a distal metatarsal osteotomy for more severe deformities increases the risk of recurrence, undercorrection, or malunion (see Fig. 6-136).[158] Fokter et al[158] reported that results deteriorated with time: subjective satisfaction rates of 97% at 10 years diminished to 64% with long-term follow-up.

The incidence of AVN with significant collapse of the metatarsal head is difficult to determine (Fig. 6-138). However, Meier and Kenzora[365] observed AVN in 1 of 12 patients, Das De and Hamblen[118] in 2 of 38 patients, Wu[561] in none of 100 patients, and Blum[34] in 5 of 204 patients, 1 of whom was symptomatic. Carr and Boyd[60]

*References 34, 184, 214, 370, 561, and 562.

and others* have also reported the development of AVN after distal first metatarsal osteotomy. Wu[561,562] occasionally used a lateral soft tissue release in combination with the osteotomy, whereas others have avoided lateral dissection.[60,214,371,530]

The main complication of shortening of the metatarsal is that it can lead to transfer metatarsalgia.[519] The osteotomy should be avoided in an already short first metatarsal with a concomitant hallux valgus deformity. Plantar flexion of the head fragment is essential to prevent this complication. Loss of position at the osteotomy site into

*References 188, 333, 365, 370, and 463.

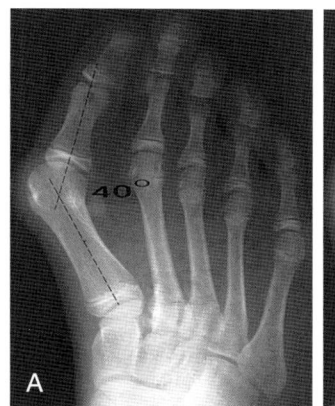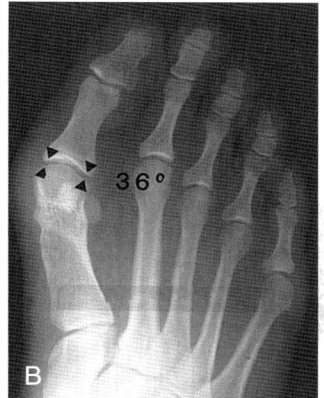

Figure 6-137 Complications after distal osteotomy. **A,** Preoperative radiograph of severe juvenile hallux valgus deformity with a congruent metatarsophalangeal joint (preoperative hallux valgus angle, 40 degrees). **B,** After a Mitchell osteotomy, the 1–2 intermetatarsal angle, hallux valgus angle, and distal metatarsal articular angle are uncorrected (postoperative hallux valgus angle, 36 degrees).

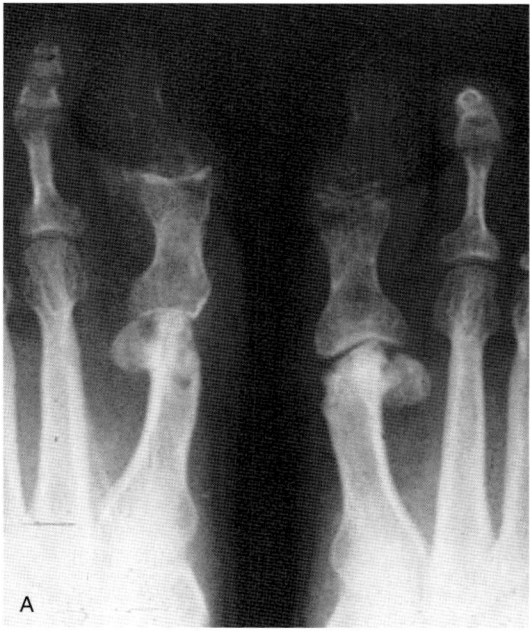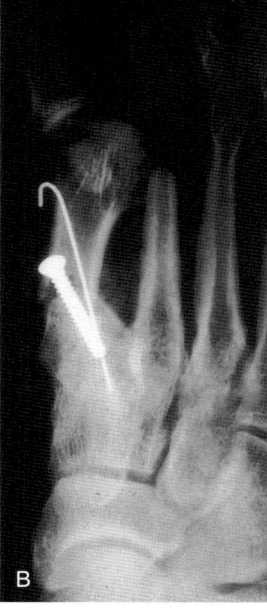

Figure 6-138 A, Avascular necrosis after a Mitchell-type osteotomy with loss of the entire head and collapse and severe shortening of the first ray. **B,** Malunion after a distal midshaft osteotomy is associated with very difficult salvage.

dorsal angulation or excessive medial or lateral deviation can result in a significant complication if not promptly recognized and corrected (see Fig. 6-138). Arthrofibrosis, though not common, may occur as well because of the extensive soft tissue dissection.

The design of this type of transverse osteotomy renders it relatively unstable and not very amenable to variations of internal fixation. Loss of correction,[276] delayed union,[366,369,370] nonunion,[366] and malunion[49,561,562] are all noted complications. The demanding technique with the high incidence of complications is the reason for the less frequent use of these types of procedures. If the hallux valgus deformity is mild, a distal chevron osteotomy, which is significantly more stable, is preferable; if the deformity is more severe, a distal soft tissue procedure with a proximal osteotomy may be advantageous. The Mitchell procedure is therefore used less commonly as more "user-friendly" proximal metatarsal osteotomies have become refined.

SCARF OSTEOTOMY

Meyer,[249,286] in 1926, is credited with first describing the longitudinal Z-type first metatarsal osteotomy, although both Burutaran[55] and Gudas[570] are also noted for early descriptions of this technique. However, Weil[40,546] and Barouk[22-24] popularized the procedure, and it was Weil who coined the name *scarf*.[40] *Scarf* is a carpentry term that describes a joint made by notching or cutting the ends of two pieces of wood and then securely fastening them together in one continuous piece so that they lap over each other (Video Clip 59).

Weil[546] described three different types of scarf osteotomy determined by the length of the longitudinal osteotomy: a short scarf osteotomy (25 mm long) used to treat hallux valgus with an IM angle of 13 degrees or less, also used for those with a higher DMAA[24]; a medium-length scarf osteotomy to treat an IM angle of 14 to 16 degrees; and a long scarf osteotomy to treat an IM angle of 17 to 23 degrees.

Many authors have recommended the use of a mid-shaft osteotomy combined with a distal soft tissue procedure as a primary procedure to correct moderate or severe hallux valgus, although an upper limit of a 20 degree IM angle has been recommended.[1,7] Several others have added an Akin osteotomy to the technique.[298,557]

The rationale for the procedure is in its versatility: the shaft of the first metatarsal is lateralized, thereby reducing the IM angle; plantar displacement is achieved to increase load on the first ray; the metatarsal can be shortened or lengthened; and a DMAA of up to 10 degrees can be addressed as well.[546]

Indications

A scarf osteotomy is indicated for the treatment of a symptomatic hallux valgus deformity of moderate or severe nature characterized by a 1–2 IM angle of 14 to 20 degrees,[23,130,286,491] a normal or slightly increased DMAA,[130] and adequate bone stock.[78]

Contraindications

Although there is apparently no age limit to the procedure, osteopenia in an elderly patient may be a relative contraindication.[78] Good bone density is important for stability of the osteotomy.[546] A scarf osteotomy is contraindicated for mild hallux valgus, for which a simpler, less complicated procedure is possible,[126] and in the presence of joint arthrosis,[286,546] restricted MTP range of motion,[546] or an open epiphysis.[286]

Technique

The surgical technique is divided into the surgical approach, osteotomy and fixation, and postoperative care.

Surgical Approach

1. A 5- to 8-cm medial longitudinal incision is made at the junction of the dorsal and plantar skin (Fig. 6-139A). It is started from a point just proximal to the IP joint and carried proximal to almost the MTC joint. The actual length of the proposed osteotomy determines the length of the actual skin incision.

2. A horizontal elliptic incision is used to excise redundant medial MTP joint capsule. The capsular flaps are developed with care taken to protect the dorsal and plantar sensory nerves. The small capillary network of plantar vessels just proximal to the sesamoids is protected, and release of the lateral metatarsal sesamoid ligament and lateral capsule is performed from the medial aspect. Rarely is the fibular sesamoid removed.

3. Alternatively, a separate interspace incision can be used for lateral capsular release. Care is taken to release the metatarsal sesamoid ligament and the lateral capsule as well.[278]

Preparation for the Osteotomy

1. A 0.045-inch K-wire is drilled in a lateral direction into the upper third of the distal first metatarsal, 2 to 3 mm from the dorsal metatarsal surface and 5 mm from the proximal dorsal metatarsal articular surface. It is also directed 15 degrees plantarward and slightly proximal as well. A second guide pin is drilled at the proximal extent of the proposed osteotomy, 2 to 3 mm from the plantar surface of the first metatarsal, at a distance approximately 1 cm from the MTC joint. It is also directed slightly plantarward and slightly proximal (parallel to the first wire). The direction of these guidewires determines the eventual angle of the osteotomy. As the osteotomy is later displaced, it will shift laterally and plantarward (Fig. 6-139B).

2. A thin oscillating or sagittal saw blade is used to create a vertical dorsal cut in the dorsal distal metatarsal neck at a right angle to the shaft in line with the K-wires. This osteotomy is located in the dense metaphyseal bone approximately 5 mm from the distal articular surface. It is inclined slightly proximally as the cut progresses in a medial-to-lateral direction (Fig. 6-139C and D).[22]

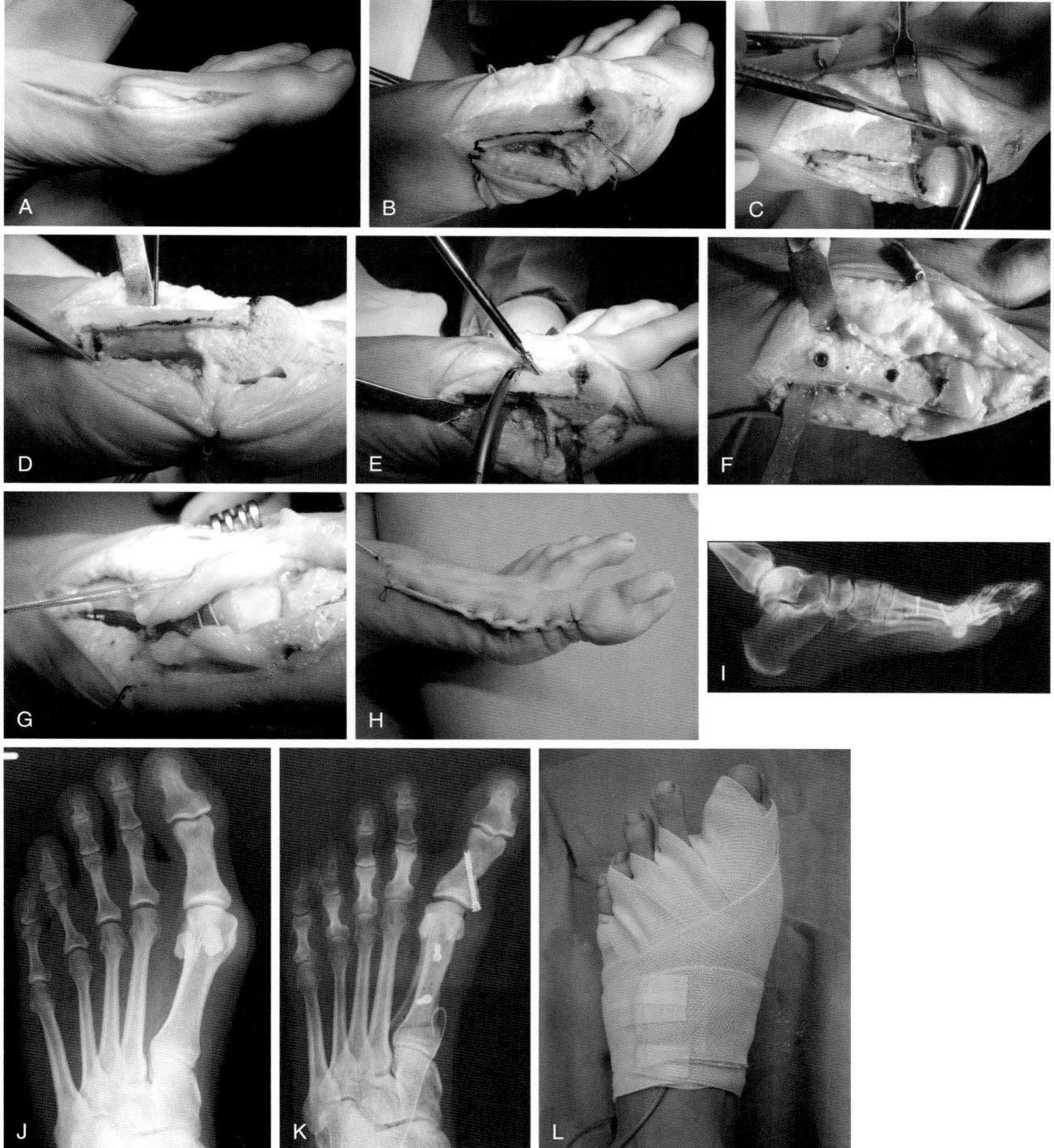

Figure 6-139 **A,** Medial longitudinal incision. **B,** Longitudinal osteotomy marked with Kirschner wires for orientation. **C,** Medial displacement and lateral release. **D,** Lateral displacement of the distal fragment. **E,** Lateral view. **F,** Dorsal view of internal fixation. **G,** Capsular closure. **H,** Skin closure. **I,** Lateral postoperative radiograph. **J,** Preoperative anteroposterior (AP) radiograph. **K,** Postoperative AP radiograph. **L,** Postoperative dressing.

3. The saw guide is then rotated on the wire so that it is parallel with the longitudinal axis of the first metatarsal but directed toward the inferior fourth of the proximal plantar cortex (where the second K-wire is located) (Fig. 6-140).

4. A longitudinal cut is made with a 20-mm sagittal saw blade. The length of the osteotomy largely depends on the desired correction.[40,546] A longer osteotomy is used to correct larger deformities. A shorter osteotomy is used to correct smaller deformities with larger DMAAs.

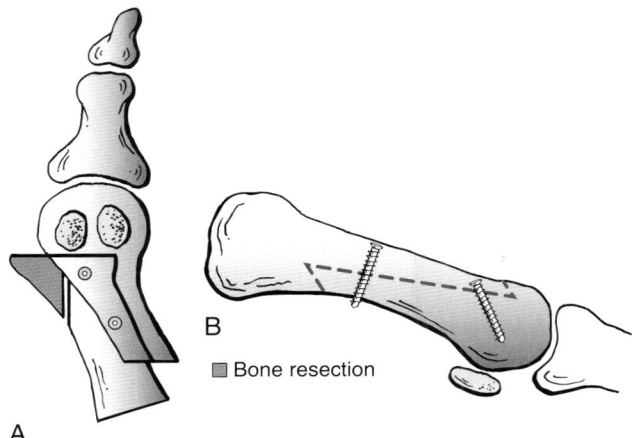

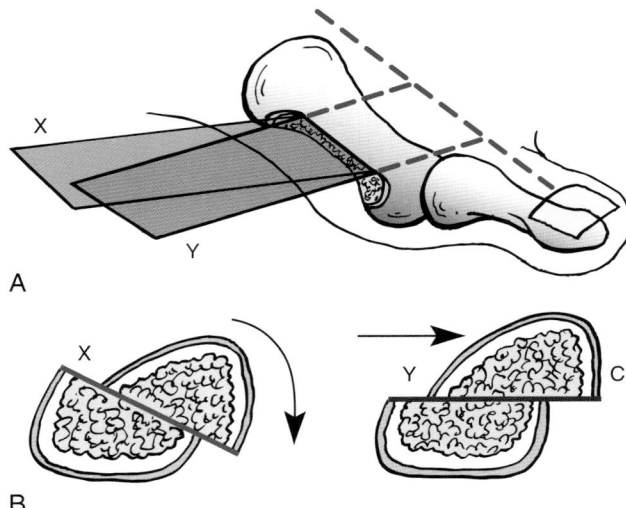

Figure 6-140 Displacement in a transverse plane. **A,** Dorsal view. **B,** Lateral view demonstrating the internal fixation.

Figure 6-142 Displacement in a frontal plane. **A,** Different planes of the cut. "Y" is from a direct medial approach that does not change the elevation C of the capital fragment; "X" shifts the capital fragment downward **(B).**

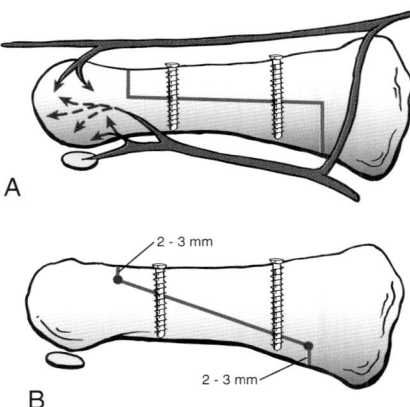

Figure 6-141 **A,** Dorsal and plantar circulation to the first metatarsal. **B,** After scarf osteotomy with internal fixation. The diagram also shows two techniques demonstrating variations in scarf osteotomy.

The typical length of the osteotomy is 30 to 35 mm, but the cut can extend almost the entire length of the metatarsal. As the osteotomy engages the lateral cortex, care is taken to avoid overpenetration into the first IM space because this may damage critical circulation to the metatarsal head and shaft. Barouk[23] suggests that the coronal level of the cut be located 2 to 3 mm from the dorsal surface distally and 2 to 3 mm from the plantar surface proximally (Fig. 6-141).

5. The third osteotomy is now performed. This cut exits the plantar aspect of the first metatarsal at a reverse 45-degree angle so that it acts as a locking mechanism as the osteotomy is translated. This cut is inclined slightly proximally as the cut progresses in a medial to lateral direction[23] so that it is parallel with the more distal cut.

6. The osteotomy is now complete, and the distal fragment should be mobile. A clamp is placed on the proximal plantar fragment to both stabilize it and pull

it medialward as the distal dorsal fragment is shifted lateralward. Lateral translation can be performed maximally to two thirds the width at the level of the metatarsal head. After displacement of the osteotomy, a bone clamp is placed to secure the reduction.

7. The osteotomy is internally stabilized with two screws directed from the dorsal medial aspect to the plantar lateral aspect of the diaphysis[198] (Fig. 6-142). Barouk[23] has advocated a self-compressing cannulated headless screw for internal fixation. Barouk suggests that an oblique distal screw should fixate the metatarsal metaphyseal-head region, and a second dorsoplantar screw should stabilize the proximal osteotomy (see Fig. 6-139E and F).

8. The excess bone remaining on the medial aspect of the metatarsal is then resected with a power saw. Although this entails removing a portion of the diaphysis and the medial eminence, care should be taken to preserve the plantar medial MTP joint articulation to avoid disturbing sesamoid function.

9. In more severe cases, an Akin osteotomy is added.[23,115,130,286,546]

Soft Tissue Repair

1. The medial capsule is repaired with interrupted absorbable suture to realign the hallux; however, overplication should be avoided (see Fig. 6-139E). The subcutaneous tissue is also approximated along the course of the exposure, and the skin is closed in routine fashion.

2. A gauze-and-tape compression dressing is applied to protect the repair (see Fig. 6-139L).

The patient is allowed to ambulate in a postoperative shoe, with weight borne as tolerated on the heel and outer aspect of the foot.

Postoperative Care

The gauze-and-tape compression dressing is removed 1 week after surgery, radiographs are obtained, and the patient is instructed in postoperative range-of-motion exercises. At 1 week after surgery, Weil[546] allows patients to progress to a roomy athletic shoe as tolerated and dressings are discontinued. At 7 weeks after surgery, if radiographs demonstrate adequate healing, the patient is allowed to resume regular activities. Coetzee et al[78] suggest treatment with a below-knee cast for 2 weeks and partial weight bearing with dressings for an additional 4 weeks. Rehabilitation is then commenced (see Fig. 6-139I and J).

Key Points in the Technique

Displacement in a transverse plane: The distal fragment can be merely translated laterally in the case of a severe deformity or rotated medially with the translation to reduce an increased DMAA. When both transverse cuts are made parallel to each other, it is a pure translational displacement (see Fig. 6-140).

Displacement in a frontal plane: To elevate the distal fragment in the case of a cavus foot, the longitudinal cut is made directly lateralward. To lower the head, the cut is made in a plantar direction, inclined approximately 15 degrees plantar-laterally (see Fig. 6-142).

Displacement in a sagittal plane: The osteotomy can be lengthened; however, lengthening may result in diminished MTP range of motion.[23] Shortening can be achieved by greater inclination of the transverse cuts, but it can also be achieved by resection of bone proximally and distally. This may have the effect of increasing range of motion of the MTP joint.

Complications

With the complexity of the scarf osteotomy come numerous possible complications,[203] including undercorrection or recurrence,[23,77,115,286,546] overcorrection, hallux varus,[23,465,546] degenerative arthritis,[115,286] loss of fixation,[79,115,286] and delayed union.[79] Schoen et al[465] reported a 20% incidence of hallux varus in their series.

AVN has been reported after a scarf osteotomy (Fig. 6-143).[465,546] Dereymaeker[130] makes the point that extensive soft tissue stripping should be avoided with this procedure. Proximally, only the medial plantar surface is elevated; distally, the dorsal aspect of the distal metatarsal is exposed. In both areas, the vascular leash supplying the first metatarsal is protected (see Fig. 6-141).

Popoff et al[424] and Newman et al[390] found in laboratory studies that a scarf osteotomy was much stronger than other types of proximal osteotomies. Adequate rigid internal fixation is necessary, and there have been multiple methods for fixation suggested.[368,389] Nonetheless, fractures can develop either acutely or in delayed fashion after surgery. Intraoperatively, if any of the cuts are not complete, twisting or translating the fragments may cause a fracture to develop[130,491]; Smith et al[491] also noted that fractures developed by overtightening the compression screws. A fracture places the osteotomy at high risk for elevatus

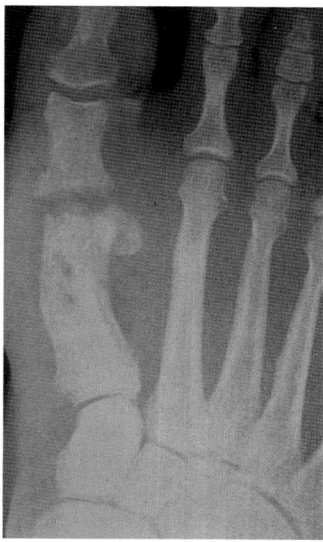

Figure 6-143 Osteonecrosis of first metatarsal head after scarf osteotomy. (Courtesy C. Coetzee, MD.)

and lateral metatarsalgia[23,546] or a subsequent stress fracture.[23,77,546] This usually occurs in the proximal metatarsal in the area of the transverse cut. If the remaining dorsal cortex is too thin, a stress fracture may occur. Weil[546] stressed the need to "plantarize" the transverse cut by placing it in the plantar third to fourth of the metatarsal. Pressure on the osteotomy leads to a fracture of the dorsal cortex, not the plantar cortex.[390,546] Barouk[23] reported a 3% incidence of stress fractures in his early experience.

Malunion of the osteotomy can develop as a result of shift and displacement of the diaphyseal segments. "Troughing" occurs when the cortices of the two halves of the metatarsal shaft wedge into the softer cancellous bone of the metatarsal shaft.[381] Troughing is like roofing tiles that fit together in an overlapping fashion and occurs with lateral shift of the distal segment. It is more common with osteopenia.[130,546] Troughing causes dorsiflexion of the first ray and can lead to lesser MTP joint metatarsalgia or overload. Also with this displacement, rotation can occur, which can be a very difficult situation to salvage.[77] To avoid this complication, the osteotomy must be kept in metaphyseal cancellous bone; the step cut should be only 2 to 3 mm into cancellous bone at the distal and proximal extent of the osteotomy (Figs. 6-144 and 6-145A-C).[77] The concept of troughing has been well described by Coetzee,[78] along with solutions on how to avoid it.[78] Coetzee has found it extremely important to create short arms (3 mm), with the distal arm close to the joint to avoid a sinking effect of the cortical ridge into the soft intramedullary cancellous bone. Others have also described modifications to avoid this complication.[381]

Weil[546] reported that diminished MTP range of motion occurs less often than in other bunion procedures, possibly because of the implementation of early exercise. Weil[546] reported average dorsiflexion of 70 degrees, but others have noted less motion.[115,465] Crevoisier et al[115]

Part II ■ Forefoot

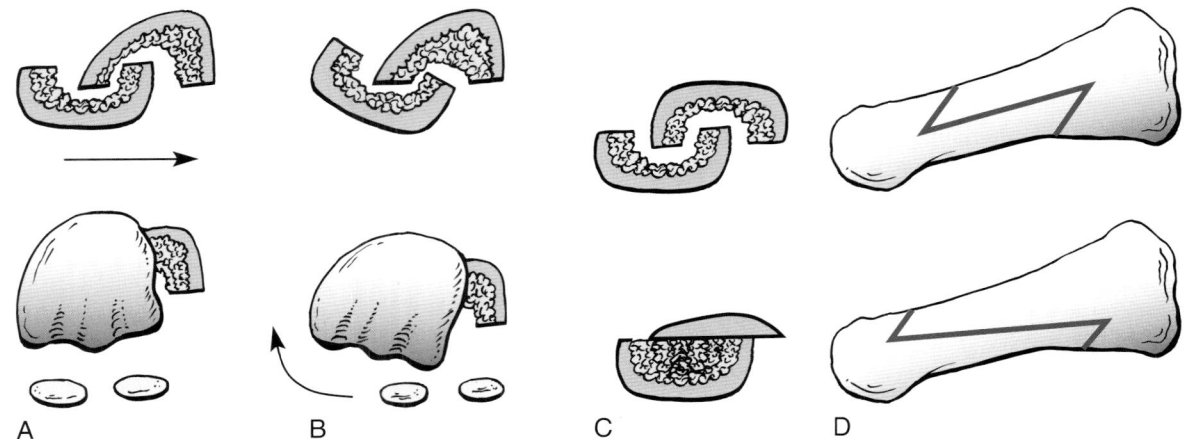

Figure 6-144 Complications of scarf osteotomy. **A,** Troughing. **B,** Troughing with malrotation. **C,** Troughing can occur as a result of making the osteotomy in the diaphyseal region. **D,** By maintaining the osteotomy in the dense bone of the metaphyses, troughing can often be avoided. (Modified from the technique of L.S. Weil, DPM, and C. Coetze, MD.)

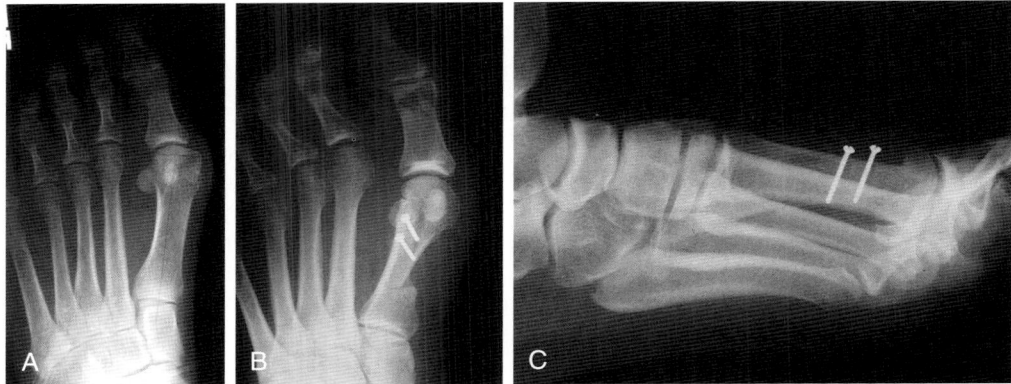

Figure 6-145 **A,** Preoperative anteroposterior standing radiograph of a moderate bunion deformity. **B** and **C,** Postoperative radiographs illustrating the troughing complication of the scarf osteotomy.

reported that 65% of patients in their series had diminished motion, which they attributed to the extensive exposure.

Results

Subjective satisfaction is reported to be routinely high and varies from 89% to 98%,[40,115,253,465,546] although Dereymaeker[130] reported that the results were slightly inferior when she compared scarf osteotomy with distal chevron osteotomy. Kundert and Fuhrmann[289] reported recurrence of the deformity in 25% of cases. Average correction of the hallux valgus angle varies from 15 to 19 degrees,[115,124,130,253,546] and average correction of the 1–2 IM angle varies from 4 to 10 degrees.* Plantar displacement of the first ray varies from 1 to 3 mm.[40,130,546]

Dereymaeker[130] found that scarf osteotomy did not achieve adequate correction of the DMAA in her series. Barouk[22] suggested that this is the ideal situation for a "short scarf" (25 mm long) because it allows lateral

rotation of the distal fragment to reduce the DMAA. A longer scarf osteotomy would not be able to rotate adequately into the IM space.

Day et al[121] subsequently reported using this technique and reduced the average DMAA from 20 to 4.5 degrees.

There is no question that the scarf technique is technically demanding,[40,286,540] and there is a difficult learning curve as well.[78,546]

DISTAL SOFT TISSUE PROCEDURE WITH PROXIMAL OSTEOTOMY

Review of the experience with the distal soft tissue procedure in a historically significant series[336] led to the conclusion that a soft tissue procedure alone was insufficient to completely and consistently correct a hallux valgus deformity when the IM angle exceeds 12 degrees. Those authors subsequently advocated a proximal crescentic metatarsal osteotomy to correct the increased IM angle. The results of the specific technique have since been reported in several studies (Video Clip 56).*

---

*References 30, 36, 40, 76, 115, 121, 124, 130, 133, 163, 169, 243, 253, 271, 284, 315, and 546.

*References 101, 136, 140, 344, 409, 516, and 535.

It is that study that has served as the foundation for the use of proximal first metatarsal osteotomies in the vast majority of moderate and severe bunion deformities.

The advantage of the crescentic osteotomy is that it minimizes the changes in first metatarsal length that is inherent to many osteotomies and also creates a broad stable osteotomy construct. A proximal chevron or long oblique osteotomy produces results quite similar to those of a proximal crescentic osteotomy.* Substantial shortening or lengthening of the first ray is rarely necessary. In a study of more than 7000 feet, Harris and Beath[211] found that the first and second metatarsals were frequently of either equal length or within a few millimeters of each other in length.

Wedge osteotomies of the proximal first metatarsal have gained popularity over recent years. Although a lateral closing-wedge osteotomy[435,472,543] has been proposed for reduction of the increased 1–2 IM angle, it does so with the risk that more bone may be removed dorsally than plantarward, which may lead to metatarsal dorsiflexion, as well as shortening, as the osteotomy is closed. This combination of shortening and dorsiflexion often leads to transfer metatarsalgia. Conversely, an opening-wedge osteotomy of the first metatarsal has also been suggested for reduction of the IM angle. This osteotomy has the inherent problem of decreased stability at the osteotomy site, one that requires open grafting and plate fixation. Furthermore, there is the concern that lengthening the first metatarsal may lead to increased tension on both soft tissues and within the first MTP joint. This is of particular concern with more severe cases of hallux valgus, as the extrinsic tendons and other soft tissue structures crossing the MTP joint are placed under greater force. Goldner and Gaines[186] concluded that an opening-wedge proximal first metatarsal osteotomy tightens the extensor mechanism and leads to postoperative recurrence of a hallux valgus deformity. A high rate of recurrence has been reported in the past with opening-wedge metatarsal osteotomies,[38,186,472] although more recent reports do show good results with newer fixation systems and modified techniques.[82,433,483,497] In addition, the lengthening effect created by the osteotomy has been found to be relatively small.[53,458] Contraindications to this technique would include those patients with a long first metatarsal or those with preoperative hallux MTP joint stiffness.[563]

Indications

A moderate or severe hallux valgus deformity with an incongruent (subluxated) MTP joint is the main indication for these procedures. As a general rule, the hallux valgus angle usually exceeds 30 degrees and the IM angle is greater than 13 degrees. Although there is no specific upper limit to the deformity that this procedure can correct, complete correction is often not possible with a hallux valgus angular deformity in excess of 55 degrees or

an IM angle greater than 25 degrees. A deformity with an IM angle less than 12 degrees will typically not require an osteotomy; if at surgery, however, there is resistance to reduction of the 1–2 IM angle or if a lateral facet is present at the base of the first metatarsal (see Fig. 6-63), an osteotomy is indicated. In addition, the proximal osteotomy may be preferred for those patients requiring an extensive soft tissue release of the hallux metatarsophalangeal joint, regardless of the IM angle. The procedure is versatile and can be performed in patients of all ages, from juvenile (assuming physeal closure) to octogenarian.

Contraindications

Contraindications to distal soft tissue reconstruction with a proximal first metatarsal osteotomy include the presence of significant arthrosis, severe metatarsus adductus,[93] and spasticity of any type. A distal soft tissue reconstruction should also be avoided in the presence of a congruous MTP joint (with a DMAA > 15 degrees)[93,312,516] because recurrence, degenerative arthrosis, or postoperative stiffness could result. Coughlin[91] reported that the final angulation of the MTP joint mirrored the magnitude of the DMAA preoperatively; thus, with substantial sloping of the metatarsal articular surface, soft tissue realignment of the MTP joint is contraindicated.

Technique: Crescentic Osteotomy

A crescentic osteotomy has been advocated as the means to correct an increased 1–2 IM angle without significantly altering the length of the first metatarsal.[93,335] The osteotomy is located in the first metatarsal metaphysis because this area provides a broad contact area, which promotes rapid healing, and a relatively large surface area, which affords stability in a dorsoplantar direction.

Initially, the crescentic osteotomy was performed with the concavity directed distally toward the great toe.[95,335] The authors noted, however, that if the osteotomy site was inadvertently displaced medially and the metatarsal head was translated too far laterally, an incongruent MTP joint and, in some cases, hallux varus resulted (Fig. 6-146). This prompted a reverse of the direction so that the concavity was directed toward the heel (Fig. 6-147), a technique now commonplace.[140,344,409] With the concavity oriented proximally, the center of the rotational axis of the osteotomy is centered at the MTC joint,[452] thus making this correction much more anatomic and biomechanically sound. This also reduces the possibility of displacing the metatarsal head too far laterally or creating a malunion.

Distal soft tissue reconstruction is performed in association with a proximal first metatarsal osteotomy and in a manner as previously described. After the lateral capsular tissues have been released, the medial capsule opened, and the medial eminence resected, the IM angle is tested to see whether an osteotomy is indicated. The first metatarsal head is pushed laterally toward the second metatarsal. A tendency for these two metatarsals to spring apart indicates insufficient mobility at the MTC joint to permit

---

*References 41, 51, 53, 82, 140, 182, 183, 348, 388, 395, 433, 454, 455, 483, 498, 510, and 558.

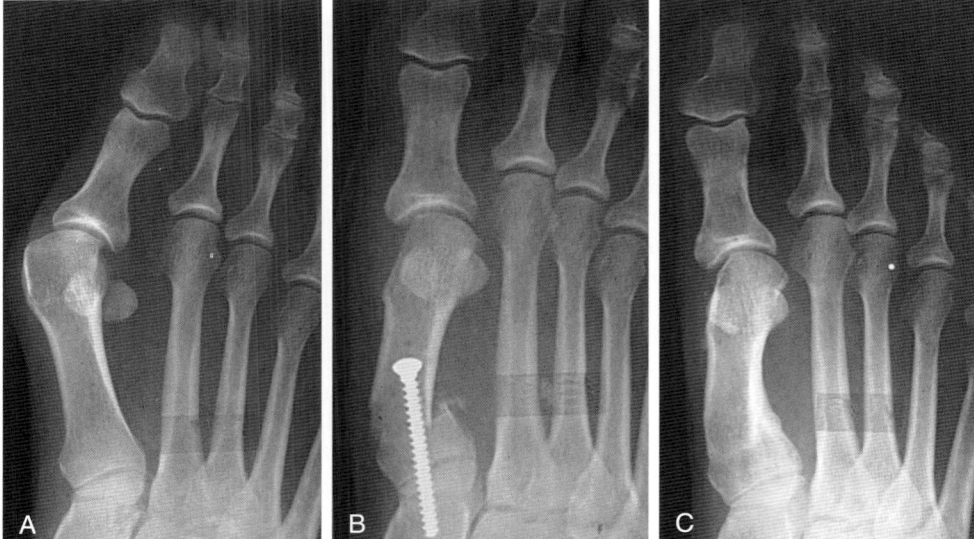

Figure 6-146 Overcorrection of a proximal osteotomy. **A,** Preoperative radiograph demonstrating a moderate hallux valgus deformity. **B,** Overcorrection of the 1–2 intermetatarsal angle with a proximal metatarsal osteotomy and resection of excessive medial eminence. **C,** Six-year follow-up radiograph demonstrating a mild hallux varus deformity. The patient had no symptoms, but progression of varus deformity is possible.

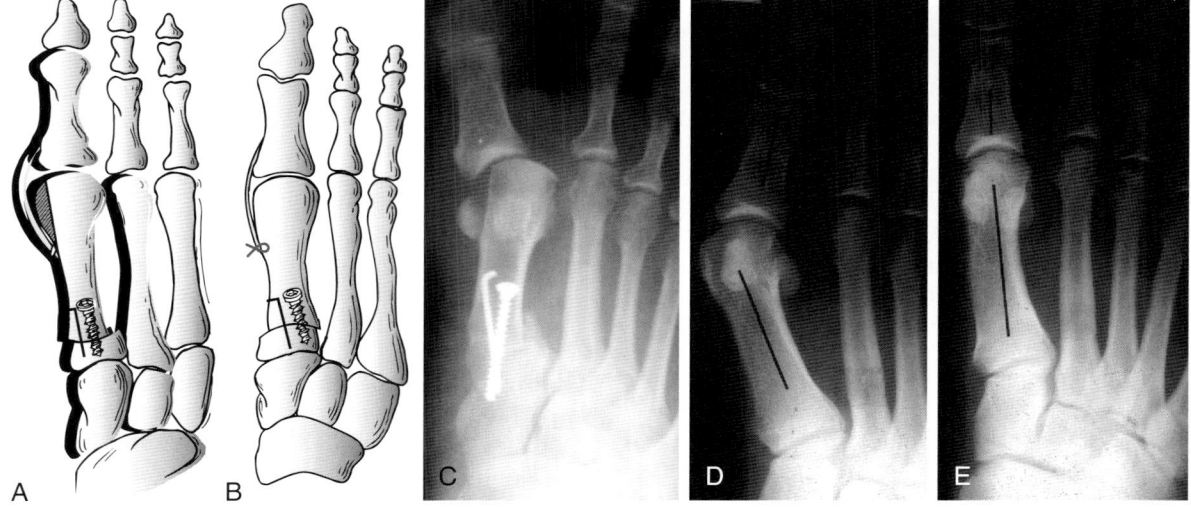

Figure 6-147 Proximal crescentic metatarsal osteotomies. **A,** With the concave surface oriented distally. **B,** With the concave surface oriented proximally. **C,** After osteotomy with the concavity oriented distally, overcorrection and hallux varus have resulted; medial displacement of the osteotomy results in excessive lateral displacement of the metatarsal head. Before **(D)** and after **(E)** osteotomy with the concavity oriented distally. Note that this orientation prevents medial displacement of the osteotomy site and therefore prevents overcorrection of the metatarsal head. For this reason, the authors now always carry out the crescentic osteotomy with the concavity directed (proximally) toward the heel.

reduction of the IM angle, and an osteotomy is indicated (see Fig. 6-93B and C).

1. Following the two distal incisions on the medial aspect of the MTP joint, and in this first inter space, a third incision is made on the dorsal aspect of the base of the first metatarsal over the extensor hallucis longus tendon. The incision starts just proximal to the MTC joint and is carried distally for about 3 cm. It is deepened through

the subcutaneous tissue to expose the extensor tendon. The extensor tendon is retracted medially or laterally to expose the metatarsal shaft (Fig. 6-148).

2. The MTC joint is identified with the tip of the knife blade, and the osteotomy site is located approximately 1 cm distal to the MTC joint (Fig. 6-148B). A screw (and K-wire) is generally used for fixation of the osteotomy site and is inserted approximately 1 cm distal to the osteotomy site.

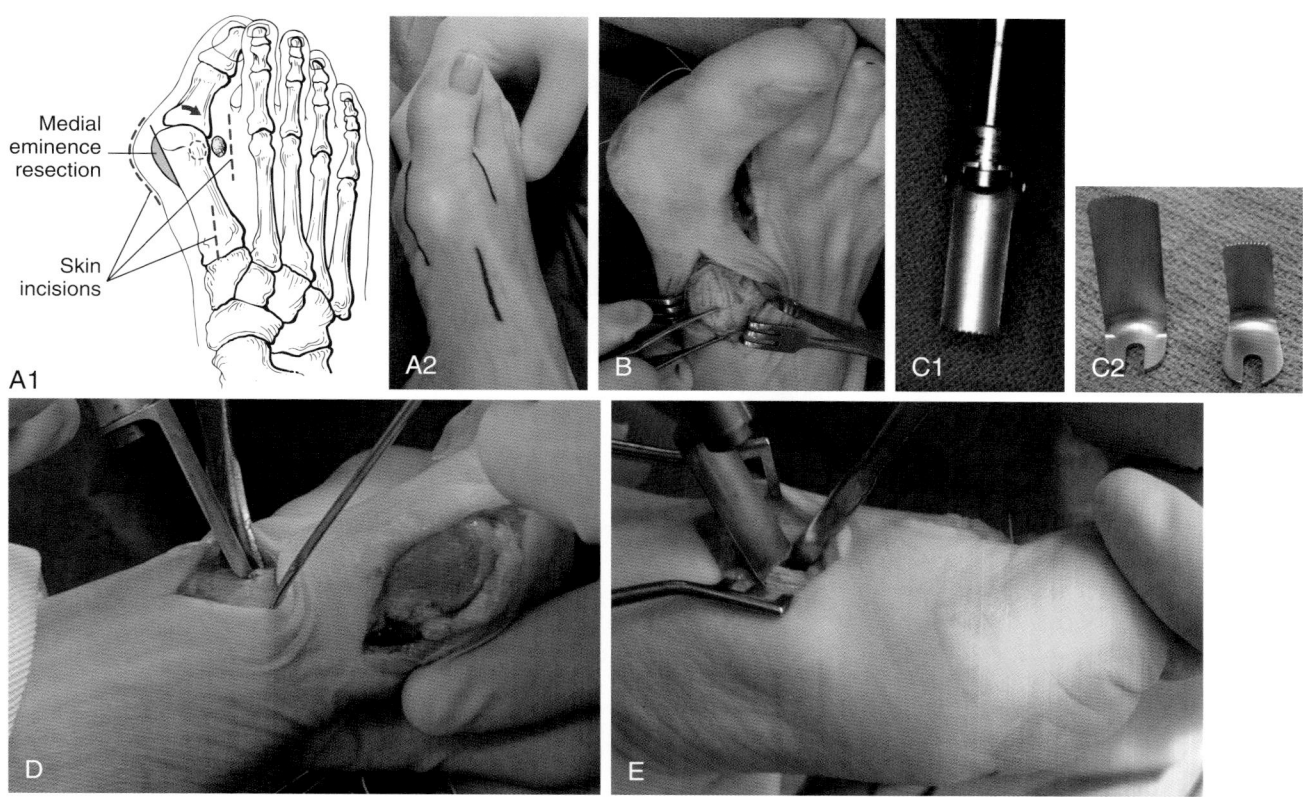

Figure 6-148 **A,** Incisions for distal soft tissue realignment with a proximal first metatarsal osteotomy. **B,** The incision for the osteotomy is made 1 cm distal to metatarsocuneiform joint. **C,** Saw blade used for crescentic osteotomy. **D,** Orientation of the saw blade with the concave surface oriented proximally. **E,** Orientation of the saw blade with the concave surface oriented distally.

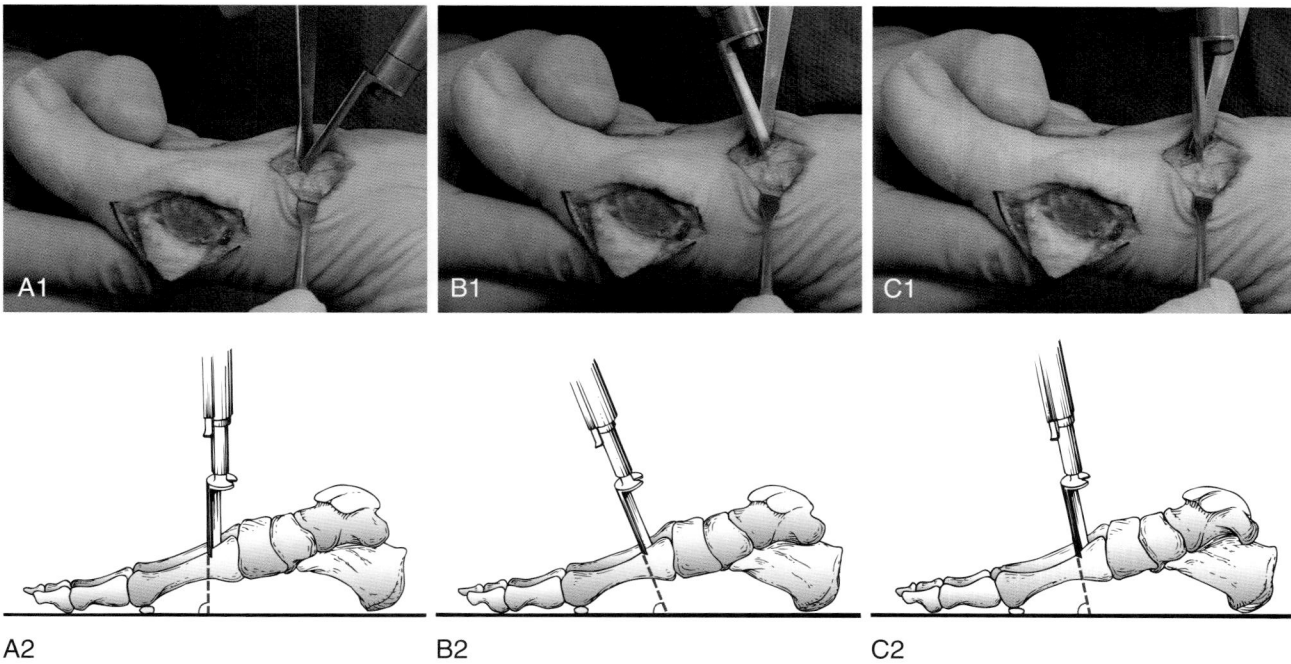

Figure 6-149 Errors in position of the saw blade. The crescentic osteotomy is placed 1 cm distal to the metatarsocuneiform joint or 8 mm distal to the open epiphysis in a juvenile. A lateral view of the osteotomy demonstrates the angle of the cut. The concave surface is proximal. **A,** This angle is incorrect because the blade is perpendicular to the floor. **B,** Incorrect angle of the osteotomy because the angle is too oblique. There is less contact at the osteotomy site. **C,** Correct angle of the osteotomy. The correct angle is neither perpendicular to the first metatarsal shaft nor perpendicular to the plantar aspect of the foot.

3. If a screw is used to fix the osteotomy, the initial glide hole is created at this time. A 3.5-mm drill bit is used to make a hole at an angle of about 45 to 50 degrees to the metatarsal shaft, with the bit passing into the metatarsal approximately 5 mm (Fig. 6-150H). A countersink is used to lower the screw head. If a 4.0-mm cannulated screw is used, the guide pin is inserted and overdrilled later in the procedure.

4. The osteotomy is created with a crescentic blade so that the concavity is directed proximally (see Fig. 6-148C-E). The plane of the osteotomy is perpendicular to neither the first metatarsal nor the bottom of the foot; rather, it is halfway between (see Fig. 6-149). In the coronal plane, it is critical that the saw blade be neither medially nor laterally rotated. Medial rotation can lead to elevatus. Often, the leg of the patient externally rotates, and if care is not taken, inadvertent medial rotation of the saw blade may occur. To help avoid this error a vertical 0.045-inch K-wire can be placed in the medial cuneiform as a guide while holding the foot in a plantigrade position (see Fig. 6-212). The saw blade is held parallel to the wire during the osteotomy, thus minimizing malrotation of the blade.[250] As the osteotomy is performed, the saw blade must exit the lateral aspect of the metatarsal shaft to ensure that the osteotomy is completed along this margin of the

metatarsal. If it is not, it is difficult to complete the osteotomy in this narrow area, and the communicating artery may be damaged. If the osteotomy is not completed along the medial side, it is simple to finish the cut with a 4-mm osteotome. Once the osteotomy is complete, a Freer elevator is used to ensure that it is completely mobile and that any periosteal hinge that might prevent displacement of the osteotomy is released. The crescentic saw blade comes in two lengths, one 4 mm longer than the other. As the osteotomy is being performed, if the shoulder of the blade impinges on the skin just proximal to the osteotomy site, the longer blade (No. 2296-31-416S7, 277-31-415, or 277-31-416S1, Stryker, Kalamazoo, Mich., or No. 5053-176, Zimmer, Wausau, Ind.) is used. The surgeon should not undertake this osteotomy without having both blades available. Again, care must be taken to avoid either medial or lateral rotation of the saw blade because such rotation may lead to plantar flexion or dorsiflexion at the osteotomy site.

5. A Freer elevator is used to displace the proximal portion of the metatarsal base in a medial direction as far as possible (Fig. 6-150B and C). The index finger is used to push the metatarsal head in a lateral direction, which displaces the osteotomy site laterally. The displacement at the osteotomy site is usually only 2 to

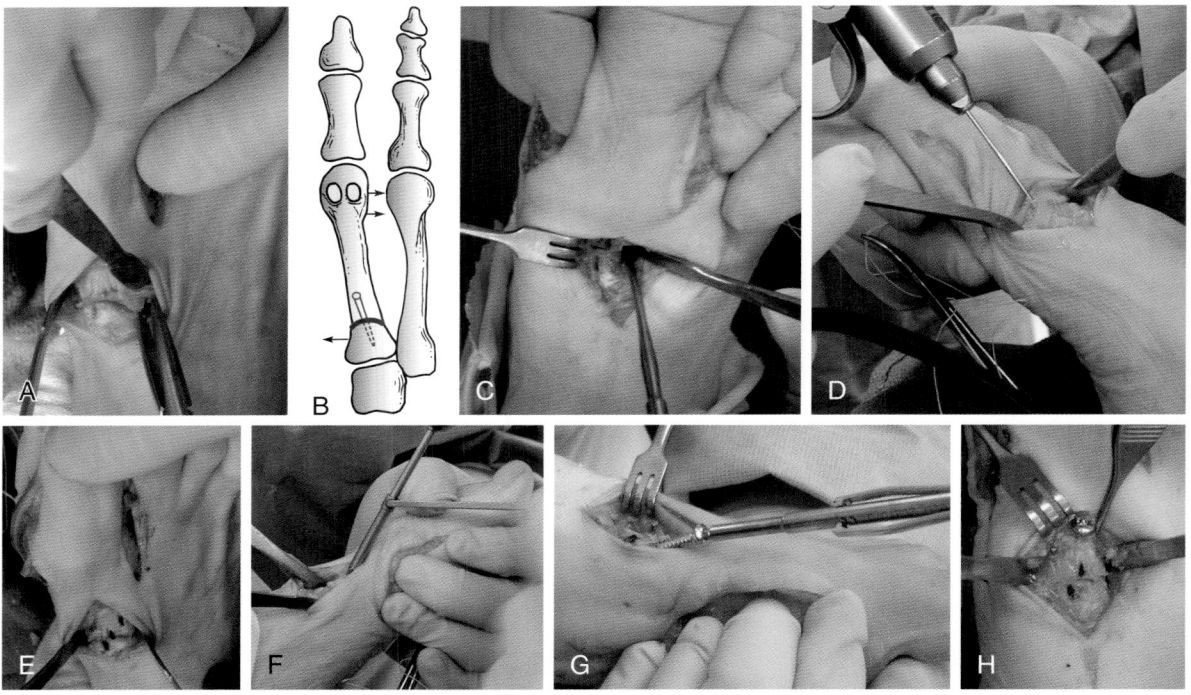

Figure 6-150 **A,** Exposure of the osteotomy site in the proximal portion of the metatarsal. A rongeur is used to remove the lateral spike of bone that frequently prevents displacement of the osteotomy. **B,** Diagram demonstrating that the proximal fragment is displaced medially as far as the metatarsocuneiform joint will permit while the metatarsal head is pushed laterally against the second metatarsal. **C,** Intraoperative photograph demonstrating the Freer elevator pushing the proximal fragment medially and the surgeon's hand pulling the first metatarsal head laterally against the second metatarsal. **D,** Kirschner wire stabilizes the osteotomy site. **E,** Note that the osteotomy site is displaced 2 to 3 mm laterally. **F,** The hole is drilled at a 45-degree angle to the long axis of the metatarsal. **G,** The screw is placed approximately 1 cm distal to the osteotomy site. **H,** After placement of the wire and screw.

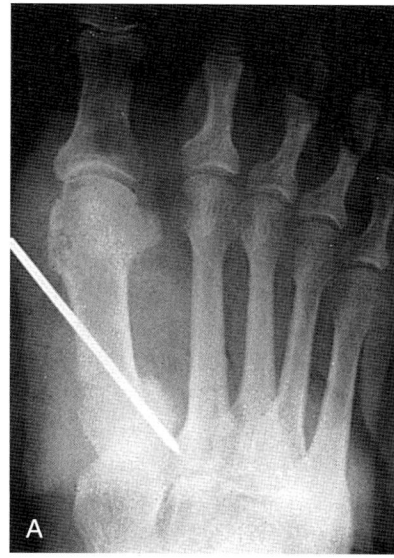 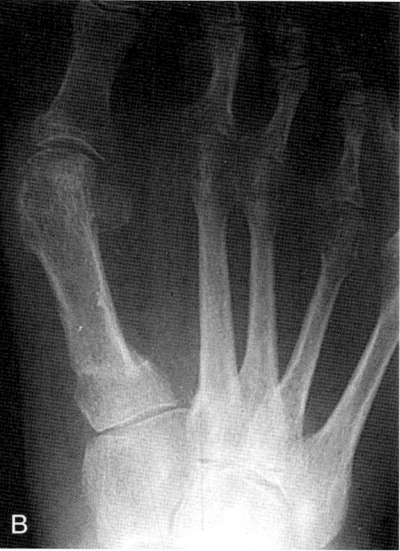

Figure 6-151 Fixation of the osteotomy site with an oblique ⁵⁄₆₄-inch Steinmann pin. Because of the high infection rate, this is rarely used except with unsuccessful internal fixation. **A,** Radiograph demonstrating the pin driven into the tarsal bones for added stability. Note that when the osteotomy site was reduced, the proximal fragment was not displaced medially on the cuneiform. **B,** After removal of the pin, the proximal fragment drifted in the medial direction on the cuneiform, which resulted in incomplete correction of the intermetatarsal angle and recurrence of the hallux valgus deformity because of the lack of medial displacement of the proximal fragment.

3 mm because a small degree of translation proximally accounts for much movement distally. Care must be taken to not overcorrect the osteotomy site. If the osteotomy site does not move freely, some medial periosteum is still attached and must be released so that the osteotomy can be rotated laterally. On occasion, a small spike of bone on the lateral aspect of the distal fragment must be removed to allow rotation of the osteotomy (Fig. 6-150A). At this point, the distal fragment can be slightly displaced plantarward (about 2 mm) to compensate for any possible dorsiflexion angulation at the osteotomy site. To ensure that the osteotomy site is not being held in a dorsiflexed position, the metatarsal head is pushed slightly plantarward until the osteotomy site just begins to open up. However, excessive plantar flexion may displace the MTC joint and should be avoided.[510]

6. While holding the osteotomy in a corrected position, the osteotomy is generally fixed with both a 0.062-inch K-wire (Fig. 6-150D and E) and a 4.0-mm small-fragment compression screw to provide rotational stability, as well as compression (Fig. 6-150F-H). The screw hole is also countersunk to lower the profile of the screw head and to prevent cracking the island of bone between the screw and osteotomy site. Other than revision cases or in patients with osteopenia, the wire may be removed before closure, which will reduce the risk of postoperative infection (Fig. 6-151). There have been recent reports of fixing the crescentic osteotomy with a plate construct as opposed to screw fixation for improved stability. The use of a plate also avoids penetration of the MTC joint.[72,532]

Technique: Medial Opening Osteotomy

Many surgeons have found the crescentic osteotomy to be a challenging technique requiring an appreciation of spatial positioning. The medial opening osteotomy is a single-plane transection and easier for the occasional bunion surgeon to conceptualize. The technique typically uses wedge-plate fixation to maintain the medial opening while providing stability for this inherently unstable osteotomy.

1. The medial based incision used for exposure of the MTP joint is extended proximally to the MTC joint, with care taken to avoid transecting superficial nerves. Periosteum is sharply reflected off of the medial aspect of the proximal one third of the metatarsal. The MTC joint does not require exposure.

2. The osteotomy is made approximately 1.5 cm distal to the MTC joint, as confirmed using fluoroscopic imaging. The angle of the bone cut is generally made perpendicular to the axis of the metatarsal, but some surgeons will make the cut oblique proximally, which will minimize the lengthening effect of the opening wedge (Fig. 6-152A).

3. Fluoroscopic imaging is used to follow the osteotomy to, but not through, the lateral cortex (Fig. 6-152B). The osteotomy is then gradually opened using a spreader device, joy stick, or osteotome (Fig. 6-152C). The soft tissues progressively stretch, and the lateral cortex fatigues as a greenstick.

4. Four hole plates, locked and nonlocked, are available with multiple options for wedge length. The wedge size is determined intraoperatively and based on the severity of the IM angle. The 3- and 4-mm sizes are the most commonly used. Larger sizes may create a distraction effect along the lateral cortex, negating the medial opening-wedge correction, and should be avoided. The plate is usually positioned directly medial on the first metatarsal (Fig. 6-153). However, in cases of metatarsalgia or overload on the lesser metatarsals (as may occur with hypermobility, pes planus), the plate can be placed more dorsal to create plantar flexion at the osteotomy.

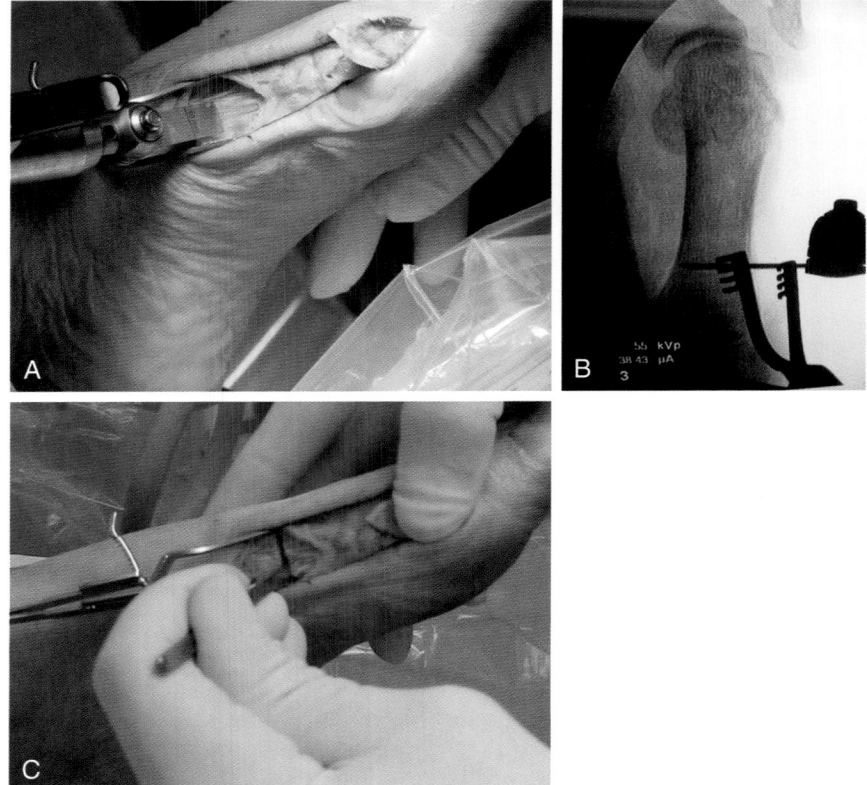

Figure 6-152 A, Medial approach to the proximal first metatarsal. Saw blade is positioned perpendicular to the long axis of the bone, approximate 15 mm from the metatarsocuneiform joint. **B,** Fluoroscopic image confirms proper level of the bone cut and is also used to advance the blade just short of the lateral cortex. **C,** An osteotome can be used to gently greenstick the lateral cortex and reduce the intermetatarsal 1–2 angle.

5. Bone graft obtained from the medial eminence previously resected is used to fill the opening in the osteotomy. In revision cases, autogenous calcaneal bone graft or allografts can be used.

Long Oblique Osteotomy (Mau, Ludloff)

In the case of a long first metatarsal, the surgeon may use a long oblique proximal osteotomy to avoid the lengthening effect of the opening-wedge technique. Multiple types and modifications have been described.[16,388,446,455,522] The modified Mau technique has been advocated by Glover et al.[183] Their medial approach is similar to the medial opening technique described previously, and the modification uses a shorter osteotomy than in the traditional Mau technique (Fig. 6-154A).

1. The periosteum is elevated in line with the osteotomy, with the proximal portion of the osteotomy placed at least 1 cm distal to the first MTC joint. The saw blade is kept parallel to the weight-bearing surface of the foot to prevent unwanted dorsal angulation of the first metatarsal head, which could occur after completion of the osteotomy (Fig. 6-154B and C).
2. To maintain complete control of the osteotomy, a guidewire for the cannulated screw is placed perpendicular in the completed proximal portion of the osteotomy. The osteotomy can then be completed dorsal-distally without fear of losing the orientation.
3. Reduction can be achieved with large reduction clamps or by using a Freer elevator on the lateral portion of the proximal fragment and placing counterpressure on the first metatarsal head. Intraoperative fluoroscopy is recommended after placing temporary fixation to achieve an IM angle less than 9 degrees (Fig. 6-154D).
4. Placing a screw too distal may cause fracture of the dorsal portion of the osteotomy site. Allow adequate space between the screws and the distal aspect of the osteotomy to prevent fracture (Fig. 6-154E-G).

Reconstruction of Hallux Valgus Deformity

1. After the proximal osteotomy is completed and before fixation, (regardless of the specific type of osteotomy chosen) attention is directed to the first web space, where two sutures are placed to approximate the adductor hallucis tendon to the lateral capsular tissues along the border of the first metatarsal head (see Fig. 6-94). If such approximation is not accomplished at this time, it is difficult to later expose the adductor tendon in the depths of the interspace after the osteotomy site has been displaced and stabilized.

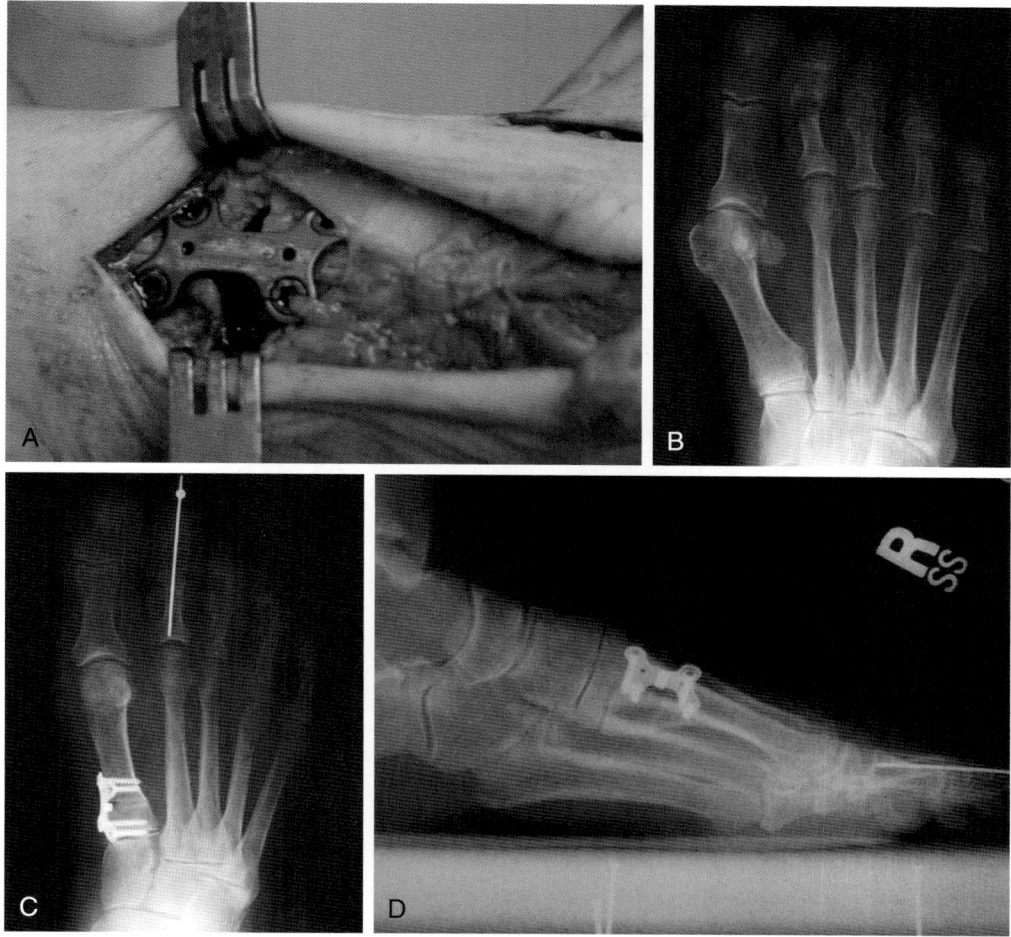

Figure 6-153 A, A 3-mm wedge plate is applied to the medial aspect of the first metatarsal, with option for locking screws. **B,** Preoperative radiograph of a 50-year-old woman with a symptomatic bunion deformity. Postoperative standing anteroposterior **(C)** and lateral **(D)** radiographs at 5 weeks, illustrating correction with medial opening-wedge technique and healing of the osteotomy.

2. Once the osteotomy site is stabilized, the sutures in the first web space are tied and the medial capsular tissue is repaired as previously described for the distal soft tissue procedure. The skin is approximated in routine manner (Fig. 6-155).

3. Intraoperative fluoroscopy may be beneficial to evaluate the correction of the IM angle, as well as to evaluate the position of the internal fixation. In addition, fluoroscopic imaging is recommended to evaluate alignment of the first MTP joint, ensuring that there is no overcorrection into varus.

4. Postoperatively, the foot is wrapped in a gauze-and-tape compression dressing to hold the hallux in correct alignment or in slight overcorrection if a severe deformity has been corrected (Fig. 6-156A).

Postoperative Care

As previously described for the distal soft tissue procedure, the foot is re-dressed weekly for 6 to 8 weeks (Fig. 6-156B). It is unusual to cast the foot postoperatively,

although a cast may be necessary in an unreliable patient or one with precarious internal fixation. Radiographs are obtained at the first office visit after surgery. Based on this radiograph, the toe is dressed in a neutral position, varus, or valgus. The patient is allowed to ambulate in a stiff-soled postoperative shoe, with weight bearing mainly on the heel and outer aspect of the foot for 8 weeks after surgery. After the final dressings are removed, the patient is permitted to ambulate, as tolerated, in a sandal or soft, wide shoe. Sutures are removed 2 to 3 weeks after surgery. MTP joint range-of-motion exercises are initiated 3 to 4 weeks after surgery, while the foot is still maintained in a postoperative dressing. An intensive walking program is begun 7 to 8 weeks after surgery.

Should the MTC joint be penetrated with internal fixation, as with the crescentic procedure, the hardware can be removed after successful healing at the osteotomy site, typically 6 to 8 weeks after surgery. Coughlin and Shurnas[110] reported that internal fixation crossed the MTC joint in 13 of 35 proximal crescentic cases. The hardware

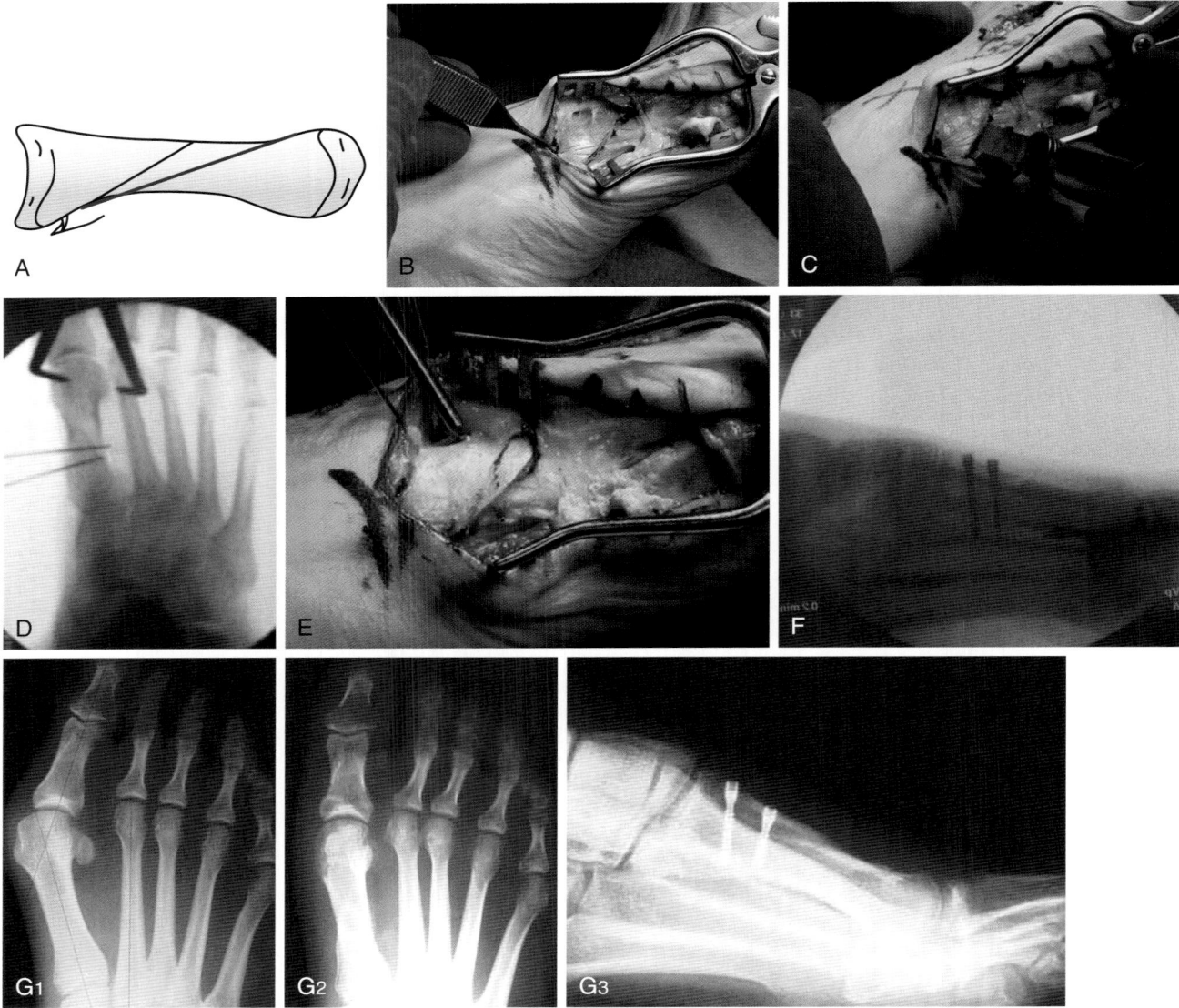

Figure 6-154   A, The modified osteotomy exits more proximal than the traditional line of the osteotomy *(in red).* **B,** Medial approach to the first metatarsal and the marking of the osteotomy, with the metatarsocuneiform (MTC) joint identified. **C,** Note that the proximal cut exits distal to the MTC joint. **D,** The correction and reduction of the intermetatarsal 1–2 angle can be obtained with a clamp while the osteotomy is temporarily secured with guide wires. **E,** The osteotomy is fixed with two screws. **F,** Screws are positioned away from the thin dorsal distal cortex to avoid fracturing. **G1,** Preoperative standing anteroposterior (AP) radiograph of a moderate bunion deformity. Postoperative standing AP **(G2)** and lateral **(G3)** showing correction obtained.

was removed 6 weeks after surgery, and at long-term follow-up, they did not identify degenerative arthritis in the MTC joint.

The degree of swelling varies among patients, but usually within 4 to 5 months after surgery, the thickening about the joint and swelling of the foot have subsided.

Results

Reported patient satisfaction rates after proximal first metatarsal osteotomy vary from 78% to 93%.* Most of what has been written has dealt with the crescentic

technique as popularized by Mann. Mann et al[344] reviewed 109 feet in which a distal soft tissue procedure and proximal crescentic osteotomy were performed. The major preoperative complaint was pain over the medial eminence in 75% of patients, around the first MTP joint or sesamoids in 7%, in the lesser toes in 7%, and from other causes in 11%. Ninety-three percent of patients were satisfied postoperatively. Of the 7% dissatisfied, half complained of pain and half complained of the varus or valgus position of the hallux. At final follow-up, 39% of patients believed that they could perform more activities on their feet, 57% thought that their level of activity was unchanged, and 4% said that their level of activity was

---

*References 63, 101, 344, 435, 452, 488, and 516.

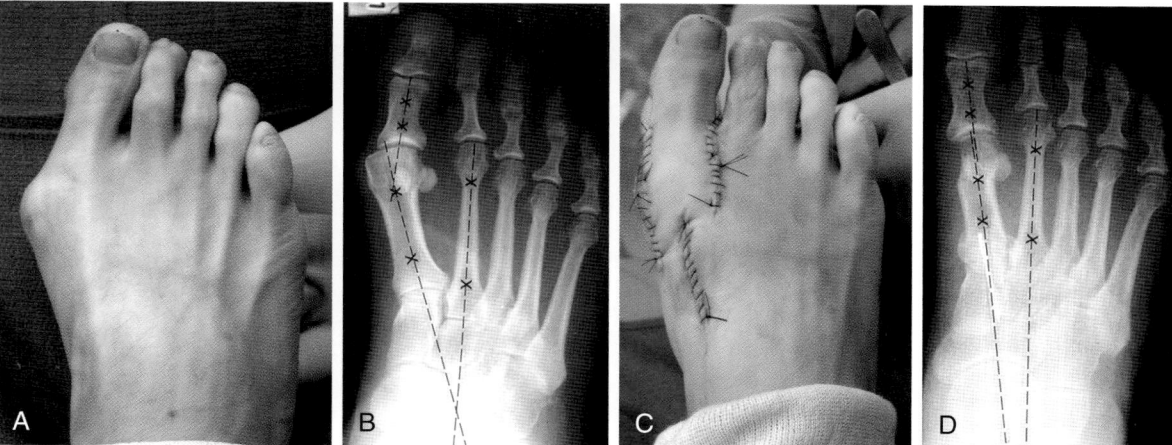

Figure 6-155 Distal soft tissue realignment with first metatarsal osteotomy. Preoperative clinical appearance **(A)** and radiograph **(B)** demonstrating a moderate hallux valgus deformity with metatarsophalangeal (MTP) subluxation (hallux valgus angle, 34 degrees; 1–2 intermetatarsal (IM) angle, 15 degrees; distal metatarsal articular angle, 10 degrees) and a subluxated MTP joint. Postoperative clinical appearance **(C)** and radiograph **(D)** 5 years after a distal soft tissue procedure with a proximal metatarsal osteotomy. The alignment has been corrected (hallux valgus angle, 5 degrees; 1–2 IM angle, 4 degrees).

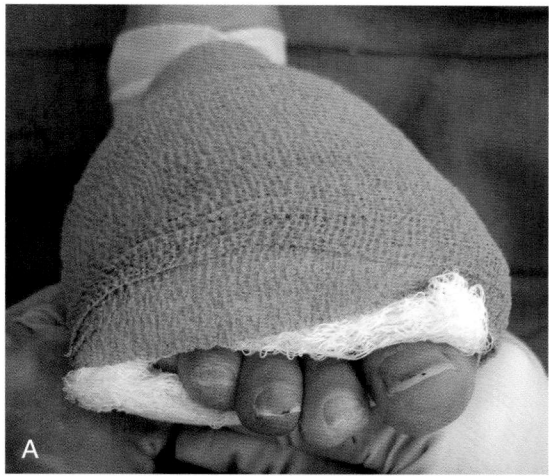
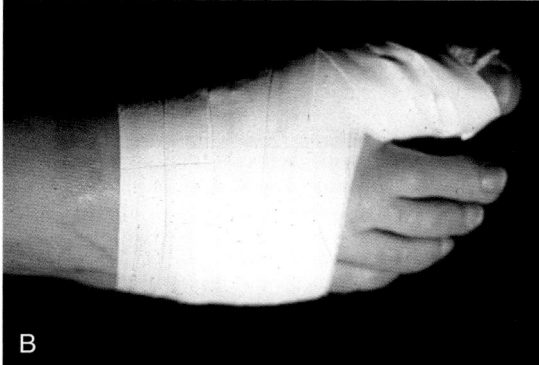

Figure 6-156 **A,** Immediate postoperative dressing. **B,** Dressing used for the remainder of treatment.

Table 6-4	Summary of 109 Feet before and after Distal Soft Tissue Procedures with Proximal Crescentic Osteotomy	
Angle	Preoperative	Postoperative
Average hallux valgus	30°	9°
Average first/second intermetatarsal	13°	5°

From reference 344.

diminished. Preoperatively, 30% of patients could wear any shoe that they desired, and postoperatively, 59% could. Still, 41% were unable to wear the shoe of their choice.

The average correction of the hallux valgus angle is consistently reported to be 23 to 24 degrees,* (Fig. 6-155) with the degree of improvement being directly proportional to the severity of the preoperative deformity (Fig. 6-157).[41,344] Mann[334] reported that with more severe deformities, an average hallux valgus correction of 30 degrees was achieved. Average correction of the 1–2 IM angle is 8 to 11 degrees after a crescentic osteotomy,[95,101,335,344,516] 3 to 6 degrees after a closing-wedge osteotomy,[435,472] and 7 degrees after an opening-wedge osteotomy.[312,488] Tables 6-4 and 6-5 summarize correction of the hallux valgus and IM angles achieved in the series and by subgroups. Reporting on 33 cases of correction of a juvenile hallux valgus deformity with distal soft tissue reconstruction and proximal first metatarsal osteotomy, Coughlin[95] noted an average 23-degree correction of the hallux valgus angle and an average 8-degree correction of the 1–2 IM angle, results identical to those reported by Mann[335] in adult patients. In the only prospective study of this procedure published, Coughlin and Jones[101]

*References 101, 136, 335, 344, 435, and 516.

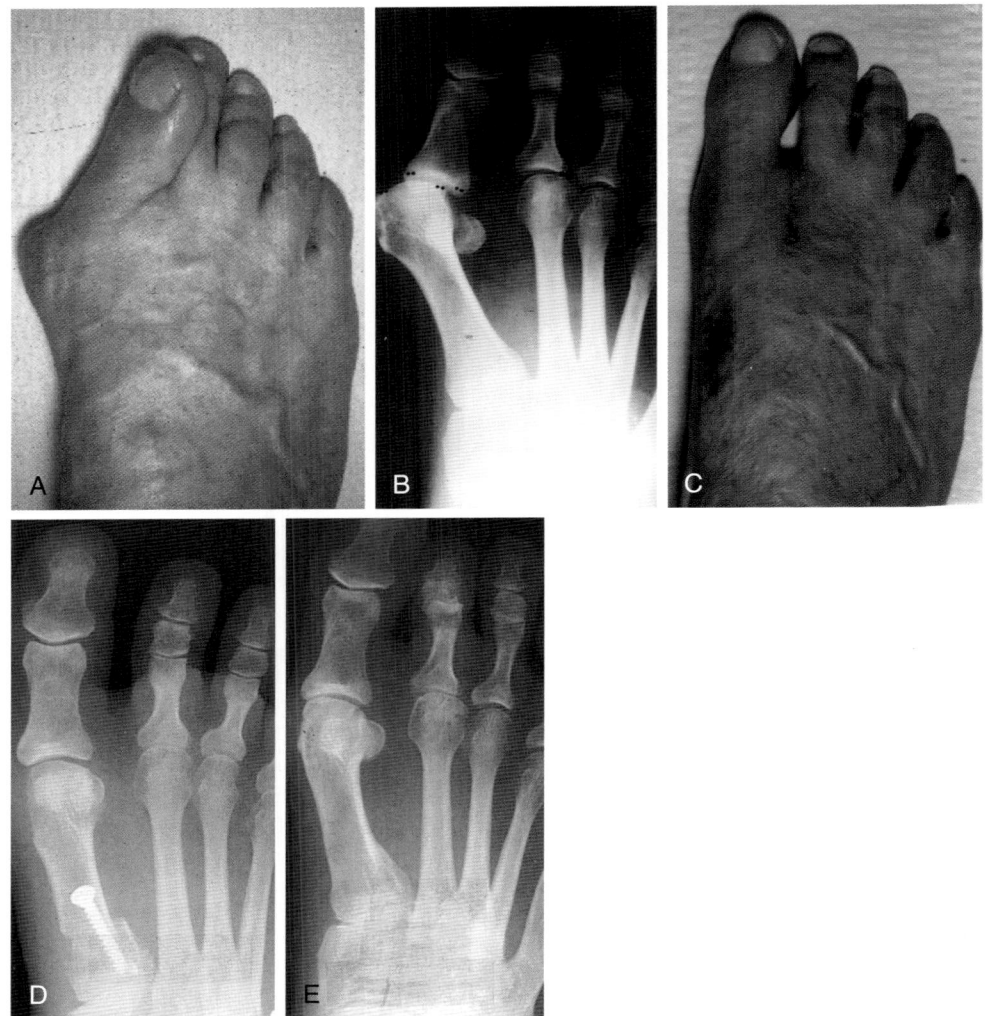

Figure 6-157 Correction of severe deformity. Preoperative clinical **(A)** and radiographic **(B)** appearance. Postoperative clinical **(C)** and radiographic **(D)** appearance. **E,** Follow-up radiograph 5 years after surgery.

Table 6-5	Summary of Results by Severity of Deformity in Distal Soft Tissue Procedures with Proximal Crescentic Osteotomy		
	Mild (< 20°)	**Moderate (21°-40°)**	**Severe (> 40°)**
Number of feet	9	87	13
Mean age (yr)	48	52	59
Mean Hallux Valgus Angle			
Preoperative	17°	30°	46°
Postoperative	3°	9°	13°
Mean First/Second Intermetatarsal Angle			
Preoperative	11°	13°	16°
Postoperative	5°	6°	5°
Hallux Varus			
Mean deformity 5.4°			
<6°, 9 cases			
>6°, 5 cases (2 dissatisfied)			

From reference 344.

reported an average 20-degree correction of the hallux valgus angle and an average 10-degree correction of the IM angle.

Mann et al[344] further observed that before surgery, 48 feet (44%) had a symptomatic callus beneath the second metatarsal head and that postoperatively, 30 of these calluses had resolved, 13 were unchanged but no longer painful, and 5 remained painful but no new lesions had developed. Coughlin and Jones[101] reported a 47% incidence of concomitant lateral metatarsalgia in patients who were scheduled to undergo surgical correction for moderate and severe hallux valgus deformities. Overall, the first metatarsal was shortened an average of 2.2 mm, a finding identical to that in other reports in the literature on proximal first metatarsal osteotomies.[309,348,409,454] Rather than shortening, there is a risk of lengthening with the opening-wedge osteotomy technique. This may alter plantar forefoot pressures as well as create increased joint surface compression at the hallux metatarsophalangeal level. Studies have shown that the lengthening effect is minimal and the risk of creating joint degeneration is minimal.[53,433,458,483,563] It is recommended that the opening-wedge technique be avoided in those patients with long first metatarsals and hallux metatarsophalangeal stiffness.[563]

As Easley et al[140] observed, in patients with moderate and severe hallux valgus deformities, evaluation of transfer lesions is hampered by the fact that forefoot problems are not isolated to the hallux and frequently involve the second and third MTP joints as well. Whereas some have suggested a relationship between first metatarsal shortening and metatarsalgia[543] or elevatus and metatarsalgia,[543] others have found no correlation.* When the metatarsal is already short before surgery, Schemitsch and Horne[463] found a positive correlation between further shortening of the first metatarsal and metatarsalgia.

Dorsiflexion at the osteotomy site should be avoided with all proximal osteotomy techniques. Brodsky et al[51] found that sagittal-plane correction is difficult with the crescentic osteotomy in particular, thus resulting in unpredictable plantar forefoot pressures. Mann et al[344] observed on lateral weight-bearing radiographs that 28% of the feet demonstrated the first metatarsal to be slightly dorsiflexed, although the magnitude was not quantified.

With the crescentic procedure, saw position and rigid internal fixation are important principles in avoiding elevatus.[88,93,313,501] Lippert and McDermott[313] found that medial or lateral rotation of the saw blade altered the eventual position of the distal first metatarsal head after the osteotomy was displaced. Medial rotation of the saw led to elevation, and lateral rotation led to plantar angulation after displacement of the osteotomy. Jones et al,[250] in a cadaveric and laboratory study, demonstrated a linear relationship between metatarsus elevatus and saw blade orientation. For every 10 degrees of saw blade angulation, a 2-mm change in the sagittal position of the distal first metatarsal was noted. They then used a K-wire to help orient the saw blade to avoid malrotation of the saw and substantially improved the accuracy of the osteotomy in a cadaveric study. Rigid fixation to prevent malunion,

*References 44, 188, 266, 344, 348, 370, 427, and 435.

preferably with locking screws, is also mandatory with the inherently unstable wedge osteotomies.[82,497]

Joseph[256] quantified MTP joint range of motion in normal subjects and reported total MTP motion of 87 degrees with an average dorsiflexion of 67 degrees and average passive plantar flexion of 20 degrees. In reports documenting postoperative MTP range of motion after proximal osteotomy and distal soft tissue repair, total passive motion ranged from 64 to 86 degrees.[91,95,535] Coughlin[95] noted an average loss of 12 degrees when compared with the nonoperated side in juveniles and an average loss of 11 degrees in adults.[91] Mann et al[344] reported that patients demonstrated 55 degrees of dorsiflexion and 9 degrees of plantar flexion for a total range of 64 degrees at midterm follow-up after surgery. Veri et al[535] reported that preoperative total range of motion averaged 86 degrees; at a minimum 1-year follow-up, range of motion averaged 69 degrees; however, at a mean follow-up of 8 years, total motion averaged 86 degrees. In a cadaver study in which range of motion was measured immediately before and after a distal soft tissue procedure and proximal metatarsal osteotomy, Coughlin et al[102] reported that the total range of MTP joint motion decreased from 85 to 62 degrees. There was a significant loss of dorsiflexion motion but not plantar flexion motion. Thus there appears to be an initial loss of motion after the realignment procedure that is probably due to intrinsic muscle tightness. Initiation of early range-of-motion activities may help diminish the eventual loss of motion, but patients should be counseled that it is not unusual to lose some motion as a consequence of the procedure (Fig. 6-158).

Two reports in the literature compared proximal crescentic osteotomy with proximal chevron osteotomy for the correction of hallux valgus (Fig. 6-159).[140,348] In both reports, the results were essentially the same with regard to correction of the hallux valgus deformity and IM angle and relief of lateral metatarsalgia. The main difference was the lack of dorsiflexion at the osteotomy site, as noted occasionally after proximal crescentic osteotomy, but statistically, it did not appear to affect either the incidence of new transfer lesions or the resolution of existing lesions. The chapter authors believe that either procedure

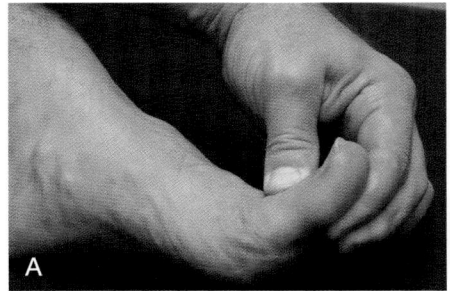
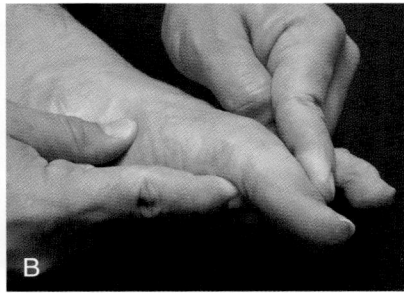
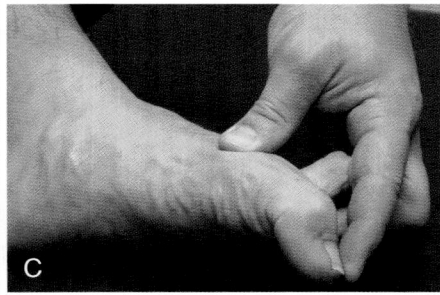

Figure 6-158 Passive dorsiflexion **(A)** and plantar-flexion **(B)** range-of-motion exercises are important in regaining motion. Pressure placed on the proximal phalanx stretches the metatarsophalangeal (MTP) joint. **C,** Incorrect stretching places stress on the interphalangeal joint instead of the MTP joint.

will result in satisfactory correction of the hallux valgus deformity, and it is the surgeon's preference which of these osteotomies should be used. Although Lian et al[311] reported proximal chevron and crescentic osteotomy to be of equal strength in resisting failure with dorsiflexion, criticism of the strength of the osteotomy and its fixation has been presented by McCluskey et al[360] and by Campbell et al.[57] These groups found both proximal chevron and oblique closing-wedge osteotomy to be stronger constructs.

Chiodo et al[66] reported the results of 70 cases in which a Ludloff oblique osteotomy was performed for moderate and severe hallux valgus deformities. The average hallux valgus angle was corrected 20 degrees, and the 1–2 IM

angle was corrected 9 degrees. In the sagittal plane, the first metatarsal was plantar flexed 1 mm. No transfer lesions were reported; varus occurred in 4 of 70 patients and delayed union in 3 of 70. The authors suggested that the plane of the osteotomy and the rigidity of the internal fixation placed the osteotomy site at minimal risk of dorsiflexion malunion. Glover et al[182] compared the modified Mau technique to the crescentic and found similar healing, correction, and patient satisfaction rates but with fewer complications.

Coughlin[95] noted that, in general, proximal osteotomy techniques are less successful in correcting a congruent joint but, with a subluxated joint, have a relatively high success rate. Mild residual deformity or degenerative arthritis may develop if one fails to appreciate the presence of an increased DMAA (see Figs. 6-56 to 6-59). Mild degenerative arthritis has been reported at both the MTP joint[344,535,543] and the MTC joint,[101,543] although it is rarely symptomatic. Correction has been found to be more reproducible in those with "moderate" as opposed to "severe" preoperative deformities.[395]

Complications

Potential complications after a distal soft tissue procedure have been listed previously. Complications after proximal osteotomy include shortening, metatarsalgia, failure of internal fixation, overcorrection (hallux varus) (Fig. 6-160), undercorrection (or recurrence) (Fig. 6-161), delayed union, and malunion (Figs. 6-162 and 6-163).

Shortening or dorsiflexion at the osteotomy site predisposes to the development of lateral metatarsalgia (Fig. 6-164), whereas lengthening the first metatarsal through an opening-wedge osteotomy may lead to stiffness and degeneration of the hallux metatarsophalangeal joint. Mann et al[344] reported a 28% incidence of dorsiflexion at the osteotomy site (although some deformities were

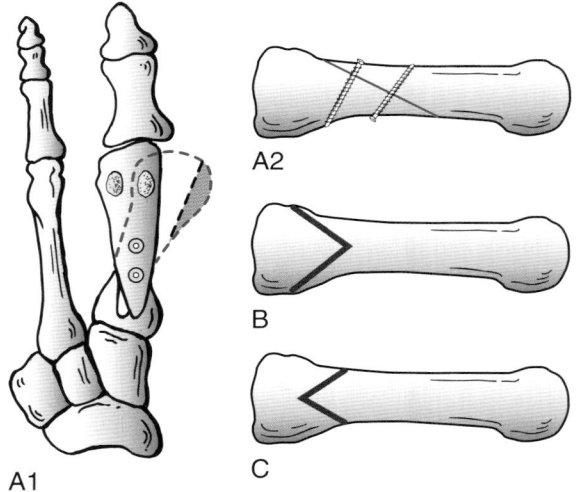

Figure 6-159 **A1** and **A2,** Ludloff osteotomy. **B,** Proximal chevron osteotomy (base proximal). **C,** Proximal chevron osteotomy (base distal).

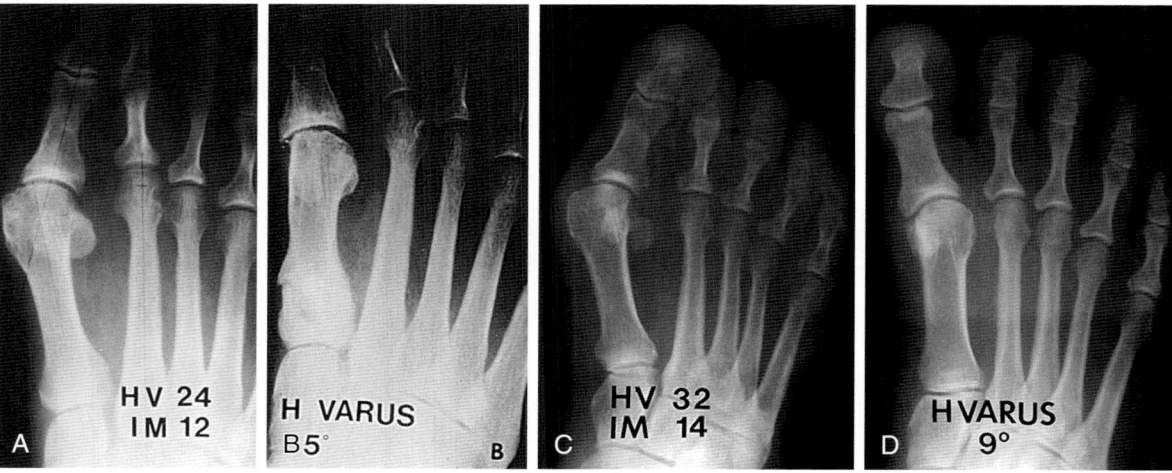

Figure 6-160 Hallux varus after a distal soft tissue procedure and proximal metatarsal osteotomy. **A** and **B,** Preoperative and postoperative radiographs, respectively, demonstrating 5 degrees of varus. **C** and **D,** Preoperative and postoperative radiographs, respectively, demonstrating 9 degrees of hallux varus. Hallux varus of this magnitude is rarely of clinical significance and represents mainly a radiographic finding.

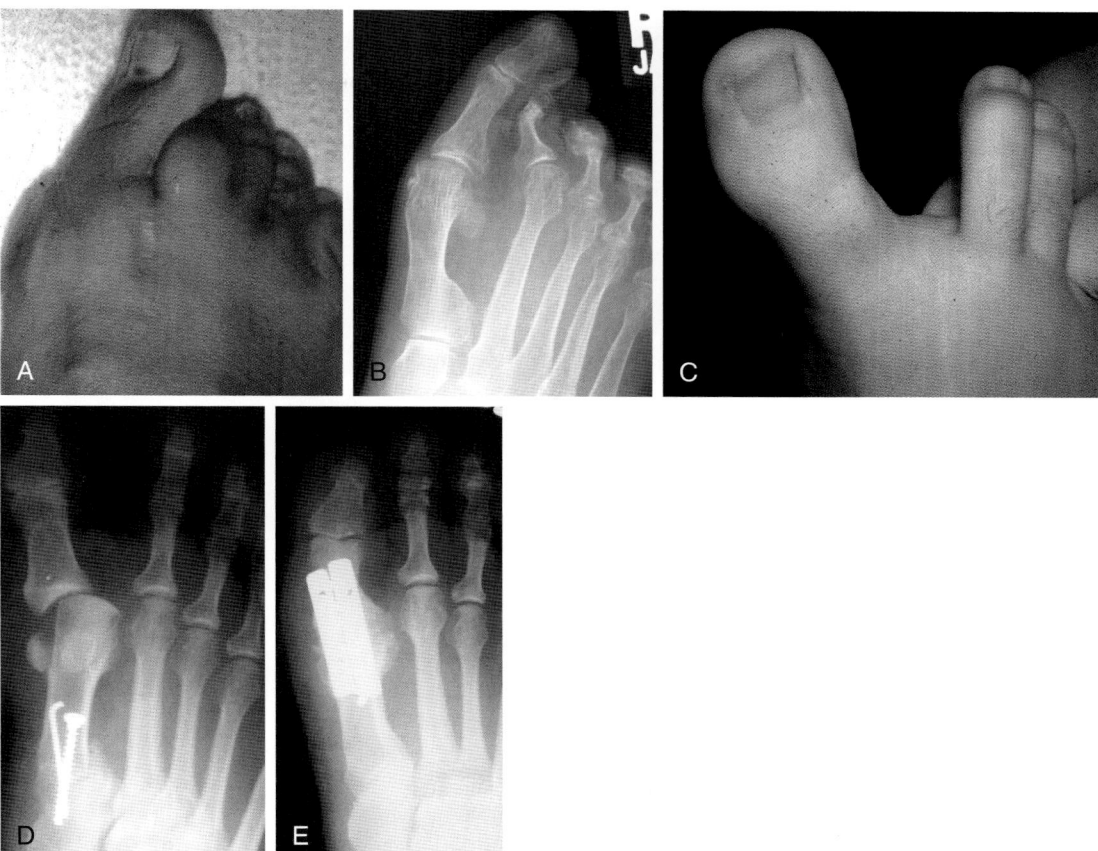

Figure 6-161 Clinical **(A)** and radiographic **(B)** examples of severe recurrence. Clinical **(C)** and radiographic **(D)** appearance of severe varus. **E,** Salvage with metatarsophalangeal joint arthrodesis.

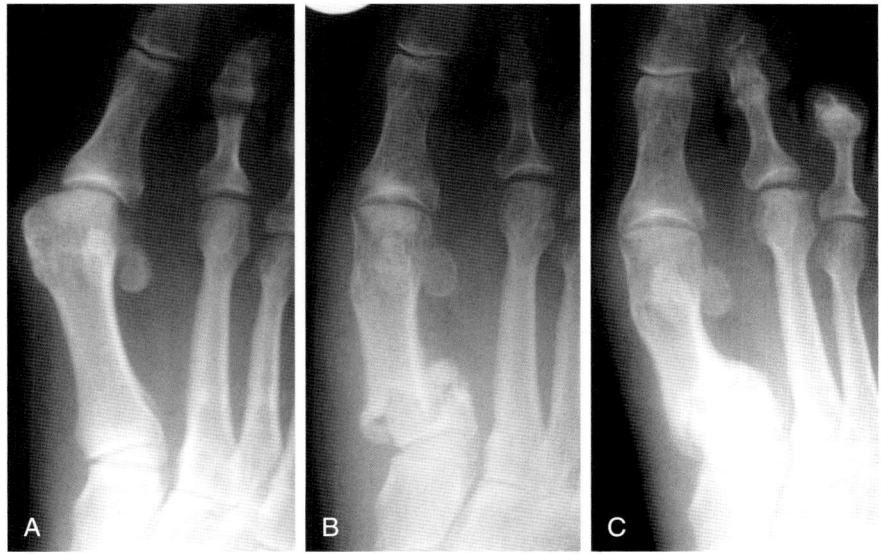

Figure 6-162 Delayed union after proximal crescentic osteotomy. **A,** Preoperative anteroposterior radiograph. **B,** Postoperative radiograph demonstrating delayed union. **C,** After below-knee casting for 6 weeks, successful union has occurred.

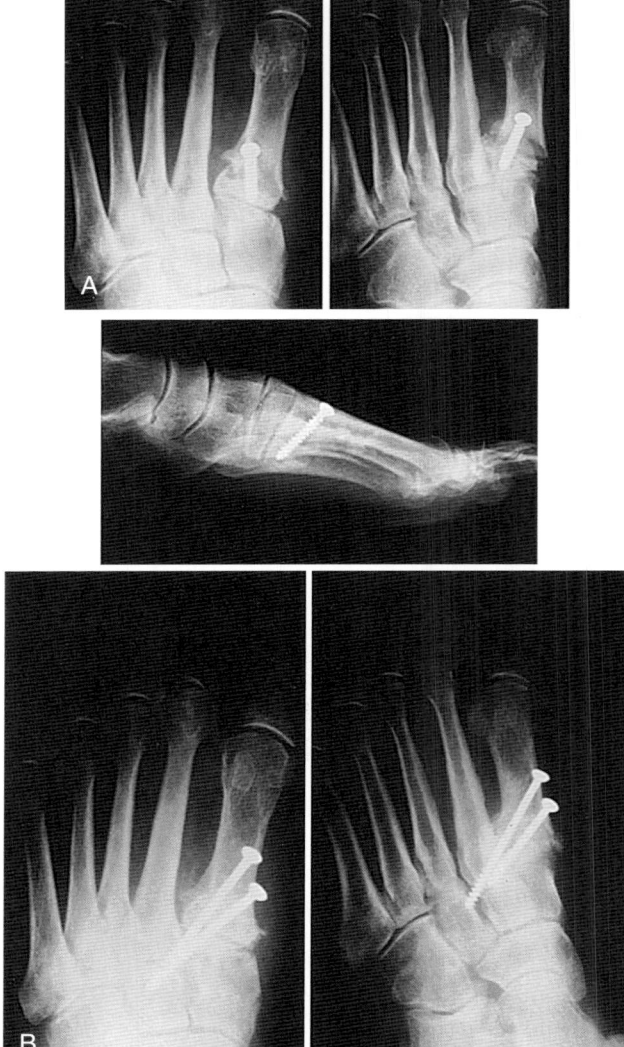

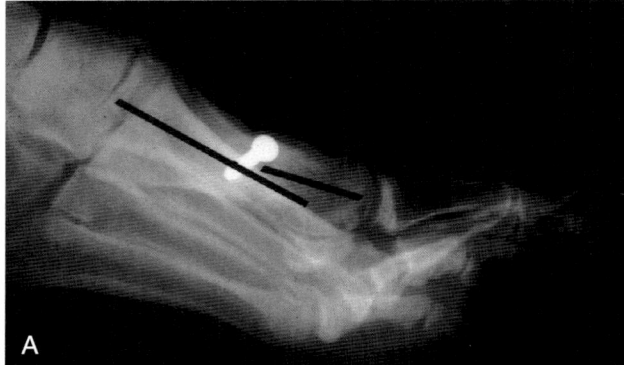

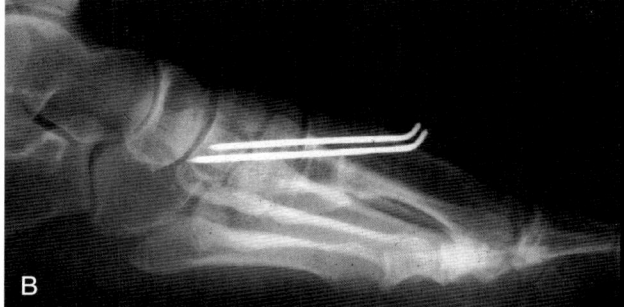

Figure 6-163 Nonunion after proximal crescentic osteotomy. **A,** Preoperative anteroposterior *(left),* oblique *(right),* and lateral *(centered)* radiographs demonstrating nonunion. **B,** Postoperative repair demonstrating satisfactory union after internal fixation and local bone graft.

Figure 6-164 **A,** Elevatus after proximal oblique. **B,** Salvage with an opening-wedge osteotomy and interposition dorsal graft.

minimal) when using a single Steinmann pin for internal fixation. Various methods of internal fixation have been used to fix proximal osteotomies, including Steinmann pins,[335,344,435,535] a single screw,[154,348,409] a screw and pin,[92,101,140] and a dorsal plate.[445,533] Mann et al[344] noted that superficial inflammation around the pin site developed in approximately 10% of patients in whom the osteotomy site was fixed with an oblique Steinmann pin, another reason why this method of fixation was discontinued (see Fig. 6-151).

Other alternatives to proximal cresecentic osteotomies include a proximal oblique osteotomy[16,66,320,384,446] and a proximal chevron osteotomy[348,452,454] (see Fig. 6-159). Markbreiter and Thompson[348] and Sammarco et al[452]

reported excellent correction with proximal chevron osteotomies of differing orientations. Complication rates were similar to those experienced with proximal crescentic osteotomy.

Rigid internal fixation appears to increase the stability at the osteotomy site. Thordarson and Leventen[516] reported less shortening with the use of a more stable internal fixation construct and emphasized that adequate internal fixation was vital to avoid dorsiflexion malunion. Malunion is an extremely difficult complication to treat and may require extensive and complex salvage techniques (see Fig. 6-164).

Mann et al[344] reported that the most frequent complication of this procedure was hallux varus, which occurred in 14 (13%) of 109 feet and averaged 5.6 degrees. None of the patients complained of pain, and none had a cock-up deformity of the first MTP joint. Three patients were dissatisfied because of the position of the toe, whereas the others had essentially no functional complaints and were satisfied with the result. Simmonds and Menelaus[488] and Mann and Coughlin[336] cautioned that a lateral sesamoid should rarely if ever be removed. This amount of varus is typically a minimal deformity and is more a radiographic finding than a clinical entity (see Fig. 6-160). Frequently, a hallux varus deformity of less than 10 degrees is asymptomatic and is considered by patients to be a subjectively satisfactory result.[516]

Easley et al[140] reported a 12% (5 of 43 patients) incidence of hallux varus after proximal chevron osteotomy. In most cases, hallux varus develops because of lateral translation of the metatarsal head after medial displacement of the proximal osteotomy. This was a much more frequent occurrence in the crescentic procedure before changing the osteotomy from being oriented concave distal to concave proximal (see Figs. 6-146 and 6-161D and E).[344] In a retrospective study, Trnka et al[525] presented a long-term follow-up of a group of patients in whom hallux varus developed (average deformity of 10 degrees of varus). In a series of 16 feet with a follow-up averaging 18 years, 12 (75%) of 16 patients still rated their result as excellent. Only those with a severe hallux varus deformity were dissatisfied or required further surgery. In most patients, the varus deformity was usually 15 degrees or less, a finding similar to that reported by Mann et al[344] (see Fig. 6-160).

Nonunion is rarely reported after osteotomy in the proximal metaphyseal region. Mann et al observed two nonunions in a series of 1500 cases.[344] Both were corrected with an interposition bone graft and internal fixation (see Fig. 6-163). Even though such treatment resulted in some shortening of the metatarsal, no symptomatic transfer lesion developed. Cedell and Astrom[63] reported a 10% nonunion rate with an opening-wedge osteotomy, and Sammarco and Russo-Alesi[454] reported three cases in a series of 72 operations involving a proximal chevron osteotomy. More recent studies evaluating the opening-wedge technique found a low nonunion rate, and several authors feel that the use of a locking plate may be beneficial.[433,483,497,563]

Epiphyseal injury can occur with a proximal first metatarsal osteotomy in the skeletally immature and lead to growth arrest and ultimately to a short first metatarsal (see Fig. 6-70). Care must be taken in an adolescent to protect the proximal first metatarsal epiphysis.

In the treatment of moderate and severe hallux valgus deformities with subluxation of the MTP joint, proximal first metatarsal osteotomy combined with distal soft tissue reconstruction can lead to a successful outcome, although it is well recognized that this procedure is technically difficult.[344,360,409]

MULTIPLE OSTEOTOMIES

The incidence of congruent hallux valgus deformities is unknown. Coughlin and Carlson[97] reviewed a series of 878 consecutive bunions over a 12-year period and determined that 18 patients (21 feet) qualified as having congruent deformities of such magnitude that they warranted extraarticular correction (2%). These authors noted that although 12 of the 18 patients underwent surgery before 20 years of age, it should be stressed that with deferred surgery, these deformities can present during the adult years. Thus congruent hallux valgus deformities, although decidedly uncommon (Fig. 6-165), may be seen and treated at any age. A soft tissue intraarticular reconstruction is contraindicated for repair of a hallux valgus deformity with a congruent MTP joint (DMAA > 15 degrees).[95] For this deformity, extraarticular correction can be achieved with either a double or triple first-ray

osteotomy.* An Akin osteotomy can diminish phalangeal angulation because of an increased PPAA. A proximal first metatarsal osteotomy or cuneiform osteotomy can decrease an increased 1–2 IM angle. In some situations, an increased DMAA requires a medial closing-wedge osteotomy of the distal first metatarsal.[164,225,407,436] Mitchell and Baxter[371] reported on the combination of a chevron osteotomy and phalangeal osteotomy to achieve an extraarticular repair. The magnitude of the DMAA and the 1–2 IM angle determines the necessity for multiple first-ray osteotomies and the magnitude of realignment. In their radiographic analysis, Richardson et al[438] reported that the average normal DMAA was 6 to 7 degrees. Coughlin[95] has observed that this angle increases as the magnitude of the congruent hallux valgus deformity increases. Likewise, he has also reported that the final hallux valgus angle closely mirrors the underlying DMAA. Thus any procedure that attempts to realign an MTP joint with an increased DMAA or lateral slope of the distal metatarsal articular surface has a substantial risk of reverting to the preoperative inclination determined by the underlying DMAA (Video Clip 58).[91,401]

First Cuneiform Osteotomy

Riedel[439] (in 1886), according to Kelikian,[263] first reported the use of a first cuneiform osteotomy for the correction of metatarsus primus varus. Young[565] used a first cuneiform osteotomy, and Bonney and Macnab[38] and Coughlin and Mann[92,105] reported on the use of a medial cuneiform osteotomy for realignment of the MTC joint to avoid disturbing an open proximal first metatarsal epiphysis. Up to now, no long-term series has been published on the use of this technique. All reports deal with individual case studies.

A medial cuneiform opening-wedge osteotomy is most commonly indicated in a juvenile patient with an open proximal first metatarsal epiphysis and a hallux valgus deformity characterized by an abnormally widened 1–2 IM angle. An opening-wedge first cuneiform osteotomy is an alternative that can effectively reduce metatarsus primus varus or an increased 1–2 IM angle without exposing the proximal first metatarsal epiphysis to an iatrogenic injury.

Jawish et al[240] reported on 63 patients (101 feet) treated with a distal soft tissue realignment combined with an opening-wedge cuneiform osteotomy by using a 5- to 10-mm–wide allograft wedge. A 16-degree correction of the hallux valgus angle and a reduction of the 1–2 IM angle of 4 degrees was achieved at an average follow-up of almost 8 years.

Technique

1. A medial longitudinal incision is centered over the first cuneiform. (The medial cuneiform is approximately 2 to 2.5 cm long, and the osteotomy is centered in the middle of the first cuneiform.)

---

*References 5, 95, 105, 123, 138, and 472.

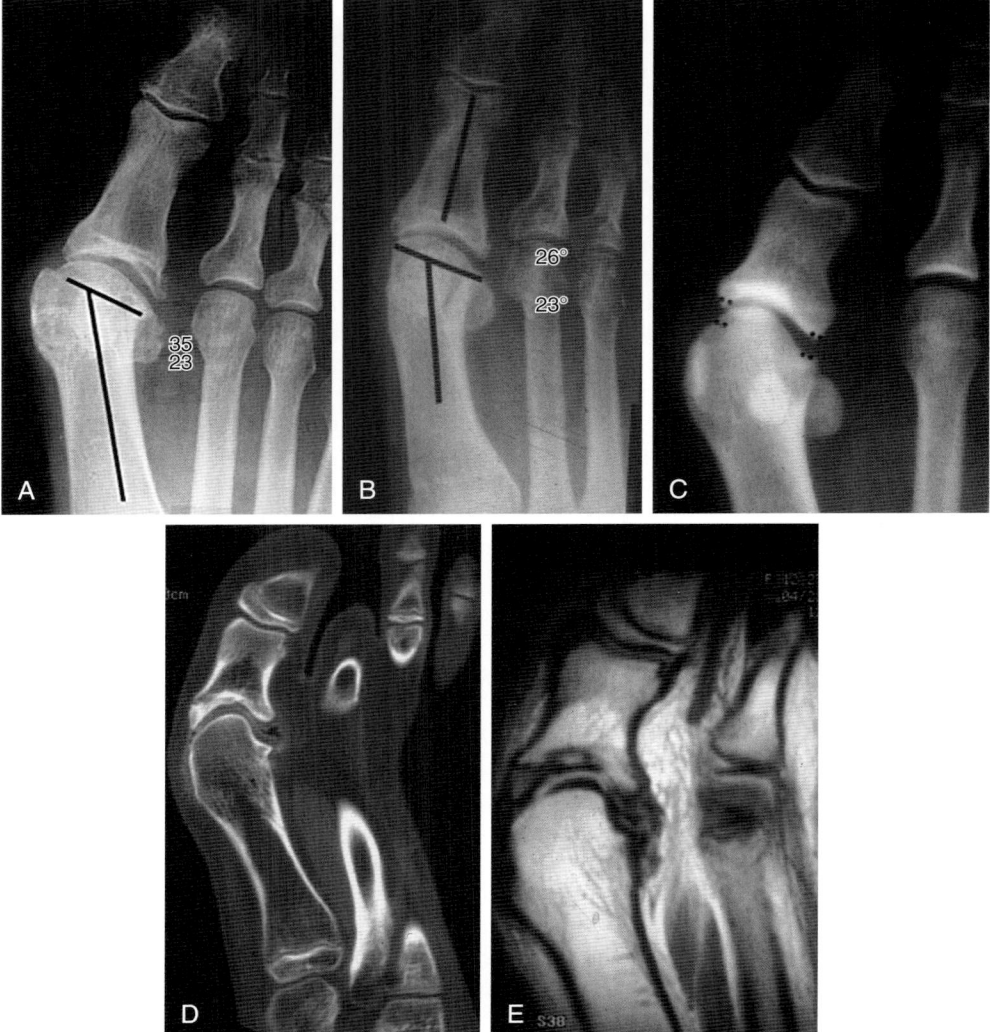

Figure 6-165 Congruent joint with a sloped distal metatarsal articular angle. **A,** Preoperative radiograph. **B,** After a distal soft tissue procedure, no improvement of the hallux valgus angle was achieved. **C,** Congruent joint as seen on a regular radiograph. **D,** Computed tomography scan. **E,** Magnetic resonance image.

2. The naviculocuneiform and the MTC joints are identified.
3. The osteotomy is directed in a medial-lateral plane and carried to a depth of 1.5 cm. The osteotomy must transect both the dorsal and the plantar cortices.

   A vertical osteotomy is positioned in the center of the first cuneiform, and the osteotomy site is opened medially (Fig. 6-166A and B).
4. Although the medial eminence can be used as an interposition graft, often little medial eminence remains with a juvenile bunion deformity. Therefore it is best to use a wedge-shaped bicortical graft from the iliac crest. The iliac crest graft is removed in a routine manner. Because of the height of the first cuneiform, a 2-cm–long graft is used. The base of the graft should be approximately 1 cm or less and should taper to a fine point at the apex. Once the osteotomy site has

been distracted, a triangular bicortical iliac crest bone graft is impacted into place and stabilized with two 0.062-inch K-wires (Fig. 6-166C).
5. With a hallux valgus deformity and a subluxated first MTP joint, a distal soft tissue realignment is performed with the cuneiform osteotomy (Fig. 6-167).
6. With a hallux valgus deformity and a congruent first MTP joint, a concomitant distal first metatarsal closing-wedge osteotomy is an option (Fig. 6-168).
7. The wound is closed routinely.

Postoperative Care
A gauze-and-tape compression dressing or a below-knee cast is applied at surgery. Frequently, the osteotomy is combined with a distal soft tissue realignment or multiple other first-ray osteotomies. The osteotomy will usually heal by 6 weeks after surgery. Internal fixation is

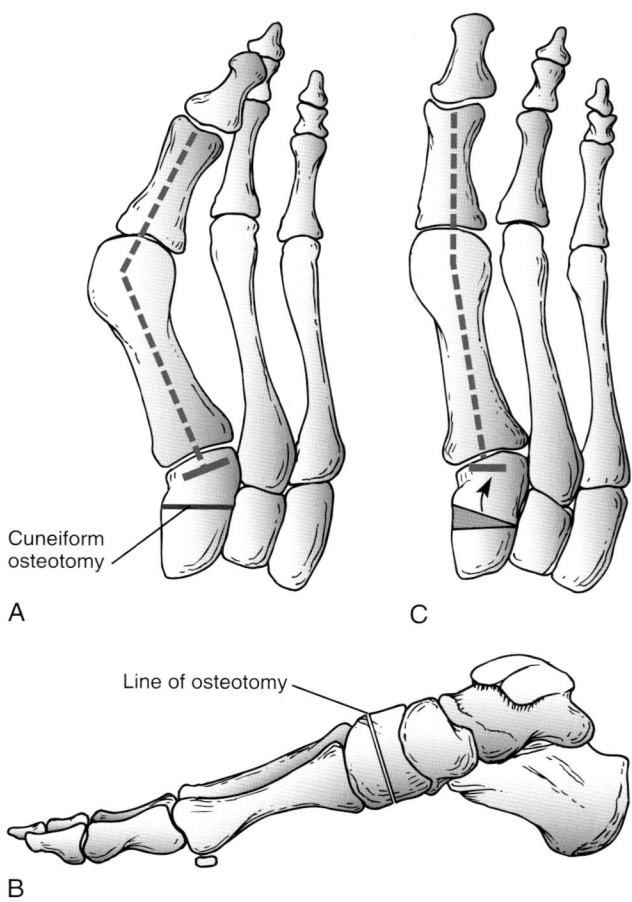

A

C

Cuneiform osteotomy

Line of osteotomy

B

Figure 6-166 Technique of cuneiform osteotomy.
A, Anteroposterior diagram of a cuneiform osteotomy before distraction. **B,** Lateral diagram of a cuneiform osteotomy.
C, After distraction of the osteotomy site and bone grafting, alignment has been improved. Internal fixation with Kirschner wires is typically used.

removed after successful healing of the osteotomy site (Fig. 6-169).

Distal First Metatarsal Closing-Wedge Osteotomy

First described by Reverdin[436] and later by Peabody[407] and others,[95,138,164,411,451] a distal first metatarsal closing-wedge osteotomy can be used for the treatment of a juvenile hallux valgus deformity or in an adult with a congruent hallux valgus deformity. It is especially useful in the presence of an increased DMAA to reorient the metatarsal articular surface more perpendicular to the longitudinal axis of the first metatarsal.

Technique

1. A medial longitudinal incision is centered over the MTP joint, beginning at the midproximal phalanx and extending 2 cm above the medial eminence.
2. The medial MTP joint capsule is released on the dorsal proximal aspect with an L-shaped, distally based capsular flap (see Fig. 6-91D).
3. At a point 1.5 cm proximal to the MTP joint, an osteotomy of the proximal metatarsal metaphysis (just proximal to the sesamoids) is performed. A second osteotomy proximal to the first is located 6 to 10 mm proximal to the initial osteotomy. It converges at its apex at the lateral cortex with the distal osteotomy. The magnitude of the medial closing-wedge osteotomy depends on the magnitude of the DMAA (1-mm resection = 5 degrees of correction of the DMAA) (Fig. 6-170).[299]
4. Care is taken to avoid injury to the sesamoid complex on the plantar aspect at the osteotomy site.
5. Once the wedge has been excised, the osteotomy site is closed. Medial translation of the capital fragment may be necessary. The osteotomy site is fixed with two oblique 0.062-inch K-wires.

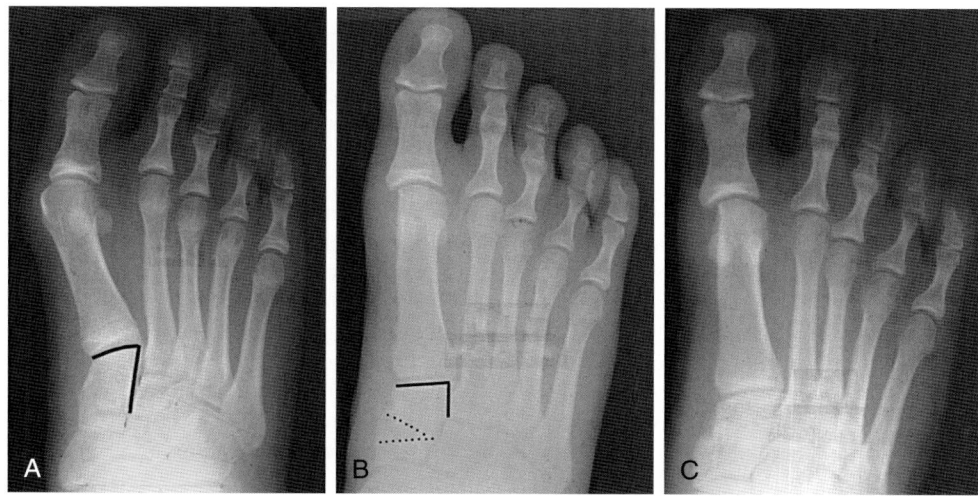

Figure 6-167 Cuneiform osteotomy technique. **A,** Preoperative radiograph demonstrating a juvenile hallux valgus deformity with metatarsus primus varus and an open epiphysis. **B,** Radiograph after opening-wedge cuneiform osteotomy and distal soft tissue repair. **C,** Two-year follow-up radiograph after cuneiform osteotomy and distal soft tissue realignment.

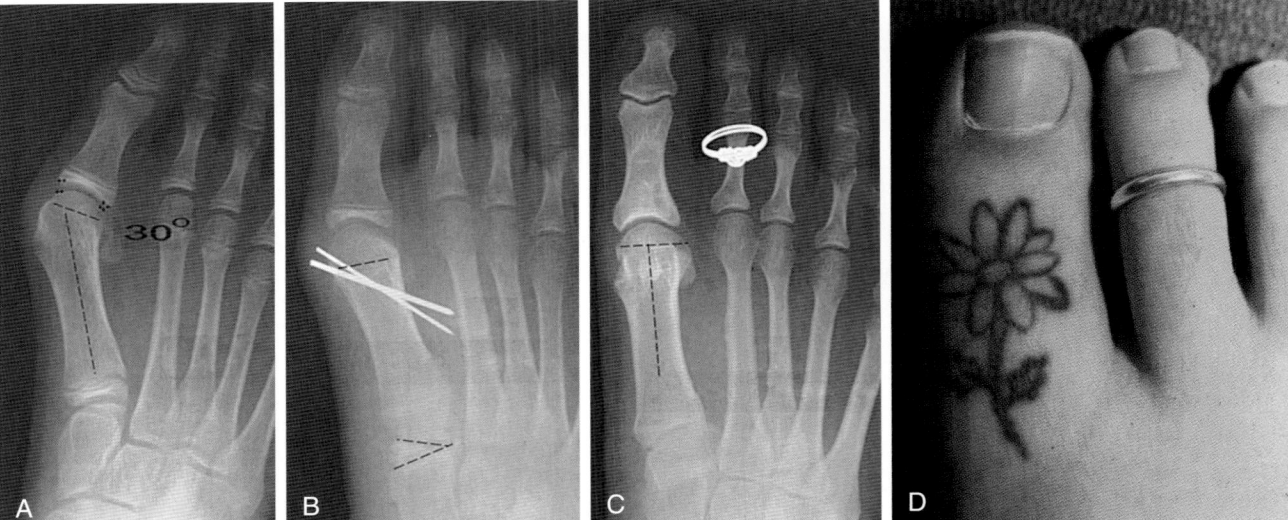

Figure 6-168 **A,** Juvenile hallux valgus with open epiphysis and distal metatarsal articular angle of 30 degrees. **B,** Radiograph after opening-wedge cuneiform osteotomy and closing-wedge distal first metatarsal osteotomy. **C,** Eight-year follow-up radiograph demonstrating successful long-term repair. **D,** Clinical photograph at 8-year follow-up.

6. The medial eminence is resected with an oscillating saw.

7. The medial capsule is approximated and secured to the first metatarsal with suture placed through a medial metaphyseal drill hole. The dorsal and proximal capsular incisions are repaired with interrupted absorbable suture.

8. After completion of this osteotomy, the hallux should be oriented in slight varus because the articular surface now closely parallels the longitudinal axis of the first metatarsal shaft. This situation creates a need for a proximal first-ray osteotomy to decrease the 1–2 IM angle. An Akin osteotomy can also be added when necessary to create a triple osteotomy (Fig. 6-171).

Other Osteotomies

Another alternative is to combine a distal first metatarsal closing-wedge osteotomy with a proximal crescentic osteotomy. Although this technique may be quite effective, careful dissection is necessary to protect the first metatarsal shaft from devascularization (Fig. 6-172). This interval may be rather small, thus increasing the risk of a vascular insult to the first metatarsal diaphysis. A better alternative may be to combine a distal first metatarsal osteotomy with a first cuneiform osteotomy, even though a first cuneiform osteotomy is more difficult. A proximal osteotomy of the first metatarsal may be considered but should be approached with caution because extensive soft tissue stripping of the first metatarsal can lead to AVN.

Alternative osteotomies have been described by Loretz et al[317] and Kramer et al.[284] Z-shaped osteotomies (scarf type) of the distal first metatarsal that both protect the sesamoid mechanism and allow realignment of the distal metatarsal articular angle are an alternative as well. Amarnek et al[5] used a crescentic distal phalangeal and

a distal metatarsal crescentic osteotomy to realign the first ray.

Results

Funk and Wells[164] and others[225,407,436] have reported success with distal first metatarsal osteotomies, as have Durman[138] and Goldner and Gaines[186] with double first-ray osteotomies. Kramer et al[284] and Day et al[121] both reported an average 15-degree correction of the DMAA with a Z-shaped rotational osteotomy, and Loretz et al[317] reported similar correction of the hallux valgus deformity with an increase in the DMAA. Funk and Wells[164] reported an average 7.2-degree correction of the 1–2 IM angle with a distal first metatarsal closing-wedge osteotomy. A biplanar and triplanar osteotomy has been used to correct an increased DMAA.[71,408] Chou et al[71] used a biplanar distal chevron osteotomy to correct the DMAA 4 degrees with this procedure.

A variety of double osteotomies have been advocated, including proximal phalangeal and first metatarsal osteotomy,[5,95,97,186] double metatarsal osteotomy,[95,97,138] phalangeal and chevron osteotomy,[371] and phalangeal and cuneiform osteotomy.[206] Reporting on the use of double and triple osteotomies for the treatment of juvenile hallux valgus with congruous MTP joints, Coughlin[95] noted an average 23-degree correction of the hallux valgus angle and an average 8.3-degree correction of the 1–2 IM angle. This correction occurred in the presence of an average DMAA of 19 degrees. These results are similar to those noted by Peterson and Newman,[411] who reported on 10 adolescent patients with an average 24-degree correction of the hallux valgus angle and an average 8-degree correction of the 1–2 IM angle after double osteotomy. A high rate of subjective satisfaction was reported in both series. Coughlin and Carlson[97] reported on the results of 21 feet

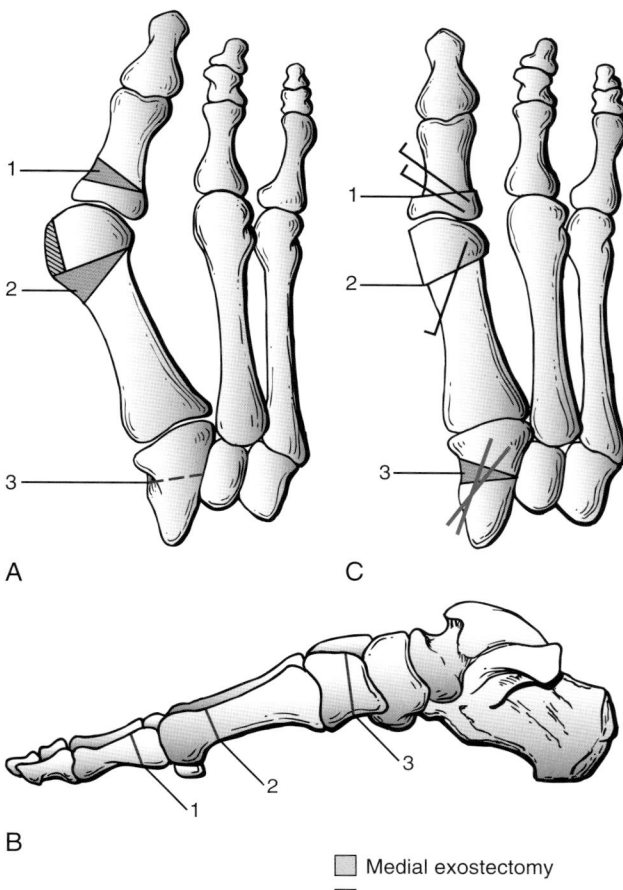

Medial exostectomy

Bone resection

Figure 6-169 Technique of multiple first-ray osteotomies. Multiple first-ray osteotomies can be used to achieve extraarticular correction of a hallux valgus deformity, especially with an increased distal metatarsal articular angle. **A, 1,** Closing-wedge osteotomy; *2,* closing-wedge osteotomy of the distal first metatarsal with resection of the medial eminence; *3,* opening-wedge osteotomy of the first cuneiform. **B,** Lateral view demonstrating the location of the osteotomies. **C,** A triple osteotomy improves the overall alignment of the first ray.

with congruent hallux valgus deformities (with an increased DMAA) treated by periarticular osteotomies. Both double and triple first-ray osteotomies were performed in the series. The average correction of the hallux valgus angle was 23 degrees, the average correction of the IM angle was 9 degrees, and the average correction of the DMAA was 14 degrees postoperatively.

In a laboratory study, Lau and Daniels[299] determined that the size of the wedge to be resected to reduce an abnormally high DMAA in a congruent hallux valgus deformity can be easily calculated preoperatively. They suggested that for every 1 mm of bone resected from the distal metaphysis in the process of performing a closing-wedge osteotomy, the DMAA was decreased by 4.7 degrees.

Complications

Complications after multiple metatarsal osteotomies may include loss of correction, malunion, loss of fixation, AVN, intraarticular injury from an associated fracture with the osteotomy, and degenerative arthrosis of the IP or MTP joints. These procedures are technically difficult and should be reserved for the occasional case of hallux valgus characterized by a congruent first MTP joint with a DMAA greater than 15 degrees. When possible, a simpler and technically easier procedure is preferable to a more complex and difficult technique. Degenerative arthritis has been reported by Bock et al,[35] who noted both metatarsal head and metatarsal sesamoid cartilaginous lesions, with increased occurrence related to the severity of the preoperative hallux valgus deformity.

METATARSOCUNEIFORM ARTHRODESIS AND DISTAL SOFT TISSUE PROCEDURE

Arthrodesis of the first MTC joint in conjunction with a distal soft tissue procedure for correction of hallux valgus was popularized by Lapidus, although it was conceived by Albrecht,[4] Kleinberg,[280] and Truslow.[527] The procedure is predicated on the principle that metatarsus primus varus must be corrected to obtain satisfactory correction of the hallux valgus deformity. Initially, Lapidus[294] specified that a suitable patient preferably should be "young and robust," with an IM angle of 15 degrees or greater and a "fixed" deformity of the MTC joint. In time, Lapidus[294] narrowed his indications substantially for the use of MTC joint fusion. If there was "adequate mobility of the first MTC joint to allow approximation of the first and second metatarsal heads," Lapidus indicated that a simple bunionectomy was sufficient treatment rather than MTC joint arthrodesis. Although Lapidus did not specifically use the procedure for the so-called hypermobile first ray, currently this appears to be one of the main indications (Video Clip 57).*

Indications

The major indication for this procedure is a moderate or severe hallux valgus deformity[79,199,204,456] (a hallux valgus angle of at least 30 degrees and a 1–2 IM angle of at least 16 degrees). Other indications include juvenile hallux valgus,[28,73,172,186,383] recurrent hallux valgus,[383,456] severe deformity,[28,45,77,383,456] a hallux valgus deformity in the presence of generalized ligamentous laxity,[28,383] and degenerative arthritis of the first MTC joint.[28,383] Hypermobility of the first ray associated with a hallux valgus deformity is probably the most frequently listed condition for which the Lapidus procedure is indicated,[†] yet none of these reports give any objective data on the preoperative or postoperative quantification of first-ray hypermobility. There remains continued difficulty in identifying patients who have substantial first-ray

---

*References 21, 54, 140, 141, 174, 218, 248, 271-273, 298, and 307.

†References 21, 33, 43, 140, 141, 174, 248, 271-273, and 298.

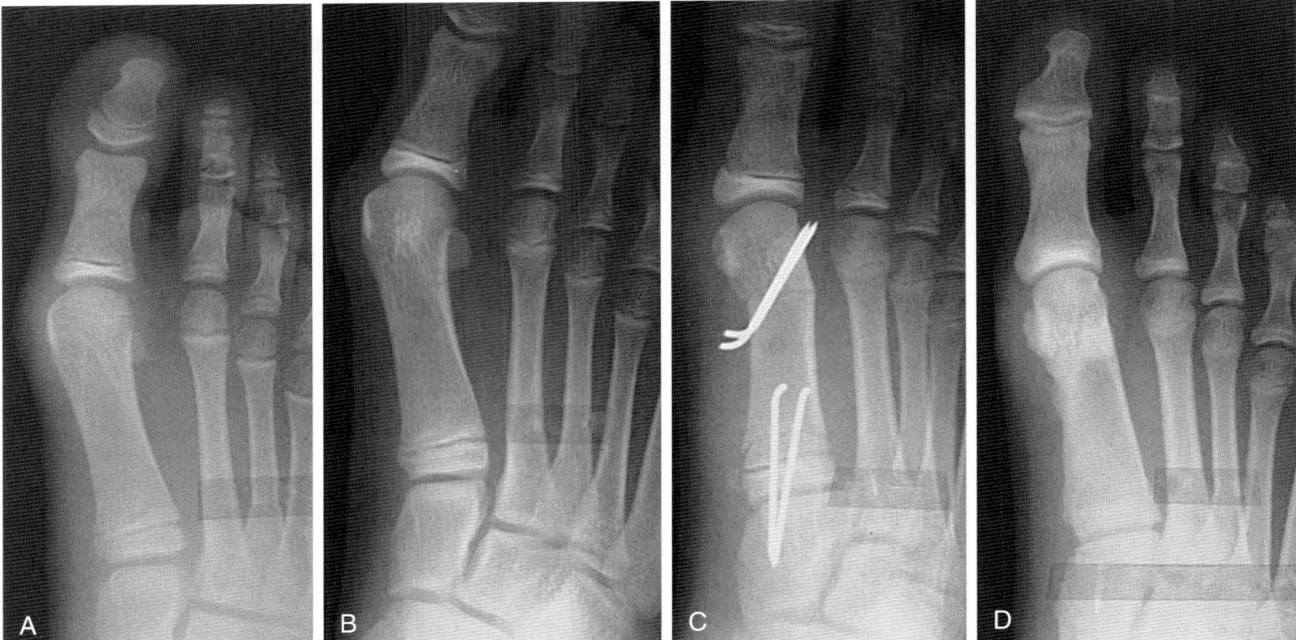

Figure 6-170 **A,** Anteroposterior (AP) radiograph demonstrating a mild hallux valgus deformity in an 11-year-old girl. **B,** AP radiograph of a 14-year-old girl demonstrating progression of the deformity. **C,** After distal first metatarsal closing-wedge osteotomy and proximal crescentic osteotomy, alignment is improved. **D,** A 2-year follow-up radiograph shows acceptable alignment.

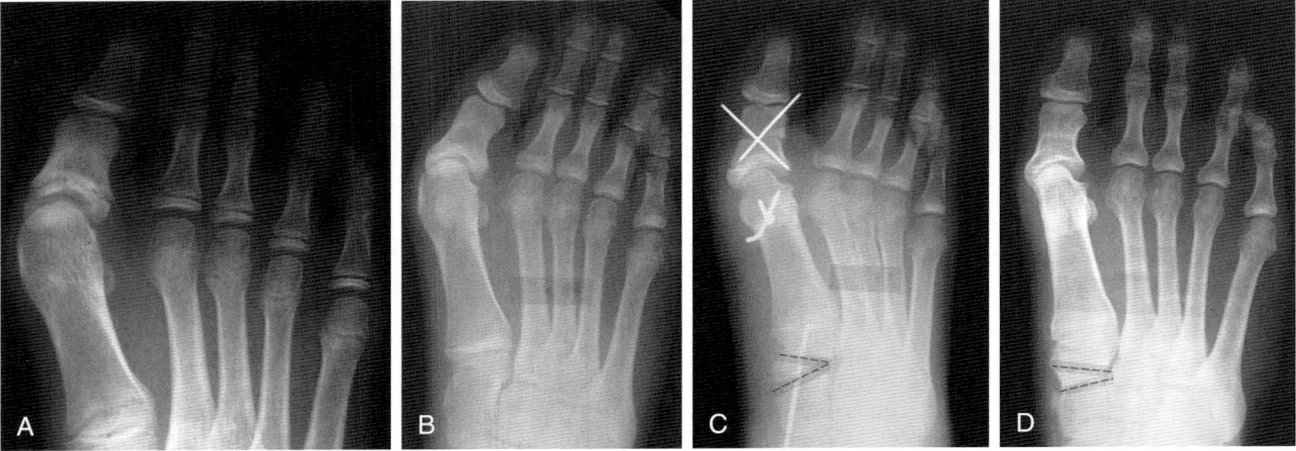

Figure 6-171 **A,** Preoperative radiograph demonstrating moderate hallux valgus deformity with a congruent metatarsophalangeal (MTP) joint (see Fig. 6-59A and B for early preoperative images when the patient was 10 years old). **B,** At skeletal maturity, a congruent MTP joint and moderate hallux valgus deformity are present. **C,** Triple osteotomy (closing-wedge phalangeal osteotomy, closing-wedge distal first metatarsal osteotomy, opening-wedge cuneiform osteotomy) has achieved realignment. **D,** Four-year follow-up radiograph demonstrating excellent correction of a juvenile hallux valgus deformity with a congruent MTP articulation.

instability[190,192] as well as the location of this instability. Recent studies by Cooper et al,[81] Ellinton et al,[144] and Kazzaz et al[262] continue to cite first-ray instability as an indication for the lapidus procedure, although it has been unequivocably demonstrated by Smith and Coughlin,[100,102,190,192,492] that the metatarsal cuneiform joint is uncommonly the site of first-ray hypermobility.

Proponents of the Lapidus procedure using it to address first metatarsocuneifrom instability have as yet failed to identify this joint as the cause of this increased mobility; the fact that it diminishes to a normal range of mobility after a distal correction without an MTC joint fusion[100] leads the chapter authors to question this particular indication. Ellington et al[144] suggested in their study that 96%

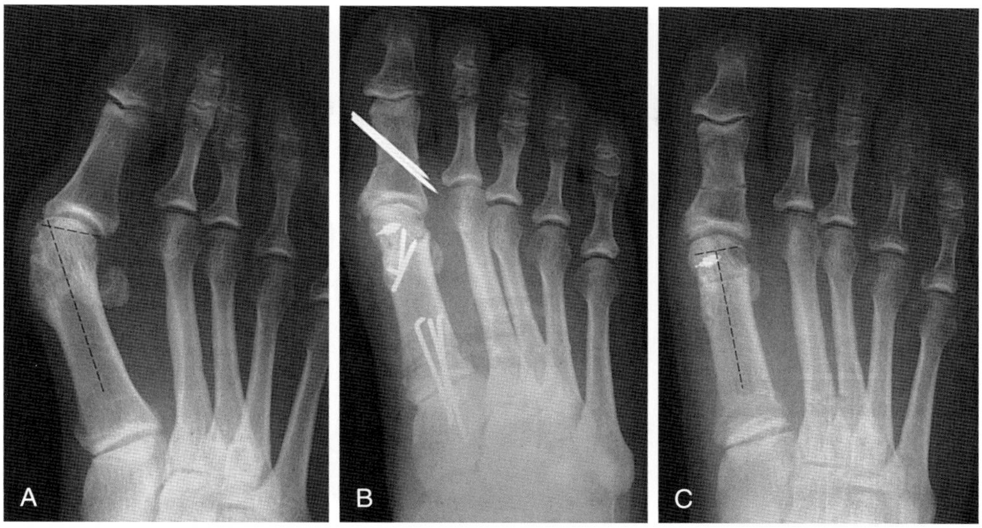

Figure 6-172 A, Preoperative radiograph in 40-year-old man who underwent unsuccessful juvenile hallux valgus correction. Note the congruent metatarsophalangeal joint (distal metatarsal articular angle of 30 degrees). **B,** Triple osteotomy (closing-wedge phalangeal osteotomy, closing-wedge distal first metatarsal osteotomy, crescentic proximal first metatarsal osteotomy) has achieved realignment of the first ray. **C,** One-year follow-up radiograph demonstrating improved alignment. (A suture anchor was used to stabilize a medial capsular disruption found at surgery.)

of subjects had first-ray hypermobility but did not quantify it. They did observe gapping of the plantar MC joint in 52% of lateral radiographs preoperatively. Of interest, Cooper et al[81] also reported on 85 feet in which they suggested clinical instability was present. They observed, as did Coughlin and Jones,[101] that radiographic plantar gapping was an inconsistent finding. Further study needs to be carried out to identify the location of increased first-ray mobility and the significance and reliability of radiographic findings, such as plantar gapping of the first MTC joint.

The authors believe that this procedure is useful in about 5% to 10% of patients with an advanced or severe hallux valgus deformity. On the other hand, for those comfortable with this procedure, it can be used for a broader spectrum of cases (in the moderate range of hallux valgus deformities) if a surgeon's results substantiate its effectiveness. The procedure is also used as a salvage procedure after failed repair of a previous hallux valgus deformity.*

Contraindication

The main contraindications are a short first metatarsal,[383] juvenile hallux valgus with an open epiphysis,[88] a mild hallux valgus deformity without excessive first-ray hypermobility (in which a lesser procedure could be performed),[88] and the presence of degenerative arthritis of the MTP joint.[325] There is probably a relative contraindication to using this procedure in a young person who is active in sports because of the stiffness that follows loss of first MTC joint function.

---

*References 28, 77, 149, 202, 383, and 456.

Technique

The surgical technique consists of a distal soft tissue procedure with lateral release of the first web space, excision of the medial eminence, and preparation of the medial joint capsule. Then the first MTC joint arthrodesis is performed, after which the first MTP joint is reconstructed.

Distal Soft Tissue Procedure

The distal soft tissue procedure is carried out in the same manner as discussed previously. (See pages 203 to 212).

Metatarsocuneiform Joint Arthrodesis

1. The MTC joint is approached through a 5-cm dorsomedial, slightly curved incision centered over the first MTC joint.[77] The joint capsule is opened dorsally and medially to expose the joint (Figs. 6-173 and 6-174A).
2. With a small curet, ring curet, or osteotome, the articular cartilage is removed in its entirety from the MTC joint (Fig. 6-174B-D). This is a sinusoidal-shaped articular surface 30 mm in height, and it is important to remove the cartilage completely from the joint's plantar lateral aspect (Fig. 6-175). The inferior lateral portion of the medial cuneiform, as well as the lateral base of the first metatarsal, is resected with an osteotomy.[28] This allows correction of both excess valgus and mild plantar flexion. The adjoining lateral surfaces of the proximal first metatarsal and medial second metatarsal are denuded as well.[77] If a facet is present on the proximal lateral aspect of the base of the first metatarsal, it is also resected.
3. The joint is gently manipulated from a dorsomedial to a plantar lateral position while bringing the first metatarsal head into a plantar lateral position (see

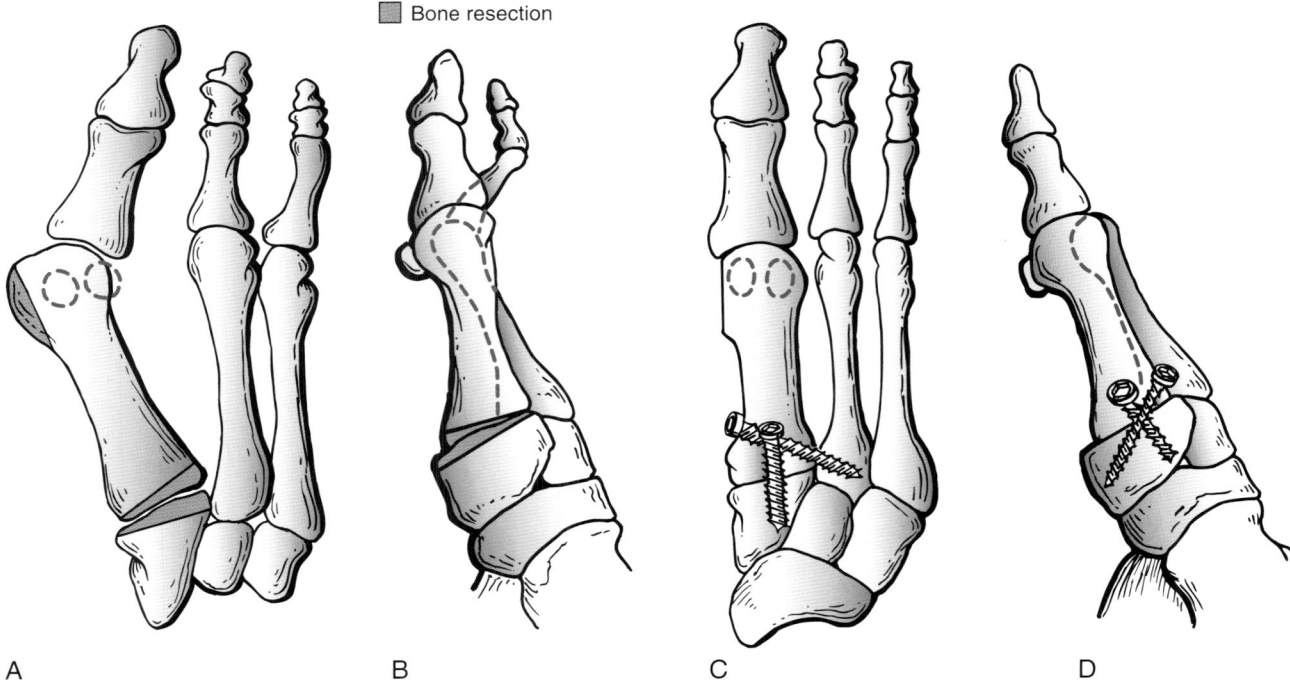

Figure 6-173   Technique of Lapidus (metatarsocuneiform [MTC] fusion). **A,** Biplanar wedge resection of the MTC joint, anteroposterior (AP) plane. **B,** The lateral view demonstrates more plantar bone resection to plantar flex the first metatarsal. The AP **(C)** and lateral **(D)** views after placement of internal fixation demonstrate plantar flexion of the osteotomy site. (A third screw can be placed from the first cuneiform through the first metatarsal in a proximal distal direction.)

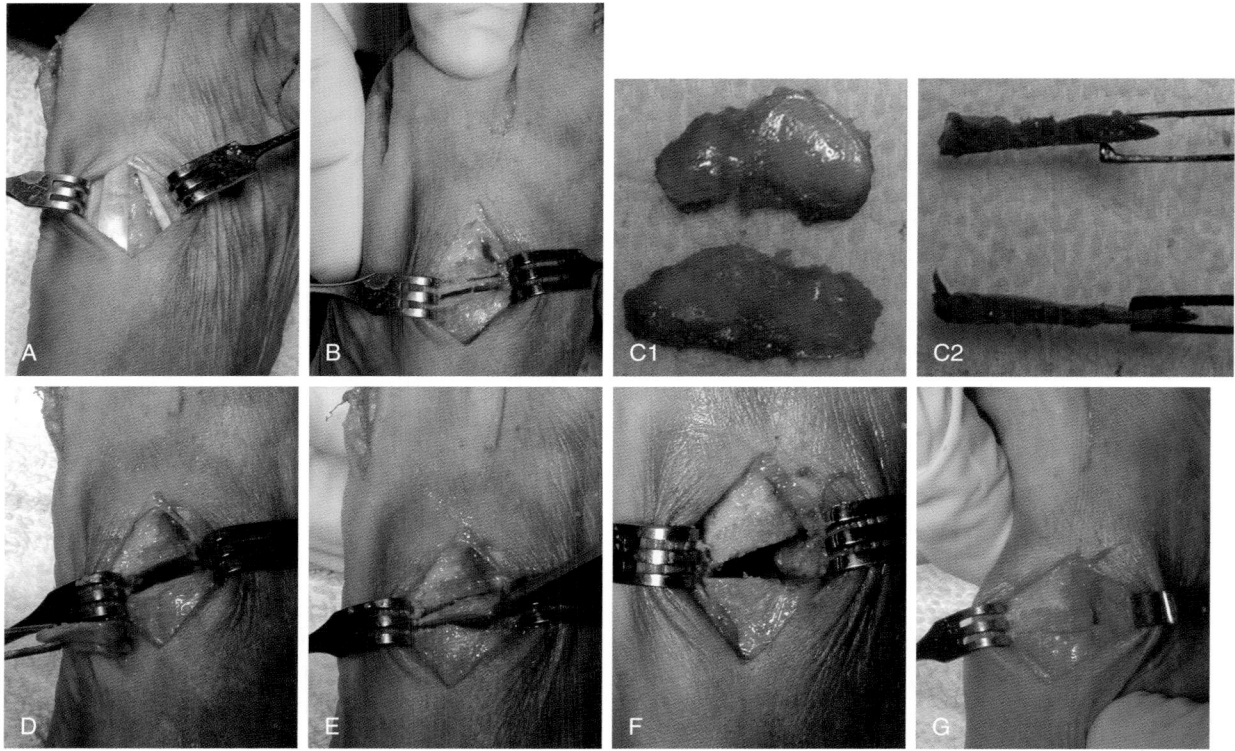

Figure 6-174   Technique for the Lapidus procedure. **A,** Operative incision. **B,** Resection of the articular surfaces. **C1, C2,** and **D,** Minimal resection of the articular surfaces. **E,** More extensive resection to reduce the intermetatarsal angle. **F,** After removal of the triangular resected segment. **G,** Closure of the arthrodesis site. (Courtesy Chris DiGiovanni, MD.)

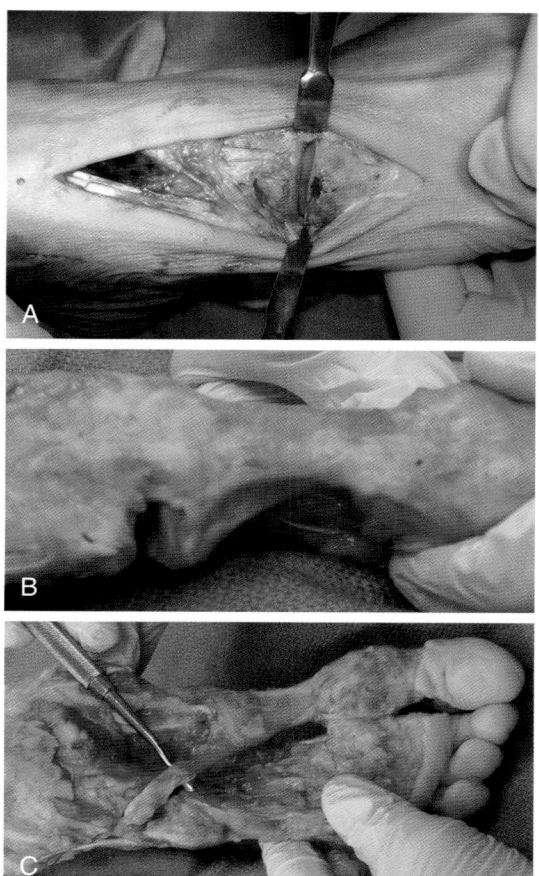

Figure 6-175 Exposure of the metatarsocuneiform joint. **A,** Wide exposure is necessary to prevent dorsiflexion malunion. **B,** Anatomic dissection demonstrates the depth of the joint. **C,** Care must be taken to avoid injury to the peroneus longus tendon on the plantar surface of the joint. (**A,** Courtesy Chris Coetzee, MD.)

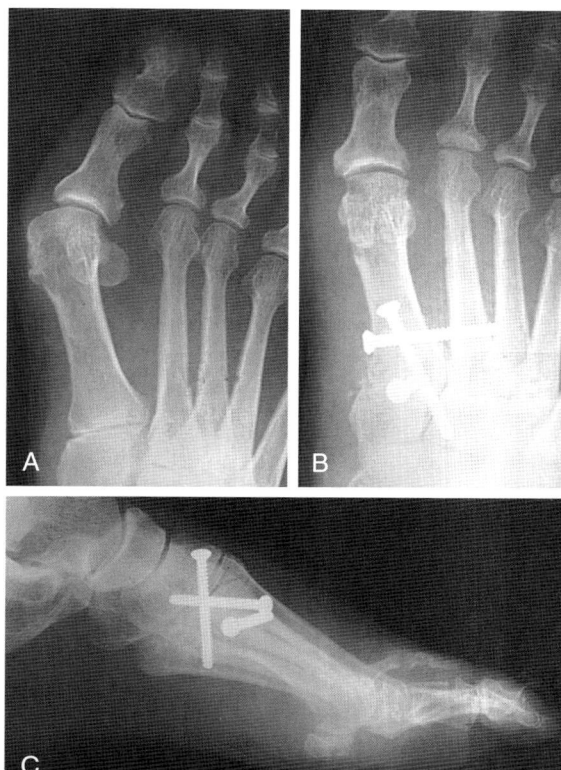

Figure 6-176 Lapidus procedure. **A,** Preoperative radiograph demonstrating a severe hallux valgus deformity. **B** and **C,** Postoperative correction has been achieved. Internal fixation is routinely removed 12 to 16 weeks after successful arthrodesis to avoid breakage of the intermetatarsal screw.

Fig. 6-174E-G). Moving the joint in this manner respects the joint's biomechanical axis. Placing the metatarsal head in a plantar lateral position corrects the IM angle so that often little if any bone needs to be resected from the joint to achieve this alignment. Although some have advocated the use of an iliac crest bone block to realign the joint, the authors believe that this is rarely necessary and technically makes the procedure much more complex. On the other hand, placement of local bone graft obtained from the medial eminence into the interval between the first and second metatarsals may be advantageous.[28,77] Likewise, cutting a small dorsal slot and filling it with local bone graft is thought by some to aid the fusion process as well.[28,204,205]

4. Sutures are placed into the first web space to secure the adductor tendon into the lateral side of the first metatarsal.

5. The first MTC joint is "feathered" with a 4-mm osteotome to increase the bony surfaces. Alternatively, multiple small holes are drilled to perforate the subchondral plate on both adjoining surfaces. The first metatarsal

is then reduced so that it is parallel with the second metatarsal to close the IM angle. As this is done, the first metatarsal can be overreduced into excess plantar direction or underreduced and excessive dorsiflexion left. This is a key maneuver, and the surgeon must continuously assess the relationship of the first to the second metatarsal when displacing the first MTC joint. When proper alignment appears to be achieved, a guide pin is placed across the MTC joint, after which a 4.0-mm cannulated self-tapping screw is inserted from the first cuneiform into the first metatarsal and a second screw is placed from the first metatarsal into the cuneiform. Usually, two[79] or three screws are used to gain rigid interfragmentary compression (Fig. 6-176). Fixation can also be achieved by placing a small plate along the joint's dorsomedial aspect that has been molded to hold the metatarsal in its corrected position. (Fig. 6-177). A derotational lag screw can be placed between the first and second metatarsals.[28] If used, it is typically removed 12 weeks after surgery.

Reconstruction of the Metatarsophalangeal Joint

1. The capsular tissues on the medial side of the MTP joint are plicated to place the hallux in satisfactory

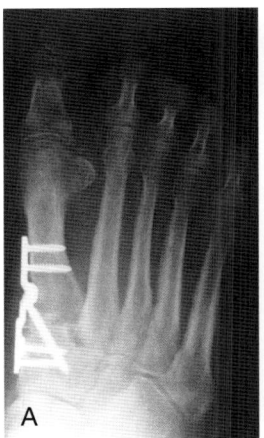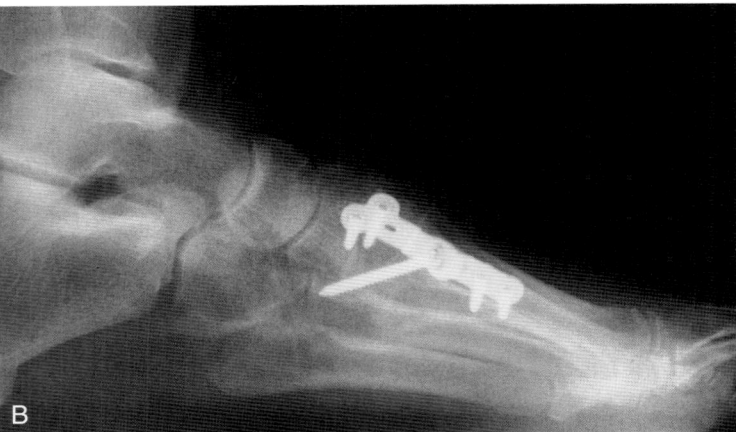

Figure 6-177 Anteroposterior **(A)** and lateral **(B)** radiographs after fixation with dorsal lateral compression plate. (Courtesy Keith Wapner, MD.)

alignment. Any pronation is corrected when the sutures are placed along the joint's medial aspect.

2. The wounds are closed with interrupted sutures, and a compression dressing is applied.

Postoperative Care

In the office, 1 to 2 days after surgery, the compression dressing is removed and another gauze-and-tape dressing applied, similar to that described for the distal soft tissue procedure. The patient is kept non–weight bearing on the affected extremity. This type of dressing is changed weekly for 8 weeks. The extremity is initially placed in a below-knee cast. Coetzee and Wickum[79] recommend a slipper cast for 6 weeks, with weight bearing only on the heel. One to 3 weeks after surgery, the sutures are removed, a radiograph is obtained, and based on alignment of the hallux, a determination is made about how to align the MTP joint with the postoperative dressings. Weight bearing is allowed 4 to 6 weeks after surgery. After 8 weeks, if adequate fusion has occurred at the MTC joint, the patient is permitted to progress to ambulation in a sandal or shoe as tolerated. If the arthrodesis is not complete, the dressings are removed from the foot so that the patient can start range-of-motion exercises for the hallux. The patient is maintained in a short-leg removable cast until the fusion is complete. More recently, Kazzaz and Singh[262] reported on 27 feet in which a postoperative shoe rather than a below-knee cast was used for immobilization. All MTC joints successfully fused.

Results

Patient satisfaction rates vary from 74% to 92%.* Many of the reports on the Lapidus procedure are marked by no or little follow-up[186,325,472,527]; short-term follow-up of less than 1 year[73,280,295]; insufficient data on the demographics, method, or criteria of assessment or radiographic information[280,294-296,383]; inclusion of patients with

varying preoperative diagnoses[28]; or use in combination with a silicon great toe implant.[14,42] The average correction of the hallux valgus angle varies from 10 to 22 degrees[28,77,352,383,385] and the 1–2 IM angle from 6 to 9 degrees.* Various nonunion rates reported include Kazzaz and Singh[262] (0%), Coetzee and Wickum[79] (6.6%), Sangeorzan and Hansen[456] and Faber et al[152] (10%), and McInnes and Bouche[362] (15.6%).

Nonetheless, Coetzee and Wickum[79] reported on their results with the Lapidus procedure. Of 105 patients, only 7 had a fibrous union. The hallux valgus angle was reduced from 37 to an average of 16 degrees; the 1–2 IM angle was reduced from 18 to 8 degrees at final follow-up. An 85% satisfaction level was reported by the cohort of patients. Hass et al[199] compared the Lapidus procedure with a proximal first metatarsal closing-wedge osteotomy and noted excellent correction with the Lapidus procedure. In another study of failed bunion procedures treated with the Lapidus procedure as a salvage reconstruction procedure.

Complications

Reported complications after the Lapidus procedure include a prolonged healing time,[456] malunion,[383,385,456] prolonged swelling,[383,456] continued pain,[456] nonunion,[†] stiffness,[28,295,383,385] recurrence,[28,77,295] and postoperative varus deformity (Fig. 6-178).[352] The pseudoarthrosis rate at the MTC joint varies from approximately 0% to 75%,[‡] with symptoms in about half these patients (Fig. 6-179). The 5% to 24% pseudoarthrosis rate reported by most authors attests to the MTC joint being a difficult joint in which to obtain a satisfactory arthrodesis; however, Mauldin et al[352] reported a 74% incidence of nonunion.

---

*References 28, 56, 73, 77, 352, 362, 383, 385, and 456.

---

*References 28, 45, 73, 204, 205, 246, 316, 383, 385, 386, and 441.
†References 28, 73, 204, 205, 246, 316, 352, 383, 385, 386, and 441.
‡References 28, 56, 73, 77, 144, 352, 362, 383, 385, and 456.

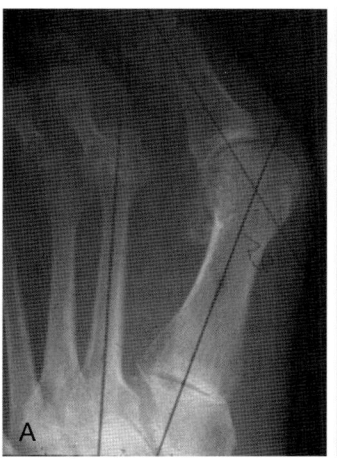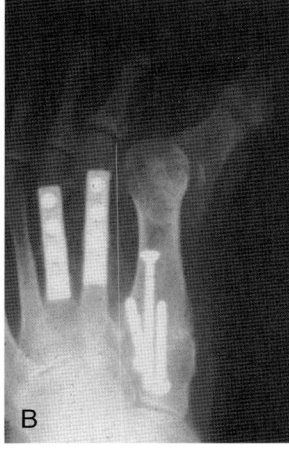

Figure 6-178 **A,** Severe hallux valgus deformity with metatarsalgia and instability of the metatarsocuneiform joint. **B,** After the Lapidus procedure, severe hallux varus deformity has resulted.

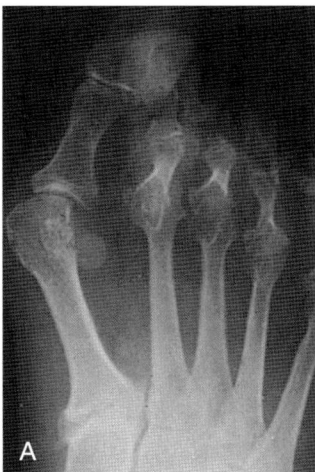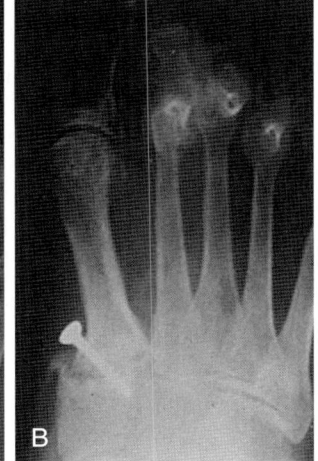

Figure 6-179 Preoperative **(A)** and postoperative **(B)** radiographs of painful nonunion after attempted metatarsocuneiform joint fusion.

Lombardi et al[316] noted a mean shortening of 8 mm after the procedure. Sangeorzan and Hansen[456] reported a 13% revision rate and a 20% overall failure rate. Mauldin et al[352] reported a 16% incidence of postoperative hallux varus, Myerson[383] and others[73,456] observed that the procedure was technically challenging, and Clark et al[73] noted a high rate of complications. More recent reports[77,79] with improved surgical technique have demonstrated a much higher level of success with this procedure.

Most authors agree that first MTC joint arthrodesis with a distal soft tissue procedure is technically difficult and should not be used in patients with the typical bunion but rather advocate it in those with marked hypermobility of the first ray and significant widening of the 1–2 IM angle or in salvage situations.[77,79] Postoperative

MTP range of motion was reported by McInnes and Bouche[362] to be 62 degrees. In a prospective study, Coetzee and Wickum[79] observed preoperative dorsiflexion of 66 degrees and no significant diminution at almost 4 years' follow-up. Plantar flexion was not affected by the procedure. Rink-Brune[441] reported that it took longer than 3 months to resolve the swelling and subjective complaints in 16% of patients. McInnes and Bouche[362] reported that only 30% of athletes returned to their preoperative level of activity, whereas 75% of more sedentary patients achieved this goal. The chapter authors believe that because of the stiffness that results after the procedure, it is less often indicated in younger and more active individuals. When the procedure results in shortening because of bone resection, the metatarsal must be placed in sufficient plantar flexion to accommodate for this shortening. Myerson[383] noted, however, that 9% of the first metatarsals in his series were dorsiflexed, half of which resulted in transfer lesions beneath the second metatarsal. More recently, the use of dorsal plating of the first MTC joint appears to have alleviated the tendency for dorsiflexion at the arthrodesis site, and can be used to increase the compression across the joint.[149,378,470] Scranton et al,[470] in a cadaveric study, found a dorsal-compression locking plate was 25% stronger than cross-compression screws in the fixation of the first MTC joint.

The use of the Lapidus procedure has gained favor in the salvaging of prior failed bunion surgery.[79,202] Hamilton et al[202] reported success in 14 of 17 (82%) feet treated for failed prior halux valgus surgery using either crossed screws or a compression plate and augmented with a bone stimulator. The three nonunions occurred in patients who smoked. Ellington et al[144] reported on successful salvage in 24 of 25 feet (96%) and at final follow-up, 87% of patients reported good or excellent results.

With an overall failure rate reported to be as high as 28%,[456] this is not the procedure of choice for the occasional foot surgeon.

METATARSOPHALANGEAL JOINT ARTHRODESIS

Arthrodesis of the first MTP joint for treatment of hallux valgus deformity was described in 1852 by Broca[50] and subsequently by Clutton.[75] Many authors have recommended the use of first MTP joint arthrodesis as a primary procedure either to correct a severe hallux valgus deformity* or for rheumatoid arthritis (Fig. 6-180 and Video Clip 36),[†] hallux rigidus (Video Clip 33),[‡] or traumatic arthritis.[96,108] It can be used as a salvage procedure for failed bunion surgery or previous infection[196] (Video Clip 34).[§]

---

*References 99, 116, 143, 187, 242, 288, 300, 314, 434, 506, and 521.
†References 27, 64, 86, 94, 96, 218, 342, 345, 346, 379, 512, 528, 529, 541, and 553.
‡References 109, 157, 175, 266, 335, 363, 453, 493, 494, 512, 528, 529, 541, 559, and 568.
§References 104, 175, 196, 215, 347, 453, 528, and 541.

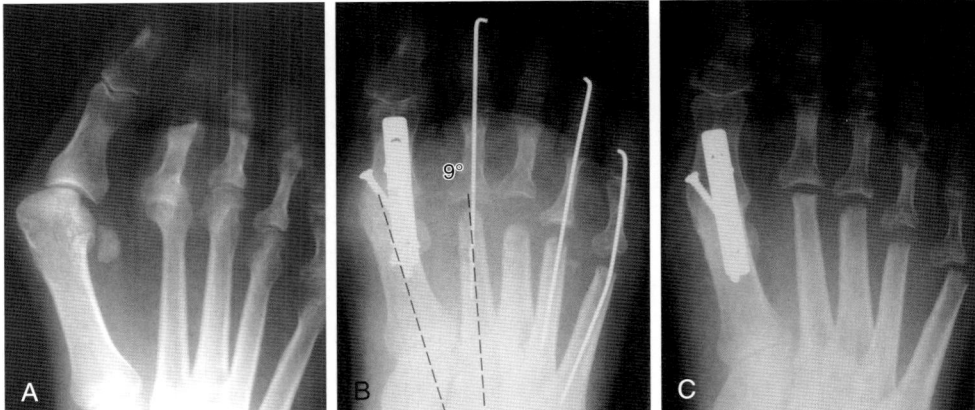

Figure 6-180 Rheumatoid arthritis with hallux valgus. **A,** Preoperative radiograph. **B,** Postoperative radiograph. **C,** Follow-up at 1 year. Note the diminution of the intermetatarsal angle as well.

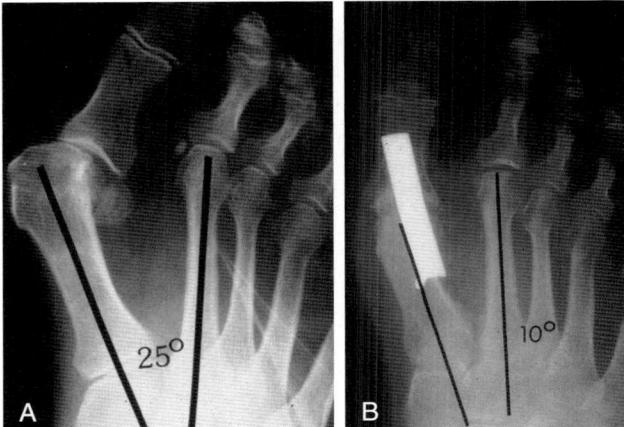

Figure 6-181 Severe hallux valgus. **A,** Preoperative radiograph with a widened intermetatarsal (IM) angle as well. **B,** After metatarsophalangeal arthrodesis, correction of both hallux valgus and the IM angle.

First MTP joint arthrodesis is also useful in a patient with neuromuscular instability secondary to a cerebral vascular accident, head injury, or cerebral palsy.[341,342,512,528] The rationale for the procedure is that the length of the first metatarsal is preserved and stability of the first ray is maintained, thereby allowing weight to be transferred to the hallux.

Indications
Arthrodesis is indicated in a patient with a severe hallux valgus deformity, usually with an angle greater than 50 degrees (Fig. 6-181), in a rheumatoid patient with hallux valgus, in an older patient with moderate or severe hallux valgus, in advanced cases of hallux rigidus, for primary arthritis or arthritis after trauma, and in a patient with a hallux valgus deformity after a CVA or head injury, or with an underlying diagnosis of cerebral palsy. As a salvage

procedure, it is indicated for a recurrent hallux valgus deformity, following a failed implant, and after an unsuccessful cheilectomy.

Contraindications
Few contraindications to arthrodesis of the first MTP joint exist. Relative contraindications include arthrosis of the IP joint or an insensate foot. Another relative contraindication is lack of motion at the MTP joint, which in some cases is annoying to patients. A thorough discussion about the trade-off between reduced MTP joint motion and realignment of the first ray is important preoperatively.

Technique
The surgical technique is divided into the surgical approach, preparation of the joint surfaces, and fixation of the arthrodesis.

Surgical Approach
1. The MTP joint is approached through a dorsal longitudinal incision just medial to the extensor hallucis longus tendon. The 5-cm incision extends from a point just proximal to the IP joint to above the MTP joint (Fig. 6-182A).
2. The incision is deepened through the extensor retinaculum, which is reflected along with the joint capsule. In this way, the dorsomedial cutaneous nerve is protected. The extensor tendon is usually retracted laterally. A complete synovectomy of the MTP joint is performed, after which the medial and lateral collateral ligaments are transected.

Preparation of Curved Concentric Surfaces
Curved concentric surfaces permit easy positioning and adjustment of the MTP joint surfaces for the arthrodesis. This process is less involved technically than cutting two flat surfaces.[490] Flat cuts may lead to excessive shortening if further resection is necessary to

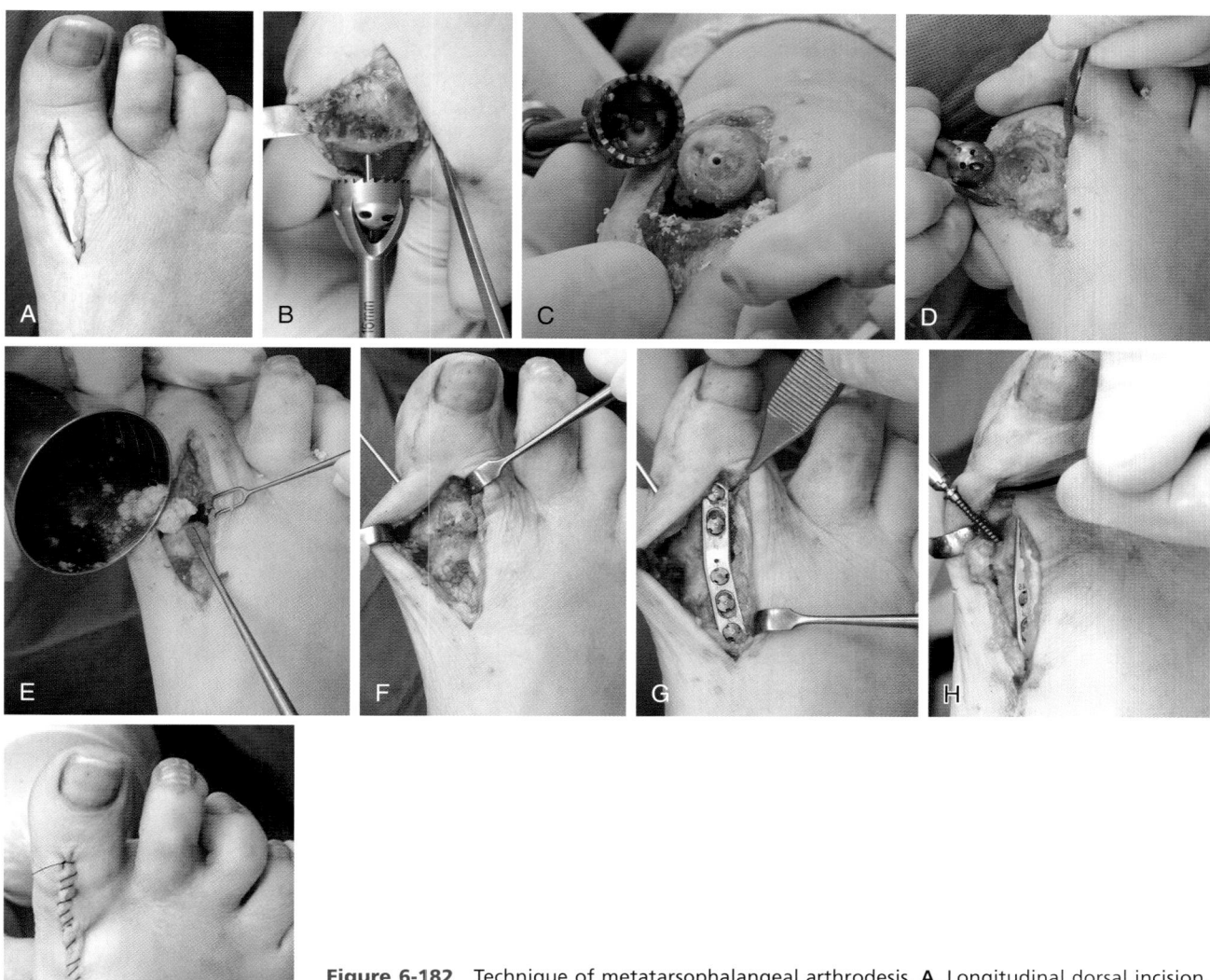

Figure 6-182 Technique of metatarsophalangeal arthrodesis. **A,** Longitudinal dorsal incision. **B,** A cannulated concave metatarsal head reamer **(C)** is used to prepare the metatarsal surface. **D,** Power-driven convex phalangeal reamers are used to prepare the phalanx. **E,** Bone slurry from the reamers is placed in the joint. **F,** Temporary fixation of the arthrodesis site with a Kirschner wire. **G,** Dorsal titanium plate fixation. **H,** Cross-screw placement. **I,** Final appearance of the foot.

achieve adequate position. The following technique for preparation of congruous curved surfaces uses cup-shaped power reamers.*

1. After soft tissue release has been performed medially and laterally, to expose the metatarsal and phalangeal articular surfaces, the medial eminence is removed with a small sagittal saw. A small wafer of bone can be resected from the base of the proximal phalanx and metatarsal head to decompress the joint or shorten the first ray if shortening is desired. If the procedure is being carried out in a rheumatoid patient

and significant shortening is necessary, more of the metatarsal head can be removed at this time. If length is to be preserved, only the articular surface should be removed. On the other hand, preparation of the joint surfaces can be accomplished without initial bone excision, and one can proceed directly to the reaming process.

2. A 0.062-inch K-wire is driven into the center of the first metatarsal head. The size of the metatarsal metaphysis is estimated and a corresponding reamer of the appropriate size is chosen (Fig. 6-182B and C). (Reamers vary from 14 to 20 mm in size, although 16 to 18 mm is the most common diameter used.) A cannulated metatarsal head reamer is used to reduce the

---

*References 87, 107, 109, 143, 187, 288, and 506.

metatarsal head and metaphysis and to shape the articular surface area into a convex cup-shaped surface, after which the wire is removed.

3. The K-wire is then driven into the base of the proximal phalanx. A convex male reamer is used to create a concave, cup-shaped surface. Typically, the smallest reamer is initially used. Reaming is continued with progressively larger reamers until the surface size matches the prepared metatarsal surface (Fig. 6-182D). The K-wire is then removed.

4. The two curved congruent surfaces are rotated into proper alignment, which is 15 degrees of valgus and 15 to 20 degrees of dorsiflexion in relation to the first metatarsal shaft (Fig. 6-182E). The hallux is derotated so that there is no pronation. A 0.062-inch K-wire is driven across the proposed arthrodesis site through a plantar medial stab wound and exits dorsolaterally (Fig. 6-182F).

Alternative Method of Joint Preparation

There are ways to create surfaces for the arthrodesis other than the curved surfaces just described.

1. The distal portion of the first metatarsal is cut with an oscillating saw, and only the articular surface is removed to create a flat surface that is angulated slightly dorsally and laterally. If the procedure is being carried out in a rheumatoid patient and significant shortening is necessary, more of the metatarsal head can be removed at this time, but if length is to be preserved, only the articular surface should be removed (Fig. 6-183A).

2. Longitudinal traction is placed on the hallux, and all the tissues inserting into the base of the proximal phalanx are released by sharp dissection.

3. The hallux is positioned with one hand holding it in approximately 15 degrees of valgus and 10 to 15 degrees of dorsiflexion in relation to the plantar aspect of the foot. The surgeon then carefully notes the relationship between the base of the proximal phalanx and the initial cut made in the metatarsal head. With

the initial cut as a guide, another cut is made parallel to it to resect the entire articular surface and subchondral bone, while leaving, if possible, the metaphyseal flare of the proximal phalanx intact (Fig. 6-183B).

4. The two parallel cuts are placed together, and their alignment is carefully observed. If the position is not correct, another cut is made, this time in the metatarsal head to adjust the alignment. If the procedure is being done in conjunction with a rheumatoid foot repair, no further shortening of the MTP joint should be undertaken until the metatarsal heads are resected and the final length of the first metatarsal can be determined.

5. The hallux is derotated so that there is no pronation. A 0.062-inch K-wire is driven across the proposed arthrodesis site through a plantar medial stab wound and exits dorsolaterally.

Internal Fixation of the Arthrodesis

1. The prepared surfaces are apposed and the alignment carefully checked. On occasion, if the lesser toes tend to deviate slightly medially, the arthrodesis site is aligned in slightly more valgus. As a general rule, the desired alignment is 15 degrees of valgus, 15 to 20 degrees of dorsiflexion, and neutral rotation. With the curved congruous surfaces, these dimensions can be easily altered by merely changing the position of the hallux. With flat surfaces, further resection of the prepared surfaces is necessary to achieve the desired alignment. A 0.062-inch K-wire is inserted as temporary fixation to hold the prepared surfaces (see Fig. 6-182F). A second cross K-wire can be placed if further stabilization is necessary before placement of internal fixation.

2. A dorsal six-hole titanium plate is then placed on the dorsal aspect of the distal first metatarsal and proximal phalanx (see Fig. 6-182G). This preformed plate has 15 degrees of valgus and 20 degrees of dorsiflexion built into it to help align the first ray in the appropriate position. It is stabilized with six dorsal plantar bicortical screws. The K-wire is removed and a cross screw

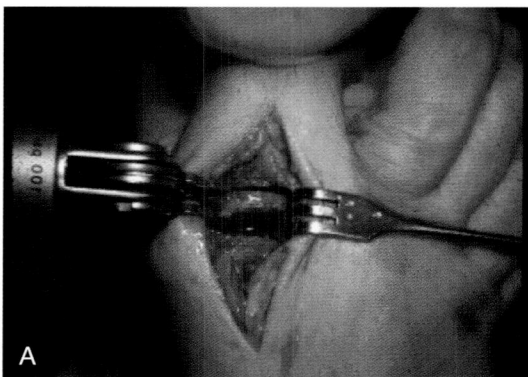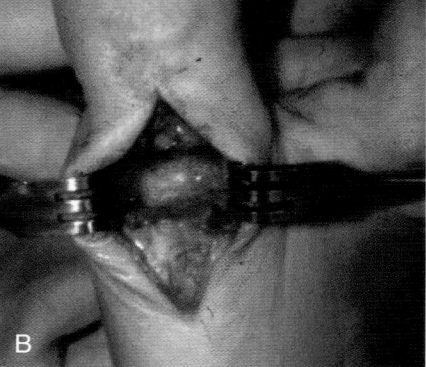

Figure 6-183 **A,** Phalangeal osteotomy to create flat surfaces. **B,** The joint is distracted before arthrodesis.

placed to further fix the arthrodesis site (see Fig. 6-182H and I).

3. Alternatively, an interfragmentary 4.0-mm cannulated screw can be inserted across the proposed arthrodesis site in a medial to lateral direction. The guide pin is placed slightly below the midline of the proximal phalanx and angled in a proximal to lateral direction. The cortex on the medial side of the phalanx is drilled and the hole countersunk. A 24- to 30-mm–long screw is inserted. As the screw is cinched down, the K-wire, which is at a right angle to the screw, is removed to permit as much interfragmentary compression as possible.

4. Any remaining prominent bone or remnants of the medial eminence are resected with a rongeur.

5. The wound is closed in two layers, with the capsule closed beneath the extensor tendon. The skin is closed with fine interrupted sutures, and a compression dressing is applied. The patient is permitted to ambulate in a postoperative shoe, with weight bearing as tolerated on the heel and other aspect of the foot.

Alternative Method of Fixation

Fixation of the arthrodesis site can be carried out in a variety of ways. The authors' philosophy is to obtain fixation that is as rigid as possible so that the patient can ambulate without a cast while achieving a satisfactory rate of fusion. At times, inadequate bone stock is present in the proximal phalanx when attempting to salvage a Keller procedure[104,536] or after removal of a prosthesis. On occasion, in a rheumatoid patient with severe osteopenia, the plate-and-screw technique cannot be used. In these circumstances, the authors prefer to use threaded Steinmann pins to gain fixation of the arthrodesis site (Video Clip 35).[86] These pins have the disadvantage of crossing the IP joint, although in two large series, this did not create a significant clinical problem.[342,346] The surgical technique follows.

1. The joint surfaces are prepared in the same manner as initially described or through the creation of congruous curved surfaces (Fig. 6-184; see also Fig. 6-183).

2. A 1/8-inch, double-pointed Steinmann pin is drilled in a proximal to distal direction out the tip of the hallux (Fig. 6-185A).

3. A second pin is drilled out parallel to the first one.

4. One of the pins protruding through the end of the proximal phalanx is cut about in half so that the chuck can be placed onto the distal end of the longest Steinmann pin.

5. The MTP joint is reduced in proper alignment (varus/valgus, dorsiflexion/plantar flexion, rotation), and with the other hand holding the handle of the drill, the Steinmann pin is slowly drilled across the arthrodesis site into the metatarsal. It should be drilled in until the surgeon feels it penetrating the cortex of the proximal first metatarsal or until it reaches the proximity of the MTC joint. The first pin is then cut off

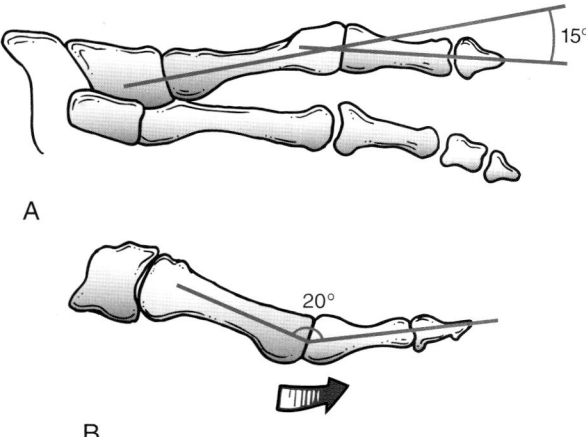

Figure 6-184 The fusion site is placed in 15 to 20 degrees of valgus **(A)**, dorsal view and about 20 degrees of dorsiflexion **(B)**, lateral view in relation to the metatarsal shaft, which is approximately 10 to 15 degrees of dorsiflexion in relation to the floor.

approximately 5 mm from the tip of the skin; the second pin is drilled across the arthrodesis site in a similar manner (Fig. 6-185B).

6. The wound is closed with interrupted sutures and a compression dressing applied. The patient is permitted to ambulate as tolerated.

7. Postoperative care is the same as for other forms of arthrodesis (Fig. 6-185C-F).

On rare occasions, because of loss of significant bone stock, it becomes necessary to add an interposition bone graft to gain more length at the first MTP joint arthrodesis site. As a general rule, a slightly shorter great toe does not create a significant problem, but if circumstances indicate that a bone graft is needed, it can be placed between the proximal phalanx and the metatarsal head as a flat piece of tricortical iliac crest or an oval "football-type" graft (Fig. 6-186 and Video Clip 34). Whenever a bone graft is added, the morbidity of the procedure increases substantially, and the healing time is usually doubled from 3 months to often 5 to 6 months. These patients should usually be kept non–weight bearing to avoid stress on the fixation device and to promote healing of the graft.

Postoperative Care

In the office, 1 or 2 days after surgery, the compression dressing is removed, and a firm 2-inch Kling gauze dressing with 1/2-inch adhesive tape is applied. The patient is permitted to ambulate in a postoperative shoe, as tolerated, with weight borne on the heel and lateral aspect of the foot.

The patient is evaluated with radiographs every 4 weeks until successful fusion occurs. At this time, the postoperative shoe is discontinued. As a general rule, 10 to 12 weeks is required for complete fusion. If longitudinal Steinmann pins have been placed, they are easily removed under a digital block in an office setting.

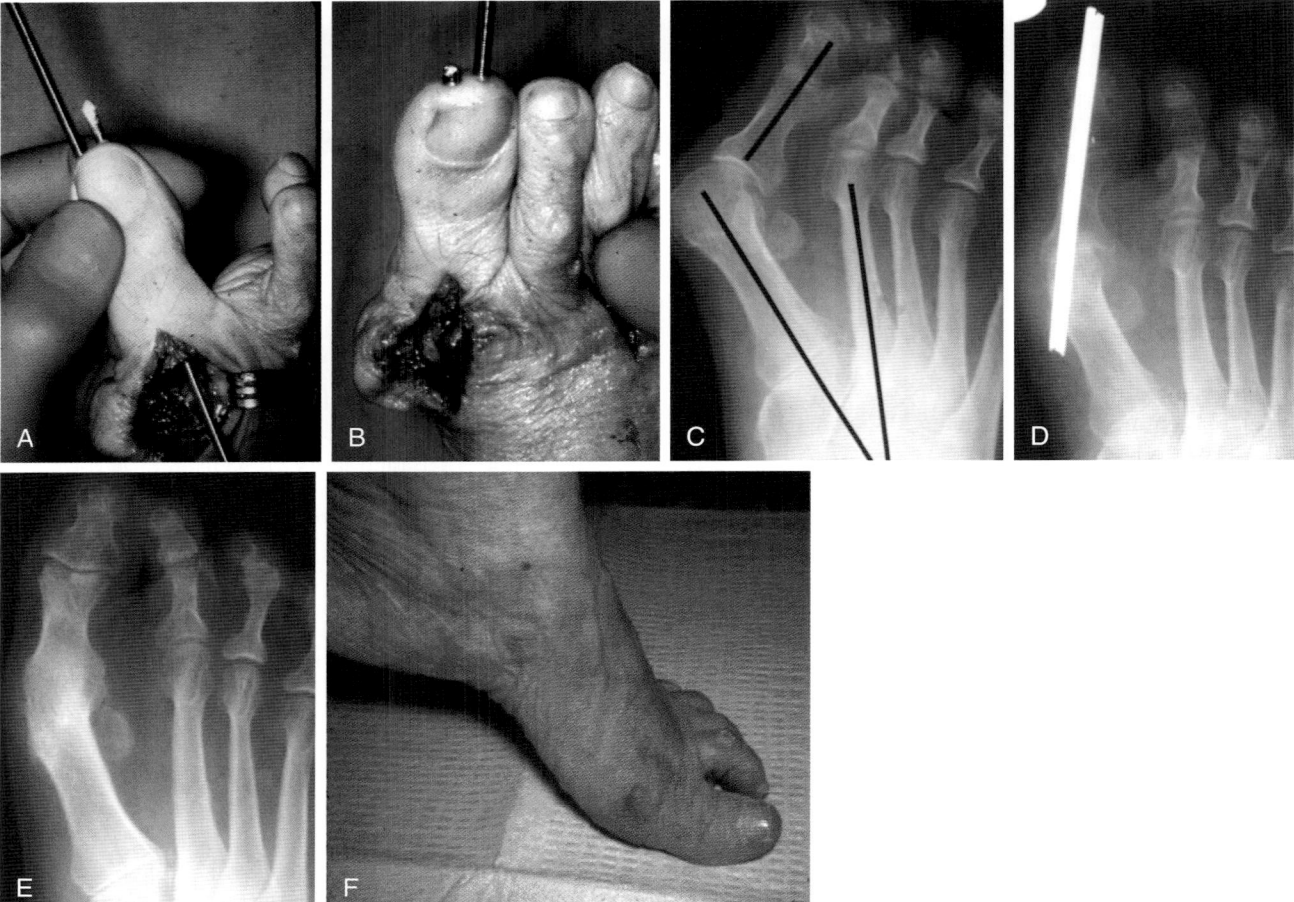

Figure 6-185 First metatarsophalangeal joint fusion technique using threaded Steinmann pins. **A,** A Steinmann pin is driven out through the tip of the great toe in retrograde manner. **B,** Pins are brought back across the attempted fusion site while manually compressing the bony surfaces together. **C,** Preoperative radiograph. **D,** After intramedullary Steinmann pin fixation. **E,** Fifteen years after surgery, a successful arthrodesis is observed. **F,** Fifteen years after surgery, the patient is able to walk on tiptoe.

Results

The reported rate of patient satisfaction after MTP arthrodesis varies from 78% to 93%.* In the only five studies reporting on the treatment of idiopathic hallux valgus by MTP arthrodesis,[99,187,231,434,521] subjective satisfaction was noted in more than 90% of patients (Fig. 6-187).

The rate of fusion varies, depending on the operative technique, the method of internal fixation, and the preoperative diagnosis. MTP joint fusion generally occurs in most patients between 10 and 12 weeks. Reported success rates vary from 77% to 100%, with an average rate of 90%[†] Coughlin[86] reported a 10% failure rate in a review of 1451 cases in the literature. In the largest series, Riggs and Johnson[440] reported a 91% fusion rate in 309 procedures. With the use of a dorsal compression plate, the reported success rate ranged from 92% to 100%.[‡]

Coughlin and Abdo[96] reported subjective good and excellent results in 93% of cases. Inadequate fixation is the more commonly cited reason for nonunion,[174,434,440,529] but true failure of fixation is uncommon.[440] As McKeever[363] noted, an unsuccessful arthrodesis or pseudoarthrosis may still give a painless and successful result (Fig. 6-188). Coughlin,[99] in a series of 21 arthrodeses, reported 3 asymptomatic nonunions (14%). In another series of 49 patients, Goucher and Coughlin[187] reported 4 nonunions (8%), three of which were asymptomatic. Hope et al[226] reported on 11 nonunions from a large series of otherwise successful arthrodeses and observed that 7 of the 11 were successfully treated with removal of the failed hardware and debridement of the wound. Only four patients required eventual redo arthrodesis or arthroplasty.

The final alignment of the fusion is very important for patient satisfaction. The recommended angle of valgus ranges from 5 to 30 degrees, with an average of 15 degrees.* Fitzgerald[157] warned that fusion in less than 20 degrees of valgus is associated with a threefold incidence

---

*References 27, 64, 87, 94, 96, 187, 218, 288, 342, 345, 346, 379, 506, 512, 528, 529, 541, and 553.
†References 99, 116, 143, 187, 288, and 506.
‡References 87, 96, 99, 116, 143, 187, 196, 288, 332, 506, and 541.

---

*References 99, 104, 157, 196, 346, 434, and 440.

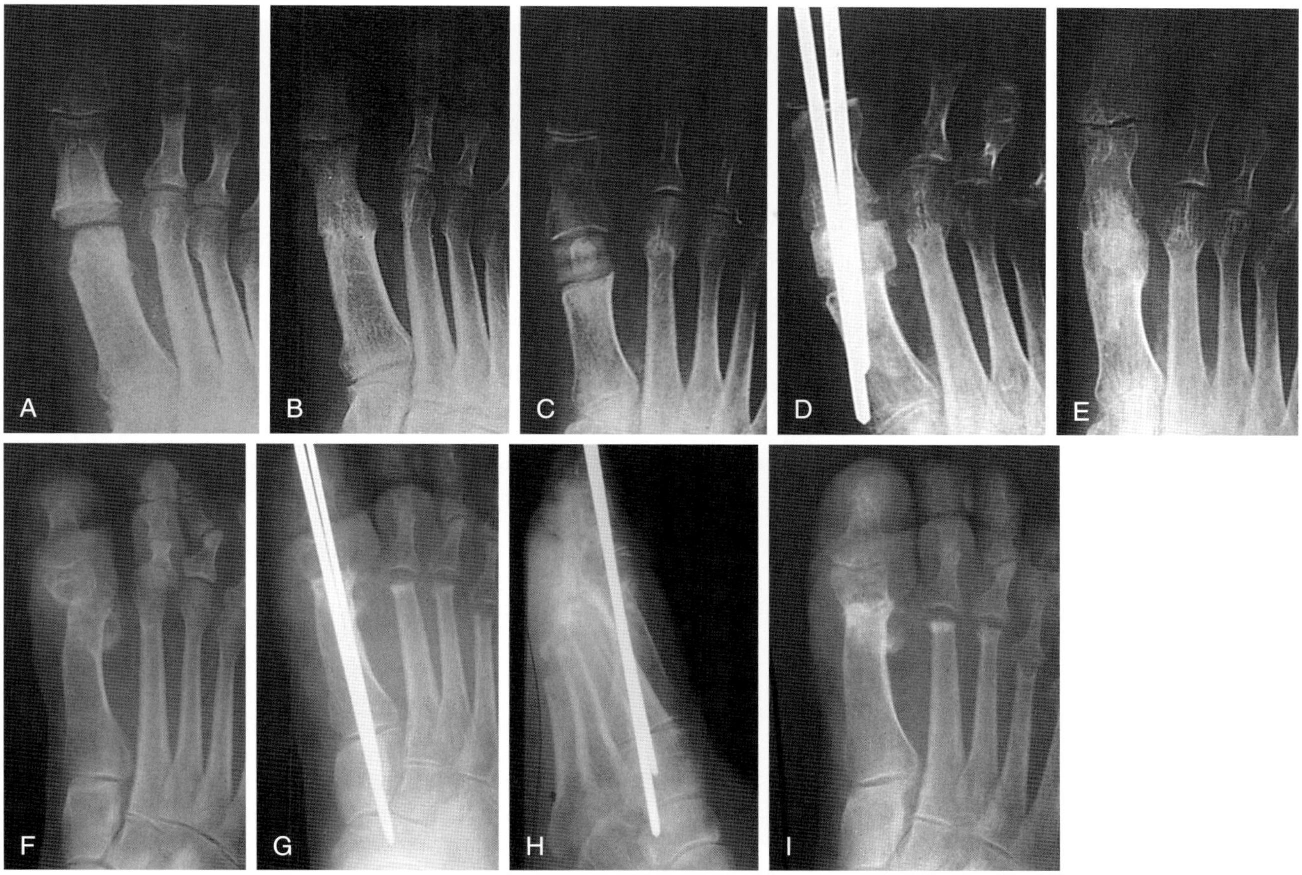

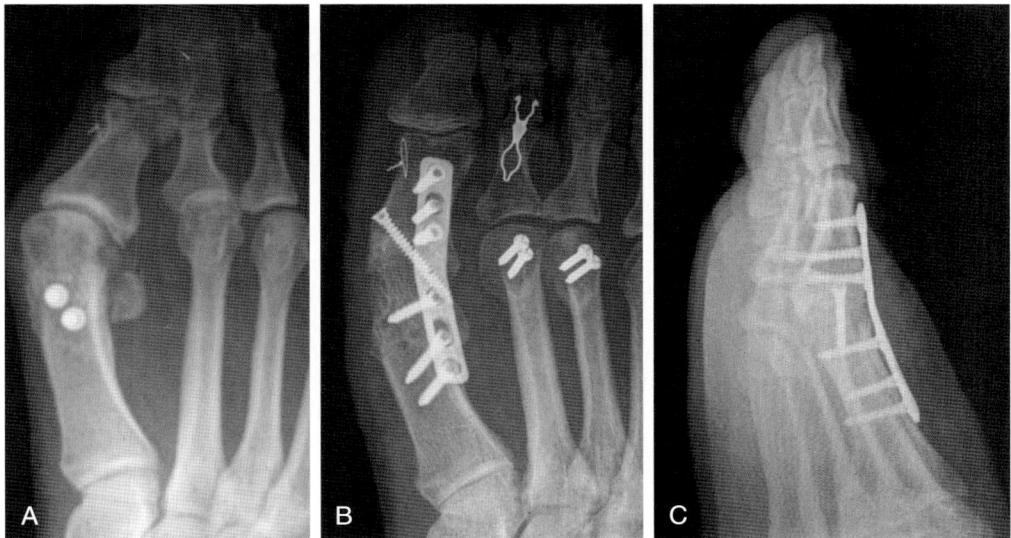

Figure 6-186 **A,** Preoperative radiograph demonstrating a failed single-stem prosthesis. **B,** Postoperative radiograph of fusion after removal of the prosthesis. **C,** Preoperative radiograph with a failed double-stemmed prosthesis. **D,** Postoperative radiograph after removal of the prosthesis and insertion of a bone graft. **E,** Successful arthrodesis. **F,** Preoperative radiograph after a failed Keller arthroplasty. **G** and **H,** After arthrodesis with the Steinmann pin technique. **I,** After removal of the pins.

Figure 6-187 **A,** Preoperative radiograph demonstrating recurrent hallux valgus deformity with increased 1–2 intermetatarsal angle. Postoperative anteroposterior **(B)** and lateral **(C)** radiographs demonstrating precontoured titanium dorsal plate.

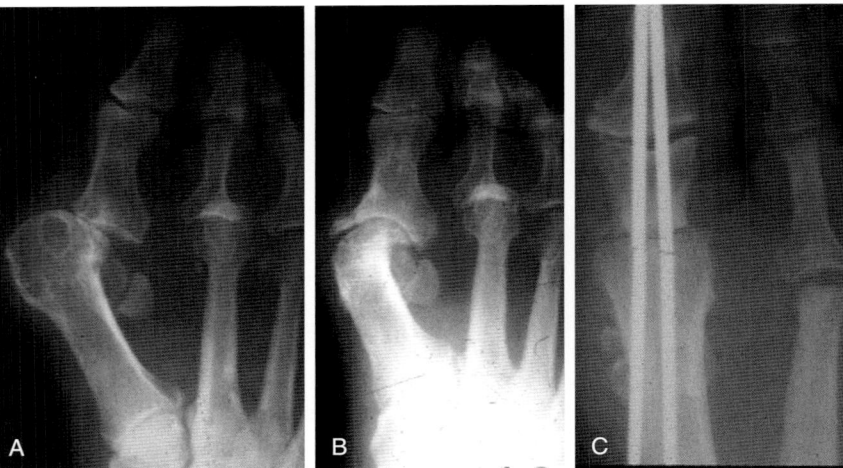

Figure 6-188 **A,** Severe hallux valgus associated with rheumatoid arthritis. **B,** Painful nonunion with a decrease in angular deformity in a satisfied patient. **C,** Broken Steinmann pins portend a nonunion.

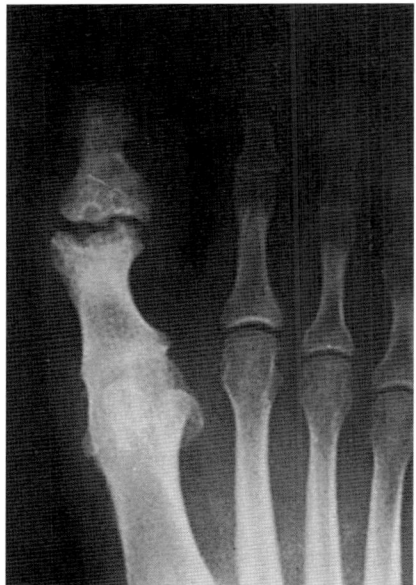

Figure 6-189 Degenerative arthritis of the interphalangeal joint is rarely symptomatic.

of IP joint arthritis. The literature reports a 6% to 33% rate of degenerative arthritis of the IP joint after arthrodesis of the MTP joint (Fig. 6-189).[99,187,218,379,440] Coughlin et al [99] reported at an average 8-year follow-up and noted little progression of IP joint arthritis and negligible IP joint pain. Grimes and Coughlin[196] reported that 8 of 33 feet showed progression of IP joint arthritis; however, in this and the previous study,[99,196] corresponding arthritis in the contralateral foot IP joint was relatively symmetric and may have been related to patient age and the long-term follow-up of each study (8 years). Mann and Oates,[342] using Steinmann pins that crossed the IP joint for internal fixation, reported a 40% incidence of degenerative changes at the IP joint. Few of these patients had any clinical symptoms at final follow-up.

Degenerative arthritis in the first MTC joint can also be a concern. Coughlin et al[99] reported on 21 feet followed for an average of 8 years after MTP arthrodesis. Four MC joints showed progression of arthritis, but four contralateral MTC joints showed similar changes. Grimes and Coughlin,[196] in a review of failed bunion surgery in which MTP joint arthrodesis was used to salvage 33 feet, noted 5 feet with degenerative changes, but 4 were observed in the contralateral foot. Thus, again, in this 8-year follow-up study, arthritic changes of the first MTC joint may have been a function of the length of follow-up as opposed to the ipsilateral MTP joint arthrodesis.

After arthrodesis, the increased 1–2 IM angle associated with a severe hallux valgus deformity is routinely reduced,* and rarely, if ever, is a first metatarsal osteotomy necessary.[212,231,341] The authors do not believe that any attempt should be made to correct the IM angle when carrying out an arthrodesis. If for some reason the IM angle is unacceptable, it can be corrected with a basal osteotomy at another time, rather than creating a situation in which, besides attempting to obtain an arthrodesis at the MTP joint, the surgeon is simultaneously attempting to heal an osteotomy at the metatarsal base. Cronin et al[116] reported an average 1–2 IM angle correction of 8.2 degrees after MTP joint arthrodesis. The average preoperative 1–2 IM angle was 17 degrees, and the average hallux valgus angle was 47 degrees. Thus the more severe the preoperative angular deformity, the more correction achieved with the arthrodesis procedure.

In the sagittal plane, the recommended angle of dorsiflexion for the fusion varies from 10 to 40 degrees† (in relation to the shaft of the first metatarsal), with 20 to 25 degrees being the most commonly recommended position.[86] The conical shape of the proximal phalanx creates a dorsal slope to the phalanx that influences the final

*References 33, 99, 104, 116, 157, 174, 187, 196, 212, 231, 242, 332, 342, 346, 363, 434, 440, 528, 553, 558, and 559.
†References 96, 99, 187, 242, 342, 346, 512, and 529.

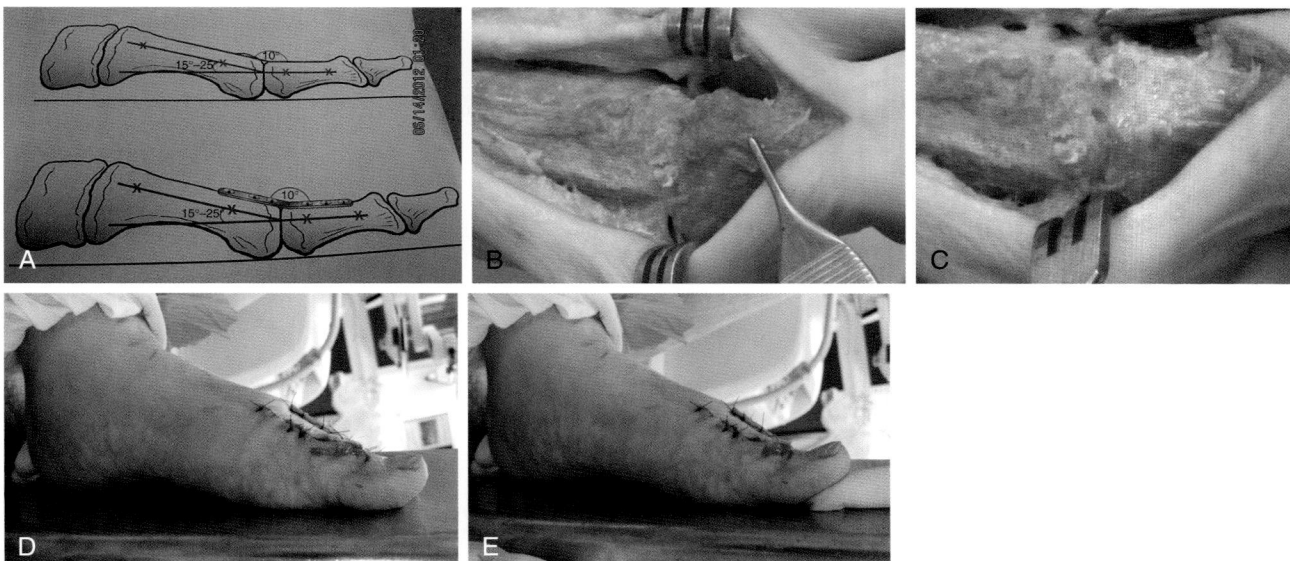

Figure 6-190 Aspects of metatarsophalangeal (MTP) joint arthrodesis. **A,** The dorsiflexion angle of arthrodesis. The dorsiflexion angle of arthrodesis is calculated using middiaphyseal reference points. These, as show in the diagram, may measure 10 to 25 degrees of dorsiflexion; the plate, to fit this angulation may only have a dorsal bend of 10 degrees. **B,** The dorsal flare of the phalanx can lead to malalignment **C,** Removal with a rongeur can assist in the alignment. **D,** Using the undersurface of an irrigation pan, or using a fingertip beneath the tip of the toe **E,** these methods allow a surgeon intraoperatively to gauge that there is adequate dorsiflexion present are both methods to avoid excessive plantar flexion at the MTP arthrodesis site.

position of the arthrodesis.[300] Precontoured plates, to a certain extent, take this into account; however, the final position of the arthrodesis is effected by the plantar inclination of the first metatarsal. A patient with a flatfoot may have much more dorsal inclination with a precontoured plate than a patient with a cavus foot. Thus, intraoperatively, a surgeon should ensure that the position of the arthrodesis is correct in a sagittal as well as a coronal plane (Fig. 6-190). Coughlin[94] reported that there was a marked increase in IP joint arthritis when the dorsiflexion angle of fusion was less than 20 degrees. Fusion in excessive dorsiflexion leads to pressure beneath the sesamoids, whereas fusion in excess plantar flexion leads to pressure beneath the tip of the great toe.

Use of a dorsal mini-fragment or titanium compression plate is relatively easy and has been associated with reasonably high success rates of fusion.[187,288] Whereas the larger and bulky small-fragment compression plates have frequently required removal,[87,332,541] the low-profile Vitallium plates[96] and titanium plates[107,109] have not required removal. Other reports on the use of compression screws for fixation have demonstrated their reliability as well and a high level of patient satisfaction.[242] The main advantage of rigid internal fixation is that it permits immediate ambulation with a postoperative shoe, thereby eliminating the need for a walking cast. However, protected ambulation is important. Ellington et al[143] reported a lower fusion rate in those who had unprotected ambulation as opposed to those who did heel weight bearing for the first 6 weeks (86% vs. 93% fusion rate, respectively). In an older patient, particularly a rheumatoid patient, the

ability to walk postoperatively without a cast is extremely important (Fig. 6-191).

The surgical technique used for MTP arthrodesis should be simple and achieve a predictable result (Fig. 6-192). Shaping of the curved congruous joint surfaces to enable the surgeon to easily adjust the metatarsal and phalanx to the desired position of valgus, extension, and rotation is a key part of this procedure. The use of rigid internal fixation is important in obtaining and maintaining the desired fusion until osseous fusion has occurred. As McKeever[363] said, however, "it is the [fusion] and its position that is important and not the method by which it is obtained."

Complications

The main complications after MTP joint arthrodesis are nonunion, malalignment, and degenerative arthrosis of the IP joint of the great toe. With the use of an interfragmentary screw and dorsal plate, the authors believe that a fusion rate of 95% can probably be achieved. In some cases of hallux rigidus in which the bone ends are extremely sclerotic, the surgeon may anticipate difficulty in obtaining fusion, and possibly weight bearing should be delayed in these patients. In some cases, the authors have found it necessary to make multiple drill holes through the sclerotic bone in an attempt to improve blood flow across the attempted arthrodesis site.

Certain situations present increased risk for a successful arthrodesis. Ellington et al[143] reported the nonunion rate for those with rheumatoid arthritis was 23%, although those without rheumatoid arthritis had a 7% nonunion

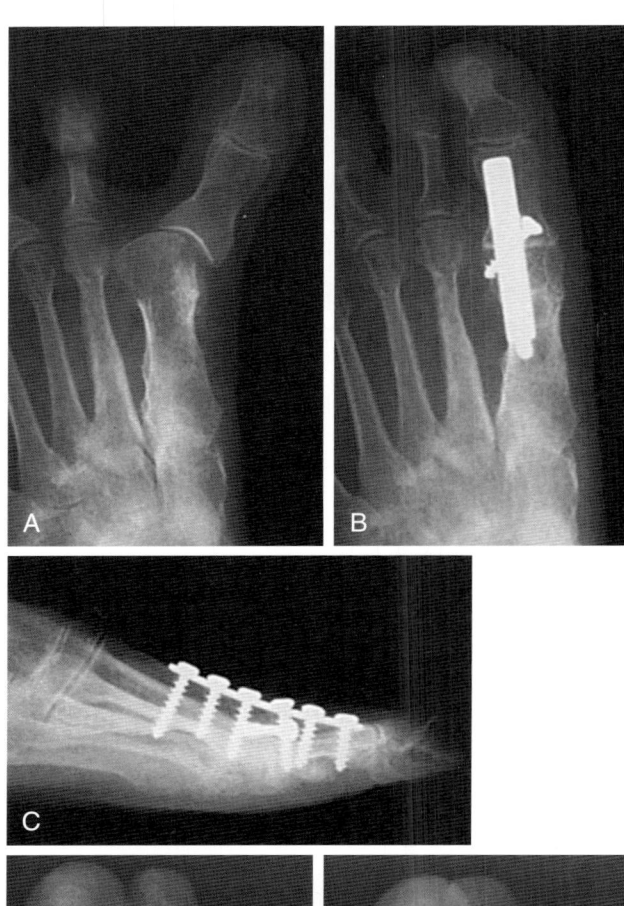

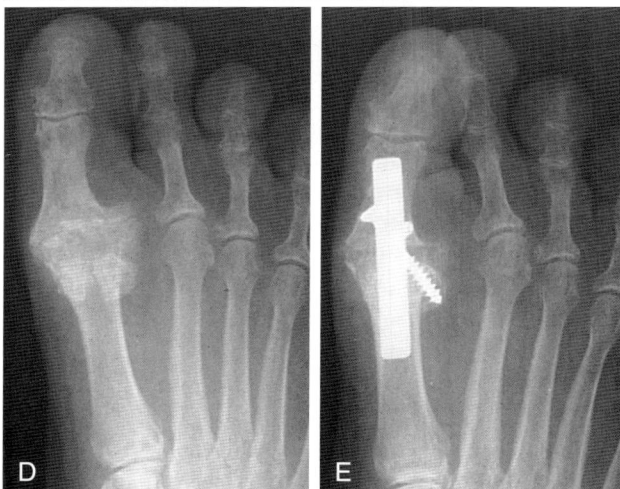

Figure 6-191 First metatarsophalangeal joint arthrodesis. **A,** Preoperative radiograph demonstrating varus with a decrease in the intermetatarsal (IM) angle. **B** and **C,** After arthrodesis, the IM angle is actually increased to a normal value. Preoperative **(D)** and postoperative **(E)** radiographs demonstrate fusion with advanced arthrosis.

rate. Hope et al[226] noted the nonunion rate in males was 19% and in females was 2.4%. They also noted that with prior failed surgery, the nonunion rate was 24%. On the other hand, Grimes and Coughlin[196] reported a successful fusion rate of 86%.

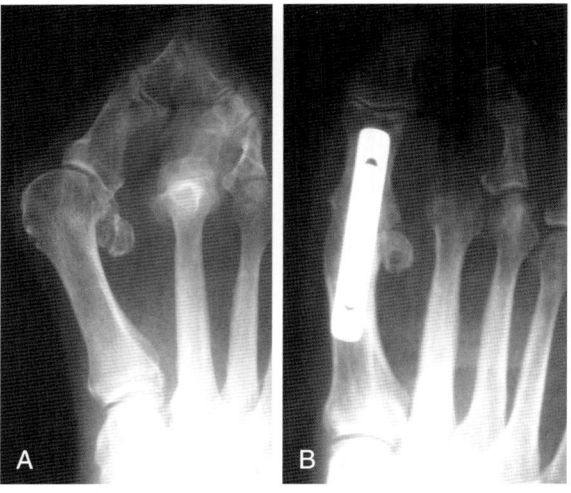

Figure 6-192 **A,** Preoperative radiograph demonstrating severe hallux valgus and a dislocated second metatarsophalangeal joint. **B,** Second toe amputation is possible with a fused hallux because there is no progression of deformity.

Nonunion, when it occurs, is often not painful.[99,187,196,226,363] If the patient has pain, repair is necessary, either by bone grafting if the fixation is adequate or by removal of the fixation device, bone grafting, and the application of new fixation if indicated.

Malunion in any plane is poorly tolerated by patients. This emphasizes the importance of close attention to the final position of the arthrodesis. As Coughlin[88] said, "no bunion procedure requires a technique that is more exacting and unforgiving than that required in arthrodesis of the first MTP joint."

KELLER PROCEDURE

Riedel,[439] in 1886, was the first to perform a resection of the base of the proximal phalanx and arthroplasty of the MTP joint as treatment of hallux valgus. Davies-Colley,[120] in 1887, described this same procedure for the treatment of hallux rigidus. It was popularized by Keller's reports in 1904 and 1912.[264] The purpose of the procedure in the treatment of hallux valgus is to decompress the MTP joint by resection of about a third of the proximal phalanx, thereby relaxing the contracted lateral structures (Video Clip 60). Although the Keller procedure was probably once the most widely used bunion procedure, with the development of other surgical techniques and critical clinical evaluation of results of the Keller procedure, its limitations and indications have been better defined.

Indications

The Keller procedure is indicated in an older patient in whom extensive surgery is contraindicated and who is essentially considered housebound ambulatory[531] or in an older patient with a severe hallux valgus deformity and marginal circulation that has resulted in chronic skin breakdown. It is often considered a salvage technique for treatment of a failed previous surgical procedure.[135,464,531,536] It is indicated for moderate hallux valgus deformities in which the hallux valgus angle is less than 30 degrees associated with degenerative arthritis of the MTP joint. The Keller procedure can also be used to treat hallux rigidus in patients in whom cheilectomy or arthrodesis cannot be performed. In this procedure, medial eminence resection, partial proximal phalangectomy, and medial capsulorrhaphy are performed to realign the hallux.*

Contraindications

This procedure is contraindicated in younger, more active individuals[318] in whom MTP joint mobility and function remain important because the stability of the first MTP joint is impaired by the Keller procedure.[104] Likewise, in older individuals in whom MTP joint function is important, who have substantial lateral metatarsalgia, or who have a severe deformity for which a subtotal correction is unacceptable, this procedure is contraindicated.

Technique

The surgical technique is divided into the surgical approach, resection of bone, and reconstruction of the MTP joint.

Surgical Approach

1. The first MTP joint is exposed through a medial approach that begins at the IP joint and extends proximally 1 cm beyond the medial eminence. A proximally based capsular flap is developed to create full-thickness dorsal and plantar skin flaps for exposure of the medial eminence (Figs. 6-193 and 6-194A; see Video Clip 60).
2. The medial eminence is exposed by sharp dissection to create a flap of medial capsule based proximally.
3. The base of the proximal phalanx is exposed subperiosteally.

Resection of Bone

1. The medial eminence is removed in line with the medial aspect of the metatarsal shaft. Any osteophytes along the dorsal aspect of the metatarsal head are removed (Fig. 6-194B).
2. The proximal third of the phalanx is removed (Fig. 6-194C; see Fig. 6–193A).
3. Resection of the lateral sesamoid is thought to release the lateral contracted structures, which aids in realignment of the hallux (Fig. 6-194D).[135]

Reconstruction of the Metatarsophalangeal Joint

1. To reestablish flexor function, an attempt is made to reapproximate the plantar aponeurosis and plantar plate to the proximal phalanx through two or three small drill holes in the remaining diaphyseal portion of the proximal phalanx.[88,542] Flexor function can also

---

*References 31, 255, 338, 437, 480, and 542.

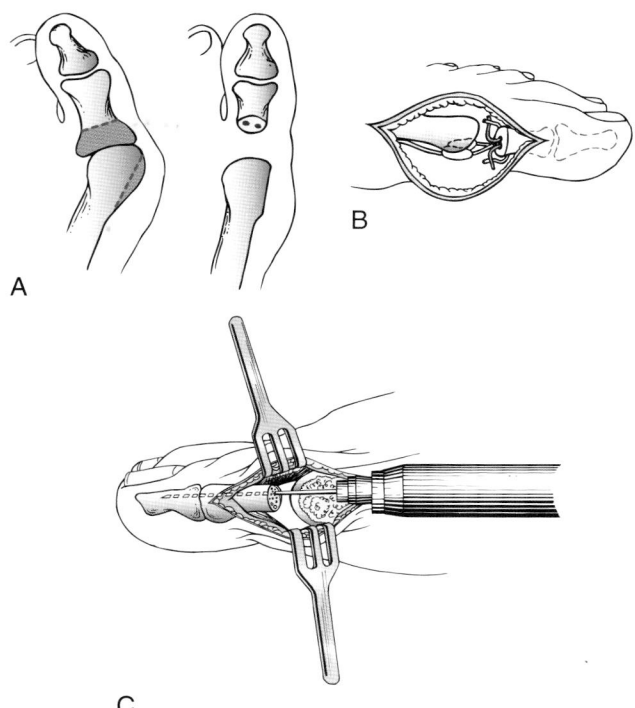

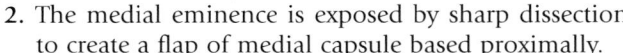

Figure 6-193 The Keller procedure. **A,** The medial eminence is removed in line with the medial aspect of the metatarsal shaft. The proximal third of the proximal phalanx is excised. **B,** An attempt is made to reapproximate the plantar and medial capsular structures to the remaining base of the proximal phalanx. **C,** Fixation of the metatarsophalangeal joint with a 5/64-inch Steinmann pin.

be enhanced by suturing the plantar aponeurosis to the flexor hallucis longus tendon, which helps prevent a cock-up deformity of the MTP joint (Fig. 6-195A).

2. A 5/64-inch Steinmann pin or two 0.062-inch K-wires[135] are introduced at the joint and driven distally; they are then drilled in a retrograde direction across the joint into the metatarsal head to provide stability in the postoperative period and to create a 5-mm gap between the base of the phalanx and the metatarsal head. The tip of the pins should be bent to prevent proximal migration (see Figs. 6-193C and 6-194E).
3. The medial capsular flap is sutured to the periosteum of the proximal phalanx and, in some cases, folded across the MTP joint to create an interposition arthroplasty (see Fig. 6-194F).
4. The skin is closed with interrupted sutures, and a compression dressing is applied.

Postoperative Care

In the office, 1 to 2 days after surgery, the compression dressing is removed and the patient placed in a firm dressing of 2-inch Kling gauze and 1/2-inch adhesive tape. The patient is permitted to ambulate in a postoperative shoe. The dressings are maintained for 6 weeks. The pins are removed 3 weeks after surgery, at which point gentle motion of the MTP joint is begun.

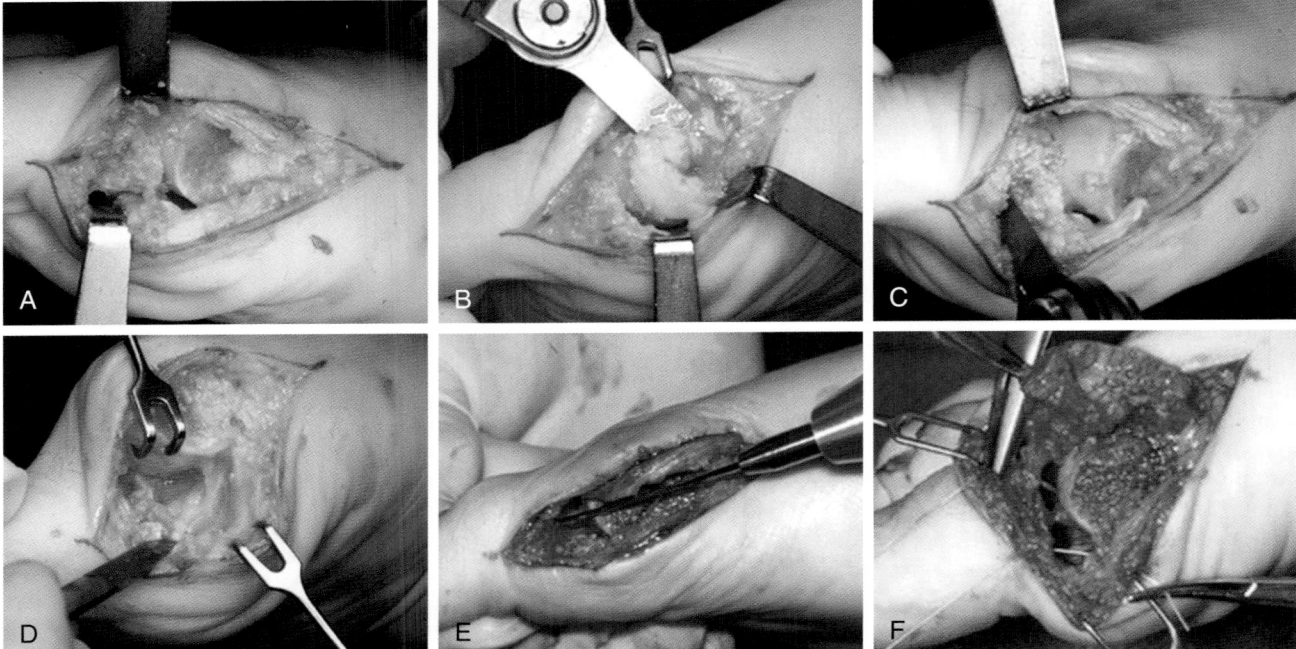

Figure 6-194 **A,** A midline incision is used to expose the medial eminence. Dorsal and plantar flaps are developed. **B,** The medial eminence is excised. **C,** The base of the proximal phalanx is resected with a power saw. **D,** The lateral sesamoid is excised. **E,** An intramedullary Kirschner wire is used to stabilize the toe. **F,** The medial capsule and intrinsics are reattached when possible to the base of the proximal phalanx. (Courtesy E. Greer Richardson, MD.)

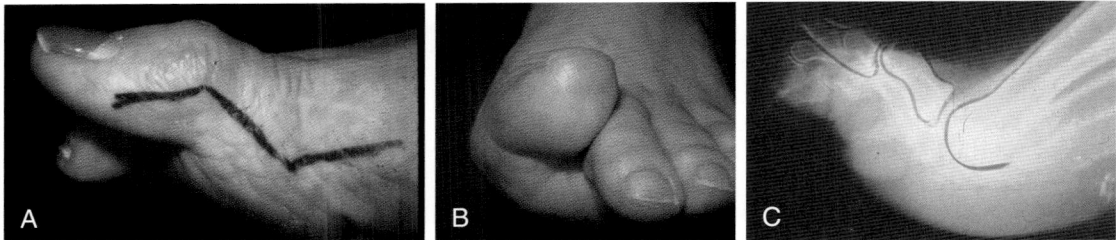

Figure 6-195 Cock-up deformity after the Keller arthroplasty. **A** and **B,** Clinical photographs. **C,** Radiographic appearance.

Results

After excisional arthroplasty, the hallux valgus angle is typically reduced approximately 50% or less,[327,530,531,536] and the 1–2 IM angle is diminished very little.[437,444,530] Satisfactory results occur more reliably when the hallux valgus angle does not exceed 30 degrees so that correction can be achieved by resection of less than a third of the base of the proximal phalanx (Fig. 6-196). Reduction of pain after the procedure can be attributed to a diminution in size of the medial eminence, which enables the use of more comfortable shoes, as well as decompression of an osteoarthritic joint. Satisfaction rates after a Keller procedure, judged mainly on the basis of relief of "bunion pain" as opposed to relief of metatarsalgia, vary from 72% to 96%.[74] Rogers and Joplin[444] reported generally poor results with this procedure: marked improvement in 9%, no change in 71%, and postoperative deterioration in 20%. Bonney and Macnab[38] observed

that the functional results tend to deteriorate with time. Henry et al[218] observed that after excisional arthroplasty, the hallux was unable to bear weight, and resultant metatarsalgia developed.

Donley et al[135] and Richardson[437] both reported an average total MTP joint range of 40 to 50 degrees, most of which was dorsiflexion. Love et al[318] reported less than 10 degrees in 18 feet. When assessing the results of a Keller procedure, the surgeon must remember that for the procedure to be successful, it should be used in older patients, who by nature are less demanding of their feet. When the procedure is used in this group, a satisfactory result can be anticipated. If, however, the procedure is used in more active persons, dissatisfaction results because of the lack of push-off of the great toe, transfer metatarsalgia (usually beneath the second metatarsal head), cock-up deformity of the first MTP joint, and recurrence of the deformity. The Keller procedure cannot correct a

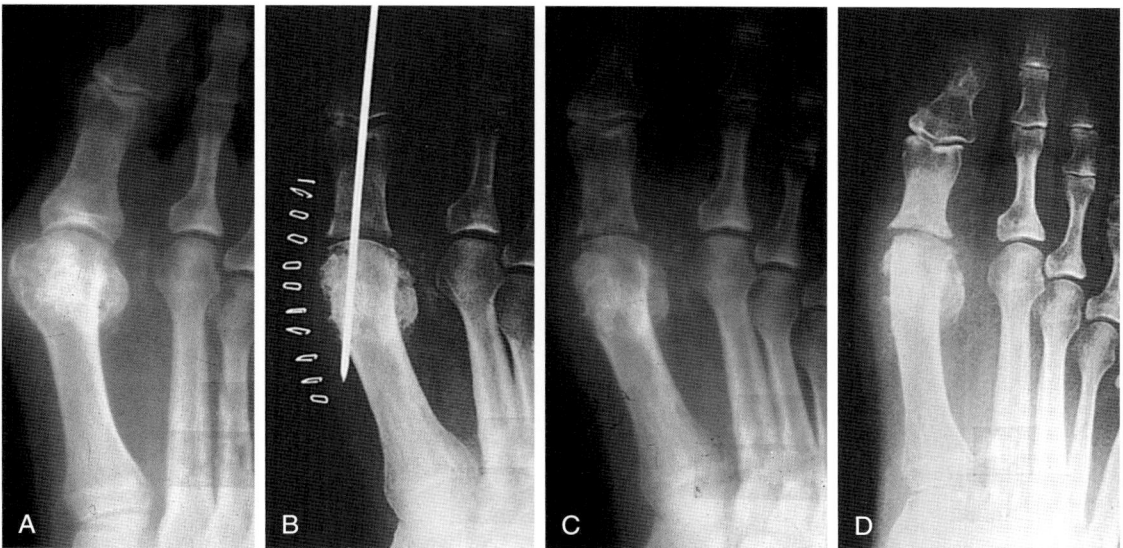

Figure 6-196 Results of the Keller procedure. **A,** Preoperative radiograph. **B,** Postoperative radiograph demonstrating pin fixation. **C,** Radiograph after pin removal. **D,** Position of the toe 9 months after surgery.

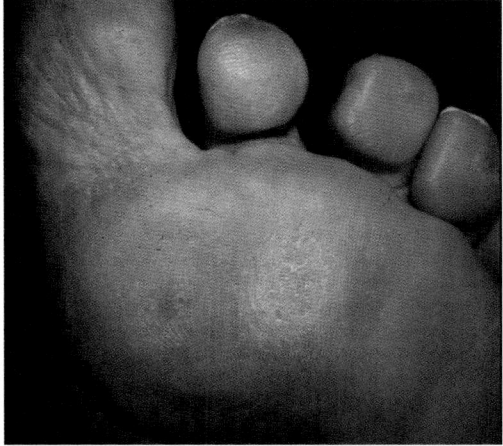

Figure 6-197 Intractable plantar keratosis beneath the second metatarsophalangeal joint after the Keller procedure.

significant hallux valgus deformity or IM angle, and other procedures should be strongly considered. Berner et al[31] have reported successful use of the Keller resection arthroplasty in the treatment of recalcitrant ulceration of the hallux in diabetic patients.

Complications
Coughlin and Mann[104] and others* have reported a high incidence of metatarsalgia after excisional arthroplasty (Fig. 6-197; see Fig. 6-195). Postoperative varus and valgus deformity may occur because of lack of intrinsic control (Figs. 6-198 and 6-199). The magnitude of phalangeal resection appears to play a role in the level of satisfaction. Although excision of half of the phalanx has

---
*References 74, 135, 218, 255, 437, 444, 530, and 536.

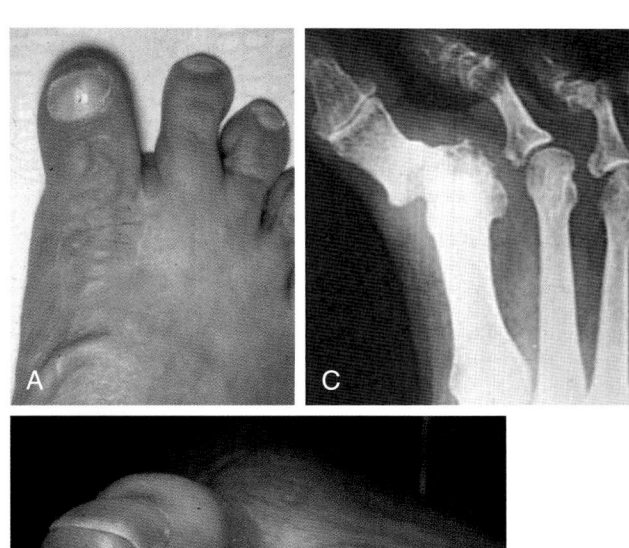

Figure 6-198 Varus deformity after the Keller procedure. **A** and **B,** Clinical photographs. **C,** Radiographic appearance.

been recommended,[38,74,255] limited phalangeal resection is associated with higher rates of postoperative satisfaction.[531] Henry et al[218] reported an association between greater phalangeal resection and increased weight bearing beneath the lateral metatarsals, as well as an increased incidence of lateral metatarsalgia. On analyzing the

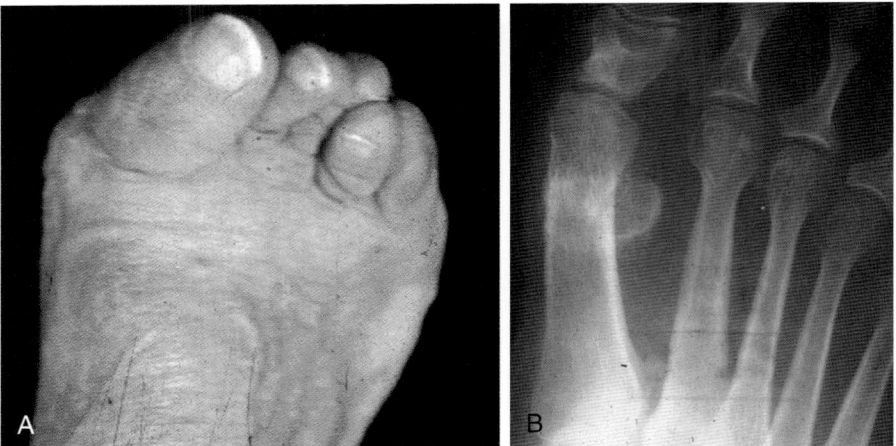

Figure 6-199 Valgus deformity after the Keller procedure. Clinical **(A)** and radiographic **(B)** appearance. (**A,** Courtesy E. Greer Richardson, MD.)

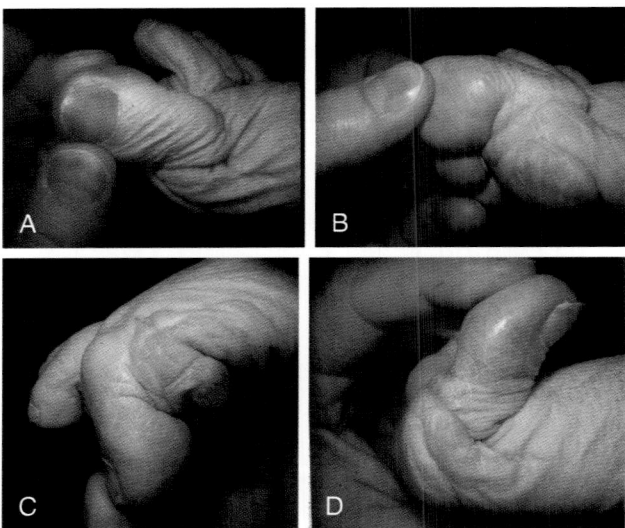

Figure 6-200 Unstable hallux after a Keller resection arthroplasty.

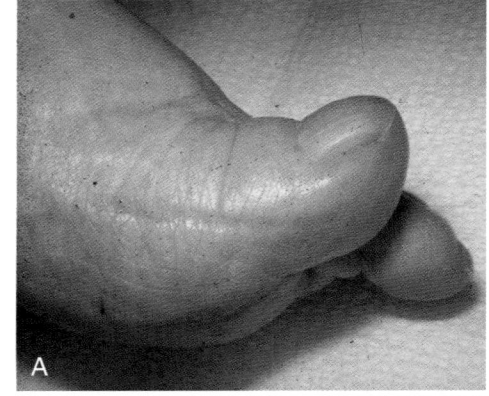

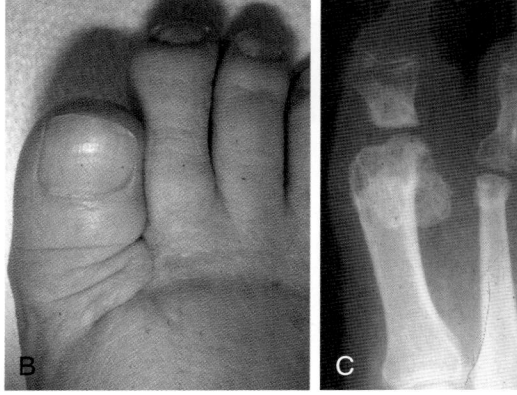

Figure 6-201 Short hallux after a Keller procedure. **A** and **B,** Clinical photographs. **C,** Radiograph.

length of the remaining phalanx, they noted that weight bearing on the hallux was present in 73% of feet, from which a third or less of the proximal phalanx had been resected, whereas it was present in only 9% when more than a third of the phalanx was resected. In patients with more severe deformities, there is a tendency to resect a greater amount of the proximal phalanx to realign the hallux. Vallier et al[531] observed that excessive resection tended to leave a short, flail, functionless great toe (Figs. 6-200 and 6-201). Donley et al[135] reported that patients lost two thirds of plantar flexion, and 40% lost plantar flexion power. Range of motion is often diminished after the Keller procedure. Postoperative metatarsalgia has been reported in most series*; other reported

complications include impaired control and function of the hallux,[104,218] diminished flexor strength,[104,327,480,530,531] marked shortening of the digit,[104,218] IP joint stiffness,[104,218] and cock-up deformity of the great toe.* Because of the high incidence of incomplete correction and the

*References 74, 218, 318, 437, 444, 480, and 531.

*References 264, 318, 327, 444, 480, and 530.

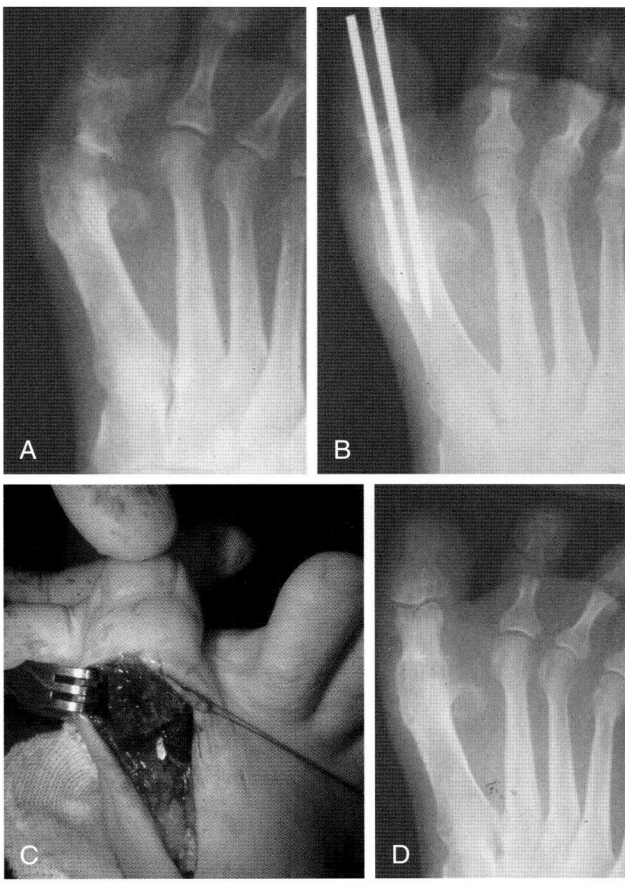

Figure 6-202 Failed Keller procedure—shortened and arthritic hallux. **A,** Clinical appearance. **B,** After arthrodesis with intramedullary Steinmann pins. **C,** Intraoperative photograph. **D,** After successful fusion.

associated postoperative lateral metatarsalgia, excisional arthroplasty is recommended only for elderly sedentary patients with osteoarthritis of the first MTP joint in the absence of metatarsalgia preoperatively.[327] As Henry et al[218] concluded, "any operation for hallux valgus should attempt to restore (or at least not destroy) the ability of the big toe to bear weight." Salvage of a failed Keller arthroplasty can be a difficult procedure and may require an interposition bone graft[104] (Figs. 6-202 and 6-203).

Coughlin and Mann[104] and Vienne et al[536] have both reported on series in which MTP joint arthrodesis was used to salvage a painful failed Keller arthroplasty. The arthrodesis led to improved weight bearing of the first ray and a correction of recurrent hallux valgus deformities. A high rate of fusion was achieved in both studies, although both authors cautioned that although salvage was successful, and pain reduction and deformity correction was achieved, function of the hallux was still impaired.

Complications of Hallux Valgus Surgery

To discuss complications of bunion surgery, the goals of treating hallux valgus deformities should first be clarified.

The main goal is to produce the most functional foot possible after surgery. This will vary, depending on the severity of the deformity and the functional capability of the patient. In a young patient with bunion pain secondary to a prominent medial eminence, a fully functional, a painless foot is the goal; in a rheumatoid patient, a foot with satisfactory overall alignment that allows reasonable footwear and an ability to walk without pain is a realistic goal.

The algorithms that are found in Figures 6-78, 6-79, and 6-82 can help the clinician decide which type of surgical procedure will produce the best surgical results. However, this does not address a patient's expectations. The patient and clinician must have the same goals in mind when surgery is being contemplated. The authors see many patients in consultation who have been misled regarding their surgery, and although the result obtained was within the normal spectrum for a specific procedure, the patient was extremely dissatisfied. If patients are made aware of the various complications associated with each specific procedure (e.g., loss of motion, residual joint pain, sensitivity about the scar), although they may not be totally satisfied, at least they face no surprises. It is important to not "sell" a patient on a procedure but rather to be sure the patient believes that all types of conservative management have been attempted and that surgery will offer a realistic solution to the problem. If the patient has no pain, it is difficult to improve the situation.

To a certain extent, each age group has specific goals for correction of a foot problem. With the wide selection of leisure and sport shoes available today, people can wear a shoe that will not place excessive pressure over the painful area. Several age groups have specific problems. For example, women in their second and third decade tend to have a ligher level of dissatisfaction with the results of bunion surgery. Their goal is usually to be able to fit into a more stylish shoe, but many of these women have a wide forefoot, so even after satisfactory correction of the deformity, they are still unable to wear their desired shoes. If they believed that the surgery would permit them to do so, they will often be quite dissatisfied. This is basically a problem in preoperative communication between the surgeon and patient. An athlete or dancer, particularly if professional, should always receive the most conservative treatment plan possible.[84] A general rule is that until such patients are significantly hampered in their ability to perform in their given profession, surgical intervention should be delayed because of the concern that after an unsuccessful surgical procedure, a painful foot will bring an end to their athletic career.

Causes of Surgical Failure

The following results represent an ideal hallux valgus repair:

- Correction of the hallux valgus and 1–2 IM angles
- Creation of a congruent MTP joint with sesamoid realignment

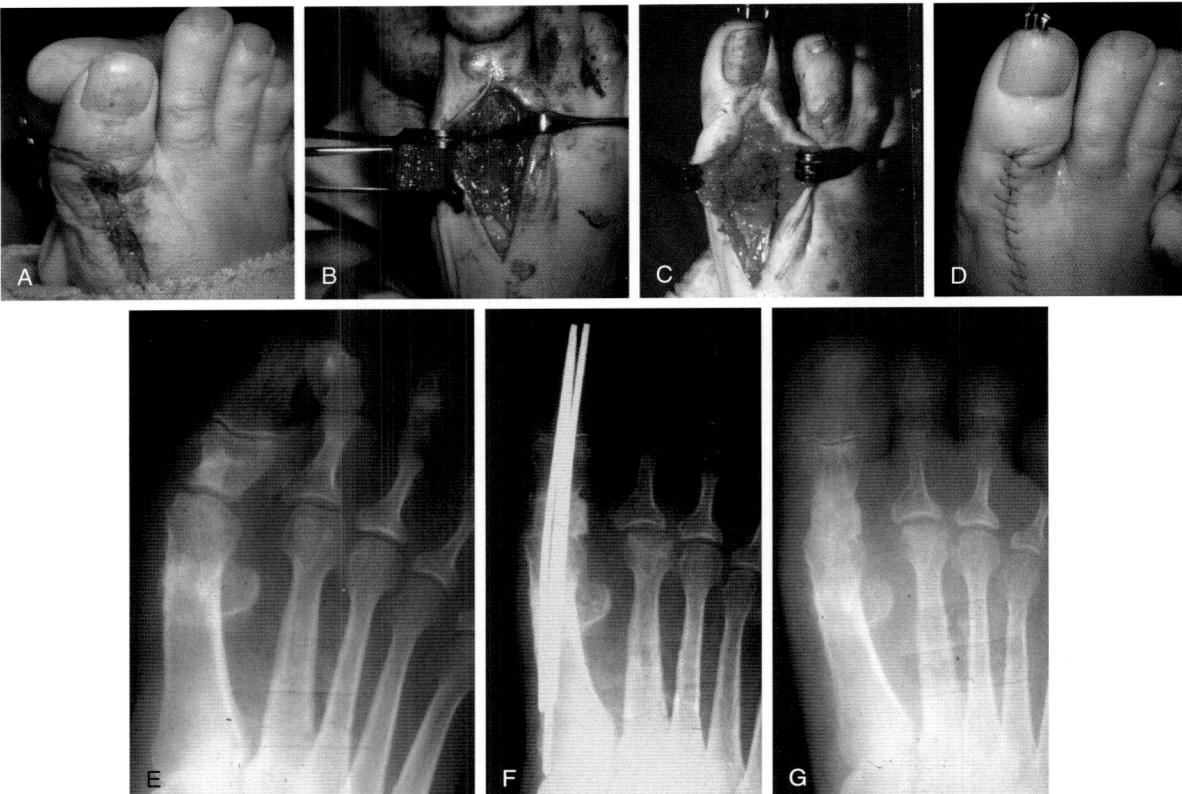

Figure 6-203 Salvage of a failed Keller procedure with an interposition bone graft. **A,** Preoperative clinical appearance. **B,** An iliac crest graft is harvested and inserted as an interposition graft. **C,** Graft is placed between prepared surfaces. **D,** Placement of Steinmann pin fixation. Preoperative **(E)** and postoperative **(F)** radiographs. **G,** After removal of internal fixation.

- Removal of the medial eminence
- Retention of functional range of motion of the MTP joint
- Maintenance of normal weight-bearing mechanics of the foot

With this ideal type of repair in mind, the authors now examine some of the factors that result in failure of a hallux valgus repair.

If an inappropriate procedure is selected for the pathologic condition present, the outcome will often be suboptimal. As pointed out in the algorithms in Figures 6-78, 6-79, and 6-82, each hallux valgus deformity needs to be carefully analyzed before selecting the appropriate surgical procedure. If a patient has a congruent joint and an attempt is made to correct the hallux valgus deformity by realigning the proximal phalanx over the metatarsal head, an incongruent joint may result. This in turn can lead to either joint stiffness, if the phalanx does not slide back into its former congruent alignment or there is recurrence of the deformity. If significant arthrosis is present in the joint and a realignment is carried out, restricted joint motion is a common result. Therefore the first step in avoiding a complication is selection of the correct surgical procedure.

If the indications for a procedure are "stretched," a suboptimal result will be obtained. This may occur when choosing a "simple bunionectomy" when a metatarsal osteotomy should be performed as well. Although the hallux is initially well aligned, recurrence of the deformity quickly results. If a chevron procedure is used to correct a severe hallux valgus deformity, full correction is rarely achieved. When performing hallux valgus surgery, a surgeon must remember that a single procedure will not result in satisfactory correction of all deformities.

Inadequate or inappropriate postoperative management may result in failure even when technically the procedure was properly performed. Soft tissues need to be carefully and meticulously supported and protected after surgery to ensure a satisfactory result. After many orthopaedic procedures, meticulous postoperative management is unnecessary, but after most hallux valgus procedures, careful follow-up is necessary to ensure a successful result.

Other causes of failure that may result from soft tissue, neurologic, or bone problems are discussed in detail next. Postoperative sepsis, though infrequent, can be a cause of failure and result in significant joint stiffness, chronic swelling, and possibly even nonunion of the osteotomy.

Finally, unrealistic patient expectations may be the cause of a failed surgical procedure. If the patient does not understand the possible limitations of the procedure preoperatively, both the patient and the surgeon may be unhappy afterward.

In selecting the surgical procedure, the surgeon must consider the options for a salvage procedure if a complication develops. The following typical complications can occur after specific procedures: soft tissue realignment resulting in a hallux varus deformity; arthrodesis resulting in nonunion; proximal first metatarsal osteotomy resulting in nonunion or malunion; and distal metatarsal osteotomy resulting in malunion, nonunion, or AVN. In the treatment of a hallux varus deformity, adequate soft tissue realignment can usually be achieved frequently, but on occasion, an arthrodesis may be necessary. After nonunion of an arthrodesis, an interposition bone grafting procedure will frequently result in successful fusion. With malunion of a metatarsal osteotomy, a corrective osteotomy can often achieve satisfactory realignment. With AVN of the metatarsal head, an arthrodesis with an interposition bone block may be necessary to achieve a satisfactory result. The authors believe that patients should have a general understanding of the type of complication that may develop so that if a second procedure is required, they will have some basic knowledge of what may be necessary.

The more common complications of hallux valgus surgery are presented here to acquaint the surgeon with the various types of problems that may arise. It is hoped that with a familiarity with these problems, the surgeon will take precautions to prevent them. A certain degree of risk is associated with any type of surgical procedure, and complications can occur regardless of the precautions taken.

Soft Tissue Problems
INFECTION
A postoperative infection may be superficial or deep. The clinician must be constantly aware of the possibility of postoperative infection and treat it vigorously if it develops. It is very important to determine as quickly as possible whether an infection is superficial to the MTP joint or whether it involves the joint itself (Fig. 6-204).

Generally speaking, a superficial infection is manifested by local cellulitis and, on occasion, evidence of ascending lymphangitis. The skin over the involved area may be red and warm, but motion of the joint will not usually cause significant pain. Attempts at aspiration of the MTP joint through an area of cellulitis are discouraged because of the risk of spreading a superficial infection into the joint space. Clinically, fever will usually develop in a patient with a superficial infection. Hematologic data may indicate an increase in the white blood cell (WBC), sedimentation rate, and C-reactive protein. Clinical judgment is important in choosing treatment, and the use of either oral or systemic antibiotics is indicated (Fig. 6-205).

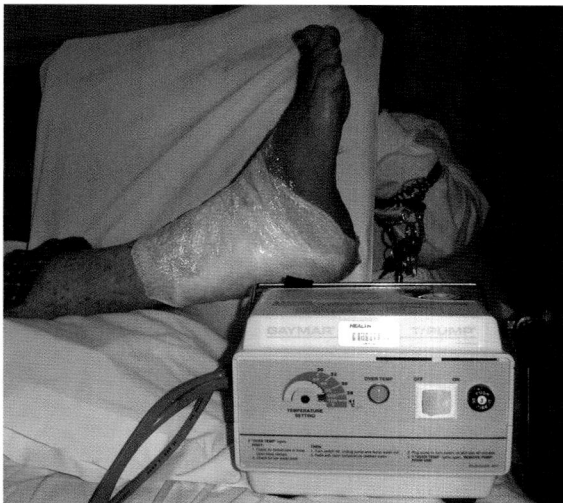

Figure 6-204 Infection after bunion surgery with ascending lymphangitis, treated with warm moist soaks and intravenous antibiotics.

A deep infection involving the MTP joint is much more severe and is usually manifested as a marked increase in pain and swelling about the MTP joint. There may be evidence of purulent discharge from the wound. MTP joint motion will typically cause discomfort, as will palpation of the joint itself. Often a fever is present, and the WBC count, C-reactive protein, and sedimentation rate are generally elevated. Management should be directed toward obtaining a specific culture and sensitivity of the offending organism. Prompt treatment with parenteral antibiotics is indicated. With purulent drainage, a decision must be made expeditiously regarding whether prompt irrigation and debridement of the joint are indicated.

After a severe joint space infection, marked intraarticular joint fibrosis and degenerative arthritis may ensue due to destruction of the articular cartilage. Changes in periarticular soft tissues after the infection may lead to recurrence of the original deformity.

DELAYED WOUND HEALING
On occasion after foot surgery, the operative wound edges appear to be locally reddened and slightly separated. There is no evidence of surrounding cellulitis or purulent drainage. The joint itself is not usually particularly swollen, and motion of the joint does not cause increased discomfort. Such cases are often caused by a superficial fungal infection. Carbolfuchsin (Carfusin) painted on the wound on one or two occasions will generally result in prompt wound healing with no further sequelae. In the presence of increasing evidence of cellulitis, a more serious problem should be suspected and treated accordingly.

SKIN SLOUGH
On occasion after surgery, a partial- or full-thickness slough about the wound may occur. Sloughing usually

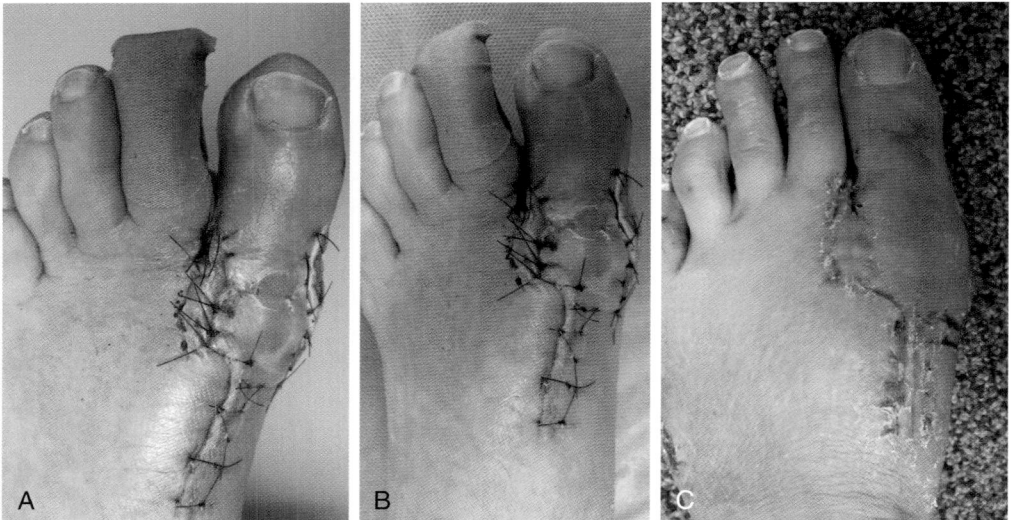

Figure 6-205 Postoperative infection. **A,** Cellulitis has developed 1 week after surgery. **B,** One week after initiation of oral antibiotics. **C,** At 3 weeks, the cellulitis is largely resolved.

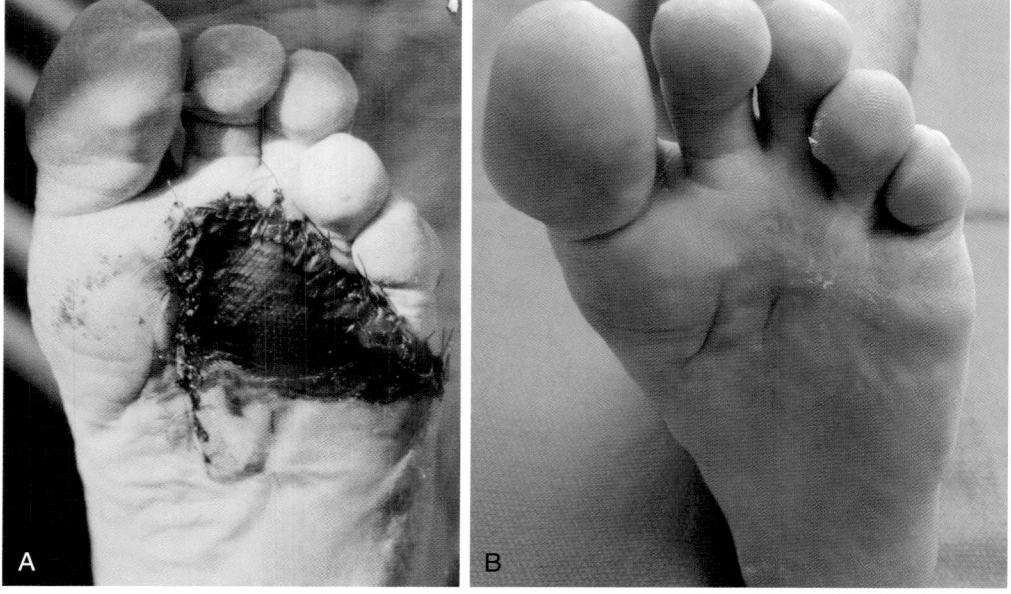

Figure 6-206 Skin slough. **A,** Full-thickness skin slough on the plantar aspect of foot covered by skin graft, which unfortunately necrosed. **B,** With time and local wound care, the area of skin loss contracted and healed.

develops 7 to 14 days after surgery and, depending on its size, may create a significant problem. The cause of the sloughing is devascularization of the involved tissue (Fig. 6-206), which can result from insufficient circulation secondary to a dysvascular foot, excessive retraction on the skin edge at surgery, placement of the skin under tension after correction of a severe deformity, or pressure from the postoperative dressing (Fig. 6-207).

Treatment varies depending on the severity of the tissue loss. In the case of a minor partial-thickness skin slough, local treatment and the passage of time usually result in a satisfactory outcome. Sloughing caused by a

dysvascular foot may require revascularization of the extremity before satisfactory wound healing can occur. Other larger, full-thickness skin sloughs may eventually require skin grafting after a satisfactory granulating bed has been achieved or could even require amputation.

ADHERENT SCAR
On occasion after a successful surgical procedure, a scar forms that is quite adherent to the underlying tissue. If a full-thickness dissection includes the underlying fatty tissue when skin flaps are developed at the time of the initial surgery, an adherent scar seldom occurs. As a

general rule, an adherent scar may actually soften over time, thus rendering it less bothersome to the patient. Soft tissue and underlying fatty tissue are generally somewhat limited on the foot, and excision of a persistent, adherent scar will not usually result in significant improvement of the situation. Persistent massage of an adherent scar may in time help mobilize the restricted tissue.

PARESTHESIAS OF THE HALLUX

Entrapment or severance (partial or complete) of a cutaneous nerve may result in either dysesthesia or anesthesia distal to the involved nerve. Protection of sensory nerves at the time of surgery is paramount; however, once a nerve injury occurs, desensitization of the involved area is managed by frequent massaging, rubbing, or tapping. This will often produce a satisfactory result over a period of several months. On occasion, it is necessary to reexplore the injured nerve and further resect the nerve proximally to an area of soft tissue to diminish the symptoms. The use of a transcutaneous nerve stimulator may be effective if surgical intervention fails. On rare occasions, a regional pain syndrome may develop (see Chapter 14).

One of the most frequently involved nerves is the dorsomedial cutaneous nerve to the great toe (Fig. 6-208A-C). An incision on the dorsomedial aspect of the first MTP joint unfortunately overlies this cutaneous nerve. On occasion, this nerve can be severed at the time of surgery or later become entrapped in scar tissue (Fig. 6-209). As a general rule, neurolysis is rarely helpful, particularly if the nerve has been partially severed. Exploration of the injured nerve through a long, dorsomedial incision enables the identification of normal and injured nerve. After carefully freeing the nerve from surrounding scar tissue and sectioning the nerve more proximally, the nerve is then transferred beneath and sutured under minimal tension to the abductor hallucis muscle. In this way, the nerve is transferred from an area of painful scar tissue to an area where there is little or no pressure. Although an area of numbness over the dorsomedial aspect of the great toe remains, the dysesthetic area is no longer present.

The plantar medial cutaneous nerve just plantar to the abductor hallucis tendon can also be injured. Symptoms develop with ambulation as the MTP joint dorsiflexes with plantar pressure over the neuroma, and often a

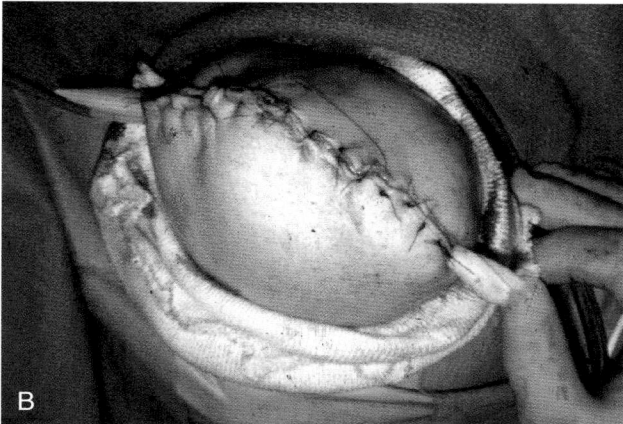

Figure 6-207 **A,** Skin slough after bunion surgery in a patient with vascular insufficiency. **B,** Above-knee amputation was eventually required.

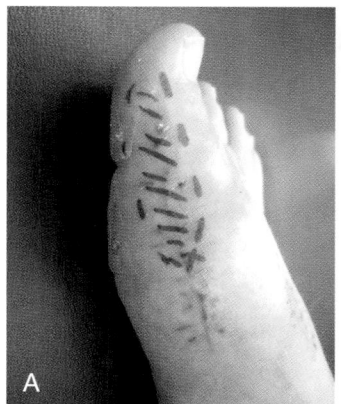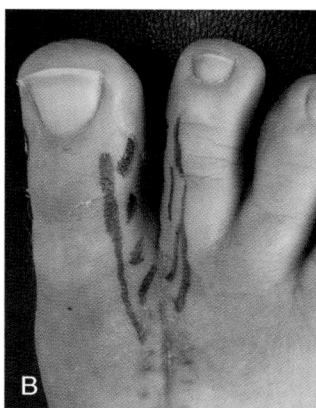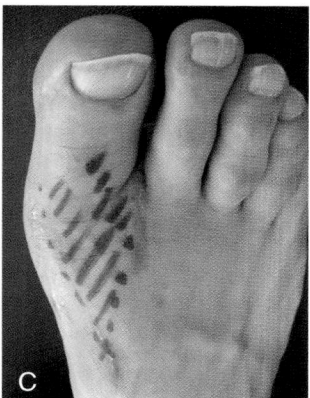

Figure 6-208 Iatrogenic injuries to nerves at surgery can lead to numbness and paresthesias. **A,** Dorsal medial cutaneous nerve to the hallux. **B,** Common digital nerve to the first web space. **C,** Injury to the superficial peroneal nerve.

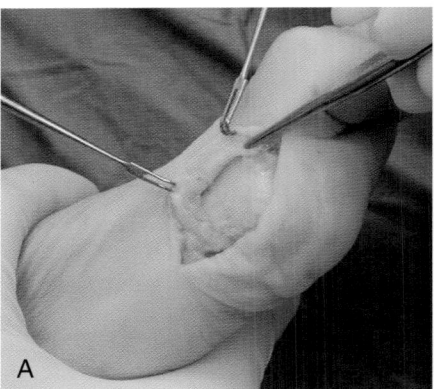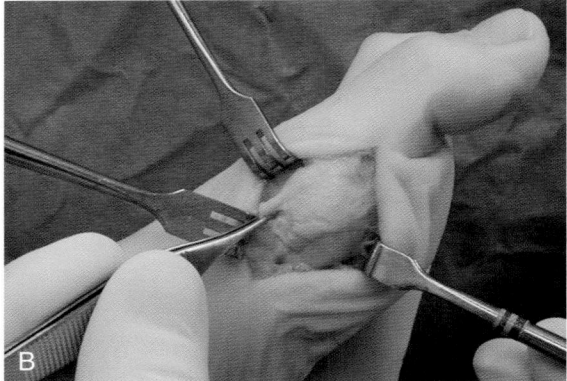

Figure 6-209 Exposure of the dorsal cutaneous nerve of the hallux. **A,** The nerve is contained in the cuff of subcutaneous tissue. **B,** The common digital nerve is identified and protected during the hallux valgus surgery but may inadvertently injured with the capsulorraphy.

patient transfers weight to the lateral border of the foot. Again, surgical treatment consists of exposing the plantar medial cutaneous nerve through a long medial incision just dorsal to the weight-bearing surface. The nerve is identified and traced proximally to normal nerve tissue. After the nerve has been freed and sectioned, it is buried proximally beneath the abductor hallucis muscle. At the time of transposition, the sectioned nerve is sutured with a minimum of tension so that as the toes are brought into dorsiflexion, symptoms will not be exacerbated. After sectioning of the injured nerve, there is residual numbness along the plantar medial aspect of the great toe.

On occasion, the common digital nerve to the first web space is partially or completely transected with exploration of the first web space. If a neuroma develops, there may be sensitivity on the plantar aspect of the foot, as well as dysesthesias on the plantar aspect of the first web space (see Fig. 6-208B). Surgical treatment involves exposure through a dorsal first web-space incision. The transverse metatarsal ligament is sectioned and the common digital nerve identified and carefully freed from surrounding tissue. If a significant neuroma is identified and transection of the nerve is necessary, it should be performed with as much length of the nerve left as possible. This ensures that the remaining stump can be elevated to an area alongside the first metatarsal so that the nerve end (where another neuroma will form) is removed from the plantar aspect of the foot. Proximal transection of the common digital nerve without elevation of the stump frequently results in a painful neuroma located more proximally in the foot. At times the common digital nerve can be freed from the adjacent soft tissue; if the nerve appears to be abnormal, it can be elevated off the plantar aspect of the foot and transferred above a portion of the adductor hallucis muscle so that the nerve is not exposed to the trauma of weight bearing.

DELAYED WOUND BREAKDOWN
On occasion after successful surgery and wound healing, the wound will once again become swollen and sensitive.

This usually occurs 4 weeks or more postoperatively but may occur many months after surgery. Frequently, the cause is a foreign body reaction to the underlying suture material. It frequently involves silk, but other suture materials (e.g., cotton, chromic, newer synthetic materials) may be involved. The area of the reaction forms a sterile abscess, the skin breaks down, and a suture granuloma develops. With time, the involved foreign material is usually extruded. On occasion, exploration of the wound may be necessary to excise the foreign material. Once removed, prompt wound healing generally occurs, although cauterization of the remaining granulation material with silver nitrate is often required.

Complications Affecting the Metatarsal Shaft
After any metatarsal osteotomy, malposition or loss of position of the osteotomy site is possible. To avoid this problem, a broad stable osteotomy, rigid internal fixation, adequate postoperative immobilization, and protected ambulation are necessary. Some osteotomies are inherently more stable than others. Surgical judgment is required to determine which sites are sufficiently stable for ambulation and which are not.

The same surgical procedure in two different patients may require a different method of fixation and postoperative weight-bearing precautions.

The following are the most common types of problems seen after metatarsal osteotomy.

SHORTENING
Shortening occurs after most metatarsal osteotomies. After the chevron procedure, an average shortening of 2.2 mm (range, 0-8) has been reported[222,430] (Fig. 6-210A). After the Mitchell procedure, even more shortening has been reported (Fig. 6-210B).* The most shortening seems to follow the Wilson procedure, with an average of 11 mm (Fig. 6-210C and D).[430] After a distal soft tissue procedure and proximal osteotomy,

*References 60, 158, 184, 214, 370, and 463.

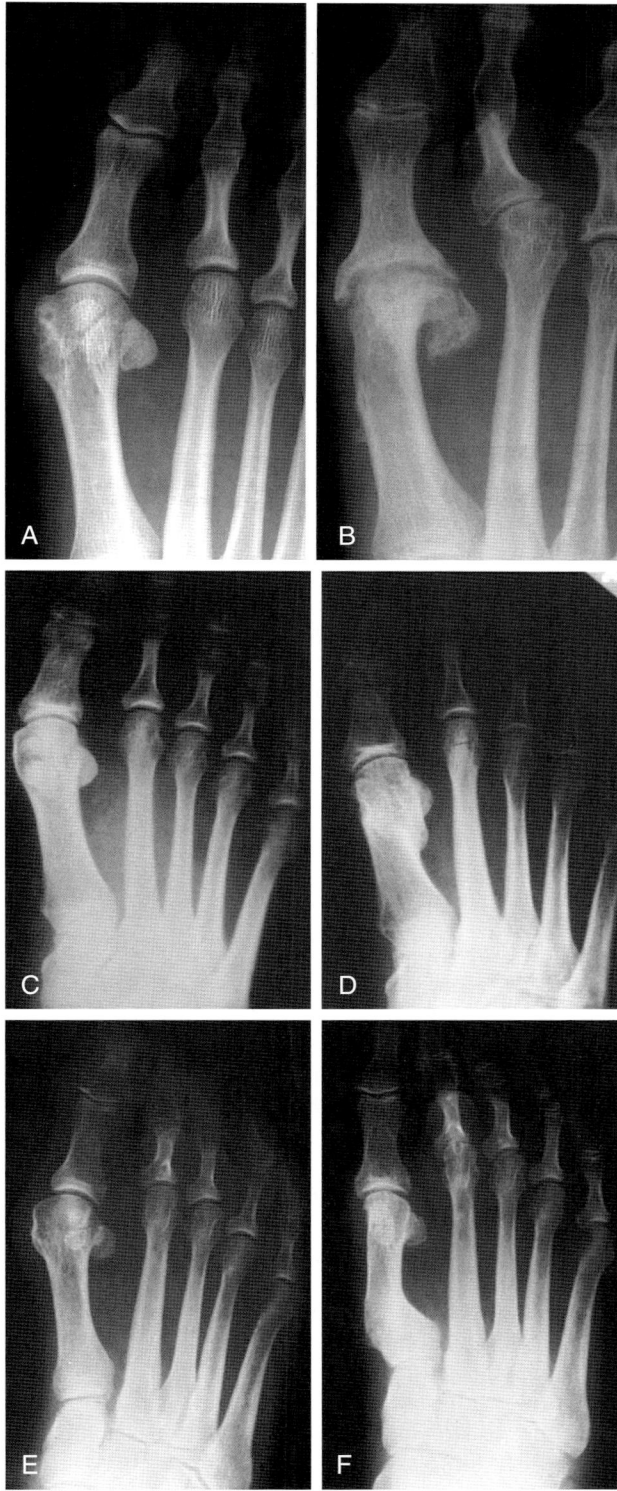

Figure 6-210 Shortening after hallux valgus surgery. **A,** Preoperative radiograph of moderate hallux valgus deformity. **B,** After chevron osteotomy. Ten years after surgery, avascular necrosis has led to substantial shortening of the first ray. **C,** Preoperative radiograph. **D,** Shortening after a Wilson or Mitchell procedure. **E,** Preoperative radiograph. **F,** Shortening after a proximal metatarsal osteotomy. Shortening of the first metatarsal may result in a transfer lesion.

approximately 2-mm shortening has been reported (Fig. 6-210E and F).[101,344] The main problem associated with shortening is the development of a transfer lesion beneath the second metatarsal head. It is difficult to assign a specific amount of shortening that will produce metatarsalgia because a number of factors play a role, including the original length of the first metatarsal and whether dorsiflexion is associated with the shortening. The degree of hallux valgus correction, range of motion, and stability of the MTP joint are factors because weight is normally transferred to the great toe at the end of stance phase. This, in turn, unloads the second metatarsal head. With insufficient stability or inadequate correction of the hallux, the first metatarsal will not carry its share of the weight. After procedures that destabilize the MTP joint, such as the Keller procedure,[218] or with a prosthesis in which significant weight bearing no longer occurs beneath the great toe, the incidence of metatarsalgia is increased.

Certain procedures (e.g., Mitchell, Wilson, closing-wedge proximal metatarsal osteotomy) have the potential for transfer metatarsalgia.[214,276,370,561] In these cases, it is imperative that the length of the first and second metatarsals be carefully assessed when planning a surgical procedure to decide whether an alternative procedure that would produce less shortening should be used.

Those experienced with the Mitchell procedure emphasize that plantar flexion of the distal fragment should be carried out to help alleviate the potential for metatarsalgia.* However, if the first metatarsal is significantly short to begin with and more shortening ensues after surgery, metatarsalgia will inevitably result. Once shortening of the first metatarsal and metatarsalgia occur, further surgical treatment is often required. Surgical treatment of this condition is difficult, and the results are often less than optimal.

Lengthening of a metatarsal is difficult to achieve both anatomically and technically. Metatarsals do not "stretch" well, and even if an interposition bone block is used, some resorption may occur and subsequent tilting of the distal portion of the metatarsal may develop. If the second metatarsal is significantly longer than the first and third, shortening of the second metatarsal to achieve a normal weight-bearing pattern can be beneficial. On rare occasions, both the second and the third metatarsals can be shortened to realign the weight-bearing pattern of the foot. On occasion, a plantar-flexion osteotomy of the first metatarsal can be used to increase its weight-bearing function.

DORSIFLEXION

Dorsiflexion of the first metatarsal can occur after a proximal osteotomy of almost any type. It can also occur distally after a chevron, Mitchell, or Wilson osteotomy. After MTC fusion, dorsiflexion of the metatarsal has been reported as well.[383,456]

---

*References 34, 184, 214, 366, 371, 561, and 562.

Dorsiflexion, as with shortening of the metatarsal, should be avoided if possible. Unfortunately, dorsiflexion of an already short metatarsal only compounds the problem of transfer metatarsalgia. At times, dorsiflexion occurs with minimal shortening, and rarely does a problem result. Exactly how much dorsiflexion versus how much shortening can be tolerated after a surgical procedure varies from foot to foot. It probably depends on the overall rigidity of a foot, the relationship of the length of the first and second metatarsals, and a patient's activity level. When substantial dorsiflexion occurs, however, it creates a difficult management problem and is probably best handled by a plantar-flexion first metatarsal osteotomy rather than by shortening or elevating the second metatarsal. Elevation of the second metatarsal often leads to a transfer lesion beneath the third metatarsal.

After a lateral closing-wedge first metatarsal osteotomy, a dorsiflexion deformity usually develops because more bone is removed dorsally than plantarward at the osteotomy site. As the osteotomy is closed, the metatarsal moves laterally and dorsally. This combination of shortening and dorsiflexion can cause significant metatarsalgia. Furthermore, internal fixation must be adequate to maintain the desired position of the osteotomy (Fig. 6-211A and B).

If dorsiflexion of the first metatarsal results in a symptomatic transfer lesion beneath the first metatarsal or results in flattening of the longitudinal arch because of loss of support by the first metatarsal head, a plantar-flexion osteotomy can be performed. There are many techniques with which to plantar flex the first metatarsal. The authors prefer to make a crescentic-shaped cut in the plantar half of the first metatarsal about 1 cm distal to the MTC joint. With this cut, the blade must exit plantarward. The top of the blade does not penetrate the dorsal surface, and the osteotomy is completed vertically with a sagittal saw (Fig. 6-211C).

In performing a proximal metatarsal ostetomy (crescentic or closing wedge), elevation of the capital fragment can occur because of malalignment of the actually osteotomy. The operative leg often externally rotates on the surgical table, and if the osteotomy is not perpendicular to the shaft of the first metatarsal (in a dorsal plantar plane), elevation can occur (Fig. 6-212). After a proximal crescentic osteotomy, dorsiflexion can occur with inadequate internal fixation. This osteotomy offers a broad cancellous surface, which is quite stable with screw fixation. At times, if the bone is osteopenic or if a screw of inadequate length is chosen, dorsal angulation may develop. Mann et al[344] reviewed a series of 109 cases and reported postoperative dorsiflexion in approximately 28% of cases, although the magnitude of the deformity was not quantified. Some of the cases of dorsiflexion were quite minor. In none of these patients, however, did a transfer lesion develop. The explanation for this is that the first MTP joint was adequately realigned, and thus the hallux continued to

bear weight in a normal manner. This appears to compensate for the dorsiflexion that developed (see Fig. 6-211D and E).

Shortening of the first metatarsal is an inherent part of the Mitchell procedure. The osteotomy is designed so that the shortening is compensated for by plantar flexion or plantar displacement (or both) of the distal fragment. Inadequate fixation of the distal fragment, however, can lead to postoperative dorsiflexion. With a dorsiflexed short first metatarsal, weight is transferred to the lesser metatarsals. Prevention of this complication is far simpler than later treatment. Salvage often entails placement of a proximal interposition bone block to both plantar flex and lengthen the first metatarsal. If only dorsiflexion ensues, correction can be achieved with a bone graft placed in the distal third of the metatarsal, closer to the apex of the deformity (see Fig. 6-211F).

After a distal oblique or Wilson-type osteotomy, both shortening and dorsiflexion occur because of inadequate fixation of the capital fragment. This presents a challenging salvage situation. Frequently, shortening of the second and, on occasion, the third metatarsal is necessary to relieve lateral metatarsalgia.

After a chevron osteotomy, dorsiflexion of the capital fragment may result in transfer metatarsalgia. Dorsal displacement of the capital fragment can be prevented by intraoperative internal fixation. When dorsiflexion of the distal fragment results in transfer metatarsalgia, it is preferable to treat the second metatarsal with a shortening osteotomy rather than attempt to realign the first metatarsal head because of the risk of AVN (see Fig. 6-211G).

After MTC joint arthrodesis, dorsiflexion may develop at the MTC joint, particularly if a bone graft has been added to the procedure. When dorsiflexion is of such magnitude that a transfer lesion develops, a plantar-flexion osteotomy of the first metatarsal can achieve realignment distal to the fused joint.

PLANTAR FLEXION
A plantar-flexion deformity of the first metatarsal occurs infrequently and is caused by inadequate internal fixation of the osteotomy site. It frequently leads to increased weight bearing beneath the first metatarsal head, with the subsequent development of a diffuse callus. An orthotic device that transfers weight laterally to the lesser metatarsal head region will often alleviate the symptoms. With a severe deformity, however, a corrective osteotomy to dorsiflex the first metatarsal can be performed (Fig. 6-213).

EXCESSIVE VALGUS (LATERAL DEVIATION) OF THE FIRST METATARSAL
On occasion, the IM angle will be overcorrected, and a negative angle will be created (Fig. 6-214). If the deformity is minimal, no significant sequelae will develop. If the overcorrection is excessive, the articular surface slopes laterally, and as the proximal phalanx is relocated on the

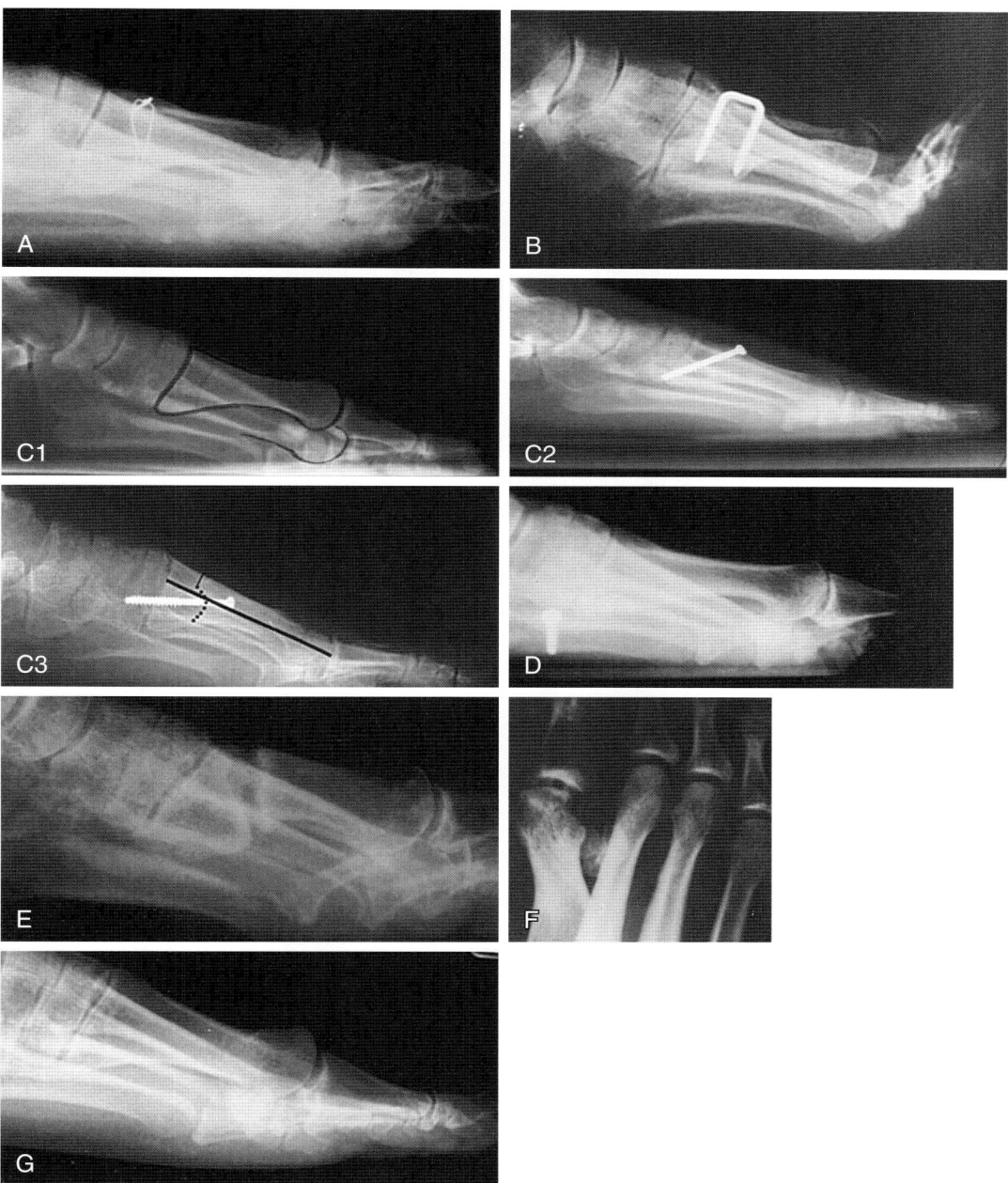

Figure 6-211 Complications resulting from dorsiflexion of a first metatarsal osteotomy. **A,** Dorsiflexion and shortening after lateral closing-wedge osteotomy. **B,** Dorsiflexion and marked shortening after lateral closing-wedge osteotomy. Preoperative **(C1)** and postoperative **(C2)** radiographs demonstrating correction of the dorsiflexion posture of the first metatarsal. **C3,** The *dotted line* demonstrates a curved plantar osteotomy with a dorsal straight cut used for this correction. **D,** Dorsiflexion of the first metatarsal after proximal crescentic osteotomy. **E,** Dorsiflexion and shortening after infection of a proximal metatarsal osteotomy. **F,** Dorsiflexion of the metatarsal head after the Mitchell procedure. **G,** Dorsiflexion of the capital fragment resulting in a transfer lesion, following a chevron osteotomy.

metatarsal head, an incongruent joint surface is created. In time, the MTP joint will become painful and degenerative arthritis may develop.

After a proximal crescentic osteotomy, if the concavity of the saw blade faces distally, there is a tendency to displace the metatarsal shaft medialward as the osteotomy is rotated. When this occurs, the metatarsal head may be translated too far laterally (Fig. 6-215). Concurrently, if the medial eminence is excessively resected, an unstable situation develops that is at risk for the development of a hallux varus deformity. Therefore, when a distal soft tissue procedure and proximal crescentic osteotomy are performed, the osteotomy to resect the medial eminence is performed 2 mm medial to the sagittal sulcus to leave

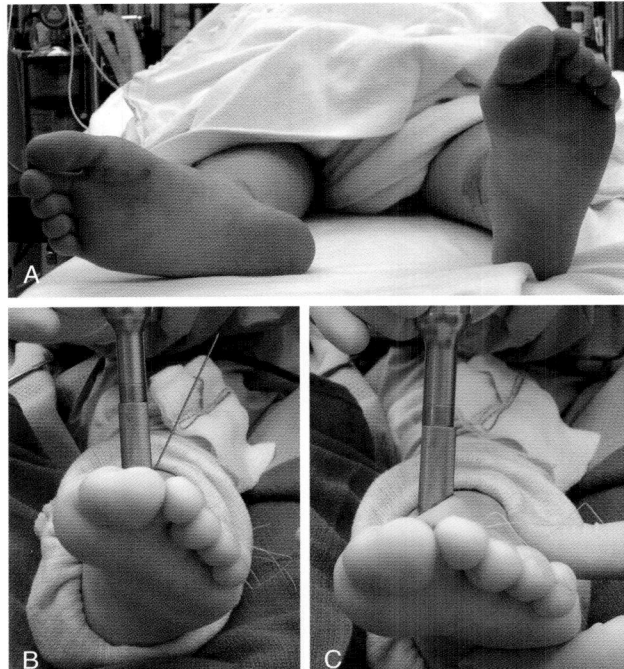

Figure 6-212 Performing a first metatarsal ostetomy may lead to elevatus because of saw position. **A,** Note lateral rotation of right leg. If a saw cut is made in this plane, displacement or closing of the ostetomy will elevate the distal fragment. **B,** A vertical Kirschner wire is placed perpendicular to the longitudinal axis of the first metatarsal. Note the saw blade in this photograph is too far medially rotated. **C,** The saw blade is rotated to parallel the Kirschner wire, and then with the osteotomy, the cut will be vertical to the shaft (neither elevating or depressing the distal fragment).[250]

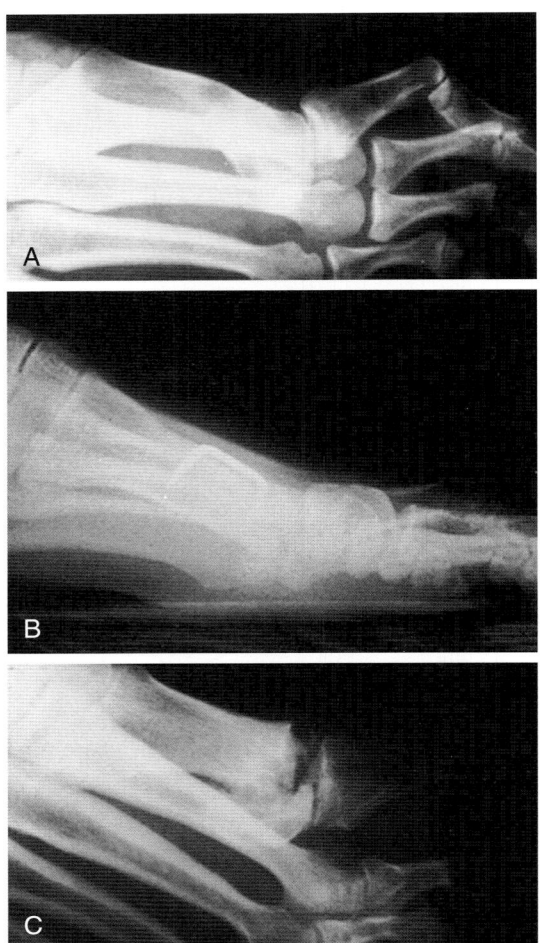

Figure 6-213 Complications after plantar flexion of a first metatarsal osteotomy. **A,** Plantar-flexion deformity after the Mitchell procedure. **B,** Correction after dorsal osteotomy. **C,** Severe plantar-flexion deformity after a chevron osteotomy.

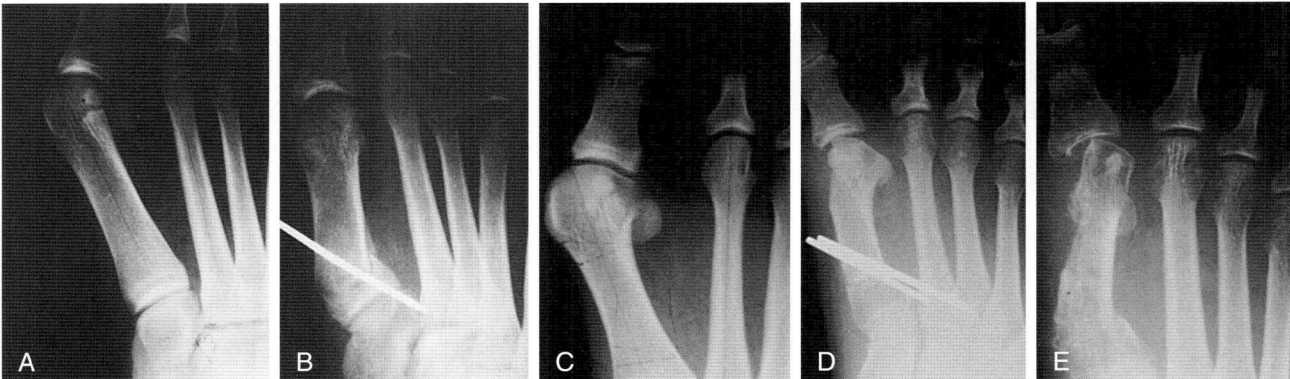

Figure 6-214 Complications associated with excessive adduction of the first metatarsal after proximal osteotomies. **A,** Hallux valgus associated with adduction of all metatarsals. **B,** Correction of hallux valgus with a proximal metatarsal osteotomy resulted in a negative intermetatarsal (IM) angle but a congruent metatarsophalangeal (MTP) joint. To gain this correction, a negative IM angle was necessary. **C,** Preoperative radiograph. **D,** Postoperative radiograph demonstrating the effects of a proximal metatarsal osteotomy with creation of an incongruent MTP joint. **E,** Creation of an incongruent joint from excessive lateral displacement of the proximal metatarsal osteotomy. When a congruent joint is present preoperatively, it must be appreciated. Any attempt to rotate the proximal phalanx on the metatarsal head will result in an incongruent joint.

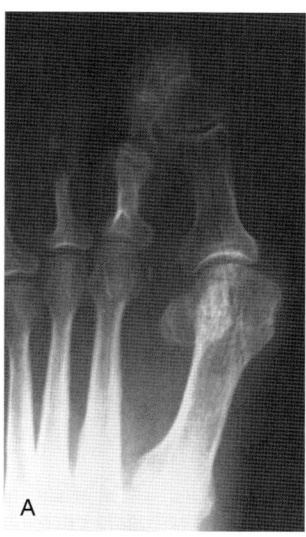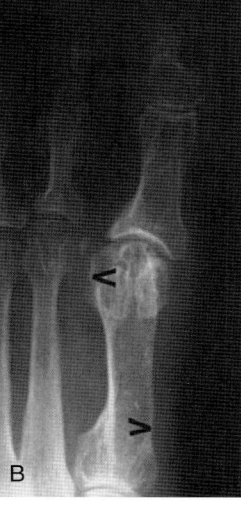

Figure 6-215 **A** and **B,** Excessive lateral displacement of the metatarsal head after a proximal crescentic osteotomy caused by medial deviation of the osteotomy site.

a "medial buttress" so that the risk of overcorrection is reduced.

Correction of this complication, if long-standing, is difficult because degenerative arthritis of the MTP joint commonly develops. Prevention, if possible, is desirable, and the use of intraoperative fluoroscopy helps minimize this complication. On occasion, it is necessary to revise the osteotomy of the metatarsal to realign the first ray. However, in most circumstances, correction of the first metatarsal must be combined with realignment of the soft tissues about the MTP joint. With advanced first MTP joint degenerative arthritis, an arthrodesis is sufficient to realign the joint and attain successful salvage.

NONUNION OF THE FIRST METATARSAL

Nonunion of the first metatarsal (proximal or distal) can occur after any osteotomy. With the improved methods of internal fixation, this complication is not common. On occasion, delayed union develops. Given sufficient time (even 4-6 months), successful healing will usually occur with adequate immobilization (see Fig. 6-162).

Nonunion can generally be prevented by adequate preparation of the bone surfaces and adequate interfragmentary compression, which promotes rapid healing.

The problem that often arises as a result of nonunion is loss of position of the metatarsal shaft, shortening, or both. Treatment of this complication is determined by the nature of the problem and may vary from bone grafting the nonunion site to performing a corrective osteotomy and rigidly fixing the nonunion site (Fig. 6-216).

Complications Affecting the Metatarsal Head
EXCESSIVE EXCISION

When most bunion procedures are performed, the medial eminence is excised. When carrying out the distal soft

tissue procedure, the authors advocate moving 1 to 2 mm medial to the sagittal sulcus to ensure that an adequate medial buttress is left in place to prevent a varus deformity. The absence of articular cartilage just lateral to the sagittal sulcus may invite further excision, but this will lead to the removal of an excessive amount of the metatarsal head and result in an unstable joint, which in turn can lead to a hallux varus deformity. Other times, excessive excision of the metatarsal head results in an incongruent articular surface, which leads to early degenerative arthritis (Fig. 6-217).

Treatment of excessive resection of the medial metatarsal head is difficult because insufficient metatarsal head remains to support the proximal phalanx. The most common means of salvage is an MTP arthrodesis to both realign the joint and eliminate the pain.

DISPLACEMENT

A distal metatarsal osteotomy can become displaced in the coronal or sagittal plane. After a distal metatarsal osteotomy, especially of the chevron type, stability is not usually an issue. Displacement of the capital fragment can occur, and most authors now advocate some form of internal fixation to prevent this complication.

The metatarsal head may shift dorsally, which can result in decreased weight bearing and a transfer lesion beneath the second metatarsal (Fig. 6-218A). Rarely does plantar displacement of the capital fragment occur after a chevron procedure (Fig. 6-218B and C). If the head deviates into excessive lateral deviation, the tibial sesamoid is often uncovered and a hallux varus deformity or MTP joint incongruity results (Fig. 6-218D and E). If the head deviates medially, the hallux valgus deformity may recur, and an incongruent joint may result as well (Fig. 6-218F). If internal fixation is not used in conjunction with a chevron procedure, serial postoperative radiographs should be obtained to ensure that displacement does not occur. If displacement does occur, it should be promptly recognized and treated.

After the Mitchell procedure, the transverse osteotomy has inherent instability that can result in displacement of the capital fragment. Although plantar displacement can occur, most commonly, dorsal displacement develops because of the dorsal pressure applied with weight bearing (see Fig. 6-218F). With dorsal displacement, metatarsalgia can result from both shortening and dorsiflexion, whereas with plantar displacement, pain usually develops beneath the first metatarsal. Lateral displacement of the capital fragment leads to a varus deformity, whereas medial displacement leads to a recurrent valgus deformity. Adequate internal fixation of the osteotomy site can prevent most of these problems.

After a distal oblique osteotomy or Wilson bunion procedure, where mild-to-moderate shortening of the first ray is permitted, the incidence of elevatus was reported to be as high as 20% in one series.[430] The pressure of weight bearing presents a significant risk to an osteotomy with inadequate internal fixation.

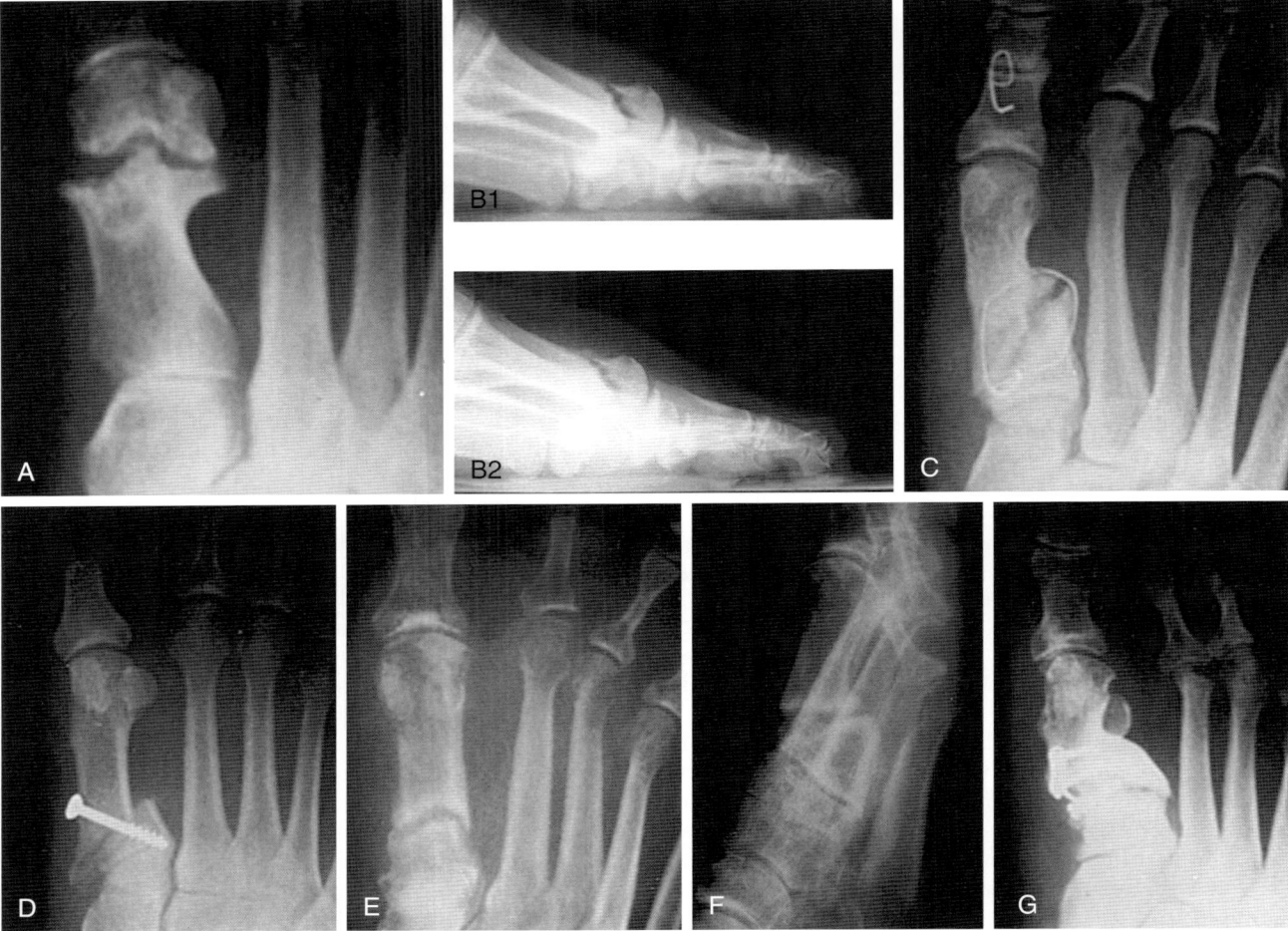

Figure 6-216 Nonunion affecting the metatarsal. **A,** Nonunion after a chevron procedure. **B,** Delayed union of a chevron osteotomy 6 months after surgery. Subsequent casting for 10 weeks resulted in union of the osteotomy site. **C,** Nonunion after an oblique proximal osteotomy. **D,** Nonunion after an oblique proximal metatarsal osteotomy. Anteroposterior **(E)** and lateral **(F)** radiographs of nonunion of a proximal crescentic osteotomy. **G,** Nonunion of a proximal metatarsal osteotomy.

Realignment of a malunited distal metatarsal osteotomy is associated with many technical difficulties. Realignment of the osteotomy site may require extensive soft tissue stripping, which increases the risk of AVN. Successful realignment can be achieved, yet significant joint arthrofibrosis may develop because of soft tissue adhesions. MTP joint arthrodesis is probably the most reliable method to salvage this condition.

AVASCULAR NECROSIS

The blood supply to the metatarsal head must be protected with a distal osteotomy (see Figs. 6-67 and 6-68). Interruption of the vascular supply to the capital fragment after extensive dissection around the MTP joint with a distal metatarsal osteotomy can result in partial or complete AVN of the metatarsal head.[477] The development of AVN does not necessarily mean that the joint will become symptomatic.

For some methods of distal osteotomy in which various techniques of internal fixation are used (i.e.,

screws instead of pins), more soft tissue stripping is necessary to gain adequate exposure for insertion of the fixation device. Although fixation is vitally important, the magnitude of soft tissue dissection should be minimized to prevent problems with AVN (Figs. 6-219 and 6-220).

The incidence of AVN, particularly after distal osteotomies, varies considerably. Meier and Kenzora[365] reported an incidence of 20% in 60 patients and pointed out that 40% of patients in whom AVN developed had also undergone some type of lateral release; however, only 15% of the patients were deemed symptomatic. Johnston[244] demonstrated cystic changes in 7 of 50 chevron procedures, along with 1 case of complete and 1 of partial AVN. Other authors of large series reported no cases of AVN.[193,213,410,421,523] Although it is difficult to determine the incidence of this complication,[333] it is probably uncommon (see Figs. 6-119 to 6-121).

Three separate studies describe a lateral soft tissue release with the chevron procedure. Peterson et al[410] reviewed 58 cases and reported 1 case of AVN. Pochatko

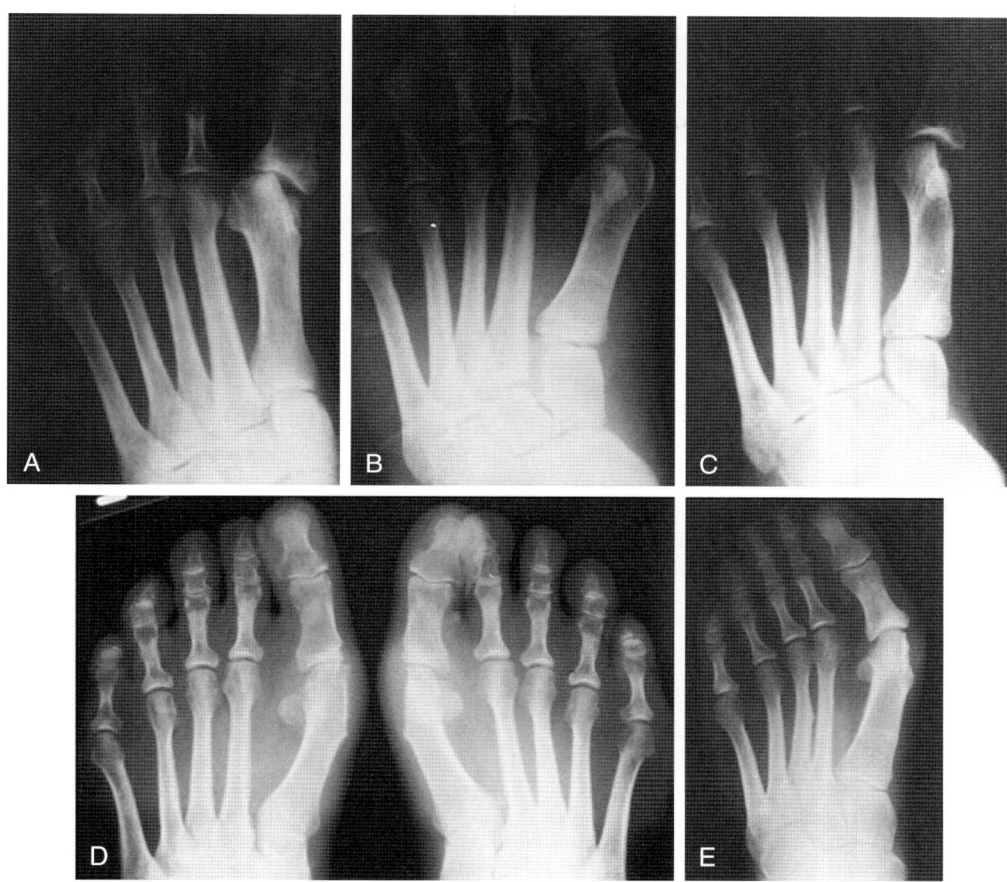

Figure 6-217 Complications after excessive excision of the metatarsal head. **A,** Excessive excision resulting in an unstable metatarsophalangeal (MTP) joint caused medial subluxation of the tibial sesamoid and a hallux varus deformity. **B,** Preoperative hallux valgus repair. **C,** Postoperative radiograph demonstrating excessive excision of the medial eminence, which resulted in a painful, unstable MTP joint. **D** and **E,** Excision of an excessive amount of metatarsal head resulted in an unstable, painful MTP joint.

et al[421] reported on 23 cases with no AVN. Thomas et al[511] reviewed 80 cases in which lateral capsular release was carried out through a plantar incision along with excision of the fibular sesamoid and found no AVN. On the basis of these studies, a careful lateral release that respects the metaphyseal and capital blood supply should avoid damage to the vascularity of the metatarsal head.

AVN may be accompanied by marked pain and arthrofibrosis of the joint. Treatment of this complication usually requires MTP arthrodesis. When the arthrodesis is performed, every effort should be made to excise the avascular portion. This may leave the toe somewhat shortened, but it is preferable to placement of an interpositional bone graft, which may take much time to unite.

AVN is reported after the Mitchell procedure (see Fig. 6-136I). Blum[34] reported a 2% incidence of AVN. Salvage with MTP joint arthrodesis is the procedure of choice.

Of historical interest, after the LeLeivre bunion procedure, a 20% incidence of AVN has been reported.[237,436] Currently, this procedure is rarely performed because of the unacceptably high incidence of AVN.

Complications Involving the Proximal Phalanx

Complications involving a proximal phalangeal osteotomy are uncommon. Some are related to placement of the osteotomy, whereas others result from inadequate fixation of the osteotomy site.[420] When malunion or nonunion occurs, a salvage procedure may be technically difficult because of the small size of the phalanx.

NONUNION

Delayed union or nonunion of the phalanx seems to occur most frequently when the osteotomy is in the midshaft or distal phalanx rather than within the proximal third of the phalanx. The diaphyseal region may be at risk for delayed healing; however, with the passage of time, most phalangeal osteotomies do heal. In the presence of phalangeal nonunion, waiting for a period of 4 to 5 months may allow healing to occur (Fig. 6-221).

MALUNION

Malunion of the proximal phalanx usually occurs as a result of loss of fixation or inadequate internal fixation at

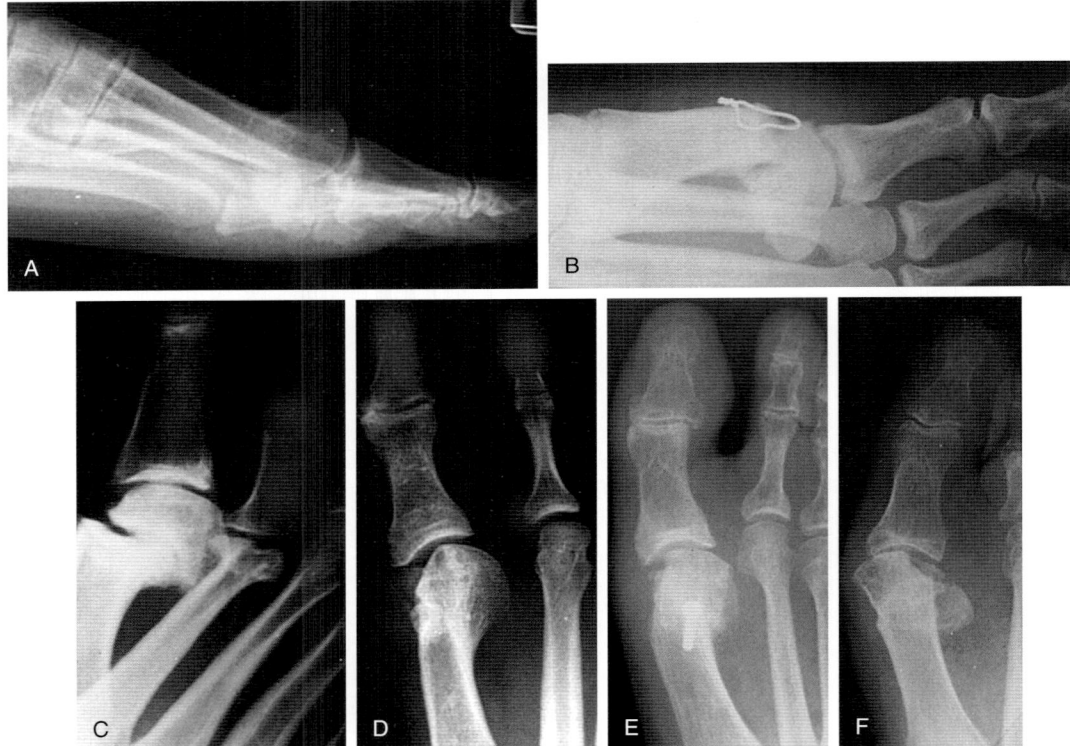

Figure 6-218 Complications secondary to displacement of the metatarsal head. **A,** Dorsal displacement after a chevron osteotomy. **B** and **C,** Plantar displacement after a distal metatarsal osteotomy. **D,** Excessive lateral deviation of the head results in an incongruent joint with a varus deformity. **E,** Lateral displacement of the metatarsal head results in recurrence of hallux valgus and an incongruent joint. **F,** Medial displacement of the capital fragment.

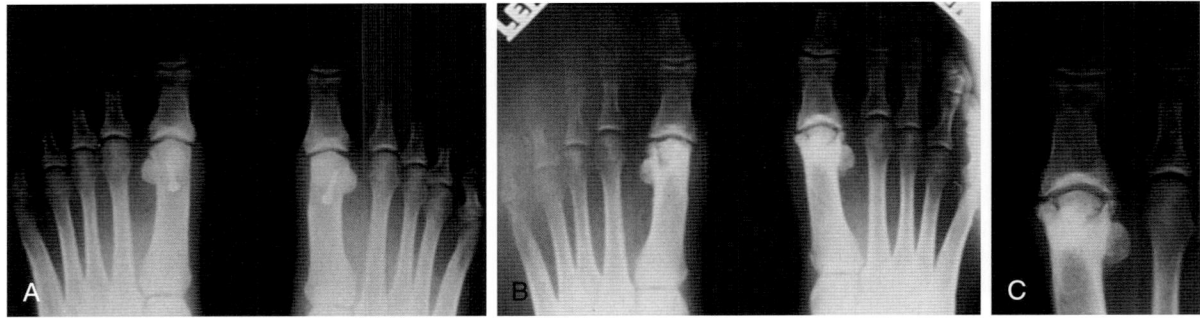

Figure 6-219 **A** and **B,** Sequence of radiographs demonstrating the development of central avascular necrosis (AVN) after placement of a screw for internal fixation. **C,** Close-up of AVN.

the osteotomy site. Loss of position is not generally of sufficient magnitude to require corrective surgery (see Fig. 6-110B).

AVASCULAR NECROSIS

Although AVN generally occurs in the metatarsal head, on occasion it occurs in the proximal phalanx. After a proximal phalangeal osteotomy, AVN may develop because of excessive soft tissue and capsular stripping or excessive manipulation of the osteotomy site. AVN presents a difficult salvage situation; typically, a Keller

procedure or arthrodesis is required to correct the problem.

ADHESIONS OF THE FLEXOR HALLUCIS LONGUS

After a proximal phalangeal osteotomy, particularly if done in the midportion of the phalanx, the flexor hallucis longus tendon may be disrupted or become adherent to the osteotomy site. Flexion of the IP joint is either absent or significantly diminished. This complication can usually be avoided by adequately mobilizing and retracting the flexor hallucis longus tendon before performing the

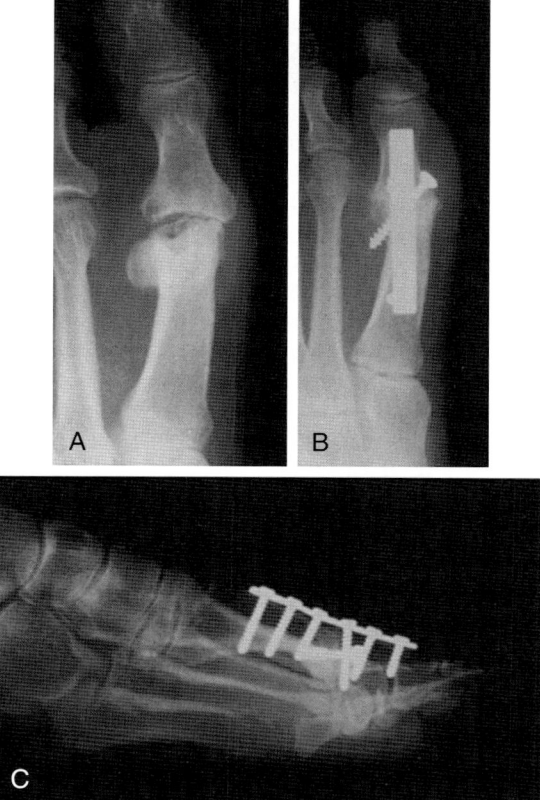

Figure 6-220 Treatment of avascular necrosis with arthrodesis of the metatarsophalangeal joint. **A–C,** Central avascular necrosis corrected by arthrodesis.

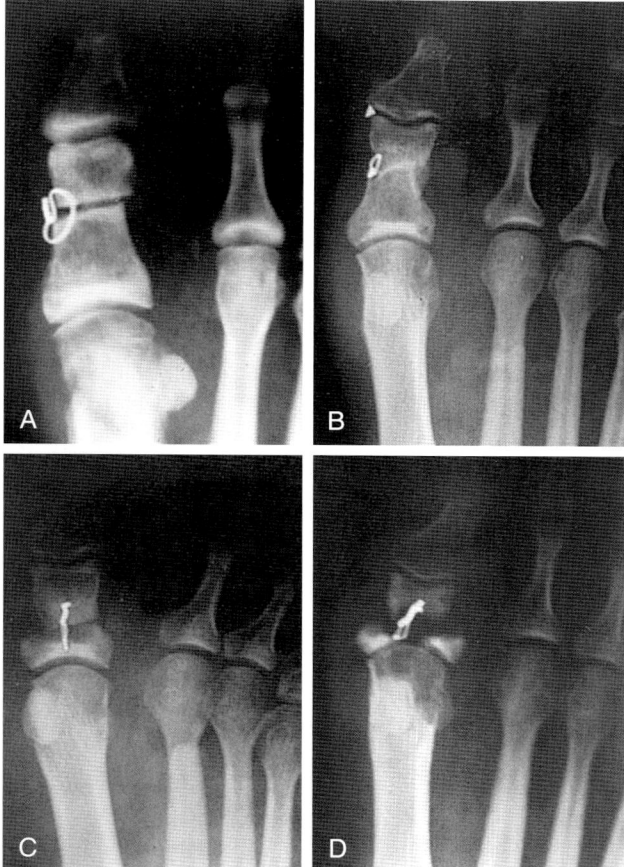

Figure 6-221 Complications after proximal phalangeal osteotomy. **A,** Radiograph demonstrating delayed union, which usually results because the osteotomy site is in the diaphysis rather than the metaphyseal portion of the bone. **B,** Sequence of radiographs demonstrating progressive avascular necrosis of the proximal phalanx after revision of the osteotomy site **(C)** and eventual complete collapse **(D).**

osteotomy to avoid inadvertent damage when the osteotomy is performed. It may be treated with an interphalangeal joint (IP) arthrodesis (see Chapter 19).

VIOLATION OF THE METATARSOPHALANGEAL JOINT

With a proximal phalangeal osteotomy, the osteotomy may inadvertently violate the MTP joint. The proximal phalanx has a concave articular surface. When the osteotomy is performed, care must be taken to ensure that the proximal cut is distal to the articular surface. With this complication, arthrofibrosis or degenerative arthritis may develop and require MTP joint arthrodesis.

INSTABILITY AFTER RESECTION OF THE BASE (KELLER PROCEDURE)

With resection of the base of the proximal phalanx after a Keller procedure, the intrinsic muscle insertion to the toe is sacrificed. Attempts to restabilize the MTP joint involve reattachment of the intrinsic muscles to the proximal phalanx stump or suturing of the flexor hallucis longus tendon to the proximal phalanx. Although some procedures do help stabilize the joint, the forces involved in walking tend, over time, to force the remaining portion of the hallux into dorsiflexion and lateral deviation. With

a fixed deformity, the toe pulp no longer strikes the ground. This creates a significant problem with footwear (Fig. 6-222; see also Figs. 6-195 to 6-199). The incidence of this complication can usually be diminished by adequate stabilization of the hallux with a Steinmann pin (for a period of 4 weeks) after the Keller procedure.

Another complication associated with instability of the proximal phalanx is that weight bearing of the great toe is greatly diminished. Weight is transferred to the lateral metatarsals, and either metatarsalgia or a transfer lesion develops (see Fig. 6-197).

Correction of instability of the hallux generally requires MTP joint arthrodesis. The authors prefer not to lengthen the toe but to accept some shortening.[104,536] The success rate of primary fusion without a bone graft is approximately 95%,[104,536] versus about 70% when a bone graft is added (see Fig. 6-202).

This salvage type of arthrodesis usually requires internal fixation with two intramedullary threaded Steinmann pins. Deficient bone stock or severe osteopenia in the proximal phalanx makes plate or screw fixation very difficult. Most patients are satisfied with the results of this salvage procedure.[104,536] The fusion increases the functional length of the first metatarsal and creates a lever arm that diminishes the stress placed on the second metatarsal head, which often relieves the metatarsalgia (see Fig. 6-203).

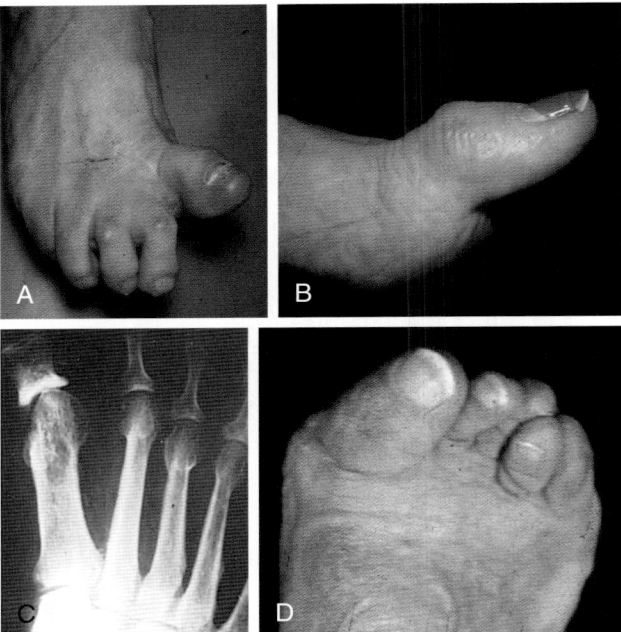

Figure 6-222 Complications after resection of the base of the proximal phalanx (the Keller procedure). **A,** Cock-up and claw toe deformity caused by loss of function of the intrinsic muscles inserting into the plantar aspect of the base of the proximal phalanx. **B,** Cock-up deformity. **C,** Hallux varus caused by excessive excision of the medial eminence. **D,** Recurrent hallux valgus after a Keller arthroplasty. (**D,** Courtesy E. Greer Richardson, MD.)

Complications Associated with Capsular Tissue of the First Metatarsophalangeal Joint
LOSS OF CORRECTION SECONDARY TO FAILURE OF MEDIAL JOINT CAPSULAR TISSUE

The etiology of recurrent hallux valgus is multifactorial. One cause is inadequate medial capsulorrhaphy, regardless of the procedure performed. This failure can result from an intrinsic problem within the capsule, such as ganglion formation or degeneration within the substance of the medial capsular tissue, or, with a very severe hallux valgus deformity, it can result from marked attenuation of the medial capsular tissue. When one of these conditions is encountered at surgery, it is preferable to imbricate the capsule rather than excise the medial capsule. A suture anchor can also be placed at the area of the defect to help stabilize the capsular deficiency (see Fig. 6-172). The formation of capsular fibrosis or scar tissue may prevent recurrence of the deformity (Fig. 6-223).

When the medial capsular flap is developed, it may be inadvertently detached at its proximal attachment. Using a capsular flap that leaves substantial attachments to both the base of the proximal phalanx and the plantar sesamoid region may reduce the frequency of this complication (see Fig. 6-91D). Anchoring the repair with metaphyseal drill holes may secure the proximal capsule. Postoperative dressings are crucial in this situation, to afford adequate support while healing takes place. Likewise, inadequate postoperative dressings may allow capsular elongation or disruption of the capsular repair. This may necessitate a revision of the capsulorrhaphy, with substantial recurrence of the deformity.

FAILURE OF LATERAL JOINT CAPSULAR TISSUE

A significant lateral MTP joint contracture develops in most patients with a severe hallux valgus deformity. After lateral capsular release, a large gap is created that can be as long as 1 cm. With a defect of this size, it is uncommon for adequate tissue to re-form across this defect. This places the hallux at increased risk for a postoperative

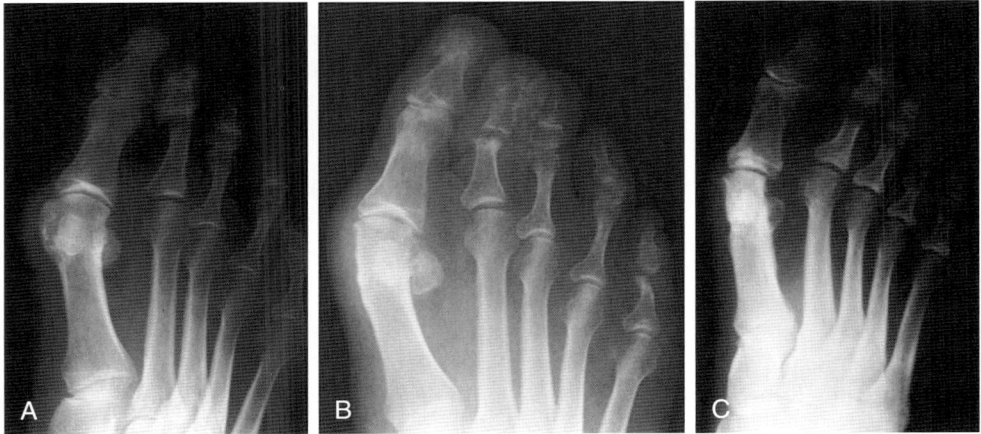

Figure 6-223 **A–C,** Recurrent hallux valgus deformity, probably caused by failure of the medial joint capsule to hold alignment of first metatarsophalangeal joint.

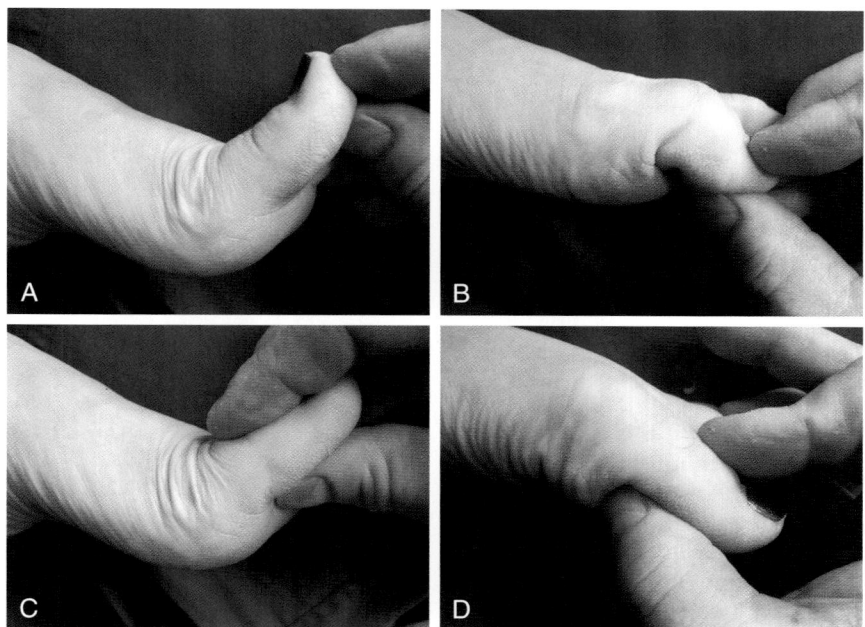

Figure 6-224 Early joint mobilization is very important to avoid restricted range of motion. **A** and **B**, Incorrect technique mobilizes the interphalangeal joint. **C** and **D**, Correct technique mobilizes the metatarsophalangeal joint.

hallux varus deformity. Mann and Coughlin[336] observed that hallux varus occurred most commonly in feet in which a more severe deformity was corrected. To avoid this complication, the lateral joint capsule can be initially perforated with multiple small puncture incisions. Next, with varus pressure on the hallux, the lateral capsule is gradually torn and the capsular tissue is "stretched out." This can lead to the formation of a large lateral capsular gap. Elevation and suturing of the adductor tendon to the lateral capsule aid in the re-formation of scar tissue in this area.

An alternative technique is to detach the capsule proximally and dorsally (L-shaped capsular release), which permits the lateral capsule to be slid distally as an entire unit, rather than incising it. The conjoined adductor tendon can actually be severed 3 cm proximal to its insertion and the stump sutured to the lateral capsule; this technique reinforces the lateral capsulorrhaphy as well.[93] Using this technique, Coughlin and Jones[100] reduced the incidence of postoperative hallux varus to a negligible amount.

ARTHROFIBROSIS OF THE METATARSOPHALANGEAL JOINT

Marked arthrofibrosis of the MTP joint can occur after a hallux valgus reconstruction of any type. Restricted joint motion can be quite disabling if the toe is fixed in marked plantar flexion or dorsiflexion. If excessive stiffness around the joint is detected early during the postoperative period, early joint mobilization is initiated. When seen late, a vigorous course of physical therapy is instituted to mobilize the MTP joint. The arthrofibrosis will usually

diminish in time and permit a functional but not normal range of motion. Joint manipulation may improve motion; however, repeat surgery in these patients rarely results in improved motion (Fig. 6-224).

Complications Involving the Sesamoids

Repositioning of the sesamoids after hallux valgus surgery is difficult when the crista (which normally divides the plantar surface of the metatarsal head into two distinct articulating surfaces) is attenuated. Constant pressure by gradual migration of the metatarsal head off the sesamoid complex leads to erosion of the metatarsosesamoidal facets and significant osteocartilagenous wear can develop (see Fig. 6-1FG).[35,449] Stabilization of the sesamoids is more difficult without a definite crista, and the sesamoids may assume a central rather than a medial position. Mann et al[344] were able to relocate the sesamoids from a medial to a normal or central location in 80% of cases; however, in the remaining cases, the sesamoids remained in a lateral position.

Mann and Donatto[340] found no significant change in the tibial sesamoid position after a chevron osteotomy. Thus a chevron procedure is contraindicated in a patient with preoperative pain attributed to the position of the tibial sesamoid beneath the metatarsal head.

Because the sesamoids are connected to the base of the proximal phalanx by the plantar plate, their location is determined in large part by the position and alignment of the proximal phalanx. If the sesamoids are not realigned adequately, more than likely the hallux valgus deformity has been undercorrected. In this situation, early recurrence is possible. Overcorrection of the position of the medial sesamoid leads to medial subluxation and a hallux varus deformity.

If the tibial sesamoid is located directly beneath the metatarsal crista, a plantar callus may develop. Shaving of the plantar half of the sesamoid will usually alleviate the problem (see Chapter 10).

UNCORRECTED SESAMOIDS

Inadequate correction of the position of the sesamoids generally results from failure to release the lateral MTP joint soft tissue contracture. This contracture is composed of several structures: the lateral joint capsule, the adductor tendon, and the transverse metatarsal ligament. The sesamoids cannot be mobilized and repositioned beneath the metatarsal head if this contracture is not released. The first metatarsal must be sufficiently mobile at the MTC joint to permit reduction of the metatarsal over the sesamoid complex. In the presence of fixed metatarsus primus varus or metatarsus adductus, unsuccessful relocation of the sesamoids requires a proximal osteotomy, or a recurrent hallux valgus deformity will develop.

MEDIAL SUBLUXATION OR DISLOCATION OF THE TIBIAL SESAMOID

Medial subluxation or complete dislocation of the tibial sesamoid may develop after a distal soft tissue procedure to correct a hallux valgus deformity. It may occur after an overcorrected proximal first metatarsal osteotomy or after lateral sesamoid excision, although it can occur even with the fibular sesamoid intact.

When the fibular sesamoid is excised, there is increased mobility of the sesamoid complex. A distal soft tissue realignment creates a situation in which medial displacement of the tibial sesamoid may occur. Subluxation or dislocation of the tibial sesamoid can also occur if the postoperative dressing holds the toe in excessive medial deviation or if a metatarsal osteotomy results in excessive lateral deviation of the metatarsal head.

Probably the most frequent cause of medial subluxation of the tibial sesamoid is excessive resection of the medial eminence. Although alignment of the sesamoids may not be too abnormal, absence of the plantar-medial metatarsal articulation allows the tibial sesamoid to displace dorsally along the medial aspect of the metatarsal head. In time, this instability can lead to further medial migration of the sesamoid and a painful hallux varus deformity (Fig. 6-225).

Treatment of this complication must be individualized. A certain amount of medial subluxation of the sesamoid is often well tolerated. However, in very active persons, the medial sesamoid may become quite painful, even if a hallux varus deformity has not developed. Excision of the tibial sesamoid can be considered if it causes irritation along the medial aspect of the metatarsal head. Although excision of both sesamoids should be avoided, on occasion, a painful tibial sesamoid is excised. If it has been a year or more since excision of the fibular

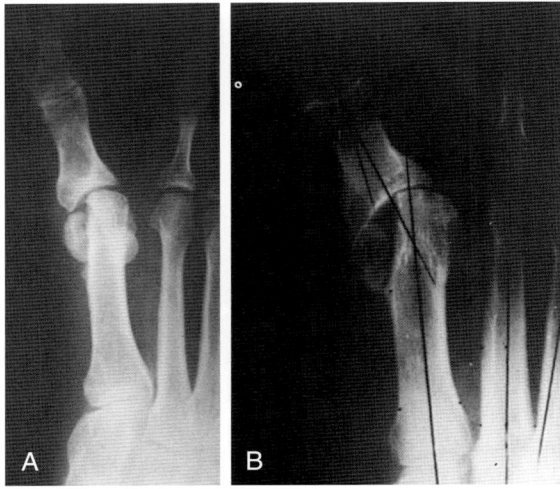

Figure 6-225 Medial subluxation of the tibial sesamoid. **A,** Excessive excision of the medial eminence and medial capsular plication resulting in medial subluxation of the sesamoid. **B,** Excessive excision of the medial eminence resulting in medial dislocation of the sesamoid.

sesamoid, the tibial sesamoid can be removed with only a small risk of a claw toe deformity developing. Medial dislocation of the tibial sesamoid is most commonly associated with a hallux varus deformity. When the hallux varus deformity is corrected, the tibial sesamoid is usually relocated beneath the metatarsal head.

With a severe hallux varus deformity, MTP joint arthrodesis is performed with excision of the dislocated tibial sesamoid.

COCK-UP DEFORMITY OF THE FIRST METATARSOPHALANGEAL JOINT

Plantar flexion of the first MTP joint is achieved primarily by the flexor hallucis brevis muscle, which inserts into the base of the proximal phalanx. With disruption of this mechanism, a muscle imbalance exists. The MTP joint is pulled into dorsiflexion by the unopposed force of the extensor hallucis brevis and the extensor hallucis longus. The flexor hallucis longus causes flexion of the IP joint. This deformity is often associated with hallux varus. After fibular sesamoid excision, the tibial sesamoid (which is the only connection between the flexor hallucis brevis and the proximal phalanx) is displaced medially. In this medially displaced position, no short flexor function is present at the MTP joint. Over time, soft tissue adhesions develop along with contracture of the abductor hallucis muscle, which leads to a fixed deformity (Fig. 6-226).

With previous tibial sesamoid excision, if a hallux valgus correction is performed with excision of the fibular sesamoid, a cock-up deformity can develop. Thus, under most circumstances, dual sesamoid excision, whether simultaneous or staged, should be avoided.

If a cock-up deformity of the hallux develops after removal of both sesamoids, treatment is tailored to the

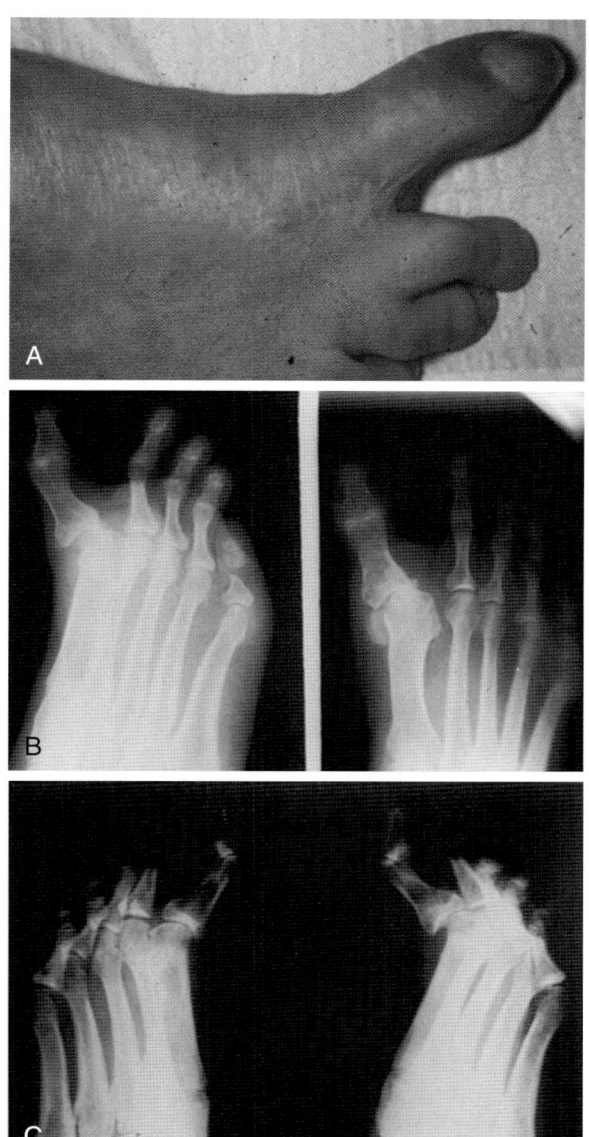

Figure 6-226 Cock-up varus deformity of the metatarsophalangeal joint after a McBride-type bunion repair. Clinical **(A)** and radiographic **(B** and **C)** views.

magnitude and rigidity of the deformity. In patients with a flexible MTP joint (with a minimum of 10 degrees of passive plantar flexion), an IP joint arthrodesis is performed. This procedure realigns the fixed flexion deformity of the IP joint and also permits the flexor hallucis longus tendon to function as a plantar flexor of the MTP joint. With a fixed extension contracture of the MTP joint, a "first-toe Jones procedure" is performed. This procedure involves transfer of the extensor hallucis longus tendon to the neck of the metatarsal. Transfer of this tendon provides the metatarsal head with a dorsiflexion force but also releases the dorsal contracture of the first MTP joint. A simultaneous IP joint arthrodesis realigns the IP joint and restores flexion power to the MTP joint (see Chapter

19). After a Keller procedure, a cock-up deformity is caused by loss of function of the flexor hallucis brevis muscle. This deformity is best treated by MTP joint arthrodesis rather than attempting to transfer a tendon to this small, unstable segment of the proximal phalanx (see Fig. 6-202).

INTRACTABLE PLANTAR KERATOSIS

After correction of a hallux valgus deformity, an intractable plantar keratosis may develop beneath the first metatarsal head. This lesion corresponds to the location of the tibial sesamoid, which at times is located in a central position directly beneath the metatarsal head. With progression of a hallux valgus deformity, the intersesamoidal ridge or crista is eroded by lateral pressure from the medial sesamoid. The crista is a major stabilizer of the sesamoid complex. With a relatively flat plantar metatarsal surface, the tibial sesamoid may be located centrally, which can be a source of pain for the patient.

Conservative treatment involves placing a metatarsal pad proximal to the sesamoid to relieve plantar pressure. Periodic trimming of the lesion is helpful. If the callosity continues to be painful, shaving the plantar half of the medial sesamoid usually produces a satisfactory clinical response (see Chapter 10). Excision of the tibial sesamoid should be avoided, especially if the lateral sesamoid has previously been removed. Dual sesamoid excision can result in a cock-up deformity of the first MTP joint because it disrupts the remaining short flexor function that stabilizes the first MTP joint. If the fibular sesamoid has not previously been removed, tibial sesamoidectomy is an option. Tibial sesamoid shaving, however, frequently alleviates the symptoms associated with a painful plantar callus in this area and is associated with much less morbidity than excision of the tibial sesamoid bone is.

Recurrent Hallux Valgus Deformity

Many factors need to be considered when evaluating a recurrent hallux valgus deformity. The characteristics of the initial deformity must be considered, as well as whether the correct surgical procedure was selected. Review of the postoperative management with the patient may provide information on the reason for failure.

The following broad categories need to be considered:

- Was selection of the surgical procedure appropriate?
- Were there technical problems during the course of the procedure that made it difficult to bring about complete correction?
- Was there a soft tissue problem, such as inadequate medial joint capsule secondary to capsular attenuation or ganglion formation within the capsule?
- Was postoperative care inadequate?

These general questions are appropriate for the review of any recurrent hallux valgus deformity. For each general group of hallux valgus procedures, certain problems arise. They are briefly discussed in the following section.

Distal Soft Tissue Procedure

For a distal soft tissue procedure to succeed, adequate release of the distal soft tissues must be performed. The lateral capsular structures, including the adductor tendon insertion into the sesamoid and proximal phalanx, must be released along with the lateral joint capsule. The transverse metatarsal ligament must also be released from the sesamoid complex to allow the sesamoids to rotate beneath the metatarsal head. The medial joint capsule must be adequately plicated. If it has deteriorated secondary to cyst formation or a ganglion involving the capsular tissue, it will have insufficient strength to stabilize the joint.

The main reason for failure of a distal soft tissue procedure is failure to recognize that significant metatarsus primus varus is present. A distal soft tissue procedure cannot be used to correct a fixed bone deformity (see Fig. 6-93). A "simple bunionectomy" fails to release the lateral joint contracture, and recurrence is common.

Chevron Procedure

A frequent cause of recurrent hallux valgus after a chevron procedure is when it is selected to correct a deformity that is of greater magnitude than the procedure was intended for. Failure to appreciate joint congruency and a lateral slope of the distal metatarsal articular surface will prevent full correction with the chevron procedure. The DMAA should be measured before a chevron procedure. If it is greater than 15 degrees, a medial closing-wedge chevron or an Akin procedure should be added (see Fig. 6-115). Inadequate capsular plication may also be another cause of recurrence. If the osteotomy is not stabilized with internal fixation, deformation may occur at the osteotomy site, with the capital fragment drifting medially and the toe laterally (see Fig. 6-121 and Fig. 6-227).

Proximal Metatarsal Osteotomy

Recurrent deformity after a crescentic, closing- or opening-wedge, or chevron-shaped proximal metatarsal osteotomy usually results from inadequate bone correction. This may be caused by failure to rotate the osteotomy site adequately or failure to remove enough bone to correct the metatarsus primus varus (Fig. 6-228). Recurrence may also be caused by failure of the associated distal soft tissue procedure. Use of a cirlage suture or wire between the first and second metatarsals may temporarily reduce the 1–2 IM angle but may be at risk for lesser metatarsal stress fracture with time (Fig. 6-229).

Akin Procedure

Recurrent deformities after an Akin procedure are generally the result of performing the procedure when it is not indicated. If there is incongruence or subluxation of the MTP joint, the Akin procedure rarely will bring about lasting correction of the deformity, and rapid recurrence

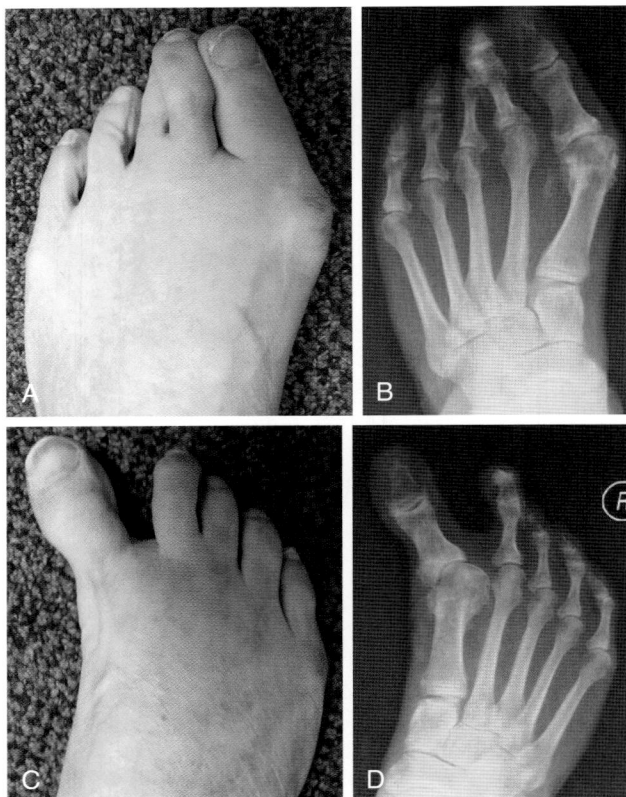

Figure 6-227 Clinical **(A)** and radiographic **(B)** views of recurrent deformity after distal metatarsal osteotomy. In the same patient, clinical **(C)** and radiographic **(D)** appearance of severe varus postoperative deformity after distal metatarsal osteotomy.

may result (see Fig. 6-112). Likewise, an increased 1–2 IM angle cannot be corrected with a phalangeal osteotomy and distal soft tissue repair.

Scarf Procedure

After a scarf osteotomy, recurrence can develop for a number of regions: pushing the procedure beyond its indications in the treatment of a severe deformity—an MTP articulator with a substantial DMAA or slope to the articular surface—or its use in osteopenic bone where fixation is tenuous and displacement or troughing occurs.

Keller Procedure

After a Keller procedure, instability often develops at the MTP joint because the base of the proximal phalanx has been resected. As a result, the proximal phalanx may drift back into a valgus deformity and result in recurrent hallux valgus (see Fig. 6-222D). Typically, a Keller procedure corrects only about 50% of the angular deformity present with hallux valgus.

Preoperative Conditions

Certain underlying conditions associated with a hallux valgus deformity may preclude a satisfactory result. It is

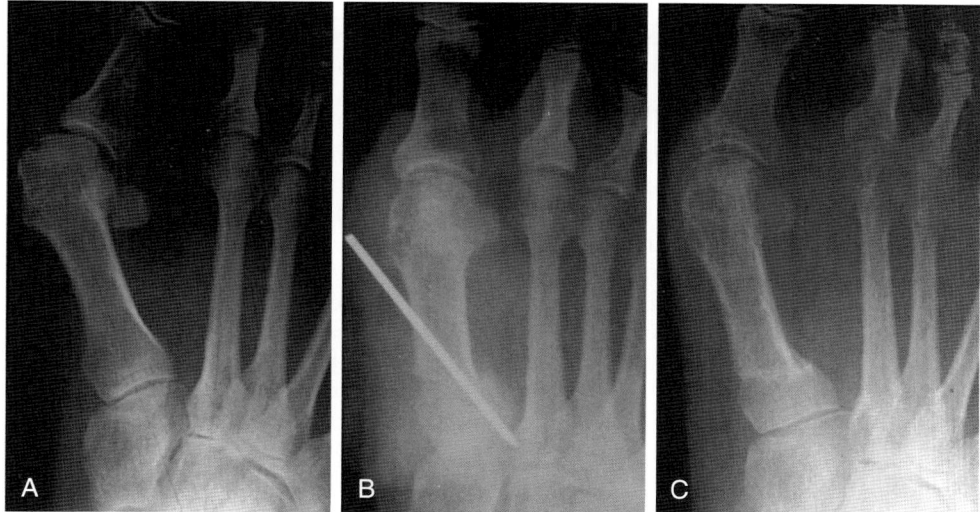

Figure 6-228   Recurrent hallux valgus deformity from inadequate medial displacement of the proximal metatarsal fragment at metatarsocuneiform joint after osteotomy. Preoperative radiograph **(A)** demonstrates lack of correction of the intermetatarsal angle after proximal metatarsal osteotomy **(B)**, and recurrent hallux valgus develops **(C)**.

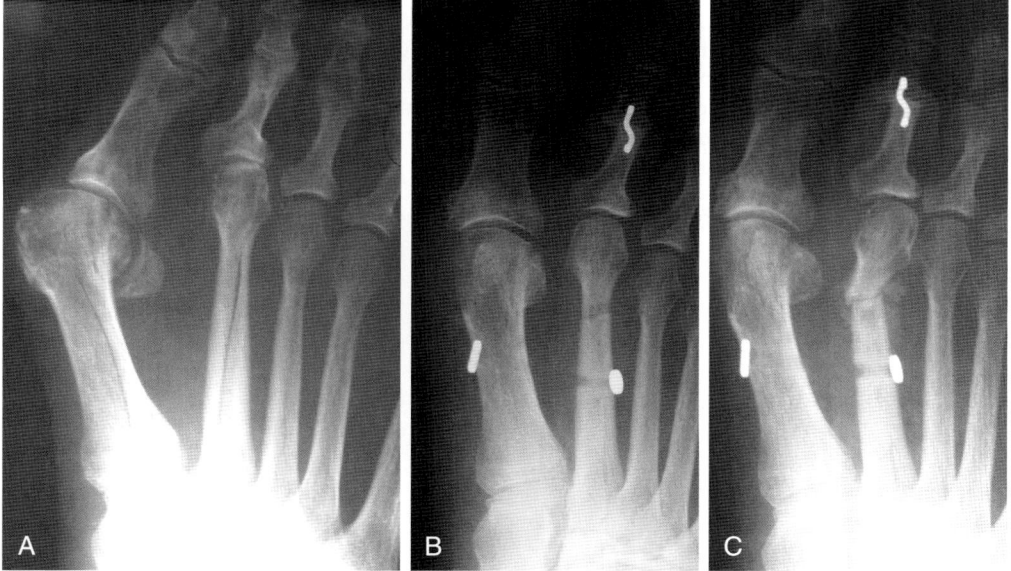

Figure 6-229   Stress fracture of the second metatarsal. **A,** Severe hallux valgus deformity. **B,** After circlage "tight rope" to reduce 1–2 intermetatarsal angle. **C,** After fracture of the second metatarsal and recurrence of the bunion deformity.

important to recognize these situations so that they can be addressed when performing the bunion procedure. At the very least, a patient should be alerted to the fact that the surgery may not be completely successful.

The following conditions, when present, may preclude obtaining a satisfactory result and should be considered in the preoperative planning:

■ Lateral deviation of the distal articular surface will preclude complete correction of the MTP joint with a distal soft tissue realignment. This problem can be corrected with a medial closing-wedge chevron procedure or a closing-wedge metatarsal or phalangeal osteotomy.

■ An underlying arthritic condition (hallux rigidus, rheumatoid arthritis) may be accompanied by inadequate capsular tissue to support a soft tissue repair. Likewise, articular cartilage degeneration may be present. In this situation, MTP joint arthrodesis should be considered for correction of the hallux valgus deformity.

■ When joint hyperelasticity is present (Ehlers-Danlos syndrome), little can be done to increase stability of the joints other than an MTP joint arthrodesis.

- With a severely pronated foot, rear foot surgery may be necessary to realign the foot and should be performed before a hallux valgus repair. If not corrected, the deformity may recur.
- While uncommon, if first-ray hypermobility is present, MTC arthrodesis is performed in conjunction with the repair if the surgeon is convinced the increased mobility occurs at the MTC joint.
- When a significant equinus deformity at the ankle joint is present in conjunction with a hallux valgus deformity, the foot must be corrected to a plantigrade position before hallux valgus repair is attempted.
- If spasticity of any cause is present, an MTP joint soft tissue realignment is at high risk for failure, and an MTP joint arthrodesis is the procedure of choice.

HALLUX VARUS

Hallux varus is medial deviation of the great toe. Similar to hallux valgus deformities, hallux varus has varying degrees of severity and causes. This condition can occur on a congenital basis, although this is quite uncommon (Fig. 6-230). More frequently, it is a deformity acquired after either a surgical procedure or trauma in which the lateral collateral ligament of the hallux is ruptured. Hallux varus may occur after a distal soft tissue or McBride type of bunionectomy,[336,343,369] but it is also observed after the chevron, Mitchell, Keller, and Lapidus procedures (see Fig. 6-227C and D).

The classic hallux varus deformity after the McBride procedure, in which excision of the fibular sesamoid is followed by MTP joint hyperextension, IP joint flexion, and medial deviation of the hallux (Video Clip 61).

Anatomically, this deformity results from a muscle imbalance caused by medial dislocation of the tibial sesamoid, although other factors are involved as well (Fig. 6-231A).

The MTP joint is flexed by the flexor hallucis brevis muscle primarily through its pull on the sesamoid complex. After fibular sesamoid excision, the MTP joint hyperextends as the metatarsal head "buttonholes" through the soft tissue defect created by the deficiency in the flexor hallucis brevis. The medial deviation is aggravated by the detachment of the adductor tendon when the medial sesamoid is removed and compounded by the unopposed pull of the abductor hallucis muscle.

With time, it becomes a fixed deformity that makes it difficult for the patient to obtain comfortable footwear. The IP joint of the great toe becomes flexed because the long extensor tendon can no longer effectively extend the IP joint. Simultaneously, the long flexor tendon is stretched around the metatarsal head, which creates a constant flexion force on the IP joint. In time, this entire deformity becomes rigid. When the metatarsal head does not buttonhole through the soft tissue defect, the hallux varus deformity consists mainly of medial deviation of the proximal phalanx without any significant cock-up deformity of the MTP joint or flexion of the IP joint (Fig. 6-231B-D). The following soft tissue factors can contribute to a hallux varus deformity:

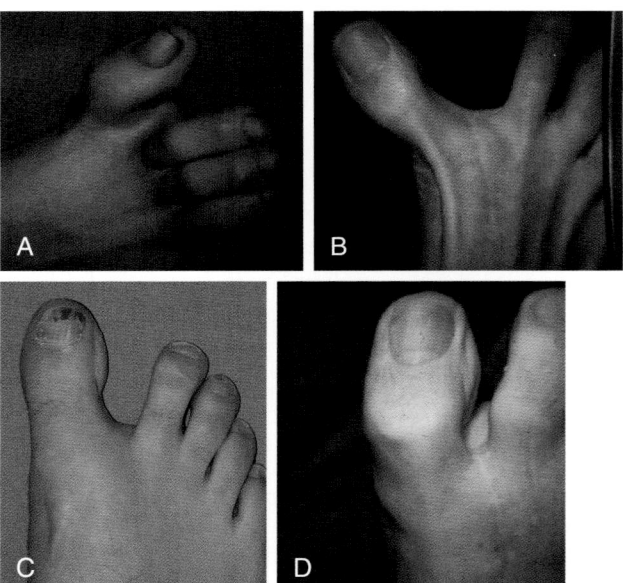

Figure 6-231 Hallux varus deformity. **A,** "Classic" hallux varus deformity with medial deviation and a cock-up deformity of the first metatarsophalangeal (MTP) joint after a distal soft tissue procedure. **B,** Hallux varus deformity with medial deviation of the MTP joint but no cock-up deformity of the joint. This type of varus may occur with both sesamoids intact. **C,** Mild hallux varus deformity. **D,** Mild varus associated with a mild cock-up deformity of the first MTP joint and flexion of the interphalangeal joint.

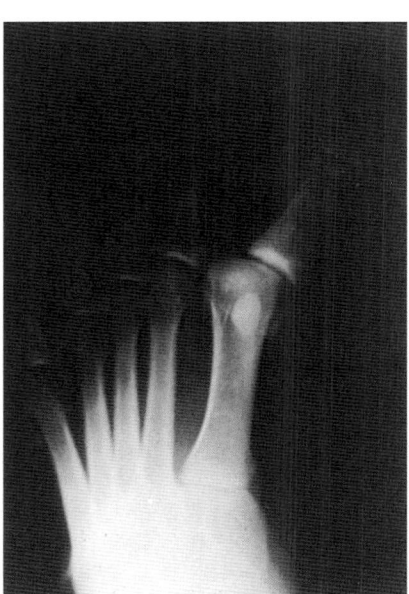

Figure 6-230 Congenital hallux varus deformity.

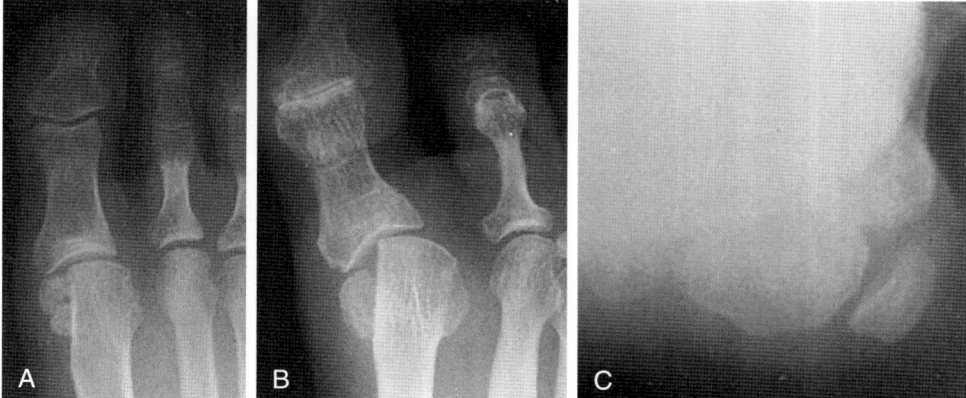

Figure 6-232 Various causes of hallux varus. **A,** Varus deformity, probably caused by overplication of the medial capsular structures. **B,** Medial displacement of the tibial sesamoid resulting in a varus deformity, probably caused by imbalance from lack of adequate lateral joint stability. **C,** Sesamoid view demonstrating medial displacement of the tibial sesamoid as a result of, or resulting in, a hallux varus deformity.

■ Overplication of the medial capsule (Fig. 6-232A)
■ Medial displacement of the tibial sesamoid (Fig. 6-232B and C)
■ Overpull of the abductor hallucis muscle against an incompetent lateral ligamentous complex (Fig. 6-233A-E)
■ Overcorrection with a postoperative dressing holding the MTP joint in a varus position
■ Excessive resection of the medial eminence (Fig. 6-233 F and G)

Hallux varus may occur after a proximal or distal metatarsal osteotomy when the metatarsal head is translated too far laterally, or if too much metatarsal head is resected, the potential exists for MTP joint instability and hallux varus.

With a chevron osteotomy, if the capital fragment is excessively displaced lateralward, a hallux varus deformity can develop (Fig. 6-234A). Likewise, with a proximal osteotomy, the distal segment can be translated too far laterally (Fig. 6-234B-G). With a crescentic osteotomy, the authors initially directed the concavity distally toward the great toe. If the metatarsal osteotomy site is translated too far medially, excessive lateral translation of the metatarsal head occurs. Once this problem was recognized, the concavity was reversed so that it faced proximally toward the heel. With this orientation, overtranslation rarely occurs because the distal metatarsal segment is locked into the proximal segment. Less commonly, a lateral closing-wedge or proximal chevron osteotomy or Lapidus procedure can be overcorrected. This can create the dual deformity of overcorrection and shortening.

A hallux varus deformity must be carefully evaluated to determine which salvage procedure is appropriate. If the varus deformity is caused by overplication of the medial capsule, release of the medial capsule may be sufficient. With a fixed deformity, however, a soft tissue capsular release is rarely effective. Plication of the lateral capsule can be added to the medial capsular release, but

this does not generally produce a lasting result. On occasion, the surgeon may encounter a mild varus deformity, and yet the sesamoids remain well aligned. In this instance, the surgeon may perform a phalangeal osteotomy to realign the hallux. This "reverse Akin" osteotomy may be performed through the prior medially based incision (Fig. 6-235A-C). These more mild and passively correctable varus deformities may also be amenable to a realignment procedure by using suture-button fixation. This minimally invasive technique allows rebalancing of the joint via medial soft tissue release and lateral fixation (Fig. 6-236A-E).[403] A tendon allograft may also be used to augment the repair.

With medial displacement of the tibial sesamoid after excision of the fibular sesamoid or excessive resection of the medial eminence, a more aggressive surgical repair may be necessary. In the initial determination, the question is whether sufficient articular surface remains to permit adequate joint function after realignment. In the presence of degenerative arthrosis, a soft tissue reconstruction is contraindicated because the MTP joint will only deteriorate further. Arthrodesis is the appropriate salvage procedure, although MTP joint motion is sacrificed.

In a hallux varus deformity with reasonable articular surface remaining, the extensor hallucis longus tendon can be used to create a dynamic correction of the deforming forces. Initially, the entire extensor hallucis longus tendon was transferred beneath the transverse metatarsal ligament and inserted into the base of the proximal phalanx of the great toe.[247] This was coupled with IP joint arthrodesis. Although this technique can produce a satisfactory result, if the IP joint does not have a fixed deformity (or can be straightened to within 10-15 degrees of full extension), it is not necessary to sacrifice IP joint function. Furthermore, if the extensor hallucis longus transfer fails and MTP joint arthrodesis is necessary, a mobile and functional IP joint is preferable. Therefore the authors modified the original procedure and split the extensor hallucis longus tendon. A portion is transferred

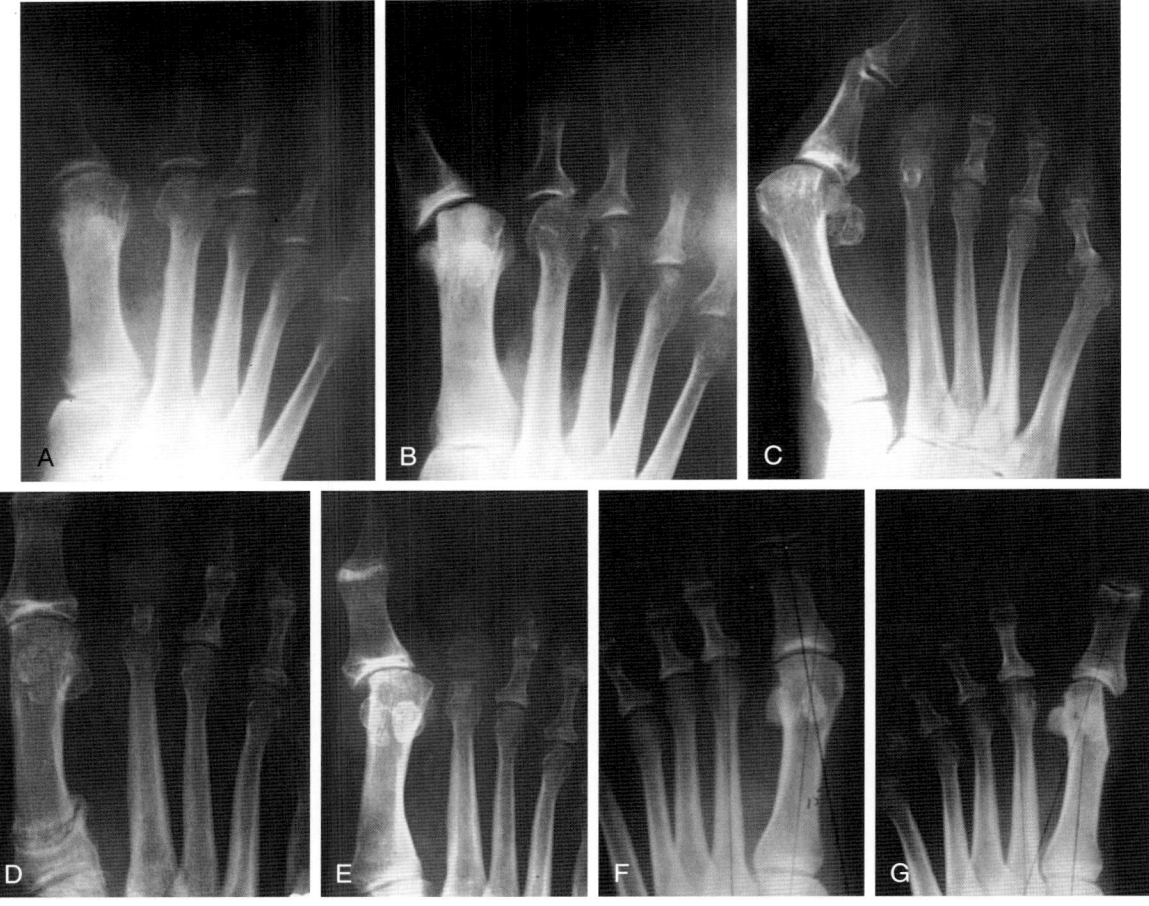

Figure 6-233 **A,** Immediately postoperatively. **B,** Progressive varus deformity developing over a period of 8 months after a distal soft tissue procedure. Note that both sesamoids are intact. This varus probably occurred because of lack of adequate lateral ligamentous stability. **C,** Preoperative radiograph. **D,** One month postoperatively, a radiograph demonstrates satisfactory alignment of the metatarsophalangeal joint. **E,** Two years postoperatively, a varus deformity has developed, probably from lack of reestablishment of the lateral ligamentous complex. Preoperative **(F)** and postoperative **(G)** radiographs demonstrate hallux varus caused by excessive excision of the medial eminence.

and a portion is left intact to control the IP joint of the hallux.

EXTENSOR HALLUCIS LONGUS TRANSFER

The surgical technique for correction of hallux varus is divided into the surgical approach and preparation for the tendon transfer, release of the medial joint contracture, and reconstruction of the MTP joint.

Surgical Approach and Preparation for Tendon Transfer

1. A dorsal curvilinear incision is made starting just lateral to the insertion of the extensor hallucis longus tendon. The incision is carried laterally toward the first web space and follows the interval between the first and second metatarsals. It is then inclined medially and ends along the lateral aspect of the extensor hallucis longus tendon in the region of the first MTC joint (Fig. 6-237A).

2. The extensor hallucis tendon is dissected free of soft tissue attachments, and the lateral two thirds of the tendon is released from its insertion. Starting with the free end, the tendon is carefully "teased out" proximally to the level of the MTC joint (Fig. 6-237B and see Video Clip 61). If when developing the lateral two thirds of the tendon the remaining portion of the tendon is inadvertently ruptured, it can be repaired by suturing the extensor hallucis brevis tendon to it.

3. The transverse metatarsal ligament is identified and a right-angle clamp or Mixner clamp is passed beneath it. Even if the transverse metatarsal ligament had been released at the time of the initial surgery, a sufficient amount of ligament usually re-forms. This remnant of the transverse metatarsal ligament is used as a pulley for the extensor tendon (Fig. 6-237C). A ligature is passed beneath the transverse metatarsal ligament to be used later in the procedure for pulling the extensor hallucis longus tendon beneath it.

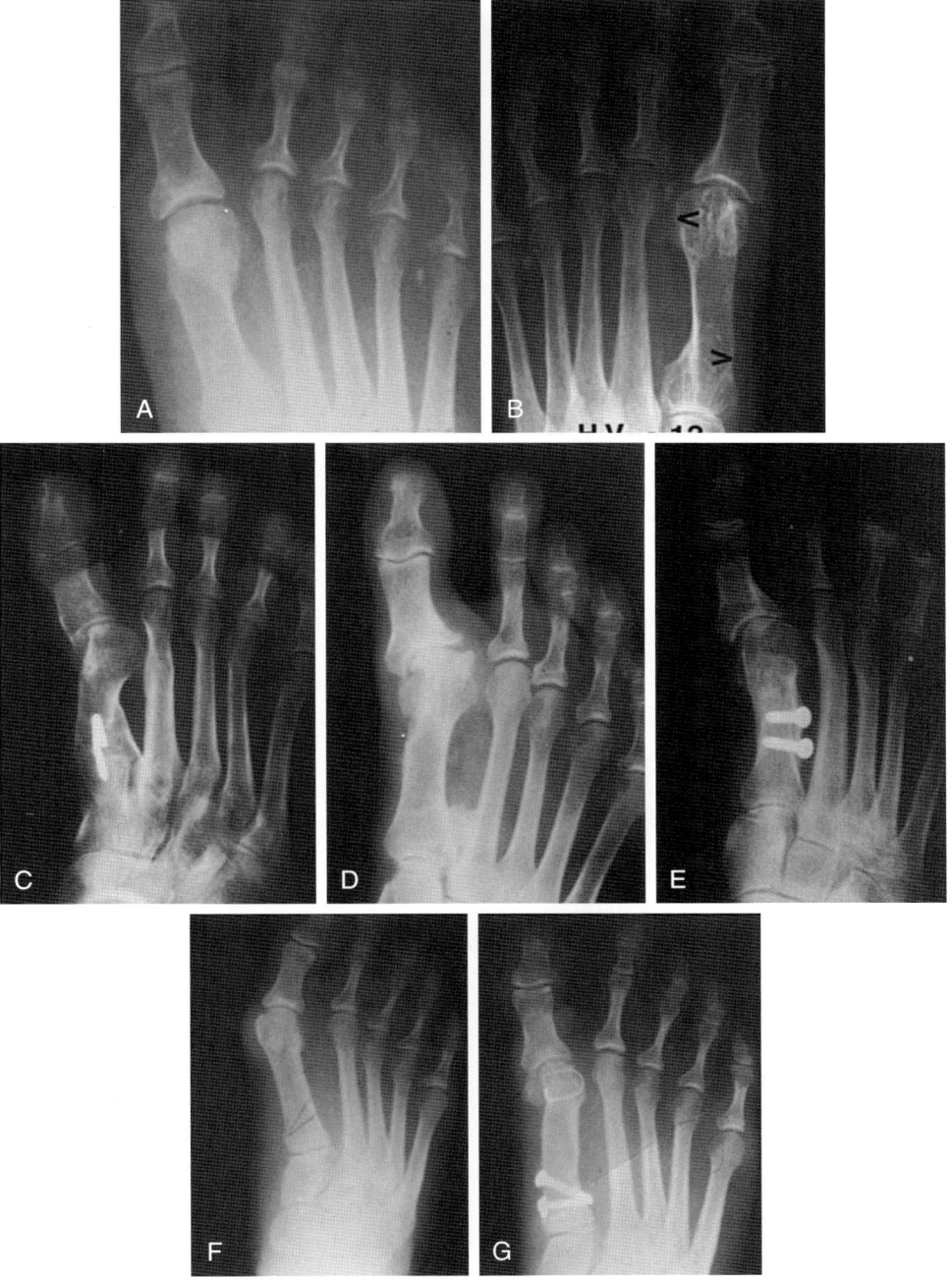

Figure 6-234 Hallux varus secondary to metatarsal osteotomies. **A,** Varus deformity after a chevron osteotomy. **B,** Varus deformity after a proximal crescentic osteotomy with excessive medial displacement of the base of the osteotomy, leading to lateral translation of the metatarsal head. **C,** Varus deformity after an oblique metatarsal osteotomy resulting in excessive lateral translation of the metatarsal head. **D,** Varus deformity after metatarsophalangeal arthrodesis secondary to lateral displacement of the metatarsal head. **E,** Varus deformity secondary to midshaft metatarsal osteotomy with excessive lateral displacement of the metatarsal head. Preoperative **(F)** and postoperative **(G)** radiographs demonstrate a hallux varus deformity after proximal and distal metatarsal osteotomy.

Medial Joint Capsule Release

1. The medial aspect of the MTP joint is approached through a long midline incision, beginning just proximal to the IP joint and ending at the midportion of the metatarsal shaft. Full-thickness dorsal and plantar skin flaps are developed, with care taken to avoid the cutaneous nerves. Too thin a skin flap can inadvertently result in sloughing of skin.

2. The medial joint capsule is cut obliquely starting at the plantar medial aspect of the base of the proximal

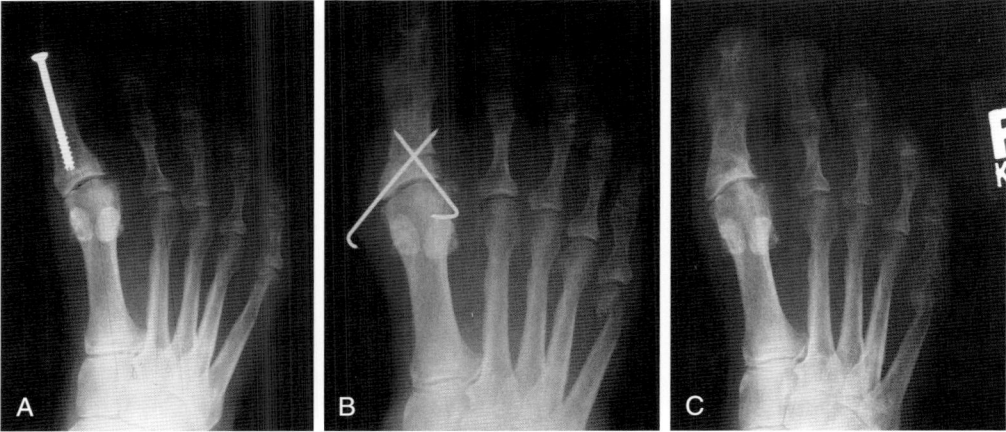

Figure 6-235 **A,** Anteroposterior (AP) standing radiograph of a patient having a prior bunionectomy and hallux interphalangeal arthrodeses complicated by hallux varus. Sesamoids are well aligned, and the joint is preserved. **B,** A lateral closing-wedge osteotomy of the proximal phalanx has been performed and secured with crossed Kirschner wires. **C,** AP radiograph at 1 year postoperatively. Note maintenance of correction.

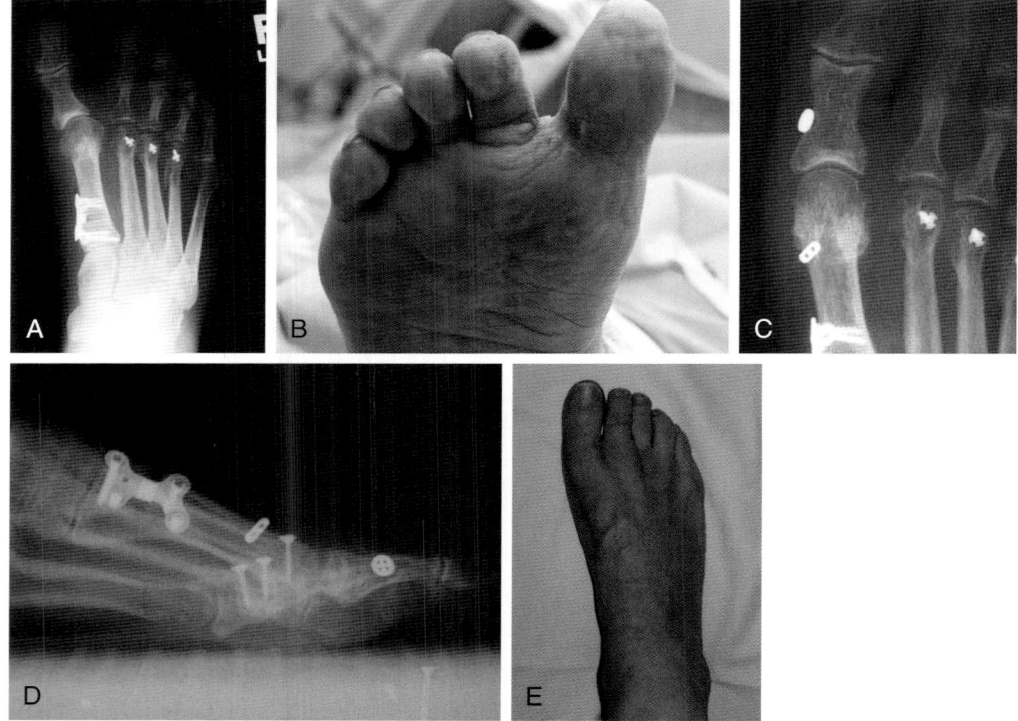

Figure 6-236 **A,** Hallux varus after prior bunion correction with proximal metatarsal osteotomy. Note absence of sesamoid displacement or degeneration. **B,** Clinical appearance of hallux varus. Anteroposterior **(C)** and lateral **(D)** radiographs at 6 months postoperative, confirming restoration of hallux alignment with suture-button technique. **E,** Clinical appearance of the foot at 1 year postoperatively.

phalanx where the abductor hallucis tendon inserts. The capsulotomy proceeds obliquely in a proximal and dorsal direction. This flap is dissected off the metatarsal head to permit the proximal phalanx to be brought out of its fixed varus deformity. A 5- to 7-mm gap is usually created in the capsular tissue.

3. The abductor hallucis tendon is identified beneath the cut in the capsule, and a long oblique cut releases the last remaining deforming force. At this point, the proximal phalanx can be brought into a valgus position with no resistance. If resistance is still present, some residual medial structure has not been adequately released.

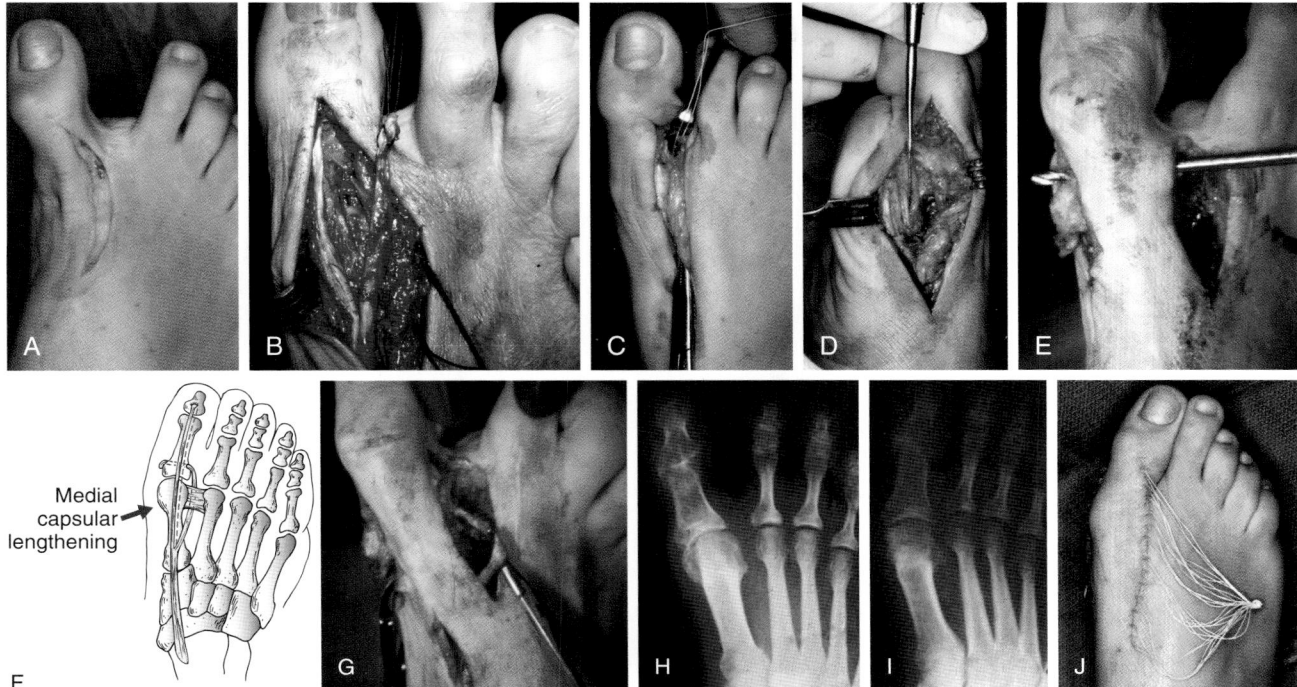

Medial capsular lengthening

Figure 6-237 Technique of hallux varus correction. **A,** Initial skin incision. **B,** Detachment of the lateral two thirds of the extensor hallucis longus tendon and proximal split of the extensor tendon. **C,** The tendon is passed beneath the transverse metatarsal ligament. The ligature is pulled through and can be used later to pull the extensor tendon beneath the transverse metatarsal ligament. **D,** The medial joint capsule is released through a longitudinal incision. **E,** A transverse drill hole is made through the base of the proximal phalanx. **F,** Diagram demonstrating passage of the lateral two thirds of the extensor hallucis longus tendon beneath the transverse metatarsal ligament and across the proximal phalanx. Note that the medial capsular structures have been lengthened. **G,** The extensor tendon is pulled through the drill hole in the proximal phalanx as the ankle joint is held in dorsiflexion to gain added length of the tendon and the hallux is held in lateral deviation and slight plantar flexion. **H,** Preoperative radiograph. **I,** Postoperative radiograph demonstrating correction of the hallux varus deformity. **J,** Postoperative clinical appearance.

4. If the tibial sesamoid is displaced medially, the abductor hallucis tendon must be freed from its attachment to it to permit the sesamoid to be placed back beneath the metatarsal head. If too much of the metatarsal head was resected at the initial surgery and the sesamoid cannot be replaced beneath the metatarsal head or if the medial sesamoid is too prominent, excision of the sesamoid should be considered (Fig. 6-237D).
5. If an MTP joint dorsiflexion contracture is present, it is treated by releasing the dorsal capsule, which enables the MTP joint to be brought into approximately 10 degrees of plantar flexion.
6. A transverse drill hole in the base of the proximal phalanx is started in the midline. It is important that the hole be drilled distal enough so that it does not inadvertently penetrate the articular surface of the proximal phalanx (Fig. 6-237E).

Reconstruction of the Metatarsophalangeal Joint
1. A ligature is placed on the end of the extensor hallucis longus tendon and is used to pass the tendon beneath the transverse metatarsal ligament.

2. With the ankle joint in dorsiflexion (which relaxes the extensor hallucis longus), the extensor hallucis longus tendon is passed through the drill hole in the base of the proximal phalanx. It is pulled taut, and the hallux is brought into valgus. The tendon is sutured into the periosteum along the medial aspect of the proximal phalanx. At this point, the toe should be aligned in approximately 10 to 15 degrees of valgus. If the toe still tends to drift into varus, either the soft tissue contracture on the medial side was inadequately released or the extensor hallucis longus tendon was not placed under sufficient tension (Fig. 6-237F and G).
3. The remaining medial third of the extensor hallucis longus tendon is plicated by weaving a suture through it to place it under tension.
4. The skin is closed with interrupted suture in routine manner, and a compression dressing is applied postoperatively (Fig. 6-123H and I).

Alternative Procedures
Alternative surgical techniques have been described to correct mild and moderate postoperative varus deformities. Lee et al[304] and Choi et al[68] have both described a

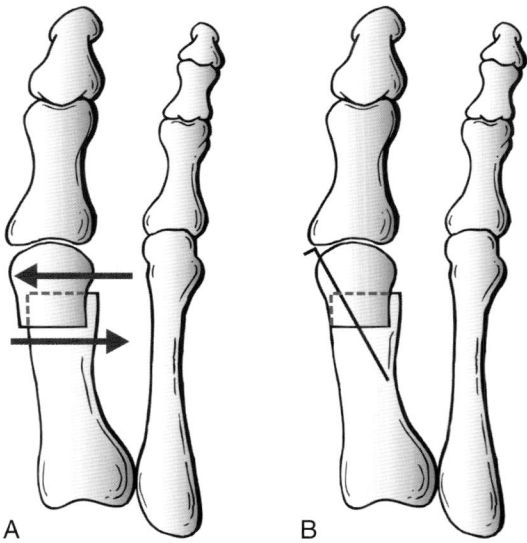

Figure 6-238 Technique of reverse chevron osteotomy to correct hallux varus deformity. **A,** Chevron osteotomy with medial displacement. **B,** After internal fixation. (Modified from Choi KJ, Lee HS, Yoon YS, et al: Distal metatarsal osteotomy for hallux varus following surgery for hallux valgus. *J Bone Joint Surg Br* 93:1079-1083, 2011.)

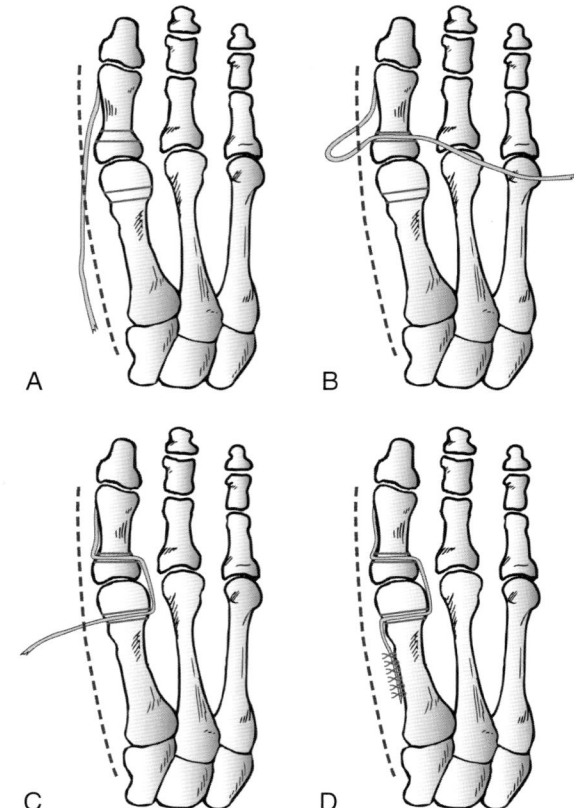

Figure 6-239 Abductor hallucis technique: technique of repair of hallux varus deformity using strip of abductor hallucis. **A,** A distally based flap of tendon of the abductor hallucis is created. Two transverse drill holes are created in the based of the proximal phalanx and in the subcapital region of the first metatarsal head. The tendon is transferred through the phalangeal drill hole **(B)** and then through the metatarsal drill hole **(C). D,** It is tightened and sewn to the periosteum of the first metatarsal shaft creating a tight lateral soft tissue cuff.[308] (Modified with permission from Leemriuse T, Hoang B, Maldague P, et al: A new surgical procedure for iatrogenic hallux varus: reverse transfer of the abductor hallucis tendon: a report of 7 cases. *Acta Orthop Belg* 74:227-234, 2008.)

distal metatarsal reverse chevron procedure in which the capital fragment is medialized to correct the varus deformity. Choi et al[68] reported on 19 patients, of which 17 of 19 had a successful realignment (Fig. 6-238). Leemrijse et al[308] have proposed developing a slip of abductor hallucis medially, and then routing in through a phalangeal drill hole and then transferring this fascial slip back through a transverse metatarsal drill hole to create a stout lateral collateral ligament (Fig. 6-239).

Postoperative Care

The postoperative dressing is removed and replaced with a snug gauze dressing and adhesive tape to hold the toe in a slightly overcorrected valgus position. The patient is permitted to ambulate in a postoperative shoe. The dressings are changed weekly for 8 weeks. A postoperative shoe should be used for another 2 weeks to allow further maturation of the tendon transfer (Fig. 6-240).

This procedure will produce a satisfactory clinical result in about 80% of patients. On occasion, slight overcorrection or undercorrection of the MTP joint occurs but is usually well tolerated. Typically, 50% to 60% of MTP joint motion is maintained after this procedure (Fig. 6-241). If little or no motion is present at the MTP joint preoperatively, the patient should be advised that this procedure will not significantly improve range of motion but will improve the overall position of the hallux. On occasion, minor skin slough develops in the skin along the medial side of the MTP joint, or delayed wound healing occurs because of the tension created by pulling the toe into a valgus position from its previous varus position. The authors do not know how to avoid this

problem because the medial incision cannot be placed in another location.

If the varus deformity develops after a resection arthroplasty (the Keller procedure), after excessive resection of the medial aspect of the metatarsal head, or in conjunction with MTP joint degenerative arthritis, MTP joint arthrodesis is the treatment of choice (see Figs. 6-202 and 6-203). Salvage with a silicone implant is contraindicated unless the deforming forces that led to the hallux varus deformity can be completely corrected. A joint replacement or silicone implant will maintain satisfactory joint alignment only if the surrounding soft tissues are well balanced.

A hallux varus deformity caused by nonunion of a metatarsal osteotomy is best corrected by MTP joint

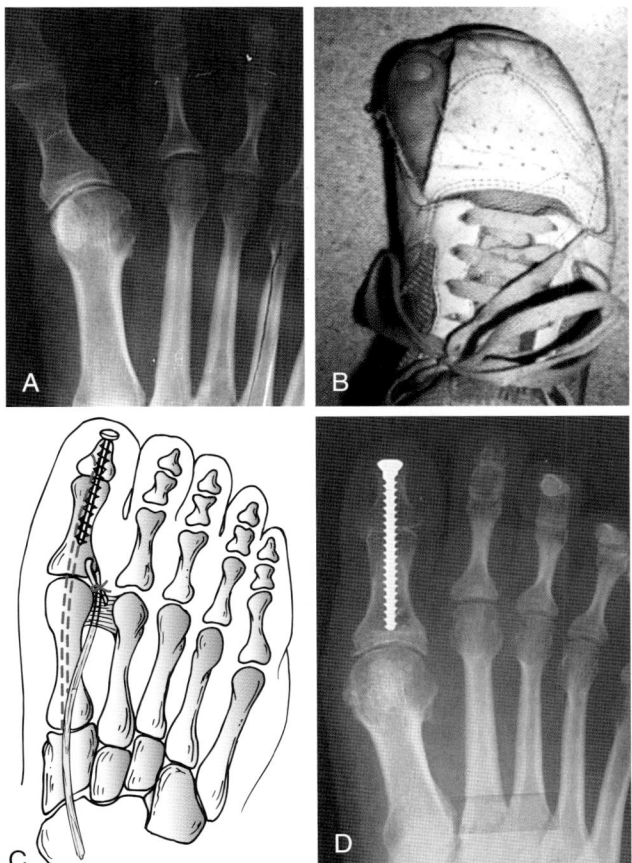

Figure 6-240 Complications after distal soft tissue repair. **A,** Hallux varus deformity after the McBride procedure. **B,** Footwear modified for the deformity. **C,** Schematic diagram of partial flexor hallucis longus transfer and interphalangeal joint fusion, which can be used to correct a hallux varus deformity. **D,** Postoperative radiograph after realignment.

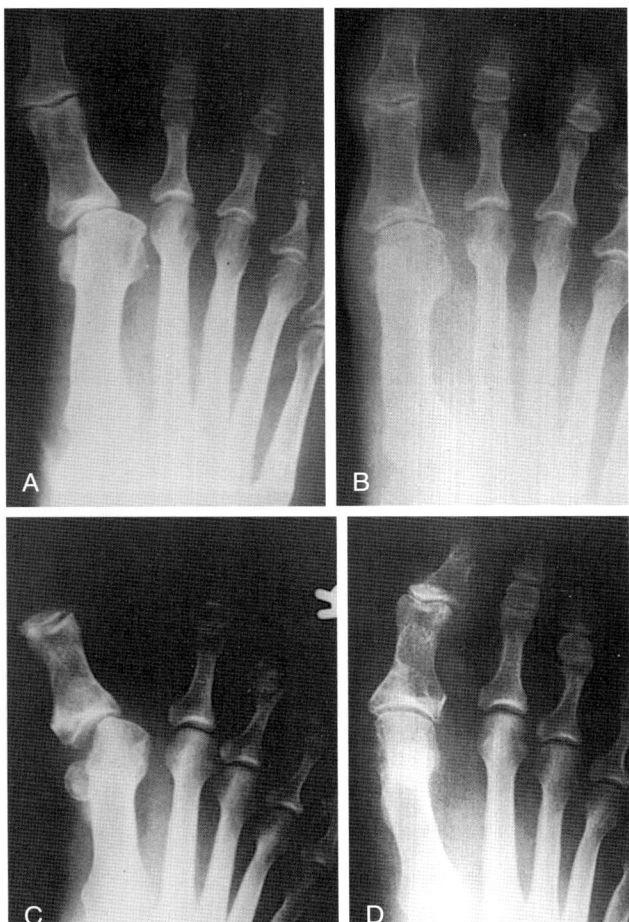

Figure 6-241 **A** and **C,** Hallux varus deformity resulting from a distal soft tissue procedure. **B** and **D,** Postoperative reconstructive procedure involving transfer of the extensor hallucis longus tendon.

arthrodesis rather than an attempt at either tendon transfer or corrective metatarsal osteotomy. Although realignment osteotomy can occasionally be performed, complete balancing of the MTP joint soft tissues is crucial to obtain a successful and long-lasting correction.

PAIN AROUND THE FIRST METATARSOPHALANGEAL JOINT AFTER BUNION SURGERY

The most common complaint before bunion surgery is pain over the medial eminence.[344] Secondary problems include sesamoid pain, pain over the medial aspect of the great toe, pain from a transfer lesion beneath a lesser metatarsal head, and, at times, pain within the MTP joint. After hallux valgus surgery, regardless of the surgical procedure, most patients are satisfied with the reduction in pain over the medial eminence. Ten percent of patients continue to complain of pain around the first MTP joint area. The causes include nerve entrapment, degenerative

MTP joint disease, sesamoid malalignment, and MTP joint arthrofibrosis. This discomfort is often poorly defined and rarely associated with clearly delineated intraarticular degenerative changes visible on radiographs. Although bone scans can define areas of arthritis, they are generally negative. Patients should be counseled preoperatively that they may have MTP joint discomfort after bunion surgery.[482]

PROSTHESES

The use of an MTP joint prosthesis in primary bunion surgery is rarely, if ever, indicated (Fig. 6-242). The occasional sedentary patient with advanced MTP joint degenerative arthritis who desires a prosthesis may be a candidate for the procedure. The use of a prosthesis in an active individual, regardless of age, is inadvisable because of the inherent problems of loosening, breakage, osteolysis, and synovitis and the high incidence of transfer metatarsalgia (Figs. 6-243 and 6-244).

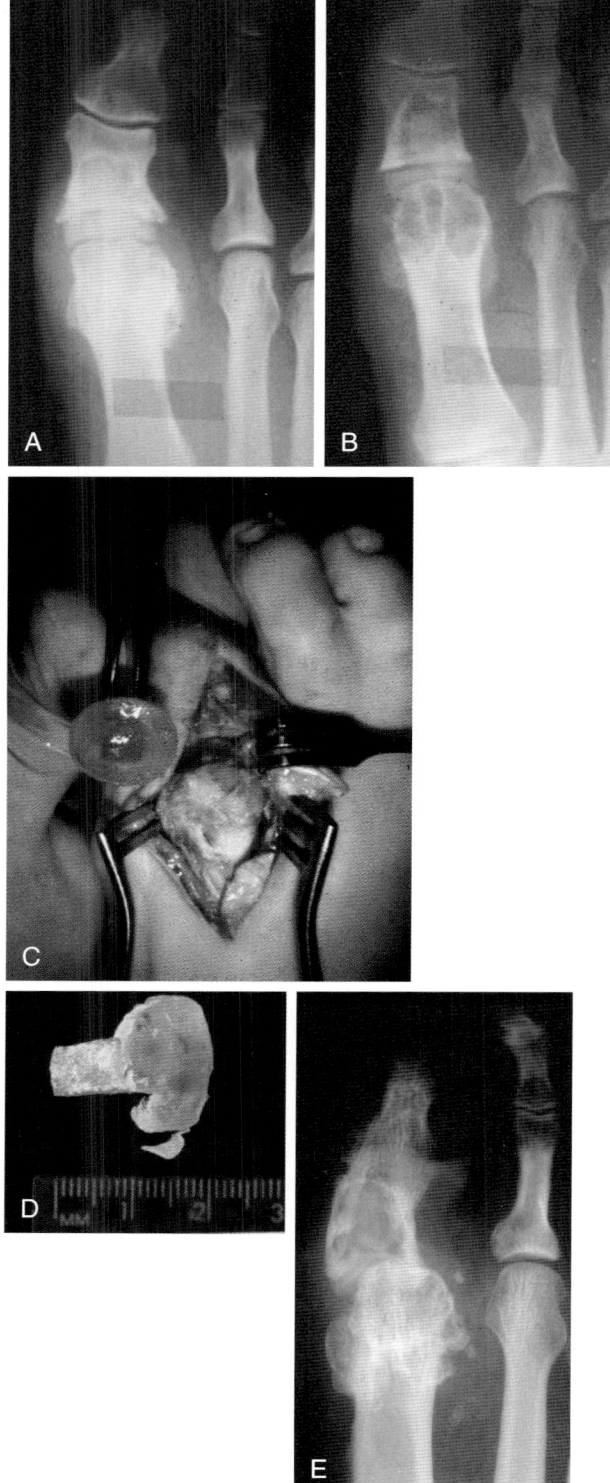

Figure 6-242 Complications of a single-stem prosthesis. **A,** One year after implantation. **B,** Five years later, severe reaction to the implant is demonstrated. **C,** At surgical removal. **D,** Eroded specimen. **E,** Severe silicone synovitis associated with a single-stem implant.

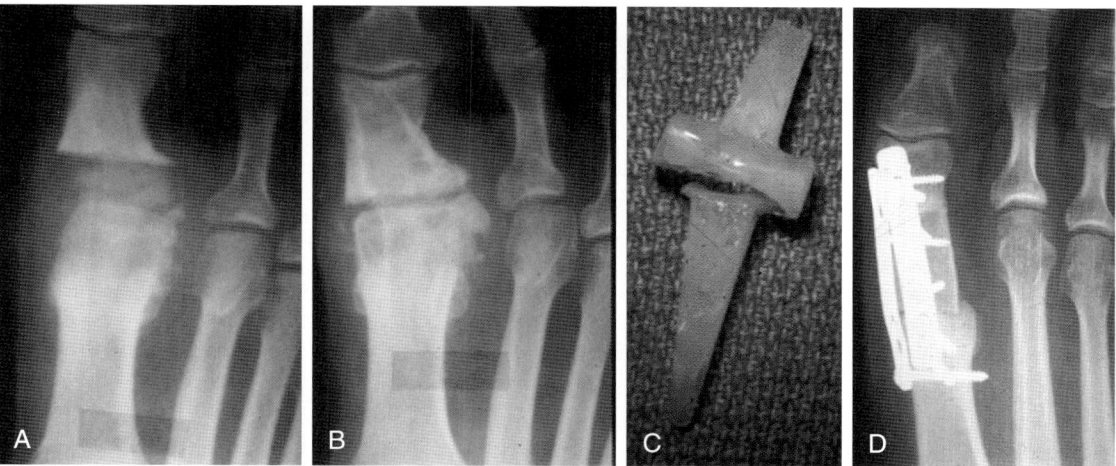

Figure 6-243 Complications of double-stem implants. **A,** Six months after implantation. **B,** Three years after surgery there is collapse and reaction surrounding the metatarsophalangeal joint. **C,** After removal later, the implant had fractured. **D,** A difficult salvage may involve an interposition bone graft. It is preferable to merely excise the reactive area and permanently remove the prosthesis when a severe reaction occurs.

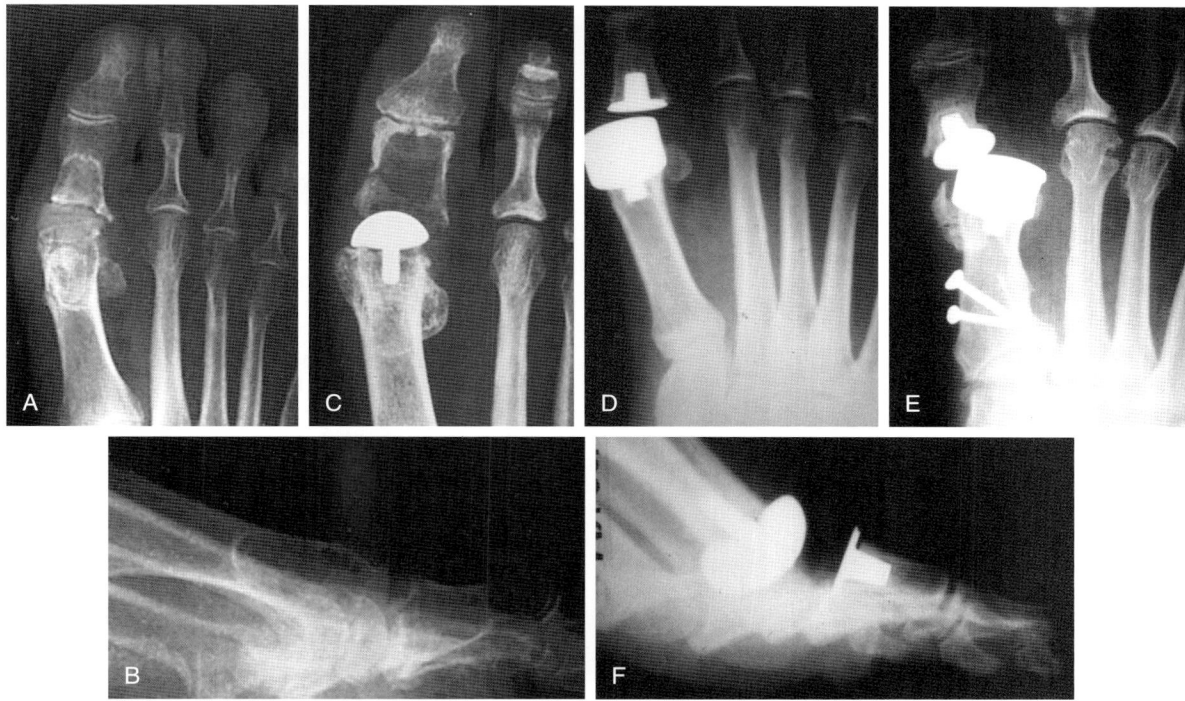

Figure 6-244 **A and B,** Lateral radiographs demonstrating settling and synovitis after implantation of a double-stemmed prosthesis. **C,** Severe osteolysis associated with loosening of components of a prosthetic replacement. **D–F,** Loosening of the metatarsal and phalangeal components with subluxation of the metatarsophalangeal joint.

The salvage procedure for a painful prosthesis entails removal of the prosthesis, complete joint synovectomy, placement of an intramedullary K-wire to stabilize the joint, and soft tissue capsulorrhaphy. The K-wire is removed 3 weeks after surgery, and range-of-motion exercises are commenced.[278] After this technique, 70% to 80% of prostheses can be removed and the first ray salvaged without performing a simple arthrodesis or a much more extensive procedure entailing arthrodesis with an interposition bone block.[189,215]

REFERENCES

1. Adam SP, Choung SC, Gu Y, O'Malley MJ: Outcomes after scarf osteotomy for treatment of adult hallux valgus deformity, *Clin Orthop Relat Res* 469:854–859, 2011.
2. Akin O: The treatment of hallux valgus: a new operative procedure and its results, *Med Sentinel* 33:678–679, 1925.
3. Akinbo S, Aiyegusi A, Owoeye O, Ogunsola M: Prevalence of hallux valgus among youth population in Lagos, Nigeria, *Nigerian Postgrad Med J* 18:51–55, 2011.
4. Albrecht G: The pathology and treatment of hallux valgus, *Tussk Vrach* 10:14–19, 1911.
5. Amarnek DL, Jacobs AM, Oloff LM: Adolescent hallux valgus: its etiology and surgical management, *J Foot Surg* 24:54–61, 1985.
6. Amarnek DL, Mollica A, Jacobs AM, Oloff LM: A statistical analysis on the reliability of the proximal articular set angle, *J Foot Surg* 25:39–43, 1986.
7. Aminian A, Kelikian A, Moen T: Scarf osteotomy for hallux valgus deformity: an intermediate followup of clinical and radiographic outcomes, *Foot Ankle Int* 27:883–886, 2006.
8. Anderson M, Blais MM, Green WT: Lengths of the growing foot, *J Bone Joint Surg Am* 38:998–1000, 1956.
9. Anderson R: Hallux valgus: Report of end results, *South Med J* 91:74–78, 1929.
10. Antrobus JN: The primary deformity in hallux valgus and metatarsus primus varus, *Clin Orthop* 184:251–255, 1984.
11. Arnold H: Die Korrektur des Hallux Valgus interphalangeus durch Closing-Wedge-Osteotomie nach Akin, *Oper Orthop Traumatol* 20:477–483, 2008.
12. Austin DW, Leventen EO: A new osteotomy for hallux valgus: a horizontally directed "V" displacement osteotomy of the metatarsal head for hallux valgus and primus varus, *Clin Orthop* 157:25–30, 1981.
13. Austin DW, Leventen EO: *Scientific exhibit: V-osteotomy of the first metatarsal head*, Chicago, 1968, American Academy of Orthopaedic Surgery.
14. Bacardi BE, Boysen TJ: Considerations for the Lapidus operation, *J Foot Surg* 25:133–138, 1986.
15. Badwey TM, Dutkowsky JP, Graves SC, Richardson EG: An anatomical basis for the degree of displacement of the distal chevron osteotomy in the treatment of hallux valgus, *Foot Ankle Int* 18:213–215, 1997.
16. Bae SY, Schon LC: Surgical strategies: Ludloff first metatarsal osteotomy, *Foot Ankle Int* 28:137–144, 2007.
17. Bai LB, Lee KB, Seo CY, et al: Distal chevron osteotomy with distal soft tissue procedure for moderate to severe hallux valgus deformity, *Foot Ankle Int* 31:683–688, 2010.
18. Banks AS, Hsu YS, Mariash S, Zirm R: Juvenile hallux abducto valgus association with metatarsus adductus, *J Am Podiatr Med Assoc* 84:219–224, 1994.
19. Barca F, Busa R: Austin/chevron osteotomy fixed with bioabsorbable poly-L-lactic acid single screw, *J Foot Ankle Surg* 36:15–20; discussion 79–80, 1997.
20. Barnett CH: Valgus deviation of the distal phalanx of the great toe, *J Anat* 96:171–177, 1962.
21. Barnicot NA, Hardy RH: The position of the hallux in West Africans, *J Anat* 89:355–361, 1955.
22. Barouk LS: Scarf osteotomy of the first metatarsal in the treatment of hallux valgus, *Foot Dis* 2:35–48, 1991.
23. Barouk LS: Osteotomie scarf du primier metarsien, *Med Surg Pied* 10:111–120, 1994.
24. Barouk LS: Scarf osteotomy for hallux valgus correction. Local anatomy, surgical technique, and combination with other forefoot procedures, *Foot Ankle Clin* 5:525–558, 2000.
25. Barouk LS, Barouk P: Joint-preserving surgery in rheumatoid forefoot: preliminary study with more-than-two-year follow-up, *Foot Ankle Clin* 12:435–454, vi, 2007.
26. Bartolozzi P, Magnan BL: *Osteotomia diatale percutanea nella chirurgia dell'alluce valgo*. Bologna, Italy, 2000, Timeo, pp 1–71.
27. Beauchamp CG, Kirby T, Rudge SR, et al: Fusion of the first metatarsophalangeal joint in forefoot arthroplasty, *Clin Orthop* 190:249–253, 1984.
28. Bednarz PA, Manoli A 2nd: Modified Lapidus procedure for the treatment of hypermobile hallux valgus, *Foot Ankle Int* 21:816–821, 2000.
29. Beighton PGR, Bird H: *Hypermobility of joints*, New York, 1983, Springer-Verlag, pp 10–12.
30. Berg RP, Olsthoorn PG, Poll RG: Scarf osteotomy in hallux valgus: a review of 72 cases, *Acta Orthop Belg* 73:219–223, 2007.
31. Berner A, Sage R, Niemela J: Keller procedure for the treatment of resistant plantar ulceration of the hallux, *J Foot Ankle Surg* 44:133–136, 2005.
32. Berntsen A: De l'hallux valgus, contribution a son étiologie et a son traitment, *Rev Orthop* 17:101–111, 1930.
33. Bingold AC: Arthrodesis of the great toe, *Proc R Soc Med* 51:435–437, 1958.
34. Blum JL: The modified Mitchell osteotomy-bunionectomy: indications and technical considerations, *Foot Ankle Int* 15:103–106, 1994.
35. Bock P, Kristen KH, Kroner A, Engel A: Hallux valgus and cartilage degeneration in the first metatarsophalangeal joint, *J Bone Joint Surg Br* 86:669–673, 2004.
36. Bock P, Lanz U, Kroner A, et al: The Scarf osteotomy: a salvage procedure for recurrent hallux valgus in selected cases, *Clin Orthop Relat Res* 468:2177–2187, 2010.
37. Bohay D, Johnson K, Manoli A: The traumatic bunion, *Foot Anle Int* 17:383–387, 1996.
38. Bonney G, Macnab I: Hallux valgus and hallux rigidus; a critical survey of operative results, *J Bone Joint Surg Br* 34:366–385, 1952.
39. Bordelon L, editor: *Surgical and conservative foot care: a unified approach to principles and practice*, Thorofare, NJ, 1988, Slack, pp 13–14.
40. Borrelli AH, Weil LS: Modified scarf bunionectomy: our experience in more than one thousand cases, *J Foot Surg* 30:609–612, 1991.
41. Borton DC, Stephens MM: Basal metatarsal osteotomy for hallux valgus, *J Bone Joint Surg Br* 76:204–209, 1994.
42. Bosch P, Markowski H, Rannicher V: Technik und erste Ergebnisse der subkutanen distalen Metatarsale-I-Osteotomie, *Orthop Praxis* 26:51–56, 1990.
43. Bosch P, Wanke S, Legenstein R: Hallux valgus correction by the method of Bosch: a new technique with a seven-to-ten-year follow-up, *Foot Ankle Clin* 5:485–498, v–vi, 2000.
44. Bouaicha S, Ehrmann C, Moor BK, et al: Radiographic analysis of metatarsus primus elevatus and hallux rigidus, *Foot Ankle Int* 31:807–814, 2010.
45. Brage ME, Holmes JR, Sangeorzan BJ: The influence of x-ray orientation on the first metatarsocuneiform joint angle, *Foot Ankle Int* 15:495–497, 1994.
46. Brahm SM: Shape of the first metatarsal head in hallux rigidus and hallux valgus, *J Am Podiatr Med Assoc* 78:300–304, 1988.
47. Brattwall M, Turan I, Jakobsson J: Pain management after elective hallux valgus surgery: a prospective randomized double-blind study comparing etoricoxib and tramadol, *Anesth Analg* 111:544–549, 2010.
48. Breslauer C, Cohen M: Effect of proximal articular set angle correcting osteotomies on the hallucal sesamoid apparatus: a cadaveric and radiographic investigation, *J Foot Ankle Surg* 40:366–373, 2001.
49. Briggs TW, Smith P, McAuliffe TB: Mitchell's osteotomy using internal fixation and early mobilisation, *J Bone Joint Surg Br* 74:137–139, 1992.

50. Broca P: Des difformities de la partie anterieure du pied produite par faction de la chaussure, *Bull Soc Anat* 27:60–67, 1852.

51. Brodsky JW, Beischer AD, Robinson AH, et al: Surgery for hallux valgus with proximal crescentic osteotomy causes variable postoperative pressure patterns, *Clin Orthop Relat Res* 443:280–286, 2006.

52. Bryant A, Tinley P, Singer K: A comparison of radiographic measurements in normal, hallux valgus, and hallux limitus feet, *J Foot Ankle Surg* 39:39–43, 2000.

53. Budny AM, Masadeh SB, Lyons MC 2nd, Frania SJ: The opening base wedge osteotomy and subsequent lengthening of the first metatarsal: an in vitro study, *J Foot Ankle Surg* 48:662–667, 2009.

54. Burns AE, Varin J: Poly-L-lactic acid rod fixation results in foot surgery, *J Foot Ankle Surg* 37:37–41, 1998.

55. Burutaran H: Hallux valgus y cortedad anatomica del primer metatarsano (correction quinrugica), *Med Chir Pied* 13:261–266, 1976.

56. Butson AR: A modification of the Lapidus operation for hallux valgus, *J Bone Joint Surg Br* 62:350–352, 1980.

57. Campbell JT, Schon LC, Parks BG, et al: Mechanical comparison of biplanar proximal closing wedge osteotomy with plantar plate fixation versus crescentic osteotomy with screw fixation for the correction of metatarsus primus varus, *Foot Ankle Int* 19:293–299, 1998.

58. Canale PB, Aronsson DD, Lamont RL, Manoli A II: The Mitchell procedure for the treatment of adolescent hallux valgus. A long-term study, *J Bone Joint Surg Am* 75:1610–1618, 1993.

59. Carl A, Ross S, Evanski P, Waugh T: Hypermobility in hallux valgus, *Foot Ankle* 8:264–270, 1988.

60. Carr CR, Boyd BM: Correctional osteotomy for metatarsus primus varus and hallux valgus, *J Bone Joint Surg Am* 50:1353–1367, 1968.

61. Catanzariti AR, Mendicino RW, Lee MS, Gallina MR: The modified Lapidus arthrodesis: a retrospective analysis, *J Foot Ankle Surg* 38:322–332, 1999.

62. Cathcart E: Physiological aspect: nature of incapacity. The feet of the industrial worker: clinical aspect; relation to footwear, *Lancet* 2:1480–1482, 1938.

63. Cedell CA, Astrom M: Proximal metatarsal osteotomy in hallux valgus, *Acta Orthop Scand* 53:1013–1018, 1982.

64. Chana GS, Andrew TA, Cotterill CP: A simple method of arthrodesis of the first metatarsophalangeal joint, *J Bone Joint Surg Br* 66:703–705, 1984.

65. Chi TD, Davitt J, Younger A, et al: Intra- and inter-observer reliability of the distal metatarsal articular angle in adult hallux valgus, *Foot Ankle Int* 23:722–726, 2002.

66. Chiodo CP, Schon LC, Myerson MS: Clinical results with the Ludloff osteotomy for correction of adult hallux valgus, *Foot Ankle Int* 25:532–536, 2004.

67. Cho NH, Kim S, Kwon DJ, Kim HA: The prevalence of hallux valgus and its association with foot pain and function in a rural Korean community, *J Bone Surg Br* 91:494–498, 2009.

68. Choi KJ, Lee HS, Yoon YS, et al: Distal metatarsal osteotomy for hallux varus following surgery for hallux valgus, *J Bone Joint Surg Br* 93:1079–1083, 2011.

69. Choi WJ, Yoon HK, Yoon HS, et al: Comparison of the proximal chevron and Ludloff osteotomies for the correction of hallux valgus, *Foot Ankle Int* 30:1154–1160, 2009.

70. Cholmeley JA: Hallux valgus in adolescents, *Proc R Soc Med* 51:903–906, 1958.

71. Chou LB, Mann RA, Casillas MM: Biplanar chevron osteotomy, *Foot Ankle Int* 19:579–584, 1998.

72. Chow FY, Lui TH, Kwok KW, Chow YY: Plate fixation for crescentic metatarsal osteotomy in the treatment of hallux valgus: an eight-year followup study, *Foot Ankle Int* 29:29–33, 2008.

73. Clark HR, Veith RG, Hansen ST Jr: Adolescent bunions treated by the modified Lapidus procedure, *Bull Hosp Jt Dis Orthop Inst* 47:109–122, 1987.

74. Cleveland M, Winant EM: An end-result study of the Keller operation, *J Bone Joint Surg Am* 32:163–175, 1950.

75. Clutton H: The treatment of hallux valgus, *St Thomas Hosp Rep* 22:1–12, 1894.

76. Coetzee JC: Scarf osteotomy for hallux valgus repair: the dark side, *Foot Ankle Int* 24:29–33, 2003.

77. Coetzee JC, Resig SG, Kuskowski M, Saleh KJ: The Lapidus procedure as salvage after failed surgical treatment of hallux valgus. Surgical technique, *J Bone Joint Surg Am* 86(Suppl 1): 30–36, 2004.

78. Coetzee JC, Rippstein P: Surgical strategies: scarf osteotomy for hallux valgus, *Foot Ankle Int* 28:529–535, 2007.

79. Coetzee JC, Wickum D: The Lapidus procedure: a prospective cohort outcome study, *Foot Ankle Int* 25:526–531, 2004.

80. Colloff B, Weitz EM: Proximal phalangeal osteotomy in hallux valgus, *Clin Orthop* 54:105–113, 1967.

81. Cooper AJ, Clifford PD, Parikh VK, et al: Instability of the first metatarsal-cuneiform joint: diagnosis and discussion of an independent pain generator in the foot, *Foot Ankle Int* 30:928–932, 2009.

82. Cooper MT, Berlet GC, Shurnas PS, Lee TH: Proximal opening-wedge osteotomy of the first metatarsal for correction of hallux valgus, *Surg Technol Int* 16:215–219, 2007.

83. Corless JR: A modification of the Mitchell procedure, *J Bone Joint Surg Br* 55/58:138, 1976.

84. Cornwall MW, Fishco WD, McPoil TG, et al: Reliability and validity of clinically assessing first-ray mobility of the foot, *J Am Podiatr Med Assoc* 94:470–476, 2004.

85. Corte-Real NM, Moreira RM: Modified biplanar chevron osteotomy, *Foot Ankle Int* 30:1149–1153, 2009.

86. Coughlin MJ: Arthrodesis of the first metatarsophalangeal joint, *Orthop Rev* 19:177–186, 1990.

87. Coughlin MJ: Arthrodesis of the first metatarsophalangeal joint with mini-fragment plate fixation, *Orthopedics* 13:1037–1044, 1990.

88. Coughlin MJ: Hallux valgus, *J Bone Joint Surg Am* 78:932–966, 1996.

89. Coughlin MJ: Hallux valgus. Causes, evaluation, and treatment, *Postgrad Med* 75:174–178, 183, 186–187, 1984.

90. Coughlin MJ: Hallux valgus in the athlete, *J Sports Med Arthrosc Rev* 2:326–340, 1994.

91. Coughlin MJ: Hallux valgus in men: effect of the distal metatarsal articular angle on hallux valgus correction, *Foot Ankle Int* 18:463–470, 1997.

92. Coughlin MJ: President's Forum: evaluation and treatment of juvenile hallux valgus, *Contemp Orthop* 21:169–203, 1990.

93. Coughlin MJ: Proximal first metatarsal osteotomy. In Kitaoka H, editor: *The foot and ankle*, 2nd ed, Philadelphia, 2002, Williams & Wilkins, pp 71–98.

94. Coughlin MJ: Rheumatoid forefoot reconstruction. A long-term follow-up study, *J Bone Joint Surg Am* 82:322–341, 2000.

95. Coughlin MJ: Roger A. Mann Award. Juvenile hallux valgus: etiology and treatment, *Foot Ankle Int* 16:682–697, 1995.

96. Coughlin MJ, Abdo RV: Arthrodesis of the first metatarsophalangeal joint with Vitallium plate fixation, *Foot Ankle Int* 15:18–28, 1994.

97. Coughlin MJ, Carlson RE: Treatment of hallux valgus with an increased distal metatarsal articular angle: evaluation of double and triple first ray osteotomies, *Foot Ankle Int* 20:762–770, 1999.

98. Coughlin MJ, Freund E: Roger A. Mann Award. The reliability of angular measurements in hallux valgus deformities, *Foot Ankle Int* 22:369–379, 2001.

99. Coughlin MJ, Grebing BR, Jones CP: Arthrodesis of the metatarsophalangeal joint for idiopathic hallux valgus: Intermediate results, *Foot Ankle Int* 26:783–792, 2005.

100. Coughlin MJ, Jones CP: Hallux valgus and first ray mobility. A prospective study, *J Bone Joint Surg Am* 89:1887–1898, 2007.

101. Coughlin MJ, Jones CP: Hallux valgus: demographics, etiology, and radiographic assessment, *Foot Ankle Int* 28:759–777, 2007.

102. Coughlin MJ, Jones CP, Viladot R, et al: Hallux valgus and first ray mobility: a cadaveric study, *Foot Ankle Int* 25:537–544, 2004.

103. Coughlin MJ, Kaz A: Correlation of Harris mats, physical exam, pictures, and radiographic measurements in adult flatfoot deformity, *Foot Ankle Int* 30:604–612, 2009.

104. Coughlin MJ, Mann RA: Arthrodesis of the first metatarsophalangeal joint as salvage for the failed Keller procedure, *J Bone Joint Surg Am* 69:68–75, 1987.

105. Coughlin MJ, Mann RA: The pathophysiology of the juvenile bunion, *Instr Course Lect* 36:123–136, 1987.

106. Coughlin MJ, Saltzman CL, Nunley JA 2nd: Angular measurements in the evaluation of hallux valgus deformities: a report of the ad hoc committee of the American Orthopaedic Foot and Ankle Society on angular measurements, *Foot Ankle Int* 23:68–74, 2002.

107. Coughlin MJ, Shurnas PS: Hallux rigidus, *J Bone Joint Surg Am* 86(Suppl 1):119–130, 2004.

108. Coughlin MJ, Shurnas PS: Hallux rigidus: demographics, etiology, and radiographic assessment, *Foot Ankle Int* 24:731–743, 2003.

109. Coughlin MJ, Shurnas PS: Hallux rigidus. Grading and long term results of operative treatment, *J Bone Joint Surg Am* 85:2072–2088, 2003.

110. Coughlin MJ, Shurnas PS: Hallux valgus in men. Part II: first ray mobility after bunionectomy and factors associated with hallux valgus deformity, *Foot Ankle Int* 24:73–78, 2003.

111. Coughlin, MJ, Smith BW: Hallux valgus and first ray mobility. Surgical technique, *J Bone Joint Surg Am* 90(Suppl 2 Pt 2):153–170, 2008.

112. Coughlin MJ, Thompson FM: The high price of high-fashion footwear, *Instr Course Lect* 44:371–377, 1995.

113. Craigmile DA: Incidence, origin, and prevention of certain foot defects, *BMJ* 4839:749–752, 1953.

114. Creer WS: The feet of the industrial worker: clinical aspect; relation to footwear, *Lancet* 2:1482–1483, 1938.

115. Crevoisier X, Mouhsine E, Ortolano V, et al: The scarf osteotomy for the treatment of hallux valgus deformity: a review of 84 cases, *Foot Ankle Int* 22:970–976, 2001.

116. Cronin JJ, Limbers JP, Kutt S, Stephens MM: Intermetatarsal angle after first metatarsophalangeal joint arthrodesis for hallux valgus, *Foot Ankle Int* 27:104–109, 2006.

117. Daniels SE, Baum DR, Clark F, et al: Diclofenac potassium liquid-filled soft gelatin capsules for the treatment of postbunionectomy pain, *Curr Med Res Opin* 26:2375–2384, 2010.

118. Das De S, Hamblen DL: Distal metatarsal osteotomy for hallux valgus in the middle-aged patient, *Clin Orthop* 218:239–246, 1987.

119. Davids JR, McBrayer D, Blackhurst DW: Juvenile hallux valgus deformity: surgical management by lateral hemiepiphyseodesis of the great toe metatarsal, *J Pediatr Orthop* 27:826–830, 2007.

120. Davies-Colley N: Contraction of the metatarsophalangeal joint of the great toe (hallux flexus), *BMJ* 1:728, 1887.

121. Day MR, White SL, DeJesus JM: The "Z" osteotomy versus the Kalish osteotomy for the correction of hallux abducto valgus deformities: a retrospective analysis, *J Foot Ankle Surg* 36:44–50; discussion 80, 1997.

122. Day T, Charlton TP, Thordarson DB: First metatarsal length change after basilar closing wedge osteotomy for hallux valgus, *Foot Ankle Int* 32:S513–S518, 2011.

123. De Lavigne C, Rasmont Q, Hoang B: Percutaneous double metatarsal osteotomy for correction of severe hallux valgus deformity, *Acta Orthop Belg* 77:516–521, 2011.

124. De Vil JJ, Van Seymortier P, Bongaerts W, et al: Scarf osteotomy for hallux valgus deformity: a prospective study with 8 years of clinical and radiologic follow-up, *J Am Podiatr Med Assoc* 100:35–40, 2010.

125. Deenik A, van Mameren H, de Visser E, et al: Equivalent correction in scarf and chevron osteotomy in moderate and severe hallux valgus: a randomized controlled trial, *Foot Ankle Int* 29:1209–1215, 2008.

126. Deenik AR, Pilot P, Brand SE, et al: Scarf versus chevron osteotomy in hallux valgus: a randomized controlled trial in 96 patients, *Foot Ankle Int* 28:537–541, 2007.

127. Dennis NZ, Das De S: Modified Mitchell's osteotomy for moderate to severe hallux valgus: an outcome study, *J Foot Ankle Surg* 50:50–54, 2011.

128. DeOrio J: Technique tip: dorsal wedge resection (uniplanar) in the chevron osteotomy for high distal metatarsal articular angle bunions, *Foot Ankle Int* 28:642–644, 2007.

129. Deorio JK, Ware AW: Single absorbable polydioxanone pin fixation for distal chevron bunion osteotomies, *Foot Ankle Int* 22:832–835, 2001.

130. Dereymaeker G: Scarf osteotomy for correction of hallux valgus. Surgical technique and results as compared to distal chevron osteotomy, *Foot Ankle Clin* 5:513–524, 2000.

131. Dermon A, Tilkeridis C, Lyras D, et al: Long-term results of Mitchell's procedure for hallux valgus deformity: a 5- to 20-year followup in 204 cases, *Foot Ankle Int* 30:16–20, 2009.

132. Devos Bevernage B, Deleu PA, Leemrijse T: The translating Weil osteotomy in the treatment of an overriding second toe: a report of 25 cases, *Foot Ankle Surg* 16:153–158, 2010.

133. Dhukaram V, Hullin MG, Senthil Kumar C: The Mitchell and Scarf osteotomies for hallux valgus correction: a retrospective, comparative analysis using plantar pressures, *J Foot Ankle Surg* 45:400–409, 2006.

134. DiGiovanni CW, Kuo R, Tejwani N, et al: Isolated gastrocnemius tightness, *J Bone Joint Surg Am* 84:962–970, 2002.

135. Donley BG, Vaughn RA, Stephenson KA, Richardson EG: Keller resection arthroplasty for treatment of hallux valgus deformity: increased correction with fibular sesamoidectomy, *Foot Ankle Int* 23:699–703, 2002.

136. Dreeben S, Mann RA: Advanced hallux valgus deformity: long-term results utilizing the distal soft tissue procedure and proximal metatarsal osteotomy, *Foot Ankle Int* 17:142–144, 1996.

137. du Plessis M, Zipfel B, Brantingham JW, et al: Manual and manipulative therapy compared to night splint for symptomatic hallux abducto valgus: an exploratory randomised clinical trial, *Foot (Edinb)* 21:71–78, 2011.

138. Durman DC: Metatarsus primus varus and hallux valgus, *AMA Arch Surg* 74:128–135, 1957.

139. DuVries H, editor: *Surgery of the foot*, St Louis, 1959, CV Mosby, pp 346–442.

140. Easley ME, Kiebzak GM, Davis WH, Anderson RB: Prospective, randomized comparison of proximal crescentic and proximal chevron osteotomies for correction of hallux valgus deformity, *Foot Ankle Int* 17:307–316, 1996.

141. Easley ME, Trnka HJ: Current concepts review: hallux valgus part 1: pathomechanics, clinical assessment, and nonoperative management, *Foot Ankle Int* 28:654–659, 2007.

142. Easley ME, Trnka HJ: Current concepts review: hallux valgus part II: operative treatment, *Foot Ankle Int* 28:748–758, 2007.

143. Ellington JK, Jones CP, Cohen BE, et al: Review of 107 hallux MTP joint arthrodesis using dome-shaped reamers and a stainless-steel dorsal plate, *Foot Ankle Int* 31:385–390, 2010.

144. Ellington JK, Myerson MS, Coetzee JC, Stone RM: The use of the Lapidus procedure for recurrent hallux valgus, *Foot Ankle Int* 32:674–680, 2011.

145. Ellis VH: A method of correcting metatarsus primus varus; preliminary report, *J Bone Joint Surg Br* 33:415–417, 1951.

146. ElSaid AG, Tisdel C, Donley B, et al: First metatarsal bone: an anatomic study, *Foot Ankle Int* 27:1041–1048, 2006.

147. Engel E, Erlick N, Krems I: A simplified metatarsus adductus angle, *J Am Podiatr Assoc* 73:620–628, 1983.

148. Engle ET, Morton DJ: Notes on foot disorders among natives of the Belgian Congo, *J Bone Joint Surg* 13:311, 1931.

149. Espinosa N, Wirth SH: Tarsometatarsal arthrodesis for management of unstable first ray and failed bunion surgery, *Foot Ankle Clin* 16:21–34, 2011.

150. Ewald P: Die Actiologie des Hallux valgus, *Dtsch Ztschr Chir* 114:90–103, 1912.

151. Fabeck L, Zekhnini C, Farrokh D, Descamps P, Delince P: Traumatic hallux valgus following rupture of the medial collateral ligament of the first metatarsalphalangeal joint: a case report, *J Foot Ankle Surg* 41:1258, 2002.

152. Faber FW, Kleinrensink GJ, Verhoog MW, et al: Mobility of the first tarsometatarsal joint in relation to hallux valgus deformity: anatomical and biomechanical aspects, *Foot Ankle Int* 20:651–656, 1999.

153. Fadel GE, Hussain SM, Sripada S, Jain AS: Fixation of first metatarsal basal osteotomy using Acutrak screw, *Foot Ankle Surg* 14:21–25, 2008.

154. Fadel GE, Rowley DI, Jain AS: Compression screw fixation for first metatarsal basal osteotomy, *Foot Ankle Int* 23:253–254, 2002.

155. Ferrari J, Malone-Lee J: The shape of the metatarsal head as a cause of hallux abductovalgus, *Foot Ankle Int* 23:236–242, 2002.

156. Ferrari J, Malone-Lee J: A radiographic study of the relationship between metatarsus adductus and hallux valgus, *J Foot Ankle Surg* 42:9–14, 2003.

157. Fitzgerald JA: A review of long-term results of arthrodesis of the first metatarso-phalangeal joint, *J Bone Joint Surg Br* 51:488–493, 1969.

158. Fokter SK, Podobnik J, Vengust V: Late results of modified Mitchell procedure for the treatment of hallux valgus, *Foot Ankle Int* 20:296–300, 1999.

159. Fox IM, Smith SD: Juvenile bunion correction by epiphysiodesis of the first metatarsal, *J Am Podiatr Assoc* 73:448–455, 1983.

160. Frey C, Zamora J: The effects of obesity on orthopaedic foot and ankle pathology, *Foot Ankle Int* 28:996–999, 2007.

161. Fridman R, Cain JD, Weil L Jr, Weil LS Sr, Ray TB: Unilateral versus bilateral first ray surgery: a prospective study of 186 consecutive cases–patient satisfaction, cost to society, and complications, *Foot Ankle Spec* 2:123–129, 2009.

162. Fritz GR, Prieskorn D: First metatarsocuneiform motion: a radiographic and statistical analysis, *Foot Ankle Int* 16:117–123, 1995.

163. Fuhrmann RA, Zollinger-Kies H, Kundert HP: Mid-term results of Scarf osteotomy in hallux valgus, *Int Orthop* 34:981–989, 2010.

164. Funk FJ Jr, Wells RE: Bunionectomy—with distal osteotomy, *Clin Orthop* 85:71–74, 1972.

165. Galland W, Jordan H: Hallux valgus, *Surg Gynecol Obstet* 66:95, 1938.

166. Gallardo J, Lagos L, Bastias C, et al: Continuous popliteaal block for postoperative analgesia in total ankle arthroplasty, *Foot Ankle Int* 33:208–212, 2112.

167. Gallentine JW, Deorio JK, Deorio MJ: Bunion surgery using locking-plate fixation of proximal metatarsal chevron osteotomies, *Foot Ankle Int* 28:361–368, 2007.

168. Garcia-Bordes L, Jimenez-Potrero M, Vega-Garcia J, Yunta-Gallo A: Opening first metatarsal osteotomy and resection arthroplasty of the first MPJ in the treatment of first ray insufficiency associated with degenerative hallux valgus, *Foot Ankle Surg* 16:132–136, 2010.

169. Garrido IM, Rubio ER, Bosch MN, et al: Scarf and Akin osteotomies for moderate and severe hallux valgus: clinical and radiographic results, *Foot Ankle Surg* 14:194–203, 2008.

170. Geissele AE, Stanton RP: Surgical treatment of adolescent hallux valgus, *J Pediatr Orthop* 10:642–648, 1990.

171. Gerbert J: The indications and techniques for utilizing preoperative templates in podiatric surgery, *J Am Podiatr Assoc* 69:139–148, 1979.

172. Giannestras N: The Giannestras modification of the Lapidus operation. In Giannestras NJ, editor: *Foot disorders: medical and surgical management*, Philadelphia, 1973, Lea & Febiger.

173. Gill LH, Martin DF, Coumas JM, Kiebzak GM: Fixation with bioabsorbable pins in chevron bunionectomy, *J Bone Joint Surg Am* 79:1510–1518, 1997.

174. Gimple K, Anspacher J, Kopta J: Metatarsophalangeal joint fusion of the great toe, *Orthopedics* 1:462–467, 1978.

175. Ginsburg AI: Arthrodesis of the first metatarsophalangeal joint: a practical procedure, *J Am Podiatr Assoc* 69:367–369, 1979.

176. Glasoe WM, Allen MK, Saltzman CL: First ray dorsal mobility in relation to hallux valgus deformity and first intermetatarsal angle, *Foot Ankle Int* 22:98–101, 2001.

177. Glasoe WM, Allen MK, Saltzman CL, et al: Comparison of two methods used to assess first-ray mobility, *Foot Ankle Int* 23:248–252, 2002.

178. Glasoe WM, Allen MK, Yack HJ: Measurement of dorsal mobility in the first ray: elimination of fat pad compression as a variable, *Foot Ankle Int* 19:542–546, 1998.

179. Glasoe WM, Grebing B, Beck S, et al: A comparison of device measures of dorsal first ray mobility, *Foot Ankle Int* 26:957–961, 2005.

180. Glasoe WM, Yack HJ, Saltzman CL: Measuring first ray mobility with a new device, *Arch Phys Med Rehabil* 80:122–124, 1999.

181. Glasoe WM, Yack HJ, Saltzman CL: The reliability and validity of a first ray measurement device, *Foot Ankle Int* 21:240–246, 2000.

182. Glover JP, Hyer CF, Berlet GC, et al: A comparison of crescentic and Mau osteotomies for correction of hallux valgus, *J Foot Ankle Surg* 47:103–111, 2008.

183. Glover JP, Hyer CF, Berlet GC, Lee TH: Early results of the Mau osteotomy for correction of moderate to severe hallux valgus: a review of 24 cases, *J Foot Ankle Surg* 47:237–242, 2008.

184. Glynn MK, Dunlop JB, Fitzpatrick D: The Mitchell distal metatarsal osteotomy for hallux valgus, *J Bone Joint Surg Br* 62:188–191, 1980.

185. Goldberg I, Bahar A, Yosipovitch Z: Late results after correction of hallux valgus deformity by basilar phalangeal osteotomy, *J Bone Joint Surg Am* 69:64–67, 1987.

186. Goldner JL, Gaines RW: Adult and juvenile hallux valgus: analysis and treatment, *Orthop Clin North Am* 7:863–887, 1976.

187. Goucher NR, Coughlin MJ: Hallux metatarsophalangeal joint arthrodesis using dome-shaped reamers and dorsal plate fixation: a prospective study, *Foot Ankle Int* 27:869–876, 2006.

188. Grace D, Hughes J, Klenerman L: A comparison of Wilson and Hohmann osteotomies in the treatment of hallux valgus, *J Bone Joint Surg Br* 70:236–241, 1988.

189. Granberry WM, Noble PC, Bishop, JO, Tullos HS: Use of a hinged silicone prosthesis for replacement arthroplasty of the

first metatarsophalangeal joint, *J Bone Joint Surg Am* 73:1453–1459, 1991.

190. Grebing BR, Coughlin MJ: The effect of ankle position on the exam for first ray mobility, *Foot Ankle Int* 25:467–475, 2004.

191. Grebing BR, Coughlin MJ: Evaluation of the Esmark bandage as a tourniquet for forefoot surgery, *Foot Ankle Int* 25:397–405, 2004.

192. Grebing BR, Coughlin MJ: Evaluation of Morton's theory of second metatarsal hypertrophy, *J Bone Joint Surg Am* 86:1375–1386, 2004.

193. Green MA, Dorris MF, Baessler TP, et al: Avascular necrosis following distal chevron osteotomy of the first metatarsal, *J Foot Ankle Surg* 32:617–622, 1993.

194. Griffiths TA, Palladino SJ: Metatarsus adductus and selected radiographic measurements of the first ray in normal feet, *J Am Podiatr Med Assoc* 82:616–622, 1992.

195. Grill F, Hetherington V, Steinbock G, Altenhuber J: Experiences with the chevron (V-) osteotomy on adolescent hallux valgus, *Arch Orthop Trauma Surg* 106:47–51, 1986.

196. Grimes JS, Coughlin MJ: First metatarsophalangeal joint arthrodesis as a treatment for failed hallux valgus surgery, *Foot Ankle Int* 27:887–893, 2006.

197. Groiso JA: Juvenile hallux valgus. A conservative approach to treatment, *J Bone Joint Surg Am* 74:1367–1374, 1992.

198. Gupta S, Fazal MA, Williams L: Minifragment screw fixation of the Scarf osteotomy, *Foot Ankle Int* 29:385–389, 2008.

199. Haas Z, Hamilton G, Sundstrom D, Ford L: Maintenance of correction of first metatarsal closing base wedge osteotomies versus modified Lapidus arthrodesis for moderate to severe hallux valgus deformity, *J Foot Ankle Surg* 46:358–365, 2007.

200. Haines RW, McDougall AM: The anatomy of hallux valgus, *J Bone Joint Surg Br* 36:272–293, 1954.

201. Halebian JD, Gaines SS: Juvenile hallux valgus, *J Foot Surg* 22:290–293, 1983.

202. Hamilton GA, Mullins S, Schuberth JM, Rush SM, Ford L: Revision lapidus arthrodesis: rate of union in 17 cases, *J Foot Ankle Surg* 46:447–450, 2007.

203. Hammel E, Abi Chala ML, Wagner T: [Complications of first ray osteotomies: a consecutive series of 475 feet with first metatarsal Scarf osteotomy and first phalanx osteotomy], *Rev Chir Orthop Reparatrice Appar Mot* 93:710–719, 2007.

204. Hansen ST: *Functional reconstruction of the foot and ankle*, Philadelphia, 2000, Lippincott Williams & Wilkins, p 221.

205. Hansen ST Jr: Hallux valgus surgery. Morton and Lapidus were right! *Clin Podiatr Med Surg* 13:347–354, 1996.

206. Hara B, Beck JC, Woo RA: First cuneiform closing abductory osteotomy for reduction of metatarsus primus adductus, *J Foot Surg* 31:434–439, 1992.

207. Hardy RH, Clapham JC: Observations on hallux valgus; based on a controlled series, *J Bone Joint Surg Br* 33:376–391, 1951.

208. Hardy RH, Clapham JC: Hallux valgus; predisposing anatomical causes, *Lancet* 1:1180–1183, 1952.

209. Harper MC: Correction of metatarsus primus varus with the chevron metatarsal osteotomy. An analysis of corrective factors, *Clin Orthop* 243:180–183, 1989.

210. Harris R, Beath T: Hypermobile flat-foot with short tendo Achilles, *J Bone Joint Surg Am* 30:116–138, 1948.

211. Harris R, Beath T: The short first metatarsal: Its incidence and clinical significance, *J Bone Joint Surg Am* 31:553–565, 1949.

212. Harrison M, Harvey F: Arthrodesis of the first metatarsophalangeal joint for hallux valgus and rigidus, *J Bone Joint Surg Am* 45:471–480, 1963.

213. Hattrup SJ, Johnson KA: Chevron osteotomy: analysis of factors in patients' dissatisfaction, *Foot Ankle* 5:327–332, 1985.

214. Hawkins F, Mitchell C, Hedrick D: Correction of hallux valgus by metatarsal osteotomy, *J Bone Joint Surg Am* 37:387–394, 1945.

215. Hecht PJ, Gibbons MJ, Wapner KL, et al: Arthrodesis of the first metatarsophalangeal joint to salvage failed silicone implant arthroplasty, *Foot Ankle Int* 18:383–390, 1997.

216. Helal B: Surgery for adolescent hallux valgus, *Clin Orthop* 157:50–63, 1981.

217. Helal B, Gupta SK, Gojaseni P: Surgery for adolescent hallux valgus, *Acta Orthop Scand* 45:271–295, 1974.

218. Henry AP, Waugh W, Wood H: The use of footprints in assessing the results of operations for hallux valgus. A comparison of Keller's operation and arthrodesis, *J Bone Joint Surg Br* 57:478–481, 1975.

219. Hernandez A, Hernandez PA, Hernandez WA: Lapidus: when and why? *Clin Podiatr Med Surg* 6:197–208, 1989.

220. Hetherington VJ, Steinbock G, LaPorta D, Gardner C: The Austin bunionectomy: a follow-up study, *J Foot Ankle Surg* 32:162–166, 1993.

221. Hewitt D, Stewart AM, Webb JW: The prevalence of foot defects among wartime recruits, *BMJ* 4839:745–749, 1953.

222. Hirvensalo E, Bostman O, Tormala P, et al: Chevron osteotomy fixed with absorbable polyglycolide pins, *Foot Ankle* 11:212–218, 1991.

223. Hiss J: Hallux valgus: its causes and simplified treatment, *Am J Surg* 11:50–57, 1931.

224. Hodor L, Hess T: Shortening Z-osteotomy for the proximal phalanx of the hallux using axial guides, *J Am Podiatr Med Assoc* 85:249–254, 1995.

225. Hohmann G: Der Hallux valgus und die uebrigen Zchenverkruemmungen, *Egerb Chir Orthop* 18:308–348, 1925.

226. Hope M, Savva N, Whitehouse S, Elliot R, Saxby TS: Is it necessary to re-fuse a non-union of a Hallux metatarsophalangeal joint arthrodesis? *Foot Ankle Int* 31:662–669, 2010.

227. Horne G, Tanze T, Ford M: Chevron osteotomy for the treatment of hallux valgus, *Clin Orthop* 183:32–36, 1984.

228. Houghton GR, Dickson RA: Hallux valgus in the younger patient: the structural abnormality, *J Bone Joint Surg Br* 61:176–177, 1979.

229. Huang PJ, Lin YC, Fu YC, et al: Radiographic evaluation of minimally invasive distal metatarsal osteotomy for hallux valgus, *Foot Ankle Int* 32:S503–S507, 2011.

230. Hueter C: *Klinik der Gelenkkrankheiten mit Einschluss der Orthopadie*, Leipzig, Germany, 1870–1871, Vogel.

231. Humbert JL, Bourbonniere C, Laurin CA: Metatarsophalangeal fusion for hallux valgus: indications and effect on the first metatarsal ray, *Can Med Assoc J* 120:937–941, 956, 1979.

232. Hurst JM, Nunley JA 2nd: Distraction osteogenesis for the shortened metatarsal after hallux valgus surgery, *Foot Ankle Int* 28:194–198, 2007.

233. Hyer CF, Glover JP, Berlet GC, et al: A comparison of the crescentic and Mau osteotomies for correction of hallux valgus, *J Foot Ankle Surg* 47:103–111, 2008.

234. Hyer CF, Philbin TM, Berlet GC, Lee TH: The incidence of the intermetatarsal facet of the first metatarsal and its relationship to metatarsus primus varus: a cadaveric study, *J Foot Ankle Surg* 44:200–202, 2005.

235. Inman VT: Hallux valgus: a review of etiologic factors, *Orthop Clin North Am* 5:59–66, 1974.

236. Ito H, Shimizu A, Miyamoto T, et al: Clinical significance of increased mobility in the sagittal plane in patients with hallux valgus, *Foot Ankle Int* 20:29–32, 1999.

237. Jahss MH: LeLeivre bunion operation, *Instr Course Lect* 21:295–309, 1972.

238. Jahss MH: Hallux valgus: Further considerations—the first metatarsal head, *Foot Ankle* 2:1–4, 1981.

239. James C: Footprints and feet of natives of Soloman Islands, *Lancet* 2:1390, 1939.

240. Jawish R, Assoum H, Saliba E: Opening wedge osteotomy of the first cuneiform for the treatment of hallux valgus, *Int Orthop* 34:361–368, 2010.

241. Johal S, Sawalha S, Pasapula C: Post-traumatic acute hallux valgus: a case report, *Foot (Edinb)* 20:87–89, 2010.

242. Johansson JE, Barrington TW: Cone arthrodesis of the first metatarsophalangeal joint, *Foot Ankle* 4:244–248, 1984.

243. John S, Weil L Jr, Weil LS Sr, Chase K: Scarf osteotomy for the correction of adolescent hallux valgus, *Foot Ankle Spec* 3:10–14, 2010.

244. Johnson JE, Clanton TO, Baxter DE, Gottlieb MS: Comparison of Chevron osteotomy and modified McBride bunionectomy for correction of mild to moderate hallux valgus deformity, *Foot Ankle* 12:61–68, 1991.

245. Johnson KA, Cofield RH, Morrey BF: Chevron osteotomy for hallux valgus, *Clin Orthop* 142:44–47, 1979.

246. Johnson KA, Kile TA: Hallux valgus due to cuneiform-metatarsal instability, *J South Orthop Assoc* 3:273–282, 1994.

247. Johnson KA, Spiegl PV: Extensor hallucis longus transfer for hallux varus deformity, *J Bone Joint Surg Am* 66:681–686, 1984.

248. Johnston O: Further studies of the inheritance of hand and foot anomalies, *Clin Orthop* 8:146–160, 1956.

249. Jones A: Hallux valgus in the adolescent, *Proc R Soc Med* 41:392–393, 1948.

250. Jones C, Coughlin M, Pierce-Villadot R, Galano P: Proximal crescentic metatarsal osteotomy: the effect of saw blade orientation on first ray elevation, *Foot Ankle Int* 26:152–157, 2005.

251. Jones CP, Coughlin MJ, Grebing BR, et al: First metatarsophalangeal joint motion after hallux valgus correction: a cadaver study, *Foot Ankle Int* 26:614–619, 2005.

252. Jones CP, Coughlin MJ, Pierce-Villadot R, et al: The validity and reliability of the Klaue device, *Foot Ankle Int* 26:951–956, 2005.

253. Jones S, Al Hussainy HA, Ali F, et al: Scarf osteotomy for hallux valgus. A prospective clinical and pedobarographic study, *J Bone Joint Surg Br* 86:830–836, 2004.

254. Joplin RJ: Sling procedure for correction of splay-foot metatarsus primus varus, and hallux valgus, *J Bone Joint Surg Am* 32:779–785, 1950.

255. Jordan HH, Bordsky AE: Keller operation for hallux valgus and hallux rigidus. An end-result study, *AMA Arch Surg* 62:586–596, 1951.

256. Joseph J: Range of movement of the great toe in men, *J Bone Joint Surg Br* 36:450–457, 1954.

257. Kadakia AR, Smerek JP, Myerson MS: Radiographic results after percutaneous distal metatarsal osteotomy for correction of hallux valgus deformity, *Foot Ankle Int* 28:355–360, 2007.

258. Kalen V, Brecher A: Relationship between adolescent bunions and flatfeet, *Foot Ankle* 8:331–336, 1988.

259. Kato T, Watanabe S: The etiology of hallux valgus in Japan, *Clin Orthop* 157:78–81, 1981.

260. Kayali C, Ozturk H, Agus H, et al: The effectiveness of distal soft tissue procedures in hallux valgus, *J Orthop Traumatol* 9:117–121, 2008.

261. Kayiaros S, Blankenhorn BD, Dehaven J, et al: Correction of metatarsus primus varus associated with hallux valgus deformity using the arthrex mini tightrope: a report of 44 cases, *Foot Ankle Spec* 4:212–217, 2011.

262. Kazzaz S, Singh D: Postoperative cast necessity after a lapidus arthrodesis, *Foot Ankle Int* 30:746–751, 2009.

263. Kelikian H: *Hallux valgus, allied deformities of the forefoot and metatarsalgia*, Philadelphia, 1965, WB Saunders, pp 136–235.

264. Keller W: Further observations on the surgical treatment of hallux valgus and bunions, *N Y Med J* 95:696, 1912.

265. Kemp TJ, Hirose CB, Coughlin MJ: Fracture of the second metatarsal following suture button fixation device in the correction of hallux valgus, *Foot Ankle Int* 31:712–716, 2010.

266. Keogh P, Nagaria J, Stephens M: Cheilectomy for hallux rigidus, *Ir J Med Sci* 161:681–683, 1992.

267. Kerr HL, Jackson R, Kothari P: Scarf-Akin osteotomy correction for hallux valgus: short-term results from a district general hospital, *J Foot Ankle Surg* 49:16–19, 2010.

268. Kilmartin TE, Barrington RL, Wallace WA: Metatarsus primus varus. A statistical study, *J Bone Joint Surg Br* 73:937–940, 1991.

269. Kilmartin TE, Barrington RL, Wallace WA: A controlled prospective trial of a foot orthosis for juvenile hallux valgus, *J Bone Joint Surg Br* 76:210–214, 1994.

270. Kilmartin TE, Flintham C: Hallux valgus surgery: a simple method for evaluating the first-second intermetatarsal angle in the presence of metatarsus adductus, *J Foot Ankle Surg* 42:165–166, 2003.

271. Kilmartin TE, O'Kane C: Combined rotation scarf and Akin osteotomies for hallux valgus: a patient focussed 9 year follow up of 50 patients, *J Foot Ankle Res* 3:2, 2010.

272. Kilmartin TE, Wallace WA: The significance of pes planus in juvenile hallux valgus, *Foot Ankle* 13:53–56, 1992.

273. Kim B, Shim D, Lee J, et al: Comparision of multi-drug injection versus placebo after hallux valgus surgery, *Foot Ankle Int* 32:856–860, 2011.

274. Kim JY, Park JS, Hwang SK, et al: Mobility changes of the first ray after hallux valgus surgery: clinical results after proximal metatarsal chevron osteotomy and distal soft tissue procedure, *Foot Ankle Int* 29:468–472, 2008.

275. King DM, Toolan BC: Associated deformities and hypermobility in hallux valgus: an investigation with weightbearing radiographs, *Foot Ankle Int* 25:251–255, 2004.

276. Kinnard P, Gordon D: A comparison between chevron and Mitchell osteotomies for hallux valgus, *Foot Ankle* 4:241–243, 1984.

277. Kitaoka HB, Franco MG, Weaver AL, Ilstrup DM: Simple bunionectomy with medial capsulorrhaphy, *Foot Ankle* 12:86–91, 1991.

278. Kitaoka HB, Holiday AD Jr, Chao EY, Cahalan TD: Salvage of failed first metatarsophalangeal joint implant arthroplasty by implant removal and synovectomy: clinical and biomechanical evaluation, *Foot Ankle* 13:243–250, 1992.

279. Klaue K, Hansen ST, Masquelet AC: Clinical, quantitative assessment of first tarsometatarsal mobility in the sagittal plane and its relation to hallux valgus deformity, *Foot Ankle Int* 15:9–13, 1994.

280. Kleinberg S: Operative cure of hallux valgus and bunions, *Am J Surg* 15:75–81, 1932.

281. Klosok JK, Pring DJ, Jessop JH, Maffulli N: Chevron or Wilson metatarsal osteotomy for hallux valgus. A prospective randomised trial, *J Bone Joint Surg Br* 75:825–829, 1993.

282. Kose O, Celiktas M, Kisin, B, et al: Is there a relationship between forefoot alignment and ingrown toenal? A case-control study, *Foot Ankle Spec* 4:14–17, 2011.

283. Kramer J: Die Kramer-Osteotomie zur Behandlung des Hallux valgus und des Digitus quintus varus, *Operat Orthop Traumatol* 2:29–38, 1990.

284. Kramer J, Barry LD, Helfman DN, et al: The modified Scarf bunionectomy, *J Foot Surg* 31:360–367, 1992.

285. Krannitz KW, Fong HW, Fallat LM, Kish J: The effect of cigarette smoking on radiographic bone healing after elective foot surgery, *J Foot Ankle Surg* 48:525–527, 2009.

286. Kristen KH, Berger C, Stelzig S, et al: The SCARF osteotomy for the correction of hallux valgus deformities, *Foot Ankle Int* 23:221–229, 2002.

287. Kuhn MA, Lippert FG 3rd, Phipps MJ, Williams C: Blood flow to the metatarsal head after chevron bunionectomy, *Foot Ankle Int* 26:526–529, 2005.

288. Kumar S, Pradhan R, Rosenfeld PF: First metatarsophalangeal arthrodesis using a dorsal plate and a compression screw, *Foot Ankle Int* 31:797–801, 2010.

289. Kundert HP, Fuhrmann R: *Personal communication*, April 21, 2005.

290. Kuo CH, Huang PJ, Cheng YM, et al: Modified Mitchell osteotomy for hallux valgus, *Foot Ankle Int* 19:585–589, 1998.

291. Lagaay PM, Hamilton GA, Ford LA, et al: Rates of revision surgery using Chevron-Austin osteotomy, Lapidus arthrodesis, and closing base wedge osteotomy for correction of hallux valgus deformity, *J Foot Ankle Surg* 47:267–272, 2008.

292. Lampropulos M, Puigdevall M, Zapozko D, Malvarez H: Treatment of first metatarsal longitudinal epiphyseal bracket by excision before closure, *J Foot Ankle Surg* 46:297–301, 2007.

293. Lane W: The causation, pathology, and physiology of several of the deformities which develop during young life, *Guy's Hosp Rep* 44:241, 1887.

294. Lapidus PW: Operative correction of metatarsus varus primus in hallux valgus, *Surg Gynecol Obstet* 58:183–191, 1934.

295. Lapidus PW: A quarter of a century of experience with the operative correction of the metatarsus varus primus in hallux valgus, *Bull Hosp Jt Dis* 17:404–421, 1956.

296. Lapidus PW: The author's bunion operation from 1931 to 1959, *Clin Orthop* 16:119–135, 1960.

297. La Reaux RL, Lee BR: Metatarsus adductus and hallux abducto valgus: their correlation, *J Foot Surg* 26:304–308, 1987.

298. Larholt J, Kilmartin TE: Rotational scarf and akin osteotomy for correction of hallux valgus associated with metatarsus adductus, *Foot Ankle Int* 31:220–228, 2010.

299. Lau JT, Daniels TR: Effect of increasing distal medial closing wedge metatarsal osteotomies on the distal metatarsal articular angle, *Foot Ankle Int* 20:771–776, 1999.

300. Leaseburg JT, DeOrio JK, Shapiro SA: Radiographic correlation of hallux MP fusion position and plate angle, *Foot Ankle Int* 30:873–876, 2009.

301. Lee HJ, Chung JW, Chu IT, Kim YC: Comparison of distal chevron osteotomy with and without lateral soft tissue release for the treatment of hallux valgus, *Foot Ankle Int* 31:291–295, 2010.

302. Lee KB, Hur CI, Chung J, Jung S: Outcome of unilateral versus siutaneous correction for hallux valgus, *Foot Ankle Int* 30:120–123, 2009.

303. Lee KB, Seo CY, Hur CI, et al: Outcome of proximal chevron osteotomy for hallux valgus with and without transverse Kirschner wire fixation, *Foot Ankle Int* 29:1101–1106, 2008.

304. Lee KT, Park YU, Young KW, et al: Reverse distal chevron osteotomy to treat iatrogenic hallux varus after overcorrection of the intermetarsal 1-2 angle: technique tip, *Foot Ankle Int* 32:89–91, 2011.

305. Lee KT, Young K: Measurement of first-ray mobility in normal vs. hallux valgus patients, *Foot Ankle Int* 22:960–964, 2001.

306. Lee WC, Kim YM: Correction of hallux valgus using lateral soft-tissue release and proximal Chevron osteotomy through a medial incision, *J Bone Joint Surg Am* 89(Suppl 3):82–89, 2007.

307. Lee WC, Kim YM: Technique tip: lateral soft-tissue release for correction of hallux valgus through a medial incision using a dorsal flap over the first metatarsal, *Foot Ankle Int* 28:949–951, 2007.

308. Leemrijse T, Hoang B, Maldague P, et al: A new surgical procedure for iatrogenic hallux varus: reverse transfer of the abductor hallucis tendon: a report of 7 cases, *Acta Orthop Belg* 74:227–234, 2008.

309. Leventen EO: The chevron procedure, *Orthopedics* 13:973–976, 1990.

310. Lewis RJ, Feffer HL: Modified chevron osteotomy of the first metatarsal, *Clin Orthop* 157:105–109, 1981.

311. Lian GJ, Markolf K, Cracchiolo A 3rd: Strength of fixation constructs for basilar osteotomies of the first metatarsal, *Foot Ankle* 13:509–514, 1992.

312. Limbird TJ, DaSilva RM, Green NE: Osteotomy of the first metatarsal base for metatarsus primus varus, *Foot Ankle* 9:158–162, 1989.

313. Lippert FG 3rd, McDermott JE: Crescentic osteotomy for hallux valgus: a biomechanical study of variables affecting the final position of the first metatarsal, *Foot Ankle* 11:204–207, 1991.

314. Lipscomb PR: Arthrodesis of the first metatarsophalangeal joint for severe bunions and hallux rigidus, *Clin Orthop* 142:48–54, 1979.

315. Lipscombe S, Molloy A, Sirikonda S, Hennessy MS: Scarf osteotomy for the correction of hallux valgus: midterm clinical outcome, *J Foot Ankle Surg* 47:273–277, 2008.

316. Lombardi CM, Silhanek AD, Connolly FG, et al: First metatarsocuneiform arthrodesis and Reverdin-Laird osteotomy for treatment of hallux valgus: an intermediate-term retrospective outcomes study, *J Foot Ankle Surg* 42:77–85, 2003.

317. Loretz L, DeValentine S, Yamaguchi K: The first metatarsal bicorrectional head osteotomy (distal "L"/Reverdin-Laird procedure) for correction of hallux abducto valgus: a retrospective study, *J Foot Ankle Surg* 32:554–568, 1993.

318. Love TR, Whynot AS, Farine I, et al: Keller arthroplasty: a prospective review, *Foot Ankle* 8:46–54, 1987.

319. Luba R, Rosman M: Bunions in children: treatment with a modified Mitchell osteotomy, *J Pediatr Orthop* 4:44–47, 1984.

320. Ludloff K: Die Beseitigung des Hallux valgus durch die schrage planta dorsale Osteotomie des Metatarsus, *Arch Klin Chir* 110:364–387, 1918.

321. Lui TH: First metatarsophalangeal joint arthroscopy in patients with hallux valgus, *Arthroscopy* 24:1122–1129, 2008.

322. Maclennan R: Prevalence of hallux valgus in a Neolithic New Guinea population, *Lancet* 1:1398–1400, 1966.

323. Mader DW, Han NM: Bilateral second metatarsal stress fractures after hallux valgus correction with the use of a tension wire and button fixation system, *J Foot Ankle Surg* 49:488. e415–e489, 2010.

324. Maffulli N, Longo UG, Oliva F, et al: Bosch osteotomy and scarf osteotomy for hallux valgus correction, *Orthop Clin North Am* 40:515–524, ix–x, 2009.

325. Maguire WB: The Lapidus procedure for hallux valgus [abstract], *J Bone Joint Surg Br* 55:221, 1973.

326. Mahan KT, Jacko J: Juvenile hallux valgus with compensated metatarsus adductus. Case report, *J Am Podiatr Med Assoc* 81:525–530, 1991.

327. Majkowski RS, Galloway S: Excision arthroplasty for hallux valgus in the elderly: a comparison between the Keller and modified Mayo operations, *Foot Ankle* 13:317–320, 1992.

328. Malal JJ, Shaw-Dunn J, Kumar CS: Blood supply to the first metatarsal head and vessels at risk with a chevron osteotomy, *J Bone Joint Surg Am* 89:2018–2022, 2007.

329. Mancuso JE, Abramow SP, Landsman MJ, et al: The zero-plus first metatarsal and its relationship to bunion deformity, *J Foot Ankle Surg* 42:319–326, 2003.

330. Magnan B, Pezze L, Rossi N, Bartolozzi P: Percutaneous distal metatarsal osteotomy for correction of hallux valgus, *J Bone Joint Surg Am* 87:1191–1199, 2005.

331. Magnan B, Fieschi S, Bragantini A, et al: Trattamento chirurgico dell'alluce del primo metatarsale, *G Ital Ortop Traumatol* 24:473–487, 1998.

332. Mankey M, Mann RA: *Arthrodesis of the first metatarsophalangeal joint utilizing a dorsal plate. Paper presented at the Summer Meeting of American Orthopaedic Foot and Ankle Society*, Boston, July 1991.

333. Mann RA: Complications associated with the Chevron osteotomy, *Foot Ankle* 3:125–129, 1982.

334. Mann RA: Decision-making in bunion surgery, *Instr Course Lect* 39:3–13, 1990.

335. Mann RA: Hallux valgus, *Instr Course Lect* 35:339–353, 1986.

336. Mann RA, Coughlin MJ: Hallux valgus—etiology, anatomy, treatment and surgical considerations, *Clin Orthop* 157:31–41, 1981.

337. Mann RA, Coughlin MJ: Hallux valgus and complications of hallux valgus. In Mann RA, editor: *Surgery of the foot*, St Louis, 1986, CV Mosby, pp 167–296.

338. Mann RA, Coughlin MJ: The great toe. In Mann RA, Coughlin MJ, editors: *Video textbook of foot and ankle surgery*, St Louis, 1991, Medical Video Productions, pp 146–184.

339. Mann RA, Coughlin MJ: Adult hallux valgus. In Coughlin MJ, Mann RA, editors: *Surgery of the foot and ankle*, 7th ed, St Louis, 1999, Mosby––Year Book, pp 150–269.

340. Mann RA, Donatto KC: The chevron osteotomy: a clinical and radiographic analysis, *Foot Ankle Int* 18:255–261, 1997.

341. Mann RA, Katcherian DA: Relationship of metatarsophalangeal joint fusion on the intermetatarsal angle, *Foot Ankle* 10:8–11, 1989.

342. Mann RA, Oates JC: Arthrodesis of the first metatarsophalangeal joint, *Foot Ankle* 1:159–166, 1980.

343. Mann RA, Pfeffinger L: Hallux valgus repair. DuVries modified McBride procedure, *Clin Orthop* 272:213–218, 1991.

344. Mann RA, Rudicel S, Graves SC: Repair of hallux valgus with a distal soft-tissue procedure and proximal metatarsal osteotomy. A long-term follow-up, *J Bone Joint Surg Am* 74:124–129, 1992.

345. Mann RA, Schakel ME 2nd: Surgical correction of rheumatoid forefoot deformities, *Foot Ankle Int* 16:1–6, 1995.

346. Mann RA, Thompson FM: Arthrodesis of the first metatarsophalangeal joint for hallux valgus in rheumatoid arthritis, *J Bone Joint Surg Am* 66:687–692, 1984.

347. Marin GA: Arthrodesis of the metatarsophalangeal joint of the big toe for hallux valgus and hallux rigidus. A new method, *Int Surg* 50:175–180, 1968.

348. Markbreiter LA, Thompson FM: Proximal metatarsal osteotomy in hallux valgus correction: a comparison of crescentic and chevron procedures, *Foot Ankle Int* 18:71–76, 1997.

349. Martinelli N, Marinozzi A, Cancilleri F, Denaro V: Hallux valgus correction in a patient with metatarsus adductus with multiple distal oblique osteotomies, *J Am Podiatr Med Assoc* 100:204–208, 2010.

350. Marwil T, Brantingham C: Foot problems of women's reserve, *Hosp Corp Q* 16:98, 1943.

351. Mattila K, Kontinen VK, Kalso E, Hynynen MJ: Dexamethasone decreases oxycodone consumption following osteotomy of the first metatarsal bone: a randomized controlled trial in day surgery, *Acta Anaesthesiol Scand* 54:268–276, 2010.

352. Mauldin DM, Sanders M, Whitmer WW: Correction of hallux valgus with metatarsocuneiform stabilization, *Foot Ankle* 11:59–66, 1990.

353. Mayo C: The surgical treatment of bunions, *Ann Surg* 48:300, 1908.

354. Mayo C: The surgical treatment of bunions, *Minn Med J* 3:326–331, 1920.

355. McBride ED: A conservative operation for bunions, *J Bone Joint Surg* 10:735–739, 1928.

356. McBride ED: The conservative operation for "bunions": end results and refinements of technic, *JAMA* 105:1164–1168, 1935.

357. McBride E: Hallux valgus, bunion deformity; its treatment in mild, moderate and severe stages, *J Int Coll Surg* 21:99–105, 1954.

358. McBride ED: The McBride bunion hallux valgus operation, *J Bone Joint Surg Am* 49:1675–1683, 1967.

359. McCluney JG, Tinley P: Radiographic measurements of patients with juvenile hallux valgus compared with age-matched controls: a cohort investigation, *J Foot Ankle Surg* 45:161–167, 2006.

360. McCluskey LC, Johnson JE, Wynarsky GT, Harris GF: Comparison of stability of proximal crescentic metatarsal osteotomy and proximal horizontal "V" osteotomy, *Foot Ankle Int* 15:263–270, 1994.

361. McHale K, McKay D: Bunions in a child: conservative versus surgical management, *J Musculoskel Med* 3:56–62, 1986.

362. McInnes BD, Bouche RT: Critical evaluation of the modified Lapidus procedure, *J Foot Ankle Surg* 40:71–90, 2001.

363. McKeever DC: Arthrodesis of the first metatarsophalangeal joint for hallux valgus, hallux rigidus, and metatarsus primus varus, *J Bone Joint Surg Am* 34:129–134, 1952.

364. Meehan PL: Adolescent bunion, *Instr Course Lect* 31:262–264, 1982.

365. Meier PJ, Kenzora JE: The risks and benefits of distal first metatarsal osteotomies, *Foot Ankle* 6:7–17, 1985.

366. Merkel KD, Katoh Y, Johnson EW Jr, Chao EY: Mitchell osteotomy for hallux valgus: long-term follow-up and gait analysis, *Foot Ankle* 3:189–196, 1983.

367. Meyer JM, Hoffmeyer P, Borst F: The treatment of hallux valgus in runners using a modified McBride procedure, *Int Orthop* 11:197–200, 1987.

368. Miller JM, Ferdowsian,VN, Collman DR: Inverted Z-scarf osteotomy for hallux valgus deformity correction: intermediate-term results in 55 patients, *J Foot Ankle Surg* 50:55–61, 2011.

369. Miller JW: Acquired hallux varus: a preventable and correctable disorder, *J Bone Joint Surg Am* 57:183–188, 1975.

370. Mitchell CL, Fleming JL, Allen R, et al: Osteotomy-bunionectomy for hallux valgus, *J Bone Joint Surg Am* 40:41–58; discussion 59–60, 1958.

371. Mitchell LA, Baxter DE: A chevron-Akin double osteotomy for correction of hallux valgus, *Foot Ankle* 12:7–14, 1991.

372. Mittal D, Anjum SN, Raja S, Raut V: The spike osteotomy for hallux valgus: a clinical and radiological evaluation, *J Foot Ankle Surg* 45:261–265, 2006.

373. Mittal D, Raja S, Geary NP: The modified McBride procedure: clinical, radiological, and pedobarographic evaluations, *J Foot Ankle Surg* 45:235–239, 2006.

374. Mizuno K, Hashimura M, Kimura M, Hirohata K: Treatment of hallux valgus by oblique osteotomy of the first metatarsal, *Foot Ankle* 13:447–452, 1992.

375. Morandi A, Dupplicato P, Sansone V: Results of distal metatarsal osteotomy using absorbable pin fixation, *Foot Ankle Int* 30:34–38, 2009.

376. Morton DJ: Hypermobility of the first metatarsal bone: the interlinking factor between metatarsalgia and longitudinal arch strains, *J Bone Joint Surg* 10:187–196, 1928.

377. Morton DJ: *The human foot*, New York, 1935, Columbia University Press.

378. Mote GA, Yarmel D, Treaster A: First metatarsal-cuneiform arthrodesis for the treatment of first ray pathology: a technical guide, *J Foot Ankle Surg* 48:593–601, 2009.

379. Moynihan FJ: Arthrodesis of the metatarso-phalangeal joint of the great toe, *J Bone Joint Surg Br* 49:544–551, 1967.

380. Munuera PV, Polo J, Rebollo J: Length of the first metatarsal and hallux in hallux valgus in the initial stage, *Int Orthop* 32:489–495, 2008.

381. Murawski CD, Egan CJ, Kennedy JG: A rotational scarf osteotomy decreases troughing when treating hallux valgus, *Clin Orthop Relat Res* 469:847–853, 2011.

382. Murawski DE, Beskin JL: Increased displacement maximizes the utility of the distal chevron osteotomy for hallux valgus deformity correction, *Foot Ankle Int* 29:155–163, 2008.

383. Myerson MS: Metatarsocuneiform arthrodesis for treatment of hallux valgus and metatarsus primus varus, *Orthopedics* 13:1025–1031, 1990.

384. Myerson MS: Hallux valgus. In Myerson MS, editor: *Foot and ankle disorders*, Philadelphia, 2000, WB Saunders, pp 213–289.

385. Myerson M, Allon S, McGarvey W: Metatarsocuneiform arthrodesis for management of hallux valgus and metatarsus primus varus, *Foot Ankle* 13:107–115, 1992.

386. Myerson MS, Badekas A: Hypermobility of the first ray, *Foot Ankle Clin* 5:469–484, 2000.

387. Nedopil A, Rudert M, Gradinger R, et al: Closed wedge osteotomy in 66 patients for the treatment of moderate to severe hallux valgus, *Foot Ankle Surg* 16:9–14, 2010.

388. Neese DJ, Zelent, ME: The modified Mau-Reverdin double osteotomy for correction of hallux valgus: a retrospective study, *J Foot Ankle Surg* 48:22–29, 2009.

389. Neven E, Vandeputte G: Technical tip: fixation of the scarf metatarsal osteotomy with a proximal buttress and a standard distal screw, *Foot Ankle Int* 30:1235–1236, 2009.

390. Newman AS, Negrine JP, Zecovic M, et al: A biomechanical comparison of the Z step-cut and basilar crescentic osteotomies of the first metatarsal, *Foot Ankle Int* 21:584–587, 2000.

391. Nicklas BJ, McEneaney PA, Lichniak JE, et al: Surgical repair of abductor hallucis muscle herniation: a case report, *J Foot Ankle Surg* 49:488.e485–e489, 2010.

392. O'Donnell T, Hogan N, Solan M, Stephens MM: Correction of severe hallux valgus using a basal chevron osteotomy and distal soft tissue release, *Foot Ankle Surg* 16:126–131, 2010.

393. Oh IS, Choi SW, Kim MK, et al: Clinical and radiological results after modified distal metatarsal osteotomy for hallux valgus, *Foot Ankle Int* 29:473–477, 2008.

394. Okuda R, Kinoshita M, Yasuda T, et al: The shape of the lateral edge of the first metatarsal head as a risk factor for recurrence of hallux valgus, *J Bone Joint Surg Am* 89:2163–2172, 2007.

395. Okuda R, Kinoshita M, Yasuda T, et al: Proximal metatarsal osteotomy for hallux valgus: comparison of outcome for moderate and severe deformities, *Foot Ankle Int* 29:664–670, 2008.

396. Opsomer G, Deleu PA, Bevernage BD, Leemrijse T: Cortical thickness of the second metatarsal after correction of hallux valgus, *Foot Ankle Int* 31:770–776, 2010.

397. Orzechowski W, Dragan S, Romaszkiewicz P, et al: Evaluation of follow-up results of McBride operative treatment for hallux valgus deformity, *Ortop Traumatol Rehabil* 10:261–273, 2008.

398. Owoeye BA, Akinbo SR, Aiyegbusi AL, Ogunsola MO: Prevalence of hallux valgus among youth population in Lagos, Nigeria, *Nigerian Postgrade Med J* 18:51–55, 2011.

399. Ozan F, Bora OA, Filiz MA, Kement Z: Interposition arthroplasty in the treatment of hallux rigidus, *Acta Orthopaedica Traumatol Turc* 44:143–151, 2010.

400. Ozkurt B, Aktekin CN, Altay M, et al: Range of motion of the first metatarsophalangeal joint after chevron procedure reinforced by a modified capsuloperiosteal flap, *Foot Ankle Int* 29:903–909, 2008.

401. Oznur A: Technical Tip: mini-fixator assisted correction of DMAA in hallux valgus surgery, *Foot Ankle Int* 27:849–850, 2006.

402. Panchbhavi VK: Technique tip: buttress Kirschner wire fixation for distal chevron osteotomy, *Foot Ankle Int* 28:133–134, 2007.

403. Pappas A, Anderson R: Management of acquired hallux varus with an endobutton, *Tech Foot Ankle Surg* 7:134–138, 2008.

404. Park J, Jung H, Kim T, Kang M: Intraoperative incidence of hallux valgus interphalangeus following basilar first metatarsal osteotomy and distal soft tissue realignment, *Foot Ankle Int* 32:962–967, 2011.

405. Patel S, Ford LA, Etcheverry J, et al: Modified Lapidus arthrodesis: rate of nonunion in 227 cases, *J Foot Ankle Surg* 43:37–42, 2004.

406. Pavlovich R Jr, Caminear D: Granuloma formation after chevron osteotomy fixation with absorbable copolymer pin: a case report, *J Foot Ankle Surg* 42:226–229, 2003.

407. Peabody D: Surgical care of hallux valgus, *J Bone Joint Surg* 13:273–282, 1931.

408. Pearce CJ, Sexton SA, Sakellariou A: The triplanar chevron osteotomy, *Foot Ankle Surg* 14:158–160, 2008.

409. Pearson SW, Kitaoka HB, Cracchiolo A, Leventen EO: Results and complications following a proximal curved osteotomy of the hallux metatarsal, *Contemp Orthop* 23:127–132, 1991.

410. Peterson DA, Zilberfarb JL, Greene MA, Colgrove RC: Avascular necrosis of the first metatarsal head: incidence in distal osteotomy combined with lateral soft tissue release, *Foot Ankle Int* 15:59–63, 1994.

411. Peterson HA, Newman SR: Adolescent bunion deformity treated with double osteotomy and longitudinal pin fixation of the first ray, *J Pediatr Orthop* 13:80–84, 1993.

412. Petratos DV, Anastasopoulos JN, Plakogiannis CV, Matsinos GS: Correction of adolescent hallux valgus by proximal crescentic osteotomy of the first metatarsal, *Acta Orthop Belg* 74:496–502, 2008

413. Phisitkul P, Sripongsai R, Chaichankul C, Femino JE: Anatomy of the plantarmedial hallucal nerve in relation to the medial approach of the first metatarsophalangeal joint, *Foot Ankle Int* 30:558–561, 2009.

414. Piggott H: The natural history of hallux valgus in adolescence and early adult life, *J Bone Joint Surg Br* 42:749–760, 1960.

415. Pinney S, Song K, Chou L: Surgical treatment of mild hallux valgus deformity: the state of practice among academic foot and ankle surgeons, *Foot Ankle Int* 27:970–973, 2006.

416. Pinney SJ, Song KR, Chou LB: Surgical treatment of severe hallux valgus: the state of practice among academic foot and ankle surgeons, *Foot Ankle Int* 27:1024–1029, 2006.

417. Pique-Vidal C: The first metatarsophalangeal arc circumference: correlation with angular measurements, *Foot Ankle Int* 28:186–193, 2007.

418. Pique-Vidal C, Maled-Garcia I, Arabi-Moreno J, Vila J: Radiographic angles in hallux valgus: differences between measurements made manually and with a computerized program, *Foot Ankle Int* 27:175–180, 2006.

419. Pique-Vidal C, Sole MT, Antich J: Hallux valgus inheritance: pedigree research in 350 patients with bunion deformity, *J Foot Ankle Surg* 46:149–154, 2007.

420. Plattner PF, Van Manen JW: Results of Akin type proximal phalangeal osteotomy for correction of hallux valgus deformity, *Orthopedics* 13:989–996, 1990.

421. Pochatko DJ, Schlehr FJ, Murphey MD, Hamilton JJ: Distal chevron osteotomy with lateral release for treatment of hallux valgus deformity, *Foot Ankle Int* 15:457–461, 1994.

422. Ponnapula P, Wittock R: Application of an interosseous suture and button device for hallux valgus correction: a review of outcomes in a small series, *J Foot Ankle Surg* 49:159.e121–e156, 2010.

423. Pontious J, Mahan KT, Carter S: Characteristics of adolescent hallux abducto valgus. A retrospective review, *J Am Podiatr Med Assoc* 84:208–218, 1994.

424. Popoff I, Negrine JP, Zecovic M, et al: The effect of screw type on the biomechanical properties of SCARF and crescentic osteotomies of the first metatarsal, *J Foot Ankle Surg* 42:161–164, 2003.

425. Portaluri M: Hallux valgus correction by the method of Bosch: a clinical evaluation, *Foot Ankle Clin* 5:499–511, vi, 2000.

426. Potenza V, Caterini R, Farsetti P, et al: Chevron osteotomy with lateral release and adductor tenotomy for hallux valgus, *Foot Ankle Int* 30:512–516, 2009.

427. Pouliart N, Haentjens P, Opdecam P: Clinical and radiographic evaluation of Wilson osteotomy for hallux valgus, *Foot Ankle Int* 17:388–394, 1996.

428. Price GF: Metatarsus primus varus: Including various clinicoradiologic features of the female foot, *Clin Orthop* 145:217–223, 1979.

429. Prieskorn DW, Mann RA, Fritz G: Radiographic assessment of the second metatarsal: measure of first ray hypermobility, *Foot Ankle Int* 17:331–333, 1996.

430. Pring DJ, Coombes RRH, Closok JK: Chevron or Wilson osteotomy: a comparison and follow-up [abstract], *J Bone Joint Surg Am* 67:671–672, 1985.

431. Radovic PA, Shah E: Nonsurgical treatment for hallux abducto valgus with botulinum toxin A, *J Am Podiatr Med Assoc* 98:61–65, 2008.

432. Rambani R, Elnaggar M, Sturdee S: Syndactyly with hallux valgus: a case report, *Foot Ankle Int* 32:641–643, 2011.

433. Randhawa S, Pepper D: Radiographic evaluation of hallux valgus treated with opening wedge osteotomy, *Foot Ankle Int* 30:427–431, 2009.

434. Raymakers R, Waugh W: The treatment of metatarsalgia with hallux valgus, *J Bone Joint Surg Br* 53:684–687, 1971.

435. Resch S, Stenstrom A, Egund N: Proximal closing wedge osteotomy and adductor tenotomy for treatment of hallux valgus, *Foot Ankle* 9:272–280, 1989.

436. Reverdin J: De la deviation en dehors du gros orteil et de son traitement chirurgical, *Trans Int Med Congr* 2:408–412, 1881.

437. Richardson EG: Keller resection arthroplasty, *Orthopedics* 13:1049–1053, 1990.

438. Richardson EG, Graves SC, McClure JT, Boone RT: First metatarsal head-shaft angle: a method of determination, *Foot Ankle* 14:181–185, 1993.

439. Riedel HL: Zur operativen Behandlung des Hallux valgus, *Zentralbl Chir* 44:573–580, 1886.

440. Riggs SA Jr, Johnson EW Jr: McKeever arthrodesis for the painful hallux, *Foot Ankle* 3:248–253, 1983.

441. Rink-Brune O: Lapidus arthrodesis for management of hallux valgus—a retrospective review of 106 cases, *J Foot Ankle Surg* 43:290–295, 2004.

442. Robinson AH, Cullen NP, Chhaya NC, et al: Variation of the distal metatarsal articular angle with axial rotation and inclination of the first metatarsal, *Foot Ankle Int* 27:1036–1040, 2006.

443. Robinson AH, Limbers JP: Modern concepts in the treatment of hallux valgus, *J Bone Joint Surg Br* 87:1038–1045, 2005.

444. Rogers WA, Joplin RJ: Hallux valgus, weak foot and the Keller operations: an end-result study, *Surg Clin North Am* 27:1295–1302, 1947.

445. Rosenberg GA, Donley BG: Plate augmentation of screw fixation of proximal crescentic osteotomy of the first metatarsal, *Foot Ankle Int* 24:570–571, 2003.

446. Ross SD: Technical tip: the crescentic shelf: a modified Ludoff osteotomy, *Foot Ankle Int* 32:452–454, 2011.

447. Roukis TS: Hallux proximal phalanx Akin-scarf osteotomy, *J Am Podiatr Med Assoc* 94:70–72, 2004.

448. Roukis TS, Landsman AS: Hypermobility of the first ray: a critical review of the literature, *J Foot Ankle Surg* 42:377–390, 2003.

449. Roukis TS, Weil L, Weil L, Landsman A: Predicting cartilage erosion in hallux valgus: clinical, radiographic analysis, *J Foot Ankle Surg* 44:13–21, 2005.

450. Rush SM, Christensen JC, Johnson CH: Biomechanics of the first ray. Part II: metatarsus primus varus as a cause of hypermobility. A three-dimensional kinematic analysis in a cadaver model, *J Foot Ankle Surg* 39:68–77, 2000.

451. Salvi AE, Mondanelli N: The Reverdin hallux valgus correction: back to the future, *J Foot Ankle Surg* 50:267–268, 2011.

452. Sammarco GJ, Brainard BJ, Sammarco VJ: Bunion correction using proximal chevron osteotomy, *Foot Ankle* 14:8–14, 1993.

453. Sammarco GJ, Idusuyi OB: Complications after surgery of the hallux, *Clin Orthop* 391:59–71, 2001.

454. Sammarco GJ, Russo-Alesi FG: Bunion correction using proximal chevron osteotomy: a single-incision technique, *Foot Ankle Int* 19:430–437, 1998.

455. Sammarco VJ: Surgical strategies: Mau osteotomy for correction of moderate and severe hallux valgus deformity, *Foot Ankle Int* 28:857–864, 2007.

456. Sangeorzan BJ, Hansen ST Jr: Modified Lapidus procedure for hallux valgus, *Foot Ankle* 9:262–266, 1989.

457. Sanhudo JA: Correction of moderate to severe hallux valgus deformity by a modified chevron shaft osteotomy, *Foot Ankle Int* 27:581–585, 2006.

458. Saragas NP: Proximal opening-wedge osteotomy of the first metatarsal for hallux valgus using a low profile plate, *Foot Ankle Int* 30:976–980, 2009.

459. Saragas NP, Becker PJ: Comparative radiographic analysis of parameters in feet with and without hallux valgus, *Foot Ankle Int* 16:139–143, 1995.

460. Sarrafian S: *Anatomy of the foot and ankle,* Philadelphia, 1983, JB Lippincott, pp 81–86.

461. Saro C, Andren B, Wildemyr Z, Fellander-Tsai L: Outcome after distal metatarsal osteotomy for hallux valgus: a prospective randomized controlled trial of two methods, *Foot Ankle Int* 28:778–787, 2007.

462. Schede F: Hallux valgus, Hallux flexus und Fussenkung, *Z Orthop Chir* 48:564–571, 1927.

463. Schemitsch E, Horne G: Wilson's osteotomy for the treatment of hallux valgus, *Clin Orthop* 240:221–225, 1989.

464. Schneider W, Knahr K: Keller procedure and chevron osteotomy in hallux valgus: five-year results of different surgical philosophies in comparable collectives, *Foot Ankle Int* 23:321–329, 2002.

465. Schoen NS, Zygmunt K, Gudas C: Z-bunionectomy: retrospective long-term study, *J Foot Ankle Surg* 35:312–317, 1996.

466. Schoenhaus HD, Cohen RS: Etiology of the bunion, *J Foot Surg* 31:25–29, 1992.

467. Schuh R, Hofstaetter SG, Adams SB Jr, et al: Rehabilitation after hallux valgus surgery: importance of physical therapy to restore weight bearing of the first ray during the stance phase, *Phys Ther* 89:934–945, 2009.

468. Schwartz N, Hurley JP: Derotational Akin osteotomy: further modification, *J Foot Surg* 26:419–421, 1987.

469. Schweitzer ME, Maheshwari S, Shabshin N: Hallux valgus and hallux rigidus: MRI findings, *Clin Imaging* 23:397–402, 1999.

470. Scranton PE, Coetzee JC, Carreira D: Arthrodesis of the first metatarsocuneiform joint: a comparative study of fixation methods, *Foot Ankle Int* 30:341–345, 2009.

471. Scranton PE Jr: Adolescent bunions: Diagnosis and management, *Pediatr Ann* 11:518–520, 1982.

472. Scranton PE Jr, Zuckerman JD: Bunion surgery in adolescents: results of surgical treatment, *J Pediatr Orthop* 4:39–43, 1984.

473. Seelenfreund M, Fried A, Tikva P: Correction of hallux valgus deformity by basal phalanx osteotomy of the big toe, *J Bone Joint Surg Am* 55:1411–1415, 1973.

474. Seiberg M, Green R, Green D: Epiphysiodesis in juvenile hallux abducto valgus. A preliminary retrospective study, *J Am Podiatr Med Assoc* 84:225–236, 1994.

475. Selner AJ, Selner MD, Tucker RA, Eirich G: Tricorrectional bunionectomy for surgical repair of juvenile hallux valgus, *J Am Podiatr Med Assoc* 82:21–24, 1992.

476. Shannak O, Sehat K, Dhar S: Analysis of the proximal phalanx size as a guide for an Akin closing wedge osteotomy, *Foot Ankle Int* 32:419–421, 2011.

477. Shariff R, Attar F, Osarumwene D, et al: The risk of avascular necrosis following chevron osteotomy: a prospective study using bone scintigraphy, *Acta Orthop Belg* 75:234–238, 2009.

478. Shereff MJ, Yang QM, Kummer FJ: Extraosseous and intraosseous arterial supply to the first metatarsal and metatarsophalangeal joint, *Foot Ankle* 8:81–93, 1987.

479. Sheridan LE: Correction of juvenile hallux valgus deformity associated with metatarsus primus adductus using epiphysiodesis technique, *Clin Podiatr Med Surg* 4:63–74, 1987.

480. Sherman KP, Douglas DL, Benson MK: Keller's arthroplasty: is distraction useful? A prospective trial, *J Bone Joint Surg Br* 66:765–769, 1984.

481. Shima H, Okuda R, Yasuda T, et al: Radiographic measurements in patients with hallux valgus before and after proximal crescentic osteotomy, *J Bone Joint Surg Am* 91:1369–1376, 2009.

482. Shurnas PS, Coughlin MJ: Recall of the risks of forefoot surgery after informed consent, *Foot Ankle Int* 24:904–908, 2003.

483. Shurnas PS, Watson TS, Crislip TW: Proximal first metatarsal opening wedge osteotomy with a low profile plate, *Foot Ankle Int* 30:865–872, 2009.

484. Siclari A, Decantis V: Arthroscopic lateral release and percutaneous distal osteotomy for hallux valgus: a preliminary report, *Foot Ankle Int* 30:675–679, 2009.

485. Silberman FS: Proximal phalangeal osteotomy for the correction of hallux valgus, *Clin Orthop* 85:98–100, 1972.

486. Silver D: The operative treatment of hallux valgus, *J Bone Joint Surg* 5:225–232, 1923.

487. Sim-Fook L, Hodgson AR: A comparison of foot forms among the non-shoe and shoe-wearing Chinese population, *J Bone Joint Surg Am* 40:1058–1062, 1958.

488. Simmonds F, Menelaus M: Hallux valgus in adolescents, *J Bone Joint Surg Br* 42:761–768, 1960.

489. Simon W: Der Hallux valgus und seine chirurgische Behandlung mit besonderer Berucksichtigung der Ludlof schen Operation, *Beitrage Klin Chir* 3:467–537, 1918.

490. Singh B, Draeger R, Del Gaizo DJ, Parekh SG: Changes in length of the first ray with two different first MTP fusion techniques: a cadaveric study, *Foot Ankle Int* 29:722–725, 2008.

491. Smith AM, Alwan T, Davies MS: Perioperative complications of the scarf osteotomy, *Foot Ankle Int* 24:222–227, 2003.

492. Smith BW, Coughlin MJ: The first metatarsocuneiform joint, hypermobility, and hallux valgus: what does it all mean? *Foot Ankle Surg* 14:138–141, 2008.

493. Smith NR: Hallux valgus and rigidus treated by arthrodesis of the metatarsophalangeal joint, *BMJ* 2:1385–1387, 1952.

494. Smith RW, Joanis TL, Maxwell PD: Great toe metatarsophalangeal joint arthrodesis: a user-friendly technique, *Foot Ankle* 13:367–377, 1992.

495. Smith RW, Reynolds JC, Stewart MJ: Hallux valgus assessment: report of research committee of American Orthopaedic Foot and Ankle Society, *Foot Ankle* 5:92–103, 1984.

496. Smith SE, Landorf KB, Gilheany MF, Menz HB: Development and reliability of an intraoperative first metatarsophalangeal joint cartilage evaluation tool for use in hallux valgus surgery, *J Foot Ankle Surg* 50:31–36, 2011.

497. Smith WB, Hyer CF, DeCarbo WT, et al: Opening wedge osteotomies for correction of hallux valgus: a review of wedge plate fixation, *Foot Ankle Spec* 2:277–282, 2009.

498. Sorto LA Jr, Balding MG, Weil LS, Smith SD: Hallux abductus interphalangeus: etiology, x-ray evaluation and treatment, *J Am Podiatr Assoc* 66:384–396, 1976.

499. Sorto LA Jr, Balding MG, Weil LS, Smith SD: Hallux abductus interphalangeus. Etiology, x-ray evaluation and treatment. 1975, *J Am Podiatr Med Assoc* 82:85–97, 1992.

500. Staheli LT: Lower positional deformity in infants and children: a review, *J Pediatr Orthop* 10:559–563, 1990.

501. Stamatis ED, Chatzikomninos IE, Karaoglanis GC: Mini locking plate as "medial buttress" for oblique osteotomy for hallux valgus, *Foot Ankle Int* 31:920–922, 2010.

502. Steel MW 3rd, Johnson KA, DeWitz MA, Ilstrup DM: Radiographic measurements of the normal adult foot, *Foot Ankle* 1:151–158, 1980.

503. Stein HC: Hallux valgus, *Surg Gynecol Obstet* 66:889–898, 1938.

504. Stephens MM: Does shortening of the first ray in the treatment of adolescent hallux valgus prejudice the outcome? *J Bone Joint Surg* 88:858–859, 2006.

505. Stienstra JJ, Lee JA, Nakadate DT: Large displacement distal chevron osteotomy for the correction of hallux valgus deformity, *J Foot Ankle Surg* 41:213–220, 2002.

506. Sung W, Kluesner AJ, Irrgang J, et al: Radiographic outcomes following primary arthrodesis of the first metatarsophalangeal joint in hallux abductovalgus deformity, *J Foot Ankle Surg* 49:446–451, 2010.

507. Szaboky GT, Raghaven VC: Modification of Mitchell's lateral displacement angulation osteotomy, *J Bone Joint Surg Am* 51:1430–1431, 1969.

508. Takao M, Komatsu F, Oae K, et al: Proximal oblique-domed osteotomy of the first metatarsal for the treatment of hallux valgus associate with flat foot: effect to the correction of the longitudinal arch of the foot, *Arch Orthop Trauma Surg* 127:685–690, 2007.

509. Tanaka Y, Takakura Y, Kumai T, et al: Radiographic analysis of hallux valgus. A two-dimensional coordinate system, *J Bone Joint Surg Am* 77:205–213, 1995.

510. Tanaka Y,Takakura Y, Kumai T, et al: Proximal spherical metatarsal osteotomy for the foot with severe hallux valgus, *Foot Ankle Int* 29:1025–1030, 2008.

511. Thomas RL, Espinosa FJ, Richardson EG: Radiographic changes in the first metatarsal head after distal chevron osteotomy combined with lateral release through a plantar approach, *Foot Ankle Int* 15:285–292, 1994.

512. Thompson F, McElveney R: Arthrodesis of the first metatarsophalangeal joint, *J Bone Joint Surg* 22:555–558, 1940.

513. Thompson FM, Coughlin MJ: The high price of high fashion footwear, *J Bone Joint Surg Am* 76:1586–1593, 1994.

514. Thompson GH: Bunions and deformities of the toes in children and adolescents, *Instr Course Lect* 45:355–367, 1996.

515. Thordarson DB, Krewer P: Medial eminence thickness with and without hallux valgus, *Foot Ankle Int* 23:48–50, 2002.

516. Thordarson DB, Leventen EO: Hallux valgus correction with proximal metatarsal osteotomy: Two-year follow-up, *Foot Ankle* 13:321–326, 1992.

517. Tonbul M, Adas M, Keris I, Zengin S: Distal first metatarsal dome (crescentic) osteotomy for repair of mild to moderate hallux valgus deformity, *J Foot Ankle Surg* 47:259–262, 2008.

518. Tonbul M, Baca E, Adas M, et al: Crescentic distal metatarsal osteotomy for the treatment of hallux valgus: a prospective, randomized, controlled studyof two different fixation methods, *Acta Orthop Traumatol Turc* 43:497–503, 2009.

519. Toth K, Huszanyik I, Boda K, et al: The influence of the length of the first metatarsal on transfer metatarsalgia after Wu's osteotomy, *Foot Ankle Int* 29:396–399, 2008.

520. Toth K, Kellermann P, Wellinger K: Fixation of Akin osteotomy for hallux abductus with absorbable suture, *Arch Orthop Trauma Surg* 130:1257–1261, 2010.

521. Tourne Y, Saragaglia D, Zattara A, et al: Hallux valgus in the elderly: metatarsophalangeal arthrodesis of the first ray, *Foot Ankle Int* 18:195–198, 1997.

522. Trnka HJ, Hofstaetter SG, Hofstaetter JG, et al: Intermediate-term results of the Ludloff osteotomy in one hundred and eleven feet, *J Bone Joint Surg Am* 90:531–539, 2008.

523. Trnka HJ, Zembsch A, Easley ME, et al: The chevron osteotomy for correction of hallux valgus. Comparison of findings after two and five years of follow-up, *J Bone Joint Surg Am* 82:1373–1378, 2000.

524. Trnka HJ, Zembsch A, Wiesauer H, et al: Modified Austin procedure for correction of hallux valgus, *Foot Ankle Int* 18:119–127, 1997.

525. Trnka HJ, Zettl R, Hungerford M, et al: Acquired hallux varus and clinical tolerability, *Foot Ankle Int* 18:593–597, 1997.

526. Trott A: Hallux valgus in adolescent, *Instr Course Lect* 21:262–268, 1972.

527. Truslow W: Metatarsus primus varus or hallux valgus? *J Bone Joint Surg* 7:98–108, 1925.

528. Tupman S: Arthrodesis of the first metatarsophalangeal joint, *J Bone Joint Surg Br* 40:826, 1958.

529. Turan I, Lindgren U: Compression-screw arthrodesis of the first metatarsophalangeal joint of the foot, *Clin Orthop* 221:292–295, 1987.

530. Turnbull T, Grange W: A comparison of Keller's arthroplasty and distal metatarsal osteotomy in the treatment of adult hallux valgus, *J Bone Joint Surg Br* 68:132–137, 1986.

531. Vallier GT, Petersen SA, LaGrone MO: The Keller resection arthroplasty: a 13-year experience, *Foot Ankle* 11:187–194, 1991.

532. Varner KE, Matt V, Alexander JW, et al: Screw versus plate fixation of proximal first metatarsal crescentic osteotomy, *Foot Ankle Int* 30:142–149, 2009.

533. Venn A, LaValette D, Harris NJ: Re: technique tip. Plate augmentation of screw fixation of proximal crescentic osteotomy of the first metatarsal, (Rosenbery GA, Donley BG: *Foot Ankle Int* 24:570–571, 2003.) *Foot Ankle Int* 25:605–606; author reply 606, 2004.

534. Verbrugge J: Pathogenie et traitement de l'hallux valgus, *Mem Bull Soc Delge Orthop* 3:40, 1933.

535. Veri JP, Pirani SP, Claridge R: Crescentic proximal metatarsal osteotomy for moderate to severe hallux valgus: a mean 12.2 year follow-up study, *Foot Ankle Int* 22:817–822, 2001.

536. Vienne P, Sukthankar A, Favre P, et al: Metatarsophalangeal joint arthrodesis after failed Keller-Brandes procedure, *Foot Ankle Int* 27:894–901, 2006.

537. Viladot A: Metatarsalgia due to biomechanical alterations of the forefoot, *Orthop Clin North Am* 4:165–178, 1973.

538. Villas C, Del Rio J, Valenti A, Alfonso M: Symptomatic medial exostosis of the great toe distal phalanx: a complication due to over-correction following akin osteotomy for hallux valgus repair, *J Foot Ankle Surg* 48:47–51, 2009.

539. Voellmicke KV, Deland JT: Manual examination technique to assess dorsal instability of the first ray, *Foot Ankle Int* 23:1040–1041, 2002.

540. Volkmann A: Ueber die sogennante Exostose der grossen Zehe, *Virchows Arch Patgol Anat* 10:297, 1856.

541. von Salis-Soglio G, Thomas W: Arthrodesis of the metatarsophalangeal joint of the great toe, *Arch Orthop Trauma Surg* 95:7–12, 1979.

542. Wagner FW Jr: Technique and rationale: Bunion surgery, *Contemp Orthop* 3:1040–1053, 1981.

543. Wanivenhaus AH, Feldner-Busztin H: Basal osteotomy of the first metatarsal for the correction of metatarsus primus varus associated with hallux valgus, *Foot Ankle* 8:337–343, 1988.

544. Wanivenhaus A, Pretterklieber M: First tarsometatarsal joint: anatomical biomechanical study, *Foot Ankle* 9:153–157, 1989.

545. Weil L Jr: Mastering the Scarf procedure for hallux valgus correction, *Foot Ankle Spec* 2:151–155, 2009.

546. Weil LS: Scarf osteotomy for correction of hallux valgus. Historical perspective, surgical technique, and results, *Foot Ankle Clin* 5:559–580, 2000.

547. Wells LH: The foot of the South African native, *Am J Phys Anthropol* 15:185, 1931.

548. West BC: Mini TightRope system for hallux abducto valgus deformity: a discussion and case report, *J Am Podiatr Med Assoc* 100:291–295, 2010.

549. Westbrook AP, Subramanian KN, Monk J, Calthorpe D: Best foot forward. Proceeding of the British Orthopaedic Foot Surgery Society, *J Bone Joint Surg Br* 85(Suppl 3):249, 2003.

550. White LE, Lucas G, Richards A, Purves D: Cerebral asymmetry and handedness, *Nature* 368:197–198, 1994.

551. White P, Issioui T, Skrivanek G, et al: The use of continuous popliteal sciatic nerve block after surgery involving the foot and ankle: does it improve the quality of recovery, *Anesth Analg* 97:1303–1309, 2003.

552. Wilkins EH: Feet with particular reference to school children, *Med Officer* 66:5, 13, 21, 29, 1941.

553. Wilkinson J: Cone arthrodesis of the first metatarsophalangeal joint, *Acta Orthop Scand* 49:627–630, 1978.

554. Wilkinson SV, Jones RO, Sisk LE, et al: Austin bunionectomy: postoperative MRI evaluation for avascular necrosis, *J Foot Surg* 31:469–477, 1992.

555. Williams WW, Barrett DS, Copeland SA: Avascular necrosis following chevron distal metatarsal osteotomy: a significant risk? *J Foot Surg* 28:414–416, 1989.

556. Wilson DW: Treatment of hallux valgus and bunions, *Br J Hosp Med* 24:548–549, 1980.

557. Wilson JD, Baines J, Siddique MS, Fleck R: The effect of sesamoid position on outcome following scarf osteotomy for hallux abducto valgus, *Foot Ankle Surg* 15:65–68, 2009.

558. Wilson JN: Oblique displacement osteotomy for hallux valgus, *J Bone Joint Surg Br* 45:552–556, 1963.

559. Wilson JN: Cone arthrodesis of the first metatarso-phalangeal joint, *J Bone Joint Surg Br* 49:98–101, 1967.

560. Wu DY: Syndesmosis procedure: a non-osteotomy approach to metatarsus primus varus correction, *Foot Ankle Int* 28:1000–1006, 2007.

561. Wu K: Mitchell's bunionectomy and Wu's bunionectomy: a comparison of 100 cases of each procedure, *Orthopedics* 13:1001–1007, 1990.

562. Wu KK: Wu's bunionectomy: a clinical analysis of 150 personal cases, *J Foot Surg* 31:288–297, 1992.

563. Wukich DK, Roussel AJ, Dial DM: Correction of metatarsus primus varus with an opening wedge plate: a review of 18 procedures, *J Foot Ankle Surg* 48:420–426, 2009.

564. Wynne-Davis R: Family studies and the causes of congenital clubfoot talipes equinovarus, talipes calcaneovalgus, and metatarsus varus, *J Bone Joint Surg Am* 46:445, 1967.

565. Young J: A new operation for adolescent hallux valgus, *Univ Penn Med Bull* 23:459, 1910.

566. Young KW, Lee KT, Kwak JJ, et al: Mass-induced unilateral hallux valgus, *Orthopedics* 33:927, 2010.

567. Yucel I, Tenekecioglu Y, Ogut T, Kesmezacar H: Treatment of hallux valgus by modified McBride procedure: a 6-year follow-up, *J Orthop Traumatol* 11:89–97, 2010.

568. Zadik FR: Arthrodesis of the great toe, *BMJ* 5212:1573–1574, 1960.

569. Zimmer TJ, Johnson KA, Klassen RA: Treatment of hallux valgus in adolescents by the chevron osteotomy, *Foot Ankle* 9:190–193, 1989.

570. Zygmunt KH, Gudas CJ, Laros GS: Z-bunionectomy with internal screw fixation, *J Am Podiatr Med Assoc* 79:322–329, 1989.

7 Chapter

Lesser Toe Deformities

Michael J. Coughlin

LESSER TOE DEFORMITIES

Lesser toe deformities can be static or dynamic. They can occur as isolated entities or be associated with deformities of the hallux, midfoot, or hindfoot. Poor footwear is the most commonly attributed cause of lesser toe deformities, but they also can be due to heritable causes or can result from congenital and neuromuscular conditions.[32,35,40,45,46,204]

The terms *hammer toe, mallet toe,* and *claw toe* have been used interchangeably by various authors in describing deformities of the toes, and their definitions have been confusing. The nomenclature adopted for this book is simple, and to a certain extent, it follows that used to

322

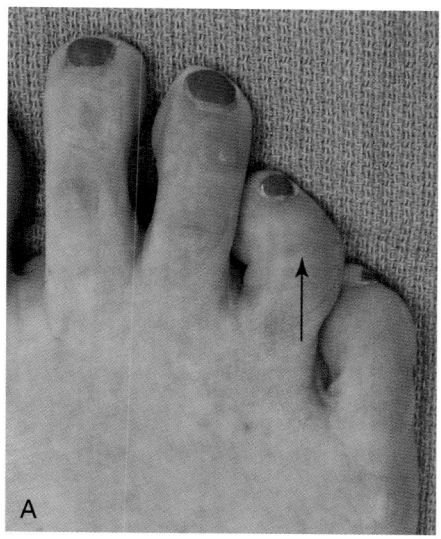
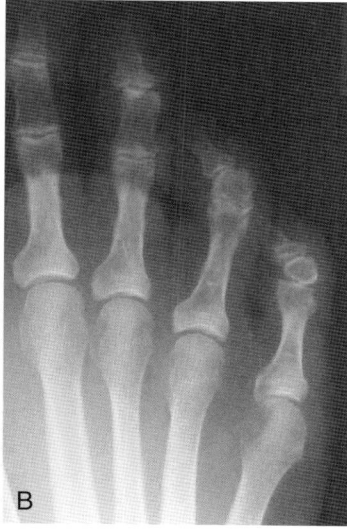

Figure 7-1 **A,** Mallet toe deformity involving distal phalangeal joint. **B,** Radiograph demonstrating mallet toe deformity.

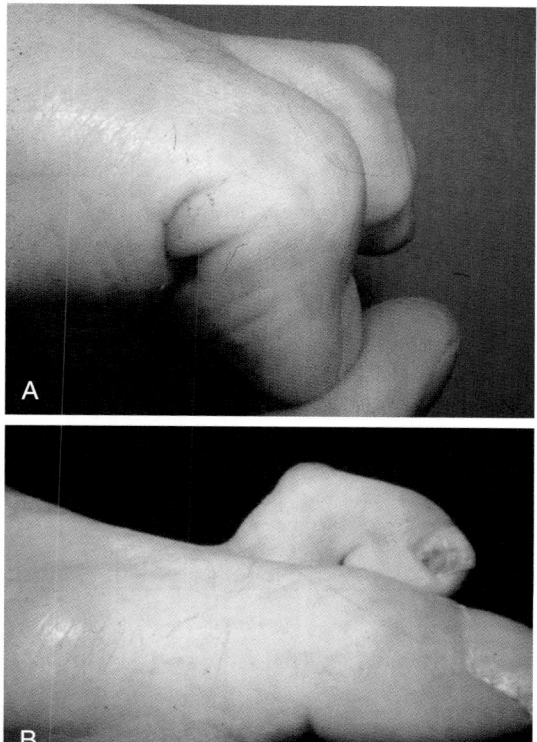
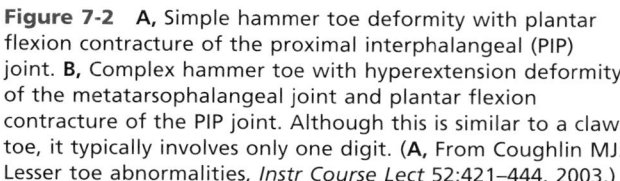

Figure 7-2 **A,** Simple hammer toe deformity with plantar flexion contracture of the proximal interphalangeal (PIP) joint. **B,** Complex hammer toe with hyperextension deformity of the metatarsophalangeal joint and plantar flexion contracture of the PIP joint. Although this is similar to a claw toe, it typically involves only one digit. (**A,** From Coughlin MJ: Lesser toe abnormalities, *Instr Course Lect* 52:421–444, 2003.)

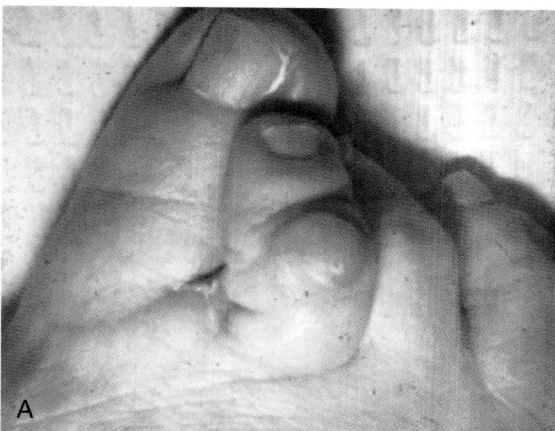
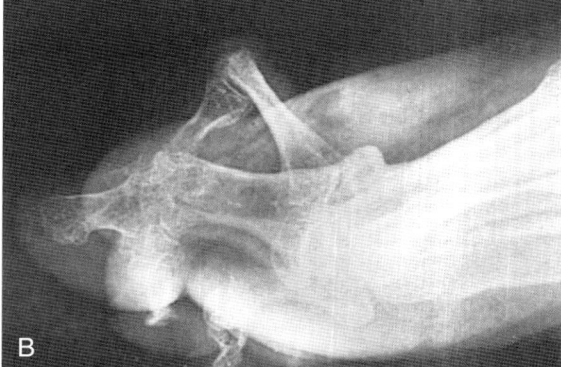

Figure 7-3 **A,** Complex hammer toe deformity involving metatarsophalangeal and proximal interphalangeal (PIP) joints. **B,** Lateral radiograph demonstrating severe flexion deformity of PIP joint.

describe deformities of the fingers. A *mallet toe* involves the distal interphalangeal (DIP) joint; the distal phalanx is flexed on the middle phalanx (Fig. 7-1). A *simple hammer toe* involves the proximal interphalangeal (PIP) joint; the middle and distal phalanges are flexed on the

proximal phalanx (Fig. 7-2A). A *complex hammer toe* typically involves one toe and consists of a flexion deformity of the PIP joint and hyperextension deformity of the metatarsophalangeal (MTP) joint (Figs. 7-2B and 7-3). A *claw toe* involves a hammer toe deformity of the

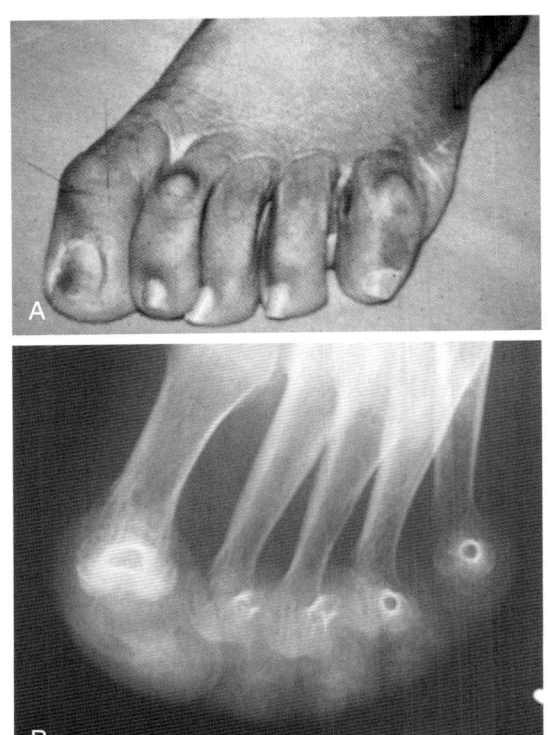

Figure 7-4 Photograph **(A)** and radiograph **(B)** of claw toe deformities involving hammer toe deformity associated with dorsiflexion of metatarsophalangeal joint.

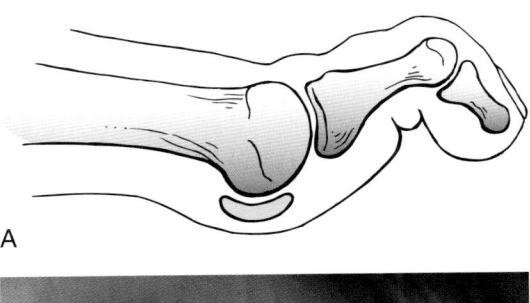

A

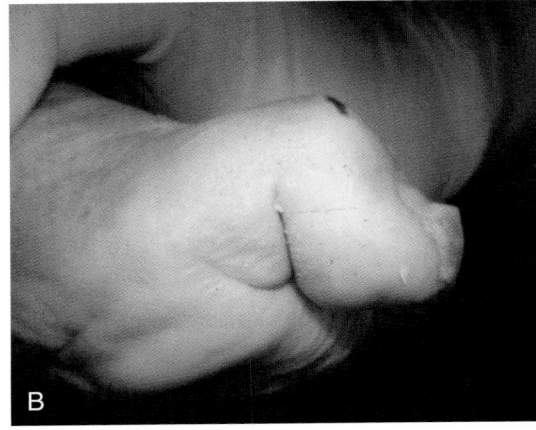

B

Figure 7-5 **A,** Hammered great toe. Note articulation of distal phalanx with plantar surface of the head of the proximal phalanx. **B,** Hammer toe deformity of hallux.

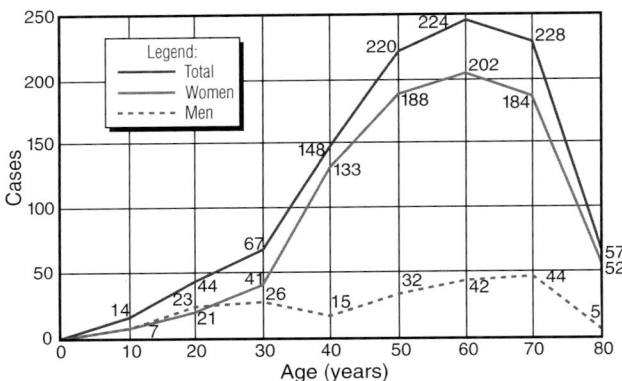

Figure 7-6 Hammer toe deformities peak during the fifth, sixth, and seventh decades in the female population. In the male population, there is no increase in the frequency of hammer toe deformities with increasing age. (From Coughlin MJ, Thompson FM: The high price of high-fashion footwear, *Instr Course Lect* 44:371–377, 1995.)

phalanges and dorsiflexion (extension) deformity at the MTP joint (Fig. 7-4).[212] To some extent, there is an overlap in the definitions of complex hammer toes and claw toes; however, claw toes usually involve all of the lesser toes and often have an underlying neuromuscular cause.

With regard to the great toe, a hammer toe can involve the interphalangeal joint. No mallet toe deformity exists in the hallux (Fig. 7-5). A claw toe deformity, which is essentially synonymous with a cock-up deformity of the great toe, occurs when there is also hyperextension of the MTP joint.

These deformities of the lesser toes range in severity from a mild and easily correctable flexible deformity to a rigid and fixed contracture. In most cases, these deformities are acquired. Both the mallet toe and the hammer toe deformities can occur in one or several toes of the same foot[35,40,45]; a claw toe deformity often involves multiple toes but can occur as an isolated entity.[39]

These deformities occur with varying frequency among different populations, but they are much more common in shoe-wearing societies. The literature dealing with deformities of the forefoot in populations that rarely wear shoes rarely mentions the mallet toe, hammer toe, or claw toe deformities.[5,71,111,233]

In various surveys regarding the incidence of these deformities among industrial workers[54,128] and military male recruits,[102,105] the incidence of hammer toe and claw toe deformities ranged from 2% to 20%. All of these

studies seem to indicate that the deformities develop slowly and insidiously and that their incidence increases almost linearly with age, peaking in the sixth and seventh decades.* These deformities occur much more commonly in women than in men (4 to 5:1).[26,40,45,46,51] A hammer toe deformity rarely is seen in infants (Fig. 7-6).[104] The incidence of forefoot surgery is unknown, but in studies of specific regional populations, Shirzad et al[210] suggested

*References 26, 37, 51, 141, and 201.

these deformities constitute between 28% and 48% of all forefoot surgery.

Etiology

Footwear is generally considered to play an important role in the etiology of hammer toe and mallet toe deformities.[32,40,45] Placing the forefoot into the constricted confines of a pointed shoe no doubt plays a major role in the onset of these deformities. The toes, to conform to a small toe box, must of necessity buckle (Fig. 7-7). This fact explains why acquired mallet toes and hammer toes are among the most common deformities of the forefoot in shoe-wearing societies (Fig. 7-8). DuVries[66] thought that shoes restrict the normal movement of the joints and impedes the actions of the intrinsic muscles of the foot. It must be kept in mind, however, that anatomic predisposing factors vary extensively, and a large number of shoe wearers do escape deformities of the forefoot.

Mallet Toe

Other than its general relationship to pressure of the toe against the shoe, the specific cause of a mallet toe is

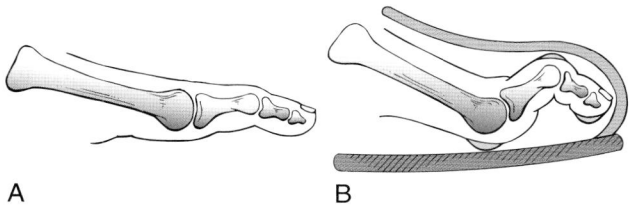

Figure 7-7 **A,** Phalanx extended to normal length. **B,** Buckling of the phalanx is caused by restriction of the toe box. The interphalangeal joints and metatarsophalangeal joints become subluxed. Over time, dislocation can occur.

unknown. Although most often idiopathic in nature, it can develop after a hammer toe repair or trauma,[40,130] or it can be associated with inflammatory arthritis.[40,41] A mallet toe can also develop after a hammer toe repair, possibly because of scarring on contracture of the long flexor tendon. The high incidence of mallet toe in the female population has led to speculation that a constricting toe box is a causative factor.[34,39,40] Female subjects constituted 84% of the patient population in one reported series,[42] the gender difference being highly significant. Brahms[21] stated that a mallet toe is often limited to one toe, although Mann and Coughlin[140] noted that the deformity can occur in more than one toe. Coughlin[40] noted in his report (60 patients, 86 toes) that although 65% of patients had single toe involvement, 18% of patients had multiple toe involvement, with three to five toes affected.

A mallet toe occurs with equal frequency in the second, third, and fourth toes,[40] but most often the involved toe is longer than the adjacent toes (Fig. 7-9). Because of pressure against the end of the shoe, the toe becomes plantar flexed at the DIP joint. Tightness of the flexor digitorum longus tendon in patients with a mallet toe deformity can be demonstrated, but whether this tightness is a primary cause or a secondary change is not known. In young children, a tight flexor tendon can result in a flexion deformity of the PIP and DIP joint. This pediatric deformity has been termed a *curly* toe* and may also be associated with a delta-shaped phalanx.[58]

The major symptoms leading to surgical repair in the adult population include discomfort because of pressure on the tip of the toe, with callus formation or dorsal pain over the DIP joint.[†]

*References 12, 98, 108, 179, 192, 210, and 214.
†References 20, 21, 24, 39, 40, 158, and 191.

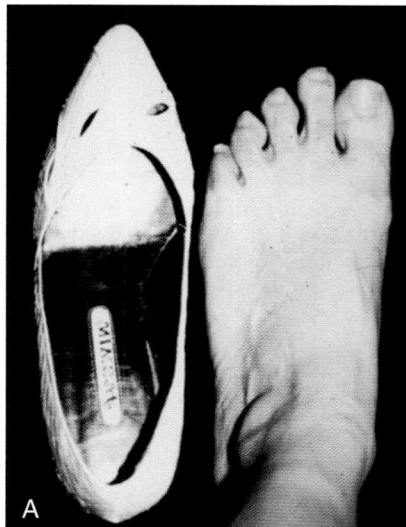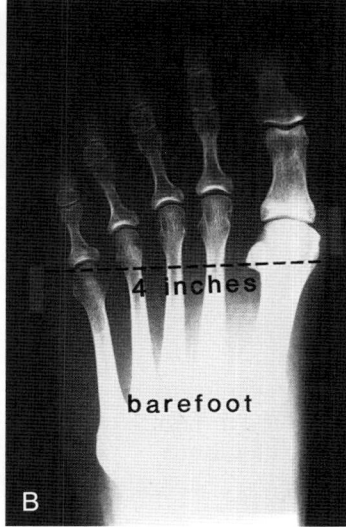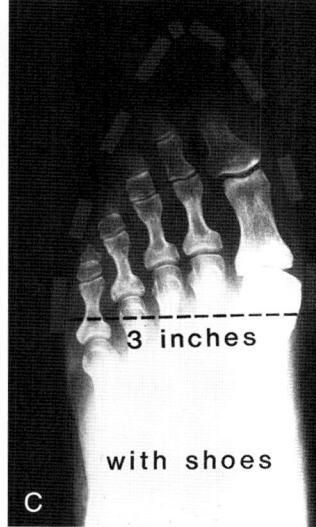

Figure 7-8 **A,** Clinical appearance of foot and pointed toe box of high-fashion shoe. **B,** Radiograph of foot without shoes showing width measuring 4 inches. **C,** Within high-fashion shoe, the forefoot width is compressed to 3 inches. Note constriction of toe box and lateral deviation of hallux.

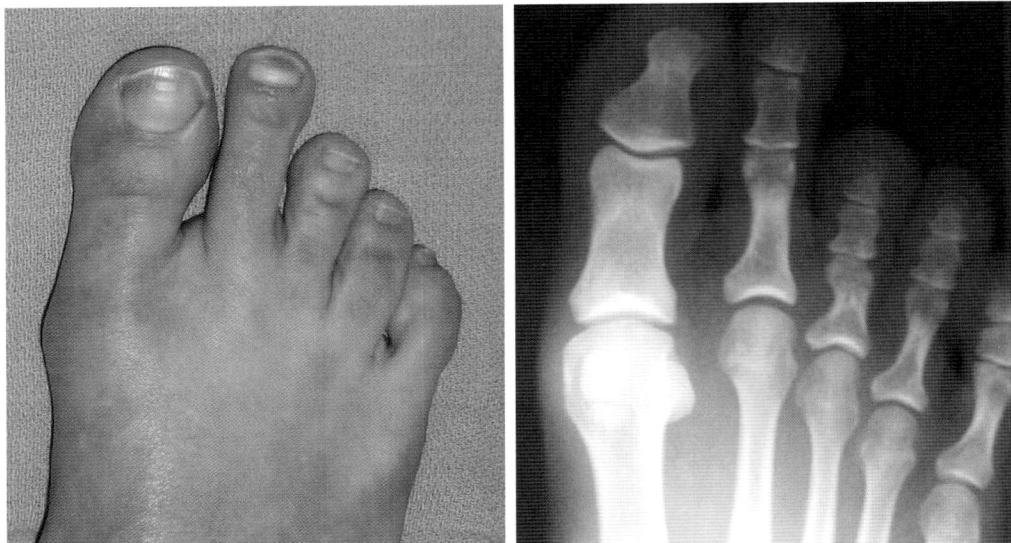

Figure 7-9 The mallet toe and hammer toe occur most often the second toe, especially when it is significantly longer than the adjacent toes.

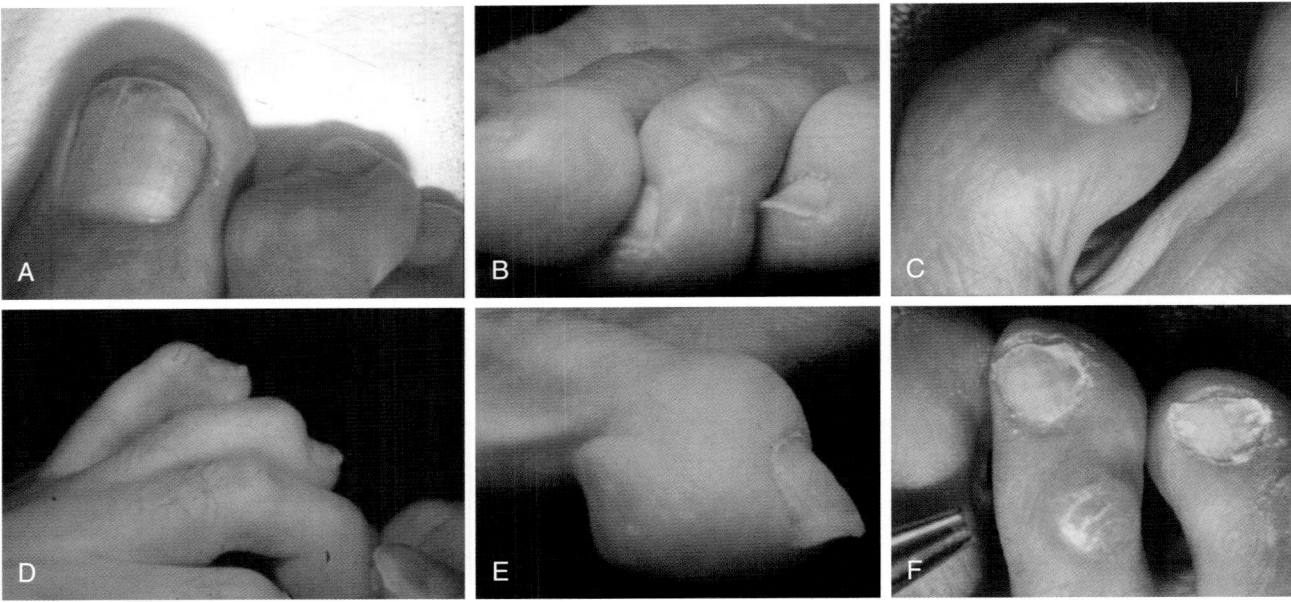

Figure 7-10 Types of mallet toe deformities. **A,** Plantar flexion and lateral deviation lead to overlapping of the third toe. **B,** Mallet toe deformity of the third toe leads to underlapping of the second toe. **C,** Curvature of the third toe impinges against the adjacent digit in the interspace. **D,** Multiple mallet toe deformities. **E,** Plantar flexion contracture of classic mallet toe. **F,** Callus formation on the dorsal aspect of the distal interphalangeal joint. (**D,** From Coughlin MJ: Lesser toe abnormalities, *Instr Course Lect* 52:421–444, 2003.)

Preoperative nail deformities occurred in 7% of mallet toes in Coughlin's series, and 93% were noted to have dorsal pain or pain at the tip of the toe, with callus formation (Figs. 7-10B and F and 7-11C and D).

Hammer Toe

The causes of a hammer toe appear to be multifactorial. The high incidence of hammer toes in the female population has led some to suggest that a constricting toe box is also a causative factor of this deformity.[17,37,51,201] Coughlin[45] reported that 62% of the patients in his series considered ill-fitting shoes to be a cause of their hammer toe deformity. The high incidence of female involvement has been previously reported[26,51,188,196,201]; females constituted 85% of the patient population in a large series,[45] the gender difference being highly significant. The

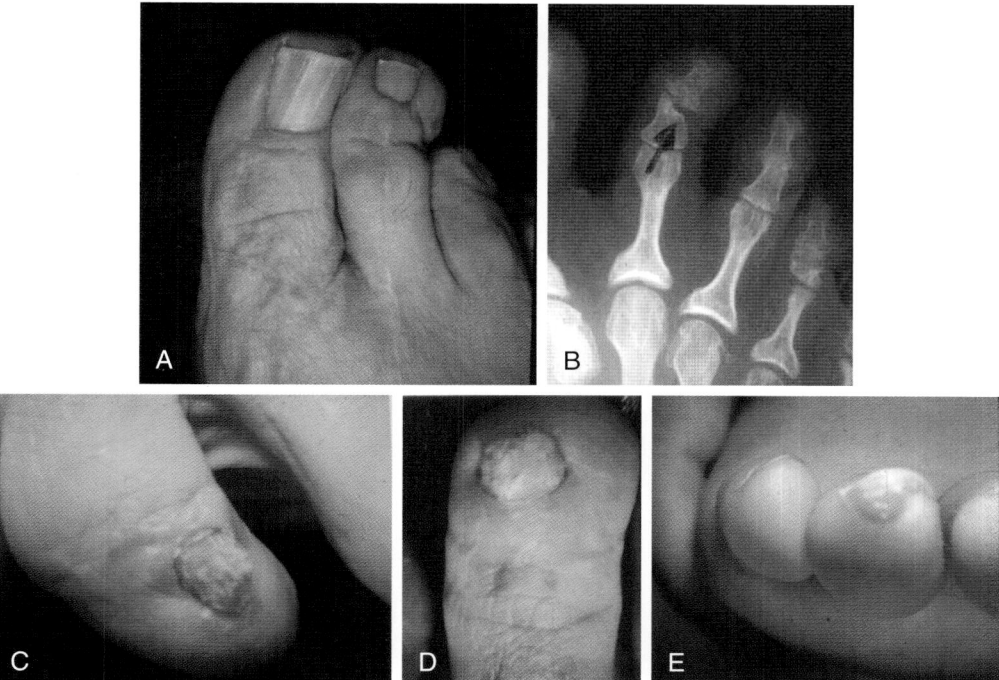

Figure 7-11 **A,** Molding of the toe after mallet toe repair. **B,** Lateral deviation after repair. **C** and **D,** Toenail deformity that preceded mallet toe repair does not improve after surgery. **E,** Callus at tip of toe usually resolves with time after surgical realignment.

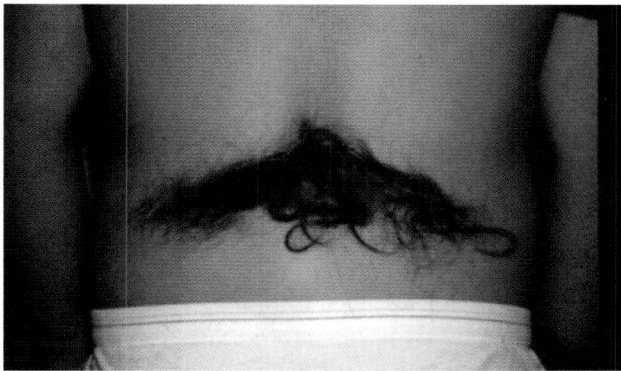

Figure 7-12 On physical examination, a patient with severe claw toe deformities is noted to have a hairy patch over the lumbosacral spine, a condition often associated with diastematomyelia.

incidence of hammer toes is reported to increase with increasing age,[26,51,201] with the peak incidence in the fifth through seventh decades. Coughlin[45] noted in his report (67 patients, 118 toes) that 30% had only single toe involvement, and 40% had three or more toes involved. Although Reece,[188] Coughlin,[45] and others[202,203,228] have reported the second toe to be the most commonly involved, Ohm[170] reported an equal frequency of occurrence in the second, third, and fourth toes. Coughlin[45] noted that increased length in comparison to adjacent digits might be a factor in hammer toe development, although this was not a factor in almost one half of cases.

A hammer toe deformity may be caused by a muscle imbalance in association with neuromuscular diseases, such as Charcot-Marie-Tooth disease, Friedreich ataxia, cerebral palsy, myelodysplasia, multiple sclerosis, and degenerative disk disease. The deformity also is seen in patients with an insensate foot associated with diabetes mellitus and Hansen disease.[43] Patients with rheumatoid arthritis, psoriatic arthritis, and other types of inflammatory arthritis also can develop a hammer toe deformity.[37,39,43] Associated hallux valgus deformities have also been implicated as a cause of hammer toe formation.[22,43,202,203] Occasionally, after fractures of the tibia or other trauma,[74,203] a progressive hammer toe deformity is observed and is likely the result of nerve or muscle injury from elevated compartment pressures in the involved leg or foot.[137]

Claw Toe

The cause of a claw toe deformity often is unclear, but it may be associated with the same neuromuscular diseases, arthritic deformities, and metabolic diseases that cause hammer toe deformities (Fig. 7-12). In many patients with a severe claw toe deformity, no cause can be identified. A claw toe is a result of muscle imbalance between the intrinsic and extrinsic musculature.[157,203] Simultaneous contracture of the long flexors and extensors of the toe, without the modifying action of the intrinsic muscles of the foot, causes the typical deformity seen in this condition (Figs. 7-13 and 7-14).[201] Taylor,[216] however, found no abnormality of the intrinsic muscles in a series of 68

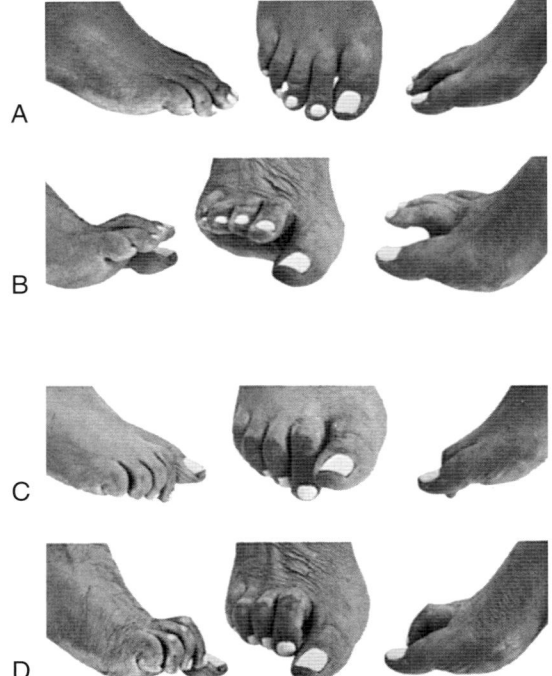

Figure 7-13 Action of muscles in claw toe deformity (from a fresh cadaver foot). **A,** At rest. **B,** Tension on the extensor digitorum longus alone. Note extension of the metatarsophalangeal joints and minimal extension of the interphalangeal joints. **C,** Tension on the flexor digitorum longus alone. Note that maximal flexion occurs at the interphalangeal joints. **D,** Tension simultaneously on the extensor digitorum longus and flexor digitorum longus. Note the resulting deformities in all but the great toe.

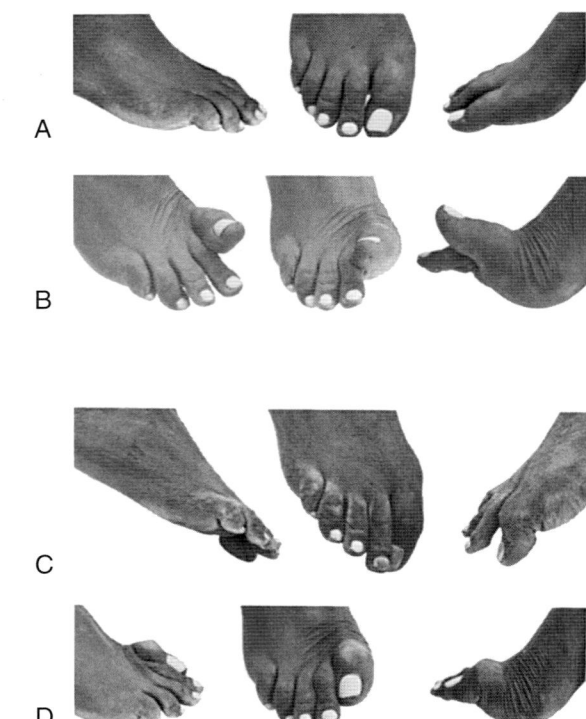

Figure 7-14 Action of muscles in a claw toe deformity of the hallux (from a fresh cadaver foot). **A,** At rest. **B,** Tension on the extensor hallucis longus alone. Note the extension of the metatarsophalangeal and interphalangeal joints. **C,** Tension on the flexor hallucis longus alone. Note the maximal flexion of the interphalangeal joints. **D,** Simultaneous tension on the extensor hallucis longus and flexor hallucis longus, with a resulting claw toe deformity.

patients who had claw toes and in whom the muscles were examined by gross inspection, stimulation, and histologic analysis.

A claw toe deformity usually involves multiple toes and often both feet (Fig. 7-15).[35] The deformity may be either rigid or flexible. It is often associated with a cavus foot, with or without a contracted Achilles tendon. Claw toes are often made worse because the patient cannot find adequate shoes, and a painful bursa develops over the PIP joint. As the claw toe deformity becomes more rigid, the toes strike the top of the shoe and the metatarsal heads are forced plantarward. As the toes subluxate dorsally, the plantar fat pad is pulled distally, and the metatarsal heads become more prominent on the plantar aspect of the foot. This deformity can result in the development of painful plantar callosities, which can ulcerate in severe cases, particularly if sensation of the foot is impaired.

Anatomy and Pathophysiology

An understanding of the anatomy and pathophysiology is helpful in selecting a treatment regimen. The most common deformity is the hammer toe, and this is used

as the prototype in discussing the pathophysiology of all three deformities.

Extensor Digitorum Longus Muscle and Tendon

The central dorsal structure of the toe is formed by the tendon of the extensor digitorum longus, which divides into three slips over the proximal phalanx; the middle slip inserts into the base of the middle phalanx, and the two lateral slips extend over the dorsolateral aspect of the middle phalanx and converge to form the terminal tendon, which inserts into the base of the distal phalanx (Fig. 7-16).[198,199] The tendon is held in a central position dorsally by a fibroaponeurotic sling that anchors the long extensor to the plantar aspect of the MTP joint and to the base of the proximal phalanx. It is surprising that there is no dorsal insertion of the extensor digitorum longus into the proximal phalanx; rather, the phalanx is virtually suspended by the extensor digitorum longus tendon and its extensor sling (Fig. 7-17).

The main function of the extensor digitorum longus is to dorsiflex the proximal phalanx (Fig. 7-18). Only when the proximal phalanx is held in flexion or in a neutral position at the MTP joint can this tendon become an extensor of the PIP joint. This concept is important

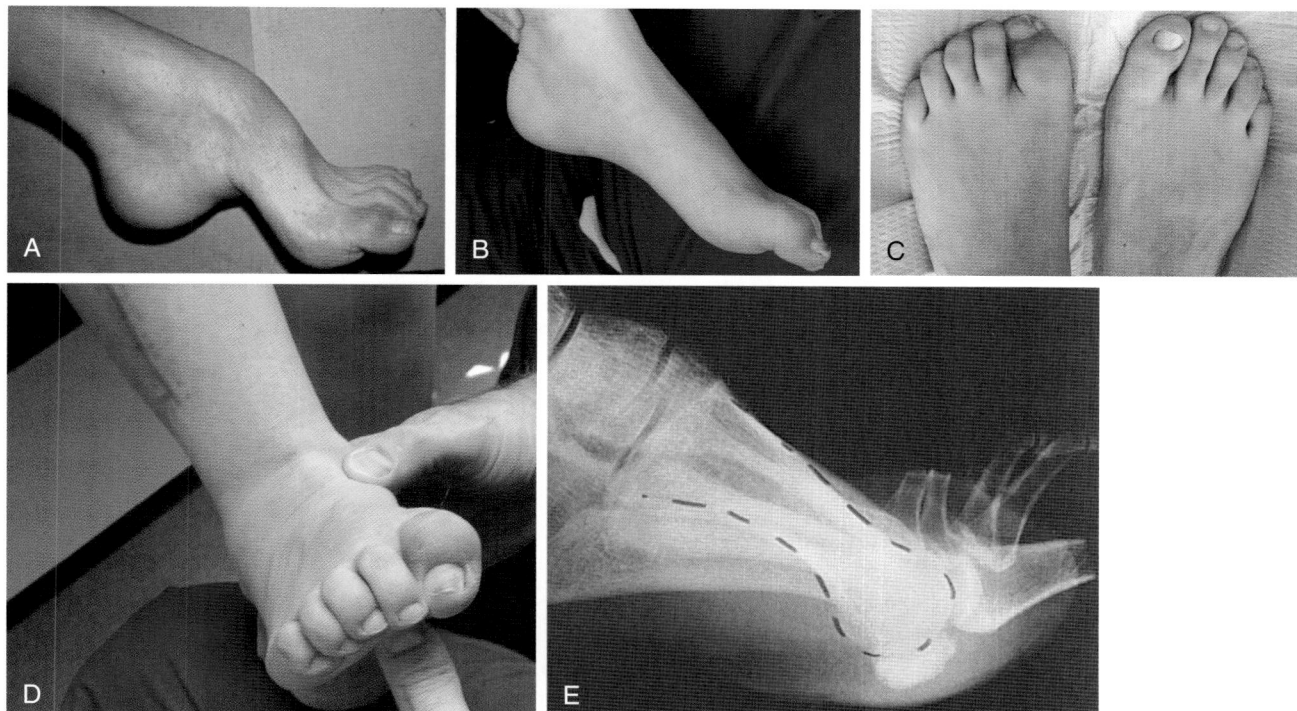

Figure 7-15 **A,** Lateral view of foot with claw toe deformities with diagnosis of Charcot-Marie-Tooth disease. **B,** Lateral view of another patient's foot; in equinus, the deformity is not obvious. The patient had a previous compartment syndrome of calf. **C,** Frontal view of both feet demonstrates claw toe deformity of right foot and normal left foot. **D,** With dorsiflexion of the ankle, the deformity substantially increases. Note scar from the previous compartment release laterally. **E,** Radiograph of claw toe deformity. Note articulation of base of lesser phalanges with dorsal aspect of metatarsal heads. Also note the plantar-flexed first metatarsal resulting from contracted extensor hallucis longus tendon.

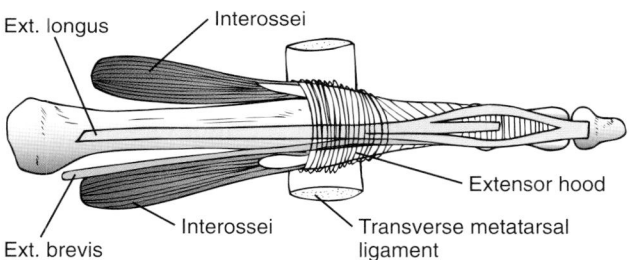

Figure 7-16 Diagram of dorsal view of the extensor mechanism of toes. (Modified from Sarrafian SK, Topouzian LK: Anatomy and physiology of the extensor apparatus of the toes, *J Bone Joint Surg Am* 51:669–679, 1969.)

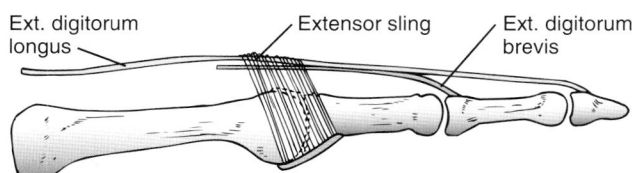

Figure 7-17 Lateral view of extensor mechanism of the lesser toe. Note that the extensor digitorum longus inserts only into the distal phalanx and secondarily suspends the metatarsophalangeal joint through the extensor sling mechanism.

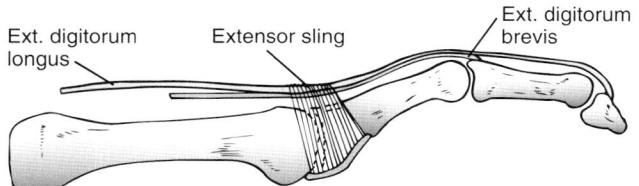

Figure 7-18 Lateral view of the extensor mechanism demonstrates the main function of the extensor digitorum longus, which is to dorsiflex the proximal phalanx.

because, with a hammer toe deformity, the long extensor tendon function on the PIP joint may be neutralized by extension of the proximal phalanx.[201]

The flexor digitorum longus tendon inserts into the distal phalanx and flexes the DIP joint, whereas the flexor digitorum brevis inserts into the middle phalanx, flexing the PIP joint. There is no insertion into the proximal phalanx, so the long flexor tendon influence on the proximal phalanx is minimal (Fig. 7-19A). Resistance to flexion at the MTP joint is maintained in the normal toe by the long extensor. Another important factor is the reactive force of the foot against the ground, which pushes the MTP joint into extension. As a result, with the proximal phalanx in an extended position, there are no major

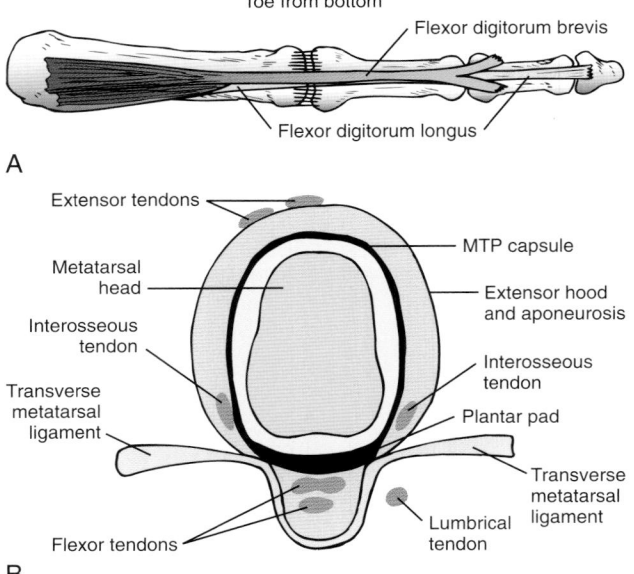

Figure 7-19 **A,** Plantar view of flexor tendon insertion. **B,** Cross section through the metatarsal head of the lesser toe demonstrates structures that pass through this region. Note that the interossei tendons are dorsal to the transverse metatarsal ligament, whereas the lumbrical is plantar to it. *MTP,* metatarsophalangeal.

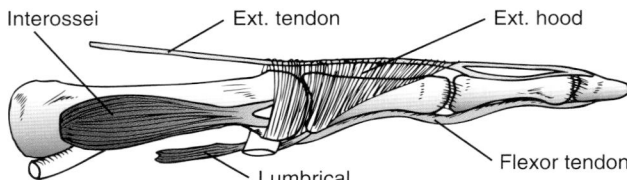

Figure 7-20 Lateral view of a lesser toe demonstrates that both tendons of the intrinsic muscles pass plantar to the axis of motion of the metatarsophalangeal joint, thereby flexing it. They pass dorsal to the axis of motion of the proximal and distal interphalangeal joints, thereby extending them. The lumbrical does not insert into the phalanx but into the extensor hood, and it is thus is a strong extensor of the interphalangeal joints.

motor antagonists to the long and short flexors; thus the toe buckles, resulting in flexion of the DIP joint and the PIP joint. Over a long period of time, if this position becomes fixed, a hammer toe deformity occurs.

Interosseous Tendons

The interosseous tendons are located dorsal to the transverse metatarsal ligament, and the lumbricals are located plantar to this ligament (Fig. 7-19B). Both tendons of the intrinsic muscles, however, pass plantar to the axis of motion of the MTP joint, flexing the MTP joint (Fig. 7-20), and pass dorsal to the axis of the PIP joint and DIP joint, extending these joints. This is an important concept to understand when performing a Weil osteotomy of the

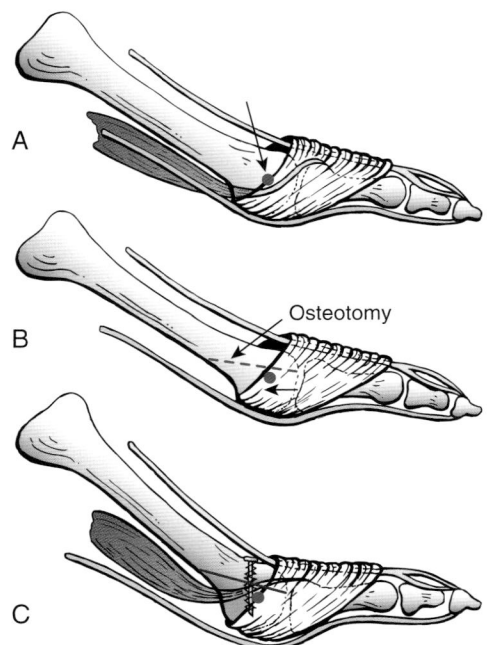

Figure 7-21 Axis of the metatarsophalangeal joint before and after Weil osteotomy. **A,** Lesser metatarsal before ostotomy; note intrinsics are plantar to the axis. **B,** Osteotomy is above the center of the metatarsal head. **C,** After the osteotomy and proximal translation of the capital fragment, the intrinsics course dorsal to the axis of rotation. This can lead to metatarsophalangeal joint dorsiflexion.

distal metatarsal; the center of MTP joint rotation is shifted plantarward, effectively making the intrinsic musculature MTP joint dorsiflex, which can lead to the development of a hyperextension deformity of the MTP joint (Fig. 7-21).[224,231,232] The plantar and dorsal interossei have only a few fibers that reach the extensor sling and therefore are weak extensors of the interphalangeal joints. The lumbrical, with all of its fibers terminating in the extensor sling, is a stronger extensor of these joints. The interossei flex the proximal phalanx by their direct attachment to the base of the proximal phalanx, whereas the lumbrical achieves flexion by placing tension on the extensor sling (Fig. 7-22). With marked dorsiflexion at the MTP joint, the lumbrical flexion power is quite limited because it is pulling at a 90-degree angle.

Plantar Plate and Collateral Ligaments

The most significant stabilizing factor of the MTP joint is the plantar plate, a combination of the plantar aponeurosis and plantar capsule.* During the walking cycle, varying degrees of dorsiflexion occur at the MTP joint. The static resistance of the plantar capsule combines with the dynamic force of the intrinsic flexors to pull the proximal phalanx back into a neutral position at the MTP joint (Fig. 7-23A). With chronic hyperextension forces on the

---

*References 43, 47, 50, 182, and 201.

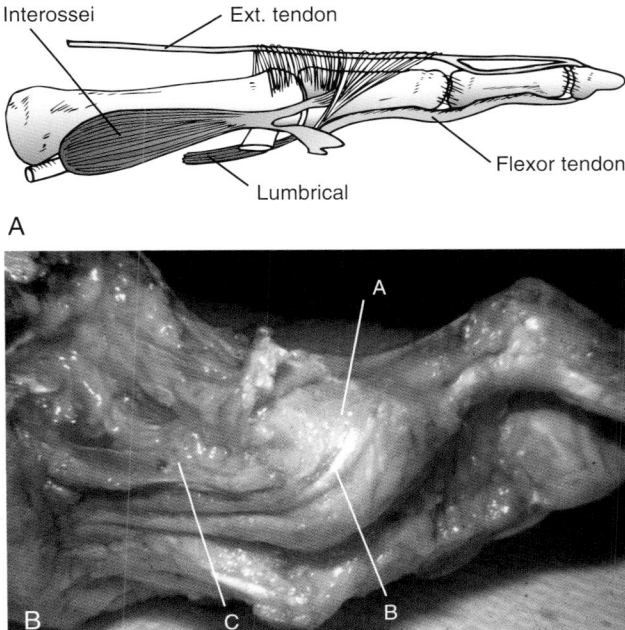

Figure 7-22 **A,** Lateral aspect of a lesser toe with portion of the extensor hood removed to demonstrate insertion of the interossei into the base of the proximal phalanx. This insertion permits the interossei to plantar flex the proximal phalanx on the metatarsal head. **B,** Anatomic dissection demonstrating extensor hood and intrinsics. *A,* central axis of metatarsophalangeal joint; *B,* lumbrical; *C,* interossei.

proximal phalanx, the plantar plate can become stretched or attenuated and rendered less efficient (Fig. 7-23B).

The lesser MTP joint is stabilized by both the collateral ligaments and the plantar plate.[8,61,62] (Fig. 7-23C and D). The plantar plate inserts on the base of the proximal phalanx, but it is attached to the metatarsal head by only a thin layer of synovial tissue that inserts just proximal to the articular surface.[61] The distal attachment of the plantar plate is composed of a medial and a lateral bundle. Proximally, the plantar plate forms the major attachment of the plantar aponeurosis. The plantar plate is the central stabilizing structure that determines the position of the flexor digitorum longus. The collateral ligaments are composed of two major structures: the phalangeal collateral ligament (PCL), which inserts onto the base of the proximal phalanx, and the accessory collateral ligament (ACL), which inserts onto the plantar plate (Fig. 7-23E).[61] The transverse metatarsal ligament attaches to the adjacent medial and lateral borders of the plantar plate.[115]

Pathophysiology

Fortin and Myerson[78] reported that the collateral ligaments were the primary stabilizers of the lesser MTP joint. When the collateral ligaments were sectioned in vitro, 48% less force was required to dislocate the lesser MTP joint. When the researchers did an isolated release of the plantar plate, 29% less force was required to dislocate the MTP joint.

The position of the proximal phalanx at the MTP joint is subject to the actions of the strong extensor digitorum

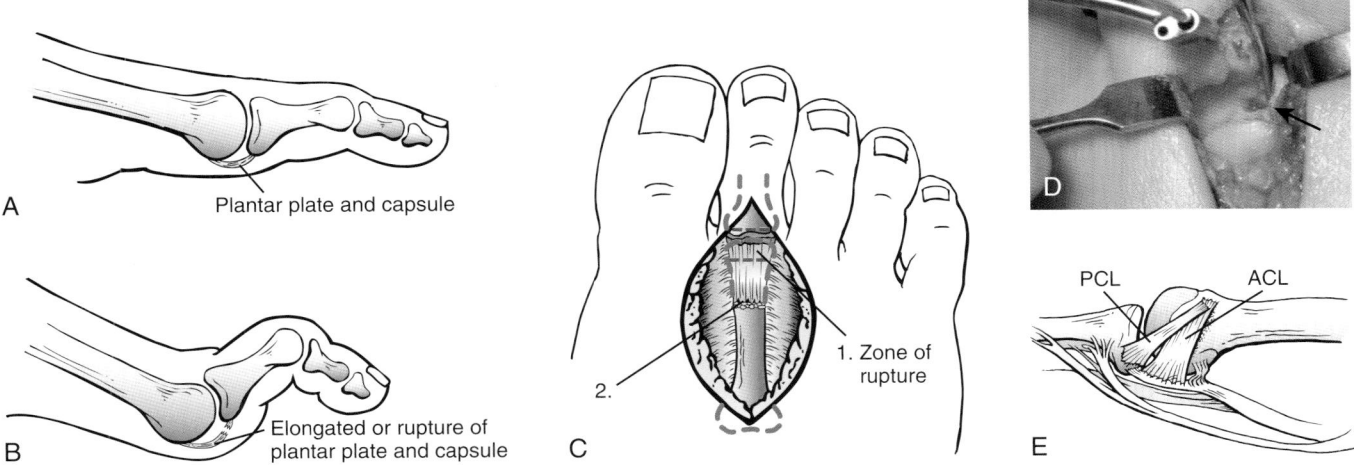

Figure 7-23 **A,** Diagram demonstrates the plantar plate and the capsule of the metatarsophalangeal (MTP) joint, which is sufficiently resilient to bring the MTP joint back into a neutral position after the joint has been dorsiflexed at lift-off. **B,** Lateral view diagram illustrates the effects of the elongated plantar plate and capsule and area of rupture. As a result of certain disease states, the capsular structures no longer are sufficient to restore the joint to its normal position after lift-off. **C,** Dorsal view with removal lesser metatarsal head; a tear or rupture off of the base of the proximal phalanx may occur. Note *1,* which is the potential zone of plantar plate rupture, and *2,* which is the proximal loose synovial attachment at proximal extent of metatarsal articular surface, where a rupture rupture rarely occurs. **D,** Clinical photograph of partial plantar plate rupture (*arrow* points to grade I rupture of lateral plantar plate). **E,** Diagram of collateral ligaments of the lesser MTP joint. The PCL inserts on the plantar tubercles of the proximal phalanx, and the ACL inserts in a broad expansion into the edge of the plantar plate. *ACL,* accessory collateral ligament; *PCL,* phalangeal collateral ligament.

longus through its sling mechanism, in opposition to the decidedly weaker antagonistic intrinsic muscles and the more static capsule and plantar aponeurosis complex. The positions of the middle and distal phalanges, on the other hand, are subject to the forces of the long and short flexors, which are directly opposed by the weaker intrinsic muscles. At each of these joints, an obvious mismatch can occur, and in each case, the extrinsic muscle overpowers the intrinsic muscle (Fig. 7-24).

The extensor digitorum longus helps extend the interphalangeal joints if the proximal phalanx is not hyperextended, and the flexor digitorum longus helps to flex the MTP joint if the proximal phalanx is not hyperextended. The hyperextended proximal phalanx, then, is definitely the key to the production of most hammer toe deformities. With a chronic hyperextended position of the proximal phalanx, maintained throughout the entire walking cycle (by wearing high-heeled shoes), the plantar structures gradually become stretched and inefficient, and thus the proximal phalanx remains in a chronically

dorsiflexed position. Therefore, with chronic extension of the proximal phalanx, the extensor digitorum longus tendon loses its tenodesing effect on the interphalangeal joints, allowing the distal phalanges to migrate into flexion. As the proximal phalanx extends, the extrinsic flexors are under greater tension, further increasing the flexion deformity at the PIP joint. The only counteracting forces to this flexion deformity are the lumbricals and the interossei, which are easily overpowered by the long flexor tendons.

Preoperative Evaluation

Physical Examination

When examining a foot with a lesser toe deformity, it is important to assess the circulatory status of the lower extremity. Although some surgical procedures require limited exposure, other procedures require extensive dissection at the MTP joint, at the interphalangeal joints, and even along both the medial and lateral aspects of the phalanges. Whether an individual digit can withstand multiple procedures and extensive surgical exposure depends on the vascular status of the digit. Preoperative evaluation is necessary to assess not only the feasibility of an individual procedure but also whether multiple procedures can be performed if necessary.

The sensory status of a foot must be evaluated as well. An impaired sensory status can indicate a systemic disease, such as diabetes, a peripheral neuropathy, or lumbar disk disease. Careful physical examination is necessary to differentiate MTP joint pain from an interdigital neuroma of the adjacent interrmetatarsal space (Fig. 7-25).[48,49] Preoperative documentation of sensation is important because a surgical dissection can diminish postoperative sensation.

The plantar aspect of the foot is examined for development of intractable plantar keratoses. Callosities can develop in association with contractures of the lesser toes,

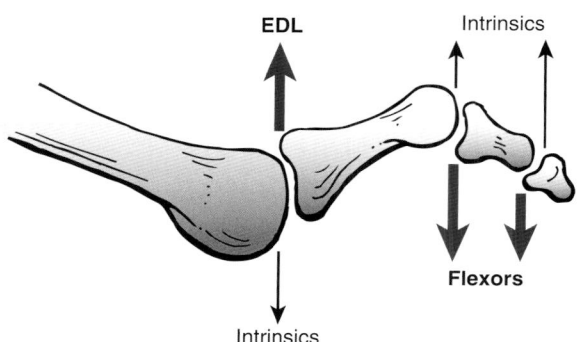

Figure 7-24 Diagram demonstrates the relationship of the intrinsic and extrinsic muscles about a lesser toe. The smaller intrinsics are overpowered by the extrinsics, leading to a hammer toe deformity. *EDL,* extensor digitorum longus.

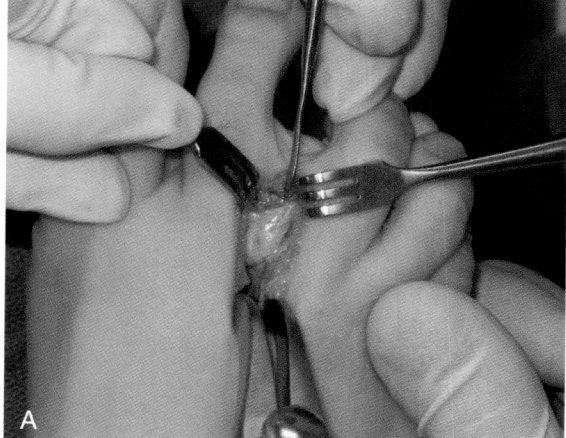
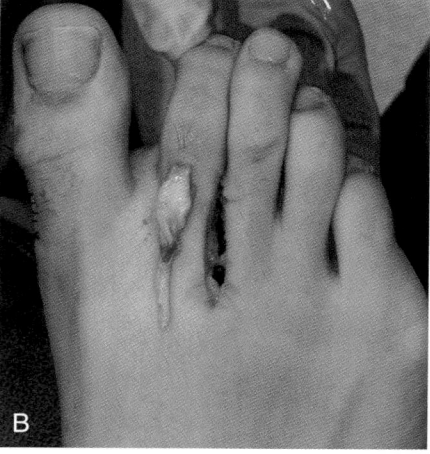

Figure 7-25 The diagnosis of combined metatarsophalangeal instability and an adjacent interdigital neuroma is uncommon and difficult to make. **A,** Medial deviation of the second toe with exposure of enlarged symptomatic interdigital neuroma. **B,** After Weil osteotomy to realign the second toe and excision of the interdigital neuroma.

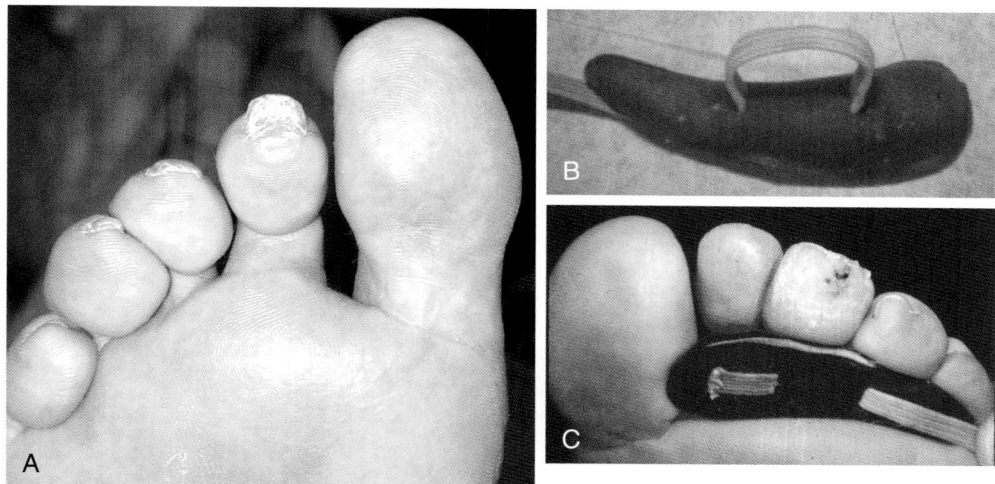

Figure 7-26 **A,** With a hammer toe deformity, a callus has developed at the tip of the second toe. **B,** A toe cradle. **C,** The cradle is used to decrease pressure beneath the tip of the lesser toe. (**C,** From Coughlin MJ: Lesser toe abnormalities, *Instr Course Lect* 52:421–444, 2003.)

the result of a buckling effect of the toes. A patient typically complains of pain caused by a callus over the distal aspect of the PIP joint but also can develop pain beneath the tip of the toe or a lesser metatarsal head (Fig. 7-26).[45,135] Realignment of the MTP joint and interphalangeal joints can decrease plantar pressure and help relieve symptomatic calluses.

The individual digits are examined for callosities on the medial and lateral aspects, as well as over the interphalangeal joint and at the tip of the toe. With a fixed hammer toe deformity, callosities can develop over the contracted PIP joint as well as at the tip of the toe. Toenail deformities can develop as well.

The alignment of the MTP joint must be evaluated.[201] Medial or lateral deviation of the toe should be noted, as well as an MTP joint hyperextension deformity. The stability of the digit is assessed by the drawer test. The digit is grasped between the thumb and index finger of the examiner, and with the digit slightly dorsiflexed, dorsal pressure is placed on the digit in an attempt to subluxate the MTP joint (Fig. 7-27). Even if the toe is not subluxed, the eliciting of pain with this maneuver is indicative of an intraarticular or periarticular abnormality. (See further discussion under subluxation second MTP joint.)

Although the evaluation of a hammer toe deformity may be seen as relatively simple, certain factors must be carefully considered to fully appreciate the nature of the deformity. These include the rigidity of the toe contractures (Fig. 7-28), the position of the MTP joint (Fig. 7-29A), and Achilles tendon tightness with the patient both sitting and standing. Tightness of the flexor digitorum longus tendon must be assessed along with examination of all of the lesser toes. Also, it is important to determine whether there is sufficient space for the involved toe when it is reduced to a normal position. The presence of prior surgical scars can influence the planned surgical exposure.

Radiographic Examination

Although a physical examination is necessary to define the extent of a lesser toe deformity, radiographic examination is necessary to evaluate the magnitude of the bone deformity (Fig. 7-29B). On an anteroposterior (AP) projection, a severe hammer toe deformity can have the appearance of a gun barrel deformity (Fig. 7-29C) when the proximal phalanx is seen end on. Assessment of the interphalangeal joints is difficult on this projection. Diminution of the MTP joint space can indicate subluxation, and overlap of the base of the proximal phalanx in relation to the metatarsal head can indicate dislocation of the MTP joint (Fig. 7-30). Medial or lateral deviation of the MTP joint can be determined as well. Subchondral erosion, flattening of the articular surfaces, or a Freiberg infraction can indicate the need for further radiographic or laboratory evaluation.

A lateral radiograph may be helpful to assess the magnitude of contracture of the interphalangeal joints (see Fig. 7-29B). Stress radiographs can help to determine subluxability of the MTP joint (see Fig. 7-27). Bone scans, computed tomography (CT), and magnetic resonance imaging (MRI) evaluation may also be used to increase information of both osseous and soft tissue abnormalties (Fig. 7-31).

FIXED HAMMER TOE DEFORMITY

Preoperative Planning

A hammer toe deformity may be flexible, semiflexible, or rigid.* If the deformity is flexible, the toe may be passively corrected to a neutral position. However, if the deformity is rigid, joint contractures preclude passive correction. The rigidity of the deformity determines

---

*References 2, 32, 35, 45, 140-142, 210, and 212.

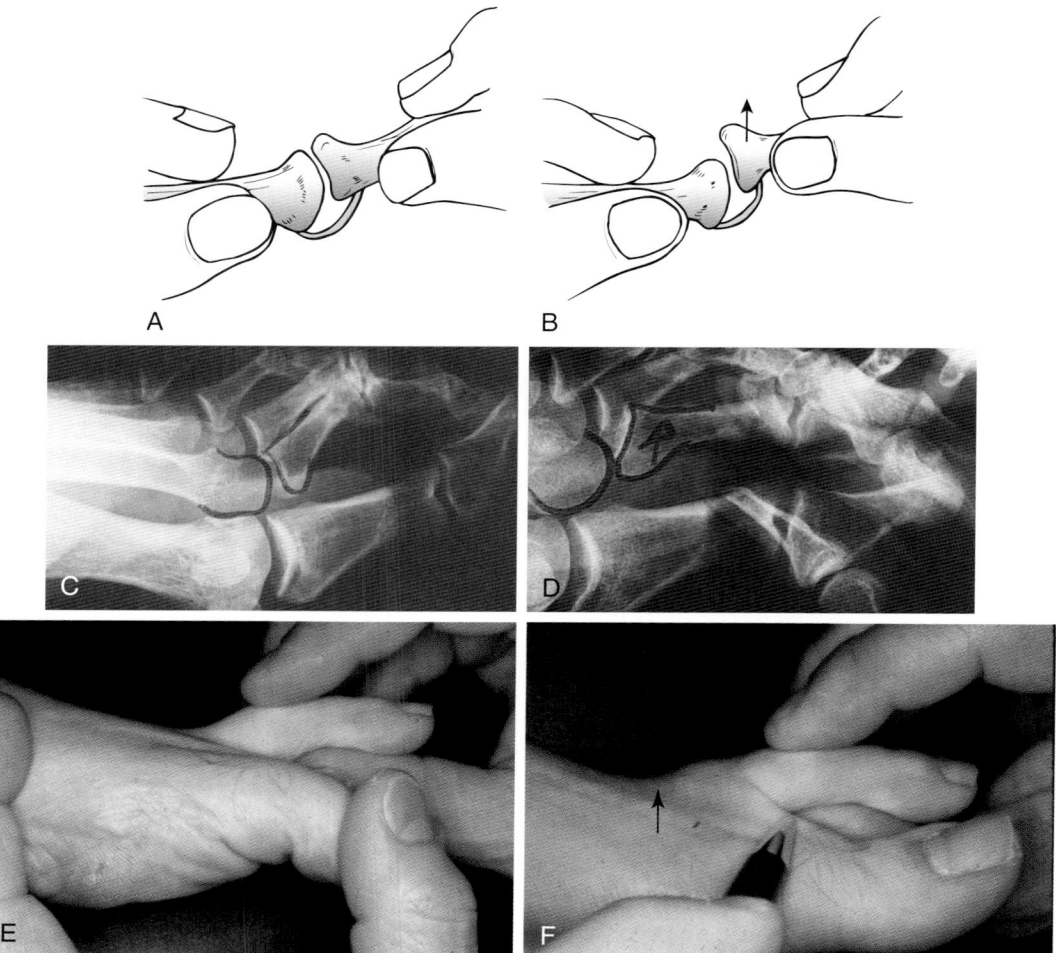

Figure 7-27 Drawer test for metatarsophalangeal (MTP) joint instability. **A,** The toe is grasped between the thumb and second finger. **B,** With dorsal force, an attempt is made to subluxate the MTP joint. With instability of the MTP joint, pain is elicited with stress on the plantar structures. **C,** Lateral radiograph of unstable second MTP joint before drawer test. **D,** Lateral radiograph after drawer test with the base of the proximal phalanx subluxed dorsally. **E,** Before dorsal subluxation of metatarsophalangeal joint with drawer test. **F,** Position of the base of the toe after dorsal subluxation.

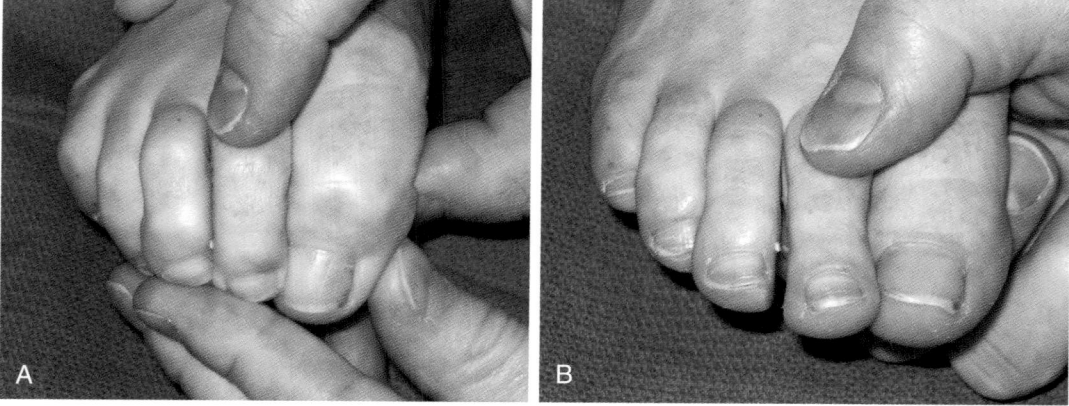

Figure 7-28 A hammer toe deformity is inspected to determine its flexibility. **A,** Fixed deformity. **B,** Flexible deformity.

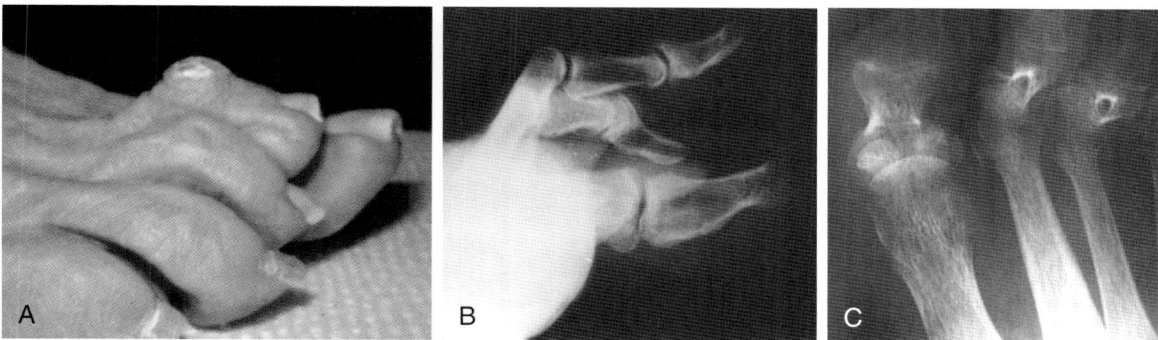

Figure 7-29 **A,** Hammer toe deformity demonstrates severe hyperextension. **B,** Lateral radiograph demonstrates hyperextension deformity of the proximal phalanx. **C,** Anteroposterior radiograph demonstrates the gun barrel sign. The proximal phalanx is seen end on, superimposed over the condyle. This conformation is pathognomonic of hyperextension deformity of the proximal phalanx.

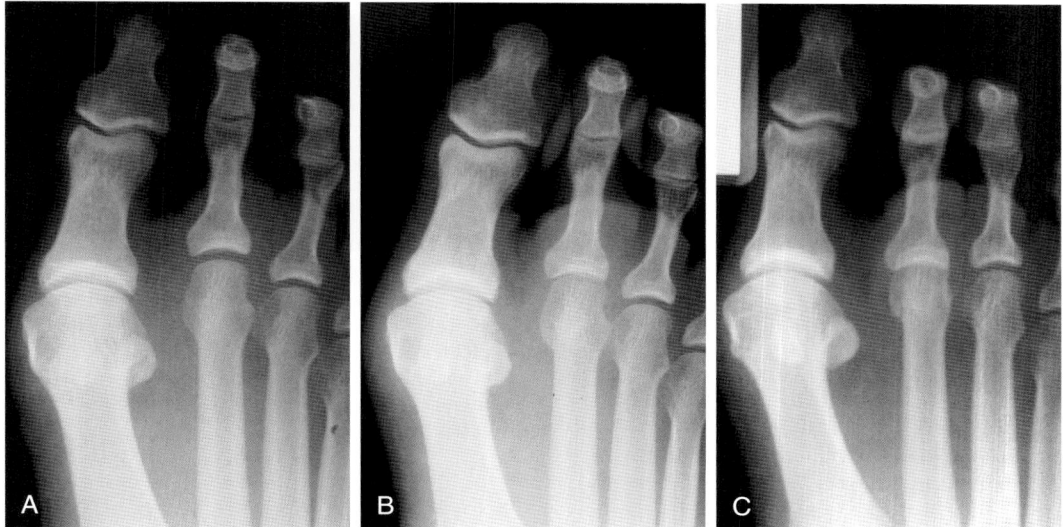

Figure 7-30 **A,** A 52-year-old man with pain at the second metatarsophalangeal (MTP) joint and a slight hallux valgus deformity. **B,** Six-month follow-up demonstrates narrowing of the joint space, pathognomonic of a hyperextension deformity. Often subluxation can occur insidiously. **C,** At 15-month follow-up, the second MTP joint has dislocated.

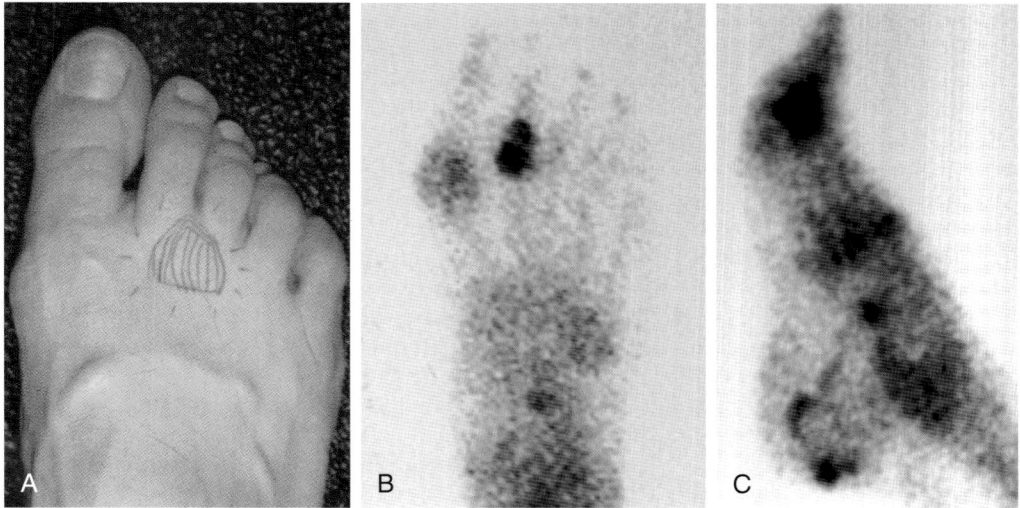

Figure 7-31 Patient with ill-defined forefoot pain. **A,** Clinical location of pain. Technetium-99m (^{99m}Tc) bone scan, anteroposterior **(B)** and lateral **(C)** views, can demonstrate pathologic changes before radiographic changes. Note the increased uptake in the area of the second metatarsophalangeal joint.

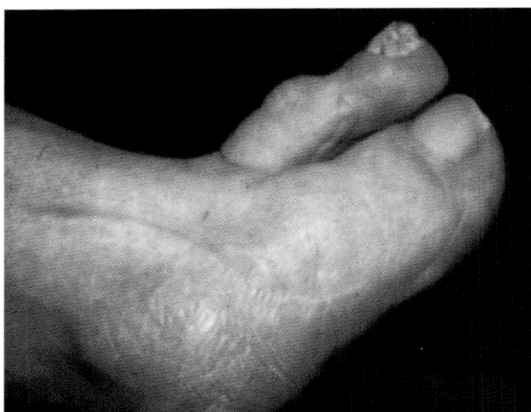

Figure 7-32 An isolated hammer toe repair or a flexor tenotomy can lead to hyperextension deformity of the involved toe.

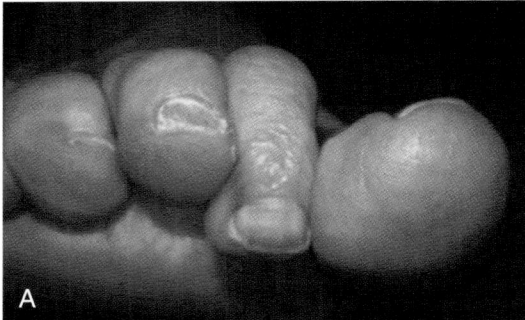

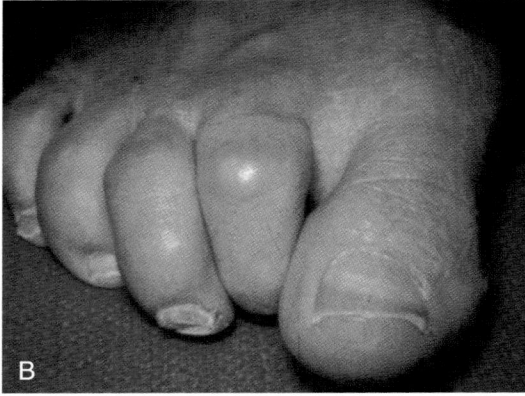

Figure 7-33 With a tight flexor tendon in an adjacent toe, a flexor tenotomy should be performed at the time of hammer toe repair. **A,** Contracture of just the second toe indicates a flexor tenotomy is possibly not necessary. **B,** A contracture is noted in all of the lesser toes. (**B,** From Chapman M, editor: *Operative orthopaedics,* Philadelphia, JB Lippincott, 1988, pp 1765–1776.)

whether conservative or surgical treatment is indicated, as well as the specific surgical procedure that should be performed.

The position of the MTP joint when the patient is standing must be carefully evaluated. If a hyperextension deformity is present, correction of only the hammer toe deformity will result in the toe sticking up in an extended position (Fig. 7-32), making shoe wearing difficult. If the MTP joint is subluxated or dislocated, this deformity should be corrected simultaneously with the hammer toe correction.[43,72,133,141,179]

Tightness of the flexor digitorum longus tendon should be carefully observed with the patient in a standing position. If the flexor digitorum longus tendon appears to be tight in the toe adjacent to the involved toe, the involved toe probably also has a contracture of the flexor digitorum longus tendon. In this case, the tendon should be released in the deformed toe at surgery or the deformity will probably recur over time (Fig. 7-33).

Another consideration in the treatment of a hammer toe is that there must be sufficient space for the corrected toe to occupy (Fig. 7-34A). If a patient has a concomitant hallux valgus deformity that has diminished the interval between the first and third toes and forced the second toe into dorsiflexion, adequate space must be obtained for the corrected lesser toe or the deformity can recur.[140] An Akin phalangeal osteotomy may be used to create room for a second toe when a hammer toe correction is performed.[179] A hallux valgus repair may be necessary to obtain sufficient space between the first and third toes to realign the second toe successfully. At times, the adjacent lesser toes can drift into medial or lateral deviation, again diminishing the interval that the corrected toe should occupy. These toes may need to be corrected to afford the corrected hammer toe adequate space.

A young patient with a flexible deformity is a candidate for conservative treatment. Likewise, an older patient with multiple medical problems may be a poor surgical candidate as well. The most important conservative measure

is for the patient to acquire roomy, well-fitted shoes.[51,212] The preferable characteristics of such shoes include a high and wide toe box and a soft sole with a soft upper portion of the toe box. This helps to prevent direct pressure against a hammer toe and subsequent development of painful callosities. Local treatment can consist of a doughnut-shaped cushion, foam toe cap (Fig. 7-34B), foam tube-gauze, or viscoelastic toe sleeves placed over the PIP joint (Fig. 7-34C-F).[2,210,212] Shoes with a stiff insole or a rocker-type outer sole may relieve pressure on the forefoot and diminish metatarsalgia (Fig. 7-35).

The shoe itself might need to be modified if the patient has pain beneath the metatarsal head. Such a modification can consist of a soft metatarsal support, a metatarsal bar, or a comfortable orthosis that relieves pressure beneath the involved metatarsal head. At times, patients modify their shoes to reduce pressure on a symptomatic hammer toe (see Fig. 7-34G and H). A toe cradle can elevate the involved digit and reduce pressure on the tip of the toe (see Fig. 7-26B and C). In more advanced cases and with multiple toe involvement, an extra-depth shoe with a polyethylene foam (Plastazote) insole can help to distribute pressure more uniformly on the plantar aspect of the foot. A program with daily manipulation of the toes should be started to try to keep the toes flexible.

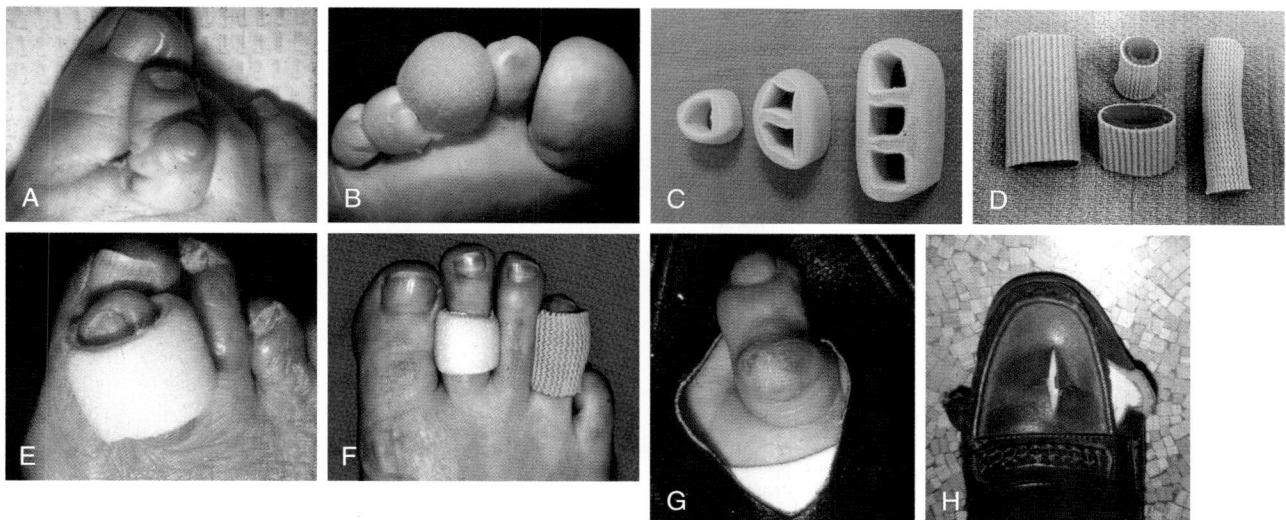

Figure 7-34 **A,** A hallux valgus deformity can reduce the space available for the second toe once the hammer toe has been corrected. **B,** A toe cap may be used to decrease pressure on the distal tip of the hammer toe. **C** and **D,** Various types of tube gauze may be used to pad a lesser toe deformity. **E** and **F,** Tube gauze is slid over the symptomatic toe to relieve pressure. **G,** Patient has modified footwear to make room for the prominent second toe. **H,** A shoe may be modified as in this case by a patient with a bunion, bunionette, and hammer toe deformity.

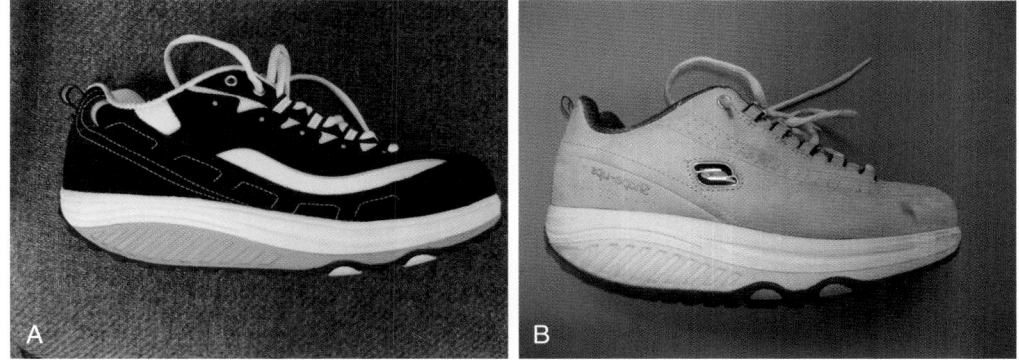

Figure 7-35 **A** and **B,** Examples of roomy shoes. Rocker sole with stiff insole may provide increased depth to the toe box and a stiff insole to diminish lesser toe joint excursion.

A traumatic boutonnière deformity can develop with a hammer toe deformity (Fig. 7-36). Rau and Manoli[187] initially reported on this rare deformity, which is caused by a rupture of the central extensor slip. As the lateral bands displace, they become flexors of the PIP joint. A flexion deformity of the PIP joint occurs and is associated with a hyperextension deformity of the DIP joint. The authors recommended a direct repair of the central slip and recentralization of the lateral bands. Quebedeaux et al[185] reported on two cases of traumatic boutonnière deformity; one developed in association with chronic rheumatoid arthritis and was treated conservatively, and the other one developed after trauma. A delayed repair and PIP arthroplasty were performed.

If a deformity of the MTP joint exists along with a hammer toe deformity (a complex hammer toe

deformity), surgical correction of this deformity also must be considered. In cases of a mild deformity, an extensor tenotomy or lengthening may be sufficient to achieve correction. In cases of a moderate hyperextension deformity of the MTP joint, an extensor tenotomy and MTP capsule release may be necessary.[64] Kirschner wire fixation also may be necessary to stabilize the arthroplasty site as well as the MTP joint. A flexor tendon transfer also may be necessary to achieve stability of the MTP joint. Where subluxation has progressed to frank dislocation of the MTP joint, the soft tissue procedures described are inadequate to achieve reduction, and a metatarsal osteotomy is necessary. (A complete discussion of the evaluation and treatment of MTP joint subluxation and dislocation is presented later in the chapter.)

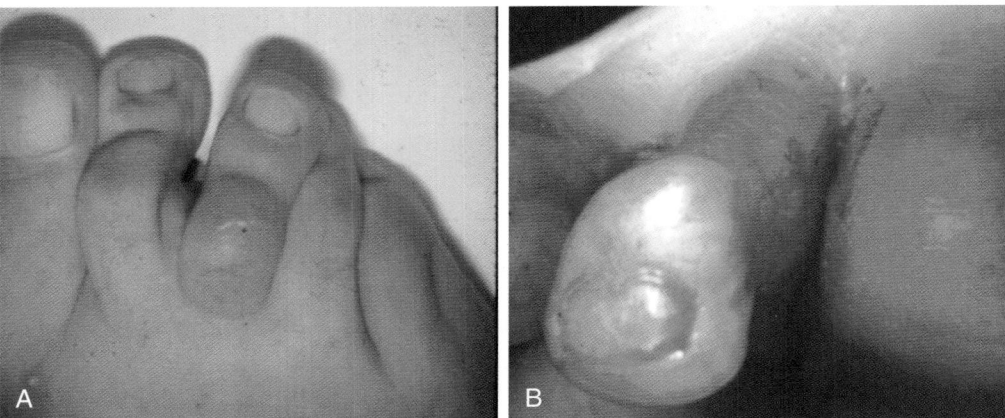

Figure 7-36 **A,** Traumatic boutonnière deformity of the second toe. **B,** A traumatic swan-neck deformity has occurred with development of a mallet toe as well as hyperextension of the proximal interphalangeal joint.

With time, and even with appropriate conservative management, most of these deformities become fixed and often require surgical correction.* The algorithm presented in Figure 7-37 is a useful guide to treatment of the hammer toe deformity. If surgery is required, it is important that the procedure be carefully selected, depending on the specific cause and type of the deformity.

Indications

The DuVries arthroplasty is recommended for reduction of a fixed hammer toe deformity involving the middle three toes. This procedure does not necessarily achieve a joint fusion; it can achieve a fibrous union that usually allows approximately 15 degrees of motion. The arthroplasty may be performed under a digital anesthetic block if there is no MTP joint involvement. If there is an MTP joint deformity, more extensive anesthesia is necessary.

Contraindications

Contraindications include acute or chronic infection, vascular insufficiency, and flexible deformities for which a resection arthroplasty is not necessary. Relative contraindications include more severe deformities involving the MTP joint, for which more extensive surgery must be combined with the DuVries arthroplasty to realign the digit completely.

DUVRIES ARTHROPLASTY PROCEDURE
Surgical Technique

1. The patient is placed in a supine position on the operating room table. The foot is cleansed and draped in the usual fashion. The use of a ¼-inch Penrose drain as a tourniquet is optional. If MTP joint surgery is

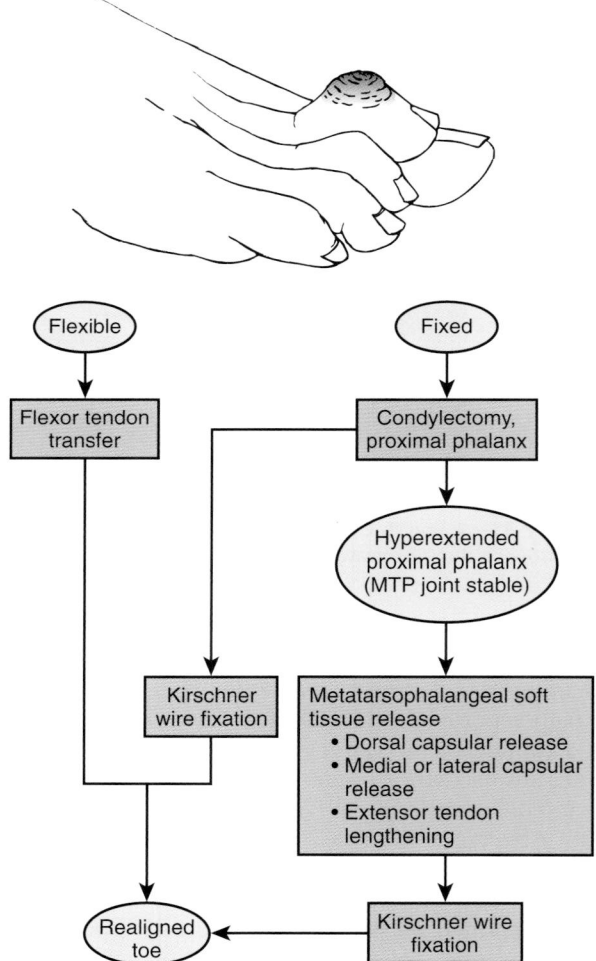

Figure 7-37 Algorithm for treatment of hammer toe deformity.

---

*References 2, 34-37, 45, 169, 210, and 212.

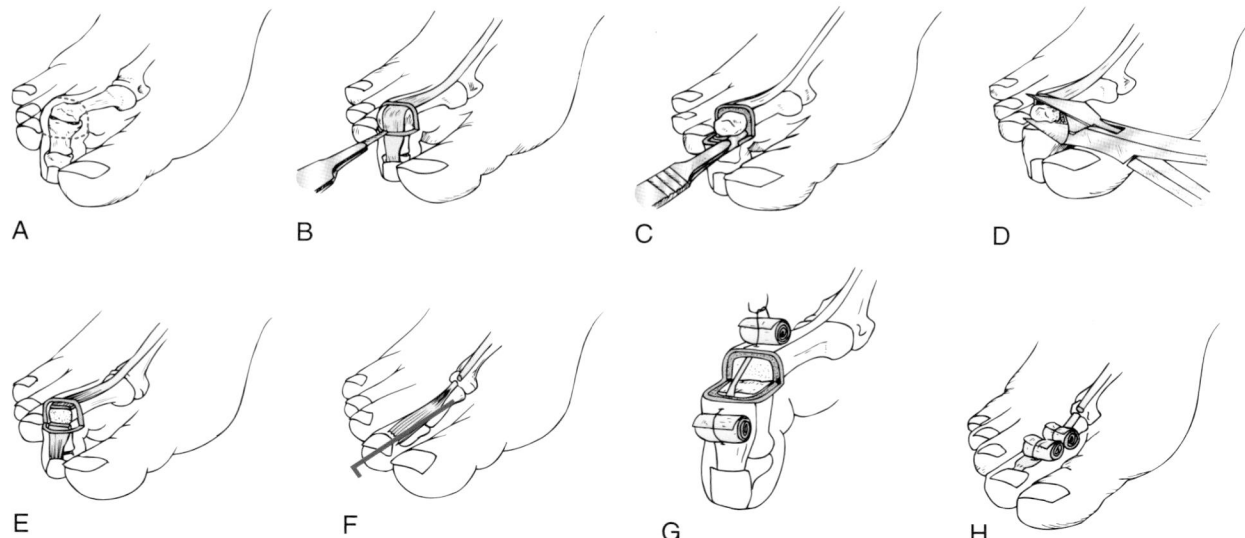

Figure 7-38 Technique for repair of a hammer toe deformity. **A,** Elliptic incision over the proximal interphalangeal (PIP) joint excises callus, if present, along with the extensor tendon and joint capsule. **B,** Removal of extensor tendon and joint capsule along lines of incision. **C,** When a knife blade is placed flat against the condyles, the collateral ligaments are cut, thereby delivering the head of the proximal phalanx into the wound. **D,** Excision of the head of the proximal phalanx proximal to the flare of the condyles. **E,** Condyles have been removed. At this time, a decision is made as to whether to perform a flexor tenotomy. If a flexor tenotomy is done, the plantar capsule is incised, and the long flexor tendon is incised in the depths of the wound. **F,** A 0.045-inch Kirschner wire is introduced at the PIP joint and driven distally, exiting the tip of the toe. The PIP joint is reduced, and the pin then is driven retrograde, stabilizing the repair. **G,** Alternative means of stabilization. Insertion of vertical mattress suture of 3-0 nylon. The deep portion of the suture approximates the extensor tendon, and the superficial portion of the suture coapts skin edges. The Telfa bolster is used to gain leverage to hold the toe in satisfactory alignment. **H,** The toe is held in satisfactory alignment after placement of sutures and bolsters.

performed, an Esmarch bandage can be used to exsanguinate the extremity and as an ankle tourniquet.[91] A digital block or regional anesthesia is used for anesthesia, depending upon the need for additional surgical procedures at the same time.

2. An elliptic or longitudinal incision[210] is centered over the dorsal aspect of the PIP joint, excising the callus, extensor tendon, and joint capsule, thereby exposing the PIP joint (Figs. 7-38A and 7-39A and Video Clip 75).

3. The collateral ligaments on the medial and lateral aspects of the proximal phalanx are severed to allow the condyles of the proximal phalanx to be delivered into the wound (see Figs. 7-38B and C and 7-39B and C). Care is taken to protect the adjacent neurovascular bundles.

4. The head of the proximal phalanx is resected just proximal to the flare of the condyles, and any prominent edges are smoothed with a rongeur (see Figs. 7-38D and 7-39D).

5. At this point, the toe should be brought into corrected alignment. If there still appears to be tension at the PIP joint, so that it is difficult to adequately correct the deformity, more bone should be resected. Also, consideration should be given to release of the flexor digitorum longus through this wound (see Figs. 7-38E and 7-33).

6. If a flexor tenotomy is performed, the plantar capsule of the PIP joint is carefully incised, and the long flexor tendon is identified in the flexor tendon sheath. The tendon is transected and allowed to retract.

7. The articular surface of the base of the middle phalanx may be resected with a rongeur.[221] This is optional.[35,45]

8. A 0.045-inch Kirschner wire is introduced at the PIP joint and driven distally, exiting the tip of the toe. With the toe held in proper alignment, the pin is driven in a retrograde fashion to stabilize and align the toe. The wire is then bent at the tip of the toe and the excess pin removed (see Figs. 7-38F and 7-39E). The Kirschner wire has enough flexibility that it can be bent at the operative site to alter the alignment when necessary.[68]

9. The wound is closed with vertical interrupted mattress sutures of 3-0 nylon (see Fig. 7-38F).

Alternative Fixation and Joint Preparation

A vertical mattress-type suture using 3-0 nylon and incorporating two Telfa bolsters is inserted. As the suture is tightened, a certain degree of leverage is placed on the toe to bring it into satisfactory alignment (Fig. 7-40, see Fig. 7-38G and H). This technique is much less commonly used. On the other hand, in an effort to secure permanent fixation without the use of Kirschner wires, several reports

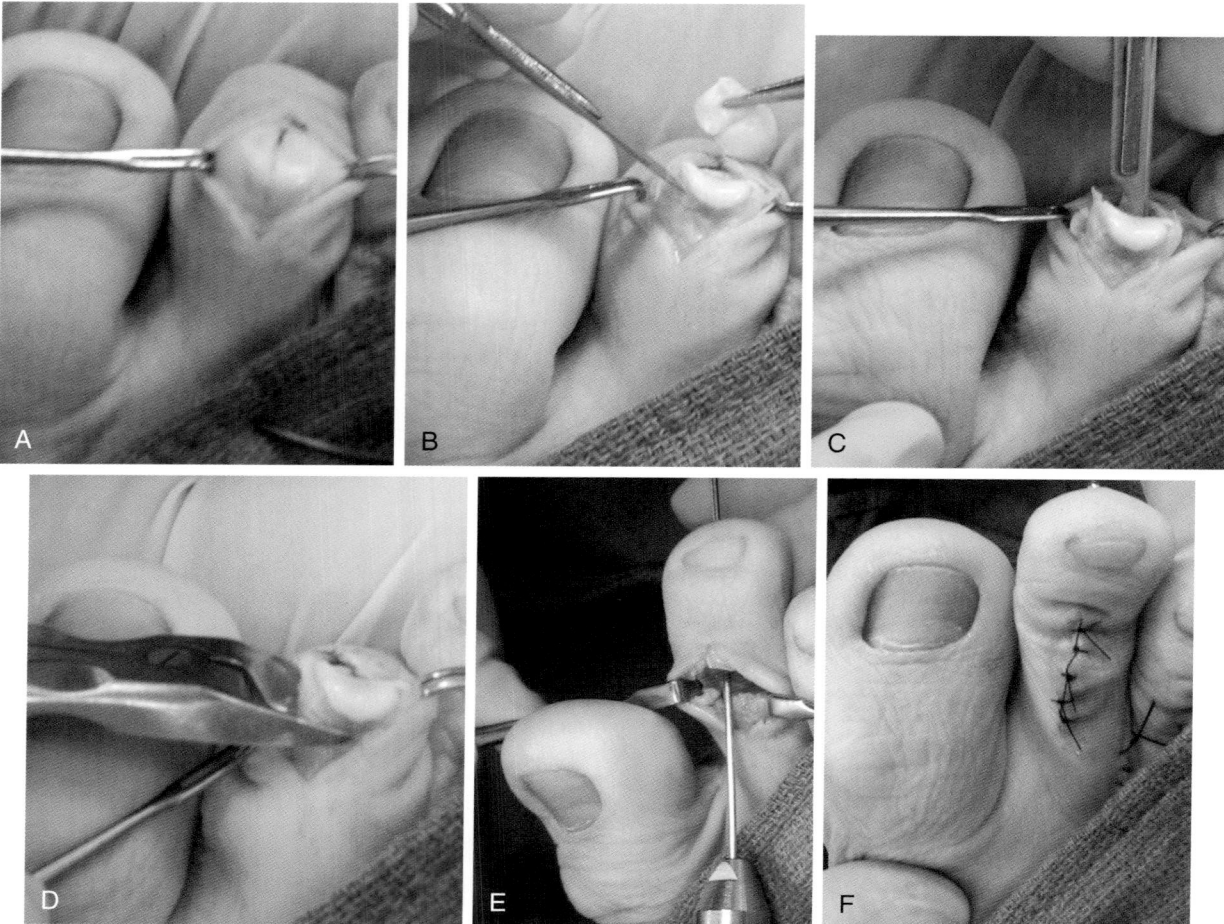

Figure 7-39 Hammer toe deformity of the second toe. **A,** After a longitudinal skin excision, the dorsal capsule and extensor tendon are exposed. **B,** Removal of extensor tendon and joint capsule along the lines of the incision. **C,** The collateral ligaments and plantar capsule are released. **D,** Exposing the condyles of the proximal phalanx, which are excised. (After excision of the head of the proximal phalanx, a flexor tenotomy may be performed; also, the articular surface of the base of the middle phalanx may be resected.) **E,** Kirschner wire fixation. **F,** After completion of repair.

have described the use of intramedullary fixation for hammer toe correction. Absorbable implants,[125,180] screw fixation[27,131,227] (Figs. 7-41 and 7-42), wire loops,[99] and other permanent intramedullary devices[2,69,193] (Fig. 7-43) have all been reported.

Weil[230] described the use of conical reamers for preparation of the joint surfaces to aid in achieving proper alignment and coaptation of the surfaces. No series have been published on this technique.

HAMMER TOE REPAIR WITH INTERMEDULLARY IMPLANT (NITINOL, SMART TOE IMPLANT)[2,193]
Surgical Technique

1. The patient is placed in a supine position on the operating room table. The foot is cleansed and draped in the usual fashion. The use of a ¼-inch Penrose drain as a tourniquet is optional. If MTP joint surgery is performed, an Esmarch bandage can be used to exsanguinate the extremity and as an ankle

tourniquet.[91] A digital block or regional anesthesia is used for anesthesia, depending upon the need for additional surgical procedures at the same time.

2. A longitudinal incision is centered over the dorsal aspect of the PIP joint. A daper elliptical incision excises the callus, extensor tendon, and joint capsule, thereby exposing the PIP joint (Fig. 7-44A and B and Video Clip 76).

3. The collateral ligaments on the medial and lateral aspects of the proximal phalanx are severed to allow the condyles of the proximal phalanx to be delivered into the wound (Fig. 7-44C). Care is taken to protect the adjacent neurovascular bundles.

4. The head of the proximal phalanx is resected at the metaphyseal–diaphyseal junction, and any prominent edges are smoothed with a rongeur (Fig. 7-44D and E).

5. If a flexor tenotomy is performed, the plantar capsule of the PIP joint is carefully incised, and the long flexor

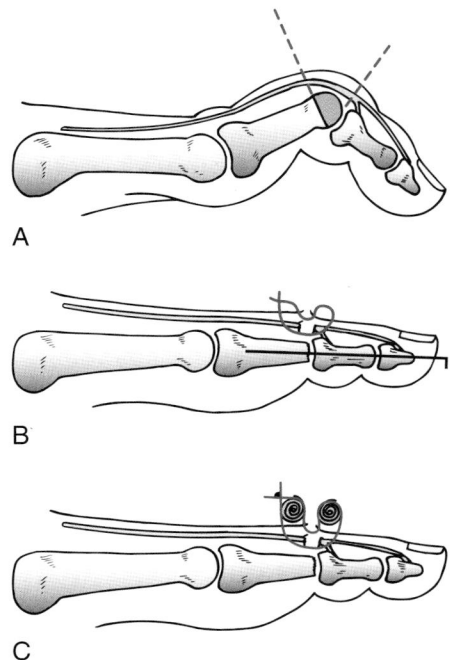

Figure 7-40 **A,** Proposed area of bone resection. **B,** After bone resection, stabilization with intramedullary Kirschner wire. **C,** Stabilization with sutures and Telfa bolsters.

tendon is identified in the flexor tendon sheath. The tendon is transected and allowed to retract.

6. The articular surface of the base of the middle phalanx may be resected with a rongeur.[193]

7. A 2-mm drill is introduced at the PIP joint and driven both proximally and distally (Figure 7-44F).

8. A broach enlarges each canal (Fig. 7-44G), and then the temperature-sensitive implant is removed from the refrgierated storage area and immediately inserted into the prepared intramedullary canal (Fig. 7-44H and I).

9. The middle phalanx is then positioned adjacent to the prepared surface of the proximal phalanx and held securely while the implant expands and stabilizes the digit. The position of the implant is verified under fluoroscopy (Fig. 7-44J).

10. The wound is closed with vertical interrupted mattress sutures of 3-0 nylon.

Postoperative Care

A small compression dressing is placed around the toe, and the patient is allowed to ambulate in a postoperative wooden shoe. If Telfa bolsters have been used, the suture and bolsters are removed 1 week after surgery. The bolsters should not be left in place for more than 1 week because of the possibility of skin necrosis developing beneath them. If a Kirschner wire has been used, the sutures and Kirschner wire are removed 3 weeks after surgery. In either case, it is important to support the toe with tape for the next 4 to 6 weeks after internal or external fixation has been removed. Localized trauma to the

digit in the first few weeks after surgery can lead to recurrent deformity and must be avoided.

Results and Complications

Ohm et al[170] reported on 25 patients (62 hammer toe repairs); hammer toes were corrected with a digital fusion technique. An equal number of corrections were performed on the second, third, and fourth toes. At short-term follow-up, a 100% fusion rate was reported. Newman and Fitton[169] reported on results in 19 patients treated with a similar technique and surprisingly noted only 40% satisfactory results.

Coughlin et al[45] reported on the results of a DuVries condylectomy in one of the largest studies (67 patients, 118 toes). Patients were evaluated at an average of 5 years after proximal phalangeal condylectomy, middle phalangeal articular resection, and intramedullary Kirschner wire fixation. Fusion of the PIP joint occurred in 81% of cases, and subjective satisfactory results were observed in 84% of cases. Pain relief in 92% of patients was no different in those with a fibrous or a bony union, although many reports suggest that a fibrous union is consistent with a successful outcome.*

O'Kane et al[171] reported their results with excisional arthroplasty in 75 patients (100 toes). They used suture fixation as opposed to intramedullary Kirschner wires and reported a high complication rate (31%). Although they did not report angular measurements, malalignment was a common occurrence (rotation, extension, axial plane malalignment), probably because of their lack of internal fixation. This lack of fixation allowed a higher rate of "toe-touch" with plantar flexion (mild recurrence) at the operative site. Suprisingly, patients were allowed, even with a lack of internal fixation, to return to regular shoes 2 weeks after surgery.

Higgs[104] stated that a fibrous union placed the digit at risk for recurrent deformity. This notion was not confirmed by Coughlin's series.[45] Although a PIP fusion is not necessarily the ultimate objective, increased stiffness or fusion of the PIP joint appears to help maintain alignment. Kelikian[121] observed that resection of both articular surfaces leads to a satisfactory result if it is followed by stiffness of the joint. The goal of surgery is to correct the deformity and maintain the correction.

Although some authors advocate attempted arthrodesis,[1,213,221,237] others have stated that a PIP joint resection suffices as treatment by achieving adequate alignment of the toe.[45,53,88,198] A fusion of the PIP joint or an arthrofibrosis succeeds by converting the pull of the flexor digitorum longus to flex the MTP joint. A fusion also gives triplanar stability to the toe. The rate of pseudoarthrosis in attempted PIP joint fusions approaches 50% in some series, although some surgeons have obtained a high fusion rate (>90%) with a peg-and-dowel technique.[1,135,202] Pichney et al and others[155,179] have used a V-type arthrodesis technique for correcting a hammer toe deformity

---

*References 53, 104, 122, 169, 170, 203, 206, and 228.

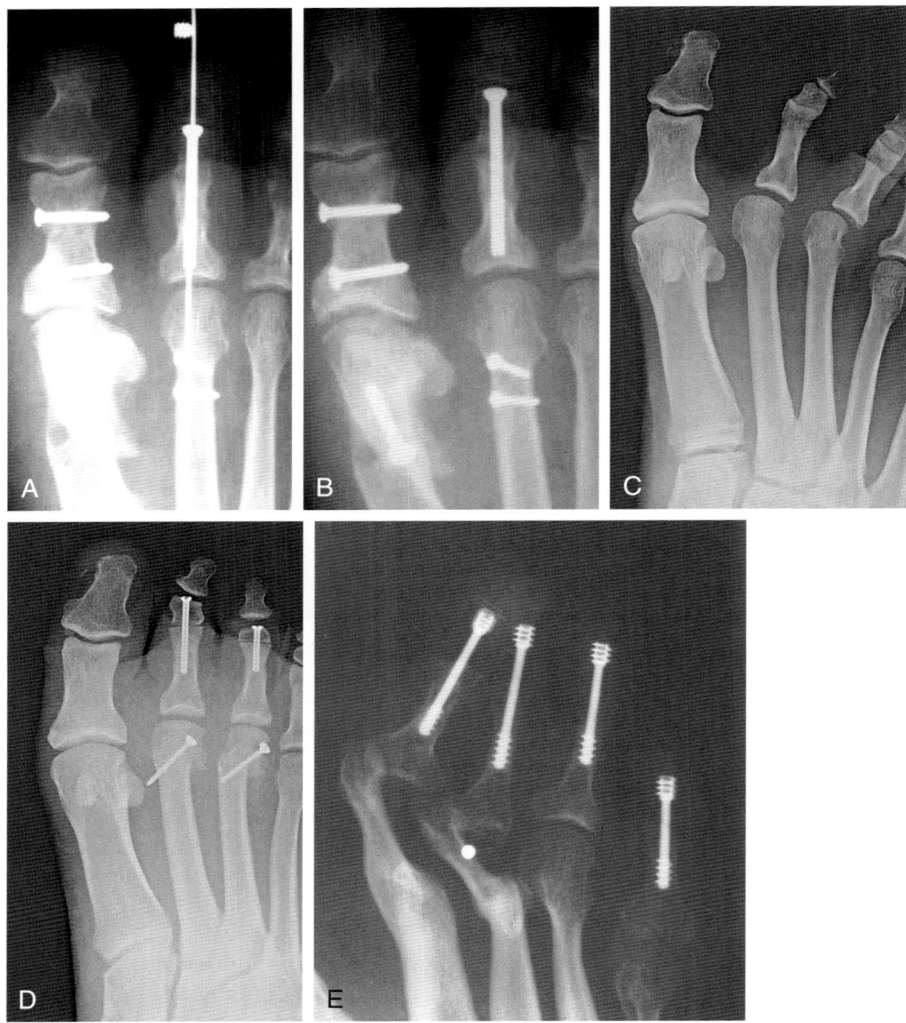

Figure 7-41 Examples on intramedullary screws for hammer toe fixation. **A,** Placement of intramedullary Kirschner wire and cannulated screw from the tip of the toe. **B,** Cannulated screw fixation. **C,** Preoperative radiograph demonstrating subluxation of second and third metatarsophalangeal (MTP) joints and hammer toes of second and third toes. **D,** After intramedullary hammer toe fixation and distal osteotomies of second and third metatarsals. **E,** Intramedullary Herbert-type screws placed from the tips of the toes for treatment of hammer toe deformities. Note marked lesser MTP joint subluxation. (**A** and **B,** From Lane G: Lesser digital fusion with a cannulated screw, *J Foot Ankle Surg* 44:172–173, 2005. Used with permission. **C** and **D,** Courtesy George Lane, DPM.)

with good success. Lehman and Smith[135] reported on PIP arthrodesis, noting a 50% satisfaction rate with a peg-and-dowel technique. Major reasons for postoperative dissatisfaction were toe angulation and incomplete relief of pain. Because of the straight nature of the fusion, toe tip elevation (a "floating toe") was noted in 14% of cases. Transverse plane angulation was observed in 11%. Forty-four percent of patients developed flexion at the DIP joint, a finding also noted by Schlefman et al[202] in their series. Ohm et al[170] and Schlefman et al[202] noted that more bone resection was necessary for a peg-and-dowel technique. Shortening, however, is a common complaint after this technique of hammer toe repair.

Any attempt at arthrodesis may place the digit in "too straight" a position. Although intramedullary devices

may increase the incidence of successful fusion, they may be predisposed to a straight toe that does not necessarily touch the ground and may be a source of dissatisfaction. On the other hand, the development of transverse plane deformities, which can occur with inadequate hammer toe fixation, are equally unpopular.

Attempts at more permanent fixation have been reported. Lane,[131] Caterini et al,[27] and Vitek[227] have reported the use of either a distally introduced intramedullary screw[27,131] or an oblique screw fixation[227] (see Figs. 7-41 to 7-43). Vitek[227] reported a 93% fusion rate. Caternini et al[27] reported a similar fusion rate; however, this technique sacrifices the DIP joint with fixation that crosses both interphalangeal joints. Konkel et al[125] reported the use of an absorbable intramedullary pin for

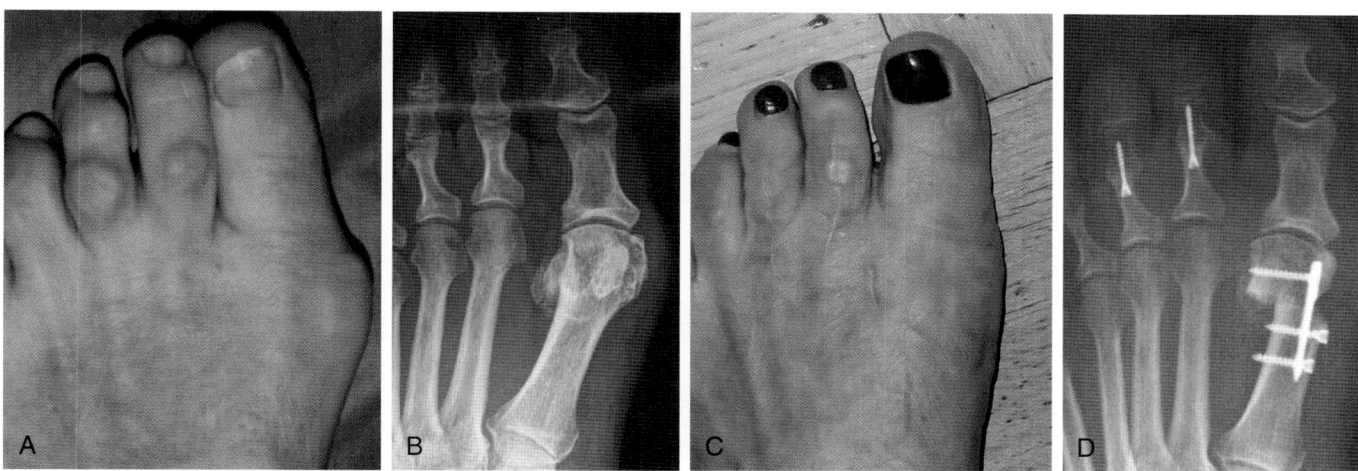

Figure-7-42 Example of screw fixation with hammer toe repair. **A,** Clinical preoperative photograph and, **B,** radiograph of hammer toe deformities of second and third toes. **C,** Postoperative clinical photograph and, **D,** radiograph after placement of oblique proximal interphalangeal joint screw fixation. (Courtesy M. Vitek, DPM.)

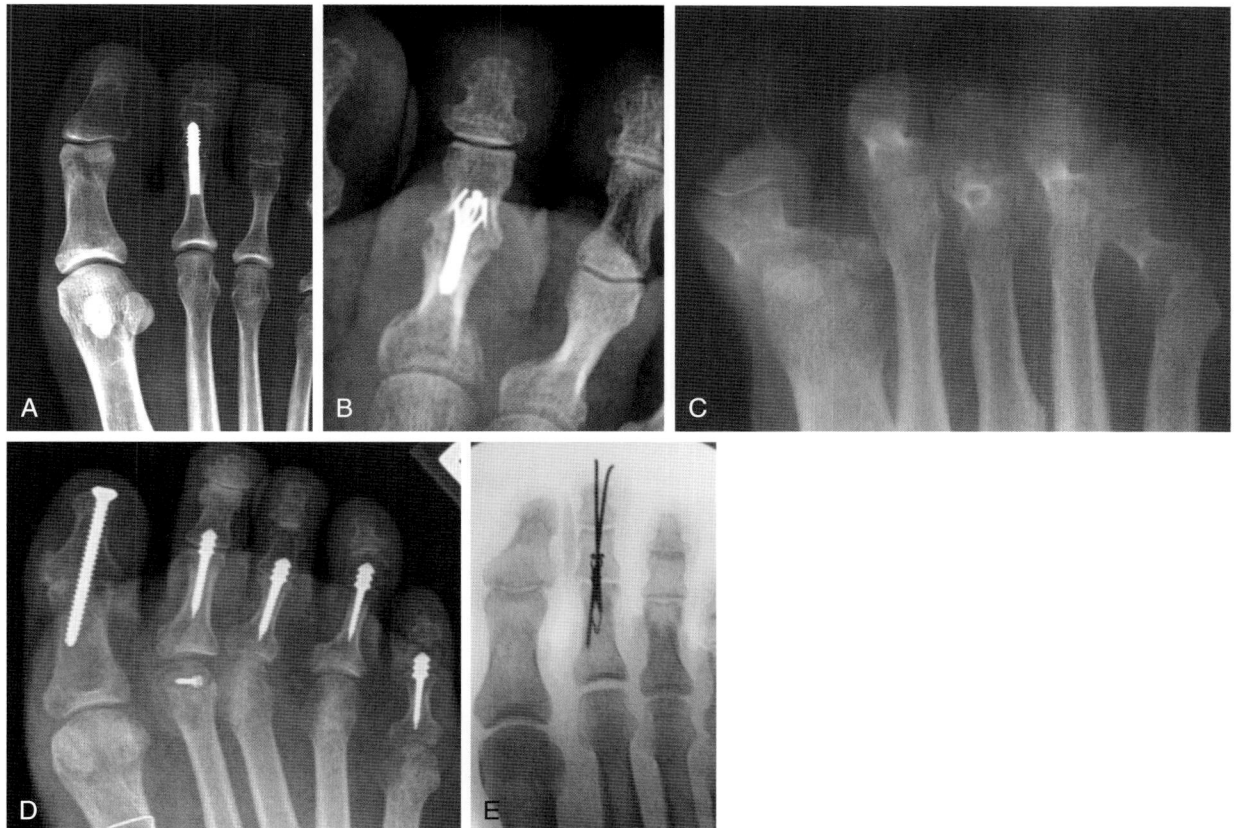

Figure 7-43 Examples of intramedullary fixation for hammer toe repairs. **A,** Stayfuse (Tornier, Minneapolis, Minn.), with correction of deformity. **B,** Ipp-On (Integra, Plainsboro, N.J.), with correction of deformity. **C,** Pro-Toe (Wright Medical, Memphis Tenn.), preoperative anteroposterior (AP) view. **D,** After implant placement in lateral four toes, with hallux interphalangeal (IP) joint arthrodesis. **E,** Smart Toe (Stryker, Kalamazoo, Mich.), with extra Kirschner wire fixation. (**A,** From Ellington JK, Anderson RB, Davis WH, et al: Radiographic analysis of proximal interphalangeal joint arthrodesis with an intramedullary fusion device for lesser toe deformities, *Foot Ankle Int* 31:372–376, 2010. Used with permission. **C,** Courtesy C. Hirose, MD. **D,** Courtesy T.J. Kemp, MD.)

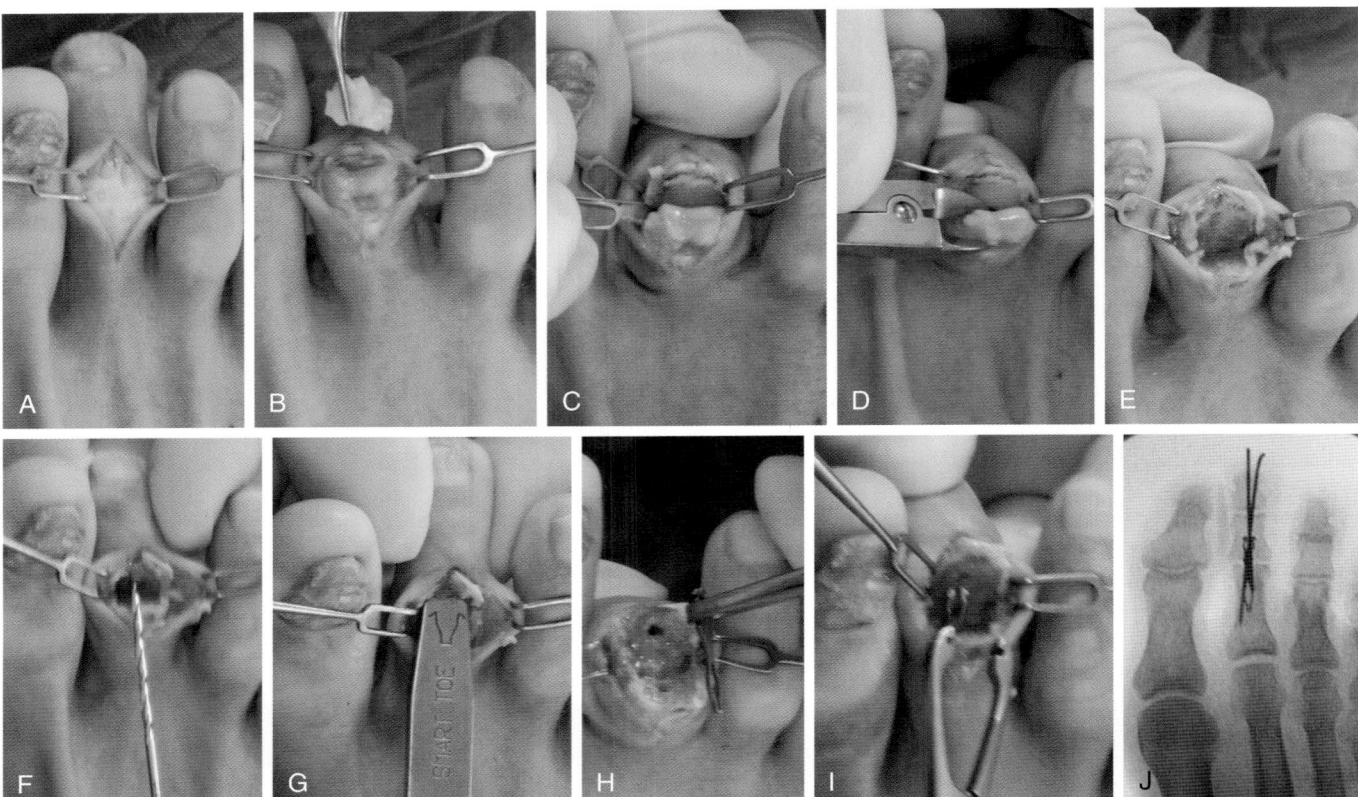

Figure 7-44 Hammer toe repair with Nitinol implant. **A,** Dorsal longitudinal incision. **B,** Excision of dorsal capsule. **C,** Release of collateral ligaments. **D,** Resection of condyles of proximal phalanx. **E,** Flat surfaces are created on both middle and proximal phalangeal surfaces. **F,** 2-mm drill hole is placed in each of the phalanges. **G,** The canals are broached. **H,** The implant is removed from refrigerated source. **I,** The implant is placed in the proximal phalanx and then placed in the middle phalanx. **J,** Postoperative fluoroscopy showing implant and additional Kirschner wire.

fixation of a hammer toe repair. A 73% union rate was noted. Three mallet toes and eight transverse plane deformities were reported, as well as a similar rate of "floating toes." Others have used an intramedullary implant placed at the operative site that does not traverse the DIP joint: the Smart Toe (Stryker, Kalamazoo, Mich.),[18,193] the Stayfuse (Tornier, Minneapolis, Minn.),[69] the Ipp-On (Integra, Plainsboro, N.J.), and the Pro-Toe (Wright Medical, Memphis, Tenn.). Ellington et al[69] reported a 60% union rate in 38 toes, and sagittal or coronal plane malalignment in 18% of cases (Fig. 7-45). Only three patients had revision surgery; the authors felt the implant assisted in maintaining alignment despite a union rate very similar to Kirschner wire fixation. Roukis[193] reported his results with the Smart Toe in 30 toes. The fusion rate was 93%; malunion occurred in 7%. No reports on the Pro-Toe have been published. The advent of intrameduallary fixation may reduce recurrence rate,* although these changes in technique and fixation will have to be weighed against the increased cost of the implants.

Malalignment is often a major reason for dissatisfaction.[45,68,125] Malalignment can occur in any one of three

planes–medial–lateral, dorsal–plantar, or rotational. Also, a hammer toe can develop in an adjacent nonoperated toe. A patient should be warned that there is a possibility of developing deformities in other toes. The development of a mallet toe deformity after a hammer toe repair is uncommon but can occur as well.[125,193] The results of hammer toe repairs are in general most gratifying, and few, if any, complications are routinely reported. Swelling of the toe can persist for 1 to 6 months after the procedure.[135,170,182] Almost invariably, however, the swelling subsides if given sufficient time (Fig. 7-46). Coughlin[45] noted that no patient had digital swelling at long-term follow-up.

Alternative treatments for hammer toe deformities include either a diaphysectomy or partial proximal phalangectomy (Fig. 7-47). McConnell[148,149] reported on a large series of patients treated with diaphysectomy of the proximal phalanx to correct a hammer toe deformity (Fig. 7-48). Satisfactory results were reported with this procedure. McConnell stated that "most cases heal by bony union." The actual alignment of the toe, complications, and rate of nonunion were not described in the report. A diaphysectomy is a useful procedure to treat a hammer toe and obtain shortening of a toe that is significantly longer than adjacent toes.

---

*References 2, 27, 69, 125, 131, 180, 193, and 227.

Partial proximal phalangectomy has been recommended by Johnson[114] and others[25,28,55,73] (Figs. 7-49 and 7-50) as a treatment for a hammer toe deformity in association with MTP joint deformity. Cahill and Connor[25] reported on 78 patients (84 toes). They noted poor objective results in 50% of patients and concluded that partial proximal phalangectomy relieved symptoms but left a cosmetically poor end result (Fig. 7-51). Conklin and Smith[30] noted a 29% postoperative dissatisfaction rate; major complaints were shortening of the ray, floppiness of the toes, metatarsalgia, weakness, and stiffness.

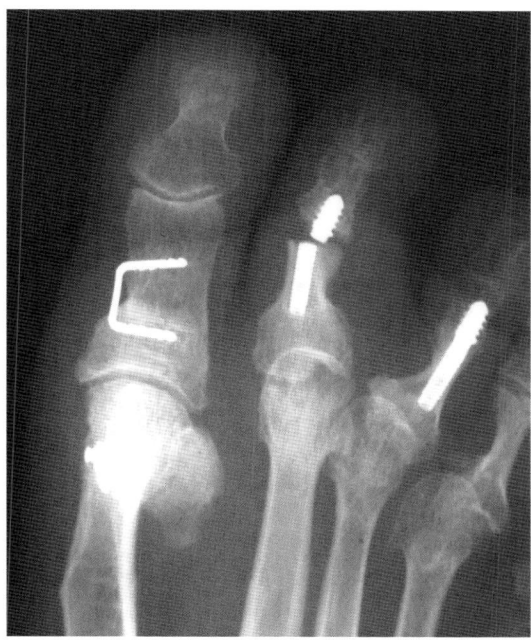

Figure 7-45 Broken implant with recurrent deformity. (From Ellington JK, Anderson RB, Davis WH, et al: Radiographic analysis of proximal interphalangeal joint arthrodesis with an intramedullary fusion device for lesser toe deformities, *Foot Ankle Int* 31:372–376, 2010. Used with permission.)

A limited syndactylization may be combined with a partial proximal phalangectomy of adjoining phalanges. Daly and Johnson[55] reported 75% patient satisfaction with this procedure; however, 43% of patients had moderate footwear restrictions, 27% reported residual pain, 28% noted moderate or severe cosmetic problems, and 18% reported a recurrent cock-up deformity. In general, the treatment of a hammer toe deformity by creating another deformity with a partial proximal phalangectomy and syndactylization should be discouraged except in a salvage situation.

Ely[70] believed a hallux valgus deformity would not progress after amputation of a second toe. Vander Wilde and Campbell[226] reported on 16 patients (22 feet) who underwent a second toe amputation. They observed mild progressive drift of the hallux but thought that it was usually not significant. Despite these reports, it is generally accepted that removal of the second toe can place the patient at risk for a progressive hallux valgus deformity in time. Amputation of the second toe may be an expeditious treatment for severe deformity in an elderly patient, but it is ill-advised in a younger patient because a hallux valgus deformity can progress (Fig. 7-52A, C, and D). Arthrodesis of the hallux MTP joint may be combined with a second toe amputation to ensure that a hallux valgus deformity will not progress with time (see Fig. 7-52E and F). Gallentine and DeOrio[82] reported on 17 amputations in patients averaging 78 years of age; 14 of 17 had a severe hallux valgus deformity, and absence of the toe was not an issue for them. They reported this to be a simple procedure with a predictable healing and recovery (Fig. 7-53).

Implants in the lesser toes have been reported by a number of authors. Shaw and Alvarez[209] reported on 672 implants placed over an 11-year period for hammer toe deformities. Several implants were removed for pain, infection, or implant failure. The authors* noted that the only true function of an implant in the lesser toe was to act as a spacer, and they found no difference between

---

*References 52, 79, 84, 151, 207-209, and 211.

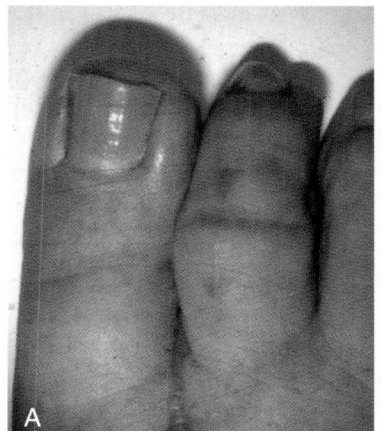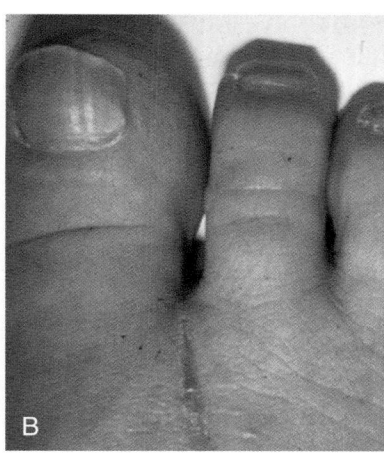

Figure 7-46 **A,** Postoperative swelling is common. **B,** With time, edema of the toe usually subsides. (From Coughlin MJ, Dorris J, Polk E: Operative repair of the hammertoe deformity, *Foot Ankle Int* 21:94–104, 2000. Copyright 2000 by the American Orthopaedic Foot and Ankle Society [AOFAS]; originally published in *Foot Ankle Int* 21:94–104, 2000. Used with permission.)

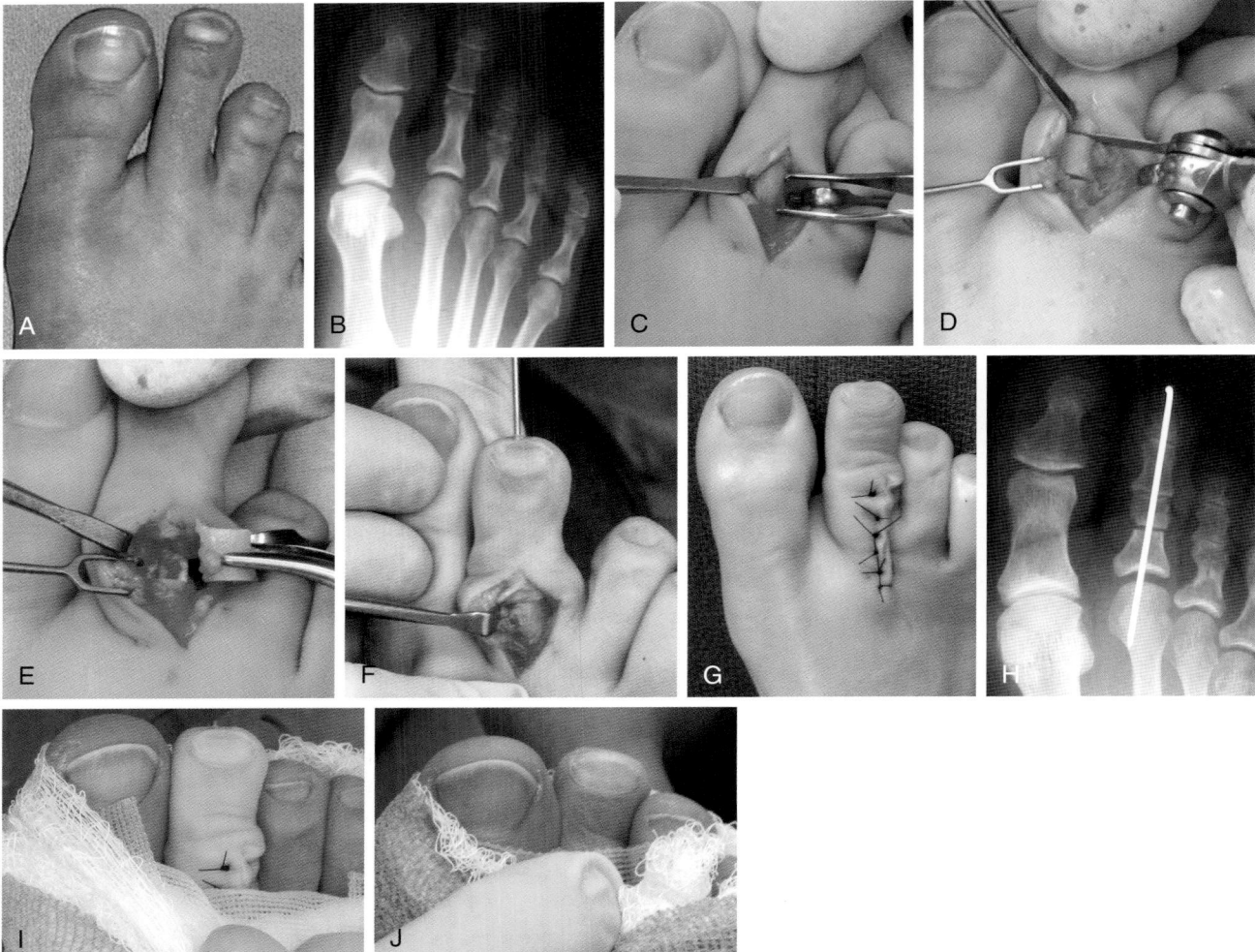

Figure 7-47 Excessively long second toe treated with diaphysectomy. Preoperative clinical **(A)** and radiographic **(B)** appearance. **C,** Dorsal phalangeal exposure with proposed excision. **D,** Sagittal saw is used for careful resection. **E,** Removal of 5-mm diaphyseal segment. **F,** Kirschner wire fixation. **G,** After skin closure. **H,** Postoperative radiograph demonstrating shortening of digit. **I** and **J,** Evaluation of postoperative vascularity is important. Capillary filling may be slow and should be monitored.

implants left in permanently and those removed at least 6 weeks after surgery.

Reports of hinged silicone joint replacement for hammer toe deformities have also been reported by Gerbert and Benedetti[84] and others.[207-209,211] Although these series reported a high level of satisfactory results, it is doubtful that the long-term results of PIP joint implants are significantly different from results of excisional arthroplasty. The risk of implant placement in this relatively subcutaneous area and the cost of the implant and surgical procedure make its use questionable when similar results are obtainable with excisional arthroplasty.

Cracchiolo et al[52] and others[79,151,208,211] have reported on the use of silicone implant arthroplasty in the lesser MTP joints (Fig. 7-54). Sgarlato[208] proposed silicone arthroplasty of the lesser MTP joints for a dislocated MTP joint, arthritis, a Freiberg infraction, congenitally shortened toes, bunionette deformity, and failed resection arthroplasty. Cracchiolo et al[52] reported on lesser MTP replacement arthroplasty in 31 feet (28 patients), noting acceptable results in 63%. Transfer metatarsalgia was the most common postoperative complication, but other complications included lesser metatarsal stress fracture, soft tissue infection, and implant failure. Cracchiolo et al[52] concluded that the implant aided in maintaining the joint in a reduced position but that there were strict limitations in the indications for silicone replacement arthroplasty. Fox and Pro[79] reported on a similar success rate (70%) with lesser MTP implant arthroplasty. Silicone replacement arthroplasty of the lesser MTP joints or lesser toes is rarely indicated and should be reserved for the occasional salvage procedure when other more standard techniques either are contraindicated or have been unsuccessful.

Recurrence of a hammer toe deformity is one of the most frustrating complications after surgery. Although excessive resection of bone should be avoided because it leads to a floppy and unstable toe (Fig. 7-55A and B), adequate bone resection is necessary to decompress the toe to obtain an adequate correction. In the face of recurrence, a flexor tenotomy may be necessary to achieve adequate correction. If sufficient bone has been excised and the flexor digitorum longus has been released when indicated, recurrent deformity rarely occurs. Placing two pins for fixation and leaving Kirchner wires for 4 to 5 weeks can help to successfully stabilize a toe after redo surgery.

After excessive bone resection, development of a flail toe is a most difficult complication to salvage.* Mahan[138,139] described a technique of bone graft stabilization of an iatrogenic flail second toe after unsuccessful hammer toe repair; however, this is an extensive reconstruction to perform on a lesser toe and should be reserved for a patient with significant symptoms (Fig. 7-55C to I). Friend[81] described a soft tissue repair using a V-Y skinplasty, soft tissue release, and partial metatarsal head resection to reconstruct an unstable flail lesser toe (Fig. 7-56).

The toe often assumes the shape of adjacent toes, a process termed *molding* (Fig. 7-57). Preoperative patient counseling about the possibility of molding usually alleviates postoperative concern on the part of the patient. If the great toe has an element of hallux valgus interphalangeus, the second toe will also probably have a slight

*References 81, 129, 138, 150, 163, and 179.

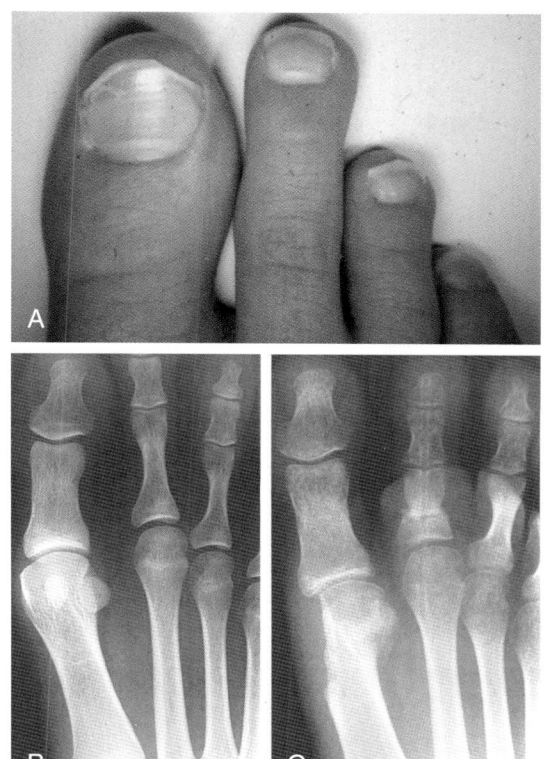

Figure 7-48 Preoperative clinical **(A)** and radiographic **(B)** views of patient with hammer toe symptoms and an unusually long second ray. **C,** Long-term radiographic follow-up.

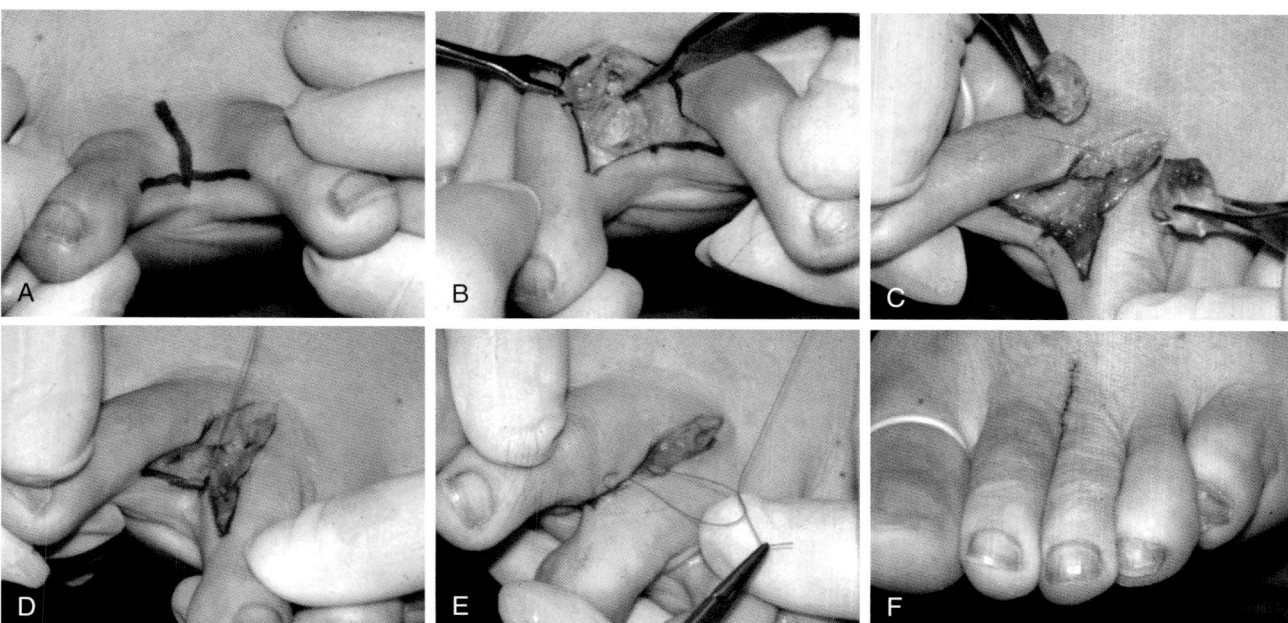

Figure 7-49 With a partial proximal phalangectomy, the base of the proximal phalanx is excised. Often, adjacent partial proximal phalangectomies are performed in combination with syndactylization. **A** and **B,** An intramedullary web space incision is made to approach the adjacent metatarsophalangeal joints. **C,** The bases of the proximal phalanges of the second and third toes have been excised. **D-F,** Closure of deep and superficial tissue. (Courtesy K. Johnson, MD.)

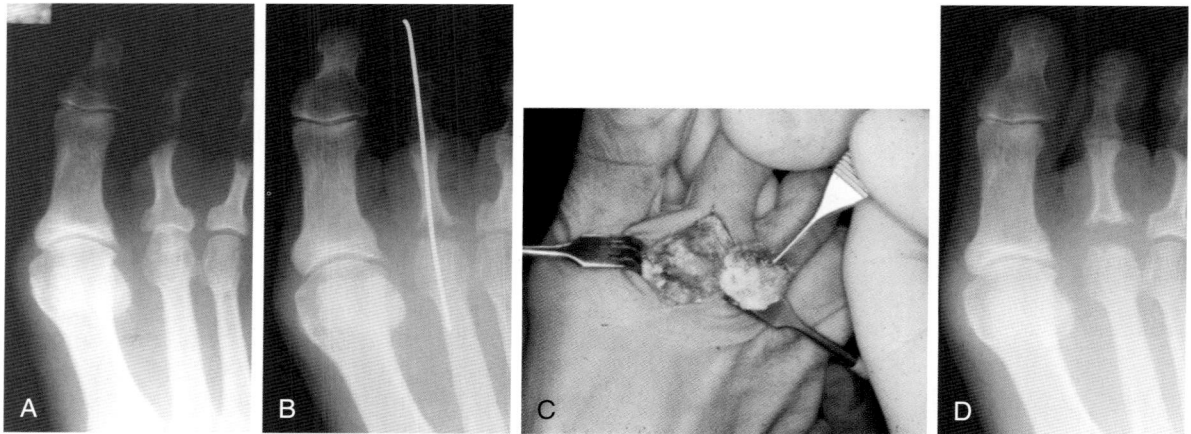

Figure 7-50 **A,** Painful degenerative arthritis of the second metatarsophalangeal joint. Radiograph demonstrates complete loss of the remaining joint space. **B,** After excision of the base of the proximal phalanx of the second toe, an intramedullary Kirschner wire is used to stabilize the repair until adequate healing is achieved. **C,** Intraoperative photograph after partial proximal phalangectomy. **D,** After removal of Kirschner wire.

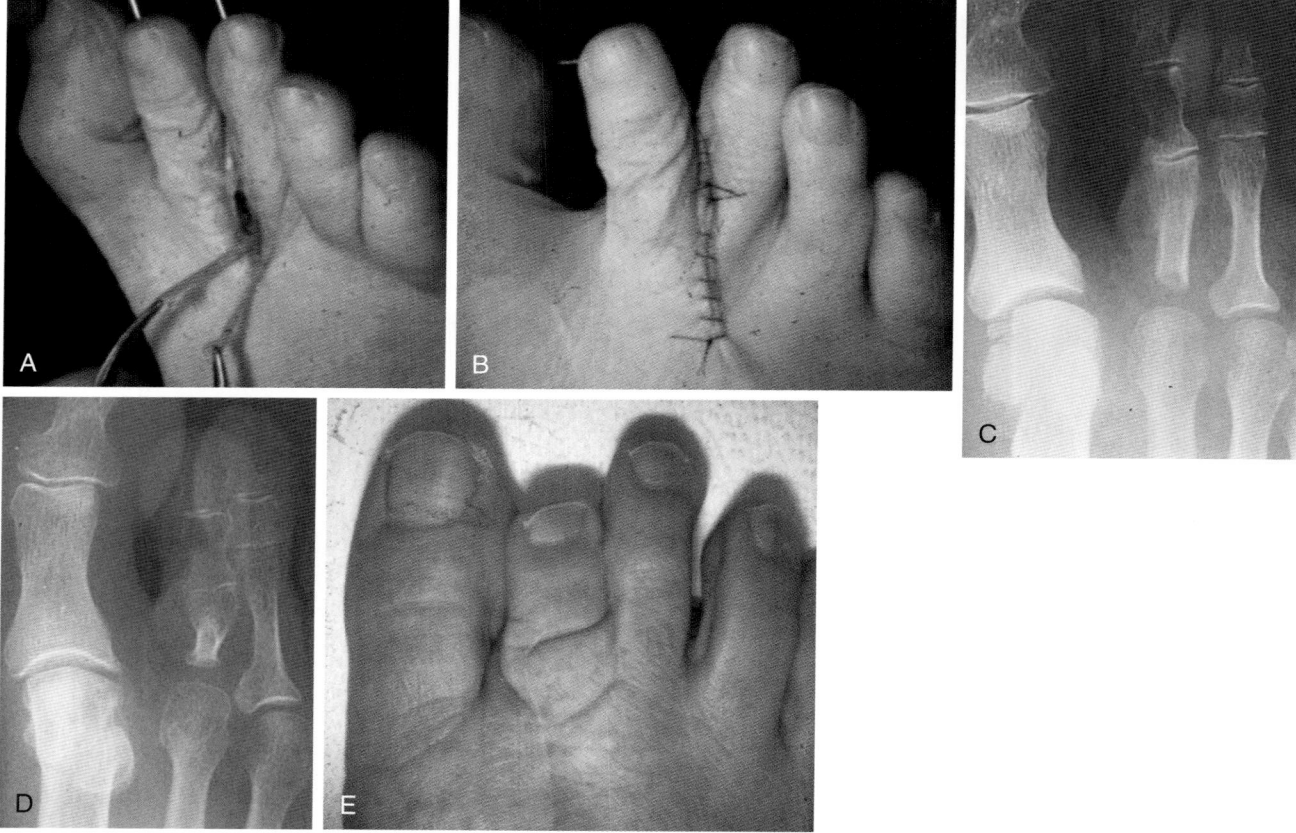

Figure 7-51 **A** and **B,** Intraoperative photographs after Kirschner wire fixation and syndactylization after partial proximal phalangectomy of the second toe deformity. **C,** Radiograph immediately after surgery. **D,** A radiograph 5 years postoperatively demonstrates severe shortening of the proximal phalanx with a varus deformity of the third toe. **E,** Cosmetically unacceptable syndactylization after partial proximal phalangectomy of only the second toe. (**E,** From Coughlin MJ: Lesser toe abnormalities, *Instr Course Lect* 52:421–444, 2003.)

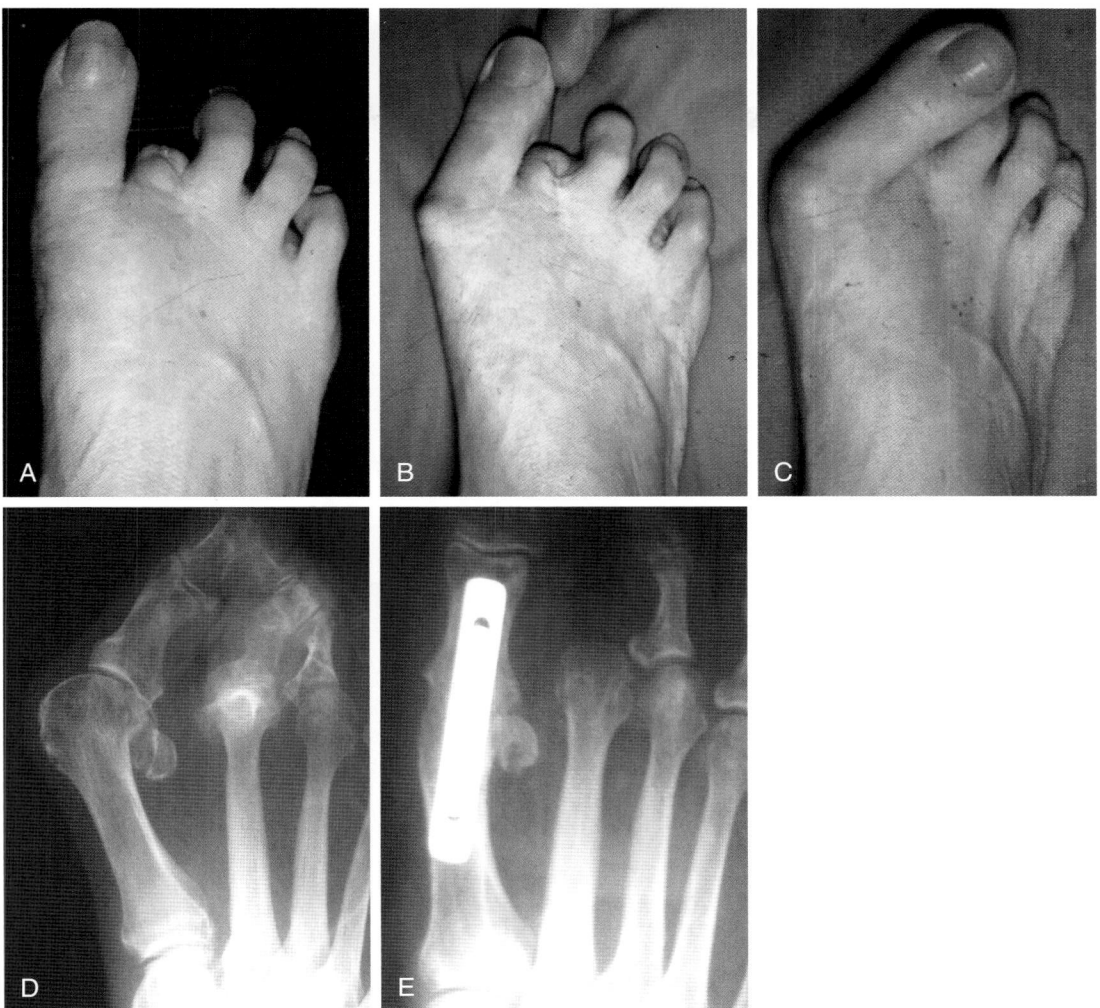

Figure 7-52 **A,** After amputation of second toe. **B** and **C,** Progressive hallux valgus after amputation of second toe. **D,** Preoperative radiograph with hallux valgus and dislocated second metatarsophalangeal (MTP) joint. **E,** After MTP fusion and second toe amputation.

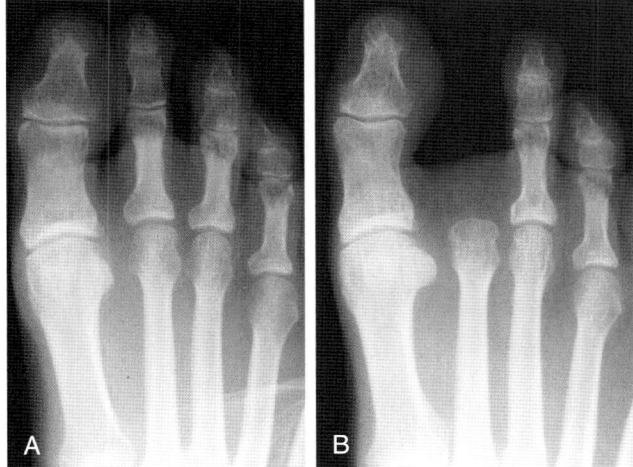

Figure 7-53 **A,** After multiple procedures to the second toe, soft tissue atrophy and chronic pain were associated with minimal metatarsophalangeal joint motion. **B,** A 3-year follow-up after second metatarsophalangeal joint disarticulation for chronic pain.

lateral curvature. It is not possible for a repaired hammer toe to remain straight when a deforming force is applied by the great toe or an adjacent toe (Fig. 7-58).

Kirschner wire fixation of hammer toe repairs was introduced by Taylor in 1940[215] to stabilize the correction. This remains the most popular technique of digital stabilization because of the ease of placement and removal, the maintenance of alignment,[189] and the increased stability after correction. Although complications such as pin tract infection (Fig. 7-59),* migration,[206,240,193] and breakage† have been observed (see Figs. 7-58G and H and Fig. 7-21), Zingas et al[240] reported a 2.5% failure rate when using 0.045-inch Kirschner wires for fixation of lesser toe deformities; however, they routinely left their Kirschner wires implanted for 6 weeks. A shorter period of implantation may in fact diminish the incidence of Kirschner wire failure. They noted the area of wire fracture

*References 1, 101, 170, 176, 177, 179, 188, 193, and 209.
†References 1, 43, 125, 170, 193, 202, and 240.

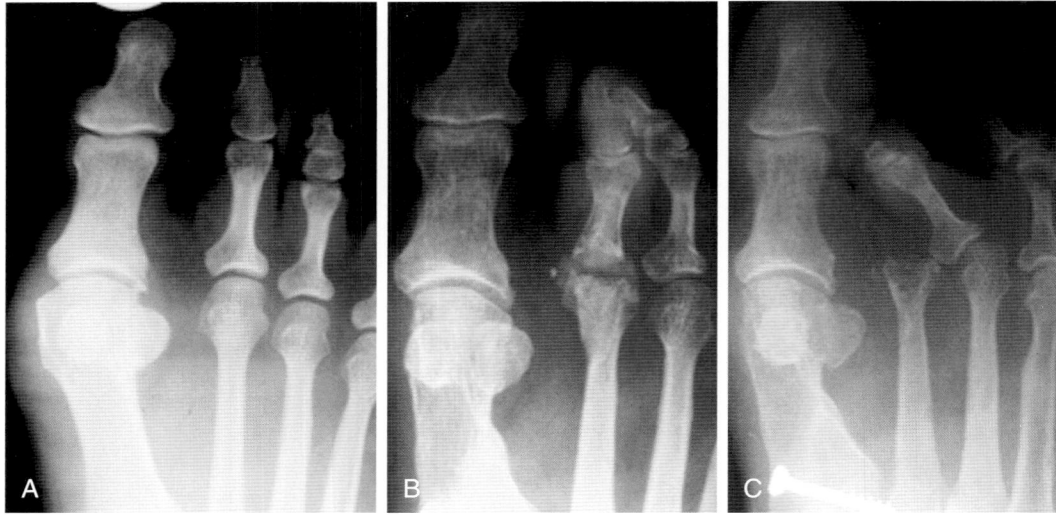

Figure 7-54 Second metatarsophalangeal (MTP) joint silicone implant arthroplasty. **A,** Mild hallux valgus deformity with painful second MTP joint. **B,** After first metatarsal osteotomy and placement of second MTP joint double-stem silicone implant. (The implant went on to failure, with eventual salvage with a second toe amputation.) **C,** At long-term follow-up, the lateral lesser toes have migrated medially.

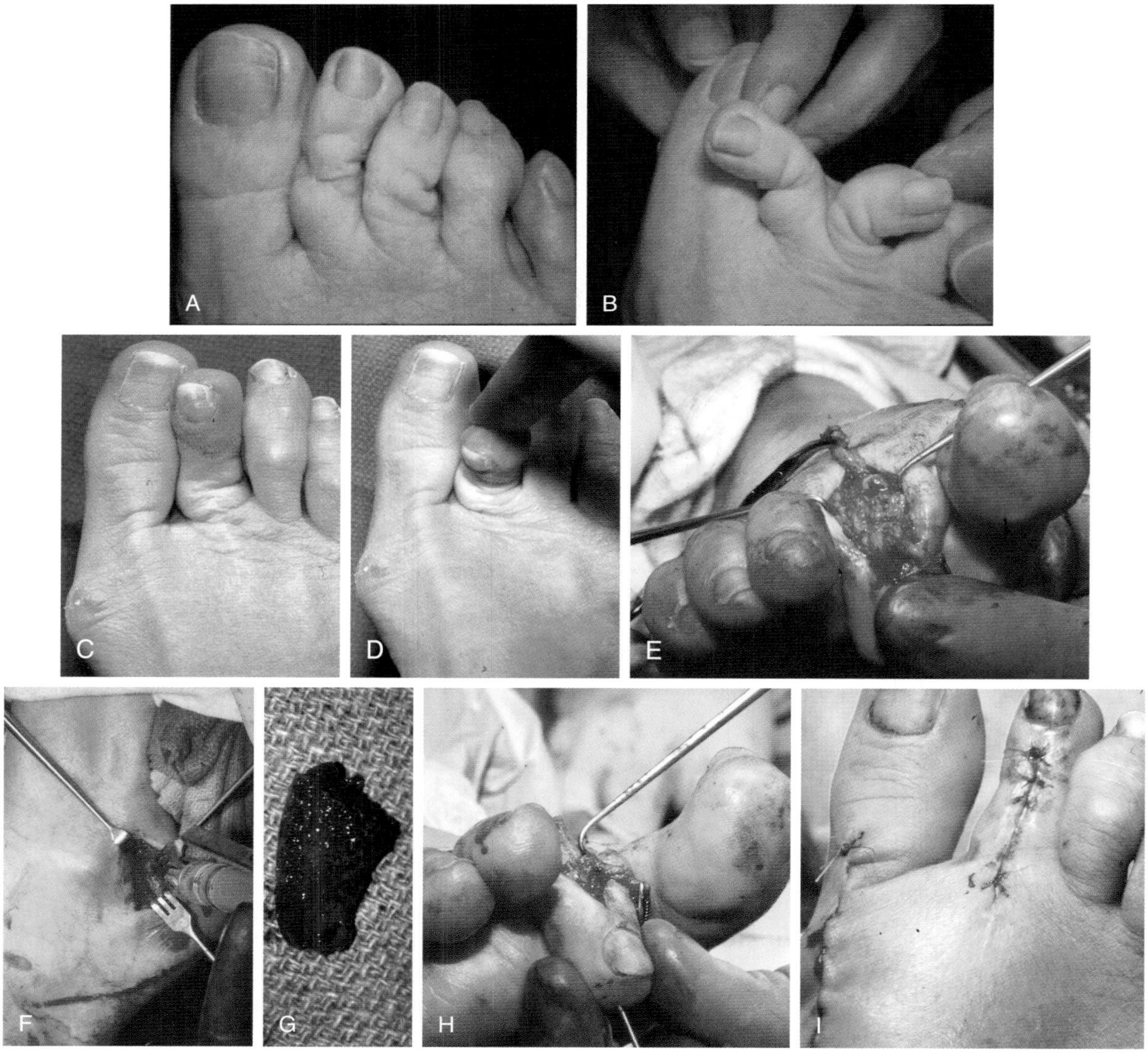

Figure 7-55 **A** and **B,** Excessive resection of bone can destabilize the lesser toes. **C** and **D,** Unstable second toe after excessive bone resection. **E,** Operative exposure of area of prior resection arthroplasty. **F,** Calcaneal exposure to obtain graft. **G,** Cylindric donor graft. **H,** Placement of graft. **I,** Final clinical appearance after interposition graft. Note adequate vascularity of digit. (**C-I,** Courtesy M.K. Mahan, DPM.)

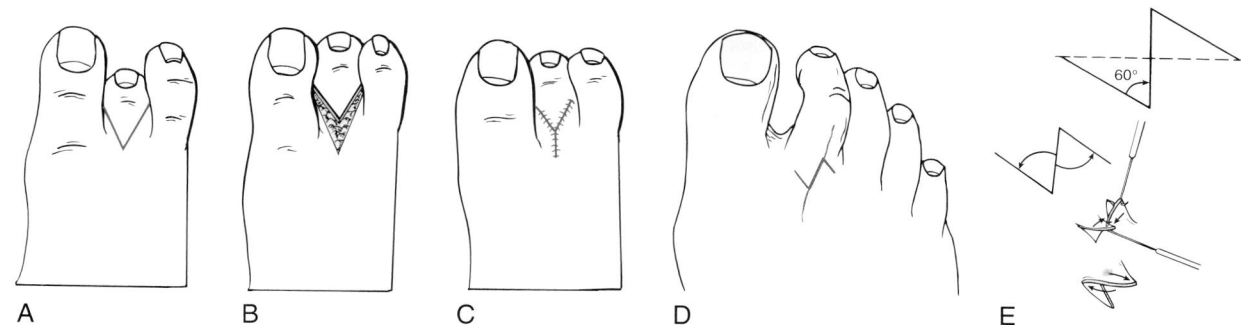

Figure 7-56 Soft tissue V-Y plasty for contracted lesser toe. **A,** Proposed V-shaped skin incision. **B,** Operative incision. **C,** Closure in Y fashion to lengthen the lesser toe. **D** and **E,** Z-plasty to correct contracted lesser toes.

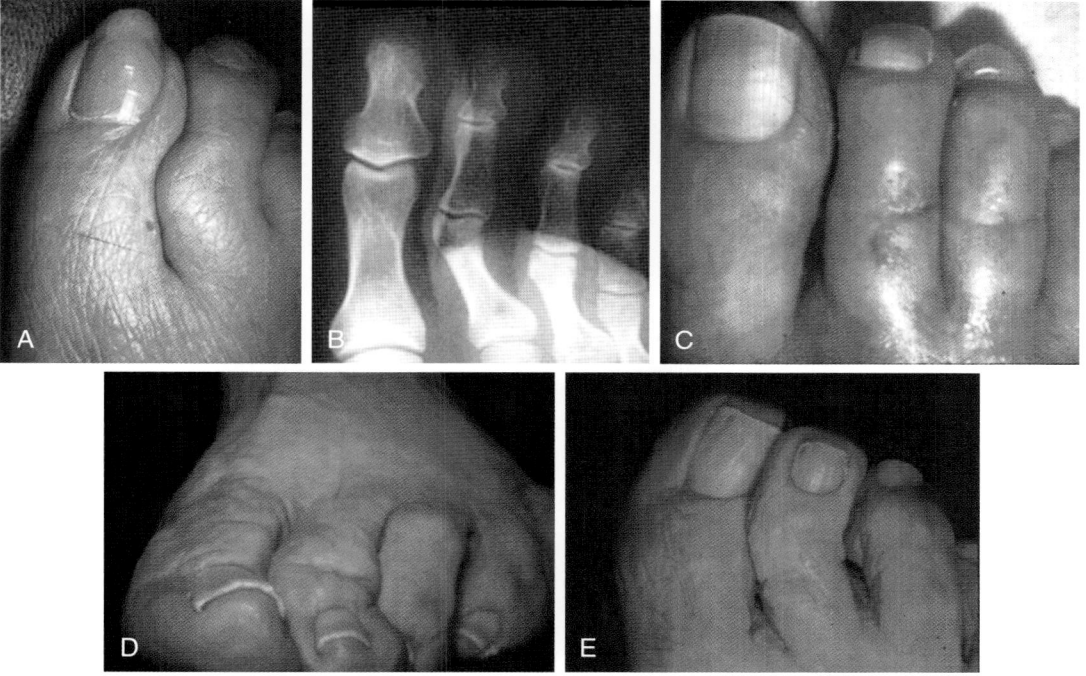

Figure 7-57 Molding of adjacent toes. Preoperative clinical examination **(A)** and radiograph **(B)** demonstrate molding of second toe. **C,** Molding of the second and third toes often occurs immediately after surgery but resolves with diminution of swelling. **D** and **E,** Molding of second toe after hammer toe repair. **(E,** From Coughlin MJ: Lesser toe abnormalities, *Instr Course Lect* 52:421–444, 2003.)

occurred a few millimeters proximal to the metatarsal head but was rarely symptomatic. Wires can be bent at the operative site after placement to improve digital alignment.[68] An 18% infection rate was reported by Reece[188] when Kirschner wires were left in place 6 weeks or more. In Coughlin's series,[45] only 3 of 118 toes developed a pin tract infection, and all resolved after pin removal. Kirschner wires were removed routinely 3 weeks after surgery. Herstik et al,[101] in a large review of lesser toes stabilized with Kirschner wires, reported an even lower infection rate (<1%). He attributed those infections mostly to skin contamination.

Other uncommon complications include postoperative numbness caused by injury of an adjacent sensory nerve,[45,170] subsequent mallet toe deformity,[2,45,125,193,202]

and decreased MTP range of motion.[170] On rare occasions, patients develop discomfort at the site where a pseudoarthrosis has developed. In these unusual cases, an injection of a corticosteroid usually gives lasting relief. If this is unsuccessful, revision hammer toe repair may be necessary to achieve bone union, with consideration of permanent intrameduallary fixation.

FLEXIBLE HAMMER TOE DEFORMITY

The patient with a flexible or dynamic hammer toe has a deformity when standing. Practically no deformity is present when the patient sits on the examining table with the foot in an equinus position. The deformity can then

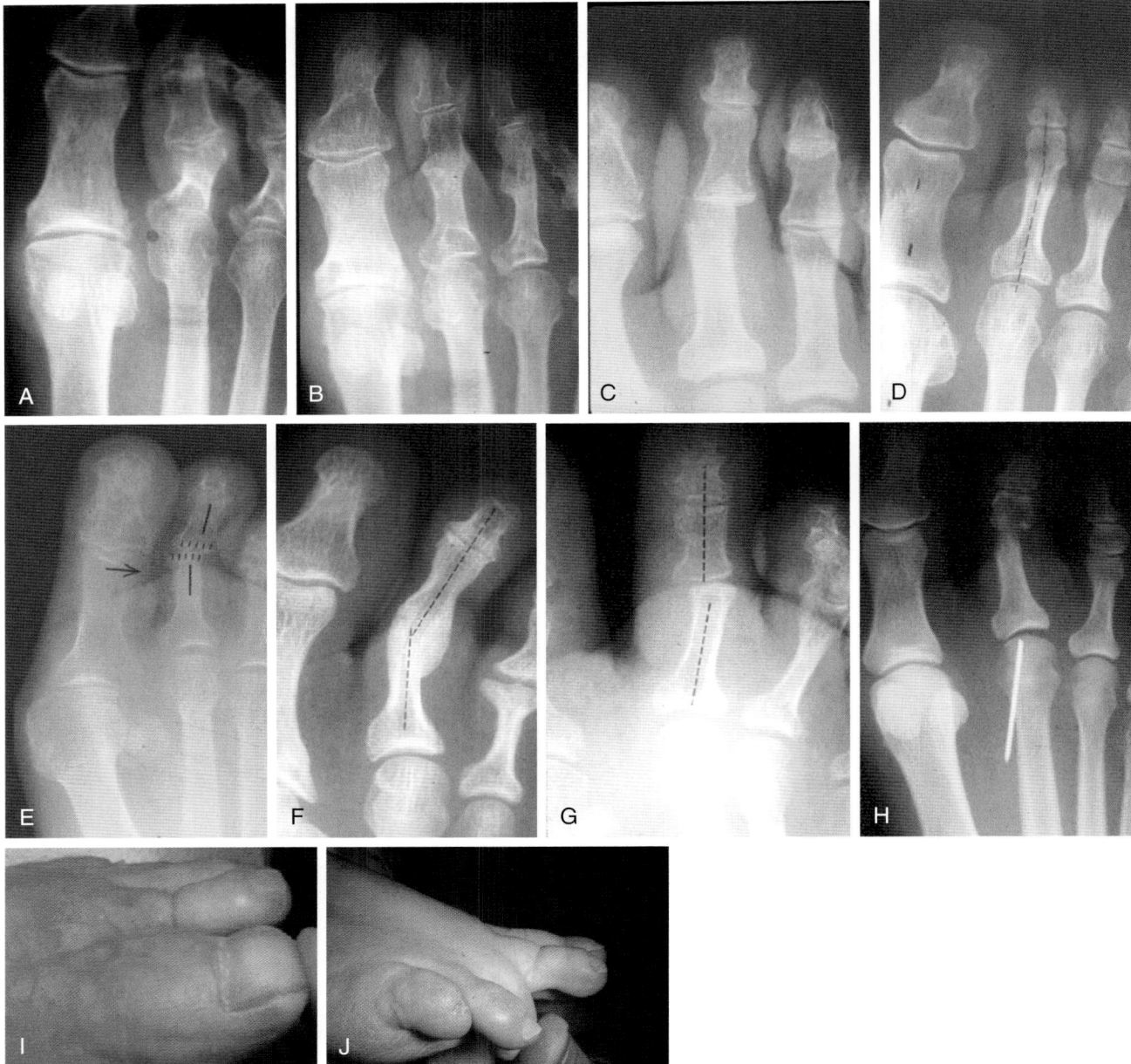

Figure 7-58 After hammer toe repair. **A,** Preoperative radiograph of second hammer toe with metatarsophalangeal joint (MTP) subluxation. **B,** After realignment. **C,** Lateral translation after hammer toe repair, with later development of interdigital corn. **D,** Mild medial angulation with satisfactory result; a successful arthrodesis resulted. **E** and **F,** Lateral deviation of the digit after hammer toe repair caused by pressure from an adjacent hallux valgus deformity. Both patients were dissatisfied. **G,** Medial deviation with fibrous union. **H,** A broken Kirschner wire at the MTP joint. Although the hammer toe repair was satisfactory, the MTP joint became malaligned. **I** and **J,** Hyperextension deformity after hammer toe repair. (**A, B, D, F, G,** and **I,** From Coughlin MJ, Dorris J, Polk E: Operative repair of the hammertoe deformity, *Foot Ankle Int* 21:94–104, 2000. Copyright 2000 by the American Orthopaedic Foot and Ankle Society [AOFAS]; originally published in *Foot Ankle Int* 21:94–104, 2000. Used with permission.)

be reproduced by dorsiflexion of the ankle joint and with pressure placed beneath the metatarsal heads. These patients do not have the classic claw toe deformity because the MTP joint is not involved. The deformity appears to be caused by a contracture of the flexor digitorum longus tendon.

This deformity may be corrected by a flexor tendon transfer. Although Girdlestone[87] is often cited as the originator of the split flexor digitorum longus tendon transfer to the dorsum of the proximal phalanx, he did not report a surgical technique to correct clawed or hammered toes; rather, he discussed the concept of a loss of intrinsic

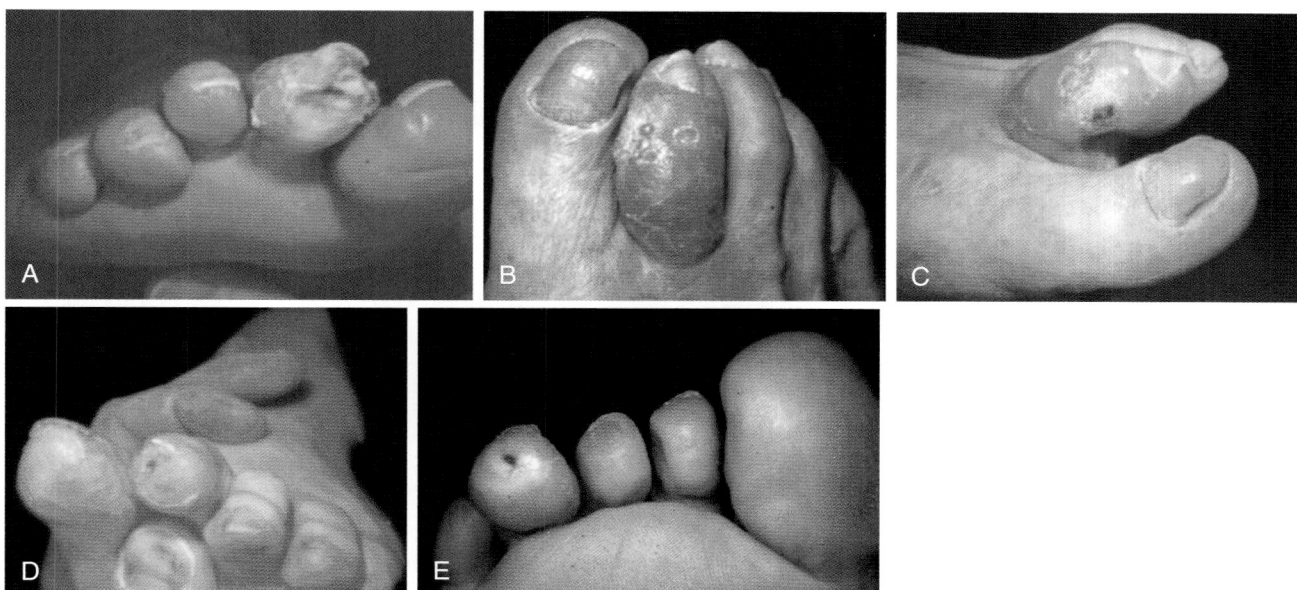

Figure 7-59 A, Severe infection in toe pulp after hammer toe repair. **B** and **C,** Infection of second toe after hammer toe repair. **D** and **E,** Pin tract infection after hammer toe repairs.

muscle function that leads to clawing of the toes. Taylor[215] also is commonly credited with describing a flexor digitorum longus transfer; however, the surgical technique that he described has evolved significantly. The use of either of the eponyms Girdlestone or Taylor to describe this procedure as it is currently used is no longer appropriate.[218]

Preoperative Planning

The theory behind the flexor tendon transfer is that the transfer enables the flexor digitorum longus tendon to assume the function of the intrinsics (i.e., plantar flexion of the MTP joint and extension of the interphalangeal joints). Merely sectioning the flexor digitorum longus usually is not sufficient to straighten the toe in these patients and sacrifices a usable tendon. The flexor tendon transfer realigns the toe at the cost of prehensile action, which has been found to be an annoying problem for some patients. Often a patient has an absence or loss of active toe flexor power at the time of the flexor tendon transfer, and the patient commonly retains passive, but not active, toe function. Major complaints include restricted interphalangeal and metatarsophalangeal joint motion and loss of active flexor digitorum longus function to the other lesser toes.

Indications

A flexor tendon transfer is indicated for primary treatment of a flexible hammer toe. It may also be used in combination with other surgical techniques in the treatment of claw toes and toes that demonstrate instability of a lesser

MTP joint. Also, it may be used as a component of the repair for MTP joint plantar plate insufficiency or a crossover second toe deformity.[168]

Contraindications

A flexor tendon transfer is contraindicated as a primary treatment of a fixed hammer toe deformity.

TENDON TRANSFER PROCEDURE[35,43]
Surgical Technique

1. The foot is cleansed and draped in the usual fashion. The foot is exsanguinated with an Esmarch bandage. An Esmarch bandage may be used as a tourniquet above the level of the ankle (Fig. 7-60A and Video Clip 77).[91]
2. Under tourniquet control, a 5-mm transverse incision is made on the plantar aspect of the foot at the level of the proximal plantar flexion crease of the toe. The soft tissue is spread, and the flexor tendon sheath is identified.
3. The flexor tendon sheath is split longitudinally. Visualization of the contents of the sheath demonstrates three tendons. The flexor digitorum longus is the central of these three tendons, is larger, and is characterized by a midline raphe (Fig. 7-60B).
4. A small curved mosquito clamp is placed into the wound, and the flexor digitorum longus tendon is brought out under tension. Percutaneously, the long flexor tendon is released from its insertion into the plantar base of the distal phalanx (Figs. 7-60C and 7-61A).

353

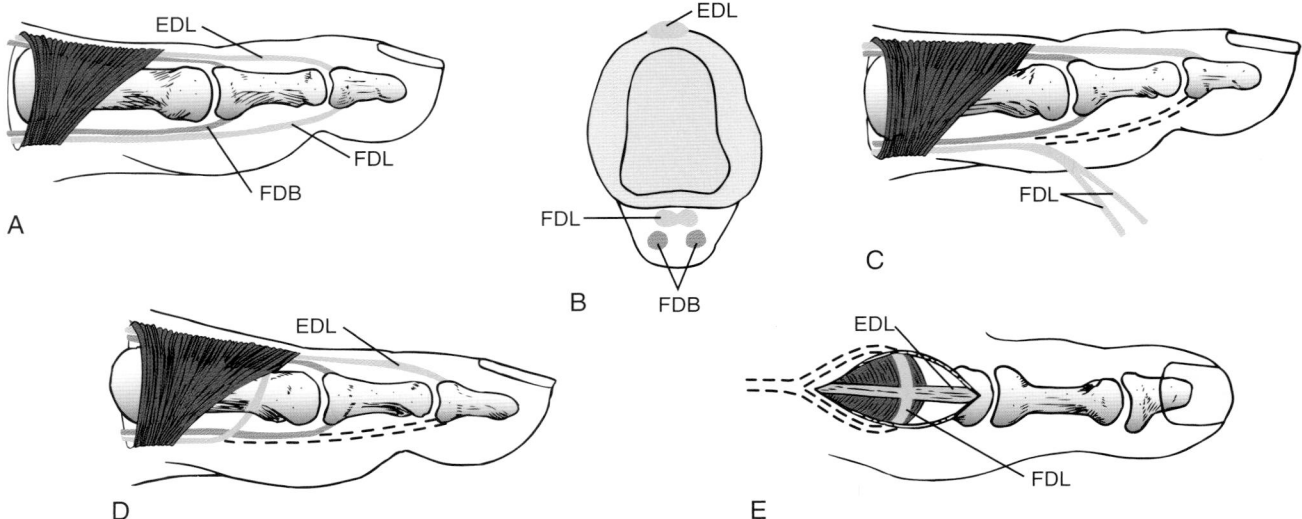

Figure 7-60 Technique for correction of dynamic hammer toe. **A,** Lateral view of lesser toe demonstrates the anatomy of flexor and extensor tendons. **B,** Cross-section anatomy through the metatarsal head region. Note that the flexor digitorum longus (FDL) is deeper than the flexor digitorum brevis (FDB). The FDL is characterized by a midline raphe. **C,** The FDL tendon has been detached from its insertion into the base of the distal phalanx and delivered into the plantar wound at the base of the toe. The tendon is then split longitudinally along its raphe, producing two tails. **D,** The FDL is delivered on either side of the extensor hood through a subcutaneous tunnel. **E,** The FDL is sutured into the extensor digitorum longus (EDL) tendon under moderate tension, and the metatarsophalangeal joint is held in approximately 20 degrees of plantar flexion.

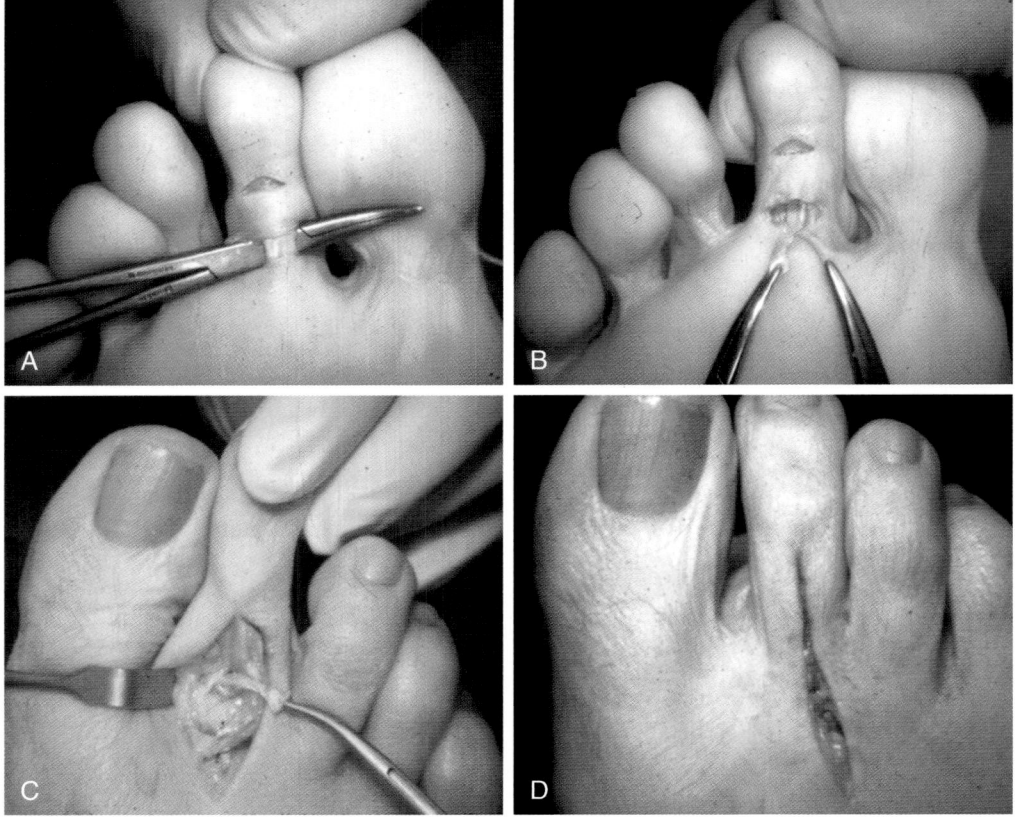

Figure 7-61 **A,** Plantar view demonstrates the flexor digitorum longus (FDL) tendon beneath the mosquito hemostat. Note the distal puncture wound releasing the long flexor tendon. **B,** The two limbs of the FDL tendon have been delivered through the more proximal plantar wound and split longitudinally. **C,** Each limb of the FDL is delivered on either side of the proximal phalanx and sutured to the extensor expansion with the toe in a corrected position. **D,** Final position of the corrected toe.

5. The raphe or decussation in the flexor digitorum longus tendon is noted, and the tendon is split longitudinally, creating two tails (see Figs. 7-60C and 7-61B).

6. Attention is directed to the dorsal aspect of the toe, where a longitudinal incision is centered over the proximal phalanx. A mosquito hemostat is passed in a dorsal to plantar direction along the extensor hood, deep to the neurovascular bundle but superficial to the extensor hood, exiting at the plantar incision.

7. The tails of the flexor digitorum longus tendon then are passed dorsally on the medial and lateral aspects of the extensor hood in the midportion of the proximal phalanx (see Figs. 7-60D and 7-61C).

8. With the toe placed in approximately 20 degrees of plantar flexion at the MTP joint, the flexor tendon is sutured to the extensor digitorum longus tendon under a slight degree of tension (see Figs. 7-60E and 7-61D).

9. If a Kirschner wire is used to stabilize the toe, it should be used only to reinforce the repair. If it is used to realign the toe, the deformity can recur when the pin is removed. If a Kirschner wire is used, it is introduced into the MTP joint through a dorsal capsule incision made to expose the base of the proximal phalanx. The pin is driven distally and exits through the tip of the toe. The pin is then driven in a retrograde fashion across the MTP joint.

10. The wounds are closed and a gauze-and-tape compression dressing is applied.

Alternative Technique

Kuwada[126,127] has described a modification of the flexor tendon transfer. After the flexor digitorum longus tendon is detached distally on the plantar aspect, it is transferred through a tunnel in the proximal phalanx and secured to the extensor digitorum longus tendon with interrupted sutures (Fig. 7-62). Gazdag and Cracchiolo[83] have reported no substantial difference between flexor tendon transfer techniques using circumferential tendon transfer or transfer through a central drill hole.

Postoperative Care

The patient is allowed to ambulate in a postoperative shoe. Dressing changes are performed weekly until the wound has healed. If a Kirschner wire has been placed, it is removed 3 weeks after surgery. Sutures are removed 3 weeks after surgery. The toe then is taped in correct alignment for an additional 3 to 6 weeks. Passive manipulation of the toe is begun 6 weeks after surgery and the patient is permitted to resume activities as tolerated.

Results and Complications

A flexor tendon transfer usually provides satisfactory correction not only for patients with an idiopathic flexible hammer toe but also for patients with cerebral palsy, patients who have had cerebral vascular accidents or a compartment syndrome, and patients with associated

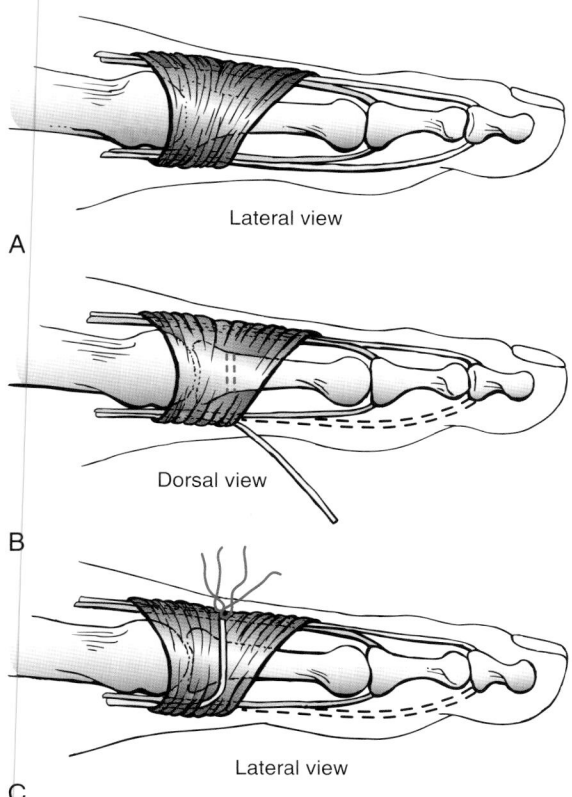

Figure 7-62 Kuwada technique. Flexor tendon transfer through a drill hole in the proximal phalanx. **A,** Lateral view. **B,** Dorsal view. **C,** After transfer of the flexor digitorum longus through a drill hole. The tendon is sutured to the extensor expansion of the extensor digitorum longus.

neuromuscular diseases such as Charcot-Marie-Tooth disease.[55] It is important for the surgeon to remember that if a fixed contracture is present, this procedure alone does not produce a satisfactory result. A flexor tendon transfer, however, may be used in association with other procedures of the lesser toe to achieve realignment of the MTP joint.

Reports by Taylor,[215,216] Pyper,[184] Boyer,[19] and others[175,218] have noted inconsistent levels of satisfaction, with results ranging from 51% to 89%. (See the discussion of claw toe repair later in this chapter.) Thompson and Deland,[218] in reporting on results of a flexor tendon transfer, observed excellent postoperative pain relief; however, only 54% of those with a subluxated MTP joint had achieved complete correction at final follow-up. Boyer and DeOrio[19] reported variable levels of satisfaction using the procedure for both fixed and flexible hammer toe deformities. Of 79 digits, those with a fixed hammer toe resulted in 64% satisfaction, while those with a flexible hammer toe noted a 55% satisfaction rate. Reasons for dissatisfaction included recurrent deformity, poor alignment, and postoperative stiffness.

Kuwada[126] and Barbari and Brevig[3] have reported a high level of satisfactory results (>90%) in patients in

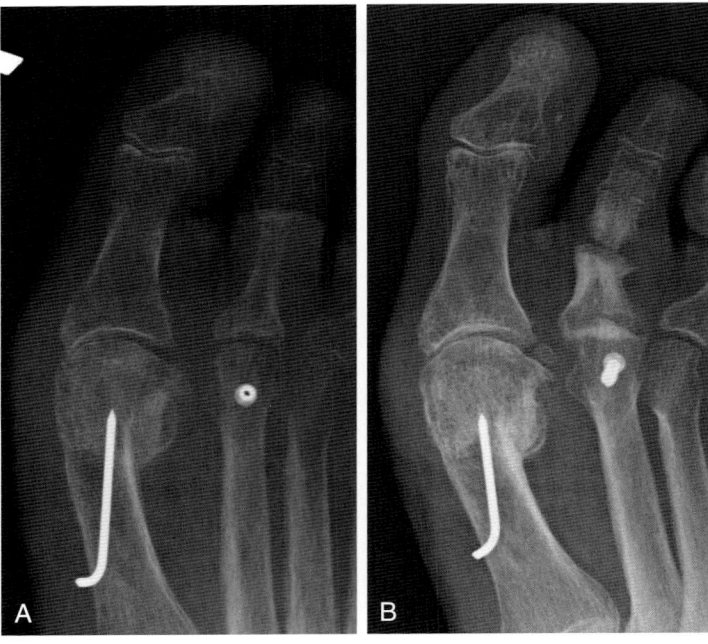

Figure 7-63 Fracture of the proximal phalanx after flexor tendon transfer **A,** After flexor tendon transfer but before phalangeal fracture. **B,** After fracture of the proximal phalanx. (From Fishco W, Roth B: Digital fracture after a flexor tendon transfer for hammertoe repair: a case report, *J Foot Ankle Surg* 49:179–181, 2010. Used with permission.)

their series after flexor tendon transfer. Barbari and Brevig[3] reported three cases where a fixed contracture of the interphalangeal joint developed postoperatively. Complications experienced after this procedure are uncommon. Occasionally, swelling of varying degrees persists for a time, but it usually subsides. Transient numbness probably caused by stretching or contusion of the adjacent neurovascular bundles can occur, but this usually improves with time. Hyperextension of the DIP joint has been noted in a few patients with concomitant spasticity and is usually associated with recurrence of flexion at the PIP joint. This may be a result of concomitant tightness of the flexor digitorum brevis. After a flexor tendon transfer, the ability to curl the toe is sacrificed. Often, at long-term follow-up after a flexor tendon transfer, stiffness develops in the PIP joint. Boyer and DeOrio[19] estimate a 50% loss of MTP and IP joint motion after a flexor tendon transfer. Myerson and Jung[165] reported that 19 of 59 patients reported serious reservations about this procedure, much of the dissatisfaction stemming from the postoperative digital stiffness. A patient should be counseled preoperatively that there will be an absence of dynamic function of the involved toe and often the other lesser toes after a flexor tendon transfer. This does not tend to cause disability, but it can be annoying to the patient. They should be alerted to the trade-off of sacrificing flexor digitorum longus function for stability and realignment of the malaligned digit.

Occasionally, the patient with a dynamic hammer toe also has an element of clawing. A release of the extensor digitorum longus tendon and simultaneous MTP capsulotomies may be performed at the same time as a flexor tendon transfer.

If a Kirschner wire has been placed across the MTP joint, the pin can break (see Fig. 7-58H).[188,240] Often, the pin fractures just proximal to the articular surface of the metatarsal head, and in this case, the distal fragment is removed and the proximal fragment is left within the metatarsal. If the distal aspect of the remaining pin penetrates the MTP joint, or if it migrates, it may be surgically removed through an MTP joint arthrotomy.

Fishco[76] has reported isolated fracture of the proximal phalanx after a flexor tendon transfer procedure (Fig. 7-63).

Postoperative vascular insufficiency of a digit can require removal of the Kirschner wire. (If the Kirschner wire has been driven across the MTP joint, sometimes just withdrawing it below this joint may improve vascularity.) Other alternatives, when there is slow capillary filling after surgery, are avoiding ice or elevation, removing and rewrapping the dressing, and temporarily dropping the extremity over the side of the bed. When these methods are unsuccessful, topical nitroglycerin ointment (Nitropaste) along the borders of the involved digit can increase the capillary filling of the digit.[19] Postoperative observation is important with this complication. Achievement of adequate alignment intraoperatively without the use of a Kirschner wire is important should the removal of internal fixation be necessary in the immediate postoperative period. Thus the Kirschner wire is used to protect a flexor tendon transfer but not to achieve further realignment of the toe.

A curly toe deformity is often associated with a mallet toe. Typically, a curly toe occurs in a younger patient, is characterized by a flexion deformity of the PIP joint and DIP joint, and is caused by a contracture of the flexor

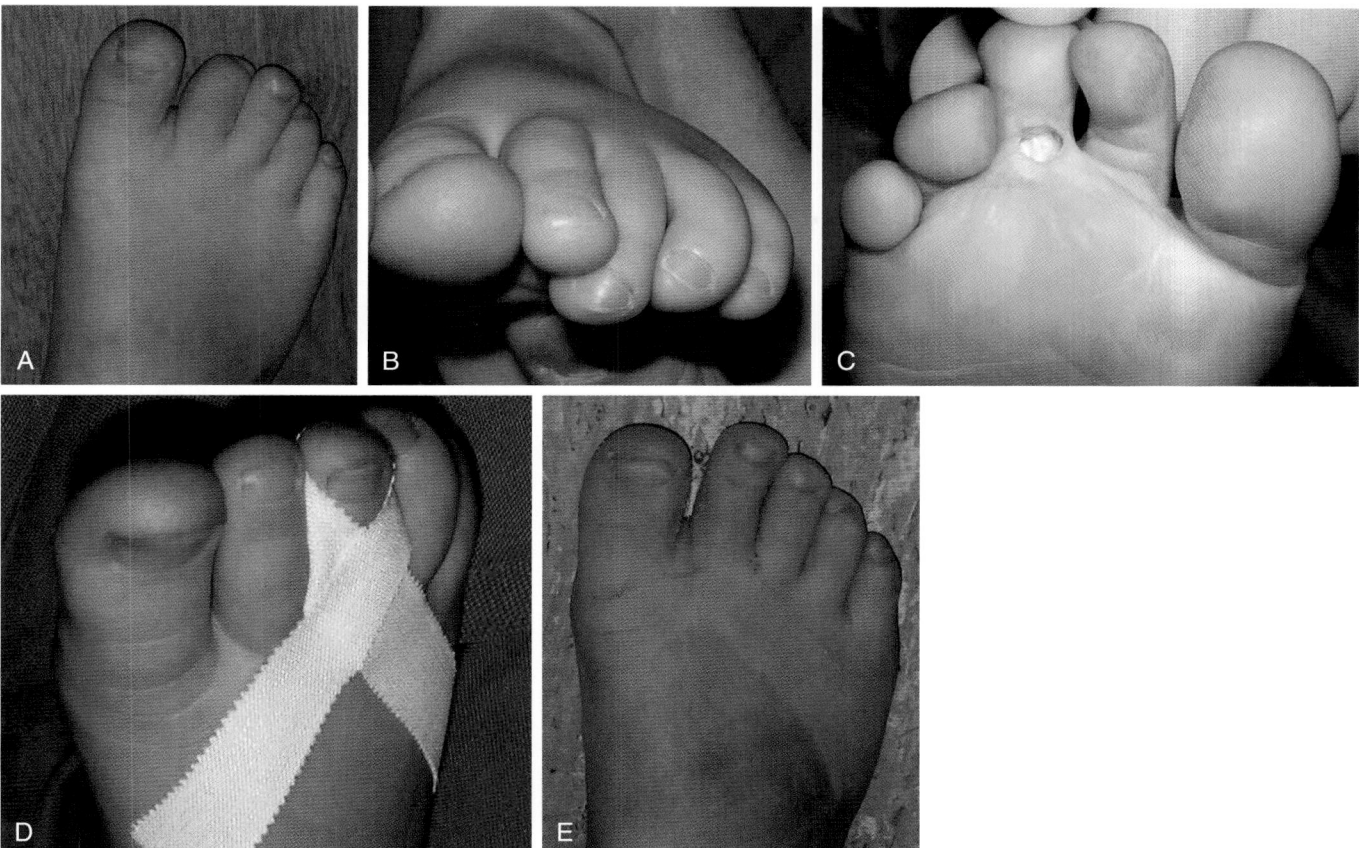

Figure 7-64 Repair of curly toe deformity. **A,** Preoperative dorsal view demonstrating curly toe or contracture of the second toe. **B,** Preoperative frontal view demonstrating contracture of the third toe of another patient. **C,** Open lengthening of long flexor tendon of third toe. **D,** Postoperative taping of third digit for 6 weeks. **E,** Final result with correction of third toe curly toe deformity (preoperative from photograph **A**). (**E,** Courtesy G. Vandeputte, MD.)

digitorum longus tendon to a specific toe (Fig. 7-64A).[167] Radiographs often demonstrate a deviation of the toe (Fig. 7-64B). Although some advocate stretching and taping to correct the deformity, Sweetnam[214] concluded that conservative treatment is rarely successful in straightening the toe. He found that there was a similar level of improvement in patients who were treated conservatively and in those who had no treatment, concluding that there was no progression or correction of deformity in either group.

A flexor tenotomy often enables complete correction of the deformity. Ross and Menelaus[192] have noted no significant weakness of the involved toe at almost 10-year follow-up after flexor tenotomy. They reported 95% successful results after flexor tenotomy. Although a flexor tendon transfer may be performed, Hamer et al[98] examined patients who had either a flexor tenotomy or flexor tendon transfer for a curly toe deformity and noted no significant postoperative difference. Thus a simple flexor tenotomy appears to be sufficient treatment. Jacobs and Vandeputte[108] reported on 11 children in whom they performed a Z-lengthening of the flexor digitorum longus

(FDL) for hammer toes and a tenotomy for mallet toes as a treatment of curly toes. A total of 15 toes (5 second, 3 third, 6 forth, and 1 fifth toes were involved). They reported excellent results in 70% of the cases (see Fig. 7-64).

Boc and Martone[12] treated an adduction deformity of the distal digit with a laterally based elliptic arthroplasty. This procedure may indeed be necessary to correct a fixed bony deformity, but in most cases, a flexor tenotomy is adequate treatment for the flexible curly toe deformity in the younger child.

MALLET TOE DEFORMITY[39,40]

A mallet toe usually is a fixed deformity, but occasionally, in a young patient, it is flexible. Symptoms develop when the tip of the toe strikes the ground. This results in development of a callosity on the tip of the involved toe. This can be treated conservatively with a small felt pad placed beneath the toe to prevent the tip of the toe from striking the ground. A shoe with an adequate toe box must be worn to accommodate the toe with a felt pad beneath it.[39]

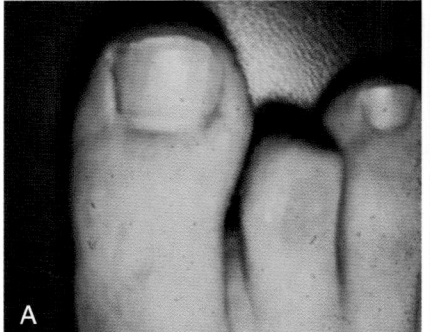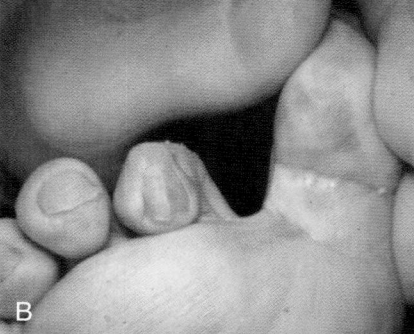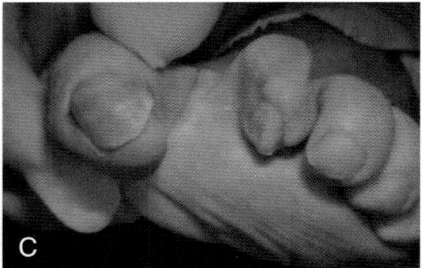

Figure 7-65 Mallet toe deformity. **A,** Dorsal view. **B,** View end on. **C,** Plantar view of another patient with severe mallet toe deformity.

A mallet toe occurs much less often than a hammer toe (ratio, 1:9).[40] It occurs in the longer toe in 75% of cases but with equal frequency in the second, third, and fourth toes (see Fig. 7-10).[40] Although excess length has been implicated as a cause of mallet toe, trauma may lead to this deformity with disruption of the extensor insertion onto the dorsal base of the proximal phalanx.[130]

Preoperative Planning

When the deformity is flexible, release of the flexor digitorum longus tendon percutaneously may be sufficient.[98,192] When the deformity is fixed (Fig. 7-65), which is more often the case, surgical intervention may be required. Bone decompression of the DIP joint, with resection of the head of the middle phalanx and release of the flexor digitorum longus tendon, results in satisfactory correction.

An algorithm, presented in Figure 7-66, describes the decision-making process for the treatment of mallet toe.

Indications

The main indication for a surgical repair is a symptomatic mallet toe. Lateral or medial deviation of the digit at the DIP joint may be corrected with a mallet toe repair as well.

Contraindications

In the presence of a combined mallet toe and hammer toe, a decision must be made as to which deformity is more severe. A combined procedure for hammer toe and mallet toe is rarely, if ever, performed.[173] When merely a flexor tenotomy is sufficient, a formal mallet toe repair can be avoided.

MALLET TOE REPAIR[34,35,40]
Surgical Technique
1. The patient is placed in a supine position on the operating room table. If MTP joint surgery is performed, an

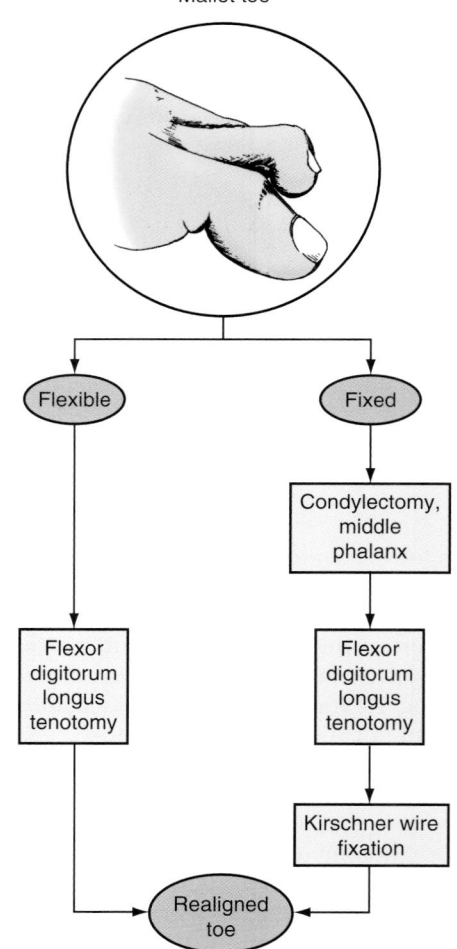

Mallet toe

Figure 7-66 Algorithm for treatment of mallet toe.

Esmarch bandage may be used to exsanguinate the extremity and may also be used as an ankle tourniquet.[91] A digital block or ankle block is administered, depending upon the necessity for additional surgical procedures.

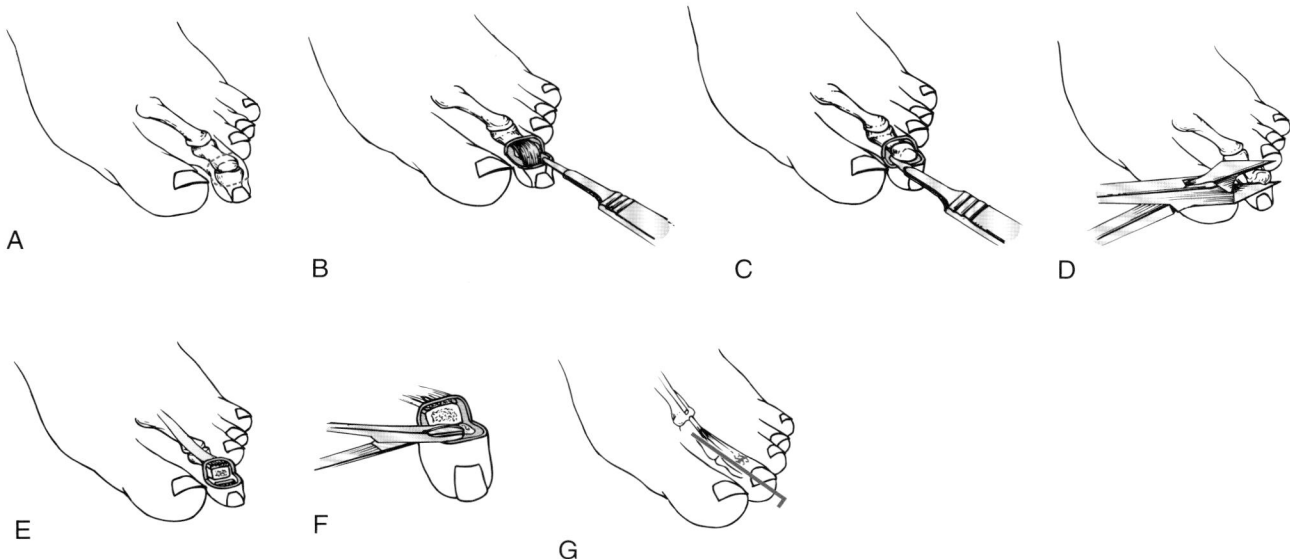

Figure 7-67 Technique for correction of mallet toe deformity. **A,** Elliptic skin incision centered over the distal interphalangeal joint. **B,** Excision of skin, extensor tendon, and capsule, exposing condyles of middle phalanx. **C,** The collateral ligaments are severed, exposing the condyles of the middle phalanx. **D,** Generous excision of the distal portion of the middle phalanx. **E,** After resection of the condyle. **F,** The articular surface of the distal phalanx is removed with a rongeur. The flexor digitorum longus tendon is identified in the base of the wound and is released. **G,** Stabilization with intramedullary Kirschner wire. Vertical mattress sutures are used to coapt the skin.

2. The foot is cleansed and draped in the usual fashion. A ¼-inch Penrose drain may be used as a tourniquet (Fig. 7-67A and Video Clip 74).
3. An elliptic incision is centered over the dorsal aspect of the interphalangeal joint. The dissection is carried down through the extensor tendon and joint capsule. The distal portion of the ellipse should be sufficiently proximal to avoid injuring the nail matrix (Figs. 7-67B and 7-68A).
4. The collateral ligaments are released on the medial and lateral aspects of the DIP joint. Care is taken to protect the adjacent neurovascular bundles (see Fig. 7-67C).
5. The condyles of the middle phalanx are delivered into the wound. The bone is transected in the supracondylar region, and the distal fragment is excised (see Fig. 7-67D and E).
6. The plantar capsule is incised in the depths of the wound, and the flexor digitorum longus is identified and released under direct vision (see Fig. 7-68B). The toe is brought into satisfactory alignment without tension. If the toe cannot be completely aligned, more bone is resected from the middle phalanx.
7. The articular cartilage is removed from the base of the distal fragment (optional) (see Figs. 7-67F and 7-68C).
8. A 0.045-inch Kirschner wire is introduced at the DIP joint and driven distally, exiting the tip of the toe (see Figs. 7-67G and 7-68D). The toe is then aligned properly, and the Kirschner wire is driven in a retrograde fashion into the middle phalanx. The pin is bent at the tip of the toe, and the remaining pin is removed (see

Fig. 7-68E-G). Often, a second pin is placed to add rotational control to the fixation construct.
9. A gauze-and-tape compression dressing is applied at surgery and changed on a weekly basis until drainage has subsided.

Alternative Fixation

Interrupted vertical mattress sutures of 3-0 nylon are used to incorporate two Telfa bolsters (Fig. 7-69). They are inserted in a similar fashion for fixation of a hammer toe. As tension is applied to the suture, leverage is created to bring the toe into satisfactory alignment. This is used quite uncommonly at this point (see technique in hammer toe section).

Postoperative Care

The patient is allowed to ambulate in a wooden-soled postoperative shoe. If bolsters have been placed, they are removed 1 week after surgery. If the bolsters are left longer than 1 week, there is risk of skin necrosis. If a Kirschner wire has been placed, the pin is removed 3 weeks after surgery. Sutures are removed at this time as well.

After removal of the pin or bolsters, the toe is held in a corrected position with a piece of tape for 6 weeks to ensure soft tissue healing.

Results and Complications

The expected results after this procedure have been routinely satisfactory. Using this procedure, with resection of the condyles of the middle phalanx and the corresponding articular surface of the distal phalanx, Coughlin[40]

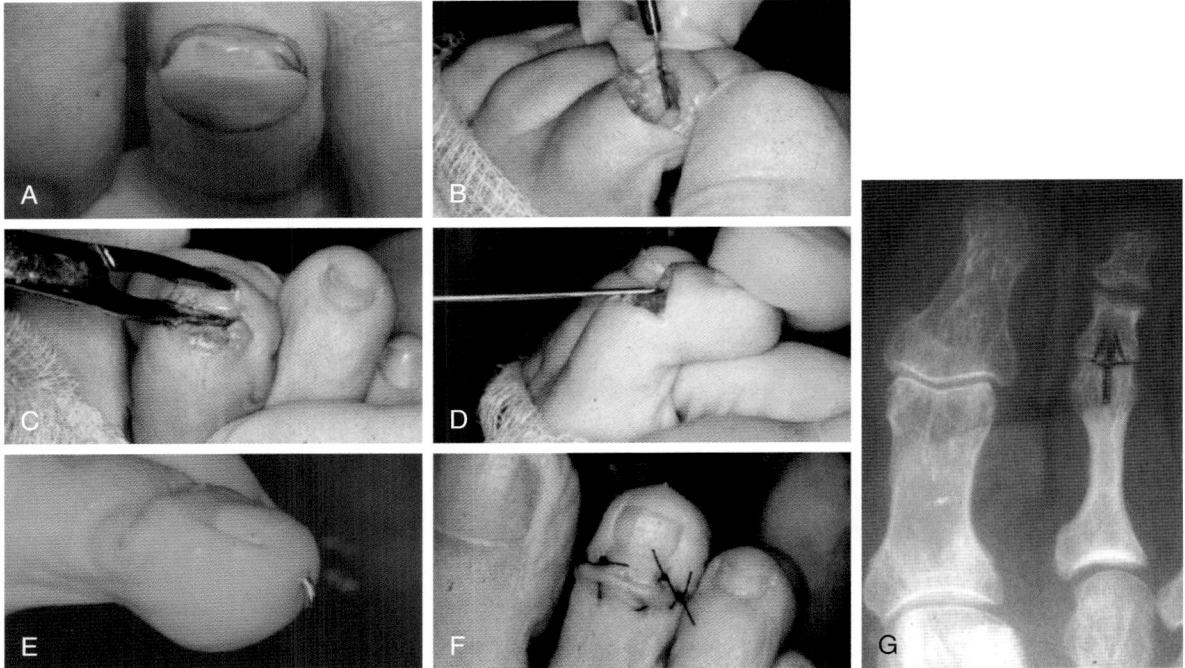

Figure 7-68 Mallet toe repair. **A,** Dorsal elliptic incision. **B,** After condyles of the middle phalanx are resected, a flexor tenotomy is performed. **C,** The articular surface of the distal phalanx is removed (optional). **D,** Insertion of Kirschner wire. **E** and **F,** After Kirschner wire insertion and closure. **G,** Radiograph with stable and painless fibrous union of corrected mallet toe deformity of the second toe.

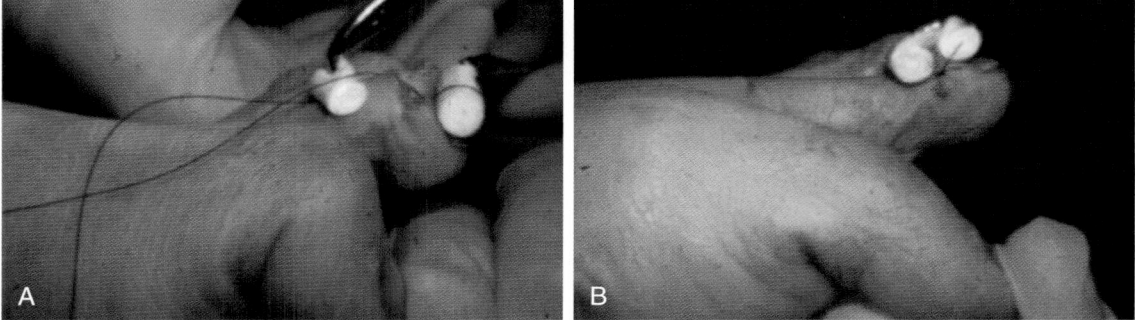

Figure 7-69 Alternative means of fixation for mallet toe repair. **A** and **B,** Placement of Telfa bolsters beneath 3-0 nylon vertical mattress suture.

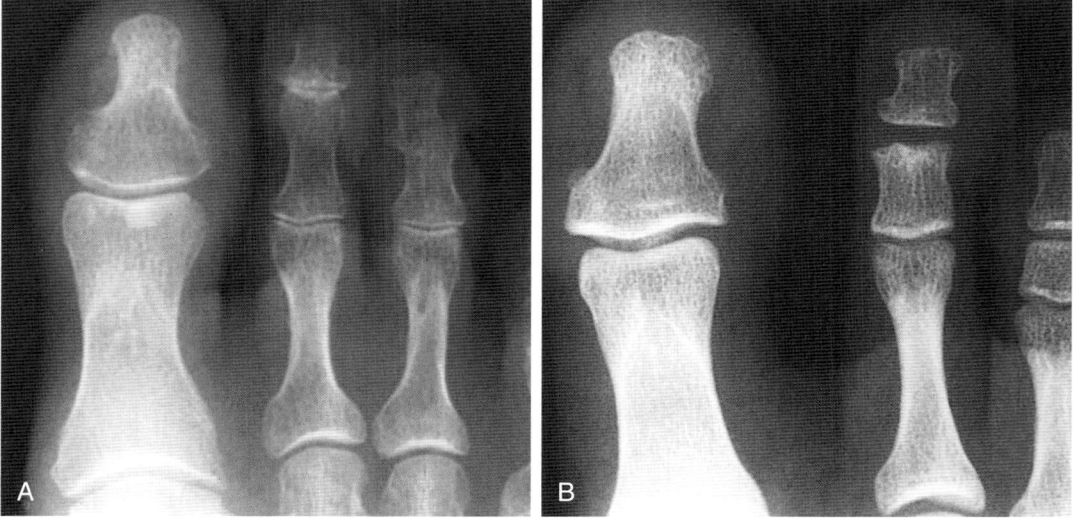

Figure 7-70 **A,** Stable fibrous union of second toe distal interphalangeal joint after mallet toe repair (distal interphalangeal [DIP]) joint after mallet toe repair. **B,** Fibrous union of DIP joint of the second toe after mallet toe repair with significant soft tissue distraction (asymptomatic).

reported successful fusion in 72% of cases (Fig. 7-70A). The satisfaction rate was only slightly higher in the group with a successful arthrodesis. Some 75% of those with a fibrous union were satisfied, although slightly less so than those with a successful DIP arthrodesis (Fig. 7-70B). Pain relief was noted by 97% and correction of the deformity by 91%. Although not performed in all cases, a flexor tenotomy appeared to be associated with a slightly higher rate of satisfaction and maintenance of the corrected position. Usually, correct alignment is maintained and complications are uncommon.

Oliver et al[173] reported on a series of 20 patients (63 toes) in which a double resection arthroplasty was performed for a dual correction of deformities at both the DIP and PIP joint (hammer toe + mallet toe). A 10% recurrence rate was noted. They used both a longitudinal incision for the proximal interphalangeal joint and a transverse incision for the DIP joint. No internal fixation was used.

The few problems that have been observed postoperatively include the following:

- Swelling often persists for several months after the procedure, but it invariably resolves with time. At long-term follow-up, no patients were noted to have swelling.[40] Molding resulting from extrinsic pressure from adjacent toes can cause angulation or malalignment (see Fig. 7-11A and B).
- Occasionally, recurrence of a mallet toe deformity is noted. This is usually because the flexor digitorum longus tendon was not released.
- Injury to an adjacent digital nerve can leave an area of numbness along either the medial or lateral border of the toe, although this is rarely a significant complaint.
- When a preoperative toenail deformity is associated with a mallet toe, this usually does not resolve after correction of the mallet toe (see Fig. 7-11C-E). The patient should be warned that although the toe can be realigned, the toenail deformity will not be corrected.

CLAW TOE DEFORMITIES

A claw toe often develops in association with neurologic conditions in which a muscle imbalance occurs[203] with weakness or loss of intrinsic muscle function.[157] It can also occur in arthritic conditions, such as rheumatoid arthritis and other collagen deficiency syndromes. At times, a claw toe deformity is associated with a cavus foot deformity.[106]

It may also be associated with the sequelae of compartment syndromes after lower-extremity trauma.[74,181]

In evaluating a claw toe deformity, every effort should be made to determine the specific diagnosis.[39] However, many of these cases are idiopathic.

What differentiates a claw toe from a hammer toe is the hyperextension deformity of the MTP joint.[167] A hammer toe may or may not be associated with hyperextension of the proximal phalanx, but a claw toe classically has a hyperextension deformity at the MTP joint.[80,103] In a claw toe, the DIP joint may be extended or flexed. The chronic hyperextended posture of the MTP joint forces the metatarsal heads plantarward and displaces the plantar fat pad, often resulting in symptomatic metatarsalgia over time. In patients with an insensate foot, ulcers can develop beneath the metatarsal heads.

Preoperative Planning

To successfully correct a claw toe deformity, the MTP joint must be brought into a neutral position so that the extensor tendon can function to extend the PIP joint and the intrinsic tendons can function as flexors of the MTP joint.

Treatment of a claw toe depends on the underlying condition. Figure 7-71 presents an algorithm for treatment of claw toe. If a significant pes cavus deformity is present, attention should be directed first to the midfoot and hindfoot deformities.[29,34,37,140,141] With a pes cavus

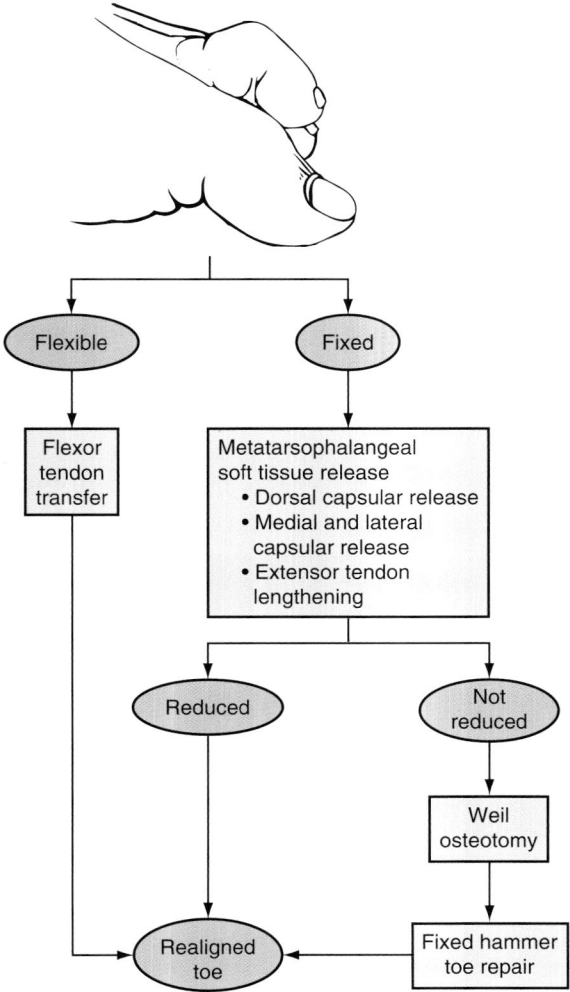

Figure 7-71 Algorithm for treatment of claw toe.

deformity, the metatarsal heads are depressed as a result of the anatomic alignment of the foot, and the toes are extended by the contracted long extensors, creating the claw toe deformity (see Fig. 7-15A).[103,104] When there is dynamic clawing without a significant cavus deformity, attention should be directed to the forefoot itself. If there is no clawing of the toes when the ankle is held in plantar flexion, and if clawing occurs with dorsiflexion of the ankle joint, a flexible claw toe deformity is present (see Fig. 7-15B-E). This may be treated with a flexor tendon transfer.[3,184,215,216] This is the same type of procedure that is used to correct a flexible or dynamic hammer toe (see Figs. 7-60 and 7-61); however, release of the MTP joints (extensor tenotomies or MTP joint capsulotomies, or both) also may be necessary.[3]

Feeney et al,[74] in treating patients with the sequelae of compartment syndromes after tibia fractures, have advocated selective proximal lengthenings of the flexor hallucis longus and flexor digitorum longus to relieve lesser toe contractures.

In the presence of a fixed contracture, a DuVries arthroplasty of the PIP joint is carried out with concomitant release of the contracted structures at the MTP joint (Fig. 7-72). In patients with severe contractures of the MTP and interphalangeal joints, release of both flexor tendons should be carried out at the time of the surgery. In patients with severe contractures, longitudinally placed Kirschner wires may be used to stabilize both the interphalangeal and MTP joints in satisfactory alignment.

Indications

In the presence of a fixed claw toe deformity, a condylectomy of the base of the proximal phalanx is performed. Release of the extensor tendon and contracted capsule at the MTP joint depends on whether a fixed contracture is present. A fixed contracture at the interphalangeal joint of the hallux is treated with an interphalangeal joint fusion. With a contracture of the extensor hallucis longus tendon, a Jones tendon transfer is performed. An extensor tendon transfer to the distal metatarsal[80,103] (Jones transfer) and the midfoot[147] also has been advocated for treatment of claw toe deformity. A distal metatarsal osteotomy may also be an alternative in the treatment regimen of a severe claw toe deformity (discussed under Weil osteotomy).

Contraindications

In the presence of a flexible claw toe deformity, a flexor tendon transfer is performed identical to that for a flexible hammer toe deformity. Transfer of a flexor tendon as sole treatment of a fixed deformity is rarely successful.

DUVRIES ARTHROPLASTY PROCEDURE
Surgical Technique

1. The patient is placed in a supine position on the operating room table. A peripheral nerve block is typically used for anesthesia. The foot is cleansed and draped in the usual fashion. The foot is exsanguinated with an Esmarch bandage, which may be used as a tourniquet above the level of the ankle.
2. A longitudinal incision is centered over the PIP joint. The skin, extensor tendon, and capsule are exposed and excised (Fig. 7-73A and B).
3. The toe is flexed and the collateral ligaments released on the medial and lateral borders of the condyle. The plantar capsule also is released (Fig. 7-73C and Video Clip 75).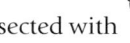
4. The condyles of the proximal phalanx are resected with a bone-cutting forceps (Fig. 7-73D).
5. If an arthrodesis is desired, a rongeur is used to remove the base of the middle phalanx (Fig. 7-73E).
6. The toe is stabilized with a 0.045-inch Kirschner wire introduced at the interphalangeal joint and driven distally (Fig. 7-73F). A release of the flexor tendons may be necessary and may be performed in the depths of the wound from a dorsal approach.
7. With the toe aligned properly, the Kirschner wire is driven proximally, stabilizing the proximal phalanx.

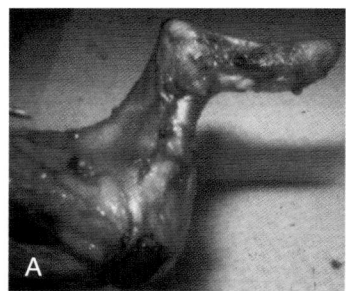
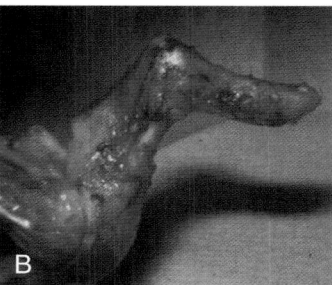
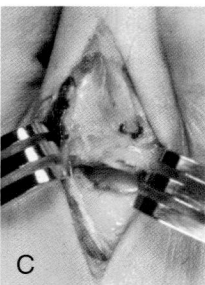
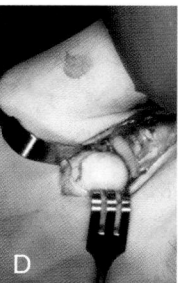
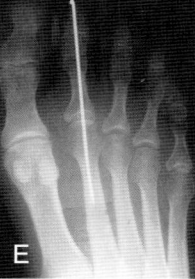

Figure 7-72 Soft tissue release and realignment. **A,** Lateral view of a cadaver dissection demonstrating a fixed hammer toe deformity and a fixed contracture of the metatarsophalangeal joint. Note the lumbrical pulling at a right angle. Also note the thickness of the lateral capsule. **B,** An extensor tenotomy and dorsal capsule release have been performed. This is an inadequate release to reduce the toe, as can be seen in this dissection. Note that a more extensive capsule release must be performed on the medial and lateral aspect to reduce the toe. **C,** Intraoperative photograph demonstrating inadequate release. **D,** An adequate capsule release has been performed. **E,** After metatarsophalangeal joint release, often intermedullary Kirschner wire fixation is used to stabilize the repair.

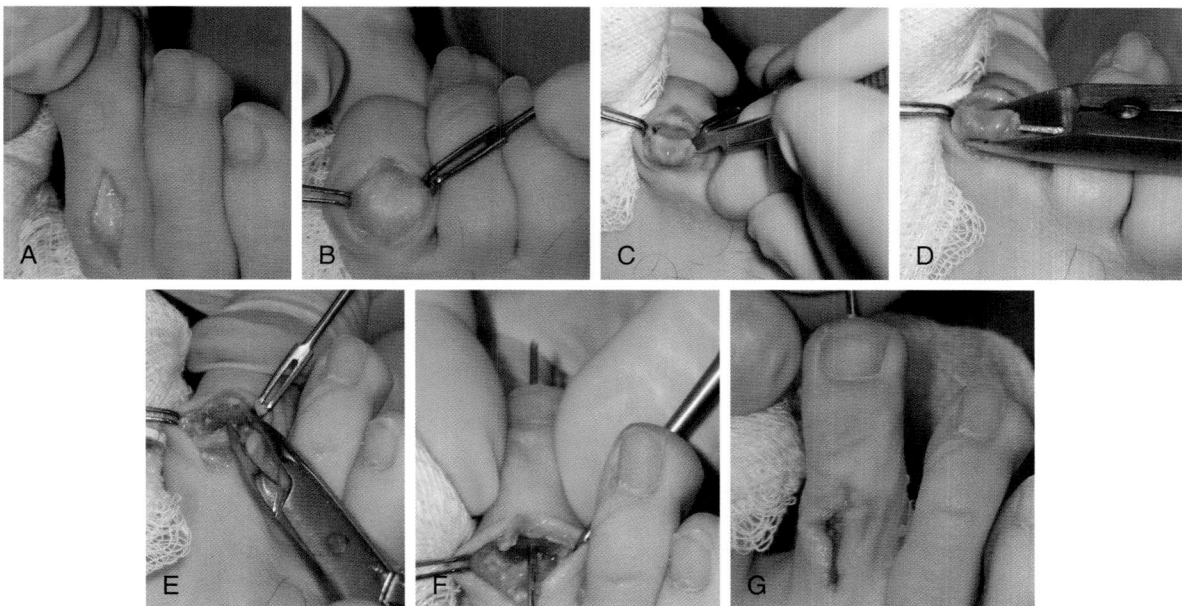

Figure 7-73 Repair of claw toe deformity. Longitudinal incision is centered over the proximal interphalangeal joint **(A)**, exposing the skin, extensor tendon, and capsule **(B)**, which is excised. **C,** The toe is flexed and the plantar capsule is released. The collateral ligaments are released from the medial and lateral border of condyles. **D,** The condyles of the proximal phalanx are removed with a bone-cutting forceps. **E,** If an arthrodesis is desired, the articular surface of the base of the middle phalanx is removed. **F,** A 0.045-inch Kirschner wire is introduced at the arthroplasty site and driven distally. **G,** With the toe reduced, the Kirschner wire is driven in a retrograde fashion, stabilizing the proximal phalanx. After skin closure, the toe is adequately aligned.

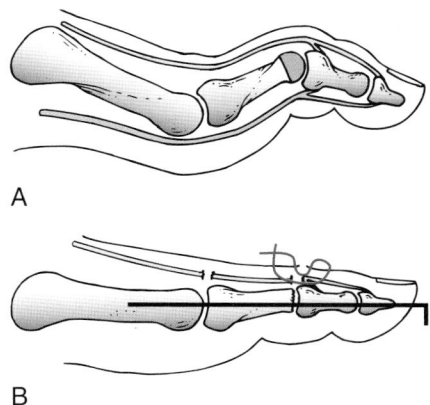

Figure 7-74 **A,** Claw toe deformity. **B,** After proximal interphalangeal joint arthroplasty, metatarsophalangeal soft tissue release, and intramedullary Kirschner wire fixation.

If an MTP joint capsule release is performed, the Kirschner wire may be driven across the MTP joint (Fig. 7-73G).

8. The skin is approximated with interrupted vertical mattress sutures.

CONTRACTURE RELEASE

In the presence of a hyperextension deformity of the MTP joint, a release of the contracted tissue and a tenotomy of the extensor tendon is performed (Fig. 7-74).

Surgical Technique

1. A 1.5-cm incision is centered over the MTP joint.
2. The dissection is deepened to the extensor tendon, which is released.
3. With retractors exposing the MTP joint capsule, the dorsal, medial, and lateral capsules and collateral ligaments are released. (This release must be carried down approximately 1 cm plantarward to allow reduction of the MTP joint.) If adhesions of the plantar plate are present, a release of the plantar capsule with a McGlamry elevator may allow reduction of the dorsiflexion contracture of the MTP joint.
4. A 0.045-inch Kirschner wire is driven retrograde across the MTP joint, stabilizing the joint.
5. The pin is bent at the tip of the toe and the remainder of the pin is cut and removed.
6. A gauze-and-tape compression dressing is applied and is changed weekly until drainage has subsided.

HALLUX/INTERPHALANGEAL JOINT ARTHRODESIS

With a fixed contracture of the interphalangeal joint of the hallux, an interphalangeal joint arthrodesis is performed.

Surgical Technique

1. The foot is cleansed and draped in the usual fashion.
2. An elliptic incision is centered over the dorsal aspect of the interphalangeal joint. The skin, extensor tendon,

and capsule are resected. The medial and lateral collateral ligaments and plantar capsule are released (Fig. 7-75A-C).

3. A power saw is used to resect the articular surface of the condyles of the proximal phalanx (Fig. 7-75D).
4. The articular surface of the distal phalanx is also resected with the power saw (Fig. 7-75E).
5. A puncture wound is created in the skin (Fig. 7-75F). A 3.5-mm gliding hole is drilled through the distal phalanx. The drill is introduced at the interphalangeal joint and driven distally through the tip of the toe.
6. A 2.5-mm fixation hole is drilled in the proximal phalanx (Fig. 7-75G).
7. A lag screw is used to stabilize the fusion. Care must be taken not to place an excessively long screw that can penetrate the MTP joint (Fig. 7-75H). A 0.062-inch Kirschner wire may be added as additional internal fixation to prevent rotation at the arthrodesis site.
8. A gauze-and-tape dressing is applied (Fig. 7-75I-K).

Postoperative Care

The patient is allowed to ambulate in a postoperative shoe. Sutures and Kirschner wires are removed 3 weeks after surgical repair of a fixed claw toe. The compression screw placed in the hallux to fuse the interphalangeal joint may be left in permanently, or if it causes discomfort, it may be removed after administration of local anesthetic.

Results and Complications

Taylor[216] performed both soft tissue release and transfer of the long and short flexor tendons to the extensor hood. He reported that the operation restores "useful function to the toe at the cost of their prehensile action." In 68 patients (112 feet), 72% good results were reported. No resection arthroplasties were performed in this series.

Pyper[184] transferred both the long and short flexors to the extensor hood and reported 51% excellent and good results and 49% fair and poor results with this procedure.

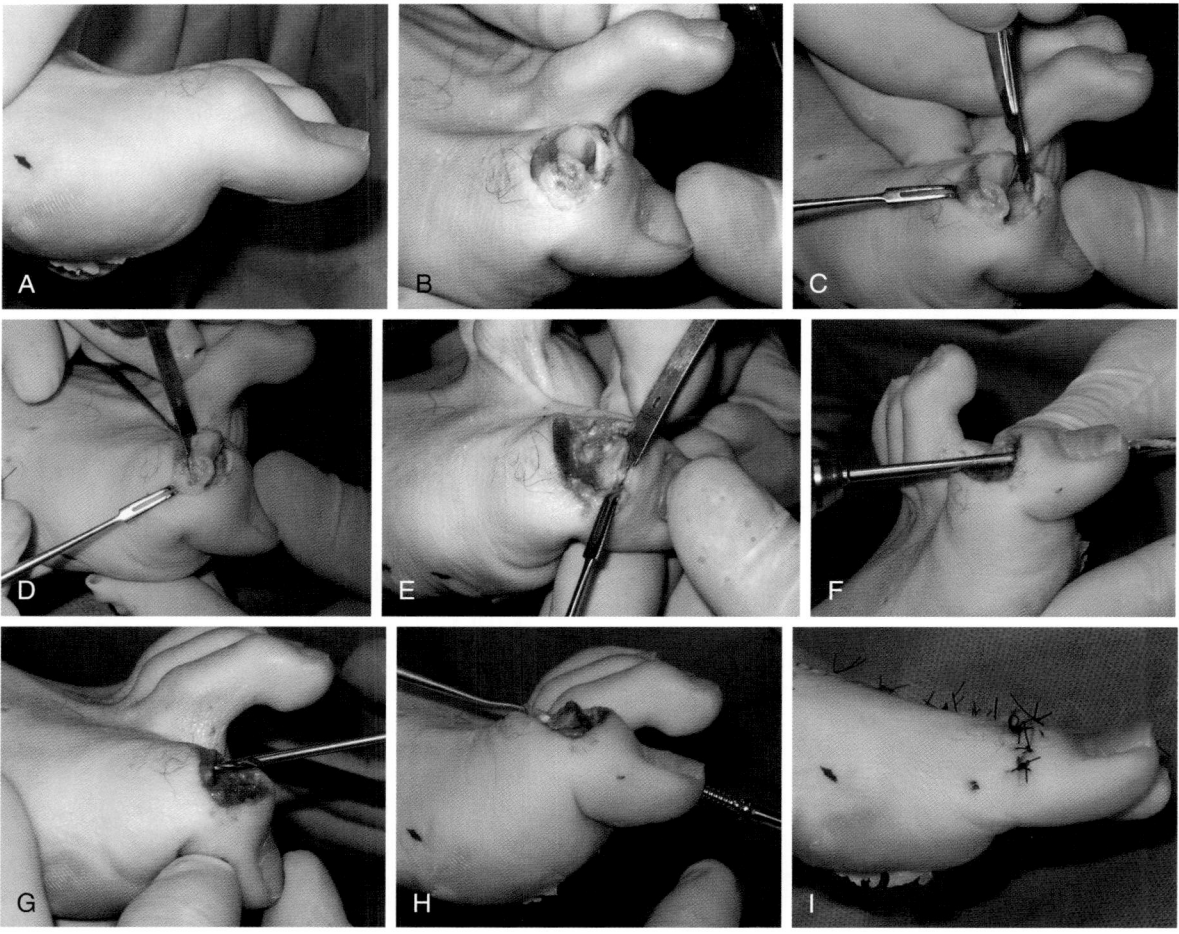

Figure 7-75 **A,** Repair of hammered great toe. After elliptical skin incision excises skin, extensor tendon, and capsule **(B)**, the collateral ligaments are released **(C). D,** A power saw is used to remove the articular surface of the condyles of the proximal phalanx. **E,** The articular surface of the distal phalanx is removed with a power saw. **F,** A gliding hole is created through the distal phalanx. **G,** A fixation hole is created in the proximal phalanx. **H,** A lag screw is placed to stabilize the repair. **I,** Result after repair of all five toes.

Suboptimal results were thought to result from uncorrected fixed flexion contractures of the lesser toes.

Parrish[175] transferred the flexor digitorum longus to the extensor hood in 23 patients. Transfer of the short flexor tendon was abandoned because of technical difficulties. Eighty-nine percent good and excellent results were reported.

Cyphers and Feiwell[54] reported their experience with flexor tendon transfer in patients with meningomyelocele and noted 60% good results.

Barbari and Brevig[3] reported on flexor tendon transfer for correction of a claw toe deformity. Satisfactory results were reported in 90% of cases, although one third of patients complained of metatarsalgia postoperatively. MTP motion was greater than 50 degrees in 33% of patients and less than 50 degrees in 6 patients. Twelve patients had no interphalangeal joint motion, 15 had reduced motion, and 12 had the same amount of motion at the interphalangeal joints. Continuing complaints were noted by patients who had a fixed claw toe deformity that might have been better treated with a resection arthroplasty. With refinement of this procedure and the use of just the flexor digitorum longus tendon, improved results have been noted, although Thompson and Deland[218] observed that only 54% of patients in their series achieved complete realignment of the MTP joint after flexor tendon transfer.

Heyman[103] advocated soft tissue release of the contracted capsular structures at the MTP and interphalangeal joints. No "excellent" results were noted, although no long-term evaluation was reported.

Lapidus[134] performed a dorsal capsule reefing at the interphalangeal joints coupled with a plantar capsulotomy and extensor tenotomy and reported uniformly good results.

Frank and Johnson[80] and McCluskey et al[147] advocated PIP joint arthroplasty to decompress the claw toe deformity and realign the toe.

Complications associated with repair of a claw toe deformity usually are related to recurrent deformity. In the presence of a flexible claw toe deformity, a flexor tendon transfer can adequately realign the deformed toes. Where a fixed contracture is present, a capital oblique osteotomy of the metatarsal may be necessary to achieve adequate realignment. (See the discussion of the Weil osteotomy later.)

MTP joint capsule releases and an extensor tenotomy or lengthening may be combined to correct a significant hyperextension deformity. Lui et al,[137] in a cadaver study, tenodesed the plantar plate to the extensor tendons. Basically, they achieved correction with both extensor and plantar releases of soft tissue contractures. They then followed up with the treatment of 23 patients with claw toe deformities using this procedure and reported satisfactory realignment. Further long-term follow-up will be necessary to assess the efficacy of this procedure.

Metatarsalgia may continue to be a complaint despite realignment of the lesser toes.[72] An algorithm is helpful in the approach to differentiating forefoot problems (Fig. 7-76). Attention to midfoot and hindfoot deformities may be necessary to relieve symptoms of metatarsalgia. Treatment of the underlying problem leading to a claw

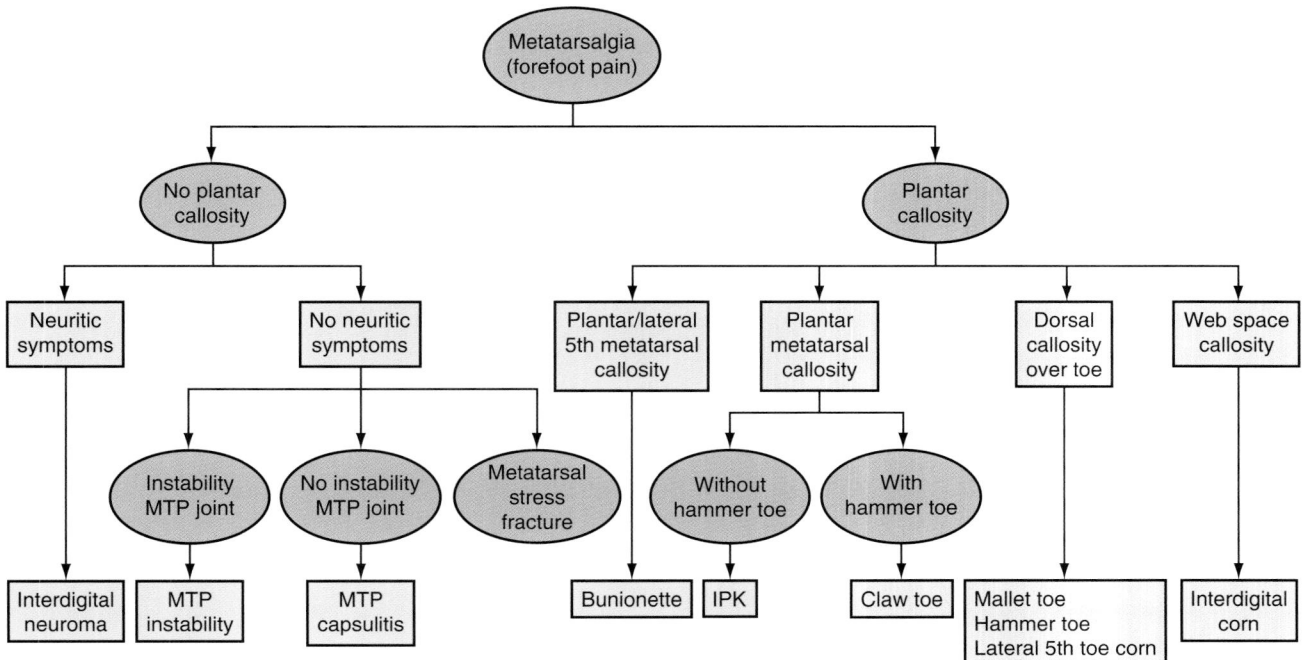

Figure 7-76 Algorithm for treatment of metatarsalgia. *IPK,* intractable plantar keratosis; *MTP,* metatarsophalangeal. (From Coughlin MJ: Common causes of pain in the forefoot in adults, *J Bone Joint Surg Br* 82:781–790, 2000.)

toe deformity should be considered before lesser toe realignment. With extensive surgery, which can include an MTP joint release, a condylectomy of the proximal phalanx, and even a flexor tendon transfer, the vascular status of the toe or toes may be compromised. The patient must be monitored closely postoperatively, because it may be necessary to remove internal fixation (e.g., Kirschner wire) in the presence of vascular compromise.

SUBLUXATION AND DISLOCATION OF THE LESSER METATARSOPHALANGEAL JOINT

Subluxation and dislocation of the lesser MTP joints can occur with relative frequency.[22,43,65] Since Coughlin[33] introduced the term *crossover toe* in 1987, several etiologies have been proposed. Certainly, a lesser MTP joint can be dislocated acutely after an injury with disruption of the plantar capsule and MTP collateral ligaments. Chronic capsular insufficiency, however, can develop in association with systemic arthritides (such as rheumatoid arthritis) and other connective tissue disorders as well as nonspecific synovitis.[143,144] Chronic synovitis eventually can lead to deterioration of the plantar plate and collateral ligaments with subsequent instability of the MTP joint.[110,144] The use of high-heel shoes is also thought to cause repetitive hyperextension forces on the lesser MTP joints, which in time may lead to attenuation or rupture of the plantar plate, and in time this can lead to subluxation or dislocation of the lesser MTP joints (Fig. 7-77).[33,120,229]

Etiology

A traumatic episode can lead to dislocation of the MTP joints (Fig. 7-78). Occasionally, after a dorsiflexion injury

to the MTP joint, the joint is irreducibly dislocated.[162,186] The typical injury mechanism occurs with forced hyperextension and axial loading of the involved toe. The postinjury radiograph often demonstrates an increased MTP joint space, and an interposed plantar plate is often identified at surgery.

Brunet and Tubin[23] reported on 27 injuries (17 patients) to the lesser MTP joint associated with sporting activities, motor vehicle accidents, and trauma. Invariably, the plantar plate and capsule were torn from the metatarsal head and become interposed, preventing successful reduction. Occasionally, the transverse metatarsal ligament had to be sectioned to allow joint reduction. Boussouga et al[16] reported a similar finding with an irreducible dislocation of the fifth MTP joint (Fig. 7-79). Dislocation of lesser MTP joints is often associated with inflammatory arthropathy,[143] and although these often

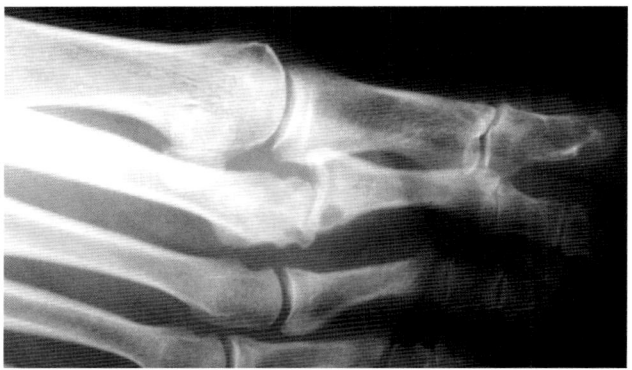

Figure 7-77 Unstable second metatarsophalangeal (MTP) joint that has developed into fully dislocated MTP joint with degenerative changes as well.

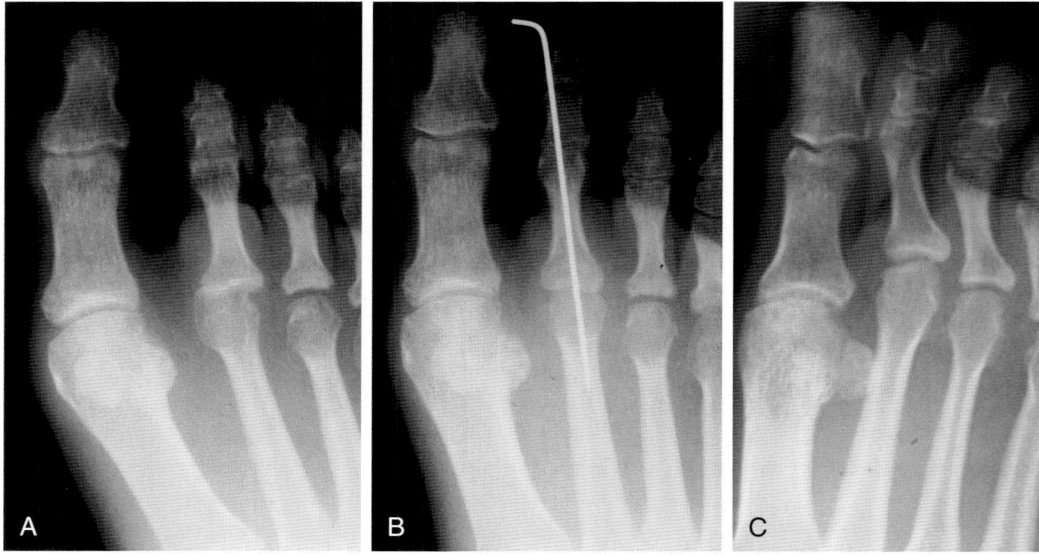

Figure 7-78 Traumatic dislocation of second metatarsophalangeal (MTP) joint after skydiving accident. **A,** Dislocated second MTP joint. **B,** After open reduction and internal fixation. **C,** Follow-up shows adequately realigned second MTP joint.

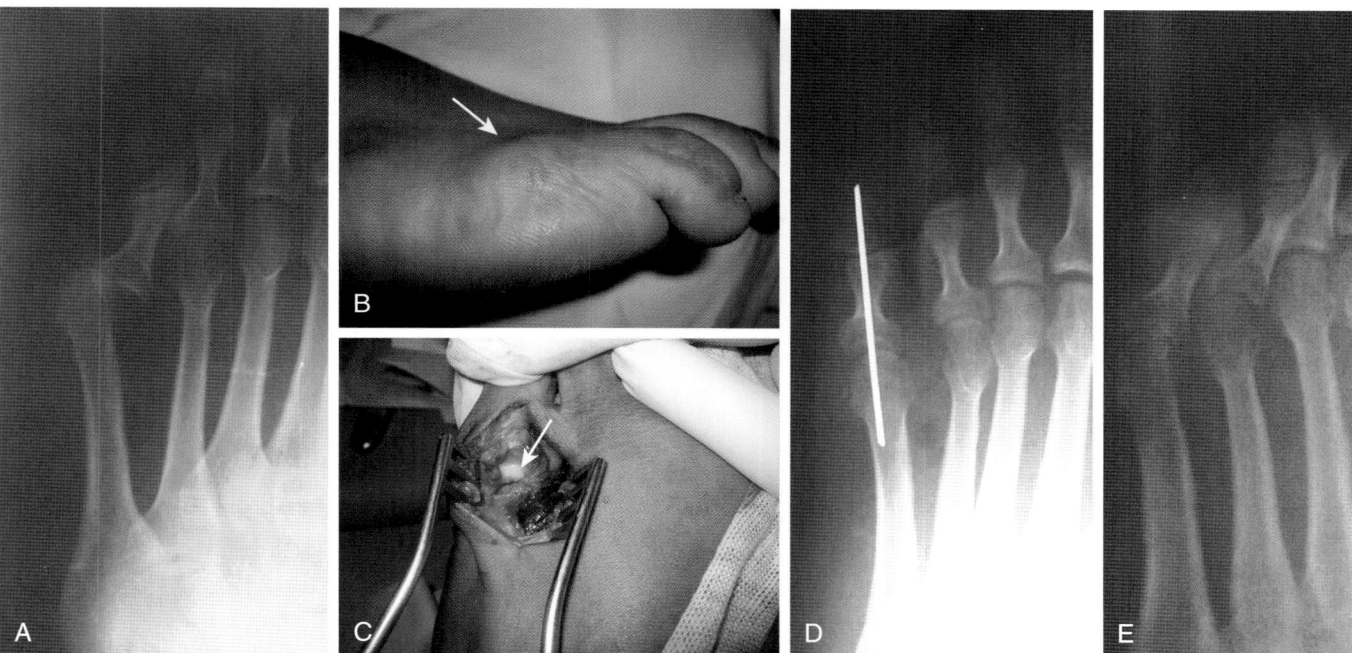

Figure 7-79 Irreducible dislocation of the fifth metatarsophalangeal (MTP) joint. **A,** Radiograph demonstrating isolated fifth MTP joint. **B,** Clinical appearance of fifth MTP joint. **C,** Intraoperative photograph demonstrating interposed plantar plate *(arrow).* **D,** After open reduction and fixation with Kirschner wire. **E,** Final result after Kirschner wire removal. (From Boussouga M, Boukhriss J, Jaafar A, Lazrak K: Irreducible dorsal metatarsophalangeal joint dislocation of the fifth toe: a case report, *J Foot Ankle Surg* 48:298 e217–220, 2010. Used with permission.)

present as multiple lesser MTP dislocations, they can develop initially as an isolated subluxtion of dislocation (Fig. 7-80).

One reason for a dislocation of the second MTP joint is that the second ray (consisting of the second metatarsal and phalanges) is usually the longest in the foot.[33-37,160] Because of the pressure of the end of the toe against the toe box, the toe buckles and the proximal phalanx have a tendency to ride up onto the dorsal aspect of the second metatarsal head. Subluxation can eventually occur, and if untreated, it can progress to dislocation. The longer period of time that the dislocation is present, the greater the degree of change noted in the surrounding soft tissue and bone. The soft tissue contractures can include shortening of the extensor tendons and contracture of the dorsal, medial, and lateral capsule. Associated with this may be a complete rupture or an attenuation of the plantar capsule. Although initially MTP joint instability was attributed to lateral collateral ligament insufficiency,[33,42-44] we now think this collateral ligament insufficiency is more commonly a later development after plantar plate deterioration.[47,50,168] Anatomic dissections of the second MTP joint suggests to us that the plantar plate is the key stabilizing structure of the joint.[8,50,120] Bhatia et al[8] and others[77] used cadaveric models to determine the anatomic restraints to dislocation of the second MTP joint and demonstrated that sectioning of the plantar plate created an unstable joint.[8] Dislocation of any of the lesser MTP joints may be caused by degeneration or

rupture of the plantar plate, which then permits the MTP joint to subluxate dorsally.[35,50,61,62] During walking, all of the forces across the MTP joint tend to hyperextend or dorsiflex the joint. Therefore any imbalance about the MTP joint (i.e., capsular or tendinous) can result in progressive dorsal subluxation. In long-standing dislocations, an accessory facet can develop on the dorsal aspect of the metatarsal head.

With a marked hallux valgus deformity (Fig. 7-81A-C; see also Fig. 7-34A), it is not uncommon to see a subluxed or dislocated second MTP joint that deviates laterally (because of pressure from the hallux) or dorsally (with the hallux crossing under the second toe). Often, however, the second toe actually deviates medially, leaving a gap between the second and third toes[174]; this deformity is termed a *crossover toe deformity.*[33] This can occur with or without a hallux valgus deformity. The toe may or may not be subluxed dorsally. Over time, erosion of the plantar plate, fibular collateral ligament of the second MTP joint, and deterioration of the lateral joint capsule allow the toe to drift in a dorsomedial direction. Less commonly, a third or fourth toe also dislocates (Fig. 7-81D and E; see Fig. 7-80). Although most prior series have reported on only instability of the second MTP joint, Nery et al[168] also reported the treatment of third and fourth MTP joint instability, although the second MTP joint was by far the most frequently involved (63%).

Hatch and Burns[100] suggested that an accessory medial head of the extensor digitorum brevis was associated with

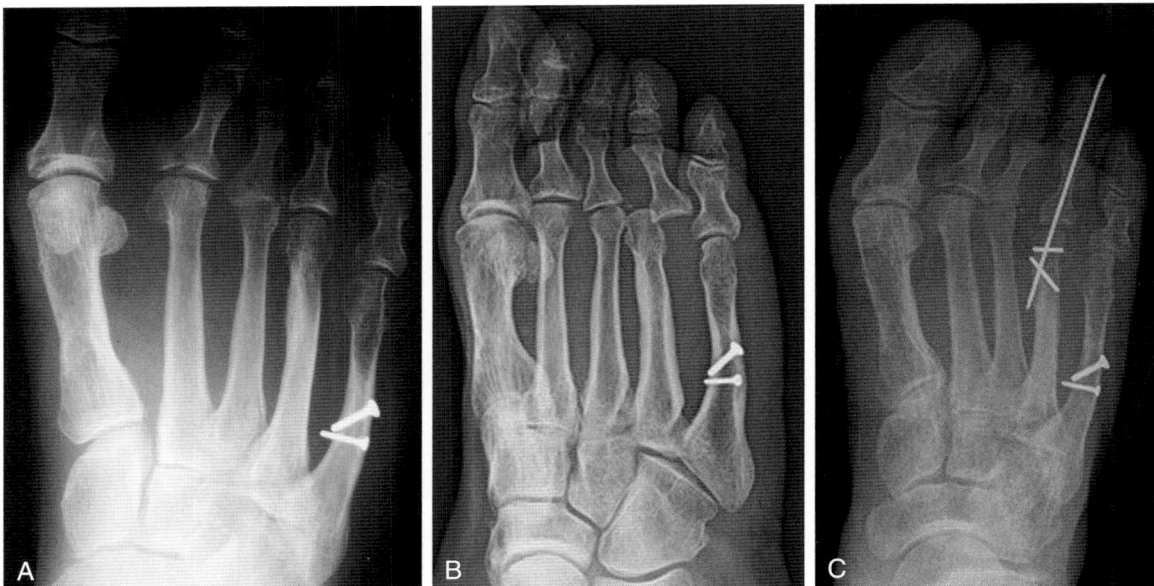

Figure 7-80 Isolated dislocation of fourth metatarsophalangeal (MTP) joint. **A,** A 62-year-old female with low-grade inflammatory arthritis, prior proximal phalanx fracture, and bunionette repair, with prodromal pain in lateral forefoot. **B,** One month later, radiographs demonstrate an isolated fourth MTP dislocation (the third MTP joint has degenerative arthritis). **C,** After open reduction internal fixation of the fourth MTP joint.

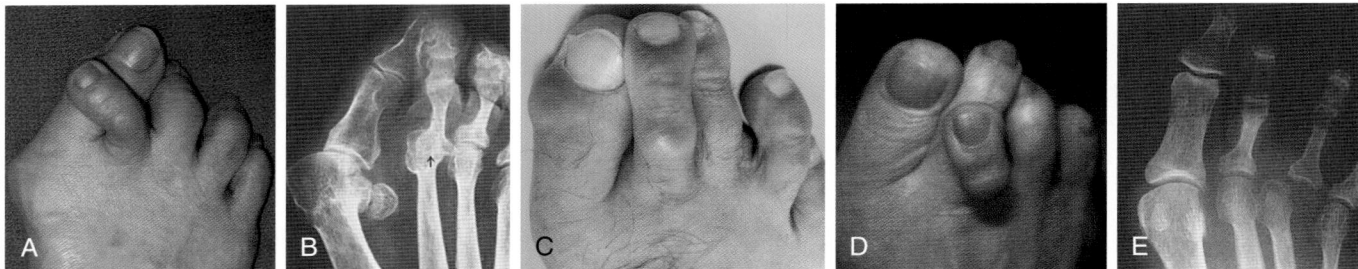

Figure 7-81 Hallux valgus deformity. Clinical **(A)** and radiographic **(B)** appearance of dislocation of second metatarsophalangeal (MTP) joint. The hallux has caused sufficient pressure against the second toe, which led to dislocation of the second MTP joint. **C,** With hallux valgus or hallux valgus interphalangeus, there is insufficient room for the adjacent second toe, necessitating realignment of the great toe. **D,** Isolated dislocation of the third MTP joint due to synovitis. **E,** Radiographic appearance of dislocated third toe in a different patient.

a crossover toe deformity and noted its presence in four of seven cadaver specimens. They speculated that the action of the extensor digitorum brevis to dorsiflex and adduct the second toe could be an underlying cause of a crossover second toe.

Anatomy of Lesser Metatarsophalangeal Joint Subluxation

The lesser MTP joints are stabilized by a combination of the static resistance provided by the collateral ligaments and plantar plate as well as the dynamic pull of the intrinsic flexors.[8,38] It is, however, mainly the plantar plate that provides this major stabilizing force.[50] The plantar plate is rectangular to trapezoidal in shape, forming a cradle beneath the metatarsal head. It originates on the metatarsal head with a thin weak synovial attachment, just proximal to the metatarsal articular surface and inserts with a stout attachment onto the plantar base of the proximal phalanx.* It also has a number of important structures that attach to it, including the distal fibers of the plantar fascia, the collateral ligaments, the transverse metatarsal ligaments, the interosseus tendons, and the fibrous sheath of the flexor tendons.[63] The overall thickness of the plantar plate can range from 2 to 5 mm. The length can range from 16 to 23 mm, and the width can range from 8 to 13 mm, depending upon the size of the metatarsal.[115] The peripheral borders of the plantar plate have been noted

---

*References 47, 50, 60, 61, 115, 168.

to be thicker than in the central region.[115] Johnson et al,[115] in a biochemical analysis of the plantar plate, observed type 1 collagen to be the most common collagen type (75%), while type 2 collagen was next most common (21%). Deland[61] also reported an analysis of the plantar plate in five normal feet and discerned that the plate was composed mainly of type 1 collagen. This collagenous composition may be a factor that affects the poor healing capability of the plantar plate tear.[77] The same healing problem has been reported to occur in the meniscus of the knee, where there is also a high level of type 1 collagen.

In the plantar plate, these collagen fibers run mostly in a longitudinal fashion, with some oblique bundles interspersed at somewhat regular intervals.[115] Biomechanically, the plantar plate functions to resist tensile loads in the longitudinal direction (particularly with dorsiflexion of the joint) as well as in an axial plane (with varus/valgus stress); it functions as well to cushion the joint and support forefoot weight-bearing forces.[61,63,115] With the application of long-term, chronic, hyperextension forces to the MTP joint, the plantar plate and the capsule may tear, stretch, or become attenuated, with eventual loss of stabilizing control of the MTP joint.[31,33,38] Recent reports have suggested a relationship between lesser MTP joint instability and the loss of plantar plate integrity.*

Haddad et al[97] observed that the weakest area of the plantar capsule is the thin synovial attachment of the plantar plate to the metatarsal neck and suggested that this tissue either lengthens or ruptures, leading to sagittal and axial deformity. It now appears, based on anatomic and surgical observation, that the initial deficiency occurs distally at the insertion of the plantar plate or in the midportion of the plantar plate.†

Deland and Sung[63] demonstrated a rupture of the lateral collateral ligament and attenuation of the lateral plantar plate in the dissection of a single specimen of a crossover second toe. Associated with this deformity was a medial subluxation of the plantar plate. As tension was applied on the medially subluxated long flexor tendon, the proximal phalanx deviated medially. The stout attachment of the plantar plate to the proximal phalanx was observed to be intact. Coughlin et al[50] reported on the anatomic dissection of 16 cadaveric specimens with second MTP joint instability and observed distal transverse plantar plate tears in all specimens, but in only 6 (38%) was disruption of a collateral ligament noted (Fig. 7-82). In a study of cadaveric specimens, Coughlin[50] reported a grading scheme to further quantify the magnitude and direction of plantar plate tears (Table 7-1). The grading of the anatomic findings (grades 0-IV) gives a means to evaluate the pathology, as well as to assist in the planning of an appropriate surgical approach, and then later to assess the results of surgical reconstruction in light of the varying magnitudes of plantar plate tears.

---

*References 14, 15, 23, 33, 42, 47, 50, 61, 168, and 229.
†References 10, 11, 15, 31, 47, 50, 83, 92-95, 168, 229, and 236.

Table 7-1	Anatomic Grading of Plantar Plate Tear[47,50,168]
Grade	**Description**
0	Plantar plate or capsular attenuation, and/or discoloration (see Fig. 7-83A)
I	Transverse distal tear (adjacent to insertion into proximal phalanx [<50%]; medial, lateral, or central area) and/or midsubstance tear (<50%) (see Figs. 7-82A, 7-83B, and 7-84A)
II	Transverse distal tear (≥50%); medial, lateral, or central area and/or midsubstance tear (≥50%) (see Figs. 7-82B, 7-83C, and 7-84B)
III	Transverse and/or longitudinal extensive tear (may involve collateral ligaments) (see Figs. 7-82C, 7-83D, and 7-84C, D)
IV	Extensive tear with button hole (dislocation) (see Figs. 7-82D, 7-83E, and 7-84E)

From Coughlin MJ, Baumfeld DS, Nery C: Second MTP joint instability: grading of the deformity and description of surgical repair of capsular insufficiency, *Phys Sportsmed* 39:132–141, 2011. Used with permission.

History and Demographics

The most common symptoms reported by patients with instability of the second MTP joint are pain and swelling on the plantar aspect of the foot, localized to the area of the distal MTP joint capsule. These symptoms may develop acutely in some cases and on a more chronic basis in others.[33,42,120,238] As the deformity progresses, the proximal phalanx can deviate in either a transverse (axial) and/or sagittal plane (Fig. 7-85).[33,42,43,120,168]

The propensity for female patient has been noted in previous clinical reports in which the frequency of female patients has varied from 71% to 86% (in series ranging in size from 18-169 patients).[33,42,15,120,168] The average age reported in series where a surgical repair has been performed has varied from 50 to 60 years.[15,42,83,120]

The differential diagnosis of pain localized to the area of the second MTP joint includes MTP joint synovitis, capsule degeneration, a Freiberg infraction (Video Clip 71), metatarsal stress fracture, degenerative arthritis, systemic arthritis localized to the second MTP joint, synovial cyst formation, and interdigital neuroma (Figs. 7-86 and 7-87 and Video Clip 86).[33,41,44,48, 34-37]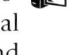

Although a synovial cyst or interdigital neuroma may be associated with pain and deviation of the toe, intrinsic capsular instability more often is the cause of malalignment of the MTP joint (Fig. 7-88).[33,42,44] It can be difficult to differentiate pain from MTP joint capsule instability and that from an adjacent interdigital neuroma[42,48,49,78,153]; however, typically a neuroma is associated with neuritic radicular pain to the involved toes as well as numbness. MTP joint instability typically is not associated with neuritic symptoms or numbness unless there is a concomitant interdigital neuroma. Likewise, reproduction of pain with a squeeze test (compression of the MT heads) and a Mulder click is typical of an interdigital neuroma.[48,161] MTP joint instability typically is not associated with numbness unless there is a concomitant interdigital neuroma. Coughlin and Schenck[49] reported

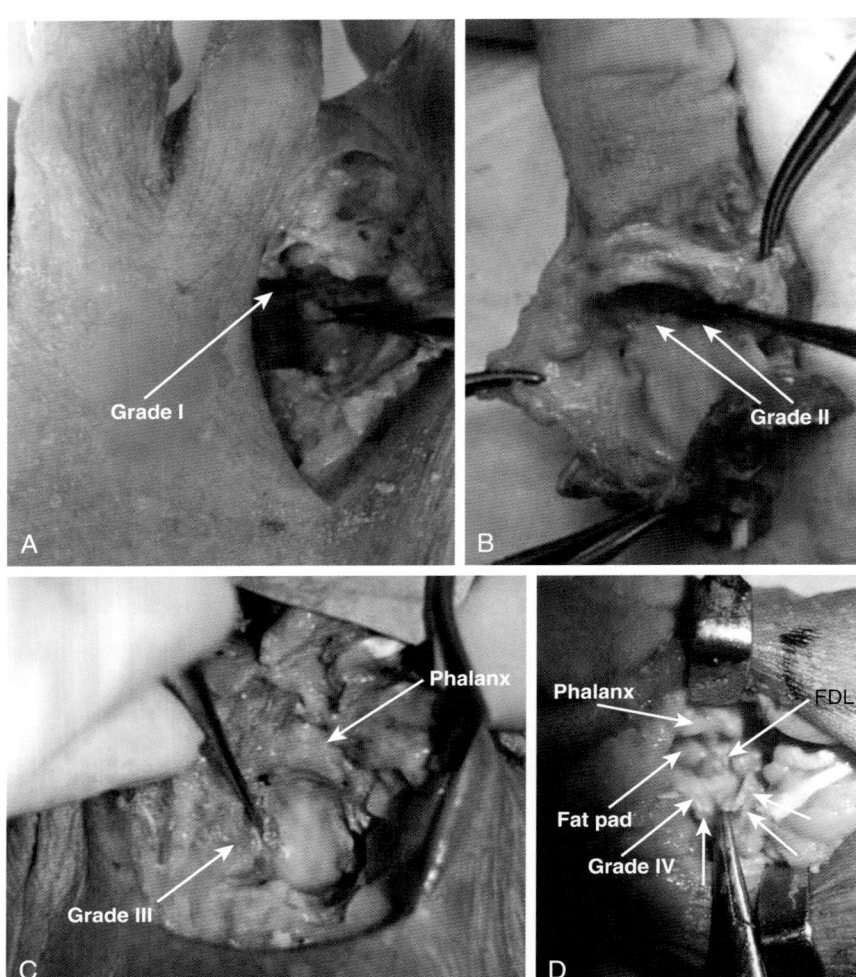

Figure 7-82 Anatomic dissection photographs demonstrating different grades of tears. **A,** Grade I tear at left base of proximal phalanx (<50% across). **B,** Grade II tear (in disarticulated specimen, phalanx at top demonstrating ≥50% tear of plantar plate insertion). **C,** Grade III tear demonstrating a pattern "7" with longitudinal midsubstance tear along the edge of the plate and also a transverse tear at the base of the proximal phalanx. **D,** Grade IV tear demonstrating complete disruption of the plantar plate (the fat pad and flexor tendon can be demonstrated in the base of the photograph). (**A, B,** and **D,** From Coughlin M, Schutt S, Hirose C, et al: Metatarsophalangeal joint pathology in crossover second toe deformity: a cadaveric study, *Foot Ankle Int* 33:133–140, 2012. Used with permission.)

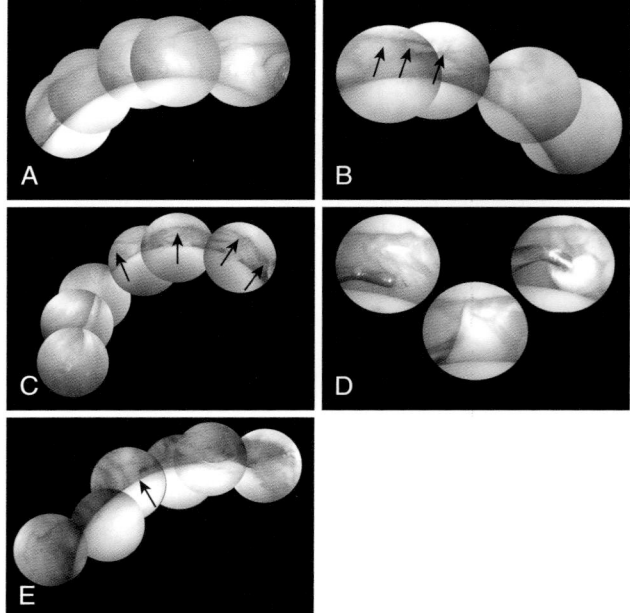

Figure 7-83 Arthroscopic photographs of grades of plantar plate tears (left foot). **A,** Grade 0: attenuation of third metatarsophalangeal (MTP) joint. In the right portion of the figure, one can see the radiofrequency instrument that was used in the treatment of this lesion. **B,** Grade I: lateral partial plantar plate tear—second MTP joint (*arrows* point to partial transverse plate tear at base of proximal phalanx). **C,** Grade II: complete transverse tear at base of proximal phalanx—second MTP joint (*arrows* point to complete transverse plantar plate tear). **D,** Grade III: transverse distal tear, with additional longitudinal component called a "7"-type tear (resembles the number 7). **E,** Grade IV: only a minimum remains of the plantar plate. The plantar fat pad surrounds the metatarsal head (the fibrous connective tissue of the plantar plate is absent). The *arrow* points to the attenuated flexor digitorum longus (FDL) tendon in the central portion of the MTP joint. (Copyright 2012 by Caio Nery, MD. Used with permission.)

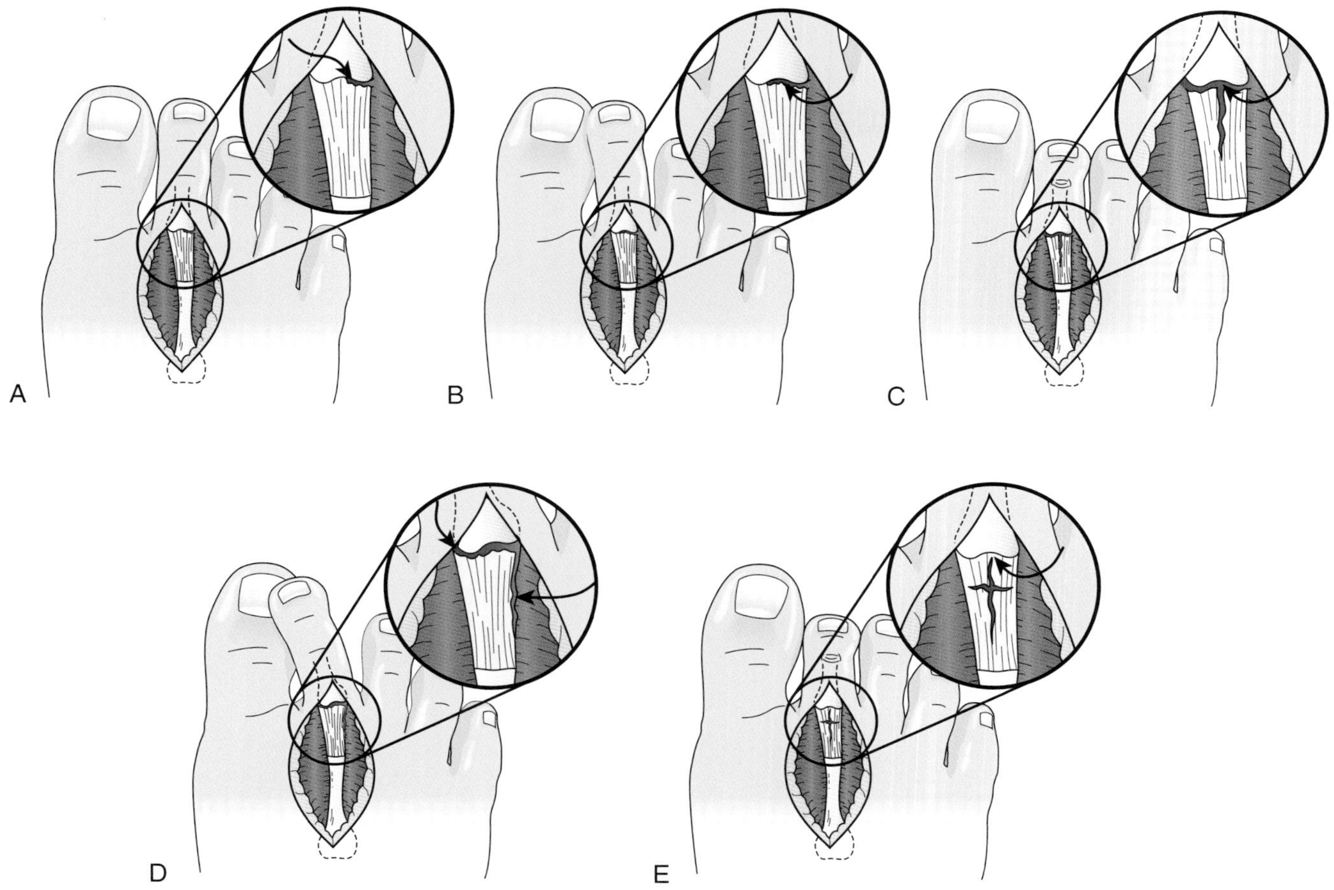

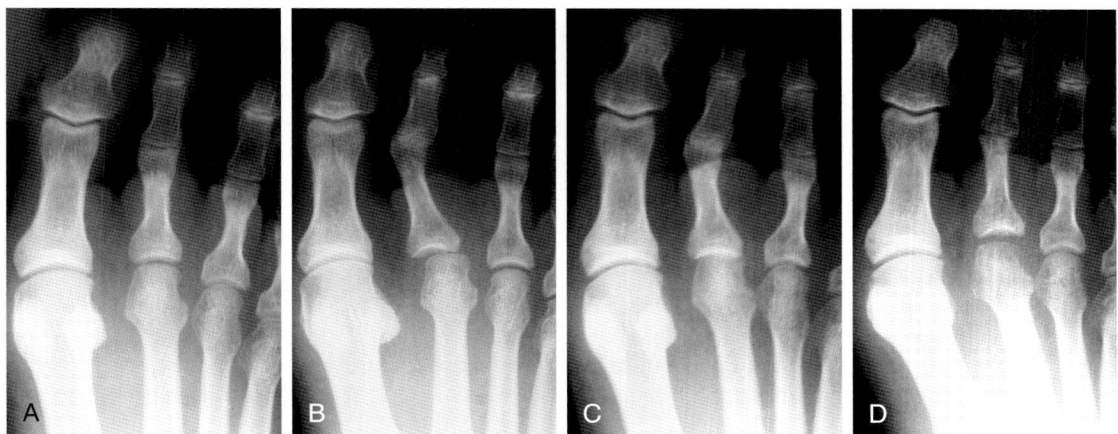

Figure 7-84 Anatomic grading of plantar plate tears. **A,** Grade I tear. **B,** Grade II tear. **C** and **D,** Two types of grade III tears. **E,** Grade IV tear: complete disruption of the plantar plate. (Used with permission from Nery C, Coughlin MJ, Baumfeld D, Mann TS. Lesser metatarsophalangeal joint instability: prospective evaluation and repair of plantar plate or capsular insufficienty. *Foot Ankle Int* 33:301-311, 2012.)

Figure 7-85 Radiographs demonstrating subluxation and dislocation of the second metatarsophalangeal (MTP) joint. **A,** Symptomatic second MTP joint without radiographic abnormality. **B,** Subluxation. **C,** Two months later, dorsal dislocation has occurred. **D,** After surgical reconstruction, the second MTP joint is relocated and stabilized.

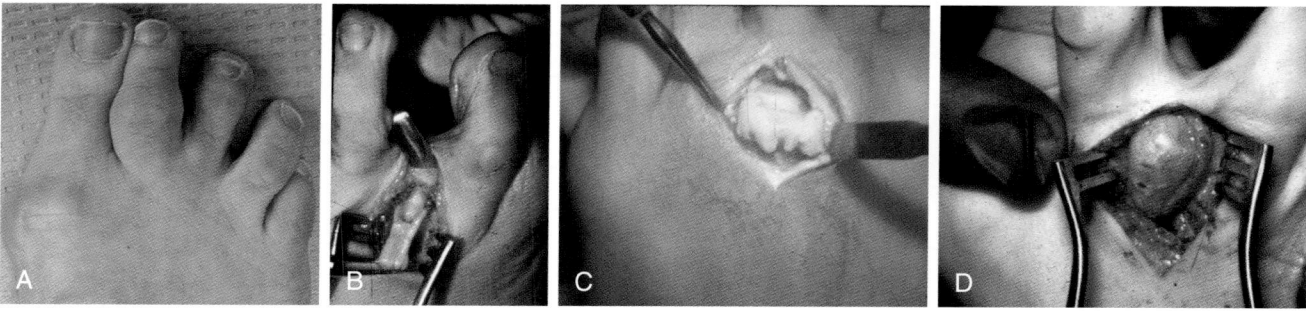

Figure 7-86 Causes of metatarsalgia. **A,** Nonspecific synovitis with swollen second toe and medial metatarsophalangeal (MTP) joint deviation. **B,** Interdigital neuroma can cause pain in this region. **C,** Freiberg infraction of the second MTP joint. **D,** Synovial cyst causing deviation of the second and third toes.

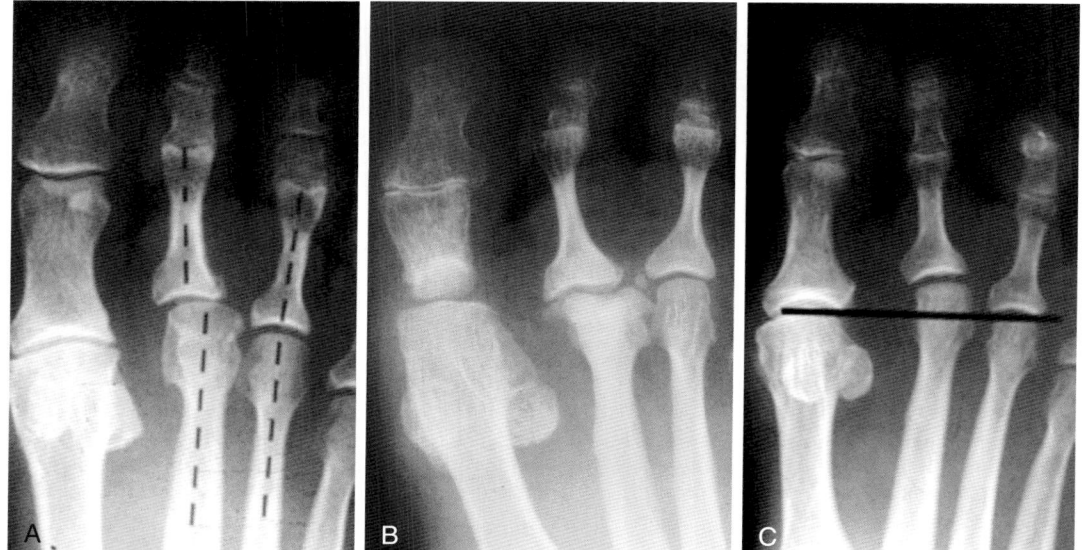

Figure 7-87 **A,** Anteroposterior radiograph demonstrating noncongruent second metatarsophalangeal (MTP) joint in early degenerative arthritis. **B,** Severe degenerative arthritis of the second MTP joint. **C,** A long second ray is often associated with a hammer toe or mallet toe deformity as well as instability of the second MTP joint.

that 20% of the cases in which an interdigital neuroma was excised also demonstrated instability of the second MTP joint (see Fig. 7-25). With the progression of deformity, patients tend to lose the ability to curl the affected toe and can lose this ability in the adjacent lesser toes (because of FDL dysfunction).

Johnson and Price[113] speculated that a pronation and adduction deformity of the midfoot and hindfoot was the contributing cause of a crossover second toe deformity; unfortunately, they failed to appreciate the significant contribution of excessive second metatarsal length, capsule instability, or plantar plate insufficiency.

Physical Examination

Synovitis of the second MTP joint on physical examination can be characterized by localized swelling in the joint or can involve the entire second toe.[144] Tenderness on palpation can be localized to either the medial or lateral aspect of the MTP joint or to the plantar aspect of the joint, depending on the exact location of the capsular disorder.

MTP joint subluxation and dislocation can lead to a subsequent hammer toe deformity.[33,42,44,140] With buckling of the second toe, an intractable plantar keratotic lesion can develop beneath the symptomatic metatarsal head. Likewise, a callus can develop over the dorsal aspect of the PIP joint as the toe impacts against the dorsal aspect of the toe box.

Often, MTP joint subluxation develops insidiously. Complaints of pain in the intermetatarsal space are not uncommon with ambulation. The patient typically does not have pain at rest. Palpation of the intermetatarsal space can cause pain, but the pain does not radiate to the toes. With dorsal dislocation of the second MTP joint, the typical symptoms result because the proximal phalanx lies dorsal to the second metatarsal, causing the toe to

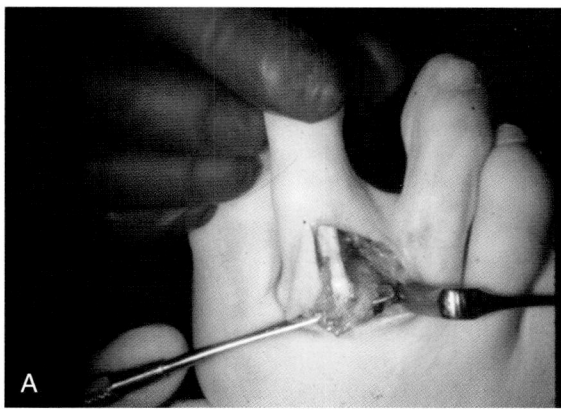

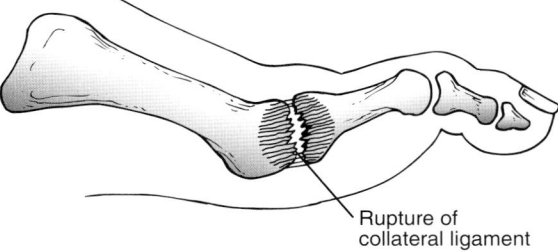

Figure 7-88 **A,** Rupture of the lateral collateral ligament of the second metatarsophalangeal (MTP) joint in foot with crossover second toe deformity. **B,** With a crossover second toe deformity, the lateral collateral ligament can rupture, with subsequent medial deviation of the toe. With time, the rupture can extend plantarward, leading to hyperextension and dislocation of the MTP joint. Note excessive length of the second metatarsal compared with adjacent metatarsals. (**A,** From Coughlin MJ: Crossover second toe deformity, *Foot Ankle* 8:29–39, 1987.)

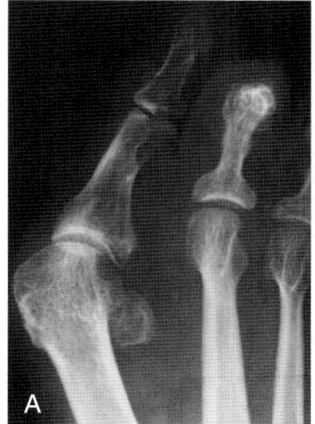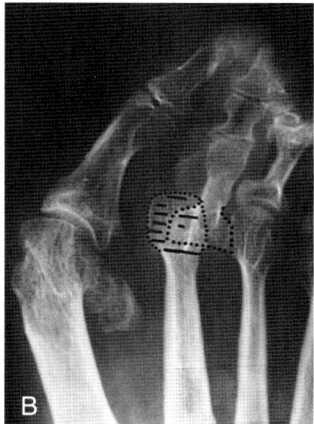

Figure 7-89 **A,** A 55-year-old woman with severe hallux valgus deformity. Note that the radiograph shows a hammer toe deformity of the second toe; however, the metatarsophalangeal (MTP) joint is well aligned. **B,** Three years after a simple bunionectomy, a recurrent hallux valgus deformity has occurred. There is now severe dislocation of the second MTP joint.

strike the top of the toe box, producing a painful lesion over the PIP joint. The shoe, in turn, forces the dislocated proximal phalanx downward against the metatarsal head, which can lead to development of a large, painful intractable plantar keratotic lesion. With dislocation of the toe, the prominent dorsal base of the proximal phalanx often is easily palpated.

The single most useful test[219] to determine the presence of a plantar plate tear and MTP joint instability is the vertical drawer test (see Fig. 7-27). Described by Thomson and Hamilton[219] and others,[32,35,42] the toe is vertically subluxated, placing pressure on the plantar plate and often eliciting characteristic pain.[43] When testing MTP joint stability, the involved toe should be dorsiflexed 25 degrees at the MTP joint before the vertical stress test is performed.[62] A positive test,[32,35,42,43] we believe, is pathognomonic for an unstable lesser MTP joint[42,120,219] (see Fig. 7-27). In more advanced stages, obvious subluxability of the involved MTP joint occurs with this stress test. This test estimates the amount of dorsal translation of the proximal phalanx base in relation to the metatarsal head when a force is applied by the examiner to the proximal

phalanx. The drawer test is rated as mild, moderate, or severe, based upon subluxability of the joint. This test may also elicit pain with dorsal/plantar stress to the symptomatic digit. The drawer test is a key component in the staging of the lesser MTP joint instability. The findings we have observed at surgery (with partial or complete disruption of the distal plantar plate) make it clear why a drawer test is positive and why the pain is localized on the plantar surface of the lesser metatarsophalangeal joint at the base of the proximal phalanx.

The specific diagnosis of MTP joint instability may be aided by local Xylocaine injections into the symptomatic areas. Differentiation of pain originating from a symptomatic interdigital neuroma or an unstable lesser MTP joint can be difficult. Coughlin[36] and others[49,156] have recommended sequential injections to help differentiate the specific area of pain.

Other physical findings may include swelling of the digit and the development of a hammer toe in more chronic situations.[120] With the patient in a standing position, the the toe is examined as to whether or not the toe pulp touches the ground. Dorsiflexion of the MTP joint leads to an inability of the digit to touch the ground (loss of toe touch, or a floating toe). The loss of digital strength (also known as toe purchase) is demonstrated by the "paper pull-out test."[15] With the patient standing, a strip of paper is placed beneath the affected toe. With the patient flexing the digit, if he or she is unable to prevent the paper from being pulled from beneath the digit, it is considered a positive test (absence of digital purchase). These physical findings are used as well to stage the level of instability. With time, a toe may subluxate (see Fig. 7-30) and finally dislocate (Fig. 7-89 and Table 7-2).

Instability of the MTP joint has previously been categorized into distinct grades[38,97,153,218,238] but typically these

Table 7-2 Clinical Staging System for Second Metatarsophalangeal Joint[47]

Grade	Alignment	Physical Examination
0	MTP joint; normal alignment. Prodromal phase with pain but no deformity	MTP joint pain, thickening or swelling of the MTP joint, reduced toe purchase, negative drawer
I	Mild malalignment at MTP joint, widening of web space, medial deviation (see Figs. 7-90A and 7-91A)	MTP joint pain, swelling of MTP joint, loss of toe purchase, mild positive drawer (<50% subluxable)
II	Moderate malalignment; medial, lateral, dorsal, or dorsomedial deformity, hyperextension of toe (see Figs. 7-90B and 7-91B)	MTP joint pain, reduced swelling, no toe purchase, moderate positive drawer (≥50% subluxable)
III	Severe malalignment; dorsal or dorsomedial deformity. Second toe can overlap the hallux. May have flexible hammer toe (see Figs. 7-90C and 7-91C)	Joint and toe pain, little swelling, no toe purchase, very positive drawer (dislocatable MTP joint), flexible hammer toe
IV	Very severe deformity: dorsomedial or dorsal dislocation, severe deformity with dislocation, fixed hammer toe (see Figs. 7-90D and 7-91D)	Joint and toe pain, little or no swelling, no toe purchase, dislocated MTP joint, fixed hammer toe

From Coughlin MJ, Baumfeld DS, Nery C: Second MTP joint instability: grading of the deformity and description of surgical repair of capsular insufficiency, *Phys Sportsmed* 39:132–141, 2011. Used with permission.

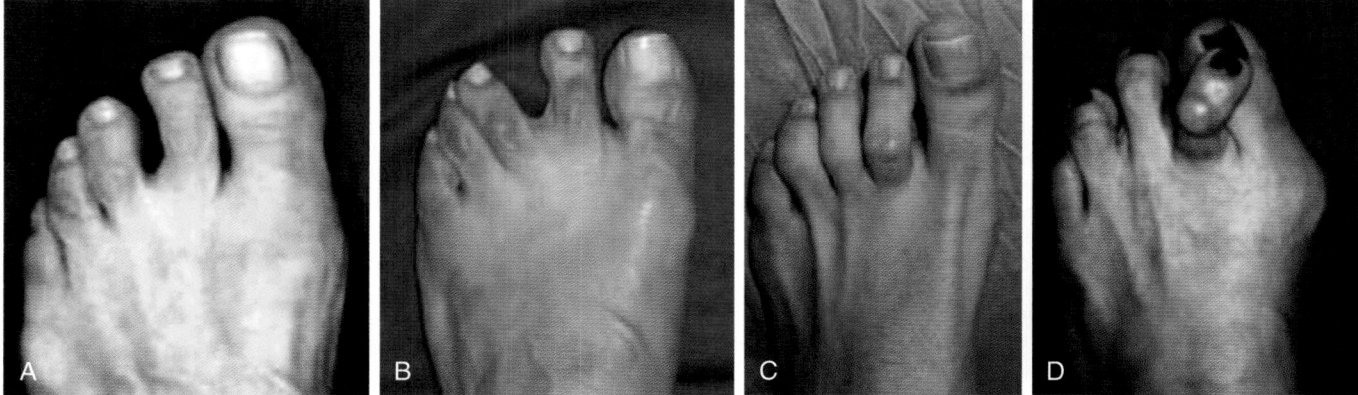

Figure 7-90 A. Stage I instability: mild medial deviation. **B,** Stage II instability: more substantial medial deviation, lateral digits remain where they have been for several years. **C,** Stage III instability: dorsal medial deviation with hammer toe formation. **D,** Stage IV instability: severe deformity with dislocation, fixed hammer toe, and chronic pain. (Copyright 2012 by Caio Nery, MD. Used with permission.)

grades have used only clinical descriptions without considering the anatomic finding of an associated plantar plate tear. Mendicino[153] and Yu[238] have both described a prodromal stage preceding subluxation, characterized by MTP joint pain and swelling.

We have developed a comprehensive staging system,[47,168] based on several of the components of these prior suggestions (see Table 7-2), to quantify findings based upon the physical examination.

Radiographic Examination

Radiographic evaluation of the MTP joint may be less important than the clinical examination.[120] Typically, the lateral inclination of the lesser toes averages approximately 12 degrees.[33,120] With progressive deviation of the MTP joint, this orientation can increase or decrease. Typically, if there is a difference of 6 degrees or more between the MTP-2 and MTP-3 angles, this is considered to be a positive radiographic examination.[120] On the AP radiograph, the diaphysis of the proximal phalanx may be hyperextended so that a gun barrel sign is seen (see Fig. 7-4B).[43] The diaphysis of the proximal phalanx projects as a round hole in the area of the distal condyle of the proximal phalanx. Radiographs may be helpful in the evaluating the magnitude of the MTP joint deformity, assessing joint congruity (see Fig. 7-87A), ascertaining the presence of MTP joint arthritis (see Figs. 7-87B and 7-77), and determining the length of the second metatarsal (see Fig. 7-87C).

On the AP radiograph, Coughlin[33] suggested, in reviewing a series of 17 patients (22 toes), that a long second metatarsal placed the second MTP joint at risk for increased intraarticular pressure and joint subluxation. Later, Kaz,[120] in reviewing the radiographs of these same 17 patients, as well as a larger series of 169 patients, concluded that the supposed increased length of the second metatarsal was largely due to the method of measurement; in cases of hallux valgus, the increased intermetatarsal angle can lead to the conclusion that the first metatarsal is shorter than the second, although, in fact, the length is virtually the same. It appears to be the "relative length" of the second metatarsal in relationship to the first metatarsal that plays a role in destabilizing the lesser MTP joints (see Fig. 7-88).

Chondrolysis of the MTP joint may be associated with degenerative arthritis[200] or a Freiberg infraction (see Fig. 7-77 and 86C). In a typical radiograph, the articular cartilage of the adjoining surface leaves a clear space of 2 to 3 mm (see Fig. 7-30).[37] As hyperextension of the MTP joint develops, this clear space diminishes as the base of the proximal phalanx subluxates dorsally over the second metatarsal head. With frank dislocation, the base of the proximal phalanx can lie dorsally over the metatarsal head and is demonstrated as an overlapping of the adjacent bone on the AP radiograph (see Fig. 7-89).

With progression of deformity, typically, the second toe deviates medially or dorsomedially and gradually comes to rest above the hallux (Fig. 7-91). A hallux valgus deformity may be identified on examination, although association with a crossover toe is disputed (see Fig. 7-91).[4,33,113]

A lateral radiograph can demonstrate dislocation or hyperextension of the MTP joint (see Fig. 7-29B). The magnitude and the chronicity of the deformity appear to be related. With time, significant contractures of adjacent soft tissues can develop, with fixed dorsal dislocation at the MTP joint.

Karpman and MacCollum[118] and others[83,153,183,236] have described arthrography of the second MTP joint, which may be helpful in assessing capsule deterioration or instability of the MTP joint. Leakage of dye into the tendon sheath of the tendon can indicate a plantar plate rupture. A bone scan can help to differentiate ill-defined pain in the forefoot. Increased uptake can signify early intraarticular MTP joint instability (see Fig. 7-31). Gregg et al[94,95] have demonstrated the use of ultrasonography in visualizing plantar plate pathology.

Magnetic resonance imaging (MRI) may be useful to assess the continuity of the plantar plate early before pronounced deformity, although in most cases, the diagnosis is made clinically. These changes may be subtle and difficult to diagnose (Fig. 7-92). Yao et al[235,236] and others[15,94,236,168] have reported MRI to be helpful in the diagnosis of plantar plate abnormalities. Nery et al[168] found MRIs to be a reliable, although an expensive, means with which to document plantar plate pathology and tears. Nery[168] observed that the most significant finding on the MRI was an area of increased signal intensity in the vicinity of the proximal phalangeal base at the location of the distal plantar plate insertion where the tears were identified.[168] MRI was helpful in identifying not only the plantar plate rupture but also longitudinal and transverse extensions of the tear in other areas of the plantar plate. (In the coronal plane, synovitis tends to distend the joint capsule with displacement of soft tissue structures.[168]) Nery[168] noted that although MRI is highly accurate in diagnosing a plantar plate tear, they had low rates of specificity because of the difficulty in defining specifically the type and extension of the plantar plate tear (Fig. 7-93).

Treatment

Conservative Treatment

A hammer toe may be managed conservatively with a comfortable, well-fitted shoe with sufficient room in the toe box to accommodate the toe deformity. Decreasing the heel height can alleviate plantar discomfort as well. A toe cradle prevents the toe tip from impacting against the ground, which also can decrease discomfort.[219] By taping the deformed toe in a neutral position, stability may be achieved over time, although this can require several months.[33,42] Prolonged taping does not correct the deformity but may achieve stabilization, with scarring at the MTP joint. However, once subluxation or dislocation has occurred, taping is not helpful. The use of taping over a long period of time can lead to ulceration of the toe or chronic edema (Fig. 7-94).

Placement of a metatarsal pad just proximal to a symptomatic metatarsal head can alleviate plantar discomfort by redistribution of weight on the plantar surface of the foot; stiffening of the insole with either a prefabricated or customized graphite or carbon fiber inlay may be advantageous (Fig. 7-95). Once an intractable plantar keratosis has developed, the use of an extra-depth shoe with a specialized liner or insert tends to relieve plantar discomfort. A roomy toe box accommodates both a fixed hammer toe deformity and a thickened insole. Padding over the tip of the contracted toe can help to decrease sensitivity of a callus either at the tip of the toe or overlying the hammer toe deformity.

The use of nonsteroidal antiinflammatory drugs (NSAIDs) can decrease discomfort from inflammation at a symptomatic MTP joint. The judicious use of an intraarticular steroid injection may be considered. Trepman and Yao[222] described nonsurgical treatment of second MTP joint synovitis with an intraarticular steroid injection and used a rocker sole to limit MTP joint dorsiflexion. At an average follow-up of 18 months, 60% of patients were asymptomatic, and an additional 33% were improved. Mizel and Michelson,[159] reporting on a similar treatment with an intraarticular steroid injection and the use of a shoe modification with an extended steel shank, noted seven of nine symptomatic feet were asymptomatic at 6-year follow-up (Fig. 7-96). The potential disadvantage of corticosteroid injections is the risk of further plantar plate attenuation with subsequent dislocation.[43,238] Reis et al[190] reported on two cases of MTP dislocation after an intraarticular steroid injection and concluded that this can cause attenuation of the plantar capsule with subsequent dislocation. More commonly, dislocation occurs in older persons who have no history of injury or injection.

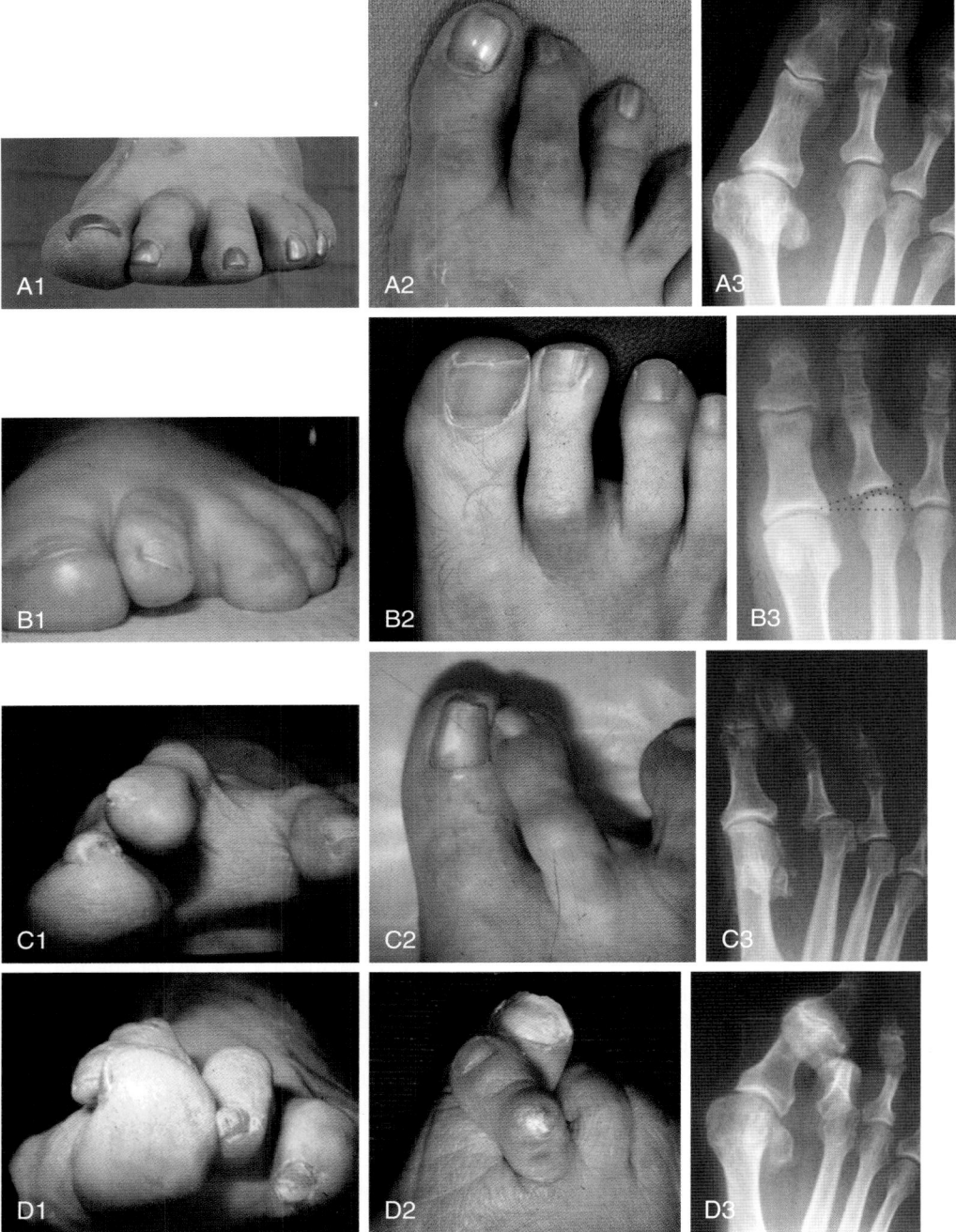

Figure 7-91   Crossover second toe deformity. **A,** Mild. **B,** Progressing deformity. **C,** Moderate deformity. **D,** Severe deformity beginning as mild subluxation of the metatarsophalangeal joint and finally progressing to frank dislocation. (**B1** and **C2,** From Coughlin MJ: Lesser toe abnormalities, *Instr Course Lect* 52:421-444, 2003.)

Fortin and Myerson[78] concluded that conservative care frequently fails and noted that an intraarticular steroid injection, in their experience, usually gave only temporary relief of 3 to 6 months, although occasionally a patient obtained permanent relief. After an intraarticular steroid injection, the affected toe is "buddy taped" to an adjacent toe for 6 to 12 weeks to reduce the incidence of MTP joint dislocation. Nonsurgical treatment of an unstable second

MTP joint deformity is often unsuccessful. Coughlin[33] reported on three patients with a mild-to-moderate crossover deformity who were treated with taping and had no progression of the deformity, but they continued to have symptoms. Reports on series of conservative treatment of this problem are conspicuously lacking in the literature. Even with lengthy nonsurgical treatment, often symptoms do not completely resolve. Residual pain is often centered on the plantar aspect of the MTP joint near the base of the proximal phalanx, the area where the positive drawer test tends to cause such dramatic pain. When chronic pain is unrelieved by conservative methods or if progressive subluxation of the second MTP joint has developed, surgical intervention may be necessary.

Surgical Treatment
PREOPERATIVE PLANNING (Fig. 7-97)
Certain factors must be appreciated in the development of the treatment plan for MTP joint subluxation or

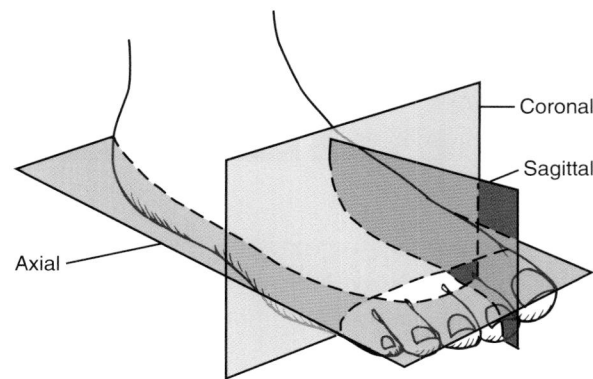

Figure 7-92 Diagram of planes used for forefoot magnetic resonance imaging.

dislocation. The presence of a hallux valgus deformity may be a cause of or may have developed subsequent to the second toe abnormality. Although a hallux valgus deformity may be asymptomatic, surgical correction often is required to obtain adequate space for the corrected second toe once it has been realigned to a normal position. Mann and Mizel[144] reported on the treatment of seven patients (average age, 57 years) with generalized thickening of the second MTP joint, increased warmth and tenderness, and decreased range of motion. They were noted to have a positive vertical stress test in all cases. Six patients were treated with a synovectomy and 50% with resection of a second interspace interdigital neuroma. They reported generally good results with this treatment.

The surgeon must determine whether a fixed or flexible hammer toe deformity is present. A fixed hammer toe deformity usually develops in the presence of a more chronic deformity and is more unusual in a mild deformity. If the hammer toe is fixed, a DuVries arthroplasty is performed (see the description of the technique of fixed hammer toe repair earlier in this chapter). If the hammer toe is flexible and is passively correctable, a flexor tendon transfer may be performed; or correction of the MTP joint with a plantar plate repair may straighten the flexible digit as well. Often a fixed contracture of the MTP joint is present. With a pure hyperextension deformity at the MTP joint, a soft tissue release is performed. A complete medial, lateral, and dorsal capsule release is performed in

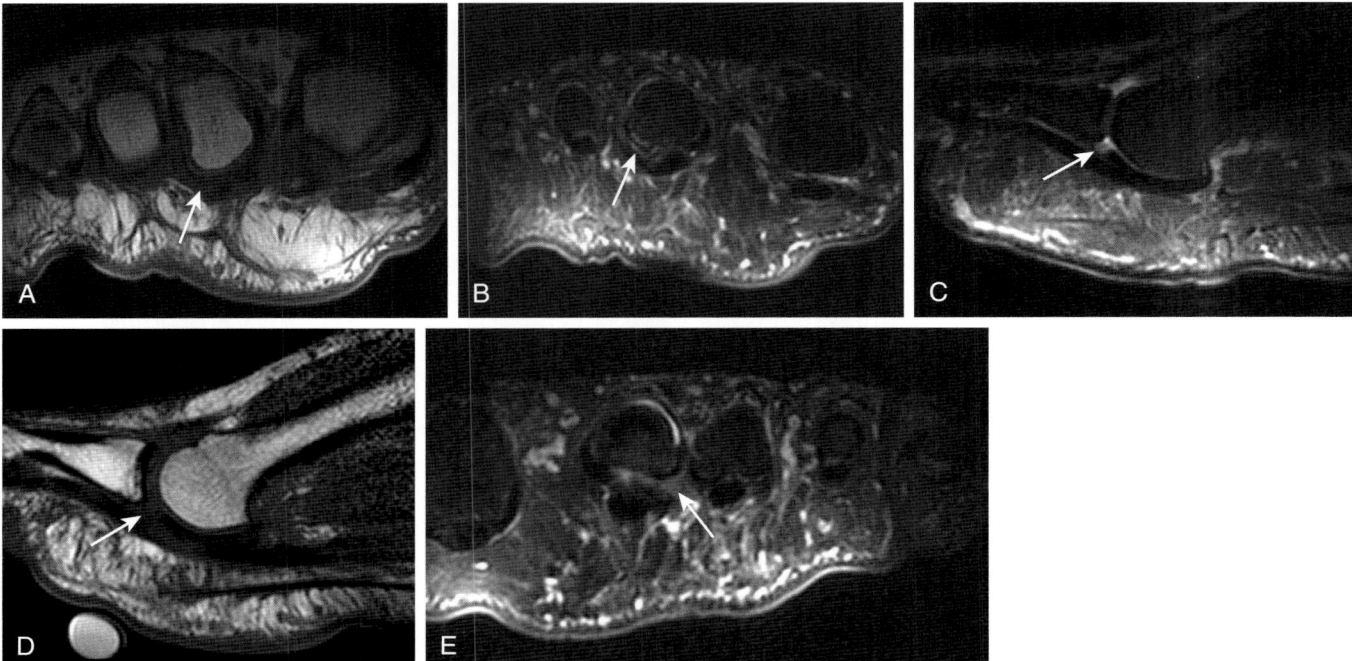

Figure 7-93 Magnetic resonance imaging (MRI) scans of plantar plate tears. **A,** Grade 0: MRI of coronal plane. Attenuation of the lateral portion of the second metatarsophalangeal (MTP) plantar plate *(arrow)*. **B,** Grade I: MRI of coronal plane. The *arrow* points to a second MTP joint plantar plate tear in the lateral portion. **C,** Grade I: MRI of sagittal plane. The *arrow* is pointing to a plantar plate tear. **D,** Grade II: MRI of sagittal plane. Complete distal transverse tear of the plantar plate *(arrow)*. **E,** Grade III: MRI of coronal plane. Lateral longitudinal tear of the second MTP plantar plate *(arrow)*. (Copyright 2012 by Caio Nery, MD. Used with permission.)

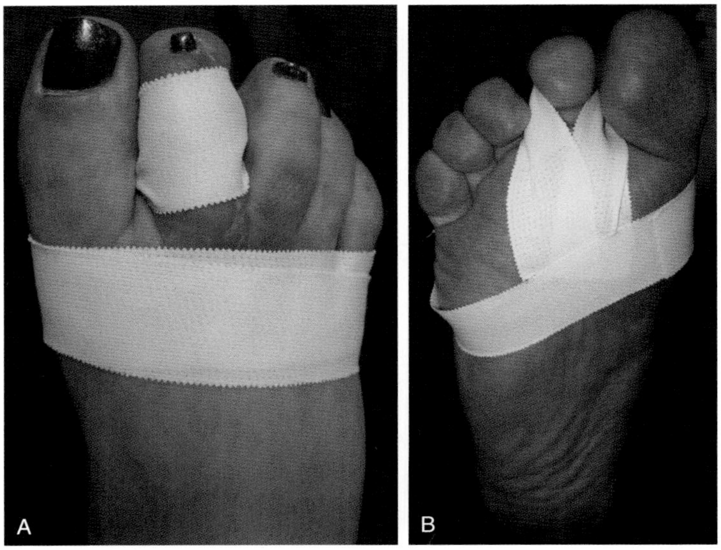

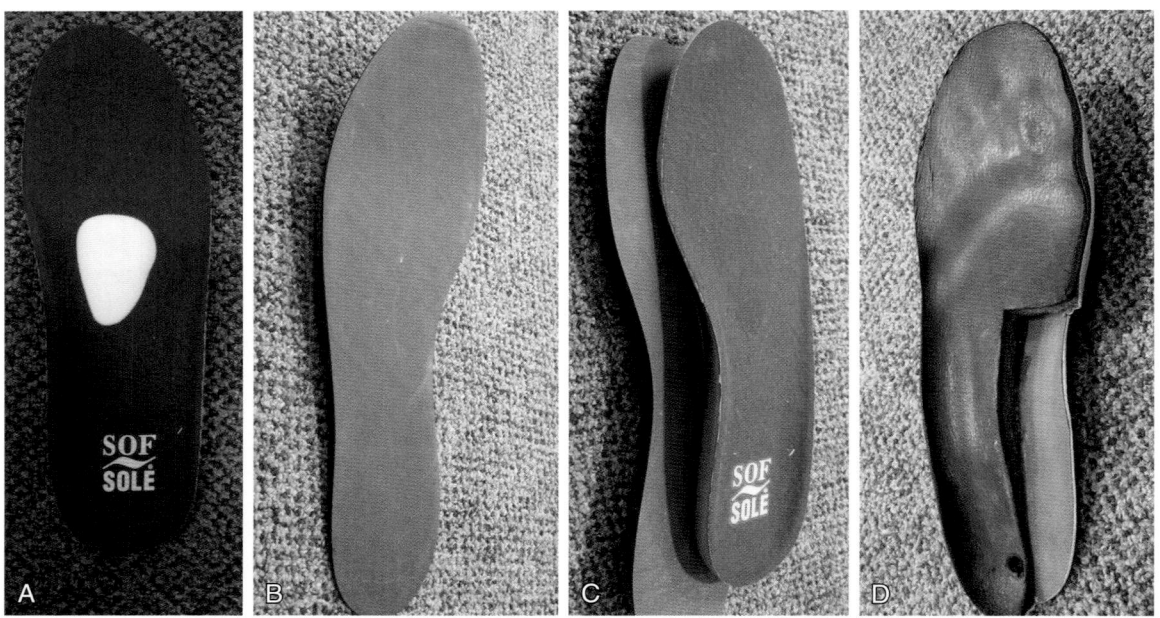

Figure 7-94 Methods of taping the second toe. **A,** Dorsal view. **B,** Plantar view.

Figure 7-95 Orthotic management of lesser metatarsophalangeal joint instability. **A,** Prefabricated graphite insole stiffens the toe box area. **B,** A graphite or carbon fiber insole can stiffen the forefoot area of the shoe. **C,** The graphite insole is combined with a prefabricated soft orthotic. **D,** A custom-made insole with carbon fiber insert within. (Courtesy Brent Hansen, Ketchum, Idaho.)

a sequential fashion to achieve complete reduction of the deformity.[78] With a hyperextension deformity, it often is necessary to release adhesions between the plantar capsule and the metatarsal head. A McGlamry elevator is used to release these contractures. If there is residual medial deviation at the MTP joint, an extensor digitorum brevis transfer may be performed[78,119] as well as a capsular reefing.

Placement of an intramedullary Kirschner wire is optional. If a fixed hammer toe repair has been performed, or if the surgeon believes increased support for the surgical repair is necessary, a Kirschner wire should be placed. This may be one of the best indications for the use of a permanent implant to stabilize the hammer toe repair. Placement of this pin may be somewhat difficult. Usually, it is driven distally from the MTP joint and exits at the tip of the toe. The wire driver then is placed on the pin distally, and the pin is driven in a retrograde fashion across the MTP joint. Occasionally, some difficulty is encountered in transfixing the MTP joint. The pin can angle into the soft tissue adjacent to the MTP joint. Even

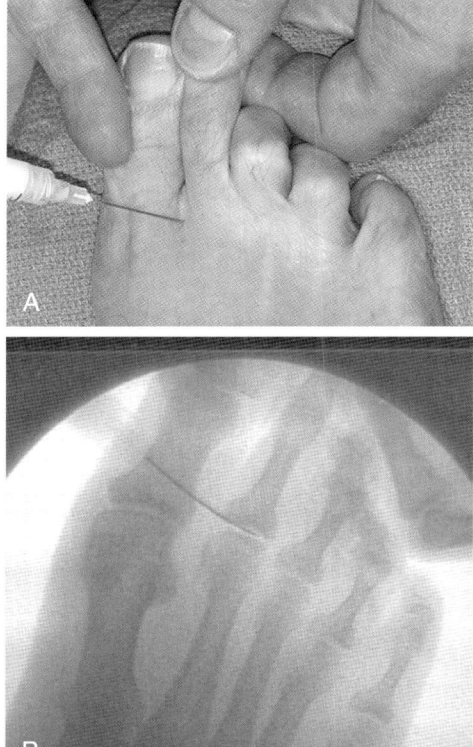

Figure 7-96 An intraarticular injection of lidocaine can temporarily relieve pain, aiding in the diagnosis of metatarsophalangeal joint instability. **A,** Injection. **B,** Fluoroscopic documentation of injection.

if the pin does not transfix the MTP joint, it can provide significant stability to the repair. A Kirschner wire should not be used to achieve additional corrective alignment because, when the wire is removed, the toe deformity can recur. The surgeon might find it easier to reef the capsule after the Kirschner wire has been advanced through the toe but before it is passed in a retrograde fashion into the metatarsal.

Despite a soft tissue release (see Fig. 7-72) and capsular reefing, often there remains an element of MTP joint hyperextension. A flexor tendon transfer may then be considered. A flexor tendon transfer removes the deforming force from the distal toe and adds a plantar flexion force to the proximal phalanx (Fig. 7-98). Whether this is a dynamic transfer or a tenodesing effect is unclear, but the transfer typically depresses the proximal phalanx and achieves adequate alignment of the MTP joint (see the earlier discussion of flexor tendon transfer). A flexor tendon transfer also adds a supporting force to an incompetent or degenerated plantar plate. To achieve stability of the second MTP joint after a soft tissue realignment, a plantar condylectomy has been advocated,[43] although it is used much less commonly at this time.

The capital oblique osteotomy was initially described by Barouk[6] and attributed by him to Weil.[231,232] The

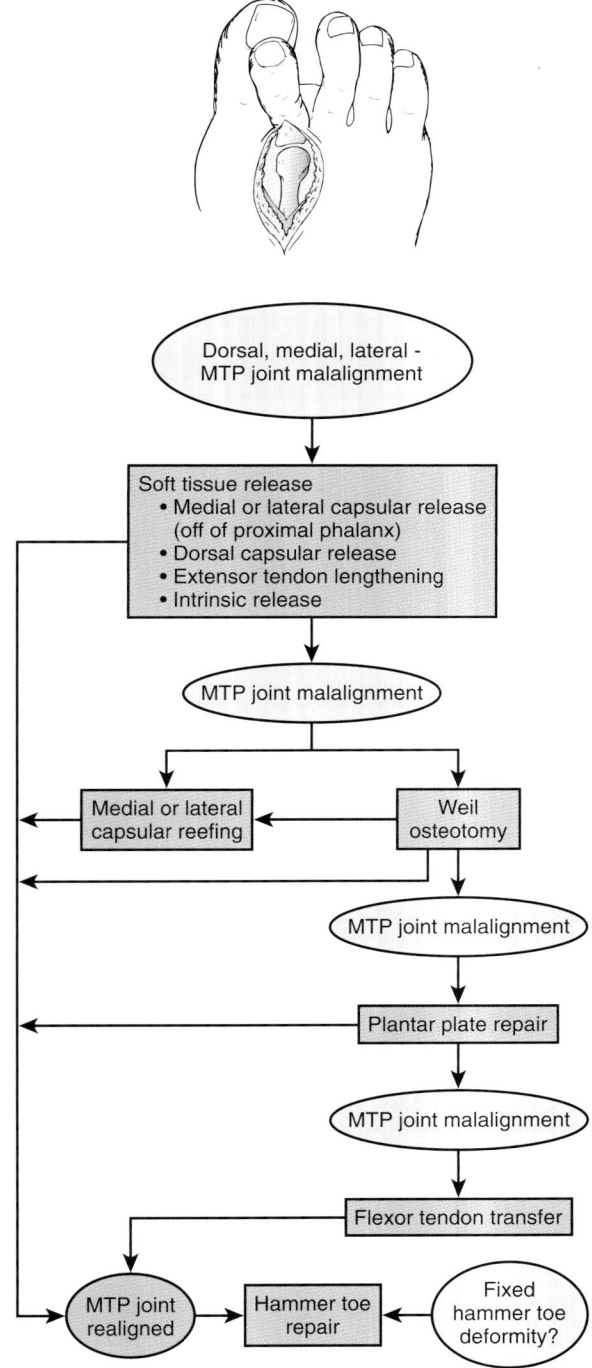

Figure 7-97 Algorithm for treatment of mild and moderate subluxation of the metatarsophalangeal joint.

technique has been described in several reports.* A Weil osteotomy is preferred to achieve access to the plantar plate as well as shortening of the metatarsal. After an osteotomy, internal fixation of the MTP joint with a Kirschner wire may be necessary after completion of any

---

*References 7, 18, 32, 36, 56, 96, 106, 123, 154, 172, 223-225, and 232.

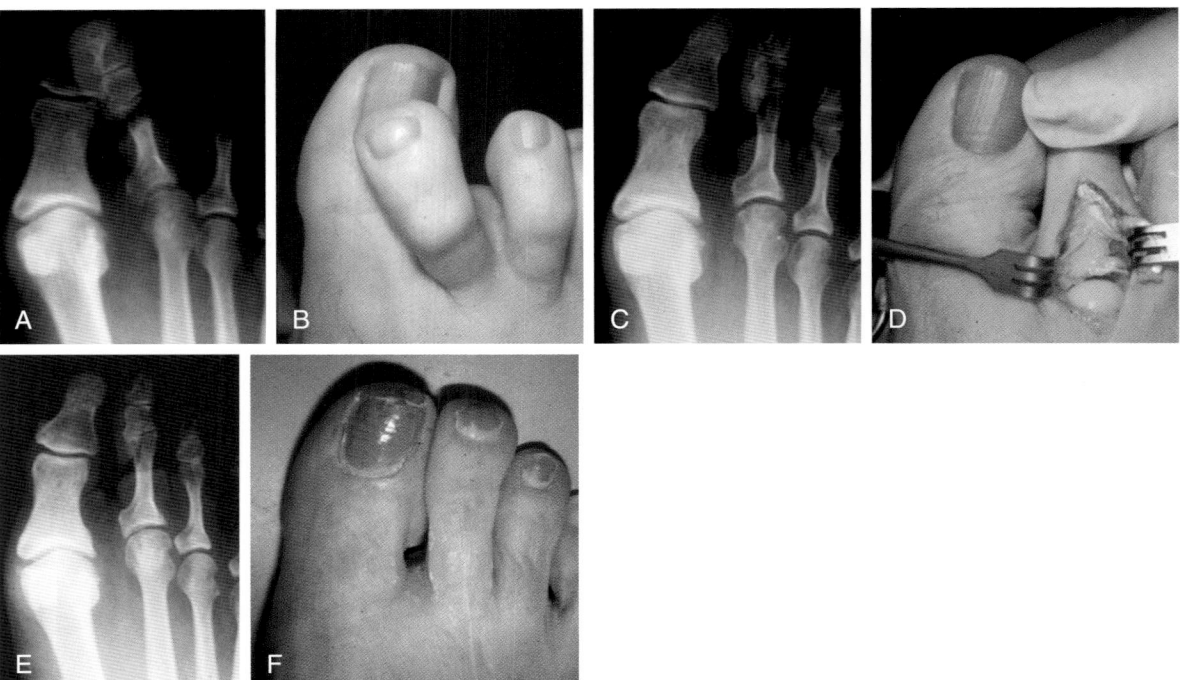

Figure 7-98 Radiograph **(A)** and clinical photograph **(B)** demonstrating a crossover second toe deformity. Radiograph **(C)** and clinical photograph **(D)** during and after a soft tissue realignment procedure for crossover second toe deformity. Radiograph **(E)** and clinical photo **(F)** at follow-up 9 years after a soft tissue release, lateral capsule reefing, and flexor tendon transfer. (From Coughlin MJ: Crossover second-toe deformity, *Foot Ankle* 8:29–39, 1987.)

of these procedures. A distal metatarsal osteotomy may be necessary if the joint cannot be reduced to an anatomic position (Fig. 7-99). An osteotomy preserves some MTP joint function and is preferable to a resection arthroplasty. The Weil osteotomy decompresses the joint, relieves pressure on the plantar plate, and likely adds an element of intraarticular scarring that stabilizes the MTP joint. In the presence of medial deviation,[61] a medial capsule release (from the proximal phalanx) may be augmented by lateral capsule reefing to align a deviated toe. Release of the proximal plantar plate has been advocated by Weil.[229] A capital oblique osteotomy is performed in the presence of more substantial deformity. In cases of moderate or severe deformity, the Weil osteotomy is performed to visualize the plantar plate.[47,168,229]

In the presence of joint instability, when the MTP joint can be successfully reduced, a plantar condylectomy may be performed in conjunction with a soft tissue release to achieve stability; this succeeds by creating scarring of the MTP joint.

Davis et al[57] and others[75,195,124] have described a proximal phalangeal osteotomy at the base of the proximal phalanx to achieve axial alignment of a malaligned toe. No long-term follow-up on patients was reported regarding the durability of this procedure (Fig. 7-100). This procedure does not stabilize or realign the MTP joint, and the toe can redeform with time (Fig. 7-101).

Many surgical procedures have been recommended when conservative treatment has failed in the treatment of lesser MTP joint instability, but some have had suboptimal results.* Most surgical procedures, previously described, indirectly treated the capsular pathology, and surgical efforts merely focused on releasing or balancing the soft tissues surrounding the MTP joint. The most frequent options were synovectomy,[144] soft tissue release,[†] tendon transfers,[‡] and bony decompression.[33,38,43,153,166,238] Results improved after the incorporation of distal metatarsal osteotomies with decompression or realignment of the involved joint, but still, this did not directly address the plantar plate degeneration or dysfunction. In fact, none of the above-mentioned methods directly treated the plantar plate tear. Although these procedures remain an important aspect of the surgical treatment, attention to the plantar plate deficiency has been recognized and is now considered as an important aspect of the surgical evaluation and treatment.[47,93,168]

Few reports have dealt with direct plantar plate repair.[77,93,153,183,238] Ford et al[77] and Jolly[116] initially suggested a technique involving a direct repair of the plantar plate (Fig. 7-102). Powless et al[183] and Bouche et al[15] reported on two series of plantar plate repairs using a plantar approach. Only recently has there been an emphasis on a dorsal approach to address plantar plate insufficiency. Cooper and Coughlin[31] found, in an

---

*References 33, 36, 42, 44, 77, 120, 153, and 165.
†References 15, 33, 42, 97, 120, and 165.
‡References 15, 33, 42, 97, 120, 153, 165, and 238.

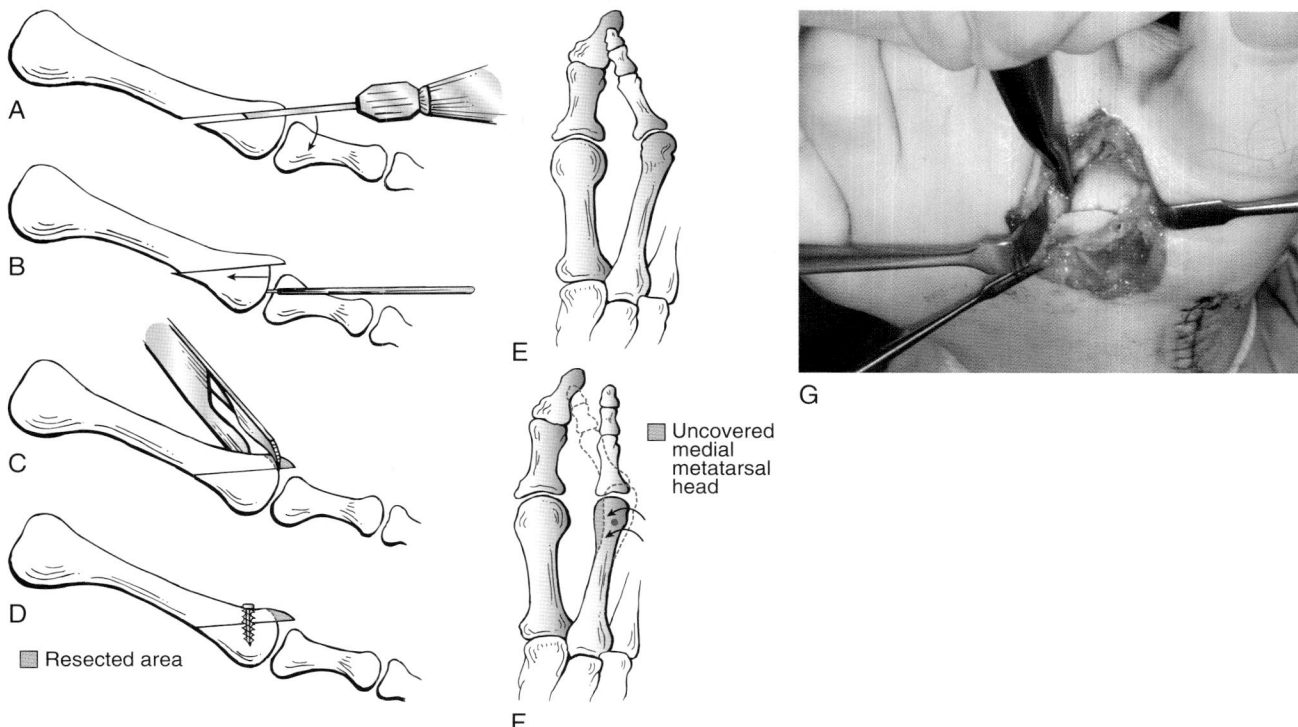

Figure 7-99 Diagram of Weil osteotomy. **A,** Saw cut is made as parallel to the plantar aspect of the foot as possible. **B,** The capital fragment is displaced proximally the appropriate amount. **C,** The dorsal flare is resected. **D,** Internal fixation. **E,** Preoperative deformity with substantial medial deviation. **F** and **G,** By shifting the head medially, the toe can be reoriented laterally.

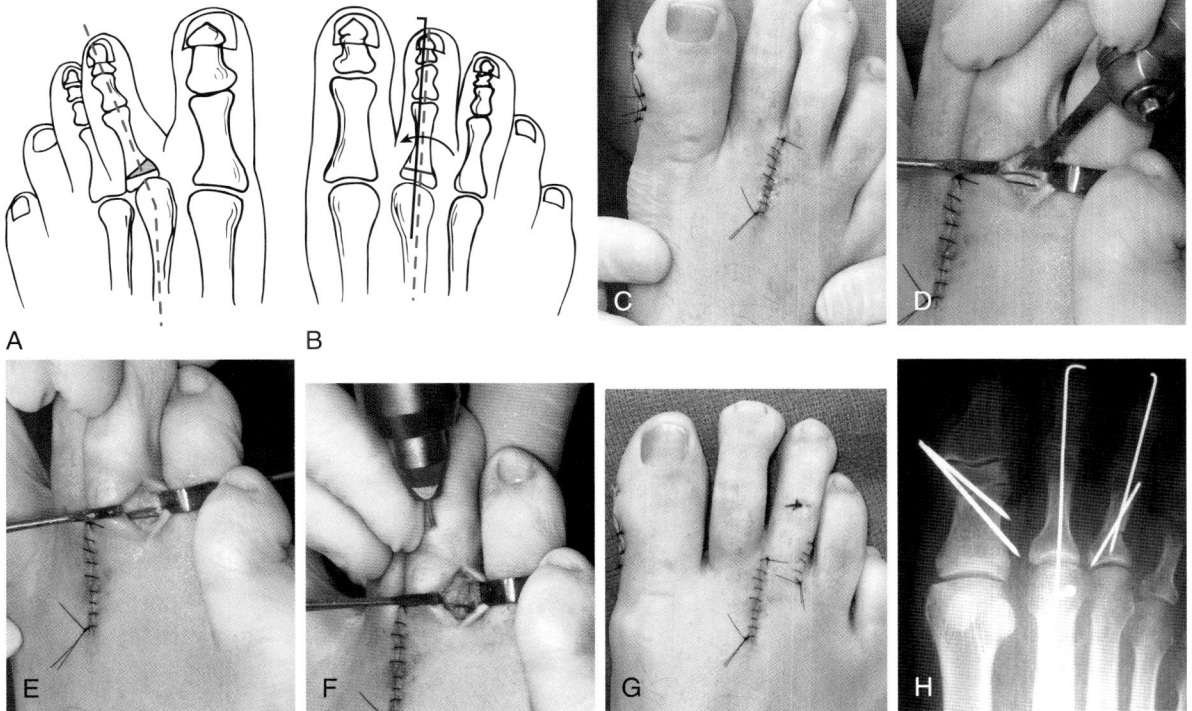

Figure 7-100 Closing-wedge phalangeal osteotomy. **A,** Proposed lateral closing-wedge proximal phalangeal osteotomy. **B,** Realignment after osteotomy. **C,** After Weil osteotomy of second metatarsal, there is residual medial deviation of the third toe. **D,** Exposure of lateral proximal phalanx and closing-wedge osteotomy. **E,** Removal of wedge. **F,** Closure of osteotomy. **G,** After wound closure. **H,** Postoperative radiograph demonstrating realignment of proximal phalanx.

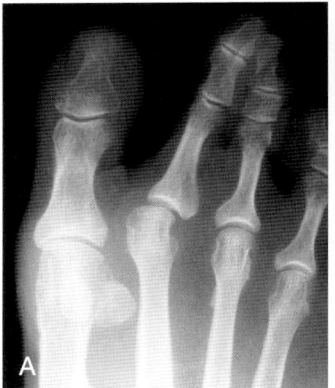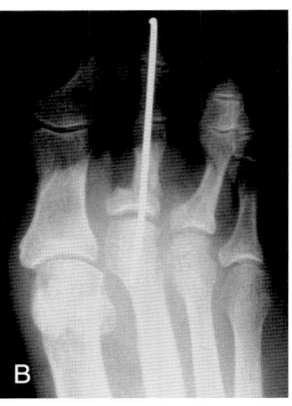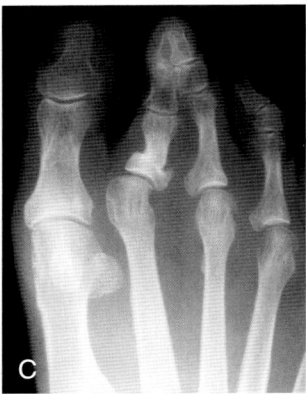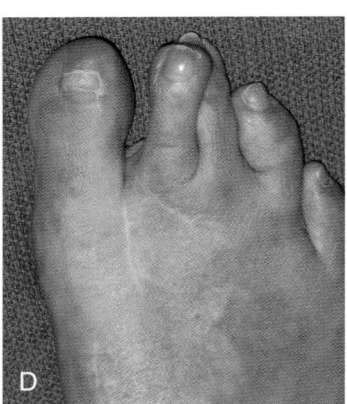

Figure 7-101 **A,** Preoperative radiograph demonstrating lateral deviation of the second toe at the metatarsophalangeal joint. **B,** After medial closing-wedge osteotomy of the proximal phalanx. Radiograph **(C)** and clinical photograph **(D)** at 8-year follow-up, demonstrating progressive lateral subluxation of metatarsophalangeal joint.

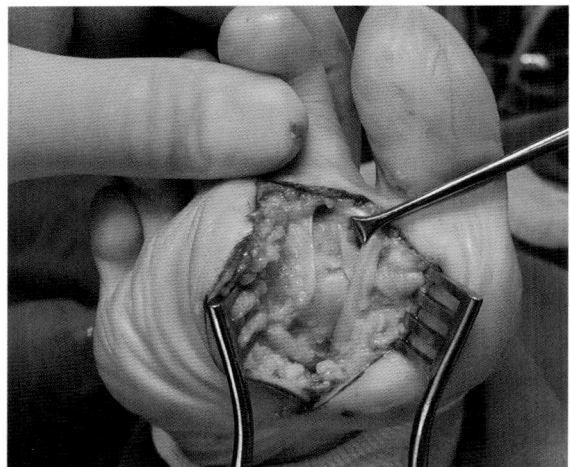

Figure 7-102 Direct repair of the plantar capsule. Note the longitudinal tear in the metatarsophalangeal capsule. (Courtesy Dr. G. Jolly.)

anatomic study on the surgical exposure of the lesser MTP joints from a dorsal approach, utilizing a Weil osteotomy, that a dorsal approach allowed adequate exposure to the MTP joint. Gregg et al,[93] Weil et al,[229] and Nery et al[168] have all reported series on plantar plate repair through a dorsal exposure.

Nery et al,[168] using arthroscopy, chose to treat grade 0 tears with radio-frequency shrinkage of the plantar plate and a Weil metatarsal osteotomy (see Fig. 7-83A). Grade 1–, 2–, and 3–type (7-83B-D) tears were treated with a Weil osteotomy (to access the torn plantar plate), followed by a direct repair of the plantar plate with reinsertion of the free border into the plantar margin of the proximal phalanx. They often combined this with a lateral collateral ligament reefing. Grade 4 tears, resulting from the extensive plantar plate damage (frequently, there was insufficient tissue to repair), were treated with a Weil osteotomy combined with the flexor-to-extensor tendon

transfer. As part of his grading and staging evaluation, Nery[168] also performed an arthroscopy of the involved joint before the open procedure.

If surgery is indicated, the MTP joint is explored. An extensor tenotomy of lengthening of the extensor digitorum longus is performed. A dorsal capsulotomy is carried out. In the presence of dorsal subluxation of the MTP joint, an aggressive medial and lateral capsular release (all of the phangeal base) must be performed. Cooper et al[31] and Peterson et al[178] cautioned that a release of the soft tissue attachments of the collaeral ligaments combined with a Weil osteotomy may compromise the circulation of the metatarsal head.

With the progression of deformity and frank dislocation, a joint decompression may be necessary. Although an MTP joint resection arthroplasty has been advocated in the past, this is rarely done now except as a salvage procedure. Dislocation of the MTP joint typically occurs insidiously (see Figs. 7-30, 7-85, and 7-89). An initial hyperextension deformity of the MTP joint can progress to severe subluxation, and over time, dislocation can result. The dislocated toe may be a pure dorsal dislocation or have a dorsomedial or dorsolateral component. In this situation, often the plantar plate has substantial disruption. Those cases that have progressed to frank dislocation require more extensive surgery. A soft tissue dissection is performed with an extensive soft tissue release (extensor tendon lengthenings and MTP capsule release are routinely necessary). Any adhesions on the plantar aspect of the metatarsal head are released as well using a McGlamry elevator. In the presence of a recent dislocation, soft tissue releases can allow relocation of the MTP joint (Fig. 7-103). Often, a flexor tendon transfer is necessary, as is Kirschner wire stabilization for the relocated toe. In this situation, postoperative treatment is identical to that outlined for less severe deformities at the MTP joint (Fig. 7-104).

The use of any of these procedures depends on the magnitude of the deformity of the MTP joint and the flexibility of the contracture of the interphalangeal joint.

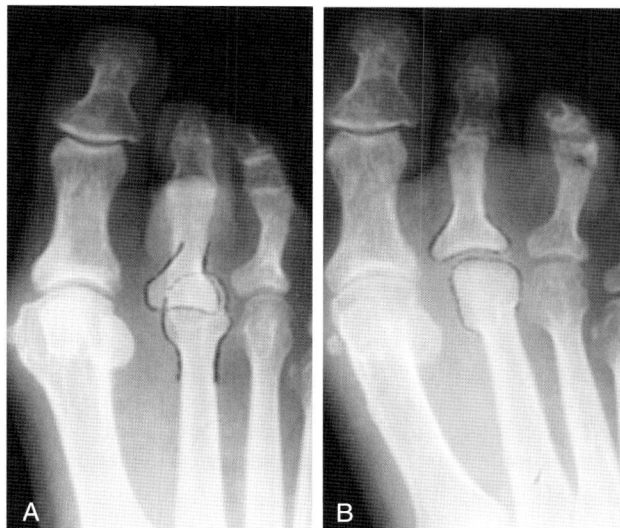

Figure 7-103 **A,** Relatively recent second metatarsophalangeal joint dislocation in a 60-year-old woman. **B,** After soft tissue release and flexor tendon transfer, adequate realignment has been achieved.

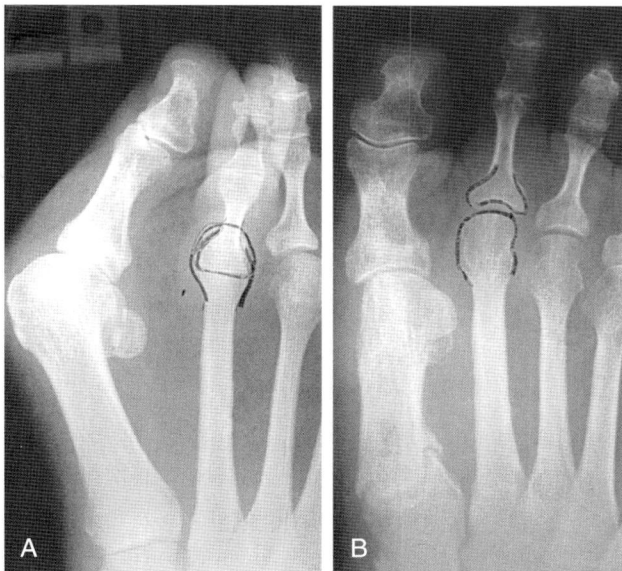

Figure 7-104 **A,** Preoperative radiograph demonstrates severe dislocation of second metatarsophalangeal joint, associated with a hallux valgus deformity. **B,** After a hallux valgus repair with a first metatarsal osteotomy, distal soft tissue release, and flexor tendon transfer, adequate realignment has been achieved.

In the presence of a rigid deformity at the PIP joint, a fixed hammer toe repair is performed. With a rigid deformity of the MTP joint, a combination of a soft tissue release (extensor tendon lengthening, MTP capsule release), bony decompression, and plantar plate repair may be necessary to realign the toe. Treatment for a hammer toe deformity usually is performed simultaneously with MTP joint realignment. Early operative intervention before dislocation of the MTP joint can allow preservation of joint function. In the presence of severe deformity, the necessity for a resection arthroplasty limits the expected functional result.

In the initial evaluation, the vascular and neurologic status of the foot and lesser toes is important when planning surgery. Often, multiple procedures are performed on the second toe to correct both a hammer toe and an MTP joint deformity. Numerous surgical procedures can impair the circulation to the toe, and occasionally, surgery must be limited if the vascular integrity is compromised. It is not always easy to ascertain whether a toe will tolerate a few or many surgical procedures, and this may be determined only at the time of surgical intervention.

The treatment of subluxation of the MTP joint should be approached in a progressive surgical fashion. Figure 7-97 presents an algorithm for treating subluxation and dislocation of the lesser MTP joint.

SOFT TISSUE RELEASE
Indications
In the presence of a mild deformity, characterized by a soft tissue contracture of the MTP joint, a soft tissue release may be sufficient to realign the toe.

Contraindications
Where more severe deformities are present, characterized by fixed contractures, soft tissue releases are commonly unsuccessful in achieving a complete realignment of the digit. Care must always be taken in the presence of a digital deformity to avoid excessive surgery that could threaten the neurologic or vascular competency of the digit.

Surgical Technique[43]
1. The patient is placed in a supine position on the operating room table. The procedure is performed under a peripheral anesthetic block. The foot is cleansed and draped in the usual fashion. The foot is exsanguinated with an Esmarch bandage. The Esmarch bandage may be used as a tourniquet above the level of the ankle.
2. Either a longitudinal second interspace incision or a dorsal lazy-S incision centered over the second MTP joint is used.
3. The extensor tendons are exposed and either retracted or released in a Z-type fashion. If a release is reformed, they are later repaired in lengthened form with interrupted sutures.
4. The MTP joint dorsal capsule is released sharply, as are the medial and lateral capsules. The capsule is released off of the base of the proximal phalanx to protect the vascular supply to the metatarsal head.[178] Care is taken to release the collateral ligaments and capsule in a plantarward direction a distance of about 6 to 8 mm in length, to avoid leaving any contracted tissue (see Fig. 7-72A-D).

5. The first lumbrical on the medial aspect of the second toe may be a significant deforming force, and it should be released with the soft tissue release. Care is taken to protect the neurovascular bundle adjacent to the lumbrical.

6. In the presence of adhesions on the plantar aspect of the MTP joint between the plantar capsule and metatarsal head, a McGlamry elevator is advanced around the metatarsal head in a dorsoplantar-proximal direction. In this way, adhesions may be released, allowing reduction of the hyperextended proximal phalanx.

7. Once the joint contractures have been released, a test for stability is performed. Repetitive passive dorsiflexion and plantar flexion of the ankle usually help determine whether the MTP joint will stay reduced. In an unstable situation, the MTP joint dislocates with intraoperative motion at the ankle (dorsoplantar flexion).

8. If the MTP joint is well aligned and stable, an intramedullary 0.045-inch Kirschner wire is introduced at the base of the proximal phalanx and driven in a distal direction exiting the tip of the toe (see Fig. 7-72E). It is then driven retrograde across the MTP joint. It is bent at the tip of the toe, and the excess pin is removed. (If a fixed hammer toe repair has been performed, the pin is introduced at the PIP joint and driven distally. It is then driven in a retrograde fashion as described.) If an intramedullary hammer toe implant has been placed, the Kirschner wire can be driven to the side of the implant and advanced into the metatarsal head.

9. After repair of the extensor tendon and routine skin closure, a compression gauze dressing is applied.

Postoperative Care

The patient is allowed to ambulate in a wooden-soled shoe. Sutures and the Kirschner wire are removed 3 weeks after surgery. The toe is then taped in a slightly plantar-flexed position for 6 weeks. Passive range-of-motion exercises are initiated 3 weeks after surgery.

REEFING OF THE SECOND METATARSOPHALANGEAL JOINT CAPSULE[142]
Surgical Technique

1. The patient is placed in a supine position on the operating room table. The procedure is performed under a peripheral anesthetic block. The foot is cleansed and draped in the usual fashion. The foot is exsanguinated with an Esmarch bandage. The Esmarch bandage may be used as a tourniquet above the level of the ankle.

2. The extensor tendons are either retracted or are lengthened with a Z-type incision and are later repaired.

3. The MTP joint dorsal capsule is released as described previously.

4. If the digit is deviated medially, the tight contracted medial capsule is released in a dorsoplantar direction off of the base of the proximal phalanx. This usually requires release of at least 6 to 8 mm of capsule to the plantar extent of the MTP joint.

5. When the second toe is deviated medially, release of the first lumbrical can remove a significant deforming force.

6. A suture is placed in the distal lateral MTP capsule then directed into the region of the plantar metatarsal capsule in a more proximal direction. Usually a figure-of-eight suture is placed (Fig. 7-105A and B).

7. One or two sutures are placed and, with the toe held in a corrected position, are tied. Usually this achieves 5 to 10 degrees of axial realignment (Fig. 7-105C-E).

8. When a paucity of tissue is present in the area of the metatarsal head or proximal phalanx, a suture anchor may be placed in either the lateral metatarsal head or proximal phalanx to secure the distal and plantar MTP capsule (Fig. 7-106).

9. Kirschner wire fixation may or may not be used depending on whether a fixed hammer toe repair has been performed or based on the stability after MTP joint capsulorrhaphy. A hammer toe implant may be used to stabilize a hammer toe repair, obviating the need for a Kirschner wire.

10. The extensor tendon is repaired and the skin is approximated in a routine fashion.

EXTENSOR DIGITORUM BREVIS TRANSFER[97,119]
Surgical Technique

1. The patient is placed in a supine position on the operating room table. The procedure is performed under a peripheral anesthetic block. The foot is exsanguinated with an Esmarch bandage. An Esmarch bandage may be used as a tourniquet above the level of the ankle. A dorsal longitudinal skin incision is centered over the MTP joint and second intermetatarsal space.

2. The MTP joint is released and the extensor digitorum brevis tendon is carefully dissected proximally (Fig. 7-107A-D).

3. Four centimeters proximal to the MTP joint, the extensor digitorum brevis tendon is severed and each end secured with an interrupted stay-suture (Fig. 7-107E-G).

4. The distal tendon stump is passed beneath the transverse metatarsal ligament from distal to proximal and passed lateral to the extensor hood. The distal attachment of the extensor digitorum brevis is carefully protected (Fig. 7-107H and I).

5. Before the tendon repair, a 0.065-inch Kirschner wire is inserted at the MTP joint and is driven distally and then retrograde across the MTP joint (Fig. 7-107J).

6. With the joint held in corrected alignment, the end of the distal stump is repaired to the proximal stump with an end-to-end suture (Fig. 7-107K and L).

7. Further reefing of the lateral capsule may be performed with interrupted 2-0 absorbable suture.

8. The soft tissue and skin are approximated in a routine fashion.

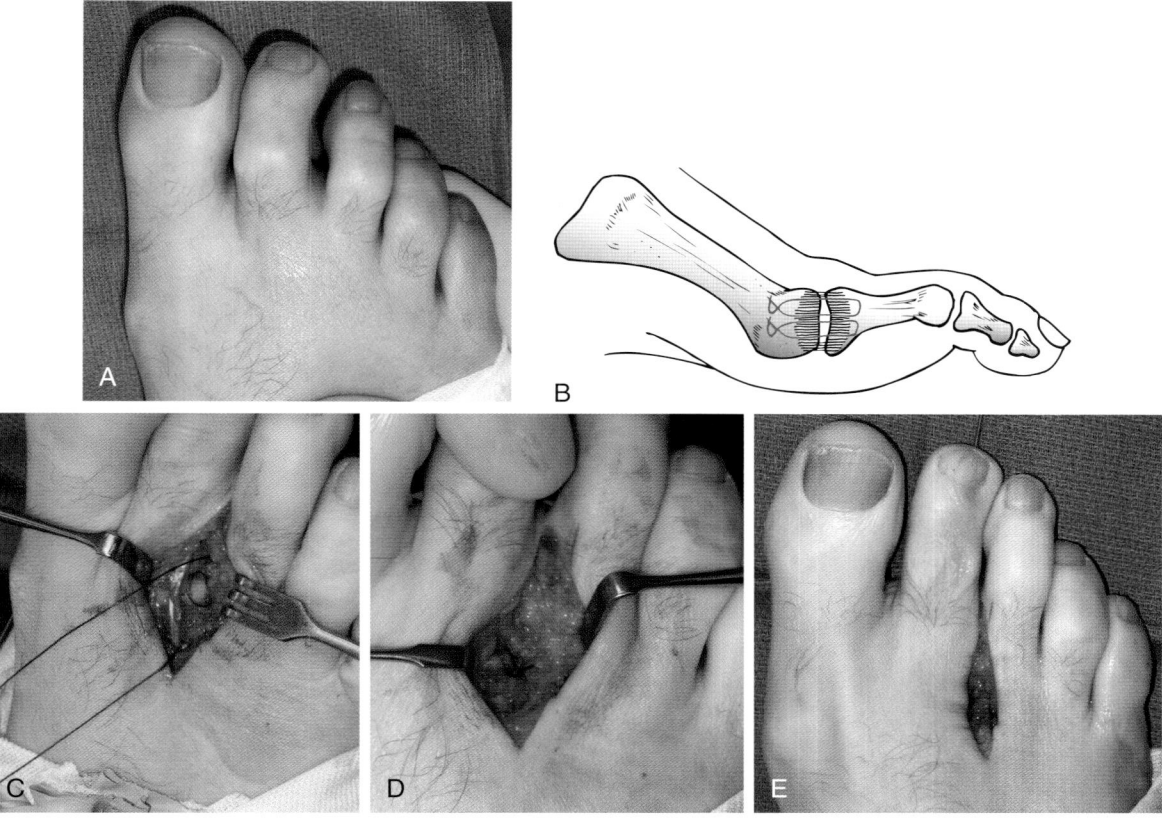

Figure 7-105 With medial or lateral metatarsophalangeal joint deviation, a release of the contracted capsule structures is performed in combination with reefing of the ligamentous structures on the contralateral or elongated side. **A,** Preoperative clinical photograph. **B,** Diagram. **C** and **D,** Intraoperative photograph in which one or two interrupted sutures are used to reef the capsule; often this allows realignment of 5 to 10 degrees in an axial plane. **E,** Clinical photograph after lateral capsule reefing to realign metatarsophalangeal joint.

Postoperative Care
A gauze-and-tape dressing is applied postoperatively and changed weekly. Sutures are removed 3 weeks after surgery, and the toe is taped in appropriate alignment for 6 weeks after surgery.

PLANTAR CONDYLECTOMY
Surgical Technique
1. The foot is cleansed and draped in the usual fashion. The foot is exsanguinated with an Esmarch bandage. The Esmarch bandage may be used as a tourniquet above the level of the ankle.
2. Either a dorsal longitudinal second interspace incision or a dorsal lazy-S incision centered over the MTP joint is used for the exposure. A soft tissue release is performed in which the extensor tendons are lengthened, and the dorsal, medial, and lateral MTP capsules are released as well (Fig. 7-108A).
3. The metatarsal head is identified, and the proximal phalanx is plantar flexed to expose the plantar condyle.

A McGlamry elevator is helpful is retracting the adjacent soft tissue.
4. A Hoke osteotomy is used to resect 3 to 4 mm of the plantar aspect of the metatarsal head. The distal metatarsal articular surface is left intact. The plantar portion is spun out from beneath the remaining metatarsal head. Care must be taken to minimize pressure on the metatarsal head to avoid a metaphyseal fracture (Fig. 7-108B-D).
5. A Kirschner wire is introduced at the MTP joint and driven distally out the tip of the toe. It is then advanced retrograde into the metatarsal to stabilize the MTP joint.
6. The extensor tendon is repaired and the skin is approximated with interrupted sutures.

Postoperative Care
A gauze-and-tape dressing is applied and changed weekly. The Kirschner wire and sutures are removed 2 to 3 weeks after surgery, and the toe is then taped in corrected position for 6 weeks.

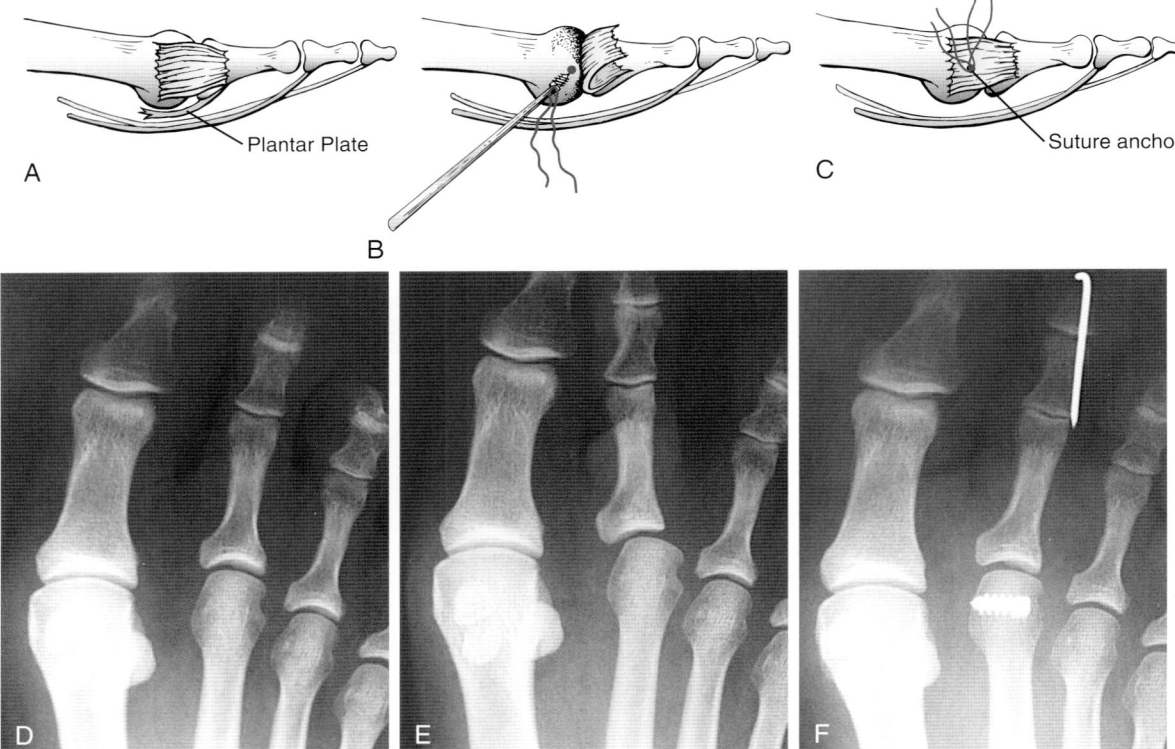

Plantar Plate

A

B

C

Suture anchor

D

E

F

Figure 7-106 A suture anchor may be helpful in reefing an elongated capsule. The capsule is detached from the metatarsal head and secured with a suture anchor. **A,** Normal lateral capsule. **B** and **C,** Lateral diagram of metatarsophalangeal (MTP) joint and plantar plate with placement of suture anchor. **D,** Radiograph demonstrating normal alignment with symptomatic second MTP joint. **E,** Preoperative radiograph demonstrating medial deviation. **F,** After flexor tendon transfer and placement of suture anchor to secure lateral MTP capsule, successful realignment is achieved.

PHALANGEAL CLOSING WEDGE OSTEOTOMY ("AKINETTE")[57,124,195]
Surgical Technique

1. The foot is cleansed and draped in the usual fashion. The foot is exsanguinated with an Esmarch bandage. The Esmarch bandage may be used as a tourniquet above the level of the ankle.
2. A longitudinal incision is centered over the dorsal aspect of the proximal phalanx of the involved digit (see Fig. 7-100A).
3. The extensor tendons are elevated, and a closing wedge phalangeal osteotomy is performed in the region of the proximal phalangeal metaphysis (see Fig. 7-100B-E).
4. The osteotomy is closed and stabilized with one or two Kirschner wires (see Fig. 7-100F-H).
5. A Kirschner wire is introduced at the MTP joint and driven distally out the tip of the toe. It is then retrograded into the metatarsal, stabilizing the MTP joint.

Postoperative Care

A gauze-and-tape dressing is applied and changed weekly. The Kirschner wire and sutures are removed 3 weeks after surgery and the toe is then taped in corrected position for 6 weeks (see Fig. 7-101).

CAPITAL OBLIQUE METATARSAL OSTEOTOMY (WEIL OSTEOTOMY)[96,231]
Indications

In the presence of an MTP joint angular deformity (whether subluxation or joint dislocation), significant soft tissue contractures preclude adequate reduction of the toe with only soft tissue procedures alone. In severe cases, bony decompression is necessary to realign the toe without creating significant tension on the neurovascular bundles. Although a partial proximal phalangectomy is an alternative, preservation of the trumpet-shaped base of the proximal phalanx affords significant stability to the MTP joint[78]; currently, a partial proximal phalangectomy is considered a salvage procedure. A DuVries arthroplasty also achieves joint decompression by excision of a small portion of the distal metatarsal articular surface. Although I have favored this method of joint decompression in the past, I now reserve a formal DuVries arthroplasty for salvage situations when other procedures have failed.

Currently, joint preservation techniques that also provide joint decompression are preferred. Joint decompression, however, is mandatory when severe contractures are present. Excessive bone resection should be avoided because it can lead to a floppy, unstable toe. A distal metatarsal osteotomy preserves some MTP joint function

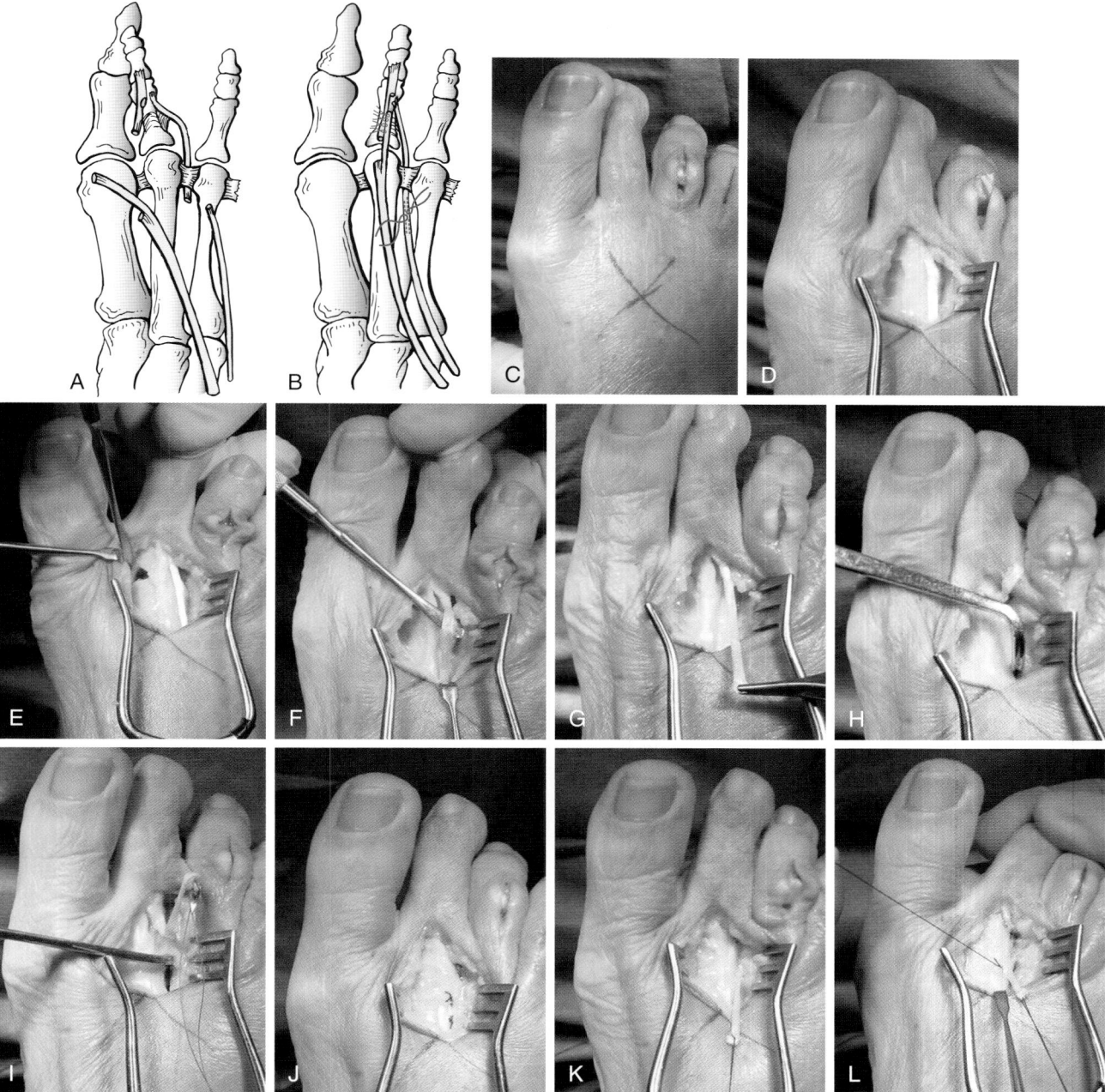

Figure 7-107 Extensor digitorum brevis transfer diagram. **A,** The distal stump of the extensor digitorum brevis is transferred beneath the transverse intermetatarsal ligament. **B,** It is reattached end to end with a Krakow suture, and the extensor digitorum longus is Z-lengthened. **C,** Preoperative clinical appearance. **D,** Dorsal exposure. **E,** Release of medial capsule. **F,** Tension on extensor digitorum brevis tendon. **G,** Tendon is released proximally. **H,** Tendon passer develops tract beneath the transverse metatarsal ligament (TML). **I** and **J,** Tendon is passed beneath ligament. **K** and **L,** Tendon is sutured with toe correctly aligned. (Courtesy L.S. Weil, DPM.)

and is preferable. It also provides access to the plantar plate. Weil[231,232] popularized a distal oblique osteotomy in the metatarsal metaphyseal region (see Fig. 7-99). Proximal displacement of the distal metatarsal segment can achieve shortening of 2 to 6 mm. Internal fixation is recommended to stabilize the osteotomy site. The osteotomy may be translated or angled medially or laterally to improve axial realignment.

Contraindications

The main contraindication for a capital oblique distal metatarsal is severe deformity for which excisional

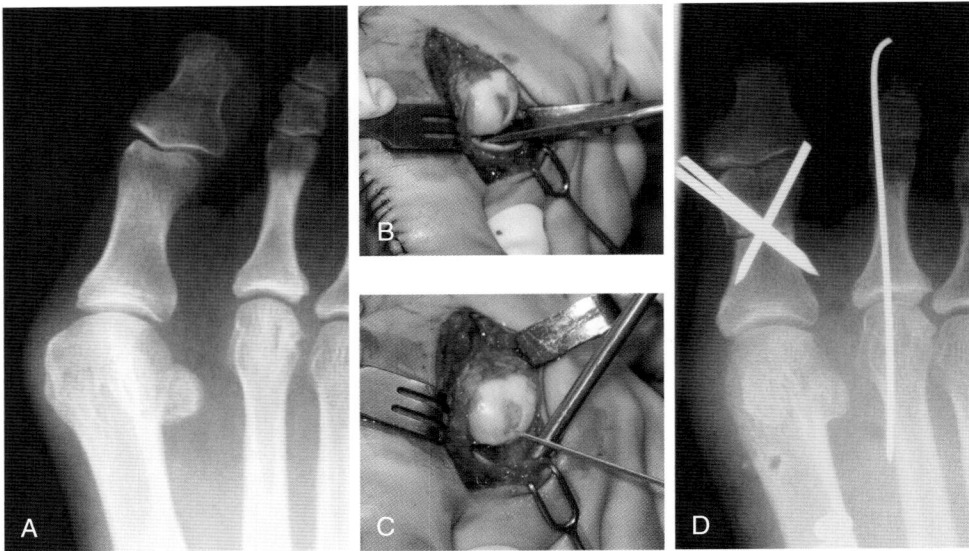

Figure 7-108 **A,** Preoperative radiograph demonstrating hallux valgus deformity with an unstable and painful second metatarsophalangeal (MTP) joint without obvious deformity. **B,** Intraoperative photograph demonstrating the osteochondral defect. The joint was unstable in the vertical plane. **C,** Plantar condylectomy. **D,** Postoperative radiograph demonstrating bunion repair and Kirschner wire stabilization of second MTP joint after plantar condylectomy. Note that an Akin procedure has been performed on the hallux.

arthroplasty is preferable. The limits of this procedure have yet to be defined, and although severe subluxation and dislocation may be reduced with a shortening osteotomy, the remaining forefoot and the possibility of transfer metatarsalgia must be considered when treating isolated metatarsophalangeal joints. The use of this osteotomy, or modifications of it, have been used successfully in moderate deformities as well.*

Surgical Technique

1. The patient is placed in a supine position on the operating room table. The procedure is typically performed under a peripheral anesthetic block. An Esmarch bandage is used to exsanguinate the extremity and may be used as an ankle tourniquet.
2. A 3- to 4-cm longitudinal incision is centered either over the distal second metatarsal or in the second intermetatarsal space (Fig. 7-109A and Video Clip 70).
3. The metatarsal head and metaphysis are identified and the ligaments are not released unless shortening of more than 3 mm is desired. If more substantial shortening is desired, the collateral ligaments are released from the phalangeal attachment (Fig. 7-109B and C). When a plantar plate repair is planned, the collateral ligaments are partially released from their phalangeal attachments.
4. The subluxated or dislocated metatarsal head is reduced and the phalanx is plantar flexed, exposing the metatarsal head. A McGlamry elevator may be used to expose the metatarsal head. It is used with

*References 10, 47, 93, 120, 168, and 229.

care to prevent devascularization of the metatarsal metaphysis (Fig. 7-109D).

5. A longitudinal oblique distal metatarsal osteotomy is performed. The saw blade penetrates the distal superior metatarsal articular surface 1 to 2 mm inferior to the dorsal metatarsal surface. The plane of the osteotomy is parallel to the plantar surface of the foot and proceeds in a proximal direction until the saw blade has penetrated the proximal phalangeal cortex (Figs. 7-109E and F and 7-110A-C; see Fig. 7-87A).
6. The distal fragment is then translated proximally the desired amount (2-6 mm) as planned preoperatively (see Figs. 7-109G and 7-99B).
7. The osteotomy site is stabilized with a plantar mini-fragment screws or spin screw. Care must be taken not to place excessively long screws, which can cause plantar symptoms.[96] Occasionally, two screws are necessary, especially when shortening of more than 4 mm is required (see Figs. 7-109H and I and 7-99D).
8. The dorsal metatarsal surface that now extends beyond the articular surface is resected and beveled with a rongeur. Occasionally, two screws are necessary, especially when shortening of more than 4 mm is required (see Figs. 7-99C and 7-109H).
9. The wound is closed in a routine fashion.
10. When shortening of more than 3 mm is required, a thin wafer of bone is removed to prevent plantar translation of the capital fragment.[231] Another alternative is to use stacked saw blades to make a thicker osteotomy (see Fig. 7-110D). The capital fragment may also be translated medially to help realign a severely angulated toe lateralward (see Fig. 7-99).

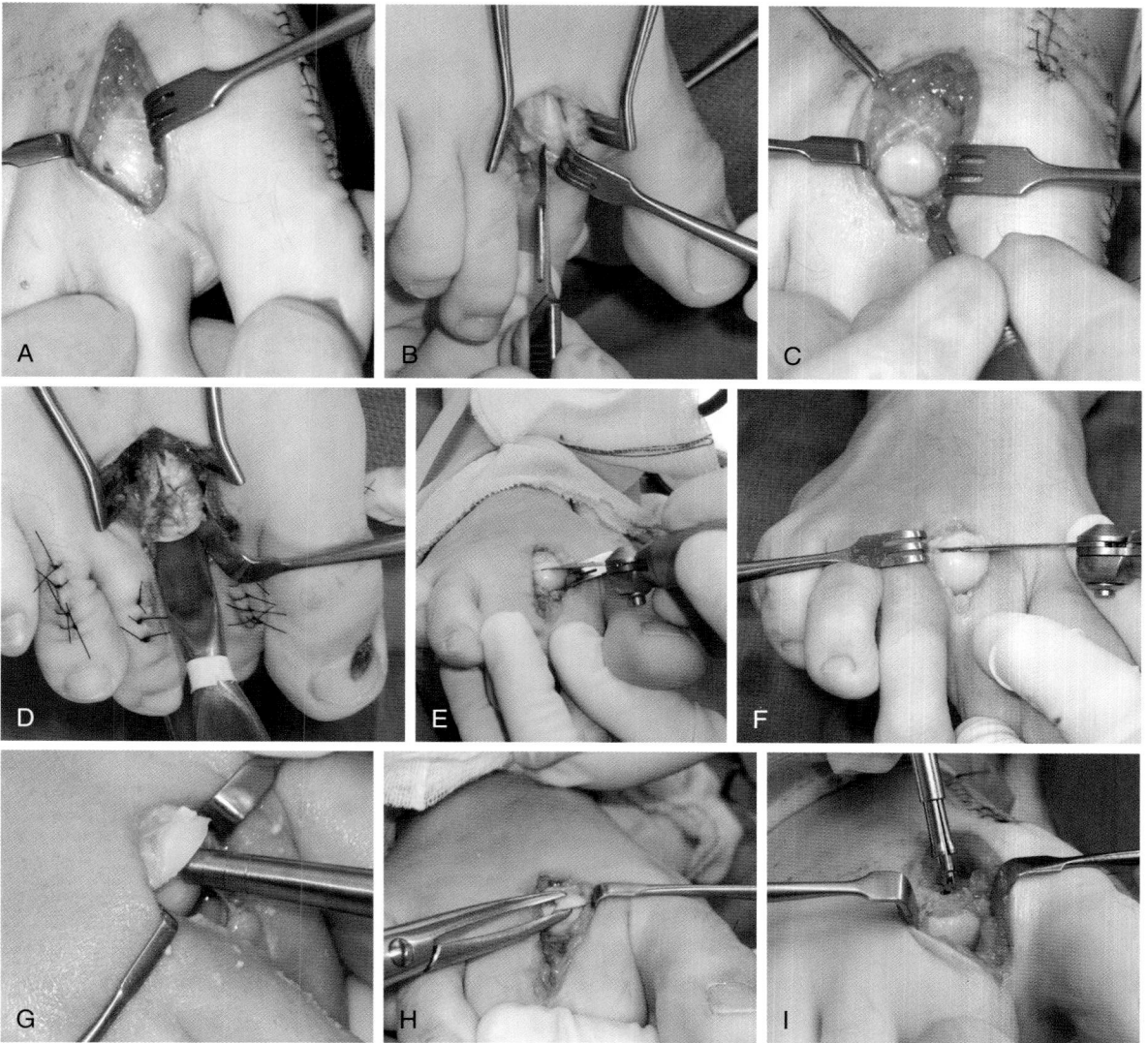

Figure 7-109 **A,** The metatarsophalangeal joint is exposed through a dorsal incision; the joint is freed up by releasing the distal ligamentous attachment and maintaining the metatarsal capsule. **B,** The capsule is released distally off of the phalanx, preserving the metatarsal head vascularity. **C,** Care must be taken when doing a proximal release not to strip the metatarsal vascular supply. **D,** An elevator may be used to free up the plantar capsule, but care must be taken to avoid disruption of the lateral capsular vascular supply. **E,** Proposed osteotomy. **F,** Stacked blades enable resection of more bone. **G,** The capital fragment is displaced proximally. A calibrated bone impactor is used to translate the capital fragment a measured amount. **H,** The dorsal ledge is resected. **I,** If a single screw does not adequately compress the ostotomy site, a second screw must be placed. (The screw must be long enough to engage the plantar fragment, but not excessively long. With shortening of more than 4 mm, two-screw fixation is often necessary.)

11. The toe is stabilized with a 0.045-inch Kirschner wire that is driven out through the tip of the toe and then retrograded into the capital fragment (see Fig. 7-110E). An alternative is to tape the toe securely to stabilize it during the postoperative period, or to use a dynamic splint to encourage active exercises of the involved digit.
12. A flexor tendon transfer is used when the MTP joint is markedly unstable after the osteotomy (Fig. 7-111).

Postoperative Care

A gauze-and-tape compression dressing is applied at surgery and changed on a weekly basis. The toe is bandaged in 5 degrees of plantar flexion. Weight-bearing ambulation is permitted with weight borne on the heel and outer aspect of the foot. If a Kirschner wire has been placed, it is removed 2 to 3 weeks after surgery. Typically, 6 weeks after surgery, successful healing has occurred at the osteotomy site. A roomy shoe or sandal is then used for ambulation. The patient is encouraged to commence

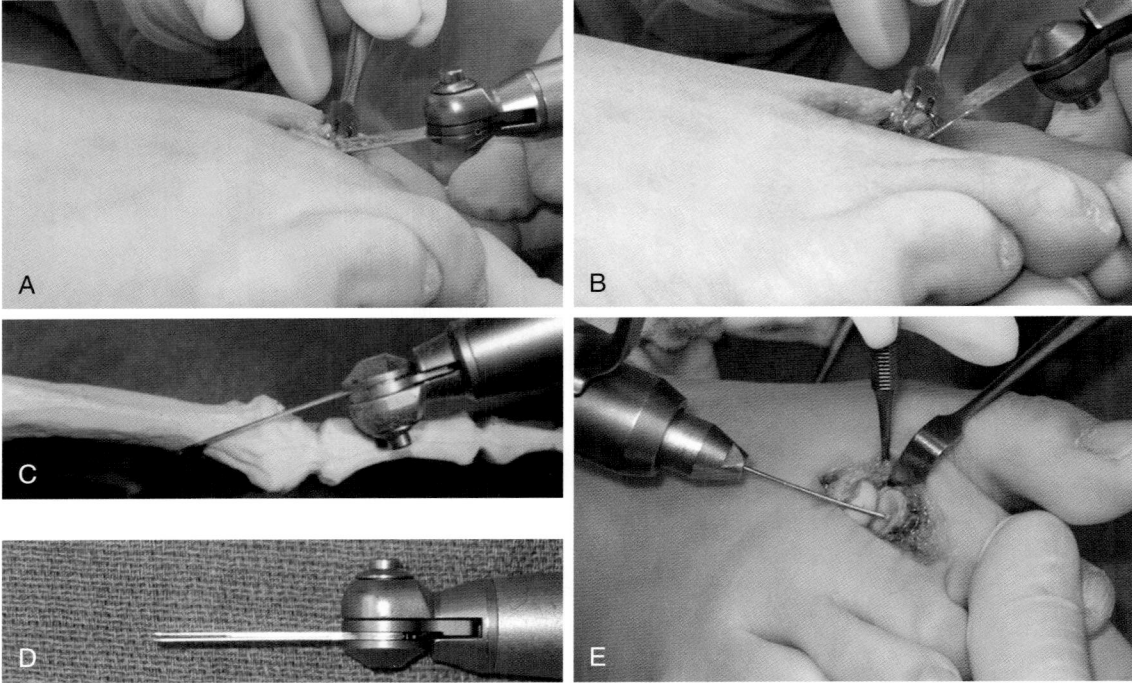

Figure 7-110 Tips for Weil osteotomy. **A,** Capital oblique osteotomy is performed with the saw plate parallel to the plantar aspect of the foot to minimize depression of the distal fragment as the osteotomy is translated proximal. **B** and **C,** Excessive plantar inclination of the saw blade can depress the translated capital fragment. (These examples show excess plantar inclination of the saw blade.) **D,** To achieve less plantar displacement, stacked blades or a thicker blade can be used for the osteotomy. Note three blades are used here, which achieves a much wider cut. **E,** On occasion, a Kirschner wire is used to stabilize the metatarsophalangeal joint, especially when substantial shortening has been achieved. Taping of the digit is another alternative.

active and passive toe exercises 2 to 3 weeks after surgery. The toe is taped to the adjacent toe or to the forefoot for another 3 to 6 weeks after the pin is removed (Fig. 7-112). Postoperative exercises (see next section on Plantar Plate Repair).

TECHNIQUE FOR PLANTAR PLATE REPAIR[47,50,168]
Indications
This technique is used for moderate MTP joint instability (grade II and III instability with malalignment of the MTP joint).

Contraindications
In the presence of degenerative arthritis of the involved MTP joint or severe deformity, a repair of the plantar plate is contraindicated. Stabilizing an arthritic joint may leave a painful stiff articulation. Insufficient capsular tissue may prevent a soft tissue repair.

Surgical Technique
1. The patient is placed in a supine position on the operating room table. The foot is cleansed and draped in the usual fashion. An Esmarch bandage is used to exsanguinate the extremity and also used as an ankle tourniquet. Regional or general anesthesia is used depending upon surgeon preference.

2. A dorsal longitudinal incision is centered over the second web space. The extensor digitorum brevis and longus are retracted medially or elongated by Z-plasty, depending on the magnitude of deformity (Figs. 7-113A and 7-114).

3. A partial collateral ligament release off of the base of the proximal phalanx of the MTP joint improves visualization.[31]

4. At this point, a McGlamry elevator may be used to release the proximal plantar plate, because this aids in proximal translation of the capital fragment.

5. A Weil osteotomy, using a sagittal saw, is performed (see Fig. 7-113B). The saw cut is made parallel to the plantar aspect of the foot, starting at a point 1 to 2 mm below the dorsal aspect of the metatarsal articular surface.[96] In the presence of a plantar keratosis beneath the metatarsal head, a small wafer of bone is removed to achieve slight elevation of the metatarsal head.[229]

6. The capital fragment is pushed proximally as much as possible (approximately 5-10 mm) (see Fig. 7-113C) and fixed temporarily with a vertical Kirschner wire to hold it in a retracted position (see Fig. 7-113D).

7. A second vertical Kirschner wire is placed in the base of the proximal phalanx. A special mini–joint distractor is placed over the vertical wires and spread to distract the MTP joint (see Fig. 7-113E).

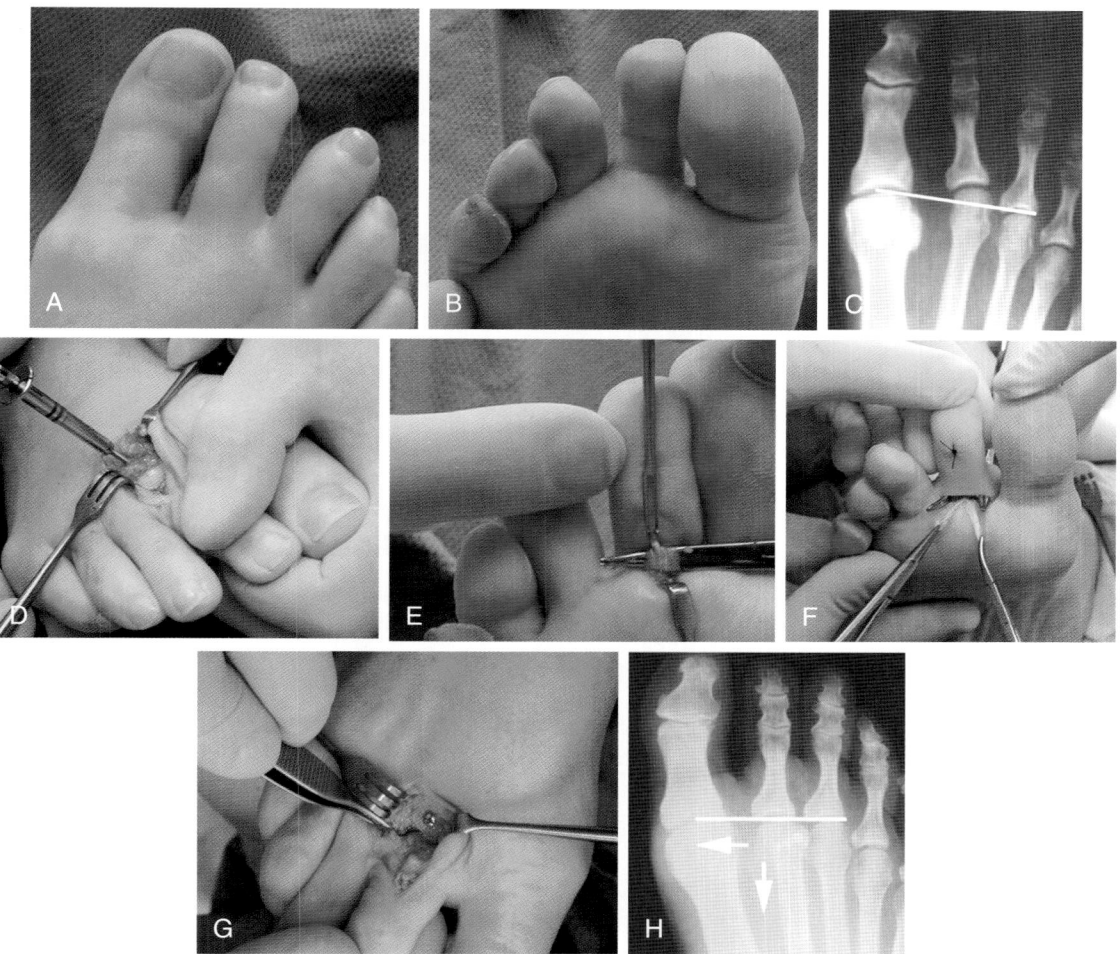

Figure 7-111 Moderate second metatarsophalangeal instability treated with flexor tendon transfer and Weil osteotomy. Preoperative clinical (**A** and **B**) and radiographic (**C**) presentation of deformity. **D,** Fixation after Weil osteotomy with shortening and medial translation. **E** and **F,** Harvest and transfer of the flexor tendon to the dorsal surface of the proximal phalanx. **G,** Dorsal view after flexor tendon transfer and Weil osteotomy. (The sutured tendon is at the inferior aspect of the wound.) **H,** Radiograph demonstrating shortening and medial translation of the capital fragment.

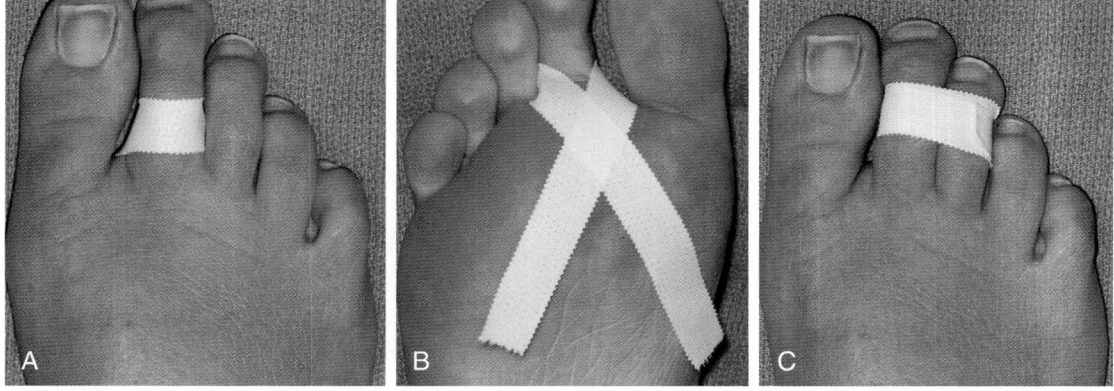

Figure 7-112 Postoperative taping technique. Taping is necessary in the postoperative period to stabilize the repair. **A,** Dorsal view. **B,** Plantar view. **C,** Buddy taping of adjacent toes can reduce pain as well.

8. The plantar plate tear is evaluated and graded (see Fig. 7-113F). Longitudinal tears in the plate (grade III) are repaired with several side-to-side interrupted non-absorbable sutures (0-Fiberwire). The more common distal transverse tears (grade I and II) are repaired by placing the same nonabsorbable sutures in the distal plantar plate.

9. The distal plantar edge of the proximal phalanx is roughened with a rongeur or curette to prepare the surface for reattachment of the plantar plate. The

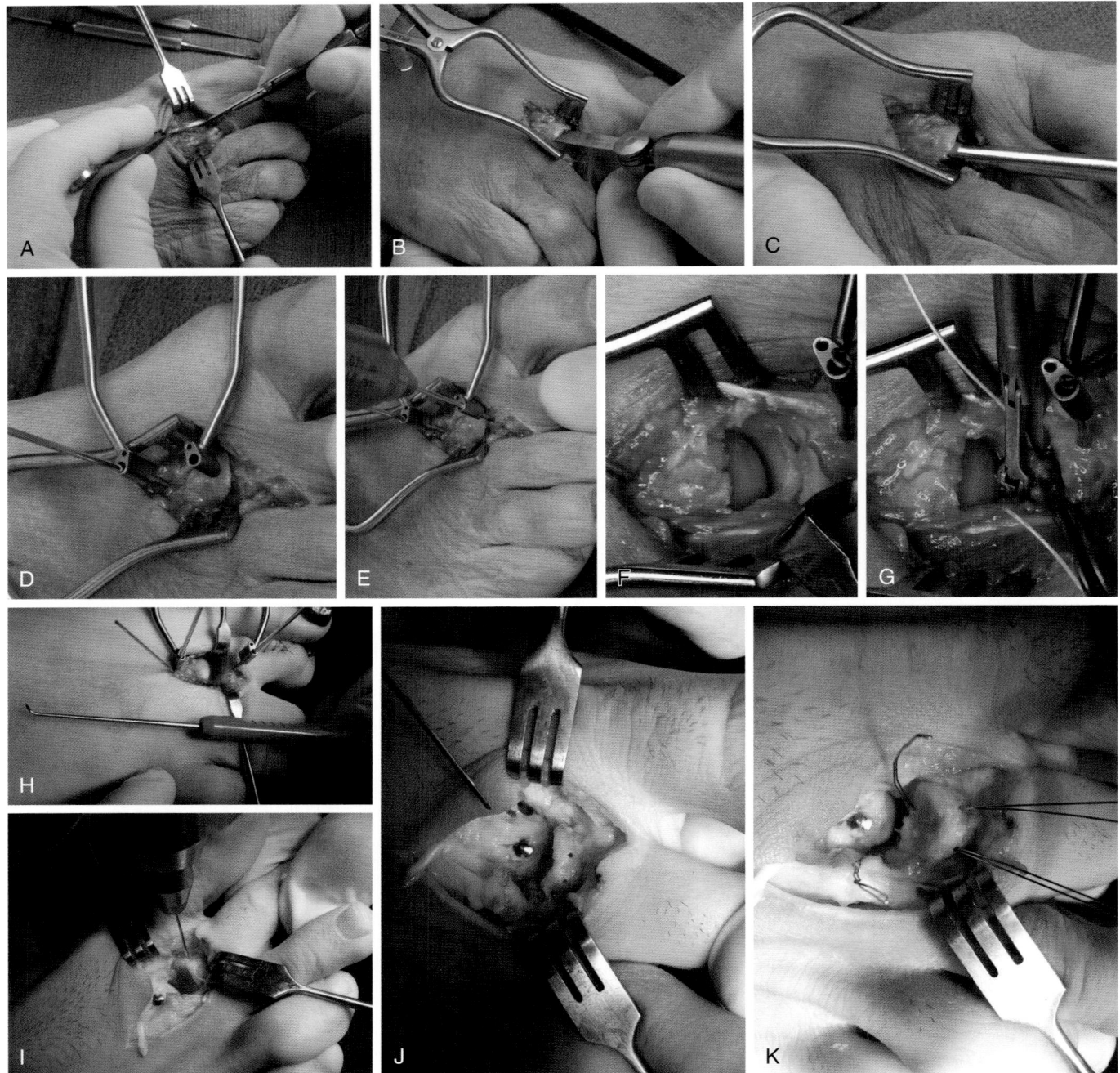

Figure 7-113 **A,** Dorsal longitudinal skin incision. **B,** Weil osteotomy. **C,** Displacing the capital fragment as far proximal as possible. **D,** The capital fragment is fixed with a vertical Kirschner wire, and the self-retaining distractor is applied. **E,** A vertical Kirschner wire is then placed in the base of the proximal phalanx, and the distractor is spread to visualize the plantar plate. **F,** Visualizing the plantar plate. **G,** Sutures are placed in the distal plantar plate. **H,** An alternative method used to pass the suture by hand. **I** and **J,** Drill holes are placed in the base of the proximal phalanx. **K** and **L,** Method of passing the sutures. (J, K; courtesy of Caio Nery, MD.)

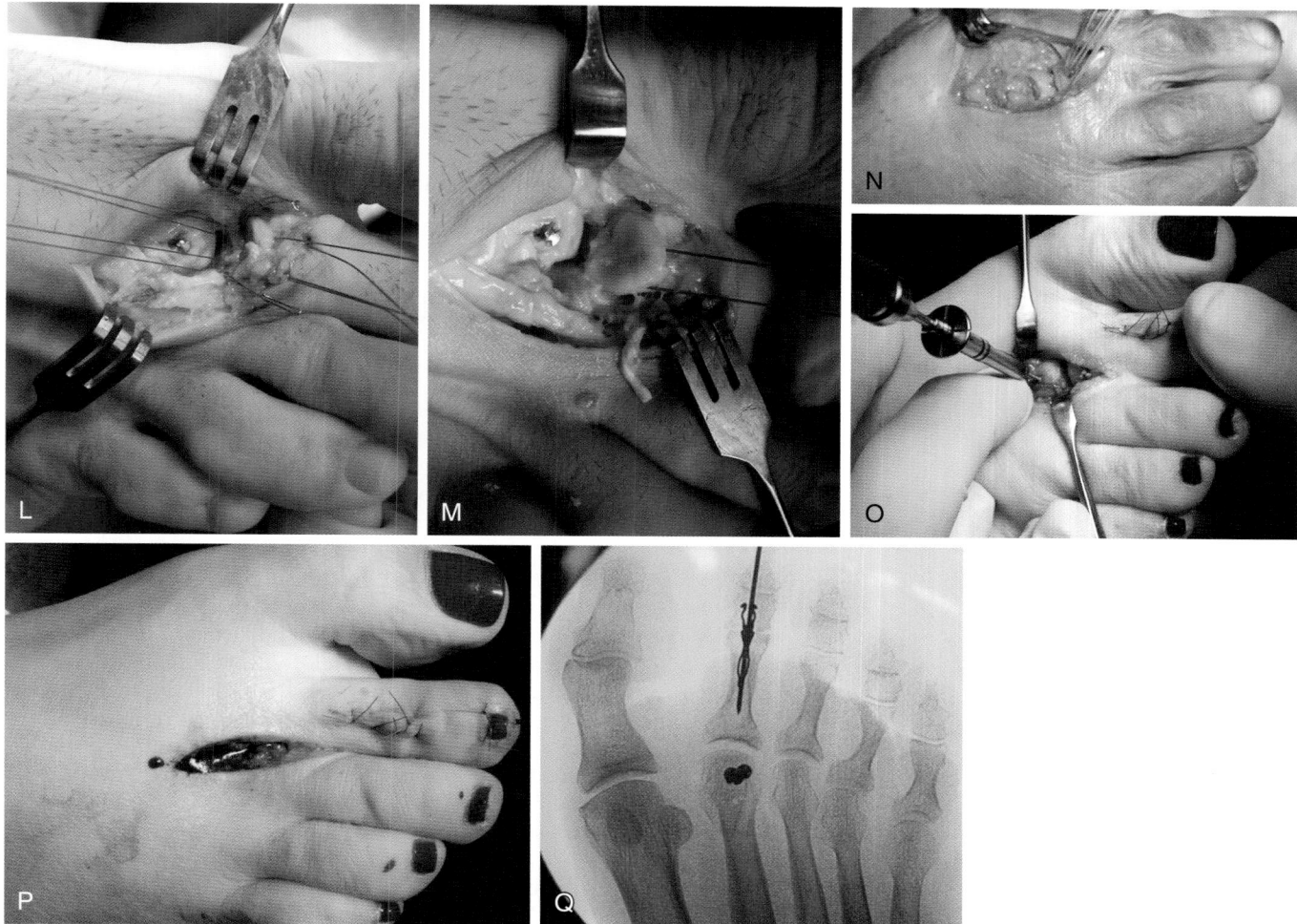

Figure 7-113, cont'd **M,** Sutures are passed through the oblique drill holes in the proximal phalanx. **N,** Suture is tied over the proximal phalanx bony bridge. **O,** Fixation of the Weil osteotomy (this may be fixed before or after tying the sutures). **P,** Clinical photograph of the repaired plantar plate and Weil osteotomy. **Q,** Radiograph after Weil osteotomy, plantar plate repair, and hammer toe repair. (L,M; courtesy of Caio Nery, MD.)

distal plantar plate is transfixed just proximal to the transverse tear using a small curved needle or a special curved Microsuture Lasso or a suture punch (Mini-Scorpion–Complete Plantar Plate Repair System, Arthrex, Naples, Fla.) (see Fig. 7-113G and H), to pass the suture within the rather restricted MTP joint surgical area of exposure.

10. After placement of these sutures, two oblique vertical drill holes (using a 1.5-mm K-wire or 1.6-mm drill) are made on the dorsal medial and dorsal lateral base of the proximal phalanx (on either side of the extensor tendon) directed from the dorsal cortex to the plantar rim of the proximal phalanx (see Fig. 7-113I and J).

11. The ends of the sutures are then passed from plantar to dorsal (with a microsuture passer) to secure the plantar plate to its insertion point on the plantar base of the phalanx (see Fig. 7-113K-N).

12. The Weil osteotomy is fixed with one or two small compression screws, typically with only 1 to 2 mm of shortening at the osteotomy site (see Fig. 7-113O). (It may be fixed either before or after the sutures are tied.)

13. Finally, with the toe held reduced on the metatarsal articular surface, in 15 to 20 degrees of plantar flexion, the sutures are tied. Tension is placed on the sutures (having been pulled through the drill holes in the proximal phalanx). They are then tied over the cortical bridge between the two drill holes on the dorsal phalangeal cortex, thereby advancing the plantar plate onto the proximal phalanx base.

14. In the presence of residual transverse plane malalignment, the lateral capsule and ligamentous complex is reefed with 2-0 nonabsorbable sutures.

15. After routine wound closure, a postoperative compression dressing is applied with the toe held in slight plantar flexion (see Fig. 7-113P and Q).

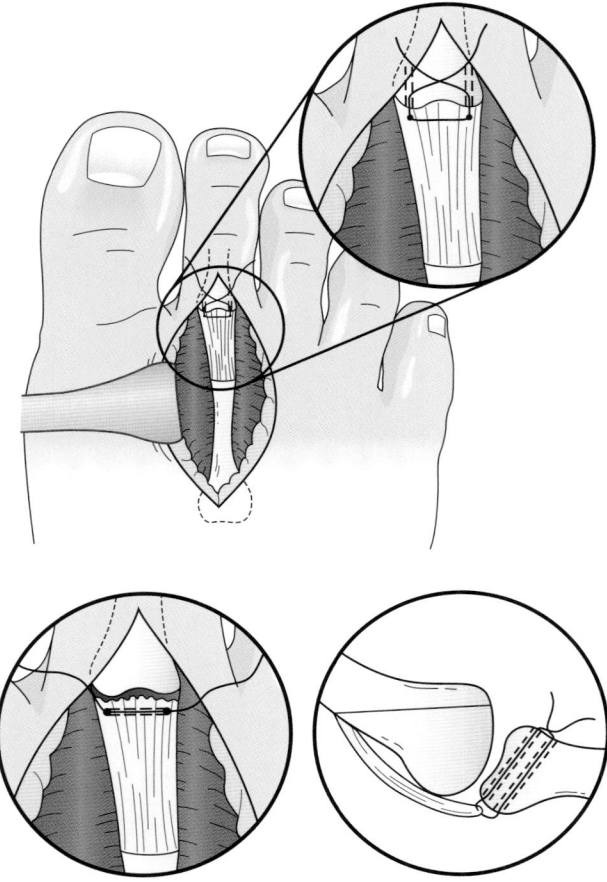

Figure 7-114 Diagram of plantar plate repair. Dorsal view of plantar plate with metatarsal head removed. *1,* Overview of suture placement. *2,* Suture placed transversely in the distal plantar plate. *3,* Suture has been passed through the base of the proximal phalanx and *4,* tied over the bony bridge. (Used with permission from Nery C, Coughlin MJ, Baumfeld D, Mann TS. Lesser metatarsophalangeal joint instability: prospective evaluation and repair of plantar plate or capsular insufficiency. *Foot Ankle Int* 33:301-311, 2012.)

Postoperative Care

After surgery, the patient is allowed to ambulate in a postoperative shoe for 6 weeks with weight bearing on the heel and lateral aspect of the foot. The dressings are changed at 1 and 2 weeks after surgery. Two to 3 weeks after the repair, postoperative dressings are discontinued, and the foot is placed in a compression wrap with a dynamic toe exercise strap (Bioskin midfoot compression wrap with Weil osteotomy strap, Cropper Medical, Ashland, Ore.) (Fig. 7-115A-D).

An exercise program is then initiated to condition the extrinsic flexors of the lesser toes. Flexion and extension passive and active range-of-motion exercises are commenced after surgery to recondition the short and long flexors and extensors of the lesser toes. A physical therapist is often included in the postoperative

regimen. One specific beneficial exercise is the use of a Thera-Band (Hypenic Corp., Akron, Ohio) sling placed over the hallux (Fig. 7-115E and F). With the ankle at neutral dorsiflexion, the hallux and lesser toes are flexed aggressively against the Thera-Band sling. Ten-minute periods of exercise three times a day compliment the exercise program of walking and isometrics for the lower extremity.

Results

Dhukaram et al[64] performed an extensive soft tissue MTP joint release and PIP joint arthroplasty for subluxated joint deformities. If a hyperextension deformity persisted after a careful soft tissue release, a Weil osteotomy was performed. In the evaluation of 69 patients (157 toes), 14% still had moderate or severe pain at the MTP joint, but only two cases demonstrated instability of the MTP joint. A patient should be forewarned that after surgery pain might not totally resolve, especially if some joint arthrosis is present.

Coughlin[33] reported on the surgical correction of 15 toes (11 patients) with a variety of methods, depending on the severity of the deformity. Extensor tenotomy or lengthening, MTP joint capsulotomy, flexor tendon transfer, Kirschner wire fixation, and occasionally metatarsal articular surface resection were used to treat these acute and chronic MTP subluxations. Findings at surgery demonstrated that 33% of second MTP joints had a rupture or complete erosion of the lateral MTP capsule, and 40% had erosion with complete rupture of the joint capsule. In 27%, a rupture could not be demonstrated, although the capsule was elongated. (In this and subsequent studies, the plantar capsule could not be visualized, so no information was obtained on the condition of the plantar plate.) Some 90% of patients were noted to have an elongated second metatarsal averaging 4 mm of increased length. Ninety-three percent good and excellent results were reported using this method of soft tissue reconstruction. Coughlin[42] later reported on a younger group of athletically active patients (9 patients, 11 toes). Using a similar soft tissue realignment procedure, 71% good and excellent results were reported.

Coughlin et al[49] reported on their experience in treating a series of 121 consecutive patients with an interdigital neuroma. Twenty percent of these patients had concurrent lesser MTP joint instability. They were treated with a correction of the joint instability and also neuroma excision. Eighty-five percent rated their result good or excellent. Those with continued symptoms isolated their pain to the symptomatic MTP joint. The authors advocated serial Xylocaine injections to isolate the area of maximal discomfort. If malalignment of the joint and a positive drawer sign were present, a joint injection was not necessary. Ill-defined forefoot pain in the area of the second MTP joint and second interspace may be difficult to differentiate, and sequential injections may be helpful in defining specific areas of pain (Fig. 7-116).

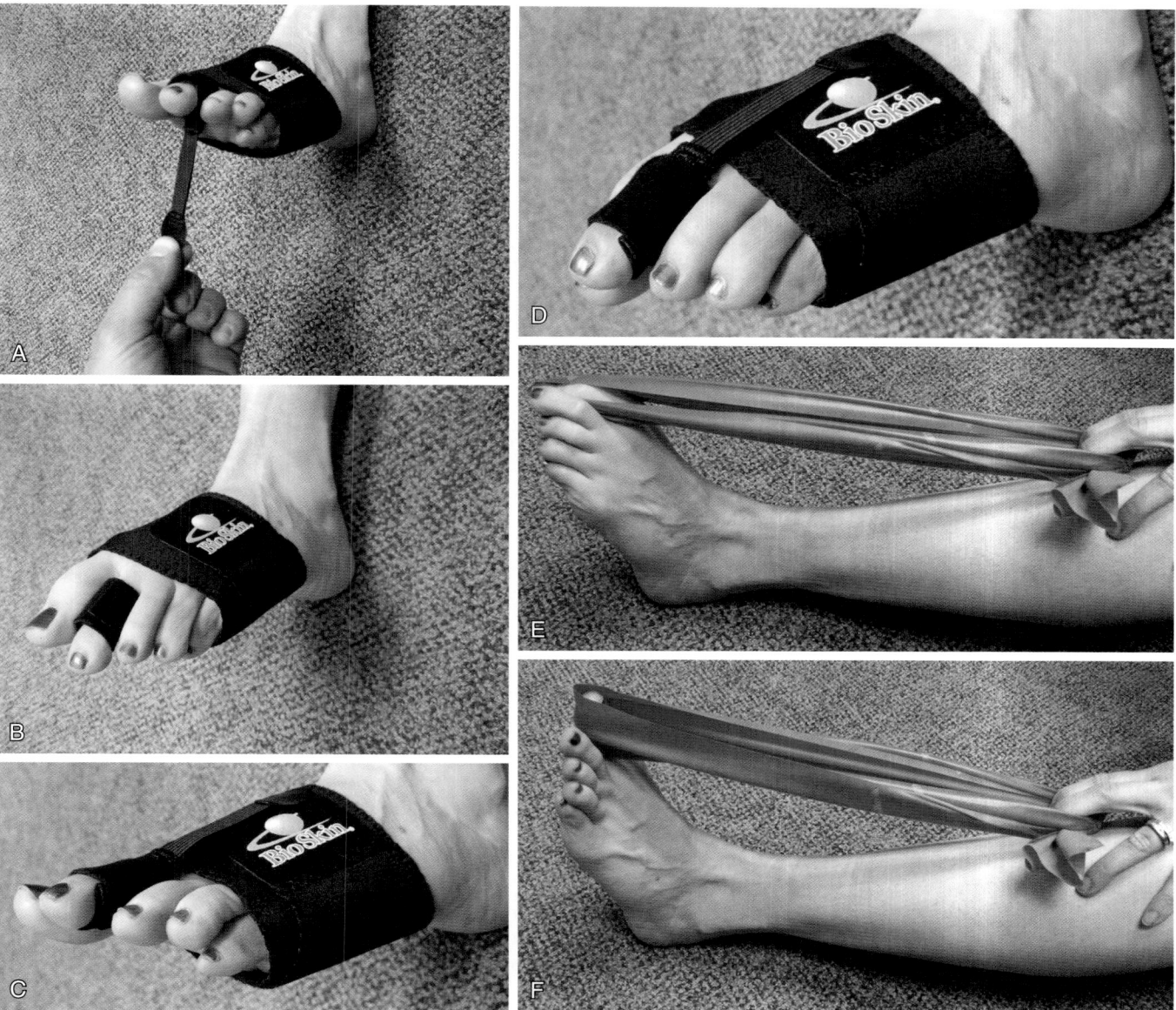

Figure 7-115 Exercises for the lesser toes. **A,** A Bioskin forefoot wrap in place, with exerciser strap on the second toe. **B,** The strap is placed under tension and this pulls the toe into a plantar-flexed position (a substitute for taping the toe downward.) **C,** The strap is now placed on the dorsal aspect under some tension. **D,** This allows the digit to be exercised to strengthen the flexor digitorum longus of the lesser toes. **E,** Thera-Band loop is placed around the great toe, and, **F,** with tension on the hallux, all the toes are plantar flexed, exercising the flexor digitorum longus and lesser toes concomitantly.

Haddad et al[97] reported on the results of 19 extensor digitorum brevis transfers for correction of mild-to-moderate crossover second toe deformity. At an average follow-up of almost 52 months, they noted successful realignment in 14 of 19 (74%) toes, two failures that were revised with a flexor digitorum longus transfer, and three toes with mild recurrent deformities that were asymptomatic. They noted an average postoperative passive range of motion of 78 degrees after flexor digitorum brevis transfer compared with a similar-sized group in their study in which a flexor digitorum longus transfer was performed where there was an average of 62 degrees of passive motion at the MTP joint. The authors suggested that stiffness might not solely be due to the tendon transfer because, in fact, deformities that were more severe were believed to develop more scarring after MTP joint realignment. However, they found that transferring the extensor digitorum brevis beneath the transverse metatarsal ligament was effective in controlling transverse plane abnormalities in the treatment of the crossover second toe

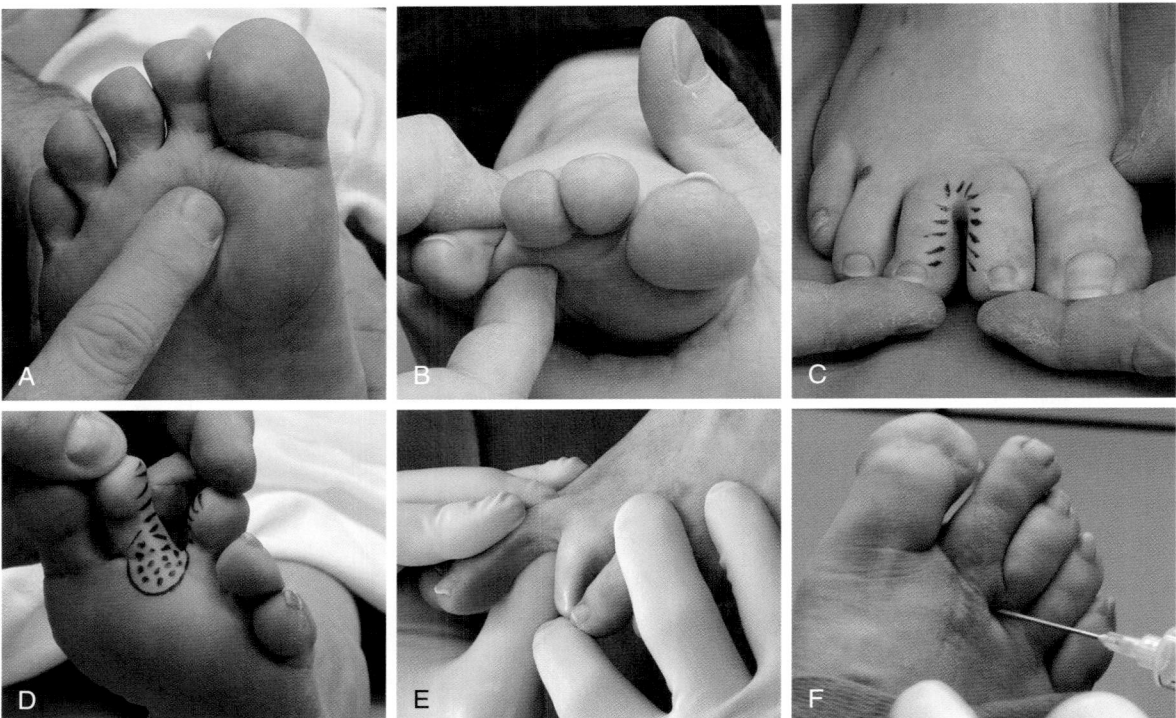

Figure 7-116 The examination to differentiate metatarsophalangeal joint pain from a neuroma can be difficult, especially in a patient who has had prior surgery. **A,** Pain is often localized to the plantar surface of the foot. **B,** Palpation for pain in the interspace can help to diagnose a neuroma. **C** and **D,** Areas of numbness or neuritic pain can occur with nerve irritation. **E,** A positive drawer sign is pathognomonic for capsular instability. **F,** Diagnostic injection may help to isolate the primary area of pain.

deformity. They recommended short extensor tendon transfer for mild and moderate deformities that were flexible; they recommended long flexor tendon transfer for more severe deformities, for rigid deformities, and for patients with combined instability and concomitant interdigital neuromas of the second intermetatarsal space. Stiffness and continued pain were common after surgery, and complete satisfaction was noted by only 69% of patients. There are no reports on the long-term efficacy of the plantar condylectomy, although it has been used in combination with other procedures in several reports.[33,42,43]

Barca and Acciaro[4] have reported on the use of an extensor digitorum longus transfer combined with a medial soft tissue release in 27 patients (30 toes) and noted 83% good or excellent results. Kaz and Coughlin[120] have described a modification of the extensor brevis transfer as a means of reefing the insufficient lateral capsular tissue.

Recently, direct plantar plate repair has been proposed, but reports remain scant.[77,93,153,183,238] Using a plantar approach, Powless et al[183] and Bouche et al[15] reported on a total of 78 plantar plate repairs in these two separate series, ranging in size from 20 to 50 cases (follow-up, 6-100 months). Gregg et al[93] published a series on 35 plantar plate repairs using a dorsal approach combined with a Weil osteotomy. At mean follow-up of 26 months, a high level of good and excellent results was reported.

Weil et al[229] reported on 15 cases in which a similar technique was used, and with an average follow-up of 22 months, they reported 77% good and excellent results. Nery et al[168] reported on the largest study to date (22 patients, 40 plantar plate repairs) using a dorsal approach and observed substantial relief of pain, correction of deformity, improved MTP joint stability, and an improvement in the mean American Orthopaedic Foot and Ankle Society (AOFAS) score from 52 to 92 points.

Nery et al[168] reported the incidence of plantar plate tears involving the second MTP joint was (64%), and the third and fourth MTP joints comprised the remaining joints. Those with a grade 0 lesion were treated with thermal shrinkage of the capsule. Twenty-two patients (40 MTP joints) underwent direct capsular repair with a Weil osteotomy used for exposure. Six patients with an unrepairable grade IV plantar plate tear underwent a Weil osteotomy and flexor tendon transfer. At an average follow-up of 17 months, an average AOFAS score of 92 points was achieved, with remarkable reduction of pain scores and improved function as well.

Davies et al[56] reported on the results of Weil osteotomies in 39 patients. Eight of 39 patients had some continued pain, but a high level of satisfactory results was reported. No cases of avascular necrosis or nonunion were observed. O'Kane et al[172] reported on 17 patients in whom a Weil osteotomy was performed. Shortening averaged 5.2 mm. After surgery, 20% of the operated toes did not contact the ground, although the authors did not find this to be a source of patient dissatisfaction.

Hofstaetter et al[106] reported intermediate term follow-up on 25 feet, with 84% excellent results. Only 32% of toes made contact with the ground. In fact, elevation of the toe tip ("floating toe") or loss of toe purchase is a commonly reported effect after Weil osteotomy, ranging in frequency from 20% to 68%.[7,106,137,154,173] On the other hand, Vandeputte et al[225] and others[47,89] who used an aggressive postoperative exercise program reported that most of patients in their series had adequate toe purchase. Boyer and DeOrio,[18] who pinned their Weil ostetomies in slight plantar flexion, reported a much lower incidence of floating toes. An aggressive exercise program postoperatively is quite important in reducing the incidence of "floating toes" (see Fig. 7-115). Restricted range of motion is probably the most common observation after this osteotomy, with estimates of 50% reduction in MTP range of motion being the common finding.[7,18,106,123,225] Trnka et al[223] reported a limitation of plantar flexion after Weil osteotomy and suggested this was caused by capsule scarring and weakening of the intrinsic musculature.

Aggressive physical therapy may be beneficial postoperatively. Early passive and active range-of-motion exercises of the involved digit help to regain toe function. Exercises should be performed several times a day. Although scarring of the plantar plate occurs after the osteotomy, vigorous manipulation does help to mobilize the joint.[224]

The healing rate after a Weil osteotomy is very high; no nonunions were reported in five different series in which 272 procedures were performed[7,18,106,123,225]

Internal fixation with a vertical mini-fragment or spin screw is common. Pain from prominent screws has been reported,[18,106] requiring removal. Grimes and Coughlin,[96] in a cadaver study, measured the vertical height of the lesser metatarsals and reported that the average height varied from 17.8 to 16.3 mm; the thinnest metatarsal head was 14.8 mm. Thus a screw of 11 to 12 mm should, in almost all cases, be acceptable for fixation of the second, third, and fourth metatarsals, and it is likely that a 14- to 15-mm long screw can be used in appropriate situations.

Grimes and Coughlin[96] noted that the average inclination of the lesser metatarsal varied from 19 to 31 degrees, a significant variation. The three varables that can be controlled when doing a Weil osteotomy are the angle of osteotomy, the thickness of the cut, and the amount of proximal displacement of the capital fragment. Grimes[96] concluded that with a plantar inclincation of 25 degrees, a 1-mm-thick saw blade provides enough bone resection to allow up to 5 mm of shortening. If it is necessary to shorten the metatarsal more than 5 mm, the possibility of increased plantar pressure necessitates bone resection at the osteotomy site to provide elevation in addition to shortening. This may be achieved by resecting a thin slice of bone at the osteotomy site (3-5 mm).[106,123] Another alternative is to stack two or three saw blades in the sagittal saw or to use a thicker saw blade to resect a greater thickness of bone (see Figs. 7-109F and 7-110D). Although the metatarsal declination angle determines the amount of plantar translation and varies from patient to patient, Weil[232] concluded that with an osteotomy angle of 25 degrees, for each 1 mm of shortening, there is 1 mm of metatarsal head depression.

Trnka et al[223] reported on a comparison of the Helal and Weil osteotomies. In 15 patients (25 osteotomies), the second, third, and/or fourth metatarsals were osteotomized with Weil's technique as treatment for dislocation of the MTP joint and then were compared with results in a similar group for which Helal osteotomies were performed. Twelve of the patients who underwent Weil osteotomies were satisfied with their results. The major reason for dissatisfaction was pain associated with a prominent plantar screw. Although some of these patients had an asymptomatic callus beneath the involved metatarsal head, the authors reported no symptomatic transfer lesions. There were no reported cases of pseudoarthrosis, avascular necrosis, nonunion, or transfer lesions after the Weil osteotomy. After the Weil procedure, 4 of the 25 dislocated MTP joints remained dislocated compared with 8 of 22 MTP joints that remained dislocated after the Helal osteotomy. The authors concluded that the Weil osteotomy provided greater accuracy in metatarsal shortening and a high level of postoperative satisfaction.

Weil et al[232] reported on the results of 69 cases in which a capital oblique osteotomy was performed. The postoperative incidence of transfer metatarsalgia was 9%, plantar flexion range of motion was limited in 17% of patients, and a hammer toe developed in 5%. There were no cases of osteonecrosis or degenerative arthritis.

Nonetheless, because of metatarsal head depression after an osteotomy, a dorsiflexion contracture can occur at the metatarsophalangeal joint after a Weil osteotomy.[154,172,224] Trnka[224] dissected two cadaver specimens and performed osteotomies at 25, 30, 35, and 40 degrees relative to the longitudinal axis of the metatarsal. Both Trnka[224] and O'Kane[172] have observed that the intrinsic tendons move dorsally with respect to the axis of the MTP joint because of depression of the plantar fragment altering the center of rotation after the osteotomy, leading to MTP joint hyperextension (see Fig. 7-21). In another laboratory study, the amount of shortening and plantar translation was evaluated.[152] Osteotomies with angles of less than 25 degrees minimize plantar translation. With a 5-mm proximal shift, the plantar displacement with a 30-degree angle was 2 mm; with a 10-mm shift, it was 5 mm. With an osteotomy less than 25 degrees, the osteotomy exits the metatarsal shaft very proximally. Metatarsals do have differing inclination angles from patient to patient and even between other lesser metatarsals in the same foot. Modifying the Weil osteotomy by inclining the blade 15 to 20 degrees in reference to the metatarsal shaft and removing a slice of bone at the osteotomy site when substantial shortening is planned can reduce plantar displacement of the metatarsal head and help to reduce hyperextension deformities as well.

Weil[232] suggests taping the toe in 5 degrees of plantar flexion after surgery to minimize MTP joint hyperextension. A flexor tendon transfer may be required if the digit remains unstable (see Fig. 7-111)[35]; however, currently, this appears to be a less popular alternative. Short-term intramedullary Kirschner wire fixation with the toe in slight plantar flexion controls alignment in both the sagittal and coronal planes and ensures an anatomic reduction. It minimizes the need for frequent dressing changes and allows early healing to stabilize the MTP joint capsule tissues, which promotes joint stability. The Kirschner wire is removed 2 to 3 weeks after the procedure, and range-of-motion exercises are commenced. With Kirschner wire stabilization, early weight bearing on the forefoot can displace the osteotomy site; a patient should be advised of the importance of protecting the forefoot region after a distal metatarsal osteotomy.

The results of distal metatarsal osteotomies performed without internal fixation have been mediocre. Idusuyi et al[107] noted a high incidence of MTP joint pain, limited motion, and unsatisfactory results. Trnka et al[223] reported a high rate of redislocation, transfer lesions, nonunions, and unsatisfactory results as well after distal metatarsal osteotomies that were not internally fixed. Davies et al[56] stressed that rigid internal fixation decreases the risk of transfer lesions. A shortening osteotomy of the second metatarsal may be performed proximal to the MTP joint. This decompresses the MTP joint by effectively lengthening the adjacent soft tissue structures. Giannestras[85] described a longitudinal oblique osteotomy of the diaphyseal portion of the metatarsal shaft (see Chapter 8). This is another technique that can be used to achieve shortening of the involved ray, but it is difficult and may be associated with delayed union, malunion, and transfer lesions (Fig. 7-117).

The obvious benefits of the Weil osteotomy are that the location affords a large area of bone contact, it is a relatively stable osteotomy, its design allows for controlled shortening, internal fixation is relatively easy to place, and the incidence of complications (other than MTP joint hyperextension) is low (see Fig. 7-21). Postoperative nonunion, avascular necrosis, and degenerative arthritis are rare (Fig. 7-118). Although a certain amount of arthrofibrosis of the MTP joint develops after a Weil osteotomy, the decreased range of motion has a stabilizing effect on the MTP joint. In general, patients with subluxation and dislocation of the MTP joint should expect a well-aligned toe that does not have normal dynamic function. The goal of surgery is to reduce plantar pain beneath the metatarsal head, to realign the toe, and to stabilize the MTP joint. Although generally there is significant improvement after these procedures, it should be explained to the patient that the involved toe will not have normal function.

With extensive surgery on a lesser toe, complications can result (see Fig 7-118). The most severe complication of surgery is vascular compromise. Although it is difficult to give guidelines regarding the extent of surgery that is feasible for a second toe, occasionally the surgeon believes that sufficient surgery has been carried out and discontinues an attempt at further correction. In this situation, a second-stage procedure may be necessary at a later date. This is certainly preferable to vascular compromise of a lesser toe.

Occasionally, the circulation to the toe is impaired after surgery. In this situation, if a Kirschner wire has been placed, it must be removed to decrease tension on the toe and relieve vascular spasm. Thus it is important to use the

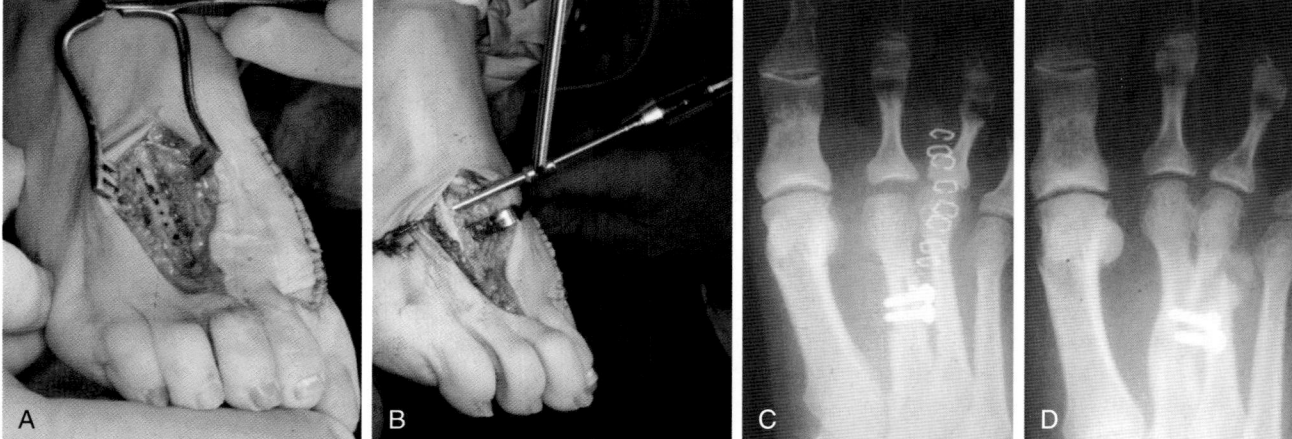

Figure 7-117 Longitudinal osteotomies require a long incision **(A)** and internal fixation with cross screws **(B). C,** Postoperative radiograph demonstrates shortening. **D,** Postoperative complications include delayed healing and stress fracture of the fourth metatarsal, with later synostosis of the adjacent metatarsals.

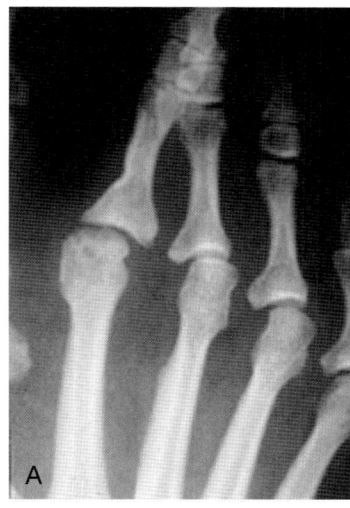
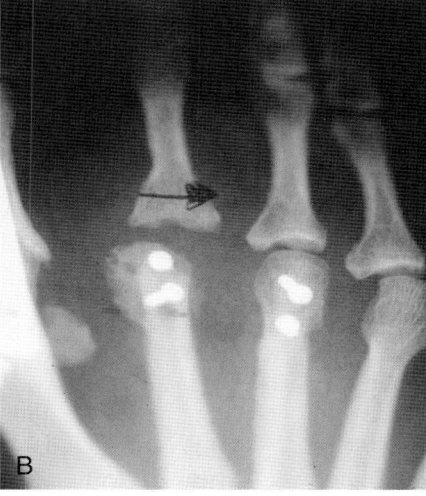

Figure 7-118 Complications of Weil osteotomy. **A,** Avascular necrosis of metatarsal head. **B,** Lateral subluxation postoperatively.

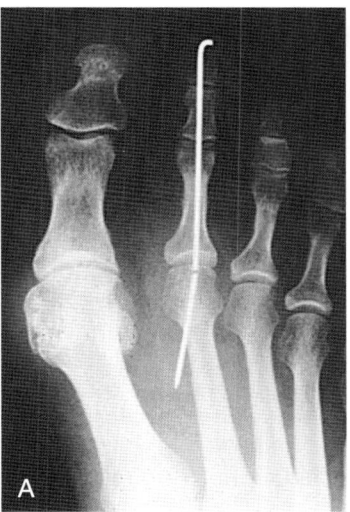
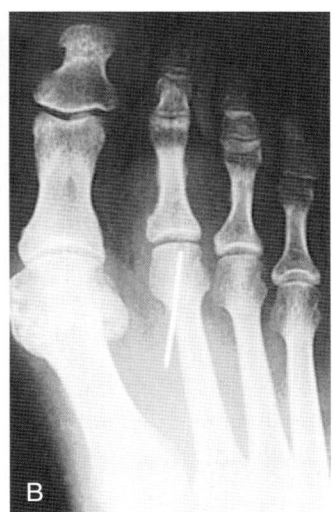
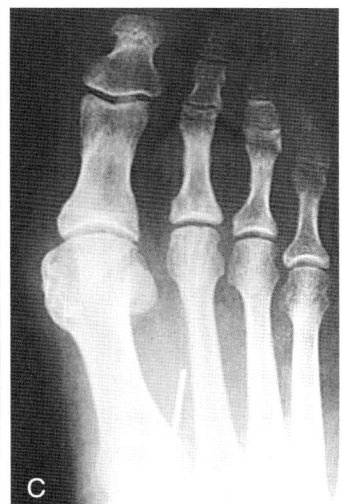

Figure 7-119 **A,** With placement of an intramedullary Kirschner wire across the metatarsophalangeal (MTP) joint, the pin can fracture. If a fractured pin compromises MTP joint function, it may be removed. **B,** Typically, the pin fractures 2 to 3 mm proximal to the articular surface, and in this case, it may be left in the metatarsal shaft. **C,** Occasionally, migration of the proximal pin necessitates removal.

Kirschner wire only as an augmentation of the surgical repair and not to achieve more alignment. If removal in the immediate postoperative period is necessary, the toe needs to be held in alignment with gauze-and-tape dressings until adequate healing has occurred. The advent of intramedullary hammer toe implants has significantly helped in this situation. A Kirschner wire used to stabilize the MTP joint may be removed where there is vascular compromise; yet, with a hammer toe implant in place, alignment of the digit is not sacrificed.

Occasionally, a Kirschner wire fatigues and breaks if the patient ambulates excessively. If a broken Kirschner wire interferes with MTP joint function, it should be removed. Typically, the wire fatigues just proximal to the joint surface, and in this situation, removal of the proximal portion is unnecessary (Fig. 7-119).

Excessive tension on the metatarsal head after relocation of a dislocated MTP joint may be complicated by avascular necrosis or degenerative arthritis. Scheck[197] has reported this occurrence after extensive soft tissue stripping in the reduction of a dislocated MTP joint.

Recurrence of an MTP joint deformity can be a complication of the subluxated and dislocated second toe. Adequate MTP soft tissue release is necessary at the initial surgery. Transfer of the long flexor tendon can remove one of the most significant deforming forces. Adequate bony decompression is necessary when a soft tissue release does not allow stable relocation of the MTP joint. The second toe must be completely realigned at surgery. Sub-total realignment that relies on the Kirschner wire to achieve the repair often results in redeformation once the Kirschner wire has been removed.

With numerous procedures being performed on the lesser toe, postoperative edema is common and can take months to subside (see Fig. 7-46). Likewise, molding of the second toe caused by extrinsic pressure from adjacent toes can occur (see Fig. 7-57). This is unavoidable, and it is important to inform the patient preoperatively about this possibility.

Postoperative pain at either the MTP joint arthroplasty site or the hammer toe site occurs occasionally. Although this pain should resolve with time, occasionally discomfort at the arthroplasty site continues. Often there is a moderate amount of restricted motion at the arthroplasty site as well. This restricted motion can afford joint stability, but it can make ambulation painful. In this situation, a revision may be performed with a partial proximal phalangectomy[88,121]; this is an alternative procedure for MTP joint dislocation.

Decreased sensation occasionally occurs in the toe as a result of extensive surgery and injury to the digital nerves. Care must be taken not to injure the nerves when soft tissue procedures and tendon transfers are performed. Usually, with the passage of time, sensation returns.

SALVAGE PROCEDURES

Indications

In the presence of severe deformities, recurrent deformity, avascular necrosis of the metatarsal head, or degenerative arthritis of the involved metatarsophalangeal joint, salvage procedures may be necessary. These include, but are not limited to, the DuVries metatarsophalangeal joint arthroplasty, partial proximal phalangectomy, and syndactylization of the lesser toes.

Contraindications

When possible, normal function of the lesser MTP joints should be preserved. Salvage procedures should be reserved for joints with severe arthritis, recurrent subluxation, or dislocation or after another unsuccessful surgical procedure, with the goal of achieving a plantigrade, less painful foot and improving the ambulatory capacity of the patient.

DUVRIES METATARSOPHALANGEAL JOINT ARTHROPLASTY
Surgical Technique[166]
1. The patient is placed in a supine position on the operating room table. The foot is cleansed and draped in the usual fashion. The foot is exsanguinated with an Esmarch bandage. The Esmarch bandage may be used as a tourniquet above the level of the ankle (Fig. 7-120A).

2. A lazy-S incision is centered over the MTP joint. A soft tissue release is performed in which the extensor tendons are lengthened, and the dorsal, medial, and lateral MTP capsules are released as well (see the discussion of soft tissue release of the MTP joint) (Fig. 7-120B).
3. The metatarsal head is identified, and the proximal phalanx is plantar flexed to expose the metatarsal articular surface. A McGlamry elevator can assist in the exposure.
4. An osteotomy is performed in a dorsoplantar direction, removing 3 to 4 mm of bone; the amount of overlap determines the amount of metatarsal head resected (Fig. 7-120C and D).
5. The dorsal, medial, and lateral edges are beveled with a rongeur (Fig. 7-120E). The plantar condyles are removed with an osteotomy (Fig. 7-120F and G), achieving a somewhat rounded head to articulate with the concave base of the proximal phalanx.
6. After bone decompression, the second toe should be reducible. The ankle is dorsiflexed and plantar flexed, and if the MTP joint is stable, the phalanx remains reduced and does not dislocate (Fig. 7-120H and I).
7. Typically, after a bone decompression, a flexor tendon transfer is performed to give stability to the proximal phalanx.
8. A Kirschner wire is introduced at the base of the proximal phalanx and driven distally, exiting the tip of the toe. It is then driven retrograde to stabilize the MTP joint. The pin is bent at the tip of the toe, and any excess pin is removed (Fig. 7-120J).
9. Myerson[121] has described a modification of the MTP arthroplasty in which the tendon of the extensor digitorum brevis and joint capsule is interposed in the joint space and anchored to the plantar aspect of the metatarsal head (Fig. 7-121). No results have been reported with this technique.

Postoperative Care
A gauze-and-tape dressing is applied and changed weekly. The patient is allowed to ambulate in a wooden-soled postoperative shoe. Sutures and the Kirschner wire are removed 3 weeks after surgery.

PARTIAL PROXIMAL PHALANGECTOMY AND SYNDACTYLIZATION[55,75]
Surgical Technique
1. The foot is cleansed and draped in the usual fashion. The foot is exsanguinated with an Esmarch bandage. With careful padding the Esmarch bandage may be used as a tourniquet above the level of the ankle.
2. The toes are distracted as a web-bisecting incision is made (see Fig. 7-49A and B).
3. The web-bisecting incision is flanked by a pair of peri-digital incisions. Plantar and dorsal flaps are developed, and small triangles of skin are resected.

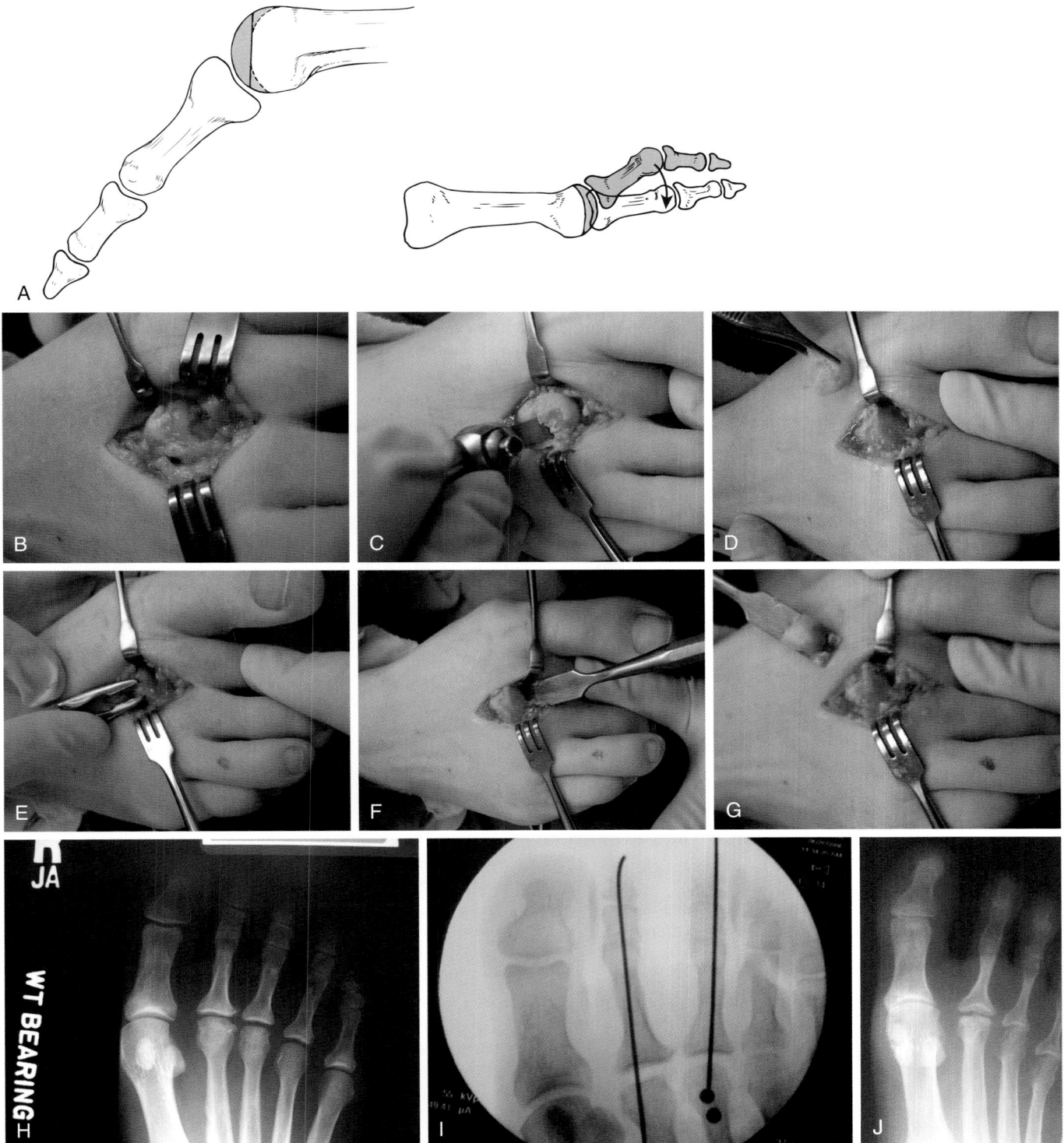

Figure 7-120 DuVries arthroplasty of the metatarsophalangeal (MTP) joint. **A,** Dorsoplantar osteotomy removes 2 to 3 mm of metatarsal head. The dorsoplantar, medial, and lateral surfaces then are beveled to create a curved surface that will articulate with the trumpet-shaped base of the proximal phalanx. **B,** Dorsal approach demonstrates endstage arthritis of the second MTP joint. **C,** Resection of distal articular surface. **D,** Removal of articular fragment. **E,** Beveling of dorsal survace. **F and G,** Resection of plantar condyle. **H and I,** Radiographs before and after arthroplasty, respectively. **J,** Five-year follow-up on another patient. Approximately 50% of joint motion is lost due to arthrofibrosis; however, this helps to maintain stability of the joint.

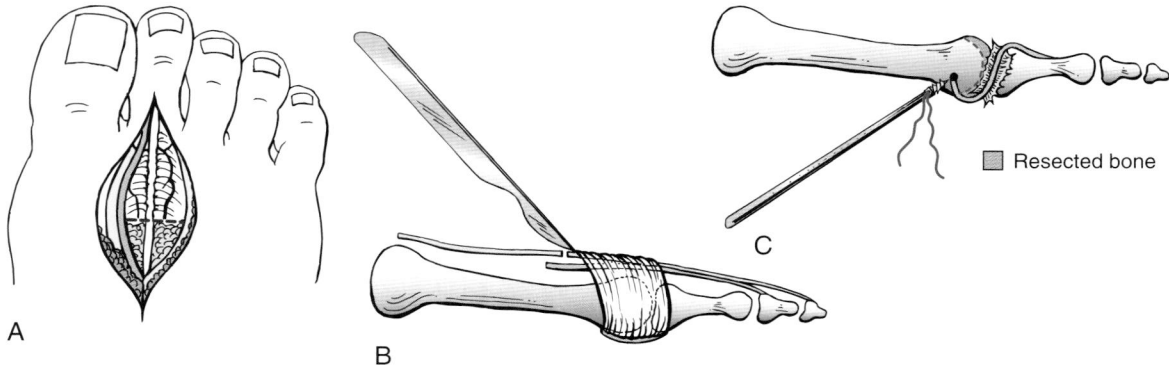

Figure 7-121 **A,** Dorsal approach with the development of an extensor hood for interposition after DuVries arthroplasty. **B,** Lateral view demonstrating area of release of extensor hood. **C,** The extensor hood is interposed between the base of the proximal phalanx and the resected surface of the metatarsal head and secured with a suture anchor (Myerson technique).

4. Adjacent partial proximal phalangectomies may be performed. Care is taken to protect the neurovascular bundles (see Fig. 7-49C).
5. Adjacent dorsal and plantar flaps are apposed and closed with a running and interrupted suture (see Fig. 7-49D-F).

Alternative Method
After excision of the base of the proximal phalanx, an intramedullary Kirschner wire may be used to stabilize the repair until adequate healing is achieved (see Fig. 7-50).

Postoperative Care
A gauze-and-tape dressing is applied and changed weekly. The patient is allowed to ambulate in a wooden-soled postoperative shoe. Sutures are removed 3 weeks after surgery. The adjacent toes are taped together for approximately 6 weeks to protect the surgical syndactylization.

Results and Complications
Conklin and Smith[30] reported 29% dissatisfaction after a proximal phalangectomy. Some 60% of patients had total relief of pain; however, shortening was the most common postoperative complaint (Fig. 7-122).

Cahill and Connor[25] reported that proximal phalangectomy for a hammer toe or claw toe deformity relieved symptoms but gave a poor cosmetic end result. Objectively, poor results occurred in 50% of cases (see Fig. 7-122).

Daly and Johnson[55] reported a series of painful lesser toes characterized by subluxation and dislocation of the second and third MTP joints that were treated with partial proximal phalangectomies and subtotal webbing. Some 28% had moderate or severe problems with cosmesis. Postoperatively, a recurrent cock-up deformity occurred in 18%, residual pain was noted in 27%, and excessive shortening was seen in 5% of cases. Some 75% of patients were satisfied or satisfied with reservations.

Feeney et al[73] reported on 28 patients who underwent hemiphalangectomy and syndactilization for end-stage arthritis or dislocation of the second MTP joint. In this series with rather short-term follow-up, more than one third of patients were lost to follow-up. Although 79% of patients reported being satisfied with the appearance, 18% had moderate or severe malalignment, and only two thirds would have the procedure performed again.

With degenerative arthritis of a lesser MTP joint, an interposition soft tissue arthroplasty can help to retain motion but diminish intractable pain (Fig. 7-123).

Karlock[117] has reported the use of second MTP joint arthrodesis to realign and stabilize a severely deformed second toe with subluxation or dislocation of the MTP joint (Fig. 7-124). In 11 patients, 10 were noted to have a good or excellent results (see Fig. 7-49). Eight of the patients also had a first MTP arthrodesis for a severe hallux valgus deformity. Karlock[117] suggested second MTP arthrodesis as a salvage alternative to amputation of the severely deformed digit. This ensures the alignment of the first ray, while avoiding a complete removal of the severely deformed second toe.

VanderWilde and Campbell[226] reported on the technique of amputation of the second toe for treatment of chronic painful deformity. Sixteen patients (23 amputations) were evaluated at long-term follow-up. Fifteen of 22 patients (68%) were satisfied. They noted that all patients experienced some progression of a preexisting hallux valgus deformity. The hallux valgus angle increased an average of 11.6 degrees on final radiographic follow-up, but only 1 patient came to first MTP arthrodesis.

Gallentine and DeOrio[82] reported on 12 patients (17 feet), with an average age of 78 years, who underwent a second toe amputation for a combined hallux valgus and severe crossover toe deformity, noting it to be a simple procedure with minimal complications and rapid healing.

After multiple procedures to the second toe, soft tissue atrophy and chronic pain can be associated with minimal MTP joint motion (see Fig. 7-53). Although a metatarsal head excision may be considered, it rarely resolves a

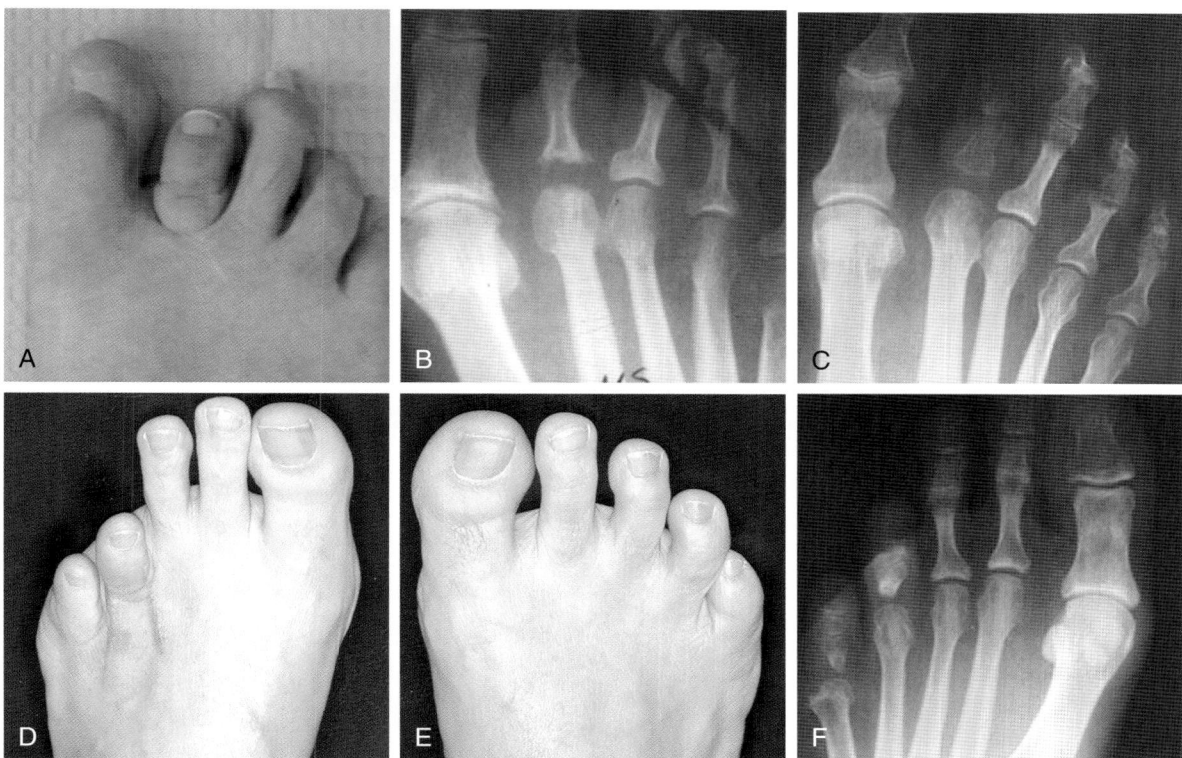

Figure 7-122 Long-term results of partial proximal phalangectomy. Clinical **(A)** and radiographic **(B)** shortening of second toe after partial proximal phalangectomy. **C,** Excessive resection of proximal phalanx. **D,** Postoperative left foot. **E,** Normal right foot. **F,** Radiographic appearance of left foot after partial proximal phalangectomy of fourth and fifth digits.

problem on a long-term basis and is associated with transfer metatarsalgia, which is quite difficult to salvage (Fig. 7-125).

FIFTH TOE DEFORMITIES

Etiology

Deformities of the fifth toe include hard corns, soft corns, and congenital or developmental MTP joint malalignment problems. Overlapping and underlapping of the fifth toe in general are congenital deformities, whereas a cock-up deformity often is associated with a hammer toe deformity. The surgical treatment of each deformity may be considerably different, and thus differentiation of the anatomic findings is important.

Anatomy

The overlapping fifth toe is a fairly common congenital deformity that can become uncomfortable because of pressure from footwear against the toe. The fifth toe is externally rotated and compressed in its AP plane. A dorsal contracture at the MTP joint is present and often is associated with a contracture of the extensor digitorum longus tendon. An underlapping fifth toe is externally rotated as it deviates beneath the fourth toe. Often, a

contracture of the flexor digitorum longus tendon is associated with an elongated extensor digitorum longus tendon. Trauma to the toenail of the fifth toe with ambulation can cause significant distortion of the toenail plate. Redundant capsule on the dorsal aspect of the MTP joint is associated with a contracted plantar medial MTP joint capsule.

With a severe cock-up deformity of the fifth toe (Fig. 7-126), the proximal phalanx articulates at nearly a right angle with the fifth metatarsal shaft. Often, this deformity is associated with a fixed hammer toe deformity. Cockin[28] has described the presence of adhesions between the plantar capsule and the plantar aspect of the metatarsal head that can limit reduction at the MTP joint unless a complete capsule release has been performed.

Preoperative Evaluation

Physical Examination

Preoperative evaluation of a deformed fifth toe necessitates appreciation of the axial rotational deformity, as well as hyperextension or flexion at the MTP joint. The degree of varus or medial deviation of the fifth toe should be observed as well as the presence of a hammer toe deformity. A severe skin contracture can necessitate bone resection rather than a soft tissue realignment procedure. Attention to the neurovascular status preoperatively is

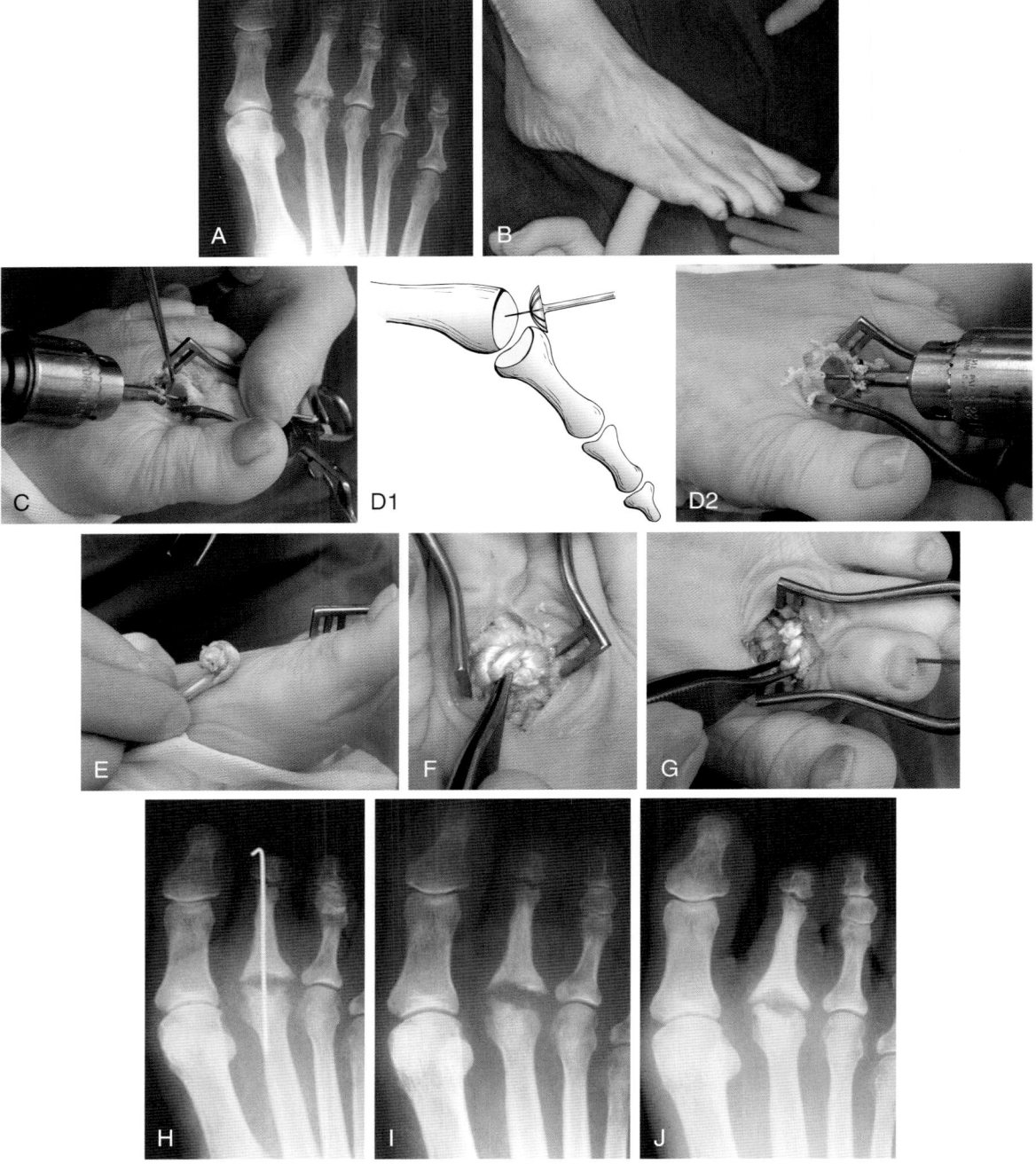

Figure 7-123 Soft tissue arthroplasty. **A** and **B,** Degenerative arthritis of the second metatarsophalangeal (MTP) joint associated with restricted range of motion. A flexion contracture of the MTP joint has occurred. Reaming of the base of the proximal phalanx **(C)** and the metatarsal head **(D). E,** Gracilis tendon bundle. **F** and **G,** Placement of an interposition tendon "anchovy." **H,** Intraoperative radiograph with Kirschner wire fixation. **I,** Postoperative radiograph after treatment with a soft tissue arthroplasty. **J,** Two years after surgery, there was a 50% reduction in range of motion.

important if a significant realignment procedure is necessary.

Conservative Treatment

When possible, shoe modifications and padding are preferable to surgical intervention. (See the section on hammer toes and padding.)

MILD OVERLAPPING FIFTH TOE DEFORMITIES

A mild overlapping fifth toe deformity may be treated in a number of ways, many of which give satisfactory results. The DuVries and the Wilson techniques are useful for a mild-to-moderate deformity; the Lapidus procedure, which involves a tendon transfer, is recommended for a more severe deformity.

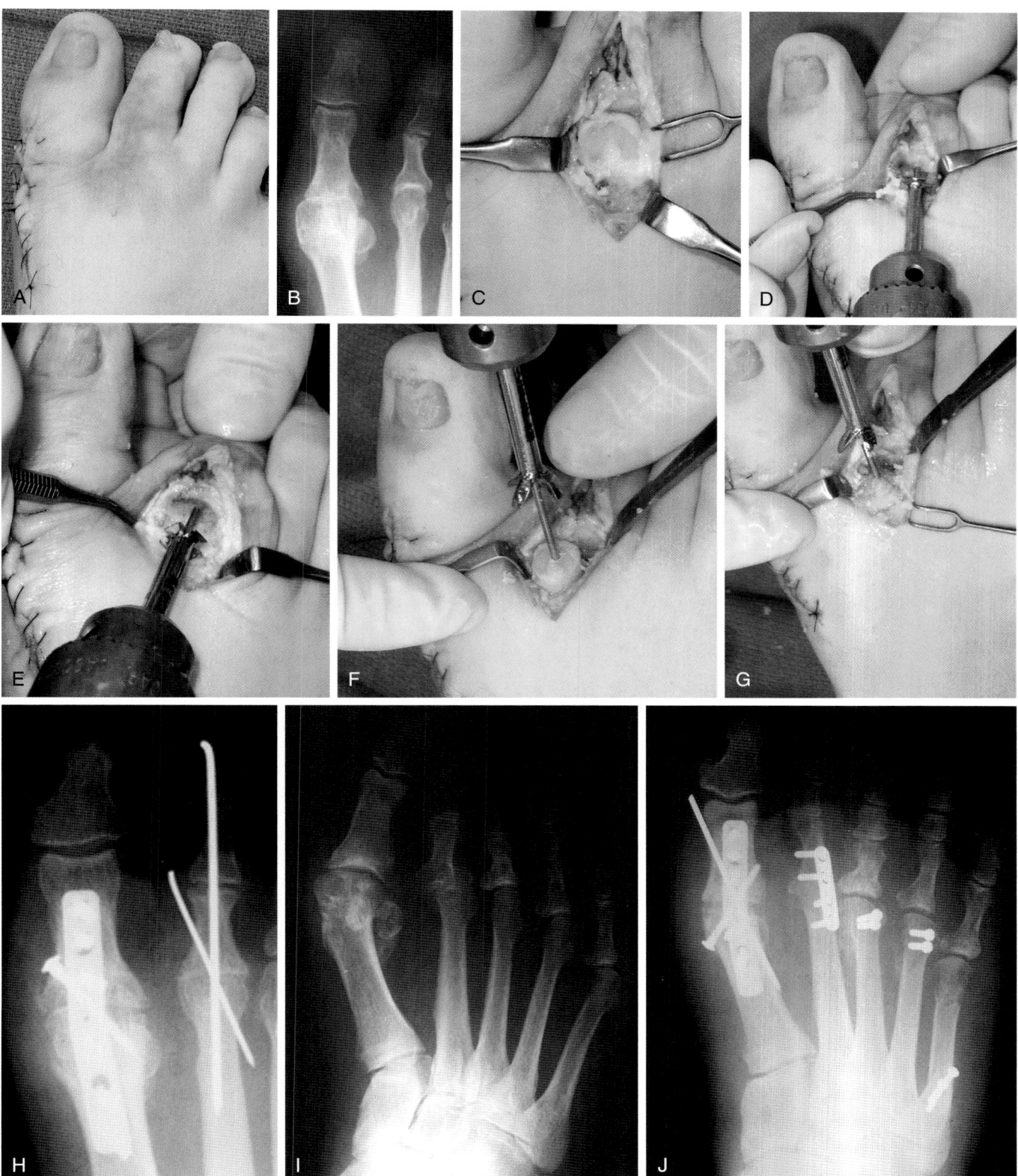

Figure 7-124 Lesser metatarsophalangeal (MTP) joint fusion. Preoperative clinical photograph **(A)** and radiograph **(B)** demonstrate end-stage arthritis of the first and second MTP joints. **C,** Clinical appearance of the metatarsal head with complete cartilage loss. **D** and **E,** Concave reaming of the base of the proximal phalanx. **F** and **G,** Convex preparation of the second metatarsal head. **H,** After arthrodesis of the first and second MTP joints. **I,** Preoperative radiograph of patient with recurrent hallux valgus, bunionette, and dislocated and degenerated second MTP joint. **J,** After first and second MTP joint arthrodeses.

DUVRIES FIFTH TOE REALIGNMENT
Surgical Technique

1. A foot block or regional anesthesia, rather than a digital block, often is used for this procedure. The foot is cleansed in a routine fashion. The foot is exsanguinated with an Esmarch bandage. The Esmarch bandage may be used as a tourniquet above the level of the ankle.
2. A longitudinal incision is centered over the fourth interspace, beginning in the web space and extending proximally just past the fifth metatarsal head (Fig. 7-127A).
3. All MTP joint contractures are released on the dorsal and medial aspect. The extensor tendon is released, as well as the medial collateral ligament and MTP joint capsule.

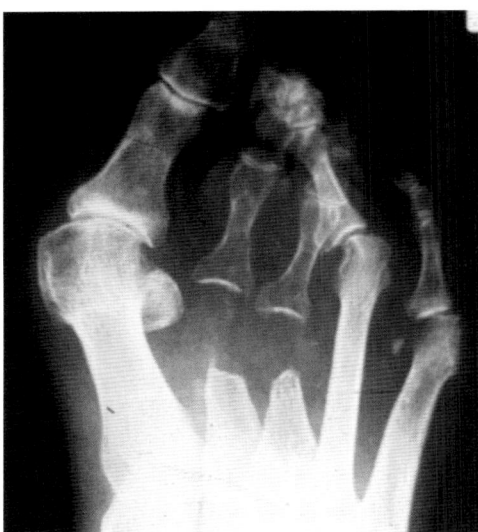

Figure 7-125 Metatarsal head excision. An isolated metatarsal head excision rarely solves a problem. After a second head excision, later the third metatarsal head was excised. Note subluxation of the fourth metatarsophalangeal joint on the radiograph, denoting increased pressure.

4. The toe is placed into an overcorrected position by bringing it into plantar flexion with slight lateral deviation. If the soft tissue contracture has been adequately released, the toe tends to stay in this position and does not redeform.
5. When the toe is brought into realignment, the skin on the fibular margin is stretched distally and skin on the tibial margin is displaced proximally. The puckered or dog-eared edges at the ends of these incisions are then excised (Fig. 7-127B).
6. The skin edges are approximated with interrupted sutures in this new position (Fig. 7-127C), and the fibular skin is advanced distally.

Postoperative Care

A gauze-and-tape compression dressing is used to hold the toe in an overcorrected position and is changed weekly for 8 weeks. The patient is allowed to ambulate in a wooden-soled shoe. Sutures are removed 3 weeks after surgery. The fifth toe is taped into plantar flexion for 3 to 6 weeks. Results are shown in Figure 7-128.

SEVERE OVERLAPPING FIFTH TOE DEFORMITIES

WILSON FIFTH TOE PROCEDURE[234]
Surgical Technique

1. A foot block or regional anesthesia, rather than a digital block, often is used for this procedure. The foot is cleansed in a routine fashion (Fig. 7-129A). The procedure is typically performed using an Esmarch ankle tourniquet with the patient in a slight lateral decubitus position.
2. A V-shaped incision is centered over the medial aspect of the fifth toe and extended into the fourth interspace (Fig. 7-129B).
3. The extensor tendons are sectioned (Fig. 7-129C), and the dorsal and medial MTP joint capsules are released. The toe is plantar flexed, which pulls the tongue of the incision distally, forming a Y-shaped skin flap. The toe

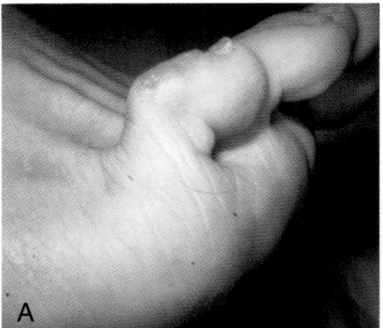
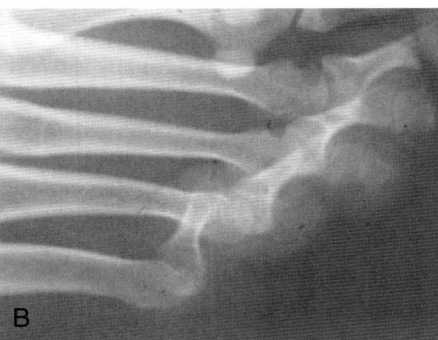
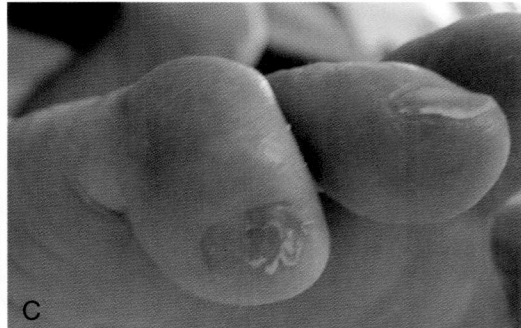

Figure 7-126 **A,** Cock-up deformity of the fifth toe. **B,** Radiograph demonstrates cock-up deformity of the fifth toe. Note that the subluxed proximal phalanx is almost at a right angle to the fifth metatarsal head. **C,** Severe fifth hammer toe without contracture of metatarsophalangeal joint.

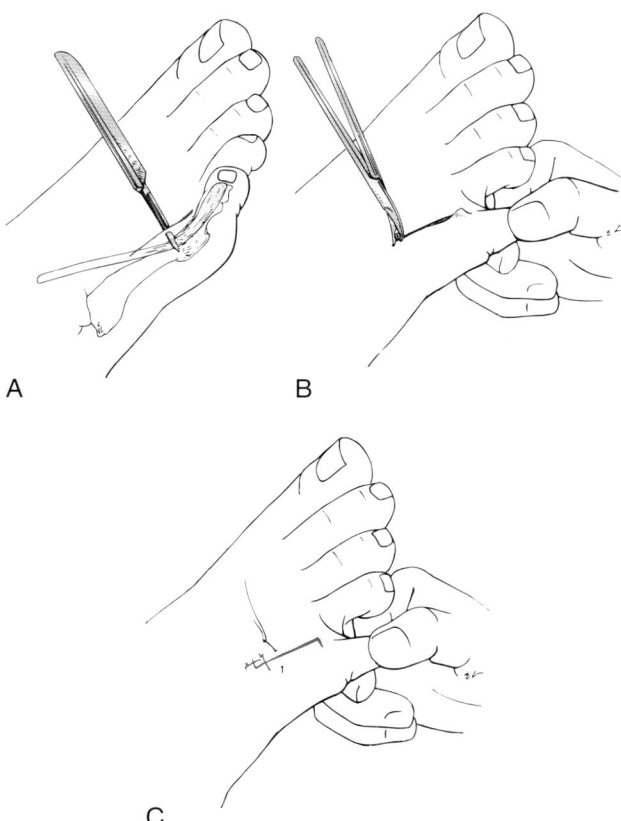

A   B

C

Figure 7-127 DuVries technique for repair of mild-to-moderate overlapping fifth toe. **A,** A longitudinal incision is made over the fourth web space. Tenotomy and capsulotomy of the fifth metatarsophalangeal joint are then performed. **B,** The fifth toe is plantar flexed to bring the fibular margin of the incision distal and the tibial margin proximal. This creates folds at each end of the incision, which are excised. **C,** The incision is sutured in the new position.

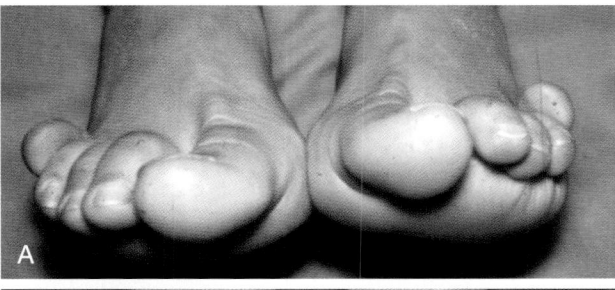
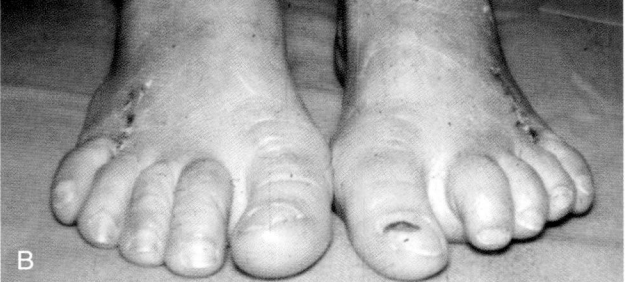

Figure 7-128 Preoperative **(A)** and postoperative **(B)** results after DuVries repair of overlapping fifth toes.

is held in an overcorrected position, and the skin is approximated with interrupted sutures (Fig. 7-129D).

Postoperative Care

A gauze-and-tape compression dressing is placed, holding the toe in an overcorrected position, and changed weekly. The patient is allowed to ambulate initially in a wooden-soled shoe and later in a sandal. Sutures are removed 3 weeks after surgery. The fifth toe is taped to the adjacent toe for 3 to 6 weeks. Results are shown in Figure 7-129G.

Results of DuVries and Wilson Procedures

In general, the results from these procedures have been satisfactory. It is important to carry out a complete soft tissue release at the time of the surgical repair. When a more severe contracture is present, recurrence is more likely, and a more aggressive surgical procedure, such as the Lapidus technique, should be considered.

LAPIDUS PROCEDURE[134] (Video Clip 73)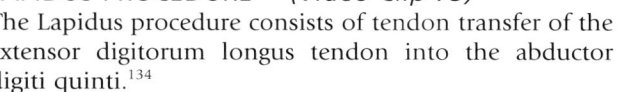

The Lapidus procedure consists of tendon transfer of the extensor digitorum longus tendon into the abductor digiti quinti.[134]

Surgical Technique

1. In general, a peripheral nerve block or regional anesthetic is used rather than a digital block. The foot is cleansed in a routine fashion. A thigh tourniquet is used with the patient placed in a lateral decubitus position.
2. A curvilinear dorsal incision extends from the medial aspect of the fifth toe over the MTP joint, then laterally over the fifth MTP joint capsule (Figs. 7-130A and 7-131A and B).
3. Another incision approximately 2 to 3 cm proximal to the MTP joint capsule is used to release the extensor digitorum longus tendon (see Figs. 7-130B and 7-131C and D).
4. With soft tissue dissection, the distal segment of the extensor tendon is preserved and is brought out through the distal wound. The dorsal, medial, and lateral MTP joint capsules are released through the distal exposure.
5. With a McGlamry elevator, any plantar adhesions between the plantar capsule and metatarsal head are released. This step is important because often there still is a hyperextension deformity of the MTP joint after the capsule is released. Adhesions on the plantar aspect may be the cause of this remaining deformity.
6. With blunt dissection, the soft tissue is spread around the medial, lateral, and plantar aspects of the proximal phalanx.
7. A suture is placed in the proximal end of the tendon stump, and the tendon is delivered circumferentially around the proximal phalanx from medial to plantar to lateral (see Fig. 7-130C). With the toe held in the corrected position, the tendon stump is sutured into the abductor digiti quinti muscle.

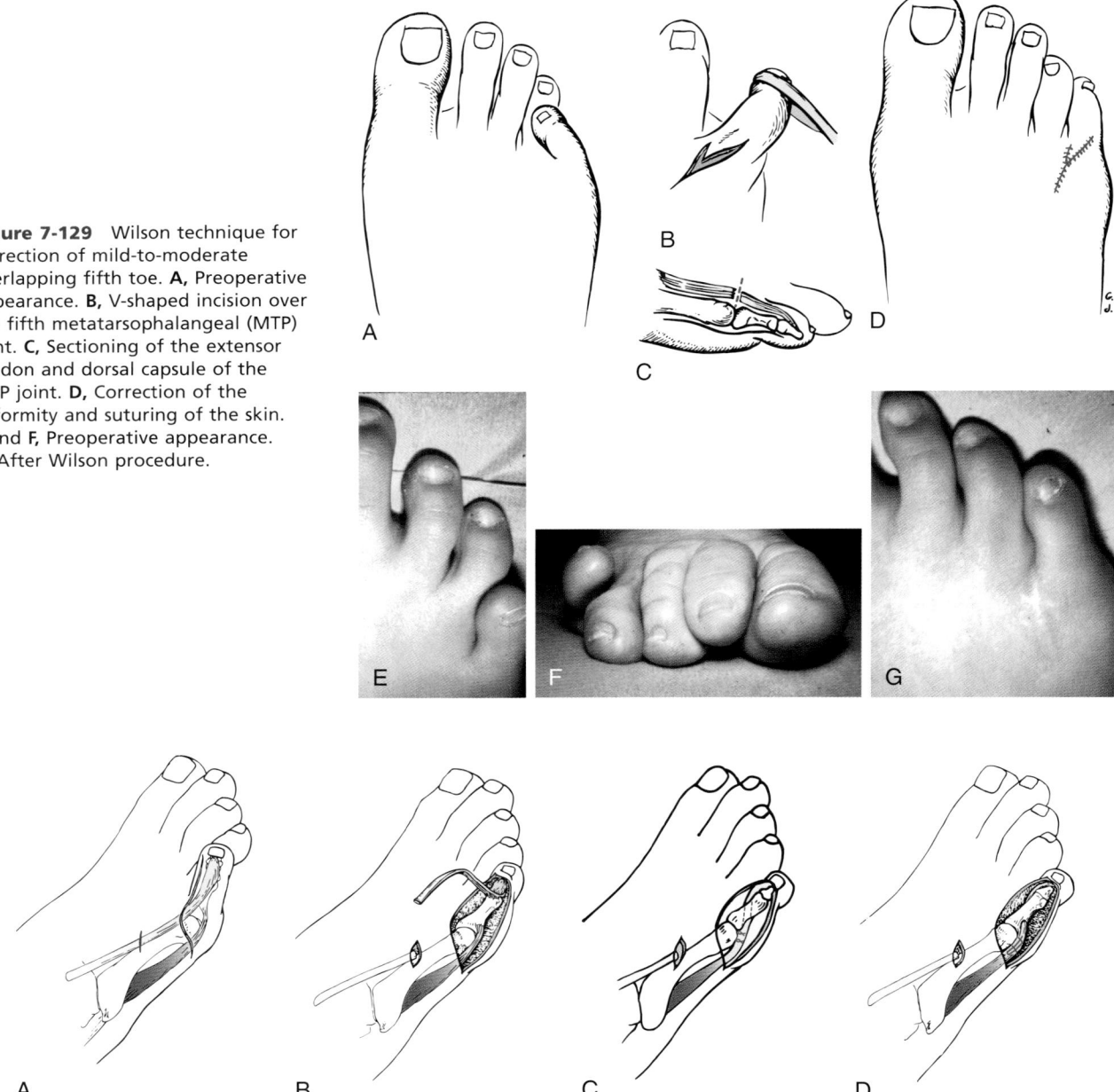

Figure 7-129 Wilson technique for correction of mild-to-moderate overlapping fifth toe. **A,** Preoperative appearance. **B,** V-shaped incision over the fifth metatarsophalangeal (MTP) joint. **C,** Sectioning of the extensor tendon and dorsal capsule of the MTP joint. **D,** Correction of the deformity and suturing of the skin. **E** and **F,** Preoperative appearance. **G,** After Wilson procedure.

Figure 7-130 Lapidus technique for correction of a severe overlapping fifth toe. **A,** Curvilinear incision is placed over the dorsum of the fifth toe metatarsophalangeal (MTP) joint and metatarsal head. A second incision is placed over the midportion of the extensor tendon to the fifth toe. **B,** The extensor tendon is brought out through the more distal wound. Dorsal, medial, and lateral MTP joint capsules are released. The plantar capsule might need to be freed up with a curved elevator if any adhesions between the metatarsal head and the plantar capsule are present. **C,** The extensor tendon is transferred around the proximal phalanx and sutured to the periosteum or soft tissue or muscle proximal to the metatarsal head. **D,** The transferred tendon may be placed through the drill hole, but more often it is transferred extraosseously. This helps to reduce the toe and to derotate it.

8. The toe is held in the corrected position, and the skin edges are approximated with interrupted sutures.

Postoperative Care
A gauze-and-tape compression dressing is applied, holding the toe in the corrected position, and is changed weekly. The patient is allowed to ambulate in a wooden-soled shoe. Sutures are removed 3 weeks after surgery. The toe is taped in the corrected position for 6 to 8 weeks after surgery (see Fig. 7-131F and G).

Results and Complications
In general, this procedure has been effective in correcting a severe overlapping fifth toe deformity. If there is any

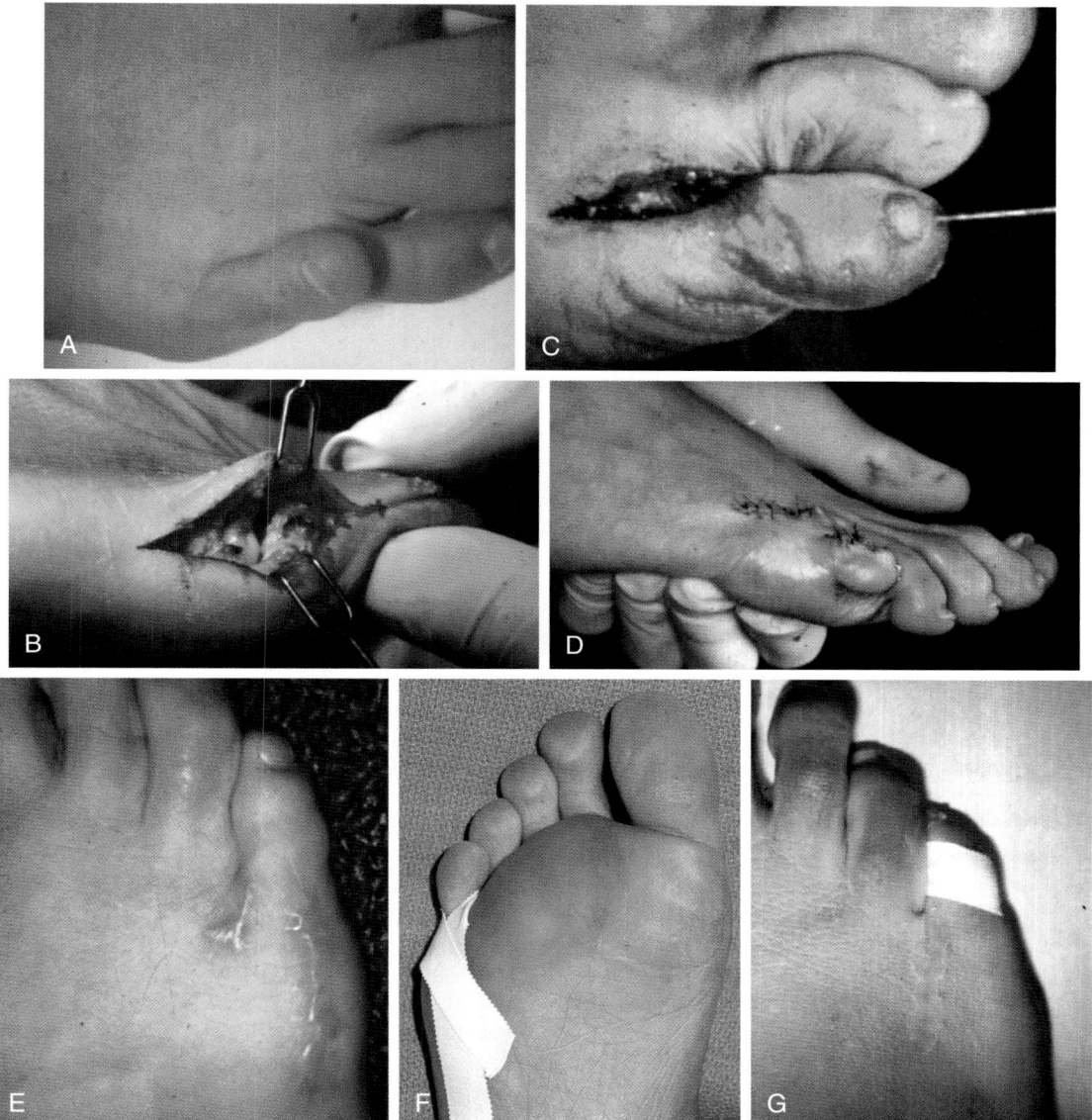

Figure 7-131 Modified Lapidus technique. **A,** Congenital overlapping fifth toe. **B,** Skin incisions are used to expose and release metatarsophalangeal joint. **C,** The extensor tendon is released through a proximal incision and brought distally into the main operative wound and transferred around the proximal phalanx, derotating and reducing the toe. Rarely a drill hole through proximal phalanx is used. **D,** At the conclusion of the procedure, the toe is adequately aligned. **E,** Postoperative alignment of the fifth toe. **F and G,** Postoperative taping is used to protect the repair. (**F,** From Coughlin MJ: Lesser toe abnormalities, *Instr Course Lect* 52:421–444, 2003.)

doubt as to whether a more extensive procedure should be performed, preservation of the extensor digitorum longus tendon gives the surgeon a means for further correction of an overlapping fifth toe deformity if soft tissue release is not sufficient to achieve adequate alignment.

Whereas DuVries[66] suggested that a drill hole be placed in the proximal phalanx to aid in the tendon transfer, Lapidus[134] suggested a soft rerouting of the tendon, and this appears to be less complicated and equally successful (see Fig. 7-130D). De Palma et al[59] have also reported a long-term follow-up on a soft tissue realignment with a

dynamic transfer of the extensor tendon in 13 patients (18 feet), with a high level of satisfactory results.

Lantzounis[132] described a soft tissue release and transfer of the extensor tendon into the fifth metatarsal neck. A soft tissue realignment was performed. Satisfactory results were reported. In general, this technique does not differ significantly from the DuVries procedure.

Cockin[28] described the Butler procedure. A dorsal racquet incision is made, and extensive soft tissue dissection is performed. A dorsal capsulotomy and extensor tenotomy are performed. Attention should be directed to the plantar capsule because often adhesions are present between the plantar metatarsal head and the plantar capsule. A curved elevator is used to release these contractures, and often the toe then can be reduced. The skin is approximated with interrupted sutures. Cockin[28] and later Black et al[9] have reported a high level of acceptable results with this procedure (greater than 91%). Although this procedure can achieve adequate realignment of the toe, the significant soft tissue dissection and required skin incisions can lead to prolonged postoperative edema. Black et al[9] reported two superficial wound infections that eventually led to unacceptable scar contractures with recurrence of the deformity.

Goodwin and Swisher,[90] Jahss,[110] Kelikian et al,[122] Leonard and Rising,[136] and Scrase[205] described a technique in which an MTP capsule release, extensor tenotomy, partial proximal phalangectomy, and syndactylization of the fourth and fifth toes were used to repair an overlapping fifth toe. Although adequate realignment may be achieved, the syndactylization procedure replaces one deformity with another. As a salvage procedure, a partial proximal phalangectomy and syndactylization may be considered.

UNDERLAPPING FIFTH TOE

In general, the deformities that occur with an underlapping fifth toe correspond to those in an overlapping fifth toe. Axial rotation, however, is associated with a redundant dorsal capsule and a contracted plantar MTP joint capsule. A redundant extensor digitorum longus is associated with a contracted flexor digitorum longus tendon. Thompson[217] has described an excisional arthroplasty to realign the underlapping fifth toe.

Surgical Treatment

THOMPSON REPAIR[217]
Surgical Technique
1. A peripheral anesthetic block or regional anesthesia is preferred to a digital block. The foot is cleansed in a routine fashion. The foot is exsanguinated with an Esmarch bandage. With careful padding, the Esmarch bandage may be used as a tourniquet above the level of the ankle (Fig. 7-132A).
2. A Z incision is centered over the proximal phalanx with the distal limb oriented laterally and the proximal Z incision oriented medially. The extensor tendon is divided, and the proximal phalanx identified (Fig. 7-132B).
3. The proximal phalanx is totally or partially excised, depending on the degree of deformity. The toe is then derotated and the capsule closed with interrupted sutures (Fig. 7-132C-E).
4. An intramedullary Kirschner wire may be used for stabilization of the toe as warranted. The Z incision is then rotated and closed with interrupted sutures (Fig. 7-132F).

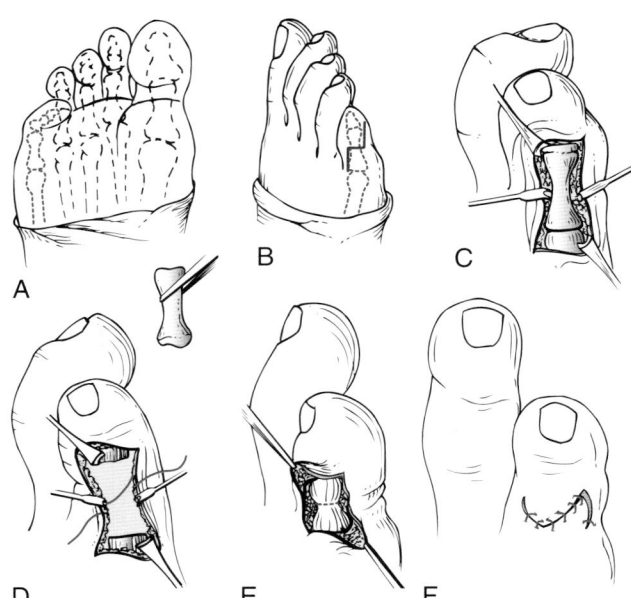

Figure 7-132 Thompson procedure. **A,** Plantar view of the preoperative deformity. **B,** Z-type incision is placed over the dorsal aspect of the proximal phalanx. **C,** The proximal phalanx is exposed. **D,** The proximal phalanx is resected in its entirety. **E,** The capsule is reefed with cerclage suture to diminish dead space. **F,** The Z-type incision is closed, with correction of deformity.

Postoperative Care
A gauze-and-tape dressing is applied and is changed weekly until drainage has subsided. The patient is allowed to ambulate in a wooden-soled shoe and later in a sandal. Sutures and the Kirschner wire are removed 3 weeks after surgery. The toe is taped to the fourth toe for approximately 6 weeks, until adequate healing has resulted.

Results and Complications
In general, results of this procedure are acceptable. Excessive resection can lead to an unstable toe or to a transfer keratotic lesion beneath the fourth metatarsal. Patients should be advised that with an excisional arthroplasty, the toe will have little if any dynamic function after the procedure. Janecki and Wilde[112] recommended a Ruiz-Mora procedure for severe cock-up deformity of the fifth toe. Although this procedure with a plantar incision has been designed for the exact opposite of the Thompson excisional arthroplasty, Janecki stressed that a subtotal phalangectomy may be advantageous in retaining fifth toe stability. The extent of resection of the proximal phalanx depends on the degree of fifth toe deformity. A flail toe might require syndactylization as a salvage procedure.

COCK-UP FIFTH TOE DEFORMITY

Often, a cock-up deformity of the MTP joint is associated with a fixed hammer toe deformity. With mild-to-moderate deformity, an extensor tenotomy or lengthening, MTP joint release, and fixed hammer toe repair may be considered. With a severe cock-up deformity, resection arthroplasty may be considered. Treatment must be directed toward bringing the toe into adequate alignment at both the MTP joint and the interphalangeal joint. The Ruiz-Mora procedure[194] as modified by Janecki and Wilde[112] is the preferred procedure.

Surgical Treatment

RUIZ-MORA PROCEDURE[67,112,194]
Surgical Technique
1. A peripheral block or regional anesthetic block is used in preference to a digital block. The foot is cleansed in a routine fashion. The foot is exsanguinated with an Esmarch bandage. The Esmarch bandage may be used as a tourniquet above the level of the ankle (Fig. 7-133A).
2. An elliptic incision is placed on the plantar aspect of the small toe and oriented along the longitudinal axis of the proximal phalanx, deviating slightly medially at the base of the toe (Fig. 7-133B).
3. An ellipse of skin is resected, after which the flexor tendon is incised. The proximal phalanx is resected (Fig. 7-134C). Janecki has recommended a subtotal resection of the proximal phalanx.
4. The skin incision is then closed at right angles to the long axis of the toe to enable the toe to be corrected

in a plantar-medial manner (see Figs. 7-133D and E and 7-134).

Postoperative Care
A gauze-and-tape compression dressing is applied and is changed weekly. The patient is allowed to ambulate in a wooden-soled postoperative shoe and later in a sandal. Sutures are removed 3 weeks after surgery.

Results and Complications
In general, acceptable results have been reported with this procedure. Janecki and Wilde,[112] however, reported a 23% incidence of bunionette formation postoperatively. They also noted a 32% incidence of a hammer toe formation in the fourth toe. These authors thus recommended a subtotal resection of the proximal phalanx to avoid floppiness of the fifth toe. If floppiness of the fifth toe results, a syndactylization procedure may be necessary.

Dyal et al[67] reported on 12 patients who underwent a Ruiz-Mora procedure for severe contraction of the fifth toe. They found average shortening of the fifth ray of 12.8 mm but observed that this presented no functional problems and found it to be an effective procedure in dealing with a cock-up deformity of the fifth toe. Nine of the patients were satisfied with the procedure. They noted that only one fourth-toe corn developed. No bunionettes were noted at long-term follow-up. A few patients were dissatisfied with severe shortening and the cosmetic result of the procedure. The authors concluded that the procedure was best reserved for iatrogenic cock-up fifth toe deformities, hard corns, and complicated cock-up fifth toe deformities (Fig. 7-135).

SYNDACTYLIZATION OF THE LESSER TOES
Surgical Technique
1. A foot block or regional anesthesia, rather than a digital block, often is used. The foot is cleansed in a

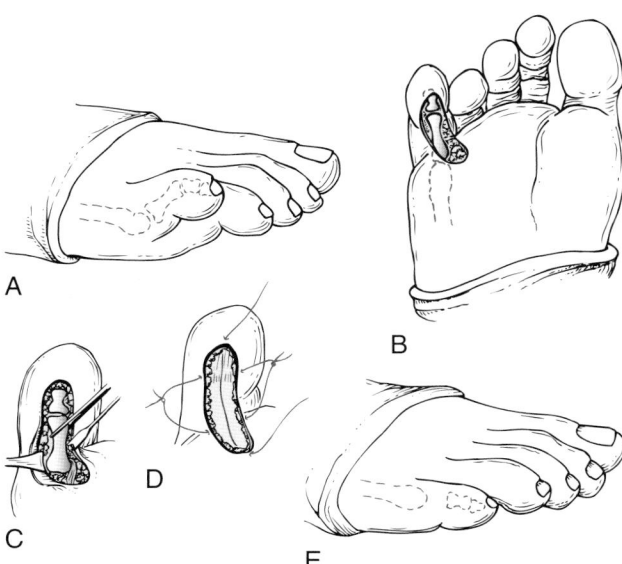

Figure 7-133 Technique for Ruiz-Mora procedure. **A,** Preoperative deformity. **B,** Radiograph of preoperative deformity. **C,** The proximal phalanx is removed through an elliptic plantar incision. **D** and **E,** Sutures are placed to reduce the skin defect, and the incision is closed so that the fifth toe is brought down into plantar flexion and slight medial deviation.

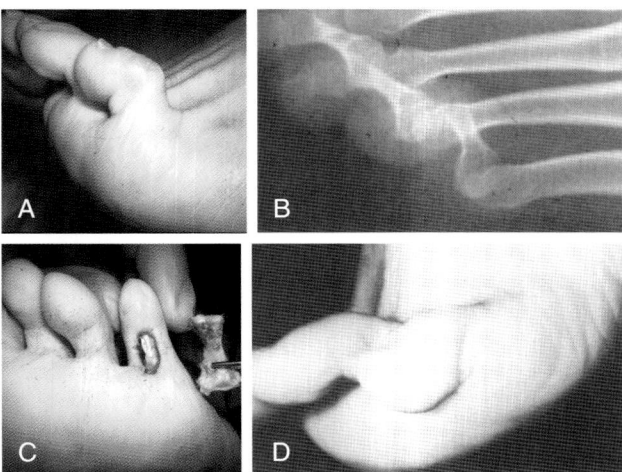

Figure 7-134 **A** and **B,** Preoperative deformity. **C,** After resection of proximal phalanx. **D,** Postoperative result.

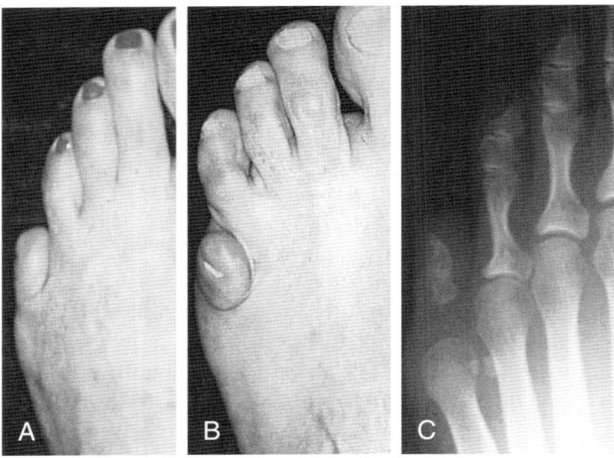

Figure 7-135 **A,** Acceptable cosmetic appearance after Ruiz-Mora procedure. **B,** Dorsal view of the foot with excessive shortening of the fifth toe. **C,** Anteroposterior radiograph after procedure. (From Dyal C, Davis W, Thompson F, Elonar SK: Clinical evaluation of the Ruiz-Mora procedure: long-term follow-up, *Foot Ankle Int* 18:94–97, 1997. Copyright 1997 by the American Orthopaedic Foot and Ankle Society [AOFAS]. Used with permission.)

routine fashion. An Esmarch bandage is used to exsanguinate the foot. The Esmarch may be used as a tourniquet as well.

2. The toes are distracted as a web-bisecting incision is made (Fig. 7-136A). The web-bisecting incision is flanked by a pair of peridigital incisions.

3. Plantar and dorsal flaps are developed, and small triangles of skin are resected (Fig. 7-136B).

4. If adjacent partial proximal phalangectomies are to be performed, the bone decompression is carried out through this incision, with care to protect the neurovascular bundles (Fig. 7-136C and D).

5. The adjacent dorsal and plantar flaps are apposed and closed with running and interrupted sutures (Fig. 7-136E).

Postoperative Care

A gauze-and-tape dressing is applied and is changed weekly. The patient is allowed to ambulate in a wooden-soled postoperative shoe. Sutures are removed 3 weeks after surgery. The adjacent toes are taped together for approximately 6 weeks to protect the surgical syndactylization.

Alternative Procedure

Thompson[217] suggested the use of a Z-plasty for a skin contracture associated with a fifth toe deformity. Myerson et al[164] have advocated this technique in treating an extension contracture of a lesser toe deformity in which mainly the skin is the contributing factor (see Fig. 7-56D and E). Thordarson[220] has recommended an MTP joint capsule release, extensor tendon lengthening, and Z-plasty of the overlying skin to correct the contracture.

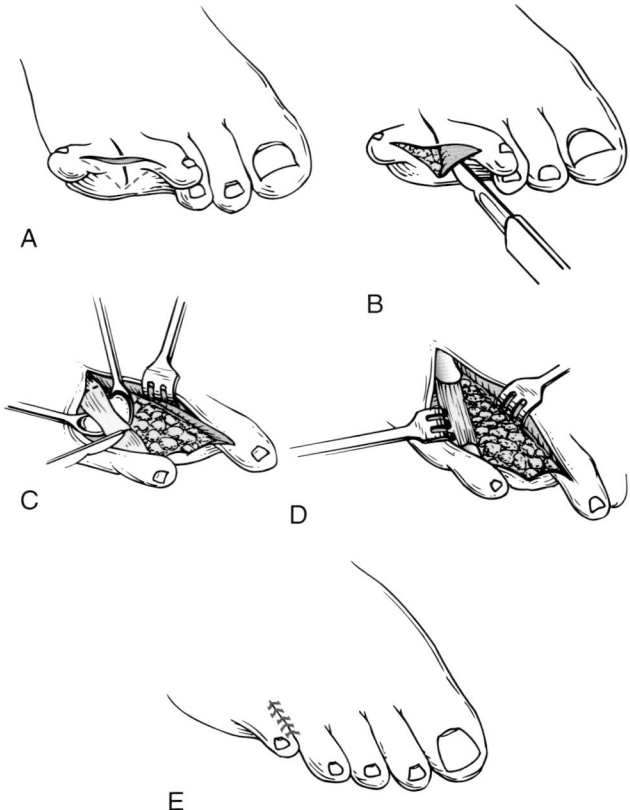

Figure 7-136 Syndactylization of fourth and fifth toes. **A,** Lines of incision for syndactylization. **B,** Skin is removed from two inferior triangles. **C,** Collateral ligaments of the proximal phalanx are incised. **D,** The proximal phalanx is resected. **E,** Skin is webbed inferiorly and superiorly.

Results and Complications

Kelikian et al[22] and others[55,146] have reported generally satisfactory results with this procedure. Although they found this to be a simple and efficient procedure, syndactylization may be cosmetically unacceptable to some patients. Correcting a deformity by creating a second deformity might not be acceptable to the patient. Daly and Johnson[55] described a relatively cosmetic syndactylization in which concomitant adjacent partial proximal phalangectomies were performed. They reported an overall 80% subjective satisfaction in 52 patients who had undergone syndactylization procedures.

Syndactylization does not always stabilize the toes. After syndactylization, a deformity can develop in an adjacent toe (see Fig. 7-120).

Surgical realignment of abnormalities of the fifth toe can be difficult. Adequate alignment must be achieved at the time of surgery. If a soft tissue release is not sufficient, either tendon transfer or bone resection must be considered. Correction of severe deformities may be complicated by skin contractures or excessive tension on the neurovascular bundles. In this situation, bone decompression of the fifth toe may be necessary to achieve acceptable alignment.

Jahss[109] reported on 10 cases of chronic and recurrent dislocation of the fifth toe with instability of the PIP or MTP joint. Recurrent dislocation developed as a result of excessive medial joint laxity and was accentuated on weight bearing. He found the simplest and most satisfactory surgical correction involved resection arthroplasty and syndactylization of the fourth and fifth toes. Marek et al[145] also advocated syndactylization as an effective and cosmetic salvage for an unstable fifth toe. Amputation of the fifth toe rarely solves a problem associated with the fifth toe on a long-term basis and can lead to a bunionette deformity or subsequent deformity of the fourth toe (Fig. 7-137).

KERATOTIC DEFORMITIES OF LESSER TOES

Etiology

A lateral fifth toe corn (Fig. 7-138) forms primarily on the exposed surfaces of the fifth toe[13] as a result of extrinsic pressure from footwear.[39,43] An interdigital corn forms over a condyle of the phalanx between the toes (Fig. 7-139).[146] It can form deep in the web space, where differentiation from a mycotic infection may be difficult, or

along the distal surface of one of the lesser toes, in which case, a firm keratosis is most common. A soft corn can become extremely painful as a result of the pressure between adjoining bony prominences.[86]

Various terms have been used to describe a lateral fifth toe corn, including *hard corn*, *heloma durum*, and *clavus durum* (Fig. 7-140). Terms used to describe a soft corn include *web space corn*, *heloma molle*, *clavus mollum*, *tyloma molle*, and *interdigital clavus*. Although it is common to refer to an interdigital corn as soft, in reality, it is often anything but soft. A *kissing corn* refers to the apposition of two prominent surfaces that have developed callosities; however, on occasion, it can develop next to an adjacent toenail rather than a bony prominence. Thus the use of Greek or Latin terminology is discouraged. Likewise, using terms that characterize the consistency and texture of the lesion is discouraged because the lesions are identical histologically. It is preferable to use the location of the callosity to describe the corn, and thus the terms *lateral fifth toe corn* and *interdigital corn* are preferred.

A corn is an accumulation of keratotic layers of epidermis over a bony prominence. The bones of the foot have numerous projections over the condyles of the heads and the bases of the metatarsals and phalanges. The shoe

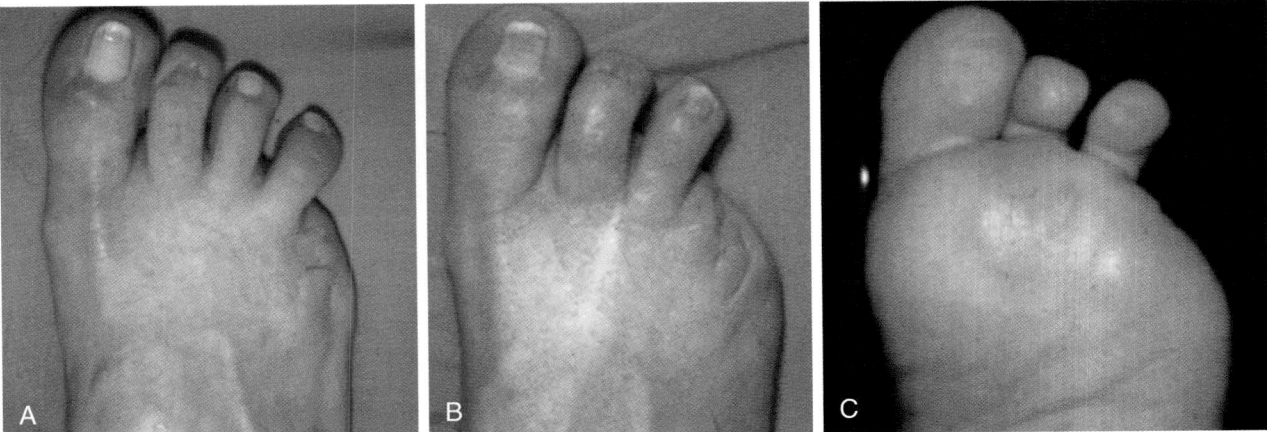

Figure 7-137 **A,** A 77-year-old woman who had an amputation of the fifth toe for a painful fifth toe hard corn. **B** and **C,** Five years later, her family physician had removed her fourth toe because of the development of a painful corn over the lateral aspect of the fourth toe.

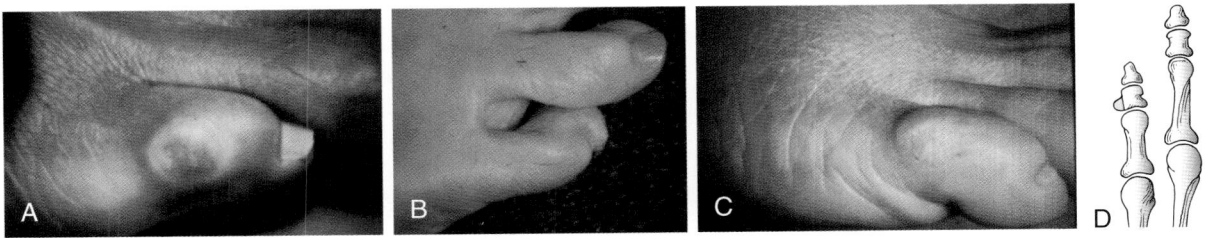

Figure 7-138 **A,** Lateral fifth toe corn over prominent condyles of the proximal phalanx. **B,** Rotation of the fifth toe can lead to a lateral fifth toe corn. **C,** Contracture of the fifth toe can lead to callus formation. **D,** Prominent condyle of either proximal or middle phalanges.

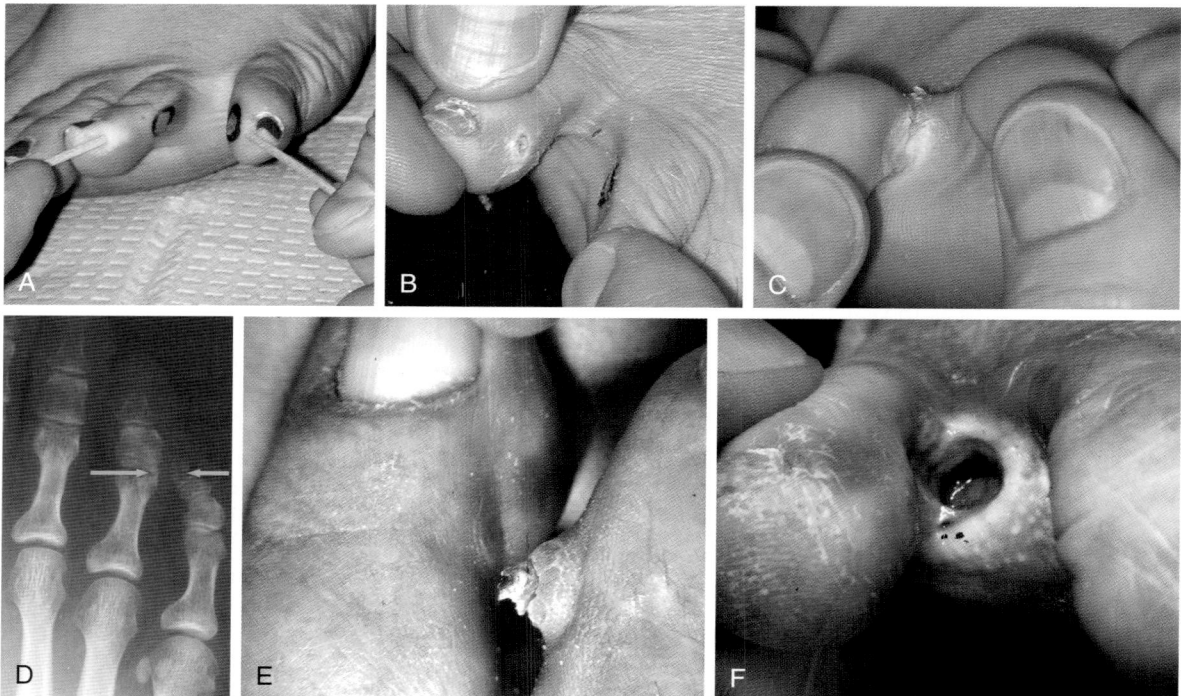

Figure 7-139 **A** and **B,** A distal interspace corn. **C,** Often a soft corn is confused with mycotic infection. **D,** Radiograph demonstrating impingement between the fourth and fifth toes. **E,** Keratotic buildup in first web space. **F,** Sinus tract in the fifth web space.

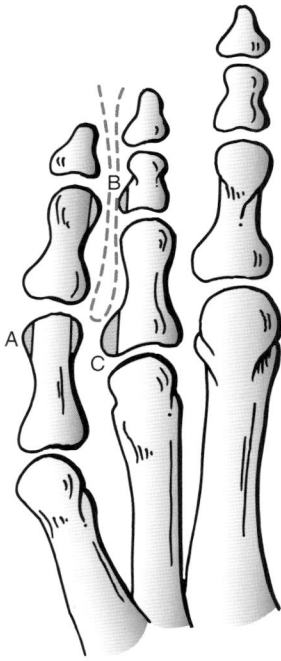

Figure 7-140 Nomenclature for corns. *A,* lateral fifth toe corn; *B,* interdigital corn; *C,* web space corn. (From Coughlin M, Kennedy M: Operative repair of fourth and fifth toe corns, *Foot Ankle Int* 24:147–157, 2003. Copyright 2003 by the American Orthopaedic Foot and Ankle Society [AOFAS]. Used with permission.)

exerts an extrinsic pressure on these prominent condylar processes, and the soft tissues over these prominences bear the brunt of the pressure and friction that the shoe exerts on the foot. Nature attempts to protect the irritated soft tissue by accumulations of thickened epithelium, but this accumulation also elevates the prominence so that the extrinsic pressure of the shoe exerts further pressure on the underlying soft tissues. With increased pressure, the skin sometimes breaks down rather than forming callus. This typically happens if pressure is applied rapidly rather than over a long period of time. In a patient with an insensate foot who is not aware of this increased pressure, often an ulceration, rather than keratotic changes, develops over a bony prominence because of the severity of pressure against the bony prominences as well. Occasionally, when a callosity becomes too thick, a cleavage plane develops between the callus and the normal skin and can become secondarily infected.

Although many authors[66,239] have suggested that an underlying exostosis is a cause of corn formation, Kelikian[122] reported that, in a review of 5000 radiographs, he rarely found evidence of osseous changes. Coughlin et al[46] observed the presence of an exostosis in only 3 of 62 cases. An enlarged condyle was not seen in any case.

Preoperative Evaluation

Physical Examination

A hard corn typically is found on the fibular aspect of the fifth toe. An obvious buildup of keratotic skin may be

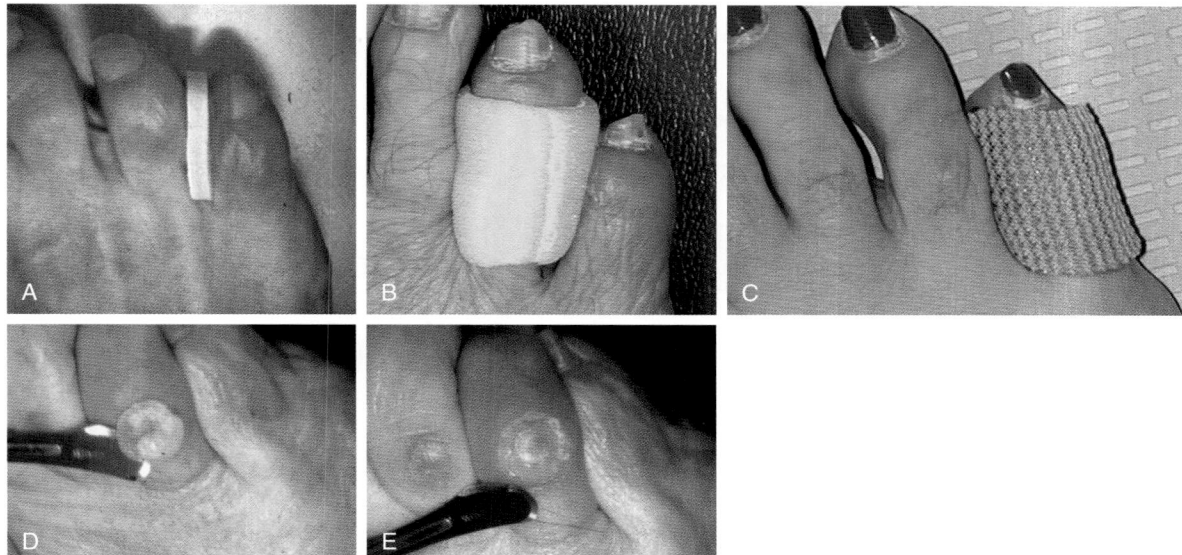

Figure 7-141 Conservative measures. Padding can alleviate symptoms of an interdigital corn **(A** and **B)** or a lateral **(C)** fifth toe corn. A corn or callus **(D)** may be trimmed **(E),** which can alleviate a significant amount of pain. **(C,** From Coughlin MJ: Lesser toe abnormalities, *Instr Course Lect* 52:421–444, 2003.)

noted.[105] The corn usually is uncomfortable but not exquisitely tender to touch. Corns are common in this region because the fifth toe receives maximal pressure from the curvature of the outer border of the toe box of standard shoes. Ordinarily, the head of the proximal phalanx of the fifth toe is the most prominent surface at this point, which is why a hard corn nearly always is located over the fibular condyle of the head of the proximal phalanx.

A corn or callus can form over the dorsal aspect of the PIP joint or DIP joint, and in this situation, it is almost indistinguishable from a hammer toe or mallet toe deformity. With a significant hammer toe or mallet toe deformity, a keratotic lesion can develop on the tip of the involved toe because of pressure exerted with ambulation. Correction of the hammer toe or mallet toe deformity often is adequate treatment for the keratotic lesion.

Although a soft corn is essentially the same as a hard corn, its location between two of the lesser toes can result in maceration of the tissue; hence the term *soft corn.* On examination, a soft corn often manifests as a medial lesion overlying the condyle of the proximal phalanx of the fifth toe, abutting a lesion on the lateral base of the proximal phalanx of the fourth toe. When found distally on the toes, this typically is a firm keratotic lesion (see Fig. 7-139A); however, when found in a web space, the degree of maceration can make it difficult to differentiate from an ulceration of the skin or a mycotic infection (see Fig. 7-139C). Occasionally, a sinus tract results, with secondary infection.

Radiographic Evaluation
Markers may be placed on the skin to identify the bony prominence associated with the keratotic lesion.

Radiographs also are helpful in the case of an ulcerated lesion, to identify areas of possible osteomyelitis (see Fig. 7-139D).

Treatment

Conservative Treatment
Palliative measures, such as reduction of the keratotic accumulation, changing the patient's footwear to broad-toed, soft-soled shoes with a larger toe box, and padding of the symptomatic area (Fig. 7-141A-C) to relieve pressure, often give relief.[86] Many patients can be taught to care for the callus themselves by shaving the area or using a pumice stone after bathing (Fig. 7-141D and E).[20]

Surgical Treatment
TREATMENT OF LATERAL FIFTH TOE CORNS
The algorithm (Fig. 7-142) for treatment of a lateral fifth toe corn is helpful in defining a successful course. For a flexible deformity, a simple flexor tenotomy (Fig. 7-143) can allow reduction of the deformity and alleviation of discomfort. The following procedure may be used for a condylectomy of the proximal phalanx[20] beneath a corn on the fibular aspect of the fifth toe. This lesion usually involves the head of the proximal phalanx, but it can involve the lateral condyle of the middle phalanx as well.

Surgical Technique
1. The patient is placed is a slight lateral decubitus position. A digital block is applied, and the foot is cleansed in the usual fashion. Typically, a tourniquet is not used.
2. A longitudinal skin incision is centered on the dorsal aspect of the fifth toe just dorsal to the hard corn

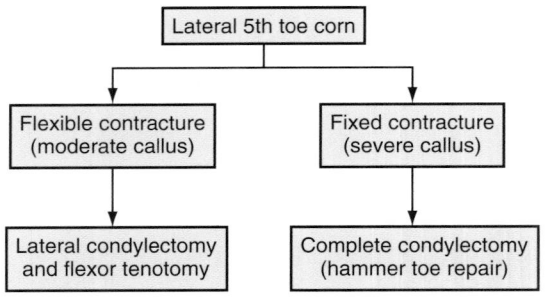

Figure 7-142 Algorithm for treatment of a lateral fifth toe corn. (Modified from Coughlin M, Kennedy M: Operative repair of fourth and fifth toe corns, *Foot Ankle Int* 24: 147–157, 2003. Copyright 2003 by the American Orthopaedic Foot and Ankle Society [AOFAS]. Used with permission.)

Flowchart:
- Lateral 5th toe corn
  - Flexible contracture (moderate callus) → Lateral condylectomy and flexor tenotomy
  - Fixed contracture (severe callus) → Complete condylectomy (hammer toe repair)

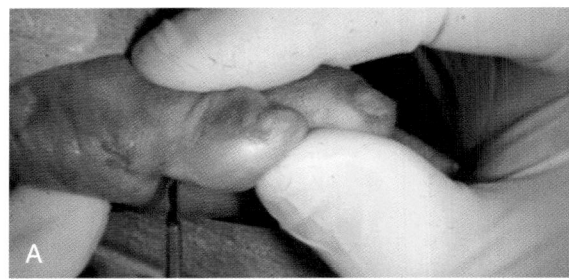
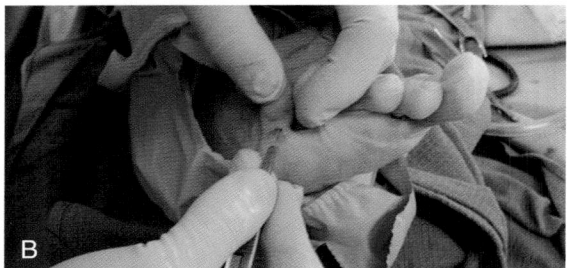

Figure 7-143 **A,** A flexor tenotomy can decrease a flexion deformity and diminish pain and callus formation for a lateral fifth toe corn. **B,** With the scalpel blade in place, hyperextension of the fifth toe simplifies the tenotomy.

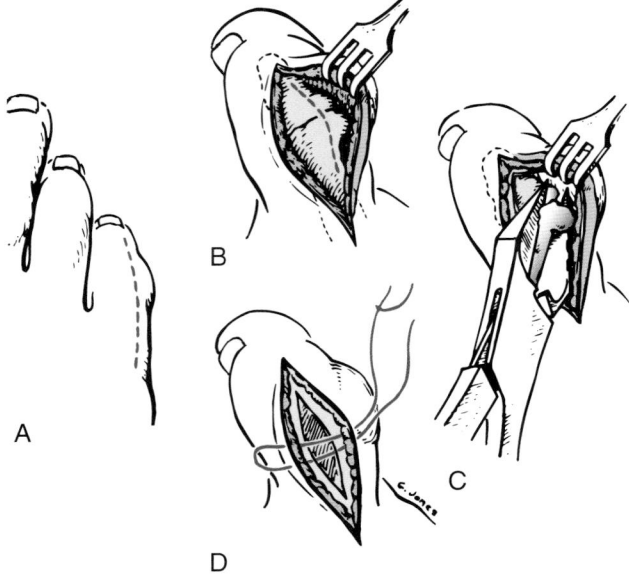

Figure 7-144 DuVries technique for condylectomy for fifth toe exostosis. **A,** Longitudinal incision over the dorsolateral aspect of the fifth toe. **B,** Skin and capsule are retracted. **C,** Fibular condyles of phalanges are excised. **D,** Skin and capsule are approximated.

6. The remaining edges are smoothed with a rongeur.
7. Interrupted capsule closure is performed to stabilize the repair (see Figs. 7-144D and 7-145D).
8. The skin is closed with interrupted nylon sutures (see Fig. 7-145E and F).

Postoperative Care
A bulky dressing is applied and changed weekly until drainage has subsided. The patient is allowed to ambulate in a wooden-soled shoe until dressings are discontinued. Sutures are removed 3 weeks after surgery. The toe is then taped to the fourth toe for approximately 6 weeks to increase stability of the soft tissues.

TREATMENT OF INTERDIGITAL CORNS
For treatment of an extremely macerated soft corn, placement of lamb's wool, soft gauze, or a pad (see Fig. 7-139C) between the toes often allows desiccation of the area so that the tissues can heal. The use of a desiccating agent, such as carbolfuchsin (Carfusin) (which is both an antifungal agent and an astringent) or rubbing alcohol, often helps the tissue to heal more rapidly. Once the tissue has healed, surgical intervention may be considered. An algorithm (Fig. 7-146) is helpful in developing a treatment plan. The treatment consists of excising the condyles of the proximal phalanx in combination with excising a corresponding condyle of the middle phalanx. Whether a single or dual excision of corresponding lesions is performed is the surgeon's preference.[20] Usually, the magnitude of the deformity helps to elucidate whether a single or double excision is necessary. A soft corn can occur

 (Figs. 7-144A and 7-145A and Video Clips 78 and 79). The incision extends from the midportion of the middle phalanx to the base of the proximal phalanx. (The corn itself is not excised, because this can lead to further friction postoperatively. The callus tends to be somewhat avascular, which can delay healing.)

3. The incision is deepened to the bone through the subcutaneous tissue and extensor tendon (Fig. 7-145B).
4. The capsule and collateral ligaments are shaved off the prominent condyle superiorly to inferiorly (see Fig. 7-144B).
5. The prominent condyle is excised with a rongeur, leaving the remainder of the joint intact (see Figs. 7-144C and 7-145C). (If both the distal portion of the proximal phalanx and the proximal portion of the middle phalanx are involved, the prominence on the middle phalanx should be excised as well.)

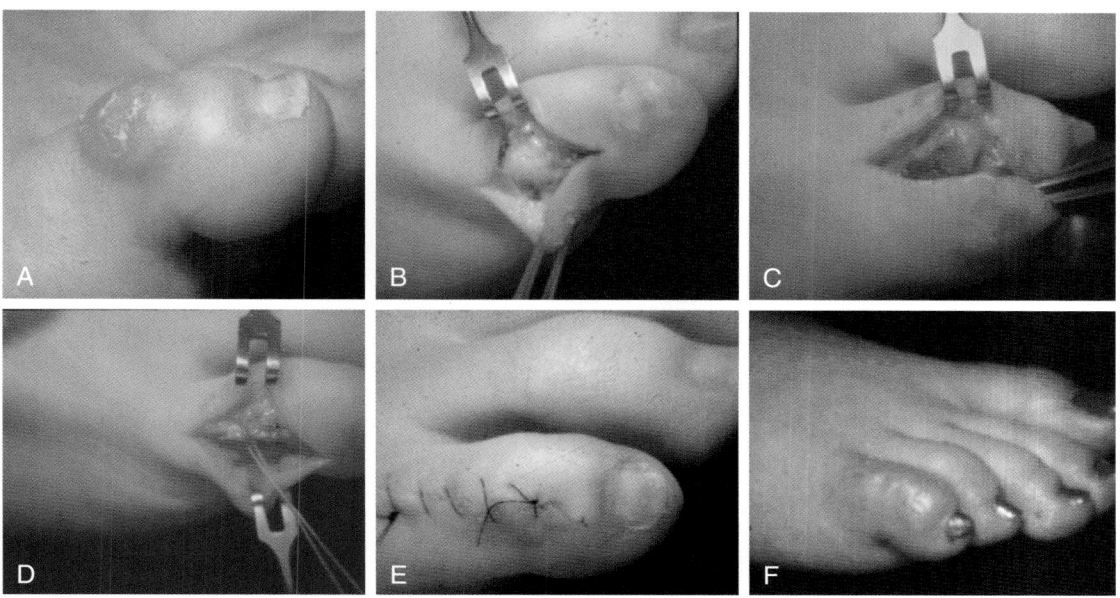

Figure 7-145 **A,** Lateral fifth toe corn. **B,** Dorsal exposure is used for resection of prominent condyle. **C,** Resection of the lateral condyle. **D,** Tight capsular closure tends to decrease the chance of later subluxation. **E,** After skin closure. **F,** Swelling diminished with time. (**A, C,** and **D,** From Coughlin MJ: Common causes of pain in the forefoot in adults, *J Bone Joint Surg Br* 82:781–790, 2000.)

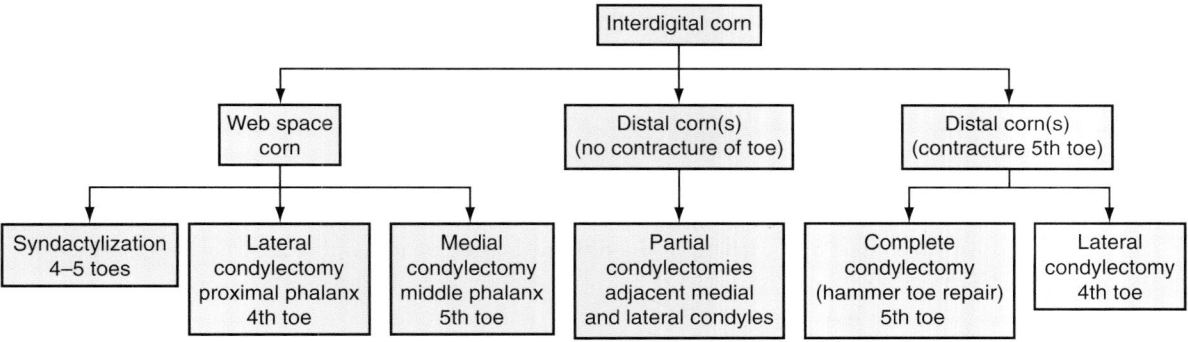

Figure 7-146 Algorithm for treatment of interdigital corn. (From Coughlin M, Kennedy M: Operative repair of fourth and fifth toe corns, *Foot Ankle Int* 24:147–157, 2003. Copyright 2003 by the American Orthopaedic Foot and Ankle Society [AOFAS]. Used with permission.)

between any of the lesser toes over any bony prominence. Although soft corns tend to be common on the medial aspect of the fifth toe, they can occur in any web space.

Surgical Technique

1. After placing a digital block, the foot is cleansed in the usual fashion. Typically, a tourniquet is not used. The patient is placed in a slightly lateral decubitus position.
2. A small incision is centered dorsally over the keratotic lesion (Fig. 7-147A and Video Clip 80).
3. The incision is deepened to the capsule overlying the prominent exostosis. The capsule is stripped off the exostosis.

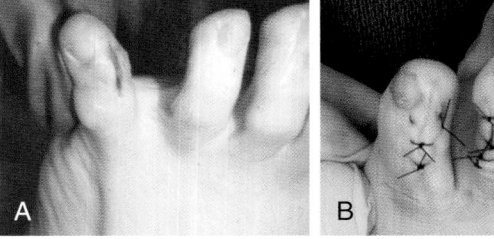

Figure 7-147 **A,** Shaving of single condyle. **B,** Shaving of adjacent condyles.

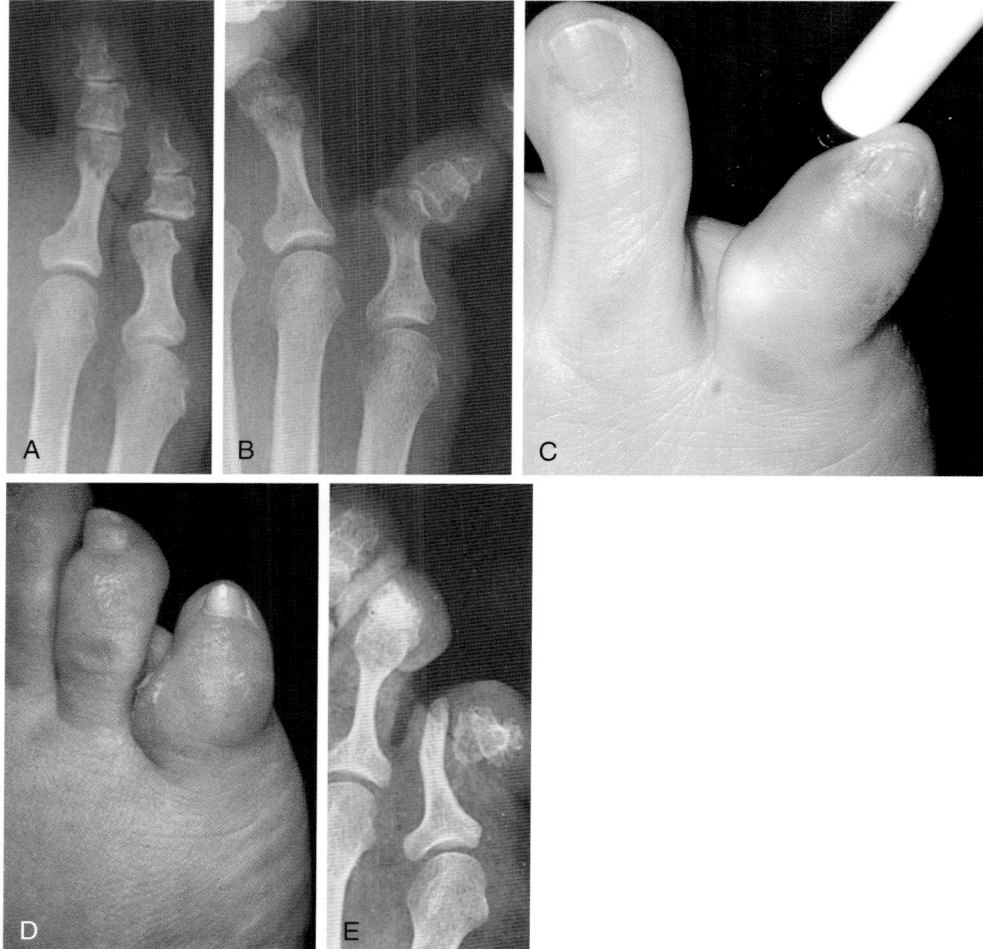

Figure 7-148 Instability of the fifth toe. **A,** Weight-bearing radiograph. **B,** With lateral stress to the fifth toe. **C,** Lateral stress applied to subluxate the toe. **D,** Fracture dislocation of the lesser toe can lead to development of a soft corn. **E,** A flail fifth toe can result from excessive bone resection. Instability of the fifth toe may be treated with a proximal interphalangeal arthroplasty with Kirschner wire fixation.

4. A rongeur is used to resect the exostosis, and roughened areas are smoothed.
5. A small concavity is produced in the area of the lesion. If possible, the interphalangeal joint capsule is repaired with interrupted sutures.
6. The skin is approximated with interrupted sutures.
7. If a simultaneous incision is made on a corresponding lesion, the exostosis is resected in a similar fashion (Fig. 7-147B).

Postoperative Care

A gauze-and-tape compression dressing is applied and changed weekly. The patient is allowed to ambulate in a postoperative shoe. Sutures are removed 3 weeks after surgery. Often padding is placed between the involved toes for 3 to 6 weeks after surgery. At approximately 4 to 6 weeks after surgery, the keratotic lesion can be gently lifted from its bed, and usually normal-appearing skin is noted beneath it.

Results and Complications

Patients generally do well after a simple condylectomy. In approximately 2% of patients, the keratotic lesion tends to persist despite relief of the bony prominence beneath it. In these cases, frequent trimming usually results in eventual reduction of the keratotic lesion to a minimally symptomatic state. Where a lateral fifth toe corn has recurred after a condylectomy, a flexor tenotomy may be used to reduce a fifth toe contracture and can alleviate symptoms. For significant recurrence or a more severe hard corn deformity, a complete condylectomy is the treatment of choice (see the section on repair of hammered fifth toe). This procedure is performed identically to a fixed hammer toe repair.

Postoperatively, it is imperative to keep the fifth toe taped to the fourth toe for 6 weeks to prevent it from becoming floppy or hanging up in stockings. An excision of a significant portion of the middle phalanx should be avoided because a floppy toe can result (see Fig. 7-122)

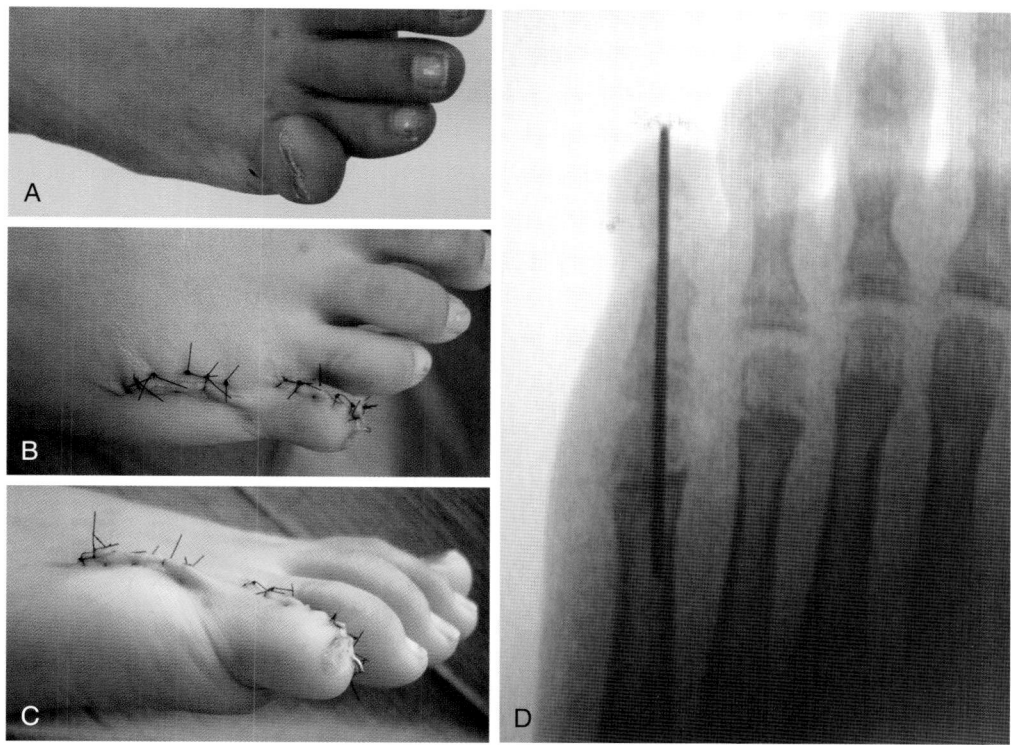

Figure 7-149 Supernumerary digit causing callus formation. **A,** Preoperative clinical appearance with accessory digit. **B** and **C,** Postoperative clinical appearance after resection of accessory digit, and condylectomy of fifth metatarsal head. **D,** Postoperative radiograph with Kirschner wire temporary fixation.

and can become dislocated over time. With instability of the fifth toe, syndactylization of the fourth and fifth toes usually alleviates symptoms (Fig. 7-148).[109]

In the only comprehensive report of surgical repair of lateral fifth toe corns and interdigital corns, Coughlin et al[46] reported on the results of treatment of 31 lateral fifth toe corns over a 20-year period and 31 interdigital corns. Indications for surgery were intractable pain that was refractory to shaving or to shoe modifications. For lateral fifth toe corns, a lateral condylectomy was performed in 20 feet, and a total condylectomy was performed in 11. For interdigital corns, a single or dual condylectomy was performed in 13, a complete condylectomy in 14, and a combination condylectomy and hammer toe repair in adjacent digits in 4 other feet for combined lateral and interdigital corns.

At an average follow-up of 92 months, overall satisfaction was excellent in 85%, good in 11%, and fair or poor in 4%. Pain was relieved in 47 of 51 patients (92%), and the average AOFAS score was 92 points. Two patients had significant callus reformation, but no chronic swelling was noted in any case. Toe stiffness was a common postoperative occurrence but was not associated with patient dissatisfaction. Subjective alignment was acceptable in 54 of 62 feet. Twenty-six of 62 feet had a hallux valgus deformity, and 25 of 62 had a bunionette deformity.

This series supports the theory that a wide foot is predisposed to develop a corn. All patients were women, and 73% associated the corn formation with constricting footwear. A lateral condylectomy was recommended for mild deformities, and a complete condylectomy was recommended for more severe deformities characterized by fixed contractures and for combined interdigital and lateral fifth toe corns on the same digit. In the interdigital-corn subgroup, a dual condylectomy was recommended for moderate deformities; when the corn was associated with a contracted fifth toe, a fifth toe complete condylectomy was preferred. In general, satisfactory results follow an interdigital corn excision. On occasion, a supernumeray digit may present with pressure and callus formation, requiring resection (Fig. 7-149).

Zeringue and Harkless[239] retrospectively evaluated 30 patients treated for a web space corn between the fourth and fifth toes. Some 94% of the affected feet were noted to have rotation of the fifth toe. They were treated with a PIP joint arthroplasty of the fifth toe, combined with a lateral-based condylectomy of the proximal phalanx of the fourth toe. A high level of satisfaction was found at an average of 33 months follow-up.

Postoperative stiffness or fibrosis of the involved interphalangeal joints is experienced by some patients. Passive manipulation can help to alleviate such stiffness. The patient should be alerted that an interphalangeal joint arthroplasty can leave residual stiffness. Recurrence of deformity, however, is the most common complaint. Where a recurrent lesion develops, a more extensive resection should be considered. A complete condylectomy (see the discussion of hammer toe repair) may be necessary in the case of recurrence or in the presence of a severe deformity.[20,46] With a soft corn, a web space incision should be avoided because it can lead to delayed healing, infection, or continued maceration.[21,46]

REFERENCES

1. Alvine FG, Garvin KL: Peg and dowel fusion of the proximal interphalangeal joint, *Foot Ankle* 1:90–94, 1980.
2. Angirasa AK, Augoyard M, Coughlin MJ, et al: Hammer toe, mallet toe, and claw toe, *Foot Ankle Spec* 4:182–187, 2011.
3. Barbari SG, Brevig K: Correction of clawtoes by the Girdlestone-Taylor flexor-extensor transfer procedure, *Foot Ankle* 5:67–73, 1984.
4. Barca F, Acciaro AL: Surgical correction of crossover deformity of the second toe: a technique for tenodesis, *Foot Ankle Int* 25:620–624, 2004.
5. Barnicot NA, Hardy RH: The position of the hallux in West Africans, *J Anat* 89:355–361, 1955.
6. Barouk LS: [Weil's metatarsal osteotomy in the treatment of metatarsalgia], *Orthopade* 25:337–344, 1996.
7. Beech I, Rees S, Tagoe M: A retrospective review of the weil metatarsal osteotomy for lesser metatarsal deformities: an intermediate follow-up analysis, *J Foot Ankle Surg* 44:358–364, 2005.
8. Bhatia D, Myerson MS, Curtis MJ, et al: Anatomical restraints to dislocation of the second metatarsophalangeal joint and assessment of a repair technique, *J Bone Joint Surg Am* 76:1371–1375, 1994.
9. Black GB, Grogan DP, Bobechko WP: Butler arthroplasty for correction of the adducted fifth toe: a retrospective study of 36 operations between 1968 and 1982, *J Pediatr Orthop* 5:439–441, 1985.
10. Blitz NM, Ford LA, Christensen JC: Plantar plate repair of the second metatarsophalangeal joint: technique and tips, *J Foot Ankle Surg* 43:266–270, 2004.
11. Blitz NM, Ford LA, Christensen JC: Second metatarsophalangeal joint arthrography: a cadaveric correlation study, *J Foot Ankle Surg* 43:231–240, 2004.
12. Boc SF, Martone JD: Varus toes: a review and case report, *J Foot Ankle Surg* 34:220–222, 1995.
13. Bonavilla EJ: Histopathology of the heloma durum: some significant features and their implications, *J Am Podiatry Assoc* 58:423–427, 1968.
14. Borne J, Bordet B, Fantino O, et al: [Plantar plate and second ray syndrome: normal and pathological US imaging features and proposed US classification], *J Radiol* 91(5 Pt 1):543–548, 2010.
15. Bouche RT, Heit EJ: Combined plantar plate and hammertoe repair with flexor digitorum longus tendon transfer for chronic, severe sagittal plane instability of the lesser metatarsophalangeal joints: preliminary observations, *J Foot Ankle Surg* 47:125–137, 2008.
16. Boussouga M, Boukhriss J, Jaafar A, et al: Irreducible dorsal metatarsophalangeal joint dislocation of the fifth toe: a case report, *J Foot Ankle Surg* 49:298 e217–e220, 2010.
17. Boyer A: *A treatise on surgical diseases, and the operations suited to them,* 2 vol, transl Alexander H. Stevens, New York, 1815-1816, T and J Swords, pp 383-385.
18. Boyer ML, DeOrio JK: Metatarsal neck osteotomy with proximal interphalangeal joint resection fixed with a single temporary pin, *Foot Ankle Int* 25:144–148, 2004.
19. Boyer ML, DeOrio JK: Transfer of the flexor digitorum longus for the correction of lesser-toe deformities, *Foot Ankle Int* 28:422–430, 2007.
20. Brahms MA: Common foot problems, *J Bone Joint Surg Am* 49:1653–1664, 1967.
21. Brahms MA: The small toes. In Jahss M, editor: *Disorders of the foot and ankle,* Philadelphia, 1991, WB Saunders, p 1187.
22. Branch H: Pathological dislocation of the second toe, *J Bone Joint Surg Am* 19:977–984, 1937.
23. Brunet JA, Tubin S: Traumatic dislocations of the lesser toes, *Foot Ankle Int* 18:406–411, 1997.
24. Buggiani FP, Biggs E: Mallet toe, *J Am Podiatry Assoc* 66:321–326, 1976.
25. Cahill BR, Connor DE: A long-term follow-up on proximal phalangectomy for hammer toes, *Clin Orthop* 86:191–192, 1972.
26. Cameron HU, Fedorkow DM: Revision rates in forefoot surgery, *Foot Ankle* 3:47–49, 1982.
27. Caterini R, Farsetti P, Tarantino U, et al: Arthrodesis of the toe joints with an intramedullary cannulated screw for correction of hammertoe deformity, *Foot Ankle Int* 25:256–261, 2004.
28. Cockin J: Butler's operation for an over-riding fifth toe, *J Bone Joint Surg Br* 50:77–81, 1968.
29. Cole WH: The classic. The treatment of claw-foot. By Wallace H. Cole. 1940, *Clin Orthop* 181:3–6, 1983.
30. Conklin MJ, Smith RW: Treatment of the atypical lesser toe deformity with basal hemiphalangectomy, *Foot Ankle Int* 15:585–594, 1994.
31. Cooper MT, Coughlin MJ: Sequential dissection for exposure of the second metatarsophalangeal joint, *Foot Ankle Int* 32:294–299, 2011.
32. Coughlin MJ: Common causes of pain in the forefoot in adults, *J Bone Joint Surg Br* 82:781–790, 2000.
33. Coughlin MJ: Crossover second toe deformity, *Foot Ankle* 8:29–39, 1987.
34. Coughlin MJ: Lesser toe abnormalities. In Chapman M, editor: *Operative orthopaedics,* Philadelphia, 1988, JB Lippincott, pp 1765–1776.
35. Coughlin MJ: Lesser toe abnormalities, *J Bone Joint Surg Am* 84:1446–1469, 2002.
36. Coughlin MJ: Lesser toe abnormalities, *Instr Course Lect* 52:421–444, 2003.
37. Coughlin MJ: Lesser toe deformities, *Orthopedics* 10:63–75, 1987.
38. Coughlin MJ: Lesser toe deformities. In Coughlin MJ, Mann CL, Saltzman CL, editors: *Surgery of the foot and ankle,* ed 8, vol 1, Philadelphia, 2007, Mosby Elsevier, pp 363–464.
39. Coughlin MJ: Mallet toes, hammer toes, claw toes, and corns. Causes and treatment of lesser-toe deformities, *Postgrad Med* 75:191–198, 1984.
40. Coughlin MJ: Operative repair of the mallet toe deformity, *Foot Ankle Int* 16:109–116, 1995.
41. Coughlin MJ: Rheumatoid forefoot reconstruction. A long-term follow-up study, *J Bone Joint Surg Am* 82:322–341, 2000.
42. Coughlin MJ: Second metatarsophalangeal joint instability in the athlete, *Foot Ankle* 14:309–319, 1993.
43. Coughlin MJ: Subluxation and dislocation of the second metatarsophalangeal joint, *Orthop Clin North Am* 20:535–551, 1989.
44. Coughlin MJ: When to suspect crossover second toe deformity, *J Musculoskel Med* 4:39–48, 1987.
45. Coughlin MJ, Dorris J, Polk E: Operative repair of the fixed hammer toe deformity, *Foot Ankle Int* 21:94–104, 2000.

46. Coughlin MJ, Kennedy MP: Operative repair of fourth and fifth toe corns, *Foot Ankle Int* 24:147–157, 2003.

47. Coughlin MJ, Nery C, Baumfeld D: Second MTP joint instability: grading of the deformity and description of surgical repair of capsular insufficiency, *Phys Sportsmed* 39:132–141, 2011.

48. Coughlin MJ, Pinsonneault T: Operative treatment of interdigital neuroma. A long-term follow-up study, *J Bone Joint Surg Am* 83:1321–1328, 2001.

49. Coughlin MJ, Schenck RC Jr, Shurnas PS, et al: Concurrent interdigital neuroma and MTP joint instability: long-term results of treatment, *Foot Ankle Int* 23:1017–1025, 2002.

50. Coughlin MJ, Schutt S, Hirose CB, et al: Plantar plate and capsular pathology in the second metatarsophalangeal joint: a cadaveric study, *Foot Ankle Int* 33:133–140, 2011.

51. Coughlin MJ, Thompson FM: The high price of high-fashion footwear, *Instr Course Lect* 44:371–377, 1995.

52. Cracchiolo A 3rd, Kitaoka HB, Leventen EO: Silicone implant arthroplasty for second metatarsophalangeal joint disorders with and without hallux valgus deformities, *Foot Ankle* 9:10–18, 1988.

53. Creer WS: Treatment of hammer toe, *BMJ* 1:527–528, 1935.

54. Cyphers SM, Feiwell E: Review of the Girdlestone-Taylor procedure for clawtoes in myelodysplasia, *Foot Ankle* 8:229–233, 1988.

55. Daly PJ, Johnson KA: Treatment of painful subluxation or dislocation at the second and third metatarsophalangeal joints by partial proximal phalanx excision and subtotal webbing, *Clin Orthop* 278:164–170, 1992.

56. Davies MS, Saxby TS: Metatarsal neck osteotomy with rigid internal fixation for the treatment of lesser toe metatarsophalangeal joint pathology, *Foot Ankle Int* 20:630–635, 1999.

57. Davis WH, Anderson RB, Thompson FM, Hamilton WG: Proximal phalanx basilar osteotomy for resistant angulation of the lesser toes, *Foot Ankle Int* 18:103–104, 1997.

58. Day MR, Hendrix CL, Gorecki GA, O'Malley D: Delta phalanx, *J Foot Ankle Surg* 35:49–53, 1996.

59. de Palma L, Zanoli G: Zanoli's procedure for overlapping fifth toe: retrospective study of 18 cases followed for 4-17 years, *Acta Orthop Scand* 69:505–507, 1998.

60. Deland JT: *Anatomy of volar plate insufficiency.* Presented at the 21st Annual Meeting of the American Orthopaedic Foot and Ankle Society, Anaheim, Calif, 1991.

61. Deland JT, Lee KT, Sobel M, DiCarlo EF: Anatomy of the plantar plate and its attachments in the lesser metatarsal phalangeal joint, *Foot Ankle Int* 16:480–486, 1995.

62. Deland JT, Sobel M, Arnoczky SP, Thompson FM: Collateral ligament reconstruction of the unstable metatarsophalangeal joint: an in vitro study, *Foot Ankle* 13:391–395, 1992.

63. Deland JT, Sung IH: The medial crossover toe: a cadaveric dissection, *Foot Ankle Int* 21:375–378, 2000.

64. Dhukaram V, Hossain S, Sampath J, Barrie JL: Correction of hammer toe with an extended release of the metatarsophalangeal joint, *J Bone Joint Surg Br* 84:986–990, 2002.

65. DuVries HL: Dislocation of the toe, *JAMA* 160:728, 1956.

66. DuVries HL, editor: *Surgery of the foot,* St Louis, 1959, Mosby, pp 359–360.

67. Dyal CM, Davis WH, Thompson FM, Elonar SK: Clinical evaluation of the Ruiz-Mora procedure: long-term follow-up, *Foot Ankle Int* 18:94–97, 1997.

68. Edwards WH, Beischer AD: Interphalangeal joint arthrodesis of the lesser toes, *Foot Ankle Clin* 7:43–48, 2002.

69. Ellington JK, Anderson RB, Davis WH, et al: Radiographic analysis of proximal interphalangeal joint arthrodesis with an intramedullary fusion device for lesser toe deformities, *Foot Ankle Int* 31:372–376, 2010.

70. Ely LW: Hammer toe, *Surg Clin North Am* 6:433–435, 1926.

71. Engle ET, Morton DJ: Notes on foot disorders among natives of the Belgian Congo, *J Bone Joint Surg Am* 13:311–319, 1931.

72. Espinosa N, Brodsky JW, Maceira E: Metatarsalgia, *J Am Acad Orthop Surg* 18:474–485, 2010.

73. Feeney S, Rees S, Tagoe M: Hemiphalangectomy and syndactylization for treatment of osteoarthritis and dislocation of the second metatarsal phalangeal joint: an outcome study, *J Foot Ankle Surg* 45:82–90, 2006.

74. Feeney MS, Williams RL, Stephens MM: Selective lengthening of the proximal flexor tendon in the management of acquired claw toes, *J Bone Joint Surg Br* 83:335–338, 2001.

75. Feeney S, Rees S, Tagoe M: Hemiphalangectomy and syndactylization for treatment of osteoarthritis and dislocation of the second metatarsal phalangeal joint: an outcome study, *J Foot Ankle Surg* 45:82–90, 2006.

76. Fishco WD, Roth BJ: Digital fracture after a flexor tendon transfer for hammertoe repair: a case report, *J Foot Ankle Surg* 49:179–181, 2010.

77. Ford LA, Collins KB, Christensen JC: Stabilization of the subluxed second metatarsophalangeal joint: flexor tendon transfer versus primary repair of the plantar plate, *J Foot Ankle Surg* 37:217–222, 1998.

78. Fortin PT, Myerson MS: Second metatarsophalangeal joint instability, *Foot Ankle Int* 16:306–313, 1995.

79. Fox IM, Pro AL: Lesser metatarsophalangeal joint implants, *J Foot Surg* 26:159–163, 1987.

80. Frank GR, Johnson WM: The extensor shift procedure in the correction of clawtoe deformities in children, *South Med J* 59:889–896, 1966.

81. Friend G: Correction of iatrogenic floating toe after resection of the base of the proximal phalanx, *Clin Podiatr Med Surg* 3:57–64, 1986.

82. Gallentine JW, DeOrio JK: Removal of the second toe for severe hammertoe deformity in elderly patients, *Foot Ankle Int* 26:353–358, 2005.

83. Gazdag A, Cracchiolo A 3rd: Surgical treatment of patients with painful instability of the second metatarsophalangeal joint, *Foot Ankle Int* 19:137–143, 1998.

84. Gerbert J, Benedetti L: Swanson design finger joint implant utilized in the proximal interphalangeal joints of the foot: a preliminary study, *J Foot Surg* 22:60–65, 1983.

85. Giannestras NJ: Shortening of the metatarsal shaft in the treatment of plantar keratosis: an end-result study, *J Bone Joint Surg Am* 40:61–71, 1958.

86. Gillet HG: Interdigital clavus: predisposition is the key factor of soft corns, *Clin Orthop* 142:103–109, 1979.

87. Girdlestone GR: Physiotherapy for hand and foot, *J Chart Soc Physiother* 32:167–169, 1947.

88. Glassman F, Wolin I, Sideman S: Phalangectomy for toe deformity, *Surg Clin North Am* 29:275–280, 1949.

89. Goforth WP, Overbeek TD, Odom RD, et al: Lesser-metatarsal medial displacement osteotomy for the treatment of digital transverse plane deformities, *J Am Podiatr Med Assoc* 95:550–555, 2005.

90. Goodwin FC, Swisher FM: The treatment of congenital hyperextension of the fifth toe, *J Bone Joint Surg Am* 25:193–196, 1943.

91. Grebing B, Coughlin MJ: Evaluation of the Esmarch bandage as a tourniquet for forefoot surgery, *Foot Ankle Int* 25:397–405, 2004.

92. Gregg J, Marks P, Silberstein M, et al: Histologic anatomy of the lesser metatarsophalangeal joint plantar plate, *Surg Radiol Anat* 29:141–147, 2007.

93. Gregg J, Silberstein M, Clark C, et al: Plantar plate repair and Weil osteotomy for metatarsophalangeal joint instability, *Foot Ankle Surg* 13:116–121, 2007.

94. Gregg J, Silberstein M, Schneider T, et al: Sonographic and MRI evaluation of the plantar plate: a prospective study, *Eur Radiol* 16:2661–2669, 2006.

95. Gregg JM, Silberstein M, Schneider T, et al: Sonography of plantar plates in cadavers: correlation with MRI and histology, *AJR Am J Roentgenol* 186:948–955, 2006.

96. Grimes J, Coughlin M: Geometric analysis of the Weil osteotomy, *Foot Ankle Int* 27:985–992, 2006.

97. Haddad SL, Sabbagh RC, Resch S, et al: Results of flexor-to-extensor and extensor brevis tendon transfer for correction of the crossover second toe deformity, *Foot Ankle Int* 20:781–788, 1999.

98. Hamer AJ, Stanley D, Smith TW: Surgery for curly toe deformity: a double-blind, randomised, prospective trial, *J Bone Joint Surg Br* 75:662–663, 1993.

99. Harris WT, Mote GA, Malay DS: Fixation of the proximal interphalangeal arthrodesis with the use of an intraosseous loop of stainless-steel wire suture, *J Foot Ankle Surg* 48:411–414, 2008.

100. Hatch DJ, Burns MJ: An anomalous tendon associated with crossover second toe deformity, *J Am Podiatr Med Assoc* 84:131–132, 1994.

101. Herstik I, Pelletier JP, Kanat IO: Pin tract infections. Incidence and management in foot surgery, *J Am Podiatr Med Assoc* 80:135–144, 1990.

102. Hewitt D, Stewart AM, Webb JW: The prevalence of foot defects among wartime recruits, *BMJ* 4839:745–749, 1953.

103. Heyman CH: The operative treatment of clawfoot, *J Bone Joint Surg* 14:335–338, 1932.

104. Higgs SL: Hammer-toe, *Postgrad Med* 6:130, 1931.

105. Hoffman P: An operation for severe grades of contracted or clawtoes, *Am J Orthop Surg* 9:441–449, 1911.

106. Hofstaetter SG, Hofstaetter JG, Petroutsas JA, et al: The Weil osteotomy: a seven-year follow-up, *J Bone Joint Surg Br* 87:1507–1511, 2005.

107. Idusuyi OB, Kitaoka HB, Patzer GL: Oblique metatarsal osteotomy for intractable plantar keratosis: 10-year follow-up, *Foot Ankle Int* 19:351–355, 1998.

108. Jacobs R, Vandeputte G: Flexor tendon lengthening for hammer toes and curly toes in paediatric patients, *Acta Orthop Belg* 73:373–376, 2007.

109. Jahss MH: Chronic and recurrent dislocations of the fifth toe, *Foot Ankle* 1:275–278, 1981.

110. Jahss MH: Miscellaneous soft tissue lesions. In Jahss M, editor: *Disorders of the foot and ankle*, Philadelphia, 1991, WB Saunders, pp 646–647, 843, 1982.

111. James CS: Footprints and feet of natives of the Solomon Islands, *Lancet* 2:1390–1393, 1939.

112. Janecki CJ, Wilde AH: Results of phalangectomy of the fifth toe for hammer toe. The Ruiz-Mora procedure, *J Bone Joint Surg Am* 58:1005–1107, 1976.

113. Johnson JB, Price TWT: Crossover second toe deformity: etiology and treatment, *J Foot Surg* 28:417–420, 1989.

114. Johnson K: Problems of the lesser toes. In Johnson K: *Surgery of the foot and ankle*, New York, 1989, Raven Press, pp 126–130.

115. Johnston RB 3rd, Smith J, Daniels T: The plantar plate of the lesser toes: an anatomical study in human cadavers, *Foot Ankle Int* 15:276–282, 1994.

116. Jolly G: *Personal communication*, San Diego, Calif, 2004.

117. Karlock LG: Second metatarsophalangeal joint fusion: a new technique for crossover hammer toe deformity. A preliminary report, *J Foot Ankle Surg* 42:177–182, 2003.

118. Karpman RR, MacCollum MS 3rd: Arthrography of the metatarsophalangeal joint, *Foot Ankle* 9:125–129, 1988.

119. Kaz A, Coughlin M: Extensor digitorum brevis transfer and Weil osteotomy for crossover second toe, *Tech Foot Ankle Surg* 9:32–36, 2010.

120. Kaz AJ, Coughlin MJ: Crossover second toe: demographics, etiology, and radiographic assessment, *Foot Ankle Int* 28:1223–1237, 2007.

121. Kelikian H: Deformities of the lesser toes. In Kelikian H: *Hallux valgus, allied deformities of the forefoot, and metatarsalgia.* Philadelphia, 1965, WB Saunders, pp 292–304.

122. Kelikian H, Clayton L, Loseff H: Surgical syndactylia of the toes, *Clin Orthop* 19:207–229, 1961.

123. Khurana A, Kadamabande S, James S, et al: Weil osteotomy: assessment of medium term results and predictive factors in recurrent metatarsalgia, *Foot Ankle Surg* 17:150–157, 2011.

124. Kilmartin TE, O'Kane C: Correction of valgus second toe by closing wedge osteotomy of the proximal phalanx, *Foot Ankle Int* 28:1260–1264, 2007.

125. Konkel KF, Menger AG, Retzlaff SA: Hammer toe correction using an absorbable intramedullary pin, *Foot Ankle Int* 28:916–920, 2007.

126. Kuwada GT: A retrospective analysis of modification of the flexor tendon transfer for correction of hammer toe, *J Foot Surg* 27:57–59, 1988.

127. Kuwada GT, Dockery GL: Modification of the flexor tendon transfer procedure for the correction of flexible hammer toes, *J Foot Surg* 19:37–40, 1980.

128. Lamberinudi C: The feet of the industrial worker, *Lancet* 2:1480–1484, 1938.

129. Lamm BM, Ades JK: Gradual digital lengthening with autologous bone graft and external fixation for correction of flail toe in a patient with Raynaud's disease, *J Foot Ankle Surg* 48:488–494, 2009.

130. Lancaster SC, Sizensky JA, Young CC: Acute mallet toe, *Clin J Sport Med* 18:298–299, 2008.

131. Lane GD: Lesser digital fusion with a cannulated screw, *J Foot Ankle Surg* 44:172–173, 2005.

132. Lantzounis LA: Congenital subluxation of the fifth toe and its correction by periosteocapsuloplasty and tendon transplantation, *J Bone Joint Surg* 22:147–150, 1940.

133. Lapidus PW: Operation for correction of hammer toe, *J Bone Joint Surg* 21:977–982, 1939.

134. Lapidus PW: Transplantation of the extensor tendon for correction of the overlapping of the fifth toe, *J Bone Joint Surg* 24:555–559, 1942.

135. Lehman DE, Smith RW: Treatment of symptomatic hammer toe with a proximal interphalangeal joint arthrodesis, *Foot Ankle Int* 16:535–541, 1995.

136. Leonard MH, Rising EE: Syndactylization to maintain correction of overlapping 5th toe, *Clin Orthop* 43:241–243, 1965.

137. Lui TH, Chan LK, Chan KB: Modified plantar plate tenodesis for correction of claw toe deformity, *Foot Ankle Int* 31:584–591, 2010.

138. Mahan KT: Bone graft reconstruction of a flail digit, *J Am Podiatr Med Assoc* 82:264–268, 1992.

139. Mahan KT, Downey MS, Weinfeld GD: Autogenous bone graft interpositional arthrodesis for the correction of flail toe. A retrospective analysis of 22 procedures, *J Am Podiatr Med Assoc* 93:167–173, 2003.

140. Mann RA, Coughlin MJ: Lesser toe deformities, *Instr Course Lect* 36:137–159, 1987.

141. Mann RA, Coughlin MJ: Lesser toe deformities. In Jahss M, editor: *Disorders of the foot and ankle*, Philadelphia, 1991, WB Saunders, pp 1207–1209.

142. Mann RA, Coughlin MJ: Lesser toe deformities. In Mann RA, Coughlin MJ, editors: *The video textbook of foot and ankle surgery.* St Louis, 1991, Medical Video Productions, pp 47–49.

143. Mann RA, Coughlin MJ: The rheumatoid foot: review of literature and method of treatment, *Orthop Rev* 8:105–112, 1979.

144. Mann RA, Mizel MS: Monarticular nontraumatic synovitis of the metatarsophalangeal joint: a new diagnosis? *Foot Ankle* 6:17–21, 1985.

145. Marek L, Giacopelli J, Granoff D: Syndactylization for the treatment of fifth toe deformities, *J Am Podiatr Med Assoc* 81:247–252, 1991.

146. Margo MK: Surgical treatment of conditions of the fore part of the foot, *J Bone Joint Surg Am* 49:1665–1674, 1967.

147. McCluskey WP, Lovell WW, Cummings RJ: The cavovarus foot deformity. Etiology and management, *Clin Orthop* 247:27–37, 1989.

148. McConnell BE: Correction of hammer toe deformity: a 10-year review of subperiosteal waist resection of the proximal phalanx, *Orthop Rev* 8:65–69, 1975.

149. McConnell BE: Hammer toe surgery: waist resection of the proximal phalanx, a more simplified procedure, *South Med J* 68:595–598, 1975.

150. McGlamry ED: Floating toe syndrome, *J Am Podiatry Assoc* 72:561–568, 1982.

151. Mednick DL, Nordgaard J, Hallwhich D, et al: Comparison of total hinged and total nonhinged implants for the lesser digits, *J Foot Surg* 24:215–218, 1985.

152. Melamed EA, Schon LC, Myerson MS, Parks BG: Two modifications of the Weil osteotomy: analysis on sawbone models, *Foot Ankle Int* 23:400–405, 2002.

153. Mendicino RW, Statler TK, Saltrick KR, Catanzariti AR: Predislocation syndrome: a review and retrospective analysis of eight patients, *J Foot Ankle Surg* 40:214–224, 2001.

154. Migues A, Slullitel G, Bilbao F, et al: Floating-toe deformity as a complication of the Weil osteotomy, *Foot Ankle Int* 25:609–613, 2004.

155. Miller JM, Blacklidge DK, Ferdowsian V, et al: Chevron arthrodesis of the interphalangeal joint for hammertoe correction, *J Foot Ankle Surg* 49:194–196, 2010.

156. Miller SD: Technique tip: forefoot pain: diagnosing metatarsophalangeal joint synovitis from interdigital neuroma, *Foot Ankle Int* 22:914–915, 2001.

157. Mills GP: The etiology and treatment of claw-foot, *J Bone Joint Surg* 6:142–149, 1924.

158. Mizel MS: Anatomy and pathophysiology of the lesser toes. In Gould J, editor: *Operative foot surgery*, Philadelphia, 1993, WB Saunders, pp 84–85.

159. Mizel MS, Michelson JD: Nonsurgical treatment of monarticular nontraumatic synovitis of the second metatarsophalangeal joint, *Foot Ankle Int* 18:424–426, 1997.

160. Morton DJ: Metatarsus atavicus: the identification of a distinctive type of foot disorder, *J Bone Joint Surg* 9:531–544, 1927.

161. Mulder JD: The causative mechanism in morton's metatarsalgia, *J Bone Joint Surg Br* 33:94–95, 1951.

162. Murphy JL: Isolated dorsal dislocation of the second metatarsophalangeal joint, *Foot Ankle* 1:30–32, 1980.

163. Myerson MS, Filippi J: Bone block lengthening of the proximal interphalangeal joint for managing the floppy toe deformity, *Foot Ankle Clin* 15:663–668, 2010.

164. Myerson MS, Fortin P, Girard P: Use of skin Z-plasty for management of extension contracture in recurrent claw- and hammertoe deformity, *Foot Ankle Int* 15:209–212, 1994.

165. Myerson MS, Jung HG: The role of toe flexor-to-extensor transfer in correcting metatarsophalangeal joint instability of the second toe, *Foot Ankle Int* 26:675–679, 2005.

166. Myerson MS, Redfern DJ: Technique tip: modification of DuVries's lesser metatarsophalangeal joint arthroplasty to improve joint mobility, *Foot Ankle Int* 25:277–279, 2004.

167. Myerson MS, Shereff MJ: The pathological anatomy of claw and hammer toes, *J Bone Joint Surg Am* 71:45–49, 1989.

168. Nery C, Coughlin M, Baumfeld D, et al: Lesser metatarsophalangeal joint instability: prospective evaluation and repair of plantar plate and capsular insufficiency, *Foot Ankle Int* 33:301–311, 2011.

169. Newman RJ, Fitton JM: An evaluation of operative procedures in the treatment of hammer toe, *Acta Orthop Scand* 50(6 Pt 1):709–712, 1979.

170. Ohm OW 2nd, McDonell M, Vetter WA: Digital arthrodesis: an alternate method for correction of hammer toe deformity, *J Foot Surg* 29:207–211, 1990.

171. O'Kane C, Kilmartin T: Review of proximal interphalangeal joint excisional arthroplasty for the correction of second hammer toe deformity in 100 cases, *Foot Ankle Int* 26:320–325, 2005.

172. O'Kane C, Kilmartin TE: The surgical management of central metatarsalgia, *Foot Ankle Int* 23:415–419, 2002.

173. Oliver TP, Armstrong DG, Harkless LB, et al: The combined hammer toe-mallet toe deformity with associated double corns: a retrospective review, *Clin Podiatr Med Surg* 13:263–268, 1996.

174. Panchbhavi VK, Trevino S: Clinical tip: a new clinical sign associated with metatarsophalangeal joint synovitis of the lesser toes, *Foot Ankle Int* 28:640–641, 2007.

175. Parrish TF: Dynamic correction of clawtoes, *Orthop Clin North Am* 4:97–102, 1973.

176. Patton GW, Shaffer MW, Kostakos DP: Absorbable pin: a new method of fixation for digital arthrodesis, *J Foot Surg* 29:122–127, 1990.

177. Petrik M, Voos K, Suthers K, Smith M: Hammer toe correction using an absorbable pin, *Oper Tech Orthop* 6:203–207, 1996.

178. Petersen WJ, Lankes JM, Paulsen F, Hassenpflug J: The arterial supply of the lesser metatarsal heads: a vascular injection study in human cadavers, *Foot Aankle Int* 23:491–495, 2002.

179. Pichney GA, Derner R, Lauf E: Digital "V" arthrodesis, *J Foot Ankle Surg* 32:473–479, 1993.

180. Pietrzak WS, Lessek TP, Perns SV: A bioabsorbable fixation implant for use in proximal interphalangeal joint (hammer toe) arthrodesis: biomechanical testing in a synthetic bone substrate, *J Foot Ankle Surg* 45:288–294, 2006.

181. Piper KJ, Yen-yi JC, Horsley M: Missed posterior deep, inferior subcompartment syndrome in a patient with an ankle fracture: a case report, *J Foot Ankle Surg* 49:398 e395–e398, 2010.

182. Pontious J, Flanigan KP, Hillstrom HJ: Role of the plantar fascia in digital stabilization. A case report, *J Am Podiatr Med Assoc* 86:43–47, 1996.

183. Powless SH, Elze ME: Metatarsophalangeal joint capsule tears: an analysis by arthrography, a new classification system and surgical management, *J Foot Ankle Surg* 40:374–389, 2001.

184. Pyper JB: The flexor-extensor transplant operation for claw toes, *J Bone Joint Surg Br* 40:527–533, 1958.

185. Quebedeaux T, Armstrong DG, Harkless LB: Acute and chronic pedal boutonniere deformity, *J Am Podiatr Med Assoc* 86:447–450, 1996.

186. Rao JP, Banzon MT: Irreducible dislocation of the metatarsophalangeal joints of the foot, *Clin Orthop* 145:224–226, 1979.

187. Rau FD, Manoli A 2nd: Traumatic boutonniere deformity as a cause of acute hammer toe: a case report, *Foot Ankle* 11:231–232, 1991.

188. Reece AT, Stone MH, Young AB: Toe fusion using Kirschner wire. A study of the postoperative infection rate and related problems, *J R Coll Surg Edinb* 32:157–159, 1987.

189. Reichert K, Caneva RG: The use of Kirschner wire fixation in forefoot surgery, *J Foot Surg* 22:217–221, 1983.

190. Reis ND, Karkabi S, Zinman C: Metatarsophalangeal joint dislocation after local steroid injection, *J Bone Joint Surg Br* 71:864, 1989.

191. Richardson E: Lesser toe abnormalities. In Crenshaw AH, editor: *Campbell's operative orthopaedics*, ed 8, St Louis, 1992, Mosby, pp 2742–2744.

192. Ross ER, Menelaus MB: Open flexor tenotomy for hammer toes and curly toes in childhood, *J Bone Joint Surg Br* 66:770–771, 1984.

193. Roukis TS: A 1-piece shape-metal nitinol intramedullary internal fixation device for arthrodesis of the proximal interphalangeal joint in neuropathic patients with diabetes, *Foot Ankle Spec* 2:130–134, 2009.

194. Ruiz-Mora J: Plastic correction of over-riding fifth toe, *Orthop Lett Club* 6, 1954.

195. Salari N, Faro FD, Miller SD: Dorsal opening wedge osteotomy of second proximal phalanx for second MTP dorsiflexion, *Foot Ankle Int* 31:1021–1024, 2010.

196. Saro C, Bengtsson AS, Lindgren U, et al: Surgical treatment of hallux valgus and forefoot deformities in Sweden: a population-based study, *Foot Ankle Int* 29:298–304, 2008.

197. Sarrafian SK: *Anatomy of the foot and ankle*, Philadelphia, 1983, JB Lippincott.

198. Sarrafian SK: Correction of fixed hammer toe deformity with resection of the head of the proximal phalanx and extensor tendon tenodesis, *Foot Ankle Int* 16:449–451, 1995.

199. Sarrafian SK, Topouzian LK: Anatomy and physiology of the extensor apparatus of the toes, *J Bone Joint Surg Am* 51:669–679, 1969.

200. Scheck M: Degenerative changes in the metatarsophalangeal joints after surgical correction of severe hammer-toe deformities. A complication associated with avascular necrosis in three cases, *J Bone Joint Surg Am* 50:727–737, 1968.

201. Scheck M: Etiology of acquired hammer toe deformity, *Clin Orthop* 123:63–67, 1977.

202. Schlefman BS, Fenton CF 3rd, McGlamry ED: Peg in hole arthrodesis, *J Am Podiatry Assoc* 73:187–195, 1983.

203. Schnepp KH: Hammer toe and claw foot, *Am J Surg* 36:351–359, 1933.

204. Schrier JC, Verheyen CC, Louwerens JW: Definitions of hammer toe and claw toe: an evaluation of the literature, *J Am Podiatr Med Assoc* 99:194–197, 2009.

205. Scrase WH: The treatment of dorsal adduction deformities of the fifth toe, *J Bone Joint Surg Br* 36:146, 1954.

206. Selig S: Hammer-toe. A new procedure for its correction, *Surg Gynecol Obstet* 72:101–105, 1941.

207. Sgarlato TE: Implants for lesser toes, *J Foot Surg* 22:247–250, 1983.

208. Sgarlato TE: Sutter double-stem silicone implant arthroplasty of the lesser metatarsophalangeal joints, *J Foot Surg* 28:410–413, 1989.

209. Shaw AH, Alvarez G: The use of digital implants for the correction of hammer toe deformity and their potential complications and management, *J Foot Surg* 31:63–74, 1992.

210. Shirzad K, Kiesau CD, DeOrio JK, et al: Lesser toe deformities, *J Am Acad Orthop Surg* 19:505–514, 2011.

211. Silberman J, Kanat IO: Total joint replacement in digits of the foot, *J Foot Surg* 23:207–212, 1984.

212. Smith BW, Coughlin MJ: Disorders of the lesser toes, *Sports Med Arthrosc* 17:167–174, 2009.

213. Soule RA: Operation for the correction of hammer toe, *N Y Med J* 91:649–650, 1910.

214. Sweetnam R: Congenital curly toes: an investigation into the value of treatment, *Lancet* 2:397–400, 1958.

215. Taylor RG: An operative procedure for the treatment of hammer toe and claw-toe, *J Bone Joint Surg* 22:607–609, 1940.

216. Taylor RG: The treatment of claw toes by multiple transfers of flexor into extensor tendons, *J Bone Joint Surg Br* 33:539–542, 1951.

217. Thompson C: Surgical treatment of disorders of the fore part of the foot, *J Bone Joint Surg Am* 46:1117–1128, 1964.

218. Thompson FM, Deland JT: Flexor tendon transfer for metatarsophalangeal instability of the second toe, *Foot Ankle* 14:385–388, 1993.

219. Thompson FM, Hamilton WG: Problems of the second metatarsophalangeal joint, *Orthopedics* 10:83–89, 1987.

220. Thordarson DB: Congenital crossover fifth toe correction with soft tissue release and cutaneous Z-plasty, *Foot Ankle Int* 22:511–512, 2001.

221. Threthowen WH: Treatment of hammer toe, *Lancet* 1:1312–1313, 1925.

222. Trepman E, Yeo SJ: Nonoperative treatment of metatarsophalangeal joint synovitis, *Foot Ankle Int* 16:771–777, 1995.

223. Trnka HJ, Muhlbauer M, Zettl R, et al: Comparison of the results of the Weil and Helal osteotomies for the treatment of metatarsalgia secondary to dislocation of the lesser metatarsophalangeal joints, *Foot Ankle Int* 20:72–79, 1999.

224. Trnka HJ, Nyska M, Parks BG, Myerson MS: Dorsiflexion contracture after the Weil osteotomy: results of cadaver study and three-dimensional analysis, *Foot Ankle Int* 22:47–50, 2001.

225. Vandeputte G, Dereymaeker G, Steenwerckx A, Peeraer L: The Weil osteotomy of the lesser metatarsals: a clinical and pedobarographic follow-up study, *Foot Ankle Int* 21:370–374, 2000.

226. VanderWilde R, Campbell D: *Second toe amputation for chronic painful deformity*. Presented at the 23rd Annual Meeting of the American Orthopaedic Foot and Ankle Society, San Francisco, Calif, 1993.

227. Vitek M: A new technique for hammertoe arthrodesis, *Foot Ankle Surg* 15:54–56, 2009.

228. Wee GC, Tucker GL: An improved procedure for the surgical correction of hammer toes, *Mo Med* 67:43–44, 1970.

229. Weil L Jr, Sung W, Weil L Sr, et al: Corrections of second MTP joint instability using a Weil osteotomy and dorsal approach plantar plate repair: a new technique, *Tech Foot Ankle Surg* 10:33–39, 2011.

230. Weil LS Jr: Hammertoe arthrodesis using conical reamers and internal pin fixation, *J Foot Ankle Surg* 38:370–371, 1999.

231. Weil LS: Personal communication, April 29, 2004.

232. Weil LS, Borrelli A, Weil L, et al: *Evaluation of the Weil metatarsal osteotomy. Long-term results*. Presented at the Summer Meeting of the American Orthopaedic Foot and Ankle Society. Boston, Mass, 1998.

233. Wells LH: The foot of the South African native, *Am J Physiol Anthropol* 15:185–289, 1931.

234. Wilson JN: V-Y correction for varus deformity of the fifth toe, *Br J Surg* 41:133–135, 1953.

235. Yao L, Cracchiolo A, Farahani K, Seeger LL: Magnetic resonance imaging of plantar plate rupture, *Foot Ankle Int* 17:33–36, 1996.

236. Yao L, Do HM, Cracchiolo A, et al: Plantar plate of the foot: findings on conventional arthrography and MR imaging, *AJR Am J Roentgenol* 163:641–644, 1994.

237. Young CS: An operation for the correction of hammer toe and clawtoe, *J Bone Joint Surg* 20:715–719, 1938.

238. Yu GV, Judge MS, Hudson JR, Seidelmann FE: Predislocation syndrome. Progressive subluxation/dislocation of the lesser metatarsophalangeal joint, *J Am Podiatr Med Assoc* 92:182–199, 2002.

239. Zeringue GN Jr, Harkless LB: Evaluation and management of the web corn involving the fourth interdigital space, *J Am Podiatr Med Assoc* 76:210–213, 1986.

240. Zingas C, Katcherian DA, Wu KK: Kirschner wire breakage after surgery of the lesser toes, *Foot Ankle Int* 16:504–509, 1995.

Chapter 8

Keratotic Disorders of the Plantar Skin

Ari J. Kaz, Roger A. Mann

This chapter discusses the etiology and treatment of keratotic lesions of the plantar skin as a result of friction, pressure, or both. These must be distinguished from the intrinsic disorders of the skin, such as verrucae and dermatosis, especially tinea infestations.

Localization of pressure along the plantar aspect of the foot illustrates the relative length of time that the center of pressure dwells beneath the metatarsal heads during normal walking (see Chapter 1). After heel strike, the center of pressure moves very rapidly to the metatarsal head area, where it dwells for more than 50% of the stance phase, after which it moves toward the toes (Fig. 8-1). Because of this extended period of weight bearing in the metatarsal area, abnormal alignment of the forefoot, either localized or generalized, can result in the formation of a keratotic lesion.

PLANTAR KERATOSES

A broad differential diagnosis (Box 8-1) must be considered in the evaluation of the patient presenting with a plantar callus. The diagnosis is usually not difficult to make, but at times the diagnosis may not be clear, and one needs to consider these various causes.

Anatomy

The predominant pattern of the metatarsal cascade demonstrates that the first metatarsal is shorter than the second approximately 60% of the time.[24] The mobility of the first metatarsocuneiform (MTC) joint or the first metatarsophalangeal (MTP) joint determines the degree of weight bearing of the first ray. The plantar aponeurosis mechanism brings about plantar flexion of the first metatarsal during the last half of stance phase and may become less functional as a hallux valgus deformity develops. As a result, plantar flexion of the first ray might not occur, which can lead to increased pressure under the second metatarsal head[57] and diffuse callus formation secondary to increased weight bearing. Hypermobility of the first MTC joint, which may be pathologic in no more than 5% of patients, can also lead to increased weight bearing by the first metatarsal. Pressure is then transferred to the lesser metatarsals, where a diffuse callus can develop

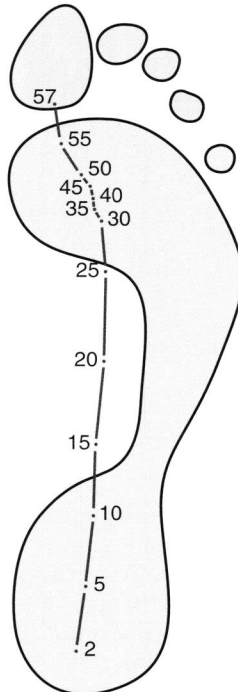

Figure 8-1 Movement of the center of pressure along the plantar aspect of the foot during walking. Note the way the center of pressure rapdly moves from the heel and dwells in the metatarsal region before moving distally to the great toe. (From Hutton WC, Stott JRR, Stokes JAF: In Klenerman L, editor: *The foot and its disorders*, Oxford, 1982, Blackwell Scientific, p 42.)

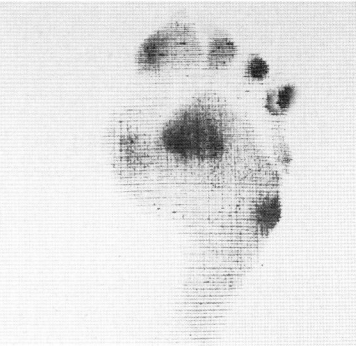

Figure 8-2 Harris mat print of a patient with hypermobility of the first metatarsal. Because the first metatarsal does not carry much weight, pressure is transferred to the second and third metatarsals as well as to the tip of the hallux.

The posture of the foot must always be considered in evaluating the patient with an intractable plantar keratosis (IPK). Abnormal callus formation can be due to an equinus deformity of the ankle joint, a cavus foot, pes planus, a varus forefoot deformity, a pes planovalgus deformity (Fig. 8-3), or abnormal alignment of the MTP joints. Unless the underlying deformity is addressed, the IPK will persist.

An equinus deformity of the ankle joint that results in increased weight bearing on the metatarsal heads can result in a diffuse callus beneath the first, second, and third metatarsal heads. This can be painful, particularly in the older patient with atrophy of the fat pad. In the patient with an insensate foot, such as the patient with diabetes or a peripheral neuropathy, ulceration of the plantar aspect of the foot can occur.

In the cavus foot, the calcaneus is usually in a dorsiflexed position and the forefoot in equinus, leading to an abnormally diminished weight-bearing area and resultant diffuse callus formation beneath the metatarsal head area. This condition often becomes more symptomatic with increasing patient age and fat pad atrophy.

The foot with pes planus does not usually develop significant callus formation beneath the metatarsal heads, unless it is associated with a hallux valgus deformity. This combination can lead to callus formation along the plantar medial aspect of the great toe at the level of the interphalangeal (IP) joint.

beneath the second and possibly third metatarsal (Fig. 8-2). The base of the second and third metatarsals is quite stable because of the rigidity of their tarsometatarsal articulations; therefore, if the first metatarsal is hypermobile or elevated from any cause, callus formation can occur beneath these metatarsal heads. The fourth and fifth metatarsals are more mobile, and therefore calluses rarely develop beneath them unless there is an abnormal foot posture or an osseous deformity.

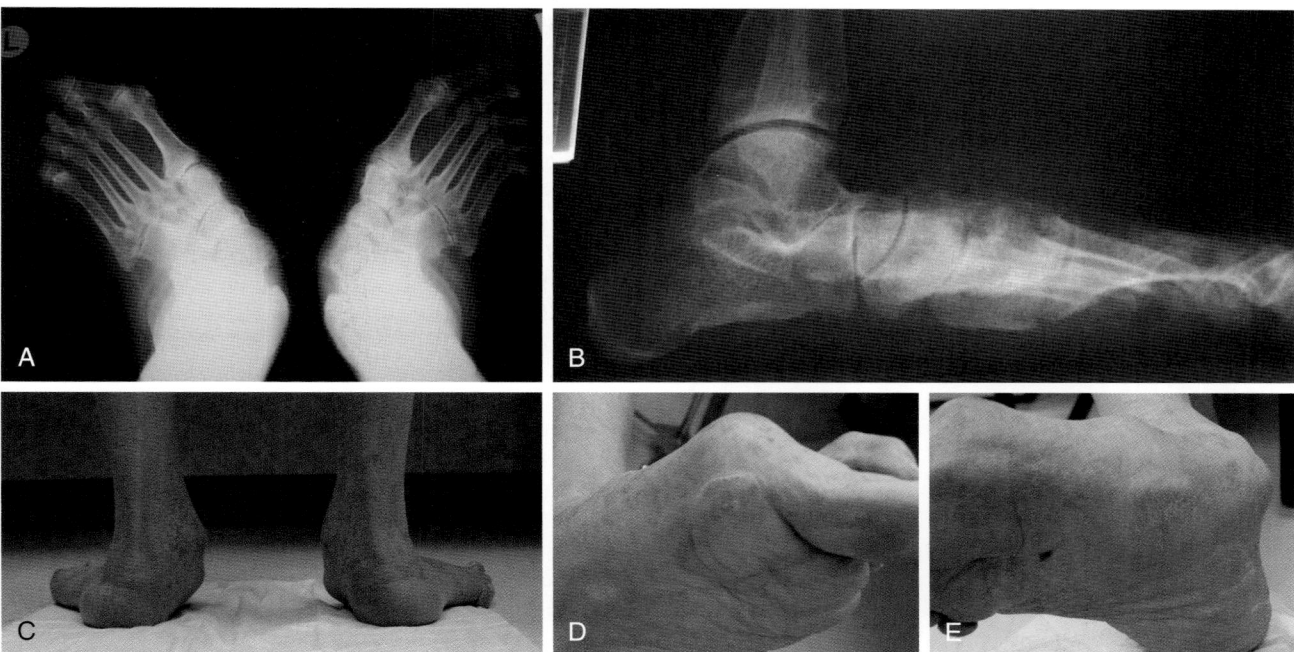

Figure 8-3 **A** and **B,** Radiographs of a patient with a severe pes planovalgus deformity. **C,** Clinical photograph of same patient demonstrating the deformity when viewed from the posterior aspect. **D,** Callus formation under first metatarsophalangeal (MTP) joint from inadequate weight bearing of medial column. **E,** Callus formation under first metatarsocuneiform (MTC) joint from collapse of medial longitudinal arch.

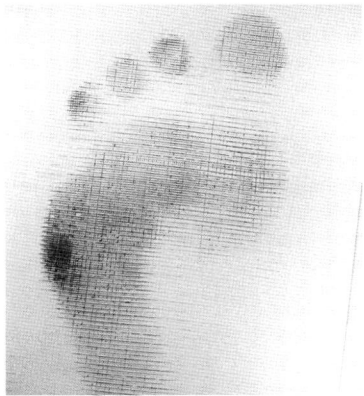

Figure 8-4 Harris mat print of patient with varus forefoot deformity. Note that pressure is borne on the lateral aspect of the foot, with significantly decreased weight bearing beneath the medial aspect of the foot.

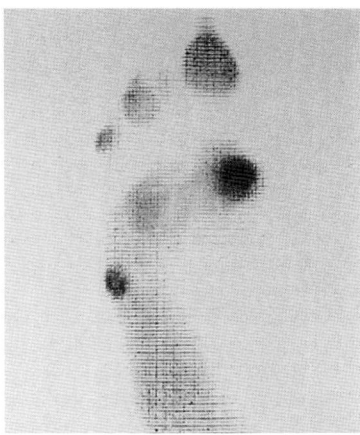

Figure 8-5 Harris mat print of patient with valgus forefoot deformity in which increased weight is borne along the medial side of the foot and, in particular, beneath the first metatarsal head.

A varus forefoot deformity, in which the lateral border of the foot is more plantar flexed than the medial border, often results in a diffuse callus beneath the fifth metatarsal head (Fig. 8-4).

A valgus forefoot deformity, in which the first metatarsal is more plantar flexed in relation to the lesser metatarsals, often results in a diffuse callus beneath the first metatarsal head region (Fig. 8-5). This is often associated with a cavus foot deformity.

Abnormal alignment of the metatarsophalangeal joints, secondary to either subluxation or dorsal dislocation, results in a plantarward force on the metatarsal head

and development of a diffuse callus beneath the involved metatarsal head. An extreme example is a patient with advanced rheumatoid arthritis (Fig. 8-6).

Diagnosis

The evaluation of a patient with a plantar keratotic lesion begins with a careful history of the condition. This should include pertinent medical conditions, history of trauma, prior surgeries, what type of footwear aggravates and relieves the pain, the wear pattern of footwear, as well as what type of treatment has been attempted in the past.

The physical examination begins with the patient standing. Careful observation should be made of the posture of the toes, characteristics of the MTP joints and longitudinal arch, and the position and posture of the hindfoot in relation to the forefoot. Strength testing of all muscle groups, a thorough neurovascular examination, and range of motion of the ankle, subtalar, transverse tarsal, and MTP joints should be noted. Hypermobility of the first ray, the presence of hallux rigidus,[22] as well as swelling, thickening, synovitis, and instability of the lesser MTP joints[57] are important diagnostic findings.

The plantar aspect of the foot is carefully evaluated. The location of the lesion and its characteristics are observed. The callus may consist of a localized seed corn, a discrete plantar keratosis beneath the fibular condyle of a metatarsal head or beneath the tibial sesamoid, a diffuse callus beneath a metatarsal head, or a diffuse callus beneath several metatarsal heads.

Weight-bearing radiographs should be obtained along with sesamoid views, if indicated. A small marker can be placed over the lesion to identify the offending structure if needed.

It is important to differentiate a wart, or plantar verruca, from a callus. Plantar verrucae are common, affecting 7% to 10% of the population.[10,37] A plantar verruca is usually localized but occasionally demonstrates a mosaic pattern and is usually not discretely located beneath a metatarsal head. Papillary lines, or rete ridges, diverge around the lesion, whereas in a callus, the rete run unchanged across the lesion.[21] To facilitate identification, the lesion is often trimmed with a No. 17 blade. Trimming enables the clinician to identify the margins of the callus, because in a well-localized plantar keratosis, the callus itself has definite circumscribed edges, as opposed to a diffuse callus, which is a generalized thickening of the plantar skin without a defined margin. A wart, on the other hand, may have a small amount of hyperkeratotic skin overlying it, but very quickly one enters the warty material, which consists of multiple end arteries that bleed vigorously, as opposed to a true plantar keratosis, which has no blood supply (Fig. 8-7). Warts are commonly caused by the human papilloma virus (HPV),[47] with the dark and moist environment within a shoe facilitating survival. Numerous treatments have been described for this often recalcitrant lesion, including chemical ablation, immunologic modifying treatments, and surgery. Common chemical ablation techniques include phenol, 10% fermaldehyde, 10% formaldehyde with monochloroacetic acid,[30] fluorouracil, and bleomycin sulfate.[53] Topical treatments include salicylic acid, fluorouracil,[64] canthadrin and podophyllotoxin,[6] formaldehyde, silver nitrate, corticosteroids, and garlic extract.[7] Cryotherapy and electrocautery have been used with varying results. Surgical excision is often required, with recurrence not uncommon.

Other rare dermatologic lesions that present as plantar callosities include keratosis palmoplantaris nummularis and epithelioma cuniculatum. If these lesions are suspected, dermatology consultation is recommended (Fig. 8-8). Keratosis palmoplantaris nummularis is an autosomal dominant skin disorder characterized by painful callus formation over areas of mechanical stress on the palms and plantar surface of the foot. It often presents upon the onset of walking in a child, with pain being the primary complaint. Physical examination

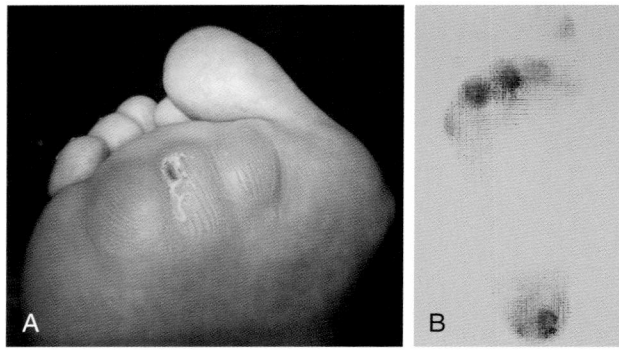

Figure 8-6 **A,** Foot in a patient with rheumatoid arthritis with large diffuse plantar calluses beneath the metatarsal heads and nonfunctional toes. **B,** Harris mat print demonstrating concentration of pressure beneath metatarsal heads and lack of weight bearing by lesser toes.

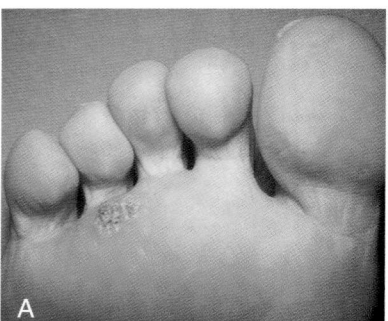
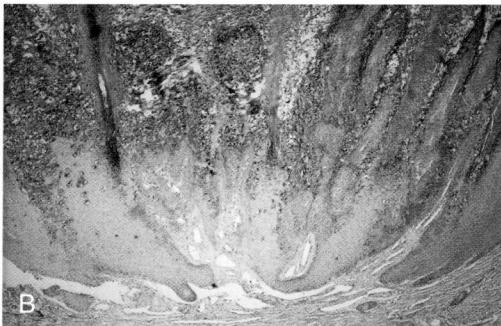
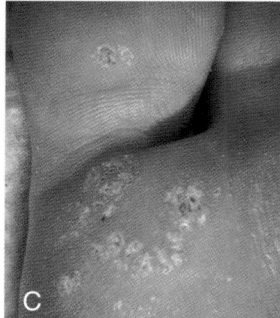

Figure 8-7 **A,** Wart on the plantar aspect of the foot does not usually occur on a weight-bearing area. **B,** Histologic features of the wart demonstrate considerable vascularity within the lesion. **C,** Mosaic wart has similar histology but is more widespread.

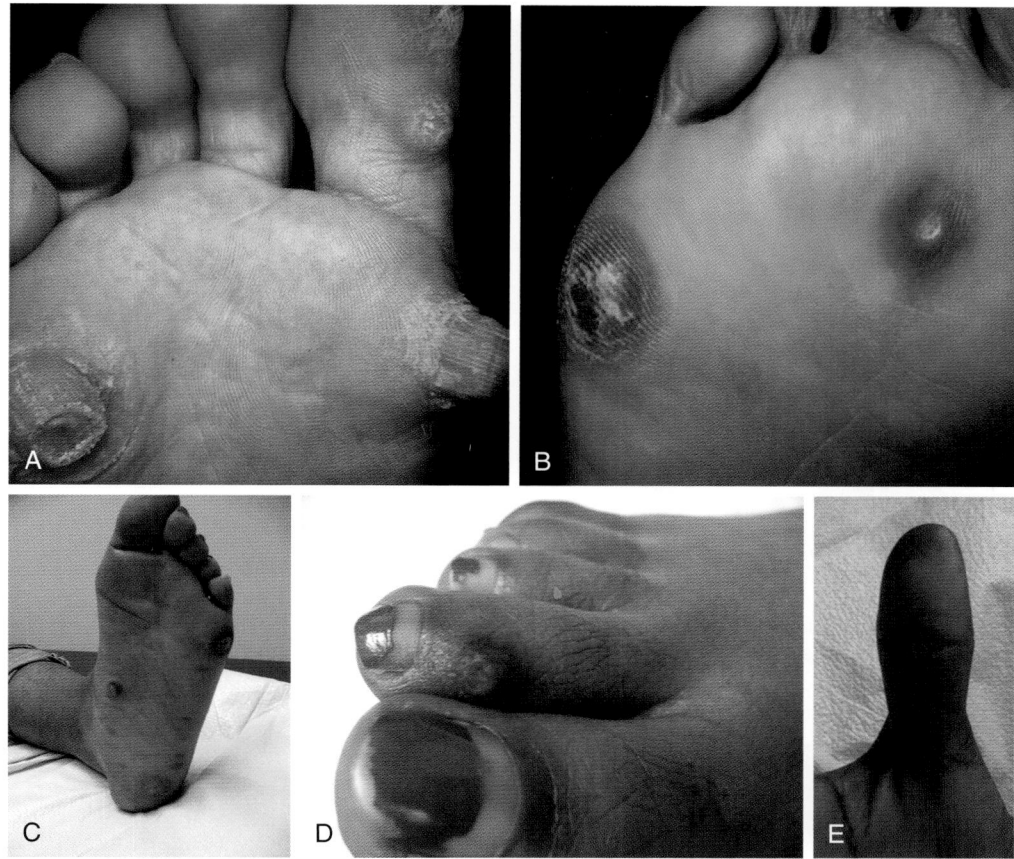

Figure 8-8 **A** and **B,** Examples of feet with hyperkeratotic skin. **C** and **D,** Plantar hyperkeratotic lesions consistent with keratosis palmoplantaris nummularis. **E,** The same patient in **C** and **D** also had painful keratotic lesions on her hands, such as this lesion on the volar interphalangeal (IP) flexion crease of the thumb.

reveals essentially normal motor and sensory function, with multiple areas of large hyperkeratotic callus formation over weight-bearing areas of the feet that are confluent with the surrounding skin.[52] Histologic evaluation is consistent with epidermolytic hyperkeratosis.[61] Operative treatment has been reported to be unsuccessful.[61] The mainstay of treatment is shaving of the callosities, orthotics, and footwear modification. The natural history and successful treatment of the disorder remain elusive.

Epithelioma cuniculatum is a form of verrucous carcinoma that affects the plantar surface of the feet.[45] It is an uncommon low-grade squamous cell carcinoma that is typically slow growing and has a tendency to local recurrence. Although metastatic disease is rare, lack of timely diagnosis can lead to its spread.[55] It can present as a painless, nonhealing ulceration on the plantar surface of the foot that slowly increases in size and is refractory to standard callus treatment.[33] Diagnosis of this rare lesion can be challenging, and deep biopsy is required. The human papilloma virus has been implicated as a causative factor, but both HPV-positive and -negative lesions have been reported.[37] Histologic analysis reveals a well-differentiated tumor composed of keratinocytes that extend the dermis

and deeper structures, forming sinuses and keratin-filled cysts. Tumor cells in the granular layer may show vacuoles.[55] There is often marked hyperkeratosis, with perakeratosis of a prominent granular layer occasionally seen.[33] Treatment options include imiquimod (a topical immune-modulating drug), carbon dioxide (CO_2) laser ablation, and surgical excision.[33]

Treatment

Conservative Treatment

The plantar callus can be trimmed with a sharp knife. A No. 17 podiatric blade is especially useful for trimming of hyperkeratotic skin. When trimming a callus, one should attempt to reduce the hyperkeratotic tissue, and if it is invaginated, this too should be trimmed. With a deep-seated lesion, however, it may not be possible to remove all of the keratotic lesion at the first trimming, and several trimmings may be necessary to permit the deep-seated portion of the callus to surface. Occasionally, a seed corn, which is a well-localized keratotic lesion, usually 2 to 3 mm in diameter, can be removed at the first sitting, although it might require a second trimming (Fig. 8-9).

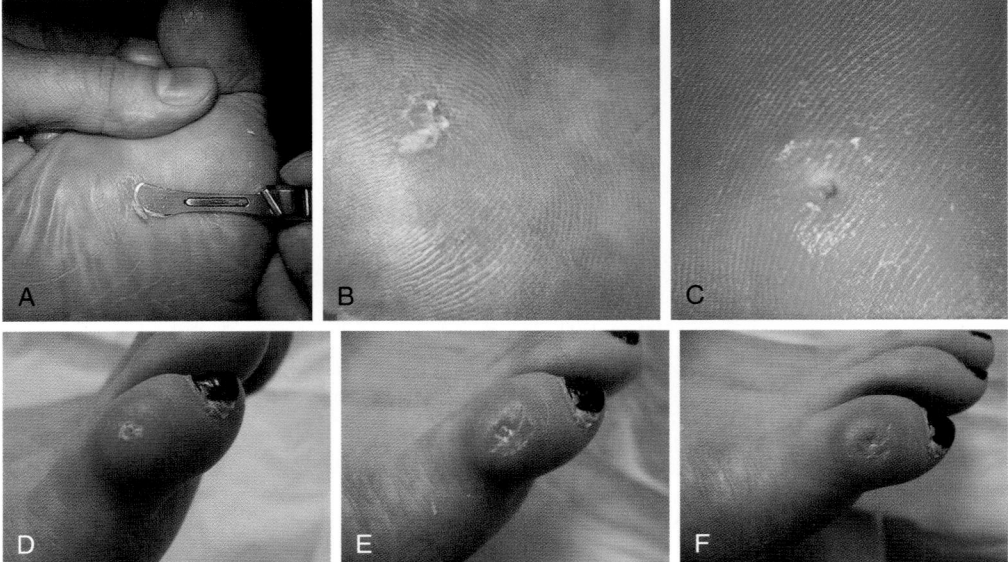

Figure 8-9 **A,** Debridement of callus with No. 17 blade. **B,** A seed corn is a small keratotic lesion on the plantar aspect of the foot that at times becomes symptomatic. **C,** Appearance of seed corn after debridement. Keratotic lesion with seed corn on dorsum of fifth proximal interphalangeal (PIP) joint. **D,** Predebridement. **E,** Debridement of callus with seed corn remaining. **F,** After debridement of seed corn.

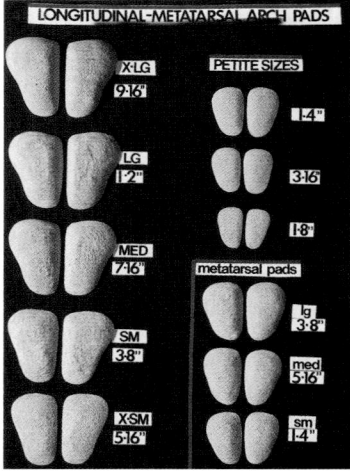

Figure 8-10 Various types of soft metatarsal supports that may be used to relieve pressure in the metatarsal area of the foot.

After debridement of the callus, a soft metatarsal support is used to relieve pressure on the involved area (Fig. 8-10). The soft support can be used, provided that the patient's shoe is of adequate size. If the patient is wearing stylish women's dress shoes, there may not be sufficient volume for the foot and the metatarsal support. The patient with a significant keratotic lesion should be encouraged to wear a broad, soft, preferably low-heeled shoe to provide more cushioning for the plantar aspect of the foot. The metatarsal support should be placed into the shoe just proximal to the area of the lesion (Fig. 8-11). It is important to instruct the patient that this support

may initially feel uncomfortable and may take a period of breaking in of a week to 10 days.

The patient is then seen periodically in the office for trimming of the lesion, adjustment of the metatarsal support, and possibly even placement of a larger one, as necessary. If the patient has a postural abnormality of the foot, such as forefoot varus or valgus, or possibly a pes planovalgus deformity or a cavus foot, a custom-made, well-molded orthotic may be of benefit.

Other footwear modification, such as a wide or tall toe box or the addition of a rocker-bottom sole, can potentially provide relief. If an equinus contracture is a contributing cause, physical therapy to stretch the gastrocsoleus complex can increase the relative length of the Achilles tendon unit, thereby increasing ankle dorsiflexion.[18]

If the callus persists and is symptomatic, surgical intervention can be considered.

Surgical Treatment: Types of Plantar Callosities
Surgical management of a plantar keratosis is based on the characteristics of the callus.

A discrete callus with a central keratotic core is observed beneath the fibular condyle of the metatarsal head and beneath the tibial sesamoid (Fig. 8-12). When the patient with a discrete, localized lesion walks over a Harris mat, the imprint created is well localized beneath the prominence that has brought about the callus (Fig. 8-13). Histologically, this lesion is a dense, keratinized lesion with a central core (Fig. 8-14).

This should be differentiated from a diffuse callus, which is often caused by deformity at the MTP joints because of instability, and usually associated with abnormal weight bearing during the third rocker portion of the

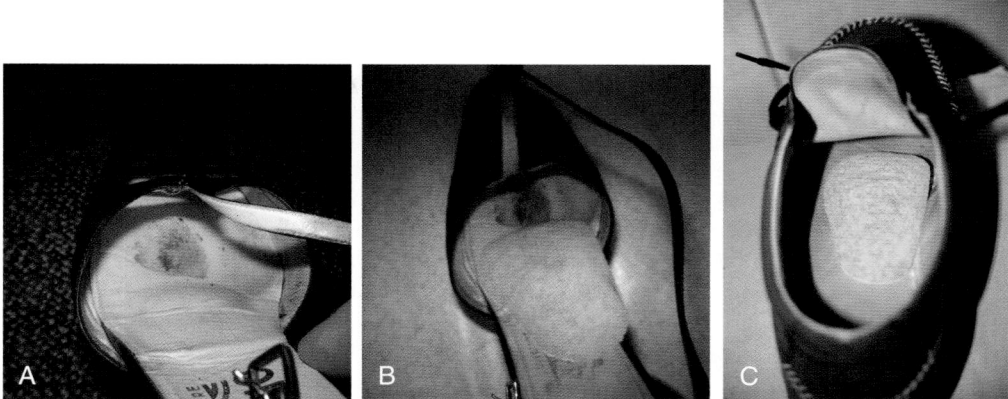

Figure 8-11 Placement of a soft metatarsal support in the shoe. **A,** Support is placed just proximal to the "smudge" on the insole. This is usually around the base of the tongue. **B** and **C,** The support can be moved medially or laterally, depending on the location of the plantar lesion.

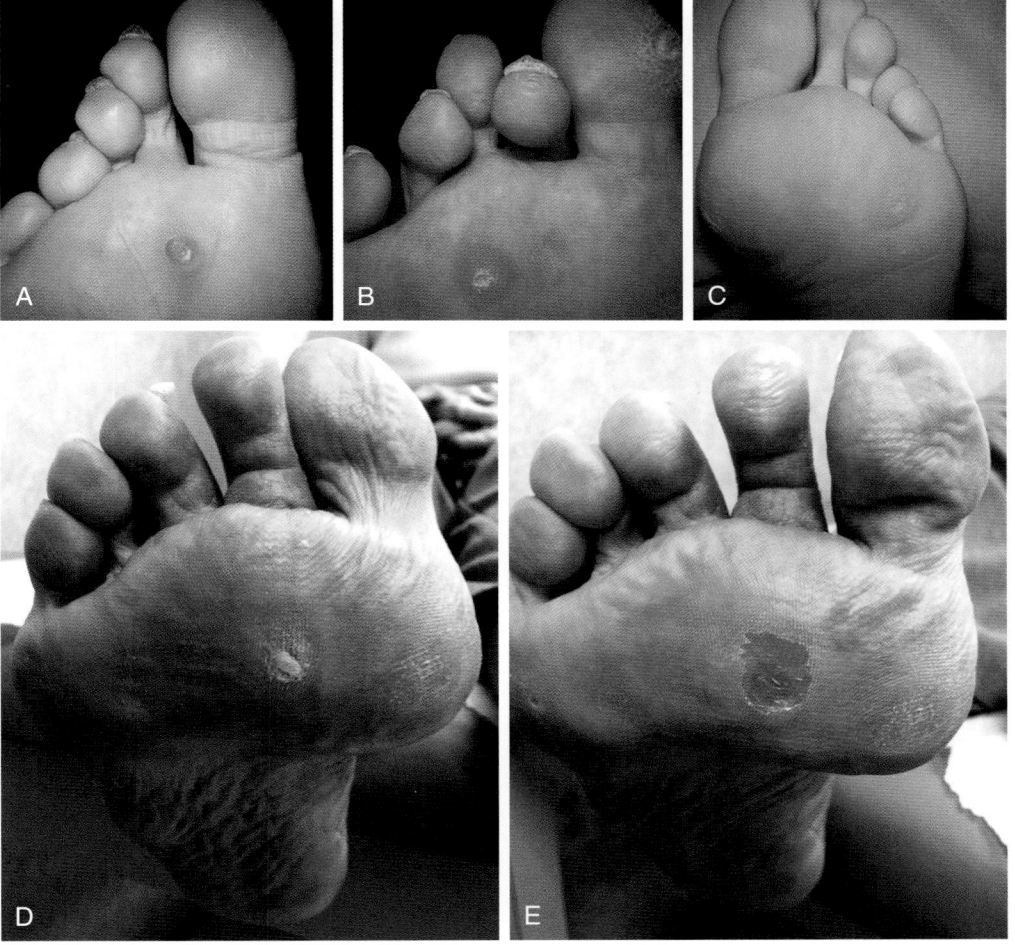

Figure 8-12 Examples of discrete intractable plantar keratoses (IPKs). **A,** Lesion beneath the second metatarsal head. **B,** Discrete keratosis beneath the third metatarsal head. **C,** Discrete keratosis beneath the fourth metatarsal head. **D,** Discrete IPK under the second metatarsal head. **E,** Same patient as in **D** after shaving of the lesion with a podiatric blade. (**B** from Mann RA: Intractable plantar keratosis *Instr Course Lect* 33:289, 1984.)

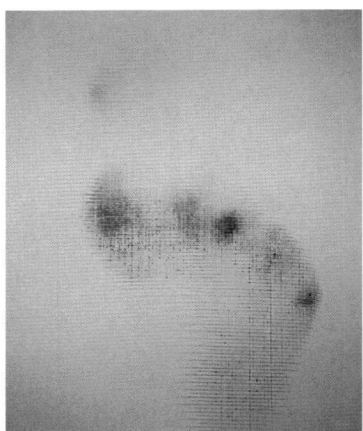

Figure 8-13 Harris mat print demonstrating well-localized area of pressure—a discrete plantar keratosis.

gait cycle, in which only the forefoot is in contact with the ground (Fig. 8-15).[15] A diffuse callus is observed beneath a metatarsal head that does not have a prominent fibular condyle and is noted most often beneath the second metatarsal head. Occasionally, a diffuse callus is noted beneath multiple metatarsal heads. When this type of callus is present and is trimmed, although the material consists of hyperkeratotic skin, there is no central core as observed in a discrete callus. When this patient walks over a Harris mat, the print that is observed is diffuse beneath the entire metatarsal head or beneath multiple metatarsal heads (Fig. 8-16). In general, a callus underneath several metatarsals is often due to forefoot overload, such as seen in ankle equinus; plantar flexion of the metatarsals, as in a cavus foot; or first-ray insufficiency. This indicates overload during the foot flat portion of the gait cycle during the

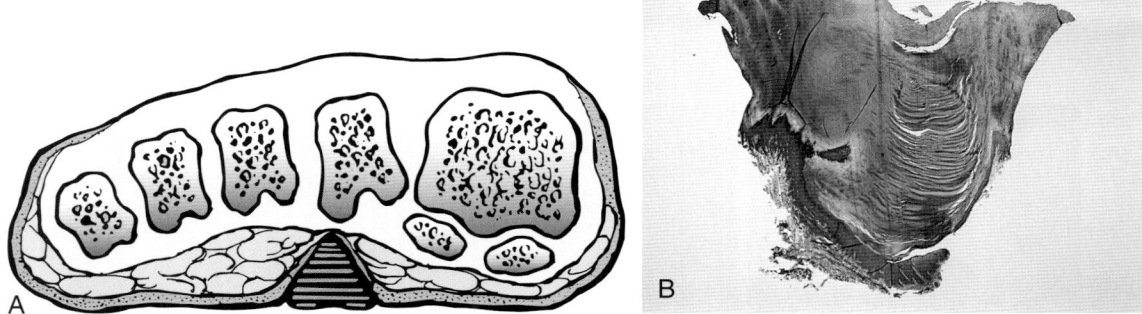

Figure 8-14 **A,** Location of a discrete plantar keratosis beneath a prominent fibular condyle. **B,** Histologic features of the keratotic lesion demonstrate layers of keratin with no blood vessels. Compare with Figure 8-7B.

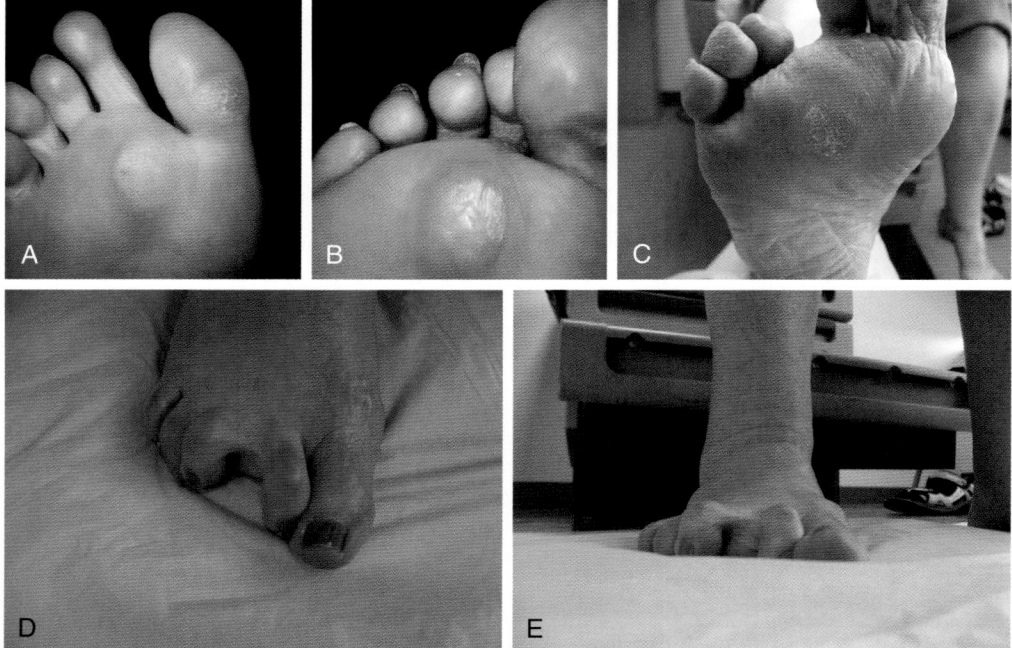

Figure 8-15 **A** and **B,** Examples of diffuse keratotic lesions. When these lesions are debrided, there is no central core, which distinguishes them from discrete keratotic lesions. **C,** Diffuse callus formation under second and third metatarsophalangeal (MTP) joints resulting from second crossover toe deformity. **D** and **E,** Clinical photographs of patient in **C** with second crossover toe deformity.

second rocker portion of swing phase.[15] This type of diffuse lesion is occasionally observed beneath the first metatarsal head if it is plantar flexed. It can be observed beneath the second metatarsal head when the first metatarsal is short, hypermobile, or due to first-ray instability brought about by an advanced hallux valgus deformity or possibly insufficiency after bunion surgery, if the joint has been destabilized. A diffuse callus beneath the second, third, and fourth

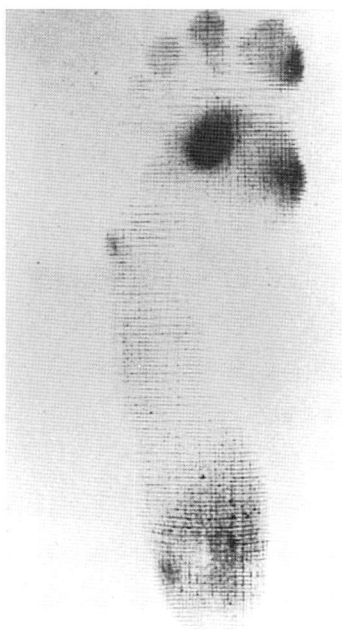

Figure 8-16 Harris mat print demonstrates diffuse keratotic lesion beneath second metatarsal head. Compare with Figure 8-15. (From Mann RA: Intractable plantar keratosis *Instr Course Lect* 33:293, 1984.)

metatarsal heads is usually observed in a patient with an extremely short first metatarsal, which results in increased weight bearing beneath the three middle metatarsals (Fig. 8-17). Occasionally, a diffuse callus is present beneath the fifth metatarsal head in patients with a varus configuration of the forefoot, or with a plantar-flexed fifth metatarsal associated with a tailor's bunion.

A diffuse type of callus can also result after trauma. A metatarsal malunion can result in a plantar-flexion deformity and resultant callus underneath the fractured metatarsal. A dorsiflexion malunion can lead to callus formation beneath an adjacent metatarsal, with the normal metatarsal left to bear increased weight.

Differentiating the type of callus is essential because the nature of the callus determines the type of surgical procedure that will give the best result. In general, a localized callus will require an elevating procedure, whereas a diffuse callus requires a shortening procedure.[15]

Localized Intractable Plantar Keratosis

A localized IPK, which is usually caused by the prominence of the fibular condyle, can be treated by a DuVries metatarsal condylectomy. DuVries[12-14] initially described the procedure in which he carried out an arthroplasty of the MTP joint by removing a portion of the distal articular surface and the plantar condyle. Coughlin[3] and Mann[41] modified the procedure by removing only the plantar condyle. Both procedures seem to lead to satisfactory clinical results.

DUVRIES METATARSAL CONDYLECTOMY
Surgical Technique
1. A hockey stick–shaped incision begins in the second web space and is carried across the metatarsal head

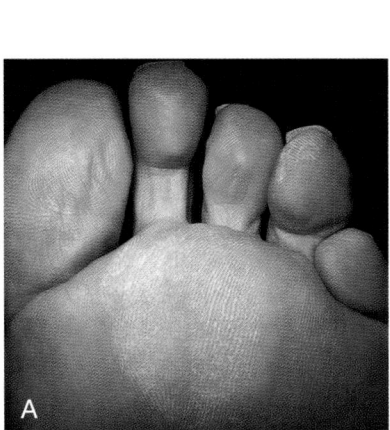
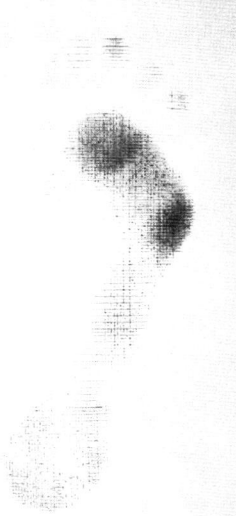
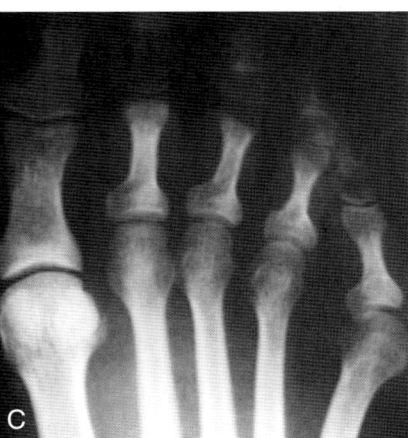

Figure 8-17 Typical findings with Morton foot (toe). **A,** Plantar aspect demonstrates diffuse callus beneath second and third metatarsal heads. **B,** Harris mat print demonstrates increased weight bearing beneath the second and third metatarsals, with little or no weight bearing beneath the first metatarsal head. **C,** Radiograph demonstrates typical Morton foot with short first metatarsal and relatively long second and third metatarsals.

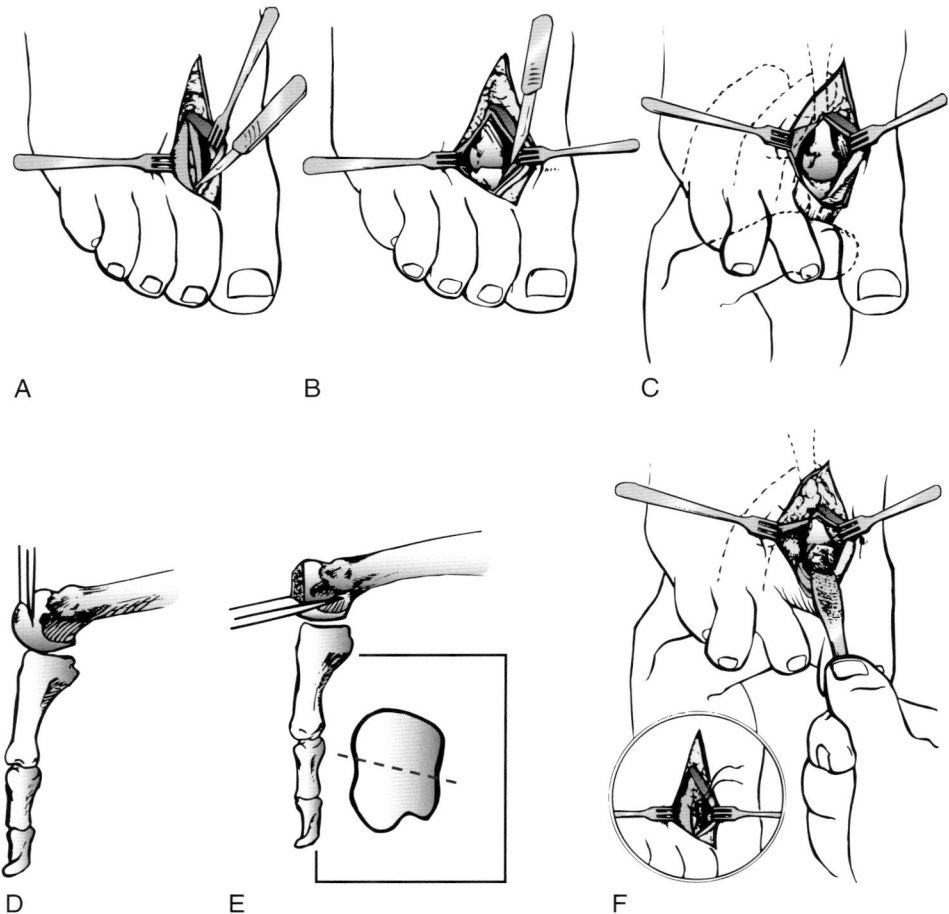

Figure 8-18 DuVries plantar metatarsal condylectomy. **A,** Hockey stick–shaped incision beginning in the web space is carried obliquely across the joint to about the middle of the metatarsal shaft. Skin and extensor tendons are retracted, and the capsule is incised longitudinally. **B,** Capsule and collateral ligaments on both sides of the metatarsal head are sectioned. **C,** The involved toe is plantar flexed with the left thumb while pressure is applied on the plantar aspect of the metatarsal shaft with the index finger. **D,** About 2 mm of articular cartilage is removed. **E,** The plantar 30% of the condyle is removed with an osteotome. Note angulation to facilitate removal of more of the fibular aspect. **F,** Edges of the metatarsal are smoothed; then the capsule and skin are closed.

proximally to about the distal third of the metatarsal shaft (Fig. 8-18A).

2. Passing medially and laterally to the extensor hood, the transverse metatarsal ligament is identified and released.

3. The interval between the long and short extensor tendons is opened and continued through the joint capsule to expose the MTP joint.

4. The collateral ligaments are transected, and the MTP joint is sharply plantar flexed while pressure is applied to the plantar aspect of the foot with the index finger of the same hand (Fig. 8-18B and C).

5. The distal 2 mm of articular cartilage is removed from the metatarsal head in a plane perpendicular to the metatarsal shaft. As this cut is made, the osteotome is angled slightly proximally; otherwise, it will skid off the cartilage and make an oblique cut (Fig. 8-18D).

6. The MTP joint is now sharply plantar flexed to bring into view the plantar condyle. The plantar 20% to 30% of the metatarsal head is removed with a 10- to 12-mm thin osteotome. The osteotome is angled slightly plantarward to avoid inadvertent splitting of the metatarsal shaft (Fig. 8-18E).

7. On completion of the osteotomy in the metatarsal head, the plantar condyle is delivered by use of a Freer elevator or thin rongeur in the adjacent interspace, and the condyle is removed. It is difficult to pull this fragment of bone out directly over the proximal phalanx, so it is pushed into the interspace and removed (Fig. 8-19).

8. The edges are carefully rongeured, and the joint is reduced (see Fig. 8-18F). The skin is closed in a routine manner.

9. A compression dressing is applied for 12 to 18 hours, and the patient is permitted to ambulate in a postoperative shoe.

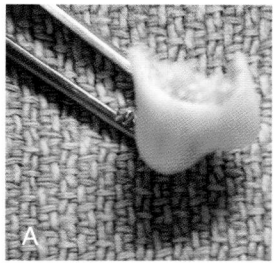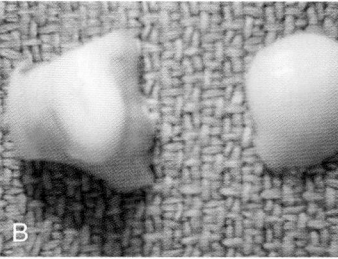

Figure 8-19 Excised plantar condyle. **A,** Note marked prominence of the fibular portion of the condyle in this specimen. **B,** Plantar view of the same specimen illustrating the large condyle. (**A** from Mann RA: Intractable plantar keratosis *Instruct Course Lect* 33:292, 1984.)

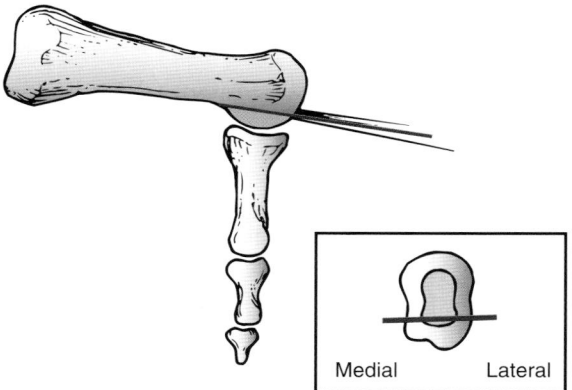

Medial   Lateral

Figure 8-20 Coughlin modification of plantar condylectomy. Plantar 20% to 30% of the condyle is removed, and the distal portion of the metatarsal head is left intact.

Postoperative Care

The bulky surgical dressing is changed after 18 to 24 hours, and the patient is placed into a snug compression dressing consisting of 2-inch conforming gauze (Kling) and adhesive tape. The patient is permitted to ambulate in the postoperative shoe, which is worn for 3 weeks. The shoe is removed, and the patient is encouraged to work on range-of-motion exercises.

Results

In a review of 100 patients surgically treated by Mann and DuVries,[42] there was 93% patient satisfaction. It was observed that 42% of the lesions were beneath the second metatarsal head, 31% beneath the third, 19% beneath the fourth, and 8% beneath the fifth. A transfer lesion occurred in 13% of the patients, and the original lesion failed to resolve in 5%.

The 5% complication rate included fracture of a metatarsal head, avascular necrosis of the metatarsal head, and clawing of the toe. There were no cases of dislocation of the MTP joint after this procedure. Postoperative range of motion of the MTP joint rarely demonstrates more than 25% loss of motion. It has always been somewhat surprising that so little motion is lost after this type of arthroplasty, whereas when a similar procedure is carried out for a dislocated MTP joint, significantly more motion is lost.

COUGHLIN MODIFIED METATARSAL CONDYLECTOMY

The modification of the condylectomy by Coughlin is carried out in the same way as the DuVries metatarsal condylectomy, except that the distal portion of the metatarsal is not removed (Fig. 8-20 and Video Clip 69).[3,41] This makes removing the plantar condyle a little more difficult. Until now, there has been no published report regarding the results of this modification of the DuVries procedure, although preliminary data indicate about a 5% incidence of transfer lesions. The use of a power rasp with which to shave down the prominent fibular condyle[46] has been described. This avoids the potential difficulty of retrieving the osteotomized plantar condyle from the

interspace. Thermal necrosis and bone debris can be avoided by use of irrigation.

Vertical Chevron Procedure

Dreeben et al[10] described a vertical chevron osteotomy of the metatarsal head for treatment of a painful callus beneath the metatarsal head. The article did not classify the callus into a localized or diffuse category. A vertical chevron osteotomy was performed in the metaphysis, and the metatarsal head was elevated approximately 3 mm.

Surgical Technique

1. A 2-cm dorsal incision is made over the metatarsal head and neck region. The extensor tendons are retracted, the metatarsal neck exposed subperiosteally, and the plantar periosteum left intact. The MTP joint is not entered.
2. A chevron-type cut with the apex based distally is produced with a power saw just proximal to the edge of the dorsal joint capsule. An attempt should be made to leave the plantar periosteum intact (Fig. 8-21).
3. The metatarsal head is displaced dorsally by plantar pressure but not more than 3 to 4 mm.
4. The osteotomy site is stabilized with a 0.045-inch Kirschner wire introduced through a separate stab wound. The skin is closed in a routine manner.

Postoperative Care

The patient walks in a postoperative shoe with weight bearing as tolerated. The Kirschner wire is removed after 3 weeks, and gentle range of motion is begun at that time. The postoperative shoe is continued for a total of 6 weeks.

Results

The series reported by Dreeben et al[10] included 45 patients. Complete relief of the symptoms was noted in 67%, 24% had residual pain, 9% demonstrated a transfer lesion, and in 4%, the callus was unchanged. The authors pointed out that the metatarsal head should be elevated at least

3 mm but not more than 4.5 mm. Kitaoka and Patzer[36] used the same procedure on 21 feet—16 women and 3 men, with a mean age of 59 years (32 to 85). They reported good results in 16, fair in 2, and poor in 3. In 4 patients (20%), the callosity persisted, and in 3 (14%), a transfer lesion developed.

Discrete Callus beneath Tibial Sesamoid

A discrete callus beneath the first metatarsal head lies under the tibial sesamoid. A localized lesion does not occur beneath the fibular sesamoid. A diffuse callus can be observed beneath the entire first metatarsal and is usually associated with a plantar-flexed metatarsal, as seen in the patient with a cavus foot or Charcot-Marie-Tooth disease.

The lesion beneath the tibial sesamoid can often be managed conservatively, although when it occurs after bunion surgery and the sesamoid is localized beneath the crista of the metatarsal head, surgical intervention is usually required (Fig. 8-22).

TIBIAL SESAMOID SHAVING

The surgical procedure we prefer is tibial sesamoid shaving, in which the plantar half of the sesamoid is removed (Video Clip 64). In the past, we advocated excision of the sesamoid for this problem, but after a review of our cases, we believe that tibial sesamoid shaving is a superior procedure with significantly less morbidity.[43]

Surgical Technique

1. The skin incision is made slightly plantar to the midline and centered over the medial aspect of the MTP joint. The incision is carried down to the capsular structures without undermining the skin (Fig. 8-23A and B).
2. Along the capsular plane, the incision is developed in a plantar direction over the medial aspect of the tibial sesamoid. Great care is taken to identify the medial plantar cutaneous nerve, which often passes with a small vessel along the plantar aspect of the abductor hallucis tendon.
3. With the nerve identified and retracted plantarward, the periosteum over the tibial sesamoid is stripped to expose the plantar two thirds of the sesamoid. The plantar half of the tibial sesamoid is removed with a small oscillating saw, and the edges are smoothed (Fig. 8-23C and D). Care must be taken to avoid injury to the flexor hallucis longus (FHL) tendon, which lies just lateral to the medial sesamoid.
4. The wound is closed in a routine manner, and a compression dressing is applied (Fig. 8-23E and F).

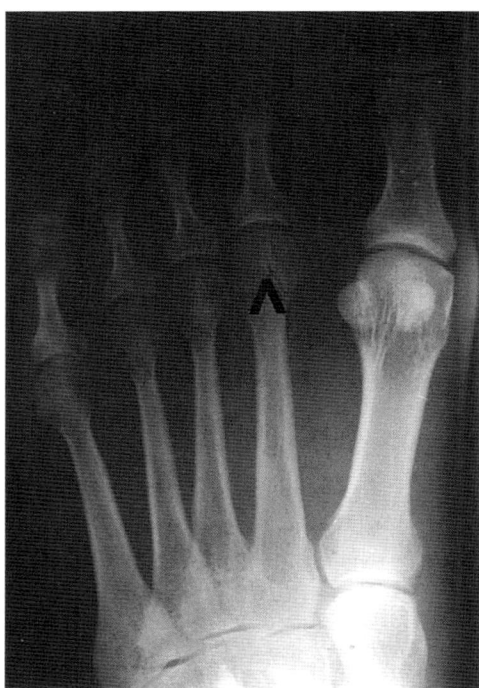
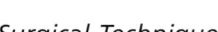

Figure 8-21 The vertical chevron procedure is carried out to create an osteotomy, as demonstrated in this radiograph. The metatarsal head should be elevated approximately 3 mm.

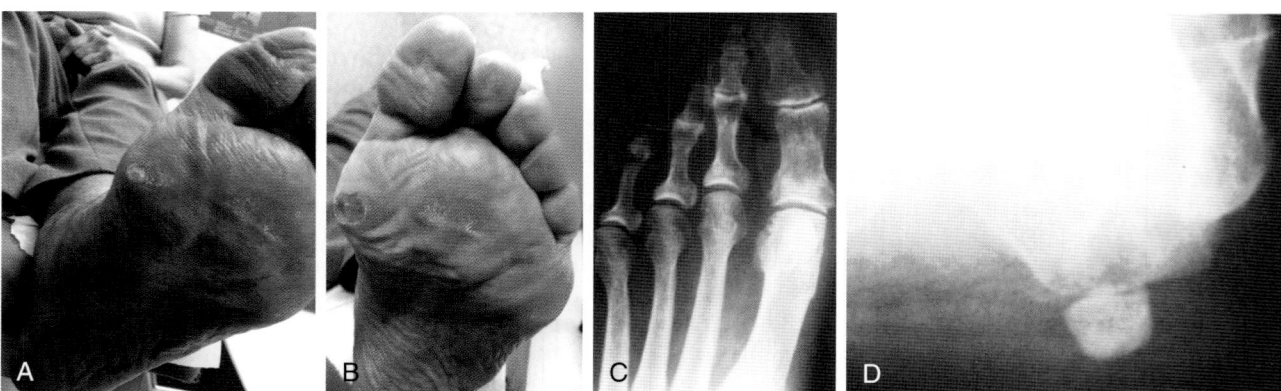

Figure 8-22 **A** and **B,** Discrete keratotic lesion beneath tibial sesamoid before and after debridement. **C,** Radiograph demonstrates a tibial sesamoid centered beneath the metatarsal head. **D,** Axial view demonstrates a sesamoid sitting beneath the crista.

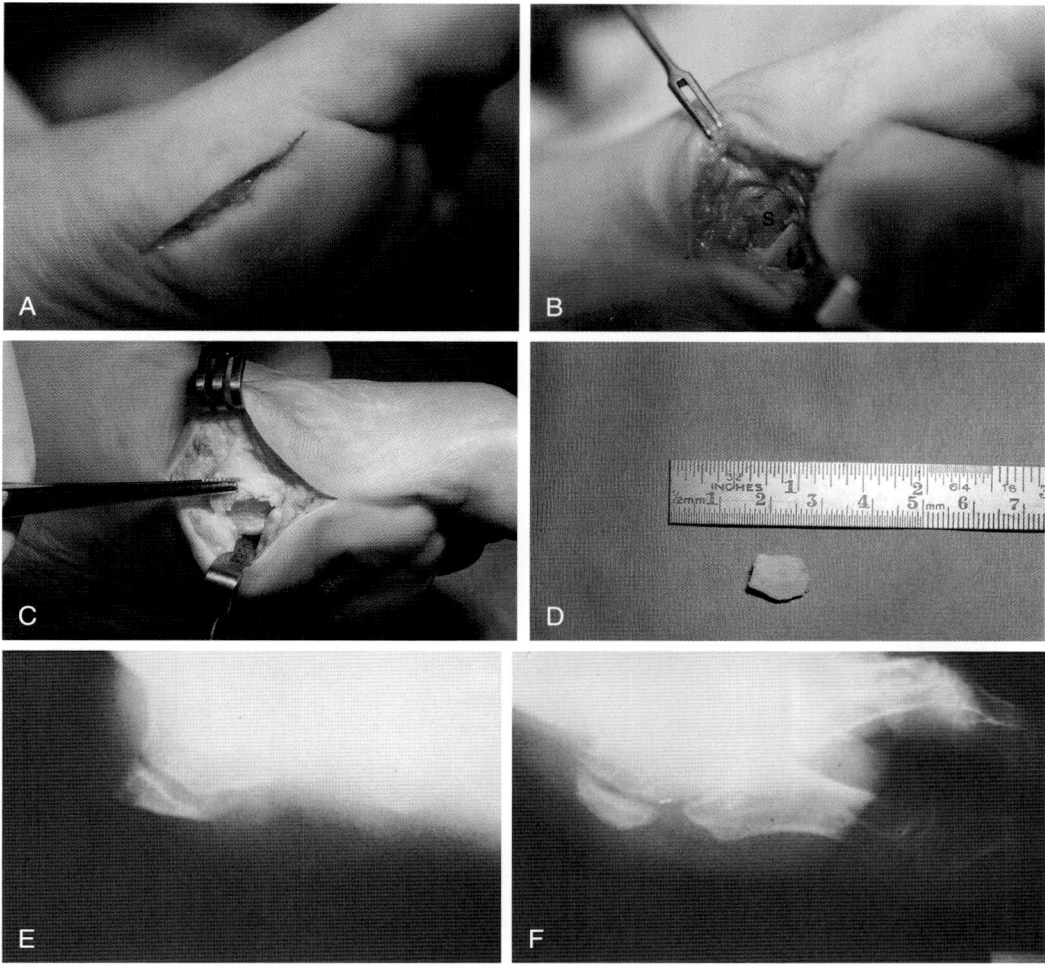

Figure 8-23 Tibial sesamoid shaving. **A,** Skin incision is made just below the midline and carried down to expose the joint capsule. The plantar medial cutaneous nerve is identified and retracted. **B,** After the tibial sesamoid is exposed, the plantar half is removed (*s,* sesamoid; *f,* flexor hallucis longus tendon). **C,** Appearance after excision of the plantar aspect of the tibial sesamoid. **D,** Excised piece of the tibial sesamoid. **E** and **F,** Axial and lateral radiographs demonstrate tibial sesamoid after removal of the plantar half. (**C** and **D** from Mann RA: Intractable plantar keratosis *Instr Course Lect* 33:289, 1984.)

Postoperative Care

The patient is kept in a postoperative shoe with the foot in a firm dressing for 3 weeks and then is permitted to ambulate as tolerated.

Results

A follow-up study of 12 of our patients demonstrated that 58% had excellent results with no recurrent callus, 33% had good results with slight recurrence of the callus, and 1 patient (9%) had a fair result and required periodic trimming of the plantar callus.[43] All patients maintained full range of motion of the first MTP joint, and none had a painful scar.

Complications

The most significant complication after this procedure is injury to the medial plantar cutaneous nerve. If this occurs and is noted at surgery, the surgeon must consider freeing up the nerve more proximally and moving it away from the plantar aspect of the foot. If the damage to the nerve appears to be too severe, the surgeon must consider whether the nerve should be sectioned and buried beneath the abductor hallucis muscle to prevent a neuroma from forming on the plantar medial aspect of the foot.

Further discussion of tibial sesamoid shaving is presented in Chapter 10.

Diffuse Intractable Plantar Keratosis

At times, the second metatarsal and/or third metatarsal are long because of the anatomic pattern of the foot. Whether a true plantar-flexed metatarsal exists, except after trauma, has not been adequately demonstrated. A diffuse IPK beneath a lesser metatarsal head may be caused by a transfer lesion as a result of an adjacent metatarsal osteotomy or trauma. A diffuse IPK beneath several

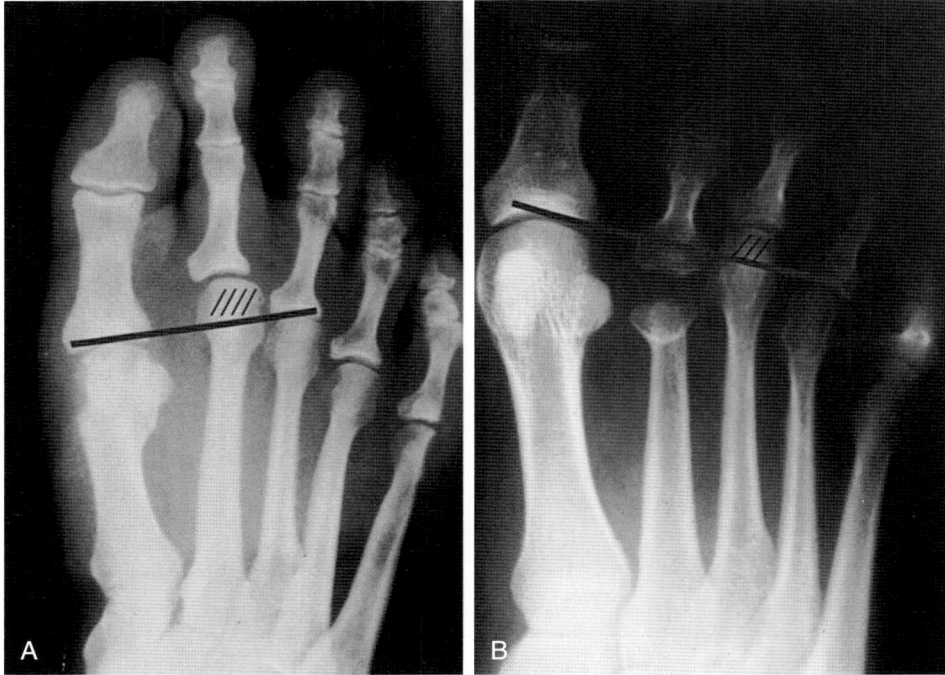

Figure 8-24 Metatarsal shortening. **A,** Line is drawn from first to third metatarsal head. This indicates the amount that the second metatarsal head needs to be shortened. **B,** Line is drawn between first and fourth metatarsal head to indicate the amount of shortening required to create a smooth metatarsal pattern.

metatarsal heads is mainly attributable to the lack of weight bearing by the first metatarsal. In support of this, there are those who believe that callosities under the lesser metatarsals will resolve if a hallux valgus deformity is corrected without performing concurrent procedures.[38]

In attempting to be as precise as possible in the treatment of a diffuse IPK, if the offending metatarsal(s) is long, it should be shortened to reestablish the metatarsal cascade (Fig. 8-24). The precise amount of desired shortening should be planned preoperatively. There are various templates available to determine the desired shortening, and digital radiographs allow precise measurements without templates. If a diffuse callus results because of a transfer lesion and the metatarsal is not long, we prefer to carry out a basal osteotomy to bring the metatarsal head to the same level as the adjacent metatarsals.

When a metatarsal osteotomy of any type is considered, it is imperative that a contracture of the MTP joint is not present. An MTP joint fixed in a dorsiflexed position can cause a painful plantar callosity that should be managed by correction of the MTP joint and not the metatarsal.

OBLIQUE METATARSAL OSTEOTOMY
The concept of the oblique metatarsal osteotomy was described by Giannestras,[20] who produced a proximal step-cut osteotomy to shorten the symptomatic

metatarsal. In his series of 40 patients, 10% developed a transfer lesion. Finding this surgical procedure technically difficult, we modified it to an oblique longitudinal osteotomy (Figs. 8-25 and 8-26). This is technically simpler and gives uniformly satisfactory results.[41]

Surgical Technique
1. The skin incision is a long dorsal incision centered over the involved metatarsal. It is developed through subcutaneous tissue and fat, with great caution taken to identify and retract the cutaneous nerves. The involved metatarsal is identified, an incision is made over its dorsal aspect down to the bone, and the metatarsal is exposed subperiosteally (Fig. 8-27A).
2. If more than 5 to 6 mm of shortening is required, the transverse metatarsal ligament needs to be sectioned, particularly when shortening the third and fourth metatarsals. This is usually not necessary for the second metatarsal.
3. Before the osteotomy is performed, a transverse mark is etched in the metatarsal at the midportion of the osteotomy so that as the osteotomy site is displaced, the surgeon can measure precisely how much shortening is occurring. With a thin saw blade, an oblique osteotomy as long as possible is produced in the metatarsal shaft. When an osteotomy is performed in the second metatarsal, the base should be directed laterally to avoid bringing the saw blade into the interspace between the base of the first and second metatarsals

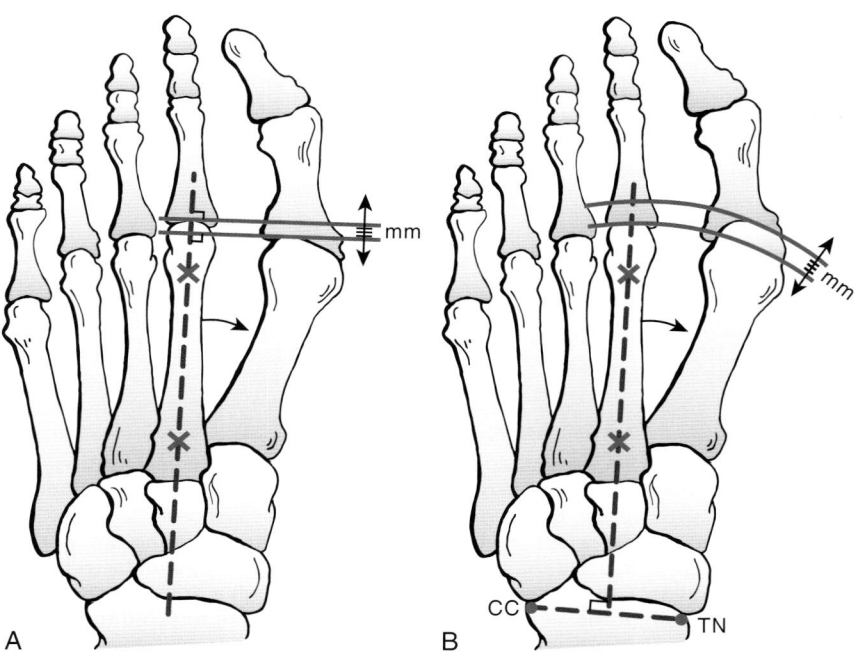

Figure 8-25   Two alternative methods of measuring metatarsal length. **A,** Morton method, or the straight-line method, compares relative length of second and third metatarsals. With increasing metatarsus primus varus, the first metatarsal "measures shorter" compared with the second. **B,** With the "arc method," alignment of the first ray does not affect the comparison of the length of the first and lesser metatarsals.

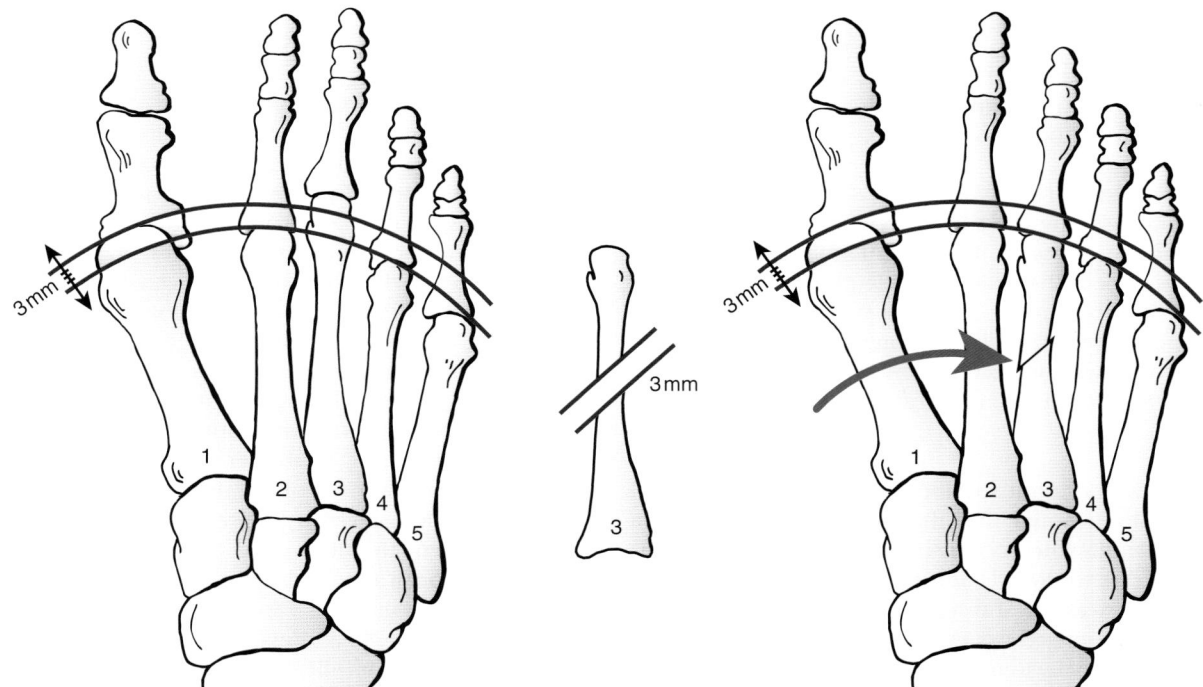

Figure 8-26   Midshaft shortening oblique osteotomy of the third metatarsal to reestablish the metatarsal cascade. The surgeon can choose from a variety of internal fixation techniques.

where the communicating artery passes (Fig. 8-27B and C).

4. The osteotomy site can be fixated with cerclage wires, small-fragment screws, or a plate. We find that two cerclage wires produce satisfactory immobilization. One of the pieces of wire passes through the bone in its corrected length to control the length of the metatarsal (Fig. 8-27D and E). Small-fragment screws can be used, but technically this is difficult, and at times the bone splinters. The use of a mini-fragment plate would seem ideal, but we found a significant nonunion rate.

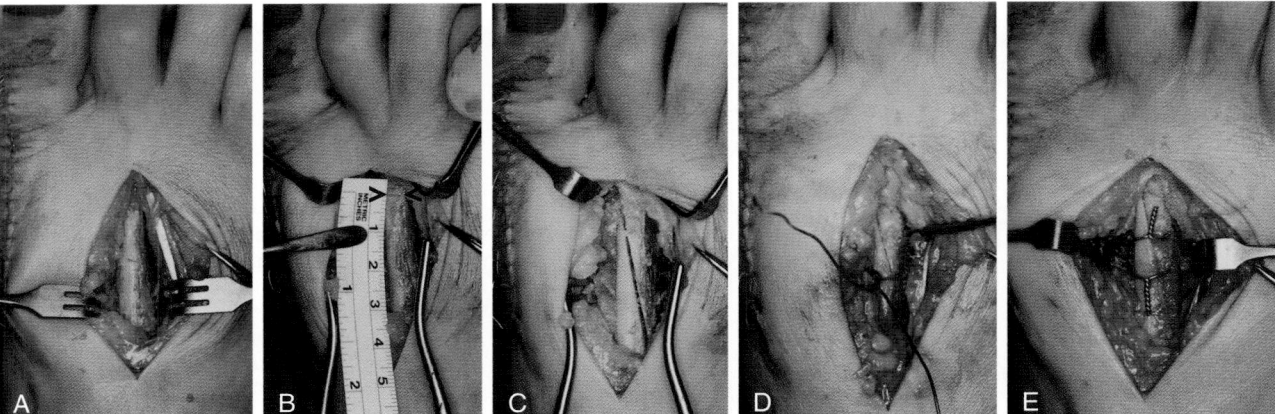

Figure 8-27 Surgical technique of oblique metatarsal osteotomy. **A,** Metatarsal is exposed through a longitudinal incision. Care is taken to avoid superficial nerves. Incision is made along the periosteum of the metatarsal, and muscle tissue is stripped from the metatarsal shaft. **B,** Mark is made on metatarsal *(arrowheads),* then a ruler is used to mark a fixed distance on the metatarsal so the bone can be shortened accurately. **C,** Long oblique osteotomy has been made. When carrying this out on the second metatarsal, the osteotomy is made on this diagonal so as to avoid the artery in the first web space. **D,** Metatarsal is accurately shortened by using the marks on the bone as a guide. First the cerclage wire is passed through a drill hole after the metatarsal has been shortened. This helps to stabilize the length of the metatarsal. **E,** Second cerclage wire is placed to help increase stability of the osteotomy site.

5. An attempt is made to repair the periosteum over the metatarsal shaft, and the skin is closed in a routine manner. A snug compression dressing is applied for the initial 18 to 24 hours.

Postoperative Care
Postoperatively, the dressing is changed to a firm 2-inch Kling and tape dressing. The patient ambulates in a postoperative shoe if the fixation is adequate, and if not, the patient is placed into a short-leg walking cast. Healing usually occurs in 8 weeks. Although at times it appears that the healing is proceeding very slowly, in reality, clinically the osteotomy site has healed (Fig. 8-28).

Results
Although we have not specifically reviewed our series of cases, we have noted that the main complication is a transfer lesion, which occurs in about 10% of cases. This is usually due to dorsiflexion of the distal fragment and not due to excessive shortening. Rigid internal fixation using two oblique screws can alleviate this problem.

A recent study by Kennedy and Deland[34] evaluated this procedure in 32 consecutive patients. Twenty-two patients had a single osteotomy of the second metatarsal, and 10 had an osteotomy of the second and third metatarsals. Pain was relieved in 31 of 32 patients, and there were no transfer lesions. The median time to radiographic union was 10 weeks. The authors pointed out that they carefully adjusted the metatarsal length radiographically, as well as carefully palpating the plantar aspect of the foot to judge whether the correct amount of shortening had been achieved. The mean radiographic shortening was 3.4 mm (range, 1 to 5 mm).

DISTAL METATARSAL OSTEOTOMY (WEIL OSTEOTOMY)
Many surgeons who utilize the Weil osteotomy report on the treatment of a subluxed or dislocated MTP joint, which, although producing metatarsalgia, might not result in an intractable plantar keratosis. Furthermore, their articles discussing this procedure do not say whether or not a keratotic lesion per se was present,[51,60,62] whereas others note that the Weil osteotomy can be very effective in resolving an IPK.[5,28] The Weil osteotomy can produce shortening of up to approximately 1 cm, which can be useful in managing the patient with a diffuse IPK beneath the second metatarsal brought about by shortening of the first metatarsal. The Weil osteotomy can also be useful for a transfer metatarsalgia problem. Whether it would be useful for the treatment of the discrete IPK beneath the fibular condyle has yet to be presented in the literature. Seventy percent to 100% good and excellent long-term results have been reported.[28,29,58,60] Advantages include a high union rate, the ability to correct significant deformities, and the ability to address adjacent metatarsals via the same incision. Complications can be significant and include stiffness, floating toe deformity,[48] transfer lesions, nonunion and malunion, recurrent deformity, plantar penetration of hardware, and vascular compromise leading to amputation.[28,48]

The maximum shortening achieved by Kennedy and Deland[34] was 5 mm, which can be easily achieved by the Weil osteotomy. Other authors report shortenings from 3 mm to 12 mm.[5,48] Based upon our experience, we believe that up to 1 cm of shortening can be obtained with the Weil osteotomy without difficulty and may be preferred to the long oblique diaphyseal osteotomy in

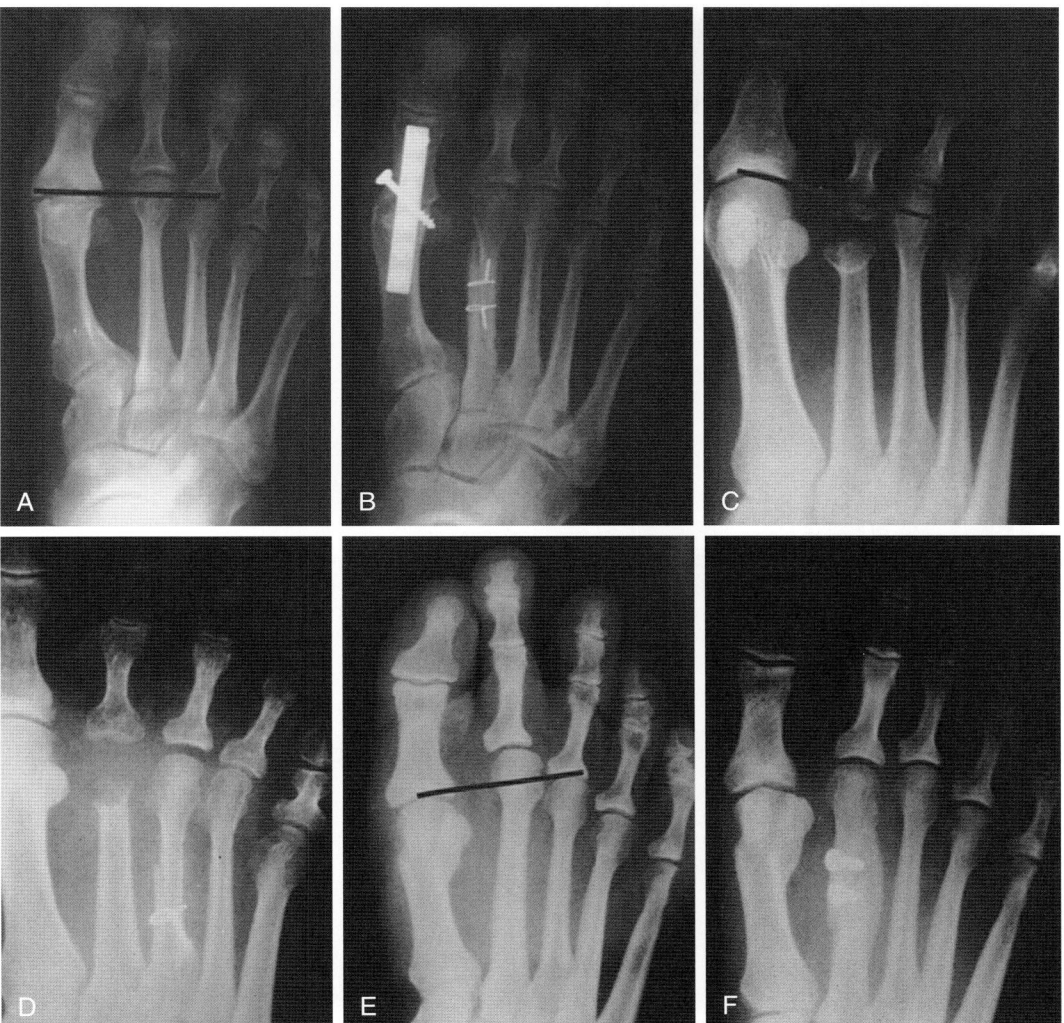

Figure 8-28 Preoperative **(A)** and postoperative **(B)** radiographs demonstrate shortening of the second metatarsal to create a smooth metatarsal arch. Preoperative **(C)** and postoperative **(D)** radiographs demonstrate shortening of the third metatarsal after resection of the second metatarsal head to create a smooth metatarsal pattern. Preoperative **(E)** and postoperative **(F)** radiographs demonstrate shortening of the second metatarsal by means of screw fixation.

cases in which a centimeter or less of shortening is necessary (Video Clip 70). The Weil osteotomy can also be done on multiple metatarsals with less chance of producing elevation of one of the metatarsal heads as compared to the diaphyseal osteotomy (Fig. 8-29). Shortening, plantar flexion, and a combination of both can be achieved with this osteotomy, depending on the angle of the saw cut.[5] A "triple" Weil osteotomy has also been reported in the literature,[15] which reportedly can minimize plantar displacement of the capital fragment and allow for shortening.

The plantar inclination of the metatarsals can greatly influence the displacement (dorsal or plantar) of the capital fragment as the fragment is displaced proximally. In the cadaveric study by Grimes and Coughlin,[23] the average plantar inclination of the second metatarsal averaged 25 degrees (however, the range of inclination was

19 to 31 degrees). Thus the angle of the osteotomy plays a significant role in whether elevation or depression of the capital fragment occurs with proximal translation. Ideally, the longitudinal saw cut should be parallel to the plantar surface of the foot to prevent plantar displacement of the capital segment (Fig. 8-30A). (A complete discussion of the Weil-type osteotomy is contained in Chapter 7.) The actual width of the saw cut ("the kerf") plays a critical role in whether the capital fragment displaces dorsally or plantarly with shortening. We have found[23] that with a longitudinal cut parallel with the plantar surface of the foot, a thin blade may be sufficient because little plantar translation occurs. With feet having a plantar inclination of the metatarsals less than 25 degrees, a thicker blade should be selected (or a small wafer of bone from the metatarsal head is removed, using two parallel saw cuts) (Fig. 8-30B). This allows up to 8 to

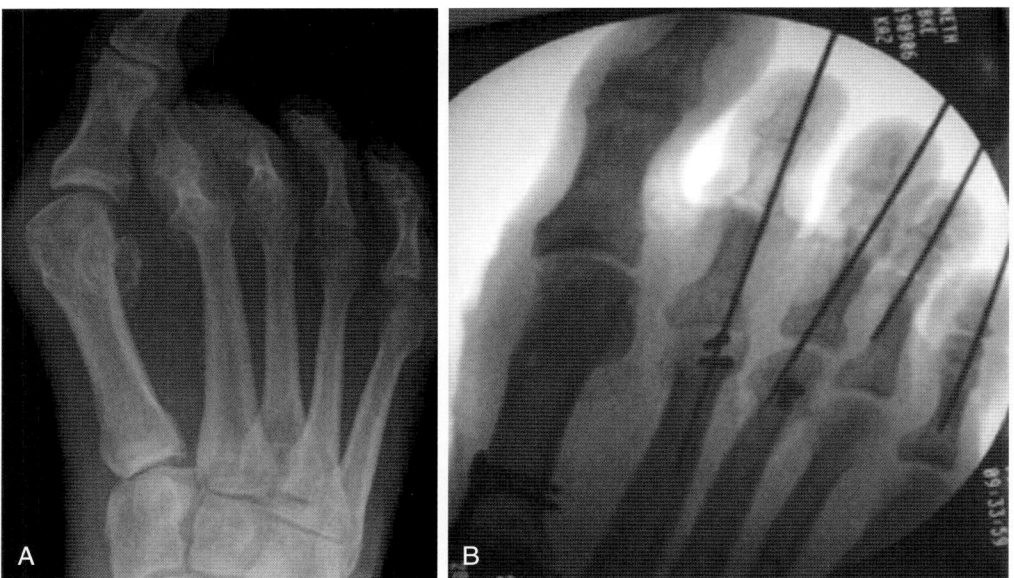

Figure 8-29 **A,** Anteroposterior (AP) radiograph of a patient with a hallux valgus deformity, dislocations of the second and third metatarsophalangeal (MTP) joints, and a second crossover toe. This patient had significant callus formation under the second and third metatarsal heads. **B,** Intraoperative fluoroscopy shot of the same patient in **A** demonstrating correction of the hallux valgus deformity, shortening of the second and third metatarsals by Weil osteotomies, and hammer toe repairs of the lesser toes. Note the re-creation of the metatarsal cascade.

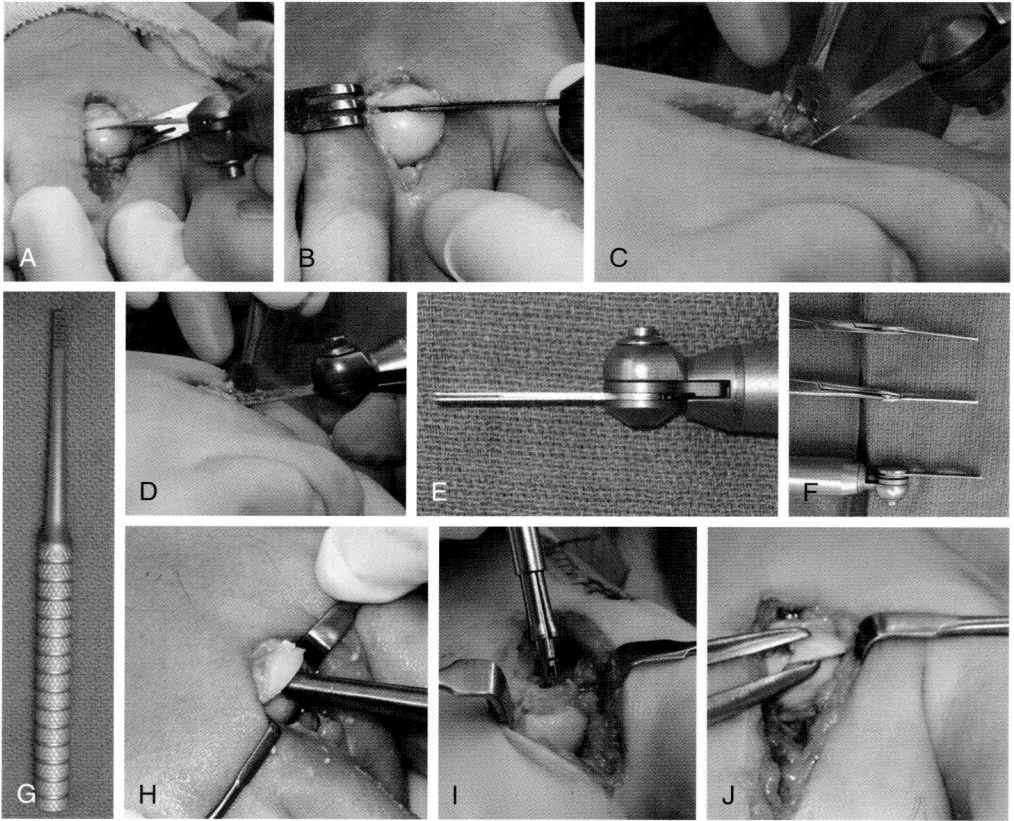

Figure 8-30 **A,** Single-blade Weil osteotomy for intractable plantar keratosis (IPK). **B,** Double-blade Weil cut with two blades to increase the "kerf" of the saw cut to elevate the capital fragment. **C,** Position of an oblique cut, which likely will cause plantar displacement of the capital fragment as it is displaced proximalward. **D,** More horizontal cut, in line with plantar surface of the foot, which likely will cause less plantar displacement of capital fragment. **E,** Close-up photograph of triple-stacked blades. **F,** Using thicker blades can increase the kerf of the saw cut. **G,** A calibrated pusher can assist in achieving the desired shortening of the osteotomy. **H** and **I,** The osteotomy is translated proximally and fixed with a vertical mini-fragment screw. **J,** The dorsal wedge of bone from the dorsal fragment is removed.

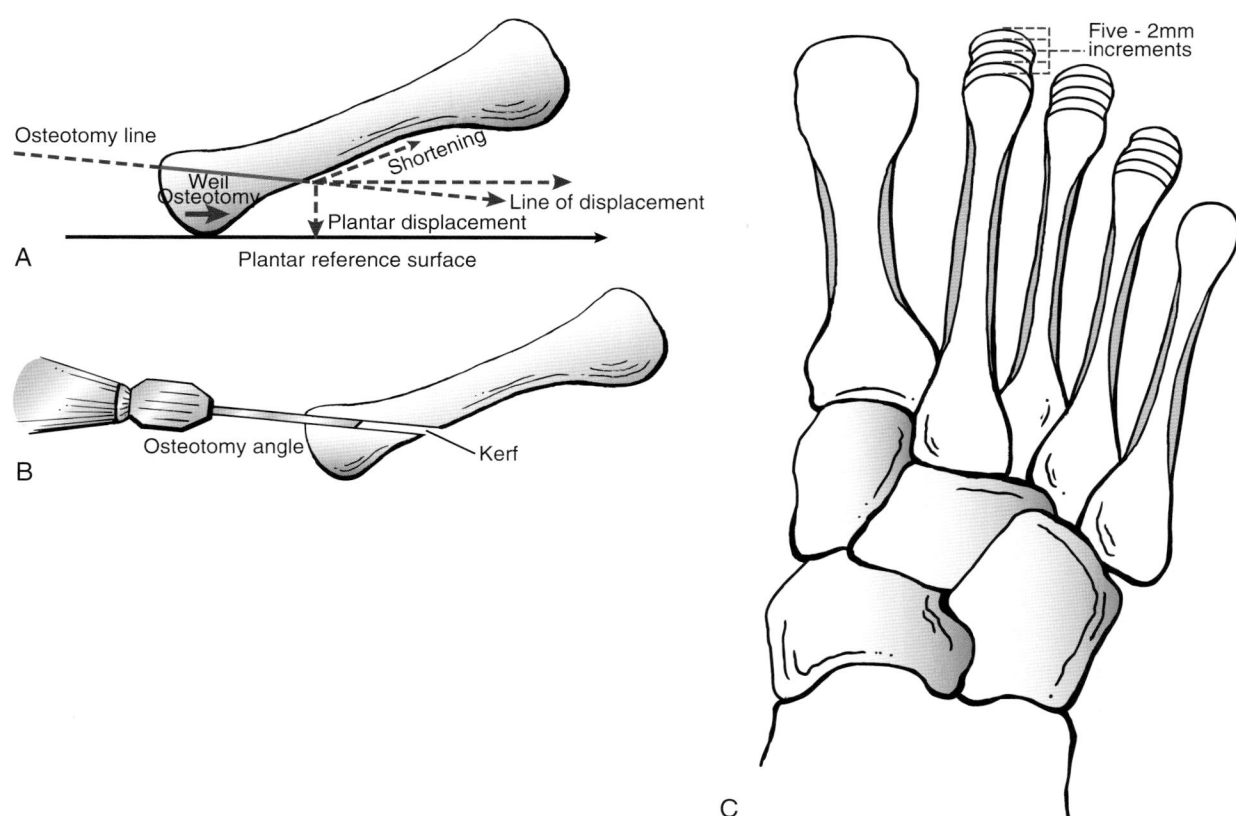

Figure 8-31 Schematic diagram of Weil osteotomy. **A,** As the osteotomy is shortened, the capital fragment is frequently depressed plantarward, increasing plantar pressure. **B,** Plantar displacement can be reduced by either the use of a thick saw blade or removing a section of bone as the Weil osteotomy is performed. **C,** Preoperative planning is helpful in deciding the amount of shortening to be achieved with each Weil osteotomy. An acetate overlay can be used to template the shortening.

10 mm of shortening without plantar displacement of the capital fragment.

The capital fragment moves along the longitudinal axis of the metatarsal bone. This movement results in both dorsal displacement of the capital fragment and shortening of the metatarsal along the plantar plane. The dorsal movement of the capital segment, resulting from the kerf of the saw blade, counteracts the depression of the capital segment (Fig. 8-31).

Surgical Technique

1. An incision is made in the web space, similar to an incision for a neuroma excision. The dissection is carried down through the subcutaneous tissue and fat. The extensor tendons are identified and retracted.
2. The MTP joint is accessed by elevating capsular tissue and periosteum off the metatarsal neck, head, and proximal aspect of the proximal phalanx. If done longitudinally, this can often be repaired after the osteotomy is completed.
3. The soft tissues are retracted medially and laterally, and the toe is plantar flexed. This exposes the metatarsal head.
4. A Weil osteotomy is then performed, with the cut beginning at the dorsal one fifth of the metatarsal head, taking care to orient the saw blade parallel to the sole of the foot (Fig. 8-30A to D).[23] If more than 6 to 7 mm of shortening is desired, a stacked saw blade can be utilized to remove a kerf of bone that will result in increased shortening. These stacked blades should be oriented with the blades converging, as opposed to diverging, to ensure control and prevent removal of too large a kerf (Fig. 8-30B, E, and F).
5. The osteotomy can be shortened precisely according to preoperative templating (Fig. 8-31C) by the use of a striated measuring device or a K-wire with an appropriately placed pen mark (see Fig. 8-30G and H). The osteotomy can be temporarily fixated with a 0.45-inch K-wire, and its position is checked with fluoroscopy. The head can be rotated around the K-wire if lateral orientation of the articular surface is desired, as when repairing a crossover toe deformity.
6. If the metatarsal cascade is re-created in acceptable alignment, the osteotomy can be permanently fixed with mini-fragment screws (see Fig. 8-30I and J). The authors' preference is to place the first screw in standard interfragmentary compression technique, drilling the near cortex with a 2.0 drill and the far cortex

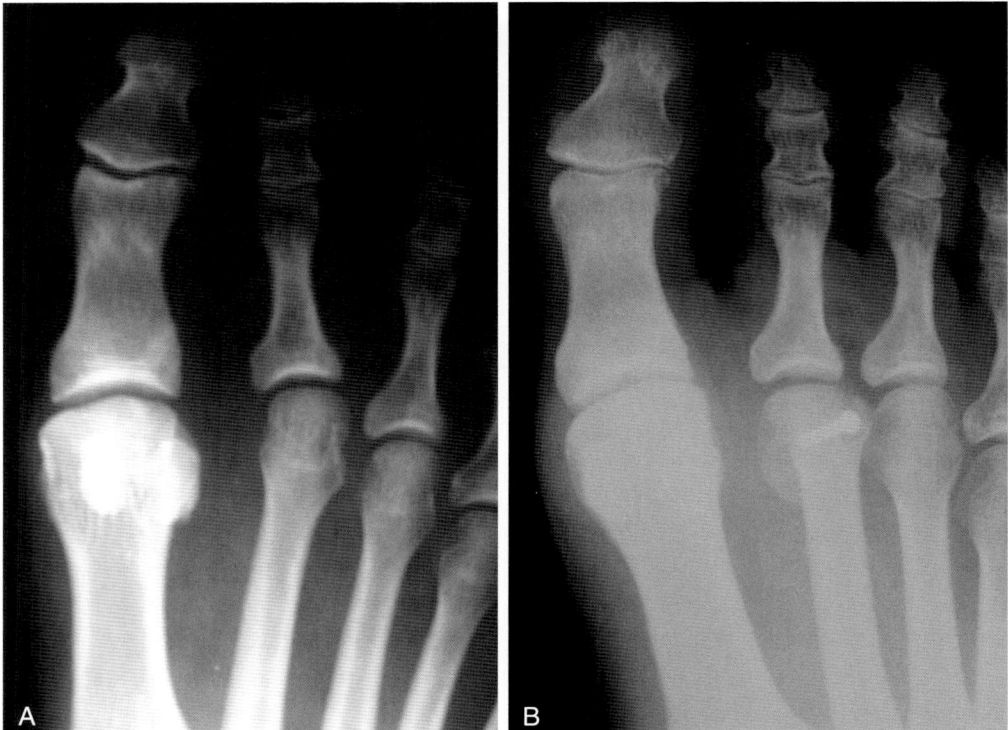

Figure 8-32 Preoperative **(A)** and postoperative **(B)** radiographs demonstrating substantial shortening of the Weil osteotomy for metatarsalgia.

with a 1.5 drill. The appropriate-length 2.0 screw is then placed (usually a 10- or 12-mm–length screw) while pushing up on the plantar surface of the distal metatarsal to aid in compression. Once this screw is tightened, the K-wire is removed, and a second screw of similar length is placed in the K-wire hole. This second screw adds stability and rotational control (Fig. 8-32). Grimes[24] found a 12-mm length of screw to be adequate in length to fix the ostetotomy in most cases, but it rarely penetrated the plantar surface of the lesser metatarsal capital fragment.

7. The protruding dorsal lip is then removed with a small rongeur.

8. A 0.45- or 0.62-inch K-wire is then driven retrograde through the middle of the articular surface of the proximal phalanx, through the middle and distal phalanges, and out the tip of the toe. The toe is then plantar flexed approximately 30 degrees and deviated laterally, and the K-wire then driven across the MTP joint and into the metatarsal head. This slightly exaggerated correction is helpful in allowing the soft tissues to scar at the correct tension, thereby minimizing the risk of excessive dorsiflexion or a floating toe after K-wire removal.

9. The joint is irrigated and capsular tissue repaired if on the side of the apex of deformity (e.g., on the lateral side of the second MTP joint with a second crossover toe). Alternatively, a tendon transfer (either an extensor digitorum brevis transfer[32] or a flexor to extensor

transfer[50]) or plantar plate repair can be used to aid in deformity correction.

10. The K-wire is bent and cut, and the skin is closed with 3-0 or 4-0 nylon. A compression dressing is then applied, and the foot is placed into a hard-soled postoperative shoe.

11. The patient is allowed to bear weight only on the heel for 6 weeks. The K-wire is removed at 3 to 4 weeks postoperatively. Range-of-motion exercises of the lesser MTP joints are begun at 6 weeks, at which time the patient is allowed to walk on the front of the foot in a postoperative shoe to simulate dorsiflexion during the push-off phase of the gait cycle. The patient then transitions into a regular shoe that can accommodate the foot, as tolerated.

Alternative Weil Osteotomy

1. When substantial shortening occurs, the capital fragment can be displaced plantarward and actually increase metatarsalgia (Fig. 8-33).

2. Alternatively, after the first cut, a parallel cut is made and a small segment of bone (2-3 mm) is removed (Fig. 8-34).

3. This allows dorsal translation of the capital fragment as shortening of the osteotomy site is achieved.

BASAL METATARSAL OSTEOTOMY

The basal metatarsal osteotomy is used when a diffuse IPK is present and there is no metatarsal shortening. This

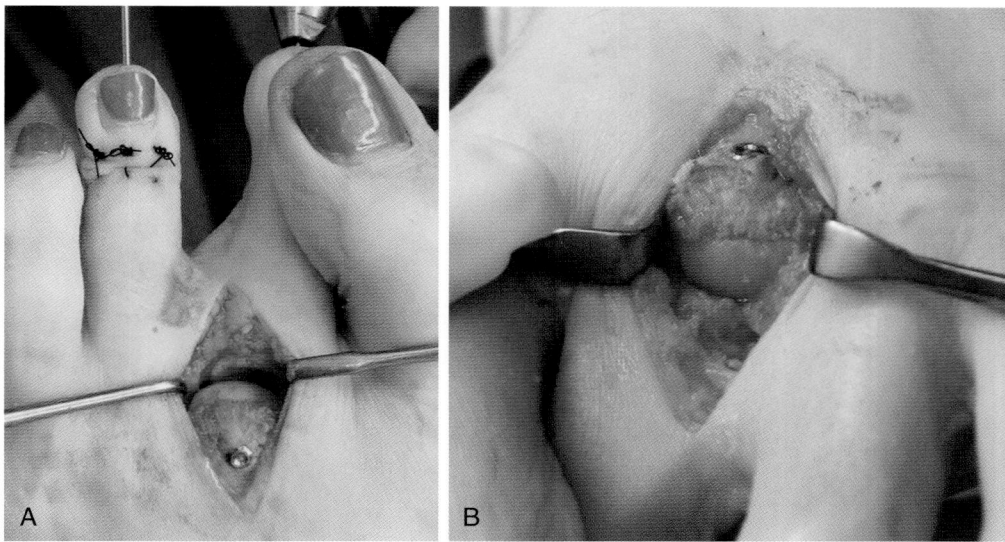

Figure 8-33 Weil osteotomy without bone resection. **A,** The final position of the osteotomy. **B,** Close-up of the end of the fixed osteotomy demonstrates how plantar displacement can occur. A resection of a wafer of bone as marked would lessen the plantar displacement of the capital fragment.

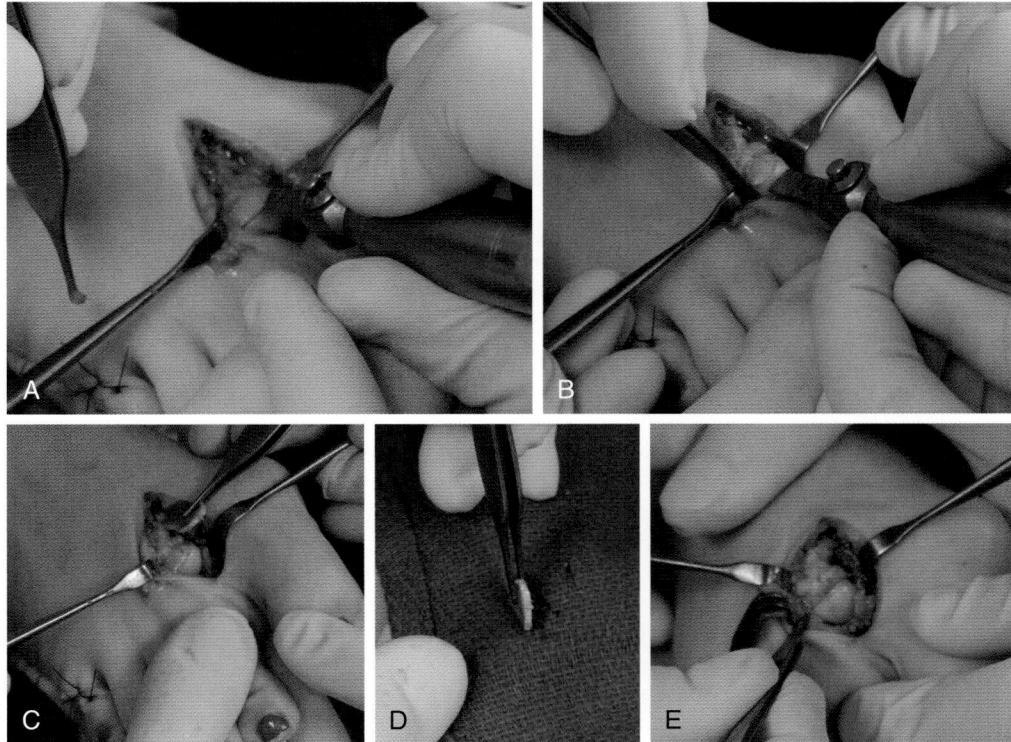

Figure 8-34 Weil osteotomy with segmental resection of bone. **A,** Initial cut for Weil osteotomy. **B,** Second cut parallel to first removing small segment of bone to allow dorsal displacement of capital fragment. **C,** The osteotomy is closed; the segment has been removed. **D,** The segment is 2 mm thick, so with the saw kerf, approximately 3 mm has been removed. **E,** Final appearance after internal fixation has been placed.

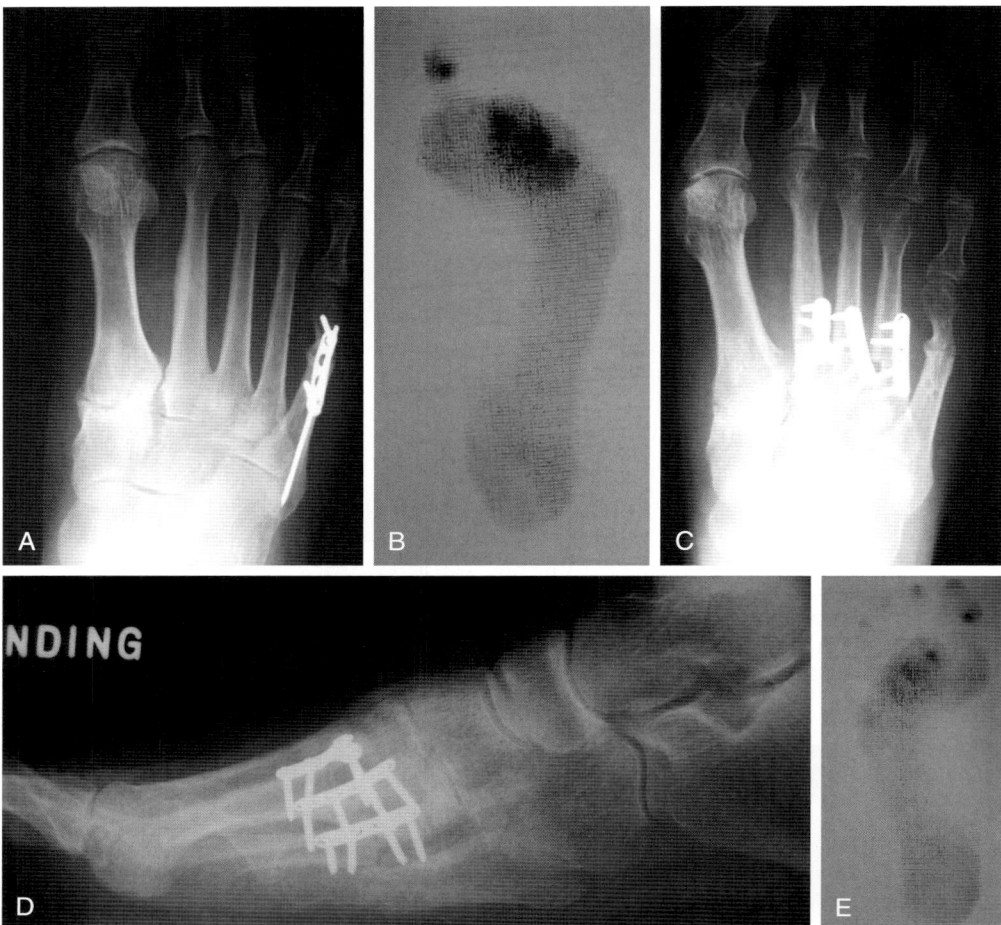

Figure 8-35 **A** and **B,** Preoperative radiograph and Harris mat of a patient who had undergone surgery on the fifth metatarsal for a bunionette correction. This led to transfer lesions under the second, third, and fourth metatarsal heads. **C** and **D,** Postoperative anteroposterior (AP) and lateral radiographs of the same patient after dorsiflexion osteotomies of the second, third, and fourth metatarsals. **E,** Note the significantly improved redistribution of weight bearing on the Harris mat.

condition usually occurs after previous metatarsal surgery or a fracture (Fig. 8-35).

Surgical Technique

1. The skin incision is made over the dorsal aspect of the proximal half of the metatarsal and carried down through subcutaneous tissue and fat, with great caution taken to avoid the cutaneous nerves.
2. The dorsal aspect of the involved metatarsal is identified, and an incision is made along the dorsal aspect of the metatarsal from about the midshaft area to the base. The periosteum is then stripped.
3. The site of the osteotomy should be just at the flare of the base of the metatarsal. If it is carried out much more proximal to this, the saw blade bounces off the adjacent metatarsals, and it is difficult to produce an accurate cut.
4. The size of the dorsally based wedge that is removed depends on the degree of depression of the metatarsal head. The involved metatarsal head usually needs to

be elevated 2 to 4 mm, and thus the size of the base of the wedge should usually not exceed 2 to 3 mm. As the osteotomy is cut, an attempt is made to leave a plantar hinge intact.

5. We prefer to fix the osteotomy site by placing a 2.7-mm screw into the proximal portion of the base of the metatarsal, drilling a transverse hole distal to the osteotomy site, and then fixing these two points with a piece of 22-gauge wire (Fig. 8-36). In this way, the osteotomy site can be completely closed, with the metatarsal held in its precise position. There are other ways to fix the osteotomy site with a screw or pin, but we have found this technique to be the most reliable (see Fig. 8-35).
6. The periosteum is closed, if possible, as is the skin. A compression dressing is applied.

Postoperative Care

The patient ambulates in a postoperative shoe until healing occurs in approximately 4 to 6 weeks. With the

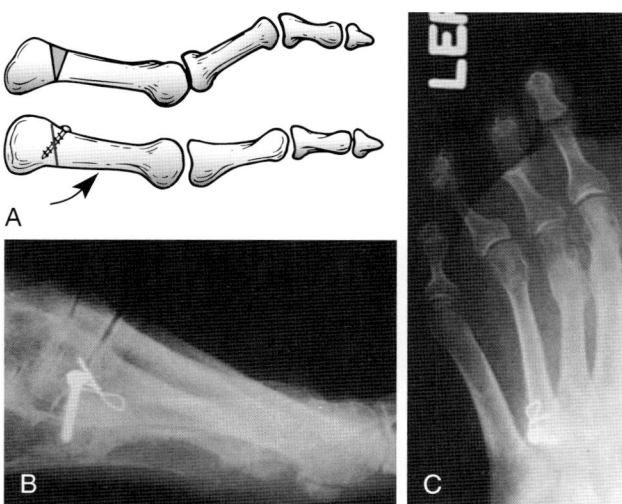

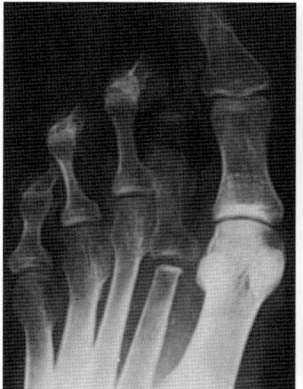
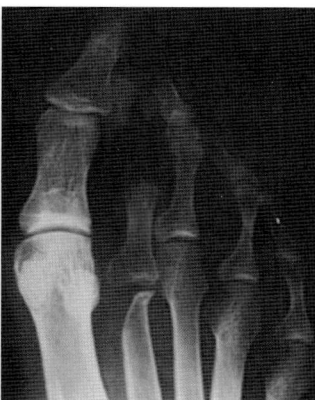

Figure 8-37 Resection of metatarsal head for intractable plantar keratosis should be avoided. After this procedure, there is significant foreshortening of the toe, and a transfer lesion develops beneath the adjacent metatarsal head.

Figure 8-36 Technique of basal metatarsal osteotomy. **A,** Diagram demonstrates basal osteotomy in which a dorsally based wedge of bone is removed from the affected metatarsal. **B** and **C,** Radiographs demonstrate basal osteotomy with fixation done by using screw-and-wire tension band.

compression obtained by this method of fixation, we have had rapid healing of the osteotomy site and no nonunions. We have not tabulated our cases, but the postoperative incidence of transfer lesions is likely less than 5%, probably because in these cases, one can accurately produce the degree of dorsiflexion necessary to correct the problem. The only other potential problem with this procedure is entrapment of a dorsal cutaneous nerve, which can usually be avoided.

Dorsiflexion Osteotomy of First Metatarsal for Plantar-Flexed First Metatarsal

This procedure is described in Chapter 20.

Other Metatarsal Osteotomies

Many types of osteotomies have been described for treating a plantar callus. Most authors have not attempted to define the type of callus (diffuse or discrete) that is being treated, as we have. The surgeon should attempt to apply the scientific method to the treatment of a plantar callus, carefully identifying the type of callus and then selecting a surgical procedure for the condition.

Helal[25] and Greiss[27] described a *distal oblique metatarsal osteotomy* of the three middle metatarsals, to relieve metatarsalgia. In theory, the osteotomy permits the metatarsal head to slide proximally, and by early ambulation, the "tread" would be leveled. In a follow-up study of this procedure, 77% of patients had good results. In a further follow-up study by Winson et al[63] of 94 patients (124 feet) who underwent this procedure, 53% had significant postoperative symptoms, including a nonunion rate of 13%, an incidence of transfer lesions of 32%, and a recurrence of the keratosis in 50% of patients. Another study of the Helal osteotomy reported only 61% good or

excellent results, with a high percentage of cases failing to find their own optimum position.[59] The authors discourage the use of floating osteotomies because the results are less than ideal.

Pedowitz,[51] using a distal oblique osteotomy and early ambulation for a single plantar callus of unspecified type, reported good results in 83% of patients. He did note a 25% incidence of either residual keratosis or transfer lesions. Treatment of a single IPK by resection of a metatarsal head should be avoided, except when an infection or chronic ulcer has occurred. Resection of a metatarsal head only leads to significant problems, including development of a transfer lesion beneath an adjacent metatarsal head, shortening and contracture of the involved toe, and, in general, significantly more problems than are solved (Fig. 8-37).

When two adjacent metatarsals are significantly longer than the others, as is occasionally noted after significant shortening of the first metatarsal with a bunion procedure, shortening of the two metatarsals may be considered. Osteotomies that allow the metatarsal heads to float or to level the tread should be discouraged (Fig. 8-38). Precise preoperative templating and internal fixation to accurately elevate or shorten a metatarsal is important.

MISCELLANEOUS CONDITIONS

Subhallux Sesamoid

At times, a midline callus is present beneath the great toe at the level of the IP joint. This callus can become quite large and can occasionally even ulcerate. The callus is caused by a subhallux sesamoid, which is a sesamoid bone lying just dorsal to the flexor hallucis longus tendon before it inserts into the base of the distal phalanx. Radiographs demonstrate the sesamoid beneath the IP joint region (Fig. 8-39).

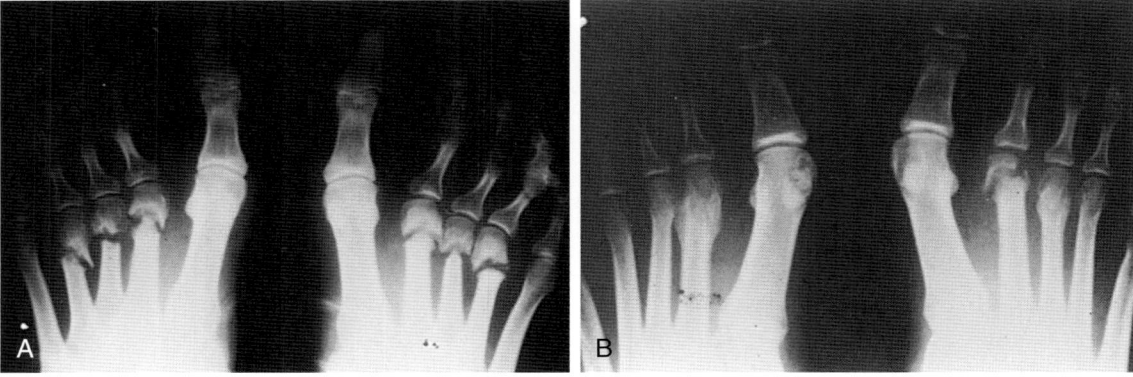

Figure 8-38 Complications after use of a high-speed bur to produce metatarsal osteotomies. **A,** Nonunions of six metatarsal necks. **B,** Radiograph of the left foot demonstrates abundance of new bone formation after the second metatarsal osteotomy. Radiograph of the right foot demonstrates nonunion through the second metatarsal head as well as joint involvement with osteotomy.

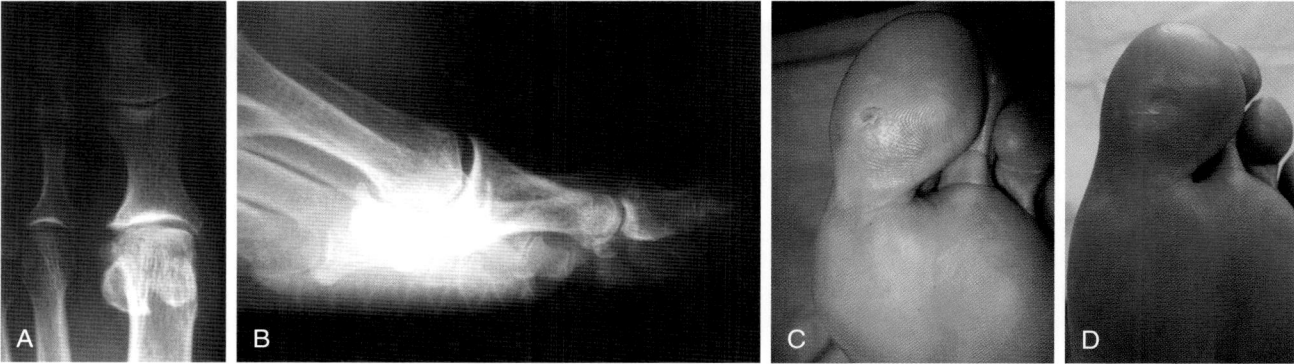

Figure 8-39 **A** and **B,** Anteroposterior (AP) and lateral radiographs of a subhallux sesamoid. This caused a painful callus under the interphalangeal (IP) joint of the hallux **(C),** which was initially treated with debridement **(D)** but eventually went on to require surgical excision.

Conservative Treatment

Nonsurgical treatment involves trimming of the callus and placing a small felt pad just proximal to the lesion to keep pressure off the callus area. If this fails, surgical intervention usually results in satisfactory resolution of the callus.

SURGICAL TREATMENT: REMOVAL OF SUBHALLUX SESAMOID

Surgical Technique

1. A longitudinal incision is made along the medial side of the hallux, starting a little plantar to the midline. The incision starts at about the level of the MTP joint and is carried distally beyond the IP joint.
2. The skin flap is reflected plantarward, to the flexor tendon sheath, with some caution used because the plantar medial cutaneous nerve is in the plantar flap. The flexor hallucis longus sheath is identified and opened to expose the flexor tendon up to its insertion into the base of the distal phalanx.
3. The flexor tendon is retracted plantarward, and the sesamoid is noted on the dorsal aspect of the tendon

just before its insertion into the phalanx. The sesamoid is carefully shelled out, with care taken not to detach the tendon from its insertion. Flexion of the IP joint will relax the flexor tendon, allowing easier removal of the sesamoid. If the flexor tendon is inadvertently detached from its insertion, it can be reattached through dorsal drill holes.
4. The wound is closed in a single layer, and a compression dressing is applied.

Postoperative Care

The patient ambulates in a postoperative shoe for approximately 3 weeks, until the soft tissue has healed, after which activities are permitted as tolerated.

Results

The results after excision of a subhallux sesamoid are uniformly satisfactory. The callus rarely, if ever, reforms. The only possible significant complication would result from inadvertently detaching the flexor hallucis longus tendon when the sesamoid is excised. This can be avoided by careful surgical technique.

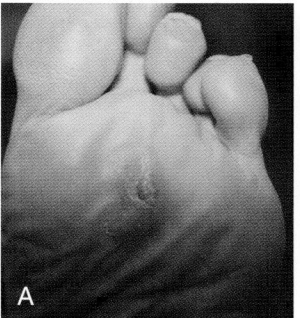 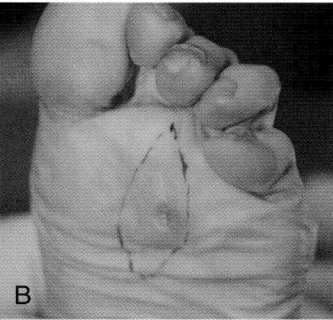 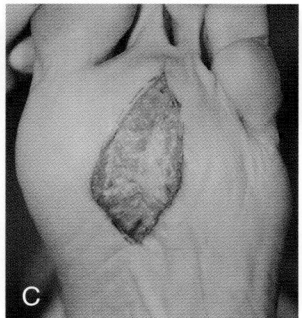 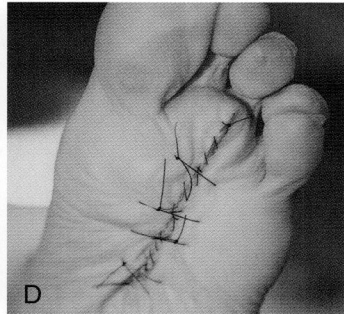

Figure 8-40 Surgical technique used to excise intractable plantar scar with callus formation. **A,** Keratotic scar. Note central hyperkeratotic lesion and surrounding adherent atrophic scar tissue. **B,** Outline of elliptic incision used to excise scar. **C,** Full-thickness removal of plantar skin, which is then undermined to mobilize it. **D,** Skin closure is carried out with retension sutures, a subdermal layer to minimize tension on the skin edge, and a fine, running cutaneous stitch to minimize scar formation.

Intractable Plantar Callus Associated with Significant Scar Tissue Formation

Occasionally, a significant scar is present on the plantar aspect of the foot. This could result from prior surgery, burning of the plantar tissue by electrocautery, treatment of a wart with acid to produce a significant burn of the subdermal layers, radiation, or an infection. Under these circumstances, occasionally a painful keratotic lesion is present with little or no subcutaneous fat left to provide a cushion between the skin and metatarsal head (Fig. 8-40A).

SURGICAL TREATMENT: SCAR EXCISION

Despite frequent trimmings and other conservative management strategies, such as custom unloading orthoses, these lesions present a significant disability for the patient. When such a problem cannot be managed effectively with nonsurgical management, an elliptic incision of the area, undermining of the surrounding tissue, and meticulous closure have been used to produce a satisfactory result.

Surgical Technique

1. The area to be excised is carefully mapped out. The criteria for the size of the lesion to be excised are based on attempting to reenter soft fatty tissue, which will provide an adequate cushion for the metatarsal region (Fig. 8-40B). A full-thickness ellipse of tissue is removed, and all the scar tissue is excised (Fig. 8-40C).
2. The skin margins are undermined, and the skin is closed in layers.
3. The initial closure is carried out with 2-0 chromic suture placed in the subdermal layers to bring the skin edges together. Then a near-far/far-near stitch is used to support the skin edge by relieving tension on either side of it. After this, a fine running stitch is used to keep the skin edges in perfect apposition and minimize scar formation. A compression dressing is then applied (Fig. 8-40D).

Postoperative Care

The patient is kept non–weight bearing for approximately 4 weeks to allow soft tissues to heal with minimal stress. Usually the sutures are left in place 2 to 3 weeks.

Results

Although this technique is used infrequently, the results have been satisfactory. Occasionally, the patient develops a minor callosity along the area of the scar tissue, but the procedure usually significantly relieves the pain created by the previous scar tissue.

Scars on the Plantar Aspect of the Foot

Although plantar incisions for excision of an interdigital neuroma, procedures on the metatarsal head, and excision of the fibular sesamoid have been advocated in the literature, if an alternative incision is possible, it is preferable. Most plantar incisions heal benignly, but if a hypertrophic scar forms or the surrounding soft tissue atrophies, it can lead to an unsolvable problem. At times, the skin incision heals benignly, but the underlying fatty tissue unfortunately atrophies over a short period and leaves the patient with inadequate cushioning on the plantar aspect of the foot (Fig. 8-41). Most foot surgery can be carried out through a dorsal approach, and we strongly advise this if at all possible. The fibular sesamoid can be removed through a dorsal incision in the first web space, which is preferable to the plantar incision. Interdigital neuromas and even recurrent neuromas can be removed through dorsal incisions rather than the plantar approach.

If a plantar incision is used, the incision must be placed between the metatarsal heads to avoid a scar directly under a metatarsal.

Osteochondrosis of a Metatarsal Head

Osteochondrosis of a metatarsal head (Freiberg infraction) most often occurs in the second metatarsal head,

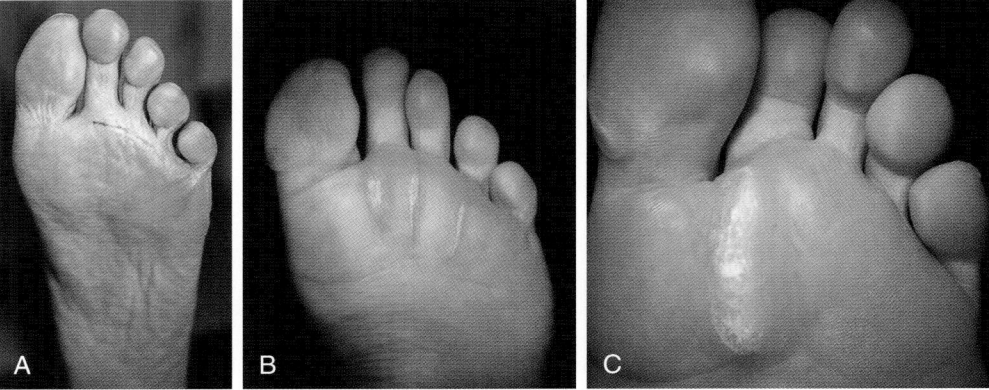

Figure 8-41 Painful plantar scars. **A** and **B,** Incisions that have been used to excise an interdigital neuroma. Unfortunately, these scars often become quite painful, sometimes from keratoses along the scar and at other times from atrophy of the fat pad. These problems make it difficult for the patient to ambulate comfortably. **C,** Hypertrophic scar after plantar incision to remove a fibular sesamoid. There is no good remedy for this situation.

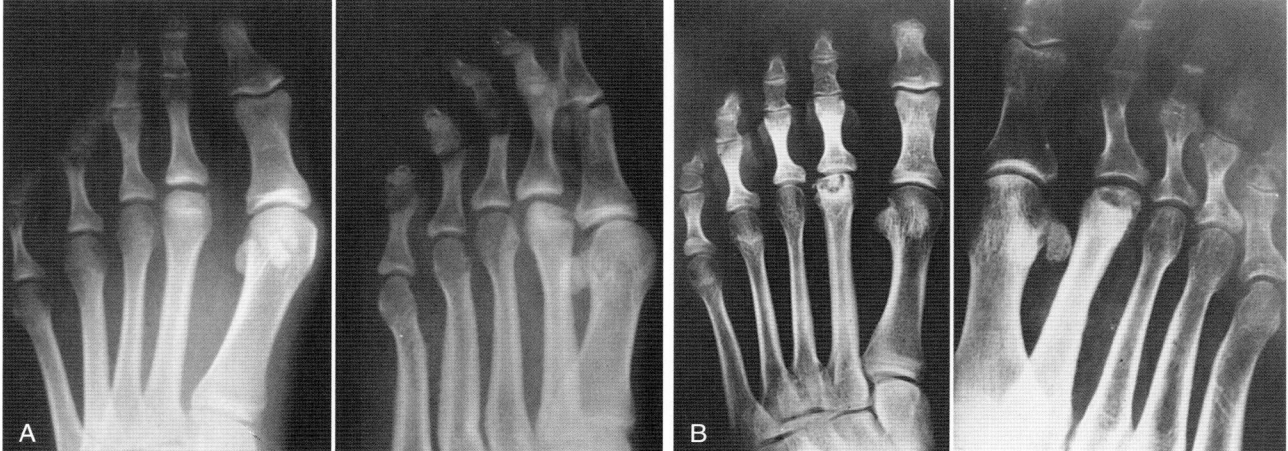

Figure 8-42 Radiographs of Freiberg infraction. **A,** Early stages demonstrate osteolysis and central collapse. **B,** Later stages of Freiberg infraction demonstrate central collapse and osteolysis.

although it can occur at the third metatarsal head in up to one quarter of cases, and less commonly in the fourth metatarsal head. It commonly presents in adolescence, with a 5:1 female:male ratio.[31] Originally described in 1914,[17] the pathogenesis of the disease process is still not fully understood. Freiberg postulated the cause to be ischemic necrosis from repetitive microtrauma resulting from the second metatarsal being longer than the other metatarsals.[11,54] This theory has been supported by several other studies.[40,56] Other authors believe the predisposition of the second metatarsal head to vascular compromise leads to a subchondral insufficiency fracture, which leads to necrosis and collapse of the osteochondral surface.[19] Other causative theories include dorsal impingement, in a mechanism similar to hallux rigidus,[26] and genetic predisposition.[1]

Smillie[56] divided the disease process into five stages based upon radiographs. In stage I, a fissure develops in the ischemic epiphysis. This can cause synovitis, which may lead to joint space widening on radiographs. In stage II, the metatarsal head flattens because of central bone resorption. Stage III is characterized by peripheral irregularities with further central collapse. The plantar cartilage usually remains intact. In stage IV, these irregular peripheral areas and the remaining plantar cartilage can fracture, leading to loose body formation. In stage V, there is marked flattening and widening of the metatarsal head, with loss of joint space and end-stage arthritic changes (Fig. 8-42).

The clinical complaint is usually pain, swelling, and limitation of motion of the affected joint. The symptom complex is aggravated by activities and often relieved by rest. Physical examination demonstrates generalized thickening about the second MTP joint secondary to synovitis. There is often increased warmth. The joint demonstrates restricted motion secondary to pain. In longstanding cases, a callus can form under the affected metatarsal head, usually from a bony deformity.

Diagnosis

The diagnosis is confirmed by radiographs demonstrating osteosclerosis in the early stages and osteolysis with collapse in the later stages. Nuclear imaging[40] and magnetic resonance imaging (MRI) can be helpful, although plain radiographs and a comprehensive history and physical examination are usually sufficient to arrive at the correct diagnosis.

Treatment

Treatment is directed initially toward protection and the alleviation of discomfort. Early in the course of the disease, particularly if no significant distortion of the head has occurred, a short-leg walking cast or a stiff post-operative shoe to decrease the stress across the involved joint is indicated. As the disease process progresses, or if the patient is seen after the acute phase has passed and the disease process has progressed to joint deterioration, surgical intervention may be of benefit.[57] Surgery in the early stage of joint involvement (typically stage II) often consists of debridement of the joint and excision of the proliferative bone (Video Clip 71).[26,56] For more severe joint involvement, numerous surgical procedures have been advocated. These include osteochondral plug transplantation,[49] osteochondral plug transplantation in combination with external fixation to unload the joint,[8] core decompression,[9,16] arthroscopic joint debridement,[44] joint surface debridement with tendon interpositional arthroplasty[4] and metatarsal osteotomies.[2,19,27, 35] These include shortening osteotomies to unload the metatarsal head,[27] and a dorsal closing wedge osteotomy to redirect the articular surface.[19,35,39] The use of shortening osteotomies is discouraged due to unsightly shortening of the toe. Although the authors do not have significant experience with the dorsiflexion osteotomy, the principle of redirecting the healthier intact plantar articular surface is sound, and the high rate of good-to-excellent results reported in the literature is encouraging.[19,35,39]

EXCISION OF PROLIFERATIVE BONE
Surgical Technique

1. The joint is approached through a hockey stick–shaped incision, starting in the second web space. The incision is carried obliquely across the metatarsal head and over the dorsal aspect of the metatarsal shaft (Fig. 8-43A).
2. The incision is deepened to expose the extensor tendons, which are split to enable dissection of the

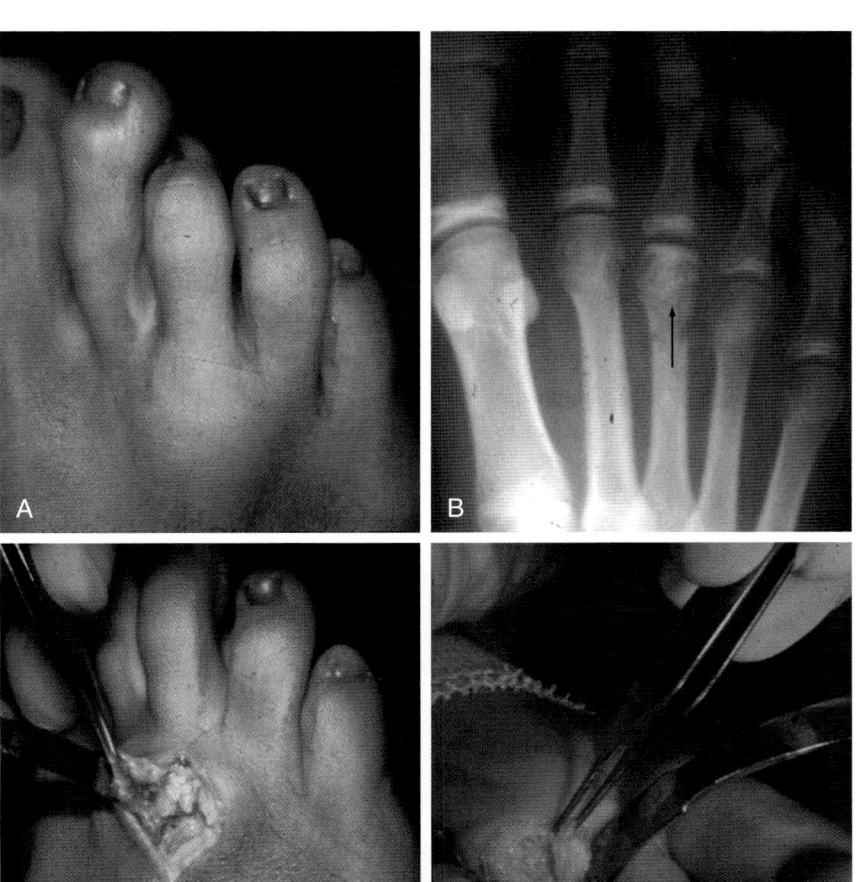

Figure 8-43 Surgical technique for debridement of Freiberg infraction. Clinical photograph **(A)** and radiograph **(B)** showing huge osteophyte formation *(arrow)* at the third metatarsophalangeal joint. **C,** Operative exposure. **D,** Removal of distal free fragment.

extensor hood off the underlying synovial tissue. By sharp dissection, the synovial tissue is removed, and the joint is inspected (Fig. 8-43B).

3. If proliferative bone is present around the metatarsal head, it is generally removed, similar to the procedure for cheilectomy to treat hallux rigidus. The medial and lateral bone is removed in line with the sides of the metatarsal, and the dorsal 20% to 30% of the metatarsal head is resected (Fig. 8-43C and D). If necessary, new bone that has formed around the base of the proximal phalanx is excised, although this occurs infrequently.

4. At this time, approximately 75 to 80 degrees of dorsiflexion should be possible at the MTP joint. If this has not been achieved, more bone probably needs to be resected.

5. The extensor mechanism is closed, the skin is closed in a single layer, and a compression dressing is applied.

Postoperative Care

The patient is maintained in a firm dressing and postoperative shoe for approximately 10 days, until the wound has healed. The patient is then started on active and passive range-of-motion exercises to gain as much motion as possible.

Results

With this technique, satisfactory symptomatic relief can usually be achieved. In general, the patient will not regain as much active motion, but passively, the MTP joint has sufficient flexibility that satisfactory function of the foot can be restored.

Although some have advocated excision of the metatarsal head or replacement with a prosthesis, we do not believe this procedure is indicated for this condition.

At times the only problem is a loose fragment, and this can be debrided without the necessity of excising any other bone.

DORSAL WEDGE OSTEOTOMY
Surgical Technique

1. A longitudinal incision is made over the metatarsal head. The extensor tendons are retracted.

2. The dorsal capsule is incised longitudinally, and the joint capsule and periosteum are elevated medially and laterally.

3. The joint is debrided and irrigated, with removal of any loose fragments.

4. A dorsally based wedge of 5 to 7 mm is removed, with the exact area of resection dependent on the area of articular damage. Care is taken to preserve soft tissue attachments to the distal fragment to prevent avascular necrosis.

5. The intact plantar portion of the metatarsal head is hinged dorsally, and fixed with either wires, bioabsorbable pins, or K-wires (Fig. 8-44).[39]

6. A below knee walking cast is applied, and the patient is allowed to bear weight on the heel only.

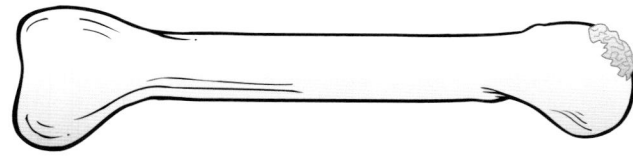
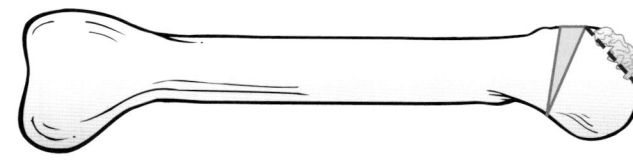
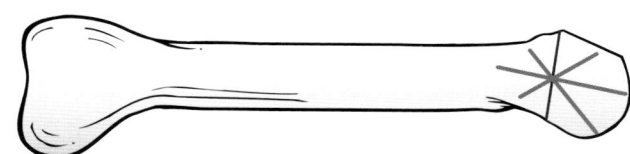

Figure 8-44 Dorsal closing wedge osteotomy. **A,** Shaded area on metatarsal head depicts articular cartilage damage. **B,** A dorsal wedge of damaged cartilage and bone is removed, the osteotomy is closed down, and **C,** two to four bioabsorbable pins can be used for internal fixation.

Postoperative Care

At 4 weeks postoperatively, the patient is transitioned into a supportive shoe, and gentle forefoot range-of-motion exercises are begun. Full weight bearing is allowed when there is radiographic evidence of union.

Results

In a series of 53 patients, Gauthier and Elbaz[19] reported only one patient had persistent pain after surgery. Other series[35,39] report similar high levels of patient satisfaction, pain relief, and return to activities with minimal complications.

INTERPOSITIONAL ARTHROPLASTY (Fig. 8-45)
Surgical Technique

1. A longitudinal incision is made over the metatarsal head. The extensor tendons are retracted.

2. The dorsal capsule is incised longitudinally, and the joint capsule and periosteum are elevated medially and laterally.

3. The joint is debrided and irrigated, with removal of any loose fragments.

4. A portion of the extensor hallucis longus (EHL) tendon can be harvested, or alternatively, an allograft tendon can be used.

5. Cylindric reamers are utilized over a centralizing guidewire to ream a concave cavity in both the metatarsal head and the proximal phalanx.

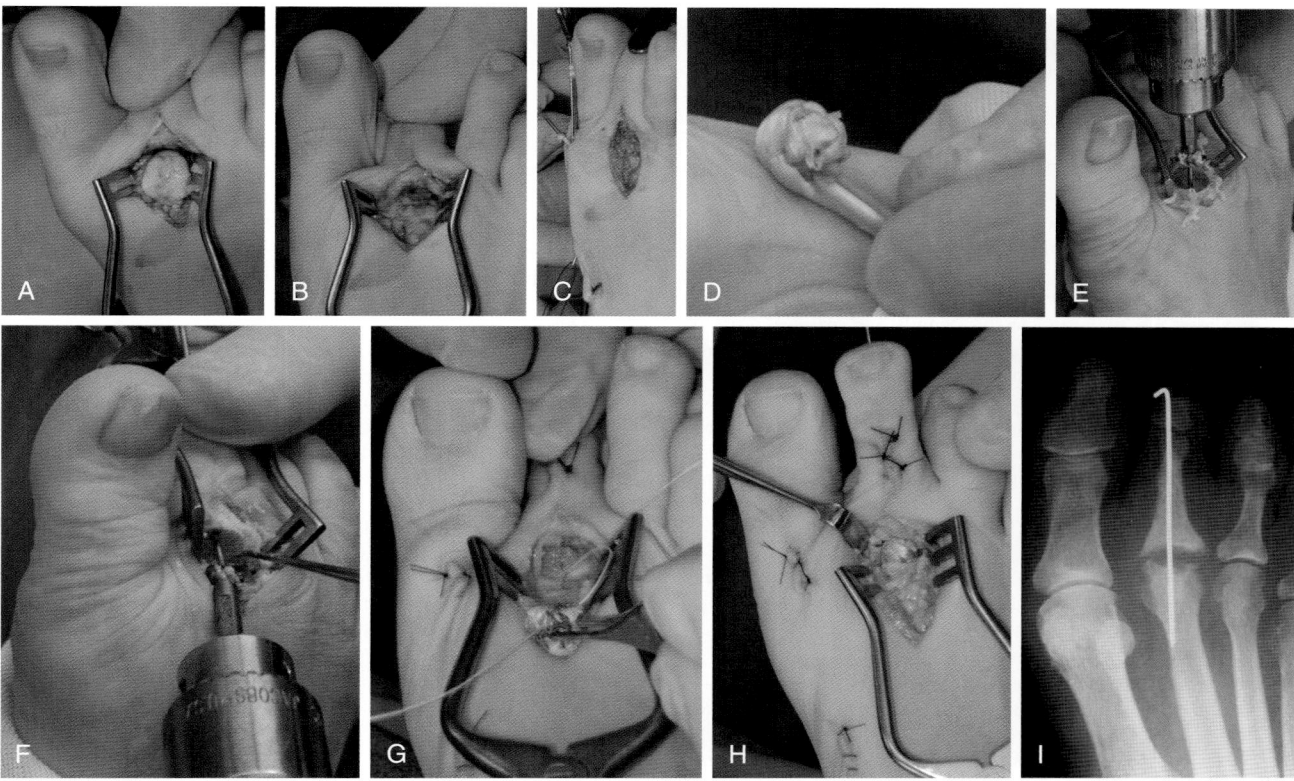

Figure 8-45 **A,** Articular cartilage damage on second metatarsal head. **B,** Articular cartilage damage on proximal phalanx. **C,** Harvesting of half of extensor hallucis longus (EHL) tendon. **D,** Harvested EHL tendon is shaped into a ball. **E and F,** The metatarsal head and proximal phalanx are prepared with concave reamers. **G,** The tendon spacer is placed into the joint and is sewn to the plantar, medial, and lateral joint capsule. **H,** A K-wire is placed across the joint for stabilization. **I,** Postoperative AP radiograph following interpositional arthroplasty and pinning.

6. The tendon is balled up into an anchovie spacer and sewn to the plantar, medial, and lateral capsular tissue for stabilization.
7. A K-wire is driven across the joint to further stabilize the construct in a reduced position.
8. The dorsal capsule is closed, as is the skin.
9. A compression dressing is applied, and a postoperative shoe, a short controlled-angle movement (CAM) walking boot, or a splint is applied.
10. Weight bearing on the heel is allowed immediately, with pin removal at approximately 4 weeks, at which time weight bearing as tolerated is allowed.

Postoperative Care

At 4 weeks postoperatively, the pin is removed, and the patient is transitioned into a supportive shoe, and gentle range-of-motion exercises are begun. Full weight bearing is allowed when pain allows and the incision has healed.

Results

There are no documented studies on this technique, but the authors and editor (MJC) have enjoyed good anecdotal results with this procedure in the younger patient who wishes to stay active and maintain motion.

REFERENCES

1. Blitz NM, Yu JH: Freiberg's infraction in identical twins, *J Foot Ankle Surg* 44:218–221, 2005.
2. Carmont MR, Rees RJ, Blundell CM: Current concepts review: Freiberg's disease, *Foot Ankle Int* 30:167–176, 2009.
3. Coughlin MJ: *Personal communication*, Boise, Idaho, 1990.
4. Coughlin MJ, Shurnas P: Soft-tissue arthroplasty for hallux rigidus, *Foot Ankle Int* 24:661–672, 2003.
5. Davies MS, Saxby TS: Metatarsal neck osteotomy with rigid internal fixation for the treatment of lesser toe metatarasophlangeal joint pathology, *Foot Ankle Int* 20:630–635, 1999.
6. de Bengoa Vallejo RB, Iglesias MEL, Gomez-Martin B, et al: Application of canthardin and podophyllotoxin for the treatemtn of plantar warts, *J Am Pod Med Assoc* 98:445–450, 2008.
7. Dehghani F, Merat A, Panjehshahin MR, et al: Healing effect of garlic extract on warts and corns, *Int J Derm* 44:612–615, 2005.
8. DeVries JG, Amiot RA, Cummings P, et al: Freiberg's infraction of the second metatarsal treated with autologous osteochondral transplantation and external fixation, *J Foot Ankle Surg* 47:565–570, 2008.
9. Dolce M, Osher L, McEneany P, et al: The use of surgical core decompression as treatment for avascular necrosis of the second and third metatarsal heads, *Foot* 17:162–166, 2006.
10. Dreeben SM, Noble PC, Hammerman S, et al: Metatarsal osteotomy for primary metatarsalgia: radiographic and pedobarographic study, *Foot Ankle* 9:214–218, 1989.
11. Drez D Jr, Young JC, Johnston RD, et al: Metatarsal stress fractures, *Am J Sports Med* 8:123–125, 1980.
12. DuVries HL: Disorders of the skin. In DuVries HL, editor: *Surgery of the foot*, ed 2, St Louis, 1965, Mosby, pp 168–169.

13. DuVries HL: New approach to the treatment of intractable verruca plantaris (plantar wart), *JAMA* 152:1202–1203, 1953.

14. DuVries HL, editor: *Surgery of the foot*, ed 2, St Louis, 1965, Mosby, pp 456–462.

15. Espinosa N, Brodsky JW, Maceira E: Metatarsalgia, *J Am Acad Orthop Surg* 18:474–485, 2010.

16. Freiberg AA, Freiberg RA: Core decompression as a novel treatment for early Freiberg's infraction of the second metatarsal head, *Orthopedics* 18:1177–1178, 1995.

17. Freiberg AH: Infraction of the second metatarsal bone, *Surg Gynecol Obstet* 19:191–193, 1914.

18. Gajdosik RL, Allred JD, Gabbert HL, et al: A stretching program increases the dynamic passive length and passive resistance properties of the calf muscle-tendon unit of unconditioned younger women, *Eur J Appl Physiol* 99:449–454, 2007.

19. Gauthier G, Elbaz R: Freiberg's infraction: a subchondral bone fatigue fracture. A new surgical treatment, *Clin Orthop Relat Res* 142:93–95, 1979.

20. Giannestras NJ: Shortening of the metatarsal shaft in the treatment of plantar keratosis, *J Bone Joint Surg* 49:61–71, 1958.

21. Glover MG: Plantar warts, *Foot Ankle* 11:172, 1990.

22. Grebing BR, Coughlin MJ: The effect of ankle position on the exam for first ray mobility, *Foot Ankle Int* 25:467–475, 2004.

23. Grimes J, Coughlin MJ: Geometric analysis of the Weil osteotomy, *Foot Ankle Int* 27:985–992, 2006.

24. Harris RI, Beath T: The short first metatarsal: its incidence and clinical significance, *J Bone Joint Surg* 31:553, 1949.

25. Helal B: Metatarsal osteotomy for metatarsalgia, *J Bone Joint Surg Br* 57:187–192, 1975.

26. Helal B, Gibb P: Freiberg's disease: a suggested pattern of management, *Foot Ankle* 8:94–102, 1987.

27. Helal B, Greiss M: Telescoping osteotomy for pressure metatarsalgia, *J Bone Joint Surg Br* 66:213–217, 1984.

28. Hofstaetter SG, Hofstaetter JG, Petroutsas JA, et al: The Weil osteotomy: a seven-year follow-up, *J Bone Joint Surg Br* 87:1507–1511, 2005.

29. Jarde O, Hussenot D, Vimont E, et al: Weil's cervicocapital osteotomy for median metatarsalgia: report of 70 cases, *Acta Orthop Belg* 67:139–148, 2001.

30. Jennings MB, Ricketti J, Guadara J, et al: Treatment for simple plantar verrucae, *J Am Pod Med Assoc* 96:53–58, 2006.

31. Katcherian DA: Treatment of Freiberg's disease, *Orthop Clin North Am* 25:69, 1994.

32. Kaz AJ, Coughlin MJ: Extensor digitorum brevis transfer and Weil osteotomy for crossover second toe, *Tech Foot Ankle Surg* 9:32–36, 2010.

33. Kelishadi SS, Wirth GA, Evans GRD: Recalcitrant verrucous lesion, *J Am Pod Med Assoc* 96:148–153, 2006.

34. Kennedy JG, Deland JT: Resolution of plantar pain following oblique osteotomy for central metatarsalgia, *Clin Orthop Relat Res* 453:309–313, 2006.

35. Kinnard P, Lirette R: Freiberg's disease and dorsiflexion osteotomy, *J Bone Joint Surg Br* 73:864–865, 1991.

36. Kitaoka HB, Patzer GL: Chevron osteotomy of lesser metatarsals for intractable plantar callosities, *J Bone Joint Surg Br* 80:516–518, 1998.

37. Laurent R, Kienzler JL: Epidemiology of HPV infections, *Clin Dermatol* 3:64, 1985.

38. Lee KB, Park JK, Park YH, et al: Prognosis of painful plantar callosity after hallux valgus correction without lesser metatarsal osteotomy, *Foot Ankle Int* 30:1048–1052, 2009.

39. Lee SK, Chung MS, Baek GH, et al: Treatment of Freiberg disease with intra-articular dorsal wedge osteotomy and absorbable pin fixation, *Foot Ankle Int* 28:43–48, 2007.

40. Mandell GA, Harcke HT: Scintigraphic manifestations of infraction of the second metatarsal (Freiberg's disease), *J Nucl Med* 28:249–251, 1987.

41. Mann RA, Coughlin MJ: Intractable plantar keratosis. In Mann RA, Coughlin MJ, editors: *Video textbook of foot and ankle surgery*, St Louis, 1991, Medical Video Productions.

42. Mann RA, DuVries MD: Intractable plantar keratosis, *Orthop Clin North Am* 4:67–73, 1973.

43. Mann RA, Wapner K: Tibial sesamoid shaving for treatment of intractable plantar keratosis under the tibial sesamoid, *Foot Ankle* 13:196–198, 1992.

44. Mareca G, Adriani E, Falez F, et al: Arthroscopic treatment of Freiberg's infraction, *Arthroscopy* 12:103–108, 1996.

45. Maron R, Grimwood RE, Siegle RJ, et al: Verrucous carcinoma arising in ulcerative lichen planus of the soles, *J Dermatol Surg Oncol* 14:547, 1988.

46. Marx R, Mizel MS: Technique tip: a modified technique for plantar DuVries condylectomy, *Foot Ankle Int* 28:1301, 2007.

47. McCarthy DJ: Therapeutic considerations in the treatment of pedal verrucae, *Clin Podiatr Med Surg* 3:433, 1986.

48. Migues A, Slullitel G, Bilbao F, et al: Floating toe deformity as a complication of the Weil osteotomy, *Foot Ankle Int* 25:609–613, 2004.

49. Miyamoto W, Takao M, Uchio Y, et al: Late-stage Freiberg disease treated by osteochondral plug transplantation: a case series, *Foot Ankle Int* 29:950–955, 2008.

50. Myerson MS, Jung HG: The role of the flexor to extensor transfer in correcting metatarsophalangeal joint instability of the second toe, *Foot Ankle Int* 26:675–679, 2005.

51. Pedowitz WJ: Distal oblique osteotomy for intractable plantar keratosis of the middle three metatarsals, *Foot Ankle* 9:7–9, 1988.

52. Ryan P, Baird G, Benfanti P: Hereditary painful callosities: case report and review of the literature, *Foot Ankle Int* 28:377–378, 2007.

53. Salk R, Douglas TS: Intralesional bleomycin sulfate injection for the treatment of verruca plantaris, *J Am Pod Med Assoc* 96:220–225, 2006.

54. Sarrafian SK: *Anatomy of the foot and ankle: descriptive, anatomical, and functional*, ed 2, Philadelphia, 1993, JB Lippincott, pp 79–85.

55. Schwartz RA: Verrucous carcinoma of the skin and mucosa, *J Am Acad Dermatol* 32:1, 1995.

56. Smillie IS: Treatment of Freiberg's infraction, *Proc R Soc Med* 60:29–31, 1969.

57. Thompson FM, Hamilton WG: Problems of the second metatarsophalangeal joint, *Orthopedics* 10:83–89, 1987.

58. Trnka HJ, Gebhard C, Mühlbauer M, et al: The weil osteotomy for treatment of dislocated lesser metatarsophalangeal joints: good outcomes in 21 patients with 42 osteotomies, *Acta Orthop Scand* 73:190–194, 2002.

59. Trnka HJ, Kabon B, Zettl R, et al: Helal osteotomy for the treatment of metatarsalgia: a critical analysis of results, *Orthopedics* 19:457–461, 1996.

60. Vandeputte G, Dereymaeker G, Steenwerckx A, et al: The Weil osteotomy of the lesser metatarsals: a clinical and pedobarographic follow-up study, *Foot Ankle Int* 21:370–374, 2000.

61. Wachters DH, Frensdorf EL, Hasuman R, et al: Keratosis palmoplantaris nummularis ("hereditary painful callosities"). Clinical and histopathologic aspects, *J Am Dermatol* 9:204–209, 1983.

62. Weil LS: *Weil head–neck oblique osteotomy: technique and fixation.* Presented at Techniques of Osteotomies of the Forefoot, Bordeaux, France, October 20–22, 1994.

63. Winson IG, Rawlinson J, Broughton NS: Treatment of metatarsalgia by sliding distal metatarsal osteotomy, *Foot Ankle* 9:2–6, 1988.

64. Young S, Cohen GE: Treatment of verruca plantaris with a combination of topical fluorouracil and salicylic acid, *J Am Pod Med Assoc* 95:366–369, 2005.

Bunionettes

Michael J. Coughlin

A bunionette deformity, or tailor's bunion, is characterized by a painful prominence of the lateral eminence of the fifth metatarsal head. Davies[16] observed that pressure over the lateral condyle of the fifth metatarsal head led to chronic irritation of the overlying bursa (Fig. 9-1). The position of a tailor sitting in a cross-legged position has given rise to the term *tailor's bunion*.[75] Friction between an underlying bony prominence and constricting footwear can lead to the development of a keratosis over the lateral aspect[22,33,42] (Fig. 9-2A) or the plantar lateral aspect[31] of the fifth metatarsal head (Figs. 9-2B and 9-3A). The fifth toe deviates in a medial direction at the fifth metatarsophalangeal (MTP) joint (Fig. 9-3B), and the fifth metatarsal deviates laterally with respect to the fourth metatarsal.

ANATOMY

Kelikian[35] described a prominent fifth metatarsal lateral eminence of a bunionette deformity as being "analogous to the medial eminence of the first metatarsal head" in a hallux valgus deformity. DuVries[22] described several anatomic variations in the fifth metatarsal head that can lead to a symptomatic bunionette. Thus the etiology and anatomic variations that occur with a bunionette deformity are much more complex than what was originally described by Kelikian[35] and Davies.[16] Although painful symptoms can be localized to the fifth MTP joint region, an abnormal alignment of the fifth metatarsal may be associated with a bunionette deformity.

Recognition of the specific anatomic variation present is important in the preoperative evaluation and can influence the specific procedure chosen to correct the bunionette deformity. The radiographic analysis of a bunionette deformity is important in defining the magnitude and type of abnormality present.

CLINICAL SYMPTOMS

The major subjective complaints of a patient with a symptomatic bunionette deformity are pain and irritation caused by friction between constricting footwear and an underlying bony abnormality. On physical examination, an inflamed bursa,[31,68,69] a lateral keratosis (see Fig. 9-2),[20] a plantar keratosis (see Fig. 9-3),[28,31,51] or a combined plantar lateral keratosis[20,33] may be present. Diebold and Bejjani[20] noted that two thirds of the patients in their series had significant pes planus. They reported that a third of the patients in their series developed a plantar keratosis, whereas half had a lateral keratotic lesion. The remaining had a combined plantar and lateral keratosis. Coughlin[14] noted that 10% of the patients in his series had developed a plantar keratosis, 70% had developed a lateral keratosis, and 20% had developed a combined plantar and lateral keratosis. Some osteotomies do not allow elevation of the capital fragment with correction of the bunionette deformity; these procedures should be avoided in the presence of a plantar keratosis.

In general, a bunionette is a static deformity. Repeated activities such as running or jogging can lead to thickening or inflammation of the overlying bursa.

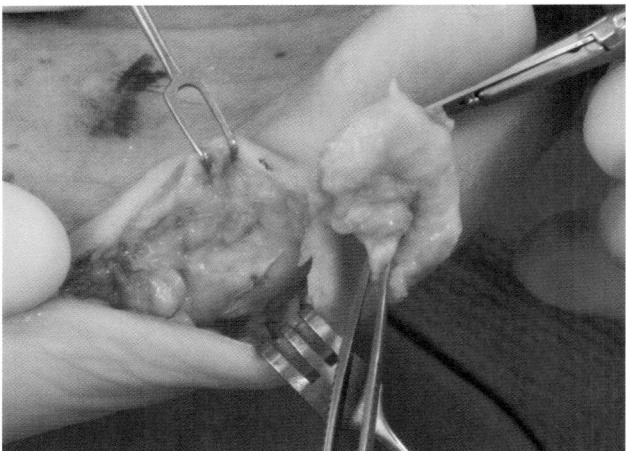

Figure 9-1 A painful bursa overlying the fifth metatarsal head is surgically excised.

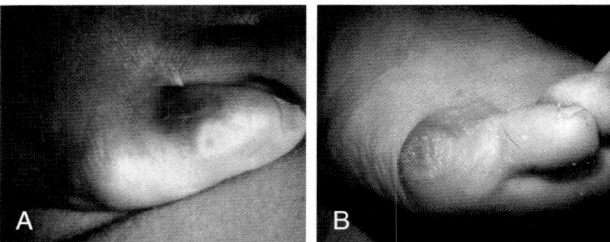

Figure 9-2 **A,** Lateral keratosis combined with lateral fifth toe corn. **B,** Plantar–lateral keratosis overlying the fifth metatarsal head. This is the most common presentation of a symptomatic bunionette.

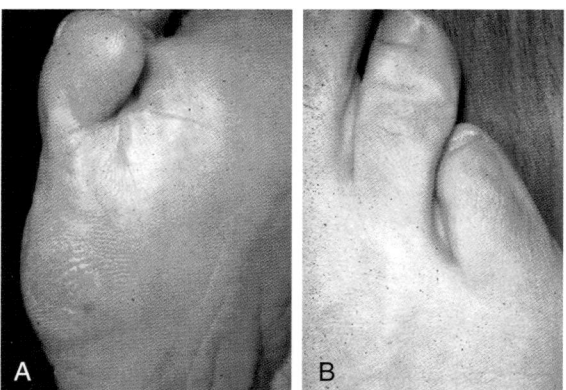

Figure 9-3 **A,** Plantar keratosis associated with bunionette deformity. **B,** Abduction deformity of the fifth toe.

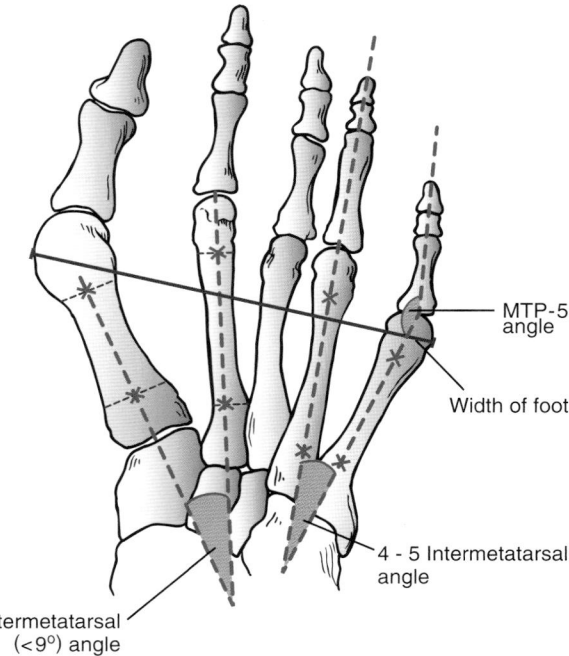

Figure 9-4 The metatarsophalangeal-5 *(MTP-5)* angle and the 4-5 intermetatarsal (IM) angle. The MTP-5 angle is that subtended by the axis of the proximal phalanx and fifth metatarsal. The 1-2 IM angle is that subtended by the axis of the first and second metatarsals. The 4-5 IM angle is that subtended by the intersecting axis of the fourth and fifth metatarsals. The width of the foot is measure with a line from the medial aspect of the first metatarsal head to the lateral aspect of the fifth metatarsal head.

keratosis in combination with a lateral keratosis because this differentiation can affect the choice of surgical procedure. In examining the bunionette deformity, an abducted fifth toe, as well as a digital rotational component to the axial deformity, must be recognized. A hammer toe deformity of the fifth toe might also be present. A bunionette can develop as an isolated deformity, but it can also develop in combination with a hallux valgus deformity. An increased angle between the fourth and fifth metatarsals (4-5 intermetatarsal [IM] angle), in combination with an increased angle between the first and second metatarsals, results in a very wide splayed-foot abnormality.[3,16,31,34,65] Likewise, the need for other forefoot surgical procedures affects the ambulatory capacity of a patient and must be considered as well. A neurovascular examination is important for determining the suitability of the patient for surgical correction.

PHYSICAL EXAMINATION

The examination of the patient with a symptomatic bunionette is performed with the patient sitting and standing. The presence of pes planus, an Achilles tendon contracture, or other forefoot abnormalities must be recognized and treated appropriately if they are symptomatic. A key to preoperative planning is the recognition of a plantar

DIAGNOSTIC AND RADIOGRAPHIC EXAMINATION

Radiographic evaluation of a symptomatic bunionette deformity includes standing anteroposterior (AP) and lateral radiographs. The significant angular measurements that define a bunionette deformity are the angle of the fifth metatarsophalangeal joint (MTP-5 angle) (Fig. 9-4)

and the 4-5 IM angle. The MTP-5 angle allows one to calculate the magnitude of medial deviation of the fifth toe in relation to the longitudinal axis of the fifth metatarsal shaft. Nestor et al[53] reported that in normal feet the MTP-5 angle averaged 10.2 degrees, and Steele et al[66] noted that in 90% of normal cases, the angle was 14 degrees or less. Nestor et al[53] and Coughlin[14] have reported that in feet with bunionettes the MTP-5 angle averaged 16 degrees.

The 4-5 IM angle is a measure of the divergence of the fourth and fifth metatarsals and is the angle measured by the intersection of lines bisecting the axis of the fourth and fifth metatarsals.[61] Divergence of the fourth and fifth metatarsals leads to pressure over the lateral eminence of the fifth metatarsal head.[18,34,39] Fallat and Buckholz[24] stated that the 4-5 IM angle in normal feet averaged 6.2 degrees (range, 3 to 11 degrees). Although some[3,4,23,34,61] have noted that a 4-5 IM angle greater than 8 degrees can be considered abnormal, Fallat[24] and Coughlin[14] have reported the 4-5 IM angle on average to be greater than 9 degrees. In general, however, angular measurements serve only to describe a bunionette deformity; it is the symptoms and not the magnitude of deformity that necessitates specific surgical treatment. The width of the foot is determined by a diagonal line drawn from the medial edge of the medial eminence of the first metatarsal to the lateral aspect of the fifth metatarsal head.

A prominent lateral condyle of the fifth metatarsal head can lead to a type 1 bunionette deformity (Fig. 9-5).[22,24,68] Hypertrophy of the lateral condyle has been reported by DuVries[22] and others.[24,69,71] The incidence of a type 1 deformity is reported to vary in incidence from 16% to 33%.[4,14,40] Zvijac et al[75] noted a variance in width

of the fifth metatarsal from 11 mm at the smallest to 14 mm at the widest, and Fallat[24] stated that the normal width of the fifth metatarsal head was 13 mm. Throckmorton and Bradlee[69] and Fallat and Buckholz[20] both reported that with excessive pronation of the foot, the lateral plantar tubercle of the fifth metatarsal head rotated laterally to create the radiographic impression of an enlarged fifth metatarsal head. Fallat and Buckholz[24] also reported a 3-degree increase in the 4-5 IM angle in the presence of a pes planus deformity. Whether true hypertrophy of the fifth metatarsal head occurs or prominence of the fifth metatarsal head results from pronation of the foot, a prominent lateral condyle of the fifth metatarsal head can become symptomatic without an increase in the 4-5 IM angle.

Lateral bowing of the diaphysis of the fifth metatarsal shaft can lead to the development of a symptomatic prominence of the lateral condyle of the fifth metatarsal head* and is classified as a type 2 bunionette deformity (Fig. 9-6). Although the proximal fifth metatarsal shaft maintains a normal IM alignment, a lateral curvature develops in the diaphysis of the fifth metatarsal, which leads to a symptomatic bunionette deformity. A prominent lateral condyle of the fifth metatarsal head can also be caused by divergence of the fourth and fifth metatarsals, which is classified as a type 3 bunionette deformity (Fig. 9-7).

Kitaoka et al,[39] in evaluating a series of patients with a symptomatic bunionette deformity, reported that an increase in the 4-5 IM angle was most often associated with a symptomatic bunionette deformity. Fifth

---

*References 4, 8, 22, 23, 24, 50, and 74.

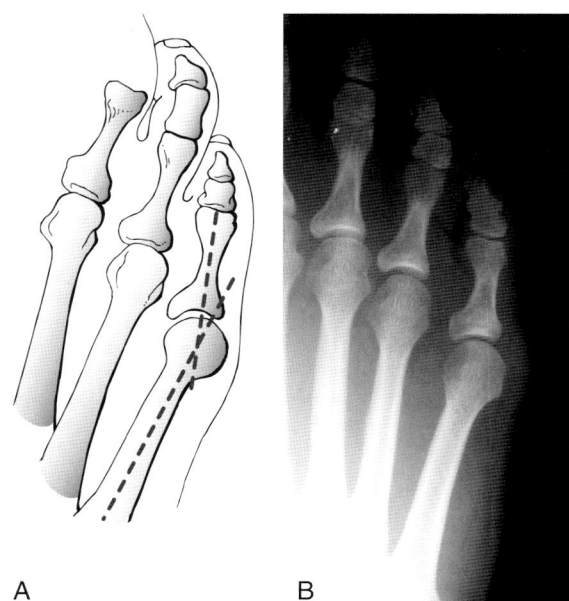

Figure 9-5 Type 1 bunionette deformity is characterized by an enlarged fifth metatarsal head.

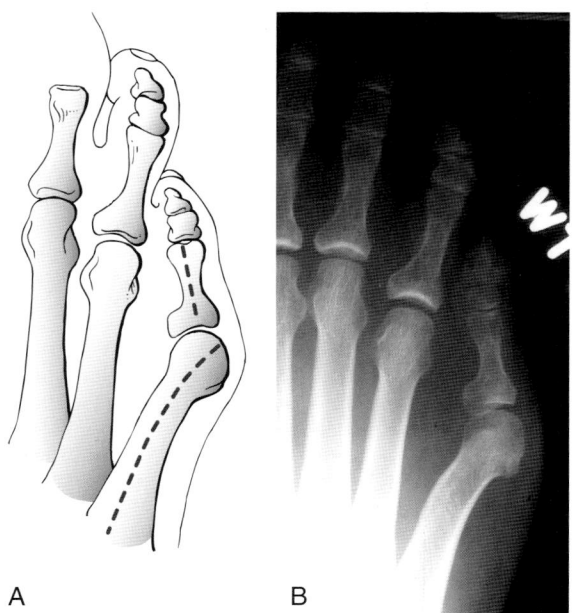

Figure 9-6 Type 2 bunionette deformity is characterized by lateral bowing of the fifth metatarsal head.

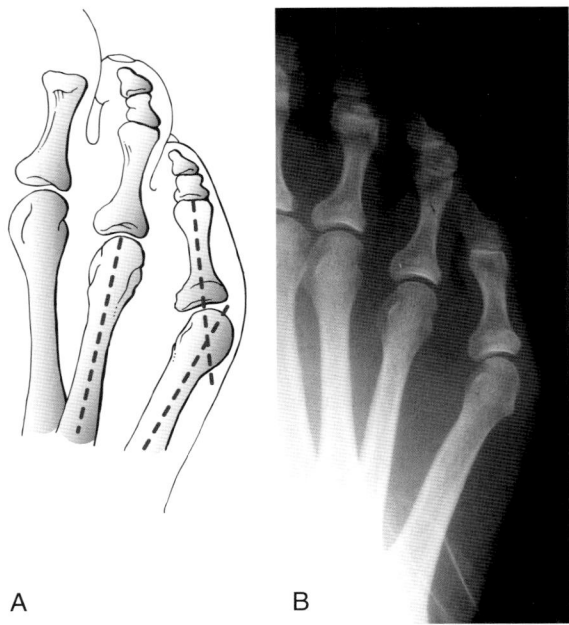

A   B

Figure 9-7 Type 3 bunionette deformity is characterized by an abnormally wide 4-5 intermetatarsal angle.

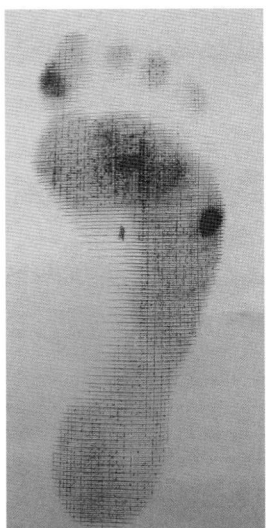

Figure 9-8 Harris mat study demonstrating increased plantar pressure beneath the fifth metatarsal head.

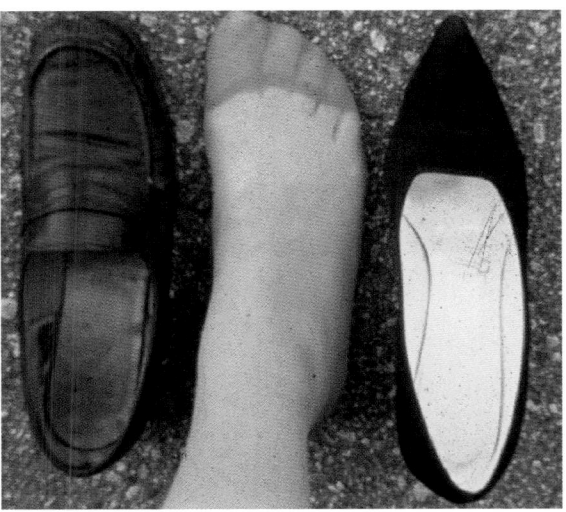

Figure 9-9 Constricting shoe *(right)* compared with roomy shoe *(left).*

metatarsal bowing or an enlarged fifth metatarsal head was observed to be a cause in less than 10% of these cases, but Coughlin[14] noted the incidence of lateral bowing of the fifth metatarsal to be 23%.

Koti[41] has suggested an additional type that involves two or more components of the other three types. This adds unnecessary complexity and does not aid in defining a treatment plan.

Regardless of the underlying MTP joint orientation and fifth metatarsal angulation, the common symptom in all patients with a bunionette deformity is increased pressure over the lateral aspect of the fifth metatarsal head caused by constricting footwear. The female-to-male ratio is reported to vary from 3 : 1 to 10 : 1[6,8,26,53] in series of patients with symptomatic bunionettes that required surgical intervention. The increased frequency of occurrence of a bunionette deformity in the female population is most likely attributable to their predilection for high-fashion footwear. With time, the development of a hypertrophic keratosis or a thickened bursa can lead to increased symptoms.

Harris mat studies can help in the assessment of increased pressure beneath a symptomatic fifth metatarsal head in association with a plantar keratosis (Fig. 9-8).

TREATMENT

Conservative Treatment

It is important for a patient to recognize that the use of constricting footwear is a significant cause of symptoms and places increased pressure on a prominent fifth metatarsal head.[15] Chronic irritation, pain, and swelling of the

bursa overlying the fifth metatarsal head can be reduced by roomy, well-fitted shoes (Fig. 9-9).*

Shaving of a hypertrophic callus (Fig. 9-10A) and padding (Fig. 9-10B-D) of a prominent fifth metatarsal head[41,53] can reduce symptoms significantly. A prefabricated or custom orthotic device may be used to diminish pronation and, as a result, reduce discomfort over a prominent fifth metatarsal head (see Chapter 4).

Conservative methods can be effective in a large number of patients. However, as painful plantar and lateral keratoses develop, surgical intervention may be necessary to relieve symptoms (Fig. 9-11). Various reported

_____

*References 10, 16, 35, 41, 42, and 58.

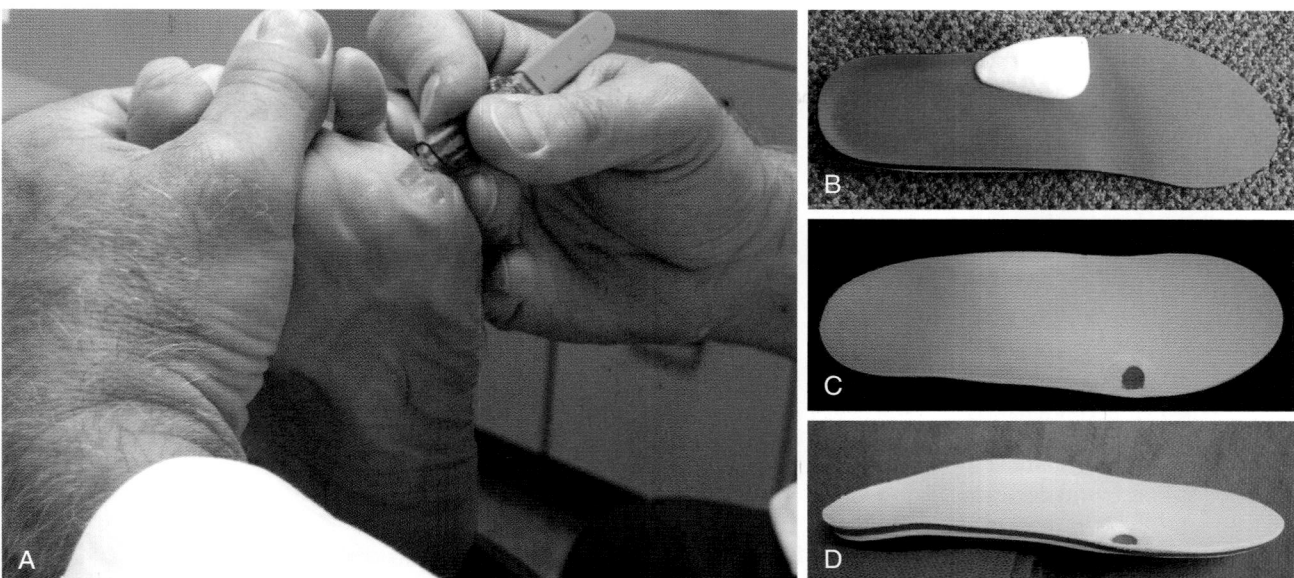

Figure 9-10 Conservative treatment may consist of relieving pressure beneath the fifth metatarsal head. **A,** Shaving of plantar callus beneath fifth metatarsal head. **B,** Customizing a prefabricated insole with a pad placed just proximal to the plantar keratosis. **C** and **D,** Orthotics, such as these modified Plastazote insoles, can be successful in alleviating symptoms.

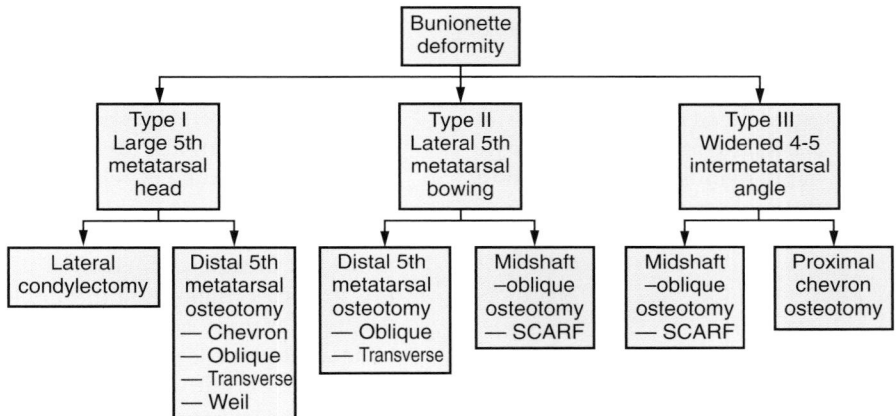

Figure 9-11 Algorithm for treatment of bunionette deformities.

techniques are presented in this section. Preferred surgical methods are noted and discussed later in the chapter.

Surgical Treatment

Preoperative Evaluation

The preoperative evaluation of a patient with a painful bunionette begins with a comprehensive history and physical examination. An AP weight-bearing radiograph typically demonstrates the characteristics of the deformity, but it also helps the surgeon to assess the status of the MTP joint. Pain and swelling of the fifth MTP joint can be caused by degenerative or inflammatory arthritis. Laboratory evaluation is occasionally helpful in diagnosing such underlying causes as gout, early rheumatoid arthritis, and infection or cellulitis.

The presence of a concomitant hammer toe deformity or a sagittal plane deformity of the MTP joint requires treatment with the correction of the bunionette.

Assessment of both the circulatory status of the involved extremity as well as the neurologic status is important, especially in those with early peripheral vascular disease, diabetes, or neuropathy. Although surgery is not necessarily contraindicated, adequate protective sensation and adequate peripheral circulation are necessary for successful healing.

Preoperative Planning

The preoperative assessment determines the underlying cause of symptoms in the patient with a painful bunionette. Likewise, the radiographic findings help to determine the preferred surgical technique. A plantar–lateral callosity requires a surgical correction that reduces the size of the lateral eminence as well as elevates the fifth metatarsal head. The radiographic findings of a mild deformity or mainly an enlarged fifth metatarsal head make a distal fifth metatarsal osteotomy a feasible alternative. A moderate or severe deformity—typically a curved fifth metatarsal shaft or a widened 4-5 IM angle—makes a midshaft diaphyseal osteotomy preferable. Thus a careful correlation of the physical findings and radiologic information allow the physician to select the appropriate surgical procedure with which to correct a bunionette deformity.

Surgical Techniques

Numerous surgical techniques have been described to correct a symptomatic bunionette deformity. These include lateral condylectomy,* fifth metatarsal head resection,[21,35,37,51,72] fifth metatarsal implant arthoplasty,[1] fifth-ray resection,[5] distal metatarsal osteotomy,† diaphyseal osteotomy,‡ and proximal fifth metatarsal osteotomy.§ Correction of the underlying disorder is necessary for preventing a recurrence of deformity. Likewise, preservation of the function of the fifth MTP joint can prevent such complications as recurrence, subluxation, dislocation, or development of a transfer lesion.

LATERAL CONDYLECTOMY

With an isolated enlargement of the fifth metatarsal head or a prominent fifth metatarsal lateral condyle without an increased 4-5 IM angle, a lateral condylectomy may be performed. The presence of pes planus or a pronated fifth ray is not necessarily a contraindication to a lateral condylectomy if the prominent lateral condyle is the only deformity present.

Indications

The main indication for a lateral condylectomy is an enlarged lateral condyle.[10,58] In this situation, a condylectomy can produce an adequate repair, although a distal metatarsal osteotomy might still be the procedure of choice. A second indication is for the treatment of localized infection overlying the lateral fifth metatarsal head.[10,41] Although lateral condylectomy might not achieve MTP joint realignment, it might alleviate the acute or chronic infection.

Contraindications

Preoperative radiographs are important in the evaluation of a bunionette deformity. With lateral angulation of the fifth metatarsal shaft in relationship to the fourth metatarsal shaft (increased 4-5 IM angle; type 3 deformity) or with lateral bowing of the fifth metatarsal shaft (type 2

---

*References 18, 22, 28, 41, 44, 50, 58, and 68.
†References 4, 7-9, 17, 18, 30-32, 34, 38-40, 47, 52, 56, 62, 65, 67, 73, and 75.
‡References 13, 14, 26, 27, 33, 46, 49, 70, and 71.
§References 3, 19, 20, 24, 33, 45, 54, and 57.

deformity), a condylectomy does not effectively reduce a prominent fifth metatarsal lateral eminence. With an enlarged 4-5 IM angle, a fifth metatarsal osteotomy is necessary to correct this divergence.[45]

The significant recurrence rate after lateral condylectomy is attributable to the use of a lateral condylectomy when a fifth metatarsal osteotomy is indicated. Kelikian[35] noted that "at best a lateral condylectomy is a temporizing measure like simple exostectomy on the medial side of the foot; in time deformity will recur."

Surgical Technique

1. The patient is positioned in a semilateral decubitus position.
2. The extremity is cleansed in a normal fashion.
3. A longitudinal skin incision is centered over the lateral condyle of the fifth metatarsal head and extends from the interphalangeal joint to 1 cm proximal to the fifth metatarsal condyle. The dorsal cutaneous nerve of the fifth toe is protected (Fig. 9-12A and B).
4. An inverted L-shaped capsular incision is used to detach the dorsal and proximal fifth metatarsal capsule. The weakest portion of the capsule is detached, and the strongest capsular attachments to the proximal phalanx and plantar capsule are maintained (Fig. 9-12C-E).
5. A sagittal saw (or osteotome) is used to resect the lateral condyle of the fifth metatarsal head (Fig. 9-12F-G).
6. The fifth metatarsal head is exposed, and with traction placed on the fifth toe, the MTP joint is distracted and the medial capsule is released with a scalpel (Fig. 9-12H and I).
7. The MTP capsule is closed by approximating it to the fifth MTP metatarsal metaphyseal periosteum and to the abductor digiti quinti muscle proximally (Fig. 9-12J). (For improved fixation, a drill hole in the fifth metatarsal dorsolateral metaphysis may be used to anchor the capsule repair.) A meticulous capsule repair is necessary to prevent recurrence of the deformity or lateral subluxation of the MTP joint.
8. The skin is closed routinely, and a compression dressing is applied.

Postoperative Care

A gauze-and-tape compression dressing is applied at surgery and is changed weekly for 6 weeks. The patient is allowed to ambulate in a postoperative shoe for 3 weeks and in a sandal for 3 weeks. Skin sutures are removed 3 weeks after surgery.

Results and Complications

Although this procedure has been frequently recommended for the repair of a bunionette deformity,* in general, only anecdotal follow-up has been published for series using a lateral condylectomy. Reported postoperative complications include recurrence of deformity

---

*References 10, 16, 18, 22, 28, 41, 44, 48, 51, and 58.

(Fig. 9-13),* subluxation of the MTP joint (Fig. 9-14),[33,38,65] and poor weight bearing with excessive resection.[42]

Kitaoka and Holiday[36] reported on 16 patients (21 feet) who had undergone a lateral condylar resection for a symptomatic bunionette (average follow-up, 6.4 years). Seventy-one percent of the patients were satisfied with their result. Twenty-three percent reported some element of forefoot pain, although half these patients considered it mild. The average preoperative 4-5 IM angle measured 12.3 degrees, and postoperatively it measured 11.1 degrees, for an average correction of 1.2 degrees. Much of this correction can be accounted for by the measurement techniques. The metatarsophalangeal-5 angle averaged

*References 29, 31, 42, 44, 51, 65, and 74.

17.0 degrees preoperatively and 14.6 degrees postoperatively. This correction was not significant on statistical analysis. Furthermore, the authors concluded that no correlation existed between the amount of correction and the level of patient satisfaction. In two feet, the MTP joint subluxated postoperatively as the fifth toe displaced medially. A tight capsule closure with excision of redundant MTP joint capsule was recommended to minimize this postoperative complication. The authors also concluded that although only a limited degree of correction of the deformity was possible with this procedure, a lateral condylectomy was often successful in relieving symptoms. No transfer lesions were reported in this series. With an intractable plantar keratotic lesion beneath the fifth metatarsal head, the authors believed that a

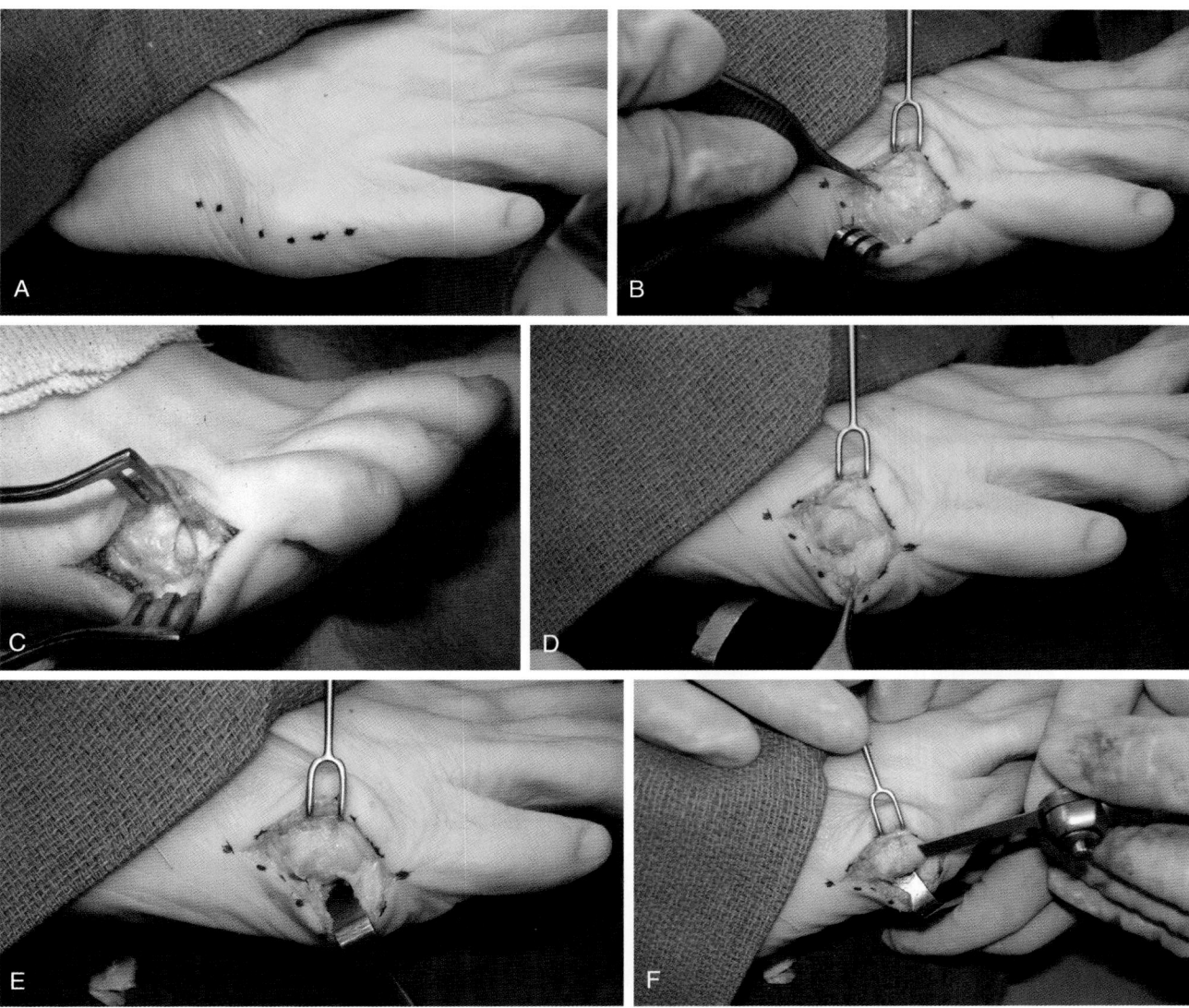

Figure 9-12 Lateral condylectomy. **A,** Skin incision. **B,** Capsular exposure. **C,** Inverted L-shaped capsular incision is used to expose the fifth metatarsal head. Dorsal and proximal capsule, the weakest area of capsular attachment, is released, and the stronger plantar and distal attachments are left intact. **D,** The L-shaped flap in turned downward. **E,** Exposing the lateral condyle of the fifth metatarsal. **F,** The lateral condyle is resected in line with the shaft of the fifth metatarsal.

Continued

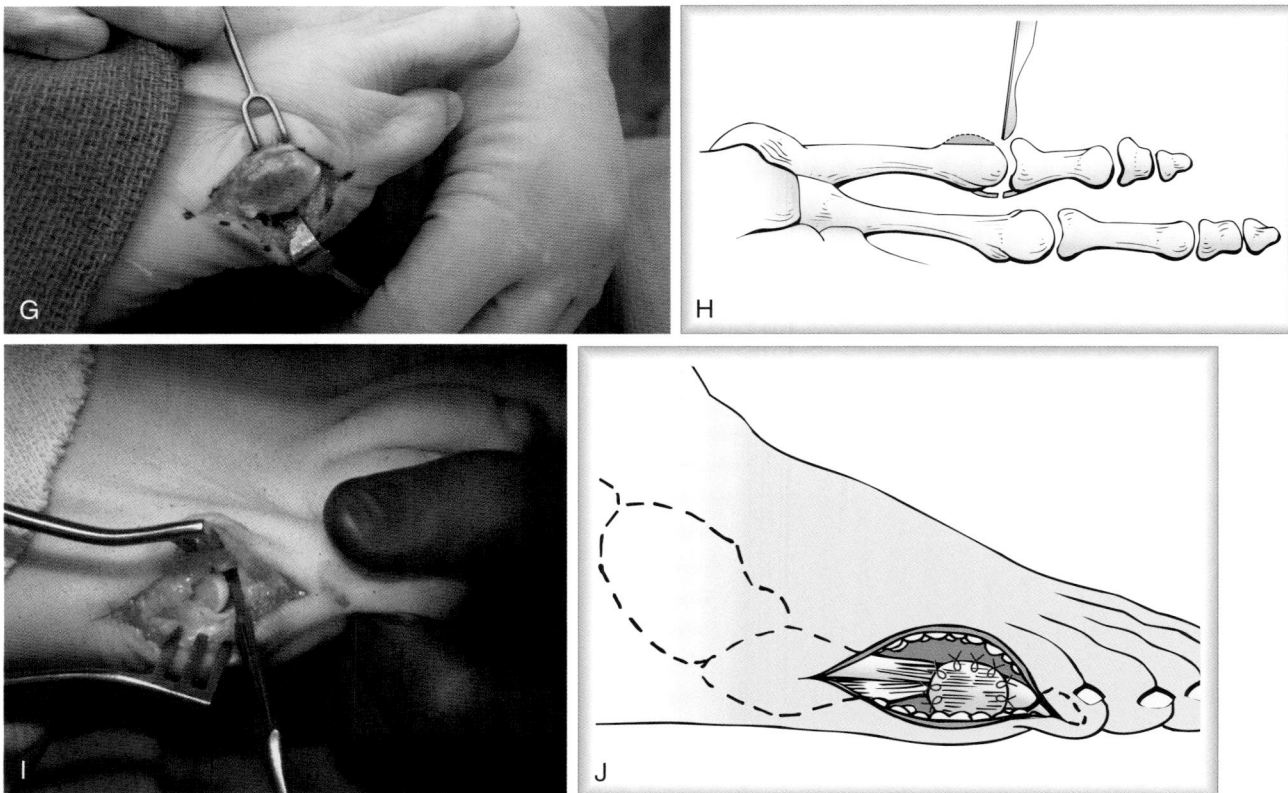

Figure 9-12, cont'd **G,** After resection of the lateral condyle. **H** and **I,** Medial capsule is released by distracting the toe and cutting the medial capsule. **J,** Lateral capsule is reefed with interrupted absorbable sutures. The proximal capsule is reefed to the abductor digiti quinti muscle, and the dorsal capsule is approximated to the dorsal periosteum. (Where insufficient tissue is present, drill holes may be placed into the metaphysis of the fifth metatarsal to secure this capsular repair.)

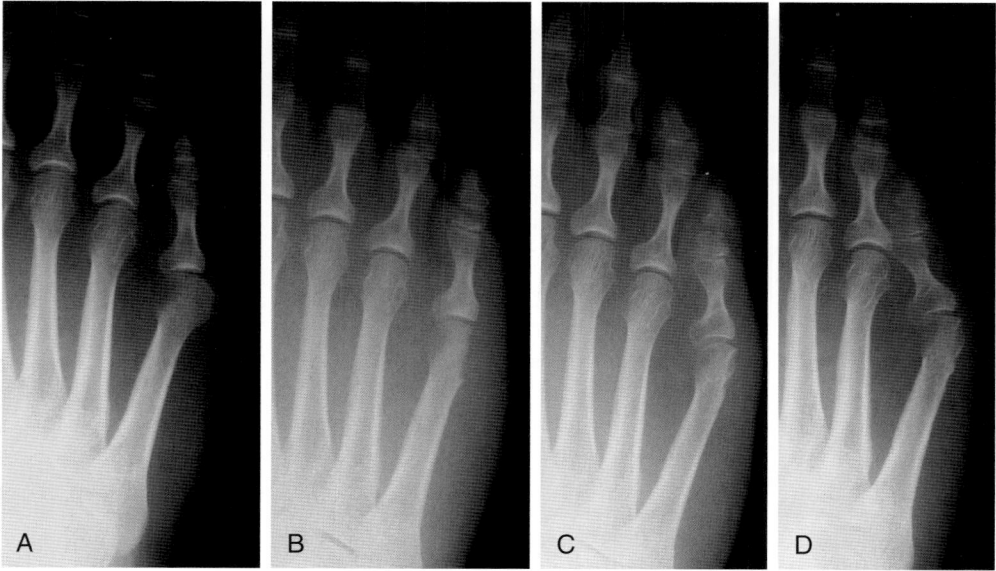

Figure 9-13 Lateral condylectomy. **A,** Preoperative radiograph demonstrating a bunionette with a type 1 deformity. **B,** After lateral condylectomy, adequate correction is achieved. **C,** Recurrence of deformity after 1 year. **D,** Recurrence of deformity after 10 years.

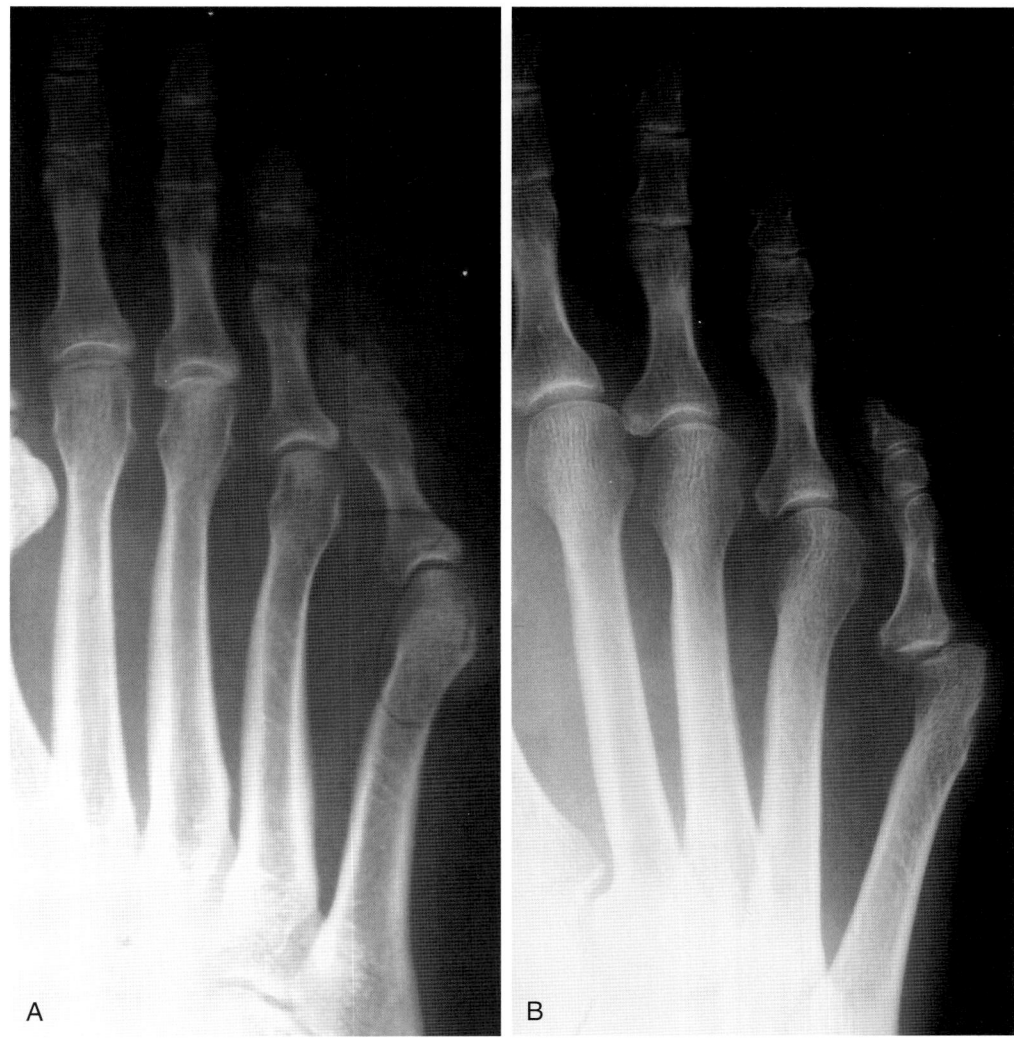

Figure 9-14 Failed lateral condylectomy. **A,** Preoperative radiograph demonstrating type 2 bunionette deformity. **B,** After lateral condylectomy, the proximal phalanx has subluxated medially.

simple condylectomy was contraindicated. Although a lateral condylar resection is a simple treatment for a bunionette deformity, the authors recognized the significant limitations of the procedure.

A meticulous fifth metatarsal capsule repair can prevent subluxation and recurrence of a bunionette deformity.[48,65] Attention to repair of the abductor digiti quinti muscle and fifth metatarsal capsule can prevent later dislocation of the MTP joint.[33]

FIFTH METATARSAL HEAD RESECTION
The failure of a lateral condylectomy as an effective treatment of a bunionette deformity has resulted in the recommendation for more extensive resection procedures. Excision of the fifth metatarsal head (Fig. 9-15),[1,21,22,37] resection of the distal half of the fifth metatarsal (Fig. 9-16),[51] and fifth-ray resection (Fig. 9-17)[5] have all been advocated as treatment for a symptomatic bunionette

deformity. McKeever[51] advocated excision of the fifth metatarsal head and one half to two thirds of the fifth metatarsal shaft; Brown[5] found that resection of almost the entire fifth ray and a fifth toe amputation adequately narrowed the foot and relieved symptoms. Kelikian[35] recommended McKeever's technique but syndactylized the fourth and fifth toes to avoid a symptomatic flail fifth toe deformity.

Indications
Ray resection, extensive fifth metatarsal diaphyseal resection, and fifth metatarsal head resection should be reserved as a salvage procedure for intractable ulceration, severe deformity, and infection, as well as in rheumatoid arthritis when multiple metatarsal head resections are performed. Fifth metatarsal head resection may also be considered in the presence of recurrent deformity with a significant soft tissue contracture.

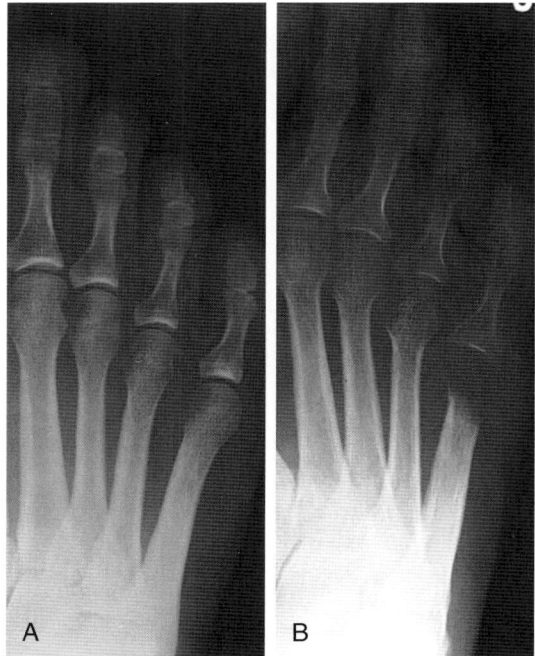

Figure 9-15 Fifth metatarsal head resection. **A,** Preoperative radiograph of 55-year-old man with diabetes and intractable ulceration beneath the fifth metatarsal head. **B,** Postoperative radiograph after fifth metatarsal head excision with successful healing of lesion.

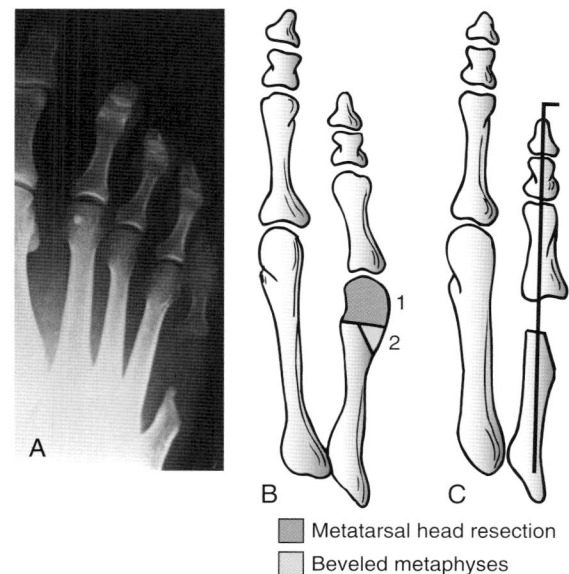

☐ Metatarsal head resection
☐ Beveled metaphyses

Figure 9-16 **A,** Fifth metatarsal head excision with resection of the distal half of the fifth metatarsal (McKeever technique) after osteomyelitis. **B,** Dorsal view of osteotomy of the fifth metatarsal. Shading denotes both resection (1) and beveling (2) necessary after osteotomy is performed. **C,** Intramedullary Kirschner wire fixation may be used to stabilize toe if neither infection nor plantar ulceration is present.

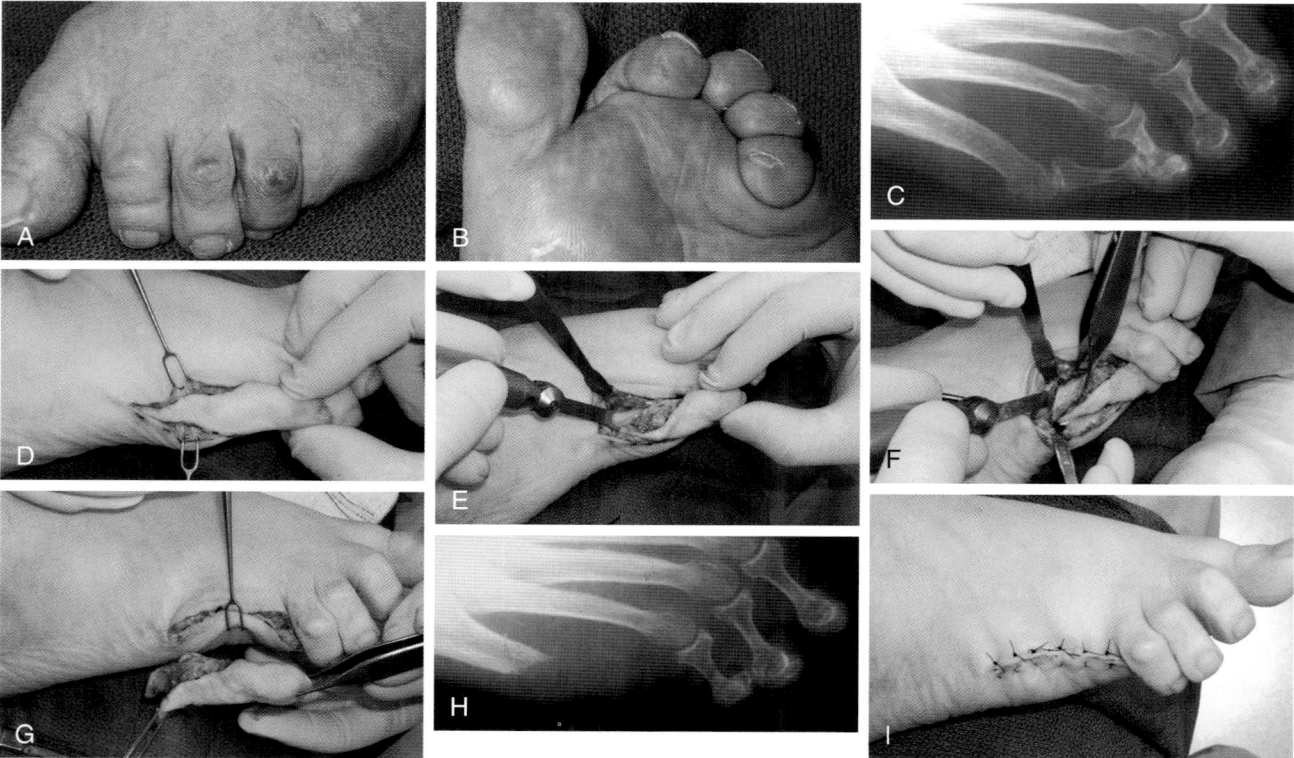

Figure 9-17 Fifth-ray resection in a patient with rheumatoid forefoot deformity. **A** and **B,** Preoperative deformity. **C,** Preoperative radiograph demonstrating subluxation of the fifth metatarsophalangeal joint. **D,** Skin incision. **E,** Oblique fifth metatarsal osteotomy. **F,** Transection of metatarsal. **G,** Specimen removed. **H,** Final postoperative radiograph. **I,** After wound closure.

Contraindications

As a primary procedure in the treatment of a bunionette deformity, less radical procedures that preserve function of the fifth ray should be considered instead of resection arthroplasty. Implant arthroplasty is to be discouraged at the fifth MTP joint. No evidence indicates that it offers improved postoperative function over resection arthroplasty, and, on occasion, significant complications are associated with this procedure.

Surgical Technique

1. The patient is positioned in a semilateral decubitus position.
2. The extremity is cleansed in a normal fashion.
3. A longitudinal incision is centered over the lateral eminence, extending from the midportion of the proximal phalanx to 1 cm above the lateral eminence. (With plantar ulceration, a dorsal incision may be used. With rheumatoid arthritis when multiple metatarsal heads are excised, a longitudinal IM incision may be placed in the fourth IM space.)
4. The capsular structures are released, and the fifth metatarsal head is exposed.
5. The fifth metatarsal shaft is transected in the metaphyseal region with a sagittal saw or a bone-cutting forceps (see Fig. 9-16A and B).
6. The prominent lateral and plantar aspects of the metatarsal shafts are beveled with a rongeur.
7. A 0.045-inch Kirschner wire is introduced at the base of the proximal phalanx and driven distally through the tip of the toe (see Fig. 9-16C). It is then driven in a retrograde manner into the metatarsal diaphysis to align and stabilize the fifth toe. With plantar ulceration or infection, Kirschner wire stabilization is contraindicated.
8. The capsule is plicated with interrupted absorbable suture. The skin edges are approximated in a routine manner.

Postoperative Care

A gauze-and-tape compression dressing is used for alignment of the fifth toe and changed weekly for 6 weeks. Ambulation is permitted in a postoperative shoe. Sutures and the Kirschner wire are removed 3 weeks after surgery.

Results and Complications

Although fifth metatarsal head resection has been recommended for treating a symptomatic bunionette deformity, in general, only anecdotal experience has been reported. McKeever[51] reported success in the treatment of 60 cases, but no specific criteria were used for the postoperative evaluation, and no complications were noted. Extensive metatarsal head resection can lead to retraction of the fifth toe,[21,37,42] subluxation of the fifth toe,[33,37] and development of a transfer lesion beneath the fourth metatarsal head.[21,37,42] The development of a flail fifth toe deformity might require syndactylization to the fourth toe.

With fifth metatarsal head resection in seven patients (11 feet), at an average 8-year follow-up, Kitaoka and Holiday[37] reported 82% fair or poor results. Complications, which occurred in 64% of cases, included severe shortening of the toe (36%), transfer lesions or unresolved plantar callosities (75%), stiffness (25%), and continued symptoms (27%). The preoperative 4-5 IM angle, which averaged 11 degrees, was noted to increase to 15.5 degrees after surgery. Fifth-ray shortening averaged 10 mm. Because of such complications as fifth-ray shortening, transfer metatarsalgia, malalignment of the fifth toe, and loss of MTP joint function of the fifth ray, Kitaoka and Holiday[37] concluded that excisional arthroplasty was not indicated as a primary procedure. In 21 patients who underwent fifth metatarsal head excision (average follow-up, 17 months), Dorris and Mandel[21] reported malalignment of the fifth toe in 59% of patients. Although 84% of patients were satisfied with the results at postoperative evaluation, limited short-term follow-up of as little as 3 months raises a question as to the long-term efficacy and durability of this procedure in light of the report of Kitaoka and Holiday.[37] Armstrong et al[2] used fifth metatarsal head resection for plantar ulcerations in patients with diabetes, and reported excellent resolution of symptoms with this technique in 22 cases.

Addante et al[1] reported on 35 patients (50 cases) after fifth metatarsal head resection and placement of silicone spheric implants. They reported an 84% success rate. Complications occurred in 16% of cases and included traumatic dislocation of the implant, chronic subluxation, silicone inflammatory reaction, wound dehiscence, abscess formation, intractable plantar keratosis (IPK), and transfer metatarsalgia.

DISTAL FIFTH METATARSAL OSTEOTOMY

An osteotomy of the fifth metatarsal may be used to correct alignment of the fifth metatarsal. Davies[16] stated that it was "unnecessary and unsatisfactory" to perform a fifth metatarsal osteotomy. Lelièvre,[44,45] however, recognized that an increased 4-5 IM angle should be corrected as a part of a bunionette repair. Kelikian[35] cautioned that delayed healing can occur after a fifth metatarsal osteotomy.

The location of the osteotomy and the surgical technique performed have a significant effect on the ultimate success of a metatarsal osteotomy. Distal, diaphyseal, and proximal metatarsal osteotomies have all been recommended in the treatment of symptomatic bunionette deformities. Many types of distal fifth metatarsal osteotomies have been recommended for the treatment of symptomatic bunionettes.* Although less correction of an increased 4-5 IM angle is achieved than with more proximal osteotomies, a distal fifth metatarsal osteotomy achieves significantly more correction than with a lateral condyle resection. Instability of some types of distal metatarsal osteotomies has caused concern regarding the

---

*References 4, 8, 9, 34, 39, 40, 46, 59, 60, and 65.

loss of alignment,[29,33] development of a subsequent transfer lesion, and recurrence of deformity.[34]

Hohmann[32] and later Steinke[67] described a distal fifth metatarsal osteotomy, reporting on the use of a transverse osteotomy of the fifth metatarsal neck. Kaplan et al[33] advocated a distal closing-wedge fifth metatarsal osteotomy that was internally fixed with a Kirschner wire. They suggested internal fixation because the distal osteotomy was unstable and might rotate postoperatively, with resulting loss of correction. Haber and Kraft[31] used a distal fifth metatarsal crescentic osteotomy. They did not use internal fixation to stabilize the osteotomy site and reported excessive callus formation at the osteotomy site and delayed healing. Catanzariti et al[9] performed a distal oblique fifth metatarsal osteotomy without internal fixation and reported a 26% recurrence rate and transfer lesions in 35% of cases.

Throckmorton and Bradlee[69] and others[4,7,13,38] described a distal fifth metatarsal transverse chevron osteotomy. Because of the stable shape of this osteotomy, Throckmorton did not use internal fixation. Boyer and DeOrio[4] have used an absorbable fixation pin for internal fixation of a chevron osteotomy. A reverse Mitchell procedure,[42,65] distal chevron osteotomy,[4,26,38,52,69] distal transverse osteotomy,[32,33,67] distal crescentic osteotomy,[31] scarf,[17,30,58,62] and distal oblique osteotomy* have all been recommended as distal fifth metatarsal osteotomy techniques. Nonetheless, a distal fifth metatarsal osteotomy might help to achieve adequate correction of a symptomatic bunionette deformity.

---

*References 8, 9, 11, 12, 39, 40, 46, 56, 59, 60, and 65.

Indications

With a type 1 deformity (enlarged head) or a moderate type 2 or type 3 deformity, a distal fifth metatarsal osteotomy may be used to achieve adequate surgical correction. The choice of a specific type of osteotomy depends on the experience of the surgeon and the anatomic variation present. Internal fixation is preferable because it stabilizes the correction obtained at surgery. Usually, a Kirschner wire, if used for internal fixation, can be removed without difficulty in an office setting a few weeks after surgery. An absorbable pin fixation has been used with success and provides an alternative to later hardware removal.[4,26] Screw fixation, may be left indefinitely because it is usually asymptomatic.

Contraindications

The main contraindication to a distal metatarsal osteotomy is a moderate or severe angular deformity for which a distal metatarsal osteotomy is inadequate to correct the angular deformity. A chevron osteotomy is not effective in correcting a bunionette deformity characterized by a plantar keratosis; in this case, a distal osteotomy that elevates the fifth metatarsal head is preferable (distal oblique osteotomy, capital oblique osteotomy).

DISTAL TRANSVERSE MEDIALIZING OSTEOTOMY WITH STEINMANN PIN FIXATION[29,43,73]
Surgical Technique
1. The patient is positioned in a semilateral decubitus position.
2. The extremity is cleansed in a normal fashion (Fig. 9-18A).

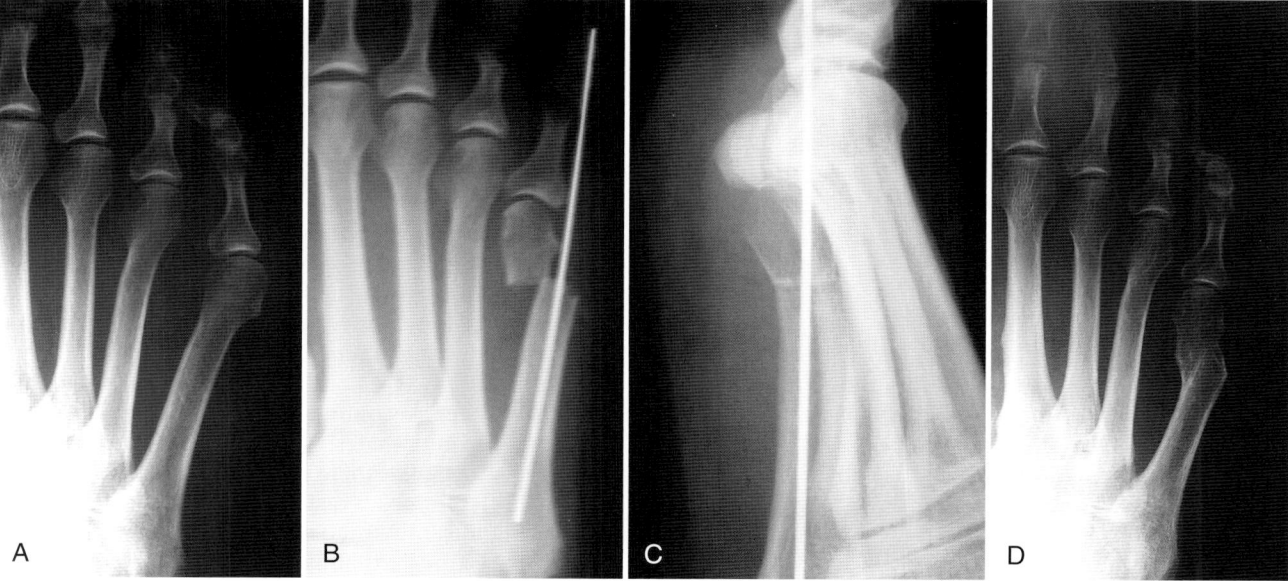

Figure 9-18 Distal transverse medializing osteotomy. **A,** Preoperative radiograph demonstrating type 3 bunionette deformity in 60-year-old female. **B** and **C,** Anteroposterior and lateral radiographs with internal fixation after osteotomy. **D,** Eight-year follow-up after osteotomy. (Courtesy Hans-Joerg Trnka, MD.)

3. A 1-cm longitudinal incision is made from a point directly proximal to the lateral eminence and directed toward the heel.

4. The soft tissues are spread, and two small retractors are placed superiorly and inferiorly to visualize the neck of the metatarsal.

5. A tranverse vertical ostetomy, perpendicular to the long axis of the fifth metatarsal, is made from lateral to medial, completely transecting the metatarsal neck.

6. If shortening is desired, the vertical direction of the ostetomy is varied so that it is inclined in a distal–proximal direction of up to 25 degrees. If lengthening is desired, the cut is inclined in a proximal–distal direction up to 15 degrees.

7. The cut creates a shelf that tends to minimize dorsal translation of the capital fragment.

8. A 1.8-mm Kirschner wire is inserted into the soft tissue adjacent to the toe on the lateral aspect and driven distally out the tip of the fifth toe. With the capital fragment displaced as far medialward as desired with a freer elevator, the Kirschner wire is then driven proximal into the diaphyseal canal until it penetrates the proximal metaphyseal region (Fig. 9-18B and C).

9. The excess pin is cut, and the skin is approximated in a routine fashion.

10. The skin is closed with interrupted sutures (Fig. 9-18D).

Postoperative Care

The foot is wrapped in a gauze-and-tape compression dressing that is changed weekly for 6 weeks. Sutures and the Kirschner wire are removed 4 weeks after surgery. The patient is allowed to ambulate in a postoperative shoe with weight bearing on the inner border of the foot for 6 weeks. At this time, use of the postoperative shoe is discontinued.

Results and Complications

Weitzel et al[73] and Giannini et al[29] have both described a transverse medial osteotomy stabilized with a longitudinal axial Steinmann pin. Weitzel et al[73] reported on 21 patients (30 feet) who were noted to have 81% good and excellent results at an average follow-up of more than 7 years. The American Orthopaedic Foot and Ankle Society (AOFAS) pain score, at this time, was 88 points, and the visual analog score (VAS) was less than 2 points. They noted an improvement in the 4-5 IM angle from 17.6 to −7.3 degrees. Complications with this limited fixation included 8 of 30 patients with dorsal displacement, 3 pin-tract infections, and 1 transfer lesion. Giannini et al[29] reported on 32 patients (50 feet) at almost 5-years follow-up. They noted an improvement in the 4-5 IM angle from 12.7 to 6.7 degrees, and the MTP-5 angle was diminished from 16.8 to 8 degrees. Two patients developed transfer lesions, but overall, 90% good and excellent results were reported in this procedure that is quite similar to a Homan osteeotomy but included axial pin stabilization.

DISTAL CHEVRON OSTEOTOMY

1. The patient is positioned in a semilateral decubitus position.

2. The extremity is cleansed in a normal fashion.

3. A longitudinal incision is centered directly over the lateral eminence and extended 1 cm above the lateral eminence. Care is taken to protect the dorsal and plantar neurovascular bundles (Figs. 9-19A and 9-20A; Video Clip 43).

4. The capsule of the MTP joint is incised along the dorsal and proximal border to create an inverted L-shaped capsule release. This flap is detached from the periosteum dorsally, as well as the abductor digiti quinti muscle proximally (see Figs. 9-19B and 9-20B).

5. The flap is turned downward to expose the lateral eminence, which is resected with a power saw (see Fig. 9-20C).

6. A 0.045-inch Kirschner wire is drilled through the center of the metatarsal head in a lateral-to-medial direction. This drill hole marks the apex of the osteotomy (see Figs. 9-19C and 9-20D).

7. A sagittal saw with in-line teeth is used to create the osteotomy. This saw blade configuration minimizes shortening at the osteotomy site (see Figs. 9-19D and 9-20E).

8. The osteotomy cut is made from a lateral-to-medial direction at an angle of approximately 60 degrees.

9. Care is taken to avoid excessive soft tissue stripping because the remaining vascular supply to the fifth metatarsal is from the medial aspect of the capital fragment.

10. The metatarsal diaphysis is grasped with a towel clip, and the capital fragment and toe are displaced in a medial direction. The displacement is approximately 33% to 50% of the width of the metaphysis (see Fig. 9-20F). The remaining metaphyseal flare is shaved with a power saw (see Fig. 9-20G).

11. The capital fragment is stabilized with a 0.045-inch Kirschner wire from a proximal or distal insertion point (see Fig. 9-19E).

12. The MTP joint capsule is repaired with interrupted absorbable suture. The capsule flap may be secured to the metatarsal metaphysis by drill holes placed in the metaphysis. The capsule is also secured to the dorsal periosteum of the fifth metatarsal and the abductor digiti quinti. A secure capsule closure helps to prevent recurrence of the deformity (see Figs. 9-19F and 9-20H).

13. The skin is closed with interrupted sutures (see Figs. 9-20I and 9-21).

Postoperative Care

The foot is wrapped with a gauze-and-tape compression dressing that is changed weekly for 6 weeks. The sutures and Kirschner wire are removed 3 weeks after surgery. The patient is allowed to ambulate in a postoperative shoe with weight bearing on the inner border of the foot for 6 weeks. The postoperative shoe is discontinued 3 weeks postoperatively (Fig. 9-21).

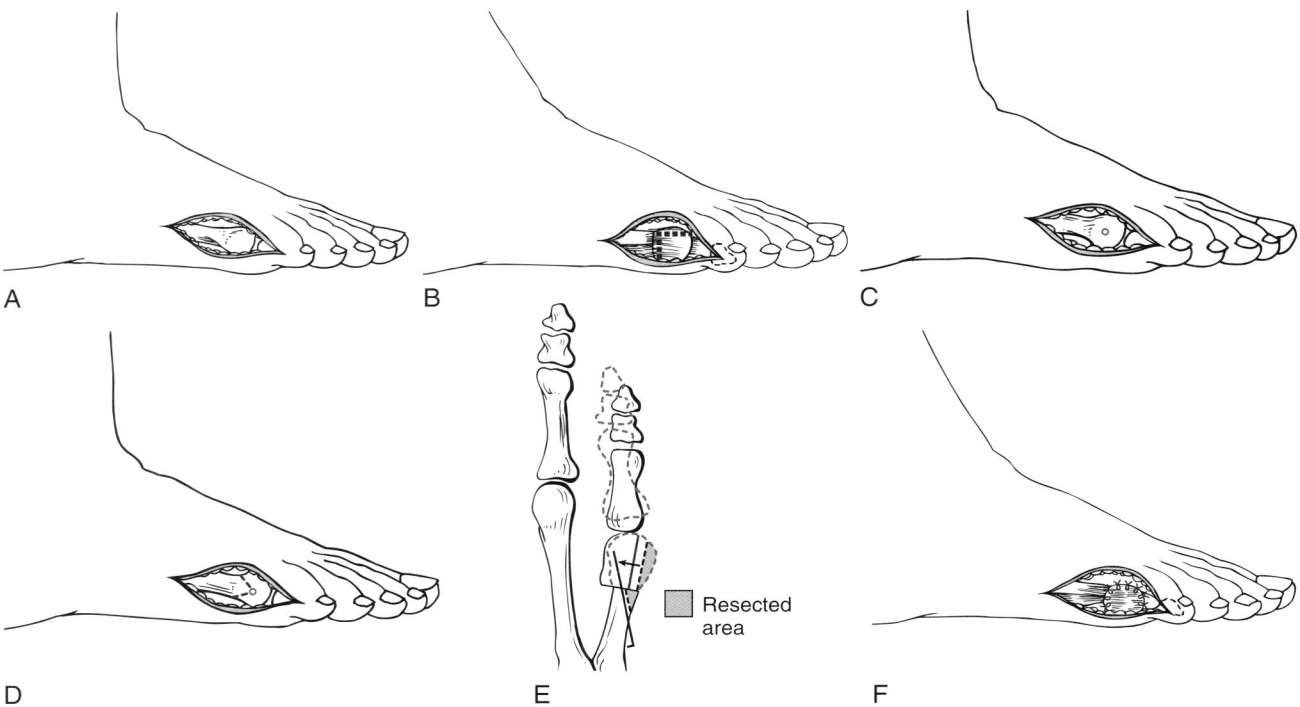

Figure 9-19 Distal chevron osteotomy. **A,** Lateral incision is centered over the fifth metatarsal head. **B,** An L-shaped capsular release is performed. Exostectomy is performed to remove the lateral condyle in line with the lateral border of the foot. **C,** Lateral-to-medial drill hole marks the apex of the chevron osteotomy. **D,** Osteotomy is performed (base proximal) at an angle of approximately 60 degrees. Distal capital fragment is displaced in a medial direction. Remaining bone is beveled around the osteotomy site. **E,** A 0.045-inch Kirschner wire is used to stabilize the capital fragment to the proximal metatarsal shaft inserted from a proximal or distal point. **F,** An interrupted capsular repair is carried out. Where insufficient capsular tissue is present, drill holes in the metaphysis may be used to secure the capsule repair.

Resected area

Results and Complications

Throckmorton and Bradlee[69] initially reported the use of a chevron osteotomy to correct a bunionette deformity. No long-term series were reported. Campbell[7] reported on 9 patients (12 chevron osteotomies) and noted that all patients were satisfied postoperatively. Leach and Igou[42] reported on a reverse Mitchell procedure on 11 feet. The average preoperative 4-5 IM angle of 11.7 degrees was corrected to 4.9 degrees; thus an average 6.8-degree correction of the IM angle was achieved. They noted no nonunions in this series.

Kitaoka et al[38] reported on the results of a distal chevron osteotomy in 13 patients (19 feet) treated for symptomatic bunionette deformities. At an average follow-up of 7.1 years, 12 of 19 feet (63%) were reported to have good or excellent results. Complications included a postoperative keratosis over the bunionette in 1 patient and transfer metatarsalgia in another. Radiographic analysis found the 4-5 IM angle preoperatively measured 11.8 degrees and postoperatively 9.2 degrees, for an average correction of 2.6 degrees. The average MTP-5 angle measured 20.7 degrees preoperatively and 12.8 degrees postoperatively, for an average correction of 7.9 degrees. The average forefoot width was decreased by 3 mm. The authors concluded that although a limited degree of correction is possible with a chevron osteotomy, this

procedure reliably achieves subjective relief of symptoms. Although they used cast immobilization for 3 weeks after surgery, they observed that immobilization with a soft compression dressing and ambulation in a postsurgical shoe was an alternative. For an unreliable patient, they suggested cast immobilization. Although Kirschner wire internal fixation was not advocated, the authors noted that it could be used if the osteotomy site was not stable.

Pontious et al[55] reported on eight chevron osteotomies and noted no dorsal displacement, indicating that this was a very stable osteotomy. Excessive soft tissue stripping on the dorsal and plantar aspect of the distal metatarsal osteotomy does, however, increase the risk of instability at the osteotomy site and also predisposes to nonunion or avascular necrosis of the fifth metatarsal head. Reporting on 12 patients (16 osteotomies), Moran and Claridge[52] stressed that there was a low margin of error with this osteotomy but also a risk of recurrence or overcorrection. They suggested that the osteotomy site be stabilized with Kirschner wire internal fixation.

Boyer and DeOrio[4] reported the results of 10 patients with 12 osteotomies fixed with an absorbable pin (Fig. 9-22). At an average follow-up of 48 months, there was no evidence of avascular necrosis, displacement of the osteotomy, or osteolysis. All osteotomies healed by 6 weeks, and the postoperative American Orthopaedic

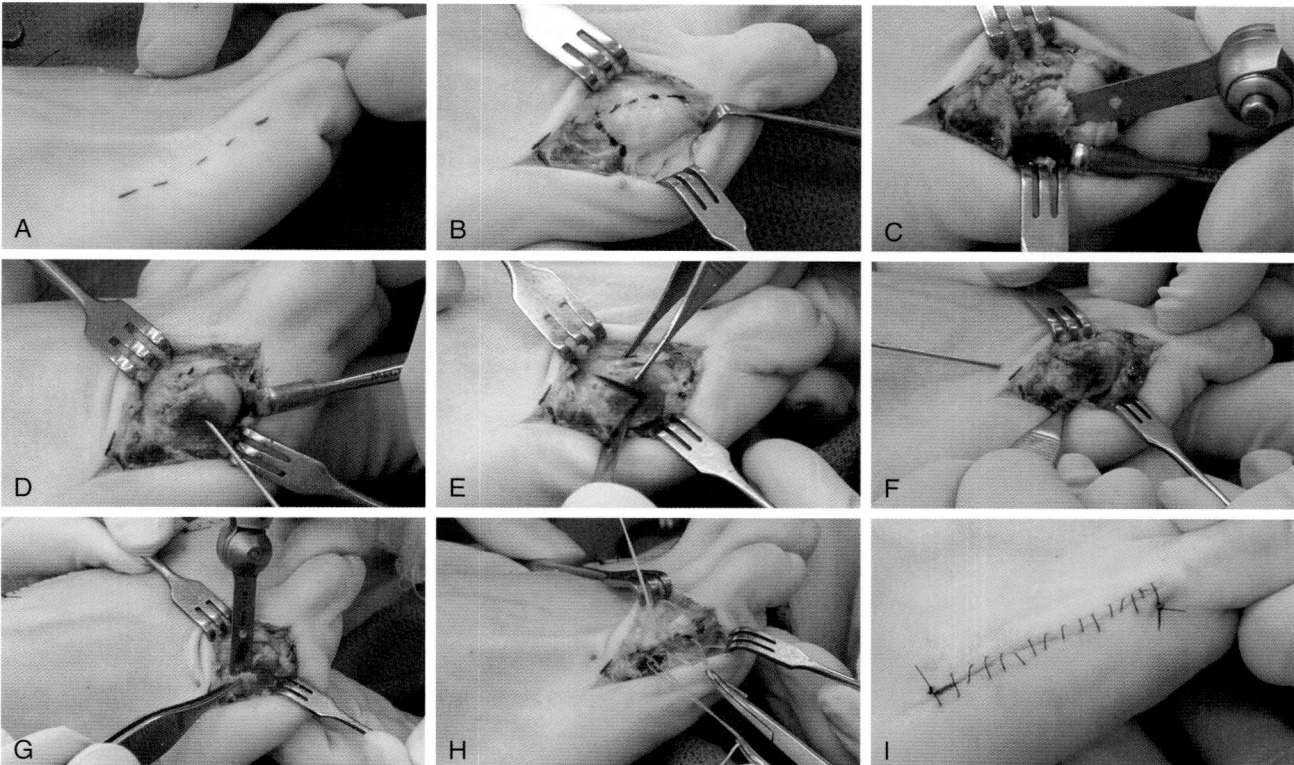

Figure 9-20 Distal chevron osteotomy. **A,** Skin incision. **B,** L-shaped capsular incision. **C,** Lateral eminence resection. **D,** Drill hole marks apex of the chevron osteotomy. **E,** After chevron osteotomy. **F,** After medial translation of capital fragment. **G,** Resection of metaphyseal flare. **H,** Capsular closure. **I,** After skin closure.

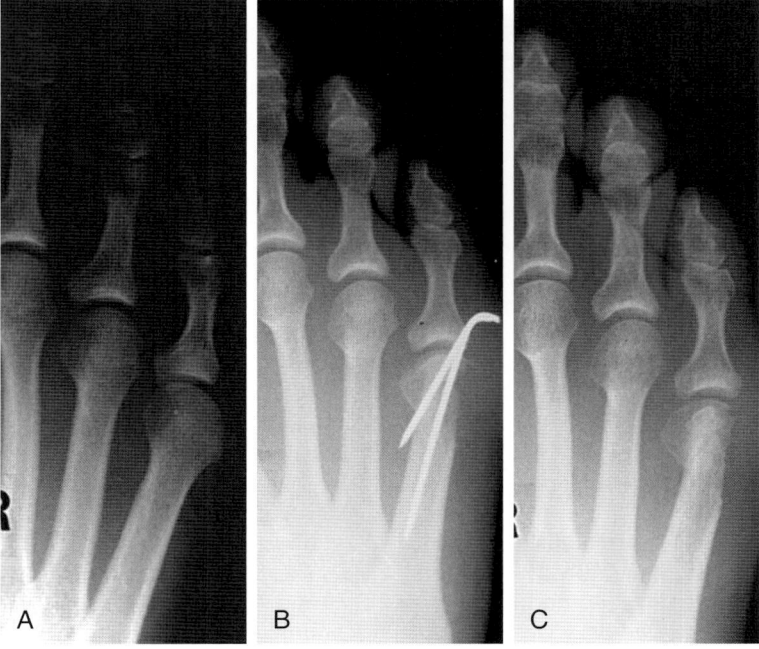

Figure 9-21 **A,** Preoperative radiograph demonstrates bunionette deformity. **B,** After chevron osteotomy with Kirschner wire fixation. **C,** Chevron osteotomy achieves adequate repair.

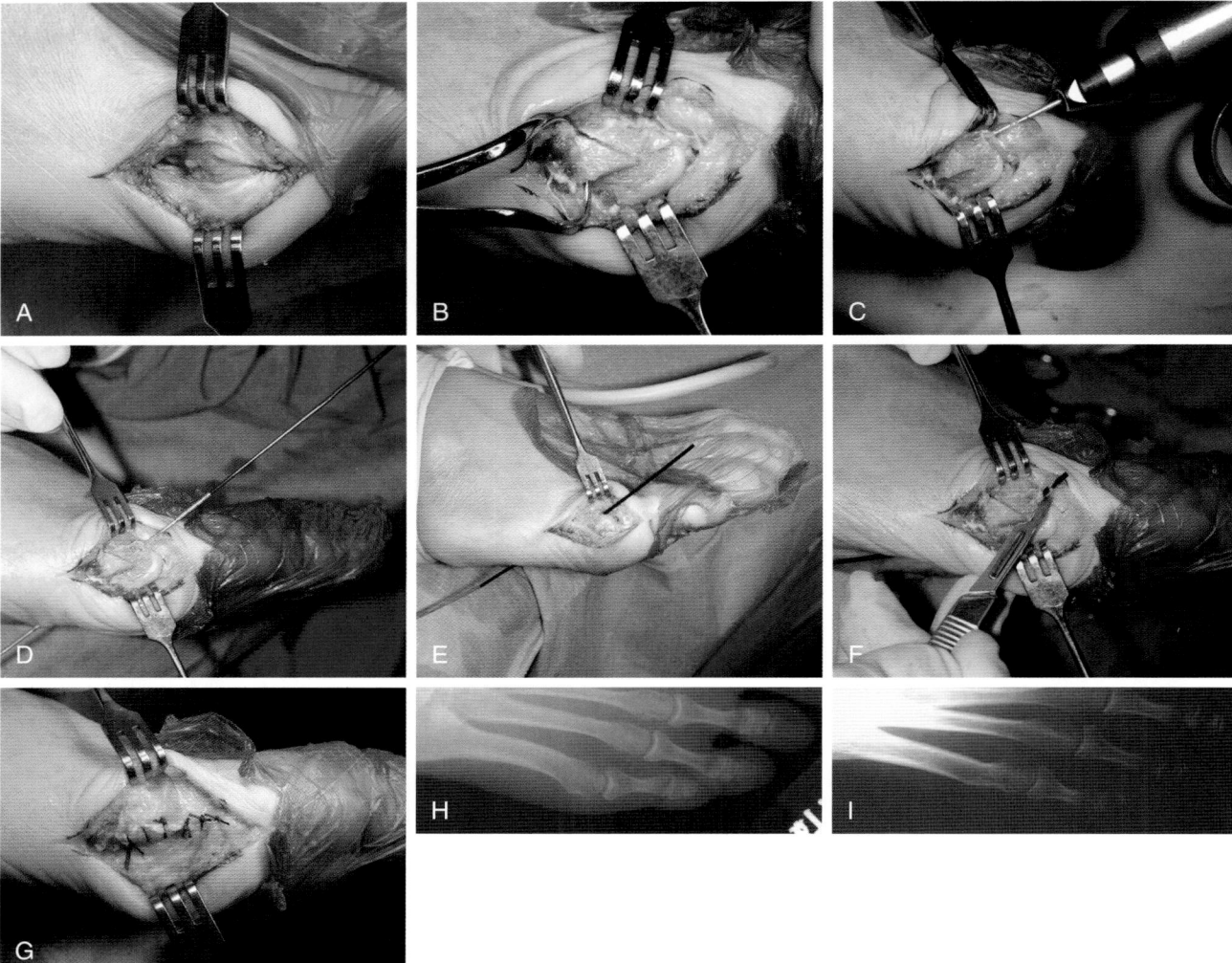

Figure 9-22 Chevron osteotomy with resorbable pin fixation (DeOrio technique). **A,** Longitudinal capsular incision. **B,** The proximal fragment is grasped with a towel clip as the capital fragment is translated medially. **C,** Fixation drill hole. **D,** Sheath with resorbable pin fixation. **E,** Sheath removed. **F,** Pin severed at the edge of the dorsal and plantar bone surfaces. **G,** Capsular closure. Preoperative **(H)** and postoperative **(I)** radiographs. (Courtesy J. DeOrio, MD.)

Foot and Ankle Society (AOFAS) score averaged 93 points. The 4-5 IM angle was diminished from 9.1 degrees to 1.4 degrees postoperatively. The MTP-5 angle was corrected from 11.8 degrees preoperatively to 6.2 degrees postoperatively. No transfer lesions were noted.

DISTAL OBLIQUE OSTEOTOMY
Surgical Technique

1. The patient is positioned in a semilateral decubitus position.
2. The extremity is cleansed in a normal fashion.
3. A longitudinal incision is made directly over the lateral eminence beginning at the midportion of the proximal phalanx and extending 1 cm above the lateral eminence. Care is taken to protect the dorsal and plantar neurovascular bundles.
4. The capsule of the MTP joint is incised along the dorsal and proximal border to create an inverted L-shaped capsular release. This flap is detached from the dorsal periosteum as well as the abductor digiti quinti muscle proximally (Fig. 9-23A).
5. After the lateral eminence of the fifth metatarsal head is exposed, the prominent condyle is resected with a sagittal saw.
6. An oblique osteotomy of the fifth metatarsal neck is carried out with the same sagittal saw. The osteotomy is oriented in a distal–lateral to proximal–medial direction (Fig. 9-23B and Video Clip 45).
7. The proximal fragment is grasped with a towel clip, and the capital fragment is displaced medially and impacted on the proximal fragment.
8. The osteotomy site is fixed with a 0.045-inch Kirschner wire, which may be left protruding through or

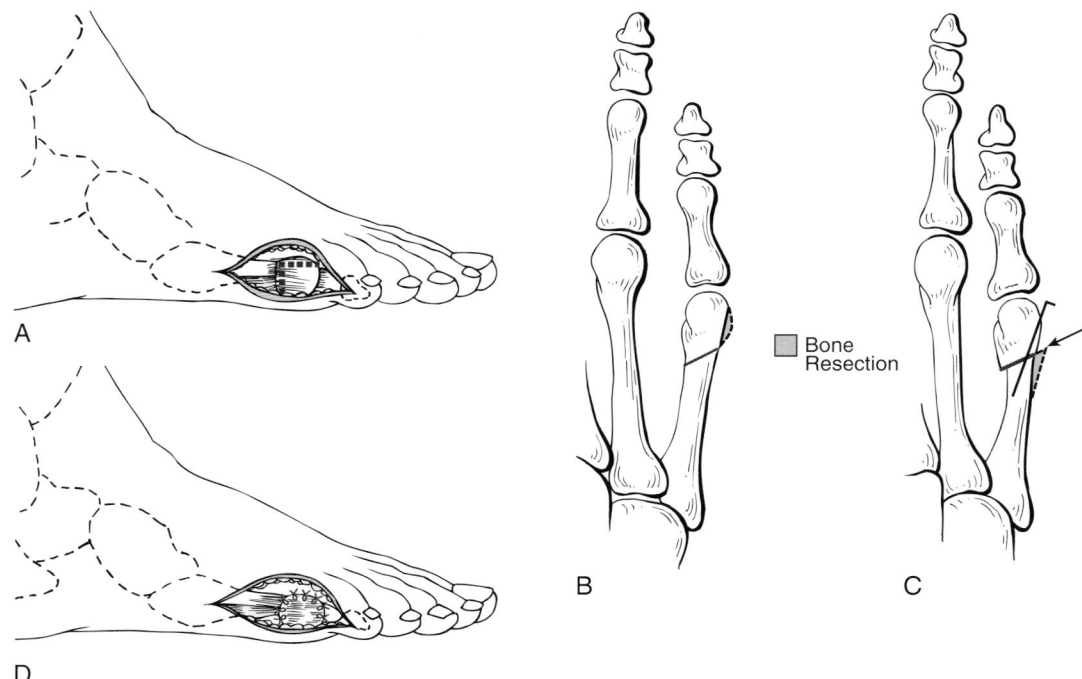

Figure 9-23 Distal oblique osteotomy. **A,** Lateral skin incision is centered over the fifth metatarsal head. L-shaped capsular release detaches the dorsal and proximal capsules (weakest area of capsular attachment). **B,** Oblique osteotomy is performed from a distal–lateral to proximal–medial direction. **C,** The capital fragment is displaced in a medial direction. Internal fixation with Kirschner wire stabilizes the osteotomy. **D,** The capsule is repaired with interrupted suture. In the presence of insufficient proximal capsule, drill holes may be placed in the metaphysis to secure the capsular repair.

buried just beneath the skin (Fig. 9-23C). Alternatively, one or two mini-fragment screws may be used to stabilize the osteotomy.[56]

9. The MTP joint capsule is repaired with interrupted absorbable suture. The capsule flap may be secured to the metatarsal metaphysis by drill holes placed in the metaphysis. The capsule is also secured to the dorsal area of the periosteum of the fifth metatarsal and the abductor digiti quinti; a secure capsule closure helps to prevent recurrence of the deformity (Fig. 9-23D).

10. The skin is closed with interrupted sutures (Fig. 9-24).

Postoperative Care

The foot is wrapped in a gauze-and-tape compression dressing that is changed weekly for 6 weeks. Sutures and the Kirschner wire are removed 3 weeks after surgery. The patient is allowed to ambulate in a postoperative shoe with weight bearing on the inner border of the foot for 6 weeks. At this time, use of the postoperative shoe is discontinued.

CAPITAL OBLIQUE OSTEOTOMY (MODIFIED WEIL) (AUTHOR'S PREFERRED TECHNIQUE)
Surgical Technique

1. The patient is positioned in a semilateral decubitus position.

2. The extremity is cleansed in a normal fashion.

3. A longitudinal incision directly over the lateral eminence is made beginning at the midportion of the proximal phalanx and extended 1 cm above the lateral eminence. Care is taken to protect the dorsal and plantar neurovascular bundles (Fig. 9-25A-C).

4. The capsule of the MTP joint is incised along the dorsal and proximal border to create an inverted L-shaped capsule release. This flap is detached from the dorsal periosteum as well as the abductor digiti quinti muscle proximally (Fig. 9-25D).

5. The lateral eminence of the fifth metatarsal head is exposed, and the prominent condyle is resected with a sagittal saw (Fig. 9-25E).

6. A longitudinal osteotomy of the fifth metatarsal is performed starting 2 to 3 mm plantar to the dorsal extent of the metatarsal articular cartilage (Video Clip 44). The osteotomy is usually parallel to the plantar aspect of the foot, although if a plantar callosity is present, the saw blade may be tipped so that the capital fragment elevates as it is translated in a medial direction (Fig. 9-25F).

7. The capital fragment is then displaced in a medial direction 2 to 4 mm; care is taken not to shorten the fifth ray at the osteotomy site (Fig. 9-25G).

8. The osteotomy site is fixed with a dorsal–plantar mini-fragment screw; the dorsal metaphyseal flare is resected with a sagittal saw (Fig. 9-25H and I).

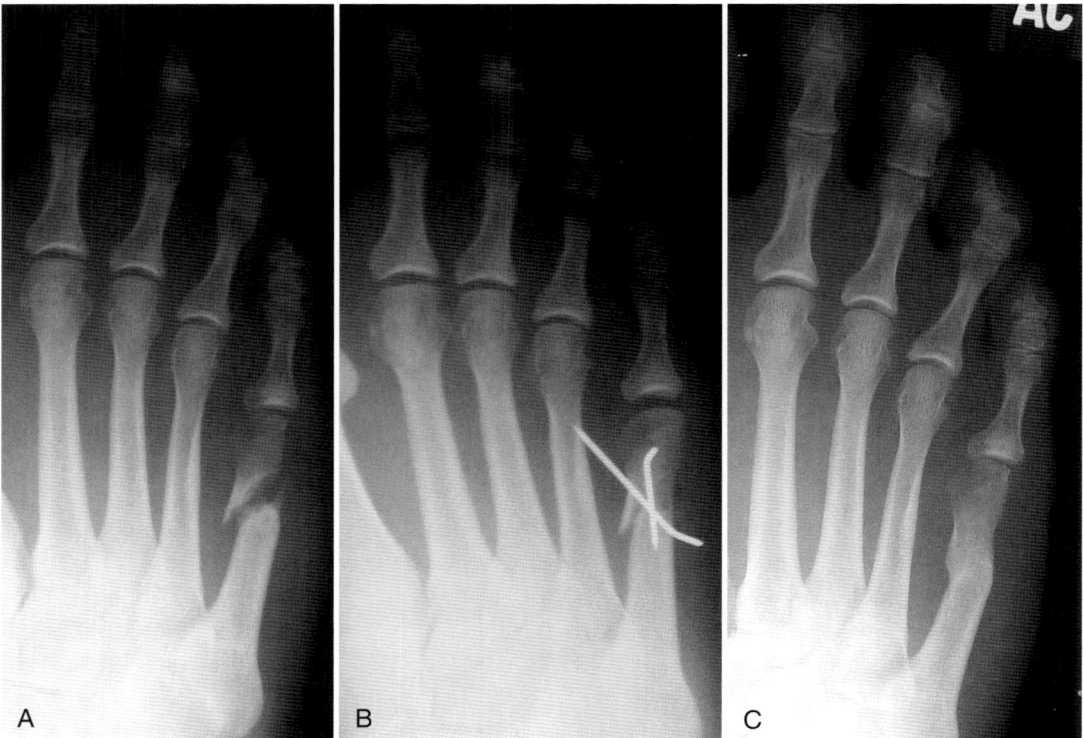

Figure 9-24 **A,** Nonunion after distal oblique osteotomy without internal fixation. **B,** Redo fixation and bone grafting. **C,** Final result with successful healing.

9. The MTP joint capsule is repaired with interrupted absorbable suture. The capsule flap may be secured to the metatarsal metaphysis by drill holes placed in the metaphysis. The capsule is also secured to the dorsal area of the periosteum of the fifth metatarsal and the abductor digiti quinti (a secure capsule closure helps to prevent recurrence of the deformity) (Fig. 9-25J).
10. The skin is closed with interrupted sutures (Fig. 9-25K-M).

Postoperative Care

The foot is wrapped in a gauze-and-tape compression dressing that is changed weekly for 6 weeks. Sutures and the Kirschner wire are removed 3 weeks after surgery. The internal fixation is rarely removed unless it becomes symptomatic. The patient is allowed to ambulate in a postoperative shoe with weight bearing on the inner border of the foot for 6 weeks. Then use of the postoperative shoe is discontinued.

Results and Complications

Sponsel[65] advocated an oblique distal fifth metatarsal osteotomy. The capital fragment was allowed to float because internal fixation was not used. An 11% delayed union rate was reported. Keating et al[34] also used an oblique distal fifth metatarsal osteotomy without internal fixation. Transfer lesions were reported in 75% of patients, and a 12% recurrence rate was noted. The authors attributed complications such as recurrent deformity and

transfer keratotic lesions to medial displacement and dorsiflexion of the distal fragment after the osteotomy. They noted a success rate of 56%. Diebold and Bejjani[20] and Frankel et al[25] suggested that, after distal fifth metatarsal osteotomies, there may be a high dissatisfaction rate because of the instability of the osteotomy site and the difficulty in obtaining adequate fixation (Figs. 9-26 and 9-27).

Pontious et al[55] compared distal fifth metatarsal osteotomies that were internally fixed to those not fixed. They stressed that internal fixation controls dorsal displacement of the capital fragment, producing less shortening and fewer complications. In a report on 46 patients (56 feet), they noted that the average healing time was 8 weeks in osteotomies that were internally fixed and 11 weeks in those that were not. They concluded that osteotomies that were internally fixed healed more predictably and that fixation prevented displacement, making it possible to maintain the corrected osteotomy position. Kitaoka and Holiday[36] and Frankel et al[25] concluded that floating fifth metatarsal osteotomies that seek their own level in an uncontrolled manner have a significant incidence of transfer metatarsalgia (Fig. 9-28).

Kitaoka and Leventen[39] performed a distal oblique osteotomy in 16 patients (23 feet) (Fig. 9-29). The orientation of this osteotomy was proximal–lateral to distal–medial. The fifth metatarsal head was displaced medially and impaled on the medial spike of the diaphyseal segment. The average 4-5 IM angle was decreased from 13

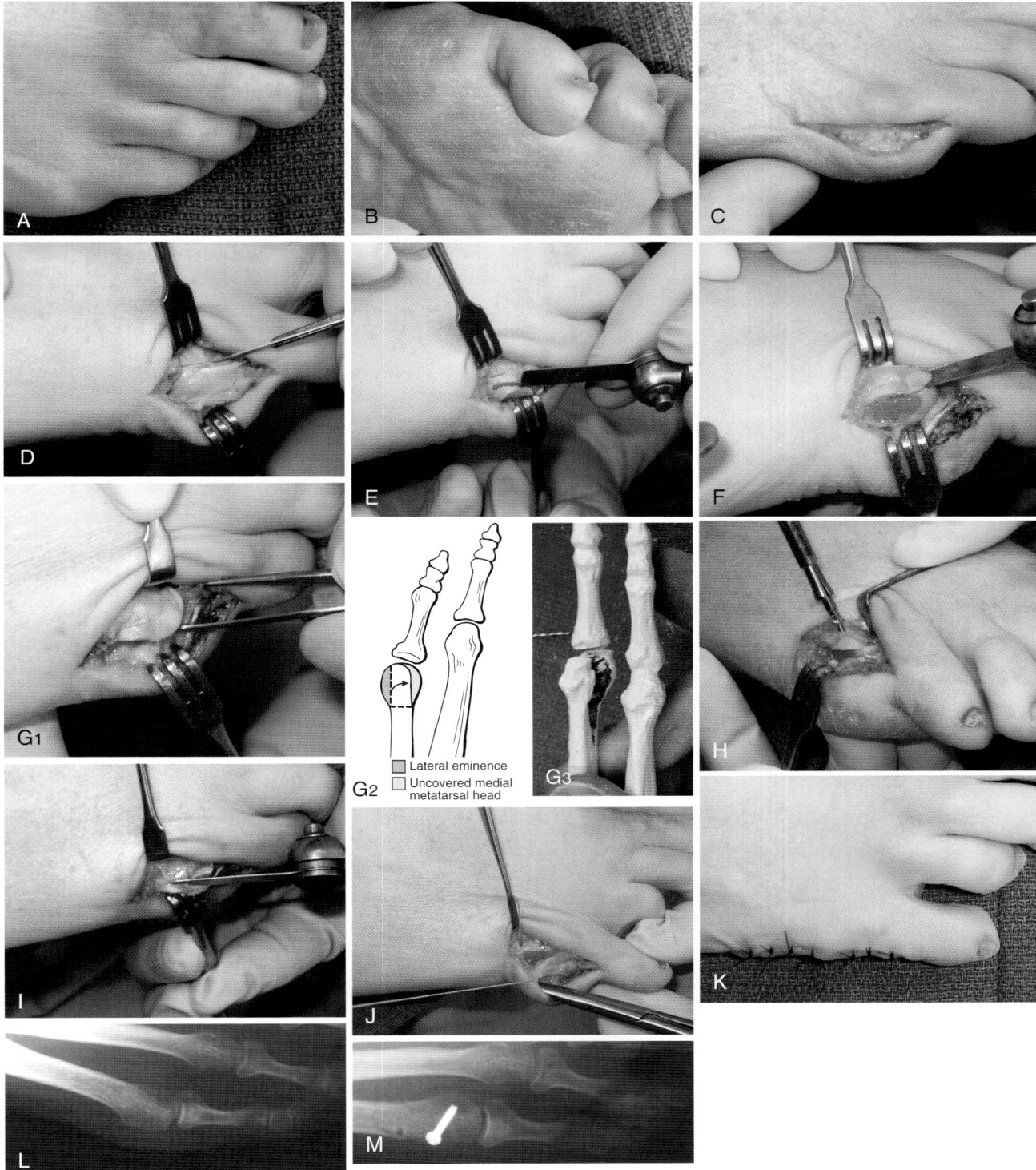

Figure 9-25 Capital oblique osteotomy. **A,** Preoperative deformity. **B,** Plantar view. **C,** Skin incision. **D,** L-shaped capsular incision. **E,** Lateral eminence resection. **F,** Capital oblique osteotomy. This cut can be rotated to elevate the capital fragment as it is translated in a medial direction. **G1,** The distal fragment is grasped with a forceps and pushed medially. **G2,** Diagram of medial translation of the capital fragment. **G3,** Demonstration of translation with sawbones model. **H,** Oblique screw fixation. **I,** Lateral flare of metaphysis is shaved. **J,** Capsule closure. **K,** Skin closure. **L,** Preoperative radiograph. **M,** Postoperative radiograph.

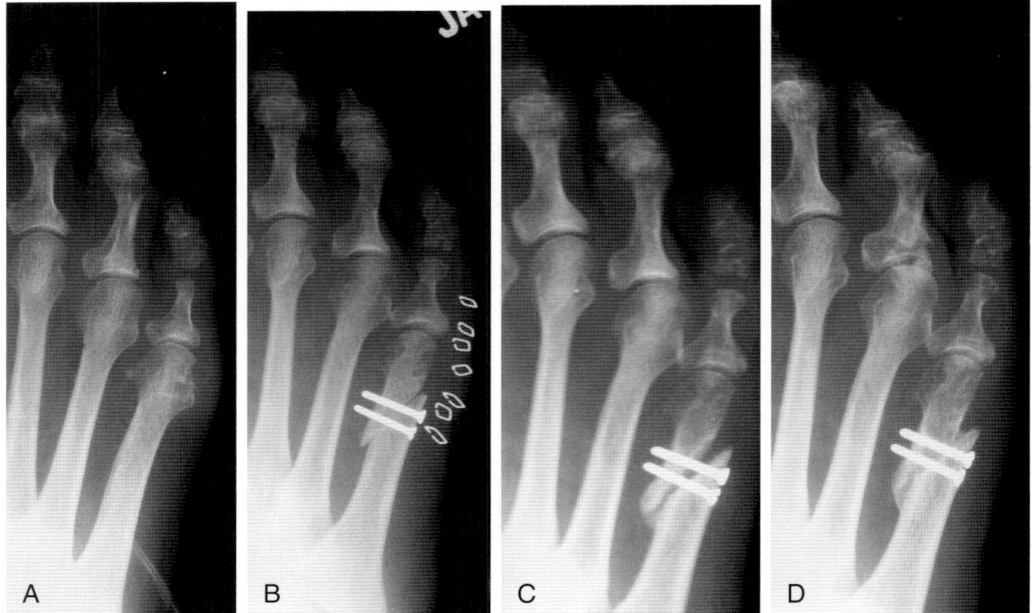

Figure 9-26 Oblique osteotomy. **A,** Preoperative radiograph. **B,** After oblique osteotomy with double screw fixation. **C,** With premature weight bearing, the patient displaced the osteotomy. **D,** With time, successful union was achieved.

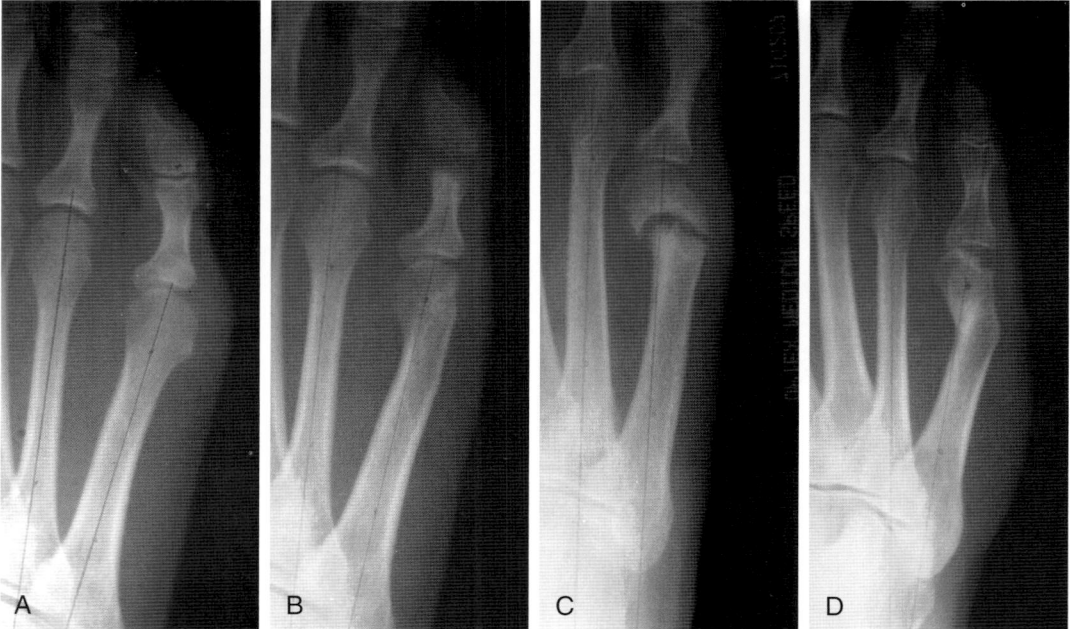

Figure 9-27 Modified L-shaped diaphyseal osteotomy. Preoperative **(A)** and postoperative **(B)** radiographs. **C,** Asymptomatic nonunion. **D,** Malunion after correction of type 3 deformity. (From Friend G, Grace K, Stone HA: L-osteotomy with absorbable fixation for correction of tailor's bunion, *J Foot Ankle Surg* 32:14–19, 1993.)

to 8 degrees (average 5 degrees of correction). Forefoot width was diminished an average of 4 mm postoperatively. Eighty-seven percent of patients reported satisfactory results. One nonunion was reported (Fig. 9-30).

Experience with distal metatarsal osteotomies demonstrates an average reduction in the 4-5 IM angle of approximately 4 to 5 degrees.[60,62,75] Whether a chevron osteotomy,[7,52,69] distal transverse osteotomy,[25,40] or oblique osteotomy[34,39,59,60,65] is performed depends on a surgeon's preference. Less correction of the 4-5 IM angle is obtained with an osteotomy located in the distal fifth metatarsal than with a more proximal osteotomy. The small area of metaphyseal bone in this region places the osteotomy at risk for delayed union, malunion, or nonunion, regardless of the specific type of procedure (Fig. 9-31).

Although a lateral condylectomy may be used to correct a bunionette deformity characterized by an enlarged fifth metatarsal head, a distal oblique osteotomy or a chevron osteotomy appears to achieve more correction than a lateral condylar resection does alone. There is a limit, however, in the amount that the capital fragment can be displaced medially; with further medial shift medially, the osseous contact gets decidedly smaller.[41] The potential complications of a distal osteotomy, such as delayed

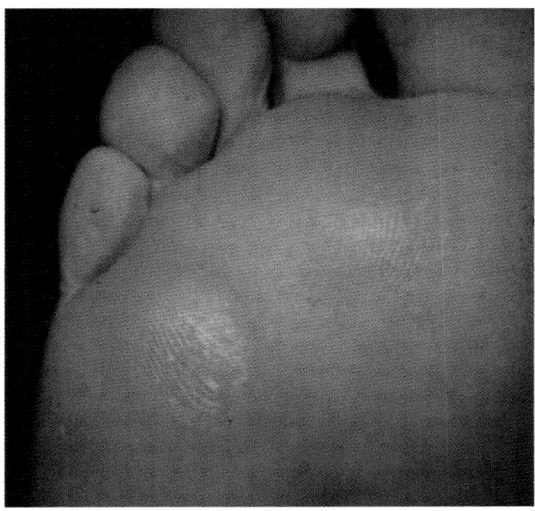

Figure 9-28 After distal fifth metatarsal osteotomy, a transfer lesion has developed beneath the fourth metatarsal.

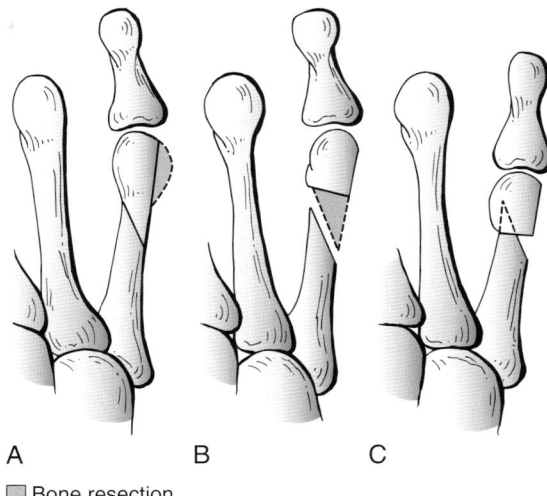

☐ Bone resection

Figure 9-29 Leventen-type osteotomy, or oblique osteotomy in reverse direction. **A,** Proposed osteotomy. **B,** Shaded area marks metaphyseal resection. **C,** Capital fragment is impaled on a spike of proximal fragment.

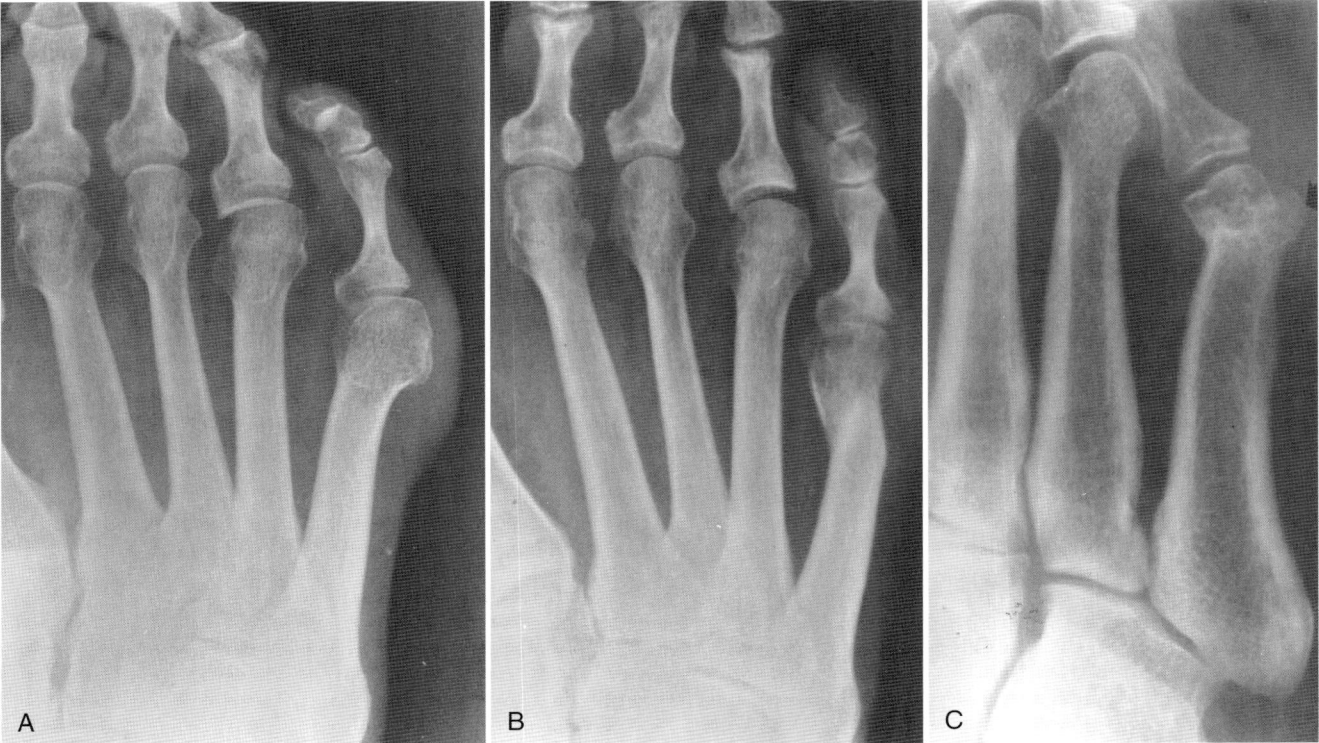

Figure 9-30 Distal oblique osteotomy. **A,** Preoperative anteroposterior radiograph with type 1 deformity. **B,** After distal oblique osteotomy. **C,** Preoperative deformity with type 2 bunionette deformity. **D,** Probably partial avascular necrosis of capital fragment with settling and prominent painful lateral spike. (Courtesy Harold Kitaoka, MD.)

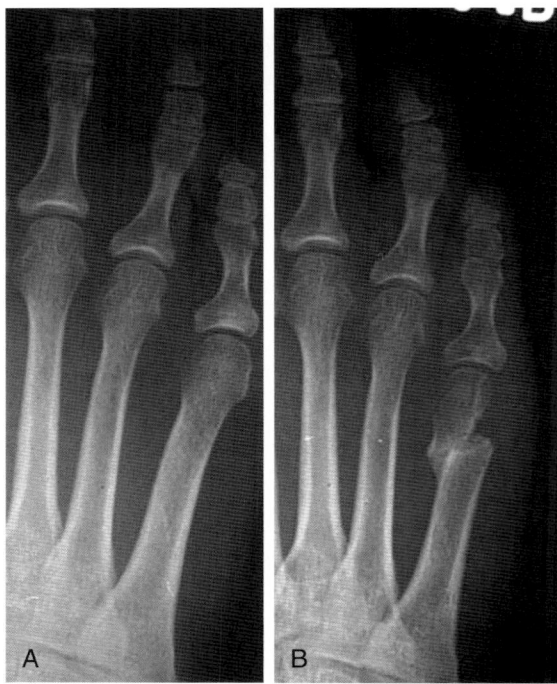

Figure 9-31 **A,** Preoperative radiograph demonstrates bunionette deformity. **B,** Postoperative radiograph demonstrates distal oblique osteotomy. **C,** Postoperative malunion after distal osteotomy.

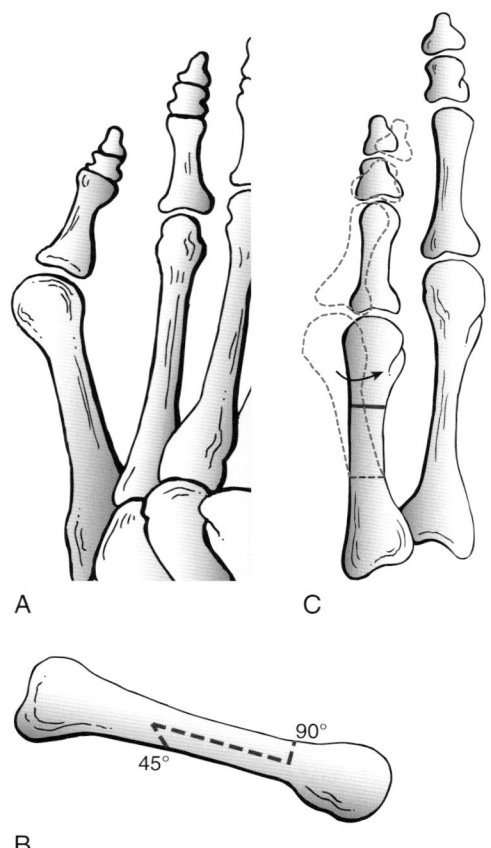

Figure 9-32 **A,** Diagram of preoperative angular deformity. **B,** Diagram of longitudinal SCARF fifth metatarsal osteotomy. **C,** After rotation and realignment of the osteotomy.

union, malunion, and development of an intractable plantar keratotic transfer lesion, make internal fixation or a stable osteotomy advisable.[9,25,60] In the presence of a bunionette deformity with formation of a lateral keratosis, either a chevron osteotomy or an oblique osteotomy, can achieve adequate correction. Because a chevron osteotomy does not allow elevation of the capital fragment, this procedure is contraindicated in the presence of a bunionette deformity with a plantar–lateral or plantar keratosis. A capital oblique or distal oblique osteotomy allows elevation by altering the plane of the osteotomy.

Radl et al[56] reported their experience with a capital oblique osteotomy. At an average follow-up of 32 months, the 14 patients (21 feet) had an improvement in their AOFAS score from 42 to 87 points, a reduction in the MTP-5 angle from 18 to 5 degrees, and a reduction in the 4-5 IM angle from 14 to 9 degrees. At final follow-up, all osteotomies had solid union, and no transfer lesions were reported.

Cooper and Coughlin[12] reported on 17 cases at an average follow-up of 21 months. Fifteen of the feet were noted to have no or mild pain, with an average decrease in the VAS from 6.5 to 1.6 points. Fifteen were noted to have excellent or good results; recurrence of one plantar and one lateral IPK was noted. We found this to be a very acceptable means of correcting type 1 and low type 2 deformities. Cooper and Coughlin[11] reported on cadaveric dissection results of 10 distal chevron and 10 distal capital oblique fifth metatarsal osteotomies. They

found almost identical angular corrections with both procedures.

MIDSHAFT SCARF OSTEOTOMY[30,47,58]
Indications
For a midshaft SCARF osteotomy, the indications are type 2 and 3 bunionettes with a moderate deformity.[30] For more severe angular deformities, a midshaft oblique osteotomy may be considered.

Contraindications
For type 1 bunionette deformities, the SCARF is definitely an alternative, although less surgery and exposure using a distal osteotomy may be sufficient to achieve an adequate correction. For a type 2 and 3 deformity of a substantial nature, a more proximal osteotomy may be considered, because the average correction noted by Maher[47] in the 4-5 IM angle was 4.2 degrees, whereas the average correction reported by Coughlin[14] with the midshaft oblique osteotomy was 10 degrees.

Surgical Technique (Fig. 9-32)
1. The patient is positioned in a semilateral decubitus position.

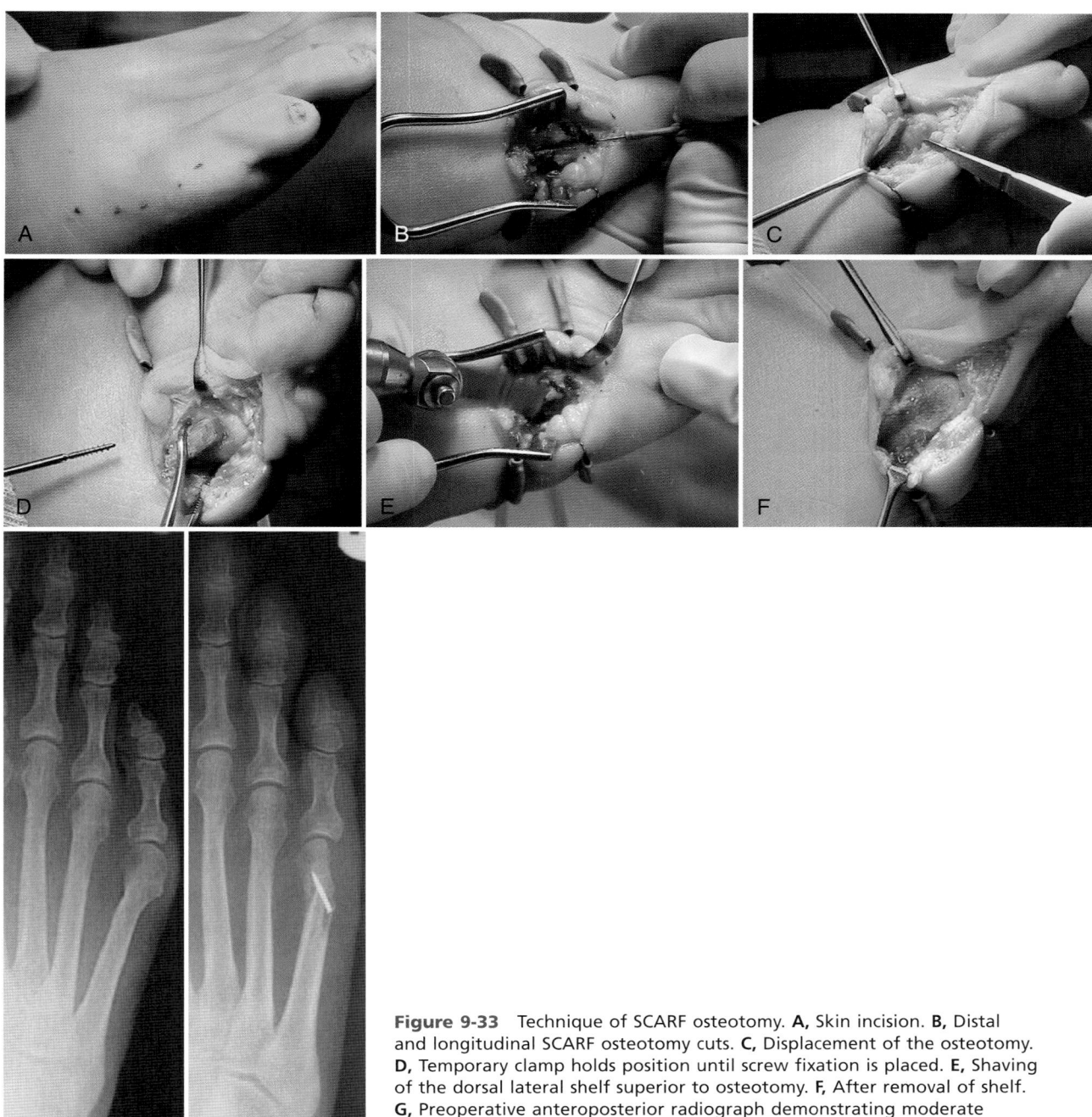

Figure 9-33 Technique of SCARF osteotomy. **A,** Skin incision. **B,** Distal and longitudinal SCARF osteotomy cuts. **C,** Displacement of the osteotomy. **D,** Temporary clamp holds position until screw fixation is placed. **E,** Shaving of the dorsal lateral shelf superior to osteotomy. **F,** After removal of shelf. **G,** Preoperative anteroposterior radiograph demonstrating moderate type 3 bunionette deformity. **H,** After SCARF osteotomy. (Courtesy L.S. Weil Jr, DPM.)

2. The extremity is cleansed in a normal fashion.
3. A 4-cm incision is centered along the lateral aspect of the fifth metatarsal head from 1 cm inferior to the joint to 3 cm proximal to the MTP joint (Fig. 9-33A).
4. The capsule is released with an inverted L-shape capsular cut, releasing the capsule both on the dorsal and proximal aspects (Fig. 9-34).

5. The SCARF osteotomy is marked from the dorsal distal metatarsal surface (within the metaphyseal cancellous bone) to the plantar proximal region of the fifth metatrsal diaphysis.
6. A sagittal saw is use to create a 60-degree angled osteotomy distal (much like a chevron), but slightly more distalward. The second cut is a longitudinal cut

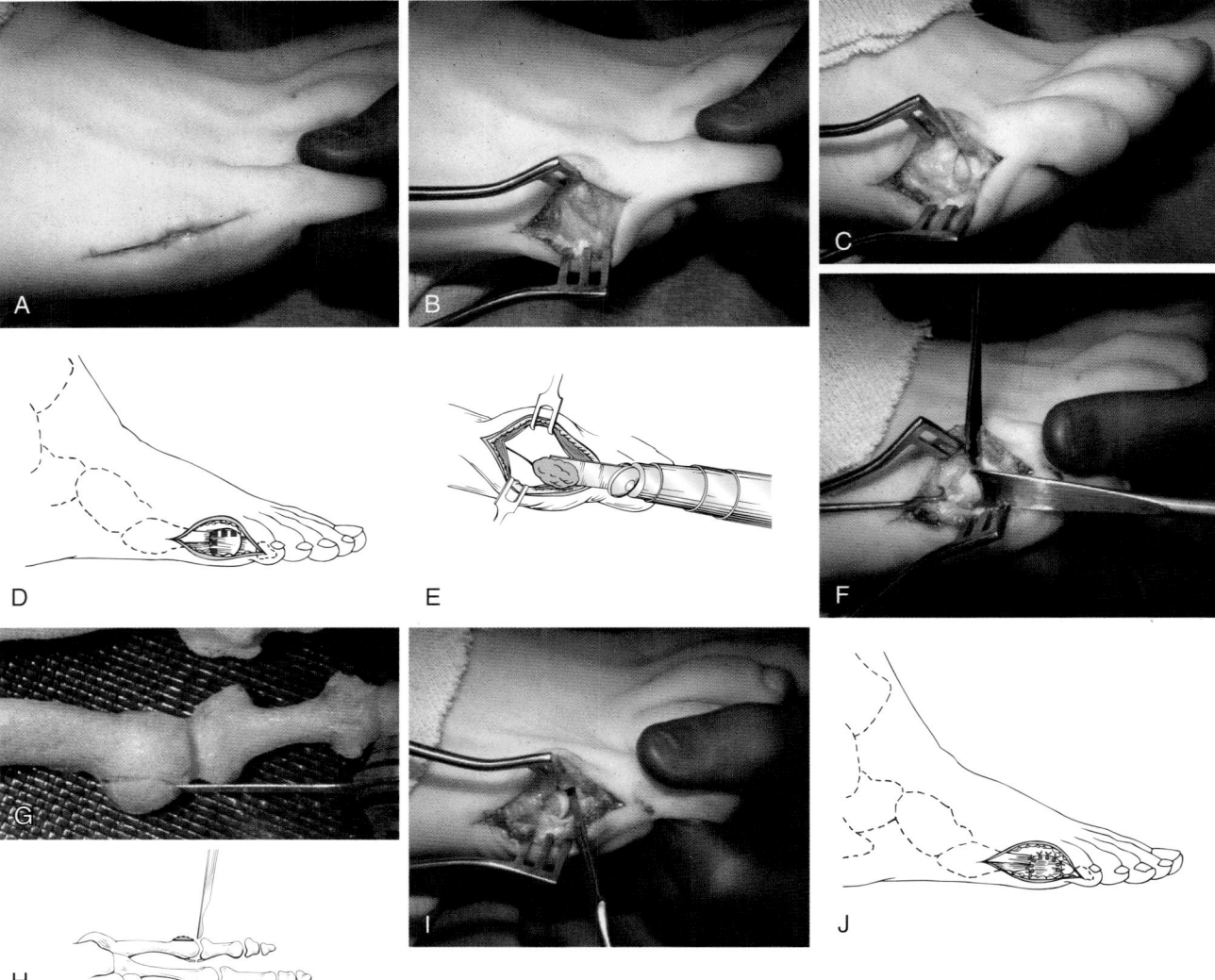

Figure 9-34 Lateral condylectomy. **A,** Skin incision. **B,** Capsular exposure. **C,** Elliptic capsular incision. **D,** Inverted L-shaped capsular incision is used to expose the fifth metatarsal head. Dorsal and proximal capsule, the weakest area of capsular attachment is released, and the stronger plantar and distal attachments are left intact. **E** and **F,** Lateral condyle is resected in line with the shaft of the fifth metatarsal. **G,** Sawbone model used to demonstrate condylar excision. **H** and **I,** Medial capsule is released by distracting the toe and cutting the medial capsule. **J,** Lateral capsule is reefed with interrupted absorbable sutures. The proximal capsule is reefed to the abductor digiti quinti muscle, and the dorsal capsule is approximated to the dorsal periosteum. (Where insufficient tissue is present, drill holes may be placed into the metaphysis of the fifth metatarsal to secure this capsular repair.)

connecting with the distal oblique cut, and extends up the shaft for 15 to 20 mm. (For a greater 4-5 IM angular deformity, a longer cut must be made [see Fig. 9-33B]).

7. If one desires to elevate the distal aspect of the metatarsal (for a plantar IPK), the saw blade for the longitudinal cut can be directed slightly cephalad so that as the osteotomy is rotated, it capital fragment is elevated (Fig. 9-35).

8. Lastly, the proximal cut is made at a 45-degree angle to the longitudinal ostetomy. The distal segment is mobilized and displaced approximately 50% the width of the metatarsal shaft. Distally, it also can be rotated medially to achieve a slightly greater correction (see Fig. 9-33C).

9. The osteotomy is held with a clamp and fixed with two vertical mini-fragment screws (see Fig. 9-33D).

10. The remaining lateral shelf of bone is resected with a sagittal saw (see Fig. 9-33E and F).

11. The lateral capsule is repaired with interrupted sutures, and the skin is approximated in a routine fashion (see Fig. 9-33G).

Postoperative Care

A gauze-and-tape compression dressing is used for alignment of the fifth toe and changed weekly for 3 weeks (see

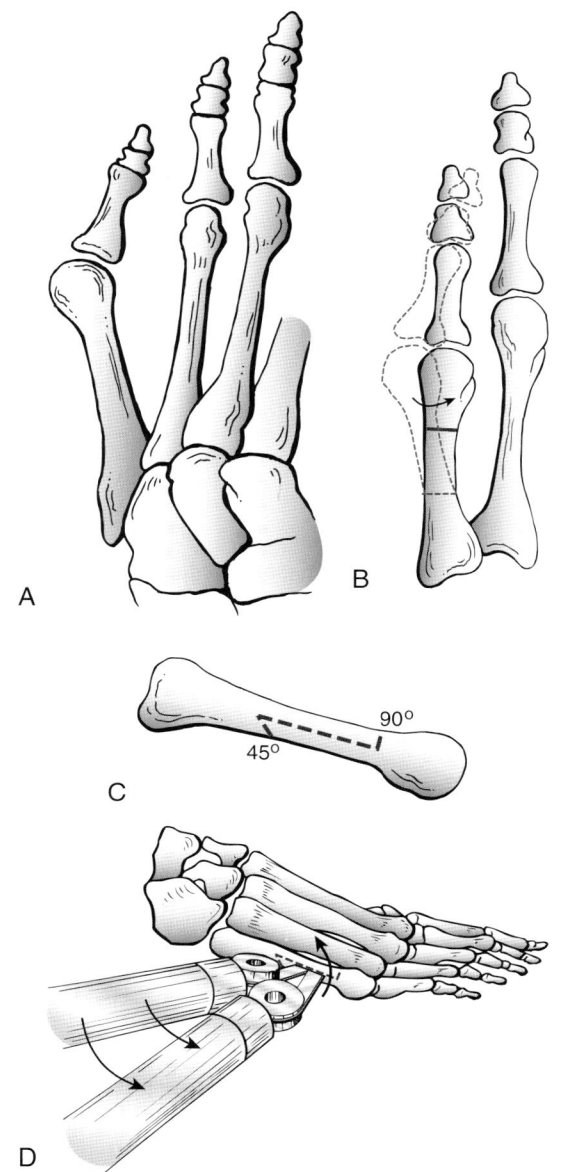

Figure 9-35 Diagram of SCARF osteotomy. **A,** Preoperative deformity. **B,** Rotation of fifth metatarsal with SCARF osteotomy. **C,** Lateral diagram of SCARF osteotomy. **D,** To elevate the distal metatarsal, dropping the hand with the saw will result in elevation of the distal segment.

Fig. 9-33H and I). Ambulation is permitted in a postoperative shoe. Sutures are removed 3 weeks after surgery. Glover et al[30] actually transitioned patients to an athletic shoe 1 week after surgery and commenced physical therapy at this point. The speed with which the patient is allowed to progress is mitigated by the quality of the repair and stability of the internal fixation.

Results and Complications

The technique of a modified chevron (SCARF) osteotomy has been described by Dayton[17] and Seide.[62] Seide and Petersen[62] reported successful results in a follow-up of 10

feet and noted an average reduction in the 4-5 IM angle of 4.5 degrees.

Maher et al[47] reported on midterm to long-term follow-up on their experience with the midshaft rotational SCARF ostetotomy. Twenty-eight patients (36 feet) were evaluated at a mean of 6.5 years. Eighty-six percent were completely satisfied. The 4-5 IM angle was reduced from 9.9 to 5.7 degrees. The mean AOFAS score was improved from 44 to 92 points. The authors stressed that, with the long arm of the SCARF, the capital fragment can be translated a substantial amount medialward, much more so than in the case of a distal osteotomy. Complications included fracture of the fifth metatarsal with subsequent metatarsalgia and seven cases (10%) with recurrent IPKs after surgery. Five patients underwent revision surgery.

Glover et al[30] reported on a retrospective review of 50 patients having undergone a SCARF bunionette repair with a minimum of 12-months of follow-up. The mean 4-5 IM angle was reduced from 10.3 to 1.8 degrees, whereas the MTP-5 angle was corrected from 15.6 to 2.4 degrees. Two cases of undercorrection and seven cases of hardware removal were necessary.

MIDSHAFT (DIAPHYSEAL) OSTEOTOMIES

An osteotomy in the diaphyseal region of the fifth metatarsal also has been recommended for the correction of a bunionette deformity. Yancy[74] described a double transverse closing-wedge osteotomy in the diaphysis to correct a type 2 bunionette deformity characterized by lateral bowing of the fifth metatarsal. Okuda et al[54] described a crescentic osteotomy in the diaphyseal region. Voutey[71] also advocated a transverse diaphyseal osteotomy but reported several complications, including delayed union, pseudarthrosis, and angulation at the osteotomy site. The transverse nature of this osteotomy rendered it relatively unstable.

Gerbert et al[27] and Shrum et al[64] described a closing-wedge diaphyseal osteotomy that was internally fixed with a cerclage wire. They suggested that with a plantar or plantar–lateral keratotic lesion, a biplanar osteotomy might be advisable to achieve medial and dorsal displacement of the distal fragment. Unfortunately, no long-term follow-up was reported in either study.

Mann[48] initially described an oblique fifth metatarsal diaphyseal osteotomy for the treatment of bunionette deformities characterized by diffuse keratotic lesions on the plantar or plantar lateral aspect of the fifth metatarsal head. The oblique nature of the metatarsal osteotomy allowed not only medial but also dorsal translation of the distal fragment, with rotation at the osteotomy site. Mann[48] advocated internal fixation with a wire loop, Kirschner wire, or small-fragment screw, or all three. The fifth MTP joint was not realigned in this procedure. Although no series was reported, Mann did report a case of nonunion. We have had extensive experience with this procedure and have encountered one other nonunion (Fig. 9-36 and Video Clip 46). London[46] suggested that if

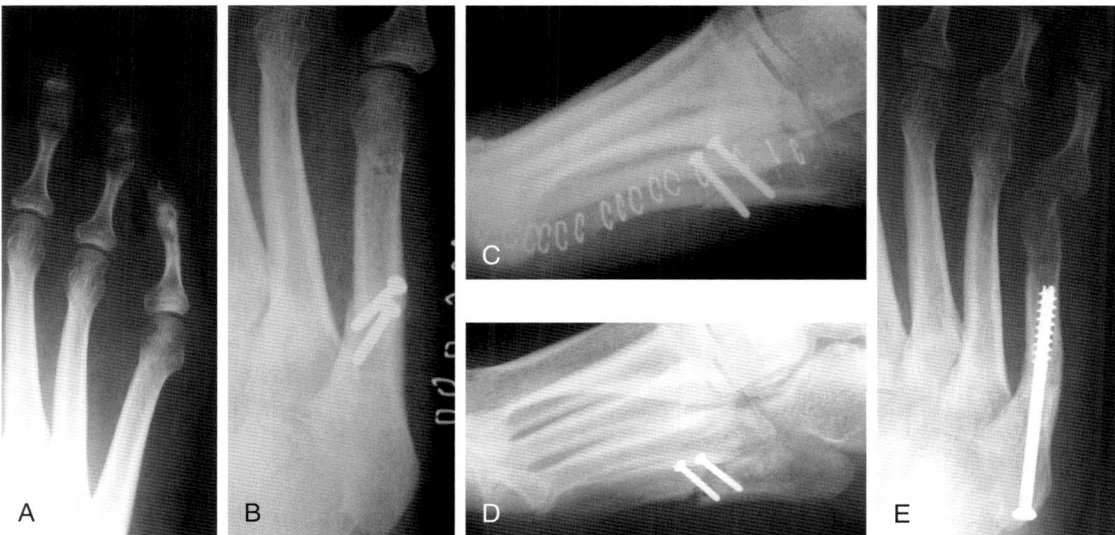

Figure 9-36 A, Preoperative radiograph demonstrates bunionette deformity with widened 4-5 intermetatarsal angle. **B,** Diaphyseal osteotomy with distal soft tissue repair achieves correction of deformity. Two mini-fragment screws are used for fixation. **C,** Lateral radiograph demonstrating fixation. **D,** Early weight bearing led to displacement and nonunion. **E,** Salvage with bone graft and intramedullary screw fixation.

the osteotomy was reversed (distal–dorsal to plantar–proximal), this would be a much more stable construct and should have a higher union rate and lower displacement rate. Unfortunately, their study was limited by some patients having only 6 weeks of follow-up; even with this limited follow-up, they did experience one nonunion. Koti and Mafulli,[41] without any evidence to corroborate their notion, suggested that midshaft oblique osteotomies were more prone to delayed or nonunion.

Indications

In the presence of a widened 4-5 IM angle associated with a bunionette deformity (type 3) or with substantial lateral bowing of the fifth metatarsal shaft (type 2), a diaphyseal osteotomy combined with a distal soft tissue realignment affords an excellent means of correction. With a combined plantar–lateral keratotic lesion, the plane of the osteotomy can be altered to achieve elevation of the distal fragment.[13,14]

Contraindications

For type 1 bunionette deformities, the magnitude of a longitudinal osteotomy is rarely necessary, and a distal osteotomy is preferable. With an unreliable patient, a more stable distal osteotomy may be preferable, although it can sacrifice some magnitude of angular correction.

Midshaft Oblique Osteotomy
(Author's Preferred Technique)

1. The patient is positioned in a semilateral decubitus position.
2. The extremity is cleansed in a normal fashion.
3. A midlateral longitudinal incision is made from the midportion of the proximal phalanx, extending in a proximal direction to the proximal aspect of the fifth metatarsal. The dorsolateral cutaneous nerve is isolated and protected (Figs. 9-37A and 9-38A).
4. The abductor digiti minimi muscle is reflected plantarward to expose the fifth metatarsal diaphysis. The periosteum on the medial aspect of the fifth metatarsal is not stripped to maintain vascular attachments.
5. The MTP joint capsule is exposed and incised along the dorsal and proximal aspect with an L-shaped incision to expose the lateral eminence (see Figs. 9-37B and 9-38B).
6. The fibular condyle of the fifth metatarsal head is resected with a sagittal saw in a line parallel with the metatarsal shaft (see Fig. 9-38C). A drill hole is placed in the metaphysis for later capsule repair (see Fig. 9-38D).
7. The fifth toe is grasped and distracted, and the fifth MTP joint is released on the medial aspect to allow its realignment at the conclusion of the procedure (see Figs. 9-37C and 9-38E).
8. With a lateral keratosis, a horizontal osteotomy is begun. The osteotomy is directed in a dorsoproximal to plantar–distal direction. The saw blade is oriented in a direct lateral-to-medial direction (see Figs. 9-37D and 9-38F).
9. Before completing the osteotomy, a 2.0-mm drill hole is placed in the distal fragment (see Fig. 9-38G). A 1.6-mm fixation drill hole is placed in the proximal fragment and tapped. The holes are drilled before completion of the osteotomy because this osteotomy can render the site quite unstable.
10. The osteotomy is completed, and the distal fragment is rotated to a point parallel with the fourth metatarsal (see Fig. 9-37E and F).

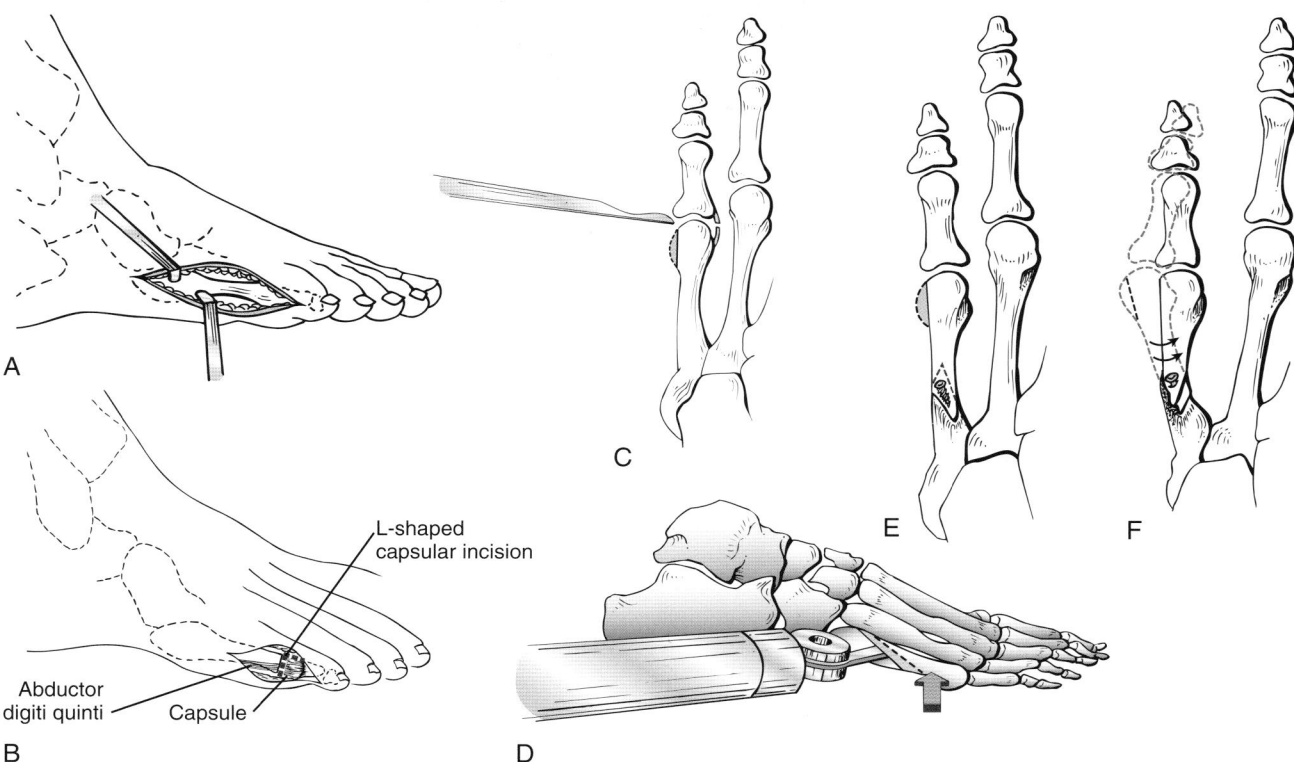

Figure 9-37 Diaphyseal oblique osteotomy. **A,** Longitudinal incision is centered over the lateral aspect of the fifth metatarsal beginning at the midportion of the proximal phalanx and extending to a point 2 cm below the base of the fifth metatarsal. **B,** L-shaped capsular incision releases dorsal and proximal aspects of the metatarsophalangeal joint capsule, the weakest area of capsular attachment. The stronger plantar and distal attachments are left intact, and the medial capsule is released. **C,** Lateral fifth metatarsal condyle is removed with a sagittal saw; the medial capsule is released with a scalpel. **D,** Orientation of diaphyseal oblique osteotomy is in a lateral-to-medial plane. **E** and **F,** Osteotomy site is rotated and fixed with a small-fragment screw. Kirschner wire fixation may be added to give rotational stability.

11. A small-fragment fixation screw is used to stabilize the osteotomy site. A Kirschner wire may be used as well to stabilize and prevent rotation around the screw (see Fig. 9-38H). (Multiple Kirschner wires may be placed as an alternative to screw fixation, although this alternative is less desirable.)
12. Prominent bone at the osteotomy site is resected with a sagittal saw.
13. The fifth MTP joint capsule is repaired, and the fifth toe is brought into proper alignment. The abductor digiti quinti muscle is approximated to the capsule proximally, and dorsally the capsule is secured to the adjacent periosteum (see Fig. 9-38I).
14. If necessary, the capsule may be attached through drill holes on the dorsoproximal aspect of the metaphysis (see Fig. 9-38D).
15. The skin is closed with interrupted sutures or staples see (Fig. 9-38J).

Postoperative Care
A gauze-and-tape compression dressing is applied at surgery and changed weekly (see Fig. 9-38K). An unreliable patient may be treated with a below-knee walking cast for 6 weeks. Sutures are removed at 3 weeks after surgery. Internal fixation may be removed at 6 weeks with radiographic proof of successful healing of the osteotomy (Fig. 9-39). The internal fixation is, however, rarely removed unless it becomes symptomatic. The patient is allowed to ambulate in a postoperative shoe with weight bearing on the inner border of the foot for 6 weeks. At this time, use of the postoperative shoe is discontinued.

Variation
If a combined plantar–lateral keratosis is present, the orientation of the oblique diaphyseal osteotomy is altered. Although a dorsal–proximal to plantar–distal cut is made, the orientation of the cut is changed from a direct lateral-to-medial direction to a more cephalad direction. The surgeon drops his or her hand and cuts in an upward direction (Fig. 9-40). Thus, as the osteotomy site is rotated, there is an elevating effect on the distal fragment. This relieves pressure on the plantar aspect of the fifth metatarsal head. The fifth MTP joint is realigned, and the osteotomy is fixed as previously described. Postoperative management is similar to that described earlier.

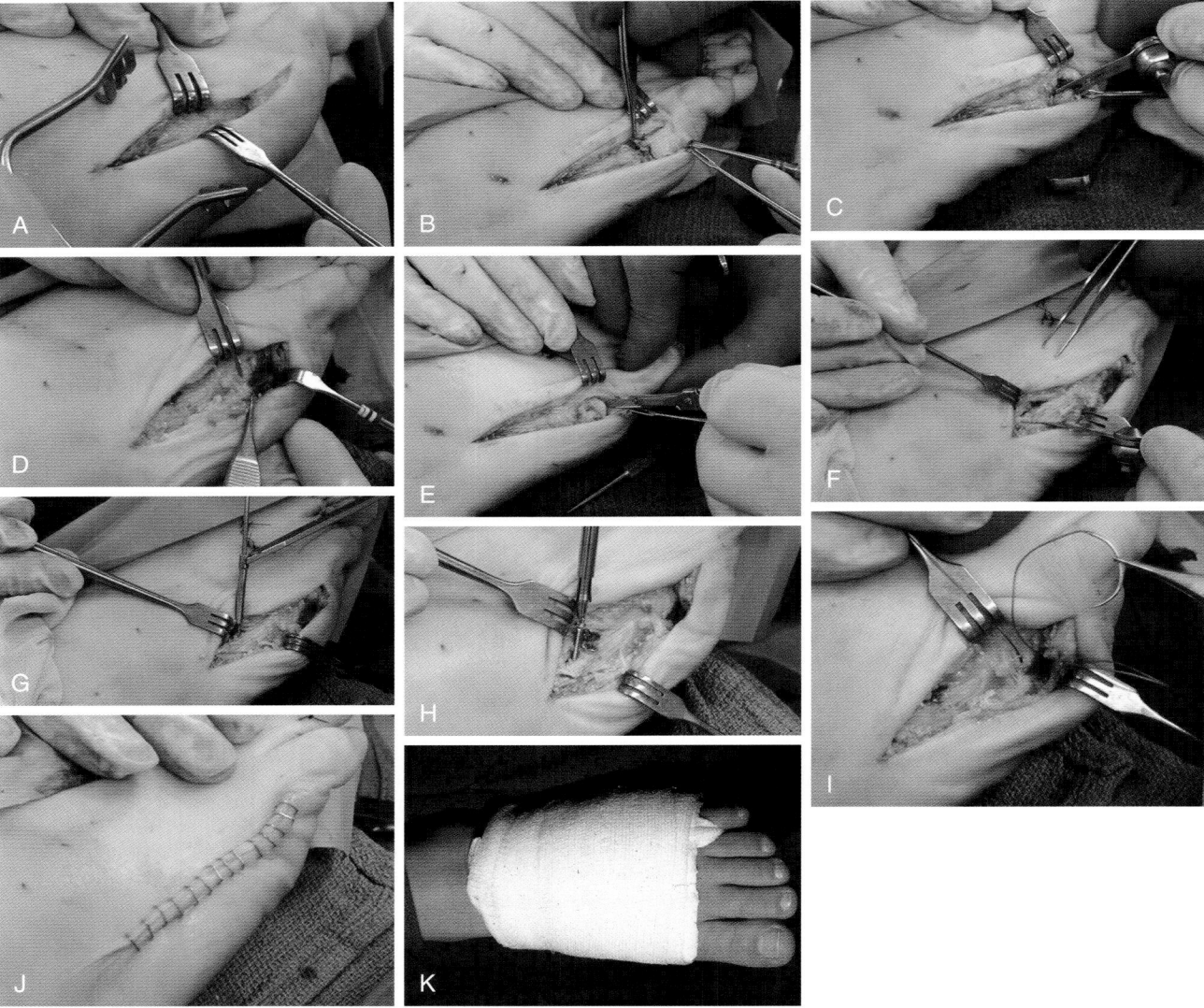

Figure 9-38 Diaphyseal oblique osteotomy. **A,** Longitudinal incision is centered over the lateral aspect of the fifth metatarsal beginning at the midportion of the proximal phalanx and extending to a point 2 cm below the base of the fifth metatarsal. **B,** L-shaped capsular incision releases the dorsal and proximal aspects of the MTP joint capsule, the weakest area of capsular attachment. **C,** Lateral eminence resection in line with the lateral cortex. **D,** Vertical drill hole in the metaphysis for later capsular repair. **E,** Medial capsular release. **F,** Longitudinal oblique osteotomy. **G,** Drill hole before completion of osteotomy is quite helpful. **H,** After rotation of osteotomy, fixation with two mini-fragment screws. **I,** Capsular repair. **J,** Skin closure. **K,** Gauze-and-tape compression dressing.

Results and Complications

Most descriptions of fifth metatarsal diaphyseal osteotomies include little long-term follow-up. Coughlin[10] reported on a longitudinal diaphyseal osteotomy with MTP joint realignment and lateral condylectomy (see Fig. 9-36). Twenty patients (30 feet) underwent surgical correction and were evaluated at an average 31 months of follow-up. No nonunions were reported. The average preoperative 4-5 IM angle of 10.6 degrees was improved to 0.8 degree, for an average correction of 9.8 degrees. The MTP-5 angle, noted to average 16 degrees preoperatively, was reduced to 0.5 degrees, for an average correction of 15.5 degrees. No symptomatic transfer lesions were

reported. Patients had a 93% satisfaction rate. The average foot width was reduced by 6 mm (range, 2-15 mm). The average fifth metatarsal shortening was 0.5 mm. No infections or incisional neuromas occurred.

Vienne et al[70] reported on the treatment of 24 patients with a Coughlin osteotomy. At an average follow-up of 24 months, they noted 97% good or excellent results and an improvement of the AOFAS score from 55 to 95 points. They reported an improvement of the MTP-5 angle of 17.3 degrees and a reduction of the 4-5 IM angle of 9.4 degrees. The width of the foot was narrowed almost 5 mm.

In a report on 11 pediatric patients with a mean follow-up of 32 months, Masquijo et al[49] noted a similar

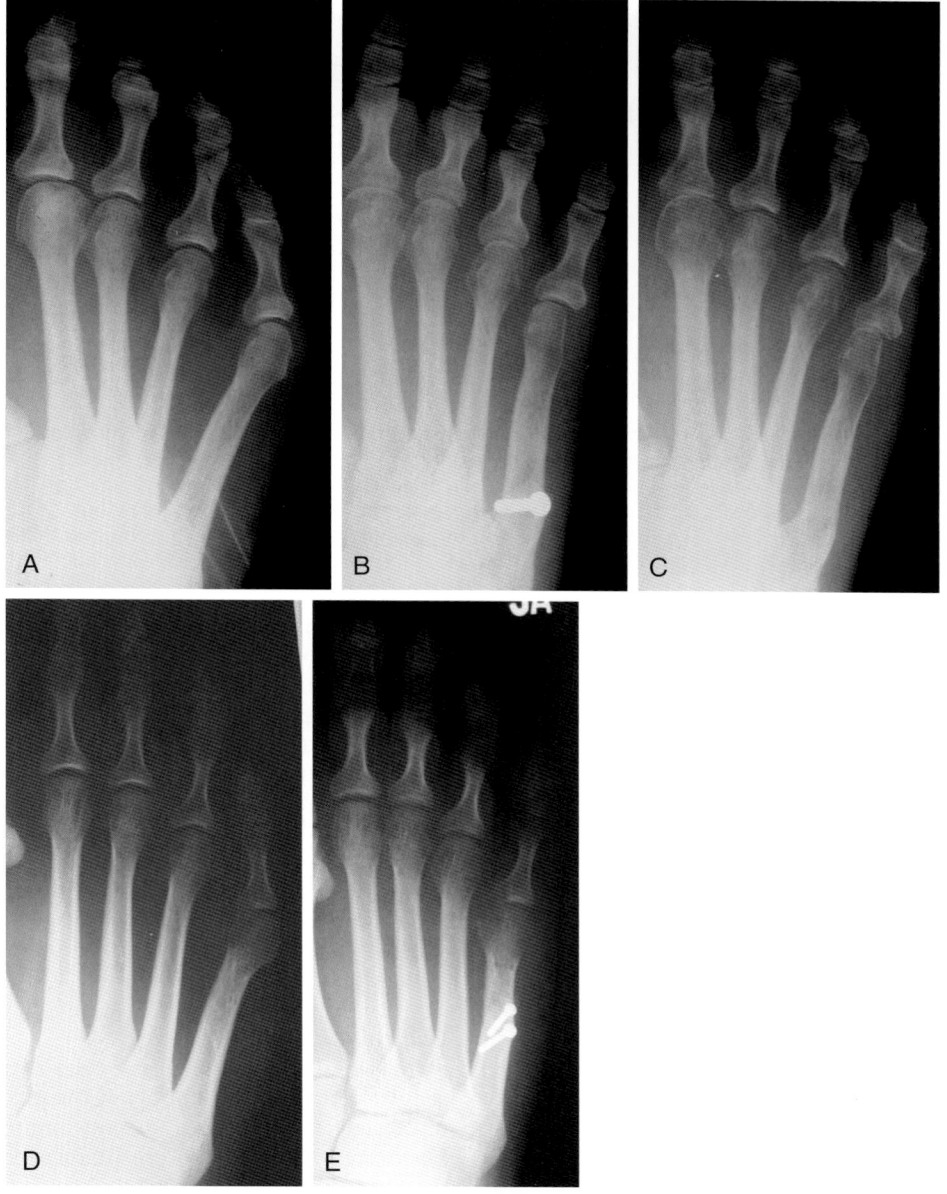

Figure 9-39 **A,** Preoperative radiograph of a type 3 deformity. **B,** After midshaft oblique osteotomy. **C,** Five-year follow-up. **D,** Type 2 preoperative deformity. **E,** After midshaft oblique osteotomy.

improvement in the MTP-5 and 4-5 intermetatarsal angle as well. All results were rated as excellent or good, and the final AOFAS score averaged 92 points.

Postoperative evaluation showed that one patient with a preoperative plantar keratosis had a mild, asymptomatic residual callus that was characterized as 75% reduced, one patient with a preoperative lateral IPK had a slight plantar keratosis, and one patient with a combined plantar and lateral keratosis had a remaining plantar keratosis that was characterized as 50% less than its preoperative size. All three patients characterized their subjective results as excellent or good. One other patient developed a mild transfer lesion that was asymptomatic, and her

result was rated excellent. Three patients developed mild fifth hammer toe deformities that did not require further treatment, and all rated their results excellent.

Internal fixation included a single screw in 4 feet and a screw and Kirschner wire in 10 feet. When screw fixation was unsuccessful, multiple Kirschner wires (6 feet) were used. No loss of fixation occurred postoperatively at the osteotomy site. Because of the subcutaneous nature of the hardware, easy removal under local anesthesia can be performed in an office setting. Eighty-seven percent of patients underwent hardware removal.[14] Currently, two mini-fragment screws are used to fix the osteotomy site. The initial screw serves as the center of rotation for the

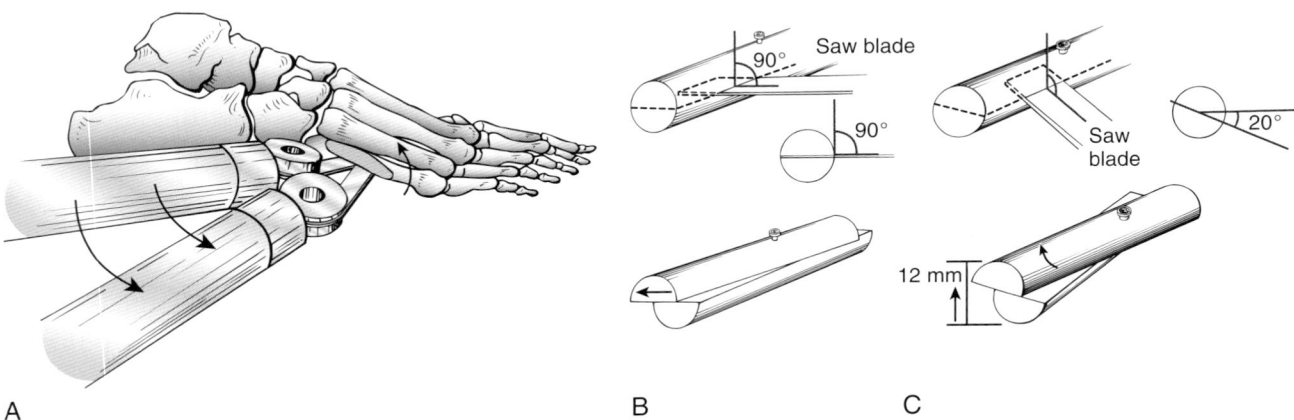

Figure 9-40 **A,** When an intractable plantar keratotic lesion is present, the saw blade is directed cephalad. The hand is dropped as the saw cut is created so that when the osteotomy site is rotated, the fifth metatarsal head is elevated. **B,** Drawing illustrating the effect of horizontal osteotomy. With the saw blade oriented in a lateral-to-medial direction, the osteotomy site is rotated and does not elevate the distal metatarsal. **C,** Drawing illustrating effect of oblique osteotomy. With the saw blade oriented medial to lateral but also superior direction, as the osteotomy site is rotated, the distal fragment elevates. (**B** and **C** modified from Lutter L, editor: *Atlas of adult foot and ankle surgery*, St Louis, 1997, Mosby, pp 110–111.)

osteotomy. Once the osteotomy has been aligned, a second screw is placed to further stabilize the osteotomy site.

London[46] performed a longitudinal oblique osteotomy at an angle reverse (dorsal–distal to plantar–proximal) to that described by Coughlin.[14] Although radiographs were only obtained up to 6 weeks after surgery, and telephone interviews were used to evaluate the clinical success, he hypothesized that this was a more stable osteotomy with this orientation. The authors reported one nonunion in their series. Masquijo[49] suggested that although London hypothesized that a reverse osteotomy angle would provide greater stability in the diaphyseal region, in the three reports by Coughlin,[14] Mosquijo et al,[49] and Vienne et al,[70] they noted all 67 cases in the three series to have healed successfully. It is likely that the midshaft oblique osteotomy can be oriented in either direction with the expectation of adequate healing in this region. Koti and Maffulli[41] suggested in their review article that delayed or nonunion of midshaft ostetomies was common, but that notion has never been substantiated in other reports in the literature.

Okuda et al[54] reported on eight patients (10 feet) in whom a crescentic diaphyseal osteotomy was performed (Fig. 9-41). Three of the 10 developed a delayed union, which occurred in those cases in which the osteotomy was more proximally located (Fig. 9-42). The authors stressed that the osteotomy should not be performed at the base of the fifth metatarsal. Radiographic healing in the series averaged 11 weeks.

PROXIMAL FIFTH METATARSAL OSTEOTOMY
Indications
The rationale for a proximal fifth metatarsal osteotomy is that it achieves correction at the actual site of the deformity, not unlike a first-ray bunion deformity. For a widened 4-5 IM angle, the theoretic advantage of a proximal fifth metatarsal osteotomy is understandable. A proximal fifth metatarsal osteotomy has been advocated as a means to correct a widened 4-5 IM angle.[19,20,24,33,41] Although a proximal osteotomy does achieve correction of the widened 4-5 IM angle at the actual site of the deformity, some controversy surrounds this procedure. Lelièvre[45] advocated a transverse osteotomy in the region of the styloid process. Diebold and Bejjani[20] noted that there was an increased "risk of disruption of the transverse metatarsal joint" with a proximally placed fifth metatarsal osteotomy.

Contraindications
Shereff et al[63] investigated the extraosseous and intraosseous arterial vascular supply of the proximal fifth metatarsal (Fig. 9-43). The intraosseous supply originates from a periosteal plexus, a nutrient artery, and metaphyseal and epiphyseal vessels. The extraosseous supply emanates from a dorsal metatarsal artery and several branches of the lateral plantar artery. The authors suggested that an osteotomy or fracture in the proximal 2 cm of the fifth metatarsal can injure both the extraosseous and the intraosseous supply, leading to delayed union or nonunion. Thus, although an osteotomy in the proximal fifth metatarsal can achieve maximal correction of a widened 4-5 IM angle, the potential for delayed union, nonunion, or tarsometatarsal joint instability makes this area somewhat less optimal for surgical correction.

Gerbert et al[27] stated that the anastomosing arterial branches in the fourth IM space may be vulnerable to injury with a proximal fifth metatarsal osteotomy. This observation is consistent with delayed healing of Jones-type fractures within the proximal 2 cm of the fifth metatarsal. Diebold and Bejjani[20] recognized that there was indeed a poor healing capacity for fractures in this region.

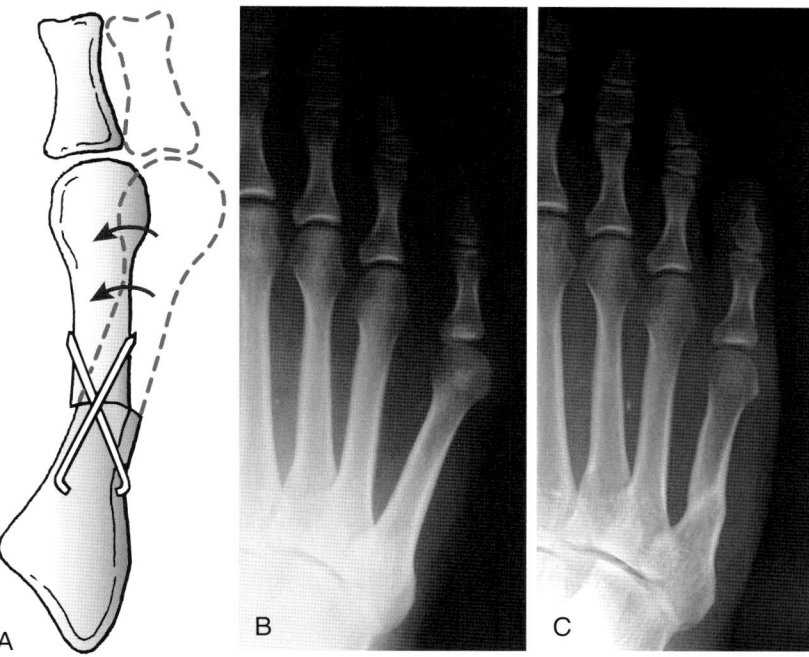

Figure 9-41 **A,** Midshaft crescentic osteotomy. **B,** Preoperative radiograph. **C,** After crescentic osteotomy and hardware removal. (From Okuda R, Kinoshita M, Morikawa J, et al: Adult hallux valgus with metatarsus adductus: a case report, *Clin Orthop* 396:179–183, 2002.)

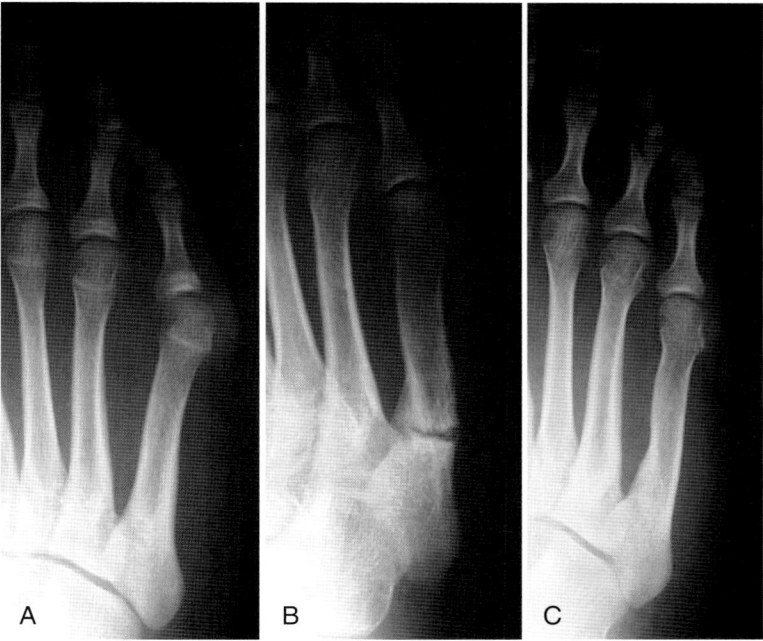

Figure 9-42 **A,** Preoperative radiograph. **B,** Delayed union after midshaft crescentic osteotomy. **C,** After successful healing. (From Okuda R, Kinoshita M, Morikawa J, et al: Adult hallux valgus with metatarsus adductus: a case report, *Clin Orthop* 396:179–183, 2002.)

Estersohn et al[23] emphasized the importance of the metaphyseal branch to the proximal fifth metatarsal region that enters on the medial aspect of the fifth metatarsal, and they cautioned that this important vascular supply should not be interrupted at surgery.

Surgical Technique
1. The patient is positioned in a semilateral decubitus position.

2. The extremity is cleansed in a normal fashion.
3. A 4-cm incision is made on the lateral aspect of the fifth metatarsal, beginning at its base and extending distally to the level of the distal metaphysis. A fifth MTP joint realignment is not usually performed (Fig. 9-44A).
4. The abductor digiti quinti muscle is retracted plantarward, taking care to protect the dorsal sensory nerve, a branch of the sural nerve.

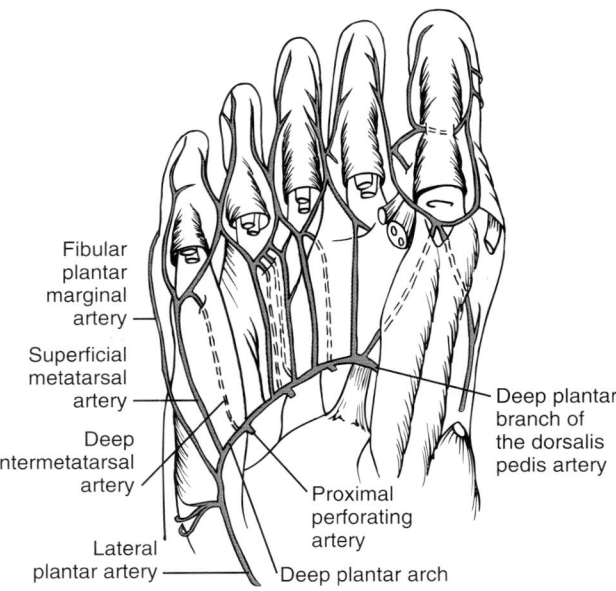

Figure 9-43 Plantar circulation is provided by the deep plantar arch, which is the source of several smaller arteries: superficial metatarsal artery, deep plantar metatarsal artery, deep plantar intermetatarsal artery, and fibular plantar marginal artery. From these vessels, numerous discrete branches supply the proximal fifth metatarsal. Area of convergence of these vessels in the proximal 1 to 2 cm of the proximal fifth metatarsal appears to be vulnerable to delayed union, with interruption of arterial circulation at this level.

5. A lateral-to-medial drill hole is created with a 0.062-inch Kirschner wire at a point 1 cm distal to the tip of the fifth metatarsal. This forms the apex of the chevron osteotomy (Fig. 9-44B).
6. A sagittal saw with "in-line" teeth is used to create the medial-to-lateral chevron with its base oriented in a distal direction (Fig. 9-44C).
7. The sagittal saw is used to create the two limbs of the chevron. The distal fifth metatarsal fragment is then rotated in a medial direction and stabilized to the fourth metatarsal with small Steinmann pins placed in the diaphysis in a lateral-to-medial direction (Fig. 9-44D and E). The pins are left extending through the skin.
8. Any prominent bone at the site of the osteotomy is beveled with a power saw.
9. The soft tissue is approximated with interrupted absorbable sutures, and the skin is closed with interrupted sutures.
10. A below-knee cast is applied.

Postoperative Care
Sutures are removed at 3 weeks, and the Steinmann pins that transfix the fourth and fifth metatarsals are removed at 6 weeks. Weight bearing is allowed in the cast at 3 weeks, and the cast is removed 6 weeks after surgery. At this time, the patient is allowed to ambulate in a roomy sandal.

Figure 9-44 Proximal fifth metatarsal osteotomy. **A,** A 4-cm incision is centered over the base of the fifth metatarsal. **B,** After exposure of the fifth metatarsal, a drill hole is placed 1 cm distal to the fifth metatarsal base, marking the apex of the osteotomy site. **C,** Lateral-to-medial chevron osteotomy is performed with a sagittal saw. **D and E,** The osteotomy site is rotated and stabilized with two Steinmann pins, which transfix the fourth and fifth metatarsals. Excess bone is shaved at the osteotomy site.

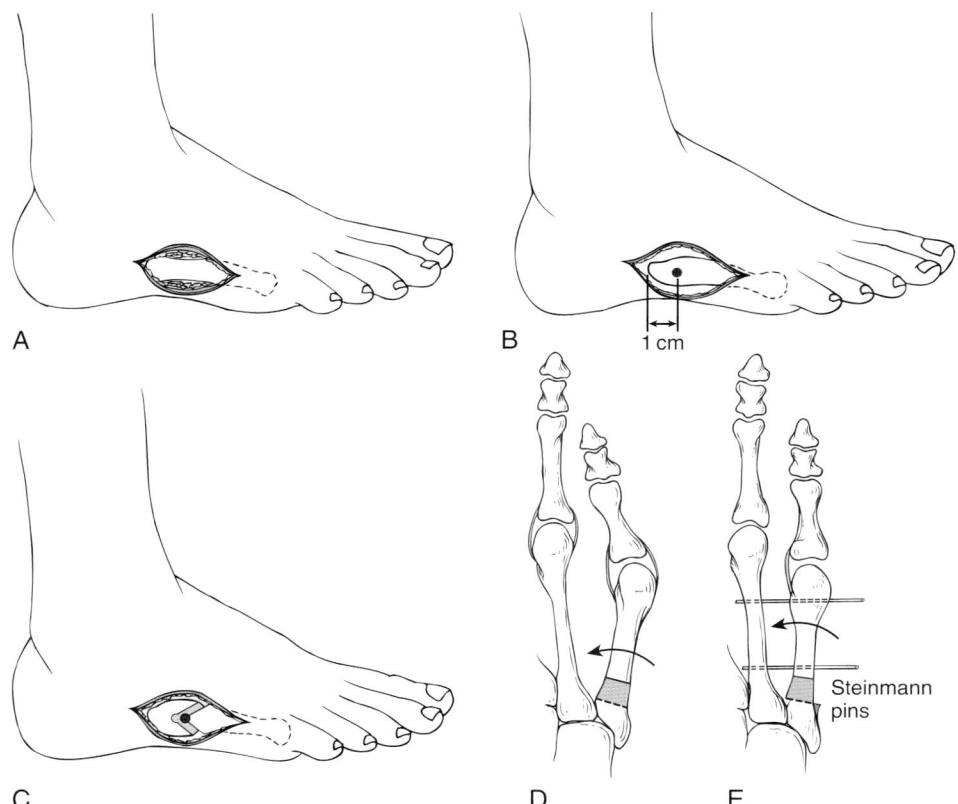

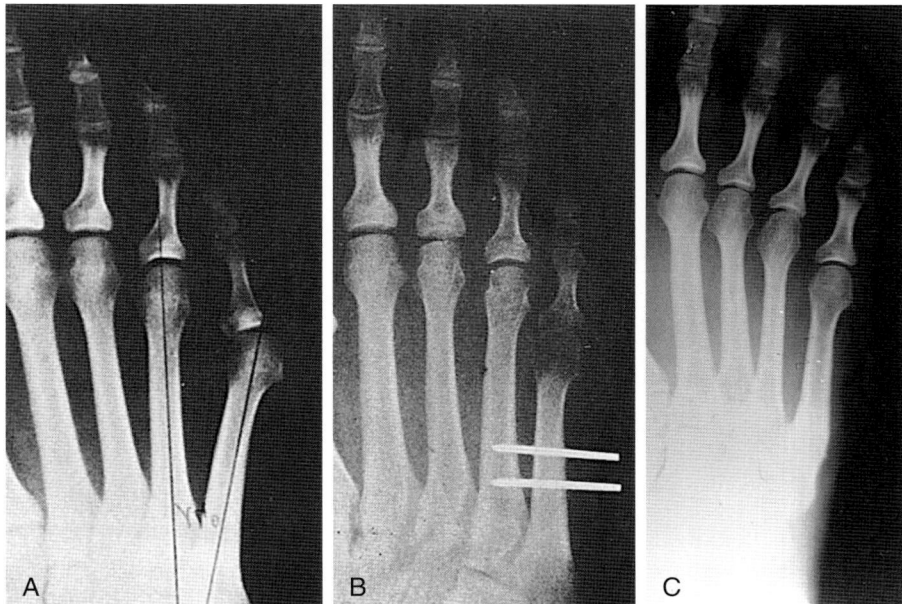

Figure 9-45 A, Preoperative radiograph demonstrates bunionette deformity. **B,** Proximal chevron osteotomy achieves correction of widened 4-5 intermetatarsal angle. **C,** After removal of internal fixation. (From Diebold PF, Bejjani FJ: Basal osteotomy of the fifth metatarsal with intermetatarsal pinning: a new approach to tailor's bunion, *Foot Ankle* 8:40–45, 1987.)

Results and Complications

In a series of 72 patients who underwent an opening-wedge osteotomy of the proximal fifth metatarsal, Bishop et al[3] reported a diminished 4-5 IM angle. Estersohn et al[23] performed a similar procedure in four cases. No long-term results were reported regarding the correction of the 4-5 IM angle or the development of complications, including delayed union, nonunion, or transfer lesions. Regnauld[57] performed a proximal closing-wedge osteotomy and stabilized it with a cerclage wire between the fourth and fifth metatarsals. Again, no results were reported.

In the only series in which significant follow-up study was reported after a proximal fifth metatarsal osteotomy, Diebold and Bejjani[20] performed a horizontal chevron osteotomy 1 cm distal to the base of the fifth metatarsal. Steinmann pin fixation was used to immobilize the osteotomy by transfixation of the fourth and fifth metatarsals for 4 to 6 weeks. In 12 patients (average follow-up, 1 year), they reported excellent results in 90% of cases. No nonunions were reported. The 4-5 IM angle was decreased from 17 to 7 degrees. Later in a follow-up report, Diebold and Bejjani[20] reported on 22 osteotomies that all successfully healed. The 4-5 IM angle was diminished from 12 degrees to 1 degree postoperatively. They recommended removing the parallel Steinmann pins 5 weeks postoperatively with evidence of radiographic healing at the osteotomy site.

Although Kaplan et al[33] observed that both proximal and distal fifth metatarsal osteotomies heal adequately because of an abundant vascular supply, the experience with delayed healing of fractures in the proximal 2 cm of

the fifth metatarsal should make the treating physician wary of an osteotomy in this area (Figs. 9-45, 9-46, and 9-47).

AUTHOR'S PREFERRED METHOD OF TREATMENT

Conservative Treatment

Early conservative management of a symptomatic bunionette includes shaving the keratotic lesion, padding the lesion, and wearing roomy footwear. Most patients with symptomatic mild bunionette deformities can be successfully treated with shoe modifications and modified insoles or orthoses that relieve pressure over a painful lateral eminence. Often, conservative methods are effective in reducing symptoms; however, in the presence of chronic bursal thickening, development of symptomatic keratoses, and intractable pain, surgical intervention may be warranted. When a bursa becomes inflamed or infection occurs, a sandal or postoperative shoe may be necessary to completely relieve pressure. Plantar pain associated with an intractable keratotic lesion can often be relieved with a prefabricated or custom insole as well.

Surgical Treatment

When intractable symptoms are refractory to nonsurgical treatment, operative intervention may be necessary. More than 30 different surgical techniques have been recommended for the surgical correction of a bunionette deformity. Excision of the lateral condyle, resection of the

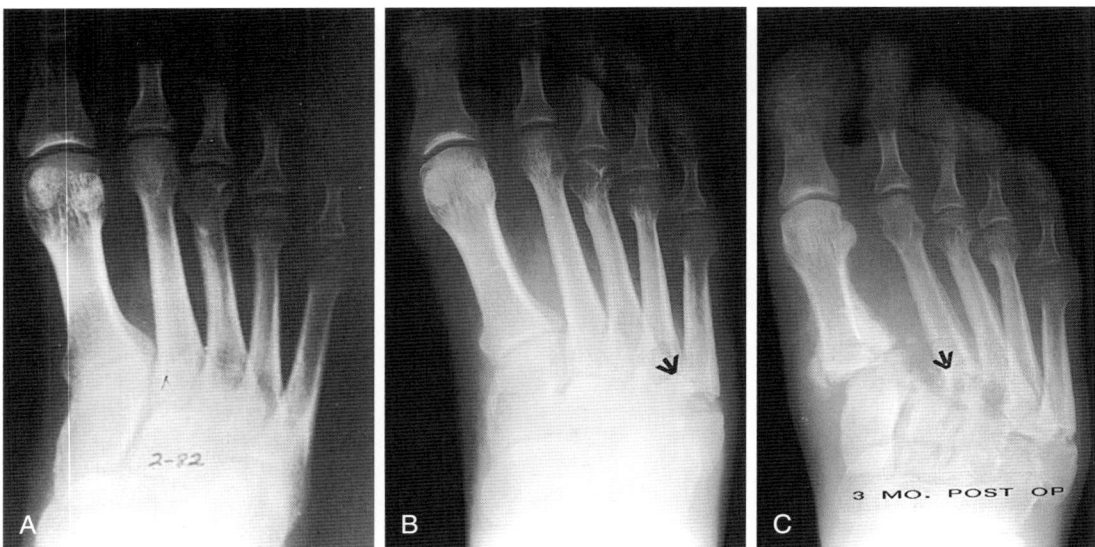

Figure 9-46 **A,** Preoperative radiograph before fifth metatarsal osteotomy. **B,** Radiograph after osteotomy demonstrates destabilization of tarsometatarsal joint. **C,** Further progression of Charcot arthropathy of the Lisfranc joint.

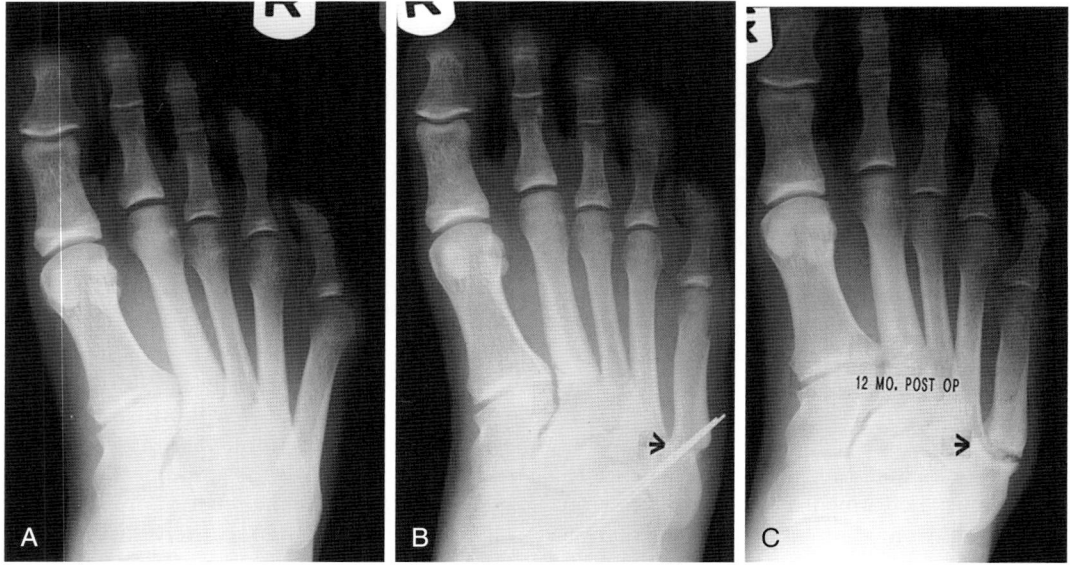

Figure 9-47 **A,** Preoperative radiograph demonstrates bunionette deformity. **B,** Radiograph after proximal fifth metatarsal osteotomy. **C,** After proximal fifth metatarsal osteotomy, delayed union has occurred. Osteotomy in this adolescent took approximately 12 months to heal.

metatarsal head and fifth ray, and osteotomies of the fifth metatarsal (distal, diaphyseal, and proximal) with or without MTP arthroplasty have been described. In most cases, the paucity of follow-up studies with these procedures and the anecdotal reports of success with various techniques should raise a question as to their long-term efficacy. Likewise, the wide range of anatomic variations manifesting with bunionette deformities tends to make the choice of technique for surgical correction somewhat complicated.

An enlarged fifth metatarsal head or lateral condyle (with or without excessive pronation of the foot) may be treated either with a lateral condyle resection and fifth MTP joint realignment or with a distal metatarsal osteotomy. Realignment of the MTP joint and meticulous closure of the capsule are important to prevent lateral subluxation or dislocation of the fifth MTP joint (Fig. 9-48). The high recurrence rate with condyle resection tends to make this technique a less desirable procedure. With a pure lateral keratotic lesion, a distal chevron

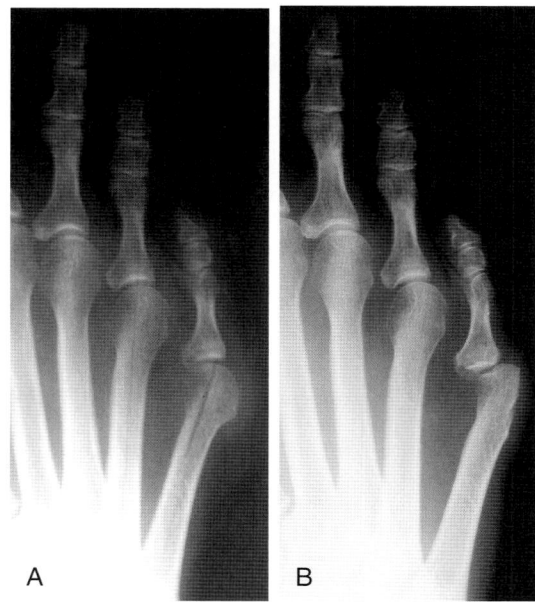

Figure 9-48 **A,** Preoperative radiograph. **B,** Dislocation of fifth metatarsophalangeal joint after lateral condylectomy.

osteotomy is an acceptable procedure, but our preferred method now is a capital oblique osteotomy. This modified Weil-type osteotomy is preferable because of its inherent stability, but it can also be modified to allow elevation of the capital fragment in the presence of a plantar keratosis. Kirschner wire or screw fixation tends to ensure stability of the osteotomy site until adequate healing has occurred. With a plantar or plantar–lateral keratosis, without an increase in the 4-5 IM angle or without lateral fifth metatarsal deviation, a capital oblique osteotomy may be the procedure of choice. A diaphyseal or distal metaphyseal biplanar osteotomy may also be considered in this situation.

In the presence of a widened 4-5 IM angle associated with a bunionette deformity (type 3) or with substantial lateral bowing of the fifth metatarsal shaft (type 2), a diaphyseal osteotomy combined with a distal soft tissue realignment affords an excellent means of correction, as does in many cases a SCARF osteotomy. Midshaft diaphyseal osteotomies allow greater correction than distal metatarsal osteotomies and do not appear to threaten the tenuous vascular supply in the region of the proximal fifth metatarsal. With internal fixation, this osteotomy appears to allow correction without a significant risk of a transfer lesion. Understanding of the extraosseous and intraosseous vascular supply to the proximal fifth metatarsal, as well as reports of delayed healing with fractures in this region, make the possibility of vascular compromise after proximal metatarsal osteotomy a worrisome complication. A diaphyseal fifth metatarsal osteotomy appears to offer a less vulnerable area for a bunionette correction. Not surprisingly, when one compares the angular correction achieved by distal and midshaft

diaphyseal osteotomies, the midshaft oblique osteotomy consistently achieved greater angular correction that other distal type osteotomies. Whether that degree of correction is needed is often the most important question to be addressed in preoperative planning.

Although considerable disagreement exists regarding the need for internal fixation after a fifth metatarsal osteotomy, the frequently reported complications of malunion, nonunion, and transfer keratotic lesions after floating osteotomies indicate the need for either internal fixation or the use of an inherently stable fifth metatarsal osteotomy (see Fig. 9-29). The principles of internal fixation where a fifth metatarsal osteotomy has been performed should be equally applied to the foot as well as elsewhere in the musculoskeletal system.

Preoperative radiographic evaluation of a bunionette deformity is important in analyzing the disorder present. Correlation of radiographic abnormalities with physical findings, including the location of the keratotic lesions, will help to define the appropriate surgical procedure.

Treatment of a symptomatic bunionette requires surgical versatility. Adapting the surgical repair to the underlying disorder will help to determine whether a condylectomy with a distal soft tissue repair, a distal metatarsal osteotomy, or a diaphyseal metatarsal osteotomy offers the best solution for a painful bunionette deformity.

REFERENCES

1. Addante JB, Chin M, Makower BL, Lescosky FA, Nowick AR: Surgical correction of tailor's bunion with resection of fifth metatarsal head and silastic sphere implant: an 8-year follow-up study, *J Foot Surg* 25:315–320, 1986.
2. Armstrong DG, Rosales MA, Gashi A: Efficacy of fifth metatarsal head resection for treatment of chronic diabetic foot ulceration, *J Am Podiatr Med Assoc* 95:353–356, 2005.
3. Bishop J, Kahn A 3rd, Turba JE: Surgical correction of the splayfoot: the Giannestras procedure, *Clin Orthop Relat Res* 146:234–238, 1980.
4. Boyer ML, Deorio JK: Bunionette deformity correction with distal chevron osteotomy and single absorbable pin fixation, *Foot Ankle Int* 24:834–837, 2003.
5. Brown JE: Functional and cosmetic correction of metatarsus latus (splay foot), *Clin Orthop* 14:166–170, 1959.
6. Buchbinder IJ: DRATO procedure for tailor's bunion, *J Foot Surg* 21:177–180, 1982.
7. Campbell D: Chevron osteotomy for bunionette deformity, *Foot Ankle Int* 2:355–356, 1982.
8. Castle JE, Cohen AH, Docks G: Fifth metatarsal distal oblique wedge osteotomy utilizing cortical screw fixation, *J Foot Surg* 31:478–485, 1992.
9. Catanzariti AR, Friedman C, DiStazio J: Oblique osteotomy of the fifth metatarsal: a five-year review, *J Foot Surg* 27:316–320, 1988.
10. Cohen BE, Nicholson CW: Bunionette deformity, *J Am Acad Orthop Surg* 15:300–307, 2007.
11. Cooper MT, Coughlin MJ: Subcapital oblique fifth metatarsal osteotomy versus distal chevron osteotomy for correction of bunionette deformity: a cadaveric study, *Foot Ankle Spec* 5:313–317, 2012.
12. Cooper MT, Coughlin MJ: Subcapital oblique osteotomy for correction of bunionette deformity—medium term results, Accepted for publication in *Foot Ankle Int* 2013.

13. Coughlin MJ: Etiology and treatment of the bunionette deformity, *Instr Course Lect* 39:37–48, 1990.

14. Coughlin MJ: Treatment of bunionette deformity with longitudinal diaphyseal osteotomy with distal soft tissue repair, *Foot Ankle* 11:195–203, 1991.

15. Coughlin MJ, Thompson FM: The high price of high-fashion footwear, *Instr Course Lect* 44:371–377, 1995.

16. Davies H: Metatarsus quintus valgus, *Br Med J* 1:664, 1949.

17. Dayton P, Glynn A, Rogers WS: Use of the Z osteotomy for tailor bunionectomy, *J Foot Ankle Surg* 42:167–169, 2003.

18. Dickson FD, Diveley RL, editors: *Functional disorders of the foot*, Philadelphia, 1953, JB Lippincott, p 230.

19. Diebold PF: Basal osteotomy of the fifth metatarsal for the bunionette, *Foot Ankle* 12:74–79, 1991.

20. Diebold PF, Bejjani FJ: Basal osteotomy of the fifth metatarsal with intermetatarsal pinning: a new approach to tailor's bunion, *Foot Ankle* 8:40–45, 1987.

21. Dorris MF, Mandel LM: Fifth metatarsal head resection for correction of tailor's bunions and sub-fifth metatarsal head keratoma: a retrospective analysis, *J Foot Surg* 30:269–275, 1991.

22. DuVries H: *Surgery of the foot*, St Louis, 1965, Mosby.

23. Estersohn F, Scherer P, Bogdan R: A preliminary report on opening wedge osteotomy of the fifth metatarsal, *Arch Podiatr Med Foot Surg* 1:317–327, 1974.

24. Fallat LM, Buckholz J: An analysis of the tailor's bunion by radiographic and anatomical display, *J Am Podiatry Assoc* 70:597–603, 1980.

25. Frankel JP, Turf RM, King BA: Tailor's bunion: clinical evaluation and correction by distal metaphyseal osteotomy with cortical screw fixation, *J Foot Surg* 28:237–243, 1989.

26. Friend G, Grace K, Stone HA: L-osteotomy with absorbable fixation for correction of tailor's bunion, *J Foot Ankle Surg* 32:14–19, 1993.

27. Gerbert J, Sgarlato TE, Subotnick SI: Preliminary study of a closing wedge osteotomy of the fifth metatarsal for correction of a tailor's bunion deformity, *J Am Podiatry Assoc* 62:212–218, 1972.

28. Giannestras NJ: Other problems of the foot. In Giannestras NJ, editor: *Foot disorders: medical and surgical management*, Philadelphia, 1973, Lea and Febiger, pp 420–421.

29. Giannini S, Faldini C, Vannini F, et al: The minimally invasive osteotomy "S.E.R.I." (simple, effective, rapid, inexpensive) for correction of bunionette deformity, *Foot Ankle Int* 29:282–286, 2008.

30. Glover JP, Weil L Jr, Weil LS Sr: Scarfette osteotomy for surgical treatment of bunionette deformity, *Foot Ankle Spec* 2:73–78, 2009.

31. Haber JH, Kraft J: Crescentic osteotomy for fifth metatarsal head lesions, *J Foot Surg* 19:66–67, 1980.

32. Hohmann F: *Fuss und Bein*, Munich, 1951, Bergman.

33. Kaplan EG, Kaplan G, Jacobs AM: Management of fifth metatarsal head lesions by biplane osteotomy, *J Foot Surg* 15:1–8, 1976.

34. Keating SE, DeVincentis A, Goller WL: Oblique fifth metatarsal osteotomy: a follow-up study, *J Foot Surg* 21:104–107, 1982.

35. Kelikian H: Deformities of the lesser toe. In Kelikian H, editor: *Hallux valgus, allied deformities of the forefoot, and metatarsalgia*, Philadelphia, 1965, WB Saunders, pp 327–330.

36. Kitaoka HB, Holiday AD Jr: Lateral condylar resection for bunionette, *Clin Orthop Relat Res* 278:183–192, 1992.

37. Kitaoka HB, Holiday AD Jr: Metatarsal head resection for bunionette: long-term follow-up, *Foot Ankle* 11:345–349, 1991.

38. Kitaoka HB, Holiday AD Jr, Campbell DC 2nd: Distal chevron metatarsal osteotomy for bunionette, *Foot Ankle* 12:80–85, 1991.

39. Kitaoka HB, Leventen EO: Medial displacement metatarsal osteotomy for treatment of painful bunionette, *Clin Orthop Relat Res* 243:172–179, 1989.

40. Konradsen L, Nielsen PT: Distal metatarsal osteotomy for bunionette deformity, *J Foot Surg* 27:493–496, 1988.

41. Koti M, Maffulli N: Bunionette, *J Bone Joint Surg Am* 83-A:1076–1082, 2001.

42. Leach RE, Igou R: Metatarsal osteotomy for bunionette deformity, *Clin Orthop* 100:171–175, 1974.

43. Legenstein R, Bonomo J, Huber W, Boesch P: Correction of tailor's bunion with the Boesch technique: a retrospective study, *Foot Ankle Int* 28:799–803, 2007.

44. Lelièvre J: [Exostosis of the head of the fifth metatarsal bone; tailor's bunion], *Concours Med* 78:4815–4816, 1956.

45. Lelièvre J, editor: *Pathologie du pied*, Paris, 1971, Masson, pp 526–528.

46. London BP, Stern SF, Quist MA, Lee RK, Picklesimer EK: Long oblique distal osteotomy of the fifth metatarsal for correction of tailor's bunion: a retrospective review, *J Foot Ankle Surg* 42:36–42, 2003.

47. Maher AJ, Kilmartin TE: Scarf osteotomy for correction of tailor's bunion: mid- to long-term followup, *Foot Ankle Int* 31:676–682, 2010.

48. Mann RA: Keratotic disorders of the plantar skin. In Mann RA, editor: *Surgery of the foot*, St Louis, 1986, Mosby, pp 194–198.

49. Masquijo JJ, Willis BR, Kontio K, Dobbs MB: Symptomatic bunionette deformity in adolescents: surgical treatment with metatarsal sliding osteotomy, *J Pediatr Orthop* 30:904–909, 2010.

50. McGlamry ED, Butlin, WE, Kitting RW: Metatarsal shortening: osteoplasty of head or osteotomy of shaft, *J Podiatry Assoc* 59:394–398, 1969.

51. McKeever DC: Excision of the fifth metatarsal head, *Clin Orthop* 13:321–322, 1959.

52. Moran MM, Claridge RJ: Chevron osteotomy for bunionette, *Foot Ankle Int* 15:684–688, 1994.

53. Nestor BJ, Kitaoka HB, Ilstrup DM, Berquist TH, Bergmann AD: Radiologic anatomy of the painful bunionette, *Foot Ankle* 11:6–11, 1990.

54. Okuda R, Kinoshita M, Morikawa J, Jotoku T, Abe M: Proximal dome-shaped osteotomy for symptomatic bunionette, *Clin Orthop Relat Res* 396:173–178, 2002.

55. Pontious J, Brook JW, Hillstrom HJ: Tailor's bunion. Is fixation necessary? *J Am Podiatr Med Assoc* 86:63–73, 1996.

56. Radl R, Leithner,A, Koehler W, Scheipl S, Windhager R: The modified distal horizontal metatarsal osteotomy for correction of bunionette deformity, *Foot Ankle Int* 26:454–457, 2005.

57. Regnauld B, editor: *Technique chirurgicales du pied*, Paris, 1974, Masson, p 23.

58. Roukis TS: The tailor's bunionette deformity: a field guide to surgical correction, *Clin Podiatr Med Surg* 22:223–245, vi, 2005.

59. Sakoff M, Levy AI, Hanft JR: Metaphyseal osteotomy for the treatment of tailor's bunions, *J Foot Surg* 28:537–541, 1989.

60. Schabler JA, Toney M, Hanft JR, Kashuk KB: Oblique metaphyseal osteotomy for the correction of tailor's bunions: a 3-year review, *J Foot Surg* 31:79–84, 1992.

61. Schoenhaus H, Rotman S, Meshon AL: A review of normal intermetatarsal angles, *J Am Podiatry Assoc* 63:88–95, 1973.

62. Seide HW, Petersen W: Tailor's bunion: results of a scarf osteotomy for the correction of an increased intermetatarsal IV/V angle. A report on ten cases with a 1-year follow-up, *Arch Orthop Trauma Surg* 121:166–169, 2001.

63. Shereff MJ, Yang QM, Kummer FJ, Frey CC, Greenidge N: Vascular anatomy of the fifth metatarsal, *Foot Ankle* 11:350–353, 1991.

64. Shrum DG, Sprandel DC, Marshall H: Triplanar closing base wedge osteotomy for tailor's bunion, *J Am Podiatr Med Assoc* 79:124–127, 1989.

65. Sponsel KH: Bunionette correction by metatarsal osteotomy: preliminary report, *Orthop Clin North Am* 7:809–819, 1976.

66. Steel MW 3rd, Johnson KA, DeWitz MA, Ilstrup DM: Radiographic measurements of the normal adult foot, *Foot Ankle* 1:151–158, 1980.
67. Steinke MS, Boll KL: Hohmann-Thomasen metatarsal osteotomy for tailor's bunion (bunionette), *J Bone Joint Surg Am* 71:423–426, 1989.
68. Stewart M: Miscellaneous affections of the foot. In Edmonson SA, Crenshaw AH, editors: *Campbell's operative orthopaedics*, St Louis, 1980, Mosby, p 1733.
69. Throckmorton JK, Bradlee N: Transverse V sliding osteotomy: a new surgical procedure for the correction of tailor's bunion deformity, *J Foot Surg* 18:117–121, 1978.
70. Vienne P, Oesselmann M, Espinosa N, Aschwanden R, Zingg P: Modified Coughlin procedure for surgical treatment of symptomatic tailor's bunion: a prospective followup study of 33 consecutive operations, *Foot Ankle Int* 27:573–580, 2006.
71. Voutey H, editor: *Manuel de chirurgie orthopédique et de rééducatioin du pied*, Paris, 1978, Mason.
72. Weisberg MH: Resection of fifth metatarsal head in lateral segment problems, *J Am Podiatry Assoc* 57:374–376, 1967.
73. Weitzel S, Trnka HJ, Petroutsas J: Transverse medial slide osteotomy for bunionette deformity: long-term results, *Foot Ankle Int* 28:794–798, 2007.
74. Yancey HA Jr: Congenital lateral bowing of the fifth metatarsal. Report of 2 cases and operative treatment, *Clin Orthop Relat Res* 62:203–205, 1969.
75. Zvijac JE, Janecki CJ, Freeling RM: Distal oblique osteotomy for tailor's bunion, *Foot Ankle* 12:171–175, 1991.

10 Chapter

Sesamoids and Accessory Bones of the Foot

Michael J. Coughlin

CHAPTER CONTENTS

SESAMOIDS

Galen is reported to have first coined the term *sesamoid* because of the resemblance of these small rounded bones to the sesame seed.[44] The anatomic location of several of the sesamoids is constant, but the frequency of occurrence of other sesamoids is quite variable.[40]

The sesamoids function to alter the direction of muscle pull, diminish friction, and modify pressure. Sesamoids occur in the substance of their corresponding tendon. They may be totally or partially contained within the tendinous structure. Some sesamoids totally ossify, some remain entirely cartilaginous, and some partially ossify with a fibrocartilaginous interface between the ossified fragments. This variability in ossification might explain the radiographic absence or presence of various sesamoids, as well as the incidence of bipartism of sesamoids.[91]

The sesamoids in the foot and ankle region are contained within the plantar plates of the interphalangeal and metatarsophalangeal (MTP) joints and in the tendons of the flexor hallucis brevis, the intrinsic tendons of the lesser toes, the tibialis anterior tendon, the tibialis posterior tendon, and the peroneus longus tendon.

The importance of this chapter is to assist the physician in recognizing both normal and pathologic variants, which may present as an uncommon or rare accessory bone of the foot and ankle, or which, on the other hand, may have developed because of trauma or an event that has caused a bony fragment to appear as an accessory bone.

SESAMOIDS OF THE FIRST METATARSOPHALANGEAL JOINT

The sesamoids of the first MTP joint play an important role in the function of the hallux. Contained within the tendons of the flexor hallucis brevis, the sesamoids of the first MTP joint have many functions: to absorb the majority of the weight of the first ray; to protect the tendon of the flexor hallucis longus, which courses over the rather exposed plantar surface of the first metatarsal head; and to help increase the mechanical advantage of the intrinsic musculature of the first ray. Although sesamoid dysfunction is uncommon, it can occur with arthritis, trauma, infection, osteochondritis, and sesamoiditis.

First MTP sesamoid abnormalities are uncommon, but degeneration or isolated injury can cause pain and significant dysfunction. To understand the nature of the clinical problems and to appreciate appropriate indications for surgical intervention, an understanding of the function of the sesamoid mechanism and of the pertinent anatomy is necessary.

Anatomy

Location, Function, and Size

The sesamoid mechanism and intrinsic musculature of the hallux differentiate the first ray from the lateral toes. The hallucal sesamoids, enveloped within the double tendon of the flexor hallucis brevis (Fig. 10-1), articulate on their dorsal surface with the plantar facets of the first metatarsal head. A crista, or intersesamoid ridge (Fig. 10-2), separates the medial and lateral metatarsal facets. This intersesamoid ridge provides intrinsic stability to the sesamoid complex. In severe cases of hallux valgus, with substantial subluxation of the sesamoid complex in relation to the first metatarsal head, the intersesamoid ridge atrophies and at times is obliterated (Fig. 10-3). Close inspection of the plantar articular surface of the first

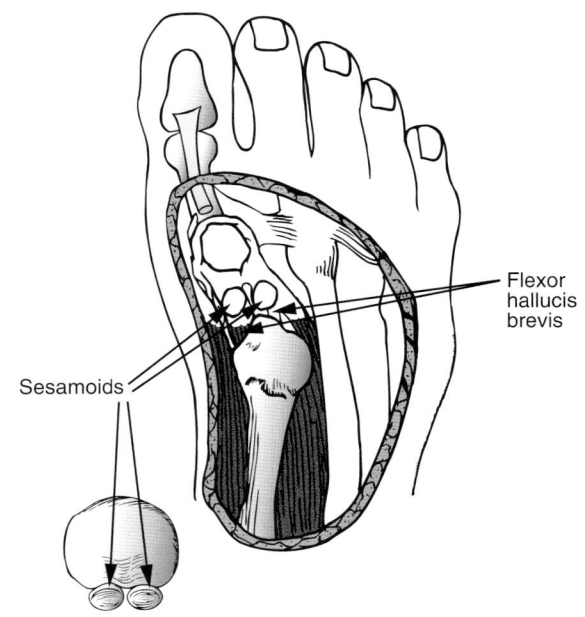

Figure 10-1 The sesamoids are enveloped within the double tendon of the flexor hallucis brevis.

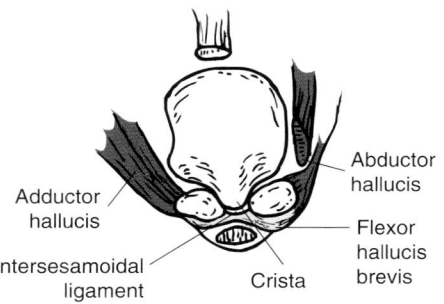

Figure 10-2 A cross section of the first metatarsal head demonstrates the sesamoid and the intersesamoidal ridge.

metatarsal frequently reveals substantial cartilage erosion and degenerative arthritis in this area (Fig. 10-4).[10]

The sesamoids are connected to the plantar base of the proximal phalanx through the plantar plate (Fig. 10-5), which is an extension of the flexor hallucis brevis tendon. The inferior surface of the sesamoids is covered by a thin layer of the flexor hallucis brevis tendon, whereas the superior surface is articular in nature. These sesamoids are entirely intratendinous, except dorsally, where they articulate with the first metatarsal head. The sesamoids are suspended by a slinglike mechanism composed of the collateral ligaments of the MTP joint and the sesamoid ligaments (Fig. 10-6) on both the medial and lateral aspects of the MTP joint. The flexor hallucis brevis,

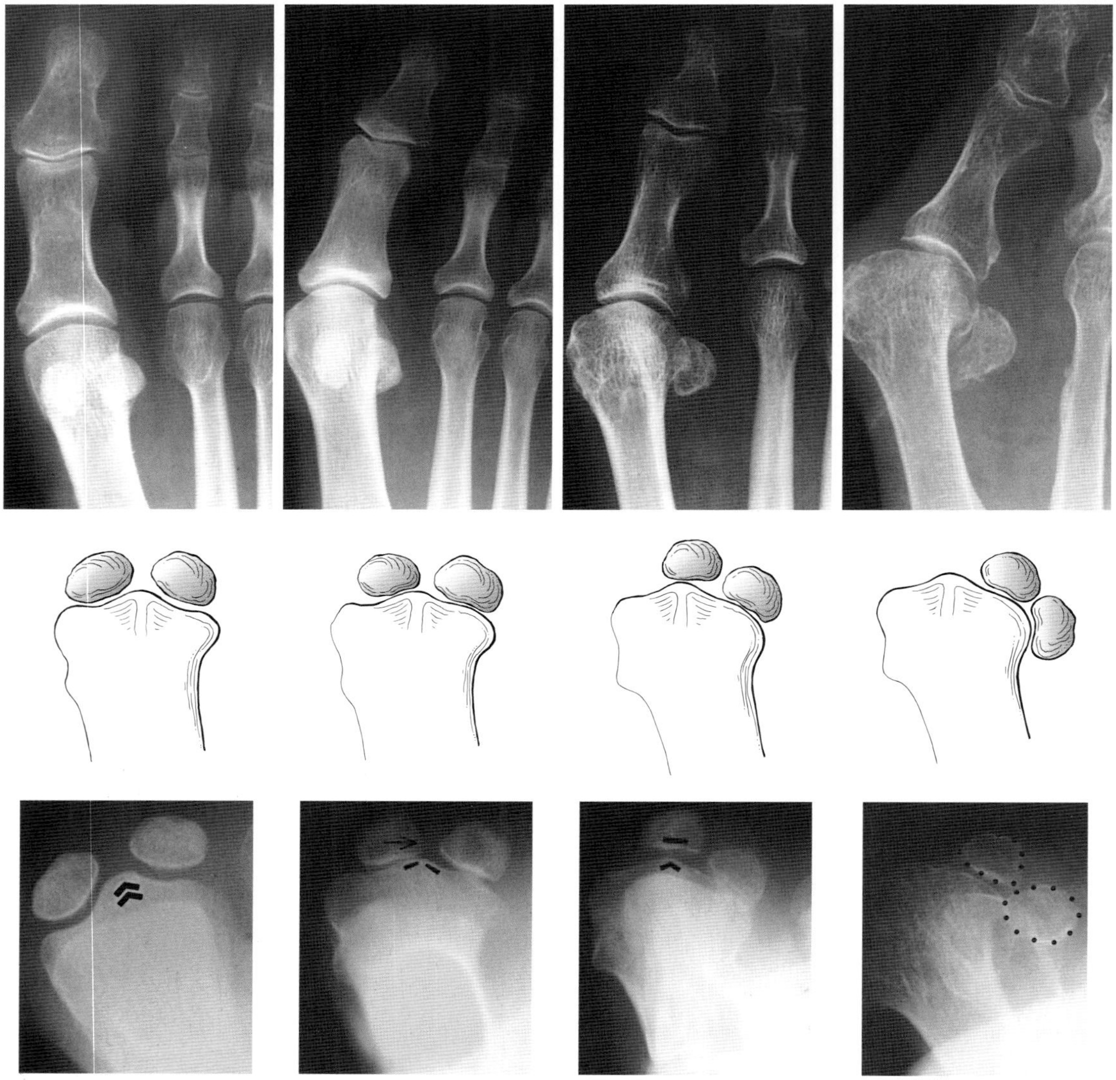

Figure 10-3 **A,** Normal axial position of the sesamoids centered on either aspect of the cristae. An anteroposterior (AP) radiograph demonstrates the normal position of the sesamoids. **B,** Mild hallux valgus deformity with mild subluxation. **C,** Moderate hallux valgus deformity associated with moderate sesamoid subluxation. AP radiograph demonstrates moderate sesamoid subluxation. **D,** Severe hallux valgus associated with severe subluxation of the sesamoids. AP radiograph demonstrates a hallux valgus angle of 60 degrees.

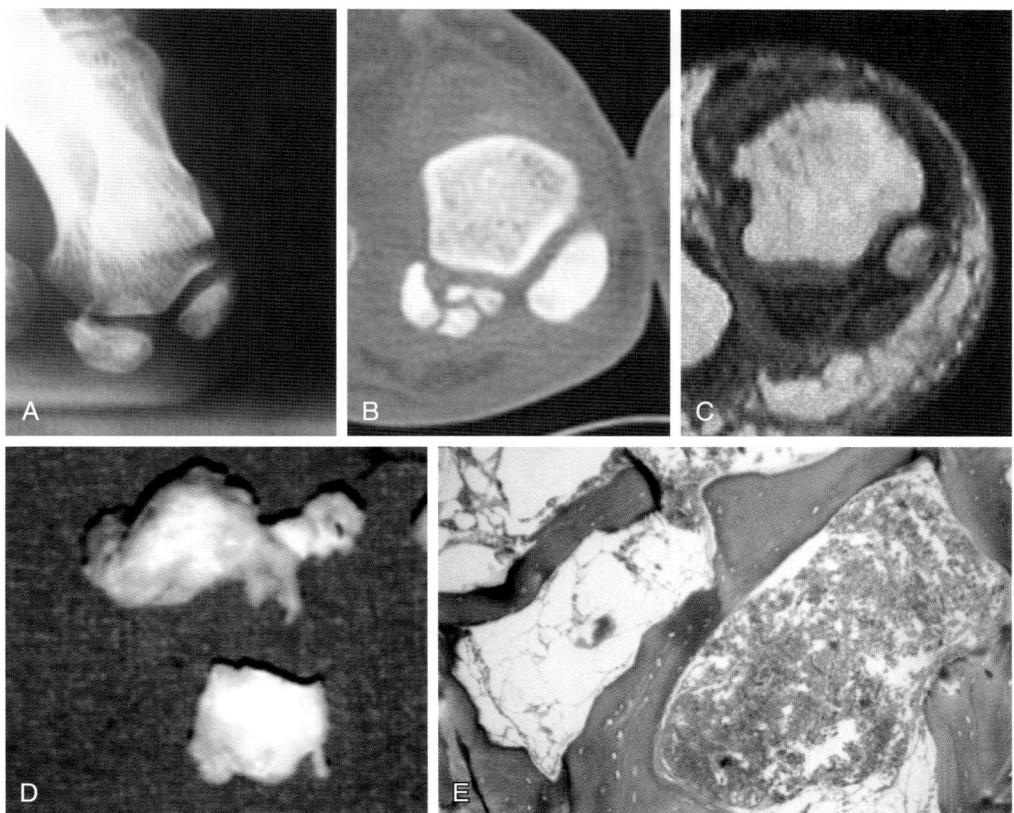

Figure 10-4 Avascular necrosis of the lateral sesamoid. **A,** Axial view demonsrating fragmented sesamoid. **B,** Computed tomography scan. **C,** Magnetic resonance imaging of lateral sesamoid fragmentation. **D,** Excised specimen. **E,** Histology section demonstrating eosinophilic infiltration of the marrow fat and necrosis of the bone trabeculae with absence of the osteocytes. (From Toussirot E, Jeunet L, Michel F, et al: Avascular necrosis of the hallucal sesamoids update with reference to two case-reports, *Joint Bone Spine* 70:307–309, 2003.)

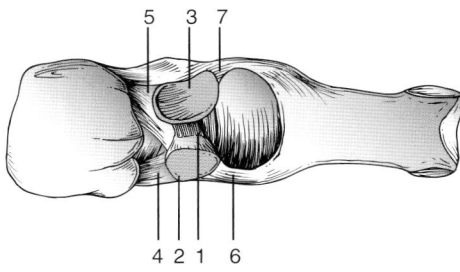

Figure 10-5 Metatarsophalangeal joint from a dorsal exposure showing the intersesamoidal ligament *(1)*, the lateral sesamoid *(2)*, medial sesamoid *(3)*, lateral metatarsosesamoid ligament (plantar plate) *(4)*, medial metatarsosesamoid ligament (plantar plate) *(5)*, lateral joint capsule *(6)*, and medial joint capsule with extension into the distal plantar plate *(7)*.

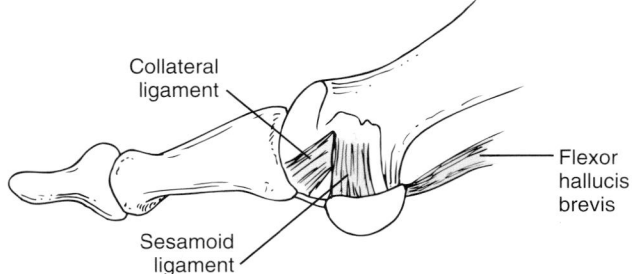

Figure 10-6 The sesamoids and collateral ligaments provide medial and lateral stability to the metatarsophalangeal joint.

through its sesamoid mechanism, provides a significant plantar flexion force at the MTP joint. The sesamoids also have an insertion into the joint capsule and the plantar aponeurosis; this provides both stabilization and a static plantar flexion force at the MTP joint.

On the medial aspect of the MTP joint, the abductor hallucis tendon (Fig. 10-7) inserts into the plantar-medial base of the proximal phalanx as well as the medial sesamoid and functions to stabilize the sesamoid mechanism medially. On the lateral aspect, the adductor hallucis tendon inserts into the lateral base of the proximal phalanx and into the lateral sesamoid to stabilize the sesamoid mechanism laterally. The medial and lateral sesamoids are connected by the intersesamoidal ligament, which forms the base of the tendinous canal enveloping the tendon of the flexor hallucis longus.

Distal to the sesamoids, the phalangeal-sesamoid ligament is a thin-layered structure that interdigitates with the collateral ligaments, extension of the plantar aponeurosis, and tendons of the flexor hallucis brevis to form the plantar plate. These structures are not individually distinguishable but, rather, coalesce to form the plantar plate. Complete or partial rupture of the plantar plate attachement may lead to a turf toe deformity with retraction of

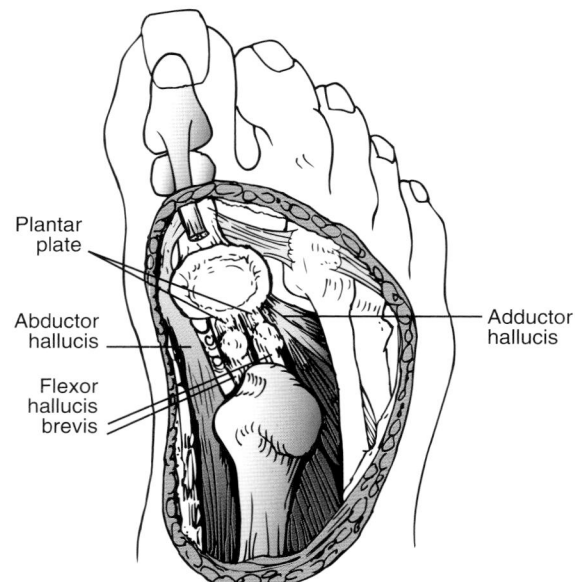

Figure 10-7 The abductor hallucis inserts into the plantar-medial base of the proximal phalanx, while the adductor hallucis inserts into the plantar-lateral base of the proximal phalanx. Both these intrinsic muscles also insert into their respective sesamoids.

the sesamoids, restricted motion, and degenerative arthritis of the first metatarsophalangeal joint.[18]

When a person is in a standing position, the sesamoids are located posterior to the metatarsal head; however, with dorsiflexion of the hallux, the sesamoids move distally, thereby protecting the otherwise exposed plantar surface of the first metatarsal head. When a person rises onto the toes, the sesamoids (especially the medial sesamoid) act as the main weight-bearing focus for the medial forefoot (Fig. 10-8).

Kewenter[54,214] noted that the medial sesamoid is located slightly more distal than the lateral sesamoid and is slightly larger. Orr[73] quantitated sesamoid size and reported that the tibial sesamoid averaged 9 to 11 mm in width and 12 to 15 mm in length. The fibular sesamoid was noted to have an average width of 7 to 9 mm and an average length of 9 to 10 mm.

Ossification

Although ossification of the hallucial sesamoids is variable, Kewenter reported that ossification usually occurs between the sixth and seventh years. Ossification of the sesamoids often occurs from multiple centers, and this may be the reason for the development of multipartite sesamoids.[54,214]

Circulation

The arterial anatomy of the first ray was evaluated in 22 anatomic specimens by Rath et al.[78] They found that the first plantar metatarsal artery provided the main arterial supply to the medial and lateral sesamoids. It anastomosed with a branch of the medial plantar artery in 90% of cases they dissected. They demonstrated both proximal and distal vessels branching off the two major arteries. Pretterklieber and Wanivenhaus,[77] in dissections of 29 cadavers, reported three different types of arterial circulation. The most common type (type A, 52%), was characterized by arterial circulation derived from the medial

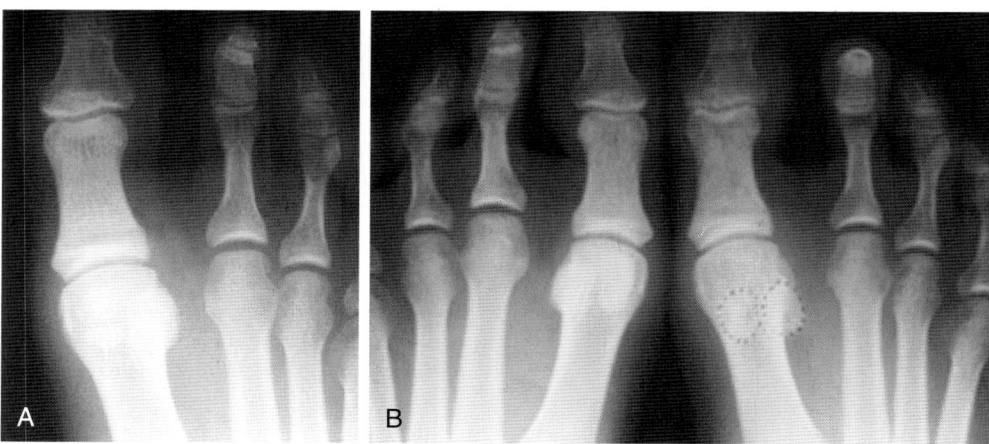

Figure 10-8 A, Anteroposterior (AP) radiograph immediately after hyperextension injury of the first metatarsophalangeal joint. B, AP radiograph of both feet 1 year later, demonstrating retraction of the sesamoid complex after disruption of the plantar plate.

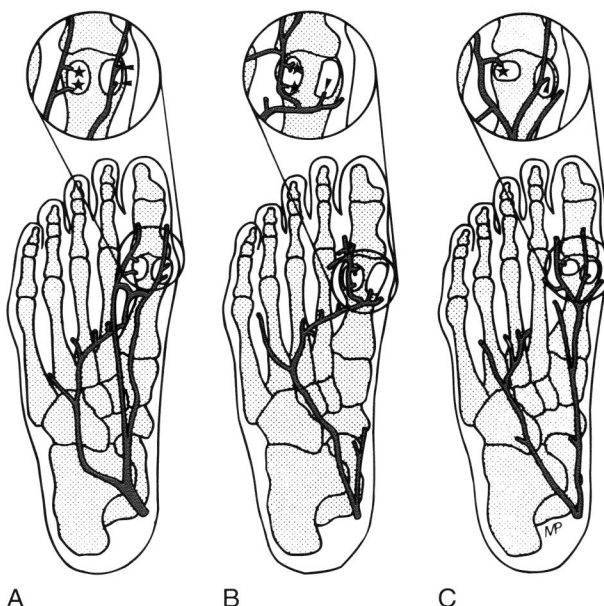

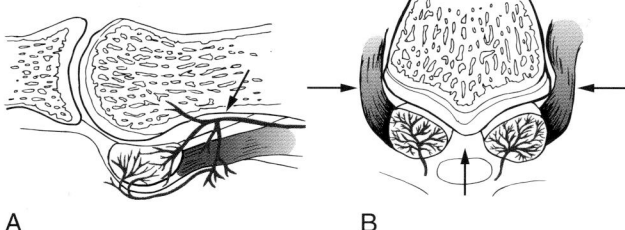

Figure 10-9 Circulation to the sesamoids. **A,** The most common pattern of arterial circulation to the sesamoids (52% of cases) involves a direct branch from both the medial plantar artery and the plantar arch. **B,** In 24% of cases, the sesamoid arterial supply is predominantly from the plantar arch. **C,** In 24% of cases, the major arterial supply is from only the medial plantar artery. When there is only one blood vessel supplying a sesamoid, a fracture may be at greater risk for avascular necrosis or nonunion. (Courtesy Michael L. Pretterklieber, MD, and Axel Wanivenhaus, MD.)

Figure 10-10 **A,** The major vascular supply enters the sesamoid proximally. An anastomosis occurs between the distal and proximal surface. **B,** The plantar vascular supply to the sesamoid is significant. (Modified from Sobel M, Hashimoto J, Amoczky SP, Bohne WH: The microvasculature of the sesamoid complex: its clinical significance, *Foot Ankle* 13:359–363, 1992.)

plantar artery and the plantar arch. In the less common types, circulation was derived mainly from either the plantar arch or only from the medial plantar artery (Fig. 10-9). Both authors concluded that the course and distribution of the arterial circulation to the sesamoids might have a significant bearing on the development of avascular necrosis after injury and possible inadvertent injury during surgical exploration of this area.

The number of arterial branches can affect healing of fractures as well as the incidence of avascular necrosis after trauma.[13] Multiple arterial branches can protect an injured sesamoid, whereas a single arterial branch to a damaged sesamoid may be interrupted by a fracture or injury and lead to delayed healing or a nonunion.

Sobel et al[97] and Rath et al,[78] in their evaluation of sesamoid vascularity, mapped the vascular supply as well of both the medial and lateral sesamoids. The major vascular supply enters the sesamoids from the proximal and plantar aspect, with a minor arterial supply entering through the distal pole of the sesamoids (Fig. 10-10A). The distal vascular supply originates through distal capsular attachments providing, in most cases, a limited arterial supply. The proximal arterial supply, through the flexor hallucis brevis, supplies one third to two thirds of the proximal sesamoid. Vascular anastomoses occur between the proximal supply and that derived from the

plantar surface to the body of the sesamoid (Fig. 10-10B). The distal portion of the sesamoid has the most tenuous vascular supply, and this can lead to delayed or unsuccessful healing after injury.

The sesamoids not only absorb weight-bearing forces on the medial aspect of the forefoot but also increase the mechanical advantage of the intrinsic musculature in plantar-flexing the proximal phalanx. The tendon of the flexor hallucis longus is protected in its tendon sheath by the medial and lateral sesamoids and provides a plantar flexion force to the distal phalanx of the great toe.

Preoperative Evaluation

Physical Examination

Patients with a symptomatic sesamoid often complain of pain and discomfort during the toe-off phase of gait. Objective clinical findings include restricted range of MTP motion, pain on direct palpation, pain with motion of the first MTP joint, swelling of the first MTP joint, and diminished plantar or dorsiflexion strength. Synovitis of the first MTP joint may be noted as well on physical examination. Occasionally, an intractable plantar keratotic lesion develops beneath either the tibial or fibular sesamoid.

The orientation of the hallux must be inspected for lateral (hallux valgus) or medial (hallux varus) deviation or for clawing of the hallux. Progressive insidious deviation of the hallux can develop with sesamoid disruption caused by trauma or fracture. Progressive hallux valgus or hallux varus can also develop as a result of a previous sesamoid resection. Hyperextension of the hallux because of discontinuity of the sesamoid complex can occur after traumatic rupture of the plantar plate (see Fig. 10-8).

Examination of the sensory nerves of the first ray is important in diagnosing a compressed digital nerve,[39] which can manifest with isolated neuritic symptoms or numbness. With compression of either the medial or lateral digital nerve by either the tibial or fibular sesamoid, a Tinel sign can be elicited along the border of the sesamoid.

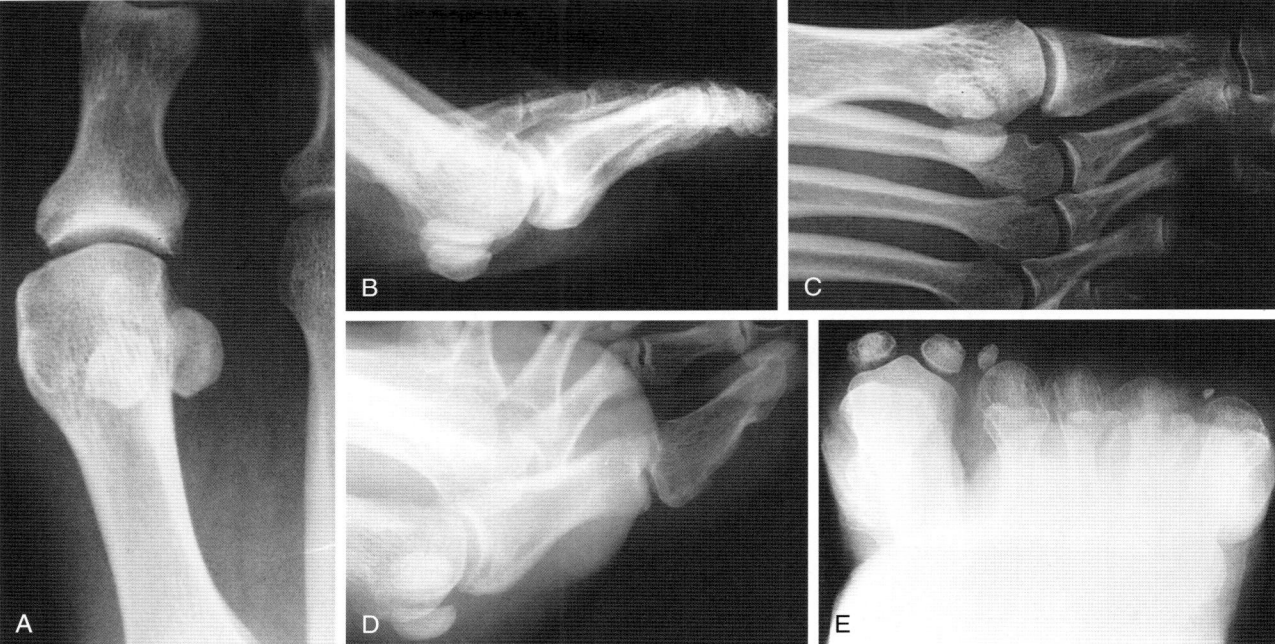

Figure 10-11 **A,** Dorsoplantar radiograph demonstrating the metatarsophalangeal sesamoids. The view is partially obstructed by the overlying metatarsal head. **B,** Lateral radiograph of the sesamoids. The medial and lateral sesamoids overlie one another and somewhat obscure the view of each individual sesamoid. **C,** A lateral oblique radiograph can best visualize the fibular sesamoid. **D,** A medial oblique radiograph shows more clearly the tibial sesamoid. **E,** An axial sesamoid radiograph presents the sesamoids without being obstructed by the overlying first metatarsal.

Radiographic Examination

Routine dorsoplantar and lateral radiographs (Fig. 10-11A and 10-11B) can provide limited information in the evaluation of a painful sesamoid. On the dorsoplantar view, the metatarsal head overlies both the medial and lateral sesamoid and often obscures detail; on the lateral projection, the medial and lateral sesamoids overlap each other. The fibular sesamoid is best demonstrated in a lateral oblique radiograph (Fig. 10-11C), where it can be seen between the first and second metatarsal heads. The tibial sesamoid is best seen on a medial oblique radiograph (Fig. 10-11D).[81] With the MTP joint dorsiflexed approximately 50 degrees, the roentgen beam is directed 15 degrees cephalad from a lateral position and is centered over the first metatarsal head. Often, however, the most useful radiograph is the axial sesamoid view (Fig. 10-11E).[43,63] Where radiographs appear normal in spite of a patient's subjective symptoms, a technetium-99m (^{99m}Tc) bone scan may be useful (Fig. 10-12A, B, and C). A bone scan can demonstrate increased uptake before the development of any significant radiographic change, such as sclerosis, fragmentation, or disintegration. Computed tomography (CT) examination can define osseous changes, such as acute fracture or fragmentation, and magnetic resonance imaging (MRI) examination may demonstrate bone edema, avascular regions, fragmentation or degeneration of a sesamoid early before radiographic changes are demonstrated on plain radiographs (see Fig. 10-4A).

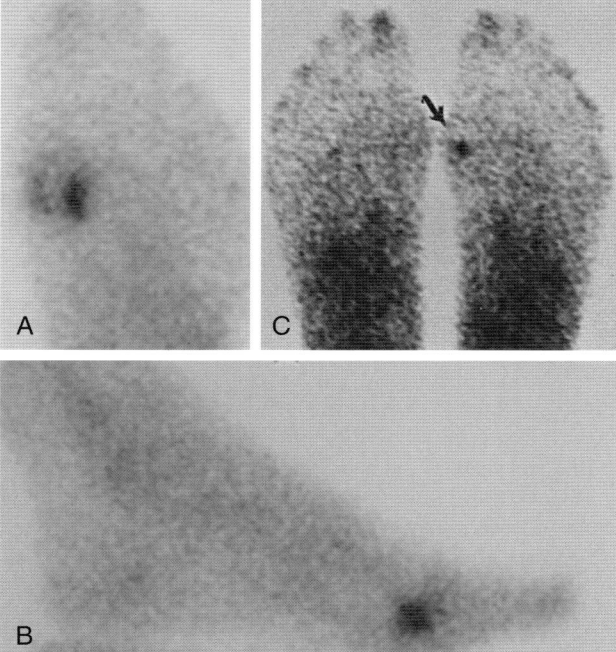

Figure 10-12 Anteroposterior **(A)** and lateral **(B)** technetium-99m (^{99m}Tc) bone scan demonstrating increased uptake in the lateral sesamoid. A fractured medial sesamoid *(arrow)* is demonstrated. **C,** A bone scan may be helpful in diagnosing an abnormality when a routine radiograph appears normal.

BIPARTITE SESAMOIDS AND FRACTURES

The incidence of partite sesamoids as well as their cause has been the subject of substantial discussion in the literature (Table 10-1). Kewenter[54,214] examined 800 feet and found a 31% incidence of bipartite tibial sesamoids (Fig. 10-13), and Dobas and Silvers[24] examined radiographs of 1000 feet and found a 19% incidence of combined tibial and fibular sesamoid bipartism (Fig. 10-14). Dobas and Silvers reported that 80% of bipartite sesamoids involve

Table 10-1 Proportion of Tibial and Fibular Division in Representative Series of Cases

Authors	Number of Cases	Tibial Division (%)	Fibular Division (%)
Kewenter[54,214]	800	30.6	1.3
Dobas and Silvers[24]	1000	16.8	2.5
Burman and Lapidus[15]	1000	7.2	0.6

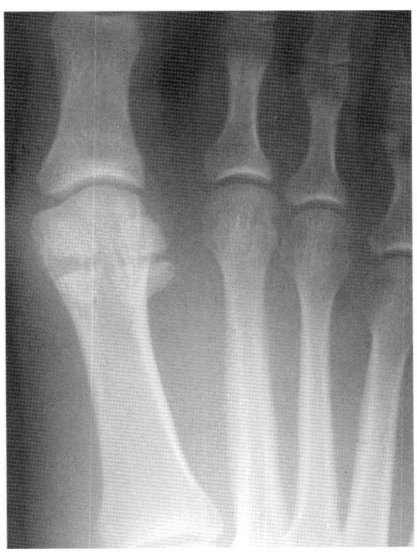

Figure 10-14 Anteroposterior radiograph demonstrating asymptomatic bipartite medial and lateral sesamoids.

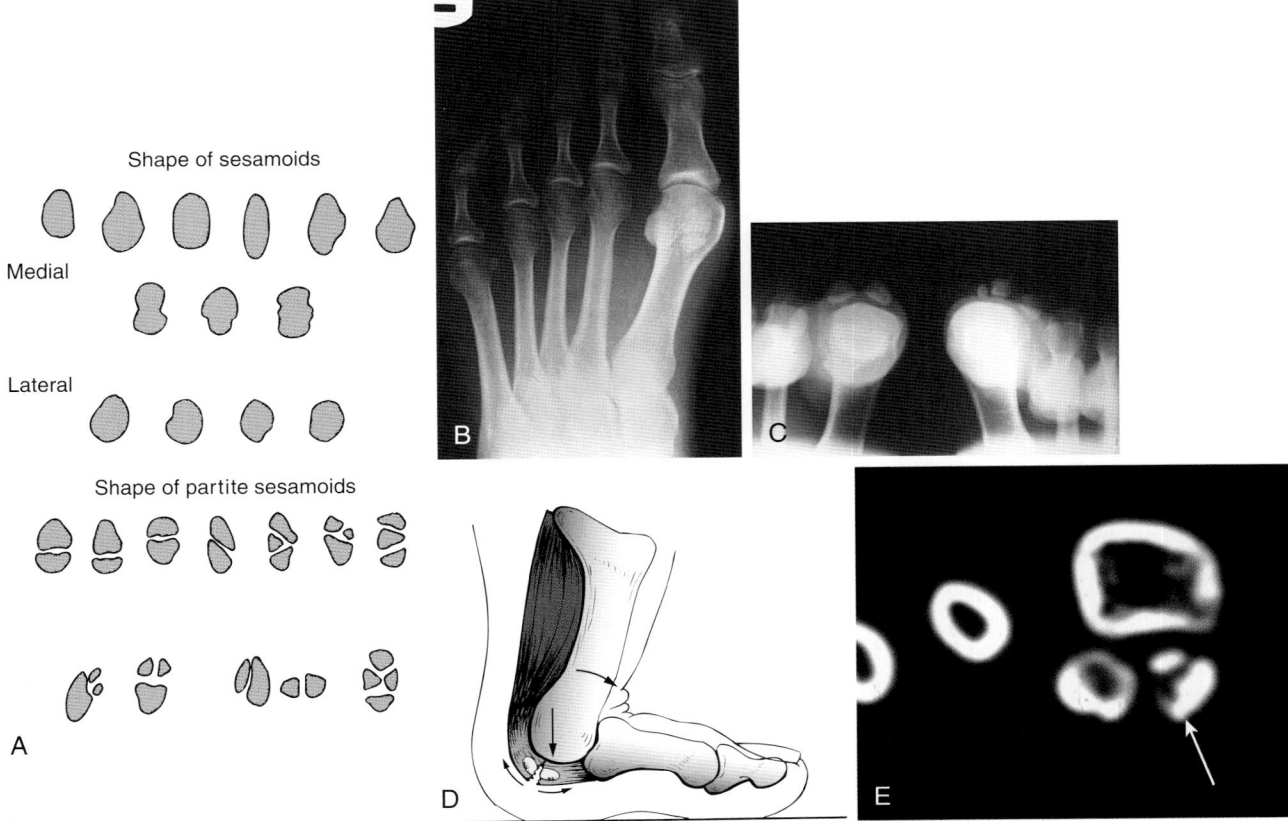

Figure 10-13 Many variations can occur in ossification of sesamoids of the metatarsophalangeal joint of the hallux. **A,** Various shapes of medial and lateral sesamoids. **B,** An anteroposterior radiograph demonstrates a bipartite medial sesamoid. **C,** An axial radiograph demonstrates a longitudinal bipartite medial sesamoid. **D,** Hyperextension injury mechanism resulting in disruption of the sesamoid complex. **E,** Computed tomography scan of multipartite sesamoid demonstrating oblique separation of medial sesamoid *(arrow).*

the tibial sesamoid. Rowe[87] noted a 6% to 8% frequency of bipartite sesamoids and stated that 90% of these were bilateral. Dobas and Silvers[24] stated that approximately 25% of partite tibial sesamoids had an identical bipartite tibial sesamoid on the contralateral side, whereas the remaining sesamoids were asymmetric when division was concerned. Jahss[46] noted that bipartism was 10 times more common in the medial sesamoid. Giannestras[32] stated that the occurrence of bipartite sesamoids was typically symmetric, but this is obviously not the case. The medial sesamoid is often divided into two, three, or four parts, whereas the lateral sesamoid is rarely divided into more than two parts (Fig. 10-15).

Inge and Ferguson[44] reported that 85% of the bilateral partite sesamoids had asymmetric divisions. They also reported that the incidence of division decreased with time, thus implying that osseous union occurs with time in the divided sesamoid. They further reported that histologic evaluation of congenital bipartite sesamoids demonstrated that articular cartilage tended to dip down between the two osseous fragments. This can predispose a bipartite sesamoid to fracture or disruption of the synchondrosis with minimal injury (see Fig. 10-13D). They speculated that the medial sesamoid has a higher frequency of bipartism than the lateral sesamoid because it is more often traumatized, a result of its greater

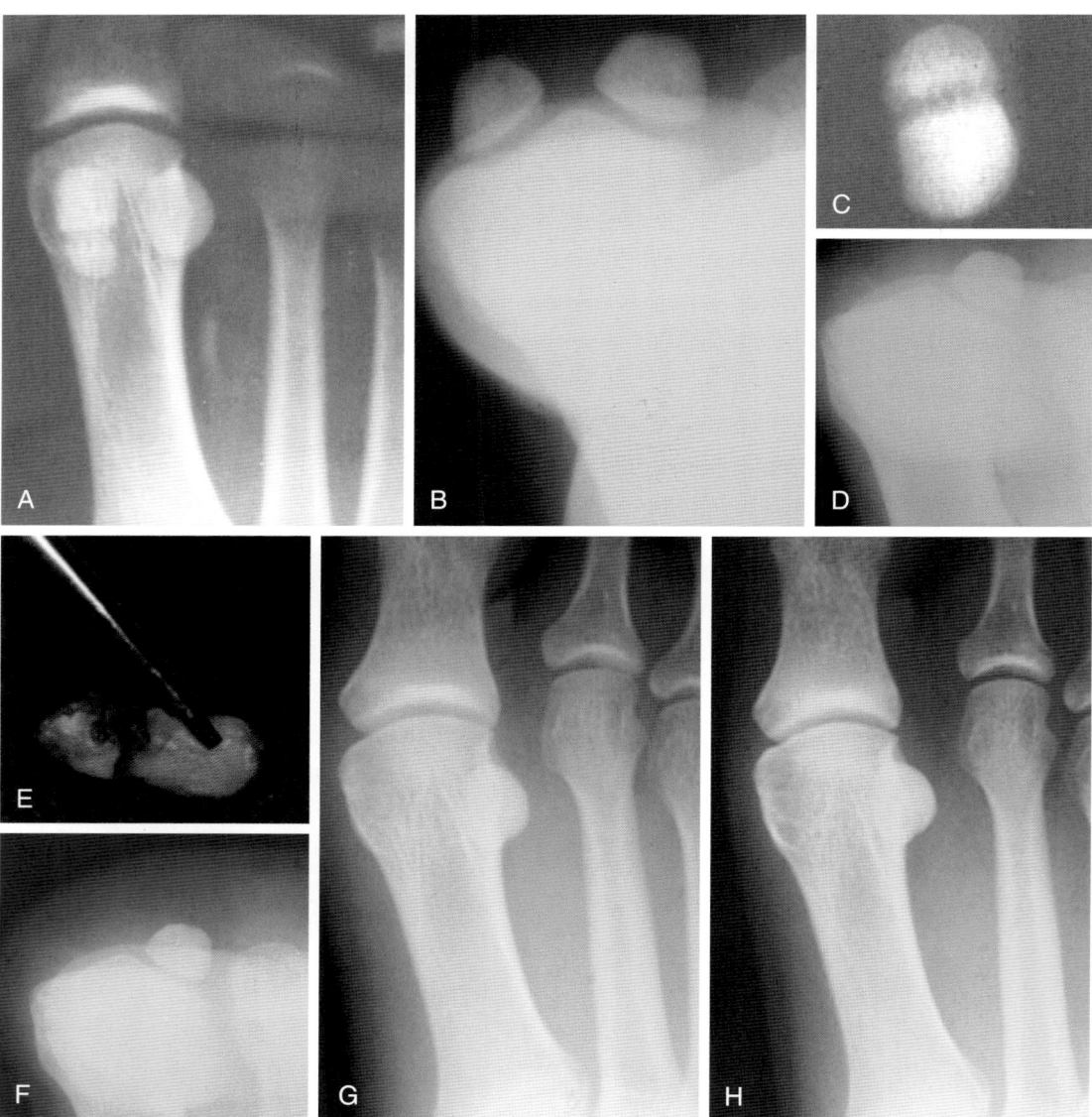

Figure 10-15 **A,** An anteroposterior radiograph demonstrates a painful bipartite sesamoid. **B,** An axial radiograph does not show evidence of a fracture or bipartite sesamoid. **C,** Radiograph of a pathology specimen showing rounded edges pathognomonic of a bipartite sesamoid. **D,** Axial view after excision of medial sesamoid. **E,** Gross pathology of a specimen. **F** and **G,** Immediately after surgery. **H,** At 19-year follow-up after medial sesamoid excision. Alignment of the first metatarsophalangeal joint is well maintained.

weight-bearing capacity. It has not been determined whether continued trauma with ambulation prevents the union of divided sesamoids or whether some of these partite sesamoids are actually nonunions of fractures.

The incidence of irregular ossification with bipartism in the medial sesamoid is well recognized. Kewenter[54,214] examined a series of sesamoids in cadavers and found that congenitally divided sesamoids fracture with much less force than normal sesamoids when experimental trauma was introduced. Although fractures of sesamoids are relatively rare, numerous cases have been reported in the literature.* Substantial trauma with MTP joint dislocation and simultaneous fractures of both sesamoids have been reported[23,103]; in general, the most frequently reported mechanism of injury is a fall onto the forefoot, sudden loading of the forefoot, or a crush injury.

It can be difficult to distinguish between a fractured sesamoid (see Fig. 10-15) and a symptomatic bipartite sesamoid.[30,104] With a divisionary line between two segments of a sesamoid, a careful physical examination and history must be correlated with radiographic findings to differentiate between a partite sesamoid and a superimposed fracture.[30] With a sesamoid fracture, pain is localized to the region of the specific sesamoid. Symptoms are typically exacerbated with ambulation and reduced with rest. Often, the patient ambulates with weight bearing on the lateral aspect of the foot to avoid motion and loading of the sesamoid complex.

On physical examination, forced passive dorsiflexion and plantar flexion can cause discomfort. Synovitis or nonspecific swelling on the plantar aspect of the sesamoid complex may be observed. The development of pain after minimal trauma in the presence of a bipartite sesamoid should alert the examiner to the possibility of a superimposed fracture of a bipartite sesamoid. An acute fracture may be noted on a radiograph with a sharp radiolucent line (Fig. 10-16); however, Inge and Ferguson[44] suggested that a fracture should not be diagnosed unless callus is present. Delay in diagnosis of a sesamoid fracture is therefore common because of the difficulty of confirming the fracture by radiography.[102,110]

Although rarely is a preinjury film available to help differentiate a partite sesamoid and a fracture, increased separation between fragments can be a definitive finding in the presence of a disruption of a partite sesamoid (Fig. 10-17). Richardson[81] recommends a bone scan to aid in diagnosis of a fracture in the presence of a bipartite sesamoid. MRIs may demonstrate increased vascularity, bone edema, or acute changes, indicating a disruption of a partite sesamoid[49] (see Fig. 10-37D). Hobart[40] recommended non–weight bearing and casting until the sesamoid fracture had healed, which usually occurred in 6 to 8 weeks (Fig. 10-18). Anderson and McBryde[2] reported on 21 patients treated with bone grafting for symptomatic tibial sesamoid nonunions (Fig. 10-19).

---

*References 1, 8, 14, 15, 30, 33, 42, 45, 56, 76, 83, 103, and 104.

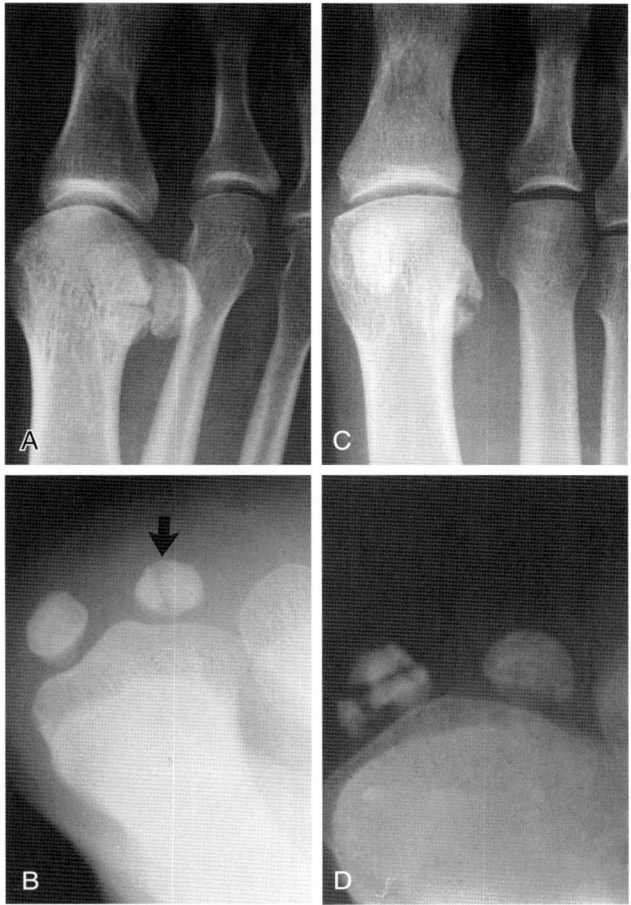

Figure 10-16 A, Oblique radiograph demonstrating an acute fracture of the medial sesamoid. **B,** Axial radiograph demonstrating a longitudinal fracture *(arrow)* of the lateral sesamoid. This fracture was only demonstrated on this particular view. **C,** Anteroposterior radiograph demonstrating a comminuted fracture of the lateral sesamoid. **D,** Axial radiograph demonstrating a comminuted fracture of the medial sesamoid.

They curetted and bone grafted the diastasis, which was typically 1 mm wide. All patients were noted to have a positive bone scan before surgery. In two cases in which articular surface deterioration was noted, a sesamoidectomy was performed. Three other patients had excessive motion at the diastasis site and were not considered candidates for bone grafting. Through an inferior extraarticular approach, they curetted and bone grafted the diastasis "nonunion site." No internal fixation was used. The patients were placed in a below-knee cast and kept non–weight bearing for 4 weeks. At final follow-up, 19 of 21 sesamoids had healed. Two patients had a persistent nonunion. Reports in which internal fixation has been used for acute sesamoid fracture[75] or chronic nonunions[9,82] have noted success. Riley and Selner[82] used a circlage wire and bone grafting in one case, and Blundell et al[9] used a percutaneous screw in nine cases and reported successful union. Pagenstert et al[75] reported two cases in which

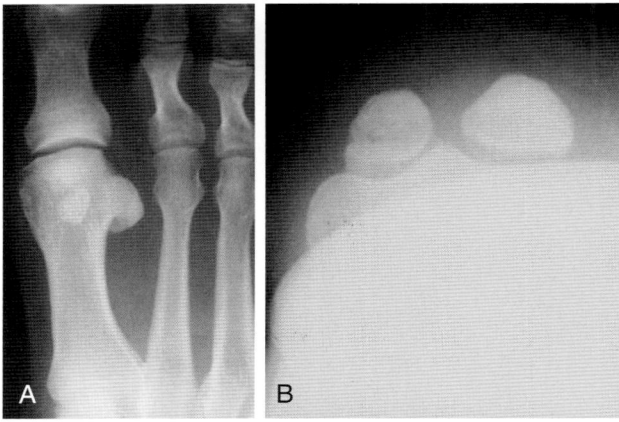

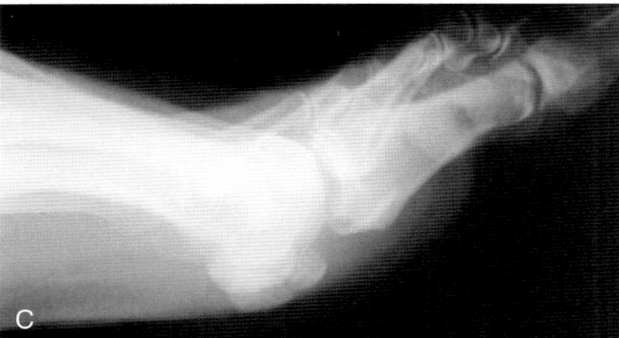

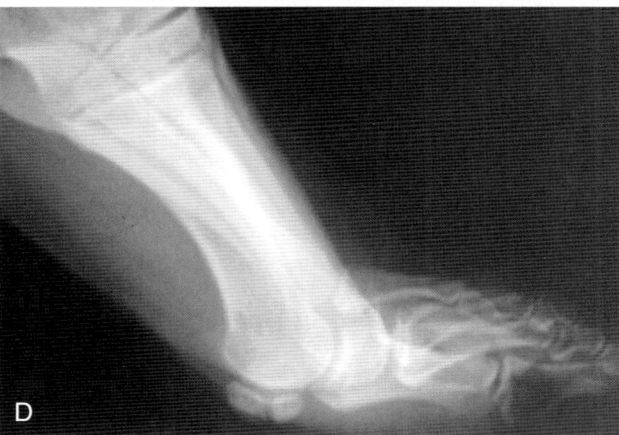

Figure 10-17 **A,** Anteroposterior radiograph demonstrating a multipartite medial sesamoid. **B,** Axial view demonstrating defect. **C,** Lateral radiograph demonstrating alignment of proximal and distal fragments. **D,** With dorsiflexion of the hallux, the alignment of the fragments changes, demonstrating motion consistent with a fracture of a partite sesamoid.

simultaneous correction of a hallux valgus deformity was combined with open reduction and internal fixation of a nonunion of a medial sesamoid.

Rodeo et al[83] reported on four cases of injuries to the hallux with progressive diastasis of bipartite sesamoids. The patients were treated with a distal resection of a smaller fragment and repair of the sesamoid mechanism.

Biedert and Hintermann[7] reported on five athletes who developed stress fractures of the medial sesamoids.

Surgical excision of the proximal fragment and repair of the flexor hallucis brevis were performed. After casting for 6 weeks after surgery, full return to sports activity was allowed at 8 weeks.

Kuo et al[57] reported a case of nonunion of the fibular sesamoid in association with chronic gout that required surgical excision.

Brodsky et al[13] retrospectively reviewed a series of 37 patients with fractured sesamoids. Avascular necrosis secondary to fracture was noted in 9 cases, 16 cases were diagnosed as stress fractures, and 12 cases were related to direct trauma. After surgical excision of the fractured sesamoid, an average postoperative American Orthopaedic Foot and Ankle Society (AOFAS) score of 93 was achieved.

Saxena and Krisdakumtorn[93] reported on 24 patients at a mean follow-up of 86 months after sesamoidectomy. There were 10 fibular and 16 tibial sesamoidectomies. Eleven patients were professional or varsity athletes and returned to activity in 7.5 weeks. The other patients returned to normal activities in 12 weeks. Complications included one varus deformity, one valgus deformity, and two cases of neuroma formation associated with fibular sesamoidectomy. Patients took longer to recover from surgery for tibial sesamoidectomy, which the authors surmised was probably due to increased weight bearing. Patients with fibular sesamoidectomies had an earlier return to activity. They noted that a dorsolateral approach may be more difficult for fibular sesamoidectomy and that the two nerve problems both occurred with a dorsolateral approach.

Custom and prefabricated orthotics and scaphoid and metatarsal pads can relieve pressure in the sesamoid region, diminishing symptoms. Taping of the toe to reduce dorsiflexion can also relieve symptoms. If conservative methods fail, surgical removal of the involved sesamoid may be necessary (see Fig. 10-20).

Rosenfield and Trepman[85] have described the use of a rocker-soled walking shoe with a full-length steel shank. An orthotic insole is added with a recess beneath the sesamoid region (Fig. 10-21).

CONGENITAL ABSENCE OF THE SESAMOIDS

Congenital variations in regard to ossification of the tibial and fibular sesamoids are common. Congenital absence of a sesamoid has been infrequently reported; however, it is probably more prevalent than is realized.[48,58] Patients are typically asymptomatic with absent sesamoids. Inge and Ferguson[44] reported two cases of congenital absence of the tibial sesamoid. Goez and DeLauro,[35] Zinsmeister and Edelman,[111] and others[21,52] have reported absence of the tibial sesamoids as well. Jeng et al[48] and others[60,108] have reported cases of an absent fibular sesamoid (Fig. 10-22).

Although absence of a sesamoid can be asymptomatic, removal of a sesamoid for painful plantar keratosis can cause postoperative pain beneath the remaining sesamoid.

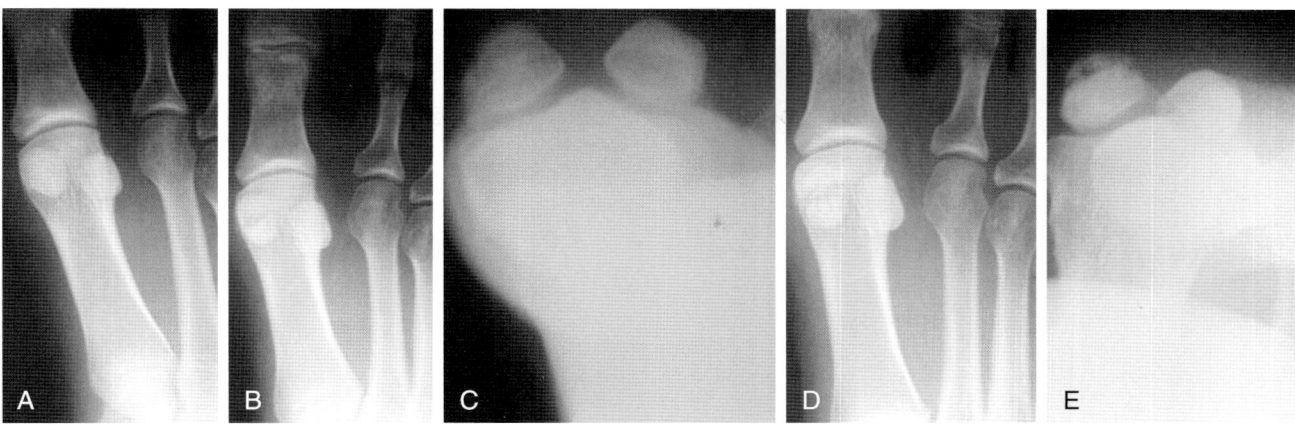

Figure 10-18 **A,** Anteroposterior (AP) radiograph of normal contralateral foot. **B,** AP radiograph of symptomatic bipartite medial sesamoid. **C,** Axial view. The patient was treated with a below-knee cast for 6 weeks, unweighting the sesamoids, and symptoms resolved. **D** and **E,** Fifteen-year follow-up. AP radiograph **(D)** and axial view **(E)** demonstrating no radiographic changes. Patient remains completely asymptomatic.

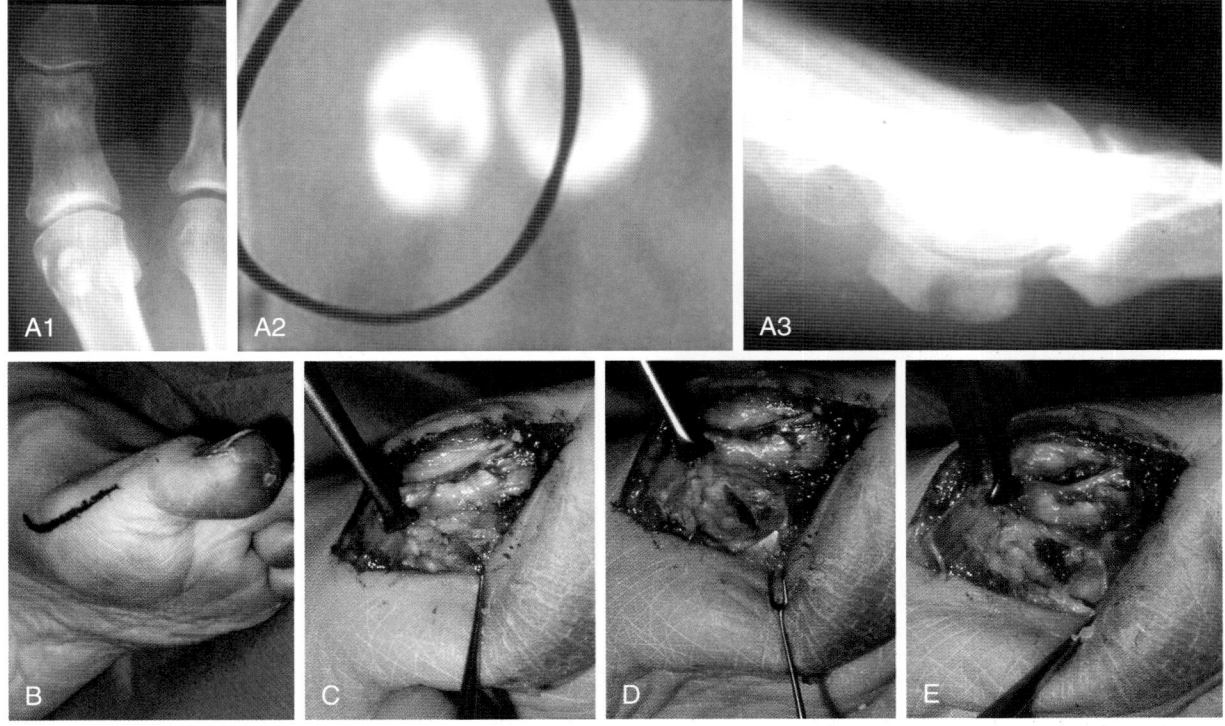

Figure 10-19 Anteroposterior radiograph **(A1),** computed tomography scan **(A2),** and lateral radiograph **(A3)** demonstrating nondisplaced fracture of tibial sesamoid. **B,** Incision used to approach metatarsal sesamoid articulation for bone grafting. **C,** Extraarticular approach exposing plantar surface of sesamoid. After curettage, the nonunion is identified, debrided **(D),** and bone grafted **(E).** (Courtesy R. Anderson, MD, Charlotte, N.C.)

The absence of a tibial sesamoid can produce a clawing of the hallux or development of a progressive postoperative hallux valgus deformity (see Fig. 10-22D).[35,108]

Jahss[47] has reported that congenital absence of both sesamoids is extremely rare (Fig. 10-23DE). Wright[107] reported one case of bilateral absence of both sesamoids associated with hallux varus deformity, and Williams et al[106] reported a case of bilateral congenitl absence with associated metatarsalgia (Fig. 10-23A, B, and C).

DISTORTED OR HYPERTROPHIED SESAMOIDS

Congenital variations of the sesamoids can lead to localized discomfort if the plantar surface of the sesamoid is

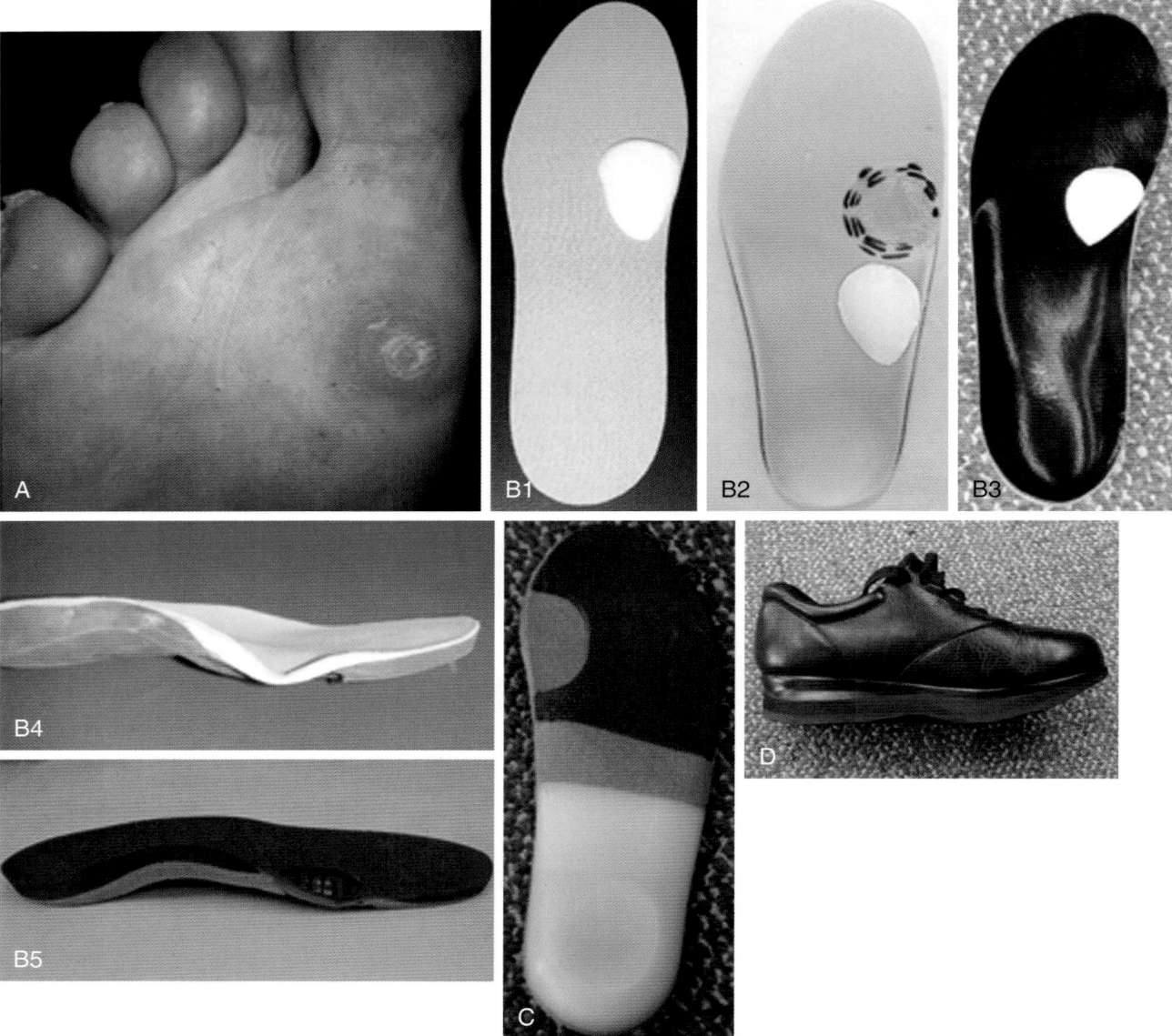

Figure 10-20 **A,** Intractable plantar keratotic lesion directly beneath the tibial sesamoid. **B1-B5,** Insoles and shoe inserts. **B1,** Insole with Hapad placed just proximal to the sesamoids, relieving pressure. **B2,** Plastazote insert with proximal Hapad and area beneath sesamoid relieved. **B3,** Custom insert with proximal Hapad. **B4** and **B5,** Custom inserts with sesamoid region molded to diminish pressure. **C,** Insert shown from plantar aspect, with area beneath sesamoids decompressed. **D,** An extra-depth shoe might be necessary to accommodate the specific insert used to relieve sesamoid pain.

irregular. Hypertrophy of a sesamoid can create an extraordinarily large or thickened projection on the plantar surface and lead to development of a hyperkeratotic lesion (Fig. 10-24). Mowad et al[70] described an osteochondroma of the tibial sesamoid manifesting with a painful plantar mass and a hypertrophic plantar keratosis (Fig. 10-25A and B).

Acquired irregularities of a sesamoid can result from a congenital anomaly in the shape of the sesamoid, from previous injury, or from a rotational deformity of the great toe. Although the sesamoids normally articulate with the plantar metatarsal facets (see Fig. 10-3),

pronation of the hallux with adduction of the first metatarsal tends to lead to a rotational deformity in the metatarsal sesamoid articulation. This distortion can lead to hypertrophy of the sesamoid. If the hypertrophy occurs in a plantar direction, excess bone formation can lead to a symptomatic keratotic lesion that can ultimately ulcerate because of weight-bearing pressure.

Unrelenting pain with ambulation is the most common presenting symptom of a hypertrophied or distorted sesamoid. Although a thickened keratotic lesion may be mistaken for a verruca plantaris, trimming of the keratosis helps to differentiate the two lesions.

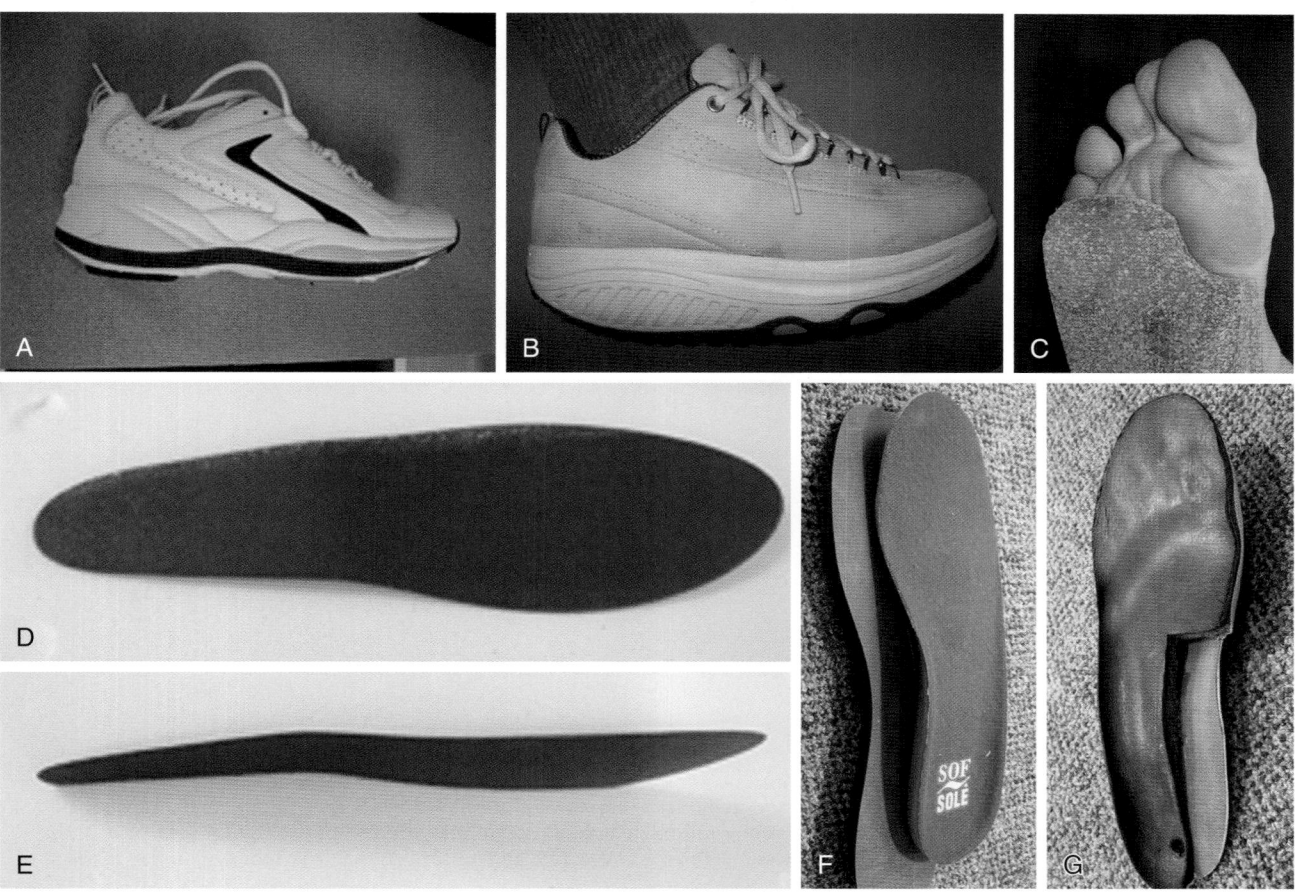

Figure 10-21 A, Rocker-soled walking shoe with a full-length steel shank and a custom orthotic insole may be used to relieve sesamoid pain. **B,** Commercially available rocker-type shoe. **C,** Custom cork insole with recessed area for sesamoids. **D,** and **E,** Graphite insole can diminish metatarsophalangeal joint motion. Top and side views. **F,** Prefabricated insert with graphite insole to stiffen the toe-box area of the shoe. **G,** Custom insole with graphite and gel-layered insole. (Courtesy Hansen Orthotics, Sun Valley, Idaho.)

The soft tissue directly beneath the sesamoids can ulcerate, leading to secondary infection and osteomyelitis. A misshapen or hypertrophied fibular sesamoid is infrequently associated with a keratotic skin lesion because normally there is minimal weight bearing on the fibular sesamoid. Nonetheless, a patient can experience pain in the first intermetatarsal space because of local irritation (Fig. 10-26A-C), and occasionally, an exostosis develops on the fibular sesamoid (see Fig. 10-22D). Saxby et al[92] have reported that a case of coalition of the tibial and fibular sesamoids with plantar pain was treated successfully with a custom orthotic device used to relieve pressure beneath the symptomatic sesamoid coalition (Fig. 10-27).

Treatment

Shaving of the symptomatic keratoses and the use of a metatarsal pad, scaphoid pad, or prefabricated or custom orthotic device can redistribute the weight-bearing pressures and relieve symptoms (see Fig. 10-20). With protracted symptoms, sesamoid shaving or sesamoidectomy may be necessary.

INTRACTABLE PLANTAR KERATOSES

An intractable plantar keratotic lesion can develop beneath the tibial sesamoid without significant hypertrophy or previous injury. Because of the position of the tibial sesamoid and its increased weight-bearing status, it is the tibial sesamoid that is often associated with an intractable plantar keratosis. A keratotic lesion can develop with a cavus foot deformity or with a plantar-flexed first ray, and this anatomy must be considered when evaluating a keratosis beneath the first metatarsal head. An osseous deformity of the sesamoid can lead to development of a symptomatic plantar keratotic lesion.

A more diffuse keratosis beneath the entire metatarsal head is usually associated with a plantar-flexed first ray or cavus deformity. A more localized callus is usually associated with a prominent sesamoid.

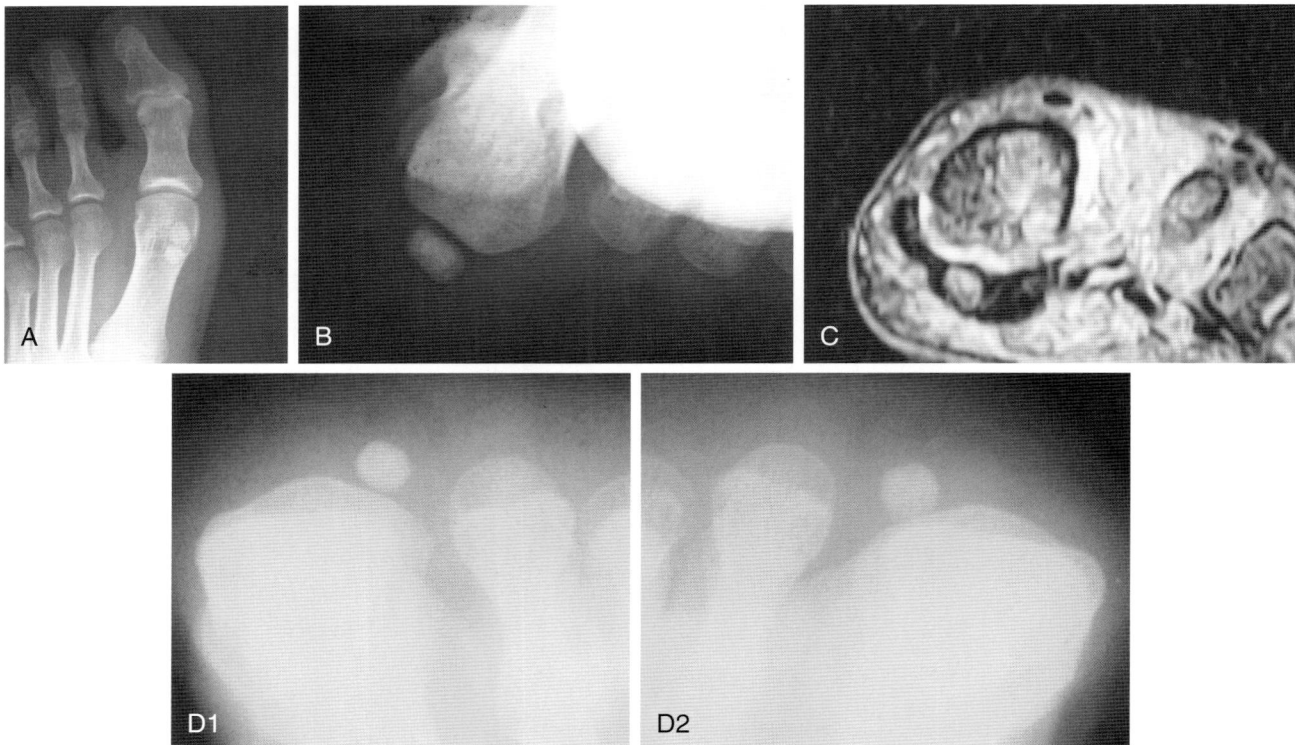

Figure 10-22 Absence of fibular sesamoid. **A,** Anteroposterior radiograph of absent fibular sesamoid with bipartite medial sesamoid. **B,** Axial view. **C,** Magnetic resonance image demonstrating absent lateral sesamoid. **D,** Axial views demonstrating congenital absence of both fibular sesamoids. (**B,** From Yildirim Y, Saygi B: Congenital absence of the lateral sesamoid, *J Am Podiatr Med Assoc* 96:78–81, 2006. Used with permission. **D,** From Jahss MS, editor: *Disorders of the foot and ankle: medical and surgical management,* ed 2, Philadelphia, 1991, WB Saunders.)

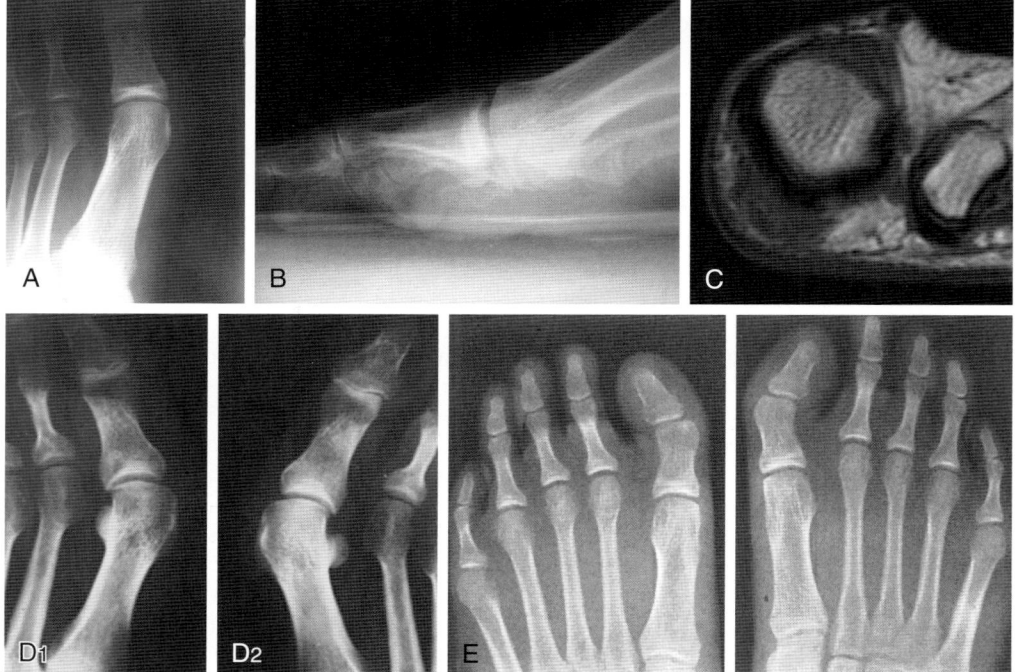

Figure 10-23 Congenital absence of both sesamoids. Anteroposterior (AP) **(A)** and lateral **(B)** radiographs of patient with absence of medial and lateral sesamoids. **C,** Computed tomography of first ray. **D** and **E,** AP radiographs of two different patients with congenital absence of both sesamoids. (**C,** From Williams TH, Pasapula C, Robinson AH: Complete sesamoid agenesis: a rare cause of first ray metatarsalgia, *Foot Ankle Int* 30:465–467, 2009. Used with permission. **D** and **E,** From Jahss MS, editor: *Disorders of the foot and ankle: medical and surgical management,* ed 2, Philadelphia, 1991, WB Saunders.)

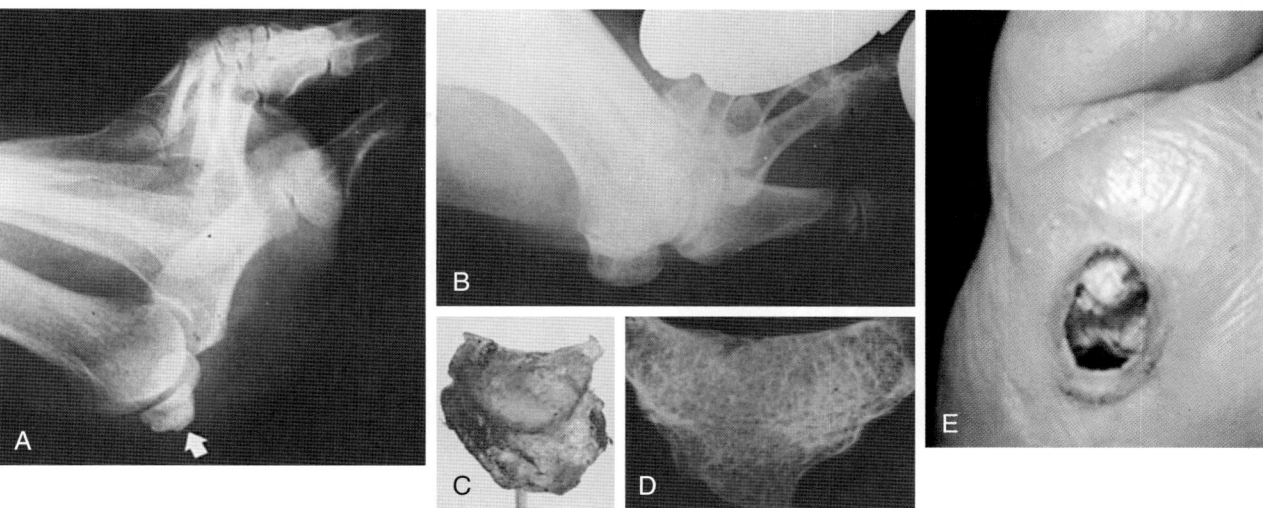

Figure 10-24 **A,** A hypertrophic ridge on the plantar surface of the tibial sesamoid is producing a hyperkeratotic skin lesion *(arrow)*. **B,** Unusually thick tibial sesamoid that induced a deep-seated callus beneath the tibial sesamoid. **C,** Extensive hypertrophy of an excised sesamoid. A chronic ulcer developed under the first metatarsal head and sesamoid. **D,** Radiograph of the medial sesamoid, demonstrating a large plantar exostosis. **E,** Plantar ulcer beneath hypertrophic sesamoid.

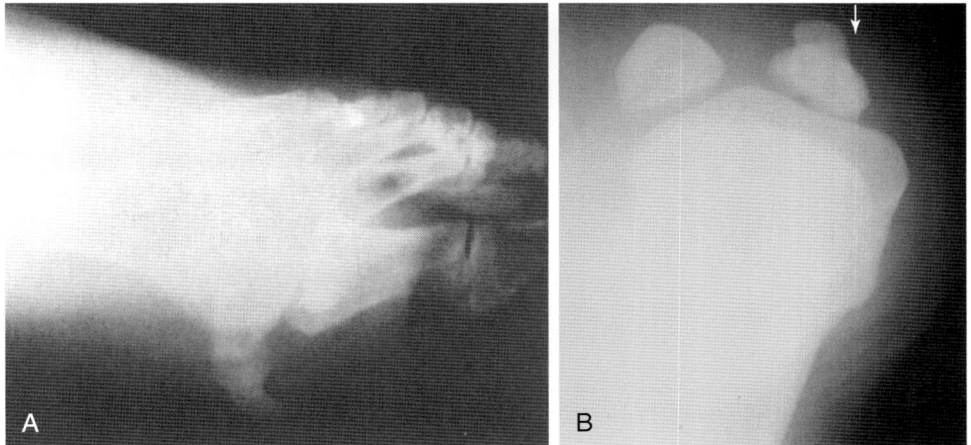

Figure 10-25 **A,** Osteochondroma of the tibial sesamoid. **B,** Plantar exostosis of the tibial sesamoid. (**A,** From Mowad S, Zichichi S, Mullin R: Osteochondroma of the tibial sesamoid, *J Am Podiatr Med Assoc* 85:765–766, 1995.)

Treatment

Often, a keratotic lesion may be debrided or shaved. A custom-molded orthosis or a soft pad placed just proximal to the symptomatic lesion often alleviates symptoms. An extra-depth shoe (increased vertical volume) with a prefabricated or custom insole can provide relief of symptoms (see Fig. 10-20D). With continued symptoms, sesamoid shaving can alleviate symptoms without impairing joint function.

Occasionally, a sesamoidectomy is necessary for an intractable lesion. Resection of a sesamoid in the presence of a cavus deformity or a plantar-flexed first ray is often associated with the recurrence of a plantar keratotic lesion. In this situation, a closing-wedge dorsiflexion metatarsal osteotomy is preferable (Fig. 10-28).

BURSITIS

Jahss[47] estimates that a bursa exists under the first metatarsal in 30% of normal feet (Fig. 10-29). With a cavus foot, a plantar-flexed metatarsal, or just excessive ambulation or standing, a subacute or chronic sesamoid bursitis can develop. Chronic bursitis may be associated with a hypertrophied or arthritic medial sesamoid as well. Kernohan et al[53] reported a case of painful calcific bursitis of the sesamoid treated successfully with surgical debridement.

Treatment

Redistribution of weight bearing with the use of a custom orthotic device or metatarsal pad placed just proximal to the symptomatic sesamoid often diminishes discomfort

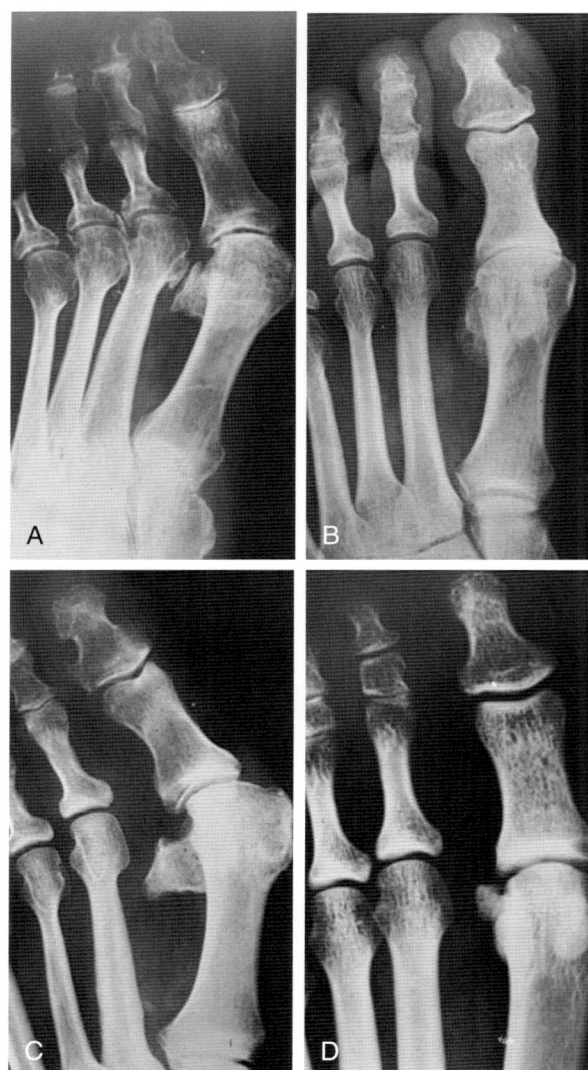

Figure 10-26 A-C, Hypertrophic changes in a fibular sesamoid with development of pain in the first intermetatarsal space. **D,** Exostosis of the fibular sesamoid.

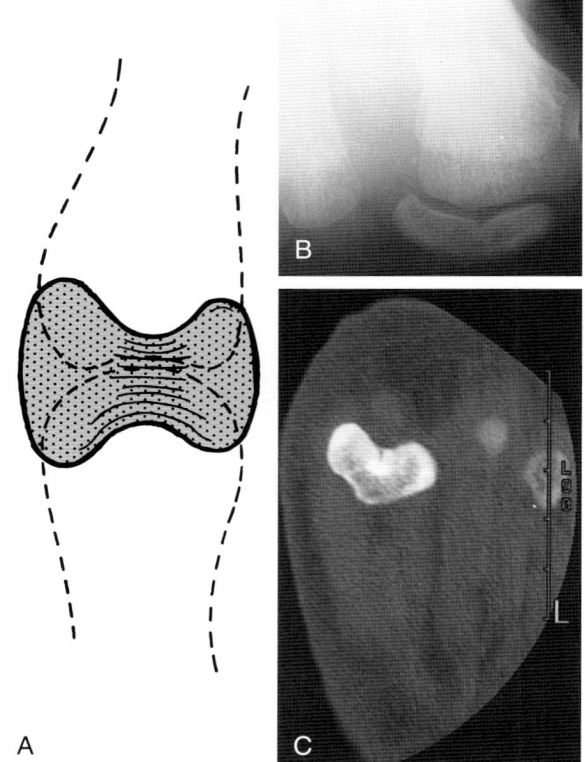

Figure 10-27 Coalition of the hallucal sesamoid. **A,** Diagram of sesamoid coalition. **B,** Axial radiograph. **C,** Computed tomography scan demonstrating coalition of tibial and fibular sesamoids. (**A** and **B,** From Saxby T, Vandemark R, Hall R: Coalition of the hallux sesamoids: a case report, *Foot Ankle* 13:355–358, 1992.)

(see Fig. 10-20). When symptoms are refractory to conservative treatment, surgery should be tailored to the underlying cause. A bursectomy sometimes gives long-lasting relief when a plantar-flexed first metatarsal or cavus foot is the underlying cause of symptoms. When the medial sesamoid is the cause of continued symptoms, surgical excision with resection of the overlying bursa often relieves symptoms.

NERVE COMPRESSION

The plantar-medial digital nerve and plantar-lateral digital nerve are located adjacent to the medial and lateral sesamoids (Fig. 10-30). Impingement of either of these branches may be a source of pain in the area of the sesamoids. Helfet[39] reported compression of the lateral plantar cutaneous nerve to the hallux. The plantar medial digital nerve can also be compressed by the medial sesamoid in a similar fashion. Often, pain is difficult to differentiate from pain localized to the adjacent sesamoid. Occasionally, a Tinel sign can be detected at the site of nerve compression. Patients might or might not appreciate decreased sensation distal to the nerve compression.

Treatment

A metatarsal pad or custom orthosis can relieve symptoms of a compressed nerve. Continued symptoms in spite of conservative care can necessitate surgical intervention. Surgical excision of the involved sesamoids may be used to relieve pain; however, a surgeon must isolate and protect the involved nerve to avoid injury. A postoperative neuroma after surgery may be more symptomatic than a patient's original complaint.

ARTHRITIS

Degenerative arthritis of the first metatarsal sesamoid articulation has been reported by several investigators.*

---

*References 37, 44, 46, 54, 62, 80, 94, 99, and 214.

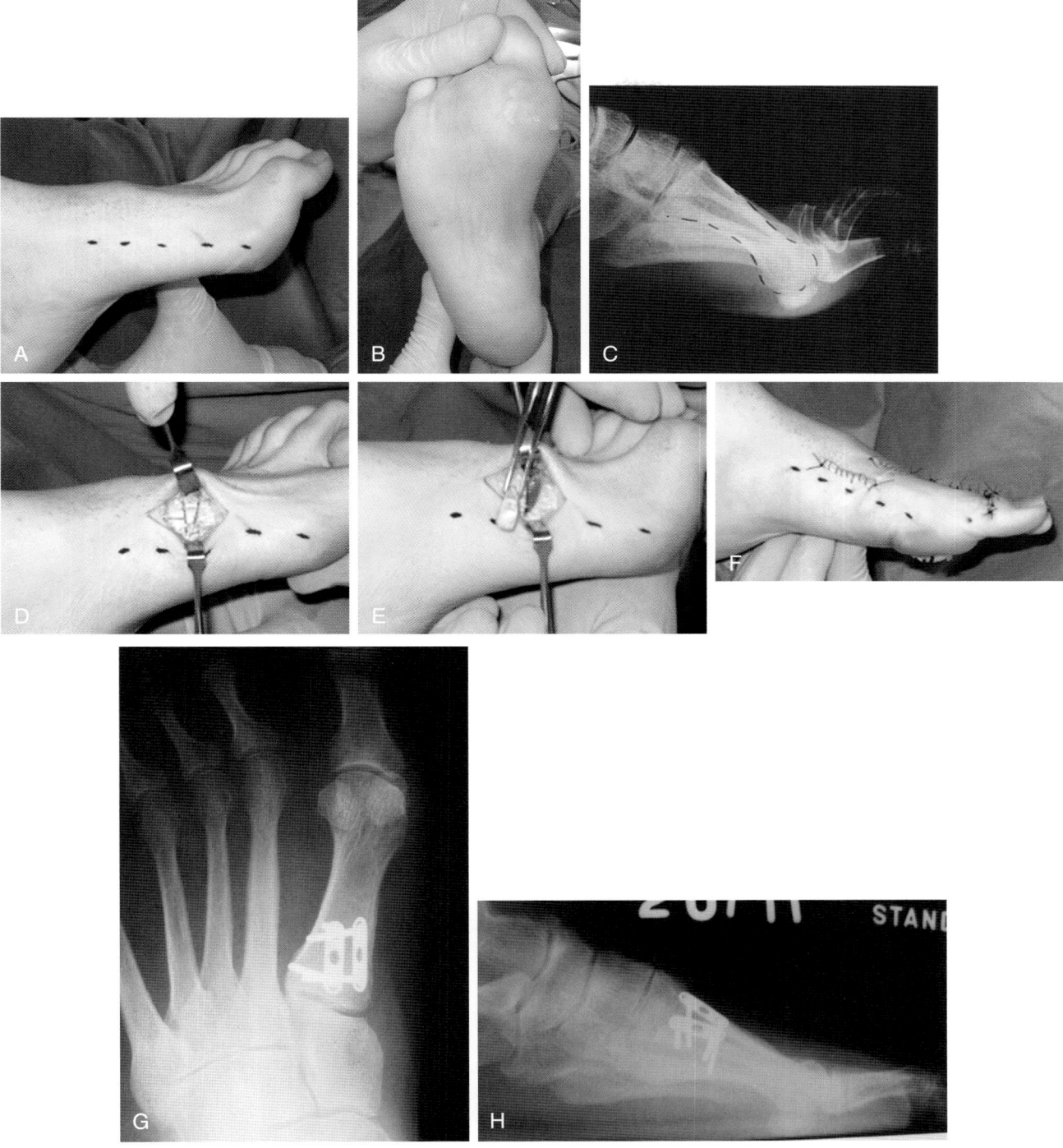

Figure 10-28 A sesamoidectomy is contraindicated with a plantar-flexed first metatarsal because symptoms usually continue postoperatively. A dorsal wedge closing osteotomy of the first metatarsal can reduce the pressure beneath the first metatarsal head. **A,** Preoperative photograph demonstrating plantar flexion of the first metatarsal. **B,** Intractable plantar keratotic lesion beneath the first metatarsal head. **C,** Lateral radiograph demonstrating a plantar-flexed first metatarsal. **D,** Outline of a closing wedge first metatarsal osteotomy. **E,** The wedge has been excised and the osteotomy closed. **F,** Appearance of the foot after closing dorsiflexion osteotomy of the first metatarsal. Anteroposterior **(G)** and lateral **(H)** radiographs after dorsiflexion closing wedge osteotomy fixed with mini-fragment plates at 90-degree orientation.

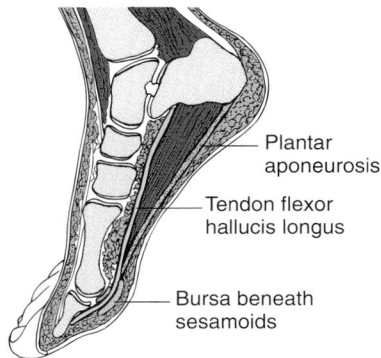

Plantar aponeurosis

Tendon flexor hallucis longus

Bursa beneath sesamoids

Figure 10-29 A bursa exists beneath the first metatarsal head and sesamoids in approximately 30% of normal feet.

Subchondral cyst formation can develop as a secondary change.[62] Symptoms may be associated with rheumatoid arthritis, hallux rigidus, psoriatic arthritis, or other systemic arthritides. Local degenerative arthritis of one or more of the sesamoids can occur. Diffuse idiopathic skeletal hyperostosis (DISH) can involve the sesamoids and lead to osteophyte formation.[47] Rupture of either the abductor hallucis or the adductor hallucis can result in the development of progressive hallux valgus or hallux varus. Complete rupture of the plantar plate can lead to clawing of the hallux.

Scranton and Rutkowski[95] reported erosion of articular cartilage in cases of progressive sesamoid chondromalacia that eventually required surgical excision. Degenerative arthritis of the metatarsal sesamoid articulation can develop as a progression of localized trauma, progressive hallux valgus,[86] chondromalacia, or sesamoiditis (Fig. 10-31).

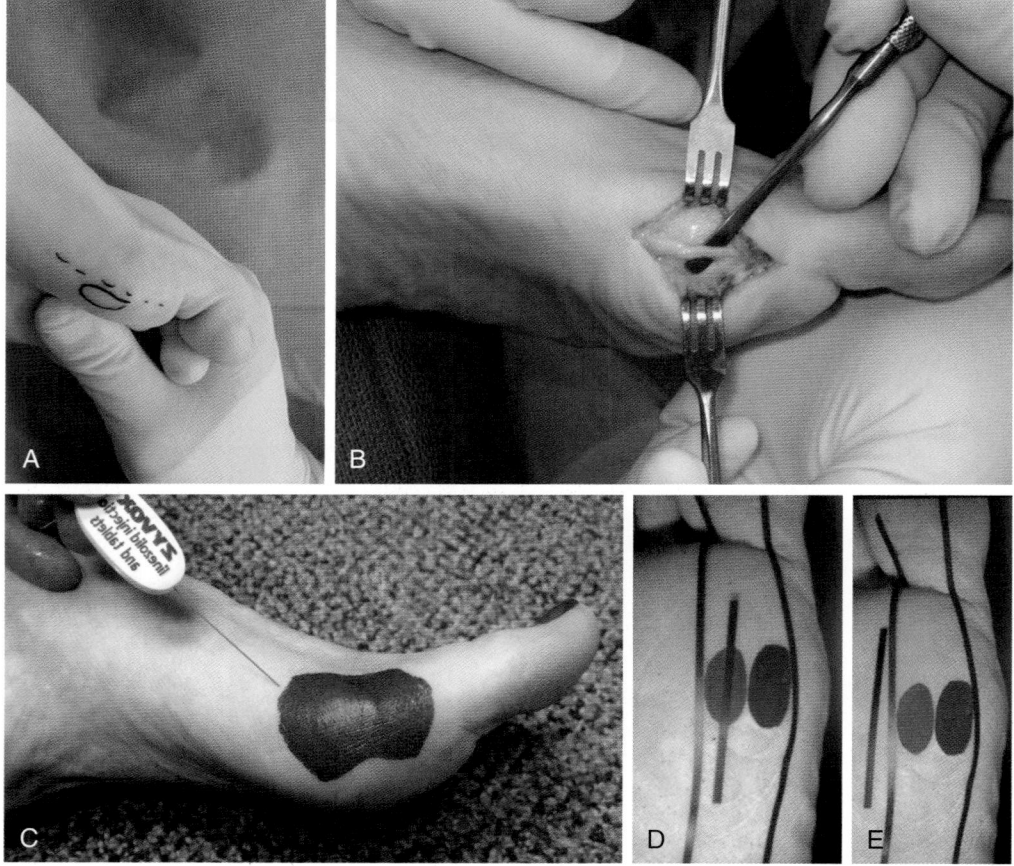

Figure 10-30 **A,** Proposed incision for excision of medial sesamoid. **B,** Medial view showing common digital nerve overlying medial sesamoid. **C,** Postoperative numbness can develop after dissection and/or injury to the sensory nerve (examination demonstrated area of numbness determined with Semmes-Weinstein monofilament testing). **D,** A plantar view of the foot demonstrating the common digital nerves to the hallux. Note the proximity of each nerve *(red lines)* to the medial and lateral sesamoids *(blue circles)*. (An incision directly over a sesamoid should be avoided.) **E,** The plantar incision *(black line)* to expose the lateral sesamoid is made between the first and second metatarsal heads just lateral to the lateral common digital nerve. *Red lines* indicate nerves, and *blue ovals* indicate the medial and lateral sesamoids.

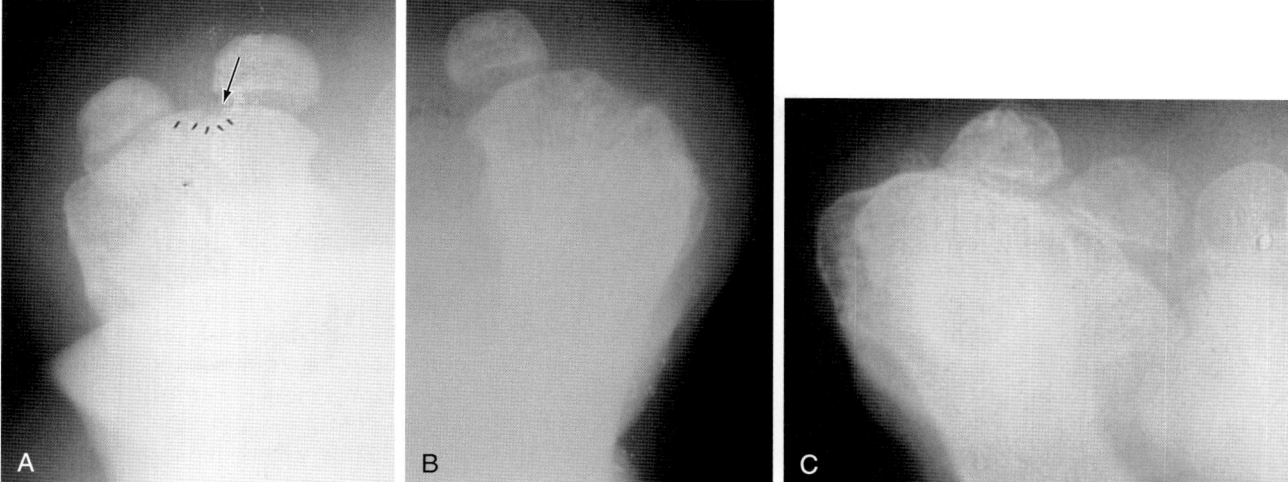

Figure 10-31 A, Axial view of a sesamoid demonstrating cystic degenerative changes in the first metatarsal head (*arrow*). **B,** One year after surgery for medial sesamoid resection, cystic changes in first metatarsal head remain present. **C,** Arthritis of the sesamoids associated with hallux valgus.

Initial symptoms include swelling, synovitis, and erythema and can be demonstrated on physical examination. Restricted MTP joint motion, pain with forced dorsiflexion, and pain on localized palpation may be noted as well.

Treatment

The goal of conservative care is to relieve discomfort with ambulation. A stiff insole, extended shank, rocker outer sole, and custom orthosis or metatarsal pad that relieves pressure beneath the first metatarsal head or reduces MTP joint motion often eliminates symptoms. Nonsteroidal antiinflammatory drugs (NSAIDs) can also decrease inflammation.

Surgical resection of the involved sesamoid may also be considered for isolated arthritis of either the lateral or medial sesamoid. In the presence of long-standing arthritis, MTP joint motion often fails to improve with surgical resection of a sesamoid, although pain may be significantly relieved.[19] When both the medial and lateral sesamoids are involved, a combined resection may be contraindicated because it will destroy the intrinsic insertion of the flexor digitorum brevis and may lead to clawing of the great toe. Julsrud[50] reported dual excision of the sesamoids with a combined IP joint fusion in the treatment of osteonecrosis of both sesamoids. Bouche[11] has suggested that with careful excision of both sesamoids, the IP joint may not require an arthrodesis. Tagoe et al,[99] however, have reported a series of 36 cases in which a dual sesamoid resection was performed. The authors reported satisfactory results when this was combined with a dorsal cheilectomy. They suggested that the reason for lack of progressive MTP or IP joint deformity postoperatively may have been related to the restricted MTP joint range of motion at the time of surgery. We suggest that an MTP joint arthrodesis may be the preferred alternative to both

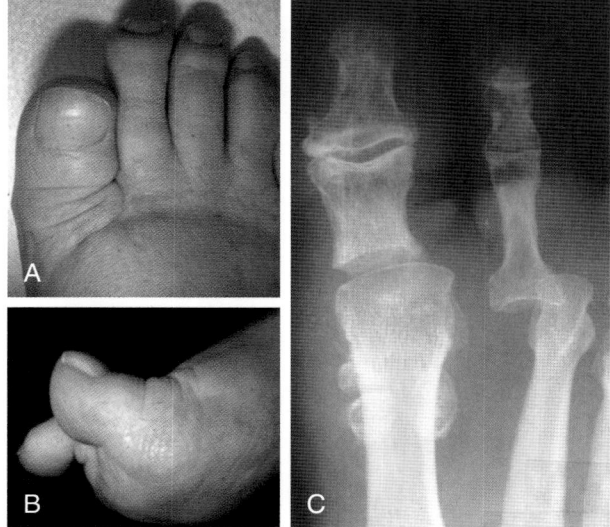

Figure 10-32 A and **B,** Photographs demonstrating postoperative clawing after the Keller procedure. **C,** Anteroposterior radiograph demonstrating postoperative retraction of the sesamoids after resection arthroplasty. Note also the dislocated second metatarsophalangeal joint.

stabilize the joint and relieve pain. A Keller resection arthroplasty is another alternative, although it can lead to postoperative clawing of the hallux as well (Fig. 10-32).[20] Dual sesamoidectomy should be considered a salvage procedure and is performed uncommonly.

SUBLUXATION AND DISLOCATION OF THE SESAMOIDS

As the magnitude of a hallux valgus deformity increases, pronation of the great toe occurs. As the hallux migrates into valgus, the first metatarsal deviates medially. As the deformity increases, the first metatarsal head progressively subluxates off of the sesamoid mechanism. Although the term "sesamoid subluxation" is associated with a hallux valgus deformity, the sesamoid migration occurs solely in relation to the first metatarsal head.[27] The sesamoid mechanism retains its relationship anatomically to the second metatarsal because it is tethered by the transverse metatarsal ligament and the conjoined adductor hallucis tendon.[48] Increased weight-bearing forces are transmitted through the first metatarsal head and tibial sesamoid. The fibular sesamoid, however, becomes displaced into the first intermetatarsal space, where weight-bearing forces are diminished.

Weil and Hill,[105] in an evaluation of 500 normal radiographs, noted a 15% incidence of bipartite tibial sesamoids in the general population. In contrast, in the examination of 500 radiographs of feet with hallux valgus, they observed a 32% incidence of hallux valgus associated with bipartite tibial sesamoids and concluded that multipartite sesamoids can predispose the first ray to a hallux valgus deformity.

As sesamoid displacement develops, the intersesamoid ridge erodes (see Fig. 10-3). There is quite often complete cartilage absence in the former loction of the cristae[10,86] (Fig. 10-33). Axial radiographs often show gradual attrition of the intersesamoid ridge with a mild and moderate hallux valgus deformity. With a severe deformity, complete erosion of the crista occurs. Insertion of the conjoined adductor tendon into the plantar-lateral base of the proximal phalanx and lateral sesamoid leads to a pronation or rotational force on the great toe as the hallux valgus deformity increases.

Treatment

After correction of a hallux valgus deformity, the alignment of the sesamoids may be undercorrected, adequately corrected, or overcorrected. Although the goal is to realign the sesamoids with the first metatarsal plantar facets, it may be necessary to achieve this correction through release of the conjoined adductor tendon and lateral capsular structures. On occasion, a lateral sesamoidectomy is performed. Although such procedures allow relocation of the tibial sesamoid to the plantar-medial facet of the first metatarsal, an unstable situation occasionally develops because of erosion of the intersesamoid ridge. In this case, the medial facet is no longer a stable articulating surface. Recurrent lateral sesamoid migration with the development of a recurrent hallux valgus deformity or medial migration of the tibial sesamoid with a resultant hallux varus deformity can occur (Fig. 10-34). The use of semirigid dressings in the acute postoperative period can help to maintain the surgical correction until the sesamoid mechanism becomes stabilized.

Although McBride[67] recommended excising the fibular sesamoid to achieve adequate release of the lateral capsular contracture, we believe a fibular sesamoid should rarely be removed in the correction of a hallux valgus deformity. After a complete lateral soft tissue release has been performed, if a significant contracture remains or if significant degenerative changes of the lateral sesamoid restrict adequate MTP joint motion with realignment of the hallux, a fibular sesamoid resection may be contemplated.

An 8% incidence of postoperative hallux varus after a McBride procedure has been reported where a fibular

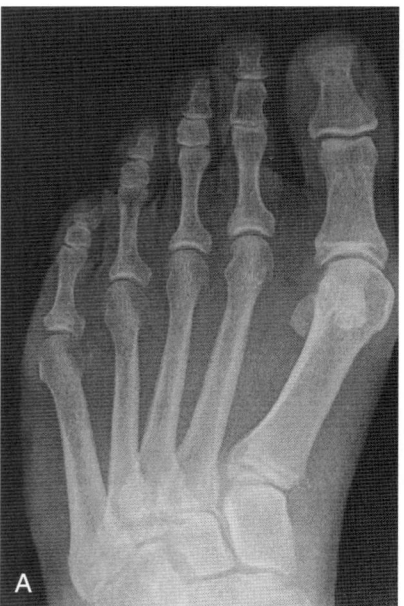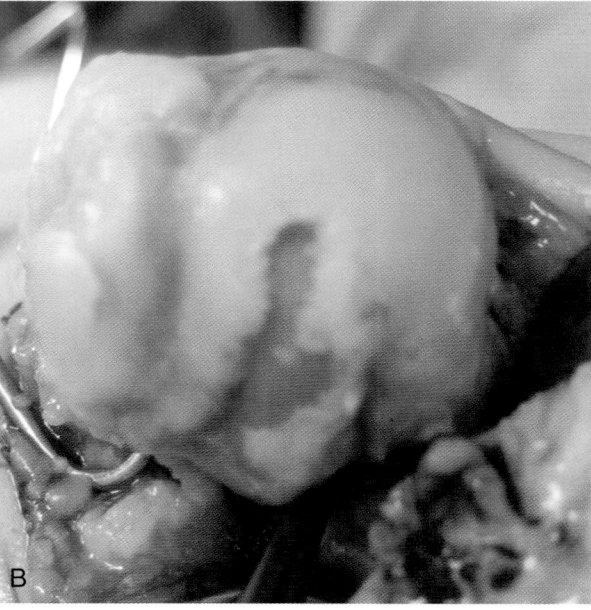

Figure 10-33 Hallux valgus deformity with erosion of sesamoids. **A,** Moderate hallux valgus deformity. **B,** Intraoperative photograph with severe erosion of medial aspect of cristae.

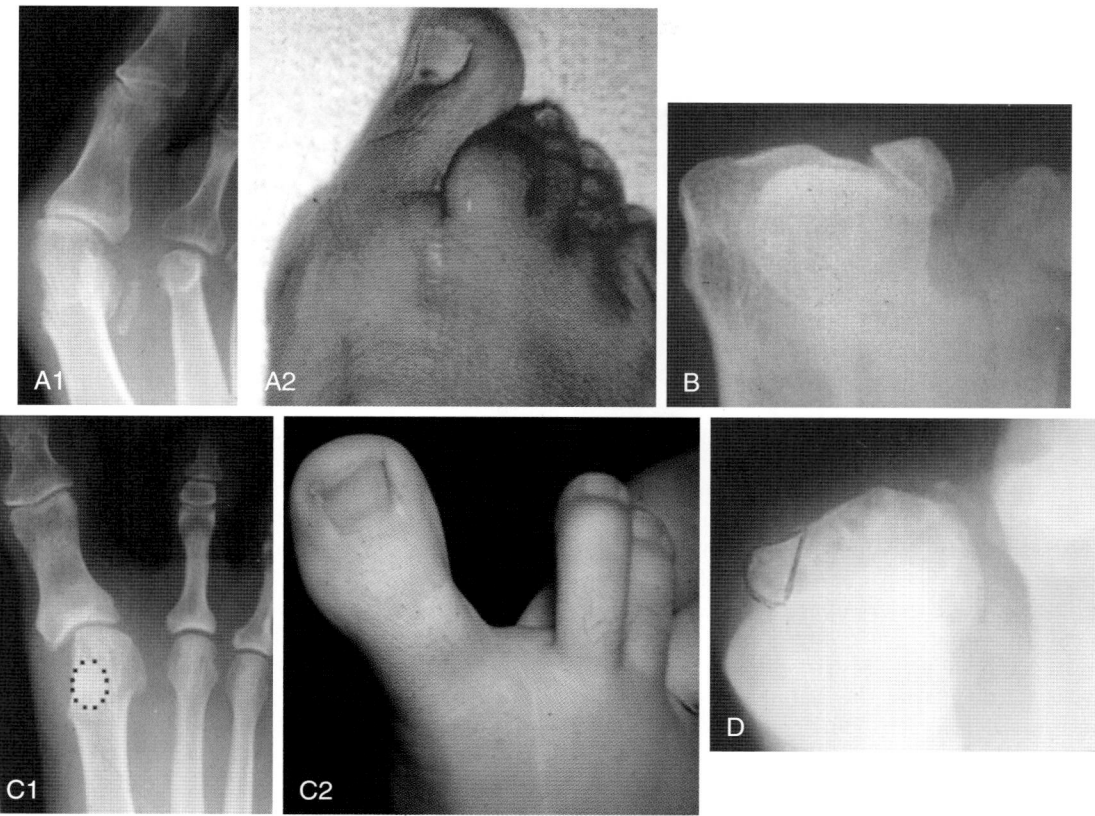

Figure 10-34 Anteroposterior radiograph **(A1)** and photograph **(A2)** demonstrating hallux valgus deformity with lateral subluxation of the lateral sesamoid after medial sesamoid excision. **B,** Axial radiograph demonstrating lateral subluxation of the lateral sesamoid. Anteroposterior radiograph **(C1)** and photograph **(C2)** demonstrating hallux varus deformity with dislocation of the medial sesamoid after lateral sesamoid excision. **D,** Axial radiograph demonstrating medial dislocation of the medial sesamoid.

sesamoid has been removed.[64] A postoperative hallux varus deformity is associated with the correction of hallux valgus deformities of a more severe nature (hallux valgus angle greater than 40 degrees).[64] Complete erosion of the intersesamoid ridge coupled with a contracted intrinsic musculature can lead to this potentially unstable situation. Overaggressive medial capsulorrhaphy and an excessive medial exostectomy can predispose to a postoperative hallux varus deformity.

Lee et al[61] reported their results after 14 cases of isolated tibial sesamoidectomy. They performed a meticulous medial capsular repair and found no change in hallux valgus or 1-to-2 intermetatarsal angles, or toe strength at an average of 62 months of follow-up.

INFECTION

Infections of the sesamoids are not common; however, several cases have been reported in the orthopaedic literature.* Osteomyelitis of the sesamoid can develop after trauma, a puncture wound, or breakdown of the plantar skin with chronic neuropathic ulceration. Often,

---

*References 17, 37, 59, 87, 96, and 100.

osteomyelitis of the sesamoid progresses to infection of the MTP joint. A gram-negative bacterial infection is often associated with chronic plantar ulceration.

On physical examination, the MTP joint becomes swollen and erythematous. Manipulation of the hallux causes pain. Often, a delay in diagnosis occurs because of the insidious nature of the infection. Radiographic changes can be very slow to develop. Patients with decreased sensation because of diabetic neuropathy, sciatic nerve injury, myelodysplasia, and peripheral neuropathy are at risk for skin breakdown and sesamoid infection. Hypertrophic callus formation beneath the sesamoids can develop because of increased pressure. Skin breakdown and trophic ulceration can develop with subsequent osteomyelitis.

Treatment

Early conservative treatment may be used to reduce pressure beneath the sesamoids. A molded insole or metatarsal pad can reduce pressure beneath the sesamoids, and paring of abundant callus can relieve symptoms (see Fig. 10-20).

In the case of a diabetic patient who has an ulcer beneath the first metatarsal head, measures to ensure that the ulceration does not recur should be undertaken after the acute infection has subsided. Use of extra-depth shoes with a polyethylene foam (Plastizote) insert (see Fig. 10-20B2) can significantly reduce the recurrence of ulceration.

Where osteomyelitis of the sesamoid has developed, surgical excision may be necessary. In the case of acute infection, an attempt should be made to make a bacteriologic diagnosis at the time of the surgical debridement of the sesamoid. Excision of either or both sesamoids may be necessary, depending upon the extent of the infection.[34] Irrigation, aggressive debridement, and localized wound care are often necessary to achieve control of the wound. Although a double sesamoidectomy should be routinely avoided, advanced osteomyelitis with involvement of both sesamoids can necessitate their removal (Fig. 10-35). Preservation of the tendons of the abductor and adductor hallucis and subperiosteal resection of the sesamoids can help to prevent a cock-up deformity of the hallux. An interphalangeal arthrodesis might eventually be necessary after dual sesamoid excision to treat a clawing of the interphalangeal joint of the hallux. Postoperatively, restricted range of motion and decreased strength of the hallux are noted after sesamoidectomy; however, often the scarring that

develops after infection prevents the claw toe deformity that typically develops after a bilateral sesamoid resection.

OSTEOCHONDRITIS/OSTEONECROSIS OF THE SESAMOIDS

Osteochondritis of the sesamoids is a rare condition that can affect either sesamoid. It is characterized by pain, tenderness to palpation, and osseous fragmentation or mottling on radiographic examination.[29,31,43,55,74,90,101] Ilfeld and Rosen[43] described osteochondritis of the sesamoid and noted it occurred infrequently. Although the cause is unclear, Helal[38] and Brodsky[13] suggested that osteochondritis develops after trauma or a crush injury. Kliman et al[55] hypothesized that the development of a sesamoid stress fracture and the subsequent reparative process lead to osteochondritis. Although trauma is likely to be the most common cause, Jahss[46] has associated osteonecrosis with diminished vascularity. He noted that osteonecrosis tends to occur in women around the age of 25 years, but it can occur in both sexes from 13 to 80 years of age. Jahss[47] reports that the tibial and fibular sesamoids are equally involved. Julsrud[50] reported simultaneous osteonecrosis in a 22-year-old woman. An

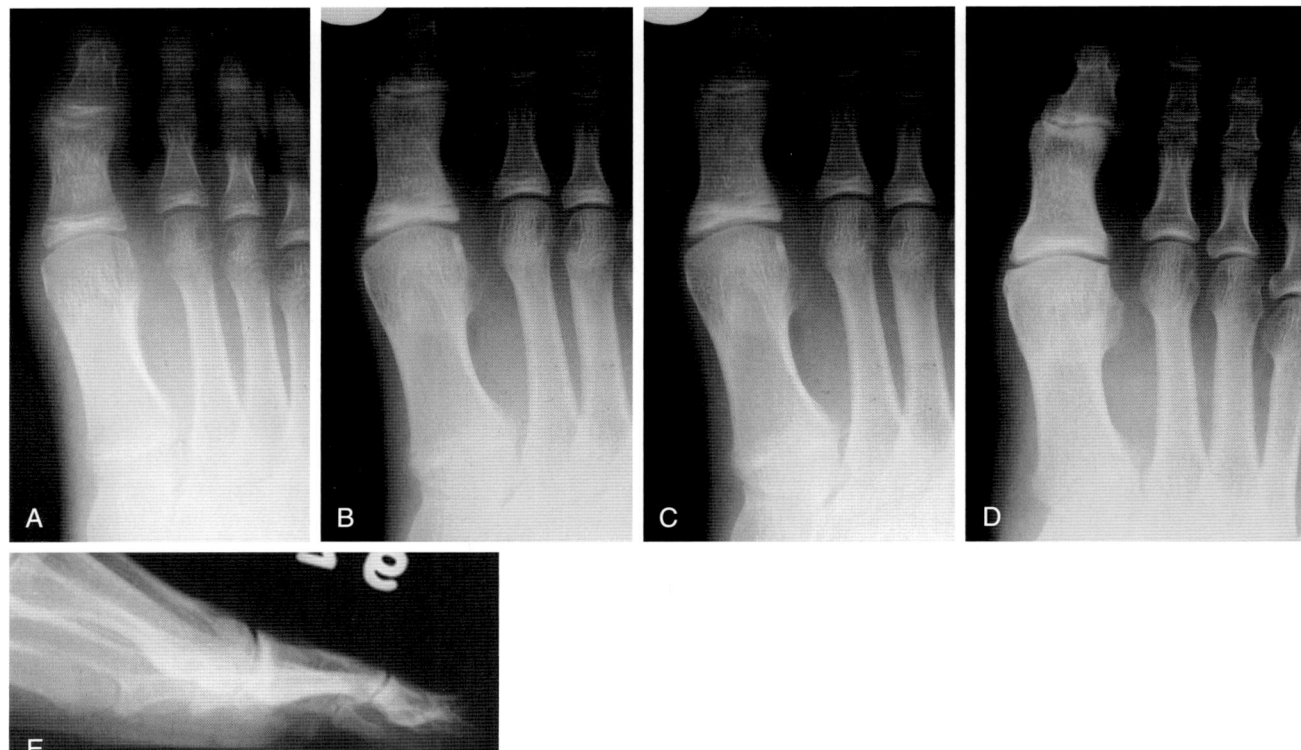

Figure 10-35 **A,** Osteomyelitis of the medial sesamoid in a skeletally immature person. **B,** After excision of both sesamoids as treatment for sesamoidal osteomyelitis. **C,** Two years after surgery, because of postoperative scarring, a cock-up deformity did not develop. Anteroposterior **(D)** and lateral **(E)** radiographs at 13-year follow-up demonstrate no subsequent deformity in spite of dual sesamoid excision.

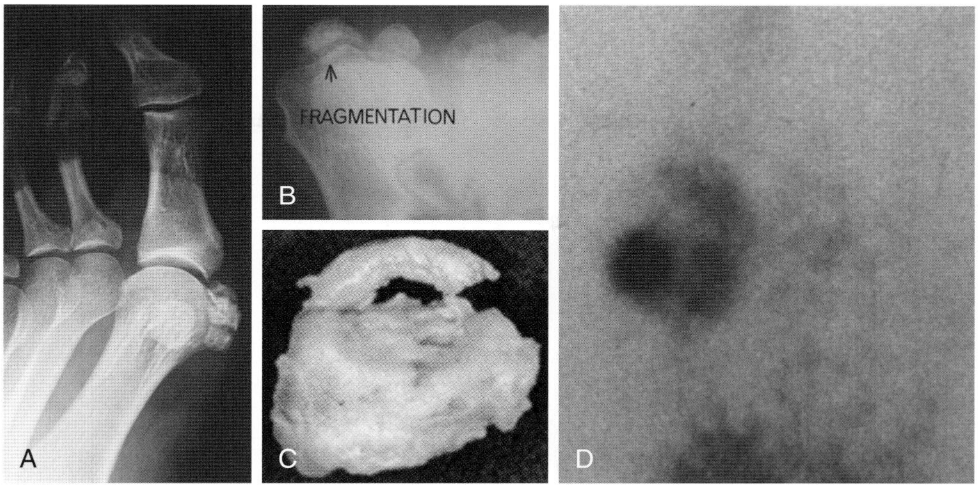

Figure 10-36 **A,** Osteochondritis is characterized by fragmentation of the medial sesamoid. **B,** Chondrolysis of the medial sesamoid as seen on an axial radiograph. **C,** Pathologic specimen demonstrating fragmentation of the sesamoid. **D,** Osteochondritis of the medial sesamoid as characterized by increased uptake on a technetium bone scan. (From Coughlin MJ: Sesamoid pain: causes and surgical treatment, *Instr Course Lect* 39:23–25, 1990.)

interphalangeal joint fusion was combined with a sesamoid excision to prevent later clawing of the hallux.

The circulation of the sesamoids can play a role in the development of osteonecrosis. Rath et al[78] and others[77,97] (see Figs. 10-9 and 10-10) have described the arterial circulation of the sesamoids. Individual arterial patterns can predispose a sesamoid to degeneration after injury. An injury pattern that disrupts the interosseous circulation can predispose an injured sesamoid to osteonecrosis. Often, however, a patient gives no history of injury. On physical examination, pain and tenderness are localized to the involved sesamoid. The metatarsal head is usually nontender.

The diagnosis of osteochondritis is usually made initially by an axial radiograph depicting the sesamoid in profile (Fig. 10-36A-C). Often, radiographic findings are negative for 9 to 12 months. In time, lysis and resorptive changes in the involved sesamoid are combined with areas of sclerosis. Mottling, fragmentation, flattening, and elongation of the sesamoid can develop. A high-resolution technetium bone scan can help to make the diagnosis of osteochondritis in the absence of radiographic findings.[50,101] With a bone scan, typically the sesamoid demonstrates increased uptake without significant involvement of the MTP joint (Fig. 10-36D). A CT scan may demonstrate the fragmentation more clearly.[29] In addition, an MRI may be helpful early, in diagnosing the acute edema in the involved sesamoid, and later, when fragmentation develops[74,101] (Figs. 10-37, 10-38, and 10-39).

Treatment

Conservative care includes reducing weight-bearing stress on the involved sesamoid. A metatarsal pad placed just proximal to the sesamoids or a custom-molded orthosis that diminishes weight bearing on the involved sesamoid might afford some relief. Although Fleischli and Cheleuitte[29] proposed casting as a treatment modality, they showed no evidence of any efficacy of this method. Indeed, it is relatively difficult to immobilize the great toe in a below-knee cast. NSAIDs can relieve symptoms.

Although conservative care can help to diminish some symptoms, fragmentation or collapse of the sesamoid usually indicates the need for surgical resection of the involved sesamoid. Fleischli and Cheleuitte[29] discussed the use of a silicone implant, which was also proposed by Helal.[38] No long-term studies have been reported on this experimental procedure, and its use should be discouraged. An intraarticular steroid injection in the presence of osteonecrosis, although not contraindicated, is unlikely to provide long-term relief and is discouraged. It can temporarily reduce swelling and discomfort, allowing increased activity, which ultimately may lead to further degeneration of the involved sesamoid.

SESAMOIDITIS

The diagnosis of sesamoiditis is a diagnosis of exclusion. Often, this condition occurs in teenagers and young adults and may be associated with trauma. Pain on weight bearing is a typical complaint. Often, there is tenderness to palpation over the involved sesamoid, which may be accompanied by inflammation or a bursal thickening on the plantar aspect of the sesamoid mechanism. The onset may be sudden or gradual, with pain on weight bearing and dorsiflexion of the great toe. Although radiographic findings are typically normal, a high-resolution technetium bone scan might demonstrate increased blood flow to the involved sesamoid.[74,81]

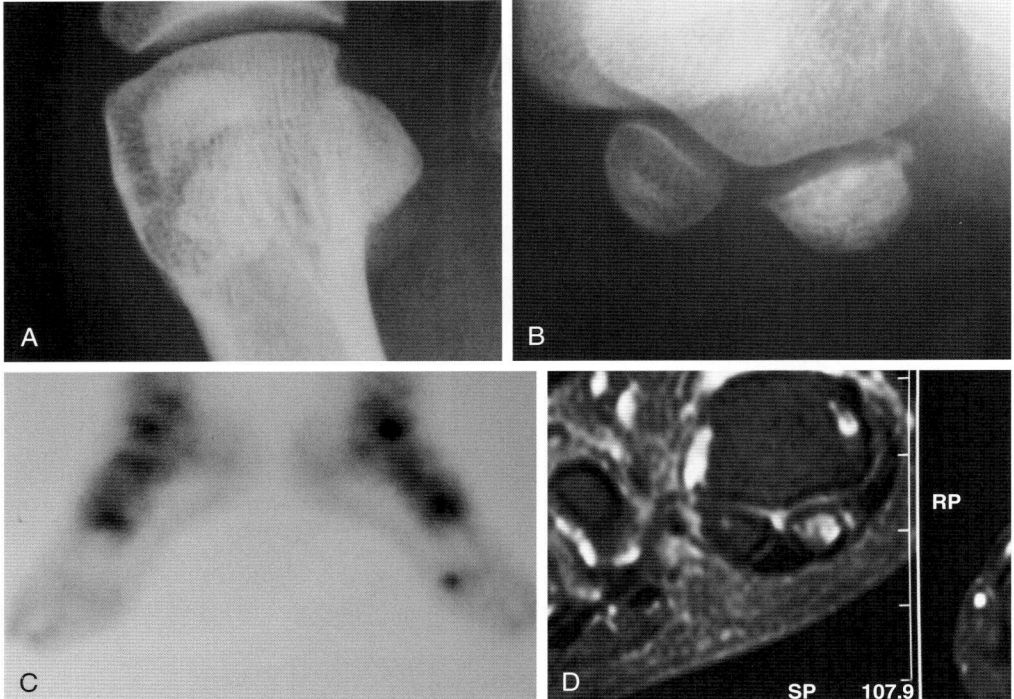

Figure 10-37 Osteonecrosis of the medial sesamoid. Anteroposterior **(A)** and axial **(B)** views of osteonecrosis of the lateral sesamoid. **C,** Technetium-99m (^{99m}Tc) bone scan demonstrating increased uptake of medial sesamoid. **D,** Magnetic resonance image demonstrating marked edema in medial sesamoid. (From Ozkoc G, Akpinar S, Ozalay M, et al: Hallucal sesamoid osteonecrosis: an overlooked cause of forefoot pain, *J Am Podiatr Med Assoc* 95:277–280, 2005. Used with permission.)

Some types of trauma associated with sesamoid injuries include jumping from a height, excessive walking or dancing, excessive dorsiflexion of the MTP joint, or the chronic use of high-fashion footwear.[88] The tibial sesamoid is more often involved because of increased weight bearing in this area of the first metatarsal head.

Dobas and Silvers[24] defined sesamoiditis as an inflammation and swelling of the peritendinous structures involving the sesamoids. Apley[5] referred to "chondromalacia of the sesamoids" and described a condition similar to sesamoiditis. Apley dissected the medial sesamoid and found remarkable similarities between the articular cartilage and the degeneration seen with sesamoiditis and that of chondromalacia of the patellofemoral joint. Hong et al[41] observed degeneration of the hyaline cartilage in surgical specimens resected with intractable pain and a diagnosis of chondromalacia or sesamoiditis.

Treatment

Decreased walking activities and the use of metatarsal pads and custom foot orthoses may reduce weight-bearing pressure and relieve symptoms. A stiff-soled shoe or a graphite insole can diminish MTP joint motion and relieve pain (see Fig. 10-21). Taping of the great toe in some degree of plantar flexion also helps to relieve pressure on the sesamoids (Fig. 10-40). Decreasing shoe heel height can reduce pressure on the involved sesamoid and relieve symptoms. NSAIDs are also efficacious at times. In the presence of continuing symptoms, surgical excision may be necessary.

Conservative Treatment

Often, sesamoid problems can be treated effectively with conservative management. A decrease in activity in both athletes and sedentary patients can help to diminish symptoms. The use of low-heeled shoes reduces pressure on the sesamoids and often relieves discomfort. When a fracture has occurred, a below-knee walking cast or wooden-soled shoe may be used to decrease stress on the sesamoid and MTP joint, although typically it is extremely difficult to control the hallux and sesamoid mechanism with a below-knee cast unless the cast is extended to the tips of the toes. A custom-molded insole or metatarsal pad placed just proximal to the symptomatic area can help to decrease pressure in the sesamoid region. Any of these modalities may be effective in treating fractures, sesamoiditis, or localized inflammation. They can also help to relieve discomfort from an intractable plantar keratotic lesion. Taping of the hallux in a neutral or slightly plantar-flexed position helps to reduce dorsiflexion with ambulation and can reduce localized irritation in the MTP joint. NSAIDs can also relieve symptoms. Infrequent judicious use of an intraarticular steroid injection can relieve inflammation or sesamoiditis (Fig. 10-41),

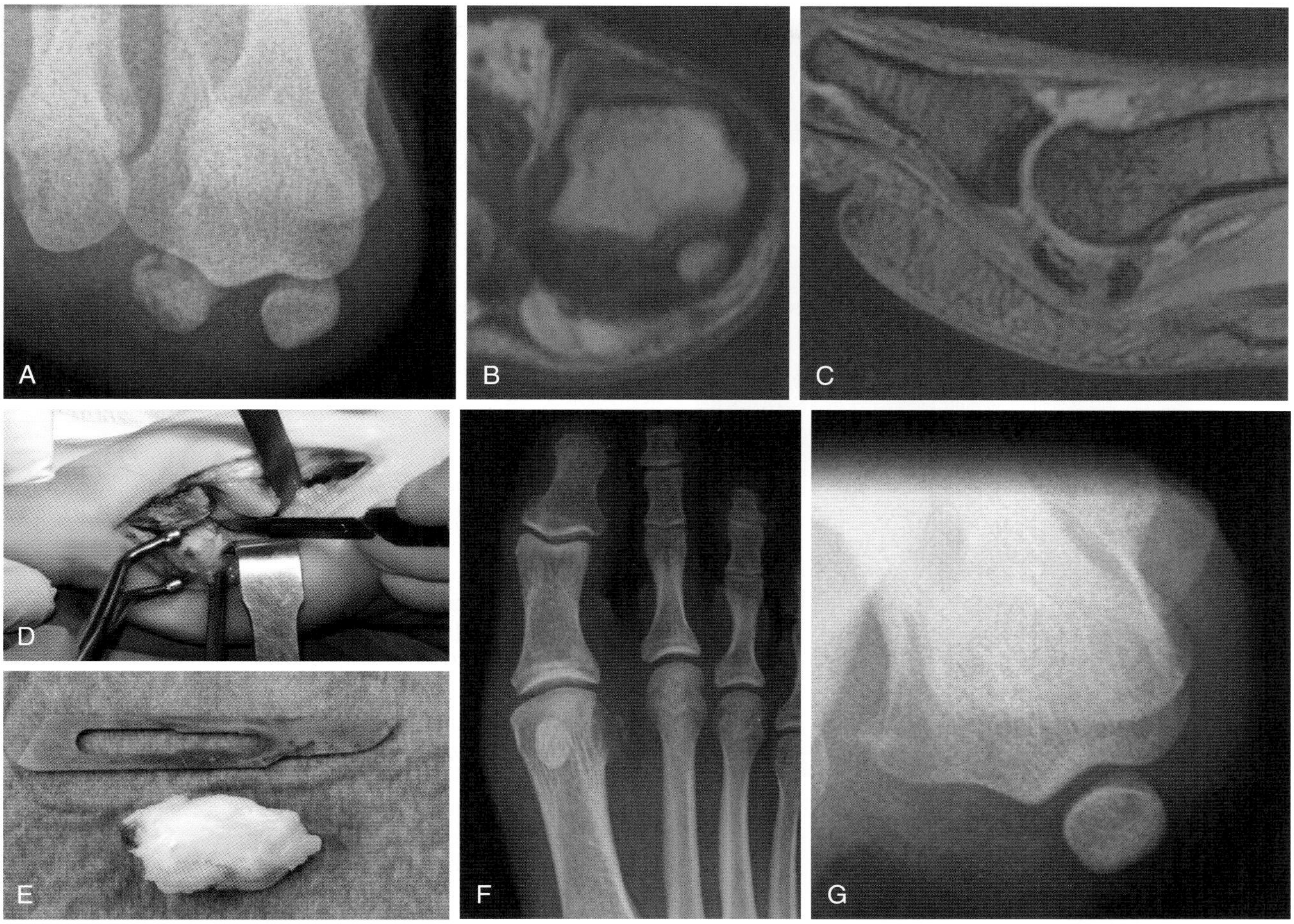

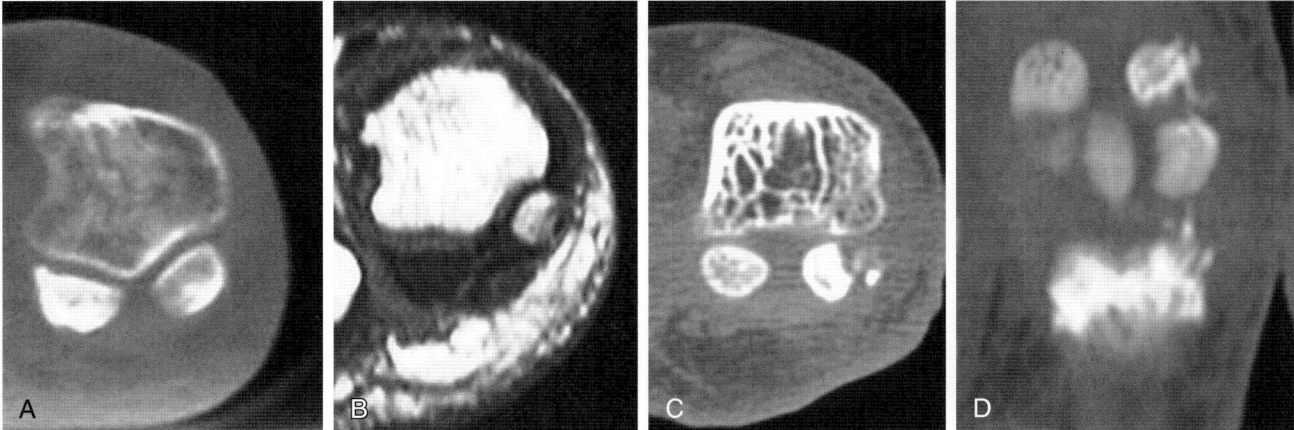

Figure 10-38 Osteonecrosis of the lateral sesamoid. **A,** Axial radiograph. Note irregularity of fragments. **B,** Axial magnetic resonance imaging (MRI) and, **C,** sagittal MRI view showing both sclerosis and fragmentation of the sesamoid. **D,** Surgical excision through an extensive medial approach. **E,** Excised specimen. Anteroposterior (**F**) and axial (**G**) postoperative radiographs showing excised lateral sesamoid. (From Rodrigues Pinto R, Muras J: Medial approach to the fibular sesamoid, *Foot Ankle Int* 31:916–919, 2010. Used with permission.)

Figure 10-39 Computed tomography (CT) and magnetic resonance imaging (MRI) scans used to define extent of osteonecrosis of the sesamoids. **A,** CT demonstrating sclerosis of the lateral sesamoid. **B,** MRI view demonstrating avascular changes in lateral sesamoid. **C,** Fragmentation of the medial sesamoid. **D,** MRI demonstrating fragmentation of both sesamoids. (All photographs courtesy Eric Toussirot, MD.)

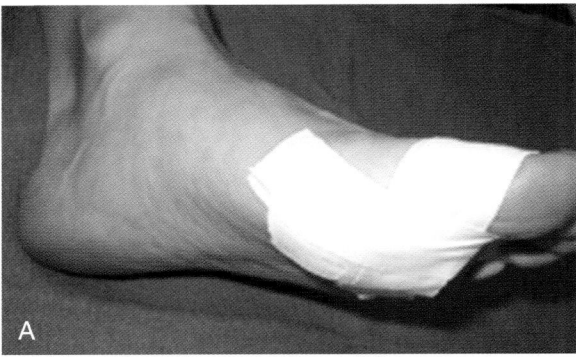

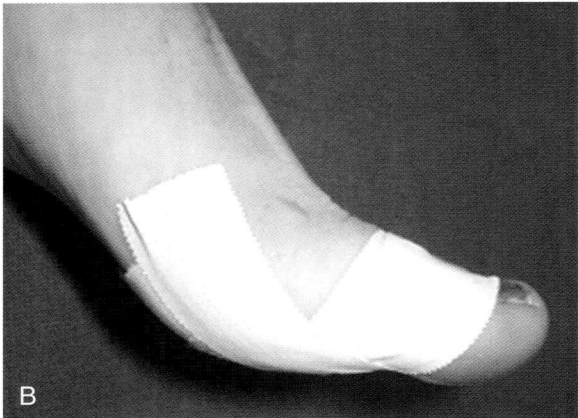

Figure 10-40 Taping of the hallux prevents excessive dorsiflexion.

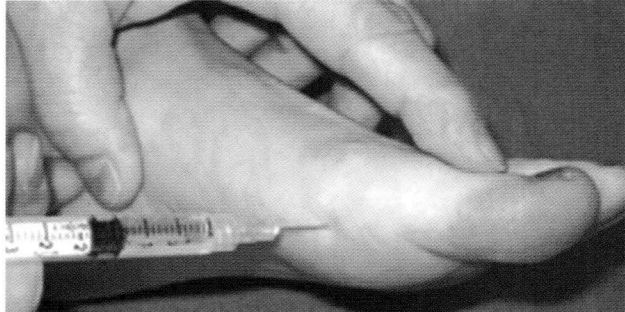

Figure 10-41 Injection for the sesamoid complex may be achieved from the medial aspect. The needle is directed between the medial sesamoid and the plantar metatarsal surface. Plantar flexion of the proximal phalanx aids in the injection by relaxing the capsular structures.

but an injection in the presence of osteonecrosis or a sesamoid fracture is contraindicated.

Decision Making in the Excision of a Sesamoid

Either a tibial or fibular sesamoid may be excised if conservative care is ineffective in relieving symptoms. It is uncommon for a significant deformity to develop after isolated excision of either of these sesamoids, assuming that the patient does not have a hallux valgus or hallux

varus deformity. Because the flexor digitorum brevis inserts into the base of the proximal phalanx after passing around the sesamoids, this attachment may be disrupted if both sesamoids are excised. Because the flexor digitorum brevis stabilizes and plantar flexes the proximal phalanx, a cock-up deformity can develop. Thus only one sesamoid should be excised. If one sesamoid has previously been resected, it is preferable that the remaining sesamoid be protected to minimize the risk of a postoperative claw toe deformity. In the presence of an isolated intractable plantar keratotic lesion beneath the remaining sesamoid, shaving the plantar half of the remaining sesamoid is preferable to resection.

Surgical excision of a chronically painful sesamoid has been advocated when conservative treatment has failed.* Giurini et al,[34] in reporting on sesamoidectomy for the treatment of chronic neuropathic ulceration beneath the first metatarsal head in diabetic patients, noted 2 of 13 patients developed clawing, although there was minimal follow-up on these patients. Abraham et al[1] reported one case of dual sesamoid excision after trauma, and Julsrud[50] reported simultaneous osteonecrosis in a 22-year-old woman. In both reports, an interphalangeal joint fusion was combined with a dual sesamoid excision. Dual sesamoid excision should in general be avoided,[19,38,44] although sometimes it is uavoidable.[99] Scranton and Rutkowski[95] reported on simultaneous medial and lateral sesamoid excision and recommended a reapproximation of the defect created by surgery to minimize postoperative disability. Jahss[46] likened the repair of the defect in the flexor hallucis brevis to a repair of the quadriceps mechanism after a patellectomy.

The surgical approach used for sesamoid excision depends on which sesamoid is to be removed. The medial sesamoid can be approached through either a plantar-medial incision or a medial approach. Kliman et al[55] cautioned against using a plantar approach because of the proximity of the plantar digital nerves, and Mann et al[65] noted the possibility of the development of a painful plantar scar (Fig. 10-42).

Mann and Coughlin[64] and others[28,90] have advocated a dorsolateral approach to resect the fibular sesamoid in cases of hallux valgus; others[19] have advocated this approach for isolated fibular sesamoidectomy as well. Pinto et al[84] described a surgical excision of the lateral sesamoid through an extensive medial approach. Van Hal et al,[102] Helal,[38] and Jahss[47] recommended a longitudinal plantar incision adjacent to the fibular sesamoid for resection of a fibular sesamoid. Jahss found the dorsal approach for sesamoidectomy "almost impossible." Indeed, the use of a direct plantar approach to excise a symptomatic lateral sesamoid makes sense; however, a painful plantar scar can be an extremely difficult complication to resolve. In the case of a normally aligned first ray, I believe a plantar approach is technically easier; however, in the

---

*References 5, 16, 17, 25, 26, 36-38, 40, 44, 46, 51, 55, 65, 72, 79, 94, 96, 98, 100, 102, and 110.

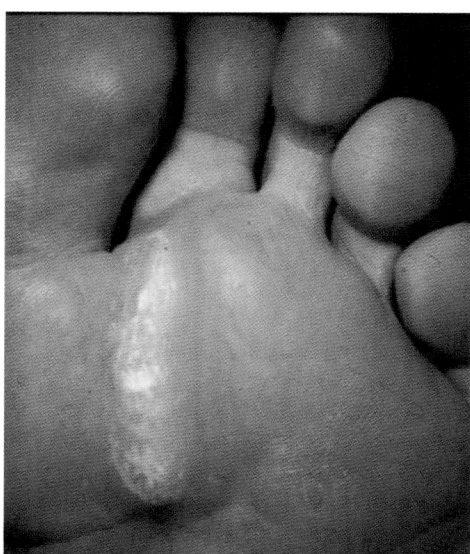

Figure 10-42 A painful plantar scar has developed after a plantar approach to resect a fibular sesamoid. (From Coughlin MJ: Sesamoid pain: causes and surgical treatment, *Instr Course Lect* 39:23–25, 1990.)

presence of a hallux valgus deformity, a dorsal approach is equally easy and avoids a plantar incision.

EXCISION OF THE TIBIAL SESAMOID

Excision of the medial sesamoid (Fig. 10-43) is much simpler than excision of the lateral sesamoid.

Surgical Technique

1. The tibial sesamoid is approached through a midmedial 3-cm incision from a point just proximal to the first metatarsal head and extending distally toward the base of the proximal phalanx (Fig. 10-44A). The incision is carried down to the joint capsule. Care is taken to isolate and protect the medial plantar cutaneous nerve, which courses just over the medial border of the tibial sesamoid (Fig. 10-44B).
2. By incising the medial capsule (Fig. 10-44C) and retracting it plantarward, the articular surface of the sesamoid can be visualized (Fig. 10-44D).
3. The tibial sesamoid is then resected subperiosteally (Fig. 10-44E). In the case of a transverse fracture of the medial sesamoid, if the surgeon chooses to resect just the proximal pole of the sesamoid, it is excised sharply along the fracture line.
4. In the depths of the wound, the tendon of the flexor hallucis longus should be identified (Fig. 10-44F). Care should be taken to avoid injury to this structure.
5. An attempt is made to close the surgical defect created by excision of the sesamoid. Usually a purse-string closure helps to approximate or reduce the remaining defect (Fig. 10-44G and H). Care must be taken to avoid injury to the adjacent sensory nerve during this dissection.

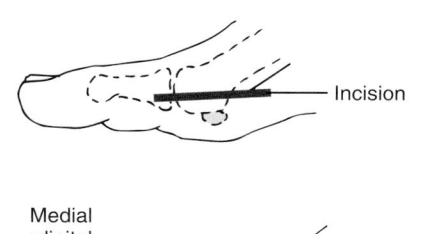
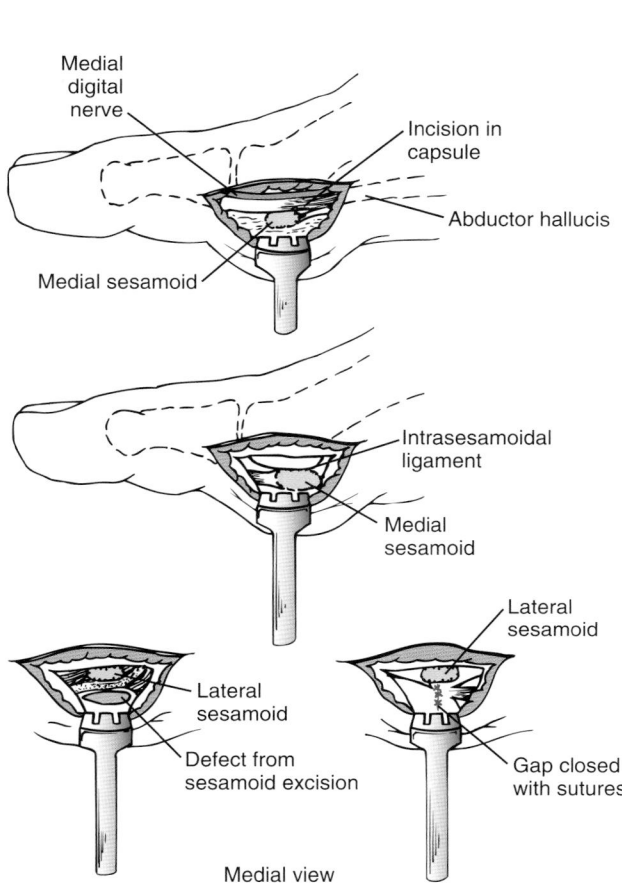

Figure 10-43 Technique of medial sesamoid excision.

6. The skin is approximated (Fig. 10-44I), and a gauze-and-tape compression dressing is applied. The patient is allowed to ambulate in a postoperative shoe for approximately 3 weeks.

SHAVING A PROMINENT TIBIAL SESAMOID[66]

Although surgical excision of a prominent tibial sesamoid may be used to treat an intractable plantar keratotic lesion, an alternative is to shave the plantar half of the tibial sesamoid. Resecting and beveling the plantar half of the tibial sesamoid can reduce a prominent tibial sesamoid enough to substantially relieve or reduce a plantar keratotic lesion.

Surgical Technique (Video Clip 64)

1. A longitudinal plantar-medial incision is made similar to that used for a medial sesamoidectomy (see Fig. 10-44A).

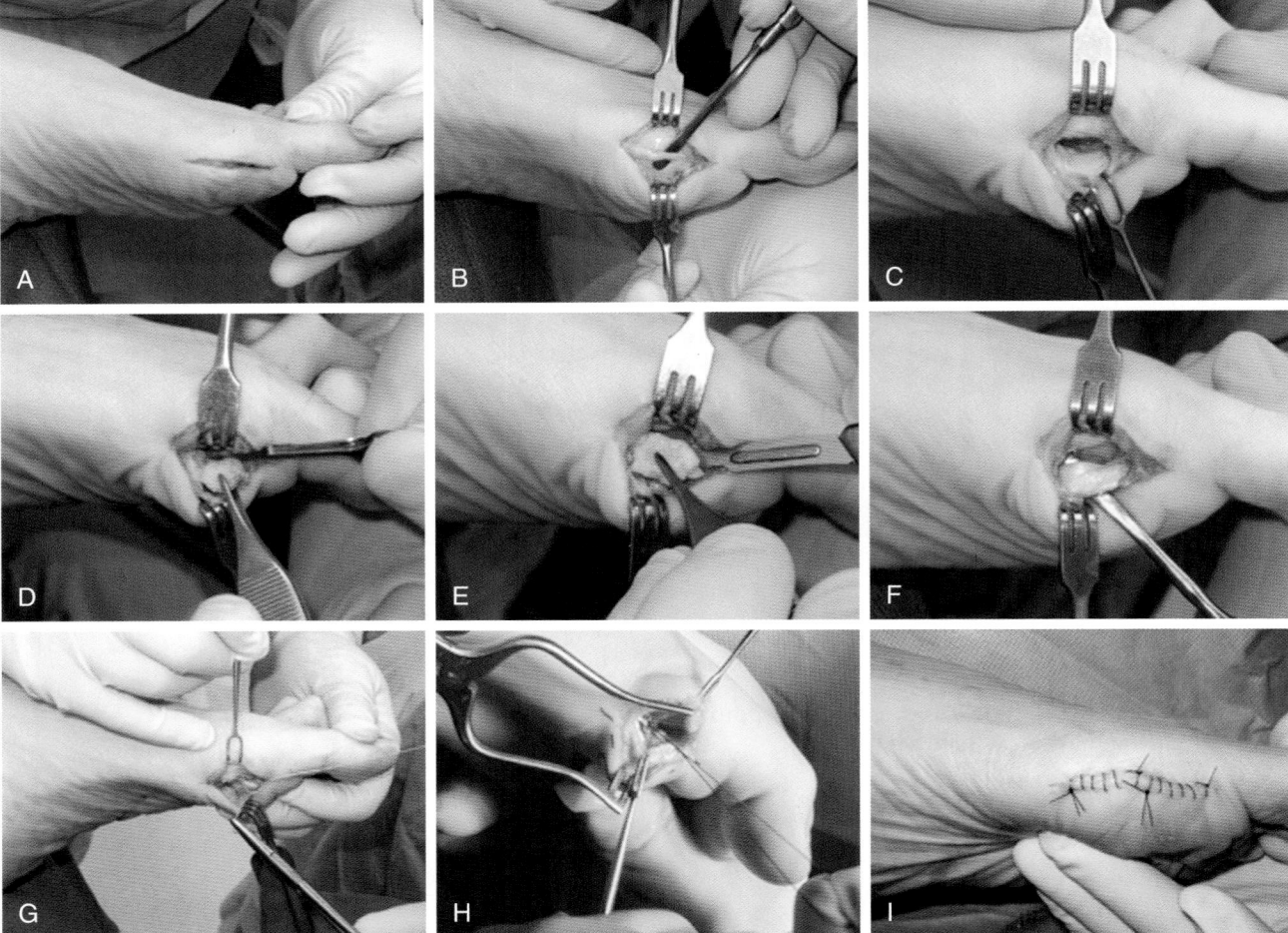

Figure 10-44 Technique of tibial sesamoid excision. **A,** A midline skin incision is made. **B,** Surgical dissection demonstrates the medial plantar sensory nerve just dorsal to the medial sesamoid. **C,** The capsule is incised just dorsal to the medial sesamoid to expose the medial sesamoid articulation. **D,** The sesamoid is retracted downward to improve visualization. **E,** The tibial sesamoid has been excised. **F,** The flexor hallucis longus tendon is inspected to ensure continuity. **G** and **H,** The defect is reduced or closed with 2-0 absorbable suture. Note the medial plantar sensory nerve overlying the repair site. **I,** Wound closure.

2. Care is taken to isolate the medial plantar digital nerve, which courses over the medial border of the tibial sesamoid (see Fig. 10-44B).
3. The metatarsal sesamoid ligament is incised to define the superior extent of the sesamoid (see Fig. 10-44C).
4. The plantar fat pad is retracted, and a sagittal saw is used to resect the plantar half of the sesamoid (Fig. 10-45A and B).
5. Care is taken to protect the flexor digitorum longus tendon, which lies immediately lateral to the tibial sesamoid.
6. Once the tibial sesamoid has been shaved, the sharp edges are beveled with a rongeur.
7. The skin is approximated in a routine fashion (see Fig. 10-44I).
8. The toe is protected in a gauze-and-tape dressing, and the patient is allowed to ambulate in a postoperative shoe for 3 weeks after surgery.

Usually, MTP motion returns quickly, and strength is unimpaired after surgery (Fig. 10-45C and D).

Postoperative Results

Aquino et al[6] reported their results in the evaluation of 26 feet that had undergone tibial sesamoid shaving for intractable plantar keratoses. An 89% subjective success rate was reported with this procedure. Because the intrinsic musculature was not disrupted, there was a negligible increase in the hallux valgus angle at final follow-up. The authors found minimal weakness at the first MTP joint postoperatively after this procedure. This procedure, however, is contraindicated in the presence of a plantar-flexed first metatarsal (see Fig. 10-28). In this situation, a dorsiflexion osteotomy is the treatment of choice for an intractable plantar keratotic lesion. If the first metatarsal is plantar flexed more than 8 degrees in relation to the lesser metatarsals, a sesamoid planing procedure is contraindicated.

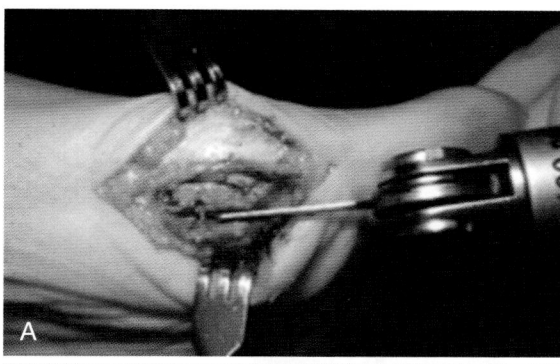

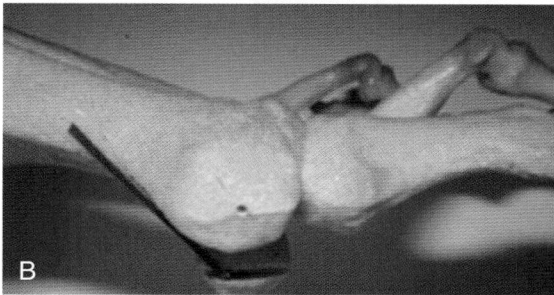

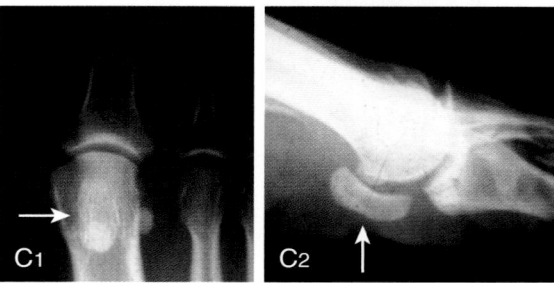

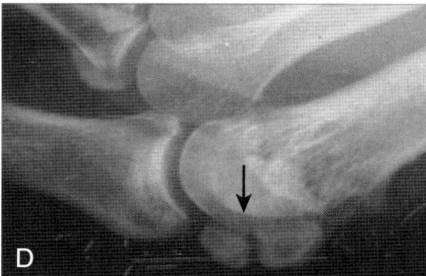

Figure 10-45 Technique of tibial shaving. **A,** A power saw is used to remove the plantar half of the tibial sesamoid. **B,** Model demonstrating 50% shaving of medial sesamoid. **C,** After shaving of the tibial sesamoid, a flat plantar surface is achieved *(arrows)*. **D,** Fracture after medial sesamoid shaving *(arrow)*.

Mann and Wapner[66] reported on 14 patients (16 feet) who underwent tibial sesamoid shaving. They noted no functional limitations, and at final follow-up, patients were reported to have a normal range of motion. Excellent or good results were reported in 15 feet. There was one case of recurrent callus formation and four cases of slight recurrence of callosity. The authors reported fracture of the remaining sesamoid as a possible complication, although none occurred.

Lee et al[61] reported on 14 cases of isolated tibial sesamoidectomy that had no angular malalignment or weakness at final follow-up. Two cases of metatarsalgia were noted postoperatively.

EXCISION OF THE FIBULAR SESAMOID
Dorsal Approach (Video Clip 65)

The fibular sesamoid may be approached through a dorsal incision in the first intermetatarsal space.

Surgical Technique
1. A 3-cm dorsal incision is made in the first intermetatarsal space (Fig. 10-46A).
2. A Weitlaner retractor or lamina spreader is used to spread the first and second metatarsals. With the tendon of the adductor hallucis as a guide, the adductor tendon is detached from the lateral joint capsule, and the fibular sesamoid is exposed. The adductor tendon is then dissected off of the lateral aspect of the sesamoid, and the intersesamoidal ligament is severed (Fig. 10-46B).
3. Care is taken to avoid damage to the common digital nerve in the first web space, which lies just beneath the transverse intermetatarsal ligament.
4. The sesamoid is firmly grasped with a toothed forceps and is excised in its entirety. Another alternative is to drill a threaded Kirschner wire into the lateral sesamoid, which can then be grasped as the sesamoid is excised.[28] It is very difficult to complete a partial sesamoid excision through a dorsal approach.
5. The plantar aspect of the wound is inspected to ensure that the flexor hallucis longus tendon has not been inadvertently severed.
6. If the adductor hallucis tendon has been detached, it should be reapproximated to the base of the proximal phalanx or the lateral MTP joint capsule.
7. The skin is approximated with interrupted sutures. A gauze-and-tape compression dressing is applied, and the patient is allowed to ambulate in a postoperative shoe for 3 weeks.

The use of a dorsal incision for excision of a fibular sesamoid may be difficult. It is somewhat more demanding than a plantar approach but avoids significant postoperative morbidity. It avoids the possibility of a painful or hypertrophic plantar scar (Fig. 10-47).

Plantar Approach
If a plantar incision is used to approach the fibular sesamoid, an intermetatarsal incision is preferred to an incision directly beneath the first metatarsal head (see Fig. 10-30C). Postoperative scarring or keloid formation directly beneath a metatarsal or sesamoid can cause intractable pain (see Fig. 10-42).

Surgical Technique
1. A slightly curved longitudinal incision is made on the lateral edge of the first metatarsal fat pad (Figs. 10-48 and 10-49A).

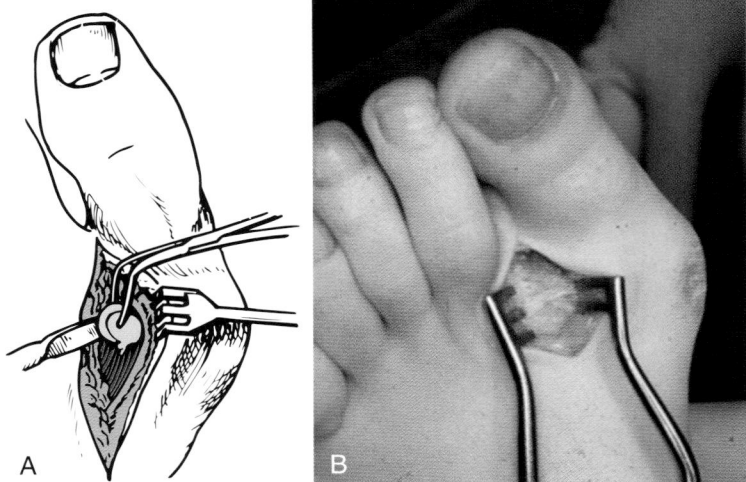

Figure 10-46 **A,** A 3-cm dorsal incision is made in the first interspace to resect the lateral sesamoid. **B,** A Weitlaner retractor aids in spreading the first and second metatarsals to expose the lateral sesamoid for resection.

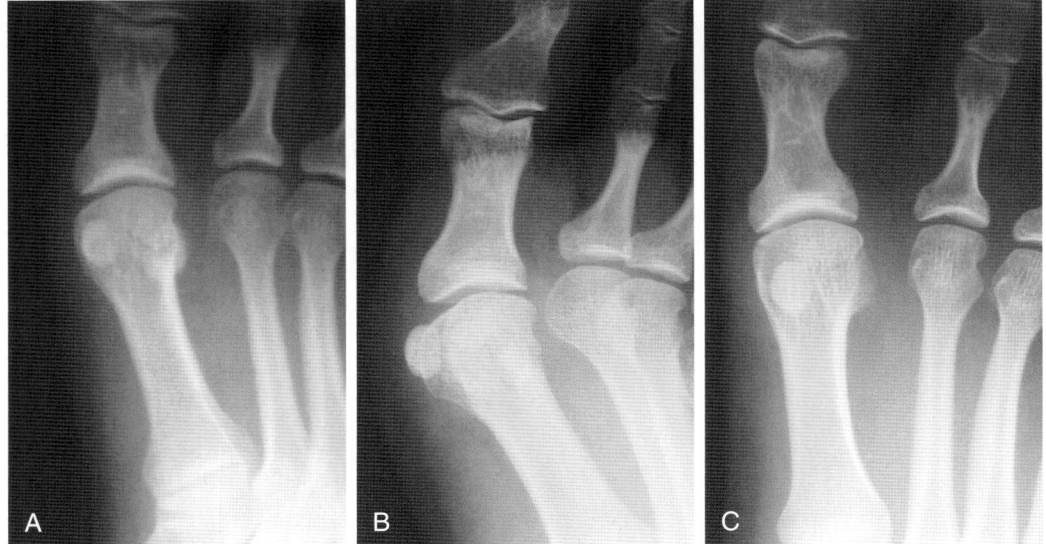

Figure 10-47 Anteroposterior **(A)** and oblique **(B)** radiographs of avascular necrosis of the lateral sesamoid. **C,** After excision of the lateral sesamoid through a dorsal interspace incision, adequate alignment is maintained.

2. Care is taken to isolate and protect the lateral plantar digital nerve to the hallux, which can course directly over the lateral edge of the fibular sesamoid.
3. The metatarsal fat pad is retracted medially with the digital nerve.
4. The lateral sesamoid is covered by a thin layer of fascia from the conjoined tendon but can be palpated in the depths of the wound. It is carefully excised with a No. 15 blade (Fig. 10-49B and C). The adductor hallucis tendon is preferably left intact.
5. The tendon of the flexor hallucis longus is inspected to ensure its continuity.

6. The fascial defect left by the excised sesamoid is approximated, if possible, with 2-0 absorbable suture and an interrupted suture technique or a purse-string closure (Fig. 10-49D and E).
7. The skin is approximated with interrupted 5-0 nylon suture, with care taken to evert the skin edges to minimize postoperative scarring (Figs. 10-49F and 10-50).

Postoperative Results

An isolated excision of a sesamoid can lead to a muscle imbalance of the MTP joint. The development of a hallux varus deformity after fibular sesamoidectomy was noted

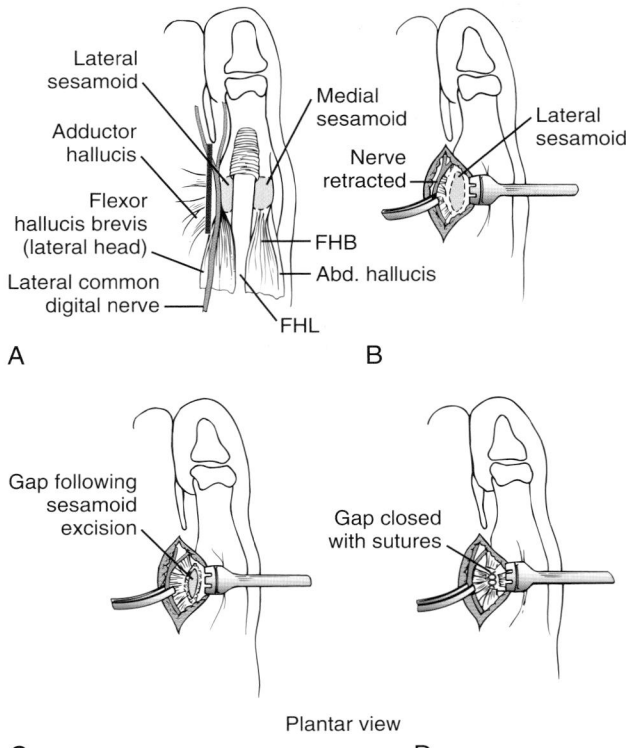

A

B

C

D

Plantar view

Figure 10-48 Technique of lateral sesamoid excision through the plantar approach. **A,** A longitudinal plantar incision is made between the first and second metatarsal heads just lateral to the common digital nerve. **B,** With the nerve retracted, the lateral sesamoid is identified and excised. **C** and **D,** The capsule is closed with 2-0 absorbable suture to minimize the surgical defect. *FHB,* flexor hallucis brevis; *FHL,* flexor hallucis longus.

by Mann and Coughlin,[64] who reported an 8% incidence of hallux varus in a postoperative review of the treatment of hallux valgus deformities with the McBride procedure. Nayfa and Sorto[72] reported a 2.2-degree increase in the intermetatarsal angle after tibial sesamoidectomy and a 6.2-degree valgus drift of the hallux after tibial sesamoidectomy. Jahss[46] noted that a wide medial excision of the tibial sesamoid could disrupt the medial MTP joint capsule and lead to a hallux valgus deformity. Likewise, a wide lateral excision with disruption of the adductor hallucis tendon can lead to a hallux varus deformity (see Fig. 10-34C and D).

Mann et al,[65] reporting on a series of sesamoidectomies, noted a valgus or varus drift of the hallux in 10% of the patients (see Fig. 10-34A and B); Saxena[93] reported varus or valgus drift in 8% of patients after sesamoidectomy. Maintenance of the integrity of the medial capsule and abductor hallucis, when a tibial sesamoidectomy is performed, and maintenance of the integrity of the adductor hallucis and lateral capsule, when a fibular sesamoidectomy is performed, are important in diminishing migration of the hallux postoperatively. When possible,

it is advantageous to repair the defect left by the sesamoid excision. After tibial sesamoidectomy, a lateral capsule release, medial capsule reefing,[19,72] and even a metatarsal osteotomy may be considered if there appears to be an increased risk of a hallux valgus deformity after tibial sesamoid excision.

Surgical excision of a sesamoid is recommended when conservative care has proved unsuccessful. Little information, however, is available regarding postoperative results. Although some[94,102,110] have reported complete relief of pain and resumption of normal activities, Inge and Ferguson[44] noted that only 41% of patients achieved complete relief (Fig. 10-51). Mann et al[65] reported complete relief of pain in 50% of their patients.

The reports from many series suggest that surgical excision can lead to significant MTP joint stiffness.* Mann et al[65] reported restricted range of motion in one third of their cases. Of 14 patients with a full range of motion, 10 had tibial and 4 had fibular sesamoidectomies. In 7 patients with restricted range of motion, three fibular sesamoidectomies and four tibial sesamoidectomies had been carried out. There does not appear to be a predilection for restricted range of motion after either tibial or fibular sesamoidectomy, although a stiff MTP joint postoperatively may be associated with preexisting arthrosis. Saxena et al[93] reported a shorter recovery period after fibular sesamoidectomy. Biedert[7] reported successful return to athletic activity in a small group of patients after excision of only the proximal pole of the symptomatic sesamoid.

Van Hal et al[102] noted no diminution in plantar flexion strength and reported no cock-up deformities of the hallux after sesamoid excision. Inge and Ferguson,[44] however, found a 17% incidence of clawing of the hallux postoperatively. They also noted that 58% of their patients had restricted MTP joint range of motion, clawing, or continued pain postoperatively. Mann et al[65] reported a 60% incidence of plantar flexion weakness. A lengthy period of preoperative conservative treatment in Mann's series may have contributed to the latter postoperative restricted motion and weakness.

Inge and Ferguson[44] reported on 31 patients (41 feet) after sesamoid excision. Twenty-five patients underwent dual sesamoidectomy. A medial sesamoid was excised in 15, and a fibular sesamoid was excised in 1. Only 41.5% of patients noted normal function and complete relief of pain after surgery. The 17% incidence of a postoperative claw toe deformity was likely due to the dual sesamoid excision.

Aper et al[3] reported their laboratory investigation regarding first-ray strength of the hallux after medial and lateral sesamoidectomy and dual sesamoidectomy. They reported that after only medial sesamoidectomy, it is unlikely that the mechanical advantage of the flexor hallucis brevis is compromised. In a follow-up study, Aper et al[4] reported that excision of either the medial or lateral

---

*References 17, 47, 65, 94, and 100.

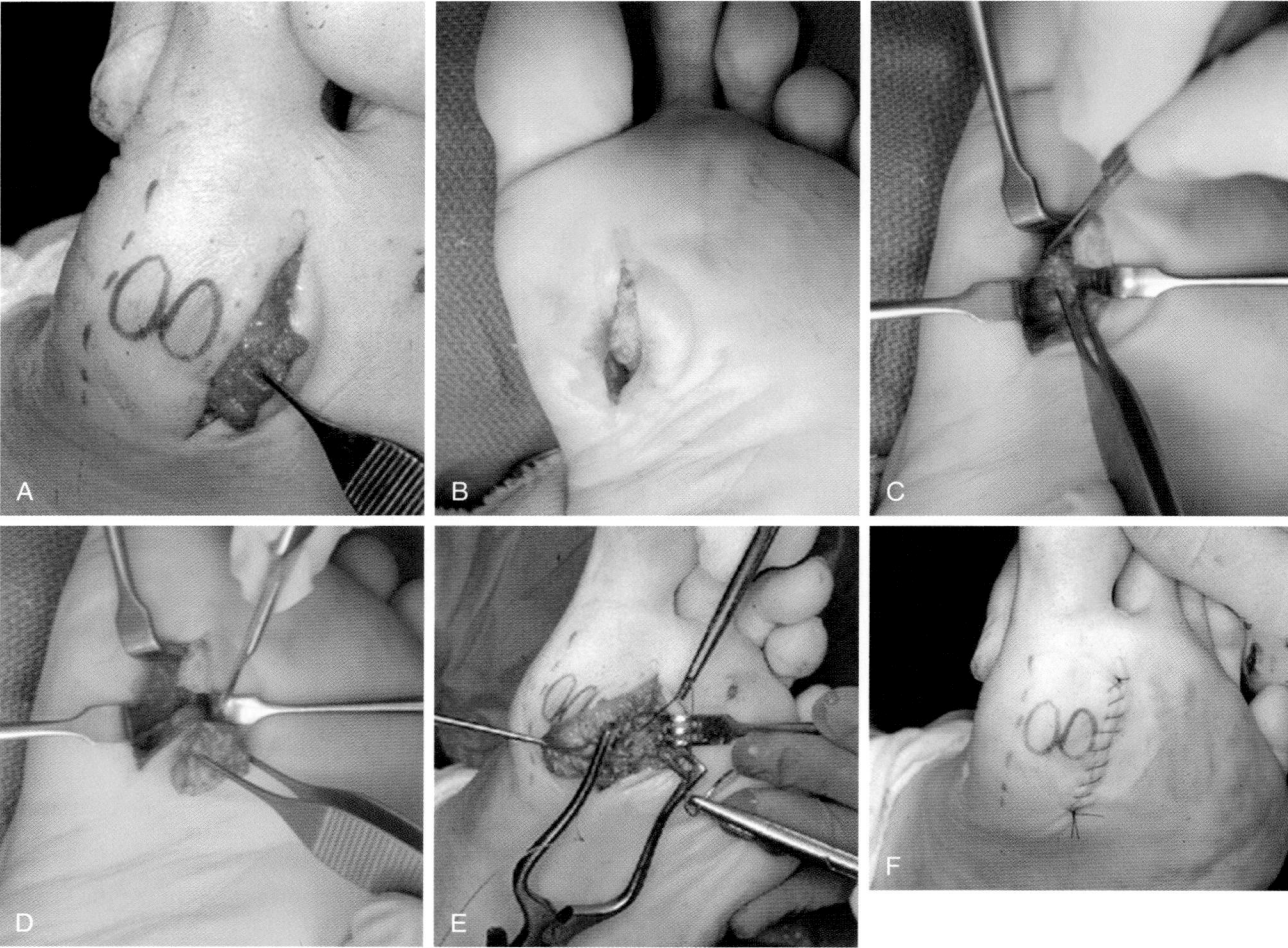

Figure 10-49 Excision of lateral sesamoid through plantar approach. **A** and **B,** Plantar longitudinal incision is centered between first and second metatarsal heads. Lateral sesamoid is freed from surrounding ligamentous attachments **(C)** and excised **(D). E,** Closure of adjacent soft tissue; care is taken to protect the common digital nerve as the defect is repaired. **F,** Skin closure.

sesamoid causes a significant decrease in the moment arm of the flexor hallucis longus. Their explanation was that removal of a sesamoid allows the flexor hallucis longus to move closer to the center of rotation, weakening the moment arm.

Mann et al,[65] reporting on the surgical excision of sesamoids in 21 patients, noted that the average age was 41 years and that 66% of their patients were women. Thirteen tibial and eight fibular sesamoids were excised. Only 50% of patients noted complete relief of pain. Of those who were still symptomatic, 75% noted only occasional or mild symptoms. Sixty percent (12 patients) noted plantar-flexion weakness. One third of the patients noted restricted range of motion. There appeared to be no difference in the postoperative results of tibial or fibular sesamoid excision. In 10% of cases, there was a mild drift of the hallux into either varus or valgus after surgery. Although the subjective level of patient satisfaction was high, the postoperative objective limitations noted were significant. Lee et al[61] reported on 20 patients who

underwent isolated tibial sesamoidectomy, with an average of more than 5 years follow-up. A meticulous soft tissue closure was performed after the sesamoidectomy, and they reported no change in the hallux valgus or 1-to-2 intermetatarsal angle. Ninety percent of patients were able to resume preoperative activities; however, 30% had difficulty or inability to stand on their tip-toes. They reported a high level of satisfaction at long-term follow-up.

Brodsky[12] reported on 23 sesamoid fractures that went on to chronic nonunion. Thirteen medial and 10 lateral sesamoids were involved. The mean time to surgery was 38.8 months. Although 21 of 23 patients had satisfactory results after surgical excision, 2 patients had postoperative weakness of the hallux, 2 had neuritic symptoms, and 6 had mild-to-moderate pain after surgery. In a follow-up report, Brodsky et al[13] reported on 37 patients (18 male and 19 female) with painful fractured sesamoids that were treated operatively. Avascular necrosis secondary to a sesamoid fracture was observed in 9 patients, 16 were noted to have sesamoid stress fractures, and 12 were

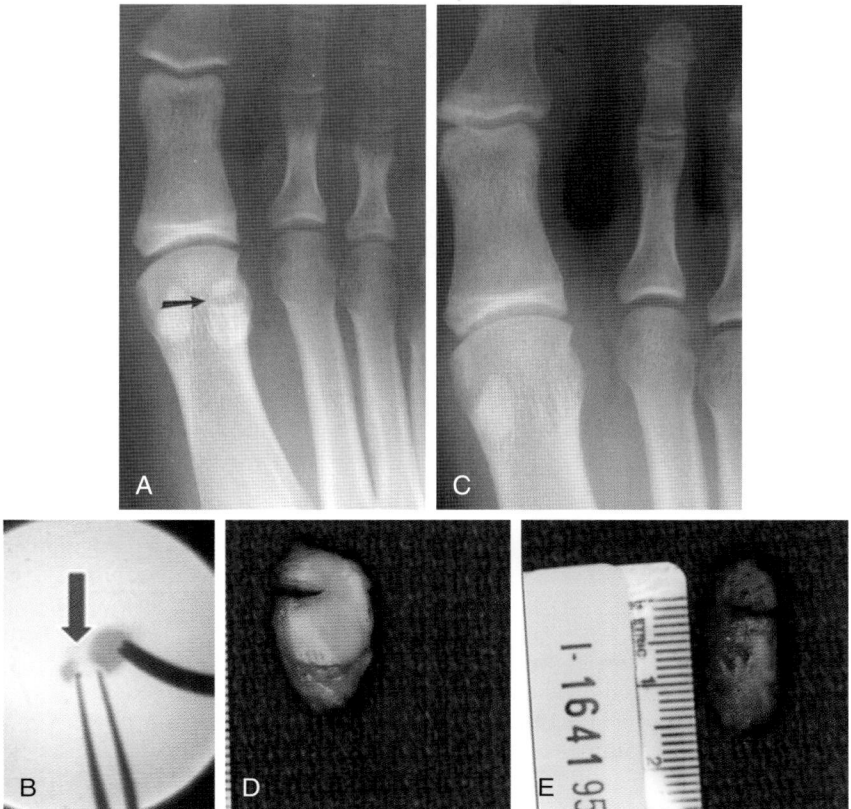

Figure 10-50 **A,** Preoperative anteroposterior radiograph demonstrating a painful lateral sesamoid suspected to be a fracture of a partite lateral sesamoid. **B,** Intraoperative fluoroscopy of resected specimen. **C,** After lateral sesamoid excision through a plantar approach. **D** and **E,** Operative specimen demonstrating evidence of disruption of the partite sesamoid.

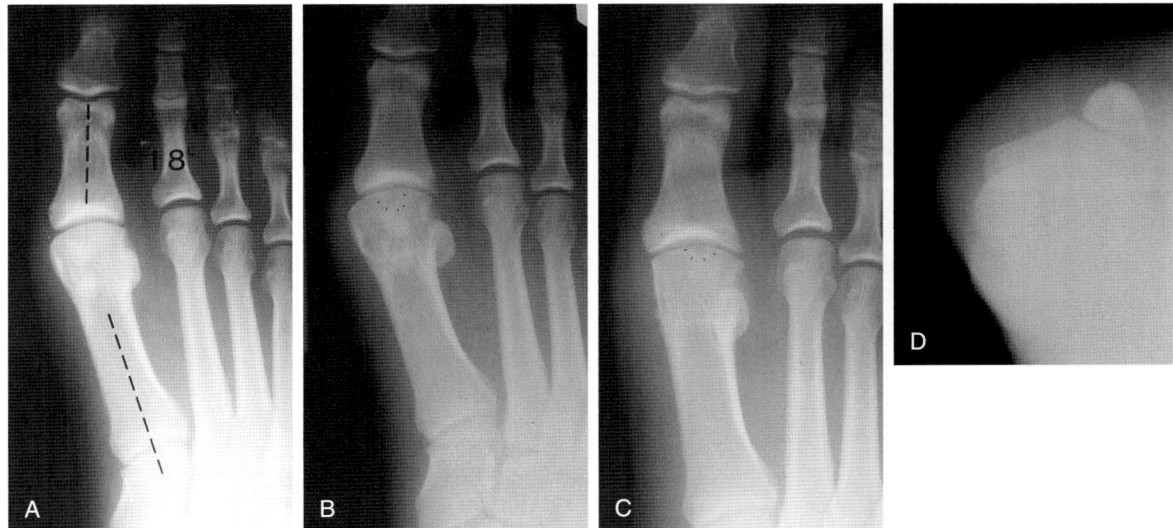

Figure 10-51 **A,** Anteroposterior radiograph of a painful bipartite medial sesamoid; 18-degree hallux valgus deformity associated with a multipartite medial sesamoid. **B,** Five years later, the valgus deformity has increased. A lengthy period of conservative care may be associated with degenerative arthritic changes of the first metatarsophalangeal (MTP) joint. Note the cyst in the first metatarsal head. There has been gradual separation of the sesamoid fragments, and increasing pain had developed. **C** and **D,** Five years after surgery, with medial capsulorrhaphy to stabilize the first MTP joint.

related to direct trauma. After surgical excision, the average AOFAS score was 93 points. Several cases of post-traumatic arthritis developed.

The first MTP joint sesamoids play an integral role in the dynamic function of the first MTP joint. Deterioration of function resulting from trauma, inflammation, fracture, or surgery can lead to significant disability. Although surgical intervention may be necessary in the treatment of a chronically painful sesamoid, the sesamoid complex should be preserved whenever possible. When conservative care is ineffectual and a sesamoidectomy is performed, care should be taken to maintain the integrity of the remaining intrinsic muscles and capsule to maintain stability and function of the first MTP joint. A single diseased sesamoid can be removed with acceptable postoperative results; however, the resection of both sesamoids should be avoided unless absolutely necessary.

INTERPHALANGEAL SESAMOID OF THE HALLUX

A subhallux sesamoid can occur as an accessory bone beneath the head of the proximal phalanx of the hallux (Fig. 10-52). This accessory bone is located on the dorsal aspect of the flexor hallucis longus tendon and articulates within the interphalangeal joint. A subhallux sesamoid is found superior to or within the tendon of the flexor hallucis longus[109] and typically is located in the midline or oriented slightly to the fibular aspect of the flexor hallucis longus tendon. It varies in size from 3 to 5 mm in diameter.[68]

Miller and Love[69] have described a cartilaginous sesamoid located in the plantar ligament of the interphalangeal joint. Trolle,[311] in sectioning 508 embryo feet, found an interphalangeal sesamoid in 56%. Typically, it is unilateral, but it can occur bilaterally. Its occurrence has been reported by Bizarro[8] to be 5% (radiographic study) and by Jahss[46] to be 13%.

If the subhallux sesamoid is large or if it is associated with hyperextension of the interphalangeal joint, pressure can be exerted against the sesamoid. Occasionally, in patients with a mild hallux flexus deformity, increased pressure is exerted on the plantar skin beneath the sesamoid. A painful hyperkeratotic lesion and, in some cases, ulceration can develop, particularly in an insensitive foot.

The diagnosis of a subhallux sesamoid is confirmed with a lateral radiograph of the hallux. The radiograph demonstrates the sesamoid just beneath the interphalangeal joint (Fig. 10-53).

Treatment

Treatment should be directed toward relieving the pressure on the subhallux sesamoid. The keratotic lesion may be shaved, and a pad may be placed just proximal to this area, which can decrease localized pressure. When conservative treatment is unsuccessful, surgical excision may be considered.

EXCISION OF A SUBHALLUX SESAMOID

Although a midline plantar incision can be used,[68,109] a medial incision is preferred.

Surgical Technique

1. Through a longitudinal medial incision centered over the interphalangeal joint, the dissection is carried plantarward to the flexor hallucis longus tendon (see Fig. 10-53D).
2. The flexor hallucis longus tendon is incised on the dorsal aspect of the tendon near its insertion. The subhallux sesamoid is embedded within the tendon. By slightly plantar flexing the interphalangeal joint, exposure is improved and the excision is made easier.
3. The subhallux sesamoid is carefully shelled out, but the flexor hallucis longus tendon is protected. If the tendon of the flexor hallucis longus is inadvertently detached from its insertion into the base of the proximal phalanx, it should be reattached by placing a suture through drill holes in the distal phalanx.
4. The wound is closed in a single layer.

Postoperative Care

A gauze-and-tape compression dressing is applied at surgery and changed on a weekly basis. The patient

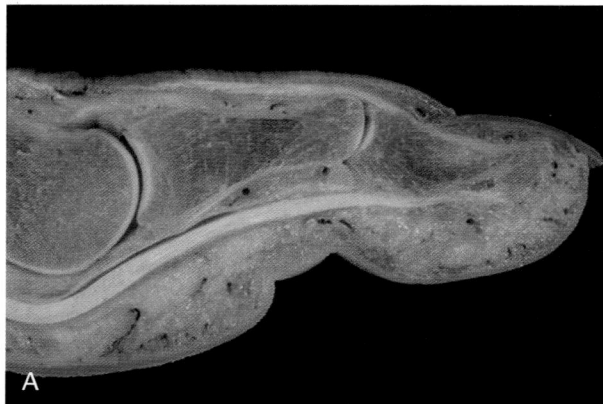
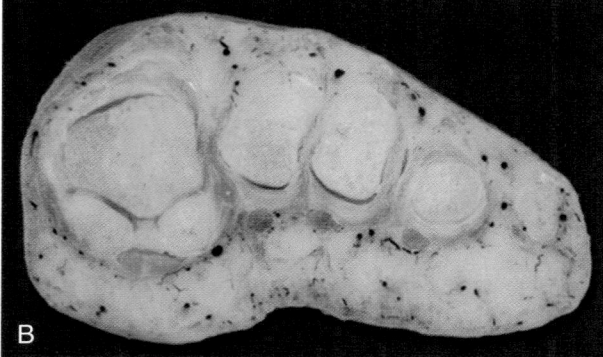

Figure 10-52 Subhallux sesamoid and metatarsophalangeal sesamoids as demonstrated in anatomic dissection. **A,** Lateral cross section. **B,** Coronal cross section. (Courtesy Pau Golano, MD, University of Barcelona, Spain.)

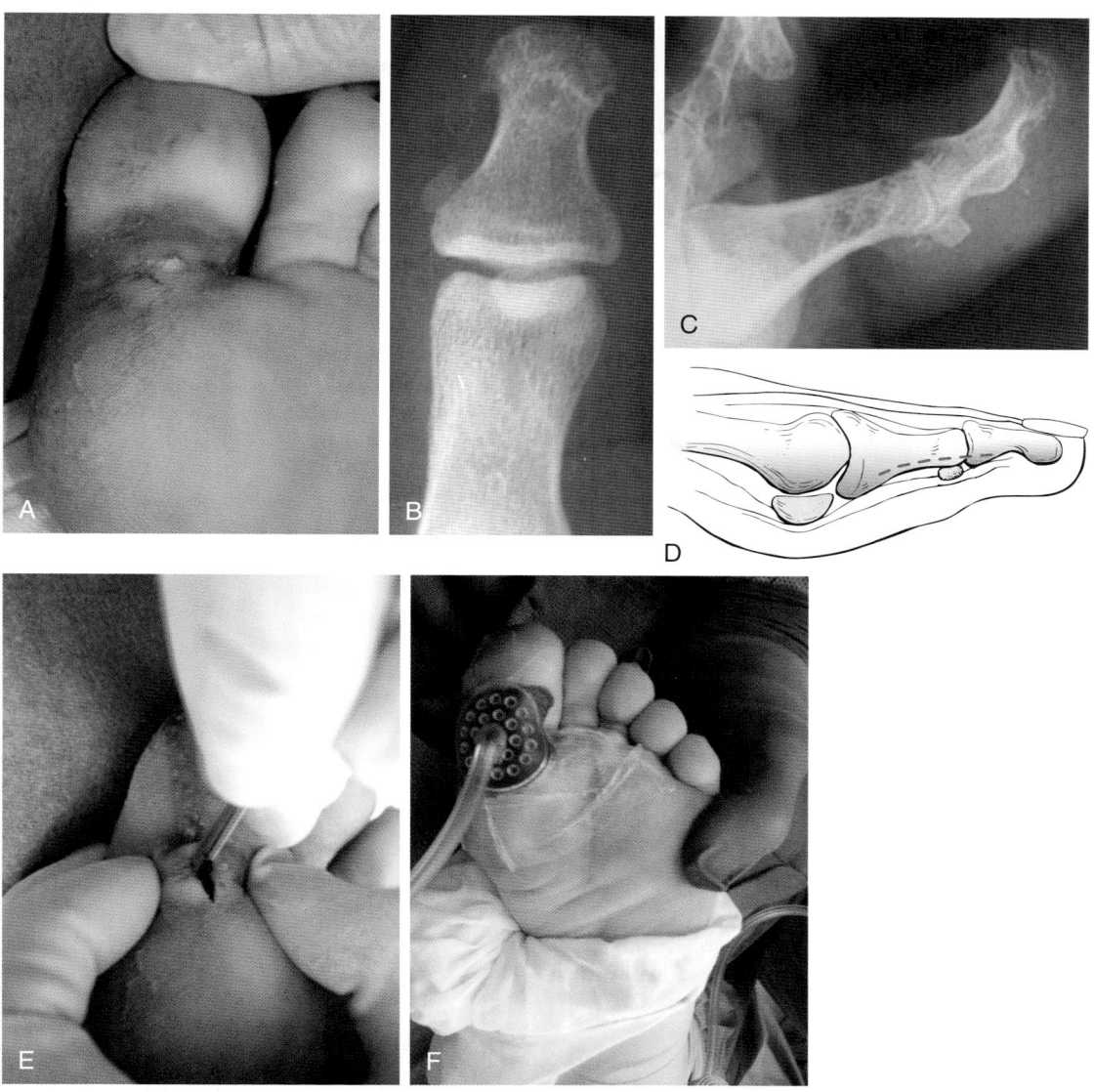

Figure 10-53 A, An interphalangeal sesamoid can produce a midline plantar callus and, in time, an infection as demonstrated here beneath the interphalangeal joint. **B,** Interphalangeal sesamoid on anteroposterior radiograph. **C,** Lateral radiograph demonstrating a large subhallux sesamoid beneath the interphalangeal joint, which, on occasion, may result in chronic ulceration. **D,** Lateral incision technique for simple excision of subhallux sesamoid. **E,** Direct plantar incision for infection. **F,** Wound vacuum-assisted closure application after infection beneath subhallux sesamoid.

ambulates in a postoperative shoe for approximately 3 weeks until soft tissue healing has occurred, after which activities are permitted as tolerated.

Results

The results after excision of a subhallux sesamoid are routinely satisfactory. The callus rarely, if ever, re-forms. The significant major complication is an inadvertent detachment of the flexor hallucis longus tendon at the time of the sesamoid excision. If detachment is recognized, repair of the tendon can be accomplished without residual deficit. A less common complaint is reduced sensation or a postoperative neuroma along the medial border of the hallux, resulting from interruption or injury

to the small sensory branches of the plantar medial digital nerve; however, this is rarely a problem.

ACCESSORY BONES OF THE FOOT AND THE UNCOMMON SESAMOIDS

Accessory bones of the foot are considered developmental anomalies.[262] Accessory bones can develop as subdivisions of normal bones or as a prominence of an ordinary tarsal bone that is abnormally separated from the main tarsal bone. Accessory ossicles can occur either bilaterally or unilaterally but are more commonly found in only one foot. Therefore comparison radiographs might not be helpful in differentiating accessory bones from trauma.

When multiple accessory bones occur in a single foot, O'Rahilly[262] has noted that they are unilateral in 50% or more of cases.

Pfitzner,[269] Dwight,[161] Trolle,[311] and O'Rahilly[262] have studied accessory bones in great detail. Trolle[311] studied serial microscopic sections from 108 feet of 254 embryos between 6 and 27 weeks of fetal age. He demonstrated that in nearly 80%, accessory bones were preformed in hyaline cartilage. The high incidence of accessory bones in embryonic feet does not correlate with their incidence in adult feet. Trolle[311] was unable to find an os trigonum in any of the embryonic feet he studied, although it is common in adults. Conversely, in 13% of embryonic feet, he found anlagen of the os paracuneiforme in spite of a much lower incidence in adult feet. He concluded that accessory bones can develop from an independent element preformed in cartilage, can develop from an independent ossification center, can be explained as tendon bones, and can be caused by unrecognized pathologic lesions. Thus it would seem that there are several explanations for the presence of these abnormalities.

O'Rahilly[262] catalogued 38 tarsal and sesamoid bones and stated that the bones may have been incomplete fusions, accessory bones, or bipartitions. Henderson[195] has shown heritable causation of accessory bones in some instances. From a clinical standpoint, only two accessory bones, the accessory navicular and the os trigonum, cause symptoms with any frequency.

INCONSTANT SESAMOIDS

Accessory or inconstant sesamoids can occur beneath any weight-bearing surface of the foot, especially beneath the lesser metatarsal heads, beneath any of the phalanges, and at times beneath all of the metatarsal heads. Accessory sesamoids vary widely in shape and size. Although ordinarily they are asymptomatic, they can become painful when an ossicle is extraordinarily large or a keratotic lesion develops. Rarely is surgery necessary to excise a symptomatic inconstant sesamoid of the forefoot.

The incidence of accessory bones of the foot varies significantly, depending on the method used to assess their individual incidence (Fig. 10-54). This information is most readily obtained by radiographic examination. Even here, however, the number, variety, and technique of the radiographic projection can influence the frequency of occurrence of accessory bones. Kewenter,[215] for example, obtained radiographs from three different aspects of the forefoot to evaluate the first MTP joint sesamoids. By correlating these views, he obtained a much higher frequency of bony abnormalities in these bones than had previously been reported. Trolle[311] used a similar method, and his work is still considered a classic in assessing the radiographic incidence of accessory bones (Fig. 10-55).

Another technique for investigating the frequency of accessory bones is through anatomic dissection or assessment of skeletal remains retained in archives. This is an

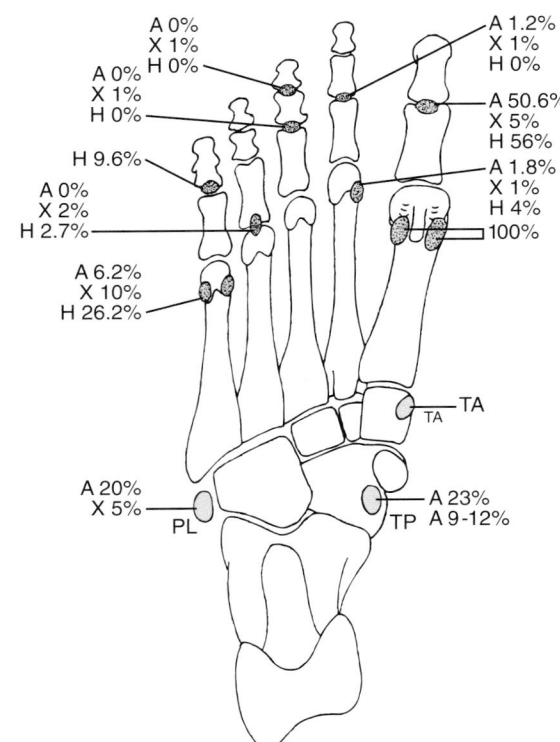

Figure 10-54 Sesamoids of the foot. Frequency of occurrence based on anatomic evaluation *(A)*, histoembryologic investigation *(H)*, and radiographic investigation *(X)*. *PL,* peroneus longus; *TP,* tibialis posterior.

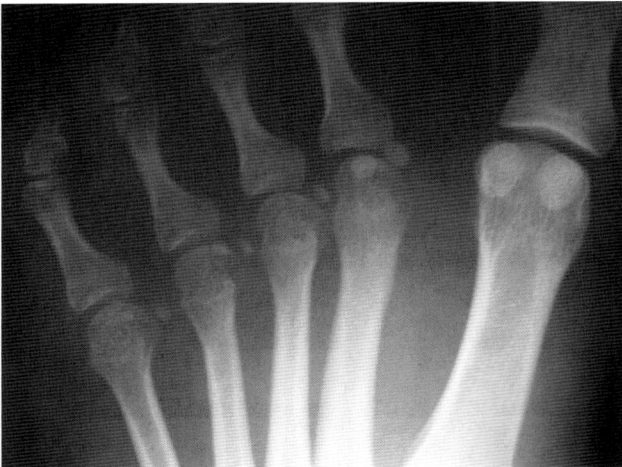

Figure 10-55 Multiple accessory sesamoids at the lesser metatarsophalangeal joints.

extremely time-consuming process. Pfitzner[269] examined 425 feet, and much of his work still forms the basis for information we use today. Mann[240,241] more recently has investigated specific bones by reviewing archive specimens as well.

Sesamoids occur uncommonly in the posterior and anterior tibial tendons, being much more common in the peroneus longus (os peroneum). Uncommon accessory bones include the os subtibiale, os subfibulare, os trigonum, os calcaneus secundarius, os calcaneus accessorius, os sustentaculi, os subcalcis, os aponeurosis plantaris, os cuboides secundarium, os talonaviculare dorsale, os supratalare, os intercuneiforme, os cuneometatarsale, os intermetatarseum, and os vesalianum.

The accessory navicular is a much more common accessory bone. Partition of the navicular and first cuneiform has also been described. Accessory bones are relatively unusual and rarely of clinical significance. Their presence can create a diagnostic dilemma, and it is important for a physician to be able to differentiate them from an acute fracture or injury. They are often identified in radiographs obtained for other reasons, such as after trauma or for complaints of pain unrelated to the accessory bone.

SESAMOID OF THE TIBIALIS POSTERIOR TENDON

Anatomy and Incidence

This sesamoid lies within the tibialis posterior tendon, where it crosses the inferior border of the spring ligament. It lies on the plantar aspect of the navicular tuberosity (Fig. 10-56).[210,311] Its occurrence has been reported to vary from 9.2%[269] to 23%[302] (Fig. 10-57). Storton, by Grant,[302] reported that a sesamoid of the posterior tibial tendon was paired in 52% and unpaired in 47% of feet examined in his anatomic study. Delfaut et al[22] demonstrated a fibrocartilaginous nonossified sesamoid in seven of eight anatomic specimens. They also reported that with magnetic resonance imaging (MRI) examination of 33 asymptomatic patients, 36% demonstrated a fibrocartilaginous sesamoid adjacent to the spring ligament. Although an ossified sesamoid of the posterior tibial tendon is uncommon, a thickening or fibrocartilaginous sesamoid appears to be relatively common.

Clinical Significance

The sesamoid of the posterior tibial tendon should be differentiated from both an accessory navicular and a

fracture (Fig. 10-58); it is often more proximal than the former, and its rounded nature should help differentiate it from the latter.

A classification scheme has been used to describe various types of accessory naviculars.[180,232,290] A type I accessory navicular is truly a sesamoid in the substance of the posterior tibial tendon. Type II is more typical of the accessory navicular commonly seen and is characterized by a synchondrosis (Fig. 10-59A). Type III is a cornuate navicular (see discussion of os tibiale externum) (Fig. 10-59B). Lepore et al[232] stated that type I (a sesamoid within the posterior tibial tendon) occurs in 30% of cases, although Grogan et al[180] noted no occurrence in 25 patients (39 feet). Bareither et al[121] examined 165

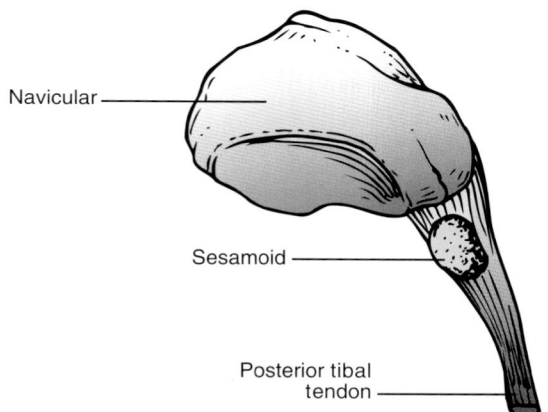

Figure 10-57 The posterior tibial tendon has a sesamoid in 23% of anatomic dissections.

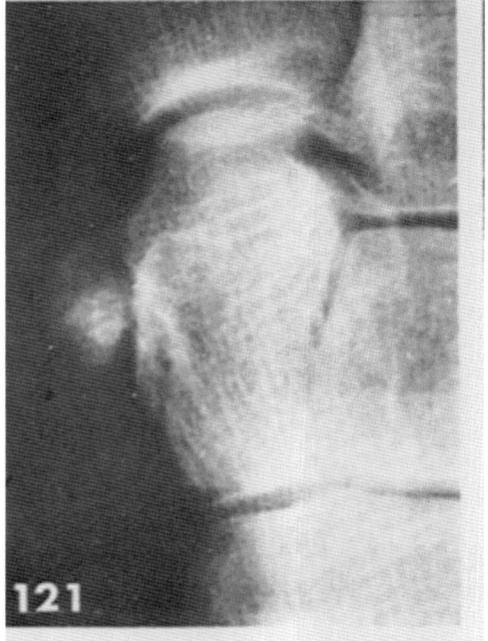

Figure 10-58 Sesamoid in the posterior tibial tendon.

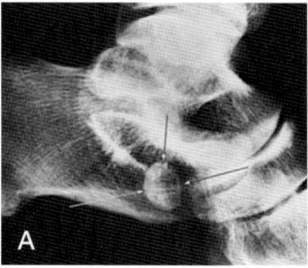 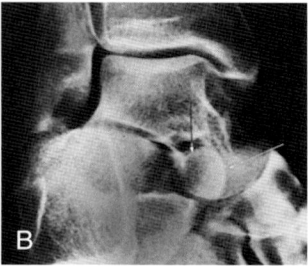

Figure 10-56 **A,** Lateral radiograph demonstrating large sesamoid in tibialis posterior tendon. **B,** Mortise view of the ankle demonstrating a sesamoid in the posterior tibial tendon. (From Keats TE: *Atlas of normal roentgen variants that simulate disease*, ed 4, St Louis, 1987, Mosby.)

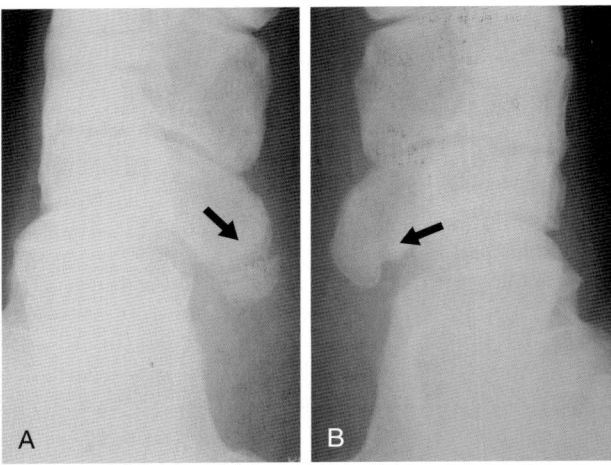

Figure 10-59 **A,** Type II accessory navicular with synchondrosis between the navicular and the accessory fragment. **B,** Type III accessory navicular with cornuate navicular. *Arrow* in both A and B denotes synchondrosis.

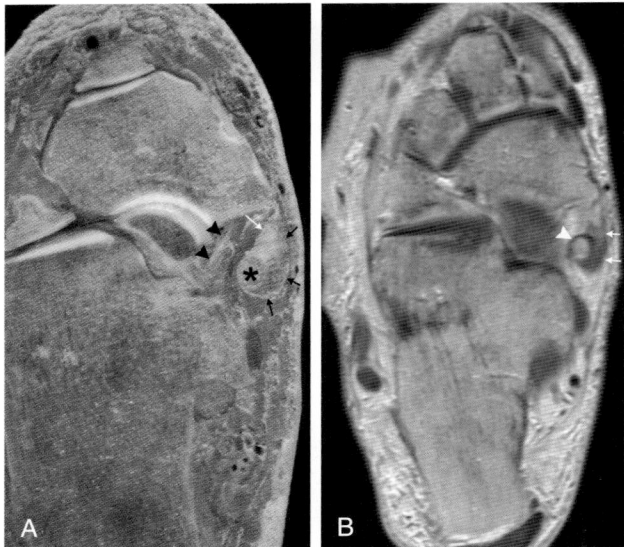

Figure 10-60 **A,** Anatomic cross section demonstrating sesamoid embedded in the posterior tibial tendon. *Arrowheads* denote synchondrosis. *denotes accessory navicular. *Small arrows* denote medial as part of accessory navicular. **B,** Magnetic resonance image demonstrating same cross section. (Courtesy A. Cotton.) *Arrows* denote accessory navicular.

cadavers. When the accessory bone was within the posterior tibial tendon (Fig. 10-60), it was separated from the navicular tuberosity by 3 to 6 mm. The accessory bone was completely or partially imbedded within the superior or deep portion, or both, of the posterior tibial tendon.

SESAMOID OF THE TIBIALIS ANTERIOR TENDON

The sesamoid of the tibialis anterior tendon is located within the substance of the tibialis anterior near the

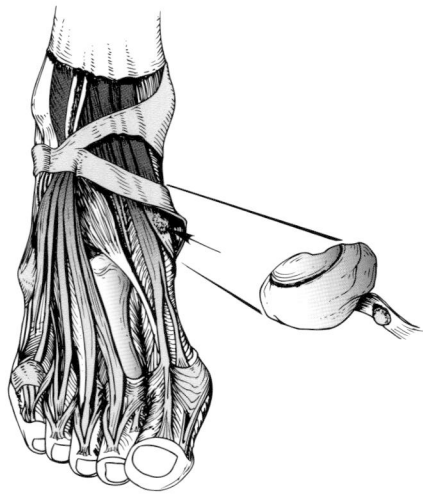

Figure 10-61 A sesamoid in the tibialis anterior tendon is located near the tendon insertion on the anterior inferior corner of the medial cuneiform.

insertion into the first cuneiform. The sesamoid lies on the anteroinferior corner of the medial surface of the first cuneiform and articulates with a facet on the medial surface of the medial cuneiform. Described by Zimmer,[335] its occurrence is very rare (Fig. 10-61).

The major clinical significance of this sesamoid is to differentiate it from a fracture on the medial aspect of the first cuneiform. A lack of tenderness in this region should alert the examiner to the possibility that this is a sesamoid within the tendon of the tibialis anterior.

OS PERONEUM

The sesamoid of the peroneus longus (the os peroneum) is located within the substance of the peroneus longus tendon and articulates with the lateral wall of the calcaneus, the calcaneocuboid joint articulation, or the inferior aspect of the cuboid in the region of the cuboid tunnel.[243,298] The sesamoid often lies where the tendon angles around the inferior cuboid on the plantar-lateral aspect of the foot (Fig. 10-62).

Sobel et al[298] described four soft tissue structures that stabilize the os peroneum: a cuboid band, a fifth metatarsal band, a plantar fascial band, and a band to the peroneus brevis, each of which attaches the sesamoid to those respective structures (Fig. 10-63). In the region of the lateral calcaneal wall, the sesamoid comes in contact with two osseous processes, the peroneal tubercle and the anterior calcaneal peroneal facet. The peroneus longus tendon is encompassed by a synovial sheath, which extends from a point proximal to the lateral malleolus to the region of the cuboid tunnel.

Sarrafian[281] notes that the sesamoid is always present but may be in an ossified, cartilaginous, or fibrocartilaginous state. Pfitzner,[269] in reporting on a series of anatomic dissections, noted its frequency to be 8.5%. Trolle,[311] in his histologic plus embryologic examination of 500 feet,

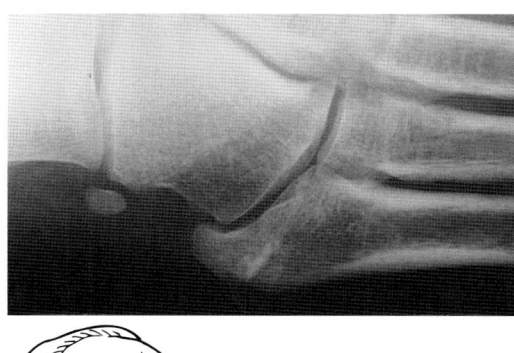

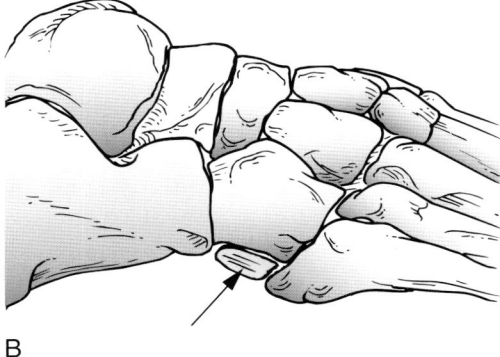

Figure 10-62 **A,** Radiograph demonstrating os peroneum. **B,** Os peroneum articulating with cuboid *(arrow)*. A more proximal location can denote a ruptured tendon.

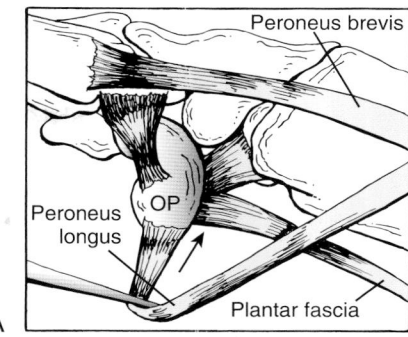

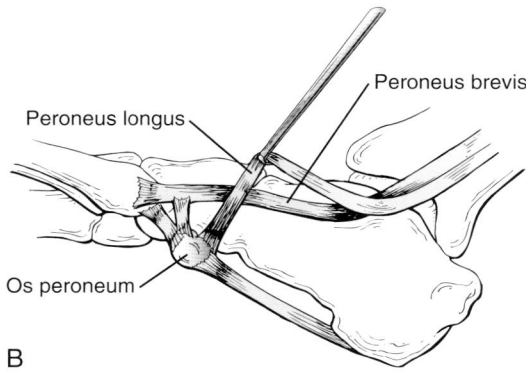

Figure 10-63 The os peroneum *(OP)* has four soft tissue attachments. **A** and **B,** The os peroneum is shown with its attachment to a plantar fascial band, a fifth metatarsal band, and a band to the peroneus brevis. The fourth band (not seen in this diagram) attaches the os peroneum to the cuboid. (Modified from Sobel M, Pavlov H, Geppert M, et al: Painful os peroneum syndrome: a spectrum of conditions responsible for plantar lateral foot pain, *Foot Ankle* 15: 112–124, 1994.)

noted the frequency to be 0.4%. Numerous radiographic studies have found the frequency to vary between 2.3% and 8.3%.* On anatomic dissection, the fully ossified os peroneum occurs in 20%, and the less-than-fully-ossified os peroneum occurs in 75%. The os peroneum may be multipartite, and this must be differentiated from an acute fracture.† A technetium bone scan may help to differentiate an acute injury[260]; an MRI may clearly define the disruption of the os perineum and tendon retraction.[132]

Occasionally, this sesamoid bone becomes symptomatic because of arthritic deterioration.[142] Osteochondritis dissecans of the os peroneum can lead to painful symptoms as well (Fig. 10-64).[208] Stropeni[301] published the first report of a fractured os perineum in 1920. Okazaki et al[260] have described a stress fracture of the os peroneum treated with excision and primary end-to-end repair (Fig. 10-65). Peterson and Stinson[268] reported on five patients with fractures through a bipartite (two feet) or multipartite (three feet). They were then treated with surgical excision of the os perineum and an in situ repair of the area of surgical excision. Thompson and Patterson[310] and others[127,132,236,264,265,324] have reported on the isolated rupture of the peroneus longus as demonstrated by the proximal migration of the os peroneum (Fig. 10-66) (see Chapter 24).

*References 114, 117, 129, 172, 193, 203, and 230.
†References 179, 199, 218, 238, 247, 265, 267, 307, 313, 324, and 329.

Clinical Significance

Awareness of the presence of the os peroneum can help the clinician to differentiate between a fracture and an accessory bone. Although this accessory bone is not common, the appearance on a radiograph of rounded edges can help to differentiate it from a fracture of the cuboid (Fig. 10-67). This accessory bone is often unilateral, and comparison films might not aid differentiating it from a fracture.

A painful os peroneum can present a diagnostic dilemma. Pain may be due to an acute fracture or disruption of a multipartite sesamoid, a chronic diastasis of a multipartite sesamoid, a degenerative tear of the peroneus longus distal or proximal to the os peroneum, an acute disruption of the peroneus longus tendon, or an enlarged peroneal tubercle (Fig. 10-68) that can entrap the peroneus longus tendon or os peroneum, limiting excursion.[298] Ruiz et al[279] described the major anatomic functions of the peroneal tubercle as providing an insertion of the inferior peroneal retinaculum, separating the tendons of the peroneus brevis and longus in a common peroneal tendon sheath and providing a fulcrum for excursion of the peroneal tendon. An enlarged

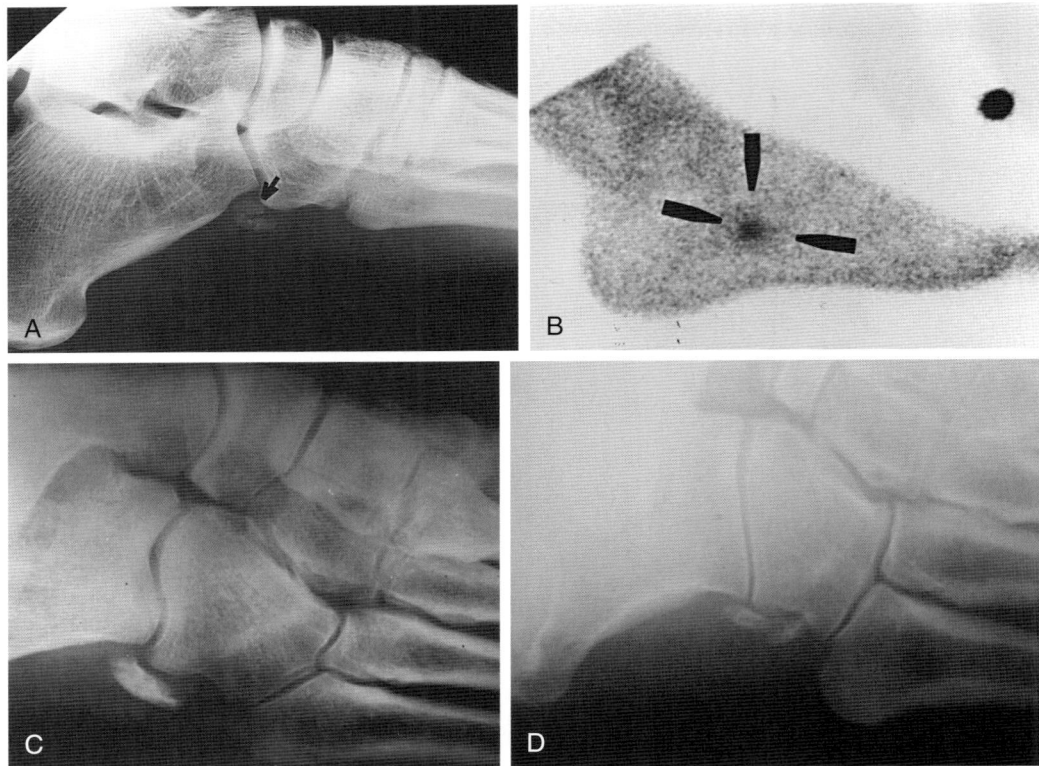

Figure 10-64 A, Osteochondritis of the sesamoid is demonstrated by fragmentation of the sesamoid. **B,** Technetium bone scan demonstrates increased uptake in the os peroneum. **C,** Osteochondritis of the os peroneum as demonstrated by a sclerotic appearance of sesamoid. **D,** Fracture of the os peroneum.

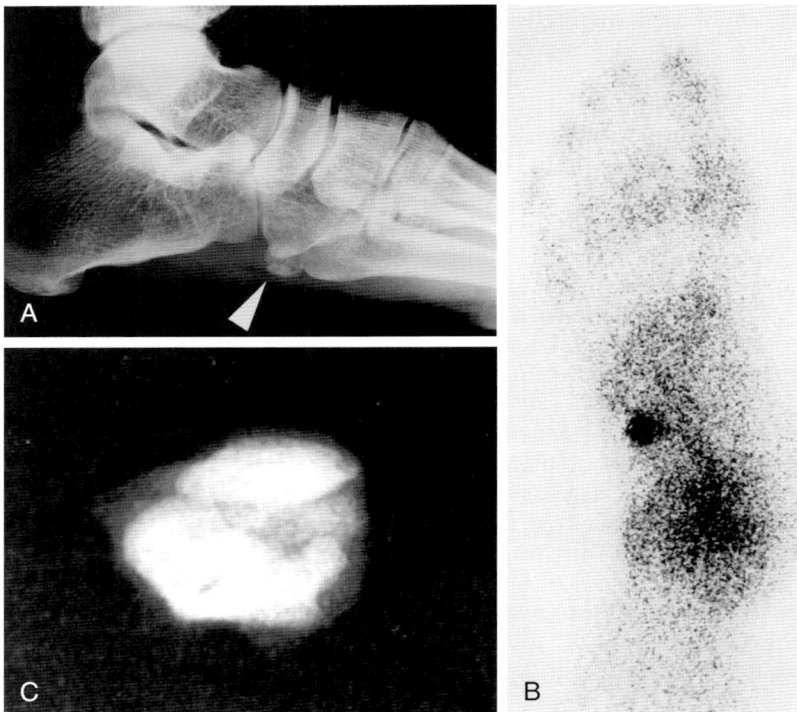

Figure 10-65 A, Lateral radiograph demonstrates fracture of the os peroneum. **B,** Increased uptake on bone scan. **C,** Radiograph of operative specimen demonstrating fractured os peroneum. (From Okazaki K, Nakashima S, Nomura S: Stress fracture of an os peroneum, *J Orthop Trauma* 17:654–656, 2003. Used with permission.)

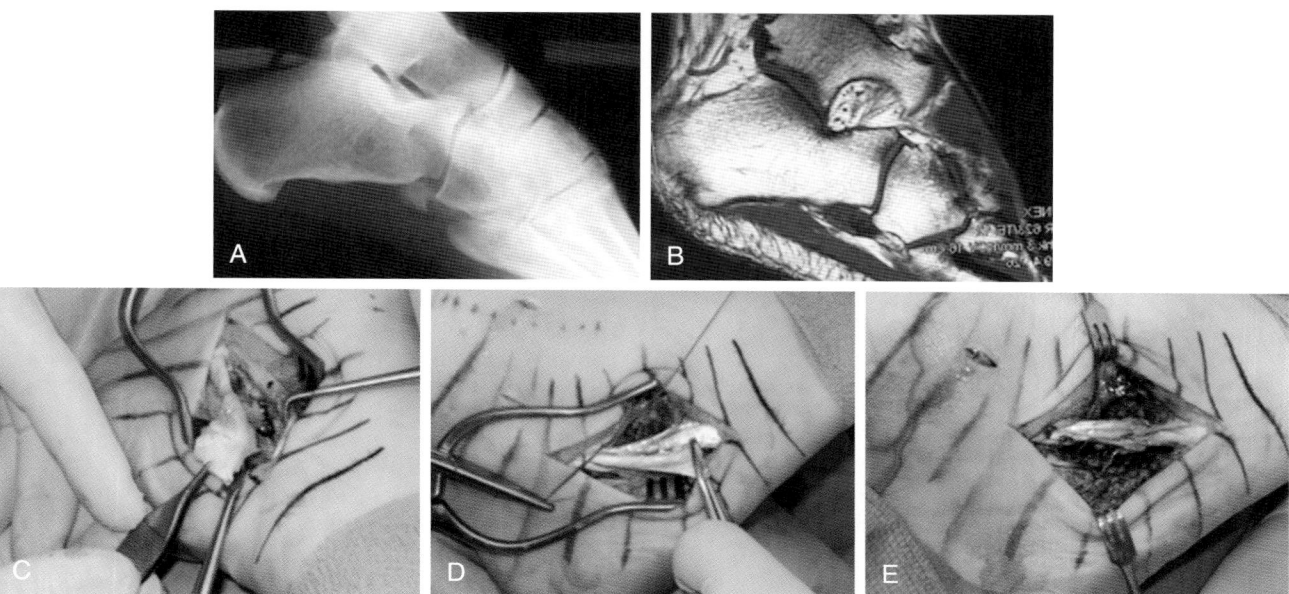

Figure 10-66 **A,** A 55-year-old woman with onset of pain on the lateral aspect of the foot and ankle, with os peroneum slightly proximal to the normal position. **B,** Magnetic resonance image of hindfoot demonstrating abnormality of the os peroneum. **C,** Intraoperative photograph demonstrating the os peroneum and discontinuity of the peroneus longus tendon. **D** and **E,** Tenodesis with Pulvertaft weave of the peroneus longus into the peroneus brevis tendon.

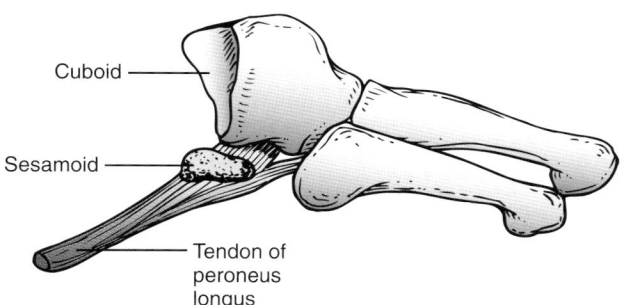

Figure 10-67 Storton[302] demonstrated a 26% incidence of an os peroneum on anatomic dissection.

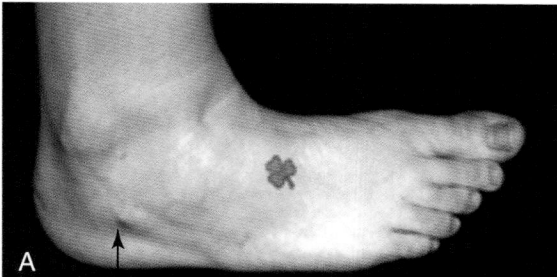

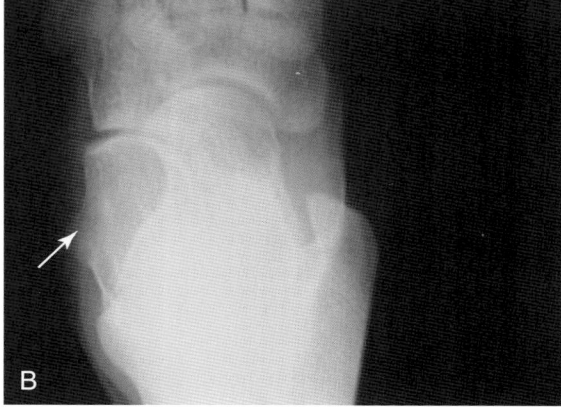

Figure 10-68 Clinical appearance **(A)** and radiographic appearance **(B)** of enlarged peroneal tubercle.

peroneal tubercle that entraps the peroneus longus tendon or os peroneum can lead to tenosynovitis[125,139,270] and require surgical excision. Berenter and Goldman[125] and Pierson and Inglis[270] described surgical resection to reduce the size of an enlarged and symptomatic peroneal tubercle.

When an os peroneum fractures, there may be disruption due to direct trauma, a violent muscle contraction, or an inversion injury associated with an ankle sprain.[126,267] Symptoms of edema and pain may be associated with either a partial or total rupture of the peroneus longus. Perlman[267] reported a case of an entrapped sural nerve associated with fracture of the os peroneum. With injury to the os peroneum and disruption of the peroneus longus at or distal to the sesamoid, proximal migration of the os peroneum or a fragment may be demonstrated on oblique radiograph[310,313] because of retraction of the tendon.[324]

Thompson and Patterson[310] reported a disruption of the peroneus longus tendon occurring distal to the os peroneum. Various treatment modalities include casting and nonsurgical treatment[127,199,236,264,313]; excision of the degenerated or fractured os perineum,[132,236,260] leaving the

533

tendon in continuity[179,267,329]; or excision and tendon repair or tenodesis with a disrupted peroneus longus (see Chapter 24).[265,310,324]

EXCISION OF THE OS PERONEUM AND TENODESIS OF THE PERONEUS LONGUS

1. The involved foot is exsanguinated, and a calf or thigh tourniquet is used for hemostasis. The foot is cleansed in the usual fashion.
2. A 4- to 6-cm longitudinal incision is centered over the lateral aspect of the cuboid and os peroneum.
3. Care is taken to identify and protect the sural nerve, which lies in close proximity to the peroneal tendon sheath.
4. The peroneus longus tendon is identified, and the os peroneum is excised. If the tendon is intact, the os peroneum may be excised and the tendon reinforced with interrupted sutures. If the tendon is ruptured and retracted, the os peroneum is excised.
5. A tenosynovectomy of the peroneus longus tendon sheath is performed.
6. The tendon sheath of the peroneus brevis is incised, and a tenodesis of the peroneus longus to the peroneus brevis is performed with the foot in dorsiflexion and eversion. The proximal segment of the peroneus longus is woven through the peroneus brevis with a Pulvertaft weave. Several interrupted nonabsorbable sutures are used to secure the tenodesis.
7. The tendon sheaths are left open to prevent constriction at the area of the tenodesis.
8. The wound is closed with interrupted sutures. Care is taken to protect the sural nerve.

Postoperative Care

A below-knee posterior splint is applied to immobilize the foot and ankle. The patient is permitted to ambulate in a non–weight-bearing cast for 2 weeks after surgery. Then a below-knee walking cast is applied, and the patient is allowed to ambulate with weight bearing, as tolerated, for 4 weeks. After this, a removable cast or ankle brace is used for another 4 weeks. Peroneal strengthening exercises are commenced after removal of the below-knee cast.

OS SUBTIBIALE

Anatomy and Incidence

The os subtibiale is located beneath the medial malleolus.* It is a rare accessory bone, appearing as a rounded, well-defined ossicle on the posterior aspect of the medial malleolus. In the younger patient, it is important to differentiate this accessory bone from a second ossification center of the medial malleolus.[202,274] Ossicles related to the anterior aspect of the medial malleolus are smaller;

---

*References 140, 166, 177, 226, 262, 280, 312, 320, 325, 327, and 333.

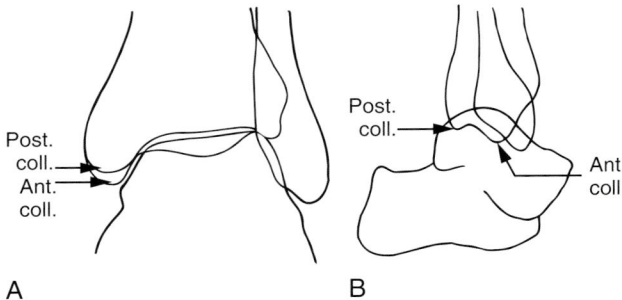

Figure 10-69 A, On an anteroposterior radiograph, the posterior colliculus is a flat line seen through the shadow of the more distal anterior colliculus. **B,** On a lateral radiograph, the anterior and posterior colliculi are seen in profile.

Coral[153,154] found them to be present in approximately 2.1% of ankle radiographs. He hypothesized that this anterior accessory bone represents an unfused secondary ossification center. Likewise, posttraumatic ossification might explain some of the other small accessory bones and less well-defined fragments in the area of the medial malleolus. Coral found accessory bones related to the medial malleolus in 4.6% of the 700 radiographs examined, but only one example was found of a true os subtibiale.

The os subtibiale was first described by Bircher in 1918,[311] and there have been isolated case reports of this accessory bone since that time. Arho[117] reported a 0.7% incidence of the os subtibiale, Holle[203] reported a 1.2% incidence, and Leimbach[230] reported a 0.2% incidence. In the area of the medial malleolus, a groove separates the anterior and posterior colliculi (Fig. 10-69). On an anteroposterior (AP) radiograph, the anterior colliculus is normally seen as the pointed tip of the medial malleolus because it extends more distally. The posterior colliculus is demonstrated as a sclerotic shadow overlying the anterior colliculus. A lateral radiograph demonstrates the anterior and posterior colliculi more clearly. Radiographs of the ankle can demonstrate abnormal ossification that may be accessory ossification centers, posttraumatic ossification, or avulsion fractures, and these should not be confused with an os subtibiale.

An accessory ossification center can occur at the distal tip of the medial malleolus (Fig. 10-70). Selby[289] evaluated serial radiographs in healthy children. He reported that in his series of 151 children, an accessory ossification center of the tip of the medial malleolus occurred more often in girls (47%) than in boys (17%). It typically appears during the 8th and 9th years (mean age for girls, 7.65 years; mean age for boys, 8.76 years). Bilaterality was reported in 90% of the girls but only 27% of the boys. The incorporation of the accessory ossification center with the medial malleolus is usually complete by the 11th year.

Powell,[273] in a radiographic study of 100 children (aged 6 to 12 years), found an accessory ossification center of the medial malleolus in 20% of cases. He also

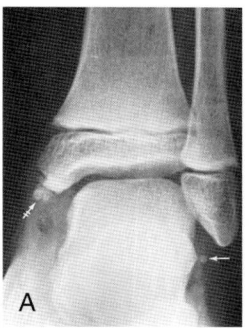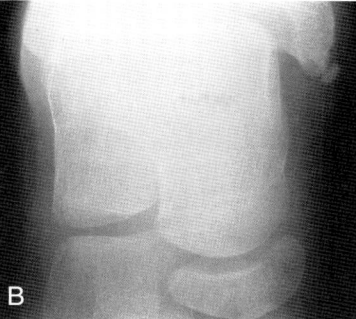

Figure 10-70 **A,** The secondary ossification center is seen at the tip of the medial malleolus. **B,** Secondary ossification center on anterior aspect of medial malleolus. (**A,** From Keats TE: *Atlas of normal roentgen variants that simulate disease*, ed 4, St Louis, 1987, Mosby.)

examined 50 adults with no previous ankle injury and found a 4% incidence of submalleolar ossicles.

In 1918, Bircher[311] described the os subtibiale as a large, rounded accessory bone with a well-defined cortex. Coral[153] reported a large os subtibiale with a diameter of 15 mm. He reported that the lateral radiograph showed this accessory bone and its relationship to the posterior colliculus. Coral[154] suggested that the characteristics of an os subtibiale are a rounded ossicle with a diameter greater than 4 mm and well-defined margins in relation to the posterior colliculus of the medial malleolus. If a rounded ossicle with well-defined margins is related to the anterior colliculus, one should suspect an unfused ossification center. An accessory bone with poorly defined margins in this region can suggest trauma and a partial or complete avulsion of the deltoid ligament.

Clinical Significance

The rounded nature of an accessory bone at the tip of the medial malleolus tends to indicate a chronic condition. Rarely is surgical excision indicated. The differentiation of an os subtibiale from an acute fracture is the major diagnostic objective, although it may be necessary to differentiate it from an unfused ossification center. The relationship to the anterior or posterior colliculus can help to differentiate an unfused ossification center from an os subtibiale. Even in the case of acute trauma overlying such an accessory bone, conservative treatment usually results in successful relief of symptoms.

OS SUBFIBULARE

Anatomy and Incidence

The os subfibulare is located beneath the lateral malleolus.* Trolle[311,312] suggested that this was a sesamoid within the peroneus longus tendon. It can be as large as 5 to

---

*References 178, 183, 239, 255, 262, and 327.

10 mm and is often well seen on an AP radiograph of the ankle joint. Trolle[311,312] reported its incidence as 0.2%, as did Leimbach,[230] who reviewed 500 radiographs of the ankle.

Abnormalities of the distal fibula, including the presence of an apophysis of the lateral malleolus are less commonly reported than those of the medial malleolus, according to Goedhard.[176] de Cuveland[158] described the apophysis of the lateral malleolus as lying anterior to the lateral malleolus (Fig. 10-71A). Goedhard[176] evaluated radiographs of 200 normal children aged 7 to 12 years to evaluate the apophysis of the lateral malleolus. He found four unilateral ununited apophyses and three bilateral ununited apophyses. He concluded that a contralateral radiograph is not necessarily helpful, because, in more than 50% of the cases, the apophysis was only unilateral. In adults, this apophysis is much less common.

Although the more common ununited apophysis is an oval accessory bone anterior to the tip of the fibula, a smaller accessory bone may be seen at the tip of the lateral malleolus (Fig. 10-71B). Bjornson[130] reported that it was rare that a persistent secondary center of ossification was present in the lateral malleolus. He noted that this persistent ossification center is quite different from the os subfibulare described by Leimbach.[230] Bowlus et al,[136] reporting on a review of 300 ankle radiographs, found 20 instances of os subfibulare, for an incidence of 6.67%. Maffulli et al[237] observed that it was one of the rarest accessory bones of the foot, and Shands and Wentz[292] reported it occurred in only two cases in 850 children (0.2%).

Bowlus et al[136] reported on two patients who presented with painful symptoms that required surgical excision. In both cases, the anterior talofibular ligament was attached to the ossicle. Mancuso et al[239] reported on a similar case of lateral ankle instability in which the anterior talofibular ligament inserted solely onto the os subfibulare. Surgical reconstruction of the lateral ankle reestablished ankle stability. The ossicle was differentiated from an avulsion fracture by its rounded, even appearance and well-defined cortical margins.

The os subfibulare is located posterior to the tip of the lateral malleolus and thus can be differentiated from the more anterior accessory ossification center (Fig. 10-71C, D, and E). Kohler and Zimmer[219] have reported several cases in adults. This accessory bone can be oval or elongated and can have a well-defined articulation with the lateral malleolus. It may be difficult to differentiate from a secondary ossification center or from a traumatic injury to the tip of the lateral malleolus. It should also be differentiated from other accessory bones on the lateral aspect of the hindfoot, such as a calcaneus secundarius and an os peroneum (see Fig. 10-62).

Champagne et al[148] had suggested the os subfibulare is contained in the tendon of the peroneal tendons based on their anatomic dissection, although most others consider the os subfibulare to be intimately associated with the distal fibula. Callanan et al[144] have described an

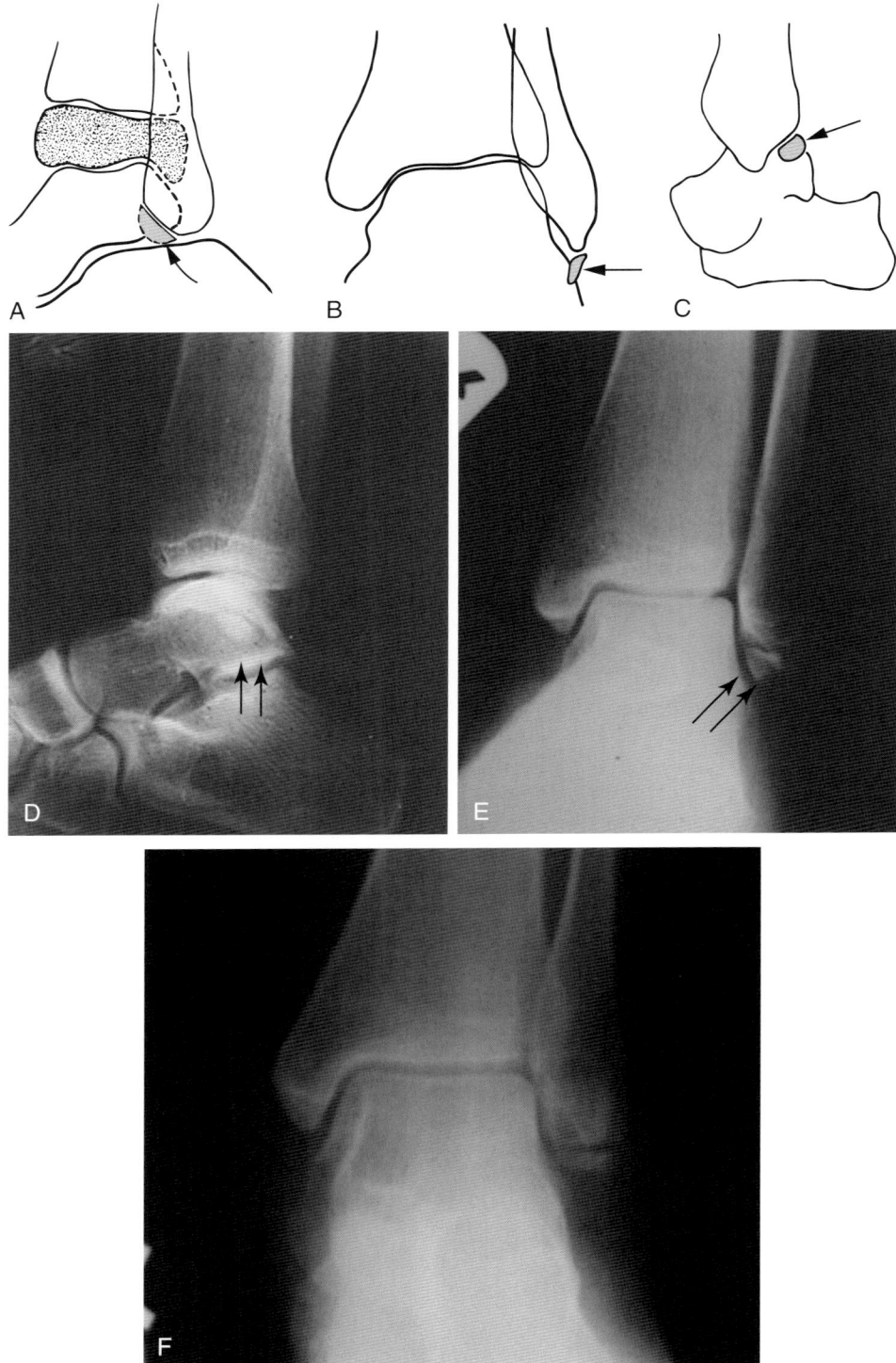

Figure 10-71 A, The more frequent ununited apophysis is seen on the anterior aspect of the distal fibula. **B,** Another accessory bone at the tip of the fibula. **C,** A true os subfibulare is located on the posterior aspect of the lateral malleolus. **D,** Lateral radiograph of ununited apophysis. **E,** True os subfibulare *(arrows).* **F,** Anteroposterior radiograph of another os subfibulare.

accessory bone on the lateral aspect of the subtalar joint, heretofore unreported, that might have been secondary to trauma or actually a true accessory subtalar ossicle.

Clinical Significance

Usually, the rounded nature of an accessory bone at the tip of the lateral malleolus indicates a chronic condition. Rarely is surgical excision indicated. Differentiation of an os subfibulare from acute trauma is a major diagnostic goal, and a bone scan may be helpful if trauma is suspected. Even in the case of acute trauma overlying an accessory bone, conservative treatment usually alleviates the symptoms.

Gruber[182] described an accessory bone in the area of the distal third of the fibula that he termed the *os retinaculi* (Fig. 10-72). This bone is found overlying the bursa of the lateral malleolus in the area of the peroneal retinaculum. This is typically a flat bone that is visible on an AP radiograph of the ankle. Although extremely rare, it should be differentiated from an accessory ossification center or trauma.

OS TRIGONUM

Anatomy and Incidence

The os trigonum was first described by Rosenmuller.[278] In 1822, Shepherd[294] described it as a fracture of the posterolateral tubercle of the talus. The os trigonum varies greatly in size and shape and appears at the posterior

process of the talus (Fig. 10-73).* It may be an actual part of the body of the talus or develop as a separate bone that may or may not be adherent to the talus by a cartilaginous articulation.

Typically, the ossicle is asymptomatic and detected only during routine radiographic examination. Often mistaken as a fracture of the posterior process of the talus,

---

*References 113, 117, 123, 124, 125, 131, 140, 165, 166, 172, 188, 190, 193, 194, 201-203, 228, 234, 248, 258, 262, 263, 269, 278, 303, 315, 322, 324, 327, and 330.

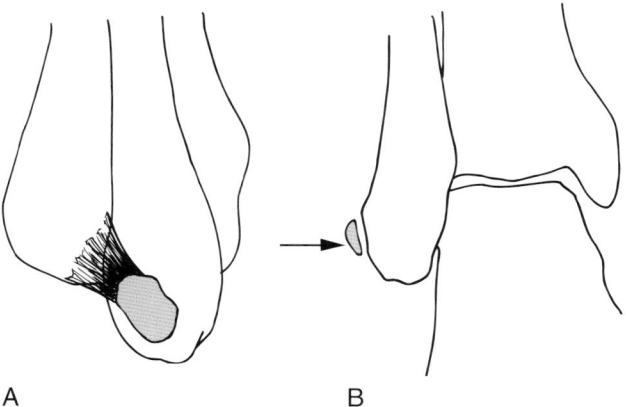

A   B

Figure 10-72   A, The os retinaculi is situated over the area of the bursa overlying the fibular malleolus. **B,** On the anteroposterior view, the os retinaculi is seen in profile.

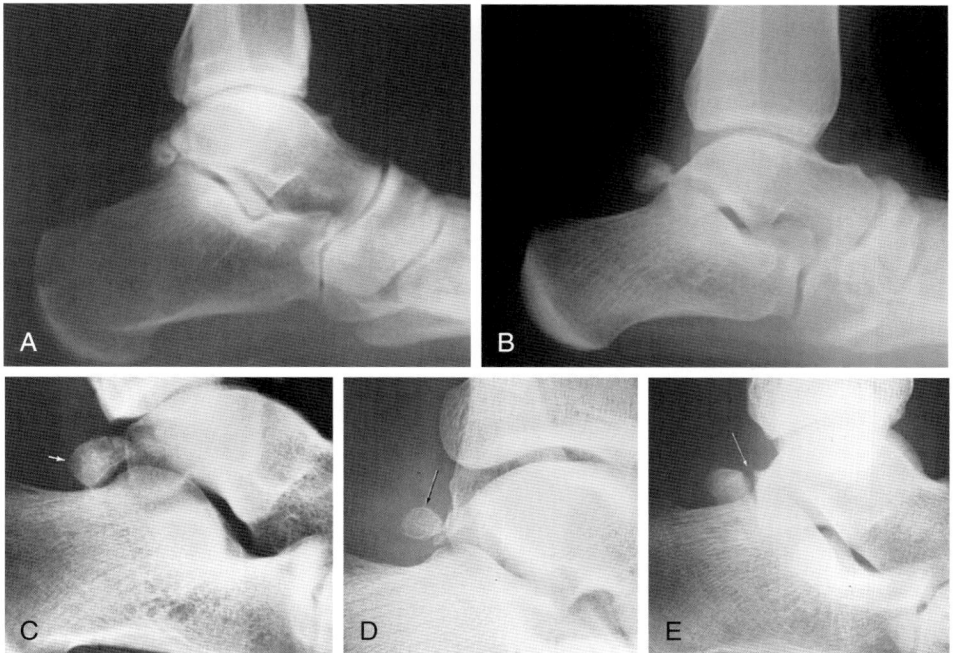

Figure 10-73   Variations in the os trigonum. **A,** This appearance may be mistaken for a fracture. **B-E,** Varying sizes and shapes of the os trigonum. (**C, D,** and **E,** From Keats TE: *Atlas of normal roentgen variants that simulate disease,* ed 4, St Louis, 1987, Mosby.)

it arises as a separate ossification center and appears between 8 and 11 years of age.[250] It is present in 1.7% to 7% of radiographs of normal feet.[129] Ossicles that are separated from the talus can become painful on plantar flexion of the foot. Distinguishing between an articulating ossicle and a fracture of the posterior process of the talus can be difficult (Fig. 10-74).

According to Mann and Owsley,[242] there was no apparent side predominance, and the lateral tubercle of the talus varied greatly in size. A free os trigonum probably represents a normal anatomic variant resulting from an unfused secondary center of ossification. The lateral tuberosity of the talus varies from a mild extension behind the posterior tubercle to an elongated thumb-shaped projection (the Stieda process) that could reach 1 cm in length, and the accessory bone occurs just lateral to the talar groove of the flexor hallucis longus tendon (Fig. 10-75).

Clinical Significance

The os trigonum can cause pain in the retrocalcaneal space; the pain is aggravated on walking and especially when the foot is placed in plantar flexion (Fig. 10-76). The os trigonum syndrome usually affects young athletes, such as ballerinas, and others whose activities involve forced plantar flexion. This forced plantar flexion can lead to a fracture of the trigonal process of the talus or impingement of the os trigonum against the posterior tibial plafond. Flexor hallucis longus tendinitis can develop because the tendon and tendon sheath can become inflamed secondary to compression in this region. When pressure is applied with the thumb and index finger

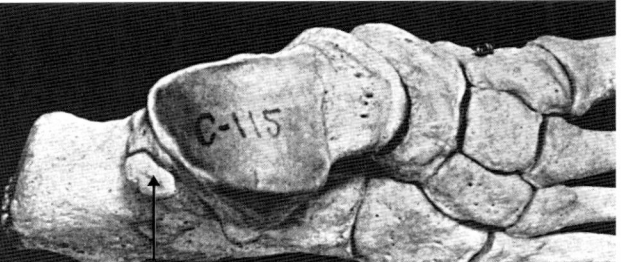
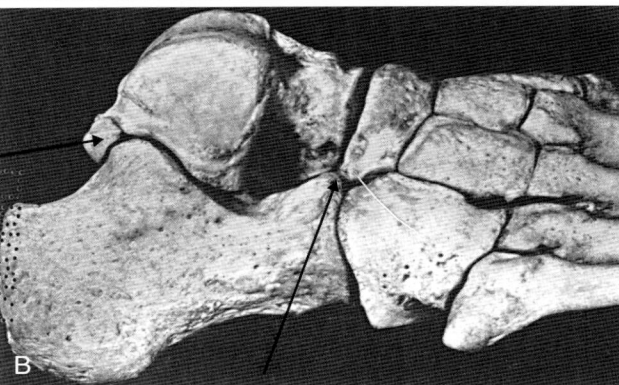

Figure 10-74 Calcaneus secundarius is demonstrated. **A,** Dorsal view demonstrating os trigonum. **B,** Lateral anatomic specimen demonstrating os trigonum. (**B,** From Dwight T: *Clinical atlas of variations of the bones of the hand and foot,* Philadelphia, 1907, JB Lippincott.)

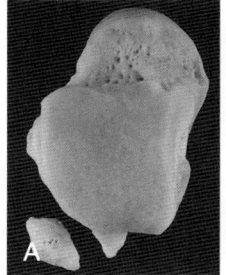
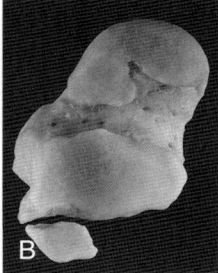
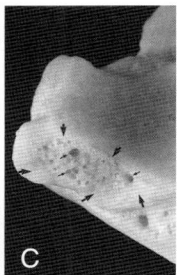

Figure 10-75 Os trigonum. **A,** Dorsal view of the left talus and free os trigonum (33-year-old white man). **B,** Plantar view of the left talus and free os trigonum. **C,** Semilunar concavity for attachment of the os trigonum (photograph taken posterolaterally). (Courtesy Robert Mann, PhD.)

Figure 10-76 Dorsal view of talus and os trigonum. *1,* Dorsal talar articular surface; *2,* os trigonum; *3,* articular interface of os trigonum; *4,* articulated os trigonum.

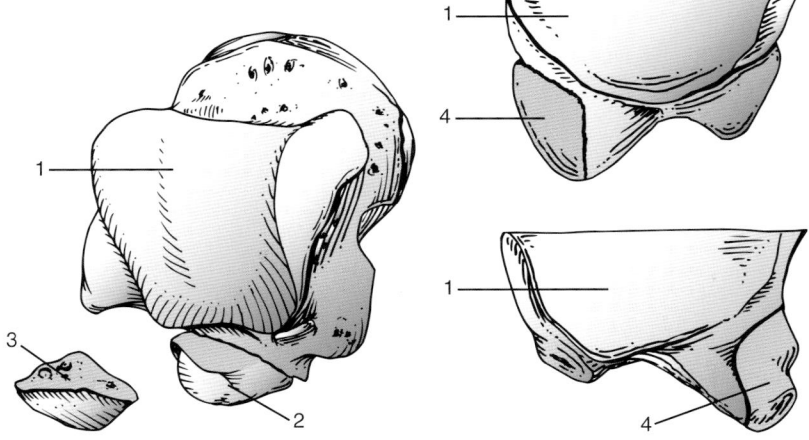

against the posterior lip of the talus, pain may be exacerbated.

Except with a sudden fracture of the os trigonum (the Shepherd fracture),[294,295] the onset of symptoms is typically gradual. The symptoms can become worse, and the condition must be differentiated from retrocalcaneal bursitis. Likewise, differentiation must be made from a fracture of the posterior facet of the talus.[328] Giuffrida et al[175] have reported six cases of a fracture of the posterior talus, several of which were misdiagnosed. A subtalar dislocation occurred with these injuries; the authors stressed that a CT scan helps to differentiate an os trigonum from a posterior process fracture. Also, with accompanying swelling and substantial pain, there should be a high index of suspicion for a talar fracture and subtalar subluxation.

With retrocalcaneal bursitis, the symptoms are acute and are generally associated with swelling and tenderness overlying the retrocalcaneal space just posterior to the insertion of the Achilles tendon instead of at the anterior

aspect of the retrocalcaneal space. Symptomatic cases can require removal of the os trigonum.

Conservative Treatment

Conservative treatment includes reduced range of motion and limitation of activity, casting,[131] and nonsteroidal antiinflammatory medications. Local steroid injection is generally discouraged because it can lead to a tendon rupture.[246]

Karasick and Schweitzer[211] have stated that pain can develop as a result of disruption of the cartilaginous synchondrosis between the os trigonum and the lateral talar tubercle. Also, part of the differential diagnosis is flexor hallucis longus tenosynovitis.

Wakeley et al[322] demonstrated that MRI was helpful in evaluating the cause of painful os trigonum syndrome. An os trigonum should be differentiated from a bipartite talus (Fig. 10-77).[285] On occasion, differentiation between

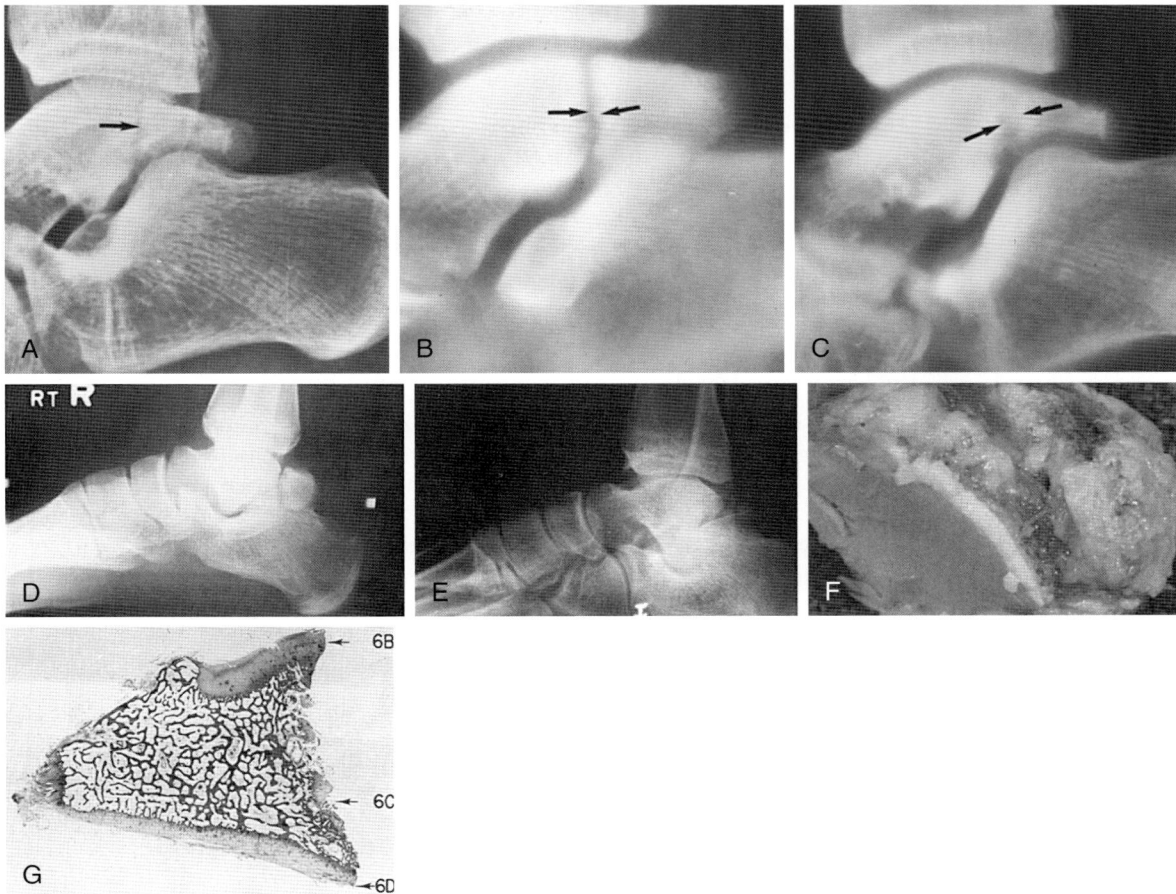

Figure 10-77 **A,** Lateral radiograph demonstrating talus partitus. This unusual anomaly is not a true os trigonum and should be appreciated and differentiated from a fracture. **B** and **C,** Tomograms of right ankle. **D,** A similar radiograph demonstrating talus partitus. **E,** Postoperative radiograph after resection of talus partitus. **F,** Surgical specimen after removal. **G,** Pathologic sectioning of resected fragment. (**A-C,** From Schreiber A, Differding P, Zollinger H: Talus partitus. A case report, *J Bone Joint Surg Br* 67:430–431, 1985. **D-G,** From Weinstein S, Bonfiglio M: Unusual accessory (bipartite) talus simulating fracture. A case report, *J Bone Joint Surg Am* 57:1161–1163, 1975.)

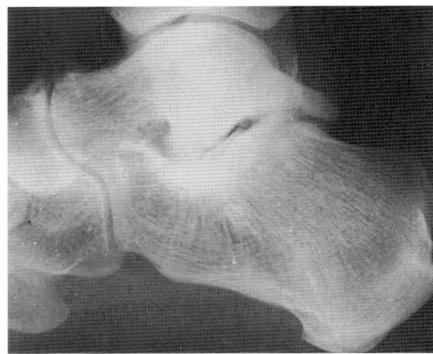

Figure 10-78 Os trigonum as an actual part of the posterior talus.

a large os trigonum and a bipartite talus[309] or talus partitus[164] may be difficult (Fig. 10-78).

Surgical Treatment (Video Clip 15)

A painful os trigonum may be approached through a medial exposure[131,190,330] or a lateral exposure.[112,131]

REMOVAL OF THE OS TRIGONUM (LATERAL APPROACH)
Surgical Technique
1. A thigh tourniquet is applied with the patient carefully positioned in a lateral decubitus position. The foot and lower part of the leg are cleansed and draped in the usual fashion.
2. A longitudinal incision approximately 5 cm in length is made over the retrocalcaneal space posterior to the distal aspect of the fibula.
3. The skin is retracted and the fascia incised. Care is taken to protect the sural nerve. The anterior margin of the fascia will be contiguous with the sheath of the peroneal tendons, which are readily retracted to expose the retrocalcaneal space.
4. The os trigonum is denuded of all attachments. A separated os trigonum can usually be delivered in one piece from the wound. An ossified os trigonum may be resected with an osteotome.
5. The remaining articular surface is smoothed with a rongeur and rasp.
6. The tendon of the flexor hallucis longus is inspected.
7. The fascia and skin are closed in layers.

Postoperative Care
A compression dressing is applied, and the patient ambulates with crutches. Touch-down weight bearing is allowed. Usually full weight bearing is tolerated within 1 week after surgery. Immobilization is usually discontinued 3 weeks after surgery.

Results
Wredmark et al[330] reported on a series of ballerinas treated for symptoms of impingement pain in the hindfoot with plantar flexion of the ankle. Surgery involved excision of the os trigonum or prominent lateral posterior process with division of the flexor hallucis longus tendon sheath. On physical examination, deep palpation in the posterior ankle region elicited pain, although only one third of patients complained of pain with passive plantar flexion. They positioned the patient supine and used a medial approach with a 5-cm vertical incision anterior to the Achilles tendon. The neurovascular bundle was identified and retracted. The tendon sheath of the flexor hallucis longus was incised longitudinally. The os trigonum was identified and excised. In half of the cases, a thickening of the flexor hallucis longus tendon or tendon sheath was observed, and the tendon sheath was released. No casting was used, and rehabilitation was started immediately with non–weight-bearing range of motion for 2 weeks. They recommended the medial approach because of the common finding of flexor hallucis longus tendon disease.

Marotta and Micheli[246] reported on 16 patients who underwent excision of an os trigonum through a posterolateral approach. Preoperative symptoms included pain localized to the posterior ankle, limitation of ankle motion, weakness, swelling, or neurologic changes associated with athletic activity. Eight of 16 still had occasional symptoms, and the postoperative recovery time averaged 3 months. Marotta and Micheli stated that this condition is twice as common unilaterally as bilaterally. Differential diagnosis included peroneal tendinitis, Achilles tendinitis, retrocalcaneal bursitis, ankle joint arthritis, or an acute fracture of the talar tuberosity.

Hedrick and McBryde[190] reported on 30 cases of os trigonum, all developing after plantar flexion injury. An os trigonum was present in 63% of cases, and an intact posterior process was symptomatic in 36%. Some 60% of cases were treated nonoperatively, and 40% required operative excision.

Abramowitz et al[112] reported on 41 patients who failed conservative treatment and underwent os trigonum excision through a lateral approach. At an average follow-up of 41 months, they reported a ligh level of patient satisfaction. Those patients who underwent surgery within 2 years of the onset of symptoms have a higher level of success than those with longer-term symptoms. Sural nerve dysfunction postoperatively was noted in 8 of 41 patients, although symptoms were temporary in 50% of patients.

Eichenbaum, Austin, and Raiken[164] reported on two cases of talus partitus. One was successfully resected; however, in the case of a very large fragment, they performed an excision of the large posterior fragment and a primary subtalar arthrodesis.

OS CALCANEUS SECUNDARIUS

Anatomy and Incidence

The os calcaneus secundarius is located on the dorsal beak of the calcaneus in an interval between the

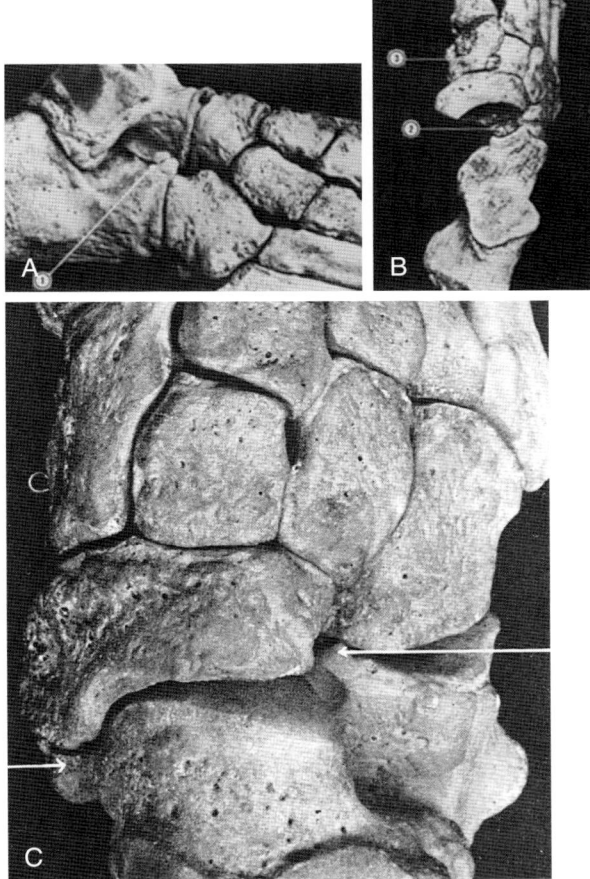

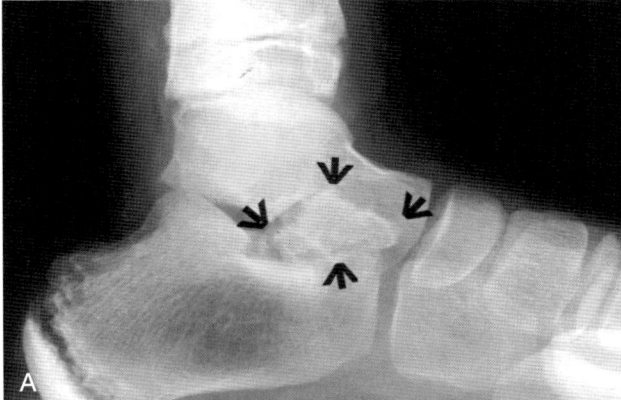

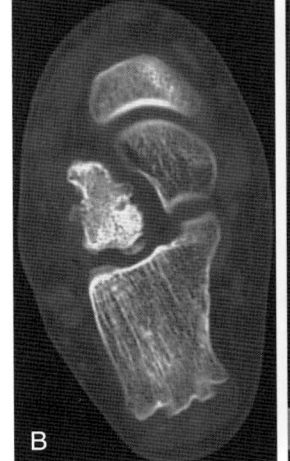

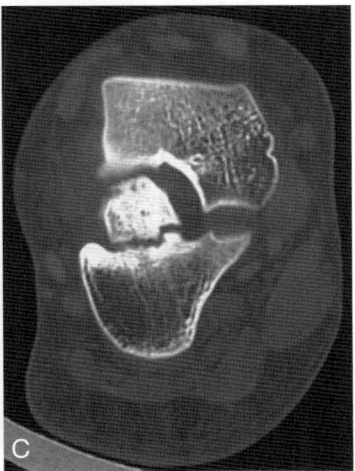

Figure 10-79 **A,** Os calcaneus secundarius, lateral view. **B,** Os calcaneus secondarius, oblique view. An os intercuneiforme is also present. **C,** Enlarged tuberosity or fused os calcaneus secondarius. This borders on being a tarsal coalition and can result in decreased subtalar motion. (From Dwight T: *Clinical atlas of variations of the bones of the hand and foot,* Philadelphia, 1907, JB Lippincott.)

Figure 10-80 Large os calcaneus secundarius. **A,** Lateral radiograph. **B** and **C,** Appearance on computed tomography examination. Restricted subtalar motion preoperatively was dramatically improved after resection. (The os calcaneus secundarius demonstrated here did not involve either the anterior or posterior subtalar facets.)

anteromedial aspect of the os calcis, the proximal aspect of the cuboid and navicular, and the head of the talus (see Fig. 10-68).* It can be round or triangular (Fig. 10-79), is typically 3 to 4 mm in diameter, and is visible on a lateral oblique radiograph of the hindfoot.

First described by Stieda,[300] the earliest known specimen of a calcaneus secundarius was reported by Holland[202] to have been found in a mummy from Thebes. Pfitzner[269] reported the first comprehensive anatomic study, and it was Dwight,[163] in 1907, who first referred to this accessory bone as the os calcaneus secundarius. Mann and Owsley[240,241] studied anatomic collections and found the incidence in early twentieth-century U.S. samples to be approximately 2%, whereas the incidence for more prehistoric groups was approximately 4.4% (Fig. 10-80). Its reported incidence in radiographic and anatomic studies varies: anatomic, 3.1% (Pfitzner[269]); anatomic (Stieda[300]), 2.5%; radiographic (Geist[172]), 2%; radiographic (Holle[203]), 1.7%; radiographic (Arho[117]), 1%; radiographic (Bizarro[129]), 1%; radiographic (Leimbach[230]), 0.4% (Fig. 10-81); and histoembryologic examination (Trolle[311]), 0%. Hoerr et al[198] evaluated radiographs in adolescents and found this accessory bone to be more frequent in boys (7%-11%) than in girls (6%-7%).

Geist[172] noted this condition to be extremely rare and observed that the calcaneus secundarius can simulate a fracture of the beak of the calcaneus. Other conditions to be differentiated are a tarsal coalition or a fibrous tarsal coalition.[186]

Clinical Significance

Differentiation of an os calcaneus secundarius from an acute fracture of the tuberosity of the calcaneus is the main objective (Fig. 10-82).[196] Some patients complain of

---

*References 115, 128, 140, 147, 166, 212, 218, 224, 225, 253, 288, and 327.

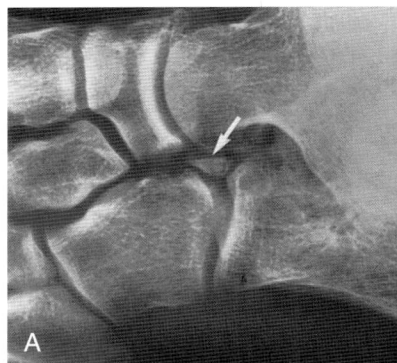

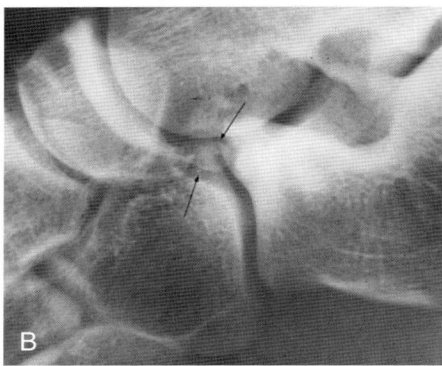

Figure 10-81 **A,** Oblique radiograph demonstrating a small os calcaneus secundarius. **B,** Lateral radiograph demonstrating a small calcaneus secundarius. (From Keats TE: *Atlas of normal roentgen variants that simulate disease,* ed 4, St Louis, 1987, Mosby.)

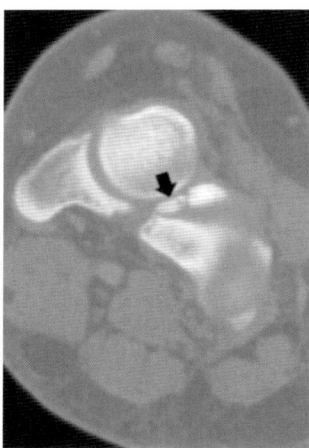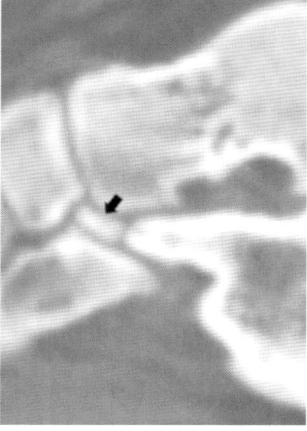

Figure 10-82 Computed tomographic scan demonstrates an os calcaneus secundarius. (From Stauss J, Connolly L, Perez-Rossello J, Treves S: Skeletal scintigraphy of possible os calcaneus secundarius, *Clin Nucl Med* 28:424–425, 2003. Used with permission.)

restricted subtalar motion and pain localized to this region (Fig. 10-83). Differentiation from a partial or fibrous calcaneonavicular coalition must be made as well because both may be associated with restricted hindfoot motion (Fig. 10-84). Wagner[321] reported excision of the

anterior tuberosity of the calcaneus for chronic pain. Krida[221] reported a case of excision of an os calcaneus secundarius for pain, with a successful outcome. The differentiation of a fracture of the anterior tuberosity of the calcaneus[223] from an os calcaneus secundarius may be delineated by a bone scan. Viana et al[318] have decribed an os talus secundarius, which may also be confused with an os calcaneus secundarius (Fig. 10-85). Callanan et al[144] have described an accessory bone in the sinus tarsi, which may be secondary to trauma or an atypical os calcaneus secundarius (Fig. 10-86).

CALCANEUS ACCESSORIUS

Anatomy and Incidence

The calcaneus accessorius was first described by Pfitzner.[269] This accessory bone approximates the trochlear process of the calcaneus on the fibular aspect just distal to the fibular malleolus.[197,202,253] At its largest extent, it is approximately 5 mm in diameter. This has also been referred to as the "os talocalcaneare laterale" by O'Rahilly (Fig. 10-87A).[262] Because it is a very rare accessory bone,[281] Trolle[311] is the only one to note its incidence and reported its incidence in his histoembryologic examination as 0.6%. He observed that it is rarely larger than "the size of a pea."

In 1860, Hyrtl[311] first described an enlarged calcaneal tuberosity in this area as the processus trochlearis (Fig. 10-87B). It had been seen radiographically on a dorsoplantar view of the foot with the ankle in hyperextension.

Clinical Significance

The calcaneus accessorius must be differentiated from an os subfibulare or an avulsion fracture. A bone scan can be used to differentiate a fracture from a calcaneus accessorius. Uhrbrand and Jensen[316] reported a large calcaneus accessorius that became symptomatic in a 5-year-old boy. This led to varus malalignment of the hindfoot, and the enlarged bone was excised with excellent results.

OS SUSTENTACULI

Anatomy and Incidence

The os sustentaculi is located on the posterior aspect of the sustentaculum tali (Fig. 10-88).* Pfitzner[269] first described this accessory bone. He noted that it occurred in less than 1% of cases and observed that it is often connected by a fibrocartilaginous or fibrous tissue interface with the sustentaculum. Neither Dwight[161] nor Trolle[311] reported this as a separate accessory bone. Holle[203] described its incidence as 1.5% in a review of 1000 radiographs. Hoerr et al[198] reported that 2% to 3% of boys and

*References 128, 133, 141, 202, 245, 252, and 262.

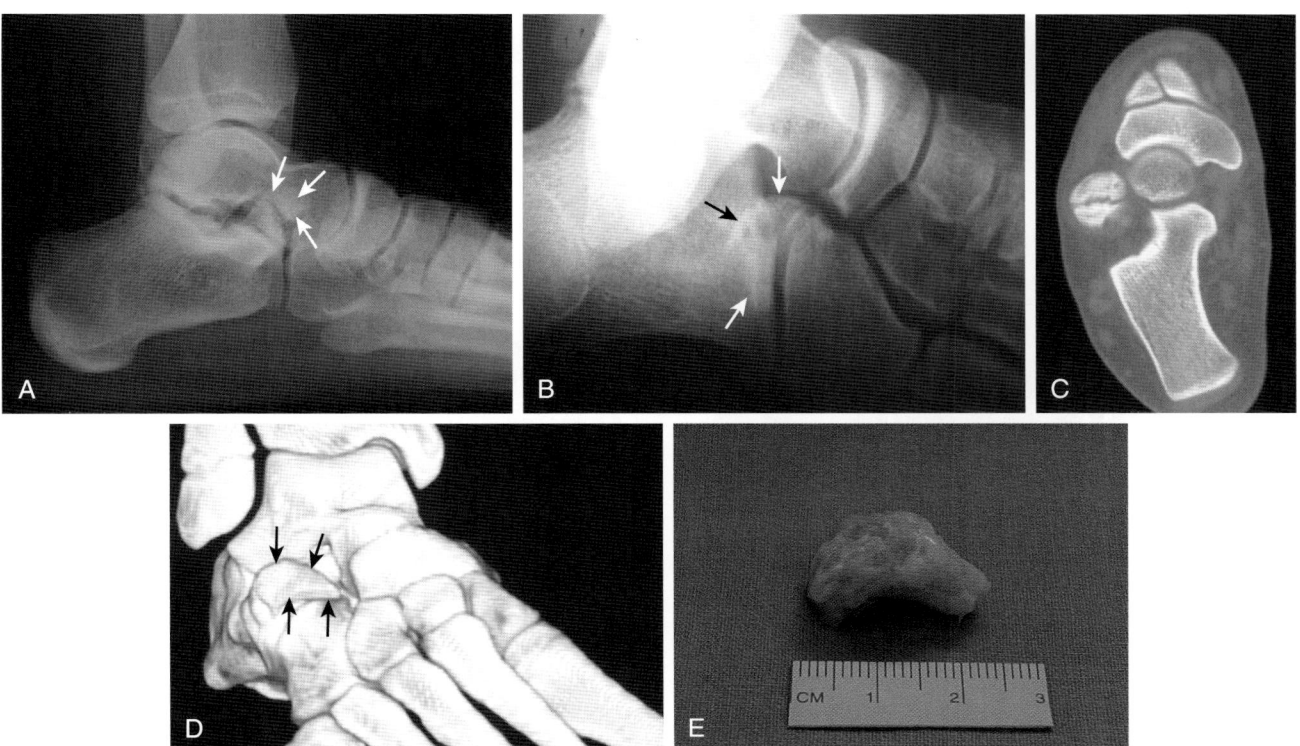

Figure 10-83 Os calcaneus secundarius. **A,** Lateral radiograph with osseous structure distinct from distal aspect of calcaneus (*arrows* encircle the os calcaneus secundarius). **B,** Oblique view of foot. A calcaneonavicular coalition is not seen; however, there is a bony formation present, overlying the anterior process of the calcaneus (*arrows* encircle the os calcaneus secundarius). **C,** Computed tomography (CT) scan showing a large accessory ossicle. **D,** Three-dimensional CT scan showing the os calcaneus secundarius (*arrows*) on the anterior aspect of the calcaneus. **E,** Excised os calcaneus secundarius. (From Ceroni D, De Coulon G, Spadola L, et al: Calcaneus secundarius presenting as calcaneonavicular coalition: a case report, *J Foot Ankle Surg* 45:25–27, 2006. Used with permission.)

0% of girls presented with this accessory bone in his radiographic review of 501 patients.

Clinical Significance

The os sustentaculi (Fig. 10-89), which is found on the medial aspect of the calcaneus, should be differentiated from the calcaneus accessorius, which is found on the lateral aspect of the talocalcaneal articulation. Harris and Beath[187] suggested that an os sustentaculi may be associated with a tarsal coalition and peroneal spastic flatfoot. Its presence may be demonstrated on routine radiography (Fig. 10-90). A CT scan of the hindfoot can help to differentiate this accessory bone from a tarsal coalition (Fig. 10-91). A tarsal coalition can require surgical intervention, whereas an os sustentaculi rarely requires surgical excision.

OS SUBCALCIS AND OS APONEUROSIS PLANTARIS

Anatomy and Incidence

Accessory bones on the plantar aspect of the calcaneus include the os subcalcis[311] (Fig. 10-92) and the os aponeurosis plantaris (Fig. 10-93).[143] O'Rahilly[262] described an accessory bone in the plantar aponeurosis close to but not adjoining the medial tubercle of the calcaneus. This should be differentiated from a calcaneal spur or a fracture of a calcaneal spur. The os aponeurosis plantaris lies enclosed in the plantar aponeurosis and can vary significantly in size. It is usually oblong and flat and can best be seen in a lateral radiograph. The os subcalcis is found on the plantar aspect of the calcaneus slightly posterior to the insertion of the plantar fascia. This bone can reach a diameter of 10 mm. There is no reported incidence of either bone.

Clinical Significance

It may be necessary to differentiate an os subcalcis from a traumatic fracture. Rarely is surgery indicated for either of these conditions unless they are associated with chronic intractable pain.

OS CUBOIDES SECUNDARIUM

Anatomy and Incidence

The os cuboides secundarium is a rare ossicle located between the calcaneus, talus, navicular, and cuboid

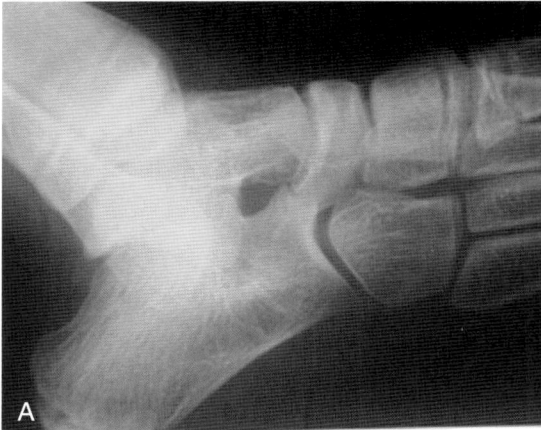

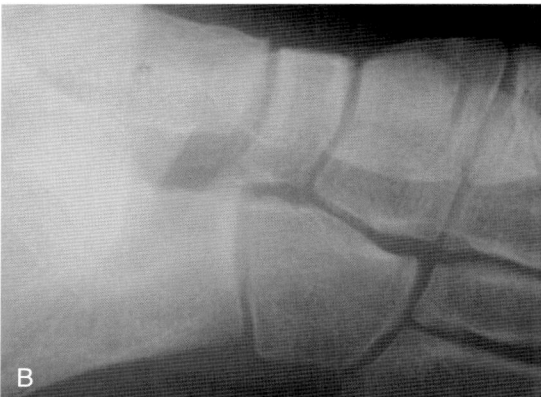

Figure 10-84 A complete **(A)** and partial **(B)** calcaneonavicular coalition must be differentiated from the os calcaneus secundarius.

(Fig. 10-94).* Located on the plantar aspect of the foot, it was first described by Pfitzner,[269] who recognized it as occurring in two different locations: fused with the cuboid and articulating with the talus (Fig. 10-95A) and fused with the navicular and articulating with the talus (Fig. 10-95B and C). This ossicle can be as large as 5 to 10 mm and is seen radiographically in both a dorsoplantar and a lateral oblique view. Although Pfitzner[269] and Dwight[161] reported the occurrence of this accessory bone, Hoerr et al,[198] in their evaluation of radiographs in 501 adolescent feet, noted this accessory bone occurred in 1% to 3% of adolescents (see Fig. 10-87D and E). Gaulke et al[171] described the excision of this bone in a 9-year-old boy and found the accessory bone bisected the tendon of the flexor digitorum brevis (Fig. 10-96).

Clinical Significance

Most commonly, this ossicle is asymptomatic and is indeed difficult to visualize on routine radiographs. Logan et al[235] demonstrated this accessory bone on both

*References 128, 161, 163, 202, 210, 311, 327, and 334.

CT scan and MRI as well. In general, it is uncommon for this accessory bone to be symptomatic.

This is a rare bone of doubtful clinical significance, except in the differentiation of it from a fracture. Although it has been suggested that an os cuboides secundarium might represent a variant of a cubonavicular coalition, the CT scan and MRI performed by Logan et al[235] demonstrated no coalition of the cuboid, the navicular, or the os cuboides secundarium.

OS TALONAVICULARE DORSALE, OS SUPRATALARE

Anatomy and Incidence

The os talonaviculare dorsale (Fig. 10-97) (also known as the Pirie bone, os supranaviculare, talonavicular ossicle, os supratalare) refers to accessory bones of varying size and shape in the area of the talonavicular joint. Pirie[271,272] reported 14 cases of an os talonaviculare dorsale, 4 of which were bilateral. Pfitzner[269] hypothesized that this accessory bone was really an avulsed exostosis. Hoerr et al,[198] in a radiographic study of 134 adolescents, reported a 15% incidence of this accessory bone in boys and an 11% incidence in girls (Figs. 10-98 and 10-99).

Osteoarthritic degeneration (Fig. 10-100) of the talonavicular joint should be differentiated from this accessory bone. The ossicle may be fused with the talus or with the navicular. The os supratalare (talus secundarius) is located on the dorsum of the talus between the ankle and talonavicular joints and may be fused with the talus or remain as a free accessory bone. It is rarely larger than 4 mm.

Clinical Significance

Accessory bones in the area of the talonavicular joint are uncommon. They should be differentiated from degenerative arthritic spurs, avulsion fractures, or other traumatic conditions. Miller and Black[256] reported a case of impingement of the deep peroneal nerve resulting from an os supranaviculare, which was treated with surgical excision. In an exploration of this area, a surgeon must protect the deep peroneal nerve and dorsalis pedis artery and vein during the dissection.

When acute pain has developed in this region, a bone scan can help to differentiate one of these accessory ossicles from an acute injury.

ACCESSORY NAVICULAR

Anatomy and Incidence

In 1605, Bauhin[172] first described the accessory navicular. Since that time, numerous names have been suggested in the literature for this accessory bone, including accessory scaphoid, accessory navicular, prehallux, and os tibiale

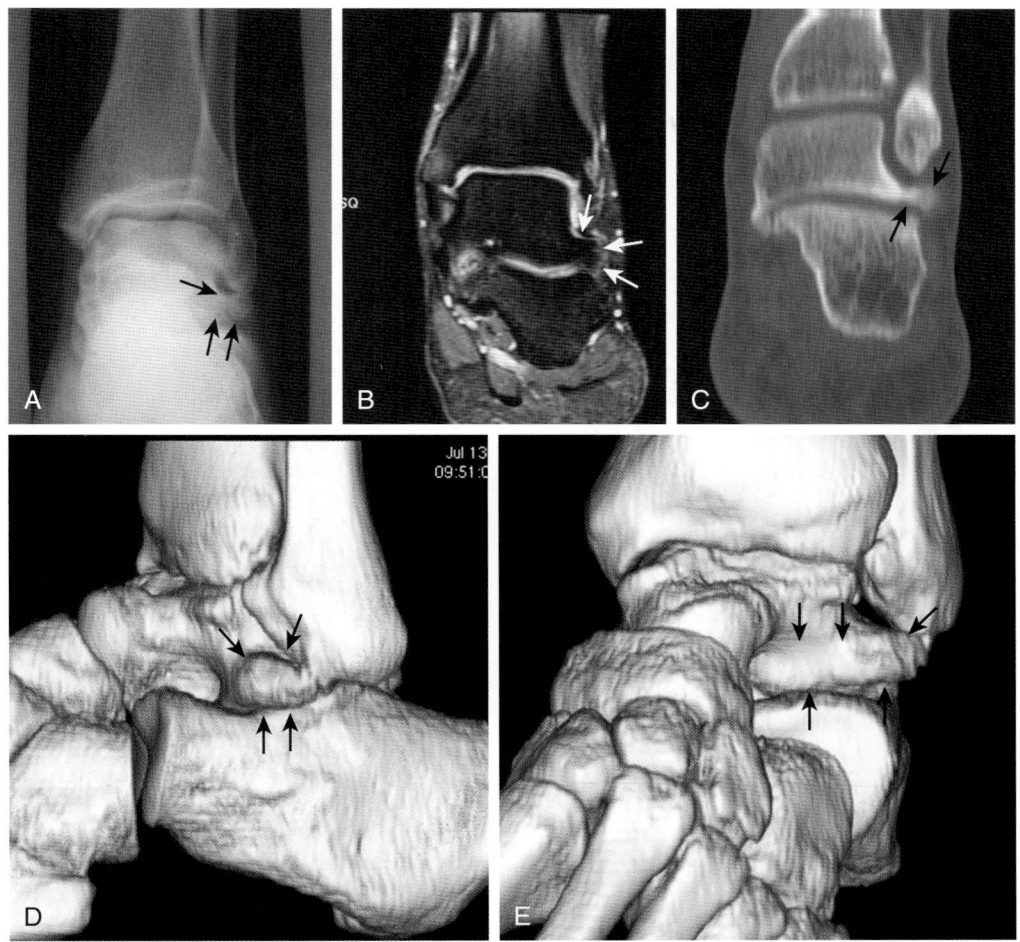

Figure 10-85 Os talus secundarius (see *arrows* in **A, B, C,** and **D**). **A,** Anteroposterior radiograph showing lateral talar exostosis. **B,** Coronal plane magnetic resonance imaging and, **C,** computed tomography (CT) scan demonstrating bony projection from lateral aspect of talus. **D** and **E,** Reconstruction CT scans showing articulation between os talus secundarius and lateral malleolus. (From Viana SL, Fernandes JL, Mendonca JL, Freitas FM: Painful os talus secundarius: a case report and imaging findings, *Foot Ankle Int* 28:624–625, 2007. Used with permission.)

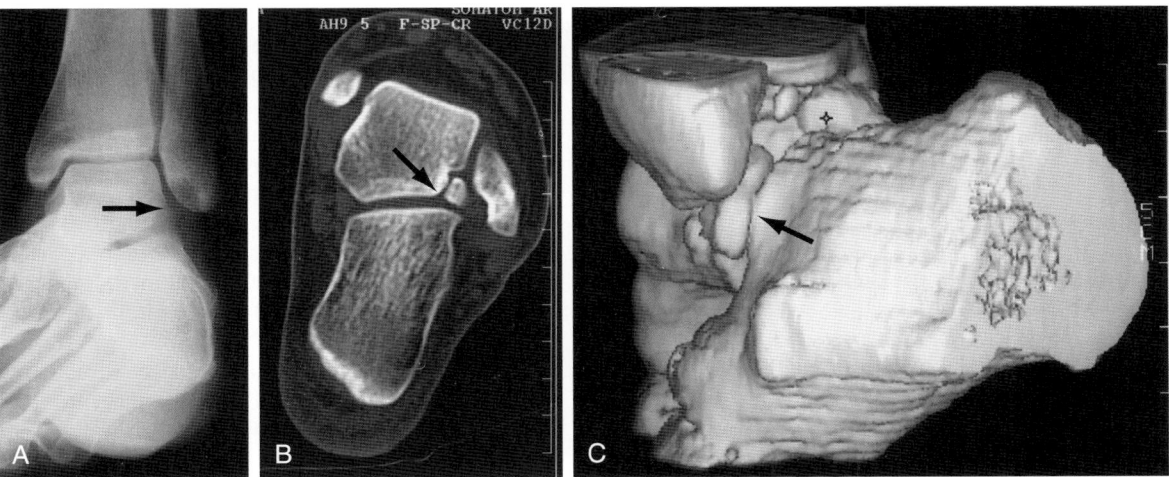

Figure 10-86 **A,** Normal anteroposterior radiograph of ankle (*arrow* points to true accessory bone). **B,** Axial computed tomography (CT) scan demonstrating accessory ossicle (*arrow*) in sinus tarsi. **C,** Reconstruction CT demonstrating what may be an old fracture of a true accessory bone (*arrow*). (From Callanan I, Williams L, Stephens M: *Foot Ankle Int* 19:475–478, 1998. Used with permission.)

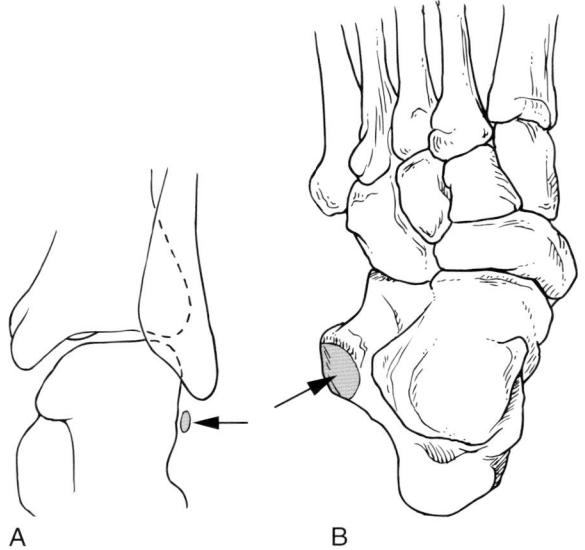

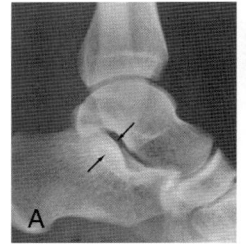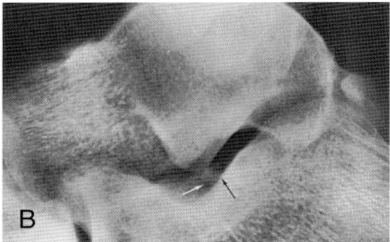

Figure 10-89 **A** and **B,** Two examples of the os sustentaculi seen in lateral projections simulating a fracture of the articular surface of the calcaneus. (From Keats TE: *Atlas of normal roentgen variants that simulate disease,* ed 4, St Louis, 1987, Mosby.)

Figure 10-87 **A,** The calcaneus accessorius is located just to the lateral aspect of the trochlear process of the calcaneus *(arrow).* **B,** The trochlear process of the calcaneus *(arrow)* may be enlarged and occasionally symptomatic.

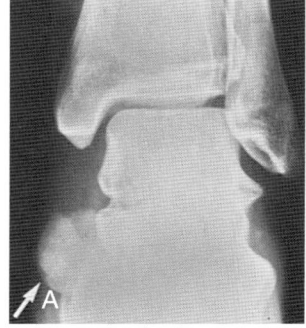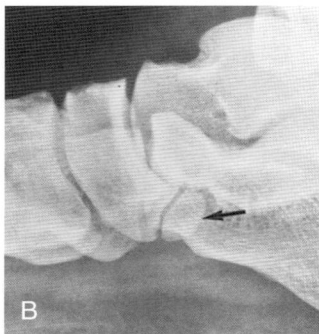

Figure 10-90 Os sustentaculi. This accessory bone is found at the posterior aspect of the sustentaculum tali on the superior aspect. **A,** Anteroposterior projection. **B,** Lateral projection. This anomalous bone may be incorporated in an accessory joint between the sustentaculum tali and the talus. (From March HC, London RI: The os sustentaculi, *AJR Am J Roentgenol* 76:1114–1118, 1956.)

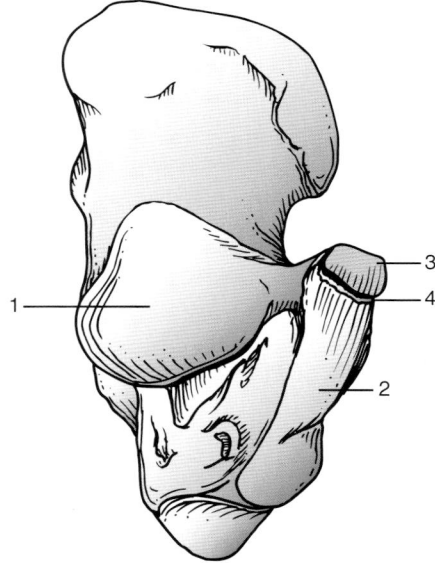

Figure 10-88 Os sustentaculi. *1,* The posterior facet of the calcaneus; *2,* the sustentaculum tali, *3,* os sustentaculi; *4,* fibrocartilaginous interface between the sustentaculum tali and os sustentaculi.

navicular.* Geist[173] reported a 14% incidence of this ossicle in supposedly normal feet, and Harris and Beath[186] reported a 4% incidence in young men; however, other authors have reported a varying frequency of occurrence. In radiographic evaluations, Hoerr et al,[198] in a study of 501 adolescents, showed an incidence of 3% to 8% in girls and 4% to 9% in boys; Bizarro[129] reported a 2% incidence, and Holland[202] demonstrated a 10% to 12% incidence. Pfitzner,[269] in an anatomic study of 425 feet, reported an 11.5% incidence, and Dwight,[163] in an anatomic study, reported a 10% incidence of an accessory navicular. Trolle,[311] in a histoembryologic study, noted a 6.4% incidence. McKusick[251] lists an accessory navicular as being inherited as an autosomal dominant trait and reports an incidence of 5%. Kiter et al[216] have suggested the accessory navicular is inherited as an autosomal dominant trait with incomplete penetrance.

*References 116, 117, 121, 128, 134, 155, 165-167, 180, 184, 185, 189, 193, 200, 201, 210, 228, 232, 234, 244, 257, 258, 263, 266, 282, 290, 304, 308, 317, 323, 327, and 334.

externum.[276] Grogan et al[180] have stated that up to 13% of the population might have an accessory navicular.

An accessory navicular is a congenital anomaly in which the tuberosity of the navicular develops from a secondary center of ossification. It is located on the medial aspect of the arch in association with the

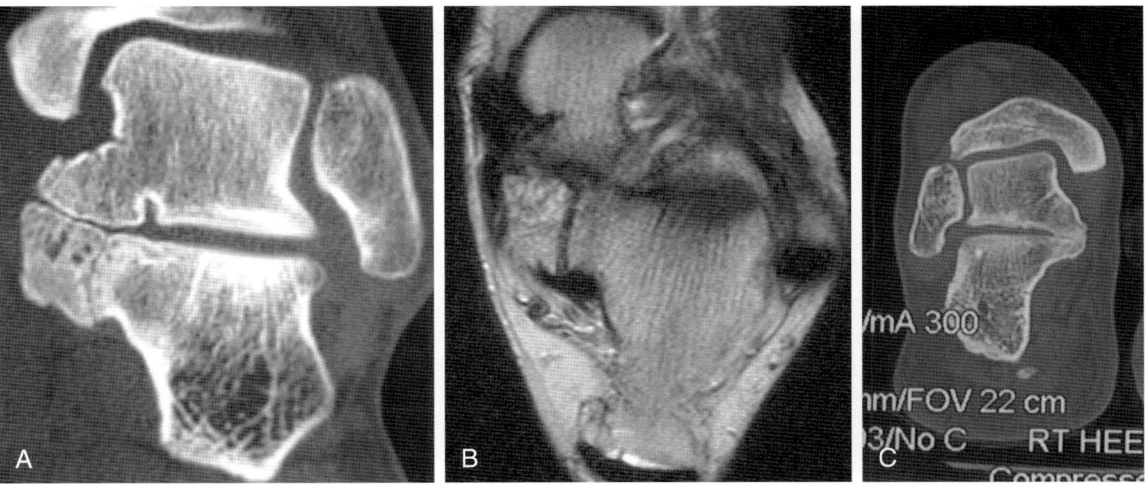

Figure 10-91 **A** and **B,** Axial scans demonstrating os sustentaculi. **C,** Talocalcaneal coalition should be differentiated from an os sustentaculi. (**A** and **B,** From Mellado J, Salvado E, Camins A, et al: Painful os sustentaculi: imaging findings of another symptomatic skeletal variant, *Skeletal Radiol* 31:53–56, 2002. Used with permission.)

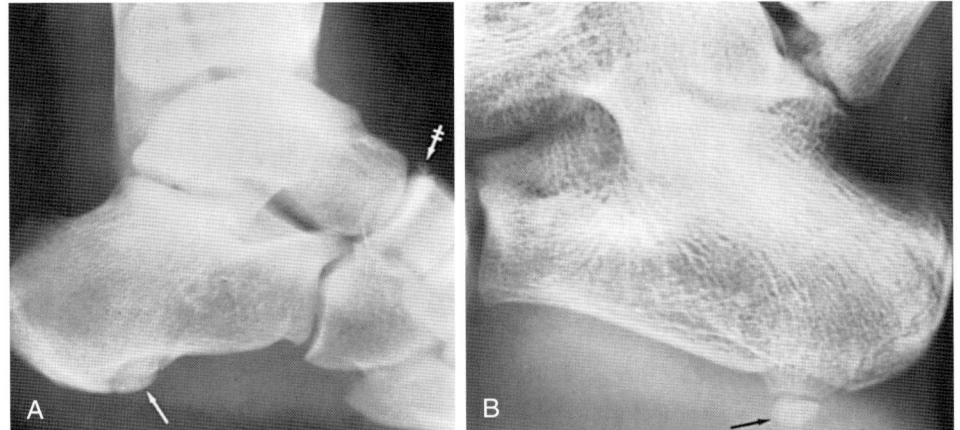

Figure 10-92 **A** and **B,** The os subcalcis occurs beneath the body of the calcaneus. (From Keats TE: *Atlas of normal roentgen variants that simulate disease,* ed 4, St Louis, 1987, Mosby.)

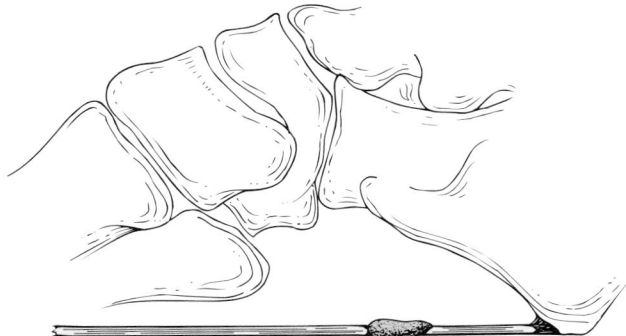

Figure 10-93 The os aponeurosis plantaris is oblong and flat and can vary significantly in size.

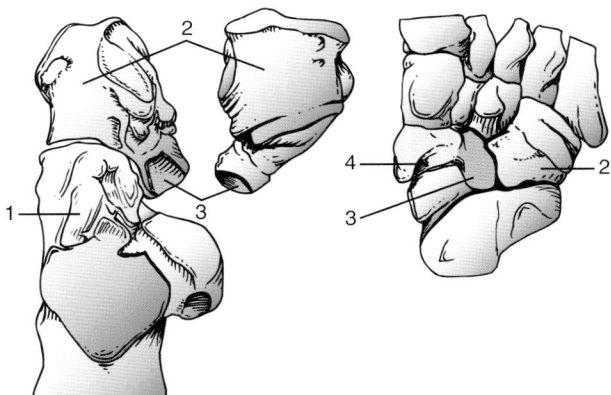

Figure 10-94 The os cuboides secundarium. *1,* The calcaneus; *2,* the cuboid; *3,* the os cuboides secundarium; *4,* the navicular.

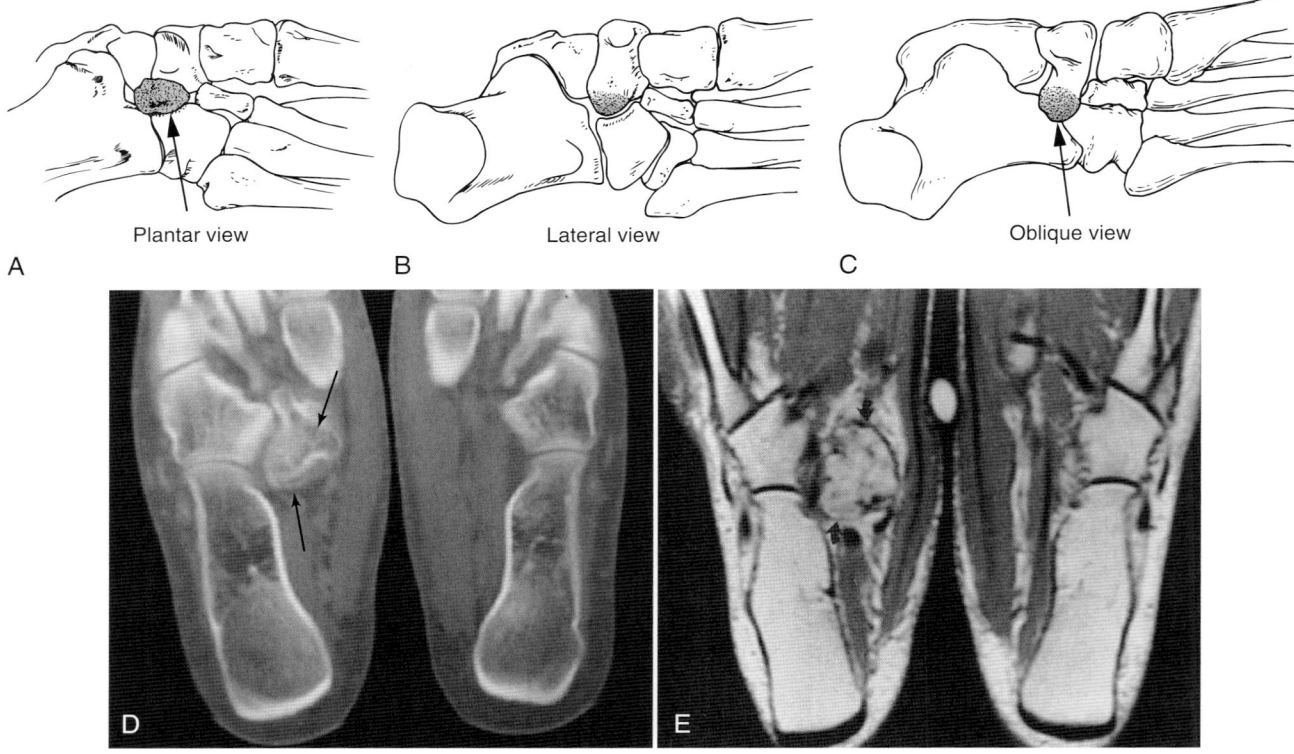

Figure 10-95 **A,** Os cuboides secundarium articulating with the cuboid and calcaneus (plantar view). **B** and **C,** Os cuboides secundarium arising from the navicular. **D,** Transverse computed tomography scan demonstrates os cuboides secundarium *(arrows).* **E,** Magnetic resonance imaging demonstrates bowing of the abductor hallucis adjacent to the os cuboides secundarium *(arrows).* (**D** and **E,** Courtesy M. Logan, MD.)

Figure 10-96 Lateral **(A)** and anteroposterior **(B)** radiographs and close-up view **(C)** demonstrating large os cuboides secundarium *(arrows).* (From Gaulke R, Schmitz H: Free os cuboideum secundarium: a case report, *J Foot Ankle Surg* 42:230–234, 2003. Used with permission.)

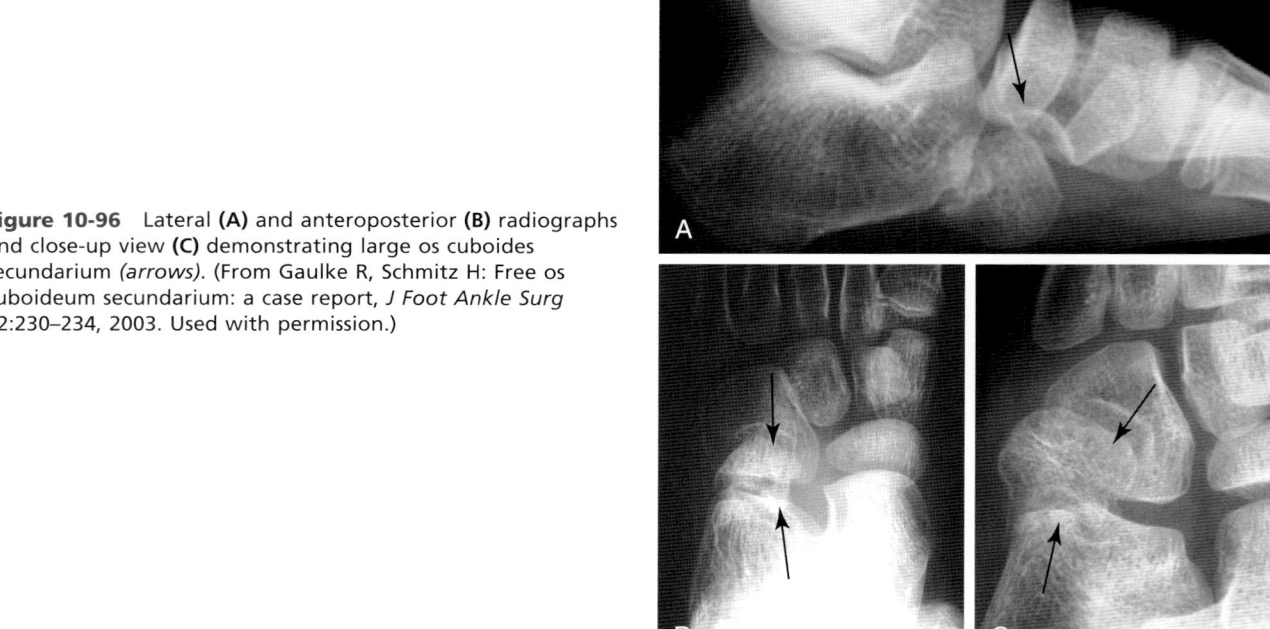

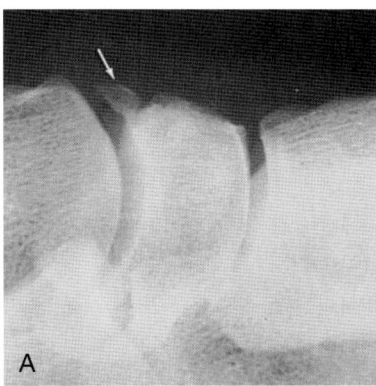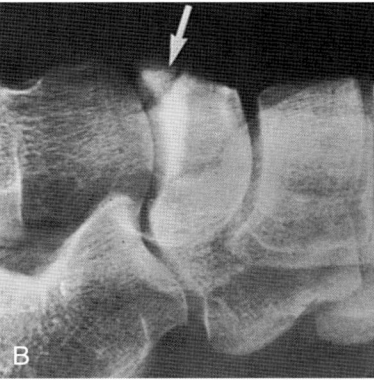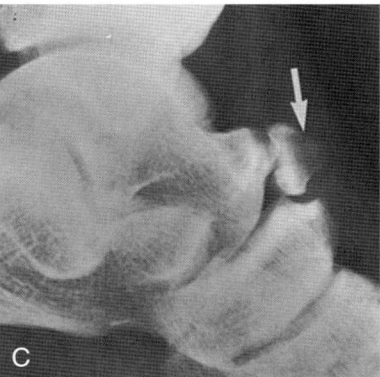

Figure 10-97 **A** and **B,** *Arrows* indicate os talonaviculare dorsale. **C,** Large os talonaviculare dorsale *(arrow)* with articulation with both the navicular and the talus. (From Keats TE: *Atlas of normal roentgen variants that simulate disease,* ed 4, St Louis, 1987, Mosby.)

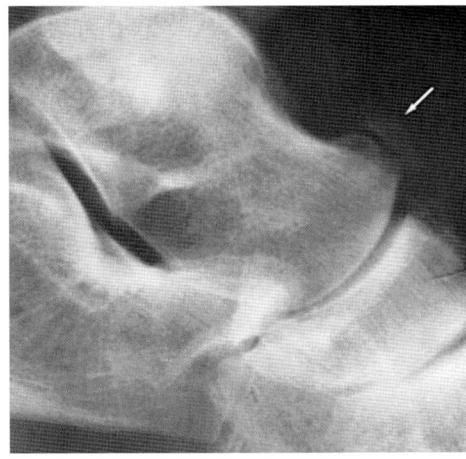

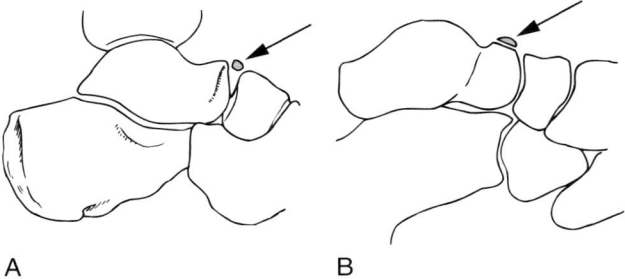

Figure 10-99 **A,** The os talonaviculare dorsale *(arrow)* can lie in the talonavicular joint on the dorsal aspect. **B,** An accessory ossicle on the dorsal surface of the talus *(arrow)* is called an *os supratalare.*

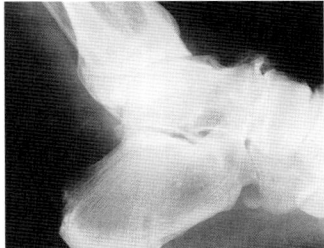

Figure 10-100 Degenerative arthritis of the talonavicular joint may be confused with an os talonaviculare dorsale or an os supratalare.

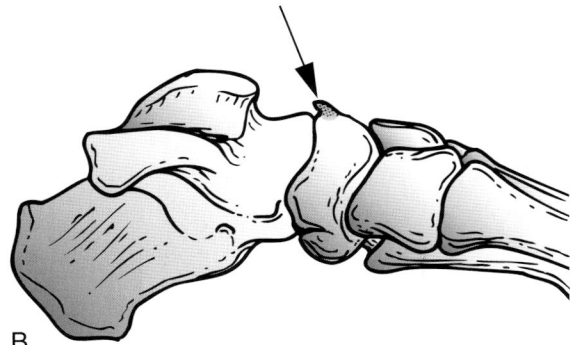

Figure 10-98 **A,** Os supratalare *(arrow).* The os supratalare emanates from the talus, whereas the os talonaviculare dorsale or supranaviculare emanates more commonly from the navicular. **B,** Diagram of os talonaviculare dorsale *(arrow).* (**B,** From Keats TE: *Atlas of normal roentgen variants that simulate disease,* ed 4, St Louis, 1987, Mosby.)

Three distinct types of accessory navicular are described.[232,276,290] Type I is a small accessory bone without attachment to the body of the navicular but formed in a well-defined round or oval shape (Fig. 10-101A). This most probably represents the sesamoid of the tibialis posterior tendon, and it is located on the plantar aspect of the tendon at the level of the inferior calcaneonavicular ligament. (See discussion on the sesamoid posterior tibial tendon.) It is almost always asymptomatic.

The second type (type II) of accessory navicular is a definite part of the body of the navicular, but the tuberosity is separated by a fibrocartilaginous plate of irregular outline (Fig. 10-101B and C) less than 2 mm in width.[121] This type often becomes symptomatic and is occasionally mistaken for a fracture of the tuberosity of the navicular

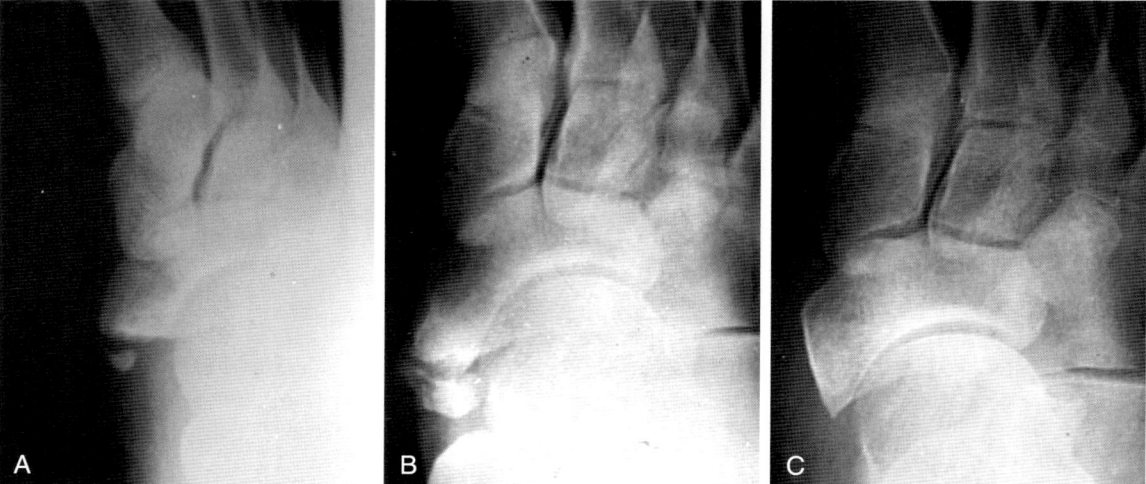

Figure 10-101 **A,** Small accessory navicular bone without attachment to the body of the navicular. Large accessory navicular seen preoperatively **(B)** and 1 year postoperatively **(C)** after excision of accessory navicular and excision of large medial tuberosity.

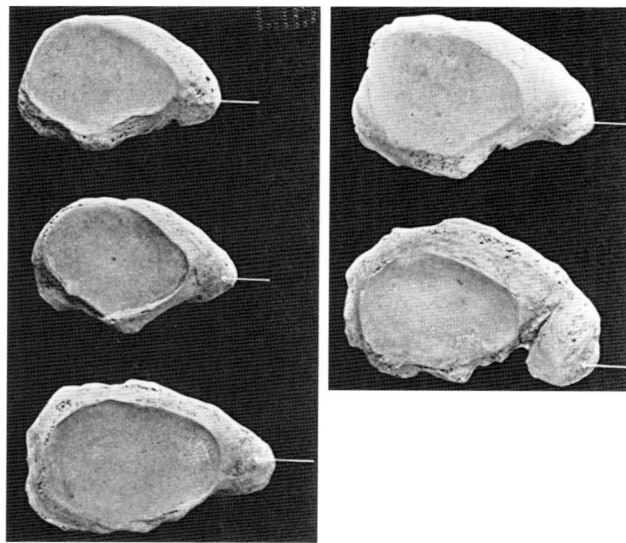

Figure 10-102 Five naviculars showing varying development of the accessory navicular. These are all characteristic of type III accessory naviculars. (From Dwight T: *Clinical atlas of variations of the bones of the hand and foot,* Philadelphia, 1907, JB Lippincott, pp 14–23.)

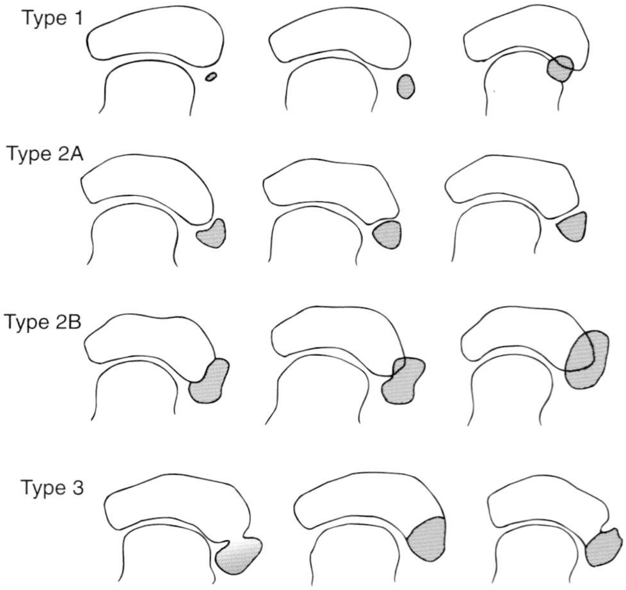

Figure 10-103 Variations in radiographic form of accessory navicular from large free fragment to small accessory fragment.

(Figs. 10-102 and 10-103). The remaining discussion concerns this type. Sella and Lawson[290] have differentiated type II accessory naviculars into two separate entities. A type IIA accessory navicular is connected with the talar process by a less acute angle, and a type IIB accessory navicular is situated more inferiorly. The main force on a type IIA is a tension force, whereas type IIB develops a shearing force. The two types can only be distinguished radiographically. Type IIA is more at risk for an avulsion injury. There is a great deal of controversy about whether an accessory navicular is the cause of a

pes planus deformity. Sella[290] has stated that increased pronation can cause more stress to the synchondrosis. Only type II accessory naviculars are characterized by a synchondrosis.

Type III accessory naviculars are united by a bony ridge, producing a cornuate navicular. Type II and type III accessory naviculars constitute 70% of these deformities.[232]

A symptomatic accessory navicular is often caused by an injury. This can be due to tension, shearing, or compression forces transmitted through the posterior tibial tendon to the fibrocartilaginous interface.

Zadek[331] studied 14 cases of symptomatic accessory navicular. On radiographs, he noted definite fusion with the body of the navicular in 5 cases, partial fusion in 3, and complete separation in 6. Zadek and Gold[332] studied the microscopic articulation of the accessory navicular to the body of the navicular. They reported that these structures were composed of hyaline cartilage, dense fibrocartilage, or both and sometimes showed ossification as well. This study of adolescents as they aged demonstrated that bony union definitely occurred in a large portion of cases. Of 14 accessory naviculars studied,[331] 5 later went on to fuse, 3 partially fused, and 6 failed to fuse. The authors concluded that many accessory naviculars do unite with the body of the navicular, but some can persist into adulthood (Figs. 10-104 and 10-105).

Kidner[215] studied the relationship of pes planus in the presence of an accessory navicular and hypothesized that flatfoot deformity had one of three causes: alteration of the line of pull of the posterior tibial tendon as a result of the prominence created by the accessory navicular; forcing of the posterior tibial tendon by the accessory navicular to become more of an adductor than a supinator of the forefoot, thereby decreasing support for the longitudinal arch; and impingement of the accessory navicular against the medial malleolus as the foot adducts, which tends to keep the foot in an abducted position and thus partially flattens the longitudinal arch.

Evaluation and Treatment

The accessory navicular should be differentiated from the os paracuneiforme (Fig. 10-106), which is found on the tibial aspect of the foot in close relationship to the naviculocuneiform joint. Also to be considered is the os cuneometatarsale-I tibiale, which is located in proximity to the first metatarsocuneiform joint. Trolle[311] reported the os paracuneiforme to have a 13% incidence.

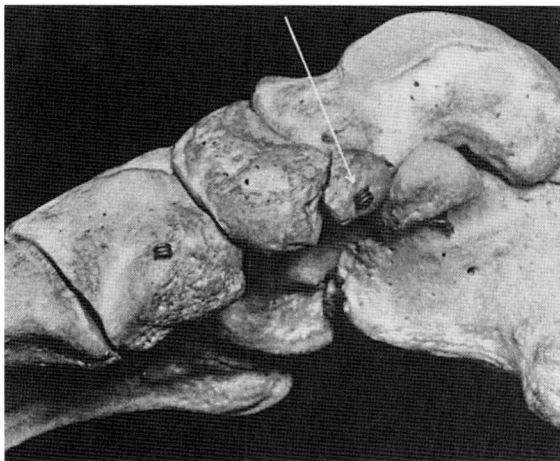

Figure 10-105 Accessory navicular demonstrated on anatomic specimen *(arrow)*. (From Dwight T: *Clinical atlas of variations of the bones of the hand and foot,* Philadelphia, 1907, JB Lippincott, pp 14–23.)

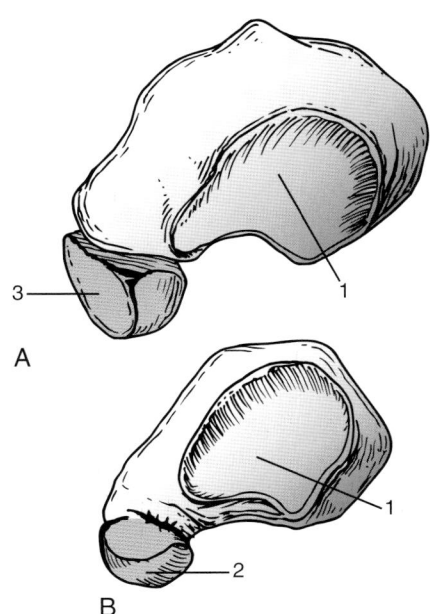

Figure 10-104 **A,** Type IIA accessory navicular. **B,** Type III accessory navicular. *1,* Proximal articular surface of navicular; *2,* incomplete segmentation of accessory navicular; *3,* accessory navicular.

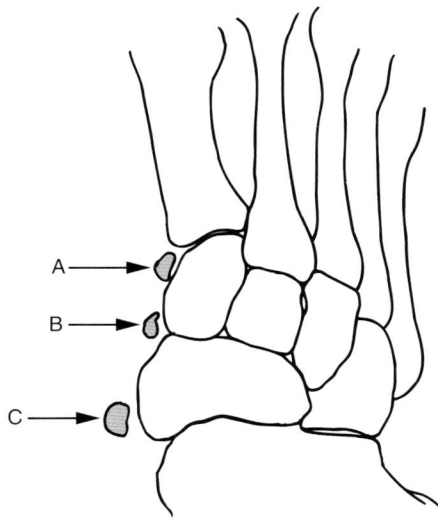

Figure 10-106 Accessory bones on the medial aspect of the boot may be confusing. An accessory bone adjacent to the first metatarsocuneiform joint is termed the *os cuneometatarsale-I tibiale (A).* An accessory bone adjacent to the naviculocuneiform joint is termed the *os paracuneiforme (B),* and a bone adjacent to the proximal pole of the navicular is termed *accessory navicular (C).* An os paracuneiforme is found just medial to the first cuneiform and distal to the location of the accessory navicular. With a larger distance between the accessory bone and the body of the navicular, a sesamoid of the anterior tibial tendon might be considered.

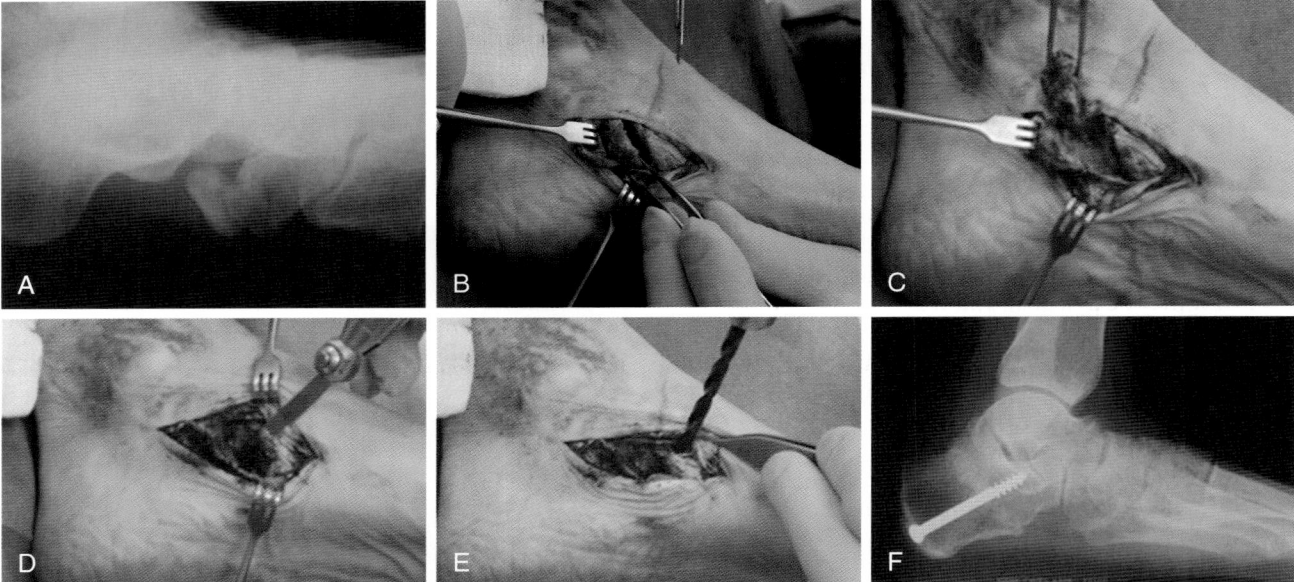

Figure 10-107 Radiograph **(A)** and intraoperative photograph **(B)** of large accessory navicular. **C,** Excision of navicular. **D,** Shaving of prominent navicular tuberosity. **E,** Drill hole for transfer of posterior tibial tendon. **F,** After calcaneal osteotomy in conjunction with modified Kidner procedure.

An accessory navicular can become symptomatic in childhood or early adulthood. In children, the symptoms are usually caused by pressure of the accessory bone against the shoe. At times, the condition is associated with progressive flattening of the longitudinal arch. In adults, symptoms usually develop after trauma to the foot, often resulting from a twisting injury. Physical examination often reveals tenderness over the prominence on the medial aspect of the instep. Radiographs demonstrate the accessory navicular. A technetium bone scan can help to differentiate a fracture from an accessory navicular.

In the asymptomatic case of an accessory navicular, reassurance of the patient is usually adequate. In cases that have become acutely symptomatic after an injury, immobilization in a below-knee walking cast, followed by the use of a longitudinal arch support, often diminishes symptoms.[180] Initial treatment should consist of casting or an orthosis, although, in the majority of cases, Grogan et al[180] have observed that nonoperative treatment is not successful, and surgical treatment is eventually necessary. When symptoms are caused by pressure over the navicular, a shoe that reduces pressure over this area should be worn. The occasional judicious use of a corticosteroid injection into the symptomatic area gives relief. When symptoms become intractable, surgical intervention may be necessary.

The Kidner procedure may be successful in alleviating symptoms. When a Kidner procedure is performed in a young patient with a pes planus deformity, excision of the accessory navicular should be accompanied by rerouting of the tibialis posterior tibial tendon through the navicular to increase the tension on the tendon. When the accessory navicular is not associated with a pes planus deformity, simple excision of the accessory navicular and plication of the tendon are sufficient. In an adult patient with a symptomatic accessory navicular with or without an associated flatfoot, the accessory navicular is excised and the tendon sutured to the side of the medial aspect of the navicular. No attempt is made to shorten or plicate the posterior tibial tendon. A calcaneal osteotomy may be performed in the presence of increased pes planus (Fig. 10-107).

KIDNER PROCEDURE
Surgical Technique

1. A thigh tourniquet is applied with the patient in a supine position. The foot is cleansed and draped in the usual fashion. The foot and leg are exsanguinated, and the tourniquet is inflated.
2. A longitudinal skin incision parallel to the upper border of the tibialis posterior tendon starts 1 cm anterior to the tip of the medial malleolus and extends to the medial cuneiform.
3. The dissection is carried down to the superior border of the tibialis posterior tendon along the length of the incision until the tendon courses plantarward beneath the navicular.
4. The accessory navicular is identified within the substance of the tendon and is excised with sharp dissection.
5. If the tibialis posterior tendon is to be rerouted through the navicular, it is detached as distally as possible.
6. If there is a significant prominence to the medial tuberosity of the navicular, it is osteotomized and resected.

7. If the tibialis posterior tendon is to be advanced, a dorsal-plantar drill hole is placed through the navicular. The foot is placed in maximal inversion and equinus. The tendon is then passed in a plantar-to-dorsal direction through the drill hole with a tendon passer, and the tendon is sutured back to itself or to the surrounding periosteal tissue.

8. If the tibialis posterior tendon is not advanced, it is sutured to the raw medial surface of the navicular with a No. 0 nonabsorbable suture. Alternatively, a suture anchor may be placed in the navicular (on the plantar-medial aspect), and the tendon is secured to the plantar aspect of the navicular. The periosteum that has been elevated from the navicular before the excision of the tuberosity is now plicated over the tendon.

Optional Procedure

In the presence of increased pes planus associated with an accessory navicular, a calcaneal slide osteotomy is performed. Through a small vertical incision inferior to the tip of the fibula and peroneal tendons, the calcaneus is exposed, with care taken to protect the sural nerve. An osteotomy of the calcaneus is performed just behind the posterior facet. The proximal calcaneal fragment is translated medially 8 to 10 mm and fixed temporarily with a Steinman pin introduced through a separate puncture incision at the tip of the heel. In the younger patient with an open calcaneal apophysis, internal fixation with a compression screw is discouraged.

Postoperative Treatment

The foot is placed in a non–weight-bearing below-knee cast for 3 weeks, and then a below-knee walking cast is used for 3 weeks. In the case of a patient on whom a tendon transfer has been performed, the foot is placed in an equinus adducted position for 4 weeks in a non–weight-bearing cast and then in a plantigrade walking cast for the final 4 weeks.

Results

Grogan et al[180] reported on 17 of 22 patients who underwent excision of an accessory navicular for a total of 39 excisions, 75% of which were type II and type III accessory naviculars. Grogan noted that excision of the accessory navicular without reimplantation of the posterior tibial tendon was routinely successful. Of 17 patients (25 feet) who underwent surgical excision, all but 1 reported excellent results and improvement from preoperative symptoms. On the other hand, Kiter et al[217] reviewed 17 patients 2 to 5 years after a simple excision of the accessory navicular, and observed that 8 of 17 had difficulty with both pes planus and a single limb heel rise test, and thought this was not an adequate means of treatment.

Ray and Goldberg[276] described management of the accessory navicular using a similar procedure in 29 feet. They excised the accessory navicular, sutured the fibers of the posterior tibial tendon to the anterior surface of the navicular, and reported good or excellent results in 26 of the cases.

In a review of 20 patients (age range, 7 to 40 years), all with an accessory navicular, Chater[149] reported similar successful results. Twelve patients were treated successfully by nonoperative means. Of the remaining 8, 6 children underwent excision of the ossicle, and 2 underwent a Kidner procedure (excision of the accessory navicular, detachment and reinsertion of the posterior tibial tendon into a drill hole into the navicular). Chater[149] noted that the Kidner technique appeared to have two advantages over a simple excision: it reinforced the spring ligament, and it helped to counteract and to correct sagging of the talonavicular joint. Leonard et al[231] reported on 13 patients (25 feet) with an accessory navicular associated with a pes planovalgus deformity treated with a Kidner procedure. They reported satisfactory restoration of the longitudinal arch and correction of heel valgus. Giannestras[174] observed, on the contrary, that pes planovalgus was only occasionally associated with an accessory navicular. He advocated simple surgical excision of the ossicle.

Chung and Chu[151] reported on a series of 31 patients with a painful type II accessory navicular treated with arthrodesis of the accessory navicular to the body of the navicular. Bony union was achieved in 82% of cases, with six nonunions. From the angular measurements of the magnitude of pes planus, it was apparent that, in few cases, the arch height improved. Scott et al[287] evaluated 20 patients who were treated for a symptomatic type II accessory navicular with either a modified Kidner procedure or arthrodesis of the accessory fragment if it was of sufficient size. In some cases, additional procedures were performed, including an Evans procedure, medial calcaneal displacement osteotomy, naviculocuneifrom arthrodesis, and a gastrocnemius recession. The authors suggested that in the small number of cases in which they performed an arthrodesis, the patients did as well as with the modified Kidner procedure. They observed two nonunions in their series of 10 fusions. With the varied procedures and small numbers of cases, it is difficult to know whether this treatment option is viable.

Harris and Beath[186] found a 4% incidence of an accessory navicular in 3619 Canadian army recruits. In a follow-up study of 77 of these men, only 4 developed significant symptoms, and the authors concluded that rarely was an accessory navicular symptomatic and that the need for surgical treatment was uncommon.

BIPARTITE NAVICULAR

Anatomy and Incidence

A bipartite navicular has also been reported by several authors.* Initially, Volk[319] reported two cases. Zimmer[334] reported a case of a bipartite navicular in a 19-year-old

---

*References 152, 200, 249, 258, 263, and 327.

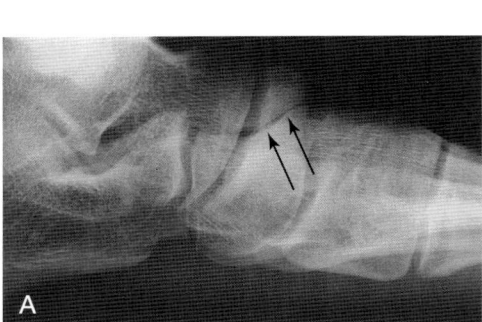
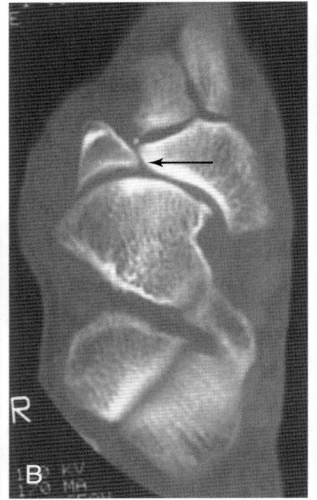
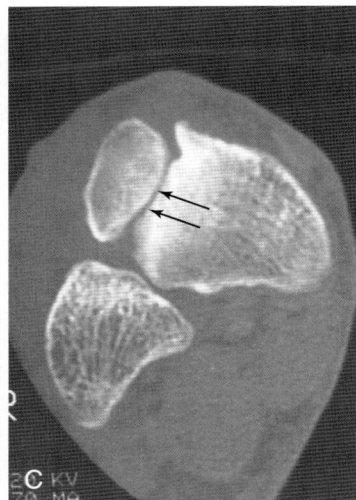

Figure 10-108 A, Lateral radiograph demonstrating bipartite navicular. **B** and **C,** Computed tomography scans demonstrating bipartite navicular. *Arrows* mark line of segmentation. (Courtesy Dr. Anik Shawdon.)

patient. Typically, the navicular is segmented into tibial and fibular segments that are well seen on a dorsoplantar radiograph. The fragments can be of varying size. Sarrafian[281] noted that, on a dorsoplantar radiograph, the smaller fragment is wedge shaped, with a medially directed base. On the lateral radiograph, the same fragment is wedge shaped in appearance, with the apex in a plantar direction. The smaller fragment is typically more dorsal in direction and may be superimposed over the first and second cuneiforms.

Shawdon et al[293] have demonstrated the bipartite navicular, on CT scanning, to be clearly evident on both axial and coronal planes. In the axial scan, the navicular appears wedge shaped, with tapering interval margins (Fig. 10-108). On CT evaluation, the appearance is distinctly different from that demonstrated with a fracture or stress fracture of the navicular. A bipartite navicular should be differentiated from an asymptomatic stress fracture or an acute fracture of the navicular. In a patient with no history of trauma, who has presented with medial midfoot pain and an abnormal but nondiagnostic radiograph, a CT scan may be helpful in differentiating the diagnosis of a bipartite navicular.

Clinical Significance

A bipartite navicular should be differentiated from an asymptomatic stress fracture or an acute fracture of the navicular.

OS INTERCUNEIFORME

Anatomy and Incidence

The os intercuneiforme is a very rare accessory bone located on the dorsum of the midfoot in an interval between the first and second cuneiforms just distal to the

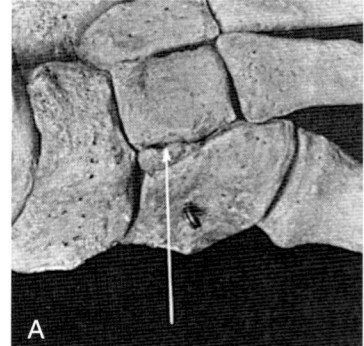
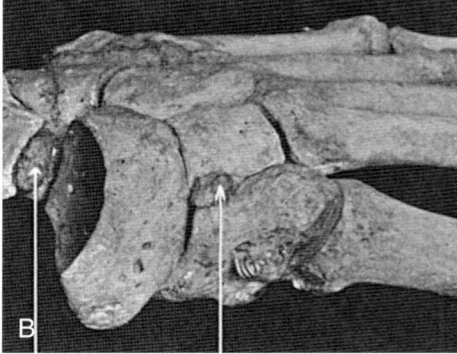

Figure 10-109 A, Dorsal view demonstrating os intercuneiforme *(arrow).* **B,** An oblique view demonstrating os intercuneiforme *(left arrow)* and os cuboides secundarium *(right arrow).* (From Dwight T: *Clinical atlas of variations of the bones of the hand and foot,* Philadelphia, 1907, JB Lippincott, pp 14–23.)

navicular (Fig. 10-109). Often an intercuneiform fossa is present. It is typically triangular in appearance. Dwight[161,162] initially reported this accessory bone, and Hoerr et al[198] stated that the incidence of the os intercuneiforme was 1% in his radiographic evaluations of 367 adolescents.

Geist[172] reported this accessory bone was present in 2% of cases.

Clinical Significance

This is a rare accessory bone, and the major clinical importance is that it should be distinguished from an acute fracture or a chronic nonunion of a fracture of the first or second cuneiforms. In the presence of pain localized to this region, a bone scan can help to differentiate this uncommon accessory bone from an acute fracture.

OS CUNEO-I METATARSALE-I PLANTARE, OS CUNEO-I METATARSALE-II DORSALE

Anatomy and Incidence

The os cuneo-I metatarsale-I plantare occurs on the plantar aspect of the foot at the base of the first metatarsal (Fig. 10-110).[262] It articulates with the plantar base of the first metatarsal and the first cuneiform. Pfitzner[269] first described this very rare accessory bone. Trolle[311] estimated its diameter as the size of a "cherrystone." It is not often seen on a dorsoplantar radiograph but can be seen in a lateral oblique view.

The os cuneo-I metatarsale-II dorsale lies on the dorsal aspect of the articulation of the second metatarsal and second cuneiform (Fig. 10-111).[284] It is wedge shaped, with the base oriented dorsally. Trolle[311] characterized it as "peppercorn" in size. This is also difficult to identify on a radiograph but can be seen in a lateral or lateral oblique view.

Clinical Significance

These are rare accessory bones that may be noted radiographically in a symptomatic or an asymptomatic patient. When present, they should be differentiated from an acute injury. Where this differentiation is difficult, a technetium bone scan can help to distinguish this from a fracture.

BIPARTITE FIRST CUNEIFORM

Anatomy and Incidence

Although first described by Morel (1797),[311] Pfitzner[269] reported the incidence of the bipartite first cuneiform as 0.5% in his series of anatomic specimens. Gruber (1877) reported an incidence of 0.33%, and Trolle[311] reported an incidence of 2.4%. Gruber (1877)[311] noted 10 complete segmentations of the first cuneiform and 5 incomplete ones in his evaluation of 2500 anatomic specimens (Fig. 10-112). Jashashvili et al[207] reported the earliest evidence of a bipartite medial cuneiform in an early homind fossil from the Early Pleistocene era.

The first cuneiform is often segmented horizontally into a larger dorsal and smaller plantar segment.*

---

*References 118, 120, 122, 128, 129, 135, 159, 169, 191, 210, 233, 258, 261, 297, and 327.

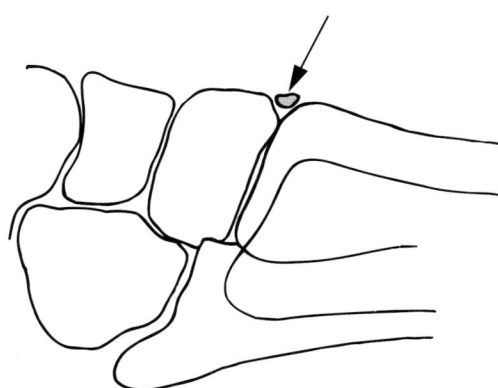

Figure 10-111 The os cuneo-I metatarsale-II dorsale *(arrow)* lies dorsally between the middle cuneiform and the second metatarsal.

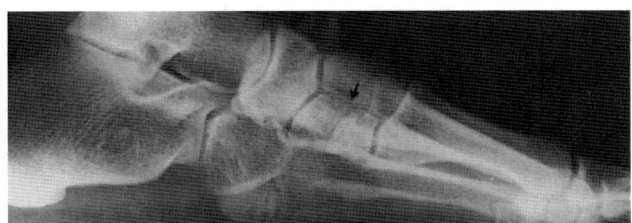

Figure 10-112 Horizontal bifurcation *(arrow)* of the first cuneiform.

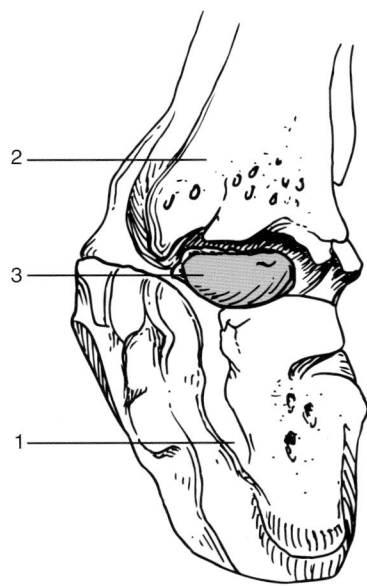

Figure 10-110 Os cuneo-I metatarsale-I plantare. *1,* First cuneiform, plantar aspect; *2,* first metatarsal, plantar aspect; *3,* os cuneo-I metatarsale-I plantare.

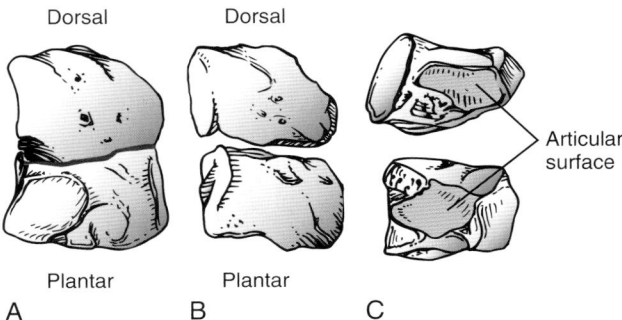

Figure 10-113 Bipartite first cuneiform. **A,** Articulated bipartite first cuneiform. **B,** Slightly separated view of first cuneiform. **C,** Disarticulated specimen showing the dorsal and plantar articular surfaces.

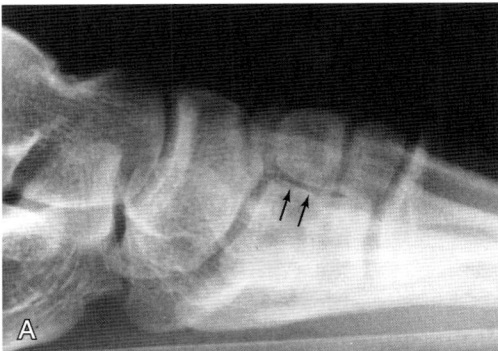

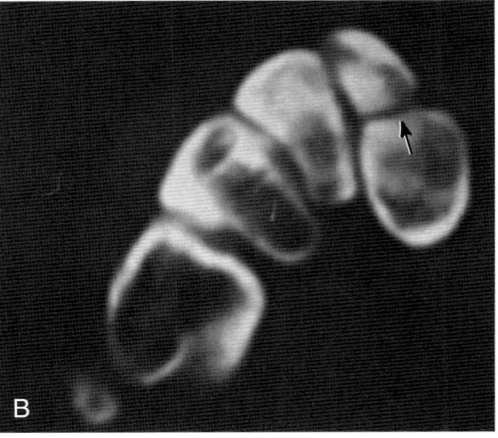

Figure 10-114 Bilateral bipartite medial cuneiform. **A,** Lateral radiograph demonstrating bipartite medial cuneiform *(arrow).* **B,** Computed tomographic scan demonstrating bilateral bipartite medial cuneiforms *(arrows).* (From Dellacorte M, Lin P, Grisafi P: Bilateral bipartite medial cuneiform. A case report, *J Am Podiatr Med Assoc* 82: 475–478, 1992.)

The dorsal segment articulates distally with the dorsal aspect of the first metatarsal base and proximally with the navicular (Fig. 10-113). The lateral surface articulates with the middle cuneiform and with the base of the second metatarsal. The plantar segment articulates as well with the base of the first metatarsal and proximally with the navicular. The inferior surface has a prominent tubercle for insertion of the posterior tibial tendon. Together, the two segments of the bipartite first cuneiform amass a volume slightly larger than the undivided medial cuneiform (Fig. 10-114). The partition can be difficult to view on a dorsoplantar radiograph and may be better visualized on an oblique radiograph or CT scan.[159]

Clinical Significance

A bipartite first cuneiform is typically nonpainful and rarely, if ever, requires surgery. With trauma to the medial aspect of the foot, it may be necessary to distinguish a fracture from a bipartite first cuneiform[261] and from a tarsal coalition (Fig. 10-115).[222] In evaluation of pain in this region, a segmented first cuneiform can be identified on CT or MRI scan. On the other hand, Kumai et al[222] have described synostosis or coalition of the medial and intermediate cuneiform, which can only be identified on CT or MRI scan. Chiodo et al[150] have described excision of the medial aspect of the bipartite medial cuneiform, and Azurza et al[118] have described internal fixation of the fragment.

METATARSOCUNEIFORM COALITION

Anatomy and Incidence

Coalitions of the first metatarsocuneiform joint are rare. Day[157] and others[170,204,305] have described osseous coalitions. Tanaka et al[306] have described a fibrous coalition in which resection was performed successfully in a 32-year-old man (Fig. 10-116), and Takakura and Nakata[305] have fused the joint to relieve pain (Fig. 10-117).

Clinical Significance

Although rare, first metatarsocuneiform coalition must be differentiated from intraarticular fractures and degenerative arthritis.

OS INTERMETATARSEUM

The os intermetatarseum is observed between the medial cuneiform and the base of the first and second metatarsals.* It was first described by Gruber in 1856,[312] but Pfitzner[269] and Dwight[163] gave the first comprehensive description of the variations of the os intermetatarseum. The os intermetatarseum (Fig. 10-118) is a spindle-shaped bone that originates from the distal corner of the medial cuneiform, tapers distally, and projects between the first and second metatarsals. It may be fused to either the first or second metatarsal or can articulate with the first and second metatarsals (Fig. 10-119) and the medial cuneiform.

*References 129, 146, 168, 220, 259, 283, 311, and 326.

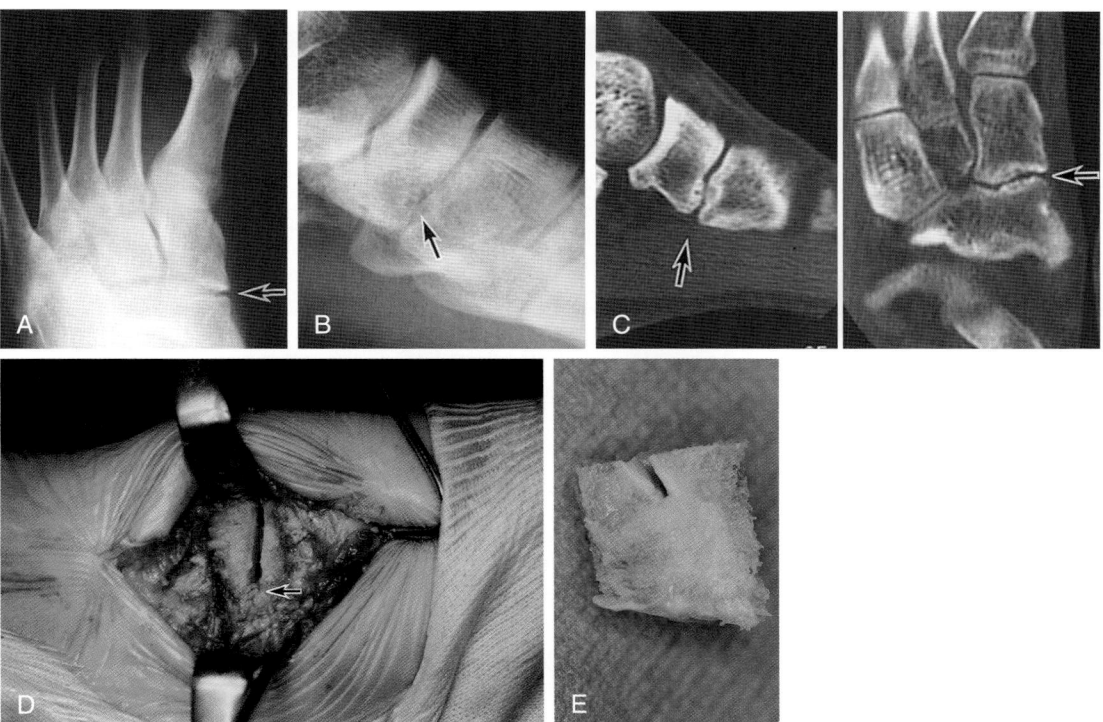

Figure 10-115 **A** and **B**, Anteroposterior and lateral radiographs demonstrating area of first naviculocuneiform joint coalition *(arrows)*. **C**, Computed tomographic scan demonstrating first naviculocuneiform joint coalition *(arrow)*. **D**, Operative appearance demonstrating coalition. **E**, Resected bone block shows fibrous and cartilaginous coalition. (From Kumai T, Tanaka Y, Takakura Y, et al: Isolated first naviculocuneiform joint coalition, *Foot Ankle Int* 17:635–640, 1996.)

Henderson[195] reported four cases of bilateral os intermetatarseum. All were associated with hallux valgus, and three cases were familial (Fig. 10-120). He noted a tendinous structure extending from the tip of the accessory bone through the muscle belly of the first dorsal interosseous that attached to the base of the proximal phalanx on the lateral aspect of the hallux. Burman and Lapidus[140] reported a 3.3% incidence of os intermetatarseum in a review of 1000 cases. Only four were reported to be painful. It was noted that the os intermetatarseum may be attached to either the first or second metatarsal (or both) or the first cuneiform or may be a completely unattached accessory bone and can appear as either a single bone or in several pieces.

Reichmister[277] reported a series of three cases in which two instances of painful os intermetatarseum were excised and one was treated conservatively. Reichmister noted that this accessory bone can cause pressure and pain by compression of the superficial peroneal nerve. Noguchi et al[259] reported on a soccer player who developed deep peroneal nerve symptoms resulting from impingement from an os intermetatarsum, with symptoms consistent to an anterior tarsal tunnel syndrome. Nakasa et al[71] reported four patients with painful os intermetarsum with paresthesias in the first web space. Surgical excision in all cases results in relief of symptoms.

Kohler and Zimmer[218] reported two cases of fracture of the os intermetatarseum, one of which healed and one of which went on to nonunion. The incidence of the os intermetatarseum has ranged from 1.2% (Trolle,[311] radiologic examination; Shands,[291] radiologic examination) to 10% (Dwight,[163] anatomic examination). Scarlet et al[284] reported this condition to be more often bilateral and to have a familial tendency.

An os intermetatarseum IV has been reported to lie between the fourth and fifth metatarsals.[311]

The differential diagnosis includes a calcified dorsalis pedis artery, a ligamentous avulsion of the adjacent metatarsal or cuneiform, and posttraumatic osteophyte formation.

Clinical Significance

Typically, this accessory bone is asymptomatic (Fig. 10-121). Its presence may be associated with hallux valgus, and in the decision-making process for correcting a hallux valgus deformity, the first metatarsocuneiform joint must be evaluated. The presence of an os intermetatarseum or a facet between the first and second metatarsal and medial cuneiform can indicate the necessity for a first metatarsal osteotomy to correct an increased angle between the first and second metatarsals. Tanaka et al[306] and others[157,204,306] have described a fibrous

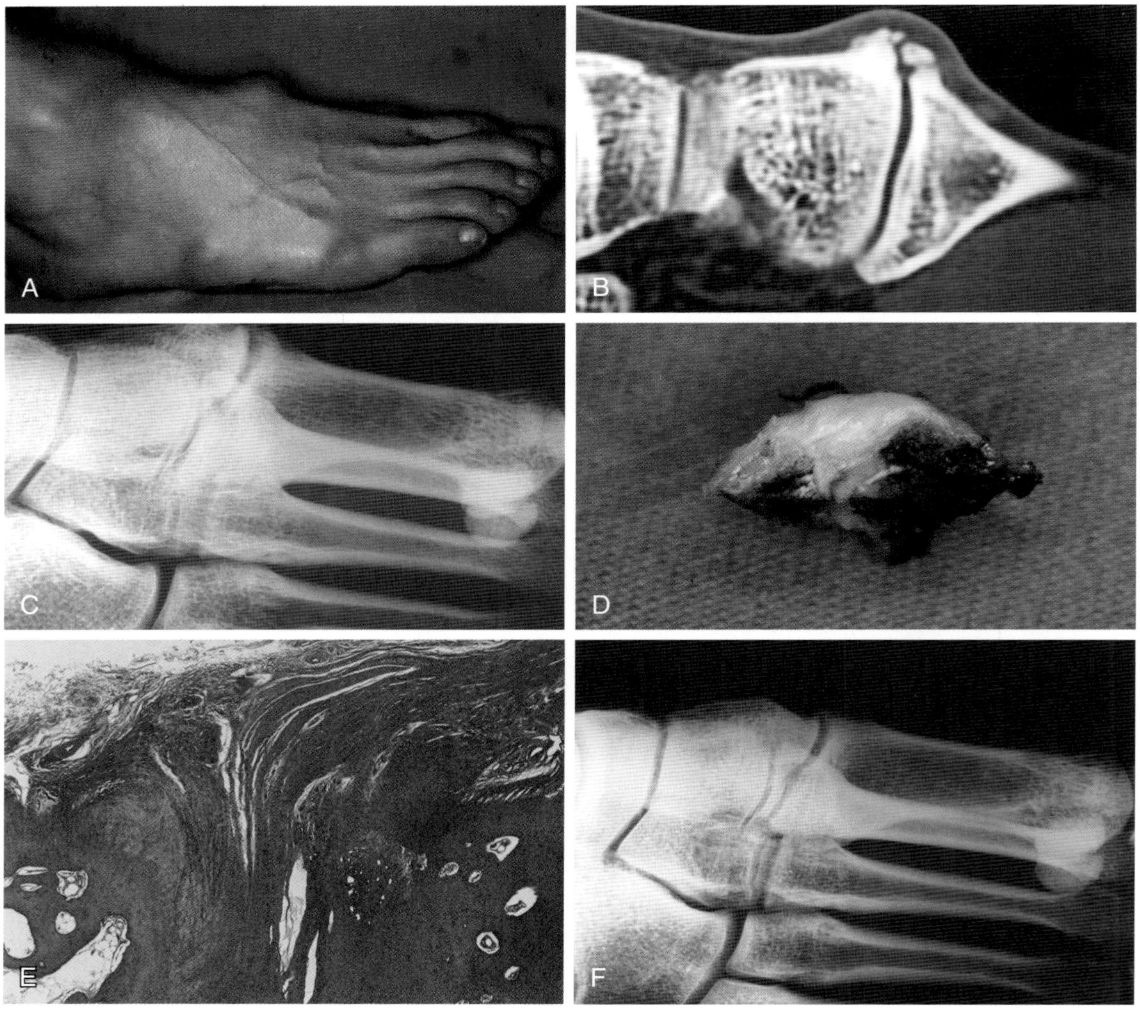

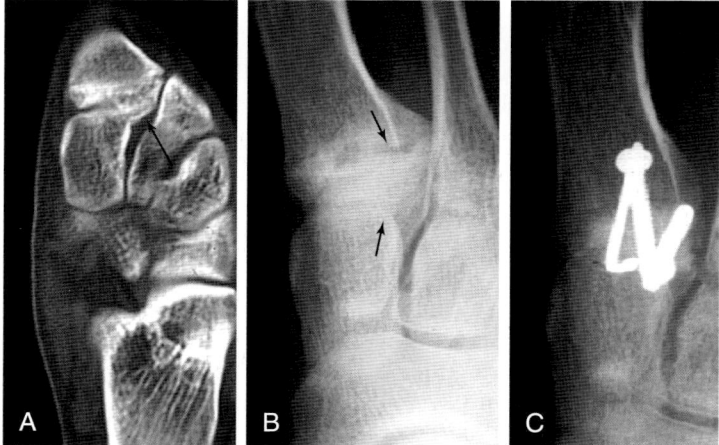

Figure 10-116   First metatarsocuneiform coalition. **A,** Clinical presentation. **B,** Lateral computed tomographic scan. **C,** Lateral radiograph. **D,** Resected dorsal coalition. **E,** Histology of resected specimen. **F,** Lateral radiograph after the resection. (From Tanaka Y, Takakura Y, Sugimoto K, Kumai T: Non-osseous coalition of the medial cuneiform-first metatarsal joint: a case report, *Foot Ankle Int* 21:1043–1046, 2000. Used with permission.)

Figure 10-117   Metatarsocuneiform coalition. Computed tomographic scan **(A)** and radiograph **(B)** demonstrating first metatarsocuneiform fibrous coalition (*arrows* in A and B point to partial joint coalition). **C,** After arthrodesis. (From Tanaka Y, Takakura Y, Sugimoto K, Kumai T: Non-osseous coalition of the medial cuneiform-first metatarsal joint: a case report, *Foot Ankle Int* 21:1043–1046, 2000. Used with permission.)

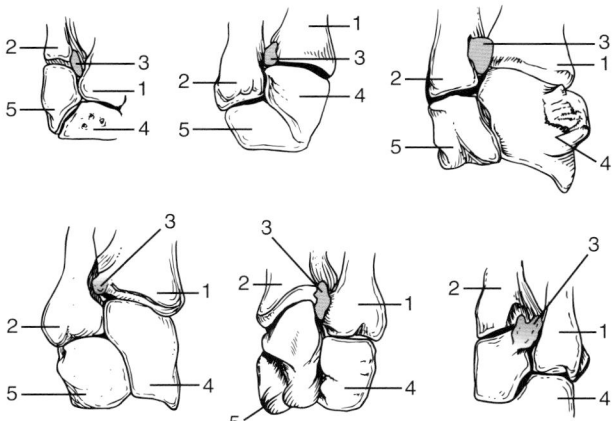

Figure 10-118 Os intermetatarseum. The os intermetatarseum may be a separate ossicle, or it can arise from the first or second metatarsal or from the first cuneiform. It may be incorporated or may be a free ossicle. *1,* First metatarsal; *2,* second metatarsal; *3,* os intermetatarseum; *4,* first cuneiform; *5,* second cuneiform.

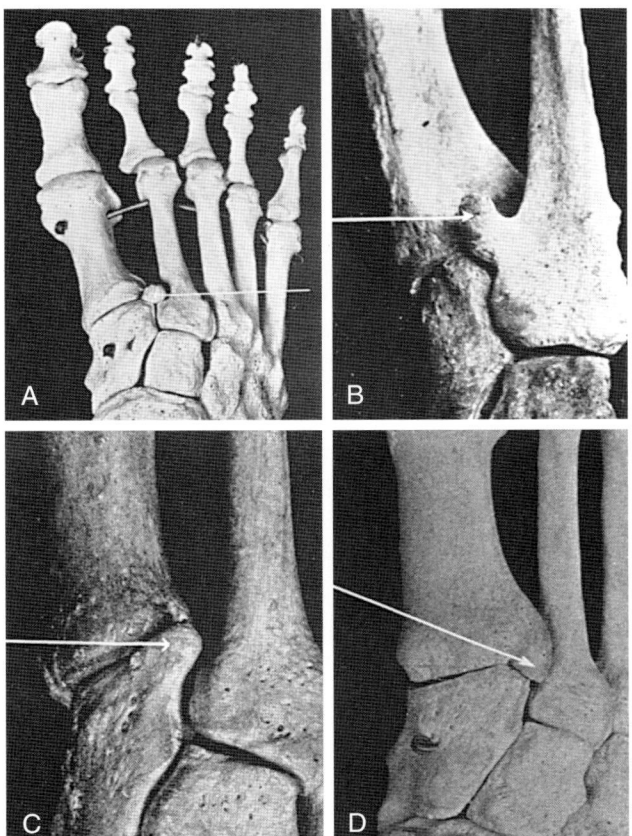

Figure 10-119 **A,** Os intermetatarseum, a separate ossicle. **B,** Os intermetatarseum *(arrow)* arising from the second metatarsal. **C,** Os intermetatarseum *(arrow)* off of first cuneiform. **D,** Os intermetatarseum *(arrow)* at the base of the first metatarsal. This can create a rigid articulation and when associated with a hallux valgus deformity may be resistant to correction without a metatarsal osteotomy. (From Dwight T: *Clinical atlas of variations of the bones of the hand and foot,* Philadelphia, 1907, JB Lippincott, pp 14–23.)

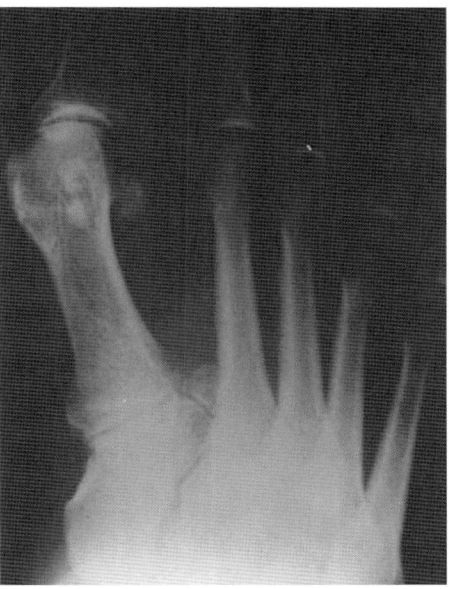

Figure 10-120 Os intermetatarseum with deviated first and second metatarsals. A first metatarsal osteotomy will be necessary to correct the intermetatarsal angle.

coalition at the first metatarsal cuneiform joint that can also restrict motion, which also may be pertinent in treating a hallux valgus deformity. Rarely, if ever, is elective surgical resection required for an os intermetatarseum. Scarlet et al[284] and Reichmister[277] have both reported cases in which a symptomatic os intermetatarseum has been excised.

OS VESALIANUM

Anatomy and Incidence

The os vesalianum is a rare accessory bone located at the proximal extent of the fifth metatarsal (Fig. 10-122).* Geist[172] found one case in 100 feet examined radiographically, and Dameron,[156] in a radiographic study of 1000 feet, noted only one case of an os vesalianum. Trolle,[311] Pfitzner,[269] and Holle,[203] in histoembryologic, anatomic, and extensive radiographic studies, found no evidence of an os vesalianum. Heimerzheim[192] found a 0.9% incidence of this accessory bone in an evaluation of 1800 radiographs.

Trolle[311] noted that the os vesalianum can attain the size of an almond and is visible on both dorsoplantar and lateral oblique radiographs (Fig. 10-123A and B). On the dorsoplantar view, a small bone can be visualized within the tuberosity of the fifth metatarsal.

Boya[137] reported a large tuberosity without any apophyseal line or lucency present and suggested it was a variant of an os vesalianum. Boya et al,[138] in another

*References 119, 128, 140, 165, 181, 182, 201, 202, 209, 213, 227, 234, 258, 263, 296, 299, and 327.

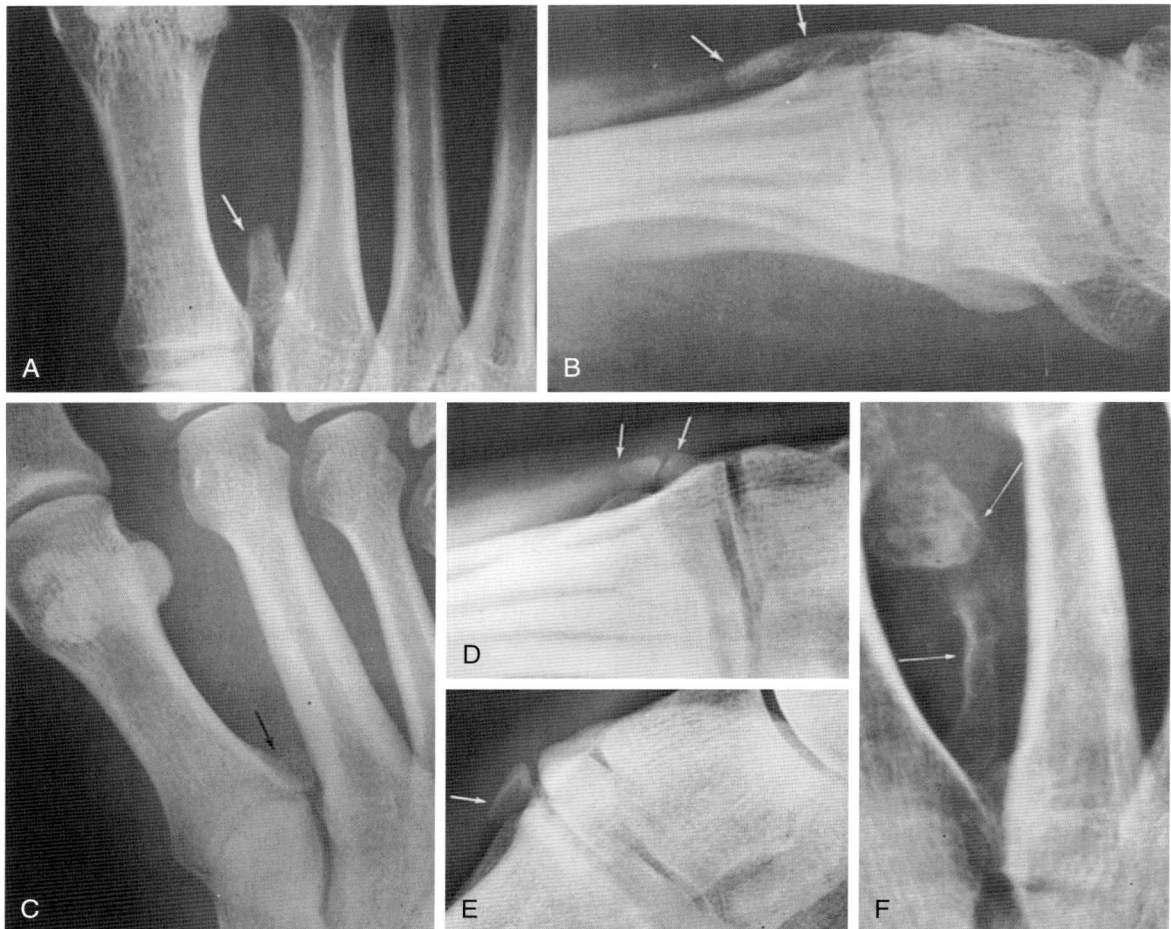

Figure 10-121 **A-F,** Examples of variable appearance of os intermetatarseum *(arrows).* Note the accessory ossicle at the distal end of the os intermetatarseum **(F).** (From Keats TE: *Atlas of normal roentgen variants that simulate disease,* ed 4, St Louis, 1987, Mosby.)

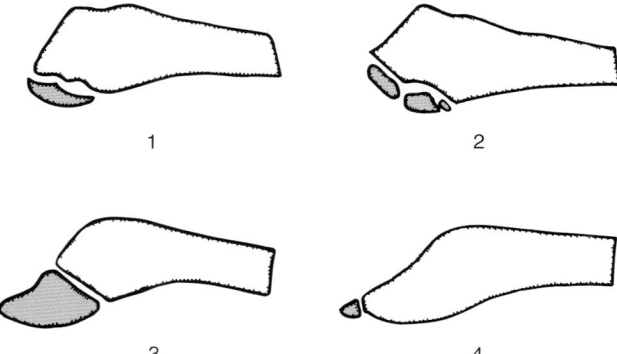

Figure 10-122 Os vesalianum. *1,* Ossification within the apophysis of the fifth metatarsal base; *2,* fragmentation within the ossification of the fifth metatarsal apophysis; *3,* ununited apophysis of the fifth metatarsal base; *4,* position of os vesalianum (note different orientation of articulation).

case, reported on a similar case with bilateral ossicles separated by a thin radiolucent line consistent with an os vesalianum.

Clinical Significance

The major objective in diagnosis is to differentiate an os vesalianum from an ossifying apophysis of the fifth metatarsal base, an apophysitis of the fifth metatarsal base,* a fracture of the tuberosity of the fifth metatarsal, a nonunion of a tuberosity fracture of the fifth metatarsal, an ununited apophysis of the fifth metatarsal base (Fig. 10-123C-E), and an os peroneum (see Fig. 10-62). Iselin[206] described an apophysitis of the base of the fifth metatarsal in teenagers. Fewer than 10 cases have been reported in the world literature. The apophysis is located within the flare of the proximal fifth metatarsal in the area where the peroneus brevis inserts.

Reported successful treatment includes rest and casting.[145,229] Canale[145] reported that bony union usually

---

*References 145, 205, 229, 254, and 275.

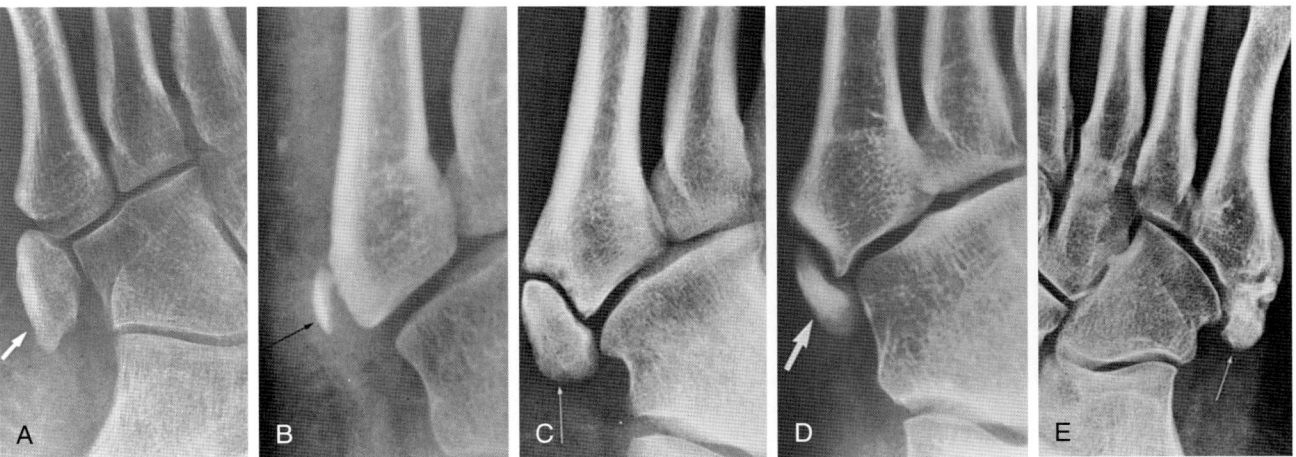

Figure 10-123 **A,** Os vesalianum. **B,** Apophysis of the base of the fifth metatarsal. **C,** Failed union of the apophysis at the base of the fifth metatarsal. **D,** Unfused apophysis of fifth metatarsal in a 19-year-old man. **E,** Failed union of the apophysis at the base of the fifth metatarsal. (From Keats TE: *Atlas of normal roentgen variants that simulate disease*, ed 4, St Louis, 1987, Mosby.)

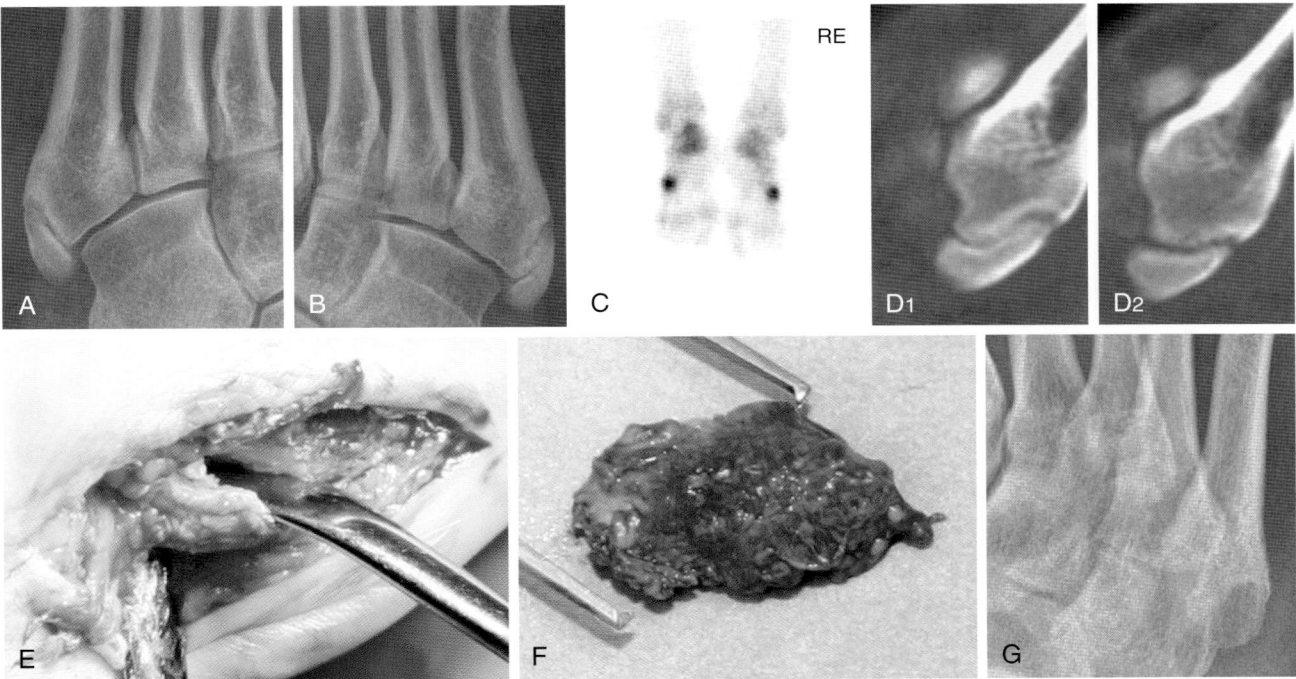

Figure 10-124 Bilateral os vesalianum. Anteroposterior radiograph of left **(A)** and right **(B)** foot. **C,** Technetium-99m (^{99m}Tc) bone scan demonstrating bilateral uptake in area of accessory bone. **D$_1$** and **D$_2$** Computed tomography scan of right foot. **E,** Surgical excision of os vesalianum. **F,** Removed ossicle. **G,** Postoperative radiograph after excision of ossicle. (From Dorrestijn O, Brouwer RW: Bilateral symptomatic os vesalianum pedis: a case report, *J Foot Ankle Surg* 50:473–475, 2011. Used with permission.)

occurs with time. Ralph et al[275] reported excision of the painful fragment without disruption of the peroneus brevis tendon with complete resolution of symptoms. Dorrestijn et al[160] reported on a bilateral case with a positive bone scan, which was treated successfully with excision on one side and conservative care on the contralateral side. Inoue et al[205] presented another bilateral case, in

which osteosynthesis was used successfully for the symptomatic side (Fig. 10-124).

Sarrafian[281] noted the following characteristics that aid in differentiating an os vesalianum: a fracture of the apophysis or base of the fifth metatarsal is transverse in direction; the ossification center of the apophysis is linear initially and longitudinally oriented parallel to the

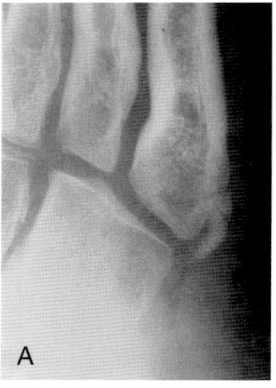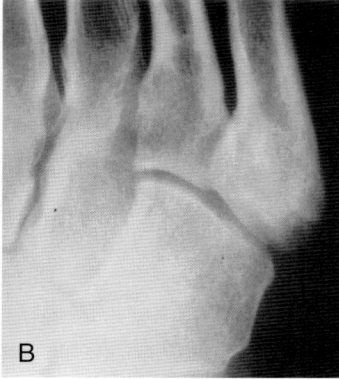

Figure 10-125 A, Iselin disease. **B,** After passage of time and consolidation of apophysis. (Courtesy S. Terry Canale, MD, Memphis, Tenn.)

metatarsal shaft; an os vesalianum is located just proximal to the tip of a well-developed fifth metatarsal tuberosity; and with an os vesalianum, the opposing surfaces may be sclerotic and denote a chronic condition.

Iselin[206] described an apophysitis of the proximal fifth metatarsal (Fig. 10-125). It has been recognized by Canale et al[145] and others[229,275] as a condition in which the ossification center undergoes aseptic necrosis, followed by gradual resorption of the fragment. It must be differentiated from a fracture and may be caused by repetitive trauma. When symptomatic, it can be successfully treated with rest, limited weight bearing, and occasionally casting. With apophysitis of the fifth metatarsal, a traumatic episode can occur, resulting in avulsion of a portion of the apophysis.

Typically, the localized pain and tenderness resolve in time because this is a self-limiting disorder in which conservative treatment can be used. After apophysitis, there may be a residual irregularity of the proximal fifth metatarsal and prominence, but this typically does not interfere with function.[286]

REFERENCES
Sesamoids

1. Abraham M, Sage R, Lorenz M: Tibial and fibular sesamoid fractures on the same metatarsal: a review of two cases, *J Foot Surg* 28:308–311, 1989.
2. Anderson R, McBryde A: Autogenous bone grafting of hallux sesamoid nonunions, *Foot Ankle Int* 18:293–296, 1997.
3. Aper R, Saltzman C, Brown T: The effect of hallux sesamoid resection on the effective moment of the flexor hallucis brevis, *Foot Ankle Int* 15:462–470, 1994.
4. Aper R, Saltzman C, Brown T: The effect of hallux sesamoid excision on the flexor hallucis longus moment arm, *Clin Orthop Relat Res* 325:209–217, 1996.
5. Apley AG: Open sesamoid: a reappraisal of the medial sesamoid of the hallux, *Proc R Soc Med* 59:120, 1966.
6. Aquino M, DeVincentis A, Keating S: Tibial sesamoid planing procedure: an appraisal of 26 feet, *J Foot Surg* 23:226–230, 1984.
7. Biedert R, Hintermann B: Stress fractures of the medial sesamoids in athletes, *Foot Ankle Int* 24:137–141, 2003.
8. Bizarro AH: On the traumatology of the sesamoid structures, *Ann Surg* 74:783–791, 1921.
9. Blundell C, Nicholson P, Blackney M: Percutaneous screw fixation for fractures of the sesamoid bones of the hallux, *J Bone Surg Br* 84B:1138–1141, 2002.
10. Bock P, Kristen K, Kroner A, Engel A: Hallux valgus and cartilage degeneration in the first metatarsophalangeal joint, *J Bone Surg Br* 86B:669–673, 2004.
11. Bouché RT: Osteonecrosis of the tibial and fibular sesamoids in an aerobic dancer [see letters to Editor], *J Foot Ankle Surg* 36:393–394, 1997.
12. Brodsky J: Sesamoid excision for chronic nonunion. 21st Annual Meeting of the American Orthopaedic Foot and Ankle Society, Anaheim, Calif, March 10, 1991.
13. Brodsky J, Krause J, Robinson A, Watkins D: Hallux sesamoidectomy for painful chronic fracture: histological and radiographic characteristics and clinical outcome. 29th Annual Meeting of the American Orthopaedic Foot and Ankle Society, Anaheim, Calif, February 7, 1999.
14. Brown TIS: Avulsion fracture of the fibular sesamoid in association with dorsal dislocation of the metatarsophalangeal joint of hallux, *Clin Orthop Relat Res* 149:229–231, 1980.
15. Burman MS, Lapidus PW: The functional disturbances caused by the inconstant bones and sesamoids of the foot, *Arch Surg* 22:960–964, 1931.
16. Cartlidge IJ, Gillespie WJ: Haematogenous osteomyelitis of the metatarsal sesamoid, *Br J Surg* 66:214–216, 1979.
17. Colwill M: Osteomyelitis of the metatarsal sesamoids, *J Bone Joint Surg Br* 51:464–468, 1969.
18. Coughlin M: Athletic injury to the first metatarsal phalangeal joint, *Med Chir Pied* 21:65–72, 2005.
19. Coughlin MJ: Sesamoid pain: causes and treatment, *Instr Course Lect* 39:23–35, 1990.
20. Coughlin MJ, Mann RA: Arthrodesis of the first metatarsophalangeal joint as a salvage for the failed Keller procedure, *J Bone Joint Surg Am* 69:68–75, 1987.
21. Day F, Jones P, Gilbert C: Congenital absence of the tibial sesamoid, *J Am Podiatr Med Assoc* 92:153–154, 2002.
22. Delfaut E, Demondion X, Bieganski A, et al: The fibrocartilaginous sesamoid: a cause of size and signal variation in the normal distal posterior tibial tendon, *Eur Radiol* 13:2642–2649, 2003.
23. DeLuca FN, Kenmore PI: Bilateral dorsal dislocation of the metatarsophalangeal joints of the great toes, *J Trauma* 15:737–739, 1975.
24. Dobas DC, Silvers MD: The frequency of the partite sesamoids of the first metatarsophalangeal joint, *J Am Podiatr Assoc* 67:880–882, 1977.
25. DuVries HL, editor: *Surgery of the foot*, ed 2, St Louis, 1965, Mosby, pp 259–278.
26. Enna CD: Observations on the hallucal sesamoid in trauma to the denervated foot, *Int Surg* 53:97–107, 1970.
27. Esemenli T, Yildirim Y, Bezer M: Lateral shifting of the first metatarsal head in hallux valgus surgery: effect on sesamoid reduction, *Foot Ankle Int* 24:922–926, 2003.
28. Ferris D, Thomas J, Owens J: Extirpation of the fibular sesamoid simplified, *J Foot Surg* 24:255–257, 1985.
29. Fleischli J, Cheleuitte E: Avascular necrosis of the hallucal sesamoids, *J Foot Ankle Surg* 34:358–365, 1995.
30. Frankel J, Harrington J: Symptomatic bipartite sesamoids, *J Foot Surg* 29:318–323, 1990.
31. Garrido IM, Bosch MN, Gonzalez MS, Carsi VV: Osteochondritis of the hallux sesamoid bones, *Foot Ankle Surg* 14:175–179, 2008.
32. Giannestras NJ: *Foot disorders: medical and surgical management*, Philadelphia, 1973, Lea & Febiger, p 426.
33. Giannikas A, Papachristou G, Papavasiliou N, et al: Dorsal dislocation of the first metatarsophalangeal joint, *J Bone Joint Surg Br* 57:384–386, 1975.

34. Giurini J, Chrzan J, Gibbons G, et al: Sesamoidectomy for the treatment of chronic neuropathic ulcerations, *J Am Podiatr Med Assoc* 81:167–173, 1991.

35. Goez J, DeLauro T: Congenital absence of the tibial sesamoid, *J Am Podiatr Med Assoc* 85:509–510, 1995.

36. Golding C: The sesamoid of the hallux, *J Bone Joint Surg Br* 42:840–843, 1960.

37. Gordon SL, Evans C, Greer RB: *Pseudomonas* osteomyelitis of the metatarsal sesamoid of the great toe, *Clin Orthop Relat Res* 99:188–189, 1974.

38. Helal B: The great toe sesamoid bone: the lus or lost souls of Ushaia, *Clin Orthop Relat Res* 157:82–87, 1981.

39. Helfet A: Pain under the head of the metatarsal bone of the big toe, *Lancet* 267:846, 1954.

40. Hobart MH: Fracture of sesamoid bones of the foot, *J Bone Joint Surg* 11:298–302, 1929.

41. Hong D, Nie L, Wang H, Zhang C: Chondromalacia of sesamoids in first metatarsal phalangeal joint, *Chin J Traumatol* 7:127–128, 2004.

42. Hubay CA: Sesamoid bones of the hands and feet, *Am J Roentgenol* 61:493–505, 1949.

43. Ilfeld FW, Rosen V: Osteochondritis of the first metatarsal sesamoid, *Clin Orthop Relat Res* 85:38–41, 1972.

44. Inge GAL, Ferguson AB: Surgery of the sesamoid bones of the great toe, *Arch Surg* 27:466–488, 1933.

45. Jahss M: Traumatic dislocations of the first metatarsophalangeal joint, *Foot Ankle* 1:15–20, 1980.

46. Jahss ML: The sesamoids of the hallux, *Clin Orthop Relat Res* 157:88–97, 1981.

47. Jahss MS, editor: *Disorders of the foot and ankle: medical and surgical management*, ed 2, Philadelphia, 1991, WB Saunders, pp 1062–1075.

48. Jeng C, Maurer A, Mizel M: Congenital absence of the hallux fibular sesamoid: a case report and review of the literature, *Foot Ankle Int* 19:329–331, 1999.

49. Jones JL, Losito JM: Tibial sesamoid fracture in a softball player, *J Am Podiatr Med Assoc* 97:85–88, 2007.

50. Julsrud M: Osteonecrosis of the tibial and fibular sesamoids in an aerobics instructor, *J Foot Ankle Surg* 36:31–35, 1997.

51. Kaiman ME, Piccora R: Tibial sesamoidectomy: a review of the literature and retrospective study, *J Foot Surg* 22:286–289, 1983.

52. Kanatli U, Ozturk AM, Ercan NG, et al: Absence of the medial sesamoid bone associated with metatarsophalangeal pain, *Clin Anat* 19:634–639, 2006.

53. Kernohan J, Dakin P, Helal B: Dolorous calcification of the lateral sesamoid bursa of the great toe, *Foot Ankle* 5:45–46, 1984.

54. Kewenter Y: Die Sesambeine des 1. Metatarsophalangealgelenks des Menschen, *Acta Orthop Scand Suppl* 2:1–113, 1936.

55. Kliman ME, Gross AE, Pritzker KP, et al: Osteochondritis of the hallux sesamoid bone, *Foot Ankle* 3:220–223, 1983.

56. Konkel KF, Muehlstein JH: Unusual fracture-dislocation of the great toe, *J Trauma* 15:733–736, 1975.

57. Kuo CC, Lee WH, Hsu HC: Nonunion of a sesamoid with tophaceous gout: a case report, *Foot Ankle Int* 28:939–941, 2007.

58. Lapidus P: Congenital unilateral absence of medial sesamoid of the great toe, *J Bone Joint Surg Am* 21:208–209, 1939.

59. Lavery L, Haase K, Krych S: Hallux hammertoe secondary to *Pseudomonas* osteomyelitis, *J Am Podiatr Med Assoc* 81:608–612, 1991.

60. Le Minor J: Congenital agsence of the lateral metatarsophalangeal sesamoid bone of the human hallux. A case report, *Surg Radiol Anat* 21:225–227, 1999.

61. Lee S, James WC, Cohen BE, Davis WH, Anderson RB: Evaluation of hallux alignment and functional outcome after isolated tibial sesamoidectomy, *Foot Ankle Int* 26:803–809, 2005.

62. Lemont H, Khoury M: Subchondral bone cysts of the sesamoids, *J Am Podiatr Med Assoc* 75:218–219, 1985.

63. Leonard MH: The sesamoids of the great toe—the pedal polemic: report of three cases, *Clin Orthop Relat Res* 16:295–301, 1960.

64. Mann RA, Coughlin MJ: Hallux valgus—etiology, anatomy, treatment, and surgical considerations, *Clin Orthop Relat Res* 151:31–41, 1981.

65. Mann RA, Coughlin MJ, Baxter D, et al: Sesamoidectomy of the great toe. 15th Annual Meeting of the American Orthopaedic Foot and Ankle Society, Las Vegas, Nev, January 24, 1985.

66. Mann RA, Wapner K: Tibial sesamoid shaving for treatment of intractable plantar keratosis, *Foot Ankle* 13:196–198, 1992.

67. McBride E: Hallux valgus bunion deformity, *J Bone Joint Surg* 9:334–346, 1952.

68. McCarthy D, Reed T, Abell N: The hallucal interphalangeal sesamoid, *J Am Podiatr Med Assoc* 76:311–319, 1986.

69. Miller W, Love B: Cartilaginous sesamoid or nodule of the interphalangeal joint of the big toe, *Foot Ankle* 2:291–293, 1982.

70. Mowad S, Zichichi S, Mullin R: Osteochondroma of the tibial sesamoid, *J Am Podiatr Med Assoc* 85:765–766, 1995.

71. Nakasa T, Fukuhara K, Adachi N, Ochi M: Painful os intermetatarseum in athletes: report of four cases and review of the literature, *Arch Orthop Trauma Surg* 127:261–264, 2007.

72. Nayfa TM, Sorto LA: The incidence of hallux abductus following tibial sesamoidectomy, *J Am Podiatr Assoc* 72:617–620, 1982.

73. Orr TG: Fracture of great toe sesamoid bones, *Ann Surg* 67:609–612, 1918.

74. Ozkoc G, Akpinar S, Ozalay M, et al: Hallucal sesamoid osteonecrosis: an overlooked cause of forefoot pain, *J Am Podiatr Med Assoc* 95:277–280, 2005.

75. Pagenstert GI, Valderrabano V, Hintermann B: Medial sesamoid nonunion combined with hallux valgus in athletes: a report of two cases, *Foot Ankle Int* 27:135–140, 2006.

76. Parra E: Stress fractures of the sesamoid, *Clin Orthop Relat Res* 18:281–285, 1960.

77. Pretterklieber M, Wanivenhaus A: The arterial supply of the sesamoid bones of the hallux: the course and source of the nutrient arteries as an anatomical basis for surgical approaches to the great toe, *Foot Ankle* 13:27–31, 1992.

78. Rath B, Notermans HP, Frank D, et al: Arterial anatomy of the hallucal sesamoids, *Clin Anat* 22:755–760, 2009.

79. Renander A: Two cases of typical osteochondropathy of the medial sesamoid bone of the first metatarsal, *Acta Radiol* 3:521–527, 1924.

80. Resnick D, Niwayama G, Feingold ML: The sesamoid bones of the hand and feet: participators in arthritis, *Diagn Radiol* 123:57–62, 1977.

81. Richardson EG: Injuries to the hallucal sesamoids in the athlete, *Foot Ankle* 7:229–244, 1987.

82. Riley J, Selner M: Internal fixation of a displaced tibial sesamoid fracture, *J Am Podiatr Med Assoc* 91:536–539, 2001.

83. Rodeo S, Warren R, O'Brien S, et al: Diastasis of bipartite sesamoids of the first metatarsophalangeal joint, *Foot Ankle* 14:425–434, 1993.

84. Rodrigues Pinto R, Muras J: Medial approach to the fibular sesamoid, *Foot Ankle Int* 31:916–919, 2010.

85. Rosenfield J, Trepman E: Technique tip: treatment of sesamoid disorders with a rocker shoe modification, *Foot Ankle Int* 21:914–915, 2000.

86. Roukis TS, Weil LS, Landsman AS: Predicting articular erosion in hallux valgus: clinical, radiographic, and intraoperative analysis, *J Foot Ankle Surg* 44:13–21, 2005.

87. Rowe MM: Osteomyelitis of metatarsal sesamoid, *BMJ* 2:1071–1072, 1963.

88. Salamon PB, Gelberman RH, Huffer JM: Dorsal dislocation of the metatarsophalangeal joint of the great toe, *J Bone Joint Surg Am* 56:1073–1075, 1974.

89. Sanhudo, JAV: The joystick technique for lateral sesamoidectomy: technique tip, *Foot Ankle Int* 3:220, 2006.

90. Salvi V, Tos L: [Osteochondrosis of the sesamoid bones of the hallux.] *Arch Ortop* 75:1294–1304, 1962.

91. Sarrafian SK: Osteology. In Sarrafian SK, editor: *Anatomy of the foot and ankle*, Philadelphia, 1983, JB Lippincott, pp 83–87.

92. Saxby T, Vandermark R, Hall R: Coalition of the hallux sesamoids: a case report, *Foot Ankle* 13:355–358, 1992.

93. Saxena A, Krisdakumtorn T: Return to activity after sesamoidectomy in athletically active individuals, *Foot Ankle Int* 24:415–419, 2003.

94. Scranton PE: Pathologic anatomic variations in the sesamoids, *Foot Ankle* 1:321–326, 1981.

95. Scranton PE, Rutkowski R: Anatomic variations in the first ray, *Clin Orthop Relat Res* 151:256–264, 1980.

96. Smith R: Osteitis of the metatarsal sesamoid, *Br J Surg* 29:19–22, 1941.

97. Sobel M, Hashimoto J, Arnoczky S, et al: The microvasculature of the sesamoid complex: its clinical significance, *Foot Ankle* 13:359–363, 1992.

98. Speed K: Injuries of the great toe sesamoids, *Ann Surg* 60:478–480, 1913.

99. Tagoe M, Brown HA, Rees SM: Total sesamoidectomy for painful hallux rigidus: a medium-term outcome study, *Foot Ankle Int* 30:640–646, 2009.

100. Torgerson WR, Hammond G: Osteomyelitis of the sesamoid bones of the first metatarsophalangeal joint, *J Bone Joint Surg Am* 51:1420–1421, 1969.

101. Toussirot E, Jeunet L, Michel F, Kantelip B, Wendling D: Avascular necrosis of the hallucal sesamoids update with reference to two case-reports, *Joint Bone Spine* 70:307–309, 2003.

102. Van Hal ME, Keene JS, Lange TA, et al: Stress fractures of the great toe sesamoids, *Am J Sports Med* 10:122–128, 1982.

103. Van Pelt M, Brown D, Doyle J, LaFontaine J: First metatarsophalangeal joint dislocation with open fracture of tibial and fibular sesamoids, *J Foot Ankle Surg* 46:124–129, 2007.

104. Ward W, Bergfeld J: Fluoroscopic demonstration of acute disruption of the fifth metatarsophalangeal sesamoid bones, *Am J Sports Med* 21:895–897, 1993.

105. Weil L, Hill M: Bipartite tibial sesamoid and hallux abducto valgus deformity: a previously unreported correlation, *J Foot Surg* 31:104–111, 1992.

106. Williams TH, Pasapula C, Robinson AH: Complete sesamoid agenesis: a rare cause of first ray metatarsalgia, *Foot Ankle Int* 30:465–467, 2009.

107. Wright SM: Congenital hallux varus deformity with bilateral absence of the hallucal sesamoids, *J Am Podiatr Med Assoc* 88:47–48, 1998.

108. Yildirim Y, Saygi B: Congenital absence of the lateral sesamoid, *J Am Podiatr Med Assoc* 96:78–81, 2006.

109. Yu G, Nagle C: Hallux interphalangeal joint sesamoidectomy, *J Am Podiatr Med Assoc* 86:105–111, 1996.

110. Zinman H, Keret D, Reis ND: Fractures of the medial sesamoid bone of the hallux, *J Trauma* 21:581–582, 1981.

111. Zinsmeister B, Edelman R: Congenital absence of the tibial sesamoid: a report of two cases, *J Foot Surg* 24:266–268, 1985.

Accessory Bones of the Foot and Uncommon Sesamoids

112. Abramowitz Y, Wollstein R, Barzilay Y, et al. Outcome of resection of a symptomatic os trigonum, *J Bone Joint Surg Am* 85-A:1051–1057, 2003.

113. Albrecht P: Das os intermedium tarsi der Saugetiere, *Zoolog Anz* 139:419–420, 1883.

114. Anatomical Society Collective Investigation: Sesamoids in the gastrocnemius and peroneus longus, *J Anat Physiol* 32:182, 1897.

115. Anderson T: Calcaneus secundarius: an osteo-archaeological note, *Am J Phys Anthropol* 77:529–531, 1988.

116. Anspach W, Wright EB: The divided navicular of the foot, *Radiology* 29:725–728, 1937.

117. Arho AO: Raajojen ylilukuiset luut rontgenkuvissa, *Duodecim* 56:399–410, 1940.

118. Azurza K, Sekellariou A: Osteosynthesis of a symptomatic bipartite medial cuneiform, *Foot Ankle Int* 22:499–501, 2001.

119. Baastrup CI: Os vesalianum tarsi and fracture of tuberositas ossis metatarsi, *Acta Radiol* 1:334–350, 1921.

120. Barclay M: A case of duplication of the internal cuneiform bone of the foot (cuneiforme bipartitum), *J Anat* 67:175–178, 1932.

121. Bareither D, Muehlman C, Feldman N: Os tibiale externum or sesamoid in the tendon of tibialis posterior, *J Foot Surg* 34:429–434, 1995.

122. Barlow TE: Os cuneiforme I bipartitum, *Am J Phys Anthropol* 29:95–111, 1942.

123. Bennett EH: On the ossicle occasionally found on the posterior border of the astragalus, *J Anat Physiol* 21:59–65, 1887.

124. Bentzon PGK: *Bilateral congenital deformity of the astragalocalcanean joint: bony coalescence between os trigonum and the calcaneus. Communication from the Orthopaedic Clinic, Copenhagen, to the Northern Orthopaedic Association*, 1930, pp 359–364.

125. Berenter J, Goldman F: Surgical approach for enlarged peroneal tubercles, *J Am Podiatr Med Assoc* 79:451–454, 1989.

126. Bessette B, Hodge J: Diagnosis of the acute os peroneum fracture, *Singapore Med J* 39:326–327, 1998.

127. Bianchi S, Abdelwahab IF, Tegaldo G: Fracture and posterior dislocation of the os peroneum associated with rupture of the peroneus longus tendon, *Can Assoc Radiol* 42:340–344, 1991.

128. Bierman MI: The supernumerary pedal bones, *Am J Roentgenol* 9:404–411, 1922.

129. Bizarro AH: On sesamoid and supernumerary bones of the limbs, *J Anat* 55:256–268, 1921.

130. Bjornson R: Developmental anomaly of the lateral malleolus simulating fracture, *J Bone Joint Surg Br* 38:128–130, 1956.

131. Blake R, Lallas P, Ferguson H: The os trigonum syndrome: a literature review, *J Am Podiatr Med Assoc* 82:154–161, 1992.

132. Blitz NM, Nemes KK: Bilateral peroneus longus tendon rupture through a bipartite os peroneum, *J Foot Ankle Surg* 46:270–277, 2007.

133. Bloom RA, Libson E, Lax E, et al: The assimilated os sustentaculi, *Skeletal Radiol* 15:455–457, 1986.

134. Bocker W: Zur Kenntnis der Varietaten des menschlichen Fußskeletts, *Berl Klin Wochenschr* 45:499–502, 1908.

135. Boker H, Muller W: Das Os cuneiform I bipartitum, eine fortschreitende Umkonstruktion des Quergewolbes im menschlichen Fuß, *Anat Anz* 83:193–204, 1936.

136. Bowlus T, Korman S, Desilvio M, et al: Accessory os fibulare avulsion secondary to the inversion ankle injury, *J Am Podiatr Assoc* 70:302–303, 1980.

137. Boya H, Ozcan O, Tandogan R, Gunal I, Arac S: Os vesalianum pedis, *J Am Podiatr Med Assoc* 95:583–585, 2005.

138. Boya H, Oztekin HH, Ozcan O: Abnormal proximal fifth metatarsal and os vesalianum pedis, *J Am Podiatr Med Assoc* 97:428–429, 2007.

139. Bruce WD, Christofersen MR, Phillips DL: Stenosing tenosynovitis and impingement of the peroneal tendons associated with hypertrophy of the peroneal tubercle, *Foot Ankle Int* 20:464–467, 1999.

140. Burman MS, Lapidus PW: The functional disturbances caused by the inconstant bones and sesamoids of the foot, *Arch Surg* 22:936–975, 1931.

141. Burman MS, Sinberg SE: An anomalous talo-calcaneal articulation: double ankle bones, *Radiology* 34:239–241, 1940.

142. Burton S, Altman M: Degenerative arthritis of the os peroneum: a case report, *J Am Podiatr Med Assoc* 76:343–345, 1986.

143. Caffey J: *Pediatric x-ray diagnosis*, ed 8, St Louis, 1985, Mosby, p 469.

144. Callanan I, Williams L, Stephens M: Os post pernei and the posterolateral nutcracker impingement, *Foot Ankle Int* 19:475–478, 1998.

145. Canale S, Williams K: Iselin's disease, *J Pediatr Orthop* 12:90–93, 1992.

146. Case D, Ossenberg N: Os intermetatarsum: a heritable accessory bone of the human foot, *Am J Phys Anthropol* 107:199–209, 1998.

147. Ceroni D, De Coulon G, Spadola L, De Rosa V, Kaelin A: Calcaneus secundarius presenting as calcaneonavicular coalition: a case report, *J Foot Ankle Surg* 45:25–27, 2006.

148. Champagne I, Cook D, Kestner S, et al: Os subfibulare. Investigation of an accessory bone, *J Am Podiatr Medical Assoc* 89:520–524, 1999.

149. Chater EH: Foot pain and the accessory navicular bone, *Ir J Med Sci* 442–471, 1962.

150. Chiodo C, Parentis M, Myerson M: Symptomatic bipartite medial cuneiform in an adult athlete: a case report, *Foot Ankle Int* 23:348–351, 2002.

151. Chung JW, Chu IT: Outcome of fusion of a painful accessory navicular to the primary navicular, *Foot Ankle Int* 30:106–109, 2009.

152. Clausen A: Os naviculare bipartitum pedis, *Nord Med* 23:1802–1804, 1944.

153. Coral A: Os subtibial mistaken for a recent fracture, *BMJ* 292:1571–1572, 1986.

154. Coral A: The radiology of skeletal elements in the subtibial region: incidence and significance, *Skeletal Radiol* 16:298–303, 1987.

155. Cravener EK, MacElroy DG: Supernumerary tarsal scaphoides, *Surg Gynecol Obstet* 71:218–221, 1940.

156. Dameron TB Jr: Fractures and anatomical variations of the proximal portion of the fifth metatarsal, *J Bone Joint Surg Am* 57:788–794, 1975.

157. Day F, Naples J, White J: Metatarsocuneiform coalition, *J Am Podiatr Med Assoc* 84:197–199, 1994.

158. de Cuveland E: Über Beziehungen zwischen vorderer Aussenknochelapophyse und Os subfibulare mit differentialdiagnostischen Erwagungen, *Fortschr Rontgenstr* 83:213–221, 1955.

159. Dellacorte M, Lin P, Grisafi P: Bilateral bipartite medial cuneiform: a case report, *J Am Podiatr Med Assoc* 82:475–478, 1992.

160. Dorrestijn O, Brouwer RW: Bilateral symptomatic os vesalianum pedis: a case report, *J Foot Ankle Surg* 50:473–475, 2011.

161. Dwight T: Description of a free cuboides secundarium, with remarks on that element and on the calcaneus secundarius, *Anat Anz* 37:218–224, 1910.

162. Dwight T: Os intercuneiforme tarsi, os paracuneiforme tarsi, calcaneus secundarius, *Anat Anz* 20:465–472, 1902.

163. Dwight T: *Variations of the bones of the hands and feet: a clinical atlas*, Philadelphia, 1907, JB Lippincott, pp 14–23.

164. Eichenbaum MD, Austin LS, Raikin SM: Chronic ankle pain secondary to talus partitus: two case reports, *Foot Ankle Int* 31:247–250, 2010.

165. Fischer H: Beitrag zur Kenntnis der Skelettvarietaten (uberzahlige Karpalia und Tarsalia, Sesambeine, Kompaktainseln), *Fortschr Nyklearmed Gebiete Rontgenstr* 19:43–66, 1912.

166. Francillon MR: Beitrag zur Klinik und Röntgenologie inkonstanter Skelettelemente des Fusses, *Dtsch Med Wochenschr* 60:1097–1100, 1934.

167. Francillon MR: Untersuchungen zur anatomischen und klinischen Bedeutung des Os tibiale externum, *Z Orthop Chir* 56:61–85, 1932.

168. Friedl E: Das Os intermetatarseum und die Epiphysenbildung am Processus Trochlearis Calcanei, *Dtsch Z Chir* 188:150–160, 1924.

169. Friedl E: Divided cuneiform I in childhood, *Rontgenpraxis* 6:193–195, 1934.

170. Fujishiro T, Nabeshima Y, Yasue S, et al: Coalition of bilateral first cuneometatarsal joints: a case report, *Foot Ankle Int* 24:793–797, 2003.

171. Gaulke R, Schmitz H: Free os cuboideum secundarium: a case report, *J Foot Ankle Surg* 42:230–234, 2003.

172. Geist ES: Supernumerary bones of the foot: a roentgen study of the feet of one hundred normal individuals, *Am J Orthop Surg* 12:403–414, 1914.

173. Geist ES: The accessory scaphoid bone, *J Bone Joint Surg* 7:570–574, 1925.

174. Giannestras NJ: *Foot disorders: medial and surgical management*, Philadelphia, 1973, Lea & Febiger, pp 233–234, 583–588.

175. Giuffrida A, Lin S, Abidi N, et al: Pseudo os trigonum sign: missed posteromedial talar facet fracture, *Foot Ankle Int* 24:642–649, 2003.

176. Goedhard G: The apophyses of the lateral malleolus, *Radiol Clin Biol* 39:330–333, 1970.

177. Grasmann M: Zur Kenntnis des Os subtibiale, *Munch Med Wochenschr* 79:824–825, 1932.

178. Griffiths J, Menelaus M: Symptomatic ossicles of the lateral malleolus in children, *J Bone Joint Surg Br* 69:317–319, 1987.

179. Grisolia A: Fracture of the os peroneum: review of literature and report of one case, *Clin Orthop Relat Res* 28:213–215, 1963.

180. Grogan D, Gasser S, Ogden J: The painful accessory navicular: a clinical and histopathological study, *Foot Ankle* 10:164–169, 1989.

181. Gruber W: Auftreten der Tuberositas des Os metatarsale V sowohl als persistirende Epiphyse, als auch mit einer an ihrem ausseren Umfange aufsitzenden persistirenden Epiphyse, *Arch Pathol Anat Physiol Klin Med* 99:460–471, 1885.

182. Gruber W: Über den Fortsatz des Seitenhockers—processus tuberositatis lateralis—des Metatarsale V und sein Auftreten als Epiphyse, *Arch Anat Physiol Wissenschaft Med* 48–58, 1875.

183. Gruber W: Über einem am Malleolus externus articulirenden Knochen, *Arch Pathol Anat Physiol Klin Med* 27:205–206, 1863.

184. Guntz E: Os tibiale and Unfall (Abriss des Os tibiale), *Arch Orthop Ungall Chir* 34:320–326, 1934.

185. Haglund P: Ueber Fraktur des Tuberculum ossis navicularis in den Jugendjahren und ihre Bedeutung als Ursache einer typischen Form von Pes valgus, *Z Orthop Chir* 16:347–353, 1906.

186. Harris RI, Beath T: *Army foot survey*, vol 1, Ottawa, 1947, National Research Council of Canada, p 52.

187. Harris RI, Beath T: Etiology of peroneal spastic flat foot, *J Bone Joint Surg Br* 30:624–634, 1948.

188. Hasselwander A: Über die Entwickelung des Processus posterior tali und des Os trigonum tarsi, *Z Morphol Anthropol* 18:553–578, 1914.

189. Hatoff A: Bipartite navicular bone as a cause of flatfoot, *Am J Dis Child* 80:991–992, 1950.

190. Hedrick M, McBryde A: Posterior ankle impingement, *Foot Ankle* 15:2–8, 1994.

191. Heidsieck E: Os cuneiforme I bipartitum, *Rontgenpraxis* 8:712–715, 1936.

192. Heimerzheim A: Über einen seltsamen Knochenbefund am Calcaneus, *Dtsch Z Chir* 187:281–283, 1924.

193. Heimerzheim A: Über einige akzessorische Fusswurzelknochen nebst ihrer chirurgischen Bedeutung, *Dtsch Z Chir* 190:96–112, 1925.

194. Henderson MS: Fractures of the bones of the foot—except the os calcis, *Surg Gynecol Obstet* 64:454–457, 1937.

195. Henderson RS: Os intermetatarseum and a possible relationship to hallux valgus, *J Bone Joint Surg Br* 45:117–121, 1963.

196. Hermann N: An unusual example of a calcaneus secundarius, *J Am Podiatr Med Assoc* 82:623–624, 1992.

197. Hirschtick AB: An anomalous tarsal bone, *J Bone Joint Surg Am* 33:907–910, 1951.

198. Hoerr NL, Pyle DI, Francis CC: *Radiographic atlas of skeletal development of the foot and ankle: a standard of reference*, Springfield, Ill, 1962, Charles C Thomas, pp 41–44.

199. Hogan J: Fractures of the os peroneum: case report and literature review, *J Am Podiatr Med Assoc* 79:201–204, 1989.

200. Hohmann G: Über Frakturen und andere traumatische Storungen am Os naviculare des Fusses, *Arch Orthop Unfall Chir* 43:12–19, 1944.

201. Holland CT: On rarer ossifications seen during x-ray examinations, *J Anat* 55:235–248, 1920.

202. Holland CT: The accessory bones of the foot. In *The Robert Jones birthday volume*, London, Oxford University Press, 1928, pp 157–182.

203. Holle F: *Über die inkonstanten Elemente am menschlichen Fussskelett (Inaugural-Dissertation)*. Munich, 1938.

204. Horinouchi T, Kinoshita M, Okuda R, et al: Coalition between the medial cuneiform and the first metatarsal. A case report, *J Jpn Soc Surg Foot* 20:93–96, 1999.

205. Inoue T, Yoshimura I, Ogata K, Emoto G: Os vesalianum as a cause of lateral foot pain: a familial case and its treatment. Abstract, *J Pediatr Orthop B* 8:56–58, 1999.

206. Iselin H: Wachstumsbeschwerden zur Zeit der Knochernen entwicklung der Tuberositas metatarsi quinti, *Deutsche Z Fur Chirurgie* 117:529–535, 1912.

207. Jashashvili T, Ponce de Leon MS, Lordkipanidze D, Zollikofer CP: First evidence of a bipartite medial cuneiform in the hominin fossil record: a case report from the Early Pleistocene site of Dmanisi, *J Anat* 216:705–716, 2010.

208. Jeppesen JB, Jensen FK, Falborg B, Madsen JL: Bone scintigraphy in painful os peroneum syndrome, *Clin Nucl Med* 36:209–211, 2011.

209. Johansson S: Os vesalianum pedis, *Z Orthop Chir* 42:301–307, 1922.

210. Jones FW: *Structure and function as seen in the foot*, ed 2, London, 1949, Bailliere, Tindall, & Cox, pp 83–100.

211. Karasick D, Schweitzer M: The os trigonum syndrome: imaging features, *AJR Am J Roentgenol* 166:125–129, 1996.

212. Kassianenko W: Calcaneus secundarius, talus accessorius und os trigonum tarsi beim Pferde, *Anat Anzeiger* 80:1–10, 1935.

213. Keats T: *An atlas of normal roentgen variants that may simulate disease*, ed 3, St Louis, 1984, Mosby.

214. Kewenter Y: Die Sesambeine des I. Metatarsophangealgelenks des Menschen, *Acta Orthop Scand Suppl* 2:1–113, 1936.

215. Kidner FC: The prehallux (accessory scaphoid) in its relation to flat foot, *J Bone Joint Surg* 11:831–837, 1929.

216. Kiter E, Erduran M, Gunal I: Inheritance of the accessory navicular bone, *Arch Orthop Trauma Surg* 120:582–583, 2000.

217. Kiter E, Gunal I, Turgut A, Kose N: Evaluation of simple excision in the treatment of symptomatic accessory navicular associated with flat feet, *J Orthop Sci* 5:333–335, 2000.

218. Kohler A, Zimmer E: *Borderlands of the normal and early pathologic in skeletal roentgenology*, ed 3, New York, 1968, Grune & Stratton, pp 245, 460, 464–468, 489, 502–527.

219. Kohler A, Zimmer E: *Grenzen des Normalen und Anfange des Pathologischen im Rontgenbilde des Skelettes*, ed 9, Stuttgart, 1953, Georg Thieme.

220. Kricun M: *Imaging of the foot and ankle*, Rockville, Md, 1988, Aspen, p 113.

221. Krida A: Secondary os calcis, *JAMA* 80:752–753, 1923.

222. Kumai T, Tanaka Y, Takakura Y, et al: Isolated first naviculocuneiform joint coalition, *Foot Ankle Int* 17:635–640, 1996.

223. Kurklu M, Kose O, Yurttas Y, Oguz E, Atesalp AS: Anterosuperior calcaneal process fracture or OS calcaneus secundarius? *Am J Phys Med Rehabil* 89:522, 2010.

224. Laidlaw PP: The os calcis. Part II, *Anat Physiol* 39:161–176, 1905.

225. Laidlaw PP: The varieties of the os calcis, *J Anat* 38:133–143, 39:161–177, 1904.

226. Lapidus PW: Os subtibale: inconstant bone over the tip of the medial malleolus, *J Bone Joint Surg* 15:766–771, 1933.

227. Laquerriere D: On the vesalian bone, *J Radiol Electrother* 21:395–400, 1916.

228. Latten W: Histologische Beziehungen zwischen Os tibiale und Kahnbein nach Untersuchungen an einem operierten Falle, *Dtsch Z Chir* 205:320–327, 1927.

229. Lehman R, Gregg J, Torg E: Iselin's disease, *Am J Sports Med* 14:494–496, 1986.

230. Leimbach G: Beitrage zur Kenntnis der Inkonstanten Skeletelemente des Tarsus, (Akzessorische Fusswurzelknochen), *Arch Orthop Trauma Surg* 38:431–448, 1938.

231. Leonard MH, Gonzalez S, Breck LW, et al: Lateral transfer of the posterior tibial tendon in certain selected cases of pes plano valgus (Kidner operation), *Clin Orthop Relat Res* 40:139–144, 1965.

232. Lepore L, Francobandiera C, Maffulli N: Fracture of the os tibiale externum in a decathlete, *J Foot Surg* 29:366–368, 1990.

233. Lichte E: On bipartite os naviculare pedis, *Acta Radiol* 22:377–382, 1941.

234. Lilienfeld A: Über die sogenannten Tarsalia, die inkonstanten accessorischen Skelettstucke des Fusses und ihre Beziehungen zu den Frakturen, im Rontgenbild, *Z Orthop Grenz Chir* 18:213–238, 1907.

235. Logan M, Connell D, Janzen D: Painful os cuboideum secundarium: cross-sectional imaging findings, *J Am Podiatr Med Assoc* 86:123–125, 1996.

236. MacDonald BD, Wertheimer SJ: Bilateral os peroneum fractures: comparison of conservative and surgical treatment and outcomes, *J Foot Ankle Surg* 36:220–225, 1997.

237. Maffulli N, Lepore L, Francobandiera C: Traumatic lesions of some accessory bones of the foot in sports activity, *J Am Podiatr Med Assoc* 80:86–90, 1990.

238. Mains D, Sullivan R: Fracture of the os peroneum, *J Bone Joint Surg Am* 55:1529–1530, 1973.

239. Mancuso J, Hutchison P, Abramow S, et al: Accessory ossicle of the lateral malleolus, *J Foot Surg* 30:52–55, 1991.

240. Mann RA, Owsley D: Os trigonum: variation of a common accessory ossicle of the talus, *J Am Podiatr Med Assoc* 80:536–539, 1990.

241. Mann RW: Calcaneus secundarius: description and frequency in six skeletal samples, *Am J Phys Anthropol* 81:17–25, 1990.

242. Mann RW: Calcaneus secundarius: variation of a common accessory ossicle, *J Am Podiatr Med Assoc* 79:363–366, 1989.

243. Manners-Smith T: A study of the cuboid and os peroneum in the primate foot, *J Anat Physiol* 42:397–414, 1908.

244. Manners-Smith T: A study of the navicular in the human and anthropod foot, *J Anat Physiol* 41:255–279, 1907.

245. March HC, London RI: The os sustentaculi, *Am J Roentgenol* 76:1114–1118, 1956.

246. Marotta J, Micheli L: Os trigonum impingement in dancers, *Am J Sports Med* 20:533–536, 1992.

247. Marti T: Die Skeletvarietaten des Fusses. Ihre klinische und unfallmedizinische Bedeutung. In Debrunner H, Francillon MR, editors: Praktische Beitrage zur Orthopädie, vol 2, Bern, 1947, H Huber, pp 27–118.

248. Martin B: Posterior triangle pain: the os trigonum, *J Foot Surg* 28:312–318, 1989.

249. Mau H: Zur Kenntnis des Naviculare bipartitum pedis, *Z Orthop* 93:404–411, 1960.

250. McDougall A: The os trigonum, *J Bone Joint Surg* 37:257–265, 1955.

251. McKusick V: *Mendelian inheritance in man: catalogs of autosomal dominant, autosomal recessive, and X-linked phenotypes*, ed 2, Baltimore, 1978, Johns Hopkins University Press, p 147.

252. Mellado J, Salvado E, Camins A, et al: Painful os sustentaculi: imaging finding of another symptomatic skeletal variant, *Skeletal Radiol* 31:53–56, 2002.

253. Mercer J: The secondary os calcis, *J Anat* 66:84–97, 1931.

254. Micheli L: The traction apophysitis, *Clin Sports Med* 6:389, 1987.

255. Michelson G: Zur Frage der sogenannten Stiedaschen Fraktur, *Rontgenpraxis* 2:896–898, 1930.

256. Miller G, Black J: Symptomatic os supra naviculare: a case report, *J Am Podiatr Med Assoc* 80:248–250, 1990.

257. Monahan JJ: The human pre-hallux, *Am J Med Sci* 160:708–720, 1920.

258. Mouchet A, Moutier G: Osselets surnumeraires du tarse, *Presse Med* 23:369–374, 1925.

259. Noguchi M, Iwata Y, Miura K, Kusaka Y: A painful os intermetatarseum in a soccer player: a case report, *Foot Ankle Int* 21:1040–1041, 2000.

260. Okazaki K, Nakashima S, Nomura S: Stress fracture of an os peroneum, *J Orthop Trauma* 17:654–656, 2003.

261. O'Neal M, Ganey T, Ogden J: Fracture of a bipartite medial cuneiform synchondrosis, *Foot Ankle Int* 16:37–40, 1995.

262. O'Rahilly R: A survey of carpal and tarsal anomalies, *J Bone Joint Surg Am* 35:626–642, 1953.

263. Paal E: Fehlbeurteilungen bei Rontgenbildern, *Arch Orthop Unfall Chir* 33:153–158, 1933.

264. Pai VS, Lawson D: Rupture of the peroneus longus tendon, *J Foot Ankle Surg* 34:475–477; discussion 510, 1995.

265. Peacock K, Resnick E, Thoder J: Fracture of the os peroneum with rupture of the peroneus longus tendon, *Clin Orthop Relat Res* 202:223–224, 1986.

266. Peh W, Gilula L: A 37-year-old man with left foot pain: symptomatic accessory navicular synchondrosis, *Ortho Rev* 23:958–961, 1994.

267. Perlman M: Os peroneum fracture with sural nerve entrapment neuritis, *J Foot Surg* 29:119–121, 1990.

268. Peterson DA, Stinson W: Excision of the fractured os peroneum: a report on five patients and review of the literature, *Foot Ankle* 13:277–281, 1992.

269. Pfitzner W: Beitrage zur Kenntmiss des Menschlichen Extremitatenskelets: VII. Die Variationen in Aufbau des Fusskelets. In Schwalbe G, editor: *Morphologische Arbeiten*, Jena, Germany, 1896, Gustav Fischer, pp 245–527.

270. Pierson J, Inglis A: Stenosing tenosynovitis of the peroneus longus tendon associated with hypertrophy of the peroneal tubercle and an os peroneum, *J Bone Joint Surg Am* 74:440–442, 1992.

271. Pirie AH: A normal ossicle in the foot frequently diagnosed as a fracture, *Arch Radiol Electrother* 24:93–95, 1919.

272. Pirie AH: Extra bones in the wrist and ankle found by roentgen rays, *AJR Am J Roentgenol* 569–573, 1921.

273. Powell HDW: Extra centre of ossification for the medial malleolus in children, *J Bone Joint Surg Br* 43:107–113, 1961.

274. Puhl H, Lindemann K: Über die Entstehung freier Körper im Talocruralgelenk, *Arch Orthop Unfall Chir* 38:726–739, 1938.

275. Ralph B, Barrett J, Kenyhercz C, DiDomenico LA: Iselin's disease: a case presentation of nonunion and review of the differential diagnosis, *J Foot Surg* 38:409–416, 1999.

276. Ray S, Goldberg V: Surgical treatment of the accessory navicular, *Clin Orthop Relat Res* 177:61–66, 1983.

277. Reichmister JP: The painful os intermetatarseum: a brief review and case reports, *Clin Orthop Relat Res* 153:201–203, 1980.

278. Rosenmuller J: De mon nullis musculorum corpus humani varietatibus, *Leipzig*, 1804.

279. Ruiz J, Christman R, Hillstrom H: Anatomical considerations of the peroneal tubercle, *J Am Podiatr Med Assoc* 83:563–575, 1993.

280. Sandor L: Zur traumatischen Genese des Os subtibiale, *Beitr Orthop Traumatol* 24:558–563, 1977.

281. Sarrafian SK: Osteology. In Sarrafian SK, editor: *Anatomy of the foot and ankle*, Philadelphia, 1983, JB Lippincott, pp 35–106.

282. Saupe E: Malazieartige Veranderungen am schmerzhaften os tibiale externum, *Rontgenpraxis* 11:533–536, 1939.

283. Scarlet JJ, Gunther R, Katz J, Schwartz H: Os intermetatarseum-one: case report and discussion, *J Am Podiatr Assoc* 68:431–434, 1978.

284. Schoen W: Seltenere akzessorische Knochen am Fussrucken, *Rontgenpraxis* 7:775–776, 1935.

285. Schreiber A, Differding P, Zollinger H: Talus partitus, *J Bone Joint Surg Br* 67:430–431, 1985.

286. Schwartz B, Jay R, Schoenhaus H: Apophysitis of the fifth metatarsal base: Iselin's disease, *J Am Podiatr Med Assoc* 81:128–130, 1991.

287. Scott AT, Sabesan VJ, Saluta JR, Wilson MA, Easley ME: Fusion versus excision of the symptomatic Type II accessory navicular: a prospective study, *Foot Ankle Int* 30:10–15, 2009.

288. Seddon HJ: Calcaneo-scaphoid coalition, *Proc R Soc Med* 26:419–424, 1932.

289. Selby S: Separate centers of ossification of the tip of the internal malleolus, *AJR Am J Roentgenol* 86:496–501, 1961.

290. Sella E, Lawson J: Biomechanics of the accessory navicular synchondrosis, *Foot Ankle* 8:156–163, 1987.

291. Shands A: Accessory bones of the foot, *South Med Surg* 93:326, 1931.

292. Shands A, Wentz I: Congenital anomalies, accessory bones, and osteochondritis in the feet of 850 children, *Surg Clin North Am* 33:1643, 1953.

293. Shawdon A, Kiss Z, Fuller P: The bipartite tarsal navicular bone: radiographic and computed tomography findings, *Australas Radiol* 39:192–194, 1995.

294. Shepherd FJ: A hitherto undescribed fracture of the astragalus, *J Anat Physiol* 17:79–81, 1883.

295. Shepherd FJ: Note on the ossicle found on the posterior border of the astragalus, *J Anat Physiol* 21:335, 1887.

296. Smith AD, Carter JR, Marus RE: The os vesalianum: an unusual cause of lateral foot pain, *Orthopedics* 7:86–89, 1984.

297. Smith T: A foot having four cuneiform bones, *Trans Pathol Soc* 17:222–223, 1865.

298. Sobel M, Pavlov H, Geppert M, et al: Painful os peroneum syndrome: a spectrum of conditions responsible for plantar lateral foot pain, *Foot Ankle* 15:112–124, 1994.

299. Spronck CH: Auftreten der ganzen Tuberositas (lateralis) des Os metatarsale V als ein für sich bestechendes, am Metatarsale und Cuboides artikulierendes Skelett-Element, *Anat Anz* 2:734–739, 1887.

300. Stieda L: Der M. peroneus longus und die Fussknochen, *Anat Anz* 4:600–607, 624–640, 1889.

301. Stropeni L: Frattura isolata di un osso soprannumernario dei tarso (os perineum externum), *Arch Ital Chir* 2:556–564, 1920.

302. Grant JCB, editor: *Grant's atlas of anatomy*, ed 5, Baltimore, 1972, Williams & Wilkins, p 356.

303. Sutton JB: A case of secondary astragalus, *J Anat Physiol* 21:333–334, 1887.

304. Swenson PC, Wilner D: Unfused ossification centers associated with pain in the adult, *AJR Am J Roentgenol* 61:341–353, 1949.

305. Takakura Y, Nakata H: Isolated first cuneometatarsal coalition: a case report, *Foot Ankle Int* 20:815–816, 1999.

306. Tanaka Y, Takakura Y, Sugimoto K, Kumai T: Non-osseous coalition of the medial cuneiform–first metatarsal joint: a case report, *Foot Ankle Int* 21:1043–1046, 2000.

307. Tehranzadeh J, Stoll D, Gabriele O: Diagnosis: posterior migration of the os peroneum of the left foot, indicating a tear of the peroneal tendon, *Skeletal Radiol* 12:44–47, 1984.

308. Thews K: Fehldeutung und behandlung auf Grund von Varietaten der Handwurzel und Fusswurzel im Rontgenbilde, *Rontgenpraxis* 11:184–186, 1939.

309. Thiel E, Feibel J, Chorey N, Gorsline R: Bipartite talus: a case report, *Foot Ankle Int* 31:552–555, 2010.

310. Thompson F, Patterson A: Rupture of the peroneus longus tendon, *J Bone Joint Surg Am* 71:293–295, 1989.

311. Trolle D: *Accessory bones of the human foot: a radiological, histoembryological, comparative anatomical and genetic study*, Copenhagen, 1948, Musksgaard, pp 20–53.

312. Trolle D: De to accessoriske knogler: os subtibiale og os subfibulare i relation til diagnosen af malleolarfracturer, *Nord Med* 25:247–249, 1945.

313. Truong T, Dussault R, Kaplan P: Fracture of the os peroneum and rupture of the peroneus longus tendon as a complication of diabetic neuropathy, *Skeletal Radiol* 24:626–628, 1995.

314. Turner W: A secondary astragalus in the human foot, *J Anat Physiol* 17:82–83, 1883.

315. Turner W: Note of another case of secondary astragalus, *J Anat Physiol* 21:334–335, 1887.

316. Uhrbrand B, Jensen T: A case of accessory calcaneus, *Acta Orthop Scand* 57:455, 1986.

317. Uhrmacher F: Varietaten des Fussskeletts als Grundlage von Fussbeschwerden, *Z Orthop Chir* 61:180–186, 1934.

318. Viana SL, Fernandes JL, Mendonca JL, Freitas FM: Painful os talus secundarius: a case report and imaging findings, *Foot Ankle Int* 28:624–625, 2007.

319. Volk C: Zwei Falle von os naviculare pedis bipartitum, *Z Orthop* 66:396–403, 1937.

320. Volkmann J: Das Os subtibiale, *Fortschr Geb Rontgenstrahlen Neven Bildgeb Verfahr Erganzungsbd* 48:225–227, 1933.

321. Wagner W: Personal communication, 1989.

322. Wakeley C, Johnson D, Watt I: The value of MR imaging in the diagnosis of the os trigonum syndrome, *Skeletal Radiol* 25:133–136, 1996.

323. Waldeyer W: Bemerkungen uber das "Tibiale externum." In *Sitzungesberichte der Königlich Preussischen Akademie der Wissenschaft*, Berlin, 1904, Deutsche Akademie der Wissenschaften, pp 1326–1332.

324. Wander D, Galli K, Ludden J, et al: Surgical management of a ruptured peroneus longus tendon with a fractured multipartite os peroneum, *J Foot Ankle Surg* 33:124–128, 1994.

325. Waschulewski H: Os subtibiale I and II. Os subfibulare, *Rontgenpraxis* 13:468, 1941.

326. Waters L: Os intermetatarseum: case study and report, *J Am Podiatr Assoc* 48:252–254, 1958.

327. Watkins WW: Anomalous bones of the wrist and foot in relation to injury, *JAMA* 108:270–274, 1937.

328. Weinstein SL, Bonfiglio M: Unusual accessory (bipartite) talus simulating fracture, *J Bone Joint Surg Am* 57:1161–1163, 1975.

329. Wilson R, Moyles B: Surgical treatment of the symptomatic os peroneum, *J Foot Surg* 26:156–158, 1987.

330. Wredmark T, Carlstedt C, Bauer H, et al: Os trigonum syndrome: a clinical entity in ballet dancers, *Foot Ankle* 11:404–406, 1991.

331. Zadek I: The significance of the accessory tarsal scaphoid, *J Bone Joint Surg* 24:618–626, 1926.

332. Zadek I, Gold AM: The accessory tarsal scaphoid, *J Bone Joint Surg Am* 30:957–968, 1948.

333. Zerna M: Das sogenannte Os subtibiale—eine seltene Anomalie, *Zentralbl Chir* 95:1481–1487, 1970.

334. Zimmer EA: Krankheiten, Verletzungen und Varietaten des Os naviculare pedis, *Arch Orthop Unfall Chir* 38:396–411, 1938.

335. Zimmer EA: Skelettelemente medial des Cuneiforme, *Acta Radiol* 34:102–114, 1950.

Chapter 11

Toenail Abnormalities

Jesse F. Doty, Michael J. Coughlin, Richard G. Alvarez

The nails are special cutaneous appendages that have the primary function of protecting the distal phalanx. Only primates have toenails, and whether the first primates with flat nails had an advantage over their peers by being able to remove parasites better from their bodies (thus promoting their evolutionary superiority) is a matter of fascinating speculation.[232]

In humans, diseases and deformities of the toenails are among the most common and disabling of foot problems. They can result from local or systemic disorders or from congenital malformations. Only a small percentage of toenail abnormalities result from systemic diseases, such as psoriasis and endocrine disorders. The majority are caused by intrinsic factors and are directly or indirectly related to tinea infections. The other deformities stem from mechanical problems and constitute some of the most common yet difficult foot problems for the treating physician.

Although few studies of physicians' reports have documented the frequency of nail disorders, Krausz[123] did examine the incidence of nail disorders (Table 11-1). During 41 years of practice, Krausz reported on 7670 patients displaying one or more nail disorders.[153]

The nail has only a few pathologic responses to disease and can demonstrate abnormalities as a manifestation of either systemic or dermatologic diseases. Before examining specific examples of nail disorders, this chapter reviews the anatomy and physiology of the toenail and

Table 11-1 Incidence of Nail Disorders	
Nail Condition	**Incidence (%)**
Onychocryptosis	26
Onychogryphosis or onychauxis	23
Onychophosis	19
Onychomycosis	8
Onychotrophia	4

Data from Krausz CE: Nail survey (1942-1970). *Br J Chir* 35:117, 1970; Nzuzi SM: Common nail disorders. *Clin Podiatr Med Surg* 6:273–294, 1989.

supporting structures, to facilitate an understanding of the pathologic conditions.

ANATOMY

The toenail or *nail plate* is composed of several layers of dense, overlapping keratinized cells. There are three layers, each originating from a different area of the nail unit. The relatively thin dorsal layer is stiff and brittle and covers the relatively thick softer middle layer. The deep layer is thought to be derived in part from the nail bed itself.[95,113,114] The nail plate differs from hair or skin in that it does not desquamate skin cells. The hardness of the nail plate can be attributed to its high sulfur content[56] and to the paucity of water within the plate. Although the nail plate is 10 times more permeable to water than the skin, the nail plate, unlike the skin, has a low fat content and thus cannot retain water.[12]

The normal nail plate grows distally approximately 0.03 to 0.05 mm/day, and it has a thickness of 0.5 to 1 mm.[107] The nail plate is supported by the nail unit,[61] or *perionychium*,[232] an area of epithelial tissue that is divided into four components (Fig. 11-1)[228]: nail bed, hyponychium, proximal nail fold, and nail matrix. Synonyms are common for various anatomic units (Box 11-1).

The nail plate lies on the *nail bed*, a roughened epithelial surface consisting of longitudinal grooves that interdigitate with corresponding grooves on the undersurface of the toenail. This interdigitation firmly bonds the nail plate to the nail bed. The nail bed or sterile matrix has only one or two layers of germinal cells, which produce the nail plate.[232] At the distal end of the nail bed, where the nail bed and the nail plate separate, a smooth border of skin called the *hyponychium* forms a seal between the distal end of the toenail and the nail bed.

On the tibial and fibular borders of the toenail, the nail plate is surrounded by epidermal skin folds termed *lateral nail folds*. The base of the toenail is covered by the *proximal nail fold*, a complex structure that has germinal cells on the proximal half of the plantar surface of the nail fold.[232] The dorsal surface of the nail fold is composed of skin on the dorsal surface of the toe. On the plantar surface of this fold, the *eponychium* forms a thin surface that attaches to the nail plate. The distal surfaces of these two components of the proximal nail fold comprise the cuticle.

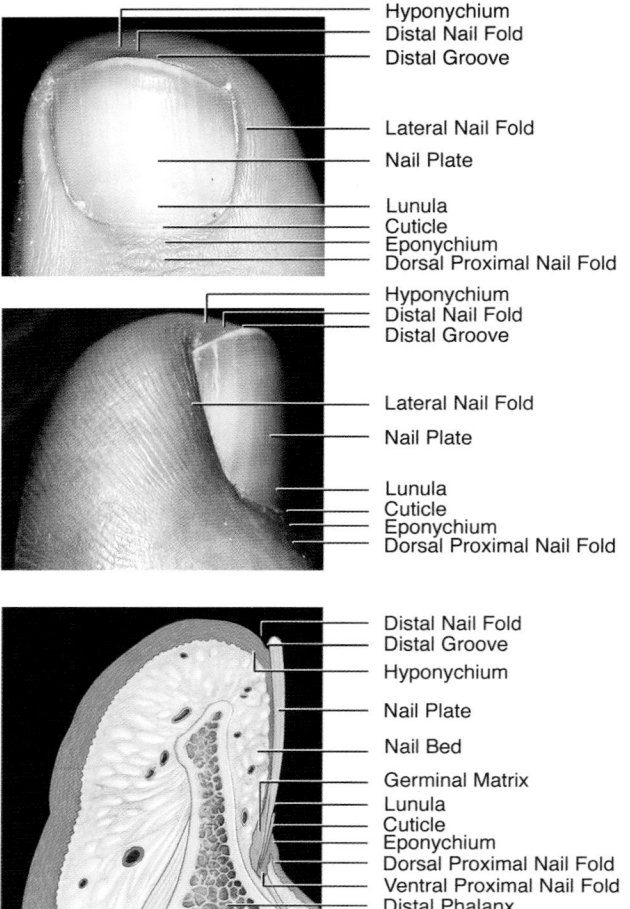

Figure 11-1 Anteroposterior *(top)* and lateral *(middle)* photographs of a toenail and a sagittal–lateral cross-sectional drawing *(bottom)* showing the various anatomic parts of the toenail unit. (Courtesy Mayo Foundation for Medical Education and Research. Used with permission.)

Box 11-1 Anatomic Synonyms
Term (Synonym)
Cuticle (eponychial fold)
Germinal matrix (nail matrix)
Nail bed (sterile matrix)

The *nail matrix* or *germinal matrix* is the main germinal area of the toenail. The germinal matrix extends from a point just distal to the lunula and as far laterally as the entire width of the nail plate,[55] and it extends 5 to 6 mm proximally to the edge of the cuticle and closely borders the insertion of the long extensor tendon and the interphalangeal joint.[95] The nail matrix is seen beneath the nail plate as the *lunula*—the opaque, crescent-shaped area at the base of the nail. It lacks color because it is less vascular than the heavily vascularized nail bed. Distally, the nail matrix is contiguous with the nail bed. The nail matrix is covered by a small epidermal surface but does not have the epidermal ridges characteristic of the nail bed. At the distal end of the lunula, the nail matrix terminates. As noted above, at the proximal margin of the matrix, a small area on the plantar surface of the proximal nail fold appears to contribute to the growth of the nail plate.[95,134,182] This is important to remember when trying to permanently ablate the nail by removing the germinal matrix from which the nail grows.

Most matrix germination occurs between the apex of the matrix and the distal border of the lunula. The area covered by the proximal nail fold forms the thin dorsal layer of the nail plate. The area of the lunula produces the thicker, softer middle portion of the nail plate and joins with the dorsal area to form the nail plate.[95] Although the germinal matrix is the major origin for toenail growth, additional microscopic germinal areas of growth may be present within the lateral nail folds and the distal nail bed.[113,114,126] These produce a thin layer of the ventral toenail plate, a factor that occasionally accounts for postoperative regrowth.[55,95,134]

The germinal matrix cells of the nail plate are oriented longitudinally. Because of pressure from the proximal nail fold, the nail plate grows distally rather than in an elevated direction. However, if the nail matrix is injured or altered because of trauma or surgery, the nail plate may grow in an abnormal direction. Likewise, the nail plate gives a certain rigidity to the soft tissue of the distal part of the toe. If the toenail is removed or ablated, the distal nail bed and soft tissue can grow in an elevated direction because of lack of dorsal pressure from the nail (Fig. 11-2). As the new nail plate begins to grow distally, it can abut these soft tissues and lead to a club nail or an ingrown toenail.

Common diseases involving the nail include infection, psoriasis, contact dermatitis and eczema, tumor, trauma, and general or systemic diseases.[216] A systematic review of nail disorders by Pardo-Castello and Pardo[165] provides a useful classification for both common and uncommon nail abnormalities and also discusses disorders caused by trauma and neoplasia. The classification includes the following:

■ Dermatologic and systemic diseases
■ Congenital and genetic nail disorders
■ Common nail abnormalities and onychodystrophies (Fig. 11-3A-E)

Nzuzi[154] presented the following logical classification of common nail disorders (onychopathies) based on the anatomic structures primarily involved (Box 11-2):

■ Nail plate disorders
■ Nail bed disorders
■ Nail fold disorders
■ Nail matrix disorders

Use of Pardo-Castello's general classification for an overview of nail disorders and Nzuzi's classification for onychopathies provides a complete and systematic approach for a discussion of toenail disorders.

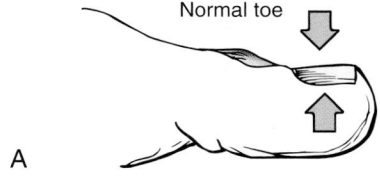

Normal toe

A

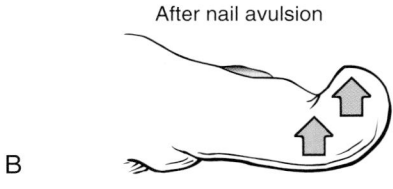

After nail avulsion

B

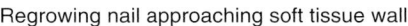

Regrowing nail approaching soft tissue wall

C

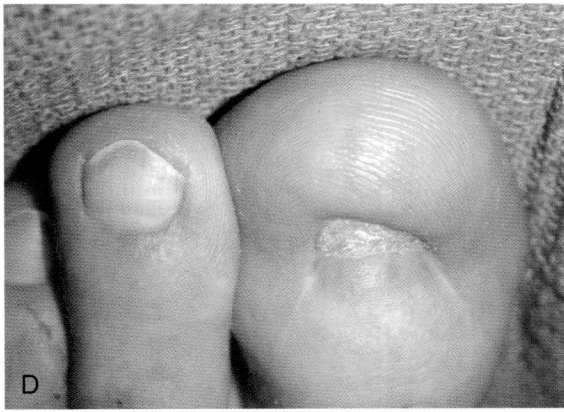

D

Figure 11-2 The toenail tends to splint the distal soft tissue of the toe. **A,** Normal configuration of the great toe. **B,** After a nail avulsion, upward pressure forces deformation of the distal nail bed. **C,** Regrowth of the nail as it approaches the soft tissue wall can cause infection. **D,** Deformity of the distal end of the toe after incomplete ablation of the nail. Without nail support, clubbing has resulted, with impingement of the growth of the remaining nail.

DERMATOLOGIC AND SYSTEMIC NAIL DISORDERS

Skin disorders involving the nails are usually within the province of the dermatologist, and systemic disorders involving the nails are typically within the internist's scope of practice. Few of these entities require localized or systemic treatment. Nonetheless, an awareness of the underlying pathologic processes and an understanding of

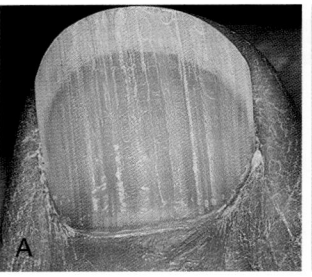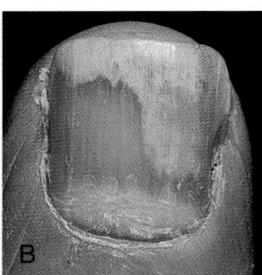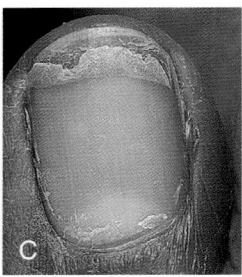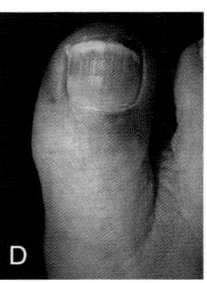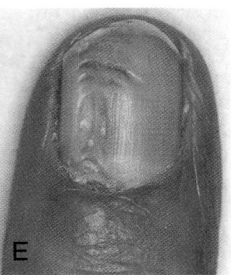

Figure 11-3 **A,** Longitudinal ridging of the nail is a change of aging. It can also be a normal variant. **B,** Onycholysis is a separation of the nail plate from the nail bed. It can occur because of repeated pressure on the distal nail plate with tight or short shoes that tend to lift the end of the nail. **C,** Onychoschizia. Distal nail fissuring or splitting occurs with dryness, and layers may peal away. **D,** Inadequate circulation may lead to rubor around the nail and thickening of the nail along with ischemic pain. **E,** Pterygium developed after myxoid cyst, leaving a longitudinal groove in the nail. (**A-C,** From Habif TP, Campbell JL Jr, Shane Chapman M, et al: *Skin disease,* ed 3, London, 2011, Elsevier. **D,** From Dockery GL: *Cutaneous disorders of the lower extremity,* Philadelphia, 1996, Elsevier. **E,** From Bolognia JL, Jorizzo JL, Rapini RP, editors: *Dermatology,* ed 2, Philadelphia, 2007, Elsevier.)

Box 11-2 Onychopathies and Other Common Toenail Abnormalities

Nail Plate
Onychocryptosis
Onychauxis
Onychogryphosis
Onychomycosis
Onychia
Onycholysis or onychomadesis
Onychopsittacus

Nail Bed
Subungual exostosis
Subungual tumor
Subungual clavus
Subungual hematoma
Subungual verruca

Nail Fold
Paronychia
Onychophosis
Pyogenic granuloma
Herpetic whitlow
Periungual verruca

Matrix
Anonychia
Pterygium
Atrophy or hypertrophy (onychauxis)

Keratinization Disorders
Psoriasis
Mycotic infections
Onychoschizia
Koilonychia
Leukonychia
Onycholysis
Onychorrhexis

Modified from Nzuzi SM: Common nail disorders. *Clin Podiatr Med Surg* 6:273–294, 1989. Used with permission.

the nail changes associated with specific dermatologic and systemic disorder assists in making a definitive diagnosis. Pathologic conditions of the toenail are defined in Box 11-3, and terms describing infections are defined in Box 11-4.

Psoriasis

Psoriasis of the toenails often accompanies cutaneous disease, and patients often mistake it for fungal involvement of the nail (Fig. 11-4A-E). Involvement of the nails is seen in 80% of patients with psoriatic arthritis and in 30% of patients who have psoriasis without arthritis.[176] The most severe form of nail involvement with psoriasis, which sometimes involves shedding and loss of the nail *(onychomadesis),* is associated with arthritic changes. Many patients without arthritic changes who have psoriasis have the following abnormal findings in either their toenails or their fingernails[225,226]:

■ *Stippling* or *geographic pitting* (tiny, often grooved depressions in the surface of the nail plate) (Fig. 11-4), which is not unique to psoriasis and is seen in alopecia areata
■ *Onycholysis,* especially laterally and distally, sometimes with yellowing and opacity of the nail plate, which separates and then detaches from the nail bed (Fig. 11-4B-D)
■ Crumbling of the nail plate
■ Staining of the nail (oil spot lesions) (Fig. 11-4B and C)
■ Subungual keratosis (Fig. 11-4E)
■ Possibly extensive skin involvement (see Fig. 11-4E).

Often these changes are confused with onychomycosis. Before therapy is instituted, scrapings of the nails should be made for microscopic examination with potassium hydroxide (KOH), and fungal cultures should be started.

Treatment of psoriatic nail changes of the feet is generally unsatisfactory. Intralesional injection of corticosteroids may be effective for treating psoriasis in fingernails,[25] but similar therapy for involved toenails is administered less often.

Eczema and Contact Dermatitis

Eczema and contact dermatitis often involve not only the skin on the dorsum of the toes but also the lateral and

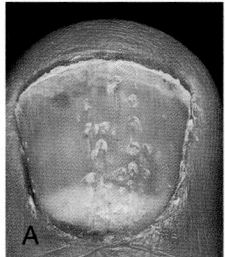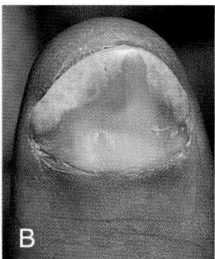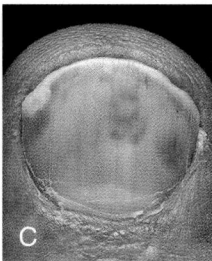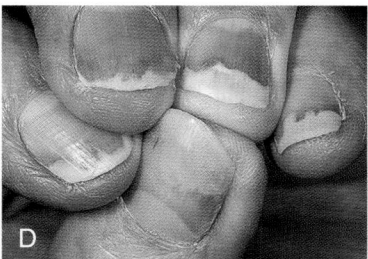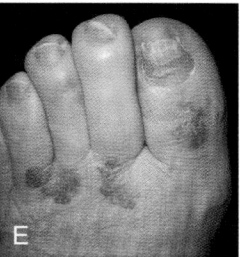

Figure 11-4 Psoriatic toenail dystrophy. The nail is thick, discolored, and distorted because of psoriasis of the nail matrix. The symmetry is striking, and the skin may also be involved. **A,** Psoriatic pits can occur in a linear fashion and may occur along longitudinal lines. **B,** Psoriasis of the nail can produce separation of the nail from the nail bed and an accumulation of subungual debris. The accumulation of serum beneath the nail may form what is called an oil spot. **C,** Oil spot lesions are brown stains seen on the nail. **D,** Separation of the nail plate and accumulation of subungual debris is common. These changes can also occur after nail trauma, and can occur with multiple nail involvement. **E,** Psoriatic involvement of both the nails and skin with several plaques on the dorsal surface. (**A-D,** From Habif TP, Campbell JL Jr, Shane Chapman M, et al: *Skin disease,* ed 3, London, 2011, Elsevier. **E,** From Dockery GL: *Cutaneous disorders of the lower extremity,* Philadelphia, 1996, Elsevier.)

Box 11-3 Glossary of Terms Describing Pathologic Conditions of the Nail

Acral: Of or belonging to the extremities of peripheral body parts.

Anonychia: Absence of nails. When anonychia is congenital, usually all the nails are absent and the condition is permanent. It can occur temporarily from trauma or systemic or local disease. Also seen in nail-patella syndrome.

Beau lines: Transverse lines or ridges marking repeated disturbances of nail growth. May be associated with trauma or a systemic disease process (see Fig. 11-7).

Clubbing: Hypertrophied, curved nail with flattened angle between the nail plate and proximal fold. Associated with chronic pulmonary and cardiac disease.

Hapalonychia: Extremely soft nails that may be prone to splitting; associated with endocrine disturbances, malnutrition, and contact with strong alkali solutions.

Hemorrhage: Bleeding. Beneath toenail, bleeding may be associated with vitamin C deficiency, subacute bacterial endocarditis, and dermatologic disorders. *Subungual hematoma* occurs after trauma to toenail bed.

Hutchinson sign: Hyperpigmentation spreading from nail to surrounding soft tissue. Pathognomonic for melanoma.

Hyperkeratosis: Thickening of the stratum corneum layer of the epidermis.

Hyperkeratosis subungualis: Hypertrophy of the nail bed. May be associated with onychomycosis, psoriasis, and other dermatologic disorders.

Koilonychia: Concavity of the nail plate in both longitudinal and transverse axes. Associated with nutritional disorders, iron deficiency anemia, and endocrine disorders.

Lentigo: A small melanotic spot without pigment, which is potentially malignant and is unrelated to sun exposure.

Leukonychia: White spots or striations in the nail resulting from trauma and systemic diseases, such as nutritional and endocrine deficiencies.

Mees lines: Horizontal striations 1 to 3 mm wide associated with growth arrest.

Melanonychia: A longitudinal streak of pigment visible in or beneath the nail.[48]

Onychauxis: Greatly thickened nail plate caused by persistent mild trauma and onychomycosis.

Onychia: Inflammation of the nail matrix, causing deformity of the nail plate and resulting from trauma, infection, and systemic diseases, such as exanthemas.

Onychitis: Inflammation of the nail.

Onychoclasis: Breakage of the nail plate.

Onychocryptosis: Ingrowing of nails or, more specifically, hypertrophy of the nail lateral fold; also referred to as *hypertrophied ungualabia* or *unguis incarnatus;* one of the most common pathologic conditions of the toenail.

Onychogryphosis: "Claw nail" or "ram's horn nail"; extreme hypertrophy of the nail gives the appearance of a claw or horn. May be congenital or a symptom of many chronic systemic diseases, such as tinea infections. See *onychauxis.*

Onycholysis: Loosening of the nail plate, beginning along the distal or free edge when trauma, injury by chemical agents, or diseases loosen the nail plate. Associated with psoriasis, onychomycosis, acute fevers, and syphilis (see Fig. 11-3B).

Onychoma: Tumor of the nail unit.

Onychomadesis: Complete loss of the nail plate.

Onychomalacia: Softening of the nail.

Onychomycosis: Fungal infection of the nail associated with fungal disease of the foot (see Fig. 11-5).

Onychophosis: Accumulation of callus within the lateral groove, involving the great toe more often than the lesser toes.

Onychoptosis defluvium: Nail shedding.

Onychorrhexis: Longitudinal ridging and splitting of nails caused by dermatoses, nail infections, systemic diseases, senility, or injury by chemical agents.

Onychoschizia: Lamination and scaling away of nails in thin layers caused by dermatoses, syphilis, or chemical agents (see Fig. 11-36).

Continued

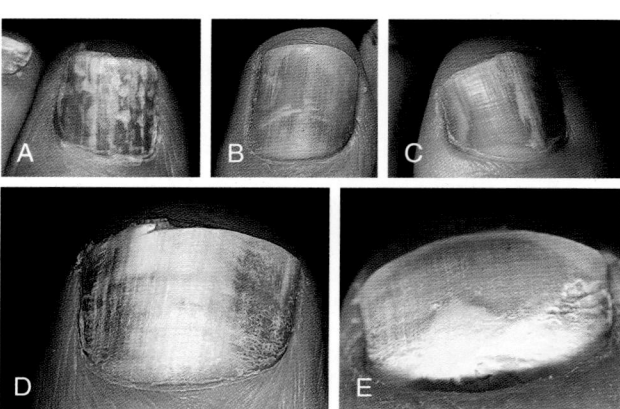

Figure 11-5 Examples of onychomycosis. **A,** Distal subungual onychomycosis. The fungal hyphae enter the nail plate distally and invade proximally into the entire plate. **B,** Distal subungual onychomycosis with extension into the entire plate. **C,** Distal subungual onychomycosis with invasion in longitudinal channels. **D,** White superficial onychomycosis occurs when fungal hyphae invade the surface of the nail plate. E, Proximal subungual onychomycoisis occurs when the fungal hyphae invade beneath the proximal nail fold. (**A-E,** From Habif TP, Campbell JL Jr, Shane Chapman M, et al: *Skin disease,* ed 3, London, 2011, Elsevier.)

proximal nail folds. With chronic inflammatory changes, transverse ridging and scaling as well as discoloration of the nail plate can develop. Accumulation of serous fluid can lead to onycholysis and subsequent onychomadesis. Allergic reaction to nail polish, resins, dyes, solvents, detergents, and other chemicals can cause eczema, and atopic dermatitis with no known cause can lead to the development of similar nail changes.

With the resolution of acute inflammation, the chronic changes of fissuring and dryness may be treated with topical corticosteroids. The primary objective of the treatment of eczema and contact dermatitis is the resolution of the acute inflammatory process surrounding the toenail unit.

Pyodermas

Bacterial infections occur commonly in the feet and are divided into primary and secondary pyodermas. *Impetigo* is a superficial skin infection that is often caused by *Staphylococcus* and/or *Streptococcus* species, and it usually affects younger children. The typical lesion consists of a thin-walled vesicle on an erythematous base. The vesicles form yellow crusts, and peripheral extension results in irregular serpiginous lesions. The lesions are common on the face but can occur anywhere on the body except the palms

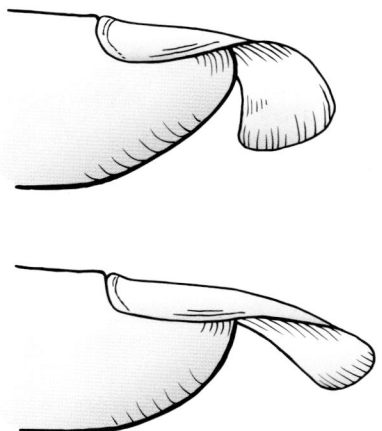

Figure 11-6 Parrot-beak nail occurs with very long nails, curling downwards. Trimming alleviates the deformity.

Box 11-5 Medicinal Solutions Used in Treatment of Cutaneous Foot Disorders

Burow solution: Aluminum sulfate in water (1 : 40 dilution)
Carbolic acid (phenol): 88% carbolic acid, 70% isopropyl alcohol
Castellani paint: Mixture of phenol, alcohol, water, resorcinol, acetone, and fuchsin
Whitfield ointment: 12% benzoic acid, 6% salicylic acid

---

and soles. *Ecthyma* is a form of pyoderma that begins as small vesicles or pustules on an erythematous base and quickly develops a purulent, irregular ulcer. These lesions are common on the lower extremities and, as with impetigo, readily respond to systemic antibiotics. Burow compresses are helpful in removing the crusts, and topical antibiotic ointment is usually applied several times a day (Box 11-5).

Secondary pyodermas that affect the feet can be grouped into three categories: infectious eczematoid dermatitis, infected intertrigo, and miscellaneous pyogenic infections of the web space.

Infectious eczematoid dermatitis results from a discharge of wet drainage seeping over the skin from underlying cellulitis or pyodermic infection. Autoinoculation often occurs, and the infection spreads by contiguous drainage.

Infected intertrigo results from friction, moisture, and sweat retention. It is common between the toes, where it is often diagnosed as a tinea infection. Treatment consists of promoting dryness with cool, drying compresses and a bland absorbent powder. Secondary infection is treated with an appropriate topical antibiotic.

Miscellaneous pyogenic infections of the web space, which are caused by gram-negative bacteria such as *Pseudomonas* and *Proteus*, produce clinical pyodermic infections that are resistant to the usual antibacterial therapy. Identification of the organisms may be difficult, and broad-spectrum antibiotic therapy may be appropriate initially.

The infection should be carefully investigated to determine the presence of any underlying systemic disorders, such as diabetes, lymphoma, or an immunodeficiency syndrome, that could predispose the patient to such cutaneous infections. Amonette and Rosenberg[5] found that the best treatment regimen was topical management with a combination of bed rest, exposure to air, and application of silver nitrate solution, Castellani paint, and gentamicin sulfate cream. *Erythrasma* is often seen in intertriginous areas, such as the web spaces. The causative organism is *Corynebacterium minutissimum*, which produces a well-demarcated, reddish brown, fine desquamation that fluoresces orange-red or coral-pink under a Wood lamp. Wearing loose stockings and shoes and using antibacterial soaps usually prevent this infection or eliminate it after it has been established. Treatment occasionally requires appropriate oral antibiotics.

Not every form of intertrigo of the web space is linked to infection by a fungal or bacterial organism. With psoriasis, the skin of the feet can be extensively involved, and usually the web space is involved as well. A therapeutic trial of a topical steroid cream can effectively eliminate this form of intertrigo.

Systemic Diseases

Diseases of the toenail can accompany many systemic disease processes, but the nail is underused as an aid in diagnosing systemic diseases. Often a provisional diagnosis of a fungal infection or trauma is made when, instead, a systemic disease process has caused changes in the color, shape, rate of growth, or texture of the toenail. Although many of these changes are nonspecific, they can give a diagnostician reason to suspect the presence of a systemic disease.

The consistency and color of the nail plate can change with systemic disease. Several eponyms are associated with these changes and, although confusing, they are in general use for specific pathologic descriptions. These include the Beau lines, Mees lines, Muehrcke lines, half-and-half nail, blue nail, and Terry nail.

With the sudden arrest in longitudinal nail growth, a transverse sulcus, a *Beau line* develops, which is 0.1 to 0.5 mm deep (Fig. 11-7). With further growth of the nail plate, the Beau line progresses distally. This is associated with severe febrile episodes, peripheral vascular disease, diabetes, trauma, Hodgkin disease, and infections such as malaria, rheumatic fever, syphilis, leprosy, typhoid fever, and various parasitic infections.

Mees lines are also associated with growth arrest of the nail plate. Mees lines are horizontal striations that typically involve more than one nail. They are usually 1 to 3 mm wide and are associated with Hodgkin disease, myocardial infarction, malaria, and arsenic and thallium poisoning.[153,154]

Muehrcke lines are white lines that occur in pairs, parallel to the lunula, and do not progress distally with nail plate growth. They occur with hypoalbuminemia and the nephrotic syndrome as well as with chronic liver disease.

Half-and-half nail is a biphasic discoloration of the nail in which the distal portion is brown, red, or pink, and

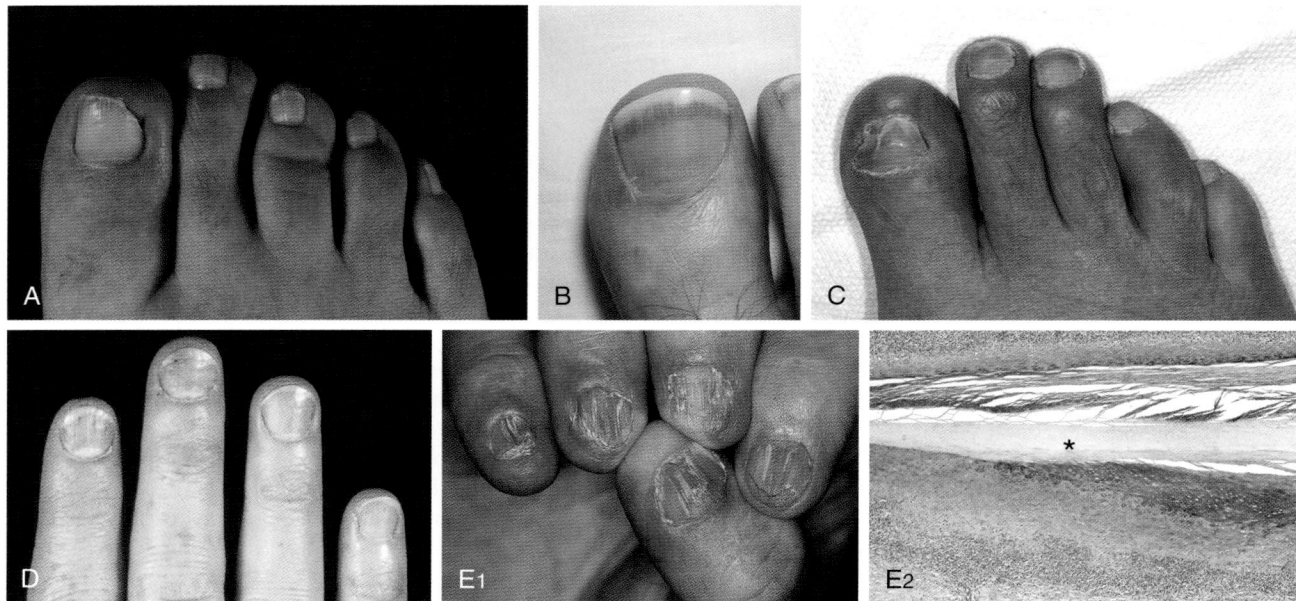

Figure 11-7 Various nail deformities. **A,** Beau lines. Horizontal troughs are apparent midway up the nail about 3 months after an illness, trauma, or in this case, chemotherapeutic treatment. B, Terry nail. Diabetes and liver disease can produce a pinkish band located at the distal edge of the nail plate. **C,** Yellow nail syndrome. The nails are discolored yellow and are often curved, particularly across the horizontal axis. **D,** Splinter hemorrhages or marks of tiny telangiectasia. Tiny subungual vessels or hemmorages occur; these are associated with a clinical case of scurvy. **E,** Nail deformity with thinning and longitudinal ridging and fissuring associated with lichen planus. (**A,** From Habif TP, Campbell JL Jr, Shane Chapman M, et al: Skin disease, ed 3, London, 2011, Elsevier. **C** and **E,** From Bolognia JL, Jorizzo JL, Rapini RP, editors: Dermatology, ed 2, Philadelphia, 2007, Elsevier. **D,** From Dockery GL: Cutaneous disorders of the lower extremity, Philadelphia, 1996, Elsevier.)

the proximal portion appears normal. Half-and-half nails are associated with chronic liver disease and chronic kidney disease.

Blue nail or *blue-gray nail* is a bluish discoloration of the nail that is associated with subungual hematoma, melanotic whitlow, and poor oxygen perfusion in methemoglobinemia, pulmonary disease, and cyanosis.

In the *Terry nail,* characteristic changes involve opacification of the nail plate with a 1- to 3-mm pinkish band at the distal edge of the nail plate. Often, this condition is connected with chronic changes associated with diabetes mellitus and liver disease (see Fig. 11-7B).

Kosinski and Stewart[122] described pathologic nail conditions that are often associated with systemic disease entities. These nail changes may be manifested in cardiovascular disorders (yellow nail syndrome or splinter hemorrhages, see Fig. 11-7C and D and Table 11-2), hematologic diseases (Table 11-3), endocrine disorders (Table 11-4), connective tissue diseases[184] (Table 11-5), local and systemic infections (Table 11-6), neoplasia (Table 11-7), and renal, hepatic, pulmonary, and gastrointestinal disorders (Table 11-8).

GENETIC DISORDERS WITH NAIL CHANGES

Heritable traits can influence the appearance of toenails. Many genetic diseases with collagen abnormalities are

Table 11-2	Cardiovascular Disorders and Associated Toenail Conditions
Disease	**Pathologic Changes**
Arterial emboli	Splinter hemorrhages
Arteriosclerosis obliterans	Leukonychia partialis
Bacterial endocarditis	Clubbing, splinter hemorrhages
Hypertension	Splinter hemorrhages
Ischemia	Onycholysis, pterygium
Mitral stenosis	Splinter hemorrhages
Myocardial infarction	Mees lines, yellow nail syndrome
Vasculitis	Splinter hemorrhages

Modified from Kosinski MA, Stewart D: Nail changes associated with systemic disease and vascular insufficiency. *Clin Podiatr Med Surg* 6:295–318, 1989. Used with permission.

associated with dermatologic abnormalities and hair and nail disorders (Table 11-9).

Darier disease (Darier-White disease or keratosis follicularis)[148] is an autosomal dominant disease characterized by distal subungual wedge-shaped keratoses, red and white longitudinal striations (Fig. 11-8A, B, and E), splinter hemorrhages, notching of the distal nail plate, subungual hyperkeratosis, and thinning of the nail plate with splintering along the edge.

Table 11-3 Hematologic Disorders and Associated Toenail Conditions

Disease	Pathologic Changes
Cryoglobulinemia	Splinter hemorrhages
Hemochromatosis	Brittleness, koilonychia, leukonychia, longitudinal striations, splinter hemorrhages
Hemophilia	Ingrown toenails,[98] pyogenic granulomata
Histiocytosis X	Onycholysis, pitting, splinter hemorrhages
Hodgkin disease	Leukonychia partialis, Mees lines, yellow nail syndrome
Hypochromic anemia	Koilonychia
Idiopathic hemochromatosis	Brittleness, koilonychia, longitudinal striations, splinter hemorrhages
Osler-Weber-Rendu disease	Splinter hemorrhages, telangiectasia
Polycythemia rubra vera	Clubbing, koilonychia
Porphyria	Onycholysis
Sickle cell anemia	Leukonychia, Mees lines, splinter hemorrhages
Thrombocytopenia	Splinter hemorrhages

Modified from Kosinski MA, Stewart D: Nail changes associated with systemic disease and vascular insufficiency. *Clin Podiatr Med Surg* 6:295–318, 1989. Used with permission.

Table 11-4 Endocrine Disorders and Associated Toenail Conditions

Disease	Pathologic Changes
Addison disease	Brown bands, diffuse hyperpigmentation, leukonychia, yellow nail syndrome, longitudinal pigmented deep yellow bands
Diabetes mellitus	Beau lines, koilonychia, leukonychia, onychauxis, onychomadesis, paronychia, pitting of nail plate, proximal nail bed telangiectasia, pterygium, splinter hemorrhages, yellow nail syndrome
Hyperthyroidism	Clubbing, increased nail growth, onycholysis, splinter hemorrhages, yellow nail syndrome
Hypothyroidism	Onycholysis, koilonychia, yellow nail syndrome
Thyroiditis	Yellow nail syndrome
Thyrotoxicosis	Koilonychia, onychomadesis, splinter hemorrhages, yellow nail syndrome

Modified from Kosinski MA, Stewart D: Nail changes associated with systemic disease and vascular insufficiency. *Clin Podiatr Med Surg* 6:295–318, 1989. Used with permission.

Table 11-5 Connective Tissue Disorders and Associated Toenail Conditions

Disease	Pathologic Changes
Alopecia areata	Leukonychia partialis, nail pitting
Atopic dermatitis/eczema	Onycholysis, onychorrhexis
Lichen planus[169,174]	Atrophy of nail plate, onycholysis, onychorrhexis, pterygium
Psoriasis	Beau lines, leukonychia, Mees lines, nail pitting, onycholysis, splinter hemorrhages
Raynaud syndrome	Koilonychia, yellow nail syndrome
Reiter syndrome	Onycholysis, nail pitting
Rheumatoid arthritis	Splinter hemorrhages, yellow nail syndrome
Scleroderma (62% of patients)[189]	Absent lunula, koilonychia, leukonychia, onycholysis, onychorrhexis, pterygium
Systemic lupus erythematosus	Clubbing, hyperpigmented periungual tissue, nail pitting, onycholysis, subungual petechiae, yellow nail syndrome

Modified from Kosinski MA, Stewart D: Nail changes associated with systemic disease and vascular insufficiency. *Clin Podiatr Med Surg* 6:295–318, 1989. Used with permission.

Table 11-6 Systemic and Localized Infections and Associated Toenail Conditions

Disease	Pathologic Changes
Bacterial endocarditis	Clubbing, splinter hemorrhages
Hansen disease	Loss of lunula, nail plate dystrophy, onychogryphosis, onychauxis, onycholysis, onychodesis, onychomadesis, onychorrhexis
Malaria	Grayish nail bed, leukonychia
Measles	Onychomadesis
Recurrent cellulitis	Yellow nail syndrome
Scarlet fever	Onychomadesis
Syphilis	Koilonychia, leukonychia partialis, onychauxis, onychia, onycholysis, onychomadesis, onychorrhexis, paronychia
Trichinosis	Splinter hemorrhages, leukonychia
Tuberculosis	Leukonychia partialis, yellow nail syndrome
Typhoid fever	Leukonychia, Mees lines
Yaws and pinta	Hypopigmentation, nail atrophy, onychia, onychauxis, paronychia, pterygium

Modified from Kosinski MA, Stewart D: Nail changes associated with systemic disease and vascular insufficiency. *Clin Podiatr Med Surg* 6:295–318, 1989. Used with permission.

Pachyonychia congenita (Jadassohn-Lewandowsky syndrome),[125,152] another autosomal dominant genetic disorder,[151,152] is characterized by hypertrophy of the nail plate, with severe thickening and yellowish-brown discoloration of the nail plate (Fig. 11-8C). The extreme thickening is more solid and more regular than with onychogryphosis and is accompanied by palmar and plantar keratoses. The thickening of the nail plate can lead to elevation of the distal nail plate and an incurved and elevated toenail. Tauber et al[202] reported a case of pachyonychia congenita and reviewed published reports of this disease.

The *nail-patella syndrome* (onychoosteodysplasia)[152,193] is an autosomal dominant disease characterized by a triangular lunula and total atrophy or hemiatrophy of the nail plate (Fig. 11-8D). Other orthopaedic conditions associated with this disease include subluxation or dislocation of the radial head, presence of iliac horns, joint hypermobility, and a subluxated or dislocated hypoplastic patella.

Dyskeratosis congenita[152] (Zinsser-Cole-Engman syndrome) can be transmitted as an autosomal dominant or X-linked recessive trait and is characterized by ridging and thinning or atrophy of the nail plate.

DOOR syndrome[152] (*d*eafness, *o*nychodystrophy, *o*steodystrophy, and mental *r*etardation) is an autosomal recessive trait characterized by mental retardation and deafness. It may also be associated with absent or atrophic nails and curved fifth digits.

Congenital malalignment of the hallux toenail may be transmitted by an autosomal dominant gene of variable expression (Fig. 11-8E). It is characterized by lateral deviation of the long axis of the nail relative to the distal phalanx. Complications of this condition are local, such as perionychium onychocryptosis. In one review, 50% of cases spontaneously improved or resolved; however, the misdirected nail matrix can be rotated surgically.[15]

Congenital nail abnormalities are errors of development that can produce other anomalies, such as *anonychia* (absence of the nails) and *polyonychia* (presence of more than one nail on a digit) or *micronychia* (small nails) (Fig. 11-9).

TRAUMA

The nail plate and nail bed can be damaged by trauma. Injury to the germinal matrix can cause abnormalities such as ridging, pitting, and grooving. After an injury to the toenail, the regrowth can be a thickened, discolored nail, and after a toenail is lost, a new nail plate can grow abnormally or normally. Trauma to the distal phalanx can cause a subungual exostosis, which often causes nail plate deformity, and an osseous injury to the distal phalanx can cause callus formation that can affect the new toenail. Thickening of the distal phalanx can cause an incurved toenail that pinches the underlying soft tissue.

Trauma to the nail plate may be caused by biomechanical abnormalities as well (see later discussion on subungual hematoma). The second toe can compress the lateral nail fold of the great toe adjacent to the second

Table 11-7 Tumors and Associated Toenail Conditions

Disease	Pathologic Changes
Breast carcinoma	Yellow nail syndrome
Bronchogenic carcinoma	Clubbing, Muehrcke lines, onycholysis
Hodgkin disease	Leukonychia partialis, Mees lines, yellow nail syndrome
Laryngeal carcinoma	Yellow nail syndrome
Metastatic malignant melanoma	Clubbing, yellow nail syndrome
Multiple myeloma	Onycholysis

Modified from Kosinski MA, Stewart D: Nail changes associated with systemic disease and vascular insufficiency. *Clin Podiatr Med Surg* 6:295–318, 1989. Used with permission.

Table 11-8 Hepatic, Renal, Pulmonary, and Gastrointestinal Disorders and Associated Toenail Conditions

Disease	Pathologic Changes
Hepatic	
Chronic hepatitis	Half-and-half nails, leukonychia
Cirrrhosis	Clubbing, Muehrcke lines, splinter hemorrhages, Terry nails
Renal	
Nephritis	Leukonychia
Nephrotic syndrome	Half-and-half nails, Muehrcke lines, yellow nail syndrome
Renal failure	Brown lunula, half-and-half nails, Mees lines
Pulmonary	
Asthma	Yellow nail syndrome
Bronchiectasis	Clubbing, inflammation of nail fold and nail bed, onychauxis, onycholysis, yellow nail syndrome
Chronic bronchitis	Clubbing, yellow nail syndrome
Interstitial pneumonia	Clubbing, yellow nail syndrome
Pleural effusion	Clubbing, onycholysis, yellow nail syndrome, leukonychia, Mees lines
Pneumonia	Clubbing, yellow nail syndrome
Pulmonary fibrosis	Cyanosis, multiple paronychia, nail pitting
Pulmonary tuberculosis	Onychauxis
Gastrointestinal	
Peptic ulcer disease	Splinter hemorrhages
Plummer-Vinson syndrome	Koilonychia
Postgastrectomy syndrome	Koilonychia
Regional enteritis	Clubbing
Ulcerative colitis	Clubbing, leukonychia

Modified from Kosinski MA, Stewart D: Nail changes associated with systemic disease and vascular insufficiency. *Clin Podiatr Med Surg* 6:295–318, 1989. Used with permission.

Table 11-9 Genetic Disorders and Associated Nail Changes

Disease or Syndrome	Genetic Inheritance	Pathologic Nail Findings
Darier disease	Autosomal dominant	Longitudinal red-and-white striations, atrophy or hypertrophy of nail plate, splinter hemorrhages, distal subungual wedge-shaped keratoses
Pachyonychia congenita	Autosomal dominant	Massive hypertrophy of nail plates, brown or yellow discoloration
Nail-patella syndrome	Autosomal dominant	Atrophy or hemiatrophy of nail, triangular-shaped lunula
Dyskeratosis congenita	X-linked recessive or autosomal dominant	Atrophy of nail plate, ridging, fusion of proximal nail fold
DOOR syndrome	Autosomal recessive	Anonychia or atrophic nails
Frizzled D 6 caused isolated nail dystrophy[78]	Autosomal recessive	Nail dysplasia, hyponychia, onycholysis, onychauxis

Modified from Norton LA: Nail disorders: a review. *J Am Acad Dermatol* 2:451–467, 1980. Used with permission.
DOOR, Deafness, onychoosteodystrophy, osteodystrophy, and mental retardation.

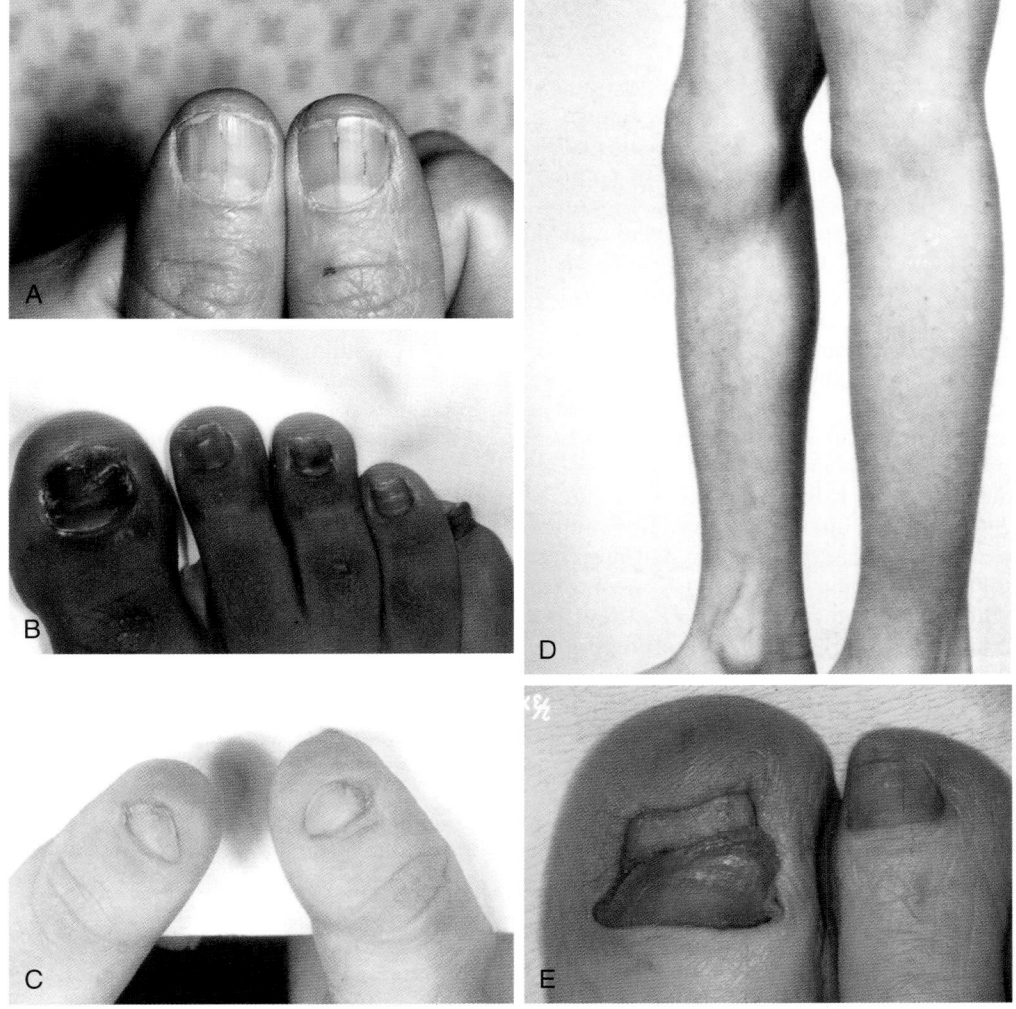

Figure 11-8   A, With Darier disease, also see distal fissuring with thin and friable nails and alternating red-and-white lines. **B,** Chronic nail changes with Darier disease of the nail, which include longitudinal ridges, subungual thickening, and notching at the distal margins. **C,** Pachyonychia congenita. Within the first year after disease onset, the nails become thickened, particularly at the tip, and wedge shaped. **D,** Nail-patella syndrome. The thumbnails and hallux toenails are either absent or partially formed. Other nails may be involved to a lesser extent. **E,** Longitudinal erythronychia (*red lines*) and notching of nail edge with Darier disease. (**A,** From Bolognia JL, Jorizzo JL, Rapini RP, editors: *Dermatology,* ed 2, Philadelphia, 2007, Elsevier. **B, D,** and **E,** From Dockery GL: *Cutaneous disorders of the lower extremity,* Philadelphia, 1996, Elsevier.)

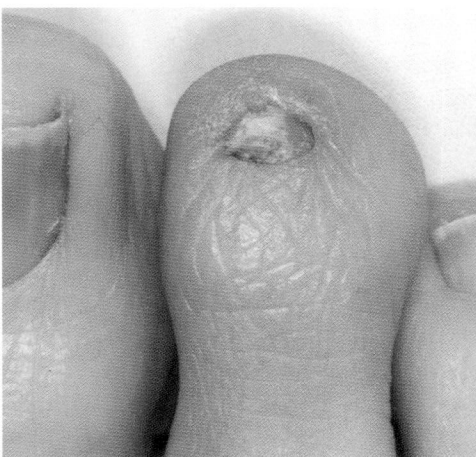

Figure 11-9 Micronychia. Nails may be totally or partially absent as the result of a congenital defect.

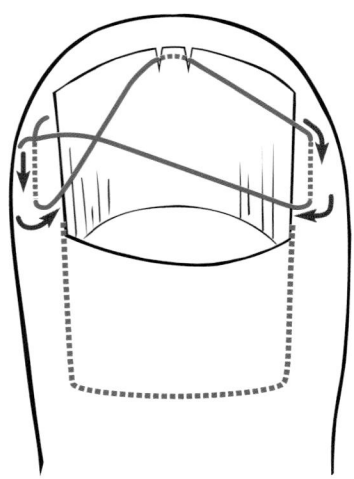

Figure 11-10 Example of placement of absorbable transverse figure-of-eight suture to the toe.

toe, causing an overgrowth of soft tissue with secondary infection. With more acute trauma, when the nail bed over the distal phalanx is crushed, after the nail bed is repaired, the fragmented nail can be replaced and secured with 2-octyl cyanoacrylate (Dermabond; Ethicon, Somerville, N.J.).[93] This material creates a bond between the nail fragments and the skin for 7 to 14 days, when the new nail pushes it off. The material serves as a rigid splint for a fracture as well as a biologic covering to minimize desiccation and hyperkeratinization of the nail matrix. It also prevents the cuticle from adhering to the underlying germinal matrix.[190]

Similar to nail plate repairs in the hand,[34] germinal matrix and nail bed repairs in the foot may be made under loupe magnification, using 7-0 absorbable suture to repair the tissue, with the intention of preventing functional or cosmetic problems. Replacing the nail prevents the eponychium from adhering to the nail bed. It may be held in place with a distal suture or two side sutures (5-0 nylon), which are removed at 7 to 10 days to prevent an epithelialized tract. If the nail is crushed too severely, similar to hand injuries, 0.020-inch silicon sheeting may be placed under the proximal nail fold to protect the nail fold. The surgeon could also remove the nail longitudinally, excise the scar tissue or lesion, and undermine the nail bed all the way to the perionychial tissues to achieve a tension-free closure, as is done for split fingernail injuries.[6] A figure-of-eight suture may be used to hold the nail in place.[112]

TRANSEVERSE FIGURE-OF-EIGHT SUTURE FOR SECURING THE TOENAIL
Surgical Technique
1. Create two small slits in the distal aspect of the nail plate.
2. Place the nail plate under the eponychial fold.
3. A 4.0 absorbable or nonabsorble suture is placed into one side of the paronychium distal to proximal.

4. The suture is passed through the notches in the distal nail plate.
5. The suture is placed in the contralateral paronychium from distal to proximal (Fig. 11-10).
6. The suture is then tied.[32]

A germinal matrix graft could also be harvested from adjacent nail tissue, and the nail narrowed as in a Winograd procedure (Fig. 11-11), or harvested from another toe.[198] Few studies are available, however, on toenail bed reconstruction. Nonetheless, it makes sense that similar procedures could be used on the toes and the fingers.

On the medial aspect of the nail plate, with excessive pronation, hypertrophy of the ungualabia can result in an ingrown toenail. Parrinello et al[166] compared the shape of the great toenail with the base of the distal phalanx and found a significant correlation between the shape of the proximal aspect of the nail plate and the shape of the phalangeal base. However, they found no correlation between the shapes of the proximal and distal portions of the nail plate. They concluded that many other factors besides trauma influence the shape of the nail, including constricting footwear, snug-fitting stockings and hosiery, inadequate or inappropriate pedicures, and heritable traits that can lead to incurvation of the nail border, with subsequent inflammation and infection.

Split-nail deformities may be treated surgically with nail removal, elliptic nail bed scar removal, and careful elevation of the matrix off the bone with extension of this dissection laterally until the nail matrix can be closed without tension.[87] Defects in the nail bed from excisional biopsy can be repaired with a free graft from the lesser toes or with split-thickness, sterile matrix grafts from the adjoining nail matrix.[50] Subungual splinters may be removed by sequential thin, sharp filings of the nail until the splinter is exposed along its entire length. This allows complete splinter removal without having to remove the entire nail.[188]

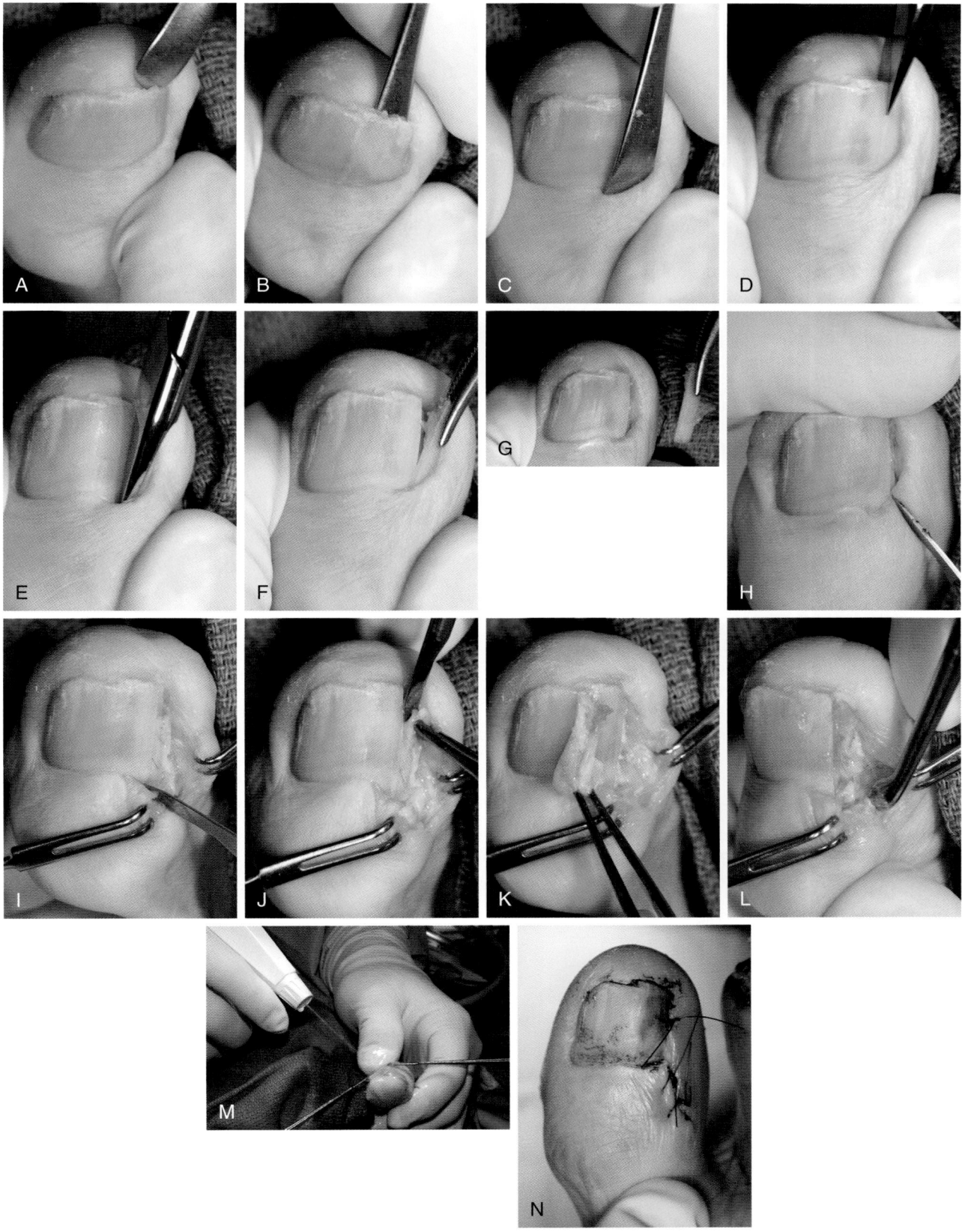

Figure 11-11 Winograd procedure for partial onychectomy. This patient had a history of repeated lateral ingrown toenail of the right great toe. Onychocryptosis is not present in these photographs. **A,** A Freer elevator is used to release the lateral nail from the nail bed. **B,** A Freer elevator is pushed past the germinal matrix. **C,** The eponychium is released from the nail. **D,** The nail is cut along the lateral border, using sharp, strong scissors or a wire cutter. **E,** Scissors are pushed proximally to cut the entire nail. **F,** The nail is grasped with a hemostat. **G,** The nail is pulled free from the nail bed. **H,** An oblique 6-mm incision is made from the corner of the eponychium. **I,** The germinal matrix is excised in line with the nail cut. **J,** The nail bed is excised from the proximal phalanx. **K,** The nail bed and germinal matrix are removed. **L,** Remaining remnants of the germinal matrix and nail bed are curetted. **M,** The wound is irrigated thoroughly. **N,** At 2 weeks, the 4-0 nylon sutures may be removed.

Crush Injuries to the Nail

The majority of these injuries occur from closing doors, dropping heavy objects, or hitting the toes on fixed objects. The most common feature will be ecchymosis with or without the presence of lacerations. A dorsal wound at the matrix region may be associated with avulsion of the base of the nail from below the proximal nail fold. This may be associated with fracture of the distal phalanx: transverse fracture of the midportion, comminuted fracture of the distal portion, or separation of the terminal tuft. In skeletally immature patients, the fracture will usually be at the physis of the proximal phalanx.

Avulsion of the nail plate can leave the nail bed open and possibly injured (Fig. 11-12). As the nail bed scars, the surface may become irregular, resulting in a deformed new nail or arrest of new nail regeneration. Wounds into the germinal matrix may result in a longitudinal groove in the nail plate or a split nail. To minimize these possible outcomes, keep the proximal fold patent with foil or the injured nail plate by placing it back under the proximal fold after fracture irrigation and nail bed repair. If the proximal portion of the germinal matrix under the proximal fold is intact, a tear in the distal germinal matrix will not necessarily prevent regrowth of the nail but may cause deformity with time. Matrix contusions may also lead to loss of nail growth. Hematomas may be evacuated to reduce pain and pressure depending on size.

In treating nail crush injuries, devitalized tissues should be excised. For fractures of the terminal phalanx, large bone fragments can be splinted or sutured. The nail often serves as a splint once the soft tissues are repaired. Damage of the matrix and periosteum requires repair with fine (6-0 or smaller) suture (Fig. 11-12).

Splinting with the nail will aid in shaping the new nail and control the scar formation of the matrix and nail bed.

TUMORS

Tumors of the soft tissue adjacent to the toenails or involving the nail unit itself can be benign or malignant (Box 11-6). Periungual and subungual warts *(verrucae)* are common soft tissue growths (Fig. 11-13). *Fibromas*[181] and *fibrokeratomas* can result from trauma to the toes, with consequent nodule formation impinging on the nail plate. These benign connective tissue lesions can also develop beneath the nail plate itself and cause elevation and deformity. Pressure on the nail matrix can create a longitudinal defect in the nail plate as well. A periungual fibroma or angiofibroma (see Fig. 11-13F) may be the first evidence of tuberous sclerosis or ectodermal dysplasia. In general, fibromas respond readily to excision or cauterization. Glomus tumors, pyogenic granulomas, and keratoacanthomas must all be considered in the differential diagnosis.

Glomus Tumor

A glomus tumor is most commonly encountered on the acral portions of the extremities. This lesion is often in the subungual area and consists of a reddish purple nodule measuring only a few millimeters in diameter. It is tender and gives rise to severe paroxysmal pain. Glomus tumors rarely ulcerate or bleed, and excision usually results in a cure, although subungual lesions are

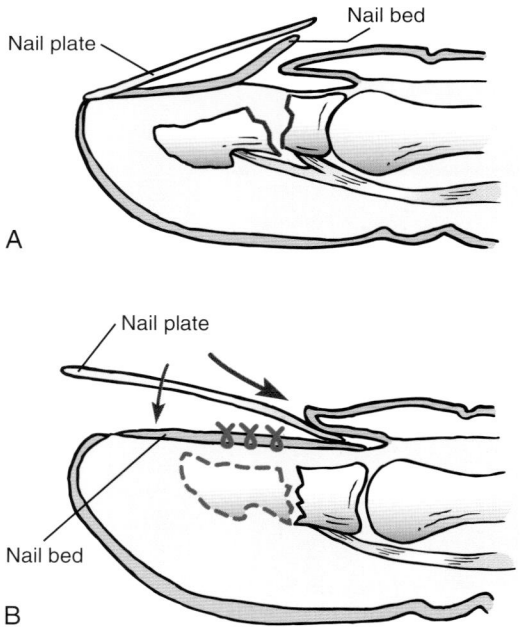

Figure 11-12 A, Avulsion of the nail plate leaves open fracture and injured nail bed. **B,** Repair of the nail bed with small absorbable suture and replacement of nail plate as a temporary splint to the fracture.

Box 11-6   Tumors Associated with Toenail Conditions
Benign Nail Tumors
Verruca
Fibroma
Fibrokeratoma
Neurofibroma
Myxoid cyst
Pyogenic granuloma
Glomus tumor
Pigmented nevus
Keratoacanthoma
Malignant Nail Tumors
Squamous cell carcinoma
Malignant melanoma
Basal cell carcinoma
Metastatic carcinoma
Bowen disease
Bone Tumors
Bone cysts (solitary or aneurysmal)
Enchondroma
Osteochondroma
Subungual exostosis

Modified from Gunnoe RE: Diseases of the nails: how to recognize and treat them. *Postgrad Med* 74:357-362, 1983. Used with permission.

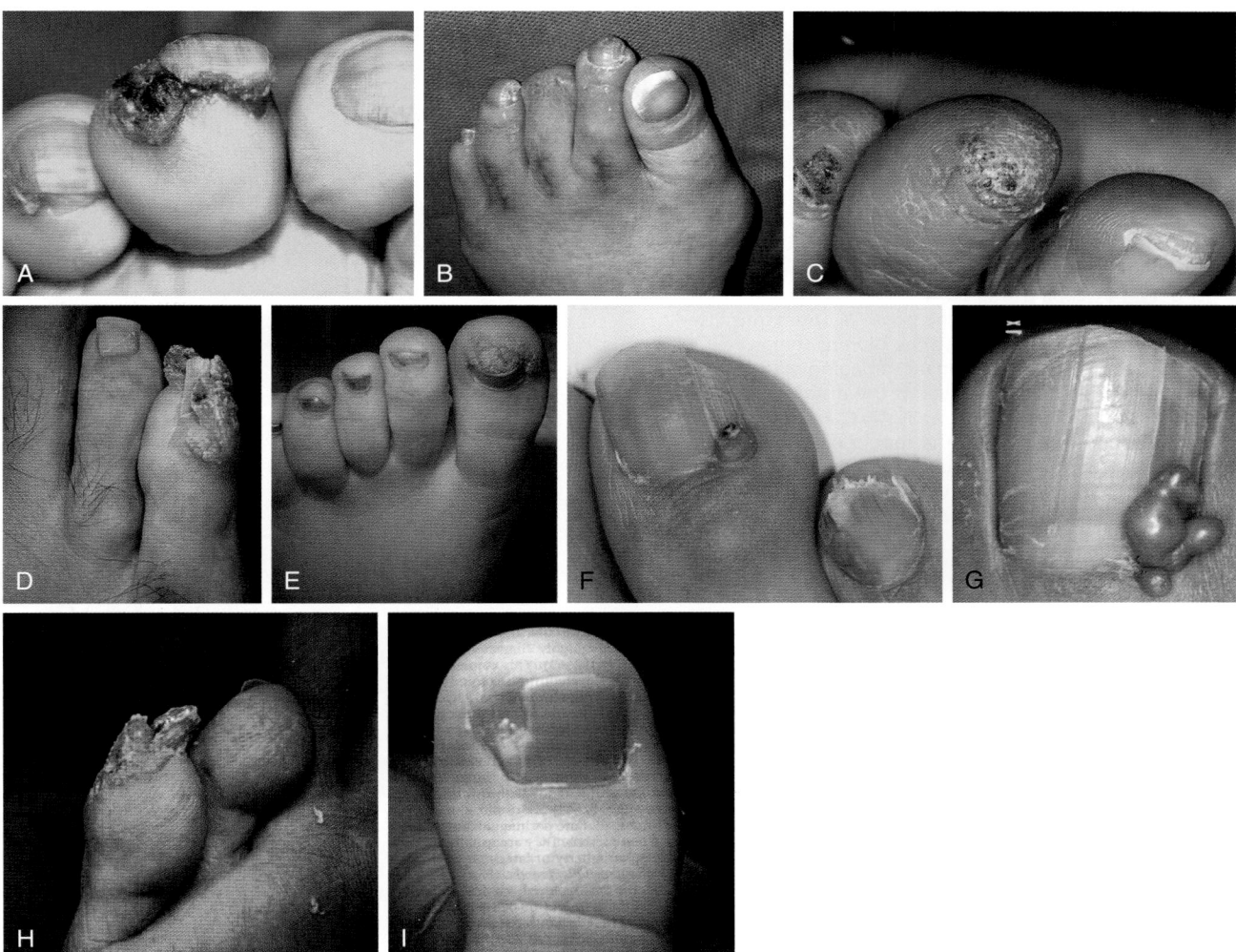

Figure 11-13 **A,** Subungual wart (verruca) on the third toe was refractory to topical treatments. **B,** Treatment of verruca on the third toe was by amputation at the distal interphalangeal joint. **C,** Verrucae on multiple toes. **D,** Filiform wart with finger-like projections around the fifth toenail. **E,** Subungual wart causes distortion of the hallux nailplate. **F,** Angiofibroma. This may be the first evidence of tuberous sclerosis or ectodermal dysplasia. **G,** Periungual fibroma producing a longitudinal deformity in the nail plate. **H,** Tuberous sclerosis. Periungual fibromas are present on the tip of the fifth toe in a patient with tuberous sclerosis. **I,** Subungual fibroma on the lateral edge of the nail plate in a patient with tuberous sclerosis. (**D, E, H,** and **I,** From Dockery GL: *Cutaneous disorders of the lower extremity,* Philadelphia, 1996, Elsevier. **G,** From Bolognia JL, Jorizzo JL, Rapini RP, editors: *Dermatology,* ed 2, Philadelphia, 2007, Elsevier.)

more difficult to eradicate. They are almost universally benign; however, because of symptoms and malignant potential, diagnosis and treatment is essential.[138] The differential diagnosis includes melanoblastoma, melanoma, neuroma, chronic perionychium, gout, arthritis, foreign body granuloma, and Kaposi sarcoma.

The glomus tumor appears to be a cutaneous arteriovenous anastomosis arising from a highly vascular compilation of epithelioid cells and glomus cells known as a glomus body.[138] This thermoregulatory structure, found densely within the fingers and toes, is responsible for temperature, vascular regulation, and sensation; hence it tends to give the patient cold insensitivity.[105,138]

The only effective treatment for a glomus tumor is complete surgical excision.[138] Excision with negative margins

results in adequate diagnosis and treatment. If malignant features are present, wide excision is needed, with close follow-up for development of metastasis.[138] Previously, it was necessary to remove the nail, incise the nail matrix, remove the tumor, and repair the nail bed. A study of seven cases,[105] however, demonstrated that creating an L-shaped incision, 5 mm distal and 5 mm medial or lateral to the nail, and lifting off the entire vascular flap allowed removal of the tumor (Fig. 11-14A-C). The flap was then sutured back to its origin after hemostasis.[105] There were no recurrences or nail irregularities. This technique might lend itself to other subungual operations as well, such as treatment of subungual exostosis. This approach has been used by others and is recommended for all noninvasive space-occupying subungual lesions, regardless of type.[180]

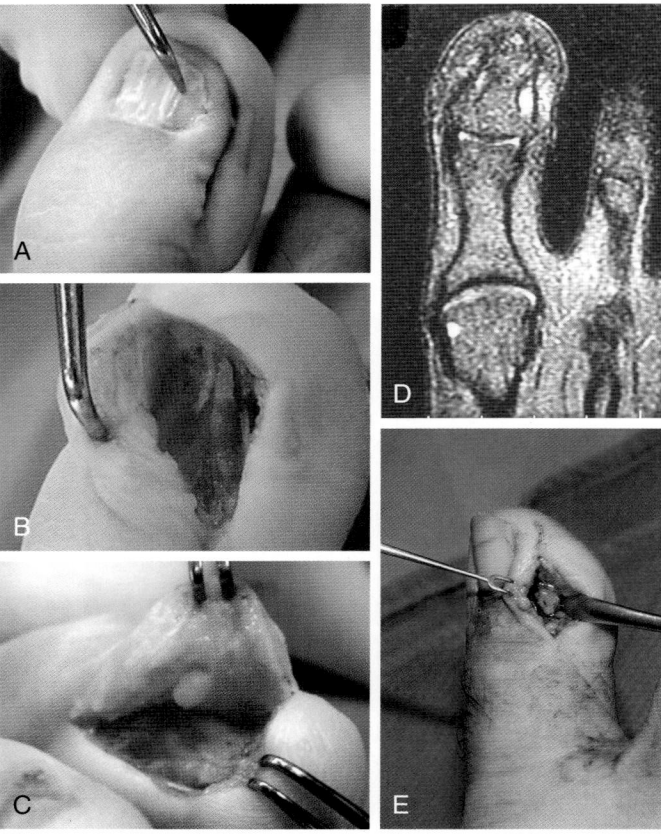

Figure 11-14 Glomus tumor. **A,** L-shaped incision to lift the entire vascular flap from the bone. **B,** The flap is lifted. **C,** The flap is elevated, showing the glomus tumor. **D,** T2-weighted magnetic resonance imaging scan with glomus tumor on the lateral side of the distal phalanx. **E,** Glomus tumor exposed surgically. (**A-C,** From Horst F, Nunley JA: Glomus tumors in the foot: a new surgical technique for removal. *Foot Ankle Int* 24:949-951, 2003; courtesy Dr. James A. Nunley. Used with permission. **D** and **E,** Courtesy Dr. Richard Marks.)

Radiographs or computed tomography (CT) scans may show small cortical abnormalities in the distal phalanx. T2-weighted magnetic resonance imaging (MRI) may be used to determine the precise location of the tumor and may show a well-circumscribed highly vascular mass (Fig. 11-14D and E).[138] Pahwa[161] described a "trap door" technique used for glomus tumor excision in which medial and lateral slits were cut in the proximal nail fold in line with the gutters. The distal plate is then carefully freed from the underlying bed and elevated from it distally, with the proximal plate and proximal fold acting as a hinge. The tumor can then be excised and then the nail plate and nail fold sutured back into position.

Another type of glomus tumor, which is different histologically and is characterized by multiple painless hemangiomas, often has an autosomal dominant familial pattern.[43,138] These multiple lesions are usually asymptomatic.

Subungual Exostosis and Osteochondroma

A subungual exostosis is a benign bony growth typically occurring on the dorsomedial aspect of the distal phalanx tuft (Fig. 11-15A-D).[37,39,52,142,145] Originally described by Dupuytren in 1817, subungual exostosis has a predilection for the hallux, although occasionally it develops in the lesser toes. A subungual exostosis typically has a

moderate growth rate, resulting in growth that rarely exceeds 0.5 cm.

Osteochondroma characteristically occurs on the dorsal aspect of the phalanx in a juxtaepiphyseal region, whereas exostosis may be closer to the tip of the phalanx (Table 11-10).[129,142,207] Osteochondroma occurs more often in adolescent boys than girls (2 : 1 ratio). In contrast, subungual exostosis is seen more commonly in young adults aged 20 to 40 years. Ippolito et al[108] found that subungual exostoses occurred more often in the female population (2 : 1 ratio), whereas Miller-Breslow and Dorfman[142] reported an equal distribution between male and female patients.

Osteochondroma is attributed to a congenital cause, although the patient may recall a traumatic event that brings a formally asymptomatic lesion to their attention.[210] Vazquez-Flores et al[210] noted in a review of 27 cases of subungual osteochondroma, trauma was recalled by 40.7% of the patients. The cause of subungual exostosis is thought to be traumatic, infectious, or from chronic irritation.[73,145,155,207] Fikry et al[73] found a history of trauma or repetitive microtrauma in 21 of 28 cases of exostosis.

In distinguishing between subungual exostosis and subungual osteochondroma, the histologic characterization of the cartilage cap is diagnostic. In a subungual osteochondroma, a hyaline cartilage cap overlies a trabeculated bony pattern. However, subungual exostosis

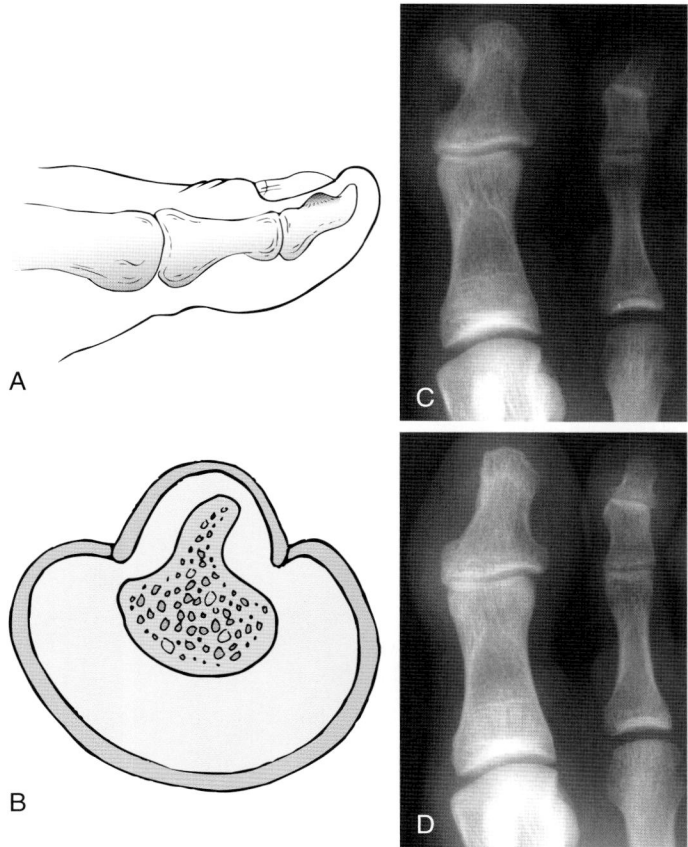

Figure 11-15 **A,** Lateral view of toe shows the effect of subungual exostosis on the configuration of the nail plate. **B,** Cross section of distal phalanx shows deformation of the nail plate by subungual exostosis. **C,** Radiograph shows subungual exostosis before excision. **D,** Radiograph after excision of exostosis.

Table 11-10 Distinguishing Features of Subungual Exostosis and Subungual Osteochondroma

Condition	Typical Age at Diagnosis (Years)	Male-to-Female Ratio	Cause	Growth Rate	Histopathology	Site	Risk of Malignancy
Exostosis	20-40	1:2	Traumatic	Moderate	Fibrocartilage	Tuft[133]	Not reported[213]
Osteochondroma	10-25	2:1	Congenital[213]	Slow	Hyaline cartilage	Juxtaepiphyseal[133]	Low[213]

Modified from Norton LA: Nail disorders: a review. *J Am Acad Dermatol* 2:457–467, 1980. Used with permission.

has a fibrocartilaginous cap that is a reactive fibrous growth with cartilage metaplasia.[142] Jahss[109] noted that a subungual exostosis is characterized histologically as chronic fibrosis caused by irritation. A trabecular bony pattern connecting with the distal phalanx can underlie the fibrocartilaginous cap.[142]

Reporting on 21 cases of subungual exostosis, Ippolito et al[108] noted that 12 patients were athletes involved in activities such as dancing, gymnastics, or football. It is believed that increased pressure against the dorsal aspect of the nail plate from a constricting toe box can cause irritation that leads to the development of a subungual exostosis. The connection between a specific traumatic incident and the subsequent development of a subungual exostosis can also explain the increased incidence of this abnormality in athletes. Many patients describe pain that is aggravated by activities such as running or walking and is most likely from the pressure of an expanding lesion against the toe box.

A subungual exostosis can be misdiagnosed or confused with other toenail abnormalities.[108] Elevation of the nail plate (Fig. 11-16A) and discoloration can resemble chronic onychomycosis or a subungual hematoma. Chinn and Jenkin[39] reported two cases of patients with pain in the proximal nail groove who had undergone an unsuccessful surgical matrixectomy and who later received a

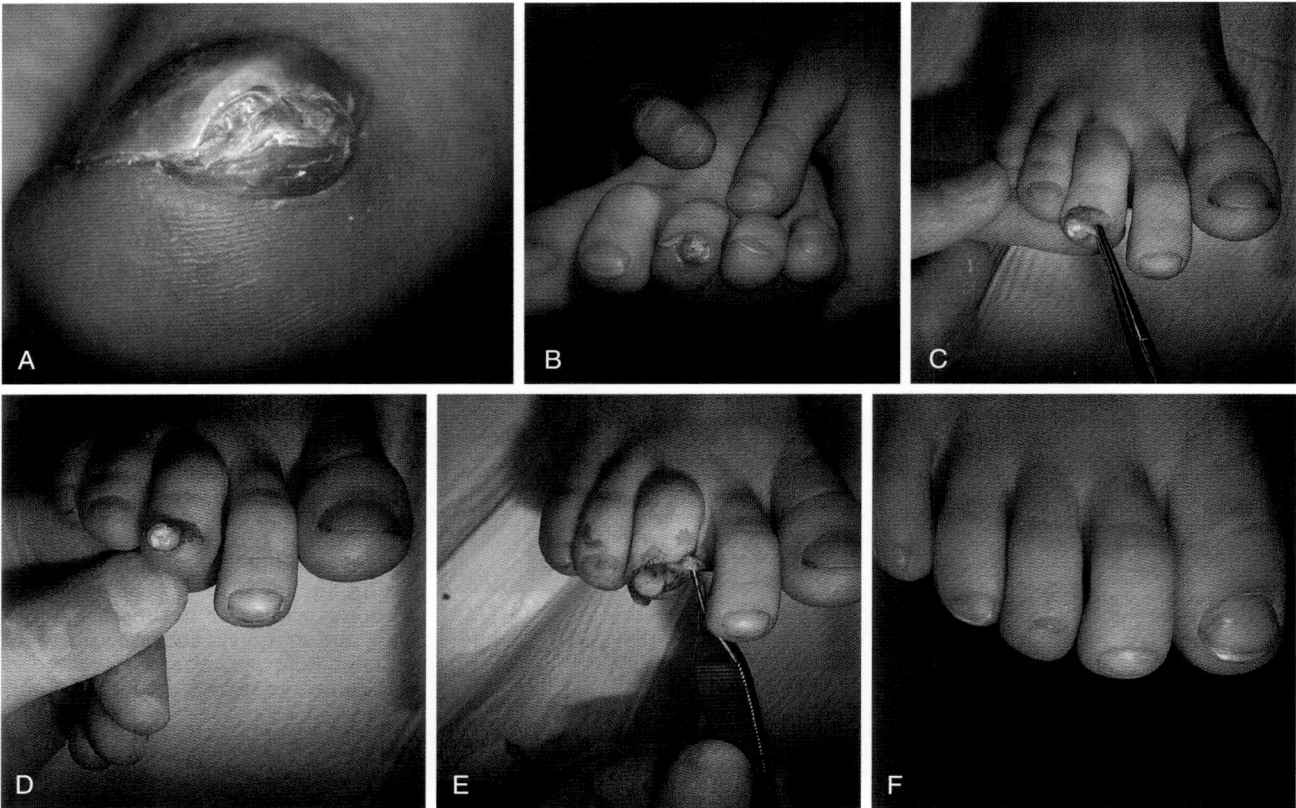

Figure 11-16 **A,** Subungual exoxtosis elevating the nail plate. **B,** Osteochondroma in 9-year-old with painful lesion of third toe previously diagnosed as a subungual wart. **C,** Surgical procedure to treat above lesion involves avulsion of the toenail. **D,** Exposure shows the osteochondroma and the cartilage cap. **E,** The lesion is surgically dissected and removed. **F,** Six weeks after excision, showing the beginning growth of a new toenail. (**A,** From Bolognia JL, Jorizzo JL, Rapini RP, editors: *Dermatology,* ed 2, Philadelphia, 2007, Elsevier. **B-F,** From Dockery GL: *Cutaneous disorders of the lower extremity,* Philadelphia, 1996, Elsevier.)

diagnosis of subungual exostosis. The differential diagnosis includes subungual verruca, pyogenic granuloma, glomus tumor, keratoacanthoma, subungual nevus, and epidermoid inclusion cyst as well as malignant lesions, such as carcinoma of the nail bed and subungual melanoma.

The diagnosis is supported by radiographic evidence of the lesion that may be seen best on a lateral or oblique radiograph. An exostosis typically appears as an exophytic bony mass on the dorsomedial tip of the distal phalanx. The lesion may appear to be growing distally away from the physis. The base is peduculated or sessile but the tip is flattened, cupped, or dome shaped.[129]

An osteochondroma appears as a sessile or pedunculated expansion of trabecular bone from the justaepiphyseal region of the distal phalanx. The base may be sessile, pedunculated, or circumscribed. The hyaline cartilage cap is not visible unless it becomes calcified. Although the lesion may be quite large, the radiographic appearance may be smaller than its actual size.[129]

De Palma et al[52] reported on 11 cases of surgical excision of a subungual exostosis with partial onychectomy. Using histochemical and immunohistochemical methods, they concluded that most subungual bony masses exhibited the characteristics of conventional osteochondromas and that the distance of the lesion from the epiphyseal line was unrelated to its histologic features (Fig. 11-16B-F).

RESECTION OF SUBUNGUAL EXOSTOSIS
Although a small asymptomatic lesion may be observed and treated conservatively, surgical resection of a subungual exostosis or subungual osteochondroma is the most common treatment of a symptomatic lesion. The operation involves either the above-described procedure for glomus tumor (see Fig. 11-14A-C) or the following procedure (Fig. 11-17A-D). A defect remaining in the nail bed after surgical excision may heal by secondary intention. However, some authors have used artificial collagen matrix substitute dermis with success.[196]

Surgical Technique
1. A digital anesthetic block is administered, and a 0.25-inch Penrose drain or a commercially available tubular tourniquet (Mara-Med, Grand Rapids, Mich.) is applied.

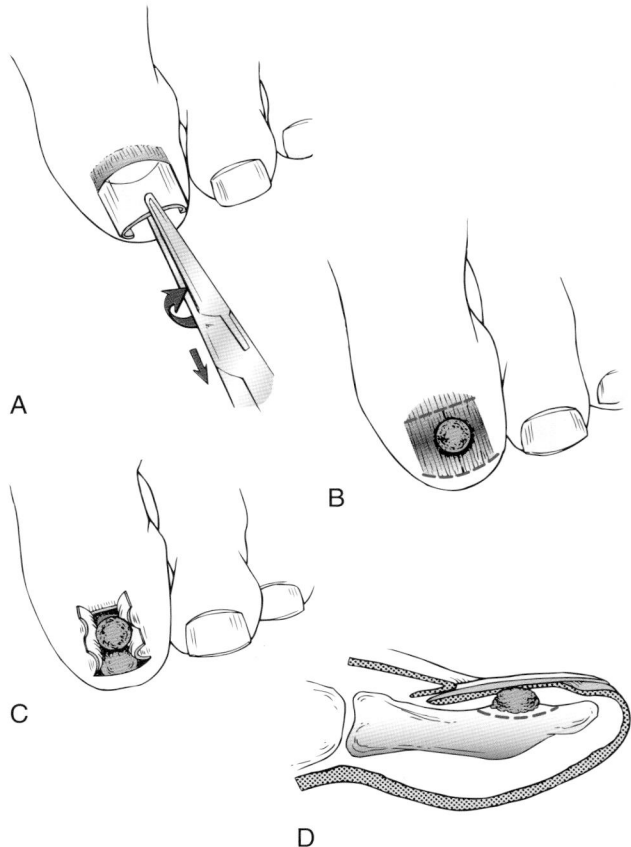

Figure 11-17 Technique for surgical excision of subungual exostosis. **A,** The toenail is completely avulsed to expose the exostosis. **B,** Longitudinal incision is made in the nail bed, avoiding injury to the nail matrix. **C,** Nail bed is reflected. **D,** Exostosis is excised with wide margins, and the nail bed is then repaired.

2. A partial or complete toenail avulsion is performed.
3. A longitudinal incision is made in the nail bed. The nail bed is reflected off the exostosis, with care to avoid damage to the nail matrix.
4. The exostosis is resected with an osteotome or bone cutter. The base of the lesion is curetted.
5. The nail bed is relocated and closed with absorbable suture.
6. A compression dressing is applied and changed 24 hours postoperatively. Dressing changes are continued until drainage subsides. The nail bed is protected with a plastic bandage strip until tenderness resolves.

Recurrence

An exostosis recurs infrequently but can develop after an incomplete resection. Recurrence may be a continuing source of irritation to the toenail. Miller-Breslow and Dorfman[142] reported a 53% incidence of recurrence when a subtotal excisional biopsy was performed. After wide local excision with curettage of the base, however, a 5% to 6% rate of recurrence is expected.[155]

Melanotic Whitlow and Malignant Melanoma

These malignant tumors are more common on the fingers than on the toes. Aulicino and Hunter[10] reported on 72 cases of subungual melanoma, of which two thirds were on the thumb or great toe. Hutchinson[107] published the first significant report on subungual melanoma in 1886. Koenig and McLaughlin[120] stated that 0.025% of all reported cancer is caused by subungual melanoma. Melanomas that involve the nails are termed *melanotic whitlows*.[83] Blackish discoloration develops, especially in the nail bed (see Fig. 11-18A), but minimal pigmentation or the absence of pigment does not exclude the diagnosis of melanoma. The Hutchinson sign (pigment spreading beyond the nail plate into the proximal or lateral nail folds, or both) is considered pathognomonic of subungual melanoma (see Fig. 11-18B).[130]

Twenty-three percent of melanomas involving the nail may be amelanotic.[14,195] Other reported colors include tan, brown, and blue.[177] A greenish tinge to the nail is most likely due to a *Pseudomonas* infection (Fig. 11-18C and D).

On physical examination, a melanoma may be accompanied by a splitting or loss of the nail, ulceration, and localized erythema. The most common cause of darkening of the nails is trauma, but other causes include Addison disease and Peutz-Jeghers syndrome. The differential diagnosis of malignant melanoma also includes glomus tumor, benign nevus, paronychia, onychomycosis, pyogenic granuloma,[120] linear melanonychia (Fig. 11-18E-G), and onychomycosis.

Often malignant melanoma is misdiagnosed as a benign condition, which can lead to long delays in diagnosis and appropriate treatment. With malignant melanoma, unlike a benign condition such as subungual hematoma (Fig. 11-18H and I), discoloration of the nail does not change as the nail grows distally and does not improve with time. A malignant melanoma might not damage the overlying nail plate, whereas a subungual hematoma can cause plate elevation. Typically, a malignant melanoma is deep black, in contrast to the less distinct color of a subungual hemorrhage. Patients are often advised to observe whether or not the pigmented area migrates distally with the growing nail plate. The patient's anxiety can be reduced with a simple and quick method of blood detection under the nail. Small scrapings of the discolored nail are obtained under the distal free edge of the nail plate. The nail plate fragments are placed on a urinalysis reagent strip (Hemostix; Bayer Medical, Newbury, United Kingdom). A drop of water is added to soak the fragments and strip. Within 1 minute, a green color may indicate blood and the likelihood of subungual hemorrhage rather than melanoma.[106]

Many patients with a subungual melanoma report the occurrence of trauma, which makes an early diagnosis difficult. Approximately 4% occur in the foot,[177] and two thirds of these appear on the hallux.[164] Melanoma occurs

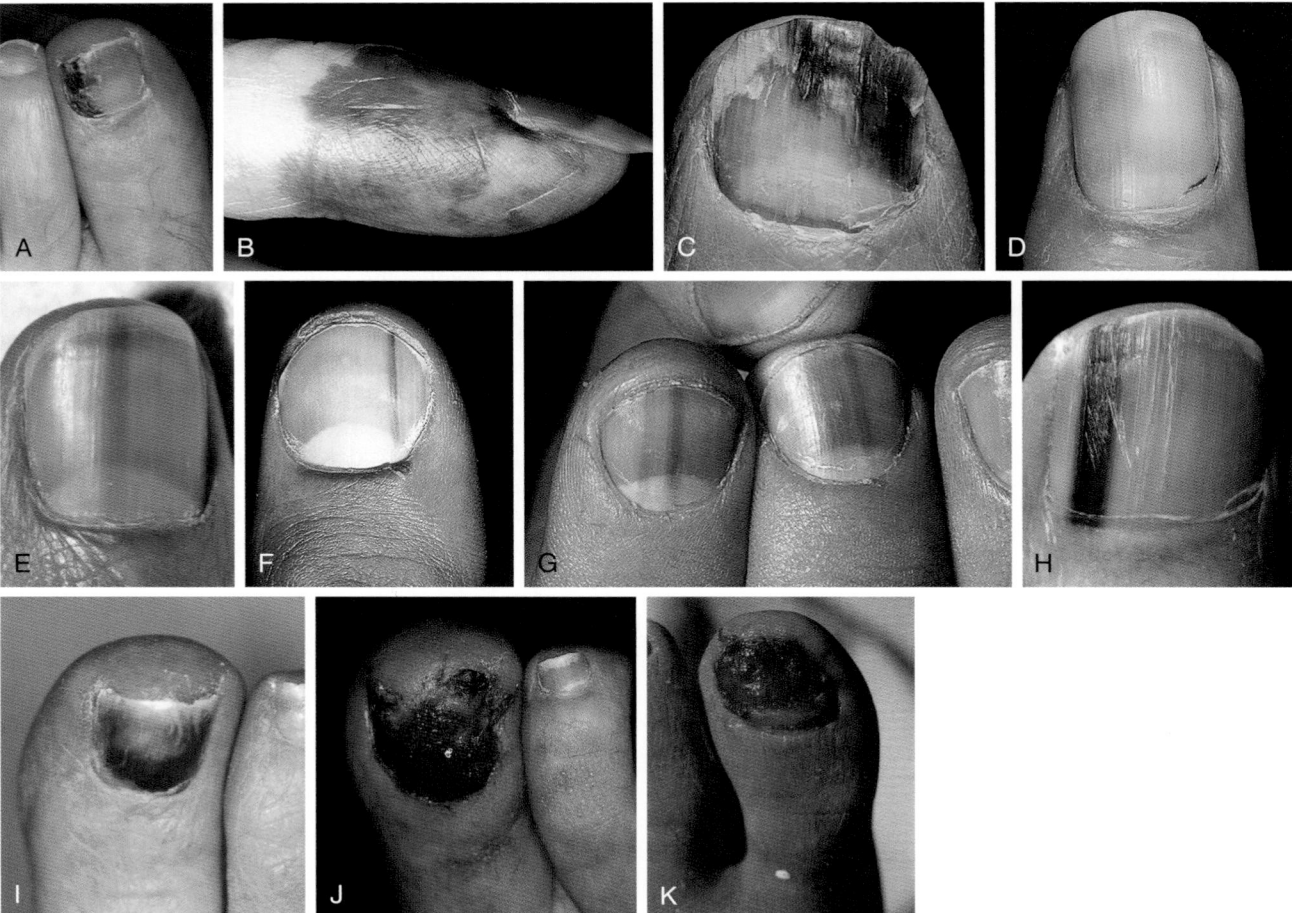

Figure 11-18 **A,** Malignant melanoma. This friable red and black tumor, is rising up the side of the nail. There is a bluish discoloration of the nail plate and pigmentation around the base of the nail. **B,** Malignant melanoma of the nail bed. There is pigmentation under the nail and around the posterior nail fold (Hutchinson sign). **C** and **D,** Pseudomonas infection. The green discoloration from the infection is distinguishable from the black of the melanoma. **E,** Linear melanonychia. A straight black line runs longitudinally from the nail fold. It is benign. Sometimes it rises from a benign mole in the nail. **F,** Longitudinal melanonychia resulting from junctional nevus of the nail matrix. **G,** Longitudinal nail bands occurred in several nails after long-term treatment with minocycline. **H,** Dark, wide, linear nail band on a single nail requires further investigation because it could be a melanoma. **I,** Trauma. The color may be black, but often there is a red-brown or russet discoloration as well. The configuration gradually grows out with time. **J,** Amelanotic melanoma with diffuse nail distruction and ulceration. **K,** Acral lentiginous melanoma with complete loss of the distal nail plate and bed. (**B-D** and **F-H,** From Habif TP, Campbell JL Jr, Shane Chapman M, et al: *Skin disease,* ed 3, London, 2011, Elsevier. **J,** From Bolognia JL, Jorizzo JL, Rapini RP, editors: *Dermatology,* ed 2, Philadelphia, 2007, Elsevier. **K,** From Dockery GL: *Cutaneous disorders of the lower extremity,* Philadelphia, 1996, Elsevier.)

more often in female patients and in white patients and has an incidence of 10% to 31% among nonwhite patients.[13,115] The typical age at presentation is 50 to 60 years. A poor prognosis is associated with lymph node involvement and nail destruction or ulceration, and the long-term survival rate varies from 18% to 40%.[71,127,132,199,215] Because the lesion is often mimicked by other conditions, it is most important to do an excisional biopsy for any suspicious lesion (such as a nonhealing ulcer, subungual discoloration, or subungual hematoma) that does not advance with the nail (Fig. 11-18J and K).

Pack and Oropeza[159] and Papachristou and Fortner[164] reported that one third of patients initially present with regional lymph node involvement and that biopsy should be done for any suspicious lesion. Early amputation is the treatment of choice, usually at the metacarpophalangeal joint, because resections more than 3 cm from the lesion are not of clinical value even for the thickest melanomas.[102] However, studies of the hand suggest that a more functional, distal removal of the affected tissue can be equally effective.[143]

Other Tumorous Conditions

Bowen disease is a relatively rare premalignant dermatologic disorder originally described by Bowen in 1912. It is typically a well-circumscribed, erythematous, papular, nodular, crusting lesion that can be mistaken for psoriasis. Bowen disease is described as a variant of squamous cell carcinoma, an in situ carcinoma that does not usually metastasize. Patients with Bowen disease are more likely to develop other primary malignancies,[21] and Graham and Helwig,[85] reporting on 35 cases, noted that 80% of patients died of primary malignancies within 9 years after the appearance of Bowen disease. Lemont and Haas[131] reported that peak occurrence is in the eighth decade, typically on the plantar aspect of the foot. Surgical excision or curettage is the treatment of choice. If the basement membrane is disrupted, however, the potential exists for distant metastases. When maximal tissue must be preserved, Mohs surgery is 90% effective,[156] and when there is no osseous involvement, Mohs surgery is considered the treatment of choice.[225] The key is to perform a biopsy of any chronic lesion involving the nail.[156]

Basal cell carcinoma is rare in the foot,[8] and squamous cell carcinoma (Fig. 11-19A and B),[9,27,47] Kaposi sarcoma, and other metastatic diseases are relatively rare malignant lesions. Patients with abnormal radiographic findings, chronic pain, swelling, inflammation, infection, or persistent splitting of the nail plate should be evaluated for an underlying tumor of the distal phalanx. A specific diagnosis is essential. After the diagnosis of a malignant tumor has been made by biopsy, amputation of the digit is the typical treatment.

Biopsies of suspicious lesions are important. With the nail removed, the recommendation is to take longitudinal biopsy specimens from the nail bed and transverse biopsy specimens from the nail matrix, with subsequent repair if possible.[174]

ONYCHOPATHIES AND OTHER COMMON NAIL ABNORMALITIES

Onychopathies[153,154] and other abnormalities of the toenails are most easily discussed by dividing them into abnormalities of the nail plate, nail bed, nail fold, and nail matrix (Boxes 11-6 and 11-7). Congenital and genetic nail disorders, traumatic nail disorders, tumors, and dermatologic and systemic nail disorders are discussed elsewhere in this chapter.

Common Nail Plate Disorders

Onychocryptosis, onychauxis, onychogryphosis, onychomycosis, onychia, onycholysis, and onychomadesis are the nail plate disorders seen most often.

Onychocryptosis

Onychocryptosis occurs when the border of the nail plate penetrates the adjacent soft tissue of the nail fold (Fig. 11-20). Synonyms for this condition include "ingrown toenail," "unguis incarnatus," and "ungualabial hypertrophy."[59,60] The differential diagnosis includes trauma, paronychia, subungual exostosis, onycholysis, and onychophosis. The term "ingrown toenail" is misleading because it implies that the side of the nail plate grows laterally and extends farther into the nail groove. All evidence indicates that the germinal matrix determines the width and growth of the nail.[22,23,165] There is no evidence that the matrix becomes wider in a person with an ingrown toenail. The incorrect assumption was that ingrown toenails were caused by an increasing width in the convexity of the nail. Thus initial attempts by

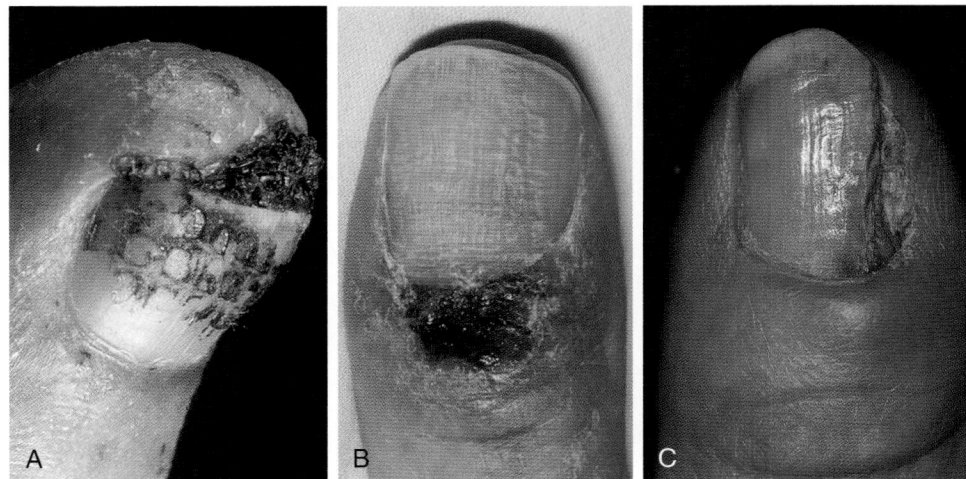

Figure 11-19 A, Squamous cell carcinoma under the nail. There is a thickening under the nail that has bled. Biopsy is indicated to establish the nature of the lesion which, in this case, is squamous cell carcinoma. **B,** Squamous cell carcinoma involving the proximal nail fold. **C,** Bowen disease. The lateral aspect of the nail plate is absent with hyperkeratosis, scaling, and fissuring of the epithelium. (**A,** From du Vivier A: *Atlas of clinical dermatology,* ed 3, Philadelphia, 2002, Elsevier. **B,** From Bolognia JL, Jorizzo JL, Rapini RP, editors: *Dermatology,* ed 2, Philadelphia, 2007, Elsevier.)

Box 11-7   Causes of Nail Deformities

External Pressure
Footwear
- Excessive tightness
- High heels
- Pointed toe box
- Short toe box

Stockings: excessive tightness
Casts extending beyond nail
Hallux rigidus
Hallux valgus
Hallux varus
Lesser toes
- Impingement on hallux
- Hammer toes
- Overlapping or underlapping toes
- Soft tissue neoplasm
- Pronation of feet

Internal Pressure
Subungual exostosis or osteoma
Subungual keratosis
Subungual hematoma
Subungual neoplasm
Onychia or paronychia
Trauma

Systemic Conditions
Cardiac disorders
Circulatory disorders
Endocrine disorders
Renal disorders
Metabolic disorders
Infection
Genetic disorders
Geriatric nail changes
Obesity

Modified from Johnson KA: *Surgery of the foot and ankle,* New York, 1989, Raven Press, p 84. Used with permission.

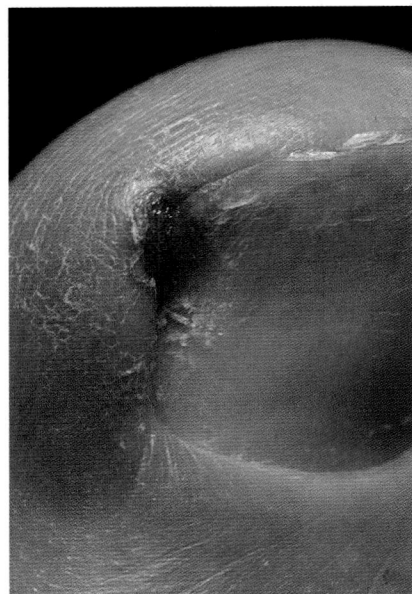

Figure 11-20   Onychocryptosis. As the skin becomes irritated, it hypertrophies, exacerbating the impingement of the nail into the soft tissue. (From Habif TP, Campbell JL Jr, Shane Chapman M, et al: *Skin disease,* ed 3, London, 2011, Elsevier.)

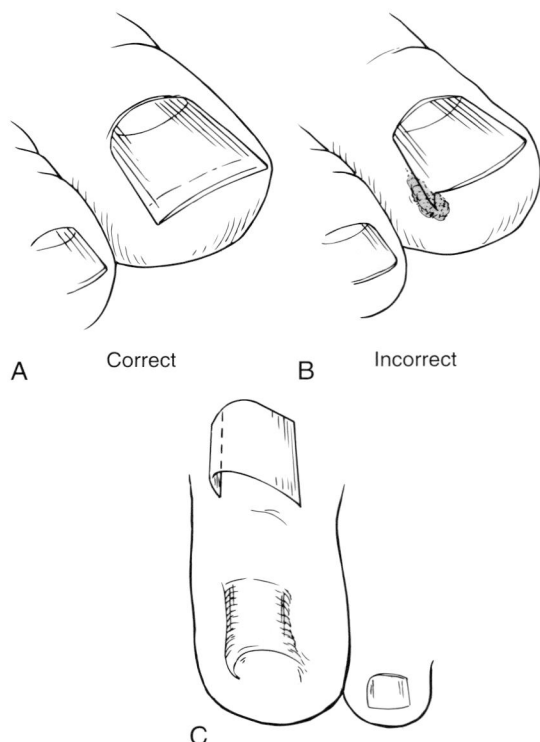

Figure 11-21   **A,** Correct nail trimming prevents in-growth into the adjacent nail fold. **B,** Incorrect trimming can lead to a fishhook-shaped spur in the lateral nail fold, with subsequent infection. **C,** Abnormal incurving of the medial border can predispose to infection.

surgeons at treating this disease were aimed at narrowing the nail margin. Frost[79] described three types of ingrown toenails: a normal nail plate that, with improper nail trimming, develops a fishhook-shaped spur in the lateral nail groove (Fig. 11-21A and B); an inward distortion of one or both of the lateral margins of the nail plate (incurved nail) (see Fig. 11-21); and a normal nail plate with soft tissue hypertrophy of the lateral border (Fig. 11-22).

Lloyd-Davies and Brill[137] stated that complete avulsion of the nail plate, which in the past was a common treatment for an ingrown toenail, probably leads to hypertrophy of the distal lip of the nail and causes the entire nail to become embedded and clubbed. If the nail of the great toe is removed, the new toenail, unlike a fingernail, often becomes deformed as it grows distally because of upward pressure placed on it during weight bearing. Elliptically excising the distal soft tissue can reduce this phenomenon[31] (Fig. 11-23A-C). Some authors have advocated excising a small portion of the dorsal distal phalanx through this same incision when treating recalcitrant ingrown toenail.[135] A similar crescent incision on the

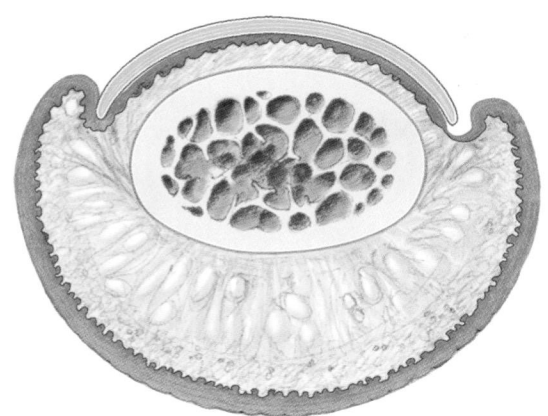

Figure 11-22 Cross-sectional view of toe through the distal phalanx. Hypertrophy of the nail leading to occlusion of the nail groove is shown on the *left*. Normal relationship between nail margin and lateral nail groove is shown on the *right*. (Courtesy Mayo Foundation for Medical Education and Research.)

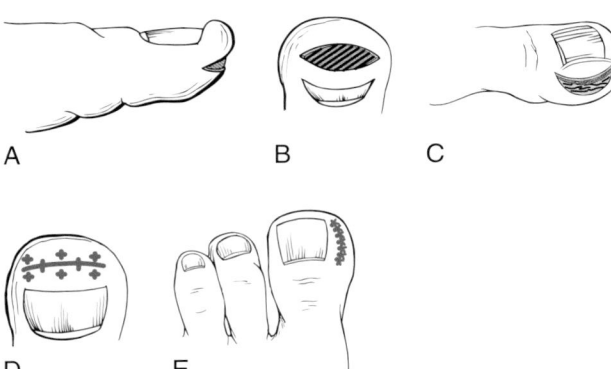

Figure 11-23 Ingrown toenail. **A-C,** Elliptic incision is used to resect redundant skin and soft tissue. **D** and **E,** Closure of the elliptic incision tends to reduce distal impingement against the advancing distal nail plate.

lateral side of the toe has been described to relieve pressure of the nail plate on the lateral nail fold for ingrown toenails[183] (Fig. 11-23D and E).

The main conditions that produce symptoms of onychocryptosis are primary hyperplasia of the nail groove in approximately 75% of cases and a deformity of the nail plate in 25% of cases. The latter is caused by an osseous malformation of the dorsum of the distal phalanx[133] or by hypertrophy and irregular thickening of the nail bed, often as a result of a tinea infection. The normal nail plate and its bed are 2 to 3 mm thick. The contour is largely determined by the dorsal shape of the distal phalanx. The shape and contour of the nail can vary widely because of secondary changes in the distal phalanx from irritation and pressure.[166] Such variations often produce nail deformities and accompanying symptoms that can all be classified as ingrown toenail. The most common type is incurvation of the nail margin.

Normally, the space between the nail margin and the nail groove is approximately 1 mm. The groove is lined with a thin layer of epithelium that lies immediately beneath and beside the nail margins. Under normal conditions, this space sufficiently protects the groove from irritation. With a narrow toe box or tight-fitting stockings, downward pressure can develop on the nail plate, the nail lip, or the lateral nail fold. This pressure obliterates the space between the nail plate margin and the nail groove and produces constant irritation. The reactive swelling in the groove leads to gradual hyperplasia of the adjacent soft tissue and ultimately to permanent hypertrophy. As this process continues, the nail groove is finally incised by the nail margin, often with ensuing secondary infection.

To temporarily relieve the acute symptoms, after using local anesthesia or a digital block, the longitudinal border of the nail may be excised (Fig. 11-24A-G).[38] A cotton packing beneath the advancing edge may elevate the nail and alleviate pressure from the nail plate. Merely excising a triangular section of the nail margin may often lead to development of a thick fishhook-shaped deformity of the lateral nail plate that will hook and drag through the nail fold as the nail grows (Fig. 11-25). However, with longitudinal or triangular excision, hypertrophy of the adjacent soft tissue can fill the space of the excised nail margin. As the nail continues to grow distally, it impinges on the elevated nail groove and gives rise to recurrent episodes of infection and formation of granulation tissue.

A congenitally broad nail plate predisposes to an ingrown toenail. This congenital factor explains why ingrown toenails sometimes occur in infants or even in neonates who have a broad nail plate or no free margin between the nail fold and nail plate. In adults, the condition is typically acquired. Sometimes the symptoms are so chronic and the nail changes are so severe that a terminal Syme amputation of the entire nail unit with shortening of the toe is appropriate (Fig. 11–26A and B).

The size, shape, and contour of the nail plate and bed are usually normal. Hyperplastic changes of the nail groove and fold are accompanied by formation of granulation tissue on the lip and groove. The granulation tissue bleeds freely with slight provocation. Hypertrophied tissue can cover a large part of the nail or most of the nail. Heifetz[96] proposed the initial classification of ingrown toenails, which has subsequently been modified to the following[141]:

Stage 1: Inflammatory stage. Swelling and erythema are present along the lateral nail fold. The edge of the nail plate may be embedded in an irritated nail fold.

Stage 2: Abscess stage. Increased pain accompanies acute or active infection. Drainage is present.
   a. <3 mm overlap of the lateral fold over the plate
   b. >3 mm overlap of the lateral fold over the plate

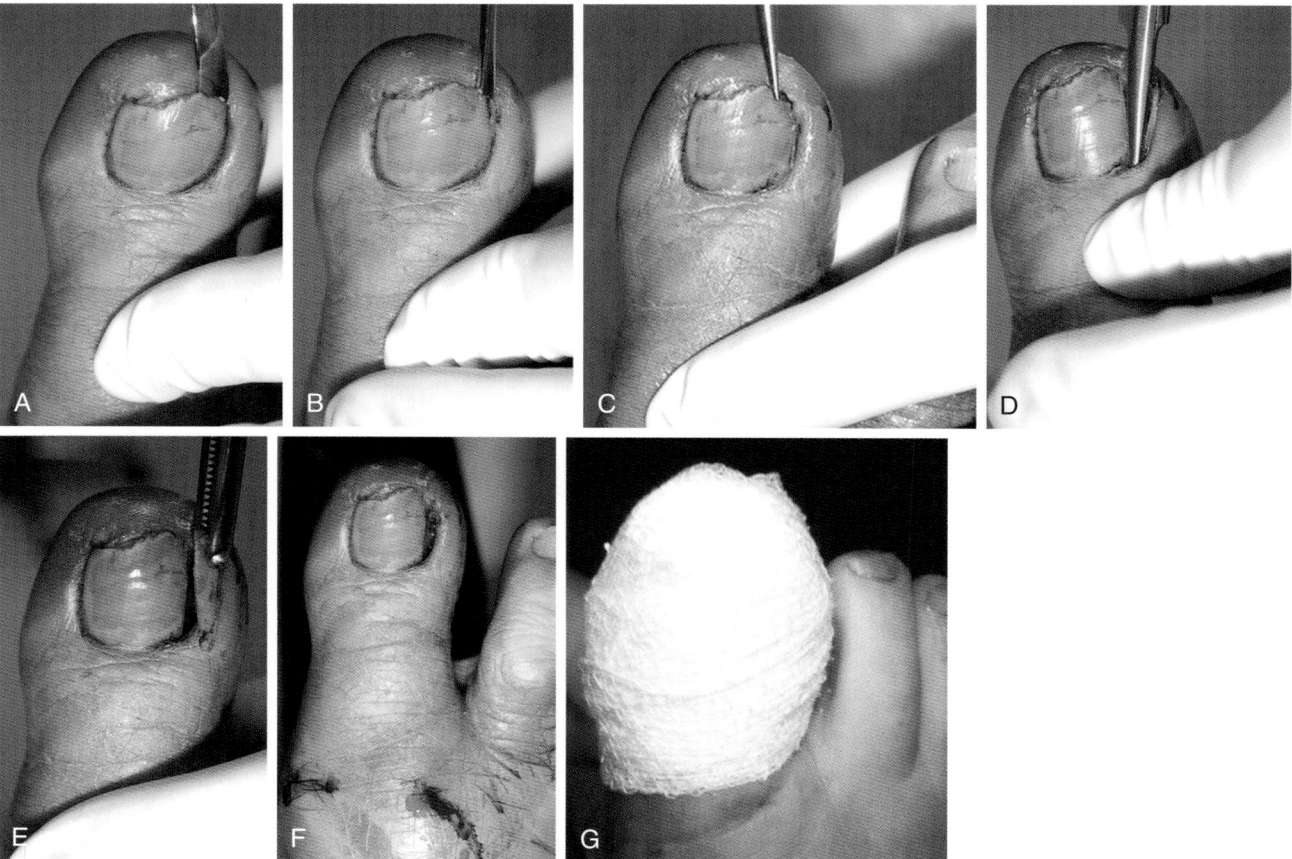

Figure 11-24 Treatment of onychocryptosis. **A** and **B,** The outer edge of the nail plate is elevated proximal to the cuticle. **C** and **D,** The nail border is incised longitudinally. **E** and **F,** A longitudinal portion of the nail is removed to relieve symptoms of acute infection. **G,** Gauze dressing is applied after the toenail procedure.

Stage 3: With chronic infection, granulation tissue develops in the lateral nail fold. The surrounding soft tissue is hypertrophied.

Stage 4: Chronic deformity of the nail plate, both nail folds, and the distal fold. It is distinguished from the other stages by distal hypertrophy.

TREATMENT

Various procedures have been reported for the cure of an ingrown toenail, but postoperative recurrence is common. Procedures generally practiced include longitudinal excision of the border of the nail plate as described above (this can temporarily resolve the infection, but a strong tendency exists for recurrent infection unless definitive treatment is performed later), reduction of the hypertrophied lateral fold, and partial or total ablation (surgical, chemical, or laser) of the germinal matrix.

There is evidence that the second type of ingrown nail, the pincer nail, is associated with broader proximal bases of the distal phalanges, which force the nail to grow broader proximally and curve tighter distally. Bisphosphonate therapy has also been implicated as a cause of this nail deformity.[68] Pincer nail is commonly associated with a dorsal distal osteophyte on the phalanx. Hence

good therapeutic results have been achieved from a combination of removing the lateral matrix horns, lifting up the nail bed from the bone, removing the distal tuft of bone,[18] and suturing the lateral dermis and subcutaneous tissue beneath the nail bed. This leaves "a flat nail bed with support on each side. The nail will then grow out straight."[87]

Unquestionably, patient education is necessary in the treatment of an ingrown toenail, both to treat an acute condition and to prevent a recurrence of infection. The patient should be instructed in proper footwear, use of loose-fitting stockings or hose, and proper nail-cutting procedures. Patients with excessive pronation may be treated with an orthotic device to decrease axial pressure on the border of the hallux. (Specific surgical procedures are discussed later in this chapter.)

Onychauxis and Onychogryphosis

Onychauxis (club nail) refers to a hypertrophied nail plate. This usually involves the great toenail, but the lesser toes may be affected as well. The deformity may be caused by systemic problems, such as nutritional deficiencies or psoriasis. The toenail may be yellow, brown, gray, or black. Most cases result from local conditions, such as

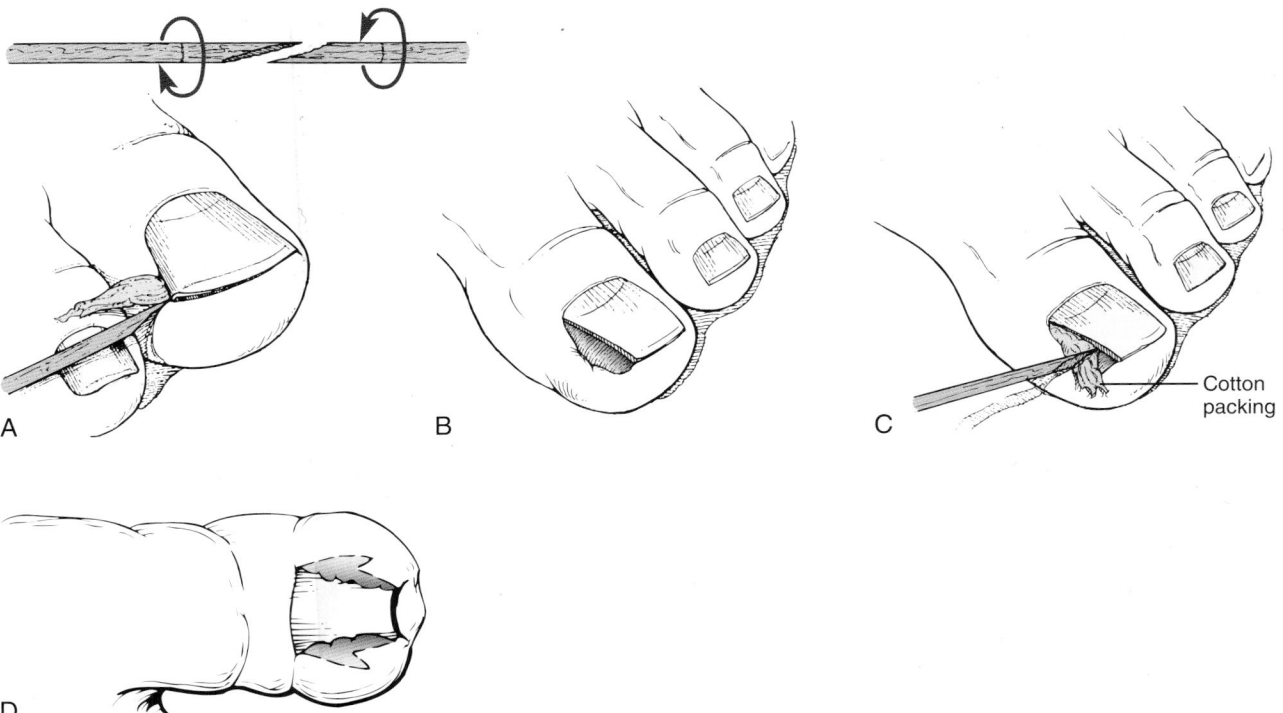

Figure 11-25 Symptoms of acute infection may be relieved by a variety of methods. **A,** A cotton packing may be placed beneath the toenail edge to elevate it. **B,** Diagonal trimming of the nail plate may remove the immediate cause of the acute infection. **C,** Cotton may be placed to elevate the toenail edge. **D,** As the nail plate regrows, infection can recur.

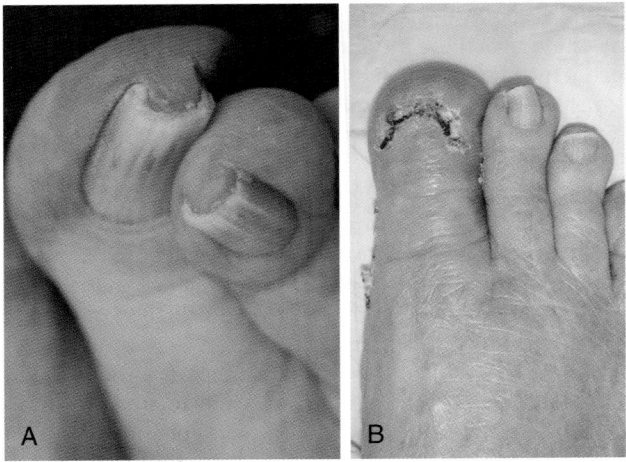

Figure 11-26 Terminal Syme amputation. **A,** Clinical example of nail incurvature in an elderly patient. Because of the chronicity of symptoms, the patient opted for a terminal Syme amputation. An osteotomy of the proximal phalanx was also performed to allow the toe to be straightened and to relieve impingement of the second toe. **B,** Three weeks postoperatively.

trauma to the nail matrix or nail bed and tinea infection, which is the most common cause. The undersurface of the nail can become tremendously thickened from the accumulation of debris from a chronic mycotic infection.[45,227] The affected nail and its bed are thickened and

deformed. When the disorder is caused by *Microsporum gypseum*, the surface of the nail might have white streaks or patches that can be excised readily. When the undersurface of the nail contains a yellowish or brown powdery substance, destruction of the nail bed has been caused by *Trichophyton purpureum*. In approximately 10% of cases of club nail, the nail bed and dorsal distal surface of the distal phalanx undergo hypertrophic changes.

Onychogryphosis refers to hypertrophy and curving of the nail plate, especially of the hallux (Fig. 11-27A and B). The nail resembles a claw or horn, and, although uncommon, its frequency in men who have tended horses has led to the appellation "hostler's toe." It has also been referred to as "ram's horn nail." The massive growth of the nail plate overlies the dorsal surface of the toe and often terminates on the plantar surface of the toe. This condition does not appear to have any relationship to a tinea infection. In most cases, it is the result of a congenital condition or repeated trauma to the nail matrix, along with poor hygiene. In some extreme cases, the nail measures several centimeters in length and curves on itself to resemble a ram's horn.

TREATMENT

To treat onychogryphosis, a strong pair of special nail clippers is used to remove the entire nail horn up to where the nail is attached securely to the nail bed (Fig. 11-27C). Subsequent trimming and debridement help the nail become asymptomatic.

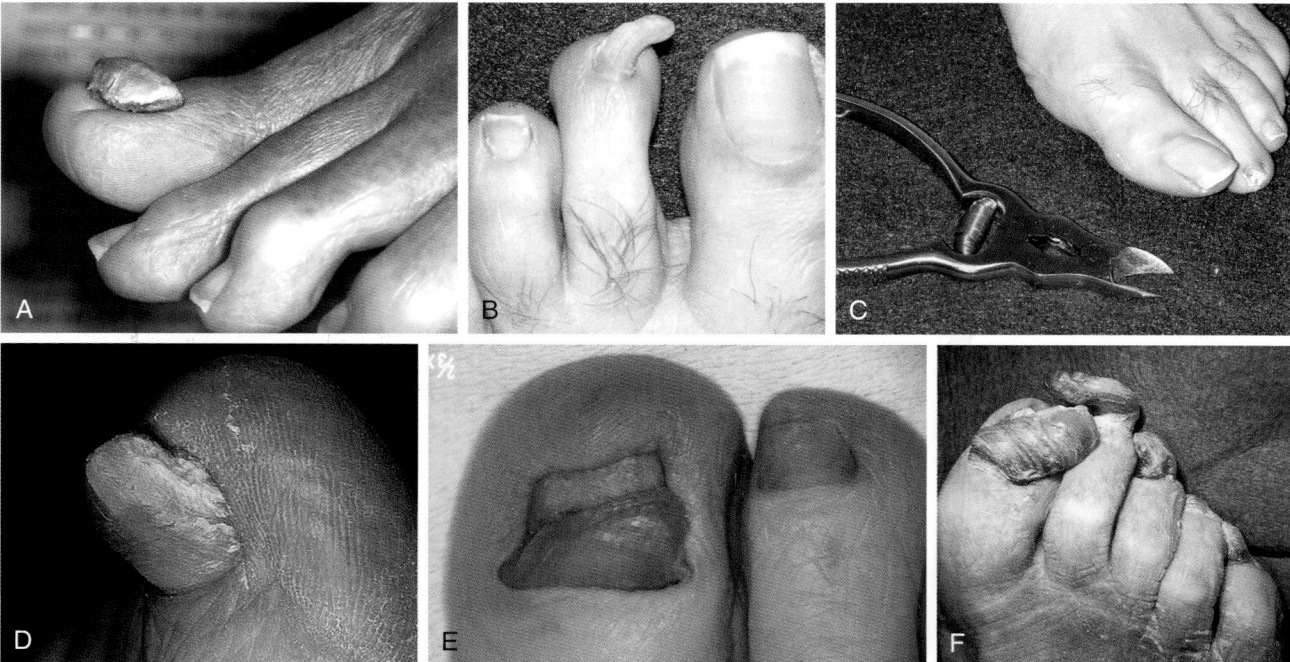

Figure 11-27 Onychogryphosis. **A** and **B,** With onychogryphosis, nails may become grossly thickened. **C,** With the use of a special nail cutter, these nails can be trimmed in the office. **D,** Thickened and elevated nail. **E,** Congenital deformity of the great toenail. **F,** Ram's horn toenail deformity from chronic infection and lack of proper care. (**D,** From Habif TP, Campbell JL Jr, Shane Chapman M, et al: *Skin disease,* ed 3, London, 2011, Elsevier. **E,** Courtesy Dr. Robert Baran. **F,** From Dockery GL: *Cutaneous disorders of the lower extremity,* Philadelphia, 1996, Elsevier.)

To treat onychauxis, the hypertrophied nail is gradually reduced by grinding it with a motorized tool. According to Frank and Freer,[77] *Current Procedural Terminology* code 11721 (debridement of six or more nails) was the most frequently used code (of 300 foot and ankle codes) in 1999. The cost to Medicare for this procedure was $245 million that year. Abramson and Wilton[2,3] advocated reducing hyperkeratotic nails with nail drills and burs. However, they noted that particles 0.5 to 5 mm can become airborne and be inhaled in the respiratory tract. Chronic exposure to nail dust aerosols can lead to conjunctivitis, rhinitis, asthma, coughing, impaired lung function, and hypersensitivity. Of the physicians with chronic exposure to nail dust from grinding hyperkeratotic nails, 31% had abnormally elevated immunoglobulin E levels on radioimmunoassay.

Antifungal medication may be applied either topically or beneath the nail plate. For severely deformed club nails, avulsion of the nail is advised. Later or concurrently, the nail matrix may be ablated with a surgical ablation technique, chemical nail plate destruction, or a terminal Syme amputation.

Onychomycosis

Onychomycosis is a progressive, recurring fungal infection that originates in the nail bed and accounts for 50% of all toenail abnormalities. Usually, the entry is between the hyponychium and the nail plate. The infection progresses to the nail, resulting in the typical appearance of yellowing and thickening of the nail. A mycotic infection of one or more of the toenails often accompanies tinea pedis (athlete's foot).[160]

Although many people consider this primarily a cosmetic problem, a portion of the patients also experience pain (36%-48%) or limited mobility (41%) as a direct result of onychomycosis[58,185,186] (Fig. 11-27D-F). Pressure necrosis from the nail bed or severe bacterial infections can even cause limb-threatening complications in older patients.[173] The greatest predisposing factors are increasing age and male sex; men are 1.7 to 3.0 times more likely to have a fungal infection than women.[88,89] Patients with vascular disease or diabetes, as well as immunocompromised patients (e.g., patients infected with human immunodeficiency virus [HIV]), also have a higher incidence of onychomycosis than the general population (see Box 11-8). With the effectiveness of the newer antifungal agents, diagnosis and treatment are more efficacious.

Zaias[227] has classified onychomycoses into four categories (Box 11-9). *Distal subungual onychomycosis* primarily involves the distal nail bed and hyponychium, with secondary involvement of the undersurface of the nail plate (Figs. 11-28A and B). *Proximal subungual onychomycosis* is rare (Fig. 11-28C). *Candidal onychomycosis* involves the entire nail plate (Fig. 11-28E) on the surface of the nail by such organisms as *Trichophyton mentagrophytes* and by *Acremonium* and *Aspergillus* species (Fig. 11-28D).

Onychomycosis is a common disorder of the nail, present in possibly 20% of the population. The prevalence

Box 11-8 Risk Factors Associated with Onychomycosis

Neurologic Disorders
Hansen disease (leprosy)
Multiple sclerosis
Peripheral neuropathy
Syphilis

Vascular Disorders
Arteriosclerotic vascular disease
Buerger disease (thromboangiitis obliterans)
Chronic thrombophlebitis
Ischemia
Venous stasis

Metabolic Disorders
Chronic alcohol abuse
Diabetes mellitus
Malabsorption syndrome
Malnutrition
Pernicious anemia
Thyroid disease

Other Systemic Disorders
Cardiac disease
Congestive heart failure
Chronic obstructive pulmonary disease
Chronic renal disease
Hypertension
Uremia

Modified from Helfand AE: Onychomycosis in the aged: an administrative perspective. *J Am Podiatr Med Assoc* 76:142–145, 1986. Used with permission.

Box 11-9 Common Organisms Cultured in Onychomycosis

Distal Subungual Onychomycosis
Dermatophytes
Epidermophyton floccosum
Trichophyton rubrum
Trichophyton mentagrophytes

Yeasts and Molds
Acremonium
Aspergillus
Candida parapsilosis
Fusarium
Scopulariopsis brevicaulis

Proximal Subungual Onychomycosis
Dermatophytes
T. rubrum
Trichophyton megninii
Trichophyton schoenleinii
Trichophyton tonsurans

White Superficial Onychomycosis
Dermatophytes
T. mentagrophytes

Yeasts and Molds
Acremonium
Aspergillus
Fusarium

Candidal Onychomycosis
Yeasts and Molds
C. parapsilosis
Candida albicans

Modified from Norton LA: Nail disorders. A review. *J Am Acad Dermatol* 2:451–467, 1980. Used with permission.

may be much higher than this, but culture or biopsy is not usually done. In patients older than 60 years, involvement can approach 75% of the population. Infection with dermatophytes, such as *Trichophyton rubrum, T. mentagrophytes,* and *Epidermophyton floccosum,* is much more common than with *Candida* species. Nondermatophytes account for less than 1% of cases of onychomycosis.[153,154] More typically, *Candida* is the cause of infection in children.

With chronic infection, the nail plate thickens and becomes discolored, brittle, and deformed. A buildup of chronic debris beneath the nail plate occurs over time. The thickened nail plate can become detached from the underlying nail bed and become painful when compressed by tight stockings or a constricting toe box.

DISTAL SUBUNGUAL ONYCHOMYCOSIS
Distal subungual onychomycosis is the most common of the four types of mycotic infections (see Fig. 11-28A and B). This deeply seated form of onychomycosis results in yellowish longitudinal streaks within the nail plate. Although the incubation period is unknown, the mode of transmission is thought to be through direct contact of a traumatized nail predisposed to mycotic infection.[99] Serologic and genetic analysis of histocompatibility leukocyte antigen (HLA) class I in a homogeneous population showed that persons lacking the HLA-DR53 phenotype were at increased risk for developing *Trichophyton rubrum* onychomycosis.[230] Therefore HLA-DR53 might

provide the immune response necessary to prevent a fungal infection.[187]

The disease often occurs before the sixth decade of life. The infectious organism invades insidiously from the free edge of the nail plate toward the base, resulting in a thickened, discolored, and deformed nail plate. The initial infection occurs in the stratum corneum, the superficial layer of the epidermis. As the inflammation continues, the response of the nail bed is cellular accumulation, nail elevation, and discoloration. With the accumulation of debris beneath the nail, further fungal and microorganism growth occurs. After invading the nail bed, the fungus penetrates the nail plate and causes delamination of the toenail.

Several dermatophytes are associated with subungual onychomycosis. *Trichophyton, Epidermophyton,* and *Microsporum* are the usual dermatophytes, and *T. rubrum* is the most common. *Trichophyton interdigitale* and *T. mentagrophytes* can also be present, and *E. floccosum* and nondermatophytes (*Scopulariopsis, Aspergillus, Fusarium,* and *Candida* species) have been reported.[139] This disease entity is not thought to be contagious.

Endonyx onychomycosis is a variant of distal subungual onychomycosis in which the fungi reach the nail via the skin but invade the nail plate directly instead of

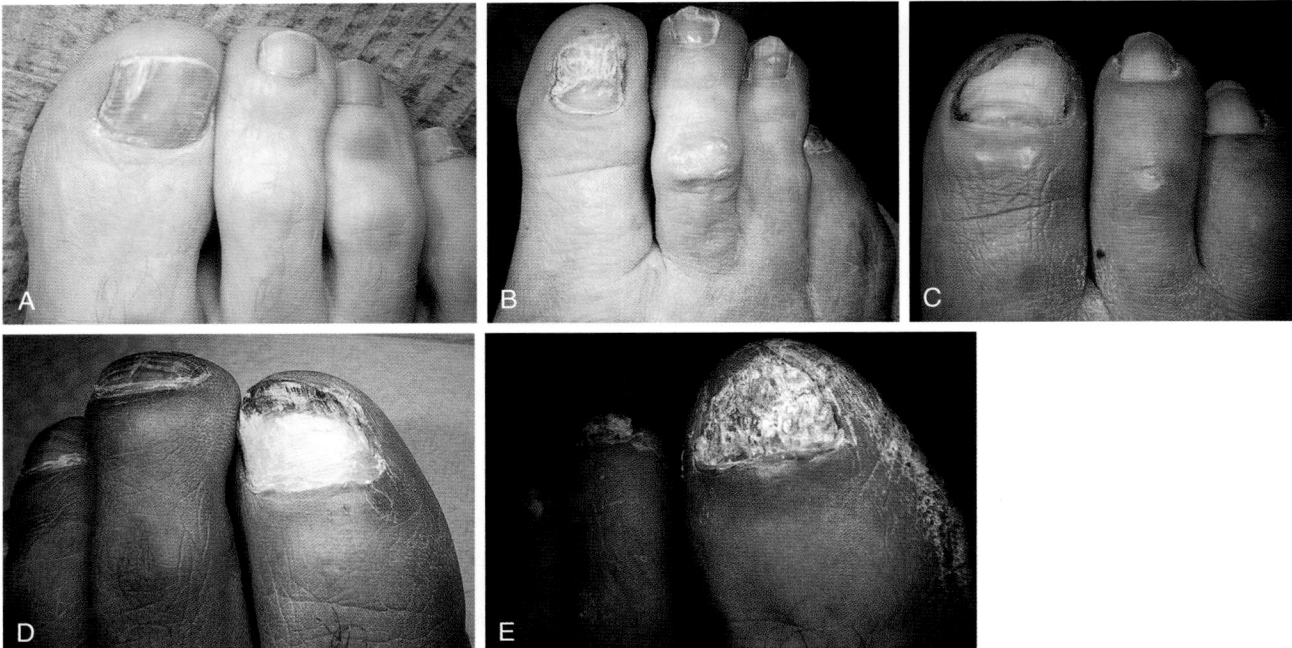

Figure 11-28 **A,** Distal subungual onychomycosis. This is the most common of the four types of mycotic infection. The nails are yellow and thickened, with hyperkeratotic material underneath. **B,** In this advanced case of distal subungual onychomycosis, the involved nail is thickened and opaque, with crumbly material distally. **C,** Proximal subungual infection of the hallux toenail. The toenail has become loosened and separated from the bed. Once separation has occurred, the nail appears white or pale, and fluid may accumulate beneath it. **D,** White superficial fungal infection. The nail is dry, brittle with a powdery consistency. **E,** Candidal infection with thickening and crumbling of the nail. (**A-E,** From Dockery GL: *Cutaneous disorders of the lower extremity,* Philadelphia, 1996, Elsevier.)

infecting the nail bed.[171] Endonyx onychomycosis does not cause hyperkeratosis. Despite the milky-white discoloration of the nail, the nail plate itself is of normal thickness and smooth.[19]

WHITE SUPERFICIAL ONYCHOMYCOSIS

White superficial onychomycosis appears as opaque, white, well-demarcated islands on the surface of the nail plate (see Fig. 11-28D). In this infection, the pathogen invades the superficial dorsal aspect of the nail plate, which results in the development of white plaques. This is the rarest form of onychomycosis and is seldom seen except in immunologically compromised patients.[28] The infection typically starts in the pericuticle nail plate and then grows distally, involving and destroying the entire nail plate. These plaques of localized fungal growth can progress to more diffuse involvement, invading the entire surface of the nail plate. The toenail can turn brownish and become roughened and pitted from chronic infection. The most common infectious organism is *T. mentagrophytes* (Table 11-11).[139] Topical antiseptics may be an effective early treatment for this type of onychomycosis.

PROXIMAL SUBUNGUAL ONYCHOMYCOSIS

Proximal subungual onychomycosis (Fig. 11-28C) occurs infrequently and is typified by whitish discoloration extending distally from underneath the proximal nail

Table 11-11	Prevalence of Infectious Organisms in White Superficial Onychomycosis
Organism	**Prevalence (%)**
Trichophyton mentagrophytes	68
Trichophyton rubrum	8
Candida albicans	4
Miscellaneous	8
No growth	12

Modified from Bodman MA, Brlan MR: Superficial white onychomycosis. *J Am Podiatr Med Assoc* 85:205–208, 1995. Used with permission.

fold. *T. rubrum* is the most usual infectious organism. This entity is more common in people infected with HIV.[57,180]

CANDIDAL ONYCHOMYCOSIS

Candidal onychomycosis, characterized by generalized thickening of the nail plate, results from *Candida albicans* or *Candida parapsilosis* infection (Fig. 11-28). Initially, longitudinal white striations appear within the nail plate. The nail bed thickens, and the distal end of the digit appears bulbous and clubbed. The nail plate can become opaque as well.

Diagnosis

An early sign of mycotic infection is thickening of the distal and lateral borders of the nail plate. The nails can become opaque, and discoloration can occur with chronic infection. The edges of the nail plate can erode, and partial or complete loss of the nail plate can occur. As time passes with advanced onychomycosis, it is difficult for the clinician to distinguish among the patterns of mycotic penetration of the nail plate. Although total dystrophic onychomycosis may be considered a separate class of onychomycosis, it is actually a progression of any of the above types, with involvement of the entire nail unit leading to possible permanent scarring of the nail matrix.[171]

When a fungal infection is suspected, diagnosis is attempted by examining a specimen under a light microscope. Vigorous scraping of the nail produces debris that can be moistened with a few drops of 10% KOH solution. Hyphae may be seen microscopically. Samples cultured on an appropriate medium can aid in the diagnosis. Although culturing finely ground nail material or debris from beneath the nail is the optimal method of making the diagnosis of onychomycosis, 30% of the results are false negatives.[49,64] Furthermore, the sensitivity of direct microscopy with KOH is not foolproof because the procedure is affected by many variables, including the skill of the slide preparer, the microscope used, and the sampling technique. Other methods of diagnosis include staining nail clippings with periodic acid–Schiff stain (PAS)[128,172] and using in vivo confocal microscopy.[104] A study to estimate and compare the cost-effectiveness and sensitivity of diagnostic tests found that PAS was the most sensitive test (99%), and KOH-CBE (chlorazol black E) was second most sensitive at 94%. However, KOH-CBE was more cost-effective.[136] It is important, but not always easy, to distinguish onychomycosis from psoriasis. Beginning antifungal medication without a confirmatory diagnosis can be both futile and expensive. A cross-sectional diagnostic study of 277 patients found that when dermatologists consider onychomycosis the most probable diagnosis and abnormal plantar desquamation (>25% of the sole) is present, treatment should be started without any further testing. Clinical diagnosis with presence of these signs was found to be as accurate as laboratory tests, with a positive predictive value of 81%. With both signs absent, the positive predictive value for predicting absence of fungi was 71%.[81]

In a review of 169 patients with nail disease, 32% had positive findings on both direct examination and culture, and 20% had positive findings on direct microscopy alone.[75] Only four historical and clinical diagnostic features significantly correlated with positive mycologic results: a history of tinea pedis in the past year; scaling on one or both soles; white, crumbly patches on the nail surface; and an abnormal color of the nail.

Systemic Treatment

In a cumulative meta-analysis that evaluated randomized, controlled trials of systemic antifungal agents for the treatment of onychomycosis, the cure rates with many antifungal drugs were similar.[91] The overall cumulative average (±standard deviation [SD]) for mycologic cure with these drugs was as follows: terbinafine (Lamisil),

76% (±3%); pulse-dosed itraconazole (Sporanox), 63% (±7%); continuous-dosed itraconazole, 59% (±5%); fluconazole (Diflucan), 48% (±5%); and griseofulvin (Fulvicin), 60% (±6%). For open studies, the rates were somewhat higher: terbinafine, 83% (±12%); pulse-dosed itraconazole, 84% (±9%); and fluconazole, 79% (±3%).

One open study[229] evaluated the use of terbinafine for the treatment of *T. rubrum* nail bed onychomycosis. With pulse-dosed oral terbinafine, 39 of 42 patients (93%) were cured. However, only 10 of 17 (59%) were cured when terbinafine was given every 4 months. It was thought that this regimen would not only save money but also lower drug-induced side effects. This use, however, is still off-label. Another study comparing intermittent terbinafine versus continuous terbinafine found that continuous dosing is better.[192] Two other studies suggest that both intermittent and continuous terbinafine treatment are better than pulsed itraconazole therapy.[90,170] Also, terbinafine may produce a lower recurrence than itraconazole.[223]

One study reported on a relatively small number of patients with onychomycosis in high-risk groups (immunocompromised patients, patients with diabetes, and patients with HIV). In these groups, terbinafine was well tolerated and equally effective in patients in all risk groups.[46] Another study supports terbinafine's safety in patients taking antidiabetic, antihypertensive, and cholesterol-lowering agents, including statins.[111]

Another study found terbinafine to be the most cost-effective drug whether used as a pulse, continuous or in combinations with other agents. However, the authors recommended 3 months of continuous treatment. The least cost-effective were itraconazole, griseofulvin, and fluconazole. The nail lacquer ciciopirox was three times more expensive than other treatments when evaluating total cost for a complete cure.[212]

With the use of all pharmacologic agents for treating onychomycosis, whether topical, oral, or parenteral, a frank discussion with the patient should cover side effects, including hypersensitivity, liver toxicity, gastrointestinal disorders, and cardiovascular effects. These drugs are contraindicated during pregnancy because of their teratogenic effects. Hepatotoxicity has been reported in patients, especially older ones, who have a history of liver dysfunction.[51] Other adverse effects include nausea and vomiting, pruritus, abdominal pain, and idiosyncratic liver dysfunction. Elevated liver enzyme levels are uncommon but have been reported in approximately 1 in 10,000 patients.[103]

A potential new treatment for onychomycosis is posaconazole. However, the low cost of generic terbinafine may limit posaconazole use to patients intolerant to terbinafine.[62,74]

Local Treatment

Local therapy includes mechanical grinding and debridement of the thickened nail plate with a motorized device, curettage of the necrotic subungual tissue, and adequate trimming of the thickened nail plate. For many patients, simple debridement adequately relieves pain and discomfort without the need for surgical or pharmacologic intervention.

Topical Treatment

The only topical brush-on treatment for onychomycosis that is approved by the U.S. Food and Drug Administration is ciclopirox (Penlac) in a lacquer solution, but its effectiveness is limited. Ciclopirox 1% cream (Loprox), terbinafine 1% cream, and ketoconazole 2% cream (Nizoral) have also been used for topical treatment. Typically, these creams are applied twice daily to the involved toenail and surrounding soft tissue.

Transungual delivery of terbinafine by iontophoresis in onychomycotic nails has been investigated. The permeation and load of drug crossing the nail plate was enhanced significantly during iontophoresis, by 37-fold, compared with passive delivery in toenails.[149]

Some clinicians prefer avulsion of the thickened nail plate, debridement of the necrotic tissue, and treatment of the matrix and nail bed twice daily. Hettinger and Valinsky[101] advocate nail avulsion to help reduce the overall duration of treatment. After nail avulsion, the area is treated with a thin layer of cream. Therapy is continued until the nail plate has regrown. The authors reported that all nails that grew back were free of mycotic infection. They reported a 96% success rate at an average of 11 months of follow-up. After removal of the infected nail plate, patient compliance was critically important to the overall success rate. Chemical nail plate destruction, surgical ablation, or a terminal Syme amputation may be considered as well. These techniques are discussed elsewhere.

In patients who are at risk of adverse kidney or liver effects and medication interactions, such as children, the elderly, and patients with systemic diseases, photodynamic therapy may be an alternative.[194,213]

A novel topical treatment of onychomycosis using Vicks VapoRub has been reported to have a positive clinical effect. This study reported 83% positive treatment effect and 27% having a mycologic and clinical cure at 48 weeks by applying the ointment to the affected nail two times a day.[44,53]

Another new alternative is the use of laser therapy to eradicate the onchomycosis. Both low-level (400-600 nM) and higher-level (800 nM) laser therapies are currently being used; the long-term results and efficacy remain to be reported.

Combination Treatment: Topical, Systemic, Debridement

A combination of oral and topical antifungal agents has also been advocated. Use of 5% nail lacquer (at publication, not approved for use in the United States) resulted in improved cure rates in severe toenail onychomycosis.[16]

Another study also promoted use of topical agents in combination with a systemic antifungal agent, advocating improved cure rates of onychomycosis compared with oral therapy alone. It further suggested a triple therapy

with the addition of debridement to improve these results.[33]

Onychia

Onychia, also known as *onychitis*, occurs with inflammation of the nail matrix and accumulation of granulation tissue around the toenail. It may be associated with poorly fitting footwear or tight socks, or it can occur after trauma to the distal phalanx, such as stubbing the toe or dropping an object onto the toe. On occasion, osteomyelitis or osteitis occurs and causes painful symptoms.

Initial treatment requires removal of the causative agent. Minimizing trauma or pressure over the toenail can alleviate symptoms. In the presence of an acute bacterial or fungal infection, culture and sensitivity testing should be performed. Appropriate antibiotic therapy may be instituted.[231] Radiography is used to identify any osseous involvement. If acute infection is present, local surgical care includes incision and drainage. Toenail avulsion and, on occasion, surgical ablation of the toenail may be necessary. Localized treatment with topical antifungal agents, such as clotrimazole (Lotrimin) or nystatin cream, may be helpful. The simultaneous use of roomy footwear or sandals might help to remove pressure from the painful toenail. Often, symptoms subside with time and aggressive conservative treatment.

Onycholysis and Onychomadesis

Onycholysis is separation of the nail plate from the nail bed along the lateral and distal borders. *Onychomadesis* is separation of the entire nail plate, beginning proximally and ending distally. Onychomadesis may be associated with drug reaction, eczema, scarlet fever, leprosy, lead poisoning, or trauma.[154] Nail ablation may be necessary to treat a chronic condition.

Onycholysis, which occurs more frequently in female patients than in male patients, seems to be associated with local trauma as well as with drug and allergic reactions, eczema, hypothyroidism, hyperthyroidism, lichen planus, bacterial and fungal infections, and vascular insufficiency. *C. albicans* and *Pseudomonas* species are the most common infectious organisms. Trimming of the separated nail plate and application of topical antifungal medication may be helpful in treating this condition. For more severe symptoms, toenail ablation may be necessary.

Onychopsittacus

Onychopsittacus or *parrot-beak nail* is a peculiar symmetric overcurvature of the free margin of the nail plate resembling a parrot's beak. The part of the nail plate attached to the nail bed is normal. If the nails are trimmed close to the nail bed, the abnormality is hidden. The occurrence rate is difficult to determine because patients hide the abnormality by keeping their nails trimmed. Conditions leading to pulp atrophy cause the parrot-beak deformity. The amount of bone and nail bed loss determines the degree of nail bed curvature. A secondary similar deformity may be seen with distal fingertip trauma, resulting

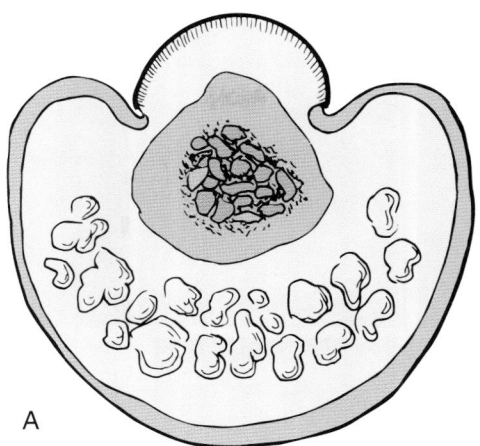
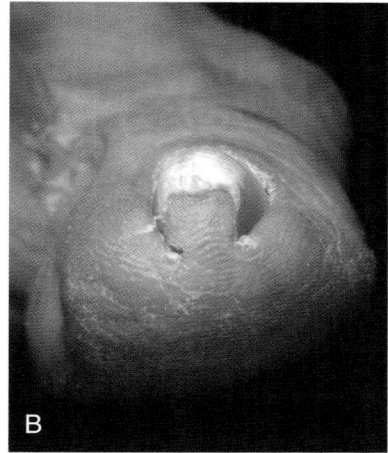

Figure 11-29 Subungual exostosis. **A,** Subungual exostosis can cause deformity of the nail plate. **B,** Clinical example of nail incurvation in an elderly patient.

in loss of nail support from the dorsal tuft of the terminal phalanx. Causes of parrot-beak nail include tight surgical closure of amputations, porphyria cutanea tarda caused by distal nail bed hemitorsion, and chronic use of crystallized freebase cocaine ("crack") Cocaine-induced vasoconstriction and digital ischemia causes pulp atrophy, resulting in loss of nail support. Soaking the nails in warm water for 30 minutes may allow the abnormality to temporarily correct (see Fig. 11-26).[54]

Nail Bed Disorders

The structure and function of the nail bed may be altered by subungual exostosis, subungual tumors, subungual clavus, subungual hematoma, or subungual verruca.

Subungual Exostosis

Abnormalities of the underlying bone can be diagnosed with the aid of a radiograph. Typically, these involve the distal phalanx. A subungual exostosis must be distinguished from an osteochondroma (see previous section on tumors). Likewise, usually when a lytic lesion is present in the distal phalanx, a benign tumor, such as an enchondroma or solitary bone cyst, should be considered.

In a patient with chronic complaints of pain, swelling, inflammation, and chronic paronychia, the physician should consider radiography to evaluate the patient for an underlying bone tumor. The development of chronic subungual ulceration should alert the clinician to the possibility of squamous cell carcinoma, probably the most common malignant tumor of the toe (Fig. 11-29, see Figs. 11-15 to 11-17).

Subungual Tumors

Subungual and periungual fibromas, exostoses, mucous cysts (Fig. 11-30, see Figs. 11-13 and 11-14), glomus tumors, enchondromas, keratoacanthomas, pyogenic

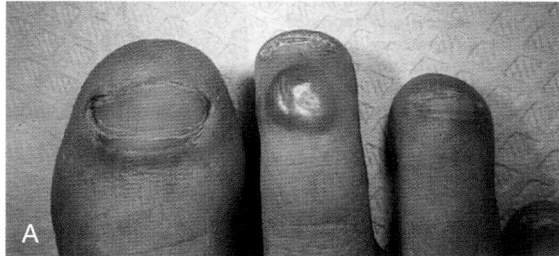
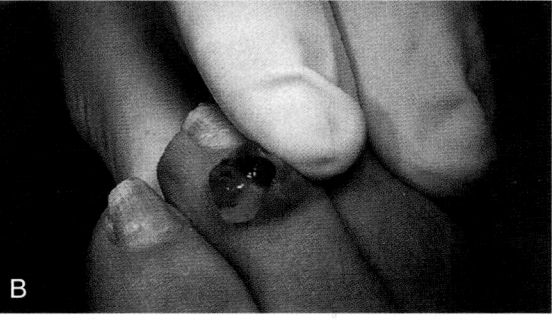

Figure 11-30 Mucous cyst. **A,** A smooth, well-circumscribed, firm, flesh-colored nodule overlies the distal interphalangeal joint of the second toe. **B,** When incised, a thick, viscous, jelly-like material can be extruded. This lesion is best treated by excision of the osteophytes at the distal interphalangeal joint or fusion of the joint. (From Dockery GL: *Cutaneous disorders of the lower extremity*, Philadelphia, 1996, Elsevier.)

granulomas, and other benign lesions occur in the area of the distal phalanx. Malignant tumors, such as squamous cell carcinoma, basal cell carcinoma, and malignant melanoma, can develop in this area as well (see previous section on tumors).

Subungual Clavus

A hyperkeratotic lesion in the subungual region is characterized by the accumulation of debris beneath the nail plate. A callus can develop in this area because of pressure

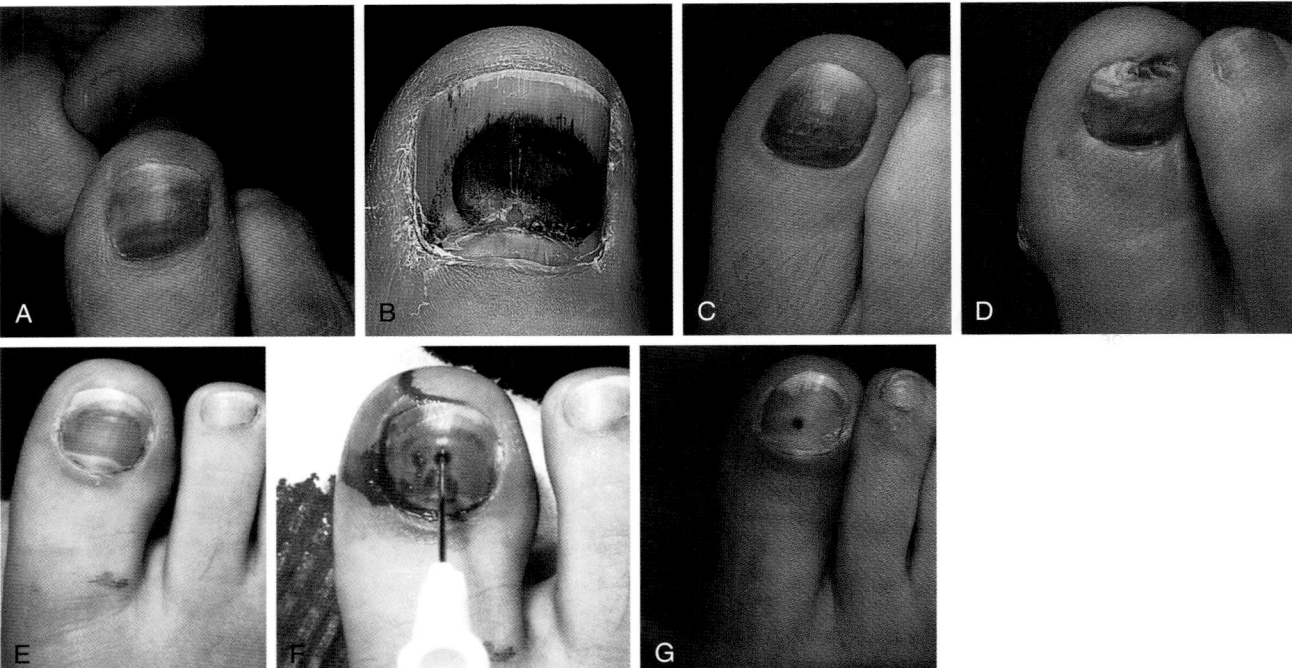

Figure 11-31 Subungual hematoma. **A,** Typical appearance of subungual hemorrhage after direct trauma to toenail. **B,** When there is considerable pain or swelling under the nail after hematoma formation, the hematoma may be released. With time, the hematoma evolves, and the subungual blood turns brown or black. This may take months to resolve. Melanoma can have a similar appearance, and the history is important. **C,** Accumulation of blood beneath the nail after trauma. The staining will persist until the nail grows out. **D,** Chronic characteristic appearance of hemorrhage with accumulation of debris beneath the nail. **E,** Acute subungual hematoma. **F,** A small hole created in the nail allows blood to drain, but the procedure must be done soon after injury because coagulated blood cannot be drained. **G,** After removal of the needle. (**A, C, D,** and **G,** From Dockery GL: *Cutaneous disorders of the lower extremity,* Philadelphia, 1996, Elsevier. **B,** From Habif TP, Campbell JL Jr, Shane Chapman M, et al: *Skin disease,* ed 3, London, 2011, Elsevier.)

from a confining toe box or long-term use of tight stockings. Vascular insufficiency, psoriasis, diabetes, localized fungal infection, and various systemic diseases also can cause subungual clavus. As the amount of debris accumulates, a yellowish-gray cast develops in the toenail. Typically, a patient complains of pain caused by external pressure from a closed-toe shoe. The differential diagnosis includes subungual exostosis, subungual osteochondroma, trauma, subungual verruca, and glomus tumor.

Debridement of the hyperkeratotic clavus is the treatment of choice. Trimming of the detached nail plate facilitates debridement of the necrotic tissue.

Subungual Hematoma

Hemorrhagic accumulation between the nail bed and the nail plate is a *subungual hematoma.* Typically, this occurs with trauma to the nail bed and rupture of small capillaries in this region. Crushing or shearing trauma to the nail produces painful subungual hemorrhage manifested by a dusky swelling of the nail plate. The differential diagnosis of a discolored nail includes subungual exostosis, malignant melanoma, Kaposi sarcoma, nevus, glomus tumor, and trauma. Within hours after injury, pressure builds up because of bleeding beneath the nail plate.

Edema, pain with movement of the digit, and blue or black discoloration under the nail can prompt the patient to seek evaluation and treatment. Fracture of the distal phalanx occurs in 25% of patients.

A syringe needle, nail drill, trephine, dental burr, fine-point scalpel blade (No. 11), heated paper clip, or carbon dioxide laser[100] may be used to penetrate the nail bed and evacuate a trapped hematoma (Fig. 11-31). Palamarchuk and Kerzner[162] describe using a handheld cautery unit to decompress a subungual hematoma. With minimal pressure on the nail, the cautery unit creates a small hole in the nail, and the hematoma is easily evacuated. Radiographs may be necessary to rule out a fracture. Further therapy may include oral antibiotics.

Tucker et al[206] studied crush injuries of the distal phalanx with concomitant nail bed injuries. In general, if the hematoma was less than 20% of the area of the nail plate, patients were not treated. Some hand surgeons suggest that less than 50% hematoma for fingernails can be neglected. A larger area of hematoma suggests the possibility of a nail bed injury and possible fracture of the distal phalanx. With an open injury, inspection of the nail bed and repair of a lacerated nail bed or matrix may be necessary. An open fracture should be treated

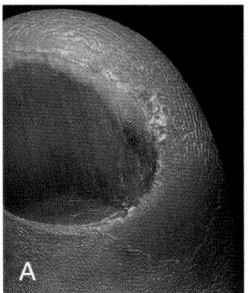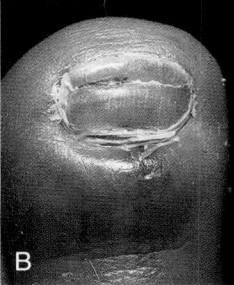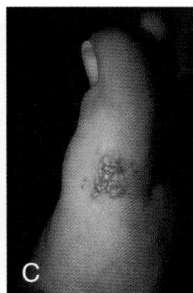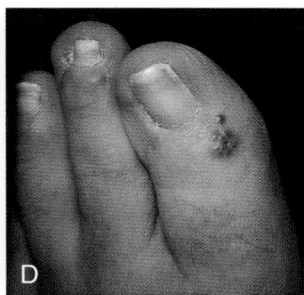

Figure 11-32 **A,** Acute paronychia. Typical appearance of *Staphylococcus* infection with localized swelling, erythema, and draining at the toenail border. Paronychia either is accompanied by an ingrown toenail or is a forerunner of an ingrown toenail. Swelling may develop with intense erythema within 24 hours. **B,** Another example of acute paronychia. **C** and **D,** Herpes simplex. The characteristic foot lesion is a cluster of minute painful red lesions on the second toe, proximal to the nail bed. This condition rarely results in herpetic whitlow or paronychia. (**A** and **B,** From Habif TP, Campbell JL Jr, Shane Chapman M, et al: *Skin disease,* ed 3, London, 2011, Elsevier. **C** and **D,** From Dockery GL: *Cutaneous disorders of the lower extremity,* Philadelphia, 1996, Elsevier.)

routinely like any open fracture. Fox[76] reported a case of osteomyelitis after an open nail bed injury and recommended aggressive irrigation and debridement and parenteral antibiotics to minimize the risk of subsequent infection.

Subungual Verruca

A subungual or periungual verruca can occur beneath the nail plate or in the nail groove (see Fig. 11-13). The appearance of a verruca is similar to that of a wart on any other part of the foot. When a verruca involves the subungual tissue, care must be taken in the treatment plan to avoid damage to the nail matrix. Usually, the wart can be ablated with chemical treatment, excision, or electrocautery or with a combination of these treatments.

Nail Fold Disorders

Nail fold disorders include paronychia, onychophosis, pyogenic granuloma, herpetic whitlow, and periungual verruca.

Paronychia

Paronychia is an inflammation of the nail groove that usually affects the hallux but can affect the lesser toes as well (Fig. 11-32A and B). It either is accompanied by an ingrown toenail or is a forerunner of an ingrown toenail. Paronychia varies in severity and can occur as a mild cellulitis. More severe cellulitis of the nail fold is characterized by swelling, erythema, pain, tenderness, and often a purulent discharge from beneath the nail fold. Secondary dystrophic changes of the nail are commonly seen, and chronic paronychia involvement with *Candida* infection can occur. At times, the infection extends to the nail matrix, in which case it is termed *onychia*. Unlike onychia, paronychia by itself is rarely caused by skin disorders such as herpes simplex. When extrinsic pressure from a confining toe box crowds the tissue on the medial aspect of the nail, a severe infection can result. Granulation tissue and

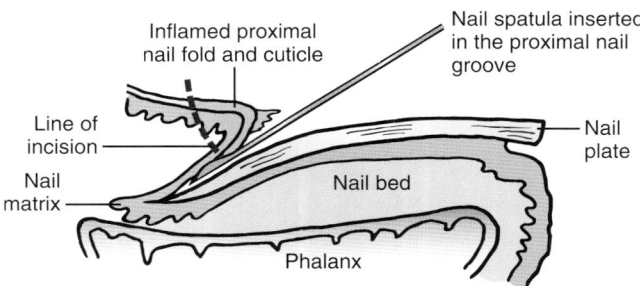

Figure 11-33 En bloc resection of proximal nail fold for chronic paronychia. The Freer Elevator is kept beneath the cuticle during the resection to protect the nail matrix from inadvertent injury.

extensive ulceration in the nail groove are characteristic of chronic changes.

TREATMENT OF PARONYCHIA
Acute
1. Relieve extrinsic pressure from footwear.
2. Excise a 2-mm linear portion of the nail margin to relieve the cutting effect of the edematous nail groove.
3. Paint the granulation tissue with a silver nitrate stick.
4. Apply a fungicidal ointment and cover with a sterile dressing.

Chronic
En Bloc Excision and Avulsion of Nail Plate[86]
1. Protect the underlying nail plate and nail matrix with a Freer or nail spatula (Fig. 11-33).
2. With the knife blade angled, obliquely excise approximately a 3-mm full-thickness section of the proximal nail fold.
3. The excision includes the indurated proximal nail fold, creating a gently sloped wound.
4. Gently remove the nail plate by a distal-to-proximal technique.

601

5. Drain any discharge, secure hemostasis and apply a nonadherent dressing.
6. Oral antibiotics are prescribed for 5 to 7 days and daily dressing changes with an antibiotic ointment are started at 1 to 2 days for approximately 1 to 2 weeks.
7. The wound is allowed to heal by secondary intention.

Onychophosis

Onychophosis occurs with an accumulation of callus within the lateral nail groove and involves the great toe more often than the lesser toes. This can occur with extrinsic pressure from a tight-fitting toe box, with pronation of the foot and abduction of the hallux, or with an incurved nail plate. Erythema and swelling typically occur in the nail groove, and this can develop into an ingrown toenail. Pain is often associated with this condition. The differential diagnosis includes subungual clavus, onychia, paronychia, and onychocryptosis.

The initial treatment involves shaving or debridement of the callus. With a purulent infection, partial avulsion

of the nail and eventual ablation of the nail matrix may be necessary. Radiographs may be helpful in ruling out a subungual exostosis, which can occur with similar symptomatic findings.

Pyogenic Granuloma

Pyogenic granuloma, first described by Hartzell[94] in 1904, is a vascular lesion that develops from connective tissue.[26,67] The cause is unknown, but trauma is often suspected. It can occur at any age, range from red to dark blue or black, and grow to be 2 to 10 mm. It grows rapidly and tends to bleed and ulcerate. It can develop secondary to trauma along the lateral nail fold (Fig. 11-34A). The differential diagnosis includes onychia, Kaposi sarcoma, glomus tumor, periungual verruca, melanoma, fibroma, hemangioma, angiosarcoma, and basal cell carcinoma. It may be pedunculated or sessile and is often complicated by a staphylococcal infection (Fig. 11-34B).

Typical treatment involves surgical excision, cauterization with silver nitrate, electrocautery, or laser. After treatment, moist dressings and antibiotics may be indicated.

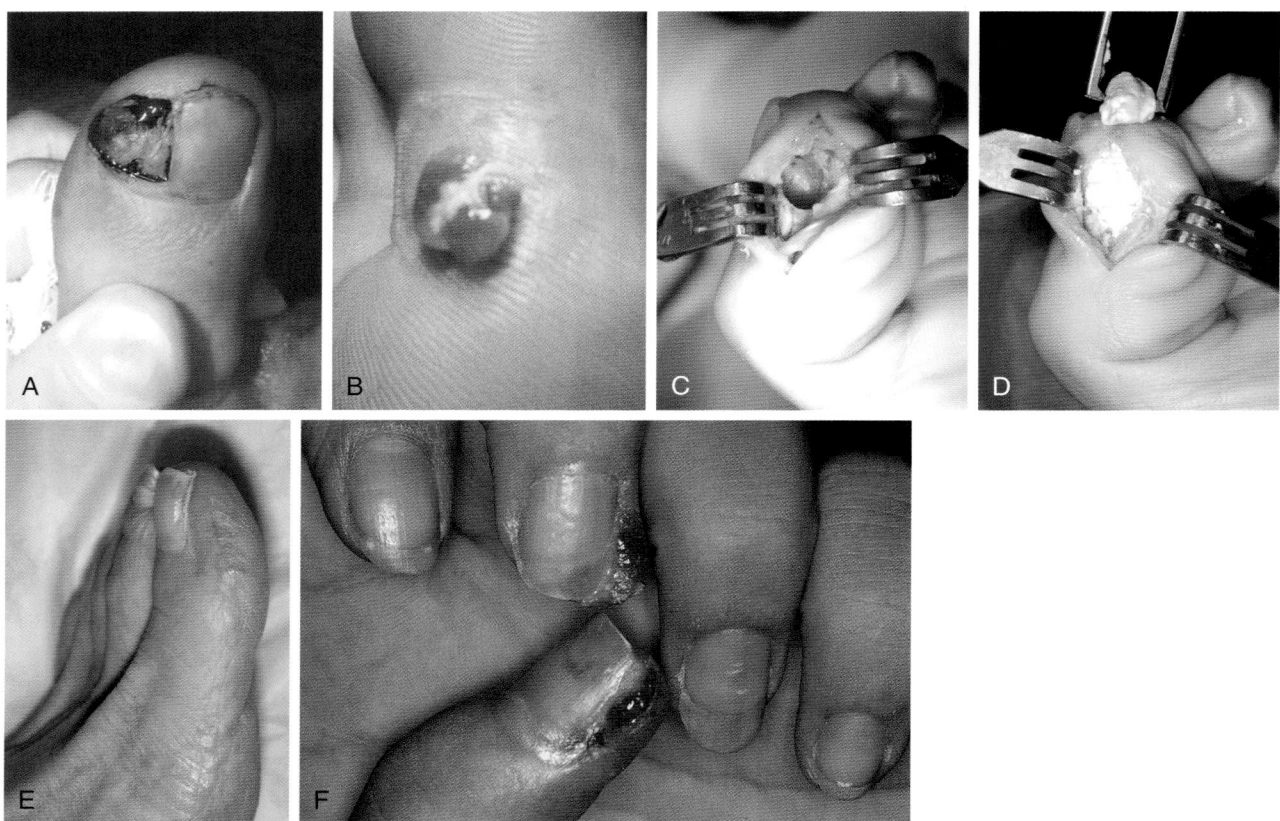

Figure 11-34 **A,** Pyogenic granuloma. A common location of this lesion is on the hallux toenail border. **B,** Pyogenic granuloma. This lesion is friable, bleeds easily, and can grow from a small stalk to a diameter of 1 cm or more. **C,** Paronychia has led to a painful burned-out cyst in the distal phalanx. **D,** Curettage of the lesion and insertion of antibiotic-impregnated calcium phosphate. **E,** Clinical result 9 months postoperatively. **F,** Multiple periungual pyogenic granulomas in a patient taking indinavir. (**A,** From Mann RA, Coughlin MJ: *The video textbook of foot and ankle surgery,* St Louis, 1990, Medical Video Productions.Used with permission. **B,** From Dockery GL: *Cutaneous disorders of the lower extremity,* Philadelphia, 1996, Elsevier. **F,** From Bolognia JL, Jorizzo JL, Rapini RP, editors: *Dermatology,* ed 2, Philadelphia, 2007, Elsevier.)

If the bone becomes infected, the lesion must be curetted and left to drain, or it can be filled with a bone graft substitute mixed with the appropriate antibiotic (Fig. 11-34C-F).

Herpetic Whitlow

Herpetic whitlow[110] is a primary infection with a herpesvirus. It often occurs symptomatically as a painful group of vesicles on one or more swollen toes (see Fig. 11-32C and D). The vesicles are often surrounded by an erythematous base. Regional lymphangitis may be associated with this condition, and the infection may be confused with bacterial infection or impetigo.

Herpetic whitlow should be distinguished from a bacterial infection, which can require systemic antibiotics and incision and drainage. A typical antibiotic regimen is not effective with a viral infection. Oral antiviral medication, such as acyclovir (Zovirax), may be successful in decreasing symptoms.

Periungual Verruca

A periungual wart is located on the margin of the nail plate and resembles warts found elsewhere on the foot (see Fig. 11-13). Of viral origin, verrucae require careful treatment to prevent trauma to the nail matrix, which can cause a permanent nail deformity. Treatment varies from chemical ablation of the wart to electrocautery or cryotherapy. Surgical excision may also be considered. If a lesion persists despite treatment, or if there is recurrence or atypia, a biopsy should be done to rule out verrucous carcinoma, the treatment of which is wide and deep surgical excision. Amputation is reserved for advanced lesions not amenable to excision.[209]

Nail Matrix Disorders

Disorders of the nail matrix can result in an abnormality of the nail plate. Ridging, atrophy, partial or complete anonychia, and pterygium formation can occur after trauma.

Anonychia

Anonychia, or the absence of toenails, may be an inherited condition,[214,231] or it can occur after surgical destruction of a germinal matrix (Fig. 11-35). It can also occur with systemic illnesses, vascular insufficiency, Raynaud disease, and frostbite. Often, the destruction of the nail matrix that leads to anonychia is surgically induced as a treatment of chronic nail conditions. No treatment is usually warranted for acquired or congenital anonychia.

Pterygium

With pterygium (see Fig. 11-3E), the cuticle grows forward on the nail plate and splits it into two or more portions. Zaias[228] noted that it occurs more often in the fourth and fifth digits. Pardo-Castello and Pardo[165] reported that it occurs more commonly in association with leprosy and peripheral neuritis. Other disease entities that can occur

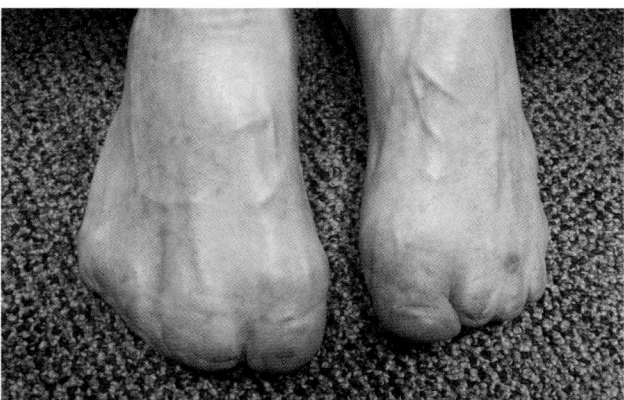

Figure 11-35 Anonychia. Anonychia may be an inherited condition or occur after trauma or surgery. In this case, a congenital absence of the digits was the cause of anonychia of all 10 toes.

with pterygium include vascular insufficiency, Raynaud disease, scleroderma, and lichen planus.

Atrophy and Hypertrophy

Hypertrophy of the nail matrix results in increased thickness of the nail plate (onychauxis) and nail bed. The nail plate can become grooved, abnormally raised, and elongated. With continued hypertrophy, onychogryphosis may develop.[231] At the other end of the spectrum, atrophy of the matrix can develop temporarily, with resultant transverse ridges or lines in the nail plate, which are called *Beau lines*. These occur when the growth of the nail matrix is suddenly arrested. As regrowth occurs, a normal nail plate develops and leaves a transverse line. This appears to be associated with increased fever, infection, and arthritis. Thinning of the nail plate can occur with anemia and lichen planus.

Pathologic Keratinization

The cells of the nail matrix can differentiate abnormally in association with a systemic disease, such as psoriasis, when keratin formation is increased in the nail bed. An abnormal rate of keratinization can occur with a fungal infection and may be associated with onychoschizia, koilonychia, and leukonychia.

Onychoschizia is a distal fissuring or splitting of the nail plate (Fig. 11-36A). Delamination can occur, with longitudinal separation of the layers of the nail plate. Hematologic disorders, trauma, infection, hypovitaminosis, and dermatologic disorders can lead to onychoschizia.

Koilonychia is a concavity of the nail plate or a spoon-shaped nail (Fig. 11-36B). Genetic factors, endocrine disorders, thyroid disease, infection, hematologic abnormalities, Raynaud disease, and nail bed tumors are all causes of koilonychia. The thickness of the nail plate varies, but it remains smooth and commonly opacifies.

Leukonychia is a whitish discoloration or spot on the nail plate (Fig. 11-36C). Several nails may be involved.

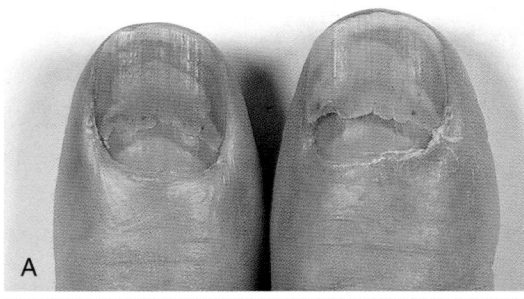

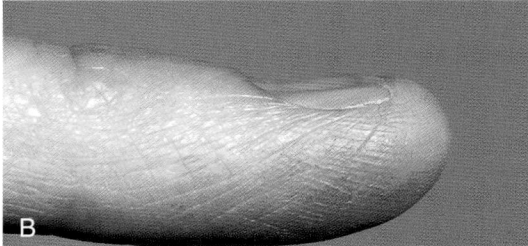

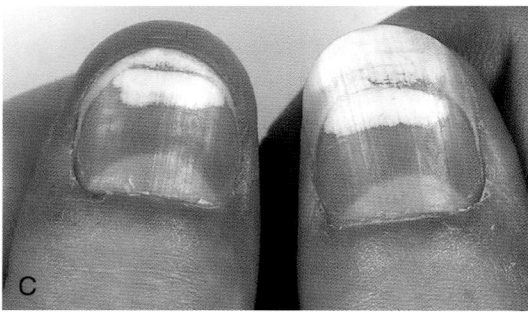

Figure 11-36 **A,** Onychoschizia. Shedding of the nails. This results from a severe illness when nail growth slows or ceases temporarily. **B,** Koilonychia. The nail is concave rather than convex and is thus spoon shaped. **C,** Leukonychia. White spots in the nails are common. Gross lesions can occur. The cause is unknown, but trauma may be relevant. (**A-C,** From du Vivier A: *Atlas of clinical dermatology*, ed 3, Philadelphia, 2002, Elsevier.)

Variations of leukonychia include punctate discoloration or transverse striations 1 to 2 mm in width that resemble Mees lines. Opacification may be partial (as in Hodgkin disease), complete (as in Hansen disease), or longitudinal (as in Darier disease). A hereditary form of leukonychia (porcelain nails or white nails) is reported to be caused by mutations in the *PLCD1* (phospholipase C delta 1) gene.[119]

Longitudinal erythronychia is a linear red band on the nail plate that originates at the proximal nail fold, traverses the lunula, and can extend to the free edge of the nail plate. Pain is the reason patients seek medical help. Longitudinal erythronychias can be clinical manifestations of underlying conditions, such as benign tumors (glomus, onychopapilloma, warty dyskeratoma), malignant conditions (malignant melanoma, squamous cell carcinoma), benign conditions (hemiplegia, postsurgical scar), genetic disorder (Darier disease), or idiopathic. Biopsy of the nail matrix and nail bed in a patient older

than 50 years should be considered to establish the diagnosis of the underlying condition (see Fig. 11-8E).[41]

Conservative and Surgical Treatment

Conservative treatment is often used with stage I (see staging under Onychocryptosis) infections of the toenail and with a prominent and painful toenail edge. Typical conservative treatment involves elevation of the lateral toenail plate from an inflamed or impinged nail fold. A wisp of cotton is carefully inserted beneath the edge of the nail plate (Fig. 11-25).[38,96,146] With elevation of the nail plate, care must be taken not to fracture the toenail when the cotton is inserted. A digital anesthetic block may be used to decrease pain when the nail plate is elevated. Collodion may be added to the cotton wisp for longevity.

The patient is encouraged to soak the toe twice daily in a tepid salt solution. The toenail region is then dried and the inflamed area coated with a desiccating solution, such as gentian violet or alcohol. Usually, the patient returns for a follow-up visit when the cotton wisp is to be removed. As the erythema diminishes, the patient is instructed to replace the cotton wisp. Desiccating agents are used until inflammation has subsided. The cotton packing must be replaced until the nail plate has grown beyond the distal extent of the nail fold. Usually, nail growth is approximately 2 mm/month, so the estimated duration of treatment can be calculated for the patient.

After the length of the nail plate is adequate, the patient is instructed in proper transverse trimming of the nail plate. Care is taken not to pick or tear the nail plate because this can cause recurrent infection.

Diagonal trimming of the nail can initially decrease the inflammation associated with acute infection, but it tends to postpone definitive treatment. Dixon[55] noted that "the nail fold tissue will quickly exploit the absence of the nail and can result in recurrence" (see Fig. 11-25D).

Treatment of ingrown toenails is individualized for each patient. Heifetz[96] observed that only during stage I can conservative methods be adequately used. When conservative care has been unsuccessful or when acute (stage II) or chronic (stage III) infection has occurred, aggressive nail care is necessary. Alternatives include partial nail plate avulsion, complete toenail avulsion, Syme toe amputation, and plastic surgery reduction of the lateral nail fold.[42,63,121] A plethora of ways exist to perform matrixectomy after partial or total nail plate avulsion, including carbon dioxide laser (83%-95% effective[69,158,222]), bipolar diathermy matrixectomy (90% effective in one study[70]), and 10% sodium hydroxide solution, which may be safer in individuals with difficult wound healing.[200] Yang[221] reported a lower recurrence rate in pediatric toenails treated with sodium hydroxide chemical matrixectomy compared with surgical matrixectomy. Some authors have reported highly successful results splinting the nail plate with various devices, including K-wires, needles, custom devices, and a hemicylindric

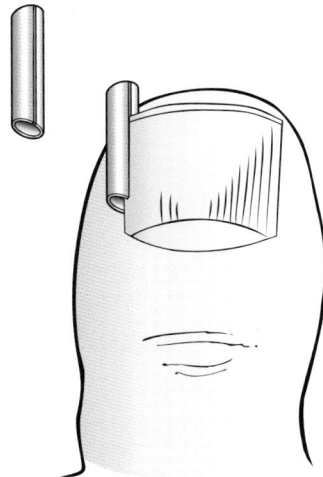

Figure 11-37 The sharp edge of the nail plate can be covered with a portion of an angiocath, split longitudinally, and placed over the border of the nail, protecting the inflamed tissue from the nail.

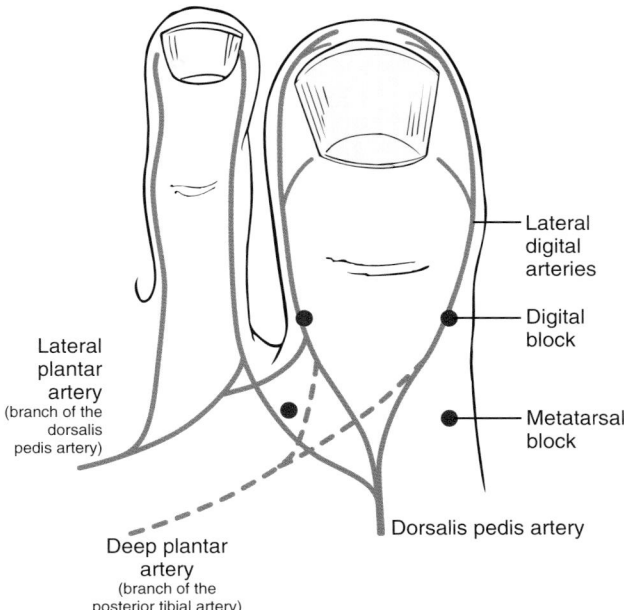

Figure 11-38 Metatarsal block. Technique of metatarsal anesthetic block with 1% lidocaine. A 25-gauge needle, 1% lidocaine anesthetic solution without epinephrine, and sodium bicarbonate (44 mEq/50 mL) are used in the digital block. A medial wheal is raised, and the needle is advanced in a dorsoplantar direction at the base of the digit, about 1 cm proximal to where a digital block is performed. The needle is then turned horizontally, and the dorsum of the toe is blocked. The needle is then inserted in a dorsoplantar direction on the lateral side of the toe to anesthetize the lateral nerve.

plastic tube cut from an angiocath (Fig. 11-37).* Often, the lateral nail fold granulation tissue is cauterized and the nail plate border exposed, followed by application of the splinting device.[65]

DIGITAL ANESTHETIC BLOCK
Technique (Video Clip 4)
A digital anesthetic block is usually sufficient anesthesia for any of the toenail procedures.[140] However, caution should be exercised to avoid ischemia. In some cases, a metatarsal block may be safer. With a metatarsal block, the risk of vascular injury is reduced by the arterial anastomotic network of the dorsalis pedis artery and posterior tibial artery (Fig. 11-38).[150]

A toe can be anesthetized within 10 minutes after injection of 1% lidocaine (4 mL in each side of the toe and 1 mL as a dorsal subcutaneous block, using a 1.5-inch 25-gauge needle and a 10-mL syringe).

Buffering 1% lidocaine with a small amount of sodium bicarbonate (in a 9 : 1 ratio with sodium bicarbonate, 44 mEq/50 mL) decreases the pain of the injection by increasing the pH of normally acidic anesthetic solutions.[20] It can also increase the effectiveness of the lidocaine and prolong its duration of action. Lidocaine (1% and 2%), 0.5% bupivacaine, and 0.5% ropivacaine have all been effective as local anesthetic agents. However, sodium bicarbonate precipitates in bupivacaine and ropivacaine, so it is best used with lidocaine. A metatarsal block can be performed in a similar manner just proximal to the metatarsophalangeal joint.

The technique involves using the anesthetic solution to raise a small skin wheal on the dorsomedial aspect of the hallux. The needle is directed in a dorsoplantar

direction to anesthetize the dorsal and plantar digital sensory nerves. After this is completed, the needle is turned horizontally and the dorsal aspect of the great toe infiltrated. The needle is then withdrawn and inserted at the lateral base of the great toe, and the dorsolateral and plantar lateral digital nerves are anesthetized (Fig. 11-39A-C, see Fig. 11-38).

A nail block can be used in some cases of onychocryptosis, onchomcosis, and paronychia. Using 0.5 mL of 2% lidocaine with or without epinephrine (1 : 100,000 concentration), inject at the midpoint of a line connecting the corner of the nail with the prominent base of the distal phalanx. Place the needle perpendicular to the skin and inject 0.25 mL under the dermis. The needle is advanced, infiltrating the solution into the deeper tissues. The contralateral side of the distal phalanx is injected in a similar fashion.[157]

PARTIAL NAIL PLATE AVULSION
After removal of the edge of the nail plate, acute or chronic infection usually subsides. Antibiotics may be used, depending on the severity of the infection.

Aftercare is important for a successful outcome after partial toenail avulsion. With distal growth of the nail

---

*References 1, 65, 66, 92, 117, 118, and 168.

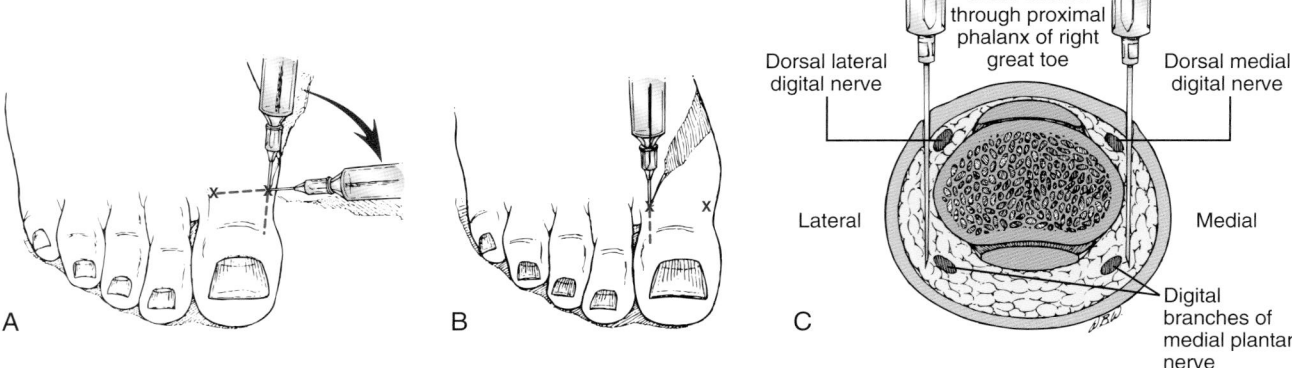

Figure 11-39 Technique of digital anesthetic block with 1% lidocaine. **A,** Initially, a medial wheal is raised, and the needle is advanced in a dorsoplantar direction. The needle is then turned horizontally, and the dorsum of the toe is blocked. **B,** A second injection is done to anesthetize the lateral aspect of the toe. **C,** A cross section shows the path of the needles.

plate, the advancing edge is at risk for recurrent infection. A cotton wisp is placed beneath the advancing edge to elevate the nail plate. A digital block may be necessary to replace subsequent packs. The patient is instructed in the technique of packing the toenail plate edge with a cotton wisp, and packing is continued until the nail edge has advanced past the distal extent of the nail groove.

Lloyd-Davies and Brill[137] reported a 47% recurrence rate of infection after partial nail plate avulsion. Another 33% of patients reported residual symptoms. Keyes[116] reported a 77% incidence of recurrence.

Surgical Technique
1. A digital anesthetic block is established, and the toe is cleansed in a routine manner.
2. A 0.25-inch Penrose drain or commercially available doughnut tubing is used as a tourniquet.
3. 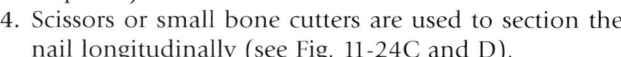 The outer edge of the toenail plate is elevated proximally to the cuticle (see Fig. 11-24A and B and Video Clip 126).
4. Scissors or small bone cutters are used to section the nail longitudinally (see Fig. 11-24C and D).
5. Care is taken to remove only as much nail as necessary. The nail is then grasped with a hemostat and avulsed (see Fig. 11-24E and F). The nail bed is examined to ensure that no spike of nail tissue remains.
6. A gauze compression dressing is applied and changed as needed until drainage subsides, usually within a few days (see Fig. 11-24G).

COMPLETE TOENAIL AVULSION
With a more extensive infection, complete toenail avulsion may be performed.

Antibiotics may be prescribed, depending on the severity of the infection. Intraoperative irrigation with 0.1% polihexanide may reduce the bacterial load and risk of recurrent infections.[24] Reepithelialization of the nail bed

occurs over 2 to 3 weeks. As the nail grows, the advancing edges should be elevated with a cotton wisp to prevent recurrence of a toenail infection.

Murray and Bedi[147] reviewed a series of 200 patients who underwent various toenail procedures. Of the 145 patients who underwent a simple toenail avulsion, 64% experienced recurrent symptoms after the initial procedure, 86% experienced recurrence after a second procedure, and 80% had recurrence after more than two avulsions.

Although toenail avulsion can give dramatic relief of not only infection but also symptoms, the rate of cure after toenail avulsion is quite low. Typically, a second procedure must be performed. Dixon[55] noted a much higher recurrence rate of infection when multiple avulsions of a single toenail were performed. Lloyd-Davies and Brill[137] reported that within 6 months, 31% of patients required further treatment after total nail plate avulsion. Palmer and Jones[163] reported a 70% recurrence of symptoms.

Surgical Technique
1. A digital anesthetic block is used and the toe cleansed as usual.
2. A 0.25-inch Penrose drain or a commercially available tubular tourniquet may be applied.
3. The nail plate is elevated from the nail bed and matrix (Fig. 11-40A and B).
4. The cuticle is incised and elevated from the nail plate.
5. The toenail is avulsed by grasping it with a hemostat (Fig. 11-40C and D). Usually, this is associated with immediate bleeding, and a compression dressing is applied. Hemostasis is usually prompt.
6. After 24 hours, daily soaking is begun in a tepid salt solution.
7. The bandage is replaced and changed daily until drainage has subsided.

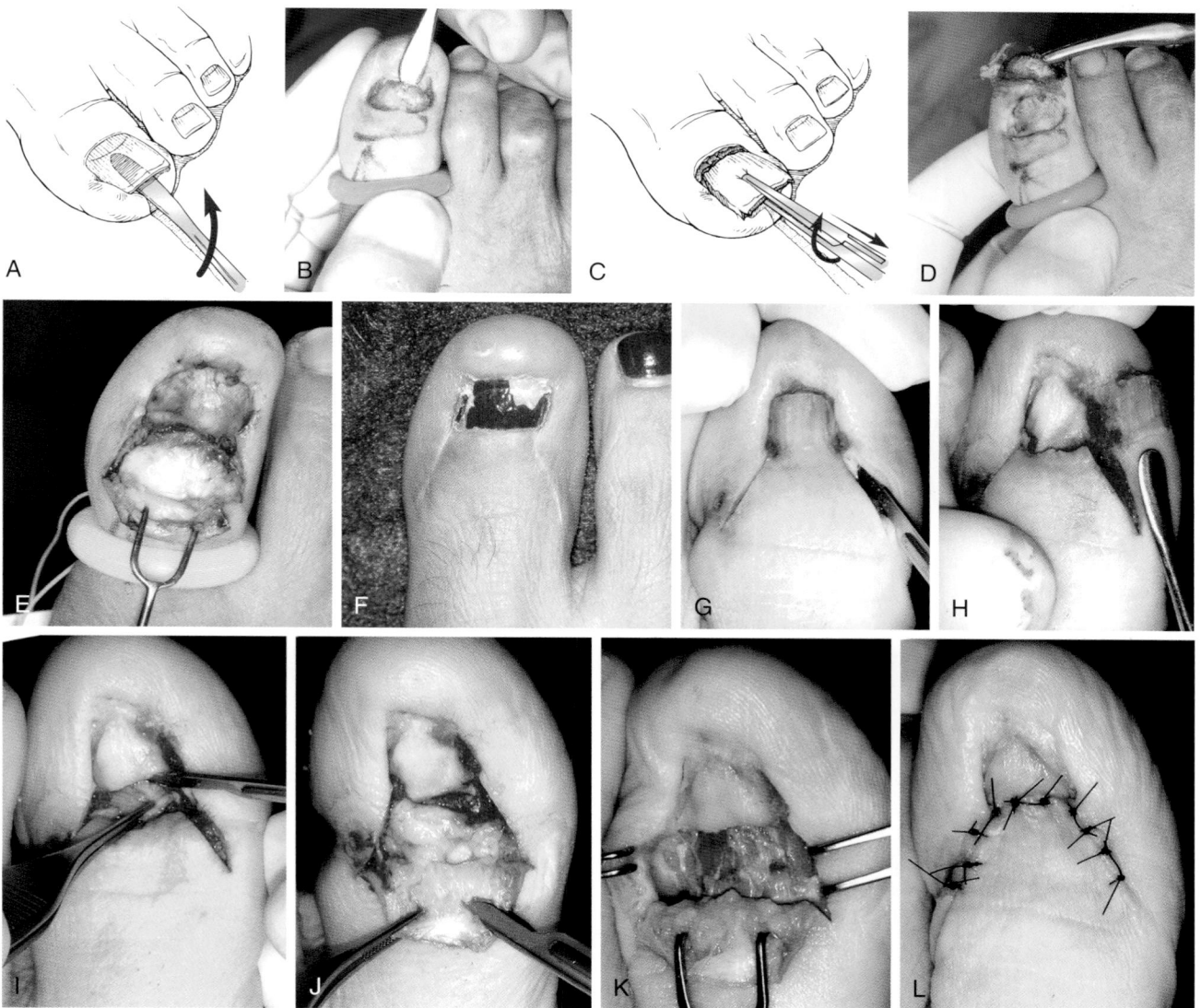

Figure 11-40 Technique of complete toenail avulsion with the Zadik procedure. **A** and **B,** Nail is freed from the nail bed. **C** and **D,** Nail is removed. **E,** Oblique cuts in soft tissue at the base of the nail allow the germinal matrix to be removed. Afterward, the proximal nail fold is repaired to the nail bed. Care is taken so that the extensor tendon is not excised from the distal phalanx. **F,** Clinical results 8 months later. **G,** Oblique cuts are made at the base of the nail plate. **H,** The nail plate is released with an elevator and removed. **I,** The germinal matrix is sharply excised from the nail bed and removed. **J,** The ventral nail fold is retracted. **K,** Complete removal of the germinal matrix. **L,** Closure of the ventral nail fold to the nail bed.

LATERAL FOLD REDUCTION

A plastic nail lip reduction may be used for a younger patient who has mild-to-moderate disease. With an acute infection, a partial toenail avulsion is performed initially. After the acute infection resolves, a plastic nail lip reduction is performed.

Surgical Technique

1. A digital anesthetic block is used, and the toe is cleansed in the usual manner.

2. A 0.25-inch Penrose drain or a commercially available tubular tourniquet is used for hemostasis.

3. A spindle-shaped section, approximately 3 mm × 1 cm and triangular in cross section, is excised from the site of the nail lip.

4. The incision extends from the distal portion of the toe to approximately 5 mm proximal to the nail fold and is located about 2 mm from the lateral nail groove (Fig. 11-41A and B).

5. Excess subdermal fat is excised.

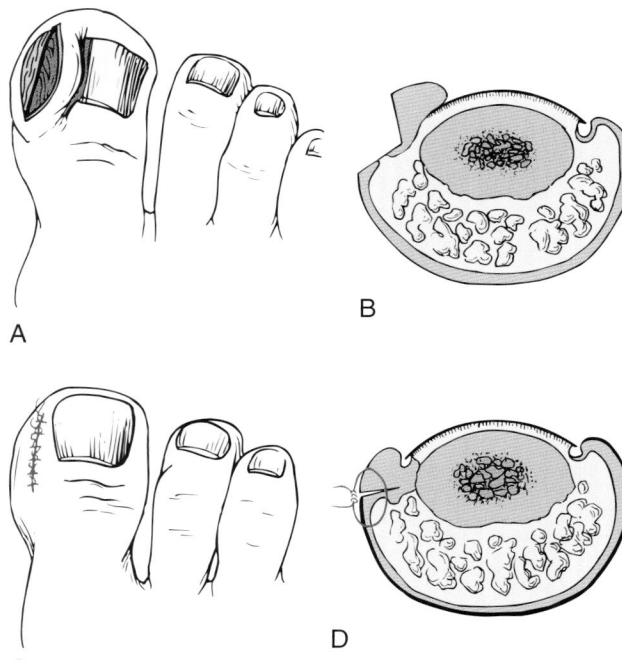

Figure 11-41 Soft tissue wedge resection for ingrown toenail. **A,** A triangular section is removed from the lateral aspect of the nail groove. **B,** Cross section after excision. **C,** The nail lip and groove are pulled down after the nail margins are sutured. **D,** Cross section after suturing.

6. The skin margins are coapted with interrupted 3-0 nylon sutures. The closure draws the nail groove laterally and downward (Fig. 11-41C and D).
7. A sterile dressing is applied and changed as needed until drainage has subsided.
8. Sutures are removed 3 weeks after the procedure.

LATERAL FOLD ADVANCEMENT FLAP

This is a similar concept to the lateral fold reduction; however, this technique allows the surgeon to excise the scarred granulation tissue. Less recurrence and better cosmesis is possibly obtained by mobilizing healthy tissue up to the nail plate.[42] El-Shaer[63] has described success with a similar laterally based V-shaped rotational flap. For the treatment of pincer nail, Kosaka[121] describes a distally based zigzag nail bed flap.

Surgical Technique

1. A digital anesthetic block is used, and the toe is cleansed as usual.
2. A 0.25-inch Penrose drain or a commercially available tubular tourniquet is used for hemostasis.
3. Granulation tissue of the lateral fold is excised down to a subperiosteal level and germinal matrixectomy is performed.
4. Two skin incisions from dorsal to plantar are made to delineate the flap. One incision is made proximally

near the eponychium, and one incision is made distally near the hyponychium. The width of the flap should equal the length of the nail fold and is usually 5 to 7 mm.
5. The flap is elevated from the periosteum and a triangular skin excision is done on each lateral side of the flap to allow mobilization of the flap dorsally.
6. The flap is advanced dorsally and sutured in position (Fig. 11-42).

Results and Complications

Cologlu[42] reported in a comparitive study on 38 cases treated with a lateral fold advancement flap. They reported no recurrences and 5.2% spicule formation rate. The reoperation rate in the lateral fold advancement group was less than in the simple wedge matrixectomy group, and they reported a higher satisfaction rate in the flap group.

PARTIAL ONYCHECTOMY (WINOGRAD OR HEIFETZ PROCEDURE)

Partial onychectomy is performed only after an acute infection has resolved, usually after a partial nail plate avulsion.[96,97,217,218] Cadaveric studies have shown that a straight needle passed proximally along the floor of the lateral nail groove defines the lateral extent of the nail matrix.[11] This helps the operator identify the lateral extent of the germinal matrix.

Surgical Technique

1. A digital anesthetic block is used, and the toe is cleansed as usual.
2. A 0.25-inch Penrose drain or a commercially available tubular tourniquet is used for hemostasis.
3. The border of the nail is freed up from surrounding tissue, as previously described, and the border of the nail is cut using heavy, strong scissors or wire cutters. The nail is then removed (see Fig. 11-11A-G).
4. With the Heifetz procedure (Video Clip 128), the resection is carried just distal to the terminal extent of the lunula (Fig. 11-43A). With the Winograd procedure (Video Clip 127), not only is the nail matrix excised, but the nail bed is resected as well (Fig. 11-43B).
5. An oblique incision is made at the apex of the nail bed (see Fig. 11-11H). The proximal nail matrix and edge of the cuticle are excised. Care is taken to avoid injury to the extensor tendon insertion and to avoid penetration of the interphalangeal joint.
6. The germinal matrix has a pearly white color and a leathery texture. It extends into the nail fold laterally, and for the Winograd procedure, it must be completely excised along with the nail bed (see Fig. 11-11I-K). Applying methylene blue to stain the nail matrix can help the surgeon identify the lateral extent of the germinal matrix.
7. In the Winograd procedure, the remaining nail bed and matrix are curetted from the cortex of the distal phalanx (see Fig. 11-11L).

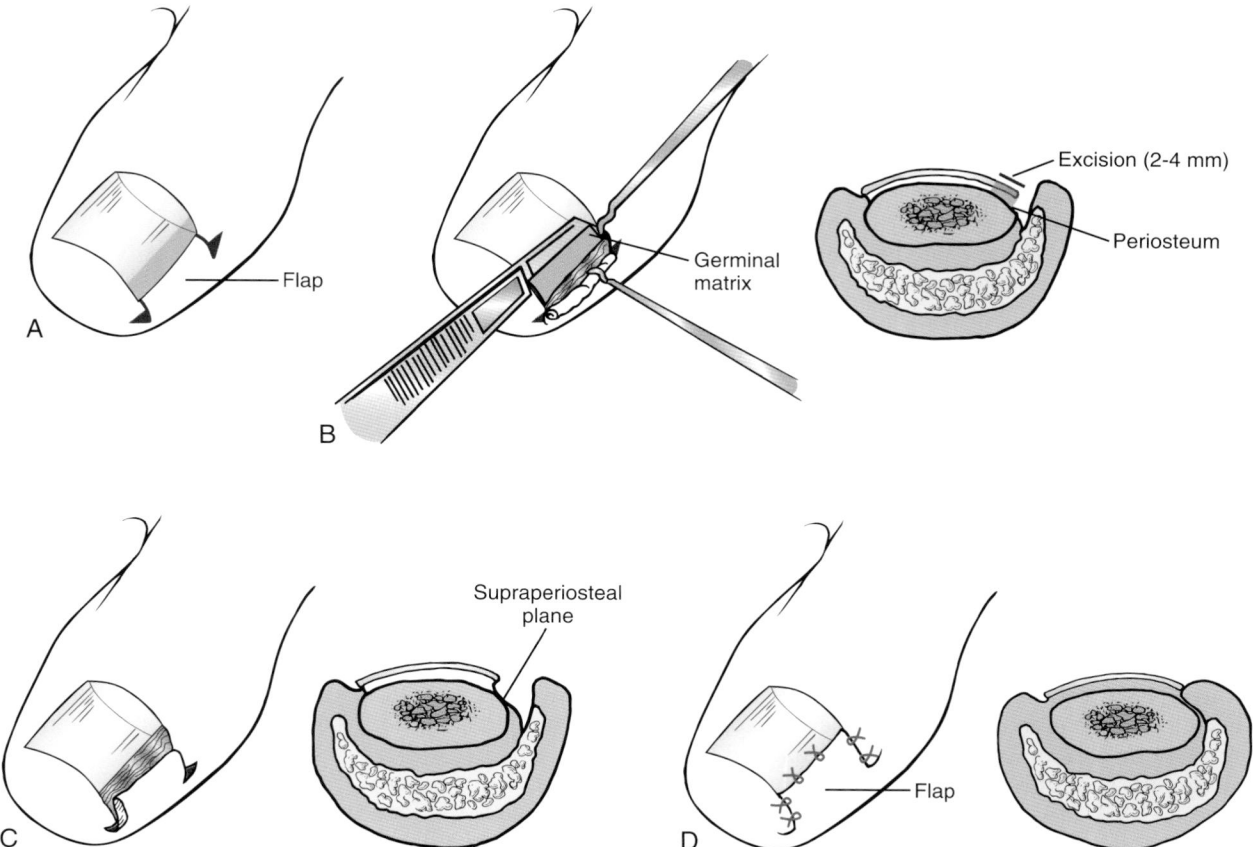

Figure 11-42 Plastic nail edge advancement. **A,** The nail edge incisions are marked. **B,** The edge of the nail plate is excised as is the germinal matrix. The skin flap is turned dorsally **(C)** and sewn in place **(D).**

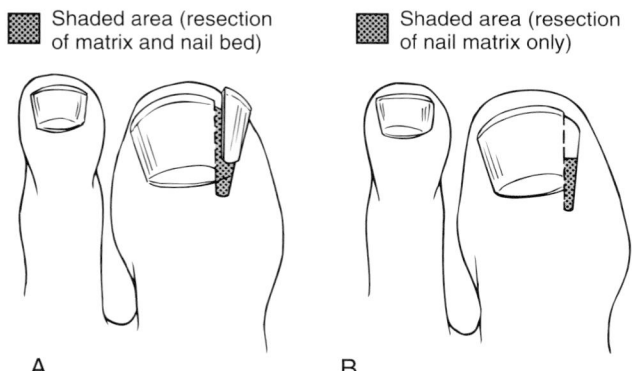

Figure 11-43 Proposed soft tissue excision for partial onychectomy (*shaded area* is excised). **A,** Winograd procedure. **B,** Heifetz procedure. (From Mann RA, Coughlin MJ: *The video textbook of foot and ankle surgery,* St Louis, 1990, Medical Video Productions.)

8. The wound is thoroughly irrigated, and the skin edges are coapted with interrupted nylon suture (see Fig. 11-11M and N).
9. A compression dressing is applied and changed at 24 hours (see Fig. 11-24G). Subsequent dressings are changed weekly until drainage resolves. Prophylactic antibiotics may be prescribed, depending on the surgeon's preference or the patient's risk of infection. Sutures are removed 2 weeks postoperatively.

Results and Complications

Murray and Bedi,[147] in a review of 200 patients, reported a 27% recurrence rate after a Winograd procedure and a 50% recurrence rate after a double Winograd procedure. Clarke and Dillinger[40] reported their experience with the Winograd procedure. Of 29 procedures evaluated, one third had unsatisfactory results, including nine recurrences and two patients who reported continued discomfort at follow-up (range, 8 to 18 months). Palmer and Jones[163] reported a 29% recurrence rate after a Winograd resection. In a series of 528 patients who had an ablation of the lateral matrix, Gabriel et al[80] reported a 1.7% recurrence rate and a 79% satisfaction rate. Winograd[218] reported a 15% recurrence rate among 20 patients. Pettine et al[167] reported that with the Heifetz procedure, the satisfaction rate was 90% and the recurrence rate was 6%. Keyes[116] reported a 12% recurrence rate with the Heifetz procedure.

Wadhams et al[211] reported the development of 10 epidermal inclusion cysts after 147 partial matrixectomies

(6.8%), typically a Winograd procedure. The average time from treatment to development of the inclusion cyst was 5.5 months. Excision of the inclusion cyst was recommended. A well-encapsulated, white, glistening mass was noted at surgery.

Alternative Procedure

Electrocautery ablation has been recommended as yet another procedure. A single-sided Teflon-coated spatula (to protect the dorsal tissues) is used to perform a lateral matrixectomy after lateral nail plate removal.[233]

COMPLETE ONYCHECTOMY (ZADIK PROCEDURE)

On occasion, a patient requires complete and permanent removal of the toenail.[224] This procedure is not performed in the presence of acute infection but usually after an initial toenail avulsion. Surgery should be delayed until infection and inflammation have subsided.

Surgical Technique

1. A digital anesthetic block is performed, and the toe is cleansed in the usual manner.
2. A 0.25-inch Penrose drain is used for hemostasis. Alternatively, commercial tourniquets are easy to use; exsanguination is accomplished as they are applied.
3. An oblique incision is made at the medial and lateral apex of the nail folds. The toenail, if present, is avulsed (Fig. 11-40E,G,H,I and Video Clip 129). Alternatively, the proximal portion of the nail is removed to explore the nail matrix.
4. The cuticle, eponychium, and proximal nail bed are completely excised.
5. The matrix is excised proximally to the cuticle, laterally into the nail folds, and distally as far as the distal extent of the lunula (see Fig. 11-40G). To assist the surgeon in identifying the lateral extent of the nail matrix, the nail matrix may be stained with methylene blue and dried.[17]
6. The nail matrix is curetted and the remaining tissue excised. Care must be taken to avoid the extensor tendon (see Fig. 11-40). In the fingers, the distance between the nail matrix and the extensor tendon averages 1.2 mm (range, 0.9-1.8 mm).[191]
7. The skin edges are approximated with interrupted 3-0 nylon sutures (see Fig. 11-40L). Excess tension should be avoided along the suture line because it can lead to sloughing of the skin.
8. A compression dressing is applied and changed 24 hours postoperatively. Further dressing changes are performed as needed, depending on the amount of drainage.

Postoperative Care

Sutures are removed 2 to 3 weeks postoperatively. The patient should be informed about possible partial regrowth of the toenail. Cosmetic results are usually better than with a Syme amputation, and the remaining nail bed accepts nail polish (see Fig. 11-40F).

Results and Complications

Murray and Bedi[147] reported a 16% recurrence rate with the Zadik procedure. Palmer and Jones[163] reported a 28% failure rate, and Townsend and Scott[204] a 50% failure rate with complete onychectomy. Eighty-nine percent of patients reported acceptable results despite the small regrowth, typically in the central region.

Alternative Procedure

The use of a carbon dioxide laser for matrixectomy has had variable success. Apfelberg et al[7] reported a 22% recurrence rate. Wright[220] reported a recurrence rate of 50% after laser toenail ablation and recommended that it not be used for either partial or complete toenail ablation.

TERMINAL SYME AMPUTATION (THOMPSON-TERWILLIGER PROCEDURE)

For symptomatic regrowth of toenail tissue or when a patient requires a more reliable excision, a terminal Syme amputation of the distal phalanx may be considered (Figs. 11-44A-C and 11-45A-D, Video Clip 130, see Fig. 11-26).[203] Nonetheless, a proximal matrixectomy is almost always preferable cosmetically to the bulbous amputation stump that is left with a Syme amputation.

Surgical Technique

1. A digital anesthetic block is used and the toe cleansed in the usual manner.
2. A 0.25-inch Penrose drain or a commercially available tubular tourniquet is used.

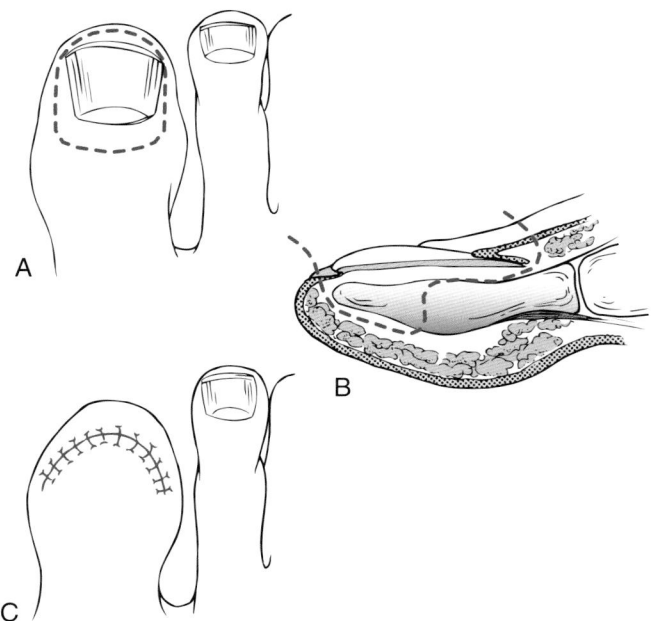

Figure 11-44 Terminal Syme amputation. **A,** An elliptic incision is used to excise all adjacent soft tissue as well as the toenail bed and matrix. **B,** Distal phalanx is excised. **C,** Excess skin is excised, and the skin edges are approximated.

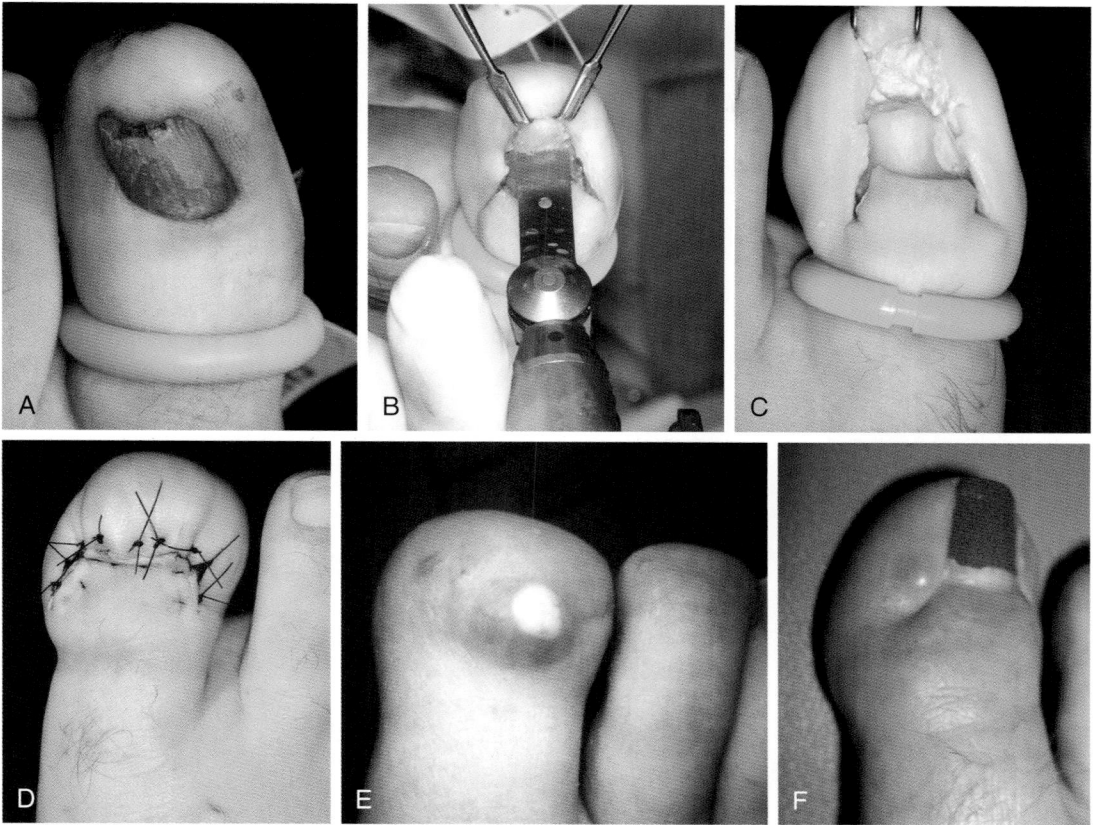

Figure 11-45 Terminal Syme amputation. **A,** Chronic onychomycosis is present with surrounding soft tissue hypertrophy that is painful. **B,** The entire nail complex has been removed. A saw is used to remove enough of the distal phalanx to close the wound without tension. **C,** A rasp has been used to round off the distal phalanx. There is ample tissue for closure of the hyponychium to the proximal nail fold. **D,** Wound closure. **E** and **F,** Regrowth of the nail after incomplete removal of the germinal matrix can produce a cyst. (**E,** From Mann RA, Coughlin MJ: *The video textbook of foot and ankle surgery,* St Louis, 1990, Medical Video Productions.)

3. An elliptic incision is used to resect the nail bed, matrix, and proximal and lateral nail folds. The cuticle and proximal border of skin are excised as well.
4. Any remaining toenail matrix and toenail bed are curetted from the dorsal surface of the distal phalanx.
5. Approximately half the distal phalanx is removed, and the remaining edges of bone are beveled with a rongeur (Fig. 11-45B and C).
6. Excess skin is removed, and the skin edges are approximated with nylon suture (Fig. 11-45).
7. A compression dressing is applied and changed 24 hours postoperatively.

Postoperative Care
Dressing changes are performed as needed until drainage has subsided. Prophylactic antibiotics may be used, depending on the surgeon's preference. Sutures are removed 3 weeks postoperatively.

Results and Complications
Murray and Bedi[147] concluded that the terminal Syme amputation is the definitive technique for recurrent nail plate growth after repeated ablation procedures. Thompson and Terwilliger,[203] in a series of 70 terminal Syme amputations, reported excellent results, with a 4% recurrence rate (Fig. 11-45E). Pettine et al[167] reported a 12% recurrence rate.

Because the cosmetic result is unsightly, some authors suggest that this procedure is appropriate only for malignant tumors invading the distal portion of the terminal phalanx.[17] Otherwise, a proximal matrixectomy (Zadik procedure) may be performed.

PHENOL-AND-ALCOHOL MATRIXECTOMY
A phenol-and-alcohol matrixectomy may be done instead of a surgical resection (Fig. 11-46A-C). Burzotta et al[35] advised that this procedure could be performed in the presence of concurrent infection. Various techniques for application of phenol, with various success rates, have been reported.

Surgical Technique
1. A digital anesthetic block is used and the toe cleansed as usual.

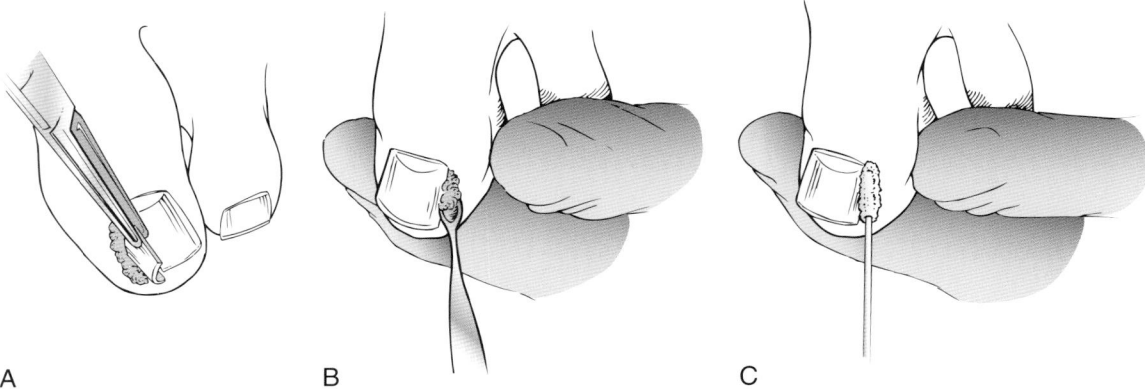

Figure 11-46 Phenol matrixectomy. **A,** The edge of the nail plate is cut with scissors and then avulsed. **B,** The lateral toenail groove and matrix are curetted. **C,** Phenol is applied to cauterize the nail matrix.

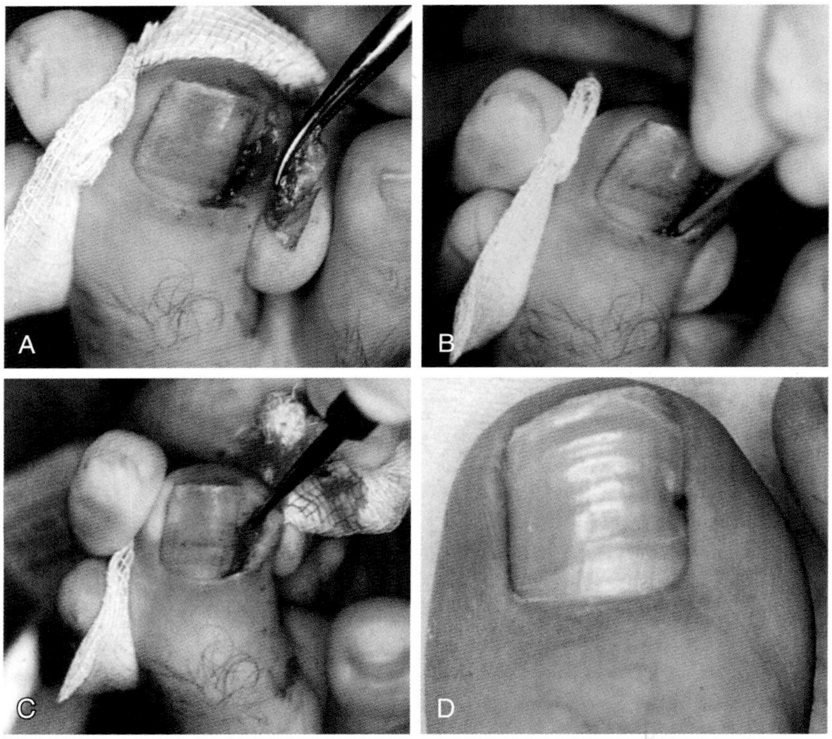

Figure 11-47 Phenol matrixectomy. **A,** The lateral edge of the nail has been removed. **B,** A sterile applicator with the cotton partially removed is used to place 88% carbolic acid on top of the germinal matrix and nail bed. **C,** The granulation tissue may be curetted. **D,** Results 6 months later. (From Salasche SJ. In Sher RK, Daniel CR 3rd, editors: *Nails: therapy, diagnosis, surgery*, ed 2, Philadelphia, 1997, WB Saunders, p 346.)

2. A 0.25-inch Penrose drain or a commercial tourniquet is applied for hemostasis.

3. The nail plate edge is avulsed (Fig. 11-47A) as previously described (see Fig. 11-24A-G).

4. The skin around the matrixectomy site may be coated with petroleum jelly to prevent injury.

5. A cotton-tipped applicator from which most of the cotton has been removed is used to apply the phenol solution. Fresh 88% carbolic acid (phenol) is used.

6. After the cotton-tipped applicator is moistened with phenol, the excess phenol is blotted on a gauze pad.

The applicator is inserted into the nail groove and matrix area for 30 seconds to 1 minute (Fig. 11-47B).[4,36,45,175,219] Bostanci et al[30] recommend rubbing the phenol into the tissue for 3 minutes.

7. After the applicator is removed, the area is flushed with alcohol to dilute the phenol and clear it from the wound. The alcohol probably acts less as a neutralizer and more as a diluter, but because the phenol is more soluble in the alcohol, its use is appropriate.

8. Two subsequent 1-minute phenol applications are performed. A tourniquet must be used to keep the

wound free of blood because blood dilutes the phenol and reduces its effectiveness.

9. After each phenol application, alcohol is used to flush the nail groove and matrix region.

10. The granulation tissue may be curetted (Fig. 11-47C).

Postoperative Care

A sterile dressing is applied and changed daily until drainage has subsided. The patient is allowed to soak the foot in a tepid salt solution. Although moderate inflammation can occur initially, good results are usually achieved (Fig. 11-47D).

Results and Complications

Regrowth of part or all of the nail plate is the most frequent complication after phenol ablation of the toenail. Chemical matrixectomies have an 80% to 95% satisfaction rate, with recurrence rates of less than 1% to 40%.[189,208]

In his long-term analysis of 733 cases, Kuwada[124] reported a recurrence rate of 4.3% after partial matrixectomy and 4.7% after complete matrixectomy. The overall reported complication rate with partial phenol matrixectomies was 9.6% and with total matrixectomies 10.9%. Mori et al,[144] in a review of 75 patients, reported a recurrence rate of 3.9% for the matrix phenolization method and 4.1% for the nail bed periosteal flap procedures. Postoperative pain was less in the matrix phenolization group, but that group had a longer duration of healing than the periosteal flap group.

However, Bostanci et al[30] concluded that phenolization was the treatment of choice for 172 patients who had 350 phenol ablations, with a recurrence rate of 0.57% (nail spikes). Bos[29] also reported a clinical trial in which he found a significantly lower recurrence rate with phenolization compared with matrix excision. This procedure has been reported to be as effective in diabetic patients as in nondiabetic patients.[72,82] Complications can occur from its use, however, including inflammation or extensive burns resulting in distal toe amputation.[179,197] Altman et al[4] found a decreased incidence of inflammation after using silver sulfadiazine and 1% hydrocortisone cream postoperatively. Although minimal postoperative pain is associated with phenol matrixectomies, prolonged healing is common because of the chemical burn induced. Duration of application of phenol is debatable, but it appears that 1 minute may be effective, and slower healing times should be expected if phenol is left in place up to 3 minutes.[201] The placement of the phenol is probably more important than the duration of contact between the phenol and tissues.

In their evaluation of phenol matrixectomies, Gilles et al[84] noted that periostitis and mixed bacterial infections developed postoperatively. Rinaldi et al[175] reported a high rate of wound cultures positive for bacteria (87.5%). However, Bos[29] was unable to detect a reduction in infection or recurrence when using local gentamycin at the surgical site. Finally, Rounding and Bloomfield[178] reported,

in a meta-analysis of nine studies, phenolization decreased the rate of recurrence of deformity but at the cost of an increased infection rate.

Alternative Procedure

Sodium hydroxide (10% solution) has been used in a manner similar to phenol. In those cases, however, neutralization of the strong base with 5% acetic acid is important.[205]

REFERENCES

1. Abby NS, Roni P, Amnon B, et al: Modified sleeve method treatment of ingrown toenail. *Dermatol Surg* 28:852–855, 2002.
2. Abramson C, Wilton J: Inhalation of nail dust from onychomycotic toenails: part I, characterization of particles. *J Am Podiatr Med Assoc* 75:563–567, 1985.
3. Abramson C, Wilton J: Nail dust aerosols from onychomycotic toenails: part II, clinical and serologic aspects. *J Am Podiatr Med Assoc* 75:631–638, 1985.
4. Altman MI, Suleskey C, Delisle R, et al: Silver sulfadiazine and hydrocortisone cream 1% in the management of phenol matricectomy. *J Am Podiatr Med Assoc* 80:545–547, 1990.
5. Amonette RA, Rosenberg EW: Infection of toe webs by gram-negative bacteria. *Arch Dermatol* 107:71–73, 1973.
6. Antony AK, Anagnos DP: Matrix-periosteal flaps for reconstruction of nail deformity. *Plast Reconstr Surg* 109:1663–1666, 2002.
7. Apfelberg DB, Rothermel E, Widtfeldt A, et al: Progress report on use of carbon dioxide laser for nail disorders. *Curr Podiatr* 32:29–31, 1983.
8. Ashby BS: Primary carcinoma of the nail-bed. *Br J Surg* 44:216–217, 1956.
9. Attiyeh FF, Shah J, Booher RJ, et al: Subungual squamous cell carcinoma. *JAMA* 241:262–263, 1979.
10. Aulicino PL, Hunter JM: Subungual melanoma: case report and literature review. *J Hand Surg Am* 7:167–169, 1982.
11. Austin RT: A method of excision of the germinal matrix. *Proc R Soc Med* 63:757–758, 1970.
12. Baden HP: The physical properties of nail. *J Invest Dermatol* 55:115–122, 1970.
13. Banfield CC, Dawber RP: Nail melanoma: a review of the literature with recommendations to improve patient management. *Br J Dermatol* 141:628–632, 1999.
14. Banfield CC, Redburn JC, Dawber RP: The incidence and prognosis of nail apparatus melanoma: a retrospective study of 105 patients in four English regions. *Br J Dermatol* 139:276–279, 1998.
15. Baran R: Significance and management of congenital malalignment of the big toenail. *Cutis* 58:181–184, 1996.
16. Baran R, Feuilhade M, Combernale P, et al: A randomized trial of amorolfine 5% solution nail lacquer combined with oral terbinafine compared with terbinafine alone in the treatment of dermatophytic toenail onychomycoses affecting the matrix region. *Br J Dermatol* 142:1177–1183, 2000. Erratum in *Br J Dermatol* 144:448, 2001.
17. Baran R, Haneke E: Matricectomy and nail ablation. *Hand Clin* 18:693–696, 2002.
18. Baran R, Haneke E, Richert B: Pincer nails: definition and surgical treatment. *Dermatol Surg* 27:261–266, 2001.
19. Baran R, Hay RJ, Tosti A, et al: A new classification of onychomycosis. *Br J Dermatol* 139:567–571, 1998.
20. Bartfield JM, Ford DT, Homer PJ: Buffered versus plain lidocaine for digital nerve blocks. *Ann Emerg Med* 22:216–219, 1993.

613

21. Bartolomei FJ, Brandwene SM, McCarthy DJ: Bowen's disease. *J Am Podiatr Med Assoc* 76:153–156, 1986.

22. Bean WB: Nail growth: a twenty-year study. *Arch Intern Med* 111:476–482, 1963.

23. Bean WB: Nail growth: 30 years of observation. *Arch Intern Med* 134:497–502, 1974.

24. Becerro de Bengoa Vallejo R, Losa Iglesias ME, Cervera LA, et al: Efficacy of intraoperative surgical irrigation with polihexanide and nitrofurazone in reducing bacterial load after nail removal surgery. *J Am Acad Dermatol* 64:328–335, 2011.

25. Bedi TR: Intradermal triamcinolone treatment of psoriatic onychodystrophy. *Dermatologica* 155:24–27, 1977.

26. Berlin SJ, Block LD, Donick II: Pyogenic granuloma of the foot: a review of the English literature and report of four cases. *J Am Podiatry Assoc* 62:94–99, 1972.

27. Berlin SJ, Stewart RC, Margolies MC, et al: Squamous cell carcinoma of the foot with particular reference to nail bed involvement: a report of three cases. *J Am Podiatry Assoc* 65:134–141, 1975.

28. Bodman MA, Brlan MR: Superficial white onychomycosis. *J Am Podiatr Med Assoc* 85:205–208, 1995.

29. Bos AM, van Tilburg MW, van Sorge AA, Klinkenbijl JH: Randomized clinical trial of surgical technique and local antibiotics for ingrowing toenail. *Br J Surg* 94:292–296, 2007.

30. Bostanci S, Ekmekci P, Gurgey E: Chemical matrixectomy with phenol for the treatment of ingrowing toenail: a review of the literature and follow-up of 172 treated patients. *Acta Derm Venereol* 81:181–183, 2001.

31. Bouche RT: Distal skin plasty of the hallux for clubbing deformity after total nail loss. *J Am Podiatr Med Assoc* 85:11–14, 1995. Erratum in *J Am Podiatr Med Assoc* 85:176, 1995.

32. Bristol SG, Verchere CG: The transverse figure-of-eight suture for securing the nail. *J Hand Surg Am* 32:124–125, 2007.

33. Bristow IR, Baran R: Topical and oral combination therapy for toenail onychomycosis: an updated review. *J Am Podiatr Med Assoc* 96:116–119, 2006.

34. Brown RE: Acute nail bed injuries. *Hand Clin* 18:561–575, 2002.

35. Burzotta JL, Turri RM, Tsouris J: Phenol and alcohol chemical matrixectomy. *Clin Podiatr Med Surg* 6:453–467, 1989.

36. Cangialosi CP, Schnall SJ: A comparison of the phenol-alcohol and Suppan nail techniques (onychectomy/matrixectomy). *Curr Podiatr* 30:25–26, 1981.

37. Cavolo DJ, D'Amelio JP, Hirsch AL, et al: Juvenile subungual osteochondroma: case presentation. *J Am Podiatry Assoc* 71:81–83, 1981.

38. Ceh SE, Pettine KA: Treatment of ingrown toenail. *J Musculoskel Med* 7:62–82, 1990.

39. Chinn S, Jenkin W: Proximal nail groove pain associated with an exostosis. *J Am Podiatr Med Assoc* 76:506–508, 1986.

40. Clarke BG, Dillinger KA: Surgical treatment of ingrown toenail. *Surgery* 21:919–924, 1946.

41. Cohen PR: Longitudinal erythronychia: individual or multiple linear red bands of the nail plate: a review of clinical features and associated conditions. *Am J Clin Dermatol* 12:217–231, 2001.

42. Cöloğlu H, Koçer U, Sungur N, et al: A new anatomical repair method for the treatment of ingrown nail: prospective comparison of wedge resection of the matrix and partial matricectomy followed by lateral fold advancement flap. *Ann Plast Surg* 54:306–311, discussion 312, 2005.

43. Conant MA, Wiesenfeld SL: Multiple glomus tumors of the skin. *Arch Dermatol* 103:481–485, 1971.

44. Vicks VapoRub might help fight toenail fungus. *Consum Rep* 71:49, 2006.

45. Coughlin M: Ingrown toenails: procedures to relieve pain and forestall recurrence. *Consultant* 35:965–975, 1995.

46. Cribier BJ, Bakshi R: Terbinafine in the treatment of onychomycosis: a review of its efficacy in high-risk populations and in patients with nondermatophyte infections. *Br J Dermatol* 150:414–420, 2004.

47. Dale SJ, Simons J: Subungual squamous cell carcinoma. *J Am Podiatry Assoc* 70:421–425, 1980.

48. Daniel CR: Longitudinal melanonychia and melanoma: an unusual case presentation. *Dermatol Surg* 27:294–295, 2001.

49. Daniel CR 3rd, Elewski BE: The diagnosis of nail fungus infection revisited. *Arch Dermatol* 136:1162–1164, 2000.

50. Das SK: Nail unit matrix transplantation: a plastic surgeon's approach. *Dermatol Surg* 27:242–245, 2001.

51. DeBenedette V: The safe and effective uses of four oral antifungal agents. *Cosm Dermatol* 7:44–46, 1994.

52. de Palma L, Gigante A, Specchia N: Subungual exostosis of the foot. *Cosm Dermatol* 17:758–763, 1996.

53. Derby R, Rohal P, Jackson C, et al: Novel treatment of onychomycosis using over-the-counter mentholated ointment: a clinical case series. *J Am Board Fam Med* 24:69–74, 2011.

54. Desai T, Magdum A, Patel T, Loghdey S: Parrot-beak nails. *Clin Exp Dermatol* 36:208–209, 2011. doi:10.1111/j.1365-2230.2010.03899.x.

55. Dixon GL Jr: Treatment of ingrown toenail. *Foot Ankle* 3:254–260, 1983.

56. Dockery GL: Nails: fundamental conditions and procedures. In McGlamry ED, editor: *Comprehensive textbook of foot surgery*, Baltimore, 1987, Williams & Wilkins, pp 3–37.

57. Dompmartin D, Dompmartin A, Deluol AM, et al: Onychomycosis and AIDS: clinical and laboratory findings in 62 patients. *Int J Dermatol* 29:337–339, 1990.

58. Drake LA, Scher RK, Smith EB, et al: Effect of onychomycosis on quality of life. *J Am Acad Dermatol* 38:702–704, 1998.

59. DuVries HL: Hypertrophy of ungual labia. *Chirop Rec* 16:11, 1933.

60. DuVries HL: Ingrown toenail. *Chirop Rec* 27:155–164, 1944.

61. Dykyj D: Anatomy of the nail. *Clin Podiatr Med Surg* 6:215–228, 1989.

62. Elewski B, Pollak R, Ashton S, et al: A randomized, placebo- and active-controlled, parallel-group, multicentre, investigator-blinded study of four treatment regimens of posaconazole in adults with toenail onychomycosis. *Br J Dermatol* 166:389–398, 2012. doi:10.1111/j.1365-2133.2011.10660.x.

63. El-Shaer WM: Lateral fold rotational flap technique for treatment of ingrown nail. *Plast Reconstr Surg* 120:2131–2133, 2007.

64. Ellis DH: Diagnosis of onychomycosis made simple. *J Am Acad Dermatol* 40:S3–S8, 1999.

65. Erdogan FG: A simple, pain-free treatment for ingrown toenails complicated with granulation tissue. *Dermatol Surg* 32:1388–1390, 2006.

66. Erdogan FG, Erdogan G: Long-term results of nail brace application in diabetic patients with ingrown nails. *Dermatol Surg* 34:84–86, discussion 86-87, 2008.

67. Estersohn HS, Stanoch JF: Pyogenic granuloma: a literature review and two case reports. *J Am Podiatry Assoc* 73:297–301, 1983.

68. Failla V, Richert BJ, Nikkels AF: Pincer nails associated with pamidronate. *Clin Exp Dermatol* 36:305–306, 2011. doi:10.1111/j.1365-2230.2010.03919.x.

69. Farley-Sakevich T, Grady J: Onychoplasty with carbon dioxide laser matrixectomy for treatment of ingrown toenails. *J Am Podiatr Med Assoc* 95:175–179, 2005.

70. Farrelly JP, J Minford J: Simple operative management of ingrown toenail using bipolar diathermy. *Eur J Pediatr Surg* 19:304–306, 2009. doi:10.1055/s-0029-1225357.

71. Feibleman CE, Stoll H, Maize JC: Melanomas of the palm, sole, and nailbed: a clinicopathologic study. *Cancer* 46:2492–2504, 1980.

72. Felton PM, Weaver TD: Phenol and alcohol chemical matrixectomy in diabetic versus nondiabetic patients: a retrospective study. *J Am Podiatr Med Assoc* 89:410–412, 1999.

73. Fikry T, Dkhissi M, Harfaoui A, et al: Subungual exostoses: a retrospective study of a series of 28 cases [French]. *Acta Orthop Belg* 64:35–40, 1998.

74. Firinu D, Massidda O, Lorrai MM, et al: Successful treatment of chronic mucocutaneous candidiasis caused by azole-resistant *Candida albicans* with posaconazole. *Clin Dev Immunol* 2011:283239, 2011. doi: 10.1155/2011/283239. [Epub Dec 1, 2010].

75. Fletcher CL, Hay RJ, Smeeton NC: Onychomycosis: the development of a clinical diagnostic aid for toenail disease: part I, establishing discriminating historical and clinical features. *Br J Dermatol* 150:701–705, 2004.

76. Fox IM: Osteomyelitis of the distal phalanx following trauma to the nail: a case report. *J Am Podiatr Med Assoc* 82:542–544, 1992.

77. Frank SC, Freer HL: Onychauxic dystrophic toenails requiring debridement in Medicare patients: prevalence and anatomical distribution. *J Am Podiatr Med Assoc* 93:388–391, 2003.

78. Fröjmark AS, Schuster J, Sobol M, et al: Mutations in Frizzled 6 cause isolated autosomal-recessive nail dysplasia. *Am J Hum Genet* 88:852–860, 2011.

79. Frost L: Root resection for incurvated nail. *J Am Podiatr Med Assoc* 40:19, 1950.

80. Gabriel SS, Dallos V, Stevenson DL: The ingrowing toenail: a modified segmental matrix excision operation. *Br J Surg* 66:285–286, 1979.

81. Garcia-Doval I, Cabo F, Monteagudo B, et al: Clinical diagnosis of toenail onychomycosis is possible in some patients: cross-sectional diagnostic study and development of a diagnostic rule. *Br J Dermatol* 163:743–751, 2010.

82. Giacalone VF: Phenol matricectomy in patients with diabetes. *J Foot Ankle Surg* 36:264–267, 1997.

83. Gibson SH, Montgomery H, Woolner LB, et al: Melanotic whitlow (subungual melanoma). *J Invest Dermatol* 29:119–129, 1957.

84. Gilles GA, Dennis KJ, Harkless LB: Periostitis associated with phenol matrixectomies. *J Am Podiatr Med Assoc* 76:469–472, 1986.

85. Graham JH, Helwig EB: Bowen's disease and its relationship to systemic cancer. *Arch Dermatol* 80:133–159, 1959.

86. Grover C, Bansal S, Nanda S, et al: En bloc excision of proximal nail fold for treatment of chronic paronychia. *Dermatol Surg* 32:393–398, discussion 398-399, 2006.

87. Gruver DI: Treatment of tubular toenail. *Plast Reconstr Surg* 112:934, 2003.

88. Gupta AK, Jain HC, Lynde CW, et al: Prevalence and epidemiology of onychomycosis in patients visiting physicians' offices: a multicenter Canadian survey of 15,000 patients. *J Am Acad Dermatol* 43:244–248, 2000.

89. Gupta AK, Konnikov N, MacDonald P, et al: Prevalence and epidemiology of toenail onychomycosis in diabetic subjects: a multicentre survey. *Br J Dermatol* 139:665–671, 1998.

90. Gupta AK, Lynch LE, Kogan N, Cooper EA: The use of an intermittent terbinafine regimen for the treatment of dermatophyte toenail onychomycosis. *J Eur Acad Dermatol Venereol* 23:256–262, 2009.

91. Gupta AK, Ryder JE, Johnson AM: Cumulative meta-analysis of systemic antifungal agents for the treatment of onychomycosis. *Br J Dermatol* 150:537–544, 2004.

92. Gupta S, Sahoo B, Kumar B: Treating ingrown toenails by nail splinting with a flexible tube: an Indian experience. *J Dermatol* 28:485–489, 2001.

93. Hallock GG, Lutz DA: Octyl-2-cyanoacrylate adhesive for rapid nail plate restoration. *J Hand Surg Am* 25:979–981, 2000.

94. Hartzell M: Granuloma pyogenicum (botryomycosis of French authors). *J Cutan Dis* 22:520–525, 1904.

95. Hashimoto K: Ultrastructure of the human toenail: cell migration, keratinization, and formation of the intercellular cement. *Arch Dermatol Res* 240:1–22, 1970.

96. Heifetz CJ: Ingrown toe-nail: A clinical study. *Am J Surg* 38:298–315, 1937.

97. Heifetz CJ: Operative management of ingrown toenail. *J Mo Med Assoc* 42:213–216, 1945.

98. Heim M, Schapiro J, Wershavski M, et al: Drug-induced and traumatic nail problems in the haemophilias. *Haemophilia* 6:191–194, 2000.

99. Helfand AE: Onychomycosis in the aged: an administrative perspective. *J Am Podiatr Med Assoc* 76:142–145, 1986.

100. Helms A, Brodell RT: Surgical pearl: prompt treatment of subungual hematoma by decompression. *J Am Acad Dermatol* 42:508–509, 2000.

101. Hettinger DF, Valinsky MS: Treatment of onychomycosis with nail avulsion and topical ketoconazole. *J Am Podiatr Med Assoc* 81:28–32, 1991.

102. Ho VC, Sober AJ: Therapy for cutaneous melanoma: an update. *J Am Acad Dermatol* 22:159–176, 1990.

103. Holub PG, Hubbard ER: Ketoconazole in the treatment of onychomycosis. *J Am Podiatr Med Assoc* 77:338–339, 1987.

104. Hongcharu W, Dwyer P, Gonzalez S, et al: Confirmation of onychomycosis by in vivo confocal microscopy. *J Am Acad Dermatol* 42:214–216, 2000.

105. Horst F, Nunley JA: Glomus tumors in the foot: a new surgical technique for removal. *Cosm Dermatol* 24:949–951, 2003.

106. Huang YH, Ohara K: Medical pearl: subungual hematoma: a simple and quick method for diagnosis. *J Am Acad Dermatol* 54:877–878, 2006.

107. Hutchinson J: Melanosis often not black: melanotic whitlow. *BMJ* 1:491–493, 1886.

108. Ippolito E, Falez F, Tudisco C, et al: Subungual exostosis: histological and clinical considerations on 30 cases. *Ital J Orthop Traumatol* 13:81–87, 1987.

109. Jahss MH: *Disorders of the foot and ankle: medical and surgical management,* ed 2, Philadelphia, 1991, WB Saunders, pp 937, 1548-1572.

110. Jarratt M: Herpes simplex infection. *Arch Dermatol* 119:99–103, 1983.

111. Jennings MB, Pollak R, Harkless LB, et al: Treatment of toenail onychomycosis with oral terbinafine plus aggressive debridement: IRON-CLAD, a large, randomized, open-label, multicenter trial. *J Am Podiatr Med Assoc* 96:465–473, 2006.

112. Jeys LM, Khafagy R: A useful technique for securing nails: the figure-of-eight suture [letter]. *Br J Plast Surg* 54:651, 2001.

113. Johnson M: The human nail and its disorders. In Lorimer DL, Neale D, editors: *Neale's common foot disorders: diagnosis and management: a general clinical guide,* ed 4, Edinburgh, 1993, Churchill Livingstone, pp 123–139.

114. Johnson M, Comaish JS, Shuster S: Nail is produced by the normal nail bed: a controversy resolved. *Br J Dermatol* 125:27–29, 1991.

115. Kato T, Suetake T, Sugiyama Y, et al: Epidemiology and prognosis of subungual melanoma in 34 Japanese patients. *Br J Dermatol* 134:383–387, 1996.

116. Keyes EL: The surgical treatment of ingrown toenails. *JAMA* 102:1458–1460, 1934.

117. Kim JY, Jung Lee Y, Sic Park J, Hyuck Lee S: A new treatment for severe incurved toenails: a case report. *Foot Ankle Int* 29:1057–1062, 2008.

118. Kim JY, Park JS: Treatment of symptomatic incurved toenail with a new device. *Foot Ankle Int* 30:1083–1087, 2009.

119. Kiuru M, Kurban M, Itoh M, et al: Hereditary leukonychia, or porcelain nails, resulting from mutations in PLCD1. *Am J Hum Genet* 88:839–844, 2011.

120. Koenig RD, McLaughlin KS: Subungual melanoma. *J Am Podiatr Med Assoc* 84:95–96, 1994.

121. Kosaka M, Asamura S, Wada Y, et al: Pincer nails treated using zigzag nail bed flap method: results of 71 toenails. *Dermatol Surg* 36:506–511, 2010.

122. Kosinski MA, Stewart D: Nail changes associated with systemic disease and vascular insufficiency. *Clin Podiatr Med Surg* 6:295–318, 1989.

123. Krausz CE: Nail survey (1942-1970). *Br J Chir* 35:117, 1970.

124. Kuwada GT: Long-term evaluation of partial and total surgical and phenol matrixectomies. *J Am Podiatr Med Assoc* 81:33–36, 1991.

125. Langford JH: Pachyonychia congenita. *J Am Podiatry Assoc* 68:587–591, 1978.

126. Lapidus P: The ingrown toenail. *Bull Hosp Joint Dis* 33:181–192, 1972.

127. Lawrence W Jr: Management of malignant melanoma. *Am Surg* 38:93–106, 1972.

128. Lawry MA, Haneke E, Strobeck K, et al: Methods for diagnosing onychomycosis: a comparative study and review of the literature. *Arch Dermatol* 136:1112–1116, 2000.

129. Lee SK, Jung MS, Lee YH, et al: Two distinctive subungual pathologies: subungual exostosis and subungual osteochondroma. *Foot Ankle Int* 28:595–601, 2007.

130. Lemon B, Burns R: Malignant melanoma: a literature review and case presentation. *J Foot Ankle Surg* 37:48–54, 1998.

131. Lemont H, Haas R: Subungual pigmented Bowen's disease in a nineteen-year-old black female. *J Am Podiatr Med Assoc* 84:39–40, 1994.

132. Leppard B, Sanderson KV, Behan F: Subungual malignant melanoma: difficulty in diagnosis. *BMJ* 1:310–312, 1974.

133. Lerner LH: Incurvated nail margin with associated osseous pathology. *Curr Podiatr* 11:26–28, 1962.

134. Lewis BL: Microscopic studies of fetal and mature nail and surrounding soft tissue. *Arch Dermatol Syphilol* 70:732–747, 1954.

135. Li J, Chen J, Hong G, et al: Clinical study of treatment for recalcitrant ingrown toenail by partial distal phalanx removal. *J Plast Reconstr Aesthet Surg* 62:1327–1330, 2009.

136. Lilly KK, Koshnick RL, Grill JP, et al: Cost-effectiveness of diagnostic tests for toenail onychomycosis: a repeated-measure, single-blinded, cross-sectional evaluation of 7 diagnostic tests. *J Am Acad Dermatol* 55:620–626, 2006.

137. Lloyd-Davies RW, Brill GC: The aetiology and out-patient management of ingrowing toe-nails. *Br J Surg* 50:592–597, 1963.

138. Luis LR Jr, Kaoru GR, Shemuel PB, Mills JL Sr: Lower extremity glomus tumors: comprehensive review for surgeons. *Vascular* 16:326–332, 2008.

139. Lundeen GW, Lundeen RO: Onychomycosis: its classification, pathophysiology and etiology. *J Am Podiatry Assoc* 68:395–401, 1978.

140. Mann RA, Coughlin MJ: Toenail abnormalities. In Mann RA, Coughlin MJ, editors: *The video textbook of foot and ankle surgery*, St Louis, 1990, Medical Video Productions, pp 56–66.

141. Martinez-Nova A, Sánchez-Rodriguez R, Alonso-Peña D: A new onchocryptosis classification and treatment plan. *J Am Podiatr Med Assoc* 97:389–393, 2007.

142. Miller-Breslow A, Dorfman HD: Dupuytren's (subungual) exostosis. *Am J Surg Pathol* 12:368–378, 1988.

143. Moehrle M, Metzger S, Schippert W, et al: "Functional" surgery in subungual melanoma. *Dermatol Surg* 29:366–374, 2003.

144. Mori H, Umeda T, Nishioka K, et al: Ingrown nails: a comparison of the nail matrix phenolization method with the elevation of the nail bed-periosteal flap procedure. *J Dermatol* 25:1–4, 1998.

145. Multhopp-Stephens H, Walling AK: Subungual exostosis: a simple technique of excision. *Cosm Dermatol* 16:88–91, 1995.

146. Murray WR: Onychocryptosis: principles of non-operative and operative care. *Clin Orthop Relat Res* 142:96–102, 1979.

147. Murray WR, Bedi BS: The surgical management of ingrowing toenail. *Br J Surg* 62:409–412, 1975.

148. Nagata F, Chu C, Phipps R: Nail involvement in Darier's disease: a case report. *J Am Podiatr Assoc* 70:635–636, 1980.

149. Nair AB, Vaka SR, Murthy SN: Transungual delivery of terbinafine by iontophoresis in onychomycotic nails. *Drug Dev Ind Pharm* 37:1253–1258, 2011.

150. Noël B: Anesthesia for ingrowing toenail surgery. *Dermatol Surg* 36:1356–1357, 2010.

151. Norton LA: Disorders of the nails. In Moschella SL, Pillsbury DM, Hurley HJ, editors: *Dermatology*, Philadelphia, 1975, WB Saunders, pp 1222–1236.

152. Norton LA: Nail disorders: a review. *J Am Acad Dermatol* 2:451–467, 1980.

153. Nzuzi SM: Common nail disorders. *Clin Podiatr Med Surg* 6:273–294, 1989.

154. Nzuzi SM: Nail entities. *Clin Podiatr Med Surg* 6:253–271, 1989.

155. Oliveira Ada S, Picoto Ada S, Verde SF, et al: Subungual exostosis: treatment as an office procedure. *J Dermatol Surg Oncol* 6:555–558, 1980.

156. Ongenae K, Van De Kerckhove M, Naeyaert JM: Bowen's disease of the nail. *Dermatology* 204:348–350, 2002.

157. Ouzounov KG: New nail block technique. *J Am Podiatr Med Assoc* 95:589–592, 2005.

158. Ozawa T, Nose K: Partial matricectomy with a CO2 laser for ingrown toenail after nail matrix staining. *Dermatol Surg* 31:302–305, 2005.

159. Pack GT, Oropeza R: Subungual melanoma. *Surg Gynecol Obstet* 124:571–582, 1967.

160. Page JC, Abramson C, Lee WL, et al: Diagnosis and treatment of tinea pedis: a review and update. *J Am Podiatr Med Assoc* 81:304–316, 1991.

161. Pahwa M, Pahwa P, Kathuria S: Glomus tumour of the nail bed treated with the "trap door" technique: a report of two patients. *J Dermatolog Treat* 21:298–300, 2010.

162. Palamarchuk HJ, Kerzner M: An improved approach to evacuation of subungual hematoma. *J Am Podiatr Med Assoc* 79:566–568, 1989.

163. Palmer BV, Jones A: Ingrowing toenails: the results of treatment. *Br J Surg* 66:575–576, 1979.

164. Papachristou DN, Fortner JG: Melanoma arising under the nail. *J Surg Oncol* 21:219–222, 1982.

165. Pardo-Castello V, Pardo OA: *Diseases of the nails*, ed 3, Springfield, Ill, 1960, Charles C Thomas, pp 19-20.

166. Parrinello JF, Japour CJ, Dykyj D: Incurvated nail: does the phalanx determine nail plate shape? *J Am Podiatr Med Assoc* 85:696–698, 1995.

167. Pettine KA, Cofield RH, Johnson KA, et al: Ingrown toenail: results of surgical treatment. *Foot Ankle* 9:130–134, 1988.

168. Peyvandi H, Robati RM, Yegane RA, et al: Comparison of two surgical methods (Winograd and sleeve method) in the treatment of ingrown toenail. *Dermatol Surg* 37:331–335, 2011. doi:10.1111/j.1524-4725.2011.01880.x.

169. Pinter A, Pätzold S, Kaufmann R: Lichen planus of nails—successful treatment with Alitretinoin. *J Dtsch Dermatol Ges* 9:1033–1034, 2011. doi:10.1111/j.1610-0387.2011.07773.x.

170. Piraccini BM, Sisti A, Tosti A: Long-term follow-up of toenail onychomycosis caused by dermatophytes after successful treatment with systemic antifungal agents. *J Am Acad Dermatol* 62:411–414, 2010.

171. Ratz J, Blumberg M: Onychomycosis. Available at http://www.emedicine.com/derm/topic300.htm. Accessed March 20, 2006.

172. Reisberger EM, Abels C, Landthaler M, et al: Histopathological diagnosis of onychomycosis by periodic acid–Schiff–stained nail clippings. *Br J Dermatol* 148:749–754, 2003.
173. Rich P: Special patient populations: onychomycosis in the diabetic patient. *J Am Acad Dermatol* 35:S10–S12, 1996.
174. Rich P: Nail biopsy: indications and methods. *Dermatol Surg* 27:229–234, 2001.
175. Rinaldi R, Sabia M, Gross J: The treatment and prevention of infection in phenol alcohol matricectomies. *J Am Podiatry Assoc* 72:453–457, 1982.
176. Rodnan GP: Psoriasis. In Rodnan GP, Schumacher HR, editors: *Primer on the rheumatic diseases*, ed 8, Atlanta, 1983, Arthritis Foundation, pp 151–152.
177. Rose J, Cohen RS, Mauro G: Subungual malignant melanoma. *J Foot Surg* 25:154–159, 1986.
178. Rounding C, Bloomfield S: Surgical treatments for ingrown toenails (review). *Cochrane Collaboration* CD001541:1–35, 2008.
179. Rounding C, Hulm S: Surgical treatments for ingrowing toenails. *Cochrane Database Syst Rev* 2:CD001541, 2000.
180. Rozmaryn LM, Schwartz AM: Treatment of subungual myxoma preserving the nail matrix: a case report. *J Hand Surg Am* 23:178–180, 1998.
181. Saltzman BS: Periungual fibroma: a case report. *J Am Podiatry Assoc* 68:696, 1978.
182. Samman PD: The human toe nail: its genesis and blood supply. *Br J Dermatol* 71:296–302, 1959.
183. Sarifakioglu E, Sarifakioglu N: Crescent excision of the nail fold with partial nail avulsion does work with ingrown toenails. *Eur J Dermatol* 20:822–823, 2010.
184. Sari-Kouzel H, Hutchinson CE, Middleton A, et al: Foot problems in patients with systemic sclerosis. *Rheumatology (Oxford)* 40:410–413, 2001.
185. Schein JR, Gause D, Stier DM, et al: Onychomycosis: baseline results of an observational study. *J Am Podiatr Med Assoc* 87:512–519, 1997.
186. Scher RK: Onychomycosis is more than a cosmetic problem. *Br J Dermatol* 130(Suppl 43):15, 1994.
187. Scher RK, Joseph W, Robbins J: Progression and recurrence of onychomycosis. Available at http://www.medscape.com/viewprogram/2334_pnt. Accessed March 20, 2006.
188. Schwartz GR, Schwen SA: Subungual splinter removal. *Am J Emerg Med* 15:330–331, 1997.
189. Shaikh H, Mansoor J: Efficacy of wedge resection with phenolization in the treatment of ingrowing toenails. *J Am Podiatr Med Assoc* 98:118–122, 2008.
190. Shepard GH: Management of acute nail bed avulsions. *Hand Clin* 6:39–56, 1990.
191. Shum C, Bruno RJ, Ristic S, et al: Examination of the anatomic relationship of the proximal germinal nail matrix to the extensor tendon insertion. *J Hand Surg Am* 25:1114–1117, 2000.
192. Sigurgeirsson B, Elewski BE, Rich PA, et al: Intermittent versus continuous terbinafine in the treatment of toenail onychomycosis: a randomized, double-blind comparison. *J Dermatolog Treat* 17:38–44, 2006.
193. Silverman ME, Goodman RM, Cuppage FE: The nail–patella syndrome: clinical findings and ultrastructural observations in the kidney. *Arch Intern Med* 120:68–74, 1967.
194. Sotiriou E, Koussidou-Eremonti T, Chaidemenos G, et al: Photodynamic therapy for distal and lateral subungual toenail onychomycosis caused by *Trichophyton rubrum*: preliminary results of a single-centre open trial. *Acta Derm Venereol* 90:216–217, 2010.
195. Spencer JM: Nail-apparatus melanoma. *Lancet* 353:84–85, 1999.
196. Suga H, Mukouda M: Subungual exostosis: a review of 16 cases focusing on postoperative deformity of the nail. *Ann Plast Surg* 55:272–275, 2005.
197. Sugden P, Levy M, Rao GS: Onychocryptosis–phenol burn fiasco. *Burns* 27:289–292, 2001.
198. Szepietowski JC, Reich A, Garlowska E, et al: Factors influencing coexistence of toenail onychomycosis with tinea pedis and other dermatomycoses: a survey of 2761 patients. *Arch Dermatol* 142:1279–1284, 2006.
199. Takematsu H, Obata M, Tomita Y, et al: Subungual melanoma: a clinicopathologic study of 16 Japanese cases. *Cancer* 55:2725–2731, 1985.
200. Tatlican S, Eren C, Yamangokturk B, et al: Chemical matricectomy with 10% sodium hydroxide for the treatment of ingrown toenails in people with diabetes. *Dermatol Surg* 36:219–222, 2010.
201. Tatlican S, Yamangokturk B: [Comparison of phenol applications of different durations for the cauterization of the germinal matrix: an efficacy and safety study]. *Acta Orthop Traumatol Turc* 43:298–302, 2009.
202. Tauber EB, Goldman L, Claassen H: Pachyonchia congenita. *JAMA* 107:29–30, 1936.
203. Thompson TC, Terwilliger C: The terminal Syme operation for ingrown toenail. *Surg Clin North Am* 31:575–584, 1950.
204. Townsend AC, Scott PJ: Ingrowing toenail and onychogryposis. *J Bone Joint Surg Br* 48:354–358, 1966.
205. Travers GR, Ammon RG: The sodium hydroxide chemical matricectomy procedure. *J Am Podiatry Assoc* 70:476–478, 1980.
206. Tucker DJ, Jules KT, Raymond F: Nailbed injuries with hallucal phalangeal fractures: evaluation and treatment. *J Am Podiatr Med Assoc* 86:170–173, 1996.
207. Tuzuner T, Kavak A, Parlak AH, Ustundag N: Subungual osteochondroma: a diagnostic dilemma. *J Am Podiatr Med Assoc* 96:154–157, 2006.
208. Vaccari S, Dika E, Balestri R: Partial excision of matrix and phenolic ablation for the treatment of ingrowing toenail: a 36 month follow-up of 197 treated patients. *Dermatol Surg* 36:1288–1293, 2010. doi:10.1111/j.1524-4725.2010.01624.x.
209. Van Geertruyden JP, Olemans C, Laporte M, et al: Verrucous carcinoma of the nail bed. *Cosm Dermatol* 19:327–328, 1998.
210. Vazquez-Flores H, Dominguez-Cherit J, Vega-Memije ME, et al: Subungual osteochondroma: clinical and radiologic features and treatment. *Dermatol Surg* 30:1031–1034, 2004.
211. Wadhams PS, McDonald JF, Jenkin WM: Epidermal inclusion cysts as a complication of nail surgery. *J Am Podiatr Med Assoc* 80:610–612, 1990.
212. Warshaw EM: Evaluating costs for onychomycosis treatments: a practitioner's perspective (review). *J Am Podiatr Med Assoc* 96:38–52, 2006.
213. Watanabe D, Kawamura C, Masuda Y, et al: Successful treatment of toenail onychomycosis with photodynamic therapy. *Arch Dermatol* 144:19–21, 2008.
214. Weiner AL: Alopecia areata with nail changes. *Arch Dermatol* 72:469, 1955.
215. Welvaart K, Schraffordt Koops H: Subungual malignant melanoma: a nail in the coffin. *Clin Oncol* 4:309–315, 1978.
216. White CJ, Laipply TC: Diseases of the nails: 792 cases: clinical and microscopial findings with resume of newer therapeutic methods. *Ind Med Surg* 27:325–327, 1958.
217. Winograd AM: Modification in technique of operation for ingrown toe-nail. *JAMA* 92:229–230, 1929.
218. Winograd AM: Results in operation for ingrown toe-nail. *Illinois Med J* 70:197–198, 1936.
219. Witt CS, Zielsdorf LM, Wysong DK: A modified partial chemical matricectomy. *J Am Podiatr Med Assoc* 76:684–685, 1986.
220. Wright G: Laser matricectomy in the toes. *Foot Ankle* 9:246–247, 1989.
221. Yang G, Yanchar NL, Lo AY, Jones SA: Treatment of ingrown toenails in the pediatric population. *J Pediatr Surg* 43:931–935, 2008.

222. Yang KC, Li YT: Treatment of recurrent ingrown great toenail associated with granulation tissue by partial nail avulsion followed by matricectomy with Sharpulse carbon dioxide laser. *Dermatol Surg* 28:419–421, 2002.

223. Yin Z, Xu J, Luo D: A meta-analysis comparing long-term recurrences of toenail onychomycosis after successful treatment with terbinafine versus itraconazole. *J Dermatolog Treat* 23:449–452, 2012. doi:10.3109/09546634.2011.579082.

224. Zadik FR: Obliteration of the nail bed of the great toe without shortening of the terminal phalanx. *J Bone Joint Surg Br* 32:66–67, 1950.

225. Zaiac MN, Weiss E: Mohs micrographic surgery of the nail unit and squamous cell carcinoma. *Dermatol Surg* 27:246–251, 2001.

226. Zaias N: Psoriasis of the nail. A clinical-pathologic study. *Arch Dermatol* 99:567–579, 1969.

227. Zaias N: Onychomycosis. *Arch Dermatol* 105:263–274, 1972.

228. Zaias N: *The nail in health and disease*, ed 1, New York, 1980, SP Medical, pp 1-43.

229. Zaias N, Rebell G: The successful treatment of *Trichophyton rubrum* nail bed (distal subungual) onychomycosis with intermittent pulse-dosed terbinafine. *Arch Dermatol* 140:691–695, 2004.

230. Zaitz C, Campbell I, Moraes JR, et al: HLA-associated susceptibility to chronic onychomycosis in Brazilian Ashkenazic Jews. *Int J Dermatol* 35:681–682, 1996.

231. Zimmerman P, Prior J, McGuire J, et al: Onychia of a macronychia in congenital aphalangia. *J Am Podiatr Med Assoc* 82:380–381, 1992.

232. Zook EG: Understanding the perionychium. *J Hand Ther* 13:269–275, 2000.

233. Zuber TJ: Ingrown toenail removal. *Am Fam Physician* 65:2547–2552, 2554, 2002.

NERVE DISORDERS

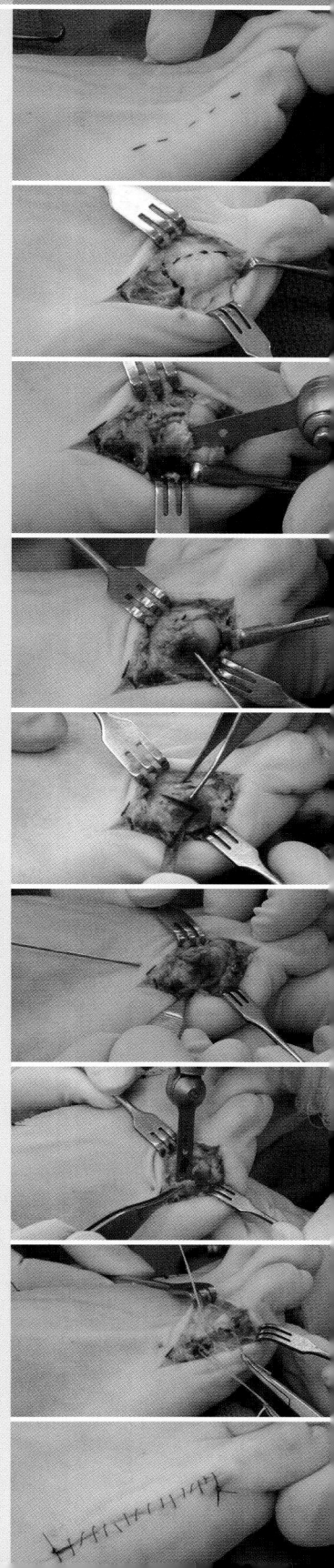

Disorders of the Nerves

Lew C. Schon, Mark A. Reed

The diagnosis and treatment of diseases of the peripheral nerves in the foot and ankle usually are quite straightforward, but, at other times, they present a very complex clinical and surgical problem. Nerve problems can result from overuse injuries (because of repetitive stresses) or from one-time traumatic events. Nerve disorders in many patients resolve uneventfully and do not require much, if any, treatment. Some nerve disorders resolve as a more recognizable condition receives treatment, such as in a patient with a grade 3 ankle sprain and a mild traction injury to the superficial peroneal nerve.

The more challenging diagnostic cases are dynamic and occur only with mechanical stresses, such as walking, running, or wearing certain shoes. Some nerve disorders occur as a *double-crush syndrome*. In the double-crush syndrome, a more proximal nerve dysfunction (radiculopathy), which may be subclinical, causes impairment of axoplasmic flow and diminishes the threshold for distal nerve symptoms from focal disease.[41,212] The role of metabolic, endocrinologic, chemical, pharmacologic, or rheumatologic conditions in nerve physiology and function must be recognized as creating or enhancing nerve dysfunction. Occasionally, the clinical problem has been aggravated by surgery, and the preoperative condition must be distinguished from the postoperative condition. The foot and ankle specialist is challenged to elucidate the differences between the symptoms from mechanical nonneurologic symptoms and those that arise from the nerves. Awareness of these features and manifestations of these conditions will help the specialist design an effective treatment plan and anticipate the outcome of the interventions.

INTERDIGITAL NEUROMA

The history of the interdigital neuroma has been long and colorful. Kelikian's detailed chronology of the history[31] is briefly summarized here. The condition was first described in 1845 by the Queen's Surgeon-Chiropodist Lewis Durlacher.[16] He described a "form of neuralgic affection" involving "the plantar nerve between the third and fourth metatarsal bones." In 1876 T.G. Morton[39] related the problem to the fourth metatarsophalangeal (MTP) joint and suspected a neuroma or some type of hypertrophy of

the digital branches of the lateral plantar nerve (LPN). In 1877 Mason[37] reported a case of pain around the second MTP joint and suspected involvement of a digital branch of the medial plantar nerve. In 1893 Hoadley[27] actually explored the digital nerves under the painful area, "found a small neuroma," excised it, and claimed that he obtained a "prompt and perfect cure." In 1912 Tubby[55] reported observing on two occasions that the plantar digital nerves were congested and thickened. In 1940 Betts[8] stated that "Morton's metatarsalgia is a neuritis of the fourth digital nerve." In 1943 McElvenny[38] stated that it was caused by a tumor involving the most lateral branch of the medial plantar nerve. In 1979 Gauthier[19] speculated that the condition was a nerve entrapment, an idea supported anatomically by others.[22,32]

Etiology

In discussions of interdigital neuroma, it must first be pointed out that the subject is not a neuroma per se, but rather a painful clinical entity involving the common digital nerve. Thus the best terminology for the condition should perhaps be *interdigital neuralgia* based on the complexity and variability of the cause. The term *neuritis* is a less favorable descriptor because the suffix "-itis" implies inflammation. Because the condition can occur as an entrapment without inflammatory cells or mediators, the suffix "-algia," used to describe pain, is more accurate.

Studies by Lassmann[32] and Graham and Graham[22] have demonstrated that most, if not all, of the histologic changes in the nerve occur beyond the transverse metatarsal ligament and that the nerve proximal to the ligament appears to be normal. These authors demonstrated quantitatively that there was a decrease in the number of thick myelinated fibers, decreased diameter in the individual nerve fibers as a result of attenuation of their myelin sheaths, and increased nerve and vesicular width. Alterations in the interdigital arteries could not be correlated with the alterations found in the nerves. Hyalinization of vessel walls has been observed in patients with interdigital neuroma, but it has also been observed in control material in patients without interdigital neuroma. In a study of 133 patients with a clinical diagnosis of Morton's syndrome, light and electron microscopic investigations revealed that in the early stages of the disease the histologic findings are dominated by certain alterations of the nerves independent of alterations of the interdigital vessels. These alterations include sclerosis and edema of the endoneurium, thickening and hyalinization of the walls of the endoneurial vessels caused by multiple layers of basement membrane, thickening of the perineurium, deposition of an amorphous eosinophilic material built up by filaments of tubular structures, demyelinization and degeneration of the nerve fibers without signs of Wallerian degeneration, and local initial hyperplasia of unmyelinated nerves, followed by degeneration. These authors concluded that Morton's syndrome is probably caused by an entrapment neuropathy predominantly characterized by the deposition of an amorphous eosinophilic material, followed by a slow degeneration of the nerve fibers.

Giannini et al[20] reported on the histopathology in 63 cases and found intraneural (epineurium and perineurium) fibrosis and sclerohyalinosis and an increase of the elastic fibers in the stroma. They also found hyperplasia of the muscle layer, very evident internal elastic lamina, and proliferation of small vessels in the muscle layer and adventitia in the vessels.

Although these studies seem to support the theory that the main cause for an interdigital neuroma is an entrapment neuropathy beneath the transverse metatarsal ligament, other factors should be considered in the origin of this condition, including anatomic, traumatic, and extrinsic factors.

Anatomic Factors

From an anatomic standpoint, the medial plantar nerve (MPN) has four digital branches (Fig. 12-1). The most medial branch is the proper digital nerve to the medial aspect of the great toe. The next three branches are the first, second, and third common digital nerves and are distributed to both the medial and the lateral aspects of the first, second, and third interspaces, respectively. The lateral plantar nerve (LPN) divides into a superficial branch (which splits into a proper digital nerve to the lateral side of the small toe) and a common digital nerve to the fourth interspace. The common digital nerve often has a communicating branch that passes to the third digital branch of the MPN in the third interspace.

Researchers have speculated that because the common digital nerve to the third interspace consists of branches from the medial and lateral plantar nerves, the common digital nerve has increased thickness and is therefore more subject to trauma and possible neuroma formation (Fig. 12-2).[30] In an anatomic dissection of 71 feet, Levitsky et al[34] observed that a communicating branch to the nerve to the third web space was present in only 27% of

specimens and was absent in 73%. This anatomic finding seems to indicate that the communicating branch has little relation to the cause of interdigital neuroma. The authors did observe, however, that the second and third interspace was significantly narrower than the first and fourth and postulated that this further indicated the possibility of an entrapment. The frequency of the communicating branch was confirmed by Govsa et al.[21] They studied the anatomy of the communicating branches of the common plantar digital nerves between the fourth and third nerves in 50 adult male cadavers and found it was present in 28% of the feet.

Some variation exists in the distribution of the common digital nerves to the plantar aspect of the foot and their relationship to the metatarsal heads. At times, when an interdigital neuroma is resected, an accessory nerve branch appears to pass obliquely beneath the metatarsal head and joins the common digital nerve before its bifurcation into the digital branches. Because these accessory branches appear to come from beneath the metatarsal head region, when they are transected, the nerve end can retract beneath the metatarsal head and result in a recurrent neuroma.

The mobility that occurs between the medial three rays and the lateral two rays may be a reason for the increased incidence of neuromas in the third web space. The medial three rays are firmly fixed at the metatarsocuneiform joints, whereas the fourth and fifth metatarsals are fixed to the cuboid, which is more mobile. This anatomic fact results in increased mobility in the third web space, and the increased motion can result in trauma to the nerve or possibly the development of an enlarged bursa, which can secondarily place pressure on the nerve. The significant number of neuromas found in the second web space in part negates this as the main cause for the development of a neuroma.[35]

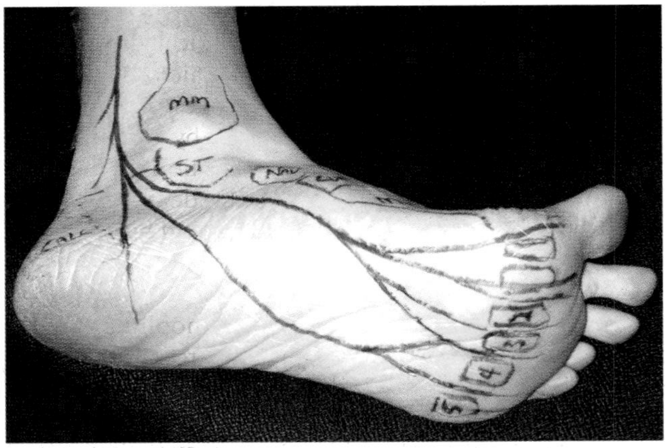

Figure 12-1 Illustration of nerves on the plantar aspect of the foot. Note the third toe has mixed innervation from the medial and lateral plantar nerves.

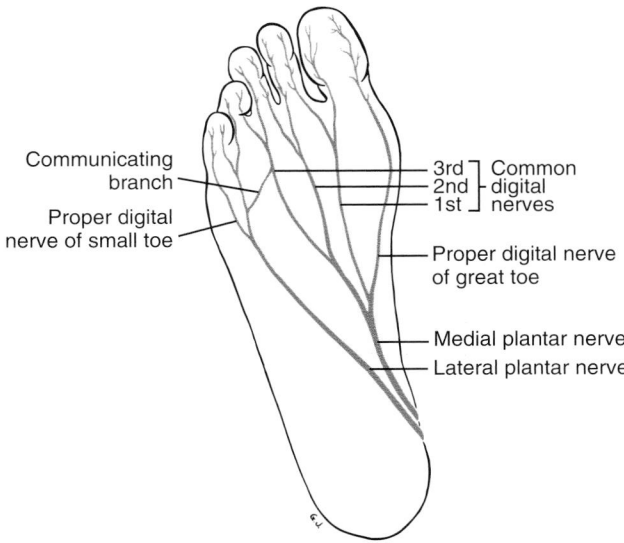

Figure 12-2 Plantar nerves of the right foot.

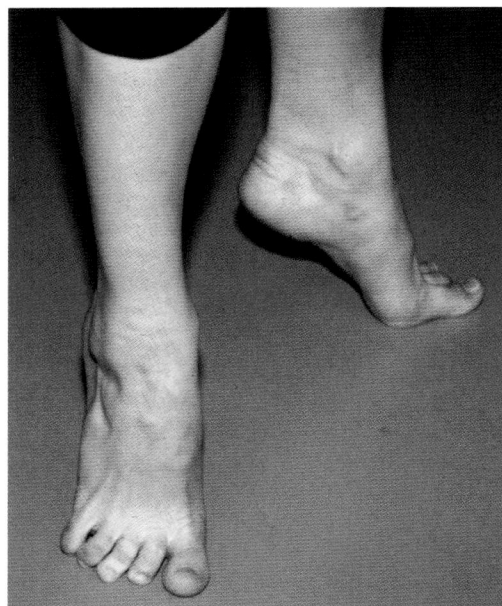

Figure 12-3   The demipointe position can increase the stretch on the common digital nerve.

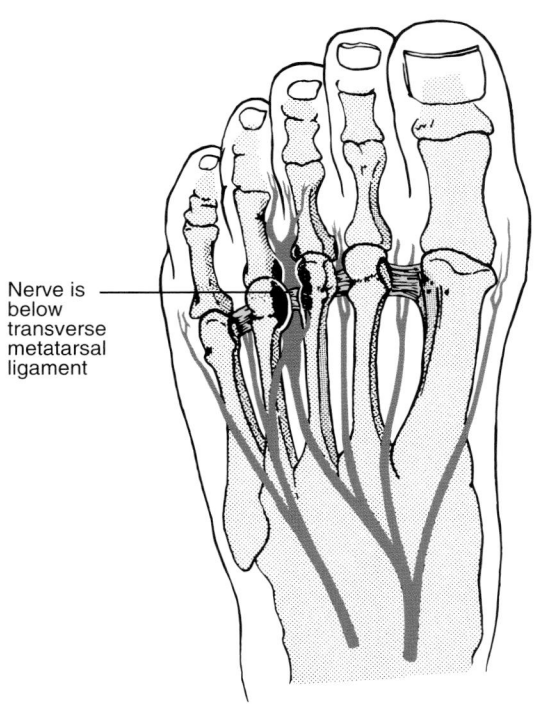

Nerve is below transverse metatarsal ligament

Figure 12-4   Illustration of the third branch of the medial plantar nerve. Note that the nerve courses plantarward, under the transverse metatarsal ligament.

During normal gait, dorsiflexion of the metatarsophalangeal (MTP) joints along with the action of the plantar aponeurosis causes plantar flexion of the metatarsal heads and, in theory, exposes the nerve to increased trauma (Fig. 12-3). The incidence of interdigital neuromas is 8 to 10 times more common in women, whose toes are often hyperextended at the MTP joint by high-fashion footwear, and this is probably a significant factor. Rather than increased trauma to the nerve itself resulting from long-term hyperextension of the MTP joints, the nerve may be tethered beneath the transverse metatarsal ligament, which results in the entrapment neuropathy previously discussed (Fig. 12-4).

Traumatic Causes

Acute trauma resulting from a fall from a height, a crush injury, or stepping on a sharp object occasionally results in a traumatic origin of an interdigital neuroma. Runners, persons who spend many hours on their feet at work, or persons who engage in certain athletic endeavors, such as racquet sports or dance, and place much stress on the metatarsal region, do not demonstrate an increased incidence of neuroma formation. The precise cause of neuroma development in one person but not in another exposed to essentially the same level of activity or inactivity remains an enigma. Even patients with atrophy of the plantar fat pad with resultant metatarsalgia rarely, if ever, report focal neuritic symptoms isolated to a single web space.

Extrinsic Factors

Extrinsic pressure against the nerve can result from a mass above the transverse metatarsal ligament or below the

ligament. Anatomically, a bursa is normally present between the metatarsal heads and is located above the transverse metatarsal ligament. Bossley and Cairney[10] studied this bursa by injecting dye in cadaver feet and demonstrated extension of the bursa distal and proximal to the transverse metatarsal ligament in the third web space. They did not observe extension of the bursa in the fourth web space. They hypothesized that the bursa can cause inflammation resulting in secondary neurofibrosis of the nerve but did not believe that the bursa caused a compressive force against the nerve. Awerbuch and Shephard[3] noted similar findings of an inflamed inter-metatarsal bursa in patients with rheumatoid arthritis, which they believed resulted in an alteration in the interdigital nerve, as well as some direct compressive effect on the nerve by the enlarged bursa.

Degeneration of the capsule of the MTP joint from unknown causes can result in a localized inflammatory response, but the nerve is not usually involved because the inflammation is above the transverse metatarsal ligament. Such deterioration of the capsule, however, can cause deviation of the proximal phalanx, usually of the third toe, in a medial direction. This in turn results in lateral deviation of the third metatarsal head against the fourth. The pressure can result in compression of bursal material present above the ligament and subsequently pressure against the underlying nerve. The deviation of the toe or instability of the MTP joint could also result in traction on the nerve, which could lead to disease

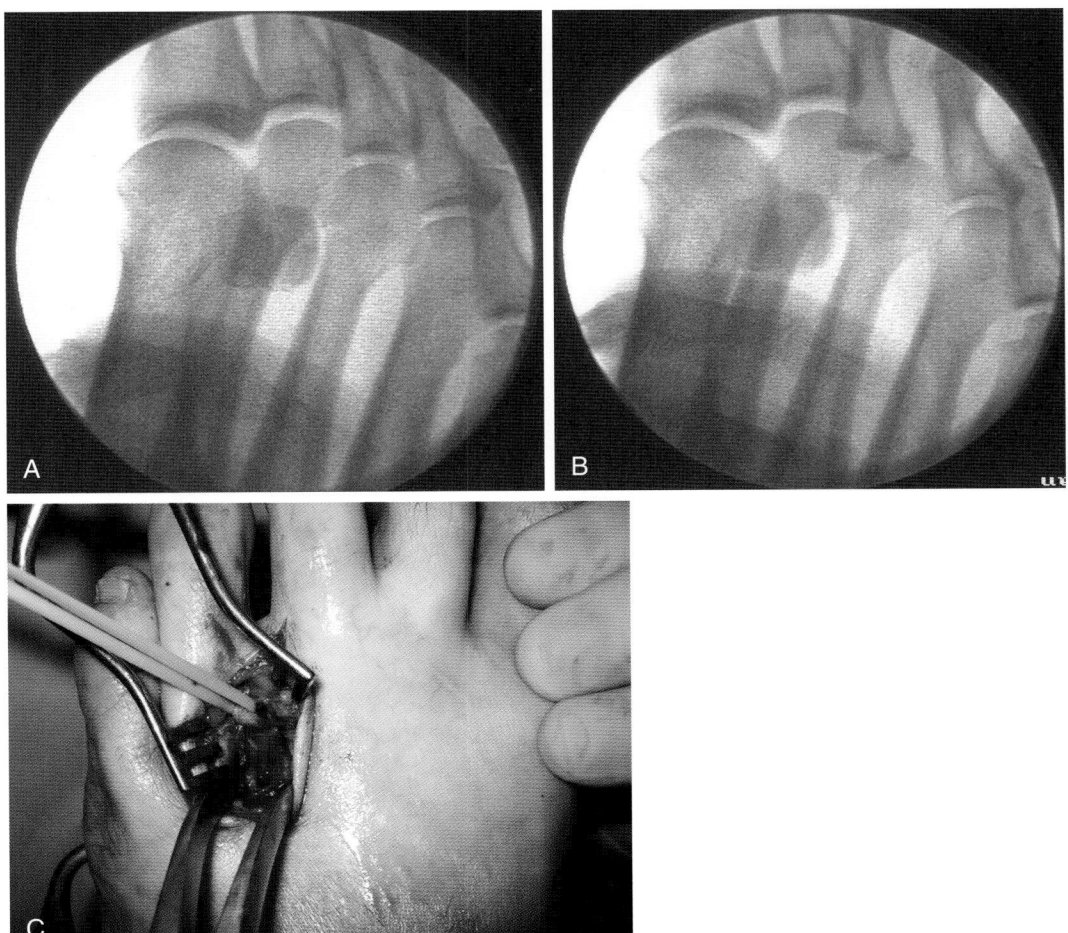

Figure 12-5   Metatarsophalangeal instability. **A,** Oblique fluoroscopy view before stressing the third metatarsophalangeal joint. **B,** Oblique fluoroscopy view after stressing the third metatarsophalangeal joint. **C,** Neuroma identified next to unstable joint.

(Fig. 12-5). Clinical symptoms of a neuroma are observed in approximately 10% to 15% of patients with deviation of the MTP joint, which may be accounted for by this anatomic malalignment (Fig. 12-6).

Occasionally, the transverse metatarsal ligament itself is thickened or contains an aberrant band that causes pressure against the common nerve. The authors have seen a few patients in whom this was present in the second web space but have not observed it in any other web space. In these cases, release of the transverse metatarsal ligament resulted in relief of the neuritic problem. A ganglion or synovial cyst can arise from the MTP joint, either as a primary entity or possibly in association with degeneration of the plantar plate. This lesion can cause direct pressure against the nerve as it passes beneath the transverse metatarsal ligament. A lipoma on the plantar aspect of the foot can result in similar compression against the nerve.

Fracture of the metatarsal from stress or a single traumatic event can result in altered loading of the metatarsal, with resultant interdigital neuralgia. In these cases, deviation of the malunion in any plane can cause traction or

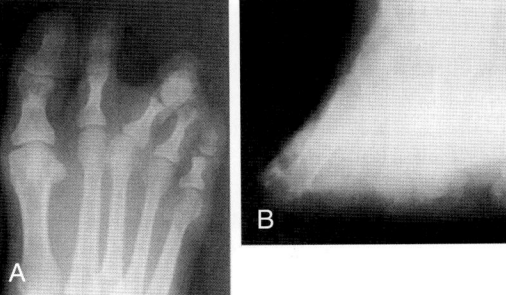

Figure 12-6   Increased pressure is created in the web space as a result of deviation of lesser toes, forcing metatarsal heads together. **A,** Anteroposterior radiograph shows lateral deviation of third toe, resulting in narrowing of second interspace. **B,** Axial view demonstrates narrowing of second interspace.

compression from the bone or any anchored soft tissues. For example, alteration in the length or function of the tendons directly from the callus or indirectly from malunion with shortening of the bone can lead to a claw toe or deviated toe with development of nerve symptoms.

This can be further complicated in a traumatically induced fracture by a direct insult to the nerve by the causative mechanism (e.g., crush, twist) at the time of bone injury.

Symptom Complex

Mann and Reynolds[35] performed a critical analysis of 56 patients in whom 76 neuromas were excised. There were 53 women and 3 men. This represents a greater female-to-male ratio than that observed by Bradley et al,[11] who reported a ratio of 4:1. The average age of the patient in the Mann and Reynolds[35] series was 55 years (range, 29-81 years).

An interdigital neuroma is usually unilateral, although bilateral neuromas were observed in 15% of the patients. The development of two neuromas simultaneously in the same foot rarely occurs; in a review of 89 neurectomies, Thompson and Deland[54] concluded that the incidence was probably less than 3%. The majority of the literature reports that the neuroma usually involves the third interspace, but an equal number of neuromas in the second and third interspaces have been noted. This same distribution was subsequently noted by Hauser[25] but was not supported by Graham et al,[23] who noted that there were twice as many neuromas in the third web space as the second. An interdigital neuroma of the first or fourth interspace is rare and probably does not exist as a clinical entity.

The most common symptom of an interdigital neuroma is pain localized to the plantar aspect of the foot between the metatarsal heads. The pain is usually characterized as burning, stabbing, tingling, or electric and radiates to the toes of the involved interspace in approximately 60% of cases. On occasion, the patient feels something "moving around" in the plantar aspect of the foot that periodically gets "caught" and results in an acute, sharp pain that radiates to the toes. This symptom complex is probably because the nerve is trapped beneath the metatarsal head, which, when body weight is applied, causes the acute pain. Occasionally, patients observe that the pain radiates toward the dorsum of the foot or more proximally along the plantar aspect of the foot.

The symptom complex is aggravated by activities on the foot, and most often the pain occurs when the patient puts on a tight-fitting high-heeled shoe. This pain is often relieved by removing the shoe and rubbing the forefoot. Often, the patient finds that the pain during gait can be limited by voluntarily curling the toes or by avoiding rolling through the ball of the feet. The patient often notes no symptoms when walking barefoot on a soft surface, only to feel pain when a high-heeled shoe is worn again. At times, wearing a broad, soft walking or jogging shoe results in a significant decrease in the symptom complex. Nonetheless, prolonged walking can induce symptoms regardless of shoe type.

Table 12-1 lists the preoperative symptoms by percentage in patients with interdigital neuroma.[35]

Table 12-1 Preoperative Symptoms of Interdigital Neuroma

Symptom	Patients Affected (%)
Plantar pain increased by walking	91
Relief of pain by resting	89
Plantar pain	77
Relief of pain by removing shoes	70
Pain radiating into toes	62
Burning pain	54
Aching or sharp pain	40
Numbness in toes or foot	40
Pain radiating up foot or leg	34
Cramping sensation	34

Diagnosis

The diagnosis of an interdigital neuroma is based on the patient's history and the physical findings. No electrodiagnostic studies are useful unless a peripheral neuropathy or radiculopathy is suspected. Radiographs are helpful to assess the foot in general and to identify an underlying bone or joint disease. Magnetic resonance imaging (MRI) may be useful in some cases to rule out other pathologies but is not warranted for establishing the diagnosis (Fig. 12-7). Similarly, ultrasound may be helpful in some situations, but the rate of false positives and negatives is too high to depend on the test. In some cases, it may be necessary to reevaluate the patient several times before one makes the diagnosis of an interdigital neuroma if the patient's symptoms are atypical.

Physical Examination

The physical examination begins by having the patient stand, with the physician carefully observing the foot for evidence of deviation of the toes, subluxation or clawing of the toes, or evidence of fullness in the involved web space or fullness of a web space not observed in the uninvolved foot. Then the range of motion of the MTP joints is observed. The MTP joints are carefully palpated on their dorsal and plantar aspects to look for evidence of synovitis of the joint, pain in the plantar pad area indicating early degeneration of the plantar pad, and evidence of pain around the joint. The patient with an interdigital neuroma does not have pain over the dorsal metatarsal heads. Typically, there is no pain over the plantar metatarsal head, but the presence of some tenderness here should be considered relative to the tenderness in the web space. Thus, if there is more pain in between the metatarsals, especially if it reproduces the character of the patient's symptoms of burning, shooting, radiating pain, then a neuroma is suspected.

Next, the physician carefully palpates the interspaces, starting just proximal to the metatarsal heads and proceeding distally into the web space. This usually reproduces the patient's pain, which often radiates out toward the tips of the toes. It is important when performing this test to ensure that there is no inadvertent compression of the dorsal tissues as a counterforce to the plantar

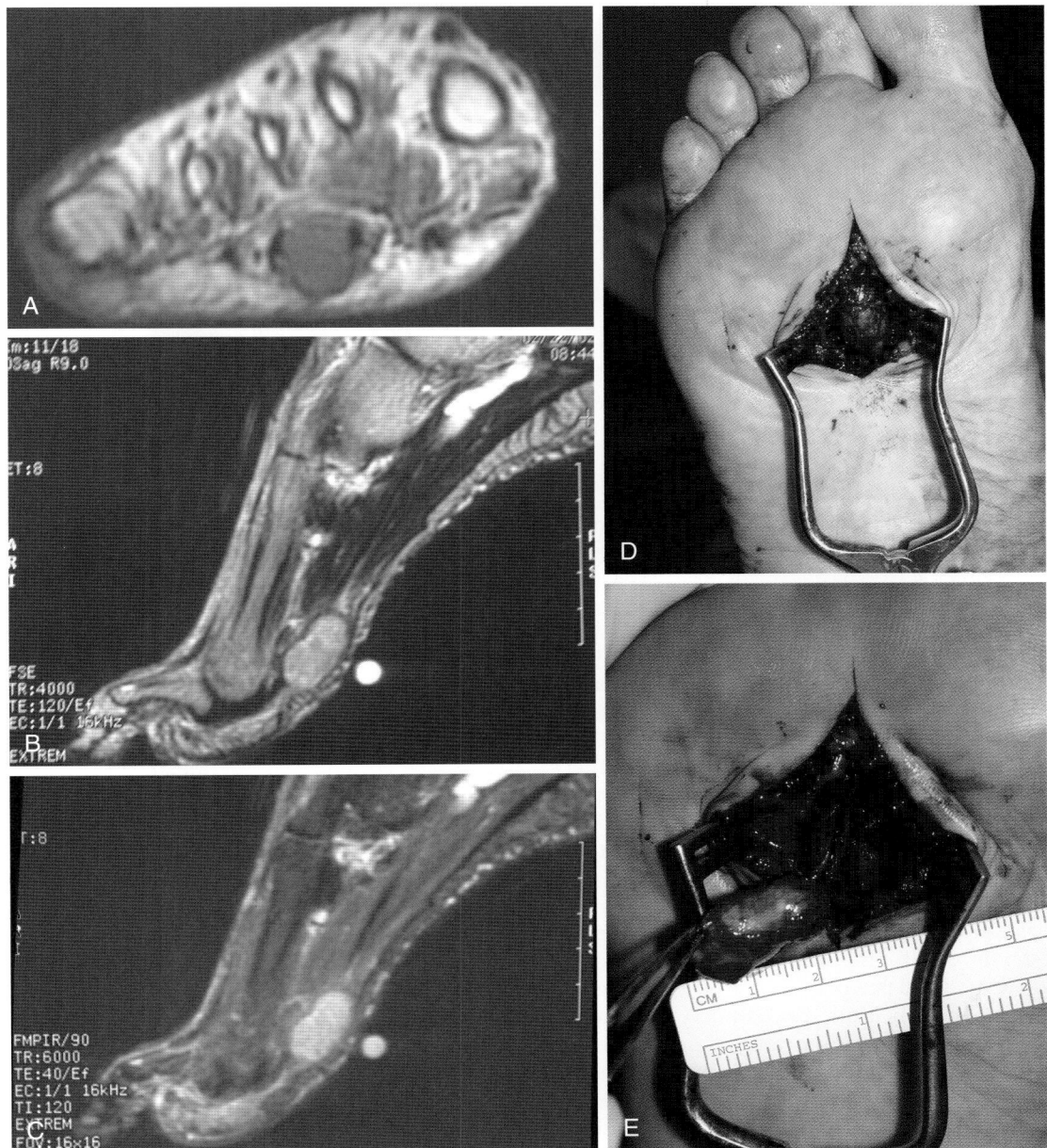

Figure 12-7 **A,** Coronal magnetic resonance image (MRI) of common digital nerve schwannoma. **B,** Sagittal MRI of schwannoma. **C,** Schwannoma has high signal intensity with fat-suppression sequences. **D,** Intraoperative exposure of schwannoma. **E,** Removal of tumor with intrafascicular dissection from the common digital nerve.

pressures that are directed dorsally. The physician should press the web space with one finger plantarly, using the other hand to stabilize the foot over a broad area of the midfoot or forefoot or against the resistance of the patient's foot alone (Fig. 12-8). Concomitant dorsal pressure can lead to discomfort from other etiologies that must be distinguished from interdigital neuralgia.

The web spaces are reexamined, and pressure is applied in a mediolateral direction with one hand to increase pressure on the tissue between the metatarsal heads. This maneuver often results in a significant crunching or

clicking feeling (the Mulder sign),[40] most often in the third web space and occasionally in the second web space. The maneuver can reproduce the patient's pain and, if so, is diagnostic of an interdigital neuroma. The presence of only a crunching or clicking feeling in the web space without reproduction of the patient's pain does not indicate a neuroma. Examination of a normal foot can demonstrate a crunching or clicking feeling, particularly in the third web space and occasionally in the second. It is unusual to elicit this crunch or click in the first and fourth web spaces. This test is not as helpful after a prior neuroma

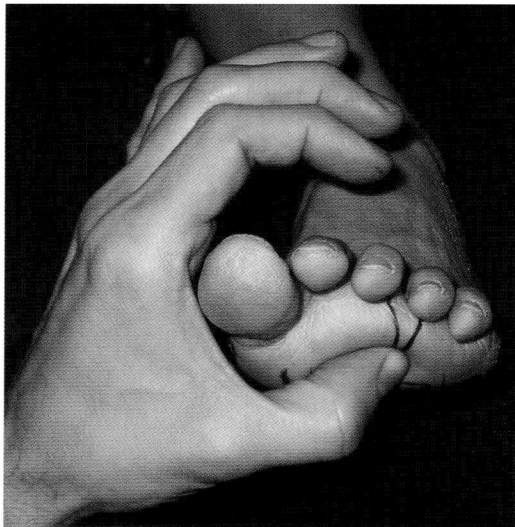

Figure 12-8 Deep palpation test for interdigital neuroma. The examiner should press from plantar to dorsal, avoiding inadvertent dorsal palpation.

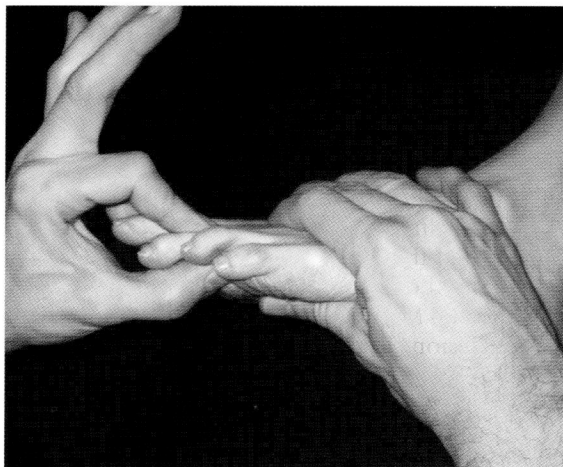

Figure 12-9 A provocative evaluation of metatarsophalangeal joint instability or inflammation is important because these can be either contributing factors or the primary cause of the patient's pain. The metatarsals are stabilized by one hand while the other secures the toe at the base of the proximal phalanx. A dorsal thrust in the sagittal plane can reveal subluxation or dislocation and can induce pain. The patient's symptoms may be either mechanical or neuritic, depending on the pathology.

resection. When the plantar aspect of the foot is palpated, occasionally a mass representing a small synovial cyst or ganglion is observed. Usually, this mass is less than 1 cm in diameter and can be rolled beneath the examiner's fingers. When the mass is associated with a web space, pressure against the mass often reproduces the patient's symptoms. A sensory examination rarely demonstrates any deficit in the patient with a neuroma.

A more complete neurologic examination should include palpation of all the web spaces and along the course of the tibial nerve branches. The tibial nerve itself should be palpated and percussed in the posterior leg, the popliteal space, and behind the femur. Other nerves should be examined, including the sural, saphenous, deep peroneal, and superficial peroneal nerves. A straight-leg maneuver should be performed to rule out radiculopathy when clinically indicated. A quick motor examination, including eversion, inversion, dorsiflexion, and plantar flexion of the toes, foot, and ankle is useful. When warranted, an examination of reflexes is performed. Checking the patient's hands for evidence of intrinsic atrophy or tremor can help identify systemic neurologic conditions.

At times, the patient's physical examination is not conclusive, and the patient needs to be reevaluated on several occasions to ensure that the symptom complex indeed indicates a neuroma. If there is pain around an MTP joint as well as in the web space, caution is advised in making the diagnosis of a neuroma because early degeneration of the plantar pad, early synovitis of the MTP joint, or some degeneration of the plantar fat may be present. It is useful to stress the MTP joint by checking for a dorsal drawer sign and instability of the MTP and induction of symptoms. When undertaking this maneuver, the physician

must secure the base of the toe at the proximal phalanx without inadvertently pressing on the nerve. With the other hand securing the foot at the metatarsals, slight traction is applied to the toe, and an attempt is made to translate the base of the proximal phalanx dorsally. The adjacent and contralateral toes should be checked to determine the baseline joint laxity for the patient (Fig. 12-9). This test may be positive with instability or synovitis, which can coexist with neuralgia, but if the pain is not reproduced with the symptoms, then instability or synovitis is not triggering the neuralgia, or the patient's forefoot pain may be coming from another condition.

Diagnostic Studies

A radiograph of the foot during weight bearing should always be obtained in an evaluation of the patient with a suspected interdigital neuroma. The purpose of the radiographic study is to observe any abnormalities within the osseous structures; subluxation, dislocation, or arthritis of the MTP joint; or possibly evidence of a foreign body.

Schon's (LCS's) opinion is that MRI has not been demonstrated as effective in the diagnosis of an interdigital neuroma. This has been substantiated by a study by Bencardino,[5] who found a lack of correlation of an MRI finding of a neuroma and symptoms in 33% of patients. If there is a question about the presence of other causes of the patient's pain, an MRI may be performed in the prone position[57] using a combination of contrast enhancement and fat suppression.[53] One study by Biasca et al[9] suggested that a more favorable result could be achieved after neuroma resection when the nerve has a transverse measurement larger than 5 mm on MRI scans.

Ultrasound is operator-dependent,[48] and although there are proponents of this imaging technique,[33,43,44] the authors and others do not find it a useful modality.[45,46] This impression has been substantiated in a report by Sharp et al.[50] These authors looked at the accuracy of preoperative clinical assessment, ultrasound, and MRI and compared these findings to intraoperative histology and the clinical outcome. They found the accuracy of the ultrasound and MRI was similar and dependent on lesion size. Small lesions were not well visualized on ultrasound. There was no correlation among the size, the pain score, or the change in pain score after surgery. Reliance on either ultrasound or MRI would have led to an inaccurate diagnosis in 18 of 29 cases. The predictive values attained by clinical assessment surpass imaging with one or both modalities.

No reliable electrodiagnostic studies are available to document the presence of an interdigital neuroma. However, these studies are useful to help identify a proximal entrapment, radiculopathy, or neuropathy when their presence is suspected.

Lidocaine can be injected into the suspected web space for diagnostic purposes. The recommended dose is 1 or 2 mL of anesthetic placed below the transverse metatarsal ligament. Although complete relief of symptoms can be obtained, caution is advised in interpreting this as confirming an interdigital neuroma because this injection may also relieve pain from local pathologic conditions, such as degeneration of the joint capsule or plantar plate. Younger and Claridge[60] performed a study to determine the role of a diagnostic block in predicting the results of surgery. In 37 patients with 41 excisions (7 patients with revisions), 24% of the primary procedures were failures despite relief with a block, and 43% of the 7 revision procedures were failures. Schon performed a recent cadaveric study comparing injection of 1 mL of fluid versus 2 mL into the third web space and found increased extravasation of fluid with the 2-mL dose. Hembree et al[26] found that injection of 1 mL of fluid was sufficient to effectively envelope the nerve but not selective enough to be used diagnostically because, even with a lower dose, there was still a high rate of extravasation into adjacent web spaces.

Administration of cortisone can be useful in about one third of patients, but cortisone can cause deterioration of the joint capsule or possibly the plantar fat. Only infrequently should more than one hydrocortisone injection be made into the web space. In some patients, medial or lateral deviation of the adjacent MTP joint has developed after multiple steroid injections, presumably from damage to a collateral ligament (Fig. 12-10). Decreasing the volume effect of the injection can help diminish the risk of damage to the MTP joint capsule, ligament, or tendon. This can be accomplished by injecting proximal to the MTP joint below the intermetatarsal ligament as opposed to more distally. In addition, if during the injection the

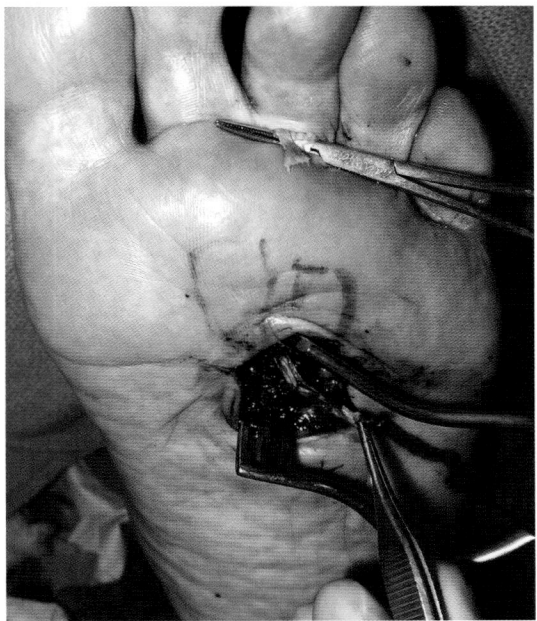

Figure 12-10 Ruptured flexor digitorum brevis tendon after cortisone injections, with resultant instability of the metatarsophalangeal (MTP) joint. The patient required neuroma excision and reconstruction of the tendon and the MTP joint.

Box 12-1	Differential Diagnosis of Interdigital Neuroma

Arthrosis of metatarsophalangeal (MTP) joint
Degeneration of plantar pad or capsule
Degenerative disk disease
Freiberg infraction
Lesion of medial or lateral plantar nerve
Lesions of plantar aspect of foot
Metatarsal stress fracture
Metatarsophalangeal joint disorders
Pain of neurogenic origin unrelated to interdigital neuroma
Peripheral neuropathy
Soft tissue tumor (e.g., lipoma)
Soft tissue tumor not involving MTP joint (e.g., ganglion, lipoma, synovial cyst)
Subluxation or dislocation of MTP joint
Synovial cysts
Synovitis of MTP joint caused by nonspecific synovitis or rheumatoid arthritis
Tarsal tunnel syndrome
Tumor of metatarsal bone

toes begin to spread apart, the injection should be stopped. If the deviation is noted after an injection, the toes should be supported by taping.

Differential Diagnosis

Many other conditions can mimic interdigital neuroma. Box 12-1 provides a differential diagnosis to assist physicians regarding this condition.

Treatment

Conservative Treatment

Conservative management consists of fitting the patient with a wide, soft, laced shoe, preferably with a low heel. This type of shoe allows the foot to spread out and thereby relieves some of the pressure on the metatarsal head region and eliminates the chronic hyperextension of the MTP joints. Thicker compressible rubber–soled shoes can also make a big difference by providing shock attenuation to the forefoot region. A soft metatarsal support is added to the shoe just proximal to the metatarsal head region, which further relieves the pressure from the involved area and helps to spread the metatarsal heads to relieve pressure on the nerves (Fig. 12-11). Occasionally, a soft metatarsal support can be added to a high-heeled shoe, provided sufficient room exists in the toe box area for both the support and the foot (Fig. 12-12). When the

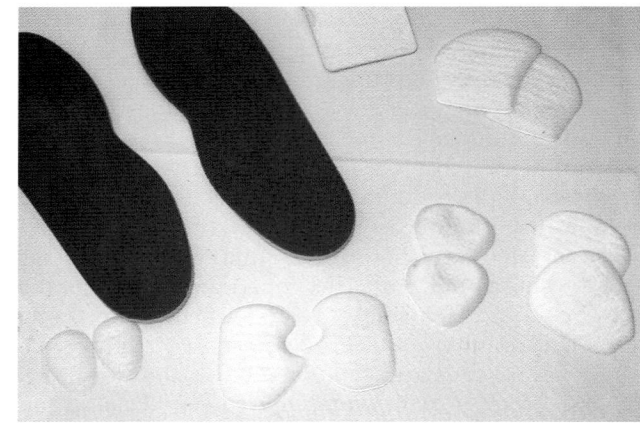

Figure 12-11   A variety of metatarsal pads are available that can be applied to the insole of the shoe or to a generic insole.

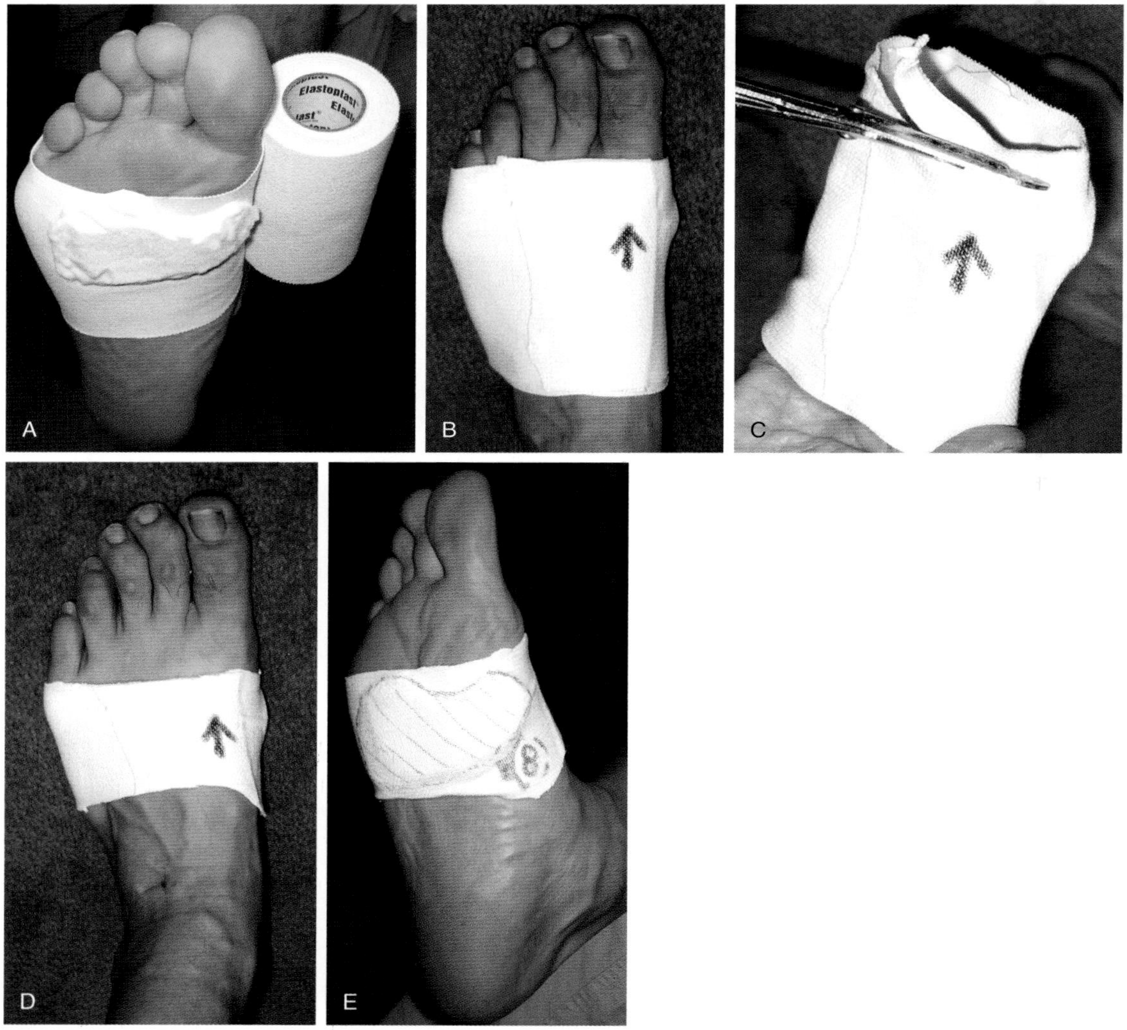

Figure 12-12   This is a useful method for making a temporary transferable metatarsal pad. **A,** The foot is wrapped with adhesive tape (Elastoplast, Johnson & Johnson, New Brunswick, N.J.) with the adhesive side away from the skin. **B,** The felt pad is cut to sit proximal to the metatarsal heads and the sesamoids. **C,** The *arrow* is drawn in line with the great toe to assist the patient in reapplying the pad. **D,** The pad is reapplied with the new trim lines. **E,** Plantar view.

patient has synovitis, instability, or deviation of the MTP, a Budin splint (Fig. 12-13) or canopy toe strapping (Fig. 12-14) can be useful to decrease secondary neuralgia. Shoe modifications, such as a metatarsal bar or rocker sole, can be also helpful (Fig. 12-15).

Injection of the interspace with a local anesthetic may be useful as a diagnostic tool, particularly if there is tenderness in two interspaces of the same foot. However, the effectiveness of the injection depends on the use of a small quantity of anesthetic agent that must be carefully directed to the common digital nerve. If the area is flooded with a large quantity of anesthetic agent, the patient

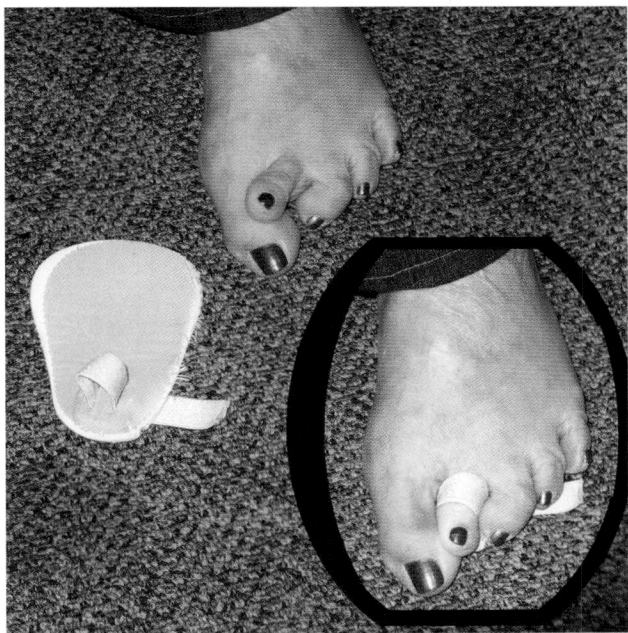

Figure 12-13 The medially deviated toe caused neuritic symptoms in this patient. The Budin splint helped secure the toe in a better position (inset) and minimized the traction on the nerve.

might feel a relief of symptoms, but the test is not very specific for pathologic conditions caused by the nerve.

Steroids can occasionally be helpful but rarely produce long-lasting relief. In a recent study of 39 interdigital neuromas treated with a single corticosteroid injection, Markovic et al[36] reported that 26 (66%) had a positive outcome (completely satisfied or satisfied with minor reservations) at 9 months. However, in a study of 76 cases of suspected interdigital neuroma, Greenfield et al[24] noted significant short-term relief with a series of steroid injections; but only 30% of patients had relief that lasted more than 2 years. Injection of corticosteroids into the area of the suspected neuroma is associated with some problems, and so the injections must be used with a certain degree of caution. Atrophy of the subcutaneous fat and discoloration of the skin can occur and be quite disturbing to the patient. If the injection is placed beyond the nerve, some atrophy of the plantar fat pad can occur. One of the more serious problems is disruption of the joint capsule adjacent to the injection site, with resultant deviation of the toe medially or laterally, depending on which capsule has been involved. This is a very unfortunate consequence of steroid injections and one that then creates a significant new problem for the patient.

Other nonsurgical management options include oral vitamin B_6 100 mg bid; antiinflammatory medications and tricyclic antidepressants (TCAs), such as imipramine (Tofranil), nortriptyline (Pamolar), desipramine (Norpramin), and amitriptyline (Elavil); selective serotonin reuptake inhibitors (SSRIs), such as sertraline (Zoloft); paroxetine (Paxil); other antidepressants, such as venlafaxin (Effexor) or duloxetine (Cymbalta); or antiseizure medications, such as gabapentin (Neurontin), pregabalin (Lyrica), topiramate (Topomax), and carbamazepine (Tegretol). This use of these drugs is off-label, but they have been shown to lessen the severity of nerve-related symptoms. For a more complete discussion of the various medications for chronic pain, consult the American Chronic Pain Association's Resource Guide to Chronic

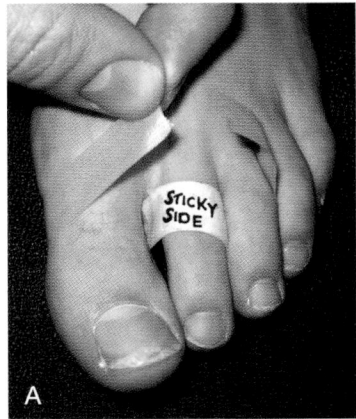 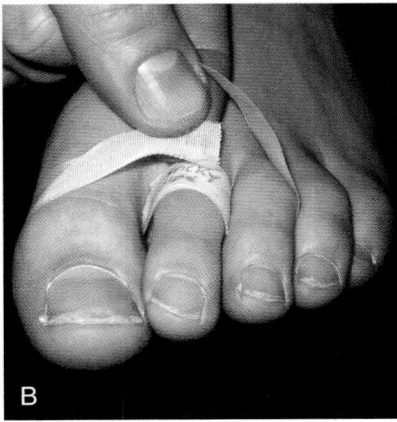 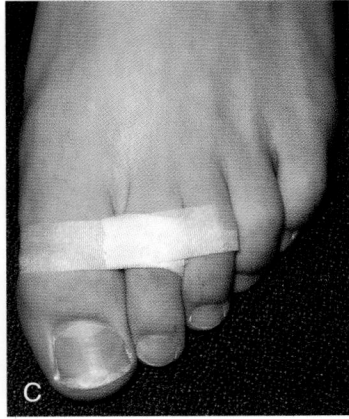

Figure 12-14 A, Canopy toe taping is applied with the adhesive side upward around the second toe. B, The tape goes underneath the first and third toes with the adhesive side against the skin. Enough tension is applied to secure the second metatarsophalangeal joint in neutral position. C, The final appearance.

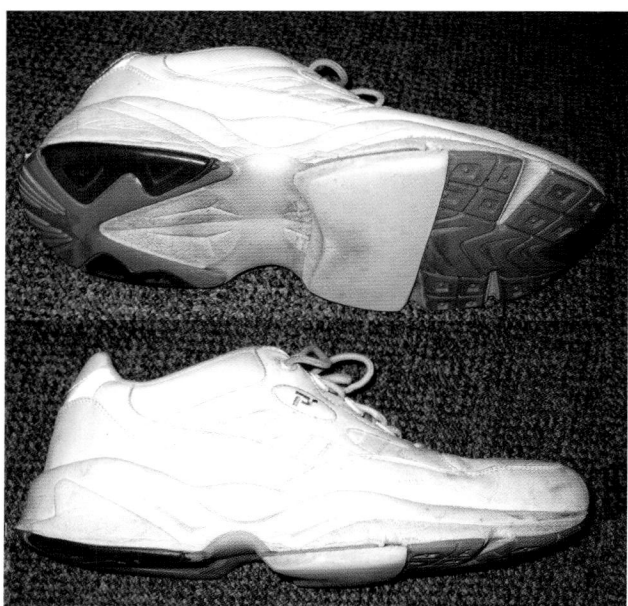

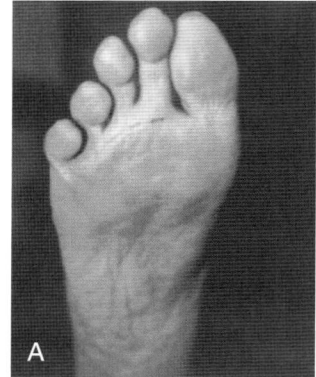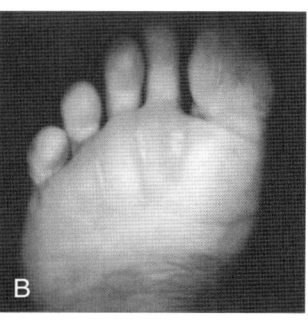

Figure 12-16   Examples of scars from plantar incisions used to excise interdigital neuroma. **A,** Transverse scar at the base of the toes can remain painful. Because of the location of the scar, the nerve is not resected proximally enough and often becomes symptomatic once again. **B,** Multiple longitudinal incisions resulted in atrophy of fat pad and some mild hyperkeratosis of scars. This results in chronic metatarsal pain.

Pain Medication & Treatment.[1] Schon recommends considering these medications for diffuse or atypical forefoot neuralgia or when there is a history of a more proximal nerve lesion.

Radiofrequency ablation and alcohol nerve injections have been proposed as less traumatic, more conservative methods of treating neuromas. Fanucci et al[18] reported their results with 40 interdigital neuroma injections with alcohol (70% carbocaine-adrenaline and 30% ethyl alcohol) under ultrasound guidance. Total or partial symptomatic relief was obtained in 90% of cases without complications. There was temporary plantar pain in 15%. Although the authors claimed the technique was feasible and cost-efficient and had high rates of therapeutic success, further investigation is warranted. In contrast, Espinosa et al[17] reported symptomatic relief in only 7 of 32 (22%) patients with MRI-confirmed interdigital neuroma who were treated with alcohol sclerosing therapy.

Most patients seem to respond fairly well to initial conservative management in that they obtain some relief of their clinical symptoms. Occasionally, the physical findings of localized pain in the involved interspace improve, but as a general rule they do not. The majority of patients continue to have symptoms, and in time, 60% to 70% elect excision of the neuroma. Not infrequently, this choice of surgical management is made because of the patient's desire to be able to wear high-heeled shoes, even though they are often comfortable in their low, soft shoes.

Surgical Treatment
SURGICAL EXCISION
An interdigital neuroma may be excised through a dorsal or a plantar approach. The main advantage of the dorsal approach is prevention of scar formation on the plantar aspect of the foot. With a dorsal approach, if the incision is not kept in the midline or is made too proximal, one of the dorsal cutaneous nerves to the web space may be disrupted or become painful, but this is an unusual complication. The plantar approach, although it sounds simple, must be accurately placed in the interspace so that it does not pass directly beneath the metatarsal head. When this incision is made, it is important that it be carried deeply down through the thick plantar fat to expose the nerve and the web space. Dissection performed medially or laterally only creates scarring of the fatty tissue; as a result, the scar can become somewhat puckered, or the fat pad beneath a metatarsal head can become atrophic (Fig 12-16).

Alternative plantar approaches include either longitudinal or transverse incisions proximal to the metatarsal head. These can avoid the painful scar in the weight-bearing area of the foot. Exposure of the nerve is usually quite easy, but for the surgeon who is unfamiliar with the anatomy from this perspective, it can be a challenge. If a keloid develops from any plantar incision, the symptoms can become very difficult to rectify. Thus, for treatment of a primary interdigital neuralgia, the dorsal approach is preferred.

A dorsal Y-incision centered over the metatarsal has been described for the treatment of adjacent interdigital neuromas, although, as discussed earlier, the presence of multiple neuromas in the same foot is exceedingly rare.[47]

Surgical Technique
1. With or without tourniquet control, an incision is made in the dorsal aspect of the foot, starting in the web space between the involved toes. The incision is carried proximally for about 3 cm to the level of the metatarsal head. It is important to keep the incision

directly in the midline because deviation to either side can result in cutting one of the dorsal digital nerves, which could cause a painful neuroma (Fig. 12-17 and Video Clip 86).

2. The incision is deepened through the soft tissue to the level of the metatarsal heads. A Weitlaner retractor or laminar spreader is placed between the metatarsal heads to gain optimal exposure (Fig. 12-18). This places the transverse metatarsal ligament under significant tension. If there is difficulty inserting the spreader

or retractor, a hemostat can be inserted between the metatarsals first to facilitate its placement.

3. Use of a neurologic Freer elevator to dissect the contents of the interspace allows the transverse metatarsal ligament to be identified and transected (Fig. 12-19).

4. The retractor or spreader is removed, set deeper between the metatarsal heads, and spread. This allows visualization of the contents of the web space. The neurologic Freer elevator allows the common digital nerve to be identified in the proximal portion of the wound, and it is traced distally to its bifurcation. Digital pressure under the web space from the plantar aspect pushes the nerve more dorsally and facilitates visualization.

5. Once the bifurcation is reached, a significant amount of soft tissue, sometimes almost appearing bursa-like, may be around the nerve. If possible, this tissue should be removed so that the nerve can be followed past the bifurcation. However, if the adhesions are too great, all this material is removed along with the nerve rather than taking the time to carefully dissect it. When the interspace is explored, the surgeon should look carefully for any accessory branches that might be coming out from beneath the adjacent metatarsal head to identify them and alter the treatment plan, if necessary. Whenever possible, preservation of the vascular structures is advantageous.

6. In the proximal portion of the wound, the common digital nerve is cut proximal to the metatarsal head, dissected out distally past the bifurcation, and excised (Fig. 12-20). As little plantar fat as possible should be removed (Fig. 12-21). If a significant accessory nerve trunk passing to the common nerve either medially or laterally is observed, the consequences of cutting this nerve and allowing it to retract under the metatarsal head area must be considered. If the nerve trunk appears to be larger than 2 mm, rather than resecting the neuroma proximal to the metatarsal heads, the common nerve should be cut just proximal to its bifurcation, which is also just proximal to the thickening

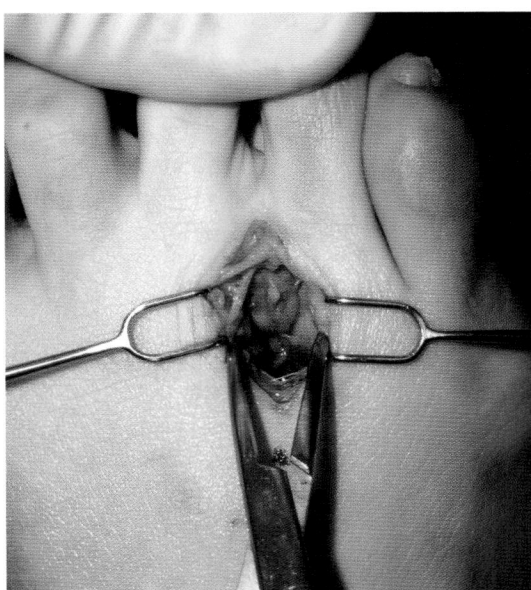

Figure 12-17   The dorsal nerve branches can be encountered—here on the medial side of the incision—during the exposure of the interdigital neuroma.

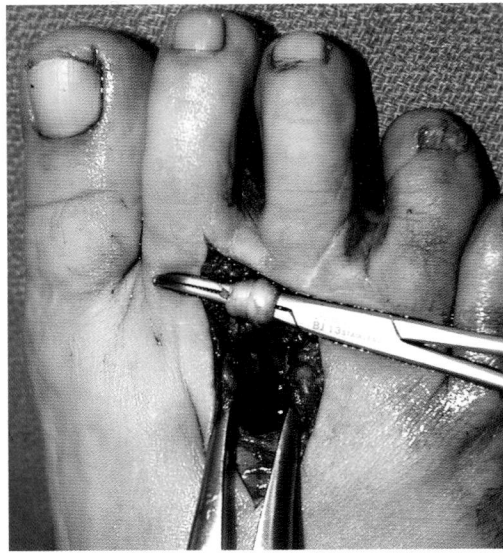

Figure 12-18   The laminar spreader between the metatarsals facilitates exposure.

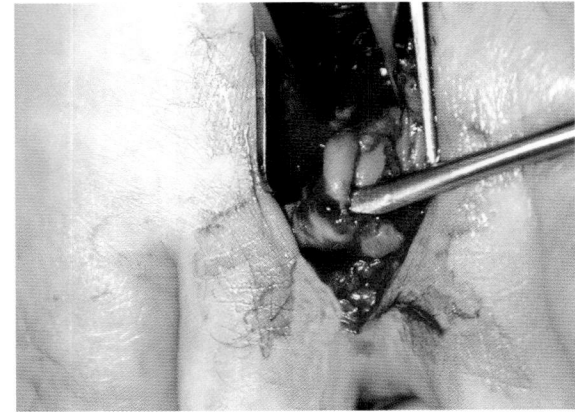

Figure 12-19   The Freer elevator is used to help identify the nerve and dissect the contents of the interspace.

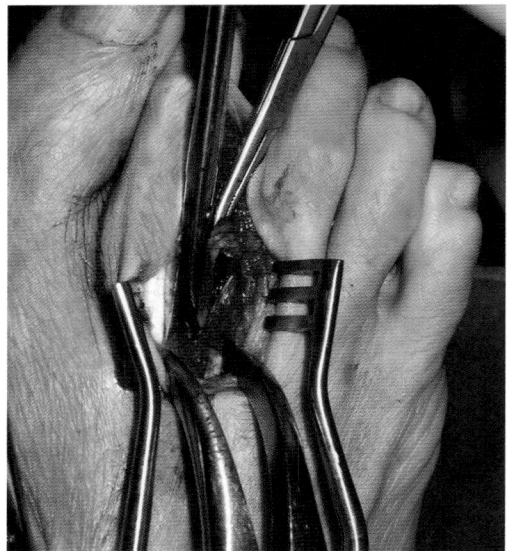

Figure 12-20 The proximal aspect of the nerve is transected beyond the metatarsal heads.

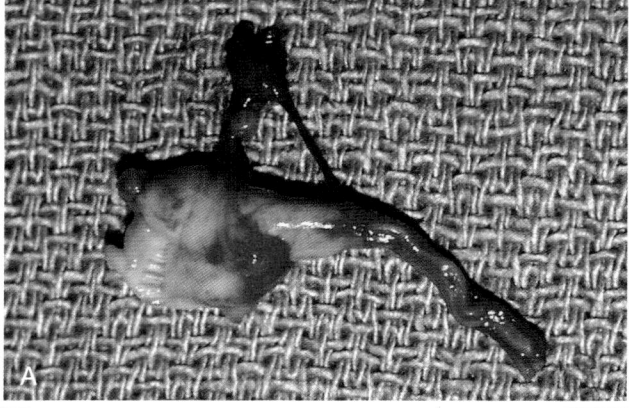

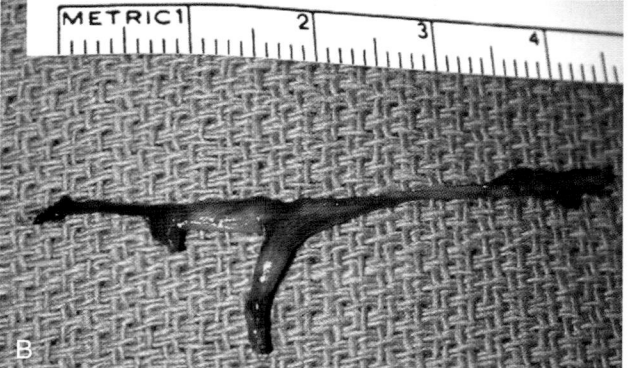

Figure 12-21 Two examples of neuromas. **A,** A thin neuroma is noted with its bifurcation. **B,** A large bulbous neuroma with a thickened bifurcation.

usually observed in the nerve distal to the transverse metatarsal ligament. The distal portion of the nerve is removed. The cut end is sutured to the side of the metatarsal or one of the intrinsic muscles so that it will not drop onto the plantar aspect of the foot. By placing

the nerve alongside the metatarsal off the bottom of the foot when the stump neuroma forms, it will not be in a weight-bearing position. When this is carried out, it is important that the nerve not be under any tension when it is sutured.

7. The skin is closed in a single layer, and a comfortable compression dressing is applied.

Postoperative Care

The patient is permitted to ambulate in a postoperative shoe. The sutures are removed between 7 and 14 days. A compressive wrap is used for 2 to 5 weeks, after which the patient is encouraged to work on active and passive range-of-motion exercises.

Uncommon Findings

Excision of an interdigital neuroma usually is a straight-forward procedure. Occasionally, a large bursa is found between the metatarsal heads, in particular in the third interspace, and must be removed to expose the underlying nerve. This is carried out by sharp dissection, with care taken not to remove any plantar fat. An accessory nerve trunk may be encountered, as mentioned earlier; if it is greater than 2 mm in diameter, the nerve distal to it can be excised and the nerve sutured to the side of the metatarsal to prevent formation of a recurrent neuroma beneath the metatarsal head. We estimate that this accessory nerve is noted in about 10% of neuromas.

Occasionally, a cyst, which usually consists of material that appears to be degenerated fat, is identified adjacent to a metatarsal head. This does not appear to be a true cyst but does have a somewhat irregular lining. When present, it should be unroofed, but again, as little fat as possible is removed to prevent atrophy of the fat pad beneath a metatarsal head.

Results

An analysis of patients in a series by Mann and Reynolds[35] after excision of an interdigital neuroma demonstrated the following results: 71% essentially asymptomatic, 9% significantly improved, 6% marginally improved, and 14% failure.

The patients who had marginal improvement with surgical failure were carefully reevaluated, with no evidence of other pathologic findings that would account for the persistent pain, such as synovitis of the MTP joint, subluxation of the MTP joint, or the presence of a neuroma in an adjacent web space. Obviously, a certain group of patients have a condition similar to an interdigital neuroma, which clinically is not fully understood at this time. The results for those patients in whom a neuroma was removed from the second web space and third web space were the same. Other follow-up studies of patients after excision of an interdigital neuroma have demonstrated similar results.[11]

Physical examination of the satisfied patient population demonstrated the following postoperative findings: local plantar pain, 65%; numbness in the interspace,

68%; and area of plantar numbness adjacent to the interspace, 51%.

Not infrequently, although the patient believed that the neuritic pain was gone, some discomfort was still noted on the plantar aspect of the foot. At times, this was described as a feeling as if a sock was wrinkled under the foot or a feeling of stepping on a piece of cotton. The fact that 32% of the patients still had normal sensation in the web space after complete excision of their interdigital neuroma indicates the degree of overlap that is present in the innervation of the area. It is also important to consider this when one is evaluating a patient with a recurrent neuroma because the presence of sensation does not necessarily mean that the neuroma has not been adequately excised. About half the patients noted some numbness on the plantar aspect of the foot adjacent to the interspace. This probably results from the plantar innervation that comes off the common digital nerve, which is disrupted when the nerve is excised.

Coughlin and Pinsonneault[13] reported on 66 patients with an average of 5.8 years' follow-up. Overall satisfaction was rated as excellent or good by 85%, but 65% were pain free, with minor or major footwear restrictions. Major activity restrictions after surgery were uncommon. Subjective numbness was present but variable in pattern in half of the patients' feet. The numbness was bothersome in 4 of 71 feet. Patients with bilateral neuroma excision or adjacent neuroma resection had a slightly lower level of satisfaction, but this difference was not significant.

Giannini et al[20] reported on 60 patients (three bilateral) who were treated with excision of interdigital neuroma. The clinical results were excellent or good in 49 (78%) feet, fair in 12 (19%), and poor in two (3%). Of these patients, 62% had normal sensation and no paresthesias, and the remaining 38% had numbness; 57% had no difficulty with footwear, and 40% had some limitation.

Womack et al[59] reported on the long-term results of 120 patients who underwent surgical excision of interdigital neuroma. At an average follow-up of 66.7 (range, 14-113) months, 61 patients (51%) had good or excellent results, indicating that long-term outcomes may be less favorable than short-term to midterm outcomes. An interesting finding was that patients with neuromas in the second web space had statistically significant worse outcomes than those with third web-space neuromas.

Benedetti et al[6] reported on 15 patients (19 feet) who underwent simultaneous surgical excision of two primary interdigital neuromas in adjacent web spaces, with an average follow-up of 68.6 months. Ten feet (53%) had complete resolution of symptoms, 6 feet (31%) had minimal residual symptoms, and 3 feet in two patients (16%) continued to have significant pain. The authors reported a dense sensory loss of the plantar aspect of the third metatarsal head to the tip of the third toe and proximal dorsal sensory loss to the second, third, and fourth toes. Although the numbness did not cause disability, the patients reported some awkwardness with nail care.

Hort and DeOrio[28] described another approach for adjacent web-space neuralgia when using a single incision, with excision of one nerve and release of the adjacent nerve. Twenty-three patients were studied, with a mean follow-up of 11 months. Of the patients, 19 (90%) had resolution of all or most of their pain, 20 (95%) had no or only minimal activity limitation, and 20 (95%) were completely satisfied with their outcome. Of 19 patients examined, none had pain with compression of the interspace of the excised nerve, although 2 (11%) had discomfort with compression of the interspace of the nerve that was only released.

A few complications deserve mention. In cases where patients had multiple steroid shots followed by surgery, there is an additional risk of wound complications, such as delayed healing or infection. When adjacent web-space neuromas have been resected, the loss of sensation in the tip of the middle toe, possibly coupled with some vascular compromise, can increase the risk of frostbite in the winter. Su et al[52] examined 674 consecutive pathologic specimens obtained after interdigital neurectomy and found that the adjacent digital artery was resected in 39% of cases. Clinically, no adverse effects were reported. Stress fracture or damage to the MTP capsule can occur if the retraction is too vigorous or the tissue or bone is incompetent. Rarely, a patient can develop complex pain syndrome type 2 (causalgia) after a neuroma resection.

PLANTAR INCISION FOR RESECTION OF THE ATYPICAL NEUROMA

When the patient has a very proximal, focal, tender trigger point for the neuralgia, Schon uses a transverse approach proximal to the metatarsal plantar fat. This permits a more direct exposure of the nerve that lies plantar to the intermetatarsal ligament and just beneath the plantar fascia and next to the flexor digitorum tendon. It allows the nerve resection to be performed off of the weight-bearing surface of the forefoot as well as resection more proximal to the level of the transverse metatarsal ligament. It permits identification of anomalous nerve branches that can anastomose with the site of the neuroma and provides easier access to adjacent digital nerves with minimal dissection through soft tissues. Finally, there is a better ability to avoid the artery and vein, which is advantageous for patients with vascular compromise. Disadvantages primarily are the potential for development of painful plantar scars or plantar keratosis.

There are two types of incisions: transverse and longitudinal. Transverse incision permits greater exposure for multiple nerve dissections. A transverse incision made 1 cm proximal to the weight-bearing region allows exposure of the adjacent interdigital nerve. It also facilitates identification of accessory or aberrant nerve branches. Avoidance of the artery, vein, and tendon is easier because the dissection is proximal to where these structures are more intermingled. The incision is within the skin fold lines, making the scar cosmetic and well tolerated. Because the exposure is proximal to the disease, the surgeon must be comfortable that nothing in the web space requires resection. Some experience is necessary to be comfortable with this approach and the orientation. The longitudinal incision is also reported to be cosmetic because it runs parallel to the lines of the connective tissue fibers. It can be continued distally between the metatarsal heads or proximally into the midfoot or hindfoot. This permits identification and resection of distal disease as well as higher transection with or without nerve burial (transposition).

Surgical Technique: Transverse Approach

1. The incision should be made 1 cm proximal to the weight-bearing area of the metatarsal heads (Fig. 12-22).
2. Dissection should be performed straight down through the subcutaneous fat and then immediately through the plantar fascia to avoid creating soft tissue planes.
3. The interdigitial nerve will be exposed immediately deep to the plantar fascia within the fatty tissue between the flexor digitorum longus tendons.
4. Aberrant or accessory nerve branches can be identified in this area.
5. The nerve can be transected proximally.
6. Adjacent interdigital neuromas can be approached by widening the incision (Fig. 12-23).
7. The wound is closed with 4-0 nylon suture.
8. A compression dressing is applied for 10 to 14 days until sutures are removed.
9. A wrap is recommended for 1 to 2 more weeks as the patient is allowed to progress with weight bearing.

Surgical Technique: Longitudinal Approach

1. The incision should be centered directly over the inter-metatarsal space so that any subsequent scarring will not take place directly under the metatarsal head. Typically, the incision should be made approximately 1 to 2 cm proximal to the proximal end of the metatarsal head.

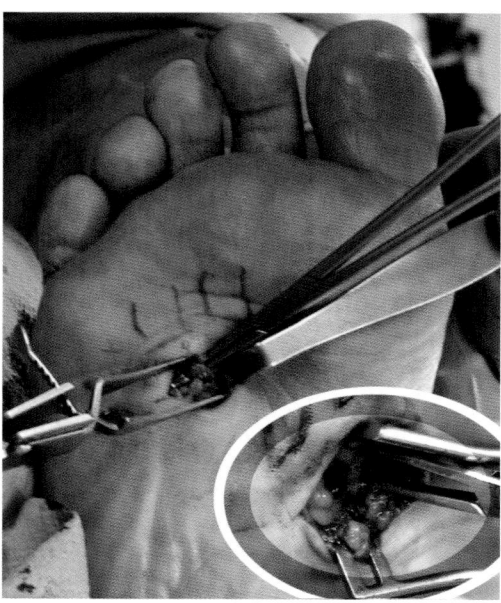

Figure 12-22 A transverse incision is made 1 cm proximal to the weight-bearing area of the metatarsal heads. The plantar fascia is cut, and the hemostat is used to spread between the long flexor tendons. As the hemostat is spread, the nerve is apparent as demonstrated in the *inset*.

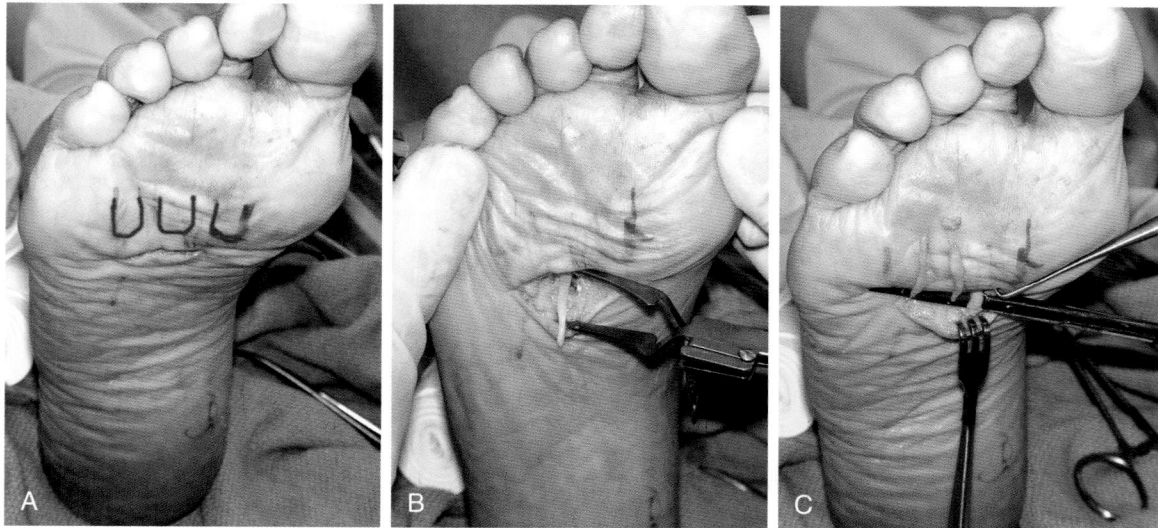

Figure 12-23 Adjacent interdigital neuroma can be approached by widening the incision. **A,** The incision is made 1 cm proximal to the metatarsal heads. **B,** A thin second web-space nerve is found distally traveling underneath the third metatarsal head. **C,** The third web-space nerve is found going between the third and fourth metatarsal heads. With further dissection in the second web space, a larger nerve is found traveling between the second and third metatarsal heads.

2. Dissection should be performed straight down through the subcutaneous fat and then immediately through the plantar fascia to avoid creating soft tissue planes.

3. The interdigitial nerve will be exposed immediately deep to the plantar fascia within the fatty tissue between the flexor digitorum longus tendons (Fig. 12-24).

4. Aberrant or accessory nerve branches can be identified in this area.

5. The nerve can be transected as proximally as possible or kept slightly longer to permit transposition into muscle (Fig. 12-25).

6. When a transposition is performed, the end of the transected nerve's epineurium can be held with a 4-0 Vicryl suture. The suture is fed through a straight needle (Keith needle), and the needle is passed through muscles between the metatarsal. It then penetrates the dorsum of the foot. With the nerve end within the muscle belly, the suture can be tied on the dorsum to help keep the nerve in place during the first 10 to 14 days.

7. The wound is closed with 4-0 nylon suture.

8. A compression dressing is applied for 10 to 14 days until sutures are removed.

9. A wrap is recommended for 1 to 2 more weeks as the patient is allowed to progress with weight bearing.

NEUROLYSIS OF THE COMMON DIGITAL NERVE AND ITS TERMINAL BRANCHES

The notion that an interdigital neuroma is caused by entrapment of the plantar digital nerve by the intermetatarsal ligament and bursa was initially discussed by Gauthier.[19] Okafor et al[42] also thought that it was a nerve entrapment and recommended neurolysis of the interdigital nerve 1 cm distal to the transverse metatarsal ligament and 3 cm proximal to it. Several other reports have discussed the techniques and outcomes of either an open or endoscopic release of the nerve. Further midterm and

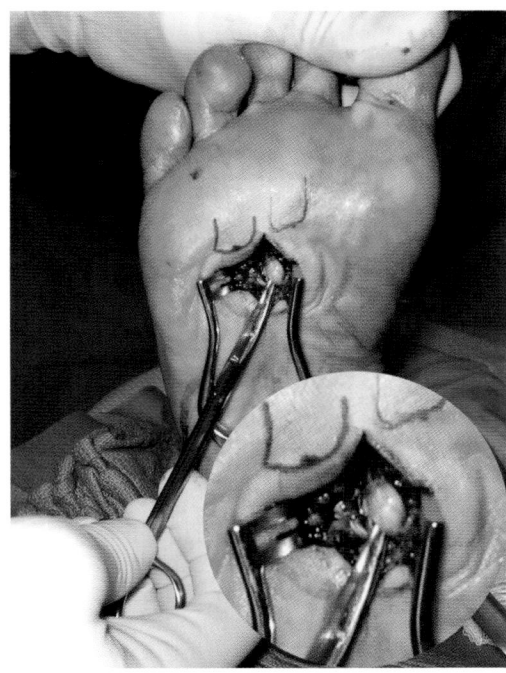

Figure 12-24 The plantar longitudinal incision is made over the intermetatarsal space so that any subsequent scarring will not take place directly under the metatarsals. *Inset,* the bulbous neuroma.

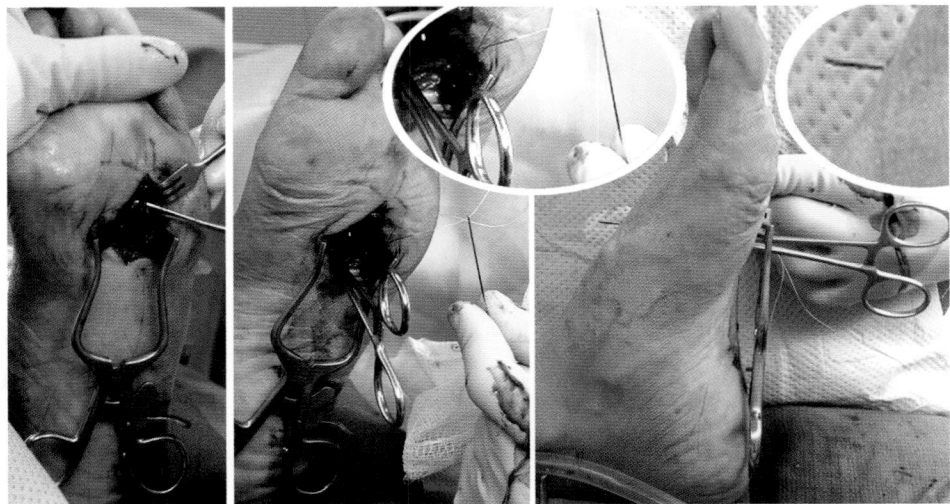

Figure 12-25 This patient had a recurrent neuroma and a history of a postoperative infection and complex regional pain syndrome type II. The nerve is transected more proximally in this operation *(left)*. The transected nerve's epineurium can be held with a 4-0 Vicryl suture. The suture is fed through a straight needle (Keith needle) *(center; inset shows close-up)*. The needle is passed through muscles between the metatarsals and out the dorsum of the foot *(right; inset shows close-up of dorsum)*. The suture is loosely tied on the dorsum to help keep the nerve ending in place within the muscles. This dorsal suture is removed in 10 to 14 days.

long-term studies are needed to determine the results and the best candidates for these procedures.[4,15,38,47,49]

Surgical Technique

1. With or without tourniquet control, an incision is made in the web space and carried proximally approximately 3 cm. It is important that the incision is made in the midline to avoid cutting one of the dorsal digital branches, which could result in a painful neuroma.
2. The incision is deepened through the soft tissues to the level of the metatarsal heads. A Weitlaner retractor or laminar spreader is placed between the metatarsal heads to spread them apart; this places the transverse metatarsal ligament under tension.
3. Using a neurologic Freer elevator to dissect out the contents of the interspace, the surgeon identifies and transects the transverse metatarsal ligament.
4. The retractor is removed and set deeper between the metatarsal heads and spread. This permits the surgeon to visualize the contents of the web space. A neurologic Freer elevator is used to identify the common digital nerve in the proximal portion of the wound and trace it distally to its bifurcation.
5. At this point, a neurolysis is performed, first by carefully excising any bursal material that may be present about the bifurcation of the common digital nerve. The presence of bursal material proximal to the transverse metatarsal ligament is rare. Then, any adhesions between the nerve and the surrounding tissues are carefully released. Caution is necessary, because plantar-directed nerve branches pass from the plantar aspect of the nerve into the tissue on the bottom of the foot.[2] Transection of these nerves can result in a painful plantar neuroma.
6. Once the nerve is freed from approximately 3 cm proximal to the intermetatarsal ligament and 1 cm distal to it, an adequate dissection has been achieved. If the nerve is inadvertently damaged during dissection, it should be excised in the usual manner as far proximal to the metatarsal heads as possible, dissected distally, and removed at the level of the bifurcation.
7. The wound is closed in a routine manner with interrupted nylon sutures.
8. A sterile compression dressing is applied, and the foot is kept wrapped for a period of 2 to 3 weeks to allow the soft tissues to heal.
9. After 3 weeks, the patient can progressively increase the level of activities.

Results

In describing their results in a series of 35 patients, Okafor et al[42] noted that if the patient had no foot disorder other than the interdigital neuroma, 13 (72%) of 18 patients noted 100% relief of symptoms after neurolysis. If the patient had a common foot disorder, such as a hallux valgus or hammer toe, 5 (30%) of 17 had complete relief, and 12 (70%) of 17 still had some symptoms. In 20 of their patients who underwent a lidocaine (Xylocaine) block before surgery with complete relief, 15 (75%) patients noted complete relief postoperatively, and 5 (25%) had significant relief.

Villas et al[56] retrospectively reviewed 69 cases of interdigital neuroma treated surgically through a dorsal approach. In cases (46 of 69) in which there was macroscopic thickening, the nerve was resected. Otherwise, a neurolysis was performed (23 of 69 cases). They noted equivalent results between the two groups.

RECURRENT INTERDIGITAL NEUROMAS

Recurrent symptoms after resection of an interdigital neuroma are very disheartening for both the patient and the surgeon. In a review of 39 patients with recurrent neuromas, Beskin and Baxter[3] noted that two thirds had symptoms within 12 months after the original surgery, and one third had symptoms 1 to 4 years after the initial surgery. The problem of a recurrent neuroma may be viewed in two ways. Patients in whom the clinical picture is similar to an interdigital neuroma, but unfortunately is not, and who continue to have symptoms in the foot after the initial surgery, probably represent the two thirds of the patients noted by Beskin and Baxter[7] who had recurrence of their symptoms within 12 months after the original surgery. In most, the initial symptoms probably never subside.

In the second group of patients, the symptoms are caused by a bulb neuroma that forms at the end of the common digital nerve. In most cases, it probably takes at least a year or more for the neuroma to be of sufficient size for symptoms to develop. This probably represents the one third of the patients in the series who had symptoms 1 to 4 years after the initial surgery. The recurrent neuroma could develop because the resection of the nerve initially was not sufficiently proximal to the metatarsal head. This could then result in a neuroma forming beneath the metatarsal head, possibly because of an aberrant branch, as noted earlier, and in some cases for reasons that are not well understood.

In discussing an anatomic basis for a recurrent neuroma, Amis et al[2] noted that plantar-directed nerve branches tether the common digital nerve to the plantar skin. These branches are concentrated about the bifurcation of the proper digital nerve, and therefore the cut end of the nerve can fail to retract. The authors observed that no plantar branches occurred 4 cm proximal to the transverse metatarsal ligament. Therefore an effort should be made to cut the nerve 4 cm proximal to the transverse metatarsal ligament to ensure that the nerve adequately retracts. Another way to ensure that the nerve will retract is to dorsiflex the ankle joint after the nerve has been transected, thereby pulling the nerve into a more proximal position. The surgical site can be examined to see whether the nerve has indeed retracted, and if not, then a more proximal resection can be considered.

In approximately three fourths of patients with a recurrent neuroma, the cause is either inadequate resection of the nerve or the formation of an adherent neuroma beneath a metatarsal head.

Johnson et al[29] reviewed a series of 39 patients with recurrent interdigital neuroma. In 67% of cases, they observed a retained primary interdigital neuroma because it was not adequately resected initially, and in 33%, a true amputation stump neuroma was the cause of the recurrent symptoms.

Clinical Symptoms

The main symptom of patients with a recurrent neuroma is pain on the plantar aspect of the foot. The pain may be similar to the initial preoperative pain, or an extremely painful area can develop that causes significant electric-like pain with weight bearing. The symptom complex is aggravated by activity and diminished by rest.

Some patients who have persistent pain after excision of a neuroma report that the pain is almost identical to what they experienced before their initial surgery. Other patients note that the new pain is different, well localized, and electric-like in quality.

Diagnosis

Physical examination in this group of patients must be carefully performed in the same manner as that for a primary neuroma. The MTP joints should be carefully palpated to look for other disorders, along with careful palpation of the web spaces. As a general rule, the patient with a recurrent neuroma demonstrates a well-localized area of tenderness, usually either beneath the metatarsal head or just adjacent to it. Palpation of this area by the examiner usually elicits a significant electric-like pain, and the patient states that this is similar to the symptomatic pain.

At times, the pain is along the medial or lateral aspect of a metatarsal head and can represent either a stump neuroma that has become adherent to the metatarsal head or possibly an accessory branch that sometimes passes obliquely beneath the metatarsal head. It is possible that the recurrent symptoms represent an activated adjacent web-space neuroma. This can be confusing to both the surgeon and the patient based on symptoms and findings and can require a nerve block for final distinction. Unfortunately, response to a nerve block is helpful but not reliably conclusive. Rarely, the neuritic symptoms are coming from a damaged dorsal nerve branch.

Patients who have well-localized findings and who demonstrate a Tinel sign in a small area usually respond best to repeat surgery. The response to the diagnostic block is also helpful to predict a success. After the physical examination, a radiographic study of the foot should be obtained to look for any osseous pathologic conditions or changes around the MTP joints.

The differential diagnosis presented for a virgin interdigital neuroma should be once again considered in a patient with a recurrent neuroma. Careful examination of the posterior tibial nerve and its terminal branches should be carried out to rule out a tarsal tunnel syndrome as the cause of the recurrent symptoms. Schon has seen several patients with growing or recurrent neurilemmomas or ganglions involving the tibial nerve or its branches incorrectly diagnosed as recurrent neuromas.

Treatment

Conservative Treatment

Conservative management of recurrent neuroma is similar to that for the virgin neuroma. The patient should wear a broad-toed, soft-soled, laced shoe with a soft metatarsal support to relieve pressure on the metatarsal head region and interspace. The medications to help diminish nerve excitation (e.g., tricyclic antidepressants, antiepilepsy medications) discussed under the conservative treatment of interdigital neuromas deserve more consideration here because a subgroup of these patients has severe symptoms and underlying nerve sensitivity. If conservative measures fail and the symptoms persist, reexploration of the interspace may be indicated.

Occasionally, the use of a transcutaneous nerve stimulator or ultrasound is useful in helping to break up the patient's pain pattern. These modalities are useful in only about 10% to 20% of cases but merit a try.

Surgical Excision

Before reexploration of an interspace, the foot should be carefully examined to attempt to localize the neuroma as accurately as possible. This helps to direct the surgeon to the area where the patient experiences maximum pain and sometimes can save needless searching in the interspace.

The question arises, at times, as to whether the recurrent neuroma should be explored from a plantar or a dorsal approach. The web space can be adequately explored from a dorsal approach, although the incision must be extended proximally slightly more (1 cm) than when removing a virgin neuroma. Advocates of a plantar approach to a recurrent neuroma think that the neuroma should be approached through a longitudinal plantar incision centered between the metatarsal heads and the nerve identified and resected proximally to the metatarsal head. They point out that it is easier to find the nerve in most cases.

The other school of thought is that because so much scarring is present around the area where the nerve had been previously excised, it is better to approach the common digital nerve proximal to the metatarsal heads and section the nerve in this region without exploring the interspace distally. In a study with this approach, 86% of 39 patients obtained significant improvement of 50% of their discomfort, but fewer than half the patients were completely symptom-free. Fifty-eight percent had difficulty wearing certain shoes, and 88% had discomfort in high heels.[3]

An analysis of seven patients with 11 recurrent neuromas excised through a dorsal incision demonstrated that 81% of the patients were essentially asymptomatic, 9% had marginal improvement, and 9% had no improvement. Conversely, Bradley et al[11] noted that only two of eight patients had improvement after surgery.

Stamatis and Myerson[51] reported on reexploration in 60 interspaces (49 patients, 49 feet) for recurrence or persistent symptoms after one or more previous procedures for excision of an interdigital neuroma, with an average follow-up of 39.7 months. Ten patients had simultaneous excision of an adjacent primary neuroma, and 19 underwent additional forefoot surgery. Fifteen patients (30.7%) were completely satisfied, 13 (26.5%) were satisfied with minor reservations, 10 (20.4%) were satisfied with major reservations, and 11 (22.4%) were dissatisfied with the outcome. Twenty-nine (59.2%) had moderate or severe restriction of footwear, and 8 (16.3%) had moderate restriction of activity after revision surgery.

Wolfort and Dellon[58] reported their results with 17 recurrent neuromas in 13 patients. At a mean of 33.8 months, 80% had excellent relief with a plantar longitudinal approach and implantation of the nerve ending into muscle. The authors also identified deficits along the tibial nerve territory by quantitative sensory examination in 54% of their patients.

Colgrove et al[12] performed a prospective, randomized study comparing the treatment of an interdigital neuroma by the standard resection operation with a transection distal to the neuroma and transposition into muscle. The follow-up was by blinded telephone interview. In the resection group, the average pain level was slightly lower through the first 6-month period, but at the 12-month review, the resection group had a slightly higher average pain level. At the 36- to 48-month review, the resection group again reported a greater average pain level and fewer asymptomatic patients. The authors concluded that it is unnecessary to excise the interdigital neuroma to obtain excellent relief of pain. They also concluded that intermuscular transposition of the neuroma produced significantly better long-term results than did the standard resection operation.

Overall, reexploration for a recurrent neuroma through either a dorsal or a plantar incision results in less than complete satisfaction in 20% to 40% of cases. This fact should be very carefully explained to the patient before surgery.

Because choosing the approach can present a dilemma for the surgeon, Schon's group recommends proceeding with the technique that is most familiar. If there is no bias based on experience, suggest the following algorithm, which is based on whether the primary neuroma excision was sufficiently proximal and whether there is an adjacent neuralgia. If there is a small dorsal incision, it is possible that the resection was not adequate and a repeat transection can be made through a longer dorsal incision. If there is an adjacent neuralgia in this scenario, either a release or resection is performed via the dorsal approach. If the incision was long enough or the primary surgeon thought that the nerve was taken back sufficiently, then a plantar approach is considered. If there is an adjacent primary neuroma as well, then a plantar transverse approach is to be considered. If the same nerve is the site of the recurrent neuroma, then a plantar longitudinal incision can permit a more proximal transection and burial.

EXCISION OF RECURRENT NEUROMA
Surgical Technique
1. The skin incision is made in the dorsal aspect of the web space, usually passing through the previous scar for a distance of 4 cm. If there is evidence of entrapment of a superficial nerve adjacent to the scar, an attempt should be made to identify it and excise it. The incision is carried down through the scar tissue in the web space by staying as much in the midline as possible.
2. A Weitlaner retractor is placed between the two metatarsals to pry them apart. In a recurrent neuroma, this is sometimes difficult to do until the dissection has been carried down through the transverse metatarsal ligament. A neurologic Freer elevator usually can be used to break up the scar tissue between the two metatarsals to identify the transverse metatarsal ligament.
3. Although the transverse metatarsal ligament might have been transected initially, it almost invariably re-forms and needs to be identified and sectioned again.
4. After the transverse metatarsal ligament is cut, the Weitlaner retractor should be reinserted more plantarward and is used to separate the metatarsal heads. If the metatarsal heads cannot be adequately separated, a portion of the transverse metatarsal ligament is still intact or some dense scar tissue has not been transected.
5. By using a neurologic Freer elevator and starting as proximal as possible in the wound, preferably in tissue that was not previously involved, one can identify the common digital nerve. As already mentioned, before surgery the examination should reveal the approximate location of the neuroma, and this is very helpful at surgery. Occasionally, if the nerve cannot be identified, the skin incision is extended proximally another centimeter, and more tissue is separated in the web space to enhance the exposure. On rare occasions, a Gelpi retractor is used to gain greater access to the web space.
6. Careful dissection allows the common digital nerve to the web space to be identified and traced distally. Once this is accomplished and the tip of the nerve is excised from the surrounding scar tissue, the nerve is cut as far proximal to the metatarsal head as possible.
7. The ankle is dorsiflexed to help pull the nerve more proximally into the foot.
8. The skin is closed with interrupted sutures and a compression dressing is applied.

For recurrent neuroma from a plantar transverse or plantar longitudinal approach, please see techniques

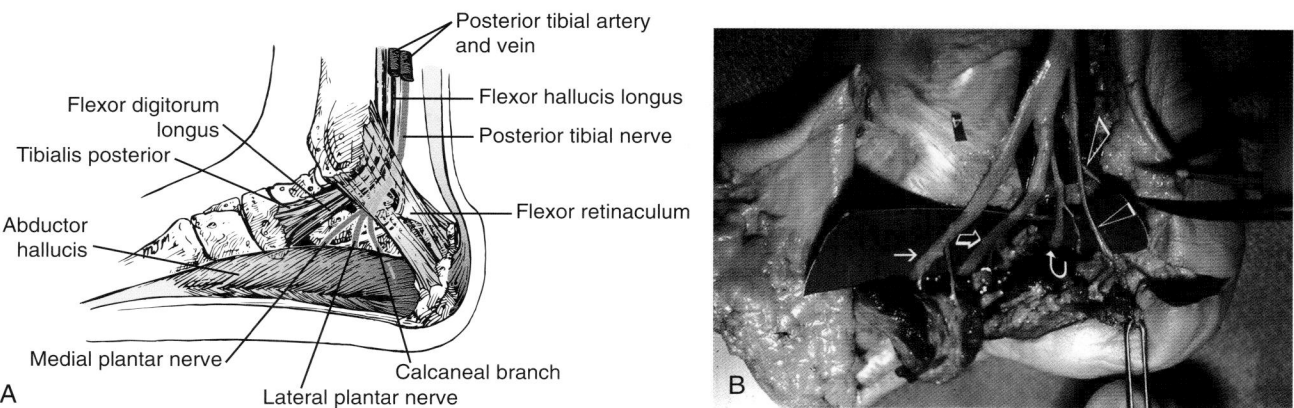

Figure 12-26 **A,** The schematic anatomy of the tibial nerve. **B,** An anatomic dissection of the tibial nerve and its branches demonstrates the medial plantar nerve *(solid arrow)*, the lateral plantar nerve *(open arrow)*, the first branch of the lateral plantar nerve *(curved arrow)*, and the calcaneal nerve *(open arrowheads)*.

under the heading for a primary resection (Surgical Technique: Transverse Approach and Surgical Technique: Longitudinal Approach).

Postoperative Care

Postoperative management consists of re-dressing the foot in 18 to 24 hours with a firm compression dressing. The foot is kept dressed for 3 weeks, during which time the patient ambulates in a postoperative shoe. After 3 weeks, the shoe is removed and the patient is started on active and passive range-of-motion exercises; the level of activity is progressively increased as tolerated. Running is restricted for approximately 2 months after excision of a recurrent neuroma to permit adequate healing to occur.

Uncommon Findings

Occasionally, reexploration of the web space reveals a quantity of thick, bursa-like material that requires excision. This material usually lies dorsal to the transverse metatarsal ligament. When the web space is explored, dense scar tissue is present about the end of the nerve, but proximal to this, the nerve appears to be almost normal. When the muscle wraps itself around the end of the nerve, identification of the nerve requires meticulous dissection of the tissues to locate it.

TARSAL TUNNEL SYNDROME

The tarsal tunnel syndrome is an entrapment neuropathy involving the posterior tibial nerve within the tarsal canal or one of its terminal branches after the nerve leaves the tarsal canal. The earliest description of the syndrome was by Kopell and Thompson[80] in 1960, and it was named "tarsal tunnel syndrome" by Keck[76] in 1962 and Lam[82] in 1967. The condition is somewhat analogous to the carpal tunnel syndrome in the wrist, but it occurs much less often.[185]

The tarsal canal is located behind the medial malleolus, and it becomes the tarsal tunnel as a result of the

flexor retinaculum passing over the structures and creating a closed space. The tarsal tunnel is a fibro-osseous structure created by the tibia anteriorly and the posterior process of the talus and calcaneus laterally. The flexor retinaculum that creates the tarsal tunnel is intimately attached to the sheaths of the posterior tibial, flexor hallucis, and flexor digitorum longus tendons (Fig. 12-26).

The posterior tibial nerve, which is a branch of the sciatic nerve, enters the canal proximally, and in 93% of cases, the nerve branches into its three terminal branches: medial plantar nerve, lateral plantar nerve, and medial calcaneal nerve within the tunnel. The medial calcaneal nerve arises off the posterior aspect of the posterior tibial nerve about 75% of the time and off the LPN about 25% of the time. It is a single branch in 79% of specimens and multiple branches in 21%. The calcaneal branches originate proximal to the tarsal tunnel in 39% of cases, within the tunnel in 34%, and distal to the tunnel in 16%.[74]

In another study, Davis and Schon[67] confirmed that the tibial nerve bifurcates within 2 cm of the medial malleolar calcaneal axis in 90% of cadaveric specimens (Fig. 12-27). In contrast to the Havel et al study,[74] they found 60% had multiple calcaneal nerve branches, and 20% of specimens had aberrant innervation of the abductor hallucis muscle. Dellon et al[69] confirmed this finding in a study of the calcaneal nerve as observed during 85 tarsal tunnel releases. In this report, 37% of feet had one calcaneal nerve, 41% had two, 19% had three, and 3% had four. They found that the MPN gave origin to a calcaneal nerve in 46% of feet. The topographic anatomy of the nerve is also useful to help understand the position of the various branches before they ramify. This helps to localize damaged nerve fascicles within the trunk of the nerve.[85]

In approximately 60% of patients with tarsal tunnel syndrome, a specific cause could be identified.[86] Some were associated with a significant specific injury, such as a severe ankle sprain, crush injury, fracture of the distal end of the tibia, dislocation of the ankle, or calcaneal fracture, and others were caused by a space-occupying

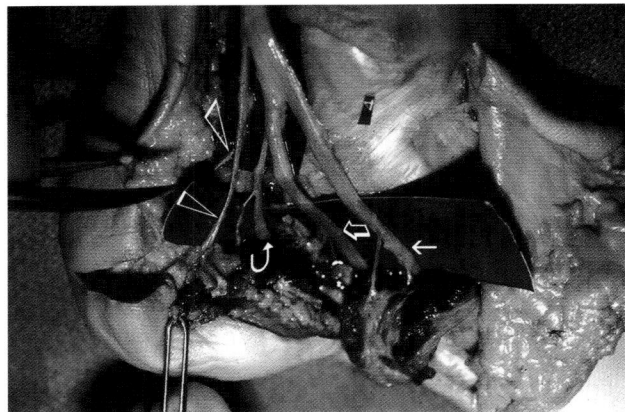

Figure 12-27 The tibial nerve is shown with its branches. The *arrowheads* indicate the calcaneal branches, the *curved arrow* indicates the first branch of the lateral plantar nerve, the *open arrow* indicates the lateral plantar nerve, and the *solid arrow* indicates the medial plantar nerve.

Table 12-2	Causes of Tarsal Tunnel Syndrome Presented in the Literature: Summary of 24 Reports
Causes	**Cases**
Idiopathic	25
Traumatic	21
Varicosities	16*
Heel varus	14
Fibrosis	11
Heel valgus	10
Ganglion	3
Diabetes	3
Obesity	3
Tight tarsal canal	3
Hypertrophic abductor hallucis	3
Rheumatoid arthritis	3
Lipoma	2
Anomalous artery	1
Acromegaly	1
Ankylosing spondylitis	1
Regional migratory osteoporosis	1
Flexor digitorum accessorius longus	1
SUBTOTAL	122
Causes not reported	64
Total	186

From Cimino WR: Tarsal tunnel syndrome: review of the literature, *Foot Ankle* 11:47–52, 1990.
*Represents 14% of the cases.

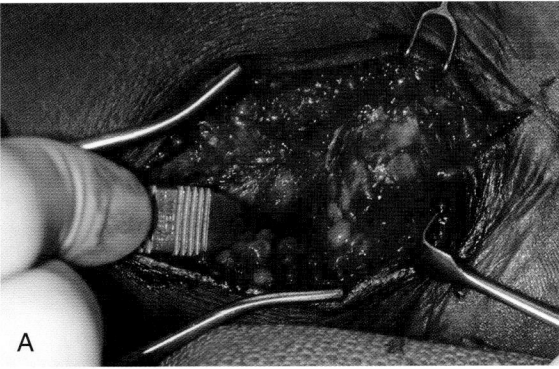

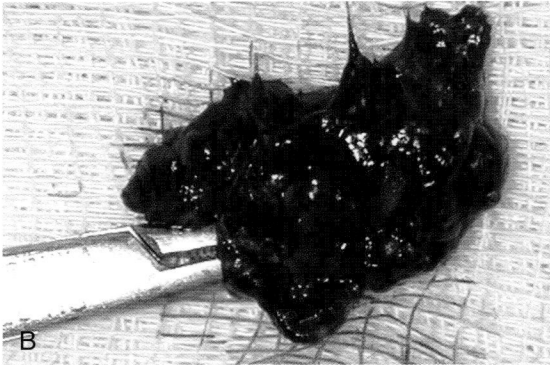

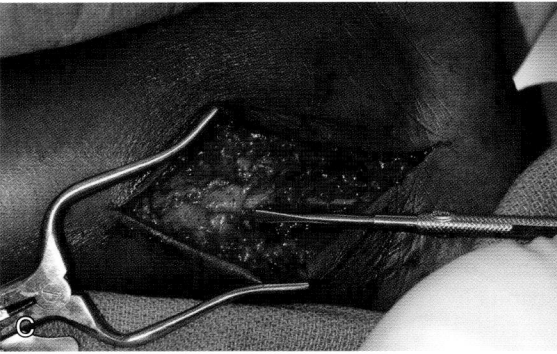

Figure 12-28 **A,** A large ganglion is noted posterior and deep to the tibial nerve. **B,** The ganglion has been removed. **C,** The tibial nerve is shown after removal but before a proximal release of the tarsal tunnel.

lesion, such as lipoma, varicosities, ganglion, synovial cyst, or exostosis. In a review of 24 reports in the literature, Cimino[65] noted that a specific cause could be identified in about 80% of patients with a tarsal tunnel syndrome (Table 12-2).

Certain local causes can result in a tarsal tunnel syndrome and include the following:

■ Ganglion of one of the tendon sheaths passing adjacent to the tarsal canal or one of the terminal branches of the posterior tibial nerve (Fig. 12-28).

■ Lipoma within the tarsal canal exerting pressure against the posterior tibial nerve.

■ Exostosis or fracture fragment from the distal end of the tibia or calcaneus.

■ Medial talocalcaneal bar that protrudes into the inferior aspect of the tarsal canal (Fig. 12-29).

■ Enlarged venous complex surrounding the posterior tibial nerve within the tarsal canal.

■ Neurilemmoma of the posterior tibial nerve within the tarsal canal (Fig. 12-30).

■ Severe pronation of the hindfoot that results in stretching or compressing of the posterior tibial nerve.

■ Accessory muscle within the tarsal tunnel, such as an accessory soleus or accessory flexor digitorum longus (Fig. 12-31).

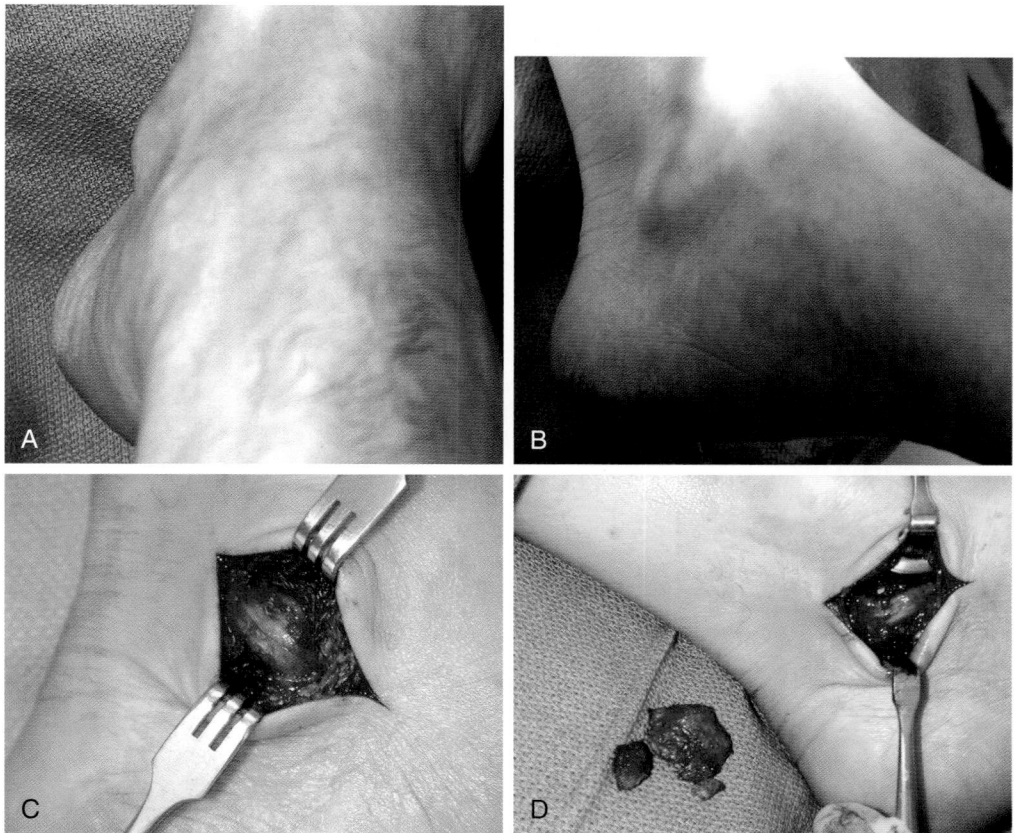

Figure 12-29 **A** and **B,** The tarsal coalition created medial bulk against the medial plantar nerve (MPN) and gave this patient tarsal tunnel symptoms. **C,** The coalition is approached, and the MPN and flexor digitorum longus tendons are exposed. **D,** The medial talocalcaneal coalition is resected, decompressing the nerve.

The role of postural deformities or mechanical abnormalities in tarsal tunnel syndrome should not be underestimated. A study of 56 feet in 28 patients with pes planus showed abnormalities in their electrodiagnostic tests.[63] Treppman et al[98] demonstrated increased pressures in the tarsal tunnel with inversion or eversion. Daniels et al[66] demonstrated increased tibial nerve tension in an unstable foot versus a stable one in eversion, dorsiflexion, and cyclic load. Lau and Daniels[83] demonstrated that tibial nerve tension was increased after a tarsal tunnel release during eversion, dorsiflexion-eversion, and cyclic load in the unstable versus the stable foot. This supported the notion that structural deformity plays a critical role in resolving tarsal tunnel syndrome in an unstable foot.

Labib et al[81] reported on the combination of plantar fasciitis, posterior tibial tendon dysfunction, and tarsal tunnel syndrome in 14 patients. They postulated that the failure of the fascia and posterior tibial tendon resulted in traction on the tibial nerve. In their series, 12 of 14 patients responded to tarsal tunnel and plantar fascia release in conjunction with correction of the hindfoot deformity. Hindfoot correction included hindfoot fusion, medial displacement osteotomy of the calcaneus, and/or tendon transfer. Schon's group has often noted that when patients with tibial neuralgia and structural deformity undergo surgical correction of the malalignments, their neuritic symptoms improve or totally resolve.

Clinical Symptoms

Whereas the patient with an interdigital neuroma is usually able to localize the area of maximum tenderness on the plantar aspect of the foot, the patient with a tarsal tunnel syndrome usually has difficulty describing the nature of the pain. When questioned, however, the patient usually states that the pain is diffuse on the plantar aspect of the foot and at the medial ankle. The pain is characterized as a burning, shooting, searing, electric, shocking, stabbing, tingling, numbing type that is usually aggravated by activities on the feet and relieved by rest. However, certain patients report that the pain is worse in bed at night, and they actually obtain relief by arising and moving around. About a third of the patients with tarsal tunnel syndrome note proximal radiation of pain along the medial aspect of the leg to the midcalf region (Valleix phenomenon).

As with all the nerve disorders, the type of activity and the specific movements or positions that exacerbate the pain should be identified. Any history of systemic disorders that can affect nerves must be noted (e.g.,

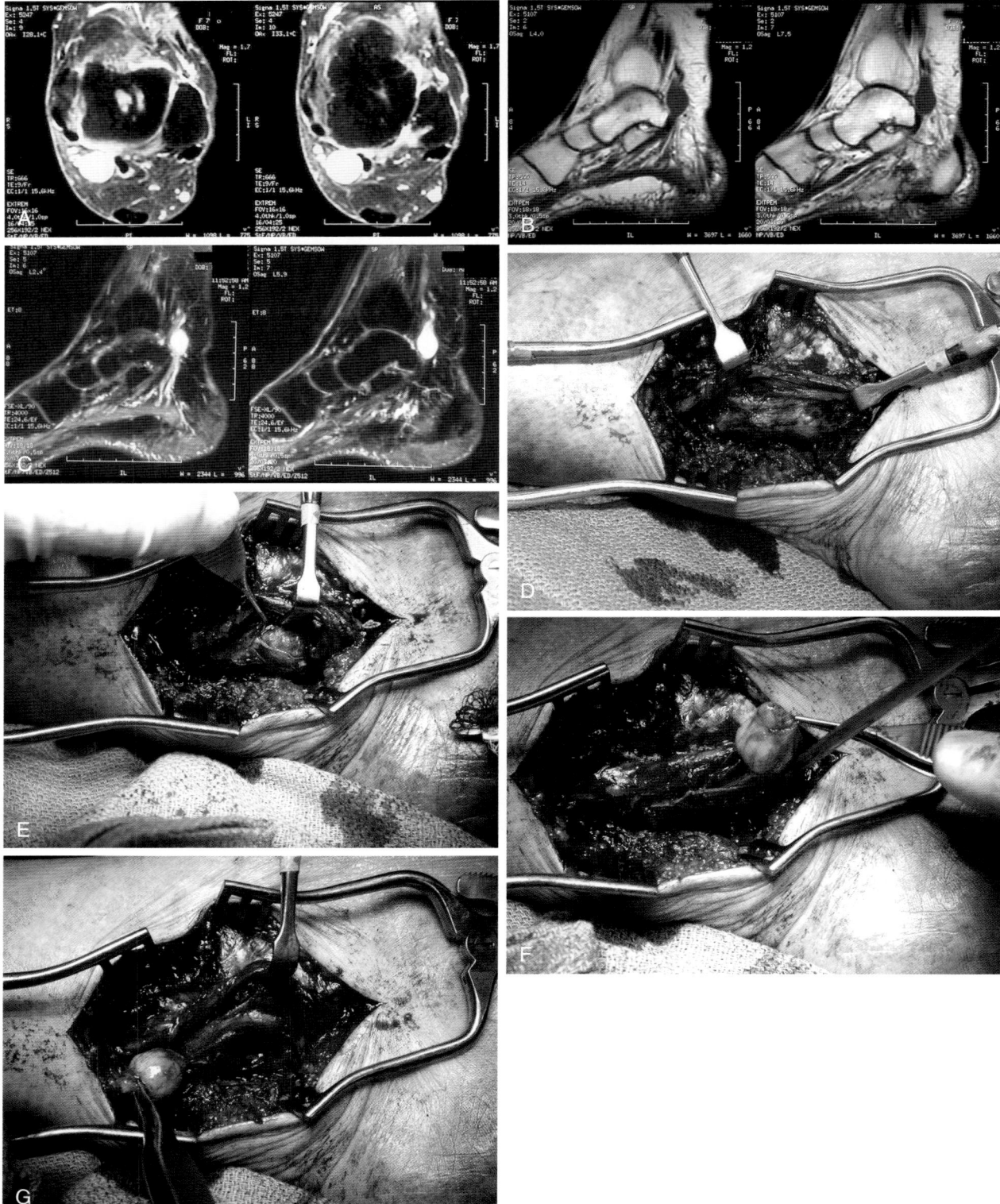

Figure 12-30 A tibial nerve schwannoma. **A,** Axial magnetic resonance image (MRI). **B,** Sagittal MRI, T1 weighted. **C,** Sagittal MRI, T2 weighted. Note the high image signal of the tumor. **D,** Intraoperative exposure. **E,** The dissection should be intrafascicular, teasing the tumor from the surrounding nerve fascicles. **F,** The tumor is peeled out of the nerve, which remains intact. **G,** The final appearance of the nerve and tumor.

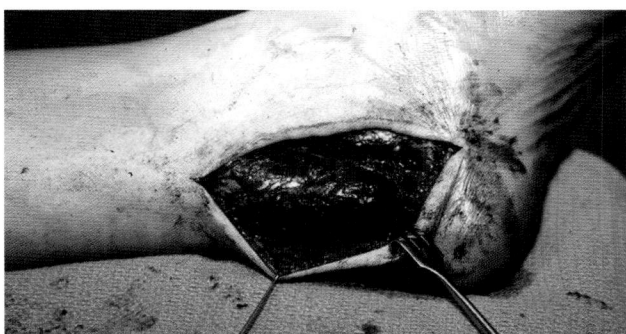

Figure 12-31 An accessory soleus is encountered during this tarsal tunnel release. A small calcaneal nerve branch is seen coursing over the muscle mass, explaining the patient's neuritic heel pain.

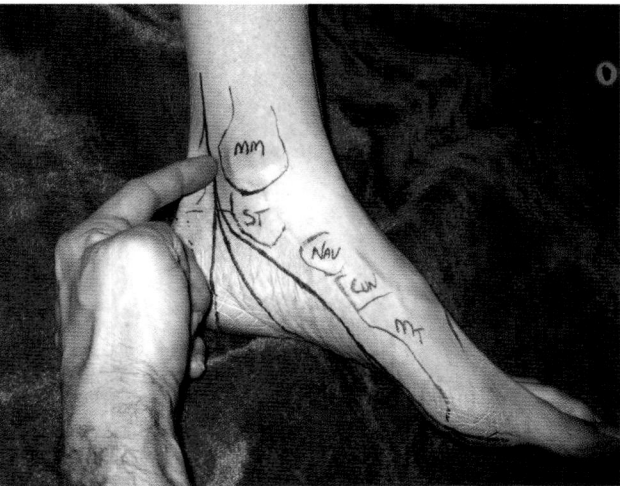

Figure 12-32 The tibial nerve and its branches are palpated and percussed.

rheumatologic disorders, Lyme disease, diabetes, thyroid disease). A review of medications, chemical exposure, alcohol abuse, or low back pain with radiculopathy should be documented to rule out other nonfocal causes of tibial neuralgia.

Diagnosis

Physical Examination

The physician begins the physical examination by having the patient stand and observing the overall posture of the foot. Any significant varus or valgus deformity of the hindfoot should be noted. Claw toe deformities or intrinsic wasting can indicate advanced nerve compromise. The range of motion of the ankle, subtalar, and transverse tarsal joints is observed next to detect any restriction of motion that could indicate a previous injury, coalition, or possibly arthrosis. The posterior tibial tendon function should be carefully tested with a side-to-side comparison of inversion power across the midline from the neutral position and from the abducted position. Watching the patient walk can also reveal subtle weaknesses, malalignments, or neurologic abnormalities. If a specific task brings on the pain, observing the patient performing that movement or simulating the provocative stresses can be helpful.

The entire course of the posterior tibial nerve is percussed, starting proximal to the tarsal tunnel and proceeding distally along its terminal branches to look for evidence of irritability of the nerve, as manifested by tingling or discomfort (Fig. 12-32). Percussion over the area of the entrapment can cause radiation of pain along the distribution of the medial or lateral plantar nerve. After percussion of the nerve, the nerve and its terminal branches should be carefully palpated to look for evidence of thickening or swelling, which can indicate a space-occupying lesion, such as a ganglion, synovial cyst, or lipoma. On rare occasions, a bony ridge is noted along the course of the posterior tibial nerve.

Sensory examination of the foot is usually not revealing. Although patients often complain of dysesthesias

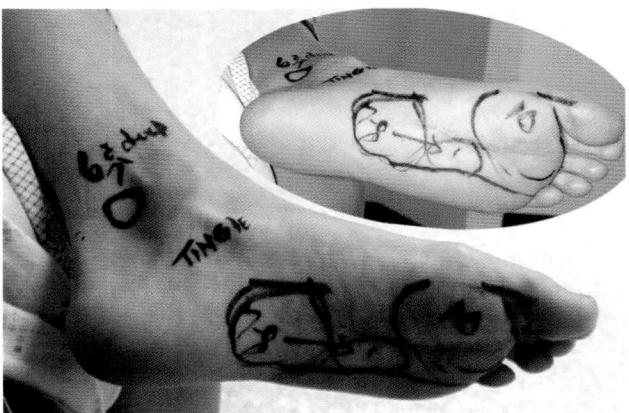

Figure 12-33 The patient had a Tinel sign at the tarsal tunnel in conjunction with severe pain and zones of subtle decreased sensation along the branch of the medial plantar nerve. The numbers indicate the level of pain in that region.

and numbness, it is difficult to demonstrate actual areas of numbness on the bottom of the foot. If there is specific involvement of the medial or lateral plantar nerve, occasionally it is possible to detect a sensory loss in the foot. Sensory testing of distal sensory branches using the Semmes-Weinstein monofilaments or two-point discrimination can reveal tibial nerve deficits (Fig. 12-33).

Motor weakness is also difficult to evaluate in such patients. Muscle weakness is difficult to detect, although at times, atrophy of the abductor hallucis or abductor digiti quinti muscle may be observed when one foot is compared with the other.

The literature has mentioned that the dysesthesias in the foot can be brought on when the hindfoot is held in an inverted or everted position, but this can be difficult to reproduce. A recent study by Kinoshita et al[78] reported success with a maneuver that passively dorsiflexed the ankle, everted the heel, and dorsiflexed all the toes. In their study, symptoms were induced after a few seconds. They also found tibial nerve tenderness and a positive percussion sign (Tinel sign).

Radiographic evaluation of the foot and ankle should be obtained to evaluate for stress fractures, fracture sequelae, bone lesions, or arthritis. If a space-occupying lesion is suspected, an MRI scan should be obtained.

Frey and Kerr[70] conducted a study in which 35 feet with suspected tarsal tunnel syndrome were evaluated with MRI. In 88% of patients, a pathologic condition was identified. The diagnosis included flexor hallucis longus tenosynovitis (11 cases), dilated veins (9), focal mass (5), fracture or soft tissue injury (5), fibrous scar tissue (3), posterior tibial tenosynovitis (1), and hypertrophied abductor hallucis muscle (1). Of the 20 patients in this group who had a positive Tinel sign, 17 (85%) had positive MRI findings. These findings included flexor hallucis longus tenosynovitis (7), venous dilation (4), focal mass (3), fibrous scar tissue (2), posterior tibial tenosynovitis (1), and negative scan (3). When an MRI scan of the contralateral limb was obtained in these 20 patients, 5 (25%) were positive. Three scans demonstrated dilated veins, and two showed flexor hallucis longus tenosynovitis. In the series, 21 patients had surgery, and the MRI finding was confirmed in 19 patients.

Ultrasound has been performed for tarsal tunnel syndrome. In a study by Nagaoka and Matsuaki,[87] 17 patients with tarsal tunnel syndrome were evaluated, and the cause of the syndrome was identified and confirmed intraoperatively. In their series, these authors reported 10 ganglia, 1 talocalcaneal coalition, 3 talocalcaneal coalitions associated with ganglia, and 3 varicose veins in patients with tarsal tunnel syndrome. Although ultrasound in experienced hands can be useful, Schon has not found it practical and prefers MRI for a more detailed analysis of soft tissue, joint, and bony abnormalities.

MR neurography has shown some promise in the diagnosis of tibial nerve entrapment syndromes in early studies. With the advent and increasing use of 3-tesla magnets, this modality is becoming more common. Although MR neurography is inferior in terms of spatial resolution when compared with ultrasound, it offers a more objective assessment of neuromuscular abnormalities and offers a higher signal-to-noise ratio and soft tissue contrast.[64]

Electrodiagnostic Studies

Electrodiagnostic testing should be performed in all patients to make the diagnosis of a tarsal tunnel syndrome or to rule out other neuropathies or proximal nerve lesions. The specific technique and the relevance of the findings have been debated in the literature.[71,90,92] In general, the electrodiagnostic tests fall into three categories: nerve conduction studies of the medial and lateral plantar nerve, measurement of the amplitude and duration of the motor evoked potentials and seeking the presence of fibrillation potentials, and sensory

conduction velocities. The conduction velocity of the common peroneal nerve should be obtained to determine whether a peripheral neuropathy is also present.

The terminal latency of the MPN to the abductor hallucis muscle should be less than 6.2 msec, and that of the LPN to the abductor digiti quinti muscle should be less than 7 msec. If the difference in terminal latency to the abductor hallucis and abductor digiti quinti is greater than 1 msec, it can indicate a tarsal tunnel syndrome. Some electromyographers believe that this is one of the less sensitive tests for this study. A study of the motor evoked potentials, which demonstrates a decreased amplitude and increased duration in patients with a tarsal tunnel syndrome, is considered more sensitive than a study of distal motor latencies.[75] When this study is performed, a search for fibrillation potentials should also be conducted. The sensory nerve conduction velocity is probably the most accurate study, although differing views exist as to the ease and reproducibility of these measurements. Proponents of this test think that the sensitivity is about 90%.[89]

Patel et al[82] recently performed an evidence-based review to evaluate the utility of nerve conduction studies (NCSs) and needle electromyography (EMG) in the diagnosis of tarsal tunnel syndrome. A total of 317 articles published in English from 1965 through April 2002 were reviewed on the basis of six selection criteria. Four articles met inclusion criteria and were considered to meet class III level of evidence. These papers examined the use of electrodiagnostic studies for the evaluation of patients with clinically suspected tarsal tunnel syndrome and found that NCSs were abnormal in some patients. Sensory NCSs were more likely to be abnormal than motor NCSs, but given the available data, the actual sensitivity and specificity could not be determined. The sensitivity of needle EMG abnormalities could not be determined. NCSs may be useful for confirming the diagnosis of tibial neuropathy at the ankle. The authors concluded that better studies are needed to more definitively evaluate electrodiagnostic techniques in tarsal tunnel syndrome.

It is obvious that the diagnosis of tarsal tunnel syndrome cannot be made solely on the basis of electrodiagnostic results, but these must be correlated with the history given by the patient and with the physical findings.

Differential Diagnosis

Box 12-2 presents the differential diagnosis of the tarsal tunnel syndrome.[100] When making the diagnosis of tarsal tunnel syndrome, the examiner must be alert to many other clinical entities that can mimic this diagnosis. For this reason, the diagnosis must be based on a strong history by the patient of neuritic symptoms in the foot in the distribution of the tibial nerve or its branches, or both, definite physical findings, as demonstrated by percussion-induced tingling along the posterior tibial nerve or its terminal branches, and supportive NCS. If all three criteria are not met, the examiner should strongly

Remote Causes
Interdigital neuroma
Intervertebral disk lesion
Plantar fasciitis
Plantar fibromatosis

Intraneural Causes
Peripheral neuritis
Peripheral vascular disease
Diabetic neuropathy
Leprosy
Neurilemmoma
Neuroma

Extraneural Causes
Ganglion
Nerve tethering
Fracture (callus, malunion, nonunion, displaced fragment)
Blunt trauma
Valgus hindfoot
Rheumatoid arthritis
Venous varicosities
Tenosynovitis
Ligament constriction
Abductor hallucis origin constriction
Tarsal coalition (middle or posterior facet)
Lipoma

Modified from Wilemon WK: Tarsal tunnel syndrome: a 50-year survey of the world literature and a report of two cases, *Orthop Rev* 8:111–117, 1979.

consider a diagnosis other than the tarsal tunnel syndrome. If only one criterion is met, the diagnosis of tarsal tunnel syndrome should be viewed with skepticism. If two of the three criteria are met, the patient is carefully monitored, and if the findings are reproducible, the diagnosis of a tarsal tunnel syndrome may be considered.

Treatment

Conservative Treatment

The conservative management of tarsal tunnel syndrome is based partially on the diagnosis. If a space-occupying lesion is present, one should excise it rather than treating the patient conservatively. If a lesion is not present, conservative management is indicated. Conservative management involves administration of nonsteroidal antiinflammatory drugs (NSAIDs), oral vitamin B_6 100 mg bid, and tricyclic antidepressants, such as imipramine, nortriptyline, desipramine, or amitriptyline. SSRIs, such as sertraline and paroxetine; other antidepressants, such as venlafaxine or duloxetine; or antiseizure medications, such as gabapentin, pregabalin, topiramate, or carbamazepine, can also be used. Topical agents, such as lidocaine or fentanyl patches, transdermal clonidine, capsaicin, and compound mixtures (TCA, ketamine), are sometimes helpful, but little data exist to support their

use.[94] Schon and Reed recommend using NSAIDs, vitamin B_6 100 mg bid, and either amitriptyline (starting at 10 or 25 mg at night and gradually increasing up to 75 mg at night over several months), pregabalin (starting at 75 mg bid and progressing to 150 mg bid over 2-3 weeks), or gabapentin (starting at 100 or 300 mg at night and progressing to a tid routine and then increasing the dose to up to 900 mg tid if not effective at the lower dosages). Vitamin B_1 (thiamine) deficiency has been implicated in peripheral neuropathy, and Schon and Reed have seen some success with vitamin B_1 supplementation for neuritic symptoms. Schon recommends a course of 300 mg bid for 6 weeks, followed by a maintenance dose of 150 mg bid for patients with recalcitrant neuritis. Occasionally, narcotic medications are warranted to enhance pain control. The dosing and increases depend on the patient's medical history, symptomatic response, and tolerance of side effects. An orthopaedist who is not comfortable with the nature of the medications, the drug interactions, their risks, or their side effects should refer the patient to a neurologist, physiatrist, or pain specialist.

Infrequently, an injection of a steroid preparation adjacent to the posterior tibial nerve can be helpful. Often, placing the extremity in a stirrup brace, off-the-shelf boot brace, or short-leg walking cast provides relief. If the patient has a postural abnormality, an orthotic device (foot orthosis or ankle–foot orthosis) to hold the foot in the neutral position may be of benefit. Gould[73] has seen success with a total-contact insert with a posteromedial nerve relief channel corresponding to the course of the lateral plantar nerve and its first branch. If the patient has edema, an elastic stocking may be used to control the swelling. If conservative management fails and the clinical symptoms are of sufficient magnitude, tarsal tunnel release should be considered.

Surgical Treatment

If the patient has a symptomatic identifiable space-occupying lesion involving the tibial nerve, surgical release should include resection of the lesion, with care taken to minimize traumatizing the nerve. When a structural deformity is identified, correction of the deformity should be adequate to resolve the symptoms. At times, the nerve release is required in addition to the realignment procedure.[81] When there is an adjacent pathologic structure that can account for the patient's tarsal tunnel symptoms, addressing the structure (debriding a synovitic tendon, fusing an arthritic joint, reconstructing a fracture malunion or nonunion, or resecting a tarsal coalition) can provide relief even without direct tibial nerve release.

When no underlying nonneurologic disease is identified, the tibial nerve release should be performed after reasonable conservative treatment as outlined above. Dellon and others have proposed tibial nerve release as well as other concurrent nerve releases for the treatment of diabetic neuropathy.[61,62,68,84] The indications for this procedure are being confirmed but include decreased sensation in the plantar aspect of the foot as determined by two-point discrimination, the presence of a positive tibial nerve percussion test (Tinel sign), and pain in the territory of the tibial nerve. The procedure is contraindicated in patients with vascular disease. At this point, there have been no reasonably designed trials conducted to support this proposed treatment.[91]

Before surgery, the patient should be advised of the complications of tibial nerve release, including, but not limited to, a lack of response of the symptoms to the release, increased symptoms, numbness, dysesthesias, persistent tenderness or paresthesias over the tarsal tunnel, swelling, nerve damage, vascular damage, infection, wound healing problems, difficulty with footwear, and causalgia or complex regional pain syndrome type 2.

TIBIAL NERVE RELEASE

The course of the tibial nerve and its branches should be determined before surgery to identify potential compression sites. Careful palpation for focal tender spots or positive percussion signs (Tinel sign) will help direct the surgeon to areas of disease. Depending on the experience of the surgeon, loupe magnification may be useful. The use of bipolar cautery assists in achieving atraumatic hemostasis.

The procedure can be performed with or without a tourniquet. Placing the patient in a mild Trendelenburg position can assist in maintaining a clear field when the tourniquet is not used. There are several advantages of not using the tourniquet: The artery and veins can be well visualized during the exposure; as the neurovascular structures are released, the surgeon can observe the unrestricted pulsations of the artery and filling of the veins; the vaso nervorum (the small vessels on the nerve) can be observed to determine adequacy of the decompression; and hemostasis can be achieved as the case proceeds, minimizing the search for random surprise bleeders.

Surgical Technique

1. The tarsal tunnel is approached through a curved incision that begins about 10 cm proximal to the tip of the medial malleolus and 2 cm posterior to the posterior margin of the tibia. It is carried distally parallel to the tibia to the level of the medial malleolus and then gently curves distally and plantarward to end at about the level of the talonavicular joint and over the midportion of the abductor hallucis muscle.
2. The incision is deepened through the subcutaneous tissue and fat to expose the flexor retinaculum. All the vessels encountered are carefully identified and cauterized (Fig. 12-34A and Video Clip 88).
3. The proximal portion of the flexor retinaculum is identified. Usually, the posterior tibial tendon is in its own sheath immediately behind the posterior margin of the tibia, after which the flexor digitorum longus and posterior tibial nerve, artery, and vein are within the next sheath. At times, however, each structure has its

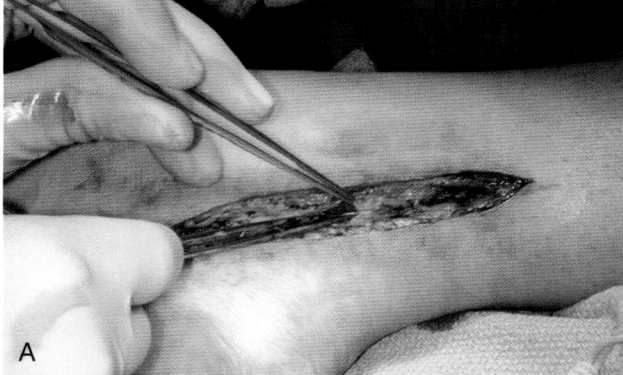

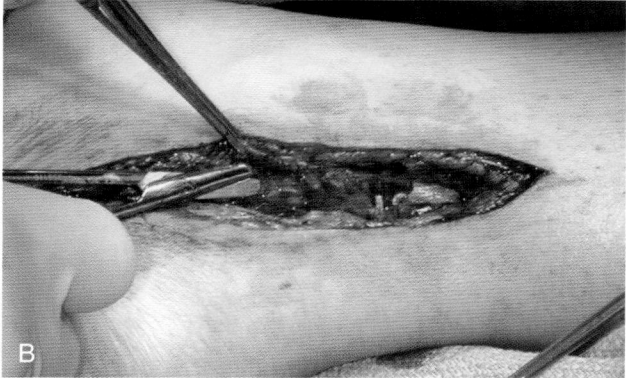

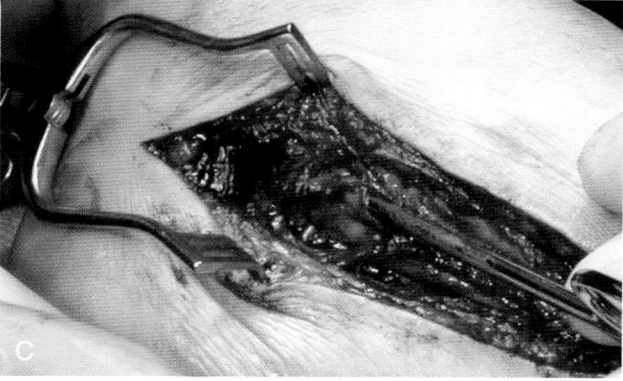

Figure 12-34 A, Tarsal tunnel release exposure of the retinaculum. **B,** The retinaculum is carefully released. **C,** The medial plantar nerve through its fibrous tunnel in the abductor hallucis should be observed and released.

own sheath. When the sheath is opened proximally, it should be carefully explored to be sure that it is the sheath containing the posterior tibial nerve. The retinaculum is then carefully released (Fig. 12-34B). Distally, around the area of the medial malleolus and distal to it, the retinaculum may be extremely taut and dense. In dissection of this area, a curved clamp should be placed between the retinaculum and the underlying tissues so as not to injure a vital structure inadvertently.

4. Once the retinaculum has been released, again, starting proximally, the posterior tibial nerve is carefully identified by blunt dissection. It is traced distally and

through the tarsal tunnel, where branching into the three terminal branches occurs.

5. The MPN is traced distally around the malleolus and is followed along beneath the abductor hallucis until it passes through a fibrous tunnel at the level of the talonavicular joint. As this dissection is carried around the medial malleolus, it may be difficult to follow the nerve, and it is sometimes necessary to identify the nerve distally and trace it back proximally underneath the leash of vessels that is covering it. Infrequently, it is necessary to ligate some of the large veins if they are regarded as a factor in compression of the nerve. The passage of the MPN through its fibrous tunnel in the abductor hallucis should be observed, and the nerve should be released (Fig. 12-34C).

6. The LPN is traced distally by blunt dissection as it passes distal to the medial malleolar calcaneal axis (a line that can be drawn between the tip of the medial malleolus and the posterior inferior aspect of the heel); it may be difficult to trace because of local vessels. The nerve can be identified more distally at the edge of the abductor hallucis. The superficial fascia over the muscle is released, and either the muscle is reflected inferiorly, or a portion of the dorsal half of the origin from the calcaneus is taken down. This exposes the deep fascia of the abductor, which can then be released. This fascia has a concave orientation and can readily compress the nerve here.

7. The first branch of the LPN is a posterior branch off the LPN that runs to the inferior aspect of the calcaneus just dorsal to the location of the typical plantar heel spur. Because it has a separate compartment distinct from the LPN, it should be released by sectioning the deep fascia of the abductor muscle.

8. By carefully following along the posterior aspect of the LPN, the medial calcaneal branch or branches should be identified. As these pass distally, care should be taken to ensure no bands of fibrous tissue are constricting them.

9. Once the posterior tibial nerve and its terminal branches have been released, the tourniquet, if one was used, should be deflated. The nerve is then carefully observed to determine whether capillary filling is adequate along the course of the nerve. Occasionally, the nerve does not "pink up" in certain areas, which can represent an area of constriction. If constriction is present, release of the epineurium overlying the nerve may be considered. This observation is made in about 5% of cases. Neurolysis is not typically performed because doing so can make the nerve more vulnerable to scarring by disrupting its surrounding bed and damaging the vaso nervosum. Any bleeding must be controlled, after which the wound is closed in layers without closing the retinaculum. If there appears to be any significant oozing around the wound, it may be closed over a drain. A compression dressing incorporating a plaster splint is applied.

Postoperative Care
Postoperative care consists of keeping the patient relatively immobilized for 2 to 3 weeks, on crutches with no weight bearing on the operated foot. If the wound is healing adequately at 10 days, the sutures can be removed and gentle range of motion is encouraged to limit adhesions. After another 2 to 3 weeks, weight bearing is permitted as tolerated, and more aggressive active and passive range-of-motion exercises are initiated.

Results
When a well-localized lesion is present, such as a ganglion, lipoma, or even a neurilemmoma, the clinical response is usually satisfactory, with complete relief of symptoms.

If no specific cause can be identified, approximately 75% of patients obtain significant relief from the surgery, and 25% obtain little or no relief. A small group of patients have increased symptoms after tarsal tunnel release. After surgery, a subgroup of patients experiences satisfactory relief of symptoms for a varying period (6-12 months) only to have their symptom complex recur.

Cimino[65] reviewed 24 articles and reported that 84 of 122 (69%) patients had good results, 27 of 122 (22%) were improved, 8 of 122 (7%) had poor results, and 3 of 122 (2%) had a recurrence of symptoms (Table 12-3). Pfeiffer and Cracchiolo[83] noted better results earlier in 32 feet but reported a decline with further follow-up at an average of 31 months. Thirty-eight percent were dissatisfied with the result and had no long-term relief of the pain. In 6 feet (19%), the pain was decreased, but the patients still had some pain and disability (a fair result). There were four wound complications (13%): three infections and one delayed healing.

Takakura et al[96] reported on 50 feet with tarsal tunnel syndrome and noted that the poorest results were in

Table 12-3	Results of Tarsal Tunnel Treatment: Summary of 24 Reports	
Results	**Number of Patients**
Surgery	
Good (resolution of symptoms)	84
Improved (mild residual symptoms)	27
Poor (symptoms unchanged or worse)	8
Recurrent (symptoms return)	3
Percentage of good and improved	91%
Orthoses	
Good (resolution of symptoms)	10
Poor	0
Refused treatment or pending	12
Other Methods	
Injection, resolution	3
Spontaneous resolution	4
Results not reported	35
Total	186

From Cimino WR: Tarsal tunnel syndrome: review of the literature, *Foot Ankle* 11:47–52, 1990.

patients who had a traumatic or idiopathic cause. The hemorrhage and crush of the nerve during the trauma can lead to more adhesions and intraneural disease. Increased duration of symptoms was also correlated with a worse outcome. In another report, Takakura et al[97] had a talocalcaneal coalition and a ganglion in six patients with pain, sensory disturbance in the sole, and a positive Tinel sign. After resection, despite early pain relief, sensory changes and paresthesias persisted. The results were excellent in one patient, good in four, and fair in one.

Better results were reported by Nagaoka and Satou,[88] who operated on 29 patients. Of these patients, 21 had excellent and 8 had good results with a ganglion excision for tarsal tunnel symptoms. Five of the patients had an associated tarsal coalition.

Kinoshita et al[79] treated 41 patients (49 feet) with tarsal tunnel syndrome. In 7 patients (8 feet), there was an accessory muscle. An accessory flexor digitorum longus muscle was identified in 6 patients and an accessory soleus muscle in 1 patient (both feet). The patients with an accessory muscle had a history of trauma or strenuous athletics. After decompression of the tibial nerve and excision of the muscle, signs and symptoms improved at an average of 4.1 months. At final follow-up (24-88 months), no functional deficit was observed.

Sammarco and Chang[93] reviewed 62 patients with tarsal tunnel findings and positive electrodiagnostic tests who underwent release. Symptom duration averaged 31 months. Postoperatively, the average time for return to usual activity was 9 months. Average length of follow-up was 58 months. The authors reported that the most common surgical findings included arterial vascular leashes indenting the nerve and scarring about the nerve. The outcome of surgery was not affected by the history of trauma. The lack of a discrete space-occupying lesion and prolonged preoperative symptoms were not associated with a poor outcome.

Gondring et al[72] studied 60 patients (68 feet) who underwent tarsal tunnel release. All of the patients demonstrated both a positive Tinel sign and an abnormal motor nerve conduction velocity measurement. Despite an objectively assessed 85% complete symptomatic relief, there was only 51% symptom relief subjectively, according to a questionnaire. There was improvement in the quality of work in 51%, in job productivity in 47%, and in interpersonal relationships in 46% of these patients.

Urguden et al[99] assessed 12 patients (13 feet) who underwent surgery for tarsal tunnel syndrome, with a mean follow-up of 83 months. The symptoms had resolved in 6 feet, were improved in 4, were unchanged in 2, and recurred after 5 years in 1. As in other studies, better results were obtained in patients with a space-occupying lesion than in those with idiopathic or post-traumatic cause. In their four cases with foot deformities (three pes planus and one splay foot), there were two good results, one fair, and one poor. It was not clear whether these patients had any additional reconstruction to correct their underlying structural issues.

Kim et al[77] performed a retrospective study of 33 years of clinical and surgical experience with 135 tibial nerve lesions, to review operative techniques and their results and to provide management guidelines for the proper selection of surgical candidates at the Louisiana State University Health Sciences Center. Of the 135 cases, traumatic injury accounted for 71, tarsal tunnel syndrome for 46, and nerve sheath tumor for 18. Of 22 lesions not in continuity, good to excellent functional recovery was achieved in 4 (67%) of 6 patients who required end-to-end suture repair and 11 (69%) of 16 patients who required graft repair. There were 113 tibial nerve lesions in continuity, which underwent primarily external or internal neurolysis or resection of the lesions. Among the 113 patients with lesions in continuity, 76 (81%) of 94 patients receiving neurolysis had good or excellent results. Five of 6 (83%) receiving suture repair, and 11 of 13 (85%) receiving graft repair recovered good to excellent function. Repair results were best in patients with recordable nerve action potentials treated by external neurolysis. Results were poor in a few patients with very lengthy lesions in continuity and in reoperated patients with tarsal tunnel syndrome.

FAILED TARSAL TUNNEL RELEASE

Overview and Etiology

Persistent or recurrent pain after previous tarsal tunnel release is a clinical challenge and a management dilemma. Failure of the patient to respond to the primary release suggests the possibilities of an incomplete release, an incorrect diagnosis (nerve not entrapped in the tarsal tunnel, more proximal cause, neuroma in continuity, true neuroma, systemic neuropathy, or radiculopathy), or poor technique (excessive nerve trauma during surgery). Analyzing what has occurred and speculating about what needs to be rectified can be difficult.

The underlying failure may be due to either intrinsic nerve damage or extrinsic nerve damage. Where there is intrinsic nerve damage, the axons have been disrupted. The failure after tarsal tunnel release occurs in this scenario when the initial nerve disease was too extensive to respond to a release (i.e., nothing was compressing or tethering the nerve to begin with or the nerve was disrupted partially or completely either initially or subsequently). When there is extrinsic nerve damage, an external process affects the nerve. In these cases, a failure to respond to release may be due to incompletely addressing the compression or tethering in the first place or that there was too much damage to the environment around the nerve to permit successful release. Occasionally, surgical intervention can result in significant scarring secondary to extensive postoperative bleeding, a wound complication, or infection. In the cases of external nerve compromise, there may be little to no primary axonal damage. Although some cases have both internal and external issues, considering these two etiologies may be helpful.

In the cases of external nerve compromise after prior release, the symptoms and signs can be labeled "adhesive neuralgia" or, as Gould prefers, "traction neuritis." In theses cases, the patient undergoes surgical release and might have temporary relief but then suffers a recurrence. The pain is typically exacerbated by movement or postural changes. On examination, there is a tender, often thickened scar that when palpated induces the patient's symptoms. Range of motion also induces the patient's pain syndrome.

In the event of internal nerve damage, there are two types of symptom complexes. The first is ectopic neuralgia, in which the patient's nerve symptoms occur spontaneously without provocation. This can be thought of as a peripheral nerve seizure and represents electrochemical imbalance within the nerve. The second type of symptom complex is nociceptive neuralgia. Here the patient experiences nerve pain with mechanical provocation. A physical event, such as a certain position of the foot or an irritation from a shoe or brace, triggers the pain. This latter situation is commonly seen with a neuroma that is lying in a vulnerable location.

It is useful to separate the cases into three categories, facilitating management and permitting a more predictable outcome. The categories (A, B, and C) are based on the presence of scar tissue around the tibial nerve and the adequacy of decompression of the trunk and the affected distal branches. The first group (A) comprises nerves encased in scar tissue but in which an adequate distal release was performed based on operative report or length of scar. This group can be subdivided into patients who never experience relief after the first surgery (A1), patients who experience temporary relief but then recurrence (A2), and patients who become worse and develop new symptoms (A3). The second group (B) consists of tibial nerve branches encased in scar tissue, combined with inadequate release of a portion of the nerve and its branches. The third group (C) has no tibial nerve scarring and an incomplete release.[95,101,104,116-118,126]

Evaluation

The history and physical examination make up the cornerstone of the evaluation. The history is usually consistent with recurrent or new symptoms or an intensification of prior manifestations of the tarsal tunnel syndrome. Knowledge of the mechanism of injury can also be helpful. If there was a space-occupying lesion (an external or nonintraneural lesion) or there had been repetitive trauma, external nerve compression or an entrapment might have been the primary diagnosis. However, if a crush or stretch injury was noted, the primary problem might not have been an external nerve problem but rather an internal nerve disorder that might never respond to a fascia release. An important component of the history is to explore the nature, duration, and intensity of the symptoms before the previous tarsal tunnel release. A review of the prior operative report may be useful in defining incomplete previous release or incorrect diagnosis. A history of wound compromise or infection after the initial release suggests new entrapment of the nerve or adhesive neuralgia.

Although pain may be poorly localized, physical examination should attempt to find foci of maximum involvement, specifically with regard to proximal or distal areas of symptoms. Percussion paresthesias over the scar of the tibial nerve release often indicate scar formation around the nerve, whereas similar findings more distal or proximal to the old incision suggest incomplete decompression. A more focal point of paresthesias might indicate a neuroma or neuroma in continuity. A zone of numbness surrounded by increased nerve sensitivity with proximal trigger points suggests a deafferentation phenomenon, a sign of nerve transection. Anesthesia dolorosa or a numb zone that is painful to touch also indicates nerve transection and neuroma. Decreased and painful range of motion and a thickened scar are consistent with adhesive neuralgia.

Occasionally, recurrent or persistent symptoms indicate complex regional pain syndrome (CRPS) type II. These include vasomotor instability; changes in extremity temperature, skin color, or hair quality; and sweating or dryness that are manifestations of sympathetically mediated pain. Other features of CRPS II include spontaneous or evoked pain, allodynia (painful response to a stimulus that is not usually painful), hyperalgesia (exaggerated response to a stimulus that is usually only mildly painful), pain that is disproportionate to the inciting event, and evidence of autonomic dysregulation (e.g., edema, alteration in blood flow, hyperhidrosis).

As in primary tarsal tunnel syndrome, electrodiagnostic studies may be of benefit, especially to localize the nerve disease, to identify transected nerve branches, and to distinguish between external nerve entrapment and internal nerve damage (especially unrecognized peripheral neuropathy or a more proximal area of disease). When conduction delays are found, the diagnosis of external entrapment is supported. Evidence of axonal damage and muscle denervation supports intraneural damage (i.e., neuroma or neuroma in continuity).[95,117] Although only limited data are available, MRI shows promise in identifying factors leading to failed tarsal tunnel release (Fig. 12-35).[129]

Injections can help isolate the involved nerve or branch. A series of injections beginning distally and progressing more proximally can find the damaged structure. It is also worthwhile to inject suspicious adjacent structures, such as tendon sheaths (e.g., posterior tibial tendon), joints (e.g., the ankle or subtalar joint), or bony sites (e.g., nonunion sites). In cases of CRPS II, medications and injections aimed at interfering with the sympathetic component of the pain can be both diagnostic and therapeutic. Perhaps the best method of blocking the autonomic dysfunction is to perform a lumbar sympathetic injection. Another useful strategy is to administer an intravenous phentolamine infusion. A patient who

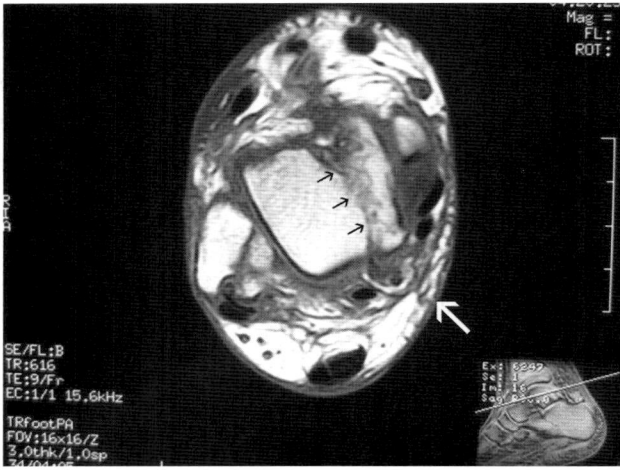

Figure 12-35 Coronal magnetic resonance image through the talus and tarsal tunnel in a patient who failed to respond to nerve release demonstrated the persistent talus nonunion *(small black arrows)*. There were signal abnormalities around the tibial nerve and changes from the previous tarsal tunnel release *(white arrow)*.

responds to the infusion may be a good candidate for trying phenoxybenzamine orally to control sympathetic dystrophy. Schon has also used intravenous lidocaine as a nerve membrane stabilizer. He has administered it under close monitoring and found it diagnostic and therapeutic. If a benefit is noted, then mexiletine, an oral version of lidocaine, can be considered to control the neuralgia.

Treatment

Conservative Treatment

Nonoperative management of persistent or recurrent tarsal tunnel syndrome may be extremely challenging. With persistent or recurrent symptoms, the patient has typically failed nonoperative measures before primary release, and thus it is unlikely that nonoperative measures will alleviate continued symptoms. However, NSAIDs, TCAs, antiepileptic medications, ketamine, an N-methyl-D-aspartate (NMDA) receptor antagonist, pain creams (e.g., Lidoderm patches), custom-compounded medications, orthotics, physical therapy, or desensitization by transcutaneous electrical nerve stimulation (TENS) should be attempted before performing revision surgery. Input by pain specialists, who can provide insight into other effective means of pain control, should be considered. A multimodality approach is often warranted.

There may be an emerging role for using vitamin C (ascorbic acid) to treat patients with continuing symptoms. A double-blinded, prospective, multicenter trial[130] evaluated three different doses of vitamin C versus placebo for patients with wrist fractures and observed the occurrence of CRPS. They found a statistically significant reduced prevalence of CRPS in patients who received vitamin C versus those in the placebo group. Based on their findings, they recommend a daily dose of 500 mg for 50 days. Although similarly well-designed studies are not currently available in the foot and ankle literature, vitamin C may show promise in the treatment of both acute and chronic nerve conditions.

Surgical Treatment

The goal of revision surgery is to achieve pain relief and improve function. Options for revision surgery include revision release, revision release with barrier procedure, revision release with transection and burial of a neuroma, and peripheral nerve stimulation (PNS) or spinal cord stimulaton. The best indications for revision release are usually limited to inadequate previous release with focal areas of nerve irritability. It is useful to separate the cases into the three categories (A, B, and C) described earlier.[95]

REVISION NEUROLYSIS

Revision neurolysis is indicated for category C patients (the prior release was inadequate based on the location of the scar, the operative record, conversation with the original surgeon, and location of the symptoms and signs). For example, if the patient had a tarsal tunnel release and did not specifically have a release of the MPN but has no symptoms and signs referable to the MPN, this tarsal tunnel release should be redone, including releasing the MPN. In this scenario, the patient has a good likelihood of a positive outcome. A revision that includes a more proximal or distal release or attention to specific branches is generally worthwhile for the patient.[95,117]

On the other hand, if the patient is in category A and has had a prior tarsal tunnel release through what appears to be an adequate surgical approach, but the patient has little or no relief of the dysesthesias and pain, reexploration of the tarsal tunnel and revision neurolysis alone has rarely been beneficial. For the patient in category B, the revision release has had some success because the nerve was not adequately released. However, in this group, the tibial nerve scarring was found to be associated with a less favorable prognosis.

Skalley et al[95] studied 12 patients (13 feet) who underwent release of a recurrent tarsal tunnel after unsuccessful surgery. They noted that 9 patients had abnormal electromyographic results, and 4 patients had normal test results. The results comprised three groups: 4 feet with encasement of the tibial nerve in scar and an adequate initial release had poor results, 5 feet with scarring and an inadequate release had equivocal results, and 4 feet with no scarring and an inadequate initial release had good results. They also concluded that the clinical history and physical examination, rather than the electromyographic studies, helped define the problem with regard to the extent of the lesion and its location.

REVISION NEUROLYSIS AND VEIN WRAP

This procedure is best indicated for patients in category B: those with histories of prior release who had temporary relief and those with adhesive neuralgia. Early on, Schon found that the revision neurolysis alone did not provide control for scar tissue recurrence. To address this problem with the tissue bed, the vein wrap was developed as a barrier method to block scar tissue from growing into the re-released nerve. The wrap has been shown to be effective in the laboratory and in several series.*

The vein is typically harvested from the ipsilateral saphenous vein in the lower leg. The vein is wrapped in a barber-pole fashion around the re-released nerve. The vein, with its endothelial side against the nerve, provides a barrier to inhibit scar tissue growth. It will not, however, provide a gliding surface for the nerve. Our study of removed sections of previously vein-wrapped nerve branches found a separable junction between the two structures,[101] with apposition of the two without any capacity for gliding. The procedure was successful in cases in which the internal nerve damage was not extreme relative to the external scarring.

Surgical Technique

Before surgery, the patient is examined to identify areas of focal increased tenderness to ensure that all affected branches are addressed (Fig. 12-36A). In addition, while the patient is standing, a rubber tourniquet is applied to the midleg, and the saphenous vein is palpated and marked for ease of subsequent intraoperative identification (Fig. 12-36B).

1. The tibial nerve and its branches are circumferentially released over the entire course of the suspected disease (determined by scarring or tenderness to palpation) (Fig. 12-36C).
2. The saphenous vein is harvested, anticipating that for every 1 cm of nerve to be wrapped, 3 cm of vein is needed (Fig. 12-36D and E).
3. The small branches of the vein are occluded with vascular clips on both sides before cutting, providing hemostasis and later permitting reinflation of the vein.
4. Care is taken not to damage the two or more associated branches of the saphenous nerve (Fig. 12-36F).
5. Once sufficient length is obtained, the vein is clamped, tied off, and removed.
6. A bulb-tipped heparin needle is inserted into the distal end of the vein and sealed with a suture to prohibit fluid leakage. The vein is then inflated with 1% lidocaine without epinephrine and maintained in a distended fashion for at least 20 minutes to block the sodium channels. This keeps the vein attenuated (wider and thinner) for greater surface area during wrapping.
7. The external surface of the vein is marked with a surgical marker to help distinguish it from the endothelial side (Fig. 12-36G).
8. The vein is cut longitudinally (Fig. 12-36H).

*References 104, 106, 111, 113, 118, 121, 125, and 128.

9. The nerve is typically wrapped in a barber-pole fashion to encase the nerve and affected branches (Fig. 12-36I). If only a portion of the nerve is scarred, the nerve is not skeletonized, and the vein can be opened and placed over the released nerve (Fig. 12-36J).
10. 6-0 Nylon is used from one edge of the graft to the other whenever a spiral is completed. This helps contour the vein covering to the surface of the nerve and keeps it from bunching up. If the procedure is done without a tourniquet, the wrap can be laid on the nerve without constriction. If the tourniquet is used, the surgeon should anticipate a 15% volume increase in the nerve and therefore wrap the nerve more loosely.
11. The wrap should cover any nerve or branch that was scarred to its bed. Any small neuromas should be included, if possible, into the wrap.
12. Meticulous hemostasis should be achieved with the tourniquet down.
13. The soft tissue is reapproximated without closing the fascia.
14. The skin is sutured.

Postoperative Care

Postoperatively, the leg is placed in a well-padded splint with the ankle in neutral. The sutures are removed at 10 to 14 days. The limb is placed into a removable off-the-shelf boot brace, and the patient is allowed to progressively apply weight during ambulation. The patient should use elastic wraps or support stockings for 3 to 12 months to minimize complications from the vein harvest.

Results

Gould et al[106] studied 64 patients at an average of 31 months of follow-up. Of those 64 patients, 63% had an excellent or good outcome, and 25% reported an increase in symptoms. However, that study had a mixed population: not all patients had primarily adhesive neuralgia.

In the Schon et al[118] series of 58 consecutive limbs (51 with tibial nerve involvement), all had adhesive neuralgia that was a result of a combination of the original nerve insult (primary compression or entrapment, traction or stretch injury, crush injury, transection, idiopathic cause, deep infection, compartment syndrome, and injection injury) and subsequent surgery (such as postoperative scarring). Duration of symptoms before vein wrapping averaged 62 months (range, 11-353 months). The number of previous surgeries for the same nerve problem averaged 2.5 (range, 1-7 procedures). All limbs had undergone at least one neurolysis procedure, which had provided a period of complete or partial pain relief. Sixteen had previous intentional or unintentional transection of a branch of the nerve. Other complications of previous surgery that might have contributed to the adhesive neuralgia included two deep-space infections and six wound dehiscences.

Retrospective follow-up was available for all patients. Follow-up averaged 48.6 months. Pain scores improved

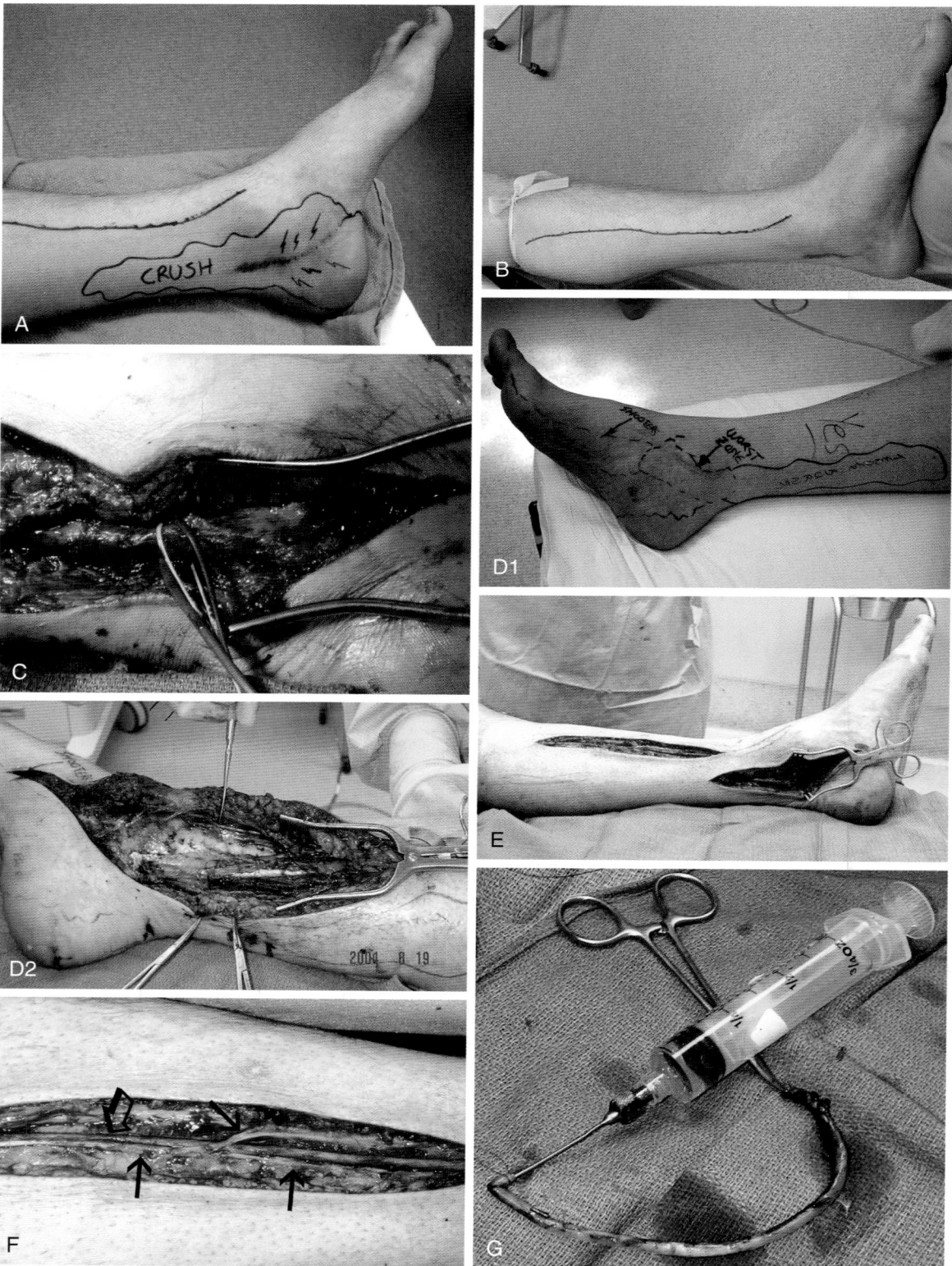

Figure 12-36 **A,** The sites of pathology are marked after inspection to identify the prior incisions and areas of pain. **B,** A tourniquet applied around the leg preoperatively facilitates tracing and marking the saphenous vein. **C,** The nerve was found to be totally encased in scar tissue. **D1** and **D2,** The vein can be harvested from the leg, beginning just proximal to the tarsal tunnel. **E,** An alternative harvest can begin anterior to the tarsal tunnel exposure as shown in this case. **F,** The saphenous vein *(open arrow)* is shown with a branching saphenous nerve *(black arrows).* **G,** The vein is distended with lidocaine and then marked to facilitate wrapping the correct side, the endothelial side, toward the nerve.

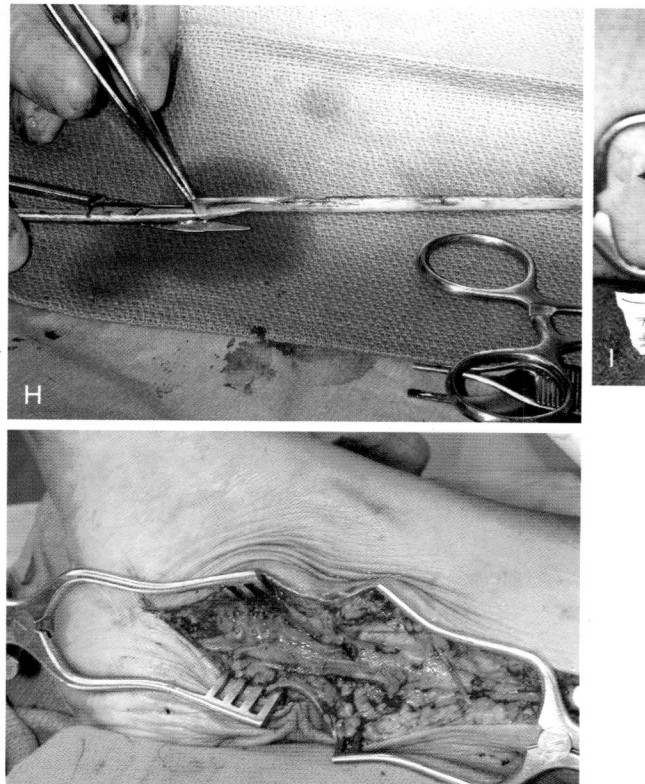

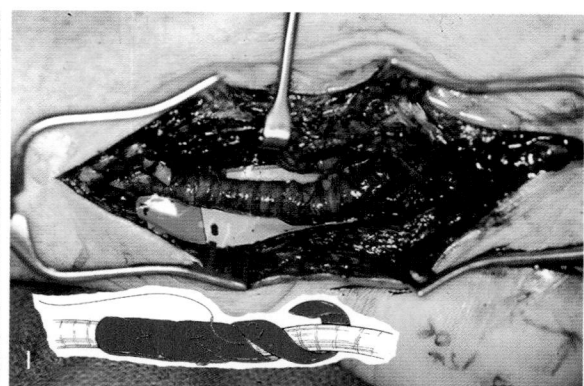

Figure 12-36, cont'd **H,** The vein is cut longitudinally. **I,** The endothelial side of the vein (unmarked) is placed on the released nerve in a barber-pole fashion. **J,** If only a portion of the nerve is scarred, then the nerve is not skeletonized, and the vein can be opened and placed over the released nerve.

from a preoperative average of 8.8 points (range, 6-10 points) to a postoperative average of 5.1 points (range, 0-10 points). Dysfunction scores improved from a preoperative average of 7.4 points (range, 3-10 points) to a postoperative average of 4.4 points (range, 0-9 points). Time to maximum improvement in this group averaged 12 months (range, 3-30 months). Fifty-five percent of the patients were satisfied, 14% were satisfied with reservations (gaining mild or minimal relief of symptoms), and 31% had unsatisfactory results. No patient reported worsening of the symptoms after a suitable recovery from the surgical procedure.

Thirty-eight of the 58 had an autograft saphenous vein, and 20 had an allograft umbilical vein (Fig. 12-37). In 7 of 38 saphenous vein patients, there were complications from the vein harvest: 3 limbs had mild saphenous nerve symptoms, 3 had mild wound healing problems, 2 had swelling from the vein harvest incisions, and 2 had prolonged donor-site pain. All but 2 of the 38 had resolution of symptoms. Of the 58 limbs with the 20 umbilical veins, there were no infections, rejections, or wound complications. Unfortunately, only 7 of 20 patients were satisfied, and 11 of 20 were dissatisfied in the umbilical vein subgroup compared with 25 of 38 satisfied and 7 of 38

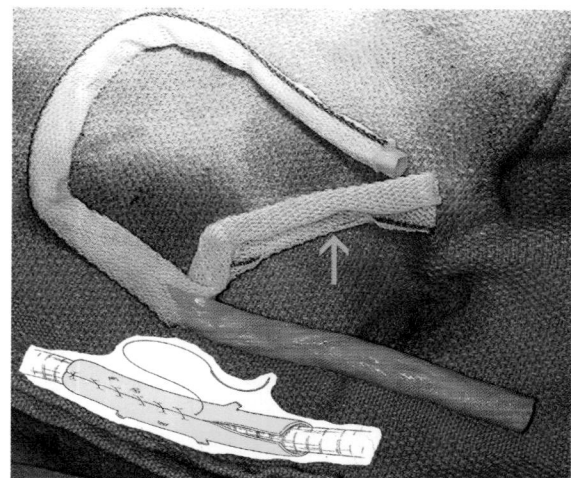

Figure 12-37 An alternative to the saphenous vein autograft is a preserved umbilical vein. The Dacron mesh *(green arrow)* that surrounds the umbilical vein is removed. The *inset* shows the method of wrapping the longitudinally split vein around the nerve.

dissatisfied in the saphenous vein subgroup. Thus Schon's group no longer uses the umbilical vein.

Interestingly, Ruch et al[115] studied 24 Sprague-Dawley rats and performed vein wraps with autograft versus glutaraldehyde-preserved allografts. They found that the allograft vein wraps incited a marked inflammatory response, with epineural scarring and adherence to the underlying nerve, whereas autograft vein wraps did not.

Varitimidis et al[125] studied the vein autogenous saphenous wrap in 19 patients with recurrent carpal tunnel and cubital tunnel syndrome. The average number of surgeries before vein wrapping was 3.3, and the mean follow-up period was 43 months. All patients reported reduction in pain, improvement in the sensory disturbances, and better electrodiagnostic findings.

A newer option is bovine collagen wrap (e.g., Neuro-Mend; Stryker, Kalamazoo Mich.), which allows wrapping of larger-diameter nerves or nerves of greater length. It is a self-curling product that coils around the nerve and maintains a self-closure. It may be used for nerves of 1.0 to 12.0 mm in diameter. Outcomes appear to be equivalent to that of allograft wrap, although more long-term studies need to be undertaken.[112] Similarly, bovine collagen tubes (e.g., NeuraWrap and NeuraGen; Integra Life Sciences, Plainsboro, N.J.) are available in up to 5-cm segments and a variety of diameters that allow nerve wrapping while avoiding the donor-site morbidity of autograft vein wraps. Again, long-term studies are sparse, but initial results show equal outcomes to autograft.[105]

PERIPHERAL NERVE STIMULATION FOR FAILED TARSAL TUNNEL RELEASE

For patients who fail to get temporary relief (group A1) or who are worse after release (group A3), especially if they have ectopic neuralgia, anesthesia dolorosa, or deafferentation phenomenon, neurostimulation should be considered. Those whose symptoms are along the tibial nerve are possible candidates for PNS. For a patient who has diffuse nerve symptomatology, with more than two nerves involved, and especially one who does not respond to a nerve block, spinal cord stimulation is preferable to peripheral neurostimulation.

Patients with a suspected combination of nerve branches encased in scar tissue and inadequate release of a portion of the nerve (group B) can undergo another revision nerve release with a vein wrap. If a major component of sympathetically mediated pain is apparent or if the patient has CRPS II, then surgery and postoperative management should include a continuous sympathetic block via epidural catheter.

Diagnostic criteria for CRPS II include

■ Continuing pain, allodynia, or hyperalgesia after a nerve injury, not necessarily limited to the distribution of the injured nerve.
■ Evidence of edema, changes in skin blood flow, or abnormal sudomotor activity in the region of the pain.

■ Diagnosis excluded by conditions that account for the degree of pain and dysfunction

All three criteria must be satisfied.[122]

Although some have suggested tibial nerve grafting for patients with traumatic tibial nerve transection,[102] we have not seen therapeutic benefit with tibial nerve transection for chronic pain. Over the course of 16 years in Schon's practice, nine patients who have had a tibial nerve transection for chronic tibial nerve pain did poorly.

The PNS procedure can be technically challenging and permanently leaves the patient with restrictions (inability to use local ultrasound, prohibition from obtaining an MRI, difficulty with electronic security systems). The device is subject to electronic malfunction (generator power depletion, alteration resulting from electromagnetic field interference) and mechanical malfunction (fluid leaks with loss of pattern of stimulation, wire breakage, lead migration, generator malposition, wire malposition with local soft tissue irritation, short circuits).

Technique for Peripheral Nerve Stimulation
When the pain is due to a lesion of one or two nerves, the procedure should be considered. Although benefit from TENS is not an indication that the patient will do well, a patient who experiences more pain with TENS is typically a poor candidate for neurostimulation. Failure of spinal cord stimulation is not a contraindication to PNS because the ability to get specific coverage in the tibial nerve territory is generally better with PNS. Previous infection or wound complications are not contraindications to PNS, but a history of recurrent infections in the extremity or elsewhere (e.g., dental or bladder infections) are a relative contraindication for PNS. Patients with idiopathic or systemic neuropathies are poor candidates for the procedure.

A meeting with the representative of the company or discussion with another patient is helpful before surgery. The patient is instructed to mark the leg, ankle, and foot with the zones of numbness, worst pain, trigger points, and so on.

1. The entire limb from the pelvis distal is prepared and draped.
2. The nerve trunk(s) proximal to the level of the disease are circumferentially exposed.
3. The wound is anesthetized, carefully avoiding nerve injection. The patient is then reversed from general anesthesia (Fig. 12-38A).
4. A trial stimulation is performed, with the patient giving feedback about the location and quality of the pain relief while the lead from an external pulse generator is moved around the nerve (Fig. 12-38B).
5. Paresthesia in the zone of pain typically indicates good placement of the lead on the nerve. If this zone can be palpated or percussed during the stimulation with reduced or absent pain, the lead placement is complete.

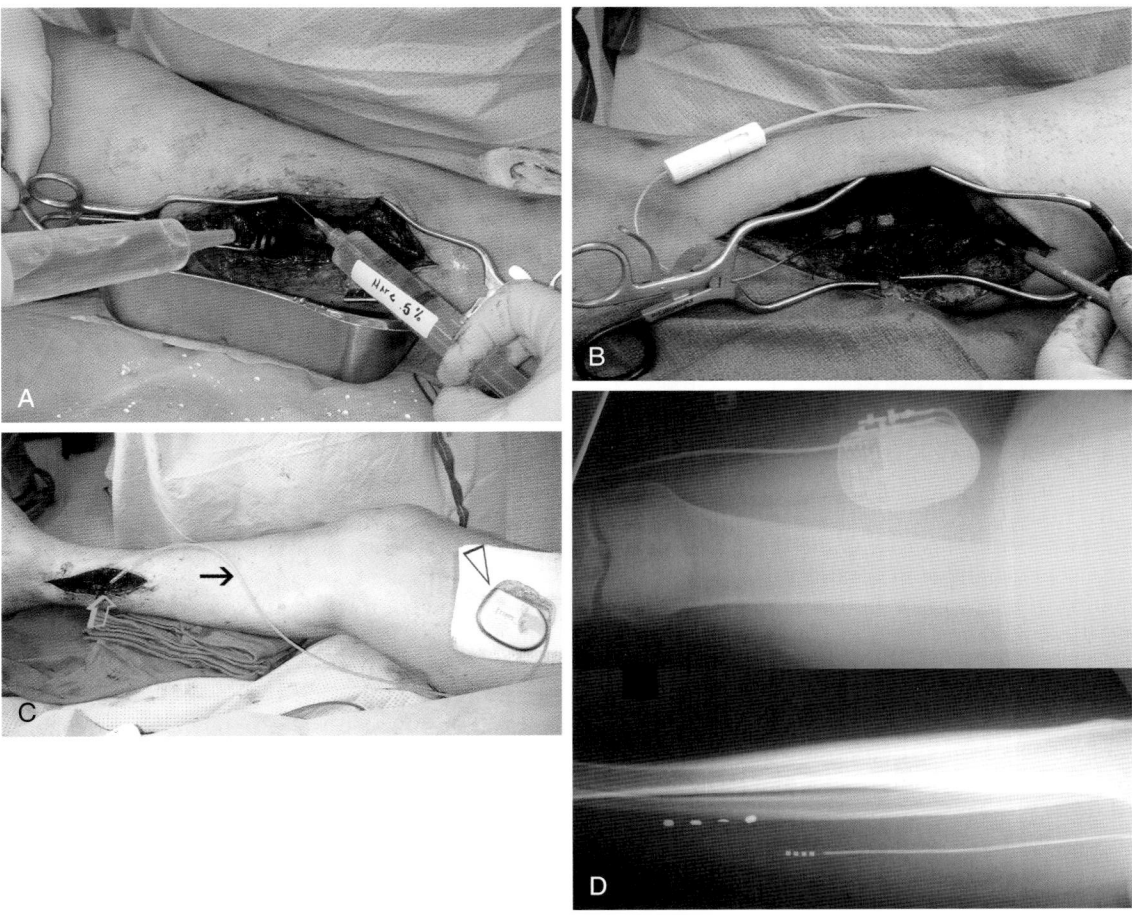

Figure 12-38 **A,** The wound is anesthetized while irrigating the tissues to avoid affecting the nerve. **B,** The lead is placed on the nerve. **C,** The lead *(green open arrow)* will be attached to the extension wire *(black solid arrow),* which is connected to the pulse generator *(red open arrowhead).* **D,** The wire will be tunneled under the tissues with special tools.

6. If there are still other zones of uncontrolled pain, the lead is moved around the nerve to improve the paresthesias and pain relief. If there are still zones of uncontrolled pain, intraoperative nerve blocks are then performed. A decision is made regarding additional nerve trunk stimulation versus additional nerve procedures (e.g., transection, transposition, or additional nerve stimulation) in conjunction with the primary stimulation.

7. Once the placement of the lead (or leads) is finalized, the lead is sutured onto the epineurium with 5-0 prolene suture. The lead should lie on the nerve without undue stress and with the four electrodes flush with its surface. The sutures should not pinch the nerve fibers because this can induce pain. Securing the lead with the patient's immediate feedback prevents creating new problems inadvertently.

8. If paresthesia (stimulation) in the zone of pain is obtained with minimal relief to palpation or percussion, a trial using a temporary external generator connected to the internal lead is then instituted. After 4 to 5 days, if the pain is controlled with adjustment of the

stimulator, an internal generator is implanted. If the pain has not decreased, a series of nerve blocks is performed to identify the nerve that produces or carries the pain signal. Once this is determined, a second-stage procedure is performed to adjust the leads, add another lead to the other nerve(s), or perform additional nerve procedures (e.g., transection, translocation, or containment procedures).

9. If the stimulation is adequate, the patient is reanesthetized with general anesthesia, and the PNS generator and extension wires are implanted. It is important to route the lead and extension wires so that they do not impinge on other structures (tendons, arteries, veins, other nerves), because mechanical stress on either the wires or the tissues can require revision. The extension wire placement is performed using special tunneling tools. The pulse generator is placed in the medial thigh (Fig. 12-38C).

Postoperative Care
The leg is placed in a splint for 2 weeks. Compression wraps are applied around the thigh. Sutures are removed

at 10 to 14 days. The compression wraps are used for 4 to 6 weeks.

Results

In 62 consecutive limbs, the duration of symptoms before PNS averaged 46 months (range, 13-96 months).[104,117,118] Of the 62 limbs, 58 (94%) had undergone at least one previous peripheral neurosurgic procedure for treatment of the neuropathic pain. The number of previous peripheral neurosurgical surgeries averaged 2.8 (range, 0-12) and included neurolysis (57), revision neurolysis (24), vein wrapping after unsuccessful neurolysis (16), transection (47), and centrocentral anastomosis (3). Thirty-eight limbs had stimulation of a single nerve trunk. The remaining had stimulation of two to four nerves. The nerves stimulated included the tibial (28 limbs), the tibial and the sural (4 limbs), the tibial and the saphenous (3 limbs), the tibial and the superficial peroneal nerves (4 limbs), the superficial peroneal and the sural nerves (2 limbs), the superficial peroneal and the deep peroneal nerves (3 limbs), the sural (3 limbs), superficial peroneal (8 limbs), the saphenous nerve (1 limb), the deep peroneal nerve (1 limb), the femoral nerve (1 limb), and the tibial nerve with at least two other nerves (4 limbs).

Pain scores improved from a preoperative average of 9 points (range, 7-10 points) to a postoperative average of 5.1 points (range, 0-8 points), and dysfunction scores improved from a preoperative average of 8 points (range, 7-10 points) to a postoperative average of 6.4 points (range, 3-10 points). The average overall percentage improvement reported by the patients was 42%. Time to maximum improvement after PNS averaged 5.2 months (range, 1-10 months). Satisfaction was reported in 38 of 62 (61%) limbs, satisfaction with reservations in 13 of 62 (21%) limbs, and dissatisfaction in 11 of 62 (18%). In the 48 (of 58, 83%) patients who were satisfied, only 1 patient had complete relief of symptoms, and at 2.5 years' follow-up no longer uses the PNS. In these 48 patients, there were improvements in hours of sleep per night, hours of uninterrupted sleep, and average walking distance. They generally felt that their quality of life and psychologic well-being had improved.

Twenty-nine of 62 limbs required revisions over the 5-year study period. Major revisions with lead replacements were performed in 21 of 29 limbs. Ten of the 21 required another nerve to be stimulated at a later surgery. Eight of the 21 had revisions of the pulse generator for battery depletion during a lead revision. New pulse generators were inserted in 2 of 29 limbs. Four of the 29 limbs have had minor hardware revisions.

Six patients had postoperative infections. Four of 29 limbs had revisions for postoperative infections (3 of these limbs are already counted in the 21 of 29 major revisions) within 6 months of implantation; one patient had a previous history of osteomyelitis. Two of 29 limbs had late infections—1 at 1.5 years and 1 at 3 years—requiring removal of some or all of the implanted components. The patient with infection at 3 years had

undergone additional lead insertion within 3 months postoperatively. Four of the six patients had resolution of the infection with intravenous antibiotics and subsequently had reimplantation of the PNS with satisfactory results. One of the patients who had had the osteomyelitis did not have adequate relief with the initial implantation and requested an amputation. The other patient, who was initially satisfied with his relief of pain for 1.3 years, did not feel that there was adequate functional improvement. This patient ultimately decided to undergo transtibial amputation. Following his amputation, he had further improvement of pain and function.[104,117,118]

Other series have reported improvement of pain symptoms in the upper extremity of 53% to 84%.*

There is a paucity of literature about the lower extremities, but Hassenbusch et al[108] reported on 30 patients who underwent PNS, 12 for lower-extremity nerve pain. In this subgroup, all had stimulation of a single nerve; 7 had stimulation of the posterior tibial nerve, and 5 had stimulation of the common peroneal nerve. Of the 12 patients, only 2 had good results; both of these had stimulation of the posterior tibial nerve. The lack of success in this study might have represented problems with inclusion criteria or technical factors.

Failure of response to re-release, vein wrap, neuroma resection and burial, or PNS does occur. The options for these patients grow more limited and include continued pain management with medications and activity modifications. Options include spinal cord stimulation (SCS), an internally implanted pain pump, and, as a last resort in select patients, amputation.

SPINAL CORD STIMULATION

SCS provides neurostimulation by direct lead application to the spinal cord and may be effective in relieving limb pain.[120,124]

Trial stimulation can be performed percutaneously, usually with only local anesthesia, and is similar to an epidural catheter insertion. The zone of stimulation tends to be broader than PNS but might not cover the distal tibial nerve territory as adequately. Regardless, if lead placement adequately covers the pain, a surgical procedure is then warranted to insert the pulse generator.

Disadvantages of the SCS include the variable acceptance by patients of the need for a spinal procedure to control limb pain. In addition, the broad coverage at times introduces abnormal sensations to normal, non-painful zones, which may be a limiting factor in the patient's ability to increase the stimulation to the painful zones. Finally, lead positional change or migration with flexion and extension of the spine can occur and can require limits in the patient's function to prevent fluctuations in stimulation intensity.

Both PNS and SCS are end-stage salvage procedures that should only be explored after all conventional treatment alternatives have been exhausted but before

*References 107, 108, 110, 114, 123, and 127.

considering amputation. Appropriate patient selection is critical to the success of PNS and SCS, and better-defined patient selection criteria are needed. Schon's prospective experience with a group of 60 patients with PNS with a minimum of 3-year follow-up has been good. Although the midterm results of PNS and SCS are encouraging, long-term follow-up is required to assess the long-term results for the management of intractable lower extremity neuropathic pain.

AMPUTATION

With intractable neurogenic pain that has failed all limb-salvage procedures, proximal amputation may be the ultimate end-stage option. Schon uses a proximal compression test to help determine if the patient might do well with an amputation. The test is performed by circumferentially squeezing the leg at the level of proposed amputation. If the patient does not experience any pain or neuralgia at this level, our experience with amputation has been good.

Schon's group carried out a prospective review[119] of patients who had a transtibial amputation and a prefabricated prosthesis, the Airlimb (Aircast, Summit, N.J.), including a subgroup of 5 patients who underwent the procedure because of chronic pain. They also have had 11 additional patients who underwent transtibial amputation for chronic nerve pain since this publication. Of these 16 patients, 12 are doing well and able to wear a custom prosthesis. One is better than before, wears a prosthesis, and no longer needs pain medication but still has a only a fair result. One is better than before surgery but is unable to tolerate a custom prosthesis, and 2 are doing poorly, with residual stump neuropathic pain and need of further revision surgery. Some of the patients had a standard recovery for a transtibial amputation, and some had resolution of their pain only after 2 to 3 years (unpublished data). This procedure is only used for situations when all other possible alternatives have been exhausted.[119]

There is little published on the results of amputation in the treatment of intractable nerve pain. Dielissen et al[103] reviewed their results from 28 patients who underwent amputations in limbs with complex regional pain syndrome (also called *reflex sympathetic dystrophy*). Amputations were performed for untenable pain (5), recurrent infection (14), or to improve residual function (15). Although only 2 patients were relieved of pain, 9 of 15 had improvement of residual function. They reported that the CRPS recurred in the stump and that only 2 patients could wear a prosthesis. Despite this, 24 patients were satisfied with their results. The authors recommended against amputation for pain relief in CRPS.

Honkamp et al[109] reported on 18 patients with chronic pain (not just from chronic nerve pain) who underwent amputation. Of these 18, 16 would have amputation again and were satisfied with the outcome. In this study, the visual analog scale (VAS) improved in pain frequency (9.8 to 1.7) and in pain intensity (8.4 to 2.6). Walking distance improved. Ten patients were able to stop their narcotics, and 7 decreased their level or dosage, or both. Before amputation, 3 patients continued to work, and 8 patients returned to work after amputation. Although this was not a select group of intractable tibial neuralgia cases, it does give some sense of potential results in select cases.

TRAUMATIC NERVE INJURIES

Nerve injuries to the foot and ankle typically occur as a result of a penetrating wound. They may be secondary to a traumatic event or, in some cases, iatrogenic after a surgical procedure. This is particularly true with arthroscopic procedures that use 3- to 5-mm incisions in areas where the small sensory nerves or branches are vulnerable. In a review of 612 arthroscopies, nerve injuries occurred in 4.4% of cases: 15 superficial peroneal, 6 sural, 5 saphenous, and 1 deep peroneal.[138]

Nerve injuries are also often seen in common foot and ankle procedures, such as open reduction and internal fixation of ankle fractures. For example, one study of 120 ankle fractures found symptomatic superficial peroneal nerve injury with (21%) and without surgery (9%), and the nerve injury was associated with worse results (Fig. 12-39).[152] Other percutaneous or minimal incision surgeries, such as a fascial compartment release, can increase the risk of nerve injury as well.[144]

When associated with significant bony and soft tissue injuries to the lower extremity, nerve injuries can often portend a poor outcome. A lack of plantar sensation in the presence of severe trauma used to be a critical factor favoring amputation over limb salvage. Newer research by the Lower Extremity Assessment Project (LEAP) study group showed that outcomes were not adversely affected by limb salvage in the presence of an insensate foot. Furthermore, they found that tibial nerve dysfunction upon presentation was often indicative of relative ischemia or neurapraxia as opposed to true nerve transection. Return of plantar sensation was seen in 67% of initially insensate feet treated with reconstruction.[134] Recovery of nerve function gives us a good rationale for not exploring the tibial nerve during reconstruction of the mangled extremity,because it often results in additional soft tissue injury.

Although the main role of most of the nerves at the level of the foot and ankle is to provide sensation, the tibial nerve and the deep peroneal nerve innervate the intrinsic musculature of the foot. Damage to these motor nerves can result in an imbalance between extrinsic and intrinsic muscles and can, over time, lead to a claw toe deformity. Sensory nerve injuries in this region can cause morbidity because of lack of distal sensation or the formation of a painful neuroma. Nerve injuries occurring in weight-bearing areas of the foot may predispose the patient to develop CRPS I.

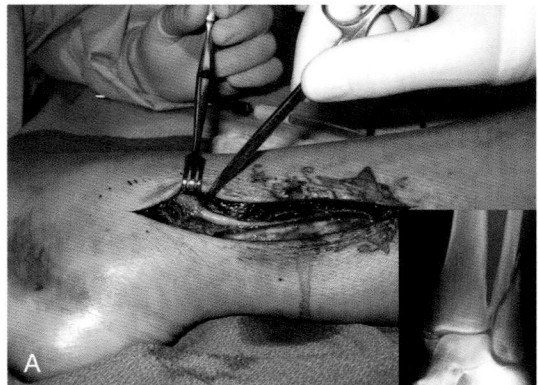
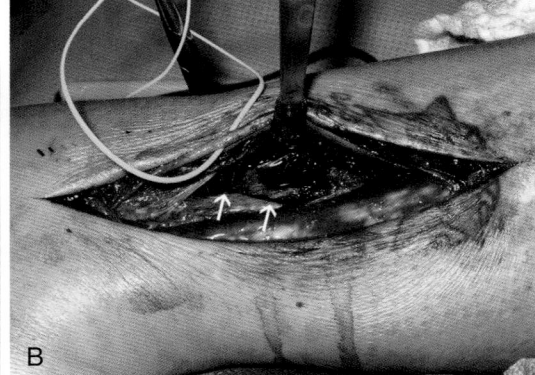

Figure 12-39 **A,** The superficial peroneal nerve is identified during exposure of this fibula fracture. *Inset,* Preoperative radiograph of fibula fracture. **B,** The nerve is released before performing open reduction and internal fixation.

Clinical Symptoms

The clinical history of the patient with a nerve injury is quite typical in that the patient either recalls the specific laceration or notices the symptoms after a surgical incision. The patient usually has fairly well-localized pain and sensory changes distally in the distribution of the affected nerve. At times, the patient is fairly comfortable when ambulating without shoes but feels significant dysesthesias and paresthesias when shoes are worn. Sometimes patients try treating themselves with various types of padding, but unfortunately, this is rarely successful in relieving pressure on the involved area.

Diagnosis

Physical examination demonstrates a scar at the site of the laceration or incision. As a general rule, there is decreased sensation distal to the area of the nerve injury, although the anatomic pattern can vary greatly because of nerve distribution variability. In the case of a neuroma, there is typically a painful area surrounding the scar.

Usually, if a neuroma has developed, it can be palpated or at least percussed (Fig. 12-40). At times, the neuroma is adjacent to the scar rather than within it. A small blunt instrument, such as the end of a pen, can be used to carefully percuss along the nerve trunk to define the involved area if palpation of the neuroma is difficult.

The diagnosis can be verified and the degree of clinical response demonstrated by injection of a small amount (2-3 mL) of local anesthetic into the area just proximal to the neuroma. At times, this also indicates whether there has been complete transection of the nerve or if it is only a neuroma in situ. If the nerve is completely transected, the area of anesthesia will be the same as when the nerve is injected, whereas in cases of neuroma in situ, the area of anesthesia will probably be greater than that mapped out during nerve percussion.

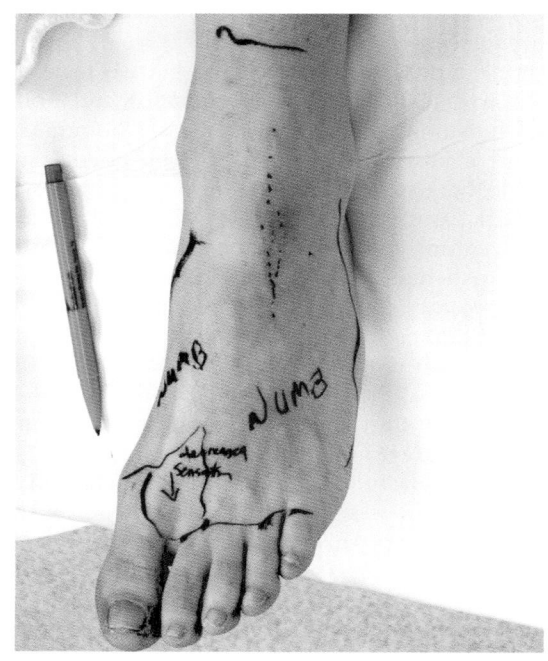

Figure 12-40 Preoperative photograph of foot with superficial and deep peroneal neuromas.

Treatment

Principles of Treatment

A paucity of literature exists to guide the treatment of nerve injuries in the foot and ankle. We have for the most part relied on the techniques that have been developed to address nerve injuries in the upper extremity.

A nerve transection encountered acutely in isolation, that is, in the absence of severe bony and soft tissue trauma, should be treated with urgent repair. This is best achieved with epineurial repair performed without undue tension. When it is not possible to perform a direct repair without significant tension, sural nerve autografts or other newer techniques must be used.

On the other hand, the presence of an insensate foot associated with severe lower-extremity trauma should be treated with either amputation or limb salvage, based on a careful assessment of patient factors and injury severity. Limb salvage should consist of surgical reconstruction of the bone and soft tissue and conservative management of the nerve injury, with expectant return of function over time.

Finally, chronic neuromas deserve an attempt at nonoperative treatment before undergoing surgical intervention.

Conservative Treatment

The conservative management of neuromas is difficult. Shoes or braces that prevent contact with the vulnerable area can be specially purchased or customized. Various types of pads may be placed, or the shoe may be expanded to help avoid pressure over the involved area. The pad or pads can be fashioned to create a channel through which the nerve can pass without pressure from the shoe.

Cortisone injections may be helpful but carry the risk of thinning the skin, making future conservative or surgical management more challenging. Other agents, such as alcohol, have been injected to damage the nerve with the hope of interrupting the pain. These agents can also cause local tissue damage that limits their effectiveness. Furthermore, at times the neurotrauma from the chemicals induces more pain. Perhaps the best treatment is lidocaine patches or various compounded pain creams. Although they have been an effective treatment in some cases, rarely do they completely improve the pain in an active patient.

Surgical Treatment
ACUTE NERVE TRANSECTIONS

For acute nerve transections of the foot and ankle, urgent epineurial repair (as opposed to grouped fascicular repair) is recommended. This minimizes the potential of further injury to the interneural elements and limits scarring at the surgical site. A successful repair requires satisfactory preparation of the nerve stumps and a tension-free approximation.[156]

When this is not possible because of gapping between the injured nerve ends, an autograft, allograft, or conduit is recommended for injured nerves with critical function, that is, the tibial nerve and the common peroneal nerve. Typically, the contralateral sural nerve is harvested for nerve grafting. Success of sural nerve autografts is based on the length of the graft; in one study, five (71%) of seven patients with grafts less than 6 cm had good results versus 0 of 5 patients with grafts longer than 6 cm.[141]

Conduits (e.g., NeuraGen, Integra Life Sciences) are becoming more popular for the reconstruction of nerves with critical-sized defects. They have the advantage of decreased morbidity compared with autografts but appear to suffer from the same limitations. Their role in the upper extremity is for gaps of less than 3 cm of small-diameter nerves (e.g., digital and radial sensory nerves).[149]

Their use in larger-diameter nerves with defects is still being defined, but preliminary findings show better results in gaps less than 3 cm.[158]

NEUROMAS

Neuromas in the foot have two forms: a bulb type of neuroma that occurs when the nerve has been transected or a spindle neuroma that results from a nerve that is still in continuity.[155]

In the treatment of neuromas on the dorsum of the foot, the surgical approach should be carefully planned to avoid placing a scar, if possible, in an area that is subject to pressure from the shoe, such as directly over the dorsum of the foot. The other area that must be carefully avoided is the anterior aspect of the ankle joint, particularly in a worker whose boot will cut across this area.

Schon's current approach is to consider transection and burial for patients with either neuromas or severe intraneural damage with nociceptive neuralgia. If the posterior tibial nerve or other major mixed motor and sensory nerve (e.g., sciatic, common peroneal) is involved, the patient is routinely offered a trial of peripheral nerve stimulation before transection. Although there have been reports of successful transection and interposition reconstruction of major nerves (e.g., tibial),[137,150] the author's group has not experienced good outcomes and does not recommend this procedure.

When performing revision transection and burial procedures, Schon suggests dissection to the affected nerve from proximal to distal toward the trigger spot. Clinically, this is more successful than an isolated proximal nerve transection and burial without distal nerve dissection. It is hypothesized that distal communication between nerves can result in the noxious stimulus coursing along an adjacent nerve, despite the proximal transection.

NERVE TRANSECTION AND BURIAL
Surgical Technique (Video Clip 87)

1. The surgery may be carried out with or without tourniquet control. Loupe magnification should be used so that excellent visualization is possible.
2. The nerve trunk must be carefully identified and dissected from the surrounding soft tissues (Fig. 12-41). As a general rule, unless one of the larger nerve trunks over the dorsum of the ankle area (e.g., intermediate dorsal cutaneous nerve, medial dorsal cutaneous nerve) is involved, resection of the nerve is recommended over attempted repair or release of the damaged nerve. Often, the resulting dysesthesias tend to be more bothersome than the anesthesia that may be created by transection of the nerve. Typically, there is sufficient overlap in the foot so that an area of anesthesia is usually not too bothersome to the patient, although an area of dysesthesia can be.
3. After the nerve has been identified and traced proximally, an adequate bed must be found for it. Any possible depression in the foot (e.g., area of the sinus tarsi)

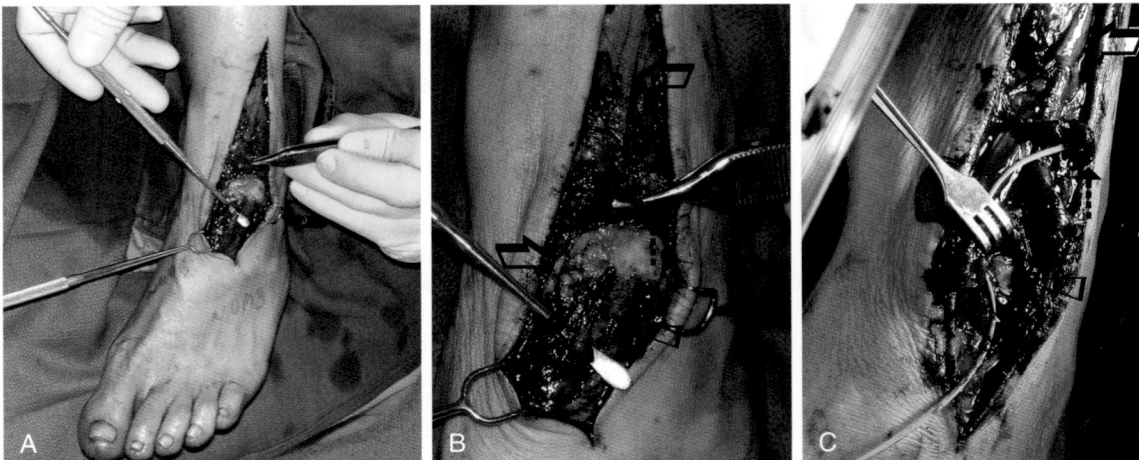

Figure 12-41 Operative photographs of patient shown in Figure 12-40. This patient had a prior ganglion resection over the anterior ankle. The patient had postoperative numbness in the territory of the superficial nerve (SPN) and decreased sensation to the deep peroneal nerve (DPN). **A,** The superficial peroneal nerve is exposed. **B,** The SPN is identified *(open arrow),* and two branches are found to be transected. The *dotted arrow* indicates the proximal end, and the *double-headed arrow* indicates the distal nerves. The deep peroneal nerve was identified over the dorsal capsule of the talonavicular joint *(open arrowhead).* **C,** The capsule of the talonavicular joint is opened, and the DPN is released *(open arrowhead).* The vessel loop is around the main trunk of the DPN *(solid arrow).* The *dotted arrow* indicates the neuroma of the SPN.

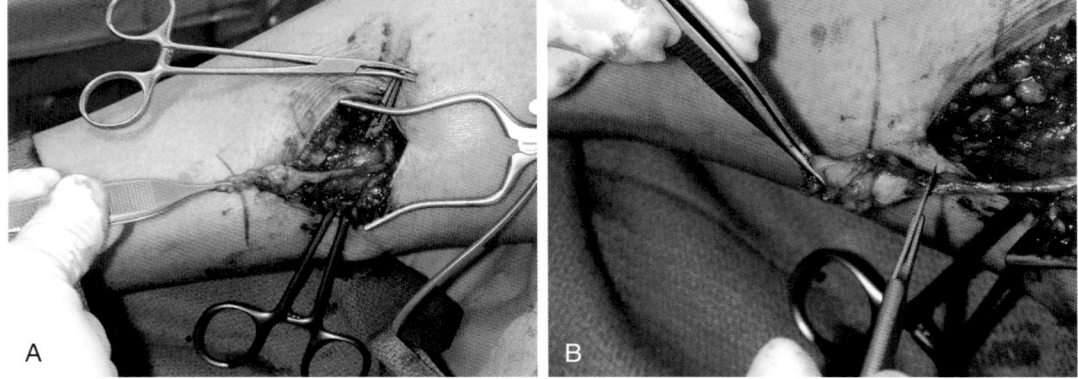

Figure 12-42 **A,** The neuroma of the sural nerve is identified in the posterior aspect of the leg. A curved hemostat is buried into the muscle and will be used to pass the nerve end once it is cut. **B,** The bulbous neuroma will be transected and then pulled through the muscle belly.

should be sought, but in other areas, the nerve needs to be traced proximally and buried beneath the extensor digitorum brevis muscle (Fig. 12-42).

4. It is useful to secure the nerve ending within the zone of protective tissue. This can be achieved by placing a 4-0 Vicryl suture in the epineureum and tying it to fascia or periosteum without undue tension. Another alternative is to bury the nerve end into bone.

Postoperative Care

The patient is treated with a compression dressing, possibly incorporating plaster splints for the first 10 days after surgery. The sutures are then removed, and a compression dressing, usually an elastic bandage, is maintained for another 3 to 4 weeks, with ambulation permitted as tolerated.

Results

Results of neurectomies *without* burial of painful neuromas in the foot have been successful in 65% to 83% of patients in primary situations.[145,157] The concern with performing simple transection is that the response of the nerve is unpredictable; occasionally, a more proximal nerve transection results in greater disability for the patients than was previously present. As described in terms of pathophysiology, disruption of the peripheral pain pathway can lead to deafferentation pain or anesthesia dolorosa. The results of revision transection are typically less favorable than those reported for primary neurectomy, with satisfactory relief of pain.

To optimize results, transection has been combined with several other procedures designed to contain or translocate the new nerve stump. The containment procedures are categorized into physical, synthetic, and physiologic types, all with the goal of limiting axonal regeneration and relocating the new stump away from noxious stimuli.

Physical containment by sealing of the distal nerve ending has been attempted by techniques involving freezing, cauterization, electrocoagulation, chemical sclerosis, mechanical crush or ligation, and nonsynthetic capping (i.e., fascia). Results of ligation techniques, chemical sclerosis, or mechanical crushing of transected nerve endings have been variable and might sometimes increase the pain.[133,157]

Synthetic containment has been attempted using methyl methacrylate, cellophane, collodium, silicone, glass, tin, tantalum, and silver and gold foils. Problems include an inability to fully seal the nerve endings with these materials and stimulation of foreign body reactions, leading to greater neuroma formation.[136,151,153,160]

Physiologic containment methods include excision and retraction into proximal normal tissue,[157] implantation into muscle,[136] and implantation into bone.*

The results of translocation of a transected nerve to limit exposure to mechanical stimuli have been variable. In a large series by Tupper and colleagues,[157] 78% of patients had a successful outcome with repeat neurectomy. Crush injuries had a better prognosis than sharp injuries. Dellon and Aszmann[136] presented an approach to the treatment of dorsal foot pain of neuroma origin with translocation of the appropriate nerves into the muscles of the anterolateral compartment away from the joint. With this approach, they reported excellent results in 9 of 11 patients, with a mean follow-up of 29 months. Miller[148] described significant pain improvement with proximal transection and burial into bone of the dorsomedial cutaneous nerve after iatrogenic primary injury. Chiodo and Miller[135] reported an average perceived pain relief of 75% with transection and burial into bone for treatment of superficial peroneal neuroma. Their study demonstrated a significant improvement in results for symptomatic superficial peroneal neuromas when treated with transection with transposition of the proximal nerve stump into bone as compared with transposition into muscle. Other physiologic containment techniques include end-to-end repair and centrocentral nerve anastomosis. These procedures decrease the likelihood of painful neuroma by containing or controlling rejuvenant nerve growth after transection.[131,132,140,146,153]

Transection and containment procedures are advantageous because of the good reported results, technical ease, and the minimal requirements for complex postoperative treatments. The ideal patient for revision transection is

one with a focal neuroma who experiences nociceptive neuralgia (severe pain with palpation or physical provocation at the trigger end of the nerve). Such patients for whom other therapies have failed are best treated with more proximal transection and burial because this method removes the irritated or irritable nerve from the zone of physical stress.

There are several potential problems with nerve transection: deafferentation pain or anesthesia dolorosa, motor denervation (which can result in muscle imbalance and deformities), vulnerability to ulcers and infections from an insensate plantar aspect of the foot, loss of essential nerve function (i.e., tibial nerve), and ectopic or spontaneous neuralgia.[106]

In patients who demonstrate ectopic neuralgia and not nociceptive neuralgia, more proximal transection and burial might not provide relief. When these cases are associated with the deafferentation phenomenon or anesthesia dolorosa, there is a particularly poor prognosis according to the authors' experience. For these patients, PNS may be a better alternative than transection and burial. In the Schon et al[118] retrospective review of patients undergoing PNS, 47 of the 62 patients had previously undergone transection and burial before PNS. Of these, 8 did not respond adequately to PNS and had poor results. The remainder all had allodynia that responded to some degree to PNS. These results suggest that for patients who fail transection techniques, PNS is still a viable option.

LATERAL PLANTAR NERVE ENTRAPMENT

First Branch

Although heel pain can occur from many conditions, such as plantar fasciitis, calcaneal stress fracture, or subcalcaneal bursitis, the diagnosis of entrapment of the first branch of the lateral plantar nerve should be entertained in chronic cases (Fig. 12-43).

Anatomy

Anatomic dissections have helped unravel the complexity of this region. The posterior tibial nerve divides into three branches: the medial calcaneal nerve, the LPN, and MPN. The medial calcaneal nerve branches off the posterior tibial nerve and penetrates or passes below the laciniate ligament to innervate the posterior and posteromedial aspect of the skin of the heel. In the retromalleolar region, the posterior tibial nerve then branches into the LPN and the MPN. The LPN is separated from the MPN by a fibrous septum originating from the calcaneus and inserting on the deep fascia of the abductor hallucis muscle. The first branch of the LPN courses between the abductor hallucis muscle and the quadratus plantae in an oblique direction. It then changes direction and courses laterally in a horizontal plane. This branch then further ramifies into three major branches. One innervates the periosteum of the medial process of the calcaneal tuberosity, one innervates the flexor digitorum brevis as it passes dorsal to this

*References 135, 139, 142, 143, 147, 148, and 159.

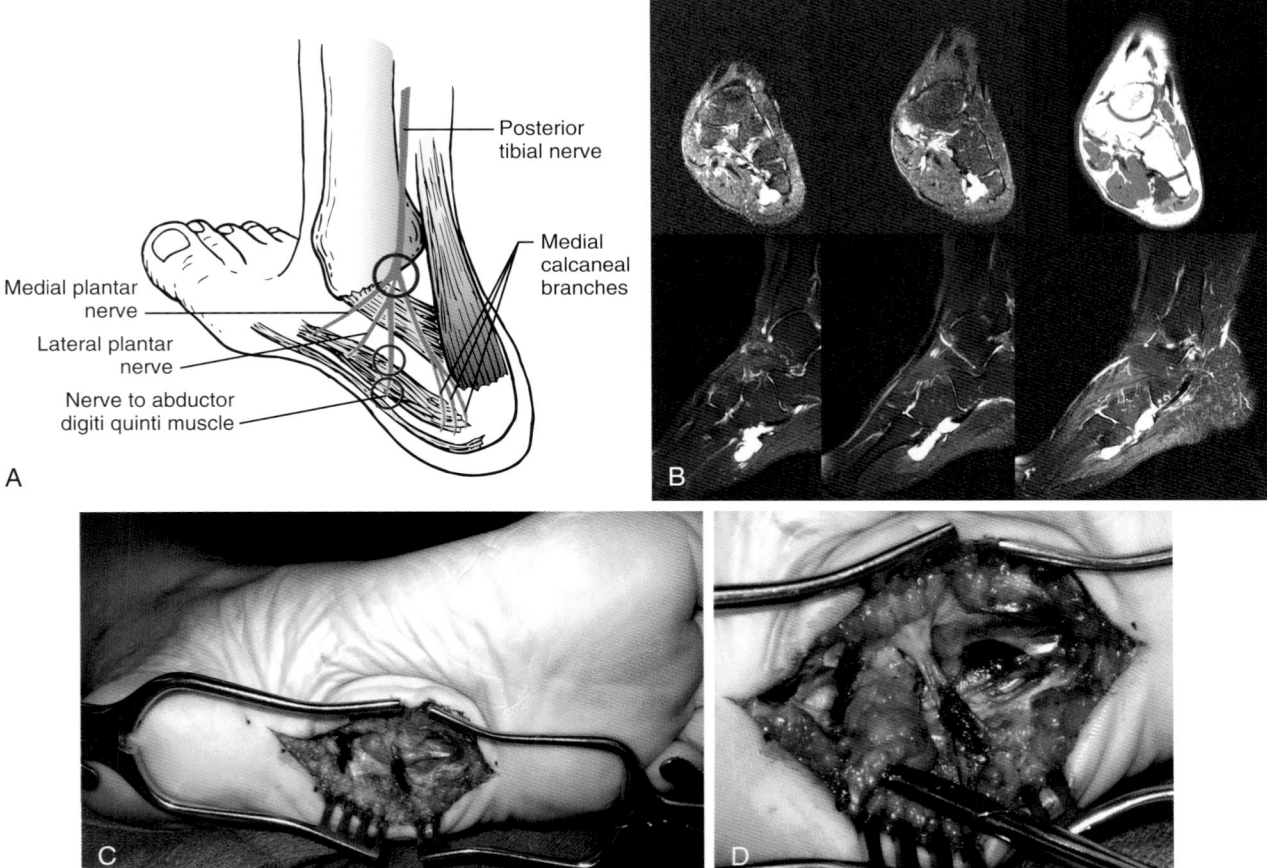

Figure 12-43 **A,** Tarsal tunnel syndrome. *Circles* indicate areas of impingement. The lateral plantar nerve can be trapped in several locations along the medial ankle: at the trifurcation of the tibial nerve, below the deep fascia of the abductor, and where the nerve changes course heading plantarly in a longitudinal fashion to traveling laterally between the quadratus plantae and the flexor digitorum brevis. **B,** The lateral plantar nerve (LPN) can be compressed in the arch of the foot after giving off the first branch of the LPN. Here the patient had numbness and tingling in the lateral aspect of the forefoot and no heel pain. The magnetic resonance image demonstrated a ganglion beneath the cuboid. **C** and **D,** At surgery, the ganglion is found and removed underneath the LPN in the midfoot region.

muscle, and the terminal branch innervates the abductor digiti minimi muscle. The branch that innervates the periosteum of the calcaneal tuberosity often supplies branches to the long plantar ligament and occasionally provides a branch that innervates the quadratus plantae muscle.[161,183]

Incidence

Approximately 5% to 15% of patients with chronic unre-solving heel pain have entrapment of the first branch of the LPN (Fig. 12-44).* The condition occurs in athletes and nonathletes. Although runners and joggers account for the majority of cases, entrapment has been reported in athletes who participate in soccer, dance, tennis, track and field events, baseball, and basketball.[161,162,181] The average age in athletes in the series reported by Baxter and Pfeffer[161] was 38 years, and 88% were men. In the

*References 81, 117, 164, 165, 167-170, 183, and 190.

Henricson and Westlin series[163] of international and national athletes, the average age was approximately 26 years, and 90% were men.

Etiology

According to several recent anatomic and clinical studies, entrapment of this branch of the LPN occurs between the deep fascia of the abductor hallucis muscle and the medial caudal margin of the quadratus plantae muscle. Inflam-mation from chronic pressure can also occur as the nerve courses over the plantar side of the long plantar ligament or the osteomuscular canal between the calcaneus and the flexor digitorum brevis. Athletes with hypermobile pro-nated feet may be particularly susceptible to chronic stretching of the nerve.[182] Hypertrophy of the abductor hallucis muscle or the quadratus plantae muscle might also explain the occurrence of this condition. Accessory muscles, abnormal bursae, and phlebitis in the calcaneal venous plexus have also been implicated.[161,182,187]

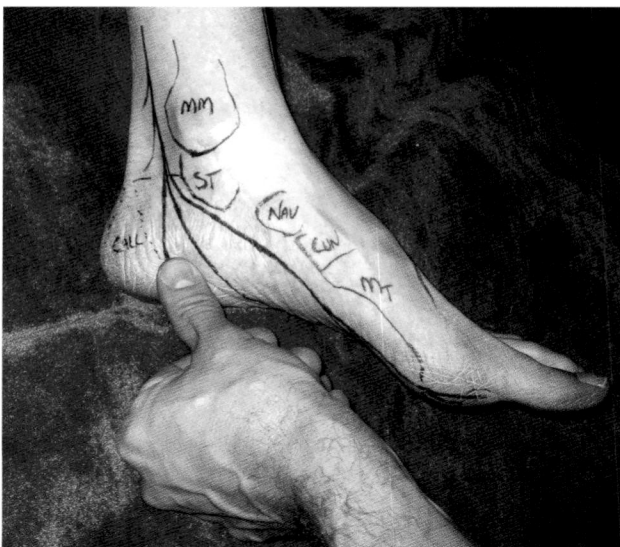

Figure 12-44 The tender spot in plantar fasciitis coincides with the first branch of the lateral plantar nerve.

Clinical Symptoms

Patients with entrapment of the first branch of the LPN report chronic heel pain. Often the pain is increased by walking or running. Pain radiates from the medial inferior aspect of the heel proximally into the medial ankle region of the foot. The pain can radiate across the plantar aspect to the lateral aspect of the foot. Often the pain is worse in the morning. Unless more proximal entrapment of the nerve occurs, patients do not usually describe numbness in the heel or the foot. The average duration of symptoms was 22 months in the Baxter and Pfeffer series.[161] The patient often gives a history of having already tried stretching programs, heel cups, NSAID administration, and injections.

Diagnosis

The physical examination must be performed with a thorough knowledge of the anatomy of this region. More proximal and distal nerve entrapments must be excluded by palpation along the entire course of the posterior tibial nerve and its branches. The pathognomonic finding in these patients is tenderness over the first branch of the LPN deep to the abductor hallucis muscle. Pressure on this point causes reproduction of the symptoms and radiation of pain proximally and distally.

Surgical Treatment
RELEASE OF THE FIRST BRANCH OF THE LATERAL PLANTAR NERVE
Surgical Technique

1. The patient should be in the supine position on the operating table. An ankle block is used most often, and no tourniquet is required, although an ankle tourniquet *may* be used.

2. A 4-cm oblique incision is made on the medial aspect of the heel over the proximal abductor hallucis muscle. The incision is centered over the course of the first branch of the LPN. The incision is oblique and placed distal to the medial calcaneal sensory nerves (Fig. 12-45A).

3. The superficial fascia of the abductor hallucis muscle is divided with a No. 15 blade, and the muscle is retracted superiorly with a small retractor (Fig. 12-45B and C).

4. The abductor muscle is reflected inferiorly, and the deep fascia is released (Fig. 12-45D). The muscle is reflected distally, and the deep fascia is released (Fig. 12-45E).

5. The abductor muscle is reflected proximally, and the deep fascia is released directly over the area where the nerve is compressed between the taut fascia and the medial border of the quadratus plantae muscle (Fig. 12-45F).

6. The muscle is reflected proximally, and the deep fascia is released. A small portion of the medial plantar fascia may be removed to facilitate exposure and clearly define the plane between the deep abductor fascia and the plantar fascia (Fig. 12-45G).

7. The heel spur, if present, is exposed with a Freer elevator, with care taken to protect the nerve that runs superiorly. The abductor hallucis muscle belly and its superficial fascia are left intact.

8. An extensive plantar fascia release is not performed unless direct visualization shows evidence of a pathologic condition in the entire proximal portion of the plantar fascia.

9. The wound is closed with interrupted sutures.

10. A bulky dressing is applied.

Postoperative Care

The sutures are removed at 10 to 14 days. The patient is allowed to bear weight on the heel at 10 days. The authors do not routinely use a boot brace or a cast, but if patients are having difficulty progressing, one can be used.

Results

Baxter and Pfeffer[161] reported on 61 heels; they had excellent or good results in 89% and complete resolution of pain in 83%. Watson et al[170] reported 88% good and excellent results. They found that MRI findings consistent with plantar fasciitis were associated with good and excellent results. The authors strongly advocated nonoperative treatment for 12 to 18 months before surgery and noted that 52% of patients required more than 6 months to reach maximum improvement.

Calcaneal Branches

Overview, Etiology, and Anatomy

The medial calcaneal branches of the tibial nerve provide sensation on the medial aspect of the heel. Anatomic studies have demonstrated a proximal origin of the

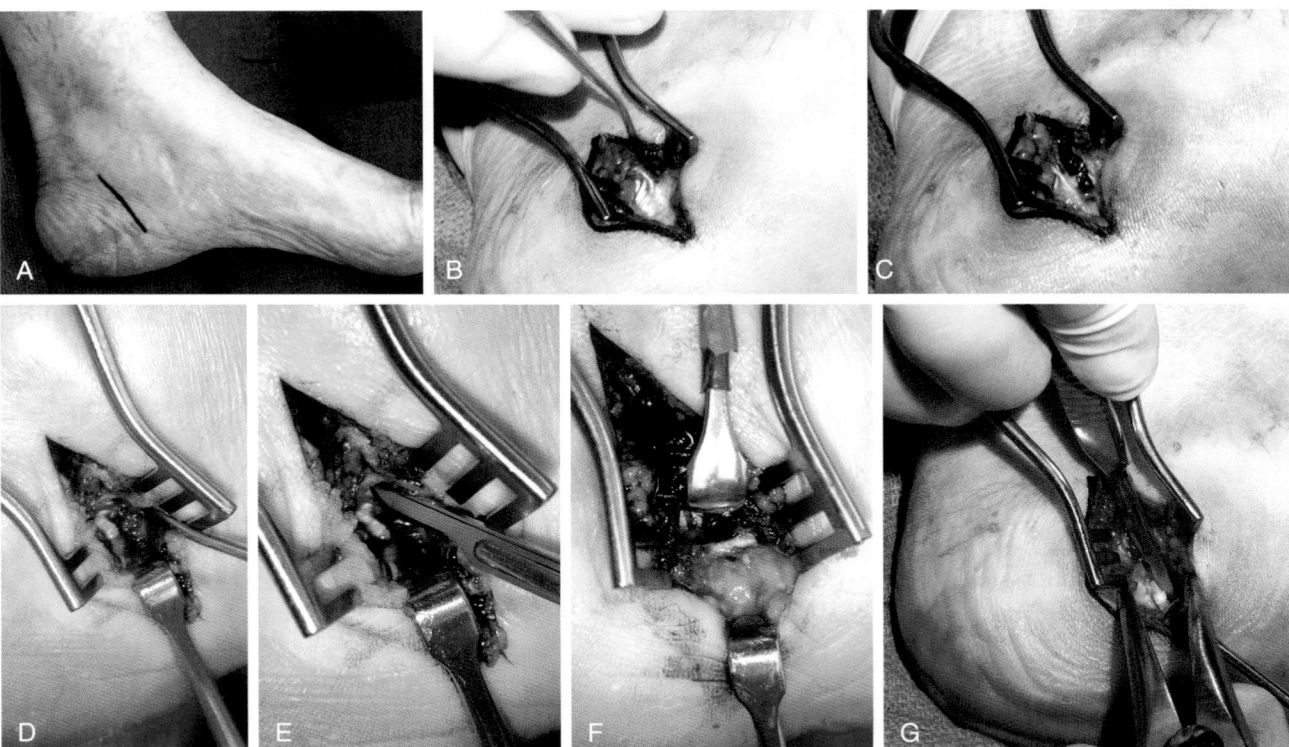

Figure 12-45 **A,** The incision is oblique along the course of the first branch of the lateral plantar nerve. **B,** The incision deepened to the superficial fascia of the abductor. **C,** The fascia is incised. **D,** The muscle is reflected distally, and the deep fascia is released. **E,** Next, the abductor muscle is reflected proximally, and the deep fascia is released directly over the area where the nerve is compressed between the taut fascia and the medial border of the quadratus plantae muscle. **F,** The muscle is reflected proximally, and the deep fascia is released. A small portion of the medial plantar fascia may be removed to facilitate exposure and clearly define the plane between the deep abductor fascia and the plantar fascia. **G,** A portion of the plantar fascia is released.

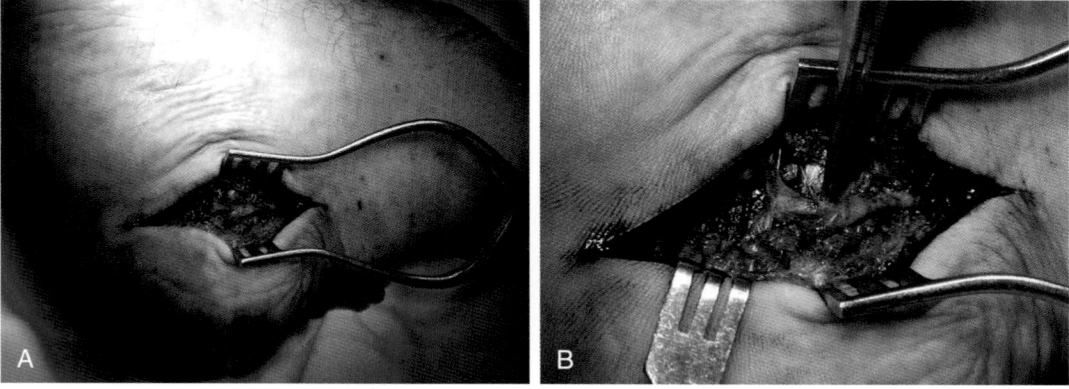

Figure 12-46 This police officer had sustained a high-energy impact injury to his medial heel with a steel bar. He had persistent pain and dysesthesias of the medial heel that did not respond to local and systemic modalities. He underwent exploration of the medial calcaneal nerves. **A,** The calcaneal nerve was enlarged and found entrapped in dense scar tissue. **B,** After release, his pain and function improved.

medial calcaneal branches from the tibial nerve and the existence of multiple medial calcaneal branches.[14,74] One study showed that 70% of medial calcaneal nerves originated proximal to the tarsal tunnel and that 60% of specimens had multiple branches.[14] Compromise of the medial calcaneal nerve branches might contribute to chronic heel pain (Fig. 12-46). The medial calcaneal nerve branches do exhibit a considerable amount of variation in terms of location, origin, and course. A medial calcaneal nerve occasionally originates from the MPN.[69,169]

Calcaneal neuromas can produce a painful heel syndrome; however, most likely such a painful heel syndrome secondary to medial calcaneal nerve compromise occurs only when a true medial calcaneal nerve neuroma results from a transection injury during previous surgery (Fig. 12-47).[169] With an accessory muscle (soleus or flexor hallucis longus), the authors have seen symptomatic tenting of the medial calcaneal nerve over the bulky muscle.

Evaluation

Confirmation of medial calcaneal nerve compression cannot be achieved by standard electrodiagnostic studies because the medial calcaneal nerve is a sensory nerve. Testing methods that rely on the patient's sensing and expressing skin sensitivity to two-point stimulation or irritation can help objectify the findings. An accessory muscle or space-occupying lesion can be appreciated on computed tomography or MRI scan.

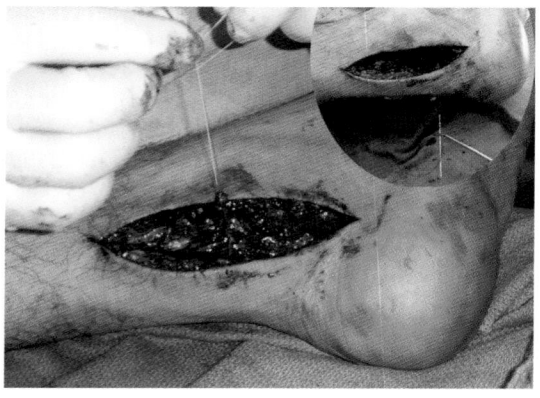

Figure 12-47 A traumatic calcaneal neuroma is identified during surgery in a patient who had a medial ankle laceration or crush. *Inset,* The neuroma is transected and buried into the posterior soft tissue with the assistance of a Keith needle.

Management

As with other syndromes, nonoperative techniques can be used. When these fail, surgical management may be considered. Typically, release of the tarsal tunnel with careful release of the medial calcaneal nerve is performed. It is advisable to identify the tibial nerve and then trace it distally into the heel. The MPN and LPN dive deep to the fascia of the abductor, and the calcaneal nerve(s) are found superficial to the muscle. Rarely, the nerve pierces the superficial fascia of the abductor and then travels in the subcutaneous fat. The nerve, which can range in diameter from 1 to 4 mm, ramifies into the skin of the medial and medial plantar heel (Fig. 12-48). When there is an accessory muscle, resection of the bulky distal portion is suggested.

Results

In the authors' experience with a limited number of cases of medial calcaneal nerve entrapment, good to excellent results have been obtained 75% of the time.[63,117,166]

MEDIAL PLANTAR NERVE ENTRAPMENT

After the MPN travels underneath the flexor retinaculum, it courses deep to the abductor hallucis muscle. The nerve runs along the plantar surface of the flexor digitorum longus tendon and passes through the knot of Henry. It continues along the medial border of the foot and ramifies into branches that lie on the medial and lateral aspects of the flexor hallucis longus tendon. The MPN is a mixed sensorimotor nerve that provides sensation to the medial sole, the plantar portions of the first through third toes, and the medial half of the fourth toe, while providing motor innervation to the abductor hallucis, flexor hallucis brevis, flexor digitorum brevis, and first lumbrical muscles. This condition should be easy to distinguish based on a typical history of a neuroma resulting from transection or severe crush injury of the MPN. Although transient neuralgia is more common than a transection

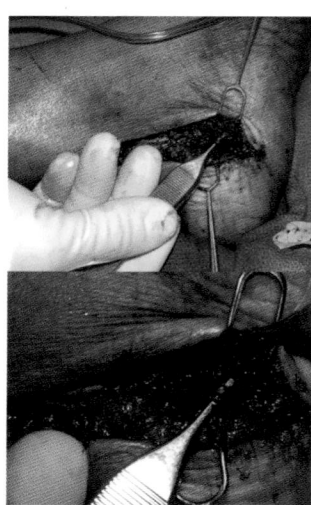

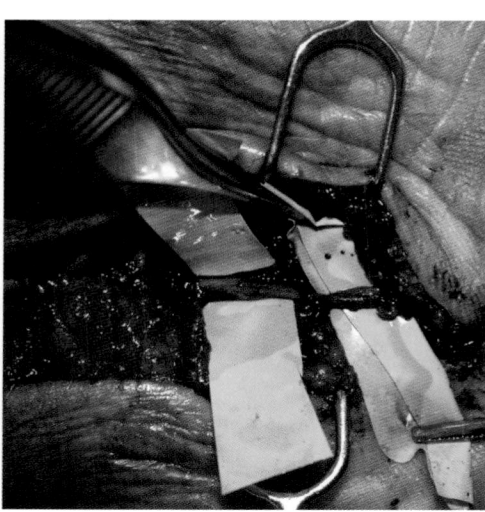

Figure 12-48 The patient had atypical medial heel neuralgia after a twisting injury. With percussion over the tibial nerve, the patient had tingling of the medial heel but not into the plantar aspect of the midfoot and forefoot. *Upper left* and *lower left* (close-up), The calcaneal nerve and two branches are identified after releasing the inferior fascia of the tarsal tunnel. The nerve was constricted by the flexor retinaculum where it penetrated the fascia. *Right,* The blue background is underneath the main trunk of the large calcaneal nerve and its more posterior branch.

injury, surgery for the jogger's foot is less common (Figs. 12-49 and 12-50).

Incidence

Medial plantar nerve entrapment classically affects joggers (jogger's foot). Although it has been reported most often in men, there is no gender predilection. No specific age distribution has been encountered.[172,198]

Etiology

Medial plantar nerve entrapment occurs in the region of the knot of Henry. Most patients are found to walk or run with excessive heel valgus or with hyperpronation of the foot. Arch supports, especially those that are built up, can compress the nerve. Kopell and Thompson[171] described the entity associated with hallux rigidus. They postulated that overactivity of the tibialis anterior, caused by the patient's attempting to lift the arch of the foot to avoid pain, contributed to the syndrome. They also believed that MPN denervation resulted in increased stress in the first MTP joint, which ultimately led to arthrosis.[171] An avid walker who had a long history of rigidus subsequently had medial plantar neuralgia. This was thought to be caused by abductor hallucis and flexor brevis muscle spasm, which was her unconscious attempt to splint the first MTP joint against dorsiflexion.

Clinical Symptoms

The patient describes aching or shooting pain in the medial aspect of the arch. The pain often radiates distally into the medial three toes and can radiate proximally into the ankle. The pain is worse with running on level ground but may be induced by workouts on stairs (Fig. 12-51). The patient might report onset of the syndrome associated with the use of a new orthosis or shoes.

Diagnosis

The patient should be examined in a weight-bearing position to identify hindfoot valgus, which can trigger this condition. The patient should also be examined standing on his or her orthotic device to identify any areas of

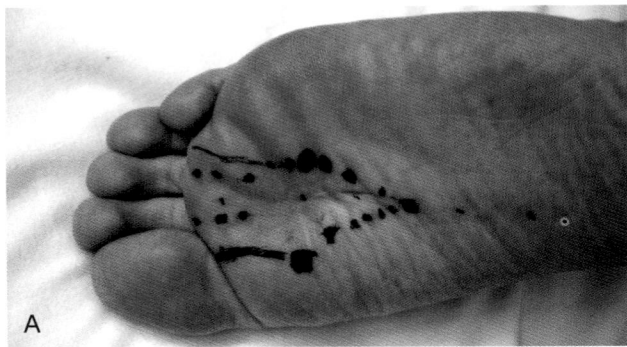
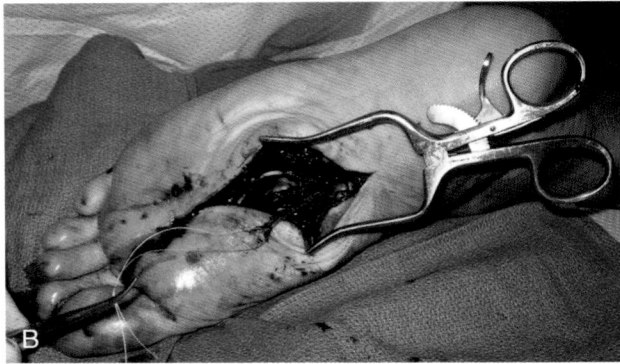

Figure 12-49 **A,** The medial plantar nerve territory was painful and had decreased sensation after a transection injury to the arch of the foot. **B,** The medial plantar nerve formed a neuroma where it was injured. This was transected more proximally and the end buried into muscle.

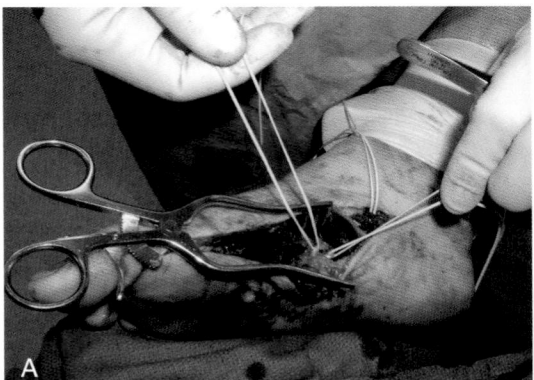
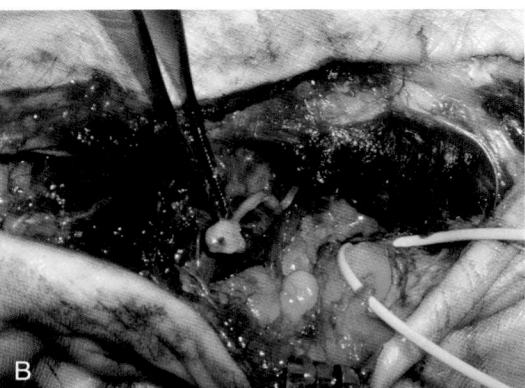
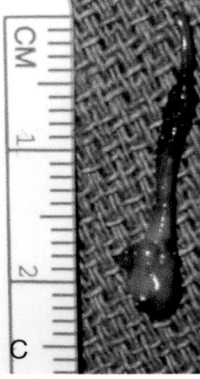

Figure 12-50 The patient complained of chronic recalcitrant medial plantar foot pain and dysesthesias after a bunion surgery with a proximal metatarsal osteotomy. The medial plantar nerve was identified proximally deep to the abductor muscle. Distally, the medial plantar nerve divides into two branches held by vessel loops inferior to the abductor muscle. **B,** The smaller branch is found to have a bulbous neuroma in the area of maximal preoperative tenderness. **C,** The neuroma is resected and the end buried into the muscle.

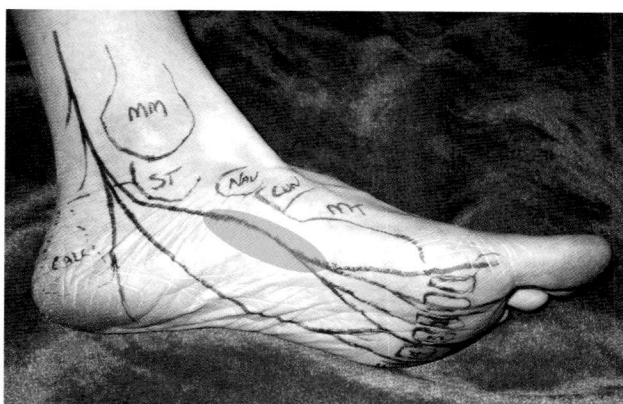

Figure 12-51 The jogger's foot with compression of the medial plantar nerve in the arch as demonstrated by the *shaded oval*.

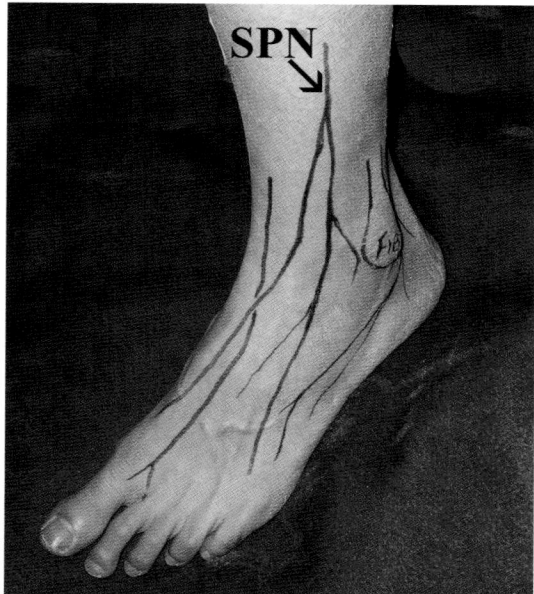

Figure 12-52 The superficial peroneal nerve *(SPN)* is drawn here after it penetrated the lateral fascial compartment.

external compression. Palpation along the MPN usually reproduces symptoms consisting of medial arch tenderness with radiation, dysesthesia, or paresthesia to the medial three toes. Symptoms may be increased with tightening of the adductor hallucis brevis muscle, which can be accomplished with a heel rise or eversion of the heel. Because of the close proximity of the MPN and the medial tendons, it can be difficult to distinguish between neuralgia and tendinitis. Occasionally, it is necessary to have a patient run on a treadmill for several minutes to identify symptoms. Decreased sensation is usually present only after the patient has been running or walking for a prolonged period.

Surgical Treatment

MEDIAL PLANTAR NERVE RELEASE
Surgical Technique
1. Under ankle block anesthetic with or without tourniquet and loupe magnification, the patient is positioned in a supine manner.
2. A 7.5-cm (3-inch) longitudinal incision is made just inferior to the talonavicular joint.
3. The superficial fascia over the abductor muscle is released, and the muscle is reflected plantarly.
4. The deep fascia is released, and the naviculocalcaneal ligament is released just inferior to the talonavicular joint (knot of Henry). In addition to the MPN, the flexor digitorum longus tendon crosses the flexor hallucis longus tendon at the location of entrapment.
5. Care is taken to avoid stripping the nerve of any fatty tissue.
6. After wound irrigation, the skin is closed with interrupted sutures and a compression dressing applied.

SUPERFICIAL PERONEAL NERVE ENTRAPMENT

The superficial peroneal nerve (SPN) is a branch of the common peroneal nerve. It courses through the anterolateral compartment and innervates the peroneus brevis and peroneus longus. Traveling between the anterior intermuscular septum and the fascia of the lateral compartment, it pierces the deep fascia approximately 8 to 12.5 cm above the tip of the lateral malleolus (Fig. 12-52). The nerve then becomes subcutaneous, and, approximately 6.4 cm above the lateral malleolus, it divides into two branches (the intermediate and the medial dorsal cutaneous nerves). The intermediate dorsal cutaneous nerve usually provides sensation to the lateral dorsal aspect of the ankle as well as the fourth toe and portions of the third and fifth toes. The medial dorsal cutaneous nerve provides sensation to the dorsomedial aspect of the ankle as it extends toward the medial aspect of the hallux as well as to the second and third toes.[185]

Incidence

The average age of patients with SPN entrapment is approximately 36 years (range, 15-79 years). Among the athletic population, the average age is 28 years. In both the general and the athletic populations, the syndrome occurs equally in men and women. Most athletes are runners, although several are soccer players. This syndrome also has been described in hockey, tennis, and racquetball players.[175,177-180,186,189]

Etiology

According to clinical and anatomic studies, the site of entrapment of the peroneal nerve occurs at its exit point from the deep fascia. In most cases, the fascial edge impinges on the exiting nerve. Fascial defects with muscle herniation exacerbate the impingement. Such herniations might only occur in the dynamic state and be part of a localized anterior exertional compartment syndrome.

Styf[188] described a short fibrous tunnel between the anterior intermuscular septum and the fascia of the lateral compartment. In almost half of his cases, he described a fibrotic, low-compliance tunnel that can predispose to a local compartment syndrome. Rosson and Dellon[184] retrospectively reviewed the location of the superficial peroneal nerve in a consecutive series of 35 limbs in 31 patients having entrapment of the superficial peroneal nerve. They found the location of the superficial peroneal nerve in the anterior compartment in 47% of the patients.

Chronic ankle sprains, a major underlying factor, subject the nerve to recurrent stretching (Fig. 12-53). A previous anterior compartment fasciotomy causes shifting of the fascia with resultant stretch and impingement of the nerve.[164,168,185] Peroneal nerve entrapment can occur idiopathically, or it can be associated with direct trauma (with ganglion) (Fig. 12-54), fibular fracture, exertional compartment syndrome (and previous fasciotomy), muscle herniation, syndesmotic sprains, lower extremity edema, and (rarely) mass effects such as tumors.[188,189,207]

Clinical Symptoms

Patients report a long history of pain over the outer border of the distal portion of the calf and the dorsum of the foot and ankle. About one third have numbness and paresthesias along the distribution. Occasionally, patients report pain only at the junction of the middle and distal thirds of the leg, with or without local swelling (Fig. 12-55). The pain is typically worse with physical activity, ranging from walking, jogging, and running to squatting. Nocturnal pain is uncommon. Relief by conservative measures is uncommon.[174,177-180,186,189]

Approximately 25% of patients with the syndrome have a history of prior trauma to the extremity, most commonly an ankle sprain. The syndrome has been reported after anterior compartment fasciotomy.

Diagnosis

Physical examination must include an evaluation of the lower back for sciatic nerve pain. The region where the common peroneal nerve sweeps around the neck of the fibula must also be examined to exclude proximal entrapment. Point tenderness is usually elicited where the nerve emerges from the deep fascia, approximately 8 to 12.5 cm above the tip of the distal end of the fibula. Paresthesias and numbness are often noted. Approximately 60% of the patients described in the literature have a palpable fascial defect.

Styf[188] describes three provocative tests to suggest a diagnosis. In the first test, the patient actively dorsiflexes and everts the foot against resistance while the nerve impingement site is palpated. In the second and third tests, the physician plantar flexes and inverts the foot, first without pressure over the nerve and then with percussion along the course of the nerve.

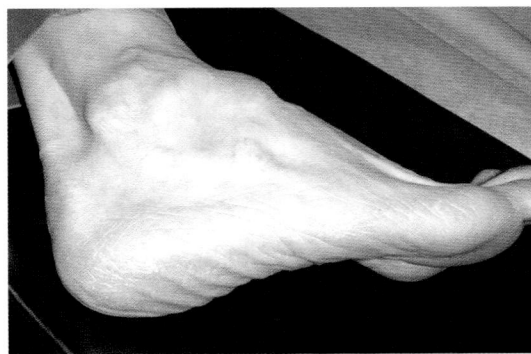

Figure 12-54 A large multilobular ganglion compresses the superficial peroneal nerve.

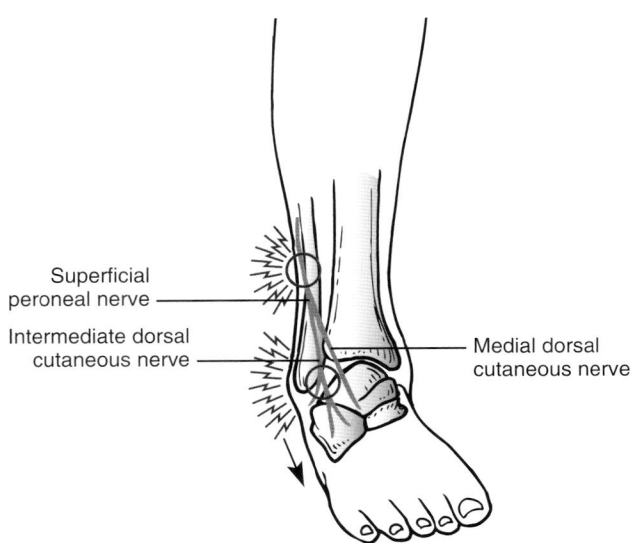

Figure 12-53 Superficial peroneal nerve entrapment. *Circles* indicate areas of impingement.

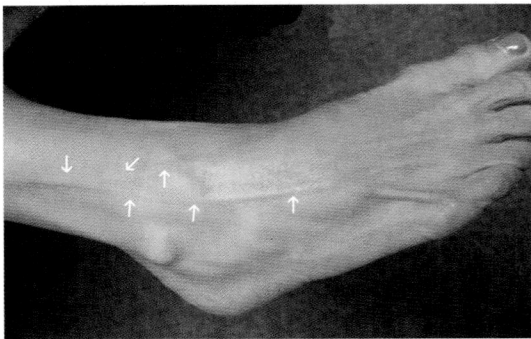

Figure 12-55 The superficial peroneal nerve is easily seen in this foot and ankle. The *white arrows* are emphasizing the course of the nerve.

Treatment

Conservative Treatment

Conservative treatment of superficial peroneal nerve injuries includes strengthening the lateral muscles of the leg, wearing a supportive ankle brace to prevent inversion of the ankle, and wearing a lateral heel and sole wedge in the shoe to prevent inversion. A boot brace may be helpful during the day. For the atypical patients who have some nocturnal symptoms, a night splint can be used to hold the ankle in dorsiflexion.

Surgical Treatment
SUPERFICIAL PERONEAL NERVE RELEASE
Surgical Technique

1. The patient is placed supine on the operating table. A beanbag or bump is useful to help tilt the patient in to a 30- to 45-degree lateral position.
2. A regional anesthetic is used to block the area proximal to the entrapment of the superficial peroneal nerve. This block needs to be carried out approximately 15 cm proximal to the distal tip of the fibula.
3. A 7.5-cm incision is made in the area of maximum symptoms.
4. Once the superficial peroneal nerve is identified, the nerve is released by incising the fascia proximal and distal to its exit point from the compartment (Fig. 12-56).
5. Often, the nerve is compressed at a localized area where the muscle herniates. No attempt is made to repair or close this hernia. When the patient had previous surgery along the course of the superficial peroneal nerve, the cause of the pain could be compression from a fascial edge or a more distal entrapment (Fig. 12-57).
6. If there is a tunnel of compression before the nerve leaves the fascia, care must be taken to release the entire fascial sheath until the nerve lies within the muscles proximally.
7. After irrigating the wound, the skin is closed with interrupted sutures and a compression dressing is applied.

In cases of extensive release, a splint might be applied as well.

Postoperative Care

Postoperatively, the patient wears a compressive wrap or splint. Ambulation is allowed as tolerated after 3 to 4 days. The sutures are removed at 2 weeks, and activities can be resumed 3 weeks after surgery if symptoms permit.

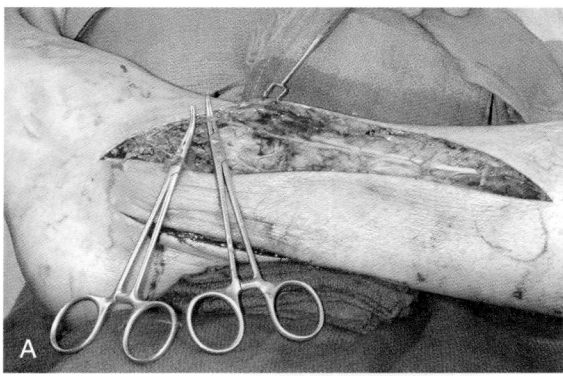
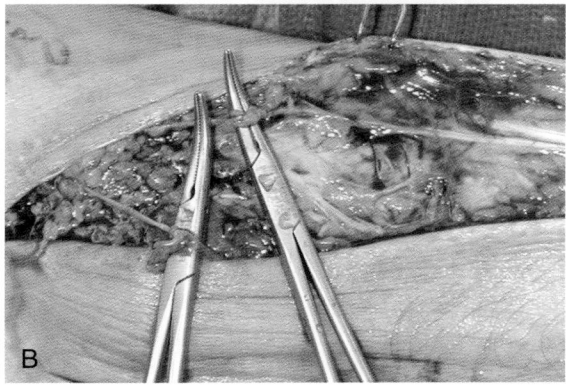

Figure 12-56 **A,** The superficial peroneal nerve is seen here, after release, piercing the lateral fascia. The nerve branches and is traced distally to the zone of trauma. **B,** The nerves become thin and are found in scar tissue in this case.

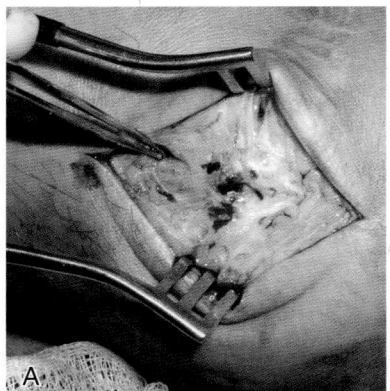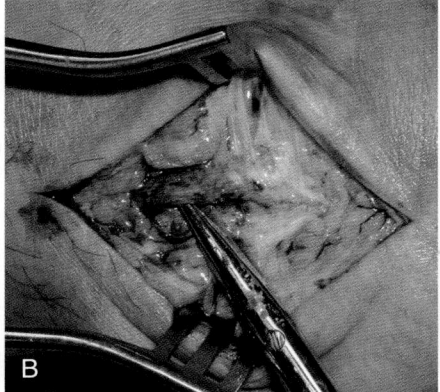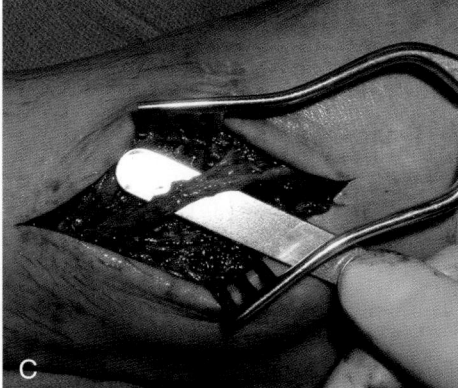

Figure 12-57 **A,** The patient had a prior fascial release and had persistent pain. The old scar is reexplored, and the superficial peroneal nerve is found encased in the tissues. **B and C,** The nerve is meticulously released.

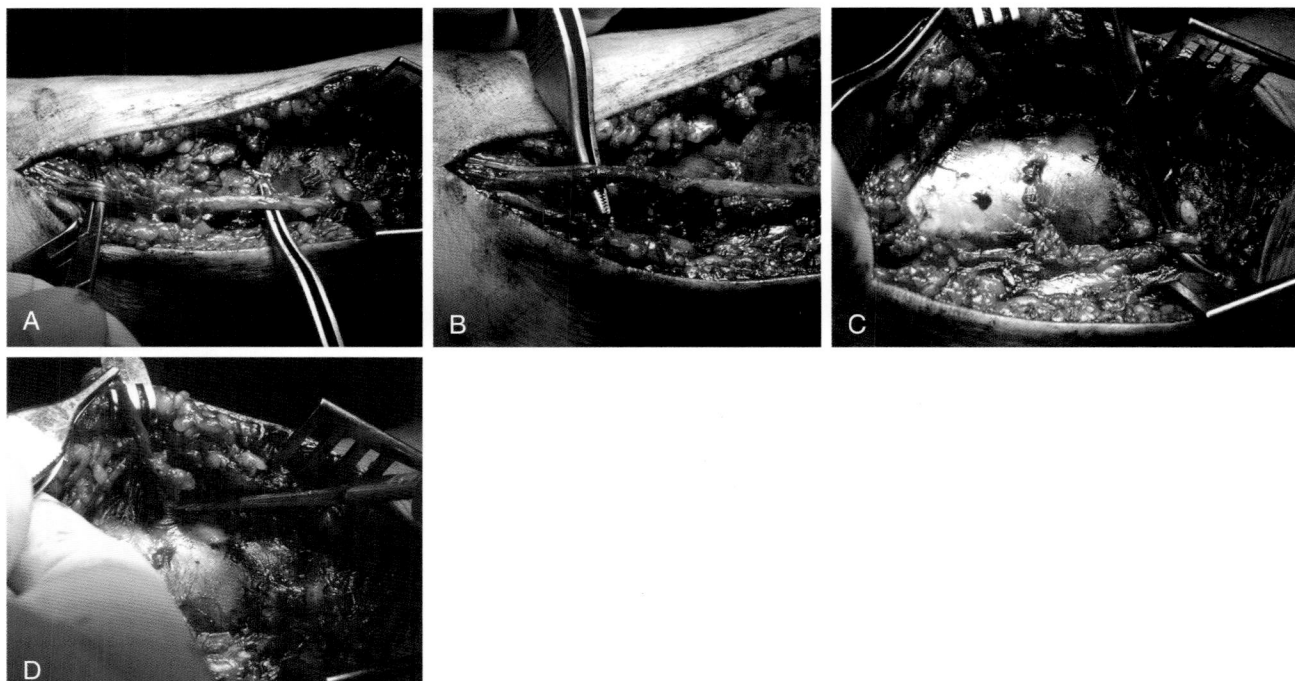

Figure 12-58   **A,** The superficial peroneal nerve is lifted by forceps more distally. The nerve was found to be frayed, flattened, and irregular in appearance in the zone of trauma. Proximal to where the nerve is lifted by the hemostat, the nerve is bound down by scar tissue. **B,** The nerve has been freed from constriction, but the amount of damage was thought to be too extensive for recovery given the magnitude of pain and the chronicity. **C,** Transection was performed, followed by transposition. The nerve, seen over the hemostat, had been passed deep into the anterior compartment and pulled out medially to ensure deep burial. **D,** The nerve is gently pulled and cut where it pierces the fascia. It is allowed to retract into the deep musculature of the anterior compartment.

Results

A larger series of superficial peroneal nerve decompressions by Styf[188] suggests that improvement of symptoms can be anticipated in 75% of cases, but the author warned that results are less predictable in athletes. Schepsis et al[186] looked at 8 of 18 (44%) patients who had symptoms, signs, and surgical findings of entrapment of the superficial peroneal nerve after surgery for exertional anterior compartment syndrome of the lower leg. All 8 patients with documented peroneal nerve entrapment had a satisfactory outcome. Other series of superficial peroneal nerve release have demonstrated effective relief of symptoms.[178,179,181,184] When the nerve has been released and the symptoms remain, the nerve can be reexplored, and transection and burial into muscle or bone may be considered (Fig. 12-58). As detailed earlier, Chiodo and Miller[135] showed better pain relief for patients treated with transection and burial into bone versus those treated with transection and burial into muscle.

DEEP PERONEAL NERVE ENTRAPMENT

The deep peroneal nerve lies between the extensor digitorum longus and the tibialis anterior muscles in the proximal third of the leg (Fig. 12-59). The nerve travels between the extensor digitorum longus and the extensor

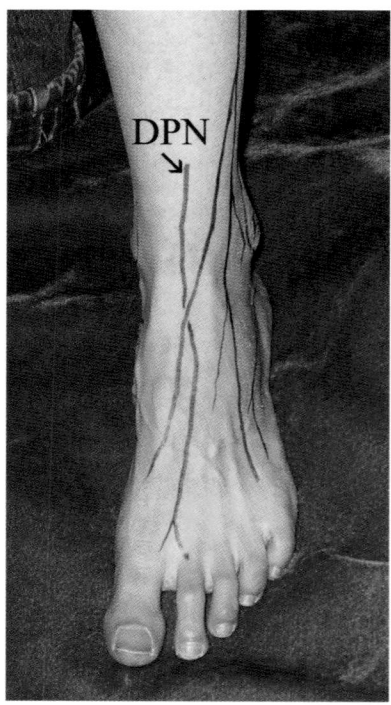

Figure 12-59   The deep peroneal nerve *(DPN)* courses along the lateral face of tibia.

hallucis longus in the region approximately 3 to 5 cm above the ankle joint, just below the inferior edge of the superior extensor retinaculum. Approximately 1 cm above the ankle joint, the nerve divides to give off a lateral branch that innervates the extensor digitorum brevis muscle. This division occurs in the region underneath the oblique superior medial band of the inferior extensor retinaculum. The medial branch of the deep peroneal nerve continues alongside the dorsalis pedis artery underneath the oblique inferior medial band of the inferior extensor retinaculum. The nerve can be compressed in this region between the retinaculum and the ridges of the talonavicular joint. The nerve continues distally between the extensor hallucis brevis and the tendon of the extensor hallucis longus. The nerve supplies sensation to the first web space in the adjacent borders of the first and second digits.[41]

Etiology

Deep peroneal nerve entrapment was initially described by Kopell and Thompson[80] in 1960 and was designated an anterior tarsal tunnel syndrome by Marinacci[172] in 1968. Krause et al[196] described a partial anterior tarsal tunnel syndrome in which only the motor or sensory component was involved.

The deep peroneal nerve can become entrapped in several locations. The most frequently described entrapment is the anterior tarsal tunnel syndrome. This syndrome refers to entrapment of the deep peroneal nerve under the inferior extensor retinaculum. Entrapment can also occur as the nerve passes under the tendon of the extensor hallucis brevis.[80] In addition, entrapment has been described under the superior edge of the inferior retinaculum, where the extensor hallucis longus tendon crosses over the nerve.[80,172,192] Compression by underlying dorsal osteophytes of the talonavicular joint and an os intermetatarseum (between the bases of the first and second metatarsals) has previously been described in runners (Fig. 12-60).[173]

Trauma often plays a role in this syndrome. Many patients have a history of recurrent ankle sprains. As the foot plantarflexes and supinates, the nerve is placed under maximum stretch, especially over the talonavicular joint.[192] Thus, with repetitive ankle sprains, nerve entrapment can occur. Tight-fitting shoes or ski boots have been implicated as an inciting factor.[172,194,196,198] Occasionally, a jogger ties a key into the lacing of the shoe, and the external compression of this key can cause localized pressure on the deep peroneal nerve. External compression can also occur in athletes who do sit-ups with their feet hooked under a metal bar. Fracture residuals or osteophytes in the region of the distal tip of the tibia, talus, navicular, cuneiforms, or metatarsal bases place undue stress on the nerve as well. Pressure from edema or a ganglion can result in a deep peroneal neuropathy.

Akyuz et al[192] reported on 14 of 300 patients with deep peroneal nerve symptoms that were correlated with

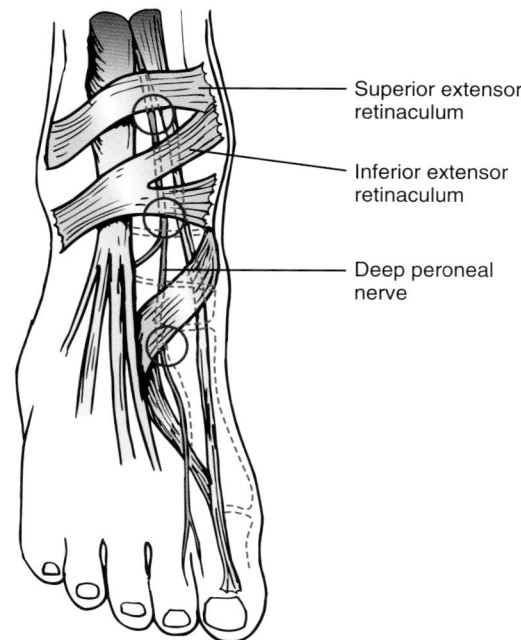

Figure 12-60 Deep peroneal nerve entrapment. *Circles* indicate areas of impingement.

- Superior extensor retinaculum
- Inferior extensor retinaculum
- Deep peroneal nerve

abnormalities on nerve conduction velocity and EMG. In their study from Turkey, they identified that *namaz*, or Islamic prayer in the kneeling position, caused prolonged stretching of the nerve.

Finally, an increasing number of deep peroneal nerve injuries have been observed with the recent increase in total ankle arthroplasty, which frequently uses an anterior approach requiring significant handling of the neurovascular bundle and deep layer closure over the DPN.[193]

Incidence

Entrapment of the deep peroneal nerve occurs most often in runners, but it can also be seen in other athletes, dancers, and people whose feet are subjected to pressure or stretch.

Evaluation

History

Patients with deep peroneal neuralgia complain of dorsal foot pain that can radiate to the first web space. As with other nerve symptoms of the foot and ankle, a history of low back pain should be documented. If the symptoms are aggravated by activity or exercise, then consideration must be given to exertional compartment syndrome. Symptoms related to tight footwear or particular activities (such as sit-ups with the anterior aspect of the ankles under a metal restraint) should be noted. A history of foot and ankle trauma or chronic ankle instability is also important. Night pain is more commonly described with

DPN entrapment than with other peripheral nerve entrapment syndromes.

Physical Examination

Palpation along the course of the deep peroneal nerve can identify an area of maximum nerve irritation, which is usually in the area of the inferior extensor retinaculum. Palpation can also locate dorsal ankle and foot osteophytes and rarely a ganglion related to previous trauma or degenerative change. Sensation in the first web space may be diminished. Areas of more proximal nerve compromise should be ruled out with examination of the lower spine, sciatic nerve, and common peroneal nerve. Weakness or atrophy, or both, of the extensor digitorum brevis muscle suggests a complete anterior tarsal syndrome or more proximal disease. However, patients can have symptoms consistent with an anterior tarsal tunnel syndrome with both motor and sensory nerve compression despite a lack of extensor digitorum brevis atrophy. This situation is secondary to an accessory extensor digitorum brevis innervation from the superficial peroneal nerve, noted in approximately 22% of patients.[195,197]

When symptoms are reported to occur in the dynamic state, the evaluation should include dorsiflexion and plantar flexion of the ankle and testing for ankle instability. If the history is consistent with an anterior compartment syndrome, then examination should also be performed after exacerbation of symptoms on a treadmill, with measurements of compartment pressures.

Diagnostic Studies and Tests

Plain radiographs are useful in identifying exostoses or osteophytes that can contribute to nerve compression. Electrodiagnostic studies can reveal areas of distal entrapment but are typically more helpful in identifying areas of more proximal nerve compression or peripheral neuropathies. Akyuz et al[191] reported prolonged distal nerve conductions velocities, distal latencies, and decreased amplitude of the deep peroneal nerve. They also had needle EMG denervation findings in the extensor digitorum brevis muscle.

Occasionally, nerve conduction studies assist in distinguishing between distal and proximal deep peroneal nerve compression within the anterior tarsal tunnel. A diagnostic nerve block can confirm clinical findings, and compartment pressures should be measured if anterior compartment syndrome is suspected.

Treatment

Conservative Treatment

Nonoperative measures include use of accommodative footwear that eliminates external compression on the dorsal ankle and foot and activity modification to avoid activities that exacerbate symptoms. As for superficial peroneal neuralgia, ankle braces can alleviate nerve pain related to ankle instability but can potentially worsen symptoms if external pressure is created. Vitamin B_6,

NSAIDs, tricyclic antidepressants, and gabapentin or other antiepileptic medications should be considered. Because the nerve is rather superficial, Lidoderm patch and topical compounded pain creams can reduce symptoms as mentioned earlier in other sections. Corticosteroid injection at the site of nerve irritation might also be beneficial.

Surgical Treatment
DEEP PERONEAL NERVE RELEASE
Surgical Technique

1. The patient is placed on the operating table in the supine position.
2. Regional anesthesia is induced at the ankle, with the anesthetic injected proximal to the area of compression.
3. The area of compression is located before surgery. This area of compression could be at the anterior ankle joint, dorsal talonavicular joint, or first metatarsal–tarsal joint area. The area is explored with a 5- to 7.5-cm incision.
4. Care is taken to release only a portion of the retinacular ligament, just in the area of compression. Preferably, only half, rather than the entire retinacular ligament, should be released to avoid bowstringing of the tendons. If more of the retinaculum needs to be released, it should be cut in a Z fashion to facilitate closure in a lengthened position.
5. The nerve and fatty tissue are retracted. If a localizing bony exostosis or an area of compression is present, this area is resected. Occasionally, when the compression is at the base of the metatarsals and there is no bony prominence to remove, the extensor hallucis brevis tendon must be released.
6. If ankle instability is diagnosed as a major contributing factor to deep peroneal neuralgia, then ankle ligament reconstruction might need to be considered. When anterior compartment syndrome has been identified, fasciotomy is also considered.
7. The wound is irrigated and the retinaculum is closed in the lengthened position if it was completely released. The skin is closed with interrupted sutures.
8. A compressive dressing is applied. If the retinacular closure was necessary a splint is recommended.

Postoperative Care

The patient uses crutches for 4 to 5 days and gradually resumes weight bearing as tolerated. If surgery is extensive, a splint is used for 2 weeks, followed by a boot brace for 2 to 4 additional weeks. If the retinaculum was not released completely, training is gradually resumed as tolerated, beginning 4 to 6 weeks postoperatively.

Results

The experience of Dellon[68] with 20 deep peroneal nerve entrapments managed with surgical decompression suggests an 80% satisfactory outcome. Poor results were typically related to internal nerve damage or neuropathies contributing to nerve compromise, in which case simple neurolysis usually proved ineffective.[68] Schon's experience with this nerve release has been best when there is a bony prominence or osteophyte. When the lesion occurred from a crush injury, the results have been less satisfactory.

SURAL NERVE ENTRAPMENT

The medial sural nerve runs between the heads of the gastrocnemius muscle and penetrates its deep aponeurosis approximately halfway up the leg. Subsequently, it anastomoses with the peroneal communicating nerve and travels along the border of the Achilles tendon next to the short saphenous veins. The nerve runs along the midline of the calf; then, at a mean distance of 9.8 cm from the calcaneus, it crosses over the edge of the Achilles tendon (Fig. 12-61).[204]

Two centimeters above the ankle, it gives off branches: one supplies sensation to the lateral aspect of the heel, and the other often anastomoses with the lateral branch of the superficial peroneal nerve. After giving off the branches to the heel, the nerve runs inferior to the peroneal sheaths in a subcutaneous position. As it reaches the tuberosity of the fifth metatarsal, the nerve ramifies to provide sensation to the lateral aspect of the fifth toe, the fourth web space, and often the third and fourth toes. Thus this network of branches supplies sensation to the posterior lateral lower leg and ankle, the lateral foot and heel, and the lateral two or three toes.[154,186,202]

Etiology

Sural nerve entrapment can occur anywhere along its course. Several cases have been described in runners who sustained fractures of the base of the fifth metatarsal after severe plantar flexion and inversion injuries.[200,201] Recurrent ankle sprains can lead to fibrosis and subsequent nerve entrapment.[201] Ganglions of the peroneal sheath or calcaneocuboid joint have also been reported.[201] An interesting case of sural nerve entrapment reported by Husson et al[177] developed after compression by an area of myositis ossificans circumscripta at the musculotendinous junction of the Achilles.

Surgery about the posterior calf, such as the Strayer procedure, can result in scarring around the sural nerve proximally. Achilles tendon reconstructions, calcaneal fracture open reduction and fixation, calcaneal osteotomy (Dwyer procedure), the approaches for lateral ligamentous reconstructions or peroneal tendon repairs, and the exposure for subtalar fusion can lead to sural nerve injury by transection, traction, or encasement in scar tissue (Fig. 12-62).

Clinical Symptoms

Most patients with sural nerve disorders recall a history of ankle injuries, typically acute or recurrent ankle sprains. Patients with persistent pain after ankle sprains might note radiating symptoms or paresthesias associated with instability. Although the pain pattern may be poorly localized, occasionally a focus of pain allows identification of a specific area of nerve compromise along the course of the sural nerve. Previous surgery on the posterior calf, lateral heel ankle, and foot should be documented, including preoperative and postoperative symptoms.[164,168]

Diagnosis

Examination of the entire course of the sural nerve should be performed from the popliteal fossa and posterior aspect of the proximal fibula to the toes. If the pain occurs only during certain activities, the patient should walk, run, or move the foot excessively before examination. Local tenderness and a positive Tinel sign are

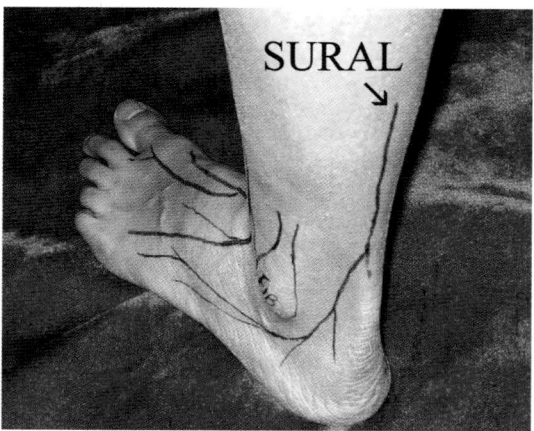

Figure 12-61 The sural nerve crosses the lateral border of the Achilles tendon.

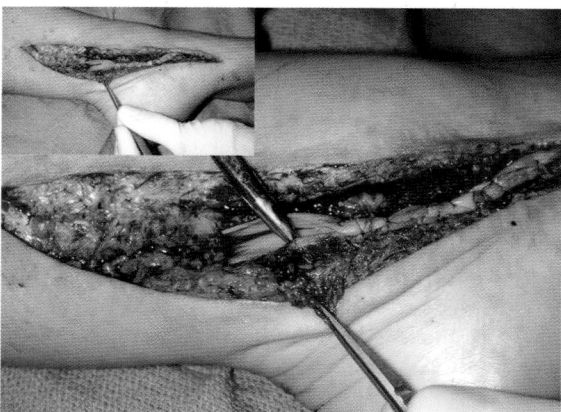

Figure 12-62 The sural nerve (draped over scissors) was released during an exposure for a peroneal tendon transfer for chronic lateral ankle ligament reconstruction. After failing re-release, the nerve was wrapped with an umbilical vein. *Inset,* Wide view of the exposure.

characteristic after running activities. Occasionally numbness is noted. The patient should be examined for coexisting disease, such as Achilles or peroneal tendinosis, ankle instability, subtalar arthritis, calcaneal fracture residua, and fifth metatarsal nonunions.

Plain radiographs should be obtained to rule out bone or joint abnormality that can contribute to nerve compression. An MRI may be helpful when soft tissue masses are suspected. Electrodiagnostic studies can occasionally confirm a clinical suspicion of limited sural nerve conduction, but these tests are typically most useful in diagnosing more proximal sites of nerve compromise. Diagnostic nerve blocks are of some use in defining sural nerve entrapment symptoms. If the nerve block fails to relieve symptoms, injection of the superficial peroneal nerve may be warranted. Selective injection into the tendon sheath or joints can also help identify contributory disease.

Treatment

Conservative Treatment

Nonoperative management of sural neuralgia requires identification of the cause of nerve compromise. Isolated sural neuralgia might respond to the medications previously discussed: vitamin B_6, NSAIDs, tricyclic antidepressants, and gabapentin or other antiepileptic medications. The Lidoderm patch and topical compounded pain creams have been particularly useful because the nerve is rather superficial. If nerve compromise is secondary to traction from chronic ankle instability, then bracing, orthotics, or shoe modifications can be effective, as for superficial peroneal neuralgia. Caution with bracing is advised because external compression can aggravate sural nerve symptoms.

Surgical Treatment
SURAL NERVE RELEASE
Surgical Technique

1. The patient is placed on the operating table in the supine position with a beanbag positioner or a roll under the hip of the affected leg. This internally rotates the leg so that the sural nerve can be better visualized.
2. A regional anesthetic is used with the block proximal to the area of compression. A tourniquet may or may not be used.
3. The area of compression is located before surgery, and only a small area of the skin is incised over the area of compression.
4. The sural nerve is identified at the area of compression and an appropriate release carried out.
5. If necessary, the nerve is moved in one direction or the other so that it will not be in an area of compression.
6. If any bony exostoses rub on the nerve, these are removed carefully, and excessive dissection or resection of fat away from the nerve is avoided.

7. Care is taken to cover the nerve and to suture the skin with interrupted suture.
8. A compressive dressing is applied.

Postoperative Care

The patient uses crutches for 3 to 4 days after surgery. If the area of release is in a joint, a boot brace is used for 2 to 4 weeks. Activity is resumed as tolerated. Usually, physical activities are not resumed until 4 weeks postoperatively.

Results

Fabre et al[199] described 13 athletes (18 limbs) who had sural nerve entrapment by the superficial sural aponeurosis in the calf. Neurolysis was performed by incising the aponeurosis and releasing the fibrous band where the nerve exited. Their results were excellent in 9 limbs (2 bilateral), good in 8 limbs (2 bilateral), and fair in 1 case.

Surgical decompression of mass effects (such as scar entrapment, ganglions, and avulsion fractures) typically results in satisfactory symptomatic relief.[164,200,201] When the cause was prior surgery, release of the nerve is not as predictable. When performing a nerve release, if a branch neuroma is encountered, resecting that damaged nerve branch with burial into a healthy bed can improve symptoms. It has been the authors' experience that sural neuralgia resulting from ankle instability is managed effectively with lateral ankle stabilization, without directly addressing the sural nerve.

For intractable pain that persists after attempted neurolysis, transection of the nerve with burial into muscle or bone has been described with good success. Many techniques have been described that typically involve tunneling the transected nerve end into muscle. Thordarson[203] has reported good results with routing the ligated nerve end deep into surrounding muscle fibers through a small incision in the fascia and tying it under slight tension, which prevents the ligated end from escaping through the fascial incision.

SAPHENOUS NERVE ENTRAPMENT

Overview, Etiology, and Anatomy

Saphenous nerve entrapment or neuralgia is not common. Typically, entrapment of this nerve occurs about the knee, but because its terminal distribution is at the medial ankle and foot, patients can present with medial distal lower-extremity pain secondary to compromise of this nerve. The saphenous nerve courses with the superficial femoral artery after originating from the femoral nerve. It penetrates the subsartorial fascia approximately 10 cm proximal to the medial femoral condyle and then divides into the infrapatellar and sartorial or distal saphenous branches. The sartorial component descends along the medial tibial border with the greater saphenous vein. Approximately 15 cm proximal to the medial malleolus, the sartorial or distal saphenous nerve separates into two branches: one that supplies sensation to the medial aspect of the ankle and one that innervates the medial foot. Although entrapment or compression can occur anywhere along the nerve's course, the most likely site of compromise is at the subsartorial fascia, just proximal to the medial femoral condyle.

Evaluation

History

Because the nerve compromise may be proximal, it is important to identify any history of knee injury, knee or bypass surgery, or pain. Direct trauma anywhere along the course of the nerve may be responsible for entrapment within scar tissue. A history of saphenous vein stripping, medial compartment release, or medial malleolar fracture may be an indication that the nerve is damaged from the injury or surgical approach.

Garland et al,[206] in a retrospective survey of patients with saphenous vein harvest after coronary bypass, found related numbness or tingling in 61%, of whom 37% improved within 3 months. There was persistent numbness beyond 2 years in 41%. Although pain was common, most improved by 3 months, and only 10% had pain persisting beyond 2 years.

In another study, Morrison et al[208] documented that 40% of patients reported symptoms of saphenous nerve injury after operation, but these symptoms affected quality of life in only 6.7%.

Hutchinson et al[207] reported on a technique of endoscopically assisted leg compartment fascial release. They found a reduced risk of saphenous vein injury (from 100% to 30%), comparing a blind percutaneous release through a 2- to 3-cm incision versus an endoscopically assisted technique.

Physical Examination

Although the patient might complain of medial ankle and foot pain, point tenderness is typically located over the subsartorial canal proximal to the medial femoral condyle. Occasionally, hyperextension of the knee produces distal symptoms. In isolated saphenous nerve compromise, no motor deficits will be present. The entire course of the nerve should be palpated to identify any other sites of possible nerve compromise. Obviously, sites of prior surgical exploration should be carefully palpated.

Diagnostic Studies

Rarely, plain radiographs can demonstrate a bony abnormality responsible for the saphenous nerve compression, but typically, physical examination will prompt radiographic evaluation. Soft tissue masses may be assessed with MRI or ultrasound. Selective injection at the site of nerve compromise in the subsartorial canal or along the medial border of the tibia or medial malleolus can be useful. Some clinicians have demonstrated that somato-

sensory evoked potentials might aid in diagnosing saphenous nerve entrapment.[194,205]

Treatment

Conservative Treatment

Nonoperative management can involve activity modification if symptoms have a dynamic component. The medications discussed earlier and the topical patches and creams can be useful, especially in a thin patient where the nerve is more superficial. Cortisone added to the diagnostic nerve block noted previously can prove therapeutic. Treating saphenous nerve entrapment with therapeutic blocks has resulted in satisfactory relief of symptoms in 38% to 80% of patients.[209,210]

Surgical Treatment

Surgical management of the more proximal entrapments requires release of the anterior aspect of the Hunter canal and dissection of the saphenous and sartorial nerve fibers from the surrounding fascia.[80,211]

For the more distal entrapments, the nerve release is performed locally. It is useful to identify the saphenous vein because the two nerve branches distally can be difficult to find.

Release of the focal entrapment can yield good results, especially when the entrapment is associated with a space-occupying lesion. Often, there has been a transection of one of the branches, and a more proximal transection and burial is needed. Rarely, patients continue to have pain and require revision nerve transection or peripheral nerve stimulation.

SUMMARY

Nerve entrapments can occur frequently, but they can be underdiagnosed when the presentation is atypical. Because pain is a subjective experience, the symptoms can be vague and may be referred. Thus the examiner must have an awareness of these syndromes in obtaining a history. A thorough knowledge of peripheral nerve anatomy is essential in establishing the diagnosis. Radiographs might reveal bony abnormalities that are causing the problems. The presence of more proximal lesions (double-crush phenomenon) and metabolic conditions should not be overlooked. Electrodiagnostic test results may be normal, but they can be useful to find these other systemic or more proximal pathologies.

In some patients, modifying footwear, wearing an orthosis, or altering activity can result in relief. Use of oral medications and topical agents can be helpful in controlling the symptoms. In certain cases, injections may be both diagnostic and therapeutic. For recalcitrant cases, surgery may be indicated and usually gives satisfactory results. In performing surgery, the risks of poor response remain. When a patient fails nerve release, revision release and transection of damaged nerves can be helpful. For those unfortunate patients who continue to suffer intractable nerve pain, the options include further nerve transection, vein wrap or other nerve-containment procedures, peripheral nerve stimulation, or spinal cord stimulation.

REFERENCES
Interdigital Neuroma

1. American Chronic Pain Association: 2013 Resource Guide to Chronic Pain Medication & Treatment. Available at http://www.theacpa.org/uploads/ACPA_Resource_Guide_2013_Final_011313.pdf. Accessed May 23, 2013.
2. Amis JA, Siverhus SW, Liwnicz BH: An anatomic basis for recurrence after Morton's neuroma excision, *Foot Ankle* 13:153–156, 1992.
3. Awerbuch MS, Shephard E, Vernon-Roberts B: Morton's metatarsalgia due to intermetatarsophalangeal bursitis as an early manifestation of rheumatoid arthritis, *Clin Orthop Relat Res* 167:214–221, 1982.
4. Barrett S, Pignetti TT: Endoscopic decompression for intermetatarsal nerve entrapment—the EDIN technique: preliminary study with cadaveric specimens and early clinical results, *J Foot Ankle Surg* 33:503–506, 1994.
5. Bencardino J, Rosenberg ZS, Beltran J, et al: Morton's neuroma: is it always symptomatic? *AJR Am J Roentgenol* 175:649–653, 2000.
6. Benedetti RS, Baxter DE, Davis PF: Clinical results of simultaneous adjacent interdigital neurectomy in the foot, *Foot Ankle Int* 17:583, 1996.
7. Beskin JL, Baxter DE: Recurrent pain following interdigital neurectomy—a plantar approach, *Foot Ankle* 9:34–39, 1988.
8. Betts LO: Morton's metatarsalgia: neuritis of the fourth digital nerve, *Med J Aust* 1:514, 1940.
9. Biasca N, Zanetti M, Zollinger H: Outcomes after partial neurectomy of Morton's neuroma related to preoperative case histories, clinical findings, and findings on magnetic resonance imaging scans, *Foot Ankle Int* 20:568–575, 1999.
10. Bossley CJ, Cairney PC: The intermetatarsophalangeal bursa: its significance in Morton's metatarsalgia, *J Bone Joint Surg Br* 62:184–187, 1980.
11. Bradley N, Miller WA, Evans JP: Plantar neuroma analysis of results following surgical excision in 145 patients, *South Med J* 69:853–854, 1976.
12. Colgrove RC, Huang EY, Barth AH, Greene MA: Interdigital neuroma: intermuscular neuroma transposition compared with resection, *Foot Ankle Int* 21:206–211, 2000.
13. Coughlin MJ, Pinsonneault T: Operative treatment of interdigital neuroma. A long-term follow-up study, *J Bone Joint Surg Am* 84:1276–1277, 2002.
14. Davis TJ, Schon LC: Branches of the tibial nerve: anatomic variations, *Foot Ankle Int* 16:21–29, 1995.
15. Dellon AL: Treatment of Morton's neuroma as a nerve compression: the role for neurolysis, *J Amer Pod Med Assoc* 82:399–402, 1992.
16. Durlacher L: *A treatise on corns, bunions, the disease of nails and the general management of the feet*, London, 1845, Simpkin, Marshall.
17. Espinosa N, Seybold JD, Jankauskas L, Erschbamer M: Alcohol sclerosing therapy is not an effective treatment for interdigital neuroma, *Foot Ankle Int* 32:576–580, 2011.
18. Fanucci E, Masala S, Fabiano S, et al: Treatment of intermetatarsal Morton's neuroma with alcohol injection under US guide: 10-month follow-up, *Eur Radiol* 14:514–518, 2004.
19. Gauthier G: Thomas Morton's disease: a nerve entrapment syndrome, *Clin Orthop Relat Res* 142:90, 1979.
20. Giannini S, Bacchini P, Ceccarelli F, Vannini F: Interdigital neuroma: clinical examination and histopathologic results in

63 cases treated with excision, *Foot Ankle Int* 25:79–84, 2004.
21. Govsa F, Bilge O, Ozer MA: Anatomical study of the communicating branches between the medial and lateral plantar nerves, *Surg Radiol Anat* 27:377–381, 2005.
22. Graham CE, Graham DM: Morton's neuroma: a microscopic evaluation, *Foot Ankle* 5:150–153, 1984.
23. Graham CE, Johnson KA, Ilstrup DM: The intermetatarsal nerve: a microscopic evaluation, *Foot Ankle* 2:150–152, 1981.
24. Greenfield J, Rea J Jr, Ilfeld FW: Morton's interdigital neuroma: indications for treatment by local injections versus surgery, *Clin Orthop Relat Res* 185:142–144, 1984.
25. Hauser ED: Interdigital neuroma of the foot, *Surg Gynecol Obstet* 133:265–267, 1971.
26. Hembree WC, Groth AT, Schon LC, Guyton GP: *Computed tomography analysis of third webspace injections for interdigital neuroma.* Submitted for publication, 2012.
27. Hoadley AE: Six cases of metatarsalgia, *Chicago Med Rec* 5:32–37, 1893.
28. Hort KR, DeOrio JK: Adjacent interdigital nerve irritation: single incision surgical treatment, *Foot Ankle Int* 23:1026–1030, 2002.
29. Johnson JD, Johnson KA, Unni KK: Persistent pain after excision of an interdigital neuroma, *J Bone Surg Am* 70:651–657, 1988.
30. Jones JR, Klenerman L: A study of the communicating branch between the medial and lateral plantar nerves, *Foot Ankle* 4:313–315, 1984.
31. Kelikian H: *Hallux valgus, allied deformities of the forefoot and metatarsalgia*, Philadelphia, 1965, WB Saunders.
32. Lassmann G: Morton's toe: clinical, light, and electron microscopic investigations in 133 cases, *Clin Orthop Relat Res* 142:73–84, 1979.
33. Levine SE, Myerson MS, Shapiro PP, et al: Ultrasonographic diagnosis of recurrence after excision of an interdigital neuroma, *Foot Ankle Int* 19:79–84, 1998.
34. Levitsky KA, Alman BA, Jesevar DS, Morehead J: Digital nerves of the foot: anatomic variations and implications regarding the pathogenesis of the interdigital neuroma, *Foot Ankle* 14:208–214, 1993.
35. Mann RA, Reynolds JD: Interdigital neuroma: a critical clinical analysis, *Foot Ankle* 3:238, 1983.
36. Markovic M, Crichton K, Read JW, Lam P, Slater HK: Effectiveness of ultrasound-guided corticosteroid injection in the treatment of Morton's neuroma, *Foot Ankle Int* 29:483–487, 2008.
37. Mason E: A case of neuralgia of the second metatarsophalangeal articulation: cured by resection of the joint, *Am J Med Sci* 74:445, 1877.
38. McElvenny RT: The etiology and surgical treatment of intractable pain about the fourth metatarsophalangeal joint (Morton's toe), *J Bone Joint Surg* 25:675–679, 1943.
39. Morton TG: A peculiar and painful affection of fourth metatarsophalangeal articulation, *Am J Med Sci* 71:37–45, 1876.
40. Mulder JD: The causative mechanism in Morton's metatarsalgia, *J Bone Joint Surg Br* 33:94–95, 1951.
41. Nemoto K, Mikasa M, Tazaki K, Mori Y: Neurolysis as a surgical procedure for Morton's neuroma, *Nippon Seikeigeka Gakkai Zasshi* 63:470–473, 1989.
42. Okafor B, Shergill G, Angel J: Treatment of Morton's neuroma by neurolysis, *Foot Ankle Int* 18:284–287, 1997.
43. Quinn TJ, Jacobson JA, Craig JG, et al: Sonography of Morton's neuromas, *AJR Am J Roentgenol* 174:1723–1728, 2000.
44. Read JW, Noakes JB, Kerr D, et al: Morton's metatarsalgia: sonographic findings and correlated histopathology, *Foot Ankle Int* 20:153–161, 1999.
45. Redd RA, Peters VJ, Emery SF, et al: Morton's neuroma: sonographic evaluation, *Radiology* 171:415–417, 1989.

46. Resch S, Stenstrom A, Jonsson A, et al: The diagnostic efficacy of magnetic resonance imaging and ultrasonography in Morton's neuroma: a radiological-surgical correlation, *Foot Ankle Int* 15:88–92, 1994.
47. Rosson G, Dellon AL: Surgical approach to multiple interdigital nerve compressions, *J Foot Ankle Surg* 44:70–73, 2005.
48. Shapiro PP, Shapiro SL: Sonographic evaluation of interdigital neuromas, *Foot Ankle Int* 16:604–606, 1995.
49. Shapiro SL: Endoscopic decompression of the intermetatarsal nerve for Morton's neuroma, *Foot Ankle Clin* 9:297–304, 2004.
50. Sharp RJ, Wade CM, Hennessy MS, Saxby TS: The role of MRI and ultrasound imaging in Morton's neuroma and the effect of size of lesion on symptoms, *J Bone Joint Surg Br* 85:999–1005, 2003.
51. Stamatis ED, Myerson MS: Treatment of recurrence of symptoms after excision of an interdigital neuroma. A retrospective review, *J Bone Joint Surg Br* 86:48–53, 2004.
52. Su E, Di Carlo E, O'Malley M, et al: The frequency of digital artery resection in Morton interdigital neurectomy, *Foot Ankle Int* 27:801–803, 2006.
53. Terk MR, Kwong PK, Suthar M, et al: Morton neuroma: evaluation with MR imaging performed with contrast enhancement and fat suppression, *Radiology* 189:239–241, 1993.
54. Thompson FM, Deland JT: Occurrence of two interdigital neuromas in one foot, *Foot Ankle* 14:15–17, 1993.
55. Tubby AH: *Deformities, including diseases of the bones and joints*, vol 1, ed 2, London, 1912, Macmillan.
56. Villas C: Neurectomy vs. neurolysis for Morton's neuroma, *Foot Ankle Int* 29:578–580, 2008.
57. Weishaupt D, Treiber K, Kundert HP, et al: Morton neuroma: MR imaging in prone, supine, and upright weight-bearing body positions, *Radiology* 226:849–856, 2003.
58. Wolfort SF, Dellon AL: Treatment of recurrent neuroma of the interdigital nerve by implantation of the proximal nerve into muscle in the arch of the foot, *J Foot Ankle Surg* 40:404–410, 2001.
59. Womack JW, Richardson DR, Murphy A, et al: Long-term evaluation of interdigital neuroma treated by surgical excision, *Foot Ankle Int* 29:574–577, 2008.
60. Younger AS, Claridge RJ: The role of diagnostic block in the management of Morton's neuroma, *Can J Surg* 41:127–130, 1998.

Tarsal Tunnel Syndrome
61. Aszmann O, Tassler PL, Dellon AL: Changing the natural history of diabetic neuropathy: incidence of ulcer/amputation in the contralateral limb of patients with a unilateral nerve decompression procedure, *Ann Plast Surg* 53:517–522, 2004.
62. Biddinger KR, Amend KJ: The role of surgical decompression for diabetic neuropathy, *Foot Ankle Clin* 9:239–254, 2004.
63. Budak F, Bamac B, Ozbek A, et al: Nerve conduction studies of lower extremities in pes planus subjects, *Electromyogr Clin Neurophysiol* 41:443–446, 2001.
64. Chalian M, Soldatos T, Faridian-Aragh N, et al: 3T magnetic resonance neurography of tibial nerve pathologies, *J Neuroimaging* 23:296–310, 2013.
65. Cimino WR: Tarsal tunnel syndrome: review of the literature, *Foot Ankle* 11:47–52, 1990.
66. Daniels TR, Lau JT, Hearn TC: The effects of foot position and load on tibial nerve tension, *Foot Ankle Int* 19:73–78, 1998.
67. Davis TJ, Schon LC: Branches of the tibial nerve: anatomic variations, *Foot Ankle Int* 16:21–29, 1995.
68. Dellon AL: Diabetic neuropathy: review of a surgical approach to restore sensation, relieve pain, and prevent ulceration and amputation, *Foot Ankle Int* 25:749–755, 2004.
69. Dellon AL, Kim J, Spaulding CM: Variations in the origin of the medial calcaneal nerve, *J Am Podiatr Med Assoc* 92:97–101, 2002.
70. Frey C, Kerr R: Magnetic resonance imaging and the evaluation of tarsal tunnel syndrome, *Foot Ankle* 14:159–164, 1993.
71. Galardi G, Amadio S, Maderna L, et al: Electrophysiologic studies in tarsal tunnel syndrome. Diagnostic reliability of motor distal latency, mixed nerve and sensory nerve conduction studies, *Am J Phys Med Rehabil* 73:193–198, 1994.
72. Gondring WH, Shields B, Wenger S: An outcomes analysis of surgical treatment of tarsal tunnel syndrome, *Foot Ankle Int* 24:545–550, 2003.
73. Gould JS: Tarsal tunnel syndrome, *Foot Ankle Clin N Am* 16:275–286, 2011.
74. Havel PE, Ebraheim NA, Clark SE, et al: Tibial branching in the tarsal tunnel, *Foot Ankle* 9:117–119, 1988.
75. Kaplan PE, Kernahan WT: Tarsal tunnel syndrome: an electrodiagnostic and surgical correlation, *J Bone Joint Surg Am* 63:96–99, 1981.
76. Keck C: The tarsal tunnel syndrome, *J Bone Joint Surg Am* 44:180–182, 1962.
77. Kim DH, Ryu S, Tiel RL, Kline DG: Surgical management and results of 135 tibial nerve lesions at the Louisiana State University Health Sciences Center, *Neurosurgery* 53:1114–1124, 2003.
78. Kinoshita M, Okuda R, Morikawa J, et al: The dorsiflexion-eversion test for diagnosis of tarsal tunnel syndrome, *J Bone Joint Surg Am* 83:1835–1839, 2001.
79. Kinoshita M, Okuda R, Morikawa J, Abe M: Tarsal tunnel syndrome associated with an accessory muscle, *Foot Ankle Int* 24:132–136, 2003.
80. Kopell HP, Thompson WAL: Peripheral entrapment neuropathies of the lower extremity, *N Engl J Med* 262:56–60, 1960.
81. Labib SA, Gould JS, Rodriguez-del-Rio FA, Lyman S: Heel pain triad (HPT): the combination of plantar fasciitis, posterior tibial tendon dysfunction and tarsal tunnel syndrome, *Foot Ankle Int* 23:212–220, 2002.
82. Lam SJS: Tarsal tunnel syndrome, *J Bone Joint Surg Am* 49:87–92, 1967.
83. Lau JT, Daniels TR: Effects of tarsal tunnel release and stabilization procedures on tibial nerve tension in a surgically created pes planus foot, *Foot Ankle Int* 19:770–777, 1998.
84. Lee CH, Dellon AL: Prognostic ability of Tinel sign in determining outcome for decompression surgery in diabetic and non-diabetic neuropathy, *Ann Plast Surg* 53:523–527, 2004.
85. Lumsden DB, Schon LC, Easley ME, et al: Topography of the distal tibial nerve and its branches, *Foot Ankle Int* 24:696–700, 2003.
86. Mann RA: Tarsal tunnel syndrome, *Orthop Clin North Am* 5:109–115, 1974.
87. Nagaoka M, Matsuzaki H: Ultrasonography in tarsal tunnel syndrome, *J Ultrasound Med* 24:1035–1040, 2005.
88. Nagaoka M, Satou K: Tarsal tunnel syndrome caused by ganglia, *J Bone Joint Surg Br* 81:607–610, 1999.
89. Oh SJ, Savaria PK, Kuba T, et al: Tarsal tunnel syndrome: electrophysiologic study, *Ann Neurol* 5:327–330, 1979.
90. Patel AT, Gaines K, Malamut R, et al: Usefulness of electrodiagnostic techniques in the evaluation of suspected tarsal tunnel syndrome: an evidence-based review, *Muscle Nerve* 32:236–240, 2005.
91. Pinzur MS: Diabetic Peripheral neuropathy, *Foot Ankle Clin N Am* 16:345–349, 2011.
92. Pfeiffer WH, Cracchiolo A 3rd: Clinical results after tarsal tunnel decompression, *J Bone Joint Surg Am* 76:1222–1230, 1994.
93. Sammarco GJ, Chang L: Outcome of surgical treatment of tarsal tunnel syndrome, *Foot Ankle Int* 24:125–131, 2003.

94. Shah A: Complex regional pain syndrome, *Foot Ankle Clin N Am* 16:351–366, 2011.

95. Skalley TC, Schon LC, Hinton RY, Myerson NS: Clinical results following revision tibial nerve release, *Foot Ankle Int* 15:360–367, 1994.

96. Takakura Y, Kitada C, Sugimoto K, et al: Tarsal tunnel syndrome. Causes and results of operative treatment, *J Bone Joint Surg Br* 73:125–128, 1991.

97. Takakura Y, Kumai T, Takaoka T, Tamai S: Tarsal tunnel syndrome caused by coalition associated with a ganglion, *J Bone Joint Surg Br* 80:130–133, 1998.

98. Trepman E, Kadel NJ, Chisholm K, Razzano L: Effect of foot and ankle position on tarsal tunnel compartment pressure, *Foot Ankle Int* 20:721–726, 1999.

99. Urguden M, Bilbasar H, Ozdemir H, et al: Tarsal tunnel syndrome—the effect of the associated features on outcome of surgery, *Int Orthop* 26:253–256, 2002.

100. Wilemon WK: Tarsal tunnel syndrome, *Orthop Rev* 8:111, 1979.

Failed Tarsal Tunnel Release

101. Campbell JT, Schon LC, Burkhardt LD: Histopathologic findings in autogenous saphenous vein graft wrapping for recurrent tarsal tunnel syndrome: a case report, *Foot Ankle Int* 19:766–769, 1998.

102. Dellon AL, Mackinnon SE: Results of posterior tibial nerve grafting at the ankle, *J Reconstr Microsurg* 7:81–83, 1991.

103. Dielissen PW, Claassen AT, Veldman PH, Goris RJ: Amputation for reflex sympathetic dystrophy, *J Bone Joint Surg Br* 77:270–273, 1995.

104. Easley ME, Schon LC: Peripheral nerve vein wrapping for intractable lower extremity pain, *Foot Ankle Int* 21:492–500, 2000.

105. Gould JS: The failed tarsal tunnel release, *Foot Ankle Clin N Am* 16: 287–293, 2011.

106. Gould JS, Hart TS, O'Brien TS, Winkler MV: Outcome analysis of vein wrapping for intractable painful nerves in continuity. Presented at the 12th Annual Summer Meeting of the American Foot and Ankle Society, Hilton Head, SC, June 28, 1996.

107. Gybels J, Van Calenbergh F: The treatment of pain due to peripheral nerve injury by electrical stimulation of the injured nerve, *Adv Pain Res Ther* 13:217–222, 1990.

108. Hassenbusch SJ, Stanton-Hicks M, Schoppa D, et al: Long-term results of peripheral nerve stimulation for reflex sympathetic dystrophy, *J Neurosurg* 84:415–423, 1996.

109. Honkamp N, Amendola A, Hurwitz S, Saltzman CL: Retrospective review of 18 patients who underwent transtibial amputation for intractable pain, *J Bone Joint Surg Am* 83:1479–1483, 2001.

110. Law JD, Swett J, Kirsch WM: Retrospective analysis of 22 patients with chronic pain treated by peripheral nerve stimulation, *J Neurosurg* 52:482–485, 1980.

111. Masear VR, Colgin S: The treatment of epineural scarring with allograft vein wrapping, *Hand Clin* 12:773–779, 1996.

112. Masear VR: Nerve wrapping, *Foot Ankle Clin N Am* 16:327–337, 2011.

113. Masear VR, Tulloss JR, St. Mary E, Meyer RD: Venous wrapping of nerves to prevent scarring [abstr], *J Hand Surg Am* 15:817–818, 1999.

114. Nashold BS Jr, Goldner JL, Mullen JB, Bright DS: Long-term pain control by direct peripheral-nerve stimulation, *J Bone Joint Surg Am* 64:1–10, 1982.

115. Ruch DS, Spinner RM, Koman LA, et al: The histological effect of barrier vein wrapping of peripheral nerves, *J Reconstr Microsurg* 12:291–295, 1996.

116. Schon LC, Anderson CD, Easley ME, et al: Surgical treatment of chronic lower extremity neuropathic pain, *Clin Orthop Relat Res* 389:156–164, 2001.

117. Schon LC, Easley ME: Chronic pain. In Myerson MS, editor: *Foot and ankle disorders*, Philadelphia, 2000, WB Saunders, pp 851–881.

118. Schon LC, Lam PW, Easley ME, et al: Complex salvage procedures for severe lower extremity nerve pain, *Clin Orthop Relat Res* 391:171–180, 2001.

119. Schon LC, Short KW, Soupiou O, et al: Benefits of early prosthetic management of transtibial amputees: a prospective clinical study of prefabricated prosthesis, *Foot Ankle Int* 23:509–514, 2002.

120. Shealy CN, Mortimer JT, Reswick JB: Electrical inhibition of pain by stimulation of the dorsal columns: preliminary clinical report, *Anesth Analg* 46:489–491, 1967.

121. Sotereanos DG, Giannkopoulos PN, Mitsionis GI, et al: Vein graft wrapping for the treatment of recurrent compression of the median nerve, *Microsurgery* 16:752–756, 1995.

122. Stanton-Hicks M, Burton AW, Bruehl SP, et al: An updated interdisciplinary clinical pathway for CRPS: report of an expert panel, *Pain Pract* 2:1–16, 2002.

123. Strege DW, Cooney WP, Wood MB, et al: Chronic peripheral nerve pain treated with direct electrical nerve stimulation, *J Hand Surg Am* 19:931–939, 1994.

124. Turner JA, Loeser JD, Bell KG: Spinal cord stimulation for chronic low back pain: a systematic literature synthesis, *Neurosurgery* 37:1088–1096, 1995.

125. Varitimidis SE, Vardakas DG, Goebel F, Sotereanos DG: Treatment of recurrent compressive neuropathy of peripheral nerves in the upper extremity with an autologous vein insulator, *J Hand Surg Am* 26:296–302, 2001.

126. Vora AM, Schon LC: Revision peripheral nerve surgery, *Foot Ankle Clin* 9:305–318, 2004.

127. Waisbrod H, Panhans C, Hansen D, Gerbershagen HU: Direct nerve stimulation for painful peripheral neuropathies, *J Bone Joint Surg Br* 67:470–472, 1985.

128. Xu J, Sotereanos DG, Moller AR, et al: Nerve wrapping with vein grafts in a rat model: a safe technique for the treatment of recurrent chronic compressive neuropathy, *J Reconstr Microsurg* 14:323–328, 1998.

129. Zeiss J, Fenton P, Ebraheim N, Coombs RJ: Magnetic resonance imaging for ineffectual tarsal tunnel surgical treatment, *Clin Orthop Relat Res* 264:264–266, 1991.

130. Zollinger PE, Tuinebreijer WE, Breederveld RS, Kreis RW: Can vitamin C prevent complex regional pain syndrome in patients with wrist fractures? A randomized, controlled, multicenter dose-response study, *J Bone Joint Surg Am* 89:1424–1431, 2007.

Traumatic Nerve Injuries

131. Barbera J, Albert-Pamplo R: Centrocentral anastomosis of the proximal nerve stump in the treatment of painful amputation neuromas of major nerves, *J Neurosurg* 79:331–334, 1993.

132. Barbers J, Gonzalez J, Gil JL: The quality and extension of nerve fibre regeneration in the centrocentral anastomosis of the peripheral nerve, *Acta Neurochir Suppl (Wien)* 43:205–209, 1988.

133. Bauer RD, Eft AL: Clinical effect of nitrogen mustard on neoplastic diseases, *Am J Med Sci* 219:216, 1950.

134. Bosse MJ: The insensate foot following severe lower extremity trauma, *J Bone Joint Surg Am* 87:2601–2608, 2005.

135. Chiodo CP, Miller SD: Surgical treatment of superficial peroneal neuromas, *Foot Ankle Int* 10:689–694, 2000.

136. Dellon AL, Aszmann OC: Treatment of superficial and deep peroneal neuromas by resection and translocation of the nerves into the anterolateral compartment, *Foot Ankle Int* 19:300–303, 1998.

137. Dellon AL, MacKinnon SE: Susceptibility of the superficial sensory branch of the radial nerve to form painful neuromas, *J Hand Surg Br* 9:42–45, 1984.

138. Ferkel RD, Heath DD, Guhl JF: Neurological complications of ankle arthroscopy, *Arthroscopy* 12:200–208, 1996.

139. Goldstein SA, Sturim HS: Intraosseoeus nerve transposition for treatment of painful neuromas, *J Hand Surg Am* 10:270–274, 1985.

140. Gorkisch K, Boese-Landgraf J, Vaubel E: Treatment and prevention of amputation neuromas in hand surgery, *Plast Reconstr Surg* 73:293–299, 1984.

141. Hattrup SJ: Delayed neural reconstruction in the lower extremity: results of interfascicular nerve grafting, *Foot Ankle* 7:105–109, 1986.

142. Herndon JH, Hess AV: Neuromas. In Green DP, Hotchkiss RN, editors: *Operative hand surgery*, New York, 1982, Churchill Livingstone, p 939.

143. Herndon JH, Hess AV: Neuromas. In Gelberman RH, editor: *Operative nerve repair and reconstruction*, Philadelphia, 1991, JB Lippincott, p 1525.

144. Hutchinson MR, Bederka B, Kopplin M: Anatomic structures at risk during minimal incision endoscopically assisted fascial compartment releases in the leg, *Am J Sports Med* 31:764–769, 2003.

145. Kenzora JE: Symptomatic incisional neuromas on the dorsum of the foot, *Foot Ankle* 5:2–15, 1984.

146. Lidor C, Hall RL, Nunley JA: Centrocentral anastomosis with autologous nerve graft treatment of foot and ankle neuromas, *Foot Ankle Int* 17:85–88, 1996.

147. Mass DP, Ciano MC, Tortosa R: Treatment of painful hand neuromas by their transfer into bone, *Plast Reconstr Surg* 74:182–185, 1984.

148. Miller SD: Dorsomedial cutaneous nerve syndrome: treatment with nerve transection and burial into bone, *Foot Ankle Int* 22:198–202, 2001.

149. Moore AM: Limitations of conduits in peripheral nerve repairs, *Hand* 4:180–186, 2009.

150. Nunley JA, Gabel GT: Tibial nerve grafting for restoration of plantar sensation, *Foot Ankle Int* 14:489–492, 1993.

151. Petropoulos PC, Stefanko S: Experimental observations on the prevention of neuroma formation. Preliminary report, *J Surg Res* 1:241–248, 1961.

152. Redfern DJ, Sauve PS, Sakellariou A: Investigation of incidence of superficial peroneal nerve injury following ankle fracture, *Foot Ankle Int* 24:771–774, 2003.

153. Robbins TH: Nerve capping in the treatment of troublesome terminal neuroma, *Br J Plast Surg* 39:239–240, 1986.

154. Solomon LB, Ferris L, Tedman R, Henneberg M: Surgical anatomy of the sural and superficial fibular nerves with an emphasis on the approach to the lateral malleolus, *J Anat* 199:717–723, 2001.

155. Sunderland S: *Nerves and nerve injuries*, ed 2, New York, 1978, Churchill Livingstone.

156. Thordarson DB: Nerve and tendon lacerations about the foot and ankle, *J Am Acad Orthop Surg* 13:186–196, 2005.

157. Tupper JW, Booth DM: Treatment of painful neuromas of sensory nerves in the hand: a comparison of traditional and newer methods, *J Hand Surg Am* 1:144–151, 1976.

158. Wagner E: The painful neuroma and the use of conduits, *Foot Ankle Clin N Am* 16:295–304, 2011.

159. Whipple RR, Unsell RS: Treatment of painful neuromas, *Orthop Clin North Am* 19:175–185, 1988.

160. White JC, Hamlin H: New uses of tantalum in nerve suture, control of neuroma formation and prevention of regeneration after thoracic sympathectomy, illustration of technical procedures, *J Neurosurg* 2:402, 1945.

Lateral Plantar Nerve Entrapment

161. Baxter DE, Pfeffer GB: Treatment of chronic heel pain by surgical release of the first branch of the lateral plantar nerve, *Clin Orthop Relat Res* 279:229–236, 1992.

162. Gould JS: Treatment of the painful injured nerve incontinuity. In Gelberman GH, editor: *Operative nerve repair and reconstruction*, Philadelphia, 1991, JB Lippincott, pp 1541–1550.

163. Henricson AS, Westlin NE: Chronic calcaneal pain in athletes: entrapment of the calcaneal nerve? *Am J Sports Med* 12:152–154, 1987.

164. Schon LC: Nerve entrapment, neuropathy, and nerve dysfunction in athletes, *Orthop Clin North Am* 25:47–59, 1994.

165. Schon LC: Plantar fascia and Baxter's nerve release. In Myerson M, editor: *Current therapy in foot and ankle surgery*, St Louis, 1993, Mosby–Year Book, pp 177–182.

166. Schon LC, Anderson CD, Easley ME, et al: Surgical treatment of chronic lower extremity neuropathic pain, *Clin Orthop Relat Res* 389:156–164, 2001.

167. Schon LC, Baxter DE: Heel pain syndrome and entrapment neuropathies about the foot and ankle. In Gould JS, editor: *Operative foot surgery*, Philadelphia, 1994, WB Saunders, pp 192–208.

168. Schon LC, Baxter DE: Neuropathies of the foot and ankle in athletes, *Clin Sports Med* 9:489–509, 1990.

169. Schon LC, Glennon TP, Baxter DE: Heel pain syndrome: electrodiagnostic support for nerve entrapment, *Foot Ankle* 14:129–135, 1993.

170. Watson TS, Anderson RB, Davis WH, Kiebzak GM: Distal tarsal tunnel release with partial plantar fasciotomy for chronic heel pain: an outcome analysis, *Foot Ankle Int* 23:530–537, 2002.

Medial Plantar Nerve Entrapment

171. Kopell HP, Thompson WAL: *Peripheral entrapment neuropathies*, ed 2, Huntington, NY, 1976, Robert E Kreiger Publications.

172. Marinacci AA: Neurological syndrome of the tarsal tunnels, *Bull L A Neurol Soc* 33:90–100, 1968.

173. Murphy PC, Baxter DE: Nerve entrapment of the foot and ankle in runners, *Clin Sports Med* 4:753–763, 1985.

174. Rask MR: Medial plantar neuropraxia (jogger's foot): report of three cases, *Clin Orthop Relat Res* 134:193–195, 1978.

Superficial Peroneal Nerve Entrapment

175. Banerjee T, Koons DD: Superficial peroneal nerve entrapment: report of two cases, *J Neurosurg* 55:991–992, 1981.

176. Cozen L: Bursitis of the heel, *Am J Orthop* 3:372–374, 1961.

177. Husson JL, Blouet JM, Massé A: Le syndrome du défilé de l'aponévrose superficielle postérieure surale, *Int Orthop* 11:245–248, 1987.

178. Kernohan J, Levack B, Wilson JN: Entrapment of the superficial peroneal nerve. Three case reports, *J Bone Joint Surg Br* 67:60–61, 1985.

179. Lowdon IM: Superficial peroneal nerve entrapment. A case report, *J Bone Joint Surg Br* 67:58–59, 1985.

180. Mackey D, Colbert DS, Chater EH: Musculocutaneous nerve entrapment, *Ir J Med Sci* 146:100–102, 1977.

181. McAuliffe TB, Fiddian NJ, Browett JP: Entrapment neuropathy of the superficial peroneal nerve. A bilateral case, *J Bone Joint Surg Br* 67:62–63, 1985.

182. Radin EL: Tarsal tunnel syndrome, *Clin Orthop Relat Res* 181:167–170, 1983.

183. Rondhuis JJ, Huson A: The first branch of the lateral plantar nerve and heel pain, *Acta Morphol Neerl Scand* 24:269–279, 1986.

184. Rosson GD, Dellon AL: Superficial peroneal nerve anatomic variability changes: surgical technique, *Clin Orthop Relat Res* 438:248–252, 2005.

185. Schepsis AA, Fitzgerald M, Nicoletta R: Revision surgery for exertional anterior compartment syndrome of the lower leg: technique, findings, and results, *Am J Sports Med* 33:1040–1047, 2005.
186. Sarrafian SK: *Anatomy of the foot and ankle: descriptive, topographic, functional*, Philadelphia, 1983, JB Lippincott.
187. Sridhara CR, Izzo KL: Terminal sensory branches of the superficial peroneal nerve: an entrapment syndrome, *Arch Phys Med Rehabil* 66:789–891, 1985.
188. Styf J: Entrapment of the superficial peroneal nerve. Diagnosis and results of decompression, *J Bone Joint Surg Br* 71:131–135, 1989.
189. Styf JR, Korner LM: Chronic anterior-compartment syndrome of the leg. Results of treatment by fasciotomy, *J Bone Joint Surg Am* 68:1338–1347, 1986.
190. Tanz SS: Heel pain, *Clin Orthop Relat Res* 288:169–178, 1963.

Deep Peroneal Nerve Entrapment
191. Akyuz G, Us O, Turan B, et al: Anterior tarsal tunnel syndrome, *Electromyogr Clin Neurophysiol* 40:123–128, 2000.
192. Borges LF, Hallett M, Selkoe DJ, Welch K: The anterior tarsal tunnel syndrome: report of two cases, *J Neurosurg* 54:89–92, 1981.
193. Flanigan RM: Peripheral nerve entrapments of the lower leg, ankle, and foot, *Foot Ankle Clin N Am* 16:255–274, 2011.
194. Gessini L, Jandolo B, Pietrangeli A: The anterior tarsal tunnel syndrome: report of four cases, *J Bone Joint Surg Am* 66:786–787, 1984.
195. Gutmann L: Atypical deep peroneal neuropathy in presence of accessory deep peroneal nerve, *J Neurol Neurosurg Psychiatry* 33:453–456, 1970.
196. Krause KH, Witt T, Ross A: The anterior tarsal tunnel syndrome, *J Neurol* 217:67–74, 1977.
197. Lambert EH: The accessory deep peroneal nerve. A common variation in innervation of extensor digitorum brevis, *Neurology* 19:1169–1176, 1969.
198. Lindenbaum BL: Ski boot compression syndrome, *Clin Orthop Relat Res* 140:109–110, 1979.

Sural Nerve Entrapment
199. Fabre T, Montero C, Gaujard E, et al: Chronic calf pain in athletes due to sural nerve entrapment. A report of 18 cases, *Am J Sports Med* 28:679–682, 2000.
200. Gould N, Trevino S: Sural nerve entrapment by avulsion fracture of the base of the fifth metatarsal bone, *Foot Ankle* 2:153–155, 1981.
201. Pringle RM, Protheroe K, Mukherjee SK: Entrapment neuropathy of the sural nerve, *J Bone Joint Surg Br* 56:465–468, 1974.
202. Solomon LB, Ferris L, Tedman R, Henneberg M: Surgical anatomy of the sural and superficial fibular nerves with an emphasis on the approach to the lateral malleolus, *J Anat* 199:717–723, 2001.
203. Thordarson DB: Burial of sural neuroma: technique tip, *Foot Ankle Int* 31:351–353, 2010.

Saphenous Nerve Entrapment
204. Webb J, Moorjani N, Radford M: Anatomy of the sural nerve and its relation to the Achilles tendon, *Foot Ankle Int* 21:475–477, 2000.
205. Dumitru D, Windsor RE: Subsartorial entrapment of the saphenous nerve of a competitive female bodybuilder, *Phys Sports Med* 17:116–125, 1989.
206. Garland R, Frizelle FA, Dobbs BR, Singh H: A retrospective audit of long-term lower limb complications following leg vein harvesting for coronary artery bypass grafting, *Eur J Cardiothorac Surg* 23:950–955, 2003.
207. Hutchinson MR, Bederka B, Kopplin M: Anatomic structures at risk during minimal-incision endoscopically assisted fascial compartment releases in the leg, *Am J Sports Med* 31:764–769, 2003.
208. Morrison C, Dalsing MC: Signs and symptoms of saphenous nerve injury after greater saphenous vein stripping: prevalence, severity, and relevance for modern practice, *J Vasc Surg* 38:886–890, 2003.
209. Mozes M, Ouaknine G, Nathan H: Saphenous nerve entrapment simulating vascular disorder, *Surgery* 77:299–303, 1975.
210. Romanoff ME, Cory PC Jr, Kalenak A, et al: Saphenous nerve entrapment at the adductor canal, *Am J Sports Med* 17:478–481, 1989.
211. Tranier S, Durey A, Chevallier B, Liot F: Value of somatosensory evoked potentials in saphenous entrapment neuropathy, *J Neurol Neurosurg Psychiatry* 55:461–465, 1992.
212. Upton RM, McComas AJ: The double crush syndrome in nerve entrapment syndromes, *Lancet* 2:359–362, 1973.

MISCELLANEOUS

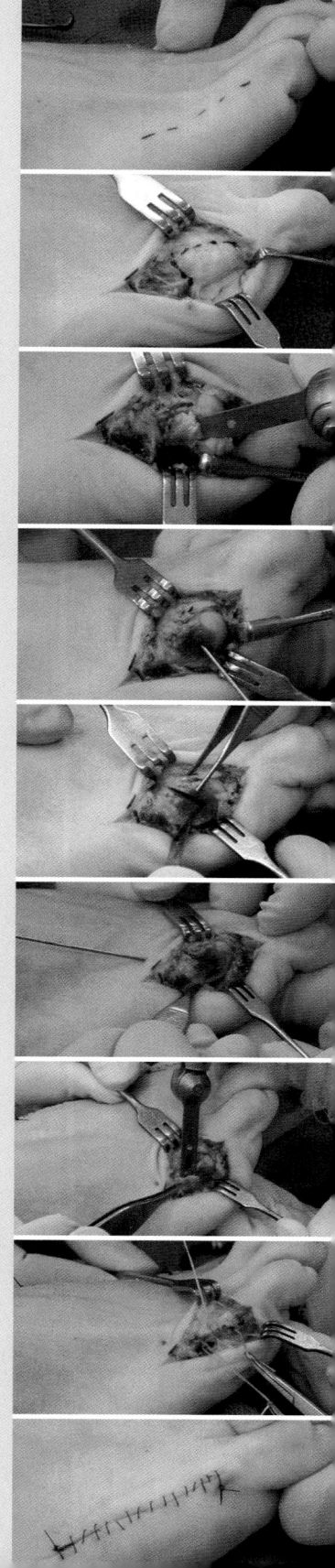

Chapter 13

Plantar Heel Pain

Benedict F. DiGiovanni, Laura K. Dawson, Judith F. Baumhauer

HISTORY

Plantar heel pain is a common disease process that continues to challenge orthopaedic surgeons. Because of the complex anatomy around the heel and the plantar surface of the foot, the function and etiology of pain have been difficult to understand.

Early examiners suggested an infectious origin for heel pain. In the 1930s, they proposed that tuberculosis, streptococcal, gonorrhea, and syphilis infections caused heel pain.[13] Dedicated research refuted the infectious etiology of heel pain, and efforts were made to find a mechanical source. With the evolution of x-ray technology, emphasis placed on the heel spur as the source of heel pain gained momentum. Steindler and Smith[66] (1938) performed rotational osteotomies to move the spur from the weight-bearing surface. In 1957, DuVries[27] categorized the different morphology of calcaneal spurs and their impact on heel pain. Contrary to these thoughts, the spurs did not lie within the plantar fascia but dorsal to it. Cadaveric studies confirmed the presence of the spur within the flexor digitorum brevis as well as within the abductor hallucis (Fig. 13-1).[30] In the 1960s, after performing a cadaveric dissection study, Tanz[67] proposed nerve entrapment as cause of heel pain (Fig. 13-2). He discovered that a branch of the lateral plantar nerve passes around the medial border of the heel and innervates the abductor digiti quinti muscle. Baxter and Thigpen later elaborated on this and demonstrated how the first branch of the lateral plantar nerve (FBLPN) becomes entrapped, resulting in plantar heel pain.[7] Although we do not often find heel pain attributed to isolated nerve pain, these early concepts and research laid the foundation of our current understanding of the anatomy, mechanisms, and causes of plantar heel pain.

EPIDEMIOLOGY

Although the exact incidence of plantar heel pain is unknown, it is estimated that more than 2 million patients receive treatment for plantar fasciitis each year in the United States.[50] Approximately 1 in 10 people will develop heel pain during their lifetime,[18] and 1% of all visits to orthopaedic surgeons are thought to be for heel pain.[56] In a 2009 study, Scher et al[61] reported a 12% incidence of plantar fasciitis in a young, active-duty military service–member population. An increased risk of plantar fasciitis has been associated with decreased ankle dorsiflexion, workers who spend prolonged periods of the day on their feet, runners, and individuals with a body mass index greater than 30 kg/m^2.[55] These studies demonstrate not only the significant number of patients impacted but also the wide range of ages within the adult population affected by plantar heel pain.

ANATOMY

Plantar Fascia

The plantar fascia is composed of bands of fibrous tissue that originate on the anteromedial aspect of the calcaneal tuberosity and insert on the bases of the proximal phalanges. Strong vertical septa divide the medial, central, and lateral portions of the plantar fascia and create three distinct compartments of intrinsic plantar muscles. The three bands of fascia spread into a broad sheet as they course distally and divide into five digital bands at the metatarsophalangeal (MTP) joints (Fig. 13-3). Each digital band divides to pass on either side of the flexor tendons and inserts into the periosteum of the base of the

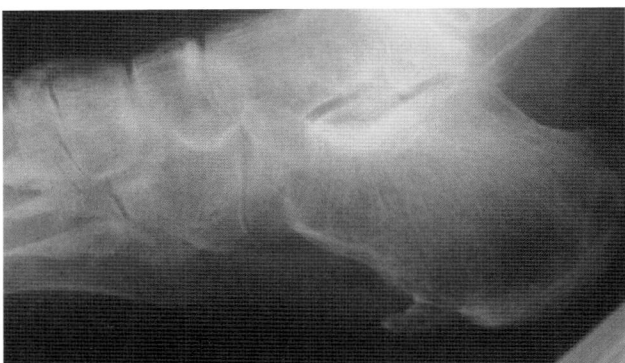

Figure 13-1 A large heel spur is seen on the calcaneus with extension into the flexor digitorum brevis.

proximal phalanges. Fibers of the plantar fascia also blend with the dermis, transverse metatarsal ligament, and flexor tendon sheath.[68,71] As the plantar fascia courses distally from its origin deep to the plantar fat pad of the heel, it becomes subcutaneous and is easily palpated beneath the longitudinal arch along the plantar aspect of the foot.

The plantar fascia is relatively inelastic. Postmortem studies found a maximum elongation of 4%, with failures in the tissue occurring at 90 kg of force at the clamp margins.[72] The fascia itself requires more than 1000 N to fail.[39] Tension along the plantar fascia develops when the toes dorsiflex during the stance phase of gait, which transmits tensile loads to its calcaneal origin. The transmission of this tensile load elevates the longitudinal arch, referred to as the windlass mechanism. Because of its inelastic properties, high tensile forces are concentrated on the origin of the plantar fascia during the push-off phase of gait, with dorsiflexion of the MTP joints via the windlass mechanism. In addition, the gastrocnemius-soleus complex pulls simultaneously and concentrates additional body weight onto the forefoot while the downward acceleration of the body concentrates an additional 20% increase in the ground reaction forces.[49] Repetitive activation of the windlass mechanism, as one might see in runners or standing workers, may result in tensile overload, microtears, inflammation, and chronic degenerative changes in the plantar fascia origin.[8,9]

Heel Fat Pad

The anatomy was first described by Teitze in 1921.[51] The structure is a honeycombed pattern of fibroelastic septa that completely enclose fat globules (Fig. 13-4). The closed-cell structure of the fat pad provides the mechanical integrity for its shock-absorbing function. The tissue septa are U-shaped around the tuberosity and anchored to the calcaneus and skin. Elastic transverse and diagonal

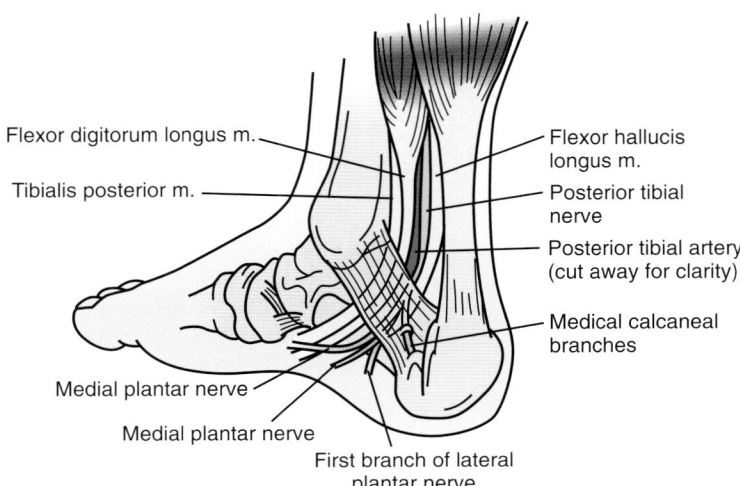

Flexor digitorum longus m.

Tibialis posterior m.

Flexor hallucis longus m.

Posterior tibial nerve

Posterior tibial artery (cut away for clarity)

Medical calcaneal branches

Medial plantar nerve

Medial plantar nerve

First branch of lateral plantar nerve

Figure 13-2 Illustration of the medial hindfoot anatomy showing the tibial nerve and its divisions.

fibers that separate the fat into compartments reinforce the chambers internally. The fat pad on the calcaneus functions as an important cushion to the hindfoot. A typical healthy man has a gait velocity of approximately 82 m/min and a cadence of 116 gait cycles/min.[59] Each heel strike generates 110% of body weight but can concentrate up to 250% of body weight with running. After approximately age 40 years, the fat pad begins to deteriorate; with the loss of collagen, elastic tissue, and water, the overall thickness and height of the fat pad decrease. These changes result in softening and thinning of the heel fat pad, decreased shock absorbency, and reduced protection of the heel tuberosity.[37]

ETIOLOGY

Heel pain can result from mechanical-related change, spondyloarthropathies, or neural-related conditions. Mechanical derangements cause classic proximal plantar fasciitis, distal plantar fasciitis, plantar fascia ruptures, and stress fractures of the calcaneus. Rheumatologic conditions cause a wide variety of presentations of pain around the heel. Finally, neurologic conditions from impingement of critical nerves about the foot and ankle cause substantial pain in the heel.

Approximately 50% of patients with heel pain have heel spurs.[65] Shmokler et al[64] found a 13.2% incidence of heel spurs in 1000 patients chosen randomly, and only 5.2% of the total patients with heel spurs reported any history of heel pain. Williams et al[71] found that 75% of patients who had heel pain also had spurs, compared with 63% of patients who had no heel pain. Although heel spurs can occur with heel pain, they are not considered the cause.

From a histologic perspective, plantar fasciitis is a fibrofatty degeneration of the plantar fascia origin with microtears and collagen necrosis.[43] This likely represents a degenerative process, more so than an inflammatory one unless the patient has an associated spondyloarthropathy, such as ankylosing spondylitis. Although some authors believe the thickness of the fat pad is the single most important determinant in heel pain,[37] other authors have actually found an increased thickness of the fat pad in patients with heel pain.[4]

The elasticity of the heel fat pad may be more important than the actual thickness. Prichasuk found that heel pad elasticity is reduced in patients with heel pain and that the elasticity decreases with increasing age and body weight.[54] More fat in a closed space, combined with loss of elasticity of septa, might increase pressure on the calcaneal tuberosity.[54]

PATIENT HISTORY AND PHYSICAL EXAMINATION

A thorough history and physical examination will most often guide the clinician to the appropriate diagnosis and treatment plan. The differential diagnosis for plantar heel pain includes proximal plantar fasciitis, calcaneal stress fractures, tumors, infections, disorders of the fat pad, midplantar fascia strain, plantar fibromatosis, flexor hallucis tendinitis, and nerve entrapment of the posterior tibial nerve (Table 13-1).

Clinicians should first review the patient's general health, including a treatment history for the heel pain (e.g., therapy, medications, injections, orthoses, or surgeries). Constitutional symptoms, such as weight loss, fevers,

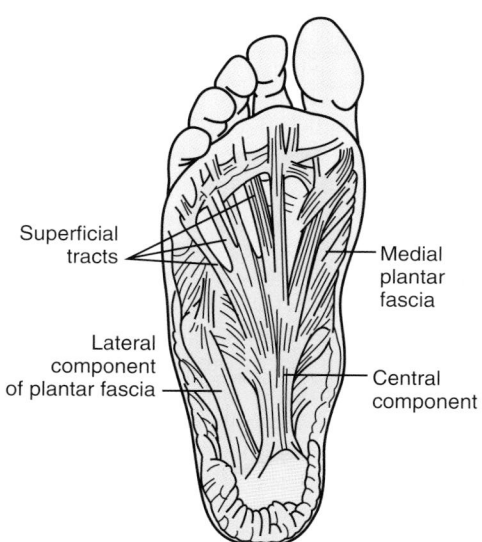

Figure 13-3 Anatomy of the plantar fascia.

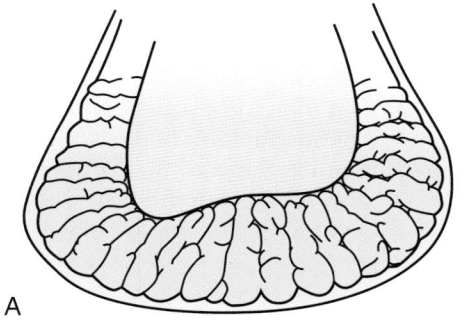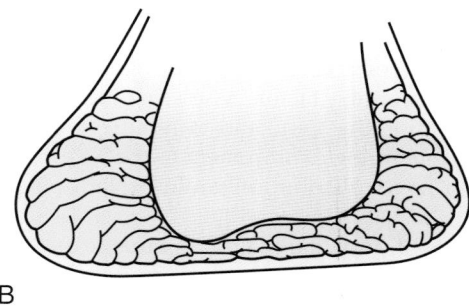

Figure 13-4 Coronal sections of a normal heel pad: non–weight bearing **(A)** and weight bearing **(B)**.

Table 13-1 Differential Diagnosis for Plantar Heel Pain

Proximal plantar fasciitis
Acute plantar fascia rupture
Entrapment of the FBLPN
Plantar fasciitis with entrapment of the FBLPN
Midplantar fascia strain
Calcaneal stress fracture
Central heel pain syndrome
Enthesitis: spondyloarthropathies
Tarsal tunnel syndrome
Plantar fibromatosis
Flexor hallucis longus tendonitis
Subcalcaneal bursitis
S1 radiculopathy

FBLPN, first branch of the lateral plantar nerve.

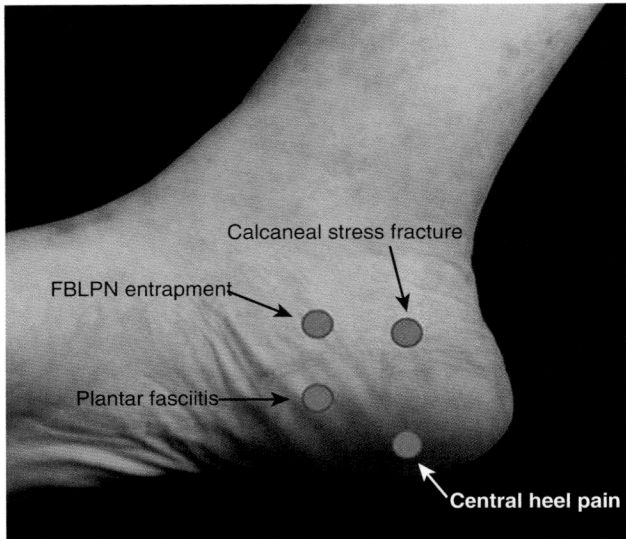

Figure 13-5 Physical examination findings of tenderness indicative of calcaneal stress fracture, first branch of the lateral plantar nerve *(FBLPN)* entrapment, proximal plantar fasciitis, and central heel pain.

chills, and night sweats, should lead the clinician to investigate a systemic condition. Further questioning should focus on the patient's activities, both recreational and occupational. Specifically, one should inquire about a change in weight or activity coincident with the onset of symptoms. In addition, the amount of time spent weight bearing throughout the day is a causative and provocative factor.[56]

Athletes who perform running and jumping activities are particularly prone to plantar heel pain. It is important to differentiate pain during heel strike versus pain with push off. In addition, pain at the onset of physical activity can differ from pain occurring during activity or after activity.

Unrelenting pain at rest or night pain is a red flag that the pain may be related to a tumor or an infectious process. Bilateral heel pain, especially in a younger patient, suggests a systemic process, such as ankylosing spondylitis, Reiter syndrome, or other seronegative spondyloarthropathies.[45] A neuritic, dysesthetic type of pain is likely caused by nerve compression and irritation that can occur at rest. Pain occurring after an acute injury is more likely a plantar fascia rupture or acute fracture within the hindfoot. Patients with ruptures of the plantar fascia often have a history of corticosteroid injection.[1,62] Paradoxically, these patients can have less pain after rupture of the plantar fascia, although there can be a subtle collapse of the longitudinal arch.

Clinicians should perform a comprehensive physical examination of the foot and ankle in search of the primary source of pain, concomitant disorder, or a locus of referred pain. A pes planus or a cavus foot deformity may be a causative or contributing factor. Assess Achilles tendon tightness. Examining the spine and extremities can help to elucidate any neurologic component to the pain; radiculopathy in an L5-S1 distribution could explain plantar heel pain.

The diagnosis of proximal plantar fasciitis is made by the patient's history of symptoms along with physical examination findings. Patients usually complain of heel pain that is most notable upon the first steps in the morning or after sitting for an extended period of time. The pain starts with a sharp shooting quality that tends to change to an ache with continued ambulation. Having patients point to the location of their greatest area of pain can be helpful. Usually, they will point to the origin of the medial longitudinal arch at the medial tubercle of the calcaneus (Fig. 13-5).

Tenderness at the plantar medial heel that is exacerbated by concomitant passive dorsiflexion of the ankle and toes is due to the increased tension placed on the origin of the plantar fascia. Continued palpation distally will usually confirm the presence of a tight fascial band or assist with diagnosing a complete or partial attenuation or rupture. Pain and tenderness confined to the middle portion of the fascial band and well distal to the origin of the plantar fascia is referred to as midplantar fascia strain by the authors.

The patient is examined in a standing position to evaluate the hindfoot alignment and longitudinal arch. Achilles tightness is also assessed, with recent studies demonstrating 83% of plantar fasciitis patients have an equinus contracture, and 57% of these patients have an isolated gastrocnemius contracture.[48]

Patients with an acute plantar fascia rupture often describe an intense tearing sensation on the plantar surface of their foot. Most patients who sustain an acute rupture had prior symptoms of plantar fasciitis. In a 2004 review of 18 athletes treated for an acute rupture, 4 had received a prior corticosteroid injection for their plantar fascia pain. Twelve of the 18 injuries took place while running, with other activities including tennis, basketball, and soccer.[60]

A plantar fascia rupture diagnosis can be made based on physical examination findings, along with the patient's

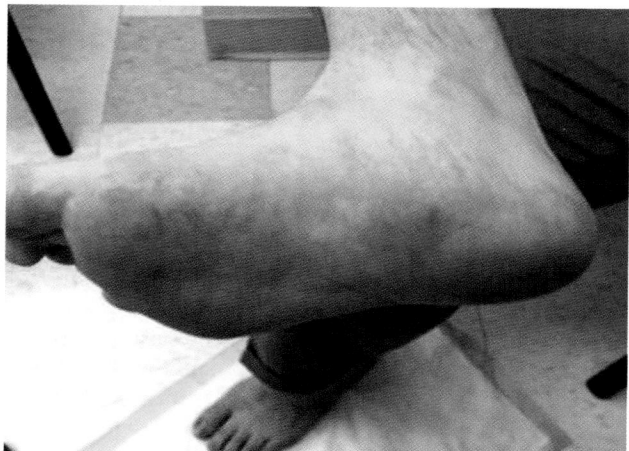

Figure 13-6 Plantar ecchymosis near the origin of the plantar fascia indicative of an acute plantar fascia rupture.

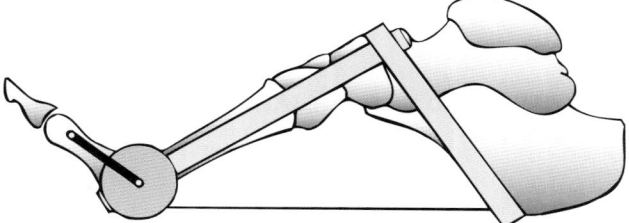

Figure 13-7 Dorsiflexion of the toes causes tension on the plantar fascia. This is the windlass effect of the plantar fascia.

description of the injury. Most patients will describe a "poplike" sensation on the bottom of their foot, with a rapid onset of intense pain. Clinical finding include the inability to perform a single-stance heel raise, pain with MTP extension, and focal plantar medial ecchymosis (Fig. 13-6). Treatment protocols vary but frequently include non–weight bearing for 2 to 3 weeks in a short-leg cast or removable cast boot. The use of ice, nonsteroidal antiinflammatory drugs (NSAIDs), orthotics, and gentle stretching is also used as the patient progresses. Although some reports describe high rates of return to activity and complete resolution of pain, other authors report a 50% rate of chronic pain and activity restriction postinjury.[1,43]

Other differential diagnoses for plantar heel pain include tarsal tunnel syndrome (TTS), entrapment of the FBLPN (also known as the "Baxter nerve"), radiculopathy, calcaneal stress fracture, central heel pain, flexor hallucis longus tendonitis, and plantar fibromatosis.

TTS can be divided into proximal and distal TTS. Proximal TTS involves a compression neuropathy of the tibial nerve under the flexor retinaculum, and distal TTS involves compression to one or more of the terminal branches of the tibial nerve. Distal TTS frequently includes involvement of the abductor hallucis muscle's deep fascia as a source of compression. With either proximal or distal TTS, patients complain of a burning or tingling element with their plantar heel pain. These symptoms can usually be reproduced by percussion over the distal course of the tibial nerve within the confines of the tarsal tunnel. An additional physical examination finding includes a pain with the "dorisflexion-eversion test" (dorsiflexion and eversion of the ankle in combination with full extension of the MTP joints). The "windlass test" (full extension of the all MTP joints, Fig. 13-7) also results in increased strain across the tibial nerve and plantar fascia, rendering both tests unreliable in determining whether plantar fasciitis or TTS is the etiology of a patient's plantar heel pain.[2]

Compression of the FBLPN is believed to be the most common neural cause of plantar heel pain. It can cause a medial plantar heel pain that is similar to or coexistent with plantar fasciitis. Entrapment of the nerve most frequently takes place between the deep fascia of the abductor hallucis and the medial border of the plantar fascia. At this location, the nerve's course changes from a vertical structure to a more horizontal position as it passes around the medial border of the calcaneus.

Lumbar radicular pain can be a source of heel pain, especially in the distribution of S1. This pain frequently lacks localized tenderness on the plantar heel and seldom demonstrates the characteristic start-up pain associated with plantar fasciitis.

Calcaneal stress fractures must be considered and evaluated in the patient presenting with plantar heel pain. The patient's history can assist in making the diagnosis by noting a significant increase in activity level after a former more sedentary lifestyle. Early on their heel pain can easily be confused with plantar fasciitis. Eventually, the pain is present throughout the day. Unlike plantar fasciitis, the pain continues to increase in intensity during weight bearing. The physical examination findings include a reproduction of pain with the calcaneal squeeze test (a medial-lateral compression of the calcaneal tuberosity, see Fig. 13-7), along with associated swelling. Confirmation of the diagnosis can usually be made with plain radiographs 2 to 3 weeks after the onset of symptoms.[32]

Plantar fibromatosis causes pain over the midportion of the fascia; the clinician can palpate nodules within the fascial substance. Flexor hallucis longus tendinitis at the level of the master knot of Henry can manifest as plantar heel pain. Tenderness with resisted flexion of the great toe can differentiate this condition from other etiologies.

Central heel pain syndrome (or calcaneal fat pad atrophy) presents with a more central and proximal location of pain than the plantar fascia's origin. Palpation of the fat pad reveals a softened and flattened surface. Erythema and inflammation can occur over the plantar aspect of the heel, a finding unique to this condition. The fat pad may be unstable from the underlying calcaneal tuberosity, with a concomitant bursitic reaction between the bone and the pad. Increased non–weight-bearing heel pad thickness and compressibility, which is equivalent to loss of heel pad elasticity, was significantly higher in the elderly population. These findings may account for the higher incidence of heel pain in older individuals.[36]

IMAGING AND OTHER DIAGNOSTIC STUDIES

Diagnostic modalities such as radiographs, bone scans, ultrasound, or magnetic resonance imaging (MRI) are not usually necessary for the diagnosis or treatment of plantar fasciitis. However, they can be useful to exclude other mechanical diagnosis of plantar heel pain. Weight-bearing foot radiographs are obtained to rule out calcaneal stress fracture or hindfoot degenerative joint disease. Consideration can be given to obtaining both foot and ankle films in patients with previous trauma to determine if external sources such as exostosis are contributing to the patient's symptoms. Computed tomography may also have a limited role in the patient with a prior history of trauma. Technetium bone scans have poor specificity and are rarely helpful in these patients. MRI is sensitive for detecting fascial ruptures, along with confirming the diagnosis of plantar fasciitis; it is most helpful in detecting space-occupying lesions of the tarsal tunnel and subtle calcaneal stress fractures or stress reactions (Figs. 13-8 and 13-9). Ultrasonography has also been used and is thought to be as reliable as MRI for the diagnosis of plantar fasciitis, but it is not as helpful with other pathologic sources of heel pain.

In the setting of a neural component to the patient's heel pain, electrodiagnostic studies can be performed to assist with ruling out associated pathology, such as radiculopathies and generalized peripheral neuropathy. Electromyographic results for the abductor hallucis or abductor digiti quinti are more likely to be abnormal in the setting of medial or lateral plantar nerve impingement than nerve conduction studies. Although a positive result adds confirmation to the clinician's diagnosis, a negative result does not rule out the diagnosis of nerve compression because these studies have an accuracy of 90%.[31] Because the neuritic component is believed to be a traction neuropathy most evident in dynamic situations, it is difficult to test with electrodiagnostic studies.[41]

Both rheumatoid arthritis and spondyloarthropathies can present with heel pain and positive findings on MRI, indicative of an inflammatory process of the plantar heel.[28] Patients with recalcitrant unilateral or bilateral heel pain might suffer from a seronegative spondyloarthropathy, such as Reiter syndrome, ankylosing spondylitis, or psoriatic arthritis. Inflammatory bowel arthritis and Behçet syndrome can also manifest as heel pain. Gerster's[33] study of 150 patients with plantar fasciitis or Achilles tendinitis showed that 22% suffered from a seronegative spondyloarthropathy, and 91% tested positive for human leukocyte antigen-B27 (HLA-B27). When comparing this group with 220 patients having rheumatoid arthritis, Gerster rarely found plantar fasciitis in the rheumatoid arthritis group. Although 20% to 30% of patients can experience bilateral plantar fasciitis, clinicians should consider HLA-B27 testing in patients with bilateral heel pain with simultaneous onset or recalcitrant heel pain. Other helpful studies include complete blood count, erythrocyte sedimentation rate, rheumatoid factor, antinuclear antibodies, and uric acid.

NONOPERATIVE TREATMENT

Proximal Plantar Fasciitis

Stretching

The overwhelming majority of patients with mechanical heel pain will respond favorably to nonoperative treatment. In plantar fasciitis, 6 to 10 months of treatment

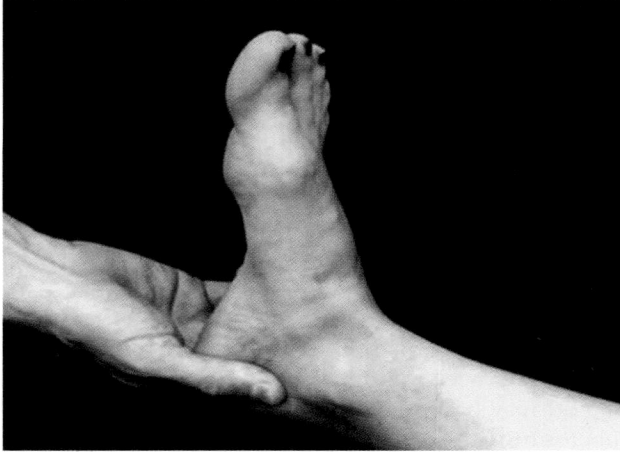

Figure 13-8 The calcaneal squeeze test: a medial-lateral compression of the calcaneal tuberosity. Pain with this test may be indicative of a calcaneal stress fracture.

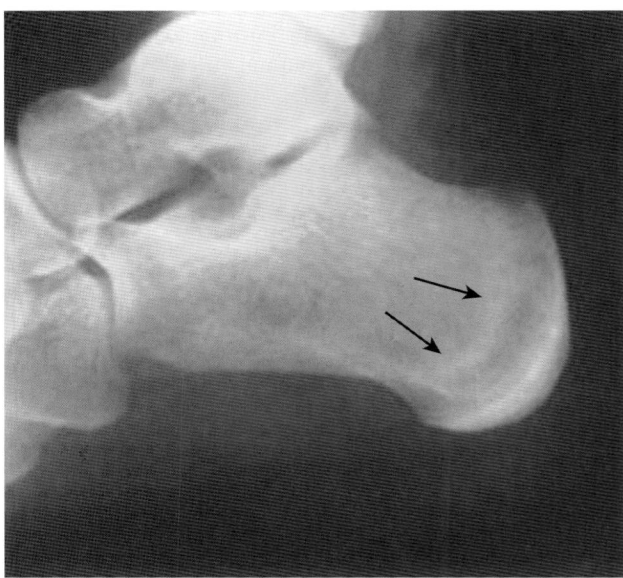

Figure 13-9 Radiograph demonstrating stress reaction of the calcaneus (arrows).

with conservative modalities results in a successful outcome for 90% of patients. As a result of the high success rate with nonoperative treatment, the American Orthopaedic Foot and Ankle Society (AOFAS) position statement recommends a minimum of 6 to 12 months of nonoperative treatment before surgical intervention is pursued for a diagnosis of plantar fasciitis.[3] The efforts of nonoperative treatment are directed toward a reduction in pain, improved function, and shortened duration of symptoms. Although the number of different treatment options for plantar fasciitis are numerous, there are level I and II evidence studies available to assist in choosing the appropriate therapy.

Isolated Achilles stretching was the primary objective of treatment for many years. There is evidence to show that 83% of patients with plantar fasciitis have an equinus contracture in either acute or chronic cases, making Achilles stretching a logical treatment choice.[48] Although Achilles stretching is still used, more recent level I and II evidence in literature outlines a plantar fascia–specific stretch (PFSS) protocol that has provided significantly better patient outcomes. As reported by DiGiovanni et al[23] in 2003, the PFSS exercise involves maintaining passive ankle and toe dosiflexion position with palpation and massage of the taunt bands of the plantar fascia on stretch (Fig. 13-10). Over a period of 8 weeks, PFSS was compared with Achilles stretching in 101 patients with plantar fasciitis of at least 10 months duration (Fig. 13-11).[23] Both groups were also treated with 3 weeks of celecoxib and prefabricated soft inserts. Eighty-two patients in this prospective randomized comparison completed the study. Statistically significant improvements were found in pain, activity limitation, and patient satisfaction in the PFSS group when compared with the Achilles group.[23] After 8 weeks of treatment, all patients were converted to the PFSS treatment. A 2-year follow-up study

with data from 66 of these patients demonstrated 75% returned to full activity without restrictions. For most patients, maximal improvement was reached within 6 months of receiving treatment, with only 16 of 66 patients seeking additional intervention later. Similar improvements in pain were found in the patients who initially started with the PFSS versus those who started with the Achilles stretching protocol and then later switched to the PFSS after 8 weeks.[24] The biomechanical impact of the PFSS was later supported by the Flanigan et al[29] cadaveric study, which investigated the foot and ankle position resulting in the greatest amount of stretch placed on the plantar fascia. Fifteen different configurations were used, with combined ankle and toe dorsiflexion producing the maximum stretch. In addition, Cheng et al[14] evaluated the finite element analysis of plantar fascia mechanics and demonstrated that toe dorsiflexion has a larger impact on plantar fascia strain than an Achilles tendon dorsiflexion force by a ratio of approximately 2 : 1. These studies assist in supporting the clinical results as well as the logic of treating patients with PFSS versus Achilles stretching alone.

Night splints keep the ankle in a dorsiflexed position (Fig. 13-12). They assist with preventing the plantar fascia from contracting during periods of inactivity, resulting in less stretch being initially placed on the fascia with the patient's first steps in the morning. High-quality studies evaluating night splints have been performed and reported. Berlet et al[10] found 75% of patients reported improvement after 1 month of use in 12 patients with recalcitrant plantar fasciitis. A level II evidence prospective crossover study of 37 patients with recalcitrant plantar fasciitis treated solely with night splints found 80% of participants had subjective improvement of statistical

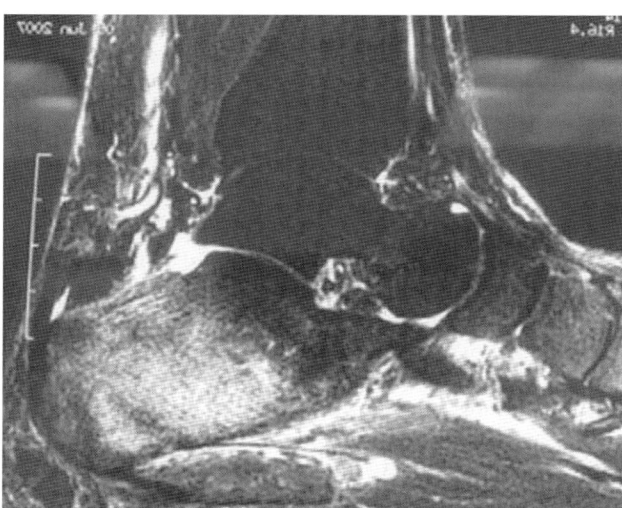

Figure 13-10 Magnetic resonance image showing significant uptake within the calcaneus indicative of a stress reaction or possible subtle stress fracture.

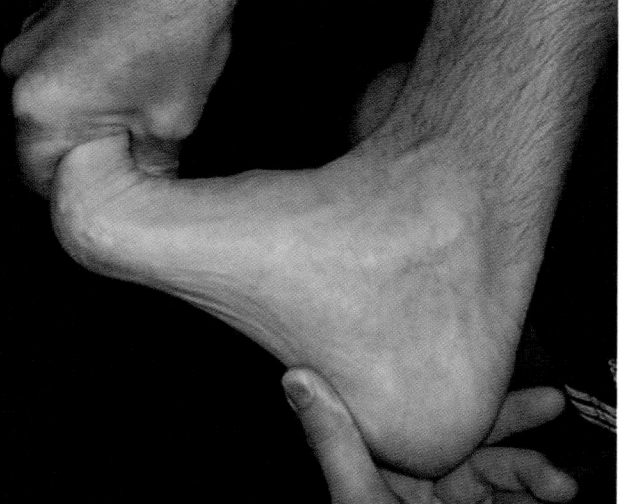

Figure 13-11 Plantar fascia–specific stretch exercise involves a maintained passive ankle and toe dorsiflexion position, with palpation and massage of the taunt bands of the plantar fascia on stretch.

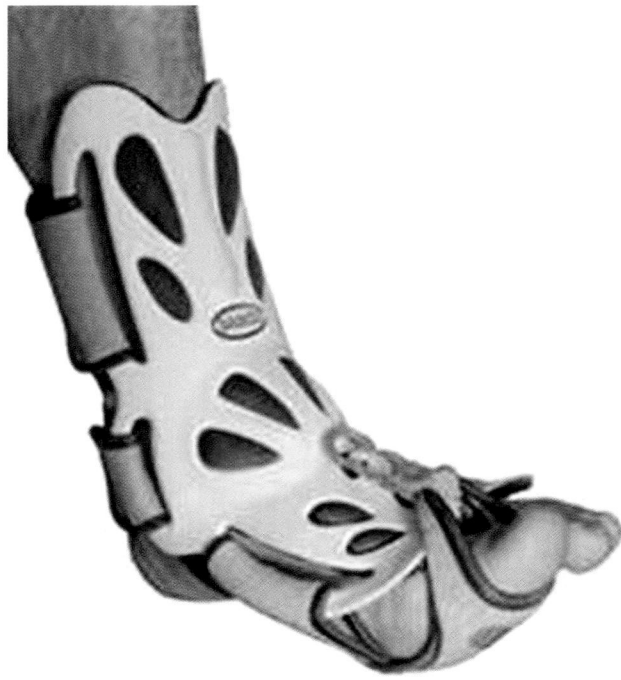

Figure 13-12 Night splints used for adjunctive treatment of plantar fasciitis.

significance in the AOFAS Ankle Hindfoot Rating System and Mayo Clinical Scoring System scores during the period of splint use. Difficulties with the use of night splints include cost, compliance, and negative impact on the patient's sleeping habits. Roos et al,[57] in a randomized trial comparing the use of night splints to orthotics for the management of plantar fasciitis, showed poorer outcomes in those patients randomized to the night splint arm of the study. Patient compliance was cited as the primary reason for inferior results. Out of 28 study patients using the night splints, only one could tolerate the use of the splints during the entire 1-year study period.

Orthotics

Orthotics are frequently used as part of a multifaceted approach in treating plantar fasciitis. They can assist with correcting mild foot deformity and provide cushioning with arch support. Their efficacy in the treatment of plantar fasciitis is difficult to determine because of their combined use with other treatments.[63] Recent studies have provided evidence that custom orthotics are not superior to often lower-cost prefabricated inserts in the treatment of plantar fasciitis. A prospective randomized blinded trial with 135 participants compared the use of sham foam inserts, firm prefabricated inserts, or semirigid custom inserts over a 12-month period. No statistically significant differences in pain at 3 or 12 months were noted between any of the treatment groups.[40] In another study that randomized 43 patients into treatment with a custom orthotic alone, anterior night splints alone, or a combination of the two, researchers found that all groups

had statistically significant improvements in their Foot and Ankle Outcome Scores at 12 and 52 weeks. After 52 weeks, those treated with orthotics alone or with orthotics and night splints had overall higher reductions in pain compared with those treated with anterior night splints alone. Patients again cited compliance as an issue with the night splints because of impacts on sleeping, pressure, and pain. Better compliance was demonstrated in the those patients treated with orthotic use.[57] Both of these recent level I evidence studies validate the 1999 study by Pfeffer et al,[50] which demonstrated that prefabricated flexible orthotics provide short-term benefits to patients with plantar fasciitis and are at least as effective as expensive custom-molded rigid orthotics.

Casting

Currently, there are no high-quality studies focused on the use of casting alone for the treatment of plantar fasciitis. However, in the recalcitrant case, casting may have a positive therapeutic impact. Placement in cast will keep the plantar fascia stretched out while improving the compliance of tissue rest for the fascia. In a review of 32 patients who had an average of 52 weeks of symptomatic plantar fasciitis unresponsive to treatments other than casting, patients were placed into a cast for an average of 6 weeks. Fifty-four percent of the patients were either satisfied or satisfied with minor reservations; 46% were dissatisfied.[68] Although immobilization may increase functional limitations and theoretically increase the risk of a deep vein thrombosis (DVT), in some patients, casting may be a reasonable treatment option for recalcitrant plantar fasciitis. The recommended duration of treatment is not clear, and further studies are warranted.

Antiinflammatories

Antiinflammatory medications used in the treatment of plantar fasciitis include various oral medications, local injections, and topical applications. Although such medications are frequently used for the inflammatory component of plantar fasciitis, reliable evidence of their therapeutic benefit is lacking. In a recent randomized control trial, the advantage of adding celecoxib versus placebo to a treatment regimen of either viscoelastic heel cups, night splints, or Achilles stretching was evaluated in 29 patients. No statistical difference was noted between the groups regarding pain or disability after 1, 2, or 6 months of treatment.[26] With insufficient data to support the use of oral nonsteroidal antiinflammatory medications alone, it is recommended that they be used sparingly as part of a more involved approach to plantar fasciitis treatment.

Corticosteroid injection for plantar fasciitis is not recommended because of lack of evidence for long-term benefit and a relatively high risk of complications. In a prospective randomized trial by Crawford et al, 106 patients were randomized into either a group receiving a local injection of lidocaine with 25 mg of corticosteroid or into a group receiving an injection with only lidocaine.

Improvements in pain were noted in the corticosteroid group after a month when compared to the lidocaine group. However, at 3 and 6 months, pain relief in the two groups was not significantly different.[19] A Cochrane review of plantar fasciitis interventions found steroid injections are typically only effective for a short duration of time, with a small therapeutic benefit of pain relief for the patient.[21] In addition, injections are associated with risk as high as 10% for plantar fascia ruptures and with plantar fat pad atrophy.[1,62]

Other described treatments using antiinflammtories include iontophoresis with corticosteroids such as dexamethasone. Osborne et al[47] published a randomized, double-blind, placebo-controlled trial of 31 patients with plantar fasciitis treated with iontophoresis, low Dye taping, and gastrocnemius stretching. Groups were broken down into treatment supplementation with placebo, acetic acid, or dexamethasone. All groups showed improvements in morning pain and morning stiffness after 2 weeks. After 4 weeks, the dexamethasone and acetic acid groups demonstrated significant pain improvements compared with placebo. The acetic acid group was the only group found to still have less morning stiffness after 4 weeks. Few complications other than minor skin irritation have been reported with the use of iontophoresis in the small sample–sized studies.[47] When added to a comprehensive approach, it may provide a small, transient benefit to the patient without the risk associated with steroid injections.

Extracorporeal Shock Wave Therapy

Multiple studies have evaluated the implementation of extracorporeal shock wave therapy (ESWT) to treat plantar fasciitis with mixed results. Multiple variables within the use of ESWT make comparison of the studies difficult. The energy density of the shock waves used for treatment are either low (<0.2 mJ/mm^2) or high (>0.2 mJ/mm^2) (Fig. 13-13).

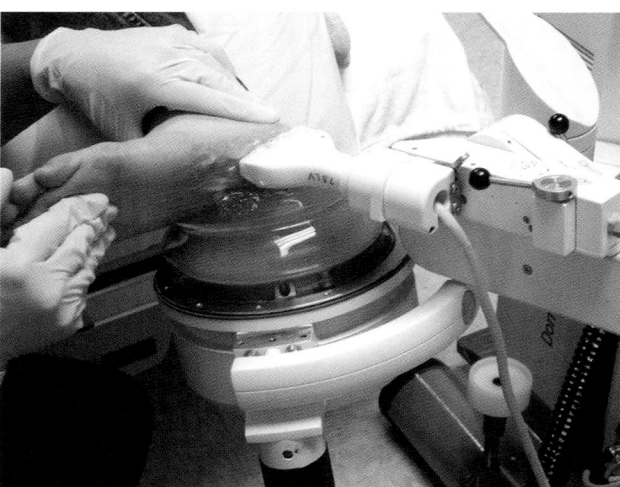

Figure 13-13 Extracorporeal shock wave treatment for plantar fasciitis.

Treatments can consist of differences in number of sessions, total number of waves given per session, length of time between sessions, and variations in the use of high- and low-energy density. Typically, high-energy ESWT requires regional or general anesthesia and is performed in one session. Low-energy ESWT does not require anesthesia and is usually performed in weekly sessions over several weeks. In a level I evidence study, 160 patients with at least 6 weeks of plantar fasciitis symptoms were randomized to treatment with three weekly low-energy ESWT or three sham treatments. Both groups at 6 and 12 weeks showed improvement in a variety of outcomes measurements, with no statistically significant differences noted. With the shorter duration of symptoms in this study population, it may be reasonable to expect most patients to improve with or without treatment. This limits our ability to generalize the study's findings for those with long-standing symptoms.[12] In a recent multicenter prospective trial, 293 patients with at least 6 months of recalcitrant plantar fasciitis were randomized to either a single high-energy ESWT or sham treatment. Improvements in pain and function were found to reach statistical significance at 3 months in the treatment group compared with the sham treatment group.[46] The mechanism of ESWT in the treatment of plantar fasciitis is not known, but it is thought that local injury is induced by the dissipation of acoustic wave energy in the tissue. This results in localized inflammation, neovascularization, and repair of the injured and degenerative plantar fascia tissue. The best available evidence suggests that both low- and high-energy EWST are safe and may provide reasonable options for the patient with at least 6 months of plantar fasciitis recalcitrant to other nonoperative treatments. However, from a cost perspective, few insurance plans cover this treatment. Out-of-pocket costs can be prohibitively expensive, rendering this an unobtainable treatment plan for most patients.

Botulinum Toxin Type A Injection

Botulinum toxin type A (trade name: Botox) injections for the treatment of plantar fasciitis have been described in several studies. In a double-blinded, placebo-controlled study (level I evidence), 27 patients with 43 treated feet were randomized into treatment with a Botox injection or placebo injection of normal saline. Clinically significant improvement in pain and foot function at 3 and 8 weeks after treatment was found in the botulinum toxin–injected group.[5] Placzek et al[53] injected 200 units of botulinum toxin type A in the plantar fascia of nine patients with an average of more than 14 months of symptoms. Pain was reduced by 50% or greater in all patients by 6 weeks, with positive effects still present at 14 weeks postinjection. All nine patients were satisfied with their treatment and required no further intervention. Although a potentially satisfactory treatment option, additional studies are necessary to further define the safety and efficacy of using botulinum toxin type A injections for the treatment of plantar fasciitis.

Heel Fat Pad Atrophy Treatment

Atrophy of the central heel is usually associated with corticosteroid injections, inflammatory diseases, and advanced age. Trauma to the heel pad, which can damage the dense strands of fibroelastic septa along with its separate nerve and vascular supply, may also lead to central heel pain and fat pad atrophy. Treatment is aimed at relieving symptoms by providing more cushioning to the heel with prefabricated heel cups or by altering the weight distribution on the plantar heel with orthotics. Use of liquid silicone subdermal injections into the heel pad to augment soft tissue cushioning has been described. Long-term post mortem examination after an average of 38 years in vivo found the product to be histologically stable and biologically well tolerated.[69] However, to our knowledge, there are no high-quality studies specifically evaluating their use to assist with describing the overall safety or efficacy of this treatment.

Rheumatologic

Systemic involvement should be considered in patients with bilateral, recalcitrant heel pain, and those who have heel pain with concurrent pain in multiple joints. For these patients, consultation with a rheumatologist is recommended. Nonoperative treatment for these patients is the same, with emphasis on stretching, prefabricated orthotics, and use of NSAIDs, which can produce a significant improvement in pain for this population.

Neurologic

Compression of the first branch of the lateral plantar nerve typically responds to the same conservative treatment protocol used for plantar fasciitis. A combined approach, using antiinflammatory medications, rest, ice, stretching, and steroid injections is usually sufficient. Prefabricated heel cups made of rubber or silicone can act as a cushion to lessen pressure over the affected area. For patients with excessive pronation, a medial longitudinal arch support can decrease compression over the area of the medial heel.

Authors' Preferred Nonoperative Treatment for Proximal Plantar Fasciitis

For a new patient presenting to our practice with a complaint of plantar heel pain, we first obtain a thorough history and a physical examination to identify the cause of the patient's complaints. Once the patient has been diagnosed with proximal plantar fasciitis, we educate the patient regarding the anatomy of the plantar fascia and the disease process. Educating the patient can allow for a better understanding and frequently leads to improved compliance with the treatment protocol. If the diagnosis of plantar fasciitis is in question, further testing with

advanced imaging, such as MRI, bone scan, or serum studies, may be indicated to guide the treatment plan. However, advanced imaging techniques are rarely ordered. Plain radiographs are not routinely obtained at the initial visit but typically obtained if the patient returns for persistent symptoms.

At our institution, a multimodal approach is taken to the nonoperative treatment of plantar fasciitis. Primary emphasis is placed on the PFSS exercise. We instruct the patient to complete these exercises at least three times daily, particularly before the first steps in the morning. Often, patients will do the stretch five to six times per day before activity for 1 month and then decrease the frequency as symptoms improve. Typically, the sharp pain with the first steps improves during the first month of treatment, with the activity-related pain taking longer to get better. A gradual improvement is most common. We inform patients that recovery is frequently 25% improvement at about 6 weeks, another 25% at 12 weeks, and then it burns itself out. Additional treatment includes the occasional use of oral NSAIDs, soft full-length shock-absorbing prefabricated orthotics, ice, and Achilles stretching. We also instruct the patient to cross train for the first 2 to 4 weeks with low-impact exercise only.

Occasionally, a patient will present with plantar fasciitis pain that is recalcitrant to the above treatment. Of the patients who are recalcitrant, about 15% to 20% present with greater than 9 months of chronic symptoms. At this point, our next most preferred treatment is cast immobilization. We place these patients in a weight-bearing fiberglass short-leg cast for 3 weeks. After 3 weeks, we bivalve the cast, and the patient is instructed to use the posterior portion as a night splint for the next 3 to 4 weeks. This treatment allows for soft tissue rest, along with maintaining a stretched position of the plantar fascia. After casting, most patients have significant pain relief and are then able to initiate the PFSS program and successfully treat their remaining plantar fasciitis symptoms without surgical intervention. A fracture boot is used for some patients who cannot tolerate casting or, because of other circumstances, may not be a candidate for a cast. In general, the authors have found boots less effective than casting for providing tissue rest and pain relief.

First Follow-up Visit

We typically inform our patients that we anticipate 25% to 50% symptomatic improvement in 6 to 8 weeks, and if not improving accordingly, they should return for repeat evaluation. At that point, we review the history and repeat the examination. An important step during this appointment is to have the patient demonstrate their PFSS technique and discuss the frequency and when performed. Often the technique and timing can be further optimized. In addition, if plain radiographs were not obtained in the past, weight-bearing views are obtained during this visit. If the diagnosis is in question or if a change in the presentation is noted, additional testing with advanced imaging may be needed. For patients who have neurogenic symptoms along with a diagnosis of plantar fasciitis, nerve conductions studies may also be obtained. If the patient is having difficulty after the prescribed treatment regimen, the initial treatment plan should be reinforced and repeated. A dorsiflexion night splint can help prevent contracture of the plantar fascia and lead to resolution of some recalcitrant cases. If symptoms persist despite these interventions, steroid injections or formal physical therapy are options. However, we seldom use these modalities of treatment for plantar fasciitis. ESWT can also be considered.

Persistent Symptoms

If the patient returns because of persistent heel pain and has had symptoms greater than 9 to 12 months, then the patient may be a surgical candidate. A thorough repeat history and examination is performed and past treatments reviewed. If nonoperative measures have been appropriately used and persistent pain and functional limitations exist, then surgical treatment options are discussed.

OPERATIVE TREATMENT

In 2012, DiGiovanni et al[22] reported the results of a cross-sectional survey study of preferred management of recalcitrant plantar fasciitis among a subgroup of orthopaedic foot and ankle surgeons. The most common surgical options include endoscopic partial plantar fascia release, open partial plantar fascia release with release of the first branch lateral plantar nerve, and gastrocnemius recession. Surgical intervention to address associated pathology can include tarsal tunnel release, complete plantar fascia release, or the addition of a gastrocnemius recession.

Open Partial Plantar Release with Release of the First Branch Lateral Plantar Nerve

In a finite element analysis, partial release of the plantar fascia is supported by showing higher stresses along the fascia medially and decreasing as it progresses laterally.[14] In 1984, Baxter and Thigpen published their successful results after an open partial plantar fascia release with release of the first branch of the lateral plantar nerve in 32 of 34 athletes.[7] However, later studies with a more diverse population of patients have produced mixed results. In a 1999 study by Davies et al,[20] less than 50% of patients were satisfied with the procedure because of continued symptoms. Conflitti et al,[17] in 2004, published their results after the same procedure, with 87% of the patients stating they were satisfied, but only 57% were without any functional limitations.

Open Plantar Release with Proximal and Distal Tarsal Tunnel Release (Video Clip 88)

Building upon the research of Baxter and his colleagues in 2009, Gould and DiGiovanni reported a modified surgical approach that combines a complete open plantar fascia release with proximal and distal tarsal tunnel release. The adaptation is based on the observation that patients undergoing plantar fascia releases, via the method described by Baxter, and who continued to be symptomatic, responded favorably to a complete plantar fascia release, with proximal and distal tarsal tunnel surgical release as a second procedure.[7,25,34] The authors described a common finding of attenuation and likely incompetence of plantar fascia appreciated on physical examination. This was noted in those who had prior partial release, history of acute rupture, and most commonly in those with chronic long-standing symptoms, often treated by multiple cortisone injections. Complete release was thought to address the chronic pathology and enable a healing response.[25,34] The authors described patients as also presenting with signs and symptoms of neurogenic pain, with after-burn pain when off their feet, and tenderness over the medial ankle and/or hindfoot. Biomechanical incompetence of the proximal plantar fascia may be associated with nerve entrapment in patients with chronic recalcitrant plantar fasciitis and heel pain, which may help to explain the therapeutic benefit of a proximal and distal tarsal tunnel release in a patient without nerve-related symptoms.[11] In a retrospective study using the procedure described by DiGiovanni et al,[21] 75% of patients were satisfied and had improved functional outcomes. The authors stressed the importance of their postoperative protocol, which included 4 weeks of weight-bearing restrictions, followed by the strict use of a preoperatively molded orthotic for a minimum of 6 months after surgery, to assist with preventing pain on the dorsal lateral border of the foot believed to result from "arch strain."[22,34]

Endoscopic Plantar Release

An advantage of endoscopic plantar release is that it is being a minimally invasive technique (Fig. 13-14). Several retrospective and case series studies suggest it may also offer a quicker recovery than an open plantar fascia release. Kinley et al[38] provided results on a comparison study of 66 endoscopic plantar fascia releases and 26 patients treated with an open release. The endoscopic group returned to activities at an average of 6.3 weeks versus 10.3 weeks for the open group. Complications included neuritis, continued or recurrent pain, and infection. Both groups sustained the noted complications, with the rate of 41% for the endoscopic group versus 34% for the open plantar release group. In a more recent study, outcomes for 16 patients (19 feet) treated with endoscopic plantar fascia release demonstrated improvement in pain and functional outcomes. Poorer results were

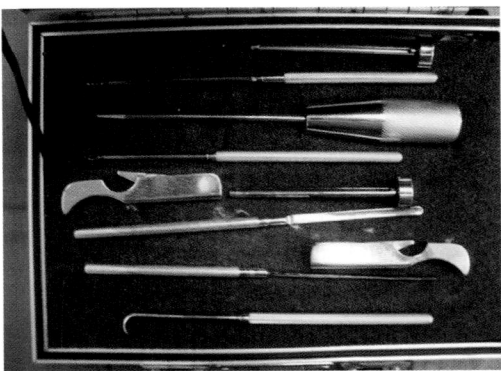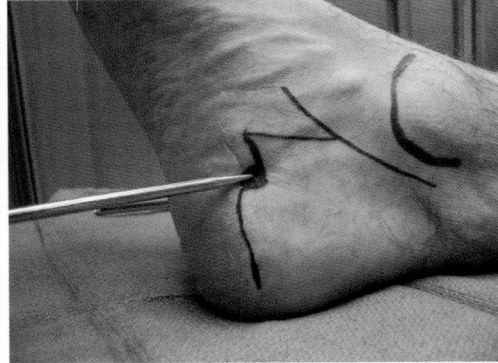

Figure 13-14 Endoscopic release of the plantar fascia.

noted in patients with symptoms of greater than 2 years of duration and patients with workmen's compensation claims.[8] Although some studies have shown the potential for quicker recovery, improved functional outcome, and pain relief, they are limited by small sample size, short follow-up, and retrospective design. In addition, endoscopic plantar fascia release does not address the related neurogenic pathology that often coexists, nor does it provide good visualization of the plantar heal structures when compared with the open release.

Gastronemius Recession

Over the last decade, gastrocnemius recession procedure has been recognized and popularized for isolated and concomitant foot and ankle pathology associated with an isolated gastrocnemius contracture (IGC). Over the last several years, published studies have reported favorable results after treating patients with recalcitrant plantar fasciitis, with an isolated contracture of the gastrocnemius, by using a gastrocnemius recession. In 2007, Chilvers et al[15] presented outcomes after performing gastrocnemius recessions on 47 feet in 39 patients with chronic plantar fasciitis and an isolated contracture of the gastrocnemius. At an average of 19 months after surgery, 27 feet had no pain, and 16 feet had reduced pain when compared with preoperative levels. In a retrospective review, Maskill et al[44] provided outcome results of gastrocnemius recessions performed on 34 feet in 29 patients with an isolated contracture of the gastrocnemius and chronic foot pain, most of whom were diagnosed with plantar fasciitis. The mean pain score decreased from a preoperative level of 8 out of 10 to a postoperative level of 2 out of 10, with an average follow-up of 19.5 months. Patient satisfaction was 93%. Advantages of an isolated gastrocnemius recession include a good chance of significant pain relief, improved ankle dorsiflexion, and preservation of the option for a plantar fascia release if the patient fails to improve with this treatment. Complications associated with this procedure include poor cosmesis, sural nerve injury, and possible weakness. Chimera et al[16] reported significant improvement in isokinetic strength at 60 degrees/sec 3 months postoperatively when compared with the patient's preoperative measurements. Sammarco et al[58] also found patients had strength improvement postoperatively but that they remained weaker than the contralateral side. Weakness is an important consideration when discussing with the patient the risks versus benefits of proceeding with this surgery. However, with the current data available, it is difficult to determine whether the weakness is exacerbated by the gastrocnemius recession or by the physiologic impact of the long-standing disease process. Although this treatment lacks high levels of evidence-based literature to support functional outcomes, it is reported to provide a consistent improvement in pain and ankle range of motion.[6,35,52,58] It is a promising option that includes a shorter recovery period for the patient and does not violate the structures of the plantar heel.

Authors' Preferred Method of Operative Treatment

The indications for operative intervention for proximal plantar fasciitis are continued pain for at least 6 months (more typically 9 months) and failure of nonoperative modalities. Other relative contraindications may include inadequate nonoperative management, failure of patient compliance with nonoperative treatment, or unrealistic expectations. Medical contraindications, such as vascular insufficiency, diabetes, and infection, are also considered in the decision to proceed with surgical intervention.

Before performing any surgical procedure, the patient must have a good understanding of the disorder, other etiologies of heel pain should be ruled out, and the patient must be presented the realistic outcomes of surgical intervention. If the patient presents with associated nerve entrapment, we consider obtaining electrodiagnostic studies or MRI before considering surgical treatment. After all of these parameters have been met, the patient is offered surgical intervention. The type of procedure is selected based upon the patient's individual presenting symptoms and signs. The authors most commonly perform a partial plantar fascia release with release of the first branch plantar nerve.

However, for those patients in whom the plantar fascia is attenuated or have had prior partial plantar release, the authors prefer a complete plantar fascia release with proximal and distal tarsal tunnel release, increasing the likelihood of addressing all associated pathology. The authors believe a key component to a successful outcome with this surgery is a postoperative protocol emphasizing limited weight bearing for 4 weeks, followed by the use of a custom premolded orthotic for approximately 6 months.

Younger Patient with Plantar Fasciitis and Associated Neurogenic Signs and Symptoms

For our younger and middle-aged patients who are physically active and have proximal plantar fasciitis with neurogenic signs and symptoms, the authors prefer an open partial plantar fascia release with release of the first branch of the lateral plantar nerve. These patients present with symptoms of neurogenic pain and tenderness at the medial hindfoot (i.e., over the proximal abductor hallucis muscle and underlying lateral plantar nerve and first branch).

OPEN PARTIAL PLANTAR FASCIA RELEASE WITH RELEASE OF FIRST BRANCH OF THE LATERAL PLANTAR NERVE
Surgical Technique

1. A regional anesthetic is placed by the anesthesia team, most often a popliteal block, and the patient is placed supine on the operating table.
2. After a surgical time-out, which includes confirmation of patient, operative site, procedure, and antibiotics, apply a well-padded pneumatic tourniquet to the calf of the affected extremity, exsanguinate with an Esmarch bandage, and inflate to 225 mm Hg.
3. Make a 5-cm curvilinear incision along the posteromedial neurovascular bundle, starting proximally from midway between the medial malleolus and the medial border of the Achilles tendon to the inferior border of the abductor hallucis muscle distally. Typically, the incision ends at the junction of the medial and plantar skin surfaces. For greater exposure, extend the incision distally approximately one quarter of the distance across the plantar aspect of the heel just anterior to the heel fat pad (Fig. 13-15).
4. The abductor hallucis brevis muscle and flexor retinaculum (laciniate ligament) will be visible. Release the superficial fascia and the flexor retinaculum over the tibial nerve. Retract the abductor hallucis muscle first dorsally, then plantarly, to fully visualize the deep fascia. Release the deep fascia of the abductor hallucis to fully decompress the bifurcation of the tibial nerve (Fig. 13-16).
5. At this level, identify the lateral plantar nerve and its first branch to the abductor digiti minimi. Gently free these nerves from the surrounding tissues, and follow

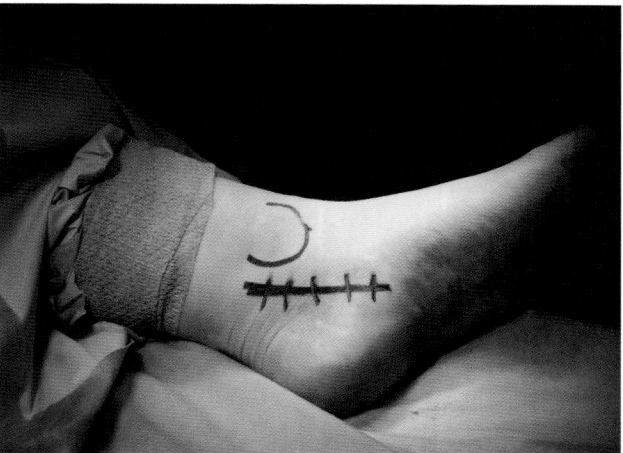

Figure 13-15 The skin incision follows the path of the posterior tibial nerve as it courses toward the plantar aspect of the foot.

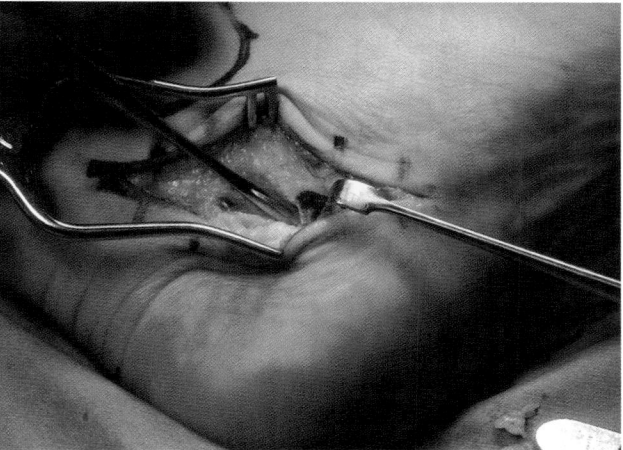

Figure 13-16 The deep fascia is seen impinging on the medial and lateral plantar nerve. Release of the deep fascia is an important component to the plantar fascia release.

with blunt dissection to verify that there is no proximal or distal impingement. Often the medial fascia of the quadratus plantae will be released.
6. Release one third to half of the plantar fascia medial band. We do not remove the plantar heel spur because of concern about associated bleeding and nerve scarring, and we have not found this necessary.
7. Irrigate the wound, deflate the tourniquet, obtain hemostasis, and close the skin with nonabsorbent sutures.
8. Apply a sterile, bulky dressing and a short-leg plaster splint with a foot plate and an ankle stirrup to maintain the ankle in neutral dorsiflexion.

Postoperative Protocol

1. The patient maintains 20% weight bearing for balance in the plaster splint for 11 to 14 days. Immobilization

aids in decreasing pain and swelling and protects the heel from scar formation.

2. At the first postoperative visit, sutures are removed, and the limb is placed in a walking boot for 3 weeks, with weight bearing as tolerated and a soft over-the-counter (OTC) insert placed within. The patient is instructed on home use of a Thera-Band ankle/foot-strengthening program and can start use of an exercise bike without a boot.

3. At the 5-week postoperative visit, the boot is discontinued, and the patient bears weight with OTC inserts, which support the heel and arch. Low-impact elliptic machine work is allowed, and at 8 weeks, progressive weight-bearing exercise is begun. Full activity is expected at 3 months postoperatively.

Trends for Surgical Treatment: Isolated Gastrocnemius Recession

For our middle-aged and older patients with an isolated contracture of the gastrocnemius and chronic proximal plantar fasciitis, a gastrocnemius recession done as a solitary procedure is being used. This subgroup of patients have plantar fascia symptoms dominating the picture, with no or minimal neurogenic signs and symptoms. When considering surgery, the patient must understand that the primary intent of this surgical intervention is pain relief and improved ankle dorsiflexion motion. We inform our patients that a decrease in plantar flexion strength has been reported and may be noted postoperatively, but it is unclear if it is associated with the procedure, underlying condition, or both.

GASTROCNEMIUS RECESSION (STRAYER)
Surgical Technique (Video Clips 101 and 102)

1. Apply a pneumatic tourniquet to the thigh of the affected extremity before placing the patient in the prone position to prevent excessive hip extension and for ease of application. Inflation of the tourniquet is not typically performed but is available if needed.

2. Position the patient in the prone position on the operating table.

3. A surgical time-out is performed, which includes confirmation of patient, operative site, procedure, and antibiotics. With a marking pen, identify the most proximal aspect of the fibular head and the most distal aspect of the lateral malleolus. Half the length of the fibula represents the typical site of the gastrocnemius muscle–tendon junction. This is based on work by Pinney et al,[52] and the authors have found this very reliable. Using a sterile tape measure, identify the midpoint between the proximal fibular head and the tip of distal fibula and place a mark. The incision will be more medially based; use the tape measure to assist with drawing a horizontal line from the lateral midpoint, marking to the more medial aspect of the posterior leg.

4. While palpating the medial side of the gastrocnemius-soleus complex, draw a vertical line 2 cm above and 2 cm below the horizontal line previously drawn. This incision is drawn over the junction of the muscle tendinous junction of the medial head of the gastrocnemius, usually about two fingerbreadths lateral to the midpoint of calf.

5. A skin incision is made (Fig. 13-17), and dissection to the first fascial layer is completed. Frequently, after the skin incision, gentle finger dissection with a laparotomy sponge is successful. Care must be taken to identify and protect the small saphenous vein branches within the superficial fat of the incision, and at times, these small veins are ligated.

6. Once the fascial layer over the gastrocnemius is identified, a small vertical incision is made with a scalpel; scissors are then used to incise the fascia layer approximately 2 cm distal and proximal. The distal muscular portion of the medial gastrocnemius can now be palpated (Fig. 13-18). Just proximal to the junction of the muscle and tendon, use finger dissection on the most medial aspect of the muscle to find the separation of the gastrocnemius and soleus muscles. Once identified, continue to bring the finger dissection in a distal direction to assist with locating the tendinous separation of the two muscles. The underlying soleus fascia should now be visible. Frequently, there is a fibrous band on the medial aspect of the gastrocnemius that makes separation of the muscles and fascia planes difficult. Release of this band with scissors may be necessary.

7. Once the tendinous portion of the gastrocnemius and soleus are identified, we use a clamp to hold up the medial edge of the gastrocnemius tendon. Then, using a sweeping action with a laparotomy sponge, palpate

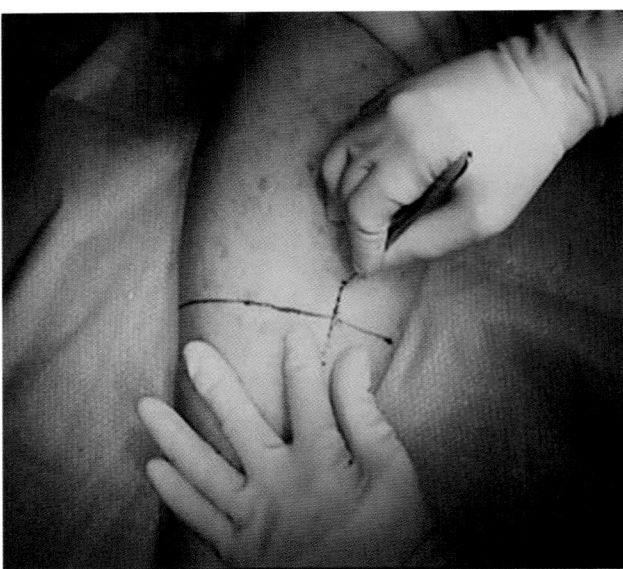

Figure 13-17 Posterior view of the leg demonstrating the skin incision for a gastrocnemius recession.

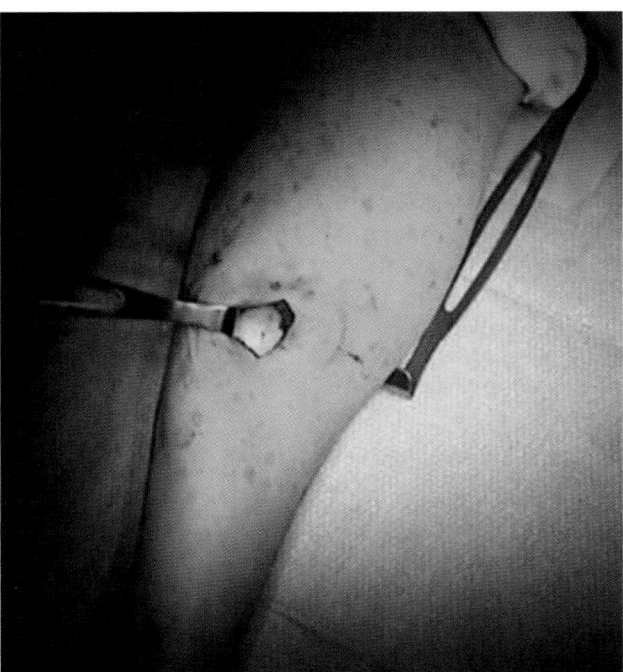

Figure 13-18 Gasctocnemius tendon with visualization of the medial gastrocnemius muscle–tendon junction in the upper right-hand corner of the incision.

the lateral edge of the tendon as well. Retractors are placed, and identification of the sural nerve is performed and care taken to confirm that the nerve is free from the underlying tendon and protected by superficial retractors. With the sural nerve protected and complete visualization of the tendinous portion appreciated, the gastrocnemius recession is completed with heavy curved Mayo scissors.

8. Dorsiflexion and plantar flexion at the ankle demonstrates the amount of lengthening. We frequently measure at least 2 cm of lengthening in a neutral dorsiflexed position.

9. We then dissect medially and identify the plantaris muscle/tendon. Often, it is contracted and contributing to the equinus contracture, and it will be released/lengthened.

10. When possible, we suture the proximal gastrocnemius fascia to the underlying soleus fascia with absorbable suture while maintaining the ankle in a neutral position. This is part of the classic Strayer procedure, and we believe this has the potential of allowing some healing and functioning of the gastrocnemius muscle. It is important to note that about one third of the time, the gastrocnemius fascia is adherent to the underlying soleus fascia, and thus the above described repair is not feasible.

11. After irrigation of the wound, closure is completed with repair of the fascia layer and reapproximation of the subcutaneous tissue. Skin closure is usually completed with absorbable monocryl suture, followed by Steri-Strips.

12. Dressings are placed over the incision, and a well-padded short-leg plaster splint with an ankle stirrup is placed to maintain the ankle in neutral dorsiflexion.

Postoperative Protocol

1. The patient is kept partial weight bearing, 20% for balance in the well-padded short-leg splint for 5 to 7 days.

2. At the first postoperative visit, the splint and dressing are taken down and the wound is inspected. If the patient is healing well, he or she is placed into a high walking boot, with weight bearing as tolerated. The patient removes the boot when not weight bearing and works on gentle active and passive ankle dorsiflexion exercises three times daily.

3. At the 4-week postoperative visit, patients are instructed to discontinue the boot and resume their plantar fascia–specific stretching as well as Achilles stretching programs. They are instructed on use of an OTC orthotic insert with heel and medial arch support. In addition, they are instructed on bilateral heel-raising exercises three times daily. They can start exercise bike work and low-impact elliptic machine work at 5 weeks postoperatively.

4. Progressive weight-bearing exercise is begun at 8 weeks postoperatively, with full activity anticipated at 3 months postoperatively.

REFERENCES

1. Acevedo J, Beskin J: Complications of plantar fascia rupture associated with corticosteroid injection, *Foot Ankle Int* 19:91–97, 1998.

2. Alshami AM, Babri AS, Souvlis T, et al: Biomechanical evaluation of two clinical tests for plantar heel pain: the dorsiflexion-eversion test for tarsal tunnel syndrome and the windlass test for plantar fasciitis, *Foot Ankle Int* 28:499–505, 2007.

3. American Orthopaedic Foot and Ankle Society. AOFAS Position statement: endoscopic and open heel surgery, http://www.aofas.org.footcaremd/conditions/ailement-of-the-heel/pages/plantar-fasciitis. Accessed October 01, 2010.

4. Amis J, Jennings L, Graham D, Graham CE: Painful heel syndrome: radiographic and treatment assessment, *Foot Ankle* 9:91–99, 1988.

5. Babcock MS, Foster L, Pasquina P, Jabbari B: Treatment of pain attributed to plantar fasciitis with botulinum toxin A: a short term, randomized, placebo-controlled, double blind study, *Am J Phys Med Rehab* 84:649–654, 2005.

6. Barske H, DiGiovanni BF: Topical review: the isolated gastrocnemius contracture and the gastrocnemius recession, *Foot Ankle Int* 10:788–791, 2012.

7. Baxter DE, Thigpen CM: Heel pain-operative results, *Foot Ankle* 5:16–25, 1984.

8. Bazaz R, Ferkel RD: Results of endoscopic plantar fascia release, *Foot Ankle Int* 28:549–556, 2007.

9. Benjamin M, Toumi H, Ralphs JR, et al: Where tendons and ligaments meet bone: attachment sites in relation to exercise and/or mechanical load, *J Anat* 208:471–490, 2006.

10. Berlet GC, Anderson RB, Davis H, et al: A prospective trial of night splinting in the treatment of recalcitrant plantar fasciitis: the Ankle Dorsiflexion Dynasplint, *Orthopedics* 25:1273–1275, 2002.

11. Brugh AM, Fallat, LM, Savoy-Moore RT: Lateral column symptomatology following plantar fascial release: a prospective study, *J Foot Ankle Surg* 41:365–371, 2002.

12. Buchbinder R, Ptasznik R, Gordon J, et al: Ultrasound-guided extracorporeal shock wave therapy for plantar fasciitis: a randomized controlled trial, *JAMA* 288:1364–1372, 2002.

13. Chang CC, Miltner LJ: Periostitis of the os calcis, *J Bone Joint Surg* 16:355–64, 1934.

14. Cheng HY, Lin CL, Wang HW, Chou SW: Finite element analysis of plantar fascia under stretch—the relative contribution of the windlass mechanism and Achilles tendon force, *J Biomech* 41:1937–1944, 2008.

15. Chilvers M, Rocco JJ, Manoli A 2nd: Gastrocnemius recession for chronic plantar fasciitis. Annual Summer Meeting of the American Orthopaedic Foot and Ankle Society, Toronto, Canada, July, 2007.

16. Chimera NJ, Castro M, Manal K: Function and strength following gastrocnemius recession ofr isolated gastrocnemius contracture, *Foot Ankle Int* 31:377–384, 2010.

17. Conflitti JM, Tarquinio TA: Operative outcome of partial plantar fasciectomy and neurolysis to the nerve of the abductor digiti minimi muscle for recalcitrant plantar fasciitis, *Foot Ankle Int* 2:482–487, 2004.

18. Crawford F, Thomson C: Interventions for treating plantar heel pain, *Cochrane Database Syst Rev* (3):CD000416, 2003.

19. Crawford F, Atkins D, Young P, Edwards J: Steroid injection for heel pain: evidence of short-term effectiveness. A randomized controlled trial, *J Rheum* 38:974–977, 1999.

20. Davies MS, Weiss GA, Saxby TS: Plantar fasciitis: how successful is surgical intervention? *Foot Ankle Int* 20:803–807, 1999.

21. DiGiovanni BF, Abuzzahab FS Jr, Gould JS: Plantar fascia release with proximal and distal tarsal tunnel release: as a surgical approach to chronic, disabling plantar fasciitis with associated nerve pain, *Tech Foot Ankle Surg* 2:254–261, 2003.

22. DiGiovanni BF, Moore AM, Zlotnicki JP, Pinney SJ: Preferred management of recalcitrant plantar fasciitis among orthopaedic foot and ankle surgeons, *Foot Ankle Int* 33:507–512, 2012.

23. DiGiovanni BF, Nawoczenski DA, Lintal ME, et al: Tissue-specific plantar fascia stretching exercise enhances outcomes in patients with chronic heel pain. A prospective, randomized study, *J Bone Joint Surg Am* 85:1270–1277, 2003.

24. DiGiovanni BF, Nawoczenski DA, Malay DP, et al: Plantar fascia specific stretching exercise improves outcomes in patients with chronic plantar fasciitis. A prospective clinical trial with two year follow-up, *J Bone Joint Surg Am* 88:1775–1781, 2006.

25. DiGiovanni BF, Rodriguez del Rio FA, Gould JS: Chronic, disabling heel pain with associated nerve pain: primary and revision surgery results. Presentation and abstract at the 17th Annual Summer Meeting of the American Orthopaedic Foot and Ankle Society, San Diego, July, 2001.

26. Donely BG, Moore T, Sferra J, et al: The efficacy of oral nonsteroidal anti-inflammatory medication in the treatment of plantar fasciitis: a randomized, prospective, placebo-controlled study, *Foot Ankle Int* 28:20–23, 2007.

27. DuVries HL: Heel spur (calcaneal spur), *Arch Surg* 74:536–542, 1957.

28. Falsetti B, Frediani B, Acciai C, et al: Heel fat pad involvement in rheumatoid arthritis and in spondyloarthropathies: an ultrasonographic study, *Scand J Rheum* 33:327–331, 2004.

29. Flanigan RM, Nawoczenski DA, Chen L, et al: The influence of foot position on stretching of the plantar fascia, *Foot Ankle Int* 27:606–611, 2006.

30. Forman WM, Green MA: The role of intrinsic musculature in the formation of inferior calcaneal exostoses, *Clin Podiatr Med Surg* 7:217–223, 1990.

31. Galardi G, Amadio S, Maderna L, et al: Electrophysiologic studies in tarsal tunnel syndrome. Diagnostic reliability of motor distal latency, mixed nerve and sensory nerve conduction studies, *Am J Phys Med Rehabil* 73:193–198, 1994.

32. Gehrmann RM, Renard RL: Current concepts review: stress fractures of the foot, *Foot Ankle Int* 27:750–757, 2006.

33. Gerster JC: Plantar fasciitis and Achilles tendinitis among 150 cases of seronegative spondarthritis, *Rheumatol Rehabil* 19:218–222, 1980.

34. Gould JS, DiGiovanni BF: Plantar fascia release in combination with proximal and distal tarsal tunnel release, *Tech Orthop Surg* 57:3385–3395, 2009.

35. Herzenberg, JE, Lamm BM, Corwin C, Sekel J: Isolated recession of the gastrocnemius muscle: the Baumann procedure, *Foot Ankle Int* 28:1154–1159, 2007.

36. Hsu TC, Wang CL, Tsao WC, et al: Comparison of the mechanical properties of the heel pad between young and elderly adults, *Arch Physical Med Rehab* 79:1101–1104, 1998.

37. Jahss MH, Kummer F, Michelson JD: Investigations into the fat pads of the sole of the foot: heel pressure studies, *Foot Ankle* 13:227–232, 1992.

38. Kinley S, Frascone S, Calderone D, et al: Endoscopic plantar fasciotomy versus traditional heel spur surgery: a prospective study, *J Foot Ankle Surg* 32:595–603, 1993.

39. Kitaoka HB, Luo ZP, Growney ES, et al: Material properties of the plantar aponeurosis, *Foot Ankle Int* 15:557–560, 1994.

40. Landorf KB, Keenan AM, Herbert RD: Effectiveness of foot orthoses to treat plantar facilities: a randomized trial, *Arch Intern Med* 166:1305–1310, 2006.

41. Lau JT, Daniels TR: Tarsal tunnel syndrome: a review of the literature, *Foot Ankle Int* 20:201–209, 1999.

42. Leach R, Jones R, Silva T: Rupture of the plantar fascia in athletes, *J Bone Joint Surg Am* 60:537–539, 1978.

43. Lemont H, Ammirati KM, Usen N: Plantar fasciitis: a degenerative process without inflammation, *J Am Podiatr Med Assoc* 93:234–237, 2003.

44. Maskill JD, Bohay D, Anderson J: Gastrocnemius recession to treat isolated foot pain, *Foot Ankle Int* 31:19–23, 2010.

45. Myerson M: *Foot and ankle disorders*, Philadelphia, 2000, WB Saunders.

46. Ogden JA, Alvarez RG, Levitt RL, et al: Electrohydraulic high-energy shock-wave treatment for chronic plantar fasciitis, *J Bone Joint Surg Am* 86:2216–2228, 2004.

47. Osborne HR, Allison GT: Treatment of plantar fasciitis by LowDye taping and iontophoresis; short term results of a double blinded, randomized, placebo controlled clinical trial of dexamethasone and acetic acid, *Br J Sports Med* 40:545–549, 2006.

48. Patel A, DiGiovanni BF: Association between plantar fasciitis and isolated contracture of the gastrocnemius, *Foot Ankle Int* 32:5–10, 2011.

49. Perry J: Anatomy and biomechanics of the hindfoot, *Clin Orthop* 177:9–15, 1983.

50. Pfeffer G, Bacchetti P, Deland J, et al: Comparison of custom and prefabricated orthoses in the initial treatment of proximal plantar fasciitis, *Foot Ankle Int* 20:214–221, 1999.

51. Pfeffer GB: Plantar heel pain. In Myerson MS, editor: *Foot and ankle disorders*, Philadelphia, 2000, WB Saunders, pp 834–850.

52. Pinney SJ, Saneorzan BJ, Hansen ST: Surgical anatomy of the gastrocnemius (Strayer procedure), *Foot Ankle Int* 25:247–250, 2004.

53. Placzek R, Deuretzbacher G, Meiss AL: Treatment of chronic plantar fasciitis with botulinum toxin A: preliminary clinical results, *Clinic J Pain* 22:190–192, 2006.

54. Prichasuk S: The heel pad in plantar heel pain, *J Bone Joint Surg Br* 76:140–142, 1994.

55. Riddle DL, Pulisic M, Pidcoe P, Johnson RE: Risk factors for plantar fasciitis: a matched case-control study, *J Bone Joint Surg Am* 85:872–877, 2003.

56. Riddle DL, Schappert SM: Volume of ambulatory care visits and patterns of care for patients diagnosed with plantar fasciitis: a national study of medical doctors, *Foot Ankle Int* 25:303–310, 2004.

57. Roos E, Engstrom M, Soderber B: Foot orthoses for the treatment of plantar fasciitis, *Foot Ankle Int* 27:606–611, 2006.

58. Sammarco GJ, Bagwe MR, Sammarco VJ, Magur EG: The effects of unilateral gastrocsoleus recession, *Foot Ankle Int* 27:508–511, 2006.

59. Sarrafian SK: *Anatomy of the foot and ankle*, ed 2, Philadelphia, 1993, JB Lippincott.

60. Saxena A, Fullem B: Plantar fascia ruptures in athletes, *Am J Sports Med* 32:662–665, 2004.

61. Scher DL, Belmont PJ Jr, Bear R, et al: The incidence of plantar fasciitis in the United States military, *J Bone Joint Surg Am* 91:2867–2872, 2009.

62. Sellman JR: Plantar fascia rupture associated with corticosteroid injection, *Foot Ankle Int* 15:376–381, 1994.

63. Shippert DW, Digiovanni BF, Baumhauer JF, et al: Recent updates in the management of plantar fasciitis, *Curr Orthop Pract* 20:130–135, 2009.

64. Shmokler RL, Bravo AA, Lynch FR, et al: A new use of instrumentation in fluoroscopy controlled heel spur surgery, *J Am Podiatr Med Assoc* 78:194–197, 1988.

65. Snook GA, Chrisman OD: The management of subcalcaneal pain, *Clin Orthop* 82:163–168, 1972.

66. Steindler A, Smith AR: Spurs of the os salcis, *Surg Gynecol* 66:663, 1938.

67. Tanz SS: Heel pain, *Clin Orthop* 28:169–178, 1963.

68. Tisdel CL, Harper MC: Chronic plantar heel pain: treatment with a short leg cast, *Foot Ankle Int*, 17:40–42, 1996.

69. Wallace DW, Balkin SW, Kaplan L, Nelson S: The histological host response to liquid silicone injections for prevention of pressure-related ulcers of the foot: a 38-year study, *J Am Podiatr Med Assoc* 94:550–557, 2004.

70. Williams PL, Warwick R, Dyson M, et al, editors: *Gray's anatomy*, ed 37, London, 1989, Churchill Livingstone, p 652.

71. Williams PL, Smibert JG, Cox R, et al: Imaging study of the painful heel syndrome, *Foot Ankle* 7:345–349, 1987.

72. Wright DG, Rennels DC: A study of the elastic properties of plantar fascia, *J Bone Joint Surg Am* 46:482–492, 1964.

SOFT TISSUE DISORDERS OF THE FOOT AND ANKLE

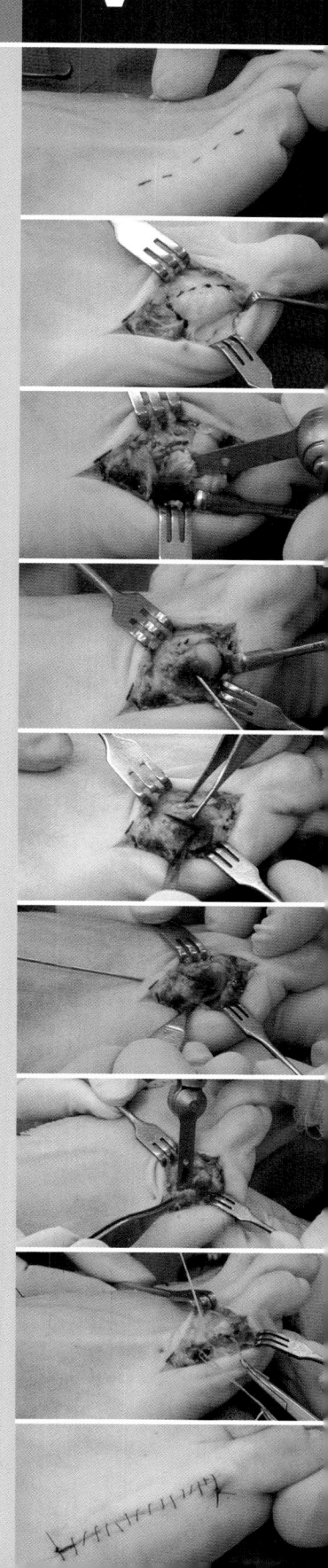

Soft Tissue Disorders of the Foot

David I. Pedowitz, Walter J. Pedowitz

CHAPTER CONTENTS

COMPLEX REGIONAL PAIN SYNDROME (REFLEX SYMPATHETIC DYSTROPHY)

Complex regional pain syndrome (CRPS) has historically gone by many names, including sympathetic trophoneurosis, minor causalgia, Sudeck atrophy, algoneurodystrophy, acute bone atrophy, peripheral trophoneurosis, painful osteoporosis, sympathalgia, and its most well-known former name—reflex sympathetic dystrophy (RSD). The term *reflex sympathetic dystrophy* (RSD), coined by Evans in 1946, was initially the popular descriptive term and remains part of the vocabulary of many treating physicians. Reflex sympathetic dystrophy describes a symptom however, and not a disease state. *Complex regional pain syndrome*, put forth by the International Association for the Study of Pain (IASP) in 1993, is now the accepted term.[9]

Historically, in the seventeenth century, the French battlefield surgeon Ambrose Paré first described this syndrome of burning pain after peripheral nerve injury. King Charles IX was treated for smallpox by Paré, who lanced his arm. After treatment, the king suffered from persistent pain, muscle contracture, and inability to flex his arm. In 1864, Mitchell, an American Civil War physician, coined the term *causalgia* for the burning pain that follows gunshot injuries to the peripheral nerves.[56] In 1900, Sudek observed spotty radiographic osteopenia in affected extremities. A little later in 1916, Leriche implicated the sympathetic nervous system, and subsequently, Livingston (1943) described the vicious circle of pain. This theory described abnormally firing self-sustaining loops in the dorsal horn. These were thought of as small irritation foci of nerve endings of major trunk nerves, which activated central projecting fibers, giving rise to pain. There is controversy about the value of the consensus process in this setting. There has been an almost complete absence of evidence-based information about this condition since it was newly defined.

According to the IASP, complex regional pain syndrome exists in two forms. CRPS I is an inappropriate nonspecific pain syndrome occurring after trauma. CRPS II develops after an injury to a specific nerve. CRPS type I (formerly RSD) develops after an initiating noxious event. It features a triad of sensory, autonomic, and motor symptoms that occur distally in the affected extremity in a generalized distribution. The symptoms are independent of the type and location of the preceding trauma. The symptoms are not limited to the distribution of a single peripheral nerve and are routinely disproportionate to the inciting event. To understand this pathologic entity thoroughly, one must become familiar with a new vocabulary of terms used to describe altered sensations (Box 14-1).

Acute nociceptive pain is the normal protective physiologic response to adverse chemical, mechanical, or thermal injury and is what most of us think of as "normal pain." The physical trauma starts a routine cascade of

BOX 14-1   Altered Sensations

Allodynia: Pain from a stimulus that does not normally evoke pain. Diabetic patients with neuropathy complain of numb extremities, yet their feet hurt when touched by a blanket or sheet.
Anesthesia dolorosa: Sensitivity to touch is absent while severe pain is present in an anesthetic area.
Hyperalgesia: Exaggerated response to a normally painful stimulus.
Dysesthesia: Unpleasant abnormal sensation, either spontaneous or evoked, that is not described as painful.
Hyperpathia: Painful syndrome characterized by an abnormally painful reaction to a stimulus, especially a repetitive stimulus, as well as an increased sensitivity. The pain usually radiates and persists after the stimulus, often with an abnormal delay between stimulus onset and sensation onset.
Hypoalgesia: Diminished pain in response to normally painful stimulus.
Hypoesthesia: Abnormally decreased sensitivity to stimulation, excluding the special senses.
Paresthesia: Abnormal sensation, either spontaneous or evoked.
Nociceptive pain: Pain caused by activity in the neural pathways in response to potentially tissue-damaging stimuli. Some examples are arthritis pain, sickle cell crisis pain, postoperative pain, and mechanical low back pain.
Neuropathic pain: Pain initiated or caused by a primary lesion or dysfunction in the nervous system. Some examples are complex regional pain syndrome, postherpetic neuralgia, and diabetic neuropathy.

chemical releases, mediated by prostaglandins, converting nociceptors in the region from high to low threshold, leading to peripheral sensitization and hyperalgesia at the damaged site. Repeated unrelieved peripheral firing causes central sensitization and hyperalgesia and allodynia distant to the damaged site. Appropriate analgesic treatment usually halts this morbid progression. In some patients however, central sensitization continues, neuronal pathways physiologically modify (plastic change), and acute pain is converted to chronic neuropathic pain.

Three prerequisites are needed to define CRPS: a painful lesion, an abnormal autonomic reflex, and an inherent tendency or predisposition that renders the patient susceptible to developing the syndrome (i.e., after trauma, burn, surgery, etc.) (Table 14-1). Onset may occur immediately (in the recovery room) or days to weeks after the initial trauma but typically is present within 1 month of the noxious event. A diagnostic delay of 6 to 12 months is not unusual in the lower limb. Classic stages of RSD are no longer used to classify the progressive development of the disease.[6,9]

Pain is present in more than 90% of patients, but CRPS goes beyond the beneficial aspect of pain (fight-or-flight response) and is pathologic. Early diagnosis is possible but not frequent. Unilateral extremity involvement is most common. Inciting causes can include athletic injury (fracture, sprain, dislocation), fasciitis, tendinitis, surgical procedure, peripheral nerve injury, immobilization in a cast or splint, infection, deep venous thrombosis, malignancy, vasculitis, herpes zoster, polymyalgia rheumatica, and cerebral vascular accident.

CRPS almost always includes inappropriate pain.[59,83] The pain is deep, spontaneous, burning, and diffuse. Pain can be triggered by a breeze, the lightest touch of a physician's hand, or even certain emotionally laden words. Patients often describe some combination of the skin feeling raw, an electric-like shooting pain, or a deep, dull bone ache. Cutaneous and deep hyperpathia are typically found. Allodynia is present, depending on the time

Table 14-1   IASP Diagnostic Criteria for Complex Regional Pain Syndrome (CRPS)*

1. The presence of an initiating noxious event or a cause of immobilization.†
2. Continuing pain, allodynia, or hyperalgesia in which the pain is disproportionate to any known inciting event.
3. Evidence at some time of edema, changes in skin blood flow, or abnormal sudomotor activity in the region of pain (can be sign or symptom).
4. This diagnosis is excluded by the existence of other conditions that would otherwise account for the degree of pain and dysfunction.

Modified from Besse JL, Gadeyne S, Galand-Desme S, et al: Effect of vitamin C on prevention of complex regional pain syndrome type I in foot and ankle surgery, *Foot Ankle Surg* 15:179–182, 2009.
IASP, International Association for the Study of Pain.
*If seen without "major nerve damage," diagnose CRPS I; if seen in the presence of "major nerve damage," diagnose CRPS II.
†Not required for diagnosis; 5%-10% of patients will not have this.

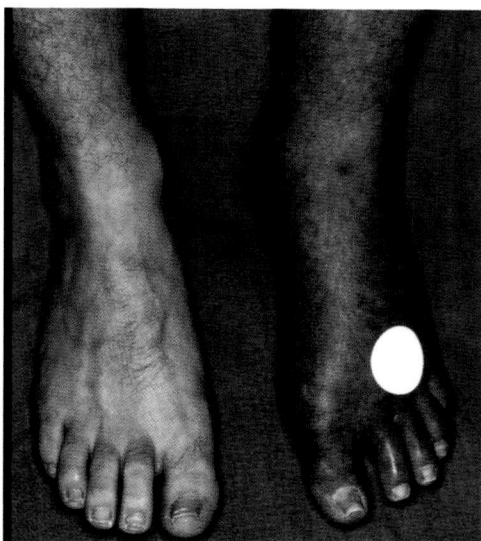

Figure 14-1 Classic complex regional pain syndrome (reflex sympathetic dystrophy): swelling, redness, and temperature change. (Courtesy Mark Myerson, MD.)

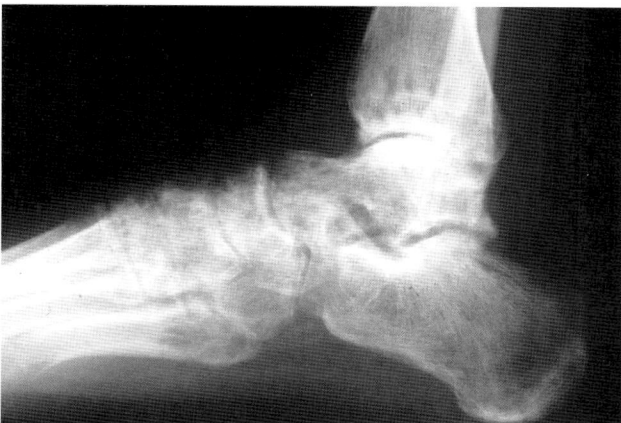

Figure 14-2 Severe osteoporosis in a lateral radiograph of a 42-year-old man with complex regional pain syndrome for 6 months.

interval from the initiating event. The pain may be sympathetically maintained, sympathetically independent, or a combination of the two. After exercise, the discomfort usually worsens.

Autonomic changes consist of swelling (edema), abnormal vasodilation, skin warming, and changes in sweating pattern (e.g., hyperhidrosis or hypohidrosis) (Fig. 14-1). Vasoconstriction with associated trophic changes come later in the disease. *Motor changes* demonstrate decreased active range of motion, decreased strength, and increased physiologic tremor (dystonia) of the distal extremity. There may be difficulty in initiating motion. *Sensory changes* include hypoesthesia, hyperesthesia, allodynia, and anesthesia dolorosa. *Trophic changes* (e.g., shiny skin, nail changes, lack of hair growth, contractures, muscle atrophy, osteoporosis, and cool, pale skin) are late findings (Fig. 14-2).

With a full-blown syndrome there is distal extremity pain and diffuse swelling; smooth, shiny skin with abnormal color and temperature is observed. Allodynia and joint pain are present. Juxtaarticular osteoporosis on radiographs and increased uptake on a three-phase bone scan may be demonstrated in the third phase. This diagnosis is excluded by the existence of conditions that would otherwise account for the degree of pain and dysfunction.

Physiology

Complex Regional Pain Syndrome Type I

A review of current literature suggests that CRPS I has a very complicated pathophysiology at several integrated levels of the entire neurologic pathway. Changes can involve the somatosensory, sympathetic, and sudomotor systems, which result in the imbalance between inhibitory and excitatory nerve function (Fig. 14-3).[70]

In the neuropathic state, peripheral areas of the nervous system not normally responsible for pain transmission are altered and now conduct pain. A-β fibers, normally pathways for touch, start to sprout and grow into the C-fiber terminals, becoming fast transmission conduits for pain.[3] Nerves outside the main area of injury may be recruited, thus explaining the late development of pain in peripheral, noninjured anatomy.

With chronic central sensitization, afferent sensory information is relayed to the cerebral cortex via the thalamus. The chemicals released from the damaged tissue (histamine, substance P, bradykinins, prostaglandins, serotonin, acetylcholine) centrally and peripherally remain elevated, and neuronal plasticity develops. At this point, the structure, function, and biochemical profile of nerves actually modify.[19]

In CRPS, the balance of glutamate (an excitatory neurotransmitter) and γ-aminobutyric acid (GABA) (an inhibitory neurotransmitter) becomes unstable. Phosphorylation of the neuropeptide N-methyl-D-aspartate receptor (NMDA) is overactivated by the glutamate and causes increased release of calcium and potassium ions, further sensitizing the NMDA receptor. The α-amino-3-hydroxy-5-methyl-4-isoxazole propionic acid (AMPA) receptors also become more active.

In addition, under these circumstances, increased substance P (a vasoactive neuropeptide causing vasodilation and extravasation) is released, and pain is processed at lower thresholds. Upregulation of sodium channels propagates nerve conduction, and the balance between inhibition and excitation is lost. This amplified response to sensory input results in allodynia.

Subsequent to these biomechanical abberations, abnormal feedback mechanisms develop. Normally dormant genes that encode ion channels, receptors, and neurotransmitters are activated,[23] causing sympathetic

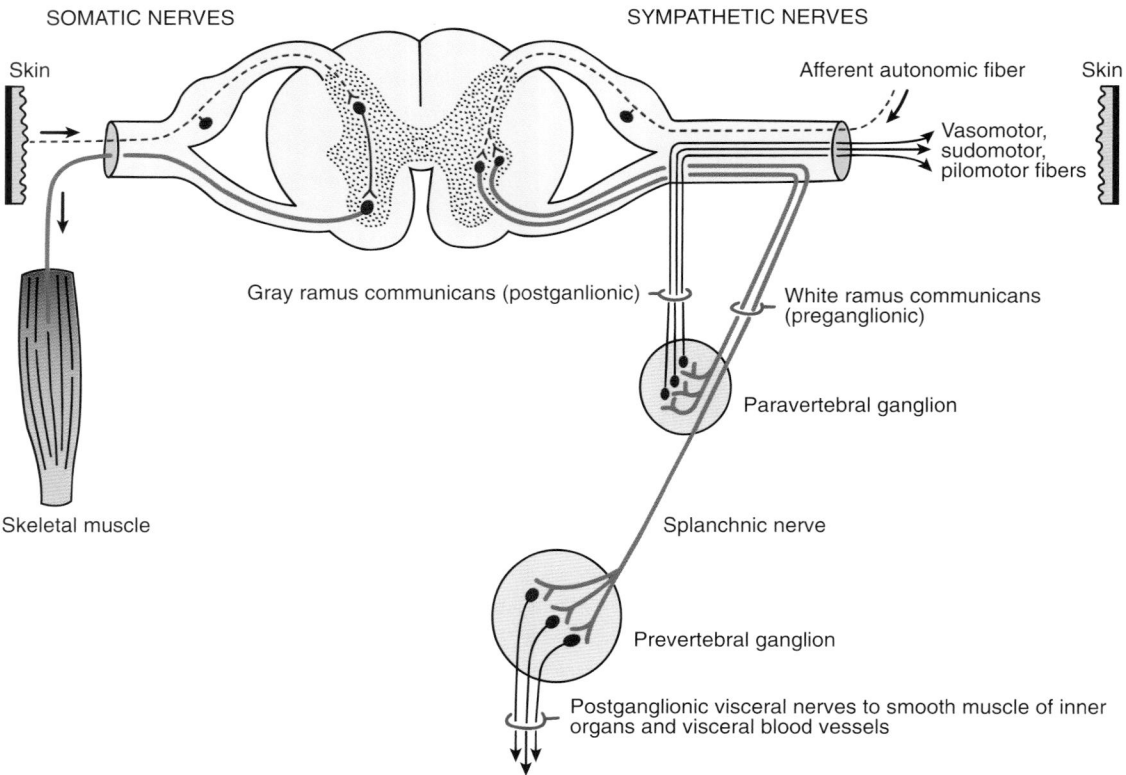

SOMATIC NERVES
SYMPATHETIC NERVES

Skin

Afferent autonomic fiber
Skin

Vasomotor, sudomotor, pilomotor fibers

Gray ramus communicans (postganlionic)

White ramus communicans (preganglionic)

Paravertebral ganglion

Skeletal muscle

Splanchnic nerve

Prevertebral ganglion

Postganglionic visceral nerves to smooth muscle of inner organs and visceral blood vessels

Figure 14-3 Systemic outflow from spinal cord and course of sympathetic fibers. *Heavy lines* indicate preganglionic fibers; *thin lines* indicate postganglionic fibers. (Modified from Pick S: *The autonomic nervous system,* Philadelphia, 1970, JB Lippincott. Reprinted with permission of Dr. Joseph Pick.)

tone to persist inappropriately.[36,43] With chronic pain, cortical reorganization of the representation of the extremity in the central nervous system (CNS) can also take place.[49]

The autonomic nervous system controls thermoregulatory and nutritional blood flow. Inappropriate arteriovenous shunting and abnormal receptor input can cause vasomotor, temperature, and trophic changes. A hot, swollen foot and a cold, ischemic, stiff foot can both be explained by this mechanism (Fig. 14-4).[42,43]

The study of neuropathic pain is still in its infancy, but we can say that normal regulatory mechanisms become impaired. At the periphery, nerves become sensitized, spontaneous ectopic discharges become common, and axonal sprouting and degeneration occur simultaneously. Centrally, there is increased sensitivity, disinhibition, and reorganization of synaptic connectivity. This response varies in different patients. If left untreated, irreversible anatomic and physiologic changes can occur, and symptoms can continue for years.

Complex Regional Pain Syndrome Type II
CRPS type II (causalgia) is a pain syndrome that develops after a distinct peripheral nerve injury. The trauma releases neurogenic inflammatory mediators, causing

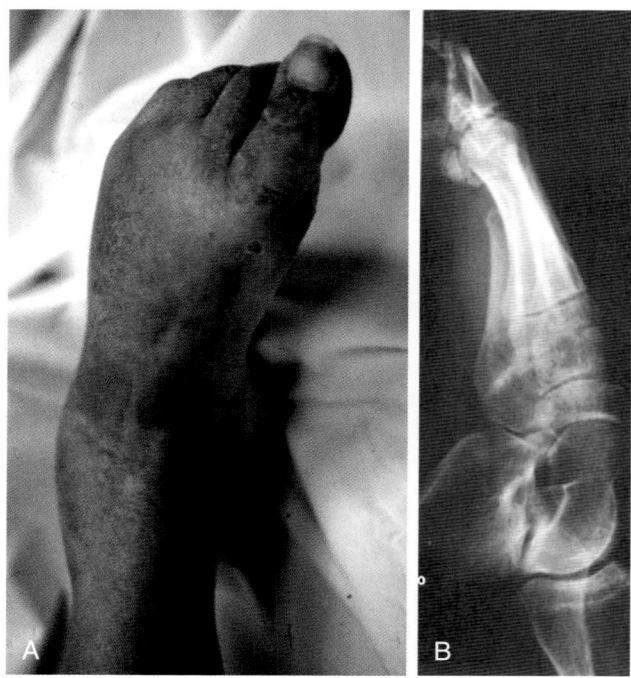

Figure 14-4 Equinus deformity after arthroscopy. **A,** Clinical view. **B,** Lateral radiograph.

spontaneous pain associated with allodynia. The sensory deficit is usually limited to the territory of the nerve but tends to spread.

Skin blood flow and sweating abnormalities are also usually restricted to the nerve territory. Motor function deficits are explained by injury to motor axons. Swelling and trophic changes are discrete. Peripheral nerve changes are responsible for the CRPS II pathophysiologic phenomena.[2]

Sympathetically maintained pain (SMP) or sympathetically independent pain (SIP) may be a component of either syndrome, and symptoms of CRPS I and CRPS II may be present in the same patient. Animal research using sympathetic blocks, α-adrenergic receptor agonists, and electrical stimulation suggests that sympathetic nervous activity can be altered to produce pain. In the diabetic patient, the neuropathic painful foot has selective sympathetic denervation, but the neuropathic painless foot does not. The degree of pain is altered by the intensity and ongoing nature of the stimulus, afferent input, efferent modulation, CNS interpretation, and physiologic adaptation.[31]

Psychiatric Manifestations

Good evidence indicates that true CRPS I or II is not psychogenic. No personality disorder is specific to CRPS. Severe pain of the disease complex is the direct cause of the psychologic suffering, not the converse.[9,17] One can often see anxiety, hopelessness, and depression in the patient. However, there is no question that other factors, such as fatigue, emotional state, stress, gender, and culture, have been shown to affect pain transmission.

In our litigious society, it is also imperative to determine whether legal issues are involved. Obviously, there are situations in which litigation influences the way a patient responds to treatment or documents symptoms.

CRPS is still clearly a diagnosis of exclusion, and the clinician must maintain a high index of suspicion. Such patients are often difficult to deal with and usually try one's patience. The evaluation is intense, the patient is often anxious, frustrated, and occasionally angry. The importance of a complete history and physical examination cannot be underscored but understandably stretches the time constraints of a busy clinical practice.

Florid cases are easy to diagnose, but most cases are confusing; many patients present with only one or two of the classic symptoms involving pain of unknown cause. No two people with this disease state have the exact same disorder. Even with the assistance of a myriad of scientific tests, the physician's role here is classic: listening, witnessing, and relieving suffering.

Incidence

Only limited information is available on the prevalence of CPRS because this process is often misdiagnosed. It can happen to anyone. Demographic studies do indicate the frequency of CRPS is three times greater in women than men. It is strongly associated with a history of cigarette smoking, suggesting a possible presensitization of receptor sites. It has been suggested that the incidence of CRPS I is 1% to 2% after fracture and 2% to 5% after peripheral nerve injuries. CRPS II (causalgia) has an incidence of 1% to 5% after injury to a peripheral nerve. It appears in all age-groups but is much less common in children younger than 10 years. With a population of 300 million, the United States may have between 150,000 and 250,000 people suffering with CRPS.

Genetics also might play a role, with the possibility that CRPS is a neuroimmune disorder linked to multiple sclerosis and narcolepsy.[25,51] Prompt recognition can prevent unnecessary investigations and lead to treatment that will shorten the course of the disease.

Differential Diagnosis

The differential diagnosis includes:

- Chronic pain syndrome
- Compartment syndrome
- Diabetic neuropathy
- Erythromelalgia
- Fibromyalgia
- Hysteria
- Ischemic monomelic neuropathy
- Malingering, worker's compensation
- Myofascial pain
- Lyme disease neuropathy
- Medicolegal status of the condition
- Personal family or sexual conflict
- Spasticity
- Tarsal tunnel syndrome

Erythromelalgia is a poorly understood clinical syndrome manifesting as hot, red, painful extremities, usually affecting the lower limbs. It is classified as primary (idiopathic) or secondary, following myeloproliferative syndrome–related thrombocytopenia. Cold, elevation, and a daily dose of aspirin usually provide relief (Fig. 14-5).

Physical Examination

The injury can be so minor and the pain so intense that a patient may be erroneously judged to be hypochondriacal or emotional.

Sensory examination is important to assess the location and distribution of the neuropathic pain and to determine if it involves a single or multiple dermatomes. One must initially establish if there allodynia (mechanical and thermal), hyperalgesia (mechanical and thermal), paresthesias, or any other pathologic neurologic signs (Fig. 14-6).

Motor evaluation must assess atrophy, muscle strength, joint motion and stability, gait, and coordination. Some

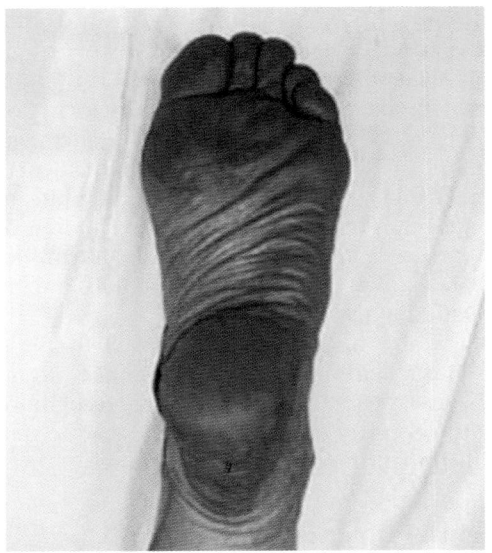

Figure 14-5 Erythromelalgia during a flare-up. (From Erythromelalgia Association. Available at http://www.erythromelalgia.org/Diagnosis.asp. Accessed June 4, 2006.)

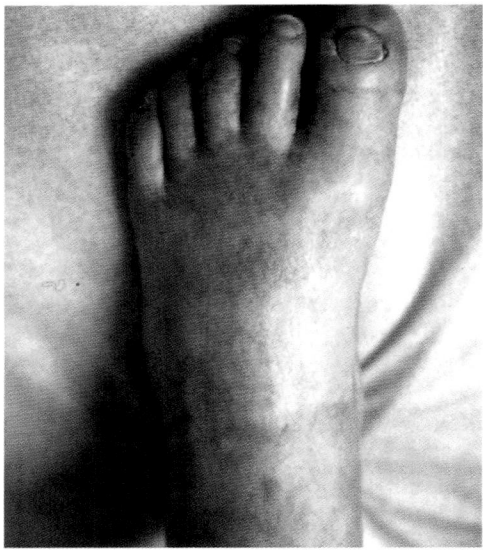

Figure 14-6 Early complex regional pain syndrome showing shiny skin.

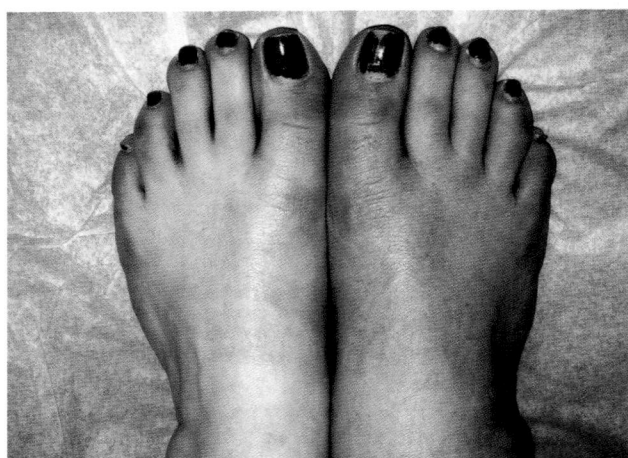

Figure 14-7 Early complex regional pain syndrome in the left foot.

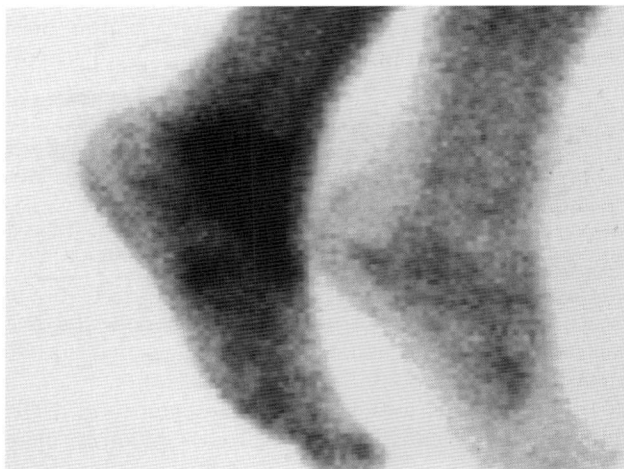

Figure 14-8 Positive bone scan in complex regional pain syndrome.

patients have edema with decreased range of motion, and the involved extremity may be warmer or colder, with or without hyperhidrosis. Changes in nail and hair growth patterns are commonly observed and should be looked for. In a study by Veldman[78] of patients with CRPS, discoloration of the skin was reported in 91%, altered skin temperature in 92%, edema in 69%, and decreased range of motion in 88% of patients (see Fig. 14-6).

The area of the body that has been exposed to chronic pain will gradually decondition. Normal symmetric coordinated motion ceases. Immobility leads to obesity, which further overloads the painful site. To compensate, the patient overuses adjacent normal areas. Further arthropathies and myopathies develop. A progression from cane to walker to wheelchair is not uncommon (Fig. 14-7).[23]

Diagnostic Evaluation

Although reliance on a single diagnostic test for CRPS can be misleading, and clinical evaluation is the mainstay of diagnosis, a three-phase technetium bone scan is the prime imaging technique for the disease. Diffuse increased tracer uptake in the delayed phase (phase 3) is said to demonstrate increased bone metabolism. Phases 1 and 2 are not specific for CRPS. Bone scan is reported to be 96% sensitive and 98% specific; other studies have shown it to be only 44% sensitive. Localized uptake might give clues to an underlying precipitating injury (Fig. 14-8).

For CRPS type I, the test seems to be more reliable when done within 6 months of the onset of symptoms and in patients older than 50 years.[7,20,28] A negative bone scan in the early phases of the disease is quite common. Despite intensive study, however, the physiologic significance of bone scanning is still unclear.

Heat, cold, and touch sensitivity can be assessed with a quantitative thermal stimulator, von Frey hairs, or electrical stimulation (Table 14-2).

Plain radiographs and computed tomography (CT) are not specific. Plain radiographs can show patchy demineralization at 3 weeks, usually more than would be expected from disuse alone. Magnetic resonance imaging (MRI) can show bone marrow stress reaction earlier than the bone scan (Fig. 14-9).

Attempts to block α-adrenergic receptor activity are not entirely reliable or reproducible and may be fraught with the problems of placebo effect and false-positive results. Despite these limitations, response to the block indicates that sympathetically maintained pain is involved. Use of blocks is therefore important for establishing the diagnosis of CRPS and planning treatment (Table 14-3).

The IASP and others no longer regard differential spinal blockade to be reliable. At best, it can be considered a screening test of sympathetic function.[71] Nerve blocks must be evaluated in terms of the entire clinical picture (e.g., decreased pain, temperature increase of 3° F or more, venous engorgement, change in skin color). Therefore sympatholysis, whether pharmacologic or by nerve conduction block, is critical in disease determination. Pain conditions without any response to sympathetic block are defined, by contrast, as sympathetically independent pain states.

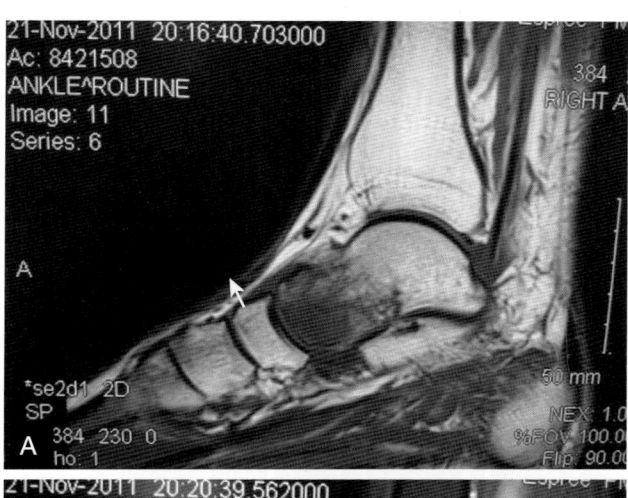

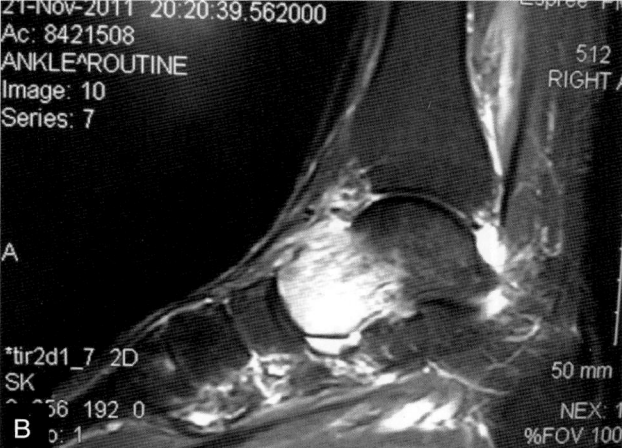

Figure 14-9 **A** and **B,** Underlying talar contusion on magnetic resonance image rules out complex regional pain syndrome.

Table 14-2 Simple Bedside Sensory Testing for Complex Regional Pain Syndrome Types I and II*

Symptom	Technique
Dynamic mechanical allodynia	Stroking with brush, gauze, or cotton applicator; hair movement Vibration by tuning fork
Static mechanical allodynia	Mechanical light pressure
Mechanical hyperalgesia	Manual pinprick by safety pin Calibrated stimulator
Mechanical summation	Apply dynamic stimuli every 2-3 sec, 3-6 times
Heat allodynia	Contact with objects kept immersed in 40°-42° C (104°-107.6° F) water
Heat hyperalgesia	Contact with objects kept immersed in 45°-47° C (113°-116.6° F) water (feels weakly painful to the clinician)
Cold allodynia	Contact with room-temperature metal object, with refrigerated object, and with coolants

From Gracely RH, Price DD, Roberts WJ, et al: In Jánig W, Stanton-Hicks M, editors: *Reflex sympathetic dystrophy: a reappraisal. Progress in pain research and management,* vol 6, Seattle, 1996, International Association for the Study of Pain, pp 151.
*Compare the opposite side for each test.

Table 14-3 Techniques for Blocking the Sympathetic Nervous System

Technique	Advantages	Disadvantages
Lumbar ganglion block	Selective with small injected volume Can monitor limb temperature	Systemic uptake of local anesthetic Possible spread to lumbar roots
Epidural local anesthetic	Allows access to torso innervation	Affects both sympathetic efferents and unmyelinated afferents Invasive

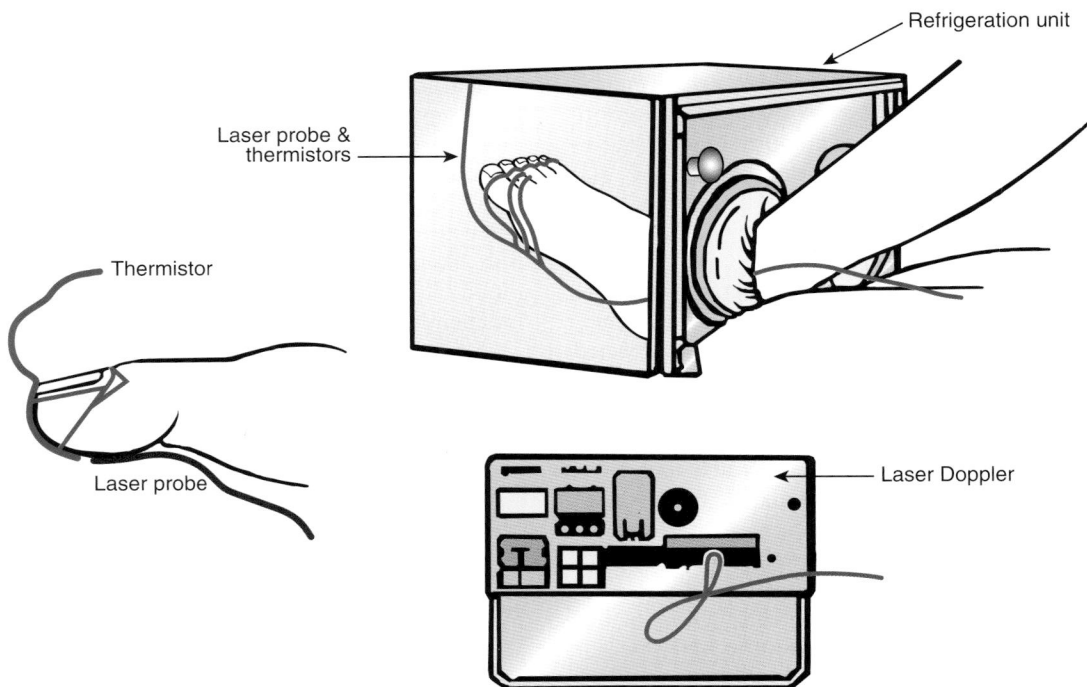

Figure 14-10   Equipment for isolated cold stress testing.

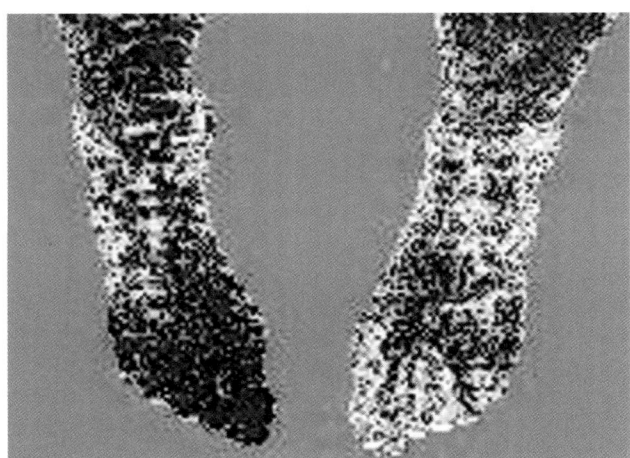

Figure 14-11   Thermogram showing differential blood flow.

Sudomotor asymmetry (resting or evoked) is thought to be significant. The quantitative sudomotor axon reflex test assesses for sweating abnormalities.

Isolated cold stress testing (cold stressor test), combined with thermographic imaging, can measure total digital (great toe) blood flow and microvascular perfusion (Fig. 14-10). The procedure combines a stressor (refrigerated environment) with a measurement technique and can provide accurate assessment of autonomic and vasomotor stability and the effectiveness of sympathetic blocks.[28,44] Limb surface temperature differential of 1° F or more is thought to be significant (Fig. 14-11).[4,25,51,70]

Laser Doppler flowmetry, with appropriate stressors, can monitor background segmental vasomotor control. It is fast, noninvasive, painless, and relatively free of artifact interference.

Electromyographic (EMG) and nerve conduction velocity (NCV) testing should be done together if an underlying discrete nerve lesion is suspected. This is critical to the diagnosis of CRPS II. Unfortunately, insurers might rule out this diagnosis because results of these studies are negative. These tests measure large-fiber disease. The critical distinction to make is that much of neuropathic pain is small-fiber (C-fiber)–mediated pain and that small-fiber abnormalities are not well tested with EMG. Therefore EMG/NCV testing has some internal inconsistencies (Fig. 14-12).

Quantitative sensory testing is used to objectively quantify perception thresholds. Precise reproducible stimuli allow comparisons between symptomatic and asymptomatic areas. Skin biopsies are being performed at selected laboratories around the country that actually show damage to the neural elements themselves in affected patients. Their clinical role is unclear.

Conservative Treatment

The main goal of treatment in CRPS is to quench the fires of the exaggerated symptoms and normalize the functioning of the extremity. Early recognition and urgent, assertive treatment are critical. Undertreatment of this pain still persists despite intense public and clinical education programs to teach about the proper use of analgesics.

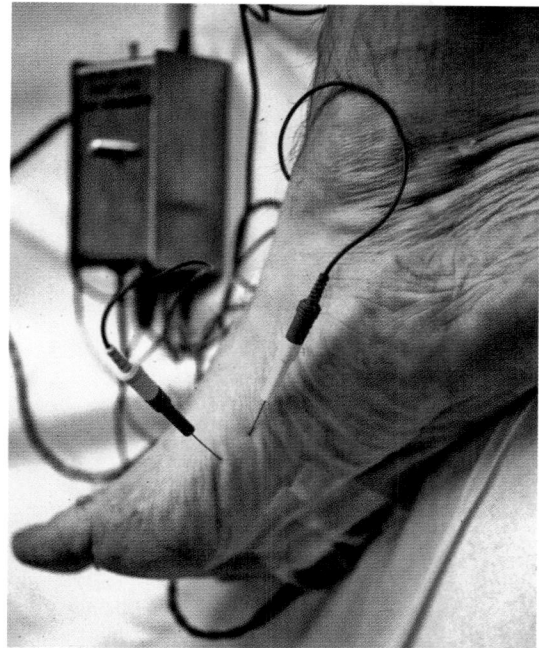

Figure 14-12 Electromyography and nerve conduction velocity testing should be done together if an underlying discrete nerve lesion is suspected.

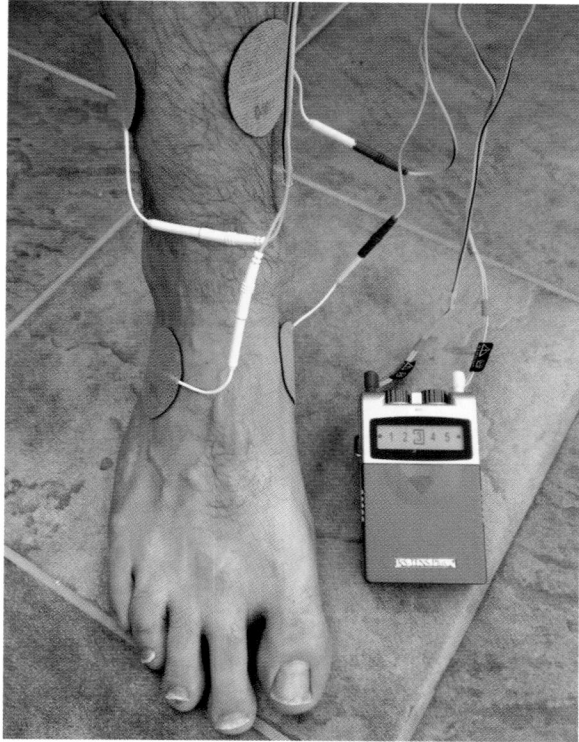

Figure 14-13 Transcutaneous nerve stimulation unit for complex regional pain syndrome.

Estimates are that half of the patients untreated in the first year have significant residual effects and risk chronicity.

Initially, CRPS I and CRPS II can manifest with the same symptoms. Physical therapy, sympathetic blocks, pharmacologic agents, and repeated careful clinical examinations are the foundations of treatment. A clinician treating this condition must take control of care management, beware of the patient's tendency to doctor shop, look out for many different physicians prescribing at the same time, and look carefully at the literature. Much of it is based on studies in failed populations.

Physical Therapy

If CRPS is diagnosed early, nonsteroidal antiinflammatory drugs (NSAIDs) should be started, mild analgesics given, and intense physical therapy initiated (desensitization; heat; whirlpool, gentle progressive range of motion). The goal of pain reduction is to facilitate function and improve the quality of life. These patients usually have intolerance to cold, and moist heat is effective.

When using physiotherapeutic maneuvers, it is best to minimize joint movement in the affected region to reduce the mechanoreceptor barrage and its increase in perceived pain.[70] One should begin with gentle gliding exercises. One should emphasize to the therapists, even by including it in the prescription, that forcing patients beyond their tolerance can worsen the syndrome.

Recreational therapy should also be part of the program. Have the patient take part in previously lost or new pleasurable activity. This increases mobility, while the socialization helps work on the often-associated depression.

Nonpharmacologic Options
TRANSCUTANEOUS NERVE STIMULATION

A transcutaneous nerve stimulator (TNS) can help reduce pain and allow the patient to progress, especially in patients in whom the pain is limited to one dermatome. This has been shown to release endorphins (naturally occurring morphine-like substances that relieve pain) and can block nerves with benign impulses, preventing their use for pain transfer (Fig. 14-13).

ACUPUNCTURE

Alternative medicine in the form of acupuncture is receiving new interest. It has been part of Chinese medicine for 2500 years and is based on the general theory that patterns of energy (*Qi*, pronounced "chee") flow through the body and are essential for health. All body parts are divided into yin and yang. In the human body, tendons and bones are yin and the skin is yang. Harmony and good health occur when the yin and yang are in perfect balance. Disruptions of this balance cause disease by changing the flow of Qi, blood, and body fluids.[47]

Acupuncture points are located where the Qi moves to the surface of the body (361 points). Insertion of the needles at the appropriate points causes a stimulus to travel to the spinal cord, releasing enkephalin and

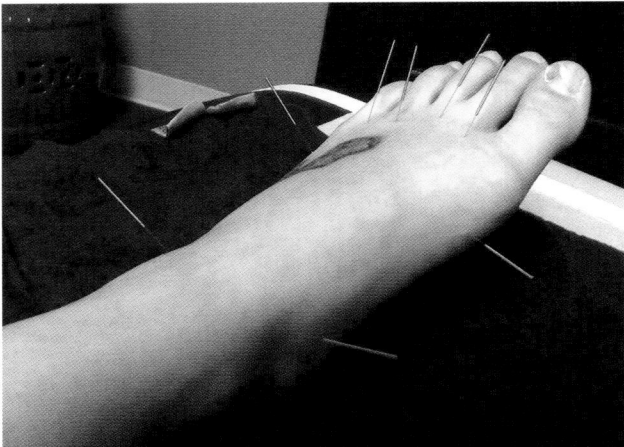

Figure 14-14 Acupuncture on the right foot to help treat allodynia resulting from tatoo removal treatments.

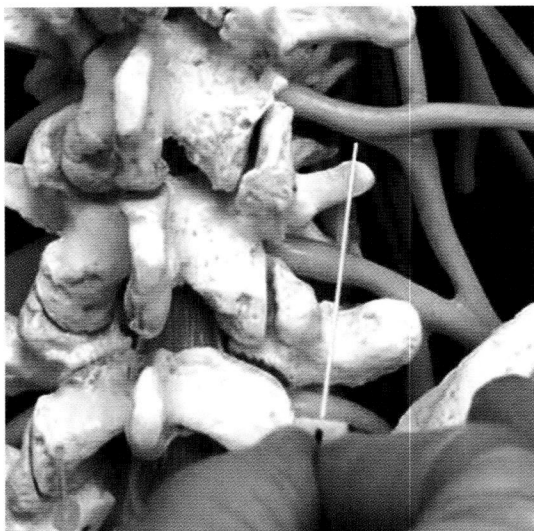

Figure 14-15 In adults with suspected complex regional pain syndrome, nerve blocks should be given early. These syndromes can partially respond to sympathetic nerve blockade. Increased limb temperature and at least 50% relief in pain after the block are good signs.

dynorphin (central neuropeptide endorphins) that attenuate pain transmission (Fig. 14-14). According to the gate control theory of pain, the stimulation of large-fiber transmission during treatment "closes the gate" to pain by overwhelming the nerve's transmission capability. Stimulation is controlled by the length and depth of insertion, the shape of the needle, and needle stimulation (heat, electricity, vibration, and rotation).

Electroacupuncture has provided relief of pain, vasodilation, and erythema, even in some refractory cases. Treatments are usually done at low frequencies (less than 10 Hz) for 20 minutes. Unfortunately, the relief from acupuncture is usually transient, and reimbursement for the procedure limits access to it.[53]

NERVE BLOCKS

In adults with suspected CRPS, nerve blocks should be given early. These syndromes can partially respond to sympathetic nerve blockade. Increased limb temperature and at least 50% relief in pain after the block are good signs (Fig. 14-15).

Neural blockade can provide sympathetic pain relief much longer than pharmacologic agents can. If associated motion loss and trophic changes are present, physical therapy, especially during the pain-free period provided during the block, is essential. Blocks may be used as often as every other day for 2 weeks to achieve long-lasting effect.[7,46]

OTHER METHODS

Trained psychologists use relaxation therapy, biofeedback, and cognitive-behavioral modification with guided imagery for selected patients. Acupuncture and these other options should not be reserved for when standard methods fail; they should also be used in conjunction with other treatments.

Pharmacologic Agents*
OPIOIDS

The use of opioids (compounds with morphine-like characteristics) for the treatment of neuropathic pain is no longer controversial and should be part of your armamentarium. Neuropathic pain is not opiate insensitive, and it was suggested at the Fourth World Congress of The World Institute of Pain, Budapest, 2007 that these drugs be titrated for therapeutic efficacy versus side effects. Opiates have the side effects of nausea, constipation, respiratory depression, urinary retention, orthostatic hypotension, confusion, and sedation, but these can be managed clinically. Opioids also inhibit rapid eye movement sleep, which can disturb sleep patterns.[18]

Lowering the dose of opioids whenever possible is advisable. However, modern pain management recognizes that there is no ceiling to the therapeutic dose of opioids. As stated by Tennant,[72] "There is no upper limit on the amount or number of different opioids prescribed for pain relief as long as the administration of the medicine does not produce physiologic abnormalities as diagnosed by face-to-face, hands on physical examination."

Current clinical practice encourages the use of opiates to cover all of the painful time as opposed to on an as-needed basis. There should be fixed doses of long-acting medication (e.g., transdermal fentanyl patch, MS Contin, OxyContin), with the ability to supplement with additional short-acting medicine for breakthrough pain (oral transmucosal fentanyl, oxycodone, hydromorphone,

---

*Please refer to the specific instructions for use for each medication mentioned in the text as dosages and precautions may change over time.

or hydrocodone).[64] In the elderly, long-acting opiates may be more efficacious than tricyclics.

When prescribing opioids, you must become comfortable with the clear clinical differences among tolerance, addiction, and dependency. Tolerance, which may be mediated through the NMDA receptor, implies that the patient has gotten used to the medication and needs a higher dose to produce the same effect. Addiction is an irrational dependence on drugs, which requires psychiatric care. Physical dependence means that the patient has to be titrated slowly off the medication to avoid withdrawal. Warnings of inappropriate opioid use include the following:

■ Impaired control over drug use
■ Refusal to participate in a medication taper
■ Reports that nothing but a specific opioid works
■ Preference for short-acting versus long-acting opioids
■ Use of multiple prescribers and pharmacies
■ Not taking medicine as prescribed
■ Loss of medication more than once
■ Use of nonprescribed psychoactive drugs in addition to prescribed medication

Because of legal ramifications, it is important to carefully document in the patient's chart your intentions in the use and administration of these substances.

Although analgesics are often used when treating patients with CRPS I, and their use is described in various treatment protocols and guidelines, the scientific support for their administration to patients with CRPS I is very limited.

One placebo-controlled randomized clinical trial (n = 43) was found that investigated the effects of sustained-release oral morphine on patients who had previously been treated with epidural spinal cord electrical stimulation (ESES).[34] No significant differences were found between the extent of pain reduction and the average time for ESES to become effective. On average, the morphine group reported 20 side effects per day, compared to 2 per day in the placebo group. An uncontrolled study with nine CRPS I and II patients evaluated the effects of continuous infusion of morphine in the axillary plexus after stellate blockade.[5] Significant pain reduction at rest and at movement and increased grip strength were found. However, the steady-state morphine concentrations were lower than the minimally effective analgesic concentration. There is little information on weak- and strong-acting opioids in patients with CRPS I. Systematic reviews on their use for neuropathic pain have found tramadol to be effective.[22]

Positive short-term effects have also been reported for strong-acting opioids administered for neuropathic and musculoskeletal pain.[35]

ATYPICAL OPIOIDS

Atypical opioids such as tramadol, an opioid receptor agonist, are clearly different from other opioids and are only minimally inhibited by naloxone. Tramadol inhibits the uptake of serotonin and norepinephrine and has been shown to be effective in some patients with neuropathic pain. It has a low potential for abuse, but it should be avoided in patients with a tendency to abuse drugs.[7]

PARACETAMOL

The use of paracetamol is described in the context of an adjuvant pain protocol in a study about the efficacy of free radical scavengers in treating CRPS I (n = 146).[63]

No studies were found evaluating paracetamol as a stand-alone treatment for CRPS I. There is no current evidence that paracetamol is effective in treating pain in CRPS I patients.

NONSTEROIDAL ANTIINFLAMMATORY DRUGS (NSAIDS)

Sixty-one CRPS I patients were retrospectively evaluated with respect to the effects of 60 mg of ketorolac administered by means of a regional intravenous blockade.[14] Twenty-six percent of patients had a complete response, 42% had a partial response, and 31% had no response. Patients with allodynia had significantly less response to the treatment. Conflicting data have been published with regard to the use of NSAIDs in patients with neuropathic pain.[58]

ANTIDEPRESSANTS

Antidepressants may be used to relieve pain by blocking presynaptic uptake of norepinephrine and serotonin. They can help lessen the global intensity of symptoms, enabling the discovery of an underlying neurologic problem (e.g., tarsal tunnel, neuroma). However, chronic pain patients might already be taking multiple medications that have significant side effects. One has to carefully watch for oversedation when adding an antidepressant to such a regimen.

In considering the use of antidepressants, four major issues must be considered:

1. Major depression and chronic pain are common conditions, and they frequently overlap.
2. Antidepressants can improve symptoms of major depression, regardless of the presence or absence of comorbid pain (although pain can reduce the chances of optimal recovery).
3. Antidepressants improve pain symptoms, regardless of the presence or absence of comorbid major depression.
4. Chronic pain and major depression have a shared neurobiology and appear to have a shared neuroanatomy (in the brain and spinal column) and neurochemistry (norepinephrine and serotonin), with similar hypothalamic-pituitary-adrenal (HPA) axis, autonomic nervous system (ANS), and inflammatory cytokine disturbances.

Tricyclic antidepressants (TCAs) and selective serotonin reuptake inhibitors (SSRIs) have more benign side-effect profiles than classic analgesics and offer the added benefit of often restoring sleep.[25,40,55] TCAs, especially amitriptyline (Elavil), work by blocking norepinephrine and serotonin reuptake, thus making more neurotransmitter available. They might also block the NMDA receptor. Amitriptyline also is a sodium channel blocker and imparts a local anesthetic-like quality.

By blocking α-adrenergic and histamine receptors, TCAs can cause postural hypotension and sedation. Their anticholinergic properties can cause dry mouth, constipation, blurry vision, and urinary retention. Desipramine and nortriptyline seem to be better tolerated than amitriptyline. However, all three seem to have a similar clinical effect. Optimal doses have not yet been established, but it is best to start at lower doses and increase until analgesia is achieved or side effects become intolerable. In the elderly, blood levels should be checked.

Selective serotonin reuptake inhibitors (SSRIs) slow the absorption of the neurotransmitter serotonin. They do not have significant cardiac effects and are generally safer than tricyclics. They can cause sedation, agitation, insomnia, and sexual dysfunction.

Multiple-action agents can often be helpful when TCAs and SSRIs fail, because these agents often affect more than one receptor or neurotransmitter system. Their exact biochemical effect on pain is not completely understood. Complications can include weight gain and sexual dysfunction.

Cymbalta, an SSRI, has been approved by the Food and Drug Administration (FDA) for both the treatment of depression and the management of pain associated with peripheral neuropathy. Cymbalta targets two chemicals, serotonin and norepinephrine, that are thought to play a role in how the brain and body affect mood and pain. Dosage for neuropathic pain is 60 mg PO QD, starting at 30 mg PO QD × 1 wk and may increase to 120 mg QD. It is not recommended in patients with impaired liver function.

Serotonin-norepinephrine reuptake inhibitors (SNRIs) are a new class of antidepressants. Like TCAs, they seem to be more effective than SSRIs for treating neuropathic pain because they also inhibit reuptake of both norepinephrine and serotonin. Venlafaxine is as effective against painful polyneuropathies (including painful diabetic neuropathy) as imipramine (the reference TCA), and both are significantly better than placebo. Like the TCAs, the SNRIs, duloxetine (Cymbalta) seem to confer benefits independent of their antidepressant effects. Side effects include sedation, confusion, hypertension, and withdrawal syndrome.

Monoamine oxidase inhibitor (MAOI) use should be reserved for experienced clinicians in special situations, because their complications are potentially fatal (Box 14-2).

SYSTEMIC STEROIDS

Oral or intravenous systemic steroids decrease capillary permeability and stabilize the basement membrane.

BOX 14-2   Commercially Available Antidepressants

Tricyclics
Clomipramine (Anafranil)
Doxepin (Sinequan)
Imipramine (Tofranil)
Trimipramine (Surmontil)
Desipramine (Norpramine)
Nortriptyline (Pamelor)
Protriptyline (Vivactil)
Amitriptyline (Elavil)

Monoamine Oxidase Inhibitors
Phenelzine (Nardil)
Tranylcypromine (Parnate)
Isocarboxazid (Marplan)

Selective Serotonin Reuptake Inhibitors
Fluoxetine (Prozac)
Paroxetine (Paxil)
Sertraline (Zoloft)
Fluvoxamine (Luvox)
Citalopram (Celexa)
Escitalopram (Lexapro)

Multiple-Action Agents
Bupropion (Wellbutrin)
Venlafaxine (Effexor)
Nefazodone (Serzone)
Mirtazapine (Remeron)
Reboxetine (Vestra)
Amoxapine (Asendin)
Maprotiline (Ludiomil)
Trazodone (Desyrel)
Duloxetine (Cymbalta)

Tapered oral methylprednisolone (Medrol Dosepak) can be effective early. With regional intravenous (IV) blocks (methylprednisolone sodium succinate and lidocaine HCl), good results were reported in 20 of 24 patients when blocks were started within 6 months of symptoms. Overall, results are mixed.[73]

Corticosteroids have been used in open trials (n = 64-69)[45] and in one controlled trial (n = 23)[12] to treat CRPS I, all of limited methodologic quality. All the studies found corticosteroids to have a very pronounced beneficial effect. Corticosteroids may have a positive effect on CRPS I, but little is known as to the duration and dosage.

ORAL SYMPATHOLYTICS

Oral sympatholytics are poorly tolerated. Fatigue, sedation, hypotension, and sexual dysfunction are major problems.[20]

Bisphosphonates

Three placebo-controlled studies have been carried out to date.[26] One study (n = 20) involved administration of alendronate 3 days in a row.[1] Another study evaluated the efficacy of clodronate (n = 32).[77] In a third study, treatment comprised alendronate (40 mg: this dose is four times as high as that given for osteoporosis) administered to 40 CRPS I patients. In the three studies, the parameters in the group of patients treated with bisphosphonates improved significantly more than in the placebo group.

It has been suggested, based on this data, that bisphosphonates have a beneficial effect on the signs of inflammation in patients with CRPS I. At present, little is known about optimum dosage, frequency, and duration of treatment.

CALCIUM CHANNEL BLOCKERS

Calcium channel blockers slow the movement of calcium ions into cells, leading to inhibition of the excitation–contraction coupling. With diminished flow, smooth muscle relaxes, peripheral blood flow increases, and discharge from hypersensitive scars can decrease. Nifedipine (Procardia) 10 to 30 mg three times daily or diltiazem (Cardizem) 30 mg four times daily (can be increased to 60 to 90 mg four times daily) can be effective. Calcium channel blockers are also helpful in the treatment of the Raynaud phenomenon.

Two studies of moderate quality and size investigated the effect of nifedipine and phenoxybenzamine in treating CRPS I.[48,49,57]

One retrospective study with 59 patients reports that nifedipine (20 mg per day) or phenoxybenzamine (up to 120 mg/day) are most effective for CRPS I in the acute phase.[57] Both studies are primarily descriptive and the outcomes are subjective, failing to describe the nature of the improvement in patients' conditions. There are indications that calcium channel blockers have some effect in the acute phase of CRPS I. Although they improve blood circulation, they also cause side effects, such as a drop in blood pressure and headache.

ANTICONVULSANTS

Anticonvulsants suppress pathologic electrical discharges in the CNS and peripheral nervous system. They raise the threshold for nerve activation and block sodium channeling. Some also facilitate γ-aminobutyric acid (GABA, an inhibitory neurotransmitter) activity. Side effects include CNS depression, drowsiness, and edema. Gabapentin (Neurontin) is the most commonly used, but lamotrigine (Lamictal), oxcarbazepine (Trileptal), phenytoin (Dilantin), and carbamazepine (Tegretol) are also reported in the literature.

Gabapentin is incorporated in a carrier protein, and there is insignificant absorption (Physicians' Desk Reference [PDR]). Interactions with other drugs are insignificant, and doses up to 3600 mg/day are well tolerated. Off-label uses of 4000 to 6000 mg/day are reported in the literature to be safe and effective.

Pregabalin (Lyrica), a new α2δ ligand (similar to gabapentin), seems to offer the benefit of more reliable dosing with fewer side effects. A calcium channel modulator, it is the latest treatment for peripheral neuropathic pain. The dose range is lower than for gabapentin: 150 to 600 mg/day divided into two or three doses. Like most drugs, it has side effects; the most commonly reported adverse reactions are dizziness and drowsiness.

Two placebo-controlled, randomized studies have been found that examined the use of gabapentin in neuropathic pain patients. The first study[69] (n = 307) shows that gabapentin causes a modest but significant reduction in neuropathic pain symptoms 8 weeks after the start of treatment. It is unclear what this means for the CRPS I patients, who made up 28% of the sample population.

In the second study (n = 58), a moderate effect on pain was found, but no significant reductions in other sensory abnormalities were found.[75] Dizziness, sleepiness, and fatigue occurred significantly more often in patients taking gabapentin than in patients taking placebo.

There are indications that gabapentin administered at doses of 600 to 1800 mg every 24 hours in the first 8 weeks can cause some reduction in pain symptoms suffered by patients with CRPS I.

There is limited evidence that gabapentin reduces sensory abnormalities such as hyperaesthesia and allodynia. The long-term effects of gabapentin on patients with CRPS I are not known.

CALCITONIN

The effects of calcitonin have been evaluated in two meta-analyses and two systematic reviews. The meta-analysis carried out by Kingery et al[41] reports conflicting findings as to the effects of calcitonin. In contrast, the meta-analysis carried out by Perez et al[62] points to calcitonin having a positive effect on pain on average, and the review carried out by Forouzanfar et al[26] also describes positive results for calcium-regulating drugs (including calcitonin) administered to CRPS I patients. There is conflicting evidence with respect to the efficacy of calcitonin for treatment of CRPS I.

TOPICAL TREATMENTS

Pain cream is recommended for treatment of superficial pain. Capsaicin, a chili pepper derivative, which depletes substance P, must be applied topically with gloves. A dose of 0.075% cream should be applied to the affected area four times a day, using only enough cream to penetrate into the skin. Doses up to 7.5% are now being tried experimentally.

EMLA is a eutectic mixture of lidocaine and prilocaine in cream form and is approved by the FDA for neuropathic pain.

Lidoderm, a 5% lidocaine patch, is applied directly over the painful site. Systemic effects are unlikely, and the primary problem is application-site sensitivity. It is FDA approved for 12 hours on and 12 hours off. However, off-label use (increased time on) is common. Quality of life has been often shown to improve after 4 weeks of treatment (Fig. 14-16).

Local Anesthetics

One quasi-experimental study with seven patients evaluated the effects of lumbar and stellate blockades with lidocaine/bupivacaine compared with placebo (follow-up 2-2.5 weeks). No significant differences were found

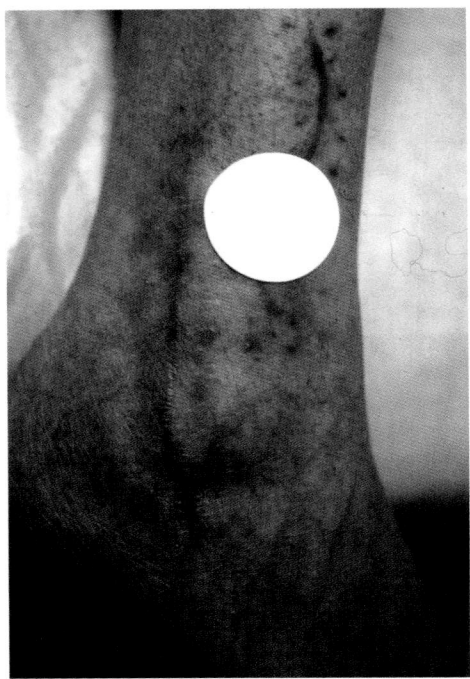

Figure 14-16 Lidoderm, a 5% lidocaine patch, is applied directly over the painful site. Systemic effects are unlikely. The primary problem is application-site sensitivity.

between active and placebo treatment with respect to initial peak pain reduction.[65]

An uncontrolled open study investigated the long-term effects (mean follow-up, 32 months; range, 7-48 months) of epidural administration of bupivacaine to 14 patients with CRPS I in the knee.[15] Treatment was continued with continuous administration of a narcotic. No pain control data were described; however, 11 patients were seen to have a complete improvement of CRPS I symptoms at the end of the follow-up.

New Treatments

Current literature suggests that some new treatments are just over the horizon. NMDA receptor–site blockers are being developed. Botulinum toxin might inhibit the release of glutamate. Pain and bone density can improve after intravenous administration of pamidronate, alendronate, or clodronate. Magnetic stimulation of the contralateral brain cortex can decrease pain.[71] Inhalation of cannabinoids (marijuana), much touted in the news for their pain-relieving qualities, does not relieve neuropathic pain, and the side effects of somnolence, fatigue, hypotension, and memory disorder make them unlikely to improve CRPS symptoms.[4]

FREE-RADICAL SCAVENGERS

Dimethylsulphoxide (DMSO), a free-radical scavenger, has been tried in patients with CRPS I. A prospective crossover study[30] with 20 patients found a positive effect of DMSO on the function of the affected limb. In addition, in 26 CRPS I patients, DMSO was found to be significantly more effective than the conventional regional ismelin block[27] in reducing pain. A randomized double-blind trial conducted with 32 CRPS I patients[86] also showed that five times daily use of topical DMSO cream provided significantly better results on CRPS I symptoms than placebo after 2 months of treatment. In general, DMSO generates lower (direct and indirect) costs than N-acetylcysteine (another available free-radical scavenger). Subgroup analysis indicates that N-acetylcysteine is more cost effective in patients with a cold form of CRPS I than DMSO. The opposite holds for warm forms of CRPS I.[76]

Robert J. Schwartzman, MD, a neurologist at Drexel University College of Medicine, is experimenting with a more radical approach. Cooperating with a group of anesthesiologists in Germany, he is treating patients who have refractory pain by injecting them with ketamine at doses high enough to induce coma for 5 days. Fifty percent improvement has been reported.[32]

The effects of a subanesthetic ketamine infusion (10 mg/hr up to 15-50 mg/hr) was assessed in a retrospective study of 33 patients with CRPS I or II.[16] Twelve patients experienced a relapse and had a second course of infusions, 3 patients had a third course, by which pain disappeared completely in 83% of patients. The average duration of pain reduction (data of 20 patients) was 9.4 months. The side effects were intoxication, hallucinations, dizziness, nausea, light-headedness, and blurred vision.

VITAMIN C

Recent investigations have suggested a role for vitamin C in the prevention of CRPS. In a double-blind, prospective, multicenter trial, 427 wrist fractures were randomly allocated to treatment with placebo or treatment with 200, 500, or 1500 mg of vitamin C daily for 50 days.[85]

The effect of gender, age, fracture type, and cast-related complaints on the occurrence of complex regional pain syndrome was analyzed. The prevalence of complex regional pain syndrome was 2.4% in the vitamin C group and 10.1% in the placebo group ($P = .002$). Early cast-related complaints predicted the development of CRPS, and based on these results, the authors recommended a daily dose of vitamin C 500 mg for 50 days to prevent CRPS. Additional investigations by the same author have yielded similar results,[84] including those which suggest a benefit from vitamin C 2 days before surgery and for 50 days after surgery for trapeziometacarpal arthritis. Thirty four patients were administered 500 mg of vitamin C and followed for a minimum of 44 months. Contrary to another published report, which demonstrated a 13% CRPS rate with this procedure, there were no cases of CRPS in this study.[84]

A similar investigation regarding the role of vitamin C in the prevention of CRPS in patients undergoing foot and ankle surgery confirmed prior studies suggesting that vitamin C may be preventative.[8]

Pain Therapies

If patients fail to respond in 1 to 2 months, they should be referred to a multidisciplinary pain center (anesthesia, orthopaedics, psychiatry, psychopharmacology, neurosurgery, neurology, physical therapy). Hospitalization may be required.

Implantable spinal electrodes for dorsal column stimulation to control intractable pain should be considered once a plateau in improvement with sympathetic blocks has been reached or in refractory cases. Based on the gate theory of pain control, a percutaneous route for implantation with low morbidity is now well developed. Long-term results are good, and late failures are primarily based on technical problems. Permanent placement should be preceded by a trial with a temporary electrode.[60]

There are numerous studies investigating these devices. Patients with chronic refractory CRPS I were randomly allocated to spinal cord stimulation (SCS) plus physiotherapy or physiotherapy alone. Trial stimulation proved successful in 24 of the 36 patients; only these patients underwent a procedure to implant a permanent SCS device. Pain intensity was reduced by 2.4 cm on a visual analogue scale after 6 months in the group receiving spinal cord stimulation plus physiotherapy compared with a group receiving only physiotherapy.[37] At 2 years follow-up, pain decrease in the SCS group was 2.1 cm more than pain decrease observed in the physiotherapy group.[39] Quality of life improved only in the patients with an implanted system; function remained unchanged. Two retrospective cohort studies have investigated effects of SCS on pain relief (n = 23-31).[11,38]

All studies relate to carefully selected patients with refractory CRPS I. There is no scientific evidence for SCS being effective in acute CRPS I. Complications requiring further surgery do occur in 25% to 50% of patients.[74]

Overall, it appears that spinal cord stimulation administered to CRPS I patients who are carefully selected and undergo successful trial stimulation experience long-term pain reduction and improvements in their quality of life but do not seem to see improved function.

Chemical or surgical lumbar sympathectomy works best in the foot and ankle. When sympathetic blocks are successful but the pain keeps returning, radiofrequency or cryoprobe lesioning could provide long-term relief. Surgical resection creates an identifiable interruption.

The efficacy of surgical sympathectomy was addressed in a systematic review,[50] based on analysis of retrospective cohort, including 7 to 73 individuals. All the studies report a clear reduction in pain resulting from sympathectomy, whereby the extent of pain relief declines over time. Long-term follow-up studies (>1 year) indicate that the chance of success is greatest if treatment is given within 3 months after the initial trauma.[68]

Chemical destruction (alcohol, phenol) of a nerve, despite excellent justification, can also have drawbacks. Further obliteration of the nerve in the background of a disease state that already affects nerves can paradoxically lead to more pain. Radiofrequency ablation, by using generated local temperatures, can be more selective in just destroying pain fibers (C fibers) while leaving the nonpain portion of the nerve alone.

Recurrence of SMP can occur secondary to upregulation of distal receptors, producing increased sensitivity to catecholamines. In some cases, postsympathectomy neuralgia in the thigh can be distressing. Sympathectomy for multiple extremities leads to problems with thermal regulation and with bowel or bladder control.[29]

Surgical Treatment

It is important that the orthopaedic surgeon maintain constant vigilance for the possibility of an underlying neurologic lesion (e.g., neuroma, tarsal tunnel syndrome) associated with CRPS II. Maximum control of the secondary hyperalgesia must be obtained before treating the peripheral nerve disease.[2,6,21,78]

The potential benefit from surgery is considerable. Classic teaching for neurolysis, repair, or resection should be carefully followed. The planned procedure should be done under epidural anesthesia, however, and the block continued using a catheter 3 to 4 days postoperatively to decrease flare-ups. Chromic suture should be avoided because chemicals released from the suture can provide a nociceptive focus.

If surgery is planned in an extremity previously involved in CRPS, conductive (spinal) anesthesia should be used. General anesthesia is associated with higher recurrence rates. At times, despite adequate planning, surgery for fixed deformity fails or symptoms recur. In this case, carefully planned bracing is often successful (Fig. 14-17).

There are several reports of amputation being used for the intractable pain of CRPS. Although there have been a few successes, the procedure is not predictable, and the literature in general does not recommend this remedy (Fig. 14-18).

In their review of uncontrolled retrospective studies, Bodde et al[9] documented "recurrence" in nearly half of the patients with CRPS I treated with amputation (including phantom-limb symptoms in 15 patients), prosthetic use by fewer than half of the patients who had been fitted with a prosthesis after amputation, and return to employment in fewer than one third of the patients. They maintain that amputation remains a "valid" treatment for resistant infection but encourage seeking other options before amputation is performed because of pain or dysfunction. The authors remark that they see no reason to alter the current guidelines put forth by Perez et al,[62] which represent the efforts of a multidisciplinary task force of the Dutch Society of Rehabilitation Specialists and the Netherlands Society of Anaesthesiologists that had been charged with the creation of evidence-based guidelines for CRPS I treatment. These guidelines state: "There is insufficient evidence that amputation positively contributes to the treatment of CRPS I."

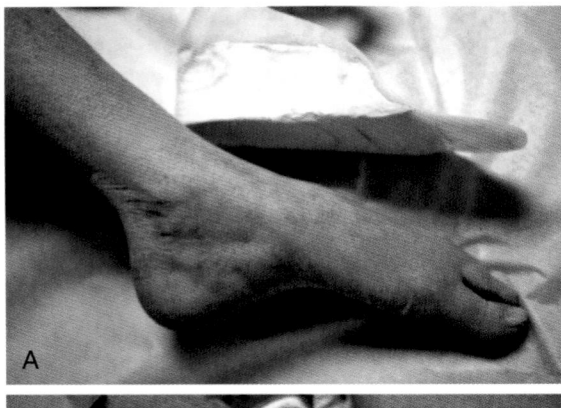

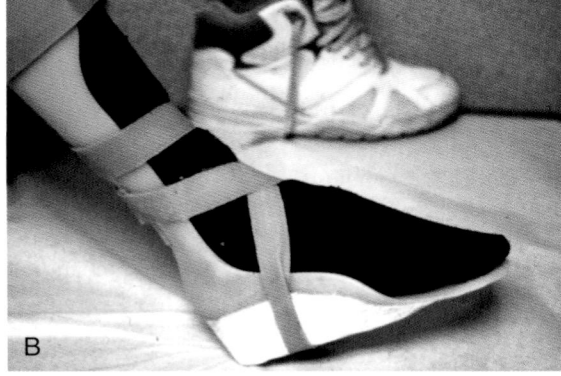

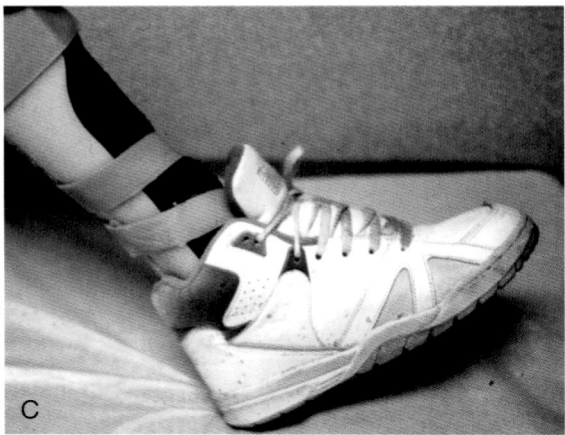

Figure 14-17 Successful bracing for fixed equinus. **A,** Fixed deformity. **B,** Custom brace. **C,** Custom brace and foot in shoe.

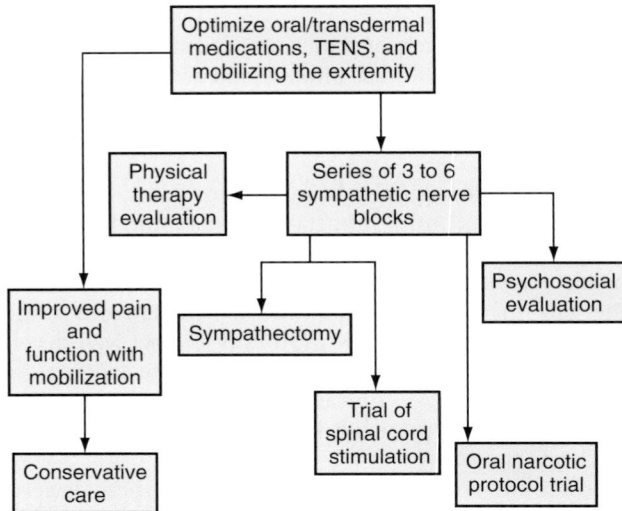

Figure 14-18 Protocol for treating complex regional pain syndrome. *TENS,* transcutaneous electrical nerve stimulation.

Pediatric Versus Adult Regimens

CRPS and SMP constitute a different syndrome in children. The incidence is increasing in children and adolescents but continues to be underdiagnosed.

Children are much less likely to have a major trauma preceding the condition, and they usually do not recall an inciting event. In adolescence, CRPS is more likely to affect girls, the lower limb is more involved than the upper, and autonomic findings are more profound.

Children are not little adults, and careful focus should be placed on personality, family and social relations, and the patient's unconscious desire to use this disease as an avoidance technique. Severity varies widely, and the disease state may be worsened from the pressures of divorce, marital conflict, and sibling rivalry or concurrent illness. Because children often deny pain, restlessness and agitation have to be carefully looked for as surrogate pain indicators.

Hospitalization with psychiatric support is often critical to resolution. Table 14-4 outlines the basic differences and pediatric and adult treatment regimens. In general, children are less disabled, and pediatric CRPS has a more favorable prognosis (Table 14-5).[31,66,81,82]

Conclusions

For pain treatment, the WHO analgesic ladder is advised, with the exception of strong opioids. For neuropathic pain, anticonvulsants and tricyclic antidepressants may be considered. For inflammatory symptoms, free-radical scavengers (dimethylsulphoxide or acetylcysteine) are advised. To promote peripheral blood flow, vasodilatory medication may be considered. Percutaneous sympathetic blockades may be used to increase blood flow in case vasodilatory medication has insufficient effect. To decrease functional limitations, standardized physiotherapy and occupational therapy are advised. To prevent the occurrence of CRPS I after wrist fractures, vitamin C is recommended, but its use in foot and ankle trauma has not fully been investigated. Adequate perioperative analgesia, limitation of operating time, limited use of tourniquet, and use of regional anesthetic techniques are recommended for secondary prevention of CRPS I.

Author's Recommendations

By no means is the treament of CRPS simple. It has a complicated etiology and often benefits from myriad

Table 14-4 Complex Regional Pain Syndrome in Children and Adults

Feature	Children	Adults
Site ratio	Lower extremity predominance 5 : 1	Upper extremity predominance
Spontaneous pain	Common	Common
Mechanical allodynia	Most patients	Most patients
Gender ratio	Marked female predominance 4 : 1	Studies mixed
Psychologic aspects	Increased tendency to CRPS with psychologic stressors	CRPS leads to secondary psychiatric pathology
Three-phase bone scan	Mixed results; used to rule out other pathology	Increased uptake in affected extremity
Treatment strategy	Resolution is often possible with physical therapy and behavioral modification Transcutaneous stimulation is helpful	Early sympathetic block
Treatment timing	Duration of disease is of little consequence	Early block is strongly advocated
Block technique	Continuous inpatient block with catheter	Multiple single outpatient blocks

CRPS, complex regional pain syndrome.

Table 14-5 Various Components of Multimodal Therapy for CRPS

	Low Risk	Medium Risk	High Risk
Functional restoration	CBT Neuro-OT/neuro-PT Vocational rehabilitation Recreational therapy CAM		
Symptom control	Topical DSMO TENS Amitriptyline, nortriptyline Oral baclofen, diazepam, clonazapam N-acetylcysteine Ca^{++} channel blocker	Sympathetic blockade Opiates, opioids GABA antagonists Carbamazepine	Sympathectomy* SCS
Disease control		Subanesthetic ketamine IV ketanserine* Corticosteroids (early)	Anesthetic ketamine Immunomodulation* Glial modulation*

Data from Moskovitz P: An overview of CRPS. *Practical Pain Management*, Jan/Feb 2010, 50-57.
Ca^{++}, calcium ion; *CAM*, complementary and alternative medicine; *CBT*, cognitive-behavioral therapy; *CRPS*, complex regional pain syndrome; *DMSO*, dimethylsulfoxide; *GABA*, γ-aminobutyric acid; *IV*, intravenous; *OT*, occupational therapy; *PT*, physical therapy; *SCS*, spinal cord stimulation; *TENS*, transcutaneous electrical nerve stimulation.
*Treatments about which there remain questions regarding their efficacy or safety.

treatment modalities by a number of actively involved clinicians. Although orthopaedic surgeons are terrific diagnosticians, the authors realize, however, that not all surgeons and practices are comfortable or suited to the long-term management of the medical aspects of this syndrome. In fact, Charles E. Argoff has coined the term *rational polypharmacy* to achieve a mix of medications that facilitates function. Our recommendation is that, if there are no contraindications, patients be started on an introductory dose of an antidepressant or anticonvulsant and be referred to the appropriate long-term care provider, which may be their primary care physician, physiatrist, or pain management specialist. We recommend starting patients on an initial dose as opposed to simply referring patients to a pain management specialist because of the unfortunate tendency for this to result in a significant delay in treatment. If their pain management physician wishes to modify the treatment strategy, one may simply defer to their expertise or negotiate a mutually agreed

strategy that all three parties think will be most effective.

Typical Case Scenarios

■ A 33-year-old black female aerobics instructor with an 8-month-old grade 2 ankle sprain had diffuse lateral foot and ankle pain. Burning paresthesias in the foot keep her up at night. She uses a cane, limps, and cannot work. A bone scan is positive, with diffuse uptake; EMG is negative. Physical therapy (PT) and NSAIDs have failed. She could not tolerate amitriptyline or desipramine. Therapy with fluoxetine 60 mg/day, intense PT, and sulindac for 5 months has helped. She now sleeps well, is off all medications, and is back at work.

■ A 27-year-old female recreational sailor badly twisted her left ankle while tacking in a race. A radiograph was negative. Two months later she could not walk without crutches. Her foot was swollen, and she had diffuse burning pain, which was worse with PT and NSAIDs. She was seen 3 months after her injury. A bone scan was positive at the medial malleolus. CT confirmed a stress fracture. She was treated with a cast for 4 weeks, then intense PT. She is now back at work and sailing. She has an occasional ache in the foot.

■ A 29-year-old white female runner sustained a stress fracture of her second metatarsal. Her left foot was swollen and osteoporotic, and she had diffuse burning pain in the entire left foot. She was non–weight bearing on crutches and failed repeated casting. A radiograph demonstrated that her fracture was healed. She was started on NSAIDs and intense PT and was fully functional and pain free 4 months later.

■ An 18-year-old white male football tackle sustained cleat injury to the dorsum of the left foot. He had progressive pain, burning, and swelling in a stocking distribution. After 2 months of rest, cast, and PT, he could not walk and was using crutches. A radiograph at 2 months showed mild juxtaarticular osteoporosis. A bone scan showed diffuse periarticular uptake in the third phase. He failed treatment with NSAIDs and amitriptyline. He had an excellent early response to sympathetic blocks. PT was given between the blocks (he had a total of five blocks). He was able to play basketball in the spring.

■ A 27-year-old woman sustained a bimalleolar fracture of the left ankle. After fracture healing, she developed residual dystrophic pain in a stocking pattern on the injured foot from the toes to the knee. She had no response to PT, NSAIDs, or tricyclic antidepressants. Her maximum response to blocks was 48 hours, but she did comment, "Wow, my leg is warm and all the pain is gone." A lumbar stimulator was implanted percutaneously with the patient under anesthesia at 8 months after injury. She walks without a limp, sleeps well, and has a minor ache in the ankle.

■ A 48-year-old man sustained a calcaneal fracture. The fracture healed, but the man developed dystrophic pain syndrome in the injured foot. He was seen 32 weeks after the fracture. He responded to sympathetic blockade but for no longer than 72 hours. EMG was positive for compression of the posterior nerve. The patient underwent an internal and external neurolysis under epidural block, with an abductor hallucis flap. He returned to work as a physician and has residual diminished light touch.

■ A 41-year-old woman, 2 months after ankle arthroscopy, had terrible neuropathic pain encompassing her leg from the knee to the toes. She had allodynia over the entire area. NSAIDs and PT failed to relieve the pain. She was started on gabapentin 900 mg/day. A repeat examination 1 month later revealed pain confined to the distribution of the superficial peroneal nerve, with the Tinel sign at the ankle. She eventually underwent resection of the nerve above the boot line, with burying of the end into muscle. She is now pain free.

■ A 22-year-old female marathon runner stepped in a pothole and sustained a Lisfranc fracture-dislocation of the right foot. She underwent an open reduction and internal fixation with screws and started weight bearing at 6 weeks. Her foot remained swollen, and the screws were removed at 4 months. The foot remained swollen, and the skin became red and shiny. Weight bearing became increasingly painful. Radiographs showed diffuse osteoporosis, and a bone scan showed diffuse uptake in the third phase. She failed NSAID therapy, tricyclic antidepressant therapy, PT, steroid therapy, and a series of epidural blocks. She was sent to a pain clinic. She has continued pain and disability 1 year later.

■ A 50-year-old male electrician was seen after removal of a 3-4 interdigital neuroma twice in the same foot, having intractable pain. After failing conservative care, he was revised through a plantar incision, and the nerve end was buried in the metatarsal base. He was excellent for 2 years, when he returned with intractable pain at the operative site. I locally injected him with a Marcaine/Xylocaine mix. He immediately stated he was pain free, and his foot was now warm. Pain is sympathetically based, and he is being considered for a stimulator.

THE POLYSURGICAL FOOT CRIPPLE5

In orthopaedic practice, the physician is often confronted with a patient whose detailed past history is filled with therapeutic misfortune, many failed surgeries, and complaints of severe foot pain. The initial clinical examination reveals no clear diagnostic choice. A large shopping bag containing numerous pairs of shoes, orthoses, and several magazine articles usually accompanies the patient. How does the physician proceed?

This is no trivial dilemma. Ultimately, all pain is perceived because of a chemical change at a neurosynaptic junction. What is the cause of pain in the patient who is now confronting the physician? Has underlying organic disease been overlooked? Is further surgery the answer? Is a psychiatric disorder present? Is the patient a malingerer? Is the patient being cared for by an unscrupulous provider?[19]

The physician's role here is to make this diagnosis and initiate proper treatment or provide appropriate referral. This is a time-consuming process that demands patience and perseverance.

Initial Evaluation

The first priority for the evaluating surgeon is to determine whether the initial diagnosis was correct, and if so, whether or not appropriate treatment was rendered. One must remember that the environment can often be altered to fit the foot, as opposed to changing the foot to fit the environment. One must also consider the possibility that an underlying systemic disease is confusing the issue. Such a situation demands that the orthopaedist proceed in a deliberate and informed manner to prevent both physician and patient confusion. Lastly, one must remain open to the idea that there has been diagnostic oversight, and that a surgical procedure may in fact be the solution to the patient's problem.

History

An adequate history is critical in dealing with the patient with multiple failed surgeries. Skillful interviewing techniques can help reveal psychosocial factors that may be playing a role in the disease process. Profiles have appeared sporadically in the literature to identify patients with a proclivity for multiple procedures, but most are based on anecdotal experience and have little objective data to support their conclusions. With this group of patients, the physician straddles the boundary between believing and knowing. The following key points, however, form a common path toward revealing the real person[19,48,61]:

- Identify the patient's motive in seeking your care. In many cases, the patient is demanding medication, hospitalization, compensation, exemption, or special status rather than seeking a rational approach to treatment based on your judgment as a physician. He or she might have a preconceived idea of what should be done and will not tolerate a differing opinion.
- Do not ignore such a demand or attempt to force a confrontation. Instead, articulate the demand openly, and engage in a neutral discussion of the pros and cons of various actions associated with it.
- If possible, obtain copies of the patient's medical records and radiographs dating back to the time of the original complaint. This information might paint a different picture than that elicited in the office history.
- Avoid "organizing" the patient's complaint by labeling it. When the name of a disease state is applied to the condition, the patient comes to believe that quality medical care depends on multiple laboratory tests, medications, and surgical procedures. He or she will expect that approach and demand this response from physicians in the future.
- Certain psychologic scales, such as the Minnesota Multiphasic Personality Inventory (MMPI) and the Waddell Equivalency Scale, have been touted as a way to identify patients with surgical proneness. They have inconsistent results, however, and are not feasible to administer because most patients in this category reject formal psychologic intervention.[19,48,61]
- In addition to multiple foot and ankle surgeries, the patient's past medical history might reveal a litany of vague pains and questionable surgeries at other sites, particularly in the pelvis and abdomen.
- Inquire how the primary complaint has changed since the patient underwent surgery. This can provide valuable clues to the source of the patient's pain or dysfunction.
- Obtain a complete list of the medications used by the patient. A retrospective study compared drug use in 23 patients who had five or more major surgeries (mean, 9.8) with that of a matched control group (mean surgeries, 1). Total drug use of polysurgical patients was 3.7 times greater than that of controls and involved narcotics, analgesics, barbiturates, and minor tranquilizers.[13]
- Carefully obtain a history of and question for signs of underlying systemic disease. Psoriasis, hypothyroidism, inflammatory bowel disease, Reiter syndrome, human immunodeficiency virus (HIV), ankylosing spondylitis, gout, and other seronegative processes can cause dactylitis, enthesopathy, and pain. Pernicious anemia, diabetes, and heavy-metal poisoning can lead to painful peripheral neuropathy.

Physical Examination

Evaluation of the patient should follow the usual guidelines for a thorough foot and ankle examination, but additional emphasis should be placed on detection of hallmarks of CRPS and RSD, factitious psychogenic pain, or underlying systemic disease. As the foot is sequentially inspected, palpated, and manipulated, awareness of these maladies should be heightened, and special tests may be implemented to better ascertain their presence.

Inspection will reveal multiple surgical scars and primary or postoperative deformities. Gait should be observed with shoes both on and off, and the entire kinetic chain of the lower extremity should be assessed (station and range of motion of hip, knee, ankle, and foot). Shoes should be scrutinized for abnormal wear patterns.

Vascular competence, temperature, color, hair growth, and sweating should be carefully noted. The clinician should inspect for abnormal nail growth, trophic changes, atrophy, extraarticular swelling, and joint contracture. Pain and sensation should be carefully charted to determine a global or a dermatomal pattern.

Palpation for areas of tenderness should proceed systematically. The clinician should check for enthesopathy (soft tissue and tendon tenderness), allodynia, hyperpathia, intolerance to cold, burning, and paresthesias.

If a careful history and physical examination plus confirmatory tests (e.g., radiographs, EMG, CT scan, MRI) demonstrate a lesion amenable to surgery, the appropriate surgical procedure should be planned. This is a multiply surgically manipulated foot, and care needs to be taken to demonstrate that it is sensate and vascularly competent and that the skin can support repeat surgical intervention. The purpose of surgery is to obtain a plantigrade, pain-free, shoeable, or braceable foot.

PSYCHIATRIC ASPECTS OF PAIN

The surgeons' need to ally themselves with their patients' needs and problems is called into question here. Although the patient and the orthopaedic surgeon must come to a mutual understanding of their roles, each listening and acknowledging the other, the physician must assume the posture of "trust but verify" to avoid deception and must remain scientifically objective. A reported 5% to 20% of foot disorders are functional.[21,24]

The patient with chronic pain is a person whose suffering is resistant to indicated medical treatment and surgical procedures. The patient might have an unnatural fear of cancer, project blame for pain on others (e.g., parent, spouse, employer), or attempt to use the pain as a means of self-punishment.[54]

Chronic pain can lead to depression. This disease process may be expressed as sadness, pessimism, a sense of failure, dissatisfaction, guilt, self-hatred, suicidal ideation, crying, irritability, social withdrawal, indecisiveness, insomnia, anorexia, weight loss, loss of libido, and somatic preoccupations. This may be a primary disease process or secondary to chronic pain.[19,54] The patient might seek to legitimize the pain by a disability payoff.

Hypochondriac Illness

The hypochondriac patient has an unrealistic interpretation of physical signs, leading to the desperate belief that the body is in imminent danger. Physical examination does not confirm significant organic disease.

The patient's complaints are vague, varying, shifting, and exaggerated and cannot be explained on an anatomic basis. Complaints of swelling reveal none present. The patient openly disagrees with the findings yet remains attached to the physician. Secondary gain from patient-physician contact seems to be the prime motivator.[54,67,79]

Hysteric Conversion

With hysteric motor disorder, the foot may be paralyzed from the knee or ankle. It can present as equinovarus with spastic or fluid weakness. The Babinski test (sign) is negative, EMG testing is normal, no clonus is present, and deep tendon reflexes are intact. The patient's leg is light, and if elevated and suddenly let go, it falls slowly to the table.[80] This disease primarily affects female patients, and a cure can be reached through psychiatric intervention.

Malingering

The malingerer is evasive and inconsistent in the history and usually has some obvious benefit to be gained from the pain (e.g., compensation payment, avoidance of unpleasant tasks). This mixed group of male and female patients has a range of mild to severe mental disturbances. Diagnostic tests are negative.

Evaluation and Referral

Psychiatric illness (e.g., hysteric conversion, depression) or factitious illness (e.g., malingering, hypochondriasis) may be mistakenly diagnosed as CRPS and treated inappropriately. Careful evaluation and psychiatric referral are critical.

COSMETIC FOOT SURGERY

The lessons taught to us by our colleagues in plastic surgery are invaluable. They have helped improve our knowledge of soft tissue handling, wound care, and graft and flap coverage. Of recent concern to our profession, however, is the emergence of purely cosmetic surgery of the foot and ankle. This practice claims to "restore" the foot and ankle to a state devoid of deformity and physically accommodating to even the most confining footwear.

One can hardly blame people for considering a cosmetic procedure on the foot. Almost every other body part is amenable to cosmetic correction, so why not the toes? Foot surgery is usually marketed to women interested in wearing the latest designer shoes. It often involves toe resections; bunionectomies, and a variety of other bony and soft tissue procedures aimed at helping patients fit into more stylish footwear, or have their feet appear more aesthetic. There are a troubling number of websites that now encourage this.

The tragedy of this practice is that it is done on feet that are pain free. In a public position statement, the American Orthopaedic Foot and Ankle Society (AOFAS) clearly states that "cosmetic foot surgery does not include surgery performed to provide pain relief, improve function, or enhance the quality of life during normal activities of daily living." The AOFAS goes on to say that purely cosmetic foot surgery "should not be considered in any circumstances." Similarly, a position statement from the podiatric surgical society, the American College of Foot and Ankle Surgeons (ACFS), states that "surgery performed solely for the purpose of improving the appearance or size of the foot or ankle carries risks without medical benefit, and therefore should not be undertaken."

Unfortunately, there are members of the foot and ankle surgery community who have adopted less strict guidelines and continue to perform these procedures, often marketing themselves and these procedures in daily newspapers and prominent urban social magazines. As physicians and orthopaedic surgeons, we will likely confront cosmetic surgery in two situations: approached by the eager patient in our office and approached by the distressed recipient of failed cosmetic procedures. The latter often presents with a painful foot, disgusted with the outcome and the prior surgeon, and unable to even don traditional footwear.

In dealing with either of these situations, the AOFAS statement, along with common sense measures as dictated by our oath to "do no harm," prevails: "In light of the risks associated with surgical procedures and the increased risk of recurrent deformity with the repetitive use of ill-fitting shoes, the AOFAS recommends that surgery not be performed simply to improve the appearance of the foot. Surgery should never be performed in the absence of pain, functional limitation, or reduced quality of life."

BURNS

Burns of the foot pose unique and difficult problems in initial management, reconstruction, and attainment of long-term functional results. The primary reconstructive goals for this region are unimpeded ambulation and pain-free weight bearing. These objectives can be achieved by strict adherence to established principles of wound management, a clear delineation of the reconstructive requirements of the foot, and a team approach toward achieving these goals.

Burns have classically been described according to depth and percentage of total body surface area (TBSA) (Table 14-6). In 1944, Lund and Browder produced a method for calculating percentage TBSA in which each foot accounts for 3.5% TBSA (for both children and adults). The relatively small contribution each foot makes to TBSA can erroneously lead to the impression that burns to the foot are minor. Because of tremendous functional risks associated with these injuries, however, all but very superficial burns of the feet should be referred to a specialized burn center for appropriate management (Fig. 14-19 and Box 14-3).

Isolated pedal burns are most often sustained at home, indoors, and in the kitchen. Even such minor burns of the lower extremities can cause severe disability, chronic pain, and loss of work.[90,93,113] These injuries can be especially troubling in patients with decreased sensory feedback resulting from peripheral neuropathy because a delay in treatment can lead to an exponential increase in morbidity. Burns to the feet must therefore be recognized early and treated expeditiously to minimize functional impairment (Fig. 14-20).

In a typical scenario, a patient sustains a minor burn on the dorsum of the foot. The local outpatient center treats the patient with an emollient and analgesics, and the patient returns to work. With the resultant dependency of the extremity and the footwear often abrading the dorsum of the foot, the patient develops secondary lymphedema and cellulitis, leading to hospitalization and the possible need for grafting and prolonged foot elevation (Fig. 14-21).

It has been estimated that more than 90% of burns can be attributed to carelessness and are therefore preventable. More than 50% of burns are related to smoking or alcohol, making burn prevention through education paramount. Diabetic neuropathy has been demonstrated to be a risk factor for foot burns (68% incidence compared with 17% in nondiabetic age-matched controls).[120] In

Table 14-6	Classification of Burns
Degree	**Description**
First	Erythema without blistering
Second	Erythema with blistering
Third	Destruction of full thickness of skin and often deeper tissues

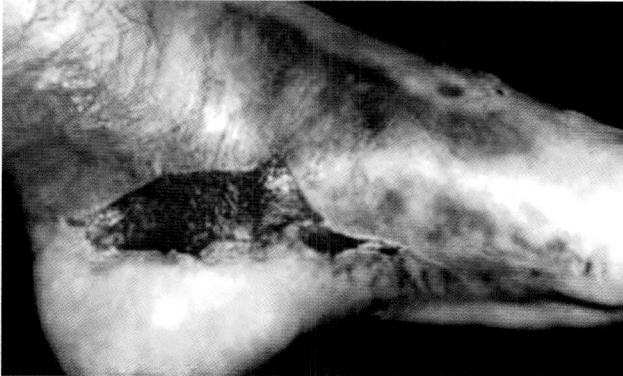

Figure 14-19 Burns of the foot pose unique and difficult problems in initial management, reconstruction, and attainment of long-term functional results.

BOX 14-3   Criteria for Transfer to Burn Center

The following types of burn injuries usually require referral to a burn center:

- Partial-thickness and full-thickness burns greater than 10% of the total body surface area (TBSA) in patients younger than 10 years or older than 50 years.
- Partial-thickness and full-thickness burns greater than 20% TBSA in other age-groups.
- Partial-thickness and full-thickness burns involving the face, eyes, ears, hands, feet, genitalia, or perineum or those that involve skin overlying major joints.
- Full-thickness burns greater than 5% TBSA in any age-group.
- Electrical burns, including lightning injury (significant volumes of tissue beneath the surface may be injured and result in acute renal failure and other complications).
- Significant chemical burns.
- Inhalation injury.
- Burn injury in patients with preexisting illness that could complicate management, prolong recovery, or affect mortality.

The following burn patients usually require referral to a burn center:

- Any burn patient in whom concomitant trauma poses an increased risk or morbidity or mortality may be treated initially in a trauma center until stable before transfer to a burn center.
- Children with burns seen in hospitals without qualified personnel or equipment for their care should be transferred to a burn center with these capabilities.
- Burn injury in patients who will require special social and emotional or long-term rehabilitative support, including cases involving suspected child abuse and neglect.

Modified from American College of Surgeons Committee on Trauma: Guidelines for the operations of burn units. In American College of Surgeons: *Resources for optimal care of the injured patient,* Chicago, 1999, American College of Surgeons, pp 55–62.

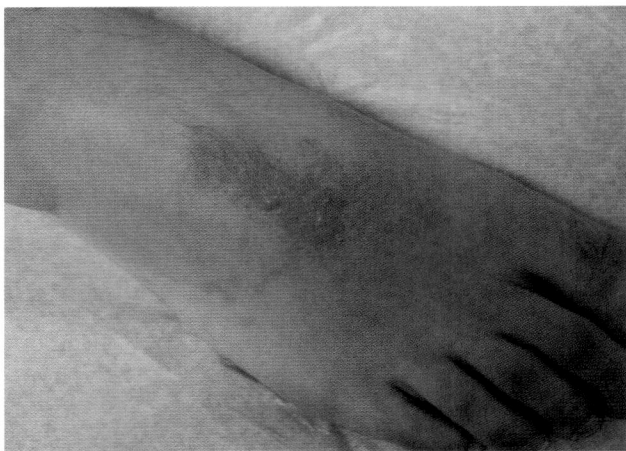

Figure 14-20 Second-degree burn on the dorsum of the foot from an ice pack.

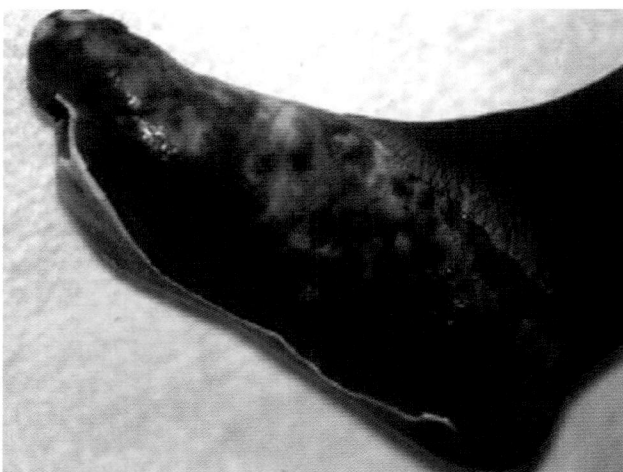

Figure 14-21 Diabetic foot burn from hot water. (From http://www.Michiganpodiatry.com.)

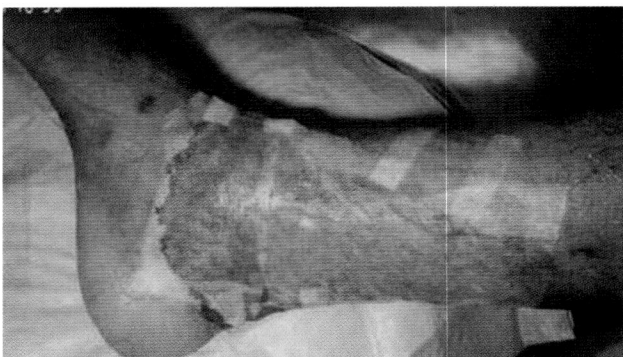

Figure 14-22 Skin substitute on a middermal burn. (From http://www.burnsurgery.org. Accessed 8/1/2012.)

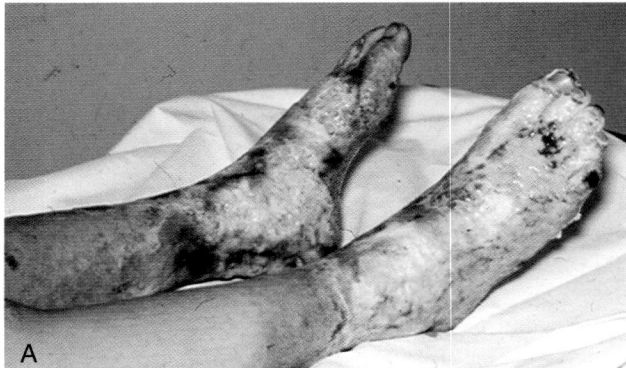

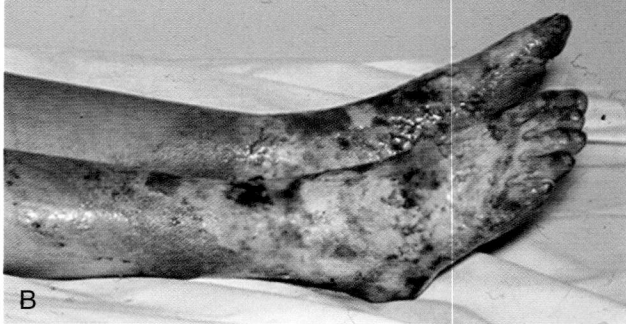

Figure 14-23 A, This 49-year-old man fell into a hot spring and sustained third-degree burns. **B,** Acute burns after lavage.

addition, diabetic patients with burns have an increased risk for nosocomial infections. This underscores the importance of educating this at-risk population.

Minor burns are common and require early and appropriate care to prevent infection and scarring. Damage can be minimized by immersing the foot in cold water as soon as possible, halting the burning process. The goals of care are then to remove dead tissue and protect viable tissue during healing. Very superficial burns require only an emollient (over-the-counter burn cream) to limit inflammation and prevent desiccation. Partial-thickness burns that are clean and superficial can benefit from a biosynthetic bilaminar membrane dressing (cultured epidermal autograft), which forms a skin substitute while protecting the wound. These materials may be a useful adjunct to burn care but are expensive ($6000 to $10,000 per 1% TBSA) (Fig. 14-22).

Most small, deep burns can be effectively excised and grafted by general or plastic surgeons in hospitals that have the proper facilities. However, burns of functionally important areas (hands and feet) should be excised by a burn specialist. Burns in excess of 10% TBSA should be excised in a burn treatment facility with specially trained support personnel, including experienced anesthesiologists, nurses, and critical care teams (Figs. 14-23 to 14-25).

Cast-Related Burns

Of particular relevance to the orthopaedic surgeon is thermal injury related to the application and removal of

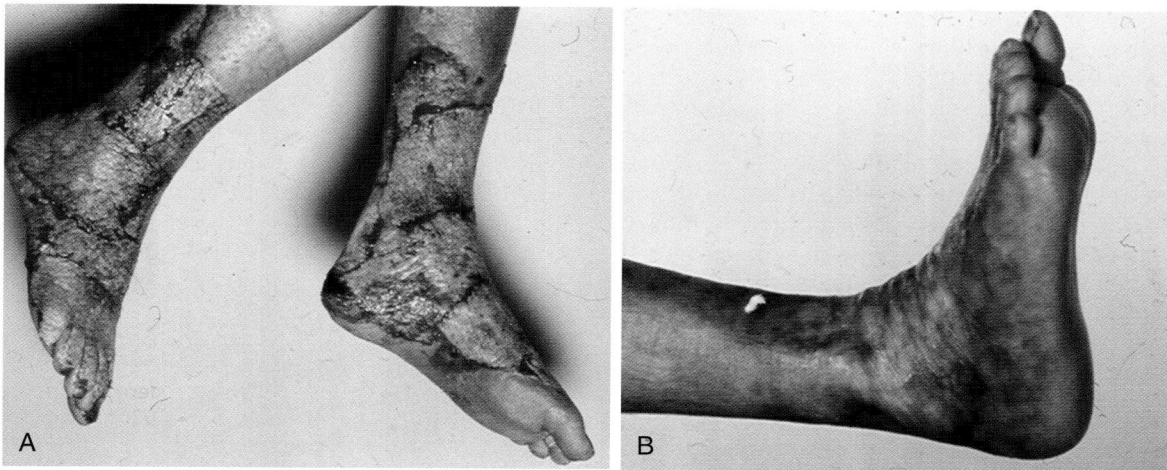

Figure 14-24 Same patient as in Figure 14-23. **A,** Feet at short-term follow-up after grafting. **B,** Motion.

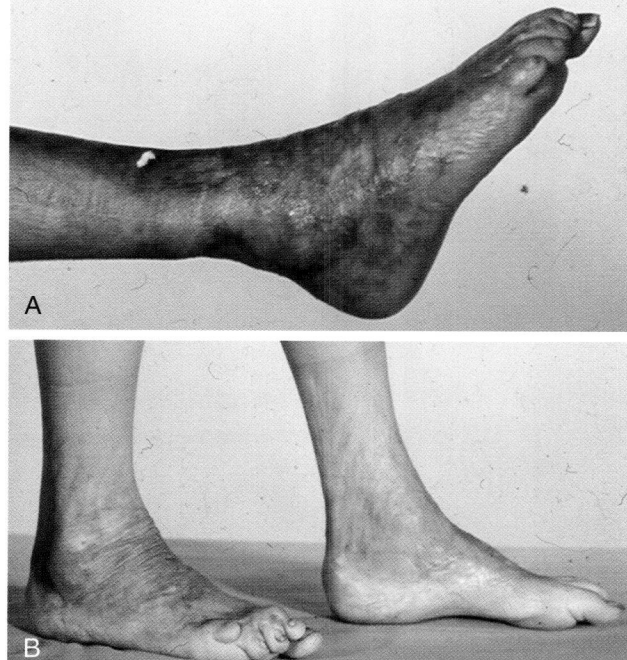

Figure 14-25 Same patient as in Figure 14-23. **A,** Motion. **B,** Clinical photograph of both feet at long-term follow-up.

over the molded area had a marked increase in temperature for approximately 6 minutes, especially when plaster was overwrapped by fiberglass. The authors recommended that care be taken when molding a plaster splint over-wrapped in fiberglass by waiting until the plaster has fully cooled.[98]

Oscillating circular saw blades have also been known to cause minor burns during cast removal. Dull blades, and specifically stainless steel blades, are more likely to consistently generate blade temperatures of 120° to 130° F. To minimize the potential morbidity of this routine in-office procedure, operators should be well trained in the proper technique and in blade maintenance (Figs. 14-26 to 14-28). In a cadaver model, Shuler and Grisafi[130] found that a poor removal technique (the cast saw blade never leaving the cast material during cutting), fiberglass casting material, and thinner cast padding resulted in significantly higher skin temperatures. The poor technique increased skin temperatures by an average of 5.0° C ($P < .05$). Fiberglass casting materials increased skin temperatures by an average of 7.4° C ($P < .05$). Four layers of cast padding compared with two layers decreased skin temperatures by 8.0° C ($P < .05$). They concluded that four layers of cast padding compared with two layers significantly reduced skin temperatures for both plaster and fiberglass casts.

Early Excision and Grafting

Small (less than 20% TBSA) full-thickness burns and indeterminate (deep partial-thickness versus full-thickness) burns, if treated by an experienced surgeon, can be excised safely and grafted. Converting such burns to a closed wound results in fewer painful debridements, decreased hospital stay, decreased cost to the patient, and less time away from school or work, with healing occurring in less than 3 weeks. Early coverage also facilitates more rapid ambulation and rehabilitation.[107] Scarring is also minimized. Women especially want cosmetically acceptable

casts. Fortunately, these are rare. Plaster and fiberglass undergo an exothermic process when combined with water. In fact, first-degree burns have been inflicted when using 30 layers of plaster dipped into water at 42° C. In general, however, when 8 or more layers of plaster are dipped into water warmer than 24° C, high enough temperatures can be reached to damage skin. Therefore judicious use of padding, lukewarm water (lower than 24° C), and adequate material are recommended.

Pressure application during casting has also been investigated as a risk factor for burn injuries. Although no burns were encountered in a recent study, the temperature

results. Split-thickness skin grafting, as opposed to secondary-intention healing with granulation tissue, is more cosmetically acceptable.[110]

If not excised, even a small burn can take 3 to 6 weeks to separate and another 2 to 3 weeks for grafting and final healing. Early excision and grafting also decrease stress, hypermetabolism, and the overall bacterial load, thus enabling the patient to resist and fight other burn complications more effectively. Because of subsequent graft contracture and extremity growth, however, early excision and grafting of foot burns in children and adolescents might not have the same advantages as seen in adults.[106] Burn tissue is also excised to remove nonviable skin as a potential source of sepsis in deep partial-thickness injuries when immediate or early excision and grafting will provide better coverage or more rapid restoration of function.

If the skin excision is to the level of the fat domes, the hair follicles and sweat glands are preserved, and graft healing can be expected in 14 to 18 days. If the bulk of

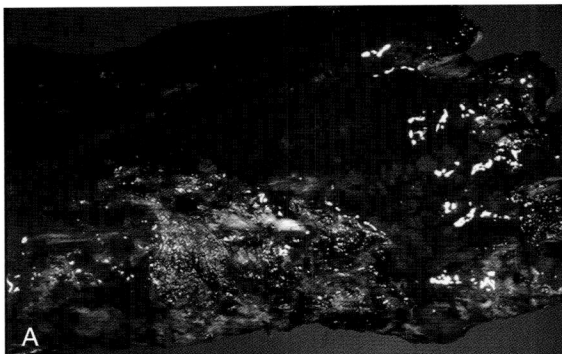

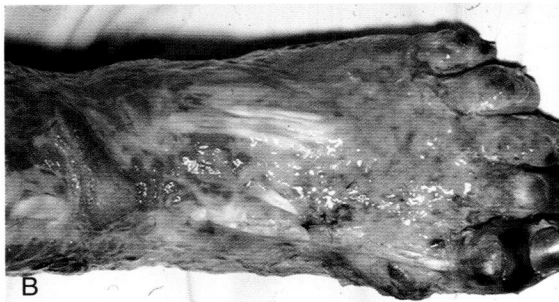

Figure 14-26 Patient with severe thermal burns of both lower extremities. **A,** Acute injury. **B,** Two weeks after injury. (Courtesy Nick Goucher, MD.)

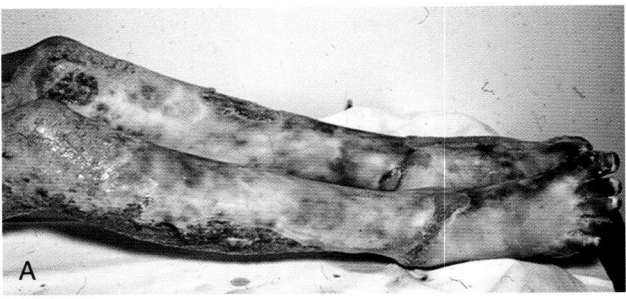

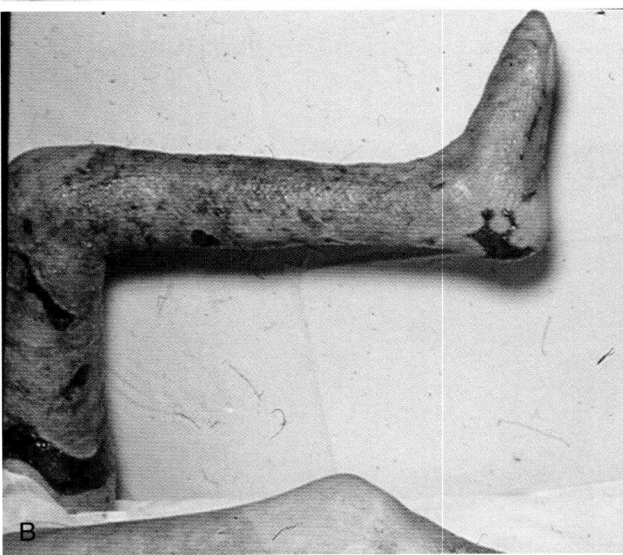

Figure 14-27 Same patient as in Figure 14-26. **A,** Before debridement. **B,** After successful split-thickness skin grafting. (Courtesy Nick Goucher, MD.)

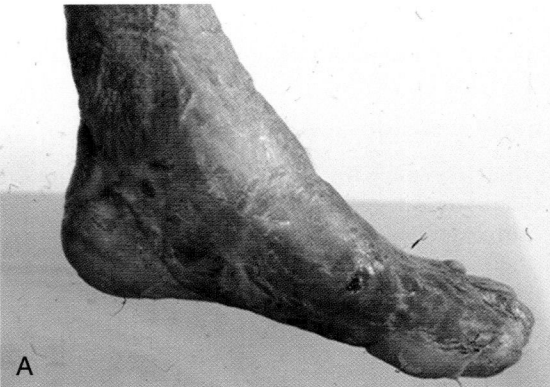

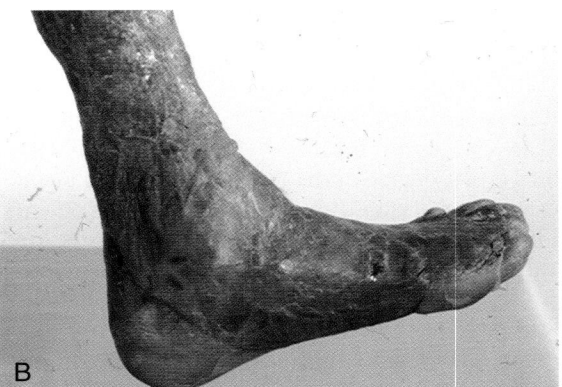

Figure 14-28 Same patient as in Figure 14-26. Early range of motion after skin grafting. **A,** Plantar flexion. **B,** Dorsiflexion. (Courtesy Nick Goucher, MD.)

the deep epithelial elements remain, healing will take 2 to 3 weeks. With deep partial-thickness burns, only meager epithelial elements remain, and healing can take 3 to 6 weeks, with poor scar formation.[101]

Traditional treatment of foot and ankle burns after excision and grafting was bed rest, limb elevation, and gradual ambulation after 5 to 10 days. Newer protocols advocate immediate application of an Unna boot in the operating room or the next day, followed by normal ambulation 4 hours later and hospital discharge. With use of sheets of narrowly meshed grafts, results were good to excellent in 95 of 100 patients. This technique avoids frequent dressing changes, permits brief or no hospital stay, and provides excellent graft take with prompt return to work.[107]

Compartment measurements should be followed in patients with significant burns because pressures can increase in time and pulses have no predictive value for ischemia. Even in noncircumferential burns, inadequate fasciotomies or escharectomies can result in footdrop, muscle necrosis, or even amputation. Patients whose hospital admission was delayed from the time of the burn showed an increased need for grafting and a longer hospitalization than those admitted on the same day. In massively burned patients, burns involving the feet are a negative predictor of survival.[95]

Wound Closure

Fasciocutaneous flaps, adipofascial reverse dorsal metatarsal artery flaps, and distally based island flaps of the dorsalis pedis artery are used to treat great toe defects. Distally based reverse island flaps of the extensor digitorum brevis muscle are harvested to cover tissue defects. Cross-leg free flaps are used to cover extensive burn wounds of the lower extremity. Full-thickness burns of the sole's plantar surface can be treated with radial forearm flaps, which are supple and adapt to the contours of the foot, preserving normal shape and making orthoses unnecessary.

Reconstruction of bilateral distal lower limb defects presents a major challenge. The problem is compounded in a large burn because of the limited availability of normal unscarred donor sites and recipient vessels. To close the wound temporarily after escharectomy, human cadaver skin or biosynthetic skin may be used. With massive burns, the patient's and family's desires must be combined with the burn team's realistic prognosis to determine the most judicious use of the available donor tissue to meet reconstructive needs.

Contractures

After healing, the initial appearance of the burn wound may appear satisfactory, but the true prognosis is uncertain until at least 4 months have elapsed, when the healing area becomes elevated and hard. Wound healing in burns is marked by increases in vascularity, fibroblasts, myofibroblasts, collagen deposition, interstitial material, and edema. These changes are conducive to the formation of hypertrophic scars and contractures.[111]

During the hypervascular phase, surgery is not indicated because of the potential for massive postoperative scarring. Constant-pressure dressings, splinting, and local injection of steroids best treat this fused mass of collagen. Once the scar has matured, local tissue response is less, and improved surgical results can be expected.[117]

Scar formation is most common on the dorsum of the foot, often resulting in hyperextension of the toes and metatarsophalangeal (MTP) joint subluxation. Prevention includes splinting and wearing shoes to maintain the toes in the straight position.

Fixed contractures in adults respond to excision of the scar over the MTP joints and application of a skin graft. The toe flexors alone are often enough to maintain correction after scar excision, but if not, toe traction is used during healing. High-top shoes with padded tongues are worn constantly in the postoperative period to maintain correction. Heel cord shortening, if present, is corrected at the same time.

In children, burn scar contractures of the feet are often treated by release of the contracture band and placement of a skin graft in the resulting defect, with an expected 85% success rate. A delay from the thermal injury to the reconstructive procedure does not affect the outcome. Immobilization postoperatively in a dynamic splint is important to prevent contracture recurrence.[88,132]

Initial positioning and splinting plus the use of serial casting and supportive tone-reducing orthoses are important. One week after the burn, equinus contractures that were not corrected with thermoplastic splints went from 45 degrees of equinus to neutral dorsiflexion over 2 months with biweekly cast changes.[115,128]

Contractures present for a long period cannot be brought into anatomic position easily because of ankylosed joints and shortened tendons, nerves, and vessels. Although tendons can be lengthened, neural and vascular structures cannot.

Complete excision of the scarred portions of involved muscles in fixed postburn equinovarus contractures is advocated.[119] External fixators (e.g., Ilizarov) associated with soft tissue procedures can be used to correct major foot deformities gradually.[96,102]

With an equinus contracture, patella tendon–bearing (PTB) orthoses are used to allow weight bearing until definitive reconstruction can be carried out.[129]

Malignant Changes

Malignant changes in burn scars have been reported in the literature. Most cases are long-standing ulcers (Marjolin ulcers), which evolve into squamous cell or some other epithelial cell carcinoma. Because malignant changes appear decades after the initial injury, residual burn scars should be routinely inspected and patients forewarned about the importance of expeditious treatment for chronic breakdown of a previously healed burn wound.[122]

Electrical Burns

The passage of electrical current through the body generates intense heat and causes tissue injury. The greater the voltage and electrical resistance of the tissue, the greater the temperature. Alternating current (AC), which causes tetany, is more dangerous than direct current (DC), and high-tension injuries (e.g., high-voltage power lines) involve contact with greater than 1000 volts.

Electrical injuries do not usually involve foot contact, but the lower extremities conduct the current to the ground, and the current exits through the foot. Although the superficial manifestation of an exit wound on the lower extremity may be small, it can overlie extensive damage to deeper structures. Additional trauma is caused by arc burn across flexion areas in the popliteal fossa and ankle, which generates heat up to 4000° F. AC-induced tetany often results in the victim's inability to release the current source, thus intensifying the destruction. The likelihood of associated injury is high. Victims often fall from high-tension wires or electrical poles, and the clothing can ignite, causing additional surface burning (Fig. 14-29).[121]

A typical lightning injury occurs in a golfer holding a golf club up high in a storm. The metal club attracts the lightning strike, and the metal-studded shoes facilitate discharge through the feet to earth.[100]

In one electrical burn case, a 25-year-old man was digging a trench with a shovel and hit a high-voltage line with the shovel (Figs. 14-30 to 14-32). Initial injury was on his finger, and the huge exit wound on his back required grafting. When he fell down, his foot kicked the high-voltage line; the electricity produced a second entrance wound in his foot, traveled through his leg, and exited through the knee. He was sick and in the intensive care unit (ICU) for a lengthy period of time. He has a residual footdrop from nerve injury, but the foot has healed.

Management guidelines for electrical injuries are similar to those for other thermal burns, but the physician needs to assess the effects of electricity on vital systems. After ensuring adequate resuscitation, the involved lower extremity should be assessed for neurovascular compromise.

The incidence of deep tissue necrosis and compartment syndrome is significant; pressures and pulses need careful monitoring. Muscle necrosis can cause myoglobinuria, requiring large fluid volumes for alkalization of the urine. High-voltage burns demand an immediate fasciotomy and escharectomy (Fig. 14-33). Survival of the extremity depends on extent of the injury, viability of the blood vessels, and management of the impending ischemia.

Tissue loss is often progressive. Muscle that is initially contractile may be nonviable on subsequent evaluation because of ongoing microvascular thrombosis; this is unique to electrical burns. Delayed gangrene is not unusual. Staged sequential exploration with conservative meticulous debridement is the best way to assess and manage the extent of the injury.

Blowout lesions can occur at the current exit wounds in the extremity and can require amputation. Closure of the amputation site is delayed until the surgeon is certain that no further progressive deep necrosis exists. Significant new bone formation at long-bone amputation sites (tibia, fibula) is common after electrical injury.[112]

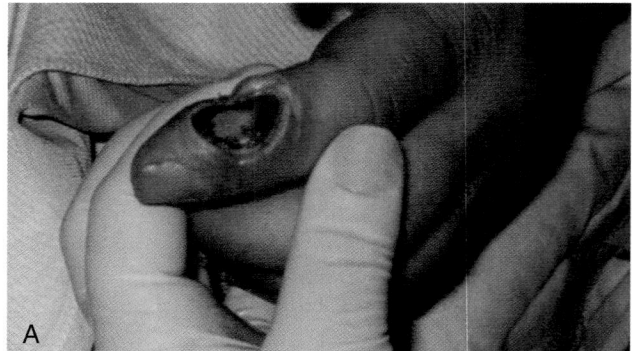
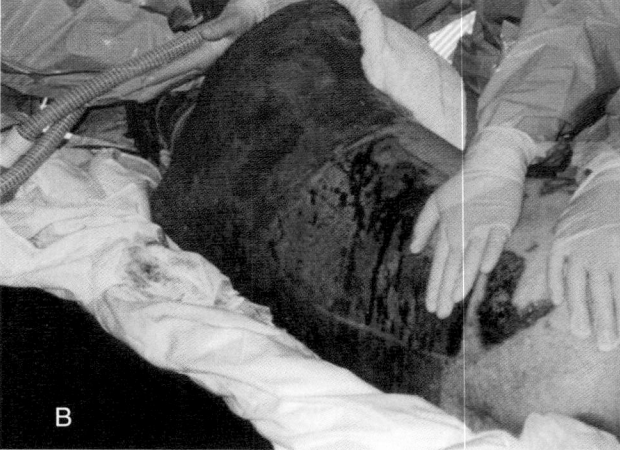
Figure 14-30 Electrical burn. **A,** Initial entry wound on hand. **B,** Severe exit wound with grafting.

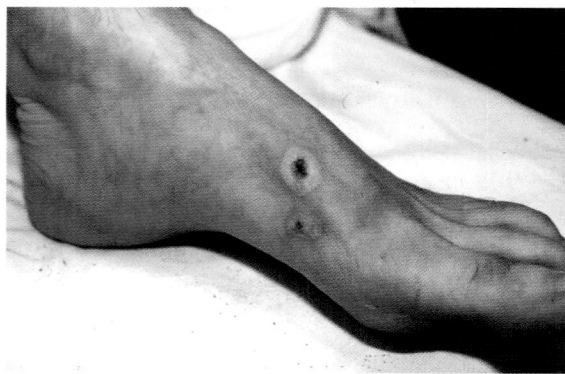
Figure 14-29 Exit wound for electrical burn.

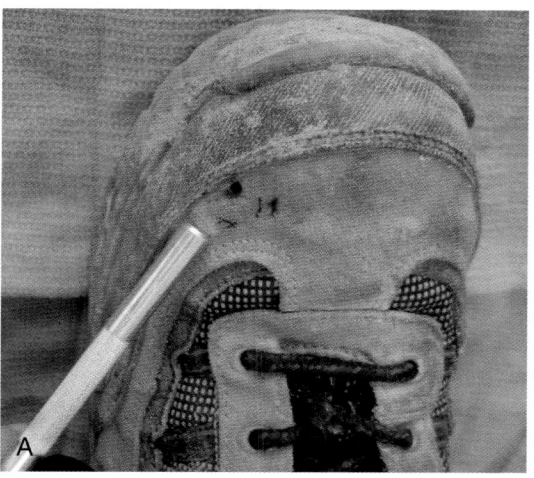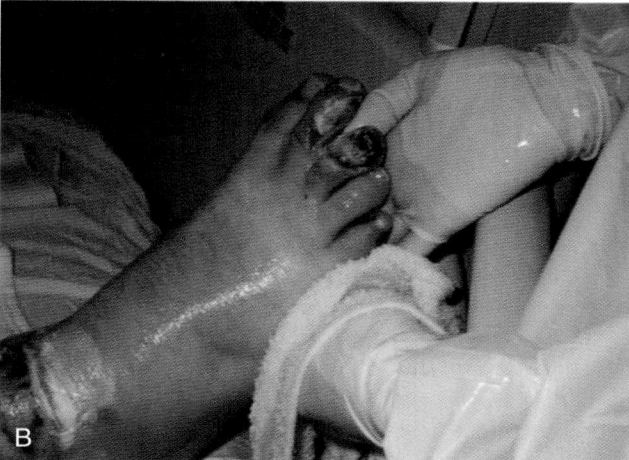

Figure 14-31 Same patient as in Figure 14-30. **A,** Second entrance area on boot. **B,** Severe exit wound on back.

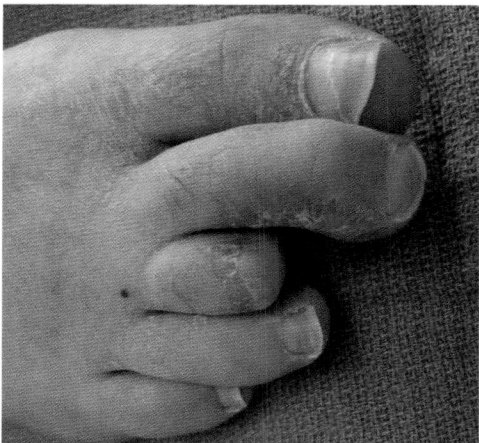

Figure 14-32 Same patient as in Figure 14-31. Healed foot 6 months later.

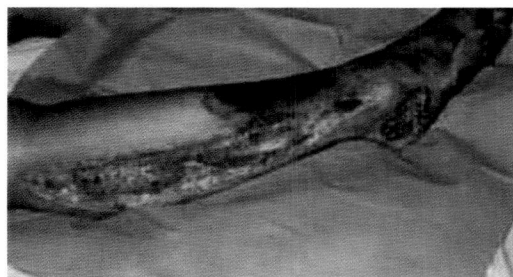

Figure 14-33 Burn fasciotomy.

The foot, often the exit site for beta current, can appear relatively benign after injury, but progressive microvascular occlusion and intraneural fibrosis have been postulated to cause intense allodynia and hyperpathia many months later. This sympathetically mediated pain is best relieved by a series of nerve blocks and intense rehabilitation (Box 14-4).[87]

BOX 14-4   Bone and Soft Tissue Changes Associated with Electrical Burns

■ Skin and subcutaneous damage may be apparent on radiographs.
■ Fractures can result from muscle cramps, mainly in the midthoracic vertebral bodies and humeral, femoral, and scapular necks. Longitudinal fractures, often after a zigzag contour (osteoschisis), can result from a direct mechanical splitting effect of the passing current.
■ Melting of bone from intense heat can result in small rounded osseous fragments resembling drips of wax (bone pearls) lying along the surface of the bone.
■ Osteonecrosis can result in osteolytic medullary lucent cystic areas in both the diaphysis and the metaphysis. Cortical sequestration, collapse of subchondral bone, epiphyseal collapse, and fragmentation have all been described.
■ Growth disturbances can result from premature fusion of the epiphysis in children.
■ Laceration of the skin can allow access of microorganisms with resulting osteomyelitis and suppurative arthritis. Suppurative arthritis can result in joint ankylosis.
■ Scars and contractures of soft tissues and periarticular calcification and ossification can cause limited joint movement.

Chemical Burns

Chemicals burn the foot through direct contact, acutely destroying tissue by a multitude of reactions that devitalize living cells. The burn can also be insidious and develop over a long time. For example, in a chemical plant worker who wears heavy socks with work boots, the socks can absorb toxic materials and burn slowly without the worker being aware.

The burns themselves do not provide any long-term management problems not previously discussed under thermal or electrical burns. The same careful attention needs to be given to prophylactic antibiotics, tetanus protection, foot elevation, pulse measurements, and compartment pressures. The key issue, however, is the acute management of the burn and obtaining the proper neutralization solutions. Lists of the solutions needed are in most emergency rooms, but the solutions themselves are often not immediately available. In general, contaminated clothing and shoes should be removed, particulate matter debrided, and vigorous water lavage commenced at once to dilute the chemical and decrease the intensity of the exposure. However, there are some notable exceptions to the use of water (Fig. 14-34).

Hydrochloric, nitric, and sulfuric acids should be neutralized with soda lime, soap, or magnesium hydroxide. Water lavage will cause ionization and increase the heat of reaction (Fig. 14-35).

Contact with white phosphorus causes extremely painful burns. Water is not harmful, but the particles are only visible under a 2% copper sulfate solution. They must be manually debrided to stop the burning.

Hydrofluoric acid is absorbed into the exposed tissues. It should be lavaged with boric acid or sodium bicarbonate. Continued pain after lavage indicates persistent chemical action. Calcium gluconate should be injected into the affected area to bind the active fluoride ion.

Phenol (carbolic acid) has limited solubility in water and should be lavaged with glycerol, polyethylene glycol, or vegetable oil.

Wet cement, a seemingly benign common material, can cause significant caustic burns of the foot and ankle in home improvement enthusiasts and the children who play in it. Professional masons are well aware of cement's toxicity.[116] Cement contains a high percentage of calcium oxide (lime). When mixed with water, lime creates a highly alkaline solution capable of burning unprotected skin. With an exposure time of 1 to 6 hours, the alkaline contact dissolves tissues, resulting in deep penetration. Early recognition and lavage are critical, but often the patient does not present until later in the day when shoes and socks are removed. Cement burns can range from superficial blistering to full-thickness necrosis and typically result in increased morbidity (Fig. 14-36).

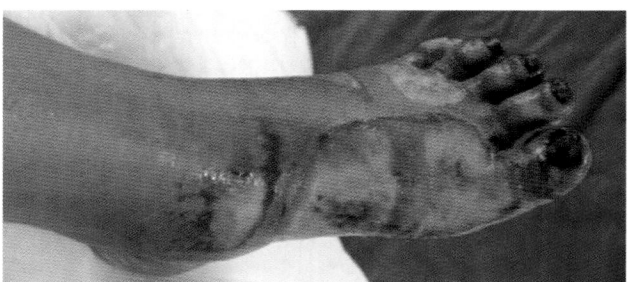

Figure 14-34 Chemical burn of foot.

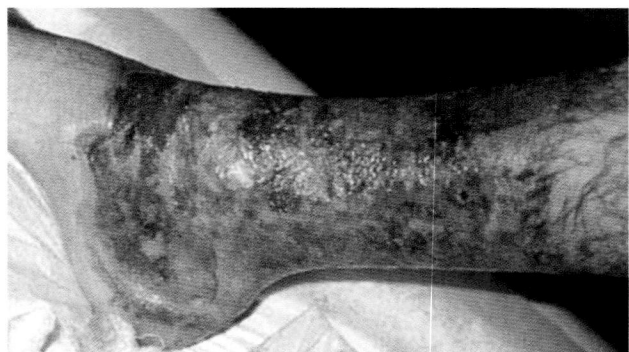

Figure 14-35 Deep alkali burn after lavage. (From http://www.burnsurgery.org. Accessed 8/1/2012.)

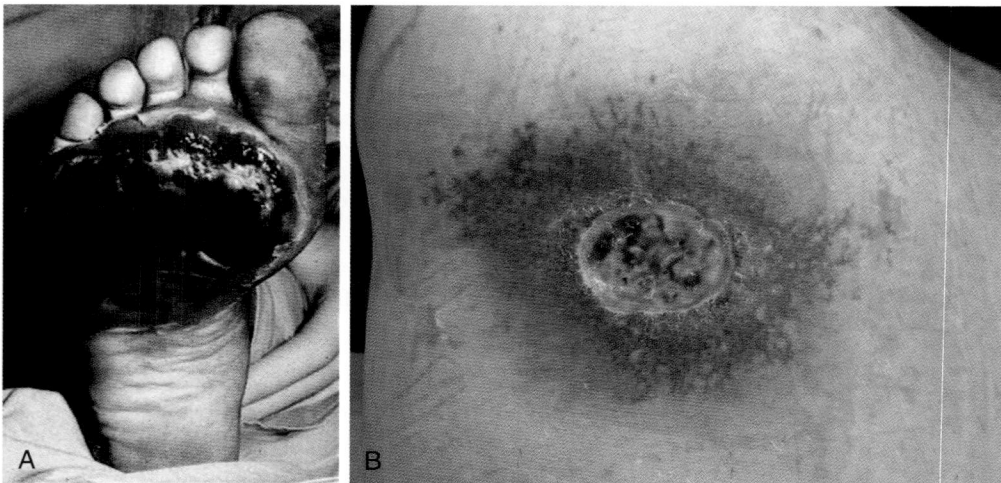

Figure 14-36 **A,** Cement burn from a hole in the sole of the shoe. **B,** Fluroscopy-induced radiation dermatitis. (**A,** From University of New South Wales, Safety School of Safety Science, Kensington, Australia. http://www.mdconsult.com/books/page.do?eid=4-u1.0-B978-0-323-03305-3..50039-1–cesec45&isbn=978-0-323-03305-3&type=bookPage&from=content&uniqId=399599533-65. Accessed June 1, 2006. **B,** Courtesy Jeffrey Callen, MD. Originally printed in Bolognia J, Jorizzo J, Rapini R: *Dermatology,* ed 2, Mosby, 2007, Edinburgh.)

Radiation Burns

Radiation burns result from exposure of tissues to ionizing radiation. Electromagnetic radiation consists of a pulse of electrical and magnetic energy of very short wavelength in the form of x-rays or gamma rays. These high-energy photons are produced in linear accelerators (x-rays) or emitted from the unstable nuclei of radioactive substances (e.g., radium, cobalt, cesium). Particulate radiation is produced by particles (e.g., electrons, protons, alpha particles, neutrons, mesons) that are capable of ionizing any tissues through which they pass.[103]

In radiation injury, deoxyribonucleic acid (DNA) is the key target. The extent of the injury depends on the type of radiation, the radiation absorbed dose (rad), and the duration of exposure.

The acute changes include erythema and subsequent ulceration of varying depth that requires a surprisingly long time to heal. The late changes, however, make this a difficult injury to reconstruct. After exposure and a prolonged latency period, parenchymal fibroblasts are gradually depleted, endarteritis obliterans and excessive tissue fibrosis develop, and the potential for cellular replication decreases. This results in radiodermatitis, radioosteonecrosis, and the increased potential for local malignant transformation.[92]

Chronic superficial ulceration secondary to radiation injury is best managed by skin grafts if the bed is well vascularized. Deeper lesions require flap coverage. Because of the high incidence of malignancy, selective biopsy should be done before surgical intervention (Table 14-7).

EXPOSURE

Frostbite

With hands and feet accounting for 90% of all recorded injuries, frostbite is a clinical entity that should not go unrecognized by those delivering orthopaedic care. Frostbite, the acute freezing of cutaneous and subcutaneous tissues, occurs when exposed skin is subjected to subfreezing temperatures. Severe overexposure and absolute low temperatures freeze human tissue, but a major cause of frostbite in the foot is central hypothermia.[131] The severity of frostbite is often closely related to the temperature gradient between intact skin and the external environment, but the most important factor remains the duration of exposure to such temperatures.

Frostbite is not a modern phenomenon. Evidence of frostbite from as early as 5000 years ago has been found in pre-Columbian mummies.[126] Clinical interest in frostbite, however, originated with problems of foot soldiers during Napoleon's Russian campaign and peaked with military experiences in World War II and the Korean War.

In modern times, frostbite has become a common problem in skiers and high-altitude climbers and in dense urban environments. The insult of cold injury seen at high altitude is so severe that heavy bomber crews during World War II sustained more injuries from frostbite than from all other causes combined.[99] Frostbite in the urban setting is also a psychosocial disease, especially among homeless, alcoholic, and schizophrenic persons. In one study investigating the occurrence of frostbite in the urban population, it was estimated that the prevalence of overt or covert psychiatric illness was 61% to 65%.[125] Unless the underlying cause of reckless, inappropriate behavior is addressed in these patients, recurrence is common (Fig. 14-37).[124,125]

Frostbite occurs more often in men, who outnumber female patients with frostbite 10 to 1.[94] Adults between 30 and 49 years of age appear to be the most commonly affected because of a delay in diagnosis and treatment, but the elderly and very young can be severely affected. Frostbite in the feet of children can have long-lasting effects, including premature fusion and abnormal growth in the epiphyseal cartilage.[114]

Homeostasis maintains a constant body temperature of 37° C (98.6° F). When external cold challenges this temperature and heat loss exceeds heat production, the body starts shivering, and flow to the peripheral extremities (hands, feet) decreases to provide warmth to the central organs. Heat loss is intensified by wet clothing, exposed

Table 14-7	Grading of Radiation Burns
Grade	**Description and Comments**
I	Clinically silent with demineralization, mainly of trabecular bone but sometimes also of inner surface of cortical bone. Repair of bone is not apparent.
II	Changes include hypertrophic bone atrophy with spongiosclerosis. Pathologic fractures can occur, especially at predisposed sites such as the femoral neck, pubic bones, ribs, and mandible. These fractures are usually associated with pain and loss of function and can heal. However, the bone never becomes completely normal.
III	Stage of osteoradionecrosis, often accompanied by fracture and infection. Infection can manifest clinically with features of osteomyelitis. The clinician must appreciate that the degree of underlying bone damage often does not correlate with overlying skin changes. Surgical intervention may be necessary to remove necrotic bone and to drain bone of infected material. Chronic sinus drainage is a common complication, and death can occur.
IV	Radiation-induced malignancy is usually osteogenic sarcoma or fibrosarcoma. Usually a latent period occurs between time of exposure and development of neoplasm, most often 10 years. Radiation dose is about 20 Gy or more. Clinical and radiologic appearances of tumors do not differ from those occurring spontaneously, and prognosis is very poor.

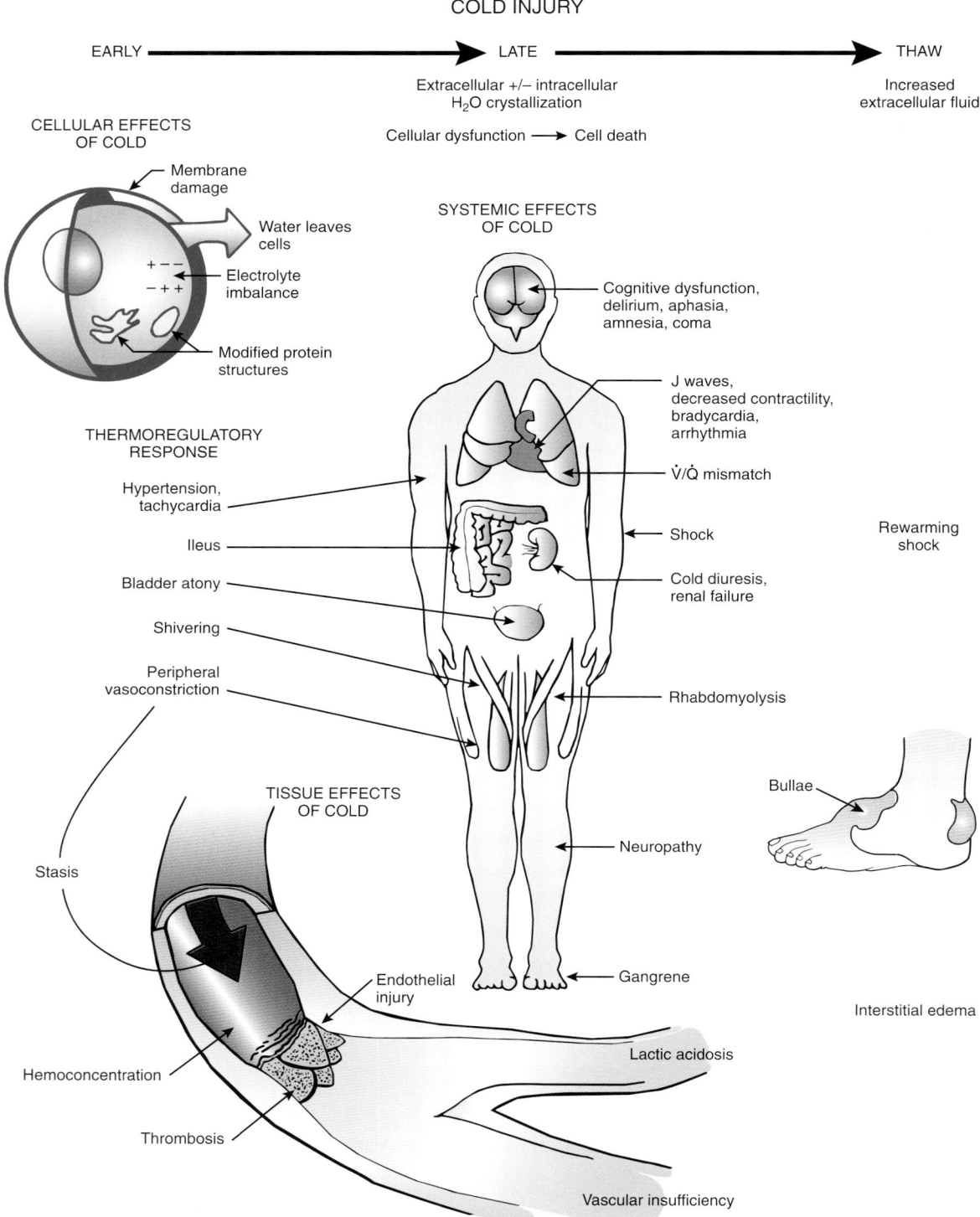

COLD INJURY

EARLY ⟶ LATE ⟶ THAW

Extracellular +/− intracellular
H₂O crystallization

Increased
extracellular fluid

Cellular dysfunction ⟶ Cell death

CELLULAR EFFECTS
OF COLD

Membrane
damage

Water leaves
cells

Electrolyte
imbalance

Modified protein
structures

SYSTEMIC EFFECTS
OF COLD

Cognitive dysfunction,
delirium, aphasia,
amnesia, coma

J waves,
decreased contractility,
bradycardia,
arrhythmia

$\dot{V}/\dot{Q}$ mismatch

Shock

Cold diuresis,
renal failure

Rhabdomyolysis

Neuropathy

Gangrene

Rewarming
shock

Bullae

Interstitial edema

THERMOREGULATORY
RESPONSE

Hypertension,
tachycardia

Ileus

Bladder atony

Shivering

Peripheral
vasoconstriction

TISSUE EFFECTS
OF COLD

Stasis

Endothelial
injury

Hemoconcentration

Thrombosis

Lactic acidosis

Vascular insufficiency

Figure 14-37 Cold-induced injuries such as hypothermia and frostbite lead to the thermoregulatory response (e.g., shivering and increased sympathetic activity), cellular and tissue effects (e.g., membrane damage, electrolyte imbalance, endothelial injury, and thrombosis), and systemic effects (e.g., shock, arrhythmia, and neuromuscular dysfunction). $\dot{V}/\dot{Q}$, (originally Latin) ventilation/perfusion.

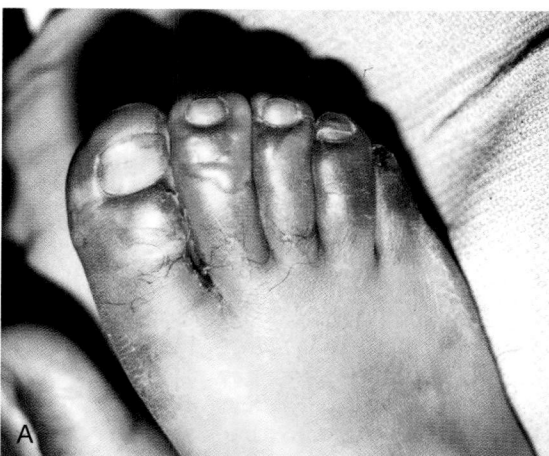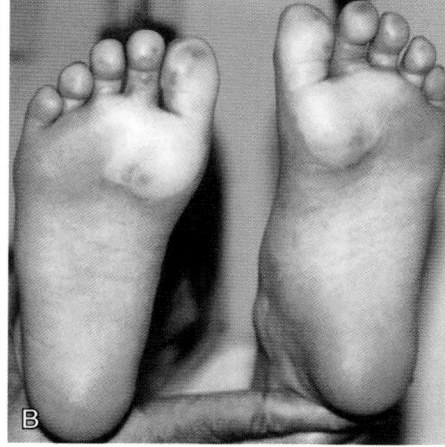

Figure 14-38 **A,** Early frostbite on toes. **B,** Bullae filled with clear fluid on the distal plantar surfaces in a second-degree frostbite. (Courtesy Timothy Givens, MD. **B,** Originally printed in Bolognia J, Jorizzo J, Rapini R: *Dermatology,* ed 2, Mosby, 2007, Edinburgh.)

BOX 14-5   Generation of Body Heat

- *Basal heat production:* Heat produced by oxidation of food at a fixed metabolic rate; maintains life processes under resting conditions; can be altered very little and is ineffective in preventing body cooling during exposure to a cold environment.
- *Muscular thermoregulatory heat:* Heat produced by shivering; increases heat production three to five times basal rate; consumes tremendous amounts of energy reserves and tends to reduce coordination and useful movement.
- *High-intensity exercise-induced heat:* Heat produced by muscular activity during vigorous walking or running; can elevate heat production up to 10 times the basal rate during very strenuous exercise; can be maintained for only a few minutes because of exhaustion of energy stores.
- *Mild- to moderate-intensity exercise-induced heat:* Same mechanism as in high-intensity exercise; can elevate to five times basal rate; can be maintained for much longer periods.

From Fritz RL, Perrin DH: Cold exposure injuries: prevention and treatment, *Clin Sports Med* 8:111–126, 1989.

BOX 14-6   Conservation of Body Heat

- *Superficial vasoconstriction:* Body heat conserved by constriction of superficial blood vessels in the skin, especially over the extremities; shunts blood away from the body surface, where blood loses heat to the cooler environment, to supply more blood flow to the brain, heart, lungs, and other internal organs.
- *Body insulation:* Insulation against heat loss by layering of subcutaneous fat and, to a lesser extent, by growing body hair.
- *External heat sources:* Insulation against heat loss through use of proper clothing and acquisition of more heat by external means, such as fire, sun exposure, hot food and drink, and contact with another body.

From Fritz RL, Perrin DH: Cold exposure injuries: prevention and treatment, *Clin Sports Med* 8:111–126, 1989.

BOX 14-7   Heat Transfer Mechanisms

- *Conduction:* Direct contact with a cold object
- *Convection:* Movement of air or water adjacent to skin
- *Radiation:* Energy emission to a cooler object
- *Evaporation:* Loss of body heat by conversion of water to gas (vapor)
- *Respiration:* Loss of heated air from lungs by exhalation

---

skin, contact with a colder object, alcohol use, evaporation, and rapid respiration (Fig. 14-38 and Boxes 14-5 to 14-7).[105]

Usually, blood flow to the extremities is abundant, even in severe cold. But if core temperature drops below 35° C (95° F), peripheral anastomoses are shut down, and the cooling of the extremities can be rapid and intense. Highly insulated footwear passively slows the rate of heat loss but does not keep the foot warm or prevent cold injury.[123] Constricting footwear intensifies the risk. Pressure on the toes decreases circulation and increases heat loss through conduction.

Gasoline and other solvents are supercooled in the cold because of their low freezing points. If they are

spilled on the foot in subfreezing conditions, frostbite can occur (Fig. 14-39).

Freezing causes vascular stasis and hypertonicity, leading to vessel occlusion, tissue hypoxia, and ischemic necrosis. On the cellular level, decreasing temperatures lead to the development of extracellular ice crystals. As the tissue fluid osmolarity increases, cellular membranes become unstable and the outflow of cellular fluid causes intracellular dehydration. The resulting elevation in

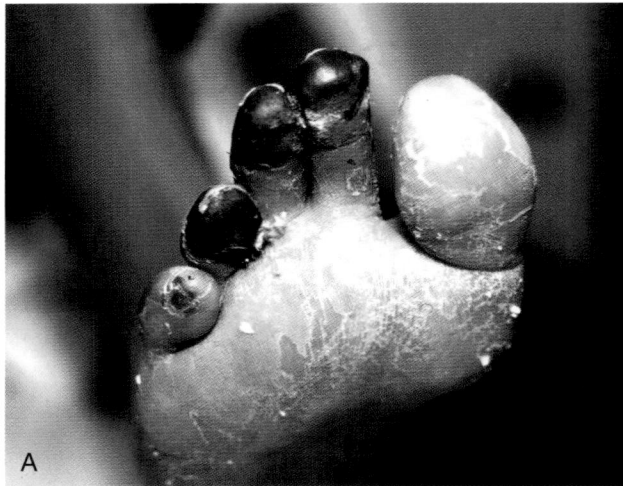

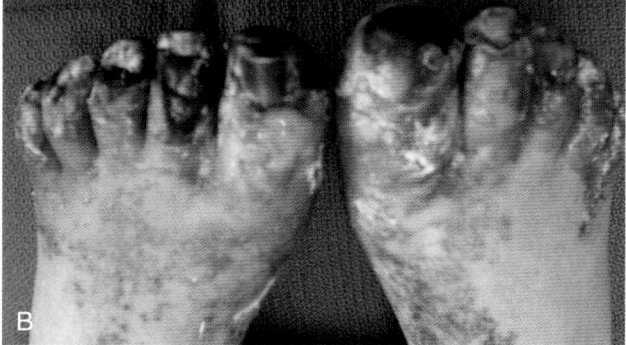

Figure 14-39 **A,** Late frostbite on toes. **B,** Large areas of partial thickness skin loss, with full-thickness loss at tips of toes.

intracellular electrolyte concentration and the formation of intracellular ice crystals cause cell death. Tendons and bone are relatively resistant to frostbite, whereas muscles, nerves, and blood vessels are very susceptible. Absolute temperature changes are predictive of the occurrence of frostbite, but the degree of irreversible damage is more closely related to the length of time that the tissue remains frozen. A delay in treatment or diagnosis is therefore detrimental (Fig. 14-40).

Frostnip, or *superficial frostbite,* is reversible ice crystal formation on the skin. On removing a boot, for example, a small, painless, blanched spot is noted on the tip of the toe. Firm pressure of a warm hand should restore color, and tingling may ensue. After rewarming, the tip may stay red, and the superficial skin layers may flake for several days. Permanent sequelae are unlikely (Fig. 14-41A). This type of cold injury can also be seen in the case of unscrupulous use of cold therapy devices (Fig. 14-41B).

True frostbite involves the actual freezing of tissue. Classically staged into four levels of increasing intensity, this is of no prognostic value in the foot, where the structures at risk are close to the surface. The sudden cessation of feeling cold and discomfort followed by a pleasant warm feeling, swelling, and a prickling sensation portends the start of this syndrome. At this early stage, rapid rewarming will reverse the frostbite, but if left untreated, it will progress to superficial blistering, deep blistering, and finally, deep tissue involvement and necrosis. The duration of freezing is directly related to the amount of tissue necrosis, and if skin temperature falls below −6.6° C (20° F), tissue loss always occurs.

Figure 14-40 **A,** Frostbitten feet. **B,** Severe case of third-degree frostbite in skier lost for several days in wilderness; the patient ended up with a below-knee amputation. (**A,** From DermIS: http://dermis.multimedica.de/dermisroot/en/43138/image.htm. Accessed June 1, 2006.)

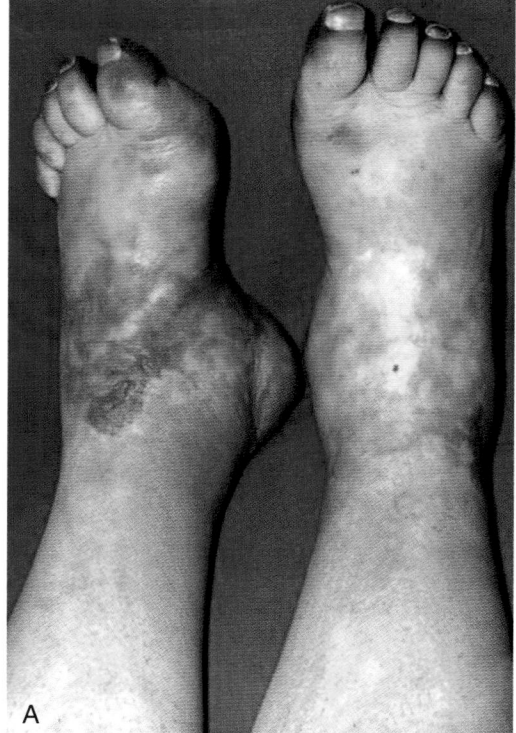

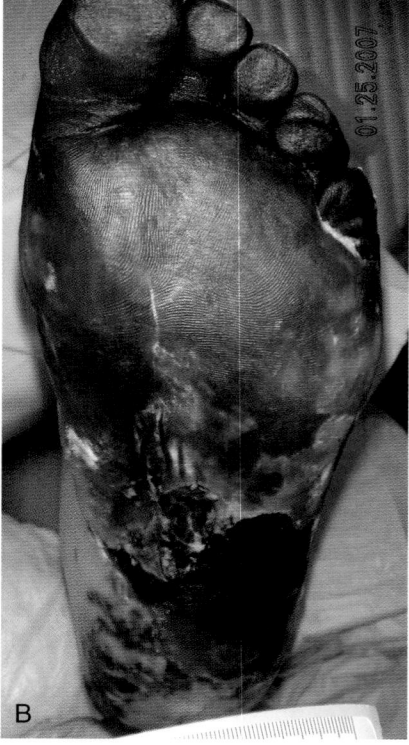

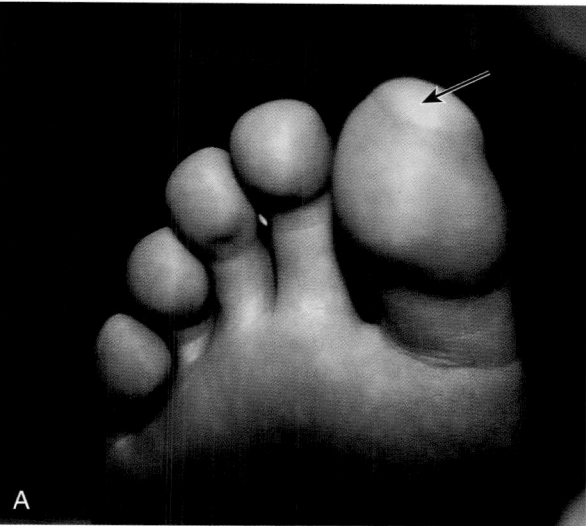
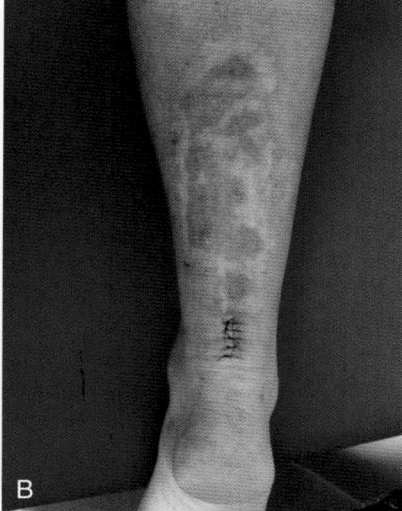

Figure 14-41 **A,** Frostnip of tip of great toe *(arrow).* **B,** Frostnip to posterior leg in patient who placed ice packs on his calf for 48 hours after an acute Achilles rupture. Local wound care was used, and surgery wasdelayed an additional week. (**A,** Courtesy Edward Dickenson, MD.)

The treatment of frostbite hinges on the principle of rapid rewarming and the identification and debridement of devitalized tissue in an effort to prevent infection. Rapid rewarming in a protected environment is the initial treatment. Refreezing of a thawed extremity will cause irreversible changes, so if a foot is rewarmed in the wilderness, for example, the patient must be kept warm and carried to a safe location (Box 14-8).

A foot bath with water at 40° to 42° C (104° to 108° F) is ideal for evenly spread rewarming and should be continued until the foot becomes warm and pliable, color returns, and sensation is near normal. Heating pads or campfires are uneven heat sources and can cause skin burn. A sock frozen to the foot should be carefully removed with additional warm water.

In the final stages of rewarming, intense pain can require parenteral analgesia. This is actually a good sign, indicating viability. Prophylactic antibiotics are indicated because infection is difficult to recognize. Tetanus protection should be given as well.

Blood flow return is accompanied by a mottled blue appearance, swelling, and large blister formation, and areas of gangrene can appear in the first 1 to 2 days. Blisters should be drained but not unroofed, antibiotic ointment should be applied, and the foot should be elevated in a bulky nonconstricting dressing. Although the extent of damage will take weeks to be revealed, initial good signs are large clear blister formation, blanching pink color, return to normal temperature, and rapid return of sensation. Hard white cyanotic areas, lack of edema, dark hemorrhagic blebs, and systemic symptoms portend poor results.[127] Although technetium scintigraphy was previously used to help define tissue viability, numerous centers are now employing MRI as the imaging modality of choice when attempting to

---

BOX 14-8 Treatment of Frostbite

Admit frostbite patient to a specialist unit, if possible.
On admission, rapidly rewarm the affected areas in warm water at 40° to 42° C (104°-108° F) for 15 to 30 minutes or until thawing is complete.
On completion of rewarming, treat the affected parts as follows:

- Debride white blisters and apply topical treatment with aloe vera every 6 hours.
- Leave hemorrhage blisters intact and apply topical aloe vera every 6 hours.
- Elevate the affected part(s) with splinting as indicated.
- Administer antitetanus prophylaxis (tetanus toxoid or tetanus immunoglobulin).
- Administer opiate analgesic IM or IV as indicated.
- Administer ibuprofen 400 mg PO q12h.
- Administer benzyl penicillin 600 mg q6h for 48 to 72 hours.
- Perform daily hydrotherapy for 30 to 45 minutes at 40° C.
  - For documentation, obtain photographic records on admission, at 24 hours, and serially every 2 to 3 days until discharge.
  - Prohibit smoking.

Modified from McCauley RL, Hing DN, Robson MC, Heggers JP: Frostbite injuries: a rational approach based on the pathophysiology, *J Trauma* 23:143–147, 1983; Murphy JV, Banwell PE, Roberts AH, McGrouther DA: Frostbite: pathogenesis and treatment, *J Trauma* 48:171–178, 2000.
IM, intramuscularly; *IV,* intravenously; *PO,* orally.

---

define lines of demarcated ischemic soft tissue after thermal injury.[91]

With the exception of circumferentially constricting eschars, surgery should be delayed 2 to 3 weeks to allow full demarcation of viable areas. Rehabilitation should be started early. Late sequelae of frostbite include cold hypersensitivity, chronic ischemic changes, hyperhidrosis, nail deformities, and SMP and/or CRPS. Nerve conduction velocity testing can indicate cold-induced neuropathy.[89] Sensory conduction velocity and distal motor delay were significantly decreased in symptomatic frostbite patients compared with control subjects. NCV measurements can provide objective findings in cold-injured patients and in those with no conspicuous signs but complaining of cold sensitivity.[97,118]

Chilblain

Chilblain (an archaic English word meaning "inflammatory swelling") is a milder form of frostbite, also called *chilblains, erythema pernio,* and *pernio.* A neurocirculatory disturbance of the foot, it is typically seen in people who work outside during the winter months. Chronic inflammation with fat necrosis is seen at the areas of the foot with the poorest cushioning: the dorsum, back of the heel, and plantar surface of the first and fifth metatarsals.

Treatment of chilblain is conservative and includes dry warm shoes and boots, frequent sock changes, and prompt removal of wet footwear. Tight shoes aggravate chilblain.

Trench Foot

When feet remain wet in the shoes and socks for prolonged periods, a condition known as *trench foot* can develop. Clinically, the manifestations of trench foot represent the effects of injury by water absorption in the stratum corneum of the skin of the feet during above-freezing temperatures of 0° to 10°C (32° to 50°F). Trench foot caused serious attrition among troops in World War I. Prolonged water immersion of feet along the 15,000 miles of trenches resulted in swollen limbs, impaired sensory nerves, inflammation, infection, and loss of tissue and limbs through gangrene (Fig. 14-42).[104,108,109]

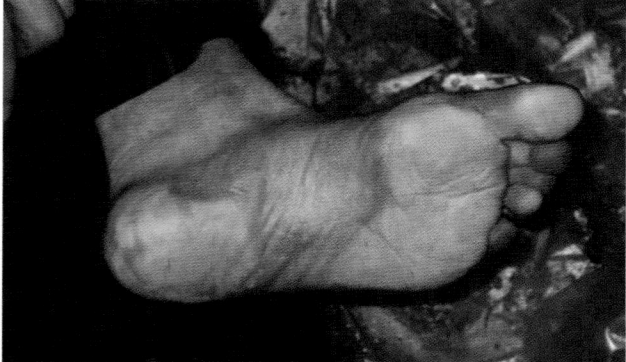

Figure 14-42 Early trench foot. (From http://www.poc.purdue.org.galleries.php?g.)

Trench foot is seen in survivors of sinking ships, downed airplanes, and military combat in wet, cold areas. It is also appearing with increasing frequency in winter among the homeless population because of the lack of shelter against the elements.[133] Cold water can increase body heat loss to a rate 25 times faster than if exposed to comparable cold air.

Symptoms of trench foot vary with the temperature of the water and duration of immersion. Removal of the wet boots and socks allows the feet to dry rapidly, leading to dusky cyanosis and blanching, followed by rapid swelling. The skin turns warm without sweating, blebs and ecchymosis form, and the foot shows obvious signs of vasodilation. Variable amounts of tissue maceration occur. Eventually, muscle necrosis with secondary arterial thrombosis can ensue.

Treatment is aimed at preserving viable tissue, preventing further tissue destruction, and avoiding infection. When uncomplicated by sepsis or ischemic injury, trench or immersion foot resolves with conservative measures. More complicated cases require use of antibiotics, surgical debridement, and possible amputation. This syndrome is exacerbated by mental confusion, peripheral neuropathy, peripheral vascular disease, or the use of tobacco and vasoconstrictor drugs such as cocaine. SMP can be a late sequela of trench or immersion foot.

FOREIGN BODY INJURIES

Puncture wounds of the foot are common presenting problems in medical offices and emergency departments. Although most seem benign, some will in fact progress to cellulitis, foreign body reaction, or even osteomyelitis. Maintaining a high index of suspicion is critical in protecting the patient's foot.

Patients presenting within 24 hours of an uncomplicated plantar puncture should have their tetanus status assessed, be treated with surface cleansing alone, and be kept non–weight bearing for 24 hours. The presence of symptoms after 48 hours is associated with a higher complication rate, and patients should be cautioned about the need for a return visit.[148]

A *foreign body reaction* can occur when external material penetrates the dermis. Granulomas from wood splinters can appear as indurated boggy nodules with no obvious site of entry. Glass, plastic, synthetic fibers, and tiny stones can provoke similar reactions.[143] Sharp metal objects can pierce the sole of the sneaker and enter the foot, often migrating after initial entry. The foreign inclusions may remain silent for a significant time before becoming symptomatic.[150]

Pieces of wood are particularly troublesome because they are often unrecognized on initial inspection and can result in significant complications. The clinical history can fail to arouse suspicion of a wooden particle, and even an apparently successful splinter excision can leave residual fragments. Clinical evidence of this retained foreign body might not appear until months or even years

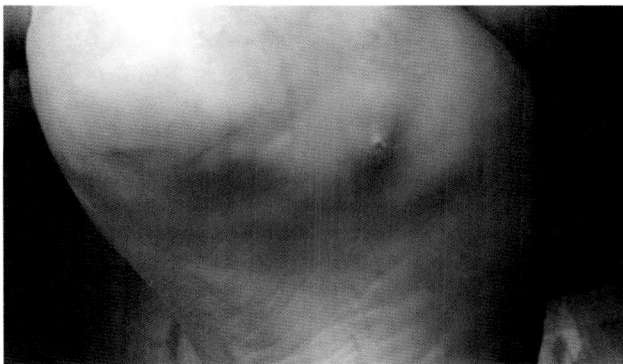

Figure 14-43 Foreign body granuloma on plantar aspect of foot.

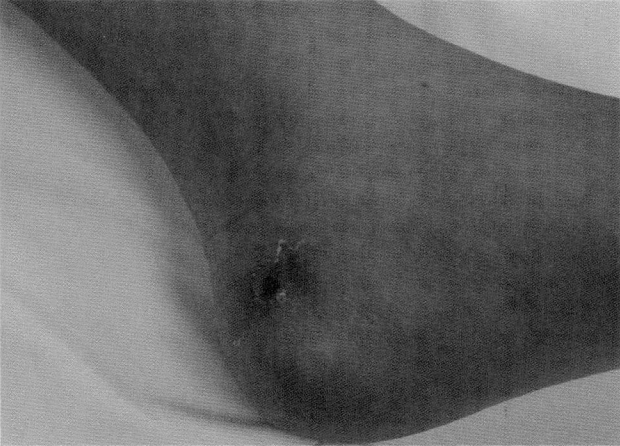

Figure 14-45 Foreign body granuloma.

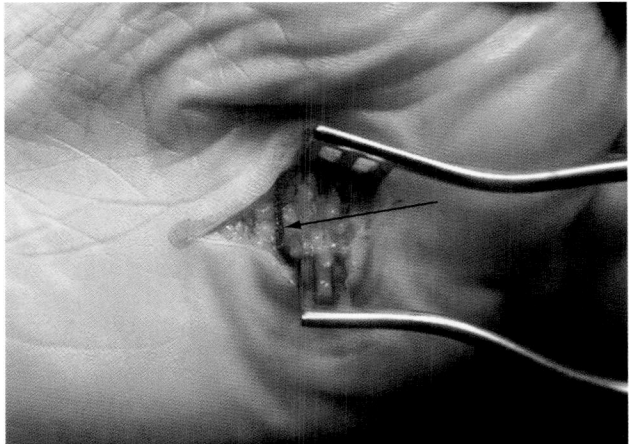
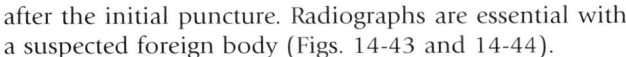

Figure 14-44 Wood splinter at base of granuloma.

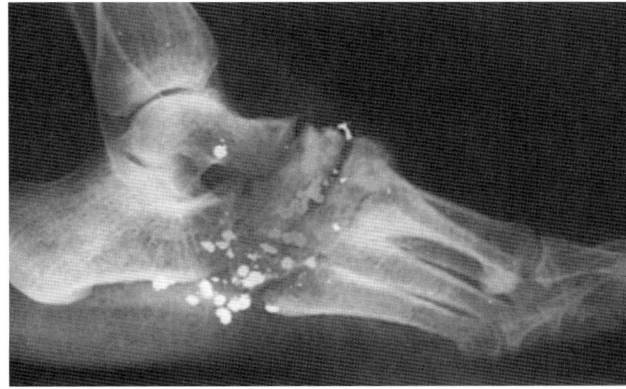

Figure 14-46 Pellets and shotgun wadding in foot.

after the initial puncture. Radiographs are essential with a suspected foreign body (Figs. 14-43 and 14-44).

Initial examination can reveal a tender chronic granulomatous reaction that may be mistaken for a plantar wart or even a skin malignancy. There may be associated drainage. Plain radiographs are negative 85% of the time in the presence of retained wooden bodies, or they can demonstrate reactive changes suggestive of tumor or infection. Direct surgical exploration is not always successful in finding these objects.

Recent studies reveal that MRI or ultrasound may be the best initial imaging modality for the clinical evaluation and localization of the suspected wooden foreign body (Figs. 14-45 and 14-46). CT is less successful because, after penetration, the wooden body absorbs water and may become radiologically indistinguishable from the surrounding tissues.[134,135,138,142,145]

Complete excision is usually required for resolution of the inflammatory mass. Fluoroscopy can aid in guiding the surgical approach. Late infection can continue to smolder with incomplete removal.[140,141] Not all foreign body penetrations need to be excised. When a deep inclusion cyst is found, close follow-up is required to determine whether the foot will become asymptomatic or if a painful mass will develop. Attempts at removal of asymptomatic foreign bodies must be weighed against potential damage to the structures of the foot with the possible creation of painful scarring.

Pseudomonas osteomyelitis should be suspected in all patients who have foot pain and swelling after sustaining a nail puncture through a sneaker. Open surgical debridement followed by a course of intravenous antibiotics is the treatment of choice.[139,140,149]

Penetrating wounds, stings, inoculation of venom, and retained animal parts are common marine and land injuries in the unwary, poorly shod recreational individual. During the summer season, it is common to see patients with snakebites, retained stingers, or embedded sea urchin spines in the emergency department.[137] These injuries vary according to global positioning, altitude, and ocean depth. It is critically important to identify the offending organism and then consult an encyclopedic text for the particular region. The increasing popular use of form-fitting mesh and neoprene "water shoes" with reinforced rubber soles may decrease the incidence of these injuries in marine environments.

It should be noted that absorbable polyglycolide pins and screws used for fracture and osteotomy fixation can produce radiologic changes resembling foreign body reactions. These require only observation because they have been shown to resolve with time. Similar but more erosive changes are seen with silicone implants. Because these are permanent devices, they may cause a chronic reaction that may necessitate removal.[136,144,146,147]

BLISTERS

Friction Blisters

Painful friction blisters can compromise athletic performance and disable otherwise healthy military personnel and athletes. Blisters result from frictional forces that mechanically separate epidermal cells at the level of the stratum spinosum. Friction blisters are more likely to form in areas that have a thick horny layer held tightly to the underlying layers (e.g., soles of the feet). Moist skin increases frictional force.[151]

Hydrostatic pressure fills the separation with plasma-like fluid with a lower protein level, followed by a sequential change in chemical content and physiologic activity. At 6 hours, the fluid contains increased amounts of amino acids and nucleosides; by 24 hours, a high level of mitotic activity occurs in the basal cells; and at 48 to 120 hours, new stratum granulosum and stratum corneum can be seen.

Speed of blister formation is increased by the magnitude of frictional force, how rapidly that force cycles, and the carrying of heavy loads. Repeated exposure of skin to low-intensity frictional forces results in epidermal thickening (calluses), which reduces the likelihood blisters will develop. Conditioning the foot to athletic or hiking footwear before intense performance also reduces blister formation.

Treatment of intact blisters by draining the fluid while maintaining the epidermal roof results in the least patient discomfort and helps to prevent secondary infection. Decompressed painful blisters feel best when they are covered with a hydrocolloid dressing, and patients can return to sports. No evidence demonstrates that antibiotics enhance blister healing.[157] Blister care seems trivial, but military recruits have died from toxic shock originating from infected pedal blisters.[152]

Acrylic socks and neoprene soles seem to result in fewer blisters in runners. Acrylic socks wick the moisture away, leaving a drier foot, drier sock, and warmer foot. Cotton and wool socks absorb twice as much moisture as acrylic socks and are associated with a damper sock and a colder and wetter foot.

A thin, polyester-lined sock, combined with a thick wool or polypropylene sock that maintains its bulk under stress and sweat, is associated with fewer blisters in military recruits. The medical community generally agrees that the double-layer sock system, especially one that uses

terry padding away from the foot surface, is superior in preventing blister formation.[150,156,158]

Before workouts, the application of a moisturizer to the foot can be helpful. Antiperspirants and drying powders can help prevent blister formation but can lead to skin irritation.[154,159]

Fracture Blisters

Fracture blisters around the foot and ankle are clinically significant in the ultimate timing of fixation of the underlying fracture. They form secondary to a stretch, stress, or torsional force, causing separation of the epidermis from the dermis, and are either clear or blood filled. The type and size of the blister are thought to be related to clinical outcome. Fractures with skin blisters or abrasions have been shown to have more than double the overall complication rate.

The skin around the foot and ankle is different from other skin, with the absence of well-formed adipose or muscle layers covering many bony structures. Also, few hair follicles are present, which are an excellent source for epithelial cells. This environment can predispose to blister formation.

Histologically, the clear fluid–filled blisters show evidence of retained epithelial cells that can aid in faster healing of the blister bed. Blood-filled blisters represent a more significant injury, which has gone into the dermis, disrupting blood supply to the overlying layers. This leads to increased time to reepithelialization and subsequent delayed wound healing (Table 14-8).[155,160]

There is no current universal consensus regarding the management of fracture blisters. Giordano et al[155] compared three methods of managing fracture blisters in the presence of ankle fractures: aspiration alone, deroofing of the blister with application of silver sulfadiazine, and leaving the blister intact. There was no advantage to any method, but they did recommend deroofing blisters that had burst (Figs. 14-47 to 14-49). Strauss and Petrucelli[176] recommend deroofing intact blisters, and treatment of with a silver sulfadiazine (Silvadene) regimen proved to be successful in minimizing soft tissue complications by promoting reepithelialization in all nondiabetic patients.

Table 14-8	Delay in Definitive Care Secondary to Fracture Blisters
Fracture Location	**Delay in Definitive Care (days)**
Ankle	6
Tibial plateau	11
Tibial shaft	3.5
Calcaneal	12
Pilon	6.75
Mean	7.7

Data from Uebbing CM, Walsh M, Miller JB: Fracture blisters, *West J Emerg Med* 12:131–133, 2011.

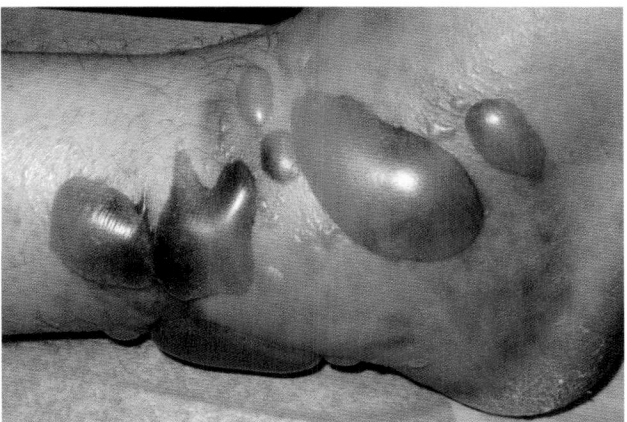

Figure 14-47 Clear blisters.

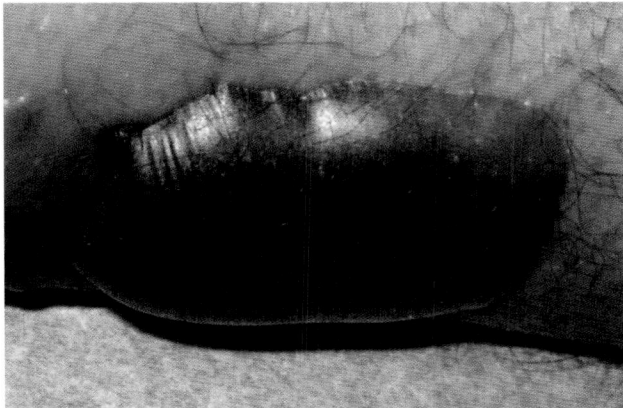

Figure 14-48 Dark blister.

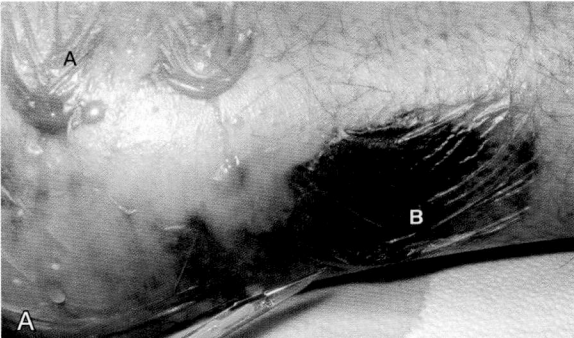

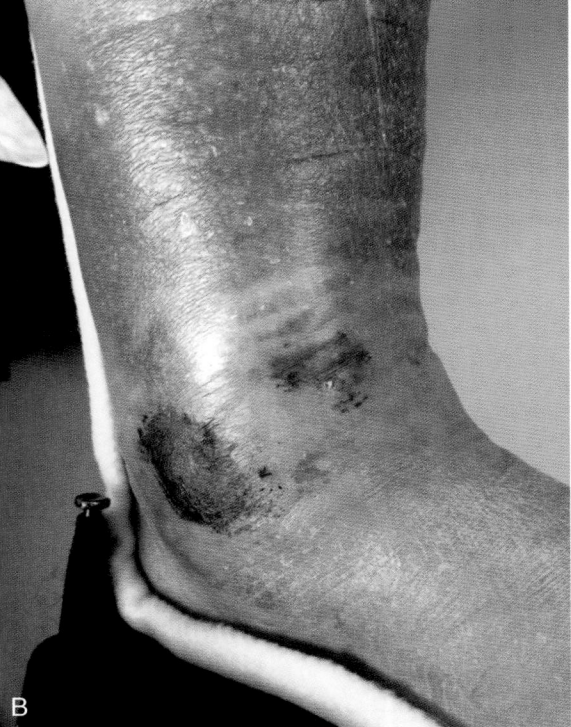

Figure 14-49 **A,** Burst clear and dark blisters. Note the quality of the skin under the clear *(A)* and dark *(B)* blisters. **B,** One week after decompression of fracture blister.

Based on our experience we feel that the blister's roof should remain intact until surgery to avoid bacterial colonization of the blister bed. If allowed to decompress on their own in a splint or cast, the blisters often become deroofed and are left sitting in a damp colonized splint lining or stockinette, which is thought to promote infection and delay healing. Aspiration with a 25-guage needle after sterile preparation of the aspiration site may help speed up the process of reepithelialization and is usually painless. If possible, the surgical incision should avoid any blister, but if necessary, it is thought to be safe to cut through a clear blister but not through a blood-filled one.

FOOT ODOR

The malodorous foot is often the subject of humor and lighthearted concern, but in reality, it can cause profound psychologic trauma and can ruin expensive shoes, socks, and stockings. Understanding the impact, cause, and care of this malady will help bring relief to many troubled patients.[173]

We are constantly bombarded with media fears that our feet are unfortunately fragrant and offensive to others.

Much plantar sweating is emotionally stimulated (e.g., love, fear, an important interview), and the subsequent odor production may be self-perpetuating. If left untreated, the pungent aroma can foul the environment, lead to social exclusion, and cause needless destruction of fashionable shoes (Fig. 14-50).

The smell itself is unique and, next to alcoholic breath, may be the most distinctive scent in the office setting. Often described as musty, amino-like, malty, cheesy, or rancid, the quality of the perceived foot odor is a direct result of the examiner's and patient's organic ability to assimilate it. Therefore special terminology is necessary.[161,164,166]

Classically referred to as *plantar bromhidrosis,* the fetid foot odor is a secondary effect of direct bacterial action on sweat-softened skin. Moisture plus heat and poor

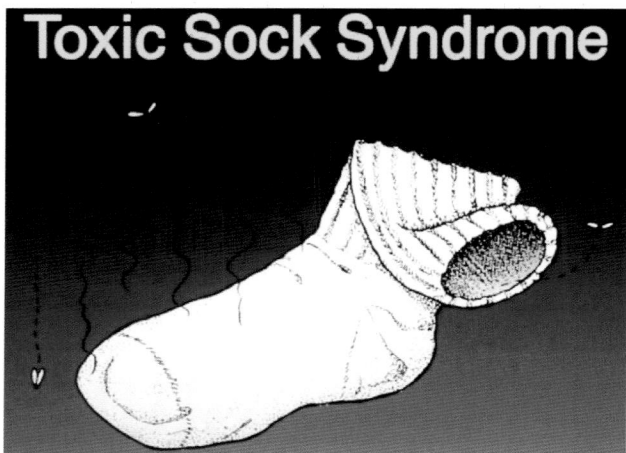

Figure 14-50 Toxic sock syndrome. The abundance of low-molecular-weight molecules is digested by common surface bacteria (e.g., micrococci, diphtheroids, *Propionibacterium* spp., *Corynebacterium* spp.) and leads to metabolic overload. The resultant anaerobic bacterial action produces isovaleric acid (thiol and thiol esters), the substance associated with foot odor.

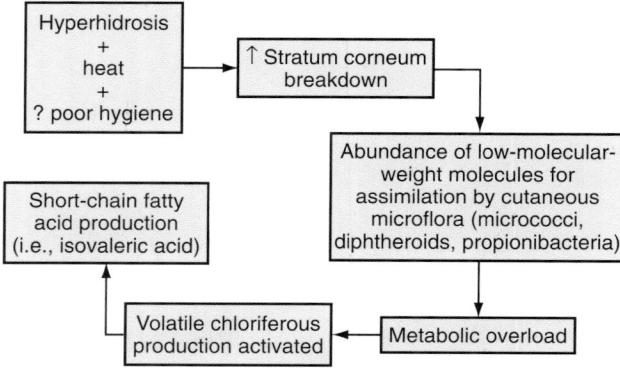

Figure 14-51 Chain of events in foot odor.

hygiene, a situation typically occurring with footwear, leads to breakdown of the stratum corneum, the outermost layer of the epidermis. Poorly constructed shoes of rubber or plastic materials allow unrelieved accumulation of sweat, which leads to skin maceration (Fig. 14-51).

This abundance of low-molecular-weight molecules is digested by common surface bacteria (e.g., micrococci, diphtheroids, *Propionibacterium* spp., *Corynebacterium* spp.) and leads to metabolic overload (Fig. 14-52). The resultant anaerobic bacterial action produces isovaleric acid (thiol and thiol esters), the substance associated with foot odor.[169,171]

Three percent of the U.S. population is unable to smell isovaleric acid. Therefore the physician who disallows patients' complaints of personal odor may be testifying only to his or her own selective anosmia. Many over-the-counter shoe inserts are available to help combat the malodorous foot. (Fig. 14-53).

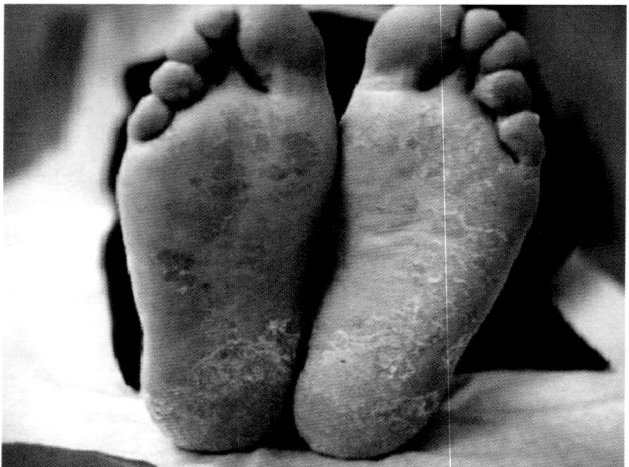

Figure 14-52 Pitted keratolysis.

PLANTAR SWEATING

Plantar sweating is a product of the eccrine glands, not the apocrine glands, of the sole of the foot. With 3000 glands per square inch in thick skin, the rate of sweat production can be greatly increased by fluid ingestion, salicylates, hyperthyroidism, hypoadrenalism, and thermoregulatory disturbances.[165,168]

Emotional hyperhidrosis is transmitted through an autosomal dominant gene. Mental, emotional, or sensory stimulation causes increased sudomotor impulses from the cortex, which leads to hypersecretion. Pools of plantar sweat form, leading to destructive sweating and staining. *Pitted keratolysis*, a foul-smelling dermatologic manifestation with discrete pits on the weight-bearing surface of the foot, may be seen in chronic cases.[175]

Plantar sweating has no known racial predilection, and it is mostly seen in young and middle-aged adults. Sweating decreases or ceases during sleep.

Treatment of plantar bromhidrosis focuses on reducing local sweating and inhibiting the growth of local bacteria. This may be accomplished by frequent washing, dusting the foot with powder to absorb perspiration (e.g., Desenex, Ammens, Efosorb), and changing shoes and socks several times during the day. Cotton absorbent hose and shoes made of materials that breathe can be helpful. Orthotics can be purchased to help keep the shoes dry. Activated-charcoal shoe inserts show brisk over-the-counter sales, but they generally do not work.

The feet should be well dried after washing, and shoes should be aired out for at least 24 hours after use. Patients should go barefoot or wear sandals. Shoes that continue to smell should be thrown out. The ingestion of garlic, onions, curries, chilies, and alcohol will add natural odor to foot sweat.

Homeopathic remedies include soaking the feet in black tea. Two tea bags are steeped in 1 pint of boiling water for 15 minutes, the tea is added to 2 quarts of cool water, and the feet are soaked for 20 to 30 minutes. Some

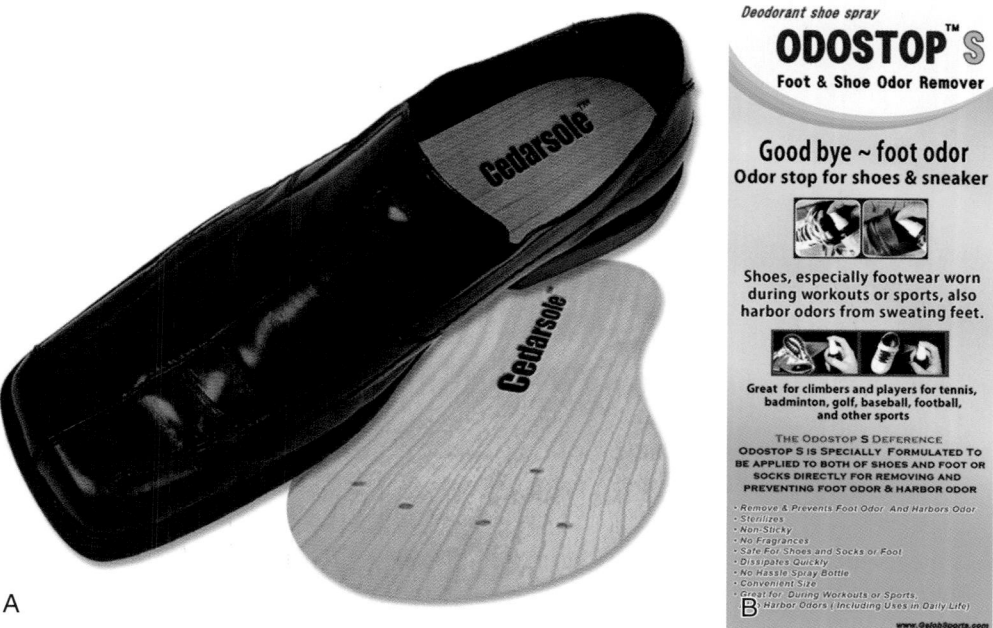

A

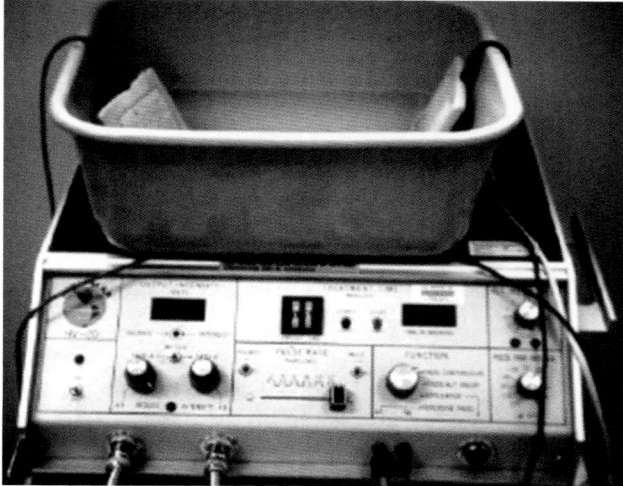

B

Figure 14-53 **A,** An example of over-the-counter inserts for the treatment of foot odor. **B,** Odor sprays are also available over the counter.

patients report improvement after 7 to 10 days of daily soaks. Similar results are reported after soaking in a solution of one part apple cider vinegar to two parts water.[174] Europeans add sage to their shoes. Use of ginger and radish rubs is reported, and there are anecdotal discussions of kosher salt soaks being helpful. After the salt water soak, feet are allowed to air dry to enhance the effect. In the southeastern United States, there are many reports of Listerine soaks neutralizing the odor.

Silver has inherent antimicrobial properties. The element binds with denatured proteins and ammonia, resulting in instant odor reduction. Emerging applications of this technology can be seen where silver has been bonded to synthetic fibers. This is now being used in manufacturing socks and diabetic shoes. The antimicrobial effect may prove effective in assuaging numerous skin-related problems.

Antiperspirants (aluminum chlorhydrate and aluminum zirconium tetrachlorohydrex glycine) can decrease moisture production but can lead to skin irritation. Burlington makes Bioguard Socks with multiple layers containing silicone quaternary amines. The amines kill bacteria and are supposed to last the life of the sock.

Topical antibiotics, topical azoles, oral erythromycin, and perhaps daily soaks with potassium permanganate (1:2000) or Burow solution (aluminum acetate, 1:40) decrease odor production. Benzoyl peroxide 5% or 10% gel is available without a prescription and can be applied in a similar manner, but it can bleach colored fabrics. Topical scented formaldehyde and topical glutaraldehyde have been used in the past to suppress plantar sweating, but they can cause allergic sensitization.

Figure 14-54 Iontophoresis machine.

If these methods fail to diminish foot odor in 3 to 4 weeks or if the skin appears abnormal, a more serious skin problem might exist. Athlete's foot with superinfection from bacteria can cause profound odor and requires referral to a dermatologist.

In emotional hyperhidrosis, atropine-like drugs (e.g., propantheline [Pro-Banthine], 15 mg three times a day) have been used, but the side effects (mouth dryness, visual disturbances, hyperthermia, convulsions) are often more troubling than the sweating itself. In some patients, tranquilizers (e.g., alprazolam [Xanax] 0.5 mg) can modify the emotional source.

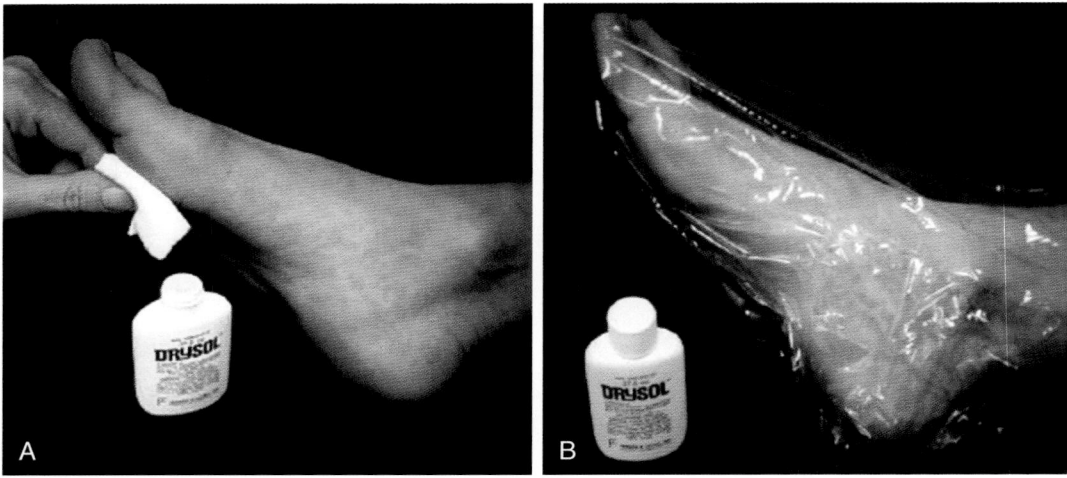

Figure 14-55 **A,** Apply Drysol. **B,** Wrap in plastic.

Iontophoresis is the use of high-voltage current through tap water to produce anhidrosis high in the sweat duct. A regimen of 15 to 20 minutes three times a week produces the desired anhidrosis, after which maintenance therapy is performed every 3 to 4 weeks. Anticholinergic drugs have been added but are thought to be too dangerous for patient use. Although this therapy is quite effective, it requires special equipment, trained personnel, and careful monitoring to ensure that burns do not occur.[167,172] General Medical Co. in Los Angeles makes a battery-operated iontophoresis device that can be used with tap water for home use (Fig. 14-54).

Drysol, a solution of 20% aluminum chloride in anhydrous ethanol, is currently the treatment of choice for plantar bromhidrosis (Fig. 14-55). Applied at bedtime and occluded with a vapor-impermeable material (e.g., plastic wrap), it is left on overnight. On rising each morning, the patient should bathe. Drysol should not be applied to broken skin.[163] This treatment should be repeated for two consecutive nights, then every three to seven nights as required. It suppresses the bacterial growth while decreasing eccrine sweating. For patients bothered by the 20% solution, a weaker 6.25% preparation is available (Xerac AC). Minor skin irritation can also be managed with weak steroid creams.

Lumbar sympathectomy can also be used to reduce plantar sweating, but it is reserved for extreme cases. When sympathectomy is complete, it produces total anhidrosis, and the soles of the feet can become excessively dry. Sweating can return years later from sympathetic regeneration, activity of extraganglionic fibers, or upregulation of distal receptors. Sympathectomy for multiple extremities leads to problems with compensatory hyperhidrosis, thermal regulation, and control of bowel or bladder function.[29]

Botulinum toxin A (Botox) has been used in recent years to halt plantar and axillary hyperhidrosis.[162,177] More recently, it has also been used to combat the effects of hyperhidrosis at the distal portion of a residual limb

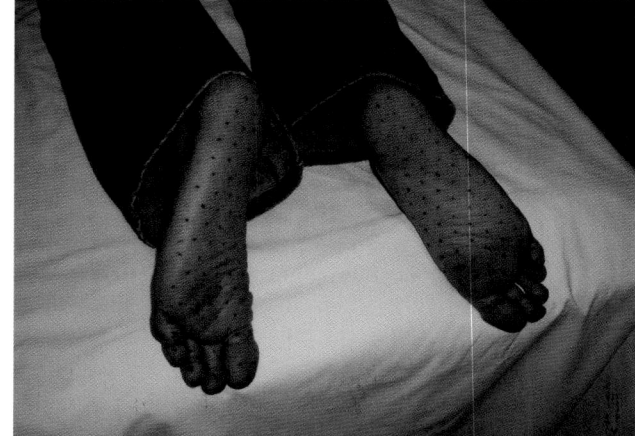

Figure 14-56 Foot marked out for botulinum toxin injections for plantar hyperhydrosis.

in amputees.[170] Although this modality may be promising, it is uncomfortable and expensive (often $1000 per foot). The frequency of treatment and expected longevity of results remain to be well defined in large groups. Nonetheless, botulinum toxin A injections appear to offer patients considerable relief from plantar hyperhidrosis (Fig. 14-56).

In summary, the physician should not initially dismiss the troublesome problem of malodorous feet. If the feet are left untreated, the course will be unaltered, but with proper care, this embarrassing problem can be controlled and its significant psychologic sequelae avoided.

REFERENCES
Complex Regional Pain Syndrome; The Polysurgical Foot Cripple

1. Adami S, Fossaluzza V, Gatti D, Fracassi E, Braga V: Bisphosphonate therapy of reflex sympathetic dystrophy syndrome, *Ann Rheum Dis* 1997 56:201–204, 1997.
2. Argoff CE: Managing neuropathic pain: new approaches for today's practice. Medscape CME [expired]. Available at

http://www.medscape.com/viewprogram/2361. Accessed June 4, 2006.

3. Argoff CE: Targeted topical peripheral analgesics in the management of pain, *Curr Pain Headache Rep* 7:34–38, 2003.
4. Attal N, Brasseur L, Guirimand D, et al: Are oral cannabinoids safe and effective in refractory neuropathic pain? *Eur J Pain* 8:173–177, 2004.
5. Azad SC, Beyer A, Römer AW, et al: Continuous axillary brachial plexus analgesia with low dose morphine in patients with complex regional pain syndromes, *Eur J Anaesthesiol* 17:185–188, 2000.
6. Baron R, Blumberg H, Jänig W: Clinical characteristics of patients with complex regional pain syndrome in Germany with special emphasis on vasomotor function. In Jänig W, Stanton-Hicks M, editors: Reflex sympathetic dystrophy: a reappraisal (Progress in pain research and management, vol 6). Seattle, 1996, International Association for the Study of Pain, p 25.
7. Beaser R: Diabetic neuropathies: Current treatment strategies. Medscape CME [expired]. Available at http://www.medscape.com/viewprogram/496065. Accessed June 5, 2006.
8. Besse JL, Gadeyne S, Galand-Desme S, Lerat JL, Moyen B: Effect of vitamin C on prevention of complex regional pain syndrome type I in foot and ankle surgery, *Foot Ankle Surg* 15:179–182, 2009.
9. Boas RA: Complex regional pain syndromes: symptoms, signs, and differential diagnosis. In Jänig W, Stanton-Hicks M, editors: *Reflex sympathetic dystrophy: a reappraisal* (*Progress in pain research and management*, vol 6). Seattle, 1996, International Association for the Study of Pain, p 79.
10. Bodde MI, Dijkstra PU, den Dunnen WF, et al: Therapy-resistant complex regional pain syndrome type I: to amputate or not? *J Bone Joint Surg Am* 93:1799–1805, 2011.
11. Calvillo O, Racz G, Didie J, Smith K: Neuroaugmentation in the treatment of complex regional pain syndrome of the upper extremity, *Acta Orthop Belg* 64:57–63, 1998.
12. Christensen K, Jensen EM, Noer I: The reflex dystrophy syndrome response to treatment with systemic corticosteroids, *Acta Chir Scand* 148:653–655, 1982.
13. Colton AM, Fallat LM: Complex regional pain syndrome, *J Foot Ankle Surg* 35:284–296, 1996.
14. Connelly NR, Reuben S, Brull SJ: Intravenous regional anesthesia with ketorolac-lidocaine for the management of sympathetically-mediated pain, *Yale J Biol Med* 68:95–99, 1995.
15. Cooper DE, DeLee JC, Ramamurthy S: Reflex sympathetic dystrophy of the knee. Treatment using continuous epidural anesthesia, *J Bone Joint Surg Am* 71:365–369, 1989.
16. Correll GE, Maleki J, Gracely EJ, Muir JJ, Harbut RE: Subanesthetic ketamine infusion therapy: a retrospective analysis of a novel therapeutic approach to complex regional pain syndrome, *Pain Med* 5:263–275, 2004.
17. Covington EC: Psychological issues in reflex sympathetic dystrophy. In Jänig W, Stanton-Hicks M, editors: Reflex sympathetic dystrophy: a reappraisal. Progress in pain research and management, vol 6, Seattle, 1996, International Association for the Study of Pain, p 191.
18. Cronin A, Keifer JC, Baghdoyan HA, et al: Opioid inhibition of rapid eye movement sleep by a specific mu receptor agonist, *Br J Anaesth* 74:188–192, 1995.
19. DeVaul RA, Faillace LA: Persistent pain and illness insistence: a medical profile of proneness to surgery, *Am J Surg* 135:828–833, 1978.
20. DeVaul RA, Hall RC, Faillace LA: Drug use by the polysurgical patient, *Am J Psychiatry* 135:682–685, 1978.
21. Dirks HF, Wunder J, Reynolds J, et al: A scale for predicting nonphysiological contributions to pain, *Psychother Psychosom* 65:153–157, 1996.
22. Duhmke RM, Cornblath DD, Hollingshead JR: Tramadol for neuropathic pain, *Cochrane Database Syst Rev* 2:CD003726, 2004.
23. Ekman EF, Koman AL: Acute pain following musculoskeletal injuries and orthopaedic surgery: mechanisms and management, *Instr Course Lect* 54:21–33, 2005.
24. Faust D: The detection of deception, *Neurol Clin* 13:255–265, 1995.
25. Forman N, Palmeri B, Menza M: Somatoform disorders: diagnosis and treatment, *N J Med* 90:119–122, 1993.
26. Forouzanfar T, Köke AJ, van Kleef M, Weber WE: Treatment of complex regional pain syndrome type I, *Eur J Pain* 6:105–122, 2002.
27. Geertzen JH, de Bruijn H, de Bruijn-Kofman AT, Arendzen JH: Reflex sympathetic dystrophy: early treatment and psychological aspects, *Arch Phys Med Rehabil* 75:442–446, 1994.
28. Gellman H, Nichols D: Reflex sympathetic dystrophy in the upper extremity, *J Am Acad Orthop Surg* 5:313–322, 1997.
29. Gillespie JA: Extent and permanence of denervation produced by lumbar sympathectomy, *BMJ* 1:79–83, 1961.
30. Goris RJ, Dongen LM, Winters HA: Are toxic oxygen radicals involved in the pathogenesis of reflex sympathetic dystrophy? *Free Radic Res Commun* 3:13–18, 1987.
31. Gracely RH, Price DD, Roberts WJ, et al: Quantitative sensory testing in patients with complex regional pain syndrome (CRPS) II and I. In Jänig W, Stanton-Hicks M, editors: Reflex sympathetic dystrophy: a reappraisal. Progress in pain research and management, vol 6, Seattle, 1996, International Association for the Study of Pain, p 151.
32. Groopman J: When pain remains, *New Yorker*, October 10, 2005, pp 36–41.
33. Grundberg AB: Reflex sympathetic dystrophy: treatment with long-acting intramuscular corticosteroids, *J Hand Surg Am* 21:667–670, 1996.
34. Harke H, Gretenkort P, Ladleif HU, Rahman S, Harke O: The response of neuropathic pain and pain in complex regional pain syndrome I to carbamazepine and sustained-release morphine in patients pretreated with spinal cord stimulation: a double-blinded randomized study, *Anesth Analg* 92:488–495, 2001.
35. Kalso E, Edwards JE, Moore RA, McQuay HJ: Opioids in chronic non-cancer pain: systematic review of efficacy and safety, *Pain* 112:372–380, 2004.
36. Katz MM, Hungerford DS: Reflex sympathetic dystrophy affecting the knee, *J Bone Joint Surg Br* 69:797–803, 1987.
37. Kemler MA, Barendse GA, van Kleef M, et al: Spinal cord stimulation in patients with chronic reflex sympathetic dystrophy, *N Engl J Med* 343:618–624, 2000.
38. Kemler MA, Barendse GA, Van Kleef M, et al: Electrical spinal cord stimulation in reflex sympathetic dystrophy: retrospective analysis of 23 patients, *J Neurosurg* 90(Suppl 1):79–83, 1999.
39. Kemler MA, De Vet HC, Barendse GA, et al: The effect of spinal cord stimulation in patients with chronic reflex sympathetic dystrophy: two years' follow-up of the randomized controlled trial, *Ann Neurol* 55:13–18, 2004.
40. King SA: Antidepressants: a valuable adjunct for musculoskeletal pain, *J Musculoskel Med* 12:51–57, 1995.
41. Kingery WS: A critical review of controlled clinical trials for peripheral neuropathic pain and complex regional pain syndromes, *Pain* 73:123–139, 1997.
42. Koban M, Leis S, Schultze-Mosgau S, Birkin F: Tissue hypoxia in complex regional pain syndrome, *Pain* 104:149–157, 2003.
43. Koltzenberg M: Afferent mechanisms mediating pain and hyperalgesias in neuralgia. In Jänig W, Stanton-Hicks M, editors: Reflex sympathetic dystrophy: a reappraisal. Progress in pain research and management, vol 6, Seattle, 1996, International Association for the Study of Pain, p 123.

44. Koman AL, Poehling GG, Smith TL: Complex regional pain syndrome: reflex sympathetic dystrophy and causalgia. In Green DP, editor: *Operative hand surgery*, ed 4, New York, 1999, Churchill Livingstone.

45. Kozin F, Ryan LM, Carerra GF, Soin JS, Wortmann RL: The reflex sympathetic dystrophy syndrome (RSDS). III. Scintigraphic studies, further evidence for the therapeutic efficacy of systemic corticosteroids, and proposed diagnostic criteria, *Am J Med* 70:23–30, 1981.

46. Law JD, Kirkpatrick AF: Update: spinal cord stimulation, *Am J Pain Manage* 2:34–43, 1992.

47. Lee BY, LaRiccia PJ, Newberg AB: Acupuncture in theory and practice, *Hosp Physician* 40:11–17, 2004.

48. Mackenzie TB: The initial patient interview: Identifying when psychosocial factors are at work, *Postgrad Med* 74:259–265, 1983.

49. Maihofner C, Handwerker HO, Neundorfer B, Birklein F: Patterns of cortical reorganization in complex regional pain syndrome, *Neurology* 61:1707–1715, 2003.

50. Mailis A, Furlan A: Sympathectomy for neuropathic pain, *Cochrane Database Syst Rev* 2:CD002918, 2003.

51. Mailis A, Wade J: Profile of caucasian women with possible genetic predisposition to reflex sympathetic dystrophy: a pilot study, *Clin J Pain* 10:210–217, 1994.

52. Manicourt DH, Brasseur JP, Boutsen Y, et al: Role of alendronate in therapy for posttraumatic complex regional pain syndrome type I of the lower extremity, *Arthritis Rheum* 50:3690–3697, 2004.

53. Marwick C: Acceptance of some acupuncture applications, *JAMA* 278:1725–1727, 1997.

54. Masterton G: Factitious disorders and the surgeon, *Br J Surg* 82:1588–1589, 1995.

55. Max MB, Lynch SA, Muir J, et al: Effects of desipramine, amitriptyline and fluoxetine on pain in diabetic neuropathy, *N Engl J Med* 326:1250–1256, 1992.

56. Mitchell SW: *Injuries of nerves and their consequences*, Philadelphia, 1872, JB Lippincott.

57. Muizelaar JP, Kleyer M, Hertogs IA, DeLange DC: Complex regional pain syndrome (reflex sympathetic dystrophy and causalgia): management with the calcium channel blocker nifedipine and/or the alpha-sympathetic blocker phenoxybenzamine in 59 patients, *Clin Neurol Neurosurg* 99:26–30, 1997.

58. Namaka M, Gramlich CR, Ruhlen D, et al: A treatment algorithm for neuropathic pain, *Clin Ther* 26:951–979, 2004.

59. Nath RK, Mackinnon SE, Stelnicki E: Reflex sympathetic dystrophy: the controversy continues, *Clin Plast Surg* 23:435–446, 1996.

60. North RB, Kidd DH, Zahurak M, et al: Spinal cord stimulation for chronic, intractable pain: experience over two decades, *Neurosurgery* 32:384–395, 1993.

61. Paar GH: Factitious disorders in the field of surgery, *Psychother Psychosom* 62:41–47, 1994.

62. Perez RS, Kwakkel G, Zuurmond WW, de Lange JJ: Treatment of reflex sympathetic dystrophy (CRPS type 1): a research synthesis of 21 randomized clinical trials, *J Pain Symptom Manage* 21:511–526, 2001.

63. Perez RS, Zuurmond WW, Bezemer PD, et al: The treatment of complex regional pain syndrome type I with free radical scavengers: a randomized controlled study, *Pain* 102:297–307, 2003.

64. Phillips WJ, Currier BL: Analgesic pharmacology: II. Specific analgesics, *J Am Acad Orthop Surg* 12:221–233, 2004.

65. Price DD, Long S, Wilsey B, Rafii A Analysis of peak magnitude and duration of analgesia produced by local anesthetics injected into sympathetic ganglia of complex regional pain syndrome patients, *Clin J Pain* 14:216–226, 1998.

66. Ruggeri SB, Athreya BH, Doughty R, et al: Reflex sympathetic dystrophy in children, *Clin Orthop Relat Res* 163:225–230, 1982.

67. Rynearson RR, Stewart WL: The dependency problem: the most common surgical risk, *Surg Clin North Am* 52:459–465, 1972.

68. Schwartzman RJ, Liu JE, Smullens SN, et al: Long-term outcome following sympathectomy for complex regional pain syndrome type 1 (RSD), *J Neurol Sci* 150:149–152, 1997.

69. Serpell MG, Neuropathic Pain Study Group: Gabapentin in neuropathic pain syndromes: a randomised, double-blind, placebo-controlled trial, *Pain* 99:557–566, 2002.

70. Stanton-Hicks M: Complex regional pain syndrome, *Anesth Clin North Am* 21:733–744, 2003.

71. Stanton-Hicks M, Raj PP, Racz GB: Use of regional anesthetics for diagnosis of reflex sympathetic dystrophy and sympathetically maintained pain: a critical evaluation. In Jänig W, Stanton-Hicks M, editors: Reflex sympathetic dystrophy: a reappraisal. Progress in pain research and management, vol 6, Seattle, 1996, International Association for the Study of Pain, p 217.

72. Tennant F: Over-prescribing and overmedicating. Diagnosis is by physical examination, not a pill, *Intractable Pain News* 2005. Available at http://www.paincare.org/phorum-3.4.8a/read.php?f=1&i=11141&t=11141&v=t. Accessed June 4, 2006.

73. Tountas AA, Noguchi A: Treatment of posttraumatic reflex sympathetic dystrophy syndrome (RSDS) with regional intravenous blocks of corticosteroid and lidocaine: a retrospective review of 17 consecutive cases, *J Orthop Trauma* 5:412–419, 1991.

74. Turner JA, Loeser JD, Bell KG: Spinal cord stimulation for chronic low back pain: a systematic literature synthesis, *Neurosurgery* 37:1088–1095, 1995; discussion 1095–1096.

75. van de Vusse AC, Stomp-van den Berg SG, Kessels AH, Weber WE: Randomised controlled trial of gabapentin in complex regional pain syndrome type 1 [ISRCTN84121379], *BMC Neurol* 4:13, 2004.

76. van Dieten HE, Perez RS, van Tulder MW, et al: Cost effectiveness and cost utility of acetylcysteine versus dimethyl sulfoxide for reflex sympathetic dystrophy, *Pharmacoeconomics* 21:139–148, 2003.

77. Varenna M, Zucchi F, Ghiringhelli D, et al: Intravenous clodronate in the treatment of reflex sympathetic dystrophy syndrome. A randomized, double blind, placebo controlled study, *J Rheumatol* 27:1477–1483, 2000.

78. Veldman PH, Goris RJ: Multiple reflex sympathetic dystrophy: which patients are at risk for developing a recurrence of reflex sympathetic dystrophy in the same or another limb? *Pain* 64:463–466, 1996.

79. Voiss DV: Occupational injury: fact, fantasy, or fraud? *Neurol Clin* 13:431–443, 1995.

80. Wallach J: Laboratory diagnosis of factitious disorders, *Arch Intern Med* 154:1690–1696, 1994.

81. Wilder RT: Reflex sympathetic dystrophy in children and adolescents: differences from adults. In Jänig W, Stanton-Hicks M, editors: Reflex sympathetic dystrophy: a reappraisal. Progress in pain research and management, vol 6, Seattle, 1996, International Association for the Study of Pain, p 67.

82. Wilder RT, Berde CB, Wolohan M, et al: Reflex sympathetic dystrophy in children. Clinical characteristics and follow-up of seventy patients, *J Bone Joint Surg Am* 74:910–919, 1992.

83. Wilson PR, Low PA, Bedder MD, et al: Diagnostic algorithm for complex regional pain syndromes. In Jänig W, Stanton-Hicks M, editors: Reflex sympathetic dystrophy: a reappraisal. Progress in pain research and management, vol 6, Seattle, 1996, International Association for the Study of Pain, p 93.

84. Zollinger PE, Kreis RW, van der Muelen HG, et al: No higher risk of CRPS after external fixation of distal radial fractures—

subgroup analysis under randomised vitamin C prophylaxis, *Open Orthop J* 4:71–75, 2010.

85. Zollinger PE, Tuinebreijer WE, Breederveld RS, Kreis RW: Can vitamin C prevent complex regional pain syndrome in patients with wrist fractures? A randomized, controlled, multicenter dose-response study, *J Bone Joint Surg Am* 89:1424–1431, 2007.

86. Zuurmond WW, Langendijk PN, Bezemer PD, et al: Treatment of acute reflex sympathetic dystrophy with DMSO 50% in a fatty cream, *Acta Anaesthesiol Scand* 40:364–367, 1996.

Burns and Exposure

87. Aldrete JA, Ghaly R: Delayed sympathetically maintained pain caused by electrical burn at the current's entry and exit sites, *J Pain Symptom Manage* 9:541–543, 1994.

88. Alison WE Jr, Moore ML, Reilly DA, et al: Reconstruction of foot burn contractures in children, *J Burn Care Rehabil* 14:34–38, 1993.

89. Arvesen A, Wilson J, Rosen L: Nerve conduction velocity in human limbs with late sequelae after local cold injury, *Eur J Clin Invest* 26:443–450, 1996.

90. Balakrishnan C, Rak TP, Meininger MS: Burns of the neuropathic foot following use of therapeutic footbaths, *Burns* 21:622–623, 1995.

91. Barker JR, Haws MJ, Brown RE, et al: Magnetic resonance imaging of severe frostbite injuries, *Ann Plast Surg* 38:275–279, 1997.

92. Bernstein EF, Sullivan FJ, Mitchell JB, et al: Biology of chronic radiation effect on tissues and wound healing, *Clin Plast Surg* 20:435–440, 1993.

93. Bill TJ, Edlich RF, Himel HN: Electric heating pad burns, *J Emerg Med* 12:819–824, 1994.

94. Boswick JA Jr, Thompson JD, Jonas RA: The epidemiology of cold injuries, *Surg Gynecol Obstet* 149:326–332, 1979.

95. Burns BF, McCauley RL, Murphy FL, et al: Reconstructive management of patients with greater than 80 per cent TBSA burns, *Burns* 19:429–433, 1993.

96. Calhoun JH, Evans EB, Herndon DN: Techniques for the management of burn contractures with the Ilizarov fixator, *Clin Orthop Relat Res* 280:117–124, 1992.

97. Crouch C, Smith WL: Long term sequelae of frostbite, *Pediatr Radiol* 20:365–366, 1990.

98. Deignan BJ, Iaquinto JM, Eskildsen SM, et al: Effect of pressure applied during casting on temperatures beneath casts, *J Pediatr Orthop* 31:791–797, 2011.

99. Dembert ML, Dean LM, Noddin EM: Cold weather morbidity among US Navy and Marine Corps personnel, *Mil Med* 146:771–775, 1991.

100. Dowling J, Barry OCD, Lennon F, et al: Lightning injury, *Ir Med J* 77:250–251, 1984.

101. Engrav LH, Dutcher KA, Nakamura D: Rating burn impairment, *Clin Plast Surg* 19:569–572, 1992.

102. Erdogan B, Gorgu M, Girgin O, et al: Application of external fixators in major foot contractures, *J Foot Ankle Surg* 35:218–221, 1996.

103. Fisher JC: Introduction to radiation injury: another silent epidemic, *Clin Plast Surg* 20:431–433, 1993.

104. Francis TJ: Non-freezing cold injury: a historical review, *J R Naval Med Serv* 70:134–139, 1984.

105. Fritz RL, Perrin DH: Cold exposure injuries: prevention and treatment, *Clin Sports Med* 8:111–126, 1989.

106. Gore D, Desai M, Herndon DN, et al: Comparison of complications during rehabilitation between conservative and early surgical management in thermal burns involving the feet of children and adolescents, *J Burn Care Rehabil* 9:92–95, 1988.

107. Grube BJ, Engrav LH, Heimbach DM: Early ambulation and discharge in 100 patients with burns of the foot treated by grafts, *J Trauma* 33:662–664, 1992.

108. Haller JS Jr: Trench foot: a study in military-medical responsiveness in the Great War, 1914–1918, *West J Med* 152:729–733, 1990.

109. Hamlet MP: An overview of medically related problems in the cold environment, *Mil Med* 152:393–396, 1987.

110. Heimbach DM: Early burn excision and grafting, *Surg Clin North Am* 67:93–107, 1987.

111. Helm PA: Burn rehabilitation: dimensions of the problem, *Clin Plast Surg* 19:551–558, 1992.

112. Helm PA, Walker SC: New bone formation at amputation sites in electrically burn-injured patients, *Arch Phys Med Rehabil* 68(5 Pt 1):284–286, 1987.

113. Hopkins RS: Consumer product–related injuries in Athens, Ohio, *Am J Prev Med* 5:104–112, 1989.

114. Inoue G, Miura T: Microgeodic disease affecting the hands and feet of children, *J Pediatr Orthop* 11:59–63, 1991.

115. Johnson J, Silverberg R: Serial casting of the lower extremity to correct contractures during the acute phase of burn care, *Phys Ther* 75:262–266, 1995.

116. Kelsey R, Alvey T: Skin burns from prolonged exposure to wet cement, *J Am Podiatr Med Assoc* 85:315–317, 1995.

117. Kucan JO, Bash D: Reconstruction of the burned foot, *Clin Plast Surg* 19:705–719, 1992.

118. Kumar VN: Intractable foot following frostbite: case report, *Arch Phys Med Rehabil* 63:284–285, 1982.

119. Manoli A 2nd, Smith DG, Hansen ST Jr: Scarred muscle excision for the treatment of established ischemic contracture of the lower extremity, *Clin Orthop Relat Res* 292:309–314, 1993.

120. Memmel H, Kowal-Vern A, Latenser BA: Infections in diabetic burn patients, *Diabetes Care* 27:229–233, 2004.

121. Moghtader JC, Himel HN, Demun EM, et al: Electrical burn injuries of workers using portable aluminum ladders near overhead power lines, *Burns* 19:441–443, 1993.

122. Nishimoto S, Matsushida T, Matsumolo K, et al: A rare case of burn scar malignancy, *Burns* 22:497–499, 1996.

123. Oakley EH: The design and function of military footwear: a review following experiences in the South Atlantic, *Ergonomics* 27:631–637, 1984.

124. Pinzur MS: Frostbite: prevention and treatment, *Biomechanics* 4:14–21, 1997.

125. Pinzur MS, Weaver FM: Is urban frostbite a psychiatric disorder? *Orthopedics* 20:43–45, 1997.

126. Post PW, Donner DD: Frostbite in a pre-Columbian mummy, *Am J Phys Anthropol* 37:187–191, 1972.

127. Pulla RJ, Pickard LJ, Carnett TS: Frostbite: an overview with case presentations, *J Foot Ankle Surg* 33:53–63, 1994.

128. Ridgway CL, Daugherty MB, Warden GD: Serial casting as a technique to correct burn scar contractures: a case report, *J Burn Care Rehabil* 12:67–72, 1991.

129. Ross BW, Krilov MA: A patellar-tendon–bearing orthosis used in pediatric burn rehabilitation, *Arch Phys Med Rehabil* 73:950–952, 1992.

130. Shuler FD, Grisafi FN: Cast-saw burns: evlauation of skin, cast, and blade temperatures generated during cast removal, *J Bone Joint Surg Am* 90:2626–2630, 2008.

131. Taylor MS: Cold weather injuries during peacetime military training, *Mil Med* 157:602–604, 1992.

132. Waymack JP, Fidler J, Warden GD: Surgical correction of burn scar contractures of the foot in children, *Burns* 14:156–160, 1988.

133. Wrenn K: Immersion foot: a problem of the homeless in the 1990s, *Arch Intern Med* 151:785–788, 1991.

Foreign Body Injuries

134. Yang ZN, Shih HR, Chao L, et al: Free transplantation of sub-axillary lateral thoraco-dorsal flap in burn surgery, *Burns* 10:164–169, 1984.

135. Banerjee B, Das RK: Sonographic detection of foreign bodies of the extremities, *Br J Radiol* 64:107–112, 1991.

136. Bostman OM: Osteolytic changes accompanying degradation of absorbable fracture fixation implants, *J Bone Joint Surg Br* 73:679–682, 1991.

137. Frey C: Marine injuries: prevention and treatment, *Orthop Rev* 23:645–649, 1994.

138. Gooding GA, Hardiman T, Sumers M, et al: Sonography of the hand and foot in foreign body detection, *J Ultrasound Med* 6:441–447, 1987.

139. Inaba AS, Zukin DD, Perro M: An update on the evaluation and management of plantar puncture wounds and *Pseudomonas* osteomyelitis, *Pediatr Emerg Care* 8:38–44, 1992.

140. Krych SM, Lavery LA: Puncture wounds and foreign body reactions, *Clin Podiatr Med Surg* 7:725–731, 1990.

141. Markiewitz AD, Karns DJ, Brooks PJ: Late infections of the foot due to incomplete removal of foreign bodies: a report of two cases, *Foot Ankle Int* 15:52–55, 1994.

142. Mizel MS, Steinmetz ND, Trepman E: Detection of wooden foreign bodies in muscle tissue: experimental comparison of computed tomography, magnetic resonance imaging, and ultrasonography, *Foot Ankle Int* 15:437–443, 1994.

143. Montano JB, Steele MT, Watson WA: Foreign body retention in glass-caused wounds, *Ann Emerg Med* 21:1360–1363, 1992.

144. Pelto-Vasenius K, Hirvensalo E, Vasenius J, et al: Osteolytic changes after polyglycolide pin fixation in chevron osteotomy, *Foot Ankle Int* 18:21–25, 1997.

145. Rockett MS, Gentile SC, Gudas SJ, et al: The use of ultrasonography for the detection of retained wooden foreign bodies in the foot, *J Foot Ankle Surg* 34:478–484, 510–511, 1995.

146. Rokkanen P, Bostman O, Vainionpaa S, et al: Absorbable devices in the fixation of fractures, *J Trauma* 40(Suppl 3):S123–S127, 1996.

147. Schneider HJ, Weiss MA, Stern PJ: Silicone-induced erosive arthritis: radiologic features in seven cases, *AJR Am J Roentgenol* 148:923–925, 1987.

148. Schwab RA, Powers RD: Conservative therapy of plantar puncture wounds, *J Emerg Med* 13:291–295, 1995.

149. Talley JH: Fluoroquinolones: new miracle drugs? *Postgrad Med* 89:101–103, 106–108, 111–113, 1991.

Blisters

150. Verdile VP, Freed HA, Gerard J: Puncture wounds to the foot, *J Emerg Med* 7:193–199, 1989.

151. Akers WA: Measurements of friction injuries in man, *Am J Ind Med* 8:473–481, 1985.

152. Berkley SF, McNeil JG, Hightower AW, et al: A cluster of blister-associated toxic shock syndrome in male military trainees and a study of staphylococcal carriage patterns, *Mil Med* 154:496–499, 1989.

153. Carragee EJ, Csongradi JJ, Bleck EE: Early complications in the operative treatment of ankle fractures. Influence of delay before operation, *J Bone Joint Surg Br* 73:79–82, 1991.

154. Darrigrand A, Reynolds K, Jackson R, et al: Efficacy of antiperspirants on feet, *Mil Med* 157:256–259, 1992.

155. Giordano CP, Koval KJ: Treatment of fracture blisters: a prospective study of 53 cases, *J Orthop Trauma* 9:171–176, 1995.

156. Knapik JJ, Hamlet MP, Thompson KJ, et al: Influence of boot-sock systems on frequency and severity of foot blisters, *Mil Med* 161:594–598, 1996.

157. Knapik JJ, Reynolds KL, Duplantis KL, et al: Friction blisters: pathophysiology, prevention and treatment, *Sports Med* 20:136–147, 1995.

158. Patterson HS, Woolley TW, Lednar WM: Foot blister risk factors in an ROTC summer camp population, *Mil Med* 159:130–135, 1994.

159. Reynolds K, Darrigrand A, Roberts D, et al: Effects of an antiperspirant with emollients on foot-sweat accumulation and blister formation while walking in the heat, *J Am Acad Dermatol* 33:626–630, 1995.

160. Varela CD, Vaughn TK, Carr JB, et al: Fracture blisters: clinical and pathological aspects, *J Orthop Trauma* 7:417–427, 1993.

Foot Odor and Sweating

161. Aluminum chloride for hyperhidrosis, *Drug Ther Bull* 19:101–102, 1981.

162. Campanati A, Bernardini ML, Gesuita R, Offidani A: Plantar focal idiopathic hyperhidrosis and botulinum toxin: a pilot study, *Eur J Dermatol* 17:52–54, 2007.

163. Critchley M: *The citadel of the senses*, New York, 1986, Raven.

164. Fitzpatrick TB, Eisen AZ, Wolff K, et al: *Dermatology in general medicine*, ed 4, New York, 1993, McGraw-Hill, pp 753–755.

165. Darrigrand A, Reynolds K, Jackson R, et al: Efficacy of antiperspirants on feet, *Mil Med* 157:256–259, 1992.

166. Gibbons B: The intimate sense of smell, *National Geographic* 170:324–361, 1986.

167. Grice K: Hyperhidrosis and its treatment by iontophoresis, *Physiotherapy* 66:43–44, 1980.

168. Hurley HJ: Disorders of the eccrine sweat gland. In Moschella SL, Pillsbury DM, Hurly HJ, editors: *Dermatology*, Philadelphia, 1975, WB Saunders, pp 1165–1190.

169. Kanda F, Yagi E, Fukada M, et al: Elucidation of chemical compounds responsible for foot odor, *Br J Dermatol* 122:771–776, 1990.

170. Kern U, Kohl M, Seifert U, Schlereth T: Botulinum toxin type B in the treatment of residual limb hyperhidrosis for lower limb amputees: a pilot study, *Am J Phys Med Rehabil* 90:321–329, 2011.

171. Kobayashi S: Relationship between an offensive smell given from human foot and *Staphylococcus epidermidis*, *Jpn J Dermatol* 45:797–800, 1990.

172. Levit F: Simple device for treatment of hyperhidrosis by iontophoresis, *Arch Dermatol* 98:505–507, 1968.

173. Pedowitz WJ: The malodorous foot, *Foot Ankle Int* 17:54–55, 1996.

174. Ramsey ML: Foot odor: how to clean the air, *Physician Sports Med* 24:91–92, 1996.

175. Rook A, editor: *Textbook of dermatology*, Boston, 1986, Blackwell Scientific, pp 1894–1895.

176. Strauss EJ, Petrucelli G, Bong M, et al: Blisters associated with lower-extremity fracture: results of a prospective treatment protocol, *J Orthop Trauma* 20:618–622, 2006.

177. Vergilis-Kalner IJ: Same-patient prospective comparison of botox versus dysport for the treatment of primary axillary hyperhidrosis and review of literature, *J Drugs Dermatol* 10:1013–1015, 2011.

Infections of the Foot

J. Speight Grimes, Jr.

The foot provides a unique environment for the development of infections. The infections can be aggressive and result in significant disability. The foot's environment is modified by footwear, trauma, systemic illness, and climate. Each of these factors can increase the susceptibility of the foot to infection. Footwear, by its nature, is occlusive and raises the temperature and humidity around the foot. The humidity can reach 100% in the interspaces of the toes. This warm, moist environment is ideal for bacteria.

CLASSIFICATION

Infections are classified to assist with treatment selection. Classification is by host type, organism, or anatomic location. Host factors are the most significant. Hosts can be classified as normal or compromised. A compromised host changes both the differential diagnosis and the treatment of a foot infection. Compromised hosts include patients with systemic illness, poor nutritional state, peripheral vascular disease, trauma, and peripheral neuropathy. Diabetes is the most common systemic host factor in a patient with foot infection. Diabetic foot infections are considered in Chapter 27.

It is convenient to separate infections by the offending organism. The organisms are broadly classified as bacterial, mycobacterial, and fungal. These broad categories are subdivided into numerous groups that determine effective treatment options. Selection of the appropriate antibiotic in particular depends on the involved organism.

Anatomic location determines access to the affected region by therapeutic agents and the body's own defenses, as well as anatomic structures at risk from the infection. The necessity of surgical intervention is often dependent on location of the infection. The location can be classified as soft tissue, joint, or bone. A localized collection of purulent material, an abscess, is a special classification by anatomic location. This isolated space is addressed surgically.

SOFT TISSUE INFECTIONS

Soft tissue infections often present secondary to trauma to the protective stratum corneum of the epidermis (Fig. 15-1). Surgery, injury, maceration, intravenous (IV) drug abuse, eczema, and constitutionally derived skin breaks can provide a portal of entry for the pathologic organism. Blisters, ulcers, and open wounds are often colonized with bacteria. In a compromised host, these bacteria can spread, resulting in a localized, and ultimately systemic, infection. More virulent organisms can use a portal to spread within a normal host. The offending organism can often be deduced from the point of entry and host status. For example, postoperative wound infections in a normal host are often group A streptococci.[5]

Breaks in the epidermis are not necessary for soft tissue to become infected. Some virulent organisms possess toxins that weaken the skin's defenses. These organisms are able to attack healthy hosts without an entry portal.[34] *Staphylococcus aureus* is the primary pathogen to penetrate intact skin. It manifests as cellulitis or an abscess.

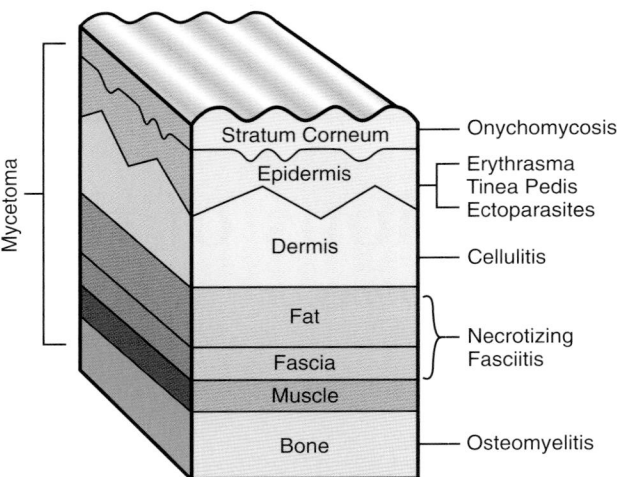

Figure 15-1 Layers of skin affected by infections.

Erythrasma

Erythrasma is a superficial infection of the skin caused by *Corynebacterium minutissimum*. Normally found in the webspaces, it can also be found in a more generalized distribution.

The scaly lesions vary from red to brown, are well defined, and have irregular borders (Fig. 15-2A). The lesions are most commonly asymptomatic but can be pruritic. The lesions can become fissured and macerated, creating breaks in the protective stratum corneum. These openings can result in more extensive infections.

Erythrasma is commonly confused with psoriasis, dermatophytosis, and candidiasis. A Wood lamp examination can help distinguish erythrasma because the colonies glow coral-red. Erythromycin (250 mg four times daily for 14 days) is the treatment of choice.[50]

Cellulitis

Cellulitis is the acute inflammatory response to a pathogen, often bacterial. Aerobic gram-positive cocci, *S. aureus* and streptococci, are the most commonly involved pathogens. Cellulitis is characterized by superficial swelling, pain, erythema, and localized warmth (Fig. 15-2B). Proximal lymphadenopathy is not uncommon. Erythema streaking along the course of lymph drainage (lymphangitis) is common with streptococcal infections, while localized pus-producing lesions are staphyloccal.[33] Cellulitis is limited to the dermis and subcutaneous tissues.

The treatment of cellulitis uses empiric antibiotics directed against *Staphylococcus* and *Streptococcus* species.[5] The affected limb should be elevated to help control swelling. Moist heat is applied to the affected area using a Koch-Mason dressing. This dressing consists of a layer of moist gauze covered with an occlusive barrier. A warming blanket is wrapped over the barrier (Fig. 15-3).

The rise of methicillin-resistant *S. aureus* (MRSA) has complicated the selection of antibiotics. This organism is resistant to the β-lactam antibiotics, including the penicillins

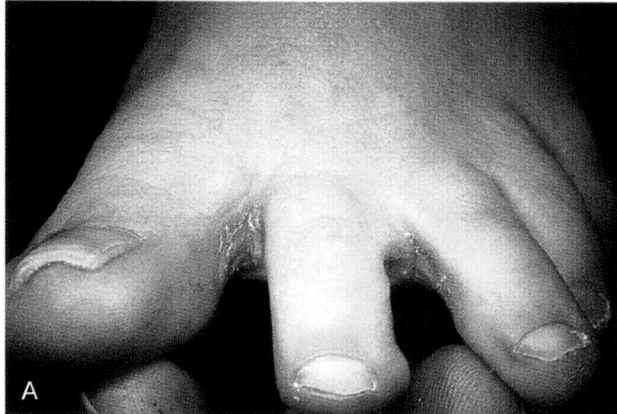

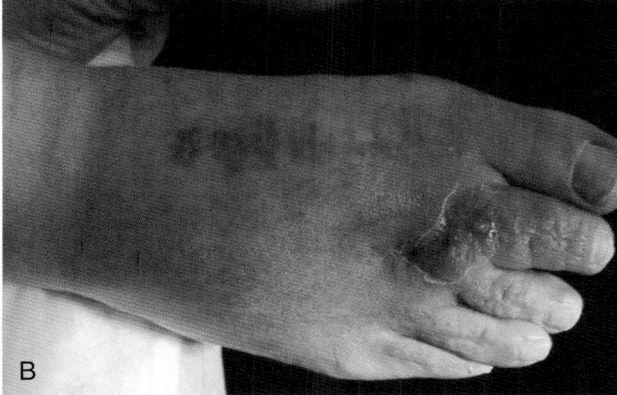

Figure 15-2 **A,** Erythrasma. In advanced cases, fissures develop in the webspaces. **B,** Cellulitis with streaking and erythema on the dorsum of the foot. (**A,** From Dockery G: *Cutaneous disorders of the lower extremity,* Philadelphia, 1997, WB Saunders, p 43. Used with permission.)

and cephalosporins. MRSA is now found in hospital-acquired and community-acquired infections. The risk factors for hospital-acquired MRSA are recent hospitalization, recent surgery, dialysis, residence in a long-term care facility, diabetes, and chronic or repeated courses of antibiotics.[33,118] Fifty-seven percent of nosocomial isolates of *S. aureus* are resistant to methicillin.[110] The risk factors for community-acquired MRSA are young age, socially disadvantaged environment, minority ethnicity, member of the armed forces, an athlete, and primary skin infections.[33,34] MRSA transmission during team sports has been documented and should be considered in the differential diagnosis of clusters of skin abscesses in athletes.[57] A community's bacterial spectrum can assist in determining the risk of community-acquired MRSA in the general population.

For patients with mild cellulitis and no risk factors for MRSA, treatment involves oral first-generation cephalosporins, such as cephalexin 50 mg/kg per day (2 g divided into 4 doses for adults) divided every 6 hours. For more severe cases, systemic involvement, or a compromised host, parenteral antibiotics are first-line agents. Cefazolin 80 mg/kg per day (4 g for adults) IV divided four times daily is often the primary agent. An aminoglycoside, gentamicin 5 mg/kg every day, should be added for diabetic patients and IV drug abusers to provide a broader coverage for possible gram-negative species.[5] Alternative medications for infections at risk for both gram-positive and gram-negative organisms are β-lactams/β-lactamase inhibitory combinations, moxifloxacin, tigecycline, or trimethoprim-sulfamethoxazole.[33]

For patients with risk factors for MRSA infections, alternatives to β-lactams should be first-line treatments. Initial treatment of MRSA infections with β-lactams can exacerbate the infection or compromise outcomes by delaying appropriate treatment. For mild cases, clindamycin, a fluoroquinolone (moxifloxacin has extended gram-positive activity), tetracycline, or trimethoprim are acceptable choices.[33] Selection of an antibiotic depends on resistance spectrums of the community and patient factors. For severe infections with suspected MRSA or failure of a β-lactam, parenteral treatment with linezolid, daptomycin, tigecycline, or vancomycin is appropriate. Because of concerns over the cost and the possibility of resistance to these agents, these antibiotics should be reserved for severe infections with a high clinical suspicion of MRSA.

The patient should be reevaluated at 48 hours after initiation of treatment. If there is poor clinical response, the antibiotic therapy should be changed. One should consider clindamycin or amoxicillin-clavulanate in these patients. The erythema can continue for days after the infection has been effectively treated. Desquamation of the skin is common as the localized edema resolves.

Necrotizing Fasciitis

Necrotizing fasciitis is a rapidly destructive infection of soft tissues with a high mortality rate. Early diagnosis is the key to effective management. This infection spreads along the fascial planes and is associated with thrombosis of the cutaneous microcirculation. It generally affects skin, subcutaneous tissues, and fascia. It is often associated with streptococcal species; however, the majority of cases are polymicrobial.[23,35,120] A portal of entry is found in only half of all patients.[120] Risk factors include diabetes, obesity, peripheral vascular disease, intravenous drug use, alcohol abuse, malnutrition, smoking, corticosteroid therapy, immune suppression, cancer, and age.[13] Nonsteroidal antiinflammatory drugs (NSAIDs) can delay the diagnosis of necrotizing fasciitis by reducing the symptoms but have not been shown to be a risk factor.[10]

The clinician should maintain a high clinical suspicion of necrotizing fasciitis. Because of the limited clinical signs, an initial diagnosis of cellulitis is common. The definitive signs of necrotizing fasciitis are hemorrhagic bullae, skin necrosis, fluctuance, crepitus, and neurologic deficits. These definitive signs are often not found until late in the disease progression.[120] Delay in treatment can significantly increase the risk of mortality. Patients with a risk factor, pain out of proportion to clinical findings, or subcutaneous air on radiographs should be considered at risk for necrotizing fasciitis. The threshold for surgical debridement should be low in these patients. Failure of

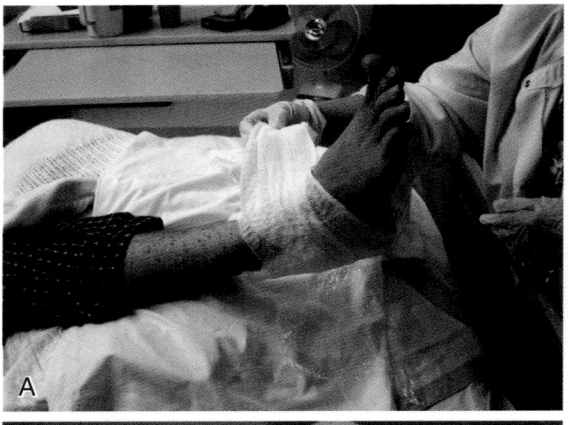
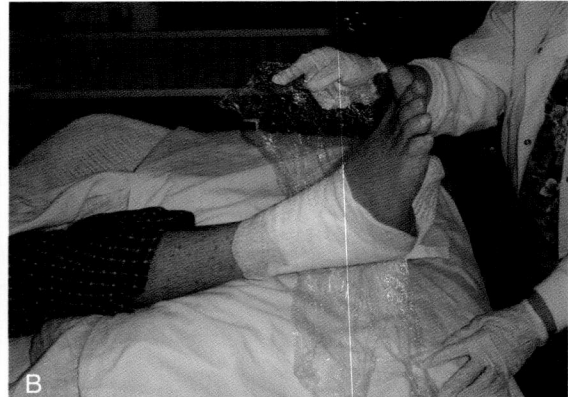
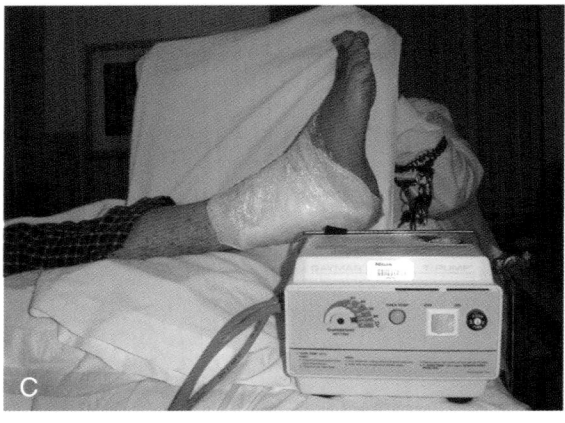

Figure 15-3 Koch-Mason dressing. **A,** Moist gauze is applied to the affected area. **B,** The gauze is covered with an occlusive barrier, plastic wrap in this instance. **C,** A warming blanket set for 40°C (104°F) is wrapped around the limb.

intravenous antibiotics in the treatment of cellulitis points to an early presentation of necrotizing fasciitis.

Laboratory data may be useful in identifying high-risk patients presenting with cellulitis but should never delay surgical treatment of patients with clinical presentation consistent with necrotizing fasciitis. Table 15-1 lists the components of the Laboratory Risk Indicator for Necrotizing Fasciitis (LRINEC). Patients with a score of 6 to 7 should be considered moderate risk, and greater than 7 should be considered high risk.[121] Interventions to correct laboratory disturbances can reduce the accuracy of the score, but an increasing score despite antibiotics may indicate the presence of necrotizing fasciitis.

The risk factors for necrotizing fasciitis include smoking, diabetes, IV drug abuse, and peripheral vascular disease.[35,119,120] The lower extremity is the most commonly affected region.[23] The foot is the second most common site in the lower extremity.[35] Patients rapidly deteriorate. Leukocytosis, weeping blisters, blue skin discoloration, sensory deficits, systemic sepsis, shock, and mental status changes are late manifestations.[23,119] Figure 15-4 shows the clinical appearance of necrotizing fasciitis.

Treatment of necrotizing fasciitis involves early surgical debridement and broad-spectrum antibiotics. Because of the thrombosis of microcirculation, antibiotics alone are ineffective. In suspicious cases, a limited biopsy is often warranted. A 2-cm incision is made under local anesthesia. The surgeon bluntly dissects down to the deep

Table 15-1 LRINEC Scoring		
Sum of the Score for the Six Components		
0-5	Low risk	<50%
6-7	Moderate risk	50%-75%
8-13	High risk	>75%
Laboratory Test	**Value**	**Score**
C-reactive protein (mg/L)	<150	0
	≥150	4
White blood cell count	<15,000	0
(cells/μL)	15,000-25,000	1
	>25,000	2
Hemoglobin (g/dL)	>13.5	0
	11-13.5	1
	<11	2
Sodium (mmol/L)	>135	0
	<135	2
Creatinine level (mg/dL)	≤1.58	0
	>1.58	2
Glucose (mg/dL)	<180	0
	>180	1

Modified from Wong C, Khin, L, Heng K, et al: The LRINEC (Laboratory Risk Indicator for Necrotizing Fasciitis) score: a tool for distinguishing necrotizing fasciitis from other soft tissue infections, *Crit Care Med* 32:1535–1541, 2004.
LRINEC, Laboratory Risk Indicator for Necrotizing Fasciitis.

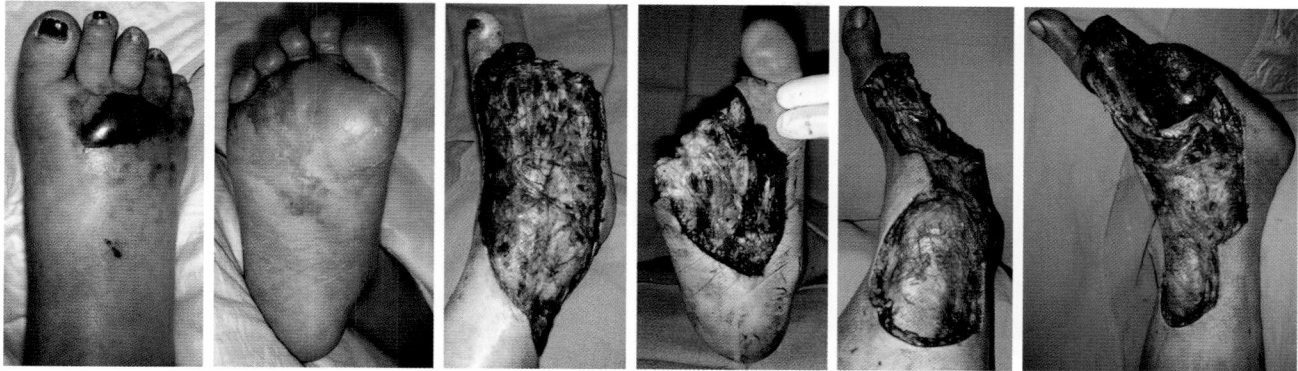

Figure 15-4 Necrotizing fasciitis of the foot. **A** and **B,** Clinical appearance on presentation. **C** and **D,** After first debridement. **E** and **F,** After final debridement. (Courtesy Thomas S. Roukis, DPM. Reproduced from Schade VL, Roukis TS, Haque M: Clostridium septicum necrotizing fasciitis of the forefoot secondary to adenocarcinoma of the colon: case report and review of the literature. *J Foot Ankle Surg.* 49(2):159.e1-8, 2010.)

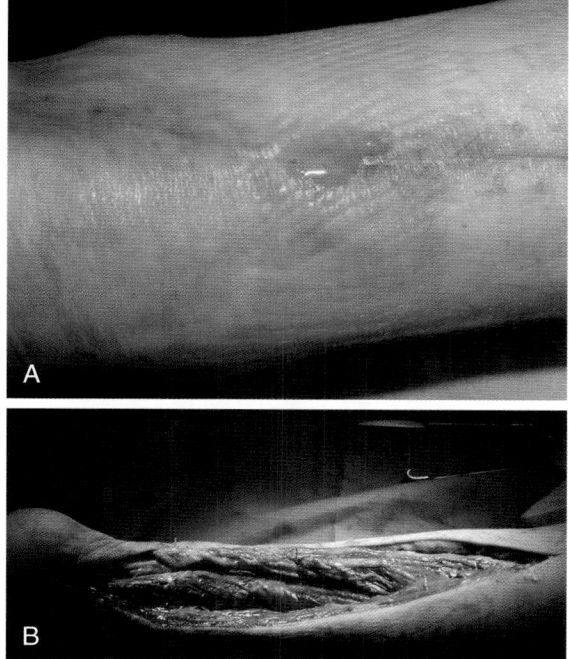

Figure 15-5 **A,** Small amount of clear exudate in postoperative incision. **B,** Wound developed into necrotizing fasciitis of the leg, seen after debridement of the necrotic tissue. (Courtesy Dr. Alister Younger.)

fascia. Biopsy specimens are sent for cultures and pathologic examination. A lack of bleeding, dishwater-colored drainage, or minimal resistance to finger dissection along the fascial plane are signs of necrotizing fasciitis.[23,120] An aggressive surgical debridement should be extended until the skin and subcutaneous tissue appear viable and firmly adherent to the underlying fascia (see Fig. 15-4). All necrotic skin, subcutaneous tissue, fascia, and muscle should be removed (Fig. 15-5). Repeat debridement should be carried out at 48-hour intervals.[35,120] Hydrogel or negative-pressure therapy dressings are used to promote granulation tissue.[13]

Medical treatment with antibiotics starts empirically with a combination of a penicillin, an aminoglycoside, and clindamycin. Clindamycin and linezolid inhibit M protein and exotoxin production, facilitating phagocytosis and suppressing the production of tumor necrosis factor-α.[13] Culture results are used to modify the antibiotic regimen. Coagulopathy, cardiopulmonary collapse, and acute renal failure are seen in the more advanced stages of necrotizing fasciitis. Blood component therapy, dialysis, and cardiopulmonary support should be used aggressively when indicated. A patient's metabolic requirements are doubled during the treatment period. Supplemental feedings or total parental nutrition should be considered.

Hyperbaric oxygen is used as an adjunctive treatment at some medical centers.[13,23] Hyperbaric chambers come in single- and multiple-place systems (Fig. 15-6). Studies have demonstrated a beneficial trend, but there is no conclusive evidence for the effectiveness of hyperbaric oxygen. Prompt surgical debridement continues to be the most important factor in reducing mortality.[23,35,119,120]

Abscesses

An abscess is a collection of purulent material and infection in a closed space. In the foot, the infection is usually an extension of a subcutaneous infection or penetrating wound. Often, abscesses involve the deep spaces of the foot (Fig. 15-7A). With a deep-space infection, the patient presents with pain and swelling along the instep. Examination demonstrates a loss of the longitudinal arch. Patients often become bedridden because of the pain of weight bearing. Loeffler and Ballard[70] described five plantar spaces (Table 15-2).

Treatment

The infection is often polymicrobial. Without treatment, the infection will spread along the flexor tendons, extending into the deep compartment of the leg (Fig. 15-7B-E).

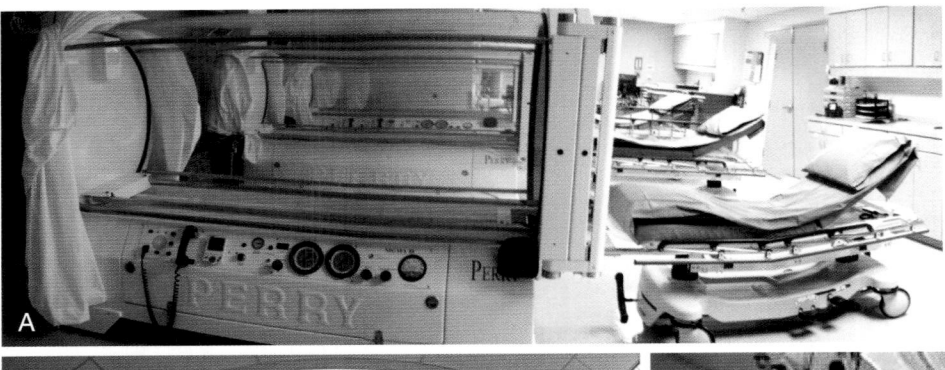
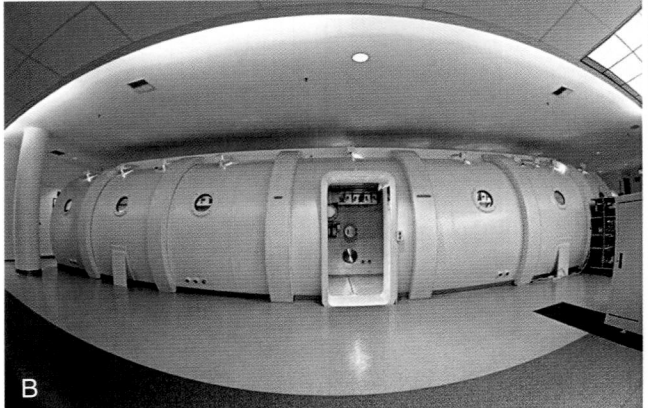
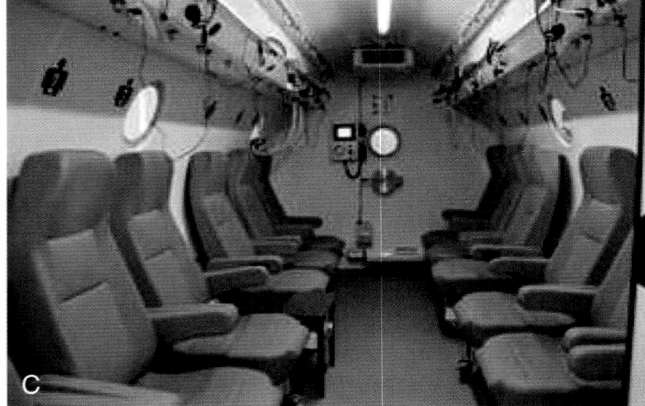

Figure 15-6 **A,** Single-place hyperbaric chambers. **B** and **C,** Multiple-place hyperbaric chamber. (**A,** Courtesy Covenant Wound Care Center, Lubbock, Tex. **B,** Courtesy Cory J. Huffine, MS, RN, NP-C.)

Table 15-2	**Plantar Fascial Spaces of the Foot**	
Number	**Name**	**Description**
1	Superficial posterior	Posterior, plantar to calcaneus and plantar aponeurosis
2	Plantar	Central, between plantar aponeurosis and flexor digitorum brevis
3	Central	Central, between flexor digitorum brevis and quadratus plantae
4	Posterior dorsal	Posterior to metatarsals, between quadratus plantae and tarsal bones
5	Dorsal	Dorsal to adductor hallucis

Surgical debridement is essential in treating the abscess. Appropriate antibiotics are based on intraoperative cultures. If the infection appears to be localized more medially, a medial single-incision fasciotomy can be used to expose the infected compartment. The majority of deep abscesses of the foot occur in the central plantar space. If the infection appears to localize more dorsally in the forefoot, a two-incision fasciotomy approach allows ready exposure to the more dorsal spaces.

DEBRIDEMENT OF PLANTAR ABSCESS
The surgical approach described by Loeffler and Ballard is as follows.[70]

Surgical Technique
1. The incision begins posterior to the medial malleolus and ends between the first and second metatarsal heads. The incision runs along the midline of the plantar surface of the foot.
2. The plantar aponeurosis is divided. This opens the superficial plantar space and the space located just dorsal to the aponeurosis.
3. The dissection continues through the interval between the abductor hallucis and flexor digitorum brevis. This exposes the large space between the flexor digitorum brevis and the quadratus plantae. The plantar arteries and nerves run in this space.
4. The abductor hallucis and flexor digitorum brevis are detached from the calcaneus and are retracted anteriorly. This exposes the quadratus plantae muscle. The flexor hallucis longus tendon is separated from the quadratus plantae, exposing the compartment dorsal to the quadratus plantae.
5. This dissection is continued distally, keeping the plantar nerves visualized. The final compartment is entered deep to the adductor hallucis muscle.
6. The wound is irrigated and left open. Delayed primary closure can usually be achieved in 48 to 72 hours.

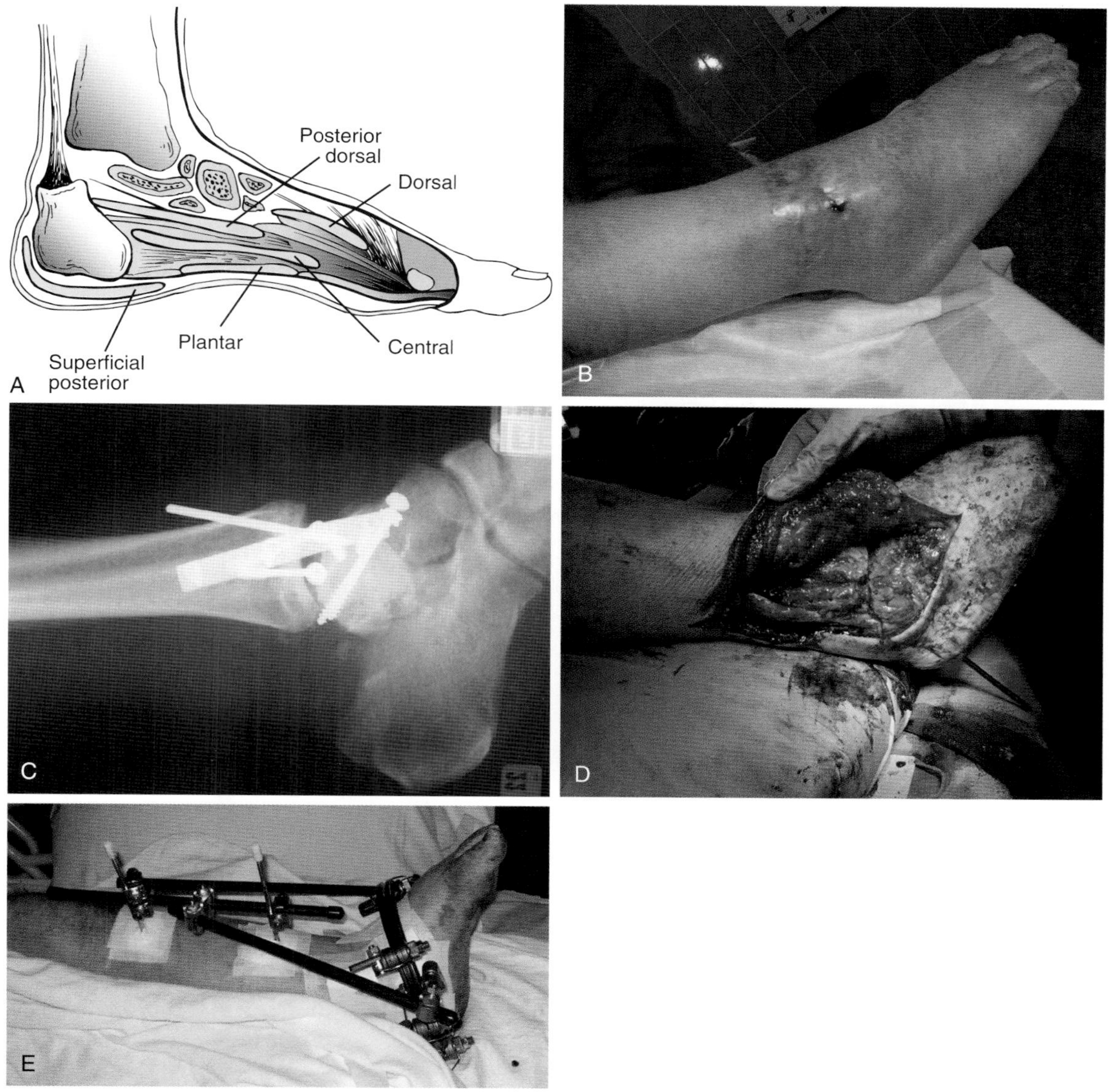

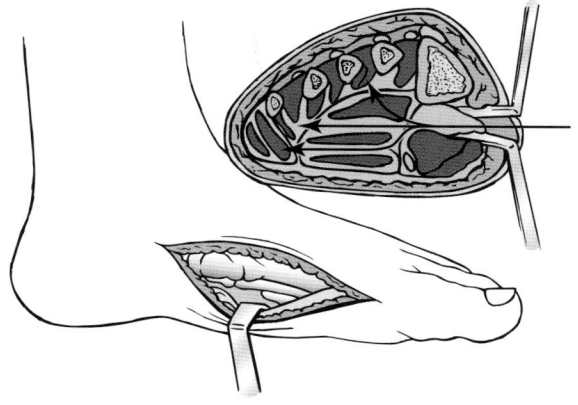

Figure 15-7 **A,** Diagram of potential spaces in the foot. **B,** Abscess in the area of the lateral ankle after surgery. **C,** Radiograph demonstrating internal fixation. **D,** Wide debridement at surgery. **E,** Soft tissue control aided by the application of an external fixator. (Courtesy Dr. Alister Younger.)

DEBRIDEMENT OF MEDIAL ABSCESS

The medial single-incision approach is as follows (Fig. 15-8).

Surgical Technique

1. The incision runs the length of the first metatarsal just along its inferior border.
2. Blunt dissection creates a plane between the first metatarsal and the abductor hallucis muscle.
3. Blunt finger dissection continues into the space dorsal to the quadratus plantae more proximally.
4. Blunt finger dissection is then directed dorsal to the adductor hallucis into the space dorsal to the adductor hallucis. Sharp dissection should be avoided because

Figure 15-8 Diagram of dorsal and medial incision forefoot fasciotomy.

of the presence of the plantar arteries and nerves in this space.

5. Blunt dissection then separates the quadratus plantae and the flexor digitorum brevis to enter this space.

DEBRIDEMENT OF DORSAL ABSCESS

The spaces plantar to the flexor digitorum brevis are difficult to reach from a medial incision. The two-incision approach is as follows.

Surgical Technique

1. Two longitudinal incisions are made directly above the second and fourth metatarsals. The incision runs from the base of metatarsal to the metatarsal neck.
2. Using a blunt instrument, spread longitudinally directly down to bone.
3. The intermetatarsal spaces are entered by blunt dissection adjacent to the metatarsals.
4. The dissection can be extended down to the quadratus plantae muscle. It is difficult to reach the medial and lateral compartments from these incisions.

Gas Gangrene

Gas gangrene can follow trauma or surgical procedures. *Clostridium* species and mixed aerobic and anaerobic infections can produce gas in the soft tissues. The mixed infections show abundant gas on radiographic or magnetic resonance imaging (MRI) studies (Fig. 15-9). Clostridial infections are characterized by muscle necrosis on MRI. Patients with gas gangrene are acutely sick, but they often do not have fever. The affected area is painful, with overlying bullae. These bullae are filled with sweet-smelling fluid if they are infected with clostridia. With mixed infections, the bullae are typically filled with foul-smelling fluid. *Clostridium septicum* is seen in nontraumatic clostridial infection associated with malignancy.[107]

Treatment requires extensive excision of all gangrenous tissue combined with intravenous antibiotics. Sufficient debridement often requires amputation. Penicillin G is the antibiotic of choice for clostridia. Hyperbaric

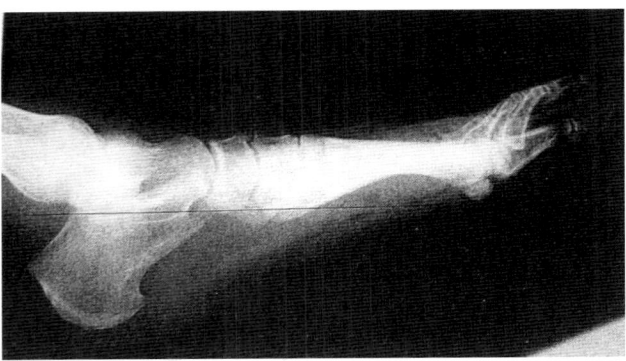

Figure 15-9 Radiograph showing gas in the superficial soft tissues. (From Finkelstein B: Autoamputation of the foot caused by untreated gas gangrene: a case report, *J Foot Ankle Surg* 42:366–670, 2003.)

oxygen can be a useful adjunct treatment when it is available. Repeated surgical debridement at 48 hours is often required.

JOINT INFECTIONS

An infected joint can develop from an adjacent infection, direct traumatic inoculation, or hematogenous spread. Septic arthritis is recognized clinically by the abrupt appearance of redness, swelling, and tenderness about the joint.[43] Fever is not a prerequisite for the diagnosis of septic arthritis.[77] Infection should be a primary consideration in any acute monoarticular arthritis, followed by crystal arthropathy, Reiter syndrome, or a neuropathic joint. Adjacent soft tissue swelling and increased joint fluid can be detected on imaging studies. The diagnosis is made by joint aspiration before antibiotic treatment. The joints most commonly affected are the knee, hip, and ankle.[58] Multiple joints are involved in 20% of cases.[77]

Treatment of suspected septic arthritis begins with aspiration of the joint. The fluid obtained is analyzed for color, Gram stain, cultures, glucose, protein, crystals, and cell count with differential. Aspiration through an area of cellulitis should be avoided.[89] Other studies to consider include peripheral blood cell count, C-reactive protein, erythrocyte sedimentation rate, uric acid, and blood cultures. Joint fluid analysis generally shows leukocyte counts greater than 100,000/mm^3, 90% polymorphonuclear leukocytes, elevated protein, and glucose level less than that of serum.[76]

The standard definition of a positive joint aspiration is a leukocyte count greater than 50,000.[43,67,89] Using that standard, the sensitivity of the examination is only 64%.[67] Any leukocyte count greater than 10,000 cells/mm^3 should be considered suspicious of a joint infection and the patient closely monitored. Gram staining has a sensitivity of 50%.[43] Cultures are generally positive unless the organism is *Neisseria gonorrhoeae* or the patient received antibiotics before the aspiration. Table 15-3 provides a guideline for interpreting laboratory studies.

The joint fluid should also be examined under polarized microscopy for crystals. Both gout and pseudogout can mimic a septic joint. Cell count alone cannot distinguish gout from a septic joint.[77] For patients with no mechanism for direct inoculation of the joint, blood cultures should be obtained. Blood cultures will return the causative agent in approximately 30% of cases.

Diabetes mellitus, joint prosthesis, inflammatory arthritis (rheumatoid), osteoarthritis, crystal arthropathy, cutaneous ulcers, and alcoholism predispose a patient to septic arthritis.[77] Antitumor necrosis factor therapy doubles the risk of septic arthritis.[42] S. aureus is the most common organism in septic joints. In children younger than 2 months, group B streptococci are the most likely pathogens. *Neisseria gonorrhoeae* is a common pathogen in the sexually active young adult. In these patients, an enriched agar with high carbon dioxide culture should be included in the joint aspirate studies. Puncture wounds

Table 15-3 Joint Fluid Analysis

Diagnosis	Cell Count	Glucose	Gram Stain	Cultures
Normal	WBC < 200, PMNs < 25%	≈Serum	Negative	Negative
Noninflammatory*	2000 < WBC < 3000; PMNs < 25%	≈Serum	Negative	Negative
Inflammatory†	5000 < WBC < 75,000; PMNs 50%-75%	<75% serum	Negative	Negative
Septic	WBCs > 50,000; PMNs > 75%	<50% serum	Positive in 50%	Positive before antibiotics

PMN, polymorphonucleocyte; WBC, white blood cell.
*Degenerative joint disease, neuropathy, systemic lupus erythematosus, rheumatic fever.
†Gout, pseudogout, systemic lupus erythematosus, psoriasis, Reiter disease, rheumatoid arthritis.

can inoculate the joint with anaerobic and gram-negative species.

Drainage of purulent material from the joint is essential in the treatment of septic arthritis. This may be by open surgical procedure or aspiration. The method chosen is controversial. There is little evidence to support open surgical drainage of an infected joint in the foot.[73] Daily aspiration of the affected joint is often sufficient. Indications for surgical intervention include failure to clinically respond within 48 hours of therapy, persistence of pyarthrosis beyond 48 hours, inaccessibility of the joint for aspiration, viscous material that defies attempts at aspiration, and radiographic changes affecting bone.[55] Many surgeons do not feel they can adequately drain the joints in the foot by aspiration alone and prefer open drainage for all septic joints in the foot.

Surgical decompression requires adequate exposure of the joint, a synovectomy, and a thorough irrigation with saline. The joint is allowed to continue to drain using suction or a Penrose drain for 24 to 48 hours. The foot should be splinted to allow relative rest and for patient comfort. If the symptoms have not resolved, repeat irrigation and debridement should be undertaken at 48 hours. The use of antibiotics in the irrigation has not been shown to have superior results to saline alone.[43]

Broad-spectrum empiric antibiotics should be administered parenterally. Nafcillin combined with third-generation cephalosporins will cover most infections. For patients with a penicillin allergy, levofloxacin is an accepted substitute. Patients at risk for MRSA (nursing home residents, recent inpatients, or those who live in areas where community-acquired MRSA is higher than 10%) should be covered by an appropriate antibiotic.[77] The choice of antibiotic is adjusted depending on the pathogen isolated from the aspirate. Therapy should continue for 4 weeks.[89]

OSTEOMYELITIS

Osteomyelitis is the infection of bone. It is characterized by acute inflammation, vascular engorgement, edema, cellular infiltration, and abscess formation. The infective agents can be bacteria, fungi, or mycobacteria. The source of the infection can be hematogenous, an adjacent infection, or direct inoculation by trauma or surgery. The infection can be acute or chronic. The clinical presentation varies based on the organism, location, and host factors.

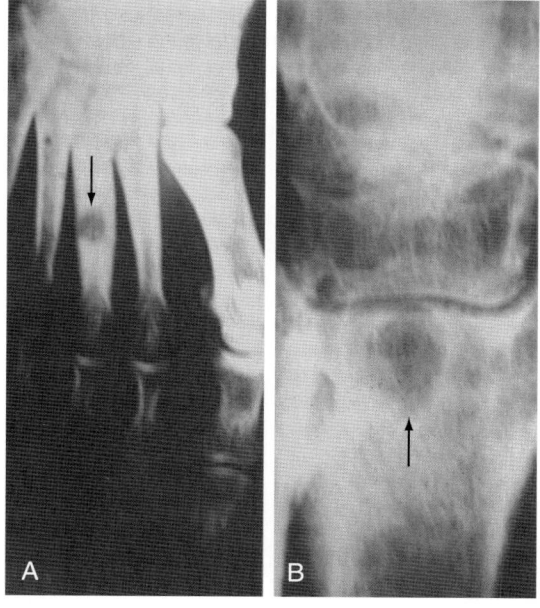

Figure 15-10 Radiographs of osteomyelitis demonstrating a Brodie abscess. **A,** Abscess in the lower end of the tibia *(arrow).* **B,** Abscess in the third metatarsal *(arrow).* Note the increased density and periosteal thickening of the entire metatarsal shaft. (From Frierson JG, Hecht PJ: Infections of the foot. In Coughlin MJ, Mann RA, editors: *Surgery of the foot and ankle,* ed 7, St Louis, 1999, Mosby, p 885.)

A conclusive diagnosis is made with a bone biopsy. The diagnosis of osteomyelitis is clinically important because of the length of therapy required for the treatment of bone infections and the necessity for surgical debridement. Sickle cell anemia, chronic granulomatous disease, and diabetes mellitus predispose a patient to develop osteomyelitis.[71]

Hematogenous infections are most common in children and can affect any of the bones of the foot. The calcaneus and talus are the most commonly involved sites in the foot, with 7% and 4% of all hematogenous infections, respectively.[6] S. aureus is the usual pathogen. A Brodie abscess is a particular form of chronic osteomyelitis found in the lower portion of the tibia, talus, or forefoot.[6,113] These abscesses have a sclerotic wall and contain purulent material. A Brodie abscess typically has no systemic symptoms, and laboratory studies are often normal. Treatment of a Brodie abscess is debridement and antibiotics (Fig. 15-10).

The clinical presentation of acute osteomyelitis includes fever, local pain, swelling, and tenderness. Laboratory studies may show an elevated white blood cell count, erythrocyte sedimentation rate, and C-reactive protein. In compromised hosts and in patients with involvement of the small bones of the foot, the laboratory studies may not be abnormal. Blood cultures are positive in half of patients.[55] Cultures obtained from sinus tracts are often unreliable. Identification of the pathogen requires bone aspiration or biopsy. Bone biopsy and culture has a sensitivity of 95% and specificity of 99% if taken before antibiotics are administered.[87]

Radiographic changes include osteolysis, periosteal reaction, cortical erosion, and formation of sequestra and involucrum[18] (Figs. 15-11 and 15-12). These changes take 10 to 14 days to appear. The early signs of soft

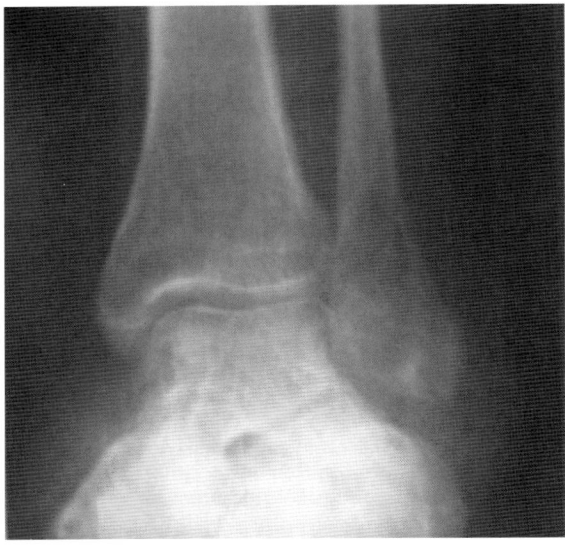

Figure 15-11 Radiograph of osteomyelitis demonstrating osteopenia of the surrounding bone. (From Marcinko DE: *Infection of the foot*, St Louis, 1998, Mosby.)

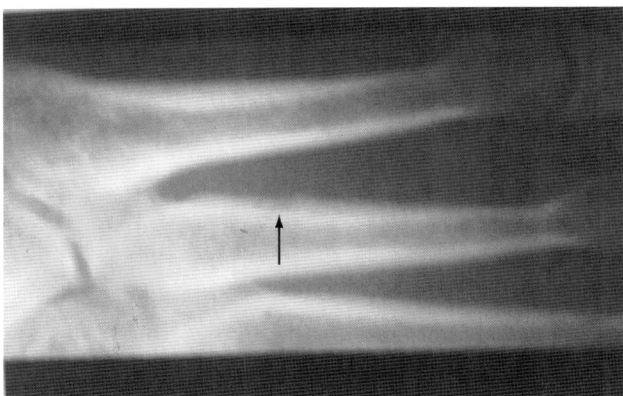

Figure 15-12 Radiograph of osteomyelitis demonstrating cortical erosion of cortical bone *(arrow)*. (From Marcinko DE: *Infection of the foot*, St Louis, 1998, Mosby.)

tissue swelling, periosteal thickening and elevation, and osteopenia are subtle and are often missed.[71] Bone mineral loss of 30% is required for radiographic change to be visible. The radiographic findings resemble malignancy, fractures, and neuropathic conditions. Because of these problems, radiographs have a sensitivity of 43% to 75% and specificity of 75% to 83%. During treatment, radiographic findings often lag behind clinical response.

MRI can detect changes in the bone earlier than plain films can. Osteomyelitis is identified by alteration of the bone marrow signal that results in a loss of the normal fatty signal on T1 and the enhancement of edema on T2 images. MRI can also demonstrate secondary signs, such as cellulitis, fluid collection, cortical interruption, and sinus tract formation. The presence of secondary signs can increase the sensitivity of a scan.[85] The scan provides precise anatomic details showing adjacent abscess formation, sinus tracts, and the extent of osseous involvement. MRI has a sensitivity of 77% to 100% and specificity of 80% to 100%.[84] Gadolinium enhancement can improve the detection of adjacent soft tissue disease.[84,86] The use of contrast is particularly helpful in the diabetic foot and postsurgery patient. The presence of surgical implants reduces the effectiveness of MRI. Neuropathic disease, altered weight bearing, and surgery can cause marrow changes consistent with osteomyelitis.

Fast spin-echo short T1 inversion recovery (FSE STIR) images are useful for initial screening. Their high sensitivity and rapidity of scan can detect small marrow changes. Patients with positive scans can then undergo additional imaging by using gadolinium-enhanced fat-suppressed T1-weighted sequences. The increased specificity of these examinations helps to eliminate false positives. In cases with discordant marrow signs, secondary signs can be used to determine the presence of osteomyelitis. The secondary signs with highest positive predictive value are cortical interruption, a cutaneous ulcer, and a sinus tract.[85]

Radionuclide bone scans are extensively used in diagnosing osteomyelitis. The three-phase bone scan changes take only 2 days to appear.[49] Osteomyelitis is characterized by accumulation of the tracer in all three phases of the scan. This relatively inexpensive test has a very low false-negative rate. Fracture, neuropathic joints, trauma, surgery, and hyperemia can result in positive test results for three-phase bone scan. The sensitivity of the study ranges from 69% to 100% and specificity from 38% to 82%.[18] Three-phase bone scans combined with labeled white blood cells increases the specificity. This combination improves the sensitivity to 73% to 100% and specificity to 55% to 100%.[117] The test is complicated and requires an additional hospital day to perform. The combined tests are generally more expensive than MRI.

A recent development in imaging for musculoskeletal infections is ^{18}F-fluorodeoxyglucose positron emission tomography (PET). PET evaluates cellular glucose metabolism to identify increased use by activated neutrophils and macrophages. The sensitivity is 91% to 100%, and specificity is 88% to 91%.[22,29] An advantage of PET is the ability to differentiate between Charcot lesions and osteomyelitis.[53] PET is particularly useful around metal implants, which limit the usefulness of MRI. The studies are limited to facilities with a PET scanner and are expensive. Elevated blood glucose can result in false-negative results. PET should be considered for differentiating Charcot lesions and osteomyelitis or for detecting osteomyelitis near metallic implants (see Chapter 3).

The treatment of osteomyelitis depends upon surgical debridement. Antibiotics are less effective in acidic, anaerobic, hypercapnic, and poorly perfused regions. Excision of necrotic bone, removal of purulent material, and elimination of any dead space is essential to the success of antibiotic treatment. The surgical debridement is more important than serum levels of antibiotics or duration of treatment.[72] Care should be taken during the debridement to ensure all dysvascular bone is removed. Punctate bleeding should be visible on all bone surfaces. An expendable bone can be completely resected and the wound treated as a soft tissue infection, substantially decreasing the duration of treatment. After debridement is completed, the dead space produced must be obliterated. A combination of local tissue closure, drains, antibiotic-impregnated spacers, and tissue transfer procedures is necessary to fill the dead space and cover exposed bone. Adequate coverage of bone is required to treat osteomyelitis.

The selection of antibiotic is initially governed by the suspected pathogen. This choice is modified by sensitivity testing. A peak minimum serum bactericidal dilution of 1:8 is the goal of therapy. Four to 6 weeks of parenteral antibiotic therapy after the last debridement is the current standard of therapy. This type of therapy is expensive and inconvenient for patients. Outpatient services, peripheral inserted central catheter (PICC), and portable infusion pumps have helped reduce the burden of parenteral therapy. For many antibiotics, the oral and parenteral forms result in similar serum concentrations. Oral antibiotics are used for osteomyelitis in children after the initial response to parenteral antibiotics. Small clinical studies have demonstrated that oral therapy is effective in adults for susceptible organisms.[36,41,70,72] Additional studies and a mechanism to ensure patient compliance are necessary before oral therapy is recommended for adult osteomyelitis therapy.

Treatment of systemic conditions and hyperbaric oxygen are adjuncts to surgery and antibiotics. Attention should be paid to good nutrition, control of diabetes, and smoking cessation. Medical interventions to improve vascular status should be implemented as well. Animal studies have demonstrated hyperbaric oxygen is as effective as antibiotics in treating bone infected with *S. aureus*. Hyperbaric oxygen increases the intramedullary oxygen tensions in models of osteomyelitis. Increased oxygen tension is toxic to anaerobic organisms and assists phagocytic processes. Experimental models have demonstrated that antibiotics are more effective in oxygen-rich environments. Treatment regimens are 60 to 120 minutes per day with 100% oxygen at 2 to 3 atm.[72,114] The use of hyperbaric oxygen is often limited by availability.

Sedimentation rate and C-reactive protein levels are used to monitor the efficacy of the treatment. The return of these studies to normal during the course of therapy is a favorable prognostic sign. The sedimentation rate, C-reactive protein, and leukocyte counts can become elevated after each surgical debridement. The use of these laboratory studies in treating chronic osteomyelitis or a host compromised by systemic disease is limited. In these patients, the studies might not be elevated before treatment.

BIOFILMS

When treating infections involving bone or surgical implants, one should consider the concept of a biofilm. A biofilm is hydrated matrix of proteins and polysaccharides that encompass a polymicrobial collection of cells. Bacterial cells can exist both in a free-floating planktonic state or as one of these polymicrobial communities (Fig. 15-13). Most bacteria exist in nature as biofilm communities adherent to inert surfaces.[46] The cells within these communities may exist in a different phenotypic state from the planktonic cells. The characteristics of a biofilm make eradicating an infection difficult.

A biofilm is closely adherent to any inert material, such as necrotic bone or surgical implants. The ability of a biofilm to adhere to a surgical implant depends on the material of the implant as well as surface characteristics. Titanium has a lower adherence rate and has been recommended over stainless steel for high-risk cases.[109] Preexisting organic material on implants increases the susceptibility of an implant to colonization by a biofilm. Once established, biofilms can last a lifetime.[115] For purposes of clinical treatment, one should consider biofilms permanent until the affected surface is removed.[25,109]

Bacteria in a biofilm are resistant to antibiotics and host defenses.[109,115] Antibiotics are much more effective against isolated free-floating, planktonic cells. The matrix itself can limit access or inactivate antibiotics.[115] The bacteria may exist in a sporelike state that is resistant to antibiotics beyond any native resistance of the organism. The host reaction to the biofilm can result in significant collateral damage to native tissues because of chronic inflammatory response.[115] Low-grade biofilm infection may be misdiagnosed as aseptic loosening.[25]

The concept of biofilms gives us a paradigm to explain clinical experience with surgical treatment of infections and loosening of surgical implants. In the presence of an infection, all structures composed of inert material should be removed. Perioperative antibiotics should be directed against the planktonic bacteria released from the biofilms by the mechanical action of removing the affected surface. Cultures will often only show one species of polymicrobial matrix.[46] Local antibiotics may be effective in preventing biofilms from being reestablished.[25]

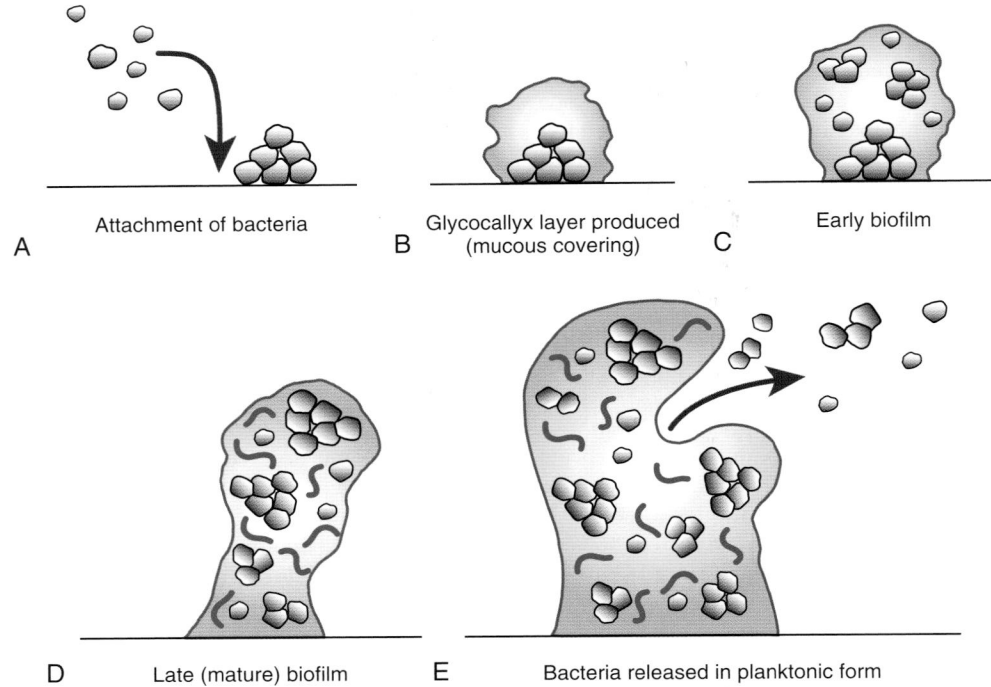

Figure 15-13   Biofilm development as a process. **A,** Attachment of cells to a surface. **B,** Production of extracellular polysaccharide irreversibly attaching cells to substrate. **C,** Development of the biofilm architecture. **D,** Maturation of the biofilm. **E,** Cells released in the planktonic state.

Table 15-4	Definitions of Staphylococcal and Streptococcal Infections
Infection	**Definition**
Cellulitis	A diffuse spreading infection of the subcutaneous tissue characterized by superficial swelling, pain, erythema, and localized warmth.
Erysipelas	Cellulitis involving the dermal lymphatics and characterized by spreading hot, erythematous, brawny, and sharply circumscribed plaques with a raised indurated border.
Folliculitis	Inflammation of a hair follicle.
Furuncle	A tender red nodule that oozes or weeps purulent material.
Hidradenitis	Inflammation of the apocrine sweat gland. Infection with multiple abscesses is called hidradenitis suppurativa.
Impetigo	A superficial cutaneous infection resulting in the inoculation of abrasions or compromised skin. It is characterized by the presence of discrete, fragile vesicles surrounded by an erythematous border. The vesicles secrete a thin, amber-colored fluid.
Osteomyelitis	An infection involving bone.
Paronychia	An infection involving the folds of skin around the nail.
Pyoderma	A skin infection with a collection of purulent material.

COMMON ORGANISMS

Bacterial Infections

Staphylococcus *Species*

Staphylococci are ubiquitous bacteria commonly associated with soft tissue and bone infections. They are divided into coagulase-positive and coagulase-negative strains. *S. aureus* is the coagulase-positive strain and is the most pathogenic. Thirty percent of the population are chronic carriers of *S. aureus*. Coagulase-negative strains are considered low-virulence nonpathogenic commensals. They are known to cause infections but are more often seen as contaminants in superficial wound and blood cultures. When found in deep wounds or multiple blood cultures, they should be considered pathogens.

Staphylococcal infections usually are associated with breaks in the skin. Trauma, dermatophyte infection, eczema, and psoriasis can provide the portal of entry. The resulting infections include impetigo, folliculitis, furuncle, hidradenitis, cellulitis, wound infection, abscess, paronychia, and osteomyelitis (Table 15-4).

Staphylococci tend to form abscesses. Toxins produced by staphylococci can result in food poisoning, toxic shock syndrome, and scalded skin syndrome. The organisms can adhere to implants, creating a glycocalyx that protects the organisms from both the body's immune system and antibiotics.

Oral agents are recommended for superficial infections. For deep or serious infections, parenteral therapy with nafcillin is recommended. If the patient is allergic to penicillin or the strain is methicillin resistant, vancomycin or linezolid are used. The addition of rifampin should be considered for serious infections. It should be pointed out that methicillin-sensitive staphylococci are more susceptible to nafcillin than to vancomycin.[116]

Streptococcus *Species*

Group A *(Streptococcus pyogenes)* and group B *(Streptococcus agalactiae)* are common organisms in human infections. Both species are β-hemolytic organisms. They are associated with pharyngitis, impetigo, pyodermas, erysipelas, cellulitis, necrotizing fasciitis, rheumatic fever, and acute glomerulonephritis. Streptococcal infections tend to cause cellulitis and lymphangitis; they usually are associated with breaks in the skin. Trauma, dermatophyte infection, eczema, and psoriasis can provide the portal of entry. Recurrent infections with streptococci are found in patients with impaired lymphatic or venous drainage.[116]

Oral agents are recommended for superficial infections. First-generation cephalosporins or clindamycin are effective. Deep infections can be difficult to distinguish from mixed infections. Broad-spectrum antibiotics, such as ampicillin-sulbactam, are recommended for initial empiric therapy. For serious infections, clindamycin should be added.

Pasteurella multocida

Pasteurella multocida is associated with animal bites. This gram-negative coccobacillus is resistant to dicloxacillin, cephalexin, clindamycin, and erythromycin. The recommended treatment is amoxicillin-clavulanate.

Clostridium *Species*

Clostridia are gas-forming organisms usually associated with penetrating trauma and with soil contamination of a wound. Plain films, computed tomography (CT), and MRI show the presence of gas. Rapid debridement is required. Extensive myonecrosis can require amputation to control the infection. The recommended treatment is a combination of clindamycin and penicillin G.[27]

Neisseria gonorrhoeae

A disseminated gonococcal infection follows the hematogenous spread of *Neisseria gonorrhoeae.* The skin and joints are often affected. The skin lesions are 1- to 5-mm macules on an erythematous base. The knee, elbow, ankle, shoulder, and hip joints are most commonly affected. Clinical symptoms include fever, migratory polyarthralgia, and tenosynovitis. Aspiration of the joint shows rare gram-negative intracellular diplococci. The antibiotic of choice is azithromycin.[81]

Aeromonas hydrophilia

Aeromonas hydrophilia is a gram-negative, β-hemolytic, facultative anaerobic bacillus. *Aeromonas* species have been found in saltwater, freshwater, sewage, canned food, fish, meats, and soil. Infections manifest with severe pain, cellulitis, edema, lymphangitis, fever, and joint pain. The organisms produce hemolysin and cytotoxin, resulting in myonecrosis. These symptoms are often confused with septic joints. *A. hydrophilia* is treated with surgical debridement and antibiotics. Appropriate antibiotics include fluoroquinolones, trimethoprim-sulfamethoxazole, or third-generation cephalosporins. Foot infections have been documented after penetrating trauma.[61]

Borrelia burgdorferi

The spirochete *Borrelia burgdorferi* is responsible for Lyme disease. The classic description of this disease begins with erythema chronicum migrans, an annular skin lesion. This erythematous lesion spreads out from a clearing center around the original bite site (Fig. 15-14). The vector, *Ixodes* ticks, is small, and the original bite is often not noticed. The cutaneous lesions are often accompanied by fever and systemic complaints. Symptoms affecting the bone and joints can begin anywhere from 1 week to several years after the bite. Sixty percent of untreated Lyme disease patients have arthritic complaints. The complaints can range from mild migratory arthralgia to erosive joint disease. The ankle is the third most commonly involved joint.

Laboratory studies may show a mild elevation of the erythrocyte sedimentation rate. The diagnosis is made by serology showing antibodies to *B. burgdorferi.* Neurologic and cardiac symptoms can develop. Appropriate antibiotic treatment is doxycycline 100 mg twice a day for 14-21 days.

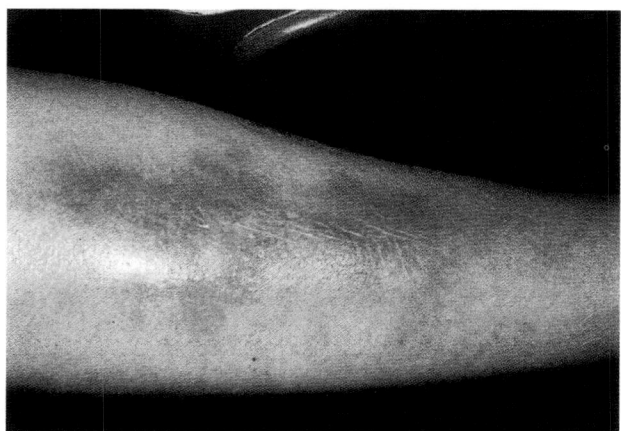

Figure 15-14 Erythema chronicum migrans skin lesion of *Borrelia burgdorferi* infection. Note the erythematous spread from the central lesion. (From España A: Erythemas. In Bolognia JL, Jorizzo JL, Rapini RP, editors: *Dermatology,* St Louis, 2003, Mosby, p 308.)

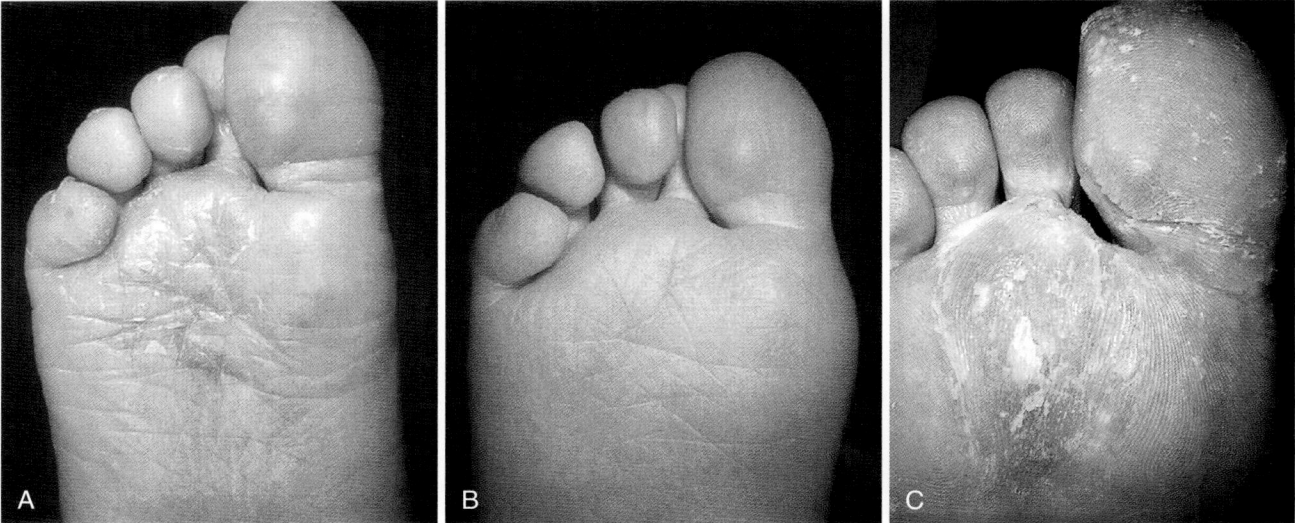

Figure 15-15   Tinea pedis. **A,** Chronic fungal infection confirmed by potassium hydroxide preparation. **B,** Resolved after treatment with antifungal cream. **C,** Severe untreated tinea pedis on plantar aspect of the foot. (From Dockery G: *Cutaneous disorders of the lower extremity,* Philadelphia, 1997, WB Saunders, pp 53, 55. Used with permission.)

Fungal Infections

Tinea Pedis

Athlete's foot is a very common infection of the foot, with an incidence of 17.7 percent.[28] This fungal infection attacks the skin and nails. The interdigital spaces are affected with itching, cracking, scaling, and blistering. *Trichophyton rubrum* and *Trichophyton mentagrophytes* are the most common organisms. Other dermatophytes and bacteria can be involved. Diagnosis is with skin scrapings in a 10% potassium hydroxide solution. Under a microscope, hyphal elements will be visible (Fig. 15-15).

Treatment of tinea pedis with topical over-the-counter clotrimazole (Lotrimin) or prescription terbinafine (Lamisil) is generally effective. These medications are available as ointments, creams, and sprays. They should be applied twice a day after washing the foot with a mild soap. It is important to keep the foot dry during the treatment period. Occlusive footwear should be avoided. Socks should be changed as often as necessary to keep the feet dry. After 4 weeks of unsuccessful topical treatment, oral ketoconazole (200 mg/day) may be considered.

Although tinea pedis is considered a benign condition, it can predispose the skin to bacterial infection. The treatment in diabetic patients can prevent bacteria from using the skin breaks as portals of entry. In severe tinea pedis infections, the host flora in the intertriginous regions changes with higher numbers of gram-negative organisms.[28] These organisms can exploit breaks in the skin to cause nonclostridial gas gangrene, myonecrosis, and crepitant cellulitis. Aggressive treatment of tinea pedis in diabetic patients can prevent more significant infections.

Onychomycosis

Onychomycosis is a fungal infection of the nail bed, matrix, or plate. It is responsible for half of all nail deformities. It is more common in patients older than 60 years, diabetic patients, patients with peripheral vascular disease, and immunocompromised patients. Its incidence in the United States is estimated to be 13%. *T. rubrum* is the most common organism (Fig. 15-16).

Patients present with hyperkeratotic discolored nails. The nail sometimes separates from the nail bed. Diagnosis is based on microscopic examination with potassium hydroxide preparation or cultures.[102] Microscopic examination is dependent on an examiner's experience, and sensitivity runs around 50%.[2] Cultures are the gold standard and allow identification of the organism. To maximize the effectiveness of the diagnostic studies, the nail should be clipped and the specimen obtained with a curette from the nail bed adjacent to the cuticle.

Treatment entails either topical or systemic antifungals. Ciclopirox lacquer is a topical medication approved by the U.S. Food and Drug Administration (FDA) for nail fungus. However, successful treatment was reported in only 30% of patients treated with ciclopirox.[3,17,48] Oral systemic therapy has been shown to be more effective, with cure rates of 70% to 80%. Continuous terbinafine 250 mg/day for 3 months has been shown to be the most effective FDA-approved regimen.[47,102] Because of the risk of hepatitis and blood dyscrasias, a complete blood count and liver enzyme levels should be drawn before starting therapy and every 4 weeks during therapy. Pulsed therapy with itraconazole has been shown to have fewer side effects and similar clinical efficacy.[102] In pulse therapy, itraconazole 400 mg daily is administered for a 1-week pulse. This is followed by a 3-week drug-free interval. A

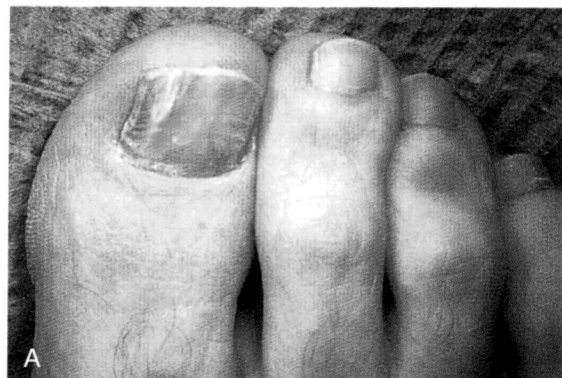

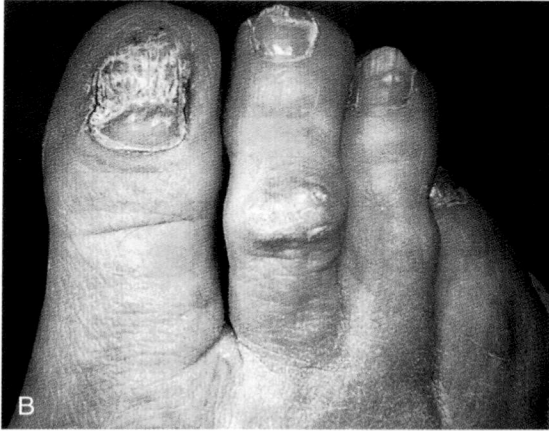

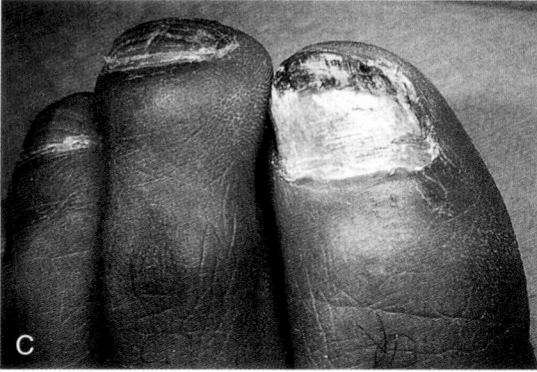

Figure 15-16 **A,** Distal subungual infection. **B,** Chronic infection with severe dystrophy. **C,** White superficial fungal infection. (From Dockery G: *Cutaneous disorders of the lower extremity,* Philadelphia, 1997, WB Saunders, pp 59, 60. Used with Permission.)

total of three or four pulses is given.[60] There are significant drug interactions for all of the systemic medications.

Coccidioides *Species*

Coccidioides immitis is endemic in California and the southwestern United States. Acquired through the respiratory tract, these fungi can affect skin, soft tissue, bone, and joints. Only 0.1% of cases progress to disseminated disease. Of those with disseminated disease, 20% develop bone and joint lesions. The symptoms can lag behind the

initial exposure by many years. Radiographs demonstrate lytic osseous changes. Diagnosis is by culture of bone or synovium. Complement fixation tests can diagnose systemic infection and evaluate the effectiveness of pharmacologic treatment. Appropriate antibiotics include itraconazole, fluconazole, and amphotericin. Surgical debridement may be required for extensive lesions or synovial involvement.[16,38]

Cryptococcus neoformans

Acquired through the respiratory tract, these fungi can affect skin, soft tissue, bone, and joints. Lymphoma, sarcoidosis, and rheumatoid arthritis are commonly associated medical conditions. The clinical symptoms can lag behind the initial exposure by many years. Radiographs demonstrate lytic osseous changes. A diagnosis is made by culture of bone or synovial biopsy. Appropriate antibiotics include amphotericin and flucytosine. Surgical debridement can be required for extensive lesions or synovial involvement. The disease commonly recurs, likely a reinfection from ubiquitous fungus in an immunocompromised patient.[24]

Mycetoma

Madura foot, caused by actinomycetes or fungi, is rare. It was first described in the Madur province of India in 1842.[123] It is generally seen in tropical regions where barefoot activity is common. The pathogens gain access by puncture wounds. Initially, small painless nodules are noted. The disease then spreads along fascial planes, and eventually draining sinuses form. Sulfur granules in the drainage are characteristic of madura foot. The infection results in a scarred mass of deformed tissue (Fig. 15-17).

Treatment involves sulfonamides or antifungal agents, local wound care, debridement, and possible amputation.[93] When radiographic evidence of bone involvement is present, surgical debridement is generally required. CT scans can identify the lesion earlier than plain radiographs. MRI images characteristically show heterogeneous low signal intensity on T1- and T2-weighted images. Biopsy specimens can identify the pathogen and help direct the choice of the appropriate antibiotic. Recurrent infection is high.[104] Genera responsible include *Madurella, Phialophora, Pyrenochaeta, Aspergillus, Fusarium, Pseudallescheria,* and *Acremonium.*[123]

Mycobacteria

Tuberculosis

Foot involvement with osteoarticular tuberculosis is rare; it affects the foot in only 0.13% of all patients with extrapulmonary disease. Despite this rarity, the disorder should be considered in endemic areas and in susceptible patients. Failure to recognize and treat the disease can result in a rigid foot and residual deformities. The disease is paucibacillary, and the diagnosis is based on a biopsy containing granulomatous tissue and caseating necrosis. The initial treatment is pharmacologic, beginning with

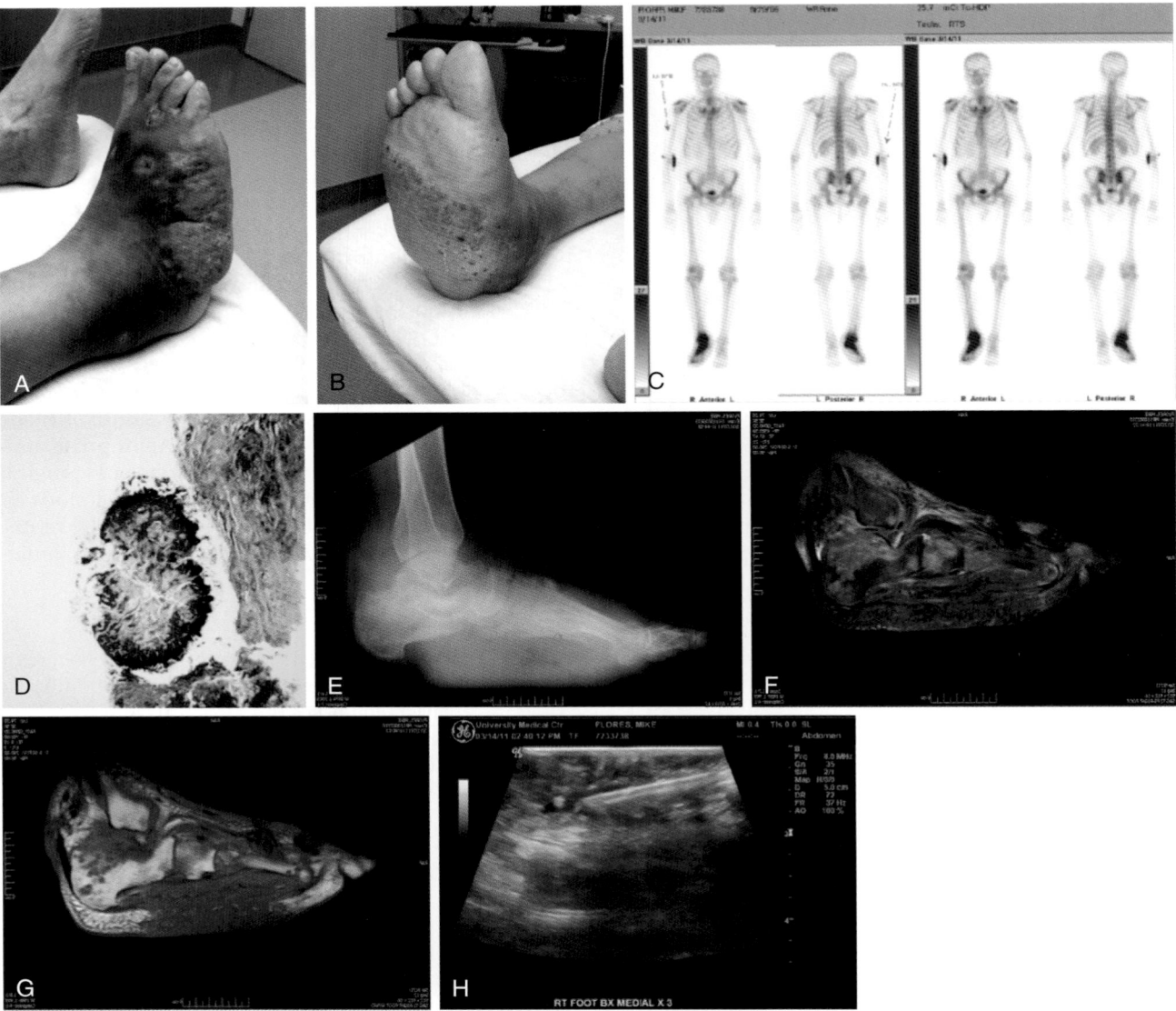

Figure 15-17 Mycetoma (madura foot) infection. **A** and **B,** Clinical appearance. **C,** Tecnetium-99 bone scan showing increased uptake around the right ankle and foot. **D,** Low-power Gram stain of sulfur granule from foot biopsy. **E,** Radiograph of the right foot showing soft tissue mass with changes in the calcaneus. **F,** Sagittal T2 magnetic resonance image (MRI) showing dot-in-ring sign. **G,** Sagittal T1 MRI of madura foot showing dot-in-ring sign, with bone involvement. **H,** Ultrasound image from needle biopsy. (Courtesy Joseph Bergman, MD.)

multidrug therapy. Surgery is limited to treating deformities resulting from the disease.

The disease manifests as a granulomatous focus adjacent to a joint or a central granuloma in the phalanges or metatarsals. The most common location is in the calcaneus. Radiographs demonstrate severe periarticular osteoporosis. A CT scan can identify the focus of the infection. The differential diagnosis includes madura foot in the tropics and Kaposi sarcoma in immunocompromised hosts (Fig. 15-18).[31]

Atypical Mycobacteria

Infection of the foot with nontuberculous mycobacteria is rare. Mycobacterial infection should be considered in

patients with indolent bone and joint infections, pathologic findings showing granulomas, negative cultures, and compromised host immunity. *Mycobacterium marinum* is associated with exposure to a marine environment. *Mycobacterium fortuitum* is a rapidly growing mycobacterium associated with soil-contaminated wounds. The diagnosis is confirmed by a biopsy with appropriate cultures. Treatment is with antituberculous drugs.

Parasitic Infections

Dermatobia hominis

Dermatobia hominis, the human botfly, is common in warm, humid lowland forests and jungles of Central and

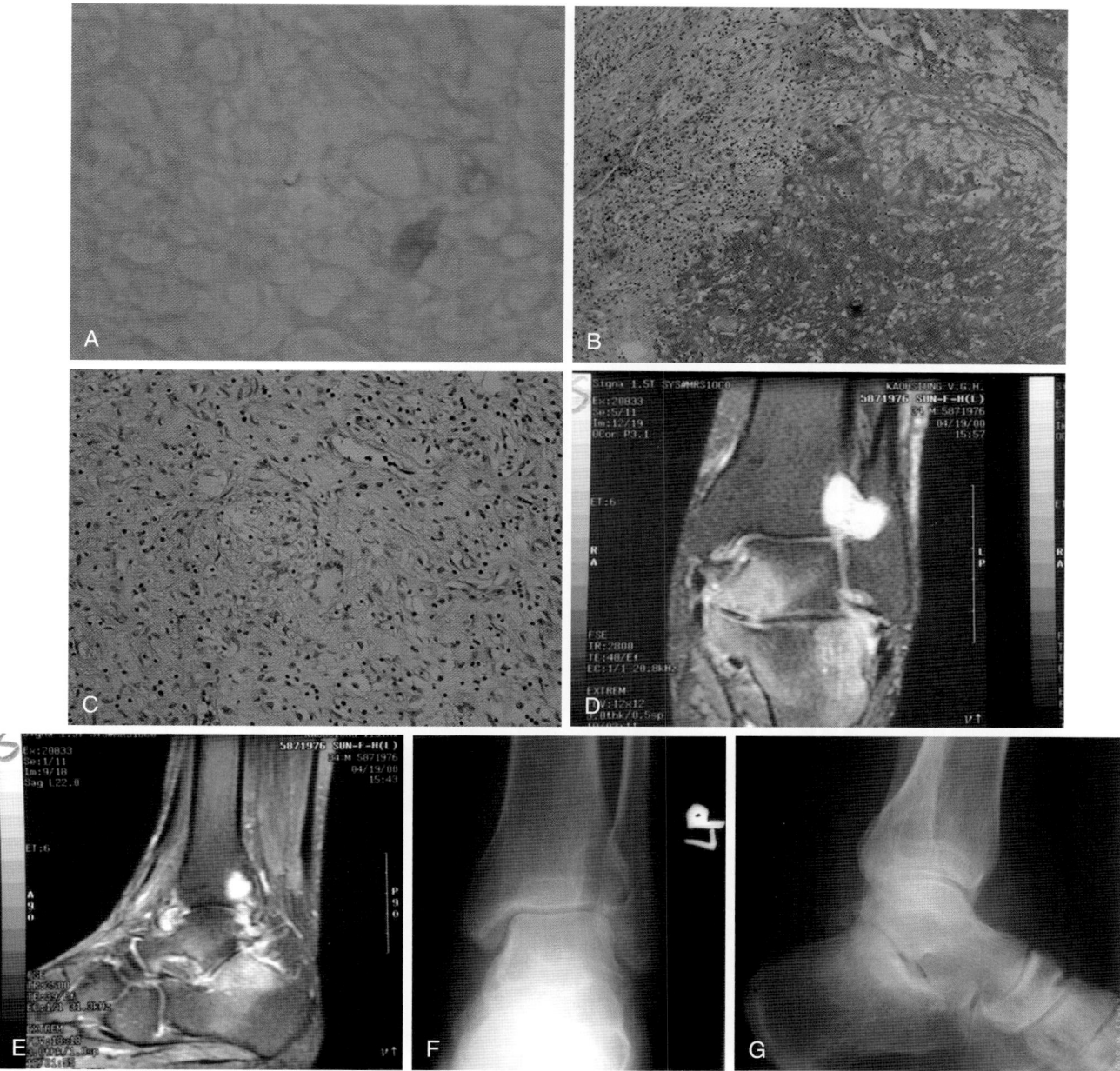

Figure 15-18 Tuberculosis of the ankle. **A,** Positive acid-fast stain. **B,** Caseous necrosis. **C,** A Langerhans cell in the center of photomicrograph. **D** and **E,** T2 magnetic resonance images of the ankle, showing proliferation of the synovium. **F** and **G,** Radiographs of the ankle. (Courtesy Yi-Jiun Chou, Department of Orthopaedic Surgery, Kaohsiung Veterans General Hospital, Taiwan.)

South America. The female deposits eggs on insects that feed on blood. When the vector insect bites an animal, the larva penetrates into the subcutaneous tissue. The larvae mature inside the host for 5 to 12 weeks. The infection manifests as furuncular myiasis, an itchy, boil-like lesion (Fig. 15-19). This is often mistaken for a staphylococcal boil. The patient may sense movement under the skin or see the larva protruding from the sinus the larva uses to breathe.[26] Treatment involves surgical removal of the larva.[1]

Cutaneous Larva Migrans

Cutaneous larva migrans results from the linear migration of helminth larvae in the epidermis. The tunneling of the parasites leaves sharply demarcated, pruritic linear or serpiginous tracks (Fig. 15-20). The tracks advance up to 2 cm per day. The most commonly affected area is the foot. The tracts can become secondarily infected.

Dog and cat hookworms, *Ancylostoma caninum* and *Ancylostoma braziliensis,* are the most frequent infestations. The eggs of these intestinal parasites are passed in stool

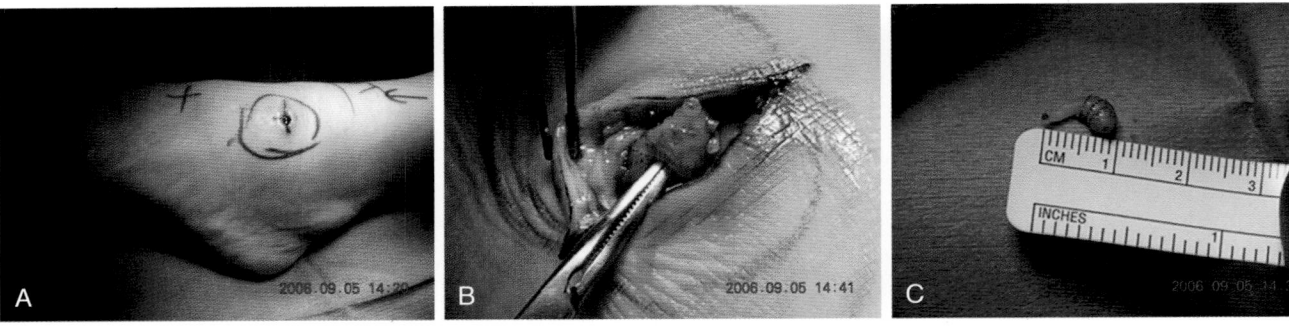

Figure 15-19 **A,** *Dermatobia hominis* (botfly) sinus tract. **B,** Moving larva in the wound. **C,** Larva noted to be more than 1 cm in length. (Photographs courtesy James M. Cottom, DPM. Reproduced from Cottom JM, Hyer CF, Lee TH: Dermatobia hominis (botfly) infestation of the lower extremity: a case report. *J Foot Ankle Surg* 47(1):51-55, 2008.)

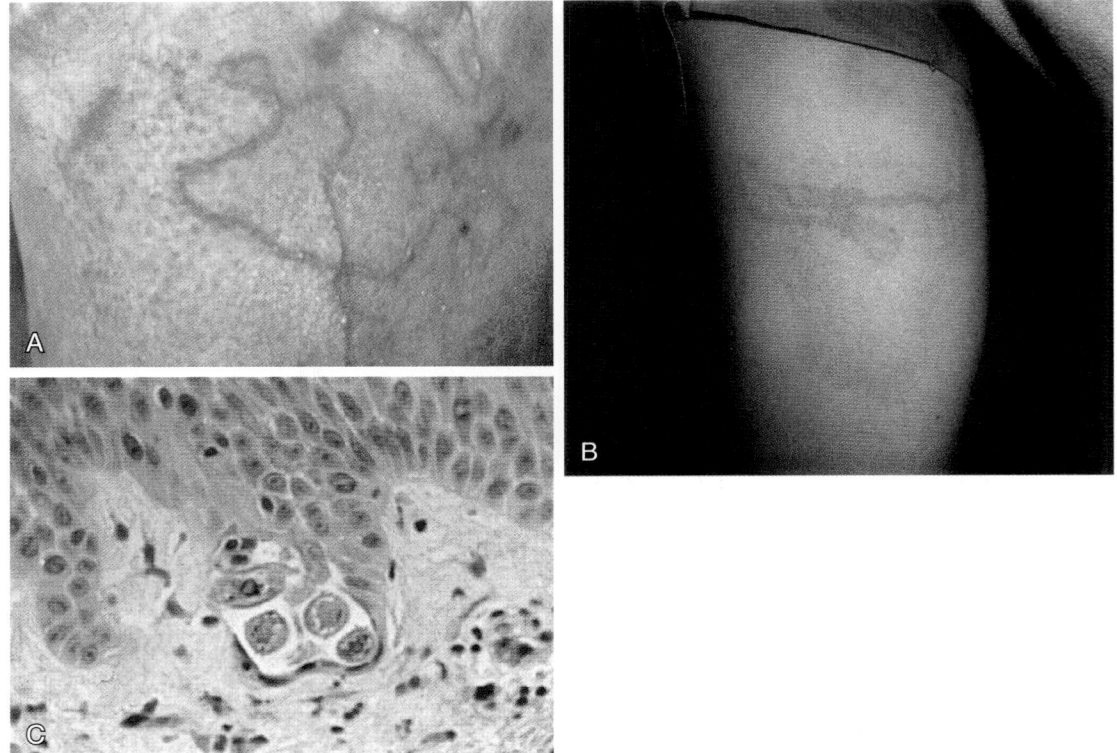

Figure 15-20 Cutaneous larva migrans of the foot. **A,** Note wandering pattern of larva beneath the skin. **B,** Hypersensitivity reaction producing an acute urticarial response. **C,** In photomicrograph, the larva is seen in cross section deep within the epidermis. (From Dockery G: *Cutaneous disorders of the lower extremity,* Philadelphia, 1997, WB Saunders. Used with permission.)

onto warm soil. The eggs mature into infectious filariform larvae. The larvae can penetrate the epidermis of intact skin, but they are unable to penetrate the dermis. They thus tunnel under the epidermis. The larvae are found in tropical regions, including the southeastern United States, the Caribbean, South and Central America, Mexico, Africa, India, and Asia. A 10-day course of topical thiabendazole is the treatment of choice. Crush a 500-mg tablet in 5 g of water-soluble cream and apply four times per day.[92] An oral alternative is albendazole 400 or 800 mg/day for 3 days.[78] Oral ivermectin is efficacious at a single dose of 12 mg.[92]

Chigger Mites

Mites of the family Trombiculidae are found in the southern United States, South America, South Pacific islands, and East Asia. They attach to the skin of the legs and secrete powerful digestive enzymes that allow them to burrow under the skin. The body's reaction to the enzymes results in intense pruritus. The excoriated lesions can become secondarily involved. The infection lasts 3 to 4 days. Treatment is with corticosteroid creams. Prevention is by using insect repellent containing *N,N*-diethyl-*m*-toluamide (DEET), wearing long-sleeved tops and long pants, and avoiding heavily infected areas (Fig. 15-21).[11]

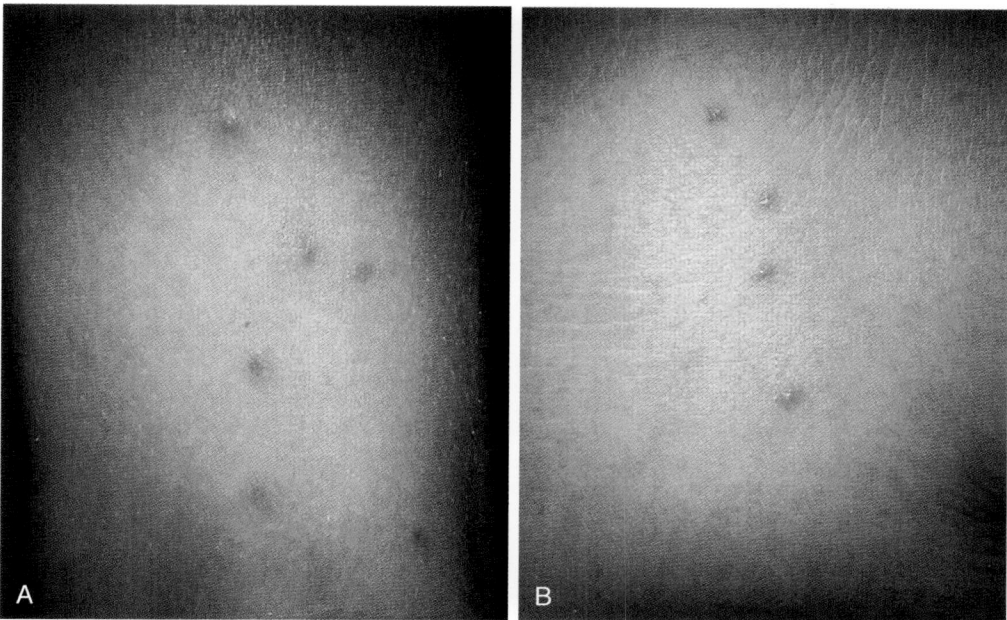

Figure 15-21 Mite bites. **A,** Cluster pattern of flea bites on lower extremity. **B,** Common distribution of bites from fleas in a breakfast, lunch, and dinner pattern. (From Dockery G: *Cutaneous disorders of the lower extremity,* Philadelphia, 1997, WB Saunders, pp 95, 96. Used with permission.)

SPECIAL CASES

Felon

A felon is a collection of purulent material in the pulp space of the distal phalanx of a toe. This infection is often near the nail. Left untreated, it can penetrate deeper and cause osteomyelitis. *S. aureus* is the usual pathogen. Lymphangitis streaks suggest the presence of streptococci or gram-negative organisms. In immunocompromised hosts, the infection is often polymicrobial.

Treatment

Treatment begins with surgical drainage of any abscess and empiric therapy with antibiotics directed against staphylococci. Cephalexin 500 mg every 6 hours is an acceptable choice. The antibiotic is adjusted based on cultures or failure to clinically respond in 48 hours. Soaking the foot in saline and elevation can help to relieve the symptoms. An ingrown toenail often precipitates a felon and should be addressed during the treatment.

DEBRIDEMENT OF A FELON
Surgical Technique
1. A digital block with local anesthetic without epinephrine is administered.
2. A Penrose drain is used as a tourniquet about the base of the digit.
3. A fish-mouth incision is created distally on the toe, running from one side of the toe to the other.
4. Blunt dissection along the plantar surface of the distal phalanx is performed using curved hemostats. Care is

taken to disrupt the numerous septations present in the distal toe pulp.
5. Any necrotic bone is debrided. Any debrided bone is sent for cultures. If no bone is available, cultures are sent of the purulent debris or soft tissue removed from the wound.
7. Light packing is placed using plain gauze. This packing is removed at 24 hours.
8. Delayed primary closure can be considered at 7 days if the infection has clinically cleared.

Puncture Wounds

Penetrating trauma to the plantar surface of the foot is a common mechanism leading to infectious complications, including amputation. Plantar puncture wounds represent 0.82% of pediatric emergency department visits.[21] The penetrating object often deposits foreign bodies along with inoculation of the pathogens. When the object is withdrawn, the injury becomes effectively a closed space. A small number (1.8%)[39] of these injuries progress to osteomyelitis. Slightly more (8%)[39] patients present or return with soft tissue infections (Fig. 15-22). The host immune status and environment of the offending object determine the course of treatment.

The initial history should note the time of the injury, footwear, object causing the injury, tetanus status, and host medical condition. Plain radiographs should be obtained to exclude foreign bodies. The physical examination should note the depth of penetration, the location over bone landmarks, and readily apparent debris. The foot should be washed with a weak povidone-iodine

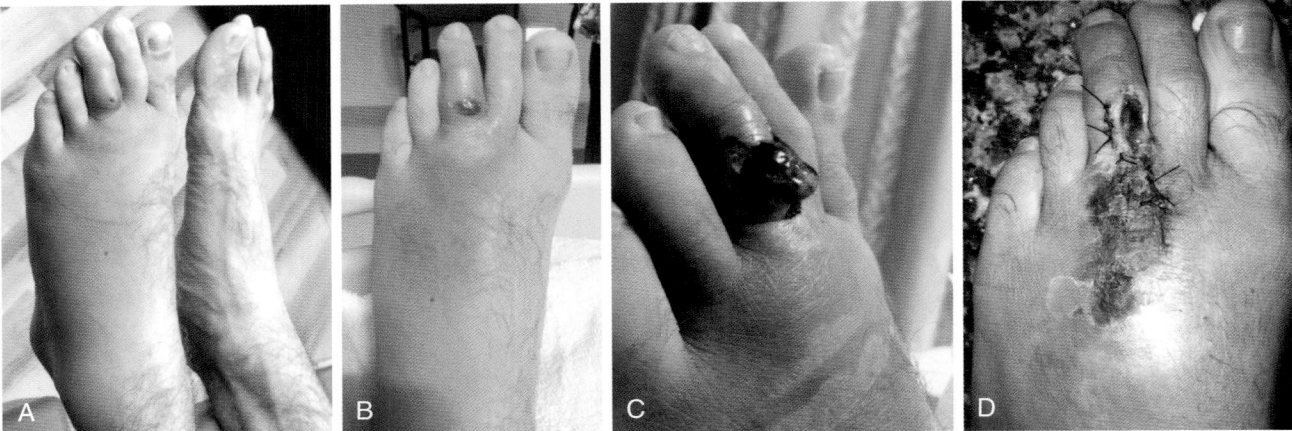

Figure 15-22 Clinical photograph of a puncture wound infection. **A,** Initial presentation. **B,** One week later, with fluctuant area. **C,** Preoperative. **D,** Three weeks out from surgical irrigation and debridement.

(Betadine) solution.[21] Open containers of hexachlorophene should not be used because they can be colonized with *Pseudomonas* species. The wound should not be blindly probed for debris and should not be closed. Prophylactic antibiotics should be administered for all immunocompromised hosts, grossly contaminated wounds, patients presenting more than 24 hours after injury, and wounds with retained debris. Surgical exploration and debridement should be undertaken for all wounds suspected of containing foreign material. Patients presenting within 24 hours of injury with clean wounds without signs of retained debris should be reexamined at 48 hours to evaluate the foot for local signs of infection.

Metal nails are the most common objects to cause plantar puncture wounds. Other commons agents are needles, glass, wood, and plastic. Puncture wounds penetrating the sole of a shoe can carry parts of the sole and sock into the wound. Wood, plastic, sock material, and foam from the shoe are not readily observed on plain radiographs. In an acute case, ultrasound can effectively resolve wooden objects such as thorns or a toothpick.[54] For patients presenting more than a few weeks after injury, MRI is the imaging modality of choice for identifying retained foreign debris.[82]

If the patient has had three doses of tetanus toxoid and no more than 5 years has elapsed since the last dose, no prophylaxis is required. For those without a recent toxoid booster, tetanus toxoid injection is indicated. Diphtheria, tetanus toxoid, and acellular pertussis vaccine (DTaP) should be given to patients younger than 7 years. Older patients receive diphtheria and tetanus toxoid (dT). For those without a history of three tetanus toxoid injections, tetanus immune globulin should be administered.

The most common pathogens for soft tissue infections are *Staphylococcus* and *Streptococcus* species. *Pseudomonas* is the most frequent cause of bone infections.[21,39,62,65] For asymptomatic patients presenting between 24 and 72 hours, oral first-generation cephalosporins or dicloxacillin are recommended. For symptomatic patients without

signs of bone involvement, parenteral antistaphylococcal and antistreptococcal antibiotics, such as nafcillin or cefazolin, should be administered. Antipseudomonal antibiotics—ceftazidime, ciprofloxacin, or piperacillin—should be considered if there is no improvement after 48 hours of treatment or bone involvement. Diabetic patients are more likely to have polymicrobial infections and should be treated with broader-spectrum antibiotics.[65] Puncture wounds sustained in an aquatic environment should be treated for organisms such as *Mycobacterium marinum*, *Vibrio* species, and *Aeromonas hydrophila*.[61] For symptoms that do not resolve within 48 hours with antibiotic treatment, a retained foreign body should be suspected.

Laboratory and systemic symptoms are generally not helpful in diagnosing osteomyelitis. Patients with plantar puncture wound infection often are nontoxic and afebrile. Patients presenting with infected puncture wounds have a normal erythrocyte sedimentation rate 36% of the time and a normal white blood cell count 57% of the time.[64] The positive predictive value of sedimentation rate to determine osteomyelitis is 35%. Soft tissue swelling, drainage, and radiographic changes should alert the clinician to osteomyelitis.

The treatment of osteomyelitis is surgical debridement followed by parenteral antibiotics. The selection of antibiotic is dependent upon the cultures obtained intraoperatively. Patients have been documented to have infections from *Pseudomonas*, *Klebsiella*, *Mycobacterium*, *Eikenella*, *Enterobacter*, *Fusobacterium*, *Proteus*, and *Escherichia* species.[39,54,62] The duration of treatment depends on host factors and the extent of debridement. Treatments from 2 to 6 weeks are documented. Forty percent amputation rates after puncture wounds in diabetic patients have been documented.[8]

Animal Bites

An estimated 2 million animal bites per year occur in the United States. Domestic dogs and cats account for 90%

of animal bites requiring medical attention. Dogs inflict crush-type injuries resulting in laceration, avulsions, and fractures. Cats inflict puncture-type inoculation wounds. Both types of bites can result in infections of the soft tissues, tendons, bones, and joint spaces. Five percent of dog bites and 25% to 50% of cat bites become infected. Bite infections are typically polymicrobial.[94] The most common pathogens include *Pasteurella multocida, S. aureus,* coagulase-negative staphylococci, streptococci, and *Corynebacterium* species. Tularemia, actinomycosis, and blastomycosis all have been reported as a result of animal bites.[88]

Treatment begins with a thorough physical examination to determine the structures affected by the bite. Radiographic studies are necessary to determine if bone is involved and if a foreign body remains in the wound. The wound is irrigated and debrided of all foreign matter and dysvascular tissue. Formal surgical irrigation and debridement is indicated for cellulitis that does not improve with antibiotics in 24 hours or if an abscess forms. Wounds are packed open to allow drainage. Tetanus prophylaxis as described for puncture wounds should be administered. Prophylactic antibiotics should also be administered.[94]

Antibiotics should be selected to treat the most common organisms. Amoxicillin combined with clavulanic acid, ampicillin combined with sulbactam, or doxycycline have been shown to be effective. Oral treatment is sufficient for prophylaxis. Parenteral administration is preferred for treatment of an established infection until clinical results indicate the effectiveness of the antibiotic therapy.

If the animal is suspected of being rabid, public health officials should be contacted. The animal is quarantined for observation or sacrificed. The wound should be irrigated with a 1% benzalkonium chloride solution. Prophylaxis with human diploid cell vaccine and human rabies immune globulin should be initiated.[88] The incubation period for rabies is from 9 to 70 days.

Human Bites

Human bites have the highest rate of infection of all animal bites. Human saliva contains 1×10^8 bacteria per milliliter. Common organisms include *Streptococcus viridans,* β-hemolytic streptococci group A, *S. aureus, Staphylococcus epidermidis, Bacteroides fragilis,* and *Eikenella corrodens.*[76] Bites have been associated with the transmission of hepatitis B, human immunodeficiency virus (HIV), and other blood-borne diseases. Treatment is the same as listed for animal bites.

Surgical Wounds

Postoperative infections are a potentially serious complication after foot and ankle surgery. Infections after surgery account for 14% to 16% of all nosocomial infections.[94] The rate of infection after foot and ankle surgery are reported to range from 1.35% to 5.3%.[32] The rate of infection is higher after traumatic injury. The associated tissue

Table 15-5	Risk Factors for Surgical Infections

Patient
Age
Nutritional status
Diabetes
Smoking
Obesity
Coexisting infections
Immune suppression
Preoperative hospitalization
Vascular status
Procedure duration
Antimicrobial prophylaxis
Duration of scrub
Shaving
Ventilation
Sterilization of instruments
Drains
Foreign material implantation
Potential space

Table 15-6	Measures to Increase Oxygenation of a Surgical Wound

Supplemental oxygenation: intraoperative and postoperative
Correction of hypovolemia
Maintain core temperature
Control pain
Avoid vasoconstrictive drugs

destruction and devascularization hinder the body's ability to defend against infection. Factors influencing the risk of surgical infection are listed in Table 15-5. These infections can range from superficial cellulitis to the deep soft tissue or bone infections.

Patient factors can be modified to reduce the risk of surgical infections. Experimental models have shown that smoking cessation for 4 weeks reduces the risk of infection to the level of nonsmokers.[112] Improved nutrition benefits both infection rate and wound healing. Concern over immune-modifying drugs used to treat rheumatoid arthritis has not been borne out in the literature. Methyltrexate, nonsteroidal antiinflammatory drugs, steroids, hydroxychloroquine, gold, and tumor necrosis factor-α inhibitors were not found to change the perioperative infections or wound complication rate in foot and ankle surgery.[14,15,83,105] Studies in general surgery have shown that aggressive postoperative glucose control in diabetic patients reduces infection rates in major surgery. Other studies have shown that measures that increase tissue perfusion and oxygenation reduce the incidence of postoperative infections (Table 15-6).[45,52,59,98]

Antibiotic prophylaxis is a controversial issue. The prophylactic use of antibiotics is widely accepted in general orthopedic procedures, especially those involving implants.[79,94,99] Studies have shown little benefit in elective foot and ankle procedures.[111,126] Infections that do develop after the prophylactic use of antibiotics tend to involve a pathogen with antibiotic resistence.[111,126] It is essential that the antibiotics be appropriately selected and used. Cefazolin is the generally recommended antibiotic for clean orthopedic procedures. It should be administered 30 to 60 minutes before incision.[74] Cefazolin should be dosed 1g for patients weighing less than 86 kg and 2 g if heavier.[99] Clindamycin is an acceptable option for patients with a significant penicillin allergy. Vancomycin is only appropriate for high-risk procedures if MRSA is a high risk.[32,94,111] Postoperative doses should be limited to less than 24 hours. Surgical-site infections with MRSA are associated with surgical drain for more than 1 day, postoperative antibiotics for more than 1 day, or discharge to a long-term care facility.[75]

Proper surgical preparation is essential. Normal skin flora exists in the follicles of glands, hair, and about the stratum corneum. A study using povidone-iodine paint or gel for lower-extremity surgery showed a 80% positive culture preoperative.[96,124] The cultures grew *S. epidermidis*, *S. aureus*, *Enterococcus faecalis*, and *Clostridium perfringens*. Povidone-iodine followed by chlorhexidine in alcohol showed a reduction to 8%, which was reduced to no positive preoperative cultures with the use of aggressive scrub technique in the toe clefts.[19] Chlorhexidine inhibits bacterial growth longer than iodine and, in an alcohol-based paint, has been shown to be the most effective surgical foot scrub.[40,97] However, even with complete elimination of the bacteria on preoperative cultures, recolonization occurred in 7.7% of cases. Despite this finding, covering the toes during foot surgery demonstrated no reduction in postoperative infections.[44]

Shaving in the preoperative period is associated with an increased rate of infection.[12,74] This is especially true for skin shaved more than 24 hours before incision. It is thought that small cuts in the dermis encourage the growth of bacteria. Surgical clippers have not been shown to cause a significant increase in infection rates.[91] If hair removal is essential for the surgical procedure, surgical clippers should be used.[74]

Despite the best efforts of surgeons and patients, infections do occur. A superficial surgical infection site is red, warm, and tender to touch (Fig. 15-23). Lymphadenopathy may be present. Fluctuant areas can indicate formation of abscess. Painful motion of the joints, pain with axial load, and changes on radiographs can indicate a deep wound infection. Patients often have increased white blood cell count, sedimentation rate, and fever with either deep or superficial infections. The most common pathogens are *S. aureus* and β-hemolytic streptococci. Superficial infections can be treated with antibiotics alone. Cephalexin or clindamycin are usually appropriate. Failure to respond to antibiotic treatment or signs of deep infection is an indication for surgical decompression. Techniques to expose the deep structures of the foot are described in the "Abscesses" section. The wounds should be allowed to drain and heal by

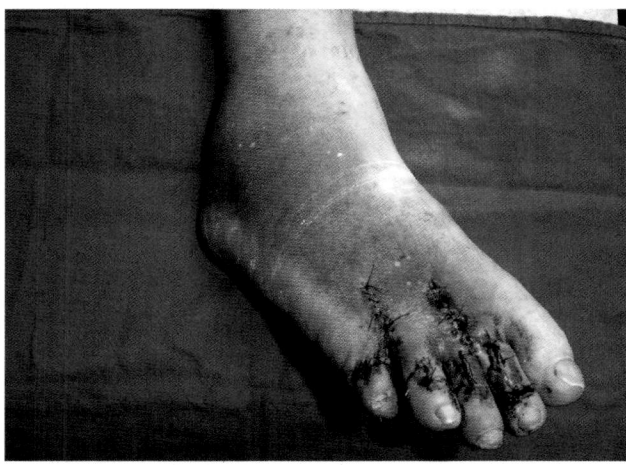

Figure 15-23 Clinical photograph of a surgical wound infection 10 days after surgery. Note the erythema spreading proximally from the wounds.

secondary intent. The choice of antibiotics is directed by intraoperative cultures.

The surgical debridement should remove all infected and necrotic tissue. If surgical debridement is planned, antibiotics should be withheld until deep tissue cultures can be obtained. Surgical implants present a difficulty for debridement. Biofilms adhere to the implant, creating a barrier to the host defense and antibiotics. With chronic infections, the implants are colonized and should be removed. In patients with acute infections, it is possible to manage the infection with the implants in place.[101] However, a high percentage of patients will need to have the implants removed to clear the infection.

Vacuum therapy can assist with wound closure. Specialized systems make this therapy convenient for the clinician and the patient. After the wound is debrided of all necrotic debris and purulent material, it is covered with polyurethane foam. Exposed nerves and vessels should be covered with a nonadherent dressing for protection. The wound is then subjected to a 125-mm Hg vacuum. The vacuum therapy decreases local edema, increases local blood flow, increases granulation tissue, and controls wound drainage better than conventional dressings. The foam dressing is changed three times per week initially. The size of the foam inserted into the wound is carefully adjusted as the wound heals to ensure no isolated pockets develop. The resulting granulating bed is often ideal for split-thickness skin grafting (Fig. 15-24).[7,30,122]

ANTIBIOTICS

No one antibiotic can be expected to be effective in all clinical settings. The type of infection, host factors, and infection location all modify the selection of the appropriate antibiotic. General references can only make broad recommendations. Local resistance patterns can change

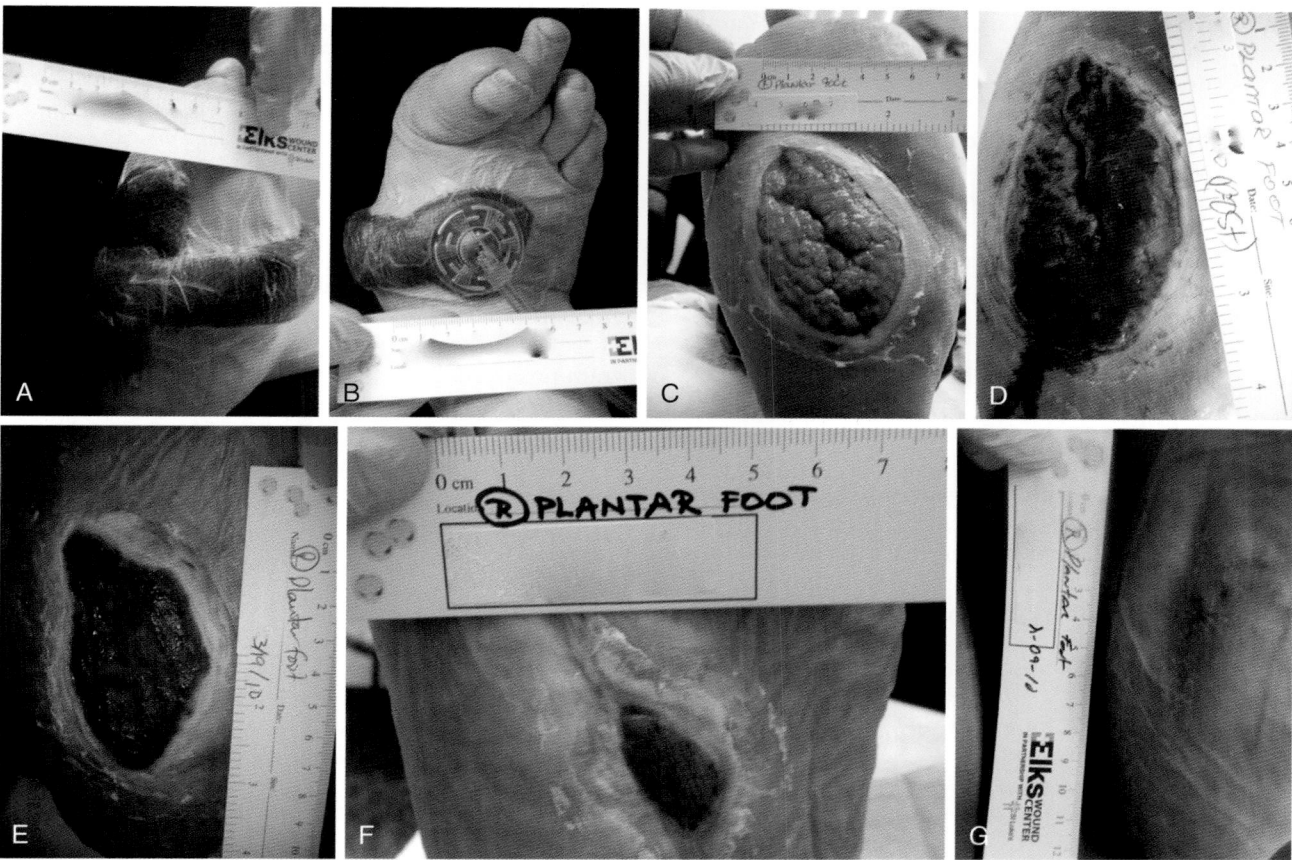

Figure 15-24 Negative pressure treatment. **A** and **B,** Application of the negative-pressure dressing. Note the bridge to the top of the foot. The hard and bulky connector for the pump is located dorsally to reduce pressure on the wound. **C,** Plantar foot ulcer at presentation. **D,** Plantar foot ulcer after debridement. **E,** Granulation tissue forming in the wound 1 month after application of the negative pressure system. **F,** Wound after 4 months of therapy. **G,** Final appearance 6 months after treatment began. (Photographs courtesy Dr. Raymond Otto, MD, Boise, Idaho.)

the recommended treatments. The suspected organism is the most important consideration in choosing an empiric antibiotic. The culture results will allow adjustments to the therapy.

A detailed description of all antibiotics is beyond the scope of this text. Key antibiotics used in orthopedics and salient information are listed as follows.

Penicillins

Natural Penicillin (Penicillin G)
Natural penicillin is inactivated by β-lactamases. It is the drug of choice for the treatment of *C. perfringens*. It has good anaerobic activity except for *B. fragilis*.

Penicillinase-Resistant Penicillins (Methicillin, Nafcillin, Dicloxacillin)
Penicillinase-resistant penicillin is resistant to β-lactamase. It is active against methicillin-sensitive *S. aureus, Streptococcus pyogenes,* and *Streptococcus pneumoniae*. It is not effective against enterococci or methicillin-resistant *S.*

aureus. Nafcillin can cause nephritis, leukopenia, and hepatic dysfunction.

Aminopenicillins (Ampicillin, Amoxicillin)
These antibiotics are effective for enterococci, *Escherichia coli, Salmonella* species, *Shigella* species, and *Proteus mirabilis.* Poor staphylococcal coverage limits their use in lower-extremity infections.

Antipseudomonal Penicillin (Ticarcillin)
Antipseudomonal penicillin is susceptible to β-lactamase. Ticarcillin is active against *Pseudomonas, Enterobacter,* and *Serratia* species and *B. fragilis.* Ticarcillin can cause sodium loading and platelet dysfunction.

Extended-Spectrum Penicillins (Piperacillin, Mezlocillin)
Extended-spectrum penicillins are susceptible to β-lactamase. These antibiotics are active against *Pseudomonas, Enterobacter, Streptococcus, Klebsiella,* and *Haemophilus* species and *B. fragilis.* These drugs are synergistic with

aminoglycosides against *Pseudomonas* and *Enterobacteriaceae* species. They can cause sodium loading and platelet dysfunction.

Aminoglycosides (Gentamicin, Tobramycin, Amikacin)

These antibiotics are active against aerobic gram-negative organisms, Enterobacteriaceae, and *Pseudomonas* species. The side effects include nephrotoxicity and ototoxicity. Amikacin is the most resistant to enzymatic inactivation.

Cephalosporins

First-Generation Cephalosporins (Cephalexin, Cefazolin)

These antibiotics are effective against methicillin-sensitive *S. aureus*, *S. epidermidis*, *Streptococcus* species, *E. coli*, *Klebsiella* species, and *P. mirabilis*. They have no activity against *Bacteroides* or *Enterococcus* species. Side effects include gastrointestinal intolerance and hypersensitivity. Their side-effect profile and relatively low cost make them ideal for superficial lower-extremity infections.[56]

Second-Generation Cephalosporins (Cefotetan, Cefoxitin)

These drugs have excellent activity against *Staphylococcus* and *Streptococcus* species, with increased activity against indole-positive *Proteus* species, *Haemophilus influenzae*, and *Klebsiella* species.

Third-Generation Cephalosporins (Cefotaxime, Ceftriaxone, Ceftizoxime, Ceftazidime)

These antibiotics are resistant to β-lactamase. They have poor activity against *Enterococcus* species. They have reduced activity against gram-positive organisms compared with first-generation cephalosporins. They have good activity against gram-negative organisms, except for *Pseudomonas* species. Ceftazidime is the exception and has anti-*Pseudomonas* activity.

Fourth-Generation Cephalosporins (Cefepime)

Cefepime is active against aerobic gram-positive organisms, gram-negative organisms, and *Pseudomonas* and *Enterobacter* species. It has no activity against *Enterococcus* species.

Fluoroquinolones

Second-Generation Fluoroquinolones (Ciprofloxacin, Ofloxacin)

These antibiotics are effective against most gram-negative organisms, including *Pseudomonas* species, *S. aureus*, and *S. epidermidis*. Skeletally immature patients should not receive fluoroquinolones. Tendon rupture can be associated with fluoroquinolones. Gram-positive organisms can develop rapid resistance. They are useful for gram-negative infections of soft tissues and bone.[56]

Third-Generation Fluoroquinolones (Levofloxacin, Sparfloxacin)

These antibiotics are effective against most gram-negative organisms, *S. aureus*, *S. epidermidis*, *Mycobacterium pneumoniae*, *Legionella* species, and *Chlamydia pneumoniae*. Skeletally immature patients should not receive fluoroquinolones. Tendon rupture can be associated with fluoroquinolones.

Fourth-Generation Fluoroquinolones (Trovafloxacin, Moxifloxacin, Gatifloxacin)

These antibiotics are effective against anaerobes, aerobic gram-positive organisms, and most gram-negative organisms. Skeletally immature patients should not receive fluoroquinolones. Tendon rupture can be associated with fluoroquinolones.

Other Antibiotics

Azithromycin

Azithromycin is a macrolide antibiotic with moderate activity against *Staphylococcus* and *Streptococcus* species and some activity against gram-negative organisms. It has good activity against *B. burgdorferi*. It is a long-acting medication dosed once per day. In the lower extremity, it can be used in patients allergic to penicillin and cephalosporins.[56]

Clindamycin

Clindamycin is active against anaerobic bacteria, *S. aureus*, *S. epidermidis*, and *Streptococcus* species. It has no activity against enterococci or gram-negative organisms. It can cause diarrhea and pseudomembranous colitis. Incidences of pseudomembranous colitis of up to 10% have been reported. Clindamycin is commonly used in diabetic foot infections.[56]

Daptomycin

Approved for complicated skin and skin structure *Staphylococcus* infections, this intravenous antibiotic has show efficacy in osteomyelitis in foot and ankle infections.[51,100] Dosed once daily at 6 mg/kg intravenous for 6 weeks, it has has similar outcomes to vancomycin. It is bactericidal against gram-positive pathogens, including MRSA. It has synergistic action with gentamicin and rifampin.[100] Adverse effects include reversible myopathy, which is monitored by measuring serum creatine phosphokinase levels.

Linezolid

Linezolid is available in both oral and intravenous form and is indicated for skin and soft tissue infections.[37] It is a bacteriostatic antibiotic effective against gram-positive pathogens, including MRSA and vancomycin-resistant *Enterococcus* species. Case reports have shown effectiveness in osteomyelitis using a 600-mg twice-daily dosage.[37] Prolonged therapy is associated with reversible anemia and irreversible peripheral and optic neuropathy. These side effects have limited its use for bone and joint infections.[100]

Rifampin

Rifampin is bactericidal against most gram-positive and negative organisms. Rapid resistance develops when it is used alone. It is often used in combination with other agents. It induces liver enzyme activity, inactivating many drugs, including oral anticoagulants and oral contraceptives. Its side effects include coloring body fluid red and inducing hepatitis and mild immunosuppression.

Tigecycline

A bacteriostatic antibiotic that is structurally similar to tetracyclines, tigecycine is approved for complicated skin and skin structure infections. It is effective against gram-positive and gram-negative bacterial pathogens, including MRSA. It is administered intravenously and commonly used for polymicrobial infections.

Trimethoprim-Sulfamethoxazole

This antibiotic combination is effective against *E. coli, P. mirabilis, H. influenzae, Klebsiella pneumoniae, Enterobacter* species, *Serratia marcescens,* and *Pseudomonas* species. *Staphylococcus* and *Streptococcus* species are often susceptible. Rifampin and trimethoprim-sulfamethoxazole may be effective for treating MRSA. Its side effects include a serum sickness–like syndrome, hemolytic anemia, and hypersensitivity reactions. It should not be administered in the last month of pregnancy.

Vancomycin

Vancomycin is active against *S. aureus, S. epidermidis,* and *Enterococcus* species. It is the antibiotic of choice for methicillin-resistant *S. aureus* and *S. epidermidis.* It can result in red man syndrome. It has been associated with nephrotoxicity and ototoxicity. It has relatively poor penetration in bone and joints.[77,100]

Local Antibiotics by Implantable Device

Local antibiotic administration in infected wounds can achieve high concentrations of antibiotic without high systemic levels. This minimizes the systemic sides effects and maximizes the effective concentration in the local wound bed. Polymethyl methacrylate beads impregnated with tobramycin have been shown to be effective in reducing the infection rates in the treatment of open fractures (Fig. 15-25).[95] The most commonly used antibiotics in beads are vancomycin, tobramycin, daptomycin, and gentamicin.[106] The same technique can be used to treat an infection. The beads can be placed into a wound and a bead pouch created by wound closure or application of an impermeable membrane. The accumulated fluid bathes the wound with a high concentration of antibiotic. Calcium sulfate–impregnated beads may also be used, but the antibiotic is rapidly released. Calcium phosphate–calcium sulfate composite beads elute the antibiotics over a longer period.[108]

When it necessary to preserve the alignment of the extremity during an extended treatment of an infection,

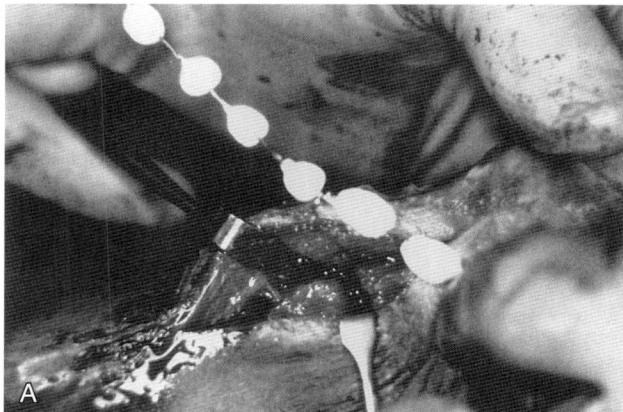
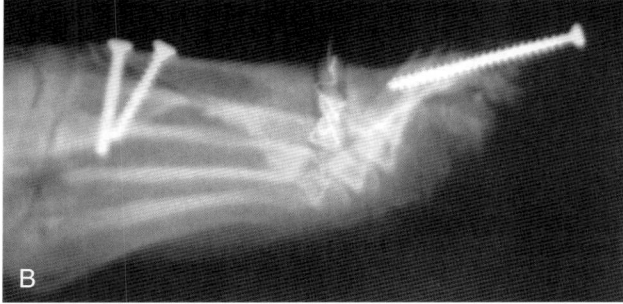

Figure 15-25 Antibiotic beads used to treat a postsurgical infection. **A,** Photograph of polymethyl methacrylate beads. **B,** Radiograph of absorbable beads in place. (From Marcinko DE: *Infection of the foot,* St Louis, 1998, Mosby, pp 179, 181.)

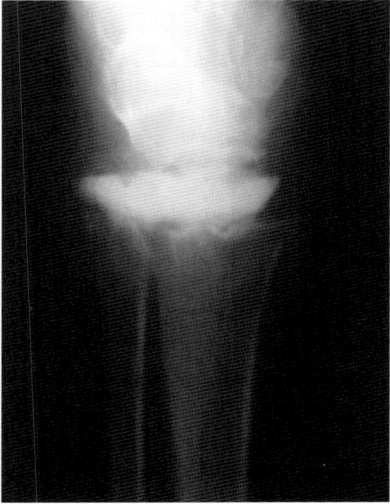

Figure 15-26 Radiograph of a polymethyl methacrylate spacer used to treat an infected total ankle arthroplasty.

an antibiotic spacer is ideal. These devices are often constructed out of polymethyl methacrylate impregnated with antibiotics. They can maintain the relationship between bones, allowing for reconstruction at a later date. Figure 15-26 shows the use of an antibiotic spacer used to treat a total ankle infection. The ankle eventually was successfully fused using external fixation.

The elution of antibiotic declines over a period of weeks, leaving a foreign body in the wound that must be removed before it can serve as a nidus for secondary infection.[63] There is concern that, as eluted antibiotics drop below the mean inhibitory concentration, selection of resistant organisms may develop.[109] This normally accompanies additional debridements in soft tissue infections. More recently, biodegradable antibiotic delivery systems have been developed.* These devices can maintain a steady elution of antibiotic for up to 3 months. These devices show great promise in the treatment of osteomyelitis.[80,90,125]

---

*References 4, 9, 20, 63, 66, 68, and 103.

REFERENCES

1. Adams DW, Cooney RT: Excision of a *Dermatobia hominis* larva from the heel of a South American traveler: a case report, *J Foot Ankle Surg* 43:260–262, 2004.
2. Alberhasky R: Laboratory diagnosis of onychomycosis, *Clin Podiatr Med Surg* 21:565–578, 2004.
3. Albert SF, Weis ZH: Management of onychomycosis with topicals, *Clin Podiatr Med Surg* 21:605–615, vii, 2004.
4. Ambrose CG, Clyburn TA, Louden K, et al: Effective treatment of osteomyelitis with biodegradable microspheres in a rabbit model, *Clin Orthop Relat Res* 421:293–299, 2004.
5. Anderson VL: Cellulitis, *Lippincotts Prim Care Pract* 3:59–64, 1999.
6. Antoniou D, Conner AN: Osteomyelitis of the calcaneus and talus, *J Bone Joint Surg Am* 56:338–345, 1974.
7. Argenta LC, Morykwas MJ: Vacuum-assisted closure: a new method for wound control and treatment: clinical experience, *Ann Plast Surg* 38:563–576; discussion 577, 1997.
8. Armstrong D, Lavery L: Surgical morbidity and the risk of amputation due to infected puncture wounds in diabetic versus nondiabetic adults, *South Med J* 90:384–390, 1997.
9. Armstrong DG, Stephan KT, Espensen EH, et al: What is the shelf life of physician-mixed antibiotic-impregnated calcium sulfate pellets? *J Foot Ankle Surg* 42:302–304, 2003.
10. Aronoff DM, Bloch KC: Assessing the relationship between the use of nonsteroidal antiinflammatory drugs and necrotizing fasciitis caused by group A *Streptococcus*, *Medicine* 82:225–235, 2003.
11. Axman WR, Brummer JJ: Chigger mite infestation, *J Am Podiatr Med Assoc* 93:399–401, 2003.
12. Balthazar ER, Colt JD, Nichols RL: Preoperative hair removal: a random prospective study of shaving versus clipping, *South Med J* 75:799–801, 1982.
13. Bellapianta JM, Ljungquist K, Tobin E, et al: Necrotizing fasciitis, *J Am Acad Orthop Surg* 17:174–182, 2009.
14. Bibbo C, Anderson RB, Davis WH, et al: The influence of rheumatoid chemotherapy, age, and presence of rheumatoid nodules on postoperative complications in rheumatoid foot and ankle surgery: analysis of 725 procedures in 104 patients [corrected], *Foot Ankle Int* 24:40–44, 2003.
15. Bibbo C, Goldberg JW: Infectious and healing complications after elective orthopaedic foot and ankle surgery during tumor necrosis factor–alpha inhibition therapy, *Foot Ankle Int* 25:331–335, 2004.
16. Bisla RS, Taber TH Jr: Coccidioidomycosis of bone and joints, *Clin Orthop Relat Res* 121:196–204, 1976.
17. Bodman MA, Feder L, Nace AM: Topical treatments for onychomycosis: a historical perspective, *J Am Podiatr Med Assoc* 93:136–141, 2003.
18. Boutin RD, Brossmann J, Sartoris DJ, et al: Update on imaging of orthopedic infections, *Orthop Clin North Am* 29:41–66, 1998.
19. Brooks RA, Hollinghurst D, Ribbans WJ, et al: Bacterial recolonization during foot surgery: a prospective randomized study of toe preparation techniques, *Foot Ankle Int* 22:347–350, 2001.
20. Buranapanitkit B, Srinilta V, Ingviga N, et al: The efficacy of a hydroxyapatite composite as a biodegradable antibiotic delivery system, *Clin Orthop Relat Res* 424:244–252, 2004.
21. Chachad S, Kamat D: Management of plantar puncture wounds in children, *Clin Pediatr (Phila)* 43:213–216, 2004.
22. Chacko TK, Zhuang H, Nakhoda KZ, et al: Applications of fluorodeoxyglucose positron emission tomography in the diagnosis of infection, *Nucl Med Commun* 24:615–624, 2003.
23. Childers BJ, Potyondy LD, Nachreiner R, et al: Necrotizing fasciitis: a fourteen-year retrospective study of 163 consecutive patients, *Am Surg* 68:109–116, 2002.
24. Chleboun J, Nade S: Skeletal cryptococcosis, *J Bone Joint Surg Am* 59:509–514, 1977.
25. Costerton JW: Biofilm theory can guide the treatment of device-related orthopaedic infections, *Clin Orthop Relat Res* 437:7–11, 2005.
26. Cottom JM, Hyer CF, Lee TH: *Dermatobia hominis* (botfly) Infestation of the lower extremity: a case report, *J Foot Ankle Surg* 47:51–55, 2008.
27. Cristofaro PA: Infection and fever in the elderly, *J Am Podiatr Med Assoc* 94:126–134, 2004.
28. Day MR, Day RD, Harkless LB: Cellulitis secondary to web space dermatophytosis, *Clin Podiatr Med Surg* 13:759–766, 1996.
29. de Winter F, van de Wiele C, Vogelaers D, et al: Fluorine-18 fluorodeoxyglucose–positron emission tomography: a highly accurate imaging modality for the diagnosis of chronic musculoskeletal infections, *J Bone Joint Surg Am* 83:651–660, 2001.
30. DeFranzo AJ, Argenta LC, Marks MW, et al: The use of vacuum-assisted closure therapy for the treatment of lower-extremity wounds with exposed bone, *Plast Reconstr Surg* 108:1184–1191, 2001.
31. Dhillon MS, Nagi ON: Tuberculosis of the foot and ankle, *Clin Orthop Relat Res* 398:107–113, 2002.
32. Donley BG, Philbin T, Tomford JW, et al: Foot and ankle infections after surgery, *Clin Orthop Relat Res* 391:162–170, 2001.
33. Dryden MS: Complicated skin and soft tissue infection, *J Antim Chem* 65(Suppl 3):iii35–iii44, 2010.
34. Eady EA, Cove JH: Staphylococcal resistance revisited: community-acquired methicillin resistant *Staphylococcus aureus*—an emerging problem for the management of skin and soft tissue infections, *Curr Opin Infect Dis* 16:103–124, 2003.
35. Elliott DC, Kufera JA, Myers RA: Necrotizing soft tissue infections. Risk factors for mortality and strategies for management, *Ann Surg* 224:672–683, 1996.
36. Embil JM, Rose G, Trepman E, et al: Oral antimicrobial therapy for diabetic foot osteomyelitis, *Foot Ankle Int* 27:771–779, 2006.
37. Falagas ME, Siempos II, Papagelopoulos PJ, et al: Linezolid for the treatment of adults with bone and joint infections, *Int J Antim Agents* 29:233–239, 2007.
38. Fishco WD, Blocher KS: Disseminated coccidioidomycosis masquerading as tendinitis, *J Am Podiatr Med Assoc* 90:508–511, 2000.
39. Fitzgerald RH Jr, Cowan JD: Puncture wounds of the foot, *Orthop Clin North Am* 6:965–972, 1975.
40. Fletcher N, Sofianos D, Berkes MB, et al: Prevention of perioperative infection, *J Bone Joint Surg Am* 89:1605–1618, 2007.

41. Galanakis N, Giamarellou H, Moussas T, et al: Chronic osteo-myelitis caused by multi-resistant gram-negative bacteria: eval-uation of treatment with newer quinolones after prolonged follow-up, *J Antimicrob Chemother* 39:241–246, 1997.
42. Galloway JB, Hyrich KL, Mercer LK: Risk of septic arthritis in patients with rheumatoid arthritis and the effect of anti-TNF therapy: results from the British Society for Rheumatology Bio-logics Register, *Ann Rheum Dis* 70:1810–1814, 2011.
43. Goldenberg DL: Septic arthritis, *Lancet* 351:197–202, 1998.
44. Goucher NR, Coughlin MJ: Covering of the toes during hind-foot and ankle surgery: a randomized controlled, clinical study, *J Foot Ankle Int* 28:413–415, 2007.
45. Greif R, Akca O, Horn EP, et al: Supplemental perioperative oxygen to reduce the incidence of surgical-wound infection. Outcomes Research Group, *N Engl J Med* 342:161–167, 2000.
46. Gristina AG, Costerton JW: Bacterial adherence to biomaterial and tissue, *J Bone Joint Surg Am* 67-A:264–273, 1985.
47. Gupta AK: Treatment of dermatophyte toenail onychomycosis in the United States. A pharmacoeconomic analysis, *J Am Podiatr Med Assoc* 92:272–286, 2002.
48. Gupta AK, Fleckman P, Baran R: Ciclopirox nail lacquer topical solution 8% in the treatment of toenail onychomycosis, *J Am Acad Dermatol* 43:S70–S80, 2000.
49. Hain SF, O'Doherty MJ, Smith MA: Functional imaging and the orthopaedic surgeon, *J Bone Joint Surg Br* 84:315–321, 2002.
50. Holdiness MR: Management of cutaneous erythrasma, *Drugs* 62:1131–1141, 2002.
51. Holtom PD, Zalavras CG, Lamp KC, et al: Clinical experience with daptomycin treatment of foot or ankle osteomyelitis, *Clin Orthop Relat Res* 461:35–39, 2007.
52. Hopf HW, Hunt TK, West JM, et al: Wound tissue oxygen tension predicts the risk of wound infection in surgical patients, *Arch Surg* 132:997–1004; discussion 1005, 1997.
53. Hopfner S, Krolak C, Kessler S, et al: Preoperative imaging of Charcot neuroarthropathy in diabetic patients: comparison of ring PET, hybrid PET, and magnetic resonance imaging, *Foot Ankle Int* 25:890–895, 2004.
54. Imoisili MA, Bonwit AM, Bulas DI: Toothpick puncture injuries of the foot in children, *Pediatr Infect Dis J* 23:80–82, 2004.
55. Jahss MH, editor: *Disorders of the foot and ankle*, Philadelphia, 1991, WB Saunders.
56. Joseph WS, Lefrock J: The use of oral antibiotics in lower-extremity infections, *Clin Podiatr Med Surg* 13:683–699, 1996.
57. Kazakova SV, Hageman JC, Matava M, et al: A clone of methicillin-resistant *Staphylococcus aureus* among professional football players, *N Engl J Med* 352:468–475, 2005.
58. Kelly PJ: Bacterial arthritis in the adult, *Orthop Clin North Am* 6:973–981, 1975.
59. Kurz A, Sessler DI, Lenhardt R: Perioperative normothermia to reduce the incidence of surgical-wound infection and shorten hospitalization. Study of Wound Infection and Temperature Group, *N Engl J Med* 334:1209–1215, 1996.
60. Lagana FJ: Curing onychomycosis: understanding the multi-tude of variables, *Clin Podiatr Med Surg* 21:555–564, vi, 2004.
61. Larka UB, Ulett D, Garrison T, et al: *Aeromonas hydrophilia* infec-tions after penetrating foot trauma, *J Foot Ankle Surg* 42:305–308, 2003.
62. Laughlin RT, Reeve F, Wright DG, et al: Calcaneal osteomyelitis caused by nail puncture wounds, *Foot Ankle Int* 18:575–577, 1997.
63. Laughlin RT, Wright DG, Mader JT, et al: Osteomyelitis, *Curr Opin Rheumatol* 7:315–321, 1995.
64. Lavery LA, Armstrong DG, Quebedeaux TL, et al: Puncture wounds: normal laboratory values in the face of severe infec-tion in diabetics and non-diabetics, *Am J Med* 101:521–525, 1996.
65. Lavery LA, Walker SC, Harkless LB, et al: Infected puncture wounds in diabetic and nondiabetic adults, *Diabetes Care* 18:1588–1591, 1995.
66. Lazarettos J, Efstathopoulos N, Papagelopoulos PJ, et al: A bioresorbable calcium phosphate delivery system with teico-planin for treating MRSA osteomyelitis, *Clin Orthop Relat Res* 423:253–258, 2004.
67. Li SF, Henderson J, Dickman E, et al: Laboratory tests in adults with monoarticular arthritis: can they rule out a septic joint? *Acad Emerg Med* 11:276–280, 2004.
68. Lin SS, Ueng SW, Liu SJ, et al: Development of a biodegradable antibiotic delivery system, *Clin Orthop Relat Res* 362:240–250, 1999.
69. Loeffler RD, Ballard A: Plantar fascial spaces of the foot and a proposed surgical approach, *Foot Ankle* 1:11–14, 1980.
70. Mader JT, Cantrell JS, Calhoun J: Oral ciprofloxacin compared with standard parenteral antibiotic therapy for chronic osteo-myelitis in adults, *J Bone Joint Surg Am* 72:104–110, 1990.
71. Mader JT, Shirtliff M, Calhoun JH: Staging and staging application in osteomyelitis, *Clin Infect Dis* 25:1303–1309, 1997.
72. Mader JT, Shirtliff ME, Bergquist SC, et al: Antimicrobial treat-ment of chronic osteomyelitis, *Clin Orthop Relat Res* 360:47–65, 1999.
73. Manadan AM, Block JA: Daily needle aspiration versus surgical lavage for the treatment of bacterial septic arthritis in adults, *Am J Ther* 11:412–415, 2004.
74. Mangram AJ, Horan TC, Pearson ML, et al: Guideline for pre-vention of surgical site infection, 1999. Centers for Disease Control and Prevention (CDC) Hospital Infection Control Practices Advisory Committee, *Am J Infect Control* 27:97–132; quiz 133–134; discussion 196, 1999.
75. Manian FA, Meyer PL, Setzer J, et al: Surgical site infections associated with methicillin-resistant *Staphylococcus aureus*: do postoperative factors play a role? *Clin Infect Dis* 36:863–868, 2003.
76. Marcinko DE, editor: *Infections of the foot*, St Louis, 1998, Mosby.
77. Mathews CJ, Weston, VC, Jones A, et al: Bacterial septic arthritis in adults, *Lancet* 375:846–855, 2010.
78. Mattone-Volpe F: Cutaneous larva migrans infection in the pediatric foot. A review and two case reports, *J Am Podiatr Med Assoc* 88:228–231, 1998.
79. Mazza A: Ceftriaxone as short-term antibiotic prophylaxis in orthopedic surgery: a cost-benefit analysis involving 808 patients, *J Chemother* 12(Suppl 3):29–33, 2000.
80. McLaren AC: Alternative materials to acrylic bone cement for delivery of depot antibiotics in orthopaedic infections, *Clin Orthop Relat Res* 427:101–106, 2004.
81. Mirmiran R, Hembree JL 3rd, Reed WP, et al: Disseminated gonococcal infection: a case of beta-lactamase–producing *Neisseria gonorrhoeae*, *J Am Podiatr Med Assoc* 90:273–275, 2000.
82. Mizel MS, Steinmetz ND, Trepman E: Detection of wooden foreign bodies in muscle tissue: experimental comparison of computed tomography, magnetic resonance imaging, and ultrasonography, *Foot Ankle Int* 15:437–443, 1994.
83. Mohan AK, Cote TR, Siegel JN, et al: Infectious complications of biologic treatments of rheumatoid arthritis, *Curr Opin Rheu-matol* 15:179–184, 2003.
84. Morrison WB, Ledermann HP, Schweitzer ME: MR imaging of inflammatory conditions of the ankle and foot, *Magn Reson Imaging Clin North Am* 9:615–637, xi–xii, 2001.
85. Morrison WB, Schweitzer ME, Batte WG, et al: Osteomyelitis of the foot: relative importance of primary and secondary MR imaging signs, *Radiology* 207:625–632, 1998.

86. Morrison WB, Schweitzer ME, Wapner KL, et al: Osteomyelitis in feet of diabetics: clinical accuracy, surgical utility, and cost-effectiveness of MR imaging, *Radiology* 196:557–564, 1995.

87. Mushlin AI, Littenberg B: Diagnosing pedal osteomyelitis: testing choices and their consequences, *J Gen Intern Med* 9:1–7, 1994.

88. Myers RA, Littel ML, Joseph WS: Bite wound infections of the lower extremity, *Clin Podiatr Med Surg* 7:501–508, 1990.

89. Nade S: Septic arthritis, *Best Pract Res Clin Rheumatol* 17:183–200, 2003.

90. Nelson CL: The current status of material used for depot delivery of drugs, *Clin Orthop Relat Res* 427:72–78, 2004.

91. Olson MM, MacCallum J, McQuarrie DG: Preoperative hair removal with clippers does not increase infection rate in clean surgical wounds, *Surg Gynecol Obstet* 162:181–182, 1986.

92. O'Quinn JC, Dushin R: Cutaneous larva migrans case report with current recommendations for treatment, *J Am Podiatr Med Assoc* 95:291–294, 2005.

93. O'Riordan E, Denton J, Taylor PM, et al: Madura foot in the U.K.: fungal osteomyelitis after renal transplantation, *Transplantation* 73:151–153, 2002.

94. Osmon DR: Antimicrobial prophylaxis in adults, *Mayo Clin Proc* 75:98–109, 2000.

95. Ostermann PA, Seligson D, Henry SL: Local antibiotic therapy for severe open fractures. A review of 1085 consecutive cases, *J Bone Joint Surg Br* 77:93–97, 1995.

96. Ostrander RV, Brage ME, Botte MJ: Bacterial skin contamination after surgical preparation in foot and ankle surgery, *Clin Orthop Relat Res* 406:246–252, 2003.

97. Ostrander RV, Botte MJ, Brage E: Efficacy of surgical preparation solutions in foot and ankle surgery, *J Bone Joint Surg Am* 87:980–985, 2005.

98. Pomposelli JJ, Baxter JK 3rd, Babineau TJ, et al: Early postoperative glucose control predicts nosocomial infection rate in diabetic patients, *JPEN J Parenter Enteral Nutr* 22:77–81, 1998.

99. Prokuski L: Prophylactic antibiotics in orthopaedic surgery, *J Am Acad Orthop Surg* 16:283–293, 2008.

100. Rice DA, Mendez-Vigo L: Daptomycin in bone and joint infections: a review of the literature, *Arch Orthop Surg* 129:1495–1504, 2009.

101. Rightmire E, Zurakowski D, Vrahas M: Acute infections after fracture repair, *Clin Orthop Relat Res* 466:466–472, 2008.

102. Rodgers P, Bassler M: Treating onychomycosis, *Am Fam Physician* 63:663–672, 677–668, 2001.

103. Rutledge B, Huyette D, Day D, et al: Treatment of osteomyelitis with local antibiotics delivered via bioabsorbable polymer, *Clin Orthop Relat Res* 411:280–287, 2003.

104. Sakayama K, Kidani T, Sugawara Y, et al: Mycetoma of foot: a rare case report and review of the literature, *Foot Ankle Int* 25:763–767, 2004.

105. Sany J, Anaya JM, Canovas F, et al: Influence of methotrexate on the frequency of postoperative infectious complications in patients with rheumatoid arthritis, *J Rheumatol* 20:1129–1132, 1993.

106. Schade VL, Roukis TS: The role of polymethylmethacrylate antibiotic-loaded cement in addition to debridement for the treatment of soft tissue and osseous infections of the foot and ankle, *J Foot Ankle Surg* 49:55–62, 2010.

107. Schade VL, Thomas SR, Haque M: *Clostridium septicum* necrotizing fasciitis of the forefoot secondary to adenocarcioma of the colon: case report and review of the literature, *J Foot Ankle Surg* 49:149.e1–159.e2, 2010.

108. Scharer BM, Sanicola SM: The in vitro elution characteristics of vancomycin from calcium phosphate-calcium sulfate beads, *J Foot Ankle Surg* 48:540–542, 2009.

109. Schildhauer TA, Robbie B, Muhr G, Koller M: Bacterial adherence to tantalum versus commonly used orthopedic metallic implant materials, *J Orthop Trauma* 20:476–484, 2006.

110. Shams WE, Rapp RP: Methicillin-resistant staphylococcal infections: an important consideration for orthopedic surgeons, *Orthopedics* 27:565–568, 2004.

111. Solomkin JS: Antibiotic resistance in postoperative infections, *Crit Care Med* 29:N97–N99, 2001.

112. Sorensen LT, Karlsmark T, Gottrup F: Abstinence from smoking reduces incisional wound infection: a randomized controlled trial, *Ann Surg* 238:1–5, 2003.

113. Stephens MM, MacAuley P: Brodie's abscess. A long-term review, *Clin Orthop Relat Res* 234:211–216, 1988.

114. Strauss MB, Bryant B: Hyperbaric oxygen, *Orthopedics* 25:303–310, 2002.

115. Stewart PS, Costerton JW: Antibiotic resistance of bacteria in biofilms, *Lancet* 358:135–138, 2001.

116. Tan JS, File TM Jr.: Management of staphylococcal and streptococcal infections, *Clin Podiatr Med Surg* 13:793–816, 1996.

117. Unal SN, Birinci H, Baktiroglu S, et al: Comparison of Tc-99m methylene diphosphonate, Tc-99m human immune globulin, and Tc-99m-labeled white blood cell scintigraphy in the diabetic foot, *Clin Nucl Med* 26:1016–1021, 2001.

118. Vinken AG, Li JZ, Balan DA, et al: Comparison of linezolid with oxacillin or vancomycin in the empiric treatment of cellulitis in US hospitals, *Am J Ther* 10:264–274, 2003.

119. Wall DB, de Virgilio C, Black S, et al: Objective criteria may assist in distinguishing necrotizing fasciitis from nonnecrotizing soft tissue infection, *Am J Surg* 179:17–21, 2000.

120. Wong CH, Chang HC, Pasupathy S, et al: Necrotizing fasciitis: clinical presentation, microbiology, and determinants of mortality, *J Bone Joint Surg Am* 85:1454–1460, 2003.

121. Wong CH, Khin, L, Heng K, et al: The LRINEC (Laboratory Risk Indicator for Necrotizing Fasciitis) score: a tool for distinguishing necrotizing fasciitis from other soft tissue infections, *Crit Care Med* 32:1535–1541, 2004.

122. Wu S, Zecha P, Feitz R, et al: Vacuum therapy as an intermediate phase in wound closure: a clinical experience, *Eur J Plast Surg* 23:174–177, 2000.

123. Young BA, Fee MJ, Giacopelli JA, et al: Mycetoma, *J Am Podiatr Med Assoc* 90:81–84, 2000.

124. Zacharias J, Largen PS, Crosby LA: Results of preprocedure and postprocedure toe cultures in orthopaedic surgery, *Foot Ankle Int* 19:166–168, 1998.

125. Zalavras CG, Patzakis MJ, Holtom P: Local antibiotic therapy in the treatment of open fractures and osteomyelitis, *Clin Orthop Relat Res* 427:86–93, 2004.

126. Zgonis T, Jolly GP, Garbalosa JC: The efficacy of prophylactic intravenous antibiotics in elective foot and ankle surgery, *J Foot Ankle Surg* 43:97–103, 2004.

Dermatology of the Foot and Lower Extremity

Douglas W. Kress

The most up-to-date dermatology textbooks describe several thousand distinct conditions. Many of these are limited to the feet. Many more involve the skin in a more widespread manner but show characteristic changes on the feet and lower extremities. This chapter defines the terms used to describe and diagnose skin lesions and discusses dermatologic conditions that affect the feet.

Dermatologic conditions are first defined by the type of primary skin lesions that occur. The most important primary skin lesions are defined as follows:

- *Bulla:* Raised, fluid-filled lesion greater than 1 cm in diameter.
- *Macule:* Flat skin lesion seen only as an area of color change on the skin surface and not palpable.
- *Nodule:* Raised solid legion with indistinct borders and a component felt deeply below the skin surface.
- *Papule:* Solid raised lesion less than 1 cm diameter.
- *Plaque:* Solid raised lesion greater than 1 cm in diameter and with distinct borders.
- *Pustule:* Papule filled with pus, giving it a yellow-white appearance.
- *Vesicle:* Raised, fluid-filled lesion less than 1 cm in diameter.

Secondary skin changes occur over time and with trauma to the skin and include the following conditions:

- *Atrophy:* Thinning of the skin seen as a shiny, wrinkled skin surface.
- *Crusting:* Dried exudate that sits on the skin surface during and after an acute dermatitis.
- *Erosion:* Depression into the skin, with the base of the lesion still within the epidermis.
- *Excoriations:* Linearly oriented crusted lesions secondary to scratching and typically seen in pruritic dermatoses.
- *Lichenification:* Thickening of the skin as manifested by accentuation of normal skin tension lines.
- *Scaling:* Excess amount of stratum corneum that appears as white plates on the skin surface.
- *Ulcer:* Depression into the skin, with the base of the lesion into the dermis.

All dermatologic conditions can be grouped into diseases that manifest with similar primary lesions. The first group discussed is *papulosquamous diseases*. The conditions in this group all manifest with redness and scaling of the skin. These lesions can show papules and plaques on the skin. The second group includes diseases expressed as isolated *papules, plaques,* and *nodules* on the skin. This group includes a number of benign and malignant tumors. The third group of diseases is defined as *purpuric eruptions*. The term *purpura* defines extravasation of red blood cells (RBCs) out of cutaneous blood vessels, which gives the skin a deep red to purplish appearance. Purpura does not blanch with pressure.

PAPULOSQUAMOUS DISEASES

Primary Skin Conditions

Atopic Dermatitis

Atopic dermatitis describes the spectrum of red, scaly pruritic rashes seen in individuals with a family history of atopy. *Atopy* describes a group of disorders that run together in families, which have historically included asthma, allergic rhinitis, food allergies, and atopic dermatitis. Most recently, a number of experts now also include eosinophillic gastroenteritis as part of the spectrum of atopy. In very young children (younger than 1 year), the characteristic rash of atopic dermatitis is limited to the face and scalp. As children get older, the rash is seen mainly on the flexors, specifically on both the popliteal and antecubital fossae. Atopic dermatitis often is manifested on the feet or hands, or both, of adults, where it is seen as a diffuse, pruritic, scaly, erythematous eruption (Fig. 16-1). Toe web spaces are usually spared, which can help differentiate atopic dermatitis from dyshidrotic eczema and tinea pedis.

Combination therapy usually works best for atopic dermatitis of the feet. This includes potent and ultrapotent topical steroid ointments to help treat the dermatitis. An oral antihistamine is often helpful to decrease the associated pruritus. In severe cases, tar derivatives can be compounded with topical steroids to increase the effectiveness of the topical preparation and to allow the use of a milder, and thus safer, topical steroid. It is important to have patients take at least 1 week off per month from the use of strong topical steroids. During this break, the best maintenance treatment is the use of over-the-counter moisturizers that contain ceramides. Ceramides are a family of proteins which help to maintain the skin's barrier function and are deficient in the skin of patients with atopic dermatitis.[4,7]

A group of agents known as topical immunomodulators (TIMs) has been approved for the treatment of atopic dermatitis. However, their poor penetration significantly limits their use on the thick skin of the soles and palms. There are several systemic treatments available for severe cases of atopic dermatitis, such as cyclosprine, methotrexate, and azothioprine; however, discussion of their use is beyond the scope of this chapter.[18]

Dyshidrotic Eczema

Dyshidrotic eczema is a common eczematous dermatitis limited to the feet and hands. The earliest clinical lesions are pruritic microvesicles along the side of the toes, fingers, feet, and hands (Fig. 16-2). However, the eruption usually progresses to take on a papulosquamous appearance. Dyshidrotic eczema was previously thought to be a response to excessive or abnormal sweating, thus the term *dyshidrosis*. Although patients with this condition often do have hyperhidrosis, this is no longer thought to be the cause. Treatment is identical to that of atopic dermatitis in most cases.

Psoriasis

Psoriasis is a common papulosquamous skin disease affecting 1% to 2% of the population. It most often

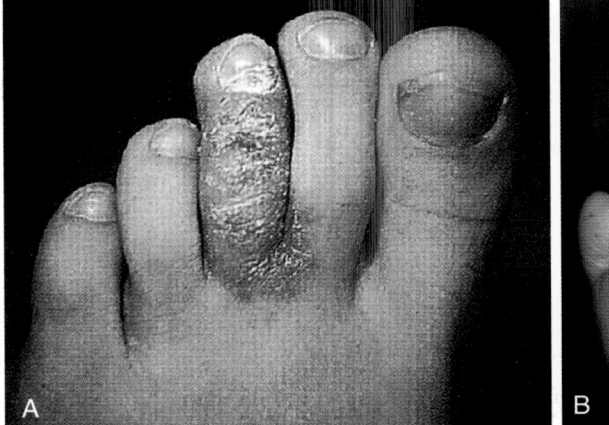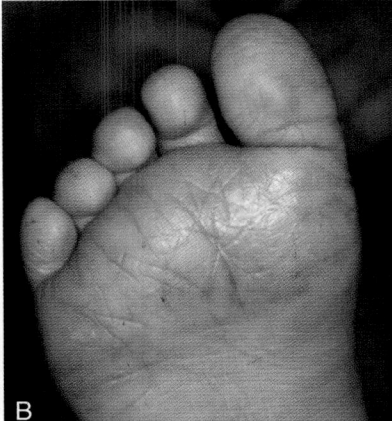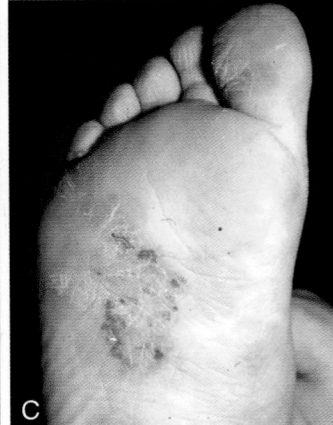

Figure 16-1 Atopic dermatitis. Note the diffuse scaling and erythema on the dorsal aspect of toes **(A)**, plantar aspect of the toes **(B)**, and plantar foot **(C)**.

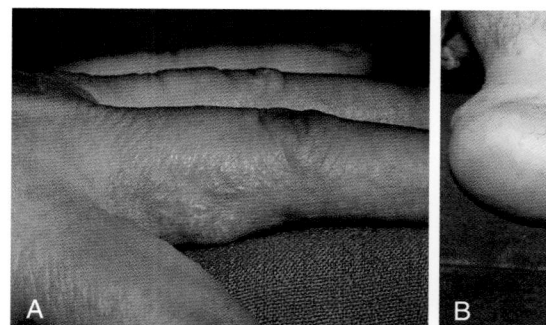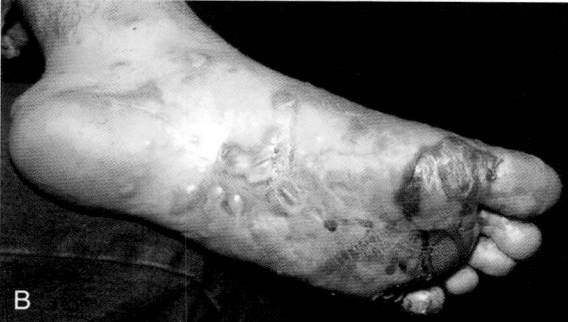

Figure 16-2 Dyshidrotic eczema. **A,** Note the areas of vesiculation on the lateral aspect of the fingers. **B,** More significant blistering and erythema can be seen in this severe case involving the plantar surface.

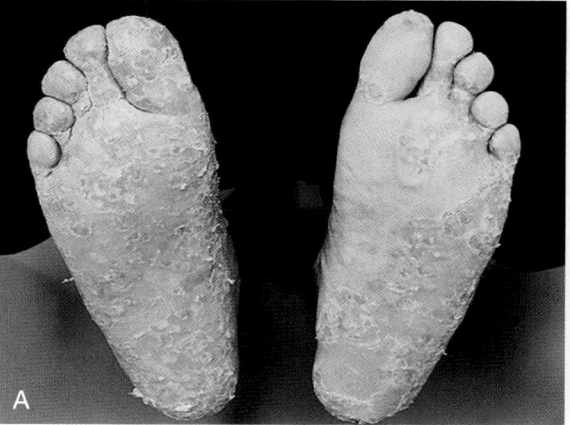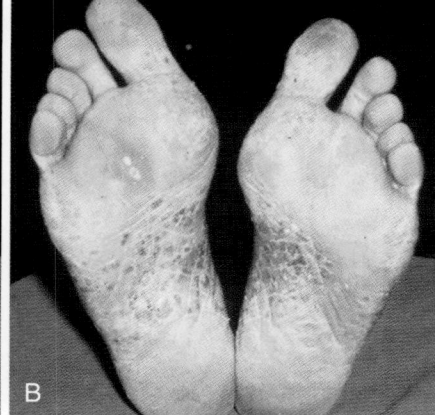

Figure 16-3 Psoriasis. **A,** Plantar psoriasis. Note the diffuse, thick, white scaling of the feet. **B,** There is also a pustular variant of psoriasis, most commonly seen on the feet as pictured here.

affects the elbows, knees, scalp, feet, and hands. The primary skin lesion of psoriasis is a well-demarcated, erythematous plaque with an overlying thick, silvery scale (Fig. 16-3). A helpful clue in diagnosing psoriasis is the finding of a pinpoint of blood when one of the overlying scales is removed. This is the *Auspitz sign*. Psoriasis lesions on the feet can be very hyperkeratotic. Pitting of the nails is seen in 35% of patients with psoriasis and up to 85% of patients with psoriatic arthritis.

Treatment for psoriasis begins with potent topical steroid ointments. If these are not effective as monotherapy, tar soaks can be used before application of the topical steroids. Several new topical preparations are also available for the treatment of plaque psoriasis, including vitamin D cream and ointment and several retinoic acid derivatives. For the most severe cases of psoriasis of the feet, treatment with either cytotoxic agents (such as methotrexate and cyclosporine) or any of the antitumor necrosis factor biologic therapies are reasonable options but are beyond the scope of this chapter.[8]

Patients with psoriasis can also manifest the Koebner phenomenon. This is psoriatic plaques within areas of skin trauma. It is commonly seen developing within surgical scars.

Contact Dermatitis

Two types of contact dermatitis can be seen on the feet: irritant and allergic. *Irritant contact dermatitis* appears as a diffuse, scaly, erythematous eruption, usually over the dorsum of the foot. It is usually only mildly itchy. This type of eruption can be caused by certain acids, soaps, or other substances that are irritating to the skin. This is a nonspecific reaction and can be seen on anyone.

Allergic contact dermatitis is a specific eruption that requires a previous exposure to an allergenic compound and is mediated by the immune system. Chronic contact dermatitis is seen as a well-demarcated area of scaling and erythema (Fig. 16-4), whereas acute contact dermatitis can also show vesiculation. Both are very pruritic. The most common causes of contact dermatitis on the feet are components used in the production of rubber or the tanning of leather.[17]

To confirm the diagnosis of irritant versus allergic contact dermatitis, patients are patch tested for the most common allergens seen in this setting. Once the irritant or allergen is determined, avoidance is recommended. If that is not possible, daily use of over-the-counter moisturizers containing dimethicone can be helpful because dimethicone creates a barrier over the skin. If those two

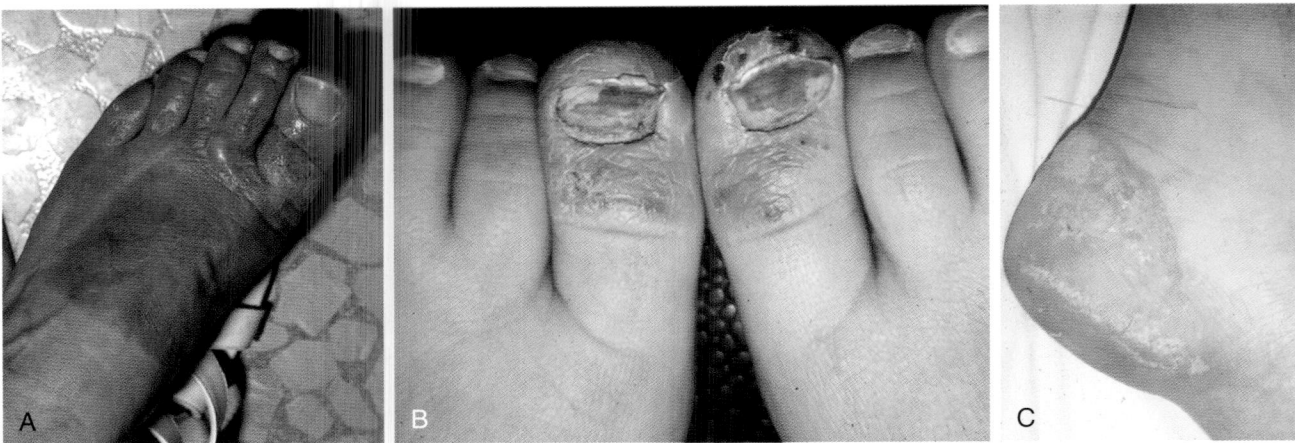

Figure 16-4 Contact dermatitis. Note the well-demarcated areas of erythema and some scaling on the dorsal foot **(A)**, the dorsal hallux bilaterally **(B)**, and the heel **(C)**.

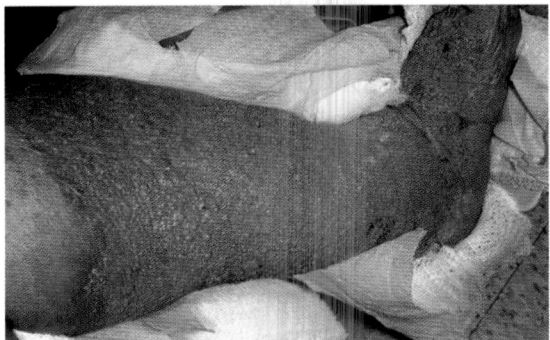

Figure 16-5 Chronic stasis dermatitis. Note the edema, erythema, and scaling of the lower extremity.

measures fail, treatment for irritant or contact dermatitis is similar to that of atopic dermatitis; a combination of potent topical steroids and oral antihistamines helps decrease the associated pruritus.

Stasis Dermatitis

Stasis dermatitis is a common papulosquamous eruption seen in elderly persons, usually those who have lower extremity edema or poor venous return. In either case, RBCs extravasate from the blood vessels of the skin into the connective tissue of the skin itself. Clinically, this is manifested as a swollen leg with overlying, pruritic scaling and erythema (Fig. 16-5). This eruption is usually limited to the anterior tibial surfaces and below, often affecting the ankles and the dorsa of the feet as well.

Treatment for stasis dermatitis begins with treating the lower extremity edema with elastic (Ace) wraps, compression therapy devices, diuretics, or any combination of these. Once the edema resolves, it is usually possible to clear the secondary stasis dermatitis with mild-to-moderately potent topical steroid ointment. It is important to keep the peripheral edema at a minimum to prevent recurrences.

The most severe and worrisome complication of stasis dermatitis is *venous stasis ulceration* (Fig. 16-6). These ulcers most often are seen on the medial aspect of the ankles. They usually result from mild trauma to an atrophied area of epidermis with compromised blood supply. The ulcers usually have a well-demarcated edge and thick, adherent yellow exudates at their bases. Most wound healing centers have found that optimum treatment includes daily application of silver sulfadiazine cream to the wound under Ace wraps. If this is not effective, Unna boots can be placed and changed weekly. Secondary infection must be treated with oral antibiotics on an as-needed basis. For severe recalcitrant ulcerations, especially in diabetics, platelet-derived growth factor is now available as a topical preparation, but it is extraordinarily expensive.

Lichen Planus

Lichen planus is a skin disease characterized by numerous polygonal, violaceous, flat-topped papules. These lesions often have very thin overlying white scales known as *Wickham striae*. The most common areas of involvement are the dorsal aspects of the ankles and wrists (Fig. 16-7). Oral and genital mucous membranes also can be involved.

An uncommon variation is *hypertrophic lichen planus.* This condition manifests with large hyperkeratotic, violaceous plaques over the anterior tibial surfaces. If left untreated, the chronic inflammation associated with this condition can predispose the affected area to a squamous cell carcinoma.[12] Lichen planus also exhibits the Koebner phenomenon (see the earlier discussion of psoriasis).

Treatment for lichen planus is usually a combination of potent topical steroid ointments and oral antihistamines because it is often quite pruritic. For more widespread cases, short pulses of systemic steroids or longer courses of systemic retinoids (derivatives of vitamin A) can be effective.

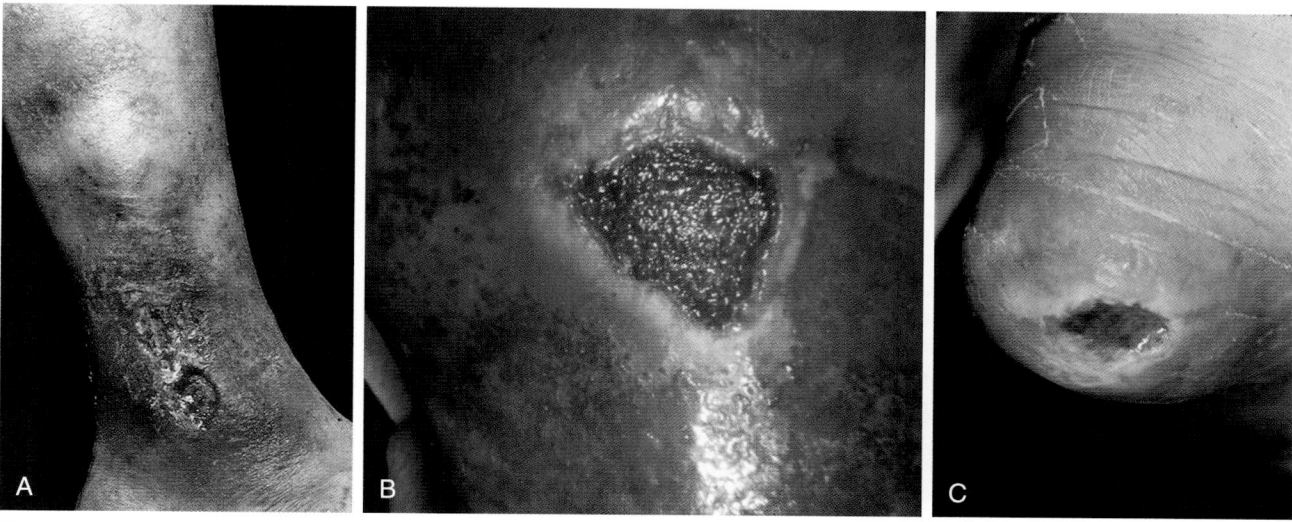

Figure 16-6 **A,** Venous stasis ulceration on the ankle. **B,** Close-up photograph of similar lesion on the calf. **C,** A similar lesion on the plantar lateral aspect of the heel.

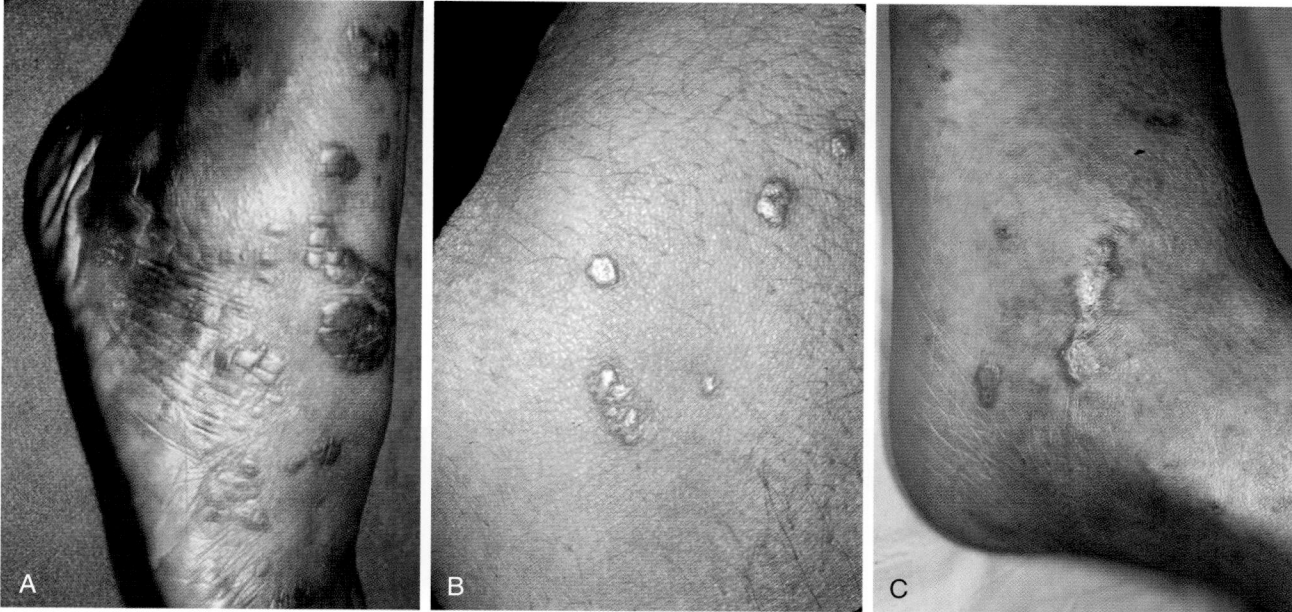

Figure 16-7 Lichen planus. **A,** Note the purple and hyperpigmented papules and plaques on the dorsal foot. **B,** Smaller papules on the foot. **C,** An example of the Koebner phenomenon.

Pityriasis Rubra Pilaris

Pityriasis rubra pilaris (PRP) is an uncommon skin condition, but it is included here because it often manifests with a characteristic eruption on the soles and palms. In its most extreme form, PRP presents as an *exfoliative erythroderma,* a condition in which patients are red and scaly from head to toe. The soles and palms of most patients with pityriasis rubra pilaris have a carnauba wax appearance (Fig. 16-8). This refers to the massive palmoplantar hyperkeratosis and its resemblance to the yellow wax

once on to treat surfboards. Pityriasis rubra pilaris can be confused with widespread psoriasis. Treatment of this condition is usually with methotrexate or etretinate, which is an oral vitamin A derivative.

Keratoderma

Keratodermas are a group of conditions associated with a thickening of the cornified layer of the epidermis. Keratodermas can be widespread or localized. Both types almost always involve the skin of the soles and palms

(Fig. 16-9). More than 20 types of keratoderma are described in the literature. Discussion of their individual features and treatment options is beyond the scope of this chapter.[21]

Skin Eruptions Caused by Infections

Tinea Pedis

Tinea pedis (athlete's foot) is a very common superficial infection affecting humans. This chronic infection is often misdiagnosed and mistreated. The warm, moist environment of the feet leads to increased maceration of the skin, which allows penetration of the causative organisms, most commonly members of the *Trichophyton* species.

Three types of tinea pedis are seen. *Interdigital tinea pedis* most often begins with involvement of the fourth interdigital web space. Clinical findings include erythema, scaling, and maceration in the web spaces. Involvement can spread to include the soles and the dorsa of the feet. When involvement of the top and bottom of the feet predominates, the term *moccasin tinea pedis* has been used to define this second type (Fig. 16-10). The somewhat more unusual third type, *bullous tinea pedis,* shows numerous small blisters and can be confused with bullous dyshidrotic eczema. The only way to confirm this diagnosis is by potassium hydroxide (KOH) examination.

For diagnosing interdigital or moccasin tinea pedis, an appropriate sample can be obtained by scraping the skin from the leading edge of scale of the lesion. This can be done by scraping one microscope slide against another or by carefully scraping with a No. 15 scalpel blade. Once a specimen has been obtained, it should be treated with 10% KOH and gently warmed. Immediate examination under the low- or high-power objective of a standard microscope should show hyphal elements (Fig. 16-11).

Many treatments are now available for uncomplicated tinea pedis. All the azole-type antifungal creams as well as ciclopirox olamine are effective in treating the most common causes of tinea pedis.[1,2,29] Creams of the allylamine class also effectively treat tinea pedis, but they are not very effective in the treatment of *Candida* infections. *Candida* can affect the toe webs and is an uncommon cause of onychomycosis. It is rarely necessary to use oral antifungal agents in the treatment of tinea pedis. Their use is discussed in the section on treatment of onychomycosis.

Onychomycosis

Onychomycosis, or fungal infection of the nails, is a common condition. Approximately 20% to 40% of

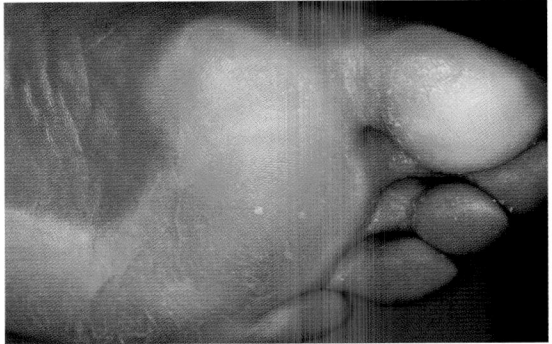

Figure 16-8 Pityriasis rubra pilaris. Plantar surface with carnauba wax–like hyperkeratosis.

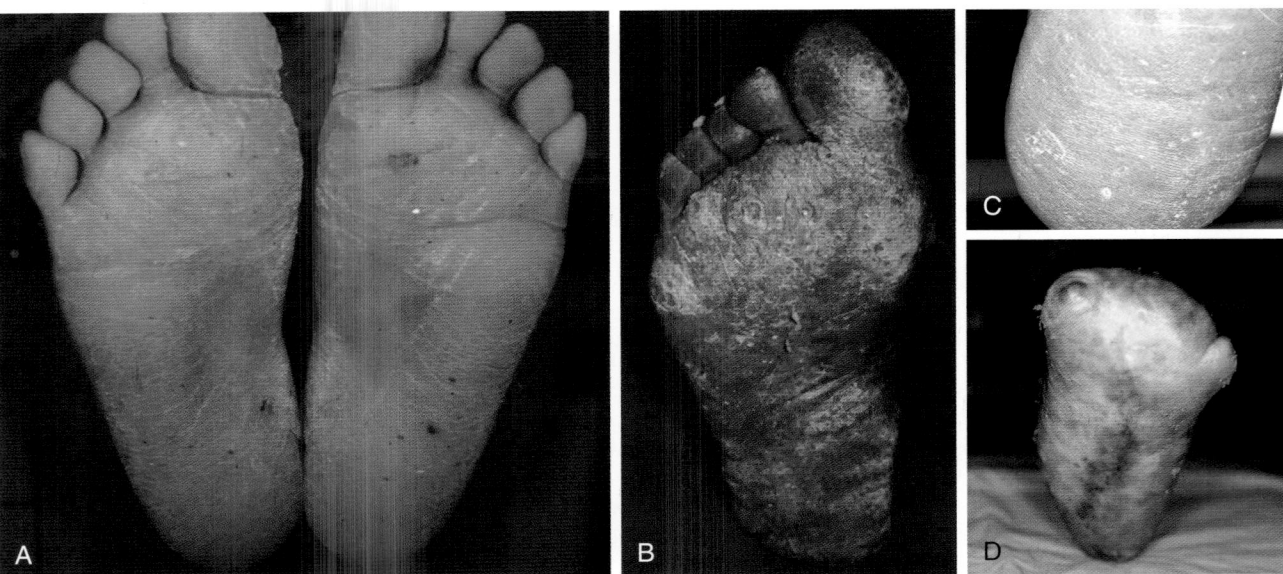

Figure 16-9 Plantar keratoderma pictured on the bilateral feet **(A)** and on one foot **(B). C,** A close-up of the thickened skin. **D,** Olmsted syndrome, a mutilating plantar keratoderma.

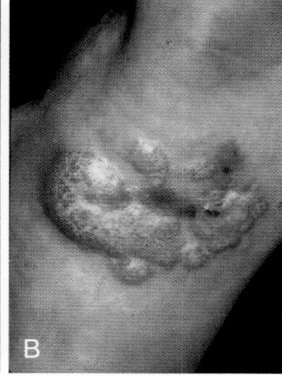

Figure 16-10 Moccasin tinea pedis. **A,** Areas of scaling and erythema with leading edge of scale. **B,** There is also a bullous variant of tinea pedis pictured here on the plantar surface. (**A,** From Dockery GL: *Cutaneous disorders of the lower extremity,* Philadelphia, 1997, WB Saunders.)

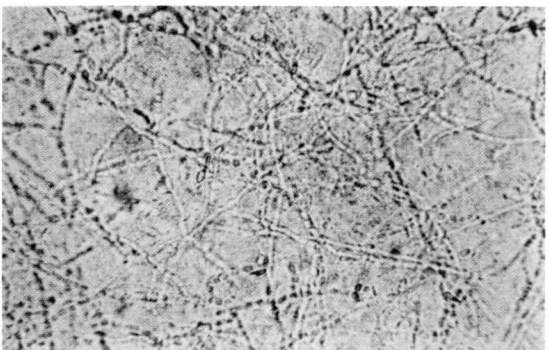

Figure 16-11 A positive potassium hydroxide examination showing the branching hyphal elements seen in all dermatophyte infections.

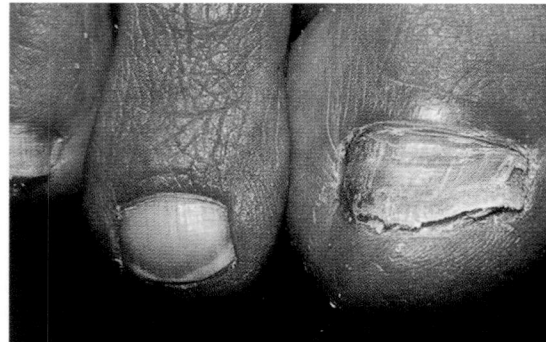

Figure 16-12 Onychomycosis. Note nail dystrophy with subungual debris.

persons older than 60 years show evidence of onychomycosis. Clinically, the most common type of onychomycosis is a progressive thickening of the nails with yellow subungual debris and overlying nail dystrophy (Fig. 16-12). Toenails are involved approximately four times more often than fingernails, and men are affected much more often than women. More than 90% of cases are caused by common dermatophytic fungi. The remaining 10% are caused by a combination of *Candida* species and other, rarer fungal organisms.

Before pursuing oral antifungal therapy for onychomycosis, it is important to confirm the diagnosis with a KOH examination or fungal culture. Only 50% of all cases of nail dystrophy are caused by fungal infection. The remaining 50% are caused by psoriasis, lichen planus, trauma, and periungual eczematous skin changes.

To obtain an appropriate sample to KOH or culture, the affected nails must be clipped back and a sample of subungual debris obtained. A KOH examination can be performed on this material as described previously, but these preparations can be very difficult to interpret. The two best ways to confirm this diagnosis are either to send the nail clippings and debris for a fungal culture or to send a large nail clipping for routine histology. The downside of sending material for a fungal culture is that final results can take as long as a month, whereas routine histology results are available within a few days.[16]

The main reason for confirming the diagnosis by biopsy or culture is that most agents effective against onychomycosis are very expensive and have several side effects and numerous drug interactions. The only oral agents currently approved by the U.S. Food and Drug Administration (FDA) for the treatment of onychomycosis in the United States are itraconazole and terbinafine.[2,14,19] Ciclopirox nail lacquer is the first topical agent to be approved for this indication.

Paronychia
Paronychia is clinically seen as painful and tender swelling and erythema of the periungual skin (Fig. 16-13). It can affect one or many fingers or toes. Historically, paronychia was thought to be a mixed infection with both a *Candida* species and either *Staphylococcus* or *Streptococcus* species. Based on that theory, treatment regimens often included both antibiotics and antifungals. The choice to use either oral or topical agents was dictated by the extent and severity of the disease state. Although this is still thought to be true in most cases of acute paronychia, some recent evidence suggests that chronic paronychia is primarily an inflammatory process, with the infection being secondary. This evidence comes from a study that showed potent topical steroids were superior to oral antifungal therapy in treating chronic paronychia.[24,26]

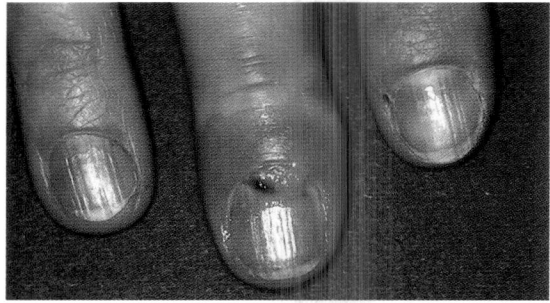

Figure 16-13 Acute paronychia. Note the periungual erythema and edema. Similar changes can be seen on the toes.

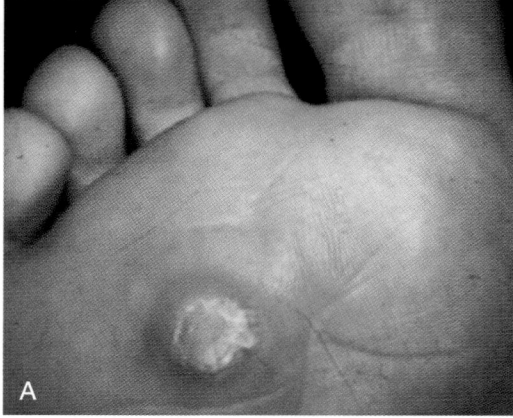

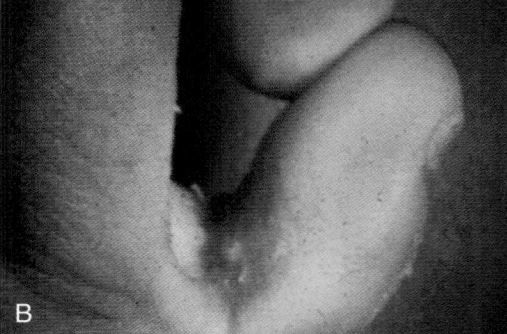

Figure 16-14 Clavi (corns). **A,** Firm, well-demarcated hyperkeratotic center of hard corn. **B,** Interdigital soft corn.

PAPULES, PLAQUES, AND NODULES

Benign Growths

Callus

Calluses are the most common hyperkeratotic skin lesions seen on the feet. They develop at sites of pressure, usually under bony prominences.[25] They tend to be among the largest lesions seen on the feet.

It is important to differentiate calluses from the other hyperkeratotic lesions that occur on the feet, such as corns and warts, because these lesions sometimes need to be treated differently. One of the best ways to differentiate all these hyperkeratotic lesions is to pare away the overlying hyperkeratosis carefully with a No. 15 scalpel blade. Several important differences can be noted as the overlying hyperkeratosis is pared away. First, the margins of calluses are rather diffuse, whereas those of corns and warts are sharply demarcated. A callus has no clinically apparent core, whereas one is usually seen with a corn. No capillary dotting is seen within a callus, and capillary dotting is almost always seen as the surface of a wart is pared down. Symptomatology can also help with diagnosis. Calluses are usually not painful, whereas both warts and corns can be very painful. Corns often show tenderness with direct pressure, whereas warts can show tenderness with lateral pressure.

Treatment of calluses usually requires removing the pressure that causes them. This can be done by having the patient wear better-fitting shoes or using special insoles made for the shoes that the patient wears most often. Some of the overlying hyperkeratosis can be removed with potent keratolytics, such as the over-the-counter or prescription-strength moisturizers containing lactic or salicylic acid. For more extreme forms of calluses, it may be necessary to use tars or urea, alone or in some combination in a moisturizing base, to help thin down the overlying hyperkeratosis. Occlusion of these keratolytic preparations can also increase their efficacy.

Clavus (Corn)

Corns, or clavi, also result from a combination of friction or localized pressure. The most common sites are on the

balls of the great toe, on the sides of the other toes, and under bony prominences, particularly in the metatarsal area (Fig. 16-14).[5,22]

The most effective treatment for corns begins with aggressive paring with a No. 15 blade. As the overlying hyperkeratosis is pared away, a small (1- to 2-mm) central core can be seen within the base of the lesion. The central core is responsible for the tenderness associated with corns. Sometimes the entire central corn can be pared away. If this is possible, paring usually provides immediate pain relief for the patient.

If care is not taken, however, the corn can recur rapidly. It is important to use corn pads to spread out the pressure on the affected area once the kernel of the lesion has been removed. If it is not possible to remove the entire core, treatment can continue with the combination of aggressive keratolytics described earlier for calluses. It is also helpful to wear shoes that do not cause so much pressure or to have special insoles or shoes made.[6]

Verruca Vulgaris (Wart)

Warts are a common infectious skin lesion seen on the feet, as well as the most common infectious skin lesions seen on the body as a whole, especially in children. Warts are benign epithelial proliferations caused by a number of different subtypes of the human papillomavirus (HPV). Different HPV subtypes are responsible for causing different clinical types of warts, as well as warts in different

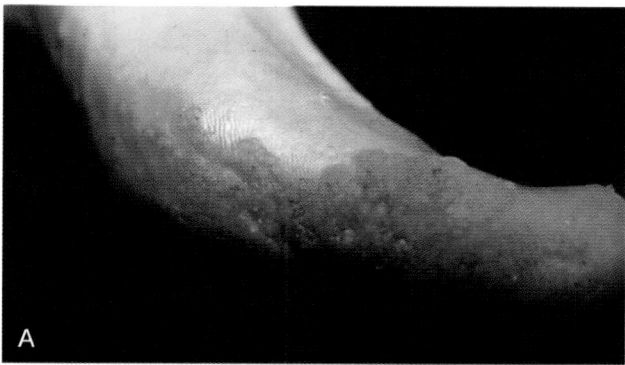

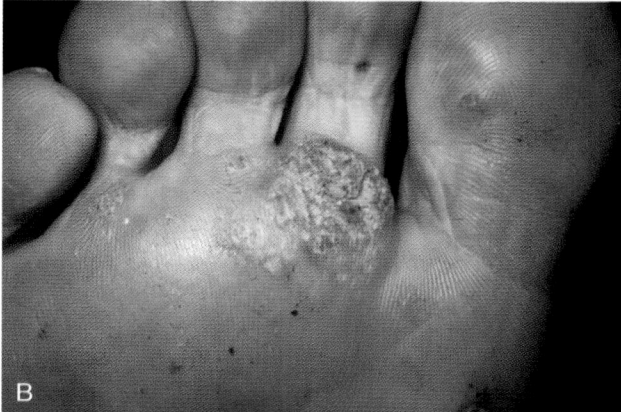

Figure 16-15 **A,** A large mosaic planter wart. **B,** A smaller wart with capillary dotting.

locations on the body. Common plantar and palmar warts are caused by HPV types 1 and 2.

Plantar warts can manifest with several different clinical patterns. The clinical spectrum ranges from small (1- to 2-mm) hyperkeratotic papules to lesions several centimeters in diameter and representing a mosaic of individual lesions (Fig. 16-15). The most useful clinical clue to identifying a wart is the presence of *capillary dotting.* Capillary dots are seen as red to brown to black speckles of less than 1 mm on the wart's surface. If these are not immediately apparent, they are often seen once some of the overlying hyperkeratosis has been pared away. It is important to pare down the lesions somewhat to differentiate warts definitively from corns and other hyperkeratotic lesions on the soles.

Numerous therapies have been reported effective in the treatment of warts.[3,9,10,15,20] Before beginning therapy for plantar warts, it is important to remember that many warts resolve without therapy, especially in children. Approximately 50% of all warts in children resolve within 2 years with no therapy. Therefore any treatment tried needs to be more successful than that high placebo effect.

I believe that the gold standard for the treatment of one or a few plantar warts is several cycles of liquid nitrogen cryotherapy. The lesion should be aggressively pared down with a No. 15 scalpel blade. Each lesion should then be treated with two 10-second cycles of liquid nitrogen cryotherapy, with a 10-second thaw between the two freezes. It is important to warn patients that after the freezing, blisters can form at the treated site. If a blister forms and is painful, simple drainage can provide significant pain relief. If the blister is not painful, it should be left intact. The lesion should be bandaged with antibiotic ointment for several days. Cryotherapy should be repeated monthly for 2 to 3 months if the lesions appear to be responding.

For numerous or extremely recalcitrant lesions, many topical therapies have been reported to be effective. These include cantharidin, salicylic acid, and podophyllotoxin applied either alone or in combination. Topical 5-fluorouracil compounded with salicylic acid has also been used. The pulse dye laser has also been reported to be effective in the treatment of plantar warts.[3] However, use of electrodesiccation or the carbon dioxide (CO_2) laser is not recommended because both can produce a smoke plume from which live virus particles can be isolated.[10]

A more recent addition to the armamentarium of topical agents includes three medicines initially designed and approved to treat genital warts in adults. These include imiquimod, podophyllotoxin, and topical sinchatecins, which is a derivative from green tea. Because these agents were initially approved for use on genital skin, an area where the skin is very thin, it is usually necessary to combine them with a topical keratolytic, such as salicylic acid, to improve their penetration and efficiacy on the thicker plantar skin.[20]

Seborrheic Keratosis

Seborrheic keratoses are one of the most common skin lesions seen as people age. They most often occur on the trunk as 0.5- to 1.5-cm tan to brown verrucous plaques that have the appearance of being stuck onto the skin. They are completely benign lesions.

A variant of seborrheic keratosis, *stucco keratosis,* is often seen in older persons below the knees and on the dorsum of the feet. These lesions appear clinically slightly different from the standard seborrheic keratosis; they are smaller and usually white to tan (Fig. 16-16). Some persons have only a few, and others have hundreds of these small keratoses scattered over their legs.

Stucco keratoses are also entirely benign lesions. If some are particularly bothersome, the treatment of choice is two short cycles of cryotherapy with liquid nitrogen.

Nevus

Pigmented melanocytic nevi are another very common skin lesion. Most persons have the majority of their nevi on the upper part of the body, but nevi also can be seen on the lower extremities and the feet. Approximately 12% of people have pigmented nevi on their soles or palms.

The main reason for being concerned about pigmented nevi is that a small percentage of them give rise to a malignant melanoma. Melanomas arising on the soles and palms are known as acral lentiginous melanomas.

Any pigmented lesion on the sole of any patient that changes significantly in size, shape, or color, or either bleeds spontaneously or develops a scab that will not heel should be biopsied. That being said, almost all plantar acral lentiginous melanomas are seen in individuals of African American descent.

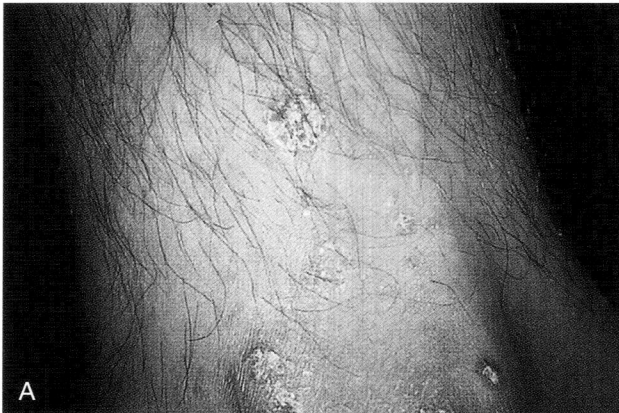

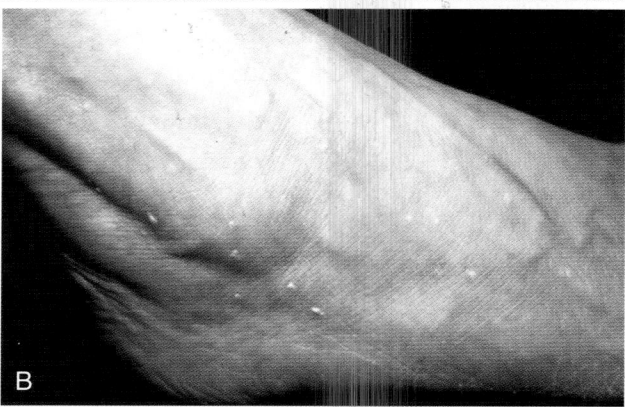

Figure 16-16 Stucco keratosis. **A,** Note numerous light tan hyperkeratotic papules on the lower leg. **B,** Another image of stucco keratosis. (**A,** From Dockery GL: *Cutaneous disorders of the lower extremity,* Philadelphia, 1997, WB Saunders.)

Black Heel

Black heel is a benign asymptomatic lesion. It was first described under the name "calcaneal petechiae." The lesion can be a look-alike for both warts and, more seriously, melanoma. Clinically, it appears as a confluent group of dark red to brown or black speckles on the heel (Fig. 16-17).

The lesion is a result of trauma to the foot and is most often seen in patients who participate in sports that involve repetitive stop-and-go action on the feet, such as basketball and tennis. The pigment is a collection of dried blood within the stratum corneum. The easiest way to confirm this diagnosis is to pare the stratum corneum above the lesion down to that layer of dried blood. The entire lesion usually can be pared out easily with a scalpel blade.

Eccrine Poroma

Eccrine poroma is a benign solitary tumor; two thirds of these lesions appear on the soles or sides of the feet. This tumor is derived from the eccrine sweat ducts and usually arises in young or middle-age adults. It is usually tender, rather firm, and often raised and slightly pedunculated (Fig. 16-18). Eccrine poroma usually measures less than 2 cm in diameter. Treatment by excision is curative.

Pyogenic Granuloma

Pyogenic granuloma is one of the many misnomers in dermatology because these lesions are neither infectious in origin nor do they produce granulomas. The more correct name is *lobulated capillary hemangioma.* They usually occur as a single erythematous, soft, slightly pedunculated papule, often with appearance of a collarette of skin surrounding the lesion (Fig. 16-19). They usually grow rapidly, up to 0.5 cm. They often bleed spontaneously or with very minimal trauma. These lesions most often occur on the face and hands of children, but they can appear on the feet as well, particularly on the lateral nail folds of the toes. These lesions are thought to occur in response to mild trauma that causes

Figure 16-17 Black heel. **A,** Numerous punctuate black speckles are seen on the heel, representing dried blood within the stratum corneum. **B,** Another image of black heel. (**A,** From Dockery GL: *Cutaneous disorders of the lower extremity,* Philadelphia, 1997, WB Saunders.)

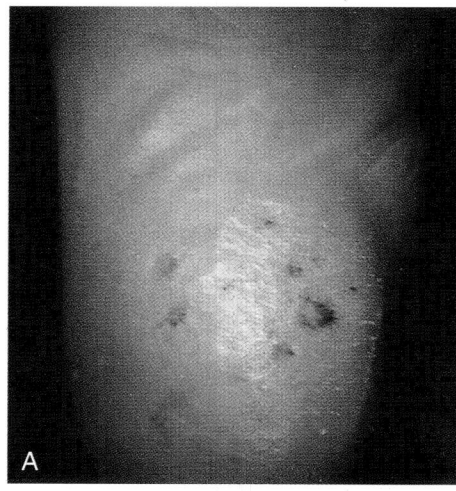

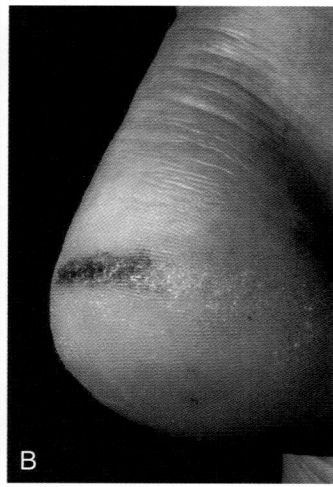

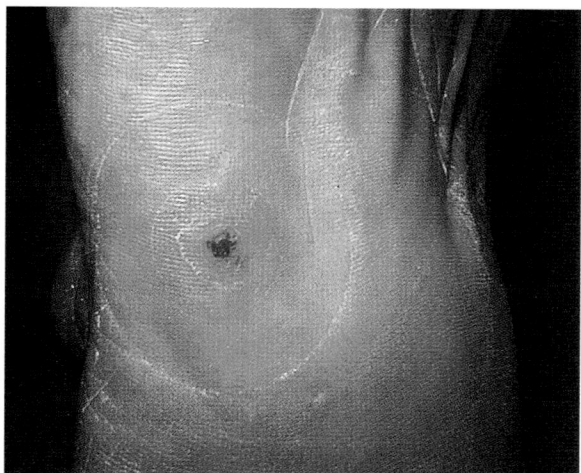

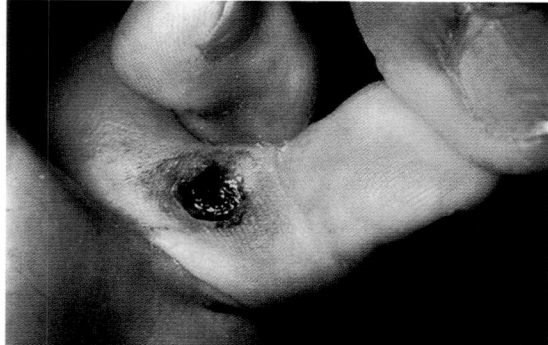

Figure 16-20 Melanoma. **A,** Note the black nodule on the toe. **B,** A close-up of a larger lesion.

Figure 16-18 Eccrine poroma. This adnexal papillomatous tumor commonly arises on the feet. Here a poroma near the heel appears almost like verrucae. It is a pedunculated, friable lesion that bleeds easily. (From Dockery GL: *Cutaneous disorders of the lower extremity,* Philadelphia, 1997, WB Saunders.)

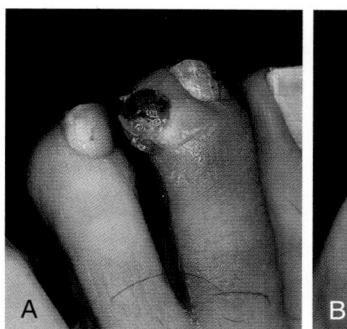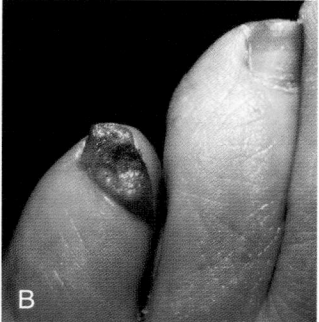

Figure 16-19 Pyogenic granuloma. **A,** Note the pedunculated vascular papule on the periungual skin with a small collarette of scale. **B,** Another pyogenic granuloma seen on the periungual skin of the fifth digit.

one of the capillaries in the skin to proliferate. One of the common causes of a pyogenic granuloma on the foot is an ingrown toenail.

The differential diagnosis of these lesions on the foot includes other types of angiomas, eccrine poroma, squamous cell carcinoma, malignant melanoma, or foreign body granuloma. The best treatment for these lesions is a shave excision, followed by destruction of the feeding blood vessel at the base with electrodesiccation.

Foreign Body

A foreign body embedded in the sole can be mistaken for any of the hyperkeratotic lesions previously discussed because the body produces a protective callus over the penetration site. This can be confused with a corn, wart, or simple callus. As previously described, it is important to pare away the overlying callus to make this diagnosis. As the callus is pared away over a foreign body, usually a small pocket of pus will be found, or the foreign body itself will become apparent, or both. Common foreign bodies found embedded in the soles include small pieces of glass and small sharp stones. Once the foreign body has been removed, the overlying skin will heal quickly without significant additional treatment.

Epidermal Inclusion Cyst

Epidermal inclusion cysts are common skin lesions mainly seen on the face, scalp, and trunk. However, they occur infrequently on the soles. When seen on the soles, they are most often a response to a penetration injury that has not left a foreign body. Epidermal inclusion cysts can be seen particularly on the feet of infants who required numerous heel sticks for blood at a very early age. No treatment is needed for epidermal inclusion cysts on the soles because they usually resolve over time. A case of an intraosseous epidermal inclusion cyst of the great toe has been reported.[28]

Malignant Growths

Melanoma

Malignant melanoma is the most dangerous lesion discussed in this chapter. The United States is currently experiencing a dramatic rise in the incidence of melanoma, with the lifetime risk being 1 in 75 for white Americans. The risk of melanoma is much lower in African Americans, but when they do have melanoma, it is on the soles and palms. Melanomas that occur at these sites are known as *acral lentiginous melanomas.*[27] Currently, almost 40,000 new cases of melanoma are reported each year, and almost 20,000 people die of melanoma each year.

The prognosis for a patient with melanoma is most closely correlated with the thickness of the melanoma when it is diagnosed. Therefore it is important for all practitioners to notice changing skin lesions that may be at risk for becoming melanoma. Most melanomas arise from a preexisting pigmented nevus that is undergoing some change, such as a dramatic increase in size, a change in pigmentation, the development of nodules within the lesion (Fig. 16-20), and either bleeding or ulceration of a previously asymptomatic pigmented lesion. A nonpigmented variant, known as *amelanotic melanoma*, can also be seen on the feet.

The differential diagnosis for either a changing or a bleeding lesion on the foot includes benign lesions, such as an irritated seborrheic keratosis, an eccrine poroma, or a pyogenic granuloma, as well as other malignant lesions, such as a Kaposi sarcoma. If melanoma is in the differential diagnosis of any lesion seen on the skin of the foot, it is absolutely necessary for that lesion to be biopsied. If a melanoma is diagnosed, surgical margins are determined by the thickness of the melanoma on histologic examination.

Squamous Cell Carcinoma

Squamous cell carcinoma (SCC) of the skin is much more common than malignant melanoma, with more than 100,000 cases of SCC reported each year. SCCs of the skin usually remain limited to the skin, but they do have metastatic potential if they are not treated in a timely and appropriate fashion. SCCs that arise on the feet are often seen in association with previously damaged or diseased skin. They can arise in old burn scars, and this type of lesion is known as a *Marjolin ulcer*. SCCs can also arise in chronically inflamed skin, such as in previous lesions of lichen planus seen on the feet or lower extremity.[12]

The clinical appearance of an SCC is usually a hyperkeratotic, erythematous papule or nodule or a crusted erosion or ulcer that will not heal. The differential diagnosis for such a lesion includes warts, foreign body granulomas, pyogenic granulomas, eccrine poromas, and in the right clinical setting, deep fungal infections. As with melanoma, if SCC is in the differential diagnosis for a lesion on the foot or lower extremity, it is imperative that the lesion be biopsied. If the histology does show an SCC, appropriate treatment would be local excision with clear margins.

Two other types of SCC can be seen on the feet. The lesions of *Bowen disease*, which is an SCC in situ, often appear clinically more similar to lesions of psoriasis, atopic dermatitis, or tinea (Fig. 16-21). Therefore, when treating someone with papulosquamous eruption, if the lesion does not respond to appropriate therapy, it must be biopsied to rule out Bowen disease. If the diagnosis of Bowen disease is made, appropriate therapy is simple excision with clear margins, superficial destruction with either electrodesiccation and curettage, deep cryotherapy, or the use of the immune response modifier imiquimod.

The second variant of SCC that should be mentioned here is *verrucous squamous cell carcinoma*. This type of SCC occurs most often on the sole, but it is very rare. Clinically, the lesion appears as a proliferating verrucous mass on the sole of the foot. Although these lesions have a very malignant superficial appearance, they do not seem to metastasize. These lesions do cause significant local tissue destruction and can infiltrate into the surrounding skin and subcutaneous tissues. Treatment is surgical excision.

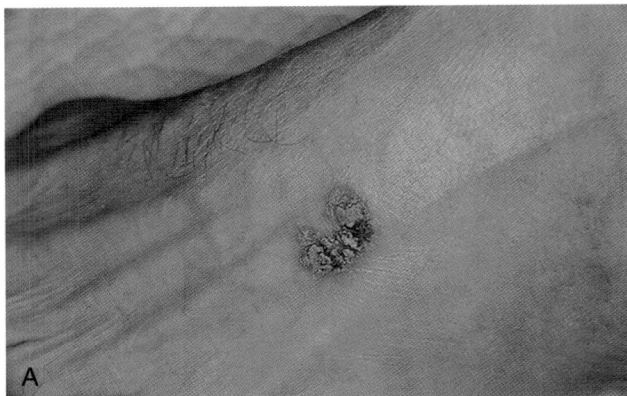

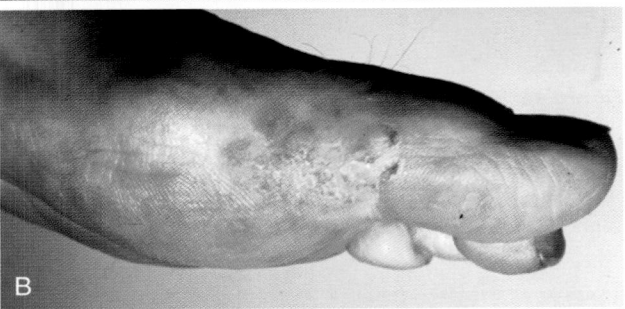

Figure 16-21 Bowen disease. **A,** This red scaly patch could easily be mistaken for psoriasis, but it is actually an early squamous cell carcinoma in situ. **B,** This lesion, also a squamous cell carcinoma in situ, is a mimic for dyshidrotic eczema.

Kaposi Sarcoma

Kaposi sarcoma is a malignant neoplasm that was well known for many years before the advent of acquired immunodeficiency syndrome (AIDS) in the early 1980s. This classic Kaposi sarcoma characteristically involved the skin of the feet. It was predominantly seen in elderly men, especially those of Mediterranean decent. The earliest clinical lesion appears very similar to a pyogenic granuloma. The clinical appearance is that of a violaceous, firm, vascular papule. As the tumor grows, it takes on the appearance of a vascular plaque (Fig. 16-22). The lesion is slow growing; untreated lesions can ulcerate and bleed. End-stage tumors usually show surrounding brawny lymphedema of the involved leg. The tumors can also metastasize, especially to the gastrointestinal tract. The differential diagnosis for the later stage includes severe stasis dermatitis (lipodermatosclerosis), hypertrophic lichen planus, and deep fungal infections.

Certainly, when Kaposi sarcoma is in the differential diagnosis, it is important to do a skin biopsy. The histology is very characteristic. Numerous therapies are available for treatment of the different stages of Kaposi sarcoma; however, the tumor appears to be particularly sensitive to radiation therapy.

Kaposi sarcoma can also be seen in immunosuppressed transplant patients, but it is most well known as it is seen in patients with AIDS. Kaposi sarcoma looks very different clinically in patients with AIDS than it does in

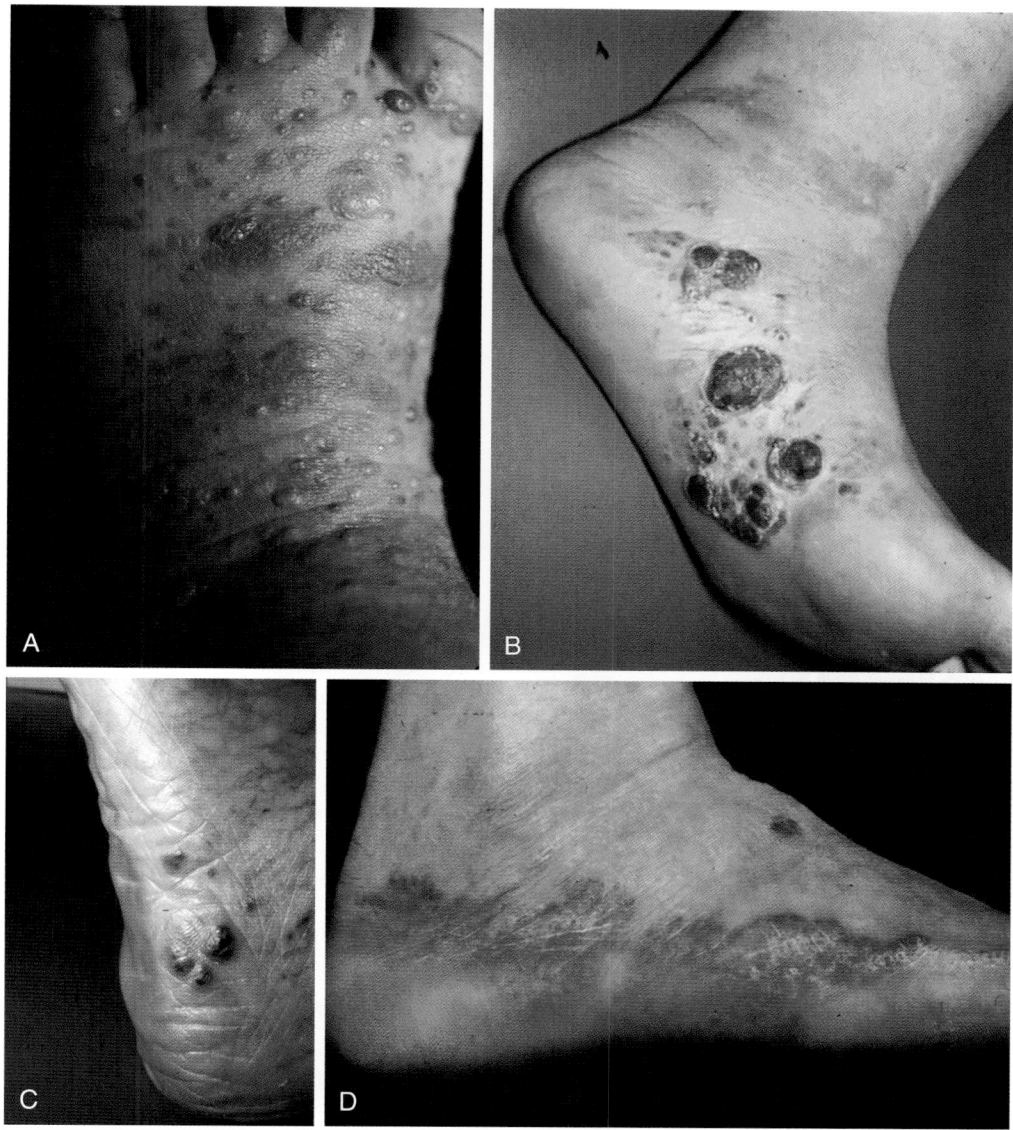

Figure 16-22 Kaposi sarcoma. **A,** Note the numerous purple papules and nodules on the dorsal foot. **B,** Larger nodules on the medial plantar surface. **C,** Purple nodules on the heel. **D,** Large purple plaques on the lateral aspect of the foot.

cases of classic Kaposi sarcoma. Lesions can be seen anywhere on the body, including the oral mucous membranes. The differential diagnosis of Kaposi sarcoma in AIDS patients includes bacillary angiomatosis. It is therefore important to confirm the diagnosis of Kaposi sarcoma by biopsy because bacillary angiomatosis is a cutaneous infection that is easily treated with oral erythromycin. It is also important to confirm the diagnosis of Kaposi sarcoma because this can be an AIDS-defining condition in patients who are positive for human immunodeficiency (HIV).[11]

PURPURIC ERUPTIONS

The spectrum of diseases that cause purpuric eruptions on the lower extremities ranges from benign forms of

capillaritis to severe forms of vasculitis that can be life threatening.

Pigmented Dermatosis

The pigmented purpuric dermatoses include several different conditions that have been separated from one another over the years. Histologically, however, all these eruptions are produced by a capillaritis. No evidence indicates a true vasculitis in any of these conditions.

The clinical spectrum of pigmented purpuric dermatoses includes *Schamberg disease,* which gives the appearance of mild scaling and erythema over the lower extremities, with numerous bright red, nonblanchable specks within its surface (Fig. 16-23). This condition has the appearance of cayenne pepper on the skin's surface. Lesions of

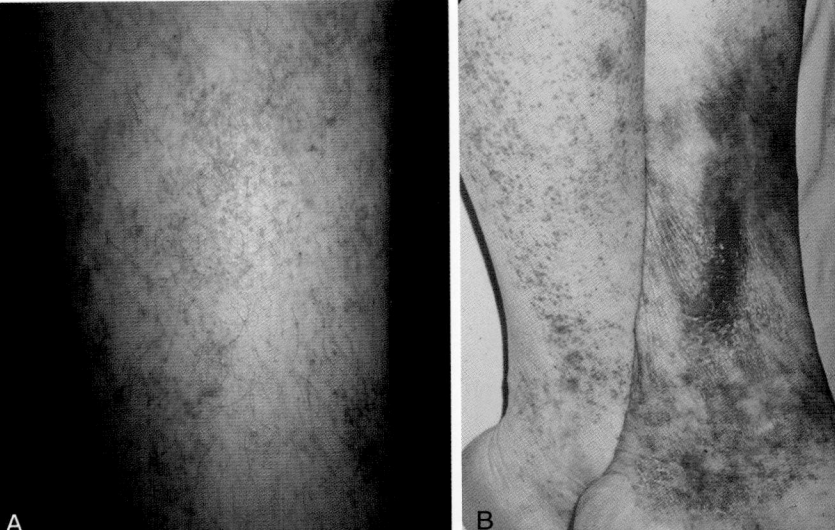

Figure 16-23 Schamberg pigmented purpura. **A,** Note the cayenne pepper–like appearance of the skin lesions. **B,** A more severe and widespread case.

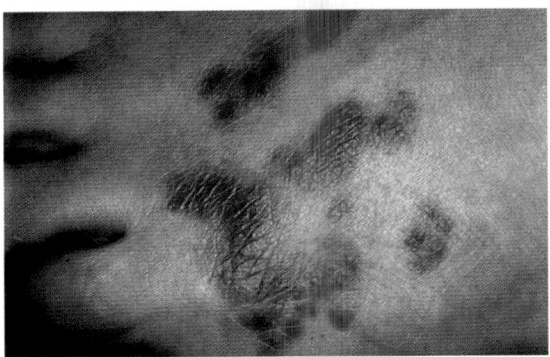

Figure 16-24 Lichenoid pigmented purpura. Violaceous, nonblanchable lesions similar in appearance to lichen planus.

lichenoid pigmented purpura can appear clinically as distinct erythematous to violaceous plaques over the lower extremities (Fig. 16-24) and can look very similar to lichen planus.

Again, on a biopsy, all these conditions show only mild extravasation of RBCs from the superficial capillaries and an extremely mild associated inflammatory response in the upper dermis. The deposition and eventual reabsorption of hemosiderin in the upper dermis is responsible for the pigmented appearance of these clinical lesions. No treatment is needed, but mild topical steroid ointment can be used if there is associated pruritus.

Atrophie Blanche

Atrophie blanche ("white atrophy") or *livedo vasculitis* is a painful eruption seen most often on the lower extremities of elderly persons. The term *vasculitis* is somewhat misleading in this condition because true vasculitis is not seen in the involved blood vessels. Engorgement and sludging occur within cutaneous blood vessels. Clinically,

this eruption produces porcelain white atrophy most often seen over the ankles (Fig. 16-25). This atrophic skin, in combination with these patients' poor blood supply, often leads to painful ulcerations.

Treatment for atrophie blanche consists of antiplatelet agents such as aspirin, dipyridamole (Persantine), and pentoxifylline (Trental). Any ulcers can be treated with silver sulfadiazine cream. Excision and split-thickness skin grafting was also reported to be effective in one case. It is often necessary to treat these patients with narcotic analgesics because the associated pain can be severe.

Leukocytoclastic Vasculitis

Leukocytoclastic vasculitis is the histologic correlate of clinical palpable purpura. These lesions show a true necrotizing vasculitis with fibrin thrombi in blood vessels, along with numerous neutrophils surrounding and invading the blood vessel walls. As the blood vessels are damaged, extravasation of RBCs occurs, producing the clinical picture of purpura. The differential diagnosis of leukocytoclastic vasculitis in adults is extensive, ranging from systemic infections to primary dermatologic and rheumatologic conditions to malignancies. The clinical spectrum of this disease ranges from palpable purpura (Fig. 16-26) to ulcerating nodules to widespread areas of livedo reticularis and necrosis (Fig. 16-27).

The pathophysiology of most types of vasculitis begins with immune complex formation. These complexes can become implanted in the walls of blood vessels, where they activate neutrophils. Blood vessel damage occurs when the neutrophils degranulate and release lytic enzymes.[13,22,23]

In addition to the skin, vasculitis can affect numerous organ systems. For example, Henoch-Schönlein purpura is most often seen in children but can occur in young adults. The classic picture is palpable purpura on the lower extremities (Fig. 16-28), with the associated

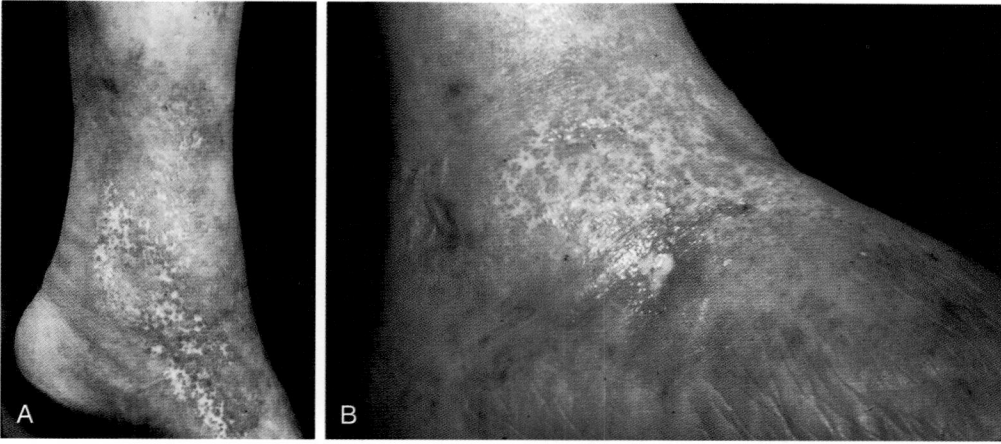

Figure 16-25   Atrophie blanche. **A,** Note the white and brown papules and atrophic patches on this chronic lesion on the lower leg. **B,** Note the erythema and small ulceration in this more active lesion, also known as lividoid vasculitis.

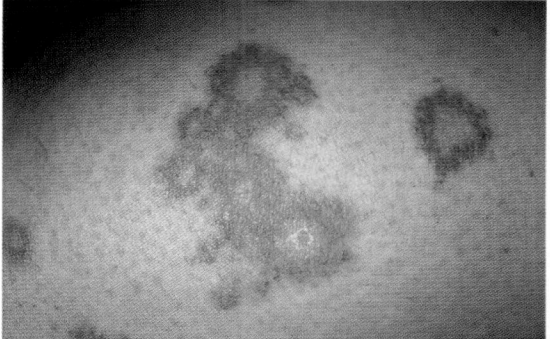

Figure 16-26   Vasculitis. This is a good clinical example of palpable purpura as seen in leukocytoclastic vasculitis.

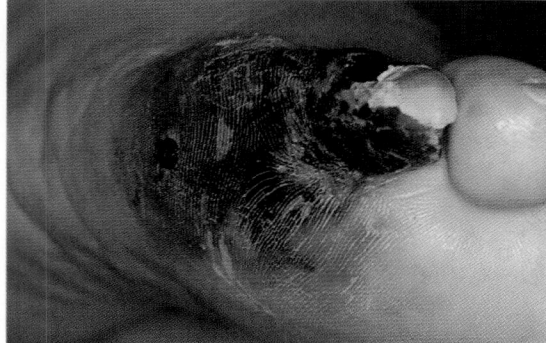

Figure 16-27   Cutaneous necrosis can be seen in severe forms of vasculitis.

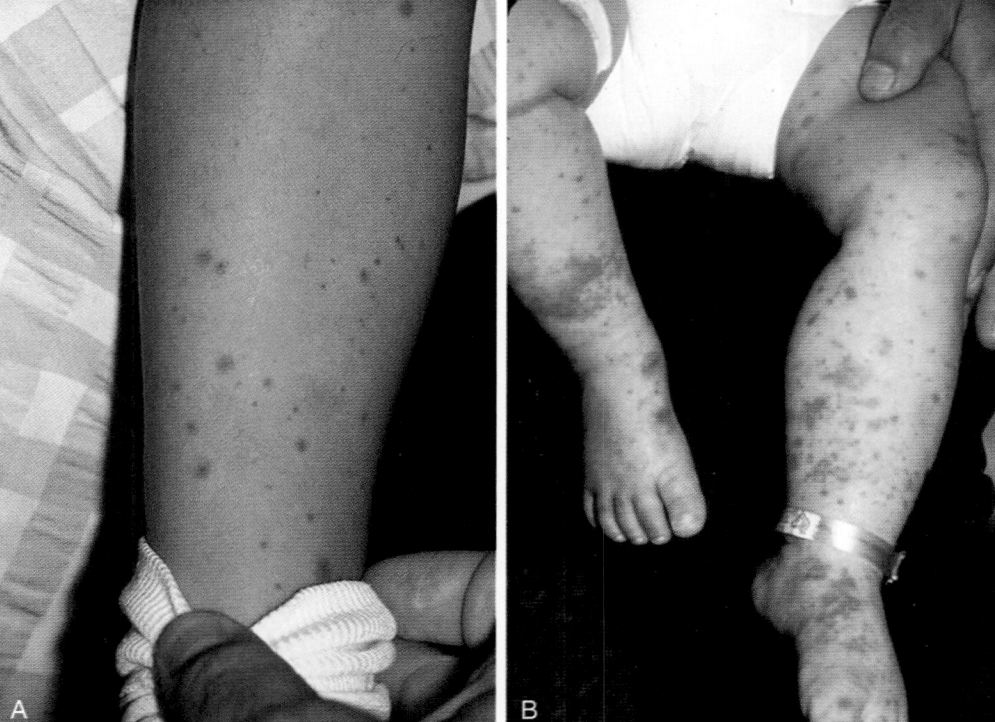

Figure 16-28   **A,** Henoch-Schönlein purpura (HSP). Characteristic lower-extremity lesions seen in a child with HSP. **B,** Another example of HSP in a younger child.

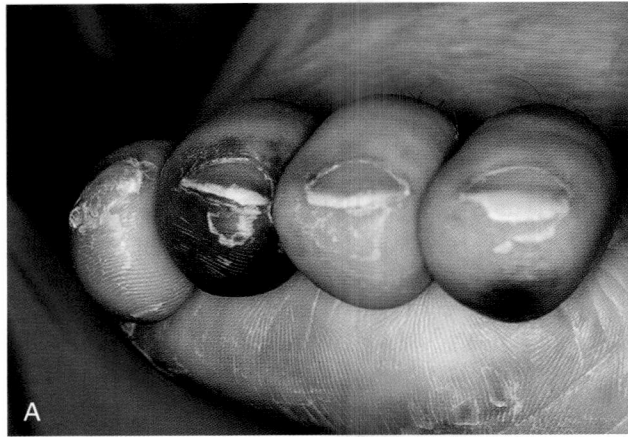

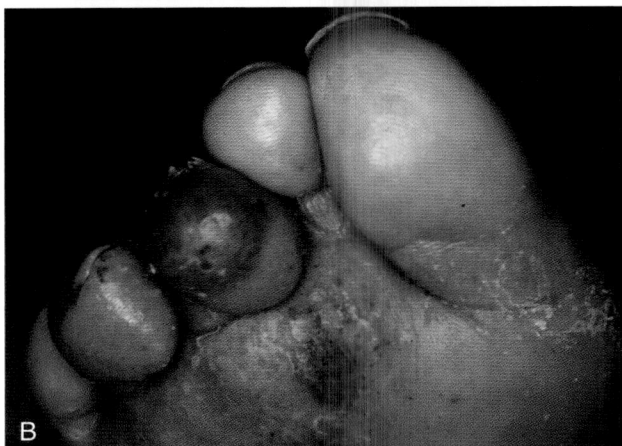

Figure 16-29 **A,** Blue or purple toe syndrome can be seen in the setting of antiphospholipid antibody syndrome, cryoglobulinemia, and other connective tissue diseases. **B,** Another example of purple toe syndrome.

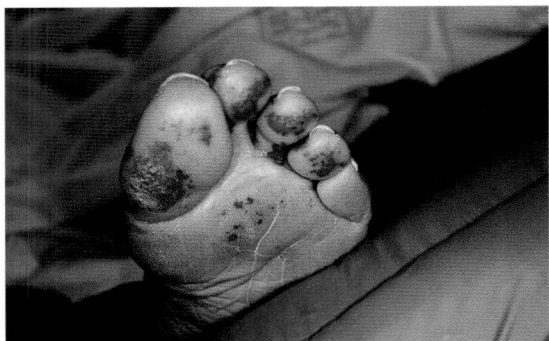

Figure 16-30 Cholesterol emboli can be seen after major cardiac or orthopaedic surgery.

leukocytoclastic vasculitis. This finding can indicate anything from an early sign of a systemic disease to a severe postoperative complication (Fig. 16-30) to a life-threatening infection.

REFERENCES

1. Bell FE, Daniel CR, Daniel MP: Ciclopirox olamine: head to foot, *J Drugs Dermatol* 2:50–51, 2003.
2. Bell-Seyer SE, Hart R, Crawford F, et al: Oral treatments for fungal infections of the skin of the foot, *Cochrane Database Syst Rev* (2):CD003584, 2002.
3. Borovoy MA, Borovoy M, Elson LM, Sage M: Flashlamp pulse dye laser (585 nm). Treatment of resistant verrucae, *J Am Podiatr Med Assoc* 86:547–550, 1996.
4. Chamlin SL, Kao J, Frieden IJ, et al: Ceramide-dominant barrier repair lipids alleviate childhood atopic dermatitis: changes in barrier function provide a sensitive indicator of disease activity, *J Am Acad Derm* 47:198–208, 2002.
5. Crawford F, Young P, Godfrey C, et al: Oral treatment for toenail onychomycosis: a systemic review, *Arch Dermatol* 138:811–816, 2002.
6. Day RT, Reyzelman AM, Harkless LB: Evaluation and management of the interdigital corn: a literature review, *Clin Podiatr Med Surg* 13:206, 1996.
7. Elias PM, Hetano Y, Williams ML: Basis for the barrier abnormality in atopic dermatitis: outside-inside-outside pathogenic mechanisms, *J All Clin Immunol* 121:1337–1343, 2008.
8. Farley E, Masrour S, McKey J, Menter A: Palmoplantar psoriasis: a phenotypical and clinical review with introduction of a new quality-of-life assessment tool, *J Am Acad Derm* 60:1024–1031, 2009.
9. Gibbs S, Harvey L, Sterling JC, Stark R: Local treatments for cutaneous warts, *Cochrane Database Syst Rev* (3):CD001781, 2003.
10. Gloster HM, Roenigk RK: Risk of acquiring human papillomavirus from the plume produced by the carbon dioxide laser in the treatment of warts, *J Am Acad Dermatol* 32:436–441, 1995.
11. Herndier B, Ganem D: The biology of Kaposi's sarcoma, *Cancer Treat Res* 104:89–126, 2001.
12. Jayaraman M, Janaki VR, Yesudian P: Squamous cell carcinoma arising from hypertrophic lichen planus, *Int J Dermatol* 34:70–71, 1995.
13. Jennette CJ, Milling DM, Falk RJ: Vasculitis affecting the skin, *Arch Dermatol* 130:899–906, 1994.
14. Jones HE, Zaias N: Double-blind, randomized comparison of itraconazole capsules and placebo in onychomycosis of toenail, *Int J Dermatol* 34:70–71, 1995.

symptom of abdominal pain. Renal and gastrointestinal vasculitis can produce blood in the urine and stool. The syndrome is usually self-limited. Other types of vasculitis can have much more severe consequences.

When evaluating a patient with possible vasculitis, it is necessary to obtain at least a skin biopsy, complete blood count, blood urea nitrogen, creatinine, and routine urinalysis. The remainder of the workup is guided by the developing clinical picture and the final biopsy report. For example, if blue or purple toe syndrome (Fig. 16-29) is noted, an antiphospholipid antibody and a more thorough rheumatologic workup should be undertaken.[13,22,23]

It is appropriate to end this discussion of dermatologic conditions of the feet with vasculitis because a discussion of vasculitis touches on everything that is important about the study of the skin. The skin is a window onto the functioning of the rest of the body. By examining it closely and defining the primary skin lesions seen, it is possible to make the correct diagnosis. In this case, purpuric papules and plaques lead to the diagnosis of

15. Kacar N, Tasli L, Korkmaz S, et al: Cantharidn-podophylotoxin-salicylic acid versus cryotherapy in the treatment of plantar warts: a randomized prospective study. *J Eur Acad Dermatol Venereol* 2011.

16. Lawry MA, Haneke E, Strobeck K, et al: Methods for diagnosing onychomycosis: a comparative study and review of the literature. *Arch Dermatol* 136:1112–1116, 2000.

17. Lazzarini R, Duarte I, Marzagao C: Contact dermatitis of the feet: a study of 53 cases. *Dermatitis* 15:125–130, 2004.

18. Leung DYM, Boguniewicz M, Howell MD, et al: New insights into atopic dermatitis. *J Clin Invest* 113:651–657, 2004.

19. Matsumoto T, Tanuma H, Kaneko S, et al: Clinical and pharmacokinetic investigations of oral terbinafine in patients with tinea unguium. *Mycoses* 38:135–144, 1995.

20. Mitsuishi T, Wakabayashi T, Kawana S: Topical imiquimod associated to a reduction of heel hyperkeratosis for the treatment of recalcitrant mosaic plantar warts. *Eur J Dermatol* 19:268–269, 2009.

21. Oji V, Tadini G, Akyiama M, et al: Revised nomenclature and classification of inherited ichthyosis: results of the first ichthyosis consensus conference in Sorèze 2009. *J Am Acad Dermatol* 63:607–641, 2010.

22. O'Keeffe ST, Woods BO, Breslin DJ, et al: Blue toe syndrome: causes and management. *Arch Intern Med* 152:2197–2202, 1992.

23. Pederson WC: Medical and surgical considerations in patients with vasculitis and Raynaud's syndrome. *Foot Ankle Clin* 6:699–713, 2001.

24. Rockwell PG: Acute and chronic paronychia. *Am Fam Physician* 63:1113–1116, 2001.

25. Saye DE: The foot corns, calluses, ingrown nails and diabetic ulcers. *Ostomy Wound Manage* 40:16–19, 22–27, 1994.

26. Tosti A, Piraccini BM, Ghetti E, Columbo MD: Topical steroids versus systemic antifungals in the treatment of chronic paronychia: an open randomized double-blind and double dummy study. *J Am Acad Dermatol* 47:73–76, 2002.

27. Walsh SM, Fisher SG, Sage RA: Survival of patients with primary pedal melanoma. *J Foot Ankle Surg* 42:193–198, 2003.

28. Wang BY, Eisler J, Springfield D, Klein MJ: Intraosseous epidermoid inclusion cyst in a great toe. A case report and review of the literature. *Arch Pathol Lab Med* 127:e298–e300, 2003.

29. Weinstein A, Berman B: Topical treatment of common superficial tinea infections. *Am Fam Physician* 65:2095–2102, 2002.

Soft Tissue Reconstruction for the Foot and Ankle

L. Scott Levin, Stephen J. Kovach

HISTORY

The evolution of extremity trauma surgery reflects the development of surgery as a specialty. The management of soft tissue injuries to the foot and ankle has evolved through major historical periods that initially included high-level amputation, regional amputation to conserve limb length, wound debridement, vascular repair, flap reconstruction, revascularization, replantation, and the current concept of acute reconstruction to save the limb and preserve function.

Open fractures have plagued surgeons since the time of Hippocrates; drawings from his original writings show crude attempts at external fixation for the purpose of examining and treating wounds.[2] Incomplete documents from the ancient Egyptian period reported that comminuted fractures were treated expectantly. "Compound fractures" were considered a fatal injury because amputation was not a part of the surgical arsenal.[3] In the sixteenth century, Ambroise Paré, one of the founding fathers of orthopaedics, warned against the potentially life-threatening condition of gangrene resulting from open fractures; he revolutionized amputation surgery by use of the tourniquet and introduced the hemostatic clamp and vascular ligatures.[68]

Important advances have taken place in the field of soft tissue reconstructive surgery, including the introduction of local flaps and free flaps as efficient methods of closing large posttraumatic soft tissue defects. A better understanding of the anatomy and physiology of free flaps, with resultant high rates of success using autologous tissue transfers, and the introduction of distally based fasciocutaneous flaps have improved the surgeon's ability to close soft tissue defects of the foot and ankle.[57]

With the evolution of operative methods for fracture fixation and the increasing incidence of high-energy trauma, the importance of concomitant soft tissue management in the treatment of open fractures of the foot and ankle cannot be underestimated. Foot and ankle surgeons treating patients who have traumatic conditions can no longer isolate their care to the bone or the reconstitution of articular surfaces. Although these goals are vital to the success of overall treatment, the foot and ankle surgeon must also accept responsibility for the management of the soft tissue surrounding the osseous structures and define a treatment plan for the soft tissues. This treatment plan can be carried out in conjunction with a reconstructive plastic surgeon or by the orthopaedic surgeon alone. The combination of soft tissue management and bone reconstruction permits optimal repair to take place in bone and soft tissue, avoiding the adverse sequelae of failed implants, failed fixation, sepsis, and ultimately amputation.

COMPLEX MUSCULOSKELETAL INJURIES

Complex foot injuries require effective coordinated care for both bone and soft tissue to achieve a successful fracture union while avoiding infection, but a variety of factors makes this difficult. These factors include compromised vascular supply at the fracture site, marginal soft tissue coverage, and wound contamination.

Initial treatment of fractures has improved significantly with the development of antibiotic therapy and aseptic surgical procedures in conjunction with improved stabilization techniques. This progress has increased limb salvage in the treatment of severe injuries to the foot and ankle at risk for amputation. Today's acute fracture management with early antibiotic treatment, irrigation and

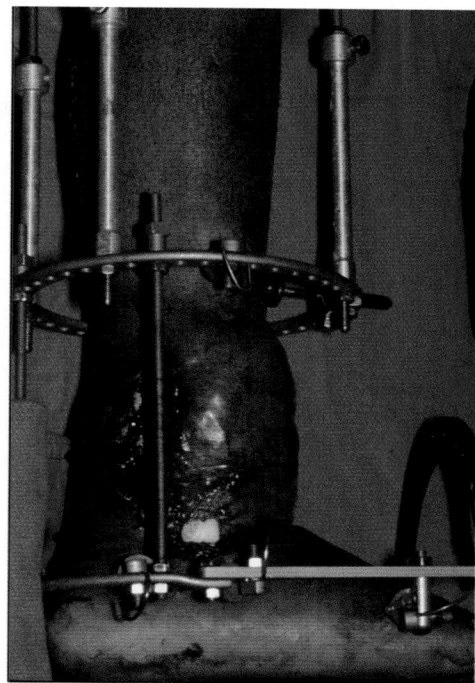

Figure 17-1 Acute fracture stabilization with an external fixator.

debridement, and acute fracture stabilization has led to a significant reduction in fracture infection rates (Fig. 17-1).

The essential elements of osseous healing of reduced fracture fragments are blood supply and stabilization. Blood supply to bone is derived from nutrient vessels as well as surrounding muscle and fascia. Compromise of a bone's soft tissue envelope or nutrient vasculature places that bone at risk for delayed union, nonunion, or the inability to fight infection if colonized with bacteria after injury.

OPEN FRACTURES

Historically, treatment of an open fracture in which soft tissue injuries have been neglected or mistreated has resulted in therapeutic disaster. It was argued that open reduction and internal fixation of closed or opened fractures was performed with significant risk. Arguments against internal fixation were that it resulted in infection, compromised bone healing, and nonunion.

The basic principles of open reduction and internal fixation, defined by the Arbeitgemeinschaft für Osteosynthesesfragen (AO) group five decades ago,[93] included anatomic reduction and stable internal fixation, careful attention to soft tissue handling, and functional rehabilitation of the injured limb—all vital to fracture management. Functional rehabilitation involves restoring muscular power and normal biomechanics.

The importance of soft tissue reconstruction has been emphasized over the last two decades. New fixation techniques, such as indirect reduction and biologic plating with implants that respect biology and avoid compromised periosteum around bone, are now being used. Compatible implants, such as the locking plates and calcaneal plates with improved metallurgy, were designed to limit the damage to soft tissue caused by overvigorous dissection and stripping of the soft tissue envelope.[85]

The surrounding soft tissue has been recognized as the vascular envelope responsible for nurturing bone back to health. The importance of its reconstruction early in the posttraumatic course cannot be overemphasized; neither can the importance of surgical anatomy, internervous planes, vascular territories, and atraumatic techniques of dissection.[69,115] Rather than dissection techniques that result in devascularization of bone and soft tissue, a keener awareness of delicate soft tissue handling and atraumatic technique by the orthopaedist contributes to the prevention of adverse iatrogenic sequelae after injury. Proper handling of soft tissue includes tools such as skin hooks that permit manipulation of skin and tissue flaps without further damage to the soft tissues.

To reconstruct the soft tissue envelope, the surgeon must identify which layers are deficient and the size of the deficiency. Subsequently, one must outline a treatment plan that simultaneously treats bone and soft tissue synergistically.

The soft tissue envelope is composed of several tissue layers, each with a specific function and its own vascular supply. Skin, which consists of epidermis and dermis, is the first soft tissue layer violated in the open injury, and its disruption defines the open fracture.

The next soft tissue layer, the subcutaneous tissue, is less vascular than the dermal plexus, yet it is important because it provides a cushion around bony prominences and may be quite specialized, such as on the plantar surface of the foot.

Fascia is the next deepest layer and surrounds muscle compartments. It contains a rich vascular plexus that can function as the basis for supporting tissue such as skin flaps, which can be transposed or transferred over adjacent, distant, or proximal soft tissue defects.

Muscles are richly vascularized structures that power the locomotor system. They have one of five blood supplies, as outlined by Mathes and Nahai.[84] Muscles can be manipulated as transposition flaps, island pedicle flaps, and free tissue transplantations (free flaps).

The deepest layer of the soft tissue envelope is a richly vascularized layer called the periosteum. This surrounds all long bones and is vital to the response of bone to injury and repair. Recent advances in anatomic dissection and free tissue transplantation have resulted in use of the periosteum, based on the medial geniculate artery case as a free flap to augment conventional methods of bone grafting.

All of the layers of soft tissue just described, including the periosteum, will accept a split-thickness skin graft (Fig. 17-2). Despite contour irregularity, if these layers are healthy and well vascularized, a skin graft can be applied to seal the open wound. This is the first goal in wound

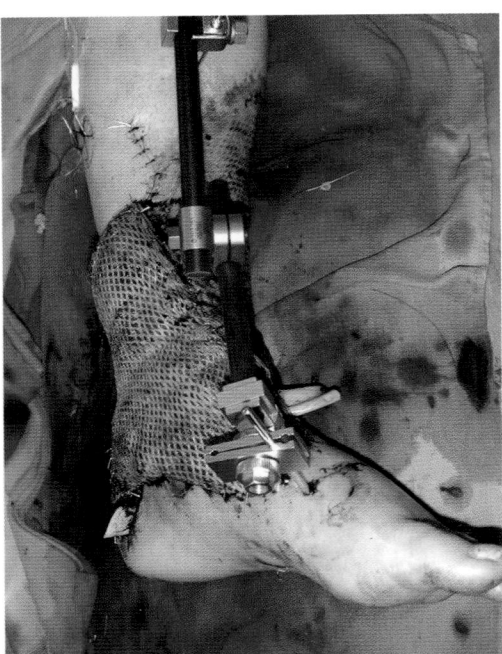

Figure 17-2 A meshed split-thickness skin graft applied over a free latissimus myocutaneous transfer.

management, that is, to reconstitute the epithelial surface of the extremity.

A logical method of reconstruction of the soft tissues must be developed to allow bone to heal and limbs to function normally. The algorithm should be capable of being used by the foot surgeon in the setting of acute or chronic soft tissue injury with or without fractures. In addition, it should be applicable to chronic conditions, such as osteomyelitis, nonunion, or tumor.[26]

In essence, the foot and ankle surgeon must acquire an understanding of the approach used by the plastic or reconstructive microsurgeon to reconstruct deficiencies in soft tissue. This approach, coupled with knowledge of treatment for bone deficiencies or deformities, serves as an *orthoplastic* philosophy of limb salvage. The reconstructive ladder represents increasingly complex solutions to correspondingly complex problems with the same goal: reconstitution of the soft tissue envelope and bone. The lowest rungs of the ladder are often as important as the highest rungs. Understanding the relationship between the needs of the wound and the various techniques offered by the reconstructive ladder is important.

THE RECONSTRUCTIVE LADDER

Patient Evaluation

Evaluation of the patient with a soft tissue injury includes determining the time of injury, mechanism of injury, energy absorption, fracture configuration, systemic injuries, damage to the soft tissue envelope, vascularity of the extremity, sensibility, ultimate ability to salvage the foot (both functional and sensate), and underlying medical conditions of the patient. The principles of evaluation of orthopaedic trauma are the same as for any basic medical evaluation. These principles apply whether in the outpatient clinic, emergency department, or trauma unit.

An evaluation of the perfusion of the traumatized limb is of paramount importance, and if vascular (arterial) injury is suspected, a vascular surgery or microsurgery consultation should be obtained. Compartment syndrome should be considered and ruled out in any injured extremity, particularly after crush injuries. A general motor examination, including the active and passive range of motion, and a detailed sensory examination should be performed. A nerve deficit may be secondary to a spinal cord injury, nerve laceration, compartment syndrome, traction injury, or entrapment between bone fragments. The radiologic evaluation starts with a standard plain radiographic examination. Computed tomography (CT) is indicated in complex foot injuries and can give valuable information regarding soft tissue damage as well.

The wound should be inspected and the wound pattern and contamination noted. The next inspection of the wound should then be in the operating room under sterile conditions. Repetitive examination of open wounds in the emergency department has led to higher rates of wound infection and osteomyelitis and should be avoided. In cases of open fractures in polytrauma patients, workup of other injuries can take several hours, not to mention the need for emergent lifesaving visceral surgery that can precede definitive care for open fractures. Prophylactic antibiotics are administered and given on a regular basis until definitive wound debridement and fracture stabilization can be performed.

Classification of Soft Tissue Injury

A classification of the soft tissue injury should allow us to evaluate the results of the treatment, to better inform our patients, and to communicate with our colleagues in a more universal language. A classification must be reproducible and easy to remember, and it should determine prognosis of the injury. The only universally accepted classification of soft tissue injuries has been a systematic injury with division into "closed" and "open."

Assessment of soft tissue injury is necessary in both open and closed fractures. The degree of soft tissue injury provides a prognosis and guides fracture management. The different classification schemes can be fairly simple or minutely detailed. The simpler schemes are noncomprehensive and inexact but are the most likely to be used.[46]

As the significance of soft tissue injuries on the influence of bone healing became more apparent, Gustilo and Anderson[43] devised a three-grade classification in 1976. Type 1 fractures have a clean wound smaller than 1 cm, type 2 wounds have a laceration greater than 1 cm and without extensive soft tissue damage, and type 3 wounds

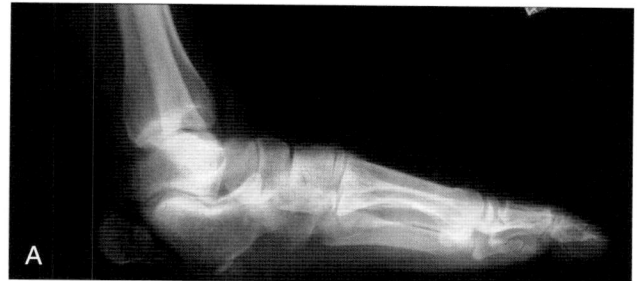
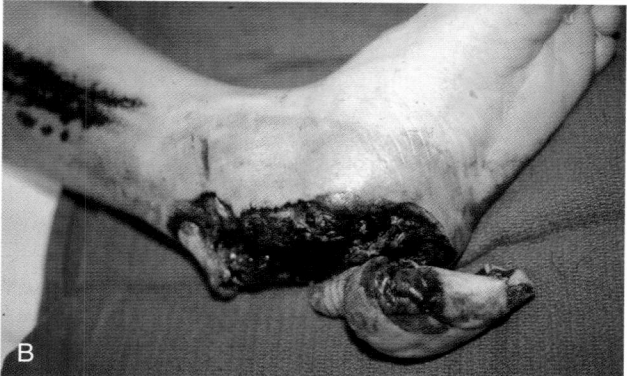

Figure 17-3 Radiographic image **(A)** and photograph **(B)** of a grade IIIB open calcaneus fracture.

are severe soft tissue lacerations with segmental or severely comminuted fractures in high-energy trauma. Because of the problems and the classification of type 3 injuries, this group was subsequently divided in three subgroups. Type 3A injury has a large soft tissue laceration or flaps but allows for adequate soft tissue coverage of bone. Also included in type 3A are fractures with severe comminution or segmental fractures, regardless of the extent of the soft tissue damage. Type 3B fractures (Fig. 17-3) are more severe, and they have extensive periosteal stripping and soft tissue loss with significant bone exposure and massive contamination. Type 3C fractures have an arterial injury requiring repair.

A more comprehensive soft tissue scale, albeit more difficult to use, is the AO soft tissue scoring system.[94] It incorporates five grades of severity and three categories of tissue. The AO classification grades the skin, muscle and tendon, and neurovascular structures. Closed fractures involving only skin are graded in four subgroups. For open fractures, four grades are given. A new feature of this classification is the evaluation for muscle and tendon injuries. Because of the prognostic value, knowledge of the extent of muscle damage and tendon involvement is essential. A common approach in all classification schemes is a determination of the length of laceration of the skin. As treatment methods have become more comprehensive and more systemic factors are taken into account when treating open fractures, the presence or absence of muscle injury, nerve injury, and vascular injury has become more important prognostically. Acute systemic factors, such as shock, associated injuries, or older age, have been recognized as important prognostic indicators also. They influence the acute treatment of fractures and the treatment of complications. For example, in osteomyelitis, debilitating factors, such as smoking and malnutrition, affect the feasibility of reconstruction.[12]

Ruedi et al[108] have developed a classification system that characterizes soft tissue injury by addressing several layers of the soft tissue envelope. This classification system determines whether the integument is open or closed. Injuries to muscle, tendon, nerve, and vessels are graded in order of severity. Although this may be more complex than the Gustilo and Anderson[43] classification of open fractures, it is an attempt similar to Tscherne's[116] classification to define in more depth the deficiency and defects of the soft tissues. Factors such as contusion or ecchymosis to skin and muscle must be identified to prevent further damage to these tissues in surgical dissection. Such damage of muscle or fascia territories can make these sites unreliable as replacement tissue.

In the limb with compromised integument and a break in the epithelial surface, underlying subcutaneous tissue, muscle, fascia, bone, and periosteum are exposed, predisposing them to desiccation with inevitable cell death and the risk of infection. To help prevent infection, a sterile moist bandage should be applied to the wound as soon as possible, bathing the damaged tissues in a physiologic medium, such as saline or lactated Ringer solution.

A biologic dressing is the first step on the reconstructive soft tissue ladder. Preventing desiccation of tissue may reduce the extent of debridement and preserves simpler options for closure, such as skin grafts.

DEBRIDEMENT

Adequate debridement of damaged tissue is paramount in the treatment of the traumatized limb. In most instances, debridement results in additional loss of tissue, depending on the degree of contamination.

The abilities of the reconstructive surgeon, particularly the ability to transplant autogenous tissue such as muscle or skin flaps, have changed the concept of debridement.[39] Surgeons treating combined injuries must accept the premise that irreversibly damaged or nonviable tissues require replacement, and the zone of injury requires expeditious reconstruction. Marginally viable tissue left behind can subsequently desiccate, infarct, and become infected, adding further delay in healing. This results in progressive dysfunction related to inflammation, fibrosis, and pain, which can be avoided if aggressive debridement is undertaken primarily. Critical vascular structures, nerves, and tendons can be cleaned, and prompt coverage can preserve their viability. Debridement may take place in the acute trauma setting or in a chronic wound that has evolved from improper handling of soft tissues.

New tools have evolved for debriding wounds. Ultrasound debridement, for example, has been used for chronic wounds. The ultrasonic methods have proved to

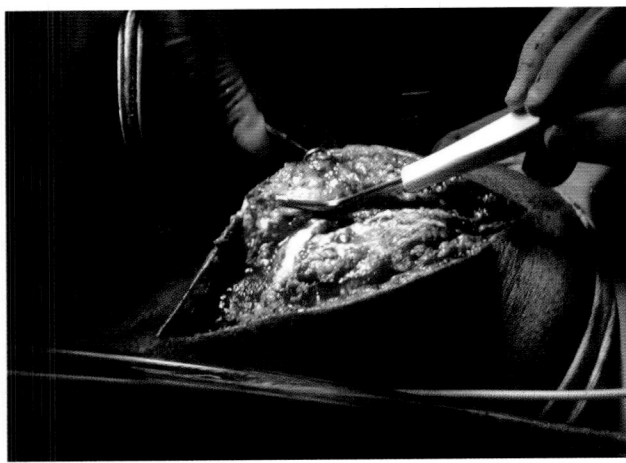

Figure 17-4 The Versajet Hydrosurgery System in use debriding a wound.

be less painful than the conventional methods of sharp debridement when used in the outpatient clinic setting. The main advantage of the technique is that debridement can be done more precisely in areas where there are patchy areas of granulation tissue that the surgeon wants to preserve.

Other devices, such as the Versajet Hydrosurgery System (Smith & Nephew, Hull, England), enables the surgeon to cut and remove damaged tissue and contaminants while simultaneously irrigating the wound. Surgical debridement is accomplished in a single step. The Versajet (Fig. 17-4) uses a high-velocity stream of sterile saline that jets across the hand piece into a vacuation collector. The Versajet requires less irrigant than traditional techniques, and it confines the irrigant to the wound area. In the acute trauma situation, this obviates the need to change large saline irrigant bags and reservoir waste canisters. This system has several power settings that can be used depending on the degree of debridement needed. One advantage of the hydrosurgery system is that there is less aerosolization of bacteria, which decreases risk to the operating room staff and surgeon based on a single wound site. Compared with conventional pulsate irrigation, the Versajet leaves significantly less bacteria in the wound.

Fresh Wounds

Debridement of the fresh wound (such as an open IIIB or IIIC pilon fracture) should be performed in an exsanguinated extremity. This permits the surgeon to carefully observe the appearance of the tissue and detect pockets in the wound, and it eliminates all foreign material. In addition, operating under tourniquet prevents unnecessary blood loss during debridement. After debridement is completed, it is relatively easy to identify major bleeders and perform proper hemostasis once the tourniquet is deflated. After release of the tourniquet, the result of debridement can also be checked by observing diffuse bleeding throughout the wound.

In the ischemic operative field, it is relatively easy to distinguish between healthy and damaged tissue. The basic elements of this judgment are the appearance and consistency of tissues. Healthy tissue in the exsanguinated limb is bright and homogeneous in color. Subcutaneous tissue is yellow, muscles are bright red, and the tendons and fascia are white and shiny. Damaged tissues are recognized by the presence of foreign bodies, irregular tissue consistency, and irregular distribution of dark red stains, which are hematomas.

All nonviable tissue is removed, preferably with a knife. It is not possible to perform exact debridement with scissors. Scissors should be used only when dissecting important structures such as nerves, vessels, or tendons.

The edge of the debridement should be in healthy tissue. Avulsed skin and muscles should be removed from the base of the avulsed flap. These tissues are contused; the anatomic pattern of the skin's vascularity is not "axial" because of avulsion of perforators, and the vascularity is therefore insufficient to maintain viability of such flaps. Denuded tendon, if not frayed, should be cleaned. Disrupted tendons can be sutured or can be fixed with a suture to surrounding tissue for later reconstruction. Exposed bones are washed with antibiotic solution and mechanically cleaned with bone rongeurs. Free bone fragments are usually removed, and if sections are quite large, they can be stored in the bone bank as bone autografts for later use when soft tissue coverage has been obtained. However, this point is controversial.

Severed vessels are ligated, provided they are not critical to the viability of the injured extremity. If vessels are vital, they are excised to normal-looking margins, and continuity is restored with interposition vein grafts.

The nerves are the only structures where debridement is not radical. Those parts that are destroyed without any doubt are removed, and major nerve stumps are anchored in the wound to prevent retraction and allow later reconstruction with nerve grafts. We prefer that a large cystoclip or hemoclip be applied to the nerve stump so it can be seen on a radiograph and appropriate secondary planning can be done in terms of surgical approach and location of the nerve stump.

Occasionally, the bed of the wound remains irregular after debridement. With additional incision, it can be made regular in shape, provided that the irregularity is not caused by tissue of functional importance. This maneuver serves to eliminate dead space by permitting the flaps, if they are to be used, close contact with the wound bed, preventing hematoma and subsequent formation of scar.

Chronic Wounds

Debridement of a chronic wound is also done with the limb exsanguinated. Superficial scar is excised completely so that the wound margins are in healthy skin and subcutaneous tissue appears normal. The goal is to treat the chronic wound like a tumor and excise it in its entirety down to normal tissue planes. All scars in the wound should be removed in the same manner as cancer surgeons operate; that is, the knife should always cut through healthy tissues. If functionally important structures are entrapped in the scar, the dissection should commence in the healthy surrounding tissue and pass toward the scar entrapment, where the structures such as nerves or tendons are carefully dissected and preserved.

This portion of the procedure is extremely difficult, and it is necessary to anticipate the changes in the anatomy caused by the injury, previous operations, and the traction exerted by scar tissue. Bone debridement is also very difficult. Although clearly necrotic parts of bone can be recognized, more experience is required to identify the viable parts of the bone callus and necrotic and inflamed areas in bone. Studies such as CT scans, bone scans, and magnetic resonance imaging (MRI) may be helpful in preoperative planning for bone and soft tissue debridement.

Swiontkowski[114] has popularized the use of the laser Doppler to determine bone blood flow in planning for debridement of infected bone. All areas of the bone not covered with periosteum are removed, and those that are exposed are burred with an iced saline bur. If punctate bleeding is encountered from the cortical bone, the bone is left behind. If not, the bone is removed until the paprika sign is identified. That is a sign of bleeding bone and live bone. This is punctate bleeding from the haversian canals that indicates bone viability. If a sequestrum is in the medullary canal, the anterior part of the bone cortex (such as the metatarsal) should be removed to provide a window for access to the medullary canal for placement of muscle flaps, which eliminates dead space and helps control infection.

DEBRIDEMENT TECHNIQUE
Surgical Technique

1. The extremity is prescrubbed to remove grime and surface dirt, and then it is prepared and draped. Nails should be cut and nail plates cleaned.
2. The leg is elevated for 5 minutes to exsanguinate it (rather than wrapping the extremity with an Esmarch bandage), and the tourniquet is inflated.
3. The wound is superficially washed with an antibiotic-saline solution to remove blood clots and superficial debris. It is advisable to use loupe magnification when debriding. The more complex the wound, the longer the debridement takes. If the patient with an open wound has been waiting for quite some time and blood is organized in muscle tissues or around fracture ends. Half-strength peroxide can be used as a first rinse solution to lyse the clot and gain access to the true depths of the wound. Half-strength peroxide has a tendency to bubble and should be washed away with normal saline solution.

4. A No. 10 or 15 scalpel blade or very sharp scissors is used to excise the skin and dermis, particularly around the edge of the wound, back to normal tissue.

5. The subcutaneous layer is inspected and debrided sharply with a No. 15 scalpel blade to the level of fascia. All fascia that is stripped, avulsed, or contaminated should be removed.

6. The next layer encountered is muscle. Muscle should be resected down to healthy tissue, regardless of the amount of muscle removed. Leaving unhealthy necrotic muscle is one of the surest ways to initiate an infection.

7. Periosteum that is elevated from bone should be excised to the level from which it is elevated. Small bone fragments devoid of periosteum or free-floating large segments, even structural ones, should be removed for fear of colonization, contamination, and infection.

8. At the conclusion of debridement, the wound is again irrigated. The tourniquet is released and all tissue planes, particularly the muscle, are observed for bleeding as the arterial pressure increases within the limb.

9. Areas that remain nonviable, particularly the dermis, skin, and muscle, are reexcised. Excision then can be done sequentially, watching for punctate bleeding from the dermis or the muscle. When large flaps have been avulsed, excision is carried out through the skin to the level of bright red blood coming from dermis on incision.

10. No attempt should be made to close the wound defect under any tension, for fear of further ischemic damage to already compromised tissue.

Special Techniques in Debridement

In the chronic bone infection, such as in the infected calcaneus, a motorized burr may be used to debride bone. Bone that is easily removed by the burr is necrotic and nonviable. At the point where there is punctate bleeding from the cortical and/or cancellous surface, indicating good viability of bone, the burring is stopped. Pulsed irrigation systems, although advocated by some, if used too vigorously with too high pressure too close to tissue planes, particularly around tendons, nerves, and vessels, can actually damage tissue and cause swelling. For this reason, we advocate copious but gentle irrigation. A wound that is appropriately debrided sharply down to all healthy tissue requires very little irrigation.

The philosophy of wound debridement should be similar to tumor resection: visualizing all normal tissue planes at the conclusion of debridement. If this is not possible, then we advocate a second-look procedure in which the debridement process is repeated, particularly if there is questionable viability of tissue. This should be done no later than 48 hours, and preferably 24 hours, after the initial debridement. If possible, during the first and not later than the second debridement, plans should be made to obtain wound coverage by one of several methods.

Within the reconstructive ladder, options are now available to reconstruct bone as well as soft tissue. No compromised tissue should be retained. The "wait and see" attitude concerning bone devoid of periosteum or muscle that is not bleeding but is covering a vital structure should be abandoned. Adequate surgical exposure is critical in the assessment of soft tissue injury as well as in its treatment.

TIMING OF RECONSTRUCTION

The optimal time for soft tissue reconstruction in severe open fractures remains controversial. The argument favoring a staged method is the need for a second-look debridement. If there is uncertainty about traumatized and devascularized tissue, a second look is performed. The main argument for early reconstruction is to reduce the nosocomial contamination and secondary necrosis of exposed tissues. Late soft tissue reconstruction is associated with a significantly higher infection rate and flap complication rate when compared with early (within 72 hours) soft tissue coverage.[20,36]

Godina[40] and other pioneers[64] changed the concept of primary repair and reconstruction of damaged tissue by advancing the phase of reconstruction from a delayed elective procedure to the day of injury. Assuming that an adequate primary debridement is feasible, the outcome should be improved by immediate soft tissue closure to avoid bone infection. Immediate reconstruction improves the time to definitive fracture union, decreases the number of operations that are performed, and reduces infection rates.[56]

Patients with IIIB and IIIC open fractures of the foot and ankle whose general condition was suitable for debridement, followed by stable internal fixation and immediate soft tissue reconstruction, demonstrated a better outcome and a shorter period of convalescence.[56] The higher incidence of infection in the delayed group may well be due to the lengthy exposure of the fracture to nosocomial contamination, the secondary damage of exposed tissue, or the necessarily incomplete nature of second-look debridement, particularly in and around a reduced fracture.

PREPARATION OF THE WOUND BEFORE RECONSTRUCTION

Wound Dressing

The standard protocol for wound management associated with fractures after surgical debridement varies with the severity of the wound. In grades I to III open fracture wounds, the gold standard technique before definitive wound coverage has been to pack the wound with saline-soaked gauze dressings, which helps eliminate dead space and prevents soft tissue desiccation. The disadvantages of saline-soaked gauze dressings include drying with soft tissue desiccation, nosocomial bacterial contamination, poor dead space management, and, often, significant patient discomfort. Similar benefits are obtained with dressings of gauze soaked in Dakin solution and half-strength povidone-iodine (Betadine). Dakin solution is bacteriostatic. Povidone-iodine, although bacteriocidal, is controversial because it is toxic to soft tissue. The advantage of all three of these dressing types is that they ensure cleanliness at the time of closure by allowing consistent monitoring of the wound site.

Fracture wounds with avulsion of the dermal surface but without damage to the underlying muscle may be treated successfully with several techniques. First is emollient coverage. Emollient-type soft tissue coverage may also be indicated to temporize a wound before soft tissue coverage. This may take the form of a hydrogel such as Vigilon (Bard Medical, Covington, Ga.), an antibiotic-impregnated occlusive dressing such as Scarlet Red (Kendall Healthcare, Mansfield, Mass.), or a simple semipermeable film such as OpSite (Smith & Nephew, Memphis, Tenn.). A copious layer of antibiotic ointment covered by a Vaseline dressing and gauze can also temporize wounds before soft tissue coverage.

There are four general types of newer wound dressings: semipermeable films (e.g., OpSite, Tegaderm [3M, St. Paul, Minn.], and bio-occlusive), hydrogels (e.g., Vigilon), occlusive hydrocolloids (e.g., Duoderm, Synthes, West Chester, Pa.), and synthetic skin substitutes (e.g., Epigard [Synthes, West Chester, Pa.] or Integra [Integra LifeSciences Corp., Plainsboro, N.J.]).[34] These newer dressings are best applied when the wound site is surrounded by a border of healthy tissue.

Semipermeable films and semiocclusive hydrogels are impermeable to water and bacteria but permeable to oxygen and water vapor. Occlusive hydrocolloids are impermeable to even water vapor and oxygen. For example, Duoderm has an inner adherent surface with an outer impermeable polyurethane foam. Epigard, one of the synthetic skin substitutes, is a nontextile open matrix polyurethane composed of two layers and backed by a microporous polytetrafluoroethylene (Teflon) film. This matrix allows new microcirculation to develop in its interstices.

Newer dressings are not without drawbacks, however, particularly the accumulation of exudate, hematoma, and seroma beneath them.[34] In addition to these wound dressings, there is an isolated report on the efficacy of honey as a broad-spectrum antimicrobial found to be effective in controlling *Staphylococcus aureus*, *Escherichia coli*, *Pseudomonas aeruginosa*, and *Klebsiella pneumoniae*. Although this finding needs further clinical verification, honey shows promise for use as a first-line wound dressing agent.[52]

Antibiotic Beads

Antibiotic beads have been used effectively to prevent or to control infection and can be used after the first debridement until the patient returns to the operating room for

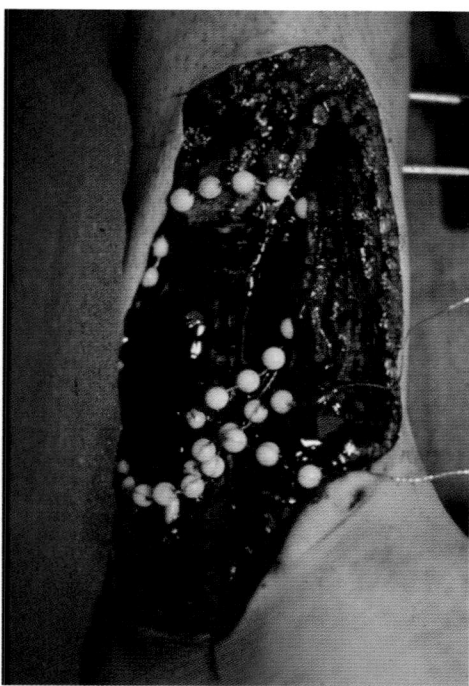

Figure 17-5 Antibiotic beads placed within an ankle wound.

a second-look debridement (Fig. 17-5). Advantages of antibiotic beads are that they can deliver antibiotics at high concentration to a compromised wound without systemic effects. The bead pouch, popularized by Henry et al,[55] seals the wound so that transudate from the wound surface is captured, bathing exposed tissues in physiologic fluids that also contain bactericidal levels of antibiotics. Wounds do not desiccate, cell death is avoided, and infection risk is reduced.

ANTIBIOTIC BEAD POUCH
The technique of local antibiotic therapy achieved via antibiotic-impregnated polymethyl methacrylate (PMMA)[54] originated with Büchholz in Germany. It was an application that used antibiotic-impregnated bone cement to treat infected arthroplasties.[53]

Antibiotic-impregnated PMMA beads are strung on steel surgical wire. A chain of medium-sized 6.3-mm PMMA beads is composed of 21 beads, each bead weighing 70 mg and containing a 5.7-mg tobramycin base. A chain of smaller beads has 20 beads that are 2 mm in diameter, each weighing 14.5 mg with a 2.2-mg tobramycin base. The surgical wire consists of three strands of size 2-0 surgical wire for the 6.3-mm beads. With the smaller size, four strands of 4-0 steel sutures are used.[123] The custom-made versus commercial fabrication processes differ in that the custom-made beads are polymerized in a mold, whereas the commercial variety is formed in a press with a corresponding increase in temperature and pressure.

The bead pouch technique is most effective for grade III open fractures. It is indicated for use in grade I fractures only if primary closure was prevented because of compartment syndrome, marked swelling, or wound edema.[54] The bead pouch technique is performed in the operating room under sterile conditions.

Surgical Technique

1. All necrotic, avascular, and contaminated tissue is removed from the fracture site during the initial irrigation and debridement. Wound margins are extended to appropriate widths.
2. A thorough lavage consisting of bacitracin and normal saline is performed.[117]
3. Depending on the severity of the fracture, reduction is accomplished with either external or internal fixation.
4. One or more chains of antibiotic beads are inserted into the wound surrounding the fracture site. Placement should be such as to fill the soft tissue cavity but leave adequate room for closure.
5. A suction drain (0.32-cm diameter) is placed in the wound. The drain should be positioned so that it exits the hematoma site through normal tissue.[117]
6. If possible, the wound should be closed with interrupted sutures. (In wounds with extensive soft tissue damage, closure may not be possible at the time of initial debridement.)
7. Wound coverage is achieved with an adhesive polyethylene wound film, such as OpSite. The semipermeable wound dressing should be stapled to the skin edges and a second layer wrapped around the entire wound area to prevent leakage of wound secretions.
8. The drain should remain in place for 48 hours. Suction is avoided because it would negate the high bactericidal dosages released by the beads into the wound hematoma.
9. The bead pouch is replaced every 48 to 72 hours in the operating room under sterile conditions. This is done to ensure adequate antibiotic concentrations in the wound environment. Aerobic and anaerobic cultures are taken at each bead change. Final wound closure is achieved through either primary suture closure or, in cases with more extensive soft tissue defects, split-thickness skin grafts or flap coverage.

Discussion

In more severe fractures, the bead pouch provides a solution to much of the debate surrounding delayed or acute soft tissue transfer. Because the bead pouch delivers high levels of antibiotics locally, the surgeon can delay definitive coverage until thorough and usually multiple debridements have been performed, a clean wound is achieved, and operative repairs of neurovascular, tendon, and ligamentous structures are made.[54] If an acute flap is indicated, the presence of the bead pouch beneath the flap serves to assuage the fears the surgeon might have that infection could occur beneath the flap.

The bead pouch technique shows significant advantages over saline-soaked gauze dressings in preventing

desiccation and subsequent soft tissue necrosis. The bead pouch provides an environment in which the bone is enveloped in a moist, protective envelope. This allows for greater infection resistance, increased wound vascularization, and a therapeutic level of antibiotics to be administered at the wound site.

Hyperbaric Oxygen

Hyperbaric oxygen (HBO) can be used to promote formation of granulation tissue and stimulate angiogenesis in wounds that are compromised, usually by impaired arterial inflow or venous outflow.[66] In addition to exposure to hyperbaric oxygen, wound dressings may be changed under sterile conditions by chamber personnel under sedation, avoiding discomfort to the patient. Patients who have gas gangrene associated with fractures require emergent debridement, hyperbaric oxygen, antibiotics, and ultimately fracture and soft tissue management.[91]

Normal tissue oxygen levels are approximately 40 mm Hg. When tissue levels fall below 30 mm Hg, normal metabolic activity is significantly impaired.[42] In infected wounds and traumatized tissue, oxygen levels often fall to less than 30 mm Hg. HBO enhances oxygen delivery to ischemic and hypoxic wounds, and even when it causes local vasoconstriction, the overall increase in blood oxygen content results in a net gain so that the net oxygen concentration at the wound increases. HBO improves neutrophil function, facilitates fibroblast cell division, increases collagen formation, and encourages new capillary budding. The promotion of angiogenesis by HBO is thought to be one of the major factors in promoting the healing of chronic hypoperfused wounds.[59]

Negative Pressure Therapy

Negative pressure therapy (NPT) exposes a wound to subatmospheric pressure. It has proved to be extremely effective in treating a wide spectrum of wounds, including traumatic wounds as well as dehisced incisions with or without exposed hardware.[6]

The wound cavity is dressed with a cell foam dressing that is connected to an adjustable vacuum source with a negative pressure of up to 125 mm Hg. The foam dressing and wound site are sealed with a thin adhesive film, converting the open wound to a controlled closed wound. Pressure is applied continuously or cyclically to the wound (Fig. 17-6). The removal of excess interstitial fluid from the wound periphery results in a decrease in the local interstitial pressure, thus restoring blood flow to compressed or collapsed vessels. Along with removal of the chronic fluid, factors that inhibit healing are also removed. An additional mechanism of action of NPT is the mechanical stimulation of cells by tensile forces placed on the tissue because of the collapse of the foam dressing by the negative pressure.

NPT closure has become an important adjunct of foot and ankle care. This device decreases edema, increases

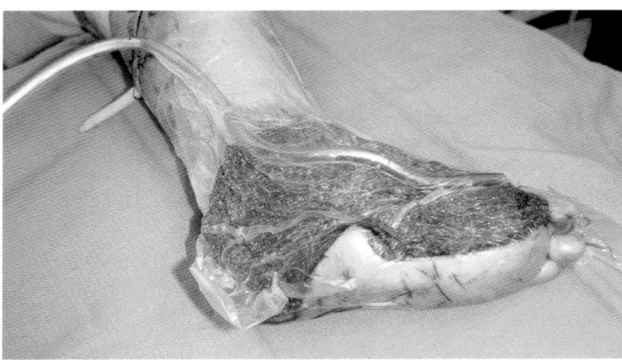

Figure 17-6 Vacuum-assisted closure was used for this traumatic foot wound before definitive coverage with a free latissimus myocutaneous transfer.

wound vascularization, fights infection, and promotes granulation tissue through proliferation of capillaries and fibroblasts.

NPT has several applications in foot and ankle surgery. It can be used for soft tissue injuries after initial debridement. If a relatively clean wound can be established, a wound vacuum-assisted closure can be applied. This device serves as a barrier dressing, and it isolates the wound from the hospital environment. Simultaneously, it encompasses all of the physiologic benefits that have been mentioned. It establishes an environment for granulation to occur.

After a second-look procedure, NPT may be used as definitive wound care treatment, usually for large cavitary wounds or wounds with irregular surface topography; a wound NPT can also stabilize the wound until definitive soft tissue treatment can occur. For example, an open calcaneus fracture that has a large cavitary soft tissue component can benefit from a wound NPT to serve as a barrier dressing from the hospital environment. When the patient is taken back to the operating room, NPT can be removed and appropriate soft tissue reconstruction can be performed with skin grafts or, more commonly, with free tissue transfer.

The advantage of NPT is similar to that of an antibiotic bead pouch in that the wound is sealed from the outside. The advantage of the bead pouch is that there is a high concentration of antibiotic that can be released into the tissue. The wound NPT relies more on physiologic rather than pharmaceutical treatment of the wound in that blood flow can be enhanced and edema can be diminished, making the wound healthier, assuming parenteral antibiotics are given.

Another application of the wound NPT has been in the treatment of fasciotomy sites. Traditionally, fasciotomy sites are covered with materials such as biosynthetic skin substitute (Biobrane, Smith & Nephew, Memphis, Tenn.) or saline dressings that require frequent dressing changes to prevent wound desiccation. In an era when hospitals are trying to diminish global costs, particularly in the trauma population, the wound NPT can remain on a

wound for 2 or 3 days, and sometimes longer, depending on the clinical circumstances. For example, the wound NPT has been a very effective stabilizer of skin grafts that are used for definitive coverage of open wounds or be skin grafted to fasciotomy sites. In those cases, the wound NPT stays on for approximately 5 days with a pressure of −75 mm Hg.

Although it is possible to definitively treat certain wounds to completion with a wound NPT, meaning complete epithelialization, a word of caution should be added regarding the use of wound NPTs with exposed hardware, such as fixation plates and screws. If the NPT is applied long enough, it is possible that a wound will granulate such that the granulation grows over exposed plates and screws. The granulation tissue contains bacteria that can colonize the plates and screws, resulting in chronic infection. In addition, the ultimate healing of soft tissue using NPT creates a healed wound, and the wound has a large degree of fibrosis associated with it. If one needed to reoperate on a foot that was treated with NPT and a skin graft, compared with supple soft tissue such as a muscle flap or regional transpositional flap, working through the scarred bed would be difficult, resulting in complications after secondary procedures, such as tendon transfers, bone grafting, or hardware exchange or removal.

Amputation versus Salvage

In complex extremity injuries, the treating physician must first determine whether limb salvage is feasible. Before complex and prolonged reconstructions are started on a limb that will ultimately function poorly or not at all, a well-fitted prosthesis should be seen as an excellent therapeutic option, and early amputation should be considered. Lange[73] and Hansen[47] have delineated a sound algorithm for these difficult cases.

If neurovascular structures are injured, are they repairable? Is normal plantar sensation possible? Does a compartment syndrome exist? Unless a compartment syndrome is recognized and treated, muscle ischemia and death will occur, converting potentially viable soft tissue to infarcted muscle and scar. This ultimately increases the need for large bloc resections and tissue replacement—a higher rung on the reconstructive ladder.

Although the evolution of sophisticated microsurgical reconstructive techniques has created the possibility of successful limb salvage in even the most extreme cases, such technical possibilities are double-edged swords. Hansen,[47] in analyzing his vast personal experience with managing open fractures, noted that protracted limb salvage attempts might destroy a patient physically, psychologically, socially, and financially, with adverse consequences for the patient's family as well. In spite of the best attempts, the functional results of limb salvage are often worse than those of an amputation. Thus enthusiasm for limb-salvage techniques, especially of the traumatized foot and ankle, must be tempered by a realistic assessment of the results, not just for the injured part but for the patient as a whole.[73] A salvaged limb must function as well as, if not better than, a prosthesis, or heroic attempts at reconstruction are not indicated. Donor-site morbidity should also be considered with free tissue transfer when considering limb reconstruction.

Indicators of a poor prognosis for limb salvage, in order of significance, are massive crush injuries, other high-energy soft tissue injuries, a warm ischemia time longer than 6 hours, severely comminuted or segmental fracture patterns, infrapopliteal arterial injury, prolonged severe hypovolemic shock, and age older than 50 years.

Occupational demands and the presence or absence of underlying diseases, such as diabetes, are also important considerations. The same anatomic injury can require a different treatment decision in a 20-year-old laborer than in a 60-year-old diabetic patient.

Similarly, a given tibial injury might need to be treated differently if there is unreconstructible ipsilateral foot trauma that precludes reasonable limb function even if the leg is salvageable. According to several authors, complete disruption of the posterior tibial nerve (in association with type IIIC tibial fracture) is also a functional liability significant enough to warrant amputation.[21,58,74] Decreased sensation on presentation is *not* an indication for amputation.

Expedient amputation of a massively traumatized limb, even if it appears salvageable, may also be necessary in the multiply injured patient who cannot tolerate the reconstructive time or metabolic demands of the reconstruction. This is an extremely difficult judgment that is highly individualized and impossible to quantitate.[77]

WOUND CLOSURE

After adequate debridement, it may be possible to close a wound primarily. This is done rarely, if ever, in cases of open fracture resulting from the danger of contamination or the need for a second-look debridement. However, approach incisions can be primarily closed after extensive aproaches for debridement.

The second rung in the reconstructive ladder is delayed primary closure. This method is considered in cases in which the adequacy of the primary debridement is uncertain; it is usually done after the initial edema subsides. Healing by second intention refers to epithelialization and wound contraction. This technique may also be applied to abrasions, avoiding the need for skin grafts.

The next level of reconstruction is use of a split-thickness skin graft (STSG), either meshed or unmeshed.

Skin Grafting

The skin is composed of dermis and epidermis. The dermis contains sebaceous glands, most of which are appendages of hair follicles.[107] Sweat glands and hair follicles are mostly located in the deep dermis. These skin appendages are lined with epithelium, thus allowing for re-epithelialization after removal of epidermis and partial removal of dermis, as in superficial burns or harvesting of split-thickness skin.

Although sebaceous glands are not under hormonal control and continue to function after skin grafting, sweat glands (both apocrine and eccrine) temporarily lose nervous control. As a result, newly grafted skin may be dry, requiring moisturizing with common over-the-counter preparations.

What type of wound can be healed with a skin graft? Any wound with a full-thickness loss of skin may be considered for skin grafting. Such defects might heal spontaneously but, because of the lack of dermal appendages, do so through the process of contraction and epithelialization from the wound periphery. When healed, these wounds have skin lacking the normal microanatomy found in native skin. Specifically, there are no rete pegs—epidermal projections into the dermis that anchor the two layers of skin together. Such a wound is relatively unstable in terms of long-term durability. Allowing spontaneous healing of a full-thickness wound is therefore only appropriate for small defects and for certain larger defects where the contraction process will not distort critical anatomy or cause a functional disturbance, such as a joint contracture.

In evaluating a wound for possible skin grafting, the surgeon must assess the adequacy of the wound bed. The process of graft healing will require ingrowth of vessels from the wound, and so relatively avascular tissue provides a poor bed for skin grafting. Exposed bone, tendon, nerve and cartilage, necrotic tissue, and devascularized fat are examples of tissues that provide a poor wound bed. Conversely, well-vascularized tissues, such as muscle, periosteum, fascia, healthy fat, and epitenon, will all accept skin grafts.

Split-thickness skin grafts (STSGs) contain less dermis than full-thickness skin grafts (FTSGs), thus allowing more of the natural wound-healing process of contraction to occur. They also have less metabolic demand relative to FTSGs and so are more likely to succeed on a vascularly compromised wound. FTSGs are thicker; more durable in the long term; can carry hair follicles, allowing future hair growth; contract less; and retain more of their natural donor-area pigmentation. In general, FTSGs retain greater sensation than do STSGs.

Because one can expect epidermis to regenerate after an STSG is harvested, donor sites can be large. Despite the spontaneous regeneration noted in these donor sites, however, there is still a permanent scar, usually noted by subtle textural changes. Therefore, in certain ethnic groups with a propensity for hypertrophic scarring, strict attention must be paid to where split-thickness skin is harvested. In some Asian or African American patients, for example, scalp skin may be preferable to thigh skin for this reason. The most common donor sites for STSGs, in order of cosmetic preference, are buttock and thigh, abdomen, back, scalp, chest wall, and arms.

Harvesting of an FTSG requires closure of the donor wound because spontaneous re-epithelialization is not possible. As a rule, FTSGs tend to be small and are usually used for reconstruction in the foot.

The healing of skin grafts has been described as a two-step process. Initially, the graft survives by imbibing wound-bed exudate. After approximately 48 hours, new blood vessels begin to sprout from the wound bed and grow up into the graft. Either capillaries from the wound bed connect with graft vessels, a process known as *inosculation,* or they form new vascular channels within the graft—*revascularization.* During these processes, fibrin and collagen are also assisting in forming a cohesive bond between graft and bed. By the fifth to seventh postgraft day, a skin graft is usually adherent and vascularized.

SPLIT-THICKNESS SKIN GRAFTING

Before skin grafting, the wound must be adequately prepared. All nonviable material must be removed sharply so that the wound bed is left with healthy, preferably bleeding, tissue. A curette is quite useful in this regard. Adequate hemostasis is imperative; however, overuse of electricocautery leaves a charred wound that is unlikely to foster inosculation and revascularization of the graft. Most often after debridement, the wound is elevated and covered with a sponge soaked in normal saline. By the time the graft has been harvested, the wound bed is usually quite dry. Topical hemostatic agents, such as thrombin, may also be used.

Equipment needed to perform an STSG consists of a dermatome, mesher, mineral oil, suture or staples, and dressings appropriate for both graft and donor site. Dermatomes have evolved from hand-held knives (e.g., Humby knife) to electric and gas-powered devices able to precisely harvest skin of various thickness. Most dermatomes require insertion of a disposable blade and have two adjustments that need to be made by the surgeon: thickness and width.

Thickness, measured in thousandths of an inch, is usually set with a dial on the dermatome itself. For most patients, graft thickness is between 0.012 and 0.017 inch. The clinical setting dictates an appropriate thickness. One must balance survival (short and long-term) of the graft with donor-site healing. Therefore, in an elderly patient with thin skin, a thinner STSG (0.012-0.013 inch) may be chosen, whereas in a younger patient a thicker STSG (0.015-0.016 inch) may be preferable. The surgeon must also choose an appropriate width of skin to harvest. This adjustment is either on the dermatome itself or dependent on an attached cover placed over the blade before harvesting.

Surgical Technique

1. The donor site is prepared by first removing any povidone-iodine and other foreign materials from the skin. Mineral oil is applied liberally to both skin and dermatome to aid in gliding.
2. The dermatome is turned on, placed at a 45-degree angle with the skin, and advanced firmly to prevent slippage. As the graft is being harvested, punctate bleeding from a white dermal bed should be seen. If subcutaneous fat is noted, harvesting should be stopped immediately, the graft replaced, a new donor site chosen, and the thickness setting on the dermatome readjusted.
3. After an adequate amount of skin has been harvested, the dermatome is lifted from the donor area.
4. The donor area is temporarily covered with a hemostatic agent (local anesthesia with epinephrine or topical thrombin is a popular choice). (Donor-site dressings are reviewed later in this discussion.)
5. The skin graft is then meshed. Meshing is necessary for two reasons. First, STSG failure is usually secondary to hematoma formation beneath it, and meshing of the skin allows drainage postoperatively. Second, when a large amount of graft is needed (e.g., for a large burn), meshing also allows the graft to expand so that a relatively small piece of skin can cover a larger area. Most popular meshers require placement of the skin on a "carrier" chosen for the ratio of mesh. Unless a paucity of STSG donor sites requires a larger ratio, most grafts are meshed at 1 to 1.5. Disadvantages of meshing mostly relate to the aesthetics of the healed meshed skin, which retains its "meshed" appearance in the long term (Fig. 17-7).
6. The STSG is placed on the graft site and held in place with skin staples or sutures. Additional fixation is often placed in central portions to encourage adherence. Absorbable or nonabsorbable suture material may be used to affix the graft to the bed, but sutures offer no advantage in terms of results, and they take significantly longer to apply. Studies have noted success using fibrin glue (derived from autologous plasma) as an aid in graft adherence.[112] The glue was found to improve graft survival, reduce blood loss, and obviate the need for meshing, thus producing a more aesthetic result (Fig. 17-8).[65]

Dressing Application

A myriad of different dressings have been used for the graft site, all with the goal of providing a moist, antimicrobial environment that facilitates ingrowth of vessels into the graft. A common technique for dressing the graft employs a mixture of acetic acid, glycerine (Bunnell solution), and benzyl chloride to soak dressings. A layer of nonadherent gauze soaked in this mixture is first placed on the graft.

The next layer applied depends on the topography of the graft bed. In a relatively concave bed, there is a natural tendency for the graft to adhere tightly to the bed, and a layer of 4 × 4 gauze soaked in modified Bunnell solution, followed by a soft, dry, noncompressible gauze wrap, is all that is required. In graft beds with "hills and valleys," cotton balls that are soaked in Bunnell solution and laid carefully in the crevices of the bed will then create a custom moulage dressing that encourages adherence of the graft throughout the bed. Additional 4 × 4 gauze

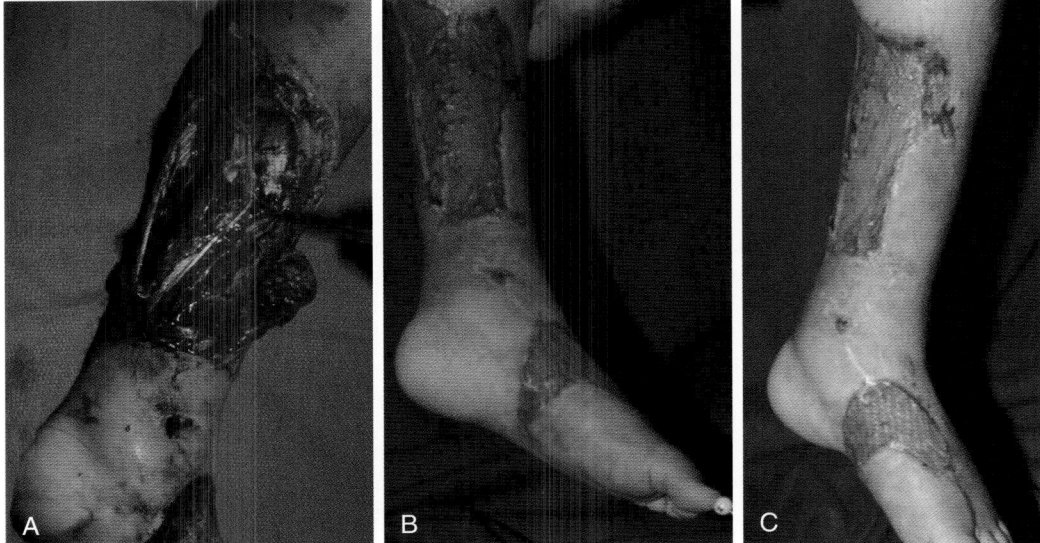

Figure 17-7 This 7-year-old boy was injured in a lawn mower accident. **A,** Wounds during debridement. **B** and **C,** The healing skin grafts several months after surgery.

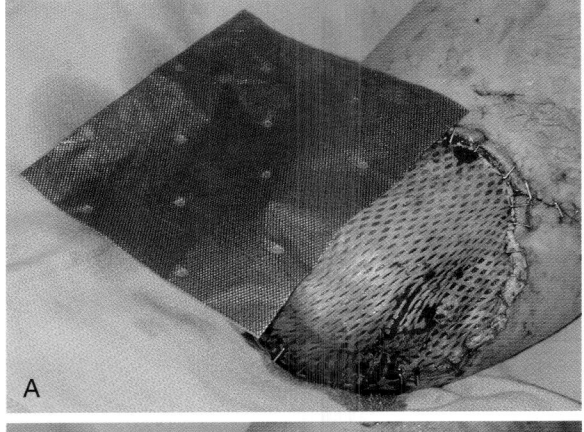

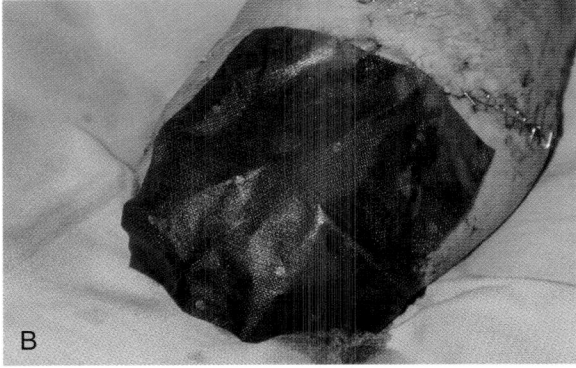

Figure 17-8 **A,** Acticoat (Smith & Nephew, Memphis, Tenn.), a silver-impregnated antimicrobial barrier dressing, can be used to cover split-thickness skin graft donor and recipient sites. **B,** Here it is placed over the skin graft of an amputation site.

layers and the dry gauze wrap are then placed over the soaked dressing.

With small grafts or grafts in areas where a gauze wrap is not logistically possible, a bolster-type bandage may be fashioned with silk or nylon sutures placed at the wound periphery and tied over the dressing to help encourage graft adherence. For grafts placed in a highly mobile area, such as the distal extremity, splinting the limb to limit movement may be appropriate as well. Care should be taken to pad the splint so as to prevent any irritation of normal skin under it.

After the graft has been properly dressed, the temporary dressing on the donor site is removed. Careful attention must be paid to the donor site because patients often complain of more discomfort in this area than at the graft site. A detailed discussion of donor-site dressings can be found in a 1991 review.[35] In certain patients, any excess STSG should be replaced on the donor site. This allows rapid (often 3-day) healing of the area of replaced graft.

In general, smaller donor sites should be dressed with semiocclusive or totally occlusive dressings. These include clear films (OpSite, Tegaderm) and hydrocolloid dressings (Duoderm) and Allovyne (Smith & Nephew, Memphis, Tenn.). These materials used on a small donor site allow relatively pain-free donor-site healing with minimal care, low cost, and low infection rates. When using a clear film, wound exudate (common to any open wound) must be aspirated for the first few days to prevent leakage. A simple way to do this involves preparing the most dependent part of the dressing with alcohol, aspirating tangentially (so as not to prick the skin surface), and then patching the dressing with a small piece of film. In larger donor sites, the amount of wound exudate becomes excessive, making these types of dressings impractical. For these wounds, semiopen dressings, such as Xeroform (Kendall

Healthcare, Mansfield, Mass.), are preferred. Although slightly more painful, they also allow donor-site healing with minimal care, low cost, and low infection rates.

FULL-THICKNESS SKIN GRAFTING

The technique for FTSG requires little in the way of instrumentation or equipment.

Surgical Technique

1. The recipient site is prepared as described for split-thickness grafting.
2. An appropriate donor site is chosen, and a template is often used to allow harvest of precisely the correct amount of skin. Because of the small size of FTSGs, local anesthesia is commonly used during harvest.
3. After hemostasis is achieved, the donor site is closed in layers.
4. The FTSG is defatted so that only dermis remains on the surface being applied to the wound bed.
5. The FTSG is placed on its recipient bed and held in place with absorbable (e.g., 5-0 chromic) or nonabsorbable (e.g., 5-0 silk or nylon) sutures. Additional sutures can be placed in the midportion.
6. FTSGs are rarely meshed. Rather, they are pie-crusted and perforated with a knife in several areas to facilitate postoperative drainage.

Dressing Application

Most FTSGs are dressed with nonadherent gauze, antibiotic ointment (e.g., bacitracin), and moistened cotton or gauze held in place with a bolster tie-over dressing.

APPLICATION OF SKIN SUBSTITUTES

In addition to autogenous STSGs, certain skin substitutes can be used to provide temporary and permanent dermal substrates for skin grafting in wounds that otherwise would have required more complex procedures, such as flaps.

Bioengineered manufactured skin substitutes, such as AlloDerm (LifeCell, Branchburg, N.J.) or Integra, have significant benefits. Alloderm is a dermal collagen matrix that can be placed on an open wound bed that might not be able to take a skin graft. The inosculation of the dermal substrate allows the dermis to regenerate for subsequent skin grafting. AlloDerm has also been used in diabetic and dysvascular feet as a way to promote healing. It has been our experience that AlloDerm does not work as well as Integra. Integra is a bilaminate skin substitute that has been very effective for wounds that are not suitable for skin grafting but would otherwise require higher rungs on the reconstructive ladder for closure, such as a local flap or free flap. Integra is an excellent tool for small wounds or wounds that almost have a dermal substrate but are not yet ready for grafting. Integra can be applied over tendons that are denuded of paratenon or in cases where dermis is required for further reconstruction.

The technique requires Integra to be placed over a debrided wound. After 14 to 21 days, the outer laminate (silicone elastic [Silastic] membrane) is removed, usually revealing a neodermis that is suitable for split-thickness skin grafting. Integra, in conjunction with NPT, has been a very effective way to promote a dermal base for skin grafting, obviating more complex procedures, such as free tissue transfer or local regional flaps. Integra is not suitable to place over large areas of exposed cortex, but if a small area requires periosteum or dermal substitution, Integra can be used. We have experience doing this with patients who were not candidates for free tissue transfer, and bone surface areas that were exposed are small enough that this technique works. Total dimensions should be no greater than 2 or 3 cm of exposed bone.

Surgical Technique

1. The cortex (bone) is burred down with a chilled high-speed burr to achieve punctate bleeding from the haversian system.
2. Integra is then applied with the intention that the bleeding vessels will result in vascular penetration into the artificial dermis.
3. After 2 to 3 weeks, the outer membrane of the Integra can be removed and the neodermis that is created can be skin grafted.

Wound-Closure Aftercare and Long-Term Issues

Patients undergoing skin grafting usually do not complain about significant amounts of pain in the grafted area. Mild analgesics, such as acetaminophen with codeine, suffice in most cases. The first 3 to 5 days after grafting are the most critical for graft survival because this is the time when inosculation and revascularization occur. Therefore it is often prudent to keep patients immobile at strict bed rest with the limb elevated during this period. Many reconstructive surgeons also give the patient prophylactic subcutaneous heparin during the time of strict immobilization.

The use of prophylactic antibiotics is controversial, but most reconstructive surgeons give them at least preoperatively and often for up to 2 to 5 days postoperatively. For a clean wound, a first-generation cephalosporin (e.g., Ancef, Kefzol) may be used. In chronic wounds that might have been previously infected, antibiotics specific for the previous cultures are appropriate.

The dressing on the graft site is usually changed on the fifth to seventh postoperative day, or earlier if there are signs or symptoms of infection or hematoma. An FTSG usually appears quite ecchymotic in the first 7 to 10 days; STSGs may appear paler. In most cases, an initial assessment of the take can be made at this point. If the graft is dry, Xeroform gauze and a light bandage are placed over the graft site. In certain situations, the graft appears moist. In this case, or if there are any signs of infection, the dressing should be changed twice a day, using 0.25% acetic acid–soaked gauze. The graft often responds favorably to this regimen, effectively saving an otherwise failing graft.

By the second week, a healthy graft may only need a dressing for protective purposes. The newly healed skin is viable but sensitive, especially to abrasive forces. Newly grafted skin is dry because of the loss of sweat glands. Application of an antibiotic ointment in the first 3 weeks, followed by any common skin moisturizer after 3 weeks, is helpful. Clips used to secure STSGs should be removed after the first 5 to 10 days to prevent overgrowth of surrounding skin. Sutures used to secure FTSGs should also be removed at this time.

In addition to moisturizing, care should be taken to keep freshly grafted areas clean. Sun exposure should be avoided, as with any fresh scar. Patients should be reassured that the initial redness of a STSG donor site will fade over time.

The most common cause of skin graft failure is hematoma beneath the graft, preventing revascularization. Other causes include inadequate immobilization, bacterial contamination, dependency, and incorrect graft orientation (placing the epidermis side down). If a hematoma or infection is identified in the first 3 to 5 days, drainage of the hematoma and local treatment of the infection may be all that is needed for partial or complete graft salvage. As always, attention to detail can help prevent most of the common causes of failure.

FLAPS

A flap is tissue transferred from one anatomic site to another. Vascularity of the transferred tissue is maintained by nutrient vessels within the flap pedicle. The pedicle may either remain attached at its origin or be divided during the transfer and reanastomosed to recipient vessels using microsurgical techniques. Microsurgical transfer of tissue is also known as a *free flap* (autologous tissue transplantation).

Flaps are useful to close defects too large for primary closure and where skin grafts are inadequate. Flaps can contain more than one type of tissue and are named based upon the tissues they contain. Examples of compound flaps are fasciocutaneous flaps, which contain skin and underlying fascia, and musculocutaneous flaps, which contain skin, fascia, and muscle. Rotation flaps, such as muscle, skin, and fascia, or a combination, can add much-needed vascularized tissue, obliterate dead space, and help to close the wound without tension. When rotational flap options are limited because of wound location or regional donor-site deficiencies, then free flaps must be considered. The most complex reconstructions often require free tissue transfer.

Muscle can be rotated into adjacent defects if the muscle's native vascular supply is preserved. The utility of any given muscle flap is limited by the size of the muscle and the length of its vascular pedicle, limiting the distance it can be rotated. The defect, both functional and cosmetic, created by the muscle transfer must also be considered. Muscle flaps can transfer richly vascularized and very

immunologically active tissue into wounds that are ischemic or infected.[60,61,109] The bulk of muscle flaps allows contour defects to be resurfaced. Skin can be transferred with the underlying muscle simultaneously or at a later date.

Bone can be also used for reconstruction as a free microvascular bone graft or a vascularized graft, alone or together with other tissues such as skin or muscle. With the development of microvascular techniques, bone grafts from various sites can be transferred with their intact blood supply. Vascularized bone grafts have proved to be advantageous in clinical settings in which nonvascularized bone grafts have been unsatisfactory, such as ischemic necrosis of the talus.

Classification of Muscle Flaps

The classification of muscle flaps is based on five patterns of muscle circulation.[84] A muscle for free tissue transfer must be able to survive on one vascular pedicle that is dominant and that will support the entire muscle mass.

Type 1: one vascular pedicle (extensor digitorum brevis, tensor fascia lata)

Type 2: dominant pedicle and minor pedicles (abductor hallucis gracilis)

Type 3: two dominant pedicles (rectus abdominis, serratus anterior)

Type 4: segmental vascular pedicles (none)

Type 5: one dominant and secondary vascular pedicles (latissimus dorsi, pectoralis major, pectoralis minor)

Pedicle muscle flaps can be locally or distally based. The flexor digitorum brevis muscle is an example of a pedicle muscle flap that can be used in heel reconstruction. Although all muscle transfers can be harvested as the muscle component alone, not all muscles can be harvested with reliable skin overlying the muscle. Examples of muscles with unreliable large skin paddles include the gracilis and pectoralis minor muscle. Including skin with the muscle transfer allows flap monitoring and provides color and texture match in an extremity that requires muscle for bulk in addition to cutaneous coverage. A musculocutaneous flap can also be used for a salvage procedure such as to repair an amputation site without further bone loss.

Fasciocutaneous Flaps

Fasciocutaneous flaps provide another option for covering defects, especially in cases in which there is no need for bulk. For example, the saphenous fasciocutaneous flap perfused by posterior medial perforators in the saphenous artery can cover defects in the distal third of the leg and can reach the foot. These flaps are often distally based (i.e., the perfusion of the flaps is from distal to proximal) (Fig. 17-9), and the flap is rotated in the more proximal position in the leg, down to the area of the foot and ankle.

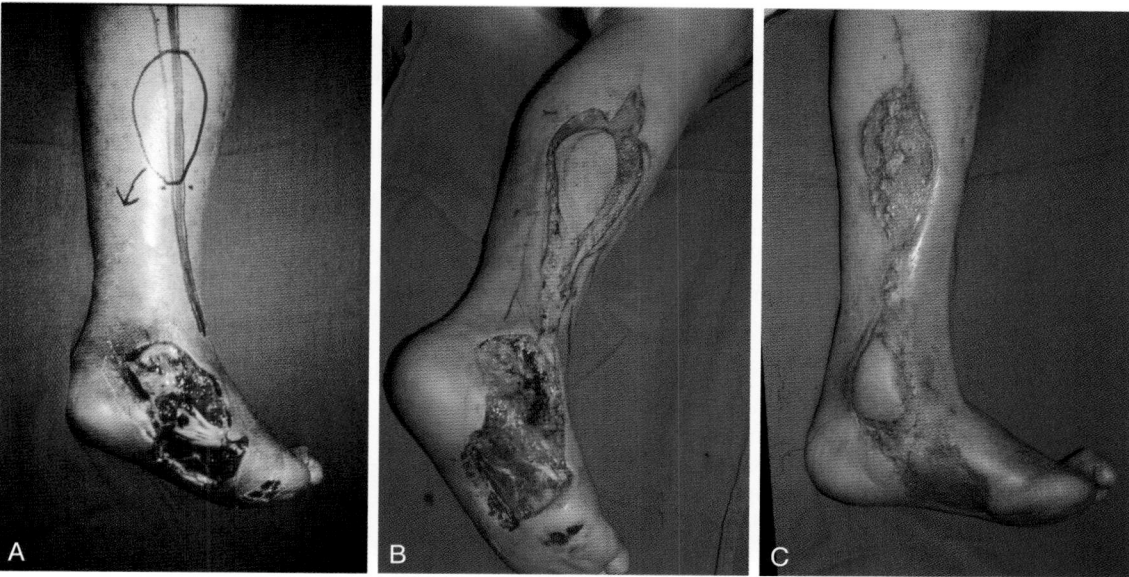

Figure 17-9 This 52-year-old diabetic man with a medial foot ulcer was treated with debridement and a saphenous vein flap.

In recent years, the sural flap has become popular and is well suited for coverage of defects around the distal ankle. The sural flap is based on perforators from the peroneal artery as well as the neurocutaneous territory of the sural nerve.

The use of fasciocutaneous flaps from the sural angiosome in the repair of soft tissue defects was first reported by Pontén in his 1981 report on the use of 23 proximally based fasciocutaneous flaps.[102] The distally based sural fasciocutaneous flap was introduced by Donski and Fogdestam 2 years later. The authors described the anatomic structure, offered a detailed description of the surgical procedure, and described their experience with the flap in three clinical cases.[31] After this report, the sural flap remained largely unmentioned in the literature, with only one publication on its anatomic aspects between 1983 and 1992.[70] Masquelet reintroduced the sural flap in 1992, with a complete, concise description of the relevant anatomy and the surgical procedure.[80] Since the work of Masquelet, the distally based sural fasciocutaneous flap has become a mainstay in the reconstruction of the lower leg, heel, and foot.

Since 1990, several flap modifications have been reported to improve flap viability and to solve a myriad of reconstructive needs.

Surgical Technique

The technical aspects of the sural flap are well described in many of the publications cited herein. The pivot point for the flap is first identified posterior and superior to the lateral malleolus. Most authors contend that the pivot point must be a minimum of approximately 5 cm proximal to the lateral malleolus, but some authors claim that a minimal distance as large as 10 to 11 cm is necessary to achieve consistent flap survival. However, a recent report

has shown that in young healthy patients, the presence of the posterior lateral malleolar artery and the lateral calcaneal artery allows the pivot point to be as close as 1.5 cm from the lateral malleolus. Doppler ultrasound may be used to identify perforating vessels to aid in the planning of a pivot point.

The skin island is then outlined to match the recipient site defect. Either of two approaches can be taken in designing the flap. If the pivot point is kept relatively low, the fascial pedicle can be kept short, and the flap can be harvested entirely from the distal two thirds of the posterior lower leg. Alternatively, if the pivot point is taken higher to preserve all potential perforating vessels, the fascial pedicle must be longer to reach the defect site. If this second approach is taken, the flap may be taken to within 1 to 2 cm of the popliteal crease. The authors of this review, however, prefer the first strategy.

The maximum size of the flap is another point of some controversy. Various case series report maximum flap sizes of 12 to 23 cm in length and 8 to 16 cm in width. The upper limits of the flap's dimensions have been best explored by Ayyappan and Chadha,[9] who report leaving as little as 1 to 2 cm of skin distal to the popliteal crease, with a pivot point only 4 to 5 cm proximal to the lateral malleolus. When outlining the flap, Doppler ultrasound may again be used to ensure inclusion of the lesser saphenous vein (LSV).

Once these preparatory steps have been taken, the skin is then incised to the level of the fascia under tourniquet control. Owing to their suprafascial location, the median sural nerve (SN), superficial sural artery (SSA), and LSV are generally transected in the course of this incision. The median SSA and LSV can then be ligated as a single unit or individually. If the proximal border of the flap is taken closer to the popliteal fossa, where the SN and LSV are located subfascially, the adipofascial connections between the fascia and the proximal portions of these structures should be carefully preserved to maintain the venocutaneous and neurocutaneous perforators that arise from their extrinsic vasculature.

Once the fascial pedicle has been elevated along with the vessels and nerve, it can be inset into the recipient defect site. The skin is then closed primarily to the extent possible, and any remaining donor site defect is closed using a split-thickness skin graft.

Surgical Indications

The sural fasciocutaneous flap can generally be used to cover any soft tissue defect of the proximal third of the foot and of the lower leg, provided that the defect is small enough to be covered by the maximal flap size and that the defect can be reached by the fascial pedicle. Because both of these two variables are highly subjective and depend on the patient's overall medical condition, the other reconstructive options available, and the surgeon's inclinations, there is no simple rule for when a defect can and cannot be covered. The sural flap has been shown to be more reliable than the lateral supramalleolar flap (another distally based fasciocutaneous flap used in the distal lower extremity) and is likely a better choice in almost all clinical situations.

The flap can be used to cover exposed vessels, bones, tendons, and hardware. As always, adequate debridement of the recipient site is the single most important step to assuring success. It has been shown that neither occlusion of the anterior and posterior tibial arteries nor varicose leg veins should be considered absolute contraindications to the use of a distally based sural flap. Most surgeons do consider an occluded peroneal artery to be a contraindication to this operation. The flap has been shown to be successful in diabetic patients, in medically compromised patients, and in the pediatric population. An anatomic study of 24 amputation specimens from patients with severe vascular disease has shown that the flap was theoretically anatomically possible in 23 of 24 specimens. The flap has also been shown by a number of authors to be useful as a cross-leg flap.

The causes of the defects needing repair that have been reported in the literature include nonhealing skin wounds or ulcers, chronic venous ulcers, soft tissue injury secondary to open fractures, chronic osteomyelitis, penetrating trauma or avulsions, contractures, gangrene, unstable scars, cancer resections, and electrical burns.

Complications

A meta-analysis of all 50 papers that report the use of the unmodified distally based sural flap was performed.[37] This analysis found that 587 of 720 flaps (82%) were reported to heal without necrosis or any other flap-related complications. Complete flap necrosis was reported as a complication in only 24 of 720 flaps (3.3%), and partial or marginal flap necrosis was reported in 76 of 720 flaps (11%). Other flap-related complications, such as venous congestion, edema, infection, and recurrent osteomyelitis, were reported in 33 of 720 flaps (4.6%).

Anterior Tibial Artery Flap

The anterior tibial artery flap can be a distally based flap similar to the radial forearm flap for coverage of the dorsum of the hand. The anterior tibial artery flap, although it does have a sound anatomic basis, should be used with caution in that the perforators of the anterior compartment are often taken, which can compromise muscle blood flow and result in necrosis or fibrosis of the anterior compartment. Because of this, donor site morbidity is high, and this flap is not recommended for routine use.

Free Flaps

Free flaps include isolated transfers, composite tissue transfers, functioning free muscle transfers, and structural transfers, such as vascularized bone grafts.

Microsurgery for extremity reconstruction began over half a century ago with the introduction of the operating microscope for anastomosis of blood vessels, described by Jacobson and Suarez.[63] Microsurgical repair of digital arteries and digital replantation began in the 1960s,[16,67] and microsurgical composite tissue transplantation began in the 1970s. Microsurgeons expanded their efforts from achieving tissue survival to include the improvement of function as well as appearance in the 1980s. In the 1990s, the emphasis shifted to outcome. Today, composite transplantation or free tissue transfer routinely not only provides coverage but also facilitates function.

A thorough understanding of free tissue transfer includes understanding the rationale for tissue transplantation, the timing of the transplant, and the transplant that should be selected. The orthopaedic surgeon should have an understanding of the current techniques of reconstructive microsurgery and should be able to obtain appropriate reconstructive consultations for patients.

Sir Harold Gillies, one of the fathers of modern reconstructive plastic surgery, used the motto "Replace like with like." The interpretation of this principle with regard to free tissue transfer is that the reconstructive microsurgeon transplants autogenously vascularizes tissue into defects that are the result of trauma, tumor, infection, or congenital defects.

Free tissue transplantation should be considered for any tissue deficit that cannot be treated by an adjacent tissue rearrangement, skin grafting, or local pedicle flaps. Free tissue transplantation is selected in instances in which there are composite deficiencies, such as skin and bone or muscle and skin.

The highest rung on the reconstructive ladder, free tissue transfer, is often used in combination with lower rungs of the ladder, such as skin closure, skin grafting, or rotational flaps.

Indications for Free Tissue Transfer in the Lower Extremity

Trauma and Sepsis

The main indication for salvage of a severely damaged limb is that the limb has potentially intact sensibility. Nerve injuries do not preclude salvage but should be distal enough to permit the return of some function (primarily sensory) within a reasonable amount of time. Conversely, complex lower limb injuries with nerve damage (transection or nerve loss) are often considered for amputation, because the return to a functional status with a good prosthesis is usually more rapid.[101] Advanced age should not be a contraindication to microvascular limb-salvage procedures. Careful preoperative patient evaluation and perioperative monitoring can effectively decrease morbidity and mortality rates to equal those for younger patients.[41]

The choice of flap to be used for wound coverage is determined by the size of the wound, the type of tissue deficit, the state of the wound (colonization, amount of cavitation), the location of the injury, and the length of the pedicle needed. The anastomosis should be done in a *safe zone* where recipient vessels have not been damaged by the initial trauma, either proximal or distal to the zone of injury. *Zone of injury* refers to the inflammatory response of the soft tissue of the traumatized lower limb, which extends beyond the gross wound and results in perivascular changes in the blood vessels. These changes include increased friability of the vessels and increased perivascular scar tissue, which can contribute to a higher failure rate, especially in lower limb free tissue transplantation, presumably because of a higher rate of microvascular thrombosis.[7]

Most surgeons avoid the zone of injury by extensive proximal dissection of the recipient vascular pedicle, and some of them use vein grafts in lower limb reconstruction. Isenberg and Sherman[62] demonstrated that clinical acceptability of the recipient pedicle (vessel wall pliability and the quality of blood from the transected end of the vessel) was more important than the distance from the wound.

Reconstruction of the traumatized leg can be challenging because both bone stabilization and soft tissue coverage are required for a successful functional outcome. Free tissue transfer using microsurgical techniques has enabled surgeons to salvage traumatized extremities that formerly would have required amputation.[44,58,74]

Osteomyelitis

Osteomyelitis is now a treatable disease. The Cierny-Mader[26] classification should be used as a guide for treatment. Management of dead space after sequestrectomy relies heavily on the technique of tissue transfer (Fig. 17-10). Free muscle flaps provide coverage for the debrided bone and soft tissue, obliterate dead space, improve vascularity, and enhance leukocyte function.[33,82,83]

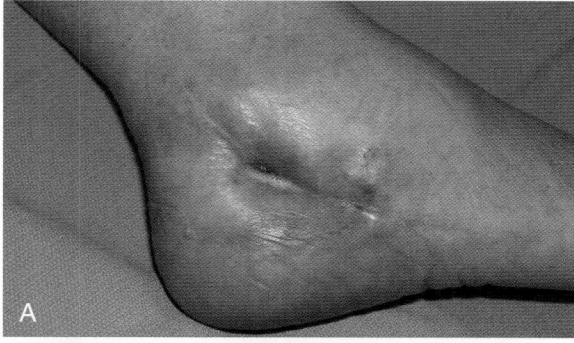
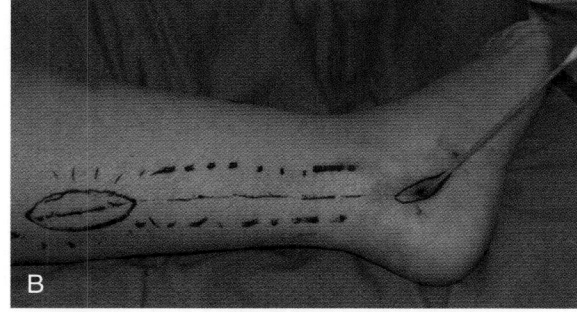
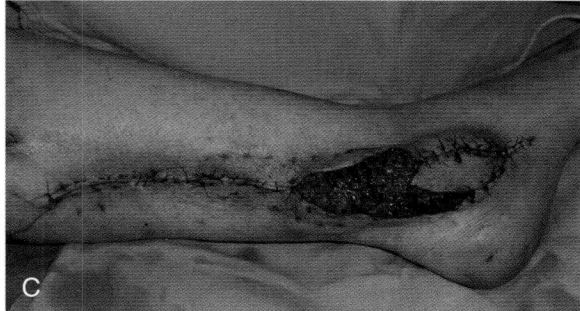

Figure 17-10 A, This 45-year-old woman with chronic osteomyelitis of the calcaneus was treated with a sequestrectomy and sural fasciocutaneous flap. **B,** Sural flap design. **C,** Initial flap inset.

Advances in skeletal reconstruction and fixation have improved the treatment of patients with osteomyelitis and large (greater than 6 cm) segmental bone defects. In the past, despite successful treatment of osteomyelitis, some patients have required amputation because of chronic nonunions. Now, once the bone infection is treated, vascularized bone transplant[86,100] or distraction osteogenesis facilitates reconstruction and provides structural stability for limb function.[4]

Local muscles traditionally were used to treat chronic osteomyelitis, and free flaps have been described more recently for this use. The advantages of using the free muscle flaps, such as latissimus dorsi,[14] serratus anterior,[48] and rectus abdominis,[18] compared with the local pedicled muscle flaps, are that they provide greater muscle bulk (filling larger wounds), have longer vascular pedicles (increasing flexibility in muscle positioning), and carry larger-diameter vessels (facilitating the microanastomosis).

TIMING OF FREE TISSUE TRANSFER

The timing of wound closure using microsurgical techniques is important. In severe injuries of the lower extremity with associated soft tissue defects, early aggressive wound debridement and soft tissue coverage with a free flap within 5 days was found to reduce postoperative infection, flap failure, bone nonunion, and chronic osteomyelitis.[19,20] Godina[40] emphasized the pathophysiology of high-energy trauma and the importance of radical debridement and early tissue coverage within the first 72 hours.

Lister and Scheker[76] reported the first case of an emergency free flap transfer to the upper extremity in 1988, and they defined the emergency free flap as a "flap transfer performed either at the end of primary debridement or within 24 hours after the injury." Yaremchuk et al[124] recommended that flaps should be transferred between 7 and 14 days after injury and several debridements. The argument in favor of this approach is that the zone of injury, which often may not be apparent at presentation, can be determined by serial debridements performed in the operating room over several days.

When deciding to perform a primary closure with a free flap, the surgeon should consider two factors: the presence of an exposed vital structure and the risk of infection. A vital structure is defined as "one that will rapidly necrose if not covered by adequate soft tissue."[22] The decision of what constitutes a vital structure depends on circumstances. Tissues such as vessels, nerves, joint surfaces, tendons, and bone denuded of periosteum can lose function and create an environment that results in infection when left exposed for long periods of time. In the decision-making process, the surgeon must consider the risk of leaving the vital structure exposed, its functional importance, and the probability of recovery of function, considering primary or delayed primary coverage.

The risk of infection is the second important factor that should be considered because it can jeopardize the limb, the quality of the functional recovery, or the free flap. As the risk of infection increases, the wisdom of primary closure with a free flap is reduced. Debridement of the wound is the surgeon's most powerful tool to reduce the risk of infection of the wound. If radical debridement is not possible, it is not considered safe to do a primary free flap transfer. Another perspective is that the ability to perform free tissue transfer allows the surgeon increased freedom to perform radical debridement and can actually reduce the risk of infection.[88] Factors such as the mechanism of injury, the elapsed time, and the degree of contamination of the wound should be considered in evaluating the risk of wound infection. In an acute, sharp, noncontaminated injury, when closure would be routinely performed if there were no skin loss, there seems to be little reason not to consider an emergency free flap.

Tissue transplants are selected with regard to donor-site morbidity, recipient-site requirements, vascular pedicle length, and anticipated aesthetic results. For example, a myocutaneous latissimus dorsi flap would not be transplanted to the dorsum of the foot because of its bulk and because the donor tissue does not match the dorsum of the foot. Other flaps, such as an isolated skin flap (radial forearm flap or lateral arm flap), would be considered a better transplant. Similarly, to fill dead space after sequestrectomy of an infected tibia, a lateral arm flap, which is a small skin flap of approximately 5 × 7 cm, would not be selected because of its lack of bulk and because muscle flaps rather than skin flaps are known to be more effective in treatment of osteomyelitis. A skin paddle with composite tissue transfers can be used either for contouring or as a monitor for perfusion of the flap.

The next consideration is whether or not dead space needs to be filled. If a flap was used purely for resurfacing, such as on the dorsum of the foot, so that secondary tendon reconstruction can be performed, a large bulky flap would not be required. However, if there is significant dead space, a large muscle flap, such as a latissimus dorsi flap, should be considered. Osseous flaps are also used for structural defects, such as intercalary bone defects resulting from trauma, tumor, or infection. If a vascularized bone flap is to be selected, the cross section of the bone defect and the available vascular supply both need to be taken into consideration.

Not all flaps are selected to replace missing tissue. In some instances, there is tissue coverage, but it is insufficient in texture or quality. For example, a soft tissue envelope may need to be augmented, such as when using a scapular flap to cover a knee as a last stage before a total ankle replacement in a knee with unstable skin. Some free flap transfers are performed for purely aesthetic reasons, such as the resurfacing of extremities. This is an unusual use of free tissue transfer, and it is only done in special cases. A combination of these selection factors is what determines free flap selection.

SELECTION OF TISSUE FOR TRANSPLANTATION

Latissimus Dorsi

The latissimus dorsi is a workhorse for extremity coverage. This flap is based on the thoracodorsal artery as the major pedicle and on branches of the intercostals and lumbar arteries as secondary segmental branches. The pedicle length is 8 to 10 cm. The latissimus is innervated by the thoracodorsal nerve, which is a direct branch of the brachial plexus and enters the muscle 10 cm from the apex of the axilla. It is important to identify the anterior border of the muscle preoperatively by having the patient contract the muscle with the hand supported on the hip in a standing position. Marking of the posterior superior iliac spine and scapular tip is helpful. It is also wise to measure 10 cm from the apex of the axilla and place a mark at this site of the pedicle entrance into the muscle.

For harvest, the patient is placed in the lateral decubitus position with an axillary roll. Dissection is most easily

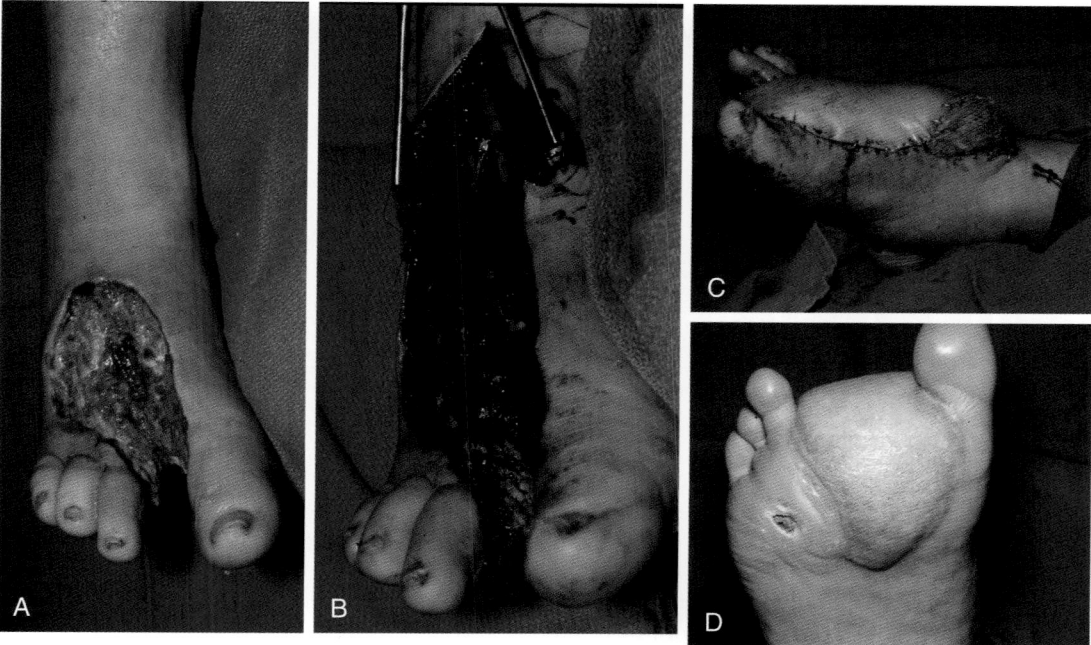

Figure 17-11 A 53-year-old diabetic man with osteomyelitis of the second toe required extensive debridement, including ray deletion (**A** and **B**). The wound was subsequently covered with a latissimus dorsi myocutaneous flap (**C** and **D**).

accomplished beginning from the anterior border of the muscle, and this method allows early pedicle identification. Elevation of the skin flaps exposes the muscle origins, which are then released from the lumbosacral fascia and iliac crest. The large secondary perforating pedicle must be carefully identified and ligated to avoid bleeding. After the pedicle is identified, the serratus branch is divided, and the entire flap is reflected toward the axilla (Fig. 17-11).

Once the flap is reflected toward the axilla and the arm is abducted, the pedicle may easily be seen entering the muscle. Proximal dissection is performed for the previously determined pedicle length, and the muscle insertion is divided. The flap is now ready for transfer. Large suction drains should be left beneath the skin flaps and in the axilla to prevent postoperative hematoma or seroma problems.

Rectus Abdominis

The rectus can be harvested with the patient in a supine position. This vertically oriented muscle extends between the costal margin and the pubic region and is enclosed by the anterior and posterior rectus sheaths. It is a type 3 muscle (two dominant pedicles) based on the superior epigastric artery and vein and inferior epigastric artery and vein. The pedicle length is 5 to 7 cm superiorly and 8 to 10 cm inferiorly.

Each of the dominant pedicles supplies just over half of the muscle. There is an anastomosis between these vessels that is usually sufficient to support the nondominant half if one of the two pedicles is ligated. Because of the larger size and easier dissection of the inferior epigastric vessel, it is usually used for free tissue transfer.

The motor innervation is supplied by segmental motor nerves from the seventh through twelfth intercostal nerves that enter the deep surface of the muscle at its middle to lateral aspects. The lateral cutaneous nerves from the 7th through 12th intercostal nerves provide sensation to the skin territory of the rectus abdominis muscle. The size of the muscle is up to 25 × 6 cm. The skin territory that can be harvested is 21 × 14 cm and is based on musculocutaneous perforators.[85]

Gracilis

The gracilis is a smaller transplant and is useful for defects requiring less bulk than the latissimus or rectus muscles. (Fig. 17-12). The gracilis muscle is a type 2 muscle (dominant pedicle and several minor pedicles). It is a thin, flat muscle that lies between the adductor longus and the sartorius anteriorly and the semimembranosus posteriorly. The dominant pedicle is the ascending branch of the medial circumflex femoral artery and venae comitantes. The length of the pedicle is 6 cm, and the diameter of the artery is 1.6 mm. The minor pedicles are one or two branches of the superficial femoral artery and venae comitantes. Their length is 2 cm, and their diameter is 0.5 mm.[38]

Motor innervation is via the anterior branch of the obturator nerve, which is located between the abductor longus and magnus muscles, and it usually enters the muscle above the level of the dominant vascular pedicle. The anterior femoral cutaneous nerve (L2-3) provides

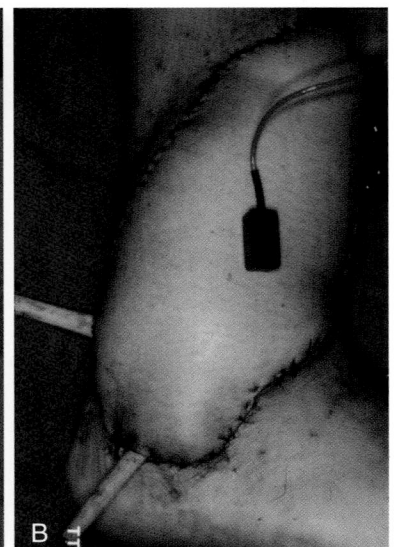

Figure 17-12 **A,** A 56-year-old woman with an open grade II tibia–fibula fracture. **B,** The wound and exposed hardware covered with a free gracilis flap.

sensory innervation to the majority of the anterior medial thigh.

This muscle functions as a thigh adductor. The presence of the adductor longus and magnus makes it an expendable muscle.

The size of the muscle is 6 × 24 cm. The skin territory is 16 × 18 cm, but the skin over the distal half of the muscle is not reliable when the flap is based on its dominant vascular pedicle, with division of the minor vascular pedicles. In obese patients, the musculocutaneous flap may be too bulky, necessitating use of a skin graft placed on the muscle.

Fibula

The free fibula transfer has revolutionized the reconstruction of long-bone defects. The segment of the fibula that can be harvested varies from 20 to 30 cm. There are two types of vascularization to the fibula, provided primarily by the peroneal artery. One source is the nutrient artery, usually unique and branching 6 to 14 cm from the origin of the peroneal artery. The nutrient artery usually enters the bone in its middle third. Periosteal vascularization comes from a series of branches from the peroneal artery and the anterior tibial artery. By isolating the peroneal artery at its origin from the posterior tibial trunk, both medullary and periosteal blood supplies are preserved. The skin on the lateral aspect of the leg gets its blood supply from four to six perforators that originate from the peroneal artery.

The harvesting of the fibula is performed under tourniquet, through a lateral approach in a patient who is supine, prone, or in a lateral position. The line of incision runs between the head of the fibula and the lateral malleolus. At the middle of the line, a point will indicate the approximate location of the nutrient vessel, and this point should be included in the graft. After incision of

the superficial aponeurosis, the dissection is directed straight toward the bone shaft, pushing the peroneal muscles and the superficial peroneal nerve forward and the soleus backward. The bone is reached quickly, and the dissection continues above the periosteum of the fibula. Dissection is continued to the interosseous membrane, which is incised to the level of the flexor hallucis longus in the posterior compartment.

The graft is measured and the bone is sectioned at both ends using a Gigli saw, although the peroneal artery has not yet been properly identified. At least 5 cm of fibula should be left intact distally to maintain ankle stability. The bundle is then located and tied at the distal portion of the graft and the dissection continued toward the peroneal–tibial bifurcation. When the recipient is ready, the pedicle is sectioned just below the bifurcation. Inclusion of the skin flap permits postoperative monitoring and simultaneous reconstruction of moderate soft tissue defects. Skin grafting of the donor site is required if the harvested skin flap is wider than 4 cm. For reconstruction of large bone and soft tissue defects, the fibular flap can be used in combination with other soft tissue flaps, such as the latissimus dorsi (Fig. 17-13).[30]

Medical Geniculate Artery Flap

In recent years, a new bone flap has been introduced for reconstruction of the foot and ankle. Based on the medial geniculate artery system, the medial geniculate artery osteocutaneous flap has become a workhorse for intractable problems of the foot and ankle involving bone and soft tissue deficiency. Traditionally, vascularized bone transfers, such as the iliac crest, the fibula, and the lateral border of the scapula, have been utilized when there is a need for vascularized bone graft. The donor site morbidity of these flaps is not insignificant. For small defects, the medial geniculate artery flap has become the treatment of

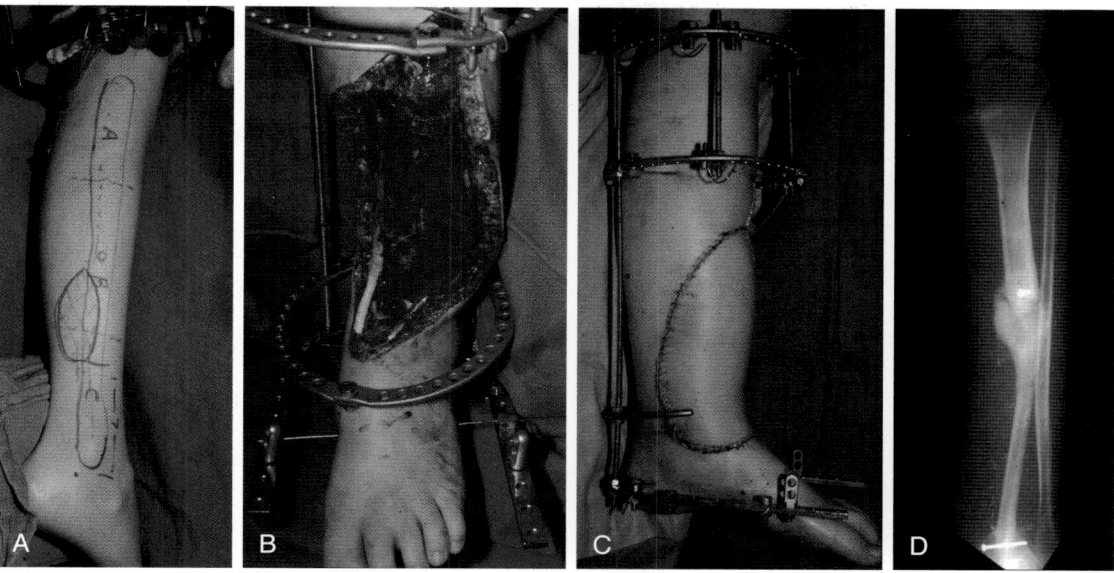

Figure 17-13 **A,** A 25-year-old woman with osteogenic sarcoma. After resection of the tumor **(B),** this patient underwent reconstruction with a vascularized free fibula graft combined with a latissimus dorsi free tissue transfer with ankle arthrodesis **(C** and **D).**

choice. The pathology addressed by this small bone flap, which can deliver cortical cancellous bone, vascularized periosteum and skin for coverage, and, often, contracted and scarred soft tissue envelopes, can be applied to problems such as talar avascular necrosis (AVN), avascular necrosis of the navicular, calcaneal nonunion, and tibial nonunion. Recently, the use of osteoarticular vascularized transfers applied in the carpus can be applied to the tarsus for areas such as cartilage injury with subsequent bone loss. The perforator flap concept can be extended to the perforating vessels that accompany the bone. These can be harvested with standard microsurgical techniques dissection. The pedicle is 8 to 10 cm in length. The vessel diameter is 1.5 to 2 mm of the artery and 2 to 3 mm of the vein. The advantage of this flap is that a long vascular pedicle can be outside the zone of injury for microvascular anastomoses. The dimensions of the bone block are approximately 2 to 3 cm × 3 cm × 3 cm. The donor site morbidity is minimal, and there is the opportunity to take vascularized periosteum to wrap, for example a nonunion of a metatarsal, or apply the periosteum with its cambium layer of pluripotential osteoprogenitor cells.

Radial Forearm Flap

The radial forearm flap is a thin, well-vascularized fasciocutaneous flap on the ventral aspect of the forearm that was widely used in China before it was popularized in the Western literature.[92,111] The flap is based on the radial artery, which can provide a 20-cm pedicle and has a diameter of 2.5 mm. This length of the pedicle facilitates the microsurgical anastomosis out of the zone of injury. The venous drainage is through the venae comitantes of

the radial artery, but the flap can include the cephalic vein, the basilic vein, or both.

The flap can contain the lateral antebrachial cutaneous nerve or the medial antebrachial cutaneous nerve and then serve as a neurosensory flap. The size of the flap can be 10 × 40 cm.

A portion of the radius can be included as a vascularized bone with this flap. The advantages of this flap are a long pedicle and potential sensory innervation. The quality of the bone from the radius is mainly cortical and not of any substantial volume.[113] Including the bone in the radial forearm flap can lead to stress fracture of the donor radius. Preliminary tissue expansion will increase the flap dimensions, and more importantly, it will allow direct closure of the donor defect (Fig. 17-14).[81]

Scapular and Parascapular Flap

The scapular flap is a workhorse of skin flaps. It is a thin, usually hairless flap from the posterior chest and can be de-epithelialized and used as a subcutaneous fascial flap, pedicled or free.

The flap is perfused by the cutaneous branches of the circumflex scapular artery and drained by its venae comitantes. The circumflex scapular artery is the main branch of the subscapular artery and the main blood supply to the scapula, the muscles that attach to the scapula, and the overlying skin. The length of the pedicle is 5 cm, and the diameter of the artery is 2.5 mm. The vascular pattern of this territory makes it possible to raise multiple skin flaps on a single vascular pedicle or to harvest the lateral border of the scapula as an osteocutaneous flap for a complex reconstruction (Fig. 17-15).

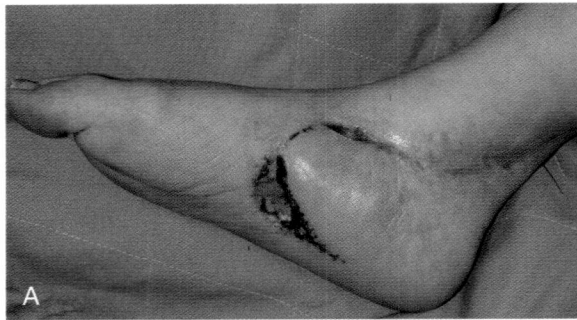
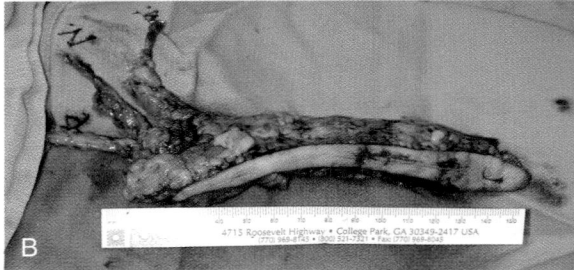
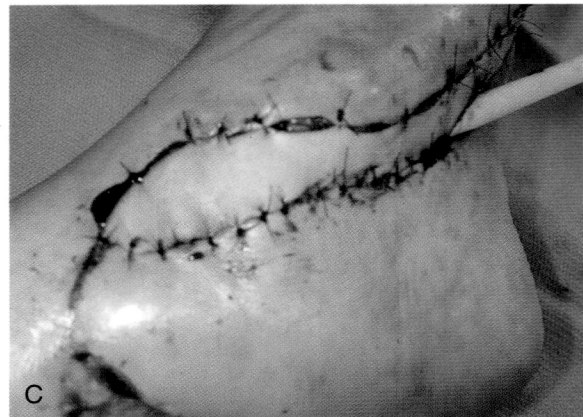

Figure 17-14 This chronic ankle wound **(A)** in a 48-year-old diabetic woman was covered with a radial forearm flap **(B and C)**.

The cutaneous territory can be 20 × 7 cm and can be divided in two components—a horizontal territory (horizontal scapular flap) and a vertical territory (parascapular flap)—based on the branches of the circumflex scapular artery after the vessel courses through the triangular space. Preliminary expansion of the territory of the scapular flap increases the flap dimensions and permits direct donor-site closure. This flap can be combined with other flaps based on subscapular blood supply and can greatly facilitate certain complex reconstructions. These include the latissimus dorsi and serratus anterior flaps, which can supply additional skin, muscle, and bone (rib) if necessary.[32,106,118] The primary indication for the scapular flap is a defect requiring a relatively thin, large cutaneous flap.[11] These kinds of defects are often found in the foot.[104] The osteoseptocutaneous free scapular flap reconstruction has been described in the lower extremity.[110]

Anterolateral Thigh Flap

The anterolateral thigh flap has become the skin flap of choice in patients that have a thin body habitus. It is one of the first perforator flaps to be popularized in the Western world, and it is based on the descending branch of the lateral femoral circumflex system. The flap does not require preoperative arteriogram. The perforators in the septum traverse between the vastus lateralis and rectus femoris are usually through the septum but most often through the rectus femoris muscle. Careful pedicle perforator identification with a Doppler probe before the procedure can help template the flap. In particularly thin patients, this is applicable in areas that require skin flaps traditionally covered by radial forearm flap, free scapular flap, or free groin flap. The anterolateral thigh flap allows for positioning of the patient in the supine position and therefore eliminating the need to position the patient, which is particularly advantageous when the patient must be supine. Vessels are quite large, anywhere from 2 to 3.5 cm for the artery, and up to 4 mm from the vein. A long vascular pedicle can be obtained. The downside of this flap is that often, in some patients, the subcutaneous layers are thick, requiring thinning of the flap, with the exception of where the perforator enters the skin. This flap has become the workhorse skin flap for reconstructive microsurgeons and has tremendous applicability for foot and ankle surgery. The flap can also be taken as a composite with vascularized nerve and muscle.

Recipient Vessels

The proper selection of recipient vessels is essential for the success of free tissue transfer, especially when the transfer is to the lower extremity. However, a general agreement on which vessels to use has not yet been reached. Conflicting data have been reported on the survival and outcome of the transferred flaps, depending on the vessel used or the location of anastomosis proximal or distal to the zone of injury. For example, the anterior tibial vessels may be preferred for their easy accessibility, whereas the posterior tibial vessels are strongly advocated by others.

Park et al[97] tried to develop an algorithm for recipient vessel selection in free tissue transfer to the lower extremity. Based on their experience, the most important factors influencing the site of recipient vessel selection were the site of the injury and the vascular status of the lower extremity. The type of flap used, method, and site of microvascular anastomosis were less important factors in determining the recipient vessels.

INFORMED CONSENT AND MEDICAL AND LEGAL ISSUES

Informed consent for free transfer should include an explanation of the principles of microsurgical tissue transplants as well as the advantages and disadvantages of

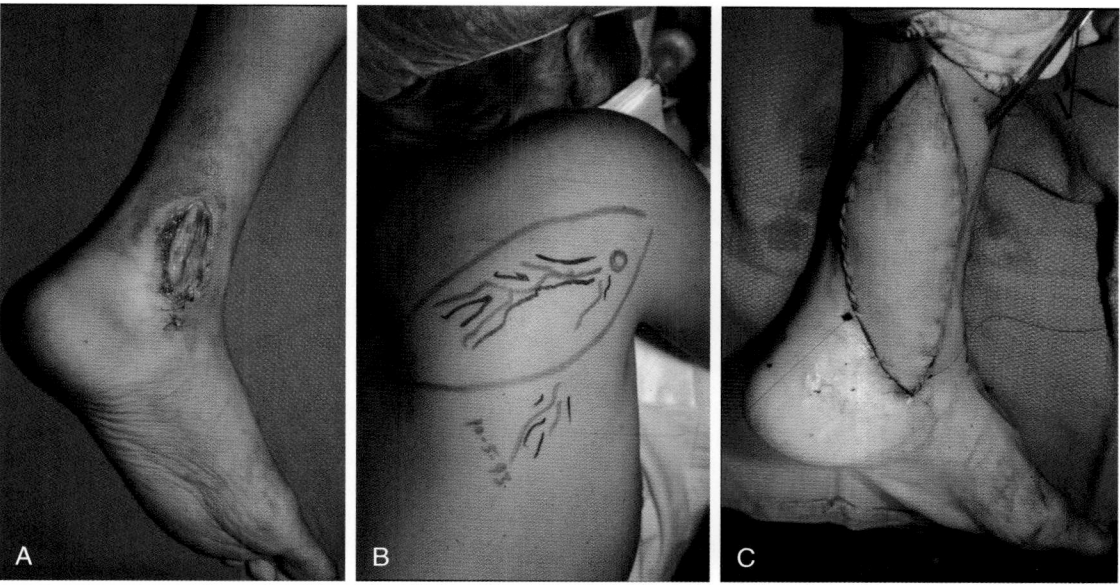

Figure 17-15 **A,** A medial ankle wound in a patient with lupus. A scapular free flap **(B)** was applied to the wound **(C).**

the procedure. The patient should understand the risk of vascular thrombosis, flap failure, loss of limb, and nerve injury. The risks include continued infection, persistent nonunion, and limb loss with or without a successful flap. No guarantees should be given regarding the surgical outcome. The possibility for salvaging a significantly compromised extremity can be offered using microsurgical techniques either with or without a successful free flap. Limb amputation after free tissue transfer may be required for pain, sepsis, or persistent bone instability.

POSTOPERATIVE CARE

Postoperative care of patients undergoing free tissue transfer requires that patients be adequately hydrated. Maintenance of proper body temperature and hematocrit is also important. Routine heparinization and anticoagulation are not used.

Flaps are usually monitored for a minimum of 5 days with an implantable Doppler probe in addition to clinical observation. The immediate postoperative period of 24 to 48 hours is critical, but there have been occasional late failures. Thus Doppler monitoring should be continued for 4 or 5 days.

Extremities should be elevated at all times to augment venous return. Patients with lower extremity flaps are not allowed to ambulate postoperatively for a minimum of 3 weeks. The inosculation and the healing of the flap to the wound bed, the selection of muscle or skin, and the take of the skin graft are factors that go into the timing to determine dependency of the lower extremity.

Patients who have reconstruction around the foot and ankle are most prone to increased venous pressure and resultant edema of the flap. This edema can result in dehiscence of the free flap from the surrounding tissue bed. For this reason, these patients are required to keep their limbs elevated and undergo bed-to-chair transfer for a minimum of 3 weeks. Some experimental data suggest that this period can be shortened. However, it is our experience that this is the amount of time it takes for the flap to mature and develop a sufficient venous return to withstand the hydrostatic pressures associated with standing.

MONITORING

Monitoring of a free tissue transfer is essential to ensure transplant success. Many different monitoring devices and techniques have been used with varying levels of success. As is true in many situations in medicine, the availability of many solutions to a problem suggests that none is superior or ideal.

Ideal flap monitoring should satisfy several criteria. It should be harmless to the patient or the flap, objective, reproducible, applicable to all types of flaps, and inexpensive. It is important that any monitor be capable of prolonged monitoring and respond rapidly to circulatory changes. Postoperative monitoring techniques can be grouped in four categories: clinical evaluation, direct vessel monitoring, indicators of tissue circulation, and metabolic parameters related to perfusion.[17]

Clinical Evaluation

Clinical evaluation remains the gold standard to which all methods of monitoring need to be compared. This involves observation of skin color, temperature, capillary refill, and bleeding characteristics. Clinical observation fulfills many of the criteria of the ideal monitoring system. It is inexpensive, readily available, and can provide a

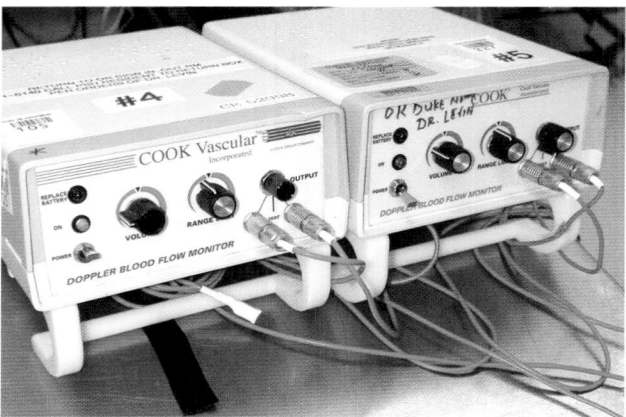

Figure 17-16 Cook Doppler units used to monitor flap circulation.

dynamic picture. The disadvantages include the need for experienced personnel and its use being confined to monitoring surface skin flaps and muscle flaps. Changes are often initially subtle, and by the time they are clinically apparent, salvage of the flap may be impossible because of irreversible tissue damage.

Direct Vessel Monitoring

Direct vessel monitoring can be done by electromagnetic flowmeters. Readings are based on measuring the electric potential induced by blood flow. The ultrasonic Doppler (Fig. 17-16) measures sound waves reflected from columns of moving blood cells. Thermocouples measure the temperature difference between preanastomotic and post-anastomotic sites on the vascular pedicle by using two microthermocouples.

Circulation Monitoring

This category of monitoring is based on measuring the change in the temperature of the skin and using it as an indicator of the blood flow in skin. Photoplethysmography is based on the change in the amount of light reflected during change in the local cutaneous blood volume, and laser Doppler flowmetry is based on the same general principles as ultrasound Doppler but measures the frequency shift of light rather than sound waves reflected from moving red blood cells. Pulse oximetry continuously monitors both pulsatility and oxygen saturation and defines blood flow from these measurements.

Metabolic Monitors

Transcutaneous oxygen monitoring and invasive measurements of PO_2 check the perfusion of tissue transplantations based on metabolic parameters. Levels of tissue oxygen tension have been monitored in flaps and have been shown to reflect the quality of capillary circulation.[1]

Monitoring is usually performed in the intensive care unit setting or a step-down setting, depending on the condition of the patient. Trends of flow can give valuable information about the dynamic perfusion range of blood flow over time. Low absolute values of perfusion, as well as relative changes from the initial flow, are alarming signs, and the flap should be clinically evaluated immediately. We prefer to use the implantable Doppler probe to monitor free flaps. The standard practice in our center is to routinely monitor patients in the intensive care unit for the first 24 hours because this is when the problems most often occur after free tissue transfer.[51]

Flap Failure and Management (Acute)

The success of free tissue transfer should be on the order of 95% to 99%. Acute complications occur usually in the first 48 hours and include venous thrombosis, arterial thrombosis, hematoma, and hemorrhage and excessive flap edema. Arterial insufficiency can be recognized by decreased capillary refill, pallor, reduced temperature, and the absence of bleeding after pinprick. This complication can be caused by arterial spasm, vessel plaque, torsion of the pedicle, pressure on the flap, technical error with injury to the pedicle, a flap that is too large for its blood supply, or small vessel disease (resulting from smoking or diabetes). Management of arterial compromise requires prompt surgical intervention to restore the blood flow.[120] Pharmacologic intervention at the time of exploration includes vasodilators, calcium channel blockers, and systemic anticoagulants for flap salvage manifesting with arterial insufficiency.[96] Ultimately, if these pharmacologic agents do not relieve spasm at the level of the arterial inflow, the anastomosis should be redone to rule out intraarterial thrombus.

Venous outflow obstruction can be suspected when the flap has a violaceous color, brisk capillary refill, normal or elevated temperature, and production of dark blood after pinprick. Venous insufficiency can occur because of torsion of the pedicle, flap edema, hematoma, or tight closure of the tissue over the pedicle. The venous outflow obstruction can result in extravasation of red blood cells, endothelial breakdown, microvascular collapse, thrombosis in the microcirculation, and flap death. Given the irreversible nature of the microcirculatory changes in venous congestion that occurs even after short periods of time, the surgeon must recognize venous compromise as early as possible.

These complications can occur alone or in any combination. The clinical observation and the monitoring of the patient (such as with implantable Doppler) should alert the surgeon, who has to decide between conservative and operative intervention. Conservative treatment may include drainage of the hematoma at the bedside, with release of a few sutures to decrease pressure. In cases of venous congestion, leeches may be helpful if insufficient venous outflow cannot be established despite a patent venous anastomosis (Fig. 17-17). The leeches inject a

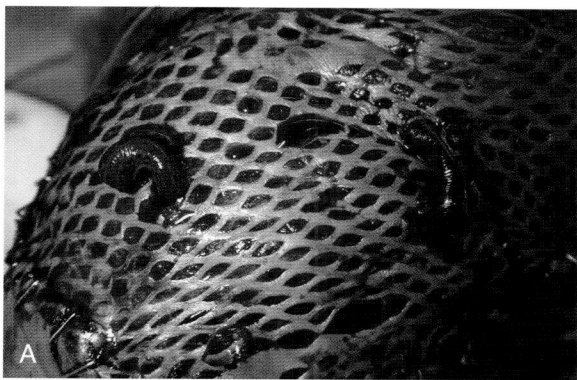
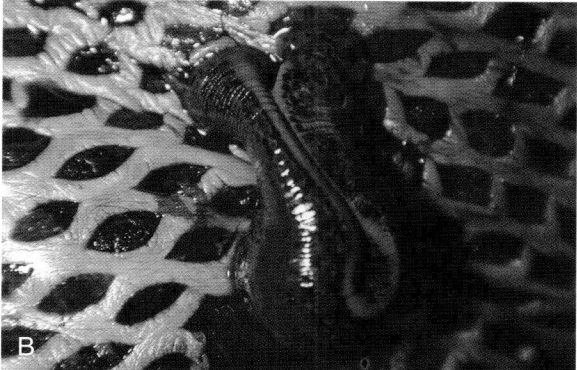

Figure 17-17 Leeches were used to attempt salvage of this free latissimus transfer to the lower extremity with venous obstruction. **A,** General view. **B,** Close-up view.

salivary component (hirudin) that inhibits platelet aggregation and the coagulation cascade. The flap is decongested initially as the leech extracts blood and is further decongested as the bite wound oozes after the leech detaches.[120]

The donor site should be given the same attention as the recipient site during the postoperative period. Complications of the donor site include hematoma, seroma, sensory nerve dysfunction, and scar formation.

Treatment of Failure (Late)

Occasionally, free flaps, despite early return to the operating room for vascular compromise, do fail. Options for management include a second free tissue transfer, noting the technical or physiologic details that led to initial failure. Most of the time, free tissue transfers fail because of technical errors in judgment, including flap harvest, compromise of the pedicle during the harvest, improper microvascular technique during anastomosis, improper insetting resulting in increased tissue tension and edema, or postoperative motion of the extremity resulting in pedicle avulsion. The next decision made by the operating surgeon as to the management of this patient is based on several factors. Obviously, if a patient required a free flap in the first place, a second free flap should be considered. If a decision is made not to redo the flap, it could be left in place based on the so-called Crane principle, in hope

that underlying granulation will be sufficient to allow skin grafting once the necrotic flap is removed.

The Crane principle can be applied in cases of a local flap or free tissue transfer that goes on to partial or total necrosis because the flap acts as a biologic dressing or eschar over a wound bed. If there is no infection, the eschar can be left on the wound bed with hope that some healing in the form of granulation can occur underneath it. Ultimately, the eschar is removed and the granulation bed is skin grafted, obviating the need for another free tissue transfer. If wound observation shows that such a bed is not produced, then a second flap must be considered.[122]

We usually prefer not to follow this course because the flap can become a source of sepsis and further compromise local tissues. Necrotic nonviable flaps should be removed, and a temporary wound dressing, such as a bead pouch or negative pressure dressing, should be used. Occasionally, when flaps fail in a severely compromised extremity, amputation should be considered because the morbidity of a second free tissue transfer, and perhaps the resultant extremity, make amputation a more reasonable choice. If a second free flap is considered, obvious errors that lead to flap compromise need to be recognized. It may be prudent to obtain an arteriogram, evaluate the coagulation profile, and investigate other issues that might have led to failure.

TEAM APPROACH TO EXTREMITY RECONSTRUCTION

Reconstruction is a coordinated effort among orthopaedic surgeons, vascular surgeons, traumatologists, and plastic surgeons. It is not uncommon in practice for an orthopaedic traumatologist to stabilize a fracture, a vascular surgeon to perform an arterial interposition graft, and a microsurgeon to do a free tissue transfer. Communication and careful preoperative planning are important to ensure successful reconstruction. The ability of the reconstructive microsurgeon to deliver the appropriate tissue at the correct time enhances limb salvage.

In instances of bone fracture, the algorithm can be followed with primary hardware placement or external fixator placement, such as an Ilizarov or an AO external fixator. If a bone graft is needed because of missing or devitalized bone, tobramycin beads or silicone spacers can be placed in the bone defect, with subsequent soft tissue coverage. This is then followed by secondary bone grafting with an iliac crest graft, allograft, vascularized graft, intercalary vascularized transplant such as the free fibular graft, or periosteal vascularized flaps.[79]

RECONSTRUCTIVE ALGORITHM BY REGION

Thus far, discussion in this chapter has focused on patient evaluation, immediate wound care, and the hierarchy of the reconstructive ladder, ranging from simple wound closure to composite tissue transplantation. The remainder of the chapter discusses reconstructive options by region.

The soft tissue coverage decision for the foot and ankle can be regionalized. Each anatomic region of the foot has certain characteristics that influence selection of the free tissue transfer for reconstruction. The foot has special requirements for shoeing and ambulation. The reconstructive ladder for injury to the foot is based on whether there is a fracture, what part of the foot is exposed, and whether the area is weight bearing or non–weight bearing. The ankle and the dorsum of the foot require thin, pliable soft tissue coverage for exposed tendons devoid of paratenon and for exposed bones or joints. The weight-bearing surface of the foot (the plantar skin) is unique with respect to its dermal-epidermal characteristics, unique subcutaneous tissue (in the heel pad), adherent dermal septa to the underlying plantar fascia, and ability to withstand constant pressure and shear forces. Coverage that provides protective sensibility can be provided with a free neurosensory flap, such as the radial forearm flap.[24] Free muscle flaps are used when bulk is necessary to obliterate dead space, such as in osteomyelitis; severe crush injuries with extensive soft tissue loss; and weight-bearing surfaces.[87] However, muscle flaps are often bulky and, if not contoured properly, can prevent the use of normal shoes.

The plantar skin has unique properties. It is thick and heavily keratinized, designed to resist high stress, and anchored to underlying bones and ligaments by thick fibrous connective tissue. The plantar surface acts as a shock-absorbing system for the foot, helping to minimize horizontal and vertical shear forces by its multidirectional fibrous septa.[121]

The forefoot includes the dorsal areas of the metatarsals and toes. The plantar aspect includes the metatarsal heads and the instep. The hindfoot can be divided into the plantar surface, instep, and lateral aspect of the calcaneus as the major regions requiring reconstruction. The ankle can be divided into the area of the Achilles tendon and the anterior aspect of the tibiotalar joint. In the forefoot, the dorsum and the area over the toes are primarily skin and subcutaneous tissue, making the exposure of tendons and joints more probable with high-energy injury. The plantar forefoot is prone to avulsion because of the vertically oriented septa that bridge from the plantar fascia to the dermal elements of the skin. The heel pad is a unique structure that contains cushion-like shock-absorbing chambers of fat that are not easily replaced.

Around the hindfoot, coverage is important to avoid scarring around the posterior tibial nerve and exposure or risk to the posterior tibial tendon. The lateral aspect of the hindfoot in the non–weight-bearing portion is often at risk after internal fixation of calcaneal fractures after an extensive lateral approach. In the ankle, the distal anterior tibia has limited subcutaneous tissue and is at risk after total ankle replacement. The skin over the Achilles tendon is also relatively devoid of subcutaneous tissue and often requires augmentation after Achilles tendon repair. It is also important to understand the specialized

skin, subcutaneous, and fat layers in each region because they guide reconstruction.

In a previous publication,[75] we have classified soft tissue reconstruction of the foot into six categories (A1, A2, B1, B2, C, and D). Each category is associated with unique problems.

Group A: Closed Fractures Treated by Open Reduction and Internal Fixation

Group A1: Inability to Close the Skin
In surgical intervention for injuries to the foot, an important factor is soft tissue swelling. Ice, elevation, and a bulky dressing will allow edema to subside, usually within 10 days of the fracture. Although indirect reduction techniques can help, if swelling is not sufficiently decreased, difficulties with wound closure will develop.

Operatively, atraumatic technique, skin hooks (rather than self-retaining retractors), loupe magnification, hemostasis during exposure, drains, and postoperative elevation with soft tissue dressings all contribute to uncomplicated wound healing. When the wound cannot be closed primarily, porcine allograft, Epigard, or split-thickness skin graft can be applied as temporary coverage. Delayed primary closure may be performed if possible.

Group A2: Postoperative Wound Breakdown
Postoperatively, surgical wound breakdown can occur. Partial-thickness defects should be managed initially with conservative measures. These include cessation of exercise, daily whirlpools and dressing changes, elevation, and oral antibiotics. This treatment usually suffices. If a plate or bone is visible, however, or if a full-thickness defect has developed, early aggressive operative soft tissue debridement should be performed.

Subsequent coverage is obtained using local or distal flaps. The decision to use a local flap to cover defects around the foot depends on the presence of acute infection, the depth of the defect, the presence of an adequate vascular supply, and damage to other areas of the foot that preclude the use of local flaps.

Recently, renewed emphasis has been placed on vascular territories (angiosomes or venosomes) that can be used as local rotation or island flaps. Choices for heel reconstruction include the medial pedis flap, dorsal pedis flap, abductor myocutaneous or fasciocutaneous flap, the peroneal flap (Fig. 17-18), supramalleolar flap, and anterior tibial artery fasciocutaneous flaps.[49,50,79,105] Muscle flaps include those from the flexor hallucis brevis or abductor hallucis, which can be rotated to cover small defects about the calcaneus; each of these muscle flaps contains its own vascular supply.

Group B: Requirements for Free Flaps for Foot Reconstruction

Arteriography and, occasionally, venography should be considered before free tissue transfer. This is especially

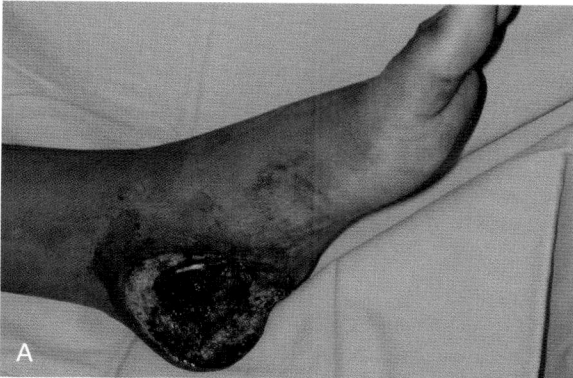

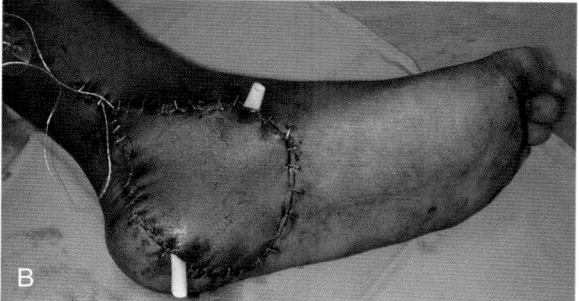

Figure 17-18 This 20-year-old man with metastatic melanoma presented for excision of tumor from the heel **(A)**, followed by reconstruction with an anterolateral thigh flap **(B)**.

important in diabetic patients and elderly patients in whom proximal lesions may preclude inflow in an area of trauma that is already compromised. Flap selection in group B reconstruction is based on need. If cutaneous coverage alone is required, the radial forearm flap provides good coverage.

A long pedicle can be obtained to enable the microsurgeon to perform vessel anastomosis out of the zone of injury, usually end-to-side on the posterior tibial artery. The lateral arm flap may be selected; however, this often produces significant donor-site morbidity. The scapular flap provides cutaneous coverage, but the skin and fat tends to be hypermobile after healing. It has less resistance to tangential shear forces if applied to the plantar surface as compared with muscle flaps. The anterolateral thigh flap in thin patients is an ideal skin flap (see Fig. 17-18).

Group B1: Traumatic Large Soft Tissue Loss with Adequate Bone Stock

Good evidence suggests that early coverage of open fractures is the treatment of choice, provided the wound environment is suitable. The type of soft tissue coverage depends on, and must be tailored to, the underlying reconstruction.

Group B2: Traumatic Loss of Soft Tissue and Bone

When both soft tissue and an osseous defect are present, a careful assessment of appropriate reconstruction must be made. If the injured bone and soft tissue are available and relatively clean, they may be debrided and reattached.

If this is not possible, reconstruction requires a free flap, structural bone block iliac crest graft, and internal fixation. Alternatively, an osteocutaneous free iliac crest, osteonecrosis or medial geniculate artery osteocutaneous flap could be considered. Careful consideration must be given to a below-knee amputation, because this might ultimately be the fastest and most efficient means of restoring function to the patient.

Group C: Osteomyelitis

Osteomyelitis of the foot usually occurs late and is commonly accompanied by marginal soft tissue overlying implants or bone.[75] Inflamed, reactive soft tissue cannot be used to close defects if a sequestrectomy is performed. Therefore distant muscle flaps should be strongly considered. Muscle flaps have been shown clinically and experimentally to aid in controlling (not curing) osteomyelitis. Studies by Cierny and Mader[26] have shown in the A host (no systemic illnesses) and B host (systemic illnesses, such as vascular disease, diabetes, history of smoking, or poor nutrition) that osteomyelitis can be controlled using free muscle flaps.

Group D: Reconstruction for Unstable Soft Tissue

Problems associated with reconstruction of the heel pad because of the lack of soft tissue support can require orthotic devices or bracing. These patients often require augmentation of unstable tissue with local or distant flaps. Although the goal of the surgeon is to replace "like with like," this is virtually impossible in heel pad reconstruction.

Patients receiving noninnervated flaps for soft tissue reconstruction of the heel must be treated in a fashion similar to patients with peripheral neuropathy. Education must be directed toward informing the patient that the foot, although restored and functional, is not normal. The patient must inspect the foot for callosities and irritations. Because of the increased mobility of flaps, particularly skin flaps, a variety of interface problems can occur, either on the flap or at the flap–skin junction. The inability to provide full sensation does not, however, preclude soft tissue reconstruction about the heel because most patients obtain some degree of proprioceptive feedback and deep sensibility from the underlying muscle, periosteum, and surrounding skin.

TRAUMA AND THE DYSVASCULAR AND DIABETIC FOOT

Nonhealing wounds of the extremities are common in patients with diabetes and peripheral vascular disease. The problem is significant, with statistics indicating that 14% of patients are hospitalized an average of 6 weeks per year for foot problems, and more than 80% of amputations are in diabetic patients. Even the contralateral limb is at risk in these patients, and there is a 50% chance of loss of the contralateral leg within 5 years.[45]

The approach to these patients involves a close collaborative effort among the orthopaedist, the peripheral vascular surgical team, and the microsurgical team to optimize the ability to obtain a rapid and accurate diagnosis and assessment of the vascular problem, the most appropriate and timely plan for wound care, and the most reliable revascularization. The results for macrovascular and microvascular anastomoses are comparable to those in nondiabetic patients undergoing the similar procedure.[72]

Diabetic patients are at risk for a high incidence of reoperation. Diabetic patients treated with cutaneous free flaps have a lower morbidity than those patients treated with muscle free flaps.[95] The cutaneous radial forearm free flap is an excellent way to treat relatively small wounds of the foot because it provides tissue with a lengthy vascular pedicle and a donor site that can often be closed primarily.

Despite the underlying medical problems in these patients, mortality is not found to be higher in cases of microsurgery reconstruction procedures done either alone or in combination with vascular reconstruction.[15] The trend today is that once the extremity has been revascularized, the most appropriate method of reconstruction can be carried out for defects of the foot. For these patients in whom the macrovascular blood supply is intact and have large, colonized wounds involving major soft tissue or bone, infection free flap coverage may be indicated. Free tissue transfer techniques are ideal in these situations because they are able to resurface any size defect; they allow aggressive resection of the wound to get rid of colonized, fibrotic, unhealthy tissue; the flap actually helps revascularize the defect; and the defect is replaced with healthy, undamaged tissue.

Diabetic and dysvascular patients require a high degree of vigilance to avoid problems both locally and systemically, with a much closer observation of the donor sites and recipient sites to prevent a higher rate of wound healing problems. Because many diabetic and dysvascular patients receiving a free flap were candidates for amputation before flap transfer (which was often offered as a last option before limb loss), these procedures do not increase the rate of limb loss but can only increase the rate of limb salvage.

It is important to analyze the result of lower extremity limb salvage as it relates to ambulatory function. Salvage of a nonuseful limb in such patients is of little value in their overall management. Likewise, heroic attempts at salvaging a limb are not indicated if the operation puts excessive stress on the patient (such as the patient with cardiovascular disease). The question of the cost-to-benefit ratio of such procedures has yet to be determined. Certainly, in this era of cost containment, the arguments against such expensive and sophisticated procedures versus straightforward amputation cannot be ignored. Although the exact cost of leg salvage in such a group of patients is difficult to determine, it may be less expensive than the combined cost of hospitalization, prosthesis fitting, rehabilitation, and disability payments.

A high degree of success can be achieved only by extremely careful patient selection. In the face of systemic difficulties, one must also exercise proper judgment and be prepared to abort attempted reconstruction to assure patient survival.

AESTHETIC CONSIDERATIONS AFTER LIMB TRAUMA

Foot appearance as well as function is important in foot and ankle surgery. Scar quality and limb contour are important considerations. A favorable scar should be a fine line and situated against a wrinkle, contour junction, or skin tension line. It should have no contour irregularities or pigmentation abnormalities and should not cause distortion or contracture. Scars can be revised or otherwise treated to improve direction, decrease their apparent length, correct distortion of anatomic units, improve surface irregularities, and correct pigment irregularities.

Hypertrophic scars and keloids constitute the unfavorable end of the scar spectrum but must be differentiated to be treated appropriately. Both demonstrate increased collagen deposition (mainly types I and III) during the fibroblastic portion of the proliferative phase of wound healing (5 days to 3 weeks).[99]

Keloids are found predominantly in black patients and, by definition, extend beyond skin wound margins. They may behave quite invasively after the most innocuous skin trauma; a mosquito bite with scratching of the skin is an example. They are familial and exhibit an autosomal dominant pattern of inheritance. Keloids may be located on any part of the body and occur in all age groups except newborns. The hallmarks of this process are greatly increased dermal collagen content, increased collagen synthesis, and decreased collagen degradation.[27] Skin levels of the degradative enzyme collagenase are higher in keloids than normal skin, normal scars, or hypertrophic scars, and they are likely blocked by α_2-macroglobulin.[29] There appears to be a poorly defined immunologic component as well, and greatly increased dermal immunoglobulin levels are measured in keloids.[28]

Hypertrophic scars are raised and, although initially quite dramatic in color and appearance, tend to regress gradually. They remain within the boundaries of the primary incision or wound and are typified by the hypertrophic burn scar. They are formed at the margins of skin grafts and in deep second- and third-degree burns that are allowed to heal by second intention. Among the reasons for unfavorable scar formation are location, tension, patient characteristics, and wound-closure techniques.

Tension across incisions or wounds is to be avoided whenever possible because it often leads to widened, prominent scars. Significant tissue loss from trauma or debridement should raise the possibility of the need for skin grafting, undermining, or flap application. Temporary use of a biologic dressing, such as porcine allograft, can allow delayed primary closure of an edematous, overly tight wound, such as an extremity fasciotomy wound.

Patient characteristics, such as age, race, skin quality, and pigmentation, also exert an influence on scar quality. Age younger than 25 years, heavily pigmented skin in any ethnic group, and thick skin predispose to unfavorable scars. Patients can serve as self-controls because the quality of previous mature scars is often readily apparent and can serve as a guide to scar outcome.

The fundamentals of good wound-closure technique remain true and should contribute to a favorable result. Wounds should be free of foreign material and necrotic tissue, closed as soon as possible after wounding, and handled with care. Skin margins should be excised when necrotic and handled with skin hooks or toothed forceps only at the dermal level. Tension should be minimized by judicious undermining if needed or by flaps, skin grafts, or delayed closure. Wound edges require accurate approximation, and closure should be in layers with eversion, using any one of a number of suture techniques. A subcuticular pull-out suture of monofilament may be considered for epidermal approximation. Whether sutures or staples are used is of less importance than having no tension at the epidermal level. Skin tension should be such that staples or sutures may be removed at 6 to 9 days and replaced by skin-closure tapes, such as Steri-Strips. Skin sutures are best tied slightly loosely rather than tightly because postoperative edema almost guarantees skin necrosis with an overly tight closure.

The postoperative treatment of new scars includes early suture removal, massage, avoiding sun exposure, and edema control. Massage reduces wound edema mechanically, can soften wound fibrosis, and helps to desensitize cutaneous reinnervation. Sun exposure after wounding causes scar hyperpigmentation for at least 6 months and should be avoided. Heavy sun block may be used if sun avoidance is impossible. Early limb edema control by elevation, limitation of dependency, and judicious use of self-adhesive wraps, such as Coban (3M, St. Paul, Minn.) is critical to minimizing wound tension and scar quality. Suture or staple removal as early as possible prevents suture tracts and improves scar quality. Skin sutures should not be used to provide wound edge approximation; dermal sutures serve this function.

Silicone sheet application to scars for up to 12 weeks provide improvement among patients with known keloid or hypertrophic scar diathesis or in unfavorable wounds, such as ungrafted superficial second-degree burns. In some cases, the improvement even in several-week-old wounds is quite dramatic. This modality is convenient, well tolerated, inexpensive, and painless.

Intralesional corticosteroid injections may also be indicated for patients with known scar diathesis. An agent such as triamcinolone at a 40 mg/mL concentration, with no more than 80 mg given in each 6-week period, often blunts the degree of collagen overdeposition seen in these patients. It inhibits the lysyl and prolyl hydroxylase necessary for collagen synthesis. The effects of steroids are reversible by vitamin A. Steroids also decrease fibroblast migration and increase collagenase activity by decreasing α_2-macroglobulin deposition.[119] This wound modulator should be used with caution because it can cause skin atrophy. It is contraindicated in pregnant patients and in patients with peptic ulcer disease.

Options for treatment of the unfavorable scar include revision and dermabrasion. Revision comprises simple excision, breakup of a long scar, and staging. The principles remain constant. Timing of revision is critical and must await scar maturation. Typically, this is 6 to 12 months in adults and up to 24 months in children. The scar's red or pink quality must fade to white. This assumes that the original wound was traumatic or closed under less-than-ideal circumstances. Scar revision may be performed earlier, weeks to months after injury, if the scar is situated perpendicular to the relaxed skin lines; a primary closure such as this will never be of good quality, regardless of the degree of maturation.[13] If a well-planned incision made by a careful surgeon in an anatomically favorable area is closed using appropriate techniques but has left an unsatisfactory scar, one should consider whether it is likely to improve with revision.

In revision, the new scar should be situated to fall within existing wrinkle or skin line complexes. A scar immediately adjacent to and parallel to a wrinkle avoids scar retraction and furrowing. Of fundamental importance is that tension be minimized. When undermining is done, the subdermal vascular supply must be preserved.

Dog-ears may be excised in a straight-line extension of the original wound. A buried dermal flap technique in which the existing scar is de-epithelialized and used for fill helps minimize scar depression. Z-plasty techniques help to correct scar contracture across joints or in areas where anatomic units are distorted.[13] The flaps must be generous for this application; they may be smaller when used to break up a long scar's vertical appearance where no distortion is present. W-plasty techniques may be used to improve scar orientation and appearance when it lies perpendicular to the relaxed skin lines. Local flaps or free flaps may be required when poor scar or soft tissue quality (especially after significant tissue loss or multiple reoperations) contributes to problems with rehabilitation or function. Full-thickness skin grafts, usually taken from the groin, may be used when attempts at revision result in gaping, tight wounds. These may be de-epithelialized and overgrafted at a later date for additional thickness. Scar massage, edema control, steroid injection, and silicone sheeting may be useful adjuncts to revision.

In patients with keloids, we have found low-dose radiation to be of benefit in conjunction with scar revision. The keloid is excised immediately within the border of the lesion, closed without tension using subcuticular sutures after dermal approximation, and injected with triamcinolone as described above. The radiation

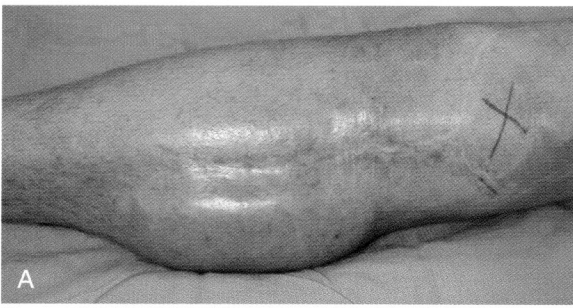
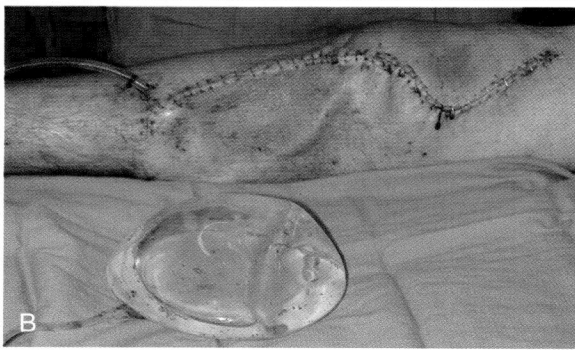

Figure 17-19 Tissue expansion in the lower extremity for scar management. **A,** With tissue expander. **B,** After removal of tissue expander.

treatment is carried out in 200-rad increments daily for 5 days and is ideally begun on the day of surgery.

Tissue expansion may be very helpful in scar management because it allows revision of large scars (Fig. 17-19) in a rapid, two-stage fashion. The expander is placed in the subcutaneous space and sequentially filled with saline, and the expanded skin is used to replace the excised scar.[103] The skin may be reexpanded as necessary. Investigation has shown[23] that large numbers of new blood vessels are formed, and mitotic activity is increased in the expanded tissue. Expansion has been used with success in extremities for trauma, tumor, congenital, and irradiation wound applications.[89] The pseudocapsule formed by expansion may be of use as a gliding surface for muscle, nerve, or tendon in the reconstructed limb. Incisions must be thoughtfully planned for later expander removal and flap advancement. Expansion must be carefully performed to avoid extrusion through old scars, exposure of an underlying prosthesis, or puncture by an implant. Filling ports are usually placed at a distance. Rare complications include transient neurapraxia after expansion and implant failure.

Dermabrasion is valuable for treating raised or irregularly contoured scars. It may be used to level high points, but it is contraindicated for depressed scars or for those in which the wound edges are stepped as a result of poor wound-closure technique. The latter wounds should be revised surgically. Dermabrasion can lead to depigmentation, and patients must be warned about this.

Finally, free tissue transfer may be used. This approach is highly unusual, but an unsightly scar can have such a bad psychologic effect that the patient wants to undergo such reconstruction. Careful selection of the flap as well as consideration of donor-scar management can result in a satisfactory aesthetic result. Tissue expanders can help by decreasing donor-site morbidity, as well as the need for debulking of flaps, which can result in an improved cosmetic result.[25]

TISSUE EXPANSION

Soft tissue expansion enjoys wide use by reconstructive plastic surgeons around the world and has been used successfully for reconstructing deformities and for removing lesions of the extremities.[6,9,78,98] Soft tissue expansion is best applied in delayed reconstruction, as well as for expansion of free flaps to be used in soft tissue reconstruction of the limbs to lower the morbidity of the donor site.[90] This technique requires adequate soft tissue for expansion, and if only skin is expanded, it should have a thickness and subcutaneous fat that will allow maintenance or restoration of contour at the site of reconstruction.

Sites such as the ankle and the foot can be suitable for tissue expansion, but expansion is difficult to use in the foot. There is a high incidence of periexpander infection if the expander is placed next to an open wound in the lower extremity. Judgment is required in all cases in deciding whether a particular patient is a good candidate for soft tissue expansion.

In the extremities, it is preferable to plan a transverse advancement of tissue instead of an axial advancement.[10] The expander should be located just above the muscle fascia. Expansion begins usually 1 to 2 weeks after implantation, is increased once a week, and is continued until the circumference of the extremity has increased by an amount equal to the width of the defect. Complications of soft tissue expansion include infection, dehiscence, seroma, dislocation of the expander, and leakage. One of the most common causes for exposure of an implant is an inadequately dissected pocket. If the pocket is small, the edge of the expander can push against the healing incision and cause a dehiscence.

The advantages of soft tissue expanders are that coverage is provided by tissue similar to the tissue that was lost, their use is cost-effective, and the procedure may be conducted on an outpatient basis. Newer techniques, such as minimally invasive placement using a balloon dissector and expanders placed through a remote access incision, can reduce the delay required for incision healing, minimize complications, and increase the amount of flap gain.[71]

REFERENCES

1. Achauer BM, Black KS, Litke DK: Transcutaneous P_{O_2} in flaps: a new method of survival prediction, *Plast Reconstr Surg* 65:738–745, 1980.
2. Adams F: *The genuine works of Hippocrates*, New York, 1891, Williams Wood.

3. Aldea PA, Shaw WW: The evolution of the surgical management of severe lower extremity trauma, *Clin Plast Surg* 13:549–569, 1986.

4. Anthony JP, Mathes SJ, Alpert BS: The muscle flap in the treatment of chronic lower extremity osteomyelitis: results in patients over 5 years after treatment, *Plast Reconstr Surg* 88:311–318, 1991.

5. Antonyshyn O, Gruss JS, Mackinnon SE, et al: Complications of soft tissue expansion, *Br J Plast Surg* 41:239–250, 1988.

6. Argenta LC, Morykwas MJ: Vacuum-assisted closure: a new method for wound control and treatment: clinical experience, *Ann Plast Surg* 38:563–576; discussion 577, 1997.

7. Arnez ZM: Immediate reconstruction of the lower extremity—an update, *Clin Plast Surg* 18:449–457, 1991.

8. Austad ED: Evolution of the concept of tissue expansion, *Fac Plast Surg* 5:277–279, 1988.

9. Ayyappan T, Chadha A: Super sural neurofasciocutaneous flaps in acute traumatic heel reconstructions, *Plast Reconstr Surg* 109:2307–2313, 2002.

10. Barfod B, Pers M: Gastrocnemius-plasty for primary closure of compound injuries of the knee, *J Bone Joint Surg Br* 52:124–127, 1970.

11. Barwick WJ, Goodkind DJ, Serafin D: The free scapular flap, *Plast Reconstr Surg* 69:779–787, 1982.

12. Bonatz E, Alonso JE: Classification of soft tissue injuries, *Tech Orthop* 10:73–78, 1995.

13. Borges AF: Timing of scar revision techniques, *Clin Plast Surg* 17:71–76, 1990.

14. Bostwick JD, Nahai F, Wallace JG, et al: Sixty latissimus dorsi flaps, *Plast Reconstr Surg* 63:31–41, 1979.

15. Briggs SE, Banis JC Jr, Kaebnick H, et al: Distal revascularization and microvascular free tissue transfer: an alternative to amputation in ischemic lesions of the lower extremity, *J Vasc Surg* 2:806–811, 1985.

16. Buncke CM, Schultz WB: Experimental digital amputation and replantation, *Plast Reconstr Surg* 36:62, 1965.

17. Bunke H: *Monitoring in microsurgery: transplantation–replantation*, Philadelphia, 1991, Lea & Febiger.

18. Bunkis J, Walton RL, Mathes SJ: The rectus abdominis free flap for lower extremity reconstruction, *Ann Plast Surg* 11:373–380, 1983.

19. Byrd HS, Cierny G 3rd, Tebbetts JB: The management of open tibial fractures with associated soft tissue loss: external pin fixation with early flap coverage, *Plast Reconstr Surg* 68:73–82, 1981.

20. Byrd HS, Spicer TE, Cierney GD: Management of open tibial fractures, *Plast Reconstr Surg* 76:719–730, 1985.

21. Caudle RJ, Stern PJ: Severe open fractures of the tibia, *J Bone Joint Surg Am* 69:801–807, 1987.

22. Chen S, Tsai YC, Wei FC, et al: Emergency free flaps to the type IIIC tibial fracture, *Ann Plast Surg* 25:223–229, 1990.

23. Cherry GW, Austad E, Pasyk K, et al: Increased survival and vascularity of random-pattern skin flaps elevated in controlled, expanded skin, *Plast Reconstr Surg* 72:680–687, 1983.

24. Chicarilli ZN, Price GJ: Complete plantar foot coverage with the free neurosensory radial forearm flap, *Plast Reconstr Surg* 78:94–101, 1986.

25. Chowdary RP, Murphy RX: Delayed debulking of free muscle flaps for aesthetic contouring debulking of free muscle flaps, *Br J Plast Surg* 45:38–41, 1992.

26. Cierny G 3rd, Mader JT: Approach to adult osteomyelitis, *Orthop Rev* 16:259–270, 1987.

27. Cohen IK, Diegelmann RF, Johnson ML: Effect of corticosteroids on collagen synthesis, *Surgery* 82:15–20, 1977.

28. Cohen IK, McCoy BJ, Mohanakumar T, et al: Immunoglobulin, complement, and histocompatibility antigen studies in keloid patients, *Plast Reconstr Surg* 63:689–695, 1979.

29. Diegelmann RF, Bryant CP, Cohen IK: Tissue alpha-globulins in keloid formation, *Plast Reconstr Surg* 59:418–423, 1977.

30. Donski PK, Buchler U, Ganz R: Combined osteocutaneous microvascular flap procedure for extensive bone and soft tissue defects in the tibia, *Ann Plast Surg* 16:386–398, 1986.

31. Donski PK, Fogdestam I: Distally based fased fasciocutaneous flap from the sural region: a preliminary report, *Scand J Plast Reconstr Surg* 17:191–196, 1983.

32. dos Santos LF: The vascular anatomy and dissection of the free scapular flap, *Plast Reconstr Surg* 73:599–604, 1984.

33. Eshima I, Mathes SJ, Paty P: Comparison of the intracellular bacterial killing activity of leukocytes in musculocutaneous and random-pattern flaps, *Plast Reconstr Surg* 86:541–547, 1990.

34. Esterhai JL Jr, Queenan J: Management of soft tissue wounds associated with type III open fractures, *Orthop Clin North Am* 22:427–432, 1991.

35. Feldman DL: Which dressing for split-thickness skin graft donor sites [see comments]? *Ann Plast Surg* 27:288–291, 1991.

36. Fischer MD, Gustilo RB, Varecka TF: The timing of flap coverage, bone-grafting, and intramedullary nailing in patients who have a fracture of the tibial shaft with extensive soft tissue injury, *J Bone Joint Surg Am* 73:1316–1322, 1991.

37. Follmar KE, Baccarani A, Baumeister S, et al: The distally based sural flap, *Plast Reconstr Surg* 119:138e–148e, 2007.

38. Giordano PA, Abbes M, Pequignot JP: Gracilis blood supply: anatomical and clinical re-evaluation, *Br J Plast Surg* 43:266–272, 1990.

39. Godina M: *A thesis on the management of injuries to the lower extremity*, Ljubljana, Slovenia, 1991, Presernova Druzba.

40. Godina M: Early microsurgical reconstruction of complex trauma of the extremities, *Plast Reconstr Surg* 78:285–292, 1986.

41. Goldberg JA, Alpert BS, Lineaweaver WC, et al: Microvascular reconstruction of the lower extremity in the elderly, *Clin Plast Surg* 18:459–465, 1991.

42. Grim PS, Gottlieb LJ, Boddie A, et al: Hyperbaric oxygen therapy [see comments], *JAMA* 263:2216–2220, 1990.

43. Gustilo RB, Anderson JT: Prevention of infection in the treatment of one thousand and twenty-five open fractures of long bones: retrospective and prospective analyses, *J Bone Joint Surg Am* 58:453–458, 1976.

44. Gustilo RB, Mendoza RM, Williams DN: Problems in the management of type III (severe) open fractures: a new classification of type III open fractures, *J Trauma* 24:742–746, 1984.

45. Gutman M, Kaplan O, Skornick Y, et al: Gangrene of the lower limbs in diabetic patients: a malignant complication, *Am J Surg* 154:305–308, 1987.

46. Hansen S: The evolution of musculoskeletal traumatology at Harborview Medical Center. In Hansen S, Swiontkowski M, editors: *Orthopaedic trauma protocols*, New York, 1993, Raven Press, pp 3–8.

47. Hansen ST Jr: The type-IIIC tibial fracture. Salvage or amputation [editorial], *J Bone Joint Surg Am* 69:799–800, 1987.

48. Harii K, Yamada A, Ishihara K, et al: A free transfer of both latissimus dorsi and serratus anterior flaps with thoracodorsal vessel anastomoses, *Plast Reconstr Surg* 70:620–629, 1982.

49. Harrison DH, Morgan BD: The instep island flap to resurface plantar defects, *Br J Plast Surg* 34:315–318, 1981.

50. Hartrampf CR Jr, Scheflan M, Bostwick JD: The flexor digitorum brevis muscle island pedicle flap: a new dimension in heel reconstruction, *Plast Reconstr Surg* 66:264–270, 1980.

51. Heller L, Levin LS, Klitzman B: Laser Doppler flowmeter monitoring of free tissue transfers: blood flow in normal and complicated cases, *Plast Reconstr Surg* 107:1739–1745, 2001.

52. Henry SL, Ostermann PA, Seligson D: The antibiotic bead pouch technique. The management of severe compound fractures, *Clin Orthop Relat Res* 295:54–62, 1993.

53. Henry SL, Ostermann PA, Seligson D: The prophylactic use of antibiotic impregnated beads in open fractures, *J Trauma Injury Infect Crit Care* 30:1231–1238, 1990.

54. Henry SL, Popham GJ, Mangino P, et al: Antibiotic impregnated beads: a production technique, *Contemp Orthop* 19:221–226, 1989.

55. Henry SL, Seligson D, Mangino P, et al: Antibiotic-impregnated beads. Part I: bead implantation versus systemic therapy, *Orthop Rev* 20:242–247, 1991.

56. Hertel R, Lambert SM, Muller S, et al: On the timing of soft tissue reconstruction for open fractures of the lower leg, *Arch Orthop Trauma Surg* 119:7–12, 1999.

57. Howard M, Court-Brown CM: Epidemiology and management of open fractures of the lower limb, *Br J Hosp Med* 57:582–587, 1997.

58. Howe HR Jr, Poole GV Jr, Hansen KJ, et al: Salvage of lower extremities following combined orthopedic and vascular trauma. A predictive salvage index, *Am Surg* 53:205–208, 1987.

59. Hunt TK, Zederfeldt B, Goldstick TK: Oxygen and healing, *Am J Surg* 118:521–525, 1969.

60. Irons GB, Fisher J, Schmitt EHD: Vascularized muscular and musculocutaneous flaps for management of osteomyelitis, *Orthop Clin North Am* 15:473–480, 1984.

61. Irons GB Jr, Wood MB: Soft tissue coverage for the treatment of osteomyelitis of the lower part of the leg, *Mayo Clin Proc* 61:382–387, 1986.

62. Isenberg JS, Sherman R: Zone of injury: a valid concept in microvascular reconstruction of the traumatized lower limb? *Ann Plast Surg* 36:270–272, 1996.

63. Jacobson JH, Suarez SE: Microsurgery and anastomosis of small vessels, *Surg Forum* 11:243–247, 1960.

64. Janzekovic Z: Early surgical treatment of the burned surface, *Panminerva Med* 14:228–232, 1972.

65. Kelton P: Skin grafts, *Sel Read Plast Surg* 7:1–20, 1992.

66. Kindwall EP, Gottlieb LJ, Larson DL: Hyperbaric oxygen therapy in plastic surgery: a review article, *Plast Reconstr Surg* 88:898–908, 1991.

67. Kleinert HE, Kasdan ML, Romero JL: Small blood-vessel anastomosis for salvage of severely injured upper extremity, *J Bone Joint Surg Am* 45:788–796, 1963.

68. Kocher MS: Early limb salvage: open tibia fractures of Ambroise Paré (1510-1590) and Percivall Pott (1714-1789), *World J Surg* 21:116–122, 1997.

69. Krettek C, Haas N, Schandelmaier P, et al: [Unreamed tibial nail in tibial shaft fractures with severe soft tissue damage. Initial clinical experiences], *Unfallchirurg* 94:579–587, 1991.

70. Le Huec JC, Midy D, Chauveaux D, et al: Anatomic basis of the sural fasciocutaneous flap: Surgical applications, *Surg Radiol Anat* 10:5–13, 1988.

71. Levin LS, Rehnke R, Eubanks S: Endoscopic surgery of the upper extremity, *Hand Clin* 11:59–70, 1995.

72. Lai CS, Lin SD, Yang CC, et al: Limb salvage of infected diabetic foot ulcers with microsurgical free-muscle transfer, *Ann Plast Surg* 26:212–220, 1991.

73. Lange RH: Limb reconstruction versus amputation decision making in massive lower extremity trauma, *Clin Orthop Relat Res* 243:92–99, 1989.

74. Lange RH, Bach AW, Hansen ST Jr, et al: Open tibial fractures with associated vascular injuries: prognosis for limb salvage, *J Trauma* 25:203–208, 1985.

75. Levin LS, Nunley JA: The management of soft tissue problems associated with calcaneal fractures, *Clin Orthop Relat Res* 290:151–156, 1993.

76. Lister G, Scheker L: Emergency free flaps to the upper extremity, *J Hand Surg Am* 13:22–28, 1988.

77. MacKenzie EJ, Bosse MJ, Pollack AN, et al: Long-term persistence of disability following severe lower limb trauma: results of a seven-year follow-up, *J Bone Joint Surg Am* 87:1801–1809, 2005.

78. Manders EK, Oaks TE, Au VK, et al: Soft tissue expansion in the lower extremities, *Plast Reconstr Surg* 81:208–219, 1988.

79. Masquelet AC, Beveridge J, Romana C, et al: The lateral supramalleolar flap, *Plast Reconstr Surg* 81:74–81, 1988.

80. Masquelet AC, Romana MC, Wolf G: Skin island flaps supplied by the vascular axis of the sensitive superficial nerves: anatomic study and clinical experience, *Plast Reconstr Surg* 89:1115–1121, 1992.

81. Masser MR: The preexpanded radial free flap [see comments], *Plast Reconstr Surg* 86:295–301, discussion 302–303, 1990.

82. Mathes SJ, Alpert BS, Chang N: Use of the muscle flap in chronic osteomyelitis: experimental and clinical correlation, *Plast Reconstr Surg* 69:815–829, 1982.

83. Mathes SJ, Feng LJ, Hunt TK: Coverage of the infected wound, *Ann Surg* 198:420–429, 1983.

84. Mathes SJ, Nahai F: Classification of the vascular anatomy of muscles: experimental and clinical correlation, *Plast Reconstr Surg* 67:177–187, 1981.

85. Mathes SJ, Nahai F: *Reconstructive surgery: principles, anatomy, and techniques*, New York, 1997, Churchill Livingstone.

86. May JW Jr, Jupiter JB, Weiland AJ, et al: Clinical classification of post-traumatic tibial osteomyelitis, *J Bone Joint Surg Am* 71:1422–1428, 1989.

87. May JW Jr, Rohrich RJ: Foot reconstruction using free microvascular muscle flaps with skin grafts, *Clin Plast Surg* 13:681–689, 1986.

88. McCabe SJ, Breidenbach WC: The role of emergency free flaps for hand trauma, *Hand Clin* 15:275–288, viii-ix, 1999.

89. Meland NB, Loessin SJ, Thimsen D, et al: Tissue expansion in the extremities using external reservoirs, *Ann Plast Surg* 29:36–39, discussion 40, 1992.

90. Moghari A, Emami A, Sheen R, et al: Lower limb reconstruction in children using expanded free flaps, *Br J Plast Surg* 42:649–652, 1989.

91. Morykwas MJ, Argenta LC: Nonsurgical modalities to enhance healing and care of soft tissue wounds, *J South Orthop Assoc* 6:279–288, 1997.

92. Muhlbauer W, Herndl E, Stock W: The forearm flap, *Plast Reconstr Surg* 70:336–344, 1982.

93. Müller ME, Allgöwer M, Schneider R, Willnegger H: *Manual of internal fixation: techniques recommended by the AO-ASIF Group*, Heidelberg, 1990, Springer-Verlag.

94. Newey ML, Ricketts D, Roberts L: The AO classification of long bone fractures: an early study of its use in clinical practice, *Injury* 24:309–312, 1993.

95. Oishi SN, Levin LS, Pederson WC: Microsurgical management of extremity wounds in diabetics with peripheral vascular disease [see comments], *Plast Reconstr Surg* 92:485–492, 1993.

96. Pang CY, Forrest CR, Morris SF: Pharmacological augmentation of skin flap viability: a hypothesis to mimic the surgical delay phenomenon or a wishful thought, *Ann Plast Surg* 22:293–306, 1989.

97. Park S, Han SH, Lee TJ: Algorithm for recipient vessel selection in free tissue transfer to the lower extremity, *Plast Reconstr Surg* 103:1937–1948, 1999.

98. Pasyk KA, Argenta LC, Austad ED: Histopathology of human expanded tissue, *Clin Plast Surg* 14:435–445, 1987.

99. Peacock EE Jr, Madden JW, Trier WC: Biologic basis for the treatment of keloids and hypertrophic scars, *South Med J* 63:755–760, 1970.

100. Peat BG, Liggins DF: Microvascular soft tissue reconstruction for acute tibial fractures—late complications and the role of bone grafting, *Ann Plast Surg* 24:517–520, 1990.

101. Pederson W: Limb salvage, *Probl Plast Reconstr Surg* 1:125–155, 1991.

102. Pontén B: The fasciocutaneous flap: Its use in soft tissue defects of the lower leg, *Br J Plast Surg* 34:215, 1981.

103. Radovan C: Tissue expansion in soft tissue reconstruction, *Plast Reconstr Surg* 74:482–492, 1984.

104. Rautio J, Asko-Seljavaara S, Laasonen L, et al: Suitability of the scapular flap for reconstructions of the foot, *Plast Reconstr Surg* 85:922–928, 1990.

105. Reiffel RS, McCarthy JG: Coverage of heel and sole defects: a new subfascial arterialized flap, *Plast Reconstr Surg* 66:250–260, 1980.

106. Roth JH, Urbaniak JR, Koman LA, et al: Free flap coverage of deep tissue defects of the foot, *Foot Ankle* 3:150–157, 1982.

107. Rudolph R, Ballantyne DL Jr: Skin grafts. In McCarthy JG, editor: *Plastic surgery*, Philadelphia, 1990, WB Saunders, pp 221–274.

108. Ruedi T, Von Hochstetter A, Schlumpf R: *Surgical approaches for internal fixation*, Heidelberg, 1984, Springer-Verlag.

109. Ruttle PE, Kelly PJ, Arnold PG, et al: Chronic osteomyelitis treated with a muscle flap, *Orthop Clin North Am* 15:451–459, 1984.

110. Sekiguchi J, Kobayashi S, Ohmori K: Use of the osteocutaneous free scapular flap on the lower extremities, *Plast Reconstr Surg* 91:103–112, 1993.

111. Song R, Gao Y, Song Y, et al: The forearm flap, *Clin Plast Surg* 9:21–26, 1982.

112. Stuart JD, Morgan RF, Kenney JG: Single-donor fibrin glue for hand burns, *Ann Plast Surg* 24:524–527, 1990.

113. Swanson E, Boyd JB, Mulholland RS: The radial forearm flap: a biomechanical study of the osteotomized radius, *Plast Reconstr Surg* 85:267–272, 1990.

114. Swiontkowski M: Criteria for bone debridement in massive lower limb trauma, *Clin Orthop Relat Res* 243:41–48, 1989.

115. Taylor GI, Palmer JH: The vascular territories (angiosomes) of the body: experimental study and clinical applications, *Br J Plast Surg* 40:113–141, 1987.

116. Tscherne H, Gotzen GL: *Fractures with soft tissue injuries*, Berlin, 1984, Springer-Verlag, pp 4–9.

117. Turen CH, DiStasio AJ: Treatment of grade IIIB and grade IIIC open tibial fractures, *Orthop Clin North Am* 25:561–571, 1994.

118. Urbaniak JR, Koman LA, Goldner RD, et al: The vascularized cutaneous scapular flap, *Plast Reconstr Surg* 69:772–778, 1982.

119. Urioste SS, Arndt KA, Dover JS: Keloids and hypertrophic scars: review and treatment strategies, *Semin Cutan Med Surg* 18:159–171, 1999.

120. Utley DS, Koch RJ, Goode RL: The failing flap in facial plastic and reconstructive surgery: role of the medicinal leech, *Laryngoscope* 108:1129–1135, 1998.

121. Weinzweig N, Davies BW: Foot and ankle reconstruction using the radial forearm flap: a review of 25 cases, *Plast Reconstr Surg* 102:1999–2005, 1998.

122. Wheatley MJ, Meltzer TR: The management of unsalvageable free flaps, *J Reconstr Microsurg* 12:227–229, 1996.

123. White M: Acute care of lower extremity trauma. In Greco RJ, editor: *Emergency plastic surgery*, Boston, 1991, Little, Brown, pp 407–434.

124. Yaremchuk MJ, Brumback RJ, Manson PN, et al: Acute and definitive management of traumatic osteocutaneous defects of the lower extremity, *Plast Reconstr Surg* 80:1–14, 1987.

Soft Tissue and Bone Tumors

George T. Calvert, R. Lor Randall

The objective of this chapter is to review elements of the history, physical examination, and diagnostic studies required to develop a differential diagnosis and treatment plan for patients presenting with tumors of the foot and ankle. Although malignant neoplasms of the foot and ankle are rare, the practicing foot and ankle surgeon must be acquainted with their presentation, staging, diagnosis, and management. The relatively frequent occurrence of benign bone and soft tissue tumors and tumor-like conditions necessitates a systematic, rational approach to facilitate differentiation between indolent, aggressive, and malignant diagnoses. Principles of imaging, staging, biopsy, treatment, and follow-up will be discussed within this framework.

CLINICAL EVALUATION

History

The importance of obtaining a thorough and accurate history in the evaluation of tumors cannot be overstated. The pervasive availability of cross-sectional imaging has regrettably diminished the perceived importance of basic history and physical examination skills in the minds of many practitioners and patients. This is truly unfortunate because proper use of history can often avoid the expense and morbidity of unnecessary testing and procedures. Furthermore, advanced diagnostic testing should not be interpreted in a vacuum. The differential diagnosis is most appropriately developed using all available information.

As with any history, the chief complaint consists of a symptom and duration. Unlike many foot pathologies, it is common for tumor patients to present with a symptom other than pain. Many note a painless mass or discomfort with footwear because of rubbing of the mass. It is important to note that pain, or lack thereof, is a poor indicator of malignancy. Many benign entities are very painful, and many if not most sarcomas fail to cause pain until they reach a large size. The character of pain is often more useful in developing a differential diagnosis. Night pain is classically associated with tumors and infection. However, a study of presenting symptoms in patients with bone sarcomas found that most reported a history of

Table 18-1 Specific History Elements Useful in Foot and Ankle Tumor Evaluation

Symptom or Complaint	Significance
Long duration with stable size	Likely benign
Waxing and waning size	Consider ganglion cyst
Burning pain or numbness	Nerve sheath tumor
Night pain	Tumor or infection
Marked relief with NSAIDs	Osteoid osteoma
History of blunt trauma	Hematoma or heterotopic ossification
History of penetrating trauma	Infection or foreign body
Personal history of malignancy	Metastatic disease

NSAIDs, nonsteroidal antiinflammatory drugs.

Table 18-2 Physical Examination Elements Useful in Foot and Ankle Tumor Evaluation

Examination Finding	Significance
Fixed to bone	Osteochondroma, osteophyte, tumor arising from bone
Transillumination	Fluid-filled cyst
Bruit on auscultation	Vascular tumor
Tinel positive	Neural tumor
Fatty consistency	Lipoma

strain or minor trauma.[188] Burning pain associated with a mass suggests nerve compression or entrapment by the mass or direct nerve involvement by a tumor such as a schwannoma. Weight-bearing pain associated with a bone lesion should alert the clinician to the possibility of pathologic fracture. Similar to pain, the duration of symptoms cannot distinguish benign from malignant entities. Masses present for many years without change in size are almost always benign. However, rapid growth can frequently occur in benign lesions, and slow, persistent growth is common in many sarcomas. Thus duration of the mass should be interpreted in light of the rate of growth and other symptoms. Table 18-1 reviews history of present illness elements, which should be addressed by the surgeon, and their association with particular pathologies. In addition, the foot and ankle surgeon should also elicit past medical and surgical history, social history (especially smoking and occupational exposures), family history (especially cancer and genetic syndromes), and review of systems relevant to the tumor complaint.

Physical Examination

Similar to history, physical examination provides critical insight for diagnosis of foot and ankle tumors. Inspection permits estimation of tumor size, alignment of the foot and ankle, discoloration, and quality of the skin and soft tissue envelope. Palpation indicates if the tumor is mobile or fixed to bone, firm or soft, warm or cold, and tender or nontender. Neurologic and vascular examination determines if the tumor is compromising either of these vital functions to the foot. Joint motion and stability is also assessed to determine if the tumor involves or adversely affects nearby joints. Physical examination tests specific to masses include auscultation and transillumination (Table 18-2). Auscultation is classically performed with a stethoscope; however, many foot and ankle surgeons routinely use ultrasound Doppler for evaluation of vascular insufficiency. Either modality can be used to identify a bruit associated with vascular malformation. Transillumination indicates that a lesion is at least partially cystic. Lymph node examination of the ipsilateral popliteal fossa and groin should also be performed.

Lymphatic spread is relatively uncommon in primary malignancies of the foot and ankle, but there are specific tumors in which it is more common.

Imaging Studies

When to order an imaging study, which test to order, and how to interpret the results are basic questions asked by the foot and ankle surgeon during the evaluation of tumors. To answer these questions, one must understand why a particular imaging study is being ordered. There are three basic reasons for which most imaging is used in the evaluation of tumors: to establish a diagnosis, to define the local anatomy and plan surgery, and to look for distant spread and stage the disease. Many modalities accomplish more than one goal. For instance, magnetic resonance imaging (MRI) may help establish a diagnosis and plan the surgery, whereas a bone scan may identify distant spread and assist with diagnosis but does not give much insight into local anatomy.

Radiographs

Plain radiographs are an essential part of the evaluation of both bone and soft tissue tumors. Radiographs should always be ordered before the other more advanced and expensive modalities. The standard anteroposterior (AP), lateral, and oblique views of either the foot or ankle, used in standard foot and ankle practice, are adequate for the evaluation of most tumors. These can be supplemented by weight-bearing radiographs or specialized views, such as the Harris axial view for lesions of the calcaneus, on a case-by-case basis. In addition, images of the contralateral side are sometimes useful in distinguishing subtle abnormalities and normal variants.

Plain radiographs are often more important in developing a differential diagnosis of bone tumors than MRI and computed tomography (CT). Table 18-3 summarizes characteristics of the images that should be assessed for all bone tumors and their significance with respect to differential diagnosis. Some key points to analyze in each set of images are the location, size, matrix, border, periosteal response, and soft tissue involvement of the lesion.[127] In addition to developing a specific radiographic differential diagnosis, the surgeon should develop a general concept of what constitutes a benign-appearing lesion as opposed to an aggressive lesion. Large size,

Table 18-3 Radiographic Features of Bone Tumors

Radiographic Finding	Description	Significance
Site within bone	Epiphyseal, metaphyseal, diaphyseal	Predilection of particular tumors for specific sites; example: chondroblastoma-epiphysis
Site within bone	Central, eccentric, periosteal	Predilection of particular tumors for specific sites; example: osteoid osteoma-periosteal
Zone of transition (border)	Sclerotic, well defined, poorly defined	Sclerotic usually slow growing; poorly defined often faster growing
Bone loss	Geographic, moth eaten, permeative	Geographic usually less aggressive; moth eaten and permeative usually more aggressive
Periosteal reaction	Present, absent	Presence suggests more aggressive lesion
Matrix	Absent, chondroid, osteoid	Suggests specific pathology
Soft tissue mass	Present, absent	Soft tissue mass associated with bone lesion typically suggests a more aggressive lesion

Table 18-4 Characteristic Imaging Findings of Specific Pathologies

Modality	Finding	Pathology
Radiograph	Phleboliths	Hemangioma
Radiograph	Fallen leaf sign	Simple bone cyst
Radiograph	Sunburst periosteal reaction	Osteosarcoma
Radiograph	Onionskin periosteal reaction	Ewing sarcoma
CT or radiograph	Cortical ridus	Osteoid osteoma or Brodie abscess
MRI	"Cluster of grapes"	Hemangioma

CT, computed tomography; MRI, magnetic resonance imaging.

periosteal response, cortical destruction, and associated soft tissue masses are all features that should alert the physician to a more aggressive lesion. Small size, sclerotic borders, and lack of soft tissue mass suggest a more indolent process.

Plain radiographs are also useful in the evaluation of soft tissue masses. They can identify or exclude underlying bone and joint abnormalities, such as osteoarthritis in the case of degenerative cysts. Soft tissue masses are often visible on radiographs, and their radiodensity may provide insight into the diagnosis. For instance, the fat of a lipoma is less radiodense than the surrounding tissues. Finally, there are some pathognomonic or at least characteristic radiographic findings associated with particular lesions. A classic example is the phlebolith, the small discrete area of soft tissue calcification seen in association with hemangiomas. Characteristic imaging findings of some specific lesions are summarized Table 18-4.

Computed Tomography

The excellent bone detail and cross-sectional imaging provided by CT can be invaluable in select cases. Advantages of CT over MRI include better bone resolution, faster image acquisition times, and lower costs. Fine cut (1 to 1.5-mm sections) CT scans can be very useful in defining the complex and irregularly shaped anatomy of the hindfoot. Cortically based lesions, such as osteoid

osteoma, are often better visualized with CT than MRI. A study comparing the diagnostic accuracy of MRI versus CT for the diagnosis of osteoid osteoma found CT to be more accurate.[86] The fast image acquisition times can be useful for patients, such as children, who cannot remain still for prolonged imaging. Fast acquisition and the ability to use metal instruments also facilitates CT-guided procedures, such as radiofrequency ablation (RFA), that would be difficult with MRI. Finally, chest CT is routinely used in the staging of malignant foot and ankle lesions to identify pulmonary metastases.

Magnetic Resonance Imaging

MRI is the imaging modality of choice for defining the local anatomy of soft tissue tumors and most bone tumors of the foot and ankle.[192] Advantages of MRI over CT include better soft tissue resolution, multiplanar imaging, and avoidance of radiation exposure. Most oncologic surgeons recommend the use of intravenous contrast with MRI when evaluating tumors of the foot and ankle. Contrast enhancement helps to better identify the maximal extent of lesions and can help with determining the differential diagnosis. Some specific tumors have a unique MRI appearance or signal pattern.[137] These are reviewed in Table 18-4. Although MRI is often very useful in the evaluation of foot and ankle tumors, the requesting surgeon should have a clear rationale for ordering this expensive test. Most asymptomatic, benign-appearing lesions can be monitored with history, physical examination, and radiographs. MRI is best used in symptomatic or aggressive-appearing lesions in which biopsy or surgical intervention is being contemplated. MRI is best understood as a planning rather than diagnostic tool.

Angiography

The role of angiography in the evaluation of foot and ankle tumors has diminished with the increased availability CT and MRI. However, it is still frequently used by interventional radiologists for embolization of highly vascular tumors. Although this is less frequently used in the foot and ankle than in more proximal locations, such interventions may be useful in the treatment of conditions such as arteriovenous malformations. Another use of angiography in foot and ankle tumor surgery is in the planning of free tissue transfer for the coverage of complex wounds after tumor resection.

Nuclear Imaging

Sarcomas have a proclivity for bone metastases, and technetium-99 bone scans are therefore a standard staging test for these tumors. Identification of distant disease before a potentially morbid resection is important as it alters prognosis and possibly the treatment plan. Dedicated bone scans of the feet can also occasionally be useful in the evaluation of local disease. Subtle stress fractures and other difficult-to-discern lesions may be identified. It is important that the ordering surgeon understands that bone scans are highly sensitive but not specific. They do not readily distinguish tumors from other causes of increased metabolic bone activity. One must also understand that bone scans do not differentiate benign from malignant lesions. Many benign lesions may have high bone scan activity, and some malignant tumors, such as myelomas, may be cold on bone scan.

A newer nuclear medicine modality is positron emission tomography (PET). The most common tracer molecule used with PET is fludeoxyglucose (FDG), an analogue of glucose. FDG-PET identifies areas of increased glucose metabolism, such as tumors. It is a standard staging modality in the evaluation of melanoma[122] and is being studied as a potentially more sensitive and specific alternative to bone scan for sarcomas.[33]

STAGING

The purpose of cancer staging is multifactorial. Staging assists in guiding treatment by determining the extent of disease. Staging also provides caregivers and patients with prognostic information about morbidity and survival. In addition, accurate staging permits investigators from different centers to communicate effectively, thus facilitating research and improved treatment. The terms *grade* and *stage* are sometimes used inappropriately. Histologic grade is determined by pathologic analysis of tumor tissue. Grade is an important component of many staging systems, but these systems use other data, such as size and anatomic spread, in addition to grade. This section will focus on the staging of bone and soft tissue sarcomas of the foot and ankle. The reader should be aware that other malignancies, such as melanoma and carcinomas, have their own staging systems. The two major staging systems used for bone and soft tissue sarcomas in North America are the Enneking system[58,59] and the American Joint Committee on Cancer (AJCC)[57] system (Tables 18-5 and 18-6).

The Enneking system uses three factors: histologic grade, compartmental involvement, and metastasis. This system was developed before the widespread availability of cross-sectional imaging. The compartment concept was deemed surgically useful as guide to the type and extent

Table 18-5 Enneking Staging System of Bone and Soft Tissue Sarcomas

Stage	Grade	Site	Metastasis
IA	G1	Intracompartmental	Absent
IB	G1	Extracompartmental	Absent
IIA	G2	Intracompartmental	Absent
IIB	G2	Extracompartmental	Absent
III	G1 or G2	Either	Present

G1, low grade; *G2*, high grade.

Table 18-6 American Joint Committee on Cancer Staging

Stage	Grade	Size	Node	Metastasis
Soft Tissue Sarcomas				
IA	G1	<5 cm	No	Absent
IB	G1	>5 cm	No	Absent
IIA	G2 or G3	<5 cm	No	Absent
IIB	G2	>5 cm	No	Absent
III	G3	>5 cm	No	Absent
	Any	Any	Yes	Absent
IV	Any	Any	Any	Present
Bone Sarcomas				
IA	G1	<8 cm		
IB	G1	>8 cm		
IIA	G2	<8 cm		
IIB	G2	>8 cm		
III	Any	Any		Skip
IV	Any	Any		Distant

G1, grade 1; *G2*, grade 2; *G3*, grade 3; *Skip* (metastasis), metastasis within the same bone.

of resection to be performed. This is less useful in the era of cross-sectional imaging because careful analysis of preoperative MRI and CT scans provide high-resolution anatomic details for surgical planning. In addition, the compartment concept is most useful in the thigh, leg, arm, and forearm. The tightly constrained anatomy of the foot and ankle mandates that all but the smallest tumors are extracompartmental.

The AJCC system uses the familiar *t*umor size–lymph *n*odes–*m*etastasis (TNM) nomenclature used in the staging of most common cancers, such as breast and lung. The staging for bone and soft tissue sarcomas differ in the AJCC system. The AJCC system is used for reporting stage data to national and international registries and is favored by most major cancer centers in North America and beyond. AJCC uses four factors in defining soft tissue sarcoma stage: histologic grade, size, lymph node involvement, and metastasis. Previous editions of the system also used location, either superficial or below the fascia, to determine stage. Location remains an important clinical consideration, but it no longer influences staging. Lymph node involvement is rare among all bone sarcomas and most soft tissue sarcomas. The five soft tissue sarcomas with relatively frequent lymphatic spread are listed in Table 18-7. Although both the AJCC and Enneking systems have been shown to accurately predict survival in retrospective cohorts of sarcoma patients, the latter's use is ever decreasing as orthopaedic oncologists further integrate into the multidisciplinary clinical oncology paradigm.

The foot and ankle surgeon should be familiar with the tests commonly ordered in the staging process. Obtaining this information is not only useful to the patient but assists the practitioner in deciding what treatments to offer and what consultations to obtain. Common staging studies are listed in Table 18-8. One must also remember that staging should be repeated before surgery if neoadjuvant chemotherapy is given or if there is any other significant delay between the initial staging and surgery.

BIOPSY

Biopsy is crucial for the effective diagnosis, staging, and treatment of foot and ankle tumors. The primary goal of biopsy is to obtain adequate tissue to establish a diagnosis without compromising the ability to perform a definitive resection if the tumor is found to be malignant. The

Table 18-7 Soft Tissue Sarcomas with Frequent Lymphatic Spread: Mnemonic CARES

Sarcoma
Clear cell sarcoma
Angiosarcoma
Rhabdomyosarcoma
Epithelioid sarcoma
Synovial sarcoma

Table 18-8 Imaging Studies Frequently Used in Sarcoma Staging

Study	Purpose
Radiographs of involved area	Diagnosis and local assessment
MRI with IV contrast of involved area	Define local extent and plan surgery
CT of involved area	Occasionally used to better define local anatomy
CT chest	Identify pulmonary metastasis
Whole body bone scan	Identify skeletal metastasis

CT, computed tomography; *IV*, intravenous; *MRI*, magnetic resonance imaging.

first decision to be made is whether biopsy is necessary. Many of the most common foot "tumors" encountered by surgeons can be excised without biopsy if the history, physical examination, and imaging are classic for a benign diagnosis. A typical example is a ganglion cyst located over a joint that waxes and wanes in size and transilluminates on examination. Most foot masses are long-standing, small, superficial lesions that can be treated by the general foot and ankle surgeon without staging and biopsy. A sound general principle is that *a biopsy should be performed if a malignant entity is included in the surgeon's preoperative differential diagnosis. Any lesion that is rapidly changing in size, larger than 5 cm, or deep should raise concern for a potentially malignant process.* It has been shown in multiple studies that sarcomas are best treated at specialized centers, and early referral should be considered for aggressive-appearing tumors.[147]

The second decision is what type of biopsy to perform. The general categories are needle and open biopsies. Needle biopsies are further subdivided into core needle biopsies and fine needle aspirations (FNA). Open biopsies are subdivided into incisional and excisional. Advantages and disadvantages of each are summarized in Table 18-9. Many needle biopsies are performed in an office setting or under image guidance in the radiology suite. If these procedures are to be performed by a radiologists or pathologist, the site of needle entry should be determined in conjunction with the surgeon, to avoid compromising future resection. A common misconception with open biopsies is the meaning of the term excisional biopsy. This refers to a biopsy technique in which the entire tumor is excised with a cuff of normal tissue (primary wide excision) for both diagnostic and definitive therapeutic effect.[6] This is best performed by experienced tumor surgeons for small, superficial masses. This type of biopsy is rarely indicated because primary wide excision is often unnecessarily morbid for benign entities. Unfortunately, many practitioners inappropriately define unplanned excisions of malignancies as excisional biopsies. These "incidentaloma" procedures are usually done without appropriate staging studies, oncologic rationale, or surgical technique. Such procedures often complicate definitive resection of the tumor and compromise the care of the patient.[145]

Although biopsies are relatively small procedures, thorough planning and meticulous surgical technique are

Table 18-9 Advantages and Disadvantages of Different Biopsy Techniques

Technique	Advantage	Disadvantage
Needle (general)	Less trauma than open	Less tissue than open
Core needle	Can show tissue architecture in addition to cytology	More traumatic than fine needle aspiration
Fine needle	Less traumatic than core	Only provides cells; no tissue architecture can be analyzed
Open (general)	More tissue than needle	More traumatic than needle
Incisional	Less extensive than excisional biopsy	Requires second operation for definitive resection
Excisional	No further surgery required if done appropriately	More traumatic; second operation is more complicated if any margins are positive

Table 18-10 Principles of Incisional Biopsy

Tourniquet optional; elevate foot and do not use Esmarch tourniquet to exanguinate; if tourniquet is used, always deflate at conclusion to confirm hemostasis

Longitudinal incision in line with foot or ankle; biopsy incision and tract must be completely excised if the lesion is malignant

Do not create skin or soft tissue flaps; cut directly down to tumor and sample; do not spread and visualize

Meticulous hemostasis is crucial; electrocautery; consider packing dead space with hemostatic material such as noncompressed Gelfoam

If drain is to be used, place in line with incision so that drain tract can be easily excised with the biopsy incision

Standard closure techniques and compressive dressing to prevent hematoma

essential to obtain adequate tissue while avoiding contamination of uninvolved tissue planes with tumor cells. Open incisional biopsy is the standard technique for most bone foot and ankle bone tumors and many soft tissue tumors. Preoperative planning involves careful review of radiographs and cross-sectional imaging. The most aggressive-appearing portion of a tumor should be targeted because it is most likely to contain diagnostic tissue. For example, in a lesion with cystic and solid components, the solid portion should be sampled. The surgeon should confirm that appropriate equipment is available, such as a C-arm intensifier and trephines for bone lesions. The pathologist should be available for frozen section analysis. Incisions should be planned to permit complete excision of the biopsy tract if definitive wide resection is necessary. This generally involves making a longitudinal incision in line with either the foot or ankle (whichever the case may be). Careful study of imaging permits selection of the most direct path to the tumor while avoiding contamination of critical neurovascular structures. Development of skin and soft tissue flaps should be avoided, and meticulous hemostasis should be maintained. Frozen section analysis permits assessment of adequacy of the sample and an initial diagnostic impression. Morbid resection or amputation should not be performed based solely upon frozen section results. The surgeon should also discuss the possible need for fresh tissue (in addition to standard fixed tissue) with the pathologist. Fresh tissue is sometimes necessary for flow cytometry or cytogenetic analysis. Drain placement in line with the incision is used only if there is significant dead space or risk of hematoma. Surgical principles of incisional biopsy are summarized in Table 18-10.[158]

RADIATION AND CHEMOTHERAPY FOR FOOT AND ANKLE TUMORS

Adjuvant treatments play an important role in the management of most malignant bone and soft tissue sarcomas as well as some benign but aggressive tumors. Detailed discussion of chemotherapy regimens and radiotherapy techniques are beyond the scope of this text. However, the foot and ankle surgeon should be aware of which tumors frequently require these treatments because it may affect surgical planning.

Bone sarcomas, specifically osteosarcoma and Ewing sarcoma, are chemotherapy responsive. They are generally treated with neoadjuvant (preoperative) chemotherapy before resection and then with additional adjuvant chemotherapy after resection. Chemotherapy is rarely used for the treatment of chondrosarcoma. Soft tissue sarcoma response to chemotherapy varies considerably with the specific pathology of the tumor. Neoadjuvant chemotherapy is used for some high-grade soft tissue sarcomas, but most are treated with radiation and surgery. Isolated limb perfusion is a special technique of chemotherapy administration in which the circulation of a limb is isolated from the rest of the body (typically with temporary vascular bypass), and high doses of chemotherapy are administered to the isolated limb.[49] This technique permits the use of chemotherapy agents and dosages that are too toxic for general systemic administration. This technique, although relatively uncommon in North America, has been frequently used in Europe and Asia with good results for the treatment of advanced soft tissue sarcomas and melanoma of the foot and ankle.[49]

Radiation therapy is part of the standard treatment for most high-grade soft tissue sarcomas. It has been shown to substantially decrease the risk of local recurrence in these tumors.[161] Preoperative and postoperative radiation each have distinct advantages and disadvantages. Preoperative radiation generally requires a smaller total dose and smaller field of radiation. This may reduce the long-term morbidity associated with radiation treatment. Some have even suggested an improved survival with preoperative radiotherapy.[155] Unfortunately, preoperative radiation may induce tissue fibrosis, making surgical resection more difficult. Preoperative radiation also has a higher wound complication and infection rate than postoperative radiation.[135] Alternatively, postoperative radiation has a lower wound complication rate but may produce greater long-term radiation–induced morbidity. There are many advocates of both strategies. In adults, for soft tissue sarcomas about the foot and ankle, strategic radiotherapy may be advocated. In children with a defined soft tissue rhabdomyosarcoma, radiation may also be chosen to avoid a major amputation if major growth plates can be spared.[96] Radiation plays a much smaller role in the treatment of bone sarcomas. Ewing sarcoma is radiosensitive, but definitive radiation is generally not advocated in the foot and ankle because definitive surgical resection is possible in this location. Furthermore, the effects of radiotherapy on the growing foot are quite devastating and compromise function compared with a below-knee amputation with a modern exoprosthesis. Radiation is also used for some benign but locally aggressive soft tissue tumors, particularly desmoid tumors. The most common method of radiation delivery to the foot ankle is external beam radiation. Brachytherapy is an alternative technique in which radiation catheters are surgically placed, and radioactive material then can be placed through them. It offers the potential advantage of administering higher local radiation doses to the tumor bed with less dosage to the adjacent healthy tissues.[11]

Metastatic disease is often treated with palliative chemotherapy and radiation. The foot and ankle surgeon should coordinate any surgical interventions for the treatment of metastatic bone disease with the patient's medical and radiation oncologists. For example, timing of prophylactic fixation may be coordinated with the patient's medical oncologist to avoid chemotherapy-induced neutropenia during the immediate perioperative period. These consultants may also be able to give valuable insight into perioperative management issues, such as pain control and end-of-life counseling.

GENERAL PRINCIPLES OF SURGICAL TREATMENT FOR SOFT TISSUE AND BONE TUMORS

Foot and ankle tumor surgery differs from most trauma and reconstructive surgery of the foot and ankle because the prevention of tumor recurrence is often more important than restoration of function. This is certainly the case for malignant tumors and is also true of many benign but locally aggressive tumors. Risk of local recurrence is largely determined by two factors: the biology of the tumor and how the tumor is treated. In addition to his staging system, Dr. Enneking provided an intellectual framework for the different types of surgical resections (Table 18-11). He defined resections as intracapsular, marginal, wide, and radical (Fig. 18-1).[58] These are roughly defined by how closely the surgical dissection plane comes to the tumor, with intracapsular resections cutting through tumor tissue and radical resection cutting far from the tumor. Within this framework, the surgeon plans the type of resection based upon the pathology of the tumor with wider resections performed for more aggressive lesions. It is very important to understand that the type of resection is not determined by the

particular type of surgery (Fig. 18-2). For example, an amputation inadvertently performed through a tumor is an intralesional resection, whereas removal of a subcutaneous tumor with a cuff of normal surrounding fat is a wide resection. Although often useful as a surgical planning tool, the Enneking definitions have been largely replaced by the residual disease classification for reporting purposes in the literature (see Table 18-11).[80a] This system is defined by pathologic analysis of the specimen

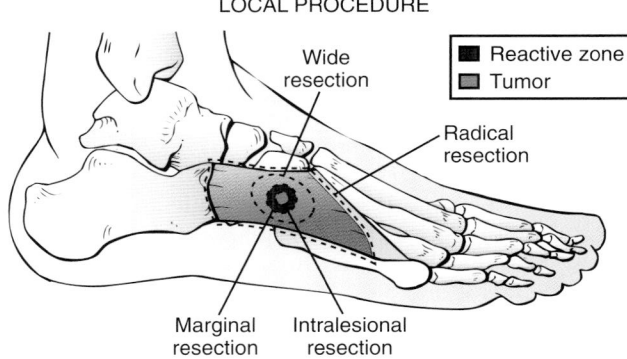

Figure 18-1 Illustration of the different types of musculoskeletal tumor resections as described by Enneking.

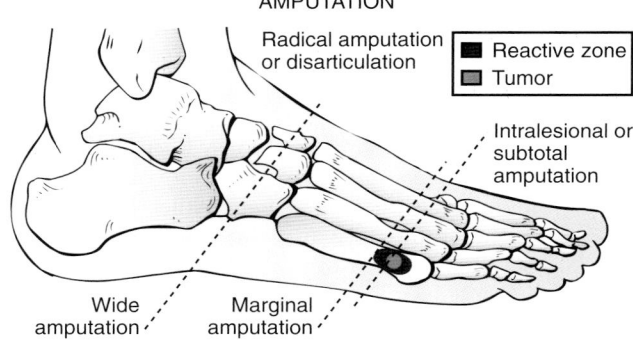

Figure 18-2 The surgical procedure does not define the type of oncologic resection. Even amputations may be intralesional if not planned appropriately.

Table 18-11 Classification of Surgical Margins: Enneking and Residual Disease Classifications		
Enneking Classification		
Type of Resection	**Plane of Dissection**	**Pathologic Goal**
Intracapsular	Within lesion	Gross tumor at margin
Marginal	Within reactive zone of tumor	Microscopic tumor at margin
Wide	Through normal tissue	No tumor at margin
Radical	Extracompartmental to tumor	No tumor at margin
Residual Disease Classification		
Type of Resection	**Pathologic Outcome**	
R0	No tumor at margin	
R1	Microscopic tumor at margin	
R2	Gross tumor at margin	

From Enneking WF: A system of staging musculoskeletal neoplasms, *Clin Orthop Relat Res* 204:9–24, 1986; Hermanek P, Wittekind C: Residual tumor (R) classification and prognosis, *Semin Surg Oncol* 10:12-20, 1994.

after resection as opposed to the preoperative plan. R0 is defined as no residual disease, R1 as microscopic residual disease, and R2 as gross residual disease. Use of these definitions for reporting ensures that investigators are defining surgical results by the same criteria.

The great heterogeneity of tumors presenting in the foot and ankle mandates an individualized surgical plan for each patient. However, some general principles warrant discussion before the succeeding descriptions of individual tumor types. All necessary staging should be completed and reviewed preoperatively, and local imaging should be carefully reviewed before surgery. Availability of any requisite special equipment and intraoperative consultants should be confirmed before surgery. Exsanguination, if performed for tourniquet inflation, should be done with elevation and not compressive wrap. Incisions should be planned such that the biopsy tract is removed with the specimen, and extensile exposure can be obtained if necessary for the present procedure or in the future in the event of recurrence. The use of sharp-toothed retractors and forceps directly upon tumor tissue should be avoided to prevent inadvertent contamination. If contamination of the wound with tumor occurs, immediate closure of the tumor defect and copious irrigation of the wound should be performed. Measures to prevent cross-contamination of separate surgical sites, such as bone graft harvest sites, should always be taken. These measures include use of separate instrument sets and regloving. Specimens should always be sent for routine pathology (and the reports later reviewed) even if the tumor has a characteristic gross appearance. The specimen should be oriented for the pathologist with long and short sutures to identify the relevant surfaces (deep, proximal, distal, medial, lateral), and the orientation should be noted in the operative report. Culture should be performed if infection is a concern. If postoperative radiation is a possibility, surgical clips should be placed to mark the extent of the resection bed. Closure of the wound under tension, especially in the setting of radiation or chemotherapy, increases the risk of dehiscence and infection. Plastic surgery consultation and flap reconstruction is more likely to succeed when performed preemptively as part of a plan rather than as a response to an established complication. Strict guidelines for the use of drains in tumor surgery do not exist, but their use when a large dead space is created by resection is prudent. Although there are exceptions to such general rules, the foot and ankle surgeon may avoid many difficulties if these are kept in mind.

Benign Soft Tissue Tumors

Benign soft tissue tumors and tumor-like conditions are the most common tumor of the foot and ankle. Incidence is difficult to define because many people with small benign tumors never seek treatment, and studies from specialized tumor centers invariably have referral bias because more complex cases are likely to be referred. A large, consecutive series (83 cases) of foot soft tissue tumors seen at the Hospital for Joint Diseases in New York found that 87% of the tumors were benign.[93] Thirty-two percent of the benign tumors were ganglion cysts, and 21% were fibromas or fibromatosis. The ganglion cysts were primarily dorsal, and the fibromas were plantar. A series of 153 foot and ankle tumors at a tertiary orthopaedic oncology unit found 61% were benign, and the most common benign soft tissue diagnosis was pigmented villonodular synovitis and giant cell tumor of the tendon sheath.[38] The discrepancy of these series likely results from referral bias because one study primarily collected cases from a foot and ankle service and the other from an orthopaedic oncology service. A wide array of pathologies accounted for the remaining diagnoses in both series. Table 18-12 lists the most common benign soft tissue tumors of the foot and ankle, their common locations, and their relative recurrence risk after excision.

Fibrous Tumors
FIBROMA AND FIBROMATOSIS
Plantar fibromas and fibromatosis are best characterized as a continuum of disease, ranging from small, isolated fibromas to extensive fibromatosis. Correspondingly, symptoms range from minimal to severe. The lesions occur most often along the medial border of the plantar fascia. The condition may present at any age, including children.[63] Males are more frequently affected than females, and the whites of northern European ancestry are more commonly affected than other races. Many patients have a family history of palmar or plantar fibromatosis. Lesions are firm and fixed to the plantar fascia and produce discomfort on weight bearing because of the irregular contour of the plantar surface in the arch of the foot (Fig 18-3). Growth is generally slow and usually

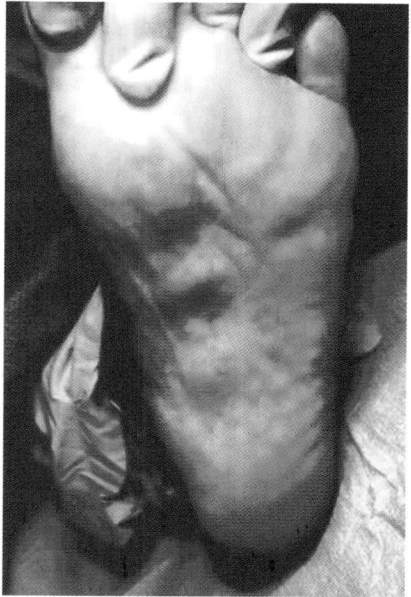

Figure 18-3 Typical size and appearance of plantar fibromatosis along the medial border of the plantar fascia.

Table 18-12 Common Benign Soft Tissue Tumors and Tumor-like Conditions of the Foot and Ankle

Tumor	Tissue of Origin	Common Location	Recurrence Risk
Fibroma (fibromatosis)	Fibrous; cutaneous or subcutaneous	Plantar foot	Low for isolated fibromas, higher for fibromatosis
Desmoid (aggressive fibromatosis)	Deep fibrous	Any	Frequent
Dermatofibroma	Skin and subcutaneous	Ankle and distal leg	Rare
Granuloma annulare	Skin and subcutaneous	Distal anterior leg and foot	Self-limited condition
Hemangioma	Vascular	Any	Rare if small and isolated; common if large and diffuse
Lymphangioma	Vascular	Any	Similar to hemangioma
Glomus tumor	Vascular	Nail bed	Rare
Pigmented villonodular synovitis	Synovial	Ankle and subtalar joints	Frequent
Giant cell tumor of the tendon sheath	Synovial	Foot tendons	Less frequent than with joint involvement
Synovial chondromatosis	Synovial	Ankle and subtalar joints	Frequent
Ganglion cysts	Synovial	Dorsal joints and tendons	Frequent
Schwannoma (neurilemoma)	Neural	Any peripheral nerve	Rare
Neurofibroma	Neural	Any peripheral nerve	Rare
Lipoma	Fat	Any	Rare
Xanthoma	Cholesterol deposition	Achilles tendon	Rare
Tophacious gout	Uric acid crystal deposition	Great toe and ankle	Common if gout is poorly controlled

stops once the lesion reaches a size of approximately 2 cm. Older patients may have an associated Dupuytren contracture of the hands or Peyronie disease of the penis. Histologically, the lesions contain myofibroblasts similar to those seen in a Dupuytren contracture.[48] The classic location of the lesion or lesions, especially in the setting of long-standing duration and personal or family history of the condition, facilitate clinical diagnosis without the need for advanced imaging or biopsy in many cases.

Asymptomatic patients require no treatment. Symptomatic patients should be given a prolonged trial of nonsurgical therapy, including footwear modification and nonsteroidal antiinflammatory drugs (NSAIDs). Because the lesions extend into dermis and skin as well as the underlying fascia, it is difficult in many cases to obtain satisfactory surgical margins. Prior series have reported relatively high recurrence rates and significant surgical morbidity. Factors associated with recurrence have included bilateral disease, multiple nodules, and positive family history.[4] Multiple different surgical techniques have been advocated, including marginal excision, subtotal fasciectomy,[4] and wide excision followed by local soft tissue reconstruction.[186] A 2000 study by Sammarco and Mangone[154] reported a operative staging system with specific surgical recommendations after review of 21 surgically treated cases of fibromatosis. Multifocal disease, adherence to the skin, and deep extension to the flexor tendon sheath were the factors associated with increasing surgical difficulty. The authors advocated incisions placed in the non–weight-bearing portion of the plantar arch, routine use of loupe magnification, avoidance of full-thickness resection of plantar skin even in cases of dermal infiltration, and initial use of local wound care with

avoidance of early skin grafting. The final point is analogous to the McKash open palm technique used by many hand surgeons in the treatment of severe Dupuytren disease. Delayed skin grafting was not associated with increased infection risk and avoided secondary procedures in many patients. Eighteen of 21 patients were satisfied with the procedure, and there were only two recurrences.

DESMOID TUMORS (AGGRESSIVE FIBROMATOSIS)

Desmoid tumor is a benign but locally aggressive fibrous tumor that may occur anywhere in the body. It bears no clinical or histologic relation to plantar fibromatosis. Most extraabdominal desmoid tumors are sporadic, but some may be associated with the familial adenomatous coli (FAP) syndrome. FAP is characterized by diffuse development of colon polyps and predilection for early colon cancer.[60] Young patients presenting with desmoids of the foot should be questioned about family history, and referral for genetic testing should be considered. A recent series from Massachusetts General Hospital identified the foot as the most common site of extraabdominal desmoids (45 of 234 cases).[114] Historically, aggressive wide resection of desmoids, including those of the foot, has been advocated because of high recurrence rates.[13] During the past decade, the understanding of this condition at many high-volume centers has shifted. Previously, desmoids were believed to have unrelenting continued local growth, but it has recently been demonstrated that many have long periods of stable size or even regression.[65] This realization has led to a more conservative approach of initial observation at many centers. Surgical treatment has also become more conservative as microscopic positive margins have not been shown to adversely influence recurrence rates.[78] Based upon these studies, acceptance of microscopically positive margins in order to preserve important neurovascular structures is appropriate in the treatment of this condition.

The foot and ankle surgeon should also be aware that desmoid tumors are one of the few benign entities in which radiation therapy and low-dose chemotherapy are used for treatment. As such, these tumors are best treated at centers that offer team-oriented multimodal treatment similar to that for malignant conditions. Early referral should therefore be considered for desmoids if these resources are not available at the presenting institution.

Dermal Tumors

Patients with common surface-based skin lesions will not generally present to foot and ankle surgeons. However, two common benign dermal lesions warrant discussion because they frequently extend subcutaneously and may present to surgeons.

DERMATOFIBROMA (BENIGN FIBROUS HISTIOCYTOMA)

This dermal-based lesion most commonly presents on the lower legs but can also be found on the feet. It is frequently painful or pruritic. Patients may relate a history of trauma or insect bite, but this association is not clearly defined in the literature. Physical examination reveals dimpling of the skin with lateral compression next to the lesion (Fitzpatrick sign).[66] As the alternative name suggests, histologic analysis reveals a fibrohistiocytic proliferation; multiple subtypes have been characterized.[201] Whether or not there is a continuum from benign dermatofibromas to dermatofibrosarcoma protuberans is debated.[84] Most patients are effectively treated with reassurance of the benign nature of the condition. Treatment with corticosteroid injection has been reported. Persistently symptomatic lesions can be resected with low recurrence rate.[201]

GRANULOMA ANNULARE

The subcutaneous form of granuloma annulare frequently presents as a superficial mass in the anterior distal leg or foot of children and adolescents.[149] Although the more common dermal form presents with characteristic papules, the subcutaneous variety often lacks surface changes on visual inspection. MRI features have been described but are not specific for the condition.[40] Histology reveals a granulomatous lesion with characteristic features best demonstrated with mucin staining. A series of 35 cases in children identified the scalp, anterior distal leg, and foot as the most common sites.[118] The condition occurs more frequently in females than males. Although surgical biopsy is often required for diagnosis, resection is not recommended because the lesions usually resolve spontaneously.

Vascular Tumors
HEMANGIOMA AND LYMPHANGIOMA

These are developmental anomalies of the vasculature rather than true clonal neoplasias. Hemangiomas typically arise in childhood and adolescence.[153] When these tumors are superficial, a noticeable bluish discoloration is observed, associated with a soft, doughy mass (Fig. 18-4). More extensive lesions can have associated localized gigantism of adjacent bone and soft tissue. Proteus syndrome and Klippel-Trénaunay syndrome may both present with vascular malformation of the leg and foot with associated gigantism.[81,171] Plain radiographs can show multiple small calcified phleboliths. MRI demonstrates a characteristic "cluster of grapes" appearance and can better define the anatomic extent of larger lesions.[137] Lymphangiomas share similar presentation and histology with hemangiomas, with the exception that the vascular channels are lymphatics rather than capillaries.[194] Hemangiomas are consequently more vascular at surgical resections. Structurally, these tumors can be of the cavernous, capillary, or mixed type; the port-wine capillary hemangiomas are most common in the foot.

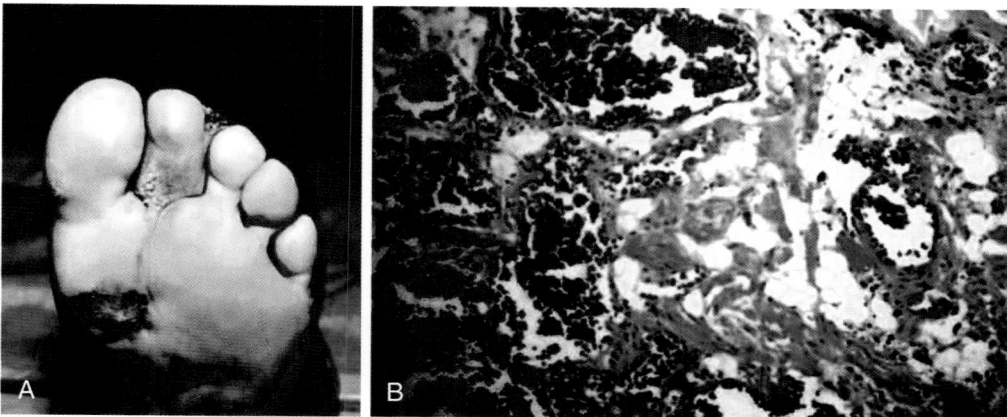

Figure 18-4 **A,** Skin and soft tissue changes in a patient with hemangioma. **B,** Histologic section demonstrating multiple vascular channels with thin endothelial lining and a benign, fibrous-supporting stroma.

Treatment is initially conservative, with observation of asymptomatic lesions and compression stockings and analgesics for symptomatic lesions. A recent randomized controlled trial of oral propranolol for infantile hemangiomas showed efficacy for children up to 5 years of age.[82] Nonsurgical procedures, specifically sclerotherapy[191] and embolization,[12] have been used with encouraging results. Symptomatic lesions in which conservative measures have failed require surgical resection. Marginal or even intralesional excision is advocated for these benign lesions. Recurrence rates reported in the literature vary widely, with discrepancies likely resulting from differences of both the tumors and techniques. A 1993 study reported a 48% recurrence rate, but many of these patients had extensive lesions.[155] A series of 89 surgically treated hemangioma patients from Harvard found an overall 19% recurrence rate and 13% rate of revision surgery for recurrence. All patients in the series were treated with marginal or intralesional resections. The role of margins in recurrence was analyzed in a 2007 study from the University of Minnesota. Recurrence rate was 7% with wide or marginal resection, 35% with intralesional resection without gross tumor remaining, and 67% with gross residual tumor.[14] Based upon these data, removal of all gross tumor at a minimum, and preferably marginal resection, is advocated when surgery is indicated. Preoperative embolization may facilitate a better resection margin in cases of large hemangiomas.

GLOMUS TUMOR

Glomus tumors, also called glomangiomas, are benign vascular tumors that have their peak incidence in the 20- to 40-year-old age range. They arise from the glomus body tissue of the dermal layer of the skin. This tissue contains an arteriovenous shunt with sympathetic innervations.[108] It is thought to shunt blood flow away from the skin in response to cold temperatures. Glomus bodies are most numerous in the tips of the fingers and toes. There are rare case reports of glomus tumors in the hindfoot,[120,144] but most occur under the nail bed. Subungual glomus tumors are associated with a female predominance of 3 : 1.[170] These tumors typically manifest with a bright red to bluish discoloration beneath the nail bed and are associated with lancinating pain that worsens with cold exposure or direct pressure. They are usually less than 1 cm in diameter. Radiographs may show well-marginated bony erosion over the dorsal surface of the distal phalanx.

Treatment consists of surgical resection of symptomatic lesions. A 2003 case series reported excellent results with subperiosteal elevation of skin, nail, and nail matrix as a single flap, followed by excision of the tumor from within the flap.[85] The authors reported complete resolution of symptoms and no recurrences in their series of seven cases. Pain relief is usually prompt, and recurrence is unusual. In any lesion found under the nail, the possibility of malignant melanoma should always be considered in the preoperative differential diagnosis.

Neural Tumors
SCHWANNOMA (NEURILEMOMA)

Schwannoma (neurilemoma, neurilemmoma, neurolemmoma) is a benign tumor of nerve sheath (Schwann cell) origin with a peak incidence in the fourth and fifth decades of life. Males were more commonly affected than females in a review of 104 cases from Scotland.[90] The tumor is usually solitary, well encapsulated, and on the surface of a peripheral nerve. Solitary Schwannomas of the foot are quite rare, with only case reports noted in the literature.[202] Schwannomas can continue growing to a very large size even in the foot.[111] Patients present with a painful nodule often associated with a positive Tinel sign in the distribution of the affected nerve. Schwannomatosis (previously called neurofibromatosis type 3) is a rare genetic disorder characterized by diffuse development of schwanomas.[109] Unlike neurofibromas, schwannomas usually have a discrete plain between the tumor and the nerve fascicles. The tumor can usually be shelled out of the nerve sheath without damage to the nerve fibers themselves (Fig. 18-5). Use of loupe magnification and microsurgical instruments may be beneficial when critical nerves are involved. Recurrence is rare, and these tumors have little malignant potential.

NEUROFIBROMA

Neurofibromas are spindle cell tumors of peripheral nerves that may be solitary or multiple. Overall, 90% are solitary, and 10% of cases are associated with neurofibromatosis. Solitary neurofibromas of the foot are rare, and their diagnosis in a child or young adult should raise the suspicion of possible neurofibromatosis.[148] Neurofibromatosis has two distinct forms: neurofibromatosis type 1 (NF1) and neurofibromatosis type 2 (NF2). NF1 is the form relevant to foot and ankle surgeons because patients with this condition develop multiple lesions throughout the body and have musculoskeletal manifestations, including scoliosis, localized gigantism, or tibial pseudoarthrosis.[182] Cutaneous manifestations evident on initial clinical examination include multiple café au lait spots and plexiform neurofibromas. Plexiform neurofibromas are large neurofibromas that can involve extensive areas of skin, subcutaneous tissue, and deep structures. They have been reported in the foot and ankle, and complete removal can be very difficult because of their permeative nature.[21] Neurofibromas permeate between nerve fibers, with no clear plane of dissection. Resection often requires removal of the affected portion of the nerve as well. Because of this, the surgeon must often choose between the disability caused by the lesion and the disability resulting from resection. The tumors can recur, and approximately 10% of patients with NF1 develop malignant peripheral nerve sheath tumors resulting from malignant transformation of a neurofibroma.

Fat Tumors: Lipoma

Lipomas are the most common benign soft tissue tumor; however, they are relatively uncommon in the foot and

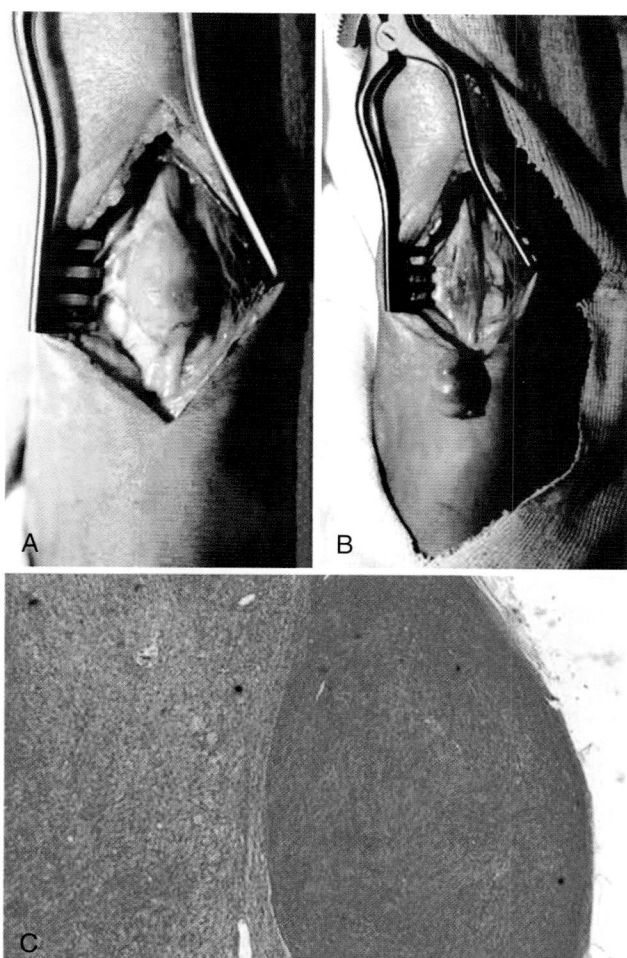

Figure 18-5 **A,** Schwannoma on the dorsal surface of the ankle. **B,** Lesion removed, leaving nerve fibers intact. **C,** Low-power photomicrograph showing admixture of spindle and round cells with palisading of the spindle cell nuclei.

ankle, likely because of the paucity of fat in this area. Lipomas can occur in the soft tissue, muscle, or bone. Most lipomas of the foot are located in the subcutaneous tissue. Those affecting bone are discussed in a later section. The lipoma mass is usually soft, nontender, mobile, and asymptomatic unless it compresses local tissue. Radiographs reveal a well-marginated, fatlike density with rare calcification secondary to fat necrosis. MRI is usually diagnostic because lipomas will be isointense to fat on all sequences, including fat suppression. Histologic analysis usually demonstrates mature fat. Numerous histologic subtypes have been described, including angiolipoma[77] and spindle cell lipoma.[117] Subtype does not affect management. Treatment consists of marginal excision of symptomatic lesions, and local recurrence is infrequent. The term "atypical lipoma" is frequently encountered in the literature and describes a lipoma with more aggressive histologic features, which does not meet the criteria for liposarcoma. This entity is still treated with marginal

excision, but clinical and, if necessary, imaging follow-up is recommended to assess for recurrence.

Synovial Tumors and Tumor-like Conditions
GANGLION
The ganglion is the product of mucoid degeneration in an area of the joint capsule or tendon sheath. They may occur at any age. As previously noted, ganglia more commonly occur on the dorsum of the foot. Ganglia can remain stable, wax and wane in size, or spontaneously rupture and resolve. Plain films are usually of little help unless underlying arthritic changes are seen in the joint adjacent to the lesion. Ultrasound and MRI of ganglion cysts have characteristic features; however, these modalities are often unnecessary to make the diagnosis. A history of waxing and waning size, location over a joint or tendon, and transillumination on physical examination may establish the diagnosis without resorting to advanced imaging. Aspiration, with identification of the typical mucinous fluid, may also be used to diagnose the lesion. The patient should be counseled that most ganglion cysts recur after aspiration.

Most ganglion cysts are treated with reassurance and observation. Symptomatic lesions are treated with marginal excision of the entire cyst and surrounding degenerative joint capsule or tendon sheath (Fig. 18-6). Patients should be advised that the ganglion cyst may recur or a new cyst may develop. A recent series of 53 operatively treated cases with minimum 2-year follow-up identified a 6% recurrence rate.[3] Thirty-five of 53 ganglia were dorsal, and 30 of the cases arose from a tendon sheath rather than a joint. All three of the recurrences occurred from tendon-based lesions. The authors cautioned that removal of all degenerative peritendinous tissue is more difficult than removal and closure of the articular-based stalk associated with joint ganglia.[3]

GIANT CELL TUMOR OF TENDON SHEATH
As its name implies, the giant cell tumor of tendon sheath (GCTTS) often arises from the synovial lining of tendon sheaths. This lesion is found more commonly in the hand than the foot.[183] An early series from the Mayo clinic found only 4 of 118 lesions in the foot.[89] The largest series studying GCTTSs in children identified 14 cases in the hand and 12 cases in the foot.[71] Most lesions manifest initially as small, painless masses that slowly enlarge (Fig. 18-7). The lesions can invade adjacent structures and produce mechanical pain and inflammation as they enlarge. There have also been case reports of associated deformity, including hallux valgus, resulting from mass effect of the lesion.[95] MRI has a characteristic appearance of low T1 and low T2 signal (dark/dark).[88] Histologically, they are composed of fibrous stroma with giant cells and cholesterol-laden histiocytes.

Surgical resection is recommended for symptomatic lesions. A 2002 series of 17 cases from England found the forefoot more commonly involved than the hindfoot; there was no predilection for plantar versus dorsal.[72]

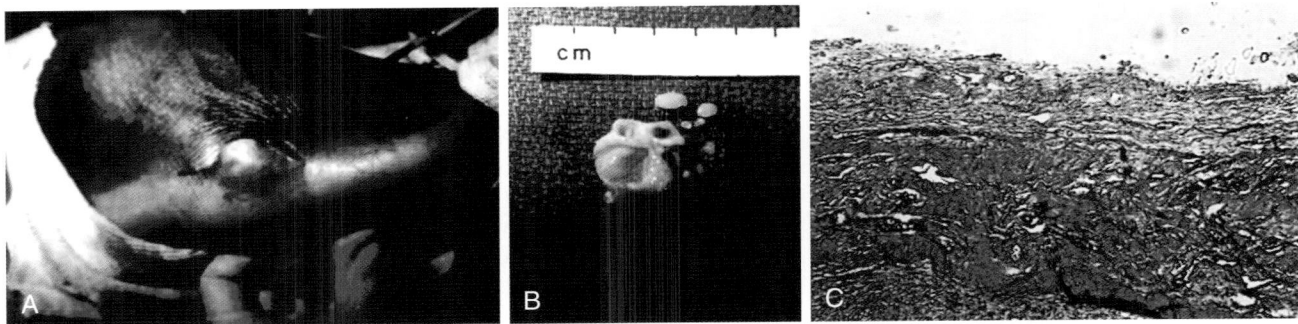

Figure 18-6 **A,** Ganglion arising from the fifth metatarsocuboid joint. **B,** Gross specimen consisting of a fibrous capsule and several "rice" bodies that were contained within the capsule. **C,** Representative section demonstrating a fibrous capsule with collagenous matrix and vascular tissue, all with benign features.

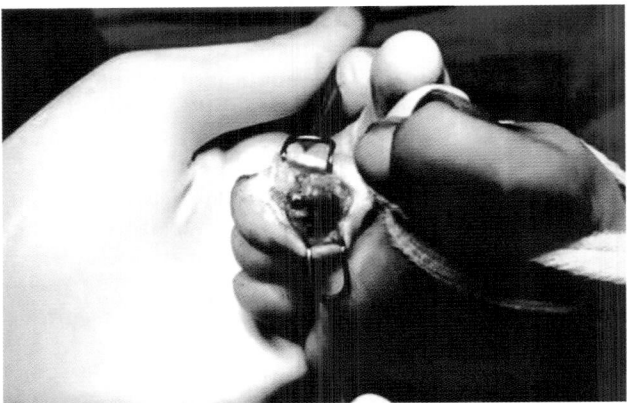

Figure 18-7 This lesion manifested as a small, painful mass on the flexor side of the third toe. Giant cell tumors of the tendon sheath have a characteristic dark red to brown color.

Fifteen cases had local excisions, one had wide excision, and one small toe was amputated. In contrast to series of GCTTS of the hand in which recurrence rates of 10% to 20% are common, the authors had no local recurrences in their foot and ankle series.[72] The authors believed that frequent use of MRI to define the extent of the GCTTS lesions was useful in obtaining complete excision and a low recurrence rate.

PIGMENTED VILLONODULAR SYNOVITIS

Pigmented villonodular synovitis (PVNS) most often occurs around joints but can also occur around periarticular tendon sheaths and bursal linings. In a recent series from the Massachusetts General Hospital, the foot and ankle were the second most common sites after the knee.[112] PVNS manifests as an intermittent swelling, often with minimal discomfort, and without a history of antecedent trauma. Joint aspiration reveals bloody or brownish fluid and frequently does not appreciably reduce the swelling because of the residual thickening of the capsule. Radiographs may demonstrate an effusion, and longstanding involvement may cause bone erosion or degenerative changes within the affected joint. Histologically,

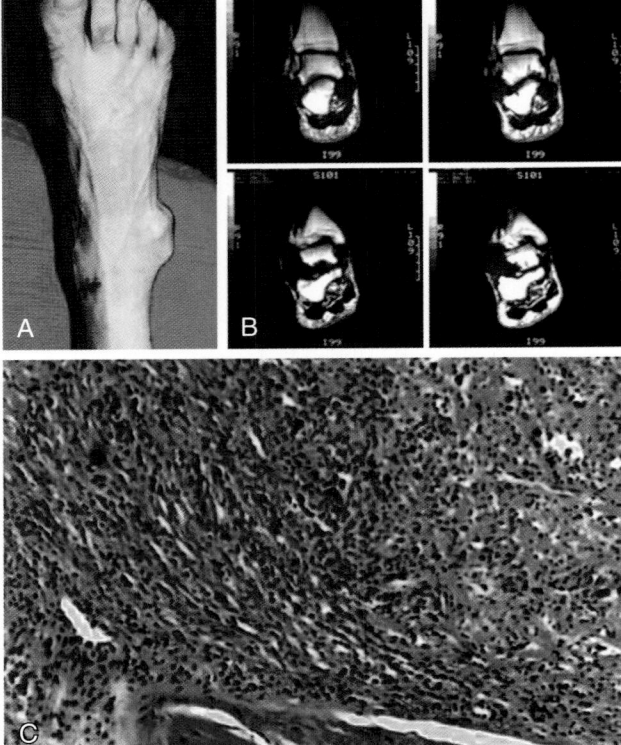

Figure 18-8 **A,** Patient presented with a mass primarily located in the area of the sinus tarsi. **B,** Magnetic resonance imaging demonstrates extension of the lesion into the ankle joint as well as unrecognized medial subtalar involvement. Surgery confirmed the presence of pigmented villonodular synovitis. **C,** Medium-power view demonstrating a dense collagenous stroma, with deeper cells containing brown pigment characteristic of hemosiderin.

PVNS is identical to GCTTS; therefore the two entities are distinguished by their anatomic locations. Similar to GCTTS, PVNS has a characteristic MRI appearance of low T1 and low T2 signal (dark/dark).[87] MRI is often diagnostic and is very useful in defining the extent of the disease (Fig. 18-8).

When the lesion is symptomatic or has radiographic evidence of progressive joint destruction, synovectomy is the treatment of choice. Synovectomy can be performed arthroscopically or open, depending on the location and extent of involvement. As one would expect, PVNS localized to one area of a joint has a lower recurrence rate than diffuse disease. A series from England reported no recurrences after seven resections of localized disease, but both cases of diffuse disease had recurrence.[18] PVNS is one of the few benign soft tissue tumors for which many authors advocate the use of radiation. A series from the Los Angeles Orthopaedic Hospital reported use of radiation for four cases of recurrent disease, with no further recurrence at an average of 3.5 years.[25] Radiation has also been advocated for treatment of severe primary PVNS.[160] Ultimately, arthroplasty or fusion may be required for severely affected joints.

SYNOVIAL CHONDROMATOSIS

Synovial chondromatosis results from chondral metaplasia within the synovial tissue. This tumor has a peak incidence in early adult life and a male-to-female ratio of 2:1. Greater than 50% of cases occur around the knee, but synovial chondromatosis can occur in the foot and ankle.[2] In a Mayo clinic series, only 8 cases of foot and ankle synovial chondromatosis were identified over 36 years.[69] On gross examination, multiple cartilaginous and osteocartilaginous nodules are embedded in the synovium, often with additional free loose bodies in the joint. Microscopically, these nodules are composed of cartilage with varying degrees of calcification. Radiographs show variable amounts of speckled calcifications, depending on the maturity of the lesions, and often more disease is present than radiographs indicate because of numerous uncalcified nodules (Fig. 18-9). MRI effectively demonstrates the uncalcified loose bodies and may better define the extent of disease.

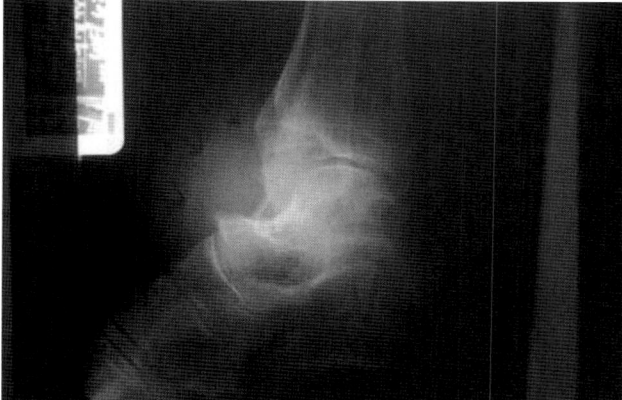

Figure 18-9 Patient with a mass over the anterior ankle. Plain radiograph demonstrates a soft tissue mass and erosion of the talus. At surgery, the ankle was filled with uncalcified nodules of synovial chondromatosis that were not apparent on radiographic examination.

Treatment of symptoms consists of synovectomy and removal of the loose bodies from the joint. This can often be accomplished arthroscopically, and use of accessory posterior portals for synovial chondromatosis resection in the ankle has been reported.[22] Recurrence occurred in four of eight patients in the Mayo Clinic series, with two patients ultimately requiring amputation for severely symptomatic recurrent disease.[69] A Massachusetts General Hospital series of five patients reported no recurrences after resection.[198] Persistent, long-standing synovial chondromatosis may lead to severe degenerative arthritis requiring arthroplasty or fusion. Isolated case reports of malignant transformation to low-grade chondrosarcoma exist, including one of the patients in the Mayo Clinic series.[69]

Metabolic Deposition Lesions
XANTHOMA OF TENDON

Tendon xanthomas result from the deposition of low-density lipoprotein in tendon tissue, where it undergoes oxidation and uptake by macrophages.[178] Xanthomatous deposits can develop in tendons as an expression of essential familial hypercholesterolemia or sporadic hypercholesterolemia. The Achilles tendon is the most commonly affected tendon. Clinically, xanthoma manifests as a painful fusiform swelling, which may be mistaken for Achilles tendinosis or tendonitis. Xanthomas have characteristic, although not pathognomonic, appearance on both ultrasound and MRI.[27] Debulking of the lesion has been reported to reduce pain but is technically difficult because of the infiltrative nature of the process, which involves the full complement of the tendon.[178] Postoperative protection to avoid rupture is recommended. Most importantly, the foot and ankle surgeon should check cholesterol levels and refer the patient for treatment of the associated hypercholesterolemia.[27] Effective treatment of the metabolic condition is not only important to treat the xanthoma but may prevent cardiac manifestations of the disease.

TOPHACEOUS GOUT

Gout results from the deposition of uric acid crystals in joints and soft tissues. The management of gouty arthritis is addressed elsewhere in this text. Gouty tophi manifest as soft tissue masses, usually adjacent to joints and bursae. They most frequently occur in patients with poorly controlled gout, but they can be the presenting manifestation of the disease. History and physical examination are often adequate for diagnosis in patients with known gout. Radiographs often demonstrate soft tissue calcification and gouty arthritis of the adjacent joint (Fig. 18-10). MRI is nonspecific,[199] and CT may be used to quantify associated bone erosion[44] but is not needed for diagnosis. A series of 45 surgically treated gouty tophi from New Zealand found the foot to be the most frequent site to require tophus excision for mechanical symptoms.[94] Eight surgeries from the series were performed to differentiate tophaceous gout from tumor. Although surgery is

Table 18-13 Malignant Soft Tissue Tumors of the Foot and Ankle

Tumor	Surgery	Radiation	Chemotherapy	Metastatic Potential
High-grade soft tissue sarcomas*	Wide margin; sentinel node biopsy if CARES tumor	Usually given; preoperative or postoperative debated	Given for metastatic and some stage 3 diagnoses	High; lung, bone, lymphatics in CARES tumors
Low-grade soft tissue sarcomas†	Wide margin; other adjuvants often unnecessary	Often given postoperative for close margins	Rarely given	Low; lung, bone
Rhabdomyosarcoma	Wide margin after neoadjuvant chemotherapy	Radiosensitive tumor but often not needed	Neoadjuvant and adjuvant routinely used	High; lung, lymphatics
Kaposi sarcoma	Surgery usually not indicated	Given for palliation of symptomatic diagnosis	Frequently used	Systemic condition
Melanoma	Wide margin and sentinel node biopsy	Rarely given in the foot	Frequently used	High; lymphatics
Squamous cell carcinoma	Wide margin	Rarely needed	Rarely needed	Low; locally aggressive
Basal cell carcinoma	Marginal excision	Unnecessary	Unnecessary	Low
Soft tissue metastases	Palliative resections only	Given for palliation of symptomatic diagnosis	Given for primary disease	Systemic condition

CARES, clear cell sarcoma, angiosarcoma, rhabdomyosarcoma, epithelioid sarcoma, synovial sarcoma.
*High-grade soft tissue sarcomas arising in the foot include synovial sarcoma, pleomorphic sarcoma, epithelioid sarcoma, clear cell sarcoma, liposarcoma (dedifferentiated, myxoid, or round cell), angiosarcoma, high-grade malignant peripheral nerve sheath tumor, and leiomyosarcoma.
†Low-grade soft tissue sarcomas arising in the foot and ankle include myxofibrosarcoma, dermatofibrosarcoma protuberans, low-grade liposarcoma, hemangioendothelioma, and low-grade malignant peripheral nerve sheath tumor.

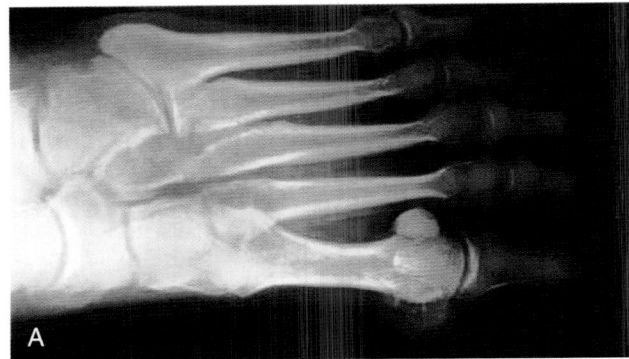

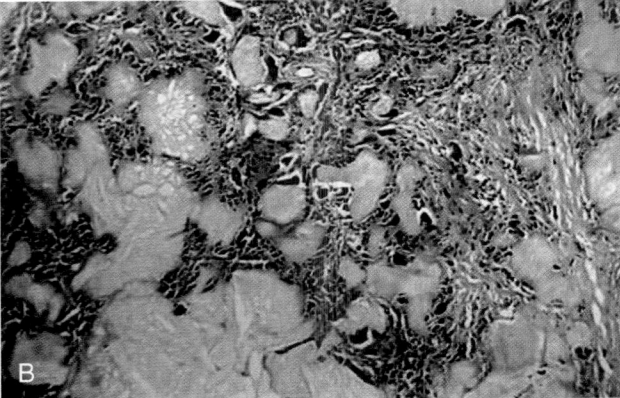

Figure 18-10 A, Subcutaneous gouty tophi. **B,** Sectioned tophus showing the urate crystals, which are lightly stained, surrounded by inflammatory cells and large macrophages, which are the most deeply stained.

beneficial for treatment of mechanically symptomatic or infected lesions, rheumatologic referral and treatment of the underlying metabolic condition is the mainstay of treatment.

Malignant Soft Tissue Tumors

Soft Tissue Sarcoma

Soft tissue sarcomas have an overall annual incidence of 5.9 per 100,000 in the United States, as measured in the Surveillance Epidemiology and End Results (SEER) database.[62] This incidence increases from 0.9 per 100,000 at age younger than 10 years to 18.2 per 100,000 at age older than 70 years.[62] Extremity soft tissue sarcomas comprise 32% of all sarcomas in the SEER database, and foot sarcomas account for only a small percentage of the extremity tumors.[62] Sarcomas are divided among numerous histologic subtypes; some of those more common in the foot are listed in Table 18-13. Synovial sarcoma is the most common soft tissue sarcoma of the foot. Epithelioid and clear cell sarcomas also disproportionately present in the foot. Rhabdomyosarcoma is overall the most common soft tissue sarcoma of children and the most common to present in the pediatric foot and ankle.[96] The more aggressive alveolar rhabdomyosarcoma subtype tends to occur in the foot and ankle and is associated with higher mortality.[152] Accordingly, in children, soft tissue masses of the foot and ankle should be discriminately evaluated with advanced imaging if they are not consistent with ganglion cysts or vascular malformations, based upon routine investigations.

Despite their rarity and varied histologic subtypes, the treatment principles for soft tissue sarcomas of the foot are relatively uniform. Suspicious lesions should be evaluated with history, physical examination, local imaging, staging studies, and biopsy, as described at the beginning of this chapter. Like other sarcomas, foot soft tissue sarcomas are best treated at centers experienced with these rare pathologies. Two recent studies have shown that unplanned excision of foot sarcomas may lead to unnecessarily morbid secondary procedures, including amputations in cases that may have otherwise been treated with limb salvage.[98,175] The need for adjuvant treatment is determined by the results of biopsy and staging. Most high-grade lesions require adjuvant radiation for local control if limb salvage is used. Chemotherapy is used for some localized high-grade soft tissue sarcomas and most metastatic soft tissue sarcomas.

The goal of soft tissue sarcoma surgery of the foot is attainment of a wide (preferably R0, but at a minimum R1) resection. Surgical resection without adjuvant treatment is often all that is required for low-grade soft tissue sarcomas (see Table 18-13). The specific surgical approach is dictated by the location and size of the tumor. Free tissue transfer is often required for coverage when limb salvage is performed.[42,98] Numerous flaps have been described for this purpose, with radial forearm fasciocutaneous, gracilis, and latissimus flaps among the most common. Although lymphatic metastases are rare among the majority of soft tissue sarcomas, several subtypes more commonly found in the foot do have lymphatic spread.[150] Sentinel lymph node biopsy should be considered in cases of synovial sarcoma, epithelioid sarcoma, rhabdomyosarcoma, and clear cell sarcoma.[5] The choice between limb salvage and amputation for soft tissue sarcomas of the foot and ankle is complex because of competing concerns, including recurrence risk, duration and intensity of treatment, function, and cosmesis.[61] Amputation often obviates the need for radiation therapy, reduces the complexity and number of surgical procedures required, and may decrease the risk of local recurrence. These advantages must be weighed against the functional and cosmetic consequences of amputation. A European study of 124 patients compared amputation with limb salvage for foot sarcomas, using a validated quality of life instrument; the study failed to identify a significant difference between the two groups.[200] The role of radiotherapy versus amputation remains contentious[96]; however, an emphasis on maximizing function without compromising the oncologic outcome should be the guiding tenet.

Kaposi sarcoma involving the foot warrants special discussion because of its unique presentation, histology, and treatment. Kaposi sarcoma is caused by human herpes virus 8 (HHV8) and most frequently presents in immunocompromised patients. It arises from endothelial tissues of blood and lymph vessels and is therefore not considered to be a true sarcoma by many.[180] It often presents on the skin of the feet as bluish skin papules. Treatment of the underlying immunosuppression is the mainstay of treatment for most patients. Kaposi sarcoma is a systemic condition, but patients may be functionally

limited because of symptomatic lesions of their feet. Foot and ankle surgeons should understand that surgical resection of these lesions is generally not beneficial. Palliative radiation therapy is efficacious for symptomatic foot involvement.[76]

Malignant Melanoma

Melanoma is more common than soft tissue sarcoma, with an incidence of 26.3 per 100,000 non-Hispanic whites in 2004.[107] Melanoma incidence is also increasing worldwide, and the rate increased by an average of 3.1% per year between 1992 and 2004 in the United States.[107] Foot and ankle melanomas are more frequent than those of the hand but still account for only a small percentage of overall melanoma incidence in white populations.[53] Foot melanomas make up a higher proportion of overall melanoma incidence among nonwhites.[53] The sole is the most common location of foot melanoma, followed by the dorsal foot and then the subungual area.[53]

Poorer survival rates have been reported for patients with foot and ankle melanomas. Fortin et al[67] identified a 60% 5-year survival for foot and ankle melanomas in a series of 60 patients. Walsh et al[184] reported a 52% 5-year survival for 37 foot and ankle melanoma patients compared with an 84% 5-year survival for 111 patients with melanomas at other lower-extremity sites. Both groups concluded that these patients tend to present with advanced tumor stage and depth. This underscores the problem of early recognition compared with melanomas at other sites. The plantar surface of the foot and the subungual areas are relatively inconspicuous to the patient. The ABCDEs of *Asymmetry*, *Border* irregularity, *Color* variegation, *Diameter*, and *Evolution* (Table 18-14) raise suspicion for melanoma in pigmented skin lesions. An even higher index of suspicion is required for foot lesions, and the mnemonic CUBED (*Color*, *Uncertain* diagnosis, *Bleeding*, *Enlargement*, and *Delay* in healing) was recently proposed to assist with identifying foot lesions more likely to be melanomas (see Table 18-14).[26]

Table 18-14 Mnemonic Devices Used to Assist in the Diagnosis of Melanoma: ABCDE and CUBED

Asymmetry	One half of lesion not identical to the other
Border	Irregular, ragged, or indistinct
Color	Multiple colors
Diameter	Greater than 6 mm
Evolution	Any change in size, shape, or color
Color	Lesion where any part is not skin colored
Uncertainty	Any lesion without definite diagnosis
Bleeding	Any bleeding including "chronic granulation tissue"
Enlargement	Lesion deteriorates or becomes larger despite treatment
Delay	Delay in healing beyond 2 months

Modified from Bristow IR, de Berker DA, Acland KM, et al: Clinical guidelines for the recognition of melanoma of the foot and nail unit, *J Foot Ankle Res* 3:25, 2010.
Biopsy or refer patient when any two CUBED criteria are present.

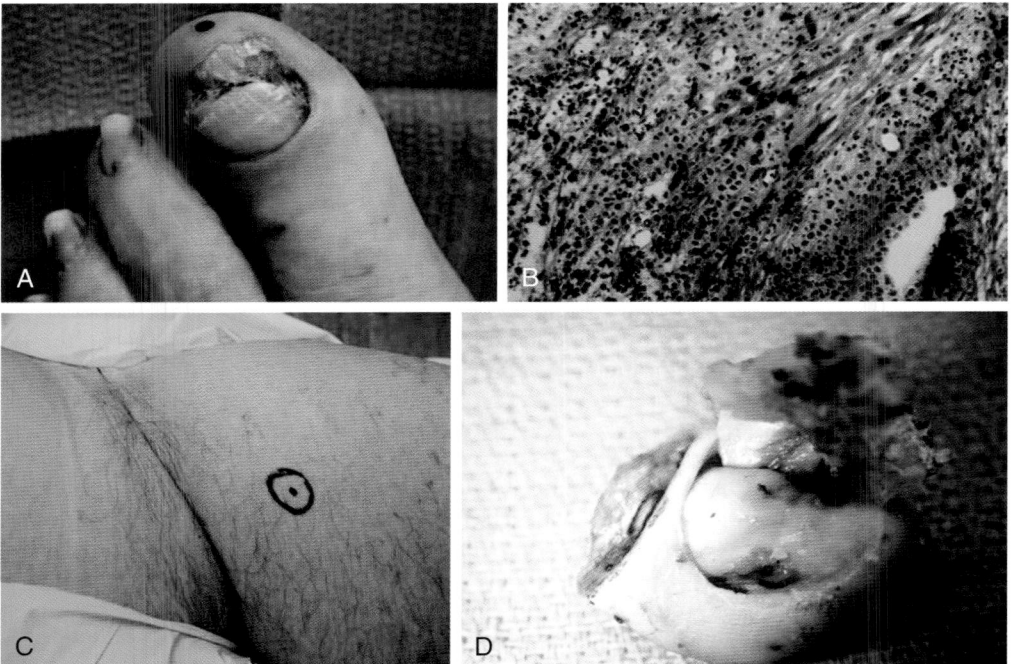

Figure 18-11 **A,** Preoperative clinical picture of a chronic nonhealing lesion of the great toe initially thought to be infection; after removal of the nail and biopsy, the lesion was consistent with melanoma. **B,** Section of tumor showing infiltration of tumor cells containing large amounts of melanin. **C,** Sentinel node biopsy site. **D,** Amputated specimen showing the lesion under the nail bed.

Subungual lesions are notoriously difficult to diagnose. Ominous features that should raise the suspicion of melanoma include spontaneous nail liftoff or nail loss attributed to trauma that fails to regenerate a new nail, nail bed pigmentation that spills into the nail fold (the Hutchinson sign), and de novo nail bed pigmentation that fails to migrate distally with time (Fig. 18-11). In addition, any nonhealing plantar ulceration in a patient without a predisposing condition (e.g., neuropathy) should be approached with a high index of suspicion, and biopsy should be the rule rather than the exception.

Surgical treatment is determined by site, depth, and stage of the lesions.[67] This can vary from wide local excision with skin grafting to amputation. The role of sentinel lymph node biopsy in the treatment of melanoma is well established.[16] Chemotherapy, radiation, isolated limb perfusion, and immunotherapy are all potential treatment options for advanced cases of melanoma. Like sarcomas, melanoma is best managed by multidisciplinary teams experienced with the condition. The foot and ankle surgeon must be familiar with the features of melanoma and its treatment.

Squamous and Basal Cell Carcinoma

Basal cell carcinoma is the most common cancer in the United States (1 in 200 individuals per year), and squamous cell carcinoma is the second most common.[141] Both occur most frequently in sun-exposed areas of the body and are more frequent in fair-skinned individuals. The

foot and ankle are less frequently affected than the face and upper extremities. Although these entities are more frequently treated by dermatologists and primary care physicians, foot and ankle surgeons may encounter these lesions in the treatment of chronic wounds or the evaluation superficial soft tissue masses. A Marjolin ulcer refers to the development of skin cancer, typically aggressive squamous cell carcinoma, in a chronic wound. Although it was initially described in burns, numerous associations, including traumatic wounds, diabetic wounds, and osteomyelitis, have been described.[92] A 1996 study from Australia identified 55 malignant skin lesions associated with chronic leg ulcers and a rate of 2.2 skin cancers per 100 leg ulcers.[195] A recent prospective study from Europe identified 10.4% skin cancer frequency among patients with chronic leg ulcers.[162] The authors of this study concluded that ulcers that fail to respond to 3 months of treatment should be biopsied.

Once the diagnosis of basal or squamous cell carcinoma of the skin is established, the treatment is excision. Squamous cell carcinoma tends to be more locally aggressive, and a wider margin is therefore advocated.[83] Skin grafting or even free tissue transfer may be required in some cases. Mohs micrographic surgery is another alternative that permits real-time microscopic analysis of the resection margins, facilitating preservation of uninvolved tissue. Basal cell carcinoma tends to be more superficial and less locally aggressive. Superficial "shave biopsies," or even topical medication treatment, have been advocated for basal cell carcinomas.[34,141]

Soft Tissue Metastases

Soft tissue metastases to the foot are very uncommon. A study from Ohio State University reviewed 118 cases of soft tissue metastases over a 30-year period and found only 2 to have occurred in the leg and 1 in the foot.[142] Radiation therapy or surgical resection of symptomatic metastatic soft tissue lesions are good palliative options in these rare cases.

Benign Bone Tumors and Tumor-like Conditions

General Principles

In addition to the previously addressed principles of biopsy and surgical technique, several special considerations specific to bone tumors merit discussion before review of individual benign bone pathologies. Curettage is a commonly used treatment for many benign bone tumors. Foot and ankle surgeons must be aware that curettage refers to several different procedures, ranging from indirect[30] or endoscopically assisted[197] curettage through small incisions to aggressive open curettage and burring through a large bone window.[20] Although debate exists as to how aggressive the curettage must be for a given pathology, there is general agreement that indolent, less locally aggressive conditions, such as simple bone cysts, require less extensive curettage, whereas more aggressive pathologies, such as giant cell tumor of bone, require more extended curettage. Appropriate instrumentation, including straight and angled curettes of various sizes, small osteotomes for creating the bone window, and a high-speed burr with multiple tip options facilitates effective curettage. Numerous adjuvant therapy techniques to

remove residual microscopic disease after curettage have been advocated. Phenol,[55] hydrogen peroxide,[10] liquid nitrogen,[17] argon beam ablation,[43] and bone cement[10] have all been advocated as methods to decrease the risks of local recurrence after curettage. Unfortunately, there is little evidence to support one technique over another. Surgeons should be aware that the phenol may burn soft tissues if they are inadvertently exposed to it, and liquid nitrogen may increase the risk of postoperative fracture.[17] Many centers advocate the use of high-speed burring without the use of additional adjuvants.[20,143]

Reconstruction after curettage is another area of considerable debate and practice variation. As previously mentioned, many advocate the use of bone cement after curettage because it provides immediate stability, and its thermal effects during curing may act as an adjuvant. However, cement has no ability to remodel and may diminish the strength of adjacent bone through stress shielding. A retrospective study of 330 giant cell tumors of bone found that cementation was associated with a higher local recurrence rate and made subsequent surgical procedures more difficult.[70] Bone graft options are numerous and covered in greater detail in the trauma section of the text. Autogenous bone marrow injection,[30] allograft cancellous chips,[123] demineralized bone matrix,[123] and calcium sulfate pellets[52] have all been advocated in the literature. Surgeons should also be aware that many small lesions, such as those common in the forefoot, will remodel without any reconstruction. Curettage without bone grafting of foot tumors has been reported in series of enchondromas[75] and aneurysmal bone cysts.[39] Table 18-15 summarizes the benign bone tumors and tumor-like conditions addressed in the following sections.

Table 18-15 Benign Bone Tumors and Tumor-Like Conditions			
Name	Matrix	Common Locations	Local Aggressiveness and Recurrence Risk
Osteochondroma	Bone	Near physes	Low
Osteoid osteoma	Bone	Hindfoot; midfoot	Low; varies with treatment
Osteoblastoma	Bone	Talus most common	Higher than osteoid osteoma
Bizarre parosteal osteochondromatous proliferation (BPOP)	Bone	Forefoot	Moderate; higher than osteochondromas and subungual exostoses
Subungual exostosis	Bone	Distal phalanges	Low
Enchondroma	Cartilage	Forefoot	Low to moderate; varies with size, location and treatment
Chondroblastoma	Cartilage	Distal tibia; distal fibula and hindfoot	Moderate to high; requires aggressive curettage or resection
Chondromyxoid fibroma	Cartilage	Any, rare	Moderate to high; requires aggressive curettage or resection
Aneurysmal bone cyst	Cystic	Any	Moderate to high; requires aggressive curettage or resection
Giant cell tumor of bone	Giant Cells	Any	Moderate to high; requires aggressive curettage or resection
Simple bone cyst	Cystic	Calcaneus	Low to moderate; varies with size and treatment
Intraosseous lipoma	Fat	Calcaneus	Low
Intraosseous ganglia	Cystic	Hindfoot, distal tibia	Low
Fibrous dysplasia	Fibrous	Any	Low to moderate
Langerhans cell histiocytosis	Histiocytes	Any	Low to moderate; may require systemic treatment for diffuse disease

Bone-Forming Tumors
OSTEOCHONDROMA

Osteochondromas are developmental anomalies that arise from the periphery of the cartilaginous growth plates. They are composed of bone and cartilage, and their cartilage cap has all the features of a physeal growth plate. The lesion increases in size and moves away from the physeal plate with age. Growth usually ceases after skeletal maturity. Very rarely, malignant transformation can occur in the cartilage cap, giving rise to a secondary chondrosarcoma. Growth of an osteochondroma in an adult should be investigated for malignant transformation. Multiple hereditary exostosis, also called multiple osteochondromatosis, is an autosomal dominant condition affecting approximately 1 in 50,000 people.[173] Affected individuals develop numerous osteochondromas, which are more likely to create skeletal deformities and undergo malignant transformation than those developing in sporadic cases.[173]

Osteochondroma symptoms are usually caused by mechanical factors, such as difficulty with shoe wear or painful bursae. Clinically, osteochondromas manifest as a hard, fixed mass. Plain radiographs are usually diagnostic because they typically reveal a confluence of the medullary canal into the stalk of the osteochondroma (Fig. 18-12). Advanced imaging is usually unnecessary. CT may be used in surgical planning to better define the adjacent anatomy and associated deformity in the hindfoot. MRI may be used to assess thickness of the cartilage cap if there is concern of malignant transformation.

Treatment of symptomatic osteochondromas consists of simple excision. Osteochondromas are one of the few

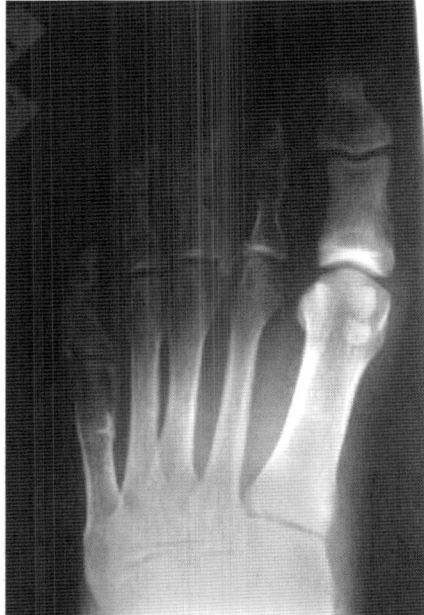

Figure 18-12 Osteochondroma of the proximal phalanx of the third toe in a patient with multiple hereditary osteochondromas.

lesions for which biopsy is generally not recommended. It is extremely difficult for pathologists to exclude low-grade chondrosarcoma based upon a small sample from the cartilage cap of an osteochondroma. A series of 23 excisions of distal tibia and fibula osteochondromas found excellent functional and symptomatic results in all patients.[36] The surgeon should ensure that the entire cartilage cap is removed and should avoid damaging the cap during excision because this may seed the surgical bed with tumor cells. Patients with multiple hereditary exostosis often develop hindfoot valgus deformities secondary to their osteochondromas.[129] Corrective osteotomies or temporary medial tibial epiphysiodesis may be required in addition to resection in order to correct the deformities.[129,164]

Extraskeletal osteochondroma is an unrelated, rare, soft tissue cartilage tumor which has a predilection for the feet and hands.[165,172] It does not arise from the physis. When symptomatic, treatment of this lesion is simple excision.

OSTEOID OSTEOMA

Osteoid osteomas account for approximately 10% of benign bone tumors and occur in males twice as frequently as in females.[8] Osteoid osteoma can occur in any bone of the foot but is more common in the hindfoot and midfoot.[166,167] It most often occurs between 5 and 25 years of age.[8] Although classically associated with a history of localized nocturnal pain relieved by NSAIDs, patients may present with activity-related pain or even an incidental traumatic episode. Radiographs often demonstrate cortical thickening but may fail to identify the small nidus at the center of the reactive bone. In a study of foot osteoid osteomas, CT was more accurate than MRI in making the diagnosis (Fig. 18-13).[167]

Although these lesions have been known to resolve spontaneously over time, most often the patient's discomfort dictates surgical intervention. The critical step in treatment is accurate identification and removal of the nidus. Traditional treatment consisted of en bloc excision, but the majority of lesions are now successfully treated with less invasive procedures, including limited curettage and radiofrequency ablation.[8] CT guidance is often a useful adjunct for these minimally invasive techniques. Some osteoid osteomas occur near the articular surface, and successful arthroscopic debridement of such lesions has been reported.[23,179] Local recurrence is rare and can be treated with repeat treatment with ablation or curettage.

OSTEOBLASTOMA

Osteoblastoma comprises approximately 3% of benign bone tumors and has a similar male predilection but slightly older age distribution than that of osteoid osteoma. Osteoblastoma is histologically identical to osteoid osteoma. It is distinguished by its larger size (greater than 1 cm) and different clinical presentation. On radiographs, osteoblastoma is larger, more radiolucent,

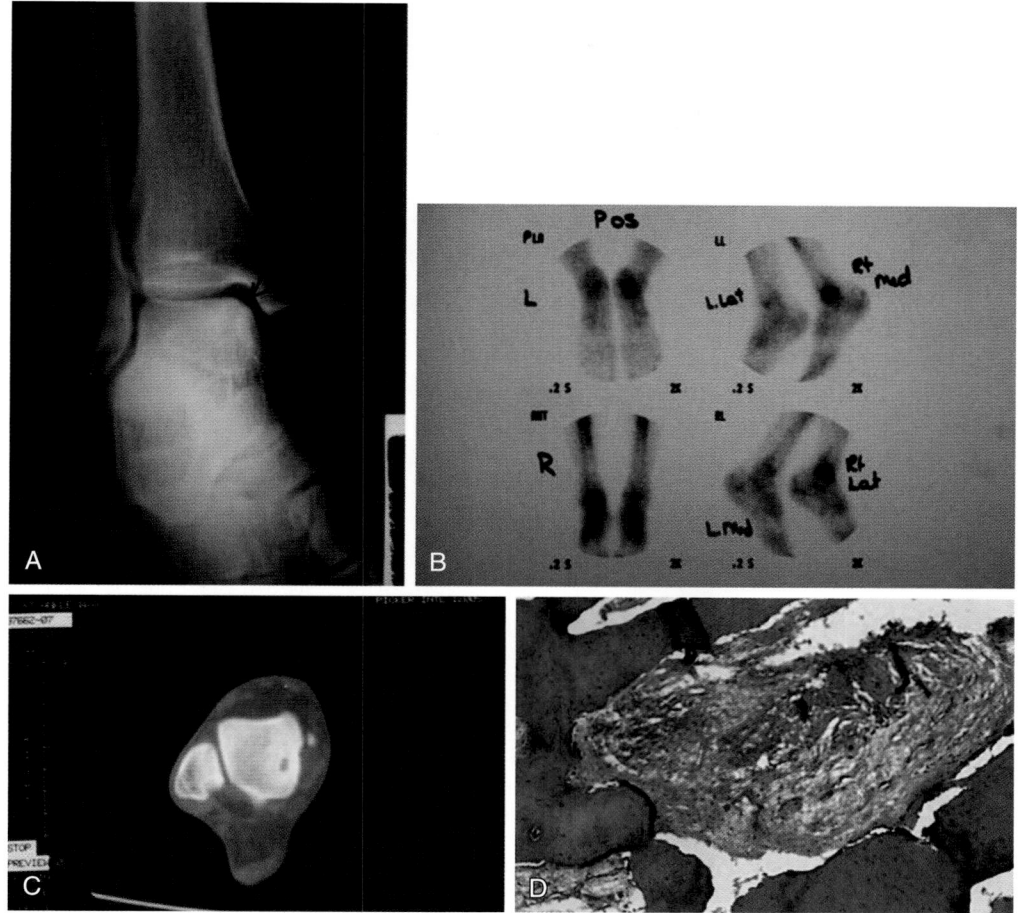

Figure 18-13 **A,** Anteroposterior radiograph shows only a faint nidus in the medial talus of an osteoid osteoma. **B,** Bone scan confirms suspicion. **C,** Computed tomography scan demonstrates nidus and adjacent halo of reactive bone. **D,** Representative histologic section showing a thickened rim of reactive bone surrounding a well-vascularized central nidus of mesenchymal tissue.

and has less reactive bone than osteoid osteoma. An Armed Forces Institute of Pathology review of 329 osteoblastomas found the foot and ankle to be the third most common site (41 cases).[174] The talus is the most common location in the foot and ankle, comprising 18 of 41 cases in the Armed Forces series.[174] Whereas osteoid osteoma is nonprogressive and may heal spontaneously, osteoblastoma is progressive and locally aggressive. Because of the larger size and more aggressive behavior, osteoblastoma treatment usually consists of extended intralesional curettage with or without bone grafting.[8] Recurrence is more common than with osteoid osteoma and may require bone resection rather than repeat curettage, depending on the extent of the disease.

BIZARRE PAROSTEAL OSTEOCHONDROMATOUS PROLIFERATION (BPOP)

BPOP (also called the Nora lesion) is a rare primary benign bone tumor with a predilection for the hands and feet. Age at presentation ranges from adolescence to the elderly; males and females are affected equally.[130] The clinical presentation often mimics that of osteochondroma with a fixed osteocartilaginous lesion of the phalanges or metatarsals. Mass effect from the lesion may cause forefoot deformities.[128] The lesion is differentiated from osteochondroma by lack of medullary continuity with the underlying bone and its distinctive histology. Bizarre, enlarged chondrocytes, which are often binucleated, differentiate BPOP lesions from osteochondromas.[119,130] Foot and ankle surgeons should be aware of this lesion because it *may be mistaken by pathologists for low-grade chondrosarcoma.* In addition, 18 of 35 (51%) BPOP lesions recurred in the original Mayo Clinic series,[130] and 6 of 22 (27%) cases recurred in a 2011 series from the United Kingdom.[15] More aggressive resection and closer clinical and radiographic follow-up than that used for osteochondromas is therefore prudent.

SUBUNGUAL EXOSTOSIS

Subungual exostosis is a benign osteochondral lesion that causes pain and nail deformity. This lesion arises from the tip of the distal phalanx and manifests as a periungual or

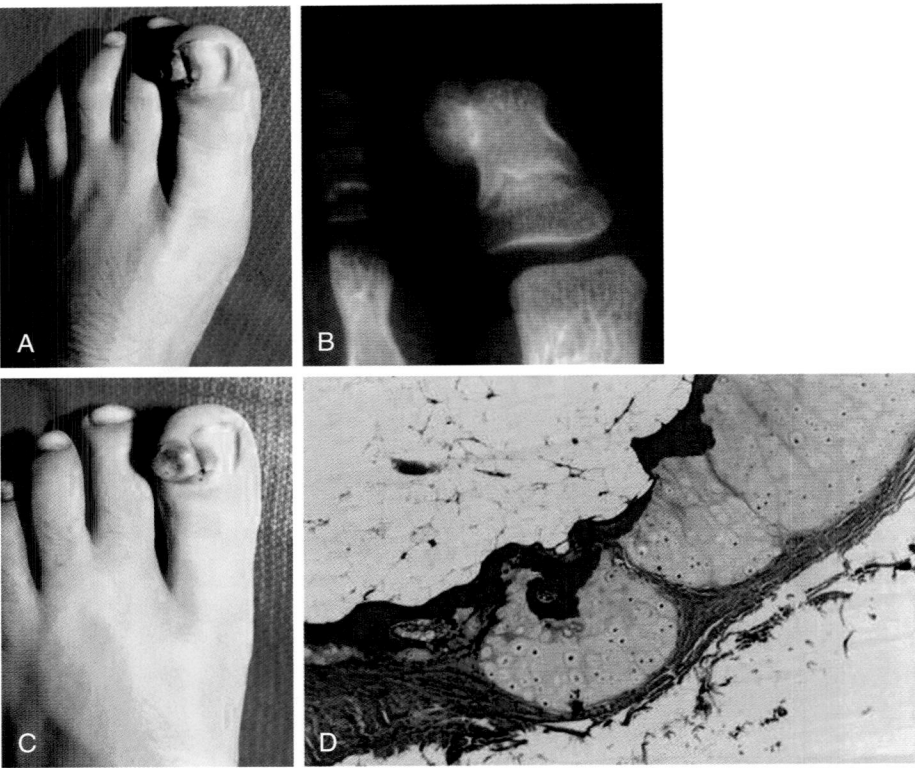

Figure 18-14 **A,** This patient had an 8-month history of pain and deformity of the lateral border of the great toe. **B,** Anteroposterior radiograph demonstrates a mature osteochondral lesion (subungual exostosis) arising from the metaphysis area of the distal phalanx. Contrast this with the radiograph of the osteochondroma in Figure 18-12. **C,** Appearance of toe after complete excision of the lesion and a portion of the overlying nail bed. **D,** Typical histopathology showing a stalk of trabecular bone with a fibrocartilaginous cap and islands of cartilage.

subungual nodule. The characteristic radiographic appearance is usually diagnostic (Fig. 18-14). Ossification varies with the maturity of the lesion. These lesions differ from osteochondromas because they are thought to be a reactive process rather than physeal growth abnormalities.[100] Excision usually requires nail removal, but recurrence rates are low, and the final cosmetic and functional results are good in the published series of these lesions.[47,100]

Cartilage-Forming Tumors
ENCHONDROMA
Enchondromas are the second most common benign bone tumor overall and the most common benign bone tumor of the foot.[134] They are often asymptomatic and incidentally identified on radiographs obtained for other reasons. When symptomatic, they are frequently associated with pathologic fractures (Fig. 18-15). Plain radiographs typically reveal a well-demarcated ovoid lesion with stippled calcifications. Advanced imaging with MRI or CT is generally unnecessary unless there is concern for malignant degeneration to low-grade chondrosarcoma. In the foot, enchondromas are most frequently located in the metatarsals. Asymptomatic lesions do not require biopsy or treatment. They should be followed with serial radiographs. One proposed follow-up regimen is repeat

radiographs at 3 months, 6 months, 1 year, and then annually.[115] Symptomatic lesions are treated by curettage and bone grafting. Small lesions do not necessarily require grafting, and reported recurrence rates are low.[75] If a pathologic fracture has occurred, immobilization until the fracture is healed, with subsequent curettage, is a common treatment. Malignant degeneration to chondrosarcoma is uncommon in general and less common in the hands and feet than in the long bones. Findings concerning for chondrosarcoma include cortical destruction, soft tissue mass, and extensive endosteal scalloping.[68] Low-grade chondrosarcoma treatment will be addressed later in the chapter.

Periosteal chondromas and extraskeletal chondromas are histologically similar to enchondromas but occur at the bone surface[140] and extraskeletal sites,[189] respectively. They are less common than enchondromas and may be excised when symptomatic. Surgeons should also be aware that there are two nonhereditary syndromes associated with development of multiple enchondromas. Ollier disease is characterized by multiple enchondromas, often most pronounced in a single extremity. Maffucci syndrome is characterized by the combination of multiple enchondromas and hemangiomas. A 2011 multicenter review from Europe identified a 40% lifetime risk of

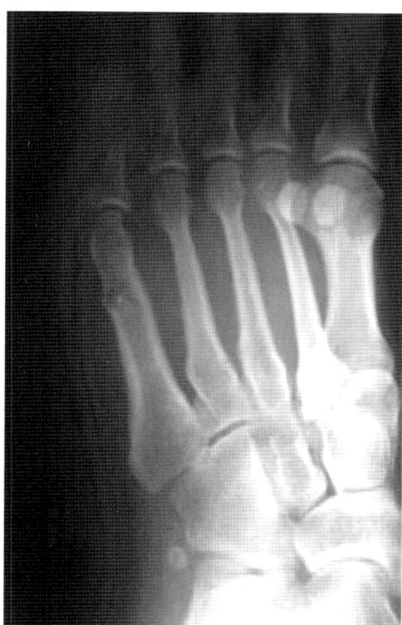

Figure 18-15 Pathologic fracture through a previously asymptomatic enchondroma of fifth metatarsal.

malignant degeneration in patients with these conditions.[181] Routine surveillance and a heightened index of suspicion for malignancy are therefore warranted in these patients.

CHONDROBLASTOMA

Chondroblastomas are cartilage-forming tumors that usually occur in the epiphyses of skeletally immature individuals. A 1997 Armed Forces Institute of Pathology review identified 35 of 322 (13%) cases as occurring in the foot.[64] Males are affected more frequently than females. The talus and calcaneus are the most commonly affected locations in the foot.[45,64,65] Oddly, chondroblastomas of the foot often present at an older age than in other locations, with the majority presenting after skeletal maturity in both the Armed Forces and Mayo Clinic series.[64,65] Presentation usually consists of pain, with associated joint discomfort and swelling secondary to the tumor's subchondral location. Radiographs reveal a subchondral lesion with a slight reactive rim that is usually radiolucent. MRI and CT provide better anatomic detail for surgical planning. MRI better delineates the articular cartilage of the adjacent joint and excludes the presence of soft tissue mass. CT better demonstrates bone detail and may be useful if there is concern for pathologic fracture. Unlike many of the previously described benign bone tumors, imaging is not diagnostic of chondroblastoma, and biopsy-proven diagnosis is essential before treatment. Curettage is the treatment of choice for most chondroblastomas. Resection and reconstruction may be technically simpler for the rare cases involving the smaller bones of the forefoot.[106,146] A 2000 review of 73 surgically treated cases from all sites of the body identified a 15%

recurrence rate; however, most recurrences were in the proximal femur.[146] Chondroblastoma, along with giant cell tumor of bone, is one of the rare benign bone tumors with metastatic potential, usually to the lung.[106] Although very rare (3 of 82 cases in the M.D. Anderson series) and usually associated with large proximal lesions, surveillance chest radiographs for 5 years are prudent.[106]

CHONDROMYXOID FIBROMA

Chondromyxoid fibromas (CMFs) are less common than enchondromas and chondroblastomas. The name is derived from the distinctive histologic appearance, which has chondroid, myxoid, and fibrous elements. The foot is reported to be the third most common site, accounting for up to 17% of cases.[131,163] CMF typically presents in adolescence and young adulthood (most cases are before age 30 years), and, like chondroblastoma, CMF affects males more than females.[163] Radiographs reveal a purely radiolucent lesion. MRI and CT may better define local anatomy for surgical planning, but no imaging findings are unique to CMF. Biopsy is required for diagnosis. Treatment usually consists of curettage, but resection with reconstruction may be considered for the smaller bones of the forefoot. Recurrence rates of 20% to 25% have been reported.[103,163] One series of 30 cases (from all sites of the body) reported that grafted lesions had a lower recurrence rate.[103]

Benign Aggressive Bone Tumors
ANEURYSMAL BONE CYST

Aneurysmal bone cysts (ABCs) have an overall annual incidence of 1.4 per million and are relatively uncommon in the foot and ankle.[102] The underlying pathophysiology of ABCs is debated, but at least some of the lesions are true neoplasms with characteristic genetic mutations.[132] Most ABCs develop in the first two decades of life and have eccentric metaphyseal locations. Females are affected slightly more often than males,[102] and the distal fibula is the most commonly affected site in the foot and ankle.[1,97] Radiographs demonstrate a radiolucent, expansile lesion with a thin shell of reactive periosteal bone (Fig. 18-16). MRI may demonstrate characteristic fluid/fluid levels within the lesion. Pathologic fractures may occur, and cortical breakthrough is often evident despite the benign nature of the tumor. Biopsy is required for diagnosis, and careful histologic examination is required to distinguish ABC from telangiectatic osteosarcoma. Treatment consists of aggressive curettage or resection if the bone is expendable (Fig. 18-17). A review of distal fibula ABCs from the Rizzoli Institute compared six curettage cases with three resections.[97] There were no recurrences in either group, and the curettage cases had fewer surgeries and complications.[97] Overall, a 20% recurrence rate has been reported for ABCs,[113] and follow-up for local recurrence is recommended.

GIANT CELL TUMOR

Giant cell tumors (GCTs) of bone usually occur in the metaphases and epiphyses or in equivalent apophysis.

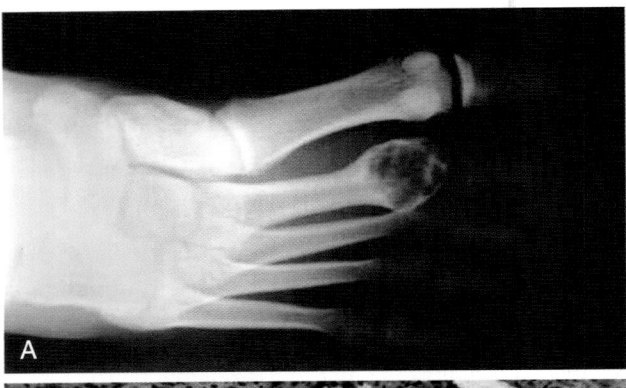

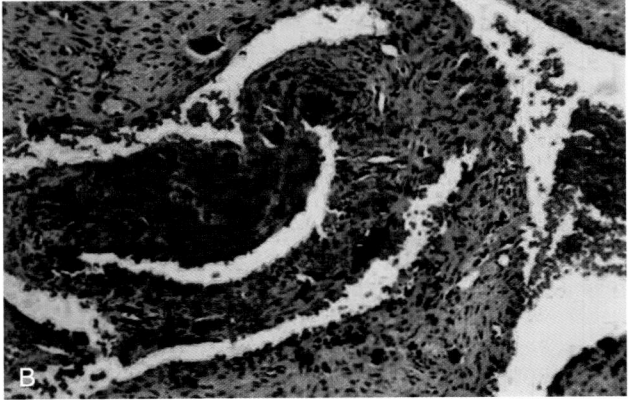

Figure 18-16 A, Aneurysmal bone cyst (ABC) derives its name from its characteristic radiographic appearance. This ABC of the second metatarsal demonstrates expansile radiolucency and shell of reactive periosteal bone typically associated with its presence. **B,** Medium-power view demonstrating vascular channels with numerous red blood cells surrounded by fibrous stroma and occasional giant cells.

Patients 20 to 40 years of age are most frequently affected, and GCTs before skeletal maturity are rare. Approximately 4% of GCTs occur in the foot and ankle; the hindfoot and distal tibia are the most commonly affected bones.[133] Localized pain and swelling are common, and pathologic fractures may occur.

Plain radiographs show a geographic, radiolucent lesion with a small rim of reactive bone. MRI and CT provide further anatomic detail (Fig. 18-18), but they are not diagnostic. Biopsy is required for diagnosis, and histologic analysis demonstrates characteristic multinucleated giant cells in a fibrous stroma. Chest radiograph or CT is recommended at presentation and in follow-up surveillance because metastatic pulmonary implantation may occur.[151,168]

Treatment is surgical with either aggressive curettage with or without adjuvants[116] or resection and reconstruction of expendable bones, such as the metatarsals.[28] As discussed previously, there is little data to support the use of specific adjuvants or grafting materials. Recurrence rates with these techniques range from 10% to 30%.[116,133] Individual cases of complex reconstructions, including the use of Illizarov frames[41] and custom tantalum

spacers,[56] have been reported. The largest series of GCT pathologic fractures reported an 84% joint salvage rate with curettage, grafting, and internal fixation.[46] This joint salvage rate was lower than patients without fracture, but the authors concluded that an attempt at joint salvage is worthwhile in most cases. Finally, the receptor activator of nuclear factor kappa-beta (RANK) ligand inhibitor denosumab has shown efficacy in a phase 2 trial of patients with giant cell tumor of bone.[176] Although not yet approved by the Food and Drug Administration (FDA) for GCT treatment, this agent may be considered for compassionate use in severe cases in which amputation or other morbid surgery is being considered.

Cystic Bone Lesions
SIMPLE BONE CYST
Simple (also called unicameral) bone cysts of the foot occur most often in the calcaneus,[139] but other locations, including the talus,[35] have been reported. Simple bone cysts are thought to be growth abnormalities rather than true neoplasms. These lesions are often incidentally found on radiographs obtained for other reasons. In contrast to unicameral cysts in long bones, which typically undergo spontaneous involution with skeletal maturity, simple bone cysts of the calcaneus often persist through adulthood (Fig. 18-19). Radiographs demonstrate a radiolucent lesion without aggressive features; SBCs frequently develop in the anterolateral aspect of the calcaneus. Advanced imaging and biopsy are usually unnecessary. Serial radiographs and clinical examination are often adequate to confirm the benign nature of the tumor. MRI, if obtained, demonstrates a homogeneous lesion with fluid signal that does not enhance with contrast.

Surgical treatment is considered for pathologic fractures and other symptomatic lesions. A wide array of treatment options, including injection of corticosteroids,[193] injection of allograft demineralized bone matrix,[51] endoscopically assisted curettage and grafting,[197] limited incision curettage and grafting,[52] and open curettage and grafting.[139] No treatment method has been shown to be clearly superior. Symptomatic relief and functional outcomes of calcaneus lesions are usually good even if there is some radiographic persistence of the cyst.[139]

INTRAOSSEOUS LIPOMA
In contrast to their soft tissue counterparts, intraosseous lipomas are very rare, but when they occur, the calcaneus is the most commonly affected bone.[29] Radiographs demonstrate a lucent lesion that frequently has central calcifications (Fig. 18-20).[29,126] Surgeons should be aware that the normal trabecular architecture of the calcaneus may be mistaken for a cyst or lipoma.[50] CT and MRI confirm the presence of fat within the lesion but are usually unnecessary. Most intraosseous lipomas are asymptomatic and identified incidentally. They can be followed with serial examinations and radiographs to confirm

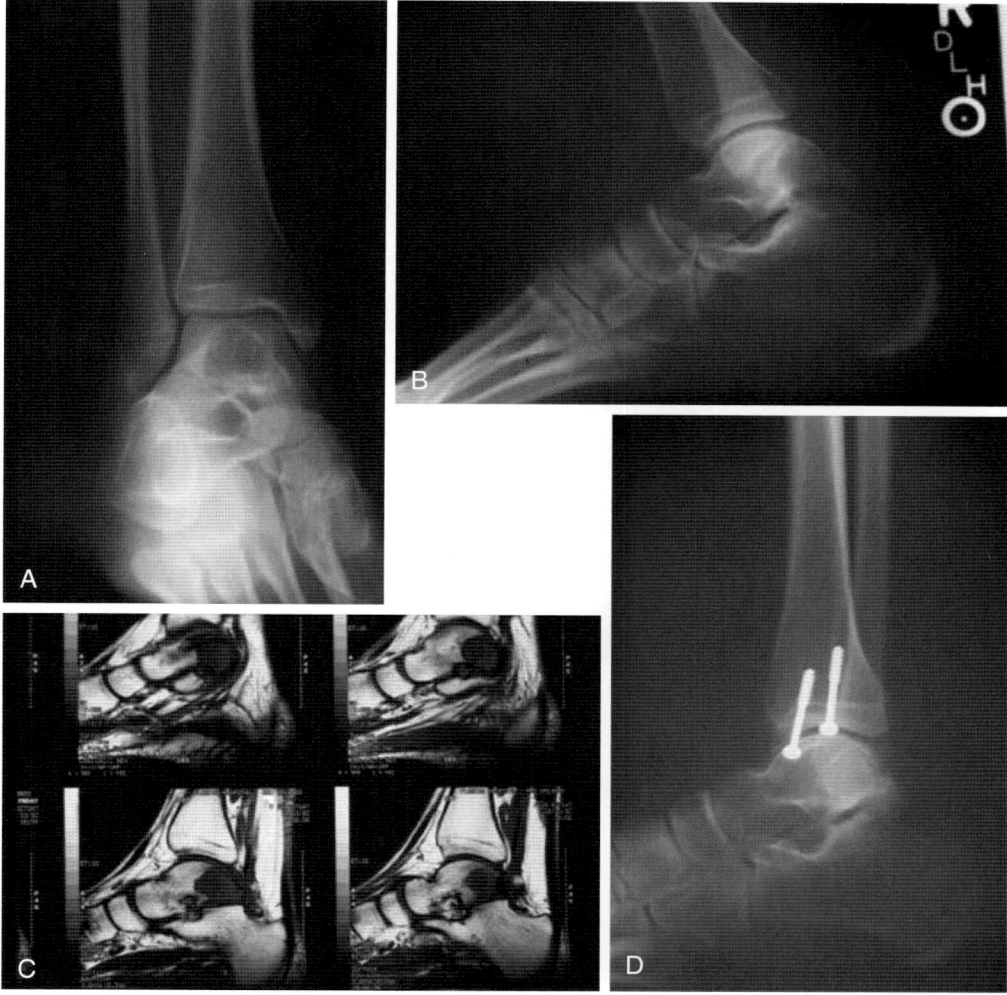

Figure 18-17 Aneurysmal bone cyst of talus. **A,** Anteroposterior radiograph. **B,** Lateral radiograph. **C,** Magnetic resonance image. **D,** Postoperative lateral radiograph demonstrates stabilization of malleolar osteotomy and appearance of the lesion after extended curettage and bone grafting.

stability. Surgery is not recommended unless there are persistent symptoms.[9] Surgical treatment consists of curettage and grafting.[74,187] Recurrence is thought to be rare, but the reported case series are too small to give an informative rate.

INTRAOSSEOUS GANGLION AND DEGENERATIVE BONE CYST

Both of these lesion occur in periarticular sites and share similar histology, defined grossly by thick, yellow cystic fluid and microscopically by a bland hypocellular fibrous lining.[80,159] Most lesions are asymptomatic and incidentally noted on radiographs, appearing as a rounded, circumscribed radiolucency with a distinct margin (Fig. 18-21). The most common site in the foot is the medial malleolus.[80,125] Historically, intraosseous ganglia have been distinguished from degenerative (subchondral) cysts based upon lack of associated degenerative joint disease and failure to communicate with the nearby joint.[80] This view has been challenged by evidence derived from modern cross-sectional imaging. A study of 45 intraosseous ganglia, diagnosed by traditional histologic and plain radiographic criteria, found that many had either articular communication or soft tissue extension when studied with MRI.[190] In addition, articular degenerative changes were far more prevalent than demonstrated by radiographs alone. The authors concluded that the distinction between these entities is semantic and based upon the clinician's impression of the degree of associated arthritis.[190]

Surgical intervention is indicated only for symptomatic lesions. Radiographs are often diagnostic, and many lesions may be followed with serial examinations and conservative treatment of the associated arthritis. Large lesions may require biopsy to rule out true neoplasms. Curettage and grafting is the preferred treatment for large intraosseous ganglia without substantial associated degenerative changes.[125] Treatment of the underlying

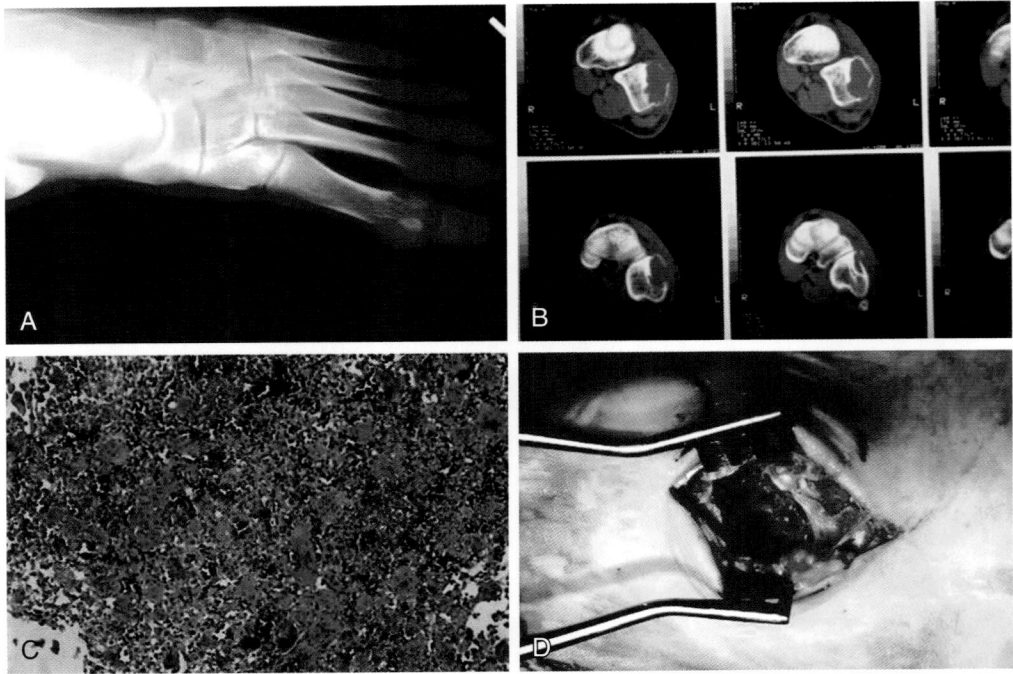

Figure 18-18 A, Radiolucent lesion of cuboid demonstrates a geographic pattern of bone loss and mild rim of reactive bone attempting to contain the lesion. This is typical of giant cell tumors. Additional differential diagnoses include aneurysmal bone cyst and cartilage lesions. **B,** Computed tomography confirms the geographic nature of the lesion and indicates loss of cortex, which should raise concern of soft tissue extension of the tumor. **C,** Low-power view of curettage showing giant cells, mononuclear stromal cells, and areas of hemorrhage. **D,** Cavity remaining after extended curettage can be treated by various methods in an attempt to decrease local recurrence.

arthritis, usually with fusion or arthroplasty, is recommended for lesions with associated degenerative disease.

EPIDERMOID INCLUSION CYST

Epidermoid inclusion cysts typically occur beneath the nail bed of the distal phalanx; they are far less common in the toes than in the fingers.[185] They are thought to result from trauma that displaces nail matrix into or adjacent to the phalanx.[185] As these ectopic cells grow, they form a keratin-lined cyst. Clinically, this cyst causes enlargement of the digit and is painful. On radiographs, it produces a radiolucency in the subungual area of the distal phalanx (Fig. 18-22). Treatment consists of confirmatory biopsy, followed by curettage with or without grafting of the lesion.[185]

Tumor-like Conditions of Bone
INFECTION

Osteomyelitis is extensively covered in Chapter 15. However, surgeons should consider bone infection in the differential of many presumed bone tumors. Classic signs and symptoms may be lacking, and radiographic changes of osteomyelitis may be subtle or nonspecific. Metaphyseal radiolucency with early periosteal elevation and a permeative radiographic appearance are good diagnostic clues (Fig. 18-23). The radiographic differential diagnosis of such lesions includes eosinophilic granuloma and Ewing sarcoma. Focal infection (Brodie abscess) may

resemble osteoid osteoma both clinically and radiographically.[169] Therefore foot and ankle surgeons are encouraged to culture presumed tumors at the time of biopsy if infection is considered a possibility. One should also remember that skin cancers may develop in chronic wounds as discussed previously.

EOSINOPHILIC GRANULOMA

Eosinophilic granuloma (Langerhans cell histiocytosis, formerly histiocytosis X) is a group of nonneoplastic proliferative disorders that most commonly affect children.[157] The precise etiology of the condition is not defined, but it is characterized histologically by the proliferation of histiocytes. Bone involvement manifests as permeative lesions affecting the skull, axial skeleton, and diaphyses of long bones.[7] Foot and ankle involvement is rare except in cases of widespread systemic disease. Treatment of isolated single-site bone involvement is usually observation because most lesions are self-limited. Treatment of systemic disease is medical, with chemotherapy or immunosuppression.

FIBROUS DYSPLASIA

Fibrous dysplasia is a developmental skeletal disease characterized by histologically immature fibrous connective tissue and poorly formed immature trabecular bone.[138] Fibrous dysplasia ranges from small, single monostotic lesions to widespread, disseminated

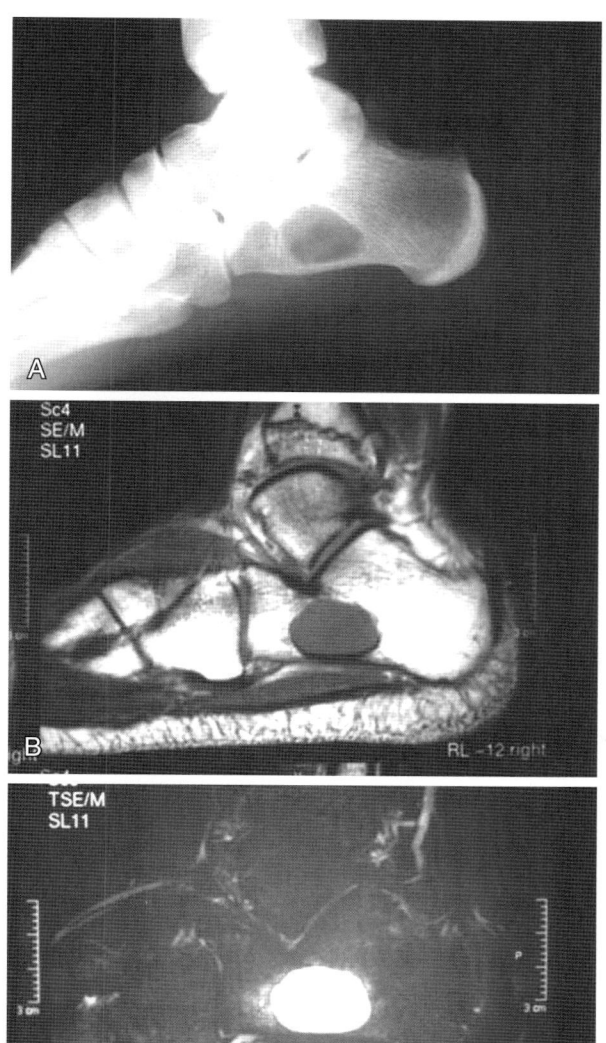

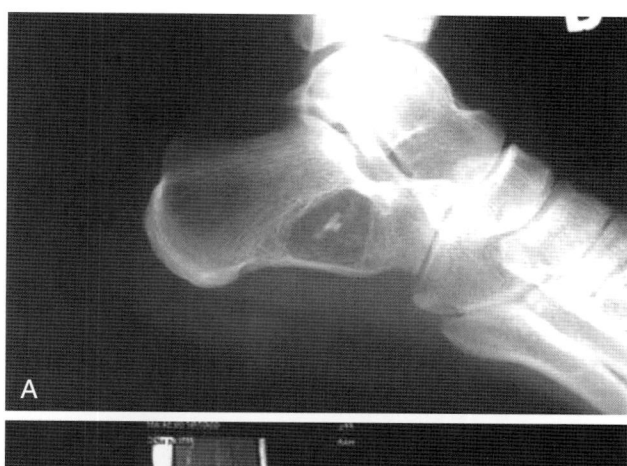

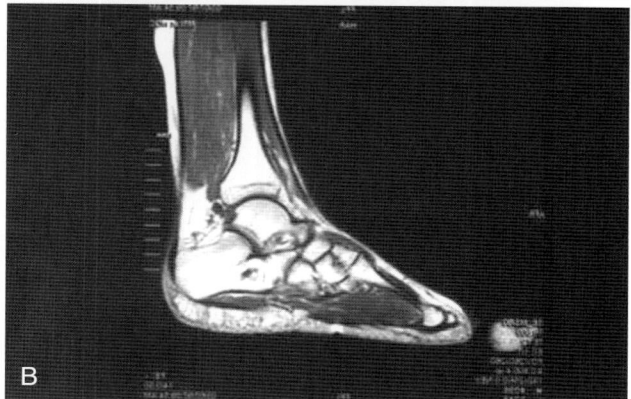

Figure 18-20 **A,** Intraosseous lipoma with central calcification. **B,** Magnetic resonance (MR) image confirms the presence of fat within the lesion. Compare this to the MR characteristics of the unicameral cyst in Figure 18-19.

Figure 18-19 **A,** Unicameral cyst of the calcaneus persisting into adulthood and discovered incidentally. **B,** T1-weighted magnetic resonance image distinguishes cyst from fat. **C,** T2-weighted image demonstrates a bright signal, confirming fluid content.

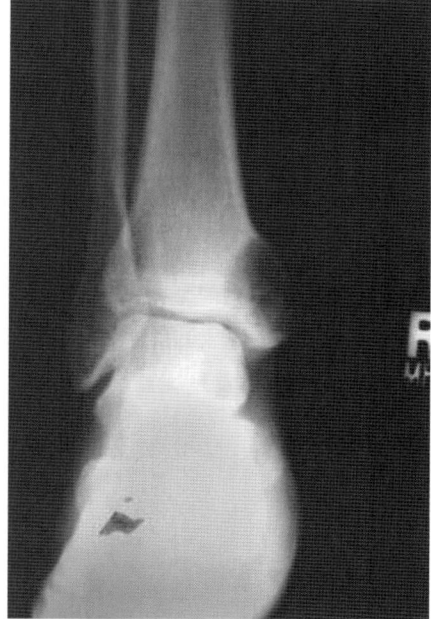

Figure 18-21 Typical location and appearance of intraosseous ganglion. In this location, giant cell tumor should be considered part of the differential diagnosis.

polyostotic lesions involving large areas of multiple bones. The characteristic radiographic picture is one of loss of trabecular detail and a homogeneous ground-glass appearance. The lesions occur most often in the metaphysis, but the changes may extend throughout the entire bone (Fig. 18-24).

The polyostotic variety is often confined to one extremity or one side of the skeleton. The lesions appear during childhood, remain active during growth, and become latent during adulthood.[138]

Clinical presentation may be incidental or secondary to pathologic fracture. It can occur as one aspect of the

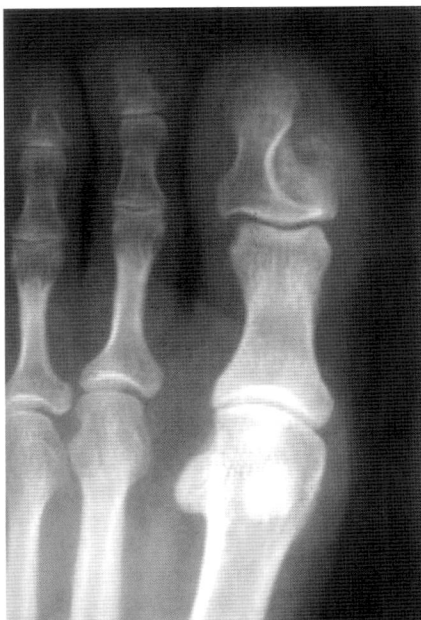

Figure 18-22 Radiograph demonstrates extrinsic erosion of the distal phalanx from an epidermoid inclusion cyst.

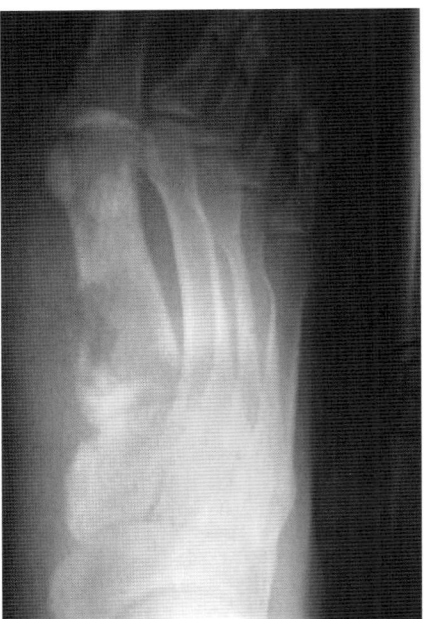

Figure 18-23 Radiograph demonstrates painful mass overlying dorsum of first metatarsal. Needle aspiration yielded gross pus, and cultures revealed *Staphylococcus aureus* infection.

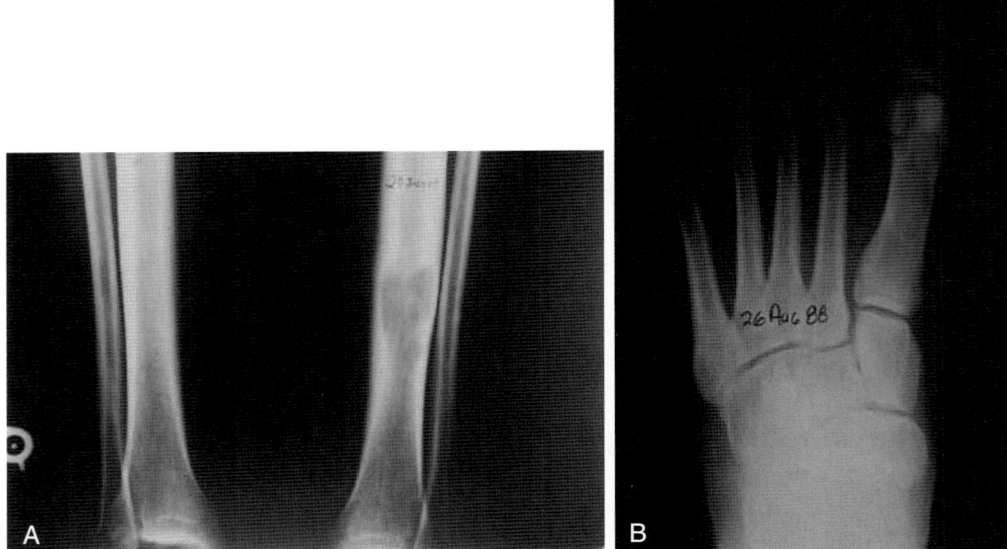

Figure 18-24 **A,** Patient with polyostotic fibrous dysplasia and involvement of the tibia. **B,** Typical ground-glass appearance in the ipsilateral first metatarsal.

Table 18-16	Malignant Bone Tumors		
Name	**Adjuvants**	**Surgical Treatment**	**Metastasis**
Chondrosarcoma	Usually None	Wide limb-sparing resection vs. amputation	Lung and bone
Osteosarcoma	Chemotherapy	Wide limb-sparing resection vs. amputation	Lung and bone
Ewing sarcoma	Chemotherapy +/− radiation	Wide limb-sparing resection vs. amputation	Lung and bone
Metastatic lesions	Dependent on primary pathology	Palliative treatment of painful lesions and fractures	−

−, Not applicable.

McCune-Albright syndrome, a combination of skeletal lesions, cutaneous lesions (café au lait spots), and precocious puberty.[138] Treatment of foot lesions is usually symptomatic, but surgery may be necessary for repetitive stress fractures or deformity. Curettage, grafting, and internal fixation are generally used.

HYPERPARATHYROIDISM (BROWN TUMOR)
Brown tumors develop as the result of bone resorption secondary to elevated levels of parathyroid hormone. These are radiolucent lesions that may be mistaken for neoplasms. Although rare in the foot and ankle,[196] surgeons should be aware of the condition and check parathyroid hormone levels if there is any clinical suspicion. Patients with known endocrinopathies or chronic renal failure are particularly at risk.[99] Treatment is medical unless a pathologic fracture requiring fixation develops.

Malignant Bone Tumors

General Principles
Primary malignant bone tumors of the foot and ankle are rare. Advances in chemotherapy have dramatically increased survival rates among patients with osteosarcoma and Ewing sarcoma. Surgery may be curative for chondrosarcomas and remains the primary method of local disease control for osteosarcoma and Ewing sarcoma. As previously discussed, all primary bone sarcomas should undergo staging preoperatively and should be followed with surveillance imaging postoperatively. Primary malignant bone tumors should be considered systemic diseases that are best treated by multidisciplinary teams. Foot and ankle surgeons should consider early referral of suspicious lesions to centers experienced with multidisciplinary management of these tumors. Table 18-16 summarizes the malignant bone tumors of the foot and ankle.

Chondrosarcoma
Chondrosarcomas are the most common primary malignant bone tumor of the foot and ankle.[38,124] A review of 2890 chondrosarcomas reported an average age of 51 years, 44.5% occurrence in the extremities, and slight male predominance.[73] In a review of 12 chondrosarcomas of the foot from the Scottish Bone Tumor Registry, 4 were hindfoot, and 8 were midfoot and forefoot. Primary chondrosarcomas present with pain or a new mass; patients with secondary chondrosarcomas may note

change in a preexisting mass. Radiographs reveal a destructive lesion, usually containing a cartilaginous matrix (Fig. 18-25). Low-grade chondrosarcoma is difficult to distinguish from enchondroma, but changing size on serial radiographs, cortical breakthrough, and prominent endosteal scalloping are indicators of more aggressive behavior.[68] MRI will demonstrate the intramedullary extent of the lesion and identify any associated soft tissue mass. Histologically, multiple subtypes of chondrosarcoma have been described. For the foot and ankle surgeon, the key distinction is the histologic grade because low-grade lesions are treated differently than intermediate- and high-grade lesions. Surgeons should also understand that secondary chondrosarcomas arise from enchondromas and osteochondromas; these lesions are usually low grade. Dedifferentiated chondrosarcoma arises from a lower-grade chondrosarcoma and is a high-grade lesion with a poor prognosis.

As with all sarcomas, treatment follows staging and diagnosis. Unlike the other primary bone sarcomas, chondrosarcoma is chemotherapy and radiotherapy resistant. Surgery is therefore the primary treatment. Wide resection is the treatment for intermediate- and high-grade chondrosarcomas. Debate exists as to whether limb salvage with reconstruction[105,177] or amputation[32,136] is the best option for large lesions. The decision is individualized, based upon anatomic factors and patient goals. Low-grade chondrosarcomas differ from other bone sarcomas in that extended curettage, rather than resection, is an acceptable treatment. Low local recurrence rates with excellent functional outcomes using curettage have been reported for low-grade chondrosarcomas in general[37,121] and phalangeal chondrosarcomas[24] specifically.

Osteosarcoma
Osteosarcoma of the foot and ankle is very rare; a review from the Rizzoli Institute found that foot osteosarcomas accounted for only 12 cases (0.6%) of the disease over an 81-year period.[19] Most osteosarcoma patients are children and adolescents; however, foot osteosarcoma patients in the Rizzoli series averaged 33 years of age.[19] The hindfoot is the most commonly affected area. Pain, swelling, and pathologic fracture are common presenting complaints. Plain radiographs reveal a destructive lesion with associated bone production (Fig. 18-26). MRI identifies the extent of marrow involvement and usually demonstrates an associated soft tissue mass. Histology reveals a malignant osteoid forming tumor.

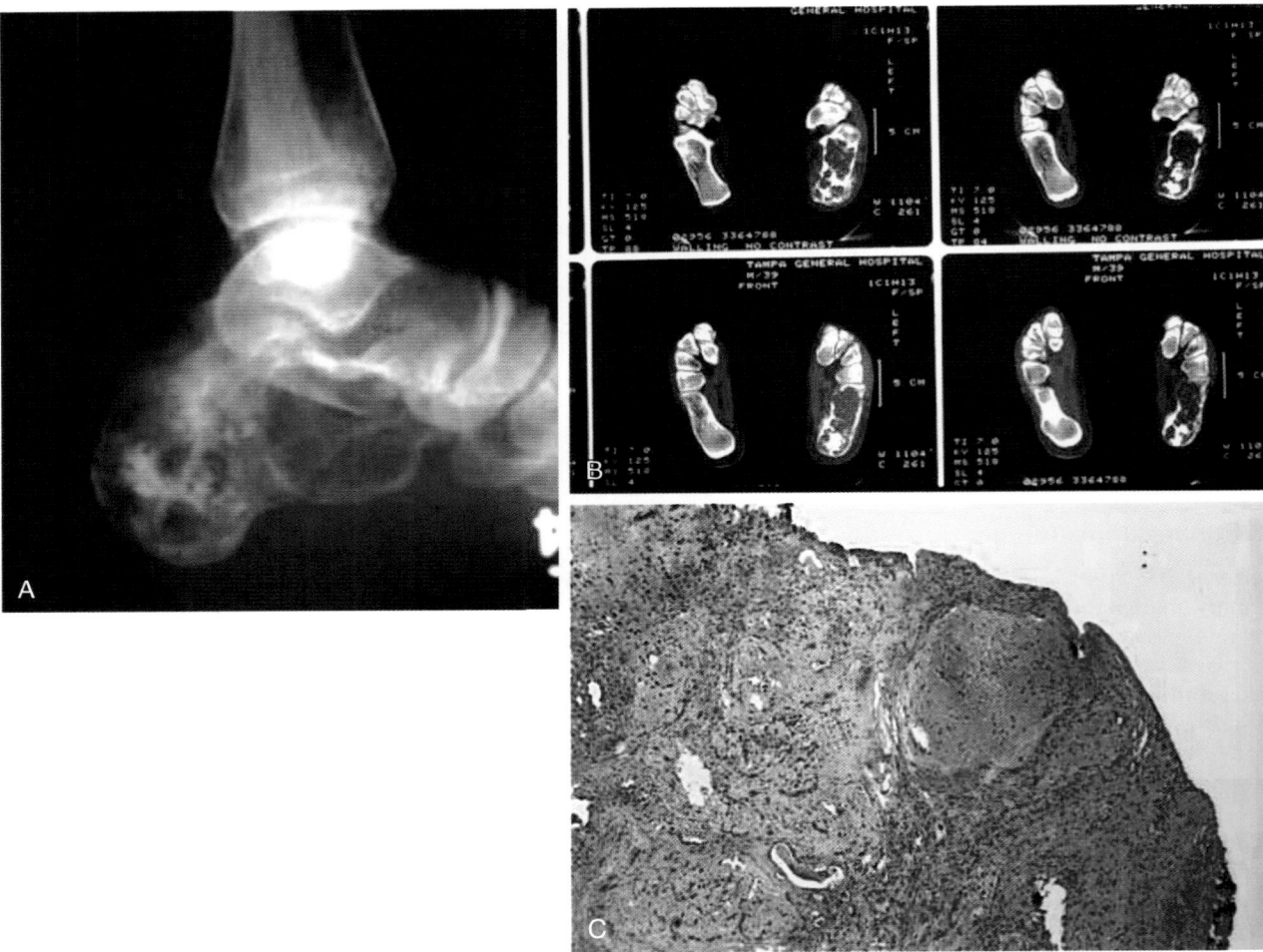

Figure 18-25 **A,** Lateral view of calcaneus demonstrates a destructive lesion with central calcification. **B,** Computed tomography confirms the destructive nature of the tumor and demonstrates both cortical breakthrough and soft tissue extension. **C,** Low-power photomicrograph of the biopsy specimen shows nodular cartilaginous tissue surrounded by vascular fibrous tissue consistent with chondrosarcoma.

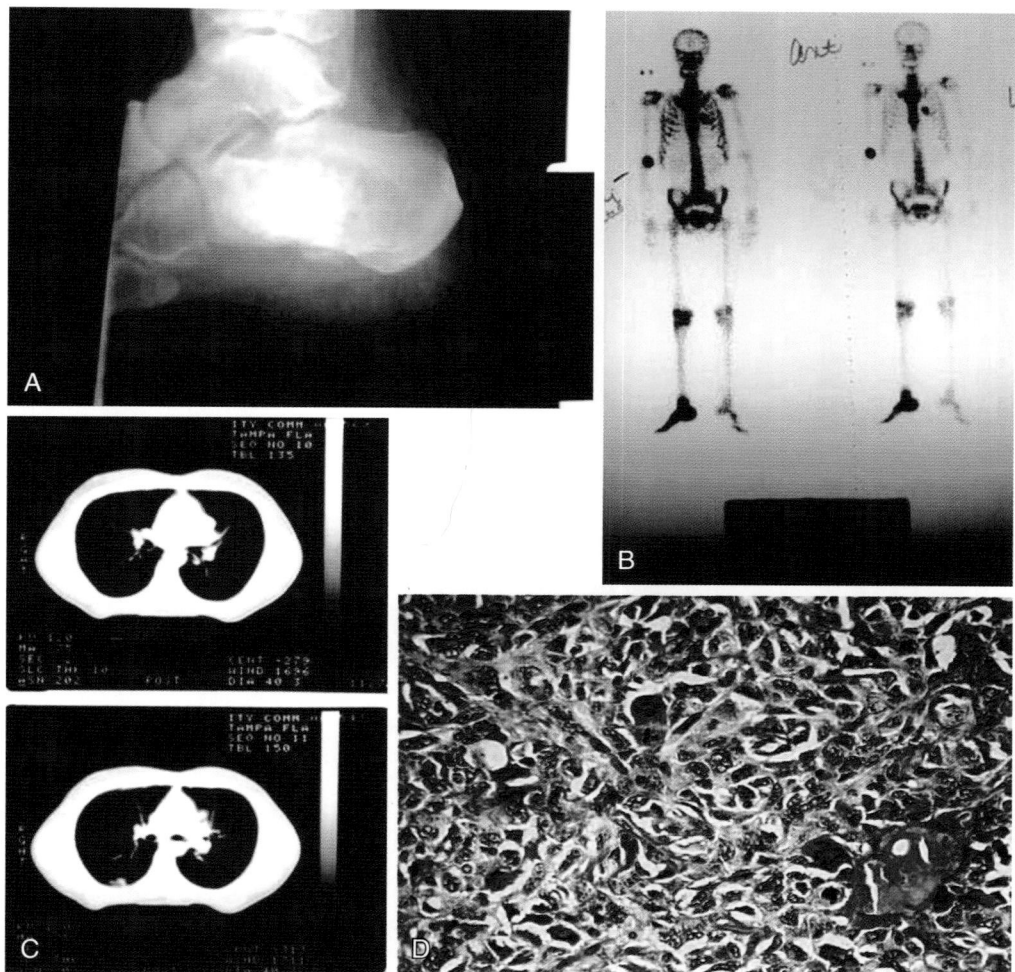

Figure 18-26 A, Lateral radiograph of the hindfoot typifies the abnormal production and destruction of bone seen in osteosarcoma. **B,** Bone scan demonstrates intense uptake in the calcaneus as well as a region of uptake in chest. **C,** Computed tomography of lung confirms the presence of lung metastasis at presentation. **D,** High-power photomicrograph of the biopsy demonstrating bizarre cellular forms, mitoses, and pink matrix consistent with osteoid production.

After staging and biopsy confirmation of the diagnosis, multidisciplinary treatment is initiated. High-grade osteosarcomas (the majority) are treated with neoadjuvant chemotherapy, followed by wide resection, and then additional chemotherapy. Hindfoot lesions often require below-knee amputation to obtain wide margins.

Ewing Sarcoma

Ewing sarcoma is less common than osteosarcoma overall, but it occurs more commonly than osteosarcoma in the foot.[31,101] It occurs most often in children and young adults. Systemic symptoms, such as fever and chills, may be present, and Ewing sarcoma may be mistaken for an infection.[54] The soft tissue component of the lesion may be quite extensive compared with the bone involvement. Radiographs often reveal only subtle radiolucency with a permeative pattern, and thus the differential diagnosis includes osteomyelitis and eosinophilic granuloma. MRI defines the local extent of the disease. Histology reveals a small, blue, round cell tumor (Fig. 18-27). More than 90% of these tumors have a characteristic translocation of chromosomes 11 and 22.[104]

After appropriate staging and biopsy confirmation of the disease, multidisciplinary treatment is initiated. Like osteosarcoma, neoadjuvant chemotherapy, wide surgical resection, and adjuvant chemotherapy are the main treatments. Unlike chondrosarcoma and osteosarcoma, Ewing sarcoma is radiosensitive, but this modality is rarely used in the foot and ankle because wide surgical resection (with amputation if necessary) is possible at this site.[101,156]

Metastatic Carcinoma

Although metastatic carcinomas are overall far more common than primary malignant tumors of bone, they are seldom found distal to the knee. A review of 694 consecutive cases of skeletal metastases from the University of Miami found that only 14 (2%) occurred in the

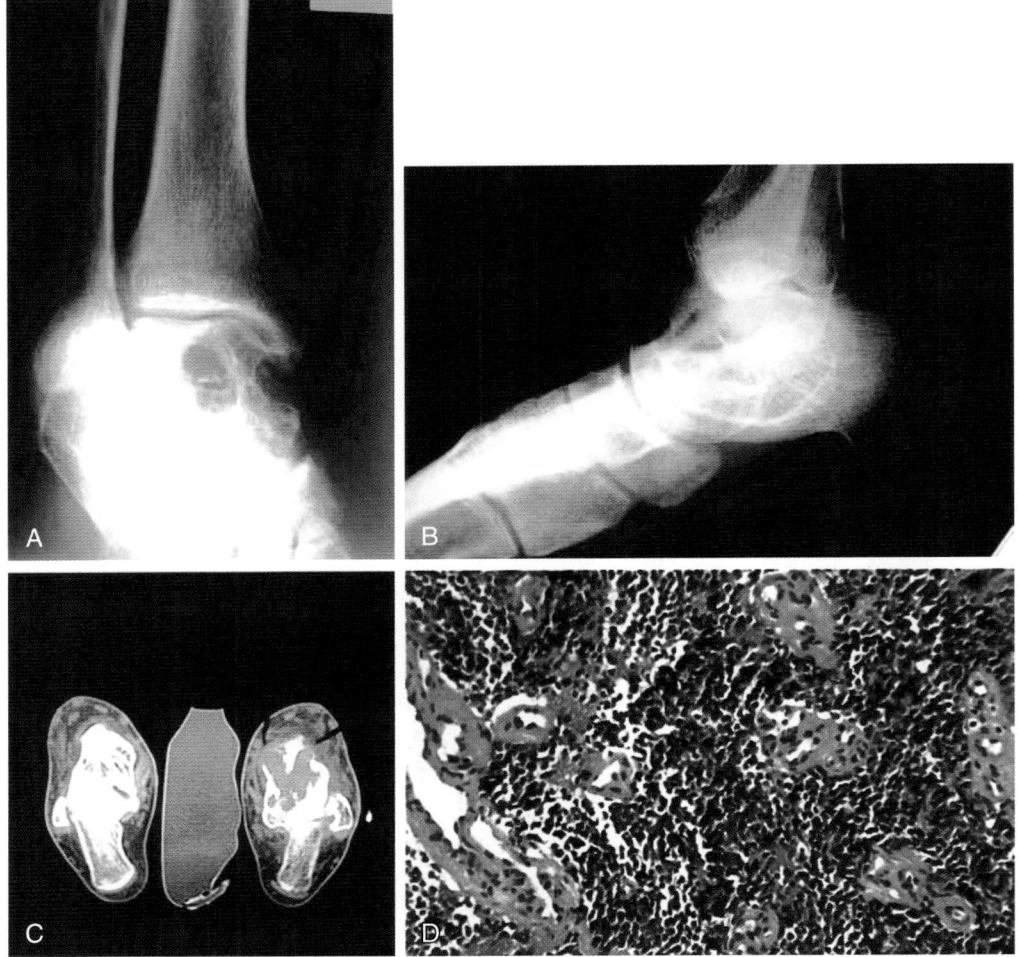

Figure 18-27 **A,** Anteroposterior radiograph of the ankle showing a lesion of the medial talus with preservation of the cortex. **B,** Lateral radiograph of the same patient. **C,** Computed tomography scan showing significantly more soft tissue extension than would have been expected based on the plain radiographs. **D,** Biopsy material demonstrating a darkly staining "blue cell" lesion, showing the poorly differentiated small round cells of Ewing sarcoma.

foot.[110] Lung carcinoma is historically believed to be the most common source of foot bone metastatses.[91] However, the Miami series found that 8 of 14 foot metastases were of genitourinary origin.[110] A series of 17 foot metastases from the Mayo Clinic found that renal cell carcinoma and colon cancer were common sources in addition to lung cancer.[79] Surgery to treat or prevent pathologic fracture may be indicated to improve quality of life. Nonsurgical treatments, including radiation therapy, bisphosphanates, and denosumab, may also improve patient symptoms and prevent fracture development.

REFERENCES

1. Abuhassan FO, Shannak AO: Subperiosteal resection of aneurysmal bone cysts of the distal fibula, *J Bone Joint Surg Br* 91:1227–1231, 2009.
2. Adelani MA, Wupperman RM, Holt GE: Benign synovial disorders, *J Am Acad Orthop Surg* 16:268–275, 2008.
3. Ahn JH, Choy W-S, Kim H-Y: Operative treatment for ganglion cysts of the foot and ankle, *J Foot Ankle Surg* 49:442–445, 2010.
4. Aluisio FV, Mair SD, Hall RL: Plantar fibromatosis: treatment of primary and recurrent lesions and factors associated with recurrence, *Foot Ankle Int* 17:672–678, 1996.
5. Andreou D, Tunn PU: Sentinel node biopsy in soft tissue sarcoma, *Recent Results Cancer Res* 179:25–36, 2009.
6. Arca MJ, Biermann JS, Johnson TM, Chang AE: Biopsy techniques for skin, soft-tissue, and bone neoplasms, *Surg Oncol Clin North Am* 4:157–174, 1995.
7. Arkader A, Glotzbecker M, Hosalkar HS, Dormans JP: Primary musculoskeletal Langerhans cell histiocytosis in children: an analysis for a 3-decade period, *J Pediatr Orthop* 29:201–207, 2009.
8. Atesok KI, Alman BA, Schemitsch EH, et al: Osteoid osteoma and osteoblastoma, *J Am Acad Orthop Surg* 19:678–689, 2011.
9. Bagatur AE, Yalcinkaya M, Dogan A, et al: Surgery is not always necessary in intraosseous lipoma, *Orthopedics* 33: 303, 2010. doi: 10.3928/01477447-20100329-13.
10. Balke M, Schremper L, Gebert C, et al: Giant cell tumor of bone: treatment and outcome of 214 cases, *J Cancer Res Clin Oncol* 134:969–978, 2008.
11. Ballo MT, Lee AK: Current results of brachytherapy for soft tissue sarcoma, *Curr Opin Oncol* 15:313–318, 2003.

12. Baptista EG, Achour H, Boccalandro F, Smalling RW: Cavernous hemangioma of the foot and antecubital fossa: an alternative therapeutic option, *Catheter Cardiovasc Interv* 58:527–531, 2003.

13. Barbella R, Fox IM: Recurring desmoid tumor of the foot: a case study, *Foot Ankle Int* 17:221–225, 1996.

14. Bella GPB, Manivel JC, Thompson RC Jr, et al: Intramuscular hemangioma: recurrence risk related to surgical margins, *Clin Orthop Relat Res* 459:186–191, 2007.

15. Berber O, Dawson-Bowling S, Jalgaonkar A, et al: Bizarre parosteal osteochondromatous proliferation of bone: clinical management of a series of 22 cases, *J Bone Joint Surg Br* 93:1118–1121, 2011.

16. Bichakjian CK, Halpern AC, Johnson TM, et al: Guidelines of care for the management of primary cutaneous melanoma. American Academy of Dermatology, *J Am Acad Dermatol* 65:1032–1047, 2011.

17. Bickels J, Meller I, Shmookler BM, Malawer MM: The role and biology of cryosurgery in the treatment of bone tumors. A review, *Acta Orthop Scand* 70:308–315, 1999.

18. Bisbinas I, De Silva U, Grimer RJ: Pigmented villonodular synovitis of the foot and ankle: a 12-year experience from a tertiary orthopedic oncology unit, *J Foot Ankle Surg* 43:407–411, 2004.

19. Biscaglia R, Gasbarrini A, Bohling T, et al: Osteosarcoma of the bones of the foot—an easily misdiagnosed malignant tumor, *Mayo Clin Proc* 73:842–847, 1998.

20. Blackley HR, Wunder JS, Davis AM, et al: Treatment of giant-cell tumors of long bones with curettage and bone-grafting, *J Bone Joint Surg Am* 81:811–820, 1999.

21. Blitz NM, Hutchinson B, Grabowski MV: Pedal plexiform neurofibroma: review of the literature and case report, *J Foot Ankle Surg* 41:117–124, 2002.

22. Bojanić I, Bergovec M, Smoljanović T: Combined anterior and posterior arthroscopic portals for loose body removal and synovectomy for synovial chondromatosis, *Foot Ankle Int* 30:1120–1123, 2009.

23. Bojanić I, Rogošić S, Mahnik A, Smoljanović T: Removal of osteoid osteoma of the tibia using two-portal posterior ankle arthroscopy, *J Foot Ankle Surg* 51:103–105, 2012.

24. Bovée JV, van der Heul RO, Taminiau AH, Hogendoorn PC: Chondrosarcoma of the phalanx: a locally aggressive lesion with minimal metastatic potential: a report of 35 cases and a review of the literature, *Cancer* 86:1724–1732, 1999.

25. Brien EW, Sacoman DM, Mirra JM: Pigmented villonodular synovitis of the foot and ankle, *Foot Ankle Int* 25:908–913, 2004.

26. Bristow IR, de Berker DA, Acland KM, et al: Clinical guidelines for the recognition of melanoma of the foot and nail unit, *J Foot Ankle Res* 3:25, 2010.

27. Bude, RO, Adler RS, Bassett DR: Diagnosis of Achilles tendon xanthoma in patients with heterozygous familial hypercholesterolemia: MR vs sonography, *AJR Am J Roentgenol* 162:913–917, 1994.

28. Burns TP, Weiss M, Snyder M, Hopson CN: Giant cell tumor of the metatarsal, *Foot Ankle* 8:223–226, 1988.

29. Campbell RSD, Grainger AJ, Mangham DC, et al: Intraosseous lipoma: report of 35 new cases and a review of the literature, *Skeletal Radiol* 32:209–222, 2003.

30. Canavese F, Wright JG, Cole WG, Hopyan S: Unicameral bone cysts: comparison of percutaneous curettage, steroid, and autologous bone marrow injections, *J Pediatr Orthop* 31:50–55, 2011.

31. Casadei R, Magnani M, Biagini R, Mercuri M: Prognostic factors in Ewing's sarcoma of the foot, *Clin Orthop Relat Res* 420:230–238, 2004.

32. Cawte TG, Steiner GC, Beltran J, Dorfman HD: Chondrosarcoma of the short tubular bones of the hands and feet, *Skeletal Radiol* 27:625–632, 1998.

33. Charest M, Hickeson M, Lisbona R, et al: FDG PET/CT imaging in primary osseous and soft tissue sarcomas: a retrospective review of 212 cases, *Eur J Nucl Med Mol Imaging* 36:1944–1951, 2009.

34. Chavis M, Jacobs AM, Demetri GJ Jr: Basal cell carcinoma: an infrequent pedal reality, *J Foot Surg* 28:346–351, 1989.

35. Chieppa WA, Shinder M: Unicameral bone cyst of the talus, *J Am Podiatr Med Assoc* 79:441–446, 1989.

36. Chin KR, Kharrazi FD, Miller BS, et al: Osteochondromas of the distal aspect of the tibia or fibula. Natural history and treatment, *J Bone Joint Surg Am* 82:1269–1278, 2000.

37. Cho WH, Song WS, Jeon DJ, et al: Oncologic impact of the curettage of grade 2 central chondrosarcoma of the extremity, *Ann Surg Oncol* 18:3755–3761, 2011.

38. Chou LB, Ho YY, Malawer MM: Tumors of the foot and ankle: experience with 153 cases, *Foot Ankle Int* 30:836–841, 2009.

39. Chowdhry M, Chandrasekar CR, Mohammed R, Grimer RJ: Curettage of aneurysmal bone cysts of the feet, *Foot Ankle Int* 31:131–135, 2010.

40. Chung S, Frush DP, Prose NS, et al: Subcutaneous granuloma annulare: MR imaging features in six children and literature review, *Radiology* 210:845–849, 1999.

41. Cribb GL, Cool P, Hill SO, Mangham DC: Distal tibial giant cell tumour treated with curettage and stabilisation with an Ilizarov frame, *Foot Ankle Surg* 15:28–32, 2009.

42. Cribb GL, Loo SC, Dickinson I: Limb salvage for soft-tissue sarcomas of the foot and ankle, *J Bone Joint Surg Br* 92:424–429, 2010.

43. Cummings JE, Smith RA, Heck RK Jr: Argon beam coagulation as adjuvant treatment after curettage of aneurysmal bone cysts: a preliminary study, *Clin Orthop Relat Res* 468:231–237, 2010.

44. Dalbeth N, Doyle A, Boyer L, et al: Development of a computed tomography method of scoring bone erosion in patients with gout: validation and clinical implications, *Rheumatology (Oxford)* 50:410–416, 2011.

45. Davila JA, Amrami KK, Sundaram M, et al: Chondroblastoma of the hands and feet, *Skeletal Radiol* 33:582–587, 2004.

46. Deheshi BM, Jaffer SN, Griffin AM, et al: Joint salvage for pathologic fracture of giant cell tumor of the lower extremity, *Clin Orthop Relat Res* 459:96–104, 2007.

47. de Palma L, Gigante A, Specchia N: Subungual exostosis of the foot, *Foot Ankle Int* 17:758–763, 1996.

48. de Palma L, Santucci A, Gigante A, et al: Plantar fibromatosis: an immunohistochemical and ultrastructural study, *Foot Ankle Int* 20:253–257, 1999.

49. Deroose JP, van Geel AN, Burger JW, et al: Isolated limb perfusion with TNF-alpha and melphalan for distal parts of the limb in soft tissue sarcoma patients, *J Surg Oncol* 105:563–569, 2011. doi:10.1002/jso.22121.

50. De Wilde V, De Maeseneer M, Lenchik L, et al: Normal osseous variants presenting as cystic or lucent areas on radiography and CT imaging: a pictorial overview, *Eur J Radiol* 51:77–84, 2004.

51. Di Bella C, Dozza B, Frisoni T, et al: Injection of demineralized bone matrix with bone marrow concentrate improves healing in unicameral bone cyst, *Clin Orthop Relat Res* 468:3047–3055, 2010.

52. Dormans JP, Sankar WN, Moroz L, Erol B: Percutaneous intramedullary decompression, curettage, and grafting with medical-grade calcium sulfate pellets for unicameral bone cysts in children: a new minimally invasive technique, *J Pediatr Orthop* 25:804–811, 2005.

53. Durbec F, Martin L, Derancourt C, Grange F: Melanoma of the hand and foot: epidemiologic, prognostic and genetic features. A systematic review, *Br J Dermatol* 166:727–739, 2012. doi:10.1111/j.1365-2133.2011.10772.x.

54. Durbin M, Randall RL, James M, et al: Ewing's sarcoma masquerading as osteomyelitis, *Clin Orthop Relat Res* 357:176–185, 1998.

55. Dürr HR, Maier M, Jansson V, et al: Phenol as an adjuvant for local control in the treatment of giant cell tumour of the bone, *Eur J Surg Oncol* 25:610–618, 1999.

56. Economopoulos K, Barker L, Beauchamp C, Claridge R: Case report: reconstruction of the distal tibia with porous tantalum spacer after resection for giant cell tumor, *Clin Orthop Relat Res* 468:1697–1701, 2010.

57. Edge SB, Byrd DR, Compton CC, et al: *AJCC Cancer Staging Manual*, 7th ed, New York, 2009, Springer.

58. Enneking WF: A system of staging musculoskeletal neoplasms, *Clin Orthop Relat Res* 204:9–24, 1986.

59. Enneking WF, Spanier SS, Goodman MA: A system for the surgical staging of musculoskeletal sarcoma, *Clin Orthop Relat Res* 153:106–120, 1980.

60. Fallen T, Wilson M, Morlan B, Lindor NM: Desmoid tumors—a characterization of patients seen at Mayo Clinic 1976-1999, *Fam Cancer* 5:191–194, 2006.

61. Ferguson PC: Surgical considerations for management of distal extremity soft tissue sarcomas, *Curr Opin Oncol* 17:366–369, 2005.

62. Ferrari A, Sultan I, Huang TT, et al: Soft tissue sarcoma across the age spectrum: a population-based study from the Surveillance Epidemiology and End Results database, *Pediatr Blood Cancer* 57:943–949, 2011.

63. Fetsch JF, Laskin WB, Miettinen M: Palmar-plantar fibromatosis in children and preadolescents: a clinicopathologic study of 56 cases with newly recognized demographics and extended follow-up information, *Am J Surg Pathol* 29:1095–1105, 2005.

64. Fink BR, Temple HT, Chiricosta FM, et al: Chondroblastoma of the foot, *Foot Ankle Int* 18, 236–242, 1997.

65. Fiore M, Rimareix F, Mariani L, et al: Desmoid-type fibromatosis: a front-line conservative approach to select patients for surgical treatment, *Ann Surg Oncol* 16:2587–2593, 2009.

66. Fitzpatrick TB, Gilchrest BA: Dimple sign to differentiate benign from malignant pigmented cutaneous lesions, *N Engl J Med* 296:1518, 1977.

67. Fortin PT, Freiberg AA, Rees R, et al: Malignant melanoma of the foot and ankle, *J Bone Joint Surg Am* 77:1396–1403, 1995.

68. Gajewski DA, Burnette JB, Murphey MD, Temple HT: Differentiating clinical and radiographic features of enchondroma and secondary chondrosarcoma in the foot, *Foot Ankle Int* 27:240–244, 2006.

69. Galat DD, Ackerman DB, Spoon D, et al: Synovial chondromatosis of the foot and ankle, *Foot Ankle Int* 29:312–317, 2008.

70. Gaston CL, Bhumbra R, Watanuki M, et al: Does the addition of cement improve the rate of local recurrence after curettage of giant cell tumours in bone? *J Bone Joint Surg Br* 93:1665–1669, 2011.

71. Gholve PA, Hosalkar HS, Kreiger PA, Dormans JP: Giant cell tumor of tendon sheath: largest single series in children, *J Pediatr Orthop* 27:67–74, 2007.

72. Gibbons C,. Khwaja HA, Cole AS, et al: Giant-cell tumour of the tendon sheath in the foot and ankle, *J Bone Joint Surg Br* 84:1000–1003, 2002.

73. Giuffrida AY, Burgueno JE, Koniaris LG, et al: Chondrosarcoma in the United States (1973 to 2003): an analysis of 2890 cases from the SEER database, *J Bone Joint Surg Am* 91:1063–1072, 2009.

74. Gonzalez JV, Stuck RM, Streit N: Intraosseous lipoma of the calcaneus: a clinicopathologic study of three cases, *J Foot Ankle Surg* 36:306–310; discussion 329, 1997.

75. Goto T, Kawano H, Yamamoto A, et al: Simple curettage without bone grafting for enchondromas of the foot, *Arch Orthop Trauma Surg* 124:301–305, 2004.

76. Gressen EL, Rosenstock JG, Xie Y, Corn BW: Palliative treatment of epidemic Kaposi sarcoma of the feet, *Am J Clin Oncol* 22:286–290, 1999.

77. Grivas TB, Savvidou OD, Psarakis SA, et al: Forefoot plantar multilobular noninfiltrating angiolipoma: a case report and review of the literature, *World J Surg Oncol* 6:11, 2008.

78. Gronchi A, Casali PG, Mariani L, et al: Quality of surgery and outcome in extra-abdominal aggressive fibromatosis: a series of patients surgically treated at a single institution, *J Clin Oncol* 21:1390–1397, 2003.

79. Hattrup SJ, Amadio PC, Sim FH, Lombardi RM: Metastatic tumors of the foot and ankle, *Foot Ankle* 8:243–247, 1988.

80. Helwig U, Lang S, Baczynski M, Windhager R: The intraosseous ganglion. A clinical-pathological report on 42 cases, *Arch Orthop Trauma Surg* 114:14–17, 1994.

80a. Hermanek P, Wittekind C: Residual tumor (R) classification and prognosis, *Semin Surg Oncol* 10:12–20, 1994.

81. Hoeger PH, Martinez A, Maerker J, Harper JI: Vascular anomalies in Proteus syndrome, *Clin Exp Dermatol* 29:222–230, 2004.

82. Hogeling M, Adams S, Wargon O: A randomized controlled trial of propranolol for infantile hemangiomas, *Pediatrics* 128:e259–e266, 2011.

83. Holgado RD, Ward SC, Suryaprasad SG: Squamous cell carcinoma of the hallux, *J Am Podiatr Med Assoc* 90:309–312, 2000.

84. Horenstein MG, Prieto VG, Nuckols JD, et al: Indeterminate fibrohistiocytic lesions of the skin: is there a spectrum between dermatofibroma and dermatofibrosarcoma protuberans? *Am J Surg Pathol* 24:996–1003, 2000.

85. Horst F, Nunley JA: Glomus tumors in the foot: a new surgical technique for removal, *Foot Ankle Int* 24:949–951, 2003.

86. Hosalkar HS, Garg S, Moroz L, et al: The diagnostic accuracy of MRI versus CT imaging for osteoid osteoma in children, *Clin Orthop Relat Res* 433:171–177, 2005.

87. Iovane A, Midiri M, Bartolotta TV, et al: Pigmented villonodular synovitis of the foot: MR findings, *Radiol Med* 106:66–73, 2003.

88. Jelinek JS, Kransdorf MJ, Shmookler BM, et al: Giant cell tumor of the tendon sheath: MR findings in nine cases, *AJR Am J Roentgenol* 162:919–922, 1994.

89. Jones FE, Soule EH, Coventry MB: Fibrous xanthoma of synovium (giant-cell tumor of tendon sheath, pigmented nodular synovitis). A study of one hundred and eighteen cases, *J Bone Joint Surg Am* 51:76–86, 1969.

90. Kehoe NJ, Reid RP, Semple JC: Solitary benign peripheral-nerve tumours. Review of 32 years' experience, *J Bone Joint Surg Br* 77:497–500, 1995.

91. Kemnitz MJ, Erdmann BB, Julsrud ME, et al: Adenocarcinoma of the lung with metatarsal metastasis, *J Foot Ankle Surg* 35:210–212, 1996.

92. Kerr-Valentic MA, Samimi K, Rohlen BH, et al: Marjolin's ulcer: modern analysis of an ancient problem, *Plast Reconstr Surg* 123:184–191, 2009.

93. Kirby EJ, Shereff MJ, Lewis MM: Soft-tissue tumors and tumor-like lesions of the foot. An analysis of eighty-three cases, *J Bone Joint Surg Am* 71:621–626, 1989.

94. Kumar S, Gow P: A survey of indications, results and complications of surgery for tophaceous gout, *N Z Med J* 115:U109, 2002.

95. Kuo C-L, Yang S-W, Chou Y-J, Wong C-Y: Giant cell tumor of the EDL tendon sheath: an unusual cause of hallux valgus, *Foot Ankle Int* 29:534–537, 2008.

96. La TH, Wolden SL, Su Z, et al: Local therapy for rhabdomyosarcoma of the hands and feet: is amputation necessary? A report from the Children's Oncology Group, *Int J Radiat Oncol Biol Phys* 80:206–212, 2011.

97. Lampasi M, Magnani M, Donzelli O: Aneurysmal bone cysts of the distal fibula in children: long-term results of curettage and

resection in nine patients, *J Bone Joint Surg Br* 89:1356–1362, 2007.

98. Latt LD, Turcotte RE, Isler MH, Wong C: Case series. Soft-tissue sarcoma of the foot, *Can J Surg* 53:424–431, 2010.

99. Lee S, Lerer DB, Dorfman HD, Coco M: Brown tumors developing in renal transplant recipients with persistent hyperparathyroidism: two case reports and review of literature, *Clin Nephrol* 61:289–294, 2004.

100. Lee SK, Jung MS, Lee YH, et al: Two distinctive subungual pathologies: subungual exostosis and subungual osteochondroma, *Foot Ankle Int* 28:595–601, 2007.

101. Leeson MC, Smith MJ: Ewing's sarcoma of the foot, *Foot Ankle* 10:147–151, 1989.

102. Leithner A, Windhager R, Lang S, et al: Aneurysmal bone cyst. A population based epidemiologic study and literature review, *Clin Orthop Relat Res* 363:176–179, 1999.

103. Lersundi A, Mankin HJ, Mourikis A, Hornicek FJ: Chondromyxoid fibroma: a rarely encountered and puzzling tumor, *Clin Orthop Relat Res* 439:171–175, 2005.

104. Lessnick SL, Dei Tos AP, Sorensen PH, et al: Small round cell sarcomas, *Semin Oncol* 36:338–346, 2009.

105. Li J, Guo Z, Pei GX, et al: Limb salvage surgery for calcaneal malignancy, *J Surg Oncol* 102:48–53, 2010.

106. Lin PP, Thenappan A, Deavers MT, et al: Treatment and prognosis of chondroblastoma, *Clin Orthop Relat Res* 438:103–109, 2005.

107. Linos E, Swetter SM, Cockburn MG, et al: Increasing burden of melanoma in the United States, *J Invest Dermatol* 129:1666–1674, 2009.

108. Luis LR Jr, Kaoru GR, Shemuel PB, Mills JL Sr: Lower extremity glomus tumors: comprehensive review for surgeons, *Vascular* 16:326–332, 2008.

109. MacCollin M, Chiocca EA, Evans DG, et al: Diagnostic criteria for schwannomatosis, *Neurology* 64:1838–1845, 2005.

110. Maheshwari AV, Chiappetta G, Kugler CD, et al: Metastatic skeletal disease of the foot: case reports and literature review, *Foot Ankle Int* 29:699–710, 2008.

111. Mangrulkar VH, Brunetti VA, Gould ES, Howell N: Unusually large pedal schwannoma, *J Foot Ankle Surg* 46:398–402, 2007.

112. Mankin H, Trahan C, Hornicek F: Pigmented villonodular synovitis of joints, *J Surg Oncol* 103:386–389, 2011.

113. Mankin HJ, Hornicek FJ, Ortiz-Cruz E, et al: Aneurysmal bone cyst: a review of 150 patients, *J Clin Oncol* 23:6756–6762, 2005.

114. Mankin HJ, Hornicek FJ, Springfield DS: Extra-abdominal desmoid tumors: a report of 234 cases, *J Surg Oncol* 102:380–384, 2010.

115. Marco RA, Gitelis S, Brebach GT, Healey JH: Cartilage tumors: evaluation and treatment, *J Am Acad Orthop Surg* 8:292–304, 2000.

116. Marcove RC, Weis LD, Vaghaiwalla MR, Pearson R: Cryosurgery in the treatment of giant cell tumors of bone: a report of 52 consecutive cases, *Clin Orthop Relat Res* 134:275–289, 1978.

117. Math KR, Pavlov H, DiCarlo E, Bohne WH: Spindle cell lipoma of the foot: a case report and literature review, *Foot Ankle Int* 16:220–226, 1995.

118. McDermott MB, Lind AC, Marley EF, Dehner LP: Deep granuloma annulare (pseudorheumatoid nodule) in children: clinicopathologic study of 35 cases, *Pediatr Dev Pathol* 1:300–308, 1998.

119. Meneses MF, Unni KK, Swee RG: Bizarre parosteal osteochondromatous proliferation of bone (Nora's lesion), *Am J Surg Pathol* 17:91–697, 1993.

120. Miyano JA, Fitzgibbons TC: Glomangioma of the ankle simulating injury to the flexor hallucis longus: a case report, *Foot Ankle Int* 17:768–770, 1996.

121. Mohler DG, Chiu R, McCall DA, Avedian RS: Curettage and cryosurgery for low-grade cartilage tumors is associated with low recurrence and high function, *Clin Orthop Relat Res* 468:2765–2773, 2010.

122. Mohr P, Eggermont AMM, Hauschild A, Buzaid A: Staging of cutaneous melanoma, *Ann Oncol* 20(Suppl 6):vi14–vi21, 2009.

123. Moretti VM, Slotcavage RL, Crawford EA, et al: Curettage and graft alleviates athletic-limiting pain in benign lytic bone lesions, *Clin Orthop Relat Res* 469:283–288, 2011.

124. Murari TM, Callaghan JJ, Berrey BH Jr, Sweet DE: Primary benign and malignant osseous neoplasms of the foot, *Foot Ankle* 10:68–80, 1989.

125. Murff R, Ashry HR: Intraosseous ganglia of the foot, *J Foot Ankle Surg* 33:396–401, 1994.

126. Narang S, Gangopadhyay M: Calcaneal intraosseous lipoma: a case report and review of the literature, *J Foot Ankle Surg* 50:216–220, 2011.

127. Nichols RE, Dixon LB: Radiographic analysis of solitary bone lesions, *Radiol Clin North Am* 49:1095–1114, v, 2011.

128. Noguchi M, Ikoma K, Matsumoto N, Nagasawa K: Bizarre parosteal osteochondromatous proliferation of the sesamoid: an unusual hallux valgus deformity, *Foot Ankle Int* 25:503–506, 2004.

129. Noonan KJ, Feinberg JR, Levenda A, et al: Natural history of multiple hereditary osteochondromatosis of the lower extremity and ankle, *J Pediatr Orthop* 22:20–124, 2002.

130. Nora FE, Dahlin DC, Beabout JW: Bizarre parosteal osteochondromatous proliferations of the hands and feet, *Am J Surg Pathol* 7:245–250, 1983.

131. O'Connor PJ, Gibbon WW, Hardy G, Butt WP: Chondromyxoid fibroma of the foot, *Skeletal Radiol* 25:143–148, 1996.

132. Oliveira AM, Perez-Atayde AR, Dal CP, et al: USP6 and CDH11 oncogenes identify the neoplastic cell in primary aneurysmal bone cysts and are absent in so-called secondary aneurysmal bone cysts, *Am J Pathol* 165:1773–1780, 2004.

133. O'Keefe RJ, O'Donnell RJ, Temple HT, et al: Giant cell tumor of bone in the foot and ankle, *Foot Ankle Int* 16:617–623, 1995.

134. Ostrowski ML, Spjut HJ: Lesions of the bones of the hands and feet, *Am J Surg Pathol* 21:676–690, 1997.

135. O'Sullivan B, Davis AM, Turcotte R, et al: Preoperative versus postoperative radiotherapy in soft-tissue sarcoma of the limbs: a randomised trial, *Lancet* 359:2235–2241, 2002.

136. Papagelopoulos PJ, Mavrogenis AF, Badekas A, Sim FH: Foot malignancies: a multidisciplinary approach, *Foot Ankle Clin* 8:751–763, 2003.

137. Papp DF, Khanna AJ, McCarthy EF, et al: Magnetic resonance imaging of soft-tissue tumors: determinate and indeterminate lesions, *J Bone Joint Surg Am* 89(Suppl 3):103–115, 2007.

138. Parekh SG, Donthineni-Rao R, Ricchetti E, Lackman RD: Fibrous dysplasia, *J Am Acad Orthop Surg* 12:305–313, 2004.

139. Park I-H, Micic ID, Jeon I-H: A study of 23 unicameral bone cysts of the calcaneus: open chip allogeneic bone graft versus percutaneous injection of bone powder with autogenous bone marrow, *Foot Ankle Int* 29:164–170, 2008.

140. Parodi KK, Farrett W, Paden MH, Stone PA: A report of a rare phalangeal periosteal chondroma of the foot, *J Foot Ankle Surg* 50:122–125, 2011.

141. Patel RV, Frankel A, Goldenberg G: An update on nonmelanoma skin cancer, *J Clin Aesthet Dermatol* 4:20–27, 2011.

142. Plaza JA, Perez-Montiel D, Mayerson J, et al: Metastases to soft tissue: a review of 118 cases over a 30-year period, *Cancer* 112:193–203, 2008.

143. Prosser GH, Baloch KG, Tillman RM, et al: Does curettage without adjuvant therapy provide low recurrence rates in giant-cell tumors of bone? *Clin Orthop Relat Res* 435:211–218, 2005.

144. Quigley JT: A glomus tumor of the heel pad. A case report, *J Bone Joint Surg Am* 61:443–444, 1979.

145. Qureshi YA, Huddy JR, Miller JD, et al: Unplanned excision of soft tissue sarcoma results in increased rates of local recurrence

despite full further oncological treatment, *Ann Surg Oncol* 19:871–877, 2012.

146. Ramappa AJ, Lee FY, Tang P, et al: Chondroblastoma of bone, *J Bone Joint Surg Am* 82-A:1140–1145, 2000.

147. Ray-Coquard I, Thiesse P, Ranchère-Vince D, et al: Conformity to clinical practice guidelines, multidisciplinary management and outcome of treatment for soft tissue sarcomas, *Ann Oncol* 15:307–315, 2004.

148. Reed TS, Marty JA: Peripheral nerve tumors. Large neurofibroma of the foot, *J Am Podiatr Med Assoc* 85:552–554, 1995.

149. Requena L, Fernández-Figueras MT: Subcutaneous granuloma annulare, *Semin Cutan Med Surg* 26:96–99, 2007.

150. Riad S, Griffin AM, Liberman B, et al: Lymph node metastasis in soft tissue sarcoma in an extremity, *Clin Orthop Relat Res* 426:129–134, 2004.

151. Rock MG, Pritchard DJ, Unni KK: Metastases from histologically benign giant-cell tumor of bone, *J Bone Joint Surg Am* 66:269–274, 1984.

152. Rodeberg DA, Stoner JA, Garcia-Henriquez N, et al: Tumor volume and patient weight as predictors of outcome in children with intermediate risk rhabdomyosarcoma: a report from the children's oncology group, *Cancer* 2010. [Epub ahead of print]. doi:10.1002/cncr.25719.

153. Rogalski R, Hensinger R, Loder R: Vascular abnormalities of the extremities: clinical findings and management, *J Pediatr Orthop* 13:9–14, 1993.

154. Sammarco GJ, Mangone PG: Classification and treatment of plantar fibromatosis, *Foot Ankle Int* 21:563–569, 2000.

155. Sampath S, Schultheiss TE, Hitchcock YJ, et al: Preoperative versus postoperative radiotherapy in soft-tissue sarcoma: multi-institutional analysis of 821 patients, *Int J Radiat Oncol Biol Phys* 81:498–505, 2011.

156. San-Julian M, Duart J, de Rada PD, Sierrasesumaga L: Limb salvage in Ewing's sarcoma of the distal lower extremity, *Foot Ankle Int* 29:22–28, 2008.

157. Satter EK, High WA: Langerhans cell histiocytosis: a review of the current recommendations of the Histiocyte Society, *Pediatr Dermatol* 25:291–295, 2008.

158. Scarborough MT: The biopsy, *Instr Course Lect* 53:639–644, 2004.

159. Schajowicz F, Clavel Sainz M, Slullitel JA: Juxta-articular bone cysts (intra-osseous ganglia): a clinicopathological study of eighty-eight cases, *J Bone Joint Surg Br* 61:107–116, 1979.

160. Schnirring-Judge M, Lin B: Pigmented villonodular synovitis of the ankle-radiation therapy as a primary treatment to reduce recurrence: a case report with 8-year follow-up, *J Foot Ankle Surg* 50:108–116, 2011.

161. Schoenfeld GS, Morris CG, Scarborough MT, Zlotecki RA: Adjuvant radiotherapy in the management of soft tissue sarcoma involving the distal extremities, *Am J Clin Oncol* 29:62–65, 2006.

162. Senet P, Combemale P, Debure C, et al: Malignancy and chronic leg ulcers: the value of systematic wound biopsies: a prospective, multicenter, cross-sectional study, *Arch Dermatol* 148:704–708, 2012. doi:10.1001/archdermatol.2011.3362.

163. Sharma H, Jane MJ, Reid R: Chondromyxoid fibroma of the foot and ankle: 40 years' Scottish bone tumour registry experience, *Int Orthop* 30:205–209, 2006.

164. Shawen SB, McHale KA, Temple HT: Correction of ankle valgus deformity secondary to multiple hereditary osteochondral exostoses with Ilizarov, *Foot Ankle Int* 21:1019–1022, 2000.

165. Sheff JS, Wang S: Extraskeletal osteochondroma of the foot, *J Foot Ankle Surg* 44:57–59, 2005.

166. Shereff MJ, Cullivan WT, Johnson KA: Osteoid-osteoma of the foot, *J Bone Joint Surg Am* 65:638–641, 1983.

167. Shukla S, Clarke AW, Saifuddin A: Imaging features of foot osteoid osteoma, *Skeletal Radiol* 39:683–689, 2010.

168. Siebenrock KA, Unni KK, Rock MG: Giant-cell tumour of bone metastasising to the lungs. A long-term follow-up, *J Bone Joint Surg Br* 80:43–47, 1998.

169. Sim FH, Dahlin CD, Beabout JW: Osteoid-osteoma: diagnostic problems, *J Bone Joint Surg Am* 57:154–159, 1975.

170. Smyth M: Glomus-cell tumors in the lower extremity. Report of two cases, *J Bone Joint Surg Am* 53:157–159, 1971.

171. Sooriakumaran S, Landham TL: The Klippel-Trenaunay syndrome, *J Bone Joint Surg Br* 73:169–170, 1991.

172. Spencer RJ, Blitz NM: Giant extraskeletal osteochondroma of the plantar midfoot arch, *J Foot Ankle Surg* 47:362–367, 2008.

173. Stieber JR, Dormans JP: Manifestations of hereditary multiple exostoses, *J Am Acad Orthop Surg* 13:110–120, 2005.

174. Temple HT, Mizel MS, Murphey MD, Sweet DE: Osteoblastoma of the foot and ankle, *Foot Ankle Int* 19:698–704, 1998.

175. Thacker MM, Potter BK, Pitcher JD, Temple HT: Soft tissue sarcomas of the foot and ankle: impact of unplanned excision, limb salvage, and multimodality therapy, *Foot Ankle Int* 29:690–698, 2008.

176. Thomas D, Henshaw R, Skubitz K, et al: Denosumab in patients with giant-cell tumour of bone: an open-label, phase 2 study, *Lancet Oncol* 11:275–280, 2010.

177. Toma CD, Dominkus M, Pfeiffer M, et al: Metatarsal reconstruction with use of free vascularized osteomyocutaneous fibular grafts after resection of malignant tumors of the midfoot. A series of six cases, *J Bone Joint Surg Am* 89:1553–1564, 2007.

178. Tsouli SG, Kiortsis DN, Argyropoulou MI, et al: Pathogenesis, detection and treatment of Achilles tendon xanthomas, *Eur J Clin Invest* 35:236–244, 2005.

179. Tüzüner S, Aydin AT: Arthroscopic removal of an osteoid osteoma at the talar neck, *Arthroscopy* 14:405–409, 1998.

180. Uldrick TS, Whitby D: Update on KSHV epidemiology, Kaposi sarcoma pathogenesis, and treatment of Kaposi sarcoma, *Cancer Lett* 305:150–162, 2011.

181. Verdegaal SH, Bovée JV, Pansuriya TC, et al: Incidence, predictive factors, and prognosis of chondrosarcoma in patients with Ollier disease and Maffucci syndrome: an international multicenter study of 161 patients, *Oncologist* 16:1771–1779, 2011.

182. Vitale MG, Guha A, Skaggs DL: Orthopaedic manifestations of neurofibromatosis in children: an update, *Clin Orthop Relat Res* 401:107–118, 2002.

183. Walsh EF, Mechrefe A, Akelman E, Schiller AL: Giant cell tumor of tendon sheath, *Am J Orthop* 34:116–121, 2005.

184. Walsh SM, Fisher SG, Sage RA: Survival of patients with primary pedal melanoma, *J Foot Ankle Surg* 42:193–198, 2003.

185. Wang BY, Eisler J, Springfield D, Klein MJ: Intraosseous epidermoid inclusion cyst in a great toe. A case report and review of the literature, *Arch Pathol Lab Med* 127:e298–e300, 2003.

186. Wapner KL, Ververeli PA, Moore JH, et al: Plantar fibromatosis: a review of primary and recurrent surgical treatment, *Foot Ankle Int* 16:548–551, 1995.

187. Weinfeld GD, Yu GV, Good JJ: Intraosseous lipoma of the calcaneus: a review and report of four cases, *J Foot Ankle Surg* 41:398–411, 2002.

188. Widhe B, Widhe T: Initial symptoms and clinical features in osteosarcoma and Ewing sarcoma, *J Bone Joint Surg Am* 82:667–674, 2000.

189. Williams DS, Zichichi S: Extraskeletal chondroma of the foot, *J Am Podiatr Med Assoc* 88:506–509, 1998.

190. Williams HJ, Davies AM, Allen G, et al: Imaging features of intraosseous ganglia: a report of 45 cases, *Eur Radiol* 14:1761–1769, 2004.

191. Winter H, Dräger E, Sterry W: Sclerotherapy for treatment of hemangiomas, *Dermatol Surg* 26:105–108, 2000.

192. Woertler K: Soft tissue masses in the foot and ankle: character-istics on MR Imaging, *Semin Musculoskelet Radiol* 9:227–242, 2005.

193. Wright JG, Yandow S, Donaldson S, Marley L: A randomized clinical trial comparing intralesional bone marrow and steroid injections for simple bone cysts, *J Bone Joint Surg Am* 90:722–730, 2008.

194. Wu KK: Lymphangioma of the ankle region, *J Foot Ankle Surg* 35:263–265, 1996.

195. Yang D, Morrison BD, Vandongen YK, et al: Malignancy in chronic leg ulcers, *Med J Aust* 164:718–720, 1996.

196. Yazgan P, Ozturk A, Orhan I, et al: Third metatarsal brown tumor with secondary hyperparathyroidism: an atypical local-ization, *J Am Podiatr Med Assoc* 98:314–317, 2008.

197. Yildirim C, Mahiroğullari M, Kuşkucu M, et al: Treatment of a unicameral bone cyst of calcaneus with endoscopic curettage and percutaneous filling with corticocancellous allograft, *J Foot Ankle Surg* 49:93–97, 2010.

198. Young-In Lee F, Hornicek FJ, Dick HM, Mankin HJ: Synovial chondromatosis of the foot, *Clin Orthop Relat Res* 423:186–190, 2004.

199. Yu JS, Chung C, Recht M, Dailiana T, Jurdi R: MR imaging of tophaceous gout, *AJR Am J Roentgenol* 168:523–527, 1997.

200. Zahlten-Hinguranage A, Bernd L, Ewerbeck V, Sabo D: Equal quality of life after limb-sparing or ablative surgery for lower extremity sarcomas, *Br J Cancer* 91:1012–1014, 2004.

201. Zelger B, Zelger BG, Burgdorf WHC: Dermatofibroma—a criti-cal evaluation, *Int J Surg Pathol* 12:333–344, 2004.

202. Zuckerman JD, Powers B, Miller JW, Lippert F: Benign solitary schwannoma of the foot. A case report and review of the litera-ture, *Clin Orthop Relat Res* 228:278–280, 1988.

ARTHRITIS, POSTURAL DISORDERS, AND TENDON DISORDERS

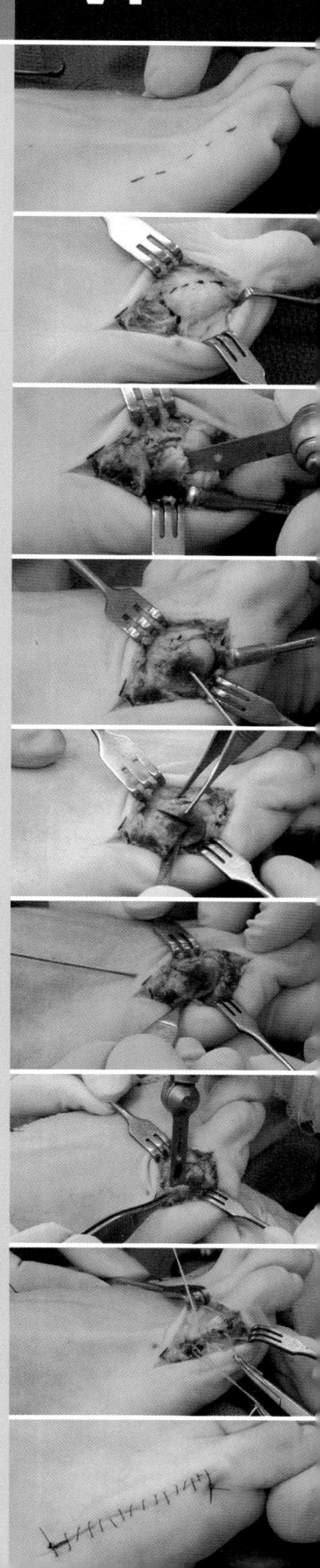

Arthritis of the Foot and Ankle

Christopher B. Hirose, Michael J. Coughlin, Faustin R. Stevens

CHAPTER CONTENTS

ARTHRITIC CONDITIONS OF THE FOOT

Overview

Arthritis is the destruction of articular cartilage, and it comprises one of the most common human diseases. Approximately one fourth of the population will develop foot pain during their lifetime, and a significant percentage of this is due to arthritis.[201,548]

Several types of arthritis exist: osteoarthritis or degenerative joint disease, posttraumatic arthritis, inflammatory arthritis, crystal-induced arthritis, seronegative arthritis, septic arthritis, and other lesser known arthritides. Osteoarthritis is, by far, the most common type.

Arthritic joint disease has affected man from the beginning. The 3300 BC Ötzi Ice Man, found high in the Alps between Austria and Italy, had arthritic joints.[250] Older human specimens dating to 4500 BC show evidence of arthritis, and even prehuman Neanderthal specimens demonstrate changes consistent with arthritic disease.

One early treatment for arthritis was made from the bark of the willow tree. The active ingredient was later isolated from the bark and named salicin. In 1853, Charles Gerhardt discovered a method to buffer salicin, forming acetylsalicylic acid, which reduced the gastrointestinal side effects; however, he had no interest in marketing the compound. While working for Bayer in 1897, Felix Hoffmann and Arthur Eichengrun[503] further purified acetylsalicylic acid, and Hoffman used it to help his father, who was suffering from arthritis. Bayer patented and successfully marketed this compound as "aspirin."

Further discoveries continue to elucidate the various causes of arthritides. Three genes have recently been linked to the degenerative form of arthritis. In addition, all cartilage degeneration appears to have a final common mechanism of chondrocyte apoptosis (programmed cell death), regardless of the type of arthritis.[291] Likewise, treatment of arthritis has gone far beyond aspirin; however, there remains much to learn in the diagnosis and treatment of this significant disease.

Degenerative Joint Disease

Osteoarthritis, or degenerative joint disease, is the most common of all the arthritides. Its prevalence increases exponentially with age; by age 65 years, 80% to 90% of our joints are affected. The prevalence of osteoarthritis is second only to cardiovascular disease.

Osteoarthritis of the foot and ankle occurs in all age groups. It occurs in middle and later years as primary idiopathic osteoarthritis (Fig. 19-1) and in a younger population after trauma—a type of secondary arthritis (Fig. 19-2A and B).

Other causes of secondary arthritis include obesity, hemochromatosis, ochronosis, and Ehlers-Danlos syndrome. Factors that can affect the onset and progression of arthritis include physical activity, occupation, and

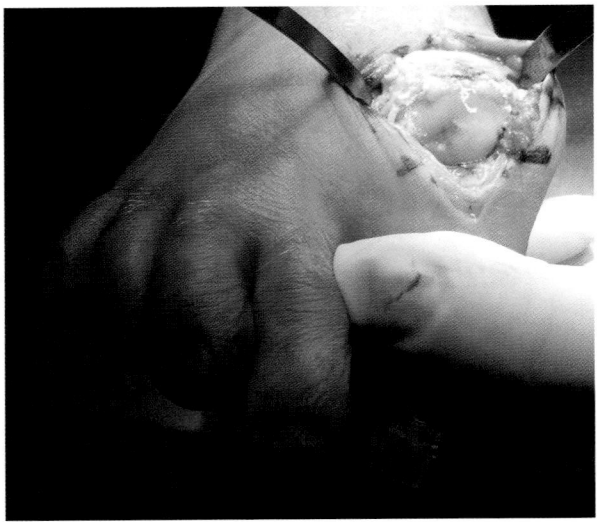

Figure 19-1 Intraoperative degenerative joint disease of the first metatarsophalangeal joint.

genetic predisposition. Despite advances in modern medicine, the precise etiology of arthritis remains unknown, and no current treatment has been shown to completely halt its progression.

The disease is characterized by an inherent defect in the chondrocytes and the cartilage matrix they produce. Early in the course of disease, chondrocytes multiply in number. Later they produce interleukin-1 (IL-1) and tumor necrosis factor (TNF), which inhibit the formation of proteoglycans and type 2 collagen. This in turn leads to degeneration and thinning of the cartilage layer. Three genes are now known to be linked to the osteoarthritic process, including GDF5 on chromosome 7 and MCF2L on chromosome 13.[124]

Despite some reports to the contrary, the cytokine production mentioned above stimulates an inflammatory cell response, and inflammatory cells are found within the joint. Once the cascade begins, water content in the cartilage layer increases and the concentration of proteoglycans decreases. Grossly, the cartilage surface becomes soft and friable, and it begins to fissure.

Microscopically, the normally smooth cartilage surface shows cracks and thinning. The synovium becomes fibrotic and hyperemic, with chronic inflammatory cell infiltratration. With repeated mechanical trauma, fragments of articular cartilage may break off into the joint, forming loose bodies (Fig. 19-3A and B).

Eventually, subchondral bone may be exposed, and a polished, eburnated bone surface is created. Crevices in the bone can form, which allows synovial fluid to penetrate the surface, forming subchondral cysts. Osteophytes form on the periphery of the joint. This cartilaginous and bony destruction results in restricted range of motion, pain, and loss of function.

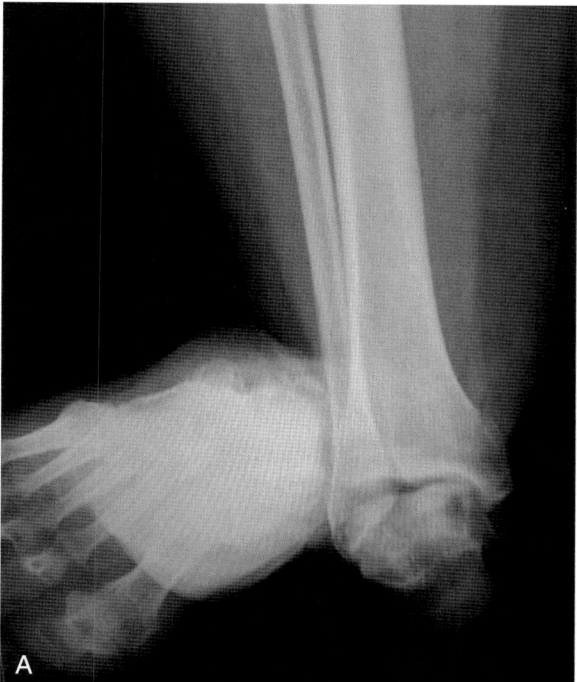

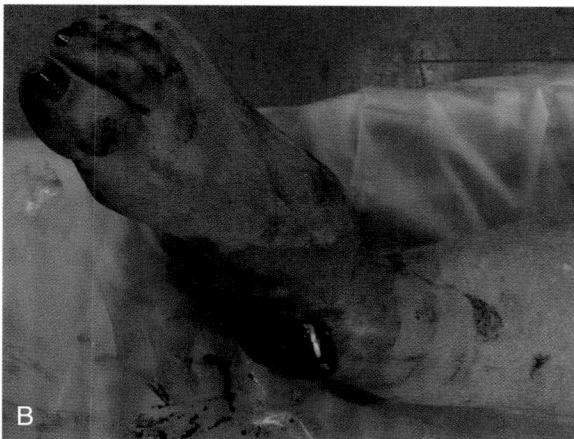

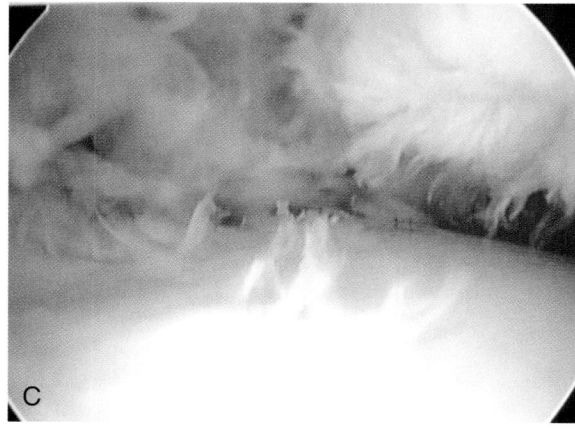

Figure 19-2 **A,** Radiograph demonstrating a traumatic open talar head fracture. **B,** Intraoperative photograph of the same traumatic open talar head fracture. **C,** Arthroscopic ankle intraarticular photograph of soft, fissuring, and friable cartilage.

History and Physical Examination

The history elicited from a patient with osteoarthritis varies depending on the number and location of joints involved. Many persons note morning stiffness with deep, dull pain. Typically, symptoms are aggravated by walking, standing, or physical activity and decrease with rest. Some report constant pain as well as muscular weakness. As the day progresses, the pain typically worsens.

Physical examination often demonstrates swelling around the affected joint with restricted motion. Surrounding bursae may be inflamed. Crepitation is sometimes present, and with forced motion, pain may be elicited. Periarticular osteophytes are often obvious to palpation and may cause numbness because of compression of an overlying nerve (e.g., deep peroneal nerve coursing over dorsal first tarsometatarsal [TMT] joint) (Fig. 19-4). Skin ulcerations may develop on the plantar tarsometatarsal joints because of longitudinal collapse of the arch of the foot.

Radiographic Examination

Typical radiographic findings include joint space narrowing, subchondral sclerosis, subchondral cyst formation, intraarticular loose bodies, periarticular osteophytes, and loss of normal foot alignment. These findings are best demonstrated on weight-bearing radiographs (Fig. 19-5A).

Brodén views are helpful for detecting arthritis of the subtalar joint. Talonavicular arthritis is often accompanied by a loss of the Meary angle (Fig. 19-5B), and calcaneocuboid arthritis is best seen on a medial oblique foot radiograph. Menz and colleagues[375] noted that osteoarthritis is readily diagnosed on anteroposterior (AP) and lateral radiographs and that these findings show good interobserver reliability. Periarticular bone loss and osteoporosis rarely occur. Magnetic resonance imaging (MRI) may show cartilage thinning and signal change on T2-weighted imaging in the subchondral bone. When subtler forms of arthritis are suspected, computed tomography (CT) is useful to document the severity and extent of the disease, although CT scans are routinely non–weight-bearing images.

Van Saase et al[573] noted the prevalence of first metatarsophalangeal (MTP) joint arthritis to be 28%, lesser MTP joints to be 8%, and the proximal interphalangeal (IP) joints to be 7%. The radiographic prevalence of midfoot and hindfoot joint arthritis has not been reported.

Treatment

Conservative treatment methods, such as weight reduction and activity modification, may reduce symptoms. Thus manual laborers who develop arthritis of the foot or ankle may see pain reduction with more sedentary occupations. Although rest is often advocated, animal studies have shown that increased activity diminishes the symptoms of arthritis and may slow its progression.[203] Cross training may also be beneficial to reduce stress on

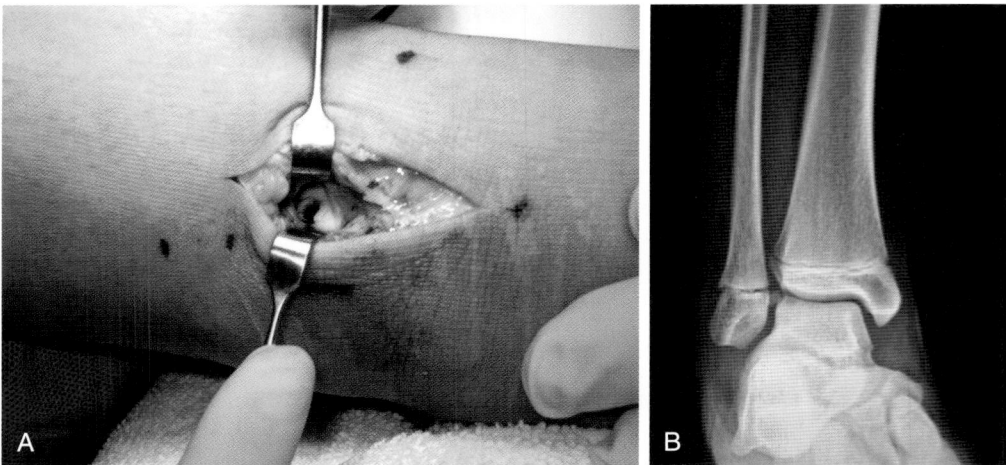

Figure 19-3   **A,** Lateral talar osteochondral defect secondary to trauma. **B,** Anteroposterior radiograph of the free-floating fragment of the talar osteochondral defect.

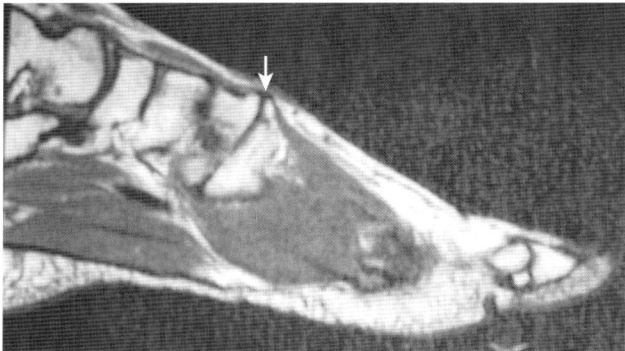

Figure 19-4   Sagittal plane magnetic resonance imaging scan demonstrating dorsal first tarsometatarsal osteophytes (*arrow*).

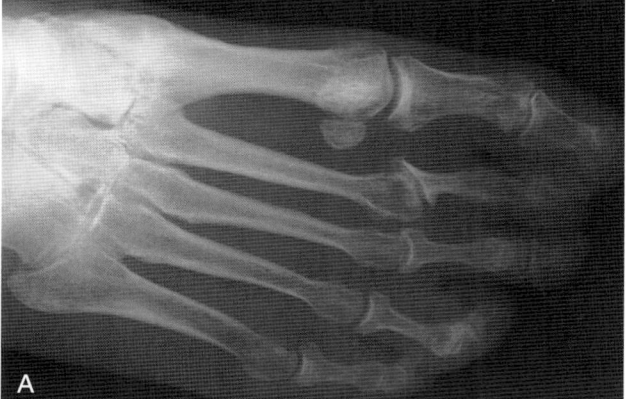

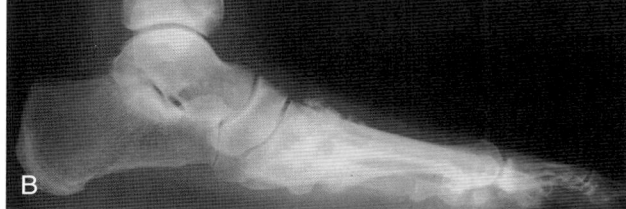

Figure 19-5   Anteroposterior weight-bearing **(A)** and lateral **(B)** radiographs demonstrate degenerative arthritis of the tarsometatarsal joints.

affected joints while maintaining joint mobility (i.e., joggers may substitute cycling or swimming).

Over-the-counter footwear or prescription footwear can reduce symptoms over bony prominences.[115] Orthoses can support unstable areas and areas with rigid deformities. Semiflexible orthoses appear to be better tolerated than rigid orthoses in treating degenerative joint disease of the hindfoot and midfoot. Orthoses that may be considered include ankle–foot orthoses (AFOs) for ankle, hindfoot, and midtarsal deformities; rocker-bottom shoe modifications for decreased ankle, hindfoot, and forefoot motion; molded-leather ankle braces for hindfoot arthritis; and custom-made and prefabricated orthoses for midfoot and forefoot problems. The University of California Biomechanics Laboratory (UCBL) brace is designed to limit the motion of the subtalar joint.

Nonsteroidal antiinflammatory drugs (NSAIDs) are often used as first-line pharmacologic treatment. However, concerns remain regarding potential gastrointestinal and cardiac side effects. All NSAIDs have been linked to an increased cardiac risk.[501]

Intraarticular corticosteroid injections can provide significant and sometimes prolonged clinical relief; however, the American College of Rheumatology recommends waiting at least 3 months between injections.[10] Several studies have noted efficacy for up to 2 years; yet some patients experience much shorter relief. This difference is poorly understood. In larger joints, synovial fluid aspiration before steroid injection may increase effectiveness and duration and may reduce clinical relapse.[584] Side effects include periinjection lipodystrophy; skin atrophy; postinjection flare-reaction (1%-10% of patients), thought to be caused by the crystalline preparation of the steroid); and facial flushing (15% more common in women).

Prolonged steroid use has many side effects, including hypothalamic-pituitary axis suppression and hepatic gluconeogenesis, which worsens glucose intolerance among diabetics. Intraarticular injections have far less systemic side effects than oral preparations, and the effect is usually transient.[425]

Contraindications to intraarticular steroid injection include preexisting septic arthritis, surrounding cellulitis, injection into a prosthetic joint, preexisting fracture, or coagulopathy. Although septic arthritis has been reported after intraarticular injection (1 in 3,000 to 1 in 50,000 in the knee[80]) the risk is small with appropriate skin preparation and technique. Cartilage degeneration after intraarticular steroid injection has been noted in animals, but similar complications in humans have not been reported. Steroids may be effective regardless of the type of arthritis. Preoperative fluoroscopic-guided injections (Fig. 19-6) may help determine which joints would be improved by arthrodesis. However, the anesthetic/steroid mixture may leak to adjacent tarsometatarsal joints in up to 20% of cases.[289]

To date, there are no pharmacologic agents known to halt cartilage destruction or restore the cartilage matrix. However, Sampson and Hilton[490] demonstrated that teriparatide (Forteo), a recombinant parathyroid hormone, increases proteoglycan content and inhibits cartilage degeneration in mice. Although this drug is used to treat osteoporosis, further studies may reveal other applications.

The primary surgical indication for degenerative arthritis of the foot or ankle is intractable pain or deformity that is not relieved with local or systemic pharmacologic treatment or biomechanical aids, such as immobilization or bracing. Surgical techniques vary from arthrodesis to excisional arthroplasty to osteotomy. Joint implants, in general, have been disappointing in the forefoot and hindfoot (see later discussion of first MTP implants).

DEGENERATIVE ARTHRITIS OF THE HINDFOOT

The hindfoot comprises the subtalar, talonavicular and calcaneocuboid joints and includes the adjacent bones and soft tissue structures. These joints are coupled to provide stability and shock-absorption. As the subtalar joint inverts, the transverse tarsal joint locks, stabilizing the hindfoot and midfoot to allow for toe-off. As the subtalar joint everts, the transverse tarsal joint is unlocked, to allow for shock absorption when the foot is planted.

Pain while walking on uneven ground is a common complaint of patients with subtalar arthritis. Many of these patients have pain directly over the sinus tarsi with deep palpation. Pain over the talonavicular joint or calcaneocuboid joint is often seen with transverse tarsal arthritis.

A prior talar neck fracture (Figs. 19-7 and 19-8) accounts for 50% to 100% of posttraumatic subtalar joint arthritis.[69]

Pennal noted that up to 60% of patients with talar fractures required subsequent subtalar arthrodesis.[433] In Sanders' series, 37% of patients with talus fractures required a second surgery; 76% went on to subtalar arthrodesis, 23% had triple arthrodesis, and 11% had pantalar arthrodesis.[491]

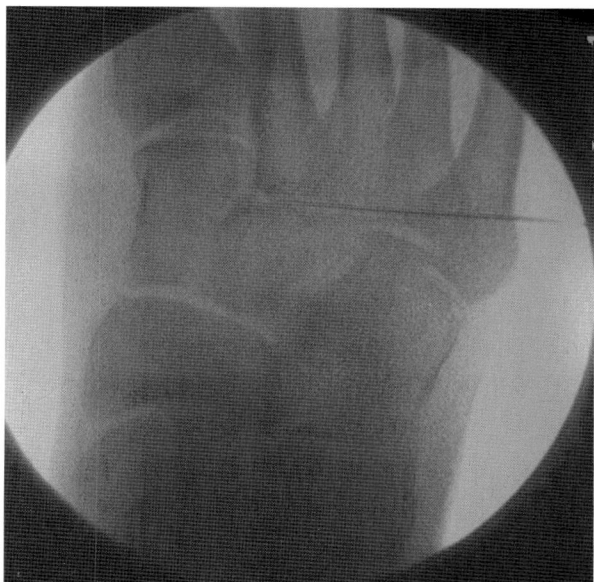

Figure 19-6 Fluoroscopy and intraarticular midfoot steroid injection.

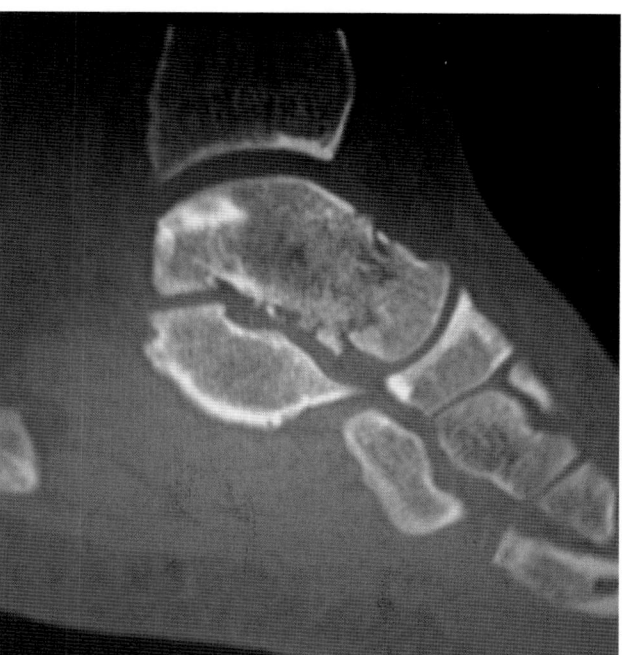

Figure 19-7 Lateral computed tomography scan of a nondisplaced talar neck fracture.

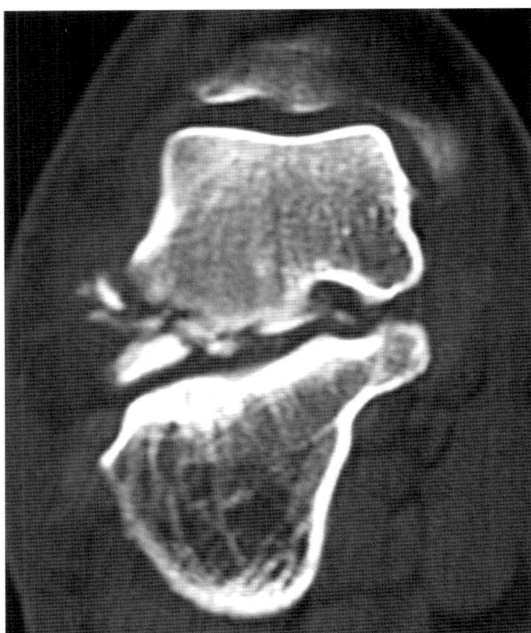

Figure 19-8 Coronal computed tomography scan demonstrating posttraumatic subtalar arthritis.

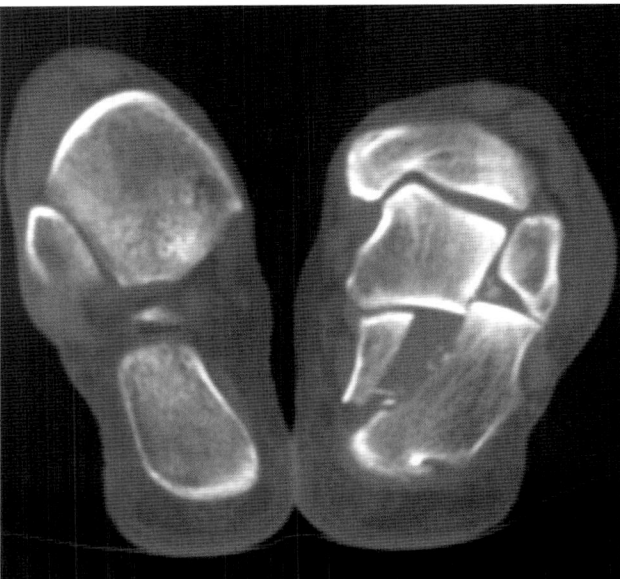

Figure 19-9 *Left,* Normal hindfoot architecture. *Right,* Sanders type II calcaneus fracture shown in a coronal computed tomography scan.

Up to 17% of intraarticular calcaneal fractures will require a second surgery because of symptomatic subtalar arthritis.[41] Sanders concluded that this is dependent upon the degree of comminution of the subtalar joint, because 23% of Sanders type II fractures, and 73% of Sanders type IV fractures required subtalar arthrodesis (Fig. 19-9).[492]

Subtalar Arthrodesis

Subtalar arthrodesis in the nontrauma setting has reported success rates of 80% to 90% good-to-excellent results.[485] Unfortunately, when performed in the setting of post-traumatic arthritis, good-to-excellent results are reported in only 50% to 60% of cases.[350] Thermann noted 41% fair-to-poor results with secondary subtalar arthrodesis after calcaneal fracture,[547] and Pennal noted poor results in his small series of early subtalar arthrodesis for talar neck fractures despite high fusion rates in both series. Flemister et al[163] noted a fusion rate of 96% in a series of 86 subtalar arthrodeses resulting from complications after calcaneal fracture, yet patients only achieved a mean American Orthopaedic Foot and Ankle Society (AOFAS) Hindfoot score of 75 at 2-year follow-up. Because of poor results with secondary arthrodesis after calcaneal fractures, Huefner et al[242] reported results of primary subtalar arthrodesis for comminuted calcaneal fractures. This team noted good-to-excellent results in 5 of 6 patients using the AOFAS scoring system. These differences in outcome between primary and secondary subtalar arthrodesis remain poorly understood.[3]

Complications after comminuted calcaneal fractures include a loss of calcaneal height, loss of talar declination, and anterior ankle impingement. For these patients, many have advocated a bone block subtalar arthrodesis to restore the calcaneal height, and talar declination. Garras et al[179] reported on the use of frozen structural allograft for this purpose and noted a 90% successful fusion rate using structural autograft.

Saville et al[496] reported using the medial approach for hindfoot arthrodesis when severe valgus deformity is present. In their series, 10 patients underwent subtalar arthrodesis, 6 underwent subtalar and talonavicular arthrodesis, and 2 had triple arthrodesis. All wounds healed, and 17 of 18 patients went on to successful fusion over 5.6 months. The authors suggested that when the hindfoot is in extreme valgus, use of a medial approach may help avoid tension-related lateral wound problems and decrease sural nerve complications.

Glanzmann and Sanhueza-Hernandez[187] reported their results of arthroscopic subtalar arthrodesis. They noted a 100% fusion rate using a posterolateral portal (just lateral to the Achilles tendon) and an anterolateral portal (centered upon the sinus tarsi). Joint preparation is done primarily through the posterolateral portal with a shaver, curette, and motorized burr. Visualization is achieved via a 3.5-mm arthroscope through the antero-lateral portal. Lee et al[328] also reported arthroscopic sub-talar arthrodesis but with prone positioning through two posterior portals (medial and lateral to the Achilles tendon). Scranton et al[505] reported on a comparison of open versus arthroscopic subtalar arthrodesis and noted that there was no large difference in operative time: 58 minutes for the open procedure versus 63 minutes for the arthroscopic procedure. The main advantage of an arthroscopic approach is decreased wound issues.

However, fusion rates and other parameters have not been shown to be superior to traditional approaches.

Regardless of approach, hindfoot positioning during subtalar arthrodesis can be challenging. Optimally, the calcaneus should be in slight valgus (approximately 5 degrees) relative to the talus. Frigg et al[172] suggested that visual inspection is inadequate to determine correct hindfoot position, and that the Saltzman-el-Khoury hindfoot alignment view should be used. This weight-bearing, posterior to anterior radiograph is aimed 20 degrees caudal, with the x-ray beam parallel to the medial border of the foot.[486] Unfortunately, this is impractical in an operative setting.[172] Thus visual inspection and fluoroscopic imaging are most commonly used to determine hindfoot position during surgery.

Graft use (autograft, allograft, or bone substitute) and hardware configuration are additional options the surgeon must consider for hindfoot arthrodesis. The authors routinely use proximal tibial or iliac crest autograft and cannulated lag screw fixation to achieve compression across the joint (Fig. 19-10).

Frigg et al[171] reported on the use of porous tantalum interposition for ankle and subtalar arthrodesis and found that fusion was successful in nine of nine patients. Tantalum has been used for spine fusions and in the setting of hip and knee surgery. The advantage appears to be rapid ingrowth into the tantalum without donor-site morbidity.

Calcaneocuboid Arthrodesis

The incidence of calcaneocuboid joint arthritis after calcaneal fracture has been reported to be between 33% and 76%, with a higher percentage in joint depression-type fractures.[142] However, those with fractures involving the actual calcaneocuboid joint are typically asymptomatic.[294] Astion and Wulker[15,599] both noted that an isolated calcaneocuboid fusion has little effect on the motion of the adjacent joints and that the motion of the calcaneocuboid is small.

Talonavicular Arthrodesis

Isolated arthritis of the talonavicular joint (either resulting from trauma or degeneration) may require isolated fusion. However, arthrodesis of the talonavicular joint has a high nonunion rate. This is likely due to the spheric shape of the joint and the resultant difficulty in exposure and preparation of the joint surfaces. Published reports demonstrate a union rate between 63% and 97%.[165,221] Chen et al[82] reported a 94% union rate using either staples or screws without bone graft for isolated talonavicular joint fusions. Jarrell et al[256] compared three methods of fixation and determined that there was no significant difference in load to failure between the three constructs. These studies support the notion that excellent joint surface preparation is more important than either fixation type or use of graft. Indications for talonavicular arthrodesis include isolated arthritis (Fig. 19-11), rheumatoid arthritis, or pes planovalgus deformity.

Astion[15] reported that isolated talonavicular joint fusion limits the subtalar joint to 8% of its native motion. In addition, fusing the talonavicular joint alone behaves similarly to the double hindfoot arthrodesis.[546]

Double Arthrodesis

The double arthrodesis (fusion of the talonavicular and calcaneocuboid joints) may be undertaken when these joints are diseased, while the subtalar joint is spared.

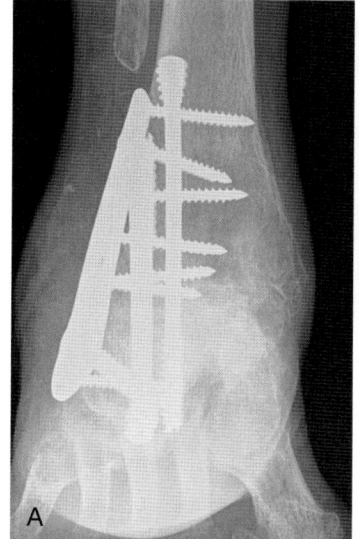
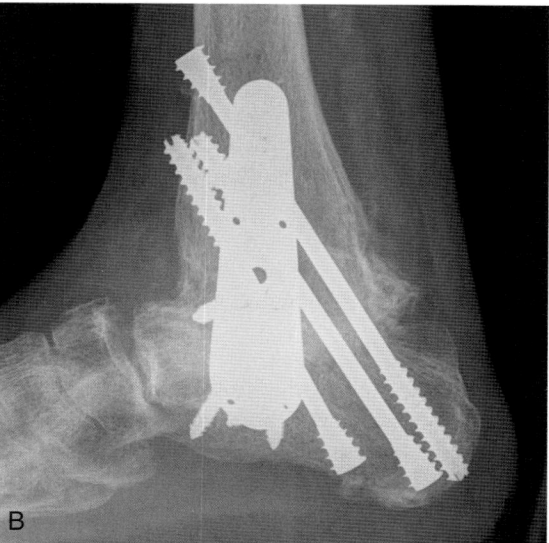

Figure 19-10 **A,** AP radiograph and **B,** lateral radiograph of primary subtalar and ankle arthrodesis for pantlar degenerative arthritis.

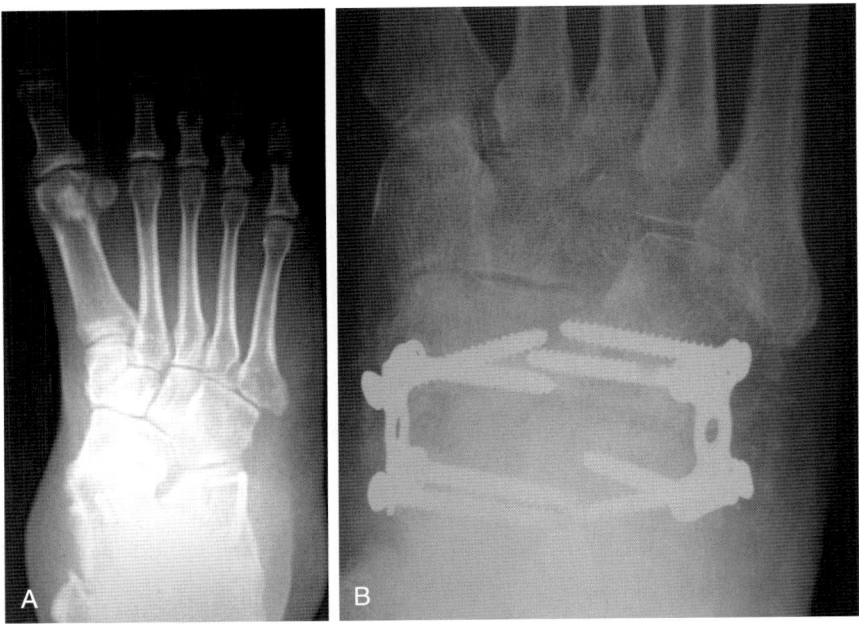

Figure 19-11 **A,** Anteroposterior (AP) radiograph demonstrating end-stage talonavicular arthritis. **B,** AP radiograph of double arthrodesis (talonavicular and calcaneocuboid joints) with plates and screws.

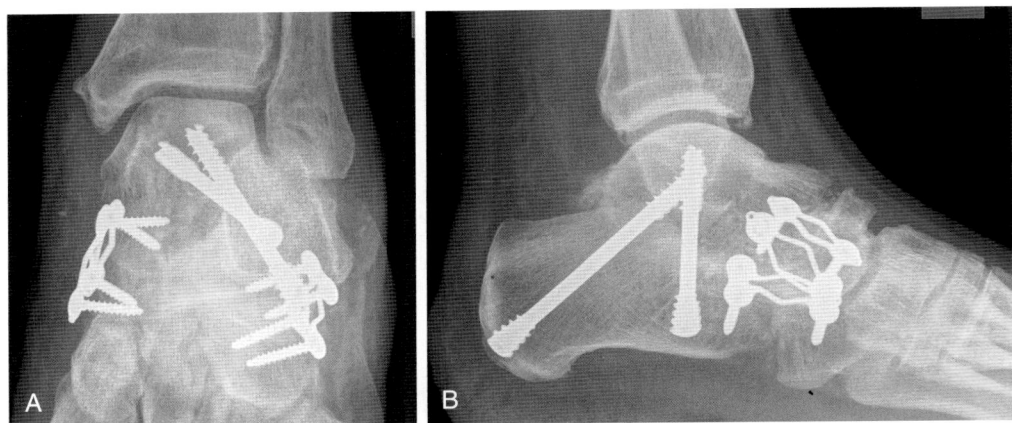

Figure 19-12 Anteroposterior **(A)** lateral **(B)** weight-bearing ankle radiographs after triple arthrodesis.

Locking of the transverse tarsal joints results in an essentially immobile subtalar joint, and this double arthrodesis functions much like a triple hindfoot arthrodesis.[89] Beischer et al[28] noted that with a double or triple joint hindfoot fusion, the ankle joint range of motion during stance decreases by 33% while the ipsilateral knee range of motion increases by 13%.

Citing less than desireable results after triple arthrodesis, Sammarco et al[489] recommended a modified double arthrodesis of the subtalar and talonavicular joints. They noted that all of their patients were satisfied with the result, and only 1 of 16 patients required revision surgery for nonunion. Advantages of this type of double versus triple arthrodesis include reduced operative time and avoidance of potential calcaneocuboid nonunion (reported as 20% with the triple arthrodesis).[24]

Triple and Pantalar Arthrodesis

The triple arthrodesis is regarded by many as a salvage procedure. Typical indications include posttraumatic hindfoot arthritis, rheumatoid arthritis, or stage III posterior tibial tendon dysfunction. It is a demanding procedure. The purpose is to restore plantigrade position of the foot, with the hindfoot in slight valgus. Not infrequently, a forefoot osteotomy is required to correct forefoot rotation in the coronal plane. Malunion is not uncommon and frequently leads to dissatisfaction for both the surgeon and patient. Resnick et al[461] demonstrated that placing the calcaneus in too much valgus (Fig. 19-12) increases the force on the deltoid ligament by 76% during weight bearing. In contrast, a varus hindfoot places pressure on the lateral column and fifth metatarsal and may lead to lateral ankle instability and ankle arthritis.

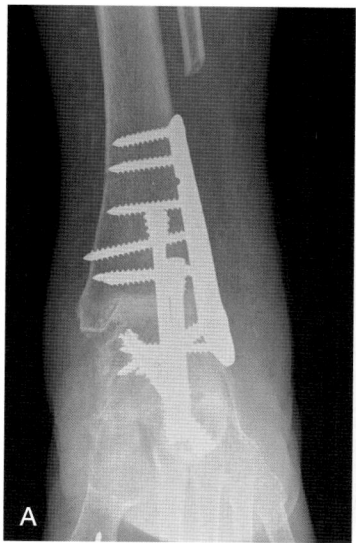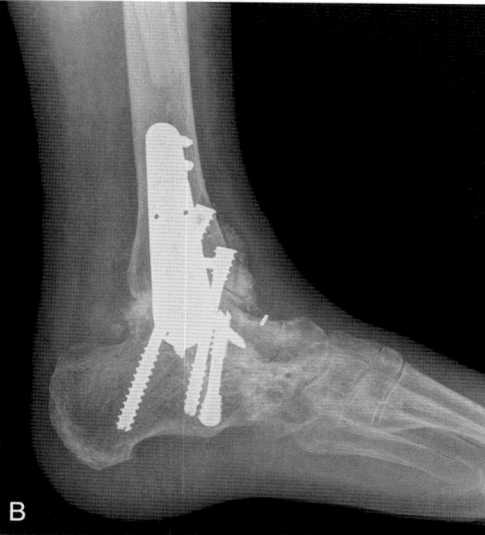

Figure 19-13 Anteroposterior **(A)** and lateral **(B)** radiographs demonstrating a pantalar arthrodesis. After a triple arthrodesis, an ankle arthrodesis was performed as a staged pantalar arthrodesis.

Arthritis in adjacent joints (ankle and tarsometatarsal joints) has been reported after triple arthrodesis in up to 58% of patients in a 21-year follow-up.[585] Nonunion and avascular necrosis have been reported. Graves[200] and Beischer[28] noted that 28% to 33% of their patients walked with a limp after triple arthrodesis despite successful fusion.

For those with disabling hindfoot and ankle arthrosis, Acosta et al[2] recommended pantalar arthrodesis involving the tibiotalar, subtalar, talonavicular, and calcaneocuboid joints (Fig. 19-13). Although 23 of 27 patients went on to solid fusion, there was a 37% complication rate, and only 5 patients had an excellent result. The authors suggested that, like the triple arthrodesis, this procedure be considered only as a salvage operation.[2]

DEGENERATIVE ARTHRITIS OF THE MIDFOOT

Midfoot arthritis frequently develops as a sequela of a fracture or dislocation through the Lisfranc joint but may also develop spontaneously because of osteoarthritis or inflammatory arthritis. Thus it generally has a bimodal presentation: those with a traumatic etiology often seek care in their thirties, while those with a nontraumatic etiology often present in their fifties.[270] Zonno and Myerson[611] suggested that most midfoot pain is due to atraumatic osteoarthritis, although others maintain that trauma is the primary cause of arthritic change in the midfoot. Davitt et al[123] hypothesized that midfoot degeneration is the result of metatarsal length differences. The authors noted that a longer second metatarsal correlated with midfoot arthritis. Wearing high-heeled shoes may also contribute to midfoot arthritis.[606]

It should also be noted that arthritis in any of the tarsometatarsal joints in the absence of a history of trauma may represent an early Charcot (joint) deformity. Charcot arthropathy can develop with diabetes as well as with peripheral neuropathy and other neurologic disorders (Fig. 19-14).

Regardless of the cause, the development of midfoot arthritis can be an extremely disabling condition because of the stress placed on the longitudinal arch with weight bearing. A bony prominence may develop on the dorsal aspect of the midfoot because of osteophyte formation, which makes wearing shoes painful. A progressive flatfoot deformity can also develop from instability of the metatarsocuneiform (MTC) joint, with development of a plantar bony prominence and subsequent callus formation. Jung et al[270] noted four presentations associated with tarsometatarsal joint arthritis: no deformity, pes planovalgus, hallux valgus, and the rocker-bottom deformity. Mann et al[357] noted that 78% of patients with midfoot arthritis had abnormal foot posture and difficulty with shoe wear.

With continued arthritic change, an abduction and dorsiflexion deformity of the midfoot occurs (Fig. 19-15). This progression of pain and deformity makes ambulation difficult.

In examination of the foot, passive manipulation of the midfoot involves abduction of the forefoot and a pronation stress test to determine the location of maximal pain. The piano-key test (Fig. 19-16) is positive when a plantarly directed force applied to the metatarsal head elicits pain in the same tarsometatarsal joint. This is a sensitive indicator of a symptomatic joint or joints.[282]

A complicating factor with midfoot arthropathy is a simultaneous hindfoot deformity. Malalignment at the

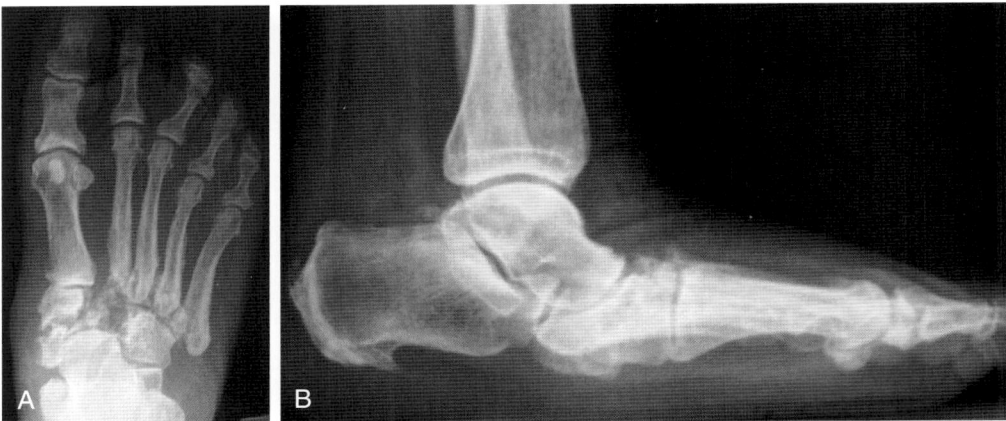

Figure 19-14 Anteroposterior **(A)** and lateral **(B)** radiographs demonstating marked midfoot arthritis with painful progressive deformity.

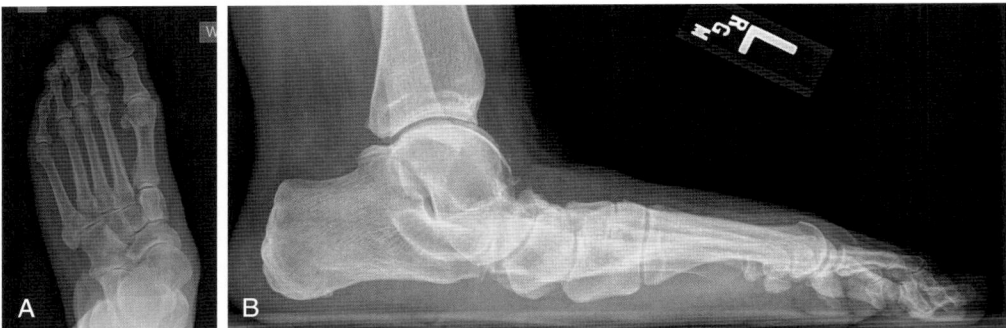

Figure 19-15 Anteroposterior **(A)** and lateral **(B)** radiographs demonstrating severe peritalar subluxation with inflammatory arthritis.

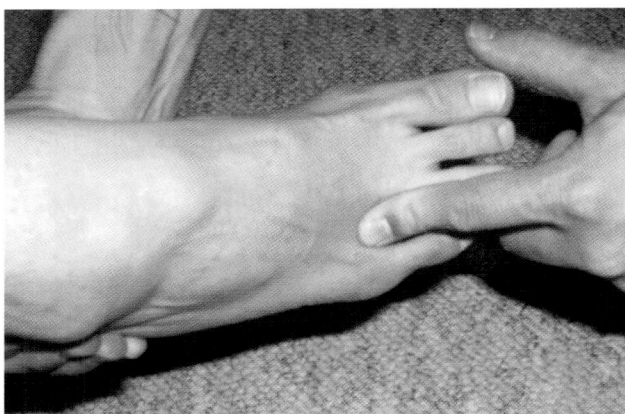

Figure 19-16 The piano-key test is positive when a patient feels pain in their tarsometatarsal joint with a plantarly directed force applied to the metatarsal head.

transverse tarsal joint and a valgus deformity of the hindfoot often are associated with severe midfoot arthritis. A careful preoperative physical examination is necessary to determine the extent of the midfoot and hindfoot malalignment. In the subtle cavus foot with degenerative

arthritis, the Coleman block test helps to determine the need for associated hindfoot procedures, such as the addition of a calcaneal osteotomy or creation of plantar flexion through the first MTC joint, with the arthrodesis or opening wedge through the medial cuneiform (Fig. 19-17).

Correctable or supple hindfoot valgus associated with medial column arthritis should reduce with proper restoration of alignment (reduction of any varus or rotational deformity, abduction, and dorsiflexion) during the midfoot arthrodesis but any fixed or residual valgus deformity without arthritis should be addressed with a medial displacement osteotomy or lateral column lengthening. Moreover, gastrocnemius recession or Achilles lengthening may be necessary after correction is achieved and bone alignment is restored to obtain a plantigrade foot.

Anatomically, the tarsometatarsal joint is divided into three columns: the medial column (first MTC joint), the middle column (second and third MTC joints), and the lateral column (fourth and fifth metatarsocuboid joints). Radiographically, the medial column is reduced when the medial border of the first metatarsal is aligned with the medial border of the medial cuneiform. The middle column is aligned when the medial border of the second

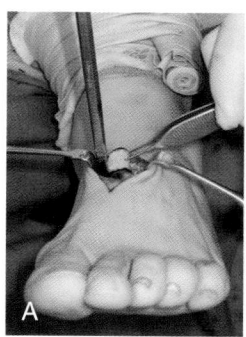
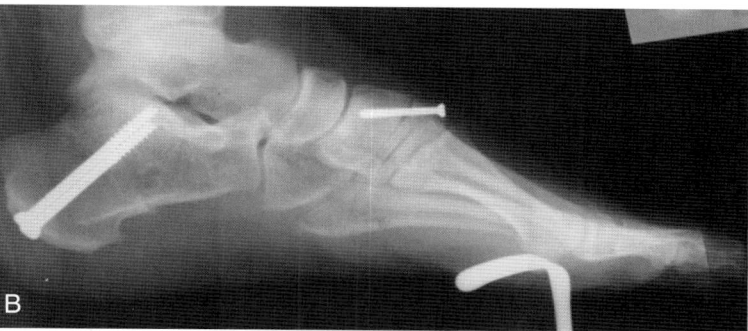

Figure 19-17 A, Cotton osteotomy and placement of dorsal bone graft into medial cuneiform to plantar flex the first ray. **B,** A lateral radiograph demonstrating the Cotton and calcaneal osteotomy. (Original photographs by J.E. Johnson, MD, and C.B. Hirose, MD.)

metatarsal is aligned with the medial border of the intermediate cuneiform. For the lateral column, reduction is achieved when the medial border of the fourth metatarsal is aligned with the medial border of the cuboid. On the lateral radiograph, restoration of the first metatarsal declination angle and arch height are imperative.

Arthritic changes such as joint space narrowing can be seen on the weight-bearing anterior posterior radiograph. On the lateral radiograph, midfoot collapse of the tarsometatarsal joints may or may not be seen. The changes may also coincide with pes planovalgus deformities (forefoot abduction with midfoot collapse). Jung et al[270] noted that with primary osteoarthritis of the tarsometatarsal joints radiographs demonstrate a lower medial cuneiform height than that of posttraumatic arthritis.

Menz et al[376] reported that foot structure differs in elderly patients with midfoot arthritis compared with those without. In those with radiographic evidence of naviculocuneiform and talonavicular joint arthritis, they noted significantly flatter feet as evidenced by a small calcaneal inclination and a larger calcaneal first-metatarsal angle.

Treatment

Conservative management of midfoot degenerative arthritis includes a soft or rigid custom-molded orthosis that provides support to the longitudinal arch. A full-length carbon fiber insert may also be used. Rao et al[450] demonstrated that these orthotics significantly lessen the load duration and the intensity borne by the midfoot. Ibuki et al[249] also reported that carbon fiber foot plates provided equivalent improvements in pain, activity levels, and walking ability when compared with custom-molded semirigid orthotics.

A polypropylene AFO may be used for more advanced degenerative arthrosis. Cast immobilization and, occasionally, a short-leg brace may be used to diminish pain. Unfortunately, as arthritis of the MTC joint progresses, with subsequent loss of the longitudinal arch and abduction of the forefoot, the use of AFOs becomes more limited. An AFO does not reorient the foot but does add

support and stability to the foot. In time and with progression of deformity, surgical intervention is indicated.

Surgery consists of an arthrodesis of the involved midfoot joints. Most often, the second and third tarsometatarsal joints are involved. The first metatarsal medial cuneiform articulation is involved less often and the fourth and fifth metatarsocuboid articulation least often.[304,447] Whether to include the intercuneiform articulations depends on inspection of these areas for arthrosis. Sangeorzan et al[493] infrequently incorporated the intercuneiform joints (1 of 16), whereas Mann et al[357] and Horton and Olney[240] incorporated them in the arthrodesis technique more often. If any doubt exists, Mann et al[357] suggest incorporating the intercuneiform joint within the arthrodesis.

In the patient with a pes planus deformity and abduction of the forefoot, it is important to reestablish the normal alignment of the midfoot at surgery. This is accomplished by bringing the medial Lisfranc joint into normal alignment with the hindfoot by adducting and plantar flexing the first, second, and third MTC articulations. Although a lateral column arthrodesis is much more difficult to achieve, on occasion, it may be necessary to realign the entire Lisfranc joint in the presence of severe deformity. Komenda et al[304] recommended reduction of the lateral column and temporary pin fixation until ambulation is initiated. They found a lateral column arthrodesis typically is unnecessary even in the presence of arthrosis (see Chapter 20).

Promising results have been obtained with interposition arthroplasty for lateral column arthritis,[36] and this procedure may be used as a second-stage procedure if needed for continued symptoms. Berlet et al[36] performed tendon interposition for fourth and fifth tarsometatarsal arthritis and noted that 6 of 8 patients were satisfied. Shawen et al[508] used ceramic sphere interposition. Their patients showed an 87% improvement in American Orthopaedic Foot and Ankle Society (AOFAS) scores and, 11 of 11 would undergo the procedure again. Alternatively, reliable results have been reported with arthrodesis of the fourth and fifth tarsometatarsal joints as isolated procedures or in combination with medial column

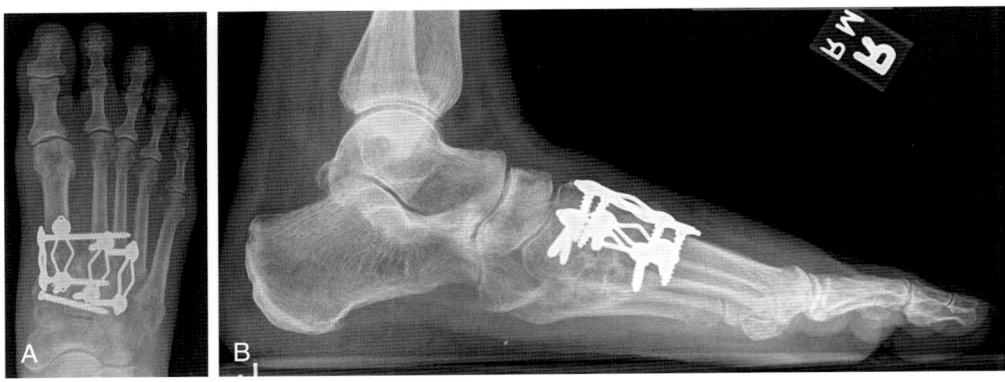

Figure 19-18 Anteroposterior **(A)** and lateral **(B)** radiographs of a first, second, and third tarsometatarsal joint arthrodesis, using dorsal locking compression plates.

arthrodesis for rocker-bottom deformities in neuropathic conditions.[447]

Multiple fixation methods have been described, including an in situ bone dowel technique,[263] slot graft technique,[298] plate and screw fixation,[304,357] as well as Kirschner (K)-wire fixation with bone grafting.[493] A plantarly placed plate and screws may offer a mechanical advantage over screws alone[362]; however, a comparison of a dorsomedial locking plate with crossed screws (Fig. 19-18) to secure the first metatarsocuneiform joint showed no significant difference in mechanical strength.[206]

The potential concern with lateral midfoot arthrodesis as part of a medial column or central column procedure is that it creates an extremely rigid midfoot. In neuropathic conditions, it may be necessary to achieve the additional stability afforded by inclusion of the lateral column joints, but in posttraumatic or inflammatory cases, the authors prefer to avoid arthrodesis of the lateral column.

Whether to perform reduction of a midfoot deformity has been a controversial topic. Johnson and Johnson[263] reported on patients with mild and moderate midfoot deformities. They performed in situ fusions using K-wire internal fixation with a supplemental autogenous iliac crest graft technique. Nine of 13 patients (70%) reported good or excellent results and three nonunions. The most often fused joints were the second and third tarsometatarsal (66%) joints.

In a review of 16 patients, Sangeorzan et al[493] advocated reduction of the pes planus and abduction deformity and noted 11 of 16 cases with satisfactory results (69%). Few patients had excellent results or a normal foot, but many "returned to work."

Horton and Olney[240] performed three in situ fusions and six realignment arthrodeses on eight patients (nine feet) for posttraumatic or degenerative arthrosis of Lisfranc joints. They used a five-hole, one-third semitubular plate that spanned the tarsometatarsal joint. An iliac crest graft was packed into the intervals between the tarsometatarsal joints and between the first and second metatarsals. The authors noted a strong correlation between reduction

of the deformity and the outcome and reported seven of nine good and excellent results.

Mann et al[357] reported that 38 of 41 patients with primary, traumatic, or inflammatory arthrosis of the midfoot were satisfied. They advocated reduction of the deformity. Eleven patients had an autogenous bone graft placed at the time of arthrodesis.

Komenda et al[304] and Sangeorzan et al[493] recommend that the lateral column not be included in the arthrodesis because this area is usually asymptomatic even with significant radiographic evidence of arthrosis. They emphasized that realignment of the midfoot contributes to a successful result. Komenda et al[304] stated that if there is 15 degrees of malalignment in the transverse or sagittal plane or greater than 2 mm of displacement, reduction of the deformity is indicated. They did use temporary internal fixation when the lateral column was realigned but did not routinely perform arthrodesis for the lateral column.

Shereff et al[333] reported 81% successful results using iliac crest bone graft and K-wire fixation in 16 patients. They found that fusion of the fourth and fifth TMT joints was associated with significantly poorer functional and subjective scores.

The use of an autogenous iliac crest graft often increases the success rate of arthrodesis. Sangeorzan et al[493] stated that an additional graft was not necessary. Komenda et al[304] used an ancillary graft in one third of cases and Mann et al[357] in one fourth of cases.

The current authors prefer to avoid using iliac crest unless structural defects require its use. However, the use of bone healing and enhancing substrates, such as platelet concentration systems, have shown promise. Han and colleagues demonstrated that platelet-rich plasma (PRP) enhances osteoinductivity.[216] Landi et al[317] noted an increase in fusion rates at 3 months as well as an increase in bone density by using a platelet gel in lumbar fusions. Hauschild[229] reported on a successful fusion in a canine tarsal joint by using PRP. Gandhi et al[176] reported on nine patients with foot and ankle nonunions. Using PRP and autologous bone graft at time of revision, the mean time to fusion was 2 months. Bibbo and colleagues[44] also used PRP for foot and ankle fusions, concluding that PRP increased the fusion rate with low complications.

Electrical, magnetic, or ultrasonographic bone stimulation can also be helpful. Several studies have reported on the positive influence of each of these modalities. Dhawan[131] reported a faster time to fusion with the use of pulsed electromagnetic field (PEMF) therapy in hindfoot fusions.

The authors believe that realignment with compression screw fixation across the respective TMT joints and a medial column plate as a neutralization or primary construct is needed to obtain a successful result in most cases. There is no consensus on the preferred approach for all midfoot arthritic problems, and the technique used must be tailored to the individual patient's problem and the surgeon's experience.

The authors' preferred approach is to incorporate the medial column joints and to leave the lateral column mobile, in general, a two-incision technique is used for the arthrodesis, with a medial and dorsal incision spaced as far apart as possible to minimize wound-healing problems.

Patient satisfaction after midfoot fusion ranges from very good to acceptable. Nemec and colleagues[410] noted 90% patient satisfaction. Mann et al[357] reported an overall satisfaction of 86%, and Jung et al[270] reported an 87% satisfaction. However, Baumhauer[430] suggested that patients may only experience 60% reduction in pain.

The magnitude of surgery requires a lengthy postoperative convalescence. After midfoot arthrodesis, most workers have difficulty returning to an occupation that requires standing for a full 8-hour day. Postoperative complications include skin slough, metatarsalgia, and incisional neuromas.[43,304,357]

Nonunion rates have been reported to be between 3% and 8%, but anecdotal evidence may point to a higher rate.[270,341,410] Moreover, in a review of complications associated with midfoot and hindfoot arthrodesis, Bibbo et al[43] reported that wound problems can be expected in 3% to 5% of nondiabetic patients undergoing elective arthrodesis procedures, but that rate increased up to 53% in diabetic patients (Fig. 19-19). Given the increasing

numbers of diabetic patients in the United States and other countries, every effort should be made to prevent complications by evaluating and treating the vascular, neurologic, and general nutritional status of the patient before arthrodesis. Hindfoot alignment must be considered before midfoot arthrodesis as well, and concomitant osteotomies of staged hindfoot reconstruction, or both, should be considered.

INFLAMMATORY ARTHROPATHIES

Rheumatoid Arthritis

Rheumatoid arthritis (RA) is a systemic autoimmune disease characterized by synovitis, periarticular bone loss, and osteoporosis. It can affect both small and large joints, is generally symmetric, and affects both the upper and lower limbs.[472] The disease affects 0.3% to 2.1% of the general population, and Rana[449] has estimated that five million people in the United States suffer from rheumatoid arthritis. RA is two to four times more common in women than in men, yet no predilection exists for any single ethnic group.[259] Onset can occur at any age, but the prevalence increases with age, peaking during the third to fifth decades. The disease course generally follows one of three pathways: (1) a relentless, destructive and aggressive course; (2) a monocyclic course notable for a single episode of synovitis without permanent cartilage damage; and (3) a polycyclic course with multiple episodes of attack followed by remissions. Up to 70% of cases follow the polycyclic course.[521]

The actual cause of the disease is unknown; however, genetic and environmental factors may play a role in etiology. Patients with an identical twin who has RA are four times more likely to develop RA than nontwin counterparts.[336] Associations have also been found with viral infections, including cytomegalovirus, rubella, Epstein-Barr virus, and parvovirus.[259] These viral agents may mimic portions of human leukocyte antigen (HLA) DR4, which stimulates the immune system to begin attacking the synovial lining of the joint in genetically susceptible individuals. Further etiologic studies are needed to fully elucidate the cause of RA.

The disease can affect all joints of the body but has a predilection for the small joints of the hand and foot. Much attention has been centered on rheumatoid deformities of the hand in terms of initial involvement of individual joints; with acute onset, however, the feet are involved slightly more often than the hand (15.7% vs. 14.7%) (Short et al cited by Calabro[65]). Foot and ankle symptoms account for more than 50% of the presenting complaints in those initially diagnosed with RA. In addition, it has been estimated that 85% to 90% of patients with RA will eventually experience foot or ankle problems.[565,569]

Moreover, persons affected with mild-to-moderate rheumatoid arthritis with concomitant foot involvement have marked reduction in mobility and functional

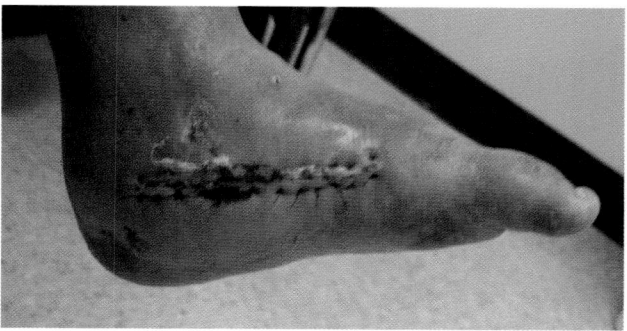

Figure 19-19 Delayed wound healing incision in a patient with diabetes.

capacity.[587] An increased incidence of foot problems occurs with duration of the disease process,[380] and in chronic RA, Michelson[380] reported that ankle and hindfoot symptoms were much more common (42%) than forefoot symptoms (28%) in a series of 99 patients followed in an outpatient setting. In chronic rheumatoid arthritis, symmetric involvement is common. Early on, however, asymmetric involvement may be observed.

History and Physical Examination

Early complaints of patients with RA involve poorly defined forefoot pain and metatarsalgia. Typically, these complaints result from synovitis and an intraarticular effusion, which lead to painful ambulation. Poorly defined metatarsalgia can indicate an interdigital neuroma; in time, however, synovitis and deformity can make the diagnosis more straightforward. Zielaskowski[610] has reported an association of rheumatoid synovitis, nodule formation, and interdigital neuroma.

A variable course of presentation occurs in the symptomatic rheumatoid foot. Nonspecific forefoot swelling is characterized by tenderness to palpation and pain on ambulation. The most common forefoot deformities are hallux valgus, subluxation or dislocation of the lesser MTP joints, and fixed hammer toe or claw toe deformities of the lesser toes (Fig. 19-20).

Rheumatoid arthritis can be divided into the following four stages based on physical examination and radiographic findings:

- *Stage I:* Discomfort and synovitis; no bone deformity or significant joint space narrowing
- *Stage II:* Early involvement with flexible deformity; minimal erosive changes
- *Stage III:* Fixed soft tissue deformity; significant erosive joint changes
- *Stage IV:* Severe hallux valgus, dislocation of the lesser MTP joints with fixed hammer toe or claw toe deformities, pes planovalgus (flatfoot), and hindfoot arthroses; articular destruction on radiographs

Forefoot

In the early stages of rheumatoid arthritis, specific changes in the foot include inflammation of the synovium, with distention of the MTP joint capsule. Synovial proliferation leads to chronic capsule distention, resulting in loss of integrity of both the MTP joint supporting capsular structures and the collateral ligaments. With continued ambulation in the presence of soft tissue instability and with constant dorsiflexion stress on the MTP joints, subluxation and eventual dislocation occur.[380,527] As the MTP joints of the lesser toes dislocate, the base of the proximal phalanx eventually comes to rest on the dorsal metatarsal metaphysis (Fig. 19-21).

Progressive contracture of the long flexor tendons and the plantar intrinsic muscles lock the base of the proximal phalanx on the dorsal metatarsal neck. The proximal phalanx becomes fixed in a dorsiflexed position, creating a plantar-directed force on the metatarsal head.[115] Simultaneously, the plantar fat pad is drawn distally, leaving only an extremely thin soft tissue covering on the plantar aspect of the metatarsal heads (Fig. 19-22). The loss of the protective plantar fat pad cushion, coupled with increased stress on the underlying skin, can lead to the development of intractable plantar keratotic (IPK) lesions and, in time, ulceration of the plantar skin (Fig. 19-23).

The rheumatoid plantar fat pad is also significantly different than those of nonrheumatoid patients. Analysis with liquid gas chromatography demonstrates that the rheumatoid fat pad has a significantly higher ratio of saturated to unsaturated fat, as well as a higher viscosity. This is thought to reduce absorption of energy with foot strike, which may contribute to development of IPK lesions.[460]

Subluxation and dislocation of the lesser toes creates an imbalance between the intrinsic and extrinsic muscles and gives rise to progressive hammering of the lesser toes. Occasionally, a swan-neck deformity of a lesser toe develops, but more often, a hyperextension deformity of the MTP joint occurs in combination with a flexion deformity of the proximal interphalangeal (PIP) and distal

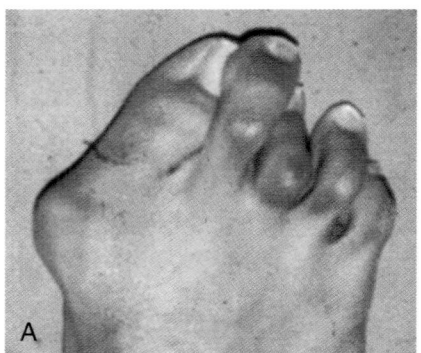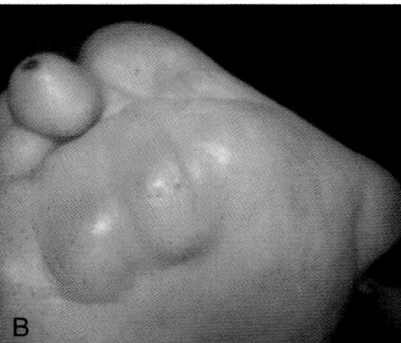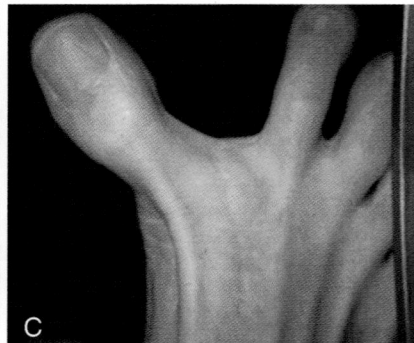

Figure 19-20 **A,** Clinical photograph of hallux valgus deformity with subluxation of the lesser metatarsophalangeal joints and complex hammer toe deformities. **B,** Plantar clinic photograph demonstrating lesser toe dislocation and plantar keratoses. **C,** Hallux varus deformity clinical photograph with lateral soft tissue attenuation and rupture.

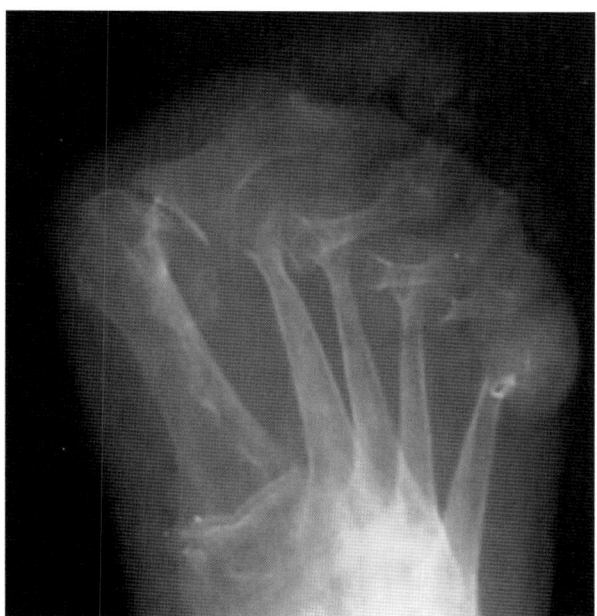

Figure 19-21 Radiograph of a patient with rheumatoid arthritis. The lesser metatarsophalangeal joints are dislocated, with proximal phalanges resting on the dorsal metatarsal necks.

interphalangeal (DIP) joints (claw toe deformity). Because of severe contracture of the lesser toes, significant shoe-fitting problems result. Callosities can develop over the dorsal aspect of the PIP joint, causing areas of pressure. Large synovial cysts or rheumatoid nodules can develop in the forefoot and, when located on weight-bearing surfaces, lead to significant difficulty with ambulation. Although, typically, the lesser toes deviate in a lateral direction, medial deviation occasionally occurs. The resultant direction depends, to a great extent, on the direction in which the hallux deviates (varus or valgus).

Michelson et al[380] reported that within the first 1 to 3 years of rheumatoid arthritis, 65% of patients are noted to have MTP synovitis. With chronic rheumatoid arthritis, Vidigal et al[575] and others[369,527] have reported that approximately two thirds of patients develop subluxation and dislocation of the lesser MTP joints (Fig. 19-24). Michelson et al[380] and others[369,565,575] have reported that the incidence of hammer toe or claw toe deformity of the lesser toes varies from 40% to 80%.

Hallux valgus increases in incidence and severity in the chronic stages of rheumatoid arthritis.[65] Michelson et al[380] and others[527,565,575] have reported a high incidence of hallux valgus in patients with chronic rheumatoid

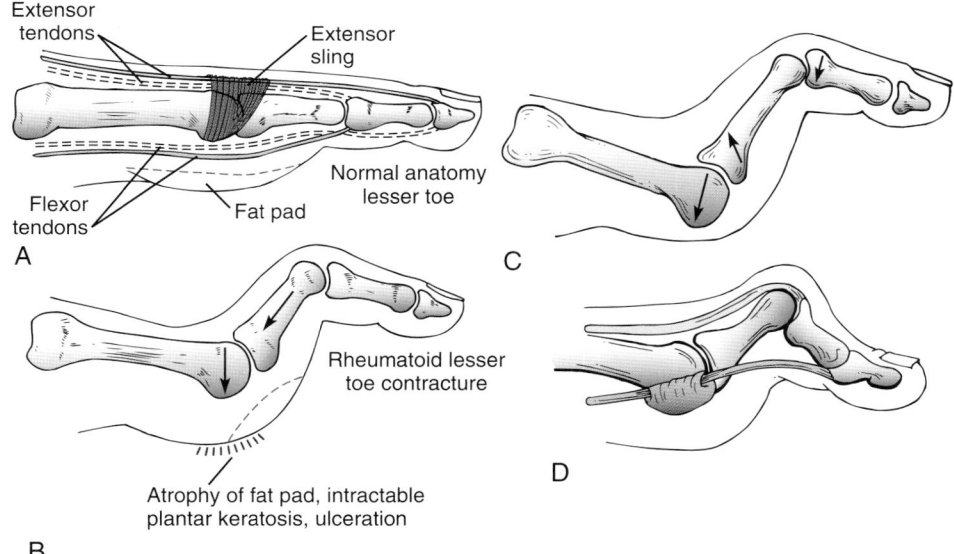

Figure 19-22 **A,** Normal alignment and balance of the metatarsophalangeal (MTP) joints and toes. Fat pad is centered beneath metatarsal heads. **B,** As rheumatoid deformity progresses, an imbalance occurs with progressive dorsal subluxation of the MTP joints and deformities of the lesser toes. The fat pad is drawn distally by the contracting lesser toes. **C,** End-stage deformity. Dislocation of the MTP joint with proximal phalanx ankylosed to the dorsal aspect of the metatarsal head. This forces the metatarsal head into the plantar aspect of the foot and results in severe callus formation. Lesser toes develop hammer toe deformities that often become severely contracted, and the fat pad is drawn distally and is no longer in a functional position. **D,** With chronic dorsiflexion deformity of the proximal phalanx at the MTP joint, flexor tendons subluxate dorsally, becoming functional extensors of the MTP joint.

arthritis (59%-90%). With progressive clawing of the lesser toes, little lateral stability is afforded to the great toe, and the hallux migrates laterally to a fixed position either under or over the second and third toes. Progression of the rheumatoid process includes destruction of articular cartilage and resorption of subchondral bone, which tends to destabilize the hallux. As the hallux valgus deformity worsens, the weight-bearing function of the first ray lessens and a greater proportion of weight is borne on the lesser metatarsal heads. Craxford et al[117] reported increased pressure beneath the second and third metatarsal heads with chronic rheumatoid arthritis.

With time, the total number of diseased forefoot joints increases, as does the severity of the disease.[244] In a longitudinal study, van der Leeden et al[569] studied newly diagnosed patients with rheumatoid arthritis over an 8-year span, specifically looking at clinical impairment and walking disability. On presentation, 67% of patients

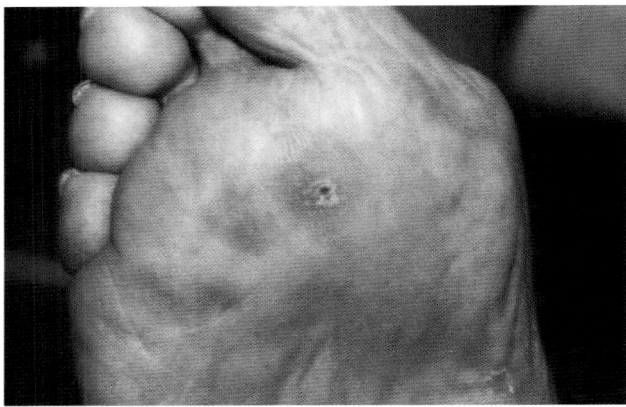

Figure 19-23 Plantar forefoot ulceration after chronic lesser metatarsophalangeal dislocation (From Firestein GS, Budd RC, Harris ED Jr, et al, editors: *Kelley's textbook of rheumatology,* ed 8, Philadelphia, 2008, Elsevier.)

had clinically painful and swollen MTP joints, which decreased to 40% to 50% over a 2-year period, while being treated medically. Even though the clinical numbers appeared to stabilize, the severity of radiologic forefoot damage increased. Once forefoot disease is present, deformity tends to progress rapidly over time, especially in the absence of pharmacologic treatment.

Midfoot

Vidigal et al[575] reported midtarsal joint involvement in approximately two thirds of patients with chronic rheumatoid arthritis. Chronic synovitis and eventual chondrolysis of the tarsometatarsal joints often occur with chronic disease. Associated with this, flattening of the longitudinal arch occurs in approximately 50% of patients.[527] With disease progression, the talar head assumes a plantar medial position (Fig. 19-25) as the soft tissue structures supporting the talar head become attenuated. This midfoot collapse may have a mutlifactorial etiology. Several reports have linked arthritis and ligamentous laxity to pes planus, although others have indicated posterior tibial tendon rupture as the source.[135,281,295] In reality, all of the above likely contribute to the clinical picture.

Often with pes planus, a valgus deformity of the hindfoot occurs. The resultant ambulatory pattern is a shuffling, flat-footed steppage gait. Fu and Scranton[173] noted that with progressive rheumatoid arthritis the foot changes to a passive weight-bearing platform for ambulation. Usually, because of the limitation of motion at the midfoot joints, a fibrous or bony ankylosis develops, but reduced motion is rarely restrictive.

Occasionally, the first MTC joint becomes extremely hypermobile, with subsequent loss of normal weight-bearing function. Resultant transfer metatarsalgia can occur from this hypermobility. Loss of the longitudinal arch on weight-bearing lateral radiographs is demonstrated by sagging at either the MTC or the naviculocuneiform articulation. Severe deformity can occur over time and make weight bearing almost impossible.

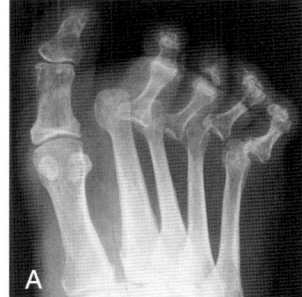
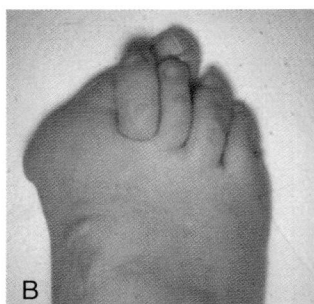
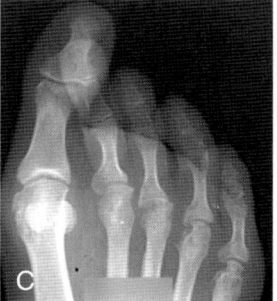
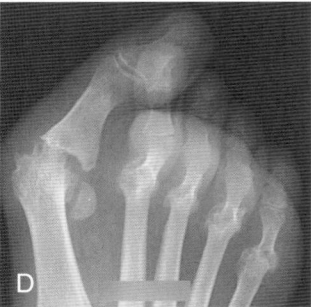

Figure 19-24 **A,** Preoperative radiograph demonstrates lesser metatarsophalangeal (MTP) joint dislocations, marginal erosions with chondrolysis, and relative sparing of the 1st MTP joint. **B,** Clinical photograph at presurgical follow-up demonstrates hallux valgus deformity with dislocation of lesser MTP joints. **C,** Thirty-year-old woman demonstrating marginal erosions of the third, fourth, and fifth MTP joints with chondrolysis.**D,** Eight years later, radiographs demonstrate severe hallux valgus, chondrolysis, and dislocation of lesser MTP joints.

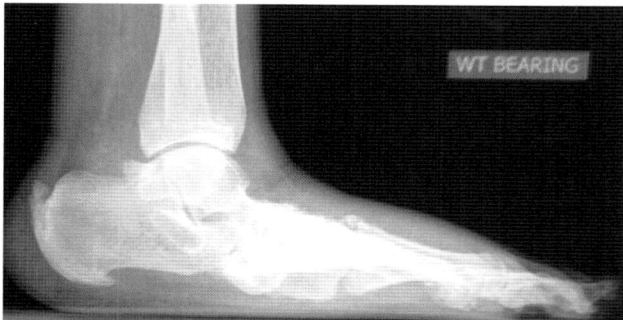

Figure 19-25 Midfoot arch collapse with migration of the talar head plantarward.

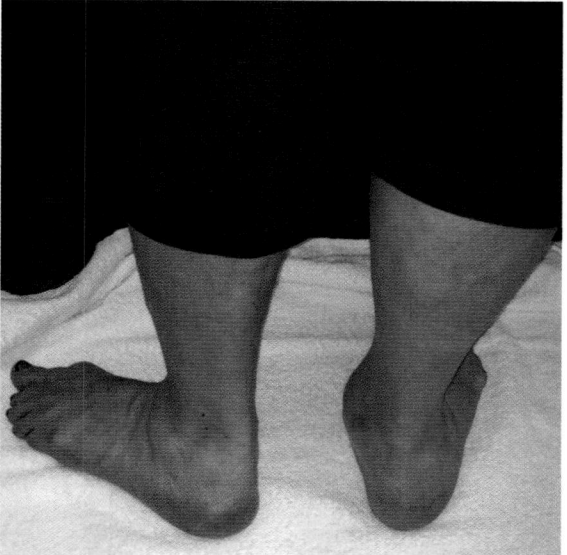

Figure 19-26 Hindfoot valgus in a patient with rheumatoid arthritis. (Courtesy A. Dingman, MD.)

Hindfoot

With hindfoot involvement, a patient might misconstrue subtalar or transverse tarsal joint pain as "ankle" pain. Careful physical examination may be necessary to differentiate these symptomatic areas. Selective injections or imaging studies, such as CT scan or MRI (or both) can provide conclusive information.

Vainio[565] reported that 72% of women and 59% of men with chronic rheumatoid arthritis had involvement of either the midtarsal or the subtalar joint but that surgical intervention was relatively infrequent. Clayton[91] reported that the forefoot was involved 10 times more often than the hindfoot. Kavlak[278] noted that patients often show an obvious hindfoot valgus position and that a varus hindfoot is seldom seen (Figs. 19-26 and 19-27).

Changes in the hindfoot occur with much longer duration of rheumatoid arthritis. Spiegel and Spiegel[527] observed that in patients with rheumatoid arthritis of less than 5 years' duration, only 8% demonstrated hindfoot arthrosis, whereas in those who had had rheumatoid arthritis longer than 5 years, 25% were symptomatic. They concluded that hindfoot arthrosis was an acquired deformity that developed from the mechanical stress of weight bearing.

The underlying pathophysiology with hindfoot involvement relates to progressive destruction of the capsular and ligamentous supporting structures of the subtalar joint. Because subtalar joint function is intimately associated with transverse tarsal joint function, instability of these joints can result in altered function and gait. Often, the end result is a progressive pes planovalgus deformity of the hindfoot (Fig. 19-28).

Posterior tibial tendon dysfunction with rheumatoid arthritis can lead to a unilateral progressive flatfoot deformity as well.[135,360]

Keenan et al[281] reported that pes planovalgus deformities in patients with rheumatoid arthritis resulted from exaggerated pronation forces on the weakened and inflamed subtalar joint. They demonstrated with electromyographic studies that an increased period of activity of the tibialis posterior muscle occurred, which was interpreted as an "attempt to stabilize" an unstable foot. Flattening of the longitudinal arch also can develop secondary to naviculocuneiform joint deterioration or first metatarsocuneiform joint collapse. In some patients, severe valgus of the hindfoot may be associated with a concomitant valgus deformity of the ankle joint as well (Fig. 19-29).

This creates a difficult management situation, with both ankle and hindfoot involvement. Bracing is difficult, and a pantalar fusion may be necessary to realign the foot but presents the patient with a difficult surgical recovery.

With severe, long-standing hindfoot deformity, an Achilles tendon contracture can develop. Although not a primary deformity, it occurs secondarily in relation to a chronic valgus deformity of the hindfoot. At the time of a triple arthrodesis, Achilles tendon lengthening may be necessary.

Gait analysis of patients with chronic rheumatoid arthritis when compared to those of nonarthritic subjects demonstrates delayed and reduced forefoot loading, resulting in a shorter stride length.[419] This effect may be related to pain in the forefoot which, in turn, causes a reduction of the functional lever arm of the foot during push-off.

Platto et al[439] reported an association between impaired ambulation and foot deformity. They observed a greater association between hindfoot disease and gait impairment compared with forefoot disease.[439] On the other hand, Shi et al[512] studied 100 feet with rheumatoid arthritis and reported no correlation between a loss of arch height and hallux valgus or forefoot splaying.

Imaging Modalities

The classic radiographic signs of rheumatoid arthritis are that of a synovial inflammatory disease. The hyperemia

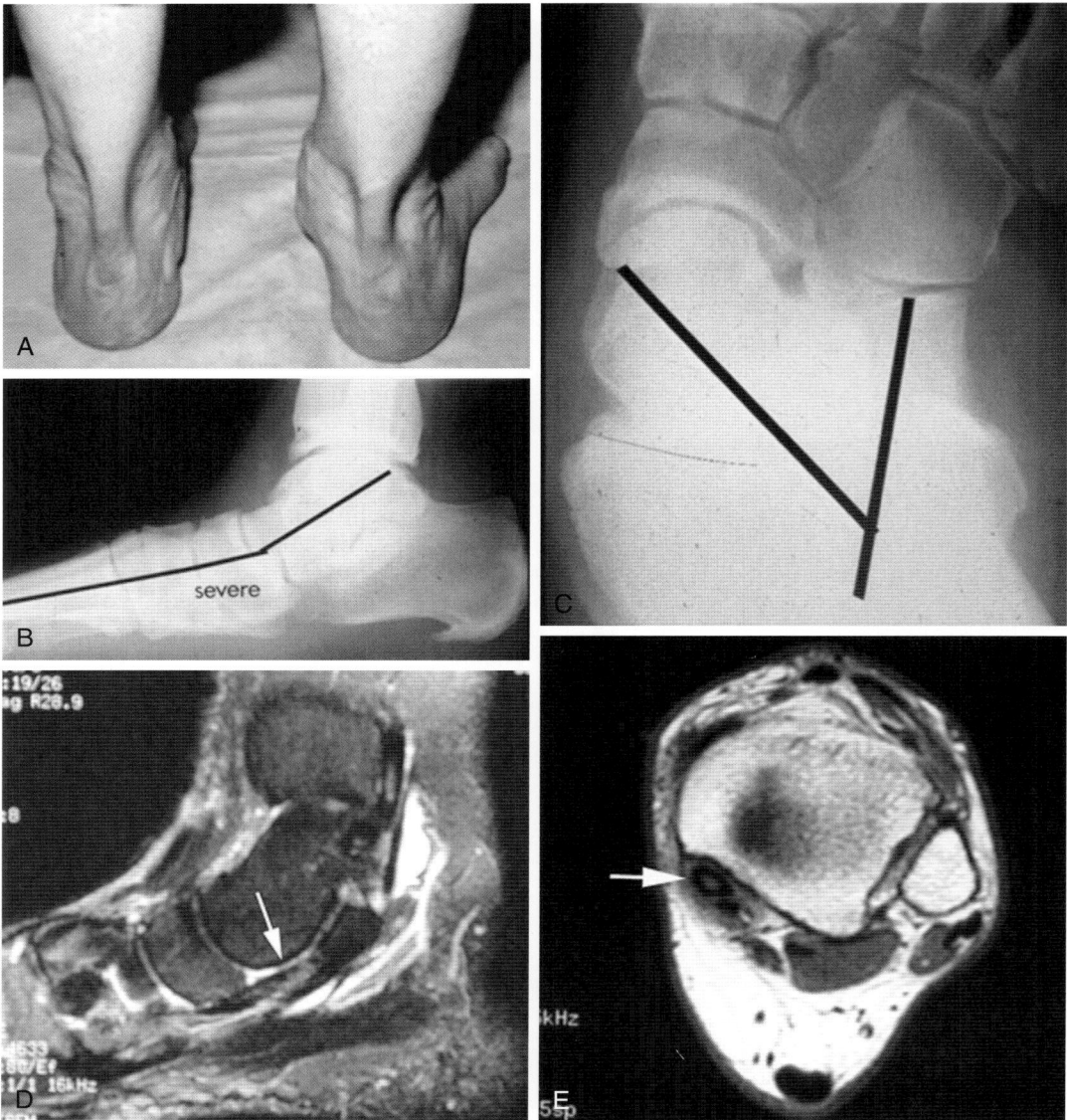

Figure 19-27 Severe hindfoot deformity secondary to rheumatoid arthritis. **A,** Clinical photograph showing hindfoot valgus position. **B,** Because of inadequate support to the talus, the talus has assumed an extremely plantar-flexed position with resultant pes planus as shown on the lateral radiograph. **C,** Peritalar subluxation is notable on the anteroposterior radiograph. **D** and **E,** Magnetic resonance images show posterior tibial tendon tendinosis and high-grade signal change within the tendon (*arrow* denotes diseased posterior tibial tendon).

involved with acute synovitis leads to periarticular osteoporosis,[207] and early radiographic examination might reveal only soft tissue swelling and diffuse juxtaarticular osteoporosis. In contrast, normal bone mineralization is usual in psoriasis, reactive arthritis, ankylosing spondylitis, and crystalline arthropathies. Synovial inflammation eventually leads to marginal cortical erosions[188] at the reflection of synovium and capsule attachment (Fig. 19-30). These peripheral erosions eventually progress to central erosions with resultant joint space narrowing, subluxation, and dislocation. Eventual destruction of the articular cartilage occurs as the rheumatoid pannus spreads around the cartilaginous surface. The articular

cartilage is thought to be destroyed by proteolytic enzymes, resulting in joint space narrowing.[64]

Gold and Bassett[188] noted that rheumatoid arthritis tends to strike earliest at the first, fourth, and fifth MTP joints. They reported that the medial aspect of the first, second, third, and fourth metatarsals and the lateral aspect of the fifth metatarsal were involved initially. The earliest visible erosions probably occur on the lateral aspect of the fifth metatarsal. The IP joints are typically spared except for the hallux.[535] Of interest, in patients with preexisting periarticular erosions, the erosions progress with time, whereas in those patients with preexisting joint space narrowing, it is the joint space narrowing that progresses with time. These two processes seem to be independent of one another.[567]

Midfoot and hindfoot changes include midfoot collapse, pes planus, and subtalar sclerosis. Localized inflammation in the areas of the retrocalcaneal bursa and at the attachment of the Achilles tendon and plantar aponeurosis are common with long-standing disease (Fig. 19-31).

Gold and Bassett[188] reported the talonavicular joint is typically the first tarsal joint to be involved. Although radiographic midfoot arthritic changes are seen in up to 62%, clinically, these are far less symptomatic (27%).[575] In a series of patients with rheumatoid arthritis who were

evaluated with CT scans, Seltzer et al[506] noted talonavicular joint involvement in 39%, calcaneocuboid involvement in 25%, and subtalar involvement in 29%.

Radiographically, the subtalar joint is involved to a lesser extent than the midfoot, with changes noted in 32% to 42% of patients. Only 21% of rheumatoid arthritis patients actually have clinical symptoms in the hindfoot.[380,575] Rarely are all three of the hindfoot joints simultaneously affected.[251]

Hattori and colleagues[227] noted two distinct patterns of pes planovalgus deformities in the rheumatoid foot. One group demonstrated degenerative changes in both the subtalar and talonavicular joints, with the talar head subluxated plantarward in relation to the navicular. A second group showed only subtalar joint involvement. Neither group demonstrated involvement of the calcaneocuboid joint.

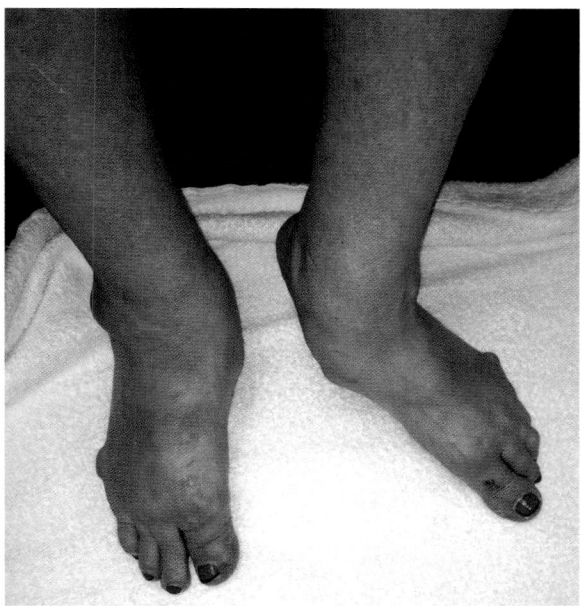

Figure 19-28 Clinical photograph of a pes planovalgus deformity with talar head subluxation plantarward. (Courtesy A. Dingman, MD.)

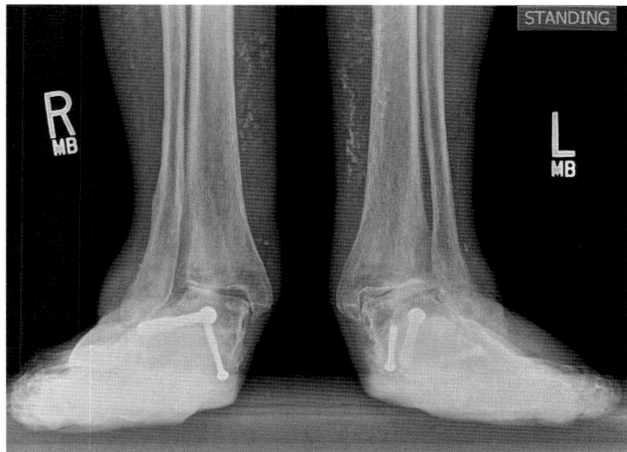

Figure 19-29 Radiographs depicting bilateral incongruent ankle valgus deformities.

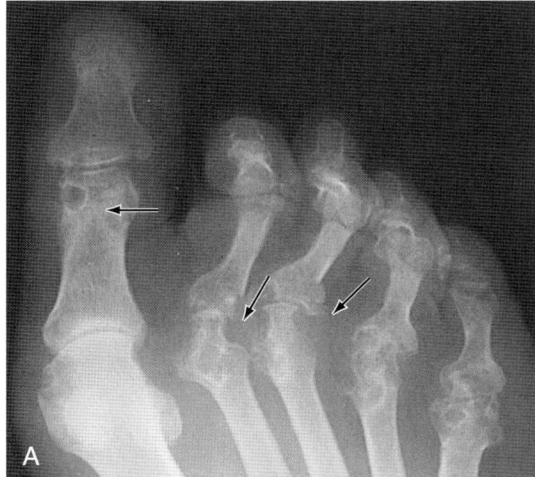
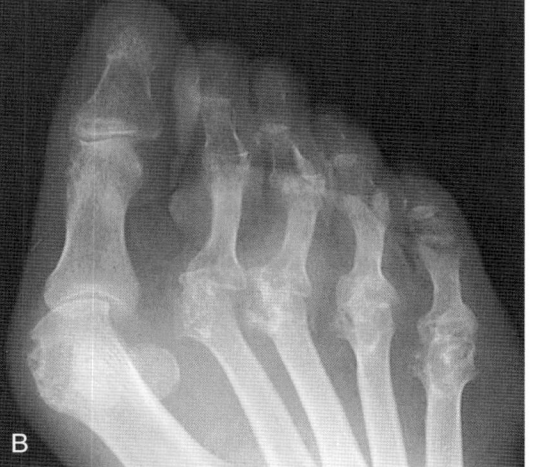

Figure 19-30 **A,** Forefoot radiograph demonstrates periarticular erosions of the lesser metatarsal heads. **B,** Subluxation, dislocation, joint space narrowing, and central erosions of the lesser metatarsophalangeal joints with hallux valgus deformity.

Radiographic progression of rheumatoid arthritis can be evaluated by various methods, but commonly used methods are those described by Larsen,[321] Rau,[451] and Steinbrocker.[533] The methods of Rau and Larsen were found to be equivalent, as reported by Tanaka et al[542] in assessing progression of early rheumatoid arthritis, which indeed affects pharmacologic treatment. Moreover, the magnitude of 5-year disability as measured by the Health Assessment Questionnaire Disability Index (HAQ-DI) was associated with joint space–narrowing scores in the first year rather than periarticular erosion.[346]

Lindqvist et al[334] noted more rapid radiographic progression in those patients with higher levels of inflammatory markers, such as sedimentation rate and rheumatoid factor. Another report suggested that 59% of 190 patients with early rheumatoid arthritis could be classified as nonprogressive based on radiographic joint changes[432] and that radiographic progression may be slowed by treatment with disease-modifying antirheumatic drugs (DMARDs) and other pharmacologic agents, including antibiotics (sulfonamides, doxycycline), salicylates, cytotoxic drugs (methotrexate, leuprolide acetate, cyclophosphamide), NSAIDs, corticosteroids, and cytokine inhibitors (etanercept, infliximab).

In patients with nonspecific pain or diffuse foot pain, or both, with no visible radiographic findings and subtle or minimal clinical findings, a technetium-99 (^{99}Tc) bone scan can help to localize disease (Fig. 19-32).[421]

Magnetic resonance imaging is increasingly used to evaluate forefoot symptoms and may be helpful in diagnosing joint erosion, chondrolysis, and other specific features of various inflammatory diseases that have characteristic MRI findings.[14] MRI is particularly sensitive early in the disease process. Boutry et al[55] noted MRI findings consistent with synovitis in up to 97% of patients with early rheumatoid arthritis (see Fig. 19-27D and E).

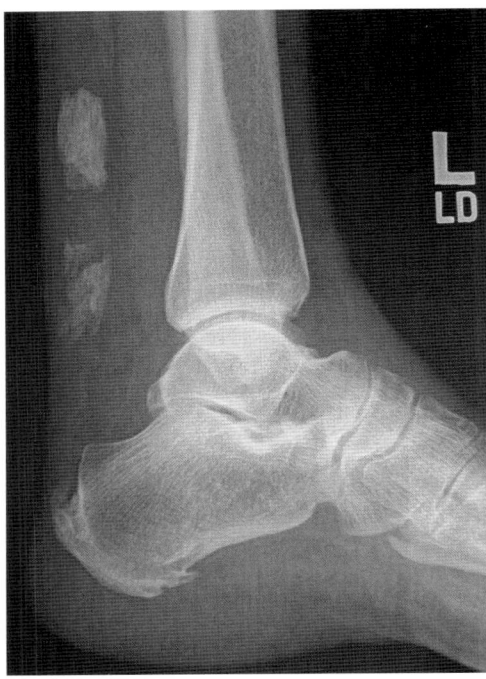

Figure 19-31 Calcification of the Achilles tendon and the Achilles insertion.

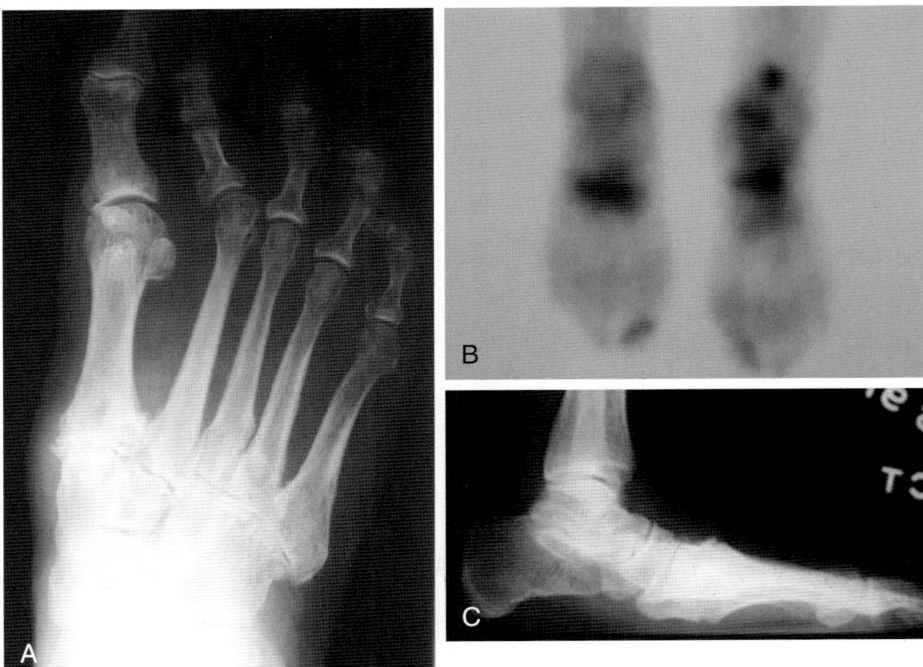

Figure 19-32 **A,** Anteroposterior (AP) radiograph demonstrates severe arthritis of the Lisfranc joint. **B,** Technetium-99 bone scan shows bilateral midfoot uptake as well as uptake in the left ankle and hindfoot. **C,** Lateral radiograph demonstrates midfoot arthritis with pes planus and rocker-sole deformity.

Microscopic Examination

The histopathology of bone lesions in rheumatoid arthritis is characterized by fibroblast proliferation; infiltration of macrophages, lymphocytes, and plasma cells; collagen deposition; and new bone formation. The hyaline cartilage surface is usually necrotic. Pannus (a collection of inflammatory cells, fibroblasts, synovium, and granulomatous tissue) is absent except at the margins of the capsular attachments. The process appears reparative in nature, but the inflammatory cell infiltrate or aggregate around small blood vessels in deeper bone marrow regions helps to confirm the diagnosis.[600] The most common soft tissue lesions are rheumatoid nodules, which often form subcutaneously and comprise lymphocytes and plasma cells. Rheumatoid nodules generally form in areas of bony prominence, such as the ulnar border of the forearm and elbow, the occiput, the lumbosacral area, and the plantar foot (Fig. 19-33); however, they can also be found in the abdominal and thoracic cavities.

In a study of 223 patients with seropositive rheumatoid arthritis, these rheumatoid nodules were histologically characterized into three classic zones: a necrotic central area, a surrounding wall of cells, and a marginal zone associated with the subcutaneous tissue or joint capsule. Such nodules appeared to develop after 4 or more years of disease duration and were associated with pain and deformity in nearly 70% of patients studied. Such necrosis or nodule formation may be an important factor that worsens the clinical prognosis in seropositive patients.[35]

At the microscopic level, the macrophage appears to play a key role. Radiologic progression of disease directly correlates with the number of macrophages lining the diseased joint within the cartilage–pannus interface (Fig. 19-34A and B). This appears to be explained by the fact that once activated, macrophages, in turn, activate osteoclasts and other "downstream" cells[293] to produce IL-1 and TNF. These cytokines stimulate osteoclasts to produce collagenase, which resorbs bone and destroys cartilage.

Rheumatoid arthritis appears to affect striated muscle as well as the joint. Using electron microscopy to evaluate muscle specimens from RA patients, de Palma et al[129] illustrated several distinct differences from normal muscle. The myofibrils demonstrated wider separation, with dilation of the sarcotubular system, and flaking of the myofibrils.

Recognition of these microscopic characteristics has led to advances in the treatment of rheumatoid arthritis, including pharmacologic agents directed against macrophage-produced cytokines.

Diagnosis

The diagnosis of rheumatoid arthritis is based on a combination of clinical evaluation, radiographic examination, and laboratory testing.

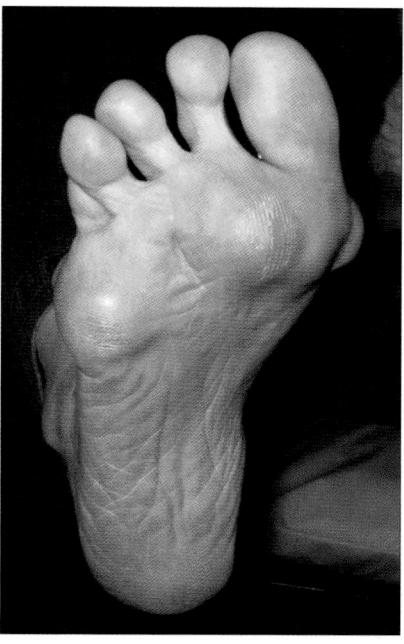

Figure 19-33 Clinical photograph of plantar rheumatoid nodules. (From Hochberg M, Silman A, Smollen J, et al, editors: *Rheumatology*, ed 5, Philadelphia, 2010, Elsevier.)

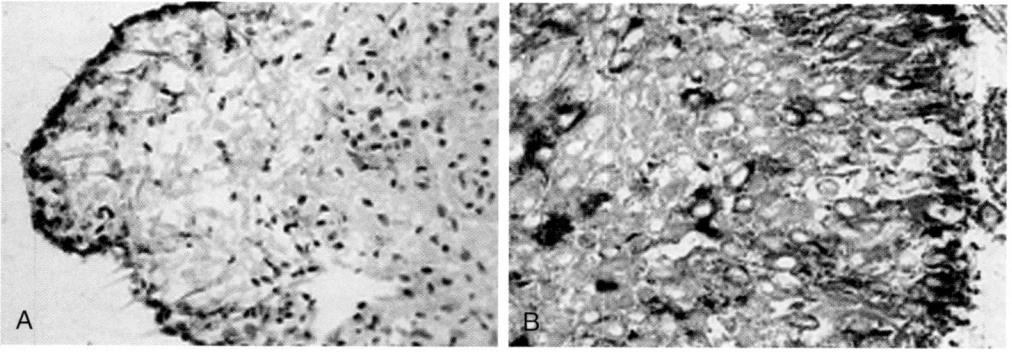

Figure 19-34 **A,** Normal synovium and stained synovial macrophages. **B,** Rheumatoid synovium with a proliferation of macrophages stained red. (Images from Hochberg M, Silman A, Smollen J, et al, editors: *Rheumatology*, ed 5, Philadelphia, 2010, Elsevier.)

The American College of Rheumatology[12] suggests that at least four of seven criteria be present (Box 19-1) to diagnose rheumatoid arthritis (the first four criteria must have been present for more than 6 weeks).

Serologic testing is positive for rheumatoid factor (RF) 70% to 90% of the time in those with rheumatoid arthritis. RF is an immunoglobulin M (IgM) antibody directed against Fc portion of the patient's own immunoglobulin G (IgG) antibodies and is thought to be part of a normal immune response that is exaggerated in rheumatoid arthritis. Elevated RF titers correlate proportionally with more severe disease. However, RF may be falsely negative, and several other diseases may have a positive RF, including systemic lupus erythematosis (SLE), Sjögren syndrome, myositis, hepatitis C, cirrhosis, syphilis, and tuberculosis. Anticitrullinated protein antibody (ACPA) is another autoantibody frequently found in patients with rheumatoid arthritis that may be even more sensitive than RF.

Treatment

An appreciation of the clinical course of rheumatoid arthritis is essential in the decision-making process of developing a treatment program. Nonetheless, initial orthopaedic treatment is directed toward pain relief, prevention of deformity, correction of deformity, preservation of function, and restoration of function. Medical management throughout the entire disease process includes pharmacologic treatment as well, which has been shown to improve ambulatory capacity.[213]

Optimal treatment for patients with rheumatoid arthritis requires cooperation of both medical and surgical interventions. With a combined approach and with newer biologic disease modifying agents, future complications may be less prevalent.

Pharmacologic Therapy

Pharmacologic agents that reduce inflammation and relieve pain facilitate the treatment of rheumatoid arthritis. For mild cases, NSAIDs are the first line of defense. The occasional judicious use of an intraarticular corticosteroid injection may be beneficial, but systemic oral steroid therapy is used less commonly because of the well-known deleterious side effects of chronic corticosteroid use. As symptoms progress, DMARDs are often added to the treatment regimen. These include methotrexate, sulfasalazine, leflunomide, and hydroxychloroquine. However, side effects may develop with chronic use. For example, cutaneous ulcers that were likely related to methotrexate toxicity have been reported to develop spontaneously in patients with rheumatoid arthritis.[395]

Biologic response modifiers (BRMs) have shown promise in moderate-to-severe cases. These modern pharmacologic agents include inflixamab (Remicade), etanercept (Embrel), and adalimumab (Humira). All three medications act as TNF-α inhibitors. Anakinra (Kineret), a novel IL-1 receptor, has also shown promising results, and several other new agents are on the horizon. Lipsky et al[337] reported that the combination of methotrexate and infliximab halted progression of joint damage over the course of 1 year. Bowen et al[56] noted improvement in foot pain and disability after 12 weeks of anti–TNF-α therapy.

Several additional studies support the beneficial effects of anti–TNF-α therapy, particularly when combined with methotrexate.[59,297,528] Smolen et al[520] also noted that the use of inflixamab with methotrexate is more effective at halting space narrowing and periarticular erosions than methotrexate therapy alone. Despite these encouraging results, 99% of patients taking anti–TNF-α therapy in a large epidemiologic study noted current foot pain.[426]

These findings could create a larger pool of patients with secondary osteoarthritis. In turn, this could lead to a change in the use of specific orthopaedic procedures from those that are typically joint destructive to those that are joint sparing[558] for many patients with rheumatoid arthritis who have nonprogressive disease.

For those patients taking long-term steroid therapy, intravenous hydrocortisone is used perioperatively to prevent adrenal crisis. The current authors follow the recommendations of Mackenzie et al,[343] administering 100 mg of hydrocortisone intravenously to those patients who have taken oral steroids for more than 2 weeks, or for those who are on steroids for adrenal insufficiency.

Jeng and Campbell[259] noted that intraarticular steroid injections appear to be beneficial for hindfoot and midfoot joints but caution that there is insufficient data to support safe use in forefoot joints.

Although a helpful part of pharmacologic therapy, DMARDs may cause bone marrow suppression and hepatotoxicity, thus laboratory screening should be done before surgical intervention in patients receiving DMARD therapy. Concerns have also been raised regarding wound healing complications.

Multiple studies have examined the effects of perioperative methotrexate use and postoperative wound complications. Although some suggest a link between methotrexate use and postoperative infection, other more powerful studies suggest that this correlation may be exaggerated.[202] The current authors do not routinely stop methotrexate use in the perioperative period.

Studies with leflunomide show contrasting results. Fuerst et al[174] reported an increased rate of wound complications (40.6% vs. 13.6%) in patients taking leflunomide compared with those taking methotrexate. In contrast, Bibbo et al[45] showed no increase in infection with the use of leflunomide.

To date, perioperative guidelines for the use of biologic response modifiers have not been established. Although increased infection rates remain a concern, a paucity of randomized controlled data prevents solid conclusions. The British Society for Rheumatologic Guidelines recommends withholding anti–TNF-α therapy for 2 to 4 weeks before surgery and reinstating it after the wound has healed.[327]

Gene therapy trials have also been conducted in patients with rheumatoid arthritis. Evans et al[149] reported on retroviral transfection of metacarpophalangeal joint synoviocytes with an IL-1 receptor antagonist. Further investigation along these lines may reveal exciting treatment options for patients with rheumatoid arthritis.

Conservative Management

The most important aspect of early nonsurgical care is wearing proper footwear. Likewise, modification of a patient's footwear may be beneficial. A carefully placed metatarsal pad just proximal to an intractable plantar keratotic lesion or an area of MTP joint tenderness can relieve discomfort associated with increased pressure. Excavating the insole beneath a pressure area can also decrease symptoms. Many patients with mild-to-moderate rheumatoid involvement of the foot can be fitted with a broad-toed, soft-soled shoe.[551] An extra-depth shoe with a Plastizote or compressible insole can help to accommodate more severe deformities. A Plastizote liner or viscoelastic insole can relieve plantar pain in a patient with an atrophied plantar fat pad. With significant lesser-toe contractures, extra-depth shoes fitted with a customized orthosis can accommodate painful plantar lesions, such as intractable plantar keratoses. Although a Plastizote liner can accommodate significant forefoot deformities, it commonly needs to be replaced every few months as the insert bottoms out. Orthotic devices and footwear that redistribute weight-bearing forces tend to decrease pressure areas, diffuse weight-bearing, decrease shearing forces, support unstable joints, and restrict motion are helpful.[114,523] Custom orthotics that incorporate a metatarsal dome pad may be more effective in reducing metatarsalgia and pressure beneath the first and second metatarsal heads.[236]

Involvement of a pedorthist and the use of orthopaedic appliances can help to prevent deformities and maintain function. There have been several studies that evaluated the use of specific custom orthotics or shoes for the treatment of rheumatoid foot deformities.[77,95,254,593] Conrad et al[95] found no benefit from posted foot orthoses compared with placebos in regard to pain relief or reduction in disability. In contrast, Woodburn et al[593] found a 19% reduction in pain, 31% reduction in disability, and 14% reduction in functional limitation with the use of custom rigid orthotics. Chalmers et al[77] reported that semirigid orthoses had a significant effect on pain reduction, and soft orthoses and supportive shoes had little or no effect. None of these orthoses had any effect on reduction of joint synovitis. Mejjad et al[374] noted that, with 1 month of use, custom orthotics reduced pain but had no effect on gait, whereas Kavlak et al[278] found that, at 3 months of use, custom orthotics not only reduced pain but improved gait and stride length. As a general rule, orthotics should conform to the patient's foot with the goal of pain reduction. Some believe that a soft orthotic should be used with an inflexible foot and that a rigid orthotic should be used for a supple one.

Moncur et al[394] studied 25 patients with rheumatoid arthritis and found that 80% improved their walking ability by using custom heat-moldable shoes. However, others have noted that wearing such shoes is distasteful and uncomfortable for these patients.

Jannink et al[254] evaluated the methodology of 11 randomized, controlled clinical trials that had studied the effect of orthopaedic shoes and orthoses. The authors reported that although all 11 studies demonstrated the effectiveness of their products, the studies evaluated did a relatively poor job of examining usability, efficiency, satisfaction, and reliability of patient use. It appears that orthoses designed to support rheumatoid arthritic foot deformities and to provide pain relief might yield some benefit, but patient satisfaction, usability, and the specific indications for a specified device remain vague, and specific indications are yet to be determined.

Metatarsalgia in the early stages of rheumatoid arthritis may be alleviated by a metatarsal arch support, over-the-counter soft insoles, metatarsal pads, or custom-made orthotic devices. Shoes with a low heel, soft leather upper, and increased depth tend to accommodate claw toes and hammer toes. Soft-soled, rocker-bottom shoes decrease stress on the metatarsal and the hindfoot region. In addition, Cho et al[86] found no difference between groups of patients wearing rocker-bottom shoes compared with those wearing custom orthotics. An over-the-counter padded insole, such as a Spenco liner (Spenco Medical, Waco, Tex.) or a molded insole, can also relieve pressure areas. Nonrigid longitudinal custom-made arch supports tend to shift pressure areas more proximally.

The reported effect of in-office plantar callosity shaving or debridement is temporary and appears to decrease substantially within a week after debridement.[594] At best, plantar callosity shaving offers temporary relief before definitive surgical treatment (Fig. 19-35).

Patients should be instructed in foot care and careful observation of skin for potential breakdown. Patients with midfoot and hindfoot pain with no fixed deformity often can be treated with a customized arch support or a polypropylene AFO. Bracing may be necessary when foot and ankle pain becomes refractory to other methods of treatment. A molded leather ankle brace or an Arizona

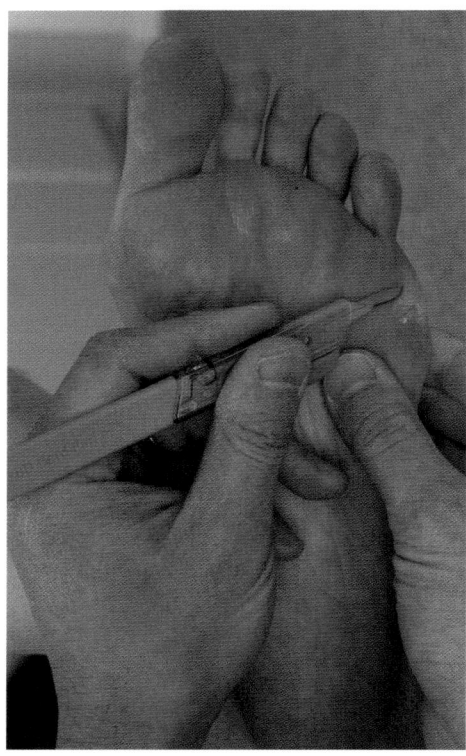

Figure 19-35 In-office shaving of plantar callus.

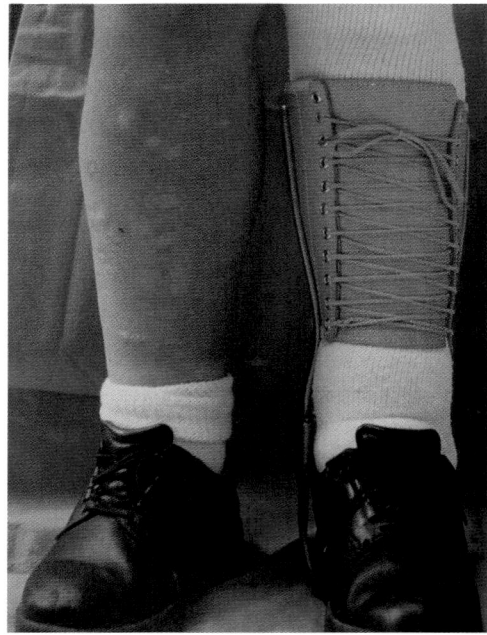

Figure 19-36 Double upright metal leather ankle–foot orthosis.

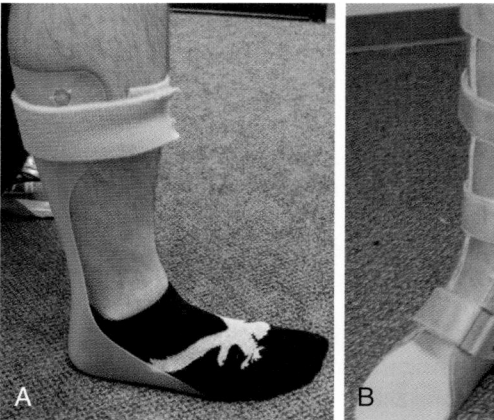

Figure 19-37 **A,** Polypropylene ankle–foot orthosis (AFO) brace. **B,** Leather AFO brace.

brace with steel stays can be worn inside a shoe and can provide significant ankle and hindfoot support (Fig. 19-36).

Conservative care for midfoot and hindfoot degeneration includes rest to relieve swollen and inflamed joints, minimizing weight bearing during acute flare-ups; cast immobilization; padding; roomy footwear; and custom-made longitudinal arch supports. With instability, a polypropylene AFO can provide some relief (Fig. 19-37A and B).

Physical therapy can be helpful in treating patients with foot problems associated with rheumatoid arthritis. Contrast baths may be used to decrease swelling and inflammation, although in the presence of the Raynaud phenomenon, they may be contraindicated. Stretching exercises for a contracted Achilles tendon and passive manipulation of the ankle and hindfoot can help to restore or maintain motion. Maintaining range of motion at the MTP joint and IP joints in the presence of acute rheumatoid arthritis may be aided by active or passive manipulation. Muscle strengthening and conditioning may be helpful in maintaining ambulatory capacity. In addition, exercise in early rheumatoid arthritis has been shown to enhance neuromuscular performance without an obvious negative effect on disease activity or joint disease.[211] Limitation of ambulation during acute episodes, exercises, and stretching of involved joints are all important physical therapy modalities in maintaining

function in the patient with chronic rheumatoid arthritis.

With the increasing involvement of numerous lower extremity joints, gait training is occasionally necessary to maintain ambulatory independence. The use of ambulatory aids, such as canes and crutches, can reduce weight-bearing stress, but this may be done at the expense of the upper extremities. With significant upper extremity involvement, platform crutches or canes with special handgrips may be necessary.

Lower extremity stress fractures may also arise as a complication of conservative treatment. In the cavus foot, the lateral metatarsals have a higher frequency of fracture,

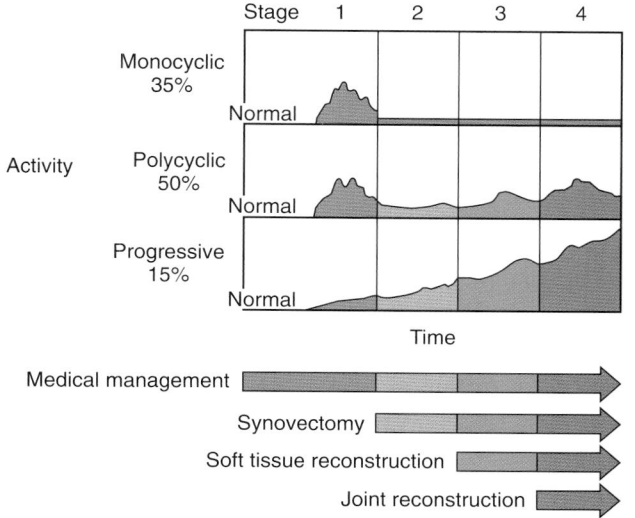

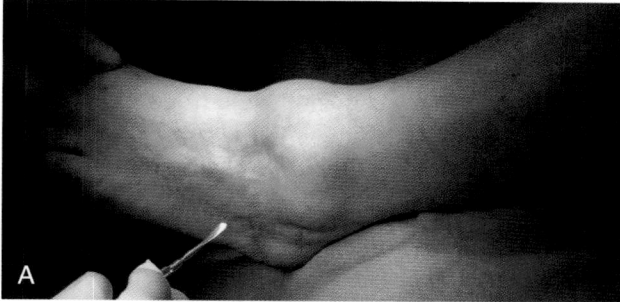

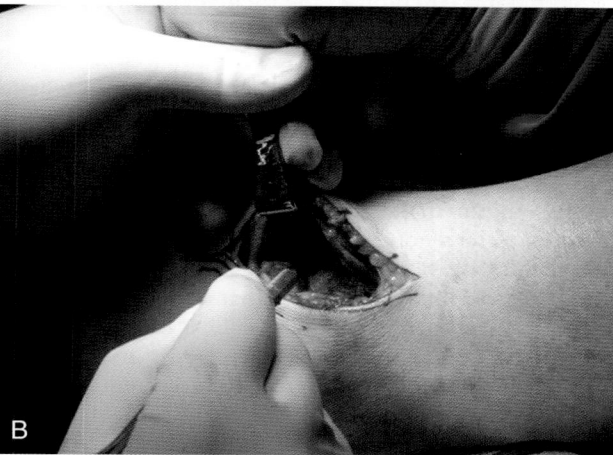

Figure 19-38 The clinical course of the three presentations of rheumatoid arthritis. Clinical flare-ups are denoted by the *y* axis. The *x* axis is time, along with initial medical management and later surgical management.

although the medial metatarsals are more likely to fracture in a planus foot. Valgus deformity of the ankle predisposes to fibular fractures. Calcaneal stress fractures may also occur.[345]

Figure 19-39 Intraoperative photographs. **A,** Preooperative. **B,** During ankle joint synovectomy.

Surgical Management

When progressive deformity occurs or unrelenting pain is refractory to conservative treatment, surgical intervention may be necessary.

Medical management should continue throughout the progression of the rheumatoid disease process. Surgical procedures may be indicated depending on the severity and progression of the inflammatory process. A monocyclic disease process infrequently requires extensive surgery, whereas a polycyclic or progressive process increases the risk of later surgical treatment (Fig. 19-38).

The precise timing of surgical intervention for the patient with rheumatoid foot and ankle deformities varies significantly and must be individualized for each patient. During the proliferative phase of synovitis, a synovectomy of an involved joint may slow the progression of the rheumatoid inflammatory process.

At other times, conservative management provides adequate relief for a patient, and no surgical intervention is warranted. With progressive collapse of the longitudinal arch, early surgical intervention can prevent significant hindfoot deformity. Furthermore, an attempt should be made to prevent loss of ambulatory capacity with progression of the disease over a long period. Surgical reconstruction to maintain ambulation is important. Surgical intervention may be interspersed with periods of conservative care so that numerous surgical procedures are not clustered during a short time.

Preoperative assessment, including attention to the vascular supply of the foot, is important. Although rheumatoid vasculitis is uncommon, it can present an increased risk to wound healing with surgery. The diagnosis of vasculitis is difficult, but nail splinter hemorrhages, neuritis or paresthesias in peripheral nerves (necrotizing vasculitis of nerve sheath vessels), skin ulcerations, poor capillary refill, and laboratory tests (antiphospholipid antibodies, RF level, C-reactive protein [CRP], erythrocite sedimentation rate [ESR]) can help facilitate the diagnosis. Anticoagulation, antiplatelet, and immunosuppressive treatment may be necessary in the treatment of this condition.[404,418,469]

For symptomatic synovitis without significant malalignment or joint disease, open or arthroscopic synovectomy of the hindfoot or transverse tarsal joints may provide temporary relief (Fig. 19-39A and B).[423]

Some patients may require lower extremity total joint replacement. In general, proximal joint surgery should precede distal joint surgery. For example, a total hip or total knee replacement usually should precede hindfoot surgery. Hindfoot surgery typically should precede forefoot surgery,[102] the rationale being that with a valgus or pronation deformity, a recurrent forefoot deformity may develop. Moreover, patients with valgus hindfoot deformities have been shown to have higher forefoot pressures compared with patients with a normal hindfoot, based on pedobarograph studies.[536] Thus the hindfoot and midfoot deformity must be addressed or forefoot reconstruction efforts can fail.[536] Limited midfoot arthrodesis can be performed concomitantly if indicated, but surgery is often staged, with the midfoot given surgical priority. Extensive bilateral forefoot surgery should be discouraged because of the magnitude of surgery as well as the decreased ambulatory capacity after surgery. In patients who are considered for total ankle arthroplasty, the authors believe that the hindfoot should be realigned before the implantation of the total ankle.

The goal for all surgeries of the midfoot and hindfoot is to obtain a plantigrade foot, with the heel positioned in approximately 5 degrees of valgus after arthrodesis or reconstruction. Surgery for rheumatoid patients mirrors hindfoot surgery for nonrheumatoid patients. For example, a subtalar arthrodesis with flexor digitorum longus tendon transfer may be performed for stage 2 posterior tibial tendon dysfunction in patients with rheumatoid arthritis.[13] Isolated disease may also be treated with isolated joint arthrodesis. Elbar and Thomas et al[144] reported complete pain relief in 75% of patients and improved ambulation in 89% of patients after isolated arthrodesis of the talonavicular joint. In subsequent studies, they noted a 5% nonunion rate and 95% good-to-excellent results.[292,120] Similarly, Chiodo et al[85] reported a 95% fusion rate at 11 weeks after isolated talonavicular joint arthrodesis.

An autogenous iliac crest graft at the time of arthrodesis depends on the magnitude of the deformity and the specific fusion that is desired. If substantial realignment is part of the surgical plan, then an iliac crest autograft or a structural allograft may be necessary. Distraction or lengthening of the medial or lateral column may be needed to reestablish alignment. Failure to perform a bone graft in the presence of a severe pes planovalgus deformity can result in undercorrection or recurrent deformity (see Chapter 25).

For those with a rigid hindfoot valgus and forefoot abduction, the triple hindfoot fusion is recommended. Results of the triple arthrodesis in patients with rheumatoid arthritis appear to be excellent, with 94% demonstrating significant pain relief in one study.[158] However, osteonecrosis of the talar dome has been reported after triple arthrodesis, and in three reported cases, a dorsally inserted screw was used for the subtalar arthrodesis.[265] Knupp et al[299] reviewed 32 consecutive cases of triple arthrodesis and noted a 100% fusion rate. No patient underwent revision surgery, but the authors did note associated midfoot arthritis in 17 patients.

Bibbo et al[45] reported no adverse affects on complication rates in 31 patients followed prospectively for 12 months after elective foot and ankle surgery. However, surgical wounds in patients with rheumatoid arthritis did not heal as rapidly when compared with patients without rheumatoid arthritis and should be monitored closely for infection, vasculitis, and other causes of delayed wound healing.[408]

Wound complications can be devastating when they occur. Niinimaki et al[414] reported on a series of 97 triple arthrodeses in patients with rheumatoid arthritis. They noted a deep infection of the sinus tarsi in 7 patients (7.2%), which required multiple debridements, intravenous antibiotics, and open cancellous bone grafting in four cases, and local muscle flap coverage in three cases. Median time to complete healing was 22 months, and the average number of operations to clear the infection was seven. The most common pathogens were *Staphylococcus epidermis* and *Staphylococcus aureus*.

Pantalar arthrodesis also appears to be an effective treatment for rheumatoid patients with severe hindfoot deformity. McKinley et al[372] reported a high level of patient satisfaction after a pantalar arthrodesis when using a lateral approach autologous bone graft.

LESSER METATARSOPHALANGEAL JOINT SYNOVECTOMY

Synovectomy of the lesser MTP joints is indicated for painful, symptomatic MTP joints early in the disease process. Subluxation or dislocation of the lesser MTP joints with formation of intractable plantar keratoses is a contraindication to simple synovectomy because surgery will achieve limited gains. Debridement of hypertrophic synovial tissue can arrest the degenerative process, reduce MTP joint distention, and decrease soft tissue deformation, which can eventually lead to subluxation and dislocation if untreated.

The duration of remission achieved with synovectomy varies from patient to patient, although Aho[7] noted good results for up to 18 months. A patient should be informed that a synovectomy may be a temporizing procedure and that eventually with progressive deformity, a forefoot arthroplasty may be necessary. Preoperatively, patients considered for synovectomy alone should have swollen and tender MTP joints with minimal deformity. Flexible or mild fixed hammering may be treated concomitantly. When planning the surgical synovectomy, dorsal interspace incisions are used so that they can be reused if later forefoot reconstruction is necessary.

Synovectomy has been recommended by Vainio[565] and others for the lesser MTP joints.*

Surgical Technique

1. The patient is placed supine on the operating table, with a well-padded bump under the hip. Either an Esmarch bandage or a well-padded thigh tourniquet is used to maintain a bloodless field for surgery.
2. The involved MTP joint is approached through a dorsal longitudinal incision made in the second web space to approach the second or third MTP joint. The incision is made in the fourth web space to approach either the fourth or fifth MTP joints.

---

*References 6, 9, 72, 114, 115, and 452.

3. Using the extensor tendon as a guide, the dissection is carried down through the extensor hood, exposing the MTP joint.
4. The proliferative synovial tissue is excised on the dorsomedial and dorsolateral aspect through sharp dissection. Care is taken to remove hypertrophic synovium beneath the collateral ligaments.
5. With longitudinal tension placed on the toe, the resection is carried as plantarward as possible. A small rongeur is used to debride any hypertrophic synovium.
6. The joint capsule is approximated with interrupted 4-0 absorbable suture. The skin is closed in an interrupted manner.
7. For a synovectomy of the first MTP joint, a dorsal longitudinal incision is centered over the first MTP joint and the dissection carried down on either side of the extensor hallucis longus (EHL) tendon. The technique otherwise is the same as that described for the lesser MTP joints.

Postoperative Care

A gauze-and-tape compression dressing is applied at surgery and changed every 10 to 14 days for 6 weeks. The patient is permitted to ambulate in a postoperative shoe with weight bearing as tolerated. Active and passive joint range-of-motion exercises are initiated 3 weeks after surgery.

Results and Complications

Raunio and Laine[452] reported on 28 patients (33 feet) who underwent MTP joint synovectomy. With short-term follow-up, they found 80% of patients satisfied and noted diminished progression of rheumatoid arthritis on both clinical and radiographic examination. Cracchiolo[115] observed that synovectomy of one or two isolated MTP joints may give temporary relief.

Vainio[565] stated that synovectomy decreased symptoms of metatarsalgia and noted reduced symptoms of interdigital neuroma in patients with synovial inflammatory disease. Higgins et al[235] reported the occurrence of interdigital neuroma associated with seronegative rheumatoid arthritis. Aho[6] reported good relief with synovectomy in 16 patients (21 feet). He noted that they were symptom free and painfree "months to years after synovectomy.

Belt et al[29] reported the results of synovectomy on 83 patients at 15 years and 68 patients at 20 years postoperatively. They concluded that synovectomy was insufficient treatment without concomitant use of immunosuppressive drugs and that 75% of joints that had undergone synovectomy alone, in their series, later went on to excisional arthroplasty. The long-term effects of newer disease-modifying agents that block the inflammatory cascade and immune signaling may be integral in eventually proving the long-term success of synovectomy and possibly obviating, with pharmacologic therapy, the need for synovectomy by disease suppression.

Care must be taken in exposing the lesser MTP joints through an intermetatarsal dissection, to avoid injury to an adjacent sensory nerve. A major complication after synovectomy is damage to a dorsal cutaneous nerve to a lesser toe or damage to a branch of the digital nerve. Either can result in postoperative numbness in a fairly confined area. Recurrence of synovial hypertrophy can develop in time, and the patient should be informed of this preoperatively.

RHEUMATOID HAMMER TOE DEFORMITY

Hammer toe and claw toe involvement of the lesser toes is common with chronic rheumatoid arthritis. Typically, the hammer toe deformity occurs in conjunction with MTP joint subluxation and dislocation. In early stages, padding of contracted lesser toes and roomy footwear can accommodate the deformed lesser toe. Surgical correction is typically deferred until a forefoot reconstruction is performed.

The surgical treatment of a hammer toe deformity depends on the severity of the deformity. A mild deformity may be treated with passive manipulation and intramedullary K-wire fixation. Closed osteoclasis in combination with forefoot arthroplasty has been advocated for a mild and moderate hammer toe deformity.[90,114,310,359,435] For more severe deformities, a proximal phalangeal condylectomy achieves realignment by bony decompression. PIP arthrodesis has been advocated by Coughlin[102] and others.[114,267,310,583] Newer methods using permanent metallic implants are now available (Smart Toe, Stryker, Kalamazoo, Mich.; Pro-Toe, Wright Medical, Arlington, Tenn.) (Figs. 19-40A and B), but these devices may be fraught with complications (Fig. 19-41B and C) and should be used carefully.

Surgical Technique (Video Clips 75 and 76)

1. An elliptic or longitudinal incision is centered over the dorsal aspect of the PIP joint, excising the callus, extensor tendon, and joint capsule, thereby exposing the PIP joint (Fig. 19-42A and B) (see Chapter 7).
2. The collateral ligaments on the medial and lateral aspect of the PIP joint of the lesser toes are severed, allowing the condyles of the proximal phalanx to be delivered into the wound. Care is taken to protect the adjacent neurovascular bundles.
3. A portion of the proximal phalanx is resected just proximal to the flare of the condyles, and any prominent remaining edges are smoothed with a rongeur (Fig. 19-42C).
4. At this point, the toe is brought into correct alignment. If tension appears to be present at the PIP joint and correcting the deformity is difficult, more bone should be resected.
5. The articular surface of the base of the middle phalanx is resected with a rongeur (this is optional).
6. A 0.045-inch K-wire is introduced at the PIP joint and driven distally, exiting the tip of the toe. With the toe

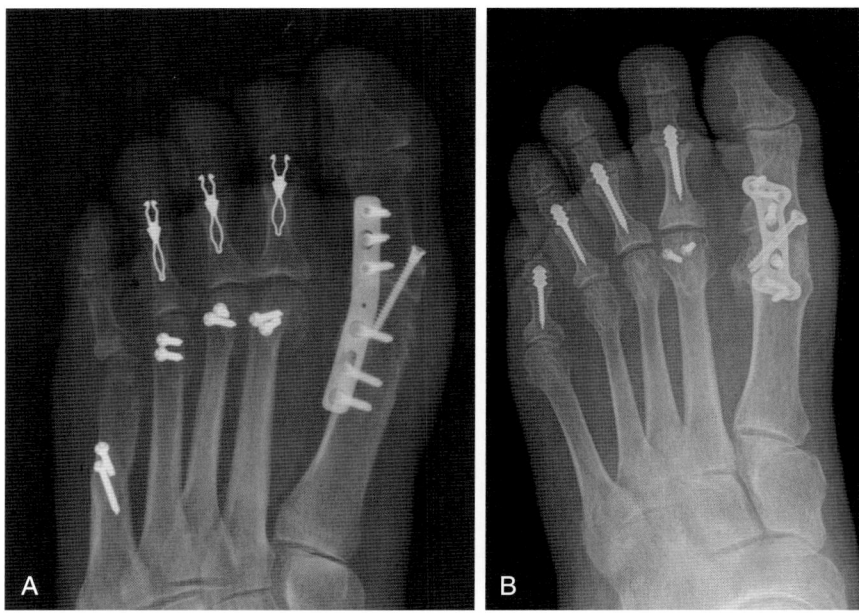

Figure 19-40 **A** and **B,** Anteroposterior radiographs after multiple hammer toe repairs, Weil osteotomies, and metatarsophalangeal joint arthrodesis.

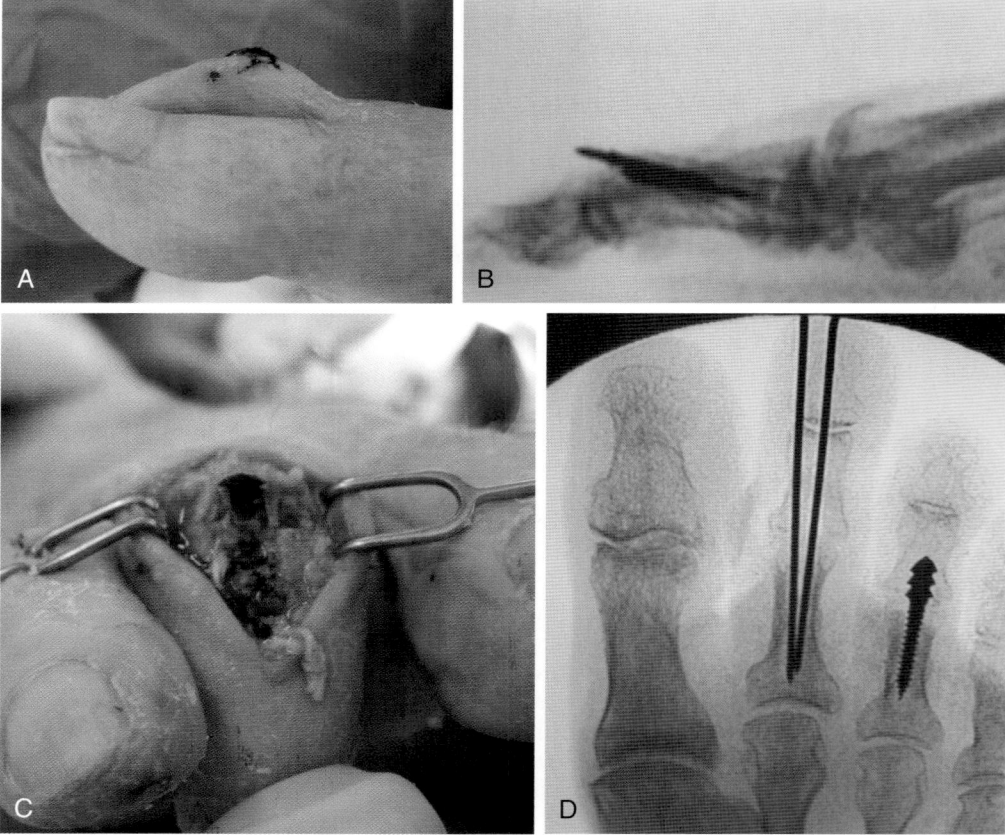

Figure 19-41 A complication with intramedullary hammer toe devices that can occur is osteopenic bone. **A,** Recurrent deformity at 6 weeks. Lateral radiograph **(B)** and clinical photograph **(C)** demonstrate dorsal cut-off of device. **D,** After intramedullary bone graft and K-wire fixation.

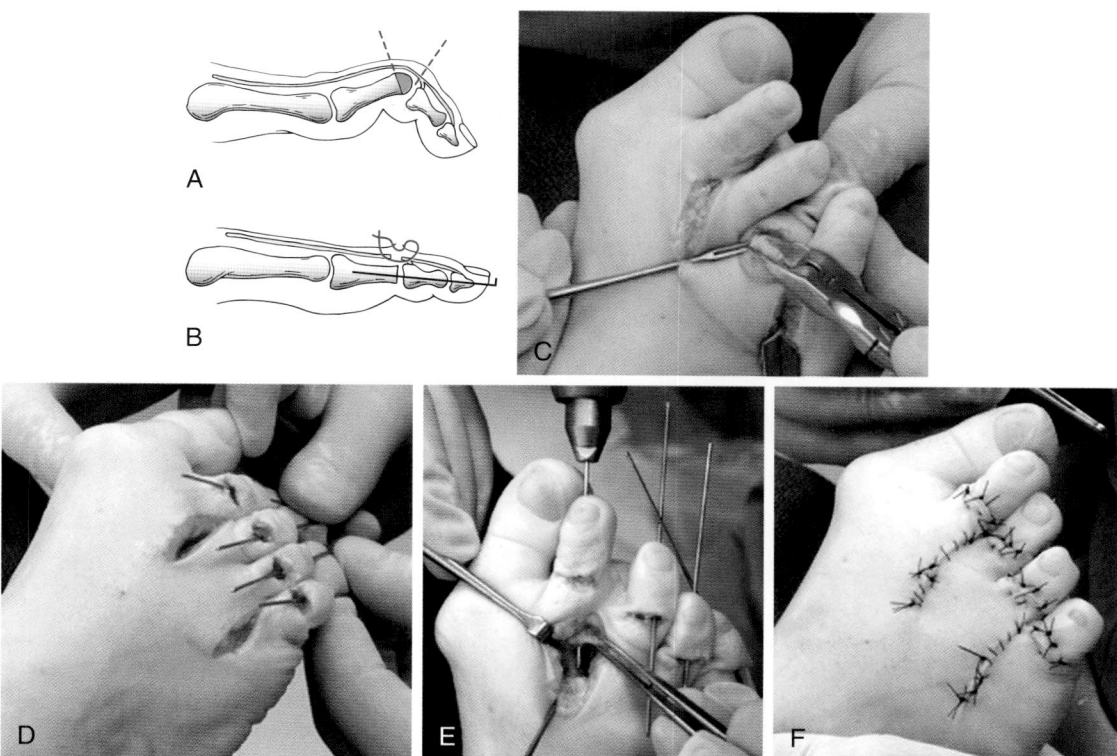

Figure 19-42 Fixed hammer toe repair. **A,** An elliptic skin incision is made to expose the condyles of the proximal phalanx, which are then resected. **B,** A K-wire is used to stabilize the proximal interphalangeal joint. **C,** Clinical photograph of a bone cutter resecting the condyles of the proximal phalanx. **D,** K-wires placed through the second through fifth toes. **E,** Retrograde drilling of the K-wires through the proximal phalanx and into the metatarsal heads. **F,** Toe alignment after suturing. (**B,** Courtesy A. Smith, MD, Prince Rupert, Canada.)

held in proper alignment, the pin is then driven in a retrograde fashion to stabilize and align the proximal phalanx (Fig. 19-42D and E). Later, after the MTP joint arthroplasty, the pin is advanced into the metatarsal diaphysis and proximal metaphysis, stabilizing the arthroplasty site. The placement of intramedullary K-wires to stabilize the surgical site depends on the surgeon's choice. K-wires have been advocated for treatment of hammer toes and lesser MTP joint excisional arthroplasty with rheumatoid foot deformities.[104,358] Internal fixation not only helps simplify dressing changes but also seems to produce a cosmetically superior result by achieving acceptable position of the toes as well as maintaining this alignment (Fig. 19-42F).

Postoperative Care
Dressings are changed every 10 days, when the rest of rheumatoid foot repair is inspected and redressed. The K-wire and sutures are removed 3 weeks after surgery.

Alternative Method: Closed Osteoclasis
An alternative to an open hammer toe repair is a closed osteoclasis. After the MTP joint forefoot arthroplasty,

passive pressure is placed on the PIP joint, and the middle and distal phalanges are brought into hyperextension (Fig. 19-43). With significant ankylosis or deformity, it may become apparent that the magnitude of pressure needed to straighten the toe can place the neurovascular status of the toe at risk. In this situation, a surgical decompression with a proximal phalangeal condylectomy is indicated.

An open arthroplasty technique of the PIP joint does enable easier placement of the intramedullary K-wire. With a closed osteoclasis, the K-wire is introduced at the base of the proximal phalanx and is driven distally out the tip of the toe. It is then retrograded in a proximal direction across the MTP joint arthroplasty site into the metatarsal diaphysis and metaphysis to stabilize the site. The skin can be protected from the K-wire by using an angiocatheter sheath during retrograde placement through the base of the proximal phalanx.

Results and Complications
Hammer Toe Repair with First MTP Joint Arthrodesis and Lesser MTP Joint Resection Arthroplasty Coughlin[104] has reported the long-term results (mean follow-up

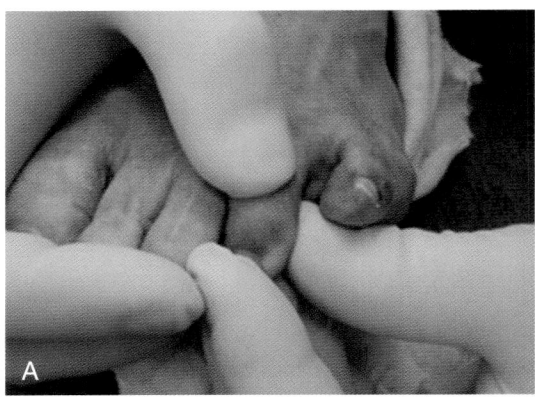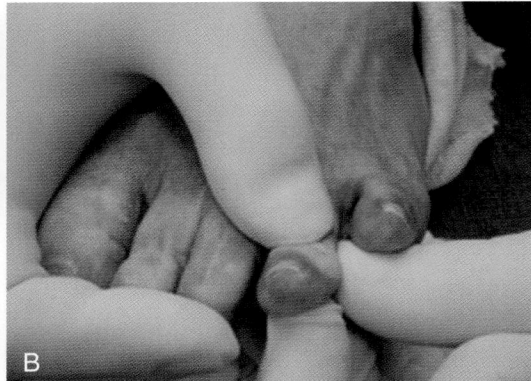

Figure 19-43 Closed osteoclasis of the fourth toe. Preoperatively **(A)** and after **(B)** osteoclasis. This toe was then fixed with an intramedullary K-wire.

of 74 months) of open hammer toe repair in combination with forefoot arthroplasty and first MTP joint arthrodesis (rheumatoid forefoot reconstruction) for rheumatoid arthritis. Of 188 toes, 142 had an open hammer toe repair, and in 76 (53%) of these, the pulp of the toe touched the ground at final follow-up. None of the lesser toes at final follow-up were reported to be a source of pain or to limit shoe choice. Successful arthrodesis of the PIP joint did not affect pain scores.

Recurrence of a hammer toe deformity places the MTP joint at risk for recurrent deformity as well. Coughlin[104] reported six postoperative mallet toe deformities (4%) (five had had a hammer toe repair) and three (2%) recurrent hammer toe deformities in 142 open hammer toe repairs associated with a complete rheumatoid forefoot reconstruction in 58 feet, with a mean follow-up of 74 months.

Recurrent clawing of a lesser toe leads to hyperextension of the MTP joint with eventual subluxation, dislocation, and redeformation of the lesser toe. Recurrence of a hammer toe or claw toe deformity is to be avoided. Redeformation can result from failed initial correction or actual recurrence. Thus a closed osteoclasis should be reserved for only mild deformities, whereas a DuVries phalangeal arthroplasty is preferred for more significant deformities (see Chapter 7). Furthermore, increased bony decompression when needed is achieved by resection arthroplasty of the lesser MTP joint.

Tanaka et al[543] reported using poly-L-lactic acid threaded pins for hammer toe correction. They noted less rigidity, yet demonstrated less deformity recurrence and no pin-tract infections in comparison with standard K-wire fixation.

The results after a hammer toe repair in the rheumatoid foot are consistently good. However, complications may occur, including persistent swelling, recurrent deformity, and skin or nail loss. Swelling of the toe can persist for 1 to 6 months postoperatively. It invariably subsides.

Occasionally, a mild deformity can recur, or a toe can deviate in either a medial or a lateral direction. This is rarely a significant problem. The lesser toe may mold to the shape of the adjacent toes. This is uncommon after a rheumatoid foot repair. Occasionally, a patient has some discomfort at the hammer toe arthroplasty site, and a painful pseudarthrosis may develop. When necessary, a corticosteroid injection provides lasting relief. After stabilization of the first ray, adjacent pressure from the hallux is uncommon. Fusion of the first MTP joint stabilizes the first ray and helps to prevent lateral pressure on the lesser toes. This has now been verified radiographically, biomechanically, and clinically in several studies. Radiographically, arthrodesis of the first MTP joint improves the first metatarsal declination and the talometatarsal and talocalcaneal angles, suggesting it achieves stabilization of the longitudinal arch.[338]

Biomechanically, arthrodesis of the first MTP joint has been associated with a decrease in measured first-ray mobility in clinical studies on patients with hallux valgus and hallux rigidus.[107,108,111] Instron testing of fixation for arthrodesis has demonstrated that the most stable construct for first MTP arthrodesis is a dorsal plate with an oblique lag screw.[440] Gait and pressure analysis before and after arthrodesis verified restoration of the weight-bearing function of the first ray. However, there was a significant change in the postoperative gait pattern, characterized by a shorter step length and a slight loss of ankle plantar flexion at toe-off, although hip and knee mechanics were not affected.[125] Clinically, Coughlin[104] has demonstrated 96% (45 of 47 feet) good or excellent results after a rheumatoid forefoot reconstruction consisting of arthrodesis of the first MTP joint, resection of the lesser metatarsal heads with preservation of the phalangeal base and extensors, and fixed hammer toe repair at a mean of 6 years of follow-up.

Surgical Reconstruction The treatment of choice for advanced rheumatoid arthritis complicated by hallux valgus, metatarsalgia, subluxation and dislocation of the

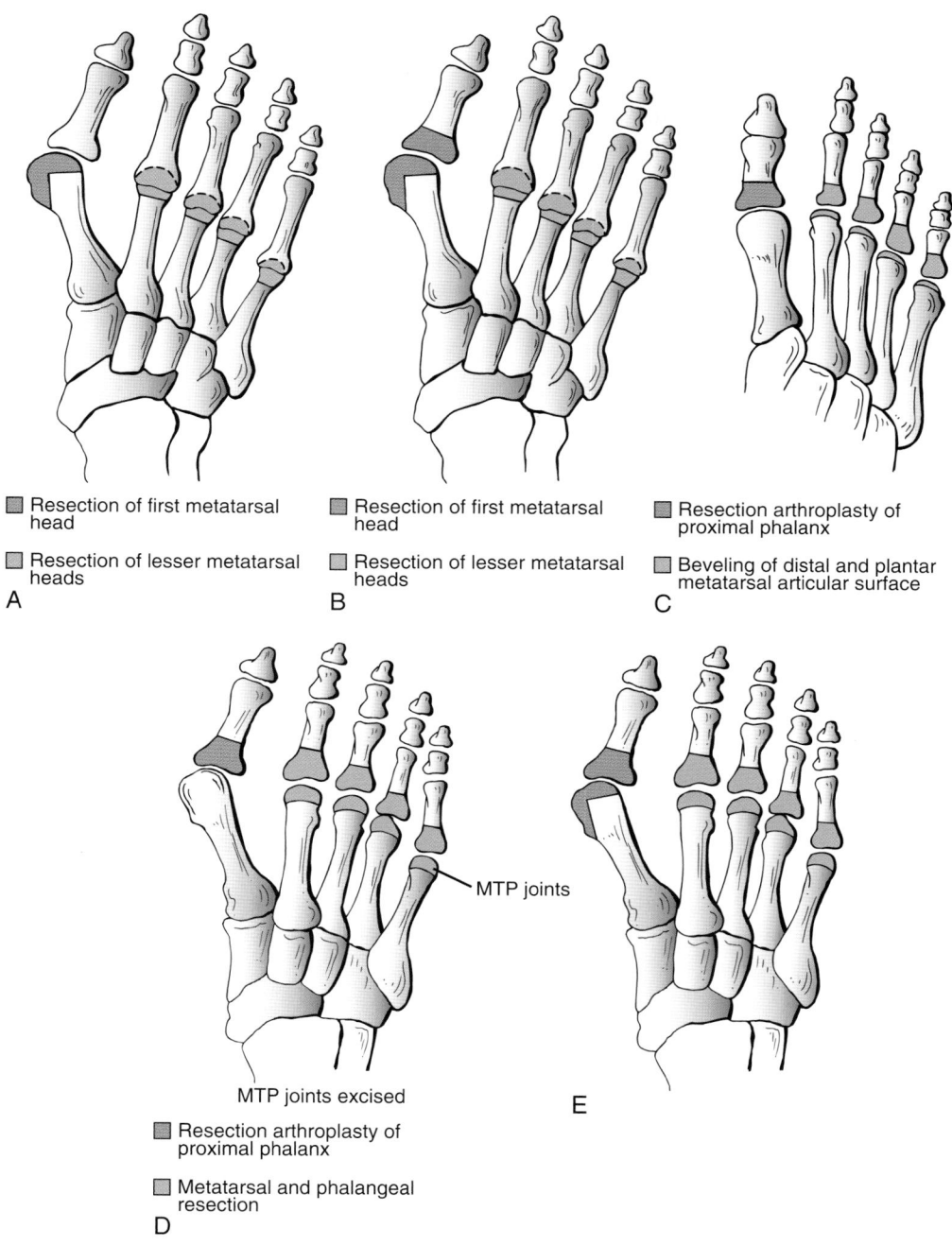

A
- ☐ Resection of first metatarsal head
- ☐ Resection of lesser metatarsal heads

B
- ☐ Resection of first metatarsal head
- ☐ Resection of lesser metatarsal heads

C
- ☐ Resection arthroplasty of proximal phalanx
- ☐ Beveling of distal and plantar metatarsal articular surface

D
MTP joints
MTP joints excised
- ☐ Resection arthroplasty of proximal phalanx
- ☐ Metatarsal and phalangeal resection

E

Figure 19-44 Treatment of the rheumatoid forefoot. **A,** The Hoffman procedure, in which the metatarsal heads are resected. **B,** The modified Hoffman procedure, as in **A,** but the base of the hallux proximal phalanx is resected for first metatarsophalangeal (MTP) arthrodesis. **C,** The Fowler procedure, in which the bases of the proximal phalanges are resected and the metatarsal heads are beveled and resected. **D,** The Clayton procedure includes metatarsal head resection with partial proximal phalangectomy. **E,** The modified Clayton procedure prepares the first MTP for arthrodesis instead of excisional arthroplasty.

lesser MTP joints, and fixed hammer toe deformities involves an arthrodesis of the MTP joint, multiple hammer toe repairs, and excisional arthroplasty of the lesser MTP joints (metatarsal head excision). Many procedures have been used to resect the lesser MTP joints (Video Clip 36). These include metatarsal head excision *(Hoffman*

procedure) (Fig. 19-44A and B), resection of the base of the proximal phalanx, resection of the base of the proximal phalanx with beveling of the plantar metatarsal surface *(Fowler procedure)*[169] (Fig. 19-44C), and partial proximal phalangectomy combined with metatarsal head resection *(Clayton procedure)* (Fig. 19-44D and E).

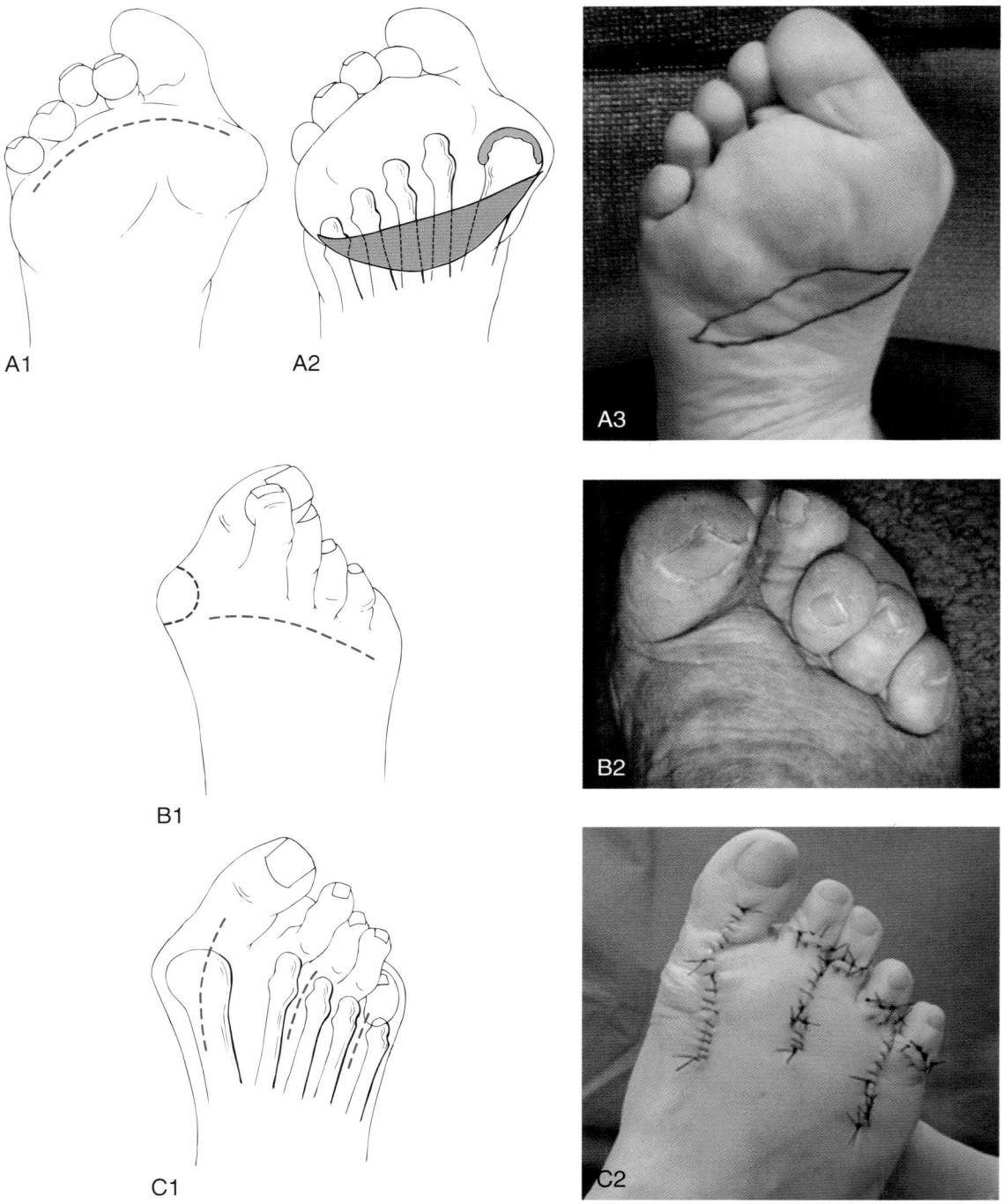

Figure 19-45 Incision type for rheumatoid forefoot reconstruction. **A1,** A transverse plantar incision. **A2** and **A3,** Elliptic plantar incision with skin resection. **B1,** Transverse dorsal incision. **B2,** The transverse dorsal incision may create toe contractures on long-term follow-up. **C1** and **C2,** Multiple dorsal longitudinal incisions.

Although the use of eponyms is discouraged, and these authors might not have recorded the initial description of their technique, their names have become associated with the individual procedure.

The choice of a particular surgical incision varies depending on the surgeon's preference. A transverse plantar incision[556] (Fig. 19-45A1), elliptic plantar incision[169,276] (Fig. 19-45A2 and A3), transverse dorsal incision (Fig. 19-45B1 and B2), and multiple dorsal longitudinal incisions (Fig. 19-45C1 and C2) have all been advocated. The current authors' preference is for three dorsal longitudinal incisions, with the medial

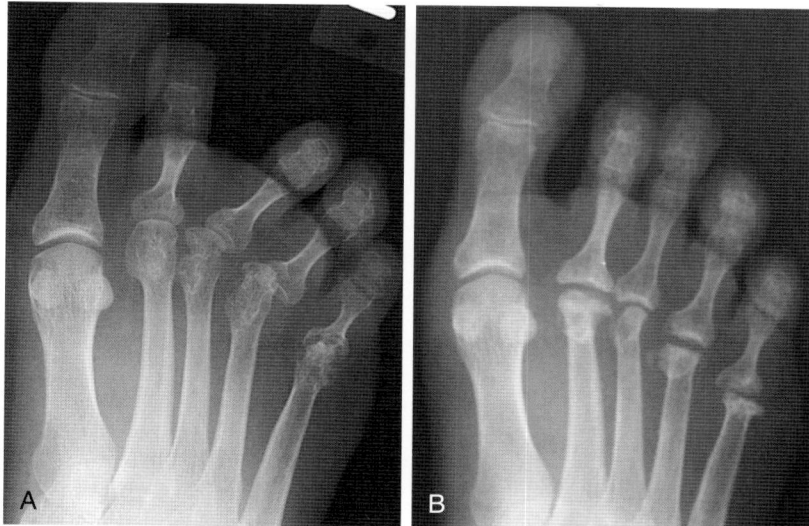

Figure 19-46 Lesser metatarsophalangeal (MTP) joint rheumatoid arthritis disease with sparing of the first MTP joint. Preoperative **(A)** and postoperative **(B)** radiographs demonstrating resection of the lesser metatarsal heads.

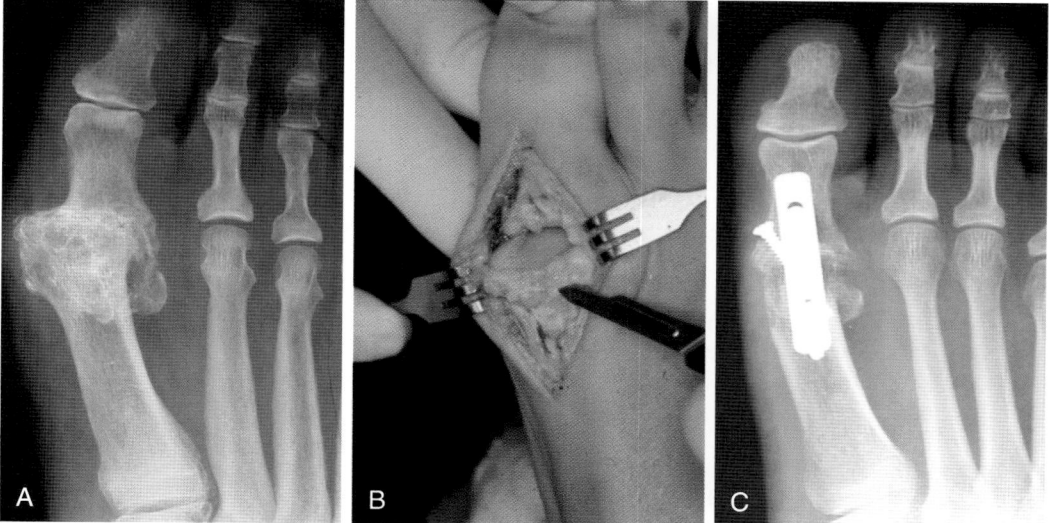

Figure 19-47 Rheumatoid disease involving only the first metatarsophalangeal joint. **A,** Preoperative radiograph demonstrating severe degenerative changes of the first metatarsophalangeal (MTP) joint. **B,** Intraoperative photograph showing first MTP joint destruction. **C,** Postoperative radiograph with first MTP arthrodesis.

incision centered over the first MTP joint and the two lateral incisions centered in the second and fourth intermetatarsal spaces.[102]

If only one or two MTP joints are affected, deciding whether an entire forefoot arthroplasty should be performed is difficult. Without first MTP joint arthrosis, an arthroplasty on the lesser MTP joints may be performed (Fig. 19-46A and B). If one or two lesser MTP joints are involved, an arthroplasty may be performed on these joints; however, a frank discussion with the patient must detail the likely progression of the disease process, with eventual involvement of the other MTP joints. Rarely is

the first MTP joint spared when all the lesser MTP joints are afflicted. And vice versa, when only the first MTP joint is involved, a fusion may be carried out and a lesser MTP resection arthroplasty is deferred (Fig. 19-47A-C). When the entire forefoot is involved, except for the fifth MTP joint, an arthroplasty of the fifth MTP joint is recommended because, over time, the fifth toe will drift medially, with resultant loss of stability of the adjacent MTP joints.

Thomas[551] recommended resection of a single symptomatic metatarsal head. If more than three joints were involved, the author recommended an entire forefoot arthroplasty, and for one or two involved lesser MTP joints—a limited resection. Morrison,[397] on the other hand, reported on limited resection in two cases and stated that such a modification was not justified. Marmor[363] reported that resection of one or two metatarsal heads "has always ended in failure." The chapter's authors support the notion of Clayton[90,91] and others[57,449,567] that if two metatarsals require resection, an entire forefoot arthroplasty is the treatment of choice. Moreover, complication rates increase with revision procedures,[104] and delaying limited procedures in favor of complete reconstruction is usually preferable.

LESSER METATARSOPHALANGEAL JOINT ARTHROPLASTY
Surgical Technique

1. The lesser MTP joints are approached through two dorsal longitudinal incisions 3 cm long. The first incision is placed between the second and third metatarsals, starting at the web space and proceeding proximally. A similar incision is placed in the fourth web space and extends proximally (Fig. 19-48A and B).
2. The skin flaps are slightly undermined, and an oblique dissection is carried out medially and laterally to identify the adjacent MTP joints. The extensor tendons are identified but are usually left intact unless a significant contracture is present. The base of the proximal phalanx can be identified by tracing the distal portion of the extensor tendon. By starting the dissection in the interspace and carrying it out obliquely, the adjacent neurovascular bundles are protected.
3. With sharp dissection, the metatarsal neck is exposed. The periosteum is stripped along the metaphysis of the metatarsal in a circumferential manner. Plantar flexion of the involved toe can often deliver the metatarsal head dorsally. A synovectomy is performed as needed. A McGlamry elevator can be useful if the deformity is not severe. However, at times, a significant MTP joint dislocation is present, and careful use of a small Hoke osteotome to strip the capsular tissue can help to expose the metatarsal head without sacrificing the extensor tendons. Once the base of the proximal phalanx is freed of its soft tissue attachments, the phalanx can be pulled somewhat distally, increasing the exposure of the metatarsal head.
4. A bone-cutting rongeur or microtooth saw blade is used to transect the metatarsal in the proximal metaphyseal region (Fig. 19-51C1 and C2). The amount of bone removed depends on the magnitude of the overlap of the proximal phalanx on the metatarsal head. An osteotome or Freer elevator can be used to release the remaining adhesions, allowing delivery of the metatarsal head. The metatarsal head is then grasped with a rongeur and pulled from the wound. Ideally, the metatarsal head is removed in one piece to avoid leaving remnants of bone, which can cause recurrence of plantar callosities (Fig. 19-48D1 and D2). Enough head is resected so that the resection

arthroplasty accommodates the tip of the surgeon's index finger with gentle longitudinal traction of the digit, or about 1 cm (Fig. 19-48G1 and G2).

5. After the metatarsal head has been removed, the plantar aspect of the remaining metatarsal shaft is beveled with a rongeur to minimize the risk of recurrent callosities.
6. Once the metatarsal head has been excised, any significant synovial cysts or plantar subcutaneous bursae are resected in the depths of the wound. Care must be taken on the plantar aspect to remove only the dorsal half of a synovial cyst to avoid excessive resection of soft tissue.
7. The procedure is repeated for the remaining metatarsal heads. Care is taken to ensure that the anatomic cascade of metatarsal length is recreated with the resections (Fig. 19-48D-F). Again, a rongeur is used to bevel the plantar aspect of the remaining metatarsal surfaces to remove any prominent plantar spikes.
8. The base of the proximal phalanx is preserved because it forms a wide concave surface that affords stability to the pseudoarticulation that has been created. (Removal of the base of the proximal phalanx leaves a greatly narrowed diaphyseal region that articulates with the remaining metatarsal diaphysis.) By removing the contracture at the MTP joint, the fat pad will realign without resection of plantar skin.[102]
9. The most important aspect of the excisional arthroplasty is achieving adequate decompression at the MTP joint. Usually a 1-cm space between the base of the proximal phalanx and the prepared metatarsal surface is sufficient (see Fig. 19-48G1 and G2). The tip of the index finger is used as a gauge to measure an adequate amount of resection. With minimal longitudinal tension on the toe, there should be a minimal amount of pressure on the tip of the index finger that has been placed in this interval.
10. With a symmetric resection of the metatarsal heads, an even distribution of pressure beneath the metatarsals should be achieved. Usually, the first and second metatarsals are of equal length, whereas the third, fourth, and fifth are progressively shorter from the medial to the lateral aspect of the forefoot. Avoiding a prominent metatarsal prevents new pressure points from developing. At this point, attention is directed toward the hammer toe deformities of the lesser toes. With a significant deformity, it is preferable to resect the condyles of the proximal phalanx in order to decompress the joint. This also aids in placement of the intramedullary K-wires. On occasion, a closed osteoclasis or manipulation of the IP joint is performed to reduce the hammer toe deformity.
11. To align the lesser toes, a 0.045-inch K-wire is introduced at the PIP joint and driven distally through the middle and distal phalanges (Fig. 19-48H and I). A K-wire of adequate length is used so that the proximal tip of the wire is eventually embedded in the proximal metatarsal base across the resection arthroplasty,

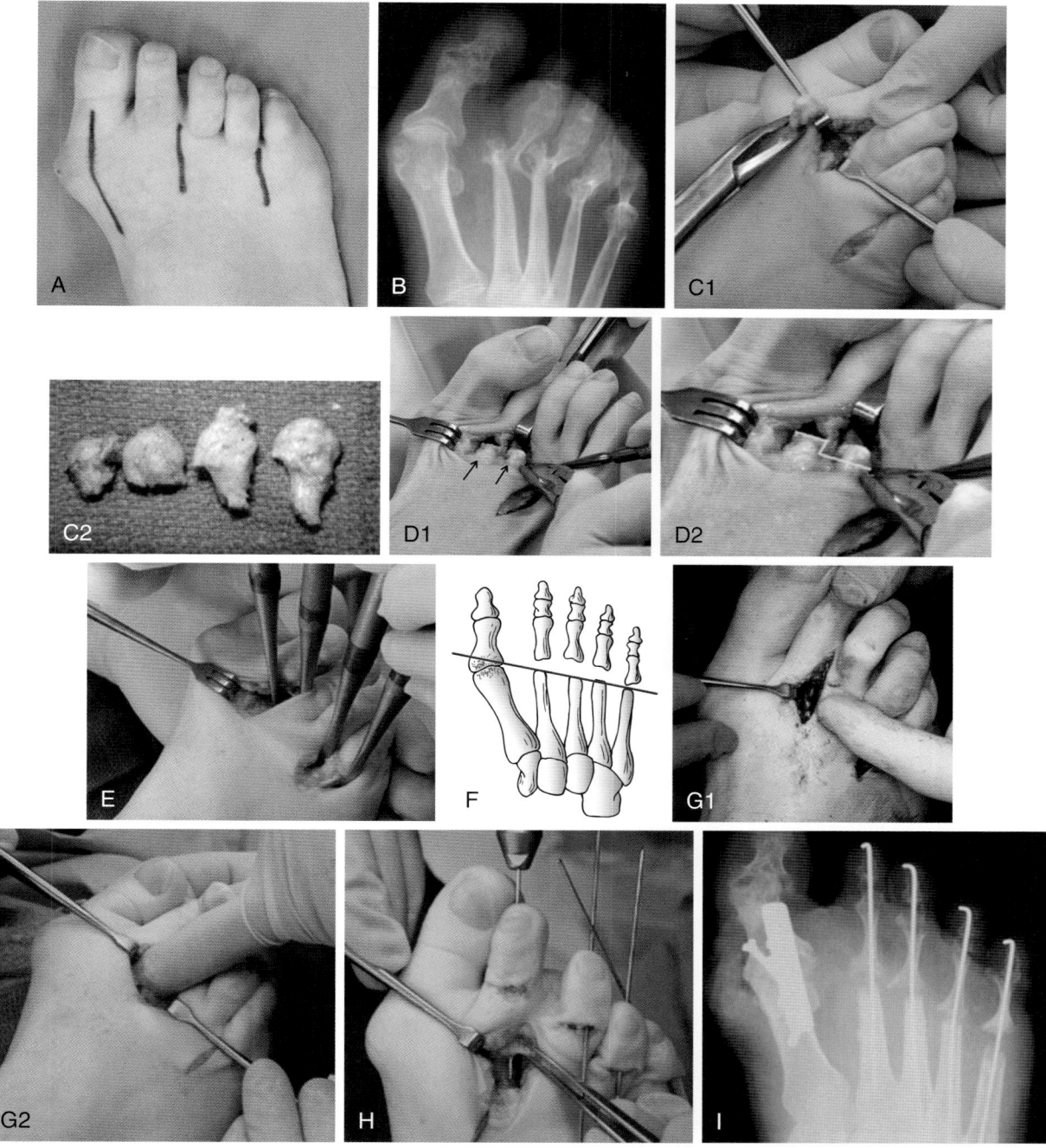

Figure 19-48 Technique of lesser metatarsophalangeal (MTP) joint arthroplasty. Preoperative clinical **(A)** and radiographic **(B)** appearance of severe rheumatoid forefoot deformity. **C1,** A bone-cutting rongeur is used to transect the metatarsal in the metaphyseal-diaphyseal region. It is grasped with a rongeur and removed. **C2,** Multiple metatarsal heads are removed. **D1,** After each metatarsal shaft is transected, the distal portion is removed. **D2,** The shaft of the third metatarsal is too long and needs to be shortened. **E,** Technique of using vertical osteotomes to gauge the cascade of metatarsal lengths when dorsal longitudinal incisions are used and direct comparison of the individual lengths is difficult. **F,** A diagram demonstrates the desirable anatomic cascade that is the goal with the resection arthroplasty so that each successive resection is a few millimeters shorter than the previous one. **G1** and **G2,** Tip of index finger (approximately 1 cm in diameter) is used to gauge the magnitude of resection. **H,** K-wires are used to stabilize hammer toe repair and lesser MTP resection arthroplasties. **I,** Radiograph demonstrates first MTP joint arthrodesis with 1-cm resection arthroplasty at each of the lesser MTP joints.

giving stability to the arthroplasty site. The pin is advanced through the proximal phalanx into the metatarsal diaphysis and proximal metaphysis. The pin is bent at the tip of the toe to prevent proximal migration. A similar technique of pin placement is carried out for all the lesser MTP joint arthroplasties (Fig. 19-49A and B).

12. The MTP joint arthroplasty sites are irrigated with an antibiotic solution, and the skin is approximated with 3-0 or 4-0 nylon sutures. The incisions for the hammer toe repairs are approximated as well.

13. Attention is then directed to the first MTP joint (discussed later in this chapter; see pages 974 to 981). Once the lesser toes have been realigned and the MTP

joint space is reduced, the surgeon has an idea of the amount the first ray needs to be shortened. Often, at least 1 cm of shortening is achieved laterally, and extra bone must be removed from the first ray to achieve its appropriate length (Fig. 19-50A-C).

14. As an alternative, the lesser toes may be fixed with permanent metallic implants at the PIP joint in addition to K-wire fixation (see Fig. 19-40). Complications may develop after the placement of intramedullary implants (see Fig. 19-41). The placement of PIP joint implants does not obviate the need for intramedullary K-wire fixation to stabilize the lesser MTP joints after resection arthroplasty.

Postoperative Care

A gauze-and-tape compression dressing is applied at surgery and changed 2 to 3 days later. The patient is permitted to ambulate in a postoperative shoe or short walking boot with weight bearing on the heel. Compression dressings are changed every 7 to 10 days for approximately 6 weeks after surgery. Typically, the K-wires are removed 3 to 5 weeks after surgery. Postoperative radiographs are obtained as necessary.

In the immediate postoperative period, circulatory status of the toes must be monitored. With severe deformities, vascular compromise can develop. Removal of intramedullary K-wires can allow revascularization of a compromised toe. If a toe remains blue or white 15 minutes after surgery, loosening the compression dressing or removing the K-wire is often necessary. Application of nitro glycerin paste to the distal aspects of the digits will improve blood flow and can allow fixation to remain in place.

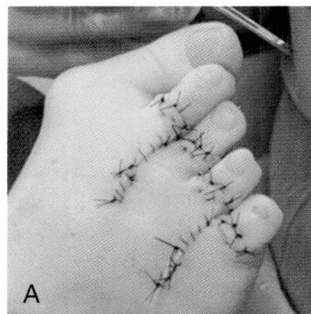
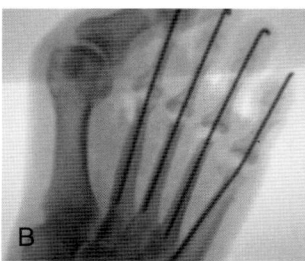

Figure 19-49 **A,** Clinical photograph shows completion of forefoot arthroplasty before the first metatarsophalangeal joint arthrodesis. **B,** Intraoperative fluoroscopy demonstrates resection of the lesser metatarsals and relative excess length of the first metatarsal, which can now be corrected during arthrodesis.

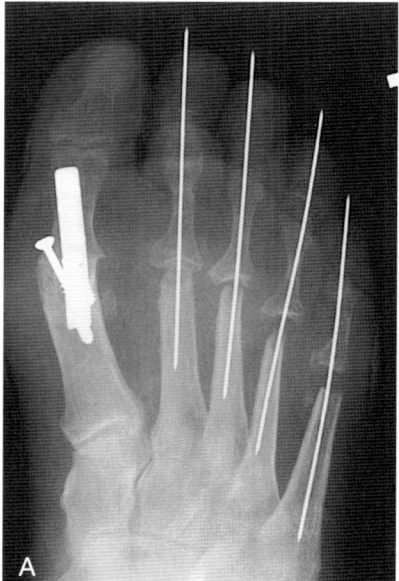
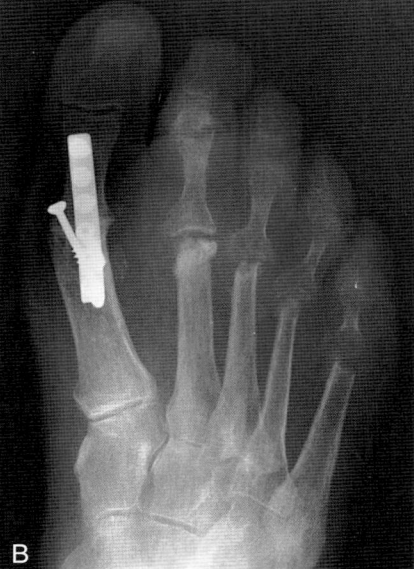
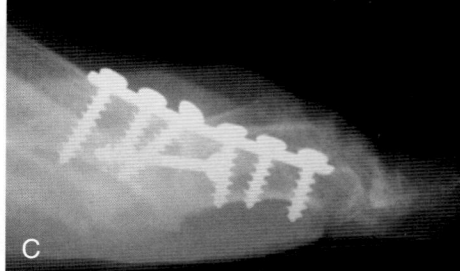

Figure 19-50 **A,** Radiograph demonstrates metatarsophalangeal (MTP) arthrodesis and multiple K-wire fixation of lesser MTP joints. **B,** After K-wire removal. **C,** Anteroposterior radiograph with contoured MTP arthrodesis plate.

Results and Complications

First MTP Joint Arthrodesis and Lesser MTP Joint Resection Arthroplasty The results after a rheumatoid forefoot repair in general are gratifying. Coughlin[104] reported 96% good or excellent results of rheumatoid forefoot reconstruction in 47 feet by using the Hoffman technique of metatarsal head resection, fixed hammer toe repair, and great toe MTP joint arthrodesis. There was a 2% to 3% recurrence rate of hammer toe and mallet toe deformities, no reported first MTP joint nonunions, and 7% redislocation of the lesser MTP joints (70% were dislocated preoperatively). Pain was absent or mild in 91% (43 of 47 feet) and moderate in 4 feet at a mean follow-up of 6 years. There were no special shoe requirements, 15 feet had no functional limitation, 28 feet had some limitation of recreational activity, and 4 had limitation of daily activity. Based on the most recent biomechanical, radiographic, and clinical data, the Coughlin rheumatoid forefoot reconstruction is the procedure of choice for chronic rheumatoid forefoot deformity.

Using first MTP arthrodesis and lesser MTP joint arthroplasty techniques, Mann and Thompson[359] reported 89% (18 cases) good and excellent results at final follow-up. Mann and Schakel[358] reported 90% good or excellent results by using a similar technique (two threaded Steinman pins for first MTP joint arthrodesis) in 28 feet, with minimal recurrence of deformity at 3.7 years of follow-up.

A major reason for dissatisfaction with many forefoot arthroplasties reported in the literature is that they were combined with first MTP joint resection arthroplasty. Watson[583] concluded that a Keller arthroplasty did not receive support from the lateral toes. Craxford et al[117] reported recurrent deformation and dissatisfaction after forefoot arthroplasty associated with resection of the first MTP joint. Indeed, progression of hallux valgus leads to redeformation of the lesser MTP joints and recurrent lesser toe deformity (Fig. 19-51A-C). Maintenance of first MTP joint alignment with an arthrodesis protects not only the hallux but also the lesser MTP joints from recurrent deformity and subsequent metatarsalgia. The relocated fat pad is maintained in a normal position after MTP arthroplasty. The lesser MTP joints do not have much motion, but this does not appear to be a problem for patients. Typically, patients no longer walk with a heel-to-toe gait but rather by placing the foot flat on the ground.

Of 1874 cases reported in several series describing various surgical techniques of lesser MTP joint arthroplasty, an overall 81% satisfactory rate has been reported. Partial proximal phalangectomy as a treatment for claw toe deformities and subluxated MTP joints achieved a satisfaction rate of 65% (180 of 278 cases).[94,139,413,487] Partial proximal phalangectomy with beveling of the metatarsal condyle, as described initially by Fowler,[169] has a lower reported success rate of 43% (116 of 177 cases). Partial proximal phalangectomy combined with metatarsal head resection, as described by Clayton[91] and others,[212] has a higher reported success rate, with 80% good and excellent results (507 of 636 cases).

In an attempt to lessen postoperative metatarsalgia, Miyamoto et al[387] described a technique of interpositional arthroplasty of the extensor digitorum longus tendon in addition to resection arthroplasty of the lesser MTP joints and noted good results without deformity at 24 months. Whether this technique improves results in comparison with simple excisional arthroplasty remains to be seen.

Saltzman[487] reported on the results of partial phalangectomy and syndactylization for mild rheumatoid forefoot deformities. Postoperatively, 64% of patients reported limitation in activity because of metatarsalgia, and 36% of patients considered the result cosmetically unsatisfactory. Some authors have used a combination of partial proximal phalangectomy with beveling of the metatarsal condyles for more moderate deformities and resorted to metatarsal head resection for more severe deformities. A metatarsal head excision, as described by Hoffman[237] and others, has the highest published success rate of 89% good and excellent results (748 of 843 cases).

Barton,[19] who compared different forefoot arthroplasty procedures, concluded that individual surgical techniques did not make a difference. However, he

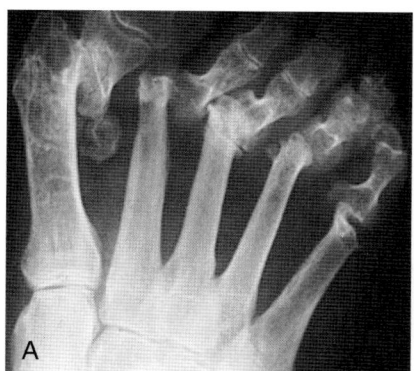
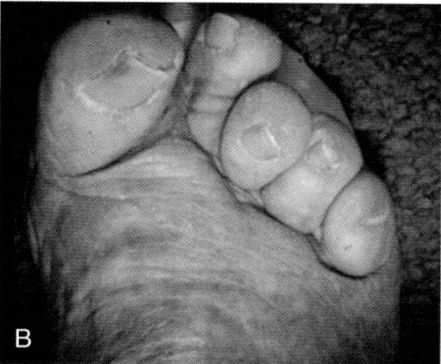
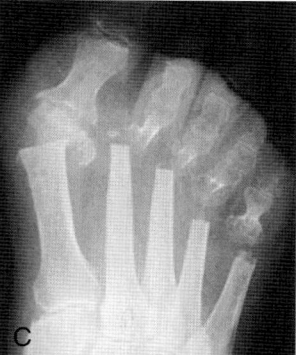

Figure 19-51 Keller resection arthroplasty. Radiographic **(A)** and clinical **(B)** appearance with hallux valgus and lesser metatarsophalangeal joint subluxation. **C,** Anteroposterior radiograph showing the lateral deviation of the toes on the metatarsals after first metatarsophalangeal (MTP) silicone implant and lesser MTP Hoffman procedure.

combined a first MTP joint excisional arthroplasty with lesser MTP arthroplasties, which likely influenced the end results. Mulcahy et al[400] reported the surgical results of two groups of patients whose treatment differed based on arthrodesis or resection of the first MTP joint and concluded that a stable first MTP joint (with an arthrodesis) and resection of the lesser metatarsal heads with K-wire fixation led to a more cosmetic forefoot and a more even distribution of forefoot pressures postoperatively.

In another study, radiographic follow-up after a Keller resection in 23 feet demonstrated first MTP joint erosive changes that continued even after the resection in more than 50% of cases.[29] Furthermore, the same authors noted that the need for revision surgery was much higher in those who underwent a Keller procedure. Raunio[452] reported a similar increase in the need for second surgery after a Keller procedure and recommended arthrodesis of the first MTP joint.

Comparing panmetatarsal forefoot resection arthroplasty techniques, Fuhrmann[175] reported better success with the Hueter-Mayo resection in 188 patients who had undergone either a Keller or a Hueter-Mayo resection arthroplasty of the first metatarsophalangeal joint, but 30% of the Hueter-Mayo group still experienced persistent metatarsalgia. Thomas et al[550] reported satisfactory results at an average follow-up of 65 months. Of the 20 patients (39 feet), 60% reported problems with their balance, and only 12% of the feet could be fitted with footwear of choice after surgery. Mild-to-severe recurrent hallux valgus was noted in 51% of cases. Thomas et al[550] reported good or excellent results in only 30% of cases.

Hasselo et al[226] reported short-term results with forefoot arthroplasty from eight surgeons who used several different reconstruction techniques for the first MTP joint, including simple bunionectomy, silicone first MTP implant, excisional arthroplasty, and arthrodesis. Little can be concluded from the long-term results because of the numerous procedures and numerous surgeons involved. Craxford et al[117] reported an initial 80% satisfaction rate after forefoot arthroplasty but noted that it diminished to 55% at 4.5 to 8.5 years of follow-up. No first MTP arthrodeses were used in this study.

Postoperative complications of resection arthroplasty techniques without first MTP arthrodesis, including claw toes, intractable plantar keratoses, metatarsalgia, and recurrent pain, have been reported in many series. Petrov et al[437] found that 28% of 15 patients who underwent panmetatarsal head resection for rheumatoid forefoot arthritis developed recurrent plantar ulceration as early as 6 months postoperatively. The most common apparent cause of re-ulceration was recurrent bone growth, most commonly under the second metatarsal head.

However, the major reason for dissatisfaction postoperatively in most series is the development of progressive hallux valgus deformity. Of note, Pastalis et al[431] found restriction of walking ability because of forefoot pain (56%), recurrent great toe deformity (72%), and recurrent painful callosities (61%), at a mean follow-up of 10.5

years. These complications can often be prevented with first MTP arthrodesis.

Vandeputte et al[566] reported the results of two separate groups of patients who were compared to evaluate the results of resection versus arthrodesis of the first MTP joint and lesser MTP resection arthroplasty. The authors concluded that when a fusion was achieved, it protected and diminished pressure beneath the lesser metatarsals more effectively than resection or pseudarthrosis. Hasselo et al[226] recommended that fusion and stability of the first ray should be the primary goal for surgical intervention of the rheumatoid forefoot.

Flint and Sweetnam[164] and Nissen[417] recommended amputation of the lesser toes as the treatment of choice for severe rheumatoid forefoot deformity (Fig. 19-52A-E). Anderson and Klaborg[11] also reported on five rheumatoid patients who underwent transmetatarsal amputation for severe forefoot pain. Four of their patients had no postoperative pain and improved gait. However, it appears that forefoot reconstruction offers better cosmetic results and improved ease in fitting footwear than do amputation procedures.

The most common complication after forefoot arthroplasty is recurrence of intractable plantar keratoses or recurrent pain from inadequate bone resection.[408] Clayton[90,91] noted a 10% repeat surgery rate after inadequate resection of the lesser metatarsal heads. Adequate decompression of the MTP joints at surgery is extremely important. If a metatarsal is significantly longer than an adjacent metatarsal, a high risk exists for the development of postoperative recurrent intractable plantar keratoses. Chronic swelling in the forefoot is a common postoperative complaint, but the swelling usually subsides with time. Isolated excision of one or two metatarsal heads is, in general, to be avoided because an intractable plantar keratotic lesion often develops beneath remaining metatarsal heads.

Repeat surgery for the rheumatoid forefoot is necessary for the following reasons:

■ Bone regrowth in the area of lesser metatarsal head resections
■ Irregular lesser metatarsal head resections
■ Limited surgery with only one or two metatarsal heads resected

A meticulous technique with attention to a regular resection of the metatarsal heads in a line in which the first and second metatarsals are of equal length and the third, fourth, and fifth metatarsals are progressively shorter helps to prevent recurrent intractable plantar keratoses (see Fig. 19-48D and F). Meticulous care in debridement of the area of the metatarsal head resection is necessary so that all bone fragments are removed because this minimizes bone regrowth. In general, all four lesser metatarsal heads should be removed. Limited surgery in which only one or two metatarsal heads are removed should be avoided.

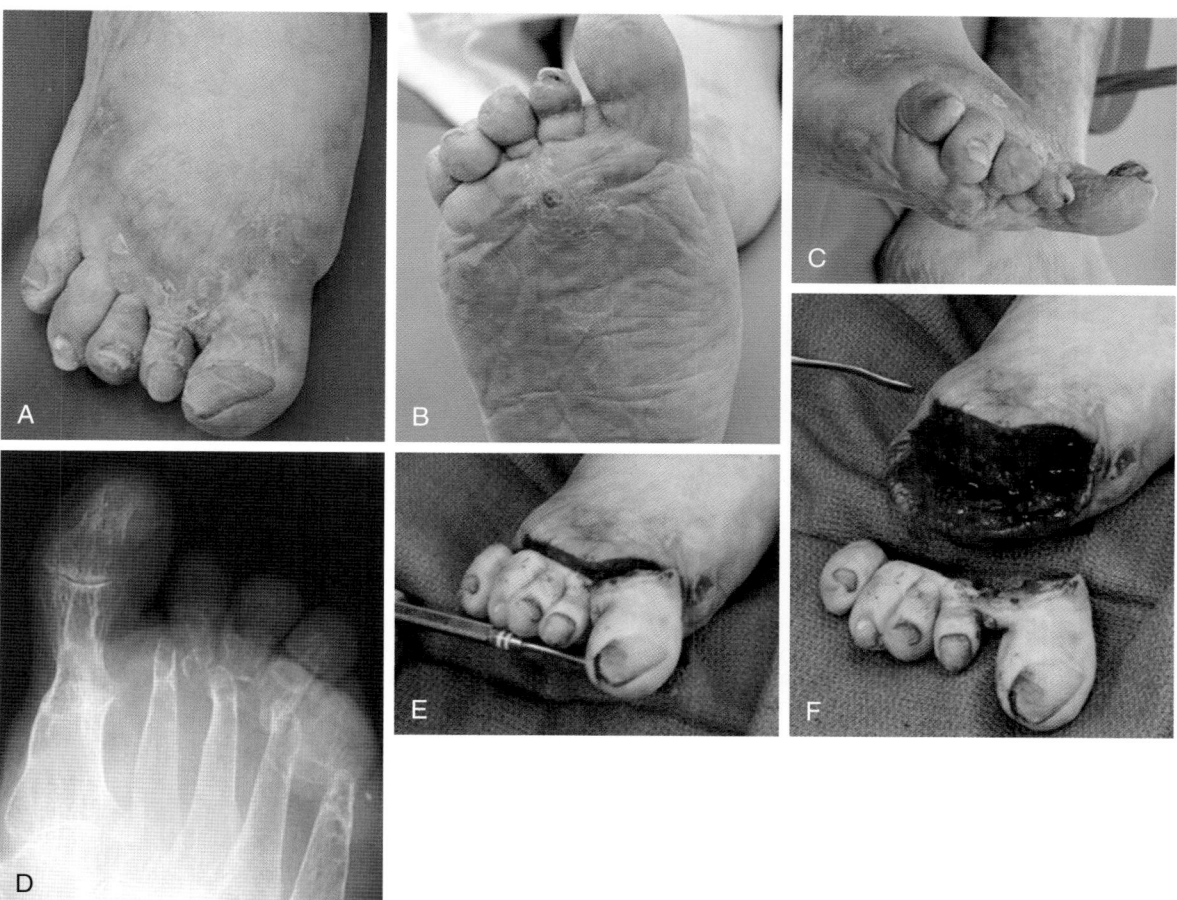

Figure 19-52 A-C, Preoperative clinical photographs showing a rheumatoid forefoot deformity with dislocated lesser metatarsophalangeal joints of a patient with poor vascularity and painful intractable plantar keratoses. **D,** Preoperative radiograph. **E,** Intraoperative photograph demonstrating surgical incision. **F,** Intraoperative photograph after disarticulation of the toes.

In a long-term report on his practice experience, Graham[198] recommended that even with minimal involvement of the first MTP joint, an arthrodesis is warranted in combination with a forefoot arthroplasty (Fig. 19-53). The author suggested that with time deterioration of the first MTP joint would likely lead to recurrent lateral forefoot deformities. Thordarson et al[554] reported similar findings in seven patients (13 feet) with initially well-preserved first MTP joints and reported that 11 of 13 feet developed recurrent hallux valgus after an attempt at joint preservation, at a mean follow-up of only 24 months.

FIRST METATARSOPHALANGEAL JOINT ARTHROPLASTY

Resection arthroplasty of the first MTP joint has been recommended in the past for reconstructing the severely deformed rheumatoid forefoot.[175] McGarvey and Johnson[369] and others[233,398] have stated that the Keller procedure in combination with forefoot arthroplasty is often unsuccessful.

McGarvey and Johnson[369] reported a 33% satisfaction rate when excisional arthroplasty was combined with lesser MTP resection arthroplasty (see Fig. 19-51). In reporting their experience with excisional arthroplasty in patients with rheumatoid arthritis, they noted recurrence of hallux valgus in 53%, recurrent metatarsalgia in 20%, and foot instability in 27%. Only one third of patients were satisfied with their postoperative result. The authors concluded that a first MTP arthrodesis was the treatment of choice in combination with forefoot resection arthroplasty. van der Heijden et al[568] reported that 29 of 41 (71%) of the resection arthroplasties of the first MTP joint were unsatisfactory (Video Clip 60).

Initially, a resection arthroplasty may give significant relief of symptoms in the treatment of a hallux valgus deformity in the rheumatoid patient. Hasselo et al[226] reported that initial acceptable results with excisional arthroplasty deteriorated rapidly, resulting in poor push-off of the first ray, recurrent deformity, unacceptable cosmetic results, and recurrent pain. Craxford et al[117] found little difference between patients who had resection arthroplasty and patients treated conservatively with

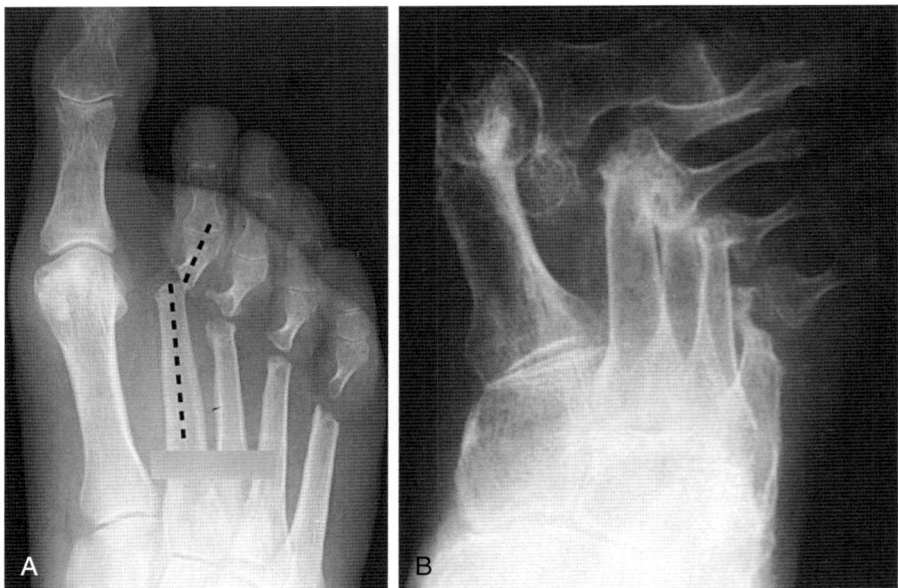

Figure 19-53 **A,** Radiograph demonstrates lateral forefoot arthroplasty (modified Clayton procedure). The first ray was uninvolved. Note the excess length of the first ray. **B,** Long-term follow-up after simple bunionectomy and lesser forefoot arthroplasty (Hoffman procedure) is complicated by severe valgus deformity of the hallux and recurrent deformity of the lesser metatarsophalangeal joints.

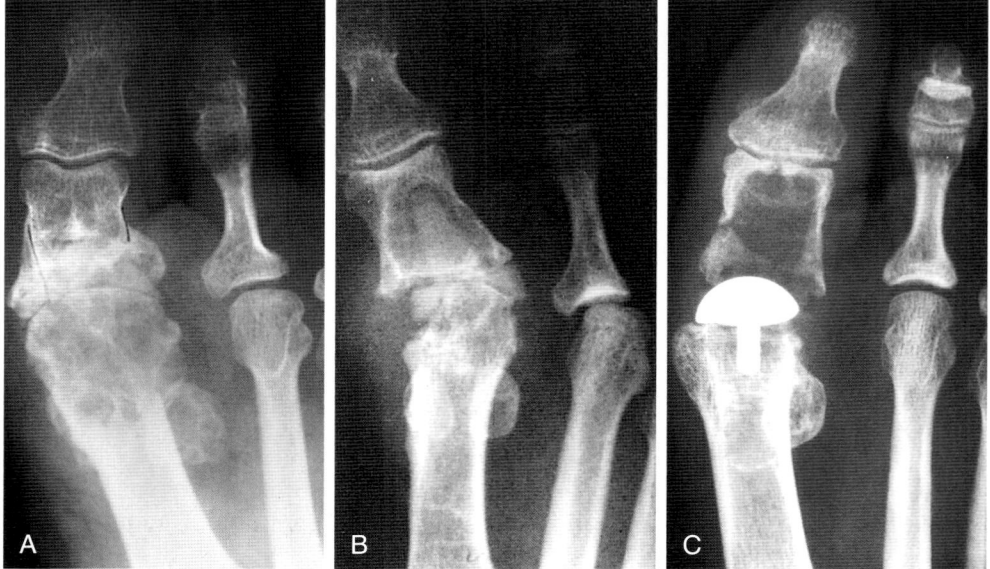

Figure 19-54 Complications after silicone implant arthroplasty. **A,** Severe osteolysis of proximal phalanx. **B,** Fragmentation, synovitis, and osteolysis after single-stem implant placement. **C,** Severe collapse, bone overgrowth, synovitis, and osteolysis after metal and silicone implant arthroplasty.

special shoes to manage their rheumatoid forefoot deformity. (For the surgical technique of excisional arthroplasty, see the later discussion under Hallux Rigidus.) Furthermore, more recent reports suggest long-term function of the foot is compromised with an unstable first ray created by the resection arthroplasty.[550] There may be a difference in extent of compromised gait postoperatively depending on the resection technique used (Keller or Mayo).[177]

Silicone elastic (Silastic) implant arthroplasty of the first MTP joint has been recommended as an alternative to resection arthroplasty (Fig. 19-54). Cracchiolo[114] and

Jenkin and Oloff[260] recommended Silastic implant replacement of the great toe and lesser MTP joints. The reported results by Hanyu et al[219] found 74% good or excellent results in 60 feet at 12 years of follow-up. However, nine implants were noted to have fractured, four were removed because of infection or recurrent deformity, and 59% had sinking of the implant with findings of silicone synovitis in 12 joints (21%).

Silastic implants have been fraught with short-term and long-term complications (see later discussion of first MTP implant arthroplasty under Hallux Rigidus). Although satisfactory results have been reported in some cases, many long-term complications have been noted, including fracture, silicone synovitis, osteolysis, and recurrent pain. Moreover, salvage of a failed implant arthroplasty is technically demanding and usually requires an interposition graft from the iliac crest or proximal tibia[231] or simultaneous arthrodesis of both the interphalangeal and MTP joint.[159] In general, silicone prosthetic replacement of the first MTP joint is rarely indicated in treatment of the rheumatoid forefoot with hallux valgus. For lesser MTP joint replacement, there appears to be little difference between resection arthroplasty and silicone implant replacement.[260] Thus the added expense and risk of implant arthroplasty in most situations are unwarranted.

Stabilization of the first ray with a first MTP arthrodesis has been recommended by DuVries[139] and others on the premise that an arthrodesed first MTP joint stabilizes the first ray. This has been verified by Coughlin et al[107,110,111] in clinical studies on hallux rigidus and hallux valgus.

A forefoot arthroplasty itself weakens support for the great toe. Consequently, during gait, the hallux and lateral toes displace dorsally and laterally. As the toes migrate dorsolaterally, weight bearing is increased on the previously resected lesser metatarsal shafts, and there is an increased incidence of metatarsalgia. After an arthrodesis, lateral translation of pressure beneath the lesser metatarsals is uncommon. After arthrodesis, in the latter half of stance phase, the foot lifts off the ground slightly earlier,[356] decreasing stress on the lesser MTP joints, decreasing metatarsalgia, and protecting the lesser toes from recurrent deformity.

Preoperative foot imprints have been compared with postoperative pressure studies. Minns and Craxford[385] reported two to three times increased pressure developing beneath the metatarsal heads before surgical resection. Also, repositioning of the plantar fat pad has been speculated to improve tolerance of pressure. Fu and Scranton[173] found significant increase of pressure developing beneath symptomatic metatarsal heads after irregular resection arthroplasty. Henry and Waugh[233] reported improved weight-bearing function of the hallux after arthrodesis and hypothesized that this accounted for the improved function.

In a long-term follow-up study after forefoot arthroplasty, Watson[583] stated that the major effect of surgical intervention was pain relief and concluded that arthrodesis was the treatment of choice for a rheumatoid forefoot deformity. After resection arthroplasty, the author noted that the valgus position of the hallux was not supported by the lesser toes. He concluded that first MTP resection arthroplasty gave mediocre results in comparison with first MTP arthrodesis.

Direct comparisons between excisional arthroplasty and arthrodesis of the first MTP joint have demonstrated that arthrodesis is superior as noted previously. Beauchamp et al[22] concluded that arthrodesis resulted in better forefoot balance, cosmesis, and shoe fitting.

Occasionally, a patient has an uninvolved first ray and significant forefoot deformity with lateral metatarsalgia. Cracchiolo[115] recommended that if the hallux was neither malaligned nor involved with MTP synovitis, it should "be left alone." With significant hallux valgus deformity without chondrolysis (Fig. 19-55), he recommended a routine hallux valgus repair, and with significant dysfunction, he recommended an arthrodesis or implant. Graham,[198] however, in a long-term report on his practice experience, recommended that with even minimal involvement of the first MTP joint, an arthrodesis was warranted in combination with a forefoot arthroplasty. He suggested that valgus angulation of the first MTP joint in time would likely necessitate forefoot realignment. Thordarson[554] reported a high failure rate after first MTP joint preservation techniques in patients with rheumatoid arthritis and concluded an arthrodesis was preferable, even with minor deformity.

Joint-Preserving Forefoot Surgery

With the advent of biologic response modifiers (BRMs), many investigators suspect that joint-preserving forefoot procedures in the rheumatoid arthritis patient may have good, if not excellent, long-term results.

Some authors have advocated such joint-sparing procedures before widespread use of BRMs. Hanyu et al[220] reported 83% satisfactory results in 75 feet (47 patients), with a mean of 6 years of follow-up using either the Mitchell osteotomy (23 feet) or first MTP joint Silastic arthroplasty (52 feet) combined with lesser metatarsal shortening oblique osteotomies. Although the authors reported that more than half of the feet appeared to look normal postoperatively, recurrent hallux valgus was observed in 15% of cases, lesser MTP joint subluxation was noted in 21%, recurrent hammer toes in 13%, and recurrent callosities in 12%. Shi et al[511] found that 17 of 21 feet with rheumatoid arthritis had great or moderate pain relief after a Lapidus procedure but found statistically significant recurrent hallux valgus (mean of 20 degrees) at a follow-up of almost 4 years. The most reliable results for reconstructive rheumatoid forefoot surgery were reported by Coughlin[104] in terms of pain relief, use of regular footwear, subjective patient satisfaction, and minimal complications.

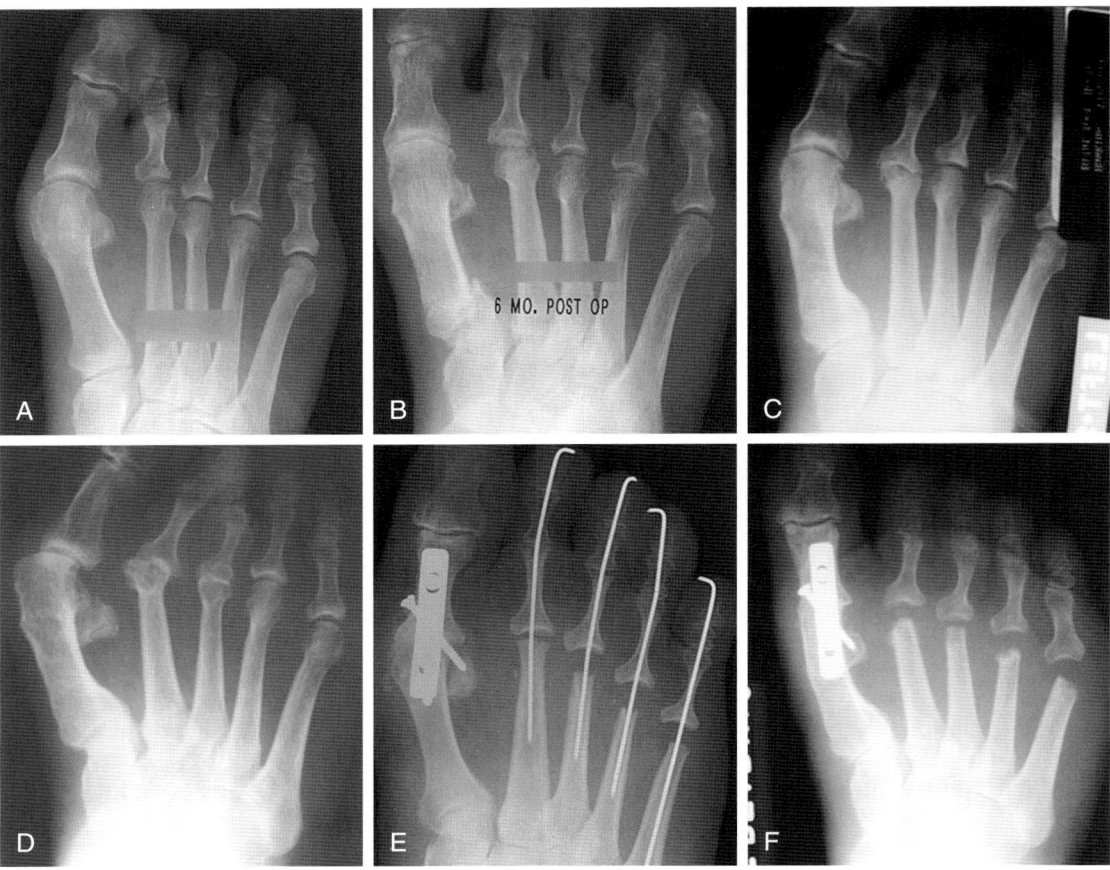

Figure 19-55 **A,** Hallux valgus deformity in a patient with mild rheumatoid arthritis. **B,** After distal soft tissue repair with a proximal first metatarsal osteotomy, realignment is achieved. **C,** Three years after surgery, mild subluxation of the first metatarsophalangeal (MTP) joint has developed. **D,** Nine years postoperatively, there is a severe recurrence of the hallux valgus deformity with dislocation of the second and third MTP joints. **E,** After MTP fusion and forefoot arthroplasty. **F,** One year postoperatively, adequate realignment is maintained.

Since the introduction of widespread BRM use, many more authors have advocated joint-preserving forefoot procedures for rheumatoid arthritis patients. Barouk and Barouk[18] and others[34,464] advocated hallux valgus correction using a SCARF osteotomy along with Weil osteotomies of the lesser metatarsals in patients with rheumatoid arthritis. Although first MTP arthrodesis could not be avoided in all patients, good results were achieved in many patients at final follow-up, although some recurrence of deformity was noted.

Bolland et al[50] performed a variation of this procedure by combining first MTP joint arthrodesis and lesser metatarsal Weil osteotomies. At a 26-month follow-up, the authors noted 88% excellent or good results, with 74% improvement in function and 70% improvement in footwear. However, they also noted a 12% recurrence rate of metatarsalgia or callosities under the lesser metatarsal heads.

Jeffries et al[258] reported their technique of pan-metatarsophalangeal joint arthrodesis. They suggest that this procedure may serve as a long-lasting deformity

correction alternative to more traditional rheumatoid forefoot procedures. However, the authors have yet to report the clinical results of this procedure.

Reize et al[459] reported their results after perfoming first through fifth metatarsal head resections. The authors reported a 30.4% attrition rate at a mean follow-up of 5.3 years. Of the patients available for follow-up, only 33% were painfree, and most (78%) had some reservations about the procedure.

Rosenbaum et al[478] compared first MTP arthrodesis and lesser metatarsal head resection with first through fifth metatarsal head resection. They concluded that arthrodesis patients had better functional results, although the resection arthroplasty patients were subjectively more satisfied. However, the arthrodesis patients were younger and more active and may have had higher expectations than the older, more sedentary resection arthroplasty group.

In a prospective randomized study, Grondal et al[205] also compared resection arthroplasty of all MTP joints versus first MTP joint arthrodesis with lesser MTP joint

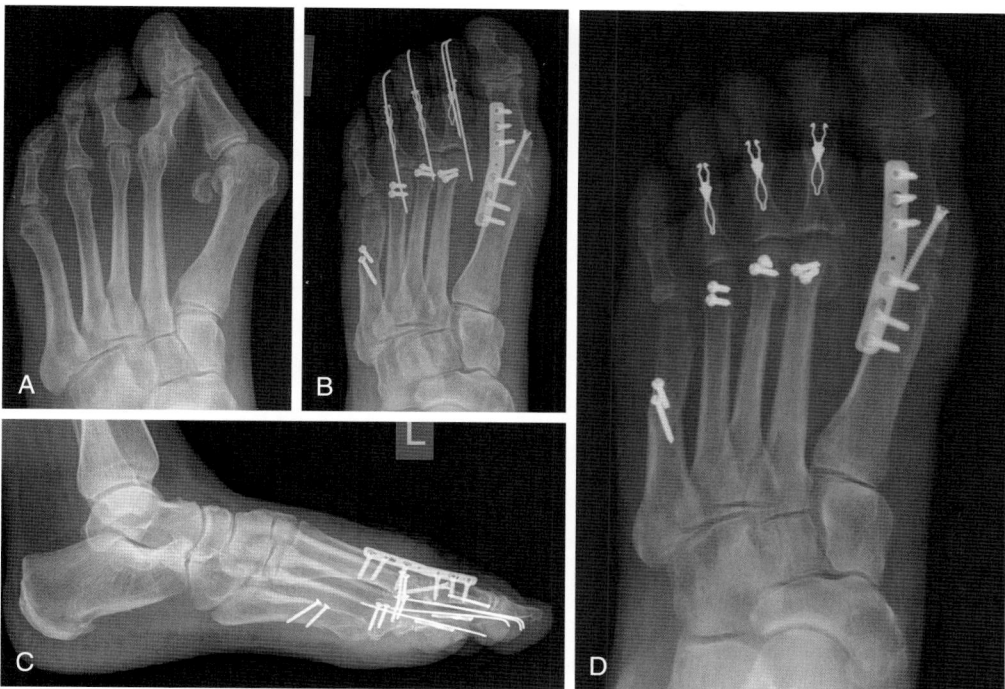

Figure 19-56 **A,** Preoperative anteroposterior radiograph showing severe hallux valgus deformity and subluxation of second metatarsophalangeal joint, and multiple hammer toe deformities. **B,** After multiple Weil osteotomies and hammer toe repairs. **C,** Postoperative lateral radiograph. **D,** After K-wire removal.

resection arthroplasty. They reported no significant differences in subjective satisfaction, activity level, or willingness to have the same procedure again. Hulse and Thomas[243] reported their results of first MTP joint preservation and lesser MTP joint resection arthroplasty compared with pan-metatarsal head resection. In those cases where the first MTP joint was initially spared because of apparent lack of disease, 44% went on to subsequent resection of the first MTP joint because of pain and deformity. Hulse and Thomas recommended a low threshold for panmetatarsal head resection in patients with rheumatoid arthritis.

Krause et al[308] compared first MTP joint arthrodesis and lesser MTP joint arthrolysis with lesser MTP joint excision and noted no significant differences between the groups in terms of subjective rating and functional capacity. They concluded that arthrolysis and preservation of the lesser MTP joints is a good alternative to traditional lesser MTP joint resection arthroplasty in mild-to-moderate cases. Nagashima et al[406] also reported that joint-sparing procedures of the hallux and lesser MTP joints may be successful. They noted pain reduction and satisfaction in 78% of their patients.

The current authors have likewise noted good results with joint-preservation techniques in patients with well-controlled rheumatoid arthritis. These patients are generally treated with BRM and/or DMARD therapy under close supervision of an experienced rheumatologist. In this population, the authors recommend

arthrodesis of the first MTP joint and preservation of the lesser MTP joints with a Weil osteotomy (Fig. 19-56).

Surgery of any type, however, should be reserved for patients with severe pain and disability because the many of these procedures are considered salvage operations, and the lesser toes postoperatively may have little active function. Surgery often does not restore functional capacity to the foot but does improve ambulatory capacity and achieves pain relief, improves cosmesis, and in general gives gratifying results.

FIRST METATARSOPHALANGEAL JOINT ARTHRODESIS

Arthrodesis of the first MTP joint provides stability to the joint and achieves permanent correction of a hallux valgus deformity. It often permits the use of ordinary footwear and, in combination with excisional arthroplasty of the lesser MTP joints, helps to achieve lasting relief of disabling pain. Arthrodesis of the first MTP joint in rheumatoid arthritis provides stability to the first ray, and the rigidity minimizes stress to the lesser MTP joints, protecting these joints from a dorsiflexion force.[359] It protects the location of the repositioned plantar fat pad beneath the lesser metatarsals and often results in a painless foot with little likelihood that further surgical intervention will be necessary. For these reasons and those mentioned previously, arthrodesis of the first MTP joint in rheumatoid arthritis is the treatment of choice for the first ray in reconstructing the rheumatoid forefoot.

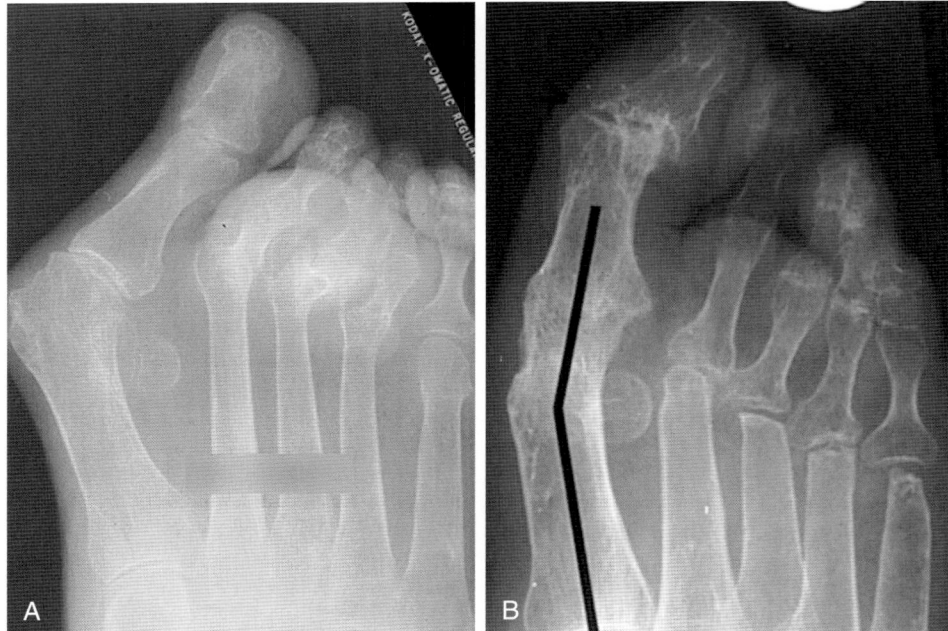

Figure 19-57 **A,** Severe hallux valgus deformity with subluxation of second, third, and fourth metatarsophalangeal joints. **B,** After arthrodesis in a relatively straight position, there is marked interphalangeal joint arthritis of the hallux 2 years after surgery.

Arthrodesis of the first MTP joint was first described by Clutton[93] in 1892. Numerous surgical techniques have been proposed describing various approaches, techniques of joint preparation, and methods of internal fixation to improve alignment capability and the success rate of fusion. First MTP arthrodesis has been recommended as a means to salvage various great toe deformities, including hallux valgus associated with rheumatoid arthritis, hallux rigidus, and severe hallux valgus, as well as recurrent hallux valgus,[184,355,562] neuromuscular instability,[184,355,356,552,562] and traumatic arthritis.[262]

The alignment of the hallux postoperatively plays a significant role in patient satisfaction. Reporting on his long-term experience with MTP arthrodesis and the relationship of first-ray alignment to later interphalangeal arthritis, Fitzgerald[160] noted a correlation between degenerative IP joint arthritis and the magnitude of MTP joint valgus. He suggested that arthrodesis in less than 20 degrees of valgus (Fig. 19-57) tripled the incidence of IP joint arthritis. Thus the magnitude of varus/valgus alignment of the arthrodesis site has been a subject of controversy. Recommendations for valgus alignment vary from 15 to 30 degrees, with 15 degrees most commonly recommended (Fig. 19-58A). If the MTP joint is fixed in a straight position (minimal valgus or a slight varus), the medial border of the hallux can impact against the medial border of the toe box, causing discomfort. In time, degenerative arthritis of the IP joint can develop.

Although Coughlin[104] could not substantiate Fitzgerald's finding of an increased incidence of IP joint arthritis

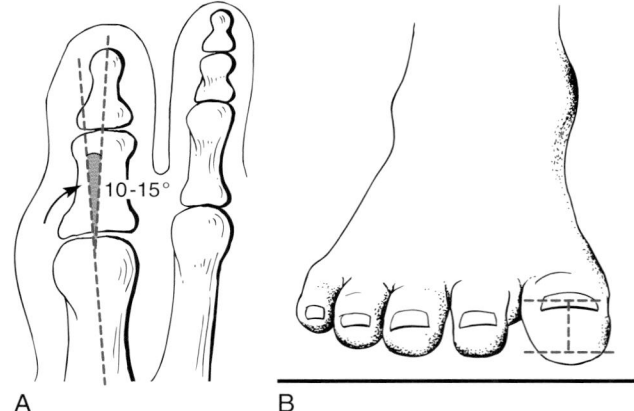

Figure 19-58 **A,** Metatarsophalangeal fusion in 15 degrees achieves acceptable alignment of the first ray. **B,** Excessive pronation or medial rotation of the hallux can lead to pressure along the medial border. Rotational malalignment should be avoided.

with decreased valgus angulation, he did observe that MTP joint dorsiflexion of less than 20 degrees was associated with IP joint degeneration in patients with rheumatoid arthritis. He recommended an MTP fusion angle between 21 and 25 degrees with respect to the metatarsal shaft.[104] Although increased valgus and dorsiflexion angles may decrease the incidence of postoperative IP joint arthritis,[104,160] first MTP arthrodesis itself increases

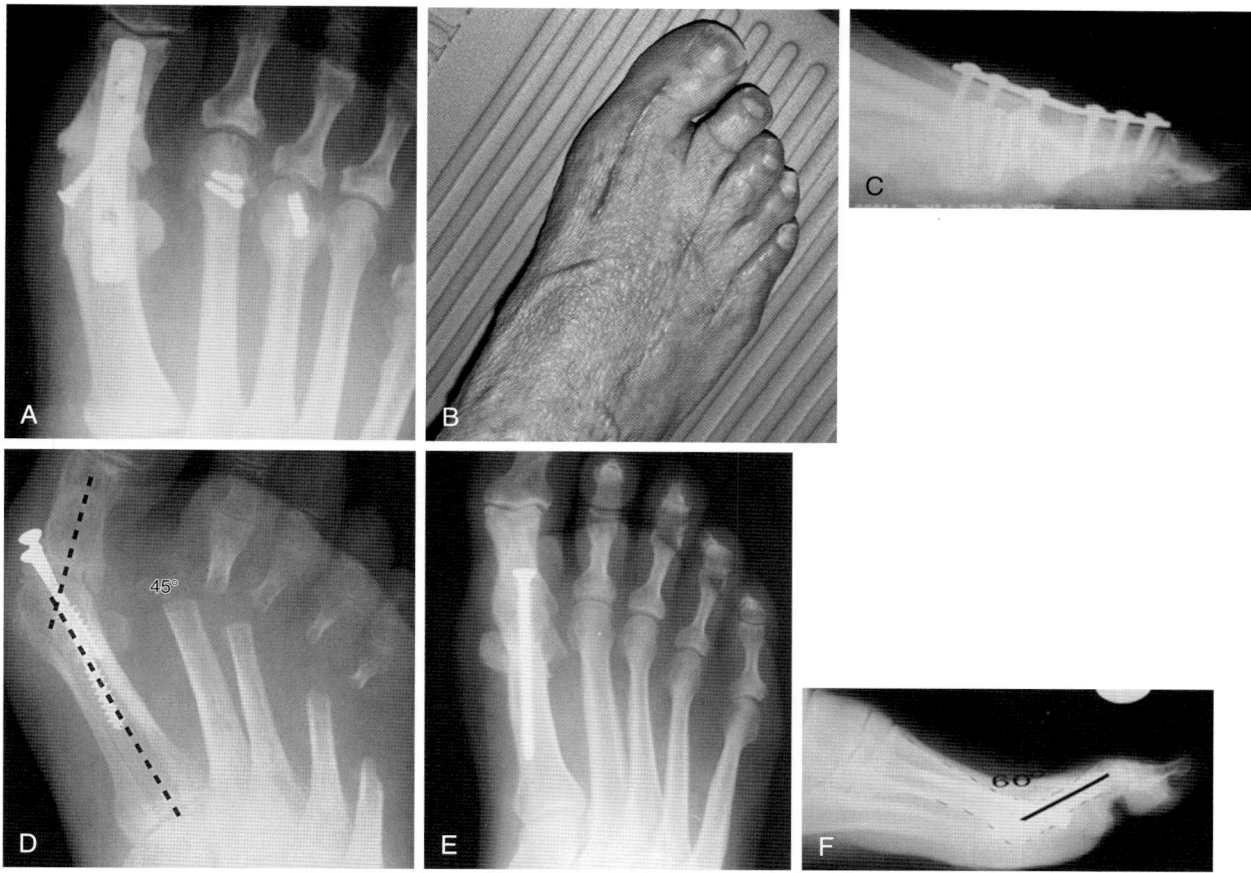

Figure 19-59 **A,** Arthrodesis in 15 to 20 degrees of valgus. **B,** Clinical appearance. **C,** Lateral radiograph. Angle of dorsiflexion may be confusing. Dorsal surface of first ray (by measurement of plate) demonstrates 10 degrees of dorsiflexion, but the axial measurement of metatarsophalangeal axis is 20 degrees. **D,** Arthrodesis in excessive valgus (hallux valgus angle 45 degrees) leaves subtotal correction of deformity. Anteroposterior **(E)** and lateral **(F)** radiographs demonstrate plantar compression-screw technique. Excess dorsiflexion (60 degrees) led to pain beneath the first metatarsal head.

stress at the IP joint. Progressive IP joint arthritis can develop over time after MTP fusion, even with significant valgus at the MTP joint, although it is rarely symptomatic.[104,359] Thus the authors recommend arthrodesis in 10 to 15 degrees of valgus (Fig. 19-59A) because it achieves a more acceptable alignment of the first ray in relationship to the lesser metatarsals. Excessive valgus at the fusion site leaves a widened forefoot and a less desirable cosmetic appearance (see Fig. 19-59B).

Recommendations for dorsiflexion (in relationship with the ground) vary from 10 to 30 degrees, with an average recommendation of slightly more than 20 degrees with respect to the metatarsal shaft axis (Fig. 19-59C). For women preferring high-heeled shoes, increased dorsiflexion at the fusion site may be desirable. Dorsiflexion of less than 10 degrees can cause a complaint of pressure at the tip of the toe,[104,398] whereas dorsiflexion greater than 40 degrees can lead to increased pressure beneath the first metatarsal head (Fig. 19-59D-F).[22]

Recommendations in the literature vary depending on the reference of measurement of dorsiflexion (first metatarsal axis, proximal phalangeal axis, plantar aspect of the foot). The plantar inclination of the first metatarsal averages 15 degrees, and with dorsiflexion of the phalanx 5 to 15 degrees, which translates into 20 to 30 degrees of angulation at the arthrodesis site.

Rotation of the hallux is important, and the toe should be placed in a neutral position.[224,335] Excessive pronation or medial rotation can lead to pressure on the medial border of the toenail, causing infection (see Fig. 19-58B).[398]

McKeever[371] and others[107,455,463] have reported that an increased angle between the first and second metatarsals (1–2 intermetatarsal angle) is not a contraindication for MTP fusion. Harrison and Harvey[224] and others[101,106,107] have reported a significant reduction in the 1–2 intermetatarsal angle after arthrodesis. Mann and Katcherian[355] and Humbert et al[245] reported an average decrease of approximately 6 degrees in the 1–2 intermetatarsal angle after arthrodesis. Coughlin[104] found a mean reduction of 3 degrees after first MTP joint arthrodesis in patients with rheumatoid arthritis. Thus a first metatarsal osteotomy is rarely, if ever, indicated in combination with first MTP arthrodesis (Fig. 19-60A-C).

Many patients express concern about their gait after MTP arthrodesis. Mann and Oates,[356] Fitzgerald,[160] and Coughlin and Grebing[107] have reported an excellent gait pattern postoperatively. Mann and Oates[356] concluded that the "foot lifts off slightly early" after an arthrodesis because dorsiflexion of the MTP joint is limited. If a first MTP arthrodesis is fixed in a proper position, Turan and Lindgren[563] stated that a patient has a "nearly normal gait." Gait analysis before and after first MTP joint arthrodesis has demonstrated restoration of the weight-bearing function of the first ray.[125] DeFrino et al,[125] however, have demonstrated a significantly shorter step length and slight loss of ankle plantar flexion at toe-off after MTP joint fusion.

The success rate of MTP arthrodesis varies significantly depending on the preoperative diagnosis, the surgical technique, and the method of internal fixation used.

The use of flat surfaces for MTP arthrodesis has been popularized because of the simplicity of creating horizontal osteotomies of the proximal phalanx and metatarsal articular surfaces (Fig. 19-61). The technique, however, requires exact precision to obtain the desired alignment. If further correction of any one of these alignment variables is necessary, the first ray must be shortened to realign the prepared surfaces. Further attempts to alter any one of these variables may have a simultaneous, undesirable affect on other alignment variables. Curved surfaces enable adjustment of one variable without necessarily altering other alignment variables (Fig. 19-62).

Preparation of first MTP joint surfaces with conical reamers was first proposed by G.K. Rose in 1950.[589] Later, Bingold[46] and Moynihan[398] advocated conical reamers to fashion the first MTP joint in preparation for fusion. Wilson[589] reported the use of a "hole-saw" to shape the metatarsal head to a cylindric shape and then used convex and concave power reamers to prepare the MTP surfaces. Marin[361] developed a handheld convex and concave reamer system. Coughlin[100,101,106] and Jeffery and Freedman[257] also have advocated power reamers.

Depending on the sclerosis of the subchondral bone, shaping of the arthrodesis site by handheld reamers can be relatively difficult.[356,361,589] Complications of the conical arthrodesis technique include loss of fixation,[463] malposition,[78,398,563] first-ray shortening,[398,589] nonunion,[23,80,363,398,563] and excess shortening at the fusion site.[398]

In an attempt to simplify the surgical technique of first MTP arthrodesis, congruous cup-shaped power reamers were designed (Fig. 19-63).[100,101] Power driven to increase torque strength in comparison with handheld reamers, all reamers were cannulated to accept a 0.062-inch K-wire to ensure precise orientation of each instrument. The concave female portion of the reamer shapes the metatarsal surface to a uniform curved hemisphere, and the convex male reamer excavates the proximal phalanx to a concave, congruous surface. The cup-shaped surfaces resect less bone, reducing ultimate first-ray shortening. The cup-shaped surface allows preparation without predetermination of the varus/valgus, rotation, and plantar flexion/dorsiflexion alignment. After joint preparation,

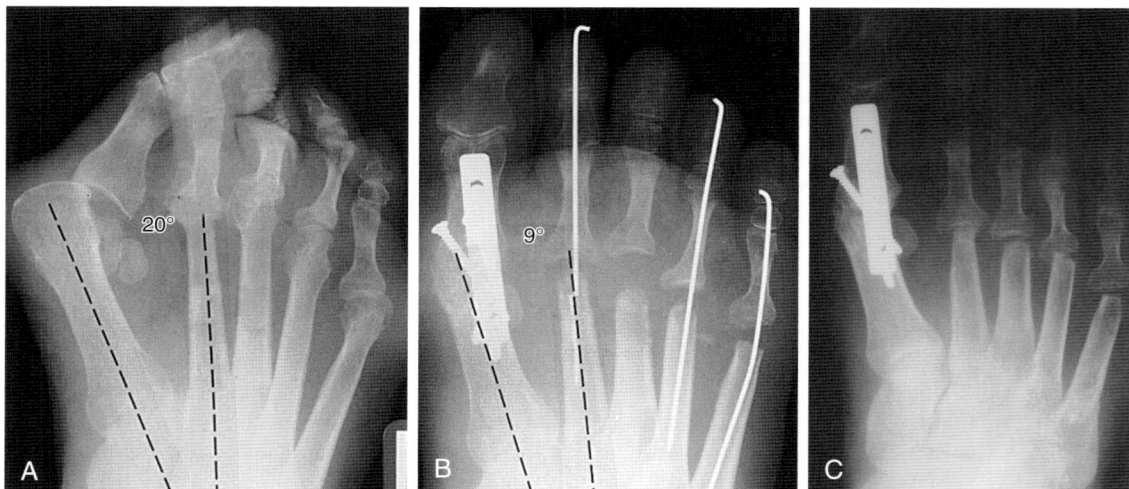

Figure 19-60 **A,** Preoperative radiograph demonstrates severe hallux valgus with dislocation of metatarsophalangeal (MTP) joint and angle of 20 degrees between first and second metatarsals. **B,** After arthrodesis and forefoot arthroplasty, angle between first and second metatarsals is reduced to 9 degrees. **C,** Final radiographs at 1 year after surgery.

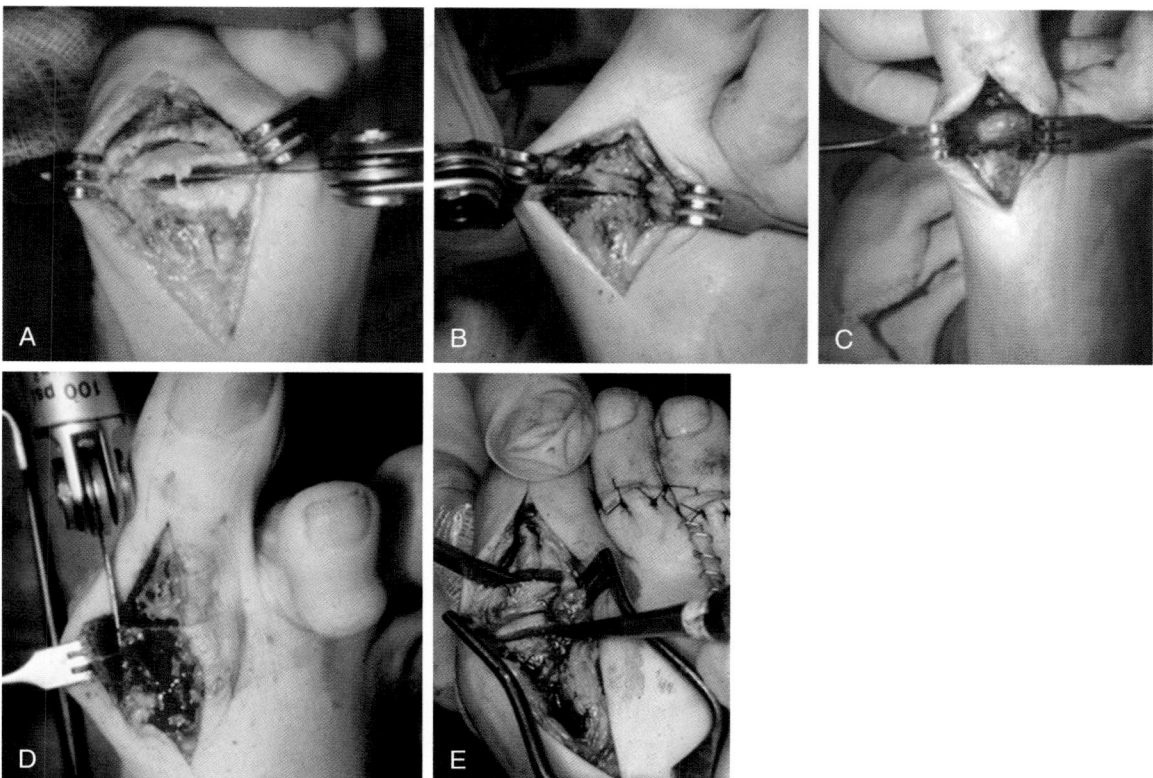

Figure 19-61 **A,** Sagittal saw is used to initially resect the arthritic metatarsal articular surfaces. **B,** Then the phalangeal surface is resected to match the metatarsal surface. **C,** Final appearance of prepared surfaces for arthrodesis. **D,** Resection of medial eminence. **E,** More extensive resection may be necessary to shorten the first ray when a forefoot arthroplasty is performed laterally.

the surgeon can then select the appropriate alignment for arthrodesis.

Various methods of internal fixation have been advocated, including screw fixation (see Fig. 19-62A, B, and E), dorsal plate (see Fig. 19-62F),[101,104,106,107] wire loop,[160,161,588,589] K-wire[160,183,184,517,607] (see Fig. 19-62C and D), cat gut suture,[563] Steinmann pin fixation* (Figs. 19-64D-F and 19-65), staples,[352] and an external fixator.[66,224] A stable construct for internal fixation is necessary. Rongstad et al[476] found that a dorsal mini-plate technique required two and a half times greater force to failure and had three times greater initial stiffness than an oblique cancellous screw. Instron testing of fixation for arthrodesis showed that the most stable construct involved machined conical reaming and a dorsal Vitallium (cobalt, chromium, and molybdenum alloy) mini-plate with an oblique lag screw,[440] which was twice as strong as an oblique lag screw alone.[440]

Curtis et al[119] evaluated crossed K-wires and flat fusion surfaces, flat surfaces with a dorsal plate and screws, flat surfaces with interfragmentary screws, and curved surfaces with lag screw fixation. They showed that the stability achieved with conical reaming "is significantly greater than that with planar joint excision." Although this study demonstrated that a single interfragmentary screw produced more stability than a plate, adding a screw to a dorsal plate further increases stability. The authors concluded that a dorsal Vitallium plate provided significantly greater bending and torsional strength than a stainless steel plate and that a power conical reaming system provided a significant advantage in obtaining fusion of the first MTP joint.[119]

Active infection is an absolute contraindication to MTP joint arthrodesis. Degenerative arthritis of the IP joint is a relative contraindication to first MTP fusion.* Marin[361] stated that at least 45 degrees of interphalangeal joint motion should be present if an MTP fusion is performed. Severe osteoporosis can make it difficult to stabilize a fusion site with routine methods of internal fixation.[100,101]

Surgical Technique

1. A dorsal longitudinal incision is centered over the first MTP joint, extending from just proximal to the interphalangeal joint to a point 3 cm proximal to the MTP joint (Fig. 19-66A and Video Clip 33).

---

*References 22, 33, 46, 262, 361, and 577.

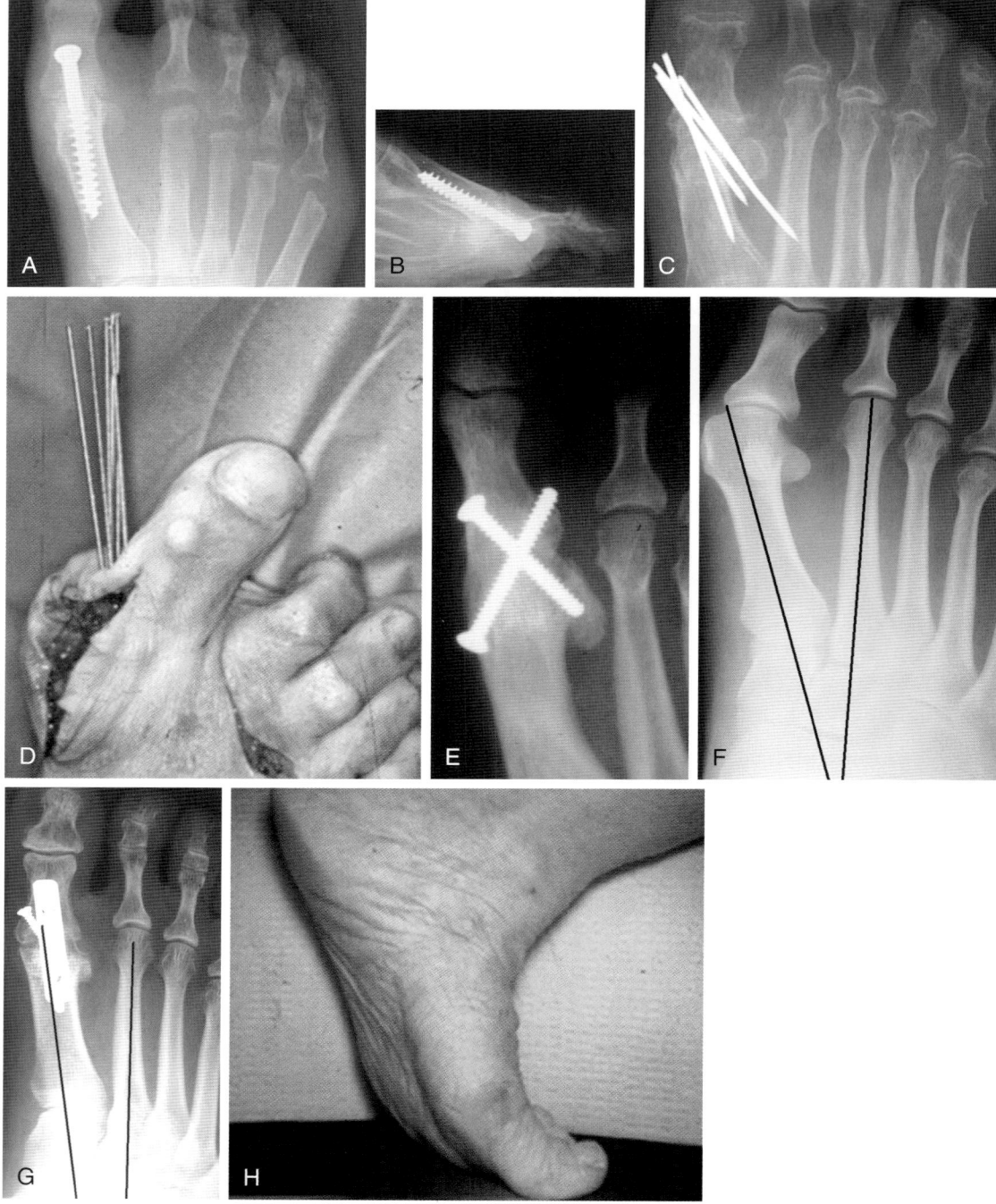

Figure 19-62 Different methods of internal fixation of the arthrodesis site. **A** and **B,** Single-screw fixation radiographs demonstrate compression-screw technique of fixation. **C** and **D,** Multiple K-wire fixation. **E,** Cross-screw fixation. **F,** Preoperative radiograph of painful hallux valgus. **G,** After arthrodesis with prebent titanium plate with cross-screw fixation as well. **H,** Twenty years after MTP joint arthrodesis, the patient is still able to stand on her tip toes. (**A,** Courtesy J. Brodksy, MD, Dallas.)

2. The dissection is deepened to the joint capsule along the medial aspect of the EHL tendon. The extensor tendon may be incised to obtain adequate exposure if necessary and is repaired at the conclusion of the procedure.

3. A sagittal saw is used to remove the medial eminence. A thin wafer of bone is removed from the metatarsal and phalangeal articular surfaces. (When further shortening is desired, more bone may be removed from the metatarsal head.) By decompressing the MTP

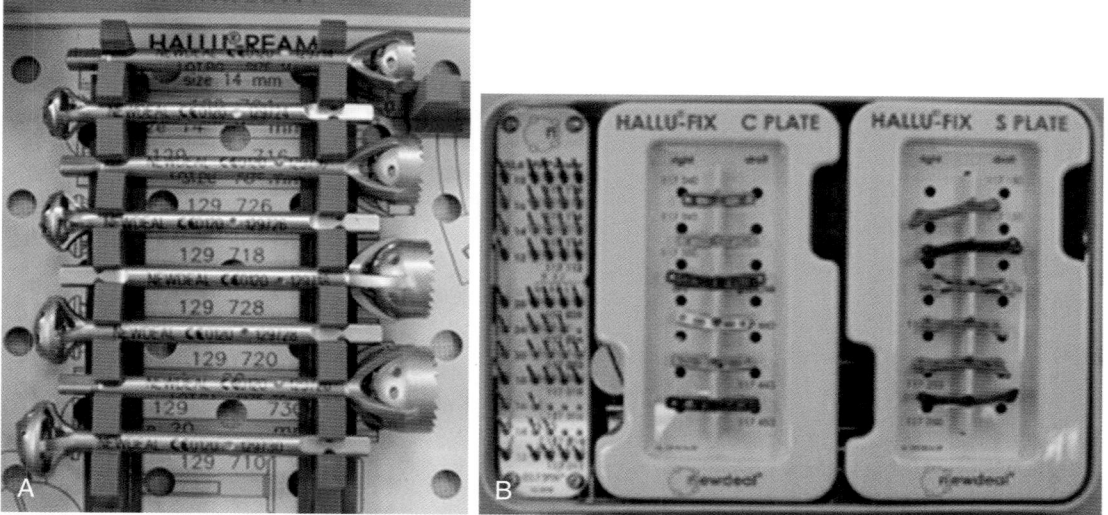

Figure 19-63 **A,** Power reamers are used to shape corresponding phalangeal and metatarsal articular surfaces for fusion. **B,** The complete set includes the reamers, plates (primary and revision), and screws.

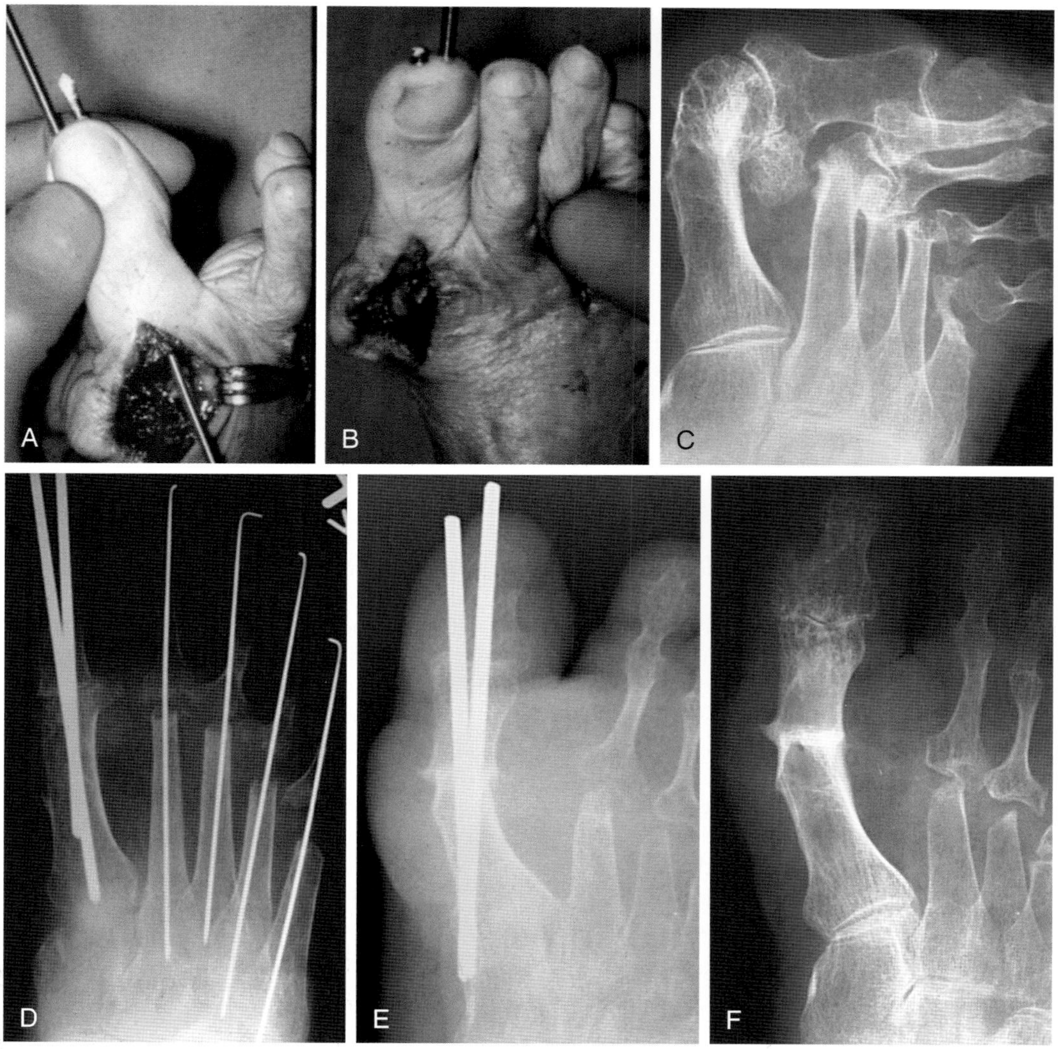

Figure 19-64 **A** and **B,** Stabilization of arthrodesis site with $\frac{1}{8}$-inch double-pointed threaded Steinmann pins. Pins are first drilled out through the tip of the toe and then are drilled back in a retrograde manner proximally across the metatarsophalangeal joint to secure the fixation. Preoperative **(C),** intraoperative **(D),** and postoperative **(E** and **F)** radiographs demonstrate repair of a recurrent rheumatoid foot deformity with severe osteoporosis. Intramedullary Steinmann pins were used for fixation.

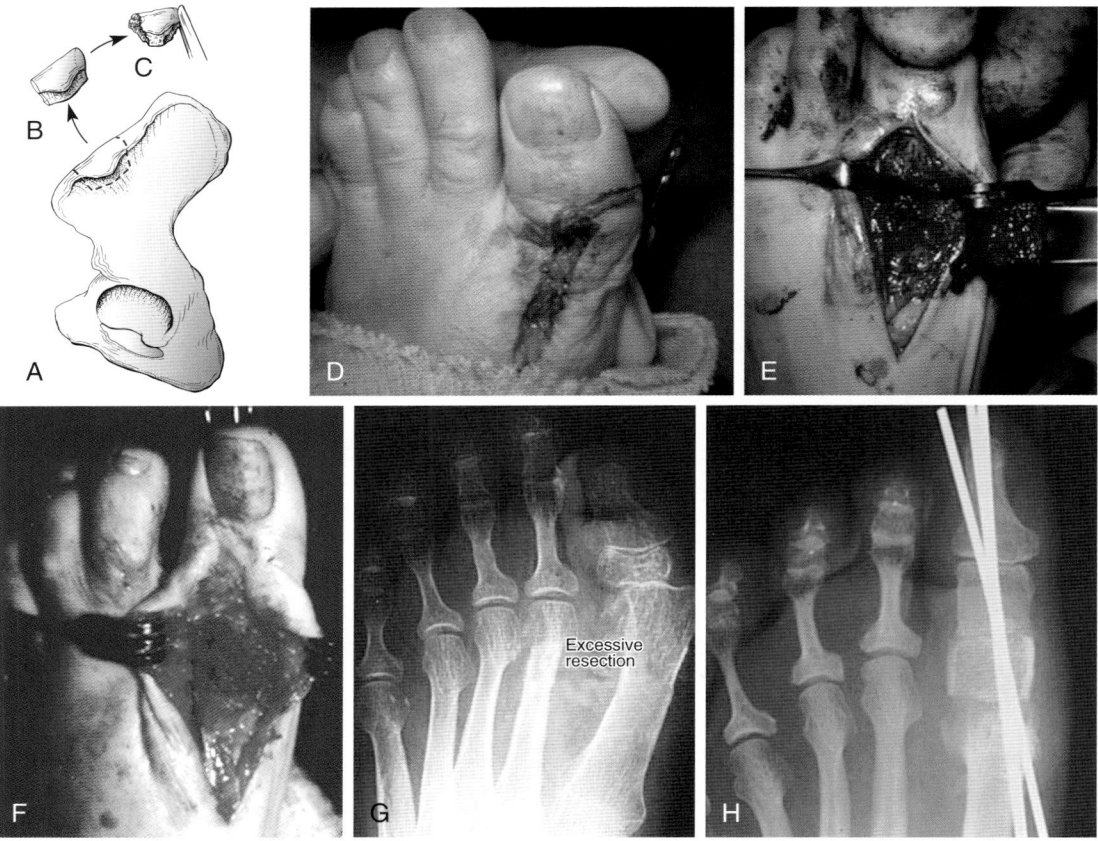

Figure 19-65 **A,** Diagram demonstrates removal of bicortical iliac crest graft. **B** and **C,** Either trapezoidal graft or football-shaped graft is used to span the defect at the metatarsophalangeal (MTP) joint. **D,** Photograph demonstrates marked shortening after debridement of the arthroplasty site. **E,** Intraoperative photograph demonstrates interposition graft before insertion. **F,** Interposition graft after insertion. It has been stabilized with three axial Steinmann pins. **G,** Radiograph demonstrates marked shortening after excisional arthroplasty. **H,** Radiograph of a different patient's foot demonstrates intercalary graft stabilized with threaded Steinmann pins.

joint, exposure is increased for preparation of the MTP joint surfaces.

4. A 0.062-inch K-wire is centered on the distal metatarsal head surface and driven in a proximal direction. A power-driven small joint reamer is then used to prepare the surfaces for arthrodesis (Fig. 19-66B and C).

5. A cannulated metatarsal barrel reamer is used to reduce the metaphysis to a cylinder of constant dimension and to create a convex cup-shaped surface. Alternatively, an osteotome can be used to shave any prominence, and a combination metatarsal barrel and head reamer can be used. Any debris or excess bone along the periphery is removed with a rongeur (Fig. 19-66D-F).

6. A K-wire is centered on the base of the proximal phalanx and driven distally.

7. A cannulated (convex) fluted phalangeal male reamer is used to prepare a concave cup-shaped surface in the proximal phalanx (Fig. 19-66G-I).

8. The K-wire is removed, and the rongeur is used to remove any remaining joint debris. Washed metatarsal reamings of cancellous bone may be used for autograft (see Fig. 19-66E).

9. The congruous cancellous joint surfaces are then coapted in the desired dorsiflexion/plantar flexion, varus/valgus, and rotation. The desired position is 15 to 25 degrees of dorsiflexion (first metatarsalphalangeal axis), 10 to 15 degrees of valgus, and neutral rotation. All angular measurements relate to the axis of the first metatarsal shaft and proximal phalanx. With the cup-shaped surfaces, rotation or any other dimension may be altered without disturbing other alignment variables.

10. After obtaining proper alignment, the fusion site is temporarily stabilized with one or two crossed 0.062-inch K-wires (Fig. 19-66J and K).

11. The fusion site is rigidly fixed with a mini-fragment six-hole plate that is precontoured in both dorsiflexion and valgus (Fig. 19-69L). A primary or revision plate

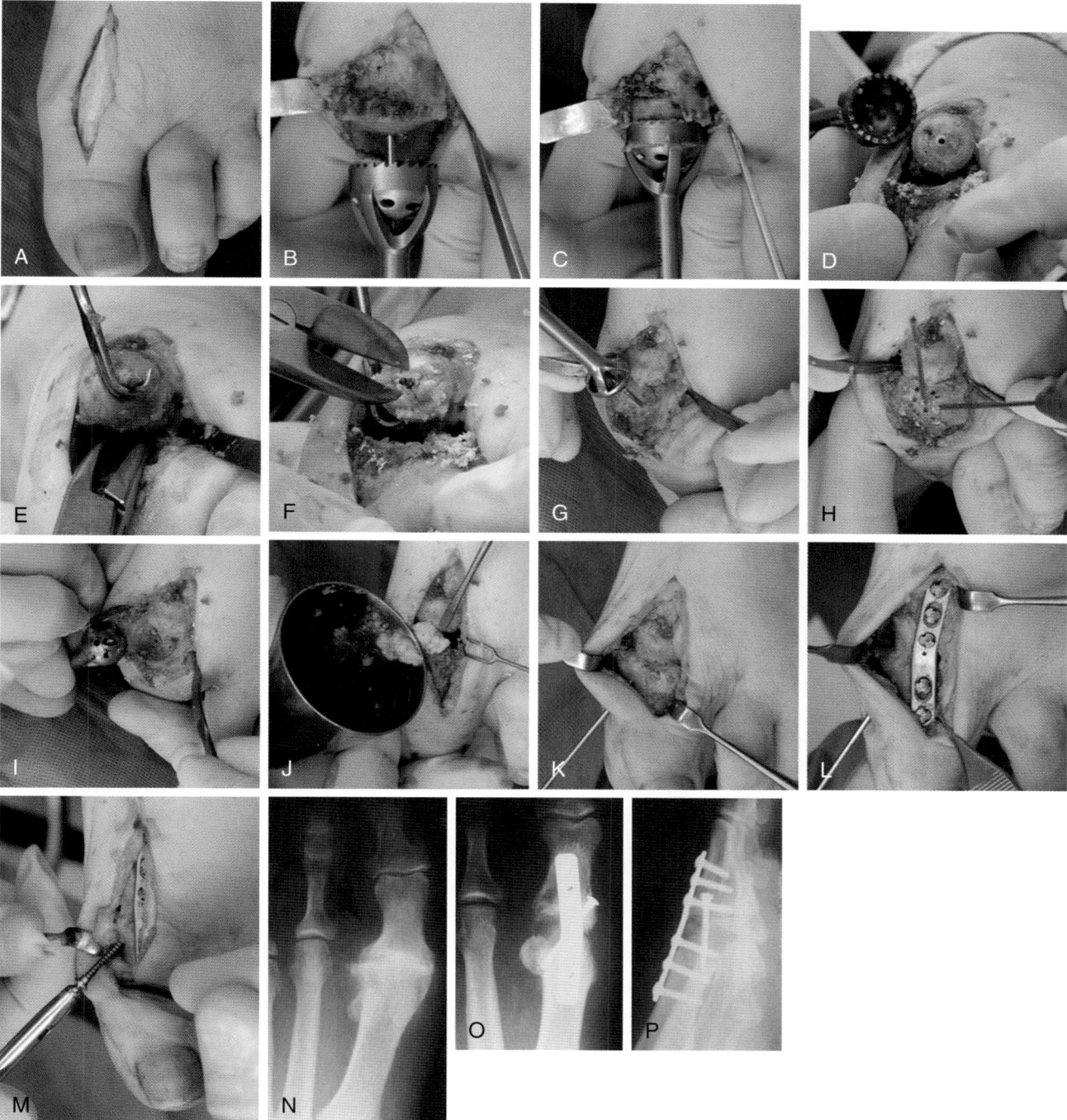

Figure 19-66 Technique of metatarsophalangeal (MTP) joint preparation. **A,** Dorsal longitudinal incision. **B,** K-wire placed in the center of the metatarsal head for control of the power reamer. **C** and **D,** Over the 0.062-inch K-wire, a cannulated reamer is used to shape the metatarsal head to a convex surface at the end of a cylinder of constant dimension. **E,** Remaining debris on the plantar aspect of the first metatarsal head is removed. **F,** When the prepared surface is sclerotic, it may be perforated with multiple drill holes or fish scaled with a bone-cutting forceps. **G,** Placement of the K-wire into the center of the phalangeal articular surface. **H,** Reaming of the phalangeal surface with a cannulated phalangeal reamer is used to create corresponding cup-shaped concave surface. **I,** If the reamed surface is sclerotic, it is perforated with several drill holes. **J,** Rinsed reamings may be used as an autologous bone graft. **K,** The phalanx is temporarily stabilized with a crossed K-wire. **L,** A prebent low-profile compression plate is placed on the dorsal aspect of the MTP joint to stabilize the fusion site. **M,** A cross screw is added for further internal fixation. **N,** Preoperative radiograph demonstrates end-stage MTP joint arthritis. **O** and **P,** Postoperative radiographs demonstrate correct alignment with 15 degrees of valgus and 20 degrees of dorsiflexion.

with more variable fixation holes can be used depending on the bone quality. The plates come prebent to set both the dorsiflexion and valgus angles and are best placed over the dorsal aspect of the prepared MTP joint surfaces. (This contour can of course be altered to a different desired position with plate benders.) Fixation with bicortical self-tapping twist-off screws is used.

12. The K-wires are removed, and a cross-compression screw is placed to augment fixation when a primary plate is used (Fig. 19-66M).

If incised, the EHL tendon is repaired. The capsule and skin are closed in a routine manner (Fig. 19-66N-P).

Postoperative Care

A gauze-and-tape compression dressing is applied at surgery and changed weekly. The patient is allowed to ambulate in a wooden-soled postoperative shoe or short walking boot, with weight initially borne on the heel and lateral aspect of the foot. If the patient is considered unreliable, a below-knee cast is applied. Dressings and casting are discontinued 8 to 12 weeks after surgery with radiographic evidence of a successful arthrodesis.

Alternative Method of Fixation

On occasion, after failure of a resection arthroplasty or with significant osteoporosis, intramedullary fixation might be needed to stabilize an arthrodesis site. Infrequently, an interposition iliac crest graft may be needed to restore length to the first ray, especially for the salvage of a failed excisional or silicone arthroplasty.

1. After the MTP joint surfaces have been prepared, a $\frac{1}{8}$-inch, double-pointed threaded Steinmann pin is centered on the base of the proximal phalanx and is driven distally across the interphalangeal joint, through the distal phalanx, and out through the tip of the toe.
2. Once the pin has been advanced out through the tip of the toe, the drill is attached to the distal end of the pin, and the pin is pulled, under power, farther distally until its tip is flush with the prepared surface of the base of the proximal phalanx. A pin cutter is used to remove 10 cm (4 inches) of the pin's distal aspect so that it will not interfere when the second pin is attached to the drill and pulled distally (Video Clip 35).
3. A second $\frac{1}{8}$-inch, double-pointed threaded Steinmann pin is then centered just to the medial aspect of the first pin and driven in a similar manner across the interphalangeal joint and out the tip of the toe. The drill is then attached to the distal end of the second pin, and this pin is pulled farther distally until its proximal point is flush with the prepared surface of the proximal phalanx (see Fig. 19-64A-C).
4. The toe is now positioned in the desired amount of rotation, valgus, and dorsiflexion.

5. With the prepared surface of the phalanx compressed on the prepared metatarsal surface, the longest pin is driven in a retrograde manner across the MTP joint into the metatarsal shaft. After the pin penetrates the proximal cortex of the first metatarsal, further advancement is not necessary. A pin cutter is then used to sever this pin, leaving approximately $\frac{1}{8}$ inch extending beyond the tip of the toe.
6. The power drill is attached to the distal aspect of the remaining pin. This pin is driven in a retrograde manner and advanced until it penetrates the metatarsal cortex. The remaining pin extending beyond the toe tip is cut, leaving $\frac{1}{8}$ inch protruding for ease in later pin removal (see Fig. 19-64D-F).
7. Routine closure of the joint capsule and skin is performed. Pins are often removed from the patient using local anesthesia in an office setting once radiographic union has been demonstrated, usually at 12 to 16 weeks after surgery.

Alternative Technique with Interpositional Graft

1. A bicortical or tricortical graft is obtained from the iliac crest graft (see Fig. 19-65A). The graft is shaped to fit the desired gap (defect) at the MTP joint (see Fig. 19-65B and C). After debridement of the MTP joint, the interposition graft is shaped and placed in the interval between the prepared surfaces of the proximal phalanx and first metatarsal. Cancellous bone is packed into any bone defects. The bicortical or tricortical graft is trapezoidal (wider plantarward and medially, narrower on the dorsolateral aspect) to allow slight valgus and dorsiflexion alignment of the arthrodesis site (see Fig. 19-65D).
2. Three doubled-pointed, $\frac{5}{64}$-inch threaded Steinmann pins are individually introduced at the MTP joint, centered on the prepared phalangeal articular surface, and driven distally, crossing the interphalangeal joint and exiting at the tip of the toe, using the technique previously described. They are then pulled distally until they are flush with the prepared surface.
3. Using a lamina spreader to distract the prepared surface, the interposition bone graft is keyed into place (see Fig. 19-65E and F).
4. After placement of the intercalary graft, the threaded Steinmann pins are individually driven across the interposed bone graft and into the metatarsal metaphysis. They are advanced in a retrograde manner until they penetrate the proximal metatarsal cortex (see Fig. 19-65G and H).

Each pin is then severed at the tip of the toe, leaving $\frac{1}{8}$ inch extending to aid in later pin removal. The subcutaneous tissue and skin are closed in a routine fashion.

Postoperative Care

A gauze-and-tape compression dressing is applied at surgery and changed weekly. Ambulation is allowed on the heel and lateral aspect of the foot in a wooden-soled postoperative shoe or short walking boot. The pins are left in place until radiographic evidence of successful arthrodesis is demonstrated, usually at a minimum of 16 weeks.

Results and Complications

In series where patients were evaluated for rate of successful postoperative arthrodesis, 1394 of 1536 arthrodeses successfully united for a 91% fusion rate (range, 77%-100%).

Coughlin[104] reported a fusion rate of 100% using power conical reamers and a mini-fragment plate in a series of 32 patients (47 feet) with rheumatoid arthritis who underwent arthrodesis as part of a rheumatoid forefoot reconstruction, with mean follow-up of 74 months. The hallux valgus deformity was corrected to a mean of 20 degrees. Subsequent IP joint arthritis correlated with an MTP dorsiflexion angle of 20 degrees or less.

Mann and Thompson[359] reported on MTP arthrodesis in 18 feet (average follow-up, 4 years). In 12 feet, a total forefoot reconstruction was performed, and in 6 feet, a subtotal forefoot reconstruction was performed. Results were classified as excellent or good in 16 feet; 17 of 18 first MTP joints went on to successful fusion, and the one fibrous ankylosis was not painful. Interphalangeal degenerative arthrosis was noted radiographically but was not found to be clinically significant.

A 92% fusion rate (1074 of 1164 feet) has been reported using conical reamers.*

Coughlin and Abdo[106] reported on 47 patients (58 feet) who underwent first MTP arthrodesis. The diagnosis in 28 cases was rheumatoid arthritis and in 16 was hallux rigidus. A 98% fusion rate was achieved. The average preoperative 1–2 intermetatarsal angle was reduced from 11.9 to 9.5 degrees and the average hallux valgus angle from 35.5 to 17.1 degrees. The average dorsiflexion was 22.6 degrees (measured on a lateral radiograph of the angle subtended by the axis of the first metatarsal and proximal phalanx). Average shortening was 4 mm. Ten patients were noted to have slight progression of interphalangeal joint arthritis, but only one was symptomatic.

Coughlin and Grebing[107] reported a similar high percentage of good and excellent clinical and radiographic results when arthrodesis was used for severe hallux valgus deformity. von Salis-Soglio and Thomas[577] reported on 48 cases with a successful fusion rate of 92%, and Mankey and Mann[349] reported on 51 cases with a similar 92% success rate. Coughlin,[101] using a relatively bulky yet flexible mini-fragment plate, reported on 35 cases with 100% fusion rate.

Chana et al[78] suggested that "subsequent procedures to remove hardware should not be necessary." Indeed, removal of hardware adds a further postoperative expense. Coughlin and Abdo[106] removed only 4 of 58 plates (6%), but Coughlin[101] removed 12 of 35 larger dorsal stainless steel plates (34%). Mankey and Mann[349] reported removal of 8 of 56 dorsal plates (14%).

When MTP fusion is combined with a lateral MTP resection arthroplasty, the first ray is often shortened to achieve an acceptable cosmetic appearance as well as to avoid an excessively long first ray, which can impact against the toe box. The comparative length of the first and second ray rarely has been analyzed after MTP arthrodesis. Mann and Oates[356] reported that three of 41 patients thought their hallux was "too short" after MTP fusion. Coughlin reported 3-mm average shortening in one series[101] and 4 mm in another series.[106]

Complications after arthrodesis are uncommon and include nonunion[245,563] and malunion.[160,161,245,563,607] Nonunion[563] can occur because of the small contact area at the fusion site (Fig. 19-67). Unsuccessful arthrodesis does not necessarily lead to painful pseudoarthrosis,[22] and McKeever[371] and others[22,78,184,245,361] have stated that a nonunion can still lead to an acceptable result. If a nonunion occurs, significant shortening can lead to metatarsalgia.[398] Results tend to vary depending on the selected method of internal fixation and the specific technique. However, an average 10% failure rate has been noted in the literature.[101] The highest rate of nonunion (23%) was reported by Gimple et al,[183] who used crossed K-wires for internal fixation. Marin[361] and Turan and Lindgren[563] observed that inadequate internal fixation was the most common cause of nonunion (Fig. 19-68).

Failure of internal fixation has been reported as well. Mankey and Mann[349] reported an 8% failure rate (4 of 51 cases) with a stainless steel plate. With a Vitallium plate and an absence of screw holes at the fusion site, Coughlin and Abdo[106] reported a 2% failure rate (1 of 58).

Malunion in any plane is poorly tolerated and underscores the need for meticulous attention to the final position of arthrodesis. Malunion can occur in any of three

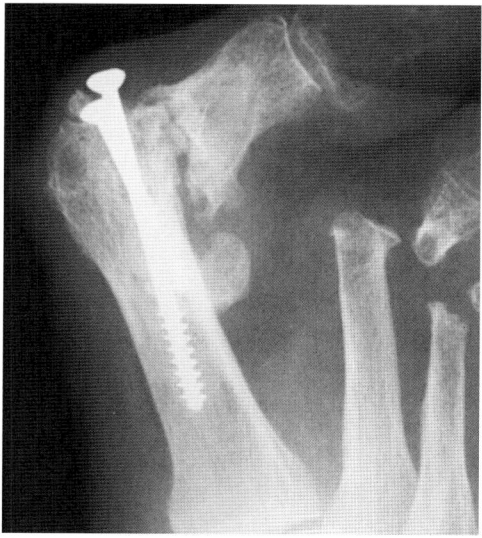

Figure 19-67 Radiograph demonstrates nonunion after compression screw fixation of arthrodesis site.

---

*References 100, 101, 104, 106, 107, 111, 112, 349, and 351.

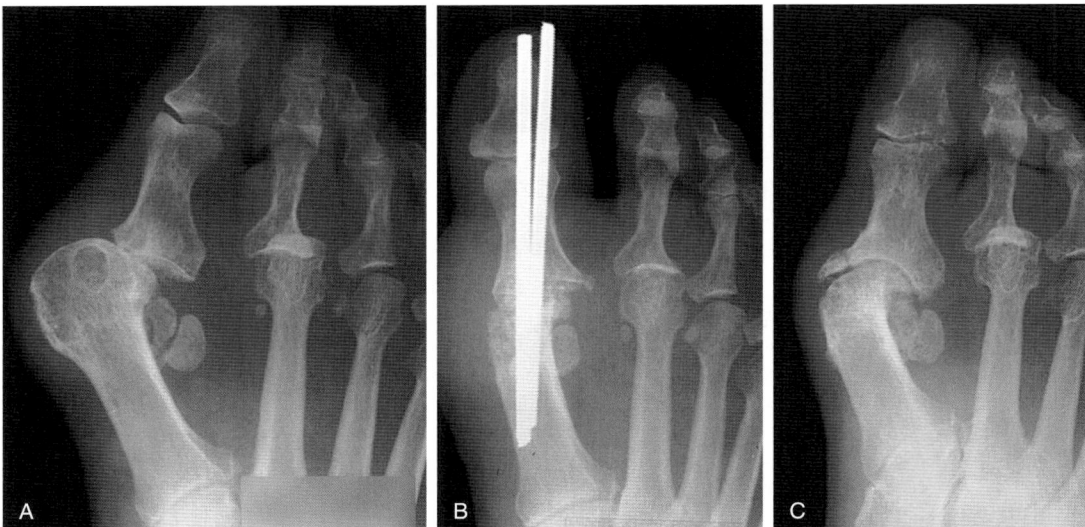

Figure 19-68 A, Radiograph demonstrates severe subluxation of the first metatarsophalangeal (MTP) joint in a steroid-dependent patient with rheumatoid arthritis. **B,** After arthrodesis with intramedullary Steinmann pin fixation. **C,** Seven years after surgery, nonunion has developed. Despite this, the patient was pleased with correction of her deformity and reported no pain.

planes: varus/valgus, dorsiflexion/plantar flexion, or rotation.

Interphalangeal joint arthritis after first MTP fusion has been reported to vary from 6% to 60% (Fig. 19-69). Coughlin and Abdo[106] reported a 10% incidence of progressive arthritis, but only 2% of cases were symptomatic. Chana et al[78] reported a 21% incidence of interphalangeal arthritis at 10-year follow-up in all joints fused in less than 20 degrees of valgus. Mann and Thompson[359] reported a 65% incidence of arthritis but did not think this was clinically significant. Mann and Schakel[358] noted a 60% incidence, but only one third of cases were symptomatic. In both series, internal fixation (threaded Steinmann pins) crossed the interphalangeal joint, which might have been a factor in the high rates of arthritis.[358,359] Interphalangeal joint hypermobility[563] can develop after fusion with inadequate dorsiflexion at the MTP joint.

Arthrodesis of the first MTP joint creates a stable medial buttress that protects the lesser toes from further deformity (Fig. 19-70A-C). Fusion tends to provide first-ray stability, preserve first-ray length, and maintain strength of the hallux. Often after a fusion, increased weight bearing on the inner aspect of the foot leads to a reduction in lateral metatarsalgia. This is in contradistinction to excisional arthroplasty, where weight bearing of the first ray is decreased and lateral metatarsalgia increased.

Reviewing their experience with the Keller procedure, Rogers and Joplin[473] noted a 63% incidence of metatarsalgia after excisional arthroplasty but only a 9% incidence after first MTP arthrodesis. Henry and Waugh[233] reported significant weight bearing on the first ray in only 40% of cases after excisional arthroplasty but in approximately 80% after MTP arthrodesis. Marin[361] and

others[160,245] reported minimal metatarsalgia after first MTP arthrodesis. Often a patient is able to wear ordinary footwear after arthrodesis.

The technique of first MTP joint arthrodesis should be simple to perform and should achieve predictable postoperative results. The ideal method of arthrodesis should allow easy adjustment of joint surfaces during surgery to vary the final arthrodesis alignment. The shaping of congruous cancellous bone surfaces that can easily be adjusted to the desired position of fusion is important in maintaining position and achieving a high rate of bony union. As McKeever[371] noted, "It is the arthrodesis and its position that [are] important and not the method by which it is produced." The ultimate goal of MTP arthrodesis is correction of a permanent deformity and creation of a stable, comfortable gait pattern that allows the patient to wear ordinary footwear.

UNCOMMON PROBLEMS ASSOCIATED WITH RHEUMATOID ARTHRITIS

Subluxation or Dislocation of a Single Metatarsophalangeal Joint

An isolated dislocation of a lesser MTP joint occurs infrequently with rheumatoid arthritis. If it develops, it typically occurs at the second or third MTP joint. When the condition is present and symptomatic, pain usually develops beneath the metatarsal head where dislocation has occurred. Pain also can occur in the area of a contracted lesser toe with hammer toe or claw toe formation. Initial treatment centers on conservative management, including an extra-depth shoe, soft insole, and metatarsal arch support.

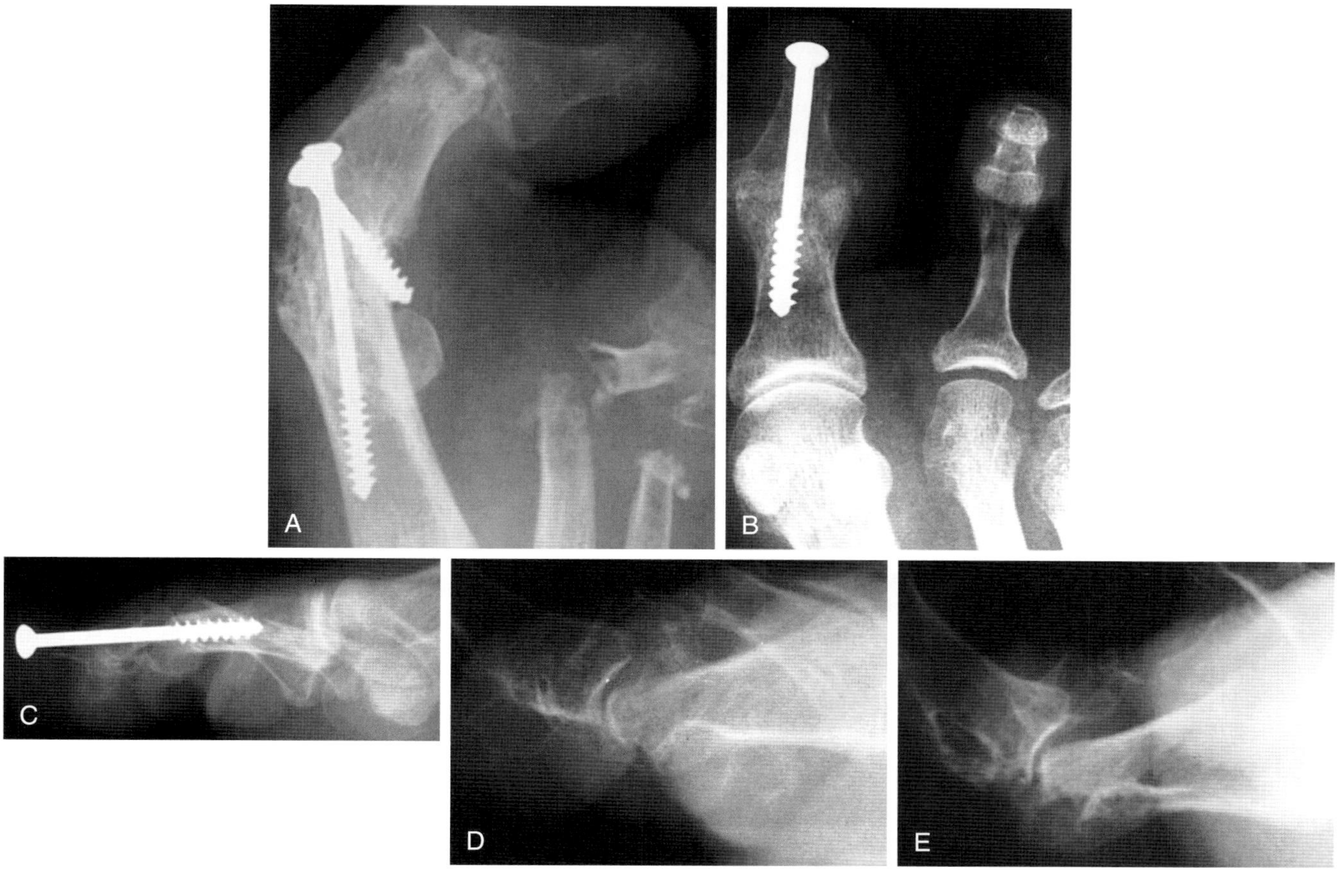

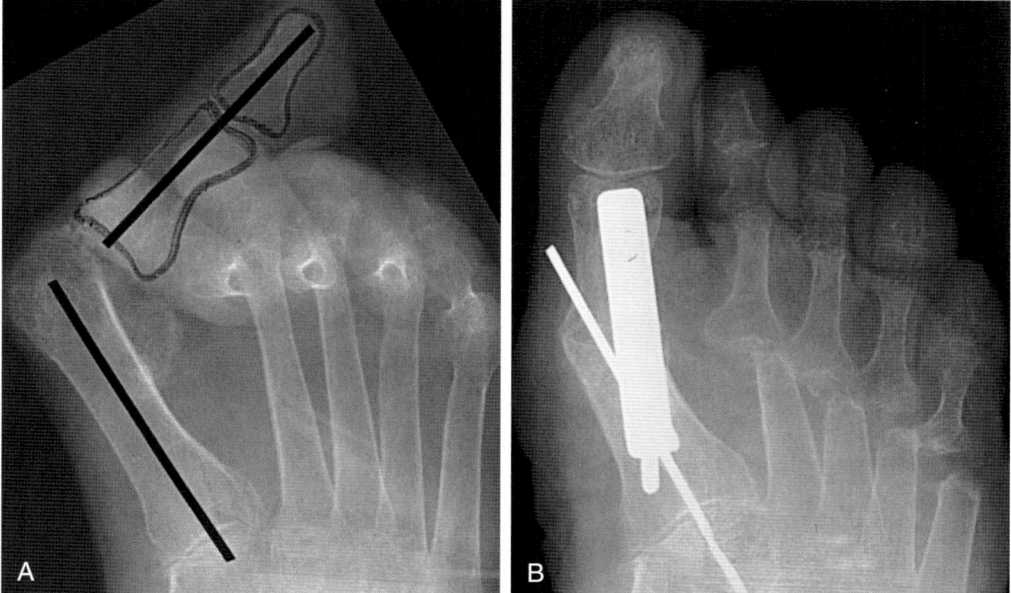

Figure 19-69 **A,** Radiograph showing severe interphalangeal joint arthritis despite first metatarsophalangeal (MTP) fusion. Anteroposterior **(B)** and lateral **(C)** radiographs demonstrating metatarsophalangeal and interphalangeal arthrodesis for arthritis. **D** and **E,** Hyperextension deformity of interphalangeal joint in time develops owing to arthrodesis of the first MTP joint in suboptimal dorsiflexion.

Figure 19-70 **A,** Preoperative radiograph demonstrates severe hallux valgus with dislocation of the metatarsophalangeal joint and angle of 20 degrees between the first and second metatarsals. **B,** After arthrodesis and forefoot arthroplasty, the angle between the first and second metatarsals is reduced to 9 degrees.

When conservative care is unsuccessful, surgical intervention can require a hammer toe repair, synovectomy, and flexor tendon transfer (see earlier discussion) and occasionally a metatarsal head excision. Isolated metatarsal head excision has been discouraged by Rana[449] and others[90,91,397,567] but recommended by Thomas.[551] A physician must explain to the patient that limited forefoot surgery can alleviate symptoms and provide short-term relief of pain, but with time and progression of the rheumatoid arthritis, the other lesser MTP joints can become malaligned. On the other hand, it is difficult for a physician to recommend a complete forefoot reconstruction based on the presence of pain and deformity at a single lesser MTP joint.

Interphalangeal Joint Arthritis of the Hallux

Occasionally, after an arthrodesis of the first MTP joint, degenerative arthritis develops at the interphalangeal joint of the hallux, possibly because of progression of the inflammatory arthritic process. Other causes of interphalangeal joint arthritis include fusion of the first ray in a relatively straight position or lack of dorsiflexion and crossing of the interphalangeal joint with internal fixation (see Fig. 19-69D and E). Valgus deviation at the interphalangeal joint can develop with a rather grotesque appearance of the tip of the toe. Occasionally, ulceration can occur on the plantar-medial aspect of the interphalangeal joint. Hyperextension of the distal phalanx can occur as well, and in these isolated cases, an arthrodesis of the first interphalangeal joint is indicated (Video Clip 63).[513] The great toe is shortened slightly to decompress the joint. Neutral rotation with minimal varus or valgus is achieved when the arthrodesis is performed. Although there may be some concern about the postoperative gait pattern, the patient with long-standing rheumatoid arthritis usually tolerates simultaneous MTP and interphalangeal joint fusion surprisingly well.

Rheumatoid Nodule or Cyst

On occasion, rheumatoid nodules or cysts form on the plantar aspect of the foot, in a weight-bearing area, or over a bony prominence. This makes wearing shoes difficult. A rheumatoid cyst or nodule should be excised, often under local anesthesia. Care should be taken to avoid superficial sensory nerves in the area of the resection.

When a cyst develops in the heel pad region, the heel pad can become unstable. This presents a difficult situation to treat because with aggressive resection there is often inadequate padding between the calcaneus and the plantar skin. Conversely, with an inadequate resection, a patient can continue to have symptoms. Thus the dorsal aspect of the cyst should be excised, leaving a portion of the plantar cyst near or in contact with the plantar skin. The area should be drained to prevent hematoma

formation. It is hoped that adhesions will form between the plantar skin and the undersurface of the calcaneus to achieve a stable plantar fat pad.[266]

Splaying of the Rheumatoid Foot

At times, significant 1–2 and 4–5 intermetatarsal angles develop with a rheumatoid forefoot deformity. The question can arise whether an osteotomy of either the first or the fifth metatarsal should be performed at the time of first MTP joint arthrodesis and lesser metatarsal head resection arthroplasty. In general, the 1–2 intermetatarsal space significantly reduces after a first MTP arthrodesis (see Fig. 19-70A and B). Likewise, the 4–5 intermetatarsal angle often reduces after resection arthroplasty. Thus it is rarely necessary to perform a first or fifth metatarsal osteotomy.

CRYSTAL-INDUCED ARTHROPATHIES

The pathogenesis of crystal deposition disease occurs with the inclusion of crystalline material within the synovium, capsule, ligaments, and osseous tissue, where an inflammatory response occurs. The common causes of crystalline deposition disease in foot and ankle disease are monosodium urate deposition disease (gout) and calcium pyrophosphate dihydrate deposition disease (pseudogout).

Gouty Arthropathy

History and Epidemiology

Gout has been known since early recorded medical history.[320] Rana[449] noted that Hippocrates described gout in the foot as "podagra" (*pous* meaning "foot," *agra* meaning "attack"), and this term is used in much of the early medical literature. Hyperuricemia occurs from an inborn error of metabolism and is the cause of *primary gout*, whereas *secondary gout* occurs as an acquired disorder or after the use of certain pharmacologic agents. A gouty attack is characterized by the precipitation of monosodium urate crystals in the synovial tissue, leading to an acute inflammatory response.

The prevalence of gout in the United States has been estimated to be as high as 6.1 million individuals.[323] The mean age of onset is 40 years and prevalence increases with age.[323,466] Gout is typically 3 to 4 times more common in men than in women, although the incidence in women increases after menopause.[411] Gout also shows a familial trend in 75% of patients.[467]

Consuming a high level of dietary purines (such as meat and seafood), alcohol, soft drinks, and fructose is associated with a higher incidence of gout, while consuming a high level of coffee, dairy products, and vitamin C is associated with a lower incidence. Acute attacks are also associated with diuretic use, hospitalization, surgery, and initiation of urate-lowering therapy.[411]

Pathophysiology

Gout usually develops as an acute episode of monoarticular arthritis. More than two thirds of patients have a second attack within a year.[412] The first MTP joint is the most commonly affected site, being reported in greater than 50% of patients in initial attacks of gout.[318,366,470] On a long-term basis, involvement of the great toe can approach 90%.[52,318] Other lower extremity joints are also commonly affected, including the midfoot (17%), followed by the ankle (14%) and knee (10%).[470]

Gout represents a complication of prolonged hyperuricemia, which can be influenced pharmacologically by decreased renal excretion or increased production of uric acid. The risk of an attack of gouty arthritis increases with higher serum levels of uric acid (greater than 7.0 mg/dL in men and greater than 6.0 mg/dL in women).[207,467] However, hyperuricemia can also be caused by psoriasis,[222] and serum uric acid levels do not always correlate with an acute attack of gout. In fact, silent hyperuricemia is present in 25% to 33% of patients,[466] although persons with uric acid levels greater than 6 mg/dL are at increased risk for gouty attacks. In a supersaturated state, monosodium urate crystals can precipitate. These precipitated crystals deposit in the synovium and capsular tissues, causing acute inflammation and pain. Over time, crystals may also be deposited in the articular cartilage and subchondral bone, presumably causing permanent damage to the joint.

It is useful to separate gout into two clinical phases: an acute phase with intermittent asymptomatic periods and a chronic tophaceous phase.[411] The acute phase of gout is characterized by the rapid onset (often within a 24-hour period) of exquisite pain and tenderness, periarticular swelling and erythema, and increased tissue temperature that mimics cellulitis. Dactylitis, or a sausage-shaped digit, has been reported to occur in patients with gout but can also occur with psoriatic arthritis, reactive arthritis, and undifferentiated spondyloarthropathy. Dactylitis is rare in rheumatoid or osteoarthritic patients unless flexor tendon sheath infection is present[480]; however, cases of concomitant gout and rheumatoid arthritis have been reported.[425] Acute gouty attacks typically resolve over a 7- to 10-day period, after which the patient may be symptom free for months or even years.[411]

If uric acid levels remain uncontrolled, a chronic phase develops. In the chronic phase of gout, urate deposits or gouty tophi develop as a chalky precipitate in the soft tissue (Fig. 19-71).[331] These tophi can produce ulceration and secondary infection and are typically seen only after several attacks.[320] Control of hyperuricemia through strict diet or medications can prevent formation of tophi.

A diagnosis of gout is made by microscopic evaluation of the crystals after an arthrocentesis or debridement of the joint. Monosodium urate crystals are typically needle shaped in appearance and range from 2 to 10 mm in length but can be significantly longer. Under polarized light, the crystals display negative birefringence (a yellowish hue), which is a characteristic finding (Fig. 19-72).

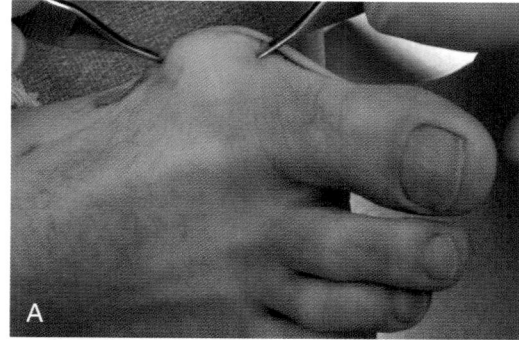
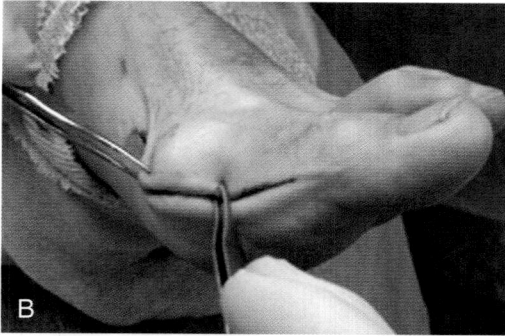
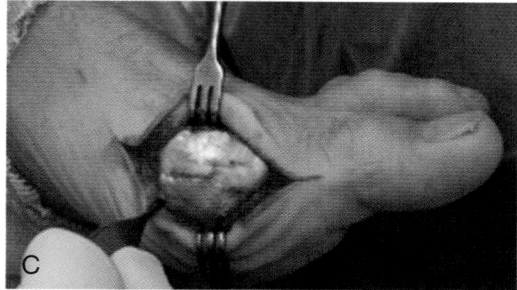

Figure 19-71 Gouty arthritis. **A** and **B,** Marked swelling and enlargement of the first metatarsophalangeal joint. **C,** Surgical debridement of white, chalky deposits.

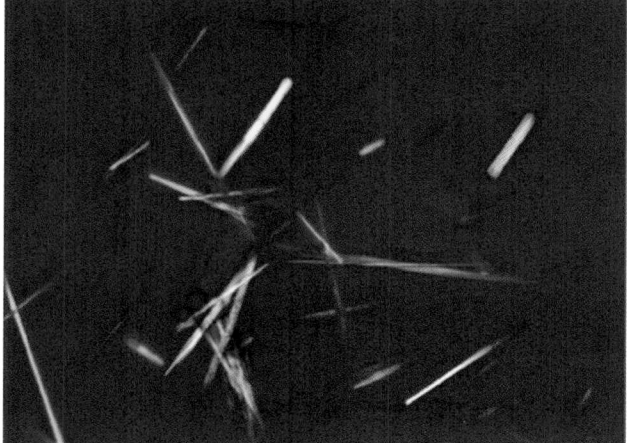

Figure 19-72 Monosodium urate crystals. Compensated polarized light micrograph (×400) depicting needle-shaped crystals with negative birefringence (yellow hue) in a specimen from a patient with gouty tophi (From Robert Terkeltaub: *Gout and other crystal arthropathies*, ed 1, Philadelphia, 2011, Saunders/Elsevier.)

The predilection of gouty attacks for the lower extremity, and specifically, the MTP joint of the hallux, has been explained as being caused by the decreased pH in the foot, decreased urate solubility with the lower temperatures exhibited in the foot, and the first MTP joint being subject to significant stress during normal gait. Landry[318] noted that at 37° C the solubility of uric acid is 6.8 mg/mL and at 30° C, 4.5 mg/mL. With decreased temperatures in peripheral tissues, decreased solubility of uric acid may be characterized by increased precipitation of monosodium urate crystals. Boss[52] noted that the intraarticular temperature of the normal knee joint is 33° C, and the intraarticular temperature of the normal ankle joint is 29° C. The temperature of a peripheral joint such as the MTP joint of the hallux is thus well below 37° C and would therefore be expected to have increased precipitation of urate crystals in relation to other parts of the body.

On radiographic examination, the initial finding merely may be soft tissue swelling. With time, crystalline deposition can cause the development of well-marginated erosions bordered by sclerotic margins at a distance from the joint (Fig. 19-73). As eventual reparative attempts are made by the adjacent bone, an elevated bony margin develops that appears to overhang the tophaceous deposit as though it were displaced by it, forming a characteristic radiographic finding (overhanging edge sign) (Fig. 19-74A).[143,364,535] The articular space is often well maintained. In the subcortical bone, a lacy pattern of bone erosion is pathognomonic of this disease process. Punched-out areas of bony lysis can grow to greater than

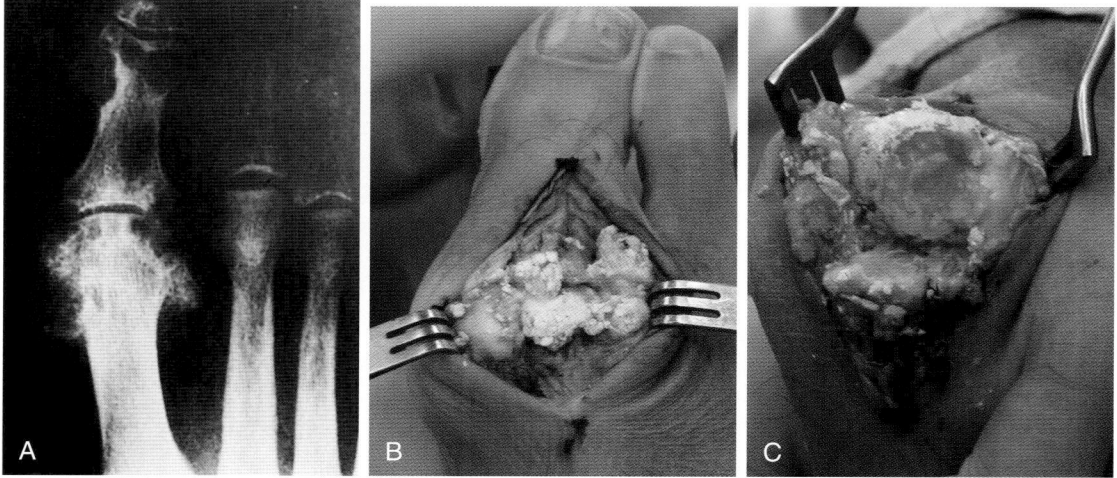

Figure 19-73 **A,** Radiograph of first metatarsophalangeal joint demonstrates periarticular erosion characteristic of gouty arthritis. **B,** Accumulation of crystalline deposits in capsular tissue. **C,** Clinical photograph shows the associated destructive joint changes of gouty arthropathy.

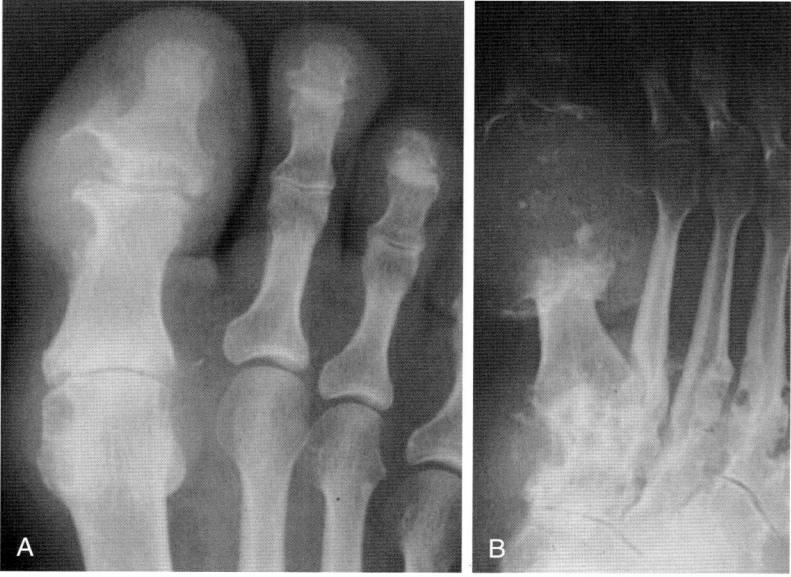

Figure 19-74 **A,** Radiograph demonstrates arthiritis of the interphalangeal joint with overhanging edge sign. **B,** Typical osseous erosion of the first metatarsophalangeal joint associated with chronic gout. (**B,** Courtesy A. Smith, MD, Prince Rupert, Canada.)

5 mm in diameter.[318,366] A distinguishable feature of gouty arthropathy is the presence of erosive lesions somewhat remote from the articular surface. Periarticular erosion just proximal to the MTP joint can occur on both the medial and the lateral aspect of the metatarsal head. Arthritic involvement of the IP joint of the great toe occurs not only in gouty arthropathy but also with psoriasis and reactive arthritis. Radiographic findings can vary from no detectable abnormality to severe destruction of foot joints. Miskew and Goldflies[386] have described avascular necrosis of the talus as a complication of gouty arthropathy.

Treatment

Several new pharmacologic agents have been developed for the treatment of gout in recent years, leading some to believe that a new era of gout treatment is beginning.[63] Pharmacologic treatment of gout should focus on decreasing acute pain and inflammation when an attack occurs, and lowering blood urate levels (by increasing excretion and decreasing formation) to prevent further attacks.

Nonsteroidal antiinflammatory drugs and colchicine are still the first-line pharmacologic agents during an acute gout attack.[411] Neogi[411] recommends naproxen 500 mg twice daily for 5 days or indomethacin 50 mg three times daily for 2 days, then 25 mg three times daily for 3 days. Both of these agents inhibit prostaglandin synthesis and thus reduce pain and inflammation. Boss[52] has recommended indomethacin 25 to 100 mg orally every 4 hours until symptomatic relief is obtained; however, 50 mg every 6 hours with gradual tapering after reduction in inflammation is a reasonable regimen.[471] Increased dosing of NSAIDs carries an increased risk of side effects, and patients must be monitored for gastritis and renal impairment.

Colchicine may be given orally or intravenously. The previously recommended oral dosage was 0.6 mg every hour until the patient experiences relief of pain or develops gastrointestinal side effects, such as nausea or diarrhea.[52,448,471] More recent recommendations suggest giving 1.2 mg orally at the first sign of a gouty flare and 0.6 mg an hour later. This regimen has shown similar pain relief to the older regimen but with fewer gastrointestinal side effects.[411] Side effects from large doses of colchicine have included alopecia, aplastic anemia, and respiratory depression,[52] and long-term effects include peripheral neuropathy. Approximately 25% of the population does not respond to colchicine.[167]

Oral glucocorticoids, such as prednisolone, may be used as a second-line treatment for acute attacks if NSAIDs or colchicine are poorly tolerated or contraindicated. Two recent randomized, double-blind studies have shown that a 5-day course of prednisolone 30 to 35 mg daily was equivalent to either naproxen or indomethacin, respectively.[255,348]

Once the acute gouty attack has subsided, pharmacologic treatment should be focused on lowering blood urate levels to prevent further attacks. Three classes of drugs are currently available for lowering uric acid levels: xanthine oxidase inhibitors, uricosuric agents, and uricase agents. Xanthine oxidase inhibitors block uric acid production and can be used whether or not there is overproduction. The most common of these agents is allopurinol. A daily oral dose of 300 to 800 mg is well tolerated by most patients.[471] Gastrointestinal discomfort occasionally is present, although serious side effects, such as hepatitis, agranulocytosis, and hypersensitivity reactions, are rare.[52] In 2009, Febuxostat was approved by the U.S. Food and Drug Administration (FDA) for the treatment of hyperuricemia. This new xanthine oxidase inhibitor has been shown to lower blood urate levels more effectively than allopurinol. However, patients were more likely to experience acute attacks during the first 8 weeks of urate-lowering therapy.[23] Colchicine is now recommended as an adjunct at a dose of 0.6 mg daily for acute flare prophylaxis during the initial period of uric acid–lowering therapy.[411]

Uricosuric agents (probenecid, sulfinpyrazone, and benzbromarone) block renal tubule urate reabsorption, thereby increasing excretion of uric acid. These drugs can be used in patients with underexcretion of uric acid (approximately 90% of patients with gout)[411] and can increase excretion by approximately 50%.[471] However, they are contraindicated in patients with a history of nephrolithiasis.

Uricase is an enzyme found in other mammalian species that converts uric acid into the much more soluble allantoin, thus lowering uric acid levels in the blood.[63] In 2010, the FDA approved Pegloticase, a modified porcine recombinant uricase, for treatment of chronic gout. In clinical trials, this new treatment rapidly lowered uric acid levels in chronic gout patients, and several patients had remarkable reduction in the size of tophi.[63] Unfortunately, Pegloticase is for refractory cases only because it must be administered intravenously, and infusion reaction rates were high in clinical testing.[411] Other agents that may be approved for use in the near future include a more selective uricosuric agent and a new, selective antiinflammatory medication.[63]

Surgery for chronic gout depends on the specific deformity and the tissues involved. As previously mentioned, the joints of the foot or ankle are the most common locations of chronic gout, and in general, debulking of the tophaceous material by curettage usually decreases symptoms.[320,597] Occasionally, however, gouty tophi can infiltrate tendons of the lower extremity rather than the joints and surrounding synovium. Jerome et al[261] recently reported a ruptured tibialis anterior tendon resulting from gouty infiltration that required primary repair. Similarly, Radice et al[444] described a case of gouty infiltration of the peroneal tendons (Fig. 19-75). Extensive debridement was required with tenodesis of peroneus brevis to the repaired peroneus longus tendon.

In the presence of long-standing gouty tophi, an ulceration or sinus tract may develop that can require debridement. After debridement, application of moist dressings and administration of parenteral antibiotics often results in the rapid resolution of lesions with minimal scarring.

The medical and surgical treatment of chronic tophaceous gout, however, can result in not only the rapid dissolution of tophi but also the destruction of bone because much of the bone matrix is replaced by monosodium urate crystals (see Fig. 19-74B). Significant shortening of the phalanges and metatarsals can occur, but Larmon and Kurtz[320] emphasized that amputation is rarely indicated.

The frequency of surgery for the treatment of chronic tophaceous gout has decreased in recent years because of improved diagnosis and medical management. Occasionally, however, an untreated patient who has had numerous attacks of chronic gout can develop tophaceous gout that requires surgical intervention (Fig. 19-76). Kurtz[315] and Larmon and Kurtz,[320] have described in detail the surgical debridement of tophaceous lesions. Kumar et al reported on their experience of 45 patients who underwent surgery for tophaceous gout. The main indication for surgery was sepsis control or prevention of ulcerated tophaceous gout. Eighty-nine percent of patients were male. Renal impairment was the most common medical problem in 38%, hypertension in 27%, heart disease in 20%, and diabetes in 18%. In the Kumar et al[311] study, 53% of patients experienced delayed wound healing, and 7% required digital amputation.

These complications can potentially be avoided using the technique described by Kemp et al.[285] They reported on the use of a vacuum-assisted wound device after debridement of chronic tophaceous gout in the first MTP joint of a patient. Despite a large skin defect (5 cm × 3 cm), the wound healed in 5 months without subsequent hallux valgus or other joint deformity (Fig. 19-77). This technique may be helpful in patients with poor healing potential and large wounds defects after debridement of tophaceous gout.

Articular degenerative changes that lead to pain, deformity, and decreased function may be treated with either excisional arthroplasty or arthrodesis. The arthrodesis and forefoot reconstructive techniques used are similar to those used for rheumatoid forefoot disease (see earlier discussion). Hindfoot or ankle joint deformities are generally treated with arthrodesis. Morino et al,[396] however, reported on a case of tophaceous gout in the dome of the talus that was treated with curettage and filling using a calcium phosphate paste (Fig. 19-78). Four years after treatment, the patient was painfree and had good range of motion at the ankle joint. Barg et al[17] reported on a series of 16 patients (19 ankles) with gouty ankle arthropathy treated with a three-component total ankle

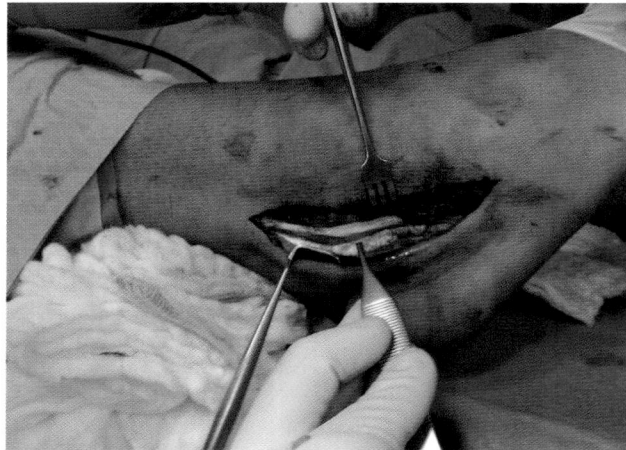

Figure 19-75 Gouty infiltration of tendon. Intraoperative photograph demonstrating gouty tophi within the substance of the peroneal tendons. (From Radice F, Monckeberg JE, Carcuro G: Longitudinal tears of peroneus longus and brevis tendons: a gouty infiltration, *J Foot Ankle Surg* 50:751–753, 2011.)

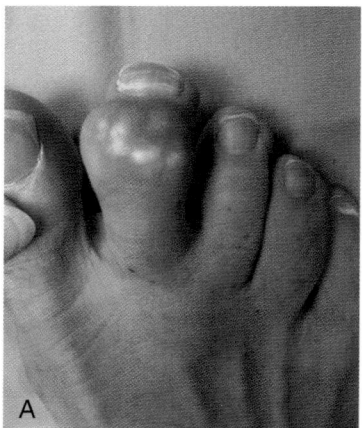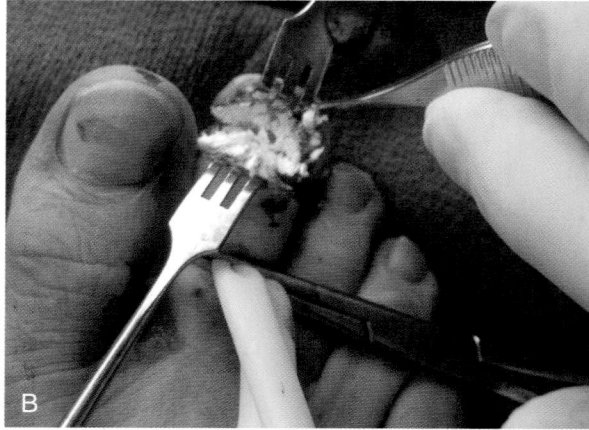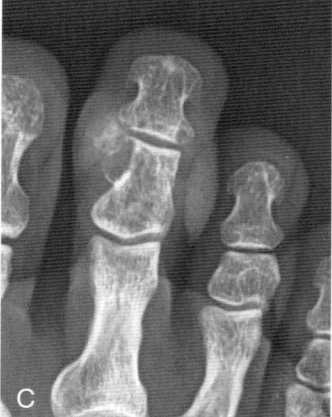

Figure 19-76 Chronic tophaceous gout. **A,** Clinical photograph of patient with long-standing gout in the second toe. Note the areas of whitish discoloration where the tophi are close to eroding through the skin. **B,** Intraoperative photograph demonstrates destruction of distal interphalangeal joint and replacement with large tophi. **C,** Radiograph of the same foot shows erosion of middle phalanx and an overhanging edge sign.

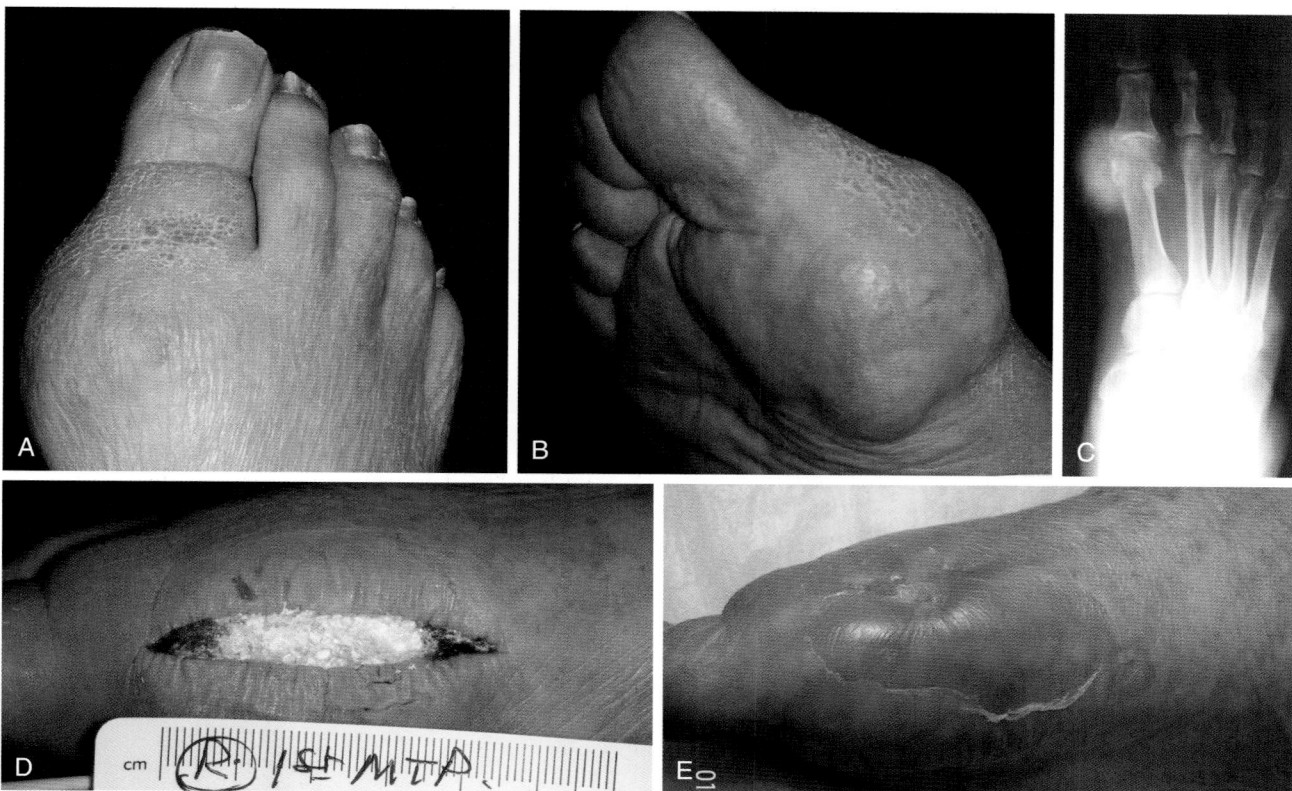

Figure 19-77 Gouty tophus. **A** and **B,** Preoperative clinical photographs demonstrate a large soft tissue mass at first metatarsophalangeal (MTP) joint. **C,** Anteroposterior radiograph of same foot with hazy, radio-dense mass consistent with gouty tophus. **D,** Postdebridement photograph shows tophaceous material recurring under vacuum sponge. **E,** Completely healed at 5 months postoperatively. (All photographs from Kemp TJ, Hirose CB, Coughlin MJ, Otto R: Treatment of chronic tophaceous gout with a wound vacuum-assisted device, *Foot Ankle Int* 31:729–731, 2010.)

arthroplasty. At mean follow-up of 5.1 years, pain and function scores had improved dramatically. One patient required revision of bilateral athroplasties 4.7 years from surgery because of painful loosening, but no other complications were reported. These two procedures represent alternatives to arthrodesis for gout of the hindfoot and ankle.

Calcium Pyrophosphate Dihydrate Deposition Disease (Pseudogout)

Incidence
Calcium pyrophosphate dihydrate (CPPD) deposition disease is also known as *chondrocalcinosis* or *pseudogout.* The incidence of pseudogout is about half the incidence of gout in the United States.[40] It occurs most often between the sixth and eighth decades of life. A familial form of pseudogout manifests at a slightly younger age.[40] Two gene locations (*CCAL1* on chromosome 8 and *CCAL2* on chromosome 5) have been identified as mutation sites that lead to familial pseudogout; however, sporadic mutations of these sites appear to be rare.[462] The male-to-female ratio is 1.5 : 1 for pseudogout.[8,40] It can have a polyarticular presentation.

Pathophysiology
CPPD crystals might be deposited in synovial and capsular tissues as well as within tendons and ligaments. The development of acute synovitis appears to develop with crystal shedding, in which crystals deposited in articular cartilage are shed into the joint. After phagocytosis of the crystals, enzymatic and lysozymal release by leukocytes leads to an intense inflammatory response. The most common areas of involvement are the MTP joints in the foot, where periarticular calcification can develop. Crystals are radiopaque and are demonstrated as linear calcifications within joint hyaline cartilage or as diffuse opacifications within soft tissues. Joint destruction, although uncommon, resembles the typical changes of osteoarthritis, including chondrolysis, subchondral sclerosis, and cyst formation. Pseudogout can be precipitated by trauma.

Chondrocalcinosis often affects the upper extremity joints and the knees, as opposed to gout, which more often involves lower extremity joints. The joints of the hindfoot are occasionally involved. Often, the knee is affected, with a linear calcification within the menisci (Fig. 19-79A).

Joint aspiration and microscopic identification of crystals are necessary to establish a diagnosis. No underlying

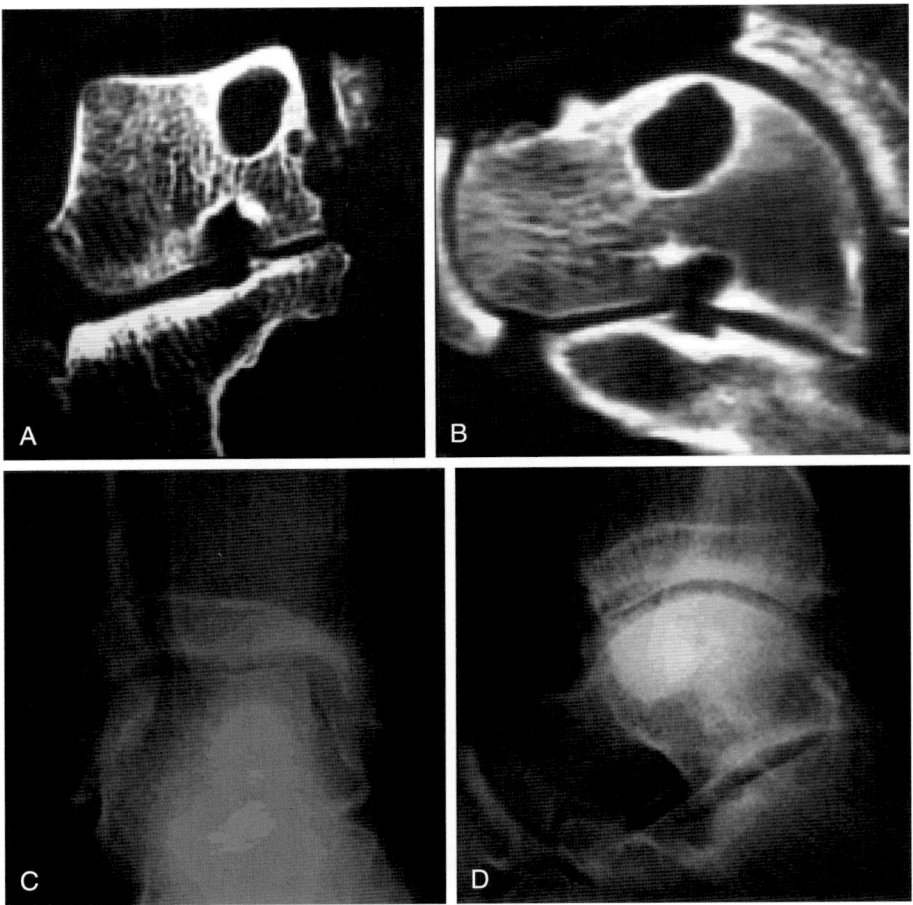

Figure 19-78 Gouty tophus in talus. **A** and **B,** Preoperative coronal and sagittal computed tomographic (CT) images showing gouty tophus lesion in the talar dome. **C** and **D,** Postoperative anteroposterior and lateral radiographs demonstrate lesion filled with calcium phosphate. (From Morino T, Fujita M, Kariyama K, et al: Intraosseous gouty tophus of the talus, treated by total curettage and calcium phosphate cement filling: a case report, *Foot Ankle Int* 28:126–128, 2007).

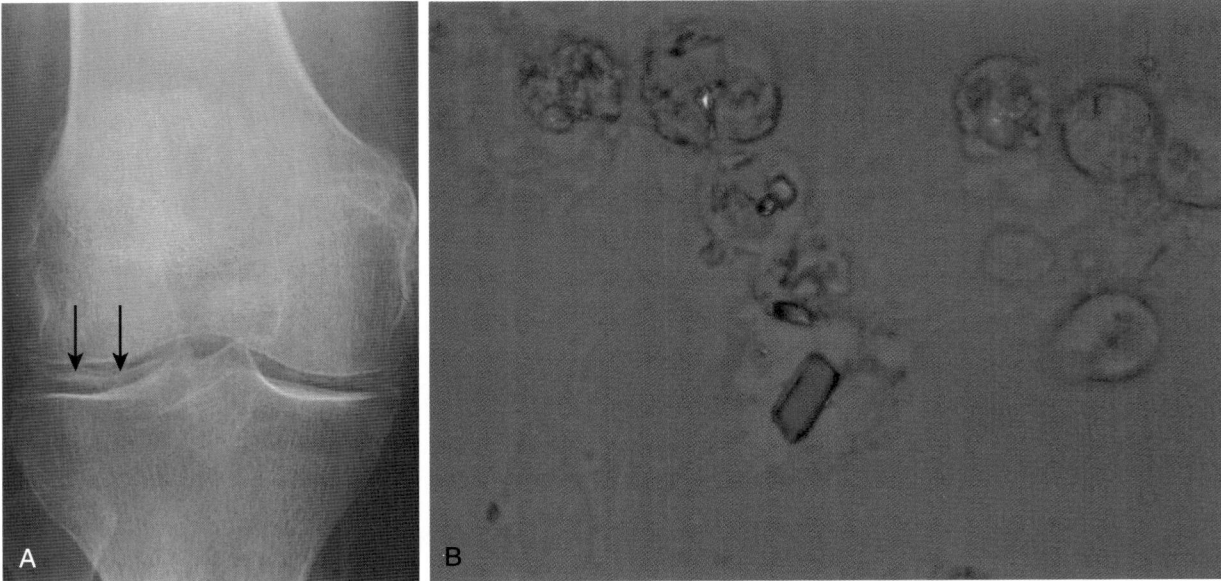

Figure 19-79 **A,** Chondrocalcinosis often affects the knee joint with calcification of menisci *(arrows).* **B,** With chondrocalcinosis, microscopic evaluation demonstrates rhomboid-shaped crystals characterized by positive birefringence (blue hue) under polarized light (compensated polarized microscopy, ×1000). (From Robert Terkeltaub: *Gout and other crystal arthropathies,* ed 1, Philadelphia, 2011, Saunders/Elsevier.)

enzymatic defect or metabolic abnormality leads to CPPD arthropathy. The disorder is typically diagnosed by the microscopic demonstration of weakly positive birefringent crystals of varying shapes under polarized light (1-20 mm in length) (Fig. 19-79B).

Treatment

Pharmacologic treatment with NSAIDs and the occasional judicious use of an intraarticular steroid injection may be warranted.[5] Colchicine is relatively inconsistent in relieving symptoms, but NSAIDs may be more helpful. Recurrent attacks separated by asymptomatic periods and eventual chronic degenerative arthropathy can develop. Recent studies have indicated that methotrexate and recombinant interleukin (IL)-1 antagonists may be effective treatments for recalcitrant cases.[87,370] Surgery, when necessary, uses techniques of arthrodesis and joint debridement typically used for osteoarthritis.

SERONEGATIVE ARTHROPATHIES

Enthesopathy is a characteristic finding of seronegative arthropathies. The site of insertion of a ligament, tendon, joint capsule, or fascia is called the *enthesis*, and inflammation of this site is called *enthesopathy*. Inflammation can lead to osteolysis, new bone formation, and capsular fibrosis. The large number of tendinous insertions and joints in the foot increases the vulnerability of this region for inflammation. Seronegative arthropathies are characterized by the absence of a positive rheumatoid factor. The arthritic process often involves the axial skeleton. Because musculoskeletal pathologic findings are often indistinguishable from rheumatoid arthritis, the presence of other findings (gastrointestinal or genitourinary disorders, dermatologic abnormalities, nail changes) may be necessary to make a conclusive diagnosis.

The three common seronegative arthropathies (psoriatic arthritis, reactive arthritis, and ankylosing spondylitis) involving the lower extremity are characterized by radiographic features that differentiate them from rheumatoid arthritis. Key radiologic features include absence of generalized osteoporosis because of a less profound synovitis, presence of whiskering or adventitious calcification around the involved joints with erosive bony changes, and intraarticular ankylosis. The seronegative arthropathies are often associated with heel pain syndrome (20% incidence).[208,471] Rheumatoid arthritis rarely manifests with initial symptoms of heel pain (see Fig. 19-80).

Psoriatic Arthritis

Definition and Incidence

Psoriatic arthritis is a member of the spondyloarthritis family and is usually seronegative, meaning serum testing for rheumatoid factor (RF) is negative. Anti–cyclic citrullinated peptide (anti-CCP) and human leukocyte antigen (HLA)-B27 testing are also infrequently positive.[277,564] It is generally characterized by skin and nail lesions and can

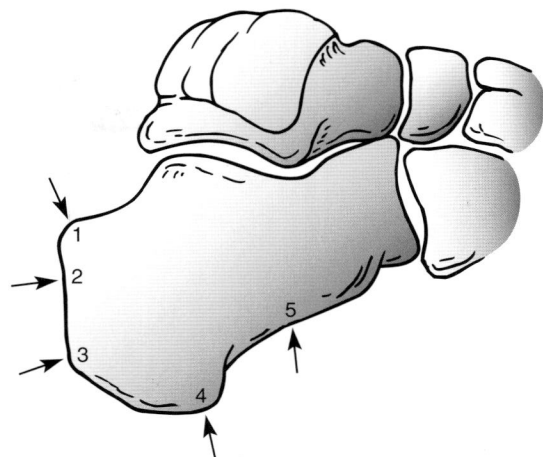

Figure 19-80 Common areas of enthesopathy associated with inflammatory arthritis. *1*, Superior aspect of calcaneus. *2* and *3*, Achilles tendon insertion. *4*, Plantar fascia insertion. *5*, Plantar aspect of calcaneus.

include enthesitis, dactylitis, iritis, peripheral arthritis (both oligoarticular asymmetric and polyarticular symmetric), spondylitis, and variations in clinical course. This heterogeneity of clinical features can make diagnosis difficult.[564]

The association of arthropathy and psoriasis was initially described by Alibert[9] in 1818, but Bazin[21] coined the term *psoriatic arthropathy* in 1860. The prevalence of psoriasis in the general population is less than 3%.[153,402,534] Onset of arthritis is typically insidious, but it can have an acute onset mimicking gout. Typically, the onset occurs in the third or fourth decade, but any age group can be affected. Unlike rheumatoid arthritis, the male-to-female ratio is 1 : 1.[81,153,162] A heritable tendency, probably polygenic in nature, has been reported.[402] Farber and Nall[153] have noted a 36% familial onset in affected subjects. Psoriatic arthritis also appears to be progressive. Despite disease-modifying pharmacologic treatment, progression occurs in almost 50% of patients.[186,274]

Two different patterns of dermatologic presentation occur with psoriasis. *Psoriasis vulgaris* (Fig. 19-81A) is characterized by silvery papules and white scaly plaques. *Psoriasis pustulosis* (Fig. 19-81B) is characterized by pustules and vesicles and commonly is found on the palms of the hands and soles of the feet.[81] Nail involvement is characterized by onycholysis, pitting, subungual hyperkeratosis, and splinter hemorrhages (Fig. 19-82). Disease with obvious nail and dermatologic disease (74%) tend to be easier to diagnose than disease with limited skin involvement.[215]

Fitzpatrick et al[162] noted arthritis associated with psoriasis in 3% to 4% of the population. Hammerschlag et al[215] reported that 14% of patients with psoriatic arthritis had skin lesions in hidden areas (gluteal fold, axilla, beneath hairlines) (Fig. 19-83). In 12% to 16%, the arthropathy precedes the onset of skin abnormalities.[215,468]

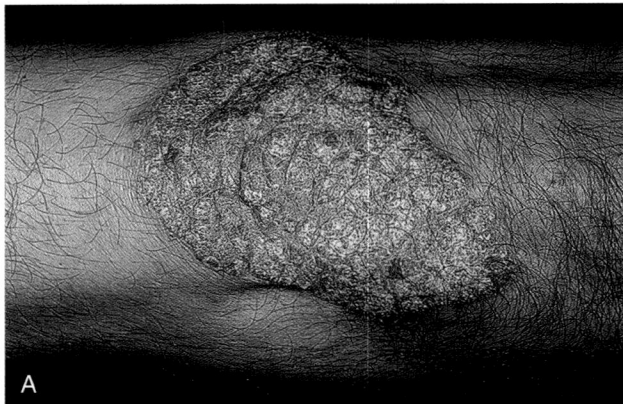

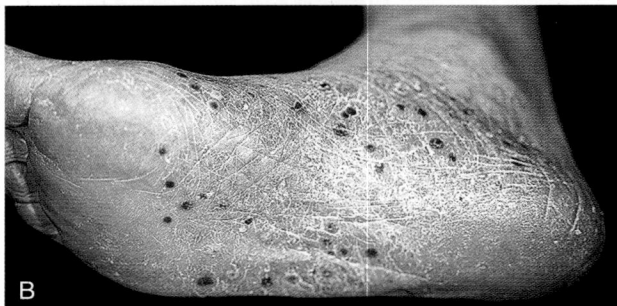

Figure 19-81 Psoriatic skin lesions. **A,** Psoriasis vulgaris is characterized by silvery papules and white scaly plaques. **B,** Psoriasis pustulosis is characterized by pustules and vesicles and is commonly found on the plantar aspect of the foot. (Images from Habif TP, Campbell JL Jr, Shane Chapman M, et al: *Skin disease: diagnosis and treatment*, ed 3, New York, 2011, Elsevier/Saunders.)

Box 19-2   CASPAR Criteria for Psoriatic Arthritis*

Inflammatory articular disease (joint, spine, or entheseal) plus the following:
Psoriasis: current (2), history of (1), family history of (1)[†]
Nail dystrophy (1)
Negative rheumatoid factor (1)
Dactylitis: current (1), history of (1)[‡]
Radiographs (hand or foot) with juxtaarticular new bone formation (1)[§]

*To meet the 2006 ClASsification criteria for Psoriatic ARthritis (CASPAR), a patient must have inflammatory articular disease and greater than or equal to 3 points from the remaining categories; the assigned scores are in parentheses. Criteria specificity is 98.7%, and sensitivity is 91.4%.
[†]Patient-reported history in a first- or second-degree relative.
[‡]As recorded by a rheumatologist.
[§]Excludes osteophyte formation.

with rheumatoid arthritis. Evaluating patients with psoriatic arthritis, Roberts et al[468] noted arthritis indistinguishable from rheumatoid arthritis in 78%, distal joint arthritis in 17%, and arthritis mutilans in 5%.

This difficulty with diagnosis led to the formation of an international research collaborative called the CASPAR (ClASsification criteria for Psoriatic ARthritis) group. In 2006, the group published their data collected on 588 consecutive patients from 30 rheumatology clinics in 13 countries.[545] Their findings outline a new set of diagnostic criteria for psoriatic arthritis (Box 19-2). These new criteria may help reduce the difficulty in diagnosing psoriatic arthritis and are supported by subsequent publications.[465,545]

Examination
Physical examination is characterized by the presentation of arthritis, with swelling, joint tenderness, and pain with erythema. The MTP joints are involved slightly more often than the ankle or interphalangeal joints. Nail dystrophy is common. Gold and Bassett[188] and others[162,215] have noted involvement of the interphalangeal joint of the hallux. Although these patients are not seriously ill, they can exhibit chronic fatigue, lymphadenopathy, fever, weight loss, and splenomegaly. Ultrasonographic evaluation of psoriatic dactylitis has demonstrated that the digital swelling is due to flexor tenosynovitis (96%) as well as articular synovitis (52%).[272]

The radiographic appearance of psoriatic arthritis is similar to that of rheumatoid arthritis.[188,207] The os calcis typically develops spurring or sclerosis on the posterior plantar surface. Erosion of the distal tuft of the terminal phalanx *(acroosteolysis)* can occur,[392] along with whittling of the phalanges and metatarsals and cupping of the proximal aspect of the phalanges and metatarsals. Whittling and cupping occurring simultaneously is termed *pencil-in-cup deformity* (Fig. 19-84B). Ankylosing of the digits can occur.

Characteristically, a predilection exists for the PIP and DIP joints with relative sparing of the MTP joint,[381] but

In one series, the average onset of psoriasis was 32 years of age, and the average onset of arthritis was 36 years.[215] Although Moll and Wright[392] reported arthritic involvement of the hands as a characteristic finding, Hammerschlag et al[215] reported that the foot and ankle were involved as the initial area of disease presentation nearly three times more often than the hand (foot and ankle 55%, hand and wrist 20%). In a series of 104 patients with psoriatic arthritis, Hyslop et al[248] reported that 62% had foot pain. In another study, the foot and ankle were reported to be the most common sites of involvement—found in 86% of patients.[215]

Psoriatic arthritis should be suspected with a familial history of psoriasis, skin and nail lesions, multiple joint arthropathy, and a sausage digit.[168] Involvement of the nails is seen in 63% of patients with psoriatic arthritis, compared with 37% of those with psoriasis without arthritic symptoms.[498] Although psoriatic arthritis characteristically has been reported to affect the DIP joints, Rodnan and Schumaker[471,472] noted that only 5% to 10% of patients exhibit classic DIP joint arthropathy (Fig. 19-84).

Patients with asymmetric arthropathy involving only two or three joints and those with a pattern of symmetric polyarthritis are clinically indistinguishable from those

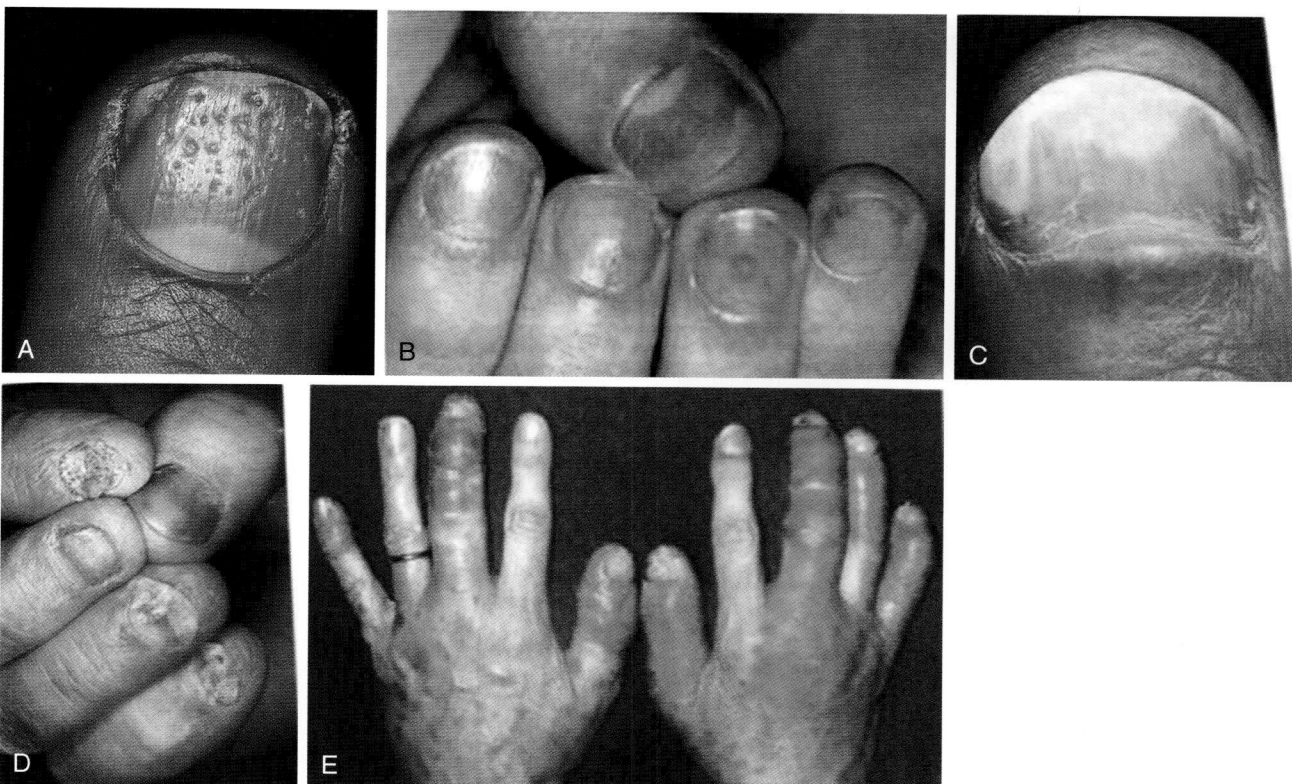

Figure 19-82 Typical nail changes in psoriasis. **A,** Nail pitting. Pits are irregularly spaced, large, and deep. **B,** Oil spot. Nails have yellow spots of discoloration called "oil spots." **C,** Onycholysis. Distal nail plate separation resulting from psoriatic inflammation at fingertip. **D,** Complex nail deformity. Nails show a combination of pitting, oil spots, and onycholysis. Differentiation from onychomycosis can be difficult. **E,** Severe psoriatic arthritis. Involvement of both the distal interphalangeal and proximal interphalangeal joints can lead to "sausage digit" seen here in bilateral thumbs and long fingers, and ring and small fingers on the *right*. Fingernails demonstrate complex changes, and skin demonstrates both psoriasis vulgaris (silvery plaques) and psoriasis pustulosis (small pustules). (**A, B,** and **E,** From Bolognia JL, Jorizzo JL, Rapini RP, editors: *Dermatology,* vol 1, ed 2, St Louis, 2008, Mosby/Elsevier. **C** and **D,** From Habif TP, Campbell JL Jr, Shane Chapman M, et al: *Skin disease: diagnosis and treatment,* ed 3, New York, 2011, Elsevier/Saunders.)

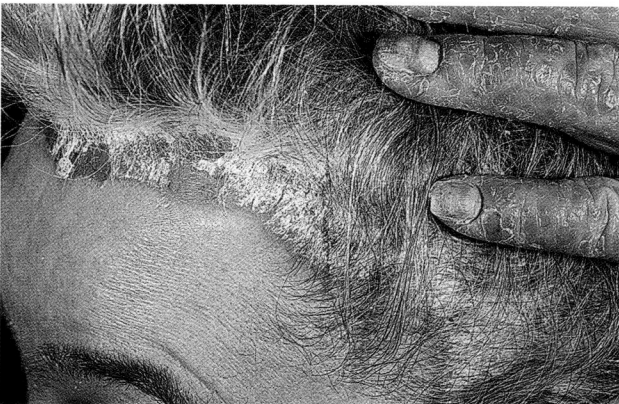

Figure 19-83 Psoriasis of the scalp. Clinical photograph demonstrates a typical psoriatic plaque beneath the hairline. (From Habif TP, Campbell JL Jr, Shane Chapman M, et al: *Skin disease: diagnosis and treatment,* ed 3, New York, 2011, Elsevier/Saunders.)

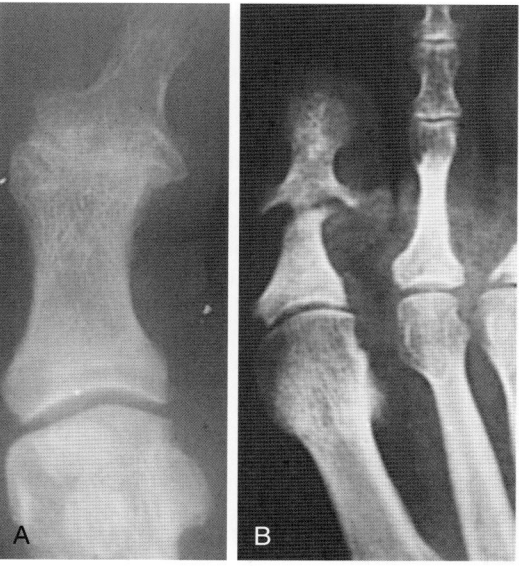

Figure 19-84 **A,** Classic distal interphalangeal joint arthropathy characteristic of psoriatic arthritis. **B,** Psoriatic arthritis with extensive destruction of the interphalangeal joint of the hallux, demonstrating "pencil-in-cup deformity." (Courtesy A. Smith, MD, Prince Rupert, Canada.)

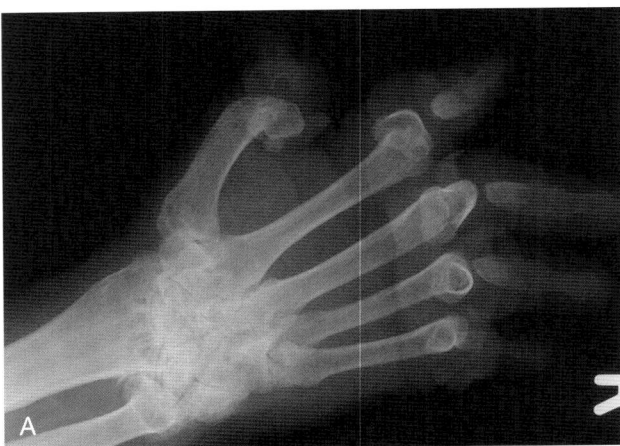

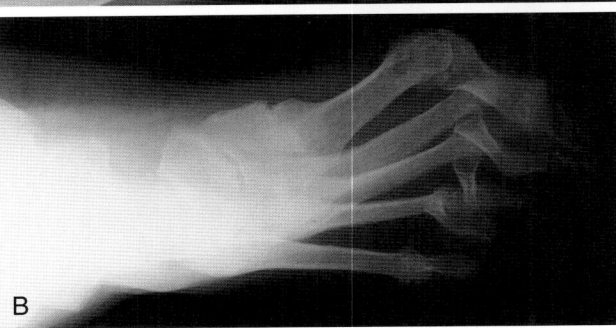

Figure 19-85 Psoriatic arthritis with arthritis mutilans. **A,** Anteroposterior radiograph of a hand with whittling of the phalanges, telescoping deformity of the fingers, and dislocation of the metacarpophalangeal joints. **B,** Anteroposterior radiograph of a foot with similar changes. (From Pope TL Jr, Bloem HL, Beltran J, Morrison WB, Wilson DJ: *Imaging of the musculoskeletal system,* vol 2, Philadelpia, 2008, Saunders/Elsevier.)

separation of patients with DIP involvement into a distinct subclass is not warranted because clinical and radiographic outcome appears to be affected by the number of joints involved (oligoarticular vs. polyarticular).[273] In 5% of patients with distal arthritis, one or more joints progress to severe osteolysis of the phalanx, with severe deformities often described as *arthritis mutilans* (complete resorption of bone), and an opera-glass or telescoping deformity of the digit can occur (Fig. 19-85). All these findings have been well described, but Moll and Wright[392] have noted that they are relatively uncommon. Erosions in the periarticular region and poorly defined periostitis can occur along the short diaphyseal regions of the phalanges.[207]

Treatment

In 2009, a landmark meta-analysis was published on the treatment of psoriatic arthritis by the Group for Research and Assessment of Psoriasis and Psoriatic Arthritis (GRAPPA).[465] According to GRAPPA recommendations, treatment should be broken down into the following categories: peripheral arthritis, skin and nail disease, axial disease, dactylitis, and enthesitis.

First-line treatment for peripheral arthritis, axial (spinal) disease, enthesitis, and dactylitis should be NSAIDs.[465,564] Patients with peripheral arthritis who have moderate-to-severe disease, or who have failed first-line therapy should be treated with a disease-modifying antirheumatic drug (DMARD), such as sulfasalazine, methotrexate, or leflunomide. Those patients who do not respond to a DMARD may require a TNF inhibitor (etanercept, infliximab, or adalimumab). In addition to controlling peripheral arthritis symptoms, these agents have shown some ability to halt the radiographic-evidenced progression of disease.[84,465] DMARDs have not been shown to be effective for axial disease, but TNF inhibitors have shown good results.[407,465] Physiotherapy modalities have also been shown to be helpful for spinal symptoms and enthesitis.[407] Phototherapy with or without acitretin is recommended as first-line treatment for skin manifestations, although methotrexate or a TNF inhibitor may also be necessary.[465] Retinoids, cyclosporine, and TNF inhibitors have shown some effectiveness against nail disease.[465]

Surgical treatment of forefoot deformities associated with psoriasis is uncommon but, when necessary, follows the surgical principles of rheumatoid arthritis, with MTP or interphalangeal joint fusions of the hallux, lesser MTP joint excisional arthroplasty, and hammer toe or mallet toe repairs. Kitaoka[296] has reported a high level of good and excellent results (89%) with arthrodesis procedures, forefoot arthroplasty, and rheumatoid-type surgical procedures in psoriatic arthritis patients followed over a 15-year period. However, Stern et al[534] reported an increased infection rate in patients with psoriatic arthritis who had undergone total joint arthroplasty and suggested preventive preoperative prophylactic measures, including perioperative antibiotics and localized skin care. It is preferable to have clear skin to operate through, and aggressive dermatologic efforts can reduce skin-related complications.

The priority is the identification of the disease process. Poorly defined metatarsalgia may be the first sign of psoriatic arthritis. The presentation of seronegative arthritis as poorly defined forefoot pain can initially be misdiagnosed as an interdigital neuroma, and the patient could undergo unnecessary surgery.[215]

Reactive Arthritis

Presentation and Etiology

Reactive arthritis is a catch-all term that refers to inflammation of joints and other tissues after an infection elsewhere in the body. Although originally described by several authors in the 18th century, a 1916 report by Hans Reiter[458] has become associated with this disease entity.[79] The article by Reiter described a soldier who developed a triad of conjunctivitis, urethritis, and arthritis 8 days after the onset of bloody diarrhea. Despite previous popularity of the term *Reiter syndrome,* recent literature has favored a return to the more general term *reactive arthritis.*[340,428,479,560]

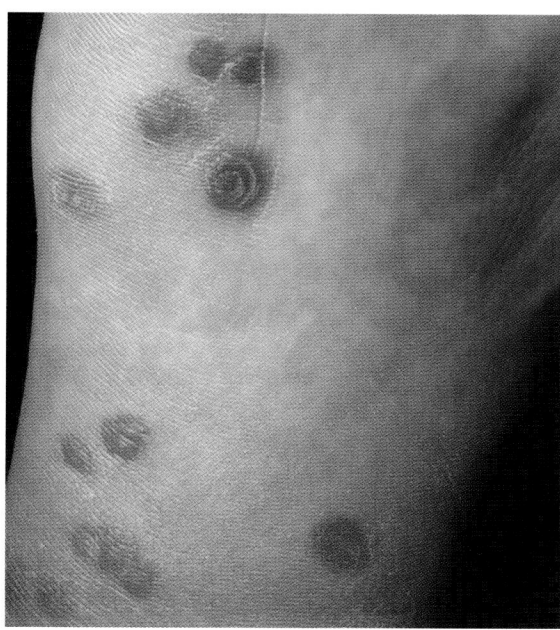

Figure 19-86 Keratoderma blennorrhagicum. Characteristic skin lesions associated with reactive arthritis have a predilection for the plantar aspect of the foot and demonstrate a thick, yellow scale that is often pustular. When the lesions occur on the penis, they are referred to as balanitis circinata. (From Bolognia JL, Jorizzo JL, Rapini RP, editors: *Dermatology*, vol 1, ed 2, St Louis, 2008, Mosby/Elsevier.)

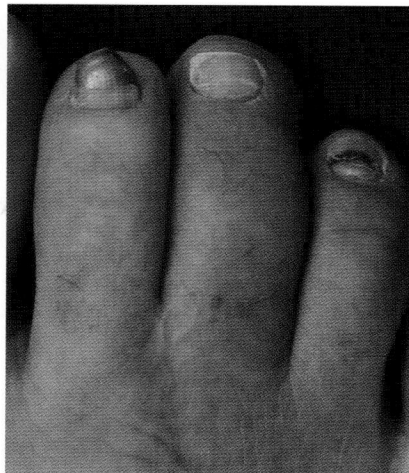

Figure 19-87 Sausage toe (third toe here) occurs in approximately one fourth of patients with psoriatic arthritis.

Reactive arthritis is generally regarded as an aseptic arthritis that is triggered by an infectious agent outside the joint.[275] Symptoms follow gastrointestinal or genitourinary tract infection,[207,275] and causative organisms include *Clamydia*, *Ureaplasma*, *Shigella*, *Salmonella*, *Yersinia*, and *Campylobacter* species.[275] Although the disease appears to be triggered by an infectious entity, 60% to 80% of patients have a positive HLA-B27 test, suggesting an immunologic predisposition.[166,279] The association between a bacterial infection and an elevated HLA-B27 led Fan and Yu[151] to propose a genetic predisposition, with arthropathy being secondarily induced by the infection.

This syndrome also frequently includes enthesitis (particularly of the calcaneus) (see Fig. 19-80), dactylitis, spondylitis, and soft tissue manifestations, such as conjunctivitis, mucosal ulceration, balanitis circinata, and keratoderma blennorrhagicum.[275] *Keratoderma blennorrhagicum* (Fig. 19-86) describes a pustular lesion on the sole of the foot that is seen in approximately 10% of those with reactive arthritis. It may be confused with psoriasis and in time can form a hyperkeratotic lesion. Keat[279] and Kataria and Brent,[275] have reported that these other symptoms can differ in frequency depending on the underlying infectious organism.

Chand and Johnson[79] reported on 120 patients with reactive arthritis at the Mayo Clinic over a 10-year period. The median age of onset was 26 years, and 50% of these patients had foot and ankle symptoms. A definite predilection for the lower extremity has been observed,* and the most frequently affected locations are the interphalangeal joints, MTP joints, ankle, and calcaneus. The knee was involved in two thirds of patients. Other physical findings are similar to those of other seronegative spondyloarthropathies.[382]

Symptoms and physical findings include pain, swelling, tenderness, mild stiffness, and erythema of the involved joints. The onset is typically acute and occurs in young men (10:1 ratio)[279] with asymmetric involvement of the lower extremity. Symptoms often occur less than 30 days after an infection of the gastrointestinal or genitourinary tract[275,279] (more than 80% of patients). Because the soft tissue manifestations may not be obvious on physical examination, and prodromal infectious illness may be considered unrelated or unimportant by the patient, reactive arthritis may be easily missed. The wary clinician, however, should suspect reactive arthritis (and look for related history and soft tissue manifestations) in a patient with asymmetric polyarticular symptoms of the lower extremity, especially if one of the areas of involvement is the calcaneus.

Significant swelling of a digit can cause a sausage toe[168,381] (Fig. 19-87). Because it is not seen exclusively in reactive arthritis, other diagnoses to be considered with a sausage toe are cellulitis, trauma, osteomyelitis, and psoriasis. Chand and Johnson[79] noted a sausage toe in 26% of patients with reactive arthritis, and Gold and Bassett[188] reported frequent involvement of the interphalangeal joint.

Although radiographic findings are not present in up to one third of patients, soft tissue swelling is often demonstrated early in the disease process, similar to rheumatoid arthritis, psoriasis, and ankylosing spondylitis. The radiographic pattern can demonstrate concomitant joint

---

*References 49, 79, 188, 207, 275, and 535.

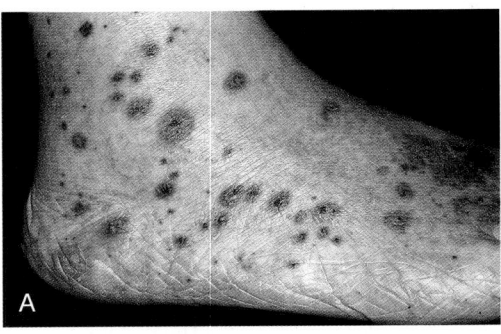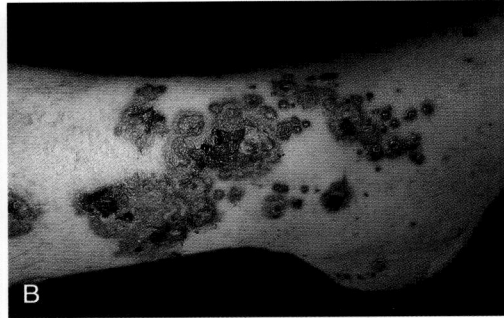

Figure 19-88 Vasculitis resulting from systemic lupus erythematosus. Lesions begin as palpable purpura and small blisters **(A)**, but may progress to bulla and eroded ulcers **(B)**. (Images from Habif TP, Campbell JL Jr, Shane Chapman M, et al: *Skin disease: diagnosis and treatment*, ed 3, New York, 2011, Elsevier/Saunders.)

involvement of the heels, sacroiliac joints, ankle, and tarsus.[514] In the presence of calcaneal pain, fluffy periostitis or exuberant new periosteal bone formation can occur at the insertion of the plantar fascia or Achilles tendon. Intraarticular and extraarticular joint erosion also may be noted, especially in the area of the interphalangeal and MTP joints. Guerra and Resnick[207] reported large, painful calcaneal spurs occurring with reactive arthritis.

Bony ankylosis and severe joint destruction are uncommon, but over time, radiographic findings can mimic psoriasis, rheumatoid arthritis, and ankylosing spondylitis.

Treatment

Reactive arthritis often has a self-limited course lasting between 3 to 12 months.[275] Complete spontaneous resolution can occur, although symptoms in some patients can linger chronically,[166] and up to 50% of patients have recurrent bouts of arthritis, with 15% to 30% developing chronic arthritis.[275] Nonsurgical treatment includes the occasional judicious use of an intraarticular corticosteroid injection and short periods of NSAID administration. DMARDs and TNF inhibitors have also been reported to be helpful in recalcitrant cases.[182,275] Because of the underlying bacterial etiology, Fan and Yu[151] have suggested a 3-month course of tetracycline to reduce the chronicity and severity of the arthritis; however, antibiotic therapy has not been effective in other trials.[329,604] Calcaneal pain may be treated with immobilization, viscoelastic heel pads or heel lifts, and dorsiflexion night splints (see Chapter 13). Surgical treatment is generally unwarranted because of the self-limited course of the disease.

Systemic Lupus Erythematosus

Presentation, Etiology, and Incidence

Systemic lupus erythematosus (SLE) is an autoimmune disease in which autoantibodies are directed against components of the cell nucleus. Its onset typically is in the second or third decade of life, and it is more common in blacks than whites and in women than men (8 : 1). The estimated incidence is 1 in 2000 in the general population.[471] Although the cause is not known, an immune complex deposition (immunoglobulins M, G, and A) occurs in the small arteries and arterioles. Osteonecrosis can occur in 5% to 8% of patients when disease duration is 5 years or longer. SLE can also be induced by pharmacologic agents, such as antibiotics, antiarrhythmics, antihypertensives, anticonvulsants, and antithyroid medications. The deposition of immune complexes in vessel walls can result not only in vasculitis but also in osteonecrosis and arthritis. Vasculitis can lead to periungual hemorrhages and punched-out cutaneous lesions forming leg ulcers (Fig. 19-88). SLE is a classic autoimmune disease with multisystem involvement.

The clinical course is variable and may be insidious or fulminant in onset. The patient can also experience repeated episodes of febrile illness, weight loss, severe fatigue, joint pain, and swelling, which can occur for months before other symptoms develop. Arthralgia and joint deformity occur because of soft tissue laxity, but rarely does bone deformity result. Arthritis and arthralgia are seen in 95% of SLE patients.[471] Involvement of the hands and feet is common. The foot may be the initial site of onset and the only site of symptoms. Sangle et al[494] reported on a series of 19 SLE patients with foot pain. They found metatarsal fractures in all 19 patients (6 bilateral) and no history of trauma in any patient.

Raynaud disease is noted in 15% of SLE patients.[27] Dermatologic changes include hyperkeratosis and atrophy of the epidermis. Peripheral neuropathy might also be noted. Musculoskeletal symptoms include myalgia secondary to myositis.

Any 4 of the following 11 criteria can indicate a diagnosis of SLE: macular rash, discoid rash, photosensitivity, oral ulcers, arthritis, serositis, renal disorders, neurologic disorders, hematologic disorders, immunologic disorders, and positive test for antinuclear antibody (ANA).[471]

Laboratory abnormalities associated with SLE include anemia and thrombocytopenia. A positive lupus erythematosus cell test occurs in 60% to 80% of patients,[27] and a positive test for ANA is present in 99%. Anti–double-stranded DNA antibodies are highly specific for SLE and are found in 70% of patients with lupus but less than 0.5% of control subjects.[445] One fifth of patients with SLE have a positive rheumatoid factor.[471]

On radiographic evaluation, the characteristic difference between SLE and rheumatoid arthritis is that although both patients experience joint pain, no erosive arthropathy is associated with SLE. However, SLE is noted as a deforming arthropathy and is a multisystem disease that can lead to myositis, polyarthritis, spontaneous tendon rupture, osteonecrosis, septic arthritis, soft tissue calcification, and osteomyelitis. Osteoporosis[535] may be present without articular erosion. Joint space narrowing can occur, as well as soft tissue calcifications. (Soft tissue calcifications can also be seen with hyperthyroidism, scleroderma, and dermatomyositis.) Periarticular cystic changes occur in 50% of patients, as does resorption of the distal tufts of the distal phalanges.[27] With repeated synovitis, subluxation, eventual dislocation, and deviation can occur in joints of the forefoot, but this joint laxity typically is painless—without swelling, synovitis, or restricted motion.

Treatment

Pharmacologic therapy is the mainstay of SLE treatment. Salicylates, NSAIDs, corticosteroids, cytotoxic drugs, and antimalarial medications are all commonly used agents to combat SLE. Glucocorticoids are generally regarded as the first-line treatment, particularly in the beginning of a flare; however, these drugs have potent side effects, which has led researchers to seek safer alternatives. Recently, several new biologic agents have been developed to target specific steps in the immune cascade triggered by SLE.[603] Ongoing clinical trials continue to show promising results with these medications, which may shape the future of SLE treatment.

Other modalities of treatment include rest during the active phases of the disease and immobilization or support with orthoses and casting. Although surgery is performed infrequently for SLE, with progressive subluxation and dislocation, arthroplasty and fusion techniques similar to those used in the treatment of rheumatoid forefoot and hindfoot deformities may be necessary. Beilstein and Hawkins[27] recommend avoiding penicillin analogues at surgery because of possible drug-induced lupus syndrome.

Ankylosing Spondylitis

Presentation and Etiology

Ankylosing spondylitis is an inflammatory arthropathy affecting the axial skeleton and peripheral joints. The sacroiliac joints are often involved. Ankylosing spondylitis is characterized by onset in the second and third decades of life, typically in the male population (male-to-female ratio, 4:1). There appears to be a strong familial tendency.[592]

Foot and ankle symptoms are uncommon,[188,535] and lower extremity symptoms infrequently lead to an initial diagnosis of ankylosing spondylitis because spine and sacroiliac symptoms are more common and more severe. Sacroiliitis and asymmetric involvement of the heel and foot, however, can herald the onset of ankylosing spondylitis. The forefoot is eventually involved in 60% of patients with chronic ankylosing spondylitis.[188] The MTP joints are affected in a way similar to that of rheumatoid arthritis, but because of less significant synovitis, less periarticular osteoporosis is present, which can help to differentiate spondylitis from rheumatoid arthritis. The overwhelming involvement of the axial skeleton with ankylosing spondylitis can make foot and ankle symptoms seem relatively insignificant. Enthesopathy is a characteristic feature of seronegative spondyloarthropathies, such as ankylosing spondylitis, and radiographic changes in the calcaneus are indistinguishable from those of reactive arthritis.[332]

Ankylosing spondylitis may be confused with *diffuse idiopathic skeletal hyperostosis* (DISH) syndrome. DISH syndrome occurs in older and middle-aged men and is characterized by stiffness of the spine and peripheral hyperostosis. It is not associated with sacroiliitis or a positive HLA-B27. The foot is often a site of ossification in DISH syndrome because of the multiple sites of ligament, tendon, and fascial attachments. More than 70% of DISH patients have radiologic abnormalities of the foot.[178] Posterior calcaneal spurring is common. Spurs are often large, vary in shape, may be multiple and bilateral, and are not associated with underlying bone erosion or sclerosis. The sesamoid bones are often involved. Treatment of DISH parallels that of degenerative arthritis, with frequent use of NSAIDs. Surgery is rarely necessary but may be done for significant bone enlargements or excision of prominent exostoses (Fig. 19-89). Radiographs of the spine can show a characteristic flowing hyperostosis or candle wax calcification adjacent to several vertebral segments.[178] In the juvenile patient, Levi et al[332] reported frequent hindfoot involvement and spontaneous arthrodesis of the tarsometatarsal joints.

Calcaneal pain at the plantar aponeurosis or the Achilles tendon insertion sites (see Fig. 19-80) is similar to enthesopathy in other forms of seronegative arthritis.

A strong association exists between HLA-B27 and ankylosing spondylitis.[500] Bluestone[49] reported a positive HLA-B27 in 75% to 100% of patients, although this test can be positive with reactive arthritis and psoriatic arthritis as well.[457] Wollheim[592] reported that 90% of patients with ankylosing spondylitis test positive for HLA-B27. Positive tests are noted more often in white and Asian populations, and the incidence is lower in the black population.

Back pain and spine stiffness might not occur until 4 to 6 months after onset of other symptoms. MTP joint involvement is similar to that of rheumatoid arthritis, but the synovitis is often less intense. Subchondral sclerosis is more evident than osteoporosis, which can help to differentiate ankylosing spondylitis from rheumatoid

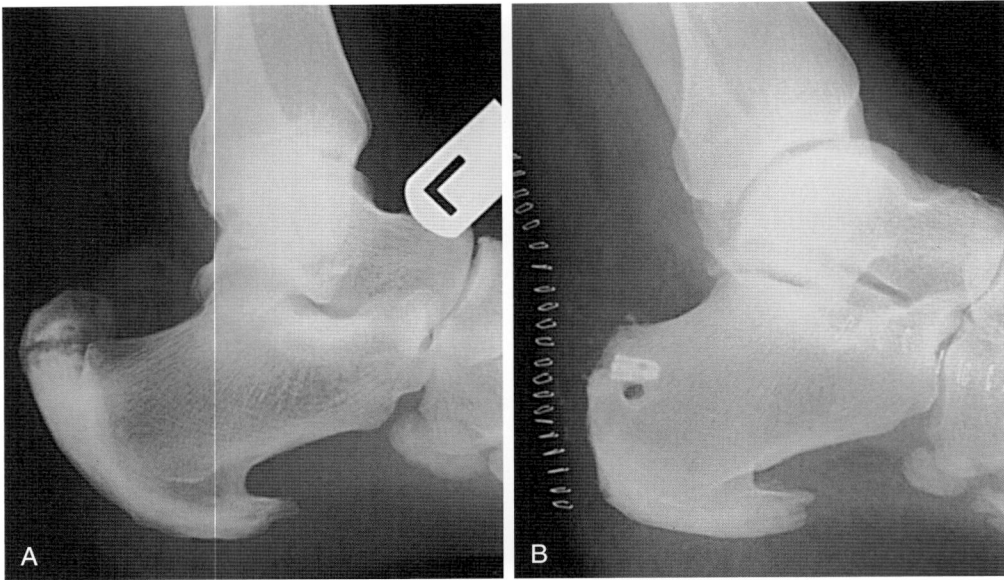

Figure 19-89 **A,** Large bone spurs occurring at the plantar fascia insertion and the Achilles tendon insertion associated with diffuse idiopathic skeletal hyperostosis (DISH) syndrome. Note fracture of the dorsal spur. **B,** After resection of a painful fractured spur and reinsertion of the Achilles tendon with a flexor hallucis longus tendon augmentation transfer.

arthritis. A more chronic inflammatory process can lead to lesser MTP joint deformities resembling rheumatoid arthritis.

Radiographic findings include periostitis and new bone formation, which can result in joint capsule ossification or bone ankylosis. A radiographic index to assess tarsal involvement in patients with possible spondyloarthropathy has shown that oblique and lateral radiographic views of the foot provide the most useful information in determining the diagnosis.[427] Bony proliferation or "whiskering" often occurs adjacent to areas of osseous erosion and is pathognomonic of ankylosing spondylitis.[207,535] Periostitis and erosions in the calcaneus along the plantar surface and in the area of Achilles tendon insertion are virtually indistinguishable from psoriasis and reactive arthritis (see Fig. 19-80).

Treatment

Pharmacologic treatment of ankylosing spondylitis involves NSAIDs and corticosteroids initially. DMARDs, such as methotrexate and sulfasalazine, have not proven effective. Newer TNF inhibitors have been particularly helpful in the treatment of spondyloarthropathies, such as ankylosis spondylitis.[58] Nonsurgical management of hindfoot enthesopathy is generally the rule and is treated the same as reactive arthritis heel pain above. Surgical treatment generally focuses on the hip and spine and most commonly involves total hip arthroplasty and spinal osteotomy with fusion.[309] Surgery for the foot in ankylosing spondylitis is uncommon, but when it is necessary, forefoot reconstruction techniques are similar to those used for rheumatoid arthritis.

Human Immunodeficiency Virus Infection and Inflammatory Arthropathies

Seronegative arthritides (reactive arthritis, psoriatic arthritis, unclassified arthritic disorders with enthesopathy) may be associated with human immunodeficiency virus (HIV) infection and acquired immunodeficiency syndrome (AIDS).[280,523,590] In a recent comprehensive review of the literature, Walker et al[579] found that HIV-infected patients have a higher prevalence of arthralgia, reactive arthritis, psoriatic arthritis, gout, osteonecrosis, rhabdomyolysis, and polymyositis than the general population. Skin and joint manifestations of psoriatic arthritis increase with worsening HIV infection, although symptoms of SLE actually improve as the CD4 count declines because less of an immune response is generated.[579]

The foot and ankle are often involved in patients with HIV and reactive arthritis, and occasionally, the enthesopathy has a fulminant course with severe limitation of ambulatory capacity. Foot and ankle involvement is reported to involve one to four sites, including the Achilles tendon (85%), MTP joint (54%), subtalar joint (23%), and the phalanges (dactylitis) (13%).[579] Radiographic changes are identical to those seen in psoriatic arthritis, with osteolysis and pencil-in-cup deformities. Inflammation, joint ankylosis, osteolysis, and periarticular erosive changes can result from severity, persistence, and recurrence of the enthesopathy.

Redfern, et al[456] reported one case of inflammatory ankle arthropathy resulting from an opportunistic infection with *Mycobacterium avium-intracellulare* in an HIV-infected man. The ankle joint was found to have extensive synovitis with an avascular talus. This patient underwent

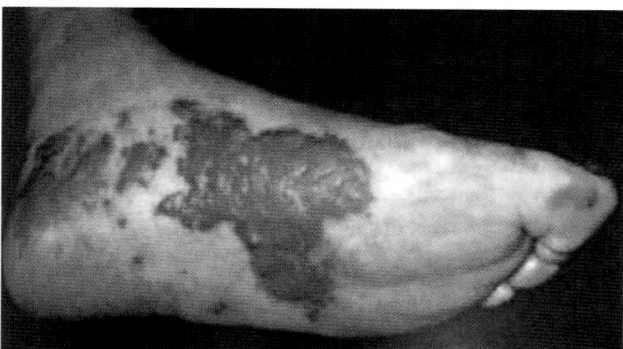

Figure 19-90 Kaposi sarcoma. Lesions are typically fleshy, reddish-purple nodules that may progress to the advanced plaque seen in this photograph. They are classically found on the feet and legs but may present on the genitalia, in the mouth, and gastrointestinal or respiratory tracts. (From Bolognia JL, Jorizzo JL, Rapini RP, editors: *Dermatology,* vol 1, ed 2, St Louis, 2008, Mosby/Elsevier.)

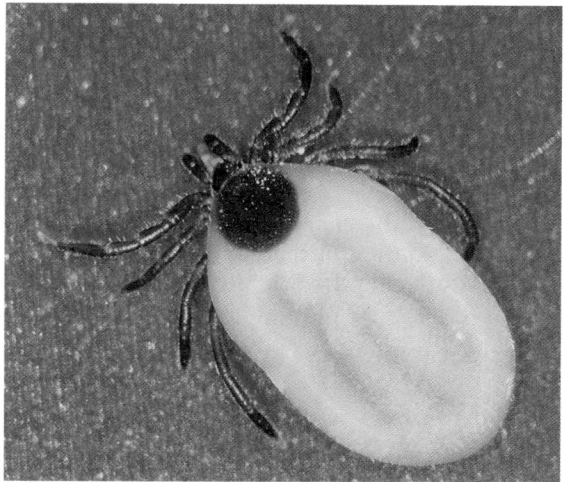

Figure 19-91 Ixodes tick. *Ixodes scapularis* (formerly known as *I. dammini*) is the best known *Ixodes* tick and frequently responsible for transmission of the spirochete *Borrelia burgdorferi*, the cause of Lyme disease. (From Bolognia JL, Jorizzo JL, Rapini RP, editors: *Dermatology,* vol 1, ed 2, St Louis, 2008, Mosby/Elsevier.)

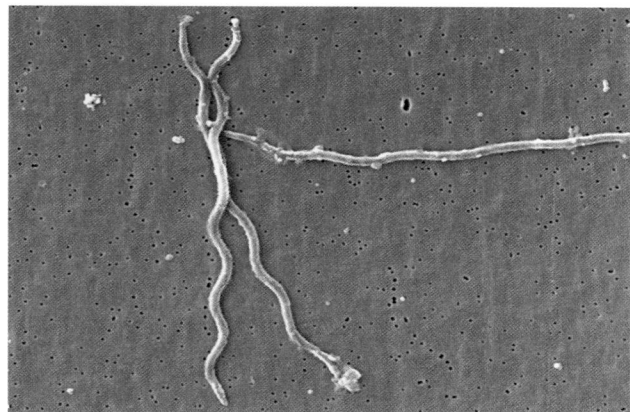

Figure 19-92 *Borrelia burgdorferi.* Digitally colorized scanning electron micrograph depicting three gram-negative, anaerobic spirochetes of the *B. burgdorferi* species. (From Centers for Disease Control and PreventionPublic Health Image Library (PHIL) #13177. Available at http://phil.cdc.gov/phil/details.asp?pid=13177. Accessed May 28, 2013.)

tibiocalcaneal fusion with an intramedullary nail and healed uneventfully after an 18-month course of triple antibiotic therapy for *Mycobacterium* infection.

NSAIDs are considered first-line therapy for musculoskeletal symptoms in HIV-infected patients and can be used according to the same guidelines as HIV-negative patients.[579] Indomethacin may have an inhibitory effect on HIV and may therefore be used preferentially in HIV patients.[54] According to Espinoza et al,[146] some patients with subclinical HIV infection and concomitant reactive arthritis treated with a DMARD (e.g., methotrexate) then develop Kaposi sarcoma (Fig. 19-90), fulminant AIDS, or an opportunistic infection (e.g., *Pneumocystis jiroveci* pneumonia). Other reports, however, show good results with sulfasalazine and methotrexate, as long as CD4 counts and viral loads are monitored carefully.[133,365] Patients who fail NSAID and DMARD therapy may require treatment with a TNF inhibitor.[579]

MISCELLANEOUS ARTHROPATHIES OF THE FOOT AND ANKLE

Lyme Disease

Presentation and Etiology

First described in 1977 after the investigation of symptoms of arthropathy in young children living near Lyme, Connecticut, this disease is now recognized in endemic areas in the Northeast, northern Midwest, and Pacific Northwest United States. Lyme disease is the most common arthropod-borne infectious disease diagnosed in the United States.[127,150] Although Lyme disease has been diagnosed in almost every state, 10 states (Md., Mass., Minn., N.J., N.Y., Conn., Pa., Wis., Del., R.I.) account for 93% of cases diagnosed each year.[515] In 2009, nearly 30,000 cases of Lyme disease were reported to the Centers for Disease Control and Prevention (CDC),

representing a 50% increase from 2006 and a 158% increase from 1995.[76]

Lyme disease is caused by a tick bite from the *Ixodes* species (Fig. 19-91) that is infected by a spirochete, *Borrelia burgdorferi* (Fig. 19-92). Deer support the adult population of the *Ixodes* ticks that transmit the disease. Mice serve as the host of immature stages of the tick and as the primary reservoir of the spirochete. Infected deer transmit the tick to humans, who then contract Lyme disease from the spirochete. However, the tick is small, and often the infectious bite is not appreciated.[150] A skin rash, fever, and general malaise may also be subclinical, and the disease can progress quietly to a secondary or tertiary phase with neurologic, cardiac, and musculoskeletal involvement similar to syphilis, another spirochete infection.

Lyme disease can be divided into three clinical stages: (I) early localized, (II) early disseminated, and (III) late.[515,595] *Stage I*, or *early localized*, disease is characterized by a typical "bulls-eye" rash called erythema chronicum migrans (ECM). The characteristic rash is an erythematous macular skin lesion that appears anywhere from 3 days to a month after the tick bite[531,532] (Fig. 19-93). The

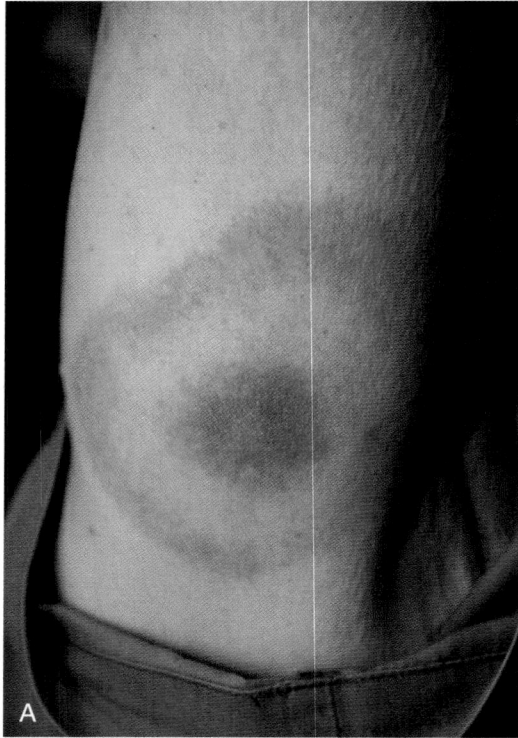

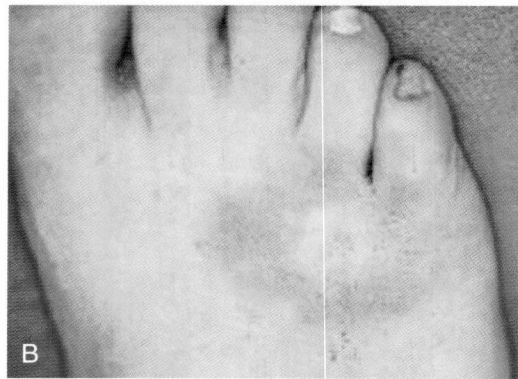

Figure 19-93 Classic erythema chronicum migrans rash associated with Lyme disease appears as "bulls-eye" lesion with enlarging borders. **A,** Posterior arm, near the axilla. **B,** Foot dorsum. (**A,** from Centers for Disease Control and Prevention Public Health Image Library (PHIL) #9874. Available at http://phil.cdc.gov/phil/details.asp?pid=9874. Accessed May 28, 2013). **B,** From Knoop K, Stack L, Storrow A, Thurman RJ, editors: *The atlas of emergency medicine*, ed 3, 2009, McGraw-Hill.)

rash is noted to have expanding edges that are characterized by a central clearing over time. It can grow to as large as 30 cm or more. Nonspecific, flu-like symptoms, such as headache, fatigue, and malaise, may accompany the rash during the early stage of disease.[529,515] However, an ECM rash is not recognized in approximately one third of patients with Lyme disease.[471]

Stage II, or *early disseminated*, disease occurs days to months later.[515] It is characterized by neurologic and cardiac manifestations, including atrioventricular block, pericarditis, congestive heart failure, neuritis, peripheral neuropathy, and aseptic meningitis.[324] Neurologic symptoms are slightly more common than cardiac symptoms and appear in approximately 15% to 20% of untreated children.[515]

Stage III, or *late*, presentation of Lyme disease includes musculoskeletal involvement and is characterized by arthropathy and tendinitis.[515] Sixty percent of untreated patients develop involvement of large joints, with the knee being most often involved.[269,515] Joint effusions are typically large and out of proportion to a patient's complaints.[324,515] Faller et al[150] reported on 10 patients with subtalar and first MTP joint pain, tendinitis, heel pain syndrome, and dysesthesias on the plantar aspect of the foot. Symptoms were present for 6 weeks to 6 years after the alleged Lyme infections, and symptoms in many patients had been misdiagnosed and treated with other modalities. Lawson and Steere[325] reported stage III developing within an average of 5 months after a tick bite (range, 1 to 32 months). If untreated initially, more than half the patients develop musculoskeletal symptoms within 2 years. Joint symptoms are often transient yet recurrent. Over time, recurrences tend to occur less often and attacks tend to be shorter.[324] Chronic arthritis develops in 10% of patients with Lyme disease,[324] and approximately 60% of untreated patients develop an intermittent arthritis.[271] Findings consistent with inflammatory arthritis are typical of the chronic stages of Lyme disease. Prolonged joint synovitis can lead to juxtaarticular osteoporosis, chondrolysis, and cortical or marginal erosions. With chronic arthritis, chondrolysis, subchondral sclerosis, juxtaarticular osteoporosis, bone erosion, and osteophyte formation can occur.[310]

Diagnosis

Lyme disease is best diagnosed by recognition of characteristic history and physical examination findings and then confirmed by serologic testing. Unfortunately, many patients do not recall a tick bite because of the tick's small size, but they may report a rash or flulike illness during the summer months,[325,515] which can indicate Lyme disease. Joint involvement may be the initial symptom and is noted by approximately one third of those infected.

Presentation of Lyme disease in this tertiary stage can mimic many other problems, including metatarsalgia and interdigital neuroma. Dennis[127] and Lawrence[324] note that there are many similarities between Lyme disease and syphilis (both of which are caused by spirochete infection). Lyme disease has been called "the great imitator" because it is difficult to diagnose clinically and is often confused with other diagnoses, including septic arthritis, juvenile arthritis in younger patients, or inflammatory arthritis in older patients. A high level of suspicion is necessary to make the correct diagnosis, which is confirmed by laboratory tests.

Once appropriate history and physical examination findings have been obtained, confirmatory, serologic testing for Lyme disease should follow a two-tiered approach.[60,515] Enzyme-linked immunosorbent assay (ELISA) is used first to screen suspected patient samples. ELISA is sensitive but not specific for Lyme antibodies and may produce false-positive results. Positive or equivocal results can then be further evaluated with Western blot analysis, which is more specific.[60,515]

Synovial fluid testing is usually not helpful because spirochetes are not readily cultured or visualized, and white blood cells may be markedly elevated, as in acute bacterial septic arthritis. Nonspecific markers of inflammation, such as erythrocyte sedimentation rate and C-reactive protein levels, may also be elevated. Polymerase chain reaction (PCR) can be done on synovial fluid to amplify and detect *Borrelia* deoxyribonucleic acid (DNA); however, serology should be regarded as the mainstay of diagnosis after appropriate history and examination findings are obtained.

Treatment (Table 19-1)

Antibiotic treatment is preferred regardless of the stage of infection. Conventional antibiotic treatment for 4 to 8 weeks is associated with clinical improvement of symptoms in most patients and with a decrease in antibody titers.[150,530,595] Early diagnosis and treatment can limit symptoms. A high index of suspicion for patients in endemic areas or who have traveled in endemic areas aids in the early diagnosis and the institution of antibiotic treatment.

For Lyme arthritis (stage III disease), current recommended treatment is doxycycline 100 mg twice daily or amoxicillin 500 mg three times a day for 28 days (Fig. 19-94).[530,595] A second round of oral therapy or intravenous therapy is recommended for persistent arthritis. If joint symptoms persist after two rounds of antibiotic therapy, arthroscopic synovectomy may be necessary.[530,595]

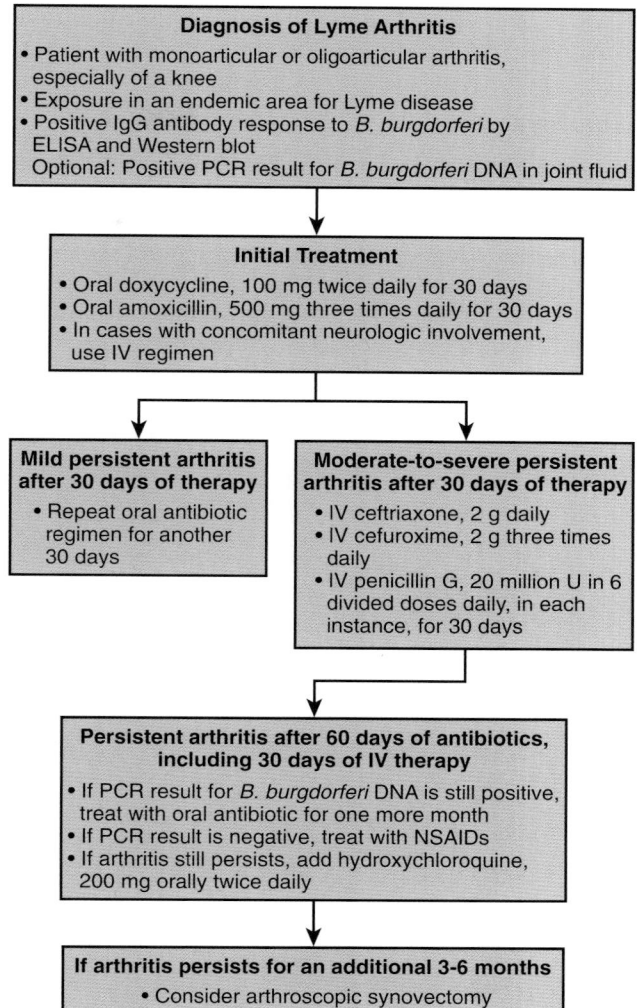

Figure 19-94 Treatment algorithm for Lyme arthritis. *B. burgdorferi, Borrelia burgdorferi;* DNA, deoxyribonucleic acid; *ELISA,* enzyme-linked immunosorbent assay; *IgG,* immunoglobulin G; *IV,* intravenous; *NSAIDs,* nonsteroidal antiinflammatory drugs; *PCR,* polymerase chain reaction. (From Steere AC, Angelis SM: Therapy for Lyme arthritis: strategies for the treatment of antibiotic-refractory arthritis. *Arthritis Rheum* 54:3079–3086, 2006).

Table 19-1	Treatment of Lyme Disease		
Stage	**Serology**	**Laboratory Data**	**Antibiotic Regimen***
I	Usually negative	Sedimentation rate 40-60 mL/hr	Doxycycline 100 mg bid or tid × 2-3 wk Amoxicillin 500-1000 mg qid × 2-3 wk
II	Usually positive		Ceftriaxone 2 g/day × 2 wk Penicillin G 20 million U qd/6 doses × 3 wk
III	Usually positive		Ceftriaxone 2 g qd × 2 wk Penicillin G 20 million U qd/6 doses × 3 wk

Modified from Lawrence S: Lyme disease: an orthopedic perspective, *Orthopaedics* 15:1331–1335, 1992.
*Erythromycin, 250-500 mg qid for 2 to 3 weeks, may be given to patients with allergies to penicillin or cephalosporins; however, this treatment might not be as effective.

NSAIDs may be of some benefit in treating joint symptoms.[60,529,595]

Fibromyalgia

The term *fibromyalgia* was coined by Hench[232] in 1976 to describe generalized musculoskeletal pain associated with a large number of localized areas that were tender to palpation. Fatigue and sleep disorders were associated with the condition as well.[225] Localized areas of tenderness (tender points) are reproducible on repeated examination[591] (Fig. 19-95), and 11 of 18 positive points must be elicited to diagnose fibromyalgia (see Table 19-2).

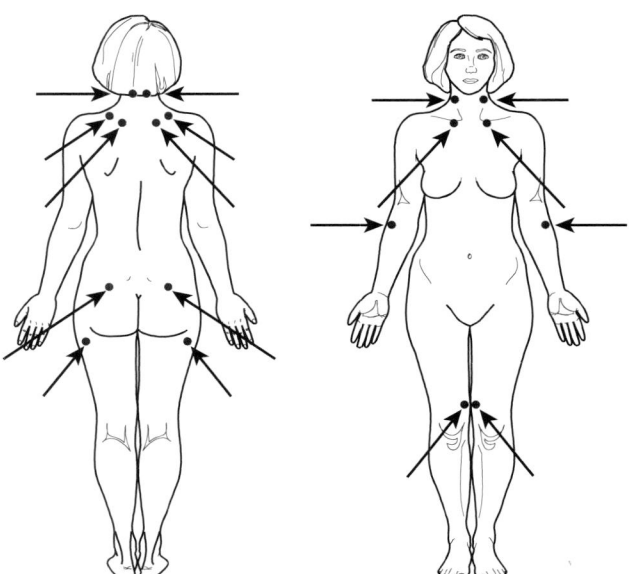

Figure 19-95 Tender points for diagnosis of fibromyalgia. Figure depicts the 18 tender points of fibromyalgia. At least 11 of these 18 points must be elicited on physical examination to establish the diagnosis of fibromyalgia.

Table 19-2	Tender Points Associated with Fibromyalgia
Location*	**Tender Points**
Knee	Medial fat pad proximal to joint line
Greater trochanter	Lateral hip region
Gluteal region	Upper outer aspect of buttocks
Lateral epicondyle	Slightly distal to epicondyle
Costochondral junction	Second costochondral junction
Supraspinatus muscle	Proximal medial border of scapular spine
Trapezius muscle	Upper border of trapezius
Lower cervical region	C5-C7 region
Occiput	Suboccipital muscle insertion

Modified from Wolfe F, Smythe H, Yunus M, et al: The American College of Rheumatology 1990 Criteria for the Classification of Fibromyalgia. Report of the Multicenter Criteria Committee, *Arthritis Rheum* 33:160–172, 1990. Copyright American College of Rheumatology.
*Each location can have bilateral involvement, for a total of 18 specific areas.

Sleep disorders include insomnia, difficulty remaining asleep, or wakening unrefreshed after sleeping.[384] Laboratory tests and radiographic evaluation do not play a role in the diagnosis of fibromyalgia but are important in ruling out other disorders, such as hypothyroidism, polymyalgia rheumatica, rheumatoid arthritis, polymyositis, SLE, metabolic myopathy, metastatic cancer, neurosis, and chronic fatigue syndrome.[31,232] Goldenberg[189] has estimated that 3 to 6 million Americans carry the diagnosis of fibromyalgia, a majority being women. The diagnosis is one of exclusion.

Fibromyalgia is unresponsive to steroids and NSAIDs alike.[31] Bennett[32] has recommended aerobic exercise as therapeutic, although fatigue and pain tend to restrict activity. Antidepressants may be helpful, as is the supportive concern of the treating physician. Many patients are relieved to receive a "diagnosis," but this obviously does not treat the symptoms. Fibromyalgia is described as a *pain syndrome* and *is not* an arthritic condition. The treating physician must differentiate it from the pain of an underlying arthritic condition.

Other symptoms often associated with fibromyalgia include the Raynaud phenomenon, headache, morning stiffness, paresthesias, depression, and anxiety. Dierick et al[132] showed that young (<30 years) and middle-aged (30-60 years) women with fibromyalgia had significantly increased stiffness in their ankles compared with healthy control subjects. Gonzalez et al[190] found that women with fibromyalgia had more pain than control subjects after knee arthroscopy.

Recognition of fibromyalgia as an entity is important because the treating physician should include it in the differential diagnosis of metatarsalgia and other areas of pain and discomfort in the foot. Although the presence of this chronic pain syndrome in other areas does not preclude surgical intervention in the area of the foot and ankle, it is unlikely that generalized foot and ankle discomfort will be relieved by surgical intervention. A frank preoperative discussion with the patient with fibromyalgia in whom foot and ankle surgery is contemplated is important regarding patient expectations and the possibility of continued pain after surgery.

Juvenile Idiopathic Arthritis

Juvenile idiopathic arthritis (JIA) refers to all forms of arthritis with onset before age 16 years.[453] Previously used terms, such as juvenile rheumatoid arthritis and juvenile psoriatic arthritis, are falling out of favor because they incorrectly suggest that that the diseases are single entities categorized by phenotypic variants.[442] Seven subtypes of disease have been established by the International League of Associations for Rheumatology based on common clinical and laboratory features.[438] Well-defined subtypes include systemic juvenile idiopathic arthritis, rheumatoid factor–positive polyarthritis, and enthesitis-related arthritis.[442] Other subtypes are less homogenous and are still being defined, suggesting the need for further investigation.[442,454]

Foot and ankle problems are common in patients with JIA. Rheumatoid factor–positive polyarthritis is thought to be much the same as adult rheumatoid arthritis and is mainly seen in adolescent girls. It usually manifests as a symmetric, polyarthritis that mainly affects the small joints of the hands and feet. Larger joints, such as ankles and knees, are also affected but usually in connection with smaller joints.[438]

Enthesitis-related arthritis is mostly seen in boys after age 6 years, and most are HLA-B27 positive. The enthesitis most commonly affects the Achilles tendon and plantar fascial insertions on the calcaneus. Associated arthritis usually affects the joints of the lower extremities.[453]

Most of the problems encountered with these patients can be treated nonoperatively. As with adult arthropathies, NSAIDS continue to play an important role in the treatment of JIA.[442,453] Intraarticular steroid injections with triamcinolone hexacetonide are frequently used to help prevent joint deformities throughout the disease course.[442,453] Systemic steroids should generally be avoided in children because of serious side effects, except for cases of systemic juvenile idiopathic arthritis that are refractory to NSAID therapy.[453]

Methotrexate has become an important second-line therapy for persistent arthritis because of its effectiveness and acceptable side effects.[453] Anti-TNF drugs have shown effectiveness against polyarticular arthritis and newer anti–interleukin-6 and anti–interleukin-1 antibody drugs have shown promising results against the systemic juvenile idiopathic arthritis.[442] More treatments may be on the horizon for JIA as genetic studies continue to define the disease and ongoing clinical trials show promising results.[442]

DEGENERATIVE ARTHRITIS OF THE INTERPHALANGEAL JOINT

Degenerative arthritis of the interphalangeal joint of the hallux can result from trauma, after arthrodesis of the MTP joint,[161] or from inflammatory arthritis (rheumatoid arthritis, psoriatic arthritis, gout). Clawing of the toe can occur as a result of contracture of the flexor hallucis longus (FHL) tendon and can lead to a fixed plantar-flexion deformity.

Conservative treatment options include an extra-depth shoe, a foam sleeve that pads both the tip of the toe and the DIP joint region, or an excavated insole to decrease pressure at the tip of the hallux. With a fixed contracture or intractable IP joint pain, arthrodesis of the IP joint of the hallux is indicated (Fig. 19-96).

The arthrodesis is performed through a dorsal L-shaped or elliptic incision. The joint surface is excised and the arthrodesis fixed with a small-fragment cancellous screw inserted at the tip of the hallux (Fig. 19-97A-C). One or two K-wires or Steinmann pins may be added to control rotation.[512] Shives and Johnson[513] reported an overall

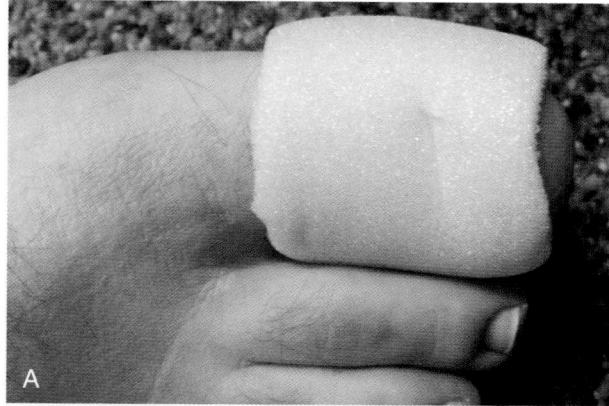

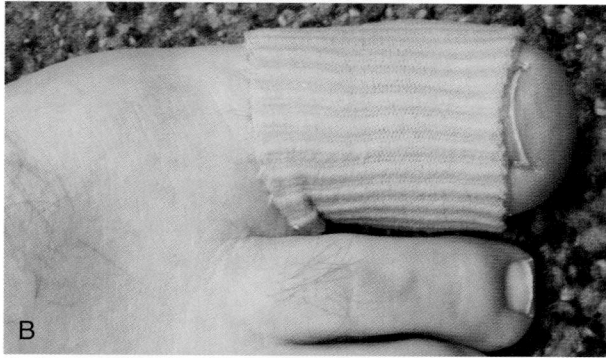

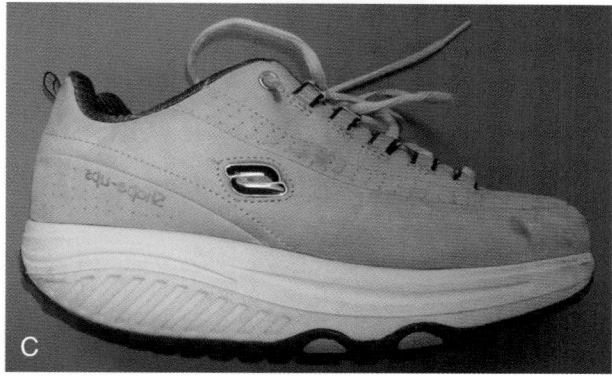

Figure 19-96 Conservative treatment of hallux rigidus. **A** and **B,** Two types of foam sleeves to wear in shoes. **C,** Rocker-soled shoe to allow more normal gait with arthritic foot and ankle.

pseudarthrosis rate of 44% with the use of only crossed K-wires for IP joint fusion. With a compression arthrodesis technique, the pseudarthrosis rate was reduced to 10% (Fig. 19-97D-F and Video Clip 63). Mizel et al[389] reported on seven patients who underwent simultaneous IP and MTP joint arthrodeses for severe arthritic rigid deformities of both joints. Using an extensile incision, the authors arthrodesed both joints and reported improved function, substantial pain relief, and successful fusion in all seven patients. Other alternatives to consider are a debridement or cheilectomy of the hallucial IP joint (Fig. 19-98), and on occasion, IP joint disarticulation (Fig. 19-99).

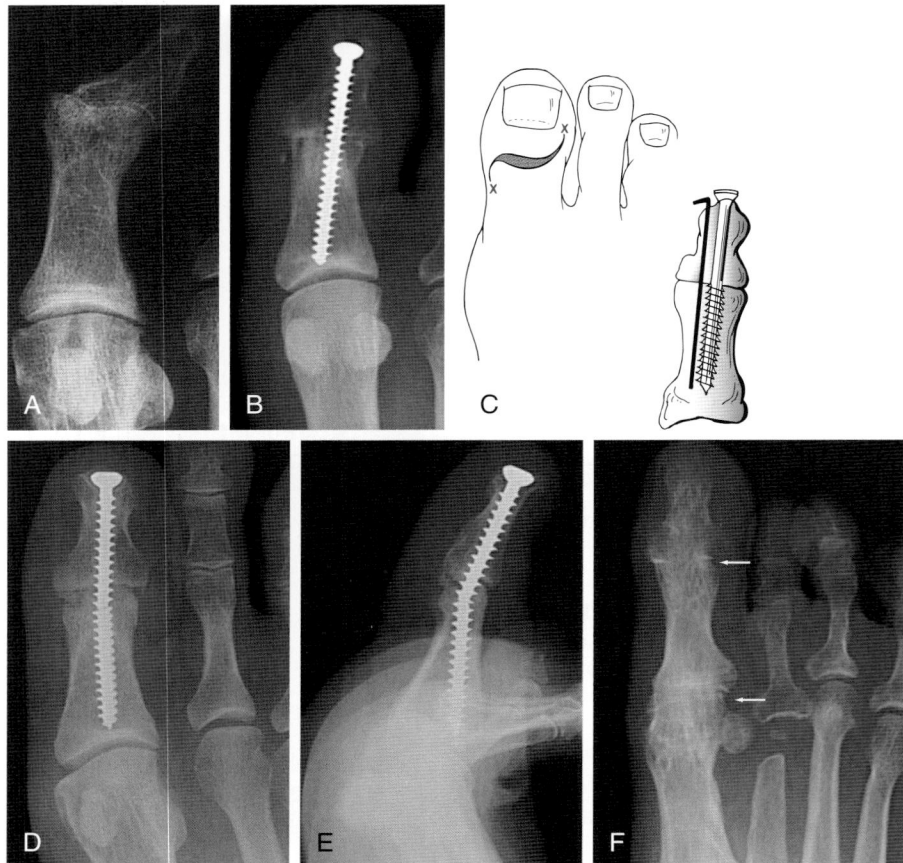

Figure 19-97   **A,** Preoperative radiograph demonstrates degenerative arthritis of interphalangeal joint. **B** and **C,** Arthrodesis after compression-screw fixation. Anteroposterior **(D)** and lateral **(E)** radiographs demonstrate failure of fixation and pseudoarthrosis after arthrodesis of the interphalangeal joint. **F,** Successful fusion of metatarsophalangeal and interphalangeal joint for degenerative arthritis.

Degenerative arthritis of the metatarsophalangeal joints of the lesser toes can occur after trauma but also may be associated with a Freiberg infraction (Figs. 19-100 and 19-101). Degenerative arthritis of the IP joints of the lesser toes may be treated with arthrodesis or excisional arthroplasty (see Chapter 7 for treatment of hammer toe deformities).

HALLUX RIGIDUS

Definition

The term *hallux rigidus* describes a painful condition of the MTP joint of the great toe characterized by restricted motion (mainly dorsiflexion) and proliferative periarticular bone formation. It was initially reported in 1887 by Davies-Colley,[122] who described a plantar-flexed position of the proximal phalanx in relationship to the first metatarsal head and proposed the name *hallux flexus.* A few months later, Cotterill[99] reported on the same condition but coined the term *hallux rigidus.* Other terms, such as *hallux limitus, dorsal bunion, hallux dolorosus, hallux malleus, and metatarsus primus elevatus* (MPE), have been

advocated.[283] The terms *hallux rigidus* and *hallux limitus* are used interchangeably, although, to some, *hallux limitus* is distinguished by a decrease in dorsiflexion, whereas hallux rigidus describes an absence of motion.[180] DuVries[140] in 1959 and Moberg[390] observed that other than hallux valgus, hallux rigidus is the most common condition to affect the first MTP joint and may be even more disabling than hallux valgus because of the limitations on ambulation that occur in more severe cases. Gould et al[195] stated that 1 in 40 patients older than 50 years develop hallux rigidus.

Incidence

Hallux rigidus was divided into two distinct age groups by Nilsonne[415]: an adolescent and an adult type. Nilsonne[415] hypothesized that hallux rigidus in the adolescent was a primary deformity, whereas in the adult, hallux rigidus was a secondary deformity resulting from the development of degenerative arthritis. Bingold and Collins[47] suggested that the two entities were merely a continuum of the same degenerative process. Goodfellow[191] reported on three patients who demonstrated classic findings

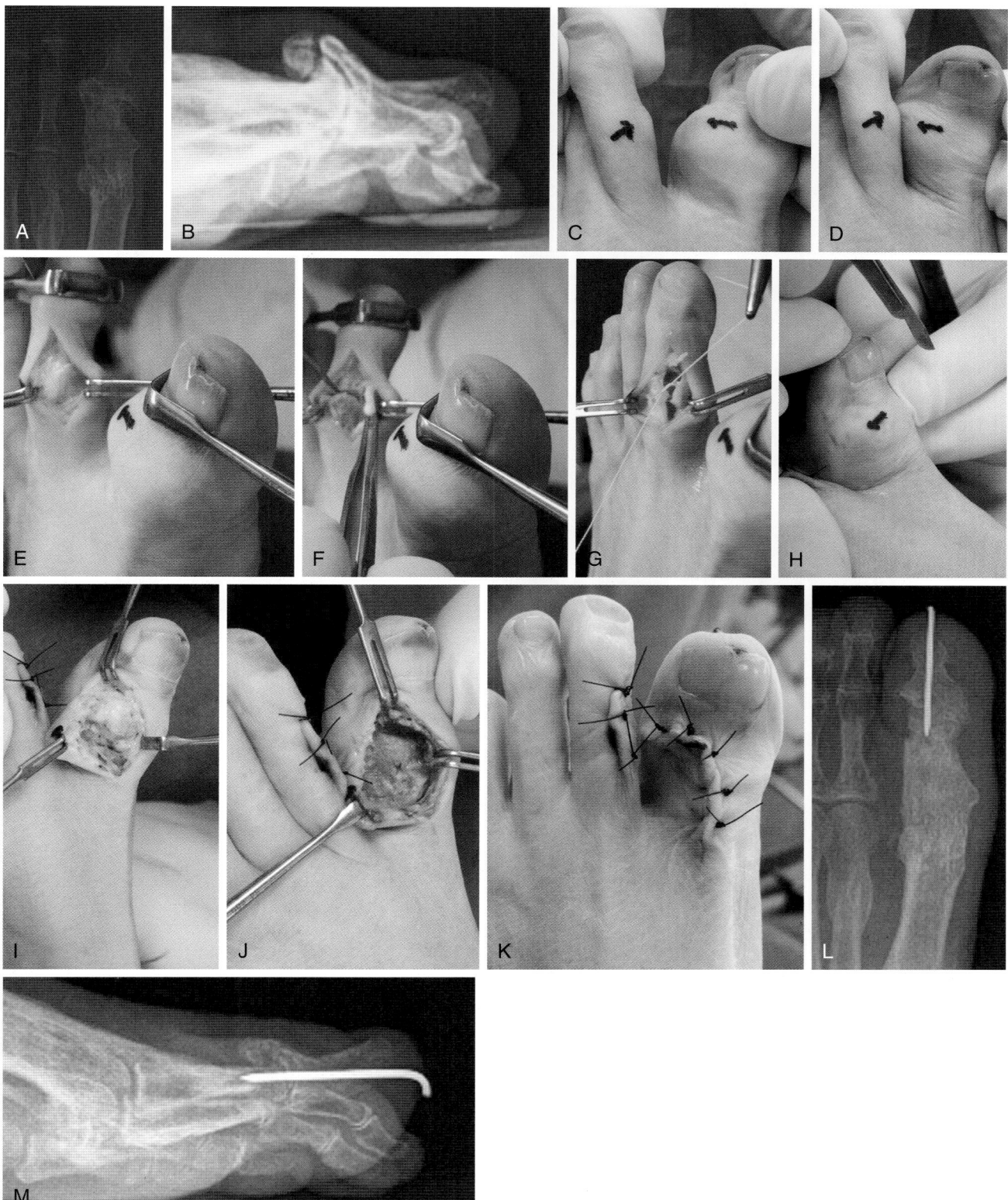

Figure 19-98 Cheilectomy of interphalangeal (IP) joint after metatarsophalangeal arthrodesis. Anteroposterior (AP) **(A)** and lateral **(B)** radiographs demonstrating severe degenerative arthritis of the IP joint of the hallux. **C** and **D,** Note "kissing exostoses" between the lateral hallux and medial second toe. **E,** Incision. **F,** Exostectomy of proximal interphalangeal joint of the second toe. **G,** Closure of capsule after exostecotmy. **H,** Exostosis of medial IP joint of the hallux. **I,** Incision. **J,** Exostectomy. **K,** Closure of wound. **L** and **M,** AP and lateral radiographs demonstrating digit after exostectomy and temporary K-wire fixation.

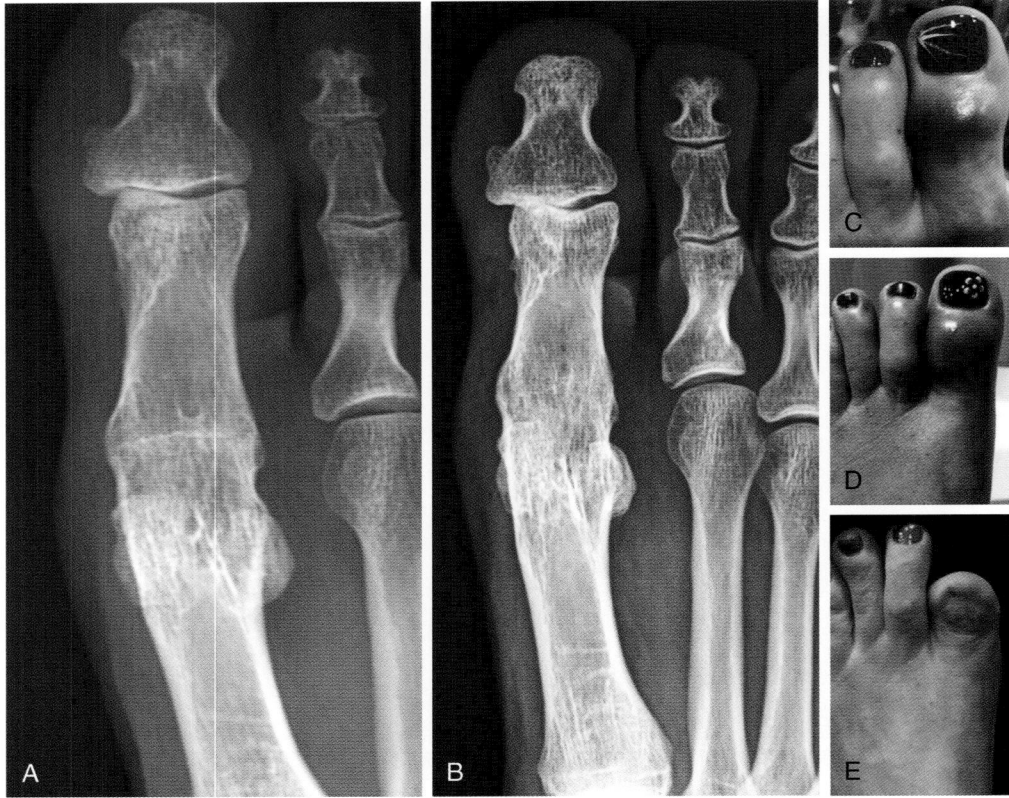

Figure 19-99 Arthritis of the interphalangeal (IP) joint of the hallux after metatarsophalangeal (MTP) arthrodesis performed 10 years earlier. **A,** Degenerative arthritis of the IP joint (note MTP fusion). **B,** Progression of painful IP joint arthritis. **C,** Swollen IP joint. **D,** More severe swelling associated with IP joint arthritis. **E,** After IP joint disarticulation.

of osteochondritis dissecans of the metatarsal articular surface, and McMaster[373] described seven patients with similar findings. Coughlin and Shurnas[110] found no evidence to support a requirement for a distinction or classification based on age.

Although Gould[194] and Nilsonne[415] suggested that hallux rigidus typically is characterized by bilateral involvement, studies reporting results of surgery have emphasized mainly unilateral involvement. However, if follow-up is continued for a long enough period, 80% or more of patients can be expected to have bilateral symptoms.[110]

Gould[194] reported a higher male involvement in those older than 30 years with complaints of hallux rigidus, but in those undergoing surgical repair, most studies have reported an overwhelmingly higher incidence of female involvement.*

Bonney and MacNab[51] also noted that in those with onset in teenage years, there was a 50% incidence of a family history. Coughlin and Shurnas[110] found in their series of patients with hallux rigidus that nearly 95% of patients with a positive family history of great toe problems had bilateral hallux rigidus and that nearly 80% of

all patients with hallux rigidus had a positive family history.

Signs and Symptoms

Although initially hallux rigidus is characterized by pain, swelling, and MTP synovitis, restricted dorsiflexion is a classic finding. As the degenerative process proceeds, proliferation of bony osteophytes on the dorsal and dorsolateral aspect of the first metatarsal head develop, creating a prominent bony ledge against which the proximal phalanx abuts (Fig. 19-102A). A substantial amount of new bone occasionally forms along the medial border of the first MTP joint. Hallux valgus is uncommon with hallux rigidus.

With time and further osteophyte formation, increased bulk around the MTP joint can lead to significant discomfort with constricting footwear (Fig. 19-102B). However, the joint space often remains reasonably well preserved despite the narrowed appearance on the AP view, as verified on the oblique radiograph (Fig. 19-102C). With enlargement of the dorsal exostosis of the first metatarsal head, the proximal phalanx can become positioned in plantar flexion with limitation of dorsiflexion, the condition for which the term *hallux flexus* was coined. With

*References 100, 109, 352, 353, 355, 356, 358, and 359.

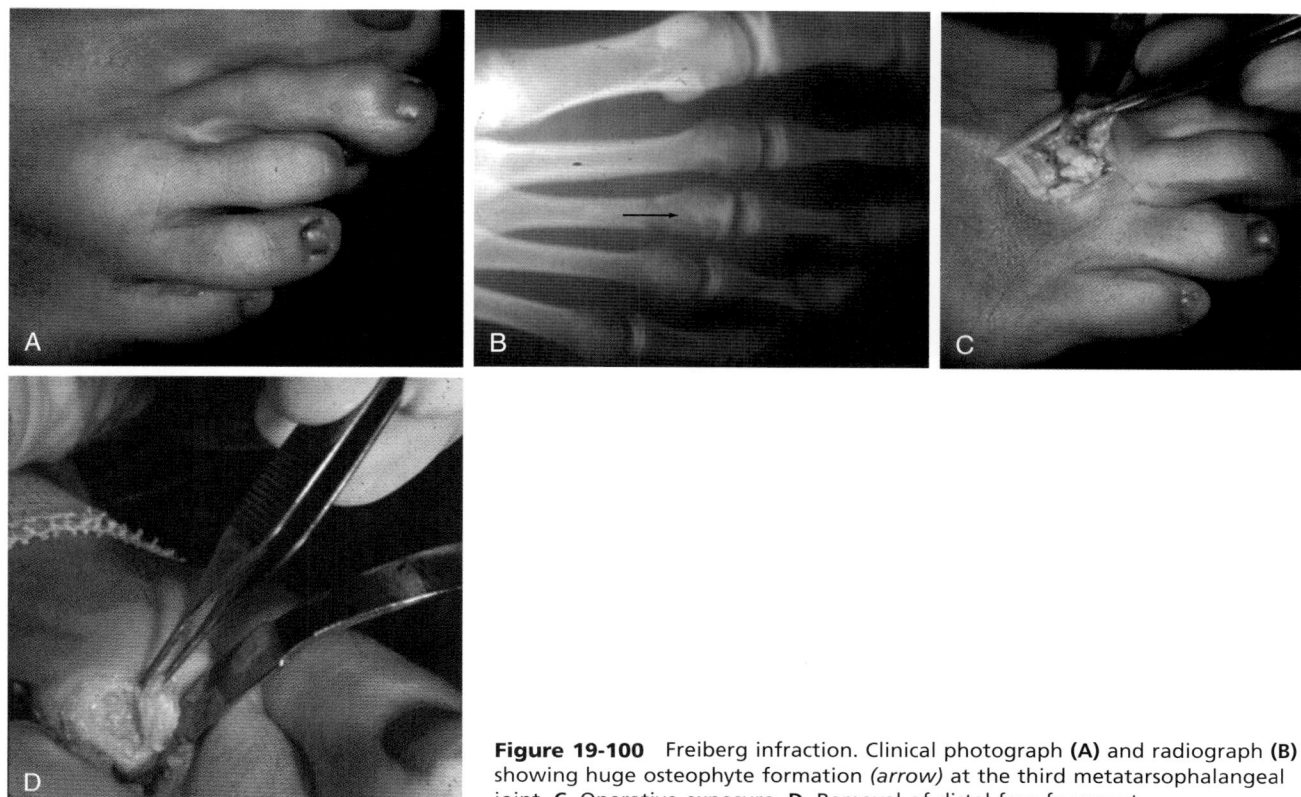

Figure 19-100 Freiberg infraction. Clinical photograph **(A)** and radiograph **(B)** showing huge osteophyte formation *(arrow)* at the third metatarsophalangeal joint. **C,** Operative exposure. **D,** Removal of distal free fragment.

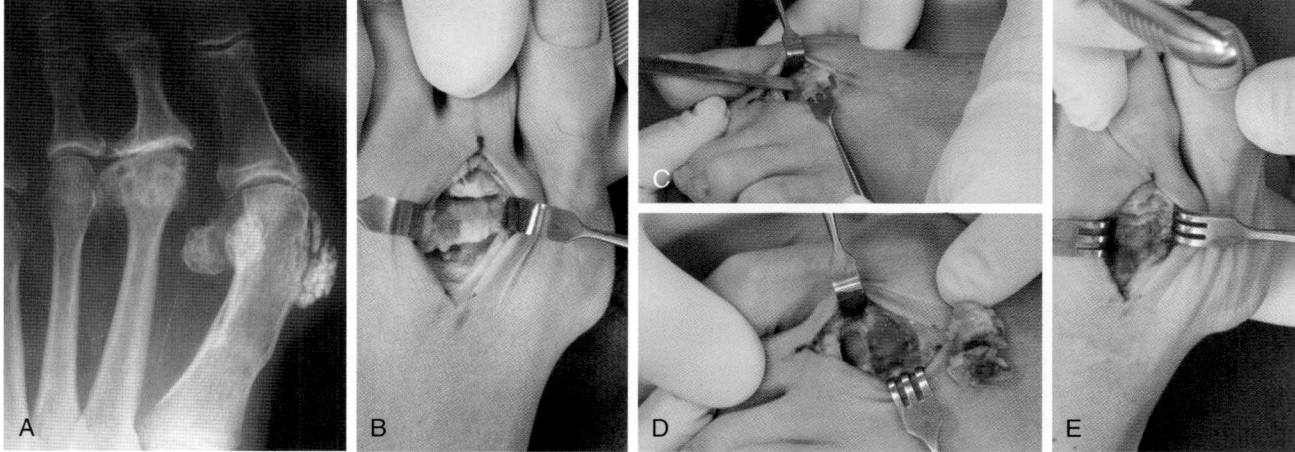

Figure 19-101 Severe degenerative arthritis of the second toe metatarsophalangeal (MTP) joint **A,** Severe degenerative joint disease (DJD) of second MTP joint, with signs of gout and DJD at hallux MTP joint. **B,** Dorsal view of operative exposure. metatarsophalangeal **C,** Proposed dorsal cheilectomy of second metatarsal head. **D,** and **E,** After cheilectomy of dorsal metatarsal head and **E,** base of proximal phalanx.

severe deformity, almost complete bony ankylosis can occur.

In adults with hallux rigidus, the basic pathologic entity is that of degenerative arthritis.[51] Mann and Clanton[351] noted that with increasing age increasing degenerative arthritis occurs. The classic location of the cartilage loss is on the dorsal half to two thirds of the metatarsal head,[228,390] often at a site between the apex of the articular surface and the dorsal margin of the proximal phalanx.

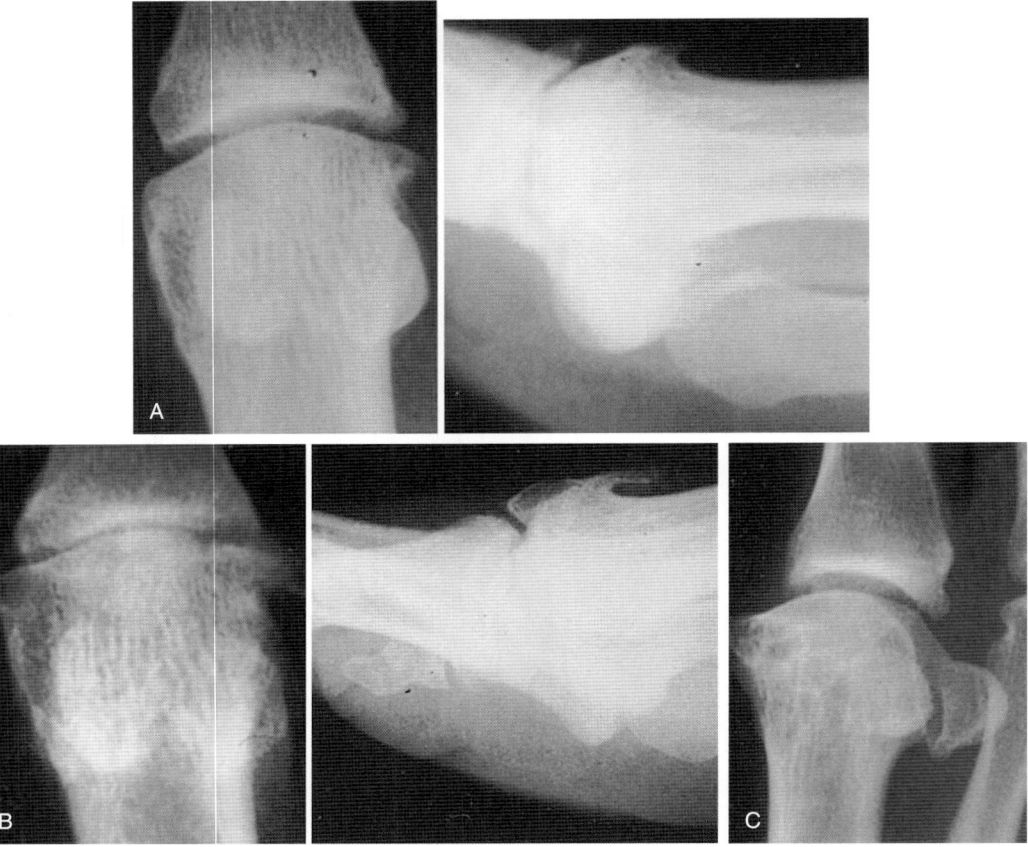

Figure 19-102 **A,** Anteroposterior (AP) and lateral radiographs demonstrate grade 1 hallux rigidus deformity. **B,** Over 10 years, significant progression of disease occurred, resulting in a grade 2 hallux rigidus deformity. **C,** Oblique radiograph demonstrates adequate joint space present, although the AP radiograph did not show an adequate joint space because of overhanging.

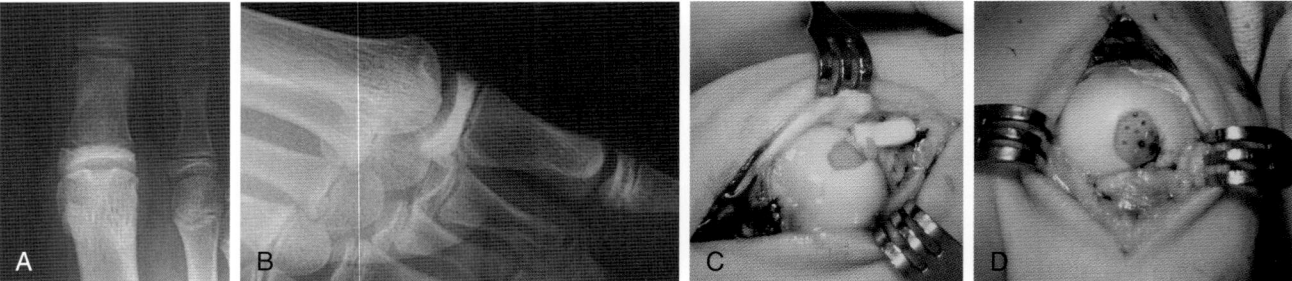

Figure 19-103 **A** and **B,** Radiographs demonstrate juvenile hallux rigidus secondary to osteochondral defect of the metatarsal head. **C** and **D,** Intraoperative photographs demonstrate osteochondral lesion. Loose fragment has been removed. The lesion was debrided and its base drilled.

Etiology

The cause of hallux rigidus or hallux limitus has not been determined, although several predisposing factors have been cited. The most common cause cited is trauma, which can occur as a single episode, such as an intraarticular fracture or crush injury, but hallux rigidus can occur with repetitive microtrauma as well. In a patient who sustains an acute injury to the MTP joint, forced hyperextension[103] or forced plantar flexion[92] can create compressive forces through jamming of the toe, with development of an acute chondral or osteochondral injury. What may begin as an acute sprain or turf toe can evolve into chronic discomfort.

An osseous injury can be diagnosed with radiographs, but with a cartilaginous injury, a diagnosis can only be made by physical examination and a high clinical index of suspicion of an intraarticular injury (Fig. 19-103A-D). A clear traumatic episode is most likely the cause of

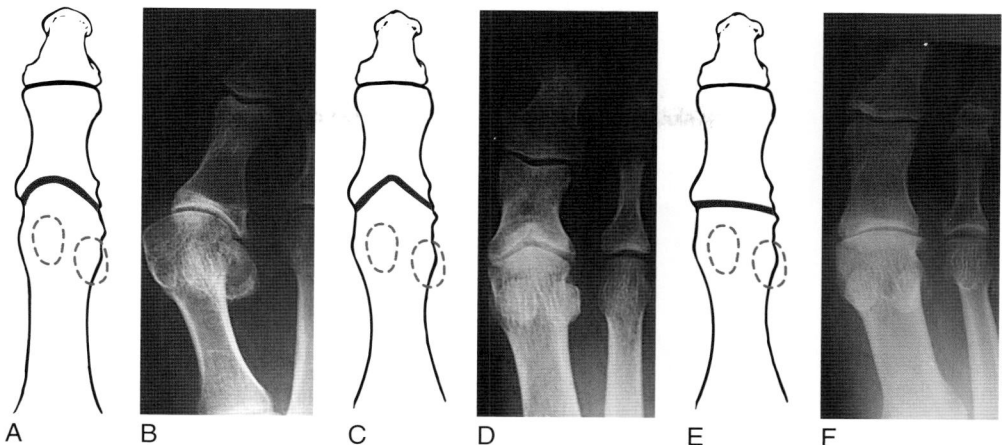

Figure 19-104 Variations in the shape of the first metatarsal articular surface, with diagrams and radiographs. **A** and **B,** Oval shape can allow valgus position to occur. Chevron surface (**C** and **D**) and flat surface (**E** and **F**) resist lateral pressure on the hallux. Although hallux valgus is uncommon, traumatic osteoarthritis can develop, resulting in hallux rigidus.

unilateral hallux rigidus, based on long-term follow-up.[110] In the adolescent patient with hallux rigidus, an osteochondral defect is often identified on radiographic examination or can be verified by MRI.[191,217,288,373,504]

Other suggested causes of hallux rigidus include a congenital flattened or squared metatarsal head,[140] a long first metatarsal, a short first metatarsal,[136,252,354] tight intrinsic muscles,[138] pes planus or hindfoot pronation, and a congruent MTP joint[140,196] (Fig. 19-104). Although investigators have hypothesized that these factors play a major role in the development of hallux rigidus, other than for osteochondritis, the only documented factors associated with the cause of hallux rigidus are a flat or chevron-shaped joint, hallux valgus interphalangeus, metatarsus adductus, bilaterality in those with a positive family history, trauma in unilateral cases, and female gender.[110,111] There have been no proven associations with first-ray mobility, metatarsal length, Achilles or gastrocnemius contracture, any type of abnormal foot posture, hallux valgus, adolescent onset, footwear, occupation, or metatarsus primus elevatus.[110,111]

The length of the proximal phalanx and first metatarsal has been implicated in the etiology of hallux rigidus.[67] Calvo et al[67] measured a series of 132 feet with hallux rigidus and concluded the length of the proximal phalanx was not associated with hallux rigidus; however, they suggested a long first metatarsal was a factor in development of first MTP joint arthritis. Coughlin and Shurnas[110] concluded a long first metatarsal (compared with the adjacent second metatarsal) was no more common in cases of hallux rigidus. Zgonis et al[609] reported similar findings in studying a control group and those with hallux rigidus, noting that the mean length of the first metatarsal was shorter than the adjacent second metatarsal, and concluded excess length was not an etiologic factor in development of hallux rigidus.

One of the more controversial areas regarding etiology is the condition known as *metatarsus primus elevatus* (Fig. 19-105), which describes a dorsal elevation of the first metatarsal in relationship to the lesser metatarsals. Although Lambrinudi[316] in 1938 and Jack[252] in 1940 initially called attention to hyperextension of the first ray, Root et al[477] advanced a popularly accepted concept that hypermobility of the first ray "is the most frequent cause of hallux limitus." Numerous other authors have supported the notion that an elevated first metatarsal is causally related to hallux rigidus or hallux limitus, but others[241,378] dispute the relevance of this claim.

Bingold and Collins[47] and others[136,477] have distinguished between a structural (fixed) and a functional (flexible) elevation of the first metatarsal. Both conditions are believed to lead to restricted dorsiflexion of the first MTP joint, but with a flexible deformity, range of motion is decreased only with weight bearing. A fixed elevation of the first metatarsal is present whether the foot is weight bearing or not. (Examples of a fixed metatarsus primus elevatus deformity are a dorsiflexed malunion of a first metatarsal osteotomy or fracture; a flexible elevation might occur with posterior tibial tendon insufficiency, muscle weakness, spasticity, or paralysis.)

Elevation can occur anywhere along the axis of the first ray (MTC, cuneiform–navicular, or talonavicular joints). As the first metatarsal elevates, the hallux impacts or jams into the dorsal metatarsal articular surface, leading initially to limited or restricted dorsiflexion and eventually to injury to the metatarsal articular surface.[136,477]

Smith[519] and others[75,154,155,477] have implicated subtalar joint pronation as the cause of first-ray hypermobility. Some investigators[241,378] have questioned the frequency and significance of metatarsus primus elevatus in relationship to hallux rigidus, and the current authors think it occurs uncommonly in association with hallux rigidus. Reporting on nine patients, Kessel and Bonney[288] noted two adults with acquired metatarsus primus elevatus after surgery and one patient who developed an elevated first metatarsal after developing MTP joint synovitis. Whether

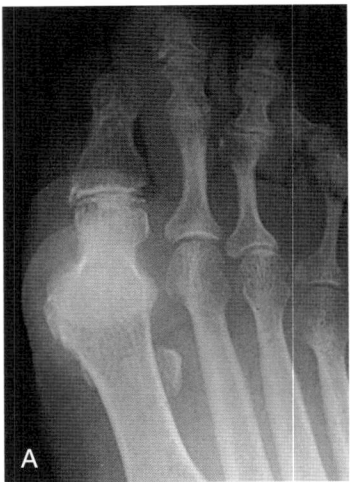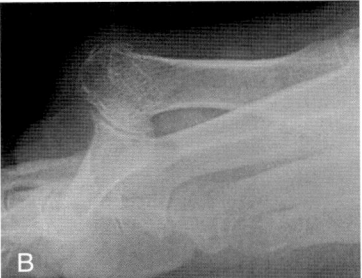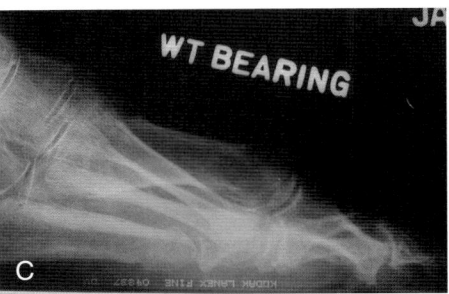

Figure 19-105 Anteroposterior **(A)** and lateral **(B)** radiographs of a severe case of hallux flexus with metatarsus primus elevatus. **C,** Severe postsurgical elevatus.

the primary cause was hallux rigidus or metatarsus primus elevatus was not clear.

Recent studies[112] have evaluated the notion of an elevated first ray in patients with hallux rigidus and demonstrated when elevation was present, it was a secondary phenomenon most likely resulting from a malfunctioning first MTP joint. Elevatus was reduced substantially after cheilectomy or interposition arthroplasty and could be corrected preoperatively or postoperatively to neutral with a dorsiflexion stress test on the first MTP joint. If the first MTP joint was arthrodesed, then postoperative elevation was corrected to almost neutral. This reduction in elevatus was associated with a decrease in first-ray mobility.[110,111] Elevatus is most commonly a secondary change with hallux rigidus and not a primary cause. It is directly related to the severity of the disease and the restriction of MTP joint motion.

From an anatomic standpoint, Meyer et al[378] have stressed that the abnormal measurements associated with metatarsus primus elevatus can result from a combination of the increased dorsoplantar diameter of the first metatarsal, the sesamoid mechanism, and the plantar soft tissue structures, which all tend either to elevate the first metatarsal or to influence the measurement of first metatarsal elevation. Bonney and MacNab[51] and Jack[252] reported that many of their patients had an elevated first ray, but no control groups were included in these studies to suggest a relationship between hallux rigidus and metatarsus primus elevatus.[378] Moberg[390] stated, "I have not seen many adult patients in which metatarsus primus elevatus has been part of the problem." Nonetheless, once metatarsus primus elevatus was implicated as a cause of hallux rigidus, several authors devised or advocated procedures to decrease first-ray elevation.[288,316,373,390]

Meyer et al[378] reported that no statistical correlation existed between hallux rigidus and an elevated first metatarsal. In analyzing lateral weight-bearing radiographs in both normal subjects and patients with hallux rigidus, the

authors reported that two thirds of the subjects had evidence of an elevated first metatarsal greater than 5 mm. Based on this observation, the authors concluded that an elevated first ray may be "perfectly normal during midstance" and that the presence of a radiographically elevated first metatarsal "should no longer be considered a pathologic entity." They further concluded that in a large majority of patients an elevated first metatarsal did not correlate with first MTP joint disease.

Horton and Myerson[241] confirmed the study by Meyer et al, showing no difference in average elevation of the first metatarsal between a control group and those with demonstrated hallux rigidus. Coughlin and Shurnas[110,111] confirmed these findings and, as noted, these authors concluded that elevatus is most likely a secondary finding that follows first MTP joint motion restriction. These same authors suggest that procedures designed to correct elevatus are treating a secondary anatomic finding and not a primary cause of hallux rigidus. Roukis et al,[481,483] in reporting on patients with hallux rigidus treated with shortening and/or plantar-flexion distal first metatarsal osteotomies, observed both a failure to improve MTP joint range of motion as well as a failure to correct metatarsus primus elevatus. This lends support to the notion that MPE is a secondary finding, largely reliant on the underlying MTP joint dorsiflexion range of motion.

History and Physical Examination

A patient with hallux rigidus typically complains of stiffness with ambulation and pain localized to the first MTP joint that is aggravated by walking and standing and relieved by rest. Pain typically is insidious in onset.

Physical examination can reveal a variety of findings, varying from mild synovial thickening early in the disease process to significant bone hypertrophy and osteophyte formation with long-term disease. The classic finding is limitation or absence of passive MTP joint dorsiflexion,[121]

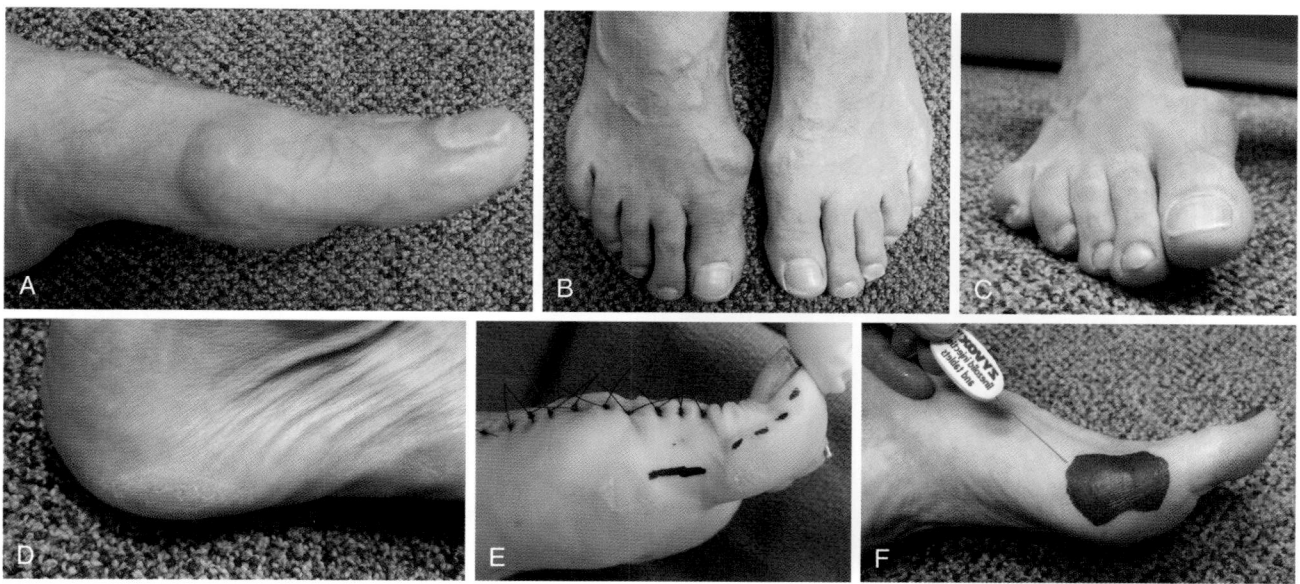

Figure 19-106 Clinical findings of hallux rigidus. **A,** Swollen hallux metatarsophalangeal (MTP) joint. **B,** Note enlarged right great toe MTP joint compared with the left foot. **C,** Everted gait develops because of stiff first MTP joint. **D,** Callus develops on lateral heel because of everted gait. **E,** Hyperextension of hallux interphalangeal joint because of restricted motion at MTP joint. **F,** Numbness develops over medial sensory nerve to the hallux because of pressure from enlarged osteophytes associated with hallux rigidus.

often in the presence of normal or adequate plantar flexion. Interphalangeal joint hyperextension can develop to compensate for restricted MTP joint dorsiflexion[155,194] (Fig. 19-106). A prominent ridge of bone on the dorsal first metatarsal head and the dorsal base of the proximal phalanx is easily palpable (Fig. 19-107). Skin irritation can develop with pressure from footwear over the dorsal exostosis.

On forced dorsiflexion, pain often is elicited with bone impingement between the base of the proximal phalanx and dorsal metatarsal osteophytes. On forced plantar flexion, pain may be elicited from stretching of the EHL, MTP joint capsule, and inflamed synovium over the dorsal osteophyte. With ambulation, the patient often directs weight bearing to the outer aspect of the foot to minimize dorsiflexion of the first MTP joint. Tingling, hyperesthesia, or a positive Tinel sign over the dorsal digital nerve in the first web space can occur from compression against the dorsolateral osteophyte.

Radiographic Evaluation

Standing AP, lateral, and sesamoid radiographs are obtained to evaluate the foot with hallux rigidus (Fig. 19-108A-C). The AP radiograph often demonstrates non-uniform joint space narrowing with widening and flattening of the first metatarsal head (Figs. 19-108D and 19-109). An oblique radiograph can demonstrate an adequate joint space, which is obscured on the AP radiograph by overlying osteophytes. Subchondral cysts and sclerosis in the first metatarsal head, widening of the base of the proximal phalanx, and hypertrophy of the sesamoids can develop in more advanced stages.

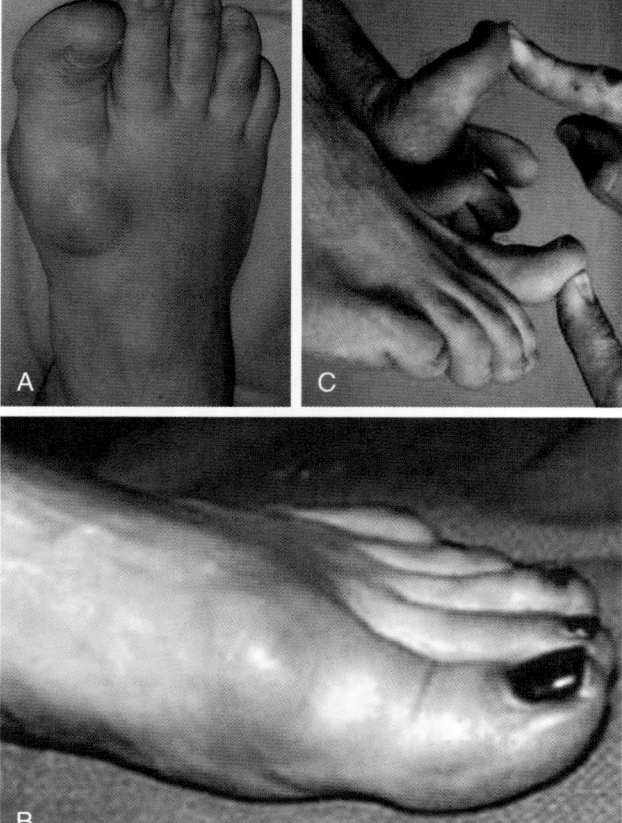

Figure 19-107 First metatarsophalangeal joint of a patient with hallux rigidus. Note increased bulk dorsally **(A)** and medially **(B)**. **C,** There is restricted dorsiflexion compared with the contralateral side.

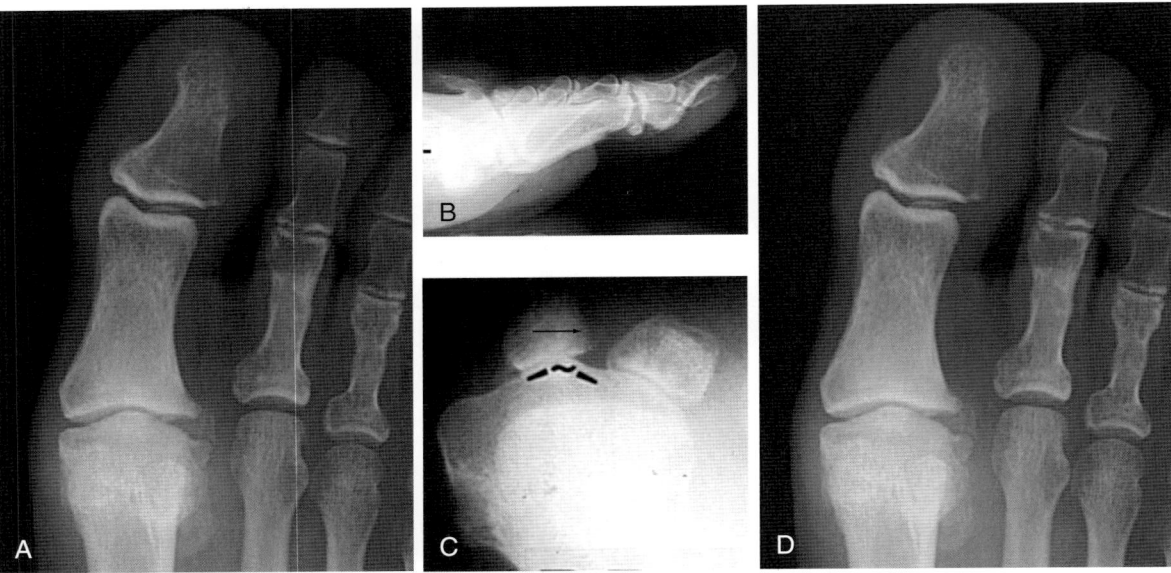

Figure 19-108 Grade II hallux rigidus. **A,** Anteroposterior radiograph. **B,** Lateral radiograph demonstrates a large dorsal osteophyte resembling dripping candle wax. **C,** Axial view demonstrates unusual occurrence of osteoarthritis of the medial sesamoid *(arrow)* associated with hallux valgus. **D,** Nonuniform narrowing of the articular surface of metatarsophalangeal joint. More chondrolysis occurs medially.

Osteophyte formation on the AP radiographs occurs more often on the lateral than the medial aspect of the metatarsal head. An osteochondral defect may be visualized in the central metatarsal articular surface area (see Figs. 19-103 and 19-109). On the lateral radiograph, in advanced cases, the dorsal metatarsal osteophyte can resemble dripping candle wax (Fig. 19-108) as the osteophyte courses proximally along the dorsal first metatarsal metaphyseal shaft. Dorsophalangeal osteophytes and loose bodies may be present, and on a dorsiflexion stress view dorsal impingement may be observed and confirms that extension is blocked.

Lateral weight-bearing radiographs are also used to evaluate the presence of an elevated first metatarsal in relationship to the lesser metatarsals. With a true lateral radiograph, the central diaphyseal axes of the first and second metatarsals are marked. Meyer et al[378] noted that in normal feet, up to 5 mm of elevation is normal (Fig. 19-111).

Evaluation of the metatarsal–sesamoid articulation with axial radiographs is important, although involvement of the sesamoid complex occurs infrequently except with severe arthroses (Fig. 19-108C).

Several different attempts have been made to classify hallux rigidus.[26] A classification scheme is helpful in standardizing terminology both for describing the magnitude of the arthritic process and for recommending treatment. Table 19-3 outlines the recommended clinical and radiographic classification of hallux rigidus based on long-term evaluation and follow-up.

Conservative Treatment

Conservative management of symptomatic hallux rigidus depends on a patient's symptoms and the magnitude of the degenerative process. Early disease (characterized by synovial irritation) is treated with NSAIDs and a stiff insole to reduce excursion of the MTP joint (Fig. 19-110). Several commercially available orthoses provide rigidity to the forepart of the shoe. Orthoses have been shown to provide greater and longer-term pain relief than NSAIDs alone (Fig. 19-113).[553]

An insole with a Morton extension can also reduce MTP range of motion and can be moved from shoe to shoe. The addition of an extended steel or fiberglass shank between the inner and outer sole may be effective in reducing MTP motion. Prefabricated and custom-made orthoses can reduce midfoot pronation, which can reduce symptoms. Unfortunately, many orthoses decrease available room in the toe box, which can increase pressure on the dorsal exostosis. A shoe with a low heel and roomy upper can accommodate the enlarged MTP joint associated with a more advanced hallux rigidus deformity. Taping of the hallux (Fig. 19-114) to decrease dorsiflexion excursion may be effective as well. Symptoms often subside if the first MTP joint is protected.

On occasion, the judicious use of an intraarticular steroid injection provides temporary relief. Repeated injections can accelerate the degenerative process and are discouraged. When symptoms restrict activity, surgical intervention may be considered.

The results of nonoperative treatment have been evaluated. Solan et al[522] noted approximately 6 months of benefit using intraarticular steroid injection and joint manipulation for mild-to-moderate hallux rigidus but found limited benefit for its use in more advanced grades of disease.[522] Pons et al[441] reported on the use of intraarticular sodium hyaluronate in a comparison with intraarticular corticosteroid injections in the treatment of painful

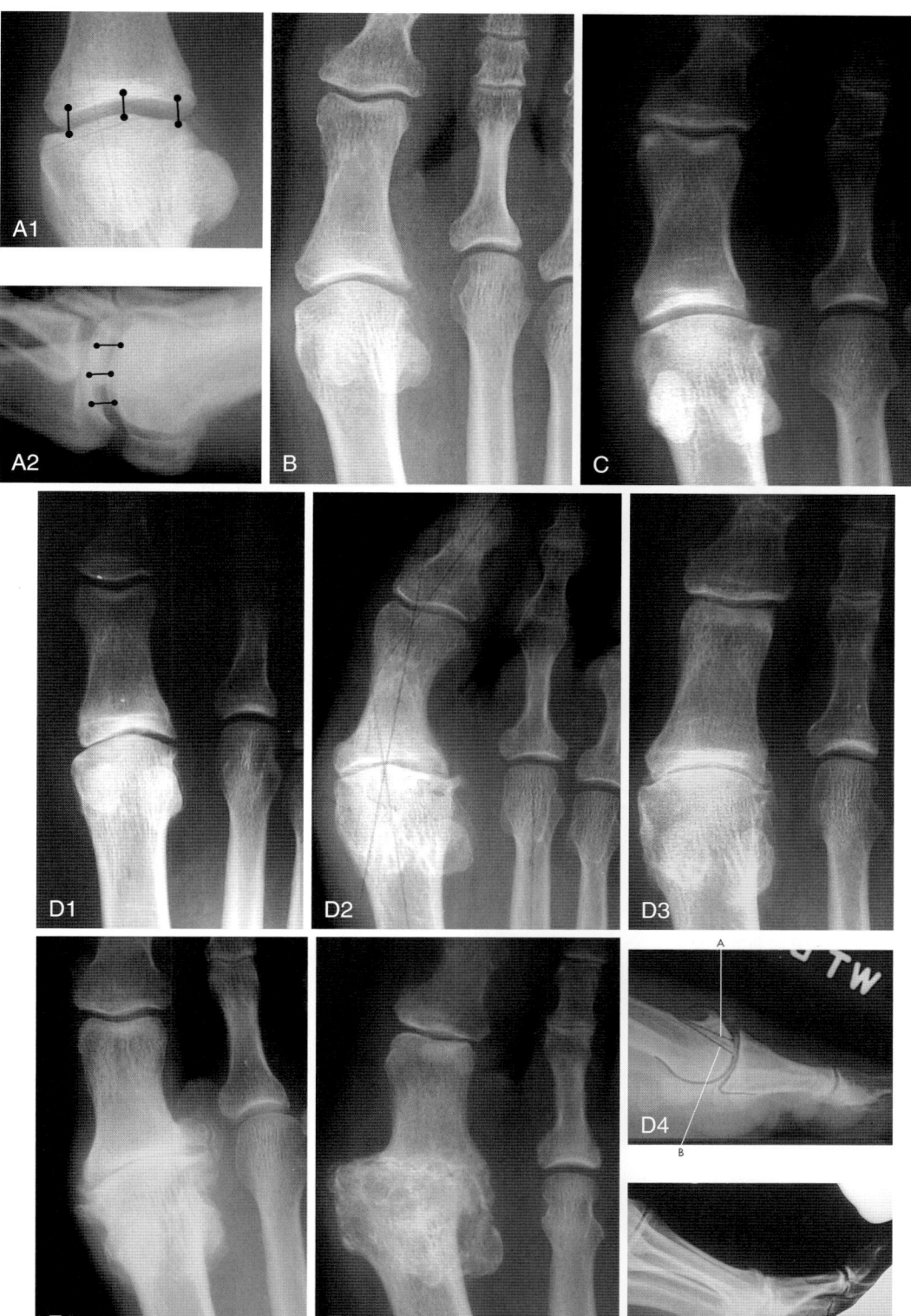

Figure 19-109 Anteroposterior (AP) **(A1)** and lateral **(A2)** radiographs demonstrating the authors' technique of measuring the width of the metatarsophalangeal (MTP) joint space. Marks are made medially, centrally, and laterally along the joint surface on both the AP and lateral radiographs. The distance between the marks is measured with a ruler corrected for magnification. The measurements are averaged and compared with the contralateral side or a normal articular length if there is bilateral disease. In this example, this is grade 0 hallux rigidus; the radiograph demonstrates essentially a normal joint on both AP and lateral views. **B,** Grade 1 hallux rigidus. The radiograph shows mild periarticular osteophyte formation, but notable loss of passive motion is detected clinically. **C,** Grade 2 hallux rigidus with notable increase in periarticular osteophytes. **D1-D3,** Grade 3 hallux rigidus with progressive chondrolysis and osteophyte formation. **D4,** Lateral radiograph shows substantial cartilage space remaining in the joint. Line *A* is a flat cut of the osteophyte, and line *B* demonstrates a more aggressive cheilectomy, which typically results in greater postoperative range of motion. **E1** and **E2,** Grade 4 hallux rigidus with pain in the midrange of motion and substantial or complete chondrolysis of the MTP joint. **E3,** Grade 3 is distinguished clinically from grade 4 by the absence of pain at the midrange of motion, but the two can be identical radiographically.

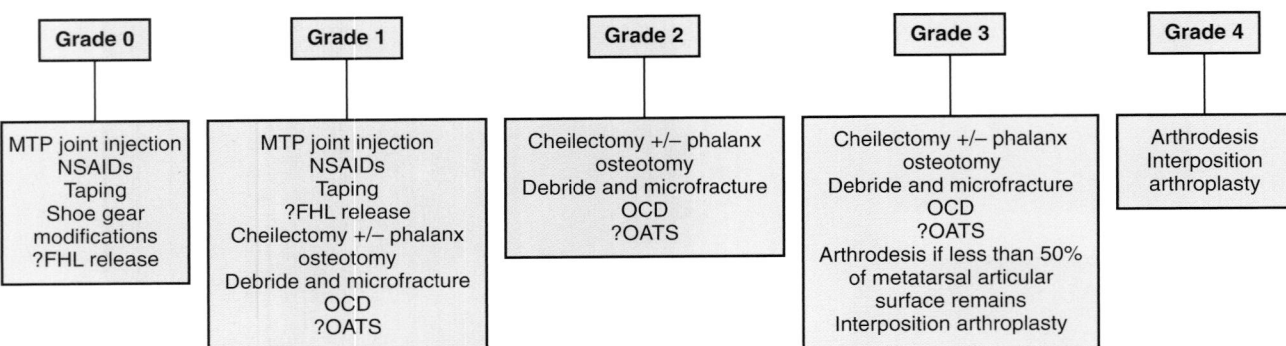

Figure 19-110 Algorithm indicating options for treatment of hallux rigidus. *FHL,* flexor hallucis longus; *MTP,* metatarsophalangeal; *NSAIDs,* nonsteroidal antiinflammatory drugs; *OCD,* osteochondral defects; *OATS,* osteochondral autograft transfer system.

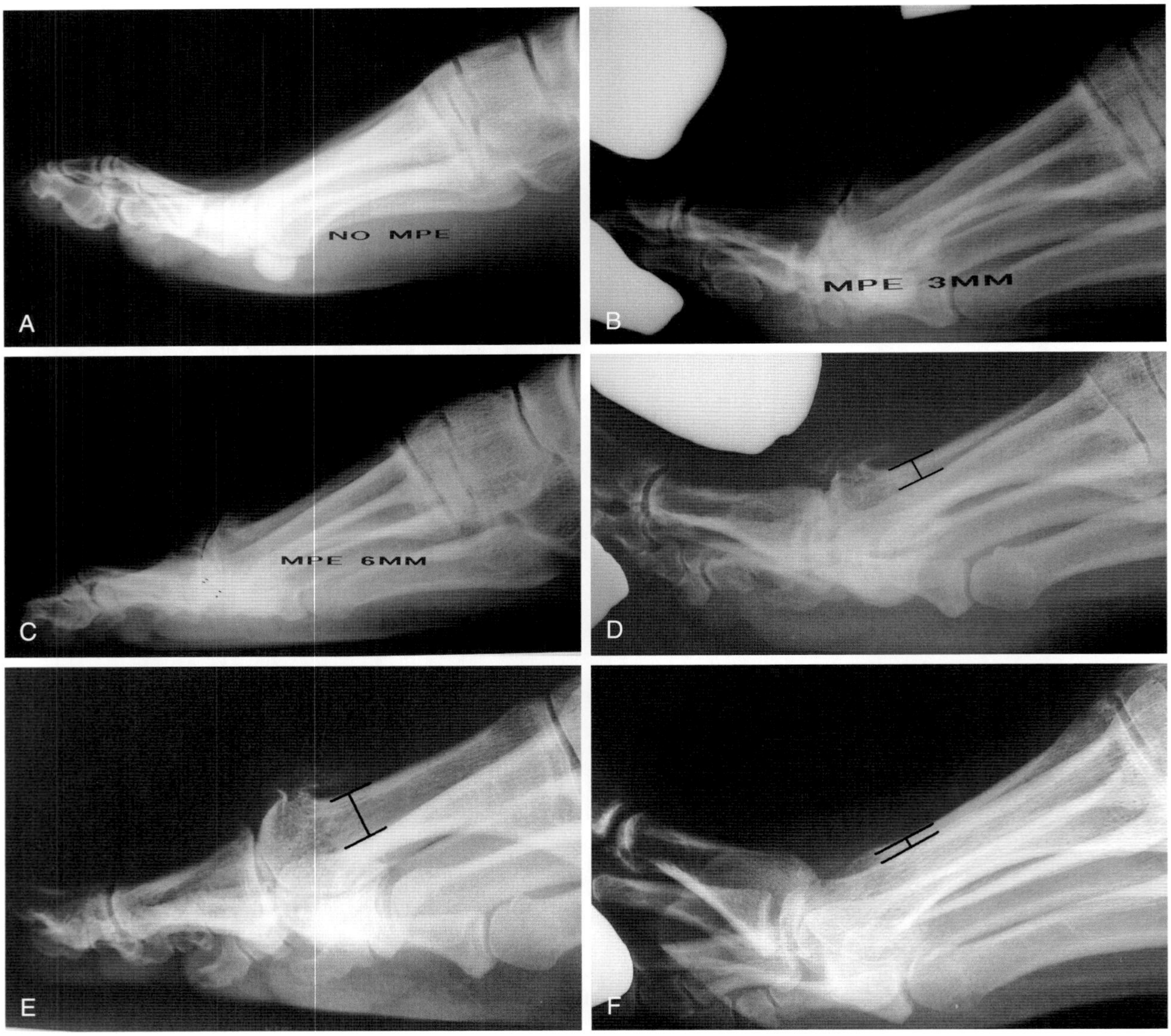

Figure 19-111 The effect of dorsiflexion stress on the first metatarsophalangeal (MTP) joint with hallux rigidus. Metatarsus primus elevatus correlates with MTP joint arthrosis noted in sequential radiographs taken over an 11-year period. **A,** Early grade 1 hallux rigidus with no metatarsus elevatus. **B,** Six years later, elevatus is 3 mm with or without stress test. **C,** Eleven years later, elevatus is 6 mm. **D,** Dorsiflexion stress reduces elevatus to 3 mm. **E,** Elevatus does increase with increasing grade of hallux rigidus. **F,** Elevatus is often reduced after either a cheilectomy or MTP arthrodesis.

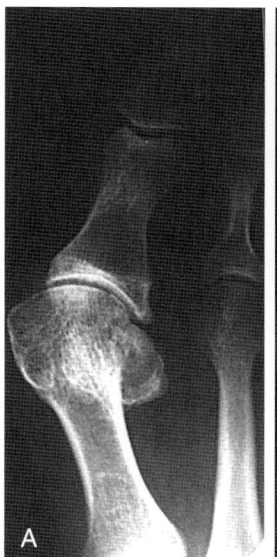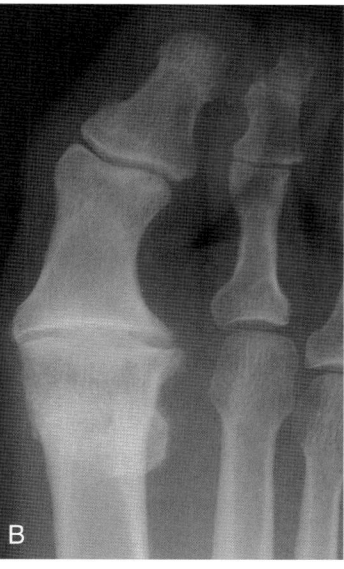

Figure 19-112 **A,** Hallux valgus is rarely seen in association with hallux rigidus. **B,** Hallux valgus interphalangeus is commonly seen. An average hallux valgus interphalangeus angle angle of 17 degrees is reported. (From Coughlin MJ, Shurnas PS: Hallux rigidus. Grading and long-term results of operative treatment, *J Bone Joint Surg Am* 85:2072–2088, 2003.)

hallux rigidus. Pain decreased significantly in both treatment groups. However, the effect was transitory, and at 1-year follow-up, a high percentage of patients in both groups had eventually required surgery.

Smith et al[518] reported the long-term results of 22 patients (24 feet), with a mean follow-up of 14 years, who were treated nonoperatively for hallux rigidus. The authors found that 75% of patients still chose not to have surgery. The intensity of pain remained similar in 22 feet, improved with time in 1, and worsened in 1. Most patients were able to minimize pain by wearing a roomy, stiff-soled shoe. Others[197] have reported successful treatment in nearly 60% of patients treated nonoperatively with footwear modifications, orthoses, injections, and taping. Follow-up ranged from 1 to 7 years (see Fig. 19-110).

The geriatric patient deserves special consideration because the mortality rate in patients older than 90 years who undergo elective surgery has been reported to be 2.3%.[4] Age alone is not the sole determinant of whether elective procedures should be considered,[74] but the severity of diseases and comorbidities are good predictors of surgical outcome.[137] Cardiovascular complications account for nearly 50% of mortality.[209] With the increase in the aging population, many geriatric patients benefit

Table 19-3	Clinical and Radiographic Classification of Hallux Rigidus		
Grade	Range of Motion	Radiograph	Clinical
0	Dorsiflexion 40-60 degrees and/or 10%-20% loss compared to normal side	Normal or minimal findings	No subjective pain, only stiffness; loss of passive motion on examination
1	Dorsiflexion 30-40 degrees and/or 20%-50% loss compared with normal side	Dorsal spur is main finding, minimal joint narrowing, minimal periarticular sclerosis, minimal flattening of metatarsal head	Mild or occasional subjective pain and stiffness; pain at extremes of dorsiflexion and/or plantar flexion on exam
2	Dorsiflexion 10-30 degrees and/or 50%-75% loss compared with normal side	Dorsal, lateral, and possibly medial osteophytes give flattened appearance to metatarsal head, no more than 25% dorsal joint space involvement on lateral radiograph, mild-to-moderate joint narrowing and sclerosis, sesamoids not usually involved but may be irregular in appearance	Moderate-to-severe subjective pain and stiffness that may be constant; pain just before maximal dorsiflexion and/or plantar flexion on examination
3	Dorsiflexion of 10 degrees or less and/or 75%-100% loss compared with normal side and notable loss of plantar flexion (often 10 degrees or less plantar flexion)	As in grade 2 but with substantial narrowing, possibly periarticular cystic changes, more than 25% dorsal joint may be involved on lateral side, sesamoids are enlarged and/or cystic and/or irregular	Nearly constant subjective pain and substantial stiffness; pain throughout range of motion on examination (but not at midrange)
4	Dorsiflexion of 10 degrees or less and/or 75%-100% loss compared with normal side and notable loss of plantar flexion (often 10 degrees or less plantar flexion)	As in grade 2 but with substantial narrowing, possibly periarticular cystic changes, more than 25% dorsal joint may be involved on lateral, sesamoids are enlarged and/or cystic and/or irregular	Nearly constant subjective pain and substantial stiffness; pain throughout range of motion on examination plus definite pain at midrange of motion

From Coughlin MJ, Shurnas PS: Hallux rigidus. Grading and long-term results of operative treatment, *J Bone Joint Surg Am* 85:2072–2088, 2003.

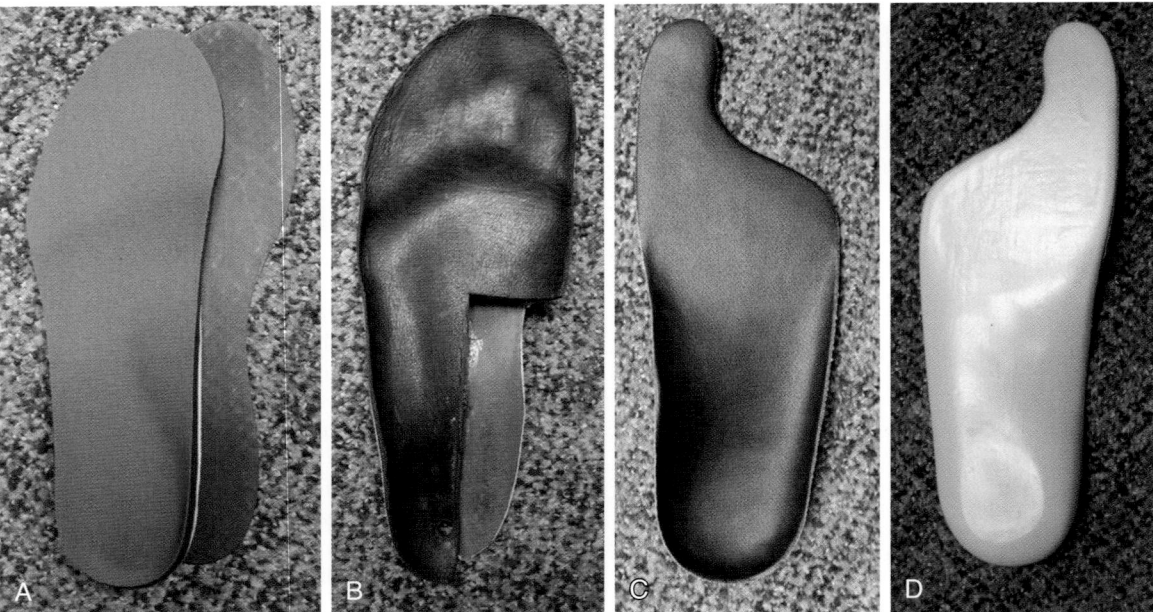

Figure 19-113 Orthoses for hallux rigidus **A,** Soft insole with graphite orthosis beneath, which stiffens entire insole, restricting metatarsophalangeal (MTP) joint excursion. **B,** Composite orthosis with gel and graphite combined. **C,** Orthotic with "Morton extension" to restrict MTP joint motion. **D,** Same orthotic from plantar aspect. (**B,** Courtesy Hansen Orthotics, Sun Valley, Idaho.)

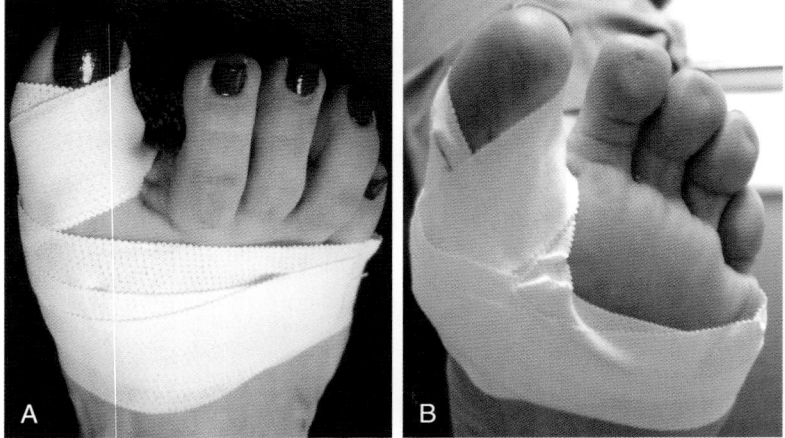

Figure 19-114 Taping of the hallux to decrease dorsiflexion excursion may reduce pain. **A,** Dorsal view. **B,** Plantar view.

from elective operative management when indicated, but they should be counseled about the increased risks.[4,52,74]

Surgical Treatment

Decision making in the surgical treatment of hallux rigidus is based on the degree of arthrosis present clinically and radiographically (Fig. 19-115). In the presence of synovial thickening without radiographic demonstration of degenerative arthritis, an MTP joint synovectomy is the treatment of choice. Moreover, synovitis and limited MTP joint motion without radiographic changes should be evaluated by ruling out an inflammatory or potentially erosive joint process (complete blood count [CBC], ESR, CRP, ANA, RF, HLA-B27, and uric acid) or considering the possibility of other causes of joint restriction. Michelson and Dunn[379] reported flexor hallucis stenosing tenosynovitis indicated by retromalleolar or arch tenderness over the FHL and increased signal on MRI as a cause of hallux limitus in patients without radiographic changes in the first MTP joint but with restricted passive joint motion.

With an osteochondral defect of the first metatarsophalangeal joint, removal of cartilaginous loose fragments and drilling of the osseous base can aid in the regeneration of a fibrocartilaginous surface (see Fig. 19-103C and D). In a younger patient, an osteochondral autogenous transfer procedure can be considered either in the first or lesser MTP joints for articular surface

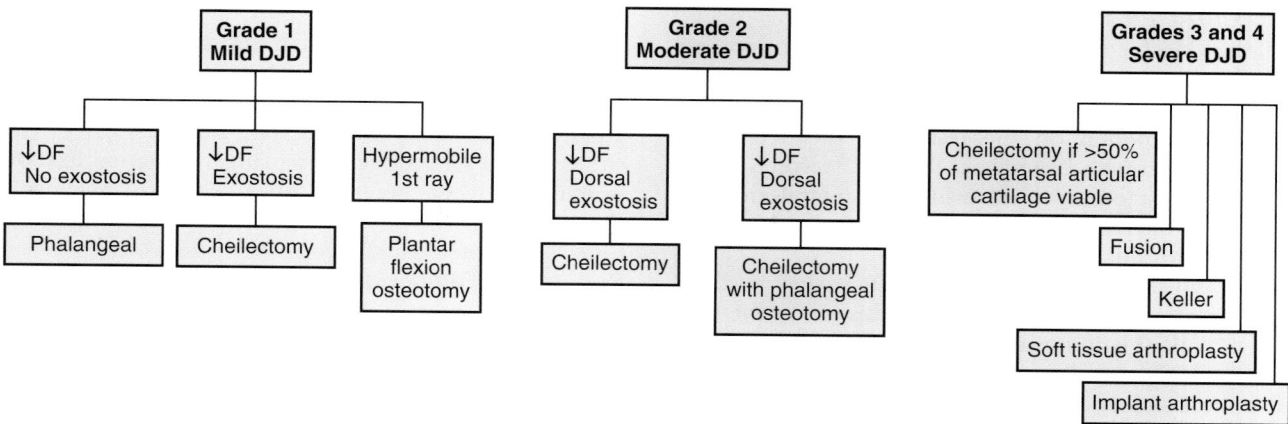

Figure 19-115 Treatment considerations for hallux rigidus. ↓, decreased; *DF,* dorsiflexion; *DJD,* degenerative joint disease; *FHL,* flexor hallucis longus; *Keller,* Keller arthroplasty.

defects.[388,608] Title et al[557] reported a case using a combined cheilectomy and osteochondral transfer as treatment for the remaining cartilaginous defect. Hopson et al[239] has also reported the use of an osteocartilaginous transfer for salvage of a failed first metatarsal head resurfacing implant.

In a juvenile or adult patient with restricted passive dorsiflexion but no significant dorsal exostosis (without clinical findings of flexor hallucis stenosis), a dorsal closing-wedge phalangeal osteotomy may improve joint function.[288,390,519,549]

In an adult patient with impingement of the proximal phalanx against a dorsal osteophyte on the metatarsal head, a cheilectomy is the preferred treatment. If an unsatisfactory result occurs, other opportunities for salvage remain. Cheilectomy is the mainstay of surgical treatment for hallux rigidus and can be combined with other procedures tailored to a specific problem, such as an osteochondral autograft transfer system (OATS) procedure for a large central defect[239] or microfracture for smaller defects, phalangeal osteotomy for severe interphalangeus or to enhance dorsiflexion, or soft tissue interposition for end-stage hallux rigidus in a patient who is opposed to an arthrodesis (Fig. 19-112).

Typically, with grade 0 or 1 hallux rigidus, careful examination for FHL stenosing tenosynovitis is performed. If FHL stenosing tenosynovitis is diagnosed, then an FHL release is performed, and a MTP joint synovectomy or phalangeal osteotomy may be added depending on the individual case. In grade 2 or 3 hallux rigidus, a cheilectomy or, occasionally, a cheilectomy combined with a phalangeal osteotomy,[552] may be considered, although reported success rates after phalangeal osteotomy are variable; Waisy et al[578] reported improved MTP joint motion, whereas Kilmartin[290] and Thomas[549]reported little or no increase in motion after a dorsal closing-wedge phalangeal ostotomy. With grade 4 hallux rigidus (severe degenerative arthritis), salvage procedures include arthrodesis, excisional arthroplasty, soft tissue interpositional arthroplasty, or prosthetic replacement.

Preoperative planning includes careful inspection of the preoperative AP and, especially, the lateral radiograph for loss of joint space. A careful physical examination is performed to assess pain with gentle loading of the hallux in a neutral position with respect to dorsiflexion and plantar flexion.[141] If this maneuver elicits pain at the midrange of motion, the remaining cartilage surface is inadequate and portends a poor prognosis for the success of cheilectomy.[111]

To establish, in general, a painfree MTP joint, an arthrodesis, interposition arthroplasty, or joint resection arthroplasty may be necessary. The authors do not advocate a Keller resection arthroplasty; rather, if an arthrodesis is not an acceptable alternative to the patient, a soft tissue interposition arthroplasty as described by Coughlin[112] or Hamilton[214] is recommended.

Although many activities are possible after an arthrodesis, many younger patients often prefer to preserve motion. Procedures to reestablish motion at the MTP joint often do so at the expense of stability.[481] Resection arthroplasty has been favored for hallux rigidus,[122,268,343,415,516] but not in the younger patient. Often, with an excisional arthroplasty, weakness of plantar flexion at the MTP joint occurs and can lead to transfer metatarsalgia.[109,322] In an older, less active patient, a resection arthroplasty or resection arthroplasty with interposition of soft tissue may be considered.[502]

For patients who want moderate physical activity, resection arthroplasty should be discouraged. However, less destructive resection arthroplasties, such as the Valenti procedure (resection of the dorsal proximal phalanx and metatarsal head in a V-shaped cut), have reported a high proportion of good and excellent results (33 of 36 procedures) in younger patients (mean age, 50.6 years) with a mean follow-up of 4.2 years.[314] Implant arthroplasty has been advocated for treatment of hallux rigidus,[537,539,540] but reported complications and severe difficulty with revision procedures have made this procedure less popular (see later discussion of implants for the first MTP joint).

PROXIMAL PHALANGEAL OSTEOTOMY

A dorsal closing-wedge proximal phalangeal osteotomy was initially proposed by Bonney and MacNab[51] for the treatment of adolescents with hallux rigidus. Kessel and Bonney[288] reported on the results of this technique. Heaney,[230] Harrison,[223] and later Moberg[390] recommended phalangeal osteotomy to use available plantar flexion and create a "functional transfer of plantar flexion to dorsiflexion" with this osteotomy.[443]

The indications for a dorsal closing-wedge proximal phalangeal osteotomy for hallux rigidus are in the adolescent patient with no significant osteophyte formation. This may be used in combination with an FHL release when indicated and less often in combination with cheilectomy in the skeletally mature patient.[549]

Surgical Technique

1. A medial longitudinal incision extending from the interphalangeal joint to a point 1 cm proximal to the first MTP joint exposes the proximal phalanx.[288,390]
2. The MTP joint is identified. A dorsal closing-wedge osteotomy is performed just distal to the MTP joint space. In the adolescent patient, care must be taken to avoid injury to an open proximal phalangeal epiphysis. The size of the resected wedge is determined by the degree of plantar flexion at the MTP joint. This osteotomy should permit the toe to be dorsiflexed to 35 degrees in relationship to the metatarsal shaft (15 degrees in relationship to the plantar surface of the foot) (Fig. 19-116A).
3. The osteotomy is firmly secured with crossed or parallel K-wires, screws, compression staples, or sutures placed through drill holes at the osteotomy site (Fig. 19-119B). If a phalangeal osteotomy is combined with a cheilectomy, stable internal fixation is mandatory because early motion is necessary for a successful cheilectomy. The wound is closed in a routine manner.

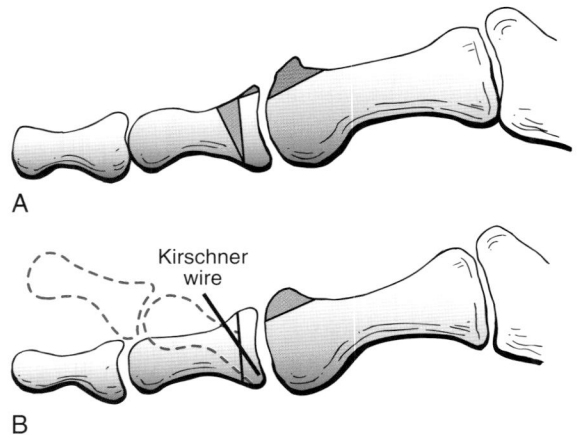

Figure 19-116 Moberg procedure. Dorsal and closing-wedge osteotomy of proximal phalanx is used to correct hallux rigidus. This exchanges plantar flexion for dorsiflexion. **A,** Proposed osteotomy and cheilectomy. **B,** After closing-wedge osteotomy.

Postoperative Care

A gauze-and-tape compression dressing is applied at surgery and changed weekly. The patient is allowed to ambulate in a postoperative shoe. Dressing changes and guarded ambulation are necessary until the osteotomy site is healed 4 to 6 weeks after surgery. Internal fixation is removed when necessary after successful healing is demonstrated.

Results and Complications

Kessell and Bonney[288] reported on nine adolescents with short-term follow-up (average, 14 months), noting pain relief in more than 90% and an average increase in dorsiflexion of 39 degrees. Although this procedure was originally recommended for adolescent patients, Moberg[390] extended the indications to the adult population. Unfortunately, the author reported no follow-up of results. In a long-term follow-up of phalangeal osteotomies (average follow-up, 11 years), Citron[88] reported that 50% of patients had complete relief of pain, although further degenerative arthrosis was noted. Waisy[578] reported midterm and long-term follow-up on 60 patients who underwent a cheilectomy and phalangeal osteotomy, and suggested that for substantial arthritis, the phalangeal osteotomy likely improved satisfaction. However, Kilmartin,[290] in a report on 49 patients who underwent a phalangeal osteotomy and cheilectomy, reported only 65% satisfaction and a loss of 1 degree of dorsiflexion at more than 1-year follow-up in his series.

Thomas and Smith[549] reported on 17 patients who underwent a combination cheilectomy and phalangeal osteotomy for grades 1 and 2 hallux rigidus. All osteotomies healed. Although the average increase in dorsiflexion was only 7 degrees, 96% of patients were satisfied with their surgical result. Southgate et al[525] reported similarly good results after proximal phalangeal osteotomy and found comparable results to arthrodesis in terms of pain relief in 10 patients with osteotomies compared with 20 patients with arthrodeses, with a mean of 12 years of follow-up.[525]

The indications for phalangeal osteotomy in relationship to hallux rigidus remain to be clearly delineated. For an adolescent with hallux rigidus, a phalangeal osteotomy appears to be advantageous, but the osteotomy must avoid an open phalangeal physis when present. In an adolescent, a cheilectomy might not be necessary because there is rarely significant arthrosis or osteophyte formation; however, inspection of the metatarsal articular surface is important because an osteochondral defect should be treated. For an adult with grade 1 hallux rigidus, a phalangeal osteotomy may be sufficient treatment. With significant MTP arthrosis, an isolated phalangeal osteotomy might not be sufficient treatment and occasionally may be combined with a cheilectomy for grades 2 and 3 disease. Whether the studies of Thomas and Smith[549] and Southgate[525] will be confirmed with greater numbers of longer-term positive results remains to be determined. Although the osteotomy may improve the static position of the hallux, marked increased dorsiflexion range of motion is rarely achieved.[290,549] It appears with only a cheilectomy, and early motion may be aggressively pursued; with a cheilectomy and phalangeal osteotomy, pain or cautious implementation of range of motion activities (because of the osteotomy) may compromise the ultimate goal of an increase in dorsiflexion.

CHEILECTOMY

Cheilectomy, or excision of the dorsal exostosis of the metatarsal head, was first proposed by Nilsonne,[415] who attempted the procedure in two cases but thought it offered only temporary relief. Bonney and Macnab[51] later used this technique for cases of "polyarthritis" and noted poor results. In 1959, DuVries[140] advocated removal of the proliferative bone at the MTP joint to enable dorsiflexion. Although he noted 90% satisfactory results, no long-term follow-up was reported. In 1979, Mann, Coughlin, and DuVries[354] described their technique of cheilectomy and reported successful results at long-term follow-up. Later, Coughlin and Shurnas[111] reported 92% successful results using Mann's technique of cheilectomy in 80 patients, with more than 9 years of follow-up. This study clearly defined the role of cheilectomy in treating all grades of hallux rigidus and proposed a clinical and radiographic classification to help select appropriate surgical treatment (see Table 19-3).

Although some have stressed the temporary nature of the procedure[48,138] or limited indications,[519] the current authors perform cheilectomy for grades 1 and 2 hallux rigidus, in younger athletic patients, and in patients with more advanced degenerative arthrosis (grade 3 hallux rigidus with more than 50% of the metatarsal articular surface remaining) who wish to avoid the risk and morbidity of a more extensive procedure. Geldwert et al[180] and others[25] have demonstrated that, for grades 1 and 2 hallux rigidus (using a different classification scheme), a cheilectomy relieved pain significantly in 93% of patients, but for grade 3 hallux rigidus, the success rate fell to 29%. A cheilectomy is a simple procedure that leaves a stable joint, has low morbidity,[180] and preserves strength and joint motion.[155,180,228]

Surgical Technique

1. A dorsal longitudinal incision extends from the middle of the proximal phalanx to 3 cm proximal to the MTP joint. The extensor hood and joint capsule are incised, and the dissection is deepened on the medial or lateral aspect of the EHL tendon (Fig. 19-117A and Video Clip 31).
2. A thorough synovectomy is carried out, and the MTP joint is inspected to locate osteophytes or loose bodies and to assess the extent of the articular cartilage damage (Fig. 19-117B). The proximal phalanx is plantar flexed to aid in exposure, and any dorsal phalangeal osteophyte is resected (Fig. 19-117C and H).
3. The joint is inspected to determine the amount and location of cartilage loss (Fig. 19-117D). If a

cheilectomy is indicated (more than 50% of metatarsal articular cartilage is viable), then the metatarsal osteophyte is generously resected on the dorsal, dorsomedial, and dorsolateral aspects using a 6-mm osteotome (Fig. 19-117E). It is critical that at least 20% to 30% of the dorsal metatarsal head is removed with this oblique osteotomy. The decision regarding the extent of bone resection depends on the size of the dorsal exostosis, the amount of articular cartilage destruction, and the need to establish adequate dorsiflexion at the conclusion of the procedure.

4. The resection is initiated just dorsal to the edge of the remaining viable metatarsal articular cartilage. (Thus, with more severe arthrosis, more metatarsal head is resected.) However, more extensive resection can increase the risk of MTP subluxation, and greater than 30% to 40% resection is discouraged. Any remaining eburnated bone or defects can be microfractured or drilled, and if less than 50% of the metatarsal articular surface is viable, an arthrodesis is recommended (Fig. 19-117F and Video Clip 32).
5. Any articular cartilage irregularities are removed, including loose cartilaginous fragments. Dorsiflexion of approximately 60 degrees is desirable after an extensive cheilectomy. Any dorsal or medial osteophytes are removed from the base of the proximal phalanx and along the upper border of the metatarsal head.
6. The raw bone surfaces are smoothed with a rasp or rongeur and may be coated with a thin layer of bone wax to impede further bleeding. The joint capsule is closed in a routine manner. A gauze-and-tape compression dressing is applied and changed weekly (Fig. 19-117G).

Postoperative Care

At 7 to 10 days after surgery, aggressive active and passive range-of-motion exercises are initiated. The patient is allowed to ambulate in a postoperative shoe with weight bearing on the heel and along the outer border of the foot. Patients are encouraged to mobilize the MTP joint 5 minutes of every hour. Weekly office visits are scheduled to monitor the patient's progress with range of motion. At 2 to 3 months after surgery, most swelling and thickening of the periarticular tissue subside. Maximal improvement in motion is usually achieved at this point.

Physical therapy can be scheduled depending on a patient's compliance and success with joint mobilization. On occasion, chronic thickening and swelling can take several months to subside, and the use of a short course of oral steroid may be useful in resolving this problem.

Results and Complications

Mann, Coughlin, and DuVries[354] reported on their experience with 20 patients and noted 85% pain relief with cheilectomy. The remaining patients had only mild discomfort. Postoperative dorsiflexion averaged 30 degrees, with minimal progression of arthrosis.

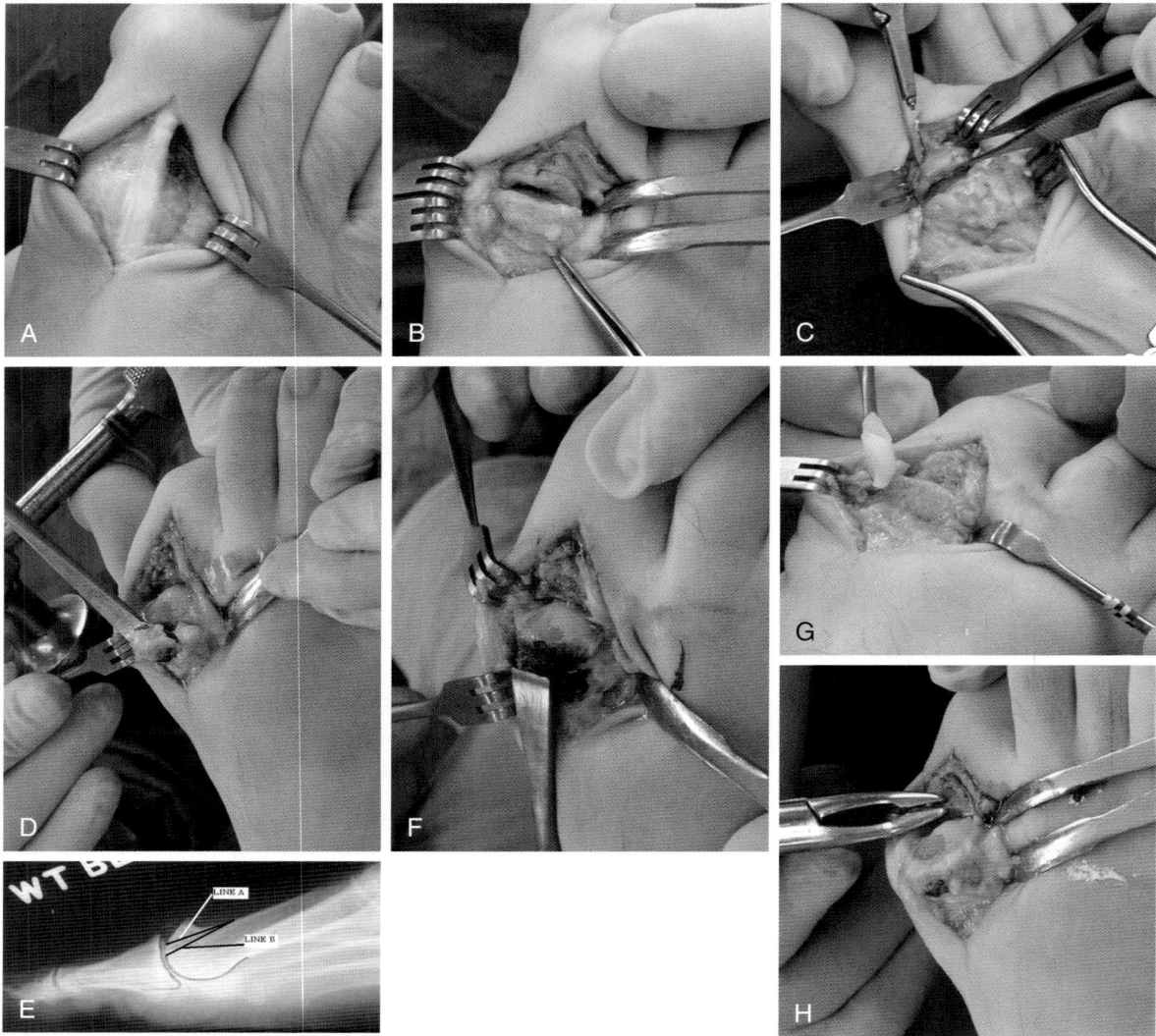

Figure 19-117 **A,** A dorsomedial skin incision is used to expose the metatarsophalangeal joint. **B,** The extensor hood is incised, the extensor tendon is retracted laterally (or medially), and the joint space is exposed. **C,** A synovectomy is performed, the joint is inspected, and any loose bodies are removed. **D,** A cheilectomy is performed to include any cartilage defect if possible. **E,** About 25% to 30% of the dorsal metatarsal head is resected. **F,** The osteotome denotes the dorsal axis of the first metatarsal; thus actually more bone is removed below this level. **G,** Bone wax is used to decrease postoperative bleeding. **H,** Any osteophytes on the dorsal base of the proximal phalanx are removed with a rongeur.

Mann and Clanton[351] later reported an average increase in postoperative range of motion of 19 degrees (average dorsiflexion, 48 degrees) after cheilectomy; 74% of patients had improvement in joint motion, and 25% had no change or lost motion. Complete or considerable relief of pain was noted by 90% of patients. Only one patient noted recurrence of a dorsal osteophyte. The authors stressed that a patient must be counseled that after surgery, some will continue to have pain, some do not gain MTP joint motion, and some actually lose MTP motion.

This concept was well demonstrated by Mulier et al[401] in 20 athletes (22 feet), at a mean age of 31 years, who underwent the Mann cheilectomy for all grades of hallux rigidus, with a mean follow-up of 5.1 years. Subjectively, 14 feet were rated excellent, 7 good, and 1 fair, but only 13 athletes were able to play at the same or higher level, and 7 played at a lower level. Two patients had symptoms clearly related to persistent symptoms of hallux rigidus.

A cheilectomy resects bone and removes bony impingement but does not repair the intraarticular damage. Thus some pain or aching might remain after surgery. Over time, the results of cheilectomy can deteriorate, depending on the severity of the degenerative process.[549] Ultimately, even with failure, a cheilectomy does not "burn bridges" and leaves options for other salvage techniques available. Likewise, it does not trade one problem for another.[141]

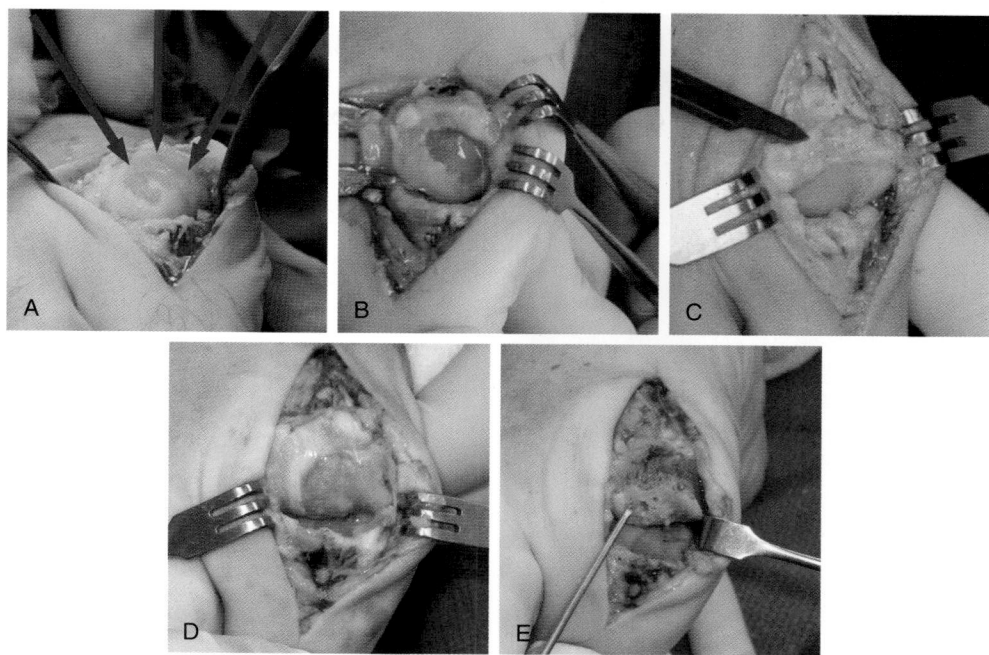

Figure 19-118 Various patterns of chondrolysis associated with hallux rigidus. **A,** Central articular lesion. *Arrows* indicate complete loss of cartilage. **B,** A dorsocentral articular lesion can often be resected with the cheilectomy; in this case, some full-loss area remains and can lead to postoperative pain. **C,** Complete lateral articular chondrolysis of this magnitude is best treated by arthrodesis. **D,** V-shaped central articular chondrolysis that extends plantarward for 50% of the height of the metatarsal head. **E,** It may be resected with cheilectomy and drilling of remaining articular defect.

Feltham[156] reported on cheilectomy results using the Mann technique on 67 patients, with a mean of 65 months of follow-up and noted a 91% satisfaction rate, with four failures. Better results were observed in patients older than 60 years; the technique was used for all grades of hallux rigidus. Lin and Murphy[332a] reported on 20 patients, with an average increase in total range of motion improving from 45 to 58 degrees. Coughlin and Shurnas[111] recommended cheilectomy for grades 1, 2, and 3 hallux rigidus (with more than 50% metatarsal articular cartilage remaining at the time of surgery). They reported 97% good and excellent subjective results (mean follow-up, 9.6 years) and 92% long-term successful results for pain relief and function after cheilectomy, Although Easley et al[141] and others[332a] hypothesized that a dorsal approach would potentially risk scarring of the extensor hallucis longus (EHL) and lead to restricted first MTP range of motion, Lin[332a] and Coughlin and Shurnas[111] both showed that there was little disadvantage to a dorsal approach. However, Lin, using a dorsolateral approach, did observe a large number of patients with postoperative numbness on the lateral aspect of the hallux, possibly because of a traction neuritis. Canseco et al[71] analyzed the gait pattern of patients before and after cheilectomy and noted a longer stride length, increased walking speed, and a shift toward a normal swing/stance ratio after cheilectomy.

It is critical that patients with more advanced clinical and radiographic disease (grades 3 [<50% metatarsal cartilage surface remaining at surgery] and 4 [end-stage disease]) understand that a cheilectomy is very likely to fail based on the results of the study. Such patients would be better served with an arthrodesis or interposition arthroplasty depending on the individual patient's needs (Fig. 19-118). Moreover, the effect of microfracture performed on any remaining small (<5 mm) defect after the cheilectomy has been completed can extend the indications for a cheilectomy, but the results of this additional technique are not completely known (Fig. 19-119). Coughlin and Shurnas[111] reported no adverse effect on the long-term results of a small number of patients who underwent microfracture with cheilectomy, but any patient with less than 50% of the metatarsal articular surface remaining had a significantly increased risk of failure of the cheilectomy (Fig. 19-120), or a residual of increased pain with longer-term follow-up.

Probably the main reason for failure of cheilectomy, as reported in the literature (in appropriately selected patients), centers on inadequate bone resection (Figs. 19-121 to 19-124). Feldman et al[155] and others[136,228,342] have advocated excision of osteophytes flush with the metatarsal shaft. This might explain Hattrup and Johnson's[228] high failure rate of greater than 30%. Only 53% of their patients were satisfied after their surgery. A cheilectomy should not remove bone "in line" with the dorsal metatarsal cortex, but it should remove up to 30% to 40% of the metatarsal head in an oblique fashion. Using Mann's technique as elaborated by Coughlin,[113] predictable and reliable long-term results can be expected.

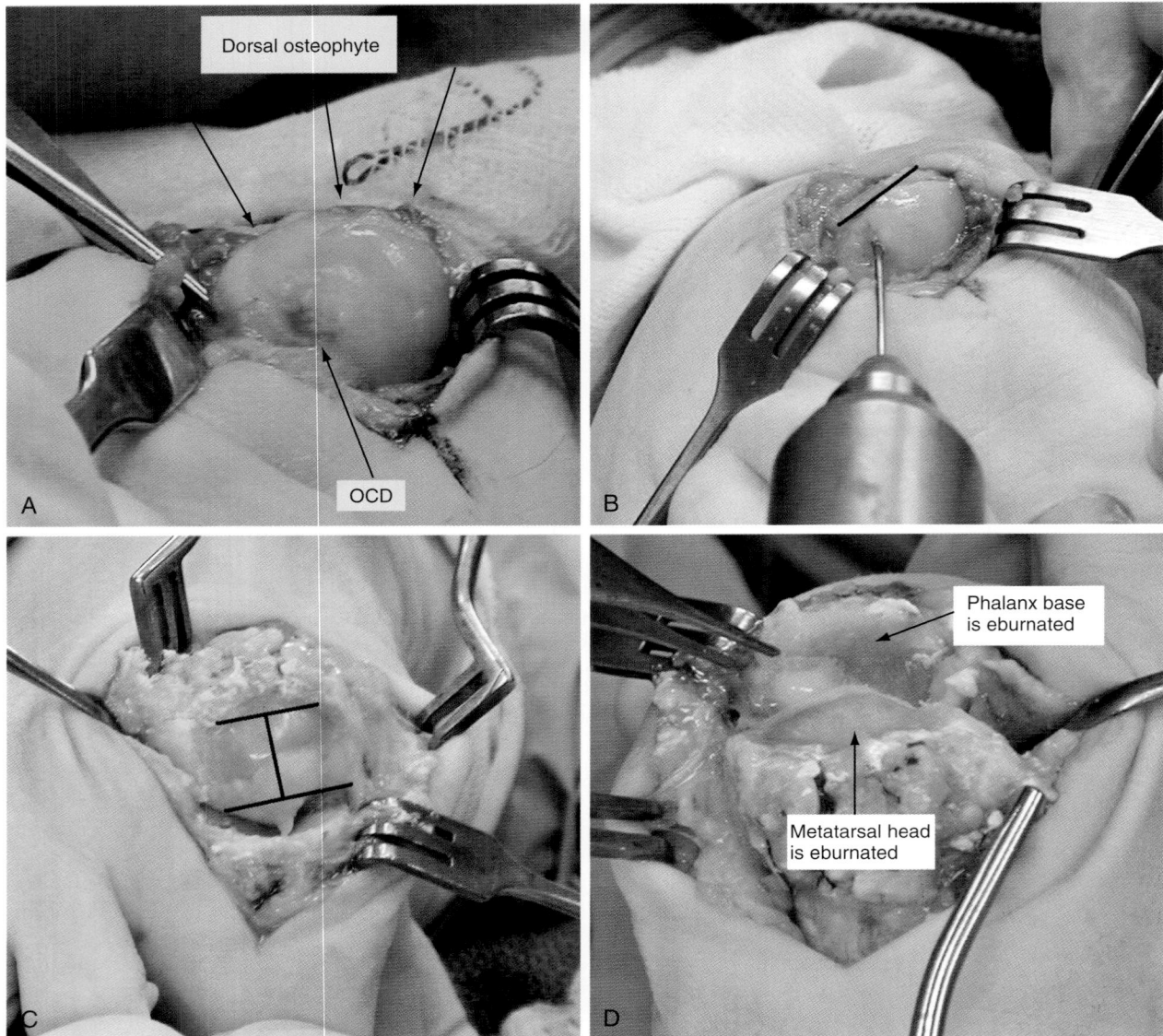

Figure 19-119 Treatment of osteochondral defect (OCD). **A** and **B,** If an area of full-thickness cartilage loss remains after a cheilectomy of up to 33% of the metatarsal head, the area may be drilled or perforated with a small K-wire after a cheilectomy (indicated by the *black line*) of up to 33% to 40% of the metatarsal head. **C,** Dorsal/plantar extent of the metatarsal head articular surface is indicated by the *black lines* before excision. Cartilaginous loss extends well into the remaining metatarsal and phalangeal articular surface. Greater than 50% loss of the cartilaginous surface portends a poorer prognosis for success after a cheilectomy. In this case, the patient was treated with a metatarsophalangeal joint arthrodesis. **D,** Substantial loss of cartilage on the phalangeal articular surface.

Unfortunately, with inadequate resection, MTP joint motion is not restored, and if impingement persists, ultimately the procedure can fail (see Figs. 19-121 and 19-122).

A more extensive bone resection has been advocated by Saxena[497] and Grady and Axe[196] by using the Valenti procedure (Fig. 19-125), which resects a sizable portion of the articular surface of the proximal phalanx and metatarsal head while retaining first-ray length and the plantar intrinsic muscle insertions. Saxena[497] reported an average

increase in dorsiflexion of 28 degrees, and Grady and Axe[196] reported an average 12-degree improvement in dorsiflexion. Excessive resection of bone, however, can lead to an unstable MTP joint with subluxation of the proximal phalanx.[228] Extensive soft tissue dissection may place the distal metatarsal at risk for partial or extensive avascular necrosis or degenerative arthritis (Fig. 19-126).[62]

Although the authors do not have experience with the Valenti procedure and do not necessarily advocate this

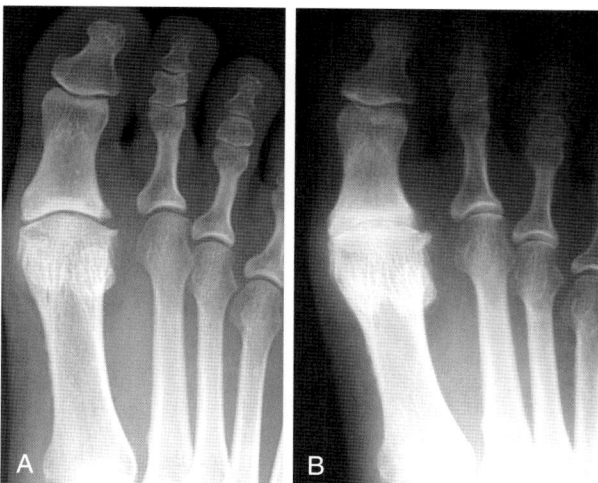

Figure 19-120 **A,** Preoperative radiograph with grade 2 hallux rigidus. **B,** After cheilectomy, complete chondrolysis has occurred. This is very unusual and can necessitate metatarsophalangeal joint arthrodesis.

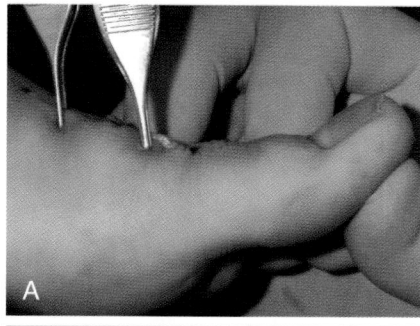

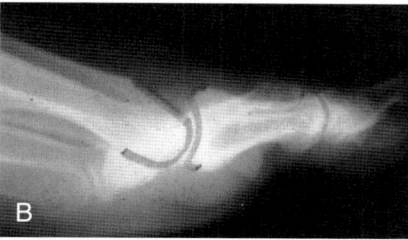

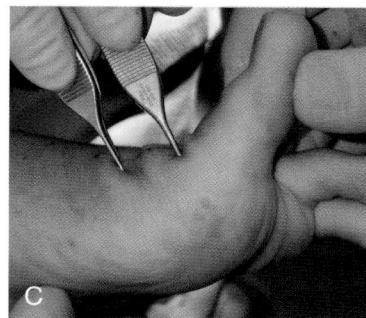

Figure 19-121 **A,** Preoperative motion. After the dorsal incision, the forceps hold the skin apposed, but marked restriction of dorsiflexion is noted. **B,** Lateral radiograph after cheilectomy. **C,** Dorsiflexion immediately after cheilectomy.

procedure, this technique supports the premise that a more extensive resection with cheilectomy improves postoperative range of motion and relieves impingement. With more advanced arthrosis, the normal gliding MTP joint motion is replaced by a rocking or hinged motion. Shereff and Baumhauer[509] noted that motion analysis of the MTP joint in hallux rigidus has demonstrated a greatly displaced center of rotation as more advanced arthritis ensues.

Although, in general, hallux rigidus is considered to be mainly a dorsal MTP joint degenerative process, occasionally substantial degenerative arthritis may develop in the metatarsal sesamoid articulation. Tagoe et al[541] reported on a series of 33 patients who underwent dual sesamoidectomies and a conservative cheilectomy. At 2- to 4-year follow-up, they reported a minimum of 75 degrees of dorsiflexion, but did not see resultant elevatus or varus/valgus malaligment. Although excision of both sesamoids is rarely necessary, the marked arthrosis present quite likely adds a stabilizing factor to the joint.

EXCISIONAL ARTHROPLASTY

Excisional arthroplasty was first described by Davies-Colley[122] in 1887 and was popularized by Keller[284] in 1904. The MTP joint is decompressed by resecting the base of the proximal phalanx, thereby relaxing contracted soft tissue structures. Excisional arthroplasty can relieve pain and has traditionally been accepted as treatment for more advanced degenerative arthritis of the first MTP joint. Gould[194] reported good relief of pain but observed that a hallux extensus deformity can occur after excisional arthroplasty. Bonney and MacNab[51] concluded that excisional arthroplasty had no place in the treatment of patients with generalized arthritis or metatarsus primus elevatus.

The Keller procedure is indicated in the older, more sedentary patient or household ambulator with grade 3 or 4 hallux rigidus in whom extensive surgery is contraindicated. It is not advocated for younger, more active patients with extensive hallux rigidus[51,295] because a flaccid, nonfunctional hallux can be a worse problem than the original hallux rigidus deformity.

Surgical Technique

1. A medial longitudinal incision is used to approach the first MTP joint. The incision extends from just proximal to the interphalangeal joint to 1 cm proximal to the medial eminence (Video Clip 60).
2. A proximally based medial capsular flap is developed, exposing the MTP joint.
3. A cheilectomy is performed, and if a prominent medial eminence is present, it is resected (see previous discussion on pages 957 to 961.). A sagittal saw is used to remove the proximal one third of the proximal phalanx (Fig. 19-127A and B).
4. To reestablish flexor power, the plantar aponeurosis and capsule are reattached to the plantar base of the proximal phalanx through several drill holes in its

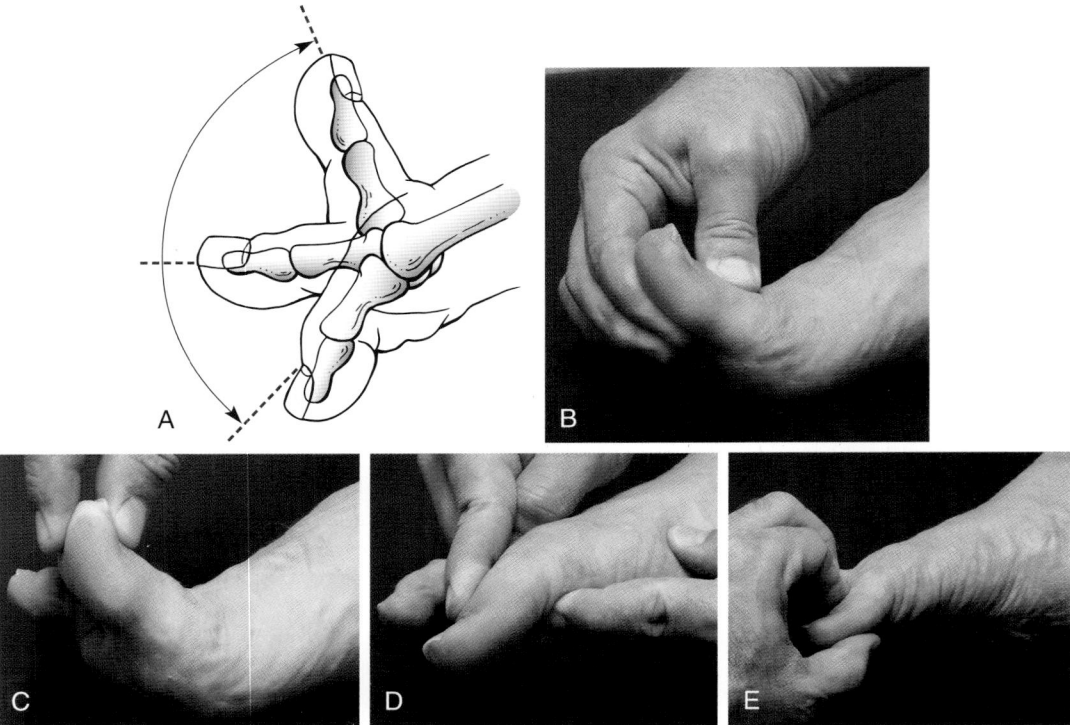

Figure 19-122 **A,** Normal range of motion of first metatarsophalangeal (MTP) joint. **B,** Technique of dorsiflexion mobilization (with plantar pressure on the proximal phalanx). **C,** Incorrect technique that places pressure on the distal interphalangeal joint. **D,** Technique of plantar-flexion mobilization. **E,** Although the surgeon can grasp the distal phalanx, better pressure can be applied to the MTP joint by grasping the proximal phalanx and pushing downward.

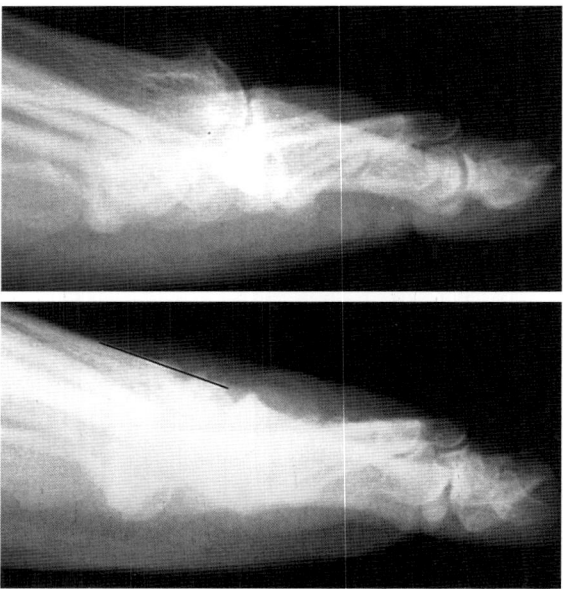

Figure 19-123 Preoperative **(A)** and postoperative **(B)** radiographs demonstrate inadequate resection of bone from metatarsal head. For a successful cheilectomy, at least 20% to 30% of dorsal metatarsal head should be excised.

base. This can also prevent a cock-up deformity at the MTP joint (Fig. 19-127C).

5. A 0.062-inch K-wire is introduced at the MTP joint and driven in a distal direction, exiting the tip of the toe. It is then retrograded proximally into the metatarsal head to stabilize the MTP joint. The pin is bent at the tip of the toe to prevent proximal migration.

6. The medial capsular flap is sutured to the periosteum of the proximal phalanx with interrupted sutures.

7. The skin is closed in a routine manner (Fig. 19-128).

Postoperative Care

A compression dressing is applied and changed weekly. The patient is allowed to ambulate in a wooden-soled shoe. The K-wire is removed 3 weeks after surgery, and gentle passive and active range-of-motion exercises are then commenced.

SOFT TISSUE INTERPOSITIONAL ARTHROPLASTY

A modified resection arthroplasty has been advocated by Ganley et al,[177] Hamilton et al,[214] and others* for hallux

---

*References 16, 38, 68, 112, 210, 286, 303, 306, 322, 344, 399, 490, and 495.

rigidus associated with more severe degenerative arthroses. An excisional arthroplasty is combined with a capsular interpositional arthroplasty technique, with this tissue serving as a biologic spacer. Indications include grade 3 and 4 hallux rigidus and situations when an arthrodesis,

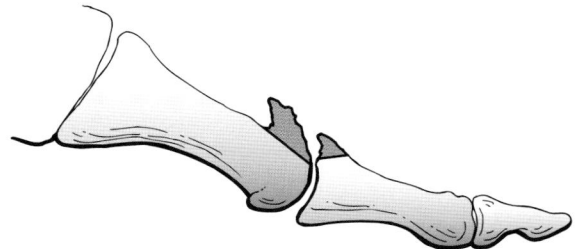

Figure 19-124 Proposed "correct" resection of the osteophyte from the base of the proximal phalanx and metatarsal head.

excisional arthroplasty, or implant might be considered. According to Hamilton et al,[214] the relative length of the first and second metatarsals should be equal. A short first metatarsal is a contraindication to this procedure because of the increased risk of a transfer lesion or lateral metatarsalgia. Coughlin and Shurnas[113] reported similar indications, using an autologous gracilis tendon biologic spacer with conical bone resection of the base of the proximal phalanx, and metatarsal head, using power reamers to create an effective joint space for placement of the tendon interposition graft. Disruption of the plantar intrinsics is avoided.

Hamilton's Surgical Technique

1. A medial longitudinal incision is centered over the first MTP joint. The MTP capsule is incised longitudinally. A periosteal elevator is used to reflect the dorsal, medial, and lateral capsule.

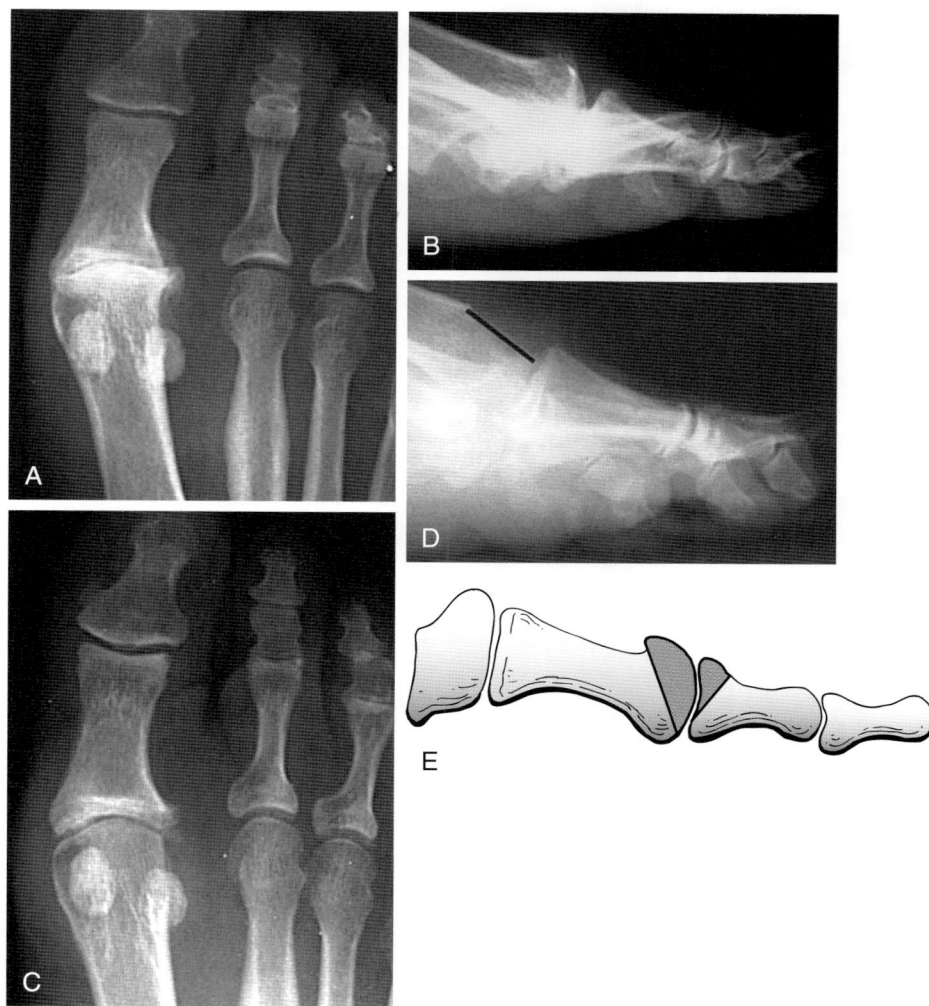

Figure 19-125 Cheilectomy. Preoperative anteroposterior (AP) **(A)** and lateral **(B)** radiographs demonstrate significant osteophyte formation. Postoperative AP **(C)** and lateral **(D)** radiographs demonstrate removal of approximately one third of the dorsal metatarsal head. **E,** Diagram of the Valenti procedure. Bone has been extensively resected from the base of the proximal phalanx and the metatarsal head.

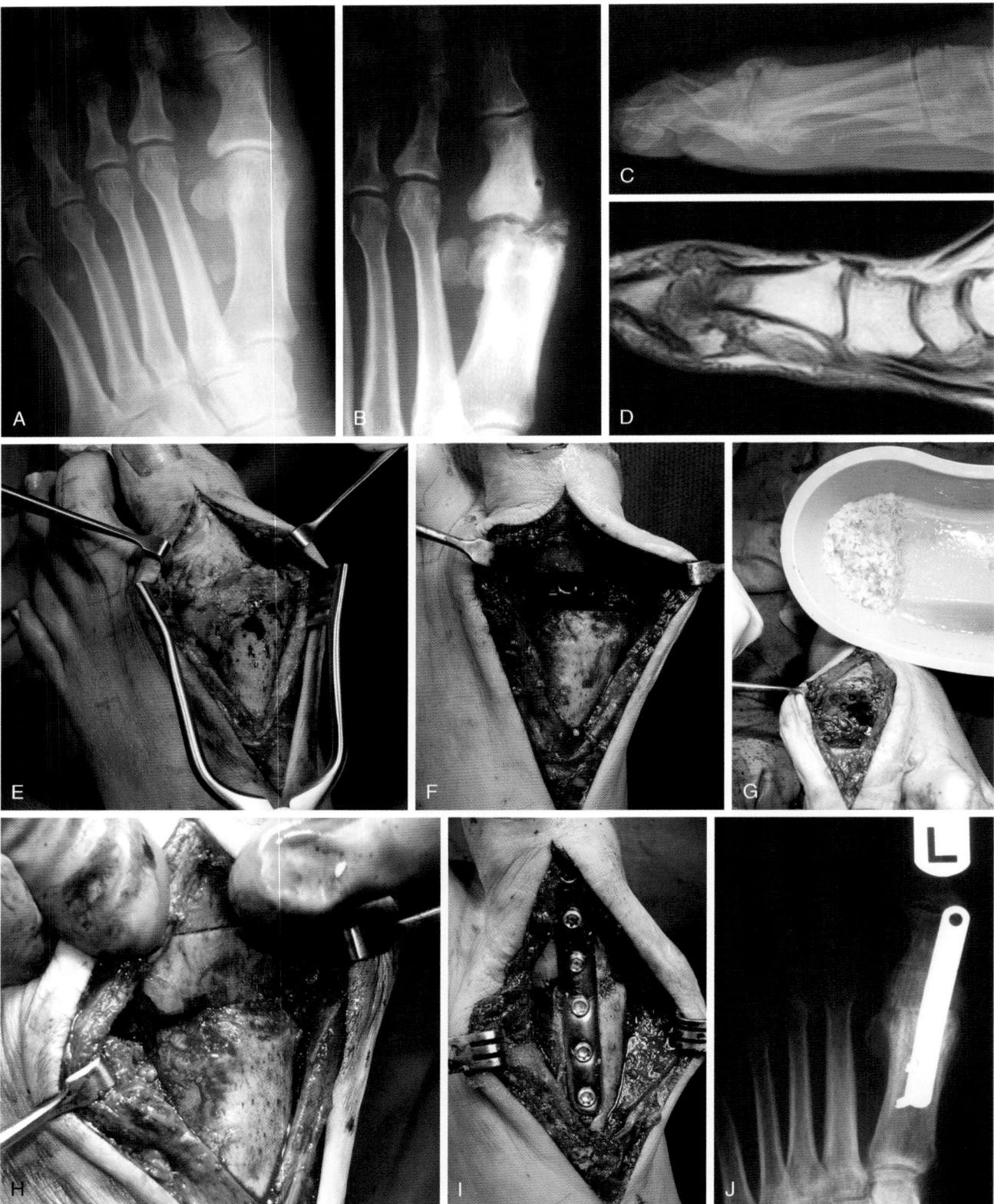

Figure 19-126   Avascular necrosis (AVN) of first metatarsal head. **A,** Preoperative radiograph demonstrating hallux rigidus. **B,** After extensive cheilectomy, AVN of the first metatarsal head has developed. **C,** Lateral radiograph. **D,** Magnetic resonance image demonstrating AVN. **E,** Intraoperative view. **F,** After resection of necrotic bone. Both granular graft **(G)** and a bulk allograft **(H)** are placed. **I,** Clinical appearance. **J,** Radiographic appearance after placement of internal fixation. (All images from Brosky TA 2nd, Menke CR, Xenos D: Reconstruction of the first metatarsophalangeal joint after post-cheilectomy avascular necrosis of the first metatarsal head: a case report, *J Foot Ankle Surg* 48:61–69, 2009.)

2. A cheilectomy is performed, and 25% or less of the proximal phalanx is resected with a transverse phalangeal osteotomy. The flexor hallucis brevis tendon is detached with this procedure and is not reattached (Fig. 19-129A).

3. The extensor hallucis brevis tendon and capsule are transversely incised approximately 3 cm proximal to the MTP joint line. The tendon and capsule are mobilized and rotated distally and plantarward and sutured to the tendon of the flexor hallucis brevis with 2-0 nonabsorbable sutures (Fig. 19-129B and C).

4. A 0.062-inch K-wire is driven distally through the proximal and distal phalanx and then advanced in a retrograde manner to stabilize the MTP joint. The pin is bent at the tip of the toe to prevent proximal migration (Fig. 19-129D).

5. The medial capsule is imbricated with interrupted absorbable sutures. The skin is approximated with a routine closure (Fig. 19-130).

6. Sanhudo et al[495] have modified this with an oblique resection of the first metatarsal head combined with a soft tissue interposition arthroplasty (Fig. 19-131).

Coughlin's Surgical Technique (Fig. 19-132)

1. A dorsomedial approach to the MTP join is made and centered over the joint. The capsule is opened longitudinally and reflected in a subperiosteal fashion to expose the metatarsal head and phalanx as described for an MTP joint arthrodesis (see Fig. 19-132A-D).

2. The osteophytes are debrided off the phalanx and metatarsal head, and concave reaming is performed on both the phalanx base and metatarsal head based on the size of the proximal phalanx base. The plantar tissues are not disturbed (see Fig. 19-132E and F).

3. A gracilis free graft is then harvested via a longitudinal incision centered over the hamstrings group insertion on the proximal medial tibia. The sartorius fascia is incised, and the gracilis tendon is identified and detached from its distal insertion. The distal end is secured with a Krakow suture and then harvested with a tendon stripper. Alternatively, an allograft tendon may be used.

4. The graft is prepared on the back table, cleaned of muscle tissue with an elevator, and rolled into a ball

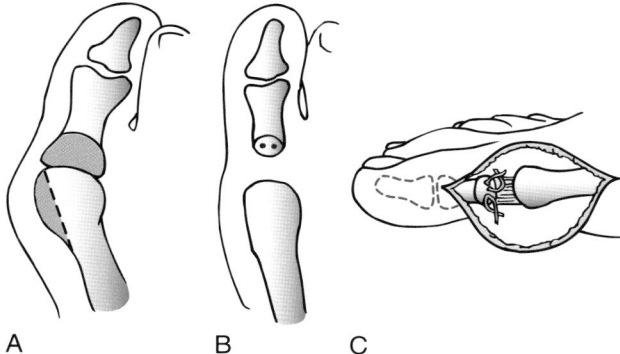

Figure 19-127 Diagram of excisional arthroplasty. **A,** Shaded area shows resected area of bone. **B,** After partial proximal phalangectomy. **C,** Reattachment of intrinsics to the base of the proximal phalanx. (With interpositional arthroplasty, intrinsics are not reattached to the base of the proximal phalanx.)

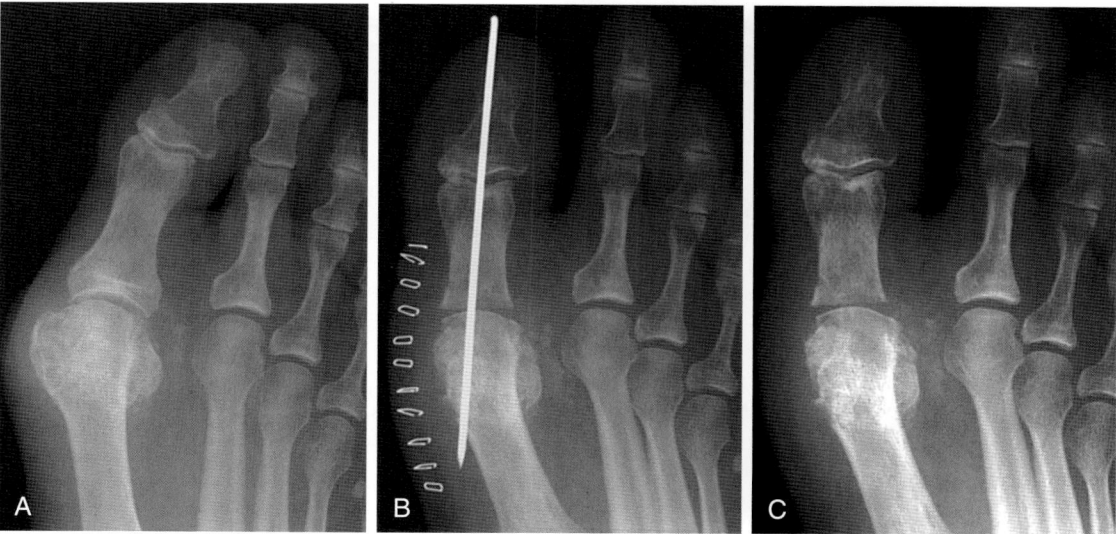

Figure 19-128 Excisional arthroplasty. **A,** Preoperative radiograph demonstrates combined hallux valgus and hallux rigidus. **B,** After excision arthroplasty with K-wire stabilization. **C,** After excisional arthroplasty.

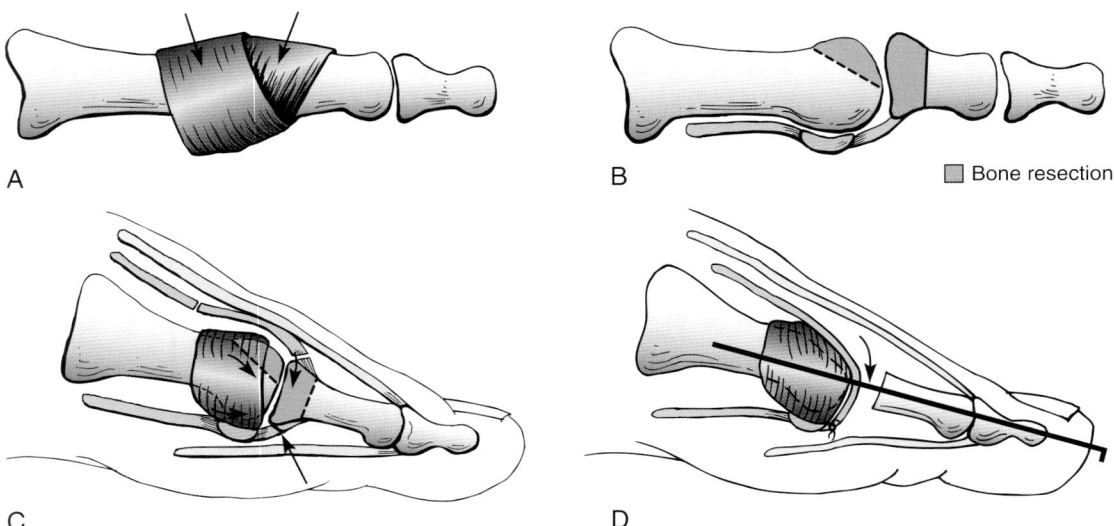

Figure 19-129 Capsular interpositional arthroplasty.[214] **A,** Anatomy of extensor expansion. **B,** Shaded area of bone marks the resection (25% of the length of the proximal phalanx is removed). Dorsal cheilectomy is performed. **C,** The extensor hallucis brevis tendon and dorsal capsule are released proximally and transposed as an interpositional arthroplasty. **D,** The tendon and capsule are sutured to the plantar plate. The flexor hallucis brevis is not reattached to the base of the proximal phalanx. A K-wire is used to stabilize the repair.

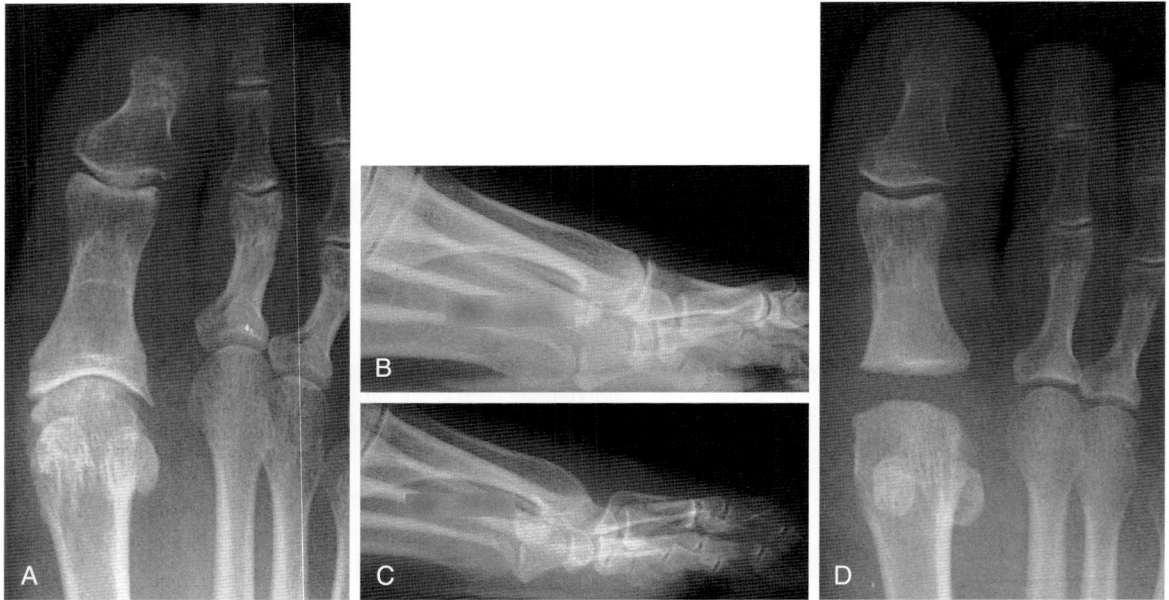

Figure 19-130 Anteroposterior (AP) **(A)** and lateral **(B)** radiographs demonstrate failed cheilectomy with chondrolysis of the first metatarsophalangeal joint. Postoperative lateral **(C)** and AP **(D)** radiographs after a Hamilton interpositional arthroplasty.

and sutured to maintain the oval shape (see Fig. 19-132G).

5. The graft is placed into the prepared joint surface, and the capsule closed over the graft and sutured into it during the closure (see Fig. 19-132H).

6. A K-wire may be used if needed for stability and is placed the same as in the resection arthroplasty, but it

is usually not required. It is removed 3 weeks postoperatively (see Fig. 19-132I).

Postoperative Care

Postoperative care is the same for both techniques. The forefoot is wrapped in a gauze-and-tape compression

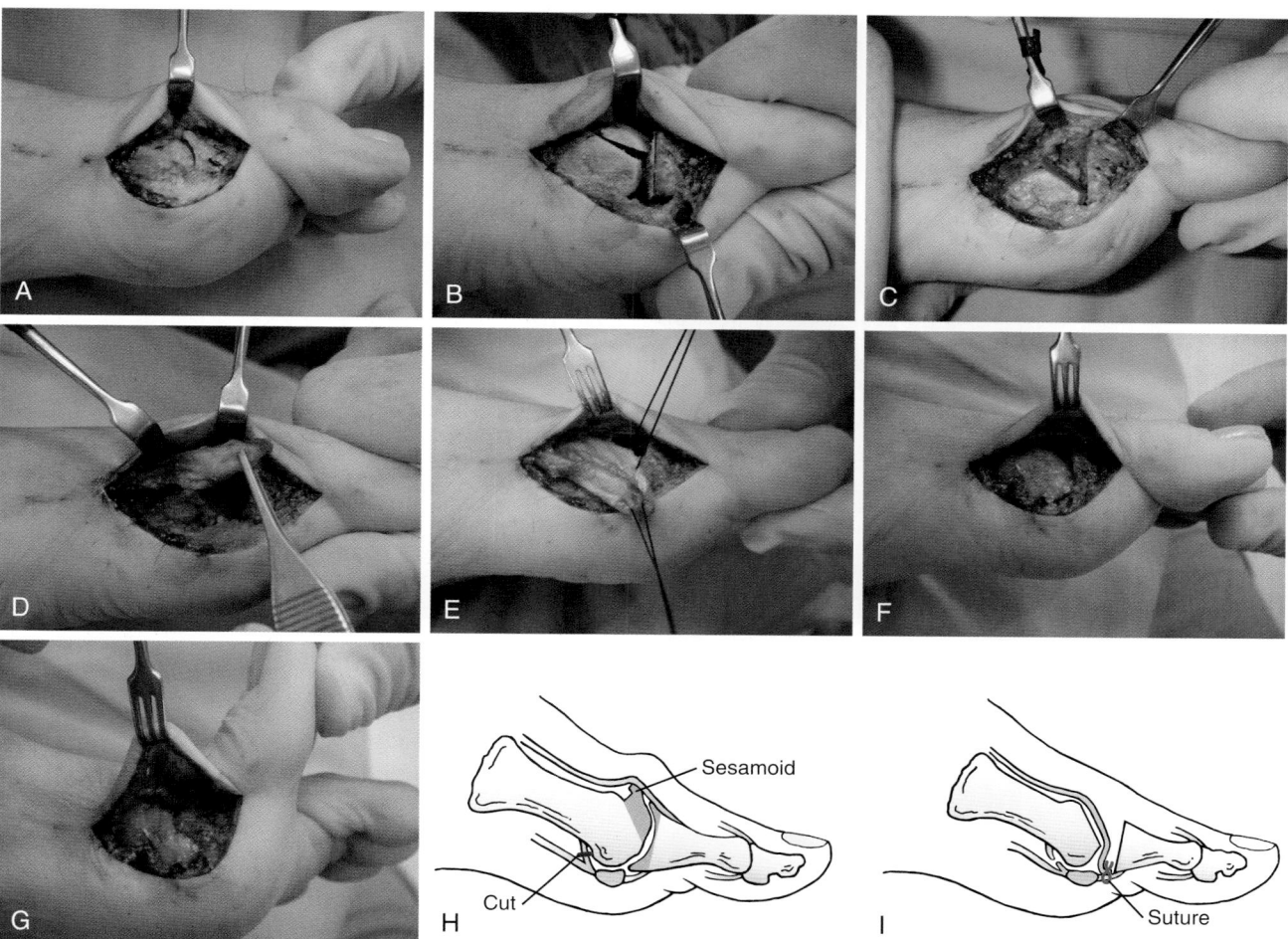

Figure 19-131   Soft tissue interposition arthroplasty. **A,** Medial longitudinal approach with medial eminence resection. **B,** Oblique resection of distal first metatarsal head and the base of the proximal phalanx to decompress the joint. **C,** After removal of bony fragments. **D,** Development of dorsal capsular flap. Sutures placed to secure the capsular flap **(E)** and tied in place **(F and G). H,** Diagram of bony resection and proximal capsular release. **I,** Suture of flap to intrinsic musculature. (Sanhudo JA, Gomes JE, Rodrigo MK: Surgical treatment of advanced hallux rigidus by interpositional arthroplasty, *Foot Ankle Int* 32:400–406, 2011. Used with permission.)

dressing at surgery and changed weekly for 6 weeks. The K-wire is removed 3 weeks after surgery. Passive range of motion in the dressing is initiated at 2 to 3 weeks after surgery when skin healing is complete. The patient is permitted to ambulate in a wooden-soled postoperative shoe, initially with weight bearing on the heel and on the outer aspect of the foot. Plantigrade ambulation is permitted 3 weeks after surgery after removal of the K-wire.

Results and Complications

Reported rates of subjective satisfaction with excisional arthroplasty vary from 76% to 96%.[92,598] Bonney and MacNab[51] observed that functional results can deteriorate over time. Rogers and Joplin[473] reported generally poor results with excisional arthroplasty and noted marked

objective improvement in only 9%, no change in 71%, and postoperative deterioration in 20% of patients after surgery. Henry and Waugh[233] noted an association between increased phalangeal resection and lateral metatarsalgia. Weight bearing on the great toe was noted in 73% of the feet from which one third or less of the proximal phalanx was resected but in only 19% of the feet from which more than one third was resected.

Beerema et al[25] reported cheielctomy was preferable for grade 1 and 2 hallux rigidus but suggested it was ineffective with more severe grades of arthrosis and that a Keller procedure was more reliable for later stages.

Schneider et al[502] reported on a 23-year follow-up on 87 cases where a resection arthroplasty was performed. The authors experienced a very low rate of final follow-up of patients, evaluating only 48% of cases. They reported

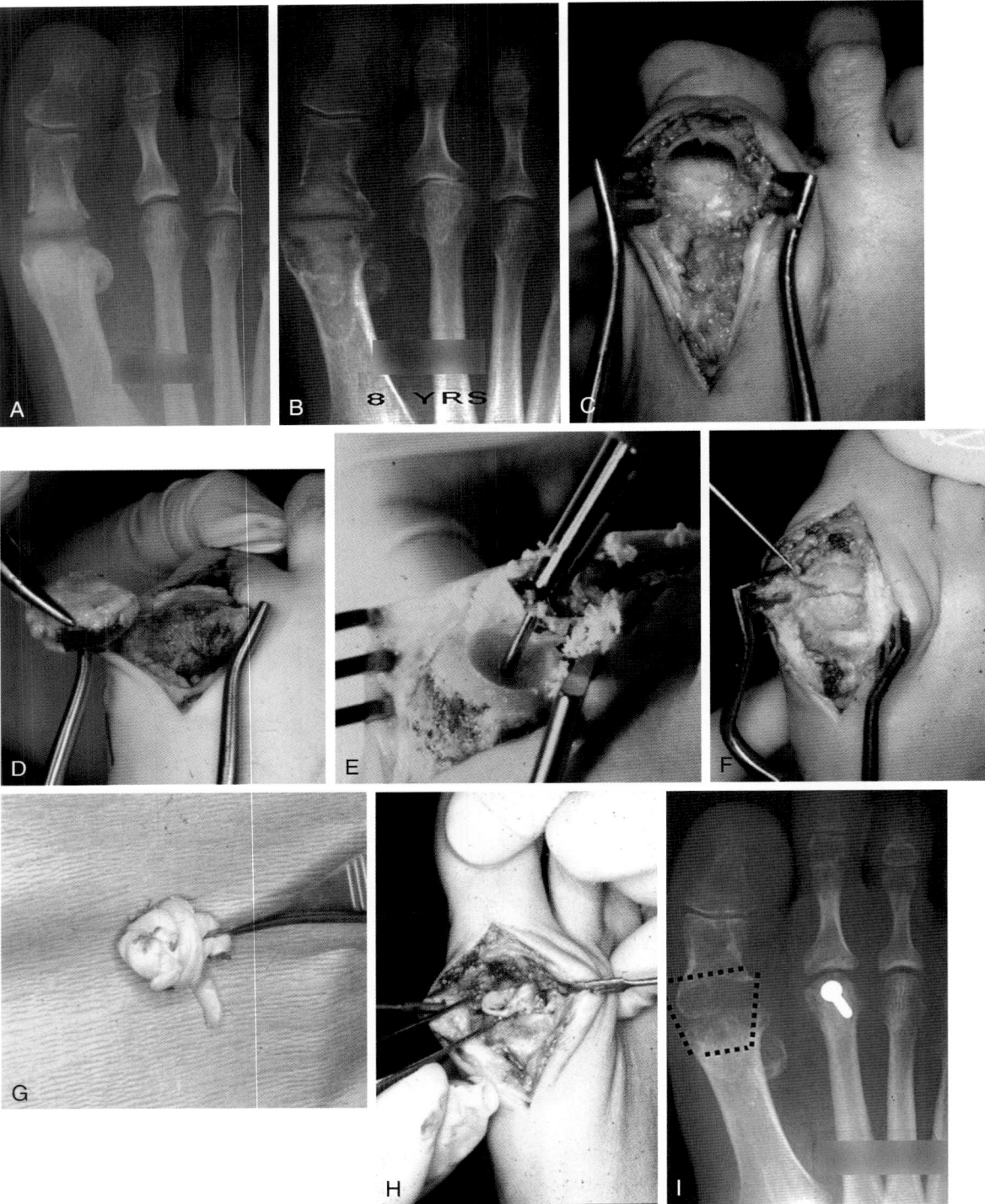

Figure 19-132 Technique of Coughlin soft tissue interposition arthroplasty. **A,** After placement of silicone double-stemmed implant for hallux rigidus. **B,** Eight years later, severe erosion has occurred around the implant. **C,** Intraoperative photograph after implant removal. **D,** After dorsal cheilectomy. **E,** Preparation of metatarsal head by reaming with power cup-shaped reamer to create a convex surface (a cannulated phalangeal reamer was used). **F,** After preparation of the phalangeal surface with a phalangeal reamer. **G,** Preparation of the tendon bundle harvested from the gracilis muscle. **H,** Placement of the tendon anchovy. **I,** Radiograph 1 year after soft tissue arthroplasty.

that of those patients seen, 63% required orthotics, 23% had metatarsalgia, and 23% demonstrated a cock-up deformity of the hallux. The average total first MTP joint motion was 30 degrees, and 26% of patients rated their subjective result as fair or poor.

An excisional arthroplasty appears to have fewer postoperative complications and improved patient satisfaction when performed for hallux rigidus in comparison with a hallux valgus deformity. Coughlin and Mann[109] reported significant postoperative metatarsalgia after excisional arthroplasty. Other complications include cock-up deformity of the great toe,[109,339,502] stiffness of the interphalangeal joint, marked shortening, impaired control and function, and decreased flexor strength of the great toe. Because of the high frequency of complications, excisional arthroplasty is recommended for elderly, low-demand patients who have no lateral metatarsalgia. It is best reserved for household ambulators who are poor candidates for any other procedure. Salvage of a failed Keller procedure is difficult to obtain as noted by Coughlin and Mann.[109] Vienne et al[576] reported on the salvage of 22 failed Keller procedures with an MTP arthrodesis. They observed successful fusion in 20 of 22 cases at an average follow-up of almost 3 years. One third required

an interposition osseous graft. Others have reported various techniques, including a peg-in-hole arthrodesis[287] and interposition bone graft, to reestablish length in a shortened first ray.[42,586]

Interposition of a flap of medial capsular tissue[97,322] or distal advancement of the dorsal capsule[399,499] has been combined with a vertical[214,306] or an oblique resection of the phalangeal base,[210] leaving the intrinsic attachments in place[344,399] or completely releasing it (Fig. 19-133).[322,499] Various techniques have been suggested to create an interposition of soft tissue, including a medial or dorsal capsule[214,306,399,499] acellular cadaver dermal tissue (AlloDerm Regenerative Tissue Matrix, Kinetic Concepts, Inc. [KCI], San Antonio, Tex.; Graft Jacket, Matrix, Wright Medical, Arlington, Tenn.)[38,303] (Fig. 19-134) allograft or autograft hamstring tendon[112,383] and allograft meniscus[126] In most cases, a cheilectomy and joint decompression has been accompanied by the interposition of various soft tissue spacers. Series ranging in size from 9 to 25 patients report an increase in the postoperative range of motion from 52 to 64 degrees and a final AOFAS score ranging from 71 to 94 points.*

*References 38, 112, 210, 286, 322, and 495.

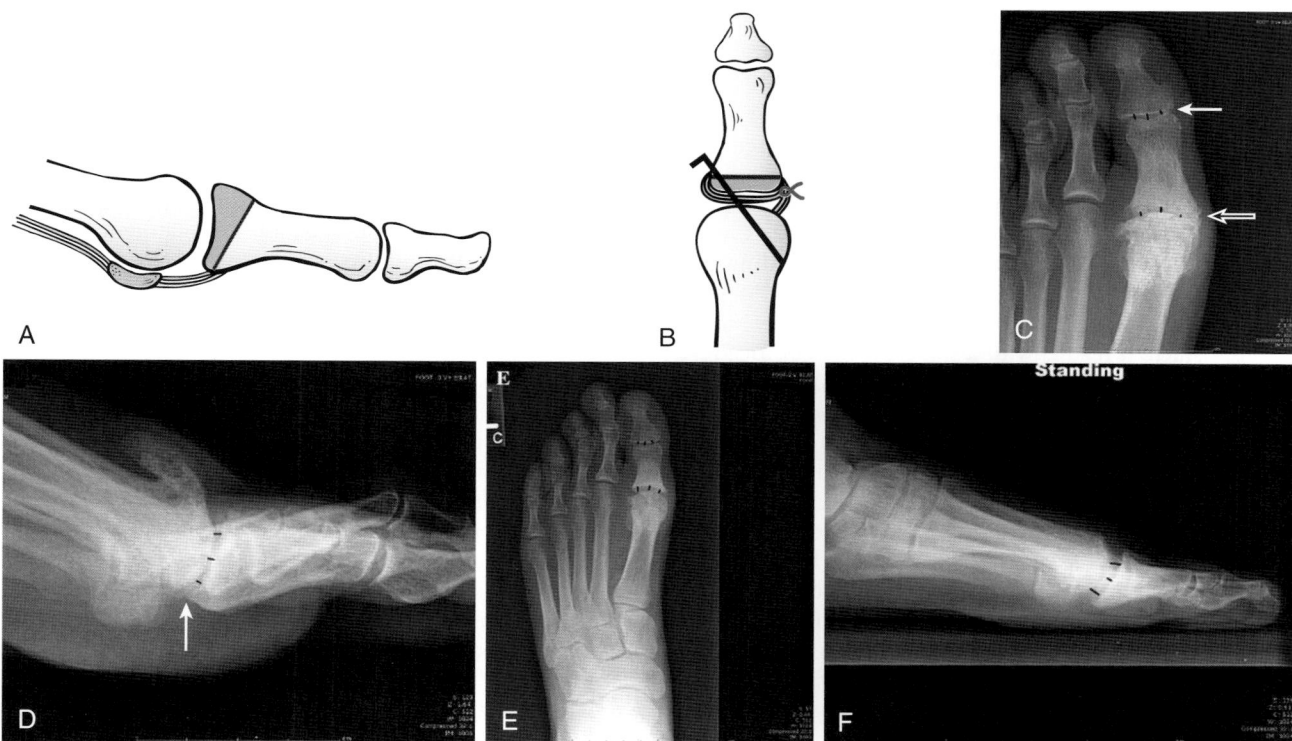

Figure 19-133 Soft tissue interposition with medial capsule. **A,** Lateral diagram showing extent of bone resection (the instrinsic insertion is left attached). **B,** Anteroposterior (AP) diagram showing suture technique of capsule and temporary K-wire fixation. **C,** AP radiograph demonstrating grade 4 hallux rigidus. The *solid arrow* points to arthritis of the interphalangeal joint. The *open arrow* points to severe first MTP joint arthritis. **D,** Lateral radiograph demonstrating complete loss of joint space with huge dorsal osteophyte. The *arrow* points to the first MTP joint. Postoperative lateral **(E)** and AP **(F)** radiographs showing increased joint space with interposition of medial capsule and minimal resection of the base of the proximal phalanx. (C and D, From Hahn MP, Gerhardt N, Thordarson DB: Medial capsular interpositional arthroplasty for severe hallux rigidus, *Foot Ankle Int* 30:494–499, 2009.)

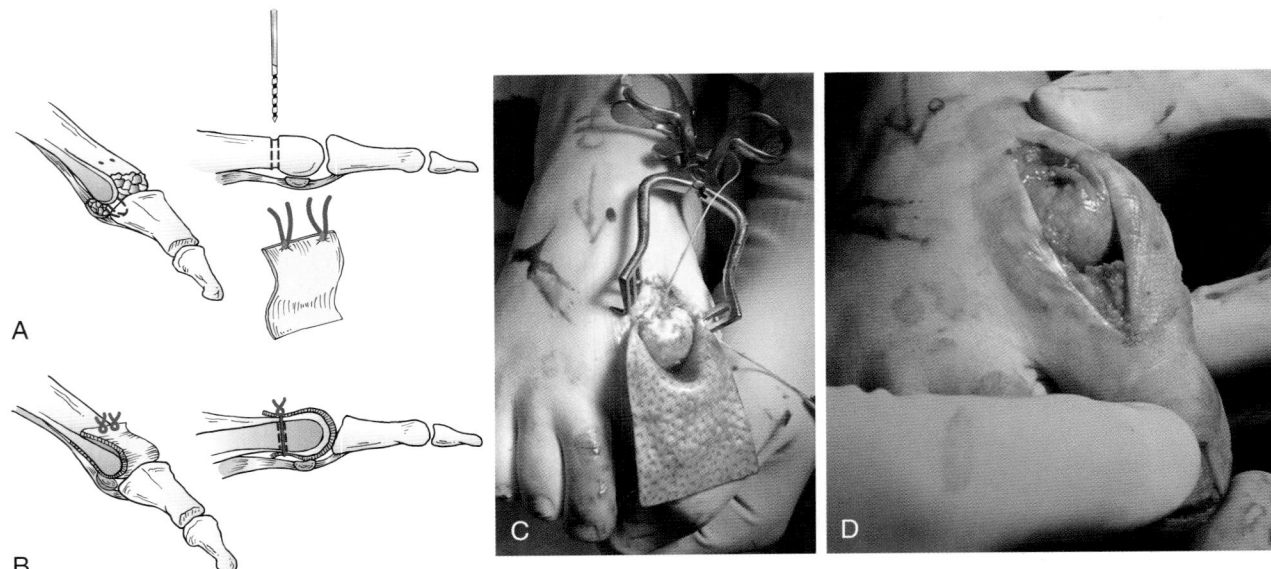

Figure 19-134 Interpositional arthroplasty with acellular graft. **A,** Drawing demonstrates end-stage degeneration of the first metatarsophalangeal (MTP) joint. After debridement, vertical drill holes are placed in the metaphysis; the acellular sheet is shown with sutures in the proximal end. **B,** After coverage of the metatarsal head dorsally, distally, and over the distal articular surface. **C,** Clinical photograph of the placement of the graft. **D,** After suturing and completion of the coverage of the first metatarsal head. (**C** and **D,** From Berlet GC, Hyer CF, Lee TH, et al: Interpositional arthroplasty of the first MTP joint using a regenerative tissue matrix for the treatment of advanced hallux rigidus, *Foot Ankle Int* 29:10–21, 2008.)

Hamilton[214] reported results on 30 patients (34 feet), all of whom had advanced degenerative arthrosis of the first MTP joint (<1 mm of joint space). A soft tissue arthroplasty was performed in these patients (see Figs. 19-129 and 19-130). Dorsiflexion increased an average of 40 degrees, and 93% of patients were satisfied with the procedure. No lateral metatarsalgia was noted. Careful selection of patients was recommended regarding first metatarsal length. Wrighton[598] reported only 59% satisfactory results with interpositional arthroplasty versus 76% satisfactory results with a standard Keller procedure. Ganley et al[177] reported on 50 patients with similar follow-up (average, 2 years) and noted 92% satisfaction. A 2% transfer lesion rate was noted. Barca[16] used a slightly different arthroplastic interpositional technique in which a rolled-up plantaris tendon was positioned at the base of the proximal phalanx. Barca[16] reported an average increase in dorsiflexion of 42 degrees (Fig. 19-135A and B).

Although Hamilton et al[214] reported generally encouraging results with interpositional arthroplasty, further follow-up is needed to document the long-term reliability of this procedure. Coughlin and Shurnas[112] reported the results of interposition arthroplasty on eight active younger patients (mean age, 40 years) with a minimum of 4 years of follow-up (Fig. 19-136, see Fig. 19-132). They reported that all patients were satisfied with the procedure, although there was slight weakness in toe flexion power in most patients. No clear transfer lesions were noted, but two patients had mild pain in the second MTP joint and increased pressure beneath the second metatarsal as demonstrated by Harris mat studies. It was not clear if these two patients had subtle second MTP joint capsular instability before the index procedure or if this problem developed subsequent to their surgery. In any case, none of the patients had limitations in activity, and no further surgeries have been performed.

Schenk et al[499] compared resection arthroplasty with and without capsular interposition for treatment of severe hallux rigidus. The authors compared 22 excisional arthroplasties with capsular interpositions with 30 simple resection arthroplasties. They found no difference in the clinical or radiographic results and concluded that interposition did not add substantial benefit. Mackay et al[344] compared interposition arthroplasty with arthrodesis. They noted an AOFAS score of 89 for excisional artroplasty and 64 points for arthrodesis. However, they had a high failure rate for the arthodesis group because of their surgical fixation, so the conclusion of this study are questionable.

Roukis,[482] in a meta-analysis of interposition arthroplasty results, reported high level of complications (31%), including plantar-flexion weakness, transfer metatarsalgia, stress fractures, arthrofibrosis, and osteonecrosis. Lau and Daniels[322] also reported great toe weakness, lateral metatarsalgia, and 73% satisfaction after interposition arthroplasty and suggested it should only be considered a salvage procedure.

FIRST METATARSAL OSTEOTOMY

Many osteotomy techniques have been described and recommended, but there are no long-term studies to substantiate their claims of successful treatment of hallux rigidus. However, there are studies that describe complications

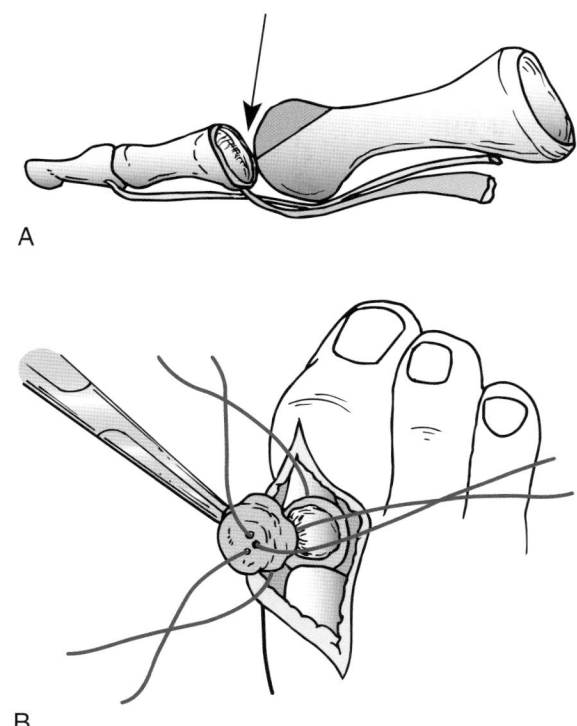

Figure 19-135 **A,** Cheilectomy and excavation of base of proximal phalanx as described by Barca.[16] **B,** Preparation of the anchovy for placement in the base of the proximal phalanx. (**A,** From Barca F: Tendon arthroplasty of the first metatarsophalangeal joint in hallux rigidus: Preliminary communication, *Foot Ankle Int* 18:222–228, 1997.)

of these procedures; salvage options are difficult at best. Osteotomies of the first metatarsal have been advocated in the treatment of hallux rigidus.[75,121,136,283,581]

Eponyms have become commonplace in describing different osteotomy techniques. The *Watermann osteotomy* uses functional articular cartilage on the plantar first metatarsal head by rotating the metatarsal articular surface dorsally[75] by means of a dorsal closing-wedge distal metatarsal osteotomy (Fig. 19-137). The *Green-Watermann osteotomy* (Fig. 19-138) plantar flexes the first metatarsal by means of a modified chevron osteotomy that can present a degenerated metatarsal cartilaginous surface to the articular base of the proximal phalanx. It can also lead to development of an intractable plantar keratosis beneath the first metatarsal head. Feldman[154] recommended the Green-Watermann osteotomy as the procedure of choice for hallux limitus, noting that it achieves success by means of a dorsal cheilectomy, plantar transposition of the first metatarsal, and shortening of the first metatarsal.

A plantar-flexion osteotomy can depress an elevated first metatarsal, and Davies[121] and Bonney and MacNab[51] have recommended this type of procedure (Fig. 19-139). Davies[121] noted "very positive results" and stated this osteotomy can "reestablish normal function and preserve the first metatarsophalangeal joint cartilage." Again, no controlled series has been presented on this technique.

A shortening osteotomy is said to relax periarticular structures[75] (Fig. 19-140) and is based upon the premise that the metatarsal protrusion or excess length of the first metatarsal is a factor in the development of hallux rigidus. In theory, these osteotomies appear to offer realignment for hallux rigidus associated with an elevated first metatarsal. However, Jahss[253] stated that limited application exists for these osteotomies. Few studies substantiate claims that these procedures are efficacious,[481,519] and Yee and Lau[601] concluded there is poor-quality or conflicting evidence to support the use of metatarsal ostetomies in the treatment of hallux rigidus. Cavalo et al[75] reported on two cases and Youngswick[605] on 10 cases but with no long-term follow-up. Feldman[154] described the surgical procedure but presented no series. The original Watermann osteotomy[581] rotates the metatarsal articular surface dorsally. If metatarsus primus elevatus is present, further dorsiflexion is contraindicated.

Mallerba et al[347] performed a Weil-type distal metatarsal ostetomy in 20 patients for grade 2 and 3 hallux rigidus combined with a cheilectomy and reported a final dorsiflexion range of motion of 44 degrees and an AOFAS score of 82 points. Ronconi et al,[475] using a similar technique for grade 1 and 2 hallux rigidus, reported final dorsiflexion motion of 45 degrees at less than 2 years of follow-up (Fig. 19-141). Oloff and Jhala-Patel[424] retrospectively reviewed 23 patients with grade 3 and 4 hallux rigidus who had undergone a cheilectomy, chondroplasty, and Youngswick-type osteotomy but made no specific conclusions based on objective data.

Derner et al[130] performed a plantar displacement osteotomy of the distal first metatarsal and achieved final total range of motion of 72 degrees (Fig. 19-142). With an average of 6 mm of shortening, although motion improved, the radiograph joint space did not improve. The authors reported 85% good and excellent results at a mean follow-up of 34 months. No mention was made of quantitative improvement in the preoperative metatarsus primus elevatus, nor in the incidence of postoperative lateral metatarsalgia. Roukis et al[483] treated 38 patients (41 feet) with a variety of distal metatarsal osteotomies for hallux rigidus (Youngwick, Green-Watermann, Weil, or SCARF) and assessed cases prospectively with clinical and radiographic analysis. They observed that the shortening of the first metatarsal contributed to instability of the medial column, reduction of the Meary angle, progressive medial drift of the second digit, and persistent metatarsus primus elevatus. Those feet with preoperative metatarsal plantar keratoses did not resolve, and an additional six feet developed second metatarsal transfer lesions. Eight other patients developed the onset of pain on the planter aspect of the hallux after surgery. *There was no significant improvement in either dorsiflexion or plantar-flexion range of motion after surgery.* Roukis et al[483] concluded that distal first metatarsal was not a "benign procedure" and observed that it could lead to iatrogenic shortening of the first metatarsal, progressive instability of the medial column, excessive plantar transpostion of the first metatarsal head,

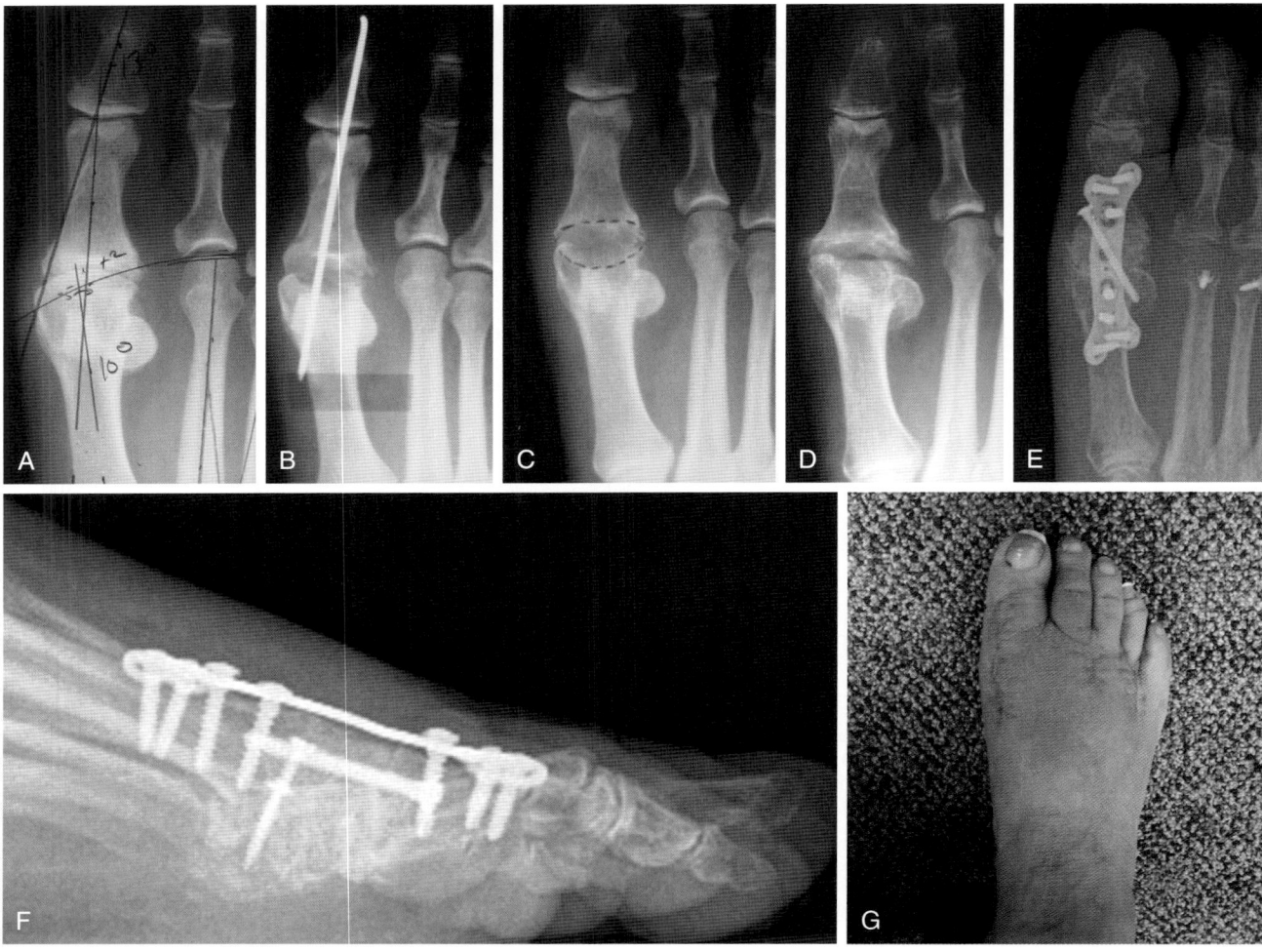

Figure 19-136 Interposition arthroplasty with later metatarsophalangeal arthrodesis salvage. **A,** Preoperative radiograph demonstrating grade 4 hallux rigidus. **B,** Intraoperative radiograph with temporary K-wire fixation and hamstring autograft interposition. **C,** Three years after surgery. **D,** Nine years after surgery patient, experienced moderate pain. **E** and **F,** Anteroposterior and lateral radiographs, respectively, demonstrating interposition graft and arthrodesis. **G,** Clinical photograph at 4 months after revision surgery.

and a paucity of improvement in range of motion or correction of metatarsus primus elevates.

Kilmartin[290] performed 59 decompression/shortening osteotomies of different types that were combined with a simple cheilectomy. Technique choice depended upon the preoperative length of the first metatarsal. At a mean of 15 months, only 54% of patients were completely satisfied. Thirty of 59 patients developed substantial postoperative transfer metatarsalgia or complications involving the lesser metatarsals, and one third of patients required subsequent lesser MTP joint corrective surgery. Dorsiflexion of only 6 degrees was achieved. Kilmartin concluded that the complications after first metatarsal decompression osteotomies were more common and more signifcant that other first-ray surgical options for the treatment of hallux rigidus. In four cases, there was significant dysfunction of the hallux postoperatively.

Coughlin and Shurnas[111,112] and Zygonis et al[609] noted that the treatment of hallux rigidus is based upon the

hypothesis that a long first metatarsal (MPD = positive metatarsal protrusion distance) is a causative factor in this etiology. Coughlin and Shurnas[111,112] concluded that a long first metatarsal was no more common in patients with hallux rigidus than in the normal population. Zygonis et al[609] measured a control group and a group with hallux rigidus. The mean first metatarsal length in the control group was 2.3 mm longer than that in the hallux rigidus group, and they concluded that these results did not support the theory that a long first metatarsal was an etiologic factor in the development of hallux rigidus. Furthermore, they could not support the use of a decompression osteotomy as definitive treatment for hallux rigidus.

Shereff and Baumhauer[509] stated, "The lack of statistical methods in small retrospective case series make the confirmation of reported good results impossible" with osteotomy techniques. Horton et al[241] concluded that a plantar-flexion osteotomy of the first metatarsal cannot

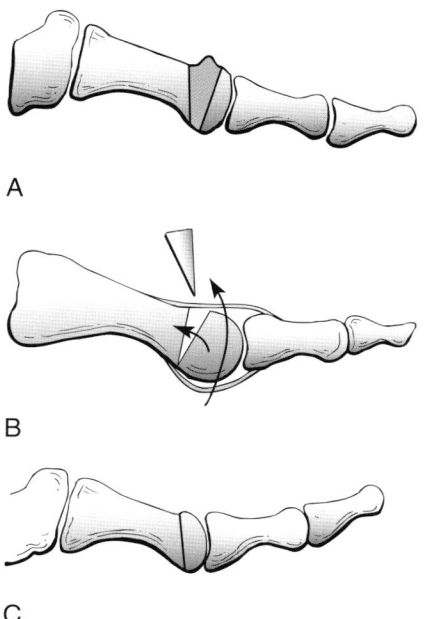

Figure 19-137 Diagram of Watermann osteotomy. **A,** Proposed closing-wedge dorsal osteotomy. **B,** Rotation of the articular surface in the dorsal direction. **C,** Modified Watermann procedure with the osteotomy located more proximally.

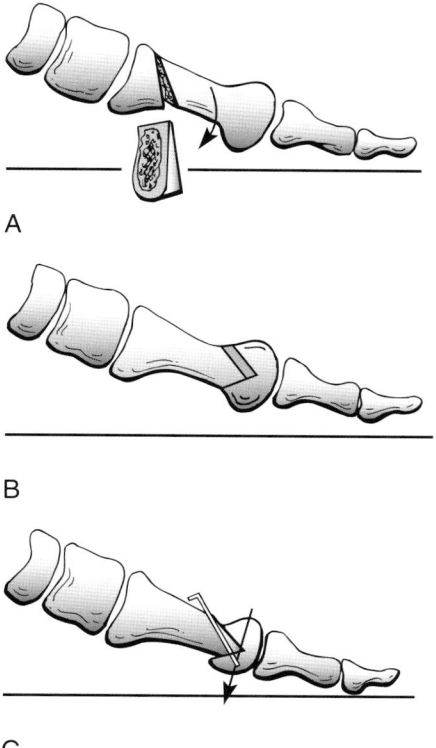

Figure 19-138 A, Plantar-flexion closing-wedge osteotomy presses first metatarsal. **B** and **C,** Green-Watermann osteotomy plantar flexes the first metatarsal by means of a modified chevron osteotomy.

be recommended based solely on the radiographic appearance of metatarsus primus elevatus. Roukis[481] performed a meta-analysis of 57 references, published and unpublished, that have been not only used as references but also used to endorse periarticular osteotomies as primary treatment techniques for hallux rigidus. He found only four studies (comprising 93 patients who were consecutively enrolled) that used appropriate methods to quantify the results and had a minimum of 18 months of follow-up). In these series, a mean increase range of motion of 10 degrees was observed, but he found little objective evidence regarding either subjective or objective outcomes to substantiate claims of efficacy. A surgical revision rate of 23% included 15% for the first ray and 8% to treat postoperative transfer lateral metatarsalgia. Three of the four studies failed to demonstrate correction of metatarsus primus elevatus, a major reason for using the technique, and 27% of patients were dissatisfied with their results. The high complication rate, combined with the difficult salvage required for either malunion of the first ray or for complications—resulting in the need for lesser metatarsal corrective surgery, led Roukis to conclude that the routine use of isolated periarticular osteotomies of the first metatarsal for hallux rigidus should be performed with caution or not at all.

Coughlin and Shurnas[111] found that any apparent elevation of the first metatarsal correlated with the grade of hallux rigidus and that it corrected to almost neutral on follow-up radiographs after either cheilectomy or arthrodesis. Therefore the current authors believe it is undesirable, in general, to perform a surgical procedure for the treatment of a secondary problem. Osteotomies designed to rotate good plantar cartilage into the joint space are done, in general, by also using a cheilectomy of the damaged cartilage surface, and thus the results of such procedures must be compared with the Mann cheilectomy alone. As previously noted, the results reported by Coughlin and Shurnas[111] with the Mann cheilectomy alone in properly selected patients yielded a high percentage of good and excellent results (97%) at long-term follow-up (9.6 years). That leaves little room for improvement but, rather, bases the selection of an osteotomy procedure on a surgeon's anecdotal experience, with potentially substantial inherent complications that leave difficult salvage options (Fig. 19-140).

Thus the results obtained with these osteotomy procedures, as published in the literature, are difficult to interpret and compare because different studies use different grading systems; different procedures are used even within individual series; the indications for some osteotomies are for low grades of severity, whereas for others, the indications are for much more severe cases of hallux rigidus. In most cases, the authors failed to documented objective results in detail. Although many more osteotomy procedures are being performed and reported at this time, more research is needed to establish the indications to quantify the complications, which in many cases are substantial, and to clearly and precisely document subjec-

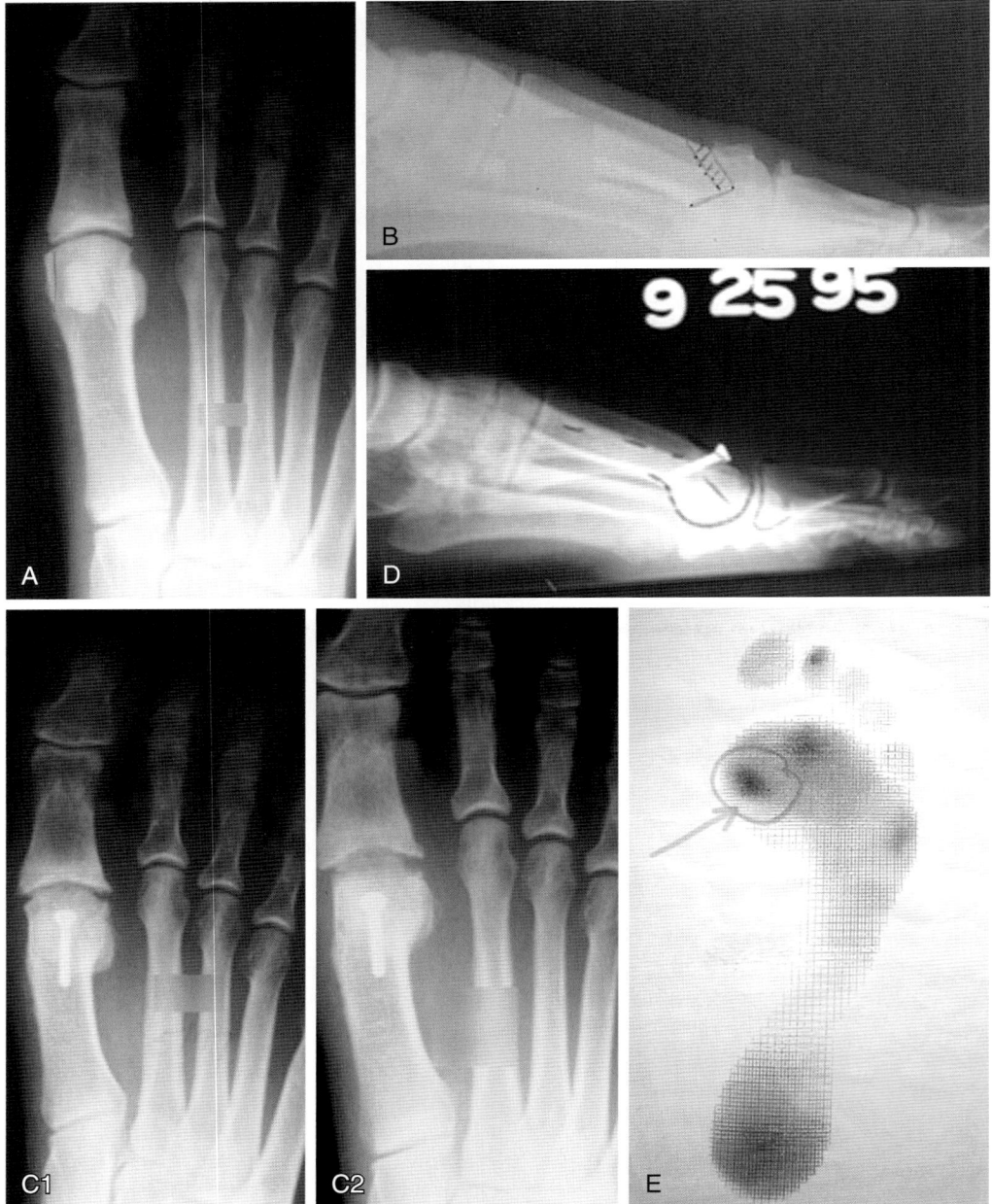

Figure 19-139   **A,** Preoperative anteroposterior (AP) radiograph demonstrates grade 1 hallux rigidus. **B,** Lateral radiograph demonstrates proposed plantar-flexion osteotomy (modified Green-Watermann procedure). Note dorsal osteophytes on phalanx and metatarsal. There is no evidence of hallux metatarsus primus elevatus. Postoperative AP radiographs immediately after **(C1)** and 2 years after **(C2)** osteotomy. **D,** Lateral radiograph 3 years after plantar-flexion osteotomy. **E,** Note the area of increased pressure beneath the first metatarsal head.

tive and objective results for each of the different proposed osteotomy techniques (Fig. 19-143).

METATARSOPHALANGEAL JOINT ARTHRODESIS
Arthrodesis of the MTP joint for hallux rigidus has been advocated in several reports. This is a salvage procedure that may be used for grade 3 or 4 severe hallux rigidus. With this procedure, the length and stability of the first metatarsal are preserved. The indications, besides hallux

rigidus, are a failed implant, failed excisional arthroplasty, or failed osteotomy. Relatively few contraindications exist for arthrodesis, although careful counseling is necessary so that patients can appreciate the restricted MTP motion that arthrodesis achieves. Brodsky et al[61] has reported that the results of gait analysis after MTP joint arthrodeses demonstrate that a fusion produces objective improvement in propulsive power, weight-bearing function of the foot, and stability during gait.

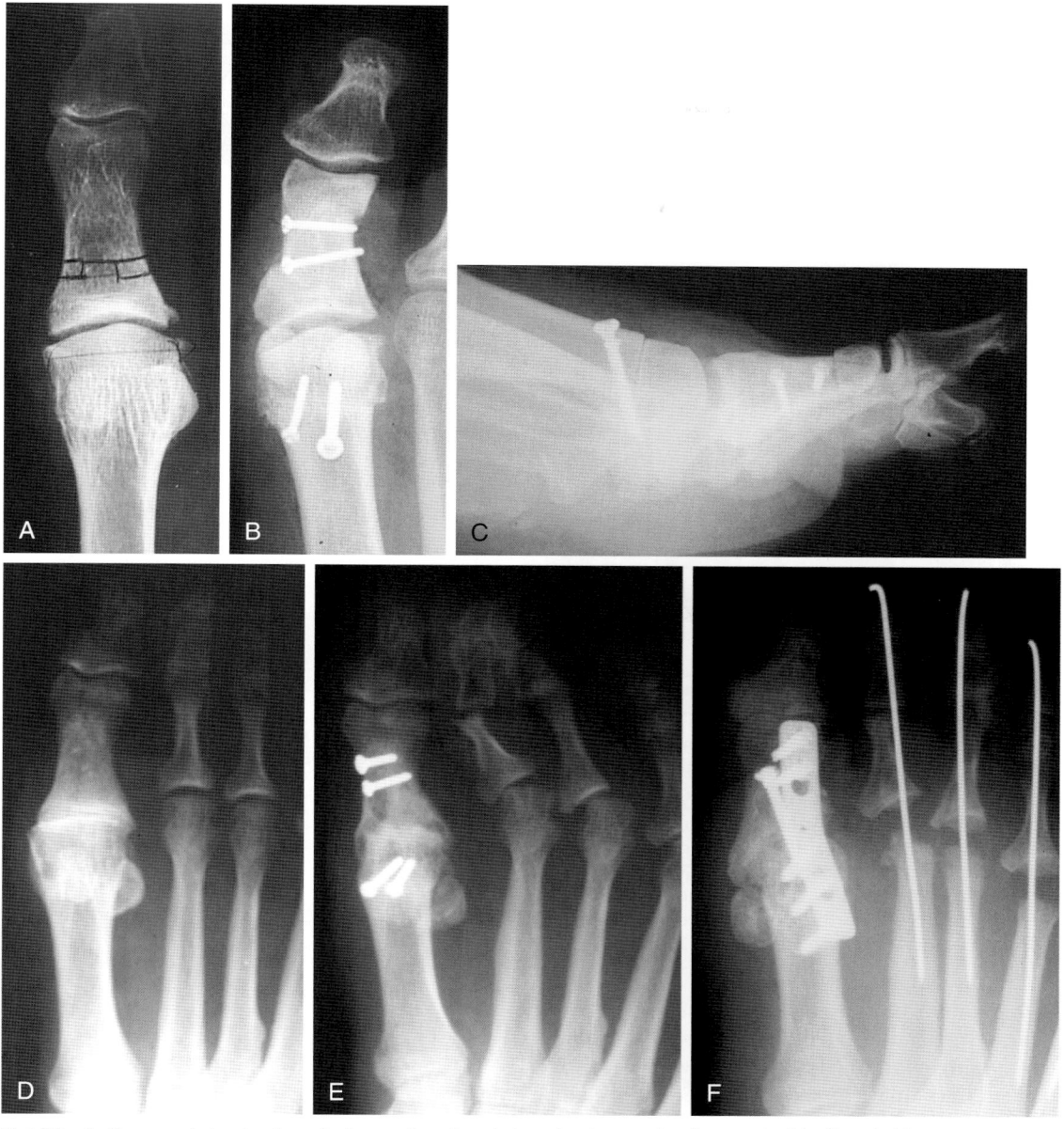

Figure 19-140 **A,** Proposed shortening phalangeal and metatarsal osteotomies for grade 1 hallux rigidus. Anteroposterior **(B)** and lateral **(C)** radiographs after shortening phalangeal and metatarsal osteotomies. **D,** Grade 4 hallux rigidus treated with attempted periarticular osteotomies. **E,** Complete chondrolysis, severe pain, and subluxation of lesser metatarsophalangeal (MTP) joints. **F,** Salvage with MTP arthrodesis and forefoot arthroplasty.

Surgical Technique

1. The MTP joint is approached through a dorsal longitudinal incision.
2. Joint surfaces are prepared for arthrodesis by resection of the remaining cartilage and subchondral bone (Fig. 19-145A, B, and C and Video Clip 33).
3. Various methods of internal fixation may be used, depending on the surgeon's preference (Fig. 19-145; see also Fig. 19-67 and Video Clip 35).

Results and Complications

The success rate for MTP arthrodesis varies significantly depending on the preoperative diagnosis, surgical technique, and method of internal fixation. Reported success rates vary from less than 77% to 100%.[*]

Methods of internal fixation for MTP joint arthrodesis vary considerably. K-wire,[1,517] circlage wire loop[1,16,420] screws,[1,152,393,580] staples,[39,157] dorsal plate,[†] and low-profile titanium plates[145,193,204,312,326] have all been advocated (see Fig. 19-144). The strength of the internal fixation construct is an important factor in maintaining the position obtained at surgery. O'Doherty[420] reported one of the highest nonunion rates (44%) (22 of 50 cases).

---

[*]References 51, 101, 103, 106, 107, 148, 183, 193, 311, 349, and 577.
[†]References 30, 37, 100, 101, 106, 111-113, 145, and 246.

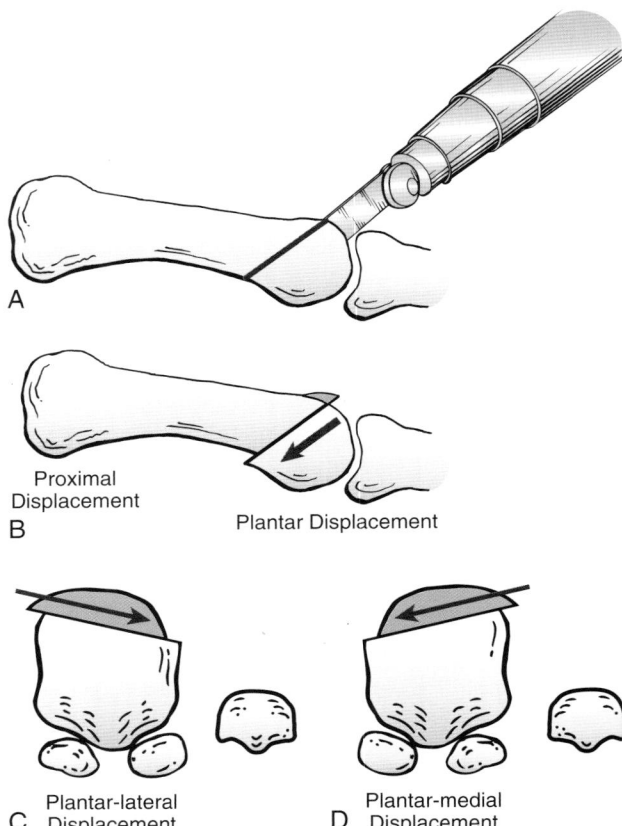

Figure 19-141 Distal first metatarsal osteotomy with capital oblique shortening osteotomy. **A,** Angle of saw cut. **B,** Plantar displacement. **C** and **D,** Modifications may allow plantar-lateral or plantar-medial displacement. (Modified from Ronconi P, Monachino P, Baleanu PM, Favilli G: Distal oblique osteotomy of the first metatarsal for the correction of hallux limitus and rigidus deformity, *J Foot Ankle Surg* 39:154–160, 2000.)

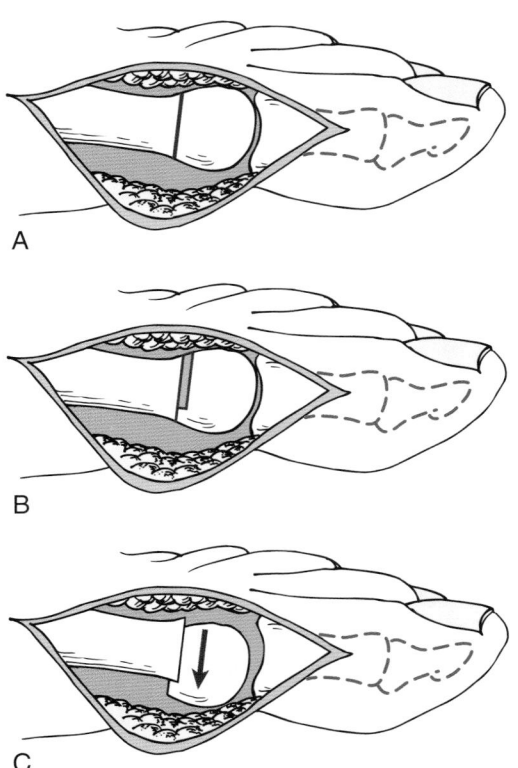

Figure 19-142 Distal vertical first metatarsal osteotomy. **A,** Angle of saw cut. **B,** Shortening achieved by wider dorsal cut. **C,** Displacement plantar and proximal to decompress the joint. (From Derner R, Goss K, Postowski HN, Parsley N: A plantar-flexor-shortening osteotomy for hallux rigidus: a retrospective analysis, *J Foot Ankle Surg* 44:377–389, 2005.)

Table 19-4	
	Relative Strength
Conical reaming and 3.5 interfragmentary screw	6
Conical reaming and crossed .062 K-wires	1
Conical reaming, mini-fragment plate, and lag screw	16
Conical reaming and only dorsal plate	1.3
Flat surfaces with single lag screw	10

Using wire loop fixation, Faraj[152] found screw fixation to be six times stronger than a wire loop, although Molloy et al[393] found a single intramedullary screw with a K-wire to be much stronger than crossed screws. Coughlin and Shurnas[111] reported 32 successful fusions of 34 (94%) and 100% good or excellent results (including the two patients with a fibrous union) and a low complication rate at a mean of 6.7 years of follow-up after arthrodesis for end-stage hallux rigidus. A low-profile Vitallium plate was used for fixation after power reaming was used to create dome-shaped arthrodesis surfaces. Only two of thirty-four patients required hardware removal. Moreover, measured first-ray mobility was significantly reduced after arthrodesis. Lombardi et al[338] have used first MTP joint arthrodesis with good results for lower grades of hallux rigidus and reported a high proportion of good and excellent results using only screws or Steinman pins (or both). They reported reliable improvement in radiographic measures of the first-ray angular deformities at a mean of 28 months. Similarly, Ettl et al[148] found a 100% union rate with screw fixation or K-wire fixation (or both) with the tension-band technique alone for end-stage hallux rigidus,

at a mean of 54 months of follow-up. The authors reported good functional results and significant pain reduction. Politi et al[440] studied the strength of diffferent MTP joint arthrodesis fixation constructs (using Kirchner wires as the baseline strength), finding conical reaming fixed with both a mini-fragment plate and a cross-lag screw to be the strongest construct (Table 19-4).

In published series on MTP arthodesis, Goucher and Coughlin[193] and others[25,30,193,312] have prepared the joint with female and male dome-shaped power reamers and used a dorsal titanium plate for internal fixation. Flat cuts have been used by some[37,580]; however, Wassink et al[580] observed that flat cuts leave little room for accurate positioning. With dome-shaped surfaces, a high rate of fusion

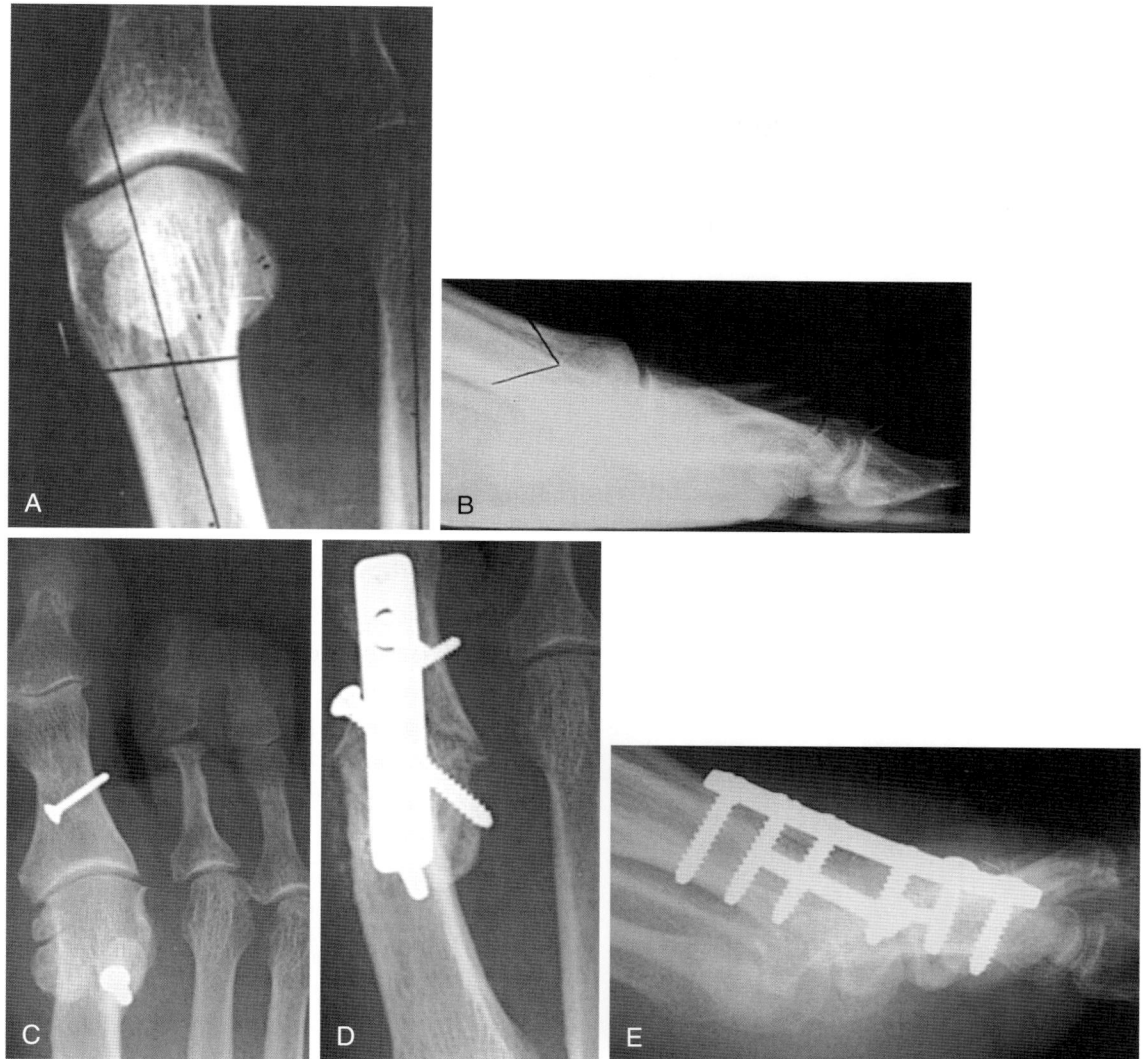

Figure 19-143 Anteroposterior (AP) **(A)** and lateral **(B)** radiographs demonstrate grade 1 hallux rigidus. **C,** After decompression shortening osteotomy of the proximal phalanx and first metatarsal. Postoperative AP **(D)** and lateral **(E)** radiographs after fusion for a painful first metatarsophalangeal joint.

has been achieved. Coughlin and Abdo[106] reported subjective good or excellent results in 93% of patients; 98% of cases went on to fusion. Other authors have reported on a dorsal compression plate for MTP arthrodesis. von Salis-Soglio and Thomas[577] reported on 48 cases with a successful fusion rate of 92%, and Mankey and Mann[349] reported on 51 cases, also with a 92% fusion rate. Coughlin[101] reported on the use of a stainless steel small-fragment plate in 35 cases with a 100% fusion rate. The main advantage of this method of rigid internal fixation is that it allows early ambulation in a postoperative shoe. Goucher[193] reported a 92% fusion rate (49 of 53 cases) and Kumar et al[312] a 98% (45 of 46) fusion rate by using a dorsal titanium plate with a cross-compression screw. Bennett and Sabetta[30] reported an 98.7% fusion rate in 200 consecutive patients who had concentrically reamed surfaces and a dorsal plate without a cross-screw and found the low-profile plate strong, and easy to use.

Ellington et al[145] reported that with locked titanium plates the nonunion rate was 16 of 23 (23%). Hunt et al,[246] in a report from the same group, used a slightly thicker precontoured unlocked stainless steel plate and reported a 12% nonunion rate. Both these series had a confounding issue that very early unprotected weight bearing was allowed in some patients (Fig. 19-146, see Fig. 19-145).

The main complications with arthrodesis are malalignment, nonunion, and degenerative arthritis of the interphalangeal joint of the hallux. Although the incidence of nonunion depends largely on the method of internal fixation, the postoperative treatment regimen has been shown to have a major effect as well. The complication rate after immediate weight bearing appears to be higher. Although Goucher and Coughlin[193] reported a 92% fusion rate with protected weight bearing for 12 weeks, Berlet et al[37] (who advocated immediate weight bearing after surgery) reported an overall complication rate of 19%, with a

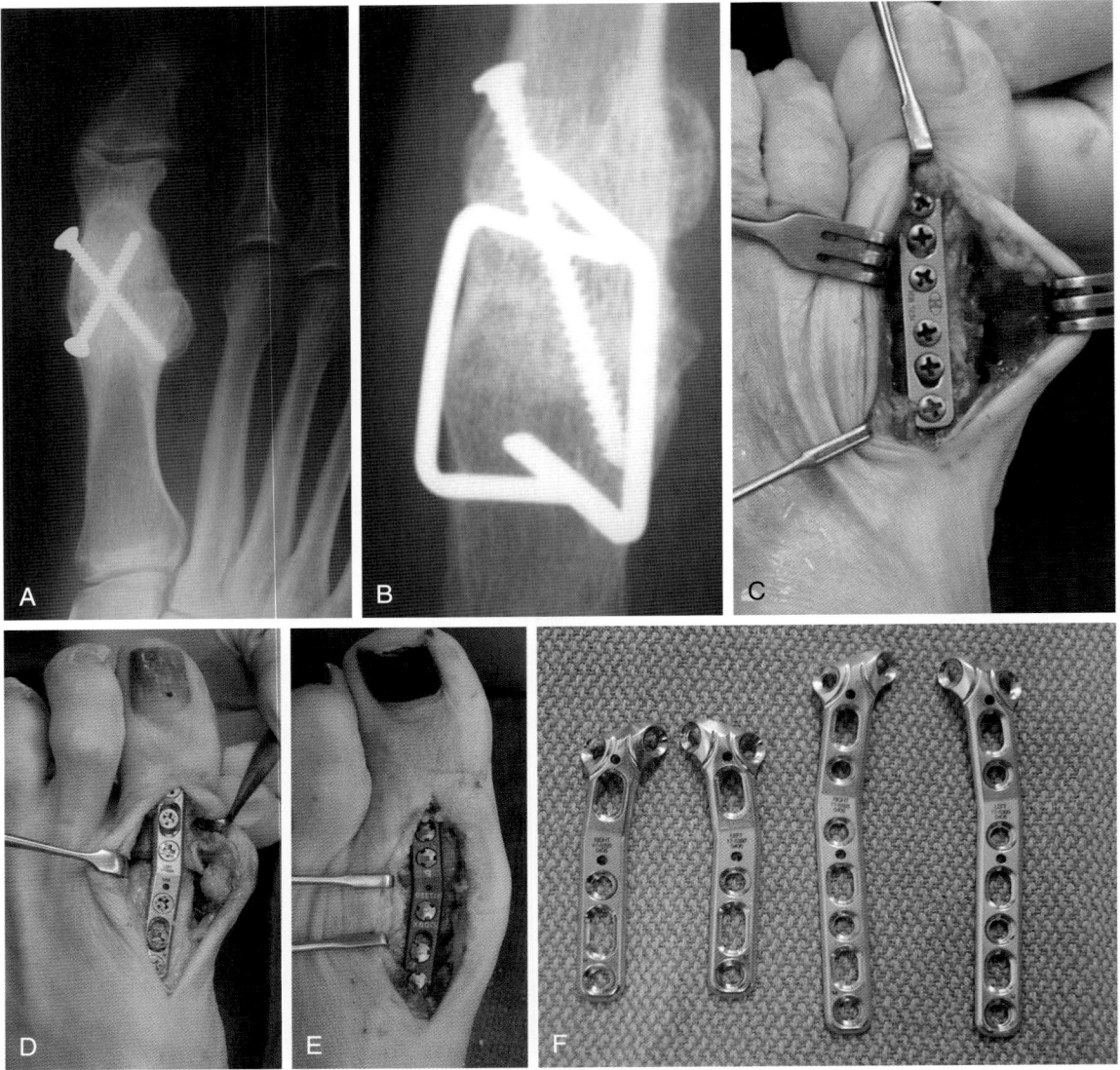

Figure 19-144 Different means of internal fixation for first metatarsophalangeal joint arthrodesis. **A,** Crossed screws. **B,** Staples and screw. **C,** Straight vitallium dorsal plate. **D,** Contoured dorsal stainless steel plate. **E,** Contoured titanium plate. **F,** Various examples of stainless steel reconstruction plates. (**B,** Courtesy Hans Peter Kundert, MD.)

13.5% rate of delayed or nonunion. Both Ellington et al[145] and Hunt et al[246] reported 13 of 107 nonunions (13.9%) for those patients for whom they started weight bearing at 2 weeks after surgery; the rate dropped to 7% when they initiated weight bearing at 6 weeks after surgery. Ellington et al[145] noted a much higher rate of nonunion in those with a diagnosis of rheumatoid arthritis—23%. Hope et al[238] found a much higher rate in males (19%) than in females (2.4%). For redo procedures, the failure rate was 24%.

In a review of 1451 cases in the literature, Coughlin[101] noted a 90% success rate of fusion. With an interfragmentary screw and dorsal plate, a fusion rate of 93% to 100% has been reported.[106] When nonunion occurs, it is often painless, and a fibrous union may be an acceptable result. Hope et al[238] noted that it is not necessary to perform a redo arthrodesis if a nonunion or fibrous union occurs.

Of 14 nonunions in their series of 139 cases, hardware was removed in 11 cases. Seven patients chose to accept the fibrous union, and the satisfaction levels were only slightly lower (AOFAS score of 72 vs. 80 points) for those with a fibrous union. Aas et al[1] and others[107,204,420] have also found that most patients with a pseudoarthrosis were minimally or asymptomatic. The current authors have also found this to be the case.[107,113,204]

Alignment of the arthrodesis site, however, is quite important. Malunion in any plane is poorly tolerated, which underscores the need for meticulous attention to the final position of the arthrodesis. Malunion can occur in any one of three planes: In the frontal plane, a varus/valgus malalignment can occur; in a sagittal plane, a dorsiflexion/plantar-flexion malalignment can develop; and in a transverse plane, a rotational deformity may be noted. With

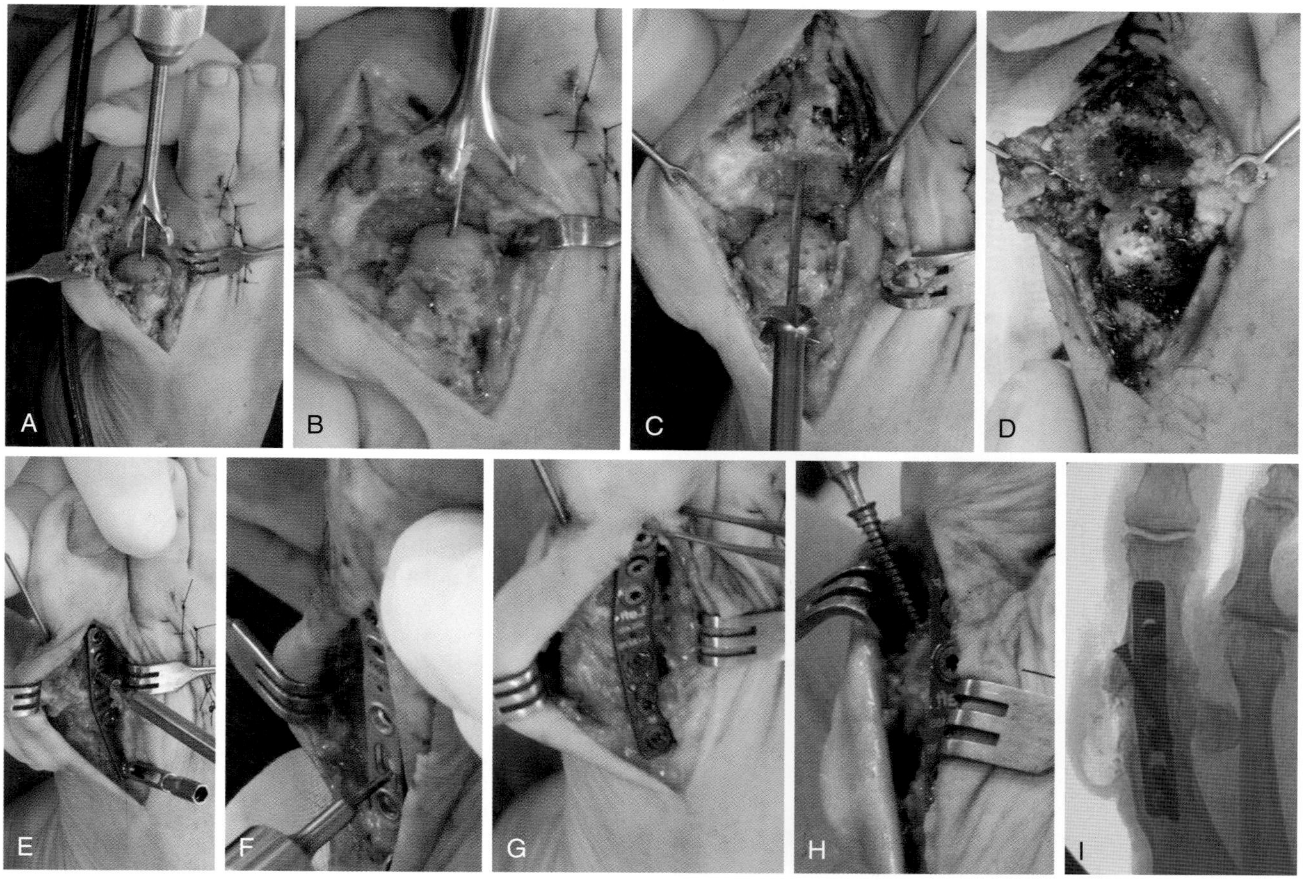

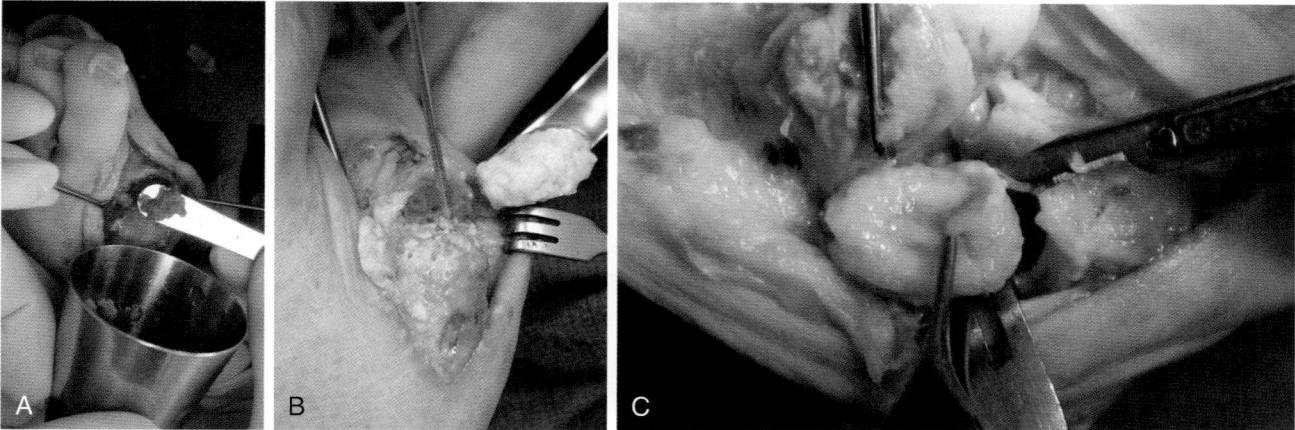

Figure 19-145 Placement of titanium locking plate. **A** and **B,** Preparation of metatarsal articular surface. **C,** Preparation of phalangeal articular surface. **D,** After perforation of both surfaces with small drill holes to increase the surface area for arthrodesis. **E,** Placement of dorsal titanium locking-plate distal screws. **F,** Placement of proximal compression screws. **G,** Final postion of plate and screws. **H,** A cross screw increases strength of the construct substantially. **I,** Final radiograph after plate and screw placement.

Figure 19-146 Technique tips for arthrodesis of the first metatarsophalangeal joint. **A,** Perforating the arthrodesis surfaces increases the surface area. **B,** Saving reamings and then creating a paste to place in and around the arthrodesis site. **C,** Removal of the medial sesamoid can relieve plantar pressure after the arthrodesis.

excessive dorsiflexion, pain can occur at the tip of the toe, over the interphalangeal joint, and beneath the first metatarsal head. With inadequate dorsiflexion, the patient might feel pressure at the tip of the toe. Varus/valgus alignment is critical as well (Figs. 19-147 and 19-148).

Accurate posititioning of the arthrodesis site is essential to a satisfactory result.[101,103,107] Coughlin, Grebing, and Jones[107] reported an 80% satisfaction rate after MTP joint arthrodesis. They did Harris mats imprints after surgery and demonstrated a clear hallux imprint in 95% of patients at final follow-up. This supports the concept that adequate weight bearing of the hallux occurs after MTP joint arthrodesis. Most frequently, the 1–2 intermetatarsal angle is reduced substantially after MTP arthrodesis without the need for proximal realignment or metatarsal osteotomy* (Riggs,[463] 4 degrees; Mann and Katcherian,[355] 4.4 degrees; Humbert et al,[245] 5.7 degrees; Coughlin et al,[107] 6 degrees; Cronin et al,[118] 6.4 degrees). This is likely because of the pull of the adductor hallucis acting on a longer level arm. Reduction of MPE occurs with MTP arthrodesis.[53,113]

The position of the arthrodesis is a key issue in ultimate patient satisfaction (Fig. 19-148). Although van Doeselaar et al[570] reported on 62 patients with MTP arthrodesis and found no correlation between foot function and the position of the hallux, they reported only one case of malalignment. Precontoured plates may assist the surgeon in obtaining a desired position of arthrodesis, but the anatomy can vary substantially from patient to patient. The conical shape of the proximal phalanx and

*References 53, 107, 118, 245, 355, and 463.

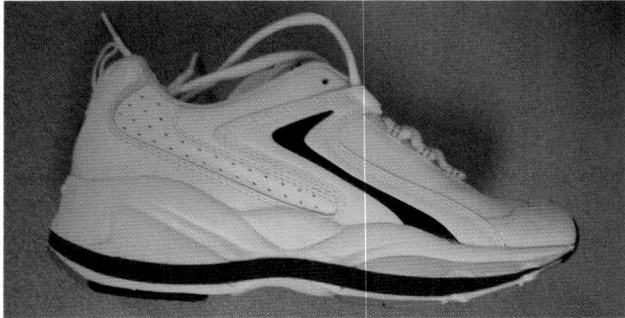

Figure 19-147 A rocker-bottom shoe can help ambulation in the patient whose first metatarsophalangeal joint was fused in inadequate dorsiflexion.

the declination of the first metatarsal can vary greatly. In a patient with pes planus, the first metatarsal declination angle can be very low. The surgeon must match a specific plate to the patient's anatomy (Fig. 19-149). Leaseburg et al[326] reported a strong coorelation between the hallux valgus angle and the plate angle but low correlation between the plate angle and the toe-to-floor distance. In a follow-up study,[128] it was suggested that excessive dorsiflexion can occur because of use of a precontoured plate or after bending the plate into excessive dorsiflexion. A plate without any dorsal bend can still achieve approximately 15 degrees of dorsiflexion because of the shape of the proximal phalanx.

Fitzgerald[160] observed an increased incidence of arthrosis at the IP joint, with MTP joint fusion in less than 20 degrees of valgus. He noted a threefold increase in the prevalence of osteoarthrosis of the IP joint with a straighter toe. Nonetheless, 10 to 20 degrees of valgus is still thought to be an acceptable position. Furthermore, Coughlin[104] found that the dorsiflexion angle was a primary determinant on the degree of IP joint arthritis and noted that 22 degrees of dorsiflexion relative to the metatarsal had the lowest correlation with subsequent IP joint arthritis, whereas less dorsiflexion was associated with an increased incidence of IP joint degenerative arthritis. Grimes and Coughlin[204] evaluated adjacent joint arthritis in 33 cases after MTP joint arthrodesis. In evaluatiing the IP joint of the hallux, there were as many joints with degenerative arthritis on the contralateral side as on the fusion side. None of these were symptomatic. In their evaluation of the first metatarsocuneiform joint, 5 of the 33 feet in the series had some element of degenerative arthritis at the metatarsocuneiform joint. In two feet, it was similar to the contralateral foot; in two other feet, there was only arthritis at the MTC joint on the operated side, but it was asymptomtic. One patient had bilateral MTP joint

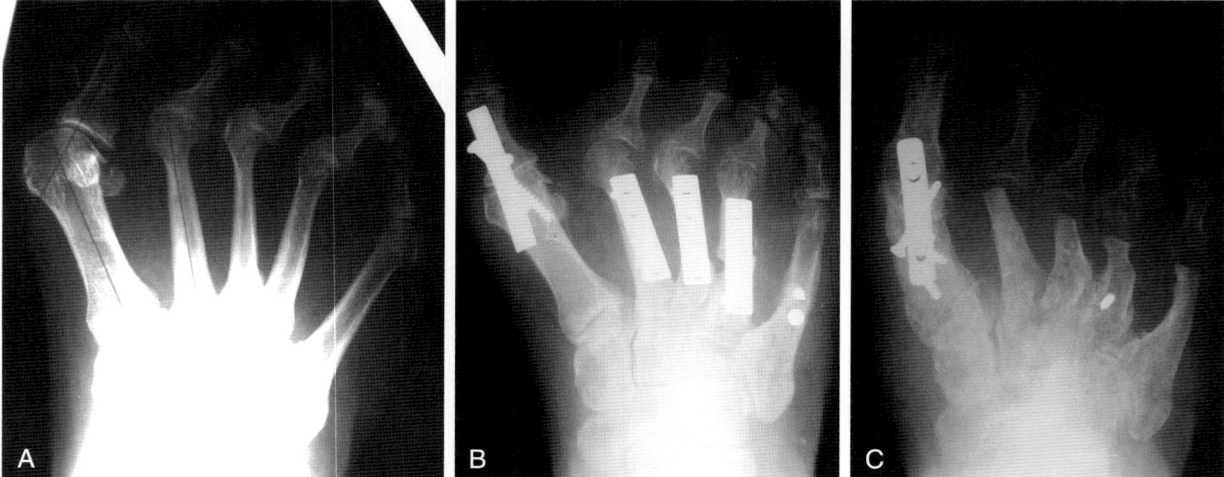

Figure 19-148 Treatment of splay foot. **A,** Preoperative radiograph showing severe splay foot. **B,** After metatarsophalangeal (MTP) joint arthrodesis, the hallux is placed excessively straight, creating a painful hallux that did not fit in a regular shoe. **C,** After redo salvage procedure, a resection arthroplasty of the lesser MTP joints and a redo arthrodesis that was shortened and placed in more valgus to achieve a foot that could now fit in a regular shoe.

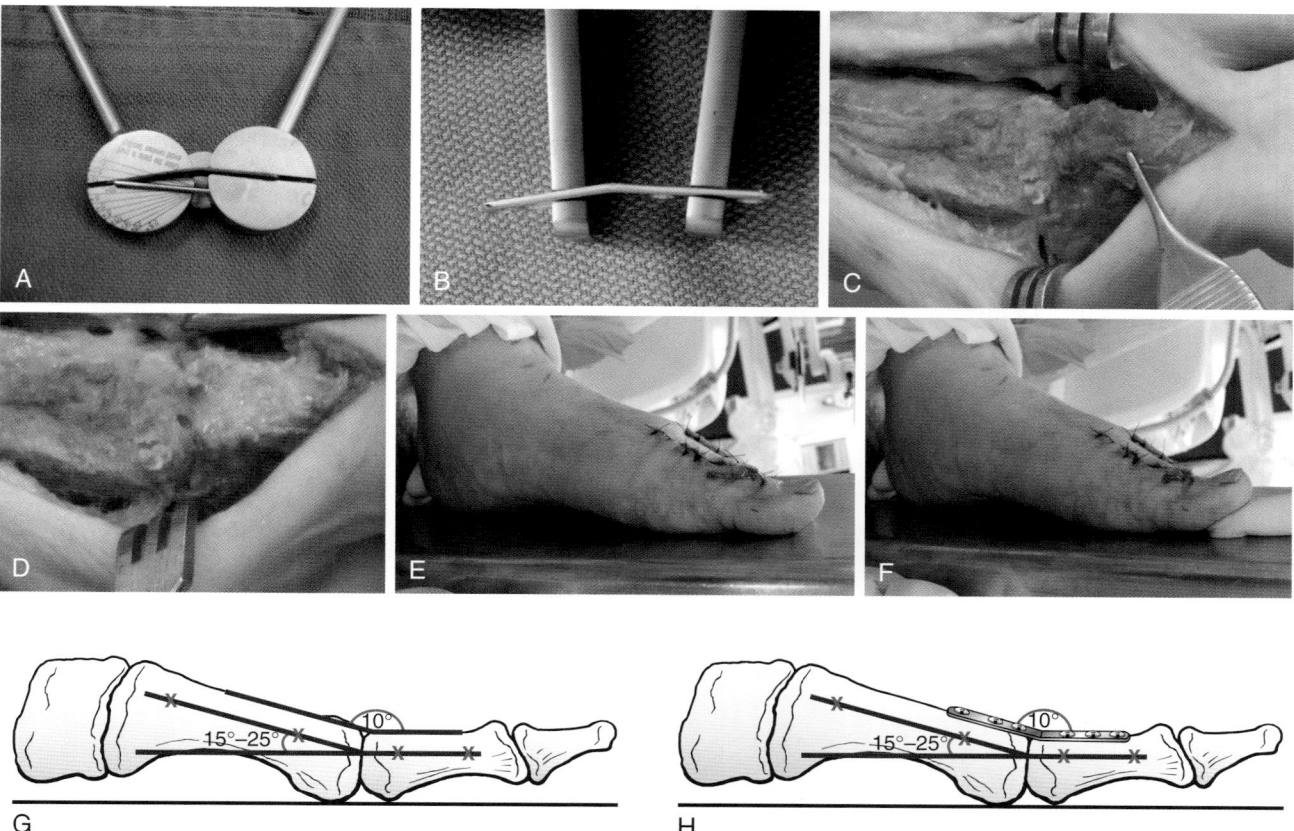

Figure 19-149 Means of adapting the dorsal plate. **A** and **B**, Plate benders to increase or decrease the dorsal angulation of the plate. **C**, The dorsal and plantar flair of the proximal phalanx makes the surface a "cone," which may increase the clinical dorsiflexion when the plate is placed. **D**, A rongeur has been used to diminish the dorsal flare, for better positioning of the plate. **E** and **F**, By using the bottom of an irrigation pan, the foot can be positioned to check the amount of dorsiflexion created by the fusion to ensure there is not excess or insufficient dorsiflexion. (Typically, if the surgeon can place a fingertip beneath the tip of the toe, the position is adequate.) **G**, The diagram shows the metatarsophalangeal joint angle as measured from the dorsal surface and with intramedullary reference points. **H**, Most precontoured dorsal plates are made with 10 degrees of dorsiflexion; however, the measured dorsiflexion angle using intramedullary reference points can vary from 15 to 25 degrees.

arthrodesis, but only developed arthritis of the MTC joint on one side. The authors concluded that arthritis of the IP or MTC joints was not an issue at an average 8-year follow-up, but arthritis was actually more a function of the age of the patients in the series. Tourne et al[559] found a 5% incidence of IP joint arthritis after MTP joint arthrodesis.

Watson and Kelikian[582] examined the cost of the MTP joint implants. The initial cost of the hardware, the time required to implant the hardware, the success rate of the arthrodesis procedure, and the necessity of eventual removal of hardware all must be considered. Watson compared Herbert screws, Association for Osteosynthesis (AO) screws, and a Vitallium plate. A 61% fusion rate of the Herbert-type screws led to a higher revision rate. The authors concluded that the plate construct eventually had the highest union rate, and the greatest clinical effectiveness, although it had a slightly higher cost because of the increased operative time needed for implantation. Hyer et al[247] also examined the cost of crossed screws in comparison with a dorsal plate.

Although the plate was decidedly higher in cost, they concluded that the dramatically higher fusion rate, higher patient satisfaction, and the control over the ultimate position of the arthrodesis had to be weighed against the cost of hardware removal, malunion, or delayed union.[312] Likewise, the cost of arthrodesis compared with a joint replacement is a factor to consider. Gibson and Thomson[181] compared 38 feet in which an arthodesis was performed with 39 feet in which a two-part joint replacement was performed. The poor range of motion obtained in the arthroplasty group, implant subsidence, continued pain, and other complications led the authors to conclude arthrodesis was the preferable procedure. Gibson and Thomson[181] also found the ultimate cost of an MTP joint arthrodesis was half that of total joint replacement arthroplasty.

Hardware removal is a definite cost consideration. The low-profile titanium plate has a low rate of removal. Goucher et al[193] reported a 4% removal rate, although Kumar et al[312] noted a 2% rate—all cases with dorsal plate fixation. One of the highest rates for hardware removal was noted after placement of a single compression screw by Wassink et al[580] (78%).

METATARSOPHALANGEAL JOINT ARTHROPLASTY

First MTP joint replacement arthroplasty has been advocated for hallux rigidus, rheumatoid arthritis, and hallux valgus and as a salvage for failed first-ray surgery.[537] Cook et al[96] presented an analysis of the different choices and advancement in joint replacement arthroplasty for the first metatrsophalangeal joint, suggesting four different categories of implants. Cook[97] and Carpenter[73] have suggested considering great toe arthroplasty implants in the following categories:

FIRST GENERATION—silicone implants (hemistem and double-stem joint replacement)

SECOND GENERATION—improved silicone implants (hemistem and double-stem replacement with grommets)

THRID GENERATION—metal (hemistem and phalangeal + metatarsal surface replacement; with press-fit fixation)

FOURTH GENERATION—metal (hemistem and phalangeal + metatarsal surface replacement; with threaded-stem fixation)

Various implants composed of different materials have been manufactured to replace the base of the proximal phalanx, distal first metatarsal articular surface, or both. Initial attempts at proximal phalangeal articular replacement using metallic prostheses involved mainly case reports with limited follow-up[83,92,267,537] (Fig. 19-150A and

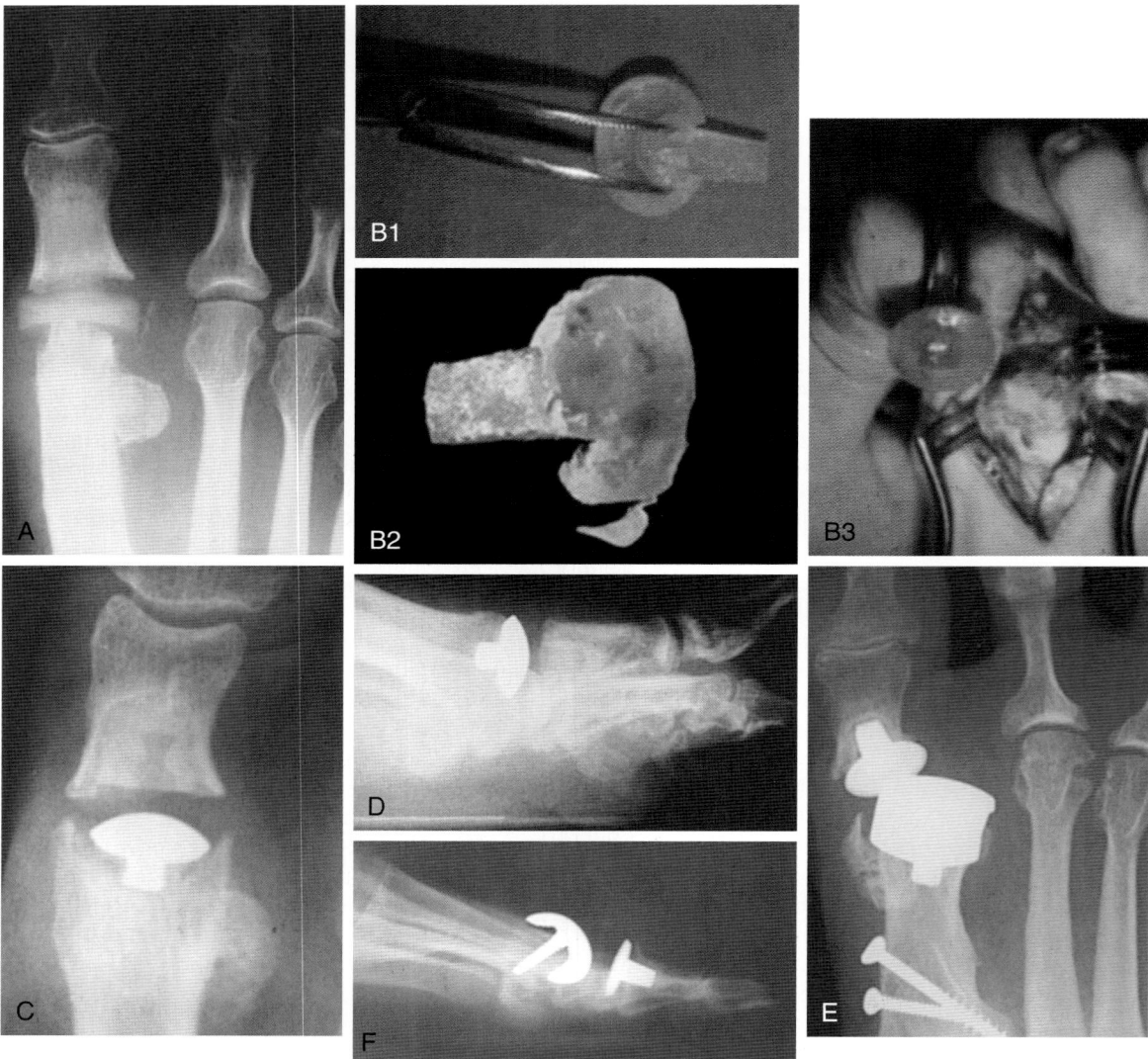

Figure 19-150 **A,** Radiograph demonstrates failed single-stem silicone arthroplasty. **B1-B3,** Failed silicone hemiarthroplasty implants. **C** and **D,** Failed cemented phalangeal and metatarsal implant with subsidence of the metatarsal component. **E** and **F,** Subluxation of the porous ingrowth component with loosening of the phalangeal implant 1 year after surgery. (**C** and **D,** Courtesy Kenneth Johnson, MD.)

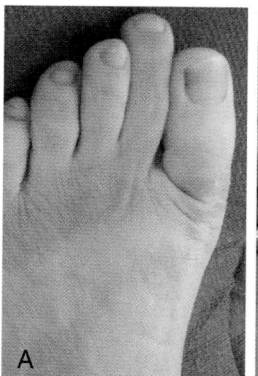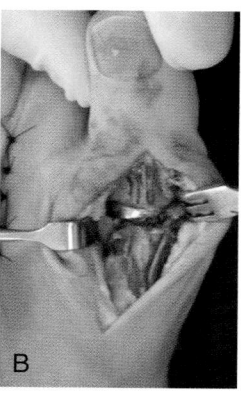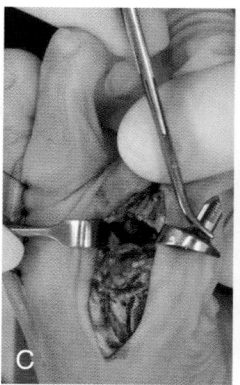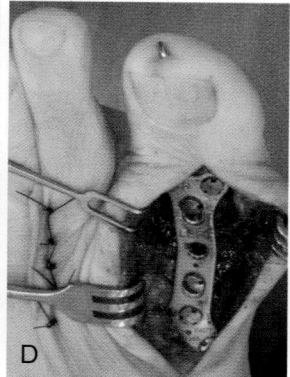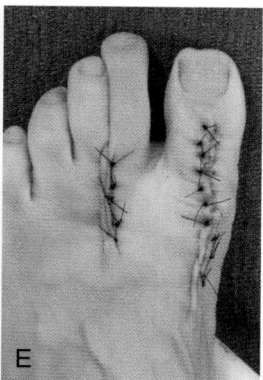

Figure 19-151 Failed hemiimplant. **A,** Clinical photograph of foot with failed hemiimplant in the proximal phalanx. **B,** Intraoperative photograph showing failed implant. **C,** Removal of the implant; no bony ingrowth had occurred. **D,** After bone grafting and placement of dorsal reconstruction titanium plate. **E,** After completion of the procedure. Ray length has been reestablished.

B). Although Townley[561] reported a large series with long-term follow-up and generally satisfactory results. Nevertheless, phalangeal base implants continue to be used.[305-307,524,544] Giza et al[185] reported on another large series of proximal phalangeal arthroplasty implants (103 cases). The gain in MTP joint motion was 4 degrees, and the average postoperative AOFAS score was 80. Reduction in pain was noted. Sorbie and Sanders[524] implanted 23 phalangeal chrome-cobalt resurfacing implants (19 of 23 were cemented) and at a mean follow-up of 34 months, noted an AOFAS score of 88 points. Konkel and Menger[305] reported on 13 titanium implants. At an average follow-up of 66 months, all prostheses had subsided to a varying degree, with definite lucencies apparent around the phalangeal implant. Complications included joint stiffness, clawing of the halllux, and transfer metatarsalgia. In subsequent reports, Konkel[306,307] noted improved results using joint implants in combination with a cheilectomy if necessary. They reported an average MTP joint range of motion of 64 degrees and a mean AOFAS score of 83 to 89 points. Eighty-five percent of patients were satisfied with their final result. The authors observed that those with grade 4 hallux rigidus did not do as well as those with lower grades (Fig. 19-151). Carpenter et al[73] used a screw in a metatarsal resurfacing replacement cap and reported a final AOFAS score of 89 points. Roukis and Townley[561] reported a 1-year follow-up on periarticular osteotomy in 16 feet compared with endoprosthetic replacement in 9 feet. The authors showed minimal improvement in first MTP joint dorsiflexion with either technique, although pain relief was good.

Raikin et al[446] compared hemiarthroplasty and MTP joint arthodeses in 48 cases. Those joints with successful fusions had lower pain scores, higher function, and satisfaction. Of 21 arthroplasties, 8 subsided though the plantar cortex, and 5 other implants subsided as well (60%). A 57% satisfactory rate was noted for the arthroplasty group. At a mean follow-up of more than 6 years, arthrodesis was considered much more predictable. Gibson and Thomson[181] in another study comparing

arthroplasty and arthrodesis, reported that 60% of the arthroplasty group at 2 years after surgery would undergo the procedure again, while 97% of the arthrodesis group would have the fusion performed again.

Finally, Ronconi et al[474] reported on their results with hemiarthroplasty compared with distal first meatatarsal decompression osteotomy for grade 3 hallux rigidus. At just more than 2 years of follow-up, only 28% of patients were very satisfied with the arthroplasty; pain, stiffness and prosthetic subluxation subsidence, and dislocation were noted complications.

Metal-Polyethylene Joint Replacements
Based on reported success with metal-polyethylene cemented total knee replacements, Johnson and Buck[264] designed a cemented nonconstraining first MTP total joint replacement. At greater than 3.5 years of follow-up of 21 feet, more than 50% implant loosening was noted, and the use of the implant was later discontinued (see Fig. 19-150C and D).[159,263a] Other reports have documented short-term experience.[48,300,302]

With short-term follow-up (18 months), Koenig[301] reported a 12% revision rate when repeat bony in-growth prostheses were implanted for revision of failed Silastic implants. In a larger study, Koenig and Horwitz[302] reported 61 implants that had been placed for a variety of indications. No information regarding long-term follow-up was provided (see Fig. 19-150E and F). Likewise, Freed[170] reported that more than 360 implants have been placed to revise failed silicone implants, but again, no information on the subjective or objective results was reported.

Ess et al[147] reported five excellent, one good, two fair, and one poor results with 2 years of follow-up after total endoprosthetic replacement (ReFlexion, Osteomed, Addison, Tex.). Radiographic loosening was noted on one cementless phalangeal component, one prosthetic subluxation, one superficial infection, and one recurrent severe valgus deformity. Only long-term follow-up will provide further information as to whether these uncemented first MTP total joint replacements will have greater success than the cemented MTP joint replacements implanted during the 1970s and 1980s. The paucity of information available with even short-term subjective and objective results makes use of these implants questionable until investigators report further information.

Kundert[313] reported on the results of a modular or total replacement of the first cases, with follow-up of 14 years; three were excluded because of the need for revision surgery. Limited MTP joint range of motion was noted in 7 of 11 patients. The authors also noted a subsidence in 12% in a larger unpublished study. Unfortunately, the scientific data on hemijoint and total joint replacement implants is unclear at best. The indications in different studies vary as to the severity of the degenerative arthritis, and the grading or staging used by authors varies as well, so it is difficult to compare different studies and different prosthetic implants (Fig. 19-152).

Cook[96] performed a meta-analysis of 47 peer-reviewed articles published on the results of MTP joint replacement arthroplasty published after 1990. The results of 3049 implants were surveyed. Patient satisfaction ranged from 85% to 94% in studies with variable indications, procedures, and follow-up—varying from minimal to midterm and, in a few cases, long-term follow-up. Despite promising initial results, Cook noted several authors had reported

on implant radiolucencies and subsidence. On the other hand, some studies have noted exceptionally high levels of satisfaction and pain relief on long-term follow-up. Yee and Lau,[601] in a meta-analysis of joint replacement for treatment of first metatarsophalangeal joint degenerative arthritis, found conflicting or poor quality of evidence to support joint replacement. Furthermore, Yee and Lau[601] observed that the long-term consequences of hemiarthroplasties (and total joint arthroplasties) that are malpositioned, have subsided, or have radiolucencies (but have yet to fail) are unknown. These projected consequences are indeed worrisome, not only from a clinical basis but from a salvage standpoint as well.

Silicone Elastomer Joint Replacement

The major experience with first MTP joint replacement was initiated with the introduction of the silicone elastomer hemiphalangeal implant by Swanson.[537] Initially described as safe and simple, it was offered as the preferred method for surgical treatment of hallux rigidus.[540] Touted as biocompatible and inert, early in vitro studies and in vivo studies by Swanson et al[540] and others[8,64] led to widespread use. Later reports of single-stem implant failure[330,574] heralded the introduction of the double-stem silicone elastomer implant,[581] which also was greeted

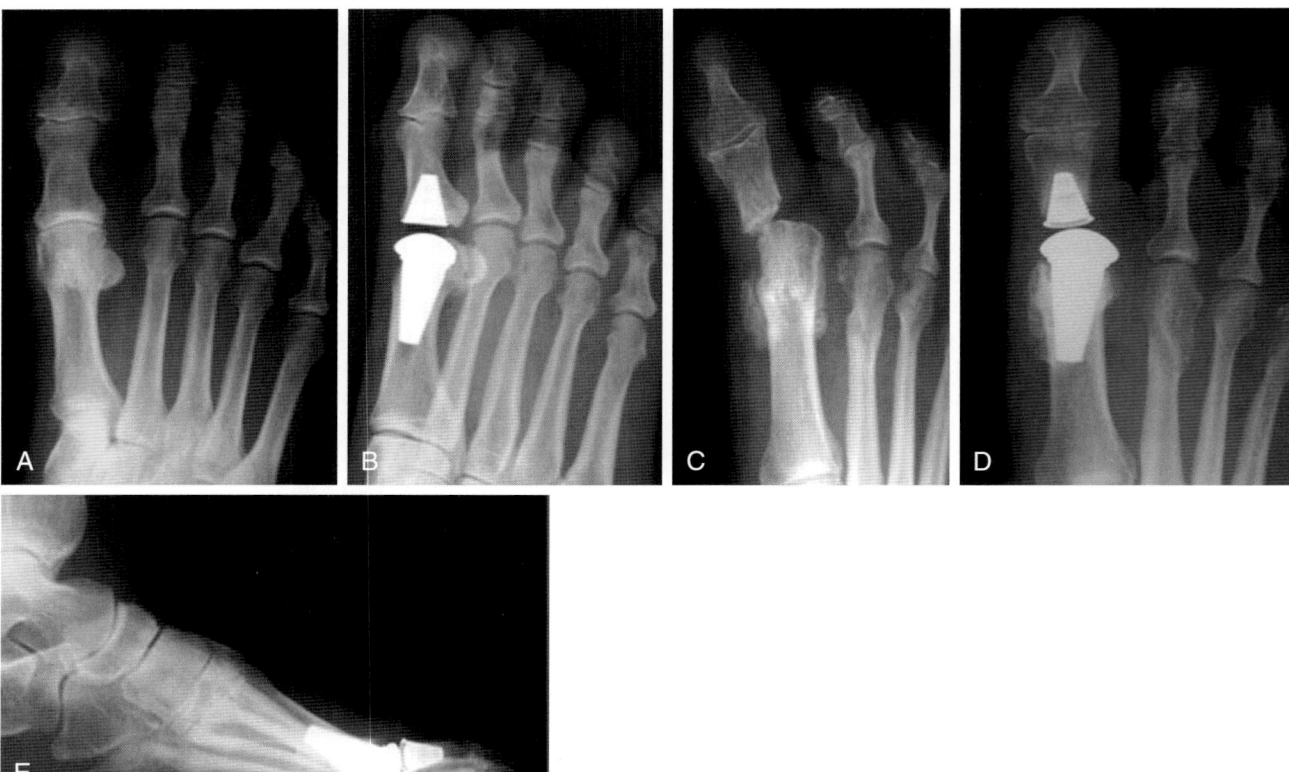

Figure 19-152 Various photographs of total toe implant. **A,** Preoperative radiograph demonstrating end-state degenerative arthritis of great toe metatarsophalangeal joint. **B,** After replacement of metatarsal and phalangeal articular surface with metal and polyethylene implants (porous ingrowth). **C,** Preoperative case after Keller resection arthroplasty. Anteroposterior **(D)** and lateral **(E)** radiographs after placement of total toe implant. (All photographs courtesy Hans Peter Kundert, MD.)

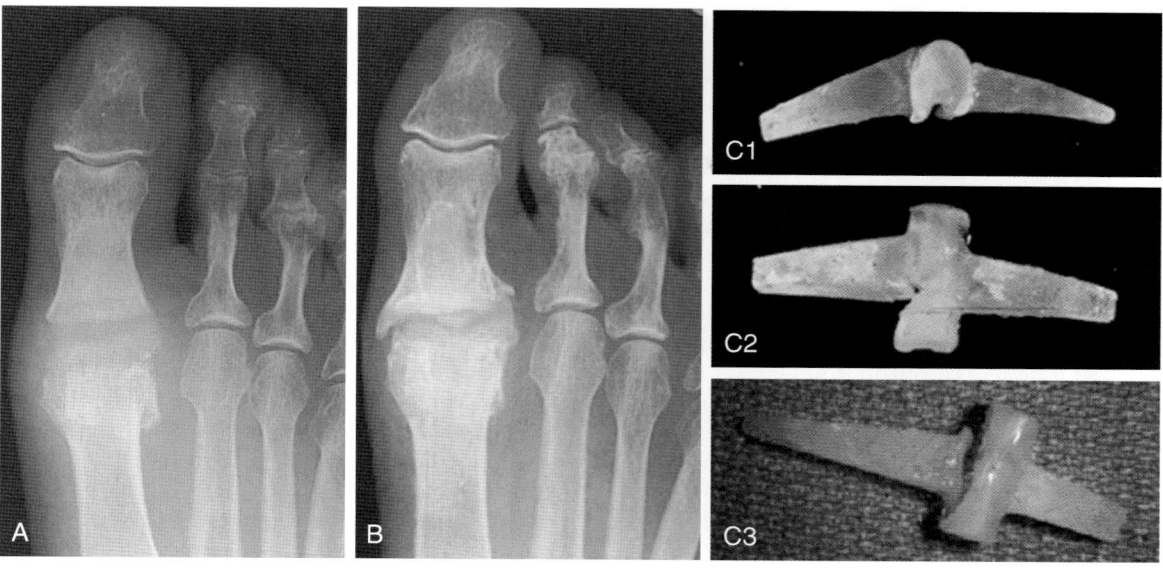

Figure 19-153   A, Radiograph demonstrates placement of double-stem silicone implant. **B,** Seven-year follow-up radiograph shows failed implant with silicone synovitis and bony resorption. **C1-C3,** Examples of failures of double-stem implants.

with great enthusiasm. Freed[170] has estimated that more than two million first MTP joint hinged silicone implants were implanted over the following two decades. Initial in vivo studies reporting few failures gave the impression that silicone elastomer implants would perform satisfactorily over a long-term period. Later studies with longer follow-up have demonstrated higher failure rates (57%-74%).[170,199]

Failure of an elastomer implant can occur for many reasons.[571,572] Intrinsic failure can result from the physical property of the materials, as evidenced by implant deformation, fatigue fracture, and microfragmentation. Intrinsic failure can occur with the use of a joint implant in a situation that exceeds the implant's design capability (e.g., younger patient, insufficient soft tissue, or bone realignment with hallux valgus deformity). When implant surgery is considered, the need for soft tissue[199,507,539] and bone balancing* cannot be overemphasized.

The viability of the silicone prosthesis appears to be directly related to the length of time it has been implanted. In early studies, Swanson[537] reported no fracture of hemistem and double-stem components, LaPorta et al[319] (average, 1 year follow-up) noted only two fractures in 536 implants, and others,[8,134,403] with relatively short-term studies, found fractures to be uncommon. Implant deformation with eventual fracture has been widely reported in other series. Granberry et al[199] hypothesized that this is caused by the cumulative effect of cyclic loading of large forces (body weight) on the implant (Fig. 19-153).

Reported complications include avascular necrosis, infection, transfer metatarsalgia,[194,199,403,488] delayed wound healing,[510] recurrent deformity,[234,377] bone proliferation, bone resorption (Fig. 19-154A), subchondral cyst

---

*References 83, 271, 301, 403, 434, and 507.

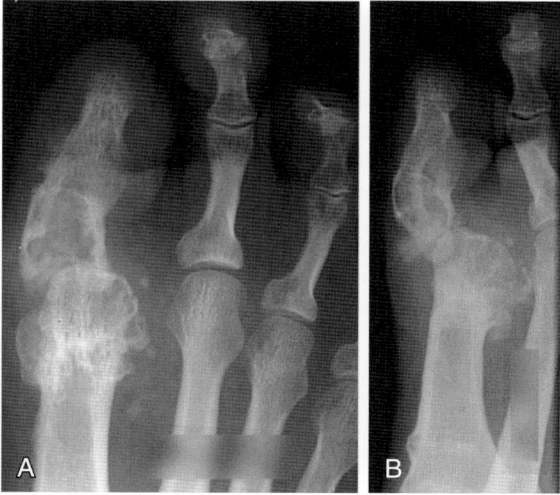

Figure 19-154   A, Anteroposterior radiograph demonstrates bone resorption. **B,** Oblique radiograph demonstrates implant displacement.

formation, implant displacement (Fig. 19-154B), and IP joint penetration of the silicone stem.[20]

Granberry et al[199] reported a twofold increase in lateral metatarsal weight bearing compared with the contralateral foot after first MTP joint replacement. Initial hopes that joint replacement would facilitate a normal gait pattern[540] were high, but the authors[199] found that normal plantar weight bearing with standing was not restored and that weakened plantar-flexion power decreased toe purchase. Pain relief,[540] as a primary indication for joint replacement, has been reported but with inconsistent results. Freed[170] reported moderate and severe first MTP pain in 16 of 51 joints (31%) after MTP arthroplasty. Based on survivorship analysis, Granberry et al[199] predicted a 50% failure rate with a hinged silicone implant component at 4 years.

Swanson et al[540] stated that MTP silicone replacement arthroplasty allowed good joint mobility, but limited range of motion of the hallux has been observed in several series.[134,170,199,218,409] Increased bony overgrowth in the periprosthetic region is associated with decreased range of motion.[134,199] Granberry et al[199] reported that 30% of cases in his series had less than 15 degrees of total MTP joint motion, and Freed[170] reported 33 of 51 (65%) had less than 20 degrees of motion.

The biocompatibility of silicone elastomer appears to be the greatest long-term problem. Initially thought to be inert and associated with little or no tissue reaction,[537,538,540] silicone elastomer in small-particle form (1 to 100 mm) leads to a significant inflammatory response. Hemiarthroplasty articulation with a degenerated incongruent metatarsal articular surface is thought to cause abrasion and microscopic particle formation.[20,70,192,330,596] Particulate synovitis has been reported with both upper- and lower-extremity implants. Gordon and Bullough[192] observed a reactive synovitis and foreign body giant cell reaction both in soft tissue and in intramedullary bone. Freed[170] has cited 64 different reports questioning the long-term viability of first MTP joint silicone elastomer implants.

Shards of silicone generated by shear and compressive forces lead to synovitis,[377,571,572] which is followed by encapsulation of these fragments both intracellularly and extracellularly. This florid synovial and periarticular soft tissue reaction is characterized by foreign body giant cell reaction.[271,422] Medical-grade silicone has been reported to be innocuous and benign,[538] but this evaluation applies to nonfragmented implants.[98] Stress and fatigue, joint overuse, poor fit, abrasion of joint surfaces, and pistoning of the prosthesis can lead to microfragmentation. Migration of these microscopic silicone fragments can occur through the lymphatic system,[192] with secondary adenopathy as a foreign body reaction. Lymphadenopathy has been reported in association with silicone elastomer failure in a number of series.

Although joint replacement has been recommended as a means of preserving great toe length,[540] Verhaar[574] and Granberry et al[199] have reported shortening of 3 to 11 mm in follow-up studies after first MTP implant placement. Granberry et al[199] observed increased shortening with longer follow-up; the shortening resulted from resorption of bone and collapse of the prosthesis.

Many implants have functioned well with little or no reactivity on a long-term basis; however, the number of complications reported raises questions regarding the viability of long-term survival of silicone elastomer first MTP implants.[234] Papagelopoulos et al[429] reported that patient age affected survivorship of the implant in 79 patients and reported 90% implant survivorship at 10 years in patients older than 57 years at the time of surgery and 82% survivorship when patients younger than 57 years of age underwent surgery. Radiographically, 40% of feet demonstrated bone resorption, 9% had cysts, 25%

had severe implant wear, and 3% had obvious implant fracture.

Townley and Taranow[561] and others[199,367] have stated that silicone possesses neither the biologic surface characteristics nor the structural durability to withstand the tension and shear stresses at the first MTP joint (associated with normal ambulatory activity). Others have noted that the implant is not durable,[199] and McCarthy and Chapman[367] reported that with the growing body of information, silicone elastomer may be unsuitable for weight-bearing joints. There is now a shift toward implantation with titanium grommets to reduce stress on the silicone elastomer, but longer-term results are pending. Likewise, long-term results with cemented MTP replacements have not been satisfactory.[377]

Freed[170] has estimated that more than two million hinged silicone implants have been placed over a two-decade period, and he estimates that three quarters of the implants in his series required removal. These estimates make it evident that revision surgery will be a common occurrence in many of these patients. Needelman et al[409] stated that a considerable number of revisions of MTP joint implants are occurring each year.

Salvage of Joint Replacement

Implants have introduced a whole new series of complications and have necessitated innovative salvage techniques.

The choices regarding surgical salvage depend on the disease present. With significant synovitis and joint reaction (characterized by swelling, pain, soft tissue thickening, infection, or radiographic evidence of bony encroachment or osteolysis), implant removal, debridement, and synovectomy may be indicated. Implant removal often leads to joint fibrosis with shortening of the first ray and decreased range of motion. Nonetheless, this can lead to a relatively stable joint and, with minimal pain, can be an acceptable result. Others have advocated revision of a failed silicone elastomer implant with a total joint revision. McDonald et al[368] and Perlman et al[434] recommended revision of a hemicomponent implant to a double-stem component but reported failure of the revision second silicone component as well. Koenig[301] reported installing a metal-polyethylene component to replace a failed silicone elastomer implant but noted a 40% failure rate. Freed[170] reported 360 metal-polyethylene implants placed for failed silicone implants but provided no follow-up.

Another option after failed MTP joint implant is first MTP arthrodesis after removal of the failed components. Fusion may be difficult to achieve because of poor bone quality. The need for supplemental bone graft and prolonged immobilization may be necessary before bony union is achieved. When successful, arthrodesis can achieve a stable first ray with improved weight-bearing function. Myerson et al[405] reported their results on 24 patients (mean age, 46 years) using interposition autograft (proximal tibia or iliac crest) or allograft interposition arthrodesis with plate and screw fixation or Steinman pins (or both), K-wires for failed metatarsal osteotomy, silicone arthroplasty, total joint replacement, and Keller resection. The authors reported two painless fibrous unions and three painful nonunions that were successfully revised to a solid fusion. The authors underscored the technical challenge of salvaging these difficult cases. Indications for first MTP joint replacement arthroplasty with a double-stem silicone elastic implant remain severe degenerative joint disease in older, more sedentary patients or household ambulators for whom excisional arthroplasty and MTP fusion are not acceptable options.

Surgical Technique[537,539,540]

1. A dorsomedial longitudinal skin incision is centered over the MTP joint.
2. A proximally based capsular flap is developed, exposing the MTP joint.
3. An oscillating saw is used to remove 3 to 4 mm of the articular surface of the metatarsal head and 2 mm of the base of the proximal phalanx (Fig. 19-155A).
4. Any osteophytes in the area of the metatarsal metaphysis are resected.
5. With a power burr, the intramedullary canal is enlarged for placement of the phalangeal and metatarsal intramedullary silicone stems.
6. A trial reduction with various-sized MTP implants is performed to choose the appropriate size. Oversized implants should be avoided. The stem of the implant should fit well into the prepared canal, allowing the transverse midsection of the implant to abut against the prepared phalangeal and metatarsal surfaces (Fig. 19-155B).

7. Some surgeons may select a titanium grommet to minimize adjacent wear at the silicone hinged-stem interface.
8. With an enlarged 1–2 intermetatarsal angle, a proximal first metatarsal osteotomy may be necessary. With significant valgus alignment of the first MTP joint, soft tissue balancing is mandatory because the double-stem implant does not provide sufficient stability to achieve joint alignment.
9. With placement of the appropriate-sized silicone prosthesis, the first MTP joint should be aligned properly in slight valgus, and the intramedullary stem should be well seated.
10. The joint capsule is closed with an interrupted absorbable suture. Sutures may be used to secure the phalangeal and metatarsal capsule, with drill holes placed in the metaphyseal region to anchor the capsular repair. The skin is approximated in a routine manner (Fig. 19-155C).

Postoperative Care

A gauze-and-tape compression dressing is applied at surgery and changed every 7 to 10 days. Mobilization of the MTP joint is important to achieve adequate dorsiflexion and plantar flexion after the surgical procedure. Physical or occupational therapy may be advantageous in regaining range of motion and strength at the first MTP joint.

FIRST METATARSOPHALANGEAL IMPLANT RESECTION ARTHROPLASTY

Indications for resection arthroplasty of the first MTP joint are a failed joint implant caused by infection, chronic synovitis, pain, and severe hallux rigidus in an older, sedentary patient in whom an arthrodesis is not an acceptable option.

Surgical Technique

1. A dorsal longitudinal incision is centered over the first MTP joint along the medial border of the extensor hallucis longus tendon. Z-plasty or lengthening of the tendon may be necessary to expose the MTP joint.
2. The hypertrophic synovium and pseudocapsule are excised, exposing the silicone implant.
3. After the implant is removed, a complete synovectomy excises thickened synovium in the periarticular area (Fig. 19-160A).
4. The intramedullary area is curetted to remove remaining synovial tissue.
5. If an excisional arthroplasty is desired, two 0.062-inch K-wires are introduced at the MTP joint and driven distally through the tip of the toe. An alternative is crossed K-wire fixation to stabilize the MTP joint (Fig. 19-160B). The wires are then driven in a retrograde manner into the first metatarsal head to stabilize the hallux. (In the presence of infection, internal fixation is not used.) The pins are bent at the tip of the toe to prevent proximal migration. Crossed K-wires are cut off level with the surface of the skin.

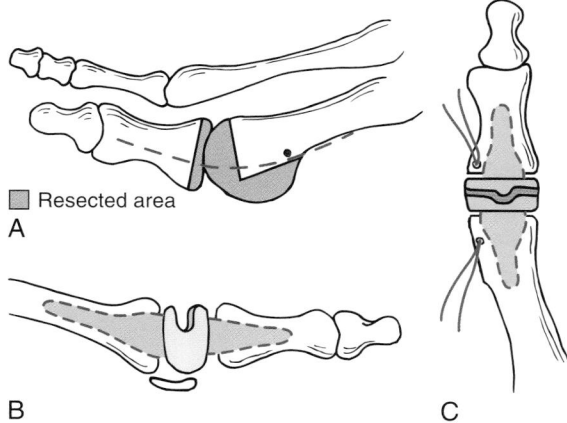

Figure 19-155 **A,** Dorsomedial longitudinal skin incision is used to approach the metatarsophalangeal joint. A sagittal saw is used to remove 2 mm of bone from the base of the proximal phalanx and medial eminence and 3 to 4 mm of distal metatarsal articular surface. **B,** After broaching of the canal, the double-stem implant is placed. **C,** Capsule is repaired with interrupted closure. Drill holes in the base of the proximal phalanx and in the metatarsal metaphysis may be used to secure the capsule closure.

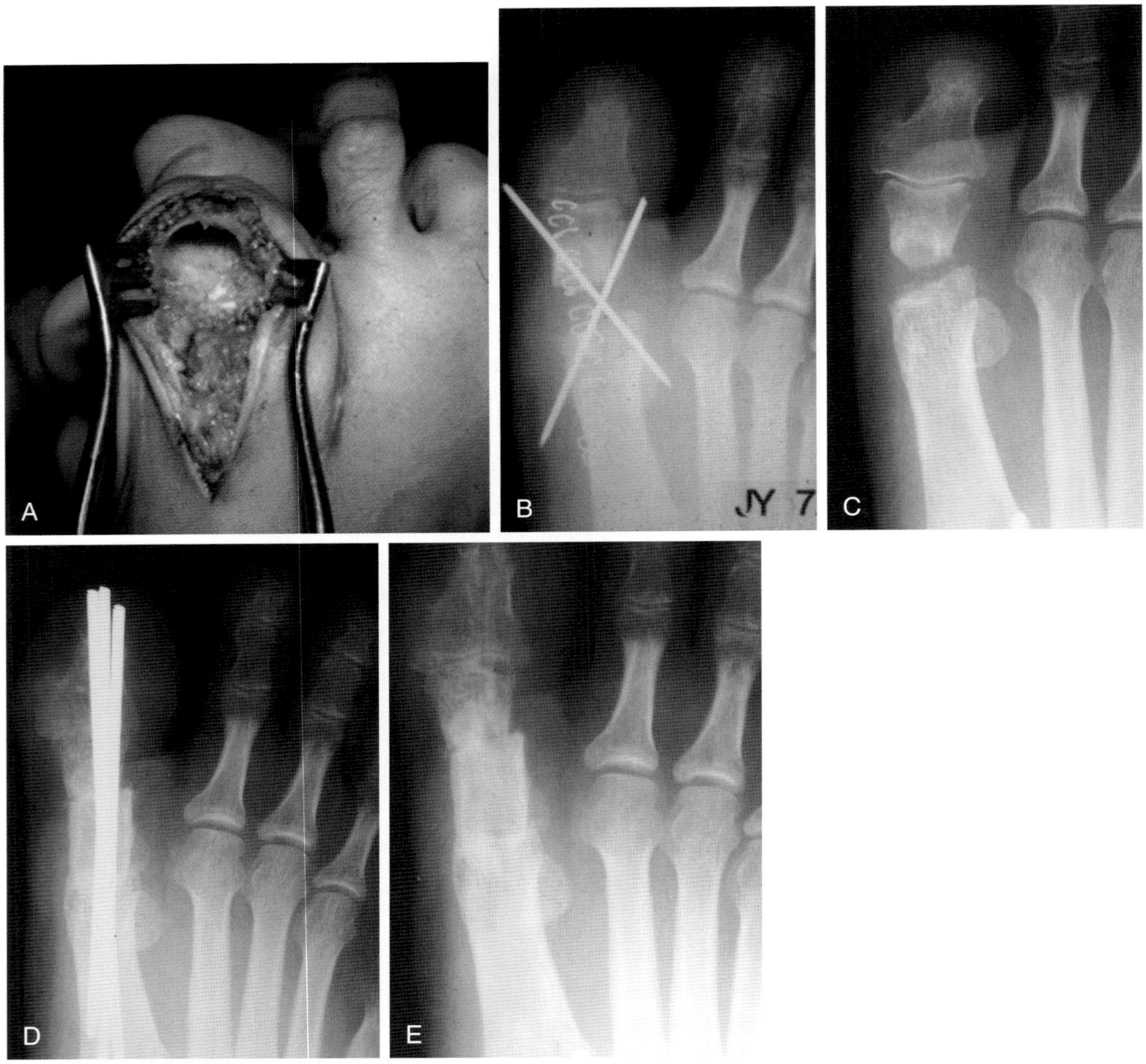

Figure 19-156 **A,** Surgical exposure demonstrates the defect after removal of a failed single-stem implant. **B,** Radiograph demonstrates crossed K-wires used to stabilize the excisional arthroplasty after removal of the implant. **C,** After removal of K-wires. **D,** Interpositional graft and arthrodesis with internal fixation. **E,** A successful fusion after removal of internal fixation.

6. The soft tissue and skin are approximated with an interrupted closure.

Postoperative Care

A gauze-and-tape compression dressing is applied at surgery and changed at 10-day intervals for 6 weeks. The patient is allowed to ambulate in the postoperative shoe. Intramedullary pins are removed 3 to 4 weeks after surgery.

FIRST METATARSOPHALANGEAL JOINT INTERPOSITIONAL ARTHRODESIS
Surgical Technique

1. Similar incision, dissection, and debridement are performed as discussed previously for excisional arthroplasty.
2. A bicortical or tricortical graft is obtained from the iliac crest (Fig. 19-157). The graft is shaped to fit the desired gap (defect) at the MTP joint. Cancellous bone is packed into defects in the intramedullary canals. Often the bicortical or tricortical shaft is trapezoidal (wider plantarward and medially, narrower on dorsolateral aspect) to allow varus/valgus and dorsiflexion/plantar flexion at the fusion site (see Fig. 19-156C-E and Video Clip 34).

3. Internal fixation is determined by the quality of the phalangeal metatarsal bone as well as the length of the bone graft (Fig. 19-158).
4. Axial Steinmann pins or mini-fragment plate fixation may be used for fixation depending on the surgeon's preference (Fig. 19-159).
5. With plate fixation, a low-profile revision plate (Integra, Integra LifeSciences, Plainsboro, N.J.) may be used and placed on the dorsomedial/dorsolateral aspect of the proximal phalanx and first metatarsal (Fig. 19-160).

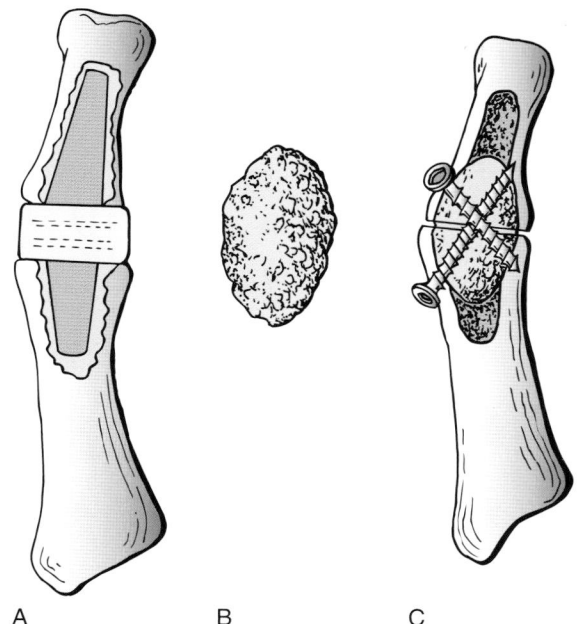

Figure 19-157 **A,** Diagram demonstrates failed Silastic arthroplasty with osteolysis. **B,** Football-shaped graft of autogenous iliac crest bone. **C,** Diagram of construct for in-site fusion with interpositional football graft and internal fixation. (Modified from Alexander I: In Myerson M, editor: *Current foot and ankle surgery,* St Louis, 1993, Mosby.)

(See the discussion of arthrodesis in the rheumatoid arthritis section earlier in this chapter.)

Postoperative Care

A gauze-and-tape dressing is applied at surgery and changed every 10 days for 8 weeks. The patient is allowed to ambulate in a wooden-soled shoe, with weight bearing on the heel and the lateral aspect of the foot. When Steinmann pins are placed, they are typically removed 16 weeks after surgery under local anesthesia and after radiographic confirmation of a successful fusion. Plates may be removed if they are symptomatic, but the use of low-profile Vitallium plates often makes this unnecessary (Fig. 19-161).

Results and Complications

Kitaoka et al[296] reported on excisional arthroplasty as a revision technique for silicone implant failure (average follow-up, 3.5 years). At surgery, the implant was removed and a joint debridement was performed. At long-term follow-up, 80% good and excellent results were reported. No significant alignment changes occurred, probably because of postoperative periarticular fibrosis. The authors noted decreased pressure beneath the tip of the hallux, decreased MTP range of motion, and a tendency toward hallux extensus.

With single-plate or dual-plate fixation, a strong mechanical construct is created to protect the intercalary

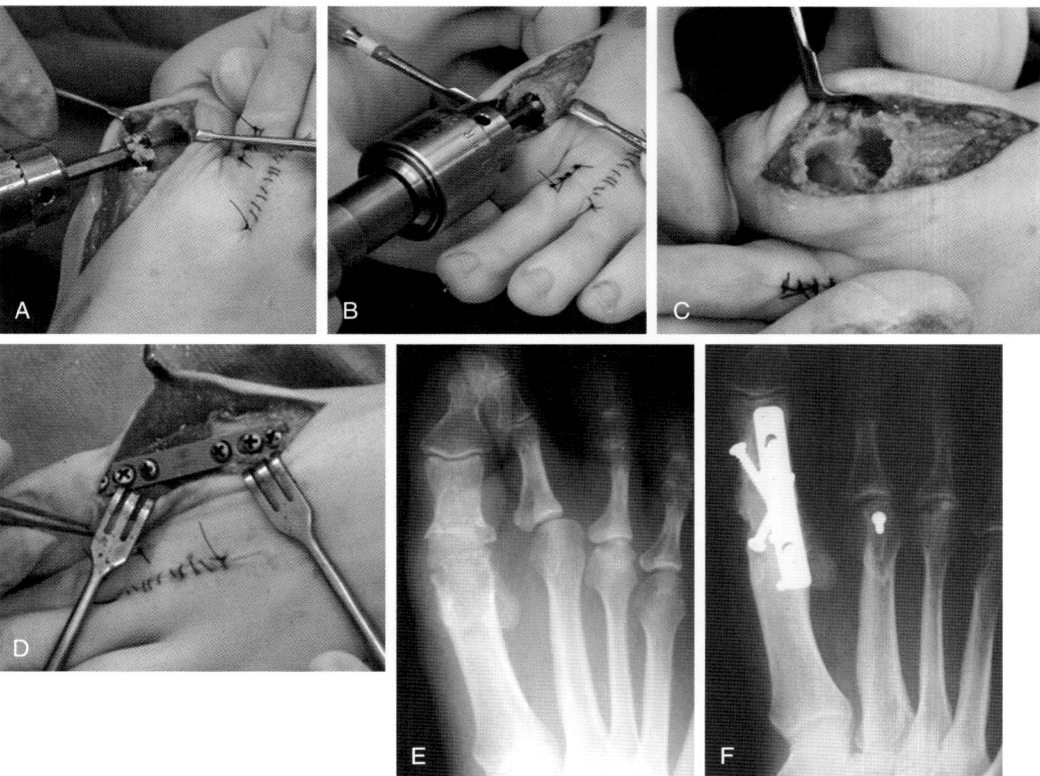

Figure 19-158 **A,** Failed double-stemmed silicone insert. Preparation of phalanx. **B,** Preparation of metatarsal head with phalangeal reamer. **C,** Both prepared surfaces. **D,** After football-shaped graft is inserted, a dorsal plate established adequate fixation of the arthrodesis site and graft. **E,** Preoperative radiograph. **F,** After arthrodesis with interposition graft.

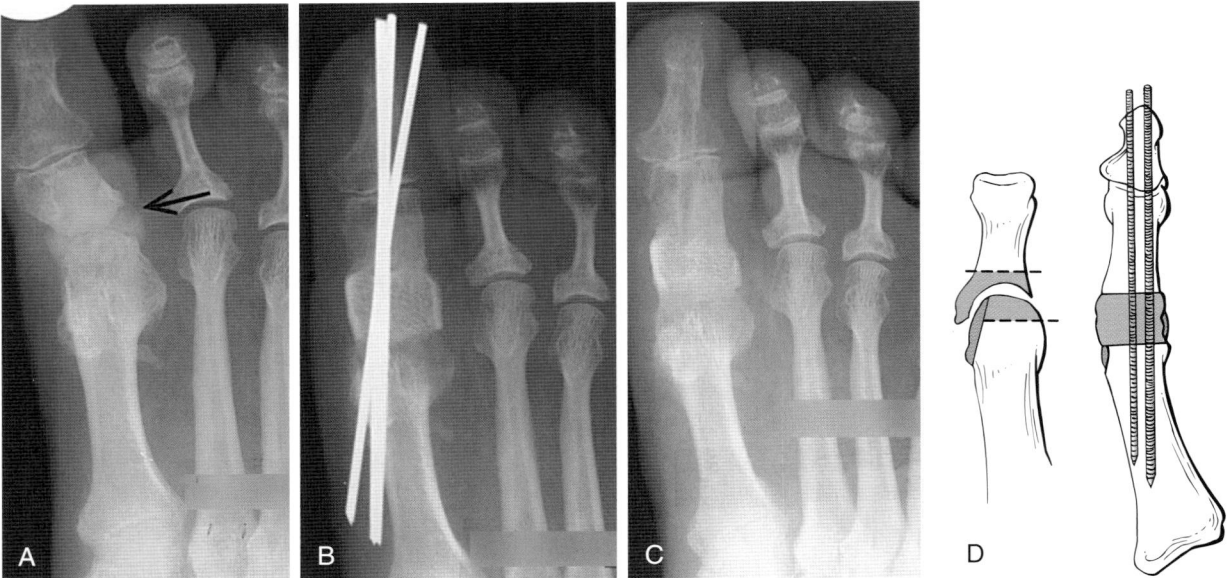

Figure 19-159 **A,** Anteroposterior radiograph demonstrates failed hemisilicone implant with shortening and extrusion of component (*arrow*). **B,** Radiograph after interpositional iliac crest arthrodesis. **C,** Radiograph 7 years after surgery demonstrates successful arthrodesis. **D,** Diagram of salvage arthrodesis.

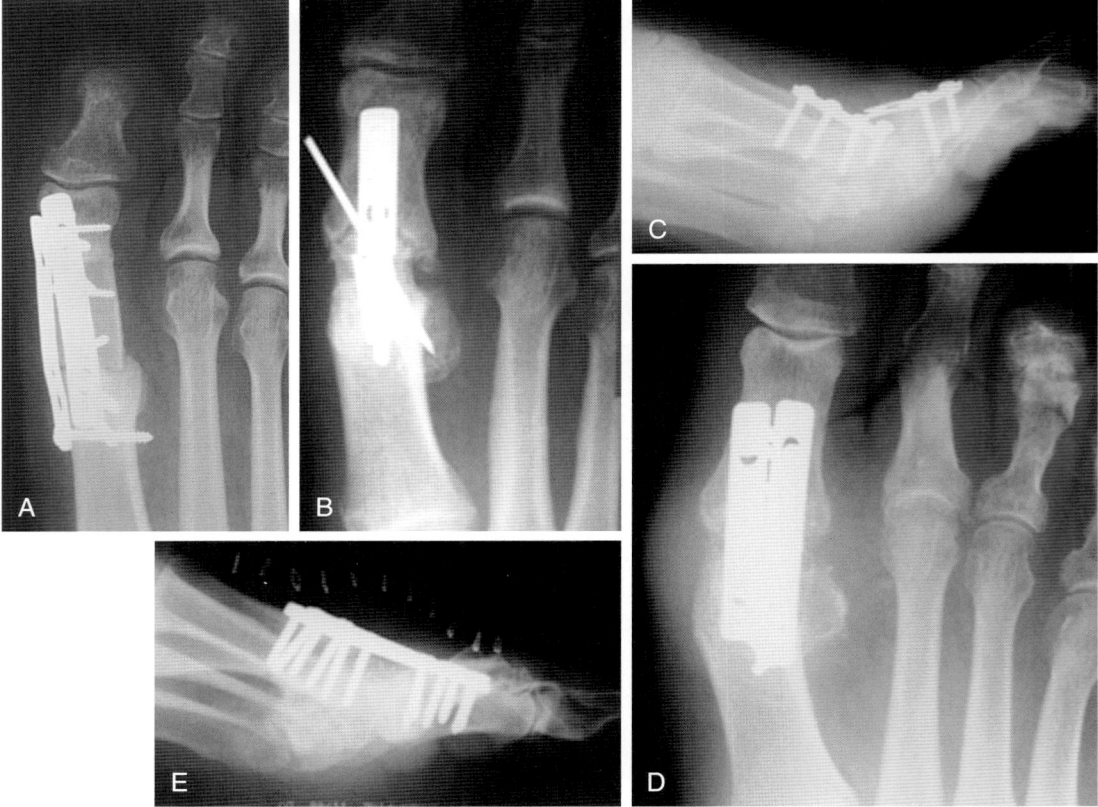

Figure 19-160 **A,** Example of arthrodesis with interpositional iliac crest graft with double-plate internal fixation to stabilize autograft. **B** and **C,** Failure of internal fixation and nonunion. **D** and **E,** Salvage with double dorsal plate technique.

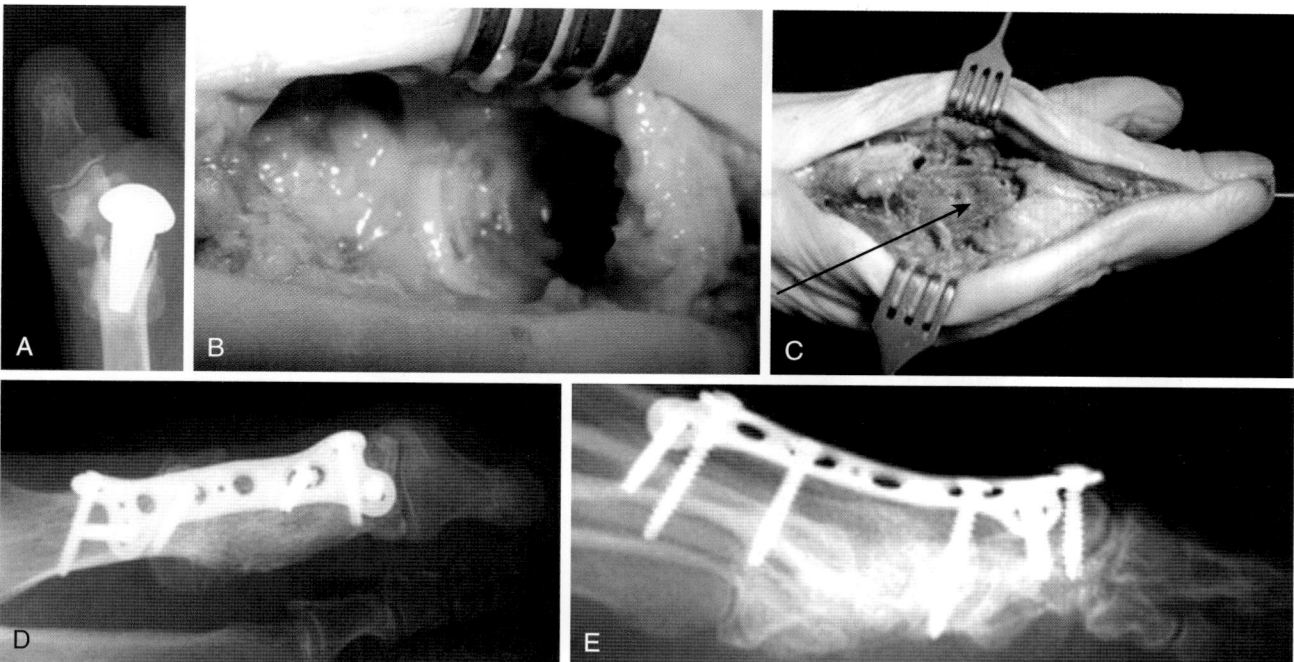

Figure 19-161 Failure of total toe implants. **A,** Subluxation of phalanx with erosion of phalanx after metatarsal head replacement. **B,** Removal of metatarsal implant. **C,** After interposition intercalary graft. Anteroposterior **(D)** and lateral **(E)** radiographs after grafting and placement of reconstruction dorsal plate. (All photographs courtesy Hans Peter Kundert, MD.)

bone graft. With Steinmann pin fixation, two or three Steinmann pins are used to "shish-kebob" the phalanx, graft, and first metatarsal (Fig. 19-162).[109] Steinmann pins are introduced at the prepared surface of the proximal phalangeal base and driven distally across the IP joint, exiting the tip of the toe. The pins are then retrograded longitudinally through the graft and into the metatarsal head and metatarsal metaphysis. The threaded pins are cut with ⅛ inch protruding from the tip of the toe to aid in later pin removal.

Arthrodesis in the salvage of a failed Keller procedure was reported both with primary fusion and with an intercalary bone graft.[109] Five cases were reported in which an interpositional graft was used for the salvage of a failed excisional arthroplasty. All five cases went on to a successful fusion. No significant complications were noted, although this extensive type of salvage carries an increased risk of failure. Wound necrosis, infection, and delayed union or nonunion of the intercalary graft can lead to failure of the salvage technique (Fig. 19-163). A fibrous union can leave an acceptable result with some residual motion. However, infection or wound healing problems can eventually lead to toe amputation or ray resection as an ultimate salvage procedure. Myerson's technique,[405] as noted earlier, produced reliable results and an acceptable union rate with autograft or allograft interposition as a salvage procedure for failed implants, resection arthroplasty, or metatarsal osteotomy. Whalen[586] described the use of an interposition graft using a patella allograft shaped to fill the osseous defect, stabilized with a dorsal plate for internal fixation. Petroutsas et al[436] have

described the use of a bone block distraction arthrodesis, using iliac crest graft shaped to interdigitate with the base of the proximal phalanx and metatarsal head by shaping the surfaces with power concentric reamers, and by using a dorsal plate and crossed screws for internal fixation (Fig. 19-164). Bhosale et al[42] also has reported a series of 10 feet treated with interposition grafting and a dorsal plate, with an 80% success rate. Vienne et al[576] described a series of 22 feet salvaged, after a failed Keller procedure, with direct arthrodesis or using an interposition graft in 7 or 22 cases. They reported a 90% fusion rate after the salvage procedure.

The placement of longitudinal Steinmann pins for stabilization of a first MTP fusion in which the threaded pins have crossed the IP joint has been associated with an inordinately high rate of radiographically observed IP joint degenerative arthritis. Nonetheless, it may be necessary to use this longitudinal pin fixation technique in the presence of significant bone loss or osteoporosis.[100] Often, when this type of fixation is necessary, minimal IP joint motion is present. Mann and Thompson[359] reported a 65% incidence of IP joint arthritis with this technique, although they did not believe the observed arthrosis was clinically significant. Mann and Schakel[358] reported a 60% incidence of interphalangeal arthritis, but only one third of patients were symptomatic.

Shereff and Jahss[510] stated that because of the high biomechanical demands placed on the first MTP joint and the complex joint interactions of the first ray, routine use of joint replacement arthroplasty cannot be recommended for the first ray until consistently good or

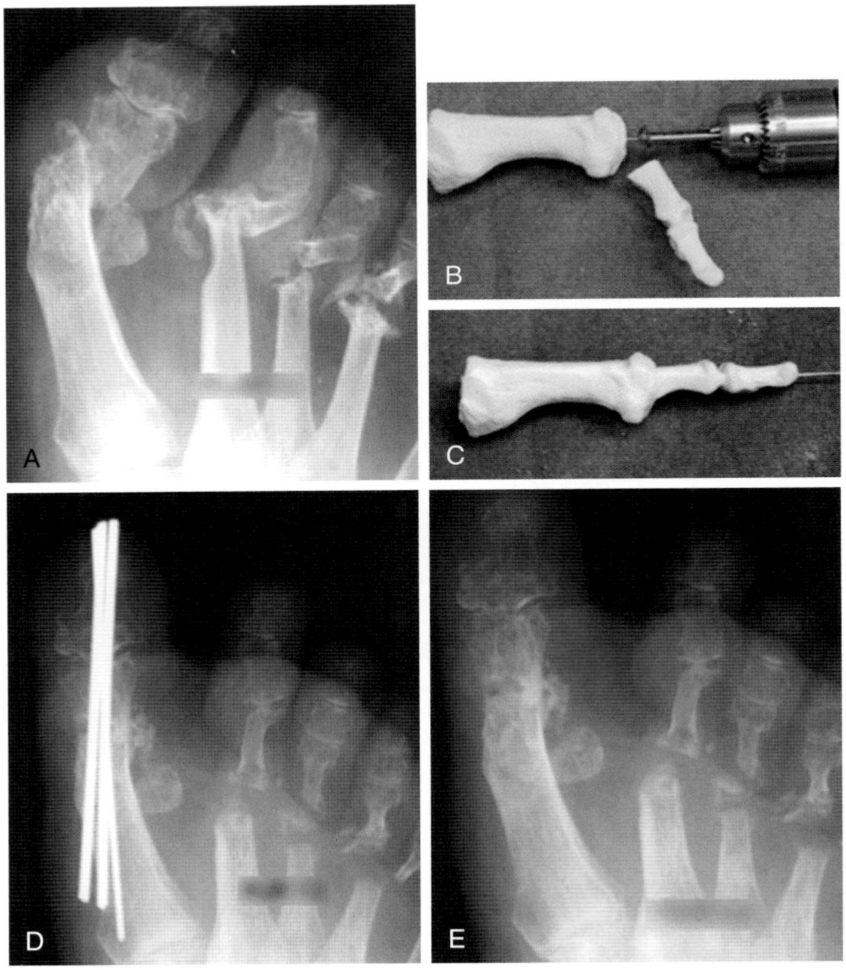

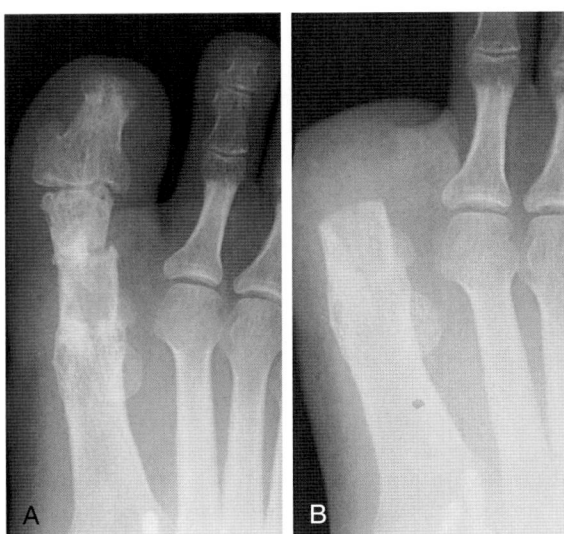

Figure 19-162 **A,** Radiograph after failed Keller resection arthroplasty. **B** and **C,** Technique of peg-in-hole arthrodesis demonstrated with sawbones model. A power phalangeal reamer is used to create a hole in the metatarsal head. **D,** Fixation with axial Steinman pins. **E,** After successful fusion of the metatarsophalangeal joint.

Figure 19-163 **A,** After removal of hardware after interposition iliac crest graft and arthrodesis. **B,** After amputation for subsequent infection after arthrodesis attempt (follow-up of case illustrated in Figure 19-150E and F). Interposition arthrodesis salvage procedures are difficult and can be fraught with significant complications.

excellent results over time are obtained. It does not appear that such results are forthcoming, and the high rate of complications associated with MTP implant surgery reported in long-term follow-up has dampened the initial enthusiasm for prosthetic replacement of the first MTP joint. This enthusiasm has been supplanted by caution in the placement of implants in younger, more active patients. Implants may still be considered in older, more sedentary patients. The options of cheilectomy and excisional arthroplasty, and even arthrodesis, appear much less onerous than the occasional significant complications associated with various implant arthroplasties.

The authors strongly recommend against implant arthroplasty and have had experiences similar to those reported by Myerson et al[405] in treating failures of implants, metatarsal osteotomies, and resection arthroplasties. The current authors conclude that such cases present a substantial surgical challenge in achieving an acceptable salvage. Appropriate use of MTP implant arthroplasty for the correct narrow indications,[218] with meticulous surgical technique, will significantly reduce the frequency of this surgery as well as the morbidity and high complication rates reported in some series.[116,391]

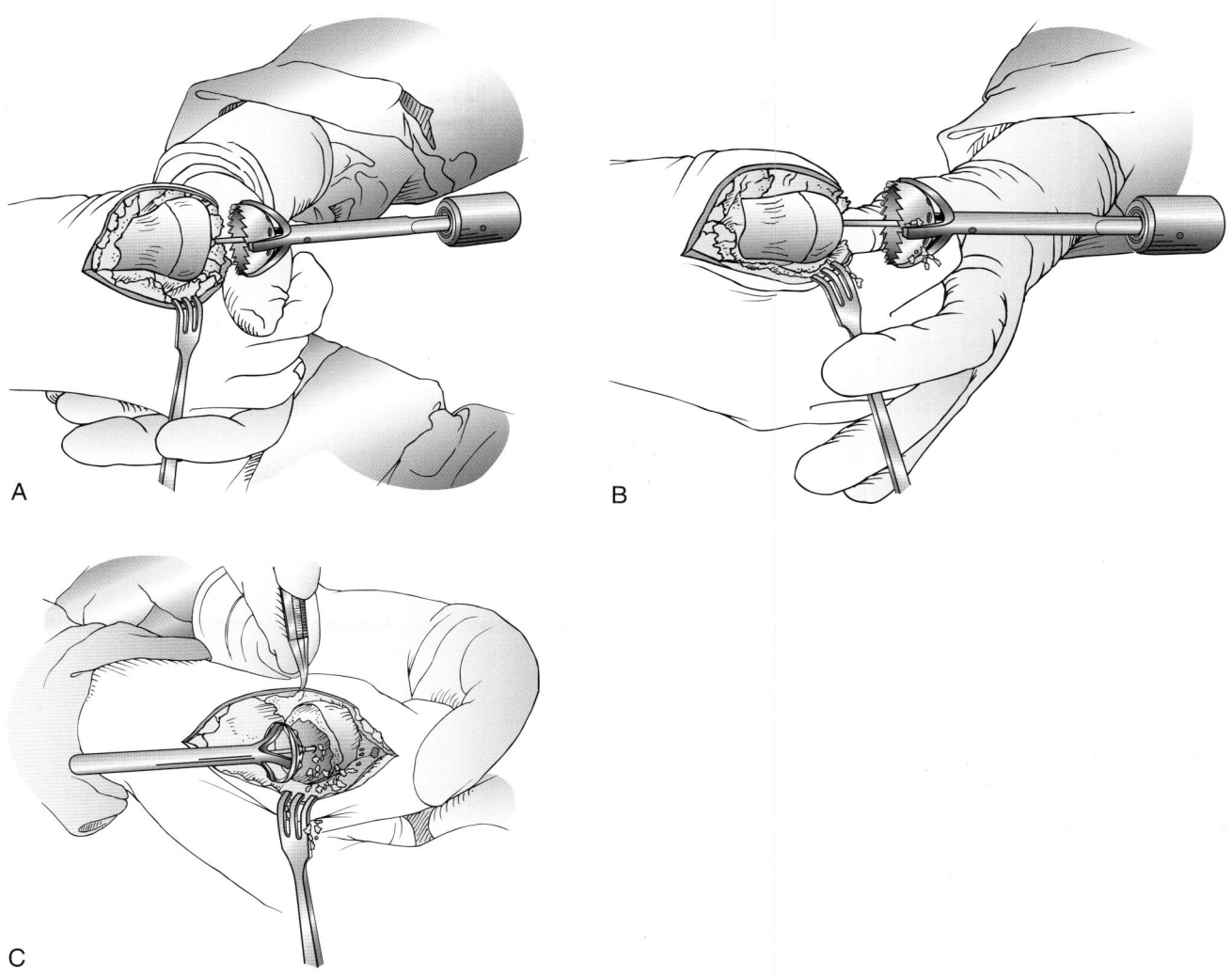

Figure 19-164 Salvage technique for interposition bone graft using reamers to prepare adjacent surfaces. **A,** Concave cannulated reamer placed on K-wire for preparation of metatarsal head. **B,** After reaming of the metatarsal head. **C,** The same reamer is used to prepare the base of the proximal phalanx. After completion of the reaming, a graft is inserted that interdigitates with each bone, and then internal fixation is placed (typically a dorsal plate is used). (All images modified from Petroutsas J, Easley M, Trnka HJ: Modified bone block distraction arthrodesis of the hallux metatarsophalangeal joint, *Foot Ankle Int* 27:299–302, 2006.)

REFERENCES

1. Aas M, Johnsen TM, Finsen V: Arthrodesis of the first metatarsophalangeal joint for hallux rigidus—optimal position of fusion, *Foot (Edinb)* 18:131–135, 2008.
2. Acosta R, Ushiba J, Cracchiolo A: The results of a primary and staged pantalar arthrodesis and tibiotalocalcaneal arthrodesis in adult patients, *Foot Ankle Int* 21:182–194, 2000.
3. Adelaar R: Changes in gait after isolated subtalar fusion, *Biomech* 4:59–65, 1997.
4. Adkins RB Jr, Scott HW et al: Surgical procedures in patients aged 90 years and older, *South Med J* 77:1357–1364, 1984.
5. Agarwal AK: Gout and pseudogout, *Prim Care* 20:839–855, 1993.
6. Aho H: Synovectomy of MTP joints in rheumatoid arthritis, *Rheumatology* 11:126–130, 1987.
7. Aho H, Halonen P: Synovectomy of the MTP joints in rheumatoid arthritis, *Acta Orthop Scand Suppl* 243:1, 1991.
8. Albin RK, Weil LS: Flexible implant arthroplasty of the great toe: An evaluation, *J Am Podiatry Assoc* 64:967–975, 1974.
9. Alibert J: *Précis théorique et pratique sur les maladies de la peau,* Paris, 1818, Calille et Revier, p 21.
10. American College of Rheumatology Subcommittee on Rheumatoid Arthritis Guidelines: Guidelines for the management of rheumatoid arthritis: 2002 update, *Arthritis Rheum* 46:328–346, 2002.
11. Andersen JA, Klaborg KE: Forefoot amputation in rheumatoid arthritis, *Acta Orthop Scand* 584:394–397, 1987.
    Anonymous: Clinical update: Lyme disease looms larger than ever, *J Musculoskel Med* 14:110–111, 1997.
    Anonymous: Treatment of Lyme disease, *Med Lett Drugs Ther* 39:47–48, 1997.
12. Arnett FC: Rheumatoid arthritis. In Wyngaarden JB, Smith LH Jr, Bennett JC, editors: *Cecil textbook of medicine,* ed 19, Philadelphia, 1992, WB Saunders, p 1508.

13. Aronow MS, Hakim-Zargar M: Management of hindfoot disease in rheumatoid arthritis, *Foot Ankle Clin N Am* 12:455–474, 2007.

14. Ashman CJ, Klecker RJ, Yu JS: Forefoot pain involving the metatarsal region: differential diagnosis with MR imaging, *Radiographics* 21:1425–1440, 2001.

15. Astion DJ, Deland JT, Otis JC, Kenneally S: Motion of the hindfoot after simulated arthrodesis, *J Bone Joint Surg Am* 79:241–246, 1997.

16. Barca F: Tendon arthroplasty of the first metatarsophalangeal joint in hallux rigidus: preliminary communication, *Foot Ankle Int* 18:222–228, 1997.

17. Barg A, Knupp M, Kapron A, Hintermann B: Total ankle replacement in patients with gouty arthritis, *J Bone Joint Surg Am* 93:357–366, 2011.

18. Barouk LS, Barouk P: Joint-preserving surgery in rheumatoid forefoot: preliminary study with more-than-two-year follow-up, *Foot Ankle Clin N Am* 12:435–454, 2007.

19. Barton NJ: Arthroplasty of the forefoot in rheumatoid arthritis, *J Bone Joint Surg Br* 55:126–133, 1973.

20. Bass SJ, Gastwirth CM, Green R, et al: Phagocytosis of Silastic material following Silastic great toe implant, *J Foot Surg* 17:70–72, 1978.

21. Bazin P: *Leçons théoriques et cliniques sur les affections cutanées de nature arthritique et dartreux*, Paris, 1860, Delahaye, pp 154–161.

22. Beauchamp CG, Kirby T, Rudge SR, et al: Fusion of the first metatarsophalangeal joint in forefoot arthroplasty, *Clin Orthop Relat Res* 190:249–253, 1984.

23. Becker MA, Schumacher HR Jr, Wortmann RL, et al: Febuxostat compared with allopurinol in patients with hyperuricemia and gout, *N Engl J Med* 353:2450–2461, 2005.

24. Bednarz PA, Monroe MT, Manoli A 2nd: Triple arthrodesis in adults using rigid internal fixation: an assessment of outcome, *Foot Ankle Int* 20:356–363, 1999.

25. Beertema W, Draijer WF, van Os, JJ; Pilot P: A retrospective analysis of surgical treatment in patients with symptomatic hallux rigidus: long-term follow-up, *J Foot Ankle Surg* 45:244–251, 2006.

26. Beeson P, Phillips C, Corr S, Ribbans W: Classification systems for hallux rigidus: a review of the literature, *Foot Ankle Int* 29:407–414, 2008.

27. Beilstein DP, Hawkins ES: Pedal manifestations of systemic lupus erythematosus, *Clin Podiatr Med Surg* 5:37–56, 1988.

28. Beischer AD, Brodsky JW, Pollo FE, Peereboom J: Functional outcome and gait analysis after triple or double arthrodesis, *Foot Ankle Int* 20:454–553 1999.

29. Belt EA, Kaarela K, Lehto MU: Destruction and arthroplasties of the metatarsophalangeal joints in seropositive rheumatoid arthritis. A 20-year follow-up study, *Scand J Rheumatol* 27:194–196, 1998.

30. Bennett GL, Sabetta J: First metatarsalphalangeal joint arthrodesis: evaluation of plate and screw fixation, *Foot Ankle Int* 30:752–757, 2009.

31. Bennett RM: Confounding features of the fibromyalgia syndrome: a current perspective of differential diagnosis, *J Rheumatol Suppl* 19:58–61, 1989.

32. Bennett RM: Physical fitness and muscle metabolism in the fibromyalgia syndrome: an overview, *J Rheumatol Suppl* 19:28–29, 1989.

33. Benson GM, Johnson EW Jr: Management of the foot in rheumatoid arthritis, *Orthop Clin North Am* 2:733–744, 1971.

34. Berg RP, Kelder W, Olsthoorn PGM, et al: Scarf and Weil osteotomies for correction of rheumatoid forefoot deformities: a review of 20 cases, *Foot Ankle Surg* 13:35–40, 2007.

35. Berger I, Martens KD, Meyer-Scholten C: Rheumatoid necroses in the forefoot, *Foot Ankle Int* 25:336–339, 2004.

36. Berlet GC, Anderson RB: Tendon arthroplasty for basal fourth and fifth metatarsal arthritis, *Foot Ankle Int* 23:440–446, 2002.

37. Berlet GC, Hyer CF, Glover JP: A retrospective review of immediate weightbearing after first metatarsophalangeal joint arthrodesis, *Foot Ankle Spec* 1:24–28, 2008.

38. Berlet GC, Hye, CF, Lee TH, et al: Interpositional arthroplasty of the first MTP joint using a regenerative tissue matrix for the treatment of advanced hallux rigidus, *Foot Ankle Int* 29:10–21, 2008.

39. Besse JL, Chouteau J; Laptoiu D: Arthrodesis of the first metatarsophalangeal joint with ball and cup reamers and osteosynthesis with pure titanium staples: radiological evaluation of a continuous series of 54 cases, *Foot Ankle Surg* 16:32–37, 2010.

40. Beutler A, Schumacher HR Jr: Gout and "pseudogout." When are arthritic symptoms caused by crystal deposition? *Postgrad Med* 95:103–106, 109, 113–116 passim, 1994.

41. Bezes H, Massart P, Delvaux D, et al: The operative treatment of intraarticular calcaneal fractures. Indications, technique, and results in 257 cases, *Clin Orthop* 290:55–59, 1993.

42. Bhosale A, Munoruth A, Blundell C, et al: Complex primary arthrodesis of the first metatarsophalangeal joint after bone loss, *Foot Ankle Int* 32:968–972, 2011.

43. Bibbo C, Anderson RB, Davis WH: Complications of midfoot and hindfoot arthrodesis, *Clin Orthop Relat Res* 391:45–58, 2001.

44. Bibbo C, Bono CM, Lin SS: Union rates using autologous platelet concentrate alone and with bone graft in high-risk foot and ankle surgery patients, *J Surg Orhtop Adv* 14:17–22, 2005.

45. Bibbo C, Goldberg JW: Infectious and healing complications after elective orthopaedic foot and ankle surgery during tumor necrosis factor-alpha inhibition therapy, *Foot Ankle Int* 25:331–335, 2004.

46. Bingold AC: Arthrodesis of the great toe, *Proc R Soc Med* 51:435–437, 1958.

47. Bingold AC, Collins DH: Hallux rigidus, *J Bone Joint Surg Br* 32:214–222, 1950.

48. Blair MP, Brown LA: Hallux limitus/rigidus deformity: a new great toe implant, *J Foot Ankle Surg* 32:257–262, 1993.

49. Bluestone R: Collagen diseases affecting the foot, *Foot Ankle* 2:311–317, 1982.

50. Bolland BJ, Sauve PS, Taylor GR: Rheumatoid forefoot reconstruction: first metatarsophalangeal joint fusion combined with Weil's metatarsal osteotomies of the lesser rays, *J Foot Ankle Surg* 47:80–88, 2008.

51. Bonney G, Macnab I: Hallux valgus and hallux rigidus; a critical survey of operative results, *J Bone Joint Surg Br* 34:366–385, 1952.

52. Boss GR, Seegmiller JE: Hyperuricemia and gout. Classification, complications and management, *N Engl J Med* 300:1459–1468, 1979.

53. Bouaicha S, Ehrmann C, Moor BK, et al: Radiographic analysis of metatarsus primus elevatus and hallux rigidus, *Foot Ankle Int* 31:807–814, 2010.

54. Bourinbaiar AS, Lee-Huang S: The non-steroidal anti-inflammatory drug, indomethacin, as an inhibitor of HIV replication, *FEBS Lett* 360:85–88, 1995.

55. Boutry N, Larde A, Lapegue F, et al: Magnetic resonance imaging appearance of the hands and feet in patients with early rheumatoid arthritis, *J Rheumatol* 30:671–679, 2003.

56. Bowen CJ, Edwards CJ, Hooper L, et al: Improvement in symptoms and signs in the forefoot of patients with rheumatoid arthritis treatedwith anti-TNF therapy, *J Foot Ankle Res* 3:10, 2010.

57. Brattstrom H, Brattstrom M: Resection of the metatarsophalangeal joints in rheumatoid arthritis, *Acta Orthop Scand* 41:213–224, 1970.

58. Braun J, Sieper J: Ankylosing spondylitis, *Lancet* 369:1379–1390, 2007.

59. Breedveld FC, Weisman MH, Kavanaugh AF, et al: The PREMIER study: a multicenter, randomized, double-blind clnical trial of combination therapy with adalimumab plus methotrexate versus methotrexate alone or adalimumab alone in patients with early, aggressive rheumatoid arthritis who had not had previous methotrexate treatment, *Arthritis Rheum* 54:26–37, 2006.

60. British Infection Association: The epidemiology, prevention, investigation and treatment of Lyme borreliosis in United Kingdom patients: a position statement by the British Infection Association, *J Infect* 62:329–338, 2011.

61. Brodsky JW, Baum BS, Pollo FE, Mehta H: Prospective gait analysis in patients with first metatarsophalangeal joint arthrodesis for hallux rigidus, *Foot Ankle Int* 28:162–165, 2007.

62. Brosky TA 2nd, Menke CR, Xenos D: Reconstruction of the first metatarsophalangeal joint following post-cheilectomy avascular necrosis of the first metatarsal head: a case report, *J Foot Ankle Surg* 48:61–69, 2009.

63. Burns CM, Wortmann RL: Gout therapeutics: new drugs for an old disease, *Lancet* 377:165–177, 2011.

64. Burra G, Katchis SD: Rheumatoid arthritis of the forefoot, *Rheum Dis Clin North Am* 24:173–180, 1998.

65. Calabro JJ: A critical evaluation of the diagnostic features of the feet in rheumatoid arthritis, *Arthritis Rheum* 5:19–29, 1962.

66. Calderone DR, Wertheimer SJ: First metatarsophalangeal joint arthrodesis utilizing a mini-Hoffman External Fixator, *J Foot Ankle Surg* 32:517–525, 1993.

67. Calvo A, Viladot R, Gine J, Alvarez F: The importance of the length of the first metatarsal and the proximal phalanx of hallux in the etiopathogeny of the hallux rigidus, *Foot Ankle Surg* 15:69–74, 2009.

68. Can Akgun R, Sahin O, Demirors H, Cengiz Tuncay I: Analysis of modified oblique Keller procedure for severe hallux rigidus, *Foot Ankle Int* 29:1203–1208, 2008.

69. Canale ST, Kelly FB Jr: Fractures of the neck of the talus. Long-term evaluation of seventy-one cases, *J Bone Joint Surg* 60:143–156, 1978.

70. Caneva RG: Postoperative degenerative changes of the metatarsal head following use of the Swanson implant: four case reports, *J Foot Surg* 16:34–37, 1977.

71. Canseco K, Long J, Marks R, et al: Quantitative motion analysis in patients with hallux rigidus before and after cheilectomy, *J Orthop Res* 27:128–134, 2009.

72. Caputi RA: Synovectomy, *Clin Podiatr Med Surg* 5:249–257, 1988.

73. Carpenter B, Smith J, Motley T, Garrett A: Surgical treatment of hallux rigidus using a metatarsal head resurfacing implant: mid-term follow-up, *J Foot Ankle Surg* 49:321–325, 2010.

74. Caselli MA, George DH: Foot deformities: biomechanical and pathomechanical changes associated with aging, part I, *Clin Podiatr Med Surg* 20:487–509, ix, 2003.

75. Cavolo DJ, Cavallaro DC, Arrington LE: The Watermann osteotomy for hallux limitus, *J Am Podiatry Assoc* 69:52–57, 1979.

76. Centers for Disease Control and Prevention: Lyme disease, updated October 1, 2012. Available at http://www.cdc.gov/lyme. Accessed May 21, 2013.

77. Chalmers AC, Busby C, Goyert J, et al: Metatarsalgia and rheumatoid arthritis-a randomized, single blind, sequential trial comparing 2 types of foot orthoses and supportive shoes, *J Rheumatol* 27:1643–1647, 2000.

78. Chana GS, Andrew TA, Cotterill CP: A simple method of arthrodesis of the first metatarsophalangeal joint, *J Bone Joint Surg Br* 66:703–705, 1984.

79. Chand Y, Johnson KA: Foot and ankle manifestations of Reiter's syndrome, *Foot Ankle* 1:167–172, 1980.

80. Charalambous CP, Tryfonides M, Sadiq S, et al: Septic arthritis following intra-articular steroid injection of the knee: a Survey of current practice regarding antiseptic technique used during intra-articular steroid injection of the knee, *Clin Rheumatol* 22:386–390, 2003.

81. Cheleuitte E, Fleischli J, Tisa L, Zombolo R: Psoriasis and elective foot surgery, *J Foot Ankle Surg* 35:297–302; discussion 371, 1996.

82. Chen CW, Huang PJ, Chen TB, et al: Isolated talonavicular arthrodesis for talonavicular arthritis, *Foot Ankle Int* 22:633–636, 2001.

83. Chen DS, Wertheimer S: The Keller arthroplasty with use of the Dow Corning titanium hemi-implant, *J Foot Surg* 30:414–418, 1991.

84. Chimenti MS, Papoutsaki M, Teoli M, et al: Radiologically significant joint improvement in a patient affected by psoriatic arthritis treated with adalimumab, *Clin Exp Rheumatol* 27:1056, 2009.

85. Chiodo CP, Martin T, Wilson MG: A technique for isolated arthrodesis for inflammatory arthritis of the talonavicular joint, *Foot Ankle Int* 21:307–310, 2000.

86. Cho NS, Hwang HJ, Chang HJ, et al: Randomized controlled trial for clinical effects of varying tpes of insoles combined with specialized shoes in patients with rheumatoid arthritis of the foot, *Clin Rehabil* 23:512–521, 2009.

87. Chollet-Janin A, Finckh A, Dudler J, Guerne PA: Methotrexate as an alternative therapy for chronic calcium pyrophosphate deposition disease: an exploratory analysis, *Arthritis Rheum* 56:688–692, 2007.

88. Citron N, Neil M: Dorsal wedge osteotomy of the proximal phalanx for hallux rigidus. Long-term results, *J Bone Joint Surg Br* 69:835–837, 1987.

89. Clain MR, Baxter, DE: Simultaneous calcaneocuboid and talonavicular fusion. Long-term follow-up study, *J Bone Joint Surg Br* 76:133–136, 1994.

90. Clayton ML: Surgery of the forefoot in rheumatoid arthritis, *Clin Orthop Relat Res* 16:136–140, 1960.

91. Clayton ML: Surgery of the lower extremity in rheumatoid arthritis, *J Bone Joint Surg Am* 45:1517–1536, 1963.

92. Cleveland M, Winant EM: An end-result study of the Keller operation, *J Bone Joint Surg Am* 32:163–175, 1950.

93. Clutton H: The treatment of hallux valgus, *St Thomas Hosp Rep* 22:1–12, 1891-1893.

94. Conklin MJ, Smith RW: Treatment of the atypical lesser toe deformity with basal hemiphalangectomy, *Foot Ankle Int* 15:585–594, 1994.

95. Conrad KJ, Budiman-Mak E, Roach KE, et al: Impacts of foot orthoses on pain and disability in rheumatoid arthritics, *J Clin Epidemiol* 49:1–7, 1996.

96. Cook E, Coo J, Rosenblum B, et al: Meta-analysis of first metatarsophalangeal joint implant arthroplasty, *J Foot Ankle Surg* 48:180–190, 2009.

97. Cook KD: Capsular interposition for the Keller bunionectomy with the use of soft-tissue anchors, *J Am Podiatr Med Assoc* 95:180–182, 2005.

98. Corrigan G, Kanat IO: Modification of the total first metatarsophalangeal joint implant arthroplasty, *J Foot Surg* 28:295–300, 1989.

99. Cotterill J: Stiffness of the great toe in adolescents, *BMJ* 1:1158, 1888.

100. Coughlin MJ: Arthrodesis of the first metatarsophalangeal joint, *Orthop Rev* 19:177–186, 1990.

101. Coughlin MJ: Arthrodesis of the first metatarsophalangeal joint with mini-fragment plate fixation, *Orthopedics* 13:1037–1044, 1990.

102. Coughlin MJ: The rheumatoid foot. In Chapman M, editor: *Operative orthopaedics*, Philadelphia, 1993, JB Lippincott, pp 2311–2322.

103. Coughlin MJ: Conditions of the forefoot. In DeLee J, Drez D, editors: *Orthopaedic sports medicine: principles and practice*, Philadelphia, 1994, WB Saunders, pp 221–244.

104. Coughlin MJ: Rheumatoid forefoot reconstruction. A long-term follow-up study, *J Bone Joint Surg Am* 82:322–341, 2000.

105. Coughlin MJ: The Scandinavian total ankle replacement prosthesis, *Instr Course Lect* 51:135–142, 2002.

106. Coughlin MJ, Abdo RV: Arthrodesis of the first metatarsophalangeal joint with vitallium plate fixation, *Foot Ankle Int* 15:18–28, 1994.

107. Coughlin MJ, Grebing BR, Jones CP: Arthrodesis of the first metatarsophalangeal joint for idiopathic hallux valgus: intermediate results, *Foot Ankle Int* 26:783–792, 2005.

108. Coughlin MJ, Jones CR: Hallux valgus: demographics, etiology, and readiographic assessment, *Foot Ankle Int* 28:759–777, 2007.

109. Coughlin MJ, Mann RA: Arthrodesis of the first metatarsophalangeal joint as salvage for the failed Keller procedure, *J Bone Joint Surg Am* 69:68–75, 1987.

110. Coughlin MJ, Shurnas PS: Hallux rigidus: demographics, etiology, and radiographic assessment, *Foot Ankle Int* 24:731–743, 2003.

111. Coughlin MJ, Shurnas PS: Hallux rigidus. Grading and long-term results of operative treatment, *J Bone Joint Surg Am* 85:2072–2088, 2003.

112. Coughlin MJ, Shurnas PS: Soft-tissue arthroplasty for hallux rigidus, *Foot Ankle Int* 24:661–672, 2003.

113. Coughlin MJ, Shurnas PS: Hallux rigidus, *J Bone Joint Surg Am* 86(Suppl 1):119–130, 2004.

114. Cracchiolo A 3rd: Management of the arthritic forefoot, *Foot Ankle* 3:17–23, 1982.

115. Cracchiolo A 3rd: Rheumatoid arthritis of the forefoot. In Gould J, editor: *Operative foot surgery*, Philadelphia, 1994, WB Saunders, pp 141–159.

116. Cracchiolo A 3rd, Weltmer JB Jr, Lian G, et al: Arthroplasty of the first metatarsophalangeal joint with a double-stem silicone implant. Results in patients who have degenerative joint disease failure of previous operations, or rheumatoid arthritis, *J Bone Joint Surg Am* 74:552–563, 1992.

117. Craxford AD, Stevens J, Park C: Management of the deformed rheumatoid forefoot. A comparison of conservative and surgical methods, *Clin Orthop Relat Res* 166:121–126, 1982.

118. Cronin JJ, Limbers JP, Kutty S, Stephens MM: Intermetatarsal angle after first metatarsophalangeal joint arthrodesis for hallux valgus, *Foot Ankle Int* 27:104–109, 2006.

119. Curtis MJ, Myerson M, Jinnah RH, et al: Arthrodesis of the first metatarsophalangeal joint: A biomechanical study of internal fixation techniques, *Foot Ankle* 14:395–399, 1993.

120. Dalziel R, Thornhill TS, Thomas WH: Isolated talonavicular fusion for hindfoot arthritis, *Orthop Trans* 6:341, 1982.

121. Davies GF: Plantarflexory base wedge osteotomy in the treatment of functional and structural metatarsus primus elevatus, *Clin Podiatr Med Surg* 6:93–102, 1989.

122. Davies-Colley M: Contraction of the metatarsophalangeal joint of the great toe, *BMJ* 1:728, 1887.

123. Davitt JS, Kadel N, Sangeorzan BJ, et al: An association between functional second metatarsal length and midfoot arthrosis, *J Bone Joint Surg Am* 87:795–800, 2005.

124. Day-Williams AG, Southam L, Panoutsopoulou K, et al: A variant in MCF2L is associated with osteoarthritis, *J Am Hum Gen* 89:446–450, 2011.

125. DeFrino PF, Brodsky JW, Pollo FE, et al: First metatarsophalangeal arthrodesis: a clinical, pedobarographic and gait analysis study, *Foot Ankle Int* 23:496–502, 2002.

126. DelaCruz, EL, Johnson AR, Clair BL: First metatarsophalangeal joint interpositional arthroplasty using a meniscus allograft for the treatment of advanced hallux rigidus: surgical technique and short-term results, *Foot Ankle Spec* 4:157–164, 2011.

127. Dennis DT: Lyme disease. Tracking an epidemic, *JAMA* 266:1269–1270, 1991.

128. DeOrio JK: Technique tip: arthrodesis of the first metatarsophalangeal joint—prevention of excessive dorsiflexion, *Foot Ankle Int* 28:746–747, 2007.

129. de Palma L, Chillemi C, Albanelli S, Rapali S: Muscle Involvement in rheumatoid arthritis: an ultrastructural study, *Ultrastruct Pathol* 2:151–156, 2000.

130. Derner R, Goss K, Postowski HN, Parsley N: A plantar-flexor-shortening osteotomy for hallux rigidus: a retrospective analysis, *J Foot Ankle Surg* 44:377–389, 2005.

131. Dhawan SK, Conti SF, Towers J, et al: The effect of pulsed electromagnetic fields on hindfoot arthrodesis: a prospective study, *J Foot Ankle Surg* 43:93–96, 2004.

132. Dierick F, Detrembleur C, Trintignac G, Masquelier E: Nature of passive musculoarticular stiffness increase of ankle in female subjects with fibromyalgia syndrome, *Eur J Physiol* 111:2163–2171, 2011.

133. Disla E, Rhim HR, Reddy A, Taranta A: Improvement in CD4 lymphocyte count in HIV-Reiter's syndrome after treatment with sulfasalazine, *J Rheumatol* 21:662–664, 1994.

134. Dobbs B: LaPorta great toe implant. Long-term study of its efficacy. Student Research Group, *J Am Podiatr Med Assoc* 80:370–373, 1990.

135. Downey DJ, Simkin PA, Mack LA, et al: Tibialis posterior tendon rupture: a cause of rheumatoid flat foot, *Arthritis Rheum* 31:441–446, 1988.

136. Drago JJ, Oloff L, Jacobs AM: A comprehensive review of hallux limitus, *J Foot Surg* 23:213–220, 1984.

137. Dunlop WE, Rosenblood L, Lawrason L, et al: Effects of age and severity of illness on outcome and length of stay in geriatric surgical patients, *Am J Surg* 165:577–580, 1993.

138. Durrant MN, Siepert KK: Role of soft tissue structures as an etiology of hallux limitus, *J Am Podiatr Med Assoc* 83:173–180, 1993.

139. DuVries H: Arthritides. In DuVries H, editor: *Surgery of the foot*, ed 2, St Louis, 1965, Mosby, pp 318–329.

140. DuVries H: Static deformities. In DuVries H, editor: *Surgery of the foot*, ed 2, St Louis, 1965, Mosby, 1959, pp 392–398.

141. Easley ME, Davis WH, Anderson RB: Intermediate to long-term follow-up of medial-approach dorsal cheilectomy for hallux rigidus, *Foot Ankle Int* 20:147–152, 1999.

142. Ebraheim NA, Biyani A, Padanilam T, Christiensen G: Calcaneocuboid joint involvement in calcaneal fractures, *Foot Ankle Int* 1996:17:563–565.

143. Egan R, Sartoris DJ, Resnick D: Radiographic features of gout in the foot, *J Foot Surg* 26:434–439, 1987.

144. Elbar JE, Thomas WH, Weinfeld MS, et al: Talonavicular arthrodesis for rheumatoid arthritis of the hindfoot, *Orthop Clin North Am* 7:821–826, 1976.

145. Ellington JK, Jones CP, Cohen BE, et al: Review of 107 hallux MTP joint arthrodesis using dome-shaped reamers and a stainless-steel dorsal plate, *Foot Ankle Int* 31:385–390, 2010.

146. Espinoza LR, Aguilar JL, Berman A, et al: Rheumatic manifestations associated with human immunodeficiency virus infection, *Arthritis Rheum* 32:1615–1622, 1989.

147. Ess P, Hamalainen M, Leppilahti J: Non-constrained titanium-polyethylene total endoprosthesis in the treatment of hallux rigidus. A prospective clinical 2-year follow-up study, *Scand J Surg* 91:202–207, 2002.

148. Ettl V, Radke S, Gaertner M, Walther M: Arthrodesis in the treatment of hallux rigidus, *Int Orthop* 27:382–385, 2003.

149. Evans CH, Robbins PD, Ghivizzani SC, et al: Clinical trial to assess the safety, feasibility, and efficacy of transferring a potentially anti-arthritic cytokine gene to human joints with rheumatoid arthritis, *Hum Gene Ther* 7:1261–1280, 1996.

150. Faller J, Thompson F, Hamilton W: Foot and ankle disorders resulting from Lyme disease, *Foot Ankle* 11:236–238, 1991.

151. Fan P, Yu D: Reiter's syndrome. In Kelley WN, Harris ED Jr, Ruddy S, Sledge CB, editors: *Textbook of rheumatology*, ed 4, Philadelphia, 1993, WB Saunders, pp 961–973.

152. Faraj AA, Naraen A, Twigg P: A comparative study of wire fixation and screw fixation in arthrodesis for the correction of hallux rigidus using an in vitro biomechanical model, *Foot Ankle Int* 28:89–91, 2007.

153. Farber EM, Nall ML: The natural history of psoriasis in 5,600 patients, *Dermatologica* 148:1–18, 1974.

154. Feldman KA: The Green-Watermann procedure: geometric analysis and preoperative radiographic template technique, *J Foot Surg* 31:182–185, 1992.

155. Feldman RS, Hutter J, Lapow L, Pour B: Cheilectomy and hallux rigidus, *J Foot Surg* 22:170–174, 1983.

156. Feltham GT, Hanks SE, Marcus RE: Age-based outcomes of cheilectomy for the treatment of hallux rigidus, *Foot Ankle Int* 22:192–197, 2001.

157. Fernandez-de-Retana P, Poggio D, Ortega JP: Technical tip: first metatarsophalangeal arthrodesis with 20-mm memory compression staples, *Foot Ankle Int* 29:613–615, 2008.

158. Figgie MP, O'Malley MJ, Ranawat C, et al: Triple arthrodesis in rheumatoid arthritis, *Clin Orthop Relat Res* 292:250–254, 1993.

159. Fink BR, Mizel MS, Temple HT: Simultaneous arthrodesis of the metatarsophalangeal and interphalangeal joints of the hallux, *Foot Ankle Int* 21:951–953, 2000.

160. Fitzgerald JA: A review of long-term results of arthrodesis of the first metatarso-phalangeal joint, *J Bone Joint Surg Br* 51:488–493, 1969.

161. Fitzgerald JA, Wilkinson JM: Arthrodesis of the metatarsophalangeal joint of the great toe, *Clin Orthop Relat Res* 157:70–77, 1981.

162. Fitzpatrick T, Johnson R, Polano M, et al: Psoriasis. In Fitzpatrick TB, Johnson RA, Polano M, et al, editors: *Color atlas and synopsis of classical dermatology*, ed 2, New York, 1992, McGraw-Hill, pp 40–53.

163. Flemister AS, Infante AF, Sanders RW, Walling AK: Subtalar arthrodesis for complications of intra-articular calcaneal fractures, *Foot Ankle Int* 21:392–399, 2000.

164. Flint M, Sweetnam R: Amputation of all toes, *J Bone Joint Surg Br* 42:90–96, 1960.

165. Fogel GR, Katoh Y, Rand J, Chao EYS: Talonavicular Arthrodesis for isolated arthritis: 9.5-year results and gait analysis, *Foot Ankle Int* 3:105–113, 1982.

166. Ford DK: The clinical spectrum of Reiter's syndrome and similar postenteric arthropathies, *Clin Orthop Relat Res* 143:59–65, 1979.

167. Ford TC: Surgical management of chronic tophaceous gout. A case report, *J Am Podiatr Med Assoc* 82:514–519, 1992.

168. Forrester DM: Radiologic vignette. The "cocktail" digit, *Arthritis Rheum* 26:664–667, 1983.

169. Fowler AW: A method of forefoot reconstruction, *J Bone Joint Surg Br* 41:507–513, 1959.

170. Freed JB: The increasing recognition of medullary lysis, cortical osteophytic proliferation, and fragmentation of implanted silicone polymer implants, *J Foot Ankle Surg* 32:171–179, 1993.

171. Frigg A, Dougall H, Boyd S, Nigg B: Can porous tantalum be used to achieve ankle and subtalar arthrodesis? *Clin Orthop Relat Res* 468:209–216, 2010.

172. Frigg A, Nigg B, Davis E, Pederson B, Valderrabano V: Does alignment in the hindfoot radiograph influence dynamic foot-floor pressures in ankle and tibiotalocalcaneal fusion? *Clin Orthop Relat Res* 468:3362–3370, 2010.

173. Fu F, Scranton P: Forefoot arthroplasty in rheumatoid arthritis: clinical appraisal and force plate analysis, *Orthopedics* 5:163–168, 1982.

174. Fuerst M, Mohl H, Baumgartel K, Ruther W: Leflunomide increases the risk of healing complications in patients with rheumatoid arthritis undergoing elective orthopaedic surgery, *Rheumatol Int* 26:1138–1142, 2006.

175. Fuhrmann RA, Anders JO: The long-term results of resection arthroplasties of the first metatarsophalangeal joint in rheumatoid arthritis, *Int Orthop* 25:312–316, 2001.

176. Gandhi A, Van Gelderen J, Berbarian WS, et al: *Platelet releasate enhances healing in patients with a non-union*. Orthopaedics Research Society 49th Annual Meeting, February 2, 2003, New Orleans, La.

177. Ganley JV, Lynch FR, Darrigan RD: Keller bunionectomy with fascia and tendon graft, *J Am Podiatr Med Assoc* 76:602–610, 1986.

178. Garber EK, Silver S: Pedal manifestations of DISH, *Foot Ankle* 3:12–16, 1982.

179. Garras DN, Santangelo JR, Wang DW, Easley ME: Subtalar distraction arthrodesis using interpositional frozen structural allograft, *Foot Ankle Int* 29:561–567, 2008.

180. Geldwert JJ, Rock GD, McGrath MP, Mancuso JE: Cheilectomy: still a useful technique for grade I and grade II hallux limitus/rigidus, *J Foot Surg* 31:154–159, 1992.

181. Gibson JN, Thomson CE: Arthrodesis or total replacement arthroplasty for hallux rigidus: a randomized controlled trial, *Foot Ankle Int* 26:680–690, 2005.

182. Gill J, Majithia V: Successful use of infliximab in the treatment of Reiter's syndrome: a case report and discussion, *Clin Rheumatol* 27:121–123, 2008.

183. Gimple K, Anspacher J, Kopta J: Metatarsophalangeal joint fusion of the great toe, *Orthopedics* 1:462–467, 1978.

184. Ginsburg AI: Arthrodesis of the first metatarsophalangeal joint: a practical procedure, *J Am Podiatry Assoc* 69:367–369, 1979.

185. Giza E, Sullivan M, Ocel D, et al: First metatarsophalangeal hemiarthroplasty for hallux rigidus, *Int Orthop* 34:1193–1198, 2010.

186. Gladman DD, Stafford-Brady F, Chang CH, et al: Longitudinal study of clinical and radiological progression in psoriatic arthritis, *J Rheumatol* 17:809–812, 1990.

187. Glanzmann MC, Sanhueza-Hernandez RS: Arthroscopic subtalar arthrodesis for symptomatic osteoarthritis of the hindfoot: a prospective study of 41 cases, *Foot Ankle Int* 28:2–7, 2007.

188. Gold RH, Bassett LW: Radiologic evaluation of the arthritic foot, *Foot Ankle* 2:332–341, 1982.

189. Goldenberg DL: Fibromyalgia and its relation to chronic fatigue syndrome, viral illness and immune abnormalities, *J Rheumatol Suppl* 19:91–93, 1989.
    Goldsmith DP, Long SS: Poststreptococcal disease of childhood: a changing syndrome, *Arthritis Rheum* 25:S18, 1982.

190. Gonzalez AC, Caballero RT, Aspiazú MB, Atrio GP: Fibromyalgia as a prognostic factor in arthroscopic surgery, *J Clin Rheumatol* 5:245, 1999.

191. Goodfellow J: Aetiology of hallux rigidus, *Proc R Soc Med* 59:821–824, 1966.

192. Gordon M, Bullough PG: Synovial and osseous inflammation in failed silicone-rubber prostheses, *J Bone Joint Surg Am* 64:574–580, 1982.

193. Goucher NR, Coughlin MJ: Hallux metatarsophalangeal joint arthrodesis using dome-shaped reamers and dorsal plate fixation: a prospective study, *Foot Ankle Int* 27:869–876, 2006.

194. Gould N: Hallux rigidus: Cheilotomy or implant? *Foot Ankle* 1:315–320, 1981.

195. Gould N, Schneider W, Ashikaga T: Epidemiological survey of foot problems in the continental United States: 1978-1979, *Foot Ankle* 1:8–10, 1980.

196. Grady JF, Axe TM: The modified Valenti procedure for the treatment of hallux limitus, *J Foot Ankle Surg* 33:365–367, 1994.

197. Grady JF, Axe TM, Zager EJ, Sheldon LA: A retrospective analysis of 772 patients with hallux limitus, *J Am Podiatr Med Assoc* 92:102–108, 2002.

198. Graham CE: Rheumatoid forefoot metatarsal head resection without first metatarsophalangeal arthrodesis, *Foot Ankle Int* 15:689–690, 1994.

199. Granberry WM, Noble PC, Bishop JO, Tullos HS: Use of a hinged silicone prosthesis for replacement arthroplasty of the first metatarsophalangeal joint, *J Bone Joint Surg Am* 73:1453–1459, 1991.

200. Graves SC, Mann RA, Graves KO: Triple arthrodesis in older adults: results after long-term follow-up, *J Bone Joint Surg Am* 75:355–362, 1993.

201. Greenberg L, Davis H: Foot problems in the US: the 1990 National Health Interview Survey, *J Am Podiatr Med Assoc* 83:475–483, 1993.

202. Grennan DM, Gray J, Loudon J, Fear S: Methotrexate and early postoperative complications in patients with rheumatoid arthritis undergoing elective orthopedic surgery, *Ann Rheum Dis* 60:214–217, 2001.

203. Griffin TM, Huebner JL, Kraus VB, et al: Induction of osteoarthritis and metabolic inflammation by a very high-fat diet in mice: effects of short-term exercise, *Arthritis Rheum* 64:443–453, 2011.

204. Grimes JS, Coughlin MJ: First metatarsophalangeal joint arthrodesis as a treatment for failed hallux valgus surgery, *Foot Ankle Int* 27:887–893, 2006.

205. Grondal L, Hedstrom M, Stark A: Arthrodesis compared to mayo resection of the first metatarsophalangeal joint in total rheumatoid forefoot reconstruction, *Foot Ankle Int* 26:135–139, 2005.

206. Gruber F, Sinkov VS, Bae SY, et al: Crossed screws versus dorsomedial locking plate with compression screw for first metatarsocuneiform arthrodesis: a cadaver study, *Foot Anke Int* 29:927–930, 2008.

207. Guerra J, Resnick D: Arthritides affecting the foot: radiographic-pathological correlation, *Foot Ankle* 2:325–331, 1982.

208. Gutierrez F, Espinoza LR: [Reactive arthritis: a review], *Rev Med Chil* 118:796–804, 1990.

209. Hackford AW: Surgical principles for the aged. In Reichel W, editor: *Care of the elderly: clinical aspects of aging*, ed 4, Baltimore, 1995, Williams & Wilkins, pp 408–415.

210. Hahn MP, Gerhardt N, Thordarso, DB: Medial capsular interpositional arthroplasty for severe hallux rigidus, *Foot Ankle Int* 30:494–499, 2009.

211. Hakkinen A, Hakkinen K, Hannonen P: Effects of strength training on neuromuscular function and disease activity in patients with recent-onset inflammatory arthritis, *Scand J Rheumatol* 23:237–242, 1994.

212. Hamalainen M, Raunio P: Long-term followup of rheumatoid forefoot surgery, *Clin Orthop Relat Res* 340:34–38, 1997.

213. Hamilton J, Brydson G, Fraser S, Grant M: Walking ability as a measure of treatment effect in early rheumatoid arthritis, *Clin Rehabil* 15:142–147, 2001.

214. Hamilton WG, O'Malley, MJ, Thompson FM, Kovatis PE: Roger Mann Award 1995. Capsular interposition arthroplasty for severe hallux rigidus, *Foot Ankle Int* 18:68–70, 1997.

215. Hammerschlag WA, Rice JR, Caldwell DS, Goldner JL: Psoriatic arthritis of the foot and ankle: analysis of joint involvement and diagnostic errors, *Foot Ankle* 12:35–39, 1991.

216. Han B, Woodell-May J, Ponticiello M, et al: The effect of thrombin activation of platelet-rich plasma on demineralized bone matrix osteoinductivity, *J Bone Joint Surg Am* 91:1459–1470, 2009.

217. Hanft JR, Mason ET, Landsman AS, Kashuk KB: A new radiographic classification for hallux limitus, *J Foot Ankle Surg* 32:397–404, 1993.

218. Hanft JR, Merrill T, Marcinko DE, et al: Grand rounds: first metatarsophalangeal joint replacement, *J Foot Ankle Surg* 35:78–85, 1996.

219. Hanyu T, Yamazaki H, Ishikawa H, et al: Flexible hinge toe implant arthroplasty for rheumatoid arthritis of the first metatarsophalangeal joint: long-term results, *J Orthop Sci* 6:141–147, 2001.

220. Hanyu T, Yamazaki H, Murasawa A, Tohyama C: Arthroplasty for rheumatoid forefoot deformities by a shortening oblique osteotomy, *Clin Orthop Relat Res* 338:131–138, 1997.

221. Harper MC, Tisdel, CL: Talonavicular arthrodesis for the painful adult acquired flatfoot, *Foot Ankle Int* 17:658–661, 1996.

222. Harris MD, Siegel LB, Alloway JA: Gout and hyperuricemia, *Am Fam Physician* 59:925–934, 1999.

223. Harrison M: Hallux limitus, *J Bone Joint Surg Br* 53:772, 1971.

224. Harrison M, Harvey F: Arthrodesis of the first metatarsophalangeal joint for hallux valgus and rigidus, *J Bone Joint Surg Am* 45:471–480, 1963.

225. Harvey CK, Cadena R, Dunlap L: Fibromyalgia. Part I. Review of the literature, *J Am Podiatr Med Assoc* 83:412–415, 1993.

226. Hasselo LG, Willkens RF, Toomey HE, et al: Forefoot surgery in rheumatoid arthritis: subjective assessment of outcome, *Foot Ankle* 8:148–151, 1987.

227. Hattori T, Hashimoto J, Tomita T, et al: Radiological study of joint destruction patterns in rheumatoid flatfoot, *Clin Rheumatol* 27:733–737, 2008.

228. Hattrup SJ, Johnson KA: Subjective results of hallux rigidus following treatment with cheilectomy, *Clin Orthop Relat Res* 226:182–191, 1988.

229. Hauschild G, Merten HA, Bader A, et al: Bioartificial bone grafting: tarsal joint fusion in a dog using a bioartificial composite bone graft consisting of beta-tricalciumphosphate and platelet rich plasma—a case report, *Vet Comp Orthop Traumatol* 18:52–54, 2005.

230. Heaney S: Phalangeal osteotomy for hallux rigidus, *J Bone Joint Surg Br* 52:799, 1970.

231. Hecht PJ, Gibbons MJ, Wapner KL, et al: Arthrodesis of the first metatarsophalangeal joint to salvage failed silicone implant arthroplasty, *Foot Ankle Int* 18:383–390, 1997.

232. Hench PK: Evaluation and differential diagnosis of fibromyalgia. Approach to diagnosis and management, *Rheum Dis Clin North Am* 15:19–29, 1989.

233. Henry AP, Waugh W, Wood H: The use of footprints in assessing the results of operations for hallux valgus. A comparison of Keller's operation and arthrodesis, *J Bone Joint Surg Br* 57:478–481, 1975.

234. Hetherington VJ, Mercado C, Karloc L, Grillo J: Silicone implant arthroplasty: a retrospective analysis, *J Foot Ankle Surg* 32:430–433, 1993.

235. Higgins KR, Burnett OE, Krych SM, Harkless LB: Seronegative rheumatoid arthritis and Morton's neuroma, *J Foot Surg* 27:404–407, 1988.

236. Hodge MC, Bach TM, Carter GM: Novel Award First Prize Paper. Orthotic management of plantar pressure and pain in rheumatoid arthritis, *Clin Biomech (Bristol, Avon)* 14:567–575, 1999.

237. Hoffman P: An operation for severe grades of contracted or clawed toes, *Am J Orthop Surg* 9:441–449, 1911.

238. Hope M, Savva N, Whitehouse S, et al: Is it necessary to re-fuse a non-union of a hallux metatarsophalangeal joint arthrodesis? *Foot Ankle Int* 31:662–669, 2010.

239. Hopson M, Stone P, Paden M: First metatarsal head osteoarticular transfer system for salvage of a failed hemicap-implant: a case report, *J Foot Ankle Surg* 48:483–487, 2009.

240. Horton GA, Olney BW: Triple arthrodesis with lateral column lengthening for treatment of severe planovalgus deformity, *Foot Ankle Int* 16:395–400, 1995.

241. Horton GA, Park YW, Myerson MS: Role of metatarsus primus elevatus in the pathogenesis of hallux rigidus, *Foot Ankle Int* 20:777–780, 1999.

242. Huefner T, Thermann H, Geerling J, et al: Primary subtalar arthrodesis of calcaneal fractures, *Foot Ankle Int* 22:9–14, 2001.

243. Hulse N, Thomas AM: Metatarsal head resection in the rheumatoid foot: 5-year follow-up with and without resection of the first metatarsal head, *J Foot Ankle Surg* 45:107–112, 2006.

244. Hulsmans HM, Jacobs JW, van der Heijde DM, et al: The course of radiologic damage during the first six years of rheumatoid arthritis, *Arthritis Rheum* 43:1927–1940, 2000.

245. Humbert JL, Bourbonniere C, Laurin CA: Metatarsophalangeal fusion for hallux valgus: Indications and effect on the first metatarsal ray, *Can Med Assoc J* 120:937–941, 956, 1979.

246. Hunt KJ, Ellington JK, Anderson RB, et al: Locked versus non-locked plate fixation for hallux MTP arthrodesis, *Foot Ankle Int* 32:704–709, 2011.

247. Hyer CF, Glover JP, Berlet GC, Lee TH: Cost comparison of crossed screws versus dorsal plate construct for first metatarsophalangeal joint arthrodesis, *J Foot Ankle Surg* 47:13–18, 2008.

248. Hyslop E, McInnes IB, Woodburn J, Turner DE: Foot problems in psoriatic arthritis: high burden and low care provision, *Ann Rheum Dis* 69:928, 2010.

249. Ibuki A, Cornoiu A, Clarke A, et al: The effect of orthotic treatment on midfoot osteoarthritis assessed using specifically designed patient evaluation questionnaires, *Prosthet Orthot Int* 34:461–471, 2010.

250. Iceman at the South Tyrol Museum of Archaeology (website). Available at http://www.iceman.it/en/the-iceman-at-the-museum. Accessed May 21, 2013.

251. Jaakkola JI, Mann RA: A review of rheumatoid arthritis affecting the foot and ankle, *Foot Ankle Int* 25:866–874, 2004.

252. Jack EA: The aetiology of hallux rigidus, *Br J Surg* 27:494–497, 1940.

253. Jahss M: Personal communication, June 26, 1997.

254. Jannink MJ, van Dijk H, de Vries J, et al: A systematic review of the methodological quality and extent to which evaluation studies measure the usability of orthopaedic shoes, *Clin Rehabil* 18:15–26, 2004.

255. Janssens HJ, Janssen M, van de Lisdonk EH, et al: Use of oral prednisolone or naproxen for the treatment of gout arthritis: a double-blind, randomised equivalence trial, *Lancet* 371:1854–1860, 2008.

256. Jarrell SE, Owen JR, Wayne JS, Adelaar RS: Biomechanical comparison of screw versus plate/screw construct for talonavicular fusion, *Foot Ankle Int* 30:150–156, 2009.

257. Jeffery JA, Freedman LF: Modified reamers for fusion of the first metatarsophalangeal joint, *J Bone Joint Surg Br* 77:328–329, 1995.

258. Jeffries LC, Rodriguez RH, Stapleton JJ, Zgonis T: Pan-metatarsophalangeal joint arthrodesis for the severe rheumatoid forefoot deformity, *Clin Podiatr Med Surg* 26:149–157, 2009.

259. Jeng C, Campbell J: Current concepts review: the rheumatoid forefoot, *Foot Ankle Int* 29:959–968, 2008.

260. Jenkin WM, Oloff LM: Implant arthroplasty in the rheumatoid arthritic patient, *Clin Podiatr Med Surg* 5:213–226, 1988.

261. Jerome JT, Varghese M, Sankaran B, et al: Tibialis anterior tendon rupture in gout: case report and literature review, *Foot Ankle Surg* 14:166–169, 2008.

262. Johansson JE, Barrington TW: Cone arthrodesis of the first metatarsophalangeal joint, *Foot Ankle* 4:244–248, 1984.

263. Johnson JE, Johnson KA: Dowel arthrodesis for degenerative arthritis of the tarsometatarsal (Lisfranc) joints, *Foot Ankle* 6:243–253, 1986.

263a. Johnson KA: Personal communication, 1994.

264. Johnson KA, Buck PG: Total replacement arthroplasty of the first metatarsophalangeal joint, *Foot Ankle* 1:307–314, 1981.

265. Jones C, Nunley J: Osteonecrosis of the lateral aspect of the talar dome after triple arthrodesis, *J Bone Joint Surg* 81:1165–1169, 1999.

266. Jones RO, Chen JB, Pitcher D, et al: Rheumatoid nodules affecting both heels with surgical debulking: a case report, *J Am Podiatr Med Assoc* 86:179–182, 1996.

267. Joplin RJ: Surgery of the forefoot in the rheumatoid arthritic patient, *Surg Clin North Am* 49:847–878, 1969.

268. Jordan HH, Bordsky AE: Keller operation for hallux valgus and hallux rigidus. An end result study, *AMA Arch Surg* 62:586–596, 1951.

269. Jouben LM, Steele RJ, Bono JV: Orthopaedic manifestations of Lyme disease, *Orthop Rev* 23:395–400, 1994.

270. Jung HG, Myerson MS, Schon LC: Spectrum of operative treatments and clinical outcomes for atraumatic osteoarthritis of the tarsometatarsal joints, *Foot Ankle Int* 28:482–489, 2007.

271. Kampner SL: Total joint prosthetic arthroplasty of the great toe—a 12-year experience, *Foot Ankle* 4:249–261, 1984.

272. Kane D, Greaney T, Bresnihan B, et al: Ultrasonography in the diagnosis and management of psoriatic dactylitis, *J Rheumatol* 26:1746–1751, 1999.

273. Kane D, Stafford L, Bresnihan B, FitzGerald O: A classification study of clinical subsets in an inception cohort of early psoriatic peripheral arthritis—"DIP or not DIP revisited." *Rheumatology (Oxford)* 42:1469–1476, 2003.

274. Kane D, Stafford L, Bresnihan B, FitzGerald O: A prospective, clinical and radiological study of early psoriatic arthritis: an early synovitis clinic experience, *Rheumatology (Oxford)* 42:1460–1468, 2003.

275. Kataria RK, Brent LH: Spondyloarthropathies, *Am Fam Physician* 69:2853–2860, 2004.

276. Kates A, Kessel, L, Kay A: Arthroplasty of the forefoot, *J Bone Joint Surg Br* 49:552–557, 1967.

277. Katz W: Psoriatic arthritis in Reiter's disease. In Katz W, editor: *Rheumatic diseases: diagnosis and management*, Philadelphia, 1977, JB Lippincott, pp 540–555.

278. Kavlak Y, Uygur F, Korkmaz C, Bek N: Outcome of orthoses intervention in the rheumatoid foot, *Foot Ankle Int* 24:494–499, 2003.

279. Keat A: Reiter's syndrome and reactive arthritis in perspective, *N Engl J Med* 309:1606–1615, 1983.

280. Keat AC: Should all patients with Reiter's syndrome be tested for HIV infection? *Br J Rheumatol* 28:409, 1989.

281. Keenan MA, Peabody TD, Gronley JK, Perry J: Valgus deformities of the feet and characteristics of gait in patients who have rheumatoid arthritis, *J Bone Joint Surg Am* 73:237–247, 1991.

282. Keiserman LS, Cassandra J, Amis JA: The piano key test: a clinical sign for the identification of subtle tarsometatarsal pathology, *Foot Ankle Int* 24:437–438, 2003.

283. Kelikian H: *Hallux valgus allied deformities of the forefoot and metatarsalgia*, Philadelphia, 1997, WB Saunders, pp 262–281.

284. Keller W: The surgical treatment of bunions and hallux valgus, *N Y Med J* 80:741–742, 1904.

285. Kemp TJ, Hirose CB, Coughlin MJ, Otto R: Treatment of chronic tophaceous gout with a wound vacuum-assist device, *Foot Ankle Int* 31:729–731, 2010.

286. Kennedy JG, Chow FY, Dines J, et al: Outcomes after interposition arthroplasty for treatment of hallux rigidus, *Clin Orthop Relat Res* 445:210–215, 2006.

287. Kennedy MP, Coughlin MJ: Peg-in-socket arthrodesis of the first metatarsophalangeal joint, *Foot Ankle Int* 23:352–354, 2002.

288. Kessel L, Bonney G: Hallux rigidus in the adolescent, *J Bone Joint Surg Br* 40:669–673, 1958.

289. Khosla ST, Thiele R, Baumauer JF: Ultrasound guidance for intra-articular injections of the foot and ankle, *Foot Ankle Int* 30:886–890, 2009.

290. Kilmartin, TE: Phalangeal osteotomy versus first metatarsal decompression osteotomy for the surgical treatment of hallux rigidus: a prospective study of age-matched and condition-matched patients, *J Foot Ankle Surg* 44:2–12, 2005.

291. Kim HA, Lee YJ, Seong SC, et al: Apoptotic chondrocyte death in human osteoarthritis, *J Rheumatol* 27:455–462, 2000.

292. Kindsfater K, Wilson MG, Thomas WH: Management of the rheumatoid hindfoot with special reference to talonavicular arthrodesis, *Clin Orthop Relat Res* 340:69–74, 1997.

293. Kinne RW, Stuhlmuller B, Burmester GR: Cells of the synovium in rheumatoid arthritis, *Arthritis Res Ther* 9:1–16, 2007.

294. Kinner B, Schieder S, Muller F, et al: Calcaneocuboid joint involvement in calcaneal fractures, *J Trauma* 68:1192–1199, 2010.

295. Kirkham BW, Gibson T: Comment on the article by Downey et al [letter], *Arthritis Rheum* 32:359, 1989.

296. Kitaoka HB, Holiday AD Jr, Chao EY, Cahalan TD: Salvage of failed first metatarsophalangeal joint implant arthroplasty by implant removal and synovectomy: clinical and biomechanical evaluation, *Foot Ankle* 13:243–250, 1992.

297. Klareskog L, van der Heijde D, de Jager JP, et al: Therapeutic effect of the combination of etanercept and methotrexate compared with each treatment alone in patients with rheumatoid arthritis, *N Engl J Med* 343:1594–1602, 2000.

298. Klein SE, Putnam RM, McCormick J, Johnson JE: The slot graft technique for foot and ankle arthrodesis in a high-risk patient group, *Foot Ankle Int* 32:686–692, 2011.

299. Knupp M, Skoog A, Tornkvist H, Ponzer S: Triple arthrodesis in rheumatoid arthritis, *Foot Ankle Int* 29:293–297, 2008.

300. Koenig RD: Koenig total great toe implant. Preliminary report, *J Am Podiatr Med Assoc* 80:462–468, 1990.

301. Koenig RD: Revision arthroplasty utilizing the Biomet Total Toe System for failed silicone elastomer implants, *J Foot Ankle Surg* 33:222–227, 1994.

302. Koenig RD, Horwitz LR: The Biomet Total Toe System utilizing the Koenig score: a five-year review, *J Foot Ankle Surg* 35:23–26, 1996.

303. Kolker D, Weinfeld S: Technique tip: a modification to the Keller arthroplasty using interposition allograft, *Foot Ankle Int* 28:266–268, 2007.

304. Komenda GA, Myerson MS, Biddinger KR: Results of arthrodesis of the tarsometatarsal joints after traumatic injury, *J Bone Joint Surg Am* 78:1665–1676, 1996.

305. Konkel KF, Menger AG: Mid-term results of titanium hemi-great toe implants, *Foot Ankle Int* 27:922–929, 2006.

306. Konkel KF, Menger AG, Retzlaff SA: Mid-term results of Futura hemi-great toe implants, *Foot Ankle Int* 29:831–837, 2008.

307. Konkel KF, Menger AG, Retzlaff SA: Results of metallic Hemi-Great Toe implant for grade III and early grade IV hallux rigidus, *Foot Ankle Int* 30:653–660, 2009.

308. Krause FG, Fehlbaum O, Huebschle LM, Weber M: Preservation of lesser metatarsophalangeal joints in rheumatoid forefoot reconstruction, *Foot Ankle Int* 32:131–140, 2011.

309. Kubiak EN, Moskovich R, Errico TJ, Di Cesare PE: Orthopaedic management of ankylosisng spondylitis, *J Am Acad Orthop Surg* 13:267–278, 2005.

310. Kuhns JG: The foot in chronic arthritis, *Clin Orthop Relat Res* 16:141–151, 1960.

311. Kumar S, Gow P: A survey of indications, results and complications of surgery for tophaceous gout, *N Z Med J* 115:U109, 2002.

312. Kumar S, Pradhan R, Rosenfeld PF: First metatarsophalangeal arthrodesis using a dorsal plate and a compression screw, *Foot Ankle Int* 31:797–801, 2010.

313. Kundert HP, Zollinger-Kies H: [Endoprosthetic replacement of hallux rigidus], *Orthopade* 34:748–757, 2005.

314. Kurtz DH, Harrill JC, Kaczander BI, Solomon MG: The Valenti procedure for hallux limitus: a long-term follow-up and analysis, *J Foot Ankle Surg* 38:123–130, 1999.

315. Kurtz J: Surgery of tophaceous gout in the lower extremity, *Surg Clin North Am* 45:217–228, 1965.

316. Lambrinudi P: Metatarsus primus elevatus, *Proc R Soc Med* 31:1273, 1938.

317. Landi A, Tarantino R, Marotta N, et al: The use of platelet gel in postero-lateral fusion: preliminary results in a series of 14 cases, *Eur Spine J* 20(Suppl 1):S61–S67, 2011.

318. Landry JR, Schilero J: The medical/surgical management of gout, *J Foot Surg* 25:160–175, 1986.

319. LaPorta GA, Pilla P Jr, Richter KP: Keller implant procedure: a report of 536 procedures using a Silastic intramedullary stemmed implant, *J Am Podiatry Assoc* 66:126–147, 1976.

320. Larmon WA, Kurtz JF: The surgical management of chronic tophaceous gout, *J Bone Joint Surg Am* 40:743–772, 1958.

321. Larsen A, Dale K, Eek M: Radiographic evaluation of rheumatoid arthritis and related conditions by standard reference films, *Acta Radiol Diagn (Stockh)* 18:481–491, 1977.

322. Lau JT, Daniels TR: Outcomes following cheilectomy and interpositional arthroplasty in hallux rigidus, *Foot Ankle Int* 22:462–470, 2001.

323. Lawrence RC, Felson DT, Helmick CG, et al: Estimates of the prevalence of arthritis and other rheumatic conditions on the United States, *Arthritis Rheum* 58:26–35, 2008.

324. Lawrence SJ: Lyme disease: An orthopedic perspective, *Orthopedics* 15:1331–1335, 1992.

325. Lawson JP, Steere AC: Lyme arthritis: Radiologic findings, *Radiology* 154:37–43, 1985.

326. Leaseburg JT, DeOrio JK, Shapiro SA: Radiographic correlation of hallux MP fusion position and plate angle, *Foot Ankle Int* 30:873–876, 2009.

327. Ledingham J, Deighton C; British Society for Rheumatology Standards, Guidelines and Audit Working Group: Update on the British Society for Rheumatology Guidelines for prescribing TNF-alpha blockers in adults with rheumatoid arthritis (update of previous guidelines of April 2001), *Rheumatology* 44:157–163, 2005.

328. Lee KB, Park CH, Seon JK, Kim MS: Arthroscopic subtalar arthrodesis using a posterior 2-portal approach in the prone position, *Arthroscopy* 26:230–238. 2010.

329. Leirisalo-Repo M: Prognosis, course of disease, and treatment of the spondyloarthropathies, *Rheum Dis Clin North Am* 24:737–751, 1998.

330. Lemon RA, Engber WD, McBeath AA: A complication of Silastic hemiarthroplasty in bunion surgery, *Foot Ankle* 4:262–266, 1984.

331. Lerman RL, Danna AT, Boykoff TJ: Tophaceous deposition in the absence of known antecedent gout, *J Am Podiatr Med Assoc* 81:273–275, 1991.

332. Levi S, Ansell BM, Klenerman L: Tarsometatarsal involvement in juvenile spondyloarthropathy, *Foot Ankle* 11:90–92, 1990.

332a. Lin J, Murphy GA: Treatment of hallux rigidus with cheilectomy using a dorsolateral approach, *Foot Ankle Int* 30:115–119, 2009.

333. Lin SS, Bono CM, Treuting R, Shereff MJ: Limited intertarsal arthrodesis using bone grafting and pin fixation, *Foot Ankle Int* 21:742–748, 2000.

334. Lindqvist E, Jonsson K, Saxne T, Eberhardt K: Course of radiographic damage over 10 years in a cohort with early rheumatoid arthritis, *Ann Rheum Dis* 62:611–616, 2003.

335. Lipscomb PR: Arthrodesis of the first metatarsophalangeal joint for severe bunions and hallux rigidus, *Clin Orthop Relat Res* 142:48–54, 1979.

336. Lipsky P: Rheumatoid arthritis. In Kasper D, editor: *Harrison's principles of internal medicine*, New York, 2005, McGraw-Hill, p, 1968.

337. Lipsky PE, van der Heijde DM, St Clair EW, et al: Infliximab and methotrexate in the treatment of rheumatoid arthritis, *N Engl J Med* 343:1594–1692, 2000.

338. Lombardi CM, Silhanek AD, Connolly FG, et al: First metatarsophalangeal arthrodesis for treatment of hallux rigidus: a retrospective study, *J Foot Ankle Surg* 40:137–143, 2001.

339. Love TR, Whynot AS, Farine I, et al: Keller arthroplasty: "a prospective review, *Foot Ankle* 8:46–54, 1987.

340. Lu DW, Katz KA: Declining use of the eponym "Reiter's syndrome" in the medical literature, 1998-2003, *J Am Acad Dermatol* 53:720–723, 2005.

341. Ly TV, Coetzee JC: Treatment of primarily ligamentous Lisfranc joint inuries: primary arthrodesis compared with open reduction and internal fixation. A prospective, randomized study, *J Bone Joint Surg Am* 88:514–520, 2006.

342. Mackay DC, Blyth M, Rymaszewski LA: The role of cheilectomy in the treatment of hallux rigidus, *J Foot Ankle Surg* 36:337–340, 1997.

343. Mackenzie CR, Sharrock NE: Trends in orthopedic surgery for rheumatoid arthritis: perioperative medical considerations in patients with rheumatoid arthritis, *Rheum Dis Clin North Am* 24:1–11, 1998.

344. Mackey RB, Thomson AB, Kwon O, et al: The modified oblique Keller capsular interpositional arthroplasty for hallux rigidus, *J Bone Joint Surg Am* 92:1938–1946, 2010.

345. Maenpaa H, Lehto MUK, Belt EA: Stress fractures of the ankle and forefoot in patients with inflammatory arthritides, *Foot Ankle Int* 23:833–837, 2002.
Maenpaa HM, Soini I, Lehto MU, Belt EA: Insufficiency fractures in patients with chronic inflammatory joint diseases, *Clin Exp Rheumatol* 20:77–79, 2002.

346. Maillefert JF, Combe B, Goupille P, et al: The 5-yr HAQ-disability is related to the first year's changes in the narrowing, rather than erosion score in patients with recent-onset rheumatoid arthritis, *Rheumatology (Oxford)* 43:79–84, 2004.

347. Malerba F, Milani R, Sartorelli E, Haddo O: Distal oblique first metatarsal osteotomy in grade 3 hallux rigidus: a long-term followup, *Foot Ankle Int* 29:677–682, 2008.

348. Man CY, Cheung IT, Cameron PA, Rainer TH: Comparison of oral prednisolone/paracetamol and oral indomethacin/paracetamol combination therapy in the treatment of acute goutlike arthritis: a double-blind, randomized, controlled trial, *Ann Emerg Med* 49:670–677, 2007.

349. Mankey M, Mann RA: *Arthrodesis of the first metatarsophalangeal utilizing a dorsal plate.* Presented at the Seventh Annual Summer Meeting of the American Orthopaedic Foot and Ankle Society, Boston, Mass, July 17, 1991.

350. Mann RA, Baumgarten M: Subtalar fusion for isolated subtalar disorders, *Clin Orthop* 146:260–265, 1988.

351. Mann RA, Clanton TO: Hallux rigidus: treatment by cheilectomy, *J Bone Joint Surg Am* 70:400–406, 1988.

352. Mann RA, Coughlin MJ: The rheumatoid foot: review of the literature and method of treatment, *Orthop Rev* 7:105–112, 1979.

353. Mann RA, Coughlin MJ: Arthrodesis of the foot and ankle. In Mann RA, Coughlin MJ, editors: *Video textbook of foot and ankle surgery*. St Louis, 1991, Medical Video Productions, pp 105–144.

354. Mann RA, Coughlin MJ, DuVries HL: Hallux rigidus: a review of the literature and a method of treatment, *Clin Orthop Relat Res* 142:57–63, 1979.

355. Mann RA, Katcherian DA: Relationship of metatarsophalangeal joint fusion on the intermetatarsal angle, *Foot Ankle* 10:8–11, 1989.

356. Mann RA, Oates JC: Arthrodesis of the first metatarsophalangeal joint, *Foot Ankle* 1:159–166, 1980.

357. Mann RA, Prieskorn D, Sobel M: Mid-tarsal and tarsometatarsal arthrodesis for primary degenerative osteoarthrosis or osteoarthrosis after trauma, *J Bone Joint Surg Am* 78:1376–1385, 1996.

358. Mann RA, Schakel ME 2nd: Surgical correction of rheumatoid forefoot deformities, *Foot Ankle Int* 16:1–6, 1995.

359. Mann RA, Thompson FM: Arthrodesis of the first metatarsophalangeal joint for hallux valgus in rheumatoid arthritis, *J Bone Joint Surg Am* 66:687–692, 1984.

360. Mann RA, Thompson FM: Rupture of the posterior tibial tendon causing flat foot. Surgical treatment, *J Bone Joint Surg Am* 67:556–561, 1985.

361. Marin GA: Arthrodesis of the metatarsophalangeal joint of the big toe for hallux valgus and hallux rigidus. A new method, *Int Surg* 50:175–180, 1968.

362. Marks RM, Parks BG, Schon LC: Midfoot fusion technique for neuroarthropathic feet: biomechanical analysis and rationale, *Foot Ankle Int* 19:507–510, 1998.

363. Marmor L: Resection of the forefoot in rheumatoid arthritis, *Clin Orthop Relat Res* 108:223–227, 1975.

364. Martel W: The overhanging margin of bone: a roentgenologic manifestation of gout, *Radiology* 91:755–756, 1968.

365. Maurer TA, Zackheim HS, Tuffanelli L, Berger TG: The use of methotrexate for treatment of psoriasis in patients with HIV infection, *J Am Acad Dermatol* 31:372–375, 1994.

366. Mauro G, Rubin RP, Kanat IO: Atypical gouty arthritis, *J Foot Surg* 24:280–282, 1985.

367. McCarthy DJ, Chapman HL: Ultrastructure of collapsed metatarsophalangeal silicone elastomer implant, *J Foot Surg* 27:418–427, 1988.

368. McDonald RJ, Griffin JM, Edelman RO: Consecutive bilateral failures of first metatarsophalangeal joint prostheses, *J Foot Surg* 25:226–233, 1986.

369. McGarvey SR, Johnson KA: Keller arthroplasty in combination with resection arthroplasty of the lesser metatarsophalangeal joints in rheumatoid arthritis, *Foot Ankle* 9:75–80, 1988.

370. McGonagle D, Tan AL, Madden J, et al: Successful treatment of resistant pseudogout with anakinra, *Arthritis Rheum* 58:631–633, 2008.

371. McKeever DC: Arthrodesis of the first metatarsophalangeal joint for hallux valgus, hallux rigidus, and metatarsus primus varus, *J Bone Joint Surg Am* 34:129–134, 1952.

372. McKinley JC, Shortt N, Arthur C, et al: Outcomes following pantalar arthrodesis in rheumatoid arthritis, *Foot Ankle Int* 32:681–685, 2011.

373. McMaster MJ: The pathogenesis of hallux rigidus, *J Bone Joint Surg Br* 60:82–87, 1978.

374. Mejjad O, Vittecoq O, Pouplin S, et al: Foot orthotics decrease pain but do not improve gait in rheumatoid arthritis patients, *Joint Bone Spine* 71:542–545, 2004.

375. Menz HB, Munteanu SE, Landorf KB, et al: Radiographic classification of osteoarthritis in commonly affected joints of the foot, *Osteoarthritis Cartilage* 15:1333–1338, 2007.

376. Menz HB, Munteanu SE, Zammit GV, Landorf KB: Foot structure and function in older people with radiographic osteoarthritis of the medial midfoot, *Osteoarthritis Cartilage* 18:317–322, 2010.

377. Merkle PF, Sculco TP: Prosthetic replacement of the first metatarsophalangeal joint, *Foot Ankle* 9:267–271, 1989.

378. Meyer JO, Nishon LR, Weiss L, Docks G: Metatarsus primus elevatus and the etiology of hallux rigidus, *J Foot Surg* 26:237–241, 1987.

379. Michelson J, Dunn L: Tenosynovitis of the flexor hallucis longus: a clinical study of the spectrum of presentation and treatment, *Foot Ankle Int* 26:291–303, 2005.

380. Michelson J, Easley M, Wigley FM, Hellmann D: Foot and ankle problems in rheumatoid arthritis, *Foot Ankle Int* 15:608–613, 1994.

381. Michet CJ: Psoriatic arthritis. In Kelley WN, Harris ED Jr, Ruddy S, Sledge CB, editors: *Textbook of rheumatology*, ed 4, Philadelphia, 1993, WB Saunders, pp 974–984.

382. Michet CJ, Machado EB, Ballard DJ, McKenna CH: Epidemiology of Reiter's syndrome in Rochester, Minnesota: 1950-1980, *Arthritis Rheum* 31:428–431, 1988.

383. Miller D, Maffulli N: Free gracilis interposition arthroplasty for severe hallux rigidus, *Bull Hosp Jt Dis* 62:121–124, 2005.

384. Millott M, Berlin R: Treating sleep disorders in patients with fibromyalgia, *J Musculoskel Med* 14:25–34, 1997.

385. Minns RJ, Craxford AD: Pressure under the forefoot in rheumatoid arthritis. A comparison of static and dynamic methods of assessment, *Clin Orthop Relat Res* 187:235–242, 1984.

386. Miskew DB, Goldflies ML: Atraumatic avascular necrosis of the talus associated with hyperuricemia, *Clin Orthop Relat Res* 148:156–159, 1980.

387. Miyamoto W, Takao M, Innami K, et al: Technique tip: interposition of extensor digitorum longus after resection arthroplasty of lesser metatarsophalangeal joints for rheumatoid forefoot deformity, *Foot Ankle Int* 32:211–214, 2011.

388. Miyamoto W, Takao M, Uchio Y, et al: Late-stage Freiberg disease treated by osteochondral plug transplantation: a case series, *Foot Ankle Int* 29:950–955, 2008.

389. Mizel MS, Alvarez RG, Fink BR, Temple HT: Ipsilateral arthrodesis of the metatarsophalangeal and interphalangeal joints of the hallux, *Foot Ankle Int* 27:804–807, 2006.

390. Moberg E: A simple operation for hallux rigidus, *Clin Orthop Relat Res* 142:55–56, 1979.

391. Moeckel BH, Sculco TP, Alexiades MM, et al: The double-stemmed silicone-rubber implant for rheumatoid arthritis of the first metatarsophalangeal joint. Long-term results, *J Bone Joint Surg Am* 74:564–570, 1992.

392. Moll JM, Wright V: Psoriatic arthritis, *Semin Arthritis Rheum* 3:55–78, 1973.

393. Molloy S, Burkhart BG, Jasper LE, et al: Biomechanical comparison of two fixation methods for first metatarsophalangeal joint arthrodesis, *Foot Ankle Int* 24:169–171, 2003.

394. Moncur C, Ward JR: Heat-moldable shoes for management of forefoot problems in rheumatoid arthritis, *Arthritis Rheum* 3:222–226, 1990.

395. Montero LC, Gomez RS, de Quiros JF: Cutaneous ulcerations in a patient with rheumatoid arthritis receiving treatment with methotrexate, *J Rheumatol* 27:2290–2291, 2000.

396. Morino T, Fujita M, Kariyama K, et al: Intraosseous gouty tophus of the talus, treated by total curettage and calcium phosphate cement filling: a case report, *Foot Ankle Int* 28:126–128, 2007.

397. Morrison P: Complications of forefoot operations in rheumatoid arthritis, *Proc R Soc Med* 67:110–111, 1974.

398. Moynihan FJ: Arthrodesis of the metatarso-phalangeal joint of the great toe, *J Bone Joint Surg Br* 49:544–551, 1967.

399. Mroczek KJ, Miller SD: The modified oblique Keller procedure: a technique for dorsal approach interposition arthroplasty sparing the flexor tendons, *Foot Ankle Int* 24:521–522, 2003.

400. Mulcahy D, Daniels TR, Lau JT, et al: Rheumatoid forefoot deformity: a comparison study of 2 functional methods of reconstruction, *J Rheumatol* 30:1440–1450, 2003.

401. Mulier T, Steenwerckx A, Thienpont E, et al: Results after cheilectomy in athletes with hallux rigidus, *Foot Ankle Int* 20:232–237, 1999.

402. Murphy G, Kwan J, Mihm M: The skin. In Robbins S, Cotran R, Kumar V, editors: *Pathologic basis of disease*, ed 3, Philadelphia, 1984, WB Saunders, pp 1291–1293.

403. Myers SR, Herndon JH: Silastic implant arthroplasty with proximal metatarsal osteotomy for painful hallux valgus, *Foot Ankle* 10:219–223, 1990.

404. Myerson MS: Adult acquired flatfoot deformity: Treatment of dysfunction of the posterior tibial tendon, *Instr Course Lect* 46:393–405, 1997.

405. Myerson MS, Schon LC, McGuigan FX, Oznur A: Result of arthrodesis of the hallux metatarsophalangeal joint using bone graft for restoration of length, *Foot Ankle Int* 21:297–306, 2000.

406. Nagashima M, Kato K, Miyamoto Y, Takenouchi K: A Modified Mohman method for hallux valgus and telescoping osteotomy for lesser toe deformities in patients with rheumatoid arthritis, *Clin Rheumatol* 26:39–43, 2007.

407. Nash P: Assessment and treatment of psoriatic spondylitis, *Curr Rheumatol Rep* 11:278–283, 2009.

408. Nassar J, Cracchiolo A 3rd: Complications in surgery of the foot and ankle in patients with rheumatoid arthritis, *Clin Orthop Relat Res* 391:140–152 2001.

409. Needelman LM, Vogler HW, Lemont H, et al: A retrospective study of the Swanson great toe hemi-prosthesis, *J Foot Ankle Surg* 32:286–290, 1993.

410. Nemec SA, Habbu RA, Anderson JG, Bohay DR: Outcomes following midfoot arthrodesis for primary arthritis, *Foot Ankle Int* 32:355–361, 2011.

411. Neogi T: Gout, *N Engl J Med* 364:443–452, 2011.

412. Neogi T, Hunter DJ, Chaisson CE, et al: Frequency and predictors of inappropriate management of recurrent gout attacks in a longitudinal study, *J Rheumatol* 33:104–109, 2006.

413. Newman RJ, Fitton JM: Conservation of metatarsal heads in surgery of rheumatoid arthritis of the forefoot, *Acta Orthop Scand* 54:417–421, 1983.

414. Niinimaki T, Yli-Luukko S, Syrjala H, et al; Deep infection in the sinus tarsi after triple arthrodesis in rheumatoid patients: a case report, *Foot Ankle Int* 29:1131–1135, 2008.

415. Nilsonne H: Hallux rigidus and its treatment, *Acta Orthop Scand* 1:295–303, 1930.

416. Nirenberg MS, Carooll MC: Atypical gout in the foot and ankle secondary to primary hyperparathyrodism, *J Am Podiatr Med Assoc* 97:245–247, 2007.

417. Nissen K: The place of amputation of all toes, *J Bone Joint Surg Br* 35:488, 1953.

418. Nousari HC, Kimyai-Asadi A, Stebbing J, Stone JH: Purple toes in a patient with end-stage rheumatoid arthritis, *Arch Dermatol* 135:648–650, 1999.

419. O'Connell PG, Lohmann Siegel K, et al: Forefoot deformity, pain, and mobility in rheumatoid and nonarthritic subjects, *J Rheumatol* 25:1681–1666, 1998.

420. O'Doherty DP, Lowrie IG, Magnussen PA, Gregg PJ: The management of the painful first metatarsophalangeal joint in the older patient. Arthrodesis or Keller's arthroplasty? *J Bone Joint Surg Br* 72:839–842, 1990.

421. O'Duffy EK, Clunie GP, Gacinovic S, et al: Foot pain: specific indications for scintigraphy, *Br J Rheumatol* 37:442–447, 1998.

422. Ognibene FA, Theodoulou MH: Long-standing reaction to a hemi-Silastic implant, *J Foot Surg* 30:156–159, 1991.

423. Oloff L, Schulhofer SD, Fanton G, et al: Arthroscopy of the calcaneocuboid and talonavicular joints, *J Foot Ankle Surg* 35:101–108, 1996.

424. Oloff LM, Jhala-Patel G: A retrospective analysis of joint salvage procedures for grades III and IV hallux rigidus, *J Foot Ankle Surg* 47:230–236, 2008.

425. O'Sullivan MM, Rumfeld WR, Jones MK, Williams BD: Cusing's syndrome with suppression of the hypothalamic-pituitary-adrenal axis after intraarticular steroid injections, *Ann Rheum Dis* 44:561–563, 1985.

426. Otter SJ, Lucas K, Springett K, et al: Comparison of foot pain and foot care among rheumatoid arthritis patients taking and not taking anti-TNF-alpha therapy: an epidemiological study, *Rheumatol Int* 31:1515–1519, 2011.

427. Pacheco-Tena C, Londono JD, Cazarin-Barrientos J, et al: Development of a radiographic index to assess the tarsal involvement in patients with spondyloarthropathies, *Ann Rheum Dis* 61:330–334, 2002.

428. Panush RS, Wallace DJ, Dorff EN, Engleman EP: Retraction of the suggestion to use the term "Reiter's syndrome" sixty-five years later: the legacy of Reiter, a war criminal, should not be eponymic honor but rather condemnation, *Arthritis Rheum* 56:693–694, 2007.

429. Papagelopoulos PJ, Kitaoka HB, Ilstrup DM: Survivorship analysis of implant arthroplasty for the first metatarsophalangeal joint, *Clin Orthop Relat Res* 302:164–172, 1994.

430. Patel A, Rao S, Nawoczenski D, et al: Midfoot arthritis, *J Am Acad Orthop Surg* 18:417–425, 2010.

431. Patsalis T, Georgousis H, Gopfert S: Long-term results of forefoot arthroplasty in patients with rheumatoid arthritis, *Orthopedics* 19:439–447, 1996.

432. Paulus HE, Oh M, Sharp JT, et al: Classifying structural joint damage in rheumatoid arthritis as progressive or nonprogressive using a composite definition of joint radiographic change: a preliminary proposal, *Arthritis Rheum* 50:1083–1096, 2004.

433. Penal GF: Fractures of the talus, *Clin Orthop* 30:53–63, 1963.

434. Perlman MD, Schor AD, Gold ML: Implant failure with particulate silicone synovitis (detritic synovitis), *J Foot Surg* 29:584–588, 1990.

435. Peterson LF: Surgery for rheumatoid arthritis-timing and techniques: the lower extremity, *J Bone Joint Surg Am* 50:587–604, 1968.

436. Petroutsas J, Easley M, Trnka HJ: Modified bone block distraction arthrodesis of the hallux metatarsophalangeal joint, *Foot Ankle Int* 27:299–302, 2006.

437. Petrov O, Pfeifer M, Flood M, et al: Recurrent plantar ulceration following pan metatarsal head resection, *J Foot Ankle Surg* 35:573–577; discussion 602, 1996.

438. Petty RE, Southwood TR, Manners P, et al: International League of Associations for Rheumatology classification of juvenile arthritis: second revision, Edmonton, 2001, *J Rheumatol* 31:390–392, 2004.

439. Platto MJ, O'Connell PG, Hicks JE, Gerber LH: The relationship of pain and deformity of the rheumatoid foot to gait and an index of functional ambulation, *J Rheumatol* 18:38–43, 1991.

440. Politi J, John H, Njus G, Bennett GL, Kay DB: First metatarsalphalangeal joint arthrodesis: a biomechanical assessment of stability, *Foot Ankle Int* 24:332–337, 2003.

441. Pons M, Alvarez F, Solana J, et al : Sodium hyaluronate in the treatment of hallux rigidus. a single-blind, randomized study, *Foot Ankle Int* 28:38–42, 2007.

442. Prakken B, Albani S, Martini A: Juvenile idiopathic arthritis, *Lancet* 377:2138–2149, 2011.

443. Purvis CG, Brown JH, Kaplan EG, Mann I: Combination Bonney-Kessel and modified Akin procedure for hallux limitus associated with hallux abductus, *J Am Podiatry Assoc* 67:236–240, 1977.

444. Radice F, Monckeberg JE, Carcuro G: Longitudinal tears of peroneus longus and brevis tendons: a gouty infiltration, *J Foot Ankle Surg* 50:751–753, 2011.

445. Rahman A, Isenberg DA: Systemic lupus erythematosus, *N Engl J Med* 358:929–939, 2008.

446. Raikin SM, Ahmad J, Pour AE, Abidi N: Comparison of arthrodesis and metallic hemiarthroplasty of the hallux metatarsophalangeal joint, *J Bone Joint Surg Am* 89:1979–1985, 2007.

447. Raikin SM, Schon LC: Arthrodesis of the fourth and fifth tarsometatarsal joints of the midfoot, *Foot Ankle Int* 24:584–590, 2003.

448. Rana NA: Gout. In Jahss M, editor: *Disorders of the foot and ankle: medical and surgical management*, ed 2, Philadelphia, 1991, WB Saunders, pp 1712–1718.
Rana NA: Juvenile rheumatoid arthritis of the foot, *Foot Ankle* 3:2–11, 1982.

449. Rana NA: Rheumatoid arthritis, other collagen diseases and psoriasis of the foot. In Jahss M, editor: *Disorders of the foot and ankle: medical and surgical management*, ed 2, Philadelphia, 1991, WB Saunders, pp 1719–1751.

450. Rao S, Baumhauer JF, Becica L, Nawoczenski DA: Shoe inserts alter plantar loading and function in patients with midfoot arthritis, *J Orthop Sports Phys Ther* 39:522–531, 2009.

451. Rau R, Wassenberg S, Herborn G, et al: A new method of scoring radiographic change in rheumatoid arthritis, *J Rheumatol* 25:2094–2107, 1998.

452. Raunio P, Laine H: Synovectomy of the metatarsophalangeal joints in rheumatoid arthritis, *Acta Rheumatol Scand* 16:12–17, 1970.

453. Ravelli A, Martini A: Juvenile idiopathic arthritis, *Lancet* 369:767–778, 2007.

454. Ravelli A, Varnier GC, Oliveira S, et al: Antinuclear antibody-positive patients should be grouped as a separate category in the classification of juvenile idiopathic arthritis, *Arthritis Rheum* 63:267–275, 2011.

455. Raymakers R, Waugh W: The treatment of metatarsalgia with hallux valgus, *J Bone Joint Surg Br* 53:684–687, 1971.

456. Redfern DJ, Coleridge SD, Bendall SP: AIDS-related ankle arthropathy: *Mycobacterium avium-intracellulare* infection, *J Bone Joint Surg Br* 86-B:279–281, 2004.

457. Reinherz RP, Sheldon DP, Kwiecinski MG: Calcaneal involvement in inflammatory disease, *Clin Podiatr Med Surg* 5:77–88, 1988.

458. Reiter H: Über eine bisher unerkannte Spirochateninfektion, *Dtsch Med Wochenschr* 42:1535–1536, 1916.

459. Reize P, Leichtle CI, Leichtle UG, Schanbacher J: Long-term results after metatarsal head resection in the treatment of rheumatoid arthritis, *Foot Ankle Int* 27:586–590, 2006.

460. Resnick RB, Hudgins LC, Buschmann WR, et al: Analysis of the heel pad fat in rheumatoid arthritis, *Foot Ankle Int* 20: 481–484, 1999.

461. Resnick RB, Jahss MH, Choueka J, et al: Deltoid ligament forces after tibialis posterior tendon rupture: effects of triple arthrodesis and calcaneal displacement osteotomies, *Foot Ankle Int* 16:14–20, 1995.

462. Richette P, Bardin T, Doherty M: An update on the epidemiology of calcium phyrophosphate dehydrate crystal deposition disease, *Rheumatology* 48:711–715, 2009.
Richter M, Wippermann B, Krettek C, et al: Fractures and fracture dislocations of the midfoot: occurrence, causes and long-term results, *Foot Ankle Int* 22:392–398, 2001.

463. Riggs SA Jr, Johnson EW Jr: McKeever arthrodesis for the painful hallux, *Foot Ankle* 3:248–253, 1983.

464. Rippstein P: Rheumatoid forefoot deformities. In *Surgical techniques in orthopedics and traumatology*. Paris, 2001, Elsevier; 55-680-B-10; p. 1–5.

465. Ritchlin CT, Kavanaugh A, Gladman DD, et al: Group for Research and Assessment of Psoriasis and Psoriatic Arthritis (GRAPPA) Treatment recommendations for psoriatic arthritis, *Ann Rheum Dis* 68:1387–1394, 2009.

466. Robbins S: Gout. In Robbins, S, Cotran R, Kumar V, editors: *Pathologic basis of disease*, ed 3, Philadelphia, 1984, WB Saunders, pp 290–295.

467. Roberton DM, Cabral DA, Malleson PN, Petty RE: Juvenile psoriatic arthritis: followup and evaluation of diagnostic criteria, *J Rheumatol* 23:166–170, 1996.

468. Roberts ME, Wright V, Hill AG, Mehra AC: Psoriatic arthritis. Follow-up study, *Ann Rheum Dis* 35:206–212, 1976.

469. Rocca PV, Siegel LB, Cupps TR: The concomitant expression of vasculitis and coagulopathy: synergy for marked tissue ischemia, *J Rheumatol* 21:556–560, 1994.

470. Roddy E, Zhang W, Doherty M: Are joints affected by gout also affected by osteoarthritis? *Ann Rheum Dis* 66:1374–1377, 2007.

471. Rodnan G, Schumacher H: Gout. In Rodnan G, Schumacher H, editors: *Primer on the rheumatic diseases*, ed 8, Atlanta, 1983, Arthritis Foundation, pp 120–127.

472. Rodnan G, Schumacher H: Psoriasis. In Rodnan G, Schumacher H, editors: *Primer on the rheumatic diseases*, ed 8, Atlanta, 1983, Arthritis Foundation, pp 49–183.

473. Rogers W, Joplin R: Hallux valgus, weak foot and the Keller operations: An end-result study, *Surg Clin North Am* 27:1295–1302, 1947.

474. Ronconi P, Martinelli N, Cancilleri F, et al.: Hemiarthroplasty and distal oblique first metatarsal osteotomy for hallux rigidus, *Foot Ankle Int* 32:148–152, 2011.

475. Ronconi P, Monachino P, Baleanu PM, Favilli G: Distal oblique osteotomy of the first metatarsal for the correction of hallux limitus and rigidus deformity, *J Foot Ankle Surg* 39:154–160, 2000.

476. Rongstad KM, Miller GJ, Vander Griend RA, Cowin D: A biomechanical comparison of four fixation methods of first metatarsophalangeal joint arthrodesis, *Foot Ankle Int* 15:415–419, 1994.

477. Root M, Orien W, Weed J: *Normal and abnormal function of the foot*, vol 2, Los Angeles, 1977, Clinical Biomechanics, pp 48, 266, 362, 367.

478. Rosenbaum D, Timte B, Schmiegel A, et al: First ray resection arthroplasty versus arthrodesis in the treatment of the rheumatoid foot, *Foot Ankle Int* 32:589–594, 2011.

479. Rosner I: Reiter's syndrome versus reactive arthritis: Naziphobia or professional concerns? *Isr Med Assoc J* 10:296–297, 2008.

480. Rothschild BM, Pingitore C, Eaton M: Dactylitis: implications for clinical practice, *Semin Arthritis Rheum* 28:41–47, 1998.

481. Roukis TS: Clinical outcomes after isolated periarticular osteotomies of the first metatarsal for hallux rigidus: a systematic review, *J Foot Ankle Surg* 49:553–560, 2010.

482. Roukis TS: Outcome following autogenous soft tissue interpositional arthroplasty for end-stage hallux rigidus: a systematic review, *J Foot Ankle Surg* 49:475–478, 2010.

483. Roukis TS, Jacobs PM, Dawson DM, et al: A prospective comparison of clinical, radiographic, and intraoperative features of hallux rigidus: short-term follow-up and analysis, *J Foot Ankle Surg* 41:158–165, 2002.

484. Roukis TS, Townley CO: BIOPRO resurfacing endoprosthesis versus periarticular osteotomy for hallux rigidus: short-term follow-up and analysis, *J Foot Ankle Surg* 42:350–358, 2003.

485. Russotti M, Cass JR, Johnson KA: Isolated talocalcaneal arthrodesis, *J Bone Joint Surg* 70A:1472–1478, 1988.

486. Saltzman CL, El-Khoury GY: The hindfoot alignment view, *Foot Ankle Int* 16:572–576, 1995.

487. Saltzman CL, Johnson KA, Donnelly RE: Surgical treatment for mild deformities of the rheumatoid forefoot by partial phalangectomy and syndactylization, *Foot Ankle* 14:325–329, 1993.

488. Sammarco GJ, Tabatowski K: Silicone lymphadenopathy associated with failed prosthesis of the hallux: a case report and literature review, *Foot Ankle* 13:273–276, 1992.

489. Sammarco VJ, Magur EG, Sammarco GJ, Bagwe MR: Arthrodesis of the subtalar and talonavicular joints for correction of symptomatic hindfoot malalignment, *Foot Ankle Int* 27:661–666, 2006.

490. Sampson ER, Hilton MJ, Tian Y, et al: Teriparatide as a chondroregenerative therapy for injury induced osteoarthritis, *Sci Transl Med* 3:101ra93, 2011.

491. Sanders DW, Busam M, Hattwick E, et al: Functional outcomes following displaced talar neck fractures, *J Orthop Trauma* 18:265–270, 2004.

492. Sanders R, Fortin P, DiPasquale T, et al: Operative treatment in 120 displaced intraarticular calcaneal fractures. Results using a prognostic computed tomography scan classification, *Clin Orthop* 290:87–95, 1993.

493. Sangeorzan BJ, Veith RG, Hansen ST Jr: Salvage of Lisfranc's tarsometatarsal joint by arthrodesis, *Foot Ankle* 10:193–200, 1990.

494. Sangle S, D'Cruz DP, Khamashta MA, Hughes GRV: Antiphospholipid antibodies, systemic lupus erythematosus, and non-traumatic metatarsal fractures, *Ann Rheum Dis* 63:1241–1243, 2004.

495. Sanhudo JA, Gomes JE, Rodrigo MK: Surgical treatment of advanced hallux rigidus by interpositional arthroplasty, *Foot Ankle Int* 32:400–406, 2011.

496. Saville P, Longman CF, Srinivasan SCM: Medial approach for hindfoot arthrodesis with a valgus deformity, *Foot Ankle Int* 32:818–821, 2011.

497. Saxena A: The Valenti procedure for hallux limitus/rigidus, *J Foot Ankle Surg* 34:485–488; discussion 511, 1995.

498. Scarpa R, Oriente P, Pucino A, et al: Psoriatic arthritis in psoriatic patients, *Br J Rheumatol* 23:246–250, 1984.

499. Schenk S, Meizer R, Kramer R, et al: Resection arthroplasty with and without capsular interposition for treatment of severe hallux rigidus, *Int Orthop* 33:145–150, 2009.

500. Scherer PR, Gordon D, Kashanian A, Belvill A: Misdiagnosed recalcitrant heel pain associated with HLA-B27 antigen, *J Am Podiatr Med Assoc* 85:538–542, 1995.

501. Schjerning Olsen AM, Fosbøl EL, Lindhardsen J, et al: Duration of treatment with nonsteroidal anti-inflammatory drugs and impact on risk of death and recurrent myocardial infarction in patients with prior myocardial infarction: a nationwide cohort study, *Circulation* 24:2226–2235, 2011.

502. Schneider W, Kadnar G, Kranzl A, Knahr K: Long-term results following keller resection arthroplasty for hallux rigidus, *Foot Ankle Int* 32:933–939, 2011.

503. Schrör K: Acetylsalicylic acid. Darmstadt, Germany, 2009, Wiley-Vch.

504. Schweitzer ME, Maheshwari S, Shabshin N: Hallux valgus and hallux rigidus: MRI findings, *Clin Imaging* 23:397–402, 1999.

505. Scranton PE Jr: Comparison of open isolated subtalar arthrodesis with autogenous bone graft versus outpatient arthroscopic subtalar arthrodesis using injectable bone morphogenic protein-enhancement graft, *Foot Ankle Int* 20:162–165, 1999.

506. Seltzer SE, Weissman BN, Braunstein EM, et al: Computed tomography of the hindfoot with rheumatoid arthritis, *Arthritis Rheum* 28:1234–1242, 1985.

507. Sethu A, D'Netto DC, Ramakrishna B: Swanson's Silastic implants in great toes, *J Bone Joint Surg Br* 62:83–85, 1980.

508. Shawen SB, Anderson RB, Cohen BE, et al: Spherical ceramic interpositional arthrooplasty for basal fourth and fifth metatarsal arthritis, *Foot Ankle Int* 28:896–901, 2007.

509. Shereff MJ, Baumhauer JF: Hallux rigidus and osteoarthrosis of the first metatarsophalangeal joint, *J Bone Joint Surg Am* 80:898–908, 1998.

510. Shereff MJ, Jahss MH: Complications of Silastic implant arthroplasty in the hallux, *Foot Ankle* 1:95–101, 1980.

511. Shi K, Hayashida K, Tomita T, et al: Surgical treatment of hallux valgus deformity in rheumatoid arthritis: clinical and radiographic evaluation of modified Lapidus technique, *J Foot Ankle Surg* 39:376–382, 2000.

512. Shi K, Tomita T, Hayashida K, et al: Foot deformities in rheumatoid arthritis and relevance of disease severity, *J Rheumatol* 27:84–89, 2000.

513. Shives TC, Johnson KA: Arthrodesis of the interphalangeal joint of the great toe-an improved technique, *Foot Ankle* 1:26–29, 1980.

514. Sholkoff SD, Glickman MG, Steinbach HL: The radiographic pattern of polyarthritis in Reiter's syndrome, *Arthritis Rheum* 14:551–555, 1971.

515. Smith BG, Cruz AI Jr, Milewski MD, Shapiro ED: Lyme disease and the orthopaedic implications of Lyme arthritis, *J Am Acad Orthop Surg* 19:91–100, 2011.

516. Smith NR: Hallux valgus and rigidus treated by arthrodesis of the metatarsophalangeal joint, *BMJ* 2:1385–1387, 1952.

517. Smith RW, Joanis TL, Maxwell PD: Great toe metatarsophalangeal joint arthrodesis: a user-friendly technique, *Foot Ankle* 13:367–377, 1992.

518. Smith RW, Katchis SD, Ayson LC: Outcomes in hallux rigidus patients treated nonoperatively: a long-term follow-up study, *Foot Ankle Int* 21:906–913, 2000.

519. Smith T, Malay O, Ruch J: Hallux limitus and rigidus. In McGlamry E, editor: *Comprehensive textbook of foot surgery.* Baltimore, 1987, Williams & Wilkins, pp 238–250.

520. Smolen JS, van der Heijde DM, Aletaha D, et al: Progression of radiographic joint damage in rheumatoid arthritis: independence of erosions and joint space narrowing, *Ann Rheum Dis* 68:1535–1540, 2009.

521. Smyth CJ, Janson RW: Rheumatologic view of the rheumatoid patient, *Clin Orthop* 340:7–17, 1997.
Sobel E, Giorgini RJ: Surgical considerations in the geriatric patient, *Clin Podiatr Med Surg* 20:607–626, 2003.

522. Solan MC, Calder JD, Bendall SP: Manipulation and injection for hallux rigidus. Is it worthwhile? *J Bone Joint Surg Br* 83:706–708, 2001.

523. Solomon G: Inflammatory arthritis. In Jahss M, editor: *Disorders of the foot and ankle: medical and surgery management,* ed 2, Philadelphia, 1991, WB Saunders, pp 1681–1702.

524. Sorbie C; Saunders GA: Hemiarthroplasty in the treatment of hallux rigidus, *Foot Ankle Int* 29:273–281, 2008.

525. Southgate JJ, Urry SR: Hallux rigidus: the long-term results of dorsal wedge osteotomy and arthrodesis in adults, *J Foot Ankle Surg* 36:136–140; discussion 161, 1997.

526. Spector AK, Christman RA: Coexistent gout and rheumatoid arthritis, *J Am Podiatr Med Assoc* 79:552–558, 1989.

527. Spiegel TM, Spiegel JS: Rheumatoid arthritis in the foot and ankle-diagnosis, pathology, and treatment. The relationship between foot and ankle deformity and disease duration in 50 patients, *Foot Ankle* 2:318–324, 1982.

528. St Clair EW, van der Heijde DM, Smolen JS, et al: Combination of infliximab and methotrexate therapy for early rheumatoid arthritis: a randomized, controlled trial, *Arthritis Rheum* 50:3432–3443, 2004.

529. Steere AC: Musculoskeletal manifestations of Lyme disease, *Am J Med* 9:44S–48S; discussion 48S–51S, 1995.

530. Steere AC, Angelis SM: Therapy for Lyme arthritis: strategies for the treatment of antibiotic-refractory arthritis, *Arthritis Rheum* 54:3079–3086, 2006.

531. Steere AC, Malawista SE, Hardin JA, et al: Erythema chronicum migrans and Lyme arthritis. The enlarging clinical spectrum, *Ann Intern Med* 86:685–698, 1977.

532. Steere AC, Malawista SE, Snydman DR, et al: Lyme arthritis: an epidemic of oligoarticular arthritis in children and adults in three Connecticut communities, *Arthritis Rheum* 20:7–17, 1977.

533. Steinbrocker O, Traeger CJ, Batterman RC: Therapeutic criteria in rheumatoid arthritis, *J Am Med Assoc* 140:659–665, 1949.

534. Stern SH, Insall JN, Windsor RE, et al: Total knee arthroplasty in patients with psoriasis, *Clin Orthop Relat Res* 248:108–110; discussion 111, 1989.

535. Stiles RG, Resnick D, Sartoris DJ: Radiologic manifestations of arthritides involving the foot, *Clin Podiatr Med Surg* 5:1–16, 1988.

536. Stockley I, Betts RP, Rowley DI, et al: The importance of the valgus hindfoot in forefoot surgery in rheumatoid arthritis, *J Bone Joint Surg Br* 72:705–708, 1990.

537. Swanson AB: Implant arthroplasty for the great toe, *Clin Orthop Relat Res* 85:75–81, 1972.

538. Swanson AB: Letter to the editor, *J Am Med Assoc* 238:939, 1977.

539. Swanson AB, de Groot Swanson G, Maupin BK, et al: The use of a grommet bone liner for flexible hinge implant arthroplasty of the great toe, *Foot Ankle* 12:149–155, 1991.

540. Swanson AB, Lumsden RM, Swanson GD: Silicone implant arthroplasty of the great toe. A review of single stem and flexible hinge implants, *Clin Orthop Relat Res* 142:30–43, 1979.

541. Tagoe M, Brown HA, Rees SM: Total sesamoidectomy for painful hallux rigidus: a medium-term outcome study, *Foot Ankle Int* 30:640–646, 2009.

542. Tanaka E, Yamanaka H, Matsuda Y, et al: Comparison of the Rau method and the Larsen method in the evaluation of radiographic progression in early rheumatoid arthritis, *J Rheumatol* 29:682–687, 2002.

543. Tanaka N, Hirose K, Sakahashi H, et al: Usefulness of bioabsorbable thread pins after reseciton arthroplasty for rheumatoid forefoot reconstruction, *Foot Ankle Int* 25:496–502, 2004.

544. Taranow WS, Moutsatson MJ, Cooper JM: Contemporary approaches to stage II and III hallux rigidus: the role of metallic hemiarthroplasty of the proximal phalanx, *Foot Ankle Clin* 10:713–728, ix–x, 2005.

545. Taylor W, Gladman D, Helliwell P, et al: CASPAR Study Group: classification criteria for psoriatic arthritis, *Arthritis Rheum* 54:2665–2673, 2006.

546. Thelen S, Rutt J, Wild M, et al: The influence of talonavicular versus double arthrodesis on load dependent motion of the midtarsal joint, *Arch Orthop Trauma Surg* 130:47–53, 47–53, 2010.

547. Thermann H, Hufner T, Schratt E, et al: Long-term results of subtalar fusions after operative versus nonoperative treatment of os calcis fractures, *Foot Ankle Int* 20:408–416, 1999.

548. Thomas MJ, Roddy E, Zhang W, et al: The population prevalence of foot and ankle pain in middle and old age: a systematic review, *Pain* 152:2870–2880, 2011.

549. Thomas PJ, Smith RW: Proximal phalanx osteotomy for the surgical treatment of hallux rigidus, *Foot Ankle Int* 20:3–12, 1999.

550. Thomas S, Kinninmonth AW, Kumar CS: Long-term results of the modified Hoffman procedure in the rheumatoid forefoot, *J Bone Joint Surg Am* 87:748–752, 2005.

551. Thomas WH: Surgery of the foot in rheumatoid arthritis, *Orthop Clin North Am* 6:831–835, 1975.

552. Thompson F, McElveney R: Arthrodesis of the first metatarsophalangeal joint, *J Bone Joint Surg Am* 22:555–558, 1940.

553. Thompson JA, Jennings MB, Hodge W: Orthotic therapy in the management of osteoarthritis, *J Am Podiatr Med Assoc* 82:136–139, 1992.

554. Thordarson DB, Aval S, Krieger L: Failure of hallux MP preservation surgery for rheumatoid arthritis, *Foot Ankle Int* 23:486–490, 2002.

555. Tiihonen R, Eerik S, Ikavalko M, et al: Comparison of bioreplaceable interposition arthroplasty with metatarsal head resection of the rheumatoid forefoot, *Foot Ankle Int* 31:505–510, 2010.

556. Tillmann K: Surgery of the rheumatoid forefoot with special reference to the plantar approach, *Clin Orthop Relat Res* 340:39–47, 1997.

557. Title CI, Zaret D, Means, KR Jr, et al: First metatarsal head OATS technique: an approach to crtilage damage, *Foot Ankle Int* 27:1000–1002, 2006.

558. Toolan BC, Hansen ST Jr: Surgery of the rheumatoid foot and ankle, *Curr Opin Rheumatol* 10:116–119, 1998.

559. Tourne Y, Saragaglia D, Zattara, A, et al: Hallux valgus in the elderly: metatarsophalangeal arthrodesis of the first ray, *Foot Ankle Int* 18:195–198, 1997.

560. Townes JM: Reactive arthritis after enteric infections in the United States: the problem of definition, *Clin Infect Dis* 50:247–254, 2010.

561. Townley CO, Taranow WS: A metallic hemiarthroplasty resurfacing prosthesis for the hallux metatarsophalangeal joint, *Foot Ankle Int* 15:575–580, 1994.

562. Tupman S: Arthrodesis of the first metatarsophalangeal joint, *J Bone Joint Surg Br* 40:826, 1958.

563. Turan I, Lindgren U: Compression-screw arthrodesis of the first metatarsophalangeal joint of the foot, *Clin Orthop Relat Res* 221:292–295, 1987.

564. Turkiewicz AM, Moreland LW: Psoriatic arthritis: current concepts on pathogenesis-oriented therapeutic options, *Arthritis Rheum* 56:1051–1066, 2007.

565. Vainio K: The rheumatoid foot; a clinical study with pathological and roentgenological comments, *Ann Chir Gynaecol Fenn* 45(Suppl 1):1–107, 1956.

566. Vandeputte G, Steenwerckx A, Mulier T, et al: Forefoot reconstruction in rheumatoid arthritis patients: Keller-Lelievre-Hoffmann versus arthrodesis MTP1-Hoffmann, *Foot Ankle Int* 20:438–443, 1999.

567. Van der Heijde D: Erosions versus joint space narrowing in rheumatoid arthritis: what do we know? *Ann Rheum Dis* 70(Suppl 1):1116–1118, 2011.

568. van der Heijden KW, Rasker JJ, Jacobs JW, Dey K: Kates forefoot arthroplasty in rheumatoid arthritis. A 5-year followup study, *J Rheumatol* 19:1545–1550, 1992.

569. Van der Leeden M, Steultjens MP, Ursum J, et al: Prevalence and course of forefoot impairments and walking disability in te first eight years of rheumatoid arthritis, *Arthritis Rheum* 59:1596–1602, 2008.

570. van Doeselaar DJ, Heesterbeek PJ, Louwerens JW, Swierstra BA: Foot function after fusion of the first metatarsophalangeal joint, *Foot Ankle Int* 31:670–675, 2010.

571. Vanore J, O'Keefe R, Pikscher I: Complications of silicone implants in foot surgery, *Clin Podiatry* 1:175–198, 1984.

572. Vanore J, O'Keefe R, Pikscher I: Silastic implant arthroplasty. Complications and their classification, *J Am Podiatry Assoc* 74:423–433, 1984.

573. Van Saase JL, van Romunde LK, Cats A, et al: Epidemiology of osteoarthritis: Zoetermeer survey. Comparison of radiological osteoarthritis in a Dutch population with that in 10 other populations, *Ann Rheum Dis* 48:271–280, 1989.

574. Verhaar J, Vermeulen A, Bulstra S, Walenkamp G: Bone reaction to silicone metatarsophalangeal joint-1 hemiprosthesis, *Clin Orthop Relat Res* 245:228–232, 1989.

575. Vidigal E, Jacoby RK, Dixon AS, et al: The foot in chronic rheumatoid arthritis, *Ann Rheum Dis* 34:292–297, 1975.

576. Vienne P, Sukthankar A, Favre P, et al.: Metatarsophalangeal joint arthrodesis after failed Keller-Brandes procedure, *Foot Ankle Int* 27:894–901, 2006.

577. von Salis-Soglio G, Thomas W: Arthrodesis of the metatarsophalangeal joint of the great toe, *Arch Orthop Trauma Surg* 95:7–12, 1979.
Wagner FW Jr: Ankle fusion for degenerative arthritis secondary to the collagen diseases, *Foot Ankle* 3:24–31, 1982.

578. Waizy H, Czardybon MA, Stukenborg-Colsman C, et al: Mid- and long-term results of the joint preserving therapy of hallux rigidus, *Arch Orthop Trauma Surg* 130:165–170, 2010.

579. Walker UA, Tyndall A, Daikeler T: Rheumatic conditions in human immunodeficiency virus infection, *Rheumatology* 47:952–959, 2008.

580. Wassink S, van den Oever M: Arthrodesis of the first metatarsophalangeal joint using a single screw: retrospective analysis of 109 feet, *J Foot Ankle Surg* 48:653–661, 2009.

581. Watermann H: Die Arthritis deformans des Großzehengrundgelenkes als selbständiges Krankheitsbild, *Z Orthop Chir* 48:346–355, 1927.

582. Watson AD, Kelikian AS: Cost-effectiveness comparison of three methods of internal fixation for arthrodesis of the first metatarsophalangeal joint, *Foot Ankle Int* 19:304–310, 1998.

583. Watson MS: A long-term follow-up of forefoot arthroplasty, *J Bone Joint Surg Br* 56B:527–533, 1974.

584. Weitoft T, Uddenfeldt P: Importance of synovial fluid aspiration when injection intra-articular corticosteroids, *Ann Rheum Dis* 59:233–235, 2000.

585. Wetmore RS, Drennan JC: Long-term results of triple arthrodesis in Charcot-Marie-Tooth disease, *J Bone Joint Surg Am* 71:417–422, 1989.

586. Whalen, JL: Clinical tip: interpositional bone graft for first MP fusion, *Foot Ankle Int* 30:160–162, 2009.

587. Wickman AM, Pinzur MS, Kadanoff R, Juknelis D: Health-related quality of life for patients with rheumatoid arthritis foot involvement, *Foot Ankle Int* 25:19–26, 2004.

588. Wilkinson J: Cone arthrodesis of the first metatarsophalangeal joint, *Acta Orthop Scand* 49:627–630, 1978.

589. Wilson JN: Cone arthrodesis of the first metatarso-phalangeal joint, *J Bone Joint Surg Br* 49:98–101, 1967.

590. Winchester R, Bernstein DH, Fischer HD, et al: The co-occurrence of Reiter's syndrome and acquired immunodeficiency, *Ann Intern Med* 106:19–26, 1987.

591. Wolfe F, Smythe HA, Yunus MB, et al: The American College of Rheumatology 1990 Criteria for the Classification of Fibromyalgia. Report of the Multicenter Criteria Committee, *Arthritis Rheum* 33:160–172, 1990.

592. Wollheim F: Ankylosing spondylitis. In Kelley WN, Harris ED Jr, Ruddy S, Sledge CB, editors: *Textbook of rheumatology*, ed 4, Philadelphia, 1993, WB Saunders, pp 943–960.

593. Woodburn J, Barker S, Helliwell PS: A randomized controlled trial of foot orthoses in rheumatoid arthritis, *J Rheumatol* 29:1377–1383, 2002.

594. Woodburn J, Stableford Z, Helliwell PS: Preliminary investigation of debridement of plantar callosities in rheumatoid arthritis, *Rheumatology (Oxford)* 39:652–654, 2000.

595. Wormser GP, Dattwyler RJ, Shapiro ED, et al: The clinical assessment, treatment, and prevention of Lyme disease, human granulocytic anaplasmosis, and babesiosis: clinical practice guidelines by the Infectious Diseases Society of America, *Clin Infect Dis* 43:1089–1134, 2006.

596. Worsing RA Jr, Engber WD, Lange TA: Reactive synovitis from particulate Silastic, *J Bone Joint Surg Am* 64:581–585, 1982.

597. Woughter HW: Surgery of tophaceous gout; a case report, *J Bone Joint Surg Am* 41:116–122, 1959.

598. Wrighton JD: A ten-year review of Keller's operation. Review of Keller's operation at the Princess Elizabeth Orthopaedic Hospital, Exeter, *Clin Orthop Relat Res* 89:207–214, 1972.

599. Wulker N, Stukenborg C, Savory K, Alfke D: Hindfoot motion after isolated and combined arthrodeses: measurements in anatomic specimens, *Foot Ankle Int* 2:921–927, 2000.

600. Wyllie JC: Histopathology of the subchondral bone lesion in rheumatoid arthritis, *J Rheumatol Suppl* 11:26–28, 1983.

601. Yee G, Lau J: Current concepts review: hallux rigidus, *Foot Ankle Int* 29:637–646, 2008.

602. YGoY Health Community: History of arthritis (website). Available at http://arthritis.ygoy.com/history-of-arthritis/.

603. Yildirim-Toruner C, Diamond B: Current and novel therapeutics in the treatment of systemic lupus erythematosus, *J Allergy Clin Immunol* 127:303–312, 2011.

604. Yli-Kerttula T, Luukkainen R, Yli-Kerttula U, et al: Effect of a three month course of ciprofloxacin on the outcome of reactive arthritis, *Ann Rheum Dis* 59:565–570, 2000.

605. Youngswick FD: Modifications of the Austin bunionectomy for treatment of metatarsus primus elevatus associated with hallux limitus, *J Foot Surg* 21:114–116, 1982.

606. Yu J, Cheung JT, Fan Y, et al: Development of a finite element model of femal foot for high-heeled shoe design, *Clin Biomech (Bristol, Avon)* 23:S31–S38, 2008.

607. Zadik FR: Arthrodesis of the great toe, *BMJ* 5212:1573–1574, 1960.

608. Zelent ME, Neese DJ: Osteochondral autograft transfer of the first metatarsal head: a case report, *J Foot Ankle Surg* 44:406–411, 2005.

609. Zgonis T, Jolly GP, Garbalosa JC, et al: The value of radiographic parameters in the surgical treatment of hallux rigidus, *J Foot Ankle Surg* 44:184–189, 2005.

610. Zielaskowski LA, Kruljac SJ, DiStazio JJ, Bastacky S: Multiple neuromas coexisting with rheumatoid synovitis and a rheumatoid nodule, *J Am Podiatr Med Assoc* 90:252–255, 2000.

611. Zonno AJ, Myerson MS: Surgical correction of midfoot arthritis with and without deformity, *Foot Ankle Clin N Am* 16:35–47, 2011.

Treatment of Hindfoot and Midfoot Arthritis

J. Chris Coetzee

Midfoot and hindfoot arthritis and deformity can cause debilitating pain and limitation in function. Unlike some other lower extremity joints, there are limited surgical options short of arthrodesis of the affected joints. Initial treatment could include shoe and activity modifications as well as the addition of orthotics. It is seldom, if ever, that these measures will halt the progression of the disease, but a fair number of patients could get by without surgery for an extended period of time.

"Conservative" surgery consists of removal of bone spurs and osteophytes from the midfoot joints. It will improve comfort in shoes, but it is questionable whether it gives good long-term pain relief. Temporary relief can be fairly reliably obtained with intermittent fluoroscopic- or ultrasound-guided cortisone injections. Intermittent injections could be a valuable alternative to surgery, especially in cases where surgery is contraindicated because of medical issues.

Arthrodesis is still the most valuable treatment option in reconstructive surgery of the foot, enabling the surgeon to create a foot that is stable, plantigrade, and relatively painfree. It is used most often to correct a painful joint secondary to arthrosis, whether it is posttraumatic, primary, or rheumatoid-related arthritis. Chronic instability of the foot and ankle from muscle dysfunction (e.g., posterior tibial tendon, poliomyelitis), or a deformity that has resulted in a nonplantigrade foot, can also be improved with selective fusions.

Arthrodesis can greatly enhance a patient's functional capacity, and there is no evidence in the literature that midfoot fusions will cause adjacent joint stress and subsequent arthrosis.

Hindfoot fusions place increased stress on the joints proximal and distal to the fusion site. After an ankle or triple arthrodesis, approximately 30% of patients demonstrate arthroses distal or proximal to the fusion site within 5 years. Although most of these findings are radiographic, their presence at 5 years raise concerns about what will happen at these joints 20 to 30 years in the future.

Many factors probably affect the onset of this arthrosis besides the increased stress. One factor is probably related to the overall stiffness or laxity of the surrounding joints. The stiffer the surrounding joints, the less the patient is able to dissipate the increased stress created by the fusion compared with a patient who has more joint laxity. Because an arthrodesis is often performed on a traumatized extremity, the adjacent joints, although not demonstrating arthrosis, might have sustained tissue damage at the time of the initial injury that makes them more vulnerable to develop arthrosis when subjected to increased stress.

Although this chapter discusses arthrodesis of the joints of the foot and ankle, the clinician should always remember that, if possible, arthrodesis should be avoided, particularly in patients younger than 50 years. This is more important in the hindfoot than the forefoot. There is little evidence that midfoot fusion results in accelerated surrounding joint arthritis. In the hindfoot, especially for posterior tibial tendon disorders, an osteotomy or a tendon transfer can be used to create a plantigrade foot without resorting to an arthrodesis. If the surgeon can offer the patient 5 to 10 years of improved quality of life from a reconstructive procedure without using an arthrodesis, this is the desired approach.

TECHNICAL CONSIDERATIONS

The two basic types of arthrodeses are an in situ fusion and one that corrects a deformity. In an *in situ fusion*, positioning the foot or ankle is usually not difficult because no deformity is present. In a *deformity-correcting fusion*, however, the surgeon must decide the precise alignment that must be obtained to produce a plantigrade foot. To determine the alignment, the surgeon first must evaluate the normal extremity. With the patient in a supine position, the patella is aligned to the ceiling, giving the surgeon a reference point from which all measurements are made. The degree of internal or external rotation, varus or valgus, and abduction or adduction is carefully noted. A particular arthrodesis is not always placed into a standard alignment; rather, it must be individualized for each patient. Using the patella as a reference point makes alignment at surgery much easier and more precise.

When evaluating the patient for an arthrodesis, the surgeon should also examine the surrounding joints as well as the limb alignment. A hindfoot arthrodesis places more stress on the surrounding joints and could accelerate degenerative changes of these joints. The most common example is acceleration of ankle arthritis after a subtalar or triple arthrodesis. This is especially true if there is valgus or varus tilt of the talus in the ankle mortise before fusion. The surgeon should consider the options and might even slightly overcorrect the fusion to unload the compromised side of the ankle joint. It is important to inform the patient who is about to undergo an arthrodesis that the surgery should render the specific joint painfree, but it might result in arthritis and pain elsewhere in the foot because of increased stress. In some cases, when multiple joints are involved, it may be more desirable to treat the patient conservatively with an orthotic device, such as an ankle–foot orthosis (AFO), rather than carry out an arthrodesis.

The surgeon should also consider correcting severe limb alignment before a hindfoot fusion. A well-aligned subtalar fusion in a patient with a severe genu varum or valgum will be malaligned when the proximal deformity is corrected with a knee replacement. It is therefore critical to establish the proper alignment of the fusion site. To do this, the surgeon must consider the entire lower extremity and not just the foot. The position of the knee or the bow of the tibia, which can occur either naturally or as a result of prior trauma, must be carefully examined when planning the arthrodesis. The alignment of the extremity distal to the fusion site is also important to be sure a plantigrade foot is created.

The biomechanics of the foot dictates its optimal alignment. When the subtalar joint is placed into an *everted (valgus) position*, it creates flexibility of the transverse tarsal joint and results in a supple forefoot. When the subtalar joint is in an *inverted (varus) position*, it locks the transverse tarsal joint. This creates a rigid forefoot and increased stress under the lateral aspect of the foot. It is therefore important to align the subtalar joint in 5 to 7 degrees of valgus when a fusion is carried out, to maintain flexibility of the forefoot. When a talonavicular arthrodesis is performed, the surgeon must remember that motion in the subtalar joint will no longer occur. Therefore the subtalar joint must be aligned into 5 degrees of valgus, after which the talonavicular joint is aligned while taking into account abduction or adduction of the

transverse tarsal joint as well as correcting any forefoot varus that might be present. This complex alignment creates a technically challenging situation for the surgeon. If the joints surrounding the talonavicular joint are not properly aligned, a plantigrade foot will not be created.

When arthrodesing the midtarsal or tarsometatarsal joints, the surgeon should always try to match the abnormal foot to the normal foot by carefully evaluating the weight-bearing posture of both feet preoperatively. The most common deformity is abduction with varying degrees of dorsiflexion. Any malalignment needs to be corrected. Once the first metatarsocuneiform joint is stabilized, the other joints need to be aligned, both in the transverse and in the dorsoplantar direction. This will align the metatarsal heads and prevent one head from being too prominent, which can result in an intractable plantar keratosis.

SOFT TISSUE CONSIDERATIONS

The soft tissue envelope of the foot and ankle often contains little or no fatty tissue. At times, this lack of soft tissue padding has been further compromised by previous surgery or trauma to the soft tissues, resulting in adherence of the soft tissue to the underlying bone. The surgical approach should be as precise as possible to avoid placing undue tension on the skin edges. If significant realignment is to be achieved, it must not be at the expense of proper wound approximation. This occasionally occurs when attempting to correct a valgus deformity of the heel in which an opening lateral-wedge osteotomy results in increased tension on the lateral skin edges, which makes closure difficult. Skin flaps should be made as full thickness as possible to diminish the possibility of a skin slough. Creating an incision down to the bone, then retracting on the deep structures and not the skin edge, is probably the best way to avoid a skin problem.

When making an incision, the surgeon must always be cognizant of the location of the cutaneous nerves about the foot and ankle. Although cutaneous nerves tend to lie in certain anatomic areas, great variation exists. Therefore, as the incision is carried down through the subcutaneous tissues, it is important to always look for an aberrant cutaneous nerve. The cutaneous nerves can be quite superficial and easily transected but sometimes become adherent within scar tissue. If this occurs, a painful scar or dysesthesias distal to the injury can result in a dissatisfied patient despite a satisfactory fusion.

Another unique problem after foot surgery is the impact of footwear, which can rub against a subcutaneous neuroma, further aggravating the problem.

If a nerve is inadvertently transected during a surgical approach, it should be carefully dissected to a more proximal level and the cut end buried beneath some fatty tissue or muscle so that it will not become symptomatic. Sometimes, although a nerve is not cut, it can be stretched as a result of retraction, which can result in a transient loss of function. Patients must be made aware of the potential for nerve injury and the area where they can experience numbness.

SURGICAL PRINCIPLES

When carrying out an arthrodesis of the foot and ankle, the following surgical principles should be carefully observed:

- A well-planned incision of adequate length should be made to avoid undue tension on the skin edges.
- An attempt should be made to create broad, congruent cancellous surfaces that can be placed into apposition to permit an arthrodesis to occur.
- The arthrodesis site should be stabilized with rigid internal fixation. This sometimes depends on the surgeon's ingenuity in creating a stable construct, particularly if poor bone stock is present. There are multiple fixation options available, including screws, staples, and locking and nonlocking plates. The most appropriate option for a specific situation should be used.
- When performing a fusion, the hindfoot must be aligned to the lower extremity and the forefoot to the hindfoot to create a plantigrade foot.

After exposure of the fusion site, the soft tissues surrounding the joints are removed. This mobilizes the joints, allowing the surgeon to realign the foot. It is most often difficult to initially visualize the joints because of dense scar tissue overgrowth and/or dorsal osteophyte formation. It is helpful to use a rongeur or osteotomes to remove the tissue and bone covering the joints.

At times, because of previous trauma or severe malalignment, mobilization of the joints is not possible, and bone resection needs to be carried out. However, alignment is possible in the majority of cases, even when a significant deformity is present, by complete mobilization of the involved joints, followed by manipulation to create a plantigrade foot.

Once the joints have been mobilized and it is determined that bone does not need to be removed, the articular surfaces are meticulously debrided of their articular cartilage and any fibrous tissue to subchondral bone. This is achieved with a curette or a small, sharp osteotome. A lamina spreader or a towel clip can facilitate distraction of the articular surfaces, making the debridement easier, but this can damage the bone if it is soft.

Once the subchondral bone is exposed, the foot is once again manipulated, placing it into the desired alignment. If this is achievable, internal fixation can be inserted. If large amounts of bone need to be removed to create a plantigrade foot, this should be done *before* removing the articular cartilage. The subchondral surfaces are heavily feathered or scaled with a 4- or 6-mm osteotome, which creates a broader, bleeding cancellous surface required for successful fusion. The articular surfaces to be arthrodesed are brought together and stabilized with provisional fixation. Several 0.62-mm Kirschner wires (K-wires) will help keep the reduction before fixation. It is also advisable to confirm reduction in all planes with fluoroscopy before definitive hardware placement. Then interfragmentary compression is achieved using appropriate definitive fixation.

By carrying out a fusion in this manner, broad bleeding surfaces of cancellous bone are brought together, which provides the best possible chance for a successful arthrodesis.

Bone graft from the iliac crest is rarely necessary when carrying out a foot or ankle arthrodesis. Sometimes bone has been lost, making a bone graft necessary, but in an in situ fusion, grafting is not usually required. If a small amount of bone is needed, it can be harvested from the calcaneus, medial malleolus, or proximal medial tibia without violating the iliac crest and causing its attendant morbidity. Likewise, bone substitutes or other materials are rarely required if the bone preparation is carried out correctly.

For internal fixation, the author prefers an interfragmentary screw that compresses the joint surfaces. With good bone quality and well-apposed bone surfaces screws or compression, staples will suffice. However, in a situation with poor bone quality or correction of severe deformities, there are several excellent midfoot plating systems available.

Although an external fixator can provide excellent fixation, if possible, a closed system without an external fixator is safer because of possible pin-tract problems with prolonged immobilization. Because of soft bone or soft tissue problems, however, it may become necessary to use an external fixator. Under these circumstances, this device provides excellent rigid fixation.

The skin closure after a fusion is very critical. The surgeon should always attempt, if possible, to obtain a soft tissue cover underneath the skin flaps, such as fat or muscle. This is important because if a superficial wound slough occurs, it will be over an underlying bed of soft tissue rather than bone. This is not always possible, particularly on the dorsum of the foot, where bone lies directly beneath the skin. If any tension is noticeable on the skin edge, some type of a relaxing skin suture should be used. A drain is useful if profuse bleeding is anticipated.

The initial postoperative dressing is very important and should support the soft tissues as well as the arthrodesis site. A heavy cotton gauze roll provides uniform compression about the extremity, supported by plaster splints. A circumferential cast should be avoided during the immediate postoperative period because it can result in undue pressure against the expanding extremity, increasing pain and possibly jeopardizing healing of the wound edges. The postoperative dressing is used for approximately 10 to 14 days before removing the sutures. The cast splint should be applied with the foot and ankle in a neutral position, and the ankle should be kept in that position while the cast hardens. Dorsiflexing or plantarflexing the ankle or foot after application and before hardening will change the pressure on the soft tissues and could result in wound issues.

A popliteal block is used for most fusions, which generally provides 18 to 36 hours of pain relief. The popliteal block may be repeated after 18 to 24 hours if the patient has too much breakthrough pain. It is much easier to prevent postoperative pain than play catch-up after the pain cycle has been established. If there are reasons not to do a popliteal block, an ankle block could give fairly similar pain relief, as long as all the nerves are included (deep and superficial peroneal, tibialis, sural, and saphaneous).

COMPLICATIONS

The main complications after an attempted arthrodesis include infection, skin slough, nerve disruption or entrapment, nonunion, and malalignment.

The possibility of *infection* is always a postsurgical concern. During surgery, antibiotic irrigation as well as parenteral antibiotics can help minimize this complication. Good surgical technique with careful handling of the tissues, removal of devitalized tissue, and prevention of hematoma formation also play an important role in minimizing the possibility of infection. If an infection occurs, it is important to recognize and treat it promptly with appropriate antibiotics.

A *skin slough* around the foot and ankle can present a difficult management problem because of the lack of adequate subcutaneous tissue. The potential for a skin slough can be minimized by creating full-thickness skin flaps, making incisions of adequate length to minimize tension on the skin edges, using postoperative drainage when appropriate, and applying a firm compression dressing postoperatively. Placing a patient into a cast without adequate padding is not advisable. When a skin slough occurs, it is important to treat it vigorously with local debridement and application of wet-to-dry dressings to promote granulation tissue, followed by coverage with a split-thickness skin graft. Vacuum-assisted closure (wound-VAC) can be extremely useful to manage a wound slough. If the slough is too large, a plastic surgeon should be consulted (Fig. 20-1).

Nerve disruption or entrapment around the foot and ankle not only creates numbness but also can cause chronic pain from footwear rubbing against the neuroma. A carefully planned surgical approach is the best treatment, but if a symptomatic neuroma occurs, it should be identified and resected into an area not subject to pressure and then buried either beneath muscle or into bone.

A *nonunion* of an attempted fusion site is always an unfortunate event. As a general rule, of the joints around the foot and ankle, the talonavicular probably has the highest incidence of nonunion. Its curved surfaces make adequate exposure difficult, and preparation of the joint surfaces may be inadequate. Even when the bone surfaces have been adequately prepared, nonunion can occur if internal fixation is inadequate. In the author's experience,

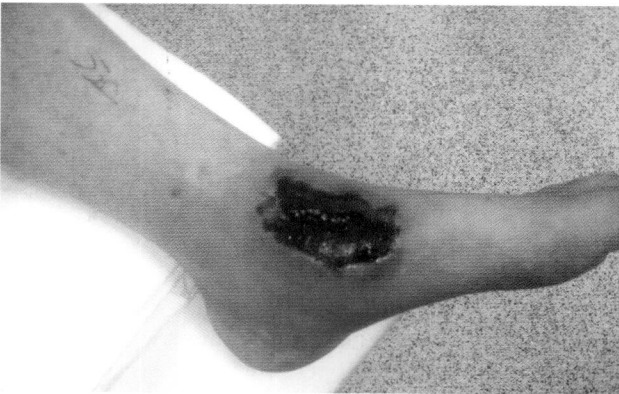

Figure 20-1 Deep skin necrosis after a medial incision in a diabetic patient. A large area of skin necrosis like this will need a thorough debridement, followed by a vacuum-assisted closure (wound-VAC) or skin flap.

more hardware is better, and thus a combination of screws, staples, and plates is recommended for the talonavicular joint.

The vascularity of the bone plays an important role in the development of a nonunion. Avascular necrosis of the talus from any cause creates a situation that is very difficult to manage. When avascular bone is present, it is often not possible to obtain a fusion to the dysvascular bone, and an attempt must be made either to bypass the avascular area or to determine the portions of the talus that still have adequate vascularity and attempt a fusion using these areas. The most common area of avascular necrosis in the midfoot is the navicular. The navicular can develop evidence of avascular changes either spontaneously (Kohlers or Mueller-Weiss syndrome) or secondary to previous injury. When this problem is encountered, the involved area needs to be resected and bone grafted. When dealing with dysvascular bone preoperatively, it is important to identify the areas of potential problems and create a surgical plan that will help solve the problem. Recognizing a dysvascular problem also helps to predict the outcome for the patient. Most often, the lateral half of the navicular is avascular, whereas the medial half still has good healthy bone. The medial healthy bone should be included in the fusion while bone graft is placed lateral between the talus and cuneiforms.

Occasionally, an asymptomatic nonunion occurs and can be treated with observation. After a triple arthrodesis, the talonavicular joint occasionally does not fuse, but because of a successful fusion of the subtalar and calcaneocuboid joints, it may not be a source of pain. If a nonunion is symptomatic, a revision of the fusion site needs to be considered. If the overall alignment of the nonunion is satisfactory, bone grafting by inlaying bone across the nonunion site often results in a fusion if internal fixation is adequate. At other times, if the nonunion site has resulted in loss of alignment, the area needs to be revised. This is done by removing the internal fixation and the fibrous tissue between the bone ends, realigning the surfaces, performing a bone graft if necessary, and inserting rigid fixation, usually with a plate-and-screw construct.

Malalignment after a fusion is a problem that usually can be avoided by meticulous bone preparation and rigid internal fixation. Malalignment after a triple arthrodesis is seen most often. The usual malalignment after a triple arthrodesis is varus of the heel and adduction or supination (or both) of the forefoot. This requires the patient to walk on the lateral aspect of the foot, causing patient dissatisfaction. When a fusion of the hindfoot is performed, it is important to evaluate the entire lower extremity preoperatively and intraoperatively to reduce the risk of malalignment. After carefully observing the normal extremity, the surgeon should always relate the foot alignment to the patella. Once the joint surfaces have been prepared and provisionally stabilized, the alignment should again be checked to be sure it is correct. Malalignment can only be prevented by careful observation of the extremity at surgery.

SPECIFIC ARTHRODESES

Much has been written about arthrodesis of the foot and ankle. Many surgical approaches, site preparations, and types of internal and external fixation have been proposed. This section presents the techniques and principles the author's group uses and believes can achieve satisfactory outcomes with careful adherence to technique. Other techniques may be equally effective, but reproducibly good results have been achieved with subtalar arthrodesis, talonavicular arthrodesis, double arthrodesis, triple arthrodesis, naviculocuneiform arthrodesis, and tarsometatarsal arthrodesis.

SUBTALAR ARTHRODESIS (Fig. 20-2A and Video Clips 26 and 27)

An isolated subtalar joint arthrodesis is the workhorse procedure of the hindfoot and results in satisfactory correction of deformity and relief of pain that enables the patient to regain the ability to perform most activities. Of the hindfoot fusions, the patient's ability to achieve a high level of function is greatest after a subtalar arthrodesis. It was previously believed that an isolated subtalar arthrodesis should not be carried out and that a triple arthrodesis would be the procedure of choice when a hindfoot fusion was indicated. The literature has demonstrated, however, that an isolated subtalar arthrodesis produces a superior result with less stress on the ankle joint than a triple arthrodesis.

The position of the subtalar joint determines the flexibility of the transverse tarsal (talonavicular–calcaneocuboid) joint, and therefore it is imperative that a subtalar arthrodesis be positioned in about 5 degrees of valgus to permit mobility of the transverse tarsal joint. If it is placed in varus, the transverse tarsal joint is locked, and the patient tends to walk on the lateral side of the foot. The posture of the forefoot also needs to be considered because if there is more than 10 to 12 degrees of fixed forefoot varus, after a subtalar arthrodesis, the patient cannot compensate for this deformity and walks on the lateral side of the foot, resulting in discomfort beneath the fifth metatarsal head or base, or both, and in severe stress on the lateral ankle ligaments. If there is a fixed forefoot varus with the hindfoot well aligned, it can be corrected by carrying out a simultaneous naviculocuneiform and/or cuneiform–first metatarsal fusion.

Indications

The most common indication for a subtalar arthrodesis is arthrosis secondary to trauma, usually a calcaneal fracture, rheumatoid arthritis, primary arthrosis, or talocalcaneal coalition that cannot be resected. It is also indicated for a muscle imbalance (e.g., loss of peroneal muscle function) or posterior tibial tendon dysfunction with an unstable subtalar joint but normal transverse tarsal joint motion and a fixed forefoot varus deformity of less than 12 degrees. A subtalar arthrodesis is indicated in patients with a neuromuscular disorder, such as Charcot-Marie-Tooth disease, poliomyelitis, or nerve injury with instability of the subtalar joint.

Although a subtalar fusion can have an excellent result, if the deformity can be corrected with a calcaneal osteotomy instead of a fusion, this should be strongly considered.

Position of Arthrodesis

The subtalar arthrodesis should be placed in approximately 5 degrees of valgus. Varus should be avoided because it results in increased stiffness of the transverse tarsal joint. Conversely, too much valgus results in an impingement against the fibula and increased stress along the medial aspect of the ankle joint.

Surgical Technique

1. The patient is placed in the supine position with a support under the ipsilateral hip to facilitate exposure of the subtalar joint.
2. A thigh tourniquet is applied.
3. The skin incision begins at the tip of the fibula and is carried distally toward the base of the fourth metatarsal. When an isolated subtalar arthrodesis is carried out, the incision usually stops at about the level of the calcaneocuboid joint (Fig. 20-2B).
4. While deepening the incision, the surgeon should be cautious, because the anterior branch of the sural nerve may be crossing the operative site plantarly and the superficial peroneal nerve dorsally.
5. The incision passes along the dorsal aspect of the peroneal tendon sheath and distally along the floor of the sinus tarsi.
6. The extensor digitorum brevis muscle origin is detached and the muscle belly reflected distally, exposing the underlying sinus tarsi, subtalar joint, and calcaneocuboid joint (Fig. 20-2C). The fat pad is dissected out of the sinus tarsi and reflected dorsally.

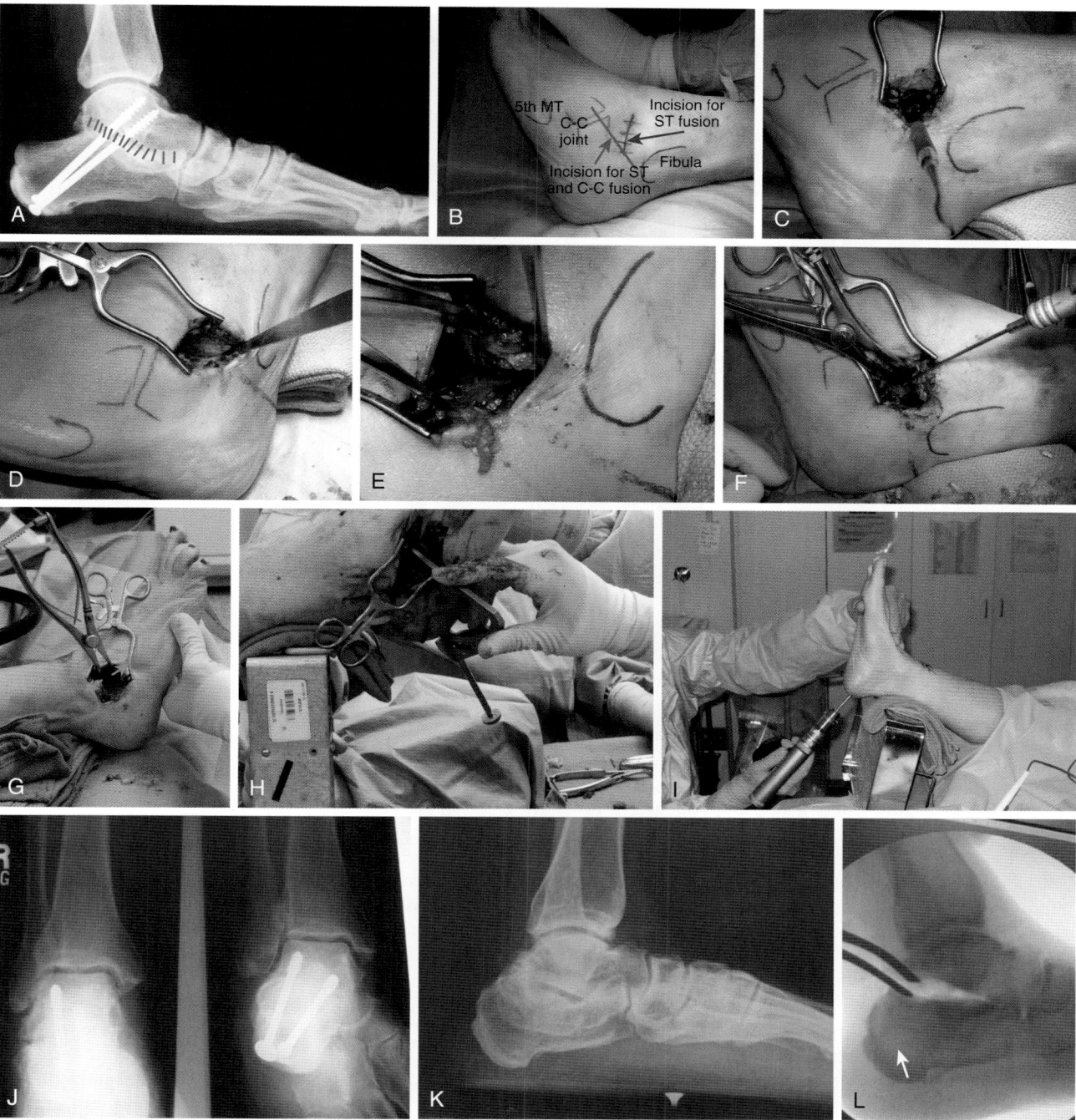

Figure 20-2 Subtalar joint fusion. **A,** Site of fusion. **B,** The universal lateral incision is made from the tip of the fibula and extends toward the base of the fourth metatarsal so as to place it in the interval between a branch of the superficial peroneal nerve dorsally and the sural nerve plantarly. This gives exposure to the subtalar *(ST)* and calcaneocuboid *(C-C)* joints. The alternative is a smaller curved sinus tarsi incision for exposure of the subtalar joint only. **C,** Exposure of subtalar joint with Weitlaner retractor. All the soft tissue is removed from the sinus tarsi and a Freer is placed in the middle facet. **D,** Also easy exposure of the posterior facet. **E,** Distraction with a lamina spreader gives excellent exposure of the subtalar joint. **F,** The opposing surfaces are deeply feathered. **G,** A lamina spreader is placed between the neck of the calcaneus and the lateral process of the talus. When distraction is applied, the talus is forced back on top of the calcaneus. **H,** The anterior cruciate guide is placed into the subtalar joint with the tine in posterior facet, as marked on the model. The guide is then set on the heel, after which a guide pin is placed across the subtalar joint. **I,** An instrument tray under the calf to allow easy access to the posterior aspect of the heel for screw placement. It also facilitates simple fluoroscopy access for a lateral view. **J,** Postoperative anteroposterior (AP) and mortise radiographs demonstrate subtalar fusion using two 6.5-mm screws. One screw goes through the anterior and medial aspect of the posterior facet into the neck of the talus. The second goes more posterior and lateral to increase two-point fixation and stability. The screw begins off the weight-bearing area of the heel. **K-M,** Preoperative, intraoperative, and postoperative radiographs demonstrate subtalar arthrodesis after calcaneal fracture. Interpositional bone graft is used to reestablish the talocalcaneal relationship.

Continued

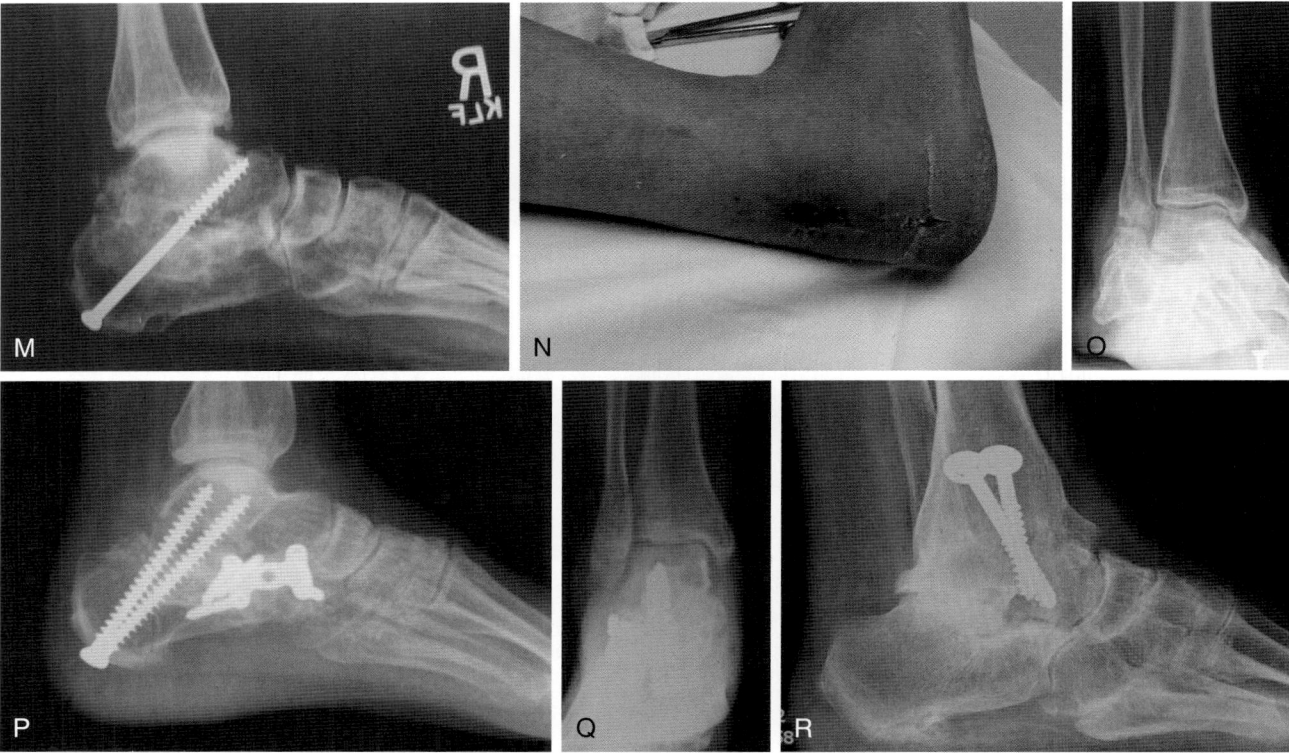

Figure 20-2, cont'd   **N,** Wound complications are not uncommon with distraction bone blocks. The incision should be straight. The usual curved incision for a calcaneal exposure have a much higher wound complication rate because of tension on the distal limb after distraction. **O,** When lateral subluxation of the subtalar joint is present, the joint must be reduced and not fused in situ. Note the calcaneus is dislocated with subfibular impingement. **P** and **Q,** Lateral and AP radiographs showing correction of the calcaneal dislocation with a combination of a subtalar bone block fusion and calcaneocuboid fusion. **R,** Preoperative radiograph demonstrating subtalar and talonavicular arthrosis in a patient with prior ankle fusion. Screw placement for the subtalar fusion is relatively simple because it can extend across the ankle joint.

The only way to visualize the middle and anterior facets of the subtalar joint is to remove all the soft tissue from the sinus tarsi. Using a curet will facilitate that.

7. A small elevator is passed along the lateral side of the posterior facet of the subtalar joint. It is not necessary to strip the peroneal tendons off the lateral side of the calcaneus unless a lateral impingement from a previous calcaneal fracture requires decompressing.

8. A lamina spreader is inserted into the sinus tarsi to visualize the posterior facet of the subtalar joint (Fig. 20-2D and E). When looking across the sinus tarsi, the surgeon can see the middle facet of the subtalar joint. If the surgery is being carried out for severe arthrosis or a talocalcaneal coalition, it is often not possible to open the subtalar joint very far. Under these circumstances, a small curet is used to remove the cartilage from the posterior facet. A thin, wide elevator then can be inserted into the joint to pry it open, after which a lamina spreader is inserted.

9. Power osteotomes are ideal to start the preparation of the posterior facet. Articular cartilage can be removed in large strips and subcondral bone exposed. Regular sharp ¼- or ½-inch osteotomes could do the same.

10. For safety, a curet of appropriate size is used to remove the cartilage posterior and posteromedial and from the middle and anterior facets. This reduces the possibility of damaging the flexor hallucis longus tendon in the posterior aspect of the joint or the neurovascular bundle along the posteromedial aspect of the joint. When removing the articular cartilage from the middle facet, it is important not to inadvertently go too far distally and damage the cartilage on the plantar aspect of the head of the talus, which lies just in front of it.

11. Once all the articular cartilage has been removed, the lamina spreader is removed and the alignment of the subtalar joint observed. If no deformity is present, the surgeon may proceed with feathering or scaling the articular surfaces (Fig 20-2F). If a varus deformity needs to be corrected, bone is removed from the lateral aspect of the posterior facet to correct the deformity. It is unusual to remove more than 3 to 5 mm of bone when correcting a deformity, although occasionally more bone needs to be removed.

12. A valgus deformity is common in posterior tibial tendon dysfunction. It is seldom necessary to remove bone from the medial side of the joint because this is

by and large a rotational deformity. There is peritalar subluxation with the navicular subluxing lateral and dorsal, while the calcaneus rotates lateral and posterior, creating a hindfoot valgus. This is corrected by placing a lamina spreader in the sinus tarsi between the lateral process of the talus and the anterior process of the calcaneus. Spreading this space open facilitates reduction around the peritalar joint. There should be caution not to overdistract because this will force the hindfoot in varus (Fig. 20-2G).

13. If a previous calcaneal fracture is present in which the lateral wall needs to be decompressed, the peroneal tendons are elevated from the lateral aspect of the calcaneus as far posteriorly and plantarward as possible. The impinging lateral wall is removed so that it is approximately in line with the lateral aspect of the talus. Sometimes, up to 7 to 10 mm of bone needs to be resected in severe cases. This bone could be morcelized and packed into the sinus tarsi.

14. The posterior and middle facets, along with the bone in the base of the sinus tarsi, are heavily scaled. The dense bone in the floor of the sinus tarsi is deeply scaled and is mobilized so that it can be packed into the tarsal canal after the internal fixation has been inserted. The bone along the lateral aspect of the calcaneus that forms the anterior process may be mobilized to within about 0.5 cm of the calcaneocuboid joint and used for bone graft. When a lateral decompression has been carried out, even more bone is available to the surgeon. Rarely is bone harvested from the iliac crest.

15. After the bone surfaces have been scaled, the subtalar joint is manipulated and placed into the desired position of 5 degrees of valgus.

16. If the calcaneus is severely collapsed, height can be restored with a bone block inserted from posterior (Fig. 20-2K-M). In this case, the incision runs along the Achilles tendon and does not curve around the plantar aspect of the foot to avoid wound problems (Fig. 20-2N).

17. The surgeon should be careful not to put too large a block in the subtalar joint. Also be careful not to force the hindfoot into varus. The larger side of the block should always go medial to create a valgus alignment.

Internal Fixation

Internal fixation is carried out with large-diameter (6.5, 7.0, or 7.3 mm) cannulated or noncannulated screws to obtain maximum interfragmentary compression. A washer is used if the bone is soft and the head is sucked into the calcaneus.

Screw patterns used for fixation of the subtalar joint include placing the screw from the neck of the talus into the calcaneus, placing a screw from the calcaneus into the talus, and placing two screws between the calcaneus and the talus. The author prefers two screws, starting off the weight-bearing surface posterior on the calcaneus, one

screw aiming a bit medial into the neck of the talus while the second screw goes across the posterior facet more lateral. This results in a rigid internal fixation with maximum purchase and interfragmentary compression across the joint. In some cases, a single screw will suffice.

18. The preferred method for stabilization is to place the screw from the heel across the subtalar joint and into the neck of the talus. Screw placement is carried out by placing an aiming guide with the sharp tine in the anterior aspect of the posterior facet of the subtalar joint (Fig. 20-2H).[2] The other end of the guide is placed on the heel pad just above the weight-bearing area. This alignment permits the screw to pass through the anterior aspect of the posterior facet and into the neck of the talus, but the screw does not penetrate the sinus tarsi area. This placement provides maximum purchase in the talar neck from the screw. If a fully threaded screw is used, the calcaneus should be overdrilled to create a gliding hole. A guide pin is drilled into the calcaneus until it is visible in the posterior facet of the subtalar joint. If placement is satisfactory, the guide is removed; if not, another attempt is made to place the guide pin correctly (Fig. 20-2I).

19. The subtalar joint is placed into 5 degrees of valgus while also correcting any peritalar rotation/subluxation, and the guide pin is drilled into the talus until it just penetrates the dorsal aspect of the neck of the talus. The pin placement is confirmed by fluoroscopy.

20. With the pin properly placed, a 2- to 3-cm transverse incision is made over the entrance of the guide pin into the heel pad. This incision must be made wide enough to accommodate the screw(s) and, if used, the washer(s) to prevent compressing the skin and fat of the heel pad. The incision is carried directly to bone, and slight stripping is done on each side of the pin to accommodate the washer. A depth gauge is used to determine the length of the screw.

21. The guide pin is advanced through the talar neck, appears on the dorsal aspect of the ankle, and is secured with a clamp. This is important so that when the holes are drilled, the guide pin cannot come out, which can result in loss of alignment. If 7.0-mm cannulated screws are used, the initial hole is drilled with a 4.5-mm bit, just penetrating the neck of the talus. A 7.0-mm drill bit is used to overdrill only the calcaneus, creating the glide hole. The hole in the talar neck is tapped, and a fully threaded, 7.0-mm cannulated screw of appropriate length is inserted. By overdrilling the calcaneus, intrafragmentary compression at the arthrodesis site is achieved. Every screw system will have a smaller and larger drill to achieve the gliding and compression holes. With a fully threaded screw, the maximum number of threads is placed in the neck of the talus, maximizing the compression. In placing the screw, the surgeon should not have more than 2 to 3 mm of screw exposed on the neck of the

talus. The position of the screw is verified with fluoroscopy.

22. If a second screw is placed, a parallel guide could be used to place the screw more lateral and posterior to the first. Fluoroscopic guidance is valuable to confirm placement and also to prevent violating the ankle joint with the drill or screw (Fig. 20-2J).

23. The guide pin is removed, and the small bone fragments that have been mobilized are packed into the tarsal canal and the sinus tarsi area. It is not necessary to fill up the sinus tarsi completely when carrying out an isolated subtalar joint fusion. If more bone is needed, it can be obtained from the calcaneus or medial malleolus by using a trephine.

Closure

24. The fat pad previously dissected from the sinus tarsi and retracted dorsally is placed back into the sinus tarsi area. The extensor digitorum brevis muscle is closed over the area, creating a cover for the arthrodesis site.

25. The subcutaneous tissue and skin are closed in a routine manner.

26. The patient is placed into a compression dressing incorporating two plaster splints.

ARTHROSCOPIC SUBTALAR FUSION

There is significant interest lately in doing the subtalar fusion arthroscopically. Several recent papers with further information on the topic are listed.[5,8] The theoretic advantages of an arthroscopic fusion are a more cosmetic approach and fewer wound complications.[1,7] In experienced hands, the results appear to be comparable to open fusions, but there are several pitfalls as well. There is a higher risk of nerve a vascular injury, and there is a very steep learning curve. There are few surgeons at present who are well enough versed in complex hindfoot arthroscopy to make this a viable mainstream alternative. That situation could theoretically change in future but is unlikely.

Postoperative Care

A preoperative popliteal block is routinely used to control postoperative pain. The patient's dressing is changed approximately 10 to 14 days after surgery, and the sutures are removed. The patient is placed into a removable cast with an elastic bandage to control swelling but is kept non–weight bearing for 6 weeks. At 6 weeks, if the radiographs demonstrate that early union is occurring, the patient is permitted to bear weight as tolerated in a removable cast. Approximately 12 weeks after surgery, radiographs are obtained, and if satisfactory union has occurred, the patient is permitted to ambulate with an elastic stocking.

Complications

The two most common complications are nonunions and varus malalignment. Nonunion of the subtalar joint occurs in 15% of cases, with a range of 1% to 45% in the reported literature. The rates of nonunion have been reported to be higher for patients with risk factors such as smoking, after high-energy injury, avascular necrosis, and diabetes. A nonunion should be repaired with bone grafting and further internal fixation.

Malalignment of the subtalar joint in too much varus results in locking of the transverse tarsal joint and increased weight bearing on the lateral side of the foot. To accommodate this, the patient often walks with the extremity in external rotation.

If the subtalar joint is placed into excessive valgus, it can impinge against the fibula, causing pain over the peroneal tendons. It can also place increased stress along the medial aspect of the ankle joint and pronation of the foot. Orthotics do not work well because the transverse tarsal joint stays locked. These are difficult to revise, and a takedown and redo of the fusion is necessary.

Sural nerve entrapment or laceration can occur and may be bothersome to the patient. Unfortunately, the anterior branch of the sural nerve can pass next to the incision, making this complication almost unavoidable, but an attempt should be made to identify it and retract it if possible. If the neuroma is too bothersome, it requires resection to a more proximal level.

Author's Experience

There are ongoing issues in getting subtalar fusions to heal. The reported nonunion rate varies from 5% to 45%. In the largest study in the literature, by Myerson and coworkers, the union rate was 84% (154 of 184) overall, 86% (134 of 156) after primary arthrodesis, and 71% (20 of 28) after revision arthrodesis.[4]

Coughlin et al[3] did a study comparing standard radiographs to computed tomography (CT) scan in evaluating subtalar fusions. The mean observed fusion of the posterior facet of the subtalar joint ranged from 41% at 6 weeks to 61% at 12 weeks and to 86% at 6 months on the radiographs; the mean fusion of the posterior facet on the CT scans ranged from 23% to 48% to 64% at the same time intervals. The agreement between the two methods was poor. The clinical results based on the American Orthopaedic Foot and Ankle Society (AOFAS) score, visual analog score (VAS), and Short Form-12 (SF-12) score were compared with the percentage of joints fused on the CT scans. Coughlin et al[3] believe the progress of the fusion cannot be determined accurately from standard radiographs. CT scanning appears to be significantly more reliable. The concept of what constitutes an adequate fusion deserves more extensive study, but it appears that fusion of more than 40% of the surface is adequate.

Mann et al[6] showed that, functionally, the patients did well, although half observed problems walking on uneven ground and climbing steps and inclines. Seventy percent participated in recreational sports (e.g., walking for pleasure, biking, skiing, swimming), and 14% were able to play sports that required running and pivoting (e.g., basketball, racquet sports). This is a much higher level of activity compared with patients who have undergone a triple arthrodesis.

The physical examination demonstrated that the alignment averaged 5.7 degrees of valgus, and the one patient with fusion in varus was dissatisfied. The range of motion demonstrated an average of 9.8 degrees of dorsiflexion compared with 14.2 degrees on the uninvolved side, for a 30% loss of motion, and plantar flexion averaged 47.2 degrees compared with 52.4 degrees, for a 9.2% loss of motion. This resulted in a 14% loss of sagittal plane motion. The transverse tarsal joint motion demonstrated 60% loss of abduction and adduction compared with the uninvolved side.[6]

Patients undergoing a subtalar arthrodesis for talocalcaneal coalition generally do very well. Talonavicular arthrosis is a rare occurrence. A triple arthrodesis is not necessary to obtain a satisfactory result, even in the presence of beaking of the talonavicular joint.

Special Considerations

Occasionally, in the patient with rheumatoid arthritis, severe subluxation occurs at the subtalar joint. It is imperative that the clinician recognizes this problem so that when a subtalar arthrodesis is carried out, the calcaneus is repositioned under the talus, restoring the normal weight-bearing alignment. Similar severe deformity is seen with a small subset of calcaneal fractures, where the tuberosity dislocates laterally and sits under the fibula. In chronic malunion/nonunion situations, the reduction could be difficult. If the surgeon fails to recognize this malalignment and places a bone block into the lateral side of the subtalar joint, wedging it open will not reposition the calcaneus into correct anatomic alignment (Fig. 20-2O-Q).

Infrequently, a subtalar fusion is required after a previous ankle fusion. It is most common after a previous talus fracture, but it could also be due to excess stress after an ankle arthrodesis. In this situation, the author's group carries out its standard type of fusion. The screw placement is a little simpler because there is no concern about penetrating the ankle joint with the screw (Fig. 20-2R). Two screws are routinely used. The subtalar joint takes longer to heal, and there is a higher nonunion rate.

TALONAVICULAR ARTHRODESIS

Although arthrodesis of the talonavicular joint involves only a single joint, biomechanically it results in almost complete loss of motion in the subtalar and transverse tarsal joints. This motion is lost because for the subtalar joint to invert and evert, the navicular must rotate over the talar head. Thus, if talonavicular movement is restricted, subtalar motion does not occur.[9,13]

An isolated talonavicular arthrodesis results in a satisfactory outcome, particularly in patients who do not place a high demand on their foot, such as rheumatoid patients. In the high-demand patient or one working at a strenuous occupation, it is probably advisable to add a calcaneocuboid or subtalar joint arthrodesis.[11,12] This creates a double arthrodesis, resulting in increased stability of the transverse tarsal joint. The addition of the calcaneocuboid or subtalar joint to the talonavicular fusion does not result in any further loss of hindfoot motion.

Indications

The most common indication for an isolated talonavicular arthrodesis is primary arthrosis, arthrosis secondary to trauma, or rheumatoid arthritis (Fig. 20-3A and B).

With instability of the talonavicular joint secondary to dysfunction of the posterior tibial tendon or collapse of the talonavicular joint from rupture of the spring ligament, an isolated talonavicular arthrodesis can be considered. In these circumstances, however, the author usually carries out a subtalar or double fusion. An unusual indication is transverse tarsal instability after a Chopart dislocation with ligamentous instability.

Alignment of the Fusion

The alignment of the normal foot is observed to determine the alignment of the affected side. The positioning of an isolated talonavicular arthrodesis is very important because the subtalar and calcaneocuboid joint motion is greatly restricted after this arthrodesis. Therefore the hindfoot and forefoot must be aligned into a plantigrade position; if not, a nonplantigrade foot will be created and may be symptomatic. The subtalar joint should be placed into 5 degrees of valgus, the talonavicular joint into neutral, and the forefoot into 0 to 5 degrees of forefoot varus (Fig. 20-4A and B).[12]

Surgical Technique

1. The patient is placed in the supine position, and a thigh tourniquet is applied. Because the extremity naturally falls into external rotation, the patient does not require turning.
2. The talonavicular joint is usually approached through a universal dorsomedial incision. If extended distally, it will allow access to the naviculocuneiform and cuneiform-metatarsal joints. The incision is started just distal to the medial malleolus and carried distally 1 cm beyond the naviculocuneiform joint (Fig. 20-4C).
3. The incision can be placed more dorsal, particularly if a large dorsal osteophyte requires removal, or in a stiff joint where debridement of the lateral half of the navicular and talus will be compromised.
4. Using a periosteal elevator or a sharp, curved osteotome, the joint capsule is stripped from the dorsal, medial, and plantar aspects of the joint.
5. If dorsal osteophytes are present, they are removed at this time, using an osteotome or a rongeur.
6. Exposure of the talonavicular joint is facilitated with a lamina spreader or by placing a towel clip into the proximal medial portion of the navicular and

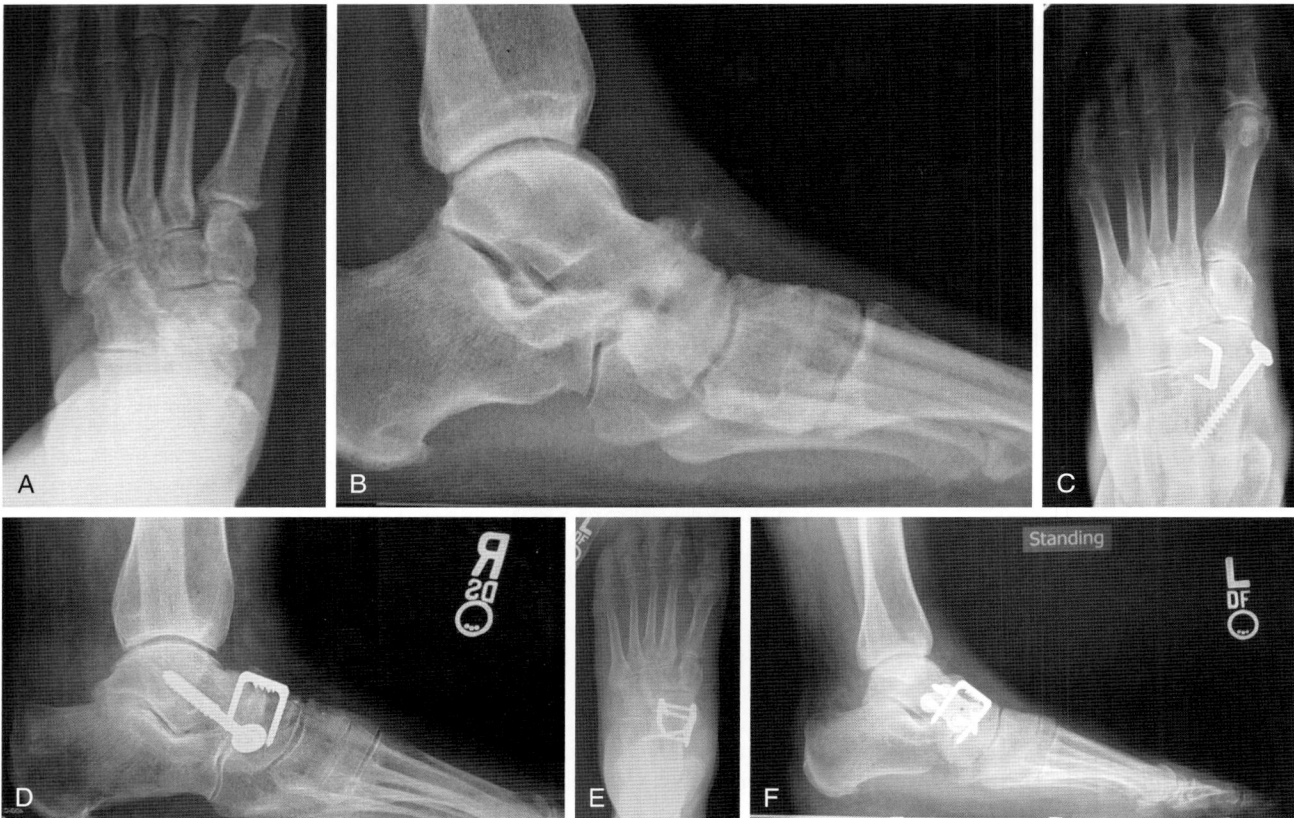

Figure 20-3 **A** and **B,** Preoperative anteroposterior (AP) and lateral radiographs demonstrate talonavicular degenerative arthritis. **C** and **D,** Postoperative AP and lateral radiographs showing screw and staple fixation of the talonavicular joint. **E** and **F,** In cases of porotic and soft bone, or if more rigid fixation is needed, a medial or dorsal plate could add stability.

applying a distracting force in a medial direction (Fig. 20-4D).

7. The articular surfaces of the talus and navicular are identified, and the articular cartilage is removed with an osteotome or curet. Power osteotomes could be very helpful.

8. A small lamina spreader sometimes can be placed into the medial side of the joint to gain better visualization. This being a curved joint, visualization of the lateral aspect is difficult but essential if satisfactory debridement is to be achieved.

9. The joint surfaces are heavily feathered, and the foot is manipulated into anatomic alignment.

10. The calcaneus is held in one hand, placing the subtalar joint in approximately 5 degrees of valgus. The talonavicular joint is manipulated, bringing the transverse tarsal joint into a few degrees of abduction and the forefoot into a plantigrade position that is perpendicular to the long axis of the tibia. If possible, the forefoot should not have a residual of more than 5 to 7 degrees of fixed forefoot varus or valgus.

11. The type of internal fixation selected depends in part on the quality of the bone. The author prefers a

4.5-mm or 6.5-mm cannulated or noncannulated compression screw inserted from the distal medial side of the navicular. A second screw could be inserted from dorsolateral, but the angle could be difficult. The author therefore prefers a large staple on the dorsolateral side. If the bone is very soft, or if there is bone loss, a locking-type plate and screws could be added to increase stability.

12. With the surgeon holding the foot in correct alignment, a guide pin is placed starting along the medial side of the navicular at the naviculocuneiform joint and drilled obliquely across the navicular into the head and neck of the talus.

13. The alignment of the foot is then once again carefully verified, and if it is satisfactory, the pin placement is checked with fluoroscopy.

14. The navicular is overdrilled, and a 40- to 50-mm–long threaded cancellous screw is inserted. The smooth shank of the screw must completely pass across the intended fusion site. If the bone is soft, a washer is used.

15. After the screw has been inserted, the stability of the arthrodesis site is checked. One or more staples are

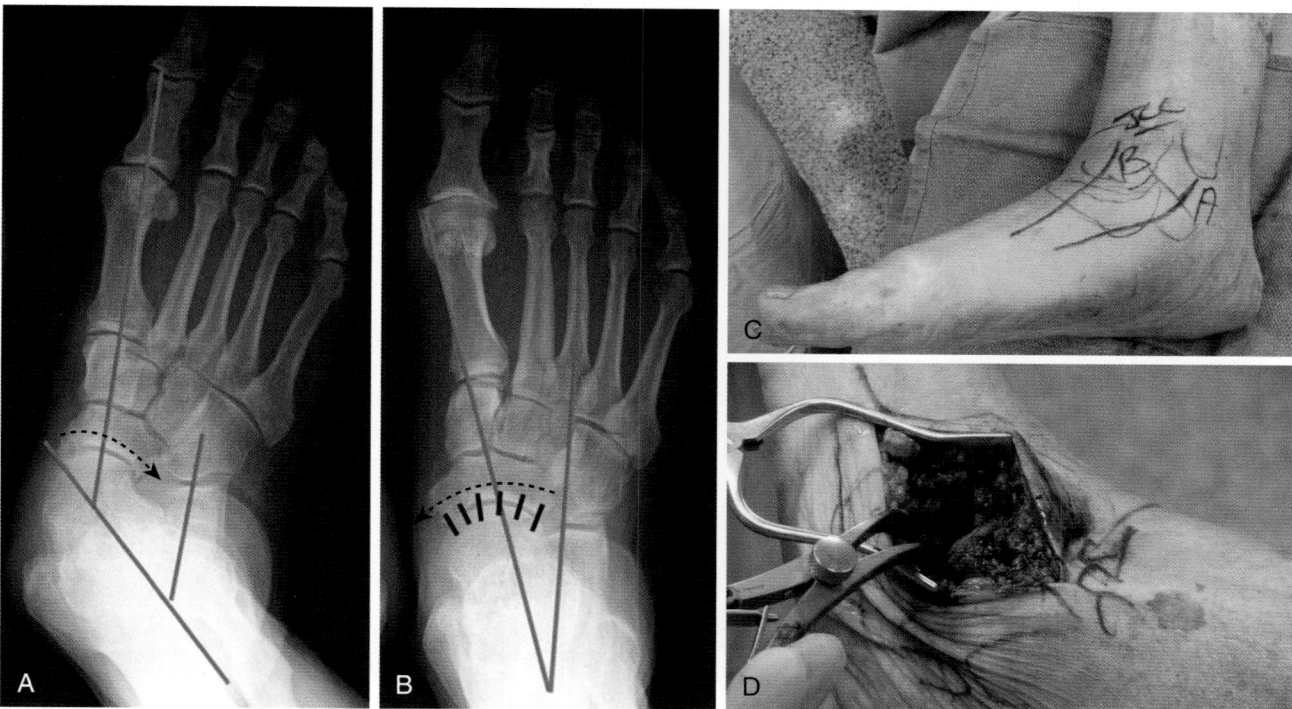

Figure 20-4 Talonavicular arthrodesis. **A,** Radiograph demonstrates changes that occur in the talonavicular joint with flatfoot deformity. The head of the talus deviates medially as the forefoot deviates laterally into abduction. It results in dorsolateral peritalar subluxation of the navicular. The talonavicular angle shows significant valgus malalignment. The talocalcaneal angle is also increased. **B,** Alignment is corrected by rotating the navicular back onto the talus in all planes. The navicular is once again centered over the head of the talus. **C,** Exposure of the talonavicular joint through a medial incision. *Line A* shows the conventional approach. This is the same incision used for a medial triple. *Line B* shows the author's preferred incision for a talonavicular fusion. This allows much better and easier access to the lateral side of the joint. **D,** Access is gained to the talonavicular joint by distracting the joint with a lamina spreader.

usually necessary to increase stability. The author uses simple Richard staples (see Fig. 20-3C and D).

16. In porotic bone, a plate construct could be used for fixation. This is also useful if the navicular fractures while inserting a screw (see Fig. 20-3E and F).

17. The wound is closed in layers, with the deep fascia being approximated over the arthrodesis site. The subcutaneous tissue and skin are closed in a routine manner. The wound over the talonavicular joint rarely breaks down.

18. The patient is placed into a compression dressing incorporating two plaster splints.

Postoperative Care

Either preoperatively or in the recovery room, a popliteal or ankle block is administered to control postoperative pain. The postoperative dressing is changed in 10 to 14 days, sutures are removed, and the patient is placed into a short-leg, removable cast with an elastic bandage to control swelling. Weight bearing is not permitted. Six weeks after surgery, radiographs are obtained, and if satisfactory union is occurring, the patient is permitted to ambulate with weight bearing as tolerated in a short-leg cast. Three months after surgery, if radiographic healing is evident, the patient is permitted to ambulate without support as tolerated.

Complications

The nonunion rate of the talonavicular joint is much higher than that of the calcaneocuboid or subtalar joint, partly because of the surgeon's inability to gain adequate exposure of the entire joint in preparation for the arthrodesis. The high nonunion rate can also result from the relative avascularity of the navicular, particularly in posttraumatic cases. If a nonunion occurs and the alignment is satisfactory, carrying out a slot-type bone graft into several areas around the talonavicular joint usually results in satisfactory union.[11]

Malalignment of the joint results in malposition of the hindfoot and forefoot. The most common malposition is a flatfoot deformity, which results from leaving the forefoot in too much abduction and the subtalar joint in valgus. This can only be corrected by revision to a triple arthrodesis.

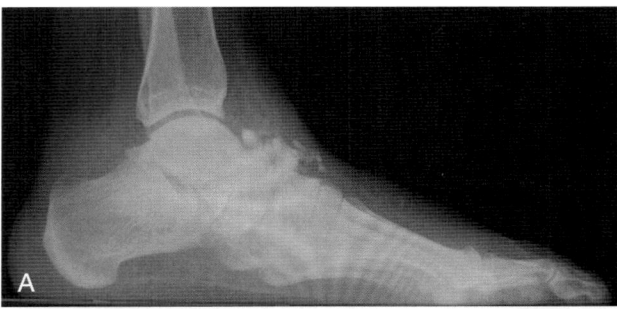

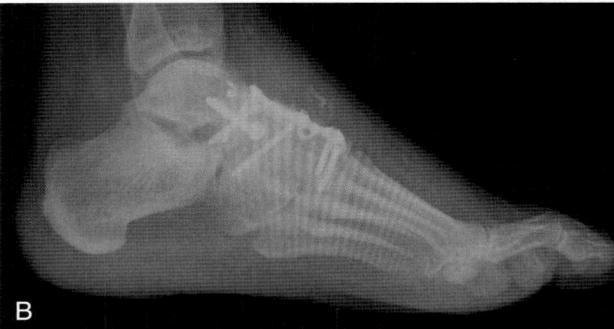

Figure 20-5 **A,** Severe destruction of the navicular. In such a situation an isolated talonavicular fusion would not be possible. **B,** Extended fusion from the talus to the cuneiforms, spanning the abnormal navicular.

Author's Experience

Isolated talonavicular fusions can be very challenging, especially in cases with avascular necrosis of the navicular, poststress fracture arthrosis, or post–Mueller-Weiss syndrome.[14] In these cases, more fixation is better than less. It is not uncommon to use a compression screw, followed by a H-type locking or nonlocking plate for added stability. If there is real concern about the vascularity of the navicular, there should be a low threshold to extend the fusion to the cuneiforms (Fig. 20-5A and B).

Special Considerations

Astion and Deland[9] showed the talonavicular joint had the greatest range of motion of the triple joints in the foot, and simulated arthrodesis of this joint essentially eliminated motion of the other joints of the complex. Fusing the talonavicular joint severely limited the motion of the remaining joints to about 2 degrees and limited the excursion of the posterior tibial tendon to 25% of the preoperative value.[9] Meanwhile, arthrodesis of the calcaneocuboid joint had little effect on the range of motion of the subtalar joint, and it reduced the range of motion of the talonavicular joint to a mean of 67% of the preoperative value, while a mean of 73% of the excursion of the posterior tibial tendon was retained. After simulated arthrodesis of the subtalar joint, a mean of 26% of the motion of the talonavicular joint, 56% of the motion of the calcaneocuboid joint, and 46% of the

excursion of the posterior tibial tendon was retained. This work confirmed that the talonavicular joint is the key joint of the triple joint complex. If possible, especially in posterior tibial tendon dysfunction in which the navicular is usually normal, the surgeon should consider a subtalar fusion in addition to other procedures to stabilize the foot.[10]

DOUBLE ARTHRODESIS (Video Clip 29)

The double arthrodesis as described by DuVries[15] consists of a fusion of the talonavicular and calcaneocuboid joints (Fig. 20-6A). It is based on the biomechanical principle that if the motion in the talonavicular and calcaneocuboid joints is eliminated, very limited motion occurs in the subtalar joint. This results in the same degree of immobilization as a triple arthrodesis, but without the necessity of completing the subtalar portion. A double arthrodesis takes less time and probably has less patient morbidity because the subtalar joint is not included in the fusion mass.[17]

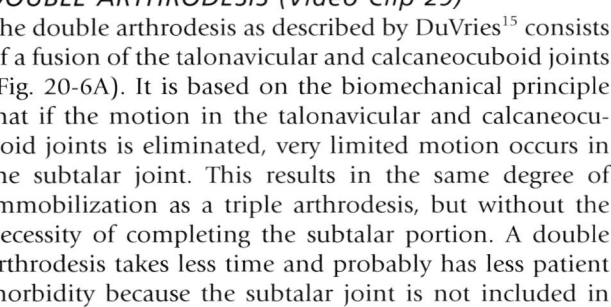

Indications

The double arthrodesis is indicated when the malalignment involves the transverse tarsal joint or forefoot, or both. It is most often carried out for patients with posterior tibial tendon dysfunction who are not candidates for a tendon reconstruction or subtalar fusion. In these patients, the subtalar joint is flexible, and no subtalar disorder is present. There is also a fixed forefoot varus, greater than 15 degrees, and abduction of the transverse tarsal joint is increased. A fusion of the talonavicular and calcaneocuboid joints is sufficient to create a plantigrade foot without including the subtalar joint. If any arthrosis is present within the subtalar joint, a triple arthrodesis is indicated.

It is also possible to have isolated talonavicular and calcaneocuboid arthritis not affecting the remainder of the foot. This is seen in rheumatoid arthritis (Fig. 20-6B-D).

Another indication for a double arthrodesis is midfoot collapse after a Chopart or peritalar dislocation. Most of these are initially treated nonsurgically, but if a recurrent collapse develops, there is no choice but to fuse the joints (Fig. 20-6E-G).

The double arthrodesis is also indicated in patients with isolated arthrosis involving the talonavicular joint who, because of their young age or high level of activity, would be placing great stress on the foot. Although an isolated talonavicular arthrodesis is excellent for the less active patient (e.g., with rheumatoid arthritis), a more active person often has some pain in the foot if the calcaneocuboid or subtalar joint is not added to the talonavicular fusion. Based on the author's experience with large patients, rather than perform a conventional double arthrodesis, a subtalar fusion is preferable. It reduces the stress on the talonavicular fusion site, which can result in fixation failure and loss of alignment. When the subtalar joint is added, creating a modified double arthrodesis, it

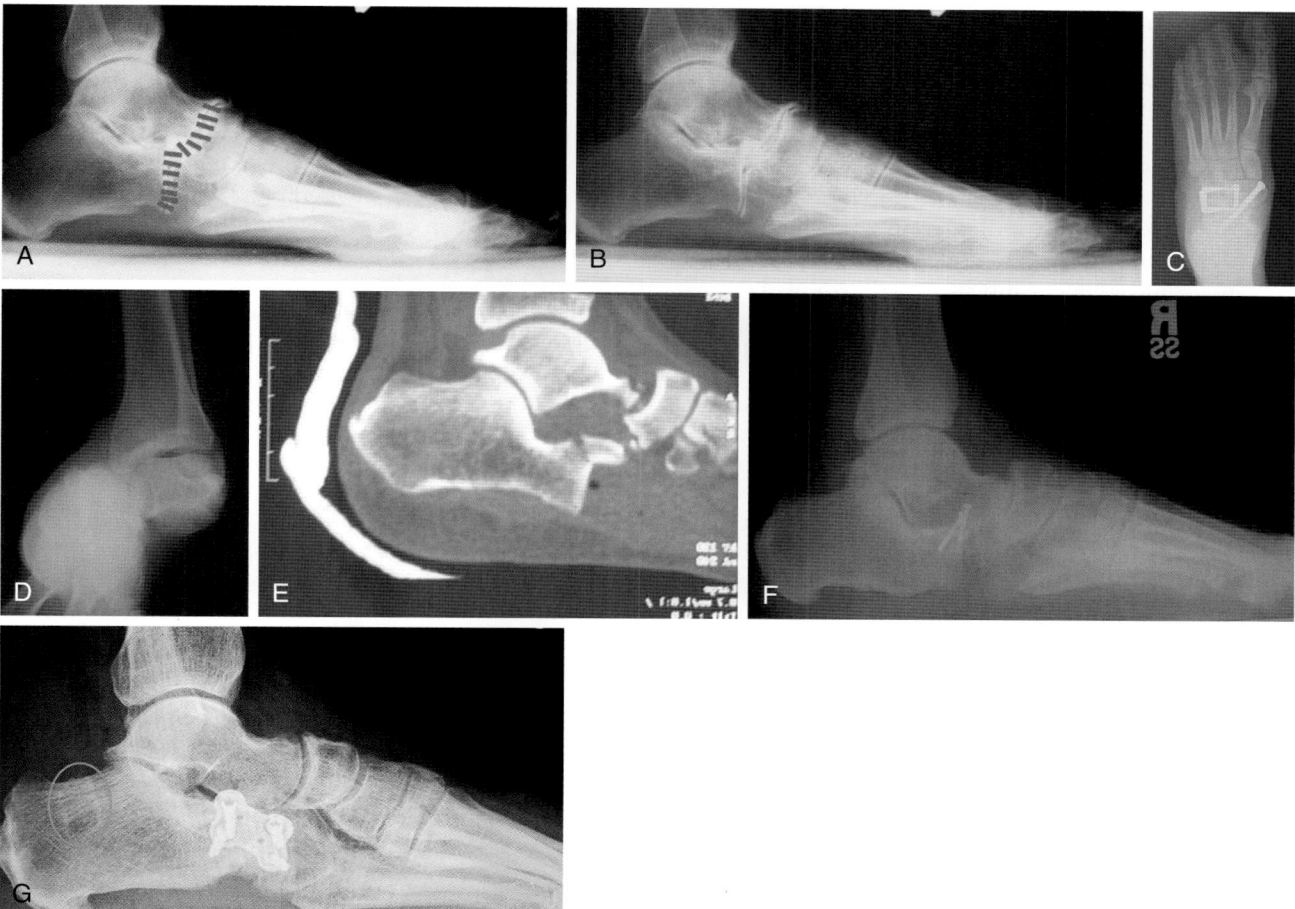

Figure 20-6 **A,** Diagram of double arthrodesis. **B** and **C,** Preoperative and postoperative radiographs demonstrating arthrodesis using the usual screw and staple for the talonavicular and two staples for the calcaneocuboid joints. **D,** Peritalar dislocation. **E,** Computed tomography scan shows fracture fragments I in the talus and calcaneus. **F,** The patient had a peritalar dislocation and a fracture of the anterior process of the calcaneus. The process fracture was reduced and screws placed, whereas the dislocation was reduced and treated in a cast for 3 months. Nine months later, there is obvious instability and collapse through the double joints. **G,** If the bone around the calcaneocuboid joint is soft, or if there are issues inserting screws, a plate construct could be used. Note the area where bone graft was taken from the calcaneus. (Corticocancellous bone was harvested from the calcaneus between the subtalar joint and Achilles insertion *[blue oval]*).

stabilizes the subtalar joint, relieving stress on the talonavicular joint. It also allows for a few degrees movement in the lateral border, which in turn helps with proprioception.

Position of Arthrodesis

The positioning of the foot for a double arthrodesis is extremely critical. The subtalar joint must be placed into 5 degrees of valgus and maintained there while the transverse tarsal joint is positioned into the same degree of abduction or adduction as the normal foot. The forefoot is placed into a plantigrade position with little or no residual fixed forefoot varus. In many patients with dysfunction of the posterior tibial tendon, one of the main components being corrected is the fixed forefoot varus of greater than 15 degrees, which precludes performing an isolated subtalar fusion.

Surgical Technique

1. The patient is placed in the supine position with a support under the ipsilateral hip to allow easy access to the medial and lateral aspects of the foot.
2. A thigh tourniquet is applied.
3. The skin incision is made along the lateral aspect of the foot, starting at the base of the fourth metatarsal, and extends proximally toward the tip of the fibula, stopping about 1 cm short of the tip.
4. The incision is deepened to the extensor digitorum brevis muscle. Care is taken to identify any anterior branch of the sural nerve that might be crossing the surgical field.
5. The capsule of the extensor digitorum brevis is opened, its origin is released, and the muscle is reflected distally about 1 cm distal to the calcaneocuboid joint.

6. The calcaneocuboid joint is identified and the soft tissue stripped plantarward and dorsally using a periosteal elevator.

7. The articular cartilage is removed from the calcaneocuboid joint as thoroughly as possible using a small, sharp osteotome or curet.

8. Placing a deep retractor into the wound along the dorsal aspect, the surgeon identifies the lateral aspect of the talonavicular joint opposite the calcaneocuboid joint and removes articular cartilage if possible. Usually, cartilage can be removed from the lateral third of the talar head and occasionally from the navicular, depending on how tight the foot is.

9. The medial approach is through a longitudinal incision, starting at the tip of the medial malleolus and carried distally 1 cm past the naviculocuneiform joint (see Fig. 20-4C).

10. The incision is deepened through the capsular tissues, after which the capsule and spring ligament are stripped from the navicular. An elevator is passed over the dorsal aspect of the talonavicular joint, completely freeing the joint.

11. Using a towel clip embedded into the proximal portion of the navicular, the surgeon distracts the talonavicular joint by pulling the foot in an adducted position and longitudinally (see Fig. 20-4D). In most cases, however, a lamina spreader is used to gain exposure.

12. The articular cartilage is removed from the talonavicular joint with an osteotome or curet. Sometimes removing the cartilage is difficult, and it is important to be sure that the joint capsule has been completely stripped from the talonavicular joint to facilitate exposure.

13. The foot is manipulated into proper alignment to determine whether any bone needs to be removed from the attempted fusion site, which generally is not necessary. However, it is important to be sure no gap is created at the calcaneocuboid joint when the foot is brought into a plantigrade position.

14. To correct a severe forefoot varus deformity (peritalar subluxation), the navicular must be rotated around the talar head in a medial and plantar direction. This is carried out by holding the hindfoot in one hand and rotating the forefoot in such a way as to plantar flex the navicular on the head of the talus while simultaneously adducting the foot. This maneuver corrects the deformity and creates a plantigrade foot.

15. With the foot held in a plantigrade position, the calcaneocuboid joint is observed because, if it is distracted, some bone needs to be removed from the talar head. This does not occur often, but again, it is important that a gap is not created between the calcaneus and cuboid.

16. Before placing the internal fixation, the bone ends are heavily scaled using a 4-mm osteotome. The talonavicular joint must be well feathered from both medial and lateral sides to ensure that the greatest amount of bone surface has been destroyed to help prevent a nonunion.

17. Many ways are available to carry out internal fixation for a double arthrodesis. If adequate bone stock exists, one or two 4.0-mm screws across the talonavicular joint provides excellent internal fixation. A single 7.0-mm screw can be used in a large patient, but in a smaller person or a person with soft bone, it can result in a fracture of the medial side of the navicular. As mentioned in the section on single talonavicular fusion, the author prefers a screw and staple combination but will use a plate in addition in porotic or poor-quality bone.

18. The foot is then manipulated into proper alignment as described earlier, and the guide pin for the 4.0-mm cannulated screw is placed across the talonavicular joint.

19. The guide pin is started at the distal end of the navicular at the naviculocuneiform joint. If the surgeon starts at the midportion of the navicular, insufficient bone may be present along the medial side of the navicular, and a fracture of the medial aspect of the navicular can occur. The surgeon should attempt to incorporate as much of the medial aspect of the navicular as possible with the screw. The placement is usually checked with fluoroscopy. The navicular is overdrilled with a 4.0-mm drill bit, after which 4.0-mm–long threaded screws are inserted. It is important that the threads cross the joint surface. If the quality of bone is not good, washers should be used.

20. The fixation of the calcaneocuboid joint is usually carried out using two 4.0-mm cannulated screws. As a general rule, the screws can be brought from proximal to distal, starting in the anterior process area and brought obliquely across into the cuboid. At times, however, the bone alignment is such that this is not possible, and the screws are brought from the cuboid into the calcaneus. Sometimes the bone is too soft, and a seam of staples is used. Again, an alternative is to use an H plate and screws (Fig. 20-6H).

21. The deep layers are closed, followed by the subcutaneous tissues and skin.

22. The wounds are instilled with 0.25% bupivacaine if no ankle or popliteal block was used, after which a compression dressing incorporating plaster splints is applied.

Postoperative Care

Before surgery or in the recovery room, a popliteal block is administered to control postoperative pain. The postoperative dressing is removed in approximately 10 days, after which the patient is placed into a removable cast with an elastic bandage to control swelling. The patient is kept non–weight bearing for 6 weeks from the time of surgery. At 6 weeks, radiographs are obtained. If satisfactory union is occurring, the patient is permitted to bear weight in a cast. Approximately 12 weeks after surgery, radiographs again are obtained. If satisfactory union has occurred, the patient is permitted to ambulate with an elastic stocking.

Author's Experience

Mann reviewed the author's experience with 32 patients (19 women, 13 men) who had undergone a double arthrodesis.[16] The average age was 62 years (range, 38-81 years), and average follow-up was 56 months (range, 24-162 months). The diagnosis was posterior tibial tendon dysfunction in 20 patients, isolated talonavicular arthrosis in 5, rheumatoid arthritis in 5, talar neck nonunion in 1, and an acquired flatfoot deformity after a spinal cord injury in 1.

The patients' satisfaction rate was 92%, and 8% were dissatisfied. Pain relief was the main benefit. The preoperative pain, assessed as 4.3 of a possible 5, diminished postoperatively to 1.4 (0 equals no pain). Functional capacity increased from 1.3 preoperatively to 3.6 (out of 4) postoperatively.

The fusion rate was 87.5% (28 of 32 cases). Four nonunions of the talonavicular joint occurred, all of which had staple fixation. Three of the four required a revision to a triple arthrodesis. As a group, the patients noted maximum recovery at about 8 months after surgery.

The patients' level of activities demonstrated that most could walk for pleasure, and five were able to run short distances; 60% played golf, biked, hiked, and swam. Seventy-five percent of the patients noted some difficulty when walking on uneven ground or inclines or when going up and down steps.

The physical examination demonstrated that the average hindfoot position was 5.8 degrees of valgus, the transverse tarsal joint had 4.4 degrees of abduction, and the forefoot varus was 9 degrees. The range of motion of the ankle joint decreased 11 degrees compared with the uninvolved side.

The radiographic evaluation demonstrated that the anteroposterior (AP) talar–second metatarsal angle improved from 30 degrees (abduction) to 14 degrees, and the lateral talar–first metatarsal angle improved from −16 degrees (indicating dorsiflexion) to −7 degrees postoperatively.

The follow-up radiographs demonstrated a slight degree of ankle arthrosis in 53% of patients, which was not present preoperatively, and 30% noted mild symptoms. Twenty percent demonstrated evidence of arthrosis in the subtalar joint, but none were symptomatic. The naviculocuneiform joint demonstrated an increase in arthrosis in 37% of patients, all of whom had slight symptoms, except for one patient, whose symptoms were severe. The tarsometatarsal joints demonstrated a 22% increased incidence, but none were symptomatic.

Special Considerations

Complex problems involving the talonavicular joint include its possible collapse secondary to fracture,

avascular necrosis, or both. At other times, involvement of the forefoot distal to the talonavicular joint occurs, with extension into the naviculocuneiform and sometimes the tarsometatarsal joints. In these situations, a modified double arthrodesis has been used to provide stability.

In many of these cases, the overall alignment of the foot is satisfactory or at least adequate for a plantigrade foot. Rather than take down the involved areas and place a large bone graft, a rectangular slot is cut from the talus to the cuneiforms or into the metatarsal bases, as indicated by the clinical circumstances. The slot is cut all the way across the foot from medial to lateral, after which a piece of iliac crest bone graft is inlaid into the slot. Fixation of the bone graft and surrounding bone is done with screws or multiple staples. At the same time, the calcaneocuboid joint is arthrodesed to provide stability to the lateral column. This is obviously an extensive procedure and is only done under certain circumstances when significant deformity within the midportion of the foot is present but no significant anatomic correction needs to be carried out. In a situation with marked destruction of the midfoot and malalignment, this procedure cannot be used. Then the surgeon would need to take down the involved area and either bone graft it or possibly collapse the lateral column to realign the midfoot. There are several midfoot-specific plating systems that allow fixation from the talus to the metatarsals if needed.

After the inlay bone graft procedure, the patient is immobilized for a prolonged period. As a general rule, weight bearing is not permitted for 3 months, after which the patient is gradually started on progressive weight bearing over the next 3 months. It is sometimes difficult to state when union has occurred, and therefore the surgeon should be very cautious in allowing patients to bear weight.

TRIPLE ARTHRODESIS (Video Clips 28 and 30)

The triple arthrodesis consists of fusion of the talonavicular, calcaneocuboid, and subtalar joints (Fig. 20-7A). Initially, the triple arthrodesis was used to treat deformities of the foot secondary to paralysis, mainly poliomyelitis, in which severe anatomic distortion was present. To correct this abnormality, large bone wedges were resected to place the foot into a plantigrade position. Little or no internal fixation was used, and at times, the patient was returned to surgery in the immediate postoperative period to remanipulate the foot into better alignment. At present, it is highly advisable to use huge rigid internal fixation under compression, not only to maintain position but also to speed up healing and increase the fusion rate.

As the number of patients with deformed feet secondary to paralysis declined, the triple arthrodesis was performed less often. It is now most often carried out for residuals of trauma, rheumatoid arthritis, and longstanding posterior tibial tendon dysfunction in which the basic bone anatomy is present. Although distorted,

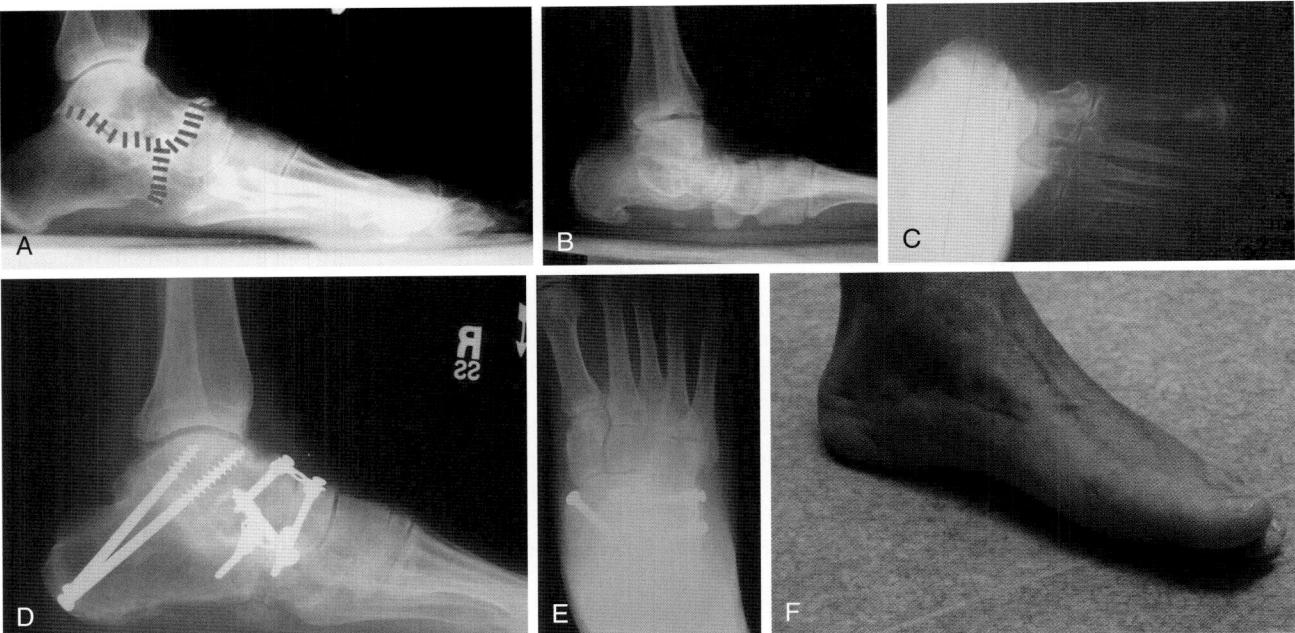

Figure 20-7 **A,** Diagram of triple arthrodesis. **B** and **C,** Very severe collapse of the foot with complete peritalar dislocation secondary to a long-standing posterior tibial tendon dysfunction. **D** and **E,** Postoperative radiograph demonstrating triple arthrodesis with anatomic restoration of foot posture using a combination of screws and plates. Note that the height of the longitudinal arch has been restored and severe abduction of the foot is corrected. **F,** Note forefoot varus with the first ray off the floor with a malunion of a triple arthrodesis.

significant bone resection is usually not necessary. This allows the procedure to be done by releasing the contracted joint capsules, removing the articular cartilage, scaling the exposed bony surfaces, and using manipulation to create a plantigrade foot (Fig. 20-7B-E).

Bone grafting from the iliac crest is rarely necessary for primary fusions, but if bone graft is needed, it can usually be obtained from the calcaneus, medial malleolus, or proximal tibia without violating the iliac crest and risking added morbidity. For revisions, especially revising a nonunion, iliac crest bone graft is advisable.

Although the triple arthrodesis is a valuable tool for the orthopaedic surgeon, it is not without postoperative complications. The literature points out that because of the added stress across the ankle joint as a result of a triple arthrodesis, approximately 30% of patients demonstrate ankle degeneration at 5 years.[25] This outcome reinforces the biomechanics of the foot and ankle complex, demonstrating that the ankle, subtalar, and transverse tarsal joints are functioning together. When a triple arthrodesis is carried out, increased stress is placed proximally on the ankle joint and distally on the midfoot. Therefore it is imperative that a more limited arthrodesis always be considered when feasible. Because of the possible ankle joint deterioration, when evaluating the patient preoperatively for a triple arthrodesis, a weight-bearing AP radiograph of the ankle must be included to ascertain if preexisting arthrosis can preclude the triple arthrodesis, or at least to predict the future for the patient.

Indications

Arthrosis involving the subtalar joint and either the talonavicular or the calcaneocuboid joint, or both, is an indication for triple arthrodesis.[23,27] Arthrosis of only the subtalar joint can usually be treated by an isolated subtalar joint fusion.

Triple arthrodesis can be used for the unstable hindfoot secondary to neuromuscular disorders, such as poliomyelitis, nerve injury, posterior tibial tendon dysfunction, or rheumatoid arthritis, in which the subtalar and transverse tarsal joints are involved. Malalignment of the foot secondary to arthrofibrosis resulting from a compartment syndrome, crush injury, or severe trauma is an indication for a triple arthrodesis. In the patient with a symptomatic, unresectable, or previously resected calcaneonavicular coalition, a triple arthrodesis is indicated. It is important to appreciate, however, that the patient with a talocalcaneal (subtalar) coalition can be treated with an isolated subtalar fusion even if there is osteophyte formation on the dorsal aspect of the talar head. The patient with a severe symptomatic pes planus deformity that is not amenable to other procedures, such as lateral column lengthening, calcaneal osteotomy, or subtalar fusion, can also be considered a candidate for a triple arthrodesis.

Untreated posterior tibial tendon dysfunction leads to a severe peritalar subluxation and valgus/abduction collapse of the foot. In severe deformities, a triple arthrodesis is advocated, but in reality, in most cases the calcaneocuboid joint does not need to be fused. When the navicular is rotated back around the talar head, the calcaneocuboid joints opens and can be the most difficult to fuse of joints.

Whenever considering a triple arthrodesis, however, the surgeon must be mindful of the consequences of the potential degeneration at the ankle joint. If a younger person can be treated with an AFO or a more limited fusion, this may be a better method of treatment.

Position of Arthrodesis

The position of a triple arthrodesis is critical because once an arthrodesis has been achieved, the foot is in a fixed position and cannot accommodate to the ground. It is therefore essential that the hindfoot be placed in about 5 degrees of valgus, the transverse tarsal joint in 0 to 5 degrees of abduction, and the forefoot in less than 10 degrees of varus. If accurate alignment is not achieved, the patient will have a nonplantigrade foot, which can cause chronic pain that requires a revision.

Surgical Technique

1. The normal foot is examined and its alignment noted. Patients have a varying degree of forefoot adduction or abduction, and the surgeon should attempt to match this with the affected extremity.
2. The patient is placed in the supine position with a support under the ipsilateral hip to improve visualization of the lateral aspect of the hindfoot. (A detailed discussion of this approach is presented in the sections on subtalar and double arthrodeses.)
3. The skin incision starts at the tip of the fibula and is carried to the base of the fourth metatarsal. Caution should be used when deepening this incision, looking for the sural nerve and possibly an anterior branch (see Fig 20-2B).
4. The extensor digitorum muscle is removed from its origin on the lateral side of the talus and calcaneus and retracted distally.
5. The subtalar and calcaneocuboid joints are visualized, and the articular cartilage is removed.
6. Through the lateral incision, the lateral aspect of the talonavicular joint is identified, and as much articular cartilage is removed as possible. (A detailed discussion of this approach is presented in the section on talonavicular arthrodesis.)
7. The skin incision begins 2 cm distal and lateral to the tip of the medial malleolus in the midline and is carried 1 cm distal to the naviculocuneiform joint (see Fig. 20-4C).
8. The incision is deepened to expose the joint capsule, which is stripped from the talonavicular joint.
9. A small lamina spreader or small osteotomes are useful in distracting the joint. Alternatively, a towel clip in the navicular can be used. All the articular cartilage is removed from the talonavicular joint.
10. At times, some articular cartilage is also removed through the lateral incision. This depends on the flexibility of the foot.
11. The foot is manipulated, first by bringing the subtalar joint into 5 degrees of valgus, then manipulating the transverse tarsal joint to eliminate the fixed forefoot varus. This is done by rotating the navicular in a plantar direction on the head of the talus and simultaneously bringing the transverse tarsal joint into about 0 to 5 degrees of abduction. This maneuver usually creates a plantigrade foot. The foot cannot be manipulated if the joints have not been completely mobilized.
12. After the manipulation, it is important to inspect the articular surfaces to be sure there is good bone apposition. If the bones are not properly apposed, it may be necessary to remove some bone, usually from the head of the talus, to shorten the medial column and close the calcaneocuboid joint.
13. In correcting the deformity of a posterior tibial tendon dysfunction, the calcaneocuboid joint might be open enough so that a fusion is not needed, thereby obviating the need for shortening the medial side.
14. Once alignment has been achieved, the joint surfaces are heavily scaled or feathered in preparation for internal fixation.
15. Temporary K-wire fixation will allow reassessing the alignment and reduction with fluoroscopy.
16. The author prefers to start internal fixation at the talonavicular joint. A guidewire is place from the medial aspect of the navicular close to the naviculocuneeoform junction, aiming for the center of the talus while using fluoroscopy. A 4.5-, 6.0-, or 6.7-mm screw is placed under compression using a gliding hole in the navicular.
17. The screw is usually 45 to 50 mm long, and a washer is used to aid compression.
18. A second point of fixation is desired across the talonavicular joint. The author prefers a large Richard staple dorsolateral, but it could also be a second screw. However, the angle is quite acute, and a second screw might be difficult to place (see Fig. 20-3C).
19. At this point, the subtalar joint is reduced in 5 degrees valgus and a screw is placed from the talar neck posterior into the calcaneus using the same principles as mentioned in the section on subtalar fusion. There is usually excellent purchase in the plantar aspect of the calcaneus, with good compression across the joint. A single screw is enough in this situation.
20. The alternative is to do the fixation in the same sequence as discussed in the section on subtalar fusion, that is, by using the anterior cruciate as a guide, a screw is placed into the posterior facet of the subtalar joint and then into the back of the heel.[20]
21. The calcaneocuboid joint is visualized and fixed with two 4.0-mm cannulated screws. The guide pin is placed from the calcaneus into the cuboid, and two partially threaded screws of appropriate length are used. If the bone is too soft, staples are used.
22. In soft bone, an H-plate construct could also be used.

23. If the surgeon is not satisfied with the coaptation of the bony surfaces, a bone graft can be used.

24. The extensor digitorum brevis muscle is closed over the lateral side of the wound, after which the subcutaneous tissue and skin are closed. On the medial side, the capsular tissue is closed over the talonavicular joint, if possible, after which the subcutaneous tissue and skin are closed.

25. Always assess at this point if there is a residual gastrocnemius contracture, and do a gastrocnemius slide if 10 degrees dorsiflexion is not achievable.

26. A compression dressing incorporating two plaster splints is applied.

MEDIAL APPROACH TO A TRIPLE ARTHRODESIS

There are situations were a single medial approach to a triple or limited triple (talonavicular and subtalar) is very useful.[22,24] The most typical indication is significant soft tissue compromise on the lateral side of the foot, which makes it high risk to place an incision in that area. Severe, but flexible peritalar subluxation can also be readily exposed, prepared, and reduced through a single medial incision.

 Surgical Technique (see medial triple video)

1. A longitudinal incision is made from the tip of the medial malleolus to the medial cuneiform.

2. The safe interval is between the tibialis posterior tendon dorsal and flexor digitorum longus plantar.

3. In most cases, the talar head is clearly visible because of long-standing subluxation, and articular cartilage is removed.

4. The sustentaculum tali is exposed, and a lamina spreader is placed between the sustentaculum and the talus. This gives a clear view of the posterior facet of the subtalar joint and also aids in reducing the talus back onto the calcaneus.

5. With a medial approach, a double fusion is preferred (subtalar and talonavicular).

6. Once the surfaces are prepared, the reduction and fixation is the same as for the surgical technique described above for triple arthrodesis.

Postoperative Care

A popliteal block is administered preoperatively or postoperatively to control the immediate postoperative pain. The patient's initial surgical cast is changed 10 to 14 days after surgery, and the sutures are removed if appropriate. The patient is placed into a short-leg removable cast with an elastic bandage to control edema and is kept non–weight bearing for 6 weeks. Then radiographs are obtained, and if satisfactory union is occurring, the patient is permitted to bear weight as tolerated in the removable cast.

Twelve weeks after surgery, radiographs are again obtained, and if a fusion has occurred, the patient wears an elastic stocking and is permitted to bear weight as tolerated. If the fusion is somewhat tenuous, the patient is asked to walk around the house without the cast and use it outside for another month.

Complications

The most frequent complication after a triple arthrodesis is a *nonunion* of one of the fusion sites, most often the talonavicular joint, probably because its exposure is more difficult and the bone may be sclerotic. If a nonunion occurs and is not symptomatic, no treatment is indicated. Occasionally, after a triple arthrodesis, if two of the three joints have fused, the joint with a nonunion is asymptomatic. If a painful nonunion is present but the alignment of the extremity is satisfactory, some type of an inlay bone block across the area of the nonunion, possibly along with reinforcement of the internal fixation, usually results in a satisfactory fusion. If the area of the nonunion is symptomatic and the alignment is unsatisfactory, revision of the arthrodesis may be necessary.

The next most common complication is *malalignment.* In my experience, the most frequent malalignment is residual varus of the calcaneus, followed by a fixed forefoot varus and then adduction of the forefoot (Fig. 20-7F). A valgus deformity of the hindfoot, although not as common as a varus deformity, is distressing for most patients and can result in an unsatisfactory outcome. In this situation, the surgeon might consider a medial displacement calcaneal osteotomy to correct the excessive valgus if the remainder of the forefoot alignment is satisfactory.

In long-standing grade 2, and more so grade 3, posterior tibial tendon dysfunction, the deltoid ligament could be dysfunctional. If the original preoperative radiographs were done non–weight bearing, this might be missed. It is also imperative to test for and treat deltoid instability, if present in this situation (Fig. 20-8A-C).

Entrapment of the sural nerve, particularly an anterior branch, giving rise to dysesthesias on the lateral side of the foot, can annoy the patient. This might need to be corrected by a neurolysis or resection of the nerve, then burying the stump under soft tissues or into bone.

Occasionally, after a triple arthrodesis in a patient with long-standing severe valgus deformity, although a plantigrade position of the foot can be achieved, the ankle cannot be brought back to neutral position because of an Achilles tendon contracture. When the triple arthrodesis is carried out, if the ankle cannot be brought into about 5 degrees of dorsiflexion, an Achilles tendon lengthening or gastrocnemius slide should be strongly considered. The surgeon must be cautious, however, not to over lengthen the tendon, but the foot should not be left in an equinus posture. Adults recover their strength very slowly, if at all, after Achilles tendon lengthening.

Revision for Malalignment

A plantigrade foot might not be achieved after a triple arthrodesis. If the patient is symptomatic, a revision of the triple arthrodesis may be indicated. Technically, these are very difficult cases and need to be carefully planned

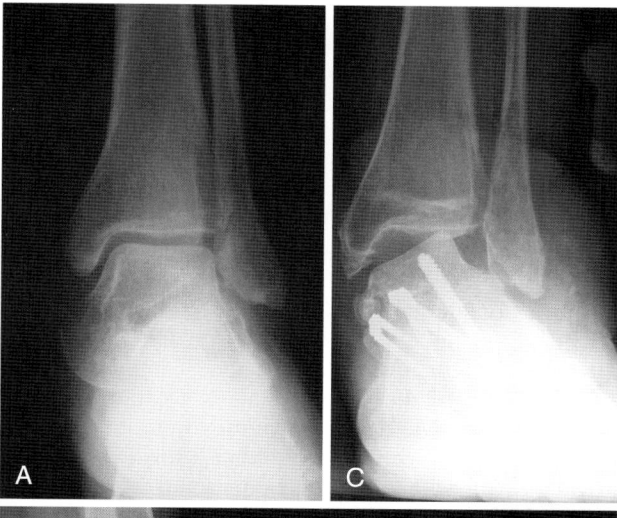
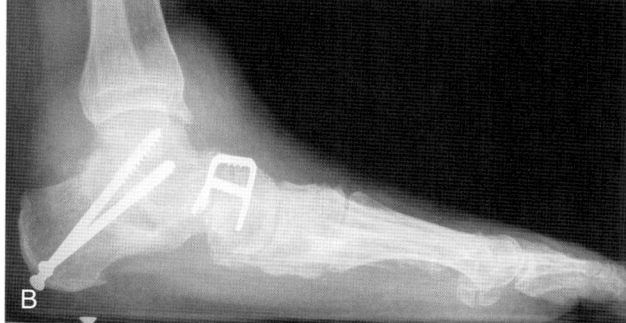

Figure 20-8 **A,** Note the significant exposure of the talus with severe peritalar subluxation. It is a non–weight-bearing radiograph, and there is no information about the ankle and deltoid ligament. **B** and **C,** Lateral and anteroposterior postoperative views show a triple arthrodesis with a secondary severe ankle varus. This is caused by a chronic deltoid insufficiency secondary to the abnormal forces on the ankle.

preoperatively to identify the precise nature and degree of the malalignment and which components of the triple arthrodesis need to be revised.[19]

If the hindfoot is malaligned and the forefoot is in a plantigrade position, the hindfoot can be corrected without revising the forefoot. If a varus deformity is present, a lateral closing-wedge Dwyer procedure can be used. Occasionally, a lateral displacement osteotomy with some rotation of the fragment from varus into valgus can produce better alignment.

When the calcaneus is in too much valgus and there is an impingement against the fibula, a calcaneal osteotomy displacing it in a medial direction can be used to correct the deformity. However, rather than create a long oblique osteotomy, as done for a Dwyer procedure, the cut is made more perpendicular just posterior to the posterior facet of the subtalar joint. The osteotomy is then displaced medially about 1 cm, and occasionally, the posterior fragment can be rotated slightly on its long axis if the degree of valgus has a rotational component. Fixation of the osteotomy is usually done with a cannulated 7.0-mm

screw placed just lateral to the Achilles tendon and driven distally across the osteotomy site into the calcaneus. If one screw is not adequate for fixation, a Steinmann pin is used for 4 weeks until the bones have become sticky.

If the hindfoot is properly aligned and the main deformity is malalignment of the forefoot, usually from residual forefoot varus, the front portion of the triple arthrodesis can be revised and the hindfoot left intact. Besides the varus deformity, an adduction deformity is also often present. This type of revision is carried out through a medial and lateral approach through the previous incisions. The soft tissues are stripped off the fusion mass around the transverse tarsal joint, which is osteotomized, and the foot is realigned. The realignment is usually carried out by rotating the forefoot block of bone into a more pronated position. If there is residual adduction or possibly abduction in the forefoot, a lateral or medial closing wedge is removed at the same time to achieve satisfactory alignment. Fixation after a revision can usually be achieved by using large screws, but if the bone is too soft, multiple staples can be useful.

The postoperative regimen after revision of a triple arthrodesis is the same as for a triple arthrodesis, that is, non–weight bearing for 6 weeks and then weight bearing for 6 weeks.

Author's Experience
Mann[21] showed that at medium-term follow-up radiographs demonstrated an increase in the arthrosis in the ankle joint in 10 of 29 cases (33%), in the naviculocuneiform joint in 5 (17%), and at the tarsometatarsal joint in 4 (14%). Saltzman[25] showed that at 45-year follow-up all patients will have radiographic signs of arthrosis at the ankle and midfoot joints. Ninety-five percent of the patients were still happy with their results, and extension of the fusion is seldom required.

Graves et al[21] studied a group consisting of 17 patients (12 women, 5 men) and 18 feet, with an average age of 66 years (range, 52-80 years). They were evaluated to determine the effect of a triple arthrodesis in the older age group because no paper had previously addressed this in the literature. The etiology was posterior tibial tendon dysfunction in 10 patients, rheumatoid arthritis in 3 (4 feet), diabetes mellitus in 1, poliomyelitis in 1, trauma in 1, and poststroke effects in 1. The follow-up was 42 months (range, 27-156 months). The procedure was carried out because of pain, deformity, or both. The pain level preoperatively was 4 on a scale of 5 and postoperatively was 1.

Fourteen patients (15 feet) were satisfied because of the improved position and diminished pain. Of interest, however, 11 patients still thought they had some pain in the foot, but it was not sufficiently symptomatic for them to be dissatisfied with the procedure. Of the 3 patients who were dissatisfied, 2 had a valgus alignment of the heel that resulted in pain. The patients observed that the time from surgery to maximum relief was about 10 months.

The level of activities improved for 9 patients (10 feet). Seven reported no change in their ambulatory capacity, and 1 believed that her ambulatory capacity was decreased. The appearance of the foot improved for 13 of 17 patients, and 2 were dissatisfied because of the valgus alignment of their heel. Twelve patients (13 feet) could wear any shoe they wanted, but 5 had some problems with footwear.

Astion and Deland[18] showed that the talonavicular joint had the greatest range of motion of the triple joints in the foot, and simulated arthrodesis of this joint essentially eliminated motion of the other joints of the complex. Fusing the talonavicular joint severely limited the motion of the remaining joints to about 2 degrees and limited the excursion of the posterior tibial tendon to 25% of the preoperative value. Meanwhile, arthrodesis of the calcaneocuboid joint had little effect on the range of motion of the subtalar joint, and it reduced the range of motion of the talonavicular joint to a mean of 67% of the preoperative value, while a mean of 73% of the excursion of the posterior tibial tendon was retained. After simulated arthrodesis of the subtalar joint, a mean of 26% of the motion of the talonavicular joint, 56% of the motion of the calcaneocuboid joint, and 46% of the excursion of the posterior tibial tendon was retained. This work confirmed that the talonavicular joint is the key joint of the triple joint complex.

Sammarco et al[26] concluded in their study that simultaneous arthrodesis of the talonavicular and subtalar joints is a reasonable treatment in the subset of patients with symptomatic hindfoot malalignment whose calcaneocuboid joints are not involved in the primary disease. This is also the author's (JCC's) experience. It is seldom, if ever, necessary to go back and fuse the calcaneocuboid joint because of symptoms.

A medial approach to a triple arthrodesis has merit in certain situations and can achieve easy exposure and reduction, especially with severe peritalar subluxation secondary to posterior tibial tendon dysfunction.

In summary, the triple arthrodesis is an excellent procedure for correcting a fixed deformity of the foot, but it should be used judiciously, particularly in the younger patient, and only when a lesser procedure cannot be used.

NAVICULOCUNEIFORM ARTHRODESIS

A naviculocuneiform arthrodesis is usually carried out for arthrosis of one or more of the articulations as a result of primary arthrosis or secondary to trauma. It is also possible to develop a collapse through the naviculocuneiform joints in a patient with posterior tibial tendon dysfunction. If the situation lends itself to a calcaneal osteotomy, whether lateral column lengthening or medializing or a combination, and a midfoot collapse is present, a naviculocuneiform fusion will preserve hindfoot motion while correcting the forefoot alignment.

In some cases, there is a significant forefoot supination/instability after a long-standing tibialis posterior dysfunction. If it is not possible to correct the alignment and medial arch stability with a naviculocuneiform fusion alone, the fusion should be extended to the first

tarsometatarsal joint. It is a fairly powerful tool to reduce the forefoot out of valgus and supination and reconstruct the medial column. It also spares the subtalar and talonavicular joints, thereby leaving a more flexible hindfoot complex (Fig. 20-9A-D).

Indications

The most common indication is isolated naviculocuneiform arthrosis secondary to trauma. The next most common indication is a midtarsal collapse secondary to posterior tibial tendon dysfunction.

Position of Arthrodesis

With arthrosis of the joint secondary to trauma, there usually is little or no deformity of the forefoot, and an in situ fusion can be carried out. Because this is a difficult articulation in which to obtain an isolated arthrodesis, the fusion mass should include the first and second and, if possible, the third naviculocuneiform joints.

When the arthrodesis is done as part of a tibialis posterior dysfunction repair, it is carried out along with either a lateral column lengthening or a medializing calcaneal osteotomy (or both) and a reconstruction of the posterior tibial tendon with a flexor digitorum longus (FDL) transfer and a gastrocnemius lengthening.

Surgical Technique

1. The patient is placed in the supine position, and a thigh tourniquet is applied. Because the extremity naturally falls into external rotation, the patient does not require turning.
2. The naviculocuneiform joint is approached through a universal dorsomedial longitudinal incision, starting just distal to the medial malleolus and carried distally halfway between the posterior tibial and anterior tibial tendon, distal enough to expose the first metatarsocuneiform joint (see Fig. 20-4C).
3. The dissection is carried down to bone. As the surgeon proceeds distally, the tibialis anterior tendon is obliquely crossing the field and needs to be mobilized so that it can be pulled somewhat distally out of harm's way.
4. By sharp and blunt dissection, the joint capsule is stripped from the medial, dorsal, and plantar aspects of the joint.
5. Using a small osteotome, the articular cartilage is removed from the first, second, and third cuneiform, as well as the corresponding surface of the navicular. Usually, it is difficult to completely denude the third naviculocuneiform joint. A small lamina spreader does help facilitate exposure of these joints.
6. It is not necessary, and probably not advisable, to fuse the intercuneiform joint. It might lead to too much soft tissue stripping and vascular compromise of the cuneiforms.
7. The articular surfaces are then feathered with a 4-mm osteotome or perforated with multiple small drill holes.

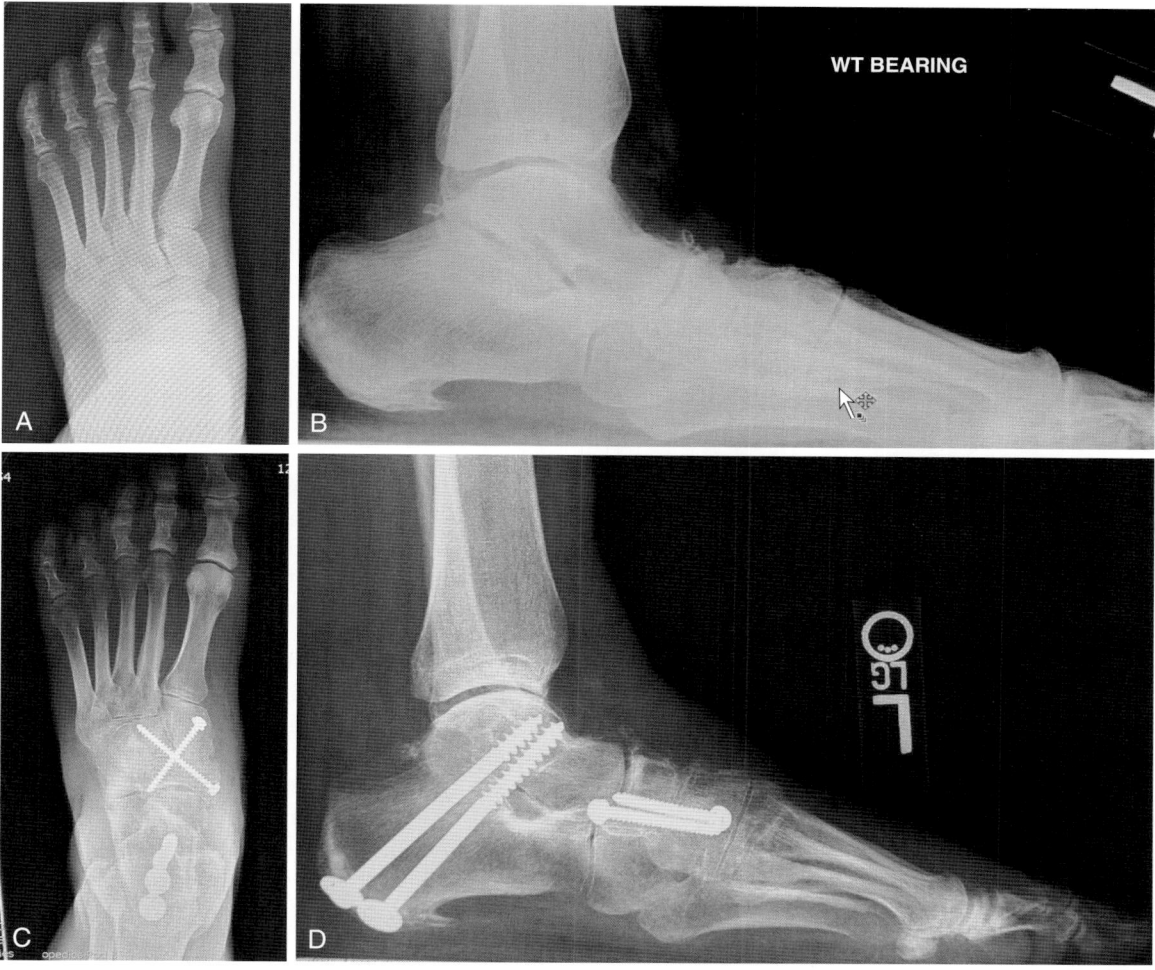

Figure 20-9 A and **B,** Anteroposterior and lateral view of naviculocuneiform collapse secondary to posterior tibial tendon dysfunction. **C** and **D,** Naviculocuneiform fusion with a screw from the navicular to middle cuneiform and a second screw from the medial cuneiform to lateral half of the navicular. Note the subtalar fusion as well. *WT,* weight.

8. The foot is corrected by rotating the distal portion of the foot medially and into plantar flexion at the fusion site while holding the hindfoot in neutral position. The goal is to restore the talo–first metatarsal angle to a straight line (0 degrees) on the anteroposterior and lateral planes.

Sometimes, it takes several manipulations in this manner to gain the necessary correction. It is important, however, that as this is carried out, the hindfoot is held in neutral position; otherwise, inadequate correction will be obtained. If correction of the deformity seems overly difficult, it is probably because of lack of adequate capsular stripping.

9. Once the foot is manipulated into satisfactory alignment, one or more 0.062-inch K-wires are placed across the dorsal aspect of the joint to stabilize it so that internal fixation can be inserted.

10. Stable fixation can be achieved by placing the screws from the tubercle of the navicular and proceeding distally into the first and second cuneiforms. A third

screw passing from the first cuneiform back into the navicular can also be used with caution. It should be placed under compression with overdrilling the cuneiform, and care should be taken to ensure the tip does not enter the talonavicular joint.

11. Usually one screw is passed from the navicular into the first cuneiform and the second from the navicular into the second cuneiform. As a rule, it is difficult to get a screw from the navicular into the third cuneiform.

12. The proliferation of compression staples makes it simpler to immobilize to the third navuculocuneiform joint without the difficulty of getting good screw placement or bone purchase.

13. There are several low-profile, midfoot-specific, locking and nonlocking plating options available for complicated naviculocuneiform fusions. It is the author's opinion that most naviculocuneiform fusions could still be done with screws and maybe the addition of a staple, and the plates should be reserved for difficult deformity corrections, situations where the added

stability and strength is preferable (diabetic feet) or if there are voids that need to be filled with graft that might delay healing. In this day and age, surgeons should be cognizant of the cost of implants and treatment and not overuse new expensive devices.

14. The wound is closed in layers, with the deep fascia being approximated over the fusion site. The subcutaneous tissue and skin are closed in a routine manner. Wounds along the medial border of the foot usually heal well.

Postoperative Care

A popliteal block is administered by anesthesia to control postoperative pain. If it is an isolated midfoot fusion, an ankle block can give equal pain relief and is easier for the patient to cope with. The postoperative dressing is changed in 10 to 14 days, sutures are removed, and the patient is placed into a short-leg removable boot with an elastic bandage to control swelling. Weight bearing is not permitted until 6 weeks after surgery. At 6 weeks after surgery, if radiographs demonstrate early union, the patient is permitted to bear weight as tolerated in a short-leg removable boot. As a general rule, the arthrodesis occurs after about 3 months. Patients should be advised not to go up on their toes for the first 3 months after surgery.

Complications

Nonunion of the naviculocuneiform joints does occur, but by including at least the first and second joints along with the internal fixation passing from the tubercle of the navicular into the cuneiforms, satisfactory union seems to occur in most cases.

Undercorrection is not uncommon in severe deformity. Before fixation, intraoperative radiographs should be done to confirm correction of the talo–first metatarsal angle on all planes.

Because of the proximity of the tibialis anterior tendon, it is occasionally damaged, and if so, should be repaired.

TARSOMETATARSAL ARTHRODESIS
(Video Clips 81-85)

Arthrodesis of the tarsometatarsal joints can involve an isolated joint, usually the second or third, or it can involve multiple joints, depending on the etiology of the arthrosis. As a general rule, patients with primary arthroses usually have fewer joints that require fusing than those with posttraumatic arthrosis.

The extent of the deformity is also variable. This depends on the number of joints involved and whether the deformity results from primary or traumatic arthrosis. The patient with primary arthrosis tends to have more pronation and a greater degree of deformity. Usually, if a single joint is involved, particularly the second or third, little or no deformity is present and therefore only an in situ fusion is necessary. If a deformity is present, however, realignment of the foot is essential to obtain a satisfactory result.

Determining the extent of the fusion site is sometimes difficult, particularly if it appears as though only one joint is involved. Besides a careful physical examination and radiographic studies consisting of weight-bearing radiographs, a CT scan or magnetic resonance image (MRI) or bone scan may be useful in determining the extent of the arthrosis and which joints should be included in the fusion mass. Even after careful physical and radiographic evaluation, if any doubt exists regarding the presence of arthrosis, the joint should be examined at surgery to be sure that arthritis is not being overlooked. Arthrosis may be seen at surgery when, even in retrospect, the radiograph appears to be normal. This is particularly true for the medial naviculocuneiform joint and the third metatarsocuneiform (MTC) joint. Although the most obvious arthrosis usually is present at the tarsometatarsal or intertarsal joints, the naviculocuneiform joints must always be carefully evaluated, particularly in the patient after trauma. If the naviculocuneiform joint does appear to be involved, at least the two medial joints should always be included in the fusion mass and, if necessary, the third. It is difficult to obtain an isolated fusion between the medial cuneiform and the navicular.

The question is often raised about whether the fourth and fifth metatarsocuboid articulations should be included in the fusion site or if they should undergo isolated fusion. As a general rule, the fourth and fifth metatarsocuboid articulations seem to be somewhat more forgiving and tend to be less symptomatic than the medial three MTC joints, despite the arthrosis. The reason may be that more flexibility exists in the two lateral rays than in the medial three rays. Motion also occurs between the third cuneiform and cuboid, which results in more motion of the two lateral rays of the foot. If clinical examination and radiographs show arthrosis at the fourth and fifth metatarsocuboid joints and a fusion is indicated, the cuboid should *not* be fused to the lateral cuneiform so that some mobility can be maintained between the medial and lateral aspects of the longitudinal arch. Not fusing the cuboid to the lateral cuneiform appears to give the foot a little more flexibility to adapt to the ground.[30] A valuable alternative to fusion of the fourth and fifth metatarsocuboid is an excision arthroplasty of the joint. It can give fairly reliable pain relief, while maintaining motion and the ability to adapt to the ground.

Indications

The main indication for arthrodesis of the tarsometatarsal joints is arthrosis resulting in pain, deformity, or both. The arthrodesis can include a single joint or multiple joints. The second most common reason for tarsometatarsal fusion is acute Lisfranc injuries, whether comminuted intraarticular fracture dislocation or completely unstable ligamentous injuries.[29,31]

Position of Arthrodesis

The arthrodesis site is positioned to correct any forefoot abduction or adduction or dorsiflexion. At times, a

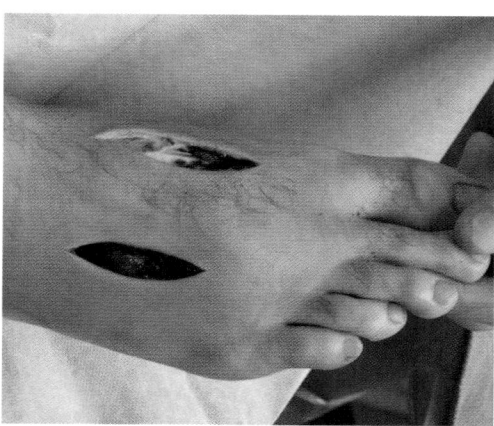

Figure 20-10 Skin incisions to expose the medial three tarsometatarsal joints.

complex deformity from trauma, particularly a crush injury, results in a deformity involving multiple planes, and it can be difficult to achieve a plantigrade foot. However, the surgeon should attempt to obtain a foot as close to plantigrade as possible.[32]

Surgical Technique
1. The patient is placed in the supine position, and a tourniquet is used about the thigh.
2. The surgical approach varies, depending on which joints are being arthrodesed. For an isolated first tarsometatarsal arthrodesis, a dorsomedial incision is used, centered over the joint. This allows satisfactory visualization of the joint as well as access to the dorsum of the foot to insert screws for internal fixation (Fig. 20-10).
3. For an isolated second MTC arthrodesis, the incision is made just lateral to the midportion of the joint. By placing the incision here, the neurovascular bundle is located medial to the incision. Subperiosteal dissection can safely mobilize and retract the neurovascular bundle medially.
4. The approach to the first, second, and third tarsometatarsal joints is carried out through two longitudinal incisions. The first is centered over the dorsomedial aspect of the first tarsometatarsal joint or possibly slightly toward the midline, compared with the isolated fusion. The second incision is made just to the lateral side of the second MTC joint. If the dorsal incision is not made sufficiently lateral, it is very difficult to visualize the third MTC joint. It is important to make long incisions to minimize traction on the skin edges (see Fig. 20-10).
5. The approach to the fourth and fifth metatarsocuboid articulations is through a dorsal incision centered between them, which provides adequate exposure.
6. When carrying out the surgical approach to the tarsometatarsal joints, the surgeon must be extremely cautious, looking for the superficial branches of the peroneal nerve that pass along the dorsum of the foot.

Along the medial aspect of the foot, the surgeon is usually working in an internervous interval, although occasionally the internal division of the superficial peroneal nerve may be encountered.
7. The approach to the second MTC joint is the most hazardous because the internal and external divisions of the superficial peroneal nerve lie in the subcutaneous tissue in a somewhat irregular pattern. As the surgeon proceeds deeper, the neurovascular bundle, containing the superficial branch of the deep peroneal nerve and dorsalis pedis artery, is encountered as the nerve and artery pass distally. The dorsalis pedis artery passes between the first and second metatarsals to the plantar aspect of the foot about 1 cm distal to the first tarsometatarsal joint. This is a common place for injury to the artery if care is not taken with dissection and retraction.
8. The incision over the fourth and fifth metatarsocuboid articulations tends to be in an internervous interval between the external division of the superficial peroneal nerve medially and the sural nerve laterally. Again, however, the nerve pattern varies greatly in this area, and nerve branches should be carefully identified and retracted.
9. When approaching tarsometatarsal joints one, two, and three, it is easier to start the subperiosteal dissection through the medial incision. From this incision, the surgeon identifies the skeletal plane and, with a sharp elevator, moves along this plane, stripping the soft tissues from the bone as far as the third MTC joint. This usually allows the surgeon to pass underneath the neurovascular bundle without causing damage to it. If the foot is severely distorted, however, this might not be safe, and the neurovascular bundle should be identified through the incision over the second MTC and carefully dissected off of the bone.
10. Once exposed, the involved joints are meticulously debrided with a curet, small osteotome, or rongeur. All the soft tissue and articular cartilage around the joints are removed, including the plantar aspects. The first tarsometatarsal joint is about 30 mm deep, and the plantar aspect can be difficult to debride without the help of a small lamina spreader.
11. In severe deformities, the first tarsometatarsal joint could be difficult to reduce, and it might be necessary to elevate part or the entire anterior tibial tendon of the cuneiform and metatarsal to remove bone prominences and allow adequate bone removal to facilitate reduction of the joint. In such a case, the anterior tibial tendon should be reattached to the metatarsal and cuneiform.
12. Once the joints are totally mobilized, it is always impressive how readily a deformity can be reduced. Occasionally, usually in the patient after trauma, some bone needs to be removed to create congruent surfaces for the fusion to occur.
13. After the joint surfaces have been debrided, the foot is realigned by first placing the first MTC joint into a

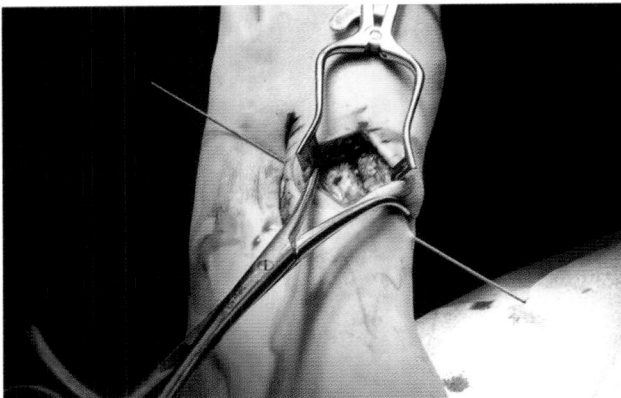

Figure 20-11 Once the tarsometatarsal joints are prepared, a reduction forceps is used to reduce and compress the joint before inserting a guide pin for a cannulated screw. In this case, the guide pin goes from the medial cuneiform into the second metatarsal.

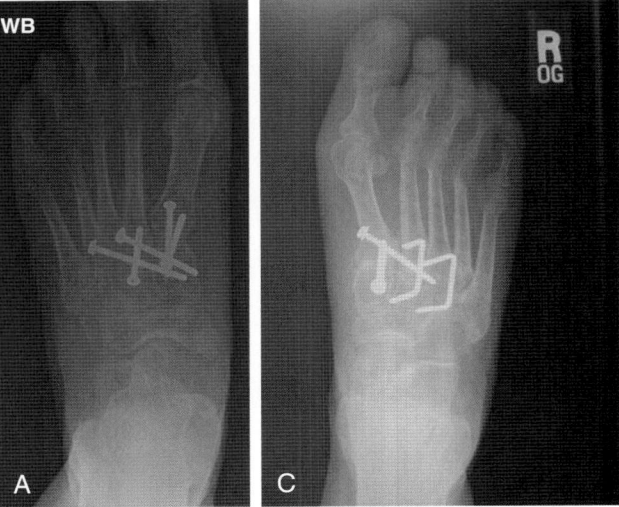

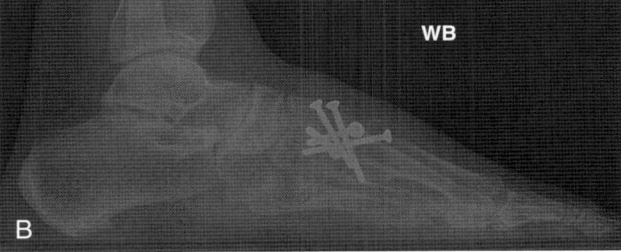

Figure 20-12 **A** and **B,** Tarsometatarsal arthrodesis with compression screws. This method gives excellent internal fixation for in situ fusion. **C,** In soft bone, or if the angle of insertion is too acute, a staple could be used instead of a screw over the second and third tarsaometatarsal joints. *WB,* weight-bearing.

plantigrade position. To help assess alignment (in particular abduction/adduction), the surgeon should always observe the normal foot before the procedure and relate it either to the alignment of the patella or to the medial side of the talus and hindfoot. As a general rule, when a deformity is present at the first MTC joint, it is usually abduction and dorsiflexion. Therefore the first metatarsal is usually manipulated into some adduction and plantar flexion. If the alignment appears correct and good bone apposition is present, the bone ends are feathered and the anticipated fusion site stabilized with the guide pin from the 4.0-mm cannulated screw set, or if solid screws are used, a temporary K-wire. If the apposition is not satisfactory, some bone is removed, feathered, and pinned (Fig. 20-11).

14. The alignment is carefully checked again, and if it is satisfactory, internal fixation can be inserted.

15. Once the first MTC joint is aligned and stabilized, the other metatarsal bases are brought over to it, which effectively realigns the deformity. The second metatarsal is adducted so that it comes to lie next to the first and then is slightly plantar flexed. As the metatarsal is plantar flexed, the surgeon palpates the first metatarsal head to be sure that the degree of plantar flexion of the second metatarsal head is not excessive. The cuneiforms usually are not very deformed and tend to fall into place as the metatarsals are manipulated into a plantigrade position.

16. If the third MTC joint is to be arthrodesed, it is aligned next in relation to the second, and in this way, the deformity is corrected (Fig. 20-12A and B).

17. The fourth and fifth MTC joints are seldom fused, but if needed, as mentioned previously, an attempt is made to carry out the fusion only to the cuboid. The surgeon must be careful not to fuse the third cuneiform–cuboid articulation.

18. The internal fixation can be carried out in many ways, but the author's group prefers to use 3.5-mm solid or 4.0-mm cannulated screws with a small head. Because the skin is thin in this area, the low-profile heads can usually be buried, so they do not require removal.

19. The first MTC joint is fixed by inserting one screw from the dorsal aspect of the first metatarsal into the medial cuneiform, after which a second screw is placed from the dorsal aspect of the medial cuneiform into the base of the first metatarsal. This gives rather rigid internal fixation to the joint. As the screws are inserted, the joint surfaces are compressed with a towel clip (see Fig. 20-11).

20. The second MTC joint is fixed by placing a long oblique screw, starting in the metatarsal, and passing it proximally across the joint into the cuneiform. The angle that this pin makes with the second metatarsal is extremely acute and at times is difficult to start because the guide pin tends to slide along the metatarsal proximally. This can sometimes be overcome by making a small vertical drill hole to identify where to start the guide pin, which is usually about 2 cm distal to the joint. The guide pin usually catches on this edge of bone and does not tend to slide up the metatarsal.

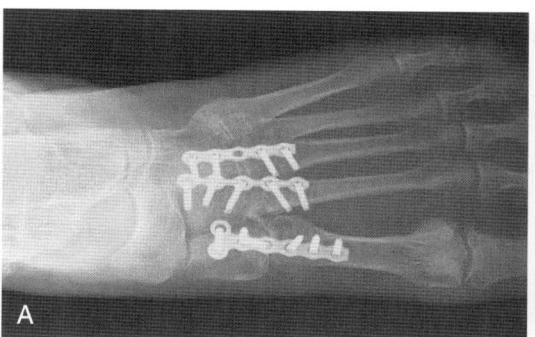
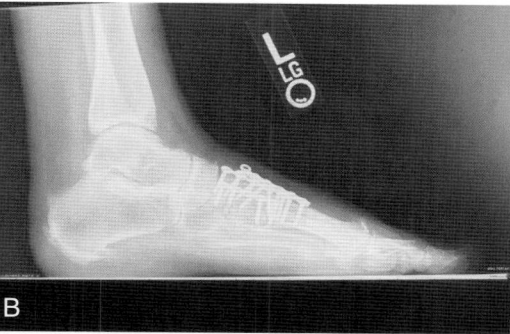
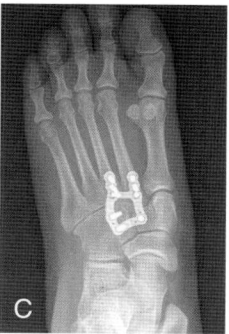

Figure 20-13 **A** and **B,** AP and lateral view in which individual plates were used over each of the medial three tarsometatarsal joints. **C,** Plate construct in which a single plate is used to fuse the second and third tarsometatarsal joints.

If this screw is not placed obliquely enough, it will not engage the cuneiform adequately, and rigid fixation will not be achieved.

21. Once the guide pin is in satisfactory position, the metatarsal is drilled with the 4.0-mm bit. The hole is countersunk to lower the profile of the head and prevent the screw head from impinging against the metatarsal when it is seated, which can fracture the dorsal portion of the metatarsal.

22. It is sometimes necessary to place the screw from the cuneiform to the metatarsal, and the same issues with the acute angle are present. In cases where it is felt the fixation is inadequate, a compression staple could be added or used as the primary fixation (Fig. 20-12C).

23. The third MTC joint is fixed in a manner similar to the second. Occasionally, the screw is placed from the lateral aspect of the base of the metatarsal obliquely into the third or occasionally the second cuneiform. A staple could be a simpler form of fixation as well.

24. In osteopenic bone, or correction of severe deformities, any combination of locking or nonlocking plates should be used to aid in the stability of the repair and thereby increase the chances of success (Fig. 20-13A-C). There are multiple systems available, each with their own pitfalls but also unique features.[28]

25. It is not always necessary to include the intercuneiform joints in the fusion. In fact, because of the shape of the intercuneiform spaces, it could be hard to fuse unless bone graft is placed. However, if there is arthrosis or instability at the intercuneiform joints, screws should be placed after preparation of the joints. A screw is placed mediolaterally across the cuneiforms to stabilize them. Another screw is then placed from the medial aspect of the first metatarsal base obliquely into the cuneiforms. This screw may also cross the second MTC joint. This screw helps to reinforce the fusion mass and ensure that rigid fixation is achieved.

26. When the naviculocuneiform joints are included in the fusion mass, a screw can be passed from the tip of the navicular into the cuneiforms, which usually provides excellent internal fixation. If the naviculocuneiform joints are to be included in the fusion site, it is imperative that at least the first and second cuneiforms be involved because an isolated fusion of the medial cuneiform and the navicular is difficult to achieve. Screws can also be placed from the cuneiforms into the navicular (Fig. 20-14A-F).

27. There will be instances with high-energy trauma where simple screw and or staple fixation will not suffice. In complex fracture dislocation of the Lisfranc joints, the surgeon should use adequate fixation to treat the fractures as well as achieve stabilization of the joints. There are several midfoot-specific plating systems available for this. The approach and management is the same, but the construct is usually initially fixed with K-wires to allow easier placement of the plate (Fig. 20-15A-E).

28. Fixation of the metatarsocuboid joint is usually achieved by placing a screw from the dorsal aspect of the fourth metatarsal into the cuboid. The fixation of the fifth metatarsocuboid joint is more difficult because the actual articulating surface is quite small. An oblique guide pin may be placed percutaneously from the lateral aspect of the metatarsal base into the cuboid and a screw inserted over it.

29. Proliferative bone over the dorsal aspect of the MTC joints is removed, morselized, and packed into any existing spaces in the fusion site. If the surgeon is not satisfied with the apposition of the bone surfaces, a bone graft, generally from the calcaneus or medial malleolus, can be used.

30. When correcting a long-standing collapsed midfoot, the surgeon should be cognizant that there could be an equinus contracture. If there is a gastrocnemius contracture after the midfoot is reduced, a Strayer lengthening should be done. It will not only increase dorsiflexion but also help to reduce the forces over the fusion sight.

31. The skin closure is very important in these cases. The skin is very fragile, and when multiple joints are arthrodesed, moderate swelling can occur.

32. The subcutaneous tissue is closed with 3-0 plain sutures and the skin with a running longitudinal near-far/far-near suture, which keeps tension off the skin edges.

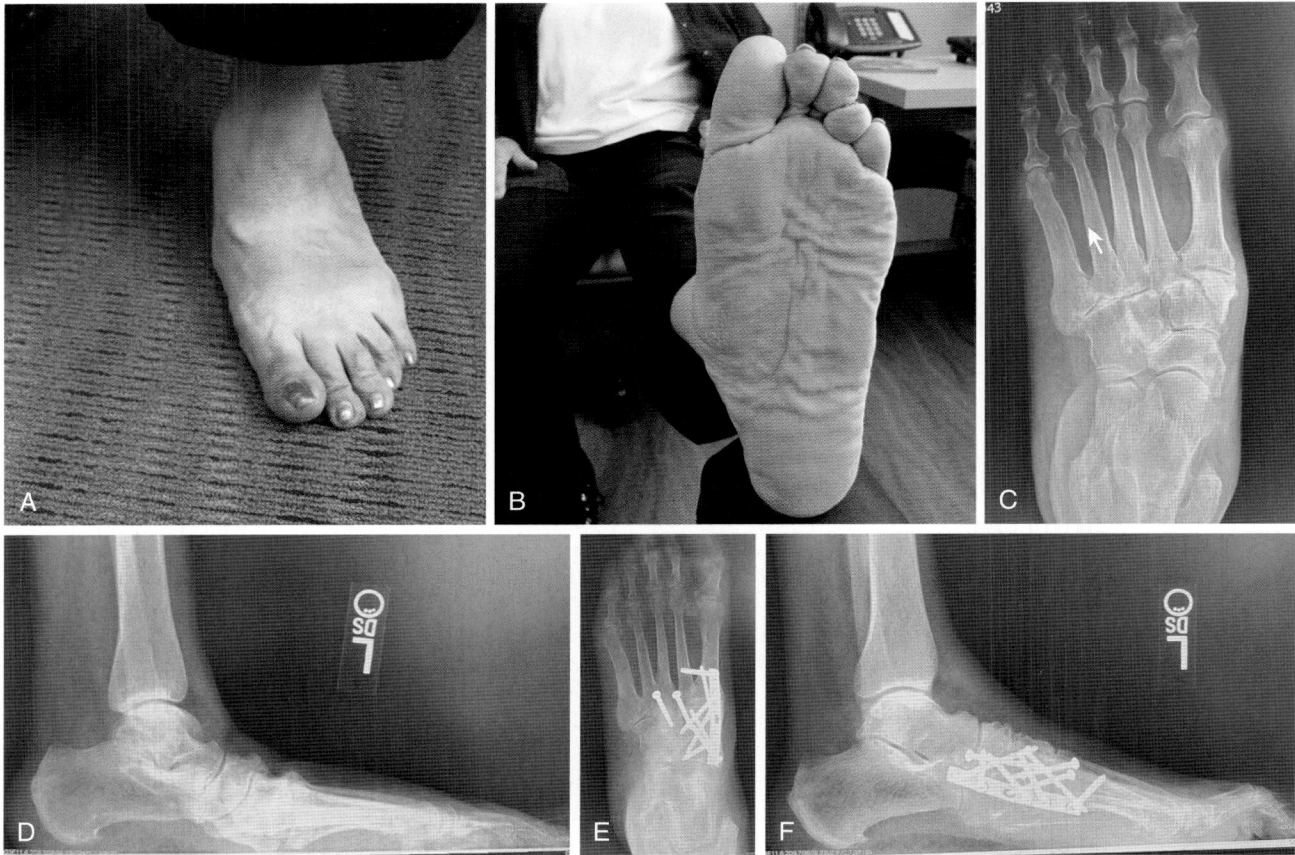

Figure 20-14 **A** and **B,** Clinical pictures of a severely collapsed midfoot with loss of the medial arch. **C** and **D,** Anteroposterior and lateral views of the same patient showing severe multijoint arthroses. **E** and **F,** Midfoot arthrodesis of multiple joints. Note that the screw pattern locks navicular to the cuneiforms; also note the intercuneiform screws. A medial plate added stability to the construct. If the tarsometatarsal joints are not involved, the arthrodesis does not need to include them.

Postoperative Care

A preoperative ankle or popliteal block is very helpful to control postoperative pain. A light compression dressing, adequate padding, and a cast splint is applied.

The patient is kept non–weight bearing or heel-only weight bearing in the postoperative cast for approximately 12 to 14 days, after which the cast is removed and the patient placed into a short-leg removable cast with an elastic bandage to control swelling. The patient is keep non–weight bearing or heel-only weight bearing for 6 weeks. At 6 weeks, radiographs are obtained, and if early union is occurring, weight bearing is permitted in the cast for another 6 weeks. Twelve weeks after surgery, radiographs are again obtained, and if satisfactory union has occurred, the patient is gradually permitted to work out of the removable cast and into a shoe. An elastic stocking is used to control swelling.

Complications

The three main complications that can occur after tarsometatarsal arthrodesis are nonunion, failure to correct a malalignment, and skin slough.

A *nonunion* of an attempted fusion site can occur, although infrequently. With meticulous preparation of the bone surfaces and rigid internal fixation, the tarsometatarsal joints have a high fusion rate. If a nonunion occurs and is symptomatic, the fibrous tissue around the involved joint needs to be excised, the bone surfaces once again scaled, the joint bone grafted if necessary, and internal fixation reapplied.

Malalignment of the foot can be a problem. The deformity usually present preoperatively is abduction and dorsiflexion, which results in a large prominence on the plantar-medial aspect of the foot in the area of the first tarsometatarsal joint. If the forefoot is not reduced by bringing the first metatarsal into adduction and plantar flexion, this prominence remains and might continue to be a source of pain for the patient. With adequate reduction, this prominence does not strike the ground, which usually provides relief for the patient. Occasionally, malalignment of a metatarsal occurs by placing it into too much dorsiflexion or plantar flexion, which can be corrected with an osteotomy and internal fixation if necessary.

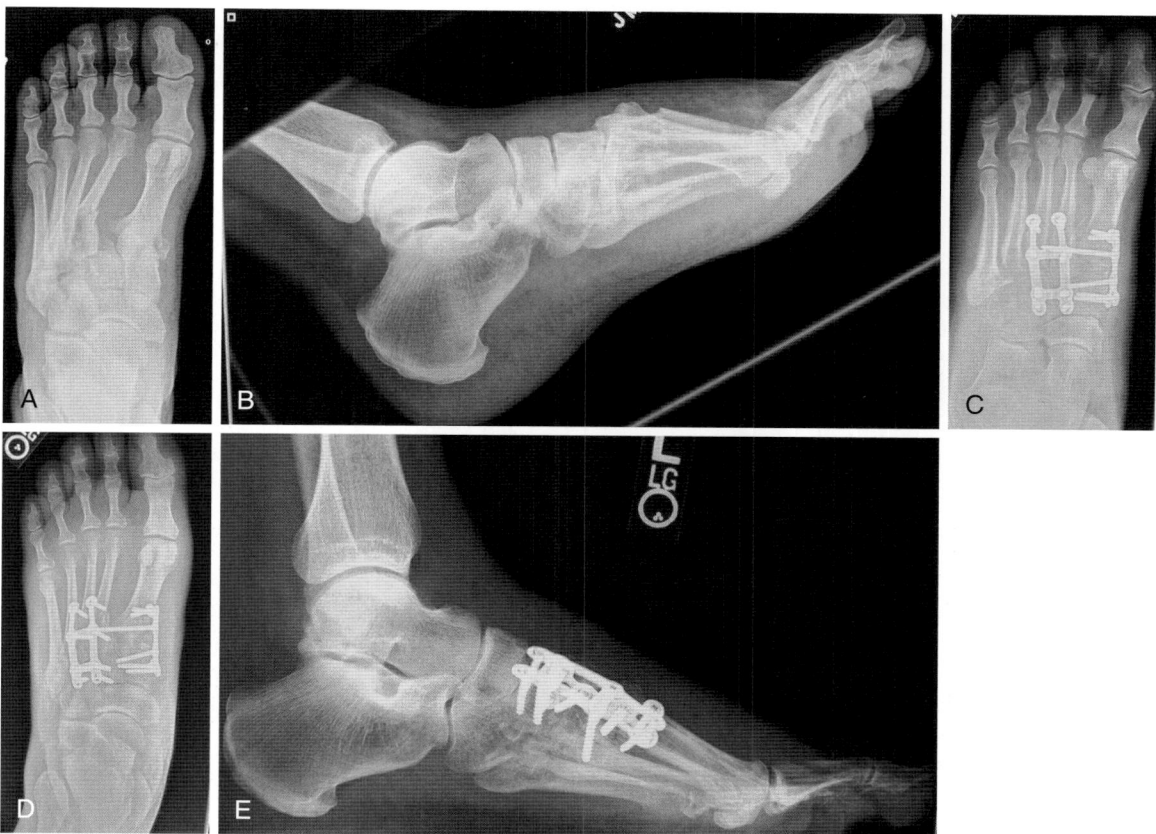

Figure 20-15 Preoperative (**A** and **B**) and postoperative (**D-F**) radiographs demonstrate arthrodesis of tarsometatarsal joints one, two, and three after a severe fracture dislocation. Note the correction of deformity in both the anteroposterior and lateral planes. Because of the complexity and comminution of the fractures, a screw construct was not applicable.

The skin on the dorsum of the foot often has little subcutaneous fat. Combined with postoperative swelling and multiple incisions, this can lead to a *skin slough*. Therefore meticulous care must be taken at surgery to obtain a good subcutaneous closure, followed by a skin closure, with a minimum amount of tension along the skin edge. The author prefers a running, horizontal mattress suture that keeps the tension off the skin edges as much as possible. If a slough occurs, local wound care usually is adequate to resolve the problem, but sometimes a skin graft or even a flap is necessary. If the slough is not too large, wound-VAC may be useful.

A *neuroma*, particularly on the dorsum of the foot, can also occur from entrapment or laceration of one of the sensory nerves on the dorsum. Usually, a small branch is involved, and although annoying to the patient, it usually is not a major problem. Occasionally, if one of the larger branches of a superficial peroneal nerve is cut, a large, painful neuroma develops and is aggravated by footwear. If this occurs and is symptomatic, the neuroma should be identified and buried either underneath the extensor digitorum brevis muscle or into a hole in the bone. The dorsum of the foot being so devoid of fatty tissue in some patients sometimes makes it difficult to bury the nerve's cut end adequately.

Author's Experience

Midfoot arthrodesis can be challenging, especially in the neglected, long-standing, rigid and severe deformities. Meticulous attention to detail is required to correct the deformities in all planes, and adequate fixation is required. The author's technique has changed over time, that is, by tending to use more fixation than before. The advent of midfoot-specific plating systems added needed choices to fixation options, but as mentioned before, simple screw fixation is still the mainstay of treatment. The union and satisfaction rate is predictably high with midfoot fusions. The fact that there is minimal movement in the midfoot joints, especially the medial column, probably contributes to sense that there is very little functional loss with a fusion.

REFERENCES
Subtalar Arthrodesis

1. Albert A, Deleu PA, Leemrijse T, Maldague P, Devos Bevernage B: Posterior arthroscopic subtalar arthrodesis: ten cases at one-year follow-up, *Orthop Traumatol Surg Res* 97:401–405, 2011.
2. Betz M, Wieser K, Vich M, Wirth SH, Espinosa N: Precision of targeting device for subtalar screw placement, *Foot Ankle Int* 33:519–523, 2012.

3. Coughlin MJ, Grimes JS, Traughber PD, Jones CP: Comparison of radiographs and CT scans in the prospective evaluation of the fusion of hindfoot arthrodesis, *Foot Ankle Int* 27:780–787, 2006.

4. Easley ME, Trnka HJ, Schon LC, Myerson MS: Isolated subtalar arthrodesis, *J Bone Joint Surg Am* 82:613–624, 2000.

5. Hungerer S, Trapp O, Augat P, Bühren V: Posttraumatic arthrodesis of the subtalar joint—outcome in workers compensation and rates of non-union, *Foot Ankle Surg* 17:277–283, 2011.

6. Mann RA, Beaman DN, Horton G: Isolated subtalar arthrodesis, *Foot Ankle Int* 19:511–519, 1998.

7. Muraro GM, Carvajal PF: Arthroscopic arthodesis of subtalar joint, *Foot Ankle Clin* 16:83–90, 2011.

8. Thaunat M, Bajard X, Boisrenoult P, et al: Computer tomography assessment of the fusion rate after posterior arthroscopic subtalar arthrodesis, *Int Orthop* 36:1005–1010, 2012.

Talonavicular Arthrodesis

9. Astion DJ, Deland JT, Otis JC, Kenneally S: Motion of the hindfoot after simulated arthrodesis, *J Bone Joint Surg Am* 79:241–246, 1997.

10. Barg A, Brunner S, Zwicky L, Hintermann B: Subtalar and naviculocuneiform fusion for extended breakdown of the medial arch, *Foot Ankle Clin* 16:69–81, 2011.

11. Chen CH, Huang PJ, Chen TB, et al: Isolated talonavicular arthrodesis for talonavicular arthritis, *Foot Ankle Int* 22:633–636, 2001.

12. Crevoisier X: The isolated talonavicular arthrodesis, *Foot Ankle Clin* 16:49–59, 2011.

13. Elftman H: The transverse tarsal joint and its control, *Clin Orthop Relat Res* 16:41, 1960.

14. Yu G, Zhao Y, Zhou J, Zhang M: Fusion of talonavicular and naviculocuneiform joints for the treatment of Müller-Weiss disease, *J Foot Ankle Surg* 51:415–419, 2012.

Double Arthrodesis

15. DuVries HL: *Surgery of the foot*, St Louis, 1959, Mosby, p 300.

16. Mann RA, Beaman DN: Double arthrodesis for posterior tibial tendon dysfunction, *Clin Orthop Relat Res* 365:74–80, 1999.

17. Thelen S, Rütt J, Wild M, et al: The influence of talonavicular versus double arthrodesis on load dependent motion of the midtarsal joint, *Arch Orthop Trauma Surg* 130:47–53, 2010.

Triple Arthrodesis

18. Astion DJ, Deland JT, Otis JC, Kenneally S: Motion of the hindfoot after simulated arthrodesis, *J Bone Joint Surg Am* 79:241–246, 1997.

19. Banerjee R, Saltzman C, Anderson RB, Nickisch F: Management of calcaneal malunion, *J Am Acad Orthop Surg* 19:27–36, 2011.

20. Betz M, Wieser K, Vich M, et al: Precision of targeting device for subtalar screw placement, *Foot Ankle Int* 33:519–523, 2012.

21. Graves SC, Mann RA, Graves KO: Triple arthrodesis in older adults: results after long-term follow-up, *J Bone Joint Surg Am* 75:355–362, 1993.

22. Jeng CL, Vora AM, Myerson MS: The medial approach to triple arthrodesis. Indications and technique for management of rigid valgus deformities in high-risk patients, *Foot Ankle Clin* 10:515–521, 2005.

23. Knupp M, Stufkens SA, Hintermann B: Triple arthrodesis, *Foot Ankle Clin* 16:61–67, 2011.

24. Philippot R, Wegrzyn J, Besse JL: Arthrodesis of the subtalar and talonavicular joints through a medial surgical approach: a series of 15 cases, *Arch Orthop Trauma Surg* 130:599–603, 2010.

25. Saltzman CL, Fehrle MJ, Cooper RR, et al: Triple arthrodesis: twenty-five and forty-four-year average follow-up of the same patients, *J Bone Joint Surg Am* 81:1391–1402, 1999.

26. Sammarco VJ, Magur EG, Sammarco GJ, Bagwe MR: Arthrodesis of the subtalar and talonavicular joints for correction of symptomatic hindfoot malalignment, *Foot Ankle Int* 27:661–666, 2006.

27. Smith RW, Shen W, DeWitt S, Reischl SF: Triple arthrodesis in adults with non-paralytic disease, *J Bone Joint Surg Am* 86:2707–2713, 2004

Tarsometatarsal Arthrodesis

28. Filippi J, Myerson MS, Scioli MW, et al: Midfoot arthrodesis following multi-joint stabilization with a novel hybrid plating system, *Foot Ankle Int* 33:220–225, 2012.

29. Ly TV, Coetzee JC: Treatment of primarily ligamentous Lisfranc joint injuries: primary arthrodesis compared with open reduction and internal fixation. A prospective, randomized study, *J Bone Joint Surg Am* 88:514–520, 2006.

30. Raikin SM, Schon LC: Arthrodesis of the fourth and fifth tarsometatarsal joints of the midfoot, *Foot Ankle Int* 24:584–590, 2003.

31. Sangeorzan BJ, Veith RG, Hansen ST Jr: Salvage of Lisfranc's tarsometatarsal joint by arthrodesis, *Foot Ankle* 10:193–200, 1990.

32. Zonno AJ, Myerson MS: Surgical correction of midfoot arthritis with and without deformity, *Foot Ankle Clin* 16:35–47, 2011.

Ankle Arthritis

Brad D. Blankenhorn, Charles L. Saltzman

Advances in the understanding of the special features of the ankle joint and the pathogenesis of degenerative joint disease have led to new approaches in the treatment of ankle arthritis. Compared with the other major lower extremity joints, the ankle joint possesses unique epidemiologic, anatomic, biomechanical, and biologic characteristics.

Unlike the hip and knee, which are prone to develop primary osteoarthritis, the ankle develops arthritis usually because of a traumatic event. Ankle articular cartilage has characteristic differences from hip or knee cartilage that might protect the ankle against developing primary osteoarthritis. Ankle articular cartilage preserves its tensile stiffness and fracture stress better than hip articular cartilage. Metabolic differences between knee and ankle articular cartilage can also help to explain the relative rarity of primary ankle osteoarthritis.

In developed nations, physicians have noted a progressive increase in the incidence of disabling ankle arthritis, which may in part be due to the combined effects of the widespread use of life-protecting thoracoabdominal level airbag restraints and the general aging of the population.[12] The increased incidence of painful posttraumatic ankle osteoarthritis has spurred interest in finding therapeutic solutions to this often disabling condition.

UNIQUE CHARACTERISTICS OF THE ANKLE JOINT

The differences in anatomy and motion between the ankle joint and the other major joints of the lower limb are readily apparent. Other differences, such as the area of contact between opposing articular surfaces and articular cartilage thickness, tensile properties, and metabolism, are less apparent. Taken together, the unique mechanical and biologic characteristics of the ankle affect the development, clinical presentation, and course of arthritis.

Anatomy and Motion

The bony anatomy of the ankle joint determines the planes and ranges of joint motion and confers a high degree of stability and congruence when the joint is loaded. The three bones that form the ankle joint—the tibia, fibula, and talus—support three sets of opposing articular surfaces. The tibial medial malleolus and the medial facet of the talus form the medial articular surfaces, the fibular lateral malleolus and the talar lateral articular surface form the lateral articular surfaces, and the

Figure 21-1 Ankle joint structure. **A,** The drawing shows how the talus fits in the mortise formed by the distal ends of the fibula and tibia. The medial malleolus and the medial surface of the talus form the opposing medial articular surfaces, the distal tibia and the superior talus form the opposing central articular surfaces, and the lateral malleolus and the lateral surface of the talus form the opposing lateral articular surfaces. Notice how the convexity of the distal tibial articular surface matches the concavity of the superior talar articular surface. The center of the matching convexity and concavity is used to divide the joint into medial and lateral compartments for the study of joint loading and joint degeneration. **B,** Standing radiograph of the ankle joint showing the features outlined in the drawing.

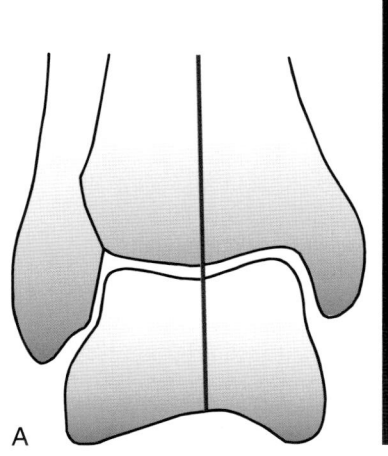

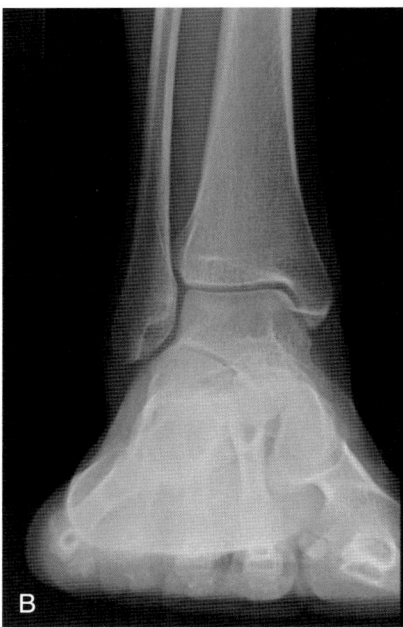

A

B

distal tibia and the superior dome of the talus form the central articular surfaces (Fig. 21-1).

The distal tibial articular surface has a longitudinal convexity that matches a concavity on the surface of the talus. The center of matching convexity and concavity divides the tibiotalar articulation into the medial and lateral compartments for evaluation of ankle loading and degenerative changes (see Fig. 21-1). The distal tibia and the medial malleolus, together with the lateral malleolus, form the ankle mortise, which contains the talus. Firm anterior and posterior ligaments bind the distal tibia and fibula together to form the distal tibiofibular syndesmosis. Medial and lateral ligamentous complexes and the ankle joint capsule stabilize the relationship between the talus and the mortise.

The bony anatomy, ligaments, and joint capsule guide and restrain movement between the talus and the mortise so that the talus has a continuously changing axis of rotation as it moves from maximum dorsiflexion to maximum plantar flexion relative to the mortise. The talus and mortise widen slightly from posterior to anterior. Thus when the talus is plantar flexed, its narrowest portion sits in the ankle mortise and allows rotatory movement between the talus and mortise. When the talus is maximally dorsiflexed, the tibiofibular syndesmosis spreads, and the wider portion of the talar articular surface locks into the ankle mortise, allowing little or no rotation between the talus and the mortise. In most normal ankles, the soft tissue structures, including joint capsule, ligaments, and muscle tendon units that cross the joint, prevent significant translation of the talus relative to the mortise.

Articular Surface Contact Area

When loaded, the human ankle joint has a smaller area of contact between the opposing articular surfaces than the knee or hip. At 500 N of load, the contact area averages 350 mm^2 for the ankle joint,[7,57] compared with 1120 mm^2 for the knee[48] and 1100 mm^2 for the hip.[9] Although in vivo contact stress has not been measured in the ankle, the smaller contact area must make the normal peak contact stress higher in the ankle than in the knee or hip.

Articular Cartilage Thickness and Tensile Properties

Ankle joint articular cartilage differs from that of the knee and hip in thickness and tensile properties. The thickness of ankle articular cartilage ranges from less than 1 mm to slightly less than 2 mm.[6] In contrast, some regions of articular cartilage in the hip or knee are more than 6 mm thick, and in most load-bearing areas, it is at least 3 mm thick.[5]

Work by Kempson[54] shows that the tensile properties of ankle and hip articular cartilage differ and that these differences increase with age (Figs. 21-2 and 21-3). In particular, the tensile fracture stress and tensile stiffness of ankle articular cartilage deteriorate less rapidly with age than those of the hip.[54] The tensile fracture stress of hip femoral articular cartilage is initially greater than that of talar articular cartilage. However, with age it declines exponentially in the hip but linearly in the ankle (see Fig. 21-2). As a result of these aging differences, ankle articular cartilage can withstand greater tensile loads than hip articular cartilage, beginning in middle age, and this

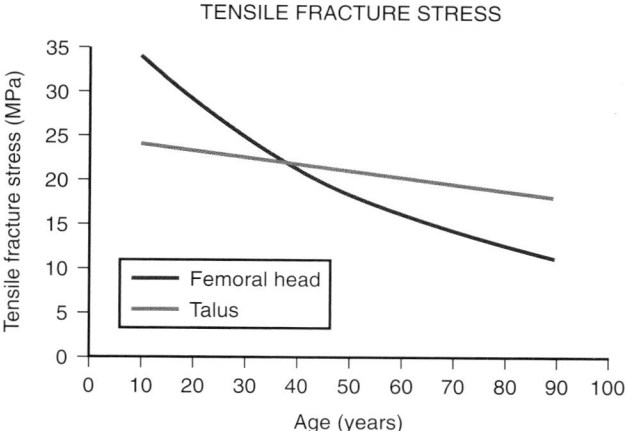

Figure 21-2 Femoral head and talus articular cartilage superficial layer tensile fracture stress versus age. Notice that the tensile fracture stress of ankle articular cartilage is greater beginning in middle age than the tensile fracture stress of femoral head articular cartilage and that the difference increases with increasing age. This illustration was developed from data reported by Kempson.[54] (Graph courtesy Joseph A. Buckwalter, MD.)

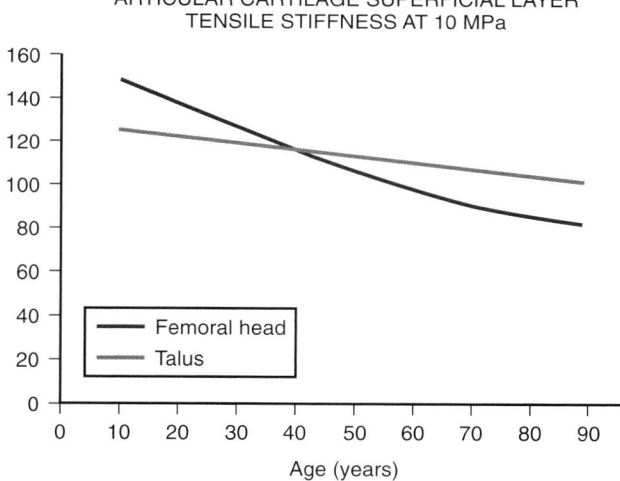

Figure 21-3 Femoral head and talus articular cartilage superficial layer tensile stiffness versus age. Notice that the tensile stiffness of ankle articular cartilage is greater beginning in middle age than the tensile fracture stress of femoral head articular cartilage and that the difference increases with increasing age. This illustration was developed from data reported by Kempson.[54] MPa, megapascals. (Graph courtesy Joseph A. Buckwalter, MD.)

difference increases with increasing age. Age-related changes in hip and ankle articular cartilage tensile stiffness follow a similar pattern (see Fig. 21-3).

Presumably, age-related declines in articular cartilage tensile properties result from progressive weakening of the collagen fibril network in articular cartilage. The cause of the age-related weakening of the articular cartilage

matrix has not been explained, but age-related changes in collagen fibril structure and collagen cross-linking have been identified that might contribute to changes in matrix tensile properties.[11,13] Kempson[54] has suggested that these differences in tensile properties might explain the apparent vulnerability of the hip and knee to degenerative changes with increasing age and the relative resistance of the ankle to development of primary osteoarthritis.

Articular Cartilage Metabolism

Ankle articular cartilage can differ from that of other joints in the expression of an enzyme that can degrade articular cartilage and in response to the catabolic cytokine interleukin-1 (IL-1). Chubinskaya and colleagues[15] detected messenger ribonucleic acid (RNA) for neutrophil collagenase (matrix metalloproteinase-8 [MMP-8]) in chondrocytes of human knee articular cartilage but not in those of ankle articular cartilage. IL-1 inhibited proteoglycan synthesis by chondrocytes in knee articular cartilage more effectively than in those of ankle articular cartilage.[47] The difference in the response to IL-1 between chondrocytes in knee and ankle articular cartilage appears to be due to a greater number of IL-1 receptors in the chondrocytes of knee articular cartilage. These observations need further study, but they suggest that metabolic differences exist between knee and ankle articular cartilage, which might help to explain the relative rarity of primary ankle osteoarthritis.

PREVALENCE OF ANKLE OSTEOARTHRITIS

Determining the prevalence of ankle osteoarthritis is more difficult than it might seem at first. As in other joints, the correlation between degenerative changes in the joint and the clinical syndrome of osteoarthritis is not consistent.[28,106] In addition, it is extremely expensive and difficult to obtain and study unbiased samples of populations to determine the prevalence of osteoarthritis. For these reasons, studies of the prevalence of osteoarthritis by examination of autopsy specimens, evaluation of radiographs of populations of patients, and evaluation of patients presenting with symptomatic osteoarthritis have significant limitations.

Autopsy Studies

Despite their limitations, including relatively small numbers of joints examined and lack of random or systematic sampling of populations, autopsy studies can provide useful information concerning differences in prevalence of degeneration among joints.

Meachim et al[66-69] examined knee, shoulder, and ankle joints at autopsies performed on adults. They found full-thickness chondral defects in 1 of 20 ankle joints from people older than 70 years.[66] Cartilage fibrillation was much more frequent than full-thickness defects in all joints.

Huch et al[47] resected 36 knees and 78 ankles from both limbs of 39 organ donors to evaluate the prevalence of ankle osteoarthritis. The joints were evaluated using a scale described by Collins.[19] Grade 0 is normal gross appearance of a joint, grade 1 is fraying or fibrillation of the articular cartilage, grade 2 is fibrillation and fissuring of the cartilage and osteophytes, grade 3 is extensive fibrillation and fissuring with frequent osteophytes and 30% or less full-thickness chondral defects, and grade 4 is frequent osteophytes and greater than 30% full-thickness chondral defects. In these studies, grades 3 and 4 were defined as osteoarthritis, and grade 2 was defined as early osteoarthritis.[47] However, the authors did not have information concerning possible symptoms associated with the joints studied, so it is not certain if the degenerative changes they identified were associated with clinical osteoarthritis. Using the Collins grading scale, Huch's group found grade 3 and 4 degenerative changes in 5 of 78 (6%) ankle joints and in 9 of 36 (25%) knee joints (Fig. 21-4). Degenerative changes were most commonly found on the medial aspect of the ankle.

In another series of investigations, Muehlman et al[74] examined seven joints, including the knee and ankle of both lower legs in 50 cadavers. The cadavers studied ranged in age from 36 to 94 years, with a mean age of 76 years. Sixty-six percent of the knee joints had grade 3 and 4 degenerative changes compared with 18% of the ankle joints (see Fig. 21-4). Ninety-five percent of the knees had grade 2, 3, or 4 degenerative changes compared with 76%

of the ankles. The authors also observed that the medial compartments of both the knees and the ankles were more commonly involved than the lateral compartments. Radiographs often showed no evidence of degenerative changes, although direct examination of the joints showed regions of full-thickness cartilage erosion. Overall, the autopsy studies demonstrate that advanced degenerative changes are at least three times more prevalent in the knee than in the ankle and that the prevalence of degenerative changes in both joints increases with increasing age (see Fig. 21-4).

Radiographic Evaluations

Although epidemiologic studies based on radiographic evaluations document a striking increase with increasing age in the prevalence of degenerative changes of all joints, including those of the foot and ankle, the reported studies have not focused on ankle osteoarthritis. Radiographic studies of ankle joint degeneration have important limitations because there is no strong correlation between formation of osteophytes and development of clinical osteoarthritis[106] and because it is difficult to evaluate the thickness of ankle articular cartilage, particularly on radiographs that were not performed in a standardized fashion. Furthermore, ankle radiographs often do not show signs of joint degeneration even when the ankle joint has regions of full-thickness erosion of articular cartilage.[74] Attempts to evaluate the prevalence of ankle degeneration and osteoarthritis by plain radiographs alone therefore have limited value.

Clinical Studies

Very few studies of the prevalence of osteoarthritis have included patients with ankle osteoarthritis. The available information suggests that knee osteoarthritis is 8 to 10 times more common than ankle osteoarthritis.[22,47] Yet the best currently available estimates suggest that knee replacements are performed more often than ankle replacements and ankle fusions combined. These observations, combined with the data from autopsy studies showing that advanced knee joint degeneration is about three to five times more common than advanced ankle joint degeneration, suggest that surgical procedures are performed less often for patients with advanced ankle osteoarthritis than for those with advanced osteoarthritis of the knee.

The reasons for this are unclear. It is possible that joint degeneration and osteoarthritis cause less severe pain and functional limitation in the ankle than in the knee. Lack of understanding of the evaluation and treatment of ankle osteoarthritis among physicians, the efficacy of nonsurgical treatments for ankle osteoarthritis, and the lack of effective and widely accepted surgical treatments for ankle osteoarthritis can also explain the apparent difference in the frequency of surgical treatment of ankle and knee osteoarthritis.

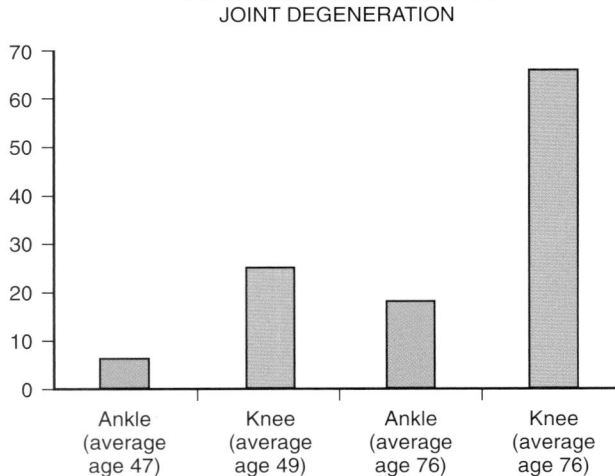

PREVALENCE OF ANKLE AND KNEE
JOINT DEGENERATION

Figure 21-4 Histogram showing the prevalence of ankle joint degeneration in autopsy studies reported by Huch and colleagues[47] and Muehlman and colleagues.[54] In these studies, the criteria for joint degeneration (osteoarthritis) were extensive articular cartilage fibrillation, osteophytes, and regions of full-thickness cartilage loss (Collins grades 3 and 4). Notice that joint degeneration was more than three times as common in the knee as in the ankle and that the prevalence of joint degeneration in the knee and the ankle increased with age. (Histogram courtesy Joseph A. Buckwalter, MD.)

PATHOGENESIS OF ANKLE OSTEOARTHRITIS

Clinical experience and published reports of the treatment of ankle osteoarthritis indicate that primary ankle osteoarthritis is rare and that posttraumatic arthritis, which develops after ankle fractures or ligamentous injury, is the most common cause of ankle osteoarthritis.[26,44,91,94,110] Over a 13-year period in the senior author's practice, 445 of 639 patients (70%) with Kellgren-Lawrence grade 3 and 4 ankle arthritis were posttraumatic cases, and only 46 (7.2%) had primary arthritis (Table 21-1).[91] The most common causes of posttraumatic arthritis were rotational ankle fractures (37%) and recurrent ankle instability (15%) (Table 21-2). Curiously, 61 patients in this group gave a history of a single major ankle sprain that never healed completely. Of the 46 patients who were classified as having primary ankle osteoarthritis, 23 (59%) had clinically significant hindfoot malalignment, which emphasizes the intrinsic resistance of the ankle joint to primary articular degeneration and the relative rarity of primary osteoarthritis of the ankle (Table 21-3).

In a similar study, Valderrabano et al[105] reviewed the etiology of symptomatic end-stage ankle arthritis for patients presenting to their clinic over a 10-year period. The results of their study were similar to ours in that they also showed that posttraumatic arthritis was the most common cause of end-stage ankle arthritis (78%). These authors also found that malleolar ankle fractures were the most common cause of posttraumatic arthritis (39%), followed by ligamentous injuries (16%) and pilon fractures (14%). Arthritis secondary to other causes was present in 13% of patients, whereas primary osteoarthritis occurred in only 9% of patients.[105]

Patients with neuropathic degenerative disease of the ankle and degenerative disease after necrosis of the talus with collapse of the articular surface make up a small portion of the patients with degenerative disease of the ankle. Primary osteoarthritis is the most common diagnosis for patients treated with hip and knee replacements. In contrast, posttraumatic osteoarthritis is the most common diagnosis in patients treated with ankle arthrodesis or replacement. This observation raises the possibility that the ankle may be at least as vulnerable as, and perhaps more vulnerable than, the hip and knee to development of severe posttraumatic osteoarthritis.

The relative rarity of primary osteoarthritis of the ankle might be the result of the congruency, stability, and restrained motion of the ankle joint, tensile properties and metabolic characteristics of ankle articular cartilage, or a combination of these factors. The thinness of ankle articular cartilage and the small contact area, leading to

Table 21-1   All Ankle Arthritis Patients* in the Senior Author's Practice over a 13-Year Period

Type of Arthritis	Number of Patients	Percentage of Total	Age Average	Age SD
Septic	10	1.6	56.7	16.94
Rheumatoid	76	11.9	58.7	12.6
Osteonecrosis	14	2.2	49.5	14.91
Neuropathic	31	4.9	53.8	13.95
Hemophiliac	12	1.9	24.3	16.86
Gouty	5	0.8	46.0	18.1
Primary	46	7.2	67.2	12.4
Post-traumatic	445	70.0	51.5	14.4

SD, standard deviation.
*Total of 639 patients.

Table 21-2   Posttraumatic Ankle Arthritis Patients in the Senior Author's Practice over a 13-Year Period

Presentation	Number	Percentage	Age Average	Age SD
Tibial and fibular shaft	18	4.0	54.9	11.5
Tibia fracture	38	8.5	49	16.3
Plafond fracture	40	9.0	43.1	11.5
Rotational ankle fracture	164	37.0	50.8	14.2
Talar fracture	38	8.3	46.9	14.5
Osteochondritis dissecans	21	4.7	44.6	12.62
Recurrent ankle instability	65	14.6	57.7	13.29
Single sprain with continued pain	61	13.7	50	16.17
TOTAL	445			

SD, standard deviation.

Table 21-3 Primary Ankle Arthritis Patients in the Senior Author's Practice over a 13-Year Period

Deformity	Number	Percentage
Congenital foot deformity	7	15
Planovalgus foot	6	13
Cavovarus foot	10	22
No foot deformity	23	50
TOTAL	46	

high peak contact stresses, can make the joint more susceptible to posttraumatic osteoarthritis. In particular, the thinner, stiffer articular cartilage of the ankle may be less able to adapt to articular surface incongruity and increased contact stresses than the thicker articular cartilage of the hip and knee, and the contact stresses may be higher in the ankle.

Joint injuries can cause damage of articular cartilage and subchondral bone that, if not repaired, creates articular surface incongruencies and decreases joint stability. Long-term incongruence or instability can increase localized contact stress. The ankle osteoarthritis that occurs after injuries appears to follow a pattern that is consistent with the hypothesis that posttraumatic ankle osteoarthritis results from elevated contact stress that exceeds the capacity of the joint to repair itself or adapt. According to this hypothesis, the development of posttraumatic ankle osteoarthritis progresses through three overlapping stages: articular cartilage injury, chondrocyte response to tissue injury, and decline in the chondrocyte response.

Neuropathies and necrosis of the talus that cause incongruity of the articular surface also lead to secondary ankle osteoarthritis. Patients with neuropathies can develop rapidly progressive joint degeneration after minimal injury or in the absence of a history of an injury. This can occur because the loss of positional sense leads to undetected ligamentous or articular surface injuries that create localized regions of increased contact stress. Articular surface incongruence resulting from necrosis of the talus can have the same effect.

Consistent with the hypothesis that excessive contact stress causes degeneration of ankle articular cartilage, the significant residual joint incongruity and severe disruption of the ankle joint articular surface predictably lead to joint degeneration, commonly within 2 years of injury. Advanced joint degeneration can also develop within 2 years after injuries that cause relatively little apparent damage to the articular surface. In some of these latter cases, the joint surface might have sustained damage that is not apparent by radiographic evaluation. In others, joint instability resulting from alterations of the anatomy of the mortise, such as spreading of the distal tibiofibular syndesmosis, shortening and rotation of the fibula, or capsular and ligamentous laxity, can cause degeneration of the joint. However, some patients develop progressive joint degeneration after ankle injuries without apparent articular surface damage, alteration of the joint anatomy, or joint instability. On the other hand, some patients with articular surface incongruity or joint instability do not develop progressive joint degeneration. The pathogenesis of posttraumatic ankle osteoarthritis is therefore more complex than it appears and needs extensive further study.

IMPACT OF ANKLE ARTHRITIS

The significant impact of knee and hip arthritis on patient function is well documented, and recent attempts have been made to better quantify the impact ankle arthritis has on the lives of patients. Several studies have established a baseline for the functional limitations on patients with end-stage arthritis of the ankle.[2,39,98] Using different measures, all of these studies have shown that ankle arthritis severely impacts the lives of patients. Glazebrook et al[39] used the Short Form-36 (SF-36) to prospectively compare patients with end-stage ankle to patients with end-stage hip arthritis. These authors showed that patients with ankle arthritis had SF-36 scores equivalent in severity to patients with end-stage hip arthritis and were two standard deviations below normal patients. Similarly, using the Musculoskeletal Functional Assessment (MFA), Agel et al[2] showed that patients with ankle arthritis scored three times worse than normal patients. In a more recent study, Segal et al[98] correlated the SF-36 and MFA scores with gait kinematics and step count. These authors found that patients with ankle arthritis had reduced function based on SF-36 and MFA scores. In addition, patients showed reduced ankle motion, ankle plantar flexion moment, peak ankle power absorbed, and peak ankle power generated in the affected limb when compared with the normal contralateral limb.

Taken together, the results of these studies show that patients are severely affected by ankle arthritis. The severity of the impact on function has been shown with different measures of functional outcomes, as well as quantified with gait analysis.

APPROACH TO THE PATIENT WITH ANKLE ARTHRITIS

History and Physical Examination

Taking a good history and performing a careful physical examination are essential. First, determine if there is a clear history of trauma contributing to the development of ankle arthritis. Although a past fracture is the most common cause of ankle degeneration, recurrent sprains (or even one major sprain without resolution) can also be responsible. Ankle arthritis is usually not the first manifestation of generalized inflammatory arthritis, but certainly it is relatively common in patients with severe multiarticular disease. Hemophilia, gout, talar avascular necrosis (AVN), or infection can all contribute to the development of end-stage arthritis.

Next, determine which activities cause ankle pain or limit function. Walking uphill causes bony impingement in the anterior ankle or the talonavicular joints. Pain caused by downhill walking suggests a problem at the back of the ankle and can include posterior soft tissue impingement, trigonal problems, or synovial chondromatosis. Pain that is primarily caused by walking on uneven ground and that is experienced in the back or lateral aspect of the ankle can indicate subtalar joint disease. Subfibular pain might not be from the ankle or subtalar joints but might be due to malalignment and secondary bony impingement of the calcaneus on the lateral process of the talus, peroneal tendons, or fibula. Posteromedial pain typically indicates a tendon problem rather than ankle arthritis.

The examination should be done with the patient sitting and standing. In the seated position, a careful vascular and neurologic assessment can be made, joint motion estimated, and points of maximal tenderness identified. The ligaments around the ankle should be tested for stability. All major extrinsic tendons need to be palpated to determine if there are associated tendinopathies. Alignment of the foot should be evaluated. Patients with recurrent instability often have a declinated first ray, whereas patients with severe flatfeet and secondary ankle disease often have clinical instability of the medial

column. In patients with rheumatoid arthritis, careful attention should be given to the skin and nails to rule out punctate infarcts suggestive of ongoing vasculitis.

The standing and walking examinations complement the seated examination. Alignment of the hindfoot is assessed from behind. Excessive varus or valgus angulation of the heel should be noted. Restriction of ankle motion can lead to early heel rise or back-knee gait. The posture of the forefoot upon striking the ground should be noted. Patients who load the lateral part of the foot might have fixed varus deformity of the ankle or transverse tarsal region.

Ankle Joint Imaging

Radiography

Plain radiographs should be taken with the patient standing whenever possible. At our center, we have a standard minimum series of radiographs taken for patients with ankle problems. These include *standing* ankle lateral, anteroposterior, mortise, and hindfoot alignment views.[89] The hindfoot alignment view is particularly important in situations where the heel is in varus or valgus and the ankle has coronal plane tilting (Fig. 21-5). If we are considering any surgery distal to the tibiotalar joint, we also obtain standing views of the entire foot.

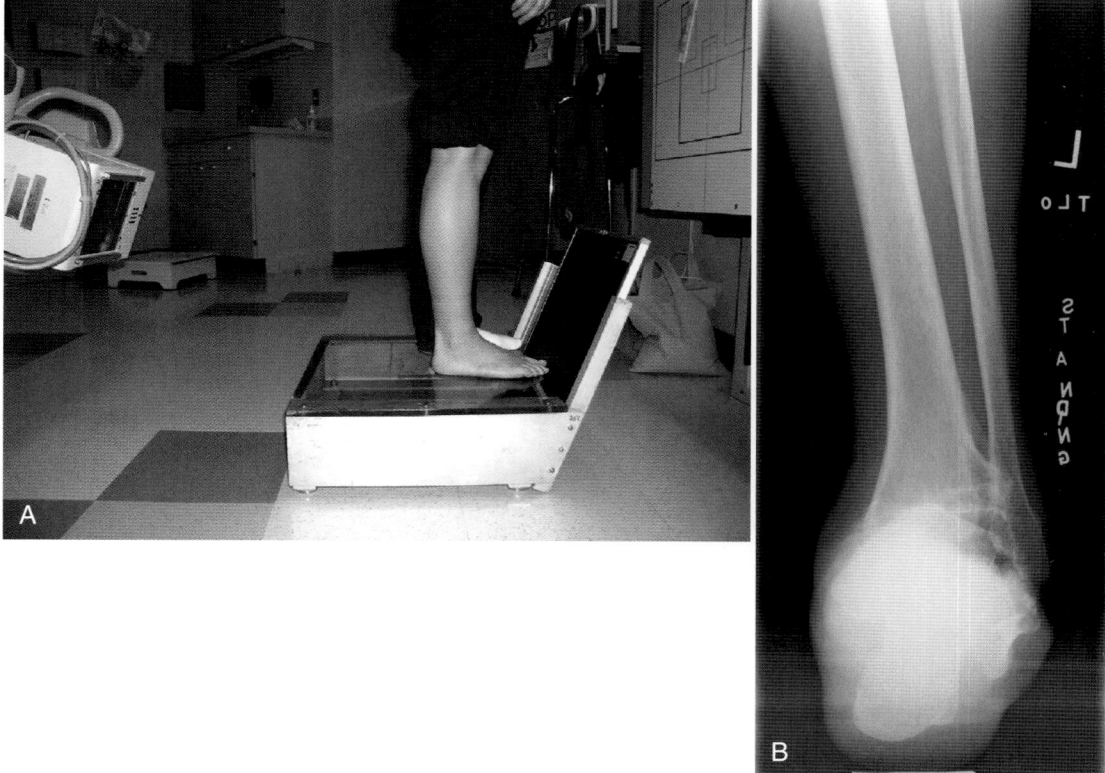

Figure 21-5   A, The hindfoot alignment view is taken with the patient standing on a platform, with the toes pointed straight ahead at the film plate. **B,** The x-ray beam is directed toward the ankle in a posterior to anterior direction, tilted 20 degrees caudad. The film is placed near the toes, also tilted 20 degrees, oriented exactly perpendicular to the beam.[89] A line passing down the central longitudinal axis of the tibia should bisect the calcaneus.

Magnetic Resonance Imaging

Magnetic resonance imaging (MRI) is a very useful adjunct for imaging the ankle. It is excellent in delineating abnormalities of soft tissues around the ankle joint. However, in assessing ankle arthritis, the value of standard MRI is often limited. First, any hardware near the ankle joint generates major artifacts that obscure visualization of articular features. Second, the articular surfaces of the ankle are naturally close packed and congruous. Unlike the knee, where joint surfaces are not congruent, there is no clear separation of articular surfaces of the tibiotalar joint. Third, the now standard, hospital-based MRI, using a 1.5-tesla (T) magnet, only captures three to four pixels across a healthy ankle articular surface. Instruments with smaller magnets (i.e., 0.50 or 0.75 T) cannot capture any articular features of normal ankles. In cases of degeneration, current standard MRI magnets cannot easily distinguish focal articular features, even with distraction.

Computed Tomography

Advances in computed tomography (CT) have revolutionized ankle imaging. The total time for scanning has been reduced to 2 to 5 minutes compared with an average capture time of 20 minutes for MRI. As a result, CT images are much less susceptible to motion artifacts. The 4- and 16-slice helical units now capture anisotropic, 1-mm[57] voxel-based data sets that can be postprocessed to show two- or three-dimensional renderings of any feature of interest (e.g., bone, tendons, cartilage). Intraarticular injection of contrast material before scanning can be used to enhance the accurate visualization of ankle articular

features (Fig. 21-6).[32] Computed tomography also has the large advantage over MRI of being able to work in an environment near retained hardware. CT arthrograms to delineate if a patient is suffering from global or focal tibiotalar arthritis or evaluate the condition of the subtalar joint have become a common adjunct to plain radiography at our center.

Selective Injections

Selective injections are used to help identify the source of pain for patients who have clinical or radiographic findings that suggest more than one focal source of pain.[55] Before the injection, the patient is asked to perform activities that cause pain in the ankle (e.g., walk on uneven ground, walk up or down stairs, run). Diagnostic injections are done under fluoroscopic control. Contrast dye is first instilled to confirm the exact location of the injection. This is followed by injecting a local anesthetic. If the pain is not reduced by at least 75%, we look for a second source. In a study of foot and ankle fusion patients, Khoury et al[55] reported that the reduction in pain after an intraarticular injection correlated to the response from surgery.

Global Ankle Arthritis Versus Focal Ankle Arthritis

When evaluating the patient with ankle pain and apparent arthritis, one of the first tasks of the clinician is to determine whether the problem is global (affects the

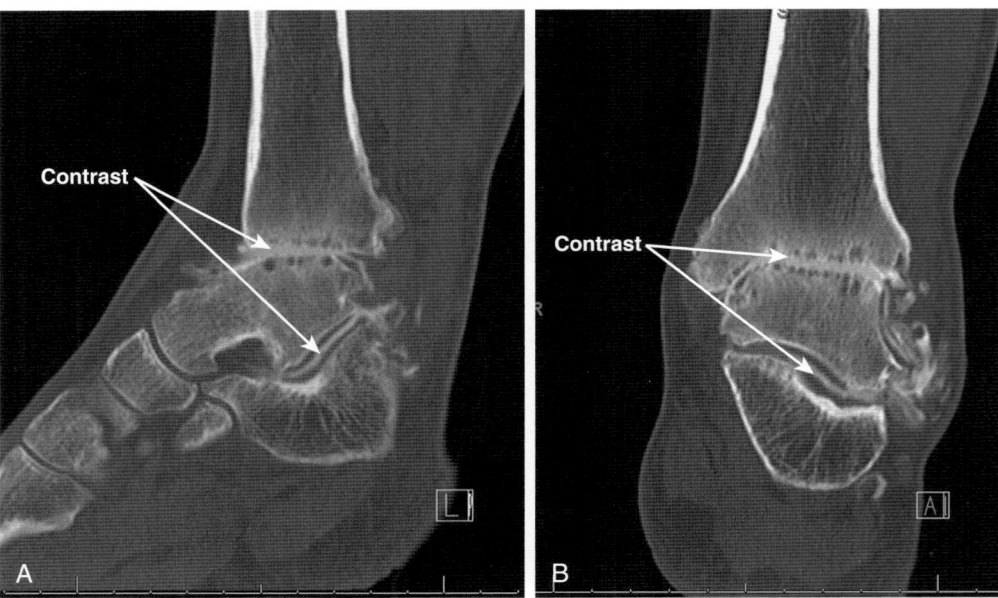

Figure 21-6 Injection of contrast media can facilitate the visualization of articular cartilage during computed tomography (CT) evaluation of a joint. If articular cartilage is present, it appears black compared with the lighter contrast material or adjacent bone. Preoperative sagittal **(A)** and coronal **(B)** CT images for a patient being evaluated for ankle arthrodesis show the ability of the technique to delineate articular cartilage. For this patient, the status of the articular cartilage for the tibiotalar and subtalar joints were evaluated.

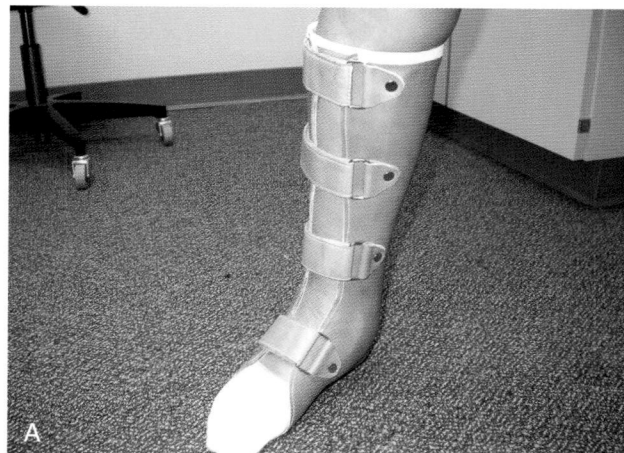
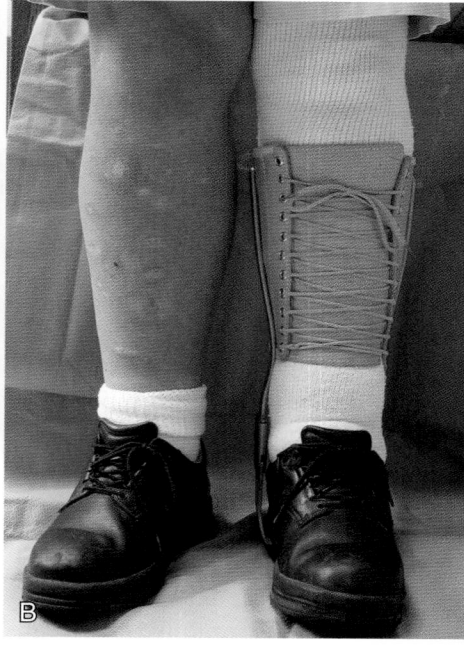

Figure 21-7 Brace treatment of ankle arthritis is directed at limiting motion and reducing axial loading. The two braces we use are a custom-made leather-lined polypropylene ankle–foot orthosis **(A)** and a calf lacer with metal drop locks fitted to a rocker-bottom shoe **(B)**. These usually are made with lace-up straps, but they can be fitted with hook-and-loop (Velcro) straps, as shown in **A,** for patients with profound loss of grip strength from end-stage rheumatoid disease.

majority of the joint), or focal (affects a specific region of the joint). Inflammatory arthritides such as rheumatoid disease and seronegative spondyloarthropathies are, by definition, global processes. Similarly, hemophiliac, gouty, crystalline deposition, and septic arthropathies are diffuse joint processes. Intraarticular pilon fractures and neuroarthropathic fractures that cause ankle arthritis generally induce a global arthritic response, especially with multiple fracture lines involving the tibiotalar joint. Conversely, tibial shaft malunions, ankle instability, and foot malalignment problems that lead to ankle cartilage loss initially often cause well-localized focal problems.

TREATMENT OF GLOBAL ANKLE ARTHRITIS

Conservative Treatment

Little has been written about the nonoperative treatment of diffuse ankle arthritis. Indeed, no retrospective or prospective clinical trials have been reported. Nonoperative treatment is based on experience and patient preferences. In our experience, the efficacy of nonsteroidal antiinflammatory drugs (NSAIDs) varies. Care must be exercised when prescribing these medications because of their sometimes substantial side effects.

A judiciously timed injection of the joint with steroids can help a patient enjoy an important life event (wedding, vacation). We do not like to give repeated injections of steroids because of the catabolic risks to soft tissues. Recently, there has been an increased interest in the use of injectable viscosupplementation for the treatment of

ankle arthritis.* Review of the studies related to this subject show a large incidence of industry support and need to be interpreted with an understanding that this might introduce bias. Studies have shown an improvement in Ankle Osteoarthritis and American Orthopaedic Foot and Ankle Society (AOFAS) scores with hyaluronic acid injection; however, this improvement was no greater than control saline injection.[18,24,88] Although the benefit of viscosupplementation beyond placebo effect is still controversial, there does not appear to be any significant adverse events associated with the injections.[99,100,109] The authors do not routinely use hyaluronic acid injections for the conservative treatment of ankle arthritis unless there is a contraindication or need to delay surgery. In these situations, viscosupplementation is considered as an alternative to repetitive corticosteroid injections.

The standard nonoperative treatment for end-stage ankle arthritis is mechanical unloading. A cane can be very helpful. If patients accept the cosmetic and functional limitations of an ankle–foot orthosis (AFO), they often obtain partial pain relief. We like to use an AFO that can be molded to the contour of the posterior calf muscles. This permits some unloading of the ankle. The two designs that appear to work best are a leather ankle lacer with an imbedded polypropylene shell for structural support or a calf lacer AFO.[92] The former fits in a shoe; the latter requires metal drop locks fixed to a single shoe (Fig. 21-7). Adding a solid ankle cushion heel (SACH)

---

*References 18, 24, 88, 99, 100, and 109.

and a rocker sole can help by further limiting ankle motion.

Operative Treatment

The decision to operate on ankle arthritis requires a clear assessment of the patient's functional needs and a complete understanding of the cause of the patient's problem. Isolated, primary global ankle osteoarthritis is relatively rare. More commonly, malalignment secondary to trauma, ligamentous instability, or foot deformity is present with painful and arthritic ankles. Regardless of treatment strategy, reestablishing normal foot alignment encourages improved foot function. With total ankle replacement, perfect coronal and anteroposterior alignment of the ankle holds the greatest promise of giving long-lasting function and low wear rates. With ankle fusion, correct alignment helps to maintain residual natural adjacent joint motion, especially in the subtalar joint, and can delay the development of secondary hind-foot arthritis.

The indications for surgery continue to evolve as techniques change and evidence for effectiveness accumulates. Since the mid-1990s, we have witnessed the emergence of several alternative strategies to treat end-stage ankle arthritis. Periankle osteotomies hold promise of prolonging ankle function by redistributing forces across joints. Ankle joint distraction with tensioned wires can similarly prolong ankle function. Ankle replacement is emerging as a viable alternative for selected patients. Of all the surgical techniques, though, ankle fusion remains the workhorse of surgical reconstruction.

Primary Ankle Fusion
SURGICAL CONSIDERATIONS

In a general sense, ankle fusion has a few clear advantages over other techniques. When the pain originates within the ankle joint, a successful arthrodesis usually eliminates it. Short-term results and complication rates have been markedly improved by modern techniques of limited periosteal stripping, rigid internal fixation, and meticulous attention to alignment and position. Pain relief is more reliable with fusion than with most other techniques. Secondary operations, other than occasional hardware removals, are relatively rare.

However, ankle fusion is not entirely without problems. First, tibiotalar bone-bridging after attempted fusion surgery is not completely reliable, and reported rates of initial fusion range from 60% to 100%.*

Second, initial pain relief can be elusive if other causes of pain are present or revealed by ankle fusion. Third, functional limitations are common, even with clinically successful fusions (Table 21-4).[75] Fourth, shoe modifications may be needed to improve the transition from heel strike and toe-off, including use of a SACH or a

---

Table 21-4 Functional Limitations after Ankle Fusion for 28 Highly Satisfied Patients[76]

Tasks	Number	Percentage
Walking on uneven ground	22	79
Difficulties with stair ascent or descent	21	75
Modify the way they pick objects up off the floor	20	71
After use of driving pedals	20	71
Aching with prolonged standing, working, or walking	18	64
Difficulty putting on boots	10	36
Difficulty getting out of a bath	6	21
Difficulty sleeping prone or supine	5	19
Swimming	3	11

---

rocker-bottom sole. Finally, accelerated degeneration of other foot joints, especially the subtalar and talonavicular joints, can occur after ankle fusion.[17] This degeneration, in turn, can lead to further bracing or fusion surgery and must be considered when contemplating an ankle arthrodesis for a young patient.

After an ankle fusion, approximately 50% of patients demonstrate arthroses distal or proximal to the fusion site within 7 years. Although most of these changes are seen on radiographs, their presence at 7 years does not bode well for what will develop at these joints over the next 20 to 30 years. Many factors probably affect the onset of this arthrosis besides the increased stress. One factor is probably related to the overall stiffness or laxity of the surrounding joints. The stiffer the surrounding joints, the less the patient is able to dissipate the increased stress created by the fusion compared with a patient with more joint laxity. Because an arthrodesis is often performed on a traumatized limb, the adjacent joints, although not demonstrating arthrosis, might have sustained tissue damage at the time of the initial injury that makes them more prone to develop arthrosis when subjected to increased stress. Patients with generalized flexibility and ample residual foot flexibility after the development of ankle arthritis tend to have improved outcomes after fusion than those who have intrinsic stiffness.

Once it has been decided to perform an arthrodesis, the next most critical factor is to establish the proper alignment of the fusion site. To do this, the surgeon must consider the entire lower leg and not just the foot. The position of the knee or the bow of the tibia, which can occur either naturally or because of prior trauma, must be carefully examined when planning the arthrodesis. The alignment of the extremity distal to the fusion site is also important to create a plantigrade foot. Sometimes when an ankle arthrodesis is being contemplated, an underlying postural deformity of the foot precludes placing the ankle in the optimal position. If a patient has a significant forefoot varus deformity, the ankle joint needs to be

---

*References 3, 4, 10, 16, 35, 49, 52, 62, 63, 72, and 87.

aligned in a little more valgus position to create a compromised plantigrade foot. Placing the ankle into its normal alignment of 5 degrees of valgus can keep the patient from placing the forefoot flat on the ground. Conversely, if the patient has a cavus foot with a fixed forefoot valgus, the ankle fusion might be placed into neutral or slight varus to create a foot that is as plantigrade as possible. Sometimes a selective osteotomy or arthrodesis of the forefoot is necessary to create a plantigrade foot after an ankle fusion if it cannot be created by the fusion alone.

The biomechanics of the foot dictates its optimal alignment. When the subtalar joint is placed into an *everted position,* it provides instability to the joint, creates flexibility of the transverse tarsal joint, and results in a supple forefoot. When the subtalar joint is in an *inverted position,* it provides stability to the joint, locks the transverse tarsal joint, and creates a rigid forefoot. It is therefore important to place the subtalar joint in 5 to 7 degrees of valgus when a fusion is done to maintain flexibility of the forefoot. A fusion in varus position creates a rigid forefoot and increased stress under the lateral aspect of the foot, which is poorly tolerated by the patient.

Soft tissue considerations are paramount to a good surgical result. Avoid making incisions through contracted, scarred skin because wound sloughs and soft tissue coverage are challenging in this anatomic region. When making an incision, the surgeon must always be cognizant of the location of the cutaneous nerves around the ankle. Although cutaneous nerves tend to lie in certain defined anatomic areas, great variation exists. It is therefore important to be always on the lookout for an aberrant cutaneous nerve as the incision is continued through the subcutaneous tissues. The most common nerves injured during ankle surgery are the medial branch of the superficial peroneal nerve, encountered in anterior longitudinal approaches, and the anterior branch of the sural nerve, encountered beneath the lateral malleolus during transfibular approaches. The cutaneous nerves can be quite superficial and easily transected or can become adherent within scar tissue. If this occurs, a painful scar or dysesthesias distal to the injury can cause the patient to be dissatisfied with an otherwise a successful fusion.

Basic Surgical Principles

Respect the soft tissues. Retract carefully. Meticulously avoid local cutaneous nerve injury or entrapment during all stages of the procedure, including closing of the wound. Remove all cartilage, and feather and penetrate into subchondral bone. Create congruent cancellous surfaces that can be placed into apposition to permit a fusion to occur. Use bone graft or bone graft substitutes only to fill defects. Stabilize the arthrodesis site with rigid fixation, if possible. Align the hindfoot to the lower extremity and the forefoot to the hindfoot to create a plantigrade foot. For really stiff feet, slight (less than 5 degrees) dorsiflexion may be preferred. Immobilize the ankle and limit weight-bearing activity until bone-bridging is certain.

Open Ankle Arthrodesis
INDICATIONS

The main indication for ankle arthrodesis is arthrosis that causes pain or deformity (or both) of the ankle joints. The arthrosis may be primary or secondary. The secondary form is caused by posttraumatic changes, postsepsis condition, avascular necrosis of the talus, failed total ankle replacement, or malalignment from a paralytic deformity. In some cases, a subtalar or transverse tarsal joint fusion (or both) is included, which results in a pantalar arthrodesis.

POSITION OF ARTHRODESIS

The desired position of the arthrodesis is as follows:

- Dorsiflexion/plantar flexion: Neutral
- Varus/valgus: 5 degrees of valgus
- Rotation: Equal or slightly more externally rotated than the opposite extremity
- Posterior displacement: Anterior aspect of the talar dome is brought to anterior aspect of tibia

Under some circumstances, such as weakness of the quadriceps muscle, the arthrodesis can be placed with the foot in 10 degrees of equinus, which will help to stabilize the knee joint. Conversely, for *really stiff feet, slight* (<5 degrees) *dorsiflexion* may be preferred. In general, however, both equinus and calcaneus positioning should be minimized to prevent a back-knee thrust with the equinus and excessive weight bearing by the calcaneus. The foot is externally rotated slightly (5 degrees) compared with the other side to allow normal knee motion. This, in turn, avoids the problem of requiring the knee to externally rotate in stance phase, which can result in gradual laxity of the medial collateral knee ligament.

MANN TECHNIQUE
Preparation

1. Alignment of the normal and abnormal limb is assessed to evaluate the degree of deformity. This is done by aligning the patella parallel to the operating table and observing the degree of rotation of the foot in relation to a perpendicular line from the patella. In this way, the surgeon can determine the degree of internal or external rotation of both the normal and the abnormal extremity. The advantage of this measurement approach is that it is relatively easy to check the alignment of the arthrodesis site at surgery.
2. A thigh tourniquet is applied, and a sandbag is placed under the ipsilateral hip to enhance the visibility of the lateral side of the foot and ankle.

Lateral Approach

3. The skin incision begins approximately 10 cm proximal to the tip of the fibula, is carried down over the shaft of the fibula, and then swings gently distally another 10 cm toward the base of the fourth metatarsal. Although this incision extends between nerves,

with the sural nerve passing posteriorly and the superficial peroneal nerve passing anteriorly, the surgeon must be aware of an anterior branch of the sural nerve that might pass through the plane of the incision (Fig. 21-8A and Video Clip 21).

4. The skin flaps are developed to create a full-thickness flap along the skeletal plane. The periosteum is stripped from the fibula anteriorly and posteriorly, and the incision is carried on distally to expose the posterior facet of the subtalar joint and the sinus tarsi.

5. The dissection is carried across the anterior aspect of the tibia and ankle joint. With a periosteal elevator, the surgeon strips soft tissue from the distal end of the tibia, ankle joint, and proximal talar neck and then medially to the medial malleolus. Care is taken not to dissect distally over the neck of the talus to protect the blood supply into the talus.

6. The fibula is osteotomized approximately 2 cm proximal to the level of the ankle joint and beveled to relieve the sharp prominence (Fig. 21-8B). The distal

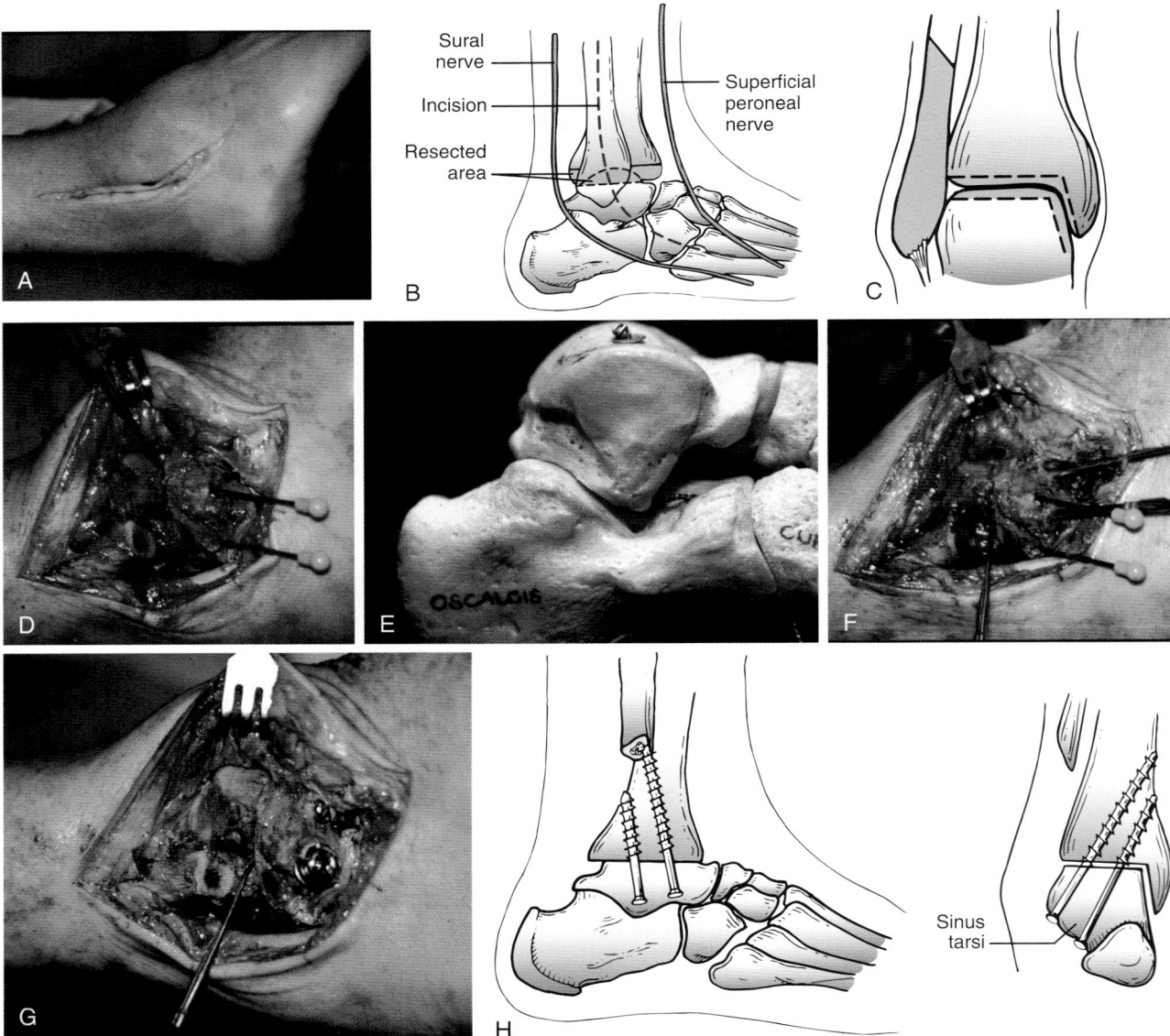

Figure 21-8 **A,** Line of skin incision. **B,** Diagram demonstrates cuts made in the fibula, distal end of tibia, and talus. Incision is between the superficial peroneal nerve and sural nerve. **C,** The cut in the tibia is made perpendicular to the long axis of the tibia. **D,** After the cut has been made in the talus, absolute bone apposition should exist without tension when the foot is in neutral position with regard to dorsiflexion/plantar flexion. **E,** Model demonstrates sites for placement of two screws across arthrodesis site: one on the plantar aspect at the junction between the neck of the talus and body and the other in the lateral process. **F,** The arthrodesis site is stabilized with two K-wires. Two 3.2-mm drill bits are placed from distal to proximal across the arthrodesis site, marking the site of screw placement. **G,** After placement of 6.5-mm screws across arthrodesis site. **H,** Placement of screws in lateral and anteroposterior projections.

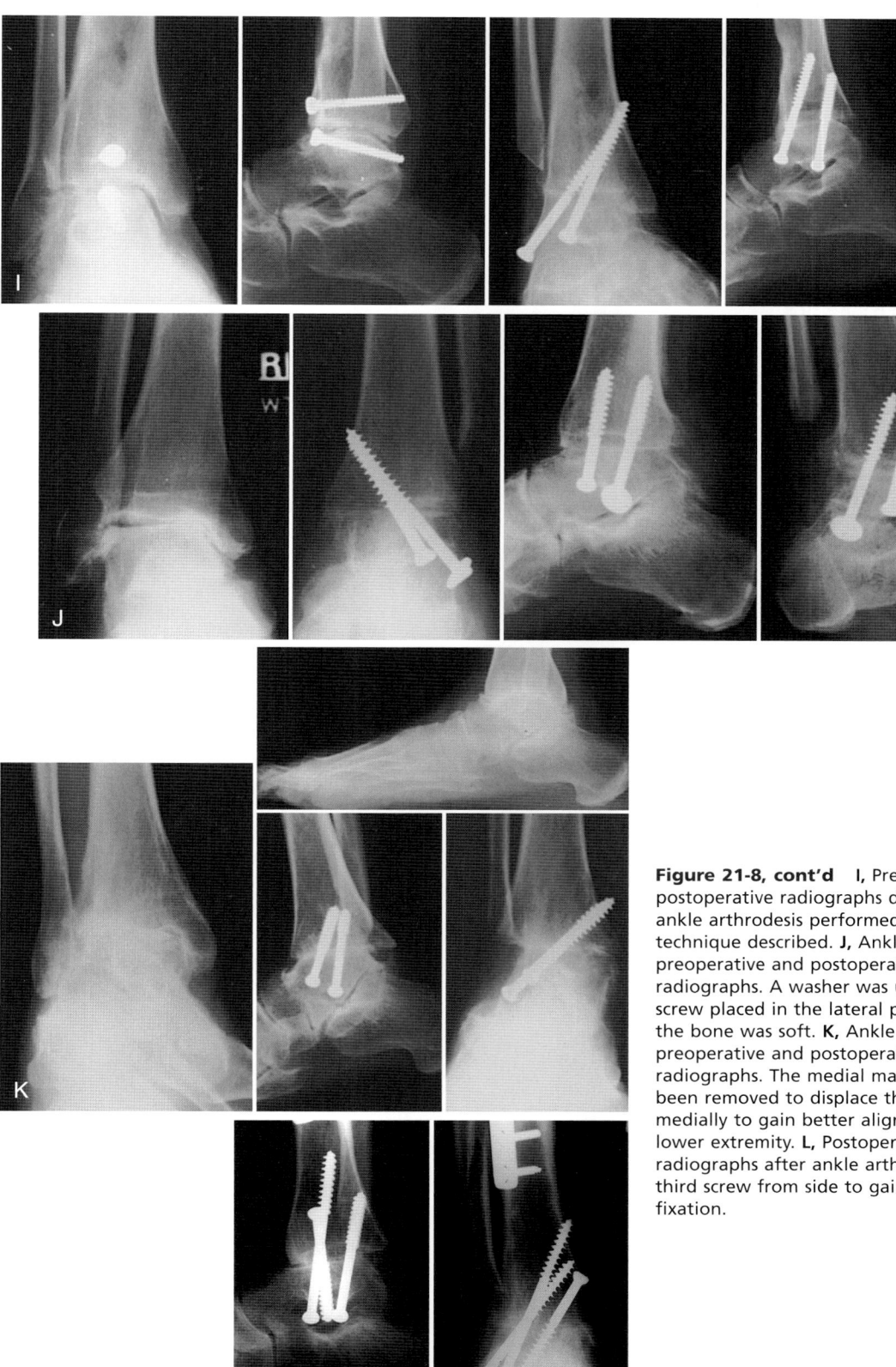

Figure 21-8, cont'd   **I,** Preoperative and postoperative radiographs demonstrate ankle arthrodesis performed with technique described. **J,** Ankle arthrodesis, preoperative and postoperative radiographs. A washer was used in the screw placed in the lateral process because the bone was soft. **K,** Ankle arthrodesis, preoperative and postoperative radiographs. The medial malleolus has been removed to displace the talus medially to gain better alignment of the lower extremity. **L,** Postoperative radiographs after ankle arthrodesis using third screw from side to gain increased fixation.

portion of the fibula is removed by sharp and blunt dissection to expose the lateral aspect of the tibia and ankle joint as well as the posterior facet of the subtalar joint. As this is carried out, the peroneal tendons are reflected posteriorly.

7. An incision is made through the deep fascia along the posterior aspect of the distal tibia, which was exposed by the removal of the fibula. A periosteal elevator is gently moved medially across the posterior aspect of the tibia and then distally toward the calcaneus. This strips the soft tissues from the posterior aspect of the tibia and ankle joint.

8. Malleable retractors are placed anteriorly and posteriorly around the distal end of the tibia, exposing the anterolateral aspect of the ankle joint.

9. The initial cut for the arthrodesis is made in the distal part of the tibia with a sagittal saw, using a short, wide blade, and the cut is completed with a deep, wide blade. This cut is made as perpendicular as possible to the long axis of the tibia, and as little bone as possible is removed from the dome of the ankle joint. This cut is brought across the ankle joint and stops just where the curve of the medial malleolus begins (Fig. 21-8C).

Medial Approach

10. A 4-cm incision is made over the anteromedial aspect of the medial malleolus over the ankle joint and swung slightly inferior around the malleolus to obtain adequate exposure of the tip of the malleolus.

11. The soft tissue is stripped anteriorly and then posteromedially around the tip of the medial malleolus, with care being taken to do as little damage to the deltoid ligament structure as possible.

12. The lateral intraarticular aspect of the medial malleolus is made visible, and the surgeon can see that the cut made in the distal tibia has not been completed. Using a 10-mm osteotome, the surgeon cuts along the lateral aspect of the medial malleolus. The articular cartilage is removed while starting to free up the initial cut that was made from the lateral side. Cutting along the lateral aspect of the medial malleolus decreases the possibility of fracturing it when mobilizing the initial cut in the distal tibia.

Lateral Approach Revisited

13. The tibial fragment is freed medially by placing a broad osteotome into the osteotomy site and gently levering it distally to break any remaining attachment to the medial malleolus, then removing it. Removal of this fragment has been facilitated by stripping the periosteum posteriorly before the cut and then making the cuts along the lateral aspect of the medial malleolus through the medial approach. Occasionally, if significant deformity exists, the entire distal end of the tibia is removed. When this is done, the tibia fragment must be split and removed in two pieces to prevent damage to the neurovascular

bundle along the posteromedial corner of the joint.

14. The foot is now placed into the desired alignment in regard to dorsiflexion/plantar flexion and varus/valgus. The superior surface of the talar dome is identified through the lateral wound, and a cut removes 3 to 4 mm from the superior aspect of the talus. The cut must be made parallel to the one that has been made in the distal end of the tibia (Fig. 21-8C and D).

Intraoperative Alignment

15. Once the talar cut has been made, the surfaces are brought together and the alignment is carefully checked. If any malalignment exists at this time, more bone is removed from the distal end of the tibia, or occasionally from the talus, to align the joint properly. As this alignment is carried out, the talus is displaced posteriorly so that the anterior aspect of the cut in the talus matches the anterior cut of the tibia. This ensures a correct amount of posterior displacement.

16. If the joint surfaces do not come together without tension, the medial malleolus is too long and needs to be shortened. Through the medial incision, sufficient bone is removed from the distal portion of the malleolus to permit the tibia and talus to come together. Usually, about 1 cm of malleolus is removed. When removing the medial malleolus, caution must be used so as not to cut the posterior tibial tendon, which can be quite adherent to the posterior aspect of the malleolus.

17. The joint surfaces can now be easily brought together and satisfactory alignment achieved (see Fig. 21-8D).

18. Holding the foot in correct alignment with the two bone surfaces approximated, the surgeon inserts provisional fixation from the lateral aspect using 0.062-inch Kirschner wires. These are placed through the lateral wound and may be driven from proximal to distal, or vice versa, but they should be placed to avoid the tract used for the fixation screws.

19. With the Kirschner wires in place, alignment is again checked for the final time by palpating the patella and checking all four planes of alignment.

Internal Fixation

20. The arthrodesis site is now further stabilized by placing two 3.2-mm drill bits across the arthrodesis site. One begins within the sinus tarsi area and the other just above the lateral process (Fig. 21-8E and F). As the initial drill hole is made in the sinus tarsi, it is important to invert the calcaneus to gain access to the undersurface of the talus. The drill bit is positioned almost parallel to the floor, aimed medially and as far proximally as possible, and inserted until the bit passes through the distal medial end of the tibia. The drill bit is disconnected from the chuck and a second drill hole placed just above the lateral process and almost parallel to the first drill bit. From a technical standpoint, if the patient has stiffness of the subtalar

joint that makes it difficult to angle the first drill bit sufficiently proximal, a small trough can be cut in the lateral aspect of the calcaneus so that the drill bit can be placed at a more oblique angle.

21. One of the drill bits is removed, the depth measured, the hole tapped, and a 6.5-mm screw inserted (Fig. 21-8G). Usually, a 60- to 70-mm screw with long threads is used. If the threads will not completely cross the arthrodesis site, a short-threaded screw is used. It is extremely important, however, for the threads to engage the medial cortex of the tibia to gain maximum interfragmentary compression. The screw placed into the lateral process area must be high enough so that it will not impinge against the posterior facet and oblique enough so that it will not crack the bone over the lateral aspect of the talus. In patients with soft bone, it is occasionally helpful to use a washer (Fig. 21-8H and I).

22. The rigidity of the arthrodesis site is now checked by stressing it. If there is any motion, the surgeon should first check for adequate apposition of the bone along the fusion site, especially medially, and if the surfaces appear to be apposed, then check that both screws are as tight as they can be without stripping them. If worrisome motion still exists, the surgeon should consider inserting a third screw through the medial incision, bringing the screw from proximal to distal into the body of the talus. If the medial malleolus has been removed, a seam of staples can be used along the medial aspect of the joint to increase the rigidity of the construct (Fig. 21-8K to M).

Closure

23. A drain is inserted and brought out proximally along the area of the anterior compartment.

24. The deep layers are closed, followed by the subcutaneous tissue and skin.

25. Approximately 20 mL of 0.25% plain bupivacaine is instilled through the drain, which is not connected to suction until after the dressing has been applied to permit it to set.

26. A compression dressing is applied and supported with two plaster splints.

27. The tourniquet is released and the drain hooked to a suction pump.

Postoperative Care

In the recovery room, when the patient begins to experience pain, the anesthesiologist performs a popliteal block. This usually provides 18 to 36 hours of pain relief. If the block is not effective for more than 12 to 16 hours, a second block can be used. The drain is removed the next day.

The postoperative dressing is left in place for 10 to 12 days, and then it is removed along with the sutures. A short-leg, non–weight-bearing cast is applied. Removable casts are not used for an ankle fusion. They do not provide enough immobilization at the arthrodesis site because of the lever arm created by the foot and the tibia.

Six weeks after surgery, the cast is removed, radiographs are taken, and if adequate healing appears to be occurring, a new short-leg fiberglass walking cast is fitted, and the patient is permitted to bear weight as tolerated.

Twelve weeks after surgery, the second cast is removed, radiographs are taken, and if healing is satisfactory, the patient is permitted to walk with an elastic stocking and to bear weight as tolerated. If the fusion site is not complete, the ankle is placed back into a cast for another month. Although in this series[19] the average time to fusion was 14 weeks, we did not hesitate to keep the ankle immobilized until adequate fusion occurred, which in some cases took 26 weeks. The patient must be made aware of this possibility before surgery to lessen the disappointment if the fusion is not complete at 12 weeks.

Clinical Experience

A review of Mann's[61] experience with the transfibular approach in 81 fusions in 77 patients (46 men and 31 women; average age, 56 years; range, 24 to 82 years) noted a chief complaint of pain in 67 of 81 (83%), deformity in 10 (12%), and instability in 4 (5%). The follow-up averaged 35 months (range, 12 to 74 months). Symptoms were present an average of 6.4 years (±1.9 years). Seventy-five percent of the patients used an AFO for approximately 1 year before surgery.

Mann's results demonstrated that 71 of 81 (88%) arthrodeses fused in an average of 13.8 weeks (±6 weeks) and that 10 (12%) failed to unite. In the subgroup of ankles treated for a nonunion, 9 of 12 healed after revision surgery. The time to union was 22.9 weeks compared with 13.8 weeks for the entire group. This compares favorably with other series in the literature: 21 weeks,[58] 54 weeks,[29] and 22 weeks.[60] Mann's technique of arthrodesis was the same as for the other cases, that is, creating fresh bone surfaces and using screws for interfragmentary compression without a bone graft.

Fusion occurred in 9 of 12 (75%) in our subgroup compared with 20 out of 26 (77%) reported by Kitaoka et al,[59] who used a bone graft and external fixation with fusion; Kirkpatrick et al,[58] who used a bone graft and internal fixation with a fusion rate of 9 of 11 (81%); and Levine et al,[60] who used bone graft and internal fixation with a fusion rate of 20 of 22 (92%). Mann's series shows that bone grafting is not necessary to obtain a union in a revision operation for nonunion, especially if a defect does not exist. If necessary, however, the surgeon should not hesitate to use a bone graft.

In the seven virgin cases in which Mann obtained a nonunion, fusion was achieved in all cases with revision surgery that consisted of opening the nonunion site, unscrewing the screws, curetting the joint surfaces to obtain fresh bleeding bone, and reinserting the internal fixation. The average time to union in this group was 16 weeks. In this subgroup, he could not identify the cause for nonunion because all his patients had been treated in a similar manner.

Ninety percent of the patients believed that the surgery helped them, 70% were satisfied without reservation, 18% were satisfied with reservation, and 12% were dissatisfied. The reason for dissatisfaction was pain in four cases, nonunion in two, a limp in one, and a wound slough in one. No shoe modification was necessary in 77%. A rocker-bottom sole was used by 16%, and 7% continued to use an AFO.

The physical examination demonstrated that the calf size was reduced an average of 3.2 cm, and shortening averaged 9 mm for the entire series. In those with primary arthrosis who had no shortening preoperatively, however, it was 4 mm. No patient had problems with the peroneal tendon, and 82% demonstrated a peroneal strength of 4+ or more. The range of motion in the sagittal plane was 23 degrees (±9), subtalar joint motion was 9 degrees (±3), and transverse tarsal joint motion was 15 degrees (±5). This represented 26%, 30%, and 70%, respectively, of these motions in the uninvolved extremity. The alignment of the fusion site was determined to be excellent in 93% of cases and poor in 7%. Those in the poor category were dissatisfied with the degree of valgus of the hindfoot.

Lateral radiographs during weight bearing demonstrated that the total motion between the talus and first metatarsal in forced plantar flexion and dorsiflexion was 24 degrees (±7 degrees); at the talonavicular joint, 14 degrees (±6 degrees); and at the talocalcaneal joint, 8 degrees (±6 degrees). This is similar to the motion observed by Abdo and Wasilewski.[1] There was a positive correlation with patient's functioning, satisfaction, and calf size with increased motion in the foot. This correlates with the gait analysis by Mazur et al,[65] who also demonstrated that increased motion permitted better compensation for an ankle fusion.[49]

Preoperative radiographs demonstrated that 56% of the patients had degenerative changes in the hindfoot, with the subtalar joint affected twice as often as the talonavicular joint and the calcaneocuboid joint rarely involved. After surgery, 20% of Mann's patients demonstrated an increase in the arthrosis, and two required a subtalar arthrodesis.[61]

In Mann's series,[61] 10 patients had no prior history of inflammatory arthritis or trauma and were classified as having primary arthrosis. The average age of this subgroup was 69 years (range, 59 to 78) compared with 52 years for the other 71 patients. The age difference was statistically significant ($P < .05$).

When the entire medial malleolus was excised to obtain alignment or translate the talus medially, or both, 41 cases with more than a 1-cm resection had an average union time of 15.4 weeks, and there were three delayed unions and seven nonunions. The time to union in this subset was significantly longer ($P < .05$) than the 40 ankles (12.9 weeks) with less than 1 cm resected. The reason for this delay in union is not apparent, but on these ankles, there had been more previous surgical procedures (1.8 vs. 1.6) and greater preoperative deformity. The procedure required greater exposure and probably more periosteal stripping. The medial malleolus can also provide greater surface area at the fusion site. From an anatomic standpoint, the blood supply to the medial malleolus can be compromised, but at surgery, special care was always taken to preserve the deltoid arterial supply to the talus.

Other authors have reported successful fusion with resection of both malleoli. Scranton[97] achieved fusion in all 13 patients using fixation with a T plate, and Marcus et al[62] achieved fusion in 12 of 13 patients using a medial onlay graft in addition to lateral fixation with staples. Myerson and Quill[77] reported two delayed unions when they used a bimalleolar resection in 16 patients. In our experience, the medial malleolus should be preserved to enhance the possibility of a more rapid union, but if it must be excised to achieve better alignment, the surgeon should not hesitate to do so.

Variations on the Transfibular Ankle Arthrodesis Technique

Several adaptations have been made to the Mann technique (Fig. 21-9).

Regional anesthetics are administered preoperatively. This reduces the need for analgesics intraoperatively and appears to reduce postoperative nausea. Indwelling nerve catheters are now available for home use and can prolong the postoperative pain-free period. Care with placing the splint is paramount when using any regional anesthetic.

A similar lateral approach is used, but the distal malleolus is rotated posteriorly on its posteriorinferior soft tissues, and its medial third is removed with a saw (Fig. 21-10A). This opens up the cancellous bone of the malleolus. All shavings from the medial third are kept for bone graft. At the end of the procedure, a small segment of fibula is removed above, and the lateral malleolar piece is moved superiorly 0.5 to 1.0 cm and placed as a lateral onlay buttress graft to the ankle arthrodeses construct.

When deformity is minimal or moderate, the distal tibia and proximal talar dome surfaces are removed to preserve the natural dome-shaped sagittal plane contour (Fig. 21-10B). This reduces the loss of limb length, which naturally results from joint preparation. We use ¼ -inch to ⅜ -inch osteotomes and side-cutting router bits to remove the joint contents. The subchondral bone is drilled with multiple small and shallow holes. The anteromedial approach described earlier is used, and the lateral surface of the medial malleolus is denuded of cartilage and subchondral bone.

Screw placement is slightly different across the tibiotalar joint because we usually try to place two large screws out of plane from each other. The first is placed from posteromedial to anterocentral in the talus (Fig. 21-10C, see Fig. 21-9D and E). The leg is arranged in the figure-of-four position. A 1-cm incision is made along the posteromedial edge of the tibia 3 cm above the joint line. Skin and soft tissues need to be retracted throughout this percutaneous approach. The screw traverses the posteromedial corner of the ankle into the talus, heading

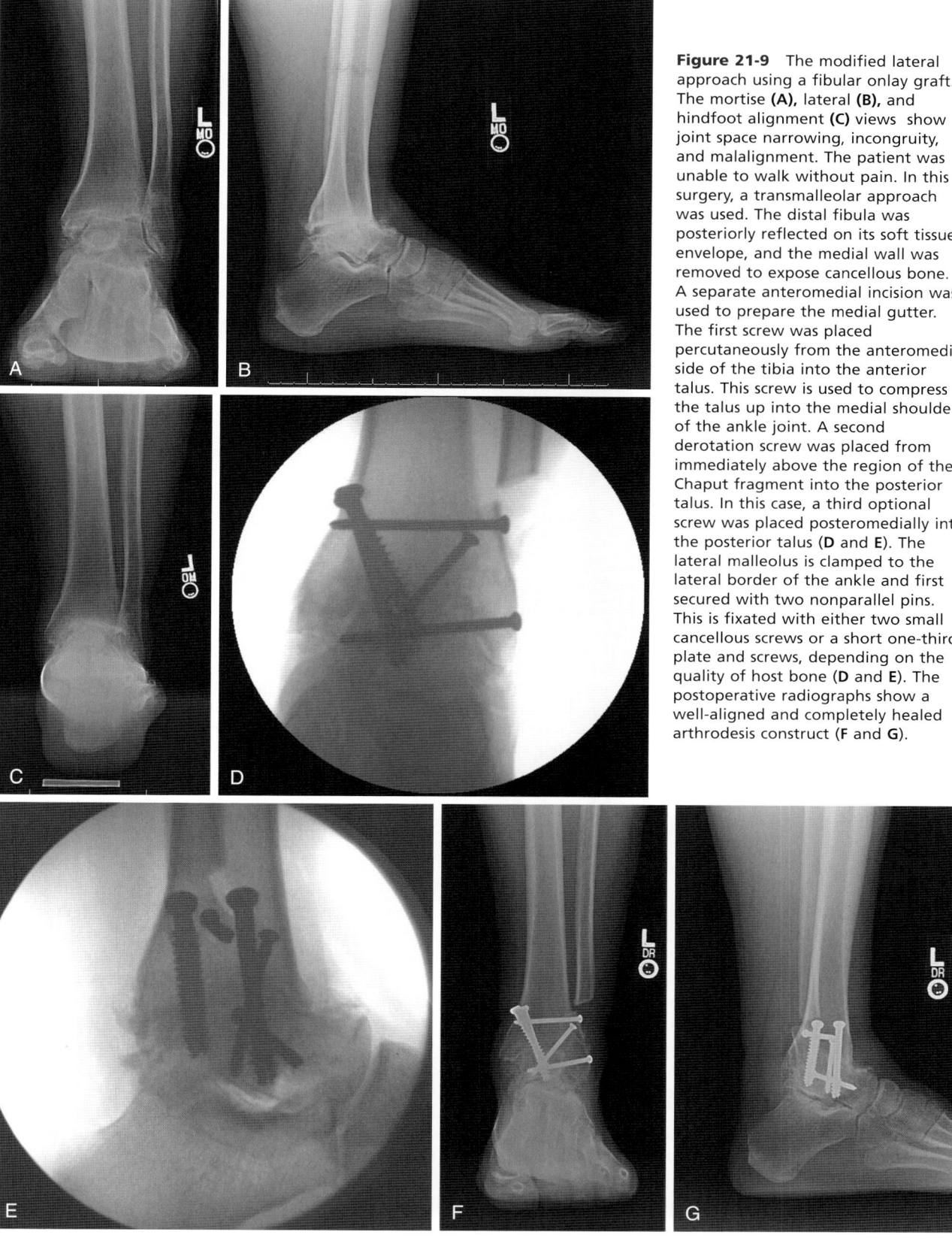

Figure 21-9 The modified lateral approach using a fibular onlay graft. The mortise (**A**), lateral (**B**), and hindfoot alignment (**C**) views show joint space narrowing, incongruity, and malalignment. The patient was unable to walk without pain. In this surgery, a transmalleolar approach was used. The distal fibula was posteriorly reflected on its soft tissue envelope, and the medial wall was removed to expose cancellous bone. A separate anteromedial incision was used to prepare the medial gutter. The first screw was placed percutaneously from the anteromedial side of the tibia into the anterior talus. This screw is used to compress the talus up into the medial shoulder of the ankle joint. A second derotation screw was placed from immediately above the region of the Chaput fragment into the posterior talus. In this case, a third optional screw was placed posteromedially into the posterior talus (**D** and **E**). The lateral malleolus is clamped to the lateral border of the ankle and first secured with two nonparallel pins. This is fixated with either two small cancellous screws or a short one-third plate and screws, depending on the quality of host bone (**D** and **E**). The postoperative radiographs show a well-aligned and completely healed arthrodesis construct (**F** and **G**).

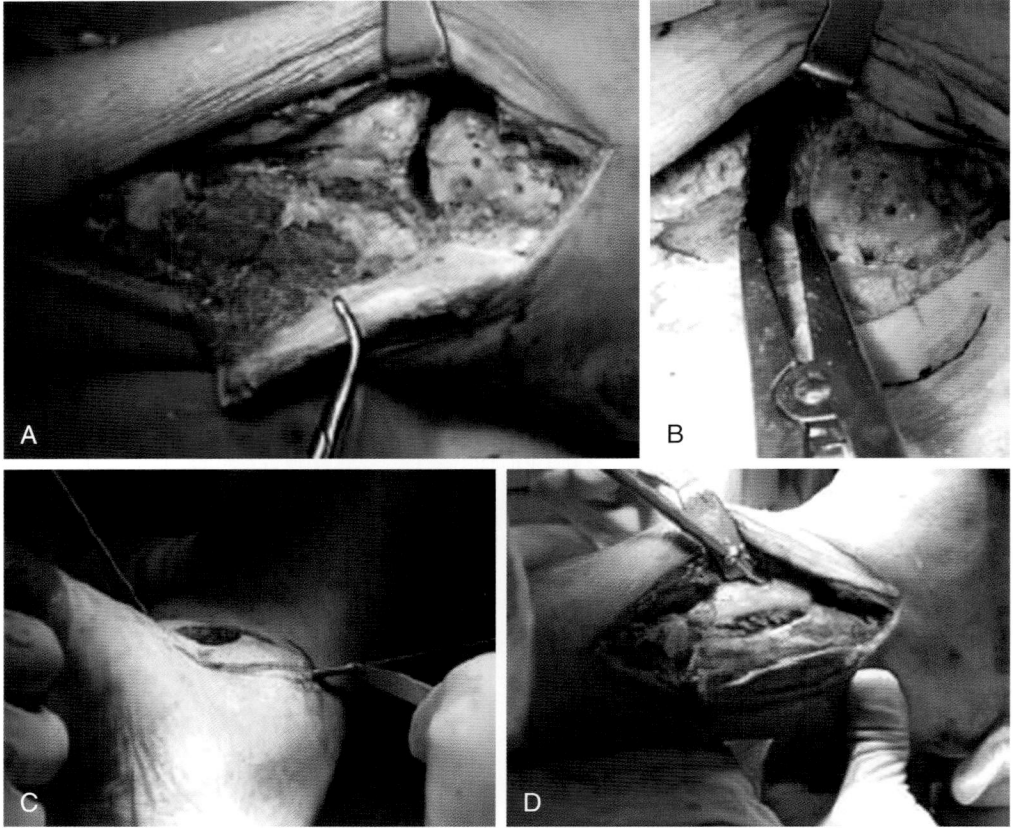

Figure 21-10 When a fibular onlay graft is used, a lateral approach over the fibula is made, and the distal fibula is posteriorly reflected on its soft tissue envelope **(A)**. The medial wall is removed to expose cancellous bone **(A)**. The matching surfaces of the talus and tibia are similarly prepared to enhance healing of the fibula as part of the fusion construct. From this approach, a laminar spreader facilitates removal of residual joint contents **(B)**. A separate anteromedial incision is often needed to prepare the medial gutter **(C)**. The first screw is placed percutaneously from the posteromedial side of the tibia, anterior to the posterior tibial tendon, into the talus **(C)**. This screw is used to compress the talus up into the medial shoulder of the ankle joint. A second derotation screw can be placed from immediately above the region of the Chaput fragment into the posterior talus **(D)**.

anteriorly. A partially threaded large cannulated screw usually compresses the construct back into the posteromedial corner.

If compression is adequate, we place one derotation screw from the anterolateral corner of the distal tibia (above the typical Chaput fragment region) into the central posterior talus (Fig. 21-10D, see Fig. 21-9D and E). This is typically a 35- to 40-mm fully threaded large (6.5- to 8.0-mm) cancellous screw. If initial compression it is not adequate, we first place another large compression screw—either as described in the Mann technique or in a straight posterior-to-anterior direction, starting lateral to the Achilles tendon—then place the fully threaded derotation screw.

The lateral malleolus is placed back onto the distal tibia and lateral talus as a vascularized lateral bone graft and to maintain the contour of the ankle. This is typically compressed first with a bone tenaculum, transfixed with nonparallel 0.062-inch Kirschner wires, and then held in place with two partially threaded 4.0-mm cancellous

screws (see Fig. 21-9D-G). In osteopenic bone, a three-hole semitubular plate is also used.

We deflate the tourniquet before closure, obtain hemostasis, and do not use a drain or bupivacaine in the wound.

Postoperative immobilization type and duration are the same as described with the Mann technique. A second alternative is to use a lateral locking plate for fixation of the tibiotalar joint (Fig. 21-11 and Video Clip 22). A lateral approach is utilized to access the tibiotalar joint. In order to place a laterally based locking plate, excision of the distal fibula is required. A fibular osteotomy is made approximately 10 cm proximal to the distal tip of the fibula. The distal fibula is then removed using blunt and/or sharp dissection. With the distal fibula excised, the tibiotalar joint is exposed. The peroneal tendons are retracted posteriorly and the tibiotalar joint is prepared for arthrodesis. If there is minimal deformity or bone loss, the contours of the articular surfaces of the tibia and talus are preserved and denuded of cartilage. The subchondral

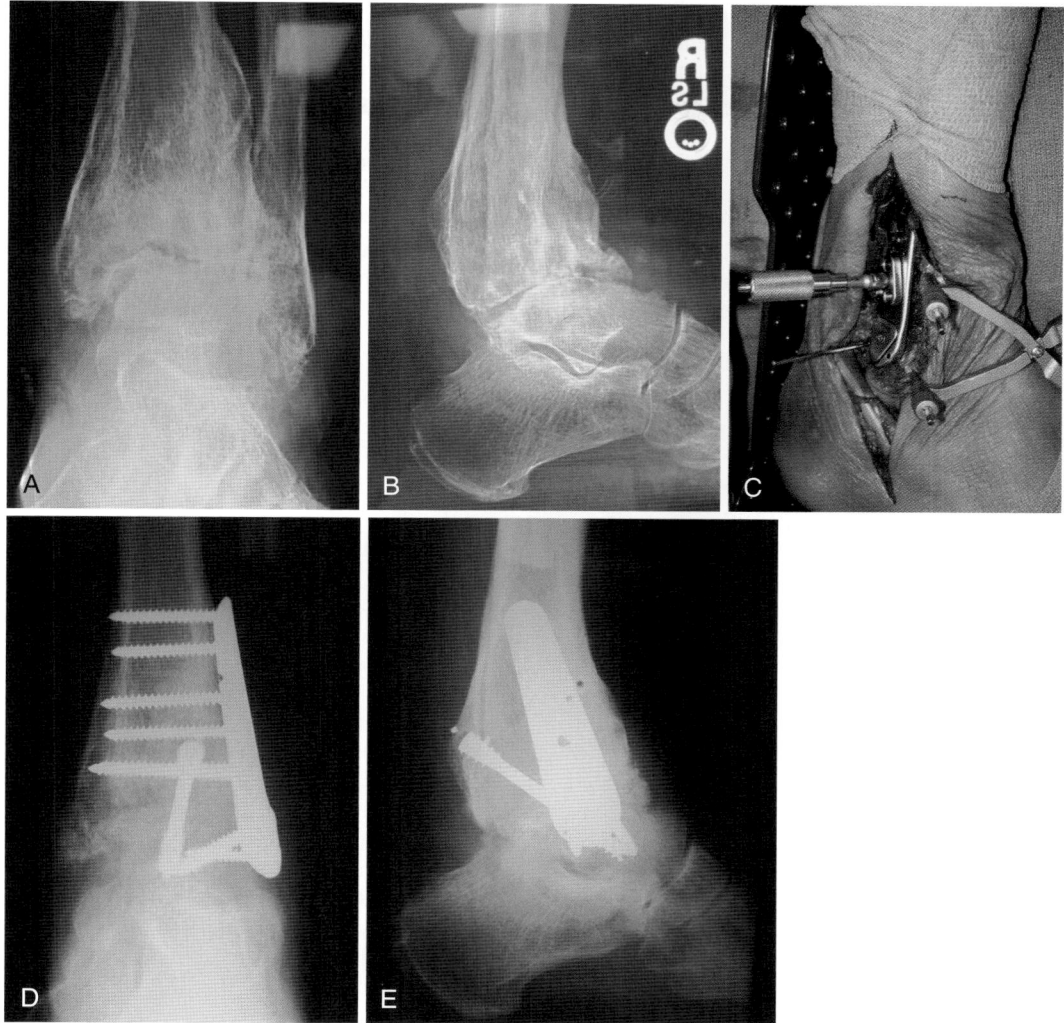

Figure 21-11 Use of a lateral approach and locking plate for tibiotalar arthrodesis. Anteroposterior **(A)** and lateral **(B)** preoperative radiographs show joint space narrowing with osteophytes and malalignment. The distal tibia is removed to give access to the tibiotalar joint **(C)**. After joint preparation, the lateral plate is applied to the talus and a compression device is used to compress the arthrodesis site **(C)**. Once compressed, the proximal tibial screws are applied. Postoperative anteroposterior **(D)** and lateral **(E)** radiographs show application of the plate with an oblique compression screws placed from posterolateral. (Case courtesy Michael Coughlin, MD.)

bone is then perforated to facilitate bony bridging. The tibiotalar joint is positioned and provisionally stabilized in the appropriate position for a tibiotalar arthrodesis using and intraoperative positioner or crossed percutaneous pins.

Once provisionally stabilized, the lateral plate is applied to the talus. The arthrodesis site is then compressed. Compression can be accomplished with a compression device, with an oblique compression screw (Fig. 21-11C) or both. An oblique screw enhances the fixation construct by adding fixation in another plane (Fig. 21-11D and E). Once compressed, the proximal tibial screws are placed. Closure and postoperative care are similar to the other lateral arthrodesis techniques.

Complications

Although malalignment after an arthrodesis was not a significant problem in Mann's series (only 4 of 81 patients were not satisfied with the position of the fusion), it can be a difficult problem for the individual patient. In the patients seen after a successful arthrodesis, the most common malalignment observed is internal rotation and varus, and the second most common is equinus. As a general rule, after fixation, when you look at the alignment if you think the heel is straight, it is still in a little varus. Malalignment after an ankle fusion can produce several gait problems.

Excessive dorsiflexion places increased stress on the heel pad, and in the patient with an insensate foot, this can cause skin breakdown. This problem can be managed with a rocker-bottom shoe.

Excessive plantar flexion can result in a back-knee thrust and a vaulting type of gait pattern. The patient often rotates the leg to be able to roll over the foot, thus placing increased stress along the medial aspect of the knee and hindfoot. The use of a SACH shoe can help to alleviate this problem.

A *varus deformity* can result in subtalar joint instability and increased stress along the lateral aspect of the foot, particularly under the base of the fifth metatarsal, and some patients develop a large callus in this area. Treatment consists of a shoe modification to redistribute pressure on the bottom of the foot.

Excessive valgus deformity produces stress along the medial aspect of the knee and hindfoot. This also results in a flatfoot posture. This deformity can be managed with an orthotic device to tilt the foot into varus.

Excessive internal or external rotation is very difficult to compensate for with any type of a shoe modification. This often results in abnormal rotation of the lower leg, sometimes giving rise to a painful hip or knee.

ARTHROSCOPIC ANKLE ARTHRODESIS

Schneider, Morgan, and others first developed techniques for arthroscopic ankle arthrodesis in the mid-1980s.[73,95] Since then, multiple studies have investigated the technique. Reported fusion rates between 89% to 100% have been reported, with the time to fusion varying from 8.9 to 12.5 weeks.[41,78]

Indications

Initial indications for arthroscopic arthrodesis included well-aligned (varus/valgus deformity < 5 degrees) arthritic ankles (Fig. 21-12A-C). However, more recently, the amount of acceptable preoperative deformity has been expanded, with reports showing excellent deformity correction and fusion rates in ankles with preoperative coronal plane deformities up to 25 degrees.[23,41] Arthroscopic arthrodesis may be favored in patients with poor soft tissue coverage or vasculopathy that have an increased risk of wound problems. In addition, patients with global inflammatory, postseptic, or hemophilic arthritis are particularly good candidates. Contraindications to this technique are ankles with active infection or Charcot arthropathy, significant focal bone loss and deformity, and very stiff immobile ankles.

Room Setup

We recommend the use of a general anesthetic, with a regional anesthetic to aid in postoperative pain control. General anesthesia aids the procedure with paralysis of all the musculature of the gastrocnemius-soleus complex to the ankle. Use of a tourniquet is optional.

Noninvasive traction is routinely applied to the ankle for portions of the arthroscopic debridement of the joint. However, use a of distractor can tighten the anterior capsule and make removal of the anterior talar dome cartilage more difficult, therefore distraction is removed for this portion of the debridement. To provide countertraction, either a well leg holder is used or the table is placed in a beach chair position with slight Trendelenburg. The break in the table at the knee allows the surgeon to put traction on the limb without moving the patient. The heel is positioned just off the edge of the table. We use a pump, large (4.0-mm) arthroscope, 4.5-mm aggressive (toothed) shaver, and 4.0-mm burr and curettes for the joint debridement.

Before the start of the surgical procedure, we draw out the palpable branches of the superficial peroneal nerve, the malleoli, and the presumed level of the tibiotalar joint space with a marking pen.

Joint Preparation

1. The limb is elevated, and the thigh tourniquet can be inflated.
2. Instill 10 to 15 mL of saline through an anteromedial approach.
3. The medial portal is then established using the nick and spread technique. A No. 15 blade is used to incise skin immediately medial to the anterior tibial tendon and 1 cm distal to the ankle. After blunt dissection is performed, the arthroscope is introduced into the anterior part of the joint.
4. If noninvasive distraction is used, it is applied now. The ankle is then distended with the arthroscopic pump. The lateral portal is then localized using an 18-gauge needle and visualized by placing the arthroscope up to the lateral margin of the peroneus tertius tendon. An incision is placed just distal to the joint, avoiding injury to any branch of the superficial peroneal nerve.
5. After blunt dissection is performed to enter the joint, the aggressive shaver is placed, and a simple anterior synovectomy is performed (Fig. 21-12D).
6. All residual cartilage in the joint is removed with a small periosteal elevator, curettes, or the shaver (Fig. 21-12E and F). If the lateral gutter does not show significant articular wear, we do not remove any cartilage from it. However, if it has degenerative changes, we remove all residual cartilage and incorporate the fibula into the fusion.
7. The burr is used to make multiple pockmarks through the subchondral cortex (Fig. 21-12G). It is critical to do this across the entire undersurface of the tibia and the anterior two thirds of the talar dome. Care is continuously taken to maintain the natural contour of the ankle joint.
8. In cases of very tight joints that are unresponsive to noninvasive distraction, we extend the incisions and place a laminar spreader in the joint to facilitate cartilage removal. (See the procedure for miniarthrotomy ankle fusion later.)
9. The tourniquet is then deflated, the pump is temporarily turned off, and the joint is inspected for adequate punctate bleeding (Fig. 21-12H).

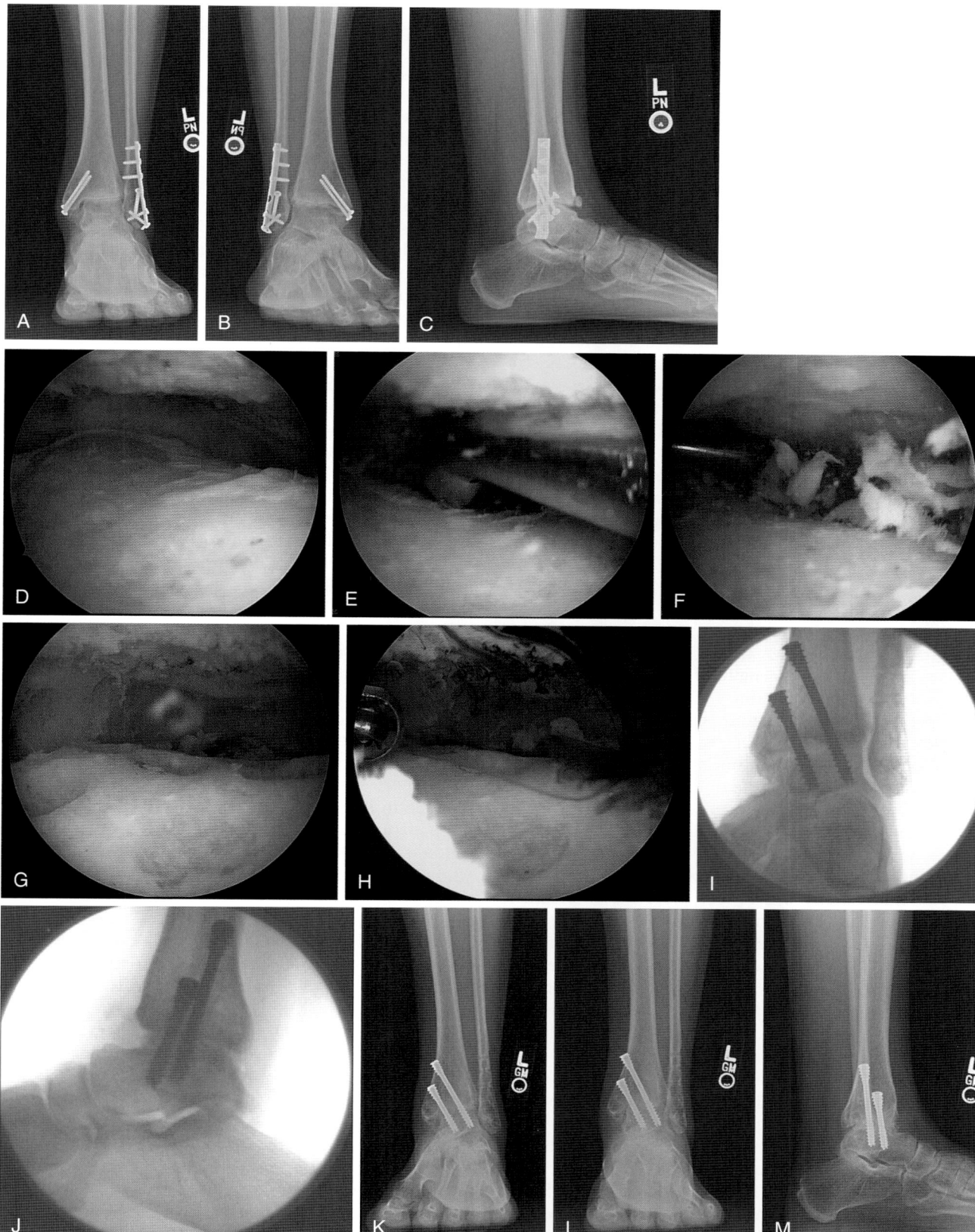

Figure 21-12 Arthroscopic ankle arthrodesis. Preoperative AP **(A)**, mortise **(B)**, and lateral **(C)** radiographs showing joint space narrowing and incongruity with normal alignment. An initial intraoperative arthroscopic view of anterior ankle shows bare bone, with some remaining damaged posterior cartilage **(D)**. After an anterior synovectomy, the remaining articular cartilage is removed using curettes, an arthroscopic shaver, and elevator **(E and F)**. The subchondral cortex is then penetrated multiple times using a small burr **(G)**. The tourniquet is then released to ensure that bleeding bone is exposed for the fusion **(H)**. Two guidewires are placed across the joint, into the talus without penetration of the subtalar or talonavicular joints. The position of the ankle is confirmed clinically before proceeding to screw fixation. In this case, two medial headless compression screws were used for fixation of the arthrodesis **(I and J)**. The distal tibiofibular joint and lateral gutter did not appear to be diseased and were left out of the construct. The postoperative radiographs show a well-aligned and completely healed arthrodesis construct **(K-M)**. (Courtesy Timothy C. Beals, MD.)

Alignment

10. The most critical step is to position the foot correctly under the tibia. With mild or minimal deformity, the focus is on getting the foot plantigrade and neutral in the sagittal plane. This seemingly easy task can befuddle even experienced surgeons. The reasons for this can relate to several factors. Some suggestions to avoid problems are as follows:
    - Place the ankle in the best position and temporarily fix it with two large Kirschner wires or cannulated pins.
    - Have your assistant hold the *leg* (not the foot) and go to the side of the room to assess the sagittal position of the ankle with the foot dorsiflexed. Do not accept anything less than perfect.
    - *Do not use fluoroscopy* to evaluate the position of the foot.
    - Always check to ensure that the foot is in a natural or slightly increased external rotation.
    - Remember the orthopaedist's "eleventh commandment": Thou shalt not varus. Varus is poorly tolerated after an ankle fusion.

Fixation

11. For a tibiotalar fusion, two to three large cannulated screws can be used. A mini–C-arm can be used to check position and length of the cannulated pins before screws are placed.
12. The first pin is placed from posteromedial to anterocentral in the talus. The leg is arranged in the figure-of-four position. A 1-cm incision is made along the posteromedial edge of the tibia 3 cm above the joint line. Skin and soft tissues need to be retracted throughout this percutaneous approach. The screw traverses the posteromedial corner of the ankle down the center of the neck of the talus. A partially threaded large cannulated screw usually compresses the construct back into the posteromedial corner.
13. A second and third screw is then placed. These can be in either compression or static. Very often, a derotation screw placed percutaneously from the anterolateral corner of the distal tibia (above the typical Chaput fragment region) into the central posterior talus is used. Care must be taken to avoid damage to local nerves with this approach. Another option is to use a second anteromedial screw, which can be placed for additional fixation (Fig. 21-12I and J).
14. When the fibulotalar joint has no apparent arthritis, it is not debrided or fixated. However if the fibulotalar joint is included in the fusion construct, a single large, partially threaded cannulated screw is used to secure the fibula to the talus. This is placed from posterolateral to inferocentral into the talar neck and body.
15. If the joint does not easily coapt, we judiciously inject a mixture of 5 to 7 mL of finely ground allograft cancellous bone and demineralized bone matrix into the regions with poor contact. This should not be done in areas of natural contact. Inclusion of the lateral malleolus increases the likelihood of grafting because the first screw tends to pull the talus over medially, leaving a small gap laterally.

Postoperative Care

The surgery can be done on an outpatient basis. This depends more on the structure of home help than medical need.

A well-padded posterior U splint is applied in the operating room. The splint and sutures are removed, and a cast is applied 7 to 14 days postoperatively. The patient is allowed 5 to 10 pounds of heel weight bearing—just enough to maintain their balance.

At 6 weeks, plain radiographs are taken. These generally show a bridging cancellous ingrowth, which appears as a hazy cloud in the joint space. As long as there is good evidence of bone-bridging, the leg is put in a removable boot. This is removed for sleeping, bathing, and sitting but is worn full time when standing. Progressive weight bearing is permitted as tolerated.

At 10 weeks postoperatively, new radiographs are taken (Fig. 21-12K-M). If the patient has no pain with standing and the radiographs are satisfactory, the patient is weaned from the boot. Although formal physical therapy is often unnecessary, we have found a 4- to 8-week course of balance and gait retraining after removal of the boot to speed recovery in elderly patients. For laborers or those who need to stand at work, the minimum total time off full duty is 4 months.

Clinical Experience

At least 18 case series, comprising 7 to 116 patients each, were reported between 1986 and 2010.* Myerson et al[77] retrospectively compared open to arthroscopic fusion in 33 patients. In patients who underwent arthroscopy, union was achieved at an average of 8.7 weeks. In patients who underwent arthrodesis by a conventional open technique using similar fixation methods, union was achieved, on average, by 14.5 weeks. Fusion rates were similar for both techniques. The two groups were not similar because patients with more deformity or extensive osteonecrosis were selectively placed in the open group. Average hospital stay was four nights for the open group and one night for the arthroscopy group. Nielsen et al[78] also compared patients undergoing open and arthroscopic ankle arthrodesis with a retrospective review. Similar to Myerson, the open arthrodesis group differed from the arthroscopic group because of having larger preoperative deformities. Patients in the arthroscopic group were discharged 2.27 days earlier than those in the open group and showed a significantly higher rate of union at 12 weeks (90% vs. 57%).[78] In a third study, O'Brien et al[79] reported the results of surgeries performed on 36 patients. Retrospectively, the two groups were matched for preoperative clinical deformity. Fusion rates of 82% in the open group and 84% in the arthroscopic group were achieved. Similar to

*References 8, 14, 20, 21, 23, 25, 31, 33, 40, 41, 51, 77, 78, 81, 82, 104, 108, and 111.

Myerson's report, hospital stays averaged three nights for the open group and one night for the arthroscopic group.

Fusion rates of 90% to 100% occurred in 11 reports,* two reported rates of 80% to 89%,[34,81] and two listed clinical fusions of 93% and 100% but radiographic evidence of fusion in 74%[27] and 50%,[27] respectively.

Six studies had average fusion times of 7 weeks or less.[†] An additional eight studies reported up to 16 weeks' average time to fusion.[‡] Another study, comprising 42 patients, had an average time for fusion based on radiographs of 5.5 months, possibly attributable to two delayed unions that required 20 months to heal. This protocol used demineralized bone matrix with autogenous bone marrow graft.[21]

Five studies listed good, very good, or excellent results in 80% to 100% of patients at follow-up ranging from 14 months to 8 years.[¶] Crosby et al[21] reported 85% satisfied at an average of 27 months. Corso and Zimmer[20] rated 88% completely satisfied at follow-up. Paremain et al[82] noted improved AOFAS scores; however, these were retrospectively assigned by the investigators. Winson et al[108] reported 80% good or excellent patient outcomes in a cohort of 104 patients at an average of 65 months of follow-up. Three further studies mentioned favorable results without using a rating scale.[14,34,104]

Complications

The most frequent complication reported has been painful hardware requiring removal.[§] The rate of this complication may be decreased with the use of headless compression screws. A recent study by Odutola et al[80] using headless compression screws in arthroscopic ankle arthrodeses showed an 88% fusion rate at 2 years in 32 patients, without the need for hardware removal in any patients. Other major sequelae were delayed union or nonunion,[8,21,108] subtalar pain or arthritis,[14,20,21,108] subtalar joint penetration,[25] cutaneous nerve injury,[20,81] infection,[14,21,51,108] malunion,[8,34,40] dorsalis pedis pseudoaneurysm,[40] broken drill bit, deep venous thrombosis,[108] stress fracture,[108] and fracture through external fixator pin site.[21] The rates of these complications are generally not higher than those reported with open techniques.

MINI-ARTHROTOMY ANKLE FUSION

Paremain et al[82] have described a method of ankle fusion that is meant to "combine the advantages of both open and arthroscopic techniques." This approach uses enlarged arthroscopic portals for exposure and removal of cartilage.

Surgical Technique

1. Two 2- to 3-cm incisions are made anterolaterally and anteromedially (Fig. 21-13).

---

*References 8, 14, 20, 23, 33, 40, 41, 78, 82, 104, and 108.
[†]References 20, 33, 34, 40, 104, and 111.
[‡]References 8, 14, 23, 25, 41, 51, 78, and 81.
[¶]References 23, 33, 40, 41, 81, 108, and 111.
[§]References 14, 20, 27, 40, 82, 104, 108, and 111.

2. A laminar spreader is alternately placed on both sides, allowing the surgeon to see the joint directly, while avoiding the soft tissue disruption of full open arthrotomy. Visibility can be less than that achieved during an arthroscopic fusion. The posterior one third of the joint is often not easily seen from this approach.
3. Autogenous bone slurry or bone substitute material can be instilled to fill gaps.

Postoperative Results

Paremain et al[82] reported early radiographic evidence of healing, which occurred at an average of 6 weeks. Radiographic evidence of fusion across the anterior two thirds of the joint as well as clinical fusion was obtained in 100% of 15 cases. The authors acknowledge that the long-term sequelae of not fusing the posterior one third of the joint are unknown.

A similar mini-open technique on the lateral side only, combined with an anteromedial portal, was described by Hartel et al.[45] They also achieved a fusion in all eight patients reported. For the occasional ankle arthroscopist, this approach can shorten operation time compared with conventional arthroscopic approaches, which can be more technically demanding. We use this approach when the insertion of arthroscopic instruments is not easy because of large anterior joint spurs or arthrofibrosis.

ANTERIOR ANKLE ARTHRODESIS WITH PLATING

An anterior approach to the ankle with rigid plate fixation offers several theoretic advantages over a lateral approach with screw fixation (Video Clip 23). The anterior approach is familiar to many foot and ankle surgeons and allows better visualization and access to the tibiotalar joint for cartilage debridement. In addition, there is less soft tissue dissection and devitalization of the bone compared with a lateral transfibular approach. The anterior approach also allows rigid plate fixation in the plane of motion of the ankle joint. This will create a more stable construct compared with crossed screw fixation. In a study comparing three crossed screws with three crossed screws supplemented with an anterior plate, Tarkin et al[101] showed a 3.5-, 1.4-, and 1.9-fold increase in the construct stiffness with anterior plating in the sagittal, coronal, and rotational planes, respectively.

One of the main disadvantages to the anterior approach to the ankle is the decreased access to the lateral gutters ankle and distal tibiofibular joint. This should be taken into account when considering this technique. Another disadvantage is the potential for difficulty with coverage of the anterior tendinous structures if a wound problem is encountered with this approach.

Indications

Current indications for anterior ankle arthrodesis include end-stage arthritis of the tibiotalar joint, with minimal deformity and without significant involvement of the distal tibiofibular joint or lateral gutter. Because the amount of soft tissue dissection is less, the authors currently recommend the technique in patients without

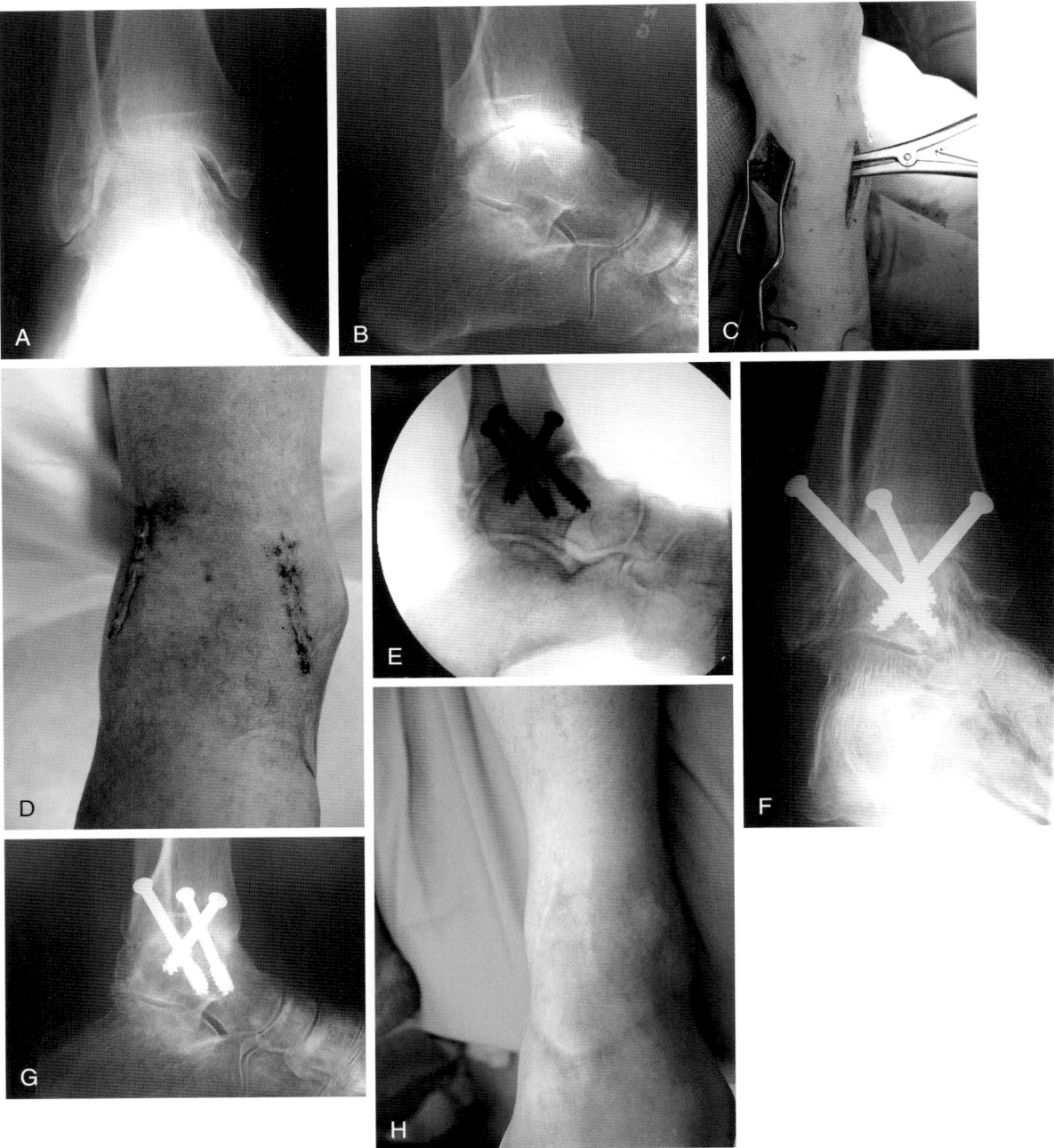

Figure 21-13 Mini-open technique of ankle fusion. Mortise **(A)** and lateral **(B)** radiographs of a 70-year-old man with painful ankle osteoarthritis. A mini-open approach was selected because his ankle moved very little and he had no deformity. The approach involves two incisions through which the joint is easily debrided of its contents. **C,** This is easily accomplished by placing a laminar spreader in one side and preparing the joint surfaces of the other side. **D,** The lateral incision can be extended to facilitate screw placement. **E,** Two or three large cannulated screws are typically used to maintain stability during the fusion process. **F** and **G,** The postoperative radiographs show a solid and well-aligned ankle. **H,** The clinical photograph shows the well-tolerated scar appearance.

significant coronal plane deformity (<5 degrees of varus/valgus). However, as with arthroscopic ankle arthrodesis, this recommendation may change as experience with the technique grows. Because of difficult soft tissue coverage of a wound problem, the anterior approach would be contraindicated in patients who have poor anterior soft tissues secondary to medical comorbidities, smoking, trauma, or previous surgery.

Room Setup

General or regional anesthesia can be used for the procedure. We recommend muscle relaxation throughout the procedure to allow for ease in plate placement and positioning of the ankle. The patient is positioned in the supine position with a bump underneath the ipsilateral hip to place the knee in a neutral position. Tourniquet use is optional. The authors find it beneficial to leave the tourniquet down during the surgical approach, to prevent postoperative hematoma formation through meticulous hemostasis. In addition, distension of the vascular structures facilitates easier identification and protection of the important anterior structures during the surgical procedure. The tourniquet is then inflated during bony preparation.

Joint Preparation

1. A midline anterior approach to the ankle is used. This is placed just lateral to the anterior tibialis tendon.

The incision extends approximately 6 cm proximal to the joint and is carried distally to allow exposure of the talar neck. The incision is carried down to the level of the fasicia of the anterior compartment, being careful to protect the branches of the superficial peroneal nerve (Figs. 21-14A and B and 21-15C).

2. The fascia of the anterior compartment is incised either over the tendon of the extensor hallicus longus or just lateral to the anterior tibialis tendon (Figs. 21-14C and 21-15D).

3. The interval between the anterior tibialis and extensor hallicus longus is developed. Care is taken to identify the anterior tibial artery, vein, and nerve. The neurovascular structures are retracted laterally after the medial vascular branches are carefully cauterized.

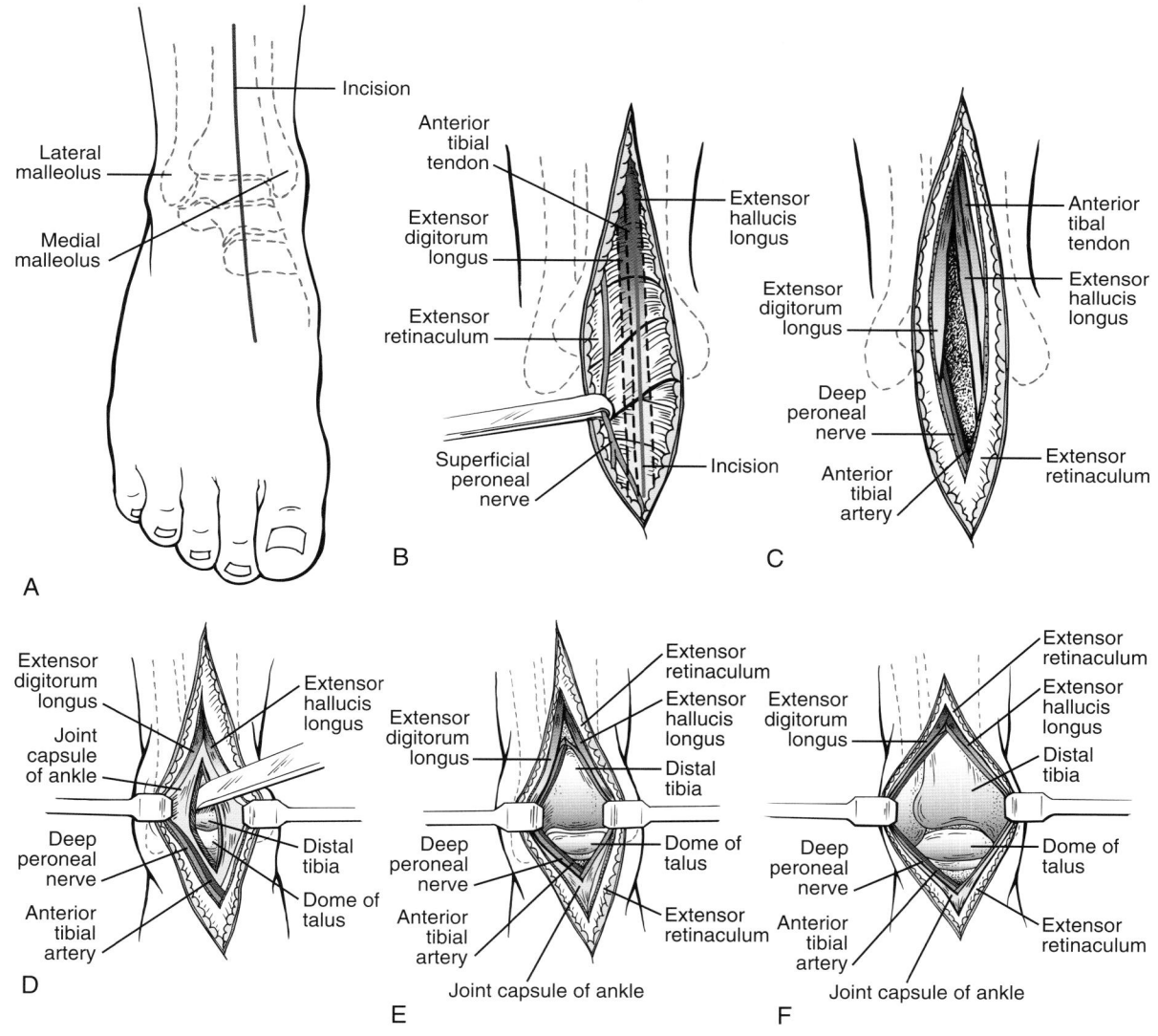

Figure 21-14 Anterior approach to the ankle. **A,** An incision is made directly anterior. **B,** The medial branch of the superficial peroneal nerve is often encountered and gently retracted laterally. **C,** The lateral bed of the extensor hallucis brevis is incised, the tendon is swept medially, and the deep neurovascular structures are retracted laterally. Often, the surgeon encounters a medially directed vascular leash that requires cautery. **D,** The capsule is incised longitudinally to preserve it for later closure. **E,** Subperiosteal dissection then allows good visualization of the anterior tibiotalar joint. **F,** Dissection is expanded to visualize the medial gutter and distal tibiofibular joint.

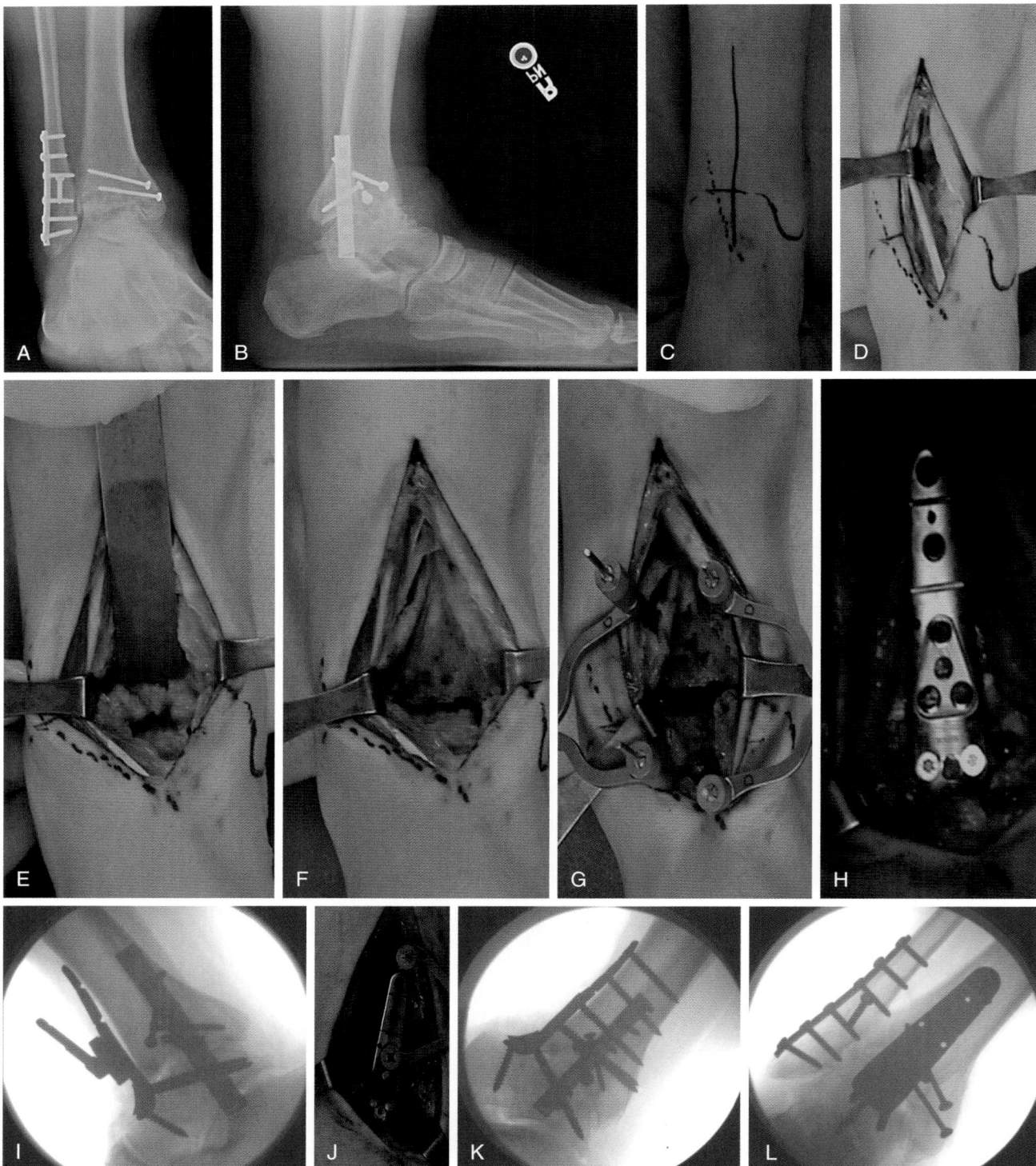

Figure 21-15 Anterior approach to the ankle and plating for tibiotalar arthrodesis. The preoperative mortise **(A)** and lateral **(B)** radiographs show tibiotalar joint space narrowing, incongruity, and malalignment. The bony landmarks as well as the path of the superficial peroneal nerve are traced out before making a direct anterior incision just lateral to the tibialis anterior **(C)**. The interval between the extensor hallicus longus and tibialis anterior is developed. The extensor hallucis longus (EHL) and neurovascular structures are retracted laterally **(D)**. An anterior arthrotomy and subperiosteal dissection expose the tibiotalar joint. An osteotome is used to remove anterior osteophytes, exposing the joint for removal of the remaining articular cartilage **(E and F)**. The joint is distracted to allow access for debridement **(G)**. The plate is positioned anteriorly along the talar neck. Some talar neck bone may need to be removed for proper plate positioning. The talar screws are inserted, taking care not to penetrate the subtalar joint **(H and I)**. The joint is compressed with a compression device **(J)**. The remaining tibial screws are then placed to secure the plate **(K and L)**.

4. An anterior arthrotomy and subperiosteal elevation is used to expose the tibiotalar joint and the talar neck. Dissection is carried medially to expose the medial gutter. To preserve vascular supply, the lateral gutter and distal tibiofibular joint are not exposed unless necessary (Fig. 21-14D-F).

5. An osteotome is used to remove anterior bone spurs from the distal tibia and talar neck (Fig. 21-15E and F).

6. Joint distraction is obtained using laminar spreaders or pin distracters (Fig. 21-15G).

7. The remaining tibiotalar joint and medial gutter cartilage is removed using curettes and osteotomes.

8. The subchondral bone is perforated using either a drill or osteotome.

9. The authors recommend the placement of bone graft into the posterior aspect of the joint space after the preparation of the joint surface is completed.

Alignment

10. The most critical step is to position the foot correctly under the tibia. The focus is on getting the foot plantigrade and neutral in the sagittal plane.

11. Place the ankle in the best position and temporarily fix it with two large Kirschner wires. Evaluate the position of the foot both clinically and with intraoperative fluoroscopy. Do not accept anything less than perfection. The goal is to have a neutral or dorsiflexed foot in the sagittal plane with a slightly valgus or neutral hindfoot. External rotation should be equivalent to the contralateral side.

12. Be sure to evaluate the fibular length after temporary fixation to ensure that excessive shortening of the tibiotalar joint has not resulted in a long fibula that could cause subfibular impingement.

Fixation

13. Once the joint has been temporarily stabilized in the appropriate position, the anterior plate is sized and temporarily pinned in place using K-wires. Resection of the talar neck and plate bending may be necessary for optimally placement.

14. The talar screws are placed being careful not to penetrate into the subtalar joint (Fig. 21-15H and I).

15. With the talar screws in place, the tibiotalar joint is compressed using a compression device or eccentric drilling of the tibial screw holes. The temporary K-wires can be withdrawn to allow for optimal joint compression (Fig. 21-15J).

16. The remaining tibial screws are placed, and fluoroscopic images are obtained to confirm hardware placement and joint reduction (Fig. 21-15K and L).

17. Bone graft is placed in the anterior joint and medial gutter.

18. Layered closure includes the fascia of the anterior compartment.

Postoperative Care

A well-padded posterior splint with side gussets is applied in the operating room. The splint and sutures are removed 2 to 3 weeks postoperatively. Once the wound has healed, the patient is placed in to a removable postoperative boot. Boot immobilization is chosen over cast immobilization because of increased stiffness of the plate fixation compared with screw stabilization. For the first 2 weeks postoperatively, the patient is allowed 5 to 10 pounds of heel weight bearing; from 2 to 6 weeks we allow up to 30 pounds of weight bearing.

At the 6-week postoperative visit, plain radiographs are taken. As long as there is good evidence of bridging bone, progressive weight bearing to tolerance is permitted. Initial weight bearing is done in the postoperative boot, and then progressive transition to a normal shoe is permitted. The patient is usually seen at 3 months after the operation for repeat radiographs and evaluation. Formal physical therapy often is not needed; however, a formalized program can help elderly patients maximize their balance and gait.

Clinical Experience

Our personal experience with this approach has been highly favorable. Interpretation of the published results of anterior plating for tibiotalar arthrodesis is difficult because of the inclusion of heterogeneous populations of patients in the clinical series to date. Most studies include patients undergoing primary arthrodesis, with patients who have had either a failed previous arthrodesis or total ankle arthroplasty. Despite the inclusion of these diverse problems, the published results to date have shown favorable results for anterior plating.

Mears et al[70] first described anterior plating for tibiotalar arthrodesis in 1991. These authors were able to obtain an 82% fusion rate in 17 patients by using a contoured 4.5-mm plate. Almost a decade later, Rowan et al[86] reported their results using an Arbeitsgemeinschaft für Osteosynthesefragen (AO) T-plate for an anterior tibiotalar arthrodesis. In this study of 33 patients, the authors were able to obtain a 94% fusion rate.[86] However, 3 patients underwent below-knee amputation despite having radiologically solid ankle fusion.[86]

Recently, there has been a renewed interest in anterior ankle arthrodesis, with three papers published in the last 3 years. These studies showed between 90% to 100% fusion rates using different plating techniques.[43,71,84] The time to fusion varied from 12.2 to 15 weeks.[43,71,84] However, these studies were hampered by the inclusion of both patients undergoing primary arthrodesis and patients undergoing arthrodesis for a failed total ankle arthroplasty.

Complications

Wound problems or infections were reported in only one study.[86] In this study, 12% of patients had superficial wound breakdown or infection. However, in half of these patients, two accessory incisions had been used to remove portions of the medial and lateral malleoli, and one patient had an arthrodesis for a previously infected ankle joint.[86]

Tibial stress fractures are a concern with this technique because of the significantly increased stiffness of the ankle with the plate. This was reported in one study,[86] and occurred in 6% of patients. Other complications included malposition (12%),[70] subtalar joint violation with hardware (21%),[86] and symptomatic hardware requiring removal (3%-14%)[71,84,86] Overall, the rate of symptomatic hardware was quite low for all published studies, and the 14% rate shown in the Mohamedean[71] study was due to the extension of the hardware across either the talonavicular or subtalar joints to improve fixation in patients with poor bone quality resulting from neurologic disorders.

Osteochondral Allograft Ankle Joint Resurfacing

Limited studies suggest the potential efficacy of fresh or freshly preserved osteochondral allografts in selected patients.[42,56,103] The development of precise cutting jigs for total ankle arthroplasty has facilitated the accurate placement of allograft parts. Anatomic matching and the relatively limited supply of donor ankles remain the limiting factors. Immunologic matching or immunosuppression has not been used for these cases, but it can have a role. Further study of this issue and risk of disease transmission is necessary.

There have been very few peer-reviewed articles related to either partial or total osteochondral allografts. None of these articles has shown remarkable success with these allografts, and some showed an alarmingly high rate of failure.

Allan Gross and his colleagues[42] in Toronto described the outcomes in nine patients treated for focal defects of the ankle articular cartilage by using fresh osteochondral allografts. All defects were greater than 1 cm in diameter. Three required fusion at 3, 5, and 7 years postoperatively. The remainder were intact at an average of 11 years postoperatively, most with good function, no pain, and patient satisfaction with the procedure (Fig. 21-16). Kim et al[56] reported on the experience of the University of California at San Diego (UCSD) group, which used shell allografts preserved at 4° C for up to 5 days. In 7 patients with global arthritis, the results at an average 12 years after operation were considered poor for 3, good for 2, and excellent for 2. Failure was primarily thought to be due to poor donor–host graft fit, and this stimulated the UCSD group to use total ankle cutting jigs in more recent cases. Their preliminary results in 12 patients (13 ankles) at an average follow-up of 21 months have been documented.[103] The group included 10 tibiotalar grafts, 1 talar graft, and 1 tibial graft. In this preliminary report, the authors revised a collapsed lateral talar dome graft to a bipolar graft and debrided two lateral gutters for impingement.

The largest peer-reviewed study to date, by Jeng et al,[50] reviewed the results of 29 patients undergoing total ankle bipolar allograft transplantation. At 2 years' follow-up, the authors showed a failure rate of 69%, and only 6 of the 9 successful patients would have undergone the operation again. The authors thought that the time to allograft implantation (23 days for their study) contributed to their high failure rate.

The limited published data regarding tibiotalar allograft transplantation suggests that the procedure must be approached with caution. The apparent high failure rate, coupled with a difficult salvage situation should limit its use to a very small number of patients. The information regarding allograft transplantation is limited, and further study is clearly needed before this procedure can become more commonly used.

SPECIAL CIRCUMSTANCES

Talar Avascular Necrosis

Avascular necrosis (AVN) of the talus is a difficult problem to treat. Fortunately, not all cases of talar AVN are clinically significant. After trauma, it is relatively common to see signs of focal talar AVN on the radiographs of asymptomatic patients. Others, though, have pain and need further evaluation.

Many treatment regimens have been devised for these patients. However, none has been subjected to rigorous testing, primarily because of the relatively low prevalence of symptomatic talar AVN. For example, in our busy tertiary clinical practice, only about 10 new patients with symptomatic talar AVN are seen each year. No one surgeon or center has had enough experience in treating these patients to provide a good scientific basis for decision-making. The following describes our personal preference in handling these unusual problems.

First, we try to determine three things: Is the AVN focal or global? Is the pain coming from a joint or from the bone? Has the talus collapsed?

If the AVN is focal and the pain is coming from the bone, treatment can be directed at the source of pain. Fluoroscopically controlled injections of the ankle and subtalar joints with a local anesthetic should help to determine the source of pain. If these injections fail to reduce it, the pain is coming from within the talus.

Typically, surgical treatment of focal and painful talar AVN involves core decompression and grafting. Mont et al[101] reported the average of 7-year follow-up results of 11 patients (17 AVN tali without collapse) treated with core decompression and grafting. Three later required fusion, but the remaining 8 patients (82%) had good results. They used autograft. Our experience mirrors theirs. Whether bone allograft is as effective as autograft has not been studied, but in our limited experience, both have provided similar positive results, suggesting that the pathogenesis of pain is related to stress fracturing and bone edema rather than osteonecrosis alone.

Gilbert et al[38] have proposed local vascularized pedicle bone grafts for treatment of these problems. In their elegant anatomic report, they show the potential for rotating a dorsal fragment of the cuboid to the ankle

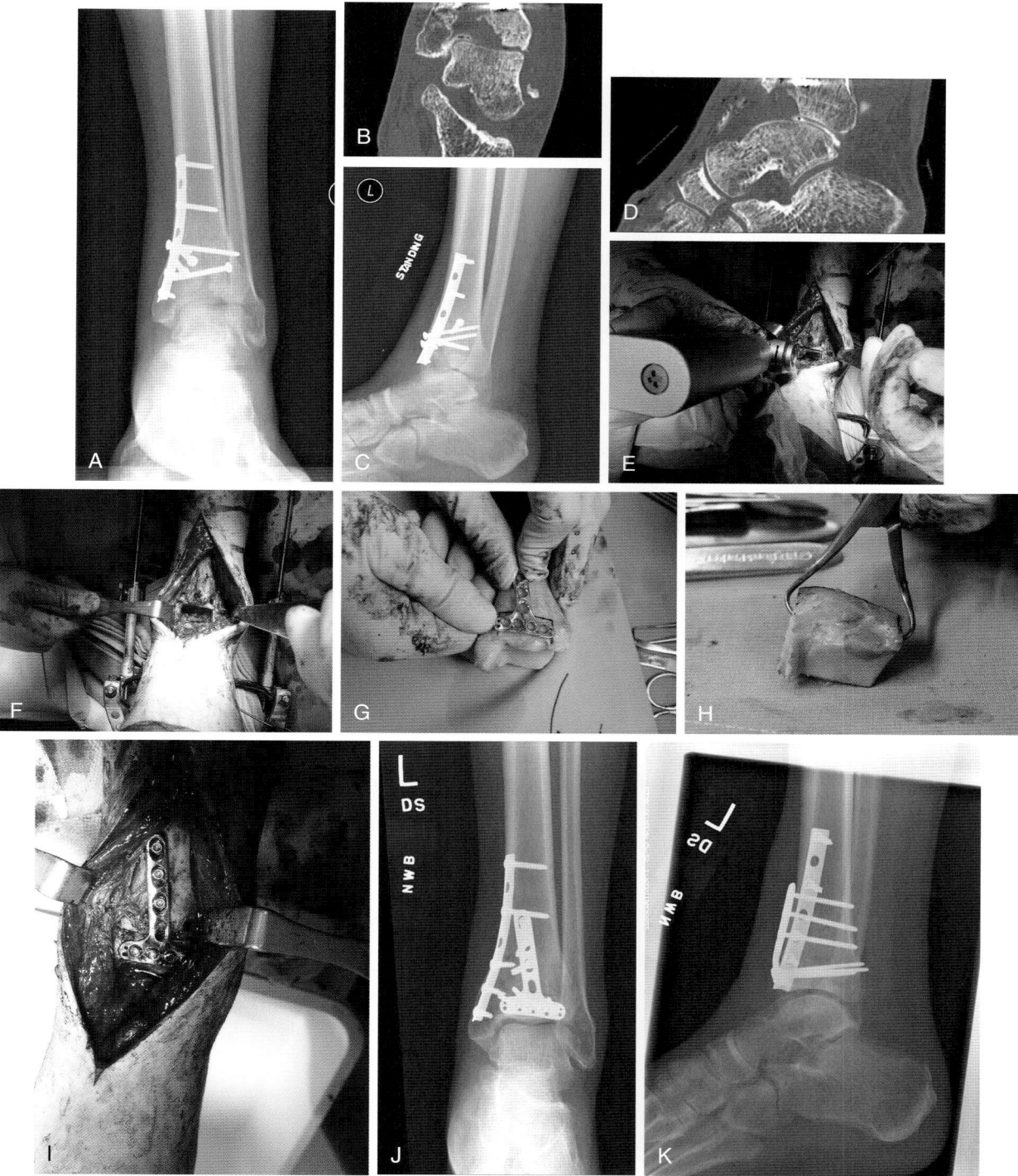

Figure 21-16 Segmental osteochondral allograft resurfacing is an option for ankles with focal posttraumatic ankle osteoarthritis and bone loss. In this case, a 24-year-old policeman sustained a pilon injury with bone loss. **A-D,** The central anterior segment of the distal tibia was completely absent when the patient was referred for definitive treatment. The dye-injected distraction computed tomographic (CT) images show preserved cartilage elsewhere. After an anatomically suitable fresh donor specimen was secured, an allograft replacement was performed. To facilitate the procedure, the joint was distracted with a simple tensioned wire frame **(E),** and a box defect was created **(F).** The allograft was prepared to fit the defect **(G),** adhering to the wise adage "measure twice, cut once" **(H). I,** After placement, we secured the allograft with a wrist plate (Zimmer Holdings, Warsaw, Ind.). **J** and **K,** The postoperative radiographs show excellent joint preservation and alignment.

region while it is still fully attached to its vascular pedicle from the lateral tarsal artery. Whether this form of treatment will help to improve the relatively good results already reported for simple decompression and grafting needs further careful clinical study.

When the AVN is focal but pain is coming from a joint, the patient is usually treated with fusion surgery. We use fluoroscopically controlled injections of the ankle and subtalar joints with a local anesthetic to determine the source of pain. These injections can also be used to help illustrate to the patient the likely response to fusion surgery.[55] The extent and location of talar collapse should be carefully evaluated. In young patients with focal problems, osteochondral autografts or allografts may be considered for partial joint resurfacing (Fig. 21-17).

If the AVN is global or diffusely distributed throughout the talar dome and body, local measures are not generally helpful. Some of these patients present with intense pain, especially with weight bearing, and no joint collapse. In the talus with MRI evidence of global or diffusely patchy AVN *and no subchondral collapse,* the AVN has the potential for resolving. In these circumstances, we simultaneously use three modalities for treatment because our experience has been positive. First, we prescribe an unloader brace, usually with a patellar tendon–bearing component or with a calf-lacer design. The ankle joint must be locked for the brace to unload. Second, we

prescribe an ultrasound bone stimulator and ask that it be used in two locations, 20 minutes per day. Third, we prescribe an oral bisphosphonate for a minimum of 4 months to tip the balance of bone resorption and deposition toward deposition. In some circumstances, where pain is unbearable on the first visit, we organize a single intravenous (IV) infusion of a longer and more immediately acting bisphosphonate. With this program, we have treated eight patients (10 tali) who have experienced near-complete resolution of their symptoms and no collapse over the past 8 years.

Most tali with subtotal AVN, however, develop subchondral collapse and secondary arthritis. This can occur at the ankle or subtalar joint or in both joints simultaneously. Often, it involves one joint at first, and typically this is the ankle joint. Fusion of the involved joint(s) is the treatment of choice. The use of uncemented, ingrowth total ankle implants is relatively contraindicated because the potential for good ingrowth and component fixation is low.

The keys to a successful fusion in the face of talar AVN are identifying the painful joint with fluoroscopically controlled injections of a local anesthetic, resecting the entire necrotic segment, adding autogenous bone graft or a substitute as a biostimulant, and obtaining and maintaining compression with fixation.

Five current methods of fixation with their advantages and disadvantages are listed in Table 21-5. The technique

Table 21-5 Advantages and Disadvantages of Fixation Methods

Fixation	Advantages	Disadvantages	Indications	Cost
Large cannulated screws	Ease of use Inexpensive Familiarity Rigid fixation	Poor axial compression Insufficient fixation of short segments Technically more demanding	Minimal bone loss Tibiotalar and/or subtalar joint involvement Primary arthrodeses Significant bone loss or instability	↑
Blade plate	Axial compression Fixed-angle construct Rigid fixation	Increased dissection Risk fracture with blade placement Difficult fit with "abnormal" anatomy	Tibiotalar and/or subtalar joint involvement Revision cases Significant bone loss or instability	↑↑↑
Locking plate	Axial compression Fixed-angle construct Anatomically contoured Familiarity Ease of use	Cost Inconsistent axial compression	Tibiotalar and/or subtalar joint involvement Revision or primary cases Complete talar body collapse	↑↑↑↑
Locked intramedullary nail	Indirect fixation Autograft from reaming Rigid axial compression	Relatively poor distal fixation Higher complication rate	Tibiotalar and subtalar joint involvement Significant bone loss Infected cases	↑↑↑↑↑
Multiplane external fixator	Early weight bearing Can tolerate noncompliance Can be used in setting of infection	Poor patient tolerance Compression across joints not being fused	Revision cases Noncompliant patients	↑↑↑↑↑↑

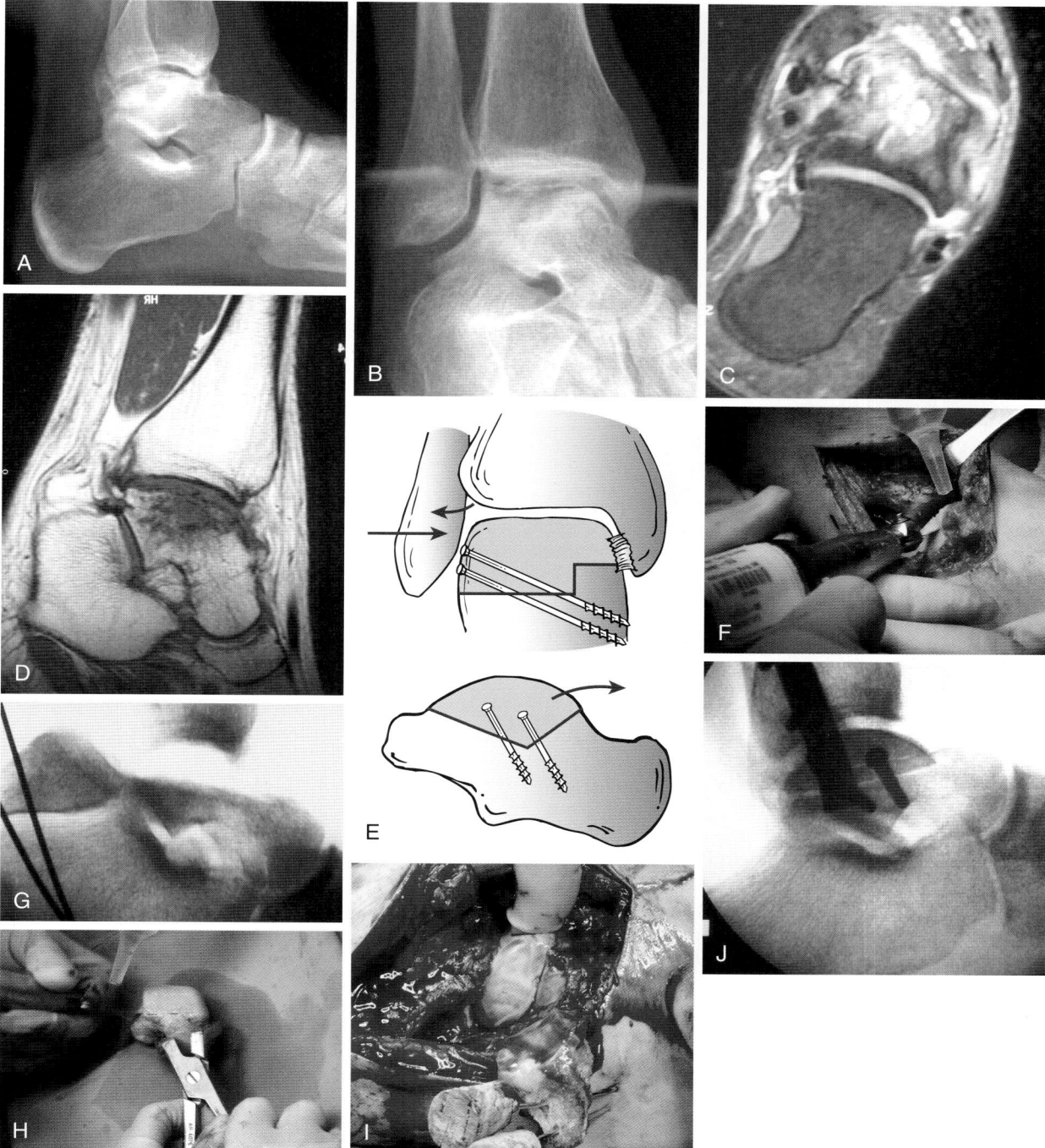

Figure 21-17 Segmental osteochondral allograft resurfacing is also an option for ankles with focal talar avascular necrosis (AVN). **A** and **B,** The preoperative radiographs of the right ankle of a 17-year-old boy with idiopathic onset of bilateral talar AVN. **C** and **D,** Magnetic resonance imaging revealed large segmental involvement. **E,** The preoperative plan for partial joint replacement. **F** and **G,** A transmalleolar approach was used, with the lateral malleolus pinned to the calcaneus. The ankle joint was opened and the defect removed with a small saw. **H** and **I,** The allograft was prepared and placed into the defect. **J,** Two buried screws were used to secure the construct, and the distal fibula was reconstructed with standard plate and screws.

Continued

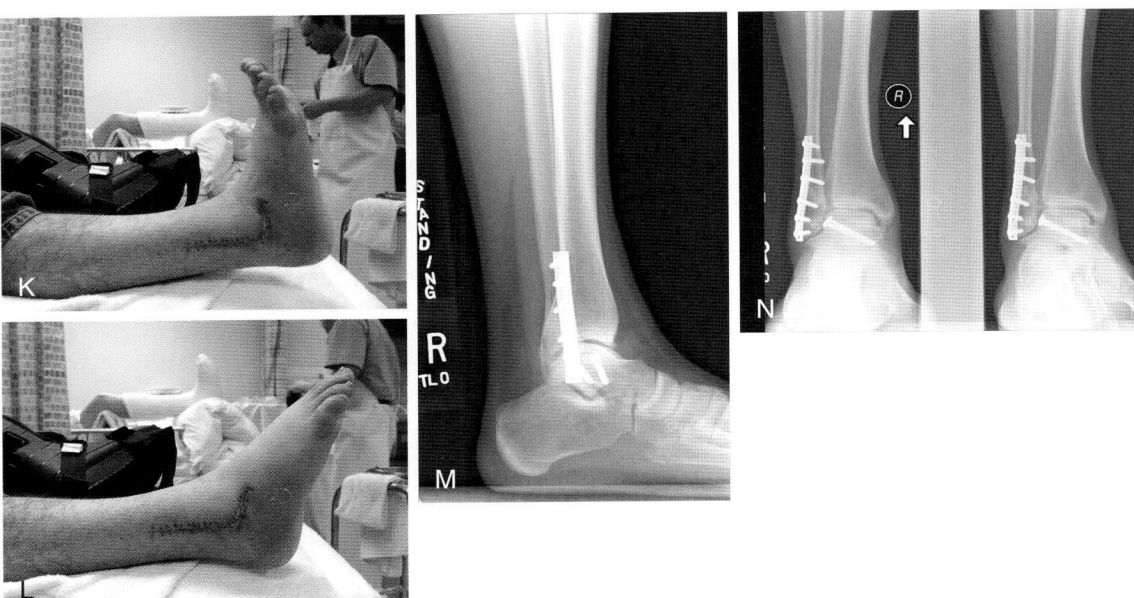

Figure 21-17, cont'd **K** and **L,** Motion when the cast was removed at 6 weeks was not painful. **M** and **N,** The patient is pain free 18 months after surgery and is planning to have the same surgery on the opposite side. (Courtesy Ned Amendola, MD.)

for each type of fixation is different. With ankle arthritis alone, these can be used with a transfibular approach as described for an open ankle arthrodesis. The following variations must be included to make the procedure successful. For fusion of the ankle and subtalar joints, lengthen the incision distally and inferiorly and avoid injury to the sural nerve. With a blade or locking plate, extend the incision slightly anteriorly and proximally 10 to 15 cm from the ankle, and identify and retract the superficial peroneal nerve. For bone resection, leave no necrotic bone. When a plate is to be applied on the lateral side, plane the incisura fibularis so that the plate adheres to the distal tibia, and remove a 7- to 10-cm segment of the distal fibula to allow the plate access to the lateral side of the tibia. With significant collapse, remove the distal half of the medial malleolus to enable compression of the ankle joint. Leaving some of the medial malleolus confers better rotational control.

In certain circumstances, a posterior approach is favored over a transfibular approach. These include revision cases with a history of anterior, lateral, or medial wound problems and severe coronal plane deformity from collapse. The theoretic advantage of the posterior approach is that it does not cause disruption of the main residual blood supply to the head and neck of the talus. The technique is described next.

SURGICAL TREATMENT OF TALAR AVASCULAR NECROSIS
Indications
Indications include talar AVN, complete body collapse with two-joint arthritis, and revision cases.

Contraindications
Contraindications include marginal vascular supply to the extremity, need for anterior ankle incisions, and simultaneous foot surgeries.

Preparation
1. The patient is positioned prone, with the foot dangling and the ankle supported by the end of the table.
2. A tourniquet is applied to the thigh. The limb is exsanguinated, and the tourniquet is inflated.
3. The preparation area includes midthigh to toes and ipsilateral posterior iliac crest if an autogenous graft is needed.

Posterior Approach and Technique of Intramedullary Nail Fixation
4. A direct longitudinal incision is made in the midline, starting 10 to 15 cm above the calcaneal tuberosity. In the proximal aspect of the wound, dissection is done meticulously to avoid injury to the sural nerve and short saphenous vein (Fig. 21-18 and Video Clip 25).
5. The Achilles tendon can be lengthened in a Z fashion with a distal medial hemisection and a proximal lateral hemisection. The flaps can be full thickness to include tendon, subcutaneous tissue, and skin. If the tendon detaches from the skin flap, it is wrapped in a moist cloth.
6. The deep crural fascia is identified and incised laterally to the midline. Mayo scissors are used to gently spread and release any attachments anterior to the fascia. The fascia is then incised while the tibial nerve and vessels are protected.

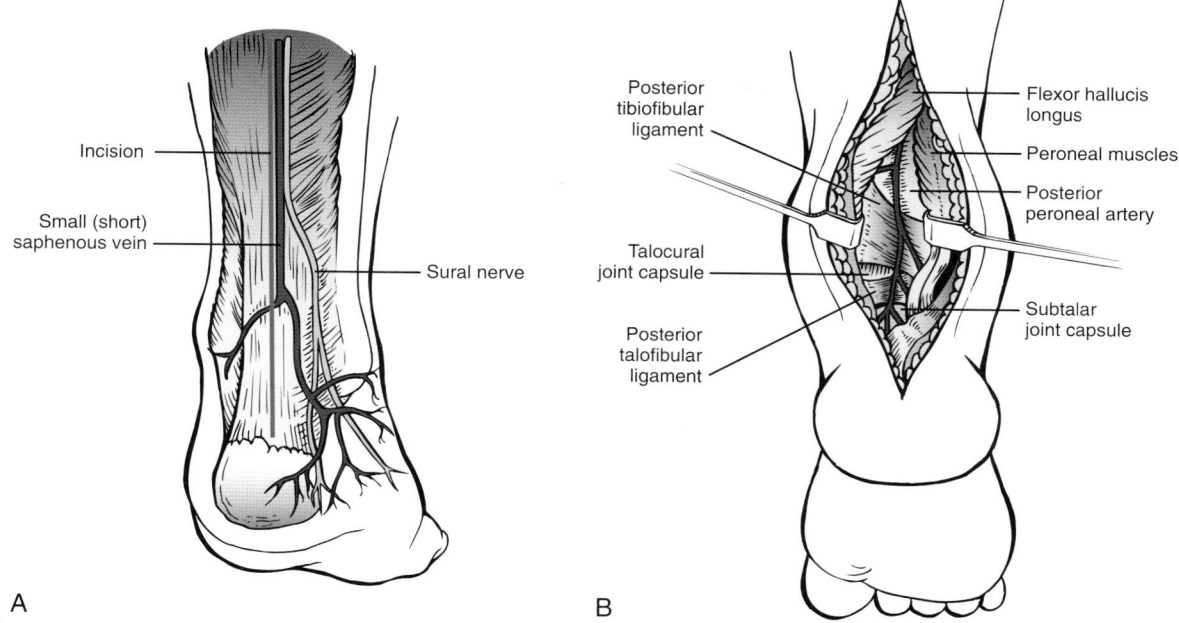

Figure 21-18   A central longitudinal approach to the posterior ankle joint respects the natural watershed area of skin blood supply. **A,** This direct central incision is well tolerated as long as the skin is not dissected free of the underlying subcutaneous tissue and is closed delicately. **B,** In the proximal part of the incision, the sural nerve is at risk for injury. The Achilles tendon is transected in a paracoronal fashion, exposing the deep crural fascia. This is incised longitudinally, exposing the belly of the flexor hallucis longus (FHL) muscle. Retracting the FHL muscle medially then exposes the investing ligaments of the posterior ankle and subtalar joints.

7. The belly of the flexor hallucis longus (FHL) muscle then becomes visible. Release part of the attachment of this muscle from the fibula and interosseous ligament to bluntly sweep the muscle and tendon medially. This protects the tibial nerve and vessels during the remainder of the operation.

8. The ligaments of the posterior aspect of the ankle and subtalar joints are removed with a rongeur. When the fibula must be shortened or removed, an inside-out technique is used. The peroneal artery is tied off or electrocoagulated, the peroneal tendons are reflected, and a subperiosteal dissection of the lateral malleolus is performed. Be careful not to buttonhole through the skin when dissecting anterior to the fibula. Any bone removed is used for grafting. Segments can be used for a structural graft, although this will need to be supplemented with more graft material.

9. Typically, a Gallie-type extraarticular fusion is attempted to supplement the direct tibiocalcaneal fusion. Preparation for this includes partial denudement of cortical bone from the posterior inferior tibia and superior calcaneal tuberosity.

10. The posterior talus is removed with fluoroscopic guidance. All necrotic bone needs to be removed. Necrotic bone often has the consistency and appearance of soft chalk with fatty infiltration. With total dome involvement, the resection needs to be extensive, usually to the anterior aspect of the ankle where healthy talar neck bone remains.

11. The four sides facing the resected dome region (tibial, lateral and medial malleolar, and calcaneal articular surfaces) are prepared by removing all cartilage and fenestrating the subchondral bone.

Bone Grafting

The choice of bone graft is made individually by the surgeon and patient. Traditionally, the posterior iliac crest was the source of graft for this operation, and it is still an excellent choice. A large structural piece can usually be fashioned from the crest for internal support. However, other options are promising and less prone to morbidity. Case series report the successful use of allograft or bone substitutes for foot or ankle fusion procedures, suggesting potential efficacy of these approaches.[76,96,102]

At present, we prefer bulk previously frozen allograft (usually femoral head) with some form of concurrent biologic adjuvant. For young, healthy, nonsmoking patients, we add bone marrow from the posterior iliac crest, admixed with demineralized bone matrix.

For older or less healthy patients, we use a limited trap-door approach to the posterior iliac crest. With a pituitary rongeur, we can usually harvest 10 to 15 mL of cancellous autograft through an 8 × 5-mm window. This is added around the interfaces of the bulk allograft, especially on the anterior part that is prepared on both sides of the neck to promote healing and on the extraarticular portion of the graft.

For patients with a high chance of nonunion (smokers, patients undergoing revision, the elderly) or those who object to the use of allograft, we use a structural posterior iliac crest graft. As with a bulk allograft, this must be cut to dovetail into the construct. The reconstruction can be limited by the amount of bone available, and height restoration is often less with an autograft than with an allograft.

Fixation

12. The anterior aspect of the graft is prepared, and autogenous bone or aspirate with demineralized bone matrix is placed deep into the wound against the exposed talar neck.
13. The structural graft is tamped into place with fluoroscopic guidance. The graft should fill the space in all six directions. The cortical surfaces on any face requiring fusion should be resected or fenestrated to promote healing.
14. An incision is made on the plantar aspect of the heel. The position of the incision is very important both in terms of proper access to the calcaneus and avoiding potential damage to the plantar nerves. We usually draw the presumed location of the nerves with a marking pen and always stay posterior to that location. The exact location for the incision is checked fluoroscopically in the sagittal plane. Typically, it is 1.5 to 2.5 cm posterior to the calcaneocuboid joint. The transverse incision starts 0.5 cm medial to the midline and courses 1.5 to 2.0 cm lateral to the midline. Dissection to the calcaneus is performed in the transverse direction with blunt curved Mayo scissors. A nasal speculum is then placed into the wound against the calcaneus while the guide pin is placed and checked and for all aspects of the reaming.
15. Under C-arm guidance, we place a guide pin onto the inferior surface of the calcaneus approximately 2 cm proximal to the calcaneocuboid joint. The pin is then drilled inferior to superior, with its tip directed slightly posteriorly and laterally. After checking that it is centered in the tibia, it is left in place, and the bone is reamed to the size of the implant.
16. Reaming usually does not have to be much wider than the implant because a scratch fit in the medullary canal is unusual with these short nails. We usually ream to the exact nail diameter and try to insert the nail. If we meet a lot of resistance, we increase reaming in 0.5-mm increments and try to insert the nail after each reaming.
17. All bone fragments from reamings are saved and placed in the medial and lateral gutters around the graft.
18. At present, the manufacturers of these nails offer two different methods for compression of the arthrodesis

site. Neither is perfect. We base the decision of which nail to use on the density of the calcaneal bone. If the patient has osteopenia from rheumatoid disease or long-standing non–weight bearing, we use a rod designed to gain compression with a temporary external fixator pin in the tibia. The compression is done against locking screws placed across the calcaneal segment of the rod. In all other cases, we use a rod with an inline compression device. This uses a worm screw mechanism pushed up against the inferior aspect of the calcaneus. With this approach, the first locking screws are placed across the tibial segment of the rod. Compression is then applied against that construct. When using the inline device, the surgeon must realize that the flange of the pusher is wider than the area previously reamed; the soft tissues must be retracted anteriorly so that the plantar nerves are not compressed (Fig. 21-19).

Closure

19. We close in two layers. A closed suction drain may be used if bleeding is excessive. The skin is closed with interrupted 4-0 nylon sutures to avoid injury to the skin.

Postoperative Care

A very well-padded posterior U splint is used. If bleeding is minimal, the splint is maintained for 10 to 14 days. In all other cases, we change the splint, on postoperative day 1 to 3, to a short-leg cast. The limb is elevated for the first 2 to 5 days.

We now frequently use long-acting peripheral nerve blocks or indwelling catheters. The rates of constipation, nausea, and other more serious complications of morphine-related analgesics have dropped significantly with this practice, and patients are more satisfied. At the first postoperative visit (10 to 14 days), it is now not uncommon for patients to tell us they had no or minimal pain with the surgery.

Weight bearing is restricted until good radiographic evidence of bridging trabeculae is obtained. Starting at 2 weeks, we allow patients to put 5 lb of weight on the heel for balance. We generally do not allow full weight bearing or heel-to-toe transfer weight bearing until we are sure the fusion is progressing. Imaging the fusion site with a large rod present is difficult, and for this reason, the average length of partial weight bearing is 3 months, average length of cast immobilization is 4 months, and average length of total immobilization is 5 to 6 months.

Rocker-bottom shoes help with initial transition to shoes. Eventually, most patients do not use them.

Pitfalls

Carefully select your pin starting point. The entry point on the calcaneus is the key. The best, and sometimes only, distal fixation screw is the posterior-to-anterior screw. The entry point must be posterior enough to allow

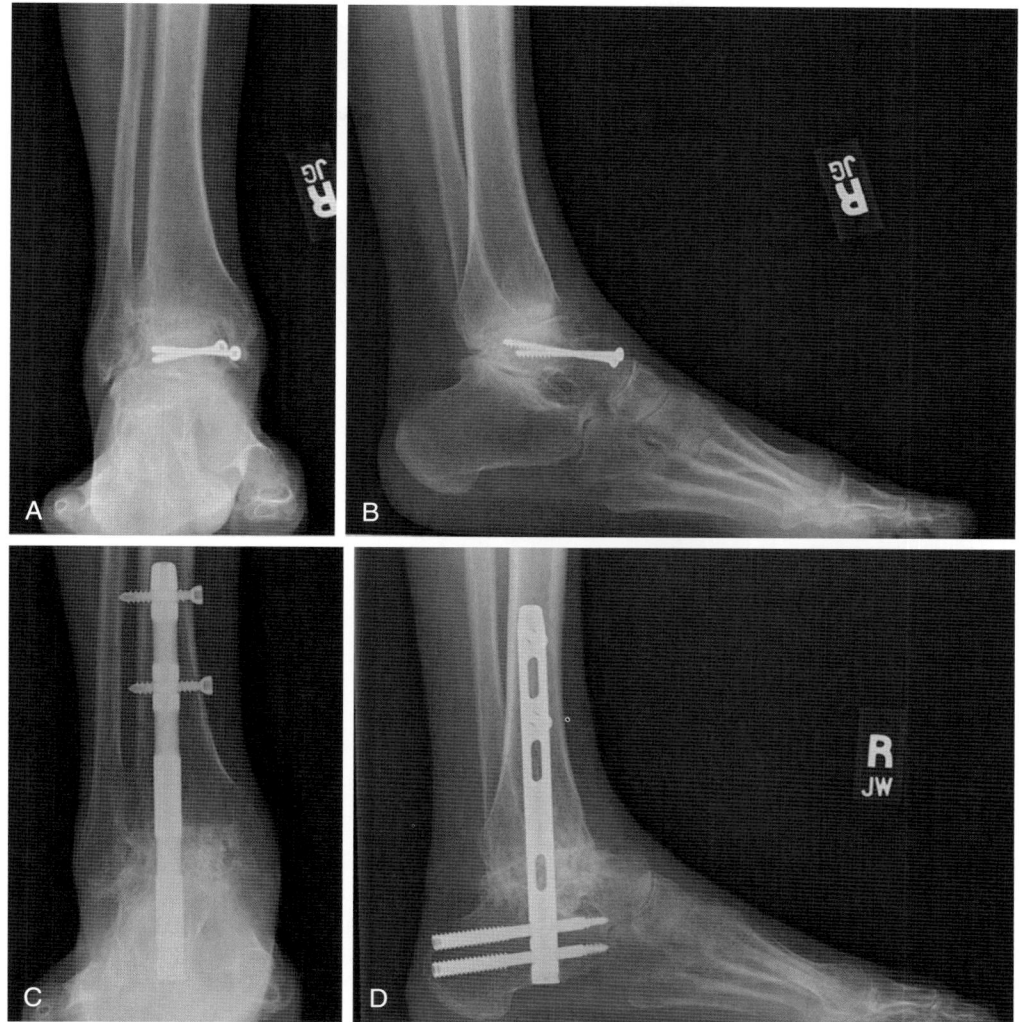

Figure 21-19 Tibiocalcaneal fusion with an intramedullary device for talar avascular necrosis. This patient had pain in the ankle and subtalar regions related to avascular bone and secondary arthritis as evidenced by the preoperative anteroposterior **(A)** and lateral **(B)** radiographs. Both the tibiotalar and subtalar joints were fused simultaneously with an intramedullary nail **(C** and **D).** (Courtesy James Brodsky, MD.)

the screw to engage 1.0 to 1.5 cm of cancellous bone anterior to the rod. The entry point must be carefully selected on a case-by-case basis. Erring in the posterior direction will translate the entire foot anteriorly, which can accelerate development of midfoot or hindfoot pain and arthritis.

Keep a very careful eye on rotation when compressing the construct and placing the locking screws. Err 5 degrees toward external rotation, and if the patient has limited hip rotation, consider erring by 10 degrees. Most patients need to rotate the limb externally to vault over the foot after a tibiocalcaneal arthrodesis.

Do not remove the locking screws to dynamize the frame. If you remove the locking screws, the construct will become rotationally unstable and will fail.

Do not allow patients to lie on their backs the whole time for the first 12 to 24 hours. Encourage them to lie on their side or prone. This will reduce the incidence of posterior wound problems.

Be patient. Some of these fusions take a long time to heal, but they will heal. The patient should expect long-term immobilization of more than 6 months. One alternative to intramedullary nail fixation for a tibiotalocalcaneal fusion can be a laterally placed locking plate (Fig. 21-20 and Video Clip 24). A lateral approach is utilized to prepare the tibiotalar and subtalar joints for arthrodesis. Similar to the posterior approach, all arthritic cartilage and bony debris are removed and any defects are filled with bone graft. After joint preparation and provisional fixation, the plate is fixed to the calcaneus

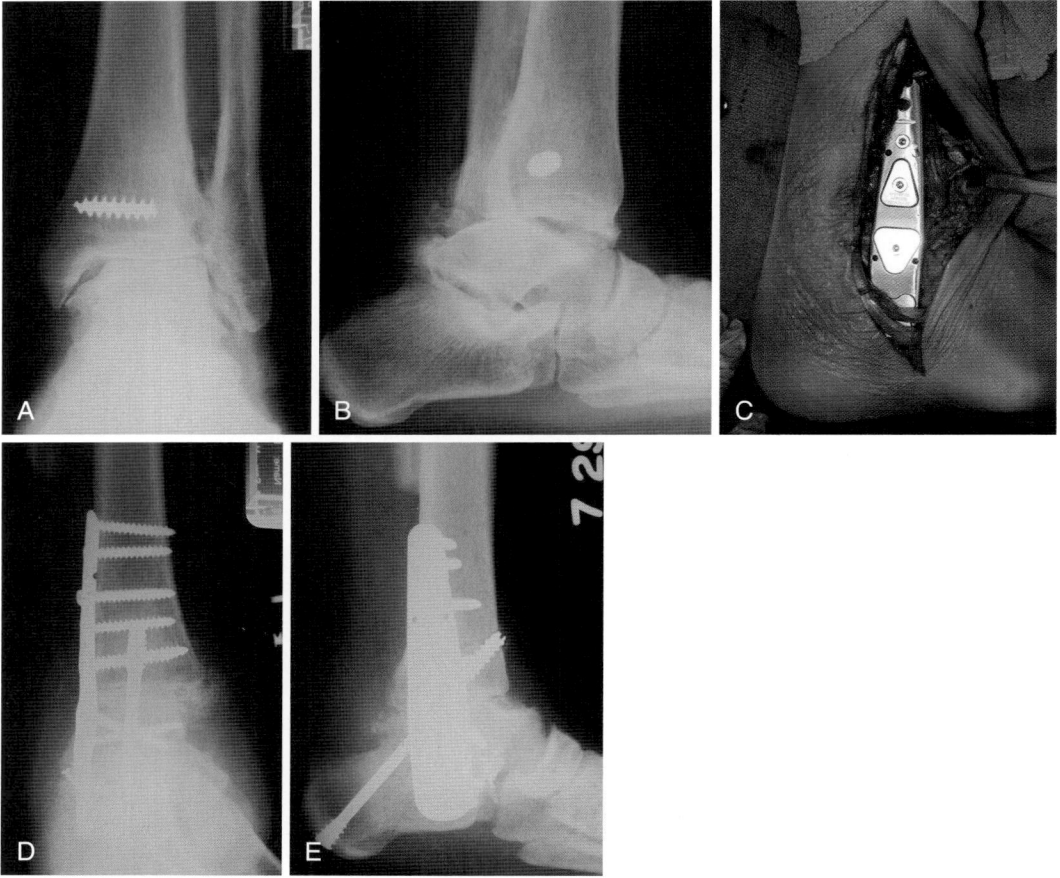

Figure 21-20 Use of a lateral approach and locking plate for a tibiotalocalcaneal arthrodesis. Preoperative anteroposterior **(A)** and lateral **(B)** radiographs showing tibiotalar and subtalar arthritis. A lateral curvilinear approach is used to access the subtalar and tibiotalar joints. The lateral locking plate is applied first to the calcaneus followed by the talus and tibia **(C)**. Compression of each joint is applied prior to fixation with the plate. Postoperative anteroposterior **(D)** and lateral **(E)** radiographs show a healed tibiotalocalcaneal arthrodesis with compression screw across the tibiotalar and subtalar joints. (Case courtesy Michael Coughlin, MD.)

first. The subtalar joint is then compressed and the plate is fixed to the talus or bone graft. Compression of the tibiotalar joint is completed prior to fixation of the plate to the tibia. A compression screw can be applied across the subtalar and tibiotalar joints prior to plate stabilization. This provides for added fixation in a plane different than the plate (Fig. 21-20D and E).

Failed Previous Fusion Surgery

Nonunion

Reported nonunion rates vary from 0% to 40%.* Nonunions appear to be more common in susceptible populations (smokers, elderly patients, noncompliant patients, and patients with neuroarthropathy, history of open trauma, or poor soft tissues)[16,83] and less common after

---

*References 29, 36, 37, 64, 65, 77, 83, 85, and 107.

minimally invasive surgeries. When to consider a nonunion a true nonunion is a controversial matter because some apparent cases of nonunion eventually unite after a year or more of immobilization.

Treatment of nonunions requires careful consideration of the patient's situation. Patients with several serious risk factors for failure or with debilitated health may be best advised not to undergo additional attempts at obtaining a solid ankle fusion. These patients should be treated with either a transtibial amputation[46] or long-term full-contact bracing.[92]

Kitaoka[59] reviewed the Mayo Clinic's experience treating ankle nonunions with external fixation. Twenty (77%) of 26 ankles successfully fused; however, at 5-year follow-up, 10 (39%) of the 26 had fair or poor results. Kirkpatrick et al[58] reported on 11 ankle nonunions primarily treated with a fibular onlay–inlay graft and internal fixation. They reported 9 of 11 successful fusions, 1 painless nonunion, and 1 below-knee amputation. Similarly, Anderson et al[4] reviewed 20 patients treated for ankle nonunions or malunions with internal fixation. In their initial series, they had 15 (75%) satisfactory fusions, with an additional 19 operations, 17 (85%) satisfied patients, and 3 (15%) below-knee amputations. Levine et al[60] described a series of 23 patients with ankle nonunions treated with either revision ankle fusions (15) or extensile fusions (9). At short follow-up, they reported fusion in 21 (91%) and satisfactory results in 19 (83%). Finally, Easley et al[31] described a review of 45 patients with tibiotalar nonunions who underwent revision surgery with either repeat internal fixation, ringed external fixator, or tibiotalocalcaneal arthrodesis. These authors obtained an 89% fusion rate for this complex set of patients.

The basic principles of successful revision surgery are essentially the same as described for primary surgery. Some caveats do apply, though. First, patient education, expectations, and ultimately compliance with postoperative protocols are essential for obtaining a successful result. It has been our experience that patients who do not want to participate in getting well are much more likely to fail. We are reluctant to consider revision surgery unless the patient shows real interest and motivation. This somewhat intangible aspect of the evaluation does require a number of discussions with the patient about the optimal time for treatment. We have treated a number of these patients in unloading braces until they are psychologically, socially, and physically ready to take on the challenge of this operation. We discuss with all of them the reported results and the possibility that a below-knee amputation might be necessary.

The technical aspects of the surgery are straightforward (Fig. 21-21). Only the minimum soft tissues are stripped to allow full access to the joint. All fibrous tissue and dead bone is removed. Infection is ruled out when indicated. Autogenous bone graft is used liberally. Fixation must be rigid. Weight bearing and smoking are restricted until full consolidation, often 4 to 5 months. CT scans can help monitor healing and give a more accurate picture of the progression of bone bridging. External electrical or ultrasound stimulation can be helpful as an adjunct to surgery,[30] but alone this is not likely to have a substantial and positive effect on the resolution of an established nonunion.[90]

Malunion

Varus or valgus malunion combined with equinus are the most common deformities that occur after ankle fusion.[53] Realignment is generally done with closing wedge procedures, although some can be treated with accurate double-plane osteotomies as described by Sangeorzan et al.[93] The advantage of closing wedges is that they do not generally stretch nerves, they are more likely to heal than opening wedges, and they offer a source of bone graft for other simultaneous foot procedures. When performing them, though, the surgeon must be aware that they often change the orientation of the foot and related joints, the two segments rarely fit and overhanging bone can irritate tendons, and they can change the length tension relationship of the musculotendinous structures that pass across the osteotomy, in effect lengthening and weakening these structures. Dome-shaped osteotomies placed around the center of rotation are less likely to have these effects, especially with single-plane deformities (e.g., equinus) (Fig. 21-22).

Arguably, the best approach to realigning the leg and foot is with Ilizarov frames. The indications, techniques, and outcomes are fully discussed elsewhere in the text. This approach is particularly useful in the circumstances of limb shortening, concomitant infection, or nonunion.

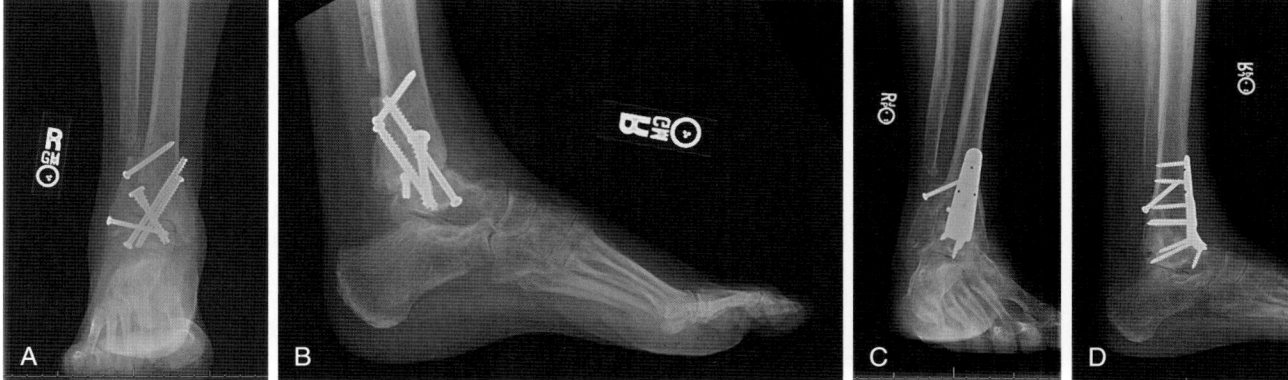

Figure 21-21 Revision of a failed transfibular tibiotalar arthrodesis with conversion to anterior plate. Preoperative anteroposterior **(A)** and lateral **(B)** radiographs show an obvious nonunion of the tibiotalar joint with use of a fibular onlay graft. The patient underwent revision tibiotalar arthrodesis through an anterior approach with removal of hardware and proximal tibial bone grafting. An anterior plate was applied similar to Figure 21-15. **C** and **D,** Radiographs taken 3 months postoperatively show a well-aligned and healed tibiotalar arthrodesis.

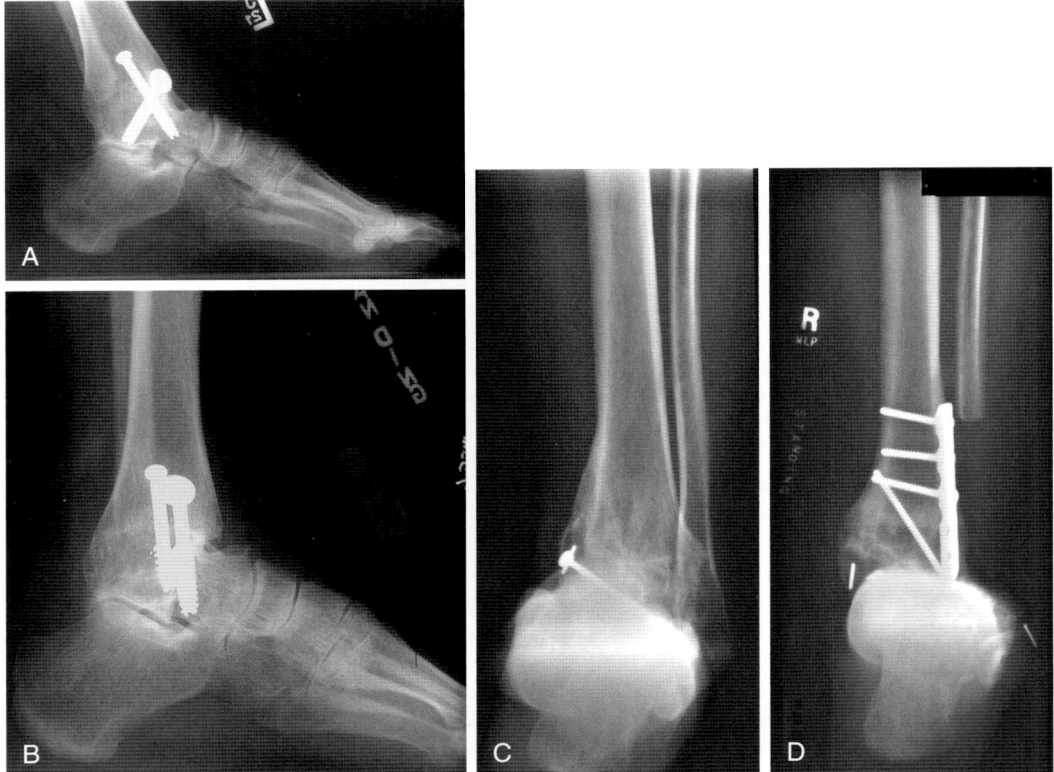

Figure 21-22 Two examples of osteotomies performed for ankle malunion. **A** and **B,** In the first, an equinus malunion after fusion involving a partial distal fibulectomy was treated by recutting the arc of the talar dome and rotating the foot into better position. Indeed, one of the original tibial screw holes was reused for fixation. **C,** In the second example, the ankle was fused in varus, as is seen on the hindfoot alignment view. **D,** The foot was reoriented under the tibia using a laterally closing wedge and blade plate fixation. Use of the plate requires partial distal fibulectomy.

However, the use of the frames carries its own inherent set of problems, including frequent (usually minor) adverse events, which are tolerated poorly by some patients, and techniques that are unfamiliar to most surgeons. The development of the Taylor Spatial Frame hardware and software (Smith & Nephew, Memphis, Tenn.) has made the application of corrective frames for malunions much more accessible to surgeons who do not subspecialize.

Secondary Subtalar Arthritis

The subtalar joint is the most common joint to develop arthritis after an ankle fusion. The rate of development of arthritis is unpredictable; however, after 20 years, essentially all patients develop radiographic evidence of subtalar joint degeneration.[17] This is thought to be the result of increased stresses across the subtalar joint. After ankle fusion, most patients walk with the foot externally rotated in order to vault over the planted foot in the terminal stages of the stance phase. In so doing, they roll through the subtalar joint in an unnatural, medial-to-lateral direction, which presumably results in focal mal-loading of articular cartilage and, ultimately, development of osteoarthritis.

Treatment of painful subtalar arthritis is fusion surgery. Because the ankle does not move, the subtalar joint is less accessible to surgical debridement than usual. We prefer to use an internervous frown-shaped incision from the tip of the fibula anterior calcaneal process to perform this surgery. After the short extensor is reflected, the entire contents of the subtalar joint are removed. For very tight joints, a Midas Rex (Medtronic, Ft. Worth, Tex.) thin router bit helps prepare the joint. Bone graft can be harvested from the distal tibia.

The key to this procedure, though, is to use either two screws or a screw and a staple to fixate the joint. After an ankle fusion and with the foot in a short-leg cast, the rotation of the foot with respect to the leg will be transmitted directly through the subtalar joint. One single large screw is not sufficient to stop that rotation (Fig. 21-23). Two screws—spaced as far apart as possible and out of plane—work well as a screw and a 90-degree out-of-plane staple. The first screw is generally put in compression; the second method of fixation (either a screw or staple) does not need compression. In complex cases, a third static screw can be used to supplement the fixation.

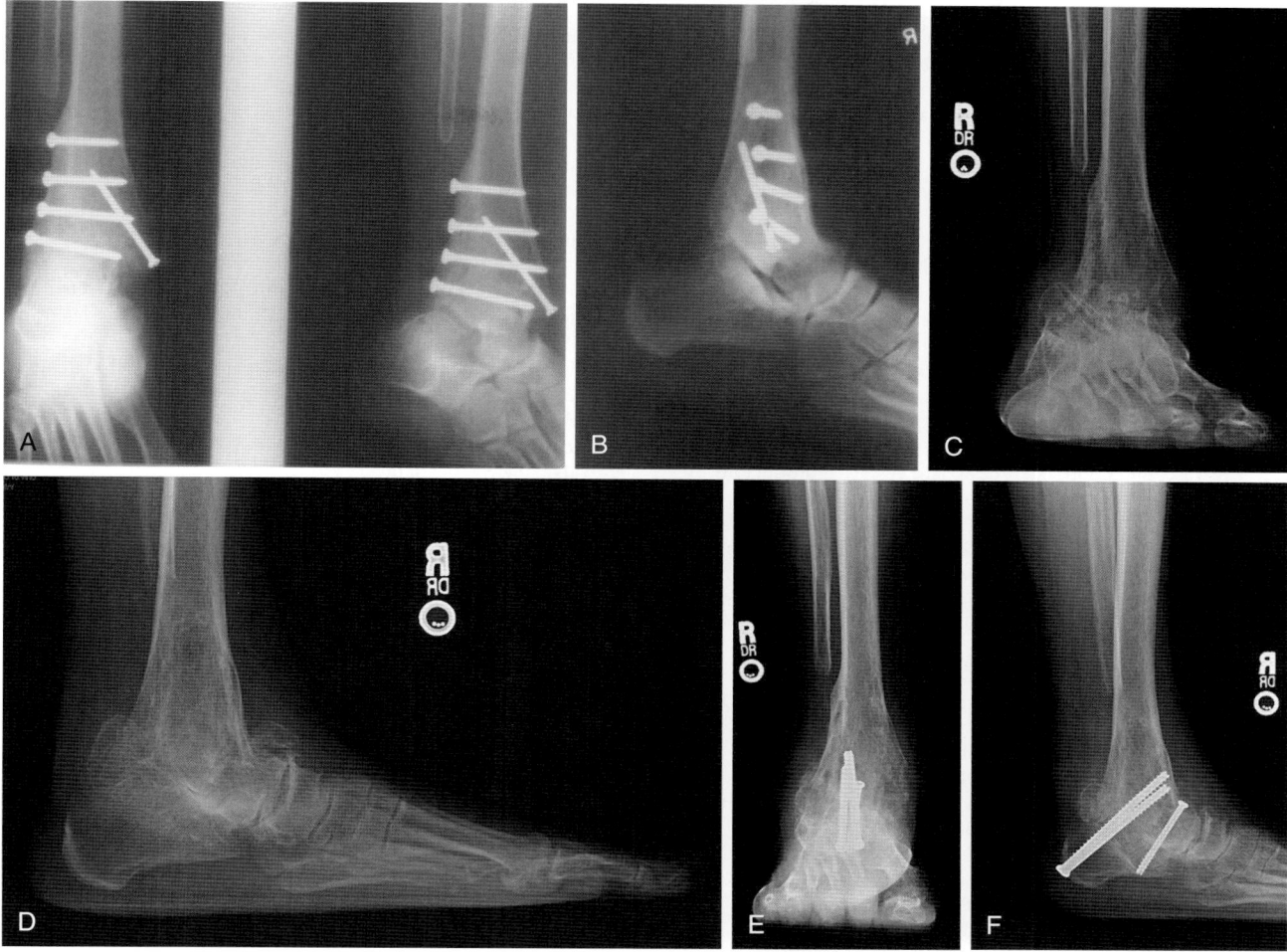

Figure 21-23 Fusion of arthritic subtalar joint after ankle fusion. The patient developed severe subtalar and talonavicular arthritis secondary to a tibiotalar arthrodesis performed approximately 40 years earlier using a Royal Airforce fibular onlay technique (**A** and **B**). The patient developed a severe valgus deformity with talonavicular and end-stage subtalar arthritis (**C** and **D**). She underwent calcaneal osteotomy to improve alignment with a subtalar arthrodesis and debridement of the talonavicular joint (**E** and **F**).

REFERENCES

1. Abdo RV, Wasilewski SA: Ankle arthrodesis: a long-term study, *Foot Ankle* 13:307–312, 1992.
2. Agel J, Coetzee JC, Sangeorzan BJ, Roberts MM, Hansen ST Jr: Functional limitations of patients with end-stage ankle arthrosis, *Foot Ankle Int* 26:537–539, 2005.
3. Ahlberg A, Henricson AS: Late results of ankle fusion, *Acta Orthop Scand* 52:103–105, 1981.
4. Anderson JG, Coetzee JC, Hansen ST: Revision ankle fusion using internal compression arthrodesis with screw fixation, *Foot Ankle Int* 18:300–309, 1997.
5. Ateshian GA, Soslowsky LJ, Mow VC: Quantitation of articular surface topography and cartilage thickness in knee joints using stereophotogrammetry, *J Biomech* 24:761–776, 1991.
6. Athanasiou KA, Niederauer GG, Schenck RC Jr: Biomechanical topography of human ankle cartilage, *Ann Biomed Eng* 23:697–704, 1995.
7. Beaudoin AJ, Fiore SM, Krause WR, Adelaar RS: Effect of isolated talocalcaneal fusion on contact in the ankle and talonavicular joints, *Foot Ankle* 12:19–25, 1991.
8. Bonnin M, Carret JP: [Arthrodesis of the ankle under arthroscopy. Apropos of 10 cases reviewed after a year], *Rev Chir Orthop Reparatrice Appar Mot* 81:128–135, 1995.
9. Brown TD, Shaw DT: In vitro contact stress distributions in the natural human hip, *J Biomech* 16:373–384, 1983.
10. Buchner M, Sabo D: Ankle fusion attributable to posttraumatic arthrosis: a long-term follow-up of 48 patients, *Clin Orthop Relat Res* 406:155–164, 2003.
11. Buckwalter JA, Mankin HJ: Articular cartilage: tissue design and chondrocyte-matrix interactions, *Instr Course Lect* 47:477–486, 1998.
12. Buckwalter JA, Saltzman C, Brown T: The impact of osteoarthritis: Implications for research, *Clin Orthop Relat Res* 427(Suppl): S6–S15, 2004.
13. Buckwalter JA, Woo SL, Goldberg VM, et al: Soft-tissue aging and musculoskeletal function, *J Bone Joint Surg Am* 75:1533–1548, 1993.
14. Cameron SE, Ullrich P: Arthroscopic arthrodesis of the ankle joint, *Arthroscopy* 16:21–26, 2000.
15. Chubinskaya S, Huch K, Mikecz K, et al: Chondrocyte matrix metalloproteinase-8: up-regulation of neutrophil collagenase by interleukin-1 beta in human cartilage from knee and ankle joints, *Lab Invest* 74:232–240, 1996.
16. Cobb TK, Gabrielsen TA, Campbell DC 2nd, et al: Cigarette smoking and nonunion after ankle arthrodesis, *Foot Ankle Int* 15:64–67, 1994.

17. Coester LM, Saltzman CL, Leupold J, Pontarelli W: Long-term results following ankle arthrodesis for post-traumatic arthritis, *J Bone Joint Surg Am* 83:219–228, 2001.

18. Cohen MM, Altman RD, Hollstrom R, et al: Safety and efficacy of intra-articular sodium hyaluronate (Hyalgan) in a randomized, double-blind study for osteoarthritis of the ankle, *Foot Ankle Int* 29:657–663, 2008.

19. Collins DH: *The pathology of articular and spinal diseases*, London, 1949, Edward Arnold, pp 23–37.

20. Corso SJ, Zimmer TJ: Technique and clinical evaluation of arthroscopic ankle arthrodesis, *Arthroscopy* 11:585–590, 1995.

21. Crosby LA, Yee TC, Formanek TS, Fitzgibbons TC: Complications following arthroscopic ankle arthrodesis, *Foot Ankle Int* 17:340–342, 1996.

22. Cushnaghan J, Dieppe P: Study of 500 patients with limb joint osteoarthritis. I. Analysis by age, sex, and distribution of symptomatic joint sites, *Ann Rheum Dis* 50:8–13, 1991.

23. Dannawi Z, Nawabi DH, Patel A, Leong JJ, Moore DJ: Arthroscopic ankle arthrodesis: are results reproducible irrespective of pre-operative deformity? *Foot Ankle Surg* 17:294–299, 2011.

24. DeGroot H 3rd, Uzunishvili S, Weir R, Al-omari A, Gomes B: Intra-articular injection of hyaluronic acid is not superior to saline solution injection for ankle arthritis: a randomized, double-blind, placebo-controlled study, *J Bone Joint Surg Am* 94:2–8, 2012.

25. De Vriese L, Dereymaeker G, Fabry G: Arthroscopic ankle arthrodesis. Preliminary report, *Acta Orthop Belg* 60:389–392, 1994.

26. Demetriades L, Strauss E, Gallina J: Osteoarthritis of the ankle, *Clin Orthop Relat Res* 349:28–42, 1998.

27. Dent CM, Patil M, Fairclough JA: Arthroscopic ankle arthrodesis, *J Bone Joint Surg Br* 75:830–832, 1993.

28. Dieppe P, Cushnaghan J, Tucker M, et al: The Bristol "OA500 study": progression and impact of the disease after 8 years, *Osteoarthritis Cartilage* 8:63–68, 2000.

29. Dohm M, Purdy BA, Benjamin J: Primary union of ankle arthrodesis: review of a single institution/multiple surgeon experience, *Foot Ankle Int* 15:293–296, 1994.

30. Donley BG, Ward DM: Implantable electrical stimulation in high-risk hindfoot fusions, *Foot Ankle Int* 23:13–18, 2002.

31. Easley ME, Montijo HE, Wilson JB, Fitch RD, Nunley JA 2nd: Revision tibiotalar arthrodesis, *J Bone Joint Surg Am* 90:1212–1223, 2008.

32. El-Khoury GY, Alliman KJ, Lundberg HJ, et al: Cartilage thickness in cadaveric ankles: measurement with double-contrast multi-detector row CT arthrography versus MR imaging, *Radiology* 233:768–773, 2004.

33. Ferkel RD, Hewitt M: Long-term results of arthroscopic ankle arthrodesis, *Foot Ankle Int* 26:275–280, 2005.

34. Fisher RL, Ryan WR, Dugdale TW, Zimmerman GA: Arthroscopic ankle fusion, *Conn Med* 61:643–646, 1997.

35. Fitzgibbons TC: Arthroscopic ankle débridement and fusion: indications, techniques, and results, *Instr Course Lect* 48:243–248, 1999.

36. Frey C, Halikus NM, Vu-Rose T, Ebramzadeh E: A review of ankle arthrodesis: predisposing factors to nonunion, *Foot Ankle Int* 15:581–584, 1994.

37. Fujimori J, Yoshino S, Koiwa M, et al: Ankle arthrodesis in rheumatoid arthritis using an intramedullary nail with fins, *Foot Ankle Int* 20:485–490, 1999.

38. Gilbert BJ, Horst F, Nunley JA: Potential donor rotational bone grafts using vascular territories in the foot and ankle, *J Bone Joint Surg Am* 86:1857–1873, 2004.

39. Glazebrook M, Daniels T, Younger A, et al: Comparison of health-related quality of life between patients with end-stage ankle and hip arthrosis, *J Bone Joint Surg Am* 90:499–505, 2008.

40. Glick JM, Morgan CD, Myerson MS, et al: Ankle arthrodesis using an arthroscopic method: long-term follow-up of 34 cases, *Arthroscopy* 12:428–434, 1996.

41. Gougoulias NE, Agathangelidis FG, Parsons SW: Arthroscopic ankle arthrodesis, *Foot Ankle Int* 28:695–706, 2007.

42. Gross AE, Agnidis Z, Hutchison CR: Osteochondral defects of the talus treated with fresh osteochondral allograft transplantation, *Foot Ankle Int* 22:385–391, 2001.

43. Guo C, Yan Z, Barfield WR, Hartsock LA: Ankle arthrodesis using anatomically contoured anterior plate, *Foot Ankle Int* 31:492–498, 2010.

44. Harrington KD: Degenerative arthritis of the ankle secondary to long-standing lateral ligament instability, *J Bone Joint Surg Am* 61:354–361, 1979.

45. Hartel RM, Van Dijk CN, Van Kampen A, De Waal Malefijt M: Arthroscopic arthrodesis of the ankle—a new technique [abstr], *Acta Orthop Scand* 64:10, 1993.

46. Honkamp N, Amendola A, Hurwitz S, Saltzman CL: Retrospective review of eighteen patients who underwent transtibial amputation for intractable pain, *J Bone Joint Surg Am* 83:1479–1483, 2001.

47. Huch K, Kuettner KE, Dieppe P: Osteoarthritis in ankle and knee joints, *Semin Arthritis Rheum* 26:667–674, 1997.

48. Ihn JC, Kim SJ, Park IH: In vitro study of contact area and pressure distribution in the human knee after partial and total meniscectomy, *Int Orthop* 17:214–218, 1993.

49. Jackson A, Glasgow M: Tarsal hypermobility after ankle fusion—fact or fiction? *J Bone Joint Surg Br* 61:470–473, 1979.

50. Jeng CL, Kadakia A, White KL, Myerson MS: Fresh osteochondral total ankle allograft transplantation for the treatment of ankle arthritis, *Foot Ankle Int* 29:554–560, 2008.

51. Jerosch J, Steinbeck J, Schroder M, Reer R: Arthroscopically assisted arthrodesis of the ankle joint, *Arch Orthop Trauma Surg* 115:182–189, 1996.

52. Kats J, van Kampen A, de Waal-Malefijt MC: Improvement in technique for arthroscopic ankle fusion: results in 15 patients, *Knee Surg Sports Traumatol Arthrosc* 11:46–49, 2003.

53. Katsenis D, Bhave A, Paley D, Herzenberg JE: Treatment of malunion and nonunion at the site of an ankle fusion with the Ilizarov apparatus, *J Bone Joint Surg Am* 87:302–309, 2005.

54. Kempson GE: Age-related changes in the tensile properties of human articular cartilage: a comparative study between the femoral head of the hip joint and the talus of the ankle joint, *Biochim Biophys Acta* 1075:223–230, 1991.

55. Khoury NJ, el-Khoury GY, Saltzman CL, Brandser EA: Intraarticular foot and ankle injections to identify source of pain before arthrodesis, *AJR Am J Roentgenol* 167:669–673, 1996.

56. Kim CW, Jamali A, Tontz W Jr, et al: Treatment of post-traumatic ankle arthrosis with bipolar tibiotalar osteochondral shell allografts, *Foot Ankle Int* 23:1091–1102, 2002.

57. Kimizuka M, Kurosawa H, Fukubayashi T: Load-bearing pattern of the ankle joint. Contact area and pressure distribution, *Arch Orthop Trauma Surg* 96:45–49, 1980.

58. Kirkpatrick JS, Goldner JL, Goldner RD: Revision arthrodesis for tibiotalar pseudarthrosis with fibular onlay–inlay graft and internal screw fixation, *Clin Orthop Relat Res* 268:29–36, 1991.

59. Kitaoka HB, Anderson PJ, Morrey BF: Revision of ankle arthrodesis with external fixation for non-union, *J Bone Joint Surg Am* 74:1191–1200, 1992.

60. Levine SE, Myerson MS, Lucas P, Schon LC: Salvage of pseudoarthrosis after tibiotalar arthrodesis, *Foot Ankle Int* 18:580–585, 1997.

61. Mann RA, Rongstad KM: Arthrodesis of the ankle: a critical analysis, *Foot Ankle Int* 19:3–9, 1998.

62. Marcus RE, Balourdas GM, Heiple KG: Ankle arthrodesis by chevron fusion with internal fixation and bone-grafting, *J Bone Joint Surg Am* 65:833–838, 1983.

63. Marsh JL, Rattay RE, Dulaney T: Results of ankle arthrodesis for treatment of supramalleolar nonunion and ankle arthrosis, *Foot Ankle Int* 18:138–143, 1997.

64. Maurer RC, Cimino WR, Cox CV, Satow GK: Transarticular cross-screw fixation. A technique of ankle arthrodesis, *Clin Orthop Relat Res* 268:56–64, 1991.

65. Mazur JM, Schwartz E, Simon SR: Ankle arthrodesis. Long-term follow-up with gait analysis, *J Bone Joint Surg Am* 61:964–975, 1979.

66. Meachim G: Cartilage fibrillation at the ankle joint in Liverpool necropsies, *J Anat* 119:601–610, 1975.

67. Meachim G: Cartilage fibrillation on the lateral tibial plateau in Liverpool necropsies, *J Anat* 121:97–106, 1976.

68. Meachim G, Emery IH: Cartilage fibrillation in shoulder and hip joints in Liverpool necropsies, *J Anat* 116:161–179, 1973.

69. Meachim G, Emery IH: Quantitative aspects of patello-femoral cartilage fibrillation in Liverpool necropsies, *Ann Rheum Dis* 33:39–47, 1974.

70. Mears DC, Gordon RG, Kann SE, Kann JN: Ankle arthrodesis with an anterior tension plate, *Clin Orthop Relat Res* 268:70–77, 1991.

71. Mohamedean A, Said HG, El-Sharkawi M, El-Adly W, Said GZ: Technique and short-term results of ankle arthrodesis using anterior plating, *Int Orthop* 34:833–837, 2010.

72. Moran CG, Pinder IM, Smith SR: Ankle arthrodesis in rheumatoid arthritis. 30 cases followed for 5 years, *Acta Orthop Scand* 62:538–543, 1991.

73. Morgan CD: Arthroscopic Tibiotalar Arthrodesis, *Jefferson Orthop J* 16:50–52, 1987.

74. Muehleman C, Bareigher D, Huch K, et al: Prevalence of degenerative morphological changes in the joints of the lower extremity, *Osteoarthritis Cartilage* 5:23–37, 1997.

75. Muir DC, Amendola A, Saltzman CL: Long-term outcome of ankle arthrodesis, *Foot Ankle Clin North Am* 7:703–708, 2002.

76. Myerson MS, Neufeld SK, Uribe J: Fresh-frozen structural allografts in the foot and ankle, *J Bone Joint Surg Am* 87:113–120, 2005.

77. Myerson MS, Quill G: Ankle arthrodesis. A comparison of an arthroscopic and an open method of treatment, *Clin Orthop Relat Res* 268:84–95, 1991.

78. Nielsen KK, Linde F, Jensen NC: The outcome of arthroscopic and open surgery ankle arthrodesis: a comparative retrospective study on 107 patients, *Foot Ankle Surg* 14:153–157, 2008.

79. O'Brien TS, Hart TS, Shereff MJ, et al: Open versus arthroscopic ankle arthrodesis: a comparative study, *Foot Ankle Int* 20:368–374, 1999.

80. Odutola AA, Sheridan BD, Kelly AJ: Headless compression screw fixation prevents symptomatic metalwork in arthroscopic ankle arthrodesis, *Foot Ankle Surg* 18:111–113, 2012.

81. Ogilvie-Harris DJ, Lieberman I, Fitsialos D: Arthroscopically assisted arthrodesis for osteoarthrotic ankles, *J Bone Joint Surg Am* 75:1167–1174, 1993.

82. Paremain GD, Miller SD, Myerson MS: Ankle arthrodesis: results after the miniarthrotomy technique, *Foot Ankle Int* 17:247–252, 1996.

83. Perlman MH, Thordarson DB: Ankle fusion in a high risk population: an assessment of nonunion risk factors, *Foot Ankle Int* 20:491–496, 1999.

84. Plaass C, Knupp M, Barg A, Hintermann B: Anterior double plating for rigid fixation of isolated tibiotalar arthrodesis, *Foot Ankle Int* 30:631–639, 2009.

85. Ross SD, Matta J: Internal compression arthrodesis of the ankle, *Clin Orthop Relat Res* 199:54–60, 1985.

86. Rowan R, Davey KJ: Ankle arthrodesis using an anterior AO T plate, *J Bone Joint Surg Br* 81:113–116, 1999.

87. Said E, Hunka L, Siller TN: Where ankle fusion stands today, *J Bone Joint Surg Br* 60:211–214, 1978.

88. Salk RS, Chang TJ, D'Costa WF, Soomekh DJ, Grogan KA: Sodium hyaluronate in the treatment of osteoarthritis of the ankle: a controlled, randomized, double-blind pilot study, *J Bone Joint Surg Am* 88:295–302, 2006.

89. Saltzman CL, el-Khoury GY: The hindfoot alignment view, *Foot Ankle Int* 16:572–576, 1995.

90. Saltzman C, Lightfoot A, Amendola A: PEMF as treatment for delayed healing of foot and ankle arthrodesis, *Foot Ankle Int* 25:771–773, 2004.

91. Saltzman CL, Salamon ML, Blanchard GM, et al: Epidemiology of ankle arthritis: report of a consecutive series of 639 patients from a tertiary orthopaedic center, *Iowa Orthop J* 25:44–46, 2005.

92. Saltzman CL, Shurr D, Kamp L, Cook TA: The leather ankle lacer, *Iowa Orthop J* 15:204–208, 1995.

93. Sangeorzan BP, Judd RP, Sangeorzan BJ: Mathematical analysis of single-cut osteotomy for complex long bone deformity, *J Biomech* 22:1271–1278, 1989.

94. Schafer D, Hintermann B: Arthroscopic assessment of the chronic unstable ankle joint, *Knee Surg Sports Traumatol Arthrosc* 4:48–52, 1996.

95. Schneider D: Arthroscopic ankle fusion, *Arth Video* 3, 1983.

96. Scranton PE Jr: Use of bone graft substitutes in lower extremity reconstructive surgery, *Foot Ankle Int* 23:689–692, 2002.

97. Scranton PE Jr: Use of internal compression in arthrodesis of the ankle, *J Bone Joint Surg Am* 67:550–555, 1985.

98. Segal AD, Shofer J, Hahn ME, et al: Functional limitations associated with end-stage ankle arthritis, *J Bone Joint Surg Am* 94:777–783, 2012.

99. Sun SF, Chou YJ, Hsu CW, et al: Efficacy of intra-articular hyaluronic acid in patients with osteoarthritis of the ankle: a prospective study, *Osteoarthritis Cartilage* 14:867–874, 2006.

100. Sun SF, Hsu CW, Sun HP, et al: The effect of three weekly intra-articular injections of hyaluronate on pain, function, and balance in patients with unilateral ankle arthritis, *J Bone Joint Surg Am* 93:1720–1726, 2011.

101. Tarkin IS, Mormino MA, Clare MP, et al: Anterior plate supplementation increases ankle arthrodesis construct rigidity, *Foot Ankle Int* 28:219–223, 2007.

102. Thordarson DB, Kuehn S: Use of demineralized bone matrix in ankle/hindfoot fusion, *Foot Ankle Int* 24:557–560, 2003.

103. Tontz WL Jr, Bugbee WD, Brage ME: Use of allografts in the management of ankle arthritis, *Foot Ankle Clin* 8:361–373, xi, 2003.

104. Turan I, Wredmark T, Fellander-Tsai L: Arthroscopic ankle arthrodesis in rheumatoid arthritis, *Clin Orthop Relat Res* 320:110–114, 1995.

105. Valderrabano V, Horisberger M, Russell I, Dougall H, Hintermann B: Etiology of ankle osteoarthritis, *Clin Orthop Relat Res* 467:1800–1806, 2009.

106. van der Schoot DK, Den Outer AJ, Bode PJ, et al: Degenerative changes at the knee and ankle related to malunion of tibial fractures. 15-year follow-up of 88 patients, *J Bone Joint Surg Br* 78:722–725, 1996.

107. Wang CJ, Tambakis AP, Fielding JW: An evaluation of ankle fusion in children, *Clin Orthop Relat Res* 98:233–238, 1974.

108. Winson IG, Robinson DE, Allen PE: Arthroscopic ankle arthrodesis, *J Bone Joint Surg Br* 87:343–347, 2005.

109. Witteveen AG, Sierevelt IN, Blankevoort L, Kerkhoffs GM, van Dijk CN: Intra-articular sodium hyaluronate injections in the osteoarthritic ankle joint: effects, safety and dose dependency, *Foot Ankle Surg* 16:159–163, 2010.

110. Wyss C, Zollinger H: The causes of subsequent arthrodesis of the ankle joint, *Acta Orthop Belg* 57(Suppl 1):22–27, 1991.

111. Zvijac JE, Lemak L, Schurhoff MR, et al: Analysis of arthroscopically assisted ankle arthrodesis, *Arthroscopy* 18:70–75, 2002.

Ankle Replacement

Alexej Barg, Charles L. Saltzman

Early results with total ankle replacement (TAR) were highly disappointing. In the search for a workable ankle design, a number of different approaches were tried. Our current ability to critically analyze design strategies from the 1970s and 1980s is limited by the paucity of published data documenting the results of total ankle arthroplasties. Most clinical series from that period included 20 to 40 patients followed for an average of 5 years or less. The length of follow-up was a major factor affecting figures for patient satisfaction because satisfaction generally declined with longer follow-up.[290] Rates of radiographic evidence for loosening with early implant designs were extremely high, ranging from 22% to 75%.*

---

*References 38, 119, 137, 143, 174, 184, and 186.

A review of the world's published data suggests that the major factors implicated in loosening were highly constrained designs and cement fixation. We do not exactly know whether the cement alone, cement plus the space needed for cement fixation, or the technique of cement fixation was the chief contributing factor in these high rates of loosening.

TAR has also been associated with a relatively high incidence of wound problems. Soft tissue around the ankle, especially in elderly patients and those with rheumatoid arthritis, provide a relatively thin envelope for arthroplasty containment. Initial problems with superficial and deep infections, resection arthroplasty, attempted reimplantation or arthrodesis, and the occasional need for below-knee amputation to control infection dampened the orthopaedic surgeon's enthusiasm for TAR.

Since the 1990s, interest in TAR has resurged with improved designs, better fixation approaches, and a new generation of optimistic surgeons. Whether the optimism is warranted is not yet fully known; however, intermediate-term results with the newer approaches appear to justify the optimism. Both fixed and mobile bearings are now available, but which of the two is better remains a matter of debate.[99,353] The fixed bearings can be highly cross-linked and are less likely to break or subluxate. The mobile bearings offer the opportunity for greater congruency and, theoretically, less wear. Head-to-head comparison of fixed- and mobile-bearing–generated wear particles show no major difference and similar overall characteristics as for total knee replacements at short term.[2,3,31,197]

In the United States, at the time of writing, the Agility implant (Depuy, Warsaw, Ind.), Scandinavian Total Ankle Replacement (STAR) (Small Bone Innovations, Morrisville, Pa.), Salto Talaris (Tornier, Amsterdam, The Netherlands), INBONE (Wright Medical, Arlington, Tenn.), and Zimmer TM Ankle (Zimmer, Warsaw, Ind.) are approved or cleared by the U.S. Foot and Drug Administration (FDA) for general use. All other implants used in the United States at this time must be prescribed on a case-by-case custom basis and fall under the scrutiny of the FDA, which regulates the use of these devices in the United States. Worldwide, many other implants are being used, most with mobile-bearing designs. The vast majority require an anterior approach for access to the joint. Modern prosthetic designs vary in area covered (some cover part of the medial or lateral recesses), contours of the articulating surfaces, materials, and fixation techniques. Limited early and intermediate results have been published for several of these implants with remarkably good results.* However, most of the clinical results with the newer implants are from inventors' initial series; further independent studies are clearly needed to determine true efficacy. Initial reports, however, show lower rates of early complications than previously published. Several issues are likely to have affected this change,

including improved surgical selection, refined indications, meticulous handling of soft tissues, less dissection for lower-profile implants, better instrumentation, and better postoperative care.

In general, TAR is continuously becoming recommended as a treatment option in patients with end-stage ankle osteoarthritis. Ankle arthrodesis cannot be accepted as the sole gold standard procedure in this patient cohort. Saltzman et al[294] reported initial findings from a prospective controlled trial of the STAR prosthesis versus ankle fusion and showed TAR led to better function and similar pain relief compared with ankles that were fused. Haddad et al[128] performed a systematic review of the literature, including 852 ankle arthroplasties and 1262 ankle fusions. Meta-analytic mean results showed 38% of the patients treated with TAR had an excellent result, 30.5% had a good result, 5.5% had a fair result, and 24% had a poor result, with the corresponding values in the ankle arthrodesis group being 31%, 37%, 13%, and 13%, respectively. The revision rate after TAR and ankle fusion was 7% and 9%, respectively.[128]

Despite the mostly favorable intermediate-term results regarding function outcomes, patient satisfaction, and implant survivorship in patients who underwent TAR, this procedure has not displaced ankle fusion for end-stage ankle osteoarthritis. Further independent studies with greater numbers of patients and longer follow-up periods are necessary to improve the postoperative outcome and to understand which factor or factors may play the substantial role in success or failure of this procedure.

SHORT HISTORY OF TOTAL ANKLE REPLACEMENT

In most articles detailing TAR history,* the study by Lord and Marotte[223] is identified as the first clinical study to report outcomes in TAR patients. However, in 2002, Muir et al[239] reported the clinical outcome in a 71-year-old male who underwent talar dome resurfacing with a custom Vitallium implant for posttraumatic osteoarthritis in 1962. The clinical examination at a 40-year follow-up showed mild hindfoot malalignment with good clinical results, including slightly decreased range of motion (35 degrees of plantar flexion), American Orthopaedic Foot and Ankle Society (AOFAS) score of 85, no pain, and no limitation of daily activities.[239]

In the aforementioned study by Lord and Morotte,[223] an inverted hip stem was implanted into the tibia. The talus had been completely removed, and a cemented acetabular cup was then implanted in the calcaneus. This procedure was performed in 25 consecutive patients, with only 7 patients reporting satisfaction postoperatively.[224] Twelve of the 25 arthroplasties failed; the authors did not recommend further use of this prosthesis design.[224] At that time, the authors recognized the complexity of ankle biomechanics and concluded that a simple hinge

---

*References 27, 35, 49, 50, 114, 157, 189, 199, 229, 253, 279, 300, 325, 326, 342, and 373.

*References 39, 98, 113, 121, 138, 147, 356, and 360.

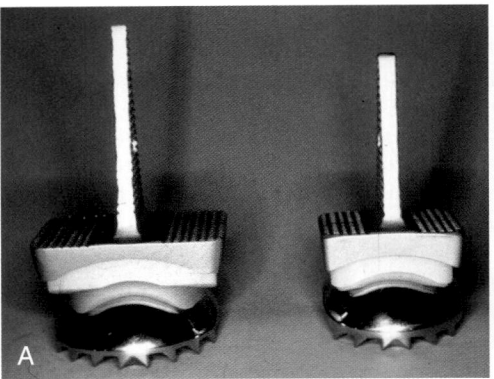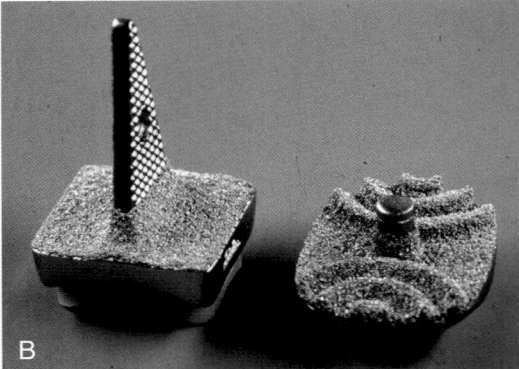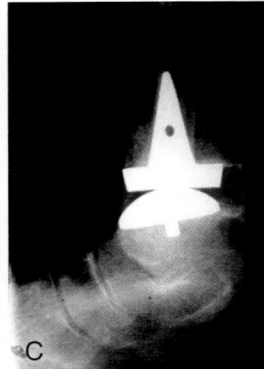

Figure 22-1 A, Irvine ankle total ankle design in two different sizes. **B,** Modification of prosthesis component with porous coating. **C,** Lateral radiograph of replaced ankle.

prosthesis system with plantar flexion and dorsiflexion would not be able to mimic the normal ankle joint.[224]

First-Generation Total Ankle Designs

St. Georg–Buchholz Ankle Prosthesis
The St. Georg–Buchholz ankle prosthesis is a semiconstrained prosthesis type introduced in 1973. However, the use of this prosthesis was abandoned after eight TARs because of the high failure rate.[48,97] Hay and Smith[135] implanted this prosthesis in 15 patients. At a mean follow-up of 10 years, 11 early and 32 late complications were reported.[135]

Imperial College of London Hospital Prosthesis
The Imperial College of London Hospital (ICLH) TAR was a two-component, constrained total ankle design with a polyethylene tibial component.[105,179] For implantation, cemented fixation with polymethyl methacrylate bone cement was used. Freeman et al[105] reported laboratory wear and fixation tests and their clinical experience of 2 years.[105] Bolton-Maggs et al[38] retrospectively reviewed midterm outcomes of 62 TARs performed between 1972 and 1981, using the ICLH ankle prosthesis Mark VII. This version of the prosthesis had a polyethylene tibial component that could be trimmed to an appropriate size at the time of operation.[297] At the mean follow-up of 5.5 years, 41 ankles were clinically reviewed. Only 13 patients had satisfactory results. The authors reported high complication rates, including wound healing problems, talar collapse, and loosening of the prosthesis components. By midterm, 13 ankles had to be revised and converted to ankle fusion. Therefore the authors suggested ankle fusion as a superior treatment option, regardless of the underlying etiology of ankle osteoarthritis (OA).[38] Samuelson et al[297] published their results obtained in 75 patients who received an ICLH prosthesis. The majority of patients (70%) reported acceptable results. The most frequently reported complication was delayed wound healing. Despite acceptable results reported by many patients, complication rates were high; thus the

authors stated that the use of this prosthesis should be approached with caution.[297] Herberts et al[143] performed 18 ICLH ankle arthroplasties in 16 patients and followed them for a mean of 36 months. In four cases, an aseptic loosening was observed; radiolucent zones greater than 2 mm were seen in another 7 ankles. Despite the acceptable results, the authors indicated that the failure rate may increase with longer follow-up.[143]

Irvine Total Ankle Replacement
The Irvine ankle design (also known as the Howmedica prosthesis) was one of the first ankle prostheses in which a special talus anatomy was closely considered (Fig. 22-1).[365]

The prosthesis designers performed anatomic measurements of 32 tali to establish the morphology of talus.[365] Evanski and Waugh[102] performed 29 cemented TARs before December 1975, using 25 Irvine ankle prostheses and 4 Smith prostheses. In all patients, significant functional improvement, including increased range of motion and pain relief, was observed. However, the mean follow-up was only 9 months, and already in this short postoperative period, malalignment occurred in two patients, one of whom needed revision surgery. In two patients, a prosthesis failure was observed (Fig. 22-2). The analysis of failures showed that the unconstrained prosthesis design in combination with its surface geometry led to increased rotation between both components, resulting in an overload of surrounding soft tissue and ligaments. Despite these poor short-term results, the authors stated that TAR would be an acceptable alternative treatment to ankle fusion.[102] However, no longer-term results in patients who underwent Irvine TAR are available in the current literature.

Richard Smith Total Ankle Replacement
Richard Smith TAR is a nonconstrained, so-called ball-and-socket (spherocentric) prosthesis that was introduced in 1975 (Fig. 22-3).[184] This prosthesis design included a metal tibial component ("socket") and polyethylene talar component ("ball"); both components

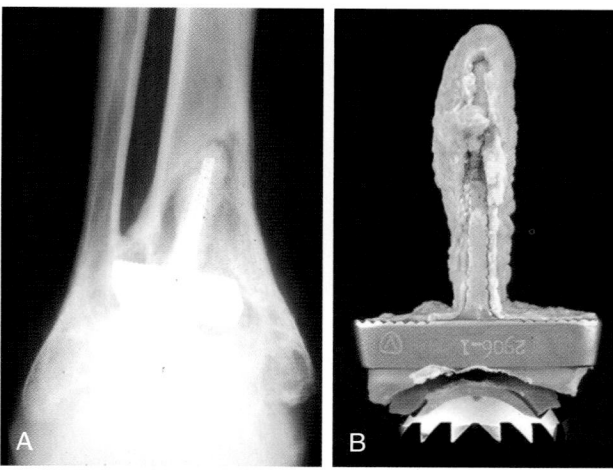

Figure 22-2 **A,** Anteroposterior radiograph of a patient who underwent total ankle replacement using Irvine prosthesis, showing significant loosening around the tibial stem. **B,** Explanted Irvine prosthesis with some cement-bone mantle around the tibial stem.

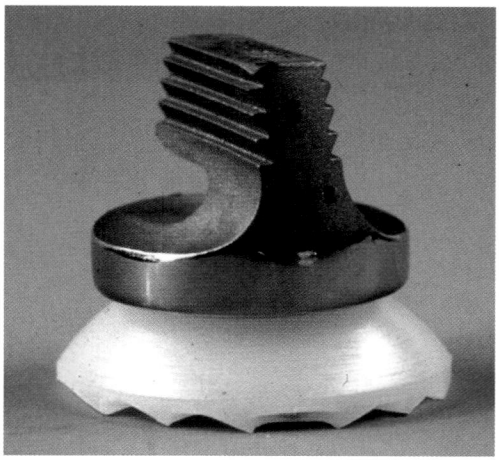

Figure 22-3 A nonconstrained spherocentric Richard Smith total ankle prosthesis.

were fixed with cement. Besides the aforementioned study by Evanski and Waugh,[102] only a few studies have been published addressing the outcome in patients who underwent Richard Smith TAR. Kirkup[184] performed 24 Richard Smith TARs in 21 patients (three cases were bilateral). Eighteen ankles were available for a mean follow-up of 7 years. Seven patients developed loosening of the tibial component, requiring revision arthroplasties using Bath-Wessex TAR in three cases at 4.1, 4.3, and 6.8 years, respectively. In one case with loosening, a deep infection occurred, resulting in ankle arthrodesis. The remaining three cases were under observation. In 7 patients, delayed wound healing was observed. Most patients in this cohort experienced substantial pain relief. Because of a high

revision rate, the recommendation was not to use this prosthesis design.[184] Dini and Bassett[88] used the Richard Smith prosthesis in 21 patients. At a mean follow-up of 27 months, failure occurred in five ankles; in other patients, significant pain relief and improved function of the ankle were observed.[88]

Conaxial Beck-Steffee Ankle Prosthesis

The Conaxial Beck-Steffee TAR is a highly constrained prosthesis type.[230] Wynn and Wilde[378] presented clinical results in 30 patients treated with Conaxial Beck-Steffee prosthesis between 1975 and 1977. All patients were reviewed at a mean follow-up of 10.8 years. Early postoperative complications were common and included wound healing problems (39%), deep infection (6%), malleoli fractures (22%), and painful talofibular impingement (14%). At 2-year follow-up, 27% of all prosthesis components already showed significant loosening. This negative tendency was confirmed at later follow-ups, resulting in a 90% loosening rate at 10 years. Therefore the authors did not recommend the further use of this prosthesis.[378]

Newton Ankle Implant

In the 1970s, St. Elmo Newton[252] reported that fused ankles may produce additional stress on the knee and midtarsus joints, thus accelerating the advancement of preexisting degenerative changes.[250,251] Therefore he performed 50 TARs since 1973, using a nonconstrained cemented prosthesis, including the high-density polyethylene tibial and Vitallium talar components (Fig. 22-4). In 75% of ankles, aseptic loosening was observed.[251] Eighteen failures occurred at a minimum follow-up of 1 year. This finding may explain related increased polyethylene wear caused by incongruency of TAR components: the tibial component was a portion of a cylinder, and the talar component was a portion of a sphere with a slightly smaller radius. Regarding the high failure rate, the following contraindications for TAR were identified: any recent infections, valgus or varus deformity of the talus of 20 degrees or greater, significant ligamentous instability of the ankle, avascular necrosis of the talus, nonunion of prior ankle fusion, and rheumatoid arthritis in patients having long-term steroid therapy.[250,251]

Bath-Wessex Total Ankle Replacement

The Bath-Wessex TAR is an unconstrained, two-component total ankle design. Carlsson et al[56] reported a 10-year survivorship analysis of 69 Bath-Wessex prostheses implanted between 1984 and 1996.[56] The initial acceptable results published in another earlier study (5-year survivorship of 81%)[55] were not maintained in this study (10-year survivorship of 66%).[56] Eighteen ankles had to be revised (12 ankle fusions and 6 revision arthroplasties). In the remaining ankles, at least one component showed radiologic loosening signs (67% of all tibial and 82% of all talar components). Therefore the authors strongly discouraged use of this prosthesis type as a standard prosthesis.[56]

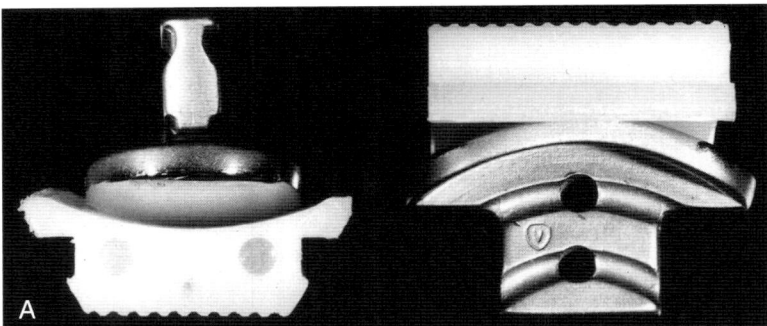
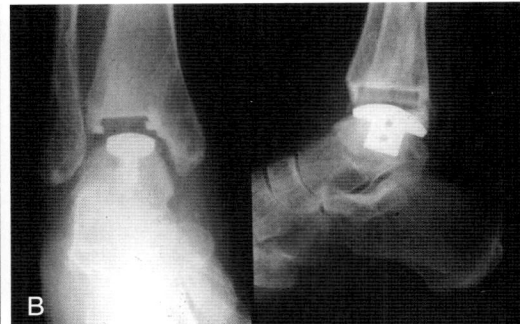

Figure 22-4 **A,** Newton ankle Implant is a nonconstrained cemented two-part prosthesis. **B,** Postoperative radiographs after implantation of a Newton ankle prosthesis.

Mayo Total Ankle Replacement

The Mayo TAR was designed as a constrained design by Stauffer in the 1970s. It was a highly congruent two-component design, including a polyethylene tibial component with cement fixation.[320,321] Stauffer and Segal[320] performed 102 TARs using the Mayo Total Ankle between 1974 and 1977. At a mean follow-up of 23 months, 53 complications were observed in 54% of ankles with post-traumatic OA and in 23% of those with rheumatoid OA. Loosening of prosthesis components in 7 ankles resulted in five revision arthroplasties and two fusions.[321] Kitaoka et al[187] reported on 204 primary Mayo TARs between 1974 and 1988 at the Mayo Clinic. The mean follow-up in this patient cohort was 9 years, with a range of 2 to 17 years. The overall 5-, 10-, and 15-year survivorship was 79%, 65%, and 61%, respectively. Because of the high failure rate, the use of this prosthesis was not recommended, especially in younger patients.[186,187] Demottaz et al[80] published a clinical gait analysis study, including 21 TARs performed between 1974 and 1977. Different prosthesis types were used in the study: 14 patients received a single-axis prosthesis (Mayo, Thompson-Parkridge-Richard [TPR], Buchholz, or Oregon) and 7 patients received a multiple-axis prosthesis (Waugh or Smith). At the mean follow-up of 15 months, pain relief and functional improvement results were disappointing. Also, the rate of progressively increasing loosening was alarmingly high at 88%. Therefore the authors suggested ankle fusion as the treatment of choice for ankle OA.[80] Lachiewicz et al[212] reviewed 17 TARs (14 Mayo ankle prostheses and 1 Buchholz ankle prosthesis) performed between 1976 and 1981.[212] The indication for the surgery in all patients was rheumatoid OA. At a mean follow-up of 39 months, all patients experienced pain relief and improved range of motion (ROM). No patients required revision surgeries; however, radiolucencies at the bone–cement interface and the subsidence of six components were observed in 11 ankles.[212] The same patient group was included in a long-term study by Unger et al.[340] Overall, 21 patients who were treated with TAR were enrolled for retrospective review at a mean follow-up of 5.6 years, with a range of 2 to 10 years. Eight from a final group of 17

available patients reported their results to be fair or poor. In 14 of 15 cases, subsidence and loosening were observed. Twelve tibial components had tilting; however, the postoperative position of the implant showed no significant correlation with radiolucency around the component.[340]

Oregon Ankle Prosthesis

The Oregon ankle is a single-axis, two-component TAR design. Groth and Fitch[126] performed 71 primary cemented TARs using Oregon ankle prosthesis between 1975 and 1985. At a mean follow-up of 6.5 years, reoperations were necessary in 19 patients, including 11 ankle fusions and 5 revision arthroplasties. The authors concluded that TAR should be limited to patients with rheumatoid arthritis and to elderly less-active patients with posttraumatic OA.[126] In 1986, McGuire et al[231] performed a retrospective comparative study addressing outcome and complication rates in patients who underwent TAR versus ankle arthrodesis. The TAR group consisted of 25 patients with six different prosthesis types (Oregon, TPR, Richard Smith, Newton, Mayo, and Buchholz). The mean follow-up was 3.8 years. Four patients with TAR had infections (vs. 5 of 18 in the arthrodesis group). Loosening occurred in 5 patients with TAR (vs. 6 nonunions in arthrodesis group). The authors concluded that TAR should not be performed in younger patients with posttraumatic OA.[231]

Thompson-Richard Prosthesis

The Thompson-Richard prosthesis (TRP) was introduced in 1976 as a two-component semiconstrained cemented implant. The prosthesis design included the polyethylene tibial component with a concave articular surface and a lip on each side designed to avoid too-excessive transversal movement of the talar component.[28,377] Wood et al[377] compared the clinical and radiologic outcome of the cemented TRP prosthesis (seven ankles replaced during 1991 and 1992) and cementless STAR prosthesis (also seven ankles). The mean follow-up for TRP and STAR groups was 7.2 and 5.4 years, respectively. In the TRP prosthesis group, four tibial components showed significant loosening, requiring ankle fusion in two cases, while all components of the STAR prosthesis remained stable at the latest follow-up.[377] A similar comparative study—TRP versus STAR prosthesis—was performed by Schill et al,[302] including 27 TRP and 22 STAR implants. At a follow-up ranging from 1 to 12 years, 37 patients with 20 TRP and 19 STAR prostheses were reviewed. In patients with TRP prostheses, a high rate of radiolucency around the tibial component (53.3%) was seen; also, in three ankles talar components were found to have significant subsidence. In patients with STAR implants, only three cases showed small radiolucent lines of the flat tibial component, while the talar components showed no signs of loosening or migration. In the TRP group, two revisions were performed, because of prosthesis loosening and malleolar fracture, resulting in a 12-year cumulative survivorship of 87%. In the STAR group, two revisions were necessary because of one meniscal-bearing breakage and correction of meniscal-bearing height, resulting in a 6-year cumulative survivorship of 94.3%.[302] Jensen and Kroner[174] observed a high rate of radiolucency around prosthesis components in 52% of 30 reviewed ankles. Revision was necessary in only two cases; however, only 69% of all patients were satisfied with the results obtained at a follow-up of 5 years.[174]

New Jersey or Cylindrical Total Ankle Replacement

The New Jersey Cylindrical Replacement design was developed in the 1970s by Michael Pappas, a bioengineer, and Frederick Buechel, an orthopaedic surgeon.[261] During the development of the design rationale, the authors recognized essential problems regarding ankle anatomy (normal ligamental function, physiologic ROM, intrinsic stability during ROM), surgical technique (component biocompatibility, minimal resection of bone, preservation of blood supply to the talus and distal tibia, postoperative rehabilitation), and mechanical objectives (optimal force transfer at bone–prosthesis interface, minimal wear, anteroposterior [AP] shear load resistance). The treatment options in case of ankle failure (ability to remove prosthesis with minimal tissue damage, revision arthroplasty vs. ankle fusion) were also thoroughly discussed.[261] Although the clinical results with the first generation of the New Jersey Cylindrical Replacement design were not satisfactory, the authors identified numerous problems regarding the design of TARs that were addressed later by other surgeons and designers.[360]

Results of First-Generation Total Ankle Designs

Most first-generation TAR designs used in 1970s and early 1980s were two-component prostheses, including both prosthesis types (constrained and unconstrained)[121,147,156] and typically included a concave polyethylene tibial component and a convex metal component for the talus, usually made of a cobalt chrome alloy. Cement fixation was used to secure the talar and tibial components. The reason for the cemented fixation was simple: in the 1970s, cementless fixation and ingrowth surfaces were rare, and cement fixation led to acceptable stability in patients who underwent total knee or hip replacement. However, first-generation TARs were recognized to have unacceptably high complication rates, including aseptic loosening on both tibial and talar sites, wide osteolysis with cyst development, subsidence, and mechanical failure of prosthesis components. Cement fixation usually required substantial bone resection to accommodate the volume of cement at the initial implantation of ankle prosthesis. Larger bone resection resulted in fixation to bone with reduced mechanical quality, especially on the tibial side.[170] This may explain some of reasons for the high failure rate. One conspicuous design feature of most first-generation ankle arthroplasty designs was a tibial component that was significantly larger than the talar component. The rationale was to achieve a physiologic range of motion of the replaced ankle as well as axial rotation. However, because of low intrinsic stability, significant shear forces occurred during the gait, which may have resulted in premature prosthesis wear and loosening, especially in patients with preexisting chronic ligamentous instability.

Interpretation of all the factors that lead to TAR failure will remain challenging because of limited data. Most clinical reports addressing outcomes in patients who underwent first-generation TAR were case reports or small case series.[290] Another critical factor limiting validity of studies were the short follow-ups of mostly 5 years or less. Patient satisfaction with this procedure was reciprocally proportional to the length of follow-up, varying between 19% and 81% of patient cohorts.[290]

In general, the clinical results of first-generation total ankle arthroplasties were highly discouraging. The alarming failure rate, along with other significant complications, including wound healing problems, inferior postoperative functional results, and so forth, led to the recommendation to use ankle fusion as the primary treatment option for ankle osteoarthritis.* In 1985, Hamblen[130] stated the following in an editorial in the British edition of *Journal of Bone and Joint Surgery*: "Clearly the answer to the question of replacing the ankle joint using current techniques must be 'no'." Failure analysis of first-generation total ankle arthroplasties showed that only significant improvements in prosthetic design, change of fixation (elimination of cemented fixation), and improved anatomic access would change the arthroplasty outcome, making this procedure a valuable treatment option in patients with end-stage ankle osteoarthritis.[290]

KINEMATICS AND BIOMECHANICS OF TOTAL ANKLE REPLACEMENT

With recent advances in biomechanics, improved materials, and surgical techniques, the newer generation of TARs tend to better reproduce the physiologic function and kinematics of the ankle, resulting in improved postoperative results and high patient satisfaction.

---

*References 56, 80, 186, 187, 251, 321, and 378.

Patients with ankle osteoarthritis usually show significant alteration of plantar pressure distribution.[163,254] Horisberger et al[163] measured plantar pressure distribution parameters in 120 patients with end-stage ankle osteoarthritis by using dynamic pedobarography. In most patients, a significant decrease of maximum force and contact area was observed. These findings might be interpreted as an attempt by patients to reduce the weight-bearing load on the arthritic ankle and to avoid pain.[163] Patients with asymmetric ankle osteoarthritis have been found to have reduced peak ground reaction forces and peak kinetic values.[254]

Valderrabano et al assessed kinematic changes after ankle fusion and TAR with regard to ROM,[344] movement transfer,[345] and talar movement.[346] All measurements were performed in native ankles, then in ankles with two-component (Agility) and three-component prostheses (HINTEGRA [Integra Life Sciences, Plainsboro, N.J.] and STAR), and finally in fused ankles. The results of the study showed near-normal kinematics after prosthesis implantation and significantly impaired measurements in fused ankles.[344-346] Komistek et al[206] used fluoroscopy to evaluate translational and rotational motions of the hindfoot in the sagittal and frontal planes in 10 subjects having a normal ankle and TAR on the opposite side (Buechel-Pappas prosthesis). The average ROM for normal versus replaced ankles was 37.4 degrees and 32.3 degrees, respectively. Furthermore, comparable kinematic patterns of motion were observed for normal and replaced ankles.[206] Yamaguchi et al[380] investigated in vivo kinematics of total ankle arthroplasty during non–weight-bearing and weight-bearing dorsiflexion and plantar flexion[381] and during the gait. In their first study, the authors measured three-dimensional (3D) kinematics and addressed the articular surface incongruency during non–weight-bearing and weight-bearing activities in 47 patients who underwent TAR using the TNK prosthesis.[381] No significant differences between non–weight-bearing and weight-bearing kinematics were detected. The observed kinematic patterns, including internal rotation during plantar flexion were similar to those observed in natural ankles. In more than 75% of all replaced ankles, incongruency of the joint surface was seen.[381] In the sequel study of the same working group, in vivo kinematics and congruency of the articular surface during the stance phase of gait were investigated in 18 ankles of 15 patients.[380] Three-dimensional–two-dimensional (3D–2D) mode image registration was performed in this study by using lateral fluoroscopic images and implant models. The mean ranges of motion for dorsiflexion/plantar flexion, inversion/eversion, and internal/external rotation were 11.1 ± 4.6 degrees, 0.8 ± 0.4 degrees, and 2.6 ± 1.5 degrees, respectively. In 8 of 18 ankles, at least one type of surface incongruency was observed during the stance phase, including anterior hinging in one ankle, medial or lateral lift-off, or excessive axial rotation. The surface incongruency, which was actually not observed in the static radiographs, has clear potential

to lead to increased contact pressure, wear, and implant loosening.[380]

Detrembleur and Leemrijse[85] addressed the effects of TAR on gait disability by analysis of energetic and mechanical variables. The study included patients who underwent TAR using three-component implant designs: Ankle Evolutive System (AES) prosthesis (Biomet, Nimes, France) (n = 16), Mobility prosthesis (Depuy, Warsaw, Ind.) (n = 3), and HINTEGRA prosthesis (n = 1). All patients were analyzed before and approximately 7 months after surgery by using instrumented motion analysis to assess spatiotemporal parameters, ankle kinematics, mechanical work, and electromyographic activity. In addition, energy expenditure was analyzed using an ergospirometer. The authors showed that TAR has a beneficial effect on locomotor function, resulting in improvement of speed, spatiotemporal parameters, ankle amplitude instance, and vertical center-of-mass displacement.[85] In a relatively large study, Brodsky et al[44] performed 3D gain analysis in 50 consecutive patients who underwent TAR using a STAR prosthesis, at a mean follow-up of 49 months, with a range of 24 to 108 months. The following kinematic and spaciotemporal parameters have been measured in this prospective study: stride length; cadence; sagittal plane range of motion of the ankle, knee, and hip; plantar flexion/dorsiflexion moment; and sagittal plane ankle power. A statistically significant improvement of range of motion from 14.2 to 17.9 degrees was observed; increased motion was also measured at the hip and knee. Furthermore, ankle power and ankle plantar-flexion moment were significantly increased. In this patient cohort, a more normal ankle function and gait were objectively observed after TAR.[44] Hahn et al[129] compared gait parameters in patients who underwent TAR and compared the results with those measured in patients with ankle arthrodesis. In addition, pain and physical function were assessed in 9 patients with TAR and ankle arthrodesis preoperative and 12 months after the surgery. Both surgical procedures provided significant pain relief and functional improvement in gait. However, patients with TAR had more natural ankle joint function with increased range of motion.[129]

Valderrabano et al[350] addressed patients' rehabilitation in the first year after TAR in a prospective study, including 15 patients with unilateral posttraumatic ankle osteoarthritis. For comparison, patients were matched to 15 healthy persons without degenerative changes, with the appropriate demographic factors as a control group. Clinical and functional status and 3D kinematic-kinetic analysis was performed preoperatively and postoperatively at 3, 6, 9, and 12 months after TAR when using a HINTEGRA prosthesis. As expected, patients with ankle osteoarthritis showed significant clinical and functional impairments preoperatively as measured using the AOFAS and Short Form-36 (SF-36) scores. Preoperatively, gait analysis revealed a significant deficiency in six of seven measured spatiotemporal variables: a decrease of the triplanar ankle movement, a decrease of the second active maximal vertical and the maximal medial ground reaction force, a reduction of the sagittal and transverse ankle joint moments, and a reduction of the ankle joint power. Three months postoperatively, patients with a replaced ankle experienced worsening of gait. However, by 12 months no differences in the spatiotemporal variables were detected with respect to normal subjects.[350] In another study, Valderrabano et al[349] addressed the muscle rehabilitation in the same patient cohort. It has been shown that TAR normalizes the muscle function (including torque and electromyographic "intensity") in OA ankles to a significant extent. However, after 1 year of rehabilitation, patients did not reach the level of the contralateral, unaffected leg.[349]

Pedobarography may be also used for measurement of plantar pressure distribution in patients after TAR.[107,156,240,284] Hintermann and Valderrabano[156] reported their preliminary results of 148 consecutive total ankle arthroplasties when using a HINTEGRA prosthesis. The normal plantar pressure distribution and a normal line of center of pressure were observed in 78.1% of all cases. An increased forefoot pressure, a discharge of the forefoot pressure, and an increased lateral pressure were found in 10.4%, 7.3%, and 4.2%, respectively, of all replaced ankles.[156] Valderrabano et al[342] analyzed results of dynamic pedobarography obtained in 65 consecutive patients with a STAR prosthesis. A normal plantar pressure distribution while walking was found in 53% of all patients. Twenty patients had an increased forefoot loading, and 6 patients had an increased lateral foot loading.[342] Frigg et al[107] assessed the hindfoot alignment in 28 consecutive patients with TAR by using visual means, radiographs (hindfoot alignment view[293]), and dynamically with pedobarography. The following pedobarographic parameters were measured: coronal index, initial heel contact on heel strike, heel index, lateral medial area index, center-of-pressure index, lateral-medial force-time integral index, and gait line integral.[107] In the opinion of the current authors, pedobarography may be helpful for detailed analysis of hindfoot analysis in patients with end-stage ankle osteoarthritis and concomitant varus (Fig. 22-5) or valgus (Fig. 22-6) deformities.

Preoperative Planning

Indications for Total Ankle Replacement

End-stage ankle arthritis is the main indication for this procedure. Unlike the hip and knee, the ankle joint is rarely affected by primary osteoarthritis. In clinical and epidemiologic studies, previous trauma has been shown to be the most common cause of ankle osteoarthritis.[295,348] Rotational ankle fractures with consecutive cartilage damage was identified as the most common reason for posttraumatic ankle osteoarthritis.[348] However, repetitive ligament injuries can also result in posttraumatic ankle osteoarthritis.[343] Other common indications for TAR are systemic (rheumatoid) arthritis[279,280,372] and secondary osteoarthritis. Secondary OA has been found to be

associated with underlying diseases and/or pathologies, such as hemophilia,[22,225,283,357] hereditary hemochromatosis,[23,77] gout,[29,207] postinfectious arthritis,[40,271] and avascular talar necrosis.[39,49,103,200] Patients with bilateral ankle osteoarthritis are good candidates for this procedure because bilateral ankle fusion generally has a detrimental influence on gait and functional outcome.[113,243,253,288] This can be particularly important in patients with secondary osteoarthritis resulting from hemochromatosis or hemophilia,[22,23] and bilateral TAR can be performed in two separate stages.[34,104,114,207,358] However, in patients with bilateral end-stage ankle osteoarthritis, simultaneous bilateral TAR has been reported,[25,28,178] resulting in significant pain relief and functional improvement comparable to the results achieved with a unilateral procedure.[25,28] Patients considered for simultaneous bilateral TAR should be informed about a prolonged initial recovery period.[28] In patients with previously performed subtalar, triple, and/or midfoot fusion, the tibiotalar fusion would completely "stiffen" the hindfoot, while the TAR may preserve the functional motion as mentioned before. The clinical outcome of TAR when combined with hindfoot fusion is comparable to that of ankle replacement alone.[183]

With increased use, an emerging indication for TAR is salvage of failed primary TAR.* A major concern in revision arthroplasty of the ankle can be anchorage of prosthesis components in deficient bone stock to ensure long-term prosthesis stability.[153,160] After removal of the prosthesis component and careful debridement, if the residual bone stock is not sufficient, ankle fusion may be a better option.†

Another special indication for total ankle arthroplasty is the salvage of painful nonunion or malunion of prior ankle fusion.[14,122,154,155] Conversion of fused ankle to TAR is a technically demanding procedure that should be performed only if remaining bone stock is sufficient and soft tissue conditions are not too compromised (especially in patients with previous long-standing ankle arthrodesis).[155] The conversion ankle arthroplasty should be limited only to experienced surgeons with adequate experience in primary TAR. If performed by experienced surgeons, this procedure has shown promising early results with low intraoperative and postoperative complication rates comparable to those observed in patients with primary TAR.[122,154]

Contraindications for Total Ankle Replacement

The contraindications for TAR may be divided into two major groups: absolute and relative contraindications.

The absolute contraindications[127,151,156,290] for this procedure include acute or chronic infections. In several studies, avascular necrosis of the talus has been identified as an absolute contraindication for TAR.‡ In patients

---

*References 8, 61, 104, 139, 161, 164, 168, 177, 189, 276, 317, 373, and 375.
†References 32, 74, 100, 101, 162, 188, 208, 269, and 333.
‡References 9, 30, 62, 127, 173, 241, 245, and 251.

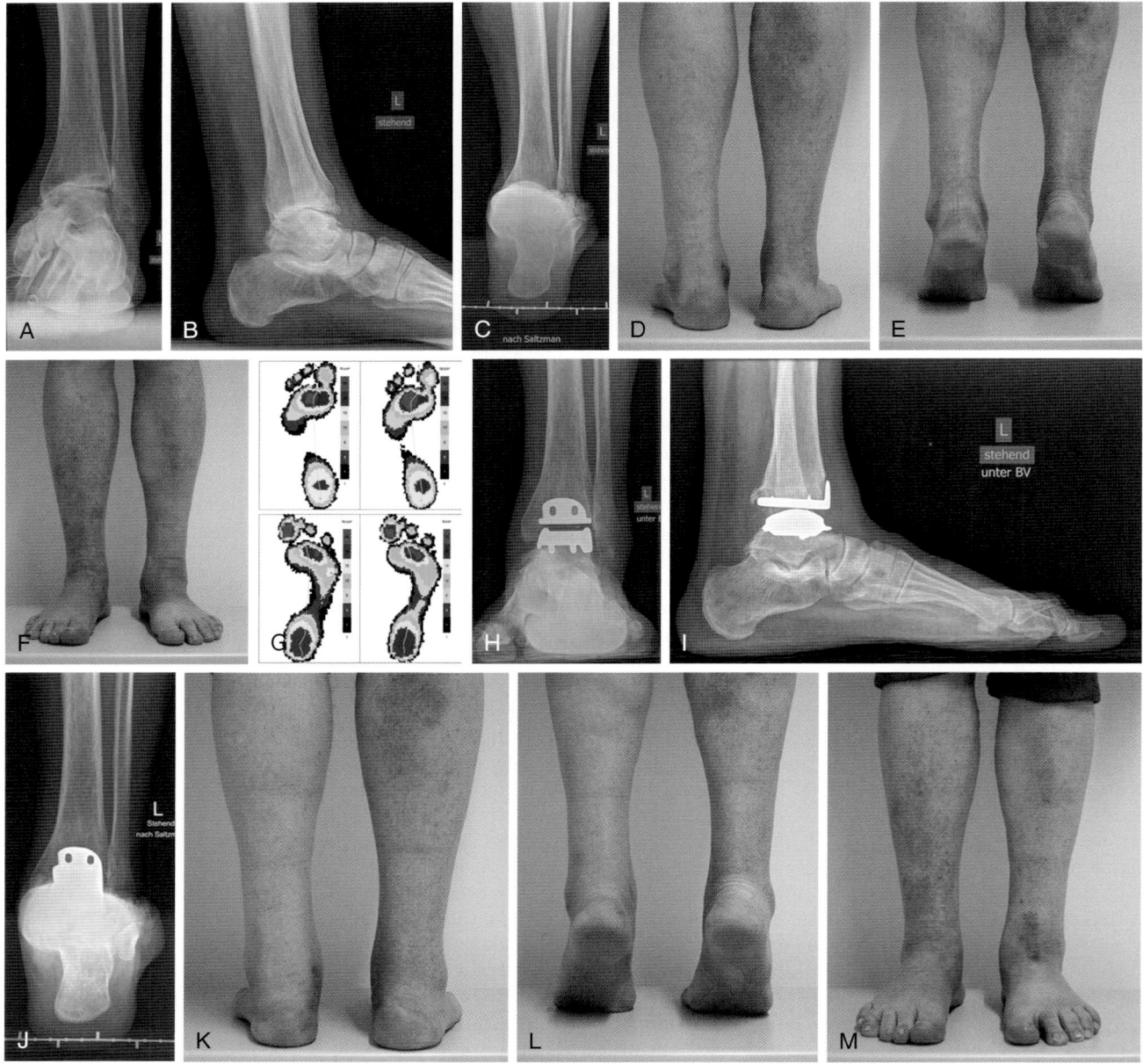

Figure 22-5 A 62-year-old male patient with varus osteoarthritic ankle. Preoperative anteroposterior **(A)** and lateral **(B)** weight-bearing radiographs show degenerative changes of the tibiotalar joint with varus tilting of the talus. **C,** Hindfoot alignment view shows slight varus malalignment of the hindfoot. **D-F,** Clinical pictures show some swelling and varus appearance of the left hindfoot. **G,** Dynamic pedobarography shows lateral overloading of the left foot *(lower row).* Postoperative (1-year follow-up) anteroposterior **(H)** and lateral **(I)** weight-bearing radiographs show well-aligned position of prosthesis components with good osseous integration. **J,** Hindfoot alignment view as well as clinical pictures **(K-M)** show physiologic alignment of the hindfoot. (Images courtesy Beat Hintermann, MD, Liestal, Switzerland.)

with avascular necrosis of more than one third of the talus, the use of a standard prosthesis component may lead to significant subsidence and loosening of the talar component and failure.* In these patients, a revision talar component[160] or a custom-made talar prosthesis[132,214,330] should be used. Patients with neuromuscular

disorders, neuroarthropathy (e.g., Charcot arthropathy of the midfoot and/or hindfoot), massive joint laxity (e.g., patients with Marfan disease), or diabetes with clinically significant distal polyneuropathy should be excluded. Patients with severe instability and/or lower-leg malalignment that cannot be surgically corrected (e.g., by corrective osteotomies[194,195,259]) should not be considered for TAR. At present, there is no concensus

---

*References 6, 39, 84, 127, 173, and 294.

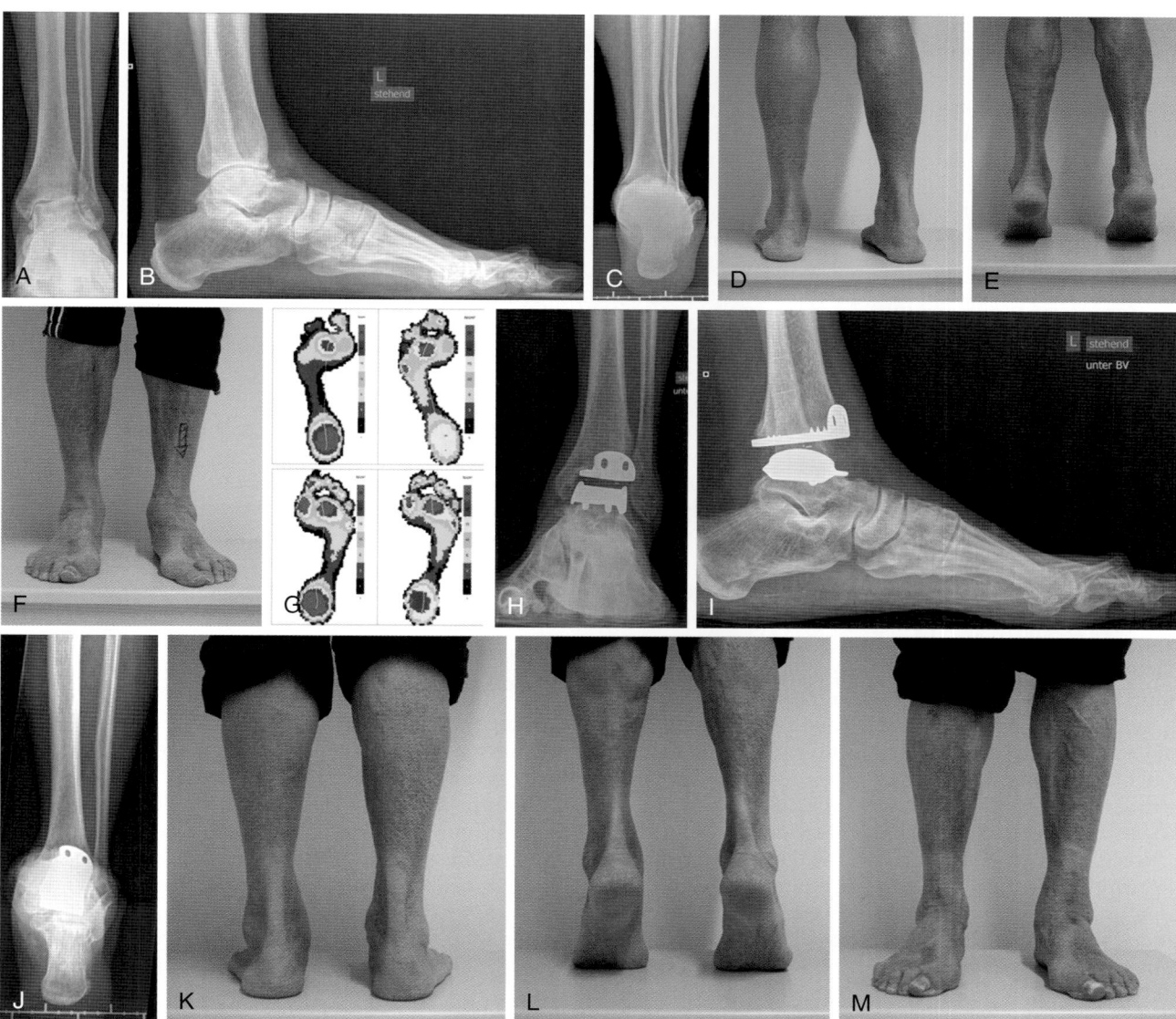

Figure 22-6 A 66-year-old male patient with valgus osteoarthritic ankle. Preoperative anteroposterior **(A)** and lateral **(B)** weight-bearing radiographs show degenerative changes of the tibiotalar joint with valgus tilting of the talus. **C,** Hindfoot alignment view shows valgus malalignment of the hindfoot. **D-F,** Clinical pictures show some swelling and valgus appearance of the left hindfoot. **G,** Dynamic pedobarography shows medial overloading of the left forefoot *(lower row)*. Postoperative (2-year follow-up) anteroposterior **(H)** and lateral **(I)** weight-bearing radiographs show well-aligned position of prosthesis components with good osseous integration. **J,** Hindfoot alignment view as well as clinical pictures **(K-M)** show physiologic alignment of the hindfoot. (Images courtesy Beat Hintermann, MD, Liestal, Switzerland.)

for a clinically relevant cut-off for the degree of coronal deformity that can be corrected at the implantation of TAR. In general, a moderate preoperative coronal deformity of less than 10 degrees can be corrected intraoperatively by modification of bone cuts (especially on the talar side). In patients with a coronal deformity of more than 10 degrees, the deformity should be corrected before the implantation of the prosthesis component (as a one- or two-stage procedure). Suspected or documented metal allergy or intolerance is rarely observed; however, these patients should be excluded preoperatively.

Although many authors suggest that previous ankle infection is an absolute contraindication for TAR,* the current authors cannot fully embrace this opinion. In a series of 17 consecutive patients with this history, who underwent HINTEGRA total ankle arthroplasty, Dr. Hintermann achieved good functional results and did not observe any recurrence of infection (unpublished data). Eichinger et al[93] and Espinosa and Klammer[98] also recommend TAR in patients with ankle OA resulting from previous infection.

*References 127, 252, 332, 356, and 368.

The relative contraindications[127,151,156,290] for this procedure include significantly reduced bone quality (e.g., resulting from severe osteoporosis, immunosuppressive therapy, or long-term therapy with steroids) and diabetes without clinically significant polyneuropathy. Smoking is another relative contraindication because it is associated with higher risk of perioperative complications, including wound breakdown.[368] Patients with high (e.g., contact sports, jumping) or increased (e.g., jogging, tennis, downhill skiing) demands for physical activities should be informed about possible mechanical failure caused by edge loading with increased wear and a potentially higher rate of aseptic loosening.[246,351]

Significant preoperative varus or valgus deformity (more than 10 degrees) has also been seen as a contraindication for TAR. With three-part ankle replacements, Doets et al[89] found that preoperative deformity in the frontal plane is difficult to correct, causing instability and subluxation of the mobile bearing, which may result in the prosthesis failure.[89] In their study of 200 STAR implants, Wood and Deakin[373] observed that preoperative varus or valgus deformity of more than 15 degrees may cause edge loading of the mobile bearing. Therefore the authors stated that this may be a relative contraindication for TAR.[372,373] However, the preoperative hindfoot deformity should not be an absolute contraindication, as long as additional realignment procedures (supramalleolar and/or calcaneal osteotomies, ligament reconstruction, subtalar fusion) can correct the deformity.[47,82,183,195] Karantana et al[177] did not observe any differences in functional outcome and prosthesis component survivorship between the patients with and without preoperative deformities, as long the deformity is addressed at the time of prosthesis implantation. Daniels et al[76] demonstrated that correction of moderate-to-severe varus deformities is possible and results in good functional outcome and stability of prosthesis components. Kim et al[183] reported that the clinical outcome of TAR performed in ankles with preoperative varus deformity of more than 10 degrees is comparable to that of neutrally aligned ankles. However, simultaneous surgical procedures addressing the preoperative deformity are necessary to achieve good results.[183]

Finally, and perhaps most importantly, the patient and the surgeon must have realistic expectations of this surgery.[34,96,213] The high satisfaction of rheumatoid osteoarthritis patients after total ankle arthroplasty likely reflects the low demands and low expectations of this patient cohort.[298] On the other hand, the expectations of patients with posttraumatic ankle osteoarthritis are generally higher than those of patients with non-posttraumatic ankle osteoarthritis.[246] In particular, predictions regarding postoperative improvement in range of motion should be made carefully; as with current implants (all with an anterior approach), postoperative improvement in ankle range of motion is relatively small (generally <10 degrees) and therefore is not one of the expected benefits from this procedure.[20,120]

"Ideal Candidate" for Total Ankle Replacement

Based on the authors' clinical experience[27,290] and results published in the current literature, these are criteria for the "ideal candidate" with end-stage ankle osteoarthritis when assessing for TAR:

■ Middle aged or older (sixth decade or older and , in general, the older the better)
■ Low demands for physical and sports activities (e.g., hiking, swimming, biking, golfing)
■ No significant comorbidities
■ No smoking
■ No obesity/overweight (normal or slightly increased body mass index; however, obesity is not a contraindication for this procedure)[17,26]
■ Good bone stock with no risk factors for impaired bone quality
■ Well-aligned and stable hindfoot
■ Good soft tissue (e.g., no previous surgeries of foot/ankle)
■ Well-preserved preoperative range of motion
■ No neurovascular impairment of the lower extremity
■ Reasonable expectations

Preoperative Examination

Clinical Examination

All previous medical reports (e.g., surgery reports) and imaging data are collected and carefully analyzed. Especially in patients with posttraumatic ankle osteoarthritis and previously performed surgeries (e.g., open reduction and internal fixation), the exact type of hardware should be identified to ensure the hardware can be removed without any difficulty before implantation of prosthetic components. Actual the patients' history is carefully assessed to specifically address the following aspects: actual pain (e.g., using a visual analog scale ranging from 0 = no pain to 10 = maximal pain),[169] limitations in daily activities and quality of life (e.g., using the SF-36 questionnaire),[363] sports activities (e.g., using the following scoring: 0 = none, 1 = moderate, 2 = normal, 3 = high, 4 = elite),[351] and current and previous treatment. Patients with any of the aforementioned absolute contraindications are excluded. Especially in patients with significant comorbidities, a consultation in neurology and/or internal medicine should be arranged before planning TAR.

The routine physical examination starts with careful inspection of the foot and ankle while sitting, standing, and walking, allowing dynamic comparison of changes at weight bearing versus non–weight bearing. The eventually observed pathologic findings should be compared with the contralateral nonaffected limb. Skin and soft tissue are carefully evaluated, with special attention given to previous surgical scars. Hindfoot stability is assessed manually, with the patient sitting (e.g., using the anterior drawer test).[15,69,70] Ankle alignment, including supramalleolar deformities and the position of heel in relation to the longitudinal axis of the lower leg, is assessed with the patient standing. However, clinical assessment of the ankle and hindfoot alignment should be interpreted carefully because visual alignment assessment is often not accurate enough.[107] Range of motion of the tibiotalar joint is determined using a goniometer placed along the lateral border of the leg and foot. All goniometric measurement should be performed in the weight-bearing position according to the method described by Lindsjö et al.[222] Intrarater and interrater reliability of the goniometric measurements is usually not very high.[382] However, the accuracy of the goniometric measurements of the tibiotalar joint range of motion was assessed by direct comparison with ankle range-of-motion measurements obtained from radiographs.[20,66,154,157] Another alternative for assessing ankle dorsiflexion and stiffness is the Iowa Ankle Range of Motion (IAROM) device, which provided valid and reliable measurements (Fig. 22-7).[369] Because many patients with end-stage osteoarthritis present with lower leg muscular atrophy,[349] basic muscle function should be assessed (e.g., the function of tibial and peroneal muscles).

Radiographic Examination

Radiographic examination of affected ankles includes weight-bearing radiographs with anteroposterior and lateral views of the foot and an anteroposterior view of the ankle. All radiographs should be performed in the weight-bearing manner for appropriate evaluation of foot and ankle alignment, statics, and biomechanics because non–weight-bearing radiographs are often misleading

(Fig. 22-8).[95,167,237] Furthermore, the standing position of patients at radiographic examination may standardize the radiographic technique, resulting in a more reliable comparison between preoperative and postoperative radiographs. All possible coexisting degenerative changes in the adjacent joints as well as any deformities (e.g., flattening of the longitudinal arch of the foot) should be identified and carefully analyzed.

Concomitant deformities in the osteoarthritic ankles may occur on the supramalleolar, intraarticular, and/or

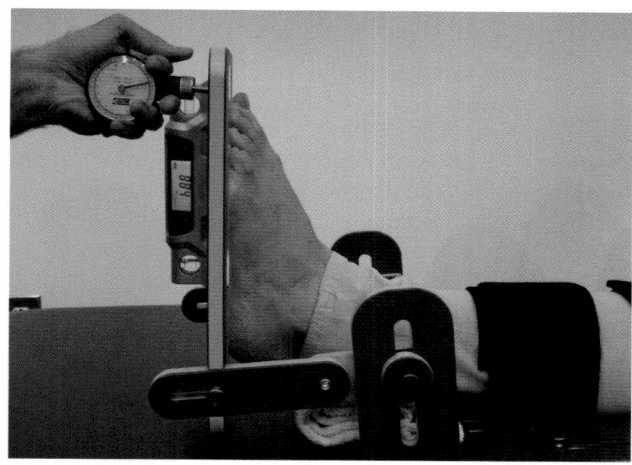

Figure 22-7 Iowa ankle range-of-motion (IAROM) device.

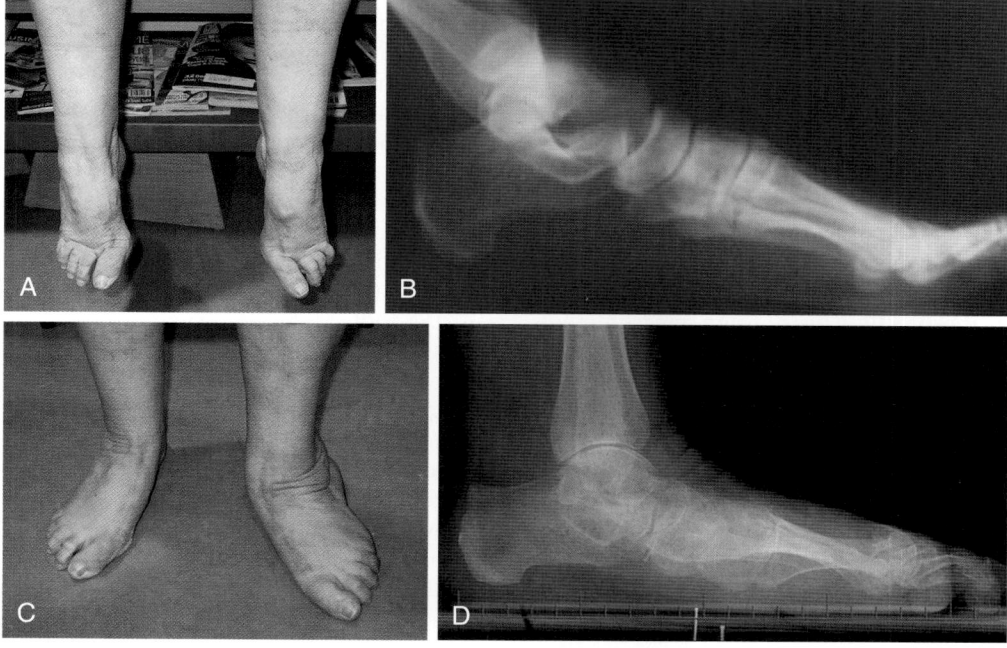

Figure 22-8 A 72-year-old female with severe flatfoot deformity resulting from third-degree posterior tibial tendon insufficiency. Without weight-bearing, breakdown of the medial arch cannot be observed clinically **(A)** or radiologically **(B)**. While in a weight-bearing position, significant flattening of the medial arch is observed clinically **(C)** and radiologically **(D)** on the lateral radiograph. The sagittal plane radiograph allows the surgeon to quantify the actual range of motion of the tibiotalar joint versus motion coming from the entire foot.

inframalleolar level. Supramalleolar ankle alignment is measured in coronal and sagittal planes by measurement of the medial distal tibial angle and the anterior distal tibial angle, respectively.[192,227,323] The medial distal tibial angle has been measured to be 92.4 ± 3.1 degrees (range, 88-100 degrees) in a radiographic study[192] and 93.3 ± 3.2 degrees (range, 88-100 degrees) in a cadaver study.[172,192] The measurement of the medial distal tibial angle depends on radiograph technique.[24,323] The anterior distal tibial angle has been measured to be 83.0 ± 3.6 degrees (range, 76-97 degrees).[227] The inframalleolar ankle alignment (especially the heel position in relation to the longitudinal axis of the lower leg) is measured using the hindfoot alignment view.[293] The hindfoot alignment view is taken at a 20-degree angle to the floor, with the foot placed with its medial border parallel to the radiographic beam.[293] As already mentioned, the visual assessment of the hindfoot alignment is not accurate; therefore the hindfoot alignment view should be performed routinely for appropriate measurement of inframalleolar hindfoot deformities.[106,107] A computed tomography (CT) scan may be helpful to assess the bony defects and to analyze the joint incongruency. In patients with degenerative changes of the adjacent joint, single photon emission computed tomography (SPECT-CT) may help to evaluate the morphologic changes and their biologic activities.[193,258] Preoperative magnetic resonance imaging (MRI) may help to assess the concomitant ligamental injuries,[136,149] pathologic changes of tendons,[60,149] and avascular necrosis of osseous structures.[136,149]

Pedobarography

One of the most widely measured parameters for gait analysis is assessment of plantar pressure distribution. In patients with ankle osteoarthritis, the following variables usually are specifically assessed: maximum force, contact time, peak pressure, contact area, and center of pressure index.[163,176] The patients are asked to walk at their own preferred speed because prescribed speed may influence and change the normal gait pattern.[242] For sufficient reliability of the pressure measurement, at least five dynamic trials of each foot should be recorded.[165] For reliable and easier analysis, the pressure distribution measurements are commonly divided into four regions, including hindfoot, midfoot, forefoot, and toes.[163]

Outcome Instruments in Studies on Total Ankle Arthroplasty

Reliable and accurate assessment of preoperative and postoperative patients' functional outcomes is crucial in monitoring the effectiveness of TAR. Naal et al[247] performed a systematic literature review including 79 original studies. Authors identified a total of 15 outcome instruments. The most commonly used ones were the AOFAS hindfoot score (n = 41),[185] the Kofoed ankle score (n = 15),[198] the visual analog scale assessing pain (n = 15),[169] and the generic SF-36 (n = 6).[363] The use of the very popular AOFAS hindfoot score is not without

problems because this score has not been validated. This questionnaire has been shown to have enough discriminatory capacity to assess postoperative improvement in patients who underwent TAR.[263] However, the research committee of the AOFAS published a policy statement recommending not to use this outcome assessment instrument.[264]

Hung et al[166] developed a lower-extremity physical-function computerized adaptive testing instrument based on the Patient Reported Outcomes Measurement Information System (PROMIS) physical function items. This novel outcome instrument had high reliability and content and construct validity; therefore it should be used in patients with lower-extremity problems, including degenerative changes of the ankle joint.[166]

SURGICAL TECHNIQUE

Surgical Technique Using an Anterior Approach

1. General or regional anesthesia can be used for TAR.
2. The patient is positioned supine with the feet on the edge of the table. A bump is placed under the ipsilateral hip until a strictly upward position of the lower extremity is obtained.
3. A pneumatic thigh tourniquet is applied.
4. If significant concomitant deformity has to be corrected, the unaffected lower extremity should be also draped to allow intraoperative comparison.
5. The surgical site is prepared in a sterile manner; in addition, a skin drape may be used.
6. After exsanguination by elevation, the thigh tourniquet is inflated. In most cases, a pressure of 250 to 350 mm Hg is sufficient. A total tourniquet time of 2 hours should not be exceeded.
7. A standard anterior ankle approach is used (Fig. 22-9). An anterior longitudinal incision (10-15 cm) is made in line with the extensor hallucis tendon (EHL) tendon.
8. The incision is brought down through the skin only. The medial fascicles of the superficial peroneal nerve's medial branch are identified and dissected free into the foot. These are usually retracted laterally. Occasionally, the authors intentionally transect a fine fascicle, coursing medially across the neck of the talus to gain more exposure. Before the operation, the authors tell the patient not to be surprised postoperatively by areas of numbness along the medial aspect of the foot.
9. After the nerve has been carefully retracted and the anterior tibial tendon is identified, the authors open the extensor retinaculum in line with EHL tendon sheath and retract the EHL medially. The retinaculum is the thickening of the deep fascia above the ankle, running from tibia to fibula.[1,255]
10. During preparation of the soft tissue envelope, special attention is paid to the tibialis anterior vascular bundle, which is located behind the extensor hallucis

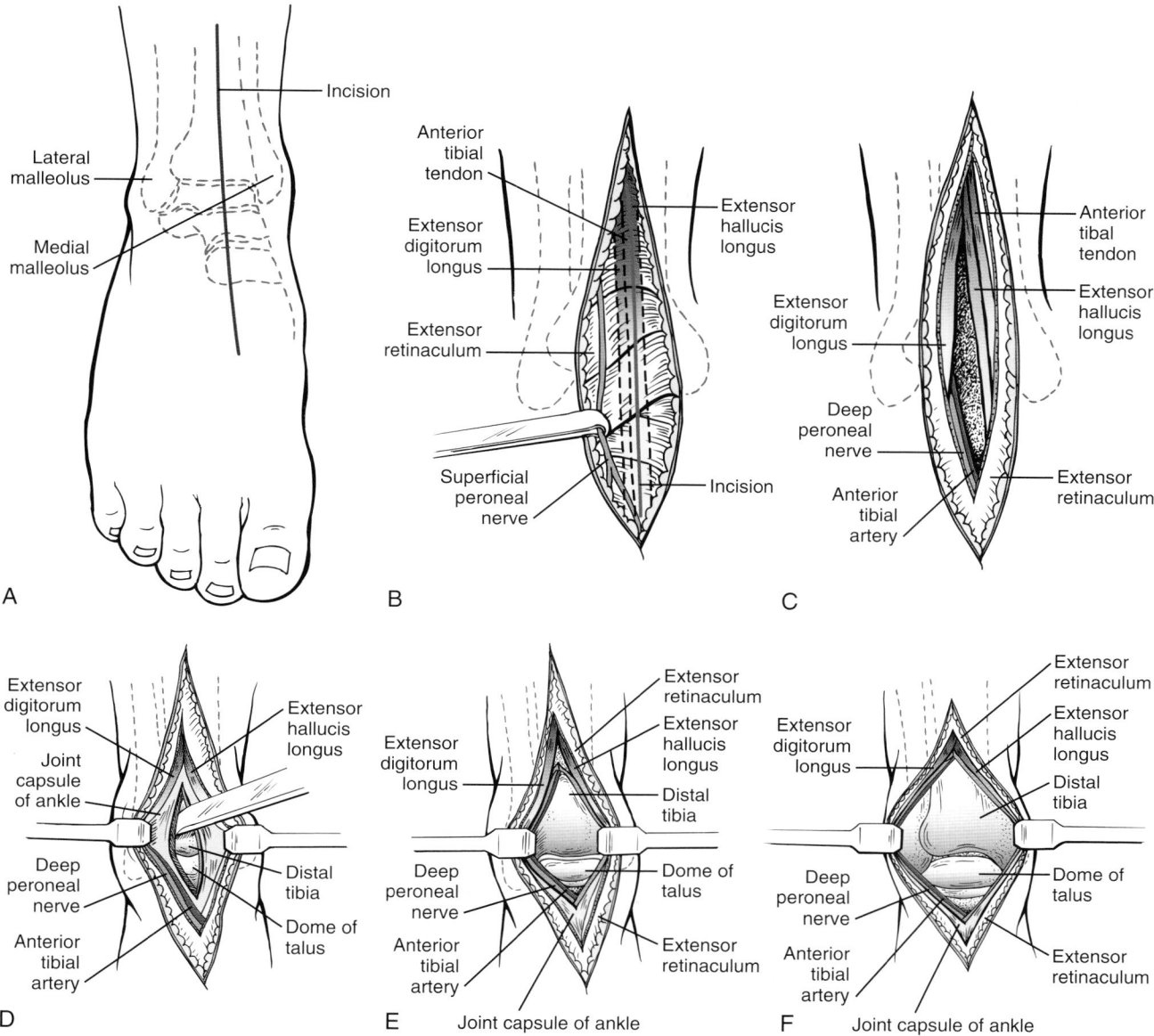

Figure 22-9 Anterior approach to the ankle. **A,** An incision is made directly anterior. **B,** The medial branch of the superficial peroneal nerve is often encountered and gently retracted laterally. **C,** The lateral bed of the extensor hallucis brevis is incised, the tendon is swept medially, and the deep neurovascular structures are retracted laterally. Often, the surgeon encounters a medially directed vascular leash that requires cautery. **D,** The capsule is incised longitudinally to preserve it for later closure. **E,** Subperiosteal dissection then allows good visualization of the anterior tibiotalar joint. **F,** Complete visualization of the the anterior tibiotalar joint including lateral and medial gutters.

longus or between the extensor hallucis longus and the extensor digitorum longus.[314]

11. The deep neurovascular bundle is gently teased free and retracted laterally. This preserves the lateral branch of the dorsalis pedis. This vessel supports the extensor digitorum brevis muscle, which is the best local muscle for the salvage of soft tissue coverage for anterior wound dehiscence.

12. The incision is deepened to the level of the joint. The authors to try to preserve the periosteum for later closure. In patients with rheumatoid arthritis or soft

bones, the subperiosteal dissection can result in inadvertent malleolar avulsions. Care must be taken to do this gently in those at risk for bone injury. The EHL interval allows the surgeon to see into the lower lateral recessus with reflection of the anterior talofibular ligament.

13. After the ankle joint is sufficiently exposed, a capsulotomy is performed.

14. If a self-retaining retractor is applied to control the soft tissue envelope, it must be relieved when not necessary. Skin hooks should not be used much so as

not to disturb wound healing. A deep blunt retractor used strategically at critical times for exposure may protect the tissues best.

15. After the joint is sufficiently exposed, the first step is to remove osteophytes on the tibia (especially on the anterolateral aspect) and the talar neck; however, the bone cortex should not be destroyed.
16. Implantation is performed by following the guidelines of the manufacturer. Every effort must be made to avoid injury to the "shoulder" region of the medial malleolus because this can cause intraoperative or postoperative malleolar fracture, a common intraoperative complication of TAR. Because the lateral malleolus in some patients is relatively more posterior, it can be inadvertently cut with approaches from front to back.
17. All distractors are removed, and the stability and motion of the ankle is checked.
18. The position of prosthesis components is checked and documented using fluoroscopy.
19. Wound closure is performed sequentially in layers, starting with the periosteum, then the extensor retinaculum, subcutaneous tissue, and skin. Skin is usually closed using 4-0 nylon. Drainage with suction may be used but is generally not necessary.
20. Soft wound dressing is used to avoid any pressure so as not to compromise wound healing. A splint is used to keep the foot in a neutral position.
21. Elevation for the first 2 days is absolutely critical. Some surgeons permit early motion.
22. The anterior approach can be used for ankle fusion procedures. It gives excellent visibility of the joint. Anterior plating (single plate or double plates)[269] can be used to secure fixation. In some cases, a more limited incision than described here works very well and limits operative time and morbidity.

Surgical Technique Using a Lateral Approach

1. General or regional anesthesia can be used for TAR.
2. The patient is placed supine on a radiolucent table with a bump placed under the ipsilateral hip to internally rotate the foot.
3. A pneumatic thigh tourniquet is applied.
4. The surgical site is prepared in a sterile manner; in addition, a skin drape may be used.
5. After exsanguination by elevation, the thigh tourniquet is inflated. In most cases, a pressure of 250 to 350 mm Hg is sufficient. Total tourniquet time of 2 hours should not be exceeded.
6. A midline incision of the fibula of about 20 cm is used, with full exposure of the lateral distal fibula (Fig. 22-10).
7. The anterior talofibular ligament (ATFL) is identified and transected for the exposure and is repaired at the end of the procedure.
8. An oblique osteotomy of the distal fibula is then performed, ending 10 to 15 mm above the joint line.
9. The tibiofibular ligaments are released from the distal fibular segment to allow the segment to be reflected and pinned to the calcaneus, while maintaining the calcaneofibular ligament (CFL) and (posterior talofibular ligament) PTFL attachments to the fibula.
10. A secondary exposure is performed over the medial gutter to allow osteophytes to be cleared, to aid in alignment of the foot into the bone preparation system, and to allow for retractors to protect the medial malleolus during bone resection.
11. The above described approach is similar to classic approaches for ankle fusion.

Total Ankle Replacement in the Valgus Osteoarthritis Ankle

In general, TAR can be performed in any patient with valgus deformity of the hindfoot, as long as the valgus malalignment can be sufficiently corrected by additional procedures. Many patients with valgus deformity show significant concomitant instability. This means that instability also has to be properly addressed at the time of prosthesis implantation.

Morphologic Types of the Valgus Osteoarthritic Ankle

Arthritic ankles with concomitant valgus deformity can be divided into two distinct morphologic types.[47] In patients with type I valgus deformity, severe pes planovalgus deformity and, generally, insufficiency of the medial ligaments and advanced tibial tendon insufficiency are observed. Usually, the tibiotalar joint shows no incongruency on anteroposterior weight-bearing radiographs. Type II valgus deformity is primarily characterized by osseous deformities with significant talus tilting within the mortise. Because of talar tilting, a significant gapping (>5 mm) of the medial ankle joint is observed on anteroposterior weight-bearing radiographs. According to the talar tilt, this morphologic entity may be divided into two subgroups: type IIA with up to 10 degrees tilting and type IIB with more than 10 degrees tilting.[47]

Surgical Technique of Total Ankle Replacement in the Valgus Osteoarthritic Ankle

A standardized surgical technique is used for implantation of the prosthesis components. The general treatment algorithm is shown in Figure 22-11. A valgus deformity of less than 10 degrees can be corrected by modification of bone cut on the tibial side. In an ankle with more than 10 degrees deformity, additional surgeries should be performed depending on the localization (supramalleolar vs. inframalleolar) and the degree of the valgus deformity:

■ Supramalleolar osteotomy (e.g., medial closing-wedge osteotomy or lateral opening-wedge osteotomy)[194,195,257,259]
■ Lengthening and (if necessary) rotational osteotomy of the distal fibula[45,152]

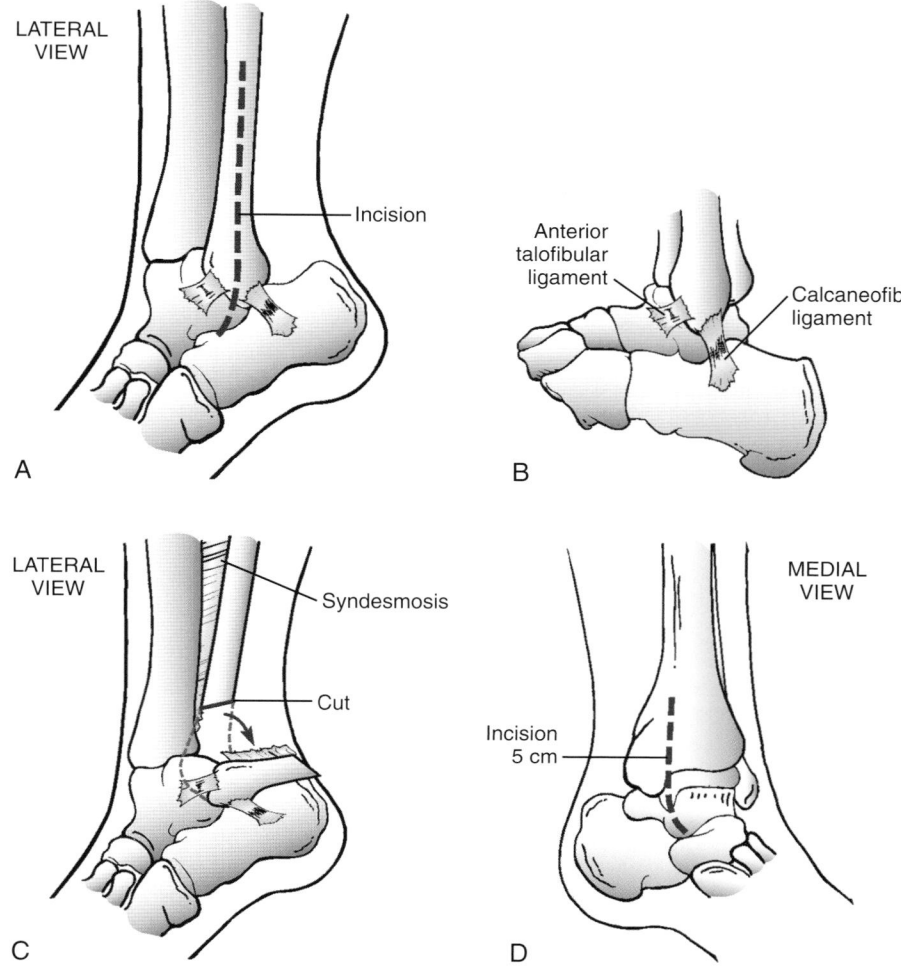

Figure 22-10 Lateral approach to the ankle. **A,** A midline incision of the fibula of about 20 cm is used. **B,** The anterior talofibular ligament is identified and transected for the exposure. **C,** An oblique osteotomy of the distal fibula ending 10 to 15 mm above the joint. **D,** A secondary medial approach over the medial gutter.

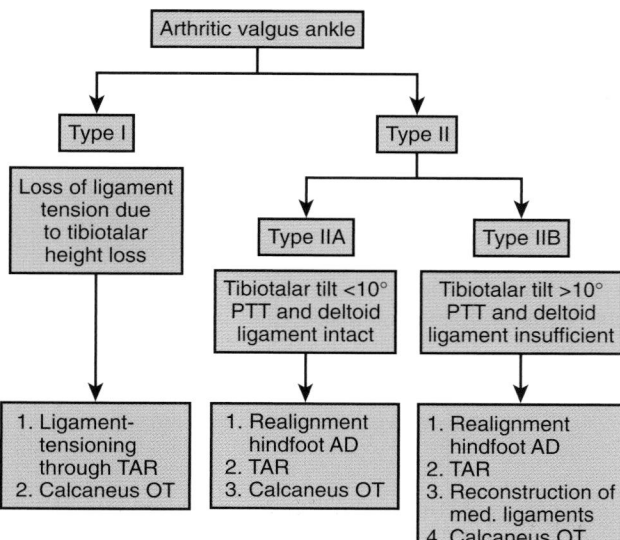

Figure 22-11 Treatment algorithm in patients with end-stage arthritic valgus ankle. *AD,* arthrodesis; *med.,* medial; *OT,* osteotomy; *PTT,* posterior tibial tendon; *TAR,* total ankle replacement.

- Corrective osteotomies of the calcaneus (Fig. 22-12): medial displacement calcaneal osteotomy[282,324] or lateral column lengthening osteotomy of the calcaneus (especially in patients with an abductus deformity of the midfoot and forefoot)[37,159,257,299]
- Reconstruction and repair of the medial ligaments[145,355]
- Corrective subtalar fusion, subtalar, and talonavicular fusion, or triple arthrodesis (Fig. 22-13)[78,196]

In patients with severe hindfoot valgus malalignment resulting from significant valgus deformity and defects of the tibial plafond, the authors suggest the following chronologic sequence of surgical procedures. First, the supramalleolar deformity should be corrected by supramalleolar osteotomy, followed by TAR as a one-stage procedure. In patients with a remaining valgus position of the heel, a calcaneal osteotomy or subtalar, subtalar and talonavicular, or triple arthrodesis (especially in patients with degenerative changes of the involved joint[s]) should be performed. Finally, ligamentous instability should be addressed by reconstruction and repair of the ligaments.

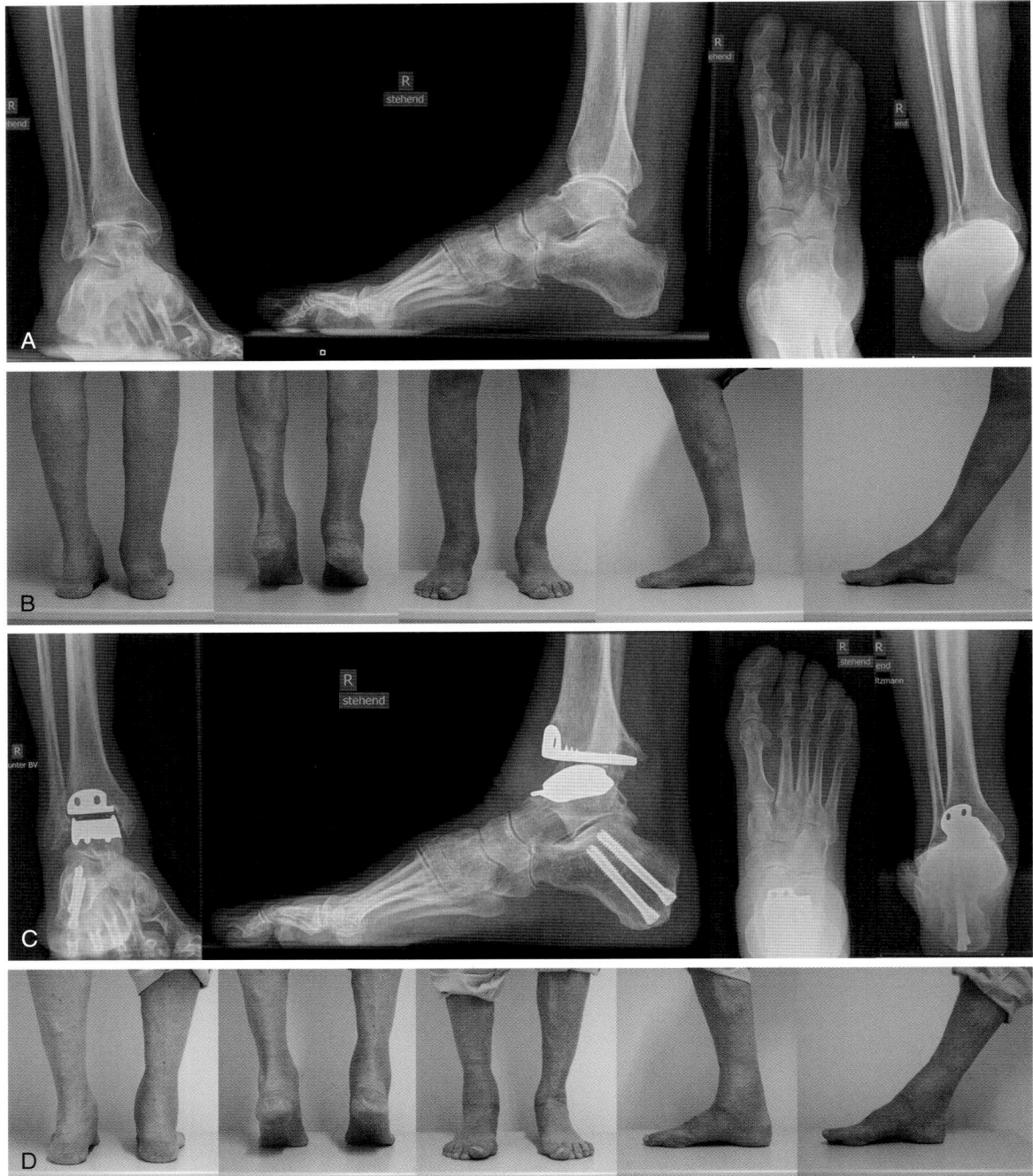

Figure 22-12 **A,** Preoperative radiographs, including hindfoot alignment view, show valgus osteoarthritic ankle with substantial valgus tilting of the talus within the mortise and valgus position of the hindfoot in a 62-year-old male. **B,** Clinical photographs show valgus malalignment of the hindfoot with only slight varization tendency of the heel at tiptoeing. **C,** Postoperative radiographs show proper position and osseous integration of both prosthetic components and osseous union of medial displacement calcaneal osteotomy at the follow-up of 4 years. Hindfoot alignment view shows well-aligned hindfoot. **D,** Clinically, nearly neutral alignment of the hindfoot is observed. (Images courtesy Beat Hintermann, MD, Liestal, Switzerland.)

In patients with severe hindfoot valgus resulting from pes planovalgus deformity with insufficiency of the medial ligaments and/or posterior tibial tendon, the authors first suggest corrective calcaneal osteotomy and/or an arthrodesis (subtalar, subtalar and talonavicular, or triple arthrodesis) before implantation of prosthesis components. At the end of the ankle replacement surgery, ligamentous reconstruction and a fibula lengthening through an osteotomy should be performed if necessary.

In patients with moderate hindfoot valgus, the authors first implant prosthesis components and then address the

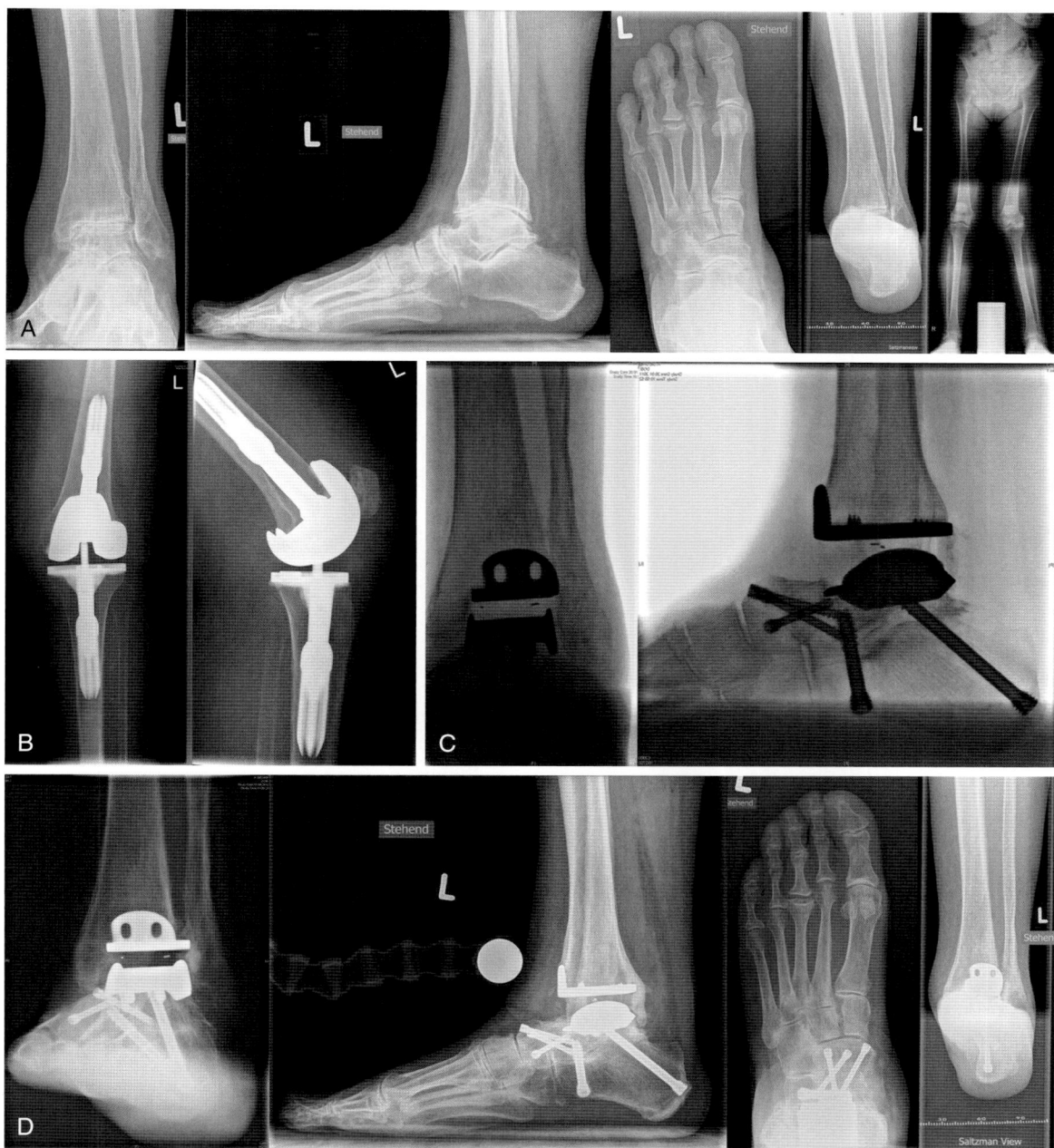

Figure 22-13 A, Preoperative radiographs, including hindfoot alignment view, show valgus osteoarthritic ankle with valgus malalignment of the hindfoot. The whole-leg radiograph additionally shows knee osteoarthritis with valgus axis. **B,** Therefore the first total knee replacement was performed. **C,** Three months later, a total ankle replacement and subtalar and talonavicular arthrodesis were performed as a one-stage procedure. **D,** Postoperative radiographs show proper position of prosthesis component with normal alignment of the hindfoot at the follow-up of 3.5 years. (Images courtesy Victor Valderrabano, MD, PhD, Basel, Switzerland.)

inframalleolar valgus malalignment by one or several of the procedures described immediately above.

Total Ankle Replacement in the Varus Osteoarthritis Ankle

The main treatment principles in patients with varus osteoarthritic ankles are the same as in patients with valgus osteoarthritic ankles: as long the varus deformity can be corrected by realignment surgeries, TAR is not contraindicated in this patient cohort.

Morphologic Types of the Varus Osteoarthritic Ankle

Two distinct morphologic types of the varus osteoarthritic ankles are described.[190] In patients with type I varus

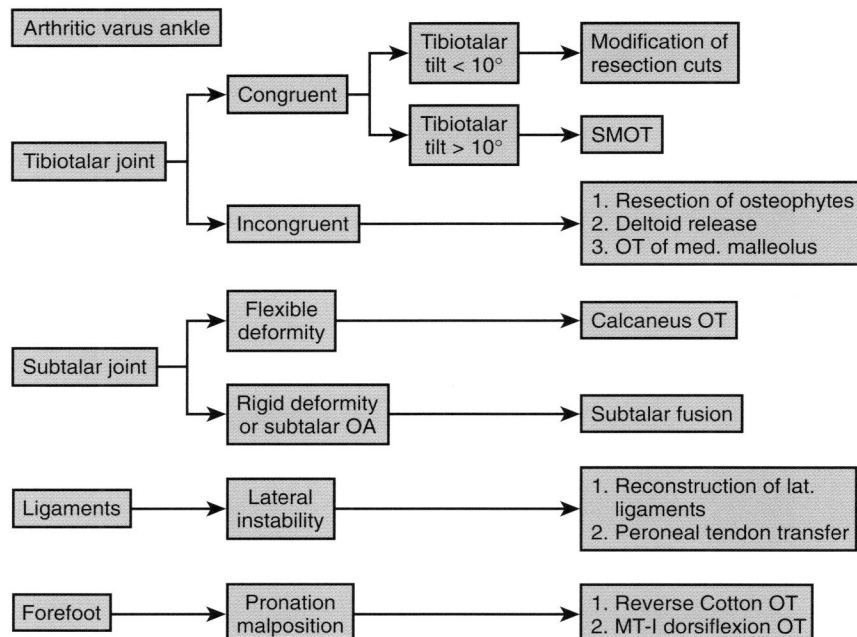

Figure 22-14 Treatment algorithm in patients with end-stage arthritic varus ankle. *lat.,* lateral; *med.,* medial; *MT,* metatarsal; *OA,* osteoarthritis; *OT,* osteotomy; *SMOT,* supramalleolar osteotomy.

deformity, there is no incongruency of the tibiotalar joint, with no talar tilting. The varus deformity is localized in the distal tibia. In type II varus deformity, substantial talar tilting within the ankle mortise is observed.[190]

Surgical Technique of Total Ankle Replacement in the Varus Osteoarthritic Ankle

A standardized surgical technique is used for implantation of the prosthesis components. The general treatment algorithm is shown in Figure 22-14. There are different methods to address the contracted medial ligaments often observed in patients with varus deformity. First, resection of osteophytes on the medial side may resolve the contraction. Second, Bonnin et al[41] suggest a complete subperiosteal release of deltoid ligament. The lengthening osteotomy of the medial malleolus, as described by Doets et al,[90] may also improve ligamentous balancing of the ankle (Fig. 22-15). In patients with a "congruent" tibiotalar joint with slight varus, the deformity can be corrected intraoperatively by adjusting the bone cuts during the preparation of implantation surfaces. In patients with inframalleolar varus deformity, a calcaneal osteotomy (e.g., Dwyer osteotomy[19,91,367] or Z-shaped osteotomy[191]) should be performed to realign the hindfoot. In patients with significant lateral instability, reconstruction of lateral ligaments should be performed: in some cases, other transfers can be considered, such as a peroneus longus to brevis tendon transfer.[182]

CLASSIFICATION OF TOTAL ANKLE REPLACEMENT

The authors suggest a classification of TAR with consideration of the following factors:

- Surgical approach (anterior, medial, lateral, posterior)
- Bearing type (fixed, mobile bearing)
- Articulation resurfaced (superior, medial, lateral)
- External surface (hydroxyapatite, beaded, porous metal)
- Bearing surface (ceramic, ultra-high-molecular-weight polyethylene [UHMWPE], highly cross-linked UHMWPE)
- Sulcus type (none vs. normal vs. deep)
- Surface morphology (cylindric, conical, ellipsoid, spheroid)

Clinical Results after Total Ankle Replacement

Agility Ankle Prosthesis

The Agility prosthesis was the first of a new generation of ankle prostheses, being designed with ingrowth for fixation. It was designed by Dr. Frank Alvine and has been used since 1984 (Fig. 22-16).[6]

For almost two decades, the Agility prosthesis was the most widely used ankle prosthesis in the United States, and with more than 20 years of implantations, it has the longest follow-up of any fixed-bearing total ankle prosthesis.[59] The Agility ankle prosthesis is a semiconstrained, two-component prosthesis consisting of a titanium tibial and cobalt-chromium talar component (Fig. 22-17). For improved osseous integration, both components have a sintered titanium bead surface. Because this prosthesis is a two-component system, a modular polyethylene insert is locked into the tibial component. The surgical technique of Agility prosthesis implantation includes an arthrodesis of the tibiofibular syndesmosis performed by using screws or fibular plating.[175] The arthrodesis of the tibiofibular syndesmosis is thought to balance the load

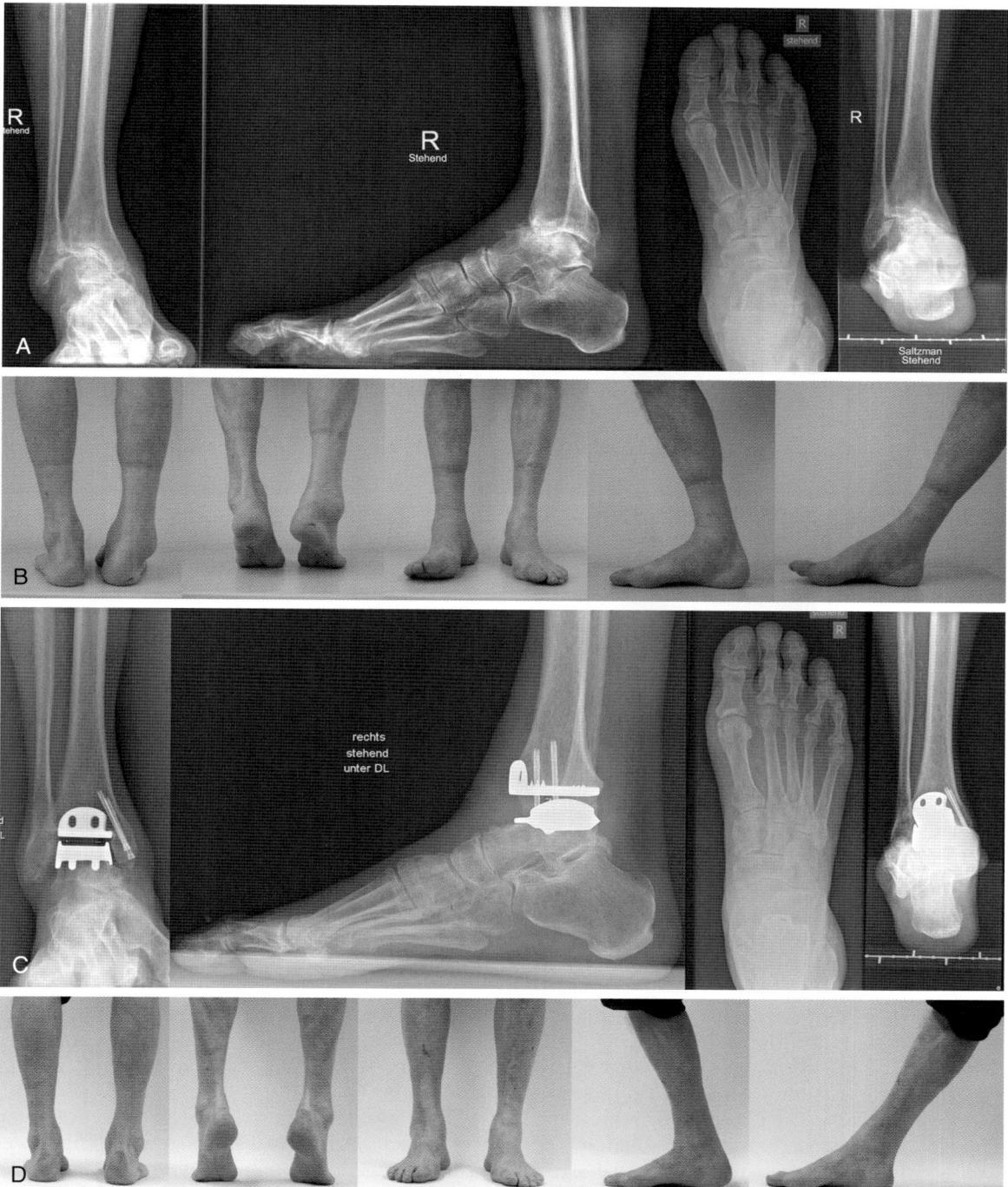

Figure 22-15 **A,** Preoperative radiographs, including hindfoot alignment, show severe varus osteoarthritic ankle with severe varus tilting of the talus in a 64-year-old male. **B,** Clinical photographs correspond with radiographs and show varus malalignment of the hindfoot. **C,** Corrective osteotomy of the medial malleolus was performed to restore the anatomic ankle mortise. Then total ankle replacement was performed using a three-component ankle prosthesis. Postoperative radiographs show neutrally aligned replaced ankle and good osseous integration of both prosthetic components at the follow-up of 3.5 years. **D,** Clinically, neutrally aligned hindfoot is observed. (Images courtesy Beat Hintermann, MD, Liestal, Switzerland.)

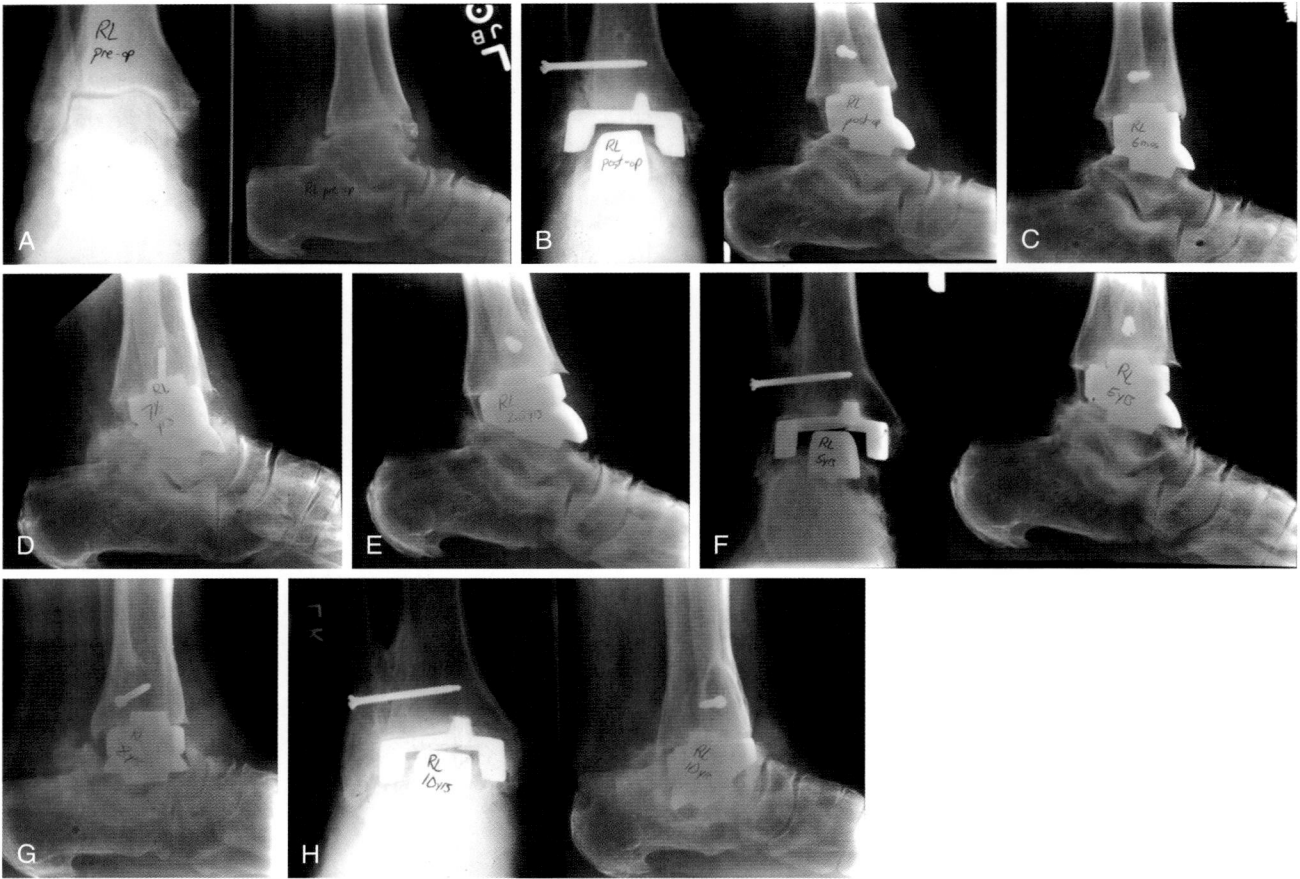

Figure 22-16 **A,** Preoperative radiographs showing end-stage ankle osteoarthritis. **B,** Agility prosthesis with thin tibial plate was implanted in 1980s. Postoperative radiographs at the follow-up of 6 months **(C)**, 1.5 years **(D)**, 2.5 years **(E)**, 5 years **(F)**, 8 years **(G)**, and 10 years **(H)**.

transfer between fibula and tibia, while fibula physiologically transfers only up to 17% of body weight.[308,328,362]

Pyevich et al[271] independently reviewed the first 100 Agility arthroplasties performed by the designer between 1984 and 1993 (Fig. 22-18). Eighty-six implants were available for a mean follow-up of 4.8 years. Only five prostheses had to be revised. It was shown, that delayed union (28 ankles) or nonunion (9 ankles) of the tibiofibular syndesmosis was associated with migration of and circumferential radiolucency around the tibial component. Postoperatively, most patients experienced significant pain relief and were satisfied with obtained results.[271] The same 100 ankle arthroplasties and an additional 32 ankle arthroplasties were included into the study by Knecht et al,[189] with a mean follow-up of 9 years. Fourteen patients had to undergo a conversion procedure to ankle fusion. More than 90% of followed patients were satisfied with their arthroplasty results. However, in 89 of 117 ankles, some radiolucency around prosthesis components was seen, confirming the previous findings that arthrodesis of tibiofibular syndesmosis impacts the clinical and radiographic outcome of this prosthesis type (Fig. 22-19).[271] Furthermore, the authors found that

progressive degenerative changes in adjacent joints occurred in less than 25% of all patients. This is approximately half of that expected (and reported) for patients with ankle arthrodesis and similar follow-up.[64,108] These findings support the claim that TAR may preserve the range of motion of the ankle and prevent development of degenerative changes in the hindfoot and midfoot joints.

Lagaay and Schuberth[213] analyzed range of motion and functional outcome in 124 patients who underwent TAR using the Agility prosthesis between 2000 and 2006. Fluoroscopy was used to measure ankle kinematics at 3, 6, and 12 months. In this study, the amount of postoperative range of motion did not correlate with patient satisfaction.[213] Kopp et al[207] reported similar results in their retrospective study, including 41 patients who underwent 43 total ankle arthroplasties using the Agility prosthesis. At a mean follow-up of 44.5 months, all patients experienced significant pain relief, and 97% were very satisfied with the surgical results and stated that they wound undergo this surgery again. In 29 ankles, radiolucency was observed, with migration or subsidence of components noted in 18 ankles. No remarkable progression of degenerative changes in adjacent joints was observed radiographically. This finding is comparable to other aforementioned studies.[189,271] To avoid the loosening of prosthesis components, the authors suggested the use of fibular plating for tibiofibular syndesmosis as described by Jung et al[175] and the routine use of the revision talar component.[207] Hurowitz et al[168] showed that the use of a prosthesis larger than size 1 is a predictive factor for better outcome. Hurowitz et al[168] further found that, among 65 studied Agility arthroplasties, patients with rheumatoid osteoarthritis had a significantly lower rate of prosthesis failure.[168] In addition to prosthesis loosening and nonunion or delayed union of tibiofibular arthrodesis, surgeons should be aware of the following complications when using the Agility prosthesis: delayed wound healing, wound infection, painful hardware, iatrogenic malleolar fracture, and neurovascular injuries.[63] Also, fracture of the polyethylene component may occur because of improper component placement and failure to correct hindfoot deformity, which induces tilt of the talar component.[11] Vaupel et al[359] performed a macroscopic and microscopic study on 10 retrieved Agility prostheses. All prosthesis components showed extensive damage, especially the polyethylene liner of the tibial component. Edge loading of the polyethylene may increase contact stresses and pathologically increase wear. This wear debris may ultimately progress to component loosening and ankle replacement failure.[359]

In 2007, the Agility LP Total Ankle System was introduced with some modification of its design.[59] All improvements were stated to have been designed after careful analysis of previously published data, to improve the outcome and to avoid the midterm and long-term complications. The new prosthesis features include a redesigned broad-based talar component (this should avoid the subsidence of the tibial component, especially in patients with nonunion of tibiofibular syndesmosis), the ability to mix and match component sizes, and a front-loading polyethylene insert (easier surgical technique for exchange of the insert).[59] Myerson and Won[245] presented their surgical technique of primary and revision TAR using custom-designed prostheses based on the Agility LP design. Their modifications to the Agility LP design included stems of the talar and tibial components that were made using standardized anteroposterior and lateral views.[245] Ketz et al[180] retrospectively reviewed data of 32

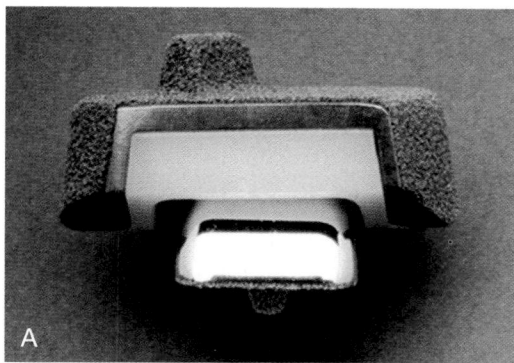

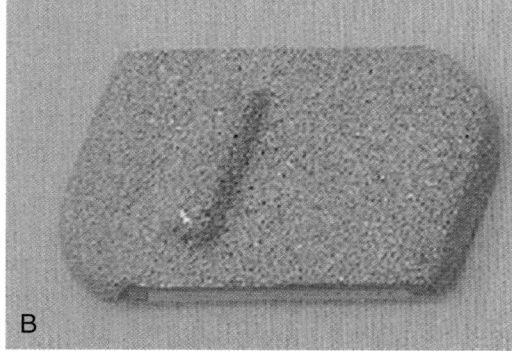

Figure 22-17 **A,** Agility prosthesis is a semiconstrained, two-component prosthesis. **B,** Superior view of the tibial component showing porous coating.

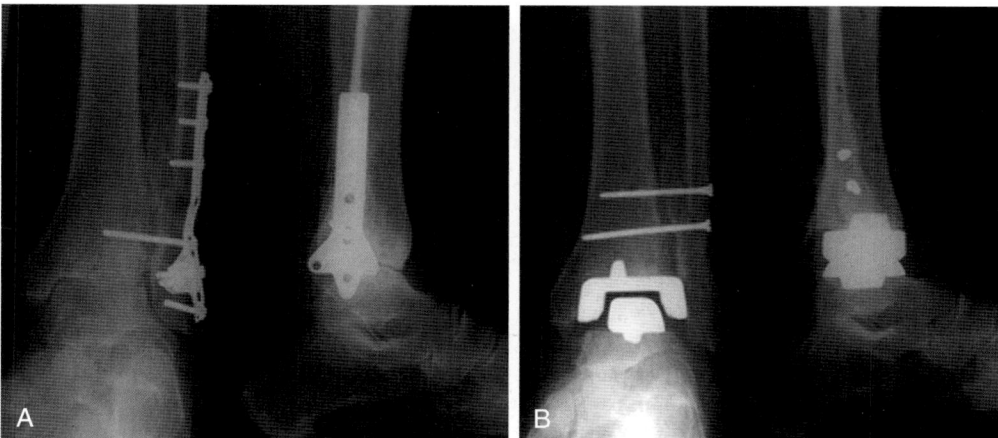

Figure 22-18 **A,** Preoperative radiographs of a 61-year-old male suffering from posttraumatic ankle osteoarthritis. **B,** Postoperative radiographs show proper position and osseous integration of both prosthetic components at a follow-up of 4 years.

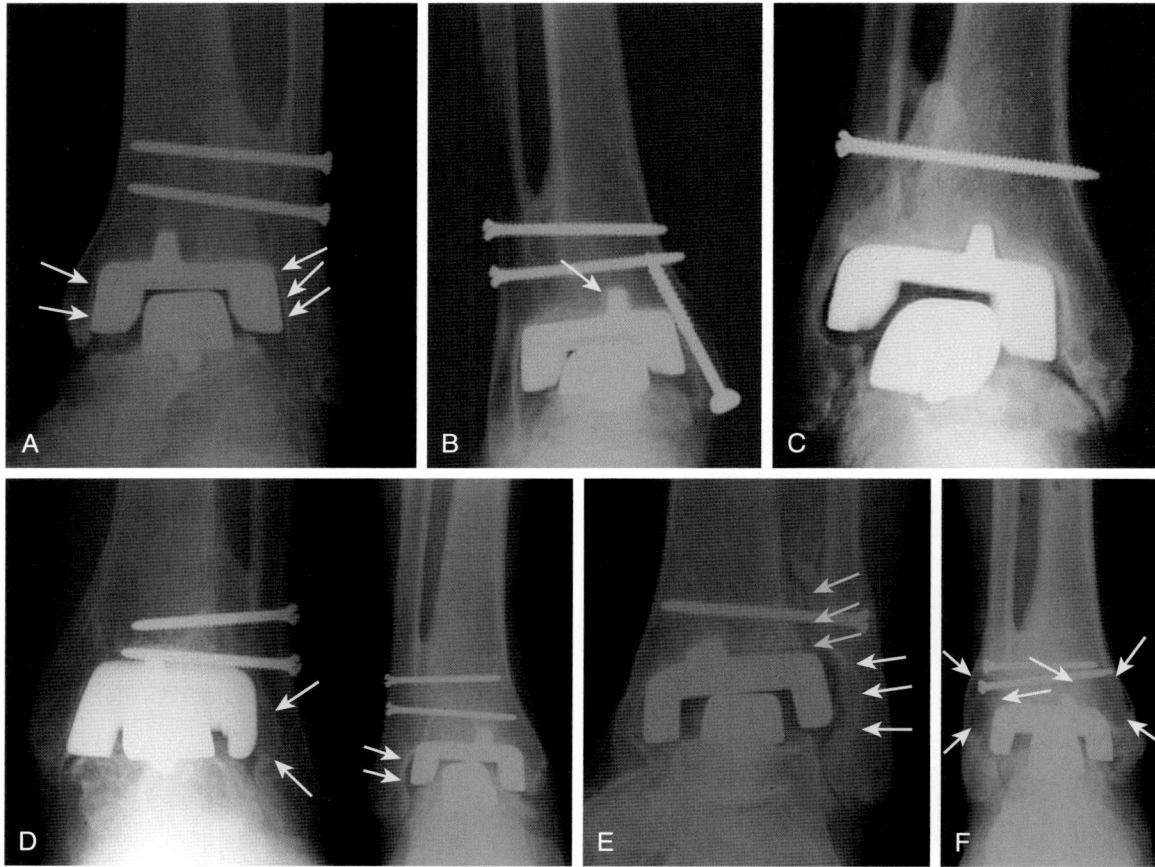

Figure 22-19 Radiolucency problems in Agility total ankle replacement. In all figures *arrows* indicate periprosthetic radiolucency. **A,** Incomplete lucency. **B,** Lucency at tibial keel. **C,** Circumferential lucency. **D,** Syndesmosis union with stable mechanical lysis. **E,** Syndesmosis nonunion with progressive lysis. **F,** Expansile lysis.

patients who underwent 33 complex and/or revision total ankle arthroplasties using a custom Agility long-stemmed talar prosthesis. All patients were available for the mean follow-up of 4.9 years. A significant functional improvement was observed, including increased range of motion and AOFAS hindfoot score. Three patients had subsequent failure of the stemmed talar prosthesis, which was treated by removal of the prosthesis and ankle arthrodesis by using an intramedullary device and a femoral head allograft.[180]

In conclusion, the Agility prosthesis is the most widely used ankle prosthesis in the United States and has the longest follow-up data available for any fixed-bearing device.[59,127,278] Since its introduction in the late 1970s, the prosthesis design has undergone several design modifications and is now available as the Agility LP Total Ankle System.[59] Published results in patients receiving the Agility TAR are consistently good and encouraging with regard to functional outcome, patient satisfaction, and implant survivorship.

Buechel-Pappas Ankle Prosthesis

As already mentioned, the first generation of the New Jersey ankle prosthesis had discouraging results.[261] This led to development of the Buechel-Pappas ankle prosthesis, which was the first reported three-component prosthesis with a mobile bearing (Fig. 22-20).[360]

In the first Buechel-Pappas design (Mark I), the anterior–posterior constraint between the tibial and mobile-bearing components has been removed. This so-called shallow sulcus design allowed more range of motion without compromising the intrinsic sagittal stability of replaced ankle. In 1988, Buechel et al[52] presented their initial results of 23 cementless ankle arthroplasties performed in 21 patients between 1981 and 1984. All patients were reviewed at a mean follow-up of 2.9 years. Postoperative complications included delayed wound healing in 4 ankles, reflex sympathetic dystrophy in 2 ankles, deep infection in 1 ankle, and 1 case of mobile-bearing subluxation. No revision surgeries regarding exchange or removal of metallic prosthesis components were necessary at the latest follow-up.[52] The same patient cohort was included in a later study with a total of 40 ankle arthroplasties performed between 1981 and 1988.[51] The mean follow-up in this patient group was 12 years. Overall clinical results were 28 ankles (70%) good to excellent, 2 ankles (5%) fair, and 10 ankles (25%) poor. The mean postoperative range of motion of replaced

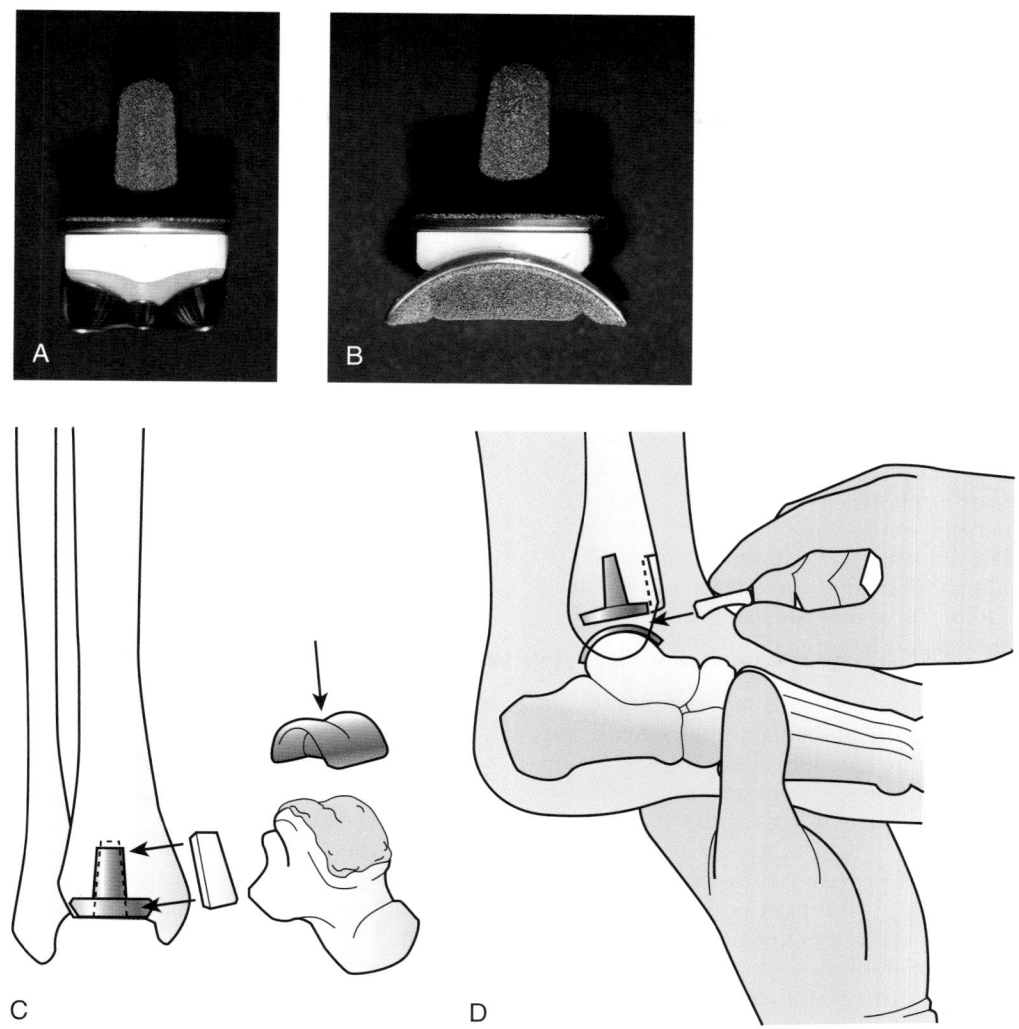

Figure 22-20 Anterior **(A)** and lateral **(B)** views of the Buechel-Pappas deep sulcus, meniscal-bearing total ankle prosthesis. **C,** Surgical technique of prosthesis implantation includes creation of an anterior tibial window by using a special window osteotome *(left)* and talar preparation *(right).* **D,** Manual insertion of meniscal bearing.

ankles was 25 degrees. The following complications were observed: delayed wound healing (9 ankles), talar component subsidence (6 ankles), bearing subluxation (4 ankles), severe bearing wear (5 ankles), malleolar fracture (3 ankles), and osteolysis (4 ankles). The 20-year overall survivorship was 74.2%.[51]

Analysis of complications from using this prosthesis design led to modifications resulting in the Mark II Buechel-Pappas prosthesis. This new design (also known as the deep sulcus design) included two fins, a thicker meniscal component, and deeper sulcus with a gap in the plastic. This modified prosthesis was used in a second patient group consisting of 75 ankle arthroplasties performed between 1991 and 2000, with a mean follow-up of 5 years.[51] The overall clinical results after 2 to 12 years were 66 ankles (88%) good to excellent, 4 ankles (5%) fair, and 5 (7%) poor. The mean postoperative range of motion was 29 degrees. The following complications with

the Mark II were observed: delayed wound healing (11 ankles), talar component subsidence (3 ankles), severe bearing wear (3 ankles), malleolar fracture (6 ankles), and osteolysis (10 ankles). Because of improved design, the rate of talar component subsidence was been significantly reduced. Also, previously observed problems with mobile-bearing wear did not occur. The 12-year overall survivorship was 92%.[51] Based on these results, the authors advocated the use of the three-component prosthesis in properly selected patients.[49,51] Nelissen et al[249] performed a radiostereometric analysis in 15 patients who underwent Buechel-Pappas ankle replacement. The authors addressed the early migration of the tibial component by using a radiostereometric setup consisting of two synchronized roentgen tubes and a uniplanar calibration box. The component migration was 0.8 mm (lateral–medial), 0.9 mm (distal–proximal), and −0.5 mm (posterior–anterior). However, migration stabilized at

6 months postoperatively in all ankles.[249] Ali et al[5] implanted 35 Buechel-Pappas ankle arthroplasties between 1990 and 2005. Thirty-four ankles have been reviewed at a mean follow-up of 5 years. Postoperatively, all patients reported significant pain relief and functional improvement as assessed by the AOFAS score. One tibial component had to be revised. Examination of radiographs in the remaining patients demonstrated no evidence of significant subsidence or radiolucency. In one patient, avascular necrosis of talus was observed; however, this patient was asymptomatic. The overall 5-year survivorship was 97%. In conclusion, the authors achieved favorable midterm results comparable to data published by the designer.[5] Kurup and Taylor[211] reviewed all Buechel-Pappas implantations performed in the first 5 years of their use of this prosthesis. The study included 34 consecutive ankle arthroplasties performed between 1999 and 2004; all patients were reviewed at a mean follow-up of 2.8 years. Five patients had intraoperative malleolar fractures, including four medial and one lateral, which all healed uneventfully. Three patients had injury to cutaneous nerves. Three patients had superficial infection treated with antibiotics; however, no deep infection was observed in this patient cohort. Eight patients had significant pain on the medial side because of medial impingement; revision surgery was required in four cases. Most patients experienced significant pain relief and functional improvement, resulting in high patient satisfaction (90.5% very happy or satisfactory).[211]

San Giovanni et al[298] reviewed a consecutive series of 31 Buechel-Pappas ankle arthroplasties performed in 23 patients with rheumatoid osteoarthritis treated between 1990 and 1997. Intraoperatively, 10 medial malleolar fractures occurred (32%). Nine postoperative complications were detected: four wound healing problems, four stress fractures, and one medial malleolar nonunion after intraoperative fracture. Two implants failed and were converted to ankle fusion, resulting in 8-year survivorship of 93%. The remaining patients were evaluated clinically and radiographically at a mean follow-up of 8.3 years. Most patients experienced substantial pain relief and functional improvement with a high satisfaction rate of 89%.[298]

Bourke and Gomez[43] reviewed CT scans and conventional radiographs of 55 consecutive patients (57 ankles) who underwent TAR using the Buechel-Pappas prosthesis between 2001 and 2010. The mean follow-up of radiographic assessment was 5 years, with a range of 18 months to 10 years. A 10-zone classification system (previously used by Besse et al[33] for conventional radiograph evaluation) was adapted for evaluation of CT scans. The majority of patients (98%) had some form of osteolysis, with 77% of patients having tibial and 80% talar lesions (Fig. 22-21). The observed talar lesions were larger than on the tibial side. The vast majority of these lesions were progressive; however, rates of progression were highly variable. Early and progressive periprosthetic osteolysis was a commonly observed in this patient cohort. CT scans have been shown to be more sensitive at detection and more accurate in quantification of such lesions. *Therefore the authors suggest that CT scanning of replaced ankles should be a routine part of the postoperative surveillance for osteolysis, loosening, and subsidence.*[43] Similar findings were observed in the study by Hanna et al.[131] Seventeen patients with 19 replaced ankles were included in this study to compare helical CT scan with conventional radiography for evaluation of periprosthetic lucency. Of the 19 ankles, a total of 29 lesions were detected by CT scanning, whereas conventional radiographs detected 18 lesions.[131]

Dhawan et al[87] retrospectively reviewed functional outcome and survivorship of prosthesis components in 29 patients with 30 Buechel-Pappas implants, with a follow-up of up to 13 years (Fig. 22-22). In three patients, revision surgeries, including two revision arthroplasties and one ankle arthrodesis were performed because of malpositioned talar components, resulting in a 5-year survivorship rate of 87.6%.[87]

The most recent follow-up study performed in patients with the Buechel-Pappas prosthesis found 12- and 20-year survivorship rates of 92% and 74.2%, respectively.[51] The Buechel-Pappas prosthesis is one of the most successful TAR prostheses reported in the literature; however, it, like most other mobile-bearing ankle designs, is not currently available in U.S. market.

Scandinavian Total Ankle Replacement (STAR) (Video Clip 16)

The STAR was developed by Danish orthopaedic surgeon Hakon Kofoed in 1978 as a two-component, anatomic, unconstrained, resurfacing ankle prosthesis with congruent parts covering the medial and lateral facet joints.[199] The first-generation design with cement fixation was used in 28 patients, with 12-year survivorship of 70% published by the designer.[198] Since 1986, the tibial part of the STAR prosthesis has included a polyethylene component (Fig. 22-23).[199] This modification was introduced to minimize rotational stress at the implant–bone interface.

A prospective study by Kofoed and Sørensen[201] addressed the survivorship differences between STAR patients with painful osteoarthritis and rheumatoid osteoarthritis. Fifty-two patients underwent cemented STAR between 1981 and 1989. The survivorship analysis of the two groups showed no significant differences, with 14-year survivorship of 72.7% for painful osteoarthritis and 75.5% for rheumatoid osteoarthritis.[201] In 1990, an additional modification was introduced—a bioactive surface for uncemented fixation technique.[199] The current design of the STAR prosthesis is a congruent, cylindric, three-component prosthesis. Initial osseous integration of the prosthesis is secured by a single fin on the talar side and by two cylindric fins on the tibial side. As already mentioned, both metallic components have hydroxyapatite-coated surfaces. The surgical technique of uncemented STAR prosthesis (Fig. 22-24) has been described in detail by Anderson et al.[9]

The designer performed a short-term clinical study addressing the biologic fixation of the STAR prosthesis,

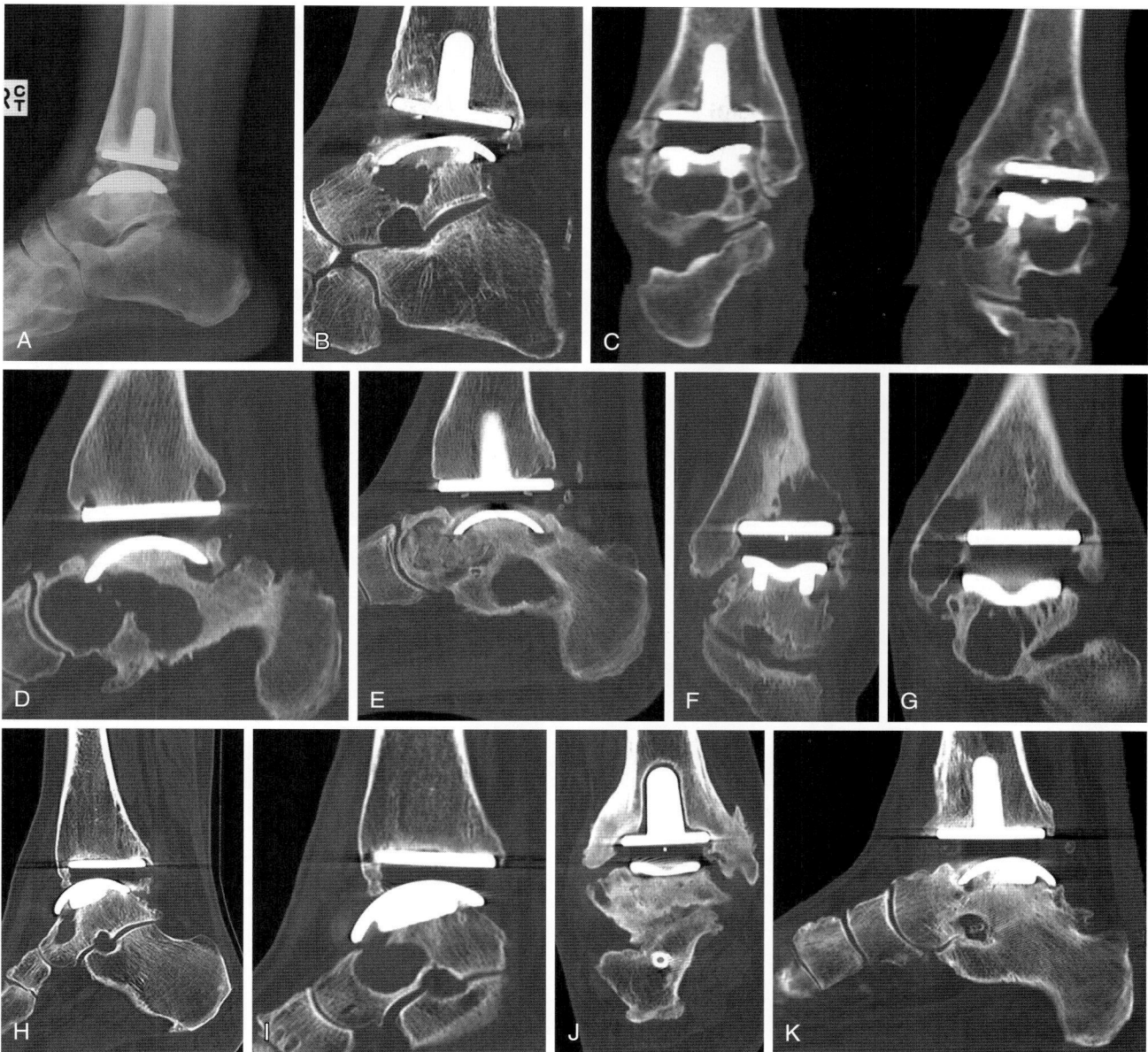

Figure 22-21 Lateral radiograph **(A)** and computed tomography (CT) scan **(B)** of a 58-year-old male with asymptomatic talar cyst. **C,** CT scan of a 61-year-old female who underwent total ankle replacement because of rheumatoid arthritis with large cystic lesion underneath both talar components. **D,** CT scan of a 42-year-old male with asymptomatic large cyst on the talar side. **E,** Bone grafting was performed to prevent the prosthesis component from collapsing. **F,** CT scan of a 52-year-old male with pain caused by fracture through a tibial cyst. Bone grafting resolved the pain immediately. **G,** A 56-year-old male with large cysts on both the tibial and talar sides. **H** and **I,** An asymptomatic 53-year-old female with substantial progression of talar cystic lesion within 3 years. CT scans showing aseptic loosening of both prosthesis components **(J)** and talar subsidence **(K)** in a 63-year-old male and a 55-year-old female, respectively. In all cases, the Buechel-Pappas prosthesis was used. (Images courtesy Gerard Bourke, MD, Melbourne, Victoria, Australia.)

with 20 ankle arthroplasties in 18 consecutive patients between 1990 and 1993.[200] At the latest follow-up, 17 patients reported excellent, 1 patient good, and 2 patients unacceptable clinical results. One ankle was revised before the 1-year follow-up for component subsidence requiring a change of the meniscal bearing.[200] The same author performed a comparative study addressing results

in patients who underwent STAR implantation with and without cement fixation.[199] The study cohort included 33 patients who had surgery between 1986 and 1989 (with cement fixation) and 25 similar patients who were treated with uncemented STAR between 1990 and 1995. The mean follow-up was 9.4 years, with a range of up to 12 years. The 12-year survivorship in the first group was 70%

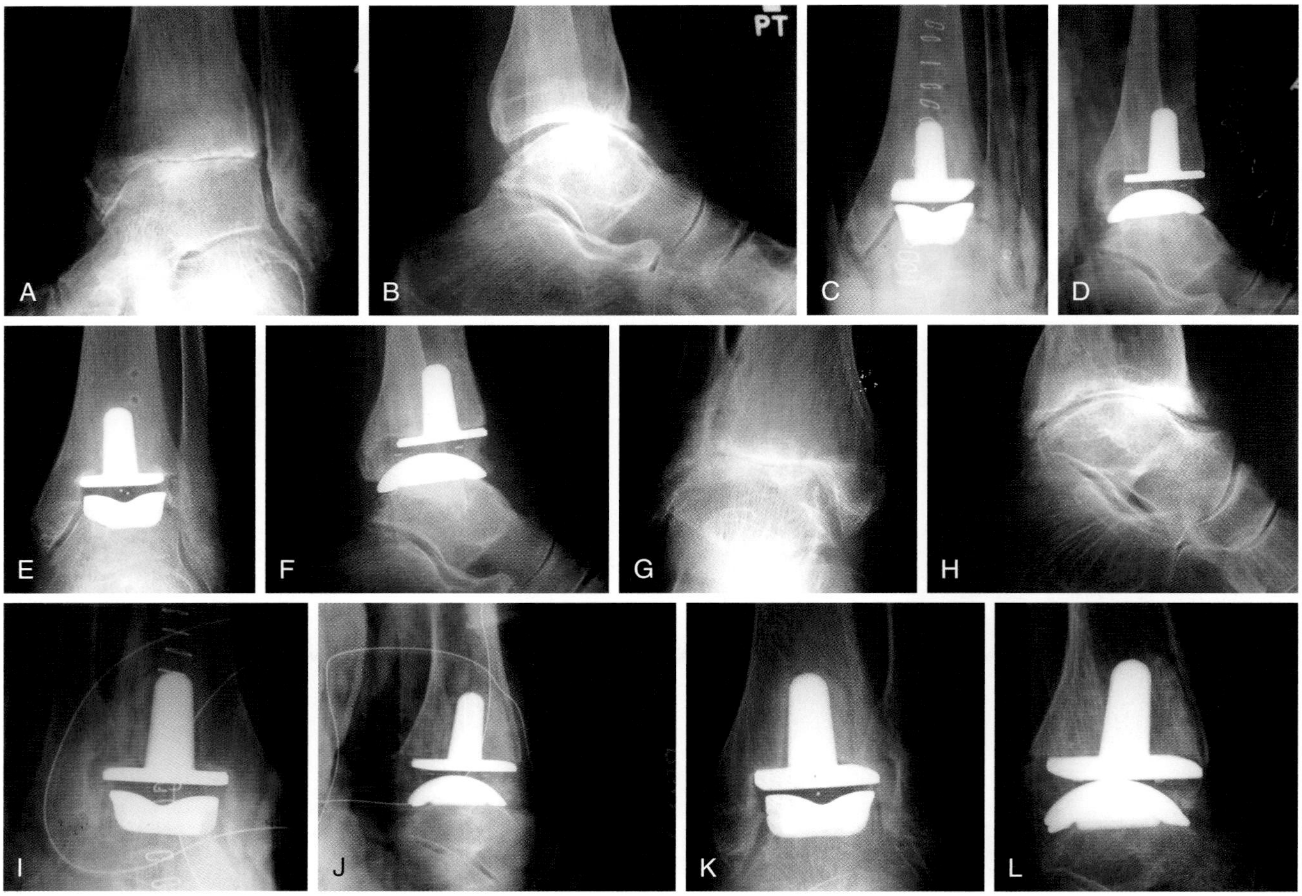

Figure 22-22 Preoperative anteroposterior **(A)** and lateral **(B)** radiographs of a 62-year-old female suffering from primary osteoarthritis. **C** and **D,** Regular Buechel-Pappas prosthesis has been used. Postoperative anteroposterior **(E)** and lateral **(F)** radiographs show some anterior radiolucency around the tibial component at a follow-up of 4 years. Preoperative anteroposterior **(G)** and lateral **(H)** radiographs of a 68-year-old male suffering from secondary osteoarthritis. **I** and **J,** Regular Buechel-Pappas prosthesis has been used. Postoperative anteroposterior **(K)** and lateral **(L)** radiographs show appropriate position of tibial and talar components at a follow-up of 11 years. (Images courtesy Ramesh K. Nayak, FRCS, Lincoln, United Kingdom.)

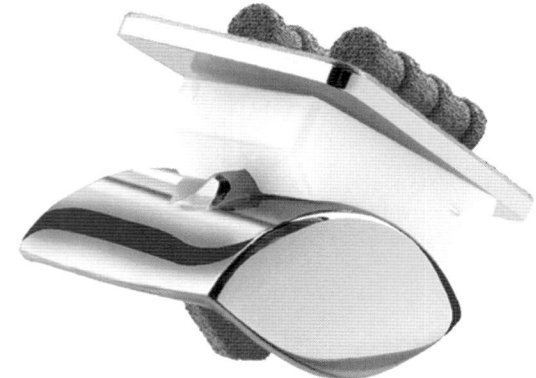

Figure 22-23 Scandinavian Total Ankle Replacement (STAR)—a three-component total ankle system.

(95% CI, 60.3%-78.5%) and in the second group 95.4% (95% CI, 91.0%-99.9%). Therefore the author suggested that modern unconstrained meniscal-bearing prostheses should be fixed without cement.[199] Garde and Kofoed[111] addressed the in vivo stability of prosthesis components in 8 consecutive patients who were treated with unilateral uncemented STAR prostheses between 1990 and 1992. In this study, stabilometry in the standing phase was assessed as a one-legged balance test, with and without shoes, and with open and closed eyes. A force plate was used to register the area used to keep balance, the length and direction of the corrective movements, and their velocity. All results were compared with those obtained from the contralateral ankle free of degenerative changes. The only significant difference detected was between velocities of corrective movements, demonstrating the biomechanical stability of the replaced ankle.[111]

The STAR prosthesis is one of the most popular in Europe and is also one of the few total ankle designs

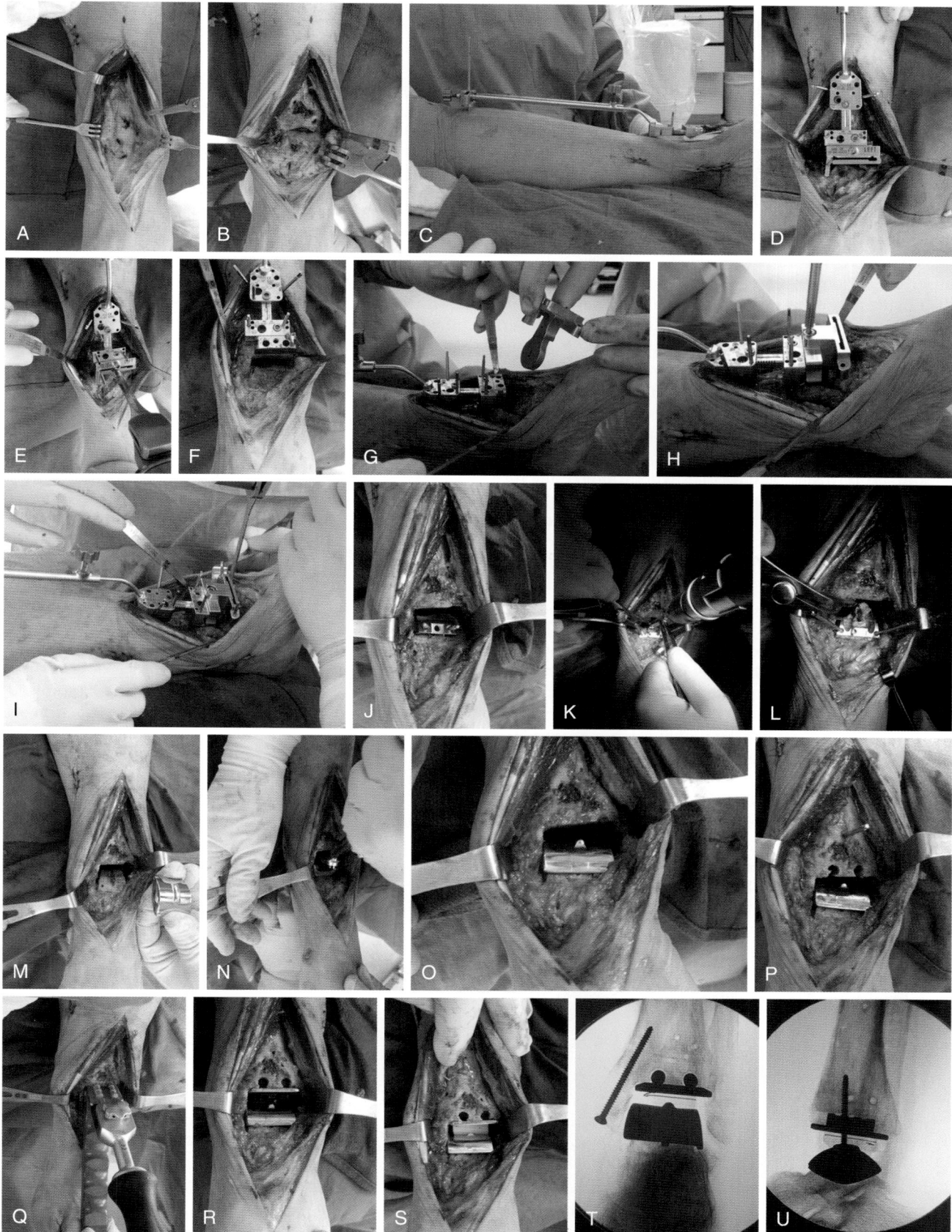

Figure 22-24 **A,** The anterior surgical approach is used. **B,** The ankle joint is exposed. The osteophytes on the anterior aspect of the tibia and the talar neck are to be removed. **C,** The guide is centered at the tuberosity of the tibia and the center of the ankle joint. **D,** The adjustable cutting block is applied in the correct position and tibial cut **(E** and **F)** is performed. **G** and **H,** Talar cutting block is applied in the correct position and horizontal talar cut **(I)** is performed. **J,** Separate guide block is applied and fixed to the top of the talus for removal of the medial and lateral sides of the talar body. **K** and **L,** The groove for anchoring the keel of the talar component is prepared with a drill. **M-O,** First, the talar component is positioned in press-fit technique. **P-R,** Then, the tibial component is positioned. **S,** Finally, an inlay is inserted between both metallic components. **T** and **U,** Final fluoroscopic check shows appropriate position of prosthesis components.

where the efficacy and safety have been shown in studies not reported by only the designer. Goldberg et al[118] reported that the STAR is the second most commonly used prosthesis in United Kingdom, after the Mobility prosthesis. Hintermann[144] reported the short-term and midterm results of 50 STAR implantations between 1996 and 1999 in 47 consecutive patients. Forty-eight ankles were reviewed and showed mostly satisfactory clinical outcomes. No prosthesis loosening or subsidence was observed, although in 1 patient, a 12-degree dorsal tilt of the tibial component occurred.[144] The same patients were included in a clinical observational study with a mean follow-up of 3.7 years (range, 2.4-6.2 years).[342] Altogether, 74 ankle arthroplasties in 71 patients were reviewed, with 54% of them being found completely painfree. Most patients showed significant functional improvement as assessed by the AOFAS score. In 3 patients, a ballooning bone lysis was observed around the tibial component. Despite prophylaxis, periarticular hypertrophic bone formation occurred in 43 ankles associated with decreased ROM. A significant tilting of the tibial component (at least 5.1 degrees) was seen in 9 ankles. Nine patients had to undergo revision surgery because of problems with prosthesis components.[342]

Brunner et al[46] reported long-term, 11 to 15 years, survivorship analysis in 72 consecutive patients (Fig. 22-25). The long-term survivorship rate of prosthesis components was substantially lower than that reported in the previous study at short-term to midterm.[342] The probability of implant survivorship was 70.7% and 45.6% at 10 and 14 years, respectively, with the following main reasons for revision: aseptic loosening, subsidence of the talar component, and progressive cyst formation. Furthermore, polyethylene insert fractures were observed in 11 ankles.[46] The STAR prosthesis was used for the first time in the United Kingdom in 1993 at Wrightington Hospital and since then has been used very frequently.[370] Wood and Deakin[373] reported the largest series—200 consecutive STAR prostheses performed between 1993 and 2000. All patients were reviewed at a mean follow-up of 46 months. In 14 patients, prosthesis failures occurred, requiring ankle fusion or revision arthroplasty. The 5-year cumulative survivorship was 92.7% (95% CI, 86.6%-98.8%). Additional surgeries were necessary in 8 ankles to treat complications such as malleolus fracture, major delay of wound healing, edge loading of the bearing, or arthrofibrosis. Overall, patients presented with satisfactory results and experienced significant functional improvement.[373]

The same patient cohort has been reviewed by Wood et al[375] at a mean follow-up of 88 months with a minimum of 60 months. One-hundred forty-three patients were available for this clinical study. A total of 24 ankles had been revised, 20 by ankle fusion and 4 by revision arthroplasty, resulting in 5- and 10-year survivorship of 93.3% (95% CI, 89.8%-96.8%) and 80.3% (95% CI, 71.0%-89.6%), respectively. Wood et al[372] addressed the clinical and radiologic outcome in patients who underwent TAR caused by rheumatoid ankle OA. The authors reviewed 211 ankle arthroplasties, including 171 STAR and 40 Buechel-Pappas implants used between 1993 and 2003. The results of 119 ankles were already published in the previous study.[373] In this study, 20 ankles failed, resulting in the 8-year cumulative survivorship of 88% (95% CI, 77%-99%). The authors found that 8-year cumulative survivorship in patients with preoperative normal ankle alignment was significantly higher (97%, 95% CI, 80%-100%).[372]

The same working group performed a randomized, controlled study of two mobile-bearing ankle designs, including 100 STAR prostheses and 100 Buechel-Pappas implants.[376] The minimum follow-up in both patient groups was 36 months. In both groups, a total of 16 ankles underwent revision surgery, of which 12 were in the Buechel-Pappas group and 4 in the STAR group. The 6-year survivorship rates in the Buechel-Pappas and STAR groups were 79% (95% CI, 63.4%-88.5%) and 95% (95% CI, 87.2%-98.1%), respectively. However, the survivorship difference did not reach statistical significance.

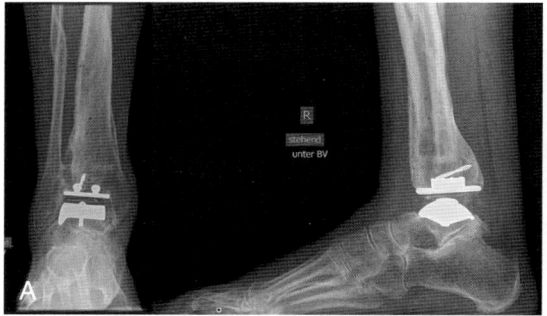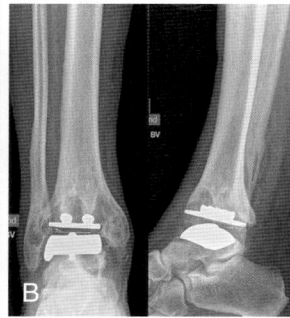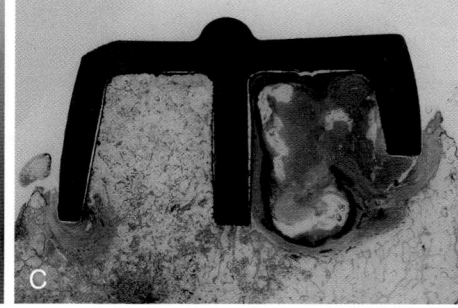

Figure 22-25 **A,** Postoperative radiographs of a 74-year-old male show proper position and osseous integration of Scandinavian Total Ankle Replacement (STAR) prosthesis at a follow-up of 12 years. **B,** Substantial loosening of both prosthesis components in a 61-year-old female at a follow-up of 5 years. **C,** Histologic examination (toluidine blue stain): cut through talar component's bone-prosthesis interface showing a large cyst beneath the talus and debonding of the single hydroxyapatite coating of the prosthesis. The 71-year-old female patient with primary instability osteoarthritis of the ankle joint died for a reason unrelated to the total ankle replacement 11 years after implantation. (Images courtesy Beat Hintermann, MD, Liestal, Switzerland.)

The authors again found that severe varus of valgus deformity significantly influences the midterm survivorship of the prosthesis.[376]

The initially published high survivorship of STAR prostheses was not confirmed in a study by Anderson et al.[8] In this study, 51 ankles were reviewed at a follow-up of 3 to 8 years. Twelve ankles had to undergo revision surgery (seven ankle fusions and five revision arthroplasties). The most common reasons for revision were loosening of at least one of the components or fracture of the meniscal bearing. Significant loosening was seen radiographically in an additional eight ankles.[8]

Murnaghan et al[241] reported their short-term experiences with the STAR prosthesis in 20 patients (22 ankles). Intraoperatively, 5 patients suffered malleolar fractures. At a mean follow-up of 26 months, 75% of all patients were painfree. Three patients required secondary surgery, with 2 of these requiring revisions of the prosthesis.[241] Christ and Hagena[61] reviewed complications and revision surgery rates in their patient cohort, including 147 STAR implants in 144 patients treated between 1997 and 2003. Intraoperatively, four malleolar fractures and one talar fissure occurred. The authors observed a high rate of wound healing problems (31 ankles), with deep infection in three cases. Also, the medial impingement was seen in four cases.[61]

Carlsson et al[54] used radiostereometric methods to address micromotion of implanted STAR prostheses in 10 patients. An initial migration was observed for the tibial components at 6 weeks, but thereafter all, but one ankle, were stable. All tibial components experienced rotation around the three axes at 6 weeks but not thereafter. The authors concluded that a stable midterm fixation of double-coated STAR implants had been proved.[54] In another study, Carlsson[53] analyzed survivorship of STAR prostheses in two groups: with single or double hydroxyapatite coating. The first group included 51 STAR implants performed between 1993 and 1999, using a single hydroxyapatite coating; the second group included 58 STAR implants performed between 1999 and 2005, using a double hydroxyapatite coating. The results of the study showed that the improvement of having a coating may improve survivorship of prosthesis components. However, the differences were not very large, showing that other factors (e.g., better patient selection for TAR) may also play an important role.[53]

Schönherr et al[304] retrospectively reviewed 49 patients who underwent TAR using the STAR prosthesis between 2000 and 2004 and presented their short-term results, with a mean follow-up of 2.5 years. All patients experienced significant pain relief and functional improvement, resulting in a high patient satisfaction grade. In the initial phase using this prosthesis, three malleolar fractures occurred intraoperatively, all of which healed. In one case, ankle arthrodesis was performed because of aseptic loosening. In another case, the tibial component was revised.[304]

The use of a mobile bearing in the STAR prosthesis design is not entirely unproblematic. Harris et al[133]

presented a case of a 65-year-old male who underwent STAR implantation. The patient required a revision surgery after developing edge loading and a polymer wear cyst within the fibula 4 years after the initial surgery. Also, polyethylene fracture in patients after STAR ankle arthroplasty may occur and require the revision surgery, as shown by Scott and Nunley.[307] Hobson et al[161] addressed the question of whether TAR can be successfully performed in patients with significant preoperative hindfoot deformity. Between 1999 and 2006, a total of 123 consecutive ankle arthroplasties using the STAR prosthesis were performed and reviewed at a mean follow-up of 4 years. All patients were divided into two groups: with hindfoot deformity less than 10 degrees (91 ankles) or with hindfoot deformity from 11 to 30 degrees (32 ankles). In both groups, comparable postoperative range of motion and complication rates were observed. In the second group, an alignment within 5 degrees of normal was achieved for most patients (84%). Gross instability was the most common reason for implant failure. Therefore the authors stated that TAR is a feasible treatment option in patients with significant preoperative hindfoot deformity when alignment and instability are adequately corrected.[161]

Rzesacz and Gosse[289] described the surgical technique of STAR prosthesis implantation in detail and reported their results of 13 patients with posttraumatic osteoarthritis who underwent TAR between 2004 and 2005. The authors stated that significant preoperative deformity in the horizontal and/or sagittal planes of more than 20 degrees may be a relative contraindication for TAR. However, the favorable short-term results of this study show that TAR may be a useful alternative to fusion for this patient group.[289] Karantana et al[177] retrospectively reviewed 52 STAR implants at a minimum follow-up of 5 years. Postoperatively, all patients showed functional improvement as assessed by the AOFAS score. Six of 52 ankles had component revision, and 2 were converted to ankle fusion, resulting in 5- and 8-year survivorship of 90% (95% CI, 76.8%-95.5%) and 84% (95% CI, 68.9%-92.2%), respectively.[177]

Saltzman et al[294] performed a prospective controlled comparative surgical trial to evaluate the safety and efficacy of a mobile-bearing TAR in treatment of end-stage ankle osteoarthritis. This nonrandomized multicentered prospective study included the Pivotal Study (158 TARs and 66 ankle arthrodeses) and the Continued Access Study (448 TARs). By 24 months, ankles treated with the STAR prosthesis had better function and comparable pain relief compared with ankles treated with arthrodesis.[294] Mann et al[229] published their results of a prospective cohort of 84 STAR ankles, 78 of which were followed for an average of 9.1 years. Nine revisions of a metallic component were observed, resulting in a cumulative survival rate of 90% at 10 years.[229]

In conclusion, the STAR prosthesis has one of the longest histories in ankle replacement surgery, with several modifications made during its clinical use.[116]

This prosthesis is one of the most popular total ankle designs in Europe and, furthermore, is the only mobile-bearing ankle prosthesis in the United States with FDA approval.[229,294] The initial satisfactory results in the studies performed by designers have been mostly confirmed by studies performed independently. Also, several national arthroplasty registries reported favorable midterm results.[104,142,164,311]

Salto Total Ankle Replacement (Video Clip 18)

The Salto Total Ankle Prosthesis was developed between 1994 and 1996 by Michel Bonnin.[41] This total ankle design belongs to the newer generation of cementless meniscal-bearing designs. The tibial component has a flat surface toward the mobile bearing, allowing its free translation and rotation. The 3-mm medial rim is designed to avoid insert impingement against the medial malleolus. For osseous integration, the tibial component has a keel and a fixation peg. The specific shape of the talar component mimics the natural talar geometry. The anterior width is wider than the posterior, and the lateral flange has a larger curvature radius than the medial. The mobile bearing is manufactured from UHMWPE and has full congruency with the talar component in flexion and extension. All components are available in three different sizes.[41] In 2008, Leszko et al[221] performed an in vivo kinematics study of the Salto Total Ankle Prosthesis in 20 patients by using fluoroscopy and a 3D–2D registration technique. The motion of the prosthesis was described in terms of clinical rotations and as rotation about the helical axis. Among the clinical rotations, the dorsiplantar flexion was the most dominant, with a mean range of motion of 9.2 degrees. The anterior–posterior translation of the mobile bearing was measured at 1.5 mm and 2.3 mm for gait and step-up, respectively.[221]

The first clinical study on the Salto prosthesis was published in 2004 by the prosthesis designer.[41] Bonnin et al[41] implanted 98 consecutive Salto prostheses between 1997 and 2000. Ninety-three implants in 91 patients were reviewed clinically and radiographically at a mean follow-up of 2.9 years. Most patients were painfree and showed a significant functional improvement as assessed by the AOFAS score (32.2-83.1 points). Two prostheses had to be converted to ankle fusions, resulting in survivorship of greater than 95% at 68 months.[41] In the next 2 years, 22 additional Salto implantations were performed as reported in another study by Weber et al,[366] including a total of 115 implants. At a mean follow-up of 1.8 years, 4 ankles had to undergo revision surgery.[366] In another study, the same working group presented survivorship at 7 to 11 years in a retrospective review of 98 TARs performed between 1997 and 2000.[40] Six replaced ankles had to be converted to ankle fusions, and an additional 18 ankles underwent reoperation without ankle fusion (10-year survivorship of 65% (95% CI, 50%-80%). The most common complications requiring additional surgeries were bone cysts (11 ankles), fracture of the polyethylene insert (5 ankles), and unexplained pain (3 ankles).[40]

Furthermore, Bonnin et al[42] addressed the sports activity level in 145 patients who underwent Salto TAR between 1997 and 2005. Ankle function was assessed using the Foot Function Index (FFI) and the Foot and Ankle Ability Measurement. In most cases, replaced ankles were reported to have normal (15.2%) or nearly normal (60.7%) function. Participation in sports and recreational activities was analyzed only in the osteoarthritis group (100 patients) but not in patients with rheumatoid osteoarthritis. Most patients participated in some sport activities; however, a return to impact sports was rarely possible.[42]

The Salto Anatomic Ankle replacement—a three part mobile-bearing design—is not available for use in the United States. In their information for surgeons, Tornier, the manufacturer of the Salto line of TARs, explains the evolution of the two-part "Salto Talaris" as follows: "Improvement in the precision of the instrumentation to achieve accurate and reproducible tibiotalar alignment enables the simplification of the implant system to a fixed-bearing design. A key principle is that the mobile-bearing concept has been moved from the implant to the instrumentation at the stage of the trial reduction. First, a measured resection with equal implant replacement is applied to the talus and distal tibia. Then, the trial tibial base, featuring a highly polished surface that remains mobile against the resected distal tibia, is allowed to rotate into proper position during ankle range of motion through a securely fixed, highly conforming articulating insert. Only after this intrinsic tibiotalar alignment is achieved are the bone cuts for the tibial keel and plug completed, fixing the tibial base and insert assembly into the optimized position."

Mehta et al[233] performed a review on the Salto Anatomic Ankle design. The authors described their preoperative planning and surgical technique and reported their initial experience with this prosthesis type, including nine patients treated from 2007 through 2008 because of end-stage rheumatoid (Fig. 22-26) or posttraumatic osteoarthritis (Fig. 22-27).[233]

In conclusion, the midterm results of the Salto TAR are promising.[40] However, the only clinical reports come from the prosthesis designer. In the United States, a modified design of the Salto TAR is approved for use in patients with ankle OA.[379] This fixed-bearing design includes a titanium tibial component with a highly conforming polyethylene articulating insert.[379] However, to date, there are no clinical studies reporting results of this prosthesis available.

HINTEGRA Total Ankle Replacement (Video Clip 20)

The HINTEGRA total ankle design (Fig. 22-28) is an unconstrained, three-component system that provides inversion-eversion stability and was designed in 2000 by Beat Hintermann, Greta Dereymaeker, Ramon Viladot, and Patrice Diebold. The mobile bearing provides axial rotation and normal flexion–extension mobility.[148,151,352] The HINTEGRA total ankle includes two metallic

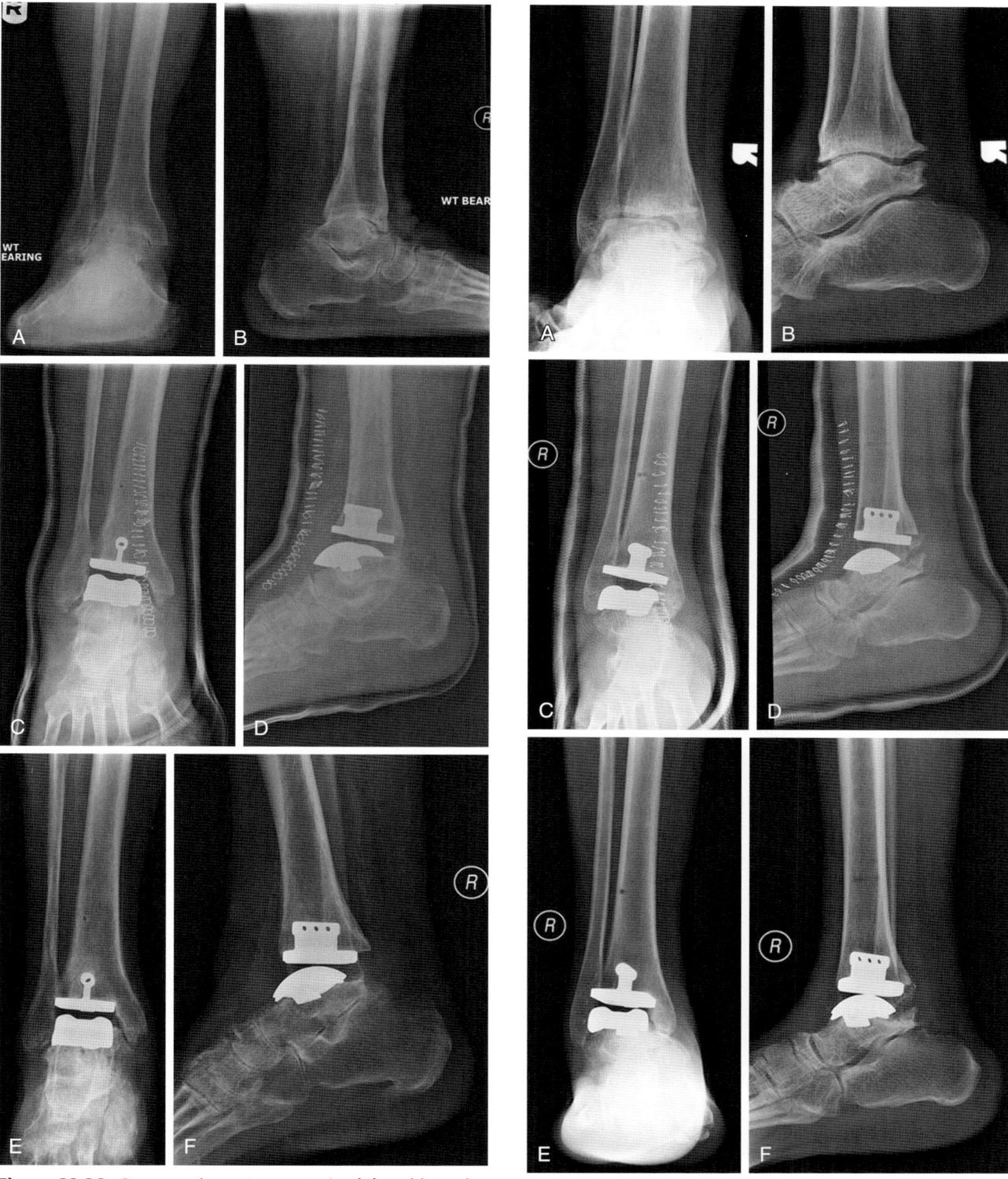

Figure 22-26 Preoperative anteroposterior **(A)** and lateral **(B)** radiographs of a 53-year-old male suffering from rheumatoid arthritis with previously performed triple arthrodesis. **C** and **D,** Regular Salto Talaris ankle prosthesis has been used. Postoperative anteroposterior **(E)** and lateral **(F)** radiographs show proper position and osseous integration of both prosthetic components at a follow-up of 7.5 months. (Images courtesy Siddant K. Mehta and Sheldon S. Lin, MD, Newark, N.J.)

Figure 22-27 Preoperative anteroposterior **(A)** and lateral **(B)** radiographs of a 38-year-old female suffering from posttraumatic arthritis. **C** and **D,** Regular Salto Talaris ankle prosthesis has been used. Postoperative anteroposterior **(E)** and lateral **(F)** radiographs show proper position and osseous integration of both prosthetic components at a follow-up of 5 months. (Images courtesy Siddant K. Mehta and Sheldon S. Lin, MD, Newark, N.J.)

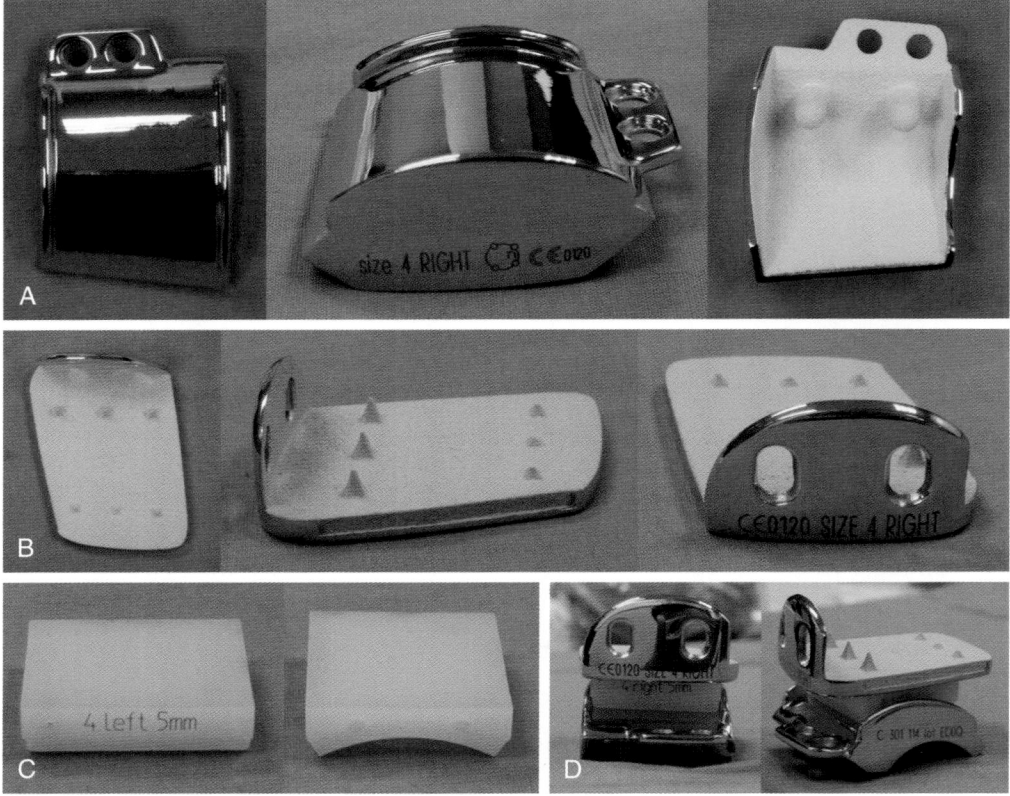

Figure 22-28 A, The talar component is conical like the native talus and has a smaller radius of curvature on the medial side. Two pegs are used for fixation. **B,** The tibial component is anatomically shaped and has a 4-mm-thick flat plate with six pyramidal peaks and an anterior shield. **C,** The ultra-high-molecular-weight polyethylene mobile bearing has a flat surface on the tibial side and a concave conical surface on the talar side. **D,** A 2.5-mm-high rim on both sides of the talar component provides mediolateral stability to the polyethylene bearing.

components and an ultrahigh-density polyethylene mobile bearing. The nonarticulating surfaces have a porous coating with 20% porosity and are covered by titanium fluid and hydroxyapatite. The tibial component has a flat, 4-mm-thick loading plate with pyramidal peaks against the tibia. Additional stability may be achieved by fixation with two screws. The talar component is conically shaped, with a smaller radius medially than laterally, mimicking the normal anatomy of talus. It has 2.5-mm-high rims on each side that ensure stable positioning and guide the anteroposterior translation of the mobile bearing. The anterior shield of this component increases primary bone support, especially in cases with weaker bone, and may prevent the adherence of scar tissue and avoid restriction of range of motion in cases with arthrofibrosis.[151]

Barg et al[21] analyzed 368 ankles treated with HINTEGRA total ankle arthroplasty to assess the mobile-bearing position by measurement of the anteroposterior offset ratio. The mean anteroposterior offset ratio was 0.0 ± 0.06 and remained constant over time during the mean follow-up of 4.3 years. This study has shown that the polyethylene mobile bearing aligned very well with the longitudinal tibial axis.[21]

The HINTEGRA TAR has been extensively used since 2000 in Europe, since 2004 in Canada and Korea, and since 2005 in Peru, Panama, and Costa Rica.[33,40,118,121,183] The use of this prosthesis is also documented in the national arthroplasty registries of Finland,[311] Sweden,[142] Norway,[104] and New Zealand.[164] In the current literature, there are numerous studies published by designer and his working group that address the clinical outcome and biomechanical properties of the HINTEGRA total ankle. In 2004, Hintermann et al[157] published the first study reporting the HINTEGRA design rationale, surgical technique, and short-term results of the first consecutive 122 ankles in 166 patients. All patients were reviewed at a mean follow-up of 1.6 years. Eight ankles had to undergo revision surgery: 4 because of loosening of at least one component, 1 because of dislocation of the mobile bearing, and 3 for other reasons. All revisions were successful. Most patients experienced significant functional improvement postoperatively as assessed by the AOFAS score; 68% were painfree at the latest follow-up. The clinically and radiographically measured ROM was 39 and 37 degrees, respectively. Tibial components were stable in all reviewed ankles; in 2 ankles, a slight migration of the talar component was observed.[157]

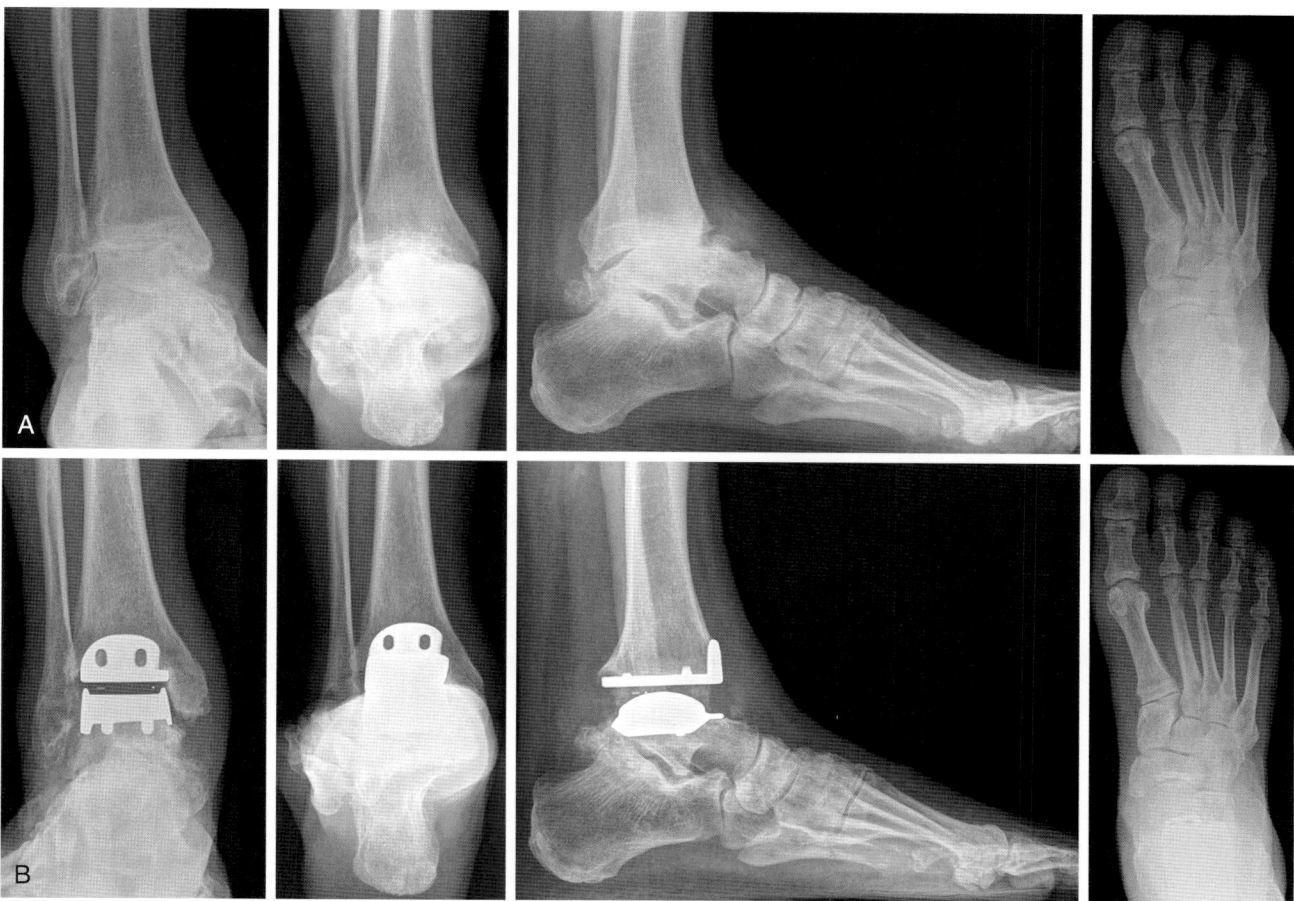

Figure 22-29 **A,** Preoperative weight-bearing radiographs of a 62-year-old male suffering from posttraumatic arthritis. Regular HINTEGRA ankle prosthesis (third generation) has been used. **B,** Postoperative weight-bearing radiographs including hindfoot alignment view show proper position and osseous integration of both prosthetic components and physiologic hindfoot alignment at a follow-up of 2 years. (Images courtesy Beat Hintermann, MD, Liestal, Switzerland.)

Similar results were published in a study by Valderrabano and Hintermann,[341] including 125 HINTEGRA implants. In 2006, Hintermann et al[158] presented midterm results of 271 HINTEGRA total ankle replacements performed in 261 patients between 2000 and 2004 (Fig. 22-29). The mean follow-up was 3 years, with a range of 1 to 5.3 years. Intraoperatively, four malleolar fractures occurred, which all healed within 6 weeks. Five ankles (1.8%) had to be converted to ankle fusions. Thirteen talar and two tibial components were later revised. In total, 39 revision surgeries (e.g., open arthrolysis, lengthening of the Achilles tendon, ligament reconstruction) were necessary to address late postoperative complications.[158] Kim et al[183] compared the outcome and complications of HINTEGRA total ankle replacements with versus without hindfoot fusion. A total of 60 ankles treated with HINTEGRA implants and subtalar or triple fusion were compared with a control group of 288 ankles treated with TAR alone. The mean follow-up was 3.3 years. The authors found that the clinical outcome of TAR when combined with hindfoot fusion (subtalar or triple

fusion) is comparable to that of ankle replacement alone. Therefore the authors recommended that hindfoot fusion should be performed simultaneously with TAR in cases when indicated.[183]

Barg et al published clinical observation studies addressing clinical and radiologic outcomes in patients who underwent HINTEGRA TAR because of end-stage OA resulting from hemophilia,[22] hemochromatosis,[23] or gout.[29] In all three patient cohorts, favorable outcomes with significant pain relief and functional improvement were observed, demonstrating TAR as a reliable option treatment.[22,23,29] Valderrabano et al[351] addressed the sporting and recreational activities of patients with end-stage ankle arthritis before and after ankle TAR. A clinical evaluation was performed preoperatively and at a mean follow-up of 2.8 years in 147 patients (152 ankles). All patients experienced significant functional improvement as assessed by the AOFAS score. After TAR, patients with sports activities had a higher AOFAS score. The three most frequent sports activities after this procedure were hiking, biking, and swimming.[351]

Daniels et al[76] published their results for 32 TARs in patients with significant preoperative varus talar deformities. In all patients, cementless, mobile-bearing, three-component prostheses had been used: 26 HINTEGRA, 4 Mobility, and 2 STAR implants. Satisfactory radiographic correction was obtained in most cases (30 ankles) at a mean follow-up of 1.4 years. In 24 ankles, additional procedures after total ankle arthroplasty were required to obtain a plantigrade foot.[76] Lee et al[217] addressed perioperative complications of HINTEGRA TAR in their 50 initial cases The same author presented two case reports addressing HINTEGRA TAR in patients after revascularization of avascular necrosis of the talar body.[218] The authors stated that in patients with avascular necrosis of the talus, healing of necrotic bone by creeping substitution TAR is a valuable option.[218]

Kim et al[183] described clinical outcomes of TAR in 23 patients with moderate-to-severe varus deformity and compared the results with those in 22 patients with neutral alignment. All patients were reviewed at a mean follow-up of 2.25 years and showed substantial pain relief and functional improvement in both groups as assessed by the visual analog score (VAS) and AOFAS score, respectively. Failure of the implant, with conversion to ankle fusion, occurred in one case in each group. The authors stated that the TAR is a valuable treatment for severe ankle osteoarthritis, including patients with hindfoot misalignment. However, the appropriate additional procedures to address the deformity were necessary to obtain good clinical results, including prosthesis stability and range of motion.[183]

Bai et al[16] compared clinical outcomes and revision rates after TAR among patients with posttraumatic and primary osteoarthritis. Sixty-seven consecutive total ankle arthroplasties were performed between 2005 and 2007 using the HINTEGRA prosthesis in 65 patients. The patients were divided into two groups: posttraumatic osteoarthritis group (37 ankles) and primary osteoarthritis group (30 ankles). At a mean follow-up of 38 months, the clinical (AOFAS score, range of motion) and radiographic outcomes were comparable. However, the incidence of postoperative complications was significantly higher in the posttraumatic osteoarthritis group.[16]

Valderrabano et al[347,349,350,354] published a series of studies addressing muscle biomechanics and muscle rehabilitation in patients with severe ankle osteoarthritis who underwent TAR. A prospective study was performed, including 15 patients who were reviewed preoperatively and postoperatively at 3-month intervals up to 1 year, and showed that TAR surgery may improve muscle biomechanics as assessed by torque measurement and electromyographic (EMG) intensity.[349] However, in most patients, the muscle rehabilitation was not complete at a follow-up of 1 year.[349]

Müller et al[240] used a Heidelberger foot and ankle analysis model to address the 3D kinematics and foot and ankle shape in 12 patients who underwent HINTEGRA TAR. The authors detected some decreased range of motion after ankle replacement compared with contralateral ankles free of degenerative changes. However, these differences did not affect the gait kinematics, showing that TAR may be able to preserve range of motion, which in turn may avoid, or at least decelerate, the degenerative changes in adjacent joints.[240]

Lee et al[219] investigated static and dynamic postural balance after TAR using HINTEGRA in 30 patients and compared the results to an age- and sex-matched control group. The authors showed that patients who underwent TAR have a higher degree of dynamic postural imbalance. Also, some motor control deficits were detected in the total ankle arthroplasty group. The authors stated that more intensive postoperative balance training may decrease the observed deficits.[219] In a retrospective cohort study that included 317 HINTEGRA ankle arthroplasties, Barg et al[20] assessed the effect of talar component malposition on clinical results, including pain relief and functional outcome. The talar position has been assessed by measuring the anteroposterior offset ratio using standard, lateral, weight-bearing radiographs at a mean follow-up of 4.3 years. The postoperative pain relief and functional results were better in patients with a neutrally aligned talar component than in both subgroups with the talar component placed more anteriorly or posteriorly.[20]

In conclusion, the midterm results in patients with HINTEGRA total ankle arthroplasty are favorable.[157,158] However, most clinical studies have been published by the designer. Comparable studies by independent authors and studies with longer follow-ups should be performed.

Mobility Ankle System

The Mobility Ankle System has been developed by Pascal Rippstein, Peter Wood, and Chris Coetzee. This is a three-component, unconstrained Buechel-Pappas–type prosthesis with a short, conical tibial stem (Fig. 22-30). The talar component of the Mobility implant resurfaces the superior dome of the talus, while the medial and lateral aspects of the talus remain untreated (unlike the Buechel-Pappas prosthesis). The talar component has a central, longitudinal sulcus and two fins enhancing its intrinsic stability. The nonarticulating surfaces are porous, coated with a titanium spray to provide osseous ingrowth after press-fit implantation.[279]

Goldberg et al[118] reported results of their questionnaire-based survey sent to all consultant members of the British Orthopaedic Foot and Ankle Society. The Mobility prosthesis was the most commonly used prosthesis among 62% of all surgeons in the United Kingdom.[118] The use of this prosthesis has also been documented in the Swedish[142] and New Zealand Ankle Arthroplasty Registries.[164] The Swedish Ankle Arthroplasty Registry included a total of 531 TARs, with 23 Mobility prostheses implanted since 2005.[142] No perioperative or postoperative complications with the Mobility prosthesis were observed in the Swedish cohort.[142] The New Zealand National Joint Registry included a total of 202 TARs, with a mean follow-up of

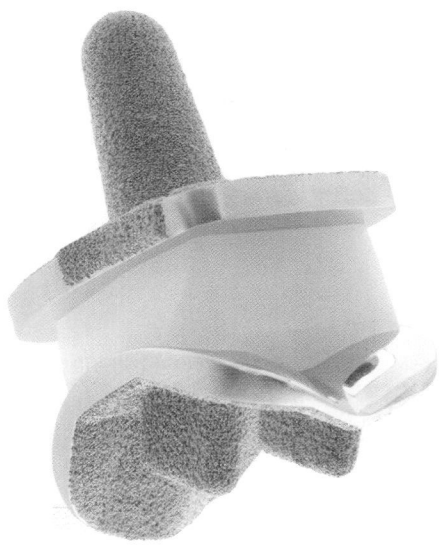

Figure 22-30 Mobility prosthesis—an unconstrained, three-component system consisting of a tibial component, a talar component, and a mobile-bearing, highly cross-linked polyethylene inlay. (Images courtesy Pascal Rippstein, MD, Zurich, Switzerland.)

6 years.[164] Twenty-nine patients in this registry underwent Mobility prosthesis implantation, with no failures observed in this study.[164] Wood et al[373] published early results from their prospective study, including 100 Mobility implantations performed in 96 patients between 2003 and 2005. At a minimum follow-up of 5 years, a total of 5 ankles (5%) had to undergo revision surgery: two ankle fusions and three revision arthroplasties, resulting in 3- and 4-year survivorship of 97% (95% CI, 91%-99%) and 93.6% (95% CI, 84.7%-97.4%), respectively. In 14 ankles, a radiolucent line or osteolytic cavity was observed. However, in only 5 ankles, it was more than 10 mm in width. The authors presented encouraging short-term results that are comparable to those obtained using other modern three-component prostheses.[373]

Naal et al[246] addressed habitual physical activity and sports participation before and after TAR in 137 consecutive patients with 155 implants. One hundred one ankles were available for the review at a mean follow-up of 3.7 years; 54 had Mobility implants. The percentage of patients who were active in sports did not change after the TAR (62.4% preoperatively and 66.3% postoperatively). The most common sports activities after total ankle arthroplasty were swimming, cycling, and fitness/weight training. The authors registered high functional improvement in their patient cohort as assessed by AOFAS scores. No association was found between sports participation, increased physical activity level, and the appearance of periprosthetic radiolucencies.[246] Thermann et al[331] reported a single case of a 58-year-old patient who underwent Mobility TAR and tibialis posterior tendon transfer for ankle osteoarthritis and footdrop deformity.

Postoperative radiographs showed a medial malleolus fracture despite intraoperative pinning with the Kirschner wires. However, the fracture completely healed after 8 weeks. Three years after the primary procedure, the patient was asymptomatic and had a stable ankle joint with 5-degree dorsiflexion and 20-degree plantar flexion.[331] Goldberg et al[117] reported two cases of early failure in patients who underwent Mobility TAR because of component malposition. In both cases, the talar component was inserted back to front, as was the polyethylene insert, requiring ankle fusion in the first case and revision arthroplasty in the second case. The authors emphasized the need for adequate training of foot and ankle surgeons in performing total ankle arthroplasty. They also suggested that designers have a responsibility to improve marketing and education for surgeons using their products, to minimize incidents of incorrect use.[117]

Espinosa et al[99] generated two finite-element models of total ankle prostheses (Agility and Mobility) to investigate the misalignment of prosthesis components on joint contact pressures (Fig. 22-31). The authors have shown that the highly congruent mobile-bearing design of the Mobility prosthesis may result in more evenly distributed contact pressures than the less-congruent two-component Agility prosthesis. However, in both designs, the misalignment of prosthesis components may lead to pathologically increased contact stresses.[99] Bell and Fisher[31] investigated polyethylene wear in Mobility and Buechel-Pappas prostheses by using a modified knee prosthesis simulator. The authors showed that wear in the two models was comparable and that the wear rate for both designs significantly increases with the inclusion of an anterior/posterior displacement in the kinematic inputs, simulating malalignment of prosthesis components.[31]

Rippstein et al[279] analyzed the clinical and radiographic results in 233 consecutive patients with 240 Mobility ankle arthroplasties. There were 10 intraoperative complications (4.2%) and 20 postoperative complications (8.6%), resulting in 18 secondary surgeries. Significant pain relief and functional improvement were observed at a mean follow-up of 2.7 years (Fig. 22-32).[279]

In conclusion, the Mobility TAR has been in general use since 2003 in Europe, Australia, New Zealand, South Africa, and Canada. In the United States, a multicenter FDA trial including this prosthesis type was started but not completed, probably because of inadequate funding.[84] Similar to the other three-component ankle prosthesis, the studies with higher and adequate numbers of patients are mostly published by the designers of the prosthesis.

TNK Total Ankle Replacement

The TNK prosthesis was developed by Dr. Takakura in Japan in 1975. In 1988, Takakura et al[327] reported a comparative study of cemented metal and uncemented ceramic TNK ankle prostheses. Both types were two-component prostheses with high-density polyethylene fixed to the tibial component. Before 1980, the authors

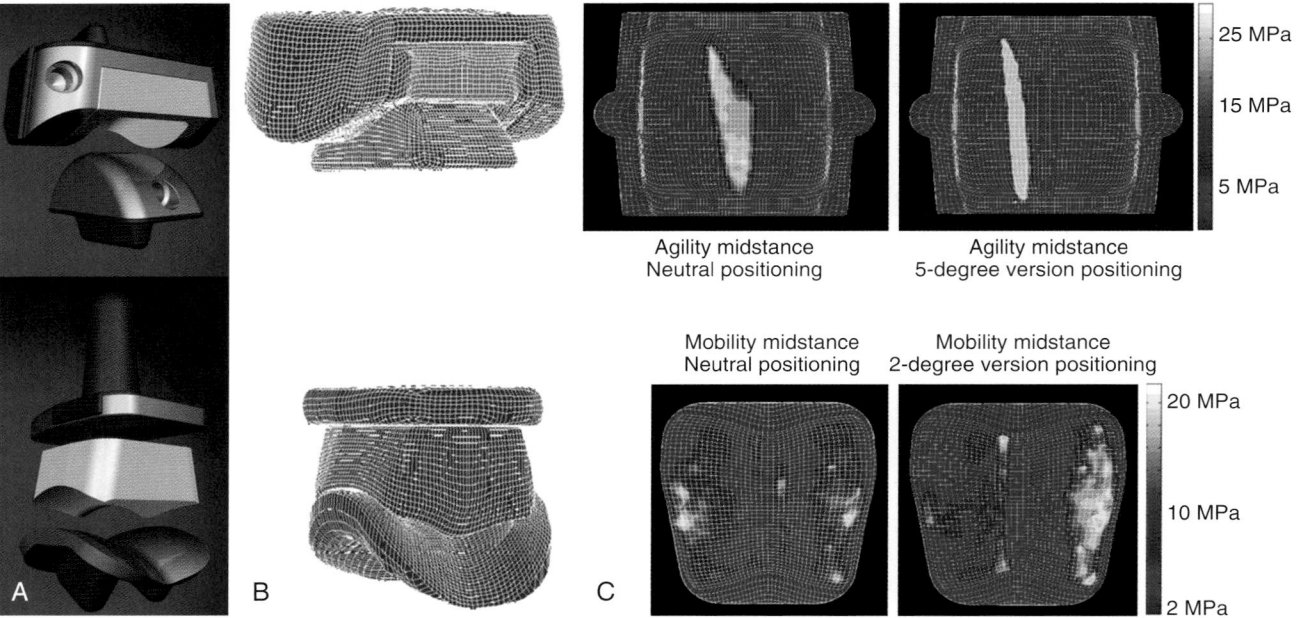

Figure 22-31 **A,** Schematic representation of the Agility *(upper row)* and Mobility *(lower row)* total ankle replacements. **B,** Computer-aided design renderings of the Agility and Mobility total ankle replacements. **C,** Finite-element evolution of the polyethylene contact pressure distribution at the midstance in the finite-element–simulated alignment. *MPa,* Megapascal. (Images courtesy Norman Espinosa, MD, and Jess Snedeker, PhD, Zurich, Switzerland.)

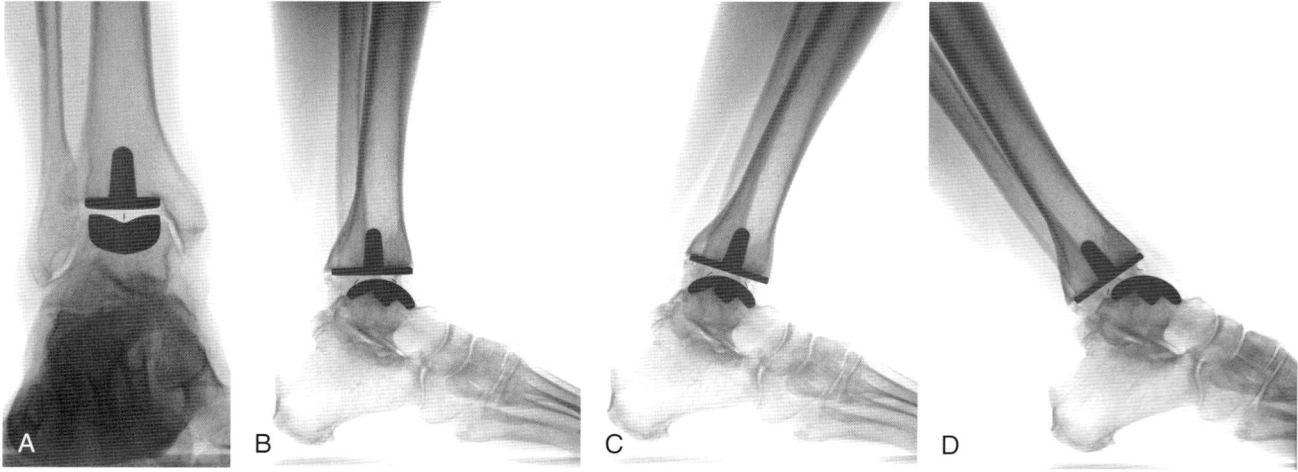

Figure 22-32 Anteroposterior **(A)** and lateral **(B)** weight-bearing radiographs in 54-year-old male who underwent total ankle replacement, using a Mobility prosthesis, 5 years earlier. Radiographs show appropriate position of tibial and talar components and polyethylene insert with no evidence of aseptic loosening or subsidence of metallic components. Lateral radiograph shows degenerative changes of subtalar joint; however, the patient is completely painfree. **C** and **D,** Lateral radiographs in dorsiflexion and plantar flexion show excellent functional results with nearly physiologic range of motion of replaced ankles (26 degrees dorsiflexion/36 degrees plantar flexion). (Images courtesy Pascal Rippstein, MD, Zurich, Switzerland.)

implanted 30 cemented stainless steel prostheses (first generation) (Fig. 22-33); after 1980, they used 9 cemented and 30 uncemented ceramic prostheses (second generation). The mean follow-up time for cemented and uncemented TARs was 8.1 and 4.1 years, respectively. Patients who underwent TAR with an uncemented prosthesis were 67% more satisfied than the other patients (27%). Five

metal ankle arthroplasties and one ceramic ankle arthroplasty had to be revised (five arthrodeses and one revision arthroplasty).[327]

The initial encouraging results were not maintained in another study by the same working group, published in 2004.[326] Significant loosening and subsidence of the prosthesis were observed in most patients with first-generation

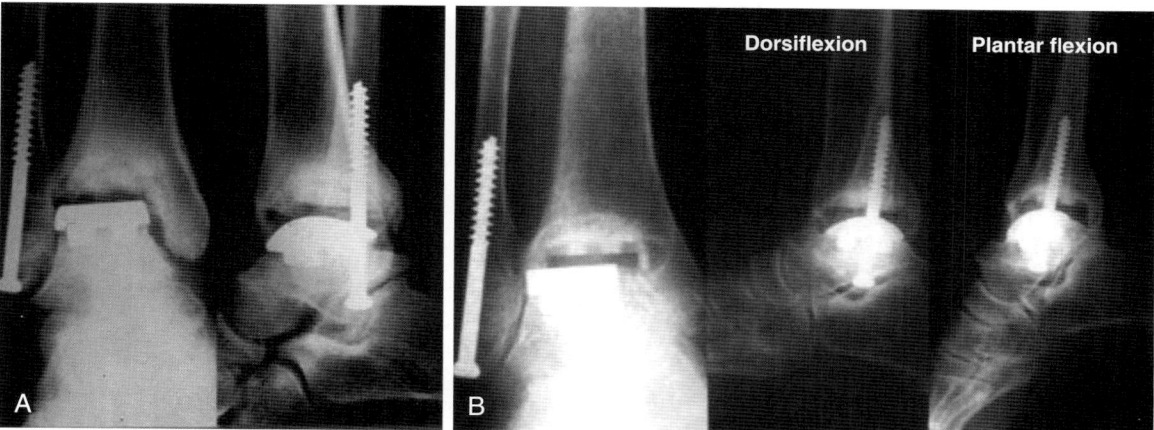

Figure 22-33 First-generation TNK prosthesis (stainless steel prosthesis) total ankle replacement (TAR) was performed in a 50-year-old female because of end-stage ankle osteoarthritis. **A,** Anteroposterior and lateral radiographs 8 years after TAR show no evidence of aseptic loosening or prosthesis subsidence. **B,** Anteroposterior radiograph 19 years after initial surgery shows a slight lateral tilting of talus within the ankle mortise. However, very good functional outcome (8 degrees dorsiflexion/37 degrees plantar flexion) and no pain were observed at the last follow-up. (Images courtesy Yasuhito Tanaka, MD, PhD, Nara, Japan.)

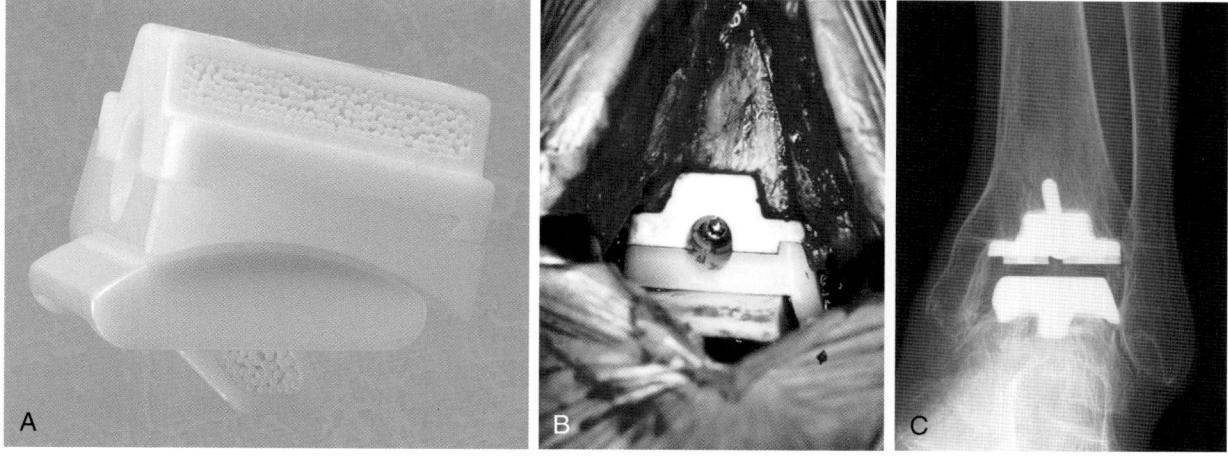

Figure 22-34 **A,** Third-generation TNK total ankle prosthesis coated with beads and hydroxyapatite as introduced in 1991. **B,** Third-generation TNK prosthesis in situ with fixation using a screw. **C,** Anteroposterior weight-bearing ankle radiograph shows appropriate position of prosthesis component with no evidence of aseptic loosening in a 64-year-old female 8 years after implantation of TNK prosthesis. (Images courtesy Yasuhito Tanaka, MD, PhD, Nara, Japan.)

TAR (stainless steel prosthesis). The second-generation TAR (ceramic prosthesis) was implanted in 60 ankles between 1980 and 1991 (cement fixation was used in 12 ankles). However, loosening and significant subsidence occurred in most patients within 5 years after the surgery. In 1991, the ceramic prosthesis (second generation) was modified by adding bead-formed alumina coated with hydroxyapatite (third generation) (Fig. 22-34).

Between 1991 and 2001, the third-generation TNK prosthesis was used in 70 ankles.[326,329] The mean follow-up in this patient group was 5 years. In three patients, the replaced ankle had to be fused (one case with deep infection, two cases with severe subsidence of talar

component). Overall results were excellent or good in the most patients (52 ankles) and significantly better than those observed in patients with a second-generation TNK prosthesis (Fig. 22-35). Patient satisfaction rate was higher in patients with osteoarthritis compared with patients with rheumatoid osteoarthritis.[326,329]

The TNK prosthesis has been used for treatment of rheumatoid osteoarthritis, with poor clinical and radiographic outcomes as shown in two studies.[248,253] Nishikawa et al[253] reviewed 26 patients (6 patients received bilateral TAR) with rheumatoid osteoarthritis who were treated with a TNK prosthesis between 1984 and 2000. At a mean follow-up of 72 months, 27 ankles in 21

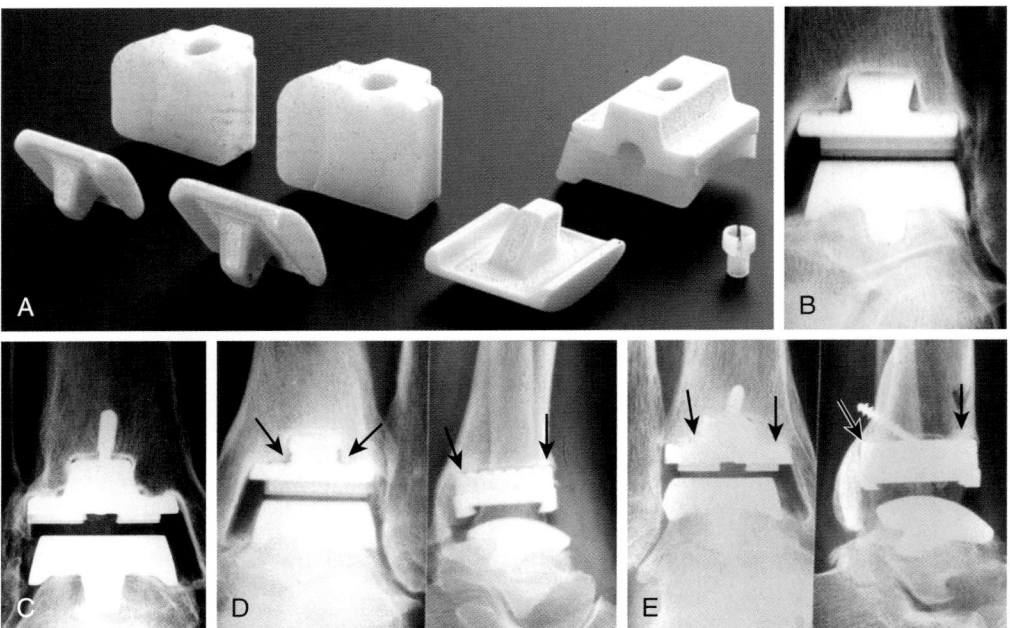

Figure 22-35   A, Second- *(left)* and third-generation *(right)* TNK total ankle prosthesis. **B,** Anteroposterior radiograph of a 67-year-old male who underwent second-generation TNK prosthesis implantation showing significant loosening around the tibial component 4.5 years after the implantation. **C,** Anteroposterior radiograph of a 62-year-old male who underwent third-generation TNK prosthesis implantation without any evidence for aseptic loosening 5 years after the implantation. **D,** Anteroposterior and lateral radiographs of a 63-year-old female with second-generation TNK prosthesis 1 year after implantation. Wide aseptic loosening is observed around the tibial component. **E,** Anteroposterior and lateral radiographs of a 68-year-old male with third-generation TNK prosthesis 1 year after implantation, with no evidence for aseptic loosening. (Images courtesy Yasuhito Tanaka, MD, PhD, Nara, Japan.)

patients were reviewed. Three ankles had to undergo revision surgery. Nine patients reported their outcome as excellent or good, but patients complained about residual pain in 13 ankles. A high rate of radiolucency was observed in this patient cohort: migration of the tibial component in 13 ankles and collapse of the talus in 9.[253] Nagashima et al[248] reported results of 21 ankle arthroplasties performed between 1998 and 2002, using the TNK prosthesis in 19 patients. Hybrid-type fixation (talus component cemented, tibial component not cemented) was used in 15 of 21 cases, while both components were cemented in the remaining cases. Early postoperative complications included 2 patients with delayed wound healing and 1 patient with deep infection. In 11 of 21 ankles, significant radiolucency lines were observed. Most patients experienced pain relief and functional improvement; however, postoperative improvement in range of motion directly correlated with preoperative range of motion.[248]

Shinomiya et al[310] performed 20 ankle arthroplasties between 1988 and 1996, using a TNK prosthesis in 18 selected patients with rheumatoid osteoarthritis. All patients were reviewed at a mean follow-up of 8 years, with a range of 5 to 12 years. All patients experienced substantial pain relief and showed functional improvement superior to those who underwent ankle arthrodesis in the same period. No conversions to ankle fusion or

revision arthroplasties were necessary in this cohort. However, a radiolucent line was observed in all replaced ankles at the final follow-up. The authors stated that TAR may be useful in young patients with rheumatoid osteoarthritis, considering their better postoperative quality of life.[310]

Shi et al[309] developed a special hydroxyapatite augmentation for bone atrophy in TAR for rheumatoid patients receiving a TNK prosthesis. This specially designed hydroxyapatite coating was used in 16 ankles (14 patients), and results were reviewed at a mean follow-up of 1.9 years. More than half of all ankles showed a radiolucency zone between the hydroxyapatite and tibial component on radiographs at the final follow-up. However, no significant changes of coating position were registered; also, no significant subsidence was noted. In conclusion, the authors suggested that this new technique using hydroxyapatite may increase the primary implant fixation to the bone, especially in patients with rheumatoid osteoarthritis and significant bone atrophy.[309]

Tsukamoto et al[339] reported a case in which a custom-made alumina ceramic total talar component was used for treatment of the collapse of the talar body in one patient who had received a TNK prosthesis. The revision surgery was performed in a 56-year-old female patient

4 years after the initial TAR. The authors achieved substantial pain relief and functional improvement, especially regarding walking ability. This case report demonstrated a feasible revision treatment in patients with failed TAR.[339]

In summary, since its introduction in 1975, the TNK prosthesis has undergone many modifications, including the material of the components (stainless steel, polyethylene, alumina ceramic), a coating (with or without hydroxyapatite), and fixation (cemented or cementless fixation). Currently, this is the only TAR design using alumina ceramic components. Although the studies by the designer reported favorable results using the third-generation TNK prosthesis,[326,329] independent studies addressing TAR results in patients with rheumatoid arthritis show less-promising results.[248,253]

Ramses Total Ankle Replacement

The Ramses TAR was developed in 1987 and first implanted in 1989 by a French designer group.[234,235] The Ramses TAR is a three-component semiconstrained prosthesis with a high-density mobile bearing.[234] Initially, between 1980 and 2000, cemented fixation of the prosthesis was used. A total of approximately 350 ankle arthroplasties using the Ramses total ankle design have been performed by the designer group. Mendolia et al[234] reported long-term results in 69 patients who underwent Ramses TAR between 1989 and 1993. In seven cases, the replaced ankle had to be converted to ankle arthrodesis (four ankles for pain without loosening and three ankles for clinical and radiographic loosening). In an additional five cases, a second surgery was performed (two cases with mobile-bearing replacement and three cases with revision arthroplasties).[234]

Delagoutte[79] performed a retrospective analysis of 110 ankle arthroplasties performed between 1991 and 1998. This was a multicenter study including 22 hospitals. Three different TAR total ankle designs were used: Ramses (n = 66, 60%), low-contact stress (LCS; Depuy, Warsaw, Ind.) (n = 36, 33%), and STAR (n = 8, 7%) prosthesis. The follow-up varied in this study from 3 to 37 months. In general, the postoperative functional results were less favorable, with no postoperative improvement in dorsiflexion. In two patients with Ramses prostheses, revision surgery was necessary to address prosthesis loosening.[79] Use of the Ramses prosthesis has been listed in 11 of 202 ankle arthroplasties mentioned in the New Zealand National Joint Registry.[164] Two failures of this prosthesis type in this patient cohort were reported.[164]

In conclusion, the midterm and long-term results in patients who underwent Ramses TAR are not satisfactory because of high revision rates of 18% and 34% at 2 and 10 years, respectively. Also, the number of painfree patients has equaled the number of patients with pain remaining.[236]

AES Total Ankle Replacement

The Ankle Evolutive System (AES) TAR is a further development of the Buechel-Pappas–type prosthesis. This

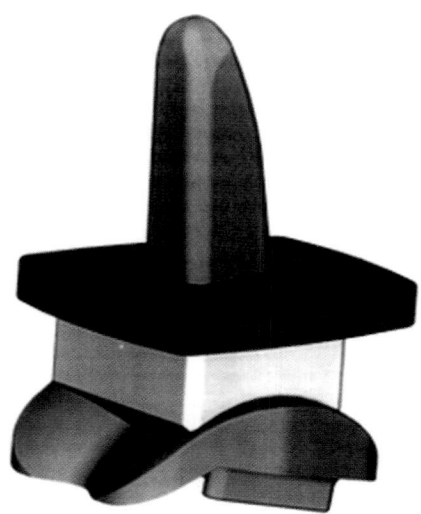

Figure 22-36 Ankle Evolutive System (AES) ankle prosthesis is a newer-generation, three-component, unconstrained, meniscal-bearing prosthesis. (Images courtesy Jean-Luc Besse, MD, PhD, Lyon, France.)

design has a modular stem and allows hemireplacement of the medial tibiotalar and talofibular joints (Fig. 22-36).[146]

This prosthesis type has been widely used in England and France[34,118] and has also been introduced in Norway.[104] One of the first reports addressing the outcome in patients who underwent AES TAR is a study by Patsalis.[262] This study included 15 AES ankle arthroplasties, with an average short-term follow-up of 8.5 months. Three malleolar fractures were observed intraoperatively. Two replaced ankles had to be revised, while the remaining 13 patients showed significant functional improvement as assessed by the AOFAS score.[262] In 2005, a short-term study by the designers of the AES prosthesis outlined the suggested surgical technique and reported good preliminary results.[10]

Henricson and Ågren[139] addressed the influence of preoperative hindfoot alignment on secondary surgery after TAR. The patient cohort included 109 STAR, 62 Buechel-Pappas, and 22 AES ankle arthroplasties. The mean follow-up time in the whole patient group was 4.2 years. In the AES TAR group, they observed two cases with instability requiring additional surgery (one case with preoperative varus and one case with preoperative valgus deformity). No revision surgeries addressing prosthesis loosening were necessary.[139] The same working group analyzed midterm survivorship of 93 AES ankle arthroplasties at a mean follow-up of 3.5 years.[140] The authors found the midterm results of AES total ankle design promising, with a 5-year survivorship with revision for any reason as an end-point of 90%.[140]

Popelka et al[270] shared their experience with 51 consecutive AES implantations carried out between 2003 and 2008. At the follow-up between 4 months and 5 years, authors observed substantial pain relief and functional improvement in their study.[270] Brooke et al[45] presented two cases with valgus malalignment after TAR using an AES prosthesis. They performed a fibula lengthening osteotomy to regain the anatomic alignment and to avoid pathologic increases in wear. In both cases, good clinical and radiographic results were achieved.[45] Kharwadkar and Harris[181] published a report of two cases using the AES tibial component as a revision component in patients with failed STAR prostheses. The hybrid AES-STAR revision procedures were performed 4 and 7 years after the primary STAR prosthesis implantation. The midterm results were satisfactory, with no restriction of daily activities.[181] Dahabreh et al[75] published a case report with a patient having revision surgery resulting from extrusion of a metal radiologic marker.[75] The exchange of the polyethylene insert was performed 9 months after the initial TAR by using an AES implant. During revision surgery, the insert was found to be intact without fracture.[75] Morgan et al[238] presented 2.5-years follow-up results in a female patient who had poliomyelitis as a child and had been treated with the AES prosthesis because of a painful degenerate ankle with preoperatively significant varus deformity. The patient showed a satisfactory functional outcome with a well-aligned replacement ankle and no evidence of loosening or osteolysis around prosthesis components.[238]

Anders et al[7] reported their midterm results in 94 patients who underwent AES TAR between 2002 and 2007. One patient died, leaving 93 ankles for evaluation at a mean follow-up of 3.5 years. There were five intraoperative malleolar fractures, which were all secured with screws. One patient was revised after 5.5 years because of loosening of both metallic components, and two patients with loosening of the tibial component were pending revisions. In three additional cases, osteolysis was seen around the component. Two ankles were revised because of fixed varus or valgus deformity. In one patient, an ankle fusion was performed because of a fracture of the distal tibia. Two patients were revised for deep infection. Overall, the cumulative 5-year survivorship with revision for any reason was 90%. In summary, the authors stated

that midterm results in their patient cohort were promising.[7]

Morgan et al[238] presented the outcomes of 38 consecutive patients who were treated with AES TAR between 2002 and 2004. All patients were reviewed clinically and radiographically at a minimum follow-up of 4 years. Most patients presented with significantly improved function and pain relief. Two replaced ankles were converted to ankle fusion, resulting in a cumulative 6-year survivorship of 94.7% (95% CI, 80.3%-98.7%). Ten patients presented with edge loading, of whom 9 had corrective surgery. In 9 patients, significant osteolysis around prosthesis components was seen. Because of nonprogressive symptoms, no further revision surgeries were suggested. Despite high patient satisfaction, the authors reported some concerns about an observed high rate of osteolysis.[238] The reported high rate of osteolysis in patients who underwent AES TAR has been confirmed by other studies. Besse et al[33] reported midterm results of their prospective study, including 51 AES implantations performed from 2003 to 2006. All patients were reviewed at a mean follow-up of 3.3 years. Eighty-two percent of all patients had good functional outcomes, showing a significant postoperative improvement of the AOFAS score. In 2 patients, replaced ankles were converted to ankle fusion because of talar component subsidence and mechanical dislocation. Although the functional outcome and patient satisfaction were comparable to other results published in studies using other third-generation prostheses (Fig. 22-37), significant osteolysis with the AES TAR was more frequent, with risk of subsidence (Figs. 22-38 to 22-40). As a consequence, the authors stopped implantation of this prosthesis type and recommended a preventive grafting for severe osteolysis.[33]

The comparably high osteolysis rate was also seen in a study by Koivu et al[203] that reviewed 130 consecutive AES implantations performed between 2002 and 2008. Radiolucent lines or osteolytic lesions were seen on plain radiographs in 48 ankles (37%). Marked osteolytic lesions were found in 27 ankles (21%). The talar component migrated in 9 ankles; in an additional 2 ankles, a shift of the tibial component was observed. Of the 27 ankles with

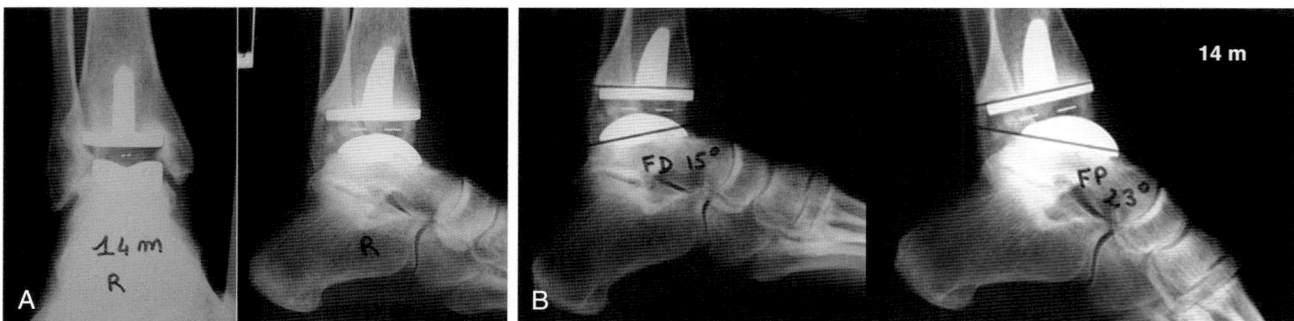

Figure 22-37   A, Postoperative radiographs of a 66-year-old male who underwent total ankle replacement using Ankle Evolutive System prosthesis 14 months ago. **B,** Good functional outcome was observed, including range of motion of 38 degrees. (Images courtesy Jean-Luc Besse, MD, PhD, Lyon, France.)

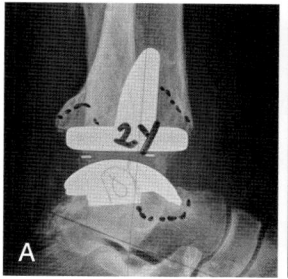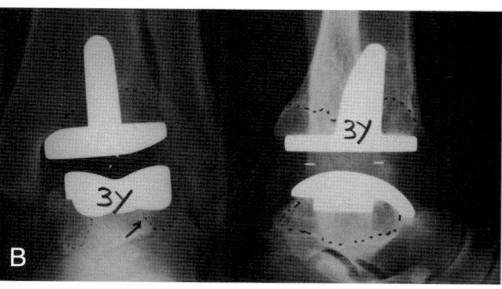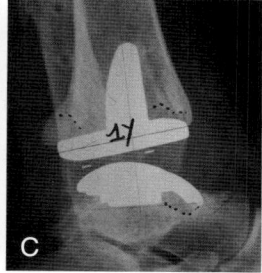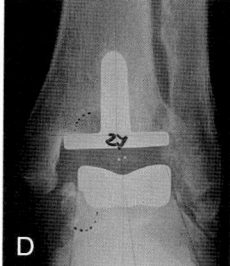

Figure 22-38 Radiographic examples of severe periprosthetic cyst formation and osteolysis 2 years **(A)**, 3 years **(B)**, 1 year **(C)**, and 2 years **(D)** after the initial Ankle Evolutive System prosthesis implantation. (Images courtesy Jean-Luc Besse, MD, PhD, Lyon, France.)

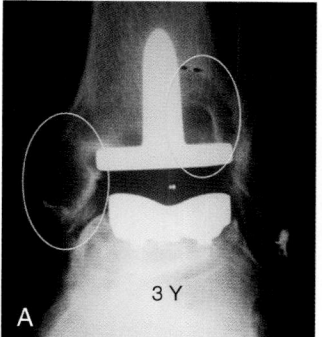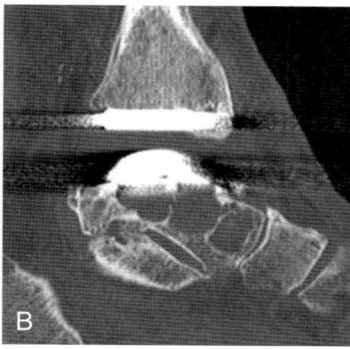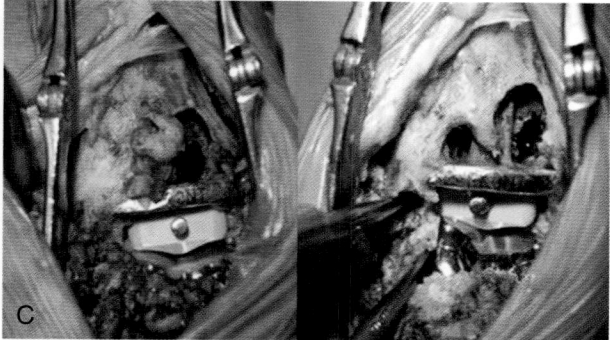

Figure 22-39 **A,** Postoperative anteroposterior radiograph of a 77-year-old male shows large cysts *(yellow ovals)* on the tibial side at the follow-up of 3 years. **B,** Computed tomography scan additionally shows large osteolysis on the talar side. **C,** All granulomas were removed and filled with cancellous bone autograft; implants were well fixed. (Images courtesy Jean-Luc Besse, MD, PhD, Lyon, France.)

marked osteolysis, 16 underwent revision surgery, resulting in a revision rate of 15.5% (Fig. 22-41). The contents of the osteolysis cavities were used for microbiologic and histologic analysis. The histologic findings were interpreted as a foreign body reaction. The authors concluded that the use of AES implants should be avoided until the reason for and extent of the osteolysis problem has been solved.[203]

The same working group performed histologic and histochemical analyses of samples of periprosthetic tissues from failed AES implants (Fig. 22-42).[204] The tissue obtained during the revision surgery, after a mean time of 4.2 years, was stained for macrophages, receptor activator of nuclear factor kappa B ligand (RANKL), its receptor RANK, and osteoprotegerin. The findings were compared with control samples. The results of this study showed that the periimplant osteolysis in early AES implant failures seems to be caused by the RANKL-driven chronic foreign body inflammation against necrotic autologous tissues (see Fig. 22-42).[204] Rodriguez et al[281] observed a high frequency of delayed appearance of osteolysis (77%) in 18 ankles replaced with AES prosthesis at the mean follow-up of 3.3 years.[281] Kokkonen et al[205] reported the midterm results of 38 AES implantations carried out between 2003 and 2007. At a mean follow-up of 2.3 years, 89% of all ankle arthroplasties were preserved, resulting in a 2-year survivorship rate of 79% (95% CI, 56%-98%). At the latest radiographic evaluation, radiolucent lines or osteolysis were detected in 11 (100%) hydroxylapatite (HA)-coated prostheses and in 19 (74%) dual-coated prostheses. Because of a high frequency of osteolysis in medium-term follow-up, many surgeons have discontinued use of this prosthesis type.[205]

In summary, recent studies of the AES TAR reported a high rate of osteolytic lesions.[33,203,238,281] It is still unclear whether the osteolysis process is a result of failure of the hydroxyapatite coating of the metal components or failure of the mobile bearing. As a result of independently published results showing high osteolysis rates, the AES prosthesis has been withdrawn from the market.[313] The AES prosthesis is a good example showing that despite positive progress in TAR development and increasing acceptance of this surgical procedure as a treatment option in patients with end-stage ankle osteoarthritis, new developments in this area should be carefully analyzed. The most obvious theory for the unacceptable high incidence of osteolysis in patients who underwent AES TAR may be polyethylene wear, third-body wear resulting from a hydroxyapatite coating, and/or the direct interaction of metal particles produced by pathologic stress shielding. Furthermore, the nonanatomic spheric shape of the talar component, which disrespects the natural shape of the

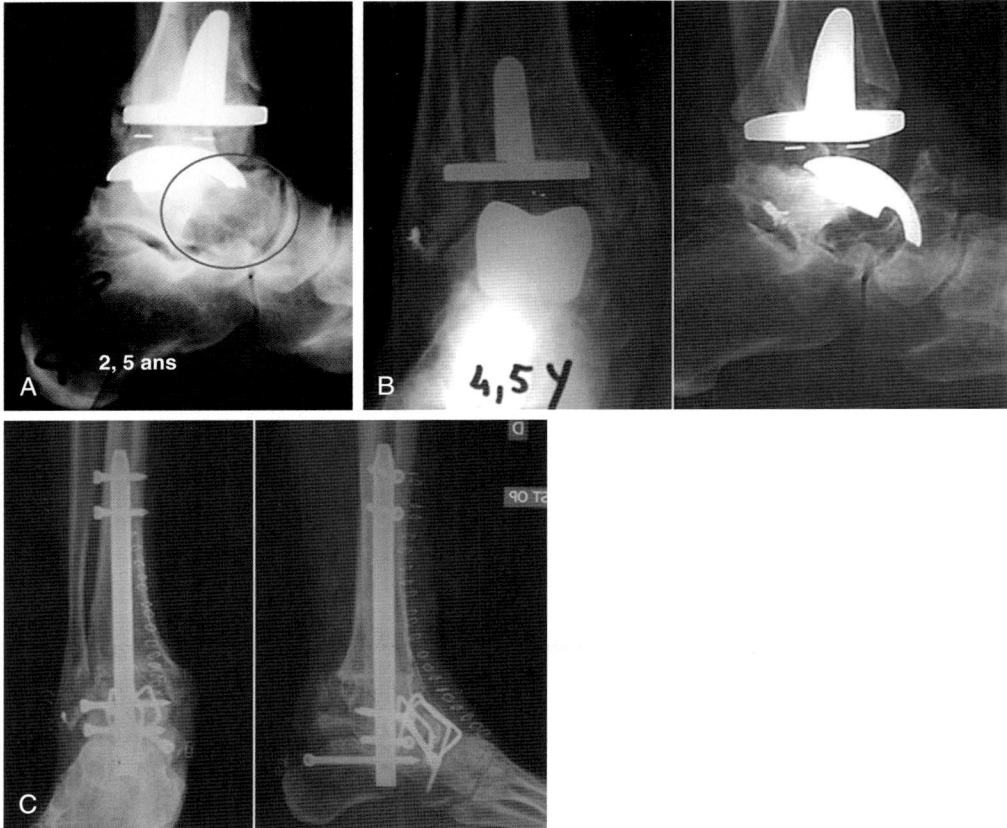

Figure 22-40 A, Postoperative lateral radiograph of 55-year-old male shows cyst formation *(circle)* on the talar side at a follow-up of 2.5 years. The patient was asymptomatic with an American Orthopaedic Foot and Ankle Society (AOFAS) score of 100. **B,** Two years later, mechanical failure with talar implant subsidence occurred; therefore revision by tibiotalocalcaneal arthrodesis with massive bone allograft and autograft plus fixation by intramedullary retrograde nail was performed **(C).** (Images courtesy Jean-Luc Besse, MD, PhD, Lyon, France.)

talus (e.g., two different curve radii) may be responsible for higher rotational and anteroposterior stress on the mobile bearing with respect to the metallic tibial component. Finally, the surgical technique of AES prosthesis required larger bone resection because of the thickness of the tibial component (5 mm), the flat cut on the talar site, and additional anchoring in the talar neck. This cancellous anchorage, in contrast to the subchondral anchorage,[4,170] may result in pathologically increased wear-particle migration.[33,383] In conclusion, it seems that complex interactions of different factors have led to a high incidence of periprosthetic osteolysis with catastrophic clinical and radiographic results resulting in the cessation of using this prosthesis.

BOX Total Ankle Replacement

The Bologna-Oxford (BOX) TAR was developed in the late 1990s by Leardini et al.[216] This prosthesis is a three-component implant with metal components fixed to the proximal talus and the distal tibia and an interposed UHMWPE meniscal bearing. The biomechanical development of this prosthesis type has been well documented in the literature by its designers.[215,216,273] In 2001,

Leardini[215] developed a geometric model of the intact human ankle complex that established the basic principles for design of new total ankle prostheses. Seven lower-leg specimens were prepared for passive non–weight-bearing flexion analysis using a stereophotogrammetric system. It was shown that the geometry of the articular surface of the ankle is strictly related to that of the ligaments (Fig. 22-43). Therefore the author stated that the ideal TAR design should be based on ligament/shape compatibility, and the careful reconstruction of ligaments should be performed in any foot/ankle surgery to recreate the normal kinematics and mechanics of the ankle.[215] In 2004, Leardini et al[216] described the BOX TAR design and rationale, including compatibility to the physiologic function of surrounding ligaments. The designers hoped to reproduce physiologic ankle mobility with the following design features: a spheric convex tibial component, a talar component with a radius of curvature in the sagittal plane longer than that of the natural talus, and a fully conforming meniscal bearing.

Preliminary results from their study of two female patients demonstrated the feasibility of their surgical technique.[216] Reggiani et al[273] developed a finite-element

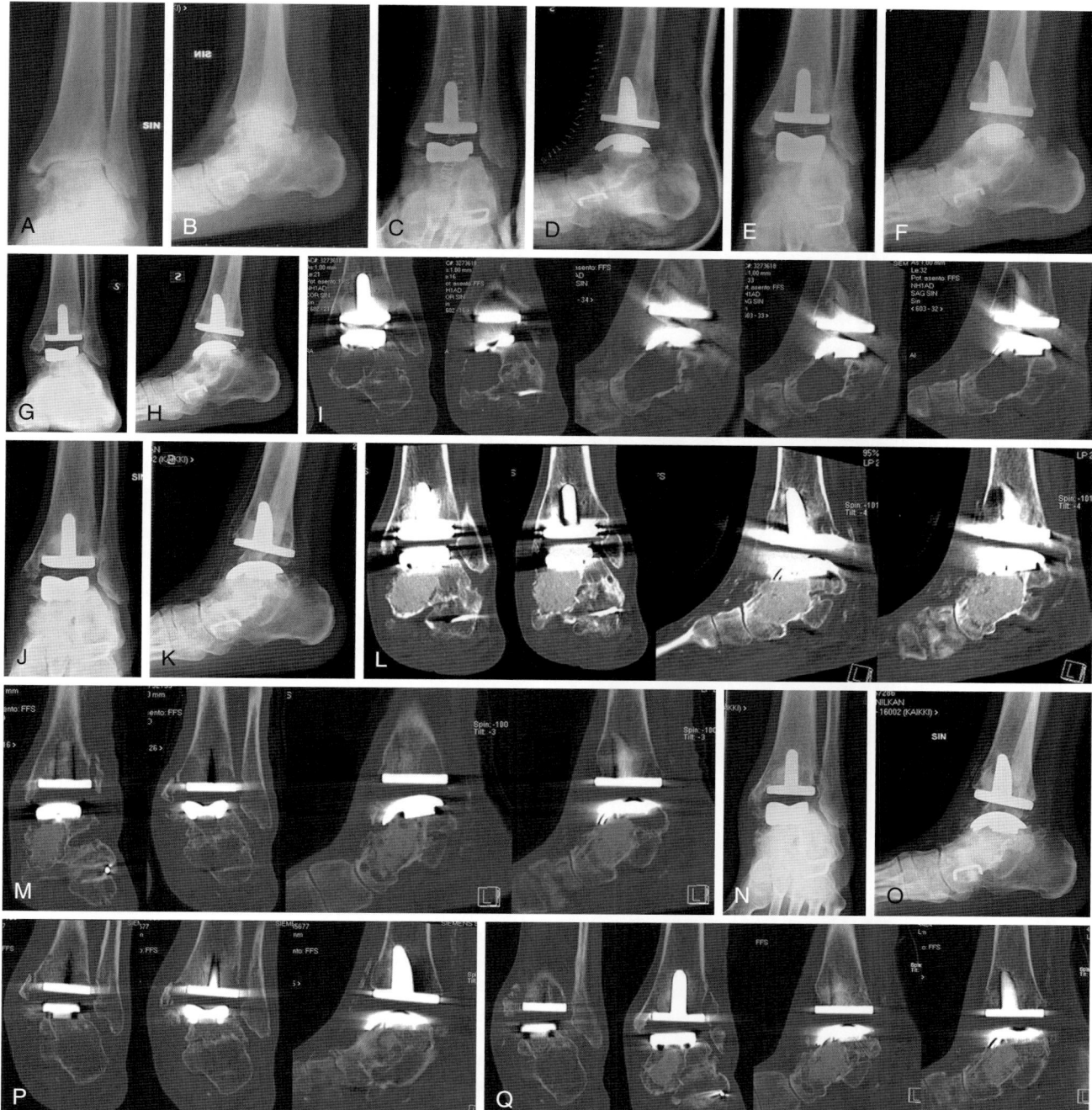

Figure 22-41 Preoperative anteroposterior **(A)** and lateral **(B)** radiographs of a 67-year-old male suffering from rheumatoid arthritis for 21 years. Previously, subtalar fusion was performed because of painful subtalar arthritis. Medications included methotrexate and folic acid. **C** and **D,** Regular Ankle Evolutive System prosthesis has been used. One year after total ankle replacement (TAR), anteroposterior **(E)** and lateral **(F)** radiographs showed proper position and osseous integration of both prosthetic components, with no evidence of loosening or osteolysis. Patient had no pain and good clinical results, including range of motion of 45 degrees. **G** and **H,** One year later (22 months after initial surgery), osteolysis underneath the talar component was visible for the first time; however, the patient had no pain. **I,** One year later (34 months after initial surgery), a computed tomography (CT) scan was performed, showing large cavities, especially under the talar component. **J** and **K,** Thirty-eight months after TAR, a revision surgery was performed: debridement of cavities and filling with allogenic bone. Both prosthesis components were intraoperatively stable. Periprosthetic tissues were used for immunohistopathologic analysis (see Fig. 22-42). **L,** A one-year control CT scan was performed. **M,** Two years later, a CT scan was performed, showing new cavities in the posterior part of the tibia and talus. **O** and **N,** A second revision was performed (26 and 64 months after the first revision surgery and initial TAR, respectively). **P,** Two months later, a control CT scan was performed. **Q,** The last CT scan was performed 1 year after the second revision surgery. The patient has been asymptomatic and painfree all the time, regardless of large cavities. (Images courtesy Helka Koivu, MD, Turku, Finland.)

1121

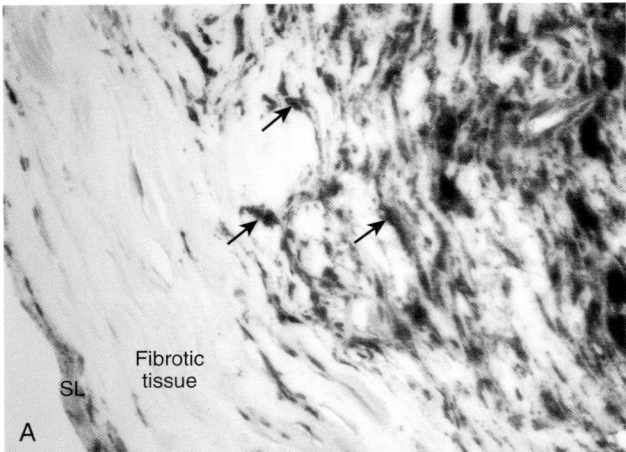

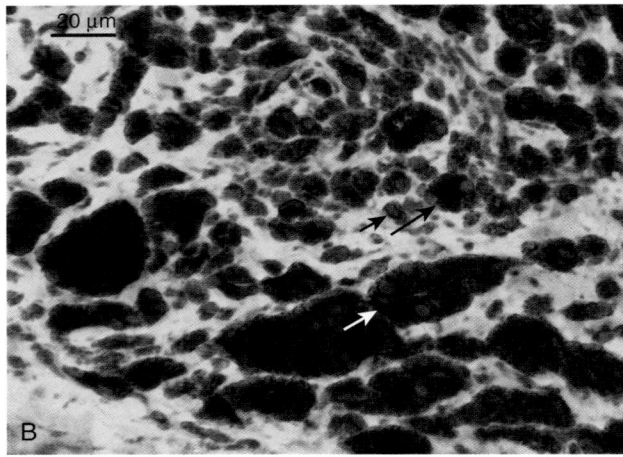

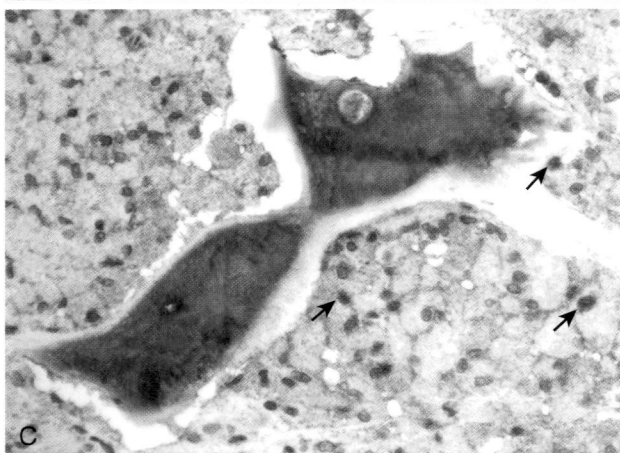

Figure 22-42 Immunohistopathologic analysis of the periprosthetic tissues obtained at implant revision in a 71-year-old male (radiographs in Fig. 22-41). **A,** CD163 in this microphotograph is a monocyte and macrophage scavenger receptor, belonging to the scavenger receptor cysteine-rich (SRCR)-family. CD163 has been stained brown using the avidin-biotin-peroxidase complex staining method. This image of the interface membrane surrounding a loosened total ankle replacement implant shows macrophage-like cells in a lining-like layer to the lower left surrounding layer *(SL)* and below it a capsule of fibrotic tissue with several aligned CD163-negative fibroblast-like cells. This fibrous tissue zone surrounds a macrophage-like cell-rich core, containing many CD163+ macrophages (some of which are marked with *short arrows*). **B,** RANK is a receptor activator of nuclear factor kappa B, which is capable of binding the RANK-ligand (RANKL). Many RANK immunoreactive mononuclear *(short arrow)*, binuclear *(long arrow)*, and multinuclear cells (foreign body giant cells, *white arrow*) are shown in this image in different stages of fusion. This indicates an ongoing chronic foreign body reaction. Avidin-biotin-peroxidase complex staining was used. **C,** RANKL is expressed in the spindle-shaped mesenchymal cells (some of which are marked with *short arrows*) in the interface membrane, with a necrotic piece of bone embedded in it, around a loosening total ankle replacement implant. Avidin-biotin-peroxidase complex staining was used. All micrographs were taken at the same magnification, with the scale bar indicating 20 μm. (Images courtesy Helka Koivu, MD, Turku, Finland.)

wear of the BOX TAR mobile bearing. The knee-wear simulator was able to reproduce load-motion patterns comparable to those of a replaced ankle. Tests of three specimens showed a linear penetration of 0.0178, 0.0081, and 0.0339 mm per million-cycle, respectively. The linear penetration observed in this study was comparable to that found in ceramic-to-polyethylene or metal-to-polyethylene couplings.[2] Two years later, Affatato et al[3] performed a comparative study of wear behavior in the BOX TAR between an in vitro simulation and retrieved prostheses. Three retrieved mobile bearings were available from revision surgeries performed 24, 24, and 9 months, respectively, after the initial total ankle implantation. Visual and microscopic observations, analyses, and Raman crystallinity-based measurements showed a similarity between the patterns generated experimentally using a four-station knee-joint simulator and those seen in retrievals with similar wear duration.[3] Ingrosso et al[171] performed gait analysis in patients with BOX ankle arthroplasties by using a stereophotogrammetric system with eight M2-cameras. The study included 10 patients, with a follow-up of 6 and 12 months after the surgery. Normal kinematics and range of motion were observed in all 10 patients at both follow-ups.[171]

Giannini et al[115] presented short-term results in 51 patients who were treated with a BOX total ankle arthroplasty (Fig. 22-44 to 22-45). The minimum follow-up in this study was 2 years. All patients showed significant functional improvement as assessed by the AOFAS score.

model to address the BOX TAR analysis during the stance phase of gait. Overall kinematics, contact pressures, and ligament forces were analyzed during both passive (e.g., virtually unloaded) and active (e.g., stance phase of gait) conditions. The authors showed that this prosthesis design was able to allow the necessary ROM and to constrain the motion of the prosthetic components, especially the mobile bearing.[273] Affatato et al[2] have used a four-station knee-joint simulator to address meniscal

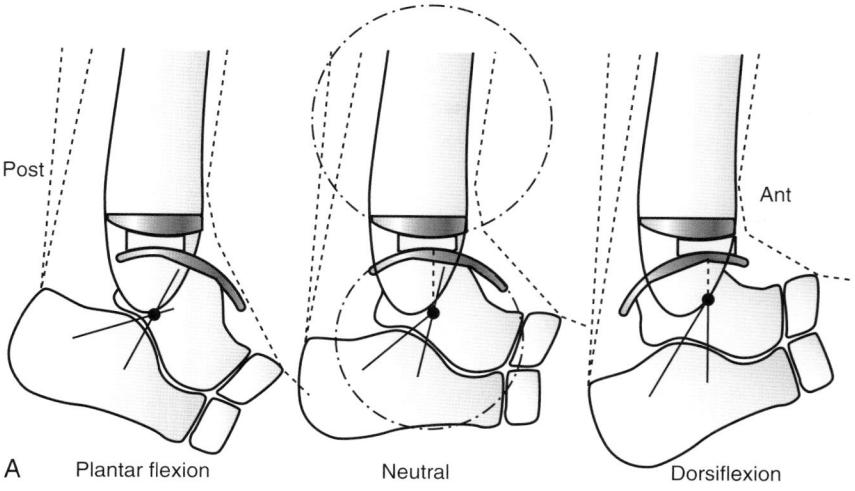

Post

Ant

A Plantar flexion   Neutral   Dorsiflexion

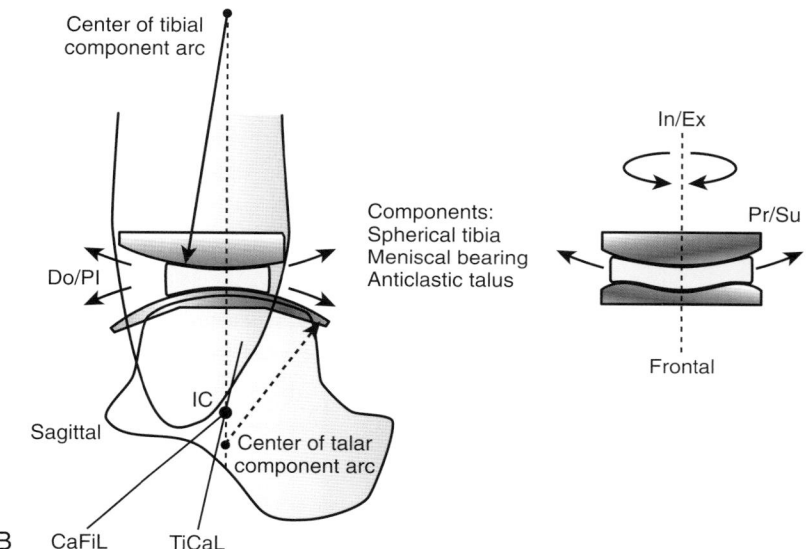

Center of tibial
component arc

In/Ex

Components:
Spherical tibia
Meniscal bearing
Anticlastic talus

Pr/Su

Do/Pl

Frontal

Sagittal

IC

Center of talar
component arc

B CaFiL   TiCaL

Figure 22-43 Bologna-Oxford (BOX) ankle is a three-part implant. **A,** Model-based diagram of the mobility of the replaced ankle in the sagittal plane. **B,** Three-part ankle replacement system including metal components fixed to the proximal talus and the distal tibia and an interposed ultrahigh-molecular-weight polyethylene meniscal bearing. **C,** Motion of the meniscal bearing in plantar flexion *(upper row)* and in dorsiflexion *(lower row)* as shown schematically *(left),* clinically *(middle),* and radiographically *(right). Ant,* anterior; *CaFiL,* calcaneofibular ligament; *Do,* dorsiflexion; *IC,* instantaneous center of rotation; *In/Ex,* internal and external rotation; *Max,* maximum; *Post,* posterior; *Pr/Su,* pronation and supination; *TiCaL,* tibiocalcaneal ligament. (Images courtesy Alberto Leardini, PhD, and Sandro Giannini, MD, Bologna, Italy.)

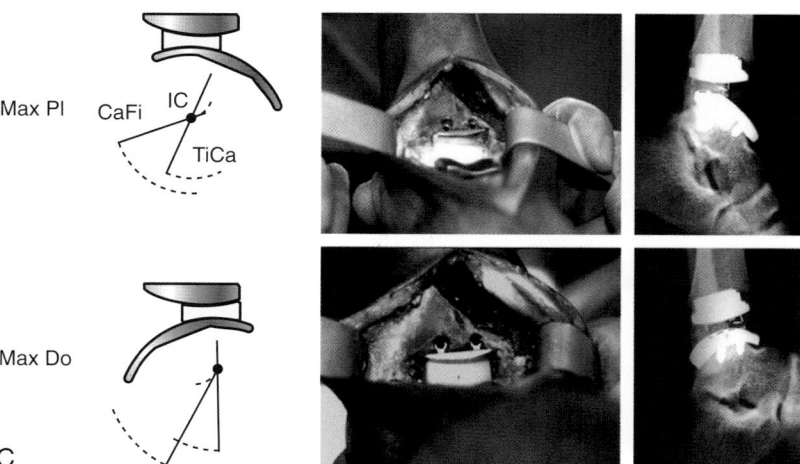

Max Pl   CaFi   IC
                  TiCa

Max Do

C

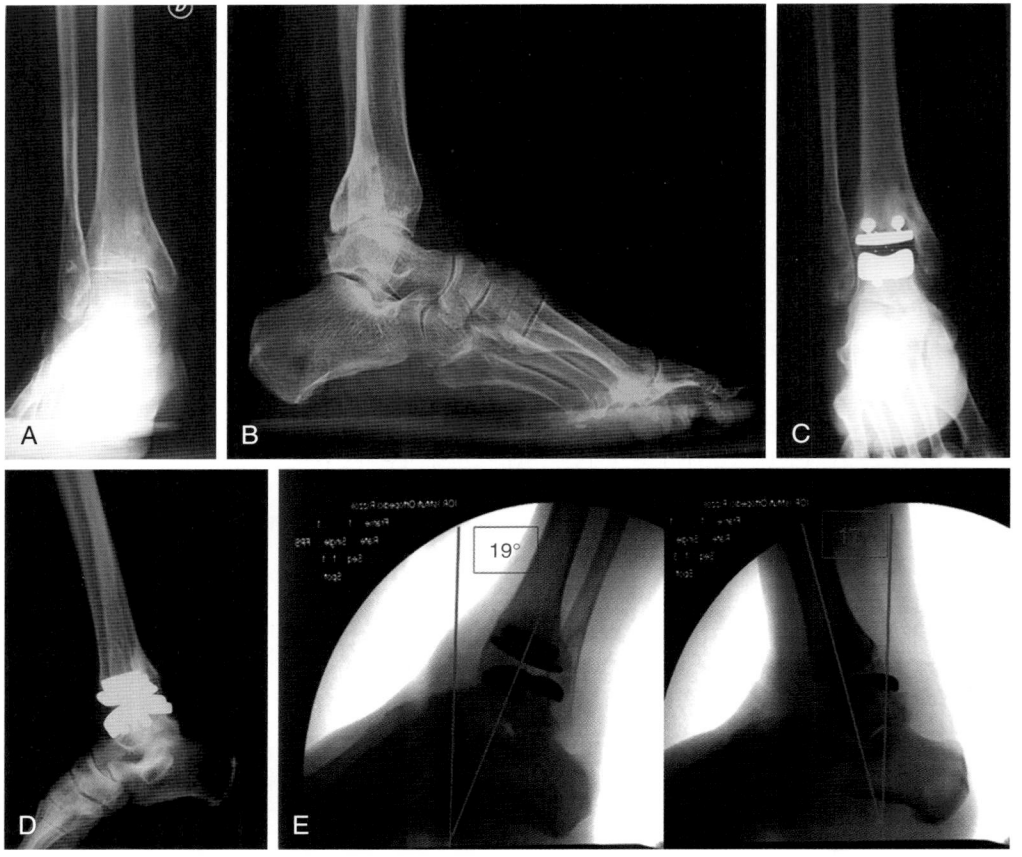

Figure 22-44 Preoperative anteroposterior **(A)** and lateral **(B)** radiographs of a 59-year-old female suffering from end-stage ankle osteoarthritis. Postoperative anteroposterior **(C)** and lateral **(D)** radiographs show proper position and osseous integration of both prosthetic components at the follow-up of 5 years. **E,** Good functional results, including ankle range of motion of 36 degrees were observed. (Images courtesy Sandro Giannini, MD, Bologna, Italy.)

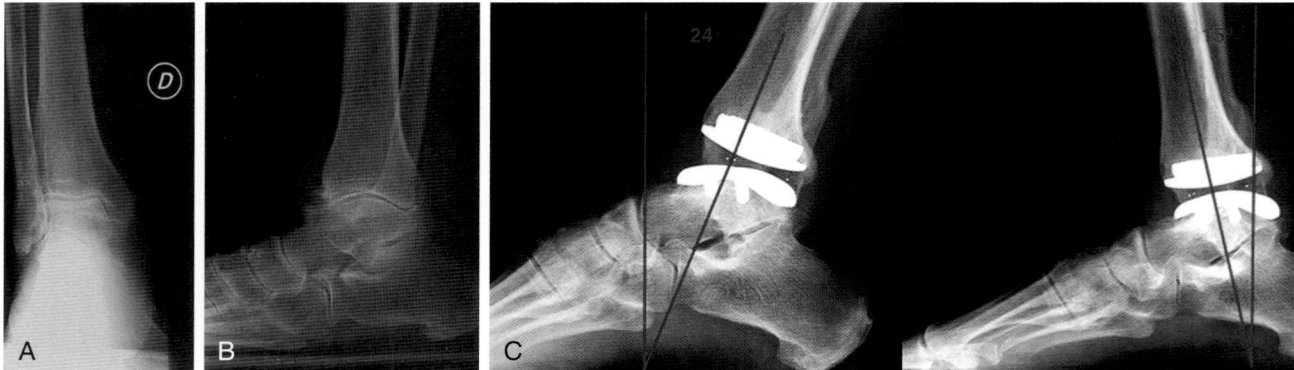

Figure 22-45 Preoperative anteroposterior **(A)** and lateral **(B)** radiographs of a 38-year-old male suffering from end-stage ankle osteoarthritis. **C,** Postoperative radiographs show proper position and osseous integration of both prosthetic components and good functional results, including ankle range of motion of 39 degrees at a follow-up of 4 years. (Images courtesy Sandro Giannini, MD, Bologna, Italy.)

In 1 patient, a revision arthroplasty had to be performed because of lateral impingement, resulting in a 3-year cumulative survivorship of 97%.[115] The main indication for this procedure was stage III ankle osteoarthritis (with subtotal or total disappearance or deformation of joint space) with preserved or restored ankle anatomy.[112] In a multicenter study including 156 patients with 158 BOX ankle arthroplasties, promising clinical results were observed at a mean follow-up of 1.4 years.[114] Two revisions and seven further second surgeries were performed.[114]

Bianchi et al[35] retrospectively reviewed 60 consecutive patients who underwent 62 ankle arthroplasties using BOX implants between 2004 and 2008. No patient was lost to the mean follow-up of 3.5 years. The overall 3.5-year survivorship was 91.9%. Radiolucencies of more than 2 mm were seen around tibial and talar components in 16 and 4 ankles, respectively. A significant functional improvement was observed at the latest follow-up, resulting in a high patient satisfaction rate of 78.3%.[35]

Cenni et al[58] addressed the position of BOX prosthesis component in 14 patients and its effect on motion at the replaced joint. Radiographs of the ankle were taken in static double-leg stance at 7 and 13 months postoperatively. The mean range of motion was about 34 degrees at both follow-ups. A weak correlation was observed between motion at the replaced ankle and possible residual subluxation and inclination of the components.[58] The same working group performed in vivo fluoroscopic analysis of kinematics in 12 patients who underwent BOX TAR.[57] A series of images were acquired by videofluoroscopy at 6, 12, and 24 months follow-up. Motion between the three components was calculated and subsequently analyzed. Over the three follow-ups, the flexion/extension range of motion was 17.6, 17.7, and 16.2 degrees, respectively. The corresponding anterior–posterior translation of the polyethylene insert with respect to the tibial component was 3.3, 3.3, and 3.2 mm, respectively, with statistically significant correlation with joint flexion.[57]

In summary, the design process and biomechanical properties of the BOX TAR have been documented in detail.[215,216,273] Also, studies addressing the wear behavior of this prosthesis design have significantly contributed to the understanding of modern three-part prostheses.[2,3] The short-term results are promising, with high satisfaction among treated patients, good functional results, and a low revision rate.[115] However, most of the aforementioned studies were performed by one of the designers of this prosthesis; therefore further study by independent groups should be performed.

ESKA Ankle Prosthesis

The ESKA ankle (ESKA Orthodynamics, Lubeck, Germany) is a two-component prosthesis designed between 1985 and 1989 for cementless implantation.[285,287] The following features were included to improve biomechanics of the replaced ankle: cementless implantation and porous-structured implant surface for faster osteointegration, shear force reduction by shape design of both metallic components, and easy replacement of the polyethylene insert without disturbing prosthesis anchoring.[285,287] Because of the ridge-like shaping and its transverse anchoring peg in both metallic components, a lateral or, in special cases, medial malleolar approach has to be used for implantation.[285] In 2001, the designer published short-term results of 56 patients treated with the ESKA prosthesis since 1990.[286] Forty of 56 patients were reviewed at a minimum follow-up of 1 year. All patients experienced significant pain relief and showed functional improvement as assessed by the Kofoed ankle score. In two cases, deep infection led to prosthesis removal and conversion to ankle fusion. Another patient showed painful progressive ossification of the joint capsule, resulting in ankle fusion.[286] The same patient cohort was again reviewed at a longer follow-up, and the results were published in another two studies.[285,287] The authors reported a significant improvement of the Kofoed ankle score from 37.6 points preoperatively to 90.4 points postoperatively.[287]

In summary, the limited studies performed by ESKA prosthesis designers reported favorable midterm results with improved ankle range of motion, pain relief, and ability to walk long distances postoperatively.[285-287] However, the authors stated that this surgery should be limited to only highly experienced foot and ankle surgeons because of the lateral approach. As with the BOX TAR, published results have come from only the prosthesis designers. Thus additional, independent analyses of ESKA efficacy should be completed.

German Ankle System

The German Ankle System is a three-component prosthesis allowing rotation around each of the three possible movement axes (Fig. 22-46).[277]

The talar component of this prosthesis includes side borders to keep the mobile bearing in position, which may prevent inlay dislocation. Both metallic components have a BONIT coating (a porous coating with a titanium plasma sprayed surface and an additional layer of calcium phosphate) to encourage osteointegration. The system includes an option for computer-assisted implantation surgery. Richter et al[277] performed the robotic-guided surgical approach on a cadaver and compared the results with those obtained using a HINTEGRA prosthesis (Fig. 22-47).

The authors found that the German ankle prosthesis had a smaller effect on resulting forces and torques during partial weight-bearing passive ankle motion than the HINTEGRA prosthesis.[277] However, to date, this prosthesis type has not received clinical approval.

Alphanorm Total Ankle Replacement

The Alphanorm TAR was developed by Tilmann in Germany and has been used since 1996.[334] The Alphanorm prosthesis is a nonconstrained Buechel-Pappas–type design with a 90-degree tibial stem without inclination.[121] Before developing the Alphanorm TAR for use, the designer had experience with the TRP prosthesis, New Jersey prosthesis, and STAR prosthesis between 1976 and 1998.[335] To date, there are no studies available addressing clinical outcomes or the surgical technique of the Alphanorm TAR.

TARIC Total Ankle Replacement

The TARIC TAR was developed by Schill in Germany and has been used since 2006.[303] The TARIC prosthesis has a

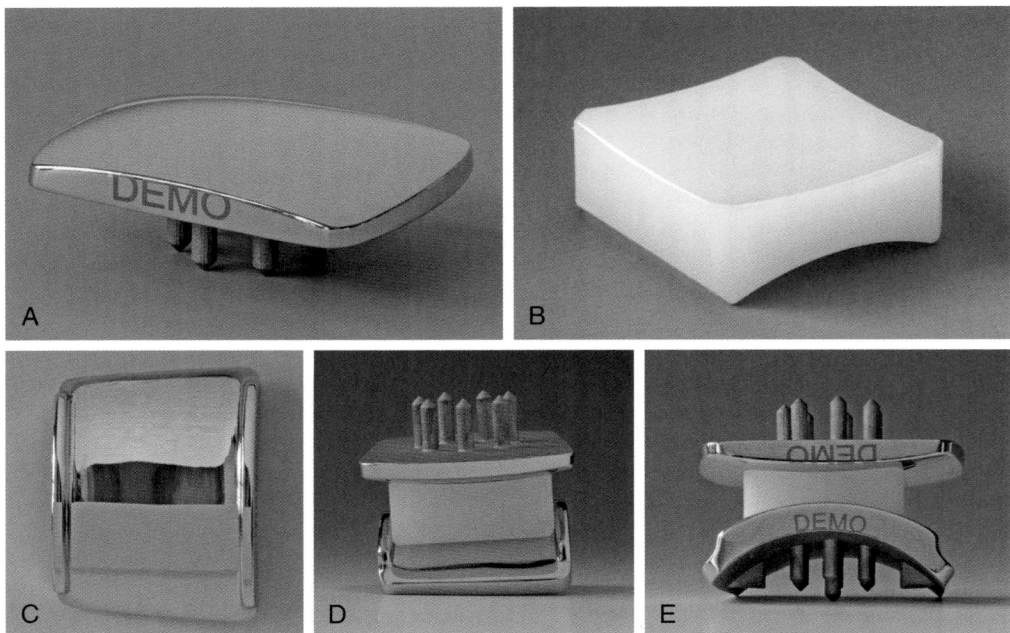

Figure 22-46 German Ankle System (R-Innovation, Coburg, Germany). **A,** Tibial component. **B,** Mobile bearing. **C,** Talar component. **D,** Three-component prosthesis anterior view. **E,** Three-component prosthesis lateral view. (Images courtesy Martinus Richter, MD, PhD, Schwarzenbruck, Germany.)

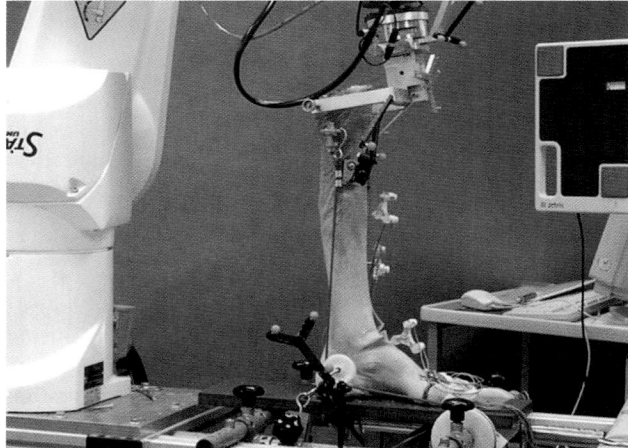

Figure 22-47 Robotic testing with robot (RX 90, Stäubli Tec-Systems, Bayreuth, Germany), ankle specimen, and motion analysis system. Specimen is mounted on the robot and footplate. Triaxial transducers of the motion analysis system were fixed to the foot plate and to the specimen. (Image courtesy Martinus Richter, MD, PhD, Schwarzenbruck, Germany.)

titanium coating and is optionally available with an additional hydroxyapatite coating. The tibial component has two fixation pegs.[121] Before creating the TARIC TAR, the designer had experience with the TRP and STAR prostheses.[302] Currently, there are no studies available addressing clinical outcomes or the surgical technique of the TARIC TAR.

INBONE Total Ankle Replacement (Video Clip 17)

The INBONE TAR is a modular, fixed-bearing, two-component total ankle system (Fig. 22-48).[72,84] It was designed by Dr. Mark Reiley and engineered by Garret Mauldin.[81] The polyethylene insert is available in different sizes, from 7 to 15 mm, and is locked into the tibial component as a two-component TAR design. The surgical technique of this prosthesis uses an intramedullary fluoroscopic guidance.[81] A special feature of this ankle design is a modular stem system for both metallic components. The tibial stem has the ability to be extended by adding additional modular segments. The stem of the talar component may be short and limited to the talar body. However, in cases where subtalar fusion has to be performed or for greater stability, the talar stem may be extended across the subtalar joint.

To date, there are limited reports in the literature reporting clinical and radiographic outcomes in patients who received INBONE TAR.[274,275] The designer team for the prosthesis has performed more than 240 INBONE ankle arthroplasties, and data have been collected in preparation for publication (Fig. 22-49 and 22-50).[94] DeOrio[81-83] described the surgical technique using INBONE total ankle arthroplasty, including his strategies on how to address the concomitant lower-leg deformities and degenerative changes of the subtalar joint. Furthermore, the following contraindications for TAR using INBONE prosthesis were mentioned, including patients with poor vascular supply, poor skin, neuropathy, and complete avascular necrosis of the talus.[81] Devries et al[86] reported the use of INBONE TAR as revision arthroplasty

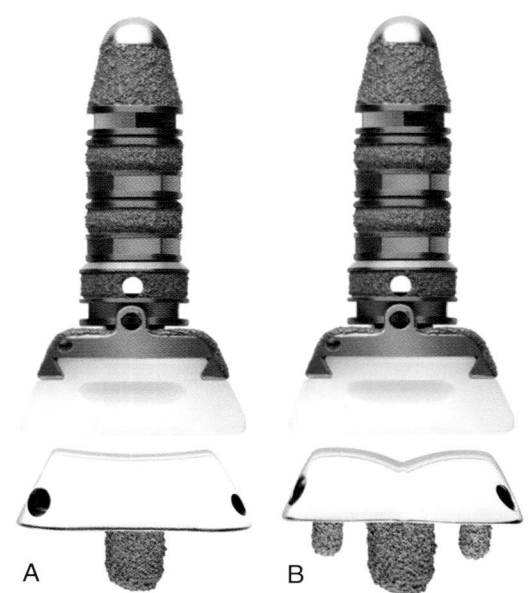

Figure 22-48 A, First generation of the INBONE prosthesis—a modular, fixed-bearing, two-component total ankle system. **B,** Second generation of the INBONE prosthesis (INBONE II) with some modifications of the talar component—a new optional talar sulcus prosthesis with a matching polyethylene component for better stability in the coronal plane.

in five patients with failed Agility ankle arthroplasties. At a mean follow-up of 1.4 years, three patients required secondary surgery, including one patient with transtibial amputation and one patient with tibiotalocalcaneal arthrodesis.[86]

Two new versions of this basic design have recently been introduced. The bearing surface has been changed to a more constrained geometry (INBONE II) (Fig. 22-51). In addition, a patient-specific surgical jig system based on CT data is used. To date, there is only limited information addressing clinical results in patients who underwent INBONE TAR. There are also no biomechanical studies available that address the kinematics and biomechanical properties of this prosthesis design.

Trabecular Metal Total Ankle (Video Clip 19)

The "Trabecular Metal" Total Ankle, introduced in 2012, is the most recent design of a lateral approach total ankle replacement. The device was developed by Drs. Chris Chiodo, Jonathan Deland, Sandro Giannini, Steve Herbst, Johnny Lau, Charles Saltzman, and Lew Schon. The engineering of the device was led by Drs. Al Burstein, Brent Parks, Yuki Tochigi, Thomas Baer, and Duane Gillard. Like some predecessors (St. George and ESKA), this device uses a transfibular lateral approach, with some distinct differences. The device is intended to reduce wound healing risks associated with anterior approaches to the ankle.

The device uses a two-piece, semiconstrained construct (Fig. 22-52). The bone-apposing surfaces of the device use Trabecular Metal material (tantalum porous structure)

and are curved to increase surface area. This curved design aligns the implant to the stress patterns evident in the trabecular architecture of the talus, thereby offering the potential for the joint reaction forces to be better aligned to the bone in hope of reducing subsidence in the talus. Stabilization rails are oriented mediolaterally to allow implant insertion from the lateral side and are designed to provide an interference fit relative to the prepared bone, orthogonal to the primary direction of the implant gliding motion, to aid in stability.

The talar component is bicondylar and designed in site-specific orientations, using a conical articulation with a larger lateral condylar sagittal radius of curvature. The articular radii of curvature increases with each increase in the size of the product, thus intending to mimic the natural ankle architecture. Similarly, anteroposterior coverage and mediolateral (ML) width also increase with each increase in size. The articular is manufactured from a cobalt-chromium (CoCr) alloy diffusion bonded to Trabecular Metal via a titanium substrate. The tibial component is designed to be used in either left or right operative sites and is made from Ti6Al4Nb (titanium + aluminum + niobium) alloy diffusion-bonded to Trabecular Metal material. The bearing surface comprises highly cross-linked polyethylene and is assembled to the tibial base at the time of surgery. The highly cross-linked polyethylene is intended to enhance longevity of the bearing material by reducing free radicals in the polyethylene chains so as to resist subsurface fatigue, delamination, and volumetric wear.

The surgical technique uses a standard transfibular approach that is similar to classic approaches for ankle fusion (Fig. 22-53). The patient is then assessed to determine the largest size that can be implanted without a lateral overhang of the implant. Once the size is determined, the patient is placed into the system alignment and fixation frame. The principle of this alignment frame is to ensure that the bone resection is perpendicular to the mechanical axis of the tibia and parallel to the floor of a plantigrade foot. The foot is placed into a translucent foot plate, with the foot placed in a neutral position. The tibia is rotated internally such that the tibial tubercle is vertical. The alignment of the foot is then determined by placing the foot in a position such that the medial gutter is at an angle of 5 to 10 degrees internal from vertical. With this confirmed, the foot is fixed to the alignment frame with a transcalcaneal pin and a half-pin into the talar neck. The tibia is aligned such that the tibial crest is parallel to alignment rods in the sagittal view. The coronal alignment is achieved using fluoroscopy to confirm that the lateral border of the tibia is parallel to an alignment rod in the frame. Once aligned, the tibia is fixed to the frame using external fixation pins.

With the patient fixed to the frame, the bone resection is performed using a pivoting cutting guide and burr driven by a medium-speed burr. This pivot is positioned at the lateral center of rotation before resection. This allows the curved bone-apposing surfaces of the implant

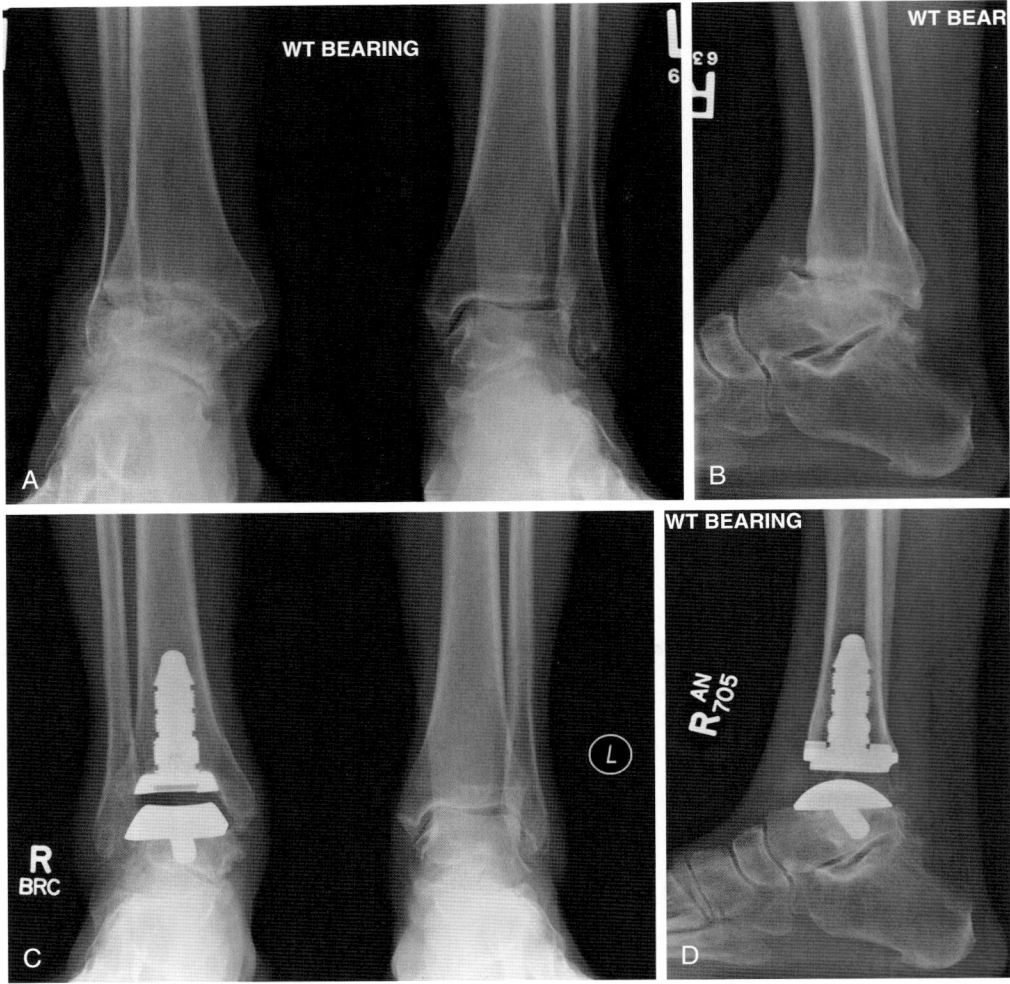

Figure 22-49 Preoperative anteroposterior **(A)** and lateral **(B)** radiographs of a 63-year-old male suffering from end-stage ankle osteoarthritis. Note severe anterior subluxation of the tibiotalar joint. The first generation of the INBONE prosthesis was used. Postoperative anteroposterior **(C)** and lateral **(D)** radiographs show proper position and osseous integration of both prosthetic components at the follow-up of 2 years and 5 months. *WT,* weight. (Images courtesy James K. DeOrio, MD, Durham, N.C.)

to be precisely prepared in the bone. Rail holes are then drilled to establish the proper position for the implant from AP, ML and axial perspectives. Provisional implants are then used to determine the appropriate polyethylene thickness by assessing the range of motion achieved and by application of a valgus stress to assess deltoid engagement. If laxity is noted in the deltoid, a thicker component is used. Implants are then inserted from the lateral side until reaching a stop depth determined by the stabilization rails, which is confirmed via fluoroscopy. If appropriate, for additional primary stability, methyl methacrylate can be inserted between the stabilization rails and the host bone without lifting the implant surface off the bone.

With the implants in their final position, external fixation pins are removed, and the frame is removed from the operative site. Fibular repair is then performed, with the fibular length adjusted based on CFL engagement. Once the position is established, the fibula is repaired using internal fixation plating. The ATFL is then repaired and

followed by an external rotation stress test of the ankle joint to assess any syndesmotic diastasis requiring repair. The wounds are then closed in a routine fashion. Weight bearing is progressed over the first 6 to 8 weeks.

Learning Curve in Total Ankle Replacement

A learning curve affects all new procedures, and TAR is not immune to this worry. To date, numerous clinical studies have demonstrated a steep learning curve associated with performing TAR. Intraoperative complications are common and include medial and/or lateral malleolar fractures, laceration to the tendons (posterior tibial tendon, flexor digitorum/hallucis longus), and nerve injures (deep/superficial peroneal nerve).[217,244,292,306] The influence of surgeon experience on complication rates in patients receiving the Agility prosthesis was examined by Saltzman et al.[292] The number of minor and major complications was worrisome. In a further study from nine contributing surgeons who documented complications in

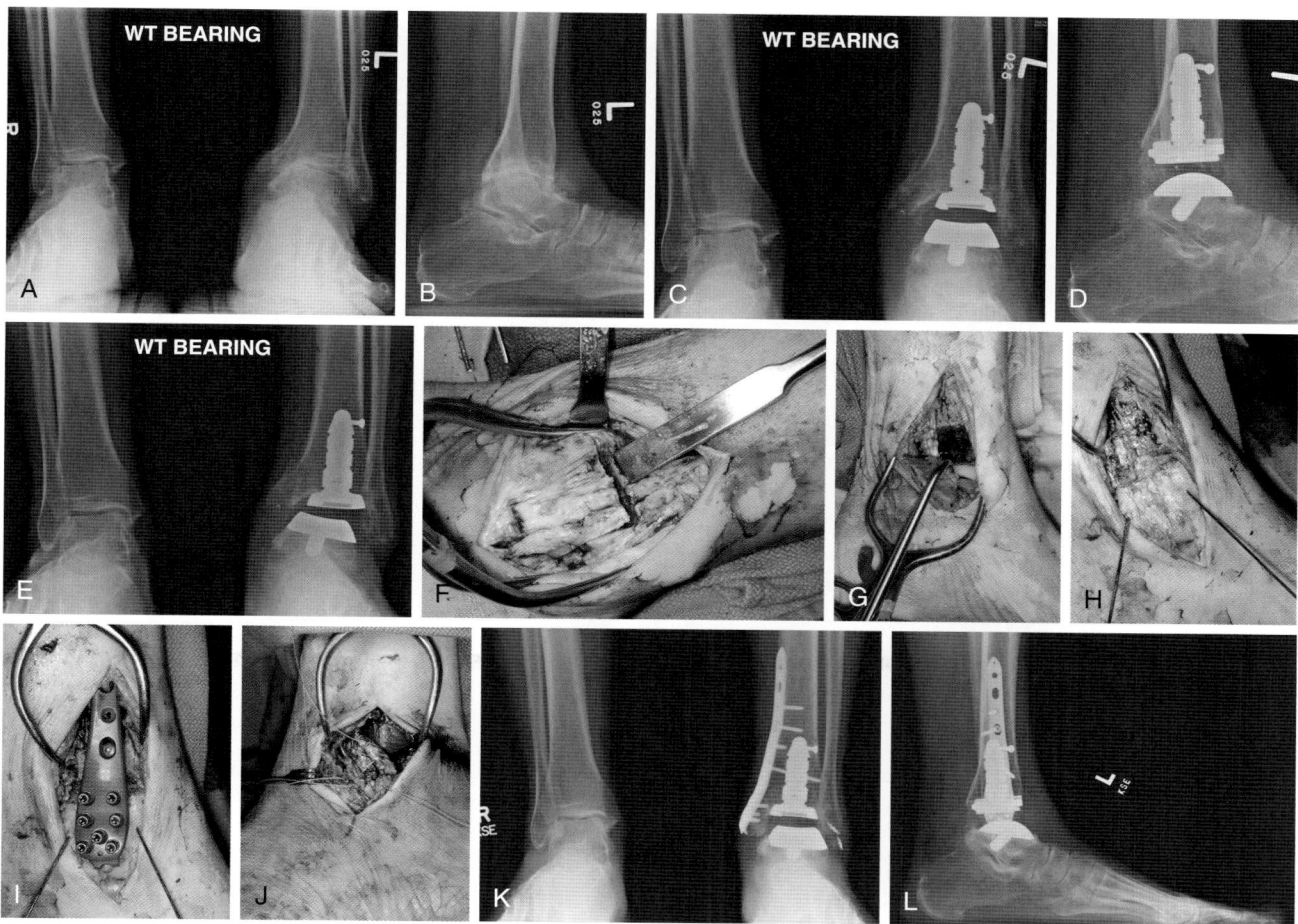

Figure 22-50 Preoperative anteroposterior **(A)** and lateral **(B)** radiographs of a 63-year-old male suffering from end-stage ankle osteoarthritis with "horizontal medial malleolus" (term coined by Dr. DeOrio). The first generation of the INBONE prosthesis was used. Postoperative anteroposterior **(C)** and lateral **(D)** radiographs show well-aligned prosthesis components at the first follow-up of 6 weeks. **E,** One year after the initial surgery, the talus has slid over to medial malleolus and is in recurrent varus. **F-J,** Patient is minimally uncomfortable; however, because severe wear may occur later, a decision was made to perform revision surgery: medial malleolus osteotomy, iliac crest graft insertion, and plate fixation. **K** and **L,** One year after medial opening-wedge osteotomy of the medial malleolus with iliac crest bone graft and plating, a normally aligned hindfoot and proper position and osseous integration of both prosthetic components were observed. *WT,* weight. (Images courtesy James K. DeOrio, MD, Durham, N.C.)

their first 10 ankle replacements (90 ankles total), these authors reported 19 intraoperative complications and 7 major revision surgeries within 2 years. The authors did not identify any specific training method that would significantly decrease complication rates.[292]

Similar initial findings were reported by Myerson and Mroczek.[244] The authors performed a retrospective radiographic and chart review of 50 arthroplasties performed by the same surgeon using the Agility prosthesis. Patients were divided into two groups based on the surgeon's experience, each including 25 patients. The number of minor wound complications decreased from six in the first group to two in the second group. Also, the number of intraoperative fractures differed and favored the second group (five vs. two fractures). All nerve or tendon lacerations (n = 4) occurred in the first group. Regarding the overall decreased complication rate in the

second group with the subsequent 25 patients, the authors stated that there is a notable learning curve in TAR performance.[244] A similar study with 50 patients who underwent Agility TAR was performed by Schuberth et al.[305] In this study, also, all patients were divided into two 25-patient groups and showed a significantly decreased rate of the following complications: medial and lateral fractures, major revisions, and malpositioning of prosthesis components.[305]

Schutte and Louwerens[306] reported their initial results obtained in 49 patients who received a STAR prosthesis. The following intraoperative complications were observed: six fractures of the medial and two of the lateral malleolus, three fractures of the distal tibia, one injury of the peroneal nerve, and two malpositions of the tibial and two of talar components. Based on these numbers, the authors concluded that TAR should be limited only to

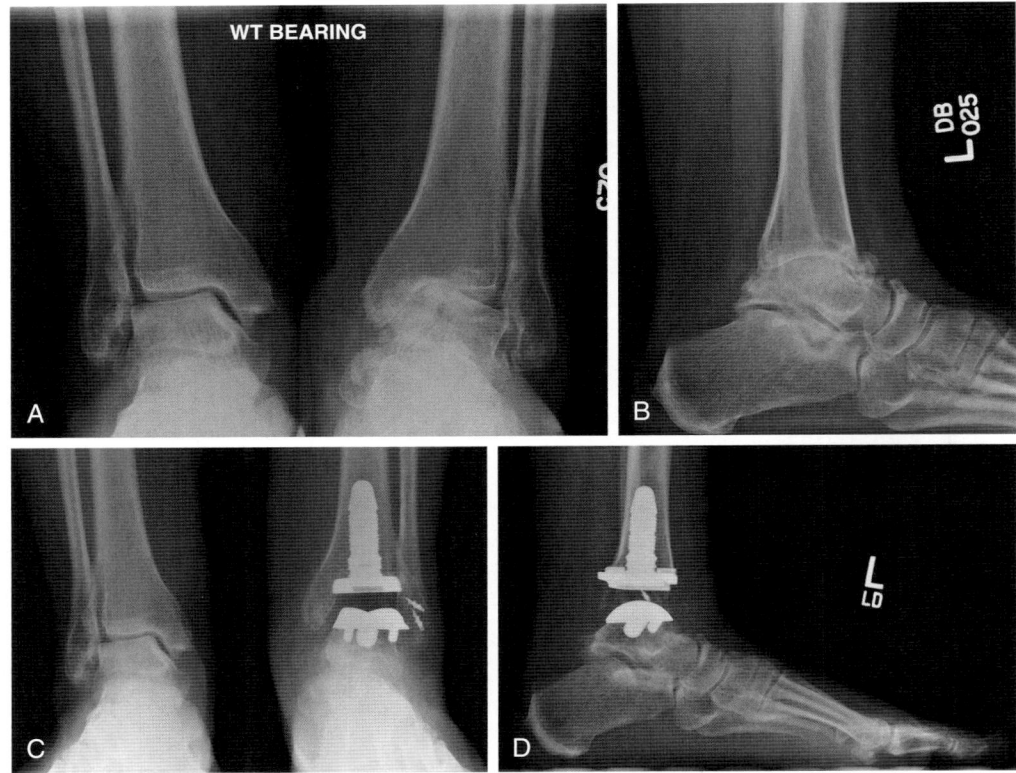

Figure 22-51 Preoperative anteroposterior **(A)** and lateral **(B)** radiographs of a 49-year-old female suffering from end-stage ankle osteoarthritis. The second generation of the INBONE prosthesis was used (INBONE II); in addition, a lateral ligament reconstruction and gastrocnemius recession were performed. Postoperative anteroposterior **(C)** and lateral **(D)** radiographs show proper position and osseous integration of both prosthetic components at the follow-up of 9 months. *WT,* weight. (Images courtesy James K. DeOrio, MD, Durham, N.C.)

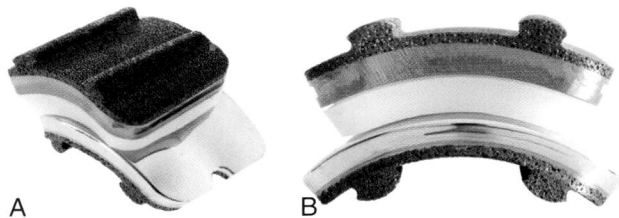

Figure 22-52 Trabecular Metal Total Ankle, a two-part, semiconstrained total ankle construct. **A,** Top view. **B,** Lateral view.

an experienced orthopaedic foot and ankle surgeon.[306] Lee et al[217] addressed the perioperative complications in the 25 initial patients who received the HINTEGRA prosthesis and compared these results with those from the subsequent 25 cases. In the first group, perioperative complications occurred in 60% of cases, while in the second group, only five complications (20%) were observed. All major complications (deep infection and aseptic loosening) occurred in the first group. The rate of minor complications (fractures, minor wound problem, nerve/tendon injuries, and heterotopic ossifications) significantly decreased in the second group. However, the

authors were unable to show a decrease in the number of malpositions of prosthesis components as a result of increased surgeon experience.[217]

The same working group compared the perioperative complications of the HINTEGRA total ankle system with the Mobility total ankle system.[220] The authors did not find any differences in perioperative complications between the two total ankle systems, but medial malleolar fractures did occur more frequently when using the Mobility prosthesis.[220] Reuver et al[276] addressed short-term results of TAR performed in low-volume centers. In total, 64 total ankle arthroplasties were performed using Salto implants between 2003 and 2007 at four low-volume centers. Fifty-five patients (59 ankles) were reviewed at a mean follow-up of 36 months. Seven ankles had to undergo revision surgery: two revision arthroplasties and five fusions because of loosening, and two cases of deep infection, resulting in a survivorship of 86% at the final follow-up. Significant pain relief and functional improvement were observed in this review as assessed by the VAS and AOFAS scores. The authors were confident that results of TAR performed in low-volume centers are comparable to most high-volume centers. However, the survival of implanted components was significantly lower, especially regarding the relatively short follow-up.[276]

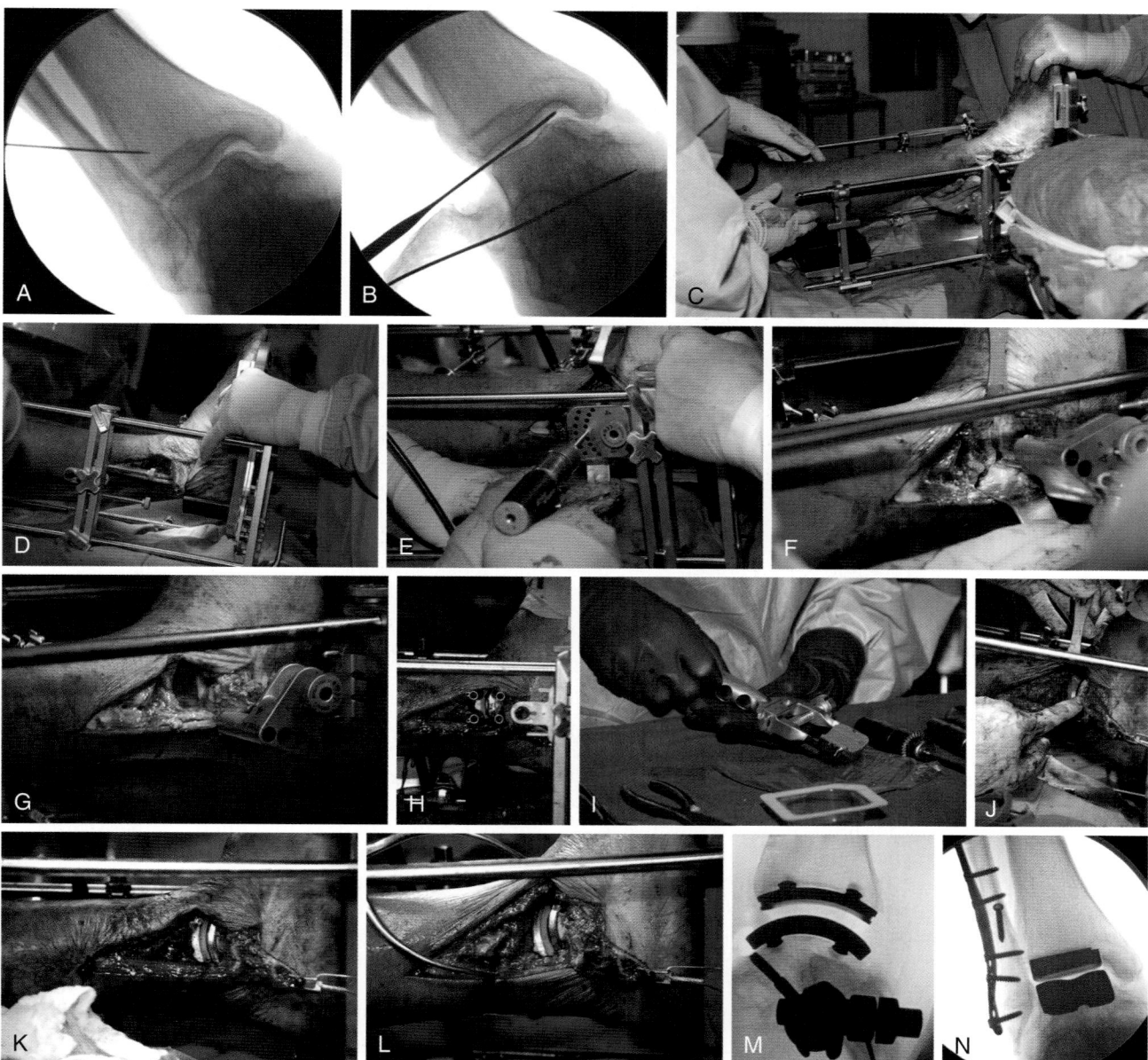

Figure 22-53 Operative technique for placement of Zimmer ankle is detailed in these images. The approach and technique is novel. **A,** An oblique transfibular osteotomy, starting above the syndesmosis and exiting medially within the syndesmosis approximately 1.5 cm above the joint line, is used. **B,** The lateral malleolus is retained on its distal ligaments, reflected distally, and held in place with a smooth Kirschner wire, exposing the lateral surface of the ankle joint. The mediolateral distance is measured and used to determine implant size. **C** and **D,** The leg is lowered onto the alignment stand and secured. **E,** After proper alignment is established, the bone cuts are first prepared with multiple perforations matched to the outer surface of the selected implant size. **F** and **G,** The bone surface is finished with a side-cutting burr. **H,** Rail holes are prepared for rail insertion, using independent tibial and talar guides. After trials with "provisional" plastic implants, the permanent implants are grasped with an insertor, extractor tool **(I)** and placed into the joint with the rails aligned with the rail holes **(J). K,** After the tibial component is placed, low-viscosity bone cement can be placed into the rail holes with a stylet, using a retrograde filling technique. **L,** The final clinical appearance after cementation shows no lift-off of the implants from the bone surface. **M** and **N,** Fluoroscopic image shows good bone fill of cement adjacent to the rails, minimal bone resection, and a well-aligned implant. The fibular osteotomy is then secured with standard fracture technique. (Images courtesy Lew Schon, MD, Baltimore, Md.)

Many surgeons have commented on the need to perform enough total ankle arthroplasties to get over the learning curve. This is partially borne out by the study of Haskell and Mann,[134] who looked at the initial and later cases from surgeons implanting a STAR prosthesis. The volume of surgery has an impact on the technical ease and reliability of TAR. To some extent, this is likely due to the nature of the implant because all present implants have different designs, each with its own problems to be mastered.

One of the most demanding steps of the TAR procedure is the correct positioning of the talar component. First, the original center of rotation of the tibiotalar joint may have changed because of joint degeneration and/or concomitant deformities. Second, even normal ankles have been shown to have a moving axis of rotation, which changes during the arc of motion.[226] In consequence, sagittal malposition of the talar component is a common intraoperative complication of TAR.[217,305] Positioning of prosthesis components, especially the talus, has been shown to strongly affect the resulting kinematics.

Tochigi et al[337] investigated the effect of talar component sagittal positioning on range of motion by using a specially modified STAR prosthesis. They found that anterior talar component displacement significantly decreased the plantar flexion, which was associated with bearing lift-off, while posterior displacement of the talar component significantly decreased the dorsiflexion.[337]

Saltzman et al[296] addressed the effect of ankle prosthesis misalignment on the periankle ligament by using an in vitro Agility prosthesis model.[296] The anterior talofibular ligament was sensitive to transverse plane displacements, while the tibiocalcaneal ligament was sensitive to coronal plane displacements.[296] Furthermore, it has been shown that not only sagittal misalignment has a negative influence on the biomechanics of the ankle but also other factors such as malrotation.

Espinosa et al[99] reported on two finite-element models of Agility and Mobility ankles (see Fig. 22-31).[99] They modeled potential misalignments with respect to the version of the tibial component, version of the talar component, and relative component rotation of the two-component design. Measured pressures consistently increased with misalignment, suggesting that accurate positioning of prosthesis components is one of the most important requirements for the success of procedure.[99]

Fukuda et al[109] reported in an in vitro study on the effect of talar component malrotation of Agility prosthesis. They found that the talar component malrotation leads to increased peak pressure, decreased contact area, and increased rotational torque, further supporting the need for accurate component placement.[109]

More informed preoperative planning and the emergence of improved instrumentation should reduce the variability in implantation to which initial use is particularly susceptible. Among the improvements seen in the current TAR generation as compared with the previous TAR generation are far better cutting guides, bone-based cutting jigs, and the use of a greater range of implant sizes.

Results of Second-Generation Total Ankle Designs

The main failure reasons of the first-generation TAR designs informed the development of the second-generation ankle prostheses. More conservative and bone-sparing cuts and the elimination of bone cement have helped to reduce the problems of component loosening. In second-generation TARs, new biologic interfaces with special porous coatings and/or the addition of hydroxyapatite were investigated as a method to ensure primary prosthesis fixation.[384,385] To reduce subsidence, the second-generation ankle prostheses were designed to increase the surface area of the metallic components, thus aiming to decrease the average local contact pressure and pressure peaks during gait. All four main second-generation TAR designs—Agility, Buechel-Pappas, HINTEGRA, and STAR prostheses—have been implanted with encouraging midterm and long-term results.[278] Positive clinical results, high patient satisfaction, and acceptable survivorship of prosthesis components presented at national meetings and published in the orthopaedic literature led to the thought that ankle fusion may not be the only reasonable treatment option for patients with severe ankle osteoarthritis. The continued critical review of second-generation implant failures and biomechanical studies provided important data that will continue to lead to the development of newer TAR designs.

Stengel et al[322] performed a systematic review and meta-analysis to address the efficacy of TAR with meniscal-bearing implants. The following inclusion criteria were defined for this study: a minimum sample size of 20 subjects, at least 1 year of follow-up, and a clinically relevant study end point. In total, 18 studies with 1086 patients were included in the review. Most patients experienced significant functional improvement (average, 45.2 points using standardized 100-point ankle and hindfoot scores) and a slight increase of range of motion (mean increase, 6.3% (95% CI, 2.2%-10.5%)). Weighted complication rates ranged from 1.6% (deep infection) to 14.7% (impingement). Secondary surgeries were necessary in 12.5% of all patients. Ankle fusions were required in 6.3% of patients because of implant failure, resulting in 1- and 5-year survivorship of 96.9% (95% CI, 94.9%-98.8%) and 90.6% (95% CI, 84.1%-97.1%), respectively. The data of this meta-analysis showed that TAR using current three-component designs provides an acceptable benefit-to-risk ratio. However, the results should be interpreted with caution because of nonoptimal methodologic quality, sample sizes, and short follow-ups.[322]

SooHoo et al[316] compared reoperation rates after ankle fusion and TAR by using California's hospital discharge database. A total of 4705 ankle fusions and 480 ankle arthroplasties were included in the review during the 10-year study period from 1995 through 2004. It was shown that patients who underwent TAR had an increased risk of device-related infection. The rates of major revision surgery after TAR were 9% at 1 year and 23% at

5 years compared with 5% and 11%, respectively, after ankle fusion. However, TAR was shown to have potential advantages in terms of functional results.[316]

In another study from 2004, SooHoo and Kominski[315] performed cost analyses of TAR compared with ankle fusion. The authors performed a thorough literature review to identify possible outcomes and their probabilities after ankle fusion versus TAR. They found that TAR generated total expected lifetime treatment costs of $16,568, which is $6,990 more than costs after ankle fusion. Furthermore, in the reference case, TAR had an incremental cost-effectiveness ratio of $18,419 for each quality-adjusted life-year gained.[315] Courville et al[71] used a Markov model and evaluated expected costs and quality-adjusted life-years for a hypothetical cohort of 60-year-old patients having end-stage ankle osteoarthritis treated with either TAR or ankle arthrodesis. Total ankle arthroplasty was associated with $20,200 more cost than was ankle arthrodesis. However, total ankle arthroplasty resulted in 1.7 additional quality-adjusted life-years, with an incremental cost-effectiveness ratio of $11,800 per year gained. Therefore, despite more expensive implants and longer follow-up, TAR remains a cost-effective alternative treatment to ankle arthrodesis in a 60-year-old cohort with end-stage ankle osteoarthritis.[71]

In 2007, Haddad et al[128] performed a systematic literature review addressing the intermediate and long-term outcomes in TAR and ankle fusion. In total, 10 studies, including 852 ankle arthroplasties, and 39 studies, including 1262 with ankle fusion, were analyzed. The authors showed that 38% of patients with TAR had excellent postoperative results, 30.5% had good results, 5.5% had fair results, and 24% had poor results. The corresponding values in patients who underwent ankle fusion were 31%, 37%, 13%, and 13%, respectively. The 5- and 10-year survivorship for TAR was 78% (95% CI, 69.0%-87.6%) and 77% (95% CI, 63.3%-90.8%), respectively. The revision rate in patients with TAR and ankle fusion was 7% (95% CI, 3.5%-10.9%) and 9% (95% CI, 5.5%-11.6%), respectively. The main reasons for revision surgery were loosening/subsidence in the total ankle arthroplasty group and nonunion in fusion group. The results of this study suggest that the intermediate outcome is comparable for both procedures.[128]

In 2010, Gougoulias et al[120] performed a systematic review of the literature to address the outcomes of total ankle arthroplasties currently in use. In total, 13 level IV peer-reviewed studies were included, reporting the outcomes of 1105 ankle arthroplasties: 234 Agility, 344 STAR, 153 Buechel-Pappas, 152 HINTEGRA, 98 Salto, 70 TNK, and 54 Mobility implants. Postoperatively, a remarkable portion of patients still had some pain (range, 27%-60%). Also, superficial wound complications and deep infection were often reported at up to 14.7% and 4.6%, respectively. The overall failure rate at 5 years had a wide range, from 0% to 32%. In general, most patients experienced significant functional improvement as assessed by the AOFAS score. However, the postoperative improvement of ROM

was relatively small (0-14 dgrees). Therefore the patients should be informed that significantly improved range of motion is not one of the postoperatively expected benefits of TAR.[120]

Slobogean et al[312] compared preference-based quality of life in patients with end-stage ankle osteoarthritis treated with TAR or ankle fusion. The quality of life of 107 subjects was assessed using health-state values derived from SF-36 (SF-6D transformation). The mean baseline SF-6D health-state value in the total ankle arthroplasty group was 0.67 (95% CI, 0.64-0.69) and 0.66 (95% CI, 0.63-0.68) in the ankle fusion group. At 1-year follow-up, both groups had significant and comparable improvements, with 0.73 for the total ankle arthroplasty group (95% CI, 0.71-0.76) and 0.73 for the ankle fusion group (95% CI, 0.70-0.76).[312]

To date, no clear advantage or superiority of the three-component versus two-component design has been determined in the literature.[75,353,383] Also, the high-quality comparative studies addressing postoperative outcomes in patients who underwent TAR versus ankle fusion are rare. Only one prospective controlled comparative surgical trial has been performed including both patient cohorts.[294] Additional high-quality prospective and independent clinical studies would significantly help to establish the clinical practice guidelines needed for surgeons to make a correct decision about treatment choice.[265-268]

FAILED PREVIOUS REPLACEMENT SURGERY

TAR is becoming an increasingly recommended treatment for patients with painful end-stage ankle osteoarthritis.[92,120,150,291,294] With increased availability, the indications for this procedure also increased, including consideration of younger and more active patients. The survivorship of ankle arthroplasties is substantially lower that what is expected from replacement of other lower-extremity joints—the hip and knee joints.[120,121] Therefore every foot and ankle surgeon practicing TAR, sooner or later, may face the problems of failed previous replacement surgery. Little has been written on the treatment of failed previous TAR. Indeed, some series have been published specifically on ankle arthrodesis as a salvage procedure for failed ankle arthroplasties. At the time of writing this chapter, only one clinical study addresses the feasibility of revision ankle arthroplasty in this patient cohort.[153] Most information is anecdotal or can be gleaned from larger reports of primary surgeries (Table 22-1).

Four major problems warrant specific discussion: infection, progressive intracomponent instability and deformity, subsidence and aseptic loosening, and polyethylene failure.

Infection

Data on wound problems and infection with ankle replacement are scarce (Table 22-2). Raikin et al[272]

Text continued on p. 1140

Table 22-1 Literature Review Addressing Clinical Outcome of Patients with Failed Primary Ankle Arthroplasties Treated with Revision Ankle Arthroplasty

Reference	Study	TAR	Prosthesis	FU (Years)	Failures	Reasons for Failures	Time until Revision	Treatment of Failures	Results of Revision
Ali et al, 2007[5]	RS, SC	35	Buechel-Pappas	5 (0.3-12.5)	1 (3%)	Pain (1)	3 years	Revision TAR (1)	Converted to ankle fusion 1 year later because of CRPS
Anders et al, 2010[7]	RS, SC	93	AES	3.5 (1.1-6.1)	7 (8%)	Loosening (1), infection (2), instability (2), Fx (2)	NA	Revision TAR (1), ankle fusion (6)	NA
Anderson et al, 2003[8]	RS, SC	51	STAR	4.3 (3-8)	12	Loosening (7), Fx of PE (2), others (3)	2.8 (0.1-5.3)	Revision TAR (5), ankle fusion (5), PE exchange (2)	3 revision TARs with excellent function, 1 with good function, 1 died
Bonnin et al, 2010[40]	PS, SC	98	Salto	8.9 (6.8-11.1)	12 (12%)	Loosening (6), PE Fx (5), malposition (1)	NA	Revision TAR (1), ankle fusion (6), PE exchange (5)	NA
Buechel et al, 2003[49]	RS, SC	50	Buechel-Pappas Total Ankle	5 (2-10)	2 (4%)	Malposition of talar component (1), talar subsidence (1)	NA	Revision TAR (2)	NA
Carlsson et al, 2001[56]	RS, SC	69	Bath-Wessex	NA	12 (17%)	Painful loosening (12)	4.3 (2.3-8.7)	Revision TAR (6), ankle fusion (12)	NA
Christ and Hagena, 2005[61]	RS, SC	144	STAR	4.8	9 (6%)	Malalignment (2), loosening (1), impingement (1), instability (1), fracture (1), deep infection (2)	NA	Revision TAR (7), aAnkle fusion (2)	NA
Doets et al, 2006[89]	PS, MC	93	LCS (19), Buechel-Pappas (74)	7.2 (0.4-16.3)	15 (16%)	Aseptic loosening (6), malalignment (6), deep infection (2), severe wound-healing problem (1)	NA	Revision TAR (1), ankle fusion (14)	Revision TAR showed loosening, requiring eventual conversion to fusion
Fevang et al, 2007[104]	RS, MC	257	Norwegian TPR (32), STAR (216), AES (3), HINTEGRA (6)	4 (0-12)	27 (11%)	Aseptic loosening (13), instability (3), malalignment (7), deep infection (2), fracture (1), pain (5), defect/wear PE (2), others (2)	2.3 (0.1-8)	Revision TAR (15), PE insert exchange (6), fusion (6)	NA
Giannini et al, 2010[115]	PS, MC	51	BOX	2.5 (2-4)	1 (2%)	Lateral impingement (1)	2	Revision TAR (1)	NA
Henricson and Ågren, 2007[139]	RS, SC	193	STAR (109), Buechel-Pappas (62), AES (22)	4.2 (1-8)	41 (21%)	Infection (5), technical error (8), loosening (11), pain (4), instability (13)	(1.0-6.6)	Revision TAR (23), ankle fusion (15), extraction of prostheses without fusion (3)	2 good results, 19 fairly good, 2 poor with persistent pain and use of two crutches
Hobson et al, 2009[161]	RS, SC	123	STAR	4 (2-8)	18 (15%)	NA	NA	Revision TAR (16), ankle fusion (2)	NA

Study		N	Implant						
Hosman et al, 2007[164]	RS, MC	202	Agility (117), STAR (45), Mobility (29), Ramses (11)	2.3 (0.6-6.3)	14 (7%)	Loosening (10), varus malalignment (1), pain (1), deep infection (2)	1.9 (0.1-5.4)	Revision TAR (10), ankle fusion (3), BKA (1)	NA
Hurowitz et al, 2007[168]	RS, SC	65	Agility	3.3 (2.0-5.9)	21 (32%)	Loosening (8), subsidence (5), malalignment (3), infection (3), osteolysis (1), post impingement (1)	NA	Revision TAR (17), ankle fusion (2), osteochondral allograft (1), BKA (1)	NA
Karantana et al, 2010[177]	RS, SC	52	STAR	6.7 (5.0-9.2)	8 (15%)	Stress fracture (2), stiffness (2), insert fractures (2), talar subsidence (1), loosening (1)	NA	Revision TAR (6), ankle fusion (2)	NA
Kitaoka and Patzer, 1996[186]	RS, SC	160	Mayo	9 (2-17)	57 (36%)	Persistent pain and loosening (all)	4.4 (0.1-13.1)	Revision TAR (10), ankle fusion (45), BKA (2)	NA
Knecht et al, 2004[189]	RS, SC	132	Agility	7.2 (2-14)	14 (11%)	Component Fx (2), loosening (4), deep infection (1), talar collapse (2), varus malpositioning (1), subsidence/migration (3), others (1)	5.8 (0.5-11.3)	Revision TAR (7), ankle fusion (7)	NA
Kofoed and Sørensen, 1998[201]	PS, SC	52	STAR	9 (6-14)	11 (21%)	Loosening (10), deep infection (1)	4.5 (0.8-8.8)	Revision TAR (5), ankle fusion (6)	NA
Kopp et al, 2006[207]	RS, SC	43	Agility	3.7 (2.2-5.3)	1 (2%)	Aseptic loosening (1)	NA	Revision TAR (1)	NA
Kumar and Dhar, 2007[209]	RS, SC	50	STAR	3 (1.5-5)	3 (6%)	Malalignment (2), pain (1)	NA	Revision TAR (3)	Good results in 2 pat, in 1 fusion using ring fixator
Mendolia et al, 2005[235]	RS, SC	69	Ramses	12 (10-14)	12 (10%)	Malalignment (4), loosening (3), instability (5)	NA	Revision TAR (5), ankle fusion (7)	NA
Morgan et al, 2010[238]	RS, SC	45	AES	4.8 (4.0-6.7)	2 (4%)	Loosening (2)	NA	Revision TAR (1), ankle fusion (1)	NA
Murnaghan et al, 2005[241]	RS, SC	22	STAR	2.2 (0.7-3.8)	2 (9%)	Malalignment (2)	NA	Revision TAR (2)	Good results
Nishikawa et al, 2004[253]	RS, SC	21	TNK	6.0 (1.3-14.1)	3 (14%)	Loosening (3)	NA	Revision TAR (1), ankle fusion (2)	Revision TAR was fused 2 years later because of loosening

Continued

Table 22-1 Literature Review Addressing Clinical Outcome of Patients with Failed Primary Ankle Arthroplasties Treated with Revision Ankle Arthroplasty

Reference	Study	TAR	Prosthesis	FU (Years)	Failures	Reasons for Failures	Time until Revision	Treatment of Failures	Results of Revision
Nunley et al, 2012[256]	RS, SC	82	STAR	5.1 (2.0-9.0)	5 (6%)	Loosening (5)	NA	Revision TAR (3), ankle fusion (2)	NA
Reuver et al, 2010[276]	RS, MC	59	Salto	3.0 (1.0-5.4)	7 (12%)	Loosening (5), deep infection (2)	NA	Revision TAR (3), ankle fusion (4)	NA
Rodriguez et al, 2009[281]	RS, SC	18	AES	3.3 (1.7-5.1)	1	Loosening with cysts (1)	NA	Revision TAR (1)	NA
Rudiger et al, 2004[287]	RS, MC	117	ESKA	(0-10)	8 (7%)	Deep infection (4), talus necrosis (1), prosthesis breakage (1), prosthesis malalignment (1), loosening with cysts (1)	NA	Revision TAR (4), fusion (4)	NA
Schutte and Louwerens, 2008[306]	PS, SC	49	STAR	2.3 (1.0-5.6)	4 (8%)	Septic (2) and aseptic (2) loosening	NA	Revision TAR (1), ankle fusion (3)	NA
Spirt et al, 2004	RS, SC	306	DePuy Agility TAR	2.8 (0.3-6.3)	33 (10.8%)	NA	NA	Revision TAR (24), BKA (8), ankle fusion (1)	NA
Vienne and Nothdurft, 2004[361]	RS, SC	66	Agility	2.4 (1.5-3.6)	2 (3%)	NA	NA	Revision TAR (1), ankle fusion (1)	NA
Wood and Deakin, 2003[373]	PS, SC	200	STAR	3.8 (2.0-8.4)	14 (7%)	NA	NA	Revision TAR (3), ankle fusion (11)	NA
Wood et al, 2008[375]	PS, SC	200	STAR	7.3 (5-13)	24 (12%)	Major delay to wound healing (1), intraop Fx (1), postop Fx (2), aseptic loosening (14), edge loading (5), broken PE (1)	NA	Revision TAR (4), ankle fusion (20)	1 revision TAR failed after 5 years and was converted to ankle fusion
Wood et al, 2010[374]	PS, SC	100	Mobility	3.6 (0.3-5.3)	5 (5%)	Insert luxation (1), Loosening (1), talar subsidence (1), pain (1), varus deformity (1)	2.6 (0.5-3.8)	Revision TAR (1), ankle fusion (2), insert exchange (2)	NA

AES, Ankle Evolutive System; BKA, below-knee amputation; BOX, Bologna-Oxford; CRPS, complex regional pain syndrome; FU, follow-up; Fx, fracture; intraop, intraoperative; MC, multicenter; NA, not applicable; PE, polyethylene; postop, postoperative; PS, prospective; RS, retrospective; SC, single center; STAR, Scandinavian Total Ankle Replacement; TAR, total ankle replacement; TPR, Thompson-Parkridge-Richard.

Table 22-2 Literature Review Addressing Infection and Wound Healing Problems in Studies Including Patients with Primary Total Ankle Replacement

Reference	Study	TAR	FU (Years)	Infection n = (%)	Infection Treatment	Wound Healing Problems n = (%)	Wound Healing Problems Treatment
Ali et al, 2007[5]	RS, SC	35 (Buechel-Pappas)	5 (0.3-9.2)	0 (0%)	–	0 (0%)	–
Anders et al, 2010[7]	RS, SC	93 (AES)	3.5 (1.1-6.1)	3 (3.2%)	Ankle fusion (1), two-stage revision (1), antibiotics (1)	NA	NA
Bai et al, 2010[16]	RS, SC	67 (HINTEGRA)	3.2 (2.1-4.5)	1 (1.5%)	Revision TAR (1)	NA	NA
Bardelli and Scoccianti, 2006[18]	RS, SC	7 (STAR)	5.1 (3.0-6.8)	0 (0%)	–	NA	NA
Barg et al, 2010[22]	PS, SC	10 (HINTEGRA)	5.6 (2.7-7.6)	0 (0%)	–	0 (0%)	–
Barg et al, 2011[25]	PS, SC	26 (HINTEGRA)	5 (2-10)	0 (0%)	–	0 (0%)	–
Barg et al, 2011[23]	RS, SC	21 (HINTEGRA)	5.3 (3.1-8.6)	0 (0%)	–	0 (0%)	–
Barg et al, 2011[26]	RS, SC	123 (HINTEGRA)	5.6 (2.4-10.5)	0 (0%)	–	8 (6.5%)	Antibiotics (8)
Barg et al, 2011[29]	PS, SC	19 (HINTEGRA)	5.1 (2.1-9.1)	0 (0%)	–	0 (0%)	–
Bianchi et al, 2012[35]	RS, SC	60 (BOX)	3.5 (2.0-5.9)	1 (1.7%)	Ankle fusion (1)	NA	NA
Bolton-Maggs et al, 1985[38]	RS, SC	62 (ICLH)	5.5 (2-11)	3 (4.8%)	Ankle fusion (2), irrigation and Antibiotics (1)	25 (40.3%)	Skin graft (9), antibiotics (16)
Bonnin et al, 2009[42]	RS, SC	179 (Salto)	4.5 (1.0-10.4)	1 (0.6%)	Ankle fusion (1)	NA	NA
Bonnin et al, 2011[40]	RS, SC	96 (Salto)	8.9 (6.8-11.1)	1 (1.0%)	Irrigation and debridement (1)	NA	NA
Buechel et al, 1988[52]	PS, SC	23 (Buechel-Pappas)	2.9 (2.0-5.3)	1 (4.3%)	NA	4 (17.4%)	NA
Buechel et al, 2003[49]	PS, SC	50 (Buechel-Pappas)	5 (2-10)	2 (4.0%)	Antibiotic suppression (2)	7 (14.0%)	NA
Buechel et al, 2004[51]	PS, SC	115 (Buechel-Pappas)	2-20	4 (3.5%)	NA	20 (17.4%)	NA
Claridge and Sagherian, 2009[63]	RS, SC	28 (Agility)	5 (1.8-8.7)	2 (7.1%)	Debridement and inlay exchange (2)	3 (10.7%)	Debridement and antibiotics (1), free flap (2)
Criswell et al, 2012[73]	RS, SC	65 (Agility)	8 (0.5-11)	3 (4.6%)	Irrigation and debridement (3)	NA	NA
Delagoutte, 2002[79]	RS, SC	66 (Ramses), 36 (LCS), 8 (STAR)	3	1 (0.9%)	NA	NA	NA
Demottaz et al, 1979[80]	RS, SC	21 (Mayo, TPR, Buchholz), 7 (Waugh, Smith)	1.2 (0.3-2.1)	0 (0%)	–	0 (0%)	–
Doets et al, 2006[89]	PS, MC	19 (LCS), 74 (Buechel-Pappas)	7.6 (0.4-16.3)	3 (3.2%)	Revision (2), ankle fusion (1)	8 (8.6%)	Ankle fusion (1), antibiotics (7)
Evanski and Waugh, 1977[102]	RS, SC	25 (Howmedica), 3 (Smith)	NA	1 (3.6%)	Ankle fusion (1)	2 (7.1%)	NA
Fevang et al, 2007[104]	PS, MC	212 (STAR), 32 (TPR), HINTEGRA (6), AES (3)	4 (0-12)	2 (0.8%)	NA	NA	NA
Freeman et al, 1979[105]	RS, SC	29 (ICLH)	NA	2 (6.9%)	Ankle fusion (2)	NA	NA
Groth and Fitch, 1987[126]	RS, SC	71 (NA)	6.5 (2-11)	0 (0%)	–	0 (0%)	–
Hay and Smith, 1994[135]	RS, SC	15 (St. Georg)	10 (3-14)	0 (0%)	–	2 (13.3%)	NA
Henricson and Ågren, 2007[139]	RS, MC	109 (STAR), 62 (Buechel-Pappas), 22 (AES)	4.2 (1-8)	5 (2.6%)	NA	NA	NA
Henricson et al, 2007[142]	PS, MC	318 (STAR), 92 (Buechel-Pappas), 69 (AES), 29 (HINTEGRA), 23 (Mobility)	NA	13 (2.4%)	Prosthesis removal (13)	NA	NA
Henricson et al, 2011[141]	PS, MC	322 (STAR), 136 (Mobility), 115 (AES), 109 (Buechel-Pappas), 66 (CCI), 36 (HINTEGRA)	NA	19 (2.4%)	Prosthesis removal (19)	NA	NA

Continued

Table 22-2 Literature Review Addressing Infection and Wound Healing Problems in Studies Including Patients with Primary Total Ankle Replacement

Reference	Study	TAR	FU (Years)	Infection		Wound Healing Problems	
				n = (%)	Treatment	n = (%)	Treatment
Hintermann et al, 2004[157]	PS, SC	122 (HINTEGRA)	1.6 (1-3)	0 (0%)	—	5 (4.1%)	Dressing and antibiotics (5)
Hobson et al, 2009[161]	RS, SC	123 (STAR)	4 (2-8)	0 (0%)	—	12 (9.8%)	Local measures (12)
Hosman et al, 2007[164]	PS, MC	117 (Agility), 45 (STAR), 29 (Mobility), 11 (Ramses)	0.6-6.3	2 (1.0%)	Ankle fusion (1), BKA (1)	NA	NA
Hurowitz et al, 2007[168]	RS, SC	65 (Agility)	3.3 (2.0-5.9)	3 (4.6%)	Two-stage revision (2), BKA (1)	9 (13.8%)	NA
Karantana et al, 2010[177]	RS, SC	52 (STAR)	5.0-9.2	0 (0%)	—	3 (5.8%)	Antibiotics (3)
Karantanta et al, 2010[178]	RS, SC	10 (STAR)	3.8 (2.2-5.4)	0 (0%)	—	0 (0%)	—
Kim et al, 2009[183]	RS, SC	45 (HINTEGRA)	2.3 (1.0-3.9)	1 (2.2%)	Ankle fusion (1)	NA	NA
Kim et al, 2010[183]	PS, SC	348 (HINTEGRA)	3.3 (1.0-6.1)	3 (0.9%)	NA	2 (0.6%)	NA
Kirkup, 1985[184]	RS, SC	24 (Richard Smith)	7 (4.7-8.7)	0 (0%)	—	7 (29.2%)	NA
Kitaoka and Patzer, 1996[186]	RS, SC	204 (Majo)	9 (2-17)	10 (4.9%)	Ankle fusion (7), antibiotics (2), BKA (1)	2 (1.0%)	Wound care (2)
Knecht et al, 2004[189]	RS, SC	132 (Agility)	9 (7-16)	3 (2.3%)	Debridement (2), ankle fusion (1)	3 (2.3%)	Wound care and antibiotics (3)
Kofoed and Stürup, 1994[202]	PS, SC	14 (STAR)	7 (5.0-9.7)	0 (0%)	—	3 (2.4%)	NA
Kofoed, 1995[198]	PS, SC	28 (STAR)	NA	1 (3.6%)	NA	NA	NA
Kofoed and Danborg, 1995[200]	PS, SC	20 (STAR)	2.5 (1-4)	0 (0%)	—	0 (0%)	—
Kofoed and Sørensen, 1998[201]	PS, SC	52 (STAR)	7.5 (2-10)	1 (1.9%)	Ankle fusion (1)	NA	NA
Koivu et al, 2009[203]	RS, SC	130 (AES)	2.6 (0.3-6.2)	1 (0.8%)	NA	NA	NA
Kokkonen et al, 2011[205]	RS, SC	38 (AES)	2.3 (0.2-5.8)	1 (2.6%)	Ankle fusion (1)	NA	NA
Kumar and Dhar, 2007[210]	RS, SC	50 (STAR)	3 (1.5-5)	0 (0%)	—	7 (14.0%)	Wound debridement and antibiotics (1), antibiotics (3), dressing (3)
Kurup and Taylor, 2006[211]	RS, SC	34 (Buechel-Pappas)	2.8 (1-5.5)	0 (0%)	—	3 (8.8%)	Antibiotics (3)
Lagaay and Schuberth, 2010[213]	RS, SC	124 (Agility LP)	1-5	2 (1.6%)	Parenteral antibiotics (2)	8 (6.5%)	NA
Lee et al, 2008[217]	RS, SC	50 (HINTEGRA)	NA	1 (2.0%)	Two-stage revision (1)	3 (6.0%)	Skin graft or topical dressing changes (3)
Lee et al, 2010[220]	RS, SC	30 (Mobility)	NA	0 (0%)	—	2 (6.7%)	NA
Makwana et al, 1995[228]	RS, SC	84 (Bath-Wessex)	6.1 (3-10)	1 (1.2%)	Ankle fusion (1)	NA	NA
Mann et al, 2011[229]	PS, SC	84 (STAR)	9.1 (2.6-11)	3 (3.6%)	Revision (3)	2 (2.4%)	Local measures (2)
McGuire et al, 1988[231]	RS, SC	25 (Smith)	3.8	3 (12.0%)	BKA (3)	NA	NA
Murnaghan et al, 2005[241]	RS, SC	22 (STAR)	2.2 (0.7-3.8)	0 (0%)	—	2 (9.1%)	Antibiotics (2)
Myerson and Mroczek, 2003[244]	RS, SC	50 (Agility)	NA	0 (0%)	—	8 (16.0%)	Dressing changes and antibiotics (8)
Nelissen et al, 2006[249]	PS, SC	15 (Buechel-Pappas)	2.0	0 (0%)	—	1 (6.7%)	Antibiotics and cast immobilization (1)
Newton, 1982[251]	RS, SC	50 (Newton)	3 (2-5)	1 (2.0%)	BKA (1)	NA	NA
Nishikawa et al, 2004[253]	RS, SC	21 (TNK)	6 (1.6-5.8)	0 (0%)	—	1 (4.8%)	Local measures (1)
Nunley et al, 2012[256]	RS, SC	82 (STAR)	5.1 (2-9)	2 (2.4%)	Ankle fusion (1), two-stage revision (1)	NA	NA

Study	Type	Number (implant)	Follow-up (yr)	Failures n (%)	Treatment of failures	Complications n (%)	Treatment of complications
Patsalis, 2004[262]	PS, SC	15 (AES)	0.7 (0.3-1.3)	1 (6.7%)	Ankle fusion (1)	NA	NA
Pyevich et al, 1998[271]	RS, SC	100 (Agility)	4.8 (2.8-12.3)	0 (0%)	—	2 (2.0%)	antibiotics (2)
Reuver et al, 2010[276]	RS, MC	59 (Salto)	3 (1.0-5.4)	3 (5.1%)	Ankle fusion (2), irrigation and debridement (1)	3 (5.1%)	Antibiotics (3)
Rippstein et al, 2011[279]	RS, SC	233 (Mobility)	2.7 (1.0-5.3)	2 (0.9%)	Debridement (2)	2 (0.9%)	Flap coverage (1), local measures (1)
Rodriguez et al, 2010[281]	RS, SC	21 (AES)	3.3 (1.7-5.1)	0 (0%)	—	0 (0%)	—
Rudigier et al, 2001[286]	RS, SC	56 (ESKA)	Min. 1	2 (3.6%)	Ankle fusion (2)	—	
Rudigier, 2005[285]	RS, SC	159 (ESKA)	NA	2 (1.3%)	Ankle fusion (2)	NA	NA
Saltzman et al, 2003[292]	RS, MC	90 (Agility)	Min. 1	4 (4.4%)	Two-stage revision (1), ankle fusion (2), BKA (1)	10 (11.1%)	Flap coverage (2), local measures (8)
Saltzman et al, 2009[294]	PS, MC	593 (STAR)	2.0	7 (1.2%)	NA	12 (2.0%)	NA
San Giovanni et al, 2006[298]	RS, SC	31 (Buechel-Pappas)	8.3 (5.0-12.2)	1 (3.2%)	Ankle fusion (1)	NA	NA
Schenk et al, 2011[300]	RS, SC	413 (Salto)	2.4 (0.1-7.0)	3 (0.7%)	Two-stage revision (1), ankle fusion (2)	NA	NA
Schuberth et al, 2006[305]	RS, SC	50 (Agility)	2 (0.5-4.2)	1 (2.0%)	Two-stage revision (1)	10 (20.0%)	Flap coverage (1), wound care and antibiotics (9)
Schutte and Louwerens, 2008[306]	RS, SC	49 (STAR)	2.3 (1.0-5.6)	2 (4.9%)	Ankle fusion (2)	NA	NA
Shinomiya et al, 2003[310]	RS, SC	20 (TNK)	8 (5-12)	0 (0%)	NA	NA	NA
Skyttä et al, 2010[311]	PS, MC	298 (AES), 217 (STAR)	3.2 (0.1-9.6)	4 (0.8%)	Ankle fusion (3)	NA	NA
Spirt et al, 2004[317]	RS, SC	306 (Agility)	2.8 (0.3-6.3)	3 (1.0%)	Ankle fusion (3)	NA.	NA
Stauffer and Segal, 1981[321]	PS, SC	102 (Mayo)	1.9 (0.5-3.7)	3 (2.9%)	Ankle fusion (5)	NA	NA
Stauffer, 1982[319]	RS, SC	22 (Mayo)	2.1 (0.5-6.2)	5 (21.7%)	Irrigation, debridement, antibiotics (1)	NA	NA
Su et al, 2004[325]	RS, SC	27 (Buechel-Pappas)	6.4 (1-14.5)	1 (3.7%)	—	NA	NA
Takakura et al, 1990[327]	RS, SC	69 (TNK)	9.3 (6.5-13)	0 (0%)		3 (4.3%)	NA
Takakura et al, 2004[326]	RS, SC	160 (TNK)	2-12.5	1 (0.6%)	Ankle fusion (1)	NA	Local measures and antibiotics (1)
Valderrabano et al, 2004[342]	PS, SC	68 (STAR)	3.7 (2.4-6.2)	0 (0%)	—	1 (1.5%)	Debridement and antibiotics (2), ankle fusion (1)
van der Heide et al, 2009[358]	RS, MC	37 (STAR), 21 (Buechel-Pappas)	2.7 (1-9)	4 (6.9%)	Ankle fusion (4)	3 (5.2%)	Local measures (3), split skin graft (1)
Wood and Deakin, 2003[373]	PR, SC	200 (STAR)	3.8 (2.0-8.4)	1 (0.5%)	Ankle fusion (1)	4 (2.0%)	NA
Wood, 2007[370]	RS, SC	280 (STAR)	NA	2 (0.7%)	Ankle fusion (2)	NA	NA
Wood et al, 2009[376]	PS, SC	100 (Buechel-Pappas), 100 (STAR)	4.1 (0.1-7.1)	1 (0.5%)	Ankle fusion (1)	NA	NA
Wood et al, 2010[373]	PS, SC	100 (Mobility)	3.6 (0.3-5.3)	1 (1.0%)	Debridement and antibiotics (1)	NA	NA
Wynn and Wilde, 1992[378]	RS, SC	36 (Beck-Steffee)	10.8 (10-13)	2 (5.6%)	NA	14 (38.9%)	NA

AES, Ankle Evolutive System; BKA, below-knee amputation; BOX, Bologna-Oxford; CCI, ceramic-coated implant; Fx, fracture; ICLH, Imperial College of London Hospital; LCS, low-contact stress; MC, multicenter; Min., minimum; NA, not available; PS, prospective; RS, retrospective; SC, single center; STAR, Scandinavian Total Ankle Replacement; TAR, total ankle replacement; TPR, Thompson-Parkridge-Richard.

performed a retrospective chart review of 106 Agility ankle arthroplasties to identify risk factors for wound healing complications after this procedure. In this study, two complication groups were observed. Twenty-seven ankles (25%) required local wound care or local antibiotics without subsequent consequences (minor-complication group), while nine ankles (8.5%) required surgical irrigation and debridement of the wound (major-complication group). Only diabetes was found to have a significant association with the occurrence of minor wound complications. Female sex, inflammatory connective tissue disease, and corticosteroid use were identified as risk factors for major wound complications.[272] Whalen et al[368] retrospectively reviewed medical records of 57 consecutive ankle arthroplasties. Sixteen patients with wound breakdown were identified at a median of 17 days after TAR. Analysis of possible risk factors revealed a significant increase in rate of wound problems associated with smoking greater than 12 pack-years, peripheral vascular disease, and cardiovascular disease.[368]

In general, surgeons apply basic total joint principles derived from data on infection in the knee and hip[386] to the treatment of wound problems and infection after TAR. The key to avoiding bad problems is prevention. Proper patient selection is the first step. Any patient with a history of ankle infection, and especially with a history of osteomyelitis, needs a careful workup to rule out persistent sources of infection. Patients with concerning soft tissue conditions from previous multiple surgeries, long-standing steroid or immunosuppression dependence, pathologic dermatologic conditions, or vascular insufficiency need to be strongly considered for alternative approaches to ankle replacement to avoid the major postoperative complications. When surgical treatment is necessary to keep these patients mobile, Saltzman's group performs arthroscopic ankle fusions.[364]

Surgical technique is an equally important factor. Meticulous nondestructive handling of soft tissues should be part of every surgery. Excellent hemostasis should be followed by careful multilayered closure starting at the periosteal–capsular layer. The dressings need to have several soft layers encased in a harder carapace. During the first few postoperative days, the leg is elevated above the heart, and the toes are monitored for swelling, which indicates that a splint needs to be changed.

Despite all these measures, wound problems and infections do occur. The treatment of superficial wound breakdown with infection is local dressing changes and prophylactic oral antibiotic coverage. Superficial wound breakdown and local infection require an aspirate of the joint through uninfected tissue to rule out deep infection and to identify the possible infective organism. If deep infection is ruled out, the patient should be given parenteral antibiotics and started on local dressing changes. If the dehiscence reaches the joint and is recognized early, surgical incision and drainage is indicated with exchange of the polyethylene. If the wound cannot be primarily closed, a local flap using the extensor digitorum brevis (Fig. 22-54) should be swung over the wound and skin grafted.

Late deep infections generally require removal of all implants, placement of a cement antibiotic spacer, and generally a properly staged attempt at fusion (Fig. 22-55).

A methyl methacrylate antibiotic spacer can be used to help sterilize the wound, and the fusion can be performed either in situ or with structural bone (Fig. 22-56).

Progressive Intracomponent Instability and Deformity

Recognition and correction of intracomponent instability and deformity requires *standing* and *weight-bearing* radiographs. The authors prefer to obtain a hindfoot alignment view to help understand the force vectors across the ankle joint in quiet standing (Fig. 22-57).[293] Frigg et al[107] addressed clinical relevance of the hindfoot alignment view in TAR. In a series of 28 consecutive patients, hindfoot alignment measured by the hindfoot alignment view correlated significantly with different load parameters of dynamic pedobarography and clinical outcome assessed using the AOFAS and SF-36 scores.[107]

The problem of postoperative malalignment is well recognized. The approach to this problem depends on a number of factors, including the intrinsic design of the TAR. In the following paragraphs of this subsection, the authors describe the reported incidences and the technical solutions proposed by experienced surgeons with deep knowledge of their implants. Yet, *the importance of preoperative and intraoperative recognition of malalignment and ligamentous laxity cannot be underestimated* (Fig. 22-58).

The first clinical report addressing the feasibility and clinical outcomes of TAR recognized preoperative varus or valgus deformity as a possible source of prosthesis failure. Newton[250,252] performed 50 TARs using the Newton ankle implant (a highly nonconstrained cemented prosthesis including high-density polyethylene tibial and Vitallium talar components). Valgus or varus deformity of the talus greater than 20 degrees was noted as an absolute contraindication for TAR.[250,252] In a later study,[251] Newton stated that with his nonconstrained TAR, although valgus or varus deformity of up to 15 degrees could be corrected initially, the coronal deformity usually recurred. All replaced ankles with a talar tilt of more than 20 degrees failed during the follow-up.[251] Kirkup[184] observed, in many patients with rheumatoid OA, that severe valgus or varus deformity was common. The author recognized that these deformities could not be corrected by cutting wedges; therefore preoperative coronal deformity greater than 30 degrees was a contraindication for TAR.[184] Stauffer and Segal[321] performed 102 TARs using the Mayo Total Ankle, which is a highly congruent two-component design including a polyethylene tibial component and cement fixation. The procedure was not performed in patients with preoperative coronal deformity (varus or valgus) of more than 20 degrees.[321]

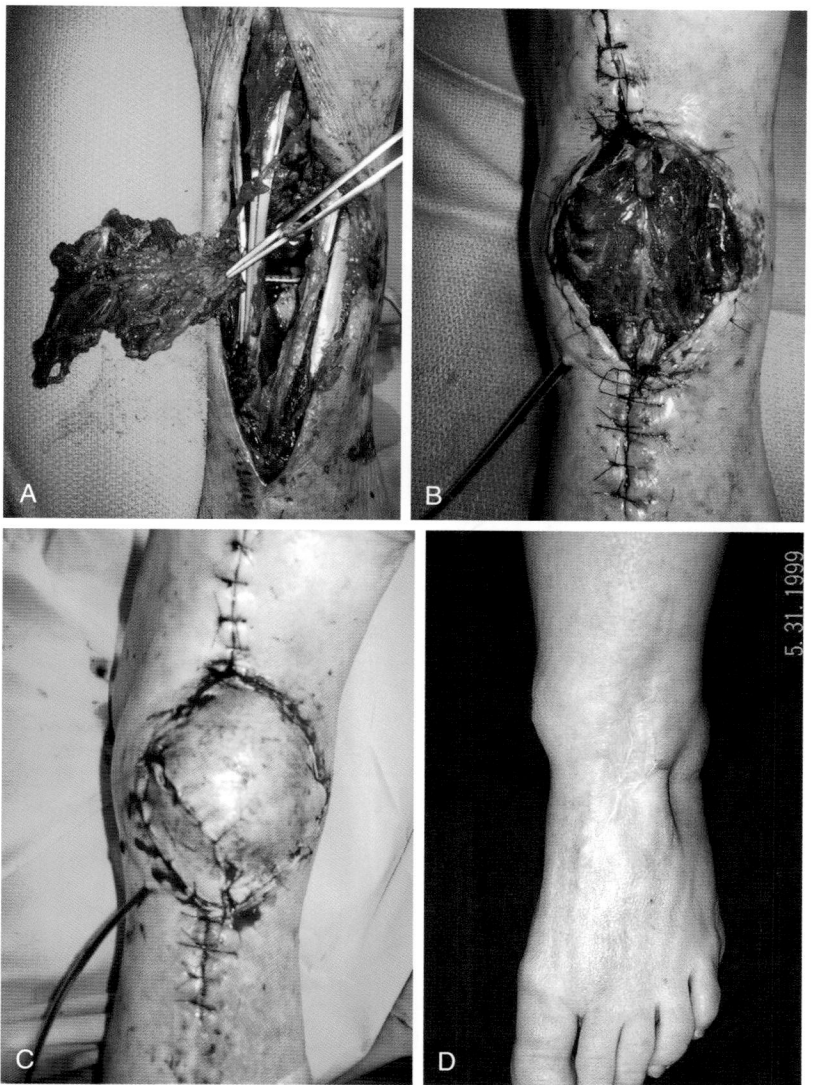

Figure 22-54 The extensor digitorum brevis is the best local muscle flap for a failed anterior ankle surgery. The deep peroneal nerve is cut to reflect the muscle on its pedicle **(A)** and then placed into the defect **(B)** and covered with skin graft **(C)**. The muscle will eventually atrophy to form a cosmetically acceptable result **(D)**.

Pyevich et al[271] analyzed the midterm results of 100 consecutive Agility TARs performed between 1984 and 1993, with a mean follow-up of 5 years. Preoperative valgus or varus malalignment was corrected using an external fixator. McIff et al[232] and Vienne and Nothdurft[361] suggested the intraoperative correction of varus or valgus deformity using the external fixator with the Agility TAR. Pyevich[271] observed that the position of the tibial component had a significant influence on the outcome: patients with tibial components placed in more than 4 degrees of valgus had significantly more postoperative pain ($P < .05$) than the patients with neutrally aligned prosthesis components.

Saltzman[290] reviewed the state of the art in using TAR in 2000 and recognized that preoperative varus or valgus deformity not sufficiently addressed during the TAR procedure may lead to loading, which accelerates the rate of polyethylene wear.[290]

Greisberg and Hansen[123,124] presented their strategies of how to address the associated deformities in patients with TAR. In patients with valgus foot caused by medial collapse, the medial column should be restored, which may also restore the appropriate tension of medial ligaments. The authors suggest placing the tibial and talar components in a slightly lateral position. If the valgus malalignment of the hindfoot persists, a medial sliding osteotomy of the calcaneus should be performed. In patients with advanced flatfoot deformity, a triple arthrodesis in addition to medial column stabilization may be performed to achieve proper alignment in the long term.

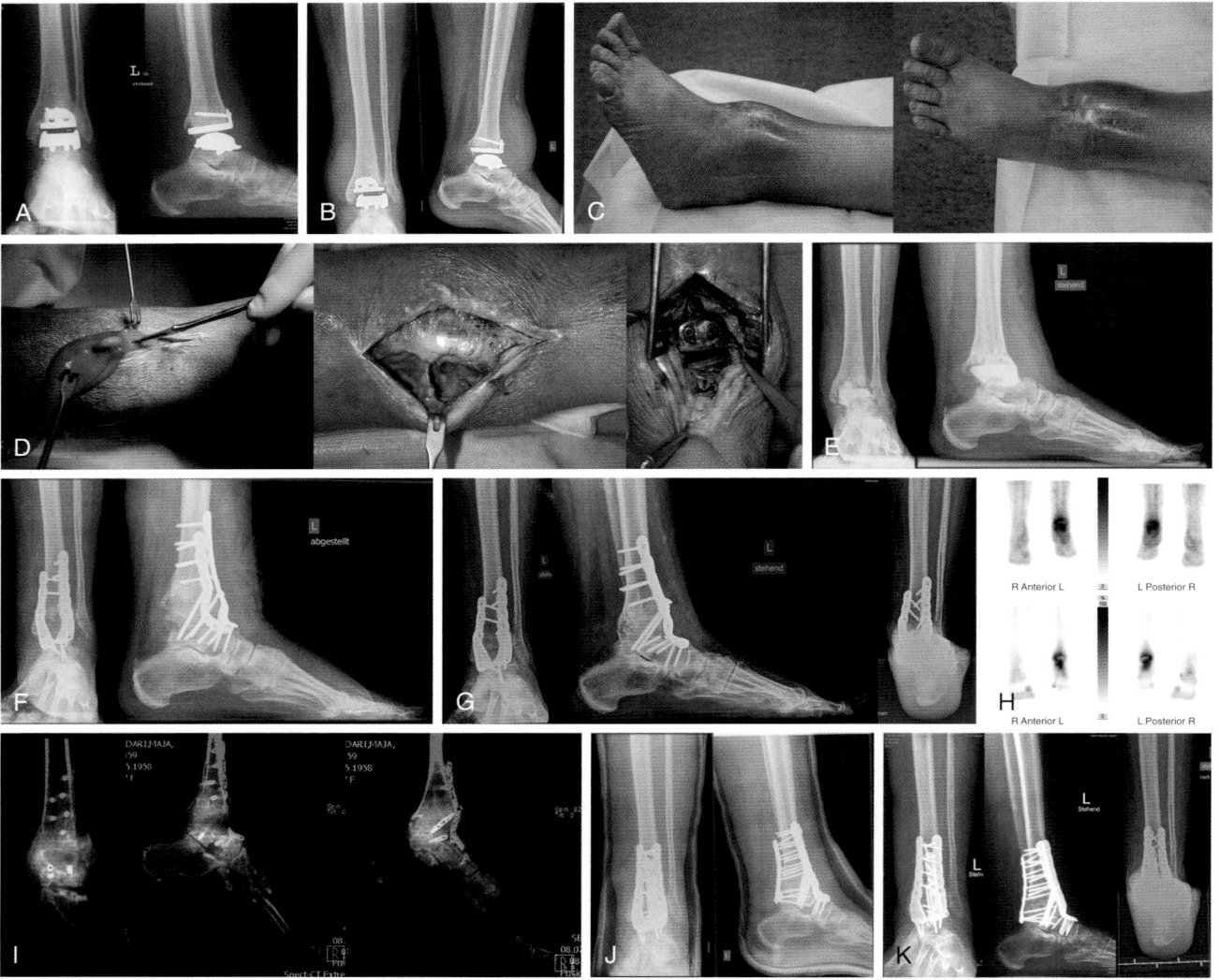

Figure 22-55 A, Postoperative radiographs of a 48-year-old female at the follow-up of 1 year after implantation; a three-component prosthesis was used because of posttraumatic osteoarthritis. **B,** Two years later, the patient was referred to the outpatient clinic for irregular clinical and radiologic follow-up because of increasing swelling and pain in the replaced ankle. **C,** Patient presented with massive swelling and fluctuation over the tibiotalar joint. **D,** During the revision surgery, 50 mL of pus was evacuated. **E,** Prosthesis has been removed and cement spacer was implanted after several biopsies were taken. **F,** Microbiologic investigation revealed a *Klebsiella* infection; therefore intravenous antibiotics were administered. One month later, isolated tibiotalar arthrodesis was performed using anterior double plating system and allograft (femoral head). **G,** Six months later, patient still complained about pain in the fused ankle. Radiographs showed progressive osseous consolidation at the site of tibiotalar arthrodesis. However, several screws were broken. **H,** Scintigraphy of the ankle showed increased activity at the site of tibiotalar arthrodesis, indicating a possible delayed union. **I,** Single photon emission computed tomography (SPECT-CT) image confirmed metabolic active delayed union at the side of tibiotalar arthrodesis. **J,** Therefore a revision surgery was performed. All hardware was removed and screws were substantially loosened. The allograft showed good integration. Re-arthrodesis of tibiotalar joint was performed using anterior double plates and an additional single plate. **K,** Six months later, radiographs showed stable positioning of allograft and neutral alignment of the hindfoot. The patient was painfree. (Images courtesy Beat Hintermann, MD, Liestal, Switzerland.)

The authors stated that patients with persistent misalignment of the replaced ankle may have a higher risk of prosthesis failure.[123,124]

Conti and Wong[67,68] reviewed the possible complications of TAR. Varus or valgus malpositioning of the prosthesis components was a possible source of TAR failure. They stated that the valgus positioning of the prosthesis component may be better tolerated than varus positioning. However, they recommended corrective osteotomy for supramalleolar deformity of more than 10 degrees and a cutting jig adjustment in ankles with any deformities of the distal tibial articular surface.[67,68]

Stamatis and Myerson[318] described how to avoid specific complications of TAR. They observed different

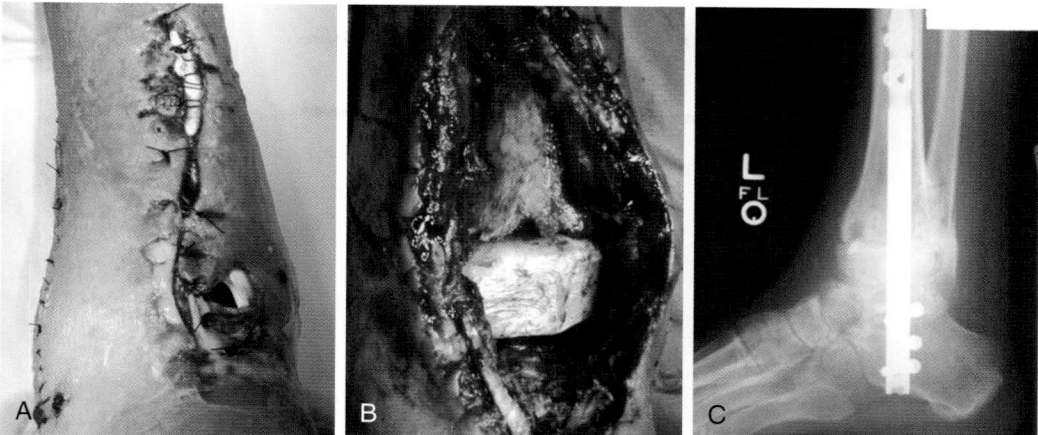

Figure 22-56 Treatment of massive ankle implant infection **(A)** with a methyl methacrylate antibiotic spacer **(B)** and staged fusion using bulk allograft **(C)**. (Photographs courtesy Chris Attinger, MD, and Paul Cooper, MD.)

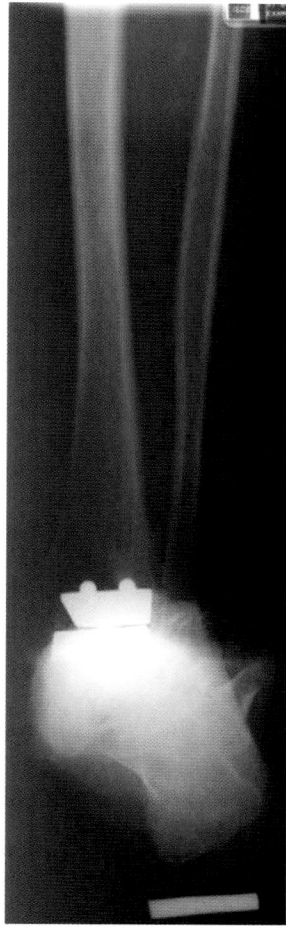

Figure 22-57 Hindfoot alignment view showing severe valgus deformity after Scandinavian Total Ankle Replacement (STAR) implant. This imbalance may lead to nonuniform mobile-bearing stress and increase the risk of bearing subluxation, wear, fracture, or component subsidence.

pathologies in valgus arthritic ankles, including ligament pathologies (contracted lateral ligaments and insufficient medial ligaments), valgus heel, shortening and deformities of the fibula causing chronic impingement, and/or rupture of the spring ligament and posterior tibial tendon. The correction of the valgus deformity included several osseous and ligament procedures.[318]

Wood and Deakin[373] reviewed results of 200 cementless, mobile-bearing STAR TARs performed between 1993 and 2000. Preoperatively, 39 ankles had a significant coronal deformity of more than 15 degrees: 17 ankles with varus and 22 ankles with valgus deformity. Seven of these 39 ankles (18%) developed edge loading, whereas only 2 of the 161 ankles with neutral alignment (1%) had comparable problems. Of the nine patients with edge loading, three had an additional surgery to improve realignment and stability of the hindfoot, and 3 ankles ended up in conversion to ankle fusion. Therefore the authors stated that the preoperative varus or valgus deformity of the talus of more than 10 degrees was a relative contraindication for TAR.[373] Similar findings were observed in a later study, including the same 200 STAR TARs.[375] Wood et al[371] performed a review and addressed the outcomes of currently available TAR designs. The authors found that the failure rate was lower in ankles that were well aligned than those ankles with more than 15 degrees of preoperative valgus or varus deformity.[371]

Assal et al[11] presented a case report describing fracture of the polyethylene component in a patient who underwent Agility TAR because of varus malalignment of the talar component. The authors stated that uncorrected foot and hindfoot deformities may induce significant valgus or varus forces resulting in pathologic polyethylene wear patterns. Therefore, especially in patients who underwent Agility TAR, normal alignment is very important because the Agility TAR system has very little intrinsic stability.[11]

Hintermann and Valderrabano[156] reviewed the use of TAR in 2003. In earlier clinical studies, the patients with significant preoperative varus or valgus deformities were

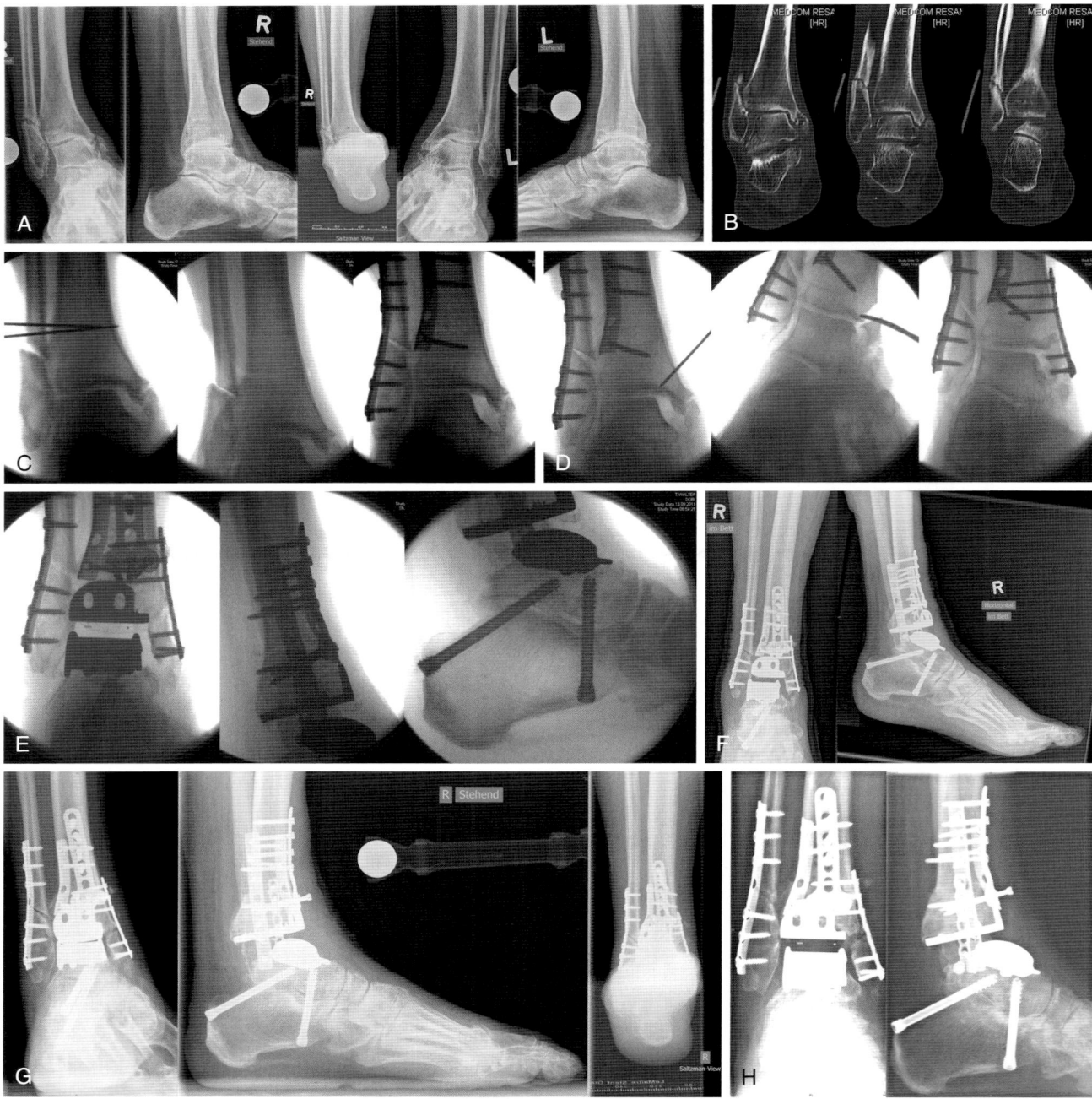

Figure 22-58   Preoperative radiographs **(A)** and computed tomography scans **(B)** of a 69-year-old male with bilateral severe varus malalignment of the hindfoot. The right ankle is painful, and the left ankle is asymptomatic. The patient suffered a fibula fracture on the right side 4 months earlier, resulting in nonunion. Ankle fusion was strictly refused by patient. **C,** First, fibula osteotomy and lateral supramalleolar osteotomies were performed to restore the fibula length and alignment of the tibiotalar joint. **D,** Then, malleolar flip-osteotomy was performed to restore the mortise. **E,** Finally, corrective subtalar fusion and implantation of a three-component ankle prosthesis were performed. **F,** Postoperative radiographs 1 week after surgery. Already, these radiographs show a too-anterior position of the talar component. **G,** Postoperative radiographs 2 months after total ankle replacement (TAR) show some anterior tilting of the tibial component with indirect signs of failure of osteosynthesis (see one screw). The Saltzman view shows neutral alignment of the hindfoot. Postoperative radiographs at 3 months **(H).**

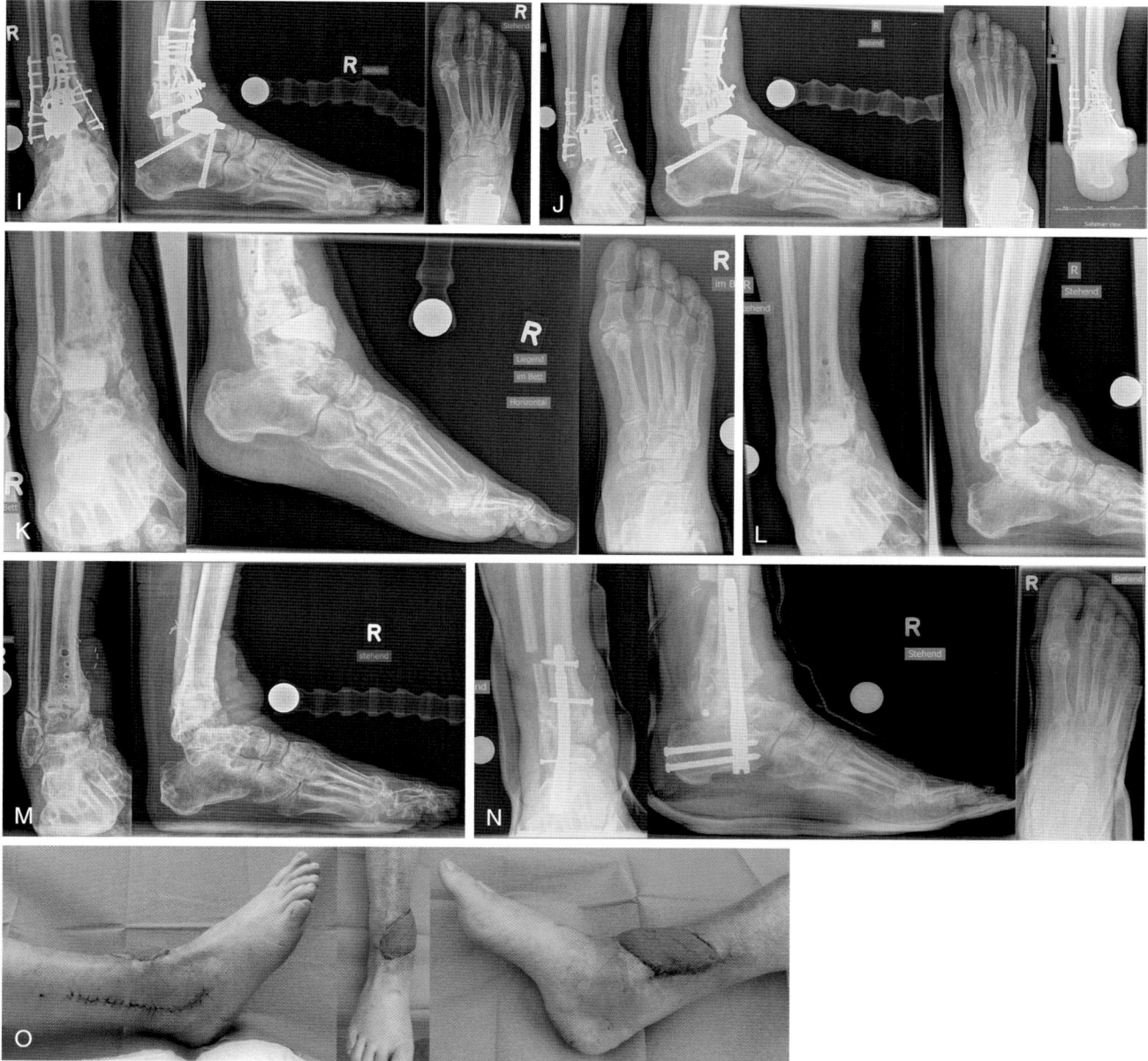

Figure 22-58, cont'd Postoperative radiographs at 4 months **(I)** and 5 months **(J)** after the surgery show progressive intracomponent instability with hardware failure. **K,** Therefore 6 months after initial TAR, removal of prosthesis component was performed with implantation of cement spacer. **L,** One month later, an increasing dislocation of the cement spacer and necrosis in the area of the anterior approach were observed. **M,** Cement spacer was removed and necrosis of skin and soft tissue was debrided. Gracilis flap from the contralateral leg with the end-to-side anastomosis of the poterior tibial artery was used for soft tissue defect. **N,** Two months later, tibiotalocalcaneal arthrodesis was performed using intramedullary nail. **O,** Clinical photographs of the operated lower extremity 10 days after surgery.

excluded from use of TAR, and ankle fusion was performed. The authors stated that as long the deformities could be corrected before or during the TAR procedure, they were not a contraindication for TAR.[156]

Takakura et al[326] reviewed 160 TARs performed between 1975 and 2000 using a TNK ceramic prosthesis that underwent three generations of development. The authors suggested not using TAR in patients with varus or valgus deformities of the tibial articular surface exceeding 15 degrees because of observed loosening and prosthesis subsidence in the early postoperative period.[326,329]

Greisberg et al[125] addressed the importance of hindfoot alignment in patients with TAR and described how to achieve a well-balanced hindfoot. Two different reasons for valgus malalignment in the ankle were described: posttraumatic arthritic ankle with loss of bone from the lateral plafond and advanced flatfoot with insufficient medial ligaments. The authors recommended medial ligament reconstruction and, if necessary, restoration of the medial column. For valgus ankles, the bone cuts were not performed too close to the medial malleolus. After implantation of final prosthesis components, the position of hindfoot and the heel were checked, and if the ankle remained in valgus, a medial sliding calcaneal osteotomy was performed.[125]

Haskell and Mann[134] presented short-term results of 86 patients who underwent STAR prosthesis, with a mean follow-up of 2 years. Thirty-five of 86 patients had a preoperative coronal plane deformity of more than 10 degrees (25 patients with varus deformity and 10 patients with valgus deformity). All patients were divided into four groups: varus-congruent, valgus-congruent, varus-incongruent, and valgus-incongruent. Ankles with talar and tibial deformities improved talar and tibial alignment toward a neutral weight-bearing axis postoperatively. The alignment was constant during the subsequent 2 years. Eight of 34 patients developed progressive edge loading, requiring four additional procedures. The patients with preoperative incongruent joints were 10 times more likely to develop postoperative edge loading.[134]

Kofoed[199] described a special sculpting technique for the talus that allows intraoperative correction of varus or valgus ankle deformity of more than 45 degrees. This technique included cutting 1- to 2-mm slices off the talus facets and the talar dome, followed by rotation of the entire hindfoot inside the ankle mortise until normal hindfoot alignment was achieved. The authors presented a case of a patient with preoperative valgus deformity of about 50 degrees, with only a slight postoperative valgus alignment of the hindfoot.[199]

Doets et al[89] performed a prospective, single-center study, including 19 LCS mobile-bearing TARs and 74 Buechel-Pappas TARs. The 8-year survivorship for both prostheses, with revision or conversion to an arthrodesis for any reason as the end point, was 85% (95% CI, 73%-93%). However, the same survivorship in 17 ankles with a preoperative varus or valgus deformity of more than 10 degrees was significantly lower ($P = .03$) with 48% (95% CI, 6%-90%), while survivorship in ankles with a neutral preoperative alignment was 90% (95% CI, 82%-98%). In two ankles with preexisting valgus deformity, a medial malleolar fracture occurred intraoperatively, with nonunion in the further course. Both ankles also developed a stress fracture of the lateral malleolus resulting in nonmanageable valgus instability that required ankle fusion. Therefore the authors defined the preoperative valgus or varus deformity of more than 10 degrees as an absolute contraindication for TAR. The authors suggested that a corrective surgery (e.g., triple arthrodesis) should be performed before the TAR to restore normal biomechanics and alignment of the hindfoot.[89]

Henricson and Ågren[139] performed 196 second-generation TARs in 186 patients, with a mean follow-up of 4 years: 109 STAR, 62 Buechel-Pappas, and 22 AES ankles.

All ankles were divided into three groups: (1) normal hindfoot alignment (normal value was set to 5-degrees valgus; n = 92); (2) varus alignment (mean, 9.6 degrees; range, 5-30 degrees; n = 55); (3) valgus alignment (mean, 11 degrees; range, 5-30 degrees; n = 46). The preoperative valgus malalignment was neutralized in 20 ankles, one was overcorrected in slight varus, and 23 ankles stayed in a valgus position (mean, 7.6 degrees; range, 5-15 degrees). The overall revision rate was 21%. In the preoperative varus group, the revision rate was 31% and in the valgus and neutral groups 17%, respectively. Therefore the authors stated that additional surgeries should be performed to achieve neutral alignment, and the TAR should be limited only to experienced foot and ankle surgeons.[139]

Coetzee[65] presented his strategies on how to perform TAR in patients with varus or valgus deformities. He identified most valgus deformities as secondary to chronic posterior tibial tendon dysfunction. A lateral release can be done to get the talus in the correct position in the mortise. A primary deltoid repair can be performed; however, it is never strong enough. The following corrective procedures were suggested: posterior tibial tendon repair with augmentation of the flexor digitorum longus tendon, gastrocnemius slide, and stabilization of the medial ray. In patients with severe and rigid valgus deformities, a triple arthrodesis was to be performed to achieve the long-term stability. The author suggested 10 degrees of varus or valgus ligamentous instability as the arbitrary cut-off point and 15 degrees as the hard cut-off point for performing an ankle fusion.[65]

Bluman and Chiodo[36] described the anatomy and biomechanics of valgus arthritic ankles and presented different therapeutic strategies. In patients with preoperative coronal deformities of more than 15 degrees, higher risk of mechanical failure existed. However, in valgus arthritic ankles, all concomitant deformities—proximal and distal to the tibiotalar joint—should be sufficiently addressed.[36]

Wood et al[376] performed a randomized, prospective, single-center study, including 200 TARs, to compare the Buechel-Pappas and STAR implants, with a minimum follow-up of 3 years. The 6-year survivorship was comparable ($P = .09$) in both groups, with 79% (95% CI, 63.4%-88.5%) and 95% (95% CI, 87.2%-98.1%) in the Buechel-Pappas and STAR groups, respectively. However, the authors observed a significantly higher ($P = .02$) incidence of prosthesis failure in ankles with preoperative varus or valgus deformity, especially when the deformity was greater than 15 degrees, resulting in a predicted failure rate at 6 years exceeding 10% for the STAR prosthesis and 25% for the Buechel-Pappas prosthesis. When the preoperative deformity was 15 degrees or less, the estimated 6-year survivorship was 86.7% for the Buechel-Pappas group and 95.5% for the STAR group.[376] Wood et al[372] also shared their experience of TAR in patients with rheumatoid ankle OA. Nearly 50% of all patients with rheumatoid OA requiring either fusion or TAR presented with valgus deformity. In patients who underwent TAR, the heel needed to be well aligned under the tibia, which can be achieved by hindfoot fusion as a one-stage procedure, or 6 or 12 weeks before the ankle replacement.[372] In some patients, the valgus deformity had been corrected without ligamental release, but an alarming gap was seen on the lateral side between the malleolus and prosthesis component.[370]

Karantana et al[177] retrospectively reviewed 45 patients with 52 TARs using the STAR prosthesis, with a minimum follow-up of 5 years. Thirteen ankles (27%) had a preoperative coronal deformity of more than 10 degrees (range, 11-25 degrees); most of the ankles were in preoperative varus. The authors believed that the preoperative hindfoot deformity was not an absolute contraindication for TAR as long the deformity was manageable by additional realignment procedures, including soft tissue releases, ligament reconstructions, calcaneal osteotomies and corrective subtalar fusion.[177]

Wood et al[374] reported short-term clinical and radiologic results of a prospective case series, including 100 Mobility TARs, with a minimum follow-up of 3 years. There were 15 ankles with a preoperative coronal deformity of 16 to 20 degrees. A varus or valgus deformity was observed in 33 (in 17 of these, it was more than 10 degrees), and in 29 (in 13 of these, it was more than 10 degrees) ankles, respectively. Postoperatively, there were five cases of edge loading of the mobile insert because of varus or valgus deformity. Of 5 ankles requiring revision surgery, 4 had significant preoperative coronal deformity: three patients with valgus deformity (11, 12, and 15 degrees, respectively) and one patient with varus deformity (19 degrees). Therefore the authors do not undertake TAR in patients with preoperative valgus or varus deformity of more than 20 degrees. In these cases, the authors recommend ankle fusion.[374]

Ellis and DeOrio[94] described in detail the surgical technique using the INBONE prosthesis. The authors described how to correct, intraoperatively, slight varus or valgus deformity by using a laminar spreader with teeth: the desired position of the talus should be 5 degrees of valgus. However, the authors stated that valgus deformity is more difficult to correct using the above-described technique.[84,94]

Skyttä et al[311] presented the survivorship analysis of the Finnish Arthroplasty Registry, including 515 TARs performed between 1982 and 2006. Nine different TAR prostheses were used: the most common TAR types were the AES, STAR, ICLH, and HINTEGRA prostheses, with 298, 217, 32, and 11 cases, respectively. The proportion of revisions done for instability in primary TAR was 39%. One of the reasons for prosthesis failure was preoperative valgus or varus deformity with insufficient ligaments.[311]

Morgan et al[238] presented the outcomes in 38 consecutive patients who underwent TAR using the AES ankle, with a minimum follow-up of 4 years. Twenty-eight patients had normal hindfoot alignment preoperatively, 10 patients had a valgus alignment ranging from 7 to 30 degrees, and 7 patients had a varus alignment ranging from 4 to 23 degrees. Postoperatively, 10 patients presented with edge loading and 5 and 2 of them had preoperative varus and valgus alignment, respectively.[238]

Kim et al[183] reported clinical and radiologic outcomes of TAR in association with hindfoot fusion. Three ankles (5%) in the hindfoot fusion group and 10 ankles (3.5%) in the control group had preoperative coronal deformity of more than 15 degrees. Significant valgus or varus deformity was not associated with worse functional outcome or higher failure rate.[183]

Bonasia et al[39] presented a review regarding indications for TAR and their surgical techniques. For small, minimal, distal tibial deformities of less than 10 degrees, realignment can be achieved by modification of the tibial cut. For more severe deformities, a dome or wedge osteotomy should be performed before TAR.[39]

Bonnin et al[40] retrospectively reviewed 98 TARs performed in 97 ankles between 1997 and 2000 by using the Salto prosthesis. The authors did not consider substantial preoperative varus or valgus deformity as a contraindication for TAR. However, all hindfoot deformities were corrected as a first step with an associated procedure (e.g., triple arthrodesis).[40] In some patients with preoperative valgus deformity, a special cemented lateral malleolar component was implanted to normalize loads transfer in this patient cohort.[41]

Recently, Trincat et al[338] presented their results from using TAR in patients with coronal plane deformities. From a total of 131 TARs, 21 TARs (16 AES ankles, 4 Salto ankles, and 1 New-Jersey ankle) were performed in ankles with preoperative coronal deformities of more than 10 degrees. There were four congruent and two incongruent valgus ankles. The following additional one-stage surgeries were performed to achieve the osseous and ligamental balancing: lateral malleolus lowering (2), Achilles tendon lengthening (4), reconstruction of medial ligaments (1), and triple arthrodesis (1). For congruent valgus ankles, surgery resulted in significant improvement of overall alignment from 14.7 ± 2.5 to 0 ± 2.5 degrees. There were no complications or failures in this subgroup. In preoperative incongruent valgus ankles, improvement of overall alignment from 19 ± 5.5 to 2 ± 4.2 degrees was observed. A failure occurred in one patient: this patient presented with a 23-degree deformity resulting from a bimalleolar fracture with insufficiency of the medial ligaments and posterior tibial tendon dysfunction. In conclusion, the short-term results of TAR in patients with preoperative coronal deformities of more than 10 degrees were satisfactory. However, several associated procedures were necessary to address the concomitant instabilities and deformities. Residual defects may compromise the longevity of prosthesis components and warrant further correction.[338]

Subsidence

Subsidence has been a problem with TAR since it was first performed. With the use of noncemented designs, subsidence of the tibial component has become less frequent,

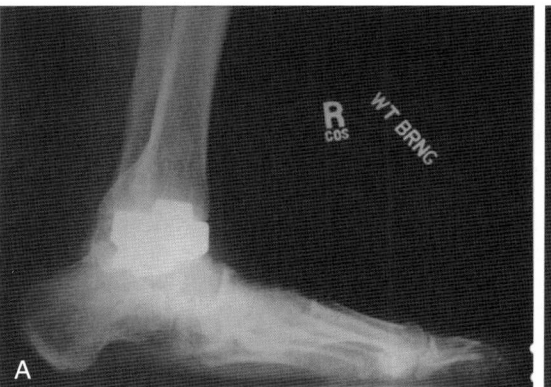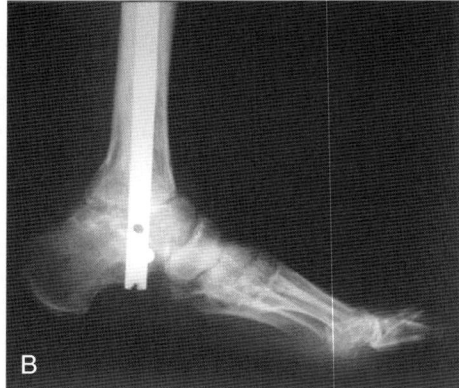

Figure 22-59 This Agility ankle was implanted in a 300-lb man who ignored his postoperative instructions and began playing golf 3 weeks after surgery. **A,** The talar component subsided deeply through the talus into the subtalar joint. **B,** This was salvaged with a tibiotalocalcaneal arthrodesis by using an intramedullary rod. *WT BRNG,* weight bearing. (Images courtesy Mark Scioli, MD, Lubbock, Tex.).

although it can still occur. There are several causes of subsidence, including insufficient bone ingrowth; insufficient bone stock; mal-loading of the ankle replacement; overstuffing of the joint, with increased stress transmitted to the bone; and overstressing the joint with high activity or weight (Fig. 22-59). In the author's laboratory, native ankle ligament strain was tested in a functional range of motion, and then the same was done with both Agility and STAR ankle replacements placed in positions of perfect and abnormal alignments.[296,336,337] These studies suggest that only the middle portion of the deltoid ligament receives any strain and, otherwise, the periankle ligaments do not strain during the stance phase of the gait cycle in a normal (nonreplaced) ankle.[336] With both the Agility and STAR ankle replacements, however, periankle ligaments are strained in the normal range of motion, and these strains are worsened by malaligned implantations.[296,337]

Together, these studies tell us that one factor influencing loosening or subsidence of total ankle components might be related to abnormal strains imposed by ligaments on the bone–implant interface. The talus is much more commonly involved with subsidence than the tibia. The reasons for this remain obscure but may include trabecular orientation and the congruency (or fit) of the outside surface of the talar component, with often complex cuts on the superior aspect of the talar dome.

The internal architecture of the talus is unique and reflects its biomechanical properties (Fig. 22-60). Compact bone in the talus is nonuniform, with thicker regions over the posterior calcaneal, medial malleolar, and lateral malleolar facets.[13] Thinner regions of compact bone exist over the trochlear surface and head of the talus.[13] The trabeculae of the talus can be resolved into two sets. The first set is deep to the medial part of the trochlear surface and from the anterior third of the lateral trochlear surface. Lamellae of this set are directed anteriorly toward the

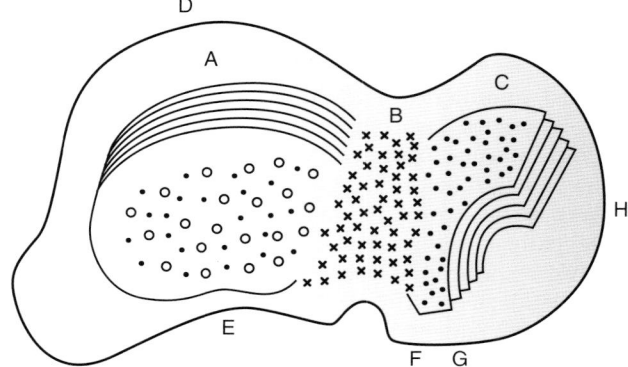

Figure 22-60 Diagrammatic representation of the trabecular architecture of the talus (right talus as seen from the medial aspect). The body of the talus consists of vertical plates *(A)*, the neck shows the trabecular meshwork of irregularly arranged plates *(B)*, and the head consists of semiarched plates *(C)*. The proximal end of the horizontal limb of semiarched plates also extends into the distal half of the neck. The distal end of the vertical and horizontal limbs of semiarched plates are shown with cut edges to demonstrate the semiarched nature. *D,* Trochlea. *E,* Posterior calcaneal facet. *F,* Middle calcaneal facet. *G,* Anterior calcaneal facet. *H,* Navicular articular surface of the head. (Modified from Pal GP, Routal RV: Architecture of the cancellous bone of the human talus. *Anat Rec* 252:185–193, 1998.)

head and neck of the talus. The second set is deep to the posterior two thirds of the trochlear surface and descend onto the posterior calcaneal facet.[13] The neck of the talus includes sagittal plates extending from the body to the head. This internal architecture may explain the distribution and transmission of forces through the talus during gait.[13,260] Furthermore, it has been shown that the internal trabecular alignment may change because of cartilage degeneration, which should be considered in ankles with degenerative changes.[301]

With many of the implants, the actual fit of the talar component to the talus is difficult or impossible to visualize intraoperatively. The exact incidence of these problems remains somewhat unclear and depends on the device being used. In an average 7-year radiographic follow-up of the Agility ankle, Knecht et al[189] reported 14% (16 of 117 ankles) had 5 mm or more of subsidence or 5 degrees or more of angular change, or both. Four percent (5 of 117 ankles) had only tibial subsidence of 5 mm or more (average, 8 mm; range, 7 to 8 mm). Eight percent (9 of 117) ankles had only talar subsidence of 5 mm or more (average, 10 mm; range, 5 to 20 mm). The survival curve on the tibial side showed stable fixation at 4 years but continued subsidence on the talar side up to 11 years.[189]

A few case series have focused on conversion of a subsided or loose ankle replacement to a fusion. In the largest of these series, Kitaoka[188] reported on the experience at the Mayo Clinic with 38 total ankles revised to fusion. A variety of different methods was used depending on the amount of bone loss and involvement of the subtalar joint. They reported 33 (89%) solid fusions for this often difficult mix of clinical problems. In a smaller series, Gabrion et al[110] reported successful fusion in 7 of 8 patients but satisfactory clinical results in only 5 patients. Culpan et al[74] treated 16 patients with failed TAR. All failed arthroplasties were converted to a fusion with internal fixation using tricortical autograft from the iliac crest to preserve the height of the ankle. In all but one ankle, a successful arthrodesis was achieved within 4.5 months.[74] Thomason and Eyres[333] used an allograft from the femoral head, with intramedullary nail fixation, in three patients with aseptic loosening of TAR. Hopgood et al[162] converted 23 failed total ankle arthroplasties to ankle fusion. Three different surgical techniques were used in this patient cohort: tibiotalar arthrodesis with screw fixation, tibiotalocalcaneal arthrodesis with screw fixation, and tibiotalocalcaneal arthrodesis with an intramedullary nail. Successful union was observed in most patients—17 of the 23 ankles. Especially in patients with rheumatoid arthritis and higher extensive destruction of the talar body, the complication rate was substantially higher.[162] Kotnis et al[208] treated 16 patients with a failed TAR. In patients with suspected infection, a two-stage procedure was planned.[208]

Not all subsided ankle replacements need conversion to fusion. Indeed, some clinical situations warrant a second attempt at an ankle replacement. If the original implant was inserted incorrectly, an early revision is often the best option. Errors related to component positioning may be seen on early radiographs, and recognizing them in an otherwise healthy and active patient should prompt a straightforward revision. If the subsidence has resulted in a substantial bone loss, then a decision needs to be made about how to handle the loss.

In general, there are two options—not mutually exclusive—for dealing with bone loss in total ankle revisions. One is to use a larger, custom or revision implant (Fig. 22-61); the other is to use bone graft. The first option works well for both tibial- and talar-sided revisions; however, the bone graft option may be best for the tibial side because the initial fixation of graft to the residual, and often very deficient, talus is technically much harder. If the subtalar joint is sacrificed, then fixation is somewhat easier because long screws can be placed through the graft into the calcaneus. When allograft is used, the component should be secured to the implant with methyl methacrylate. The authors prefer to use anatomically matched segments of allograft for this purpose (Fig. 22-62). In some cases, autograft from the iliac crest may be used to compensate the bony defect on the tibial and/or talar side. The revision procedure is then planned as two-stage procedure. First, the bony defect is corrected by iliac crest autograft. Polyethylene inlay may be used as a spacer between tibial and talus. Three or 4 months later, after osseous integration of the autograft, the implantation of ankle prosthesis is performed as a second step (Fig. 22-63). Although this approach can work, the revascularization of bulk autograft will be limited; cement use may still be required.

Polyethylene Failure

Polyethylene can fail catastrophically with fracture or slowly with generation of bioactive submicron wear particles. Catastrophic failure is relatively rare, but cases have been reported at scientific meetings.[12] Mobile bearings may be particularly prone to fracture because they can become extruded across the edge of the components (Table 22-3). Fractures have typically occurred with thin bearings because the thicker bearings are less prone to fatigue fracture (Fig. 22-64). Uncorrected deformity and secondary focal elevated internal polyethylene loading are causes for catastrophic failure.

Wear of polyethylene in total ankle arthroplasties has not yet become a major concern because long-term results are not yet available. Analyses of particles in synovial fluid from 15 TAR patients were compared with those from 11 patients with posterior-stabilized total knee arthroplasties.[197] Polyethylene particles were isolated and analyzed using scanning electron microscopy. Particle size (equivalent circle diameter) and concentration in ankles were the same as in knees after replacement surgery. These data suggest that the long-term result of total ankle arthroplasty should be as good as posterior-stabilized total knee arthroplasties in terms of polyethylene wear and the prevalence of osteolysis.

TAR polyethylene is generally not highly cross-linked. Although the benefits of this processing are becoming clear in hip replacement surgery, and may be similarly helpful after knee replacement surgery, the widespread adoption of highly cross-linked polyethylene in TARs is unlikely, especially with mobile-bearing designs. The process of cross-linking polyethylene makes the bearing more brittle and prone to fracture along crystalline lines. Three-part or mobile-bearing designs cannot fully

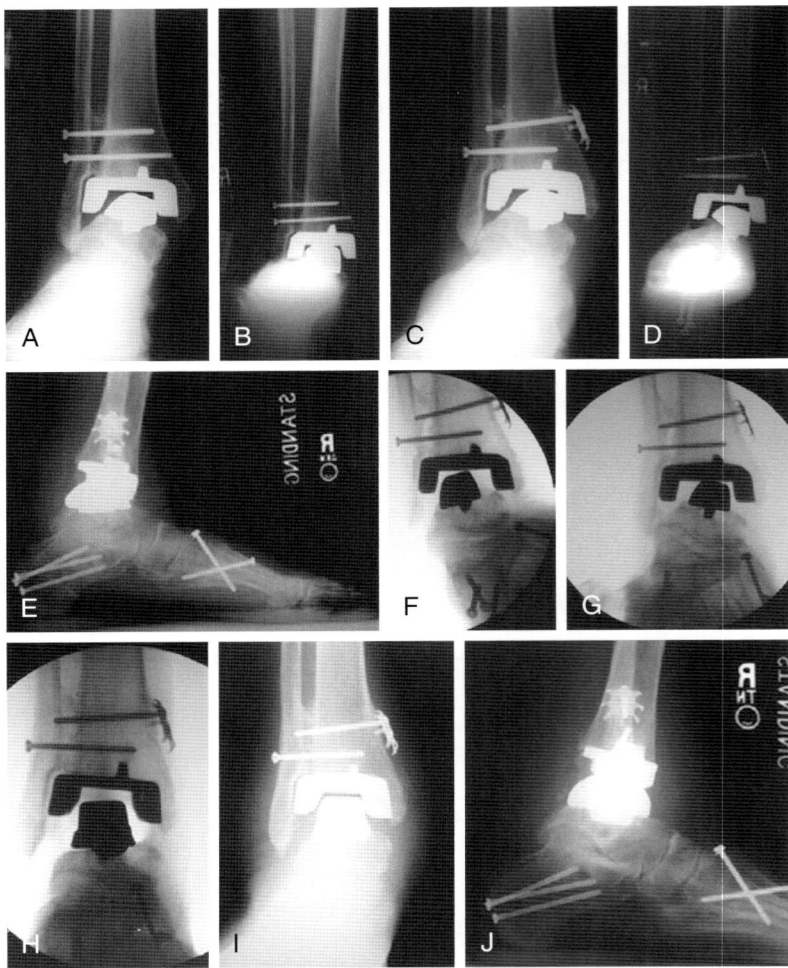

Figure 22-61 **A** and **B**, Intracomponent instability after an Agility total ankle replacement in a patient with deltoid ligament insufficiency and benign joint hypermobility syndrome. The author's (Dr. Charles Saltzman) first attempt to realign the component with extracomponent surgery failed. **C-E,** This first revision surgery involved an Achilles tendon allograft replacement of the deltoid, medialization of the calcaneal tuberosity, and first metatarsocuneiform fusion. **F** and **G,** One year later, the author's group performed a fluoroscopic evaluation of the joint with forced varus/valgus positioning. The talar component was found to easily displace in every direction, including straight distraction. A custom prosthesis was designed to reduce the extra volume between the components. **H,** Intraoperative imaging during the second revision showed excellent stability and alignment. **I** and **J,** Standing radiographs 2 years later show preservation of excellent alignment, consistent with the good clinical outcome.

preclude that the bearing will subluxate or be exposed to edge loading, so the risks of bearing fracture always remain. For that reason, the prevalence of highly cross-linked polyethylene in TAR is limited at the time of writing this chapter.

In a study of medium-term results with the Agility ankle, Knecht et al[189] reported, at an average of 7.2 years of follow-up, that 15% (18 of 117) of ankles had expansile lysis. Of these, 4 (22%) showed definite signs of progression over time on serial radiographic evaluation, and 14 appeared relatively stable on serial radiographs. Expansile lysis was a late-onset disorder appearing, on average, 35 months after TAR (range, 9 to 85 months).[189]

The extremely high incidence of severe periprosthetic osteolytic lesions in patients who underwent the AES TAR[33,203,238,281] led to this prosthesis being withdrawn from the market.

Treatment of progressive and ballooning perimplant osteolysis should be undertaken when recognized. Serial radiographs or CT scans may be needed to confirm an initial clinical suspicion (see Fig. 22-41). These lesions tend to enlarge, destroy bone, undermine stable fixation, and lead to more severe problems. At first, patients are generally asymptomatic and not willing to undergo a large revision operation. If they insist on waiting and the problem increases, painful symptoms usually arise and the reconstruction is more difficult.

In cases where the damage is limited, the initial surgery involves exchange to a thicker polyethyelene insert, complete curettage of the lesions, and bone grafting. Mobile bearings are much easier to exchange than fixed bearings. At the time of surgery, the polyethylene is inspected for signs of bearing wear, and the corresponding metal articulating surfaces are closely inspected for any surface irregularities. If irregularities are present, that surface of the implant must be replaced, or the problem will recur. If the damage to periimplant bone is extensive and has caused subsidence of the implant, the implant might need to be replaced with a new implant. With significant bone loss, a revision implantation may be necessary (Fig. 22-65).

If the wear is due to unbalanced loading of the implant, the mechanical imbalance must be corrected or the problem will recur. The surgeon must decide if this is a problem that can or will respond to revision or reconstructive surgery. In some cases, especially with severe

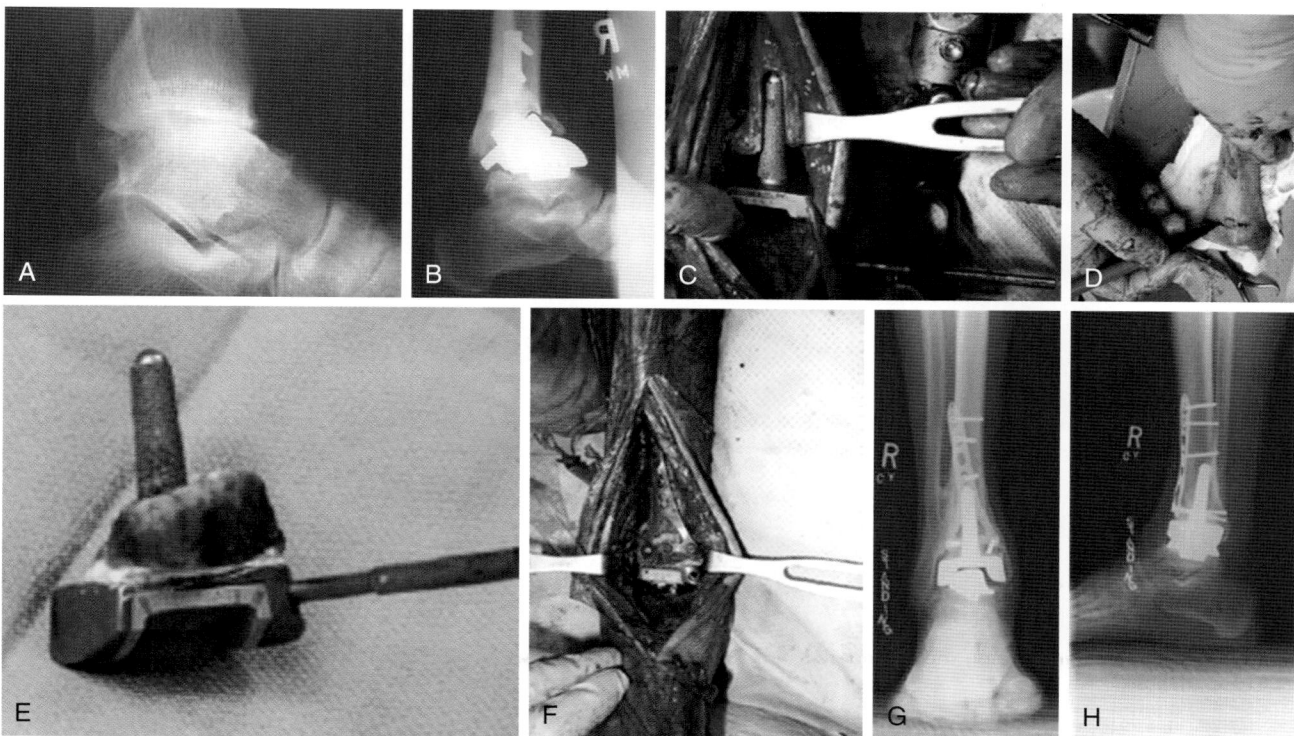

Figure 22-62 Bulk allograft bone supplementation for component subsidence. **A,** Initial preoperative lateral radiographs show anterior subluxation of the talus under the tibia. **B,** The talar implant was initially placed too anterior and never developed secure ingrowth of bone to the tibial component, ultimately resulting in anterior cortical collapse. **C,** First, the implant was removed under mechanical distraction, and a trough for the stem of a custom-designed revision tibial component was created and tested. An anatomically matched distal tibia **(D)** was cut to fill the bony defect and secured to the tibial component with methyl methacrylate **(E). F,** The allograft-component construct was fixed to the tibia with a low-profile plate, followed by insertion of a standard revision talar component. **G** and **H,** Radiographs at 3 years show bony remodeling around the allograft and stable fixation without further subsidence.

Table 22-3 Studies Reporting on Polyethylene Insert Fractures in STAR Ankle Prosthesis

Author(s)	Year	STAR-Replaced Ankles	PE-Related Complications	Revision Surgery
Anderson et al[8,9]	2003	51	Broken PE insert (n = 2)	PE replacement (n = 2)
Brunner et al[46]	2012	77	Broken PE insert (n = 11)	PE replacement (n = 9), ankle replacement (n = 2)
Harris et al[133]	2009	Case report	Edge loading and wear debris cyst, subsequent fracture of fibula	ORIF fibula, PE replacement, medial release, and lateral ligament reconstruction
Karantana et al[177]	2010	52	Broken PE insert (n = 2) with edge loading	PE replacement (n = 1), talar component and PE replacement (n = 1)
Scott and Nunley[307]	2009	93	Broken PE insert (n = 3)	PE replacement (n = 3)
Wood and Deakin[373]*	2003	200	Edge loading of PE (n = 9)	PE replacement (n = 3), ankle fusion (n = 3)
Wood et al[372]*	2007	171	Broken PE insert (n = 2)	NA
Wood et al[375]	2008	200	Broken PE insert (n = 1)	Ankle fusion (n = 1)
Wood et al[376]	2009	100	Broken PE insert (n = 2)	Ankle fusion (n = 2)

NA, not available; *ORIF,* open reduction and internal fixation; *PE,* polyethylene; *STAR,* Scandinavian Total Ankle Replacement.
* The patient cohort from the study presented in 2007 was a part of the patient cohort from the study presented in 2003.

rigid varus deformities, the surgeon might find it impossible to completely realign ankle loading to a well-balanced joint. In these circumstances, it is best to perform an ankle fusion. When reconstruction of the implant and ankle is considered feasible, the surgeon should determine if the problem has arisen from malalignment of the components or from malalignment of the ankle and foot. Treatment is then directed at the source of the problem. Revision implantations are performed to correct imbalances between components, and corrective

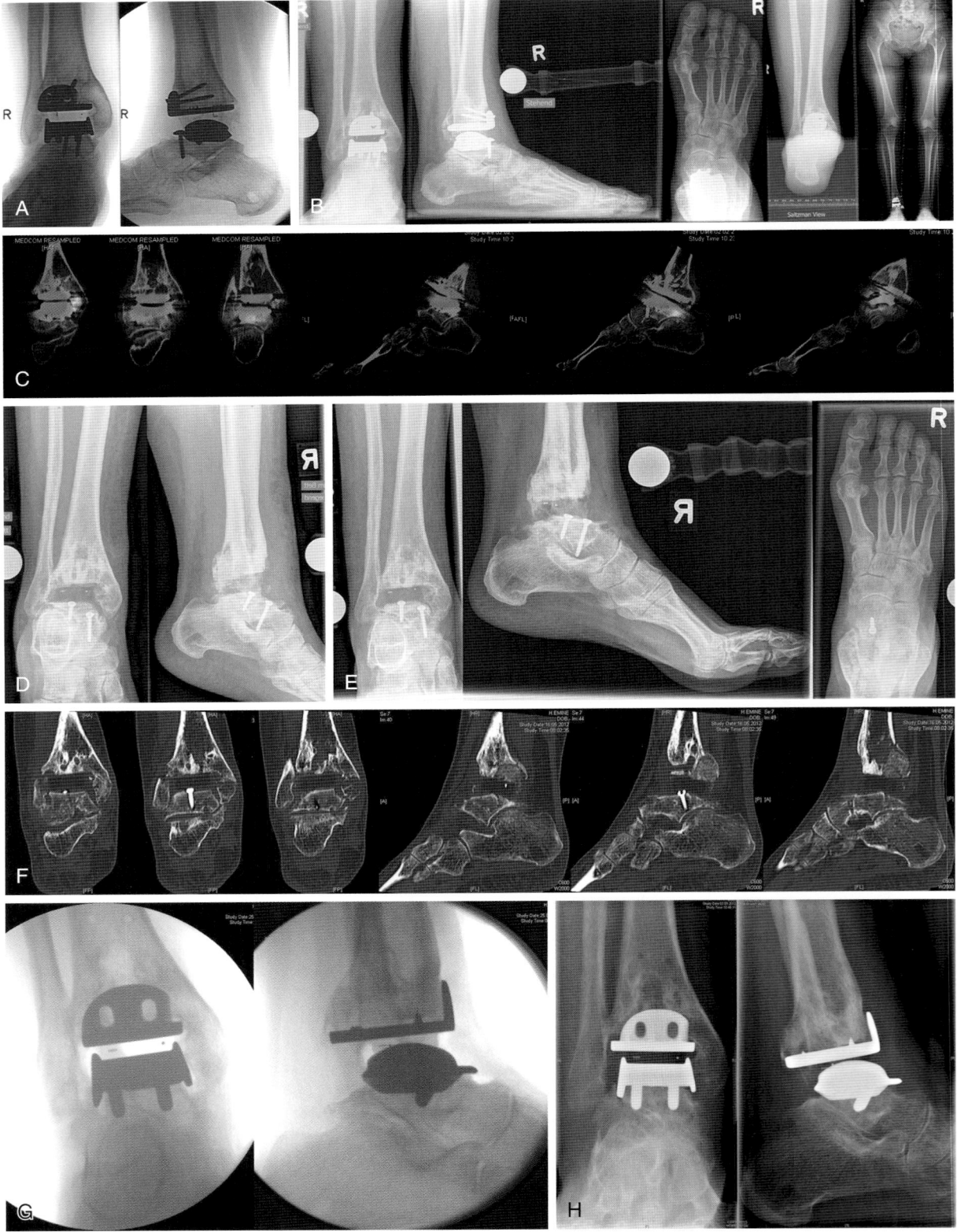

Figure 22-63 **A,** Postoperative radiographs 1 year after revision arthroplasty in a 38-year-old female. The revision surgery was performed 4 years after initial total ankle replacement because of aseptic loosening of both components. **B,** Six years later, the patient complained about severe pain in replaced ankle. Radiographs showed significant loosening of both the tibial and talar prosthesis components. **C,** Single-photon emission computed tomography (SPECT) image confirmed aseptic loosening around the tibia and talar prosthesis components. **D,** Revision surgery has been performed. The polyethylene mobile bearing and both metallic components were removed. Large cystic lesions were observed, especially underneath the talar component. After debridement, iliac crest autograft was used to fill the defect on the talar side. The autograft was fixed using two screws. Polyethylene inlay was used as a spacer. **E,** Three months later, solid integration of autograft was observed. During the 3 months, the patient was allowed to have partial weight bearing (15 kg). **F,** Solid integration of autograft was also seen on CT scans. **G,** Four months later, revision total ankle replacement was been performed. Intraoperative, solid consolidation was observed on the tibial side. **H,** Three months later, postoperative radiographs showed proper positioning of prosthesis components.

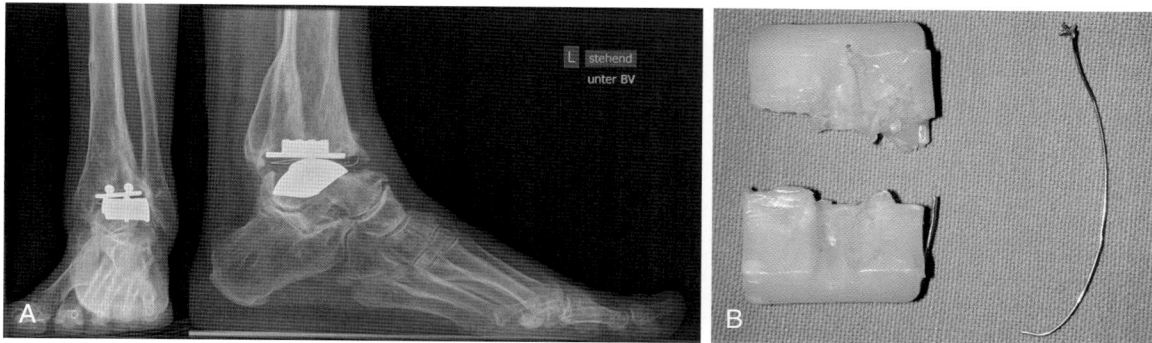

Figure 22-64 **A,** Radiographs of a 61-year-old female who underwent Scandinavian Total Ankle Replacement (STAR) 4 years earlier, showing fracture of polyethylene insert. **B,** Photograph of explanted fractured polyethylene with extruded metal marker. (Images courtesy Beat Hintermann, MD, Liestal, Switzerland.)

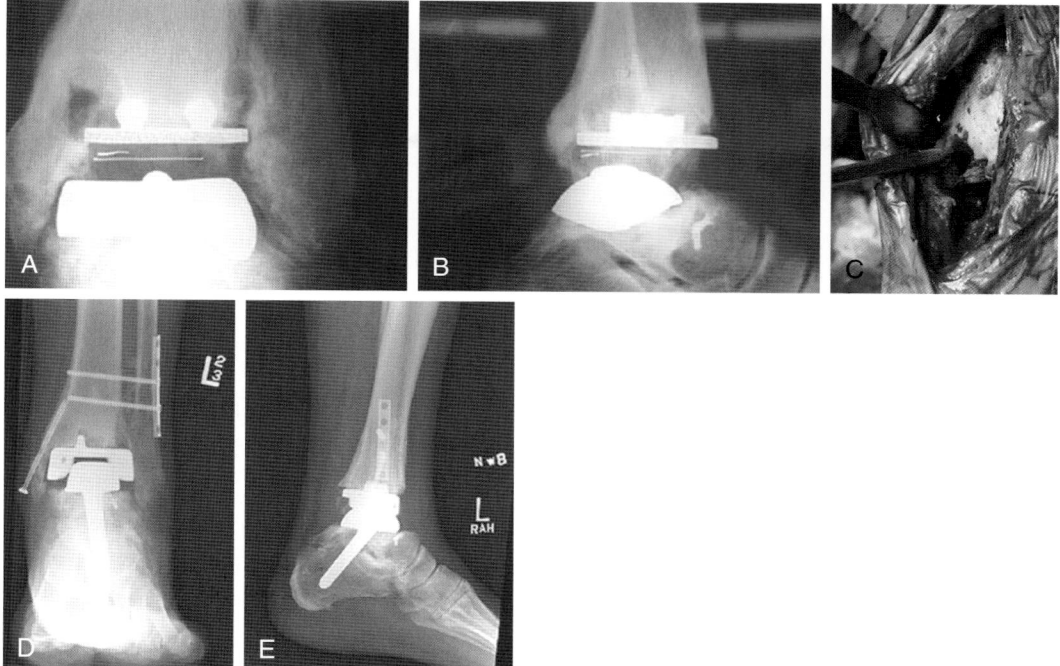

Figure 22-65 Total ankle revision for massive osteolysis. **A** and **B,** These radiographs show early polyethylene wear in a 55-year-old man 3 years after total ankle replacement. **C,** During revision surgery, large areas of osteolysis were found involving the tibial and talar sides. **D** and **E,** This ankle replacement was salvaged with the use of extra thick polyethylene and a slightly taller, stemmed talar implant for better fixation and support.

osteotomies and selective fusions are performed to balance the foot.

In the authors' opinion, the key to reconstruction is proper bone alignment, not ligament or muscle support. If the bone alignment does not ensure that the weight-bearing force goes directly through the center of the implant with quiet standing, the implant will eventually tilt and expose the ankle to the risk of host reaction to accelerated polyethylene wear. Any surgeon who performs ankle replacements needs extensive experience with total joint replacement techniques and must understand how

to align and balance the bony and articular architecture of the leg, ankle, and foot.

REFERENCES

1. Abu-Hijleh MF, Harris PF: Deep fascia on the dorsum of the ankle and foot: extensor retinacula revisited, *Clin Anat* 20:186–195, 2007.
2. Affatato S, Leardini A, Leardini W, et al: Meniscal wear at a three-component total ankle prosthesis by a knee joint simulator, *J Biomech* 40:1871–1876, 2007.
3. Affatato S, Taddei P, Leardini A, et al: Wear behaviour in total ankle replacement: a comparison between an in vitro

simulation and retrieved prostheses, *Clin Biomech (Bristol, Avon)* 24:661–669, 2009.

4. Aitken GK, Bourne RB, Finlay JB, et al: Indentation stiffness of the cancellous bone in the distal human tibia, *Clin Orthop Relat Res* 201:264–270, 1985.

5. Ali MS, Higgins GA, Mohamed M: Intermediate results of Buechel Pappas unconstrained uncemented total ankle replacement for osteoarthritis, *J Foot Ankle Surg* 46:16–20, 2007.

6. Alvine FG: The Agility ankle replacement: the good and the bad, *Foot Ankle Clin* 7:737–753, 2002.

7. Anders H, Kaj K, Johan J, Urban R: The AES total ankle replacement: a mid-term analysis of 93 cases, *Foot Ankle Surg* 16:61–64, 2010.

8. Anderson T, Montgomery F, Carlsson A: Uncemented STAR total ankle prostheses. Three to eight-year follow-up of fifty-one consecutive ankles, *J Bone Joint Surg Am* 85-A:1321–1329, 2003.

9. Anderson T, Montgomery F, Carlsson A: Uncemented STAR total ankle prostheses, *J Bone Joint Surg Am* 86-A(Suppl 1, Pt 2):103–111, 2004.

10. Asencio J, Leonardi C: Ankle Evolutive System prosthesis: a simple, accurate, and reliable specific concept for primary and revision surgery, *Tech Foot Ankle* 4:119–124, 2005.

11. Assal M, Al-Shaikh R, Reiber BH, Hansen ST: Fracture of the polyethylene component in an ankle arthroplasty: a case report, *Foot Ankle Int* 24:901–903, 2003.

12. Assal M, Greisberg J, Hansen ST Jr: Revision total ankle arthroplasty: conversion of New Jersey Low Contact Stress to Agility: surgical technique and case report, *Foot Ankle Int* 25:922–925, 2004.

13. Athavale SA, Joshi SD, Joshi SS: Internal architecture of the talus, *Foot Ankle Int* 29:82–86, 2008.

14. Atkinson HD, Daniels TR, Klejman S, et al: Pre- and postoperative gait analysis following conversion of tibiotalocalcaneal fusion to total ankle arthroplasty, *Foot Ankle Int* 31:927–932, 2010.

15. Bahr R, Pena F, Shine J, et al: Mechanics of the anterior drawer and talar tilt tests. A cadaveric study of lateral ligament injuries of the ankle, *Acta Orthop Scand* 68:435–441, 1997.

16. Bai LB, Lee KB, Song EK, et al: Total ankle arthroplasty outcome comparison for post-traumatic and primary osteoarthritis, *Foot Ankle Int* 31:1048–1056, 2010.

17. Baker JF, Perera A, Lui DF, Stephens MM: The effect of body mass index on outcomes after total ankle replacement, *Ir Med J* 102:188–190, 2009.

18. Bardelli M, Scoccianti G: Uncemented total ankle arthroplasty in post-traumatic osteoarthritis: 3- to 7-year follow-up, *J Orthopaed Traumatol* 7:93–96, 2006.

19. Barenfeld PA, Weseley MS, Munters M: Dwyer calcaneal osteotomy, *Clin Orthop Relat Res* 53:147–153, 1967.

20. Barg A, Elsner A, Anderson AE, Hintermann B: The effect of three-component total ankle replacement malalignment on clinical outcome: pain relief and functional outcome in 317 consecutive patients, *J Bone Joint Surg Am* 93:1969–1978, 2011.

21. Barg A, Elsner A, Chuckpaiwong B, Hintermann B: Insert position in three-component total ankle replacement, *Foot Ankle Int* 31:754–759, 2010.

22. Barg A, Elsner A, Hefti D, Hintermann B: Haemophilic arthropathy of the ankle treated by total ankle replacement: a case series, *Haemophilia* 16:647–655, 2010.

23. Barg A, Elsner A, Hefti D, Hintermann B: Total ankle arthroplasty in patients with hereditary hemochromatosis, *Clin Orthop Relat Res* 469:1427–1435, 2011.

24. Barg A, Harris MD, Henninger HB, et al: Medial distal tibial angle: comparison between weightbearing mortise view and hindfoot alignment view, *Foot Ankle Int* 33:655–661, 2012.

25. Barg A, Henninger HB, Knupp M, Hintermann B: Simultaneous bilateral total ankle replacement using a 3-component prosthesis: outcome in 26 patients followed for 2-10 years, *Acta Orthop* 82:704–710, 2011.

26. Barg A, Knupp M, Anderson AE, Hintermann B: Total ankle replacement in obese patients: component stability, weight change, and functional outcome in 118 consecutive patients, *Foot Ankle Int* 32:925–932, 2011.

27. Barg A, Knupp M, Henninger HB, et al: Total ankle replacement using HINTEGRA, an unconstrained, three-component system: surgical technique and pitfalls, *Foot Ankle Clin* 17:607–635, 2012. doi:10.1016/j.fcl.2012.08.006.

28. Barg A, Knupp M, Hintermann B: Simultaneous bilateral versus unilateral total ankle replacement: a patient-based comparison of pain relief, quality of life and functional outcome, *J Bone Joint Surg Br* 92:1659–1663, 2010.

29. Barg A, Knupp M, Kapron AL, Hintermann B: Total ankle replacement in patients with gouty arthritis, *J Bone Joint Surg Am* 93:357–366, 2011.

30. Bauer G, Eberhardt O, Rosenbaum D, Claes L: Total ankle replacement. Review and critical analysis of the current status, *Foot Ankle Surg* 2:119–126, 1996.

31. Bell CJ, Fisher J: Simulation of polyethylene wear in ankle joint prostheses, *J Biomed Mater Res B Appl Biomater* 81:162–167, 2007.

32. Berkowitz MJ, Clare MP, Walling AK, Sanders R: Salvage of failed total ankle arthroplasty with fusion using structural allograft and internal fixation, *Foot Ankle Int* 32:S493–S502, 2011.

33. Besse JL, Brito N, Lienhart C: Clinical evaluation and radiographic assessment of bone lysis of the AES total ankle replacement, *Foot Ankle Int* 30:964–975, 2009.

34. Besse JL, Colombier JA, Asencio J, et al: Total ankle arthroplasty in France, *Orthop Traumatol Surg Res* 96:291–303, 2010.

35. Bianchi A, Martinelli N, Sartorelli E, Malerba F: The Bologna-Oxford total ankle replacement: a mid-term follow-up study, *J Bone Joint Surg Br* 94:793–798, 2012.

36. Bluman EM, Chiodo CP: Valgus ankle deformity and arthritis, *Foot Ankle Clin* 13:443–470, 2008.

37. Bolt PM, Coy S, Toolan BC: A comparison of lateral column lengthening and medial translational osteotomy of the calcaneus for the reconstruction of adult acquired flatfoot, *Foot Ankle Int* 28:1115–1123, 2007.

38. Bolton-Maggs BG, Sudlow RA, Freeman MA: Total ankle arthroplasty. A long-term review of the London Hospital experience, *J Bone Joint Surg Br* 67:785–790, 1985.

39. Bonasia DE, Dettoni F, Femino JE, et al: Total ankle replacement: why, when and how? *Iowa Orthop J* 30:119–130, 2010.

40. Bonnin M, Gaudot F, Laurent JR, et al: The Salto total ankle arthroplasty: survivorship and analysis of failures at 7 to 11 years, *Clin Orthop Relat Res* 469:225–236, 2011.

41. Bonnin M, Judet T, Colombier JA, et al: Midterm results of the Salto Total Ankle Prosthesis, *Clin Orthop Relat Res* 424:6–18, 2004.

42. Bonnin MP, Laurent JR, Casillas M: Ankle function and sports activity after total ankle arthroplasty, *Foot Ankle Int* 30:933–944, 2009.

43. Bourke G, Gomez G: *A comparison of CT and plain film assessment of osteolysis following total ankle joint arthroplasty*. Presented at 27th Annual Summer Meeting of the American Orthopaedic Foot and Ankle Society, San Diego, California, USA, June 20-23, 2012.

44. Brodsky JW, Polo FE, Coleman SC, Bruck N: Changes in gait following the Scandinavian Total Ankle Replacement, *J Bone Joint Surg Am* 93:1890–1896, 2011.

45. Brooke BT, Harris NJ, Morgan SS: Fibula lengthening osteotomy to correct valgus mal-alignment following total ankle

arthrplasty, *Foot Ankle Surg* 18:144–147, 2012. doi:10.1016/j. fas.2009.11.002.

46. Brunner S, Barg A, Knupp M, et al: The Scandinavian Total Ankle Replacement: long-term 11 to 15 year, survivorship analysis of the prosthesis in 72 consecutive patients, *J Bone Joint Surg Am* 95:711–718, 2012.

47. Brunner S, Knupp M, Hintermann B: Total ankle replacement for the valgus unstable osteoarthritic ankle, *Tech Foot Ankle* 9:174, 2010.

48. Buchholz HW, Engelbrecht E, Siegel A: [Complete ankle joint endoprosthesis type "St. Georg"], *Chirurg* 44:241–244, 1973.

49. Buechel FF Sr, Buechel FF Jr, Pappas MJ: Ten-year evaluation of cementless Buechel-Pappas meniscal bearing total ankle replacement, *Foot Ankle Int* 24:462–472, 2003.

50. Buechel FF Sr, Buechel FF Jr, Pappas MJ: Twenty-year evaluation of cementless mobile-bearing total ankle replacements, *Clin Orthop Relat Res* 424:19–26, 2004.

51. Buechel FF Sr, Buechel FF Jr, Pappas MJ, D'Alessio J: Twenty-year evaluation of meniscal bearing and rotating platform knee replacements, *Clin Orthop Relat Res* 388:41–50, 2001.

52. Buechel FF, Pappas MJ, Iorio LJ: New Jersey low contact stress total ankle replacement: biomechanical rationale and review of 23 cementless cases, *Foot Ankle* 8:279–290, 1988.

53. Carlsson A: [Single- and double-coated star total ankle replacements: a clinical and radiographic follow-up study of 109 cases], *Orthopade* 35:527–532, 2006.

54. Carlsson A, Markusson P, Sundberg M: Radiostereometric analysis of the double-coated STAR total ankle prosthesis: a 3-5 year follow-up of 5 cases with rheumatoid arthritis and 5 cases with osteoarthrosis, *Acta Orthop* 76:573–579, 2005.

55. Carlsson AS, Henricson A, Linder L: A survival analysis of 52 Bath and Wessex ankle replacements, *Foot* 4:34–40, 1994.

56. Carlsson AS, Henricson A, Linder L, et al: A 10-year analysis of 69 Bath and Wessex ankle replacements, *Foot Ankle Surg* 7:39–44, 2001.

57. Cenni F, Leardini A, Belvedere C, et al: Kinematics of the three components of a total ankle replacement: in vivo fluoroscopic analysis, *Foot Ankle Int* 33:290–300, 2012.

58. Cenni F, Leardini A, Cheli A, et al: Position of the prosthesis components in total ankle replacement and the effect on motion at the replaced joint, *Int Orthop* 36:571–578, 2012.

59. Cerrato R, Myerson MS: Total ankle replacement: the Agility LP prosthesis, *Foot Ankle Clin* 13:485–494, 2008.

60. Chhabra A, Soldatos T, Chalian M, et al: Current concepts review: 3T magnetic resonance imaging of the ankle and foot, *Foot Ankle Int* 33:164–171, 2012.

61. Christ RM, Hagena FW: Komplikationen und Revisionseingriffe nach OSG-Totalendoprothesen, *Fuss Sprungg* 3:112–121, 2005.

62. Clare MP, Sanders RW: Preoperative considerations in ankle replacement surgery, *Foot Ankle Clin* 7:709–720, 2002.

63. Claridge RJ, Sagherian BH: Intermediate term outcome of the agility total ankle arthroplasty, *Foot Ankle Int* 30:824–835, 2009.

64. Coester LM, Saltzman CL, Leupold J, Pontarelli W: Long-term results following ankle arthrodesis for post-traumatic arthritis, *J Bone Joint Surg Am* 83-A:219–228, 2001.

65. Coetzee JC: Management of varus or valgus ankle deformity with ankle replacement, *Foot Ankle Clin* 13:509–520, 2008.

66. Coetzee JC, Castro MD: Accurate measurement of ankle range of motion after total ankle arthroplasty, *Clin Orthop Relat Res* 424:27–31, 2004.

67. Conti SF, Wong YS: Complications of total ankle replacement, *Clin Orthop Relat Res* 391:105–114, 2001.

68. Conti SF, Wong YS: Complications of total ankle replacement, *Foot Ankle Clin* 7:791–807, 2002.

69. Corazza F, Leardini A, O'Connor JJ, Parenti Castelli V: Mechanics of the anterior drawer test at the ankle: the effects of ligament viscoelasticity, *J Biomech* 38:2118–2123, 2005.

70. Corazza F, O'Connor JJ, Leardini A, Parenti Castelli V: Ligament fibre recruitment and forces for the anterior drawer test at the human ankle joint, *J Biomech* 36:363–372, 2003.

71. Courville XF, Hecht PJ, Tosteson AN: Is total ankle arthroplasty a cost-effective alternative to ankle fusion? *Clin Orthop Relat Res* 469:1721–1727, 2011.

72. Cracchiolo A 3rd, Deorio JK: Design features of current total ankle replacements: implants and instrumentation, *J Am Acad Orthop Surg* 16:530–540, 2008.

73. Criswell BJ, Douglas K, Naik R, Thomson AB: High revision and reoperation rates using the Agility Total Ankle System, *Clin Orthop Relat Res* 470:1980–1986, 2012.

74. Culpan P, Le Strat V, Piriou P, Judet T: Arthrodesis after failed total ankle replacement, *J Bone Joint Surg Br* 89:1178–1183, 2007.

75. Dahabreh Z, Gonsalves S, Monkhouse R, Harris NJ: Extrusion of metal radiological marker from a total ankle replacement insert: a case report, *J Foot Ankle Surg* 45:185–189, 2006.

76. Daniels TR, Cadden AR, Lim K: Correction of varus talar deformities in ankle joint replacement, *Oper Tech Orthop* 18:282–286, 2008.

77. Davies MB, Saxby T: Ankle arthropathy of hemochromatosis: a case series and review of the literature, *Foot Ankle Int* 27:902–906, 2006.

78. De Wachter J, Knupp M, Hintermann B: Double-hindfoot arthrodesis through a single medial approach, *Tech Foot Ankle* 6:237–242, 2007.

79. Delagoutte JP: Retrospective analysis of 110 ankle prostheses, *Eur J Orthop Surg Traumatol* 12:198–205, 2002.

80. Demottaz JD, Mazur JM, Thomas WH, et al: Clinical study of total ankle replacement with gait analysis. A preliminary report, *J Bone Joint Surg Am* 61:976–988, 1979.

81. Deorio JK: INBONE total ankle arthroplasty, *Semin Arthro* 21:288–294, 2010.

82. Deorio JK: Total ankle replacement with subtalar arthrodesis: management of combined ankle ans subtalar arthritis, *Tech Foot Ankle* 9:182–189, 2010.

83. Deorio JK: Peritalar symposium: total ankle replacements with malaligned ankles: osteotomies performed simultaneously with TAA, *Foot Ankle Int* 33:344–346, 2012.

84. Deorio JK, Easley ME: Total ankle arthroplasty, *Instr Course Lect* 57:383–413, 2008.

85. Detrembleur C, Leemrijse T: The effects of total ankle replacement on gait disability: analysis of energetic and mechanical variables, *Gait Posture* 29:270–274, 2009.

86. Devries JG, Berlet GC, Lee TH, et al: Revision total ankle replacement: an early look at agility to INBONE, *Foot Ankle Spec* 4:235–244, 2011.

87. Dhawan R, Turner J, Sharma V, Nayak RK: Tri-component, mobile bearing, total ankle replacement-mid-term functional outcome and survival, *J Foot Ankle Surg* 51:566–569, 2012. doi:10.1053/j.jfas.2012.05.002.

88. Dini AA, Bassett FH 3rd: Evaluation of the early result of Smith total ankle replacement, *Clin Orthop Relat Res* 146:228–230, 1980.

89. Doets HC, Brand R, Nelissen RG: Total ankle arthroplasty in inflammatory joint disease with use of two mobile-bearing designs, *J Bone Joint Surg Am* 88:1272–1284, 2006.

90. Doets HC, van der Plaat LW, Klein JP: Medial malleolar osteotomy for the correction of varus deformity during total ankle arthroplasty: results in 15 ankles, *Foot Ankle Int* 29:171–177, 2008.

91. Dwyer FC: Osteotomy of the calcaneum for pes cavus, *J Bone Joint Surg Br* 41:80–86, 1959.

92. Easley ME, Adams SB Jr, Hembree WC, Deorio JK: Current concepts review: results of total ankle arthroplasty, *J Bone Joint Surg Am* 93:1455–1468, 2011.

93. Eichinger S, Forst R, Kindervater M: [Indications and alternatives for arthroplasty in young patients], *Orthopade* 36:311–324, 2007.

94. Ellis S, Deorio JK: The INBONE total ankle replacement, *Oper Tech Orthop* 20:201–210, 2010.

95. Ellis SJ, Deyer T, Williams BR, et al: Assessment of lateral hindfoot pain in acquired flatfoot deformity using weightbearing multiplanar imaging, *Foot Ankle Int* 31:361–371, 2010.

96. Ellis SJ, Moril-Penalver L, Deland JT: The Scandinavian Total Ankle Replacement (STAR) system, *Semin Arthro* 21:275–281, 2010.

97. Engelbrecht E: [Ankle-joint endoprosthesis model "St. George"], *Z Orthop Ihre Grenzgeb* 113:546–548, 1975.

98. Espinosa N, Klammer G: Treatment of ankle osteoarthritis: arthrodesis versus total ankle replacement, *Eur J Trauma Emerg Surg* 36:525–535, 2010.

99. Espinosa N, Walti M, Favre P, Snedeker JG: Misalignment of total ankle components can induce high joint contact pressures, *J Bone Joint Surg Am* 92:1179–1187, 2010.

100. Espinosa N, Wirth SH: [Ankle arthrodesis after failed total ankle replacement], *Orthopade* 40:1008, 1010–1008, 1017, 2011.

101. Espinosa N, Wirth SH, Jankauskas L: Ankle fusion after failed total ankle replacement, *Tech Foot Ankle* 9:199–204, 2010.

102. Evanski PH, Waugh TR: Management of arthritis of the ankle. An alternative of arthrodesis, *Clin Orthop Relat Res* 122:110–115, 1977.

103. Feldman MH, Rockwood J: Total ankle arthroplasty: a review of 11 current ankle implants, *Clin Podiatr Med Surg* 21:393–406, vii, 2004.

104. Fevang BT, Lie SA, Havelin LI, et al: 257 ankle arthroplasties performed in Norway between 1994 and 2005, *Acta Orthop* 78:575–583, 2007.

105. Freeman MA, Kempson GE, Tuke MA: Total replacement of the ankle with the ICLH prosthesis, *Int Orthop* 2:237–331, 1979.

106. Frigg A, Nigg B, Davis E, et al: Does alignment in the hindfoot radiograph influence dynamic foot-floor pressures in ankle and tibiotalocalcaneal fusion? *Clin Orthop Relat Res* 468:3362–3370, 2010.

107. Frigg A, Nigg B, Hinz L, et al: Clinical relevance of hindfoot alignment view in total ankle replacement, *Foot Ankle Int* 31:871–879, 2010.

108. Fuchs S, Sandmann C, Skwara A, Chylarecki C: Quality of life 20 years after arthrodesis of the ankle. A study of adjacent joints, *J Bone Joint Surg Br* 85:994–998, 2003.

109. Fukuda T, Haddad SL, Ren Y, Zhang LQ: Impact of talar component rotation on contact pressure after total ankle arthroplasty: a cadaveric study, *Foot Ankle Int* 31:404–411, 2010.

110. Gabrion A, Jarde O, Havet E, et al: [Ankle arthrodesis after failure of a total ankle prosthesis. Eight cases], *Rev Chir Orthop Reparatrice Appar Mot* 90:353–359, 2004.

111. Garde L, Kofoed H: Meniscal-bearing ankle arthroplasty is stable. In vivo analysis using stabilometry, *Foot Ankle Surg* 2:137–143, 1996.

112. Giannini S, Buda R, Faldini C, et al: The treatment of severe posttraumatic arthritis of the ankle joint, *J Bone Joint Surg Am* 89(Suppl 3):15–28, 2007.

113. Giannini S, Leardini A, O'Connor JJ: Total ankle replacement: review of the design and of the current status, *Foot Ankle Surg* 6:77–88, 2000.

114. Giannini S, Romagnoli M, O'Connor JJ, et al: Early clinical results of the BOX ankle replacement are satisfactory: a multicenter feasibility study of 158 ankles, *J Foot Ankle Surg* 50:641–647, 2011.

115. Giannini S, Romagnoli M, O'Connor JJ, et al: Total ankle replacement compatible with ligament function produces mobility, good clinical scores, and low complication rates: an early clinical assessment, *Clin Orthop Relat Res* 468:2746–2753, 2010.

116. Gittins J, Mann RA: The history of the STAR total ankle arthroplasty, *Foot Ankle Clin* 7:809–816, 2002.

117. Goldberg AJ, Sharp B, Cooke P: Early failure in total ankle replacements due to component malposition: a report of two cases, *Foot Ankle Int* 30:783–787, 2009.

118. Goldberg AJ, Sharp RJ, Cooke P: Ankle replacement: current practice of foot and ankle surgeons in the United Kingdom, *Foot Ankle Int* 30:950–954, 2009.

119. Goldie IF, Herberts P: Prosthetic replacement of the ankle joint, *Reconstr Surg Traumatol* 18:205–210, 1981.

120. Gougoulias N, Khanna A, Maffulli N: How successful are current ankle replacements?: a systematic review of the literature, *Clin Orthop Relat Res* 468:199–208, 2010.

121. Gougoulias NE, Khanna A, Maffulli N: History and evolution in total ankle arthroplasty, *Br Med Bull* 89:111–151, 2009.

122. Greisberg J, Assal M, Flueckiger G, Hansen ST Jr: Takedown of ankle fusion and conversion to total ankle replacement, *Clin Orthop Relat Res* 424:80–88, 2004.

123. Greisberg J, Hansen ST Jr: Ankle replacement: management of associated deformities, *Foot Ankle Clin* 7:721–736, 2002.

124. Greisberg J, Hansen ST Jr: Total ankle arthroplasty in the advanced flatfoot, *Tech Foot Ankle* 2:152–161, 2003.

125. Greisberg J, Hansen ST, DiGiovanni C: Alignment and technique in total ankle arthroplasty, *Oper Tech Orthop* 14:21–30, 2004.

126. Groth HE, Fitch HF: Salvage procedures for complications of total ankle arthroplasty, *Clin Orthop Relat Res* 224:244–250, 1987.

127. Guyer AJ, Richardson G: Current concepts review: total ankle arthroplasty, *Foot Ankle Int* 29:256–264, 2008.

128. Haddad SL, Coetzee JC, Estok R, et al: Intermediate and long-term outcomes of total ankle arthroplasty and ankle arthrodesis. A systematic review of the literature, *J Bone Joint Surg Am* 89:1899–1905, 2007.

129. Hahn ME, Wright ES, Segal AD, et al: Comparative gait analysis of ankle arthrodesis and arthroplasty: initial findings of a prospective study, *Foot Ankle Int* 33:282–289, 2012.

130. Hamblen DL: Can the ankle joint be replaced? *J Bone Joint Surg Br* 67:689–690, 1985.

131. Hanna RS, Haddad SL, Lazarus ML: Evaluation of periprosthetic lucency after total ankle arthroplasty: helical CT versus conventional radiography, *Foot Ankle Int* 28:921–926, 2007.

132. Harnroongroj T, Vanadurongwan V: The talar body prosthesis, *J Bone Joint Surg Am* 79:1313–1322, 1997.

133. Harris NJ, Brooke BT, Sturdee S: A wear debris cyst following S.T.A.R. Total Ankle Replacement—surgical management, *Foot Ankle Surg* 15:43–45, 2009.

134. Haskell A, Mann RA: Perioperative complication rate of total ankle replacement is reduced by surgeon experience, *Foot Ankle Int* 25:283–289, 2004.

135. Hay SM, Smith TWD: Total ankle arthroplasty: a long-term review, *Foot* 4:1–5, 1994.

136. Haygood TM: Magnetic resonance imaging of the musculoskeletal system: part 7. The ankle, *Clin Orthop Relat Res* 336:318–336, 1997.

137. Helm R, Stevens J: Long-term results of total ankle replacement, *J Arthroplasty* 1:271–277, 1986.

138. Henne TD, Anderson JG: Total ankle arthroplasty: a historical perspective, *Foot Ankle Clin* 7:695–702, 2002.

139. Henricson A, Agren PH: Secondary surgery after total ankle replacement. The influence of preoperative hindfoot alignment, *Foot Ankle Surg* 13:41–44, 2007.

140. Henricson A, Knutson K, Lindahl J, Rydholm U: The AES total ankle replacement: a mid-term analysis of 93 cases, *Foot Ankle Surg* 16:61–64, 2010.

141. Henricson A, Nilsson JA, Carlsson A: 10-year survival of total ankle arthroplasties: a report on 780 cases from the Swedish Ankle Register, *Acta Orthop* 82:655–659, 2011.

142. Henricson A, Skoog A, Carlsson A: The Swedish Ankle Arthroplasty Register: an analysis of 531 arthroplasties between 1993 and 2005, *Acta Orthop* 78:569–574, 2007.

143. Herberts P, Goldie IF, Korner L, et al: Endoprosthetic arthroplasty of the ankle joint. A clinical and radiological follow-up, *Acta Orthop Scand* 53:687–696, 1982.

144. Hintermann B: [Short- and mid-term results with the STAR total ankle prosthesis], *Orthopade* 28:792–803, 1999.

145. Hintermann B: Medial ankle instability, *Foot Ankle Clin* 8:723–738, 2003.

146. Hintermann B: Current designs of total ankle prostheses. In Hintermann B, editor: *Total ankle arthroplasty: historical overview, current concepts and future perspectives*, Wien, New York, 2004, Springer, pp 69–100.

147. Hintermann B: History of total ankle arthroplasty. In Hintermann B, editor: *Total ankle arthroplasty: historical overview, current concepts and future perspectives*, Wien, New York, 2005, Springer, pp 43–57.

148. Hintermann B: Surgical techniques. In Hintermann B, editor: *Total ankle arthroplasty: historical overview, current concepts and future perspectives*, Wien, New York, 2005, Springer, pp 105–126.

149. Hintermann B: What the orthopaedic foot and ankle surgeon wants to know from MR imaging, *Semin Musculoskelet Radiol* 9:260–271, 2005.

150. Hintermann B: Ankle osteoarthritis: five take-home points regarding total ankle arthroplasty in the rest of the world. Presented at 26th Annual Summer Meeting of the American Orthopaedic Foot and Ankle Society, National Harbor, Maryland, USA, July 7-10, 2010.

151. Hintermann B, Barg A: The HINTEGRA total ankle arthroplasty. In Wiesel SW, editor: *Operative techniques in orthopaedic surgery*, Philadelphia, 2010, Lippincott Williams & Wilkins, pp 4022–4031.

152. Hintermann B, Barg A, Knupp M: Corrective supramalleolar osteotomy for malunited pronation-external rotation fractures of the ankle, *J Bone Joint Surg Br* 93:1367–1372, 2011.

153. Hintermann B, Barg A, Knupp M: [Revision arthroplasty of the ankle joint], *Orthopade* 40:1000–1007, 2011.

154. Hintermann B, Barg A, Knupp M, Valderrabano V: Conversion of painful ankle arthrodesis to total ankle arthroplasty, *J Bone Joint Surg Am* 91:850–858, 2009.

155. Hintermann B, Barg A, Knupp M, Valderrabano V: Conversion of painful ankle arthrodesis to total ankle arthroplasty. Surgical technique, *J Bone Joint Surg Am* 92(Suppl 1, Pt 1):55–66, 2010.

156. Hintermann B, Valderrabano V: Total ankle replacement, *Foot Ankle Clin* 8:375–405, 2003.

157. Hintermann B, Valderrabano V, Dereymaeker G, Dick W: The HINTEGRA ankle: rationale and short-term results of 122 consecutive ankles, *Clin Orthop Relat Res* 424:57–68, 2004.

158. Hintermann B, Valderrabano V, Knupp M, Horisberger M: [The HINTEGRA ankle: short- and mid-term results], *Orthopade* 35:533–545, 2006.

159. Hintermann B, Valderrabano V, Kundert HP: Lengthening of the lateral column and reconstruction of the medial soft tissue for treatment of acquired flatfoot deformity associated with insufficiency of the posterior tibial tendon, *Foot Ankle Int* 20:622–629, 1999.

160. Hintermann B, Zwicky L, Knupp M, et al: HINTEGRA revision arthroplasty for failed total ankle prostheses, *J Bone Joint Surg Am* 2013; accepted for publication.

161. Hobson SA, Karantana A, Dhar S: Total ankle replacement in patients with significant pre-operative deformity of the hindfoot, *J Bone Joint Surg Br* 91:481–486, 2009.

162. Hopgood P, Kumar R, Wood PL: Ankle arthrodesis for failed total ankle replacement, *J Bone Joint Surg Br* 88:1032–1038, 2006.

163. Horisberger M, Hintermann B, Valderrabano V: Alterations of plantar pressure distribution in posttraumatic end-stage ankle osteoarthritis, *Clin Biomech (Bristol, Avon)* 24:303–307, 2009.

164. Hosman AH, Mason RB, Hobbs T, Rothwell AG: A New Zealand national joint registry review of 202 total ankle replacements followed for up to 6 years, *Acta Orthop* 78:584–591, 2007.

165. Hughes J, Pratt L, Linge K, et al: Reliability of pressure measurements: the EMED F system, *Clin Biomech* 6:14–18, 1991.

166. Hung M, Clegg DO, Greene T, et al: A lower extremity physical function computerized adaptive testing instrument for orthopaedic patients, *Foot Ankle Int* 33:326–335, 2012.

167. Hunt MA, Birmingham TB, Jenkyn TR, et al: Measures of frontal plane lower limb alignment obtained from static radiographs and dynamic gait analysis, *Gait Posture* 27:635–640, 2008.

168. Hurowitz EJ, Gould JS, Fleisig GS, Fowler R: Outcome analysis of Agility total ankle replacement with prior adjunctive procedures: two to six year followup, *Foot Ankle Int* 28:308–312, 2007.

169. Huskisson EC: Measurement of pain, *Lancet* 2:1127–1131, 1974.

170. Hvid I, Rasmussen O, Jensen NC, Nielsen S: Trabecular bone strength profiles at the ankle joint, *Clin Orthop Relat Res* 199:306–312, 1985.

171. Ingrosso S, Benedetti MG, Leardini A, et al: GAIT analysis in patients operated with a novel total ankle prosthesis, *Gait Posture* 30:132–137, 2009.

172. Inman VT: *The joints of the ankle*, Baltimore, 1976, Williams & Wilkins.

173. Jackson MP, Singh D: Total ankle replacement, *Current Orthopaedics* 17:292–298, 2003.

174. Jensen NC, Kroner K: Total ankle joint replacement: a clinical follow up, *Orthopedics* 15:236–239, 1992.

175. Jung HG, Nicholson JJ, Parks B, Myerson MS: Radiographic and biomechanical support for fibular plating of the agility total ankle, *Clin Orthop Relat Res* 424:118–124, 2004.

176. Kanade RV, van Deursen RW, Harding KG, Price PE: Investigation of standing balance in patients with diabetic neuropathy at different stages of foot complications, *Clin Biomech (Bristol, Avon)* 23:1183–1191, 2008.

177. Karantana A, Hobson S, Dhar S: The Scandinavian Total Ankle Replacement: survivorship at 5 and 8 years comparable to other series, *Clin Orthop Relat Res* 468:951–957, 2010.

178. Karantana A, Martin GJ, Shandil M, Dhar S: Simultaneous bilateral total ankle replacement using the S.T.A.R.: a case series, *Foot Ankle Int* 31:86–89, 2010.

179. Kempson GE, Freeman MA, Tuke MA: Engineering considerations in the design of an ankle joint, *Biomed Eng* 10:166–171, 180, 1975.

180. Ketz J, Myerson M, Sanders R: The salvage of complex hindfoot problems with use of a custom talar total ankle prosthesis, *J Bone Joint Surg Am* 94:1194–1200, 2012.

181. Kharwadkar N, Harris NJ: Revision of STAR total ankle replacement to hybrid AES-STAR total ankle replacement-a report of two cases, *Foot Ankle Surg* 15:101–105, 2009.

182. Kilger R, Knupp M, Hintermann B: Peroneus longus to peroneus brevis tendon transfer, *Tech Foot Ankle* 8:146–149, 2009.

183. Kim BS, Choi WJ, Kim YS, Lee JW: Total ankle replacement in moderate to severe varus deformity of the ankle, *J Bone Joint Surg Br* 91:1183–1190, 2009.

184. Kirkup J: Richard Smith ankle arthroplasty, *J R Soc Med* 78:301–304, 1985.

185. Kitaoka HB, Alexander IJ, Adelaar RS, et al: Clinical rating systems for the ankle-hindfoot, midfoot, hallux, and lesser toes, *Foot Ankle Int* 15:349–353, 1994.
186. Kitaoka HB, Patzer GL: Clinical results of the Mayo total ankle arthroplasty, *J Bone Joint Surg Am* 78:1658–1664, 1996.
187. Kitaoka HB, Patzer GL, Ilstrup DM, Wallrichs SL: Survivorship analysis of the Mayo total ankle arthroplasty, *J Bone Joint Surg Am* 76:974–979, 1994.
188. Kitaoka HB, Romness DW: Arthrodesis for failed ankle arthroplasty, *J Arthroplasty* 7:277–284, 1992.
189. Knecht SI, Estin M, Callaghan JJ, et al: The Agility total ankle arthroplasty. Seven to sixteen-year follow-up, *J Bone Joint Surg Am* 86-A:1161–1171, 2004.
190. Knupp M, Bolliger L, Barg A, Hintermann B: [Total ankle replacement for varus deformity], *Orthopade* 40:964–970, 2011.
191. Knupp M, Horisberger M, Hintermann B: A new Z-shaped calcaneal osteotomy for 3-plane correction of severe varus deformity of the hindfoot, *Tech Foot Ankle* 7:90–95, 2008.
192. Knupp M, Ledermann H, Magerkurth O, Hintermann B: The surgical tibiotalar angle: a radiologic study, *Foot Ankle Int* 26:713–716, 2005.
193. Knupp M, Pagenstert GI, Barg A, et al: SPECT-CT compared with conventional imaging modalities for the assessment of the varus and valgus malaligned hindfoot, *J Orthop Res* 27:1461–1466, 2009.
194. Knupp M, Stufkens SA, Bolliger L, et al: Classification and treatment of supramalleolar deformities, *Foot Ankle Int* 32:1023–1031, 2011.
195. Knupp M, Stufkens SA, Bolliger L, et al: Total ankle replacement and supramalleolar osteotomies for malaligned osteoarthritis ankle, *Tech Foot Ankle* 9:175–181, 2010.
196. Knupp M, Stufkens SA, Hintermann B: Triple arthrodesis, *Foot Ankle Clin* 16:61–67, 2011.
197. Kobayashi A, Minoda Y, Kadoya Y, et al: Ankle arthroplasties generate wear particles similar to knee arthroplasties, *Clin Orthop Relat Res* 424:69–72, 2004.
198. Kofoed H: Cylindrical cemented ankle arthroplasty: a prospective series with long-term follow-up, *Foot Ankle Int* 16:474–479, 1995.
199. Kofoed H: Scandinavian Total Ankle Replacement (STAR), *Clin Orthop Relat Res* 424:73–79, 2004.
200. Kofoed H: Biological fixation of ankle arthroplasty: a sequential consecutive prospective clinico-radiographic series of 20 ankles with arthrosis followed for 1-4 years, *Foot* 5:27–31, 2005.
201. Kofoed H, Sorensen TS: Ankle arthroplasty for rheumatoid arthritis and osteoarthritis: prospective long-term study of cemented replacements, *J Bone Joint Surg Br* 80:328–332, 1998.
202. Kofoed H, Stürup J: Comparison of ankle arthroplasty and arthrodesis. A prospective series with long-term follow-up, *Foot* 4:6–9, 1994.
203. Koivu H, Kohonen I, Sipola E, et al: Severe periprosthetic osteolytic lesions after the Ankle Evolutive System total ankle replacement, *J Bone Joint Surg Br* 91:907–914, 2009.
204. Koivu H, Mackiewicz Z, Takakubo Y, et al: RANKL in the osteolysis of AES total ankle replacement implants, *Bone* 51:546–552, 2012. doi:10.1016/j.bone.2012.05.007.
205. Kokkonen A, Ikavalko M, Tiihonen R, et al: High rate of osteolytic lesions in medium-term followup after the AES total ankle replacement, *Foot Ankle Int* 32:168–175, 2011.
206. Komistek RD, Stiehl JB, Buechel FF, et al: A determination of ankle kinematics using fluoroscopy, *Foot Ankle Int* 21:343–350, 2000.
207. Kopp FJ, Patel MM, Deland JT, O'Malley MJ: Total ankle arthroplasty with the Agility prosthesis: clinical and radiographic evaluation, *Foot Ankle Int* 27:97–103, 2006.
208. Kotnis R, Pasapula C, Anwar F, et al: The management of failed ankle replacement, *J Bone Joint Surg Br* 88:1039–1047, 2006.
209. Kumar A, Dhar S: Total ankle replacement: early results during learning perios, *Foot Ankle Surg* 13:19–23, 2007.
210. Kumar SJ, Keret D, MacEwen GD: Corrective cosmetic supramalleolar osteotomy for valgus deformity of the ankle joint: a report of two cases, *J Pediatr Orthop* 10:124–127, 1990.
211. Kurup HV, Taylor GR: Medial impingement after ankle replacement, *Int Orthop* 32:243–246, 2008.
212. Lachiewicz PF, Inglis AE, Ranawat CS: Total ankle replacement in rheumatoid arthritis, *J Bone Joint Surg Am* 66:340–343, 1984.
213. Lagaay PM, Schuberth JM: Analysis of ankle range of motion and functional outcome following total ankle arthoplasty, *J Foot Ankle Surg* 49:147–151, 2010.
214. Lampert C: [Ankle joint prosthesis for bone defects], *Orthopade* 40:978–983, 2011.
215. Leardini A: Geometry and mechanics of the human ankle complex and ankle prosthesis design, *Clin Biomech (Bristol, Avon)* 16:706–709, 2001.
216. Leardini A, O'Connor JJ, Catani F, Giannini S: Mobility of the human ankle and the design of total ankle replacement, *Clin Orthop Relat Res* 424:39–46, 2004.
217. Lee KB, Cho SG, Hur CI, Yoon TR: Perioperative complications of HINTEGRA total ankle replacement: our initial 50 cases, *Foot Ankle Int* 29:978–984, 2008.
218. Lee KB, Cho SG, Jung ST, Kim MS: Total ankle arthroplasty following revascularization of avascular necrosis of the talar body: two case reports and literature review, *Foot Ankle Int* 29:852–858, 2008.
219. Lee KB, Park YH, Song EK, et al: Static and dynamic postural balance after successful mobile-bearing total ankle arthroplasty, *Arch Phys Med Rehabil* 91:519–522, 2010.
220. Lee KT, Lee YK, Young KW, et al: Perioperative complications of the MOBILITY total ankle system: comparison with the HINTEGRA total ankle system, *J Orthop Sci* 15:317–322, 2010.
221. Leszko F, Komistek RD, Mahfouz MR, et al: In vivo kinematics of the salto total ankle prosthesis, *Foot Ankle Int* 29:1117–1125, 2008.
222. Lindsjo U, Danckwardt-Lilliestrom G, Sahlstedt B: Measurement of the motion range in the loaded ankle, *Clin Orthop Relat Res* 199:68–71, 1985.
223. Lord G, Marotte JH: [Total ankle prosthesis. Technic and 1st results. Apropos of 12 cases], *Rev Chir Orthop Reparatrice Appar Mot* 59:139–151, 1973.
224. Lord G, Marotte JH: [Total ankle replacement (author's transl)], *Rev Chir Orthop Reparatrice Appar Mot* 66:527–530, 1980.
225. Luck JV Jr, Kasper CK: Surgical management of advanced hemophilic arthropathy. An overview of 20 years' experience, *Clin Orthop Relat Res* 242:60–82, 1989.
226. Lundberg A, Svensson OK, Nemeth G, Selvik G: The axis of rotation of the ankle joint, *J Bone Joint Surg Br* 71:94–99, 1989.
227. Magerkurth O, Knupp M, Ledermann H, Hintermann B: Evaluation of hindfoot dimensions: a radiological study, *Foot Ankle Int* 27:612–616, 2006.
228. Makwana NK, Morrison P, Jones CB, Kirkup J: Salvage operations after failed total ankle replacement, *Foot* 5:180–184, 1995.
229. Mann JA, Mann RA, Horton E: STAR ankle: Long-term results, *Foot Ankle Int* 32:473–484, 2011.
230. Matejczyk MB, Greenwald AS, Black JD: Ankle implant systems: laboratory evaluation and clinical correlation, *Orthop Trans* 3:199, 1979.
231. McGuire MR, Kyle RF, Gustilo RB, Premer RF: Comparative analysis of ankle arthroplasty versus ankle arthrodesis, *Clin Orthop Relat Res* 226:174–181, 1988.
232. McIff TE, Alvine FG, Saltzman CL, et al: Intraoperative measurement of distraction for ligament tensioning in total ankle arthroplasty, *Clin Orthop Relat Res* 424:111–117, 2004.

233. Mehta SK, Donley BG, Jockel JR, et al: The Salto Talaris total ankle arthroplasty system: a review and report of early results, *Semin Arthro* 21:282–287, 2010.

234. Mendolia G, Coillard JY, Cermolacce C, Determe P: Long-term (10 to 14 years) results of the Ramses total ankle arthroplasty, *Tech Foot Ankle* 4:160–173, 2005.

235. Mendolia G, Talus Group: The Ramses ankel replacement: design-surgical technique result, results in first 38 cases, *French Orthop Web J* 2007. Available at http://www.maitrise-orthop .com/viewPage_us.do?id=87. Accessed May 17, 2013.

236. Michael JM, Golshani A, Gargac S, Goswami T: Biomechanics of the ankle joint and clinical outcomes of total ankle replacement, *J Mech Behav Biomed Mater* 1:276–294, 2008.

237. Min W, Sanders R: The use of the mortise view of the ankle to determine hindfoot alignment: technique tip, *Foot Ankle Int* 31:823–827, 2010.

238. Morgan SS, Brooke B, Harris NJ: Total ankle replacement by the Ankle Evolution System: medium-term outcome, *J Bone Joint Surg Br* 92:61–65, 2010.

239. Muir DC, Amendola A, Saltzman CL: Forty-year outcome of ankle "cup" arthroplasty for post-traumatic arthritis, *Iowa Orthop J* 22:99–102, 2002.

240. Muller S, Wolf S, Doderlein L: [Three-dimensional analysis of the foot following implantation of a HINTEGRA ankle prosthesis: evaluation with the Heidelberg foot model], *Orthopade* 35:506–512, 2006.

241. Murnaghan JM, Warnock DS, Henderson SA: Total ankle replacement. Early experiences with STAR prosthesis, *Ulster Med J* 74:9–13, 2005.

242. Murray MP, Mollinger F, Gardner GM, Sepic SP: Comparison of free and fast speed walking patterns of normal men, *J Phys Med* 45:8–23, 1966.

243. Myerson MS, Miller SD: Salvage after complications of total ankle arthroplasty, *Foot Ankle Clin* 7:191–206, 2002.

244. Myerson MS, Mroczek K: Perioperative complications of total ankle arthroplasty, *Foot Ankle Int* 24:17–21, 2003.

245. Myerson MS, Won HY: Primary and revision total ankle replacement using custom-designed prostheses, *Foot Ankle Clin* 13:521–538, 2008.

246. Naal FD, Impellizzeri FM, Loibl M, et al: Habitual physical activity and sports participation after total ankle arthroplasty, *Am J Sports Med* 37:95–102, 2009.

247. Naal FD, Impellizzeri FM, Rippstein PF: Which are the most frequently used outcome instruments in studies on total ankle arthroplasty? *Clin Orthop Relat Res* 468:815–826, 2010.

248. Nagashima M, Takahashi H, Kakumoto S, et al: Total ankle arthroplasty for deformity of the foot in patients with rheumatoid arthritis using the TNK ankle system: clinical results of 21 cases, *Mod Rheumatol* 14:48–53, 2004.

249. Nelissen RG, Doets HC, Valstar ER: Early migration of the tibial component of the Buechel-Pappas total ankle prosthesis, *Clin Orthop Relat Res* 448:146–151, 2006.

250. Newton SE: An artificial ankle joint, *Clin Orthop Relat Res* 142:141–145, 1979.

251. Newton SE 3rd: Total ankle arthroplasty. Clinical study of fifty cases, *J Bone Joint Surg Am* 64:104–111, 1982.

252. Newton SE 3rd: An artificial ankle joint, *Clin Orthop Relat Res* 424:3–5, 2004.

253. Nishikawa M, Tomita T, Fujii M, et al: Total ankle replacement in rheumatoid arthritis, *Int Orthop* 28:123–126, 2004.

254. Nuesch C, Valderrabano V, Huber C, et al: Gait patterns of asymmetric ankle osteoarthritis patients, *Clin Biomech (Bristol, Avon)* 27:613–618, 2012.

255. Numkarunarunrote N, Malik A, Aguiar RO, et al: Retinacula of the foot and ankle: MRI with anatomic correlation in cadavers, *AJR Am J Roentgenol* 188:W348–W354, 2007.

256. Nunley JA, Caputo AM, Easley ME, Cook C: Intermediate to long-term outcomes of the STAR Total Ankle Replacement: the patient perspective, *J Bone Joint Surg Am* 94:43–48, 2012.

257. Pagenstert G, Knupp M, Valderrabano V, Hintermann B: Realignment surgery for valgus ankle osteoarthritis, *Oper Orthop Traumatol* 21:77–87, 2009.

258. Pagenstert GI, Barg A, Leumann AG, et al: SPECT-CT imaging in degenerative joint disease of the foot and ankle, *J Bone Joint Surg Br* 91:1191–1196, 2009.

259. Pagenstert GI, Hintermann B, Barg A, et al: Realignment surgery as alternative treatment of varus and valgus ankle osteoarthritis, *Clin Orthop Relat Res* 462:156–168, 2007.

260. Pal GP, Routal RV: Architecture of the cancellous bone of the human talus, *Anat Rec* 252:185–193, 1998.

261. Pappas M, Buechel FF, DePalma AF: Cylindrical total ankle joint replacement: surgical and biomechanical rationale, *Clin Orthop Relat Res* 118:82–92, 1976.

262. Patsalis T: Die AES-Sprunggelenksprothese: Indikation, Technik und erste Ergebnisse, *Fuss Sprungg* 2:38–44, 2004.

263. Pena F, Agel J, Coetzee JC: Comparison of the MFA to the AOFAS outcome tool in a population undergoing total ankle replacement, *Foot Ankle Int* 28:788–793, 2007.

264. Pinsker E, Daniels TR: AOFAS position statement regarding the future of the AOFAS clinical rating systems, *Foot Ankle Int* 32:841–842, 2011.

265. Pinzur M: FootForum: clinical practice guidelines, *Foot Ankle Int* 31:275–276, 2010.

266. Pinzur M: FootForum: experimental surgery revisited, *Foot Ankle Int* 31:102, 2010.

267. Pinzur M: FootForum: the power of evidence, *Foot Ankle Int* 31:468, 2010.

268. Pinzur MS: FootForum: experimental surgery, *Foot Ankle Int* 30:472–473, 2009.

269. Plaass C, Knupp M, Barg A, Hintermann B: Anterior double plating for rigid fixation of isolated tibiotalar arthrodesis, *Foot Ankle Int* 30:631–639, 2009.

270. Popelka S, Vavrik P, Landor I, et al: [Our experience with AES total ankle replacement], *Acta Chir Orthop Traumatol Cech* 77:24–31, 2010.

271. Pyevich MT, Saltzman CL, Callaghan JJ, Alvine FG: Total ankle arthroplasty: a unique design. Two to twelve-year follow-up, *J Bone Joint Surg Am* 80:1410–1420, 1998.

272. Raikin SM, Kane J, Ciminiello ME: Risk factors for incision-healing complications following total ankle arthroplasty, *J Bone Joint Surg Am* 92:2150–2155, 2010.

273. Reggiani B, Leardini A, Corazza F, Taylor M: Finite element analysis of a total ankle replacement during the stance phase of gait, *J Biomech* 39:1435–1443, 2006.

274. Reiley MA: INBONE total ankle replacement, *Foot Ankle Spec* 1:305–308, 2008.

275. Reiley MA: Total ankle arthroplasty with bone defects, *Foot Ankle Spec* 2:32–34, 2009.

276. Reuver JM, Dayerizadeh N, Burger B, et al: Total ankle replacement outcome in low volume centers: short-term followup, *Foot Ankle Int* 31:1064–1068, 2010.

277. Richter M, Zech S, Westphal R, et al: Robotic cadaver testing of a new total ankle prosthesis model (German Ankle System), *Foot Ankle Int* 28:1276–1286, 2007.

278. Rippstein PF: Clinical experiences with three different designs of ankle prostheses, *Foot Ankle Clin* 7:817–831, 2002.

279. Rippstein PF, Huber M, Coetzee JC, Naal FD: Total ankle replacement with use of a new three-component implant, *J Bone Joint Surg Am* 93:1426–1435, 2011.

280. Rippstein PF, Naal FD: [Total ankle replacement in rheumatoid arthritis], *Orthopade* 40:984–990, 2011.

281. Rodriguez D, Bevernage BD, Maldague P, et al: Medium term follow-up of the AES ankle prosthesis: high rate of asymptomatic osteolysis, *Foot Ankle Surg* 16:54–60, 2010.

282. Rodriguez RP: Medial displacement calcaneal tuberosity osteotomy in the treatment of posterior tibial insufficiency, *Foot Ankle Clin* 6:545–567, 2001.

283. Rodriguez-Merchan EC: Orthopedic problems about the ankle in hemophilia, *J Foot Ankle Surg* 51:772–776, 2012. doi:10.1053/j.jfas.2012.06.005.

284. Rouhani H, Crevoisier X, Favre J, Aminian K: Outcome evaluation of ankle osteoarthritis treatments: plantar pressure analysis during relatively long-distance walking, *Clin Biomech (Bristol, Avon)* 26:397–404, 2011.

285. Rudigier J: Ankle replacement by the cementless ESKA endoprosthesis, *Tech Foot Ankle* 4:125–136, 2005.

286. Rudigier J, Grundei H, Menzinger F: Prosthetic replacement of the ankle in posttraumatic arthrosis: 10-year experience with the cementless ESKA ankle prosthesis, *Eur J Trauma* 27:66–74, 2001.

287. Rudigier J, Menzinger F, Grundei H: 14 Jahre Erfahrungen mit der zementfreien ESKA-Sprunggelenksendoprothese, *Fuss Sprungg* 2:65–75, 2004.

288. Rydholm U: Is total replacement of the ankle an option? *Acta Orthop* 78:567–568, 2007.

289. Rzesacz EH, Gosse F: [Management of posttraumatic osteoarthritis of the upper ankle joint by implantation of the S.T.A.R. ankle prosthesis], *Oper Orthop Traumatol* 19:527–546, 2007.

290. Saltzman CL: Perspective on total ankle replacement, *Foot Ankle Clin* 5:761–775, 2000.

291. Saltzman CL: *Ankle osteoarthritis: five take-home points regarding total ankle arthroplasty in USA.* Presented at the 26th Annual Summer Meeting of the American Orthopaedic Foot and Ankle Society, National Harbor, Maryland, USA, July 7-10, 2010.

292. Saltzman CL, Amendola A, Anderson R, et al: Surgeon training and complications in total ankle arthroplasty, *Foot Ankle Int* 24:514–518, 2003.

293. Saltzman CL, el Khoury GY: The hindfoot alignment view, *Foot Ankle Int* 16:572–576, 1995.

294. Saltzman CL, Mann RA, Ahrens JE, et al: Prospective controlled trial of STAR total ankle replacement versus ankle fusion: initial results, *Foot Ankle Int* 30:579–596, 2009.

295. Saltzman CL, Salamon ML, Blanchard GM, et al: Epidemiology of ankle arthritis: report of a consecutive series of 639 patients from a tertiary orthopaedic center, *Iowa Orthop J* 25:44–46, 2005.

296. Saltzman CL, Tochigi Y, Rudert MJ, et al: The effect of agility ankle prosthesis misalignment on the peri-ankle ligaments, *Clin Orthop Relat Res* 424:137–142, 2004.

297. Samuelson KM, Freeman MA, Tuke MA: Development and evolution of the ICLH ankle replacement, *Foot Ankle* 3:32–36, 1982.

298. San Giovanni TP, Keblish DJ, Thomas WH, Wilson MG: Eight-year results of a minimally constrained total ankle arthroplasty, *Foot Ankle Int* 27:418–426, 2006.

299. Sands AK, Tansey JP: Lateral column lengthening, *Foot Ankle Clin* 12:301–308, 2007.

300. Schenk K, Lieske S, John M, et al: Prospective study of a cementless, mobile-bearing, third generation total ankle prosthesis, *Foot Ankle Int* 32:755–763, 2011.

301. Schiff A, Li J, Inoue N, et al: Trabecular angle of the human talus is associated with the level of cartilage degeneration, *J Musculoskelet Neuronal Interact* 7:224–230, 2007.

302. Schill S, Biehl C, Thabe H: [Ankle prostheses. Mid-term results after Thompson-Richards and STAR prostheses], *Orthopade* 27:183–187, 1998.

303. Schill S, Rehart S, Fink B: Endoprothetik am rheumatischen oberen Sprunggelenk: Historie und Zukunftsperspektive, *Fuss Sprungg* 4:98–105, 2006.

304. Schonherr R, Fuss S, Korbl M, et al: [Short-term results after STAR total ankle replacement], *Orthopade* 37:783–787, 2008.

305. Schuberth JM, Patel S, Zarutsky E: Perioperative complications of the Agility total ankle replacement in 50 initial, consecutive cases, *J Foot Ankle Surg* 45:139–146, 2006.

306. Schutte BG, Louwerens JW: Short-term results of our first 49 Scandanavian total ankle replacements (STAR), *Foot Ankle Int* 29:124–127, 2008.

307. Scott AT, Nunley JA: Polyethylene fracture following STAR ankle arthroplasty: a report of three cases, *Foot Ankle Int* 30:375–379, 2009.

308. Scranton PE Jr, McMaster JG, Kelly E: Dynamic fibular function: a new concept, *Clin Orthop Relat Res* 118:76–81, 1976.

309. Shi K, Hayashida K, Hashimoto J, et al: Hydroxyapatite augmentation for bone atrophy in total ankle replacement in rheumatoid arthritis, *J Foot Ankle Surg* 45:316–321, 2006.

310. Shinomiya F, Okada M, Hamada Y, et al: Indications of total ankle arthroplasty for rheumatoid arthritis: evaluation at 5 years or more after the operation, *Mod Rheumatol* 13:153–159, 2003.

311. Skyttä ET, Koivu H, Eskelinen A, et al: Total ankle replacement: a population-based study of 515 cases from the Finnish Arthroplasty Register, *Acta Orthop* 81:114–118, 2010.

312. Slobogean GP, Younger A, Apostle KL, et al: Preference-based quality of life of end-stage ankle arthritis treated with arthroplasty or arthrodesis, *Foot Ankle Int* 31:563–566, 2010.

313. Smith TW, Stephens M: Ankle arthroplasty, *Foot Ankle Surg* 16:53, 2010.

314. Solomon LB, Ferris L, Henneberg M: Anatomical study of the ankle with view to the anterior arthroscopic portals, *ANZ J Surg* 76:932–936, 2006.

315. SooHoo NF, Kominski G: Cost-effectiveness analysis of total ankle arthroplasty, *J Bone Joint Surg Am* 86-A:2446–2455, 2004.

316. SooHoo NF, Zingmond DS, Ko CY: Comparison of reoperation rates following ankle arthrodesis and total ankle arthroplasty, *J Bone Joint Surg Am* 89:2143–2149, 2007.

317. Spirt AA, Assal M, Hansen ST Jr: Complications and failure after total ankle arthroplasty, *J Bone Joint Surg Am* 86-A:1172–1178, 2004

318. Stamatis ED, Myerson MS: How to avoid specific complications of total ankle replacement, *Foot Ankle Clin* 7:765–789, 2002.

319. Stauffer RN: Salvage of painful total ankle arthroplasty, *Clin Orthop Relat Res* 170:184–188, 1982.

320. Stauffer RN, Chao EY, Brewster RC: Force and motion analysis of the normal, diseased, and prosthetic ankle joint, *Clin Orthop Relat Res* 127:189–196, 1977.

321. Stauffer RN, Segal NM: Total ankle arthroplasty: four years' experience, *Clin Orthop Relat Res* 160:217–221, 1981.

322. Stengel D, Bauwens K, Ekkernkamp A, Cramer J: Efficacy of total ankle replacement with meniscal-bearing devices: a systematic review and meta-analysis, *Arch Orthop Trauma Surg* 125:109–119, 2005.

323. Stufkens SA, Barg A, Bolliger L, et al: Measurement of the medial distal tibial angle, *Foot Ankle Int* 32:288–293, 2011.

324. Stufkens SA, Knupp M, Hintermann B: Medial displacement calcaneal osteotomy, *Tech Foot Ankle* 8:85–90, 2009.

325. Su EP, Kahn B, Figgie MP: Total ankle replacement in patients with rheumatoid arthritis, *Clin Orthop Relat Res* 424:32–38, 2004.

326. Takakura Y, Tanaka Y, Kumai T, et al: Ankle arthroplasty using three generations of metal and ceramic prostheses, *Clin Orthop Relat Res* 424:130–136, 2004.

327. Takakura Y, Tanaka Y, Sugimoto K, et al: Ankle arthroplasty. A comparative study of cemented metal and uncemented ceramic prostheses, *Clin Orthop Relat Res* 252:209–216, 1990.

328. Takebe K, Nakagawa A, Minami H, et al: Role of the fibula in weight-bearing, *Clin Orthop Relat Res* 184:289–292, 1984.

329. Tanaka Y, Takakura Y: [The TNK ankle: short- and mid-term results], *Orthopade* 35:546–551, 2006.

330. Tanaka Y, Takakura Y, Kadono K, et al: Alumina ceramic talar body prosthesis for idiopathic aseptic necrosis of the talus, *Key Eng Mater* 240-242:805–808, 2003.

331. Thermann H, Gavriilidis I, Longo UG, Maffulli N: Total ankle arthroplasty and tibialis posterior tendon transfer for ankle osteoarthritis and drop foot deformity, *Foot Ankle Surg* 17:203–206, 2011. doi:10.1016/j.fas.2009.10.004.

332. Thomas RH, Daniels TR: Ankle arthritis, *J Bone Joint Surg Am* 85-A:923–936, 2003.

333. Thomason K, Eyres KS: A technique of fusion for failed total replacement of the ankle: tibio-allograft-calcaneal fusion with a locked retrograde intramedullary nail, *J Bone Joint Surg Br* 90:885–888, 2008.

334. Tillmann K: [Endoprostheses of the ankle joint. Indications, development, current status and trends], *Orthopade* 32:179–186, 2003.

335. Tillmann K, Schaar M, Schaar B, Fink B: Ergebnisse von OSG-Endoprothesen bei rheumatoider Arthritis: eine klinische und pedobarographische Untersuchung, *Fuss Sprungg* 1:56–65, 2003.

336. Tochigi Y, Rudert MJ, Amendola A, et al: Tensile engagement of the peri-ankle ligaments in stance phase, *Foot Ankle Int* 26:1067–1073, 2005.

337. Tochigi Y, Rudert MJ, Brown TD, et al: The effect of accuracy of implantation on range of movement of the Scandinavian Total Ankle Replacement, *J Bone Joint Surg Br* 87:736–740, 2005.

338. Trincat S, Kouyoumdjian P, Asencio G: Total ankle arthroplasty and coronal plane deformities, *Orthop Traumatol Surg Res* 98:75–84, 2012.

339. Tsukamoto S, Tanaka Y, Maegawa N, et al: Total talar replacement following collapse of the talar body as a complication of total ankle arthroplasty: a case report, *J Bone Joint Surg Am* 92:2115–2120, 2010.

340. Unger AS, Inglis AE, Mow CS, Figgie HE 3rd: Total ankle arthroplasty in rheumatoid arthritis: a long-term follow-up study, *Foot Ankle* 8:173–179, 1988.

341. Valderrabano V, Hintermann B: HINTEGRA-Sprunggelenkprothese: Präliminäre Resultate der ersten 125 Fälle, *Fuss Sprungg* 2:7–16, 2004.

342. Valderrabano V, Hintermann B, Dick W: Scandinavian total ankle replacement: a 3.7-year average followup of 65 patients, *Clin Orthop Relat Res* 424:47–56, 2004.

343. Valderrabano V, Hintermann B, Horisberger M, Fung TS: Ligamentous posttraumatic ankle osteoarthritis, *Am J Sports Med* 34:612–620, 2006.

344. Valderrabano V, Hintermann B, Nigg BM, et al: Kinematic changes after fusion and total replacement of the ankle: part 1: range of motion, *Foot Ankle Int* 24:881–887, 2003.

345. Valderrabano V, Hintermann B, Nigg BM, et al: Kinematic changes after fusion and total replacement of the ankle: part 2: movement transfer, *Foot Ankle Int* 24:888–896, 2003.

346. Valderrabano V, Hintermann B, Nigg BM, et al: Kinematic changes after fusion and total replacement of the ankle: part 3: talar movement, *Foot Ankle Int* 24:897–900, 2003.

347. Valderrabano V, Hintermann B, von Tscharner V, et al: [Muscle biomechanics in total ankle replacement], *Orthopade* 35:513–520, 2006.

348. Valderrabano V, Horisberger M, Russell I, et al: Etiology of ankle osteoarthritis, *Clin Orthop Relat Res* 467:1800–1806, 2009.

349. Valderrabano V, Nigg BM, von Tscharner V, et al: J. Leonard Goldner Award 2006. Total ankle replacement in ankle osteoarthritis: an analysis of muscle rehabilitation, *Foot Ankle Int* 28:281–291, 2007.

350. Valderrabano V, Nigg BM, von Tschamer V, et al: Gait analysis in ankle osteoarthritis and total ankle replacement, *Clin Biomech (Bristol, Avon)* 22:894–904, 2007.

351. Valderrabano V, Pagenstert G, Horisberger M, et al: Sports and recreation activity of ankle arthritis patients before and after total ankle replacement, *Am J Sports Med* 34:993–999, 2006.

352. Valderrabano V, Pagenstert GI, Hintermann B: Total ankle replacement—three-component prosthesis, *Tech Foot Ankle* 2:84–90, 2005.

353. Valderrabano V, Pagenstert GI, Müller AM, et al: Mobile- and fixed-bearing total ankle prostheses: is there really a difference? *Foot Ankle Clin* 17:565–585, 2012.

354. Valderrabano V, von Tscharner V, Nigg BM, et al: Unterschenkel-Muskelatrophie bei Arthrose des oberen Sprunggelenks und deren Rehabilitation nach Implantation einer Sprunggelenks-prothese, *Fuss Sprungg* 5:33–43, 2007.

355. Valderrabano V, Wiewiorski M, Frigg A, et al: [Chronic ankle instability], *Unfallchirurg* 110:691–699, 2007.

356. van den Heuvel A, Van Bouwel S, Dereymaeker G: Total ankle replacement. Design evolution and results, *Acta Orthop Belg* 76:150–161, 2010.

357. van der Heide HJ, Nováková I, de Waal Malefijt MC: The feasibility of total ankle prosthesis for severe arthropathy in haemophilia and prothrombin deficiency, *Haemophilia* 12:679–682, 2006.

358. van der Heide HJ, Schutte B, Louwerens JW, et al: Total ankle prostheses in rheumatoid arthropathy: Outcome in 52 patients followed for 1-9 years, *Acta Orthop* 80:440–444, 2009.

359. Vaupel Z, Baker EA, Baker KC, et al: Analysis of retrieved agility total ankle arthroplasty systems, *Foot Ankle Int* 30:815–823, 2009.

360. Vickerstaff JA, Miles AW, Cunningham JL: A brief history of total ankle replacement and a review of the current status, *Med Eng Phys* 29:1056–1064, 2007.

361. Vienne P, Nothdurft P: OSG-Totalendoprothese Agility: Indikationen, Operationstechnik und Ergebnisse, *Fuss Sprungg* 2:17–28, 2004.

362. Wang Q, Whittle M, Cunningham J, Kenwright J: Fibula and its ligaments in load transmission and ankle joint stability, *Clin Orthop Relat Res* 330:261–270, 1996.

363. Ware JE Jr, Sherbourne CD: The MOS 36-item short-form health survey (SF-36). I. Conceptual framework and item selection, *Med Care* 30:473–483, 1992.

364. Wasserman LR, Saltzman CL, Amendola A: Minimally invasive ankle reconstruction: current scope and indications, *Orthop Clin North Am* 35:247–253, 2004.

365. Waugh TR, Evanski PM, McMaster WC: Irvine ankle arthroplasty. Prosthetic design and surgical technique, *Clin Orthop Relat Res* 114:180–184, 1976.

366. Weber M, Bonnin M, Columbier JA, Judet T: Erste Ergebnisse der SALTO-Sprunggelenkendoprothese: eine französische Multizenterstudie mit 115 Implantaten, *Fuss Sprungg* 2:29–37, 2004.

367. Weseley MS, Barenfeld PA: Mechanism of the Dwyer calcaneal osteotomy, *Clin Orthop Relat Res* 70:137–140, 1970.

368. Whalen JL, Spelsberg SC, Murray P: Wound breakdown after total ankle arthroplasty, *Foot Ankle Int* 31:301–305, 2010.

369. Wilken J, Rao S, Estin M, et al: A new device for assessing ankle dorsiflexion motion: reliability and validity, *J Orthop Sports Phys Ther* 41:274–280, 2011.

370. Wood PL: Experience with the STAR ankle arthroplasty at Wrightington Hospital, UK, *Foot Ankle Clin* 7:755–764, 2002.

371. Wood PL, Clough TM, Smith R: The present state of ankle arthroplasty, *Foot Ankle Surg* 14:115–119, 2008.

372. Wood PL, Crawford LA, Suneja R, Kenyon A: Total ankle replacement for rheumatoid ankle arthritis, *Foot Ankle Clin* 12:497–508, 2007.

373. Wood PL, Deakin S: Total ankle replacement. The results in 200 ankles, *J Bone Joint Surg Br* 85:334–341, 2003.

374. Wood PL, Karski MT, Watmough P: Total ankle replacement: the results of 100 mobility total ankle replacements, *J Bone Joint Surg Br* 92:958–962, 2010.

375. Wood PL, Prem H, Sutton C: Total ankle replacement: medium-term results in 200 Scandinavian total ankle replacements, *J Bone Joint Surg Br* 90:605–609, 2008.

376. Wood PL, Sutton C, Mishra V, Suneja R: A randomised, controlled trial of two mobile-bearing total ankle replacements, *J Bone Joint Surg Br* 91:69–74, 2009.

377. Wood PLR, Clough TM, Jari S: Clinical comparison of two total ankle replacements, *Foot Ankle Int* 21:546–550, 2000.

378. Wynn AH, Wilde AH: Long-term follow-up of the Conaxial (Beck-Steffee) total ankle arthroplasty, *Foot Ankle* 13:303–306, 1992.

379. Yalamanchili P, Donely B, Casillas M, et al: Salto Talaris total ankle replacement, *Oper Tech Orthop* 18:277–281, 2008.

380. Yamaguchi S, Tanaka Y, Banks S, et al: In vivo kinematics and articular surface congruency of total ankle arthroplasty during gait, *J Biomech* 45:2103–2108, 2012. doi:10.1016/j.jbiomech.2012.05.043.

381. Yamaguchi S, Tanaka Y, Kosugi S, et al: In vivo kinematics of two-component total ankle arthroplasty during non-weightbearing and weightbearing dorsiflexion/plantarflexion, *J Biomech* 44:995–1000, 2011.

382. Youdas JW, Bogard CL, Suman VJ: Reliability of goniometric measurements and visual estimates of ankle joint active range of motion obtained in a clinical setting, *Arch Phys Med Rehabil* 74:1113–1118, 1993.

383. Younger A, Penner M, Wing K: Mobile-bearing total ankle arthroplasty, *Foot Ankle Clin* 13:495–504, 2008.

384. Zerahn B, Kofoed H: Bone mineral density, gait analysis, and patient satisfaction, before and after ankle arthroplasty, *Foot Ankle Int* 25:208–214, 2004.

385. Zerahn B, Kofoed H, Borgwardt A: Increased bone mineral density adjacent to hydroxy-apatite-coated ankle arthroplasty, *Foot Ankle Int* 21:285–289, 2000.

386. Zimmerli W, Trampuz A, Ochsner PE: Prosthetic-joint infections, *N Engl J Med* 351:1645–1654, 2004.

Ring External Fixation in the Foot and Ankle

Douglas Beaman, Richard E. Gellman, Travis J. Kemp

PRINCIPLES OF DEFORMITY EVALUATION AND CORRECTION

Surgical techniques to correct deformity, whether performed acutely or gradually, require the treating surgeon to understand normal limb alignment and accurate deformity measurement.

Deformity within a bone segment is comprised of length, angulation, rotation, and translation measurements. Angulation and translation are present in both the coronal and sagittal planes, resulting in six measurements that are required to accurately describe a malunion deformity or displaced fracture (Fig. 23-1).

Frontal or coronal plane malalignment is commonly described as varus or valgus, whereas lateral or sagittal plane malalignment is described as either procurvatum or apex anterior and recurvatum or apex posterior. Rotational malalignment is defined as internal or external, referring to the position of the distal leg or ankle in relation to the proximal leg.

Normal Alignment and Deformity Measurement

In the frontal or coronal plane, normal alignment of the lower extremity is defined as the mechanical axis, a straight line that extends from the center of the hip joint through the knee to the center of the ankle joint (Fig. 23-2). The mechanical axis inferior to the ankle then extends down through the center of the talus and ends approximately 1 cm medial to the center vertical axis of the calcaneal tuberosity (Fig. 23-3A and B).[47]

Despite variations in body morphology, the weight-bearing mechanical axis is consistent and generally falls 10 mm medial to the center of the knee joint.[48] Significant mechanical axis deviations are associated with symptomatic joint pain and the risk of osteoarthritis from asymmetric joint loading.

Variations of the mechanical axis through the knee joint beyond 1 cm are not found in asymptomatic populations,[47] while variations in the weight-bearing line of the tibia lie within 15 mm of the lowest calcaneal point in 95% of asymptomatic populations.[56]

In the coronal plane below the knee, the mechanical axis and the anatomic axis of the tibia are parallel. An anatomic axis is a line connecting two midpoints in the diaphysis of a long bone. The anatomic axis in the tibia may fall just medial, about 3 mm, to the mechanical axis. Most radiographs to evaluate and follow patients with distal tibial deformity will not include the knee joint, so a proximal anatomic axis reference is typically used (Fig. 23-4).

SIX DEGREES OF FREEDOM

CORONAL PLANE
1) Varus/valgus angulation
2) Medial/lateral translation

SAGITTAL PLANE
3) Procurvatum/recurvatum
   angulation
4) Anterior/posterior
   translation

ROTATION
5) Internal/external

LENGTH
6) Long/short

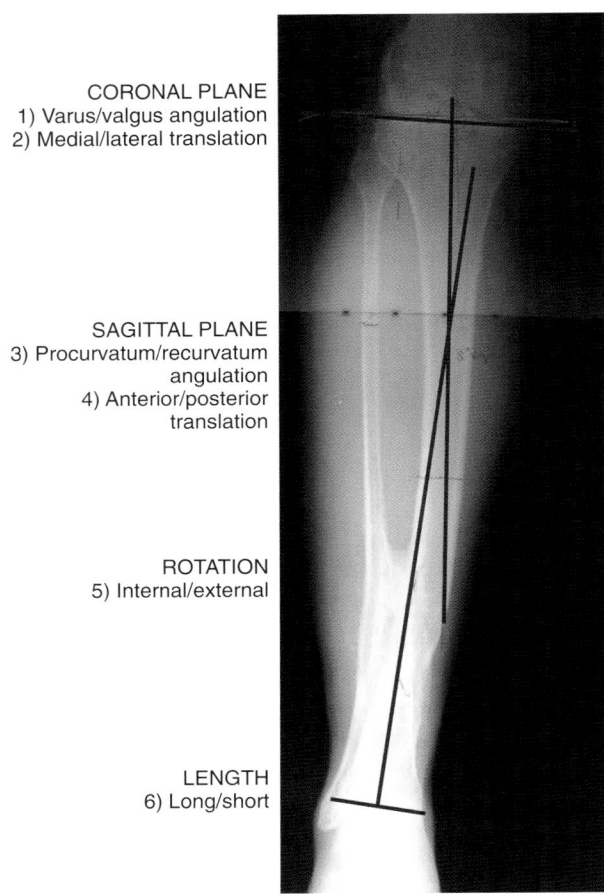

Figure 23-1 Six degrees of freedom. Deformity is described by six measurements: in the coronal plane by (1) angulation of varus or valgus and (2) medial or lateral translation, in the sagittal plane by (3) angulation of procurvatum or recurvatum and (4) anterior or posterior translation, in the axial plane by (5) rotation (internal or external), and (6) length (long or short).

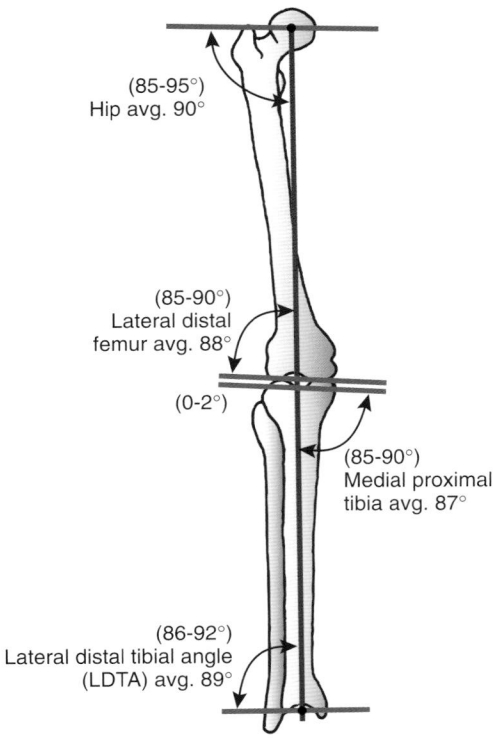

(85-95°)
Hip avg. 90°

(85-90°)
Lateral distal
femur avg. 88°

(0-2°)

(85-90°)
Medial proximal
tibia avg. 87°

(86-92°)
Lateral distal tibial angle
(LDTA) avg. 89°

Figure 23-2 Mechancial axis. The frontal or coronal plane mechanical axis of the lower extremity. The mechanical axis is the line from the center of the hip joint to the center of the ankle joint. Frontal plane joint orientation angles, average and normal range are shown for the hip, knee, and ankle. *avg.*, average.

At the ankle, the normal average lateral distal tibial angle (LDTA) is 89 degrees (normal range, 86-92 degrees). Conceptually, therefore, the goal of surgical treatment for a distal tibial coronal plane deformity is to make the distal tibial articular surface perpendicular to the tibial anatomic (or mechanical) axis.

If the deformity of the distal tibia occurs in the metaphysis and above, then the coronal plane deformity is measured by drawing the anatomic axis as the proximal reference line, and the patient's LDTA from the uninvolved limb or a standard LDTA of 89 degrees from the center of the ankle joint as the distal reference (Fig. 23-5).

In the coronal plane, if the deformity is located at the ankle joint, it is described as juxtaarticular. This occurs commonly from growth arrest or malunion collapse of a pilon fracture. In these cases, the LDTA is the intersection of the proximal anatomic axis and a line parallel to the distal tibial plafond or talar dome, assuming that they are congruent (Fig. 23-6).

To measure coronal plane alignment distal to the ankle, the hindfoot alignment view radiograph described by Saltzman[56] is used (see Fig. 23-3A and B). It is a weight-bearing radiograph that shows the distal tibial, ankle joint, and calcaneal tuberosity on a single view. This radiograph requires a specialized mounting box to angle the radiographic plate 20 degrees from the vertical plane. The long axial view is another radiograph that is non–weight bearing; it visualizes the tibia, subtalar joint, and calcaneal tuberosity and does not require a special mounting box (Fig. 23-7).

In the sagittal plane, the mechanical axis runs from the center of the hip joint to the center of the ankle, passing through the anterior portion of the knee joint. In normal alignment, the anatomic axis of the tibia in the sagittal plane will intersect the anterior fifth of the tibial plateau and bisect the distal tibia at the ankle. The normal distal tibial angle is 80 degrees, measured anteriorly and thus termed the anterior distal tibial angle (ADTA) (Fig. 23-8). The midtibial line intersects the midpoint of the talar dome and then, more distally, usually the lateral talar process, although the exact location varies with the position of ankle dorsiflexion or plantar flexion.[71,72]

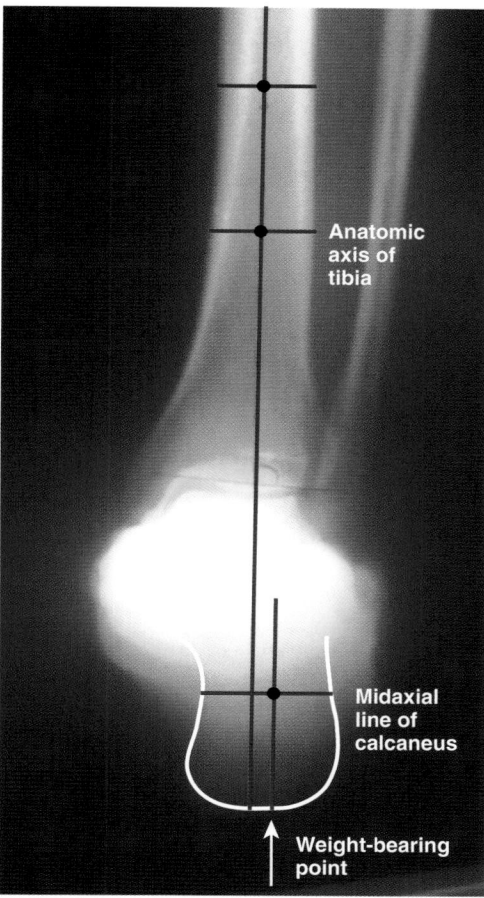

Figure 23-3 Hindfoot alignment view radiograph (Saltzman). The anatomic axis of the tibia is extended through the calcaneus, and the midaxial line of the calcaneal tuberosity is drawn. The midline of the calcaneus is usually lateral to the midline of the tibia because of the stepped articulation with the talus at the sustentaculum. The weight-bearing point on the calcaneus normally falls lateral, imparting a valgus moment on the ankle and subtalar joints.

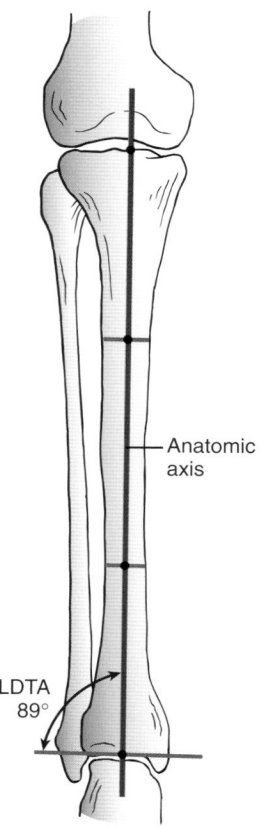

Figure 23-4 Coronal plane alignment. In a tibia with no deformity, an anatomic axis line should fall in the center of the tibial plafond or slightly medial. Next, draw a line parallel to the distal tibial articular surface or talar dome, if they are parallel. The angle described on the lateral side, the lateral distal tibial angle *(LDTA)* averages 89 degrees in large population studies.

Box 23-1

It is important to understand that malalignment in distal tibial or foot deformities can occur from three causes: malunion in the bone, intraarticular wear in the joint, or ligamentous laxity, creating tilt or asymmetric contact of the joint surface. The visualization of intraarticular wear and ligamentous laxity are best seen on weight-bearing radiographs (Fig. 23-11).

Sagittal plane deformities at or above the metaphysis are measured in a similar fashion to coronal plane deformity, using a proximal anatomic axis reference and a distal ADTA of 80 degrees or the patient's normal ADTA (Fig. 23-9). Juxtaarticular deformities are measured using the proximal anatomic axis line and a line along the distal tibial plafond (Box 23-1 and Fig. 23-10).

The rotational component of a deformity is often the most challenging to measure and treat. Measuring rotation can be performed clinically,[22,31,38,64,65] radiographically,[18,24,52] by fluoroscopy,[7] magnetic resonance imaging (MRI),[59] ultrasound,[25,26] or computed tomography (CT).[*]

Below the knee joint, a perpendicular line extending from the tibial tubercle normally matches the axis of the second toe. Clinical methods to measure rotation include the thigh-foot angle, the thigh-transmalleolar method, the second toe test,[35] and the footprint method.[22,31,64] These measurements are well established, easily performed, and can be used as estimations of rotation. However, they are only approximate because of variations in the position of the patella, the tibial tubercle, and the foot, which result in variability in measurements.[3,42]

We use the thigh-foot angle most frequently, matching rotation to the contralateral asymptomatic side. If there is significant deformity in the foot, rotation can be

---

[*]References 3, 8, 28, 29, 35, 51, 58, 61, 63, and 67.

CORONAL PLANE DEFORMITY

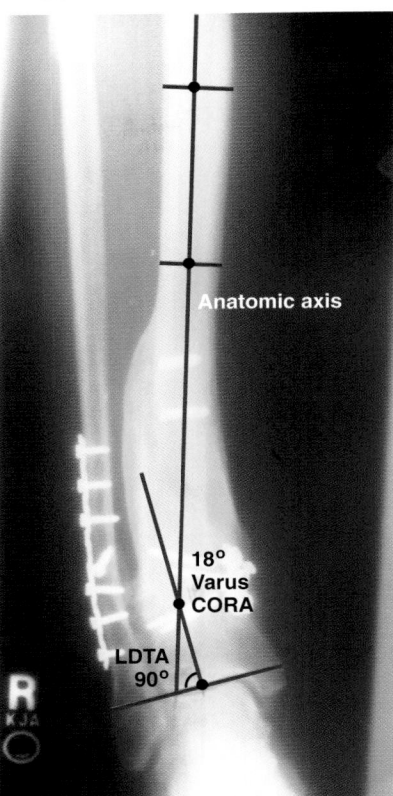

Figure 23-5 Coronal plane deformity. An example of an 18-degree varus coronal plane deformity measured as described in Figure 23-4. The proximal anatomic tibial axis and the lateral distal tibial angle are drawn. The lateral distal tibial angle *(LDTA)* of 90 degrees is normal for this patient, determined from his uninjured side. *CORA,* center of rotation of angulation.

CORONAL PLANE PERIARTICULAR

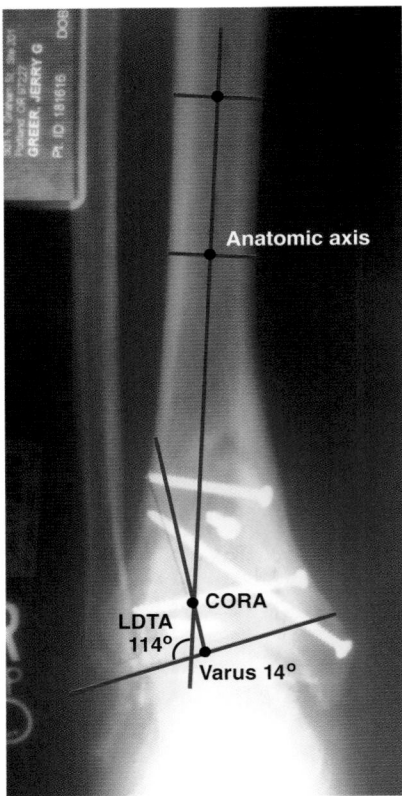

Figure 23-6 Coronal plane periarticular deformity. An example of a 14-degree periarticular varus deformity secondary to late collapse of a pilon fracture. In this case, it is easier to measure the angle formed by the proximal anatomic tibial axis and a line parallel to the talar dome. The *CORA,* center of rotation of angulation, is detailed under the section Deformity Correction.

determined by palpation of the medial and lateral malleolus at the ankle instead.

Radiographic methods of measuring tibial torsion vary among authors both in technique and reliability, and none have been widely accepted as standard. MRI and ultrasound have also been studied but not widely accepted.

Computed tomography is considered the gold standard for measuring tibial rotation.* Lee et al[35] describe the simplest method of measuring tibial torsion by using two-dimensional CT. On a CT scan, tibial rotation is defined as the angle between the transarticular axis of the proximal tibia—a line connecting both posterior condyles, and the transmalleolar axis of the ankle—a line connecting the medial and lateral malleoli (Fig. 23-12).[34]

An important factor regarding rotational deformities is their influence on the accuracy of coronal plane angular measurements on standard anteroposterior radiographs.[68]

McCann et al[41] demonstrated this in a sawbone tibia model. They found that increasing tibial rotation increased error in the angular measurement. For example, an internal rotation deformity of 25 degrees led to a false 5-degree increase in the amount of varus measured.

Appropriate radiographic techniques to prevent this error are described below.

Standing, full-length, lower-extremity, 51-inch anteroposterior (AP) radiographs from the hip to the ankle are obtained if there is a known or suspected leg-length discrepancy (LLD) or to assess possible deformity above the knee. A block placed under the shorter limb will assist in accurate measurement and determination of LLD. Deformity in the lumbar spine that creates a fixed pelvic obliquity may also create LLD (Fig. 23-13).

Foot deformity is assessed with weight-bearing radiographs that are accurately obtained perpendicular to the dorsum of the foot for AP views.

The AP foot radiograph is measured for talo–first metatarsal angle, talocalcaneal angle, navicular coverage, and

---

*References 3, 8, 28, 29, 35, 51, 58, 61, 63, and 67.

LONG AXIAL VIEW

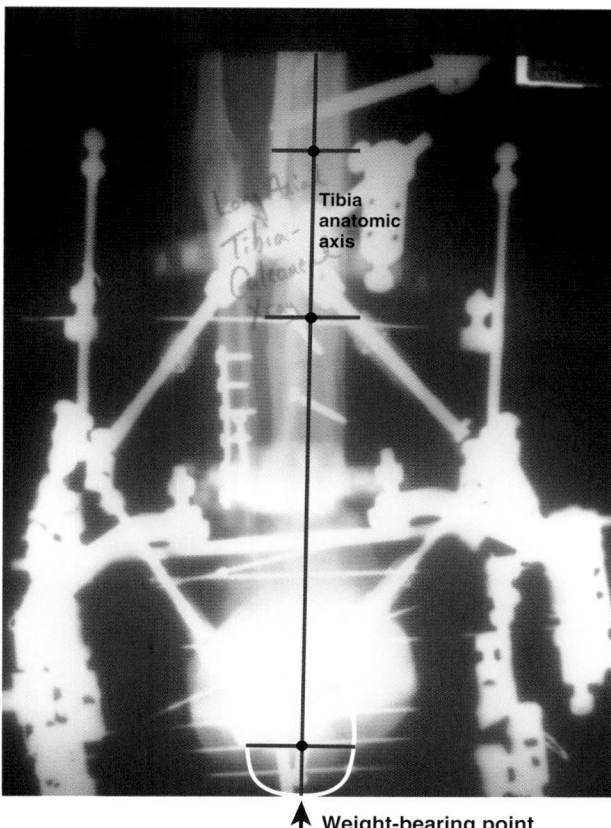

Figure 23-7 Long axial view. The long axial view of the hindfoot is a non–weight-bearing radiograph that is useful in assessing alignment when patients cannot stand on the platform for a Saltzman hindfoot alignment radiograph. It usually demonstrates the subtalar joint, unless there is obstruction by external fixation hardware or a subtalar arthrodesis, as in this case.

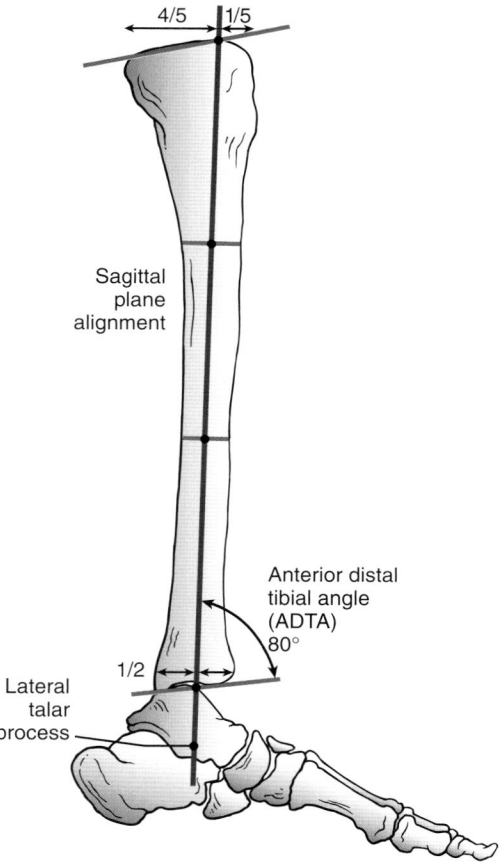

Figure 23-8 Sagittal plane alignment. In a tibia with no deformity, an anatomic axis line should fall in the center of the talar dome. Next, draw a line parallel to the distal tibial articular surface. The angle described on the anterior side, the anterior distal tibial angle (ADTA) averages 80 degrees in large population studies.

joint subluxation, fusion, coalitions, or arthritis. The lateral foot view is measured for talo–first metatarsal angle, navicular–cuneiform malalignment, talocalcaneal angle, calcaneal pitch, and the joint pathology described for the AP view. Normal foot angles have been well defined by Gentili et al.[16]

Comparison weight-bearing radiographs of the contralateral limb are usually obtained for preoperative planning.

Radiographic Evaluation

Obtaining accurate radiographs is the cornerstone of precise deformity analysis, and the radiographs must be planned to best represent the deformity.

■ First, center the beam on the region of the deformity, and include the joint proximal and distal to the deformity (Fig. 23-14).

■ Second, orient the joint toward the beam. If the knee joint is the region of interest, then the patella should be centered within the femoral condyles. The lateral view is at 90 degrees to this.[46] If the distal tibia and ankle are the location of the deformity, then the malleoli should be oriented as if taking an ankle AP radiograph, with the tibial-fibular overlap approximately 6 mm. In equinovarus foot deformity, the radiographer aligns the beam with the foot flat against the floor, angling the leg inward (Fig. 23-15).

■ Third, obtain standing radiographs whenever possible to assess intraarticular wear or ligamentous laxity contributing to the overall deformity (see Fig. 23-8).

■ Fourth, if there is a suspected leg-length discrepancy, or it is unknown whether there is deformity around the knee or hip, then obtain a 51-inch standing AP radiograph and measure the mechanical axis. If the mechanical axis falls outside of the center of

SAGITTAL PLANE DEFORMITY

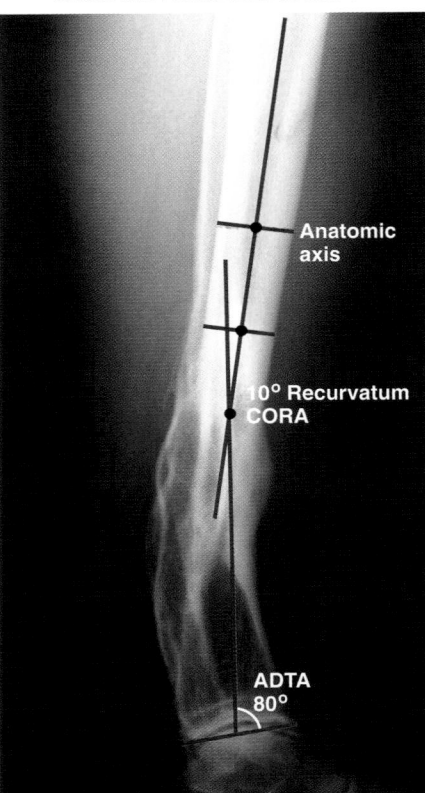

SAGITTAL PLANE PERIARTICULAR

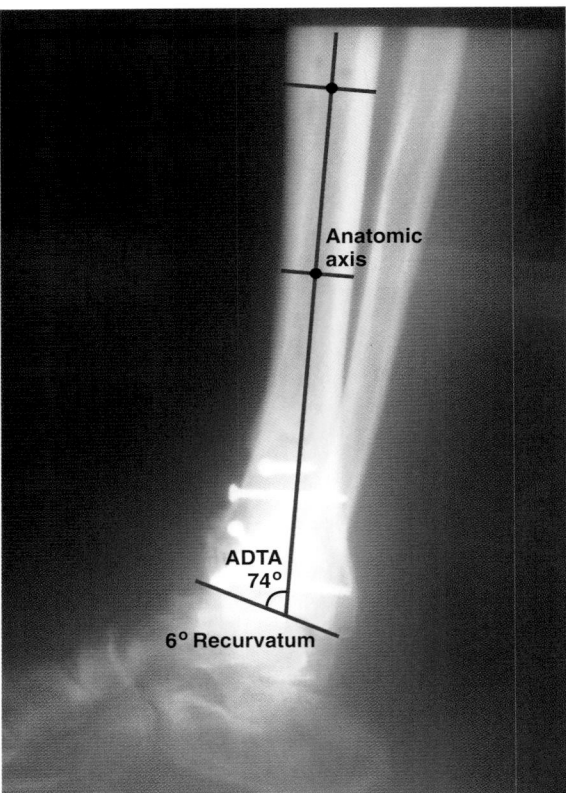

Figure 23-9 Sagittal plane deformity. An example of a 10-degree recurvatum sagittal plane deformity measured as described in Figure 23-8. The proximal anatomic tibial axis and the lateral distal tibial angles are drawn. Intersection of the two lines above the apparent apex usually indicates the presence of a translational deformity. *ADTA,* anterior distal tibial angle; *CORA,* center of rotation of angulation.

Figure 23-10 Sagittal plane periarticular deformity. An example of an approximately 6-degree periarticular varus deformity secondary to late collapse of a pilon fracture. In this case, it is easier to measure the angle formed by the proximal anatomic tibial axis and a line parallel to the talar dome. A comparison to the uninjured limb is useful with sagittal plane deformities because of variability in the anterior distal tibial angle *(ADTA).*

the knee joint, then measure the coronal plane joint orientation angles at the hip and knee to determine whether there is a deformity above the distal leg (see Fig. 23-2).

Digital versus Plain Radiographs

Digital radiographs have become the standard in many institutions. Standing anteroposterior long-leg radiographs using conventional analog printed film is being replaced by digital radiographs viewed on computer screens. Light boxes, rulers, goniometers, and grease pencils are being exchanged for computers screens that use graphics software to obtain measurements.

A wide variety of digital graphics software is available with most picture archiving and communication systems (PACS). Basic measurement tools typically include three-point angular measurements, Cobb angle measurements, digital rulers, and a calibration tool. Becoming familiar with these tools is critical to successful deformity planning.

The reliability and reproducibility of measurements obtained from digital versus conventional radiographs has been validated in multiple studies.[20,21,37,55,60] In general, digital radiographic measurements are as accurate or improve accuracy and save time compared with conventional printed radiographs.

Compensatory Deformities

Compensatory deformities can occur in the foot. Deformities of the distal tibia usually are compensated in the subtalar joint and the forefoot. The subtalar joint will compensate for a distal tibial varus deformity by moving into an everted position. Because the average eversion in the subtalar joint is 10 degrees, varus deformities greater than 10 degrees may cause symptoms on the lateral border of the foot. Further compensation occurs in the forefoot, with distal tibial varus compensated by forefoot pronation. This is seen as a valgus forefoot or a plantar flexed first ray when the patient's foot is examined in the

WEIGHT-BEARING RADIOGRAPH

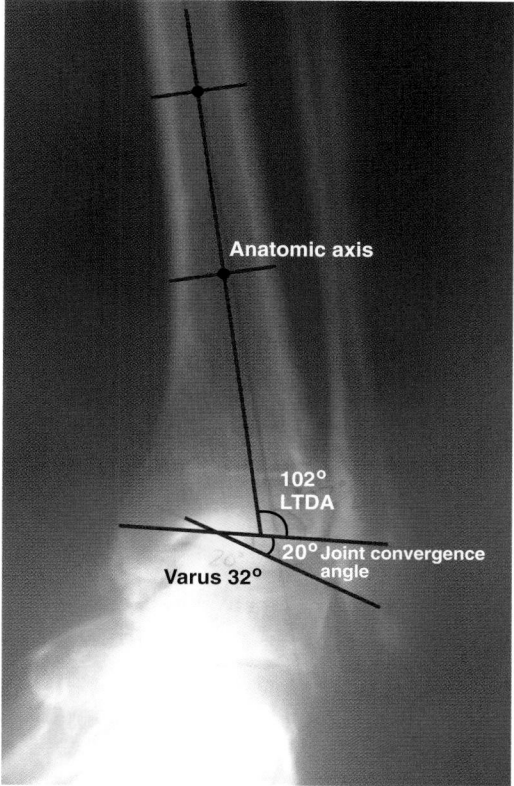

Anatomic axis

102°
LTDA

20° Joint convergence
angle

Varus 32°

Figure 23-11 Weight-bearing radiograph. The importance of weight bearing to fully assess deformity is demonstrated here. This patient has 12 degrees of varus in the distal tibia from an adolescent growth plate injury and 20 degrees of talar tilt from ligamentous laxity, which creates a total of 32 degrees of varus. A non–weight-bearing radiograph can often miss intraarticular wear and ligamentous laxity. *LDTA,* lateral distal tibial angle.

non–weight-bearing position. Distal tibial valgus will be compensated with subtalar inversion and forefoot varus (Fig. 23-16).

The need to correct the compensatory deformities depends on their extent and rigidity. The goal of correction is to create a plantigrade foot, and the compensatory deformity may be treated with arthrodesis, osteotomy, or tenotomy to achieve this goal. Muscle imbalance may also be associated with a compensatory deformity and require treatment with tendon transfer (Table 23-1).

Deformity Correction

In the tibia, the point where the proximal anatomic and the distal mechanical axes intersect is termed the apex of the deformity. Mechanically, this apex is the optimal location for an osteotomy to correct the deformity, so it also has been termed as the center of rotation of angulation (CORA). If the CORA does not fall at what appears to be

Table 23-1	Normal Joint Motions Compensatory to Different Distal Tibial Deformities	
Distal Tibial Deformity	**Compensatory Motion**	**Common Compensatory Range**
Varus	1° subtalar eversion 2° forefoot pronation	15°
Valgus	1° subtalar inversion 2° forefoot supination	30°
Procurvatum	1° ankle dorsiflexion 2° knee hyperextension	20°
Recurvatum	1° ankle plantar flexion 2° knee flexion	50°
Internal torsion	1° hip external rotation 2° forefoot pronation	Varied
External torsion	1° hip internal rotation 2° forefoot supination	Varied

the apex of the deformity, then there is a translational component of the deformity.

Once the CORA is determined, then the surgeon must decide the osteotomy location. If possible, the osteotomy is made at the CORA. After correction, the bony segment will be straight, the deformity will be corrected, and the proximal and distal mechanical axis lines will be realigned (Fig. 23-17).

Often, however, deformities in the distal tibia and foot have a CORA that does not permit an osteotomy. This may be due to insufficient distance between the joint and the CORA, as in distal tibial juxtaarticular deformities that have the CORA at or near the joint after distal tibial growth arrest or collapse after ankle pilon fractures. Other reasons include poor soft tissue or sclerotic bone that will not allow good bone healing.

In these cases, the osteotomy must be made proximal to the CORA. Correction of the angular deformity will then require translation at the osteotomy to accurately realign the distal mechanical axis to the proximal anatomic axis.

In the case of a distal tibial varus deformity, the distal tibial segment, along with angular correction will translate medially to correctly realign the limb mechanical axis (Fig. 23-18). If there is a distal valgus deformity, the distal segment is translated laterally along with the angular correction.

In summary, correction with the osteotomy at the CORA avoids secondary translations. However, it may not be feasible to perform an osteotomy at the CORA for distal tibial and foot deformities. This is an important principle and should be followed with acute or gradual corrections.

SUPRAMALLEOLAR DEFORMITY CORRECTION

Gradual correction of distal tibial deformities involves the technique of distraction osteogenesis, which is the

CT SCAN - TIBIAL ROTATION MEASUREMENT

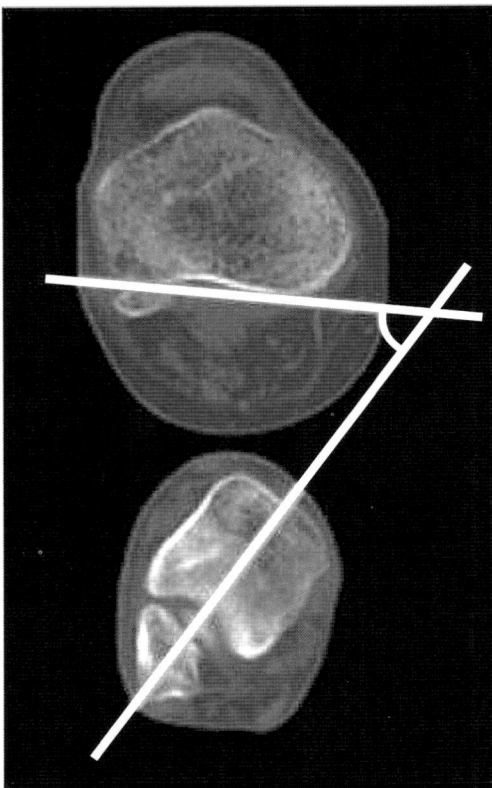

Figure 23-12 Computed tomography (CT) scan for tibial rotation measurement. Rotational alignment in the tibia is measured as the angle between a line connecting the posterior condyles of the proximal tibia and a line through the medial and lateral malleoli just above the tibial plafond. A comparison of both tibias is recommended because of significant variability in normal populations.

51-inch AP RADIOGRAPH

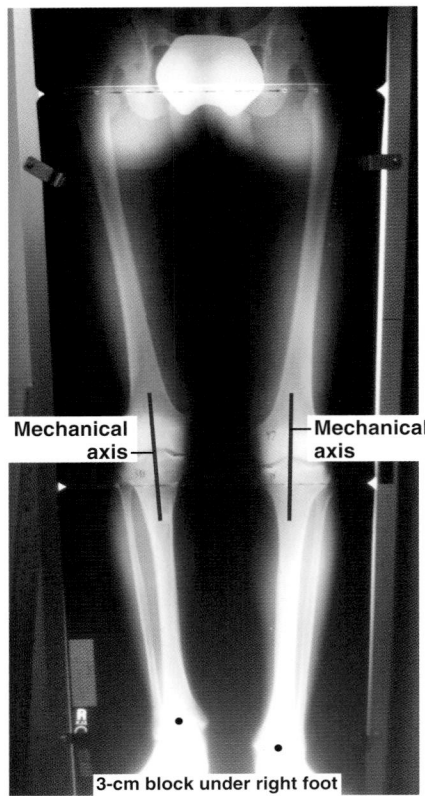

Figure 23-13 Fifty-one–inch anteroposterior (AP) standing radiograph. This view allows determination of leg-length discrepancy as well as a mechanical axis check through the center of each knee. This patient has a 3-cm block under the right foot. Individual measurements of femurs and tibias are determined to verify precise location of length discrepancy.

formation of new bone after an osteotomy using tension lengthening techniques. Distraction osteogenesis – when used with multiplanar ring external fixation techniques – is a minimally invasive method, that is important when there is a compromised soft tissue envelope or compromised bone. Ring fixation techniques allow gradual simultaneous multiplanar correction, which is difficult to obtain with acute correction. Newer ring fixation devices, such as the Taylor Spatial Frame (Smith & Nephew, Memphis, Tenn.) correct complex deformity in a more efficient and reliable manner. Gradual deformity correction allows ongoing postoperative assessment of alignment, and adjustments are continued until accurate correction is achieved.

The decision to use distraction osteogenesis or acute correction may be a difficult decision, and multiple factors are considered. These include surgeon experience and ability with the various techniques, as well as careful patient evaluation.

In our experience, distraction osteogenesis is typically chosen over acute correction when the deformity is complex, often involving an oblique plane, a rotational component, and/or limb shortening. Also, gradual correction is chosen when a deformity is particularly severe and the ability to confidently correct it acutely is compromised. Other factors include prior infection or soft tissue envelope compromise, when an acute correction is likely to result in stretch of the neurovascular structures (particularly important in the varus to valgus correction), when significant shortening would occur, or when acute correction would create an unstable osteotomy.

The use of ring fixation, with or without gradual correction of deformity, may allow the patient to be more functional during the healing period because a ring fixator will typically allow partial to full weight bearing during the recovery time. Associated ankle arthritis is another consideration because the ankle joint can be

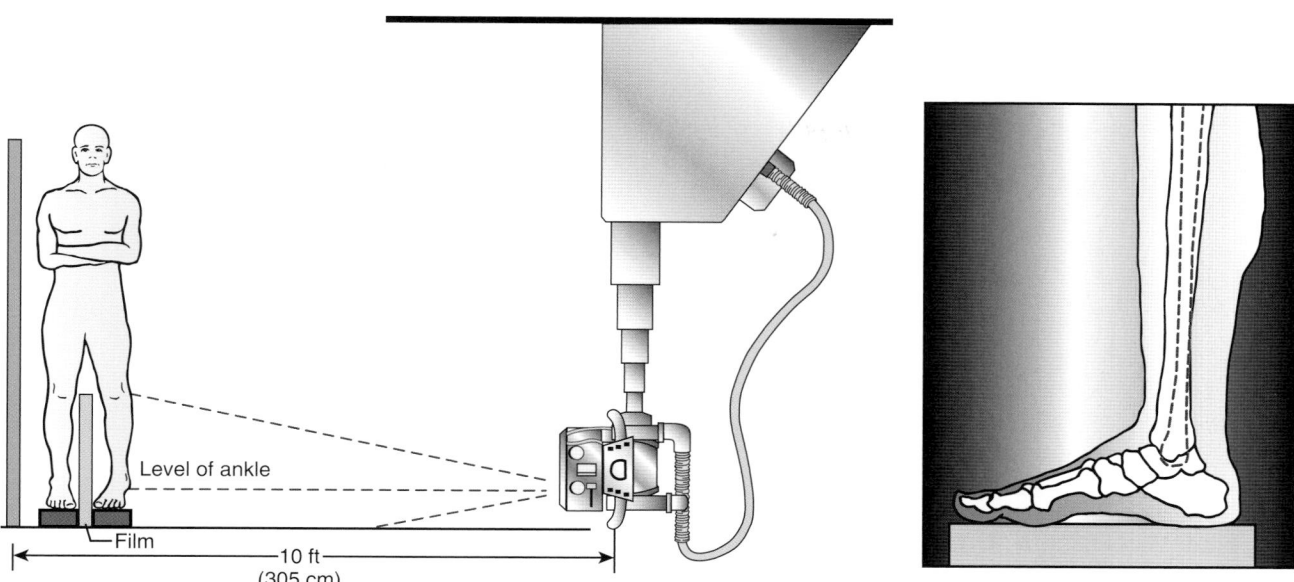

Figure 23-14 Radiograph: center beam on deformity or joint of interest. The x-ray beam is centered on the ankle or foot but includes enough of the tibial shaft to easily draw an anatomic axis line. The foot is rotated inward or outward, depending on the presence of rotational deformity and the need to visualize either the ankle or the foot.

FOOT DEFORMITY RADIOGRAPH

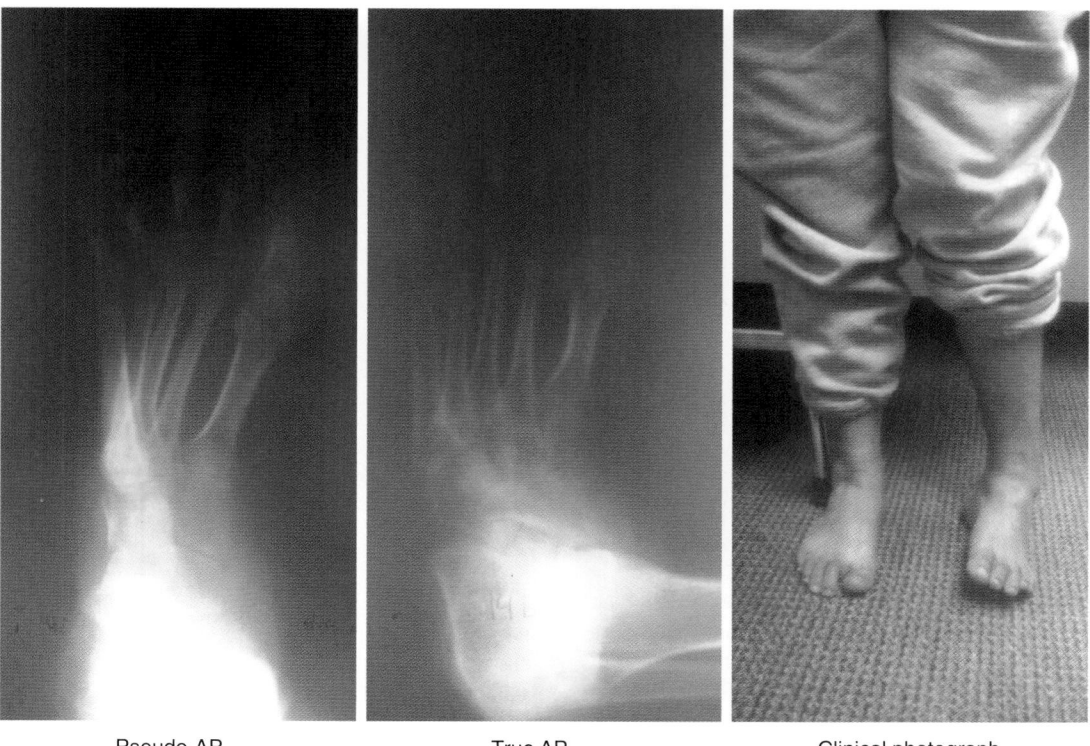

Pseudo-AP   True AP   Clinical photograph

Figure 23-15 Anteroposterior (AP) foot deformity radiograph. The two radiographs demonstrate the difference between the x-ray beam oriented perpendicular to the floor, termed the "pseudo-AP", and the beam oriented perpendicular to the dorsum of the foot for a true AP radiograph. The clinical photograph shows the foot appearance of the radiographs.

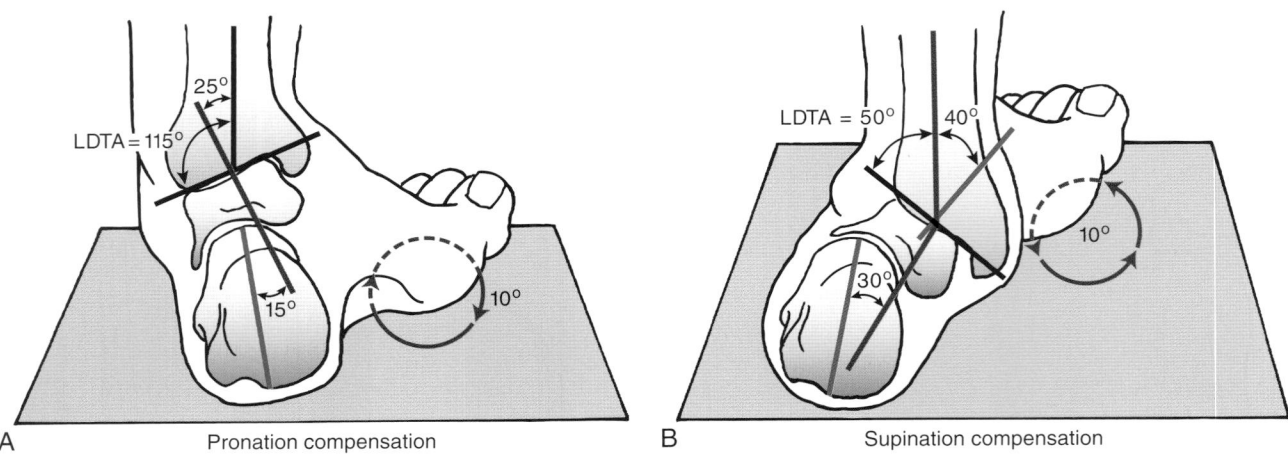

A   Pronation compensation   B   Supination compensation

Figure 23-16   Compensation for tibial varus **(A)** or valgus **(B)** deformity with subtalar motion. *LDTA,* lateral distal tibial angle.

OSTEOTOMY AT CORA

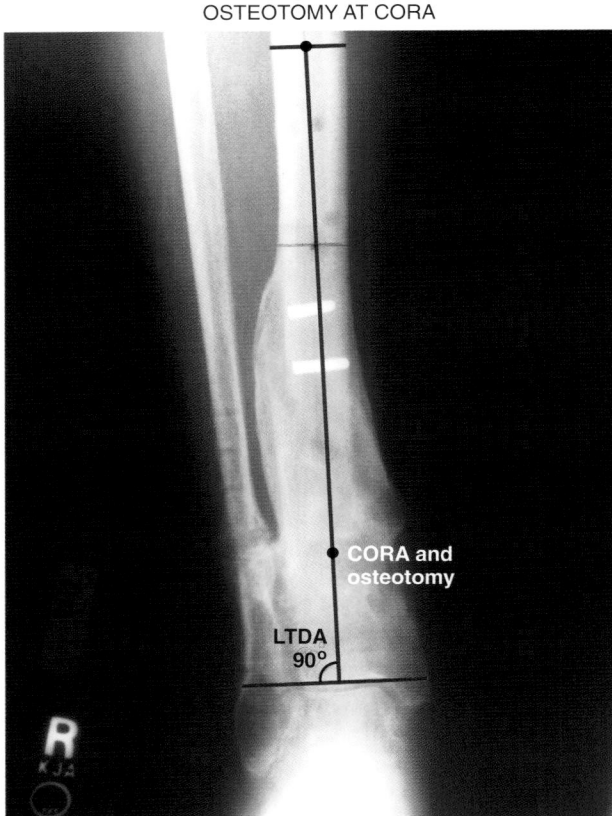

OSTEOTOMY PROXIMAL TO CORA

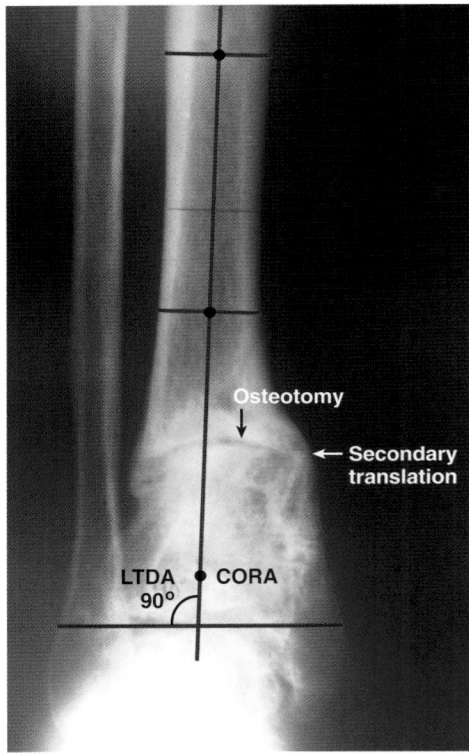

Figure 23-17   Osteotomy at center of rotation of angulation *(CORA).* Postoperative radiograph of patient shown in Figure 23-5. Osteotomy performed at CORA, followed by gradual correction with a Taylor Spatial Frame. The bone is accurately realigned with a lateral distal tibial angle *(LDTA)* of 90 degrees and no secondary translation.

Figure 23-18   Osteotomy proximal to center of rotation of angulation *(CORA).* Postoperative radiograph of patient shown in Figure 23-6. Osteotomy is performed proximal to the CORA, followed by gradual correction with a Taylor Spatial Frame. The bone is accurately realigned with a lateral distal tibial angle *(LDTA)* of 90 degrees, but there is a secondary medial translation.

distracted simultaneously with distal tibial deformity correction.

The decision to use distraction osteogenesis techniques and/or ring external fixation includes a careful evaluation of the patient and the patient's ability to care for a ring fixator. Because patient involvement is required during the treatment, we favor an organized team approach in which all people involved are familiar with the ring fixation techniques, including the orthopaedic surgeon, office staff, physical therapist, orthotist, and hospital staff, both in the operating room and patient care units.

Supramalleolar Deformity Classification

A simple method to classify and treat distal tibial and fibular deformity defines four general deformity patterns: (1) tibia only, (2) fibula only, (3) equal tibia and fibula, (4) unequal tibia and fibula. The fourth pattern, when the deformity of the fibula differs from that of the tibia, is seen after distal tibial and fibular fractures. It is usually the most difficult to analyze and to treat. Each pattern may exist with intraarticular deformity secondary to ligamentous laxity or asymmetric cartilage.

Osteotomy Location for Supramalleolar Deformity

A comprehensive deformity analysis must be performed as the first step in planning. Once the deformity pattern and CORA are defined, the location of osteotomies becomes straightforward. An osteotomy at the level of the CORA is the ideal location because only angulation is required for correction. However, as noted, the CORA may be at a suboptimal location for an osteotomy because of multiple factors. These include poor or dense bone quality, damaged soft tissue envelope, insufficient distance from the ankle joint to allow wire placements (three wires are the preferred minimum), and a deformity with significant translation, creating a CORA far away from the site of angular deformity.

Altering the location of the osteotomy from the CORA is frequently necessary, and, as previously discussed, requires translation to obtain correction.

Tibial and Fibular Osteotomy Surgical Techniques

The optimal osteotomy technique preserves periosteal blood supply and minimizes thermal bone necrosis.[56] The use of power saws should be avoided in the tibia.[15] The preferred osteotomy technique varies with the anatomic location. A multiple drill hole technique is preferred in the diaphyseal region of the tibia, whereas a Gigli saw osteotomy is preferred in the metaphyseal regions of the tibia. With gradual correction techniques, the osteotomy is usually completed after an external fixator has been applied.

Multiple Drill Hole Technique (Fig. 23-19)

1. A 1-cm, anterior tibial vertical skin incision is made. The tibia is carefully exposed medial to the tibialis anterior, and the periosteum is gently elevated along the medial and lateral borders of the tibia with a small, curved elevator.
2. A 4.8-mm drill hole is made from anterior to posterior. Through the single anterior drill hole, the drill bit is advanced carefully through several locations in the posterior cortex.
3. A 10-mm sharp osteotome is directed along medial and lateral cortices with protection of the overlying periosteum.
4. The supporting struts or rods of the fixator are removed, and the osteotome is directed into the posterior cortex

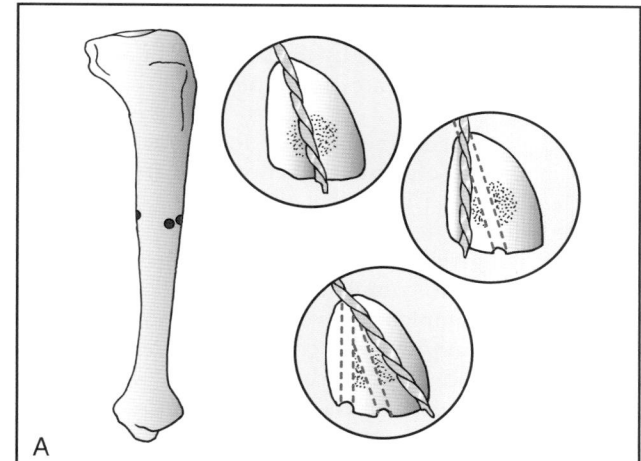

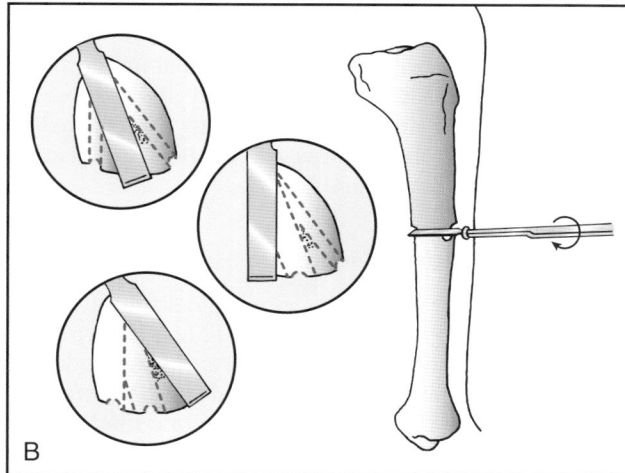

Figure 23-19 The multiple drill hole osteotomy technique is preferred in the diaphyseal region of the tibia. **A,** A 4.8-mm drill hole is made first from anterior to posterior, followed by two more drill holes placed posteromedial and posterolateral. **B,** The osteotomy is completed with an osteotome.

and twisted 90 degrees with a wrench. This typically completes the osteotomy. The distal ring may be gently rotated externally to assure completion.

5. The struts or rods are replaced at their prior lengths, reducing the osteotomy. The osteotomy is compressed 1 to 2 mm.

6. Allow a 5- to 10-day (usually 7 days) latency period before beginning corrections. This may be longer in cases with suboptimal soft tissue, bone, or other healing concerns.

Gigli Saw Technique (Fig. 23-20)

1. In the tibial metaphyseal region, two transverse incisions are used: one directly over the posteromedial edge of the bone and one anterior, just medial to the tibialis anterior.

2. Careful elevation of the periosteum is made with a small curved elevator, and a heavy suture is passed subperiorsteally anterolaterally to posteromedially under the muscle compartments of the leg by using two right-angle clamps.

3. The Gigli saw is pulled by the suture from anterior to posterior, taking care to protect all soft tissue structures.

4. The Gigli saw cuts the bone up to the medial face of the tibia, with soft tissue retraction used at all times to prevent injury. The medial tibial cortex cut is completed after the retractors have been moved to protect the medial periosteum and soft tissue. The saw is typically flattened to complete the cut.

5. Osteotomy completion is verified with the C-arm. The Gigli saw is cut with a wire cutter for easy removal. This osteotomy can generally be completed with fixator rods or struts intact, and is compressed 1 to 2 mm after completion.

Note: In the supramalleolar region (close proximity of the tibia and fibula), this technique can be modified to include the fibula, with a third longitudinal incision over the distal fibula. The suture and Gigli saw are passed sequentially from anterior to lateral to posteromedial. The osteotomy is then carried out in the same manner but includes the fibula.

Fibular Osteotomy Technique

Fibular osteotomy addresses fibular deformity at the time of tibial osteotomy. When the fibular deformity is similar to the tibial deformity in level and magnitude, the fibular and tibial osteotomies are made at the same level (osteotomy at level of CORA). An oblique fibular osteotomy is made with a small sagittal saw or the multiple drill hole technique (using a 2.0-mm drill and 8-mm osteotome).

Fibular osteotomy distal to the tibial osteotomy may be indicated if translation is required for realignment. With a fibular-only deformity, the osteotomy is generally

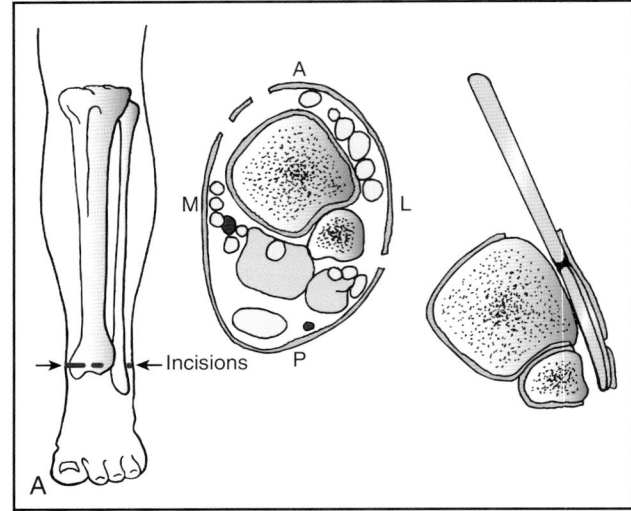

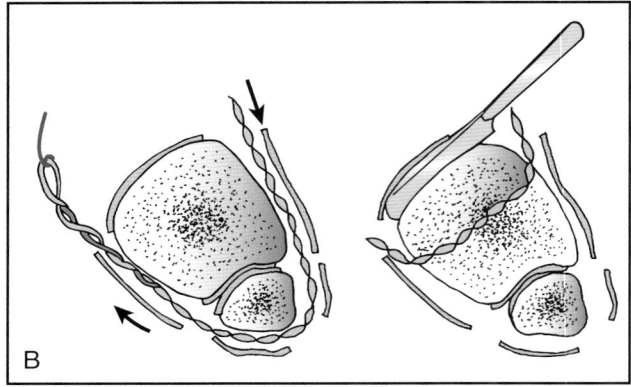

Figure 23-20 Percutaneous Gigli saw osteotomy in the supramalleolar region. At this level, there is no space between the tibia and fibula to pass the saw. The tibia and fibula are cut together. **A,** Three small incisions are used. The two medial incisions are transverse, and the lateral incision is longitudinal. The periosteum is elevated anteriorly over the tibia and fibula; then the lateral incision is made over the tip of the elevator. *A,* anterior; *L,* lateral; *M,* medial; *P,* posterior. **B,** The Gigli saw is passed with a heavy suture to the posteromedial side. The medial periosteum is elevated, and the Gigli saw is used to cut the fibula and tibia from lateral to medial.

made near the fibular CORA, leaving satisfactory distal bone for fixation.

Taylor Spatial Frame Application for Supramalleolar Deformity

Note: A thorough understanding of and training with spatial frame methodology is important before frame applications.

1. The preoperative plan should include the position of all rings, wires, half-pins, and struts or hinges. Incisions and osteotomy locations are planned based on the CORA, bone and soft tissue concerns, and goals

of the procedure. Wires and half-pins are placed to avoid neurovascular structures, poor skin or open wounds, sclerotic bone, and internal fixation. All cases have unique characteristics, demanding unique frame setups, and the following technique is based on general guidelines.

2. Position the patient with the patella facing up. This may require a bump under the ipsalateral hip and shoulder. A 9-inch C-arm image intensifier is preferred, with the base on the contralateral side.

3. Confirm the osteotomy location with the C-arm. If a Gigli osteotomy is used, pass the suture and secure it. The fibular osteotomy, when needed, is performed before frame application, unless a supramalleolar three-incision (tibia and fibula) Gigli technique is used.

4. Distal tibial fixation: An appropriate-sized full ring (1- to 2-cm soft tissue clearance) is placed orthogonal to the ankle. (*Note:* Put the proximal tibial rings on the limb before distal fixation, but secure the distal ring to the bone first). It will generally serve as the reference ring for the spatial frame software, and mounting parameters will be based on its location relative to the CORA. Fixation will vary with the individual case, but will typically include three 1.8-mm wires: transverse reference wire with medial olive; fibula-to-tibia lateral olive wire; and either a smooth medial-face tibial wire or smooth wire placed just anterior to fibula through the tibia. If sufficient bone is present (with a more proximal osteotomy location), one or two half-pins (5 or 6 mm) may be added.

5. Proximal tibial fixation: A two-ring tibial base frame is applied orthogonal to the tibial shaft in the same manner as outlined for ankle distraction. The location of the distal of these two rings is such that the majority of the spatial struts are lengthened to near the middle of the standard medium strut (approximately 145 mm). This tends to minimize the need for strut changes during correction and allows adequate placement of half-pins. It is optimal to create maximum half-pin spread and divergence. In general, one smooth transverse 1.8-mm wire and two 6-mm half-pins are placed on each ring. Attaching the proximal rings after the distal ring allows more precise placement to optimize strut lengths.

6. Spatial frame struts are applied using the appropriate ring tabs. For reconstructive purposes, the standard struts are preferred. It is important to place half-pins and wires in positions that do not interfere with the struts. This often requires careful planning, and the Taylor Spatial Frame struts may be attached before all the external fixation half-pins are placed.

7. The foot is included in the fixator in situations such as ankle arthritis, to distract the ankle; equinus contracture that requires correction; insufficient distal tibial fixation, to provide osteotomy stability; patients at risk for delayed tibial bone healing; and soft tissue concerns around the ankle. The foot ring and ankle hinges are applied in the method described for ankle distraction. Hinge placement is more difficult because of the distal location of the tibial ring. In patients without ankle arthritis or other ankle pathology, fixed holding of the foot can be achieved with four threaded rods placed between the foot ring and distal tibial ring. The foot ring in these cases is often removed in clinic after approximately 6 to 8 weeks, when early osteotomy healing is present.

8. The tibial osteotomy is completed after frame application and performed as previously described.

9. Frame mounting parameters and strut settings are determined. Deformity measurements are preoperatively planned.

   After an appropriate latency period, gradual correction is achieved using the Taylor Spacial Frame software. It is important to calculate needed length so that the osteotomy ends avoid binding. Length may be accomplished first (usually 0.5-1.0 mm/day), followed by angulation, rotation, and finally translation. The software program allows simultaneous or sequential corrections. Often, it is desirable to gain osteotomy separation before correction of deformity. Further information and experience regarding the use of Taylor Spatial Frame software and calculating deformity parameters is available through Smith & Nephew.

10. Frame management: Strut changes, when needed, are performed after stabilizing the rings with one or two threaded rods (with conical washers). After complete correction has been obtained, threaded rods (usually 4-6) are typically placed and the struts removed. This tends to improve frame stability as well as visualization on radiographs.

    Postoperative dressings remain in place for 1 to 2 weeks, and pin care begins as an outpatient. On the first postoperative day, the patient is advanced from bed to chair. Gait training begins on the second postoperative day, with weight-bearing restrictions based on frame configuration. Physical therapy is an important part of the postoperative care. This is started in the hospital and continued as an outpatient. Lower-extremity motion, conditioning, and gait are emphasized. Nonimpact activities, such as cycling and swimming, are encouraged. A stationary bicycle with modified pedals may be used.

    Pin care: At the first postoperative visit, the pin-site sponges and dressings are removed, and pin care is initiated with daily normal saline cleaning around the pin sites. After sutures are removed, the pin care is performed during a daily shower with antibacterial liquid soap and water rinse to the leg and fixator. The fixator and leg are dried with a clean towel and hair dryer set at the cool setting. Further pin care is not necessary if the pin sites remain clean and dry but is resumed if there are signs of infection about the pin sites. Pin scabs are retained unless there are signs of infection. For draining pin sites, two or more adjacent pins are wrapped together with a bulky gauze roll to decrease the motion between the skin and the pin; this may limit subsequent pin-site irritation that could progress to a pin-site infection. Lotions, ointments, or creams are generally avoided around pin sites.

When early signs of pin-site infection are noted, pin care is increased to twice daily, the pin site is wrapped with a gauze roll dressing, ankle range of motion (if present) is discontinued, and weight bearing and physical therapy are limited. If signs and symptoms of a pin-site infection do not rapidly improve, oral antibiotics are prescribed for 5 to 7 days. Recalcitrant pin-site infection is treated with intravenous antibiotic therapy with occasional pin removal.

11. Frame removal: Bony healing needs to be confirmed on at least three of four cortices by using AP and lateral radiographs. CT scanning or fluoroscopic imaging is helpful. Frames are often removed in the operating room under anesthesia but may be removed in the outpatient clinic as well. The pin sites are kept covered and dry until healed, approximately 7 to 10 days. After frame removal, a walking boot is generally used for 6 to 8 weeks, followed by a gradual return to normal activities.

ANKLE DISTRACTION

Ankle distraction arthroplasty is a component of ankle joint preservation for arthritis. Joint preservation generally includes correction of associated bony and soft tissue deformities, joint debridement, and ligament and tendon balancing. Distraction arthroplasty is based on the hypothesis that articular cartilage repair can occur when the joint is unloaded and subjected to intermittent fluid pressure changes.[75] Mechanical unloading is achieved for several months with a ring external fixator device. During this period, loading and unloading of the joint during weight bearing results in intraarticular hydrostatic pressure changes.[74,75] In vitro and animal studies have demonstrated that mechanical unloading and intermittent fluid pressure changes can alter cartilage matrix turnover.[75] Also, subchondral bone remodeling occurs with distraction and may affect cartilage repair.[53] Subchondral bone remodeling has been linked to clinical improvement.[27] Clinical studies have demonstrated improved pain and mobility, with a delay for the need of ankle arthrodesis or replacement.[27,40,50,53,70,74]

Patient evaluation for ankle distraction arthroplasty includes a thorough history and physical examination. The optimal candidate is a compliant, motivated patient, younger than 50 years—one who has posttraumatic arthritis or chronic ankle instability with arthritis, no previous history of ankle joint sepsis or ankylosis, and an appropriate psychosocial support system to facilitate recovery and in-frame care. Also, overall general good health without diabetes, vascular disease, neuropathy, or other significant medical problems affecting function is a prerequisite for ankle distraction. Furthermore, physically demanding occupations may prevent optimal clinical results, and preferred recreational activities are nonimpact ones, such as swimming and bicycling.

Ankle motion (approximately 25-30 degrees), including dorsiflexion (5-10 degrees), is preferred for successful ankle distraction arthroplasty. Ankle joint stability is assessed clinically and is confirmed with ankle stress radiographs in addition to the radiographic evaluation of any coexisting tibial, ankle, and/or foot deformity. Asymmetric loss of anterior ankle articular cartilage has been associated with less successful results in our experience.

Although clinical studies have demonstrated similar success rates for ankle distraction in all age groups,[70] older patients, in our practice, tend to have less overall capacity to tolerate the rigors of distraction arthroplasty. These include persistent pain, functional limitations, and the long recovery time (typically 1-2 years) to reach maximum improvement.

The above indications are not absolute, however, and clinical judgment must be exercised. This requires careful preoperative evaluation and counseling. For example, a 35-year-old physical laborer with severe ankle pain and ankylosis resulting from posttraumatic arthritis without deformity may best be managed with an ankle arthrodesis. Whereas a 55-year-old patient with posttraumatic arthritis and a significant distal tibial deformity with arthritic symptoms related to the deformity may best be managed with deformity correction and distraction.

FRAME APPLICATION FOR ANKLE DISTRACTION: SURGICAL TECHNIQUE

Note: A thorough understanding of cross-sectional anatomy is essential for wire and pin placement during frame applications.

Tibial Base Frame

1. A two-ring tibial base frame is applied orthogonal to the tibia. The two rings are separated by 150-mm threaded rods (the proximal ring may be a ⅔ ring).
2. For the distal ring, a transverse, smooth 1.8-mm wire is driven through the tibia from medial to lateral, 5 cm proximal to the ankle joint (this level is used for the ankle distraction procedure but is modified for other applications).
3. The distal tibial ring is connected to this wire, with the limb centered within the ring to ensure approximately 2 to 3 cm soft tissue clearance between the limb and the rings. The wire is tensioned to 110 to 130 kg.
4. The proximal ring is fixed to the tibia with two 6.0-mm half-pins placed off connecting cubes or posts, one proximal and one distal to the ring in a multiplanar fashion; the most proximal half-pin is usually placed medial (slightly anteromedial) to lateral using a

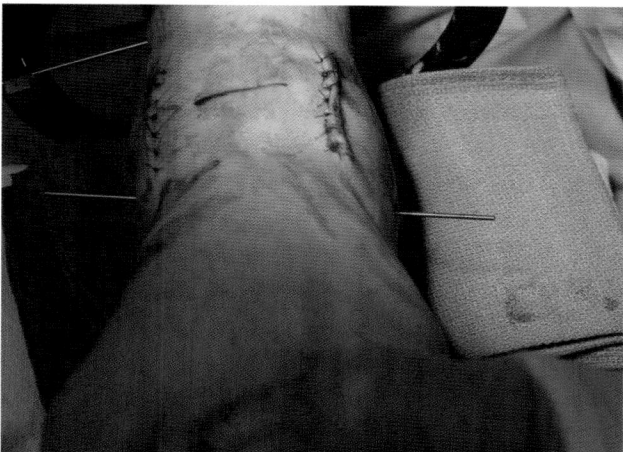

Figure 23-21 A temporary guidewire is inserted from the tip of the lateral malleolus to the tip of the medial malleolus. This wire serves as a reference for ankle hinge placement.

two-hole Rancho cube. The inferior half-pin is secured to a two-hole Rancho cube placed from anteromedial to posterolateral.

5. One or two additional 6.0-mm half-pins are then placed and secured to the distal tibial ring, also in a multiplanar orientation, one proximal and the other distal to the distal tibial ring. One is typically placed anterior to posterior. Fluoroscopic imaging is helpful to ensure appropriate half-pin length.

Ankle Hinge

1. After the tibial base frame is applied, a smooth 1.8-mm wire is placed temporarily from the tip of the lateral malleolus to the tip of the medial malleolus, using image intensification. The ends are cut approximately 2 to 3 cm from the skin edges (Fig. 23-21). This guidewire serves as a reference for hinge placement.
2. A universal Ilizarov hinge is our preferred hinge for ankle distraction. It is secured to threaded rods attached to the distal tibial ring. The hinges are aligned relative to the guidewire. The threaded rods are left 1.5 to 2.5 cm long to allow for subsequent distraction.
3. After the hinge is properly positioned, the guidewire is removed.

Foot Ring

1. It is optimal to have the foot positioned symmetrically in the foot ring, with approximately 1 to 2 cm of posterior soft tissue clearance and the ring parallel to the sole of the foot.
2. In most cases, the lateral hinge is placed directly on the ring, and a short threaded rod is used on the medial side. Typically, the hinges are connected to the foot ring, followed by wire placement. The foot ring is enclosed distally, and a movable strut may be placed from the proximal tibial ring to the ring enclosure to hold the foot in a neutral position.

3. The foot ring is secured to the foot with five smooth 1.8-mm wires: one in the talar neck, two in the calcaneal tuberosity, and two in the forefoot. The first calcaneal wire is placed from medial to posterolateral, avoiding the neurovascular structures on the medial aspect of the hindfoot, and the foot ring is secured to this wire. Then the first forefoot wire is placed proximal to the fifth metatarsal head, engaging either the fifth, fourth, and third metatarsals or the fifth and first metatarsals (plantar to the second, third, and fourth metatarsals). Care is taken to avoid distorting the normal orientation of the metatarsals relative to each other. The first two wires are connected, maintaining the foot ring parallel to the sole of the foot. The second calcaneal wire is placed from lateral to posteromedial. The second forefoot wire is placed medially to engage the first and second, and occasionally third metatarsals. The talar neck wire is then placed to avoid subtalar joint distraction, and this wire is usually not placed under tension. Tension is applied to the calcaneal wires (90 kg) and the forefoot wires (50-70 kg).

Ankle Distraction

1. After the frame is applied, the ankle joint may be acutely distracted 1 to 2 mm from the preoperative position, using the threaded rods attached to the universal hinges. This distraction usually is performed on the tibial ring attachment sites. Acute distraction is avoided if any varus or equinus deformity correction was performed to limit the risk of neurovascular compromise.
2. Multiplanar fluoroscopic ankle evaluation is performed to assess ankle range of motion and confirm absence of ankle subluxation with motion. The holding strut is removed for motion and then reapplied to hold the foot in a neutral position.
3. Two additional threaded rods are placed between the foot ring and distal tibial ring (often conical washers are needed and are used with the hinge rods for gradual distraction, which is initiated on postoperative day 1 or 2. Distraction is performed at 0.5 mm/day for 8 to 10 days to achieve approximately 5 mm increase in joint space. The holding strut may need to be lengthened as well.
4. Wounds are dressed in routine fashion, and all wires and half-pins are dressed with Ilizarov sponges, stacked from the skin to the fixation attachment to provide gentle soft tissue compression. Bulky gauze dressings are placed between the rings and the limb, especially about the ankle and posterior leg and heel, to limit swelling. The rings are overwrapped with elastic (Ace) bandages. Weight bearing as tolerated is allowed, with crutches typically used in the first 2 to 4 weeks, then intermittently. Refer to frame management in the Supramalleolar Deformity Correction section for pin care. A rocker-type walking platform is attached to the foot ring before allowing weight bearing.

5. Frame removal is performed after 12 to 14 weeks. The patient generally uses a removable cast boot for 1 to 3 months, depending on comfort level. Weight bearing as tolerated is allowed, and physical therapy is helpful to improve motion, gait, and proprioception. A modified stationary bicycle as detailed above for supramalleolar osteotomy frames is also an option.

ANKLE DISTRACTION/DEFORMITY CORRECTION: RESULTS AND COMPLICATIONS

Judet and Judet[30] published the first study in Western medical literature of ankle distraction for posttraumatic ankle arthritis with a hinged distraction apparatus. Thirteen of 16 (81%) patients had good results at 16-month follow-up.[30,47] A subsequent study of patients with hip arthrosis showed that articulated distraction of the hip yielded good results in 42 of 59 (71%) patients who were younger than 45 years but poor results in patients older than 45 years and in patients with inflammatory arthritis.[1,47]

In a prospective study of 57 patients, followed for an average of 2.8 years after ankle distraction, significant clinical improvement was noted in three fourths of the patients, improvement increased over time, and joint distraction had significantly better results than ankle joint debridement alone.[30,40,47,50,70] A subsequent review by the same researchers, at a minimum of 7 years of follow-up evaluation after ankle distraction for osteoarthritis, showed that 16 of 22 (73%) patients had significant improvement of all clinical parameters, and 6 (27%) patients had failed treatment.[50] Tellisi et al[70] reported on 23 patients at an average follow-up of 30.5 months, with 17 (74%) having significant improvement in the American Orthopaedic Foot and Ankle Society (AOFAS) score (average preoperative score was 55 and postoperative score 74). In 2012, Saltzman demonstrated, in a prospective randomized controlled trial, a significant improvement in distraction results, with motion compared with fixed distraction.[57]

Our early results with ankle distraction were presented in conjunction with osteotomy for deformity correction (Figs. 23-22 and 23-23). In 11 patients with ankle arthritis associated with deformity of the distal tibial (five deformities, most commonly valgus or recurvatum and valgus) or foot (seven deformities, most commonly cavovarus), treatment consisted of ankle joint distraction with the Ilizarov device and deformity correction.[2] Tibial deformity correction was gradual in three patients and acute in two patients, and all seven foot deformity corrections were acutely performed. Ninety percent were very satisfied or satisfied[56]; dorsiflexion range directly correlated with American Academy of Orthopaedic Surgery (AAOS) score. It was concluded that deformity correction can augment the efficacy of distraction and that dorsiflexion may be an important factor in the success of an ankle distraction procedure.[53] Our further experience with distraction has

shown that anterior asymmetric joint wear is a poor prognostic indicator.

Distal tibial deformity correction alone can also provide satisfactory results in the arthritic ankle. Several small retrospective series have shown the majority of patients with ankle arthritis who undergo distal tibial osteotomy for either varus of valgus deformity have significant improvement in their ankle pain without progression of arthritis.* In 2007, Pagenstert et al[45] reported on realignment surgery in 35 patients (average age, 43 years) with varus and valgus ankle osteoarthritis, with an average follow-up of 5 years. The AOFAS score increased from 38.5 preoperatively to 85.2 postoperatively. Slight overcorrection of deformity was believed to be optimal, and others have recommended this as well.[6,36,45,69] Whether overcorrection is necessary and to what degree is unclear.

Complications

The most common complications of ankle distraction arthroplasty include pin-site inflammation or infection, hardware failure, and failure of the procedure to relieve pain. Direct neurovascular injury resulting from pin placement can occur despite operative caution because of posttraumatic distortion of the anatomy and scarring. Other general risks include anesthetic problems, surgical wound problems and infection, and thromboembolic disease.

In patients undergoing ankle distraction with range of motion, the threaded rods attached to the universal hinges, or the hinge itself, can fail because of the major stresses placed on these portions of the fixator. If a half-pin or wire loosens, treatment includes retensioning the wires and occasionally replacing a half-pin in a new site.

Immediate correction of a deformity (especially varus and equinus) in the distal tibia or foot, especially with concomitant ankle distraction, may be complicated by traction injury of the posterior tibial nerve and tarsal tunnel syndrome. If this occurs, the deformity may be restored and traction released to remove nerve tension, and correction and traction may be reapplied gradually. Prophylactic tarsal tunnel release can limit this complication, and careful postoperative monitoring can enable early recognition and release of traction. Gradual deformity correction and ankle distraction can limit risk of traction injury to the posterior tibial nerve. Furthermore, a postoperative anesthetic nerve block is used with caution because it can mask neuropathic symptoms, and nerve recovery may be optimized by early recognition, release of traction, and tarsal tunnel release.

Tarsal tunnel release may be required in the immediate postoperative period if other measures do not restore nerve function.

Swelling and stiffness can occur after ankle distraction as a result of the underlying arthritic disorder. A period of increased pain and disability after ankle distraction can

---

*References 6, 17, 36, 45, 49, 66, and 69.

occur for 3 to 6 months after the frame is removed, occasionally persisting for up to 12 or more months. Nonimpact activities are emphasized during this time, including swimming and bicycling. Gradual improvement up to 12 to 24 months after fixator removal has been observed, and further procedures are usually deferred until this time. Patients may also experience foot pain after ring fixation of the foot. This most commonly is associated with osteopenia and resolves within 6 months; however,

wire positioning issues may lead to prolonged discomfort or arthritic changes.

Other complications that are associated with gradual correction include delayed or premature bony consolidation, malunion, fracture after or associated with frame removal, and ankle and foot stiffness, including equinus contracture. In our experience, delayed healing of the distal tibia is the most frequent significant problem encountered during gradual correction of distal tibial

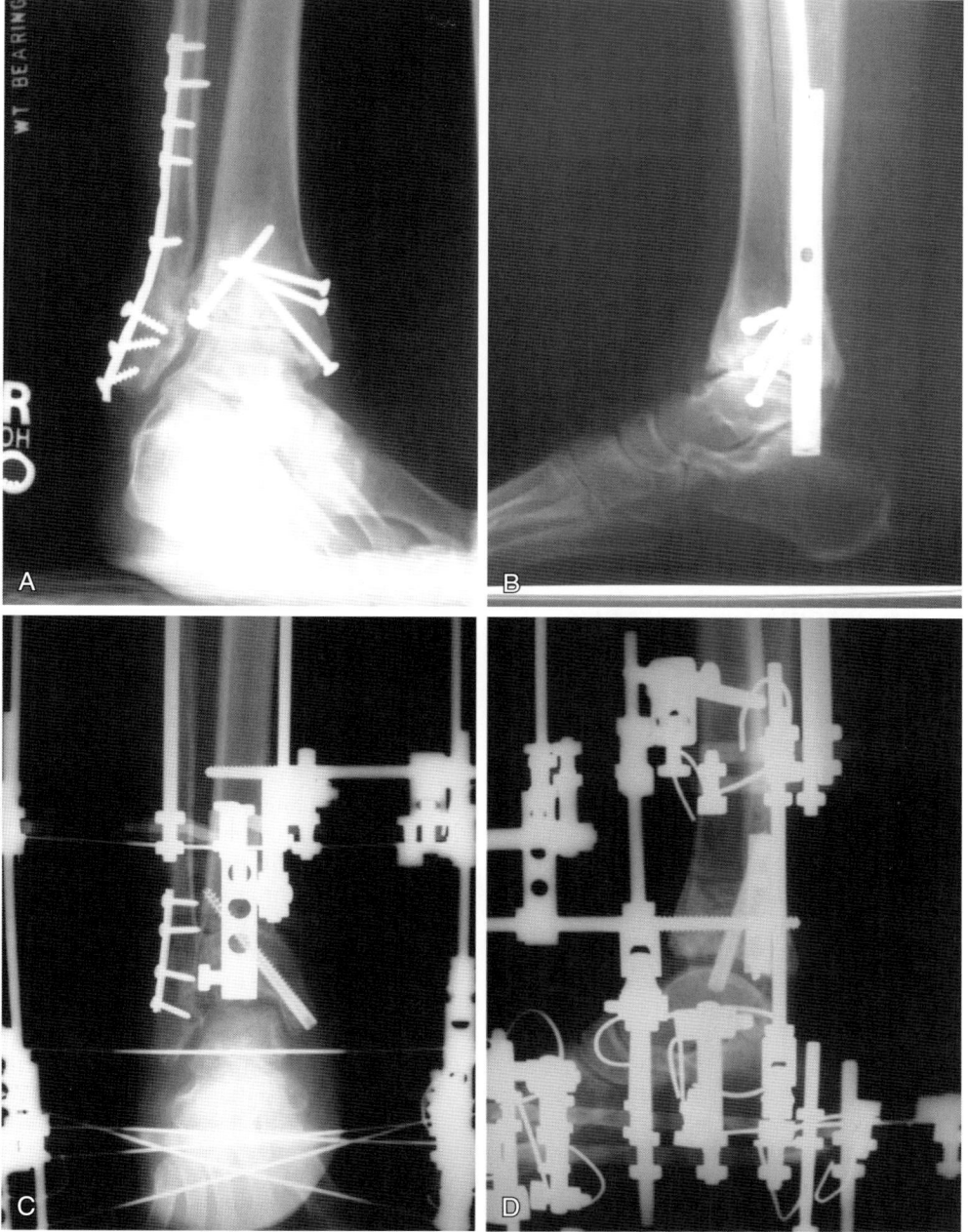

Figure 23-22 **A** and **B,** A 40-year-old woman with ankle pain was evaluated 2 years after open reduction and internal fixation of a work-related ankle fracture. Radiographs demonstrated posttraumatic arthritis and valgus deformity of the tibia and fibula. **C** and **D,** The deformity was acutely corrected with a focal dome osteotomy and internal fixation, and acute ankle distraction was applied.

Continued

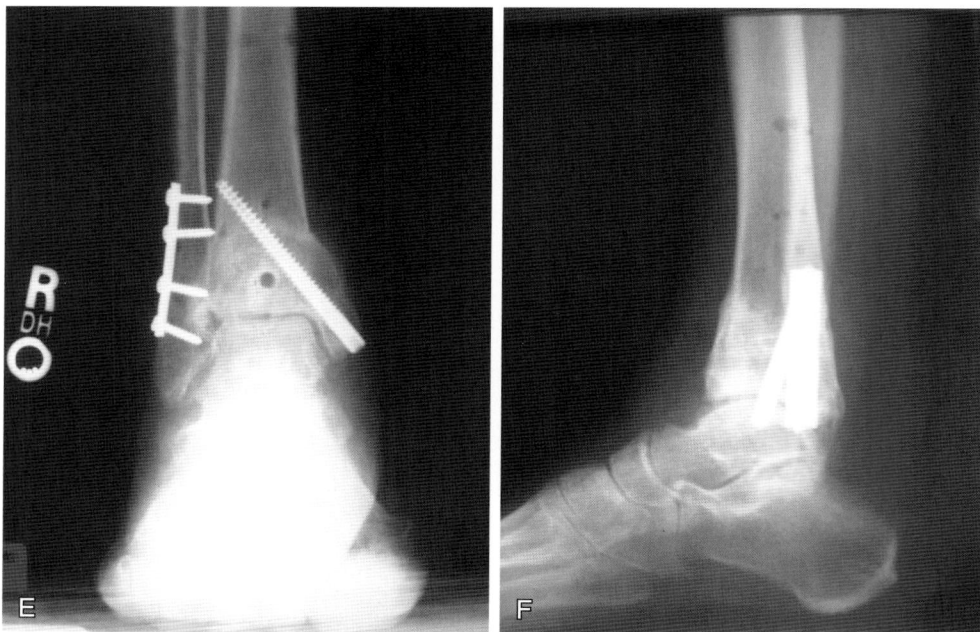

Figure 23-22, cont'd E and F, Two years after the frame was removed, radiographs show maintenance of ankle joint space. The patient had improvement of preoperative pain.

deformity. Consideration should be given for bone grafting; our preference is autologous anterior iliac crest if healing is slow or fails to progress. Also, revision of tibial fixation may be necessary if it becomes loose or inadequate.

INTRAARTICULAR DEFORMITY STRATEGIES

Intraarticular deformity may occur in conjunction with ankle arthritis. This can be associated with ligament deficiency and/or intraarticular bony deformity. Chronic deltoid or lateral ligamentous insufficiency can be isolated or associated with underlying hindfoot or distal tibial deformity. The resulting talar tilt then leads to asymmetric cartilage wear and eventually intraarticular bony deformity. Bony deformity may also be the result of an intraarticular distal tibial fracture, fibular malunion, collapse of an avascular bone region, or sequelae of a congenital condition.

The four common patterns (refer to supramalleolar deformity classification) of distal tibial and fibular deformity can exist with associated talar tilt and additional intraarticular bony wear.

The treatment strategy for joint preservation is dependent on the underlying cause. Ring fixation with ankle distraction is used to maintain mortise alignment during healing of bone and soft tissue reconstructions and to treat the arthritic joint. As the degree of talar tilt increases (especially when >10 degrees), clinical success tends to diminish.[36]

Ligamentous insufficiency is usually managed with allograft tendon ligament reconstruction, and optimization of hindfoot alignment with calcaneal osteotomy.

Considerations for managing bony deformity with joint preservation include intraarticular osteotomy, periarticular osteotomy, and optimizing fibular length. An intraarticular ankle osteotomy is best used when there is a clearly delineated fracture line or collapsed bone region. Because of the ankle anatomy, it is often difficult to regain precise intraarticular alignment after an osteotomy. Some patients develop a shallow V-shaped plafond because of asymmetric bony wear. Consideration for an intraarticular or supramalleolar osteotomy can be given in these cases, depending on the individual anatomy of the case.

A supramalleolar osteotomy is useful in conditions such as ball and socket ankle, flat-top talar deformity, and when plafond angulation is causing or exacerbating talar tilt. In these situations, a slight overcorrection (up to 5 degrees) of the distal tibial angle is acceptable.

A fibular osteotomy is useful for isolated fibular deformity. For example, posttraumatic fibular shortening can lead to valgus talar tilt and is managed with a lengthening fibular osteotomy. This can be accomplished acutely with internal fixation techniques or gradually with external fixation techniques. This deformity can progress to include lateral distal tibial wear. Joint-sparing reconstruction includes a lengthening fibular osteotomy, intraarticular distal tibial osteotomy, and joint distraction.

ANKLE AND SUBTALAR CONTRACTURE

Ring fixation techniques provide useful and powerful methods in treating soft tissue and joint contractures. Around the ankle and hindfoot, equinus and equinovarus deformities are frequently amenable to gradual correction. The primary reasons to use gradual techniques

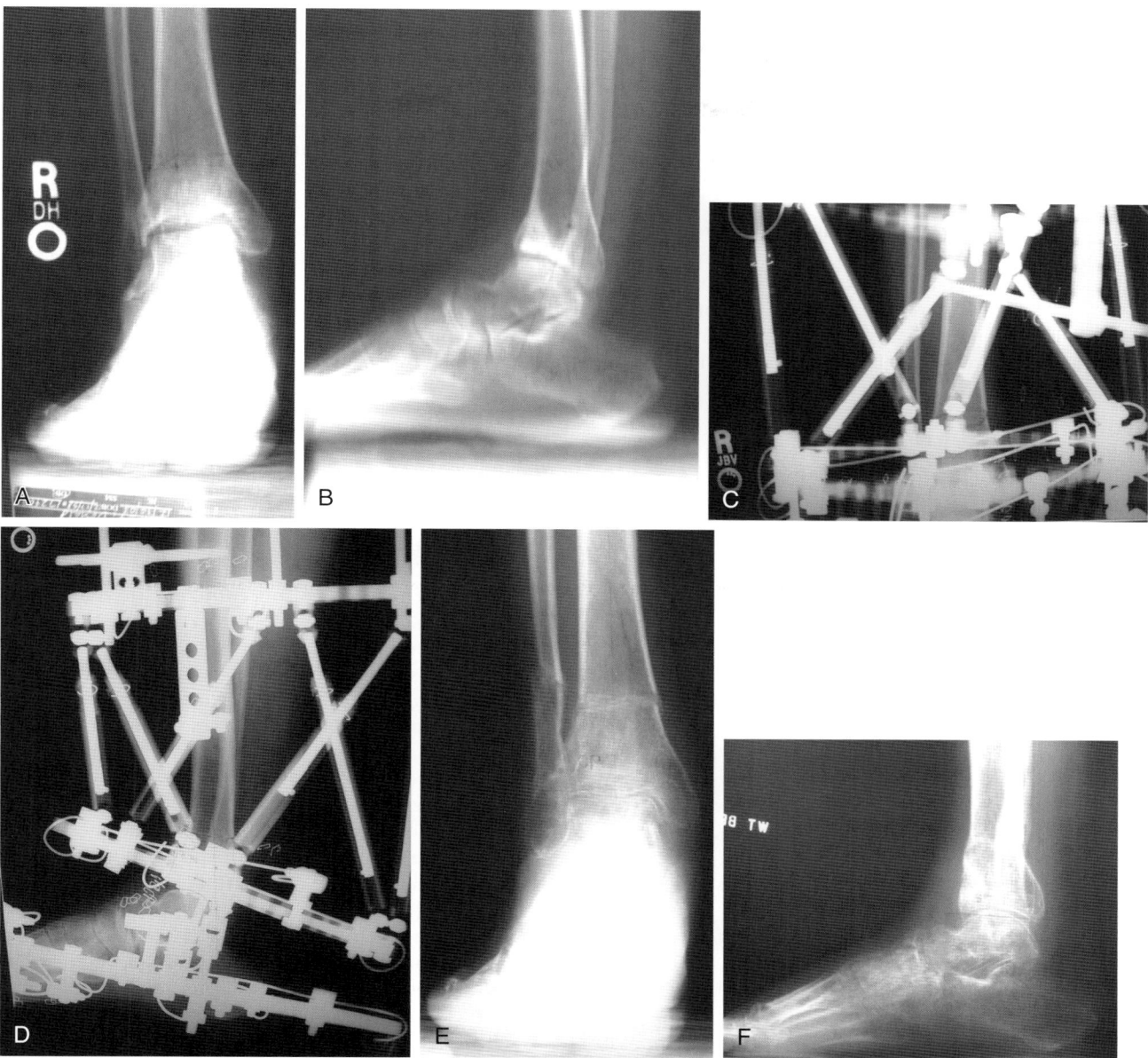

Figure 23-23 **A** and **B,** A 45-year-old man, who was a former triathlete, had had a distal tibial fracture 3 years earlier that healed with recurvatum and associated equinus compensation. **C** and **D,** The deformity was gradually corrected with a supramalleolar Gigli saw osteotomy. The fibular osteotomy was staged because the fibular deformity was unequal to the tibial deformity. Distraction was done acutely without range of motion until 6 weeks after surgery, to allow initial healing of the osteotomy. The equinus deformity was treated with physical therapy. **E** and **F,** Radiographs at 6 months after surgery showed the healed osteotomy, improved alignment, and maintenance of an ankle joint space. The patient had improvement of preoperative pain.

include less risk of compromise to the neurovascular structures and soft tissues, severe or rigid deformity that is not appropriate for acute correction, and recurrent deformity after treatment with other techniques. We also prefer ring fixation methods in patients who are at risk for cast complications (i.e., diminished sensation).

The causes of contractures include intraarticular pathology, extraarticular pathology, or a combination of both. Diagnoses include posttraumatic soft tissue contracture, joint ankylosis or arthritis; neuromuscular deformity (including cerebrovascular incident sequelae); burn contracture; congenital conditions; and contracture associated with limb lengthening.

The physical examination can be helpful in differentiating between intraarticular and extraarticular causes. This is particularly the case with extraarticular contracture of the gastrocnemius and/or soleus muscles, for which the Silfverskiold test can be used (foot dorsiflexion compared with knee extension and flexion).[62] Imaging studies can provide further information on intraarticular pathology, such as arthritis. In severe cases (>40 degrees of deformity), there tends to be contracture of most of the posterior musculotendinous structures and posterior joint capsules. These cases are typically managed with gradual techniques and selective soft tissue releases. Milder degrees of deformity may be treated with soft tissue releases alone (including tarsal tunnel release with deformity >10-20 degrees). Moderate deformity (20-40 degrees) can be treated with gradual correction alone or with partial acute correction and ring fixation methods used to correct residual deformity. Even with gradual techniques, tarsal tunnel release may be required during the correction if neurologic symptoms occur.

Equinus Gradual Correction with Ring Fixation

1. Soft tissue releases: Selective releases are performed on a case-dependent basis. As a general rule, most patients will undergo a percutaneous triple-cut Achilles tendon lengthening through three small incisions. Flexor tenotomies of the toes are included if toe contractures are present. The toes are pinned with 1.2- to 1.6-mm K-wires after frame application. The wires are then connected to the foot ring enclosure device.

2. Frame application: The foot ring is applied first in these cases to optimize the tibial ring position. The foot ring is applied in the same manner as described in ankle distraction. 1.8-mm wires are generally used except in smaller feet, where 1.5-mm wires may be used (particularly in the forefoot region). The medial to lateral calcaneal wire is an olive wire if there is a varus component to the deformity. Crossed calcaneal olive wires are used in the face of significant osteopenia. A two-ring tibial base frame (connected with 100- to 150-mm threaded rods, depending on patient size) is preferred, with the distal ring placed to allow enough room to place a posterior pushing strut or to place Taylor Spatial Frame struts. This is typically approximately 7 cm proximal to the ankle joint but may be more in more severe cases. The tibial frame is applied in a similar manner as in ankle distraction. In patients who have been nonambulatory and have significant osteopenia, we prefer to use 1.8-mm Ilizarov wires and fewer half-pins (used in more dense bone regions).

3. Hinge or strut placement: When using Taylor spatial methods, six struts are placed. The majority of equinus deformities can be corrected using a constrained hinge technique, with medial and lateral ankle hinges placed according to the ankle distraction method. With hinges, a posterior pushing strut may be used alone or in combination with an anterior pulling strut, depending on the severity and rigidity of the deformity. A slight posterior inclination (from proximal to distal) of the pushing strut helps prevent anterior talar subluxation. An unconstrained technique may be used without hinge placement for mild-to-moderate deformities, which have some flexibility. There is a greater risk for anterior talar subluxation when using unconstrained methods. The constrained hinge technique allows ankle range-of-motion exercises during and after correction is obtained. Typically, the posterior strut is replaced at the end of correction by an anterior Taylor Spatial Fast-Fix Strut (Smith & Nephew), which can be easily released for motion exercises and then relocked to maintain a dorsiflexion position.

4. Correction of deformity: Correction of the equinus deformity is accompanied by ankle joint distraction (3-5 mm) to avoid articular cartilage impaction. Gradual correction is initiated on postoperative day 2. For spatial frame applications, a distal reference is preferred, with the origin approximated by the lateral process of the talus (center of rotation of the ankle). The rate of correction is determined by the posterior skin, which can be chosen as the structure at risk, and lengthened at 1 mm/day. For the hinged technique, the posterior strut is lengthened at the rate of 1 mm/day, which also lengthens the Achilles tendon at 1 mm/day in 2 to 4 divided doses. This can be calculated using the rule of concentric circles[11]), and typically results in posterior distraction of 2 to 4 mm/day, depending on the location of the distraction rod. Correction rates can be modified based on patient tolerance and rigidity of the deformity. An overcorrection of approximately 10 to 15 degrees is preferred.

5. Frame removal: The frame is generally retained for a minimum of 6 to 8 weeks after complete correction (or if longer, the same time it took to achieve correction). At the time of removal, the patient is molded for a custom ankle–foot orthosis (AFO), and then placed in a short-leg walking cast for 4 weeks. Depending on the clinical situation, the AFO is worn full time for 6 to 12 months (longer time period with severe scarring). Nighttime bracing with an AFO or night splint is also done. Physical therapy is used for maintaining dorsiflexion motion and strength. Compliance with bracing and therapy is important to avoid recurrence. In patients without dorsiflexion motor function, tendon transfer procedures are needed to help maintain correction.

Equinovarus deformity is managed in a similar manner, with two alterations. First, the varus component is corrected before the equinus. This is accomplished by attaching the talar wire to the distal tibial ring by using plates and posts or by creating a stirrup wire construct. The varus is then corrected by using Taylor Spatial Frame technology or hinges placed along the subtalar joint axis. It is helpful to have approximately 3 mm of subtalar joint distraction to avoid cartilage impaction during correction. Because of the gliding motion of the subtalar joint, it is difficult to accurately define subtalar deformity in spatial frame terminology. Once varus is corrected, the talar wire is connected to the foot ring with posts, and the equinus is corrected as outlined above.

FOOT DEFORMITY

Deformity in the foot may be corrected through an osteotomy, arthrodesis, soft tissue procedure, or a combination of these techniques. Arthrodesis is generally recommended in the presence of arthritis, neuroarthropathy, chronic dislocations, deformity associated with loss of motor function, severe instability, and in cases of painful joint ankylosis. If these conditions are not present, it is often preferable to salvage foot motion with osteotomies to maintain as normal a gait pattern as possible and minimize the potential for progressive degenerative changes in joints adjacent to an arthrodesis. Arthrodesis and osteotomies can also be combined to correct complex deformities.

Gradual deformity correction with ring external fixation usually is performed through an osteotomy, but also can be done through deformed joints. Gradual correction through an osteotomy with distraction osteogenesis is indicated when acute correction would result in minimal bone contact at an osteotomy site, potentially increasing the risk of nonunion. A scarred, grafted, shortened, or multiply operated foot with compromised soft tissues also is an indication for gradual correction. When there is a chronic joint dislocation, gradual deformity correction through the joint can be done as the first stage of a realignment arthrodesis. Correction of severe foot deformities can be done through percutaneous or limited open osteotomies, with maintenance of foot length. Some deformities, such as residual clubfoot, may be corrected gradually through the deformed joints. This usually is performed in younger patients (younger than 8 years), but successful correction can be achieved in untreated clubfoot, and posttraumatic or neurologic deformity in older adolescents and adults.*

As with distal tibial deformity, it is useful to classify foot deformity in a simple manner that helps guide corrections. Most deformity can be divided into simple or segmental. Simple patterns in the foot refer to deformity that is isolated to the hindfoot or midfoot, or when hindfoot deformity equals that of the midfoot or forefoot. Also, a simple pattern is when compensatory deformity is flexible and completely corrects with treatment of the primary deformity. Examples include isolated hindfoot varus or valgus, forefoot valgus that is associated with flexible hindfoot varus (corrects with the Coleman block test), and a varus subtalar fusion (or coalition) with equal forefoot varus. In this latter example, correction of the hindfoot will lead to correction of the forefoot so that only one site of surgical treatment is required to achieve a plantigrade foot. Using gradual correction techniques, a simple deformity pattern will require one osteotomy or correction level. The frame design will be dependent on the type and location of the osteotomy. For example, a U-type osteotomy can be used to correct a hindfoot malunion, and a frame with a foot ring and tibial base

construct is used. Also, certain simple patterns associated with a flat-top talus or ball and socket ankle joint can be corrected through a supramalleolar osteotomy.

In contrast, a segmental pattern is when hindfoot deformity is unequal to midfoot or forefoot deformity. This can occur when the compensatory deformity becomes rigid. Segmental patterns require two or more sites of correction to achieve a plantigrade foot. Examples include rigid cavovarus deformity, requiring hindfoot correction and first metatarsal dorsiflexion osteotomy; adult-acquired flatfoot, requiring both calcaneal osteotomy and midfoot fusion (to correct forefoot varus); and a congenital foot deformity with hindfoot valgus and equinus, and forefoot varus and abduction.

When gradual correction techniques are used, segmental patterns require more complex frame designs and preoperative planning. There are several ways to approach these complex deformities: gradual correction at both levels; acute correction at one level with gradual correction at the other; staged gradual correction, with correction of the most deformed level, followed by either gradual or acute correction of the less deformed region. Whenever possible, it is preferable to perform acute correction with internal fixation at one level, which allows a less complex frame design and easier patient care for correction of the more severe deformity. This effectively turns a segmental pattern into a simple pattern with respect to frame management.

Osteotomy Types/Locations

The primary osteotomies used in the foot include the V, U, and midfoot osteotomy.[32,47] The V osteotomy is a double-limb osteotomy with an oblique calcaneal osteotomy posterior to the subtalar joint and an oblique osteotomy through the talar neck, sinus tarsi, and anterior portion of the calcaneus.[10] The two limbs of the osteotomy converge on the plantar cortex of the calcaneal body. Subtalar mobility is generally absent when this osteotomy is performed, and it is used for all types of segmental deformity patterns. The concept of the V osteotomy can be modified by moving the distal limb into the midfoot or correcting deformity through subluxed/dislocated transverse tarsal or midfoot joints (which are then typically fused in a staged manner). The posterior limb of the V osteotomy can be used alone to correct isolated hindfoot deformity. The anterior limb of the V can also be used in isolation to correct midfoot/forefoot deformity in the face of subtalar stiffness. In a similar fashion, isolated midfoot deformity can be corrected through deformed midfoot joints or with a midfoot osteotomy, which can be done through the cuboid/navicular or cuboid/cuneiforms.

The U osteotomy extends from the dorsal aspect of the talar neck, and progresses in a U shape under the subtalar joint to exit the dorsal aspect of the calcaneal tuberosity. This osteotomy can be used to correct all types of single-plane deformity (simple patterns). The hindfoot and

---

*References 4, 5, 9, 13, 14, 19, 23, 39, 43, 44, 54, and 73.

forefoot deformity must be equal when this osteotomy is used, and we prefer to use this technique with absent hindfoot motion or in the face of prior triple arthrodesis malunion. The supramalleolar osteotomy can accomplish similar corrections as the U osteotomy, with a less technically demanding osteotomy. The ankle joint will be angulated if a supramalleolar osteotomy is used to correct foot deformity, but this is acceptable in conditions such as flat-top talus and ball and socket ankle joint, with milder degrees of deformity (less than approximately 10 degrees).

Results and Complications

The results of gradual deformity correction with ring fixation in the foot are generally good for a wide range of pathology.* In most patients, a plantigrade foot posture can be achieved and maintained. Foot stiffness is common, but it is generally present preoperatively, and a stiff deformed foot is replaced with a stiff but more functional plantigrade foot. Soft tissue corrections are typically performed for equinus and equinovarus deformity in all age groups, whereas recurrent clubfoot and other similar foot deformities are typically corrected through soft tissues in younger age groups (younger than approximately 8 years old). The primary complication with all soft tissue corrections is recurrence.[5,12] This may be most common in those patients with significant precorrection scarring, such as burns, prior open surgical procedures, and other posttraumatic soft tissue compromise. Strategies to minimize recurrence include overcorrection (such as 10-15 degrees dorsiflexion in an equinus correction), soft tissue lengthening the rate of 1 mm/day, and maintaining the frame for a minimum of 6 to 8 weeks after correction (or double the time to correct the deformity if more than 8 weeks). Also, tendon transfers or arthrodesis after frame removal are occasionally necessary to maintain correction. Arthrodesis can be performed while a frame is still on, whereas tendon transfers are generally performed after or at the time of frame removal, depending on pin-site conditions.

Other complications associated with both bony and soft tissue corrections around the foot and ankle include pin-site infections, wire or frame component breakage, toe deformity, joint subluxation, arthritis or ankylosis, premature or delayed bony consolidation, overlengthening, acute and/or chronic neurovascular injury, pain, and psychologic issues.† Because of these myriad potential problems, preoperative counseling is important to make the patient aware of the need for further surgical interventions and to set realistic goals and expectations. Written information is helpful for frame management and pin care. Particularly in the foot, wires may need to be exchanged, removed, or retensioned. Occasionally, admission for intravenous antibiotic therapy and elevation is needed if outpatient oral antibiotics do not resolve a pin-site infection or if there is severe erythema and swelling. Claw toe deformity is a common reported complication and may be minimized with toe pinning during deformity correction. Frequent radiographs are taken to assess joint alignment, and subluxations should be addressed as early as possible. This may entail frame modification in the operating room.

Premature bony consolidation of an osteotomy is more common in the foot than in the tibia, and therefore the latency period after an osteotomy in the foot is shorter than that done in the tibia (3-5 days in the calcaneus and midfoot, depending on patient age, bone quality, and osteotomy technique, with a shorter period for young patients with good bone quality and percutaneous atraumatic osteotomy). Premature consolidation can be treated by increasing the distraction rate for several days if noted before significant bone formation or repeat osteotomy. It is important to confirm a foot osteotomy is complete because an incomplete osteotomy may mimic premature consolidation. Delayed consolidation can be treated with a decrease in distraction rate and bone grafting, if necessary.

Bony corrections will generally result in foot lengthening. If the foot pathology has created a short foot, lengthening is usually a desired outcome. In the face of a normal foot length, it is important to avoid overlengthening because this may create pain, claw toes and footwear difficulty. Careful radiographs or CT scan monitoring of an osteotomy may be required. Enough length must be gained to avoid bone impingement during correction, and an osteotomy may be compressed after correction to achieve optimal length. Another strategy is to resect a portion of bone at the time of osteotomy, compress, and then distract.[33]

Postcorrection arthritis and ankylosis can occur. The symptoms may be managed with bracing and the use of rocker-sole shoe. Arthrodesis is occasionally performed to manage painful joints.

Neurovascular injury is a complication associated with all ring external fixator applications. Strategies in the foot to minimize complications include the use of Doppler monitoring when performing midfoot osteotomies (especially with the Gigli saw technique), preoperative vascular studies for patients with prior vascular compromise or peripheral vascular disease, and careful postoperative monitoring. The tarsal tunnel is prone to compression even with gradual varus-to-valgus corrections, and consideration for prophylactic tarsal tunnel release should be made for varus hindfoot corrections. As discussed, tarsal tunnel release may be required during correction if clinical symptoms arise that cannot be managed with slowing of correction rate.

STATIC MODE RING FIXATION

The static mode of circular external fixation is a valuable tool in complex foot and ankle surgery. A holding frame

---

*References 4, 11, 13, 14, 19, 23, 32, 39, 44, 54, and 73.
†References 5, 11, 13, 19, 23, 32, 43, 44, 54, and 73.

can be used after an acute deformity correction and is particularly useful in cases of infection, nonunion, or infected nonunion. The advantage of using a static frame over other modes of immobilization is greater stability compared with a cast, brace, or fracture walker. The frame is rigid and strong enough to allow weight bearing. It also provides access to wounds for routine care. Ulcer complications of casting in neuropathic patients are prevented.

A holding frame can be placed to avoid existing internal fixation and, because of its stability, can allow the surgeon to limit the amount of internal fixation. In cases of compromised soft tissue, poor vascularity, or a high risk of infection, surgical approaches are performed with less dissection because internal fixation is minimized.

General principles when applying holding frames include keeping wires and half-pins away from contact with internal fixation, wounds, and infected tissue. The typical static or holding frame construct is similar to the ankle distraction or equinus frame but with multiple (4-6) threaded rods placed between the distal tibial ring and foot ring. Short plates placed off the anterior portion of the lower tibial ring (anteromedial and anterolateral) are often necessary to connect threaded rods to the foot plate for optimal stability.

An example of a patient where a static circular external fixator is indicated in our practice is a diabetic patient with neuropathy and deconditioning, who has an infected nonunion of a previous attempted ankle fusion. The frame provides stability and compression at the nonunion site for bony healing.

A holding frame may be used to stabilize complex foot and ankle reconstructions in both neuropathic and non-neuropathic patients. The frame mode may be modified during treatment in cases such as realignment of a deformed joint (gradual correction mode), followed by a staged arthrodesis (static mode, with or without internal fixation).

In our experience, the neuropathic patient will tend to have more issues with pin-site infection, loosening, and breakage. Also, we favor postframe removal bracing (AFO) for a minimum of 3 to 6 months to decrease the risks of fracture or collapse in the surrounding osteopenic bone.

REFERENCES

1. Aldegheri R, Trivella G, Saleh M: Articulated distraction of the hip. Conservative surgery for arthritis in young patients, *Clin Orthop Relat Res* 301:94–101, 1994.
2. Beaman D, Domenigoni A: *Distraction and deformity correction for ankle arthritis.* Presented at the 14th Annual Meeting of the Limb Lengthening and Reconstruction Society, Toronto, Ontario, Canada, 2004.
3. Bouchard R, Meeder PJ, Krug F, et al: [Evaluation of tibial torsion—comparison of clinical methods and computed tomography], *Rofo* 176:1278–1284, 2004.
4. Bradish CF, Noor S: The Ilizarov method in the management of relapsed club feet, *J Bone Joint Surg Br* 82:387–391, 2000.
5. Carmichae, KD, Maxwell SC, Calhoun JH: Recurrence rates of burn contracture ankle equinus and other foot deformities in children treated with Ilizarov fixation, *J Pediatr Orthop* 25:523–528, 2005.
6. Cheng YM, Chang JK, Hsu CY, et al: Lower tibial osteotomy for osteoarthritis of the ankle, *Gaoxiong Yi Xue Ke Xue Za Zhi* 10:430–437, 1994.
7. Clementz BG: Assessment of tibial torsion and rotational deformity with a new fluoroscopic technique, *Clin Orthop Relat Res* 245:199–209, 1989.
8. Eckhoff DG, Johnson KK: Three-dimensional computed tomography reconstruction of tibial torsion, *Clin Orthop Relat Res* 302:42–46, 1994.
9. El Barbary H, Abdel Ghani H, Hegazy M: Correction of relapsed or neglected clubfoot using a simple Ilizarov frame, *Int Orthop* 28:183–186, 2004.
10. El-Mowafi H: Assessment of percutaneous V osteotomy of the calcaneus with Ilizarov application for correction of complex foot deformities, *Acta Orthop Belg* 70:586–590, 2004.
11. Elomrani NF, Kasis AG, Tis JE, et al: Outcome after foot and ankle deformity correction using circular external fixation, *Foot Ankle Int* 26:1027–1032, 2005.
12. Emara KM, Allam MF, Elsayed MN, et al: Recurrence after correction of acquired ankle equinus deformity in children using Ilizarov technique, *Strategies Trauma Limb Reconstr* 3:105–108, 2008.
13. Ferreira RC, Costa MT, Frizzo GG, et al: Correction of severe recurrent clubfoot using a simplified setting of the Ilizarov device, *Foot Ankle Int* 28:557–568, 2007.
14. Franke J, Grill F, Hein G, Simon M: Correction of clubfoot relapse using Ilizarov's apparatus in children 8-15 years old, *Arch Orthop Trauma Surg* 110:33–37, 1990.
15. Frierson M, Ibrahim K, Boles M, et al: Distraction osteogenesis. A comparison of corticotomy techniques, *Clin Orthop Relat Res* 301:19–24, 1994.
16. Gentili A, Masih S, Yao L, et al: Pictorial review: foot axes and angles, *Br J Radiol* 69:968–974, 1996.
17. Graehl PM, Hersh MR, Heckman JD: Supramalleolar osteotomy for the treatment of symptomatic tibial malunion, *J Orthop Trauma* 1:281–292, 1987.
18. Güven M, Akman B, Ünay K, et al: A new radiographic measurement method for evaluation of tibial torsion: a pilot study in adults, *Clin Orthop Relat Res* 467:1807–1812, 2009.
19. Hahn SB, Park HJ, Park HW, et al: Treatment of severe equinus deformity associated with extensive scarring of the leg, *Clin Orthop Relat Res* 393:250–257, 2001.
20. Halanski MA, Noonan KJ, Hebert M, et al: Manual versus digital radiographic measurements in acetabular dysplasia, *Orthopedics* 29:724–726, 2006.
21. Hankemeier S, Hufner T, Wang G, et al: Computer-assisted analysis of lower limb geometry: higher intraobserver reliability compared to conventional method, *Comput Aided Surg* 11:81–86, 2006.
22. Hazlewood ME, Simmons AN, Johnson WT, et al: The Footprint method to assess transmalleolar axis, *Gait Posture* 25:597–603, 2007.
23. Hosny GA: Correction of foot deformities by the Ilizarov method without corrective osteotomies or soft tissue release, *J Pediatr Orthop B* 11:121–128, 2002.
24. Hutter CG Jr, Scott W: Tibial torsion, *J Bone Joint Surg Am* 31A:511–518, 1949.
25. Hudson D: A comparison of ultrasound to goniometric and inclinometer measurements of torsion in the tibia and femur, *Gait Posture* 28:708–710, 2008.
26. Hudson D, Royer T, Richards J: Ultrasound measurements of torsions in the tibia and femur, *J Bone Joint Surg Am* 88:138–143, 2006.
27. Intema F, Thomas TP, Anderson DD, et al: Subchondral bone remodeling is related to clinical improvement after joint distrac-

tion in the treatment of ankle osteoarthritis, *Osteoarthritis Cartilage* 19:668–675, 2011.

28. Jakob RP, Haertel M, Stussi E: Tibial torsion calculated by computerised tomography and compared to other methods of measurement, *J Bone Joint Surg Br* 62B:238–242, 1980.

29. Jend HH, Heller M, Dallek M, Schoettle H: Measurement of tibial torsion by computer tomography, *Acta Radiol Diagn (Stockh)* 22:271–276, 1981.

30. Judet R, Judet T: The use of a hinge distraction apparatus after arthrolysis and arthroplasty, *Rev Chir Orthop Reparatrice Appar Mot* 64:353–365, 1978.

31. King HA, Staheli LT: Torsional problems in cerebral palsy, *Foot Ankle* 4:180–184, 1984.

32. Kocaoglu M, Eralp L, Atalar AC, et al: Correction of complex foot deformities using the Ilizarov external fixator, *J Foot Ankle Surg* 41:30–39, 2002.

33. Koczewski P, Shadi M, Napiontek M: Foot lengthening using the Ilizarov device: the transverse tarsal joint resection versus osteotomy, *J Pediatr Orthop B* 11:68–72, 2002.

34. Le Damnay P: La torsion du tibia normale, pathologique, experimentale, *J Anat Physiol (Paris)* 45:598–615, 1909.

35. Lee SH, Chung CY, Park MS, et al: Tibial torsion in cerebral palsy: validity and reliability of measurement, *Clin Orthop Relat Res* 467:2098–2104, 2009.

36. Lee WC, Moon JS, Lee K, et al: Indications for supramalleolar osteotomy in patients with ankle osteoarthritis and varus deformity, *J Bone Joint Surg Am* 93:1243–1248, 2011.

37. Lohman M, Tallroth K, Kettunen JA, Remes V: Changing from analog to digital images: does it affect the accuracy of alignment measurements of the lower extremity? *Acta Orthop* 82:351–355, 2011.

38. Malekafzali S, Wood MB: Tibial torsion—a simple clinical apparatus for its measurement and its application to a normal adult population, *Clin Orthop Relat Res* 145:154–157, 1979.

39. Malizos KN, Gougoulias NE, Dailiana ZH, et al: Relapsed clubfoot correction with soft-tissue release and selective application of Ilizarov technique, *Strategies Trauma Limb Reconstr* 3:109–117, 2008.

40. Marijnissen AC, Van Roermund PM, Van Melkebeek J, et al: Clinical benefit of joint distraction in the treatment of severe osteoarthritis of the ankle: proof of concept in an open prospective study and in a randomized controlled study, *Arthritis Rheum* 46:2893–2902, 2002.

41. McCann H, Stanitski DF, Barfield WR, Leupold JA: The effect of tibial rotation on varus deformity measurement, *J Pediatr Orthop* 26:380–384, 2006.

42. Milner CE, Soames RW: A comparison of four in vivo methods of measuring tibial torsion, *J Anat* 193:139–144, 1998.

43. Nakase T, Yasui N, Ohzono K, et al: Treatment of relapsed idiopathic clubfoot by complete subtalar release combined with the Ilizarov method, *J Foot Ankle Surg* 45:337–341, 2006.

44. Oganesyan OV, Istomina IS, Kuzmin VI: Treatment of equinocavovarus deformity in adults with the use of a hinged distraction++ apparatus, *J Bone Joint Surg Am* 78:546–556, 1996.

45. Pagenstert GI, Hintermann B, Barg A, et al: Realignment surgery as alternative treatment of varus and valgus ankle osteoarthritis, *Clin Orthop Relat Res* 462:156–168, 2007.

46. Paley D: *Principles of deformity correction*, New York, 2002, Springer-Verlag.

47. Paley D: *Principles of deformity correction*, New York, 2003, Springer-Verlag.

48. Paley D, Herzenberg JE, Tetsworth K, et al: Deformity planning for frontal and sagittal plane corrective osteotomies, *Orthop Clin North Am* 25:425–465, 1994.

49. Pearce MS, Smith MA, Savidge GF: Supramalleolar tibial osteotomy for haemophilic arthropathy of the ankle, *J Bone Joint Surg Br* 76:947–950, 1994.

50. Ploegmakers JJ, van Roermund PM, van Melkebeek J, et al: Prolonged clinical benefit from joint distraction in the treatment of ankle osteoarthritis, *Osteoarthritis Cartilage* 13:582–588, 2005.

51. Rimondi E, Busacca M, Molinari M, et al: [Study of torsion defects of the lower limbs using computerized tomography], *Radiol Med* 89:22–27, 1995.

52. Rosen H, Sandick H: The measurement of tibiofibular torsion, *J Bone Joint Surg Am* 37-A:847–855, 1955.

53. Sabharwal S, Schwechter EM: Five-year followup of ankle joint distraction for post-traumatic chondrolysis in an adolescent: a case report, *Foot Ankle Int* 28:942–948, 2007.

54. Saghieh S, El Bitar Y, Berjawi G, et al: Distraction histogenesis in ankle burn deformities, *J Burn Care Res* 32:160–165, 2011.

55. Sailer J, Scharitzer M, Peloschek P, et al: Quantification of axial alignment of the lower extremity on conventional and digital total leg radiographs, *Eur Radiol* 15:170–173, 2005.

56. Saltzman CL, el-Khoury GY: The hindfoot alignment view, *Foot Ankle Int* 16:572–576, 1995.

57. Saltzman CL, Hillis SL, Stolley MP, et al: Motion versus fixed distraction of the joint in the treatment of ankle osteoarthritis: a prospective randomized controlled trial, *J Bone Joint Surg Am* 94:961–970, 2012.

58. Sayli U, Bolukbasi S, Atik OS, Gundogdu S: Determination of tibial torsion by computed tomography, *J Foot Ankle Surg* 33:144–147, 1994.

59. Schneider B, Laubenberger J, Jemlich S, et al: Measurement of femoral antetorsion and tibial torsion by magnetic resonance imaging, *Br J Radiol* 70:575–579, 1997.

60. Segev E, Hemo Y, Wientroub S, et al: Intra- and interobserver reliability analysis of digital radiographic measurements for pediatric orthopedic parameters using a novel PACS integrated computer software program, *J Child Orthop* 4:331–341, 2010.

61. Shtarker H, Volpin G, Stolero J, et al: Correction of combined angular and rotational deformities by the Ilizarov method, *Clin Orthop Relat Res* 402:184–195, 2002.

62. Silfverskiold N: Reduction of the uncrossed two-joints muscles of the leg to one-joint muscles in spastic conditions, *Acta Chir Scand* 56:315–328, 1923.

63. Song HR, Choonia AT, Hong SJ, et al: Rotational profile of the lower extremity in achondroplasia: computed tomographic examination of 25 patients, *Skeletal Radiol* 35:929–934, 2006.

64. Staheli LT, Corbett M, Wyss C, et al: Lower-extremity rotational problems in children. Normal values to guide management, *J Bone Joint Surg Am* 67:39–47, 1985.

65. Staheli LT, Engel GM: Tibial torsion: a method of assessment and a survey of normal children, *Clin Orthop Relat Res* 86:183–186, 1972.

66. Stamatis ED, Cooper PS, Myerson MS: Supramalleolar osteotomy for the treatment of distal tibial angular deformities and arthritis of the ankle joint, *Foot Ankle Int* 24:754–764, 2003.

67. Stuberg W, Temme J, Kaplan P, et al: Measurement of tibial torsion and thigh-foot angle using goniometry and computed tomography, *Clin Orthop Relat Res* 272:208–212, 1991.

68. Swanson KE, Stocks GW, Warren PD, et al: Does axial limb rotation affect the alignment measurements in deformed limbs? *Clin Orthop Relat Res* 371:246–252, 2000.

69. Tanaka Y, Takakura Y, Hayashi K, et al: Low tibial osteotomy for varus-type osteoarthritis of the ankle, *J Bone Joint Surg Br* 88:909–913, 2006.

70. Tellisi N, Fragomen AT, Kleinman D, et al: Joint preservation of the osteoarthritic ankle using distraction arthroplasty, *Foot Ankle Int* 30:318–325, 2009.

71. Tochigi Y, Suh JS, Amendola A, et al: Ankle alignment on lateral radiographs. Part 1: sensitivity of measures to perturbations of ankle positioning, *Foot Ankle Int* 27:82–87, 2006.

72. Tochigi Y, Suh JS, Amendola A, Saltzman CL: Ankle alignment on lateral radiographs. Part 2: reliability and validity of measures, *Foot Ankle Int* 27:88–92, 2006.

73. Tsuchiya H, Sakurakichi K, Uehara K, et al: Gradual closed correction of equinus contracture using the Ilizarov apparatus, *J Orthop Sci* 8:802–806, 2003.

74. van Valburg AA, van Roermund PM, Lammens J, et al: Can Ilizarov joint distraction delay the need for an arthrodesis of the ankle? A preliminary report, *J Bone Joint Surg Br* 77:720–725, 1995.

75. van Valburg AA, van Roermund PM, Marijnissen ACA, et al: Joint distraction in treatment of osteoarthritis: a two-year follow-up of the ankle, *Osteoarthritis Cartilage* 7:474–479, 1999.

Disorders of Tendons

Michael J. Coughlin, Lew C. Schon

EXTENSOR TENDONS

Extensor Tendon Injuries

The treatment of disruption of extensor tendons varies depending on whether a laceration or rupture has occurred. The first step in the treatment is an accurate diagnosis based on a careful physical examination. With an isolated rupture, typically only one tendon is involved. On the other hand, with a penetrating wound or laceration, several structures may be damaged. It is important to routinely assess the function of individual tendons and to evaluate the neurovascular status of the anterior ankle and dorsal foot. Knowledge of tendon anatomy, particularly the courses and insertions, is useful in determining the nature and extent of the pathologic process.

Anzel et al[3] evaluated 1014 cases of tendon injuries at the Mayo Clinic and noted that 21 injuries were to the extensors to the toes, a 2% incidence. They did not differentiate between injuries to the extensor hallucis longus (EHL) and extensor digitorum longus (EDL).

Extensor Digitorum Longus

Bell and Schon[4] have noted that the EDL proper can only be lacerated between the ankle and the midfoot because individual tendons are found below this level. Above the ankle, the EDL tendons are in a more centralized location, but their slips are separate, making multiple EDL lacerations possible. Obliquity of the lacerations that occur above the ankle are indicative of a common mechanism, that being the falling of a sharp object against the leg or ankle (Fig. 24-1). One may be deceived when looking at these injuries because the superficial laceration may reveal intact tendon below, only to have the deeper tendon laceration occur more distally below intact skin. The EDL is relatively superficial and easily lacerated with trauma (Fig. 24-2). Because the main function of the EDL is extension of the metatarsophalangeal (MTP) joint and the proximal and distal interphalangeal (PIP and DIP) joints of the lesser toes, when it is transected and not repaired, a claw toe deformity can develop. Patients with chronic extensor tendon lacerations report difficulty controlling the toes when attempting to put on socks or slide into shoes. During these activities, the toe tends to catch on the fabric or insole and passively flex underneath the foot. Often, because of the proximity of the anterior tibial tendon to the extensor hallucis longus and the neurovascular bundle, injury to these structures can occur simultaneously.

Anatomy

The EDL originates on the lateral tibial condyle, the anterior crest of the fibula, and the interosseous membrane, and it inserts on the base of the terminal phalanges of the four lesser toes. Innervated by the deep peroneal nerve, the EDL functions to extend the toes at the DIP joint and to dorsiflex and evert the foot.

The EDL divides into two separate tendons beneath the superior retinaculum and then further divides into two lateral tendons to the fourth and fifth toes and two

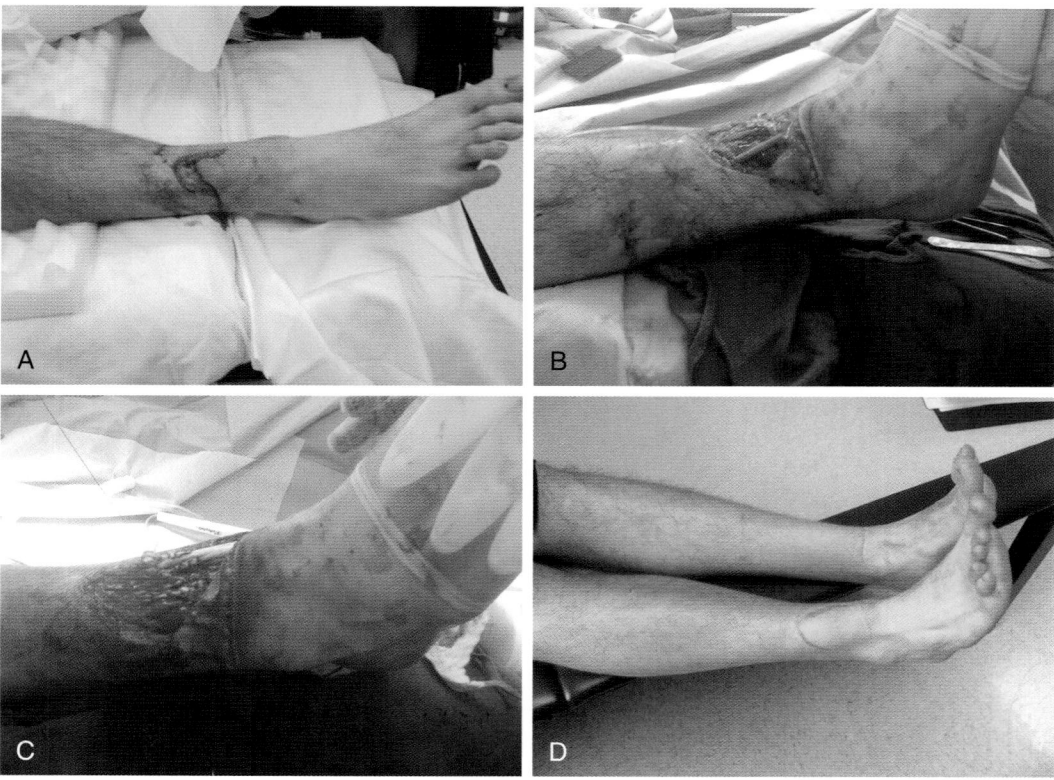

Figure 24-1 Extensor digitorum longus laceration. **A,** Oblique laceration of the lower leg. **B,** Laceration has led to transection of both the extensor digitorum longus and the extensor hallucis longus, leaving an inability to extend any of the toes. Weakness of ankle dorsiflexion is commonly observed as well. **C,** After acute repair. **D,** After repair, note identical dorsiflexion of all the toes.

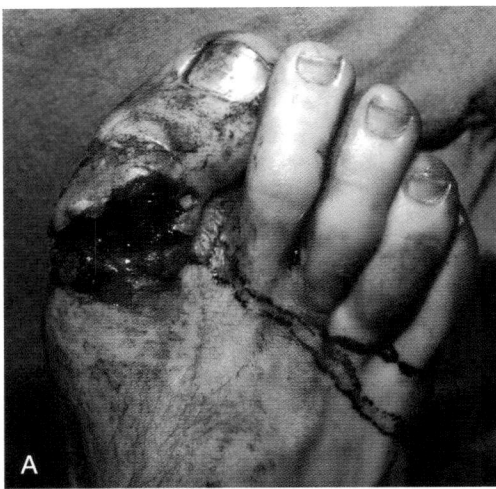

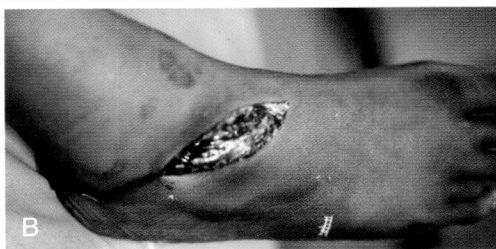

Figure 24-2 **A,** Dorsal toe laceration with distal disruption of extensor hallucis longus. After resection of the margins of the wounds, the tendon was repaired. **B,** Dorsal lateral foot laceration with disruption of the extensor tendons and preservation of the extensor hallucis longus tendon. After wound debridement, longitudinal proximal and distal extensions of the wounds permitted repair of the tendons.

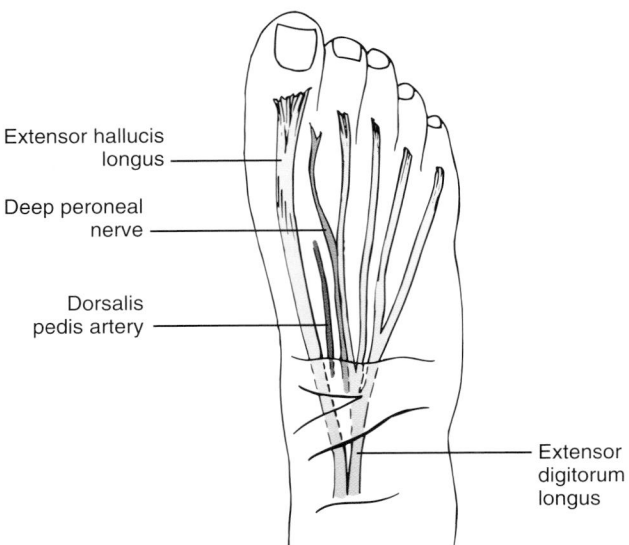

Figure 24-3 The extensor digitorum longus tendon divides into two separate tendons beneath the extensor retinaculum and then further divides into separate tendons to the four lesser toes.

medial tendons to the second and third toes (Fig. 24-3). The individual tendon of the EDL to each toe is joined on the lateral aspect by the tendon of the extensor digitorum brevis. These individual tendons are anchored at the level of the MTP joint by a fibroaponeurotic dorsal digital expansion.[24]

Physical Examination

On physical examination, an absence of extension of the lesser toes at the MTP joint is demonstrated after disruption of the EDL. Weakness of extension of the toes can also be appreciated at the PIP and DIP joints. Furthermore, because the EDL affects eversion and dorsiflexion of the foot, significant weakness of this function can be noted after tendon disruption. On palpation, a gap may be noted at the area of tendon injury. An interruption of the EDL may be diagnosed by an inability to palpate this tendon in the forefoot or ankle region as well as by weakness of lesser toe extension. The status of the superficial peroneal and deep peroneal nerves should be evaluated as well as the function of the extensor digitorum brevis.

On physical examination, difficulty can surround the diagnosis because of the ability of one tendon to substitute function for another. For example, the extensor digitorum brevis (EDB) can substitute for the EDL. On the

plantar aspect of the foot, the flexor digitorum longus (FDL) can substitute for the flexor hallucis longus (FHL) because of a crossover connection between the two flexor tendons. Comparison with unaffected contralateral toes can be useful. It is also useful to passively hold the ankle in both maximum dorsiflexion and plantar flexion and observe the positioning of the toes. In plantar flexion, the resting tension on the toes should permit them to lie in a neutral position or dorsiflexion when the tendons are intact. There should be a springiness to the toes with intact tendons that is appreciated when pushing them into plantar flexion while holding the ankle in plantar flexion. In dorsiflexion of the ankle, the toes should drop into a plantar-flexed position versus the ankle plantar-flexion position, when they should dorsiflex. Careful assessment is important to delineate a specific tendon injury.

Surgical Treatment

Bell and Schon[4] recommend that the EDL be primarily repaired using a modified Kessler suture technique. Alternatives include a modified Bunnell or Krackow technique (Fig. 24-4). Postoperatively, the foot is protected for 3 to 4 weeks with the foot and ankle in neutral position, with subsequent gradual initiation of passive range-of-motion exercises. The authors suggest night splinting after cast immobilization is discontinued.

At surgical exploration after a laceration, careful and comprehensive management is important with an open wound. All wounds should be thoroughly explored, debrided, and copiously irrigated. Any foreign bodies or materials should be removed. Inspection of adjacent neurovascular structures is important, and they should be

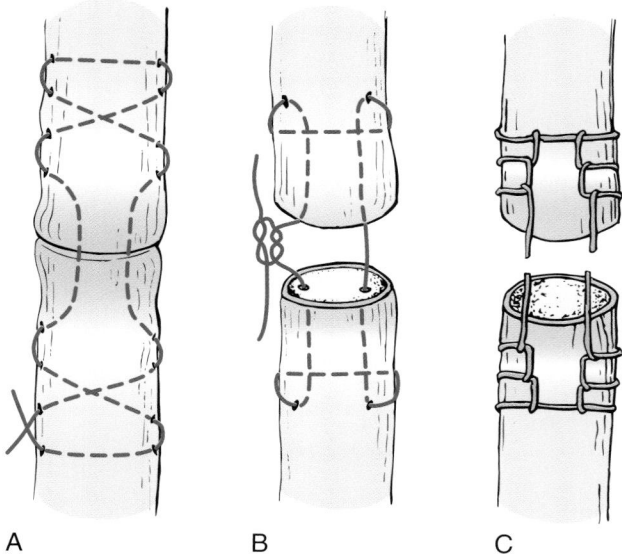

Figure 24-4 Technique of tendon repair. **A,** Modified Bunnell technique. **B,** Kessler technique. **C,** Krackow technique.

repaired or ligated as appropriate. Parenteral antibiotics, tetanus prophylaxis, and immobilization should be used depending on the specific tissue injury. A second-look operation 24 to 72 hours later should be considered for wounds with greater contamination. Postoperatively, the patient should be instructed in passive dorsiflexion of the ankle and toes, to maintain tendon gliding without straining the repair. After the wound is healed, active assistive dorsiflexion can be instituted. Resistive exercises should be avoided for 6 to 8 weeks depending upon the repair. The patient should sleep in a protective night splint to maintain neutral position. Full weight bearing in a CAM-boot can be started after the incision has healed because the boot, when standing and walking, helps maintain the tendons in a position with minimal tension.

Rooks[23] reviewed reports of EDL injuries[9,10,16,28,33] and noted 26 cases of EDL disruption. A preponderance of satisfactory results occurred after surgical repair. Lipscomb and Kelly[16] reported on six lacerations of the EDL in combination with other tendon injuries and reported 50% good results. Floyd et al[9] reported on eight EDL disruptions, seven of which were primarily repaired. The one tendon that was not repaired had a poor result. Other reports note generally good results with surgical intervention.[10,28,33] Wicks et al[33] reported on four lacerations of the EDL and concluded that those not repaired did not have a significant problem. Floyd et al[9] reported a high incidence of painful dorsal scars after laceration of the dorsum of the foot. Rooks[23] advised surgical repair of a disrupted EDL if it could be accomplished with minimal extension of the wound. He advised careful attention to associated nerve injuries as well.

Akhtar and Levine[1] reported a case of spontaneous dislocation of the EDL after a rupture of the inferior extensor retinaculum. They repaired the retinaculum and relocated the tendon successfully.

In general, injuries to the EDL tendon occur with lacerations to the dorsum of the foot or anterior ankle. In the course of surgical exploration, appropriate treatment of nerve and vessel injuries should be carried out, and repair of the disrupted EDL tendons should be done when feasible.

Extensor Digitorum Brevis

The EDB tendon originates on the distal lateral and superior surface of the calcaneus and inserts on the lateral aspect of the extensor digitorum longus tendon and also on the base of the proximal phalanx of the second through fourth toes. It is innervated by the deep peroneal nerve and provides extension at the MTP joint. The muscle is the only intrinsic muscle on the dorsum of the foot. There is no EDB tendon to the fifth toe.

The EDB is located on the lateral aspect of the forefoot and covers the lateral aspect of the subtalar joint. The tendons are quite small and are often injured after a laceration on the dorsolateral aspect of the foot. Bell and Schon[4] suggest that if the tendons are easily identified at the time of an EDL repair, an EDB repair should be performed as well. If the EDB is not repairable, EDL repair alone is adequate. No series have been reported on repairs of the EDB.

Kriza and Mushlin[13] reported an avulsion fracture of the EDB from its origin on the calcaneus. It was treated nonsurgically with a successful result. An avulsion fracture of the EDB should be distinguished from an os peroneum, a fracture of the anterior process of the calcaneus, the peroneal trochlea, a fracture of the cuboid, or a rupture of the calcaneofibular ligament.

Extensor Hallucis Longus

Anatomy
The EHL originates on the midportion of the anterior fibula and the interosseous membrane and inserts onto the base of the distal phalanx of the hallux. Innervated by the deep peroneal nerve, it extends the hallux and everts the foot. The EHL receives its motor supply much farther distally than the anterior tibial muscle and the EDL. The motor branch to the EHL travels in close proximity to the fibula for about 10 cm before penetrating the muscle belly.[25] The EHL is connected to the base of the proximal phalanx by the extensor aponeurosis, which receives contributions from the abductor and adductor hallucis. At the level of the ankle joint, the EHL becomes tendinous as it enters three successive soft tissue tunnels beneath the superior extensor retinaculum and inferior extensor retinaculum and within the extensor hood of the hallux (Fig. 24-5). These three areas play a role in a tendon entrapment or in preventing proximal retraction of the EHL tendon after injury.[12]

Lipscomb and Kelly[16] noted that as the EHL passes beneath the extensor retinacular ligaments, it is enveloped

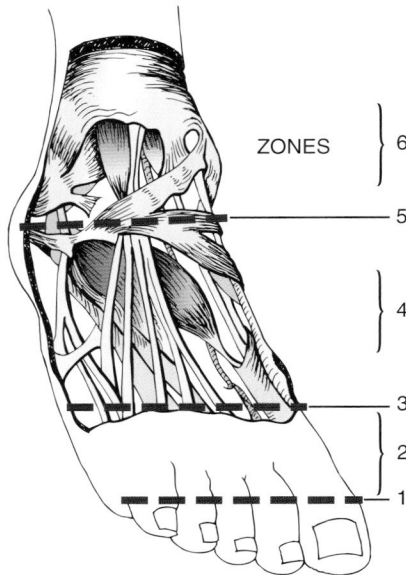

Figure 24-5 At the level of the ankle joint, the extensor hallucis longus becomes tendinous as it courses between superior and inferior extensor retinaculum. The six zones of laceration of the extensor hallucis longus are illustrated.

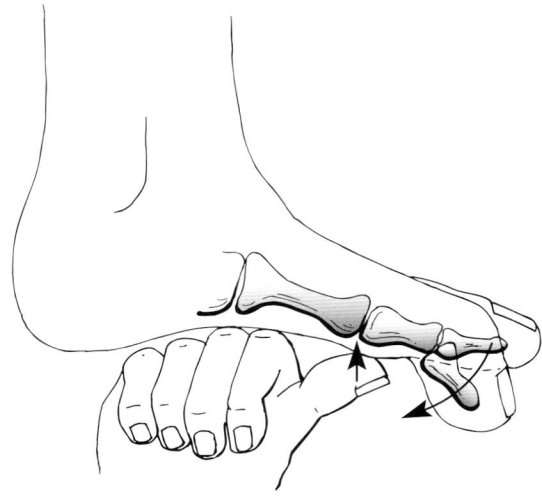

Figure 24-6 Technique of push-up test to examine function of the extensor hallucis longus (EHL). A thumb or finger is pressed on the plantar aspect of the first metatarsophalangeal joint. With unopposed function of the flexor hallucis longus, the interphalangeal joint flexes, demonstrating discontinuity or dysfunction of the EHL.

in a separate sheath, providing a gliding mechanism on the anterior aspect of the tibia and ankle.

History and Physical Examination

Attritional ruptures can occur at or around the level of the ankle joint.[19] Spontaneous ruptures of the EHL tendon occur, but lacerations are more common.[2,6] On occasion, calcification can occur with associated tendinopathy.[31]

Surgical transection of the EHL can occur during any exposure adjacent to its course, but more commonly, it can be traumatized during osteotomies when not completely protected. During cheilectomy of the first metatarsal head through a dorsal approach, the saw blade can inadvertently lacerate the EHL. Similarly, during a metatarsal osteotomy from the medial apporach, the EHL can be cut. A partial laceration can occur that may make the tendon vulnerable to late "spontaneous" rupture. An EHL rupture at the interphalangeal (IP) joint can occur in association with a violent passive plantar flexion of the IP joint with a concurrent eccentric contraction of the EHL. This can happen during soccer as the player is kicking and is blocked by another player or an object.

The patient might experience a sudden pop with a subcutaneous rupture of the EHL. Development of ecchymosis in the area of the tendon and tenderness to palpation are coupled with an inability to dorsiflex the great toe (Fig. 24-6). Tearing of the skin over the hallux IP joint may occur in association with the EHL ruptures that occur after severe IP plantar-flexion injuries. The tendon typically is not painful after rupture. An obvious defect may be present in the region of the anterior ankle with disruption of the EHL, and a gap may be noted. The tendon might not be palpable. EHB substitution can allow weak

extension of the IP joint of the hallux.[28] Patients having difficulty pulling on socks and shoes because of the weakened extension of the hallux readily experience the toe getting caught in the toe box or sock. Walking barefoot can be problematic because the patient can stub the hallux on the floor. In this situation, the toe tip has friction against the ground that, because of the forward motion and the lack of a full lift-off, results in a disruption of normal gait, making the patient vulnerable to tripping and/or falling. Depending on the location of the tendon disruption, some function might remain. Lacerations over the dorsum of the foot and the anterior ankle may be accompanied by injury to the anterior tibial or dorsalis pedis artery, deep and superficial peroneal nerves, and the anterior tibial tendon (Fig. 24-7).

Al-Qattan[2] classified the zones of injury of the extensor hallucis tendon lacerations into six areas:

Zone 1: at the insertion site on the distal phalanx
Zone 2: the area between zones 1 and 3
Zone 3: over the first metatarsophalangeal joint
Zone 4: on the dorsum of the foot between zones 3 and 5
Zone 5: laceration of the tendon beneath the extensor retinaculum
Zone 6: in the lower leg proximal to the extensor retinaculum (see Fig. 24-5).

Surgical Treatment

Extension of any laceration should be performed in a longitudinal direction to assess an injury to the EHL. Evaluation of the anterior tibial tendon, deep peroneal nerve, or other elements of the neurovascular bundle is important. The tendon is approximated and repaired with a 2-0 nonabsorbable suture with a modified Kessler or Krackow technique (Fig. 24-8; see Fig. 24-4).

If the tendon is retracted, a more proximal incision or an extension of the exposure may be necessary in the area of the anterior ankle (Fig. 24-9), and a tendon graft may be necessary to bridge a substantial defect in the case of

a delayed repair (Fig. 24-10).[8,30,32] The tendon may become caught beneath the more proximal extensor retinaculum. It is also very helpful to dorsiflex the ankle and the toes to passively deliver the tendon ends into the wound. Once the ends are found, the surgeon can insert a long 25-gauge needle perpendicularly to skewer the tendon, and this keeps it from retracting. This is a relatively atraumatic way to hold the tendon during repair.

After a primary repair, a posterior splint, brace, or cast is used for 4 weeks. Once the wound is stable, early passive and active assistive dorsiflexion of the MTP joint exercises can be initiated. Poggi and Hall[22] recommend a below-knee cast with the ankle positioned at a 90-degree angle and further plantar flexion blocked. A removable boot brace is best used in compliant patients because it permits controlled passive and active assistive dorsiflexion but not active dorsiflexion of the toe and ankle, to minimize adhesions. One should avoid passive or active plantar flexion or active dorsiflexion until 4 to 8 weeks after the repair.

Results and Complications

At the time of an EHL injury, the foot often is in a dorsiflexed position, with the EHL under tension. Significant retraction can develop depending on the level of the laceration. Laceration of the digit distal to the extensor expansion may be evidenced by no significant tendon retraction because the extensor expansion prevents proximal migration.[7,20] Scaduto and Cracchiolo[26] reviewed the world literature and noted only 43 reported cases of extensor hallucis longus tendon lacerations. Undoubtedly, there are many more cases, but experience may be diluted by the small number of cases repaired at any one institution. Al-Qattan[2] reported a large series of 15 patients treated with surgical repair of the EHL over a 12-year period. These included distal injuries as well as lacerations in zone 4 (over the dorsum of the foot). The author advocated temporary Kirschner wire fixation of both the interphalangeal and metatarsophalangeal joints for 6 weeks during the acute healing phase after the primary tendon repair. He reported a high level of

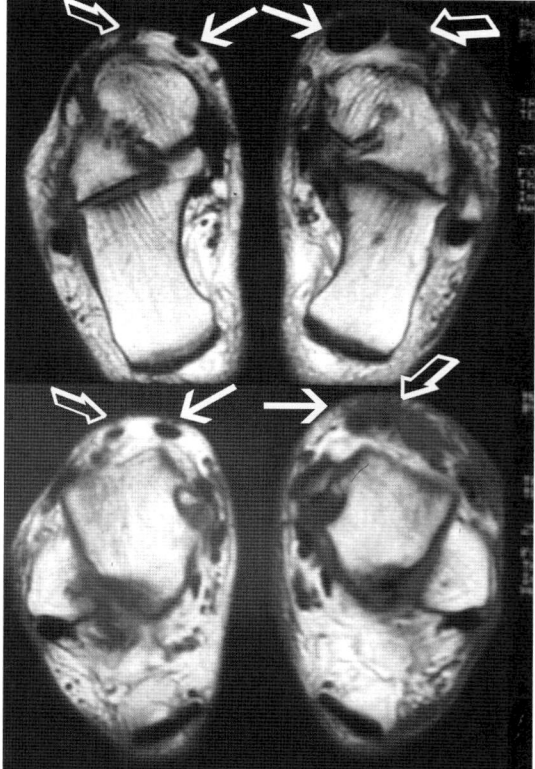

Figure 24-7 Magnetic resonance images demonstrating normal tendons on the left and injured extensor hallucis longus and anterior tibial tendon on the right after an anterior ankle deep laceration. The *solid arrows* indicate the anterior tibial tendon, and the *open arrows* indicate the extensor hallucis longus.

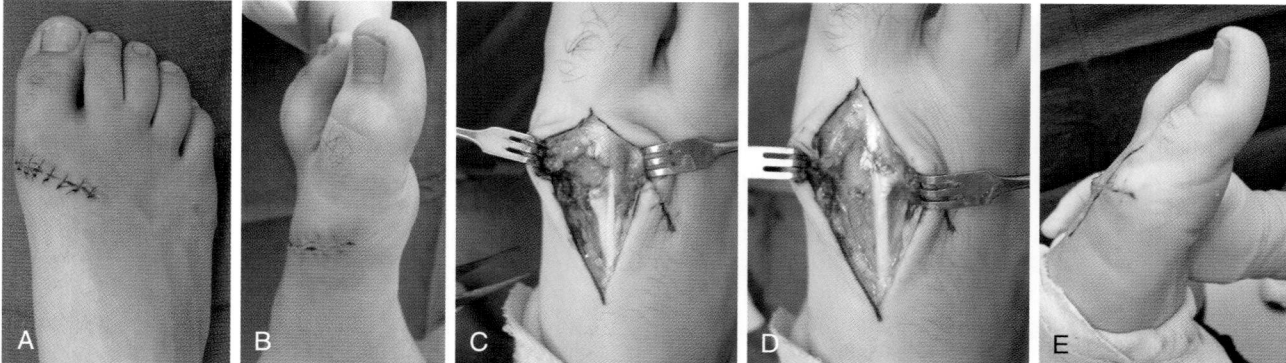

Figure 24-8 Distal laceration of extensor hallucis longus (EHL; zone 3). **A,** Laceration closed in emergency room without repair of tendon. **B,** Note extensor lag of the hallux. **C,** Exploration defining intact extensor hallucis brevis and complete laceration of extensor hallucis longus. **D,** After primary repair of EHL. **E,** Note extension of the hallux after the repair.

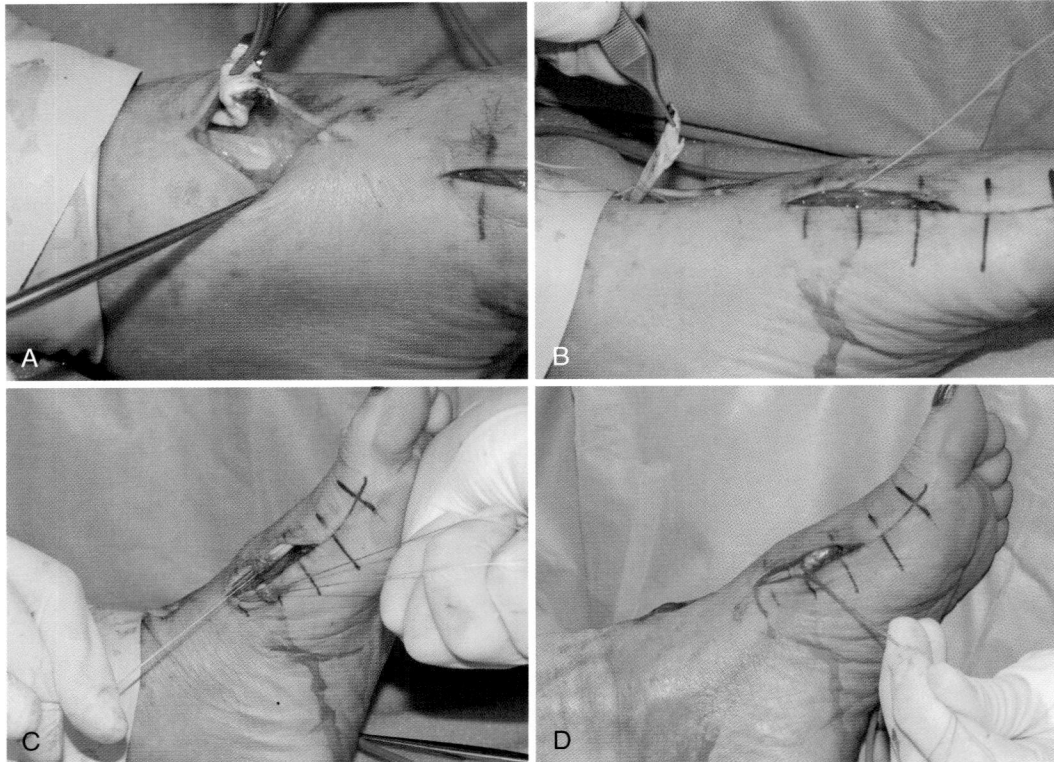

Figure 24-9   Laceration of extensor hallucis longus (zone 4). **A,** Distal laceration of extensor hallucis longus (tendon found at edge of extensor retinaculum). **B,** Preparation for transfer of tendon distally. **C,** Krakow suture placed at end of both tendons ends. **D,** After repair of tendon laceration.

satisfactory results. Duke and Greenberg[7] recommend nonsurgical treatment after a distal injury. Noonan et al[20] reported on three patients who sustained lacerations of the base of the nail with Salter fractures and concluded that these could be treated conservatively.

More proximal EHL injuries have been reported by a number of authors.[9,10,16,27-29,33] Floyd et al[9] reported on 13 EHL lacerations, of which 11 underwent a primary repair. One was not repaired, and one had a secondary repair. Using a modified Kessler suture technique or a modified Bunnell technique, they reported seven good and six fair results. They concluded that a primary repair of the disrupted EHL is indicated. Wicks et al[33] reported on 11 lacerations of the EHL, with 7 of 9 showing good results. They suggested that patients with a late, unrepaired tendon disruption may be better cared for by conservative treatment. Simonet and Sim[28] reported on 5 lacerations of the anterior ankle treated with a primary repair with satisfactory results.

Griffiths[10] reported on six cases of EHL disruption in younger patients (ages 4, 19, 21, 22, 23, and 25), five of which were repaired acutely. Based on the one patient who did not have a surgical repair, the author concluded that "formal repair of the extensor hallucis longus seems unnecessary. Its natural tendency for spontaneous repair after tenotomy is well known." Although this suggests that the EHL does not need to be repaired, Floyd et al[9] noted that the sole justification for not repairing this tendon appears to be Griffiths's one patient, who recovered spontaneously. Indeed, Griffiths did not even note the actual location of the injury.

Kass et al[12] observed that after an isolated tenotomy with the foot in a plantar-flexed position, minimal retraction occurs. On the other hand, with the EHL under tension, significant retraction can occur, and a significant gap can develop that precludes later tendon healing. Floyd et al[9] did note significant proximal retraction of the EHL in two cases. Kass et al[12] and Floyd et al[9] concluded that tenotomies are quite different from lacerations of the EHL.

Duke and Greenberg[7] reported on 75 distal tenotomies of the EHL and found no evidence of weakness of the great toe in 16 patients seen in follow-up. Bell and Schon[4] noted that the EHL, according to the literature, if left unrepaired, suffers no sequelae. They concluded, however, that these notions are based on the experience of Griffiths and thought it was imprudent to extrapolate that spontaneous recovery of EHL function routinely occurs and that EHL repair is not warranted. Since the time of that article, the authors have seen several minor chronic sequelae from a neglected laceration. The primary problems observed are clumsiness donning shoes or boots and plantar-flexion deformity of the hallux. In general, based on our clinical observations, efforts to repair the tendon should be undertaken when possible.

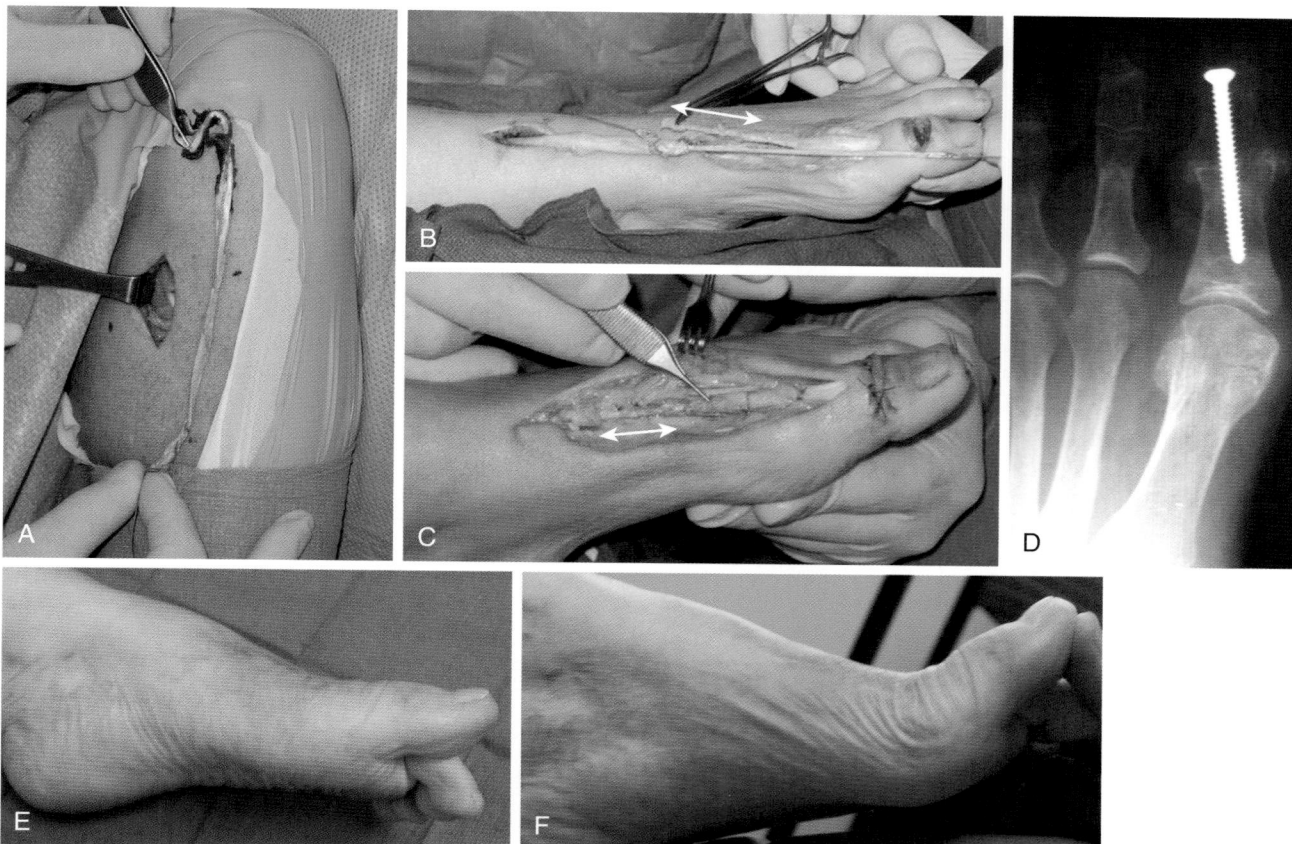

Figure 24-10 Delayed reconstruction of extensor hallucis longus (EHL) tendon with gracilis tendon allograft. **A,** The gracilis tendon is harvested from the ipsilateral knee. **B,** Tenolysis of the EHL is performed, and then a gracilis autograft is sutured to the proximal EHL stump with a Pulvertaft weave technique. *Arrow* illustrates the proliferative scar tissue attached to the distal stump of tendon that, when resected, leaves a 3-cm gap. **C,** The tendon graft has been sutured to the distal stump but also secured through a transverse drill hole in the proximal phalanx. An interphalangeal joint arthrodesis has been performed. The *arrow* denotes that the 3-cm defect has been spanned with the gracilis tendon autograft. **D,** Anteroposterior standing radiograph demonstrates the interphalangeal joint arthrodesis. **E,** Active extension of the hallux metatarsophalangeal (MTP) joint is demonstrated 6 months after reconstruction. **F,** The hallux MTP joint demonstrates 60 degrees of passive motion postoperatively. (**A** and **F,** Courtesy B. Smith, MD. **B-E,** From Smith B, Coughlin M: Reconstruction of a chronic extensor hallucis longus tendon laceration with a gracilis tendon autograft, *Orthopedics* 31:pii:orthosupersite.com/view.asp?rID=31525, 2008. Used with permission.)

Isolated rupture of the EHL occurs infrequently. Menz and Nettle[18] described a case with rupture at the musculotendinous junction. Poggi and Hall[22] reported on a closed rupture of the EHL at the level of the MTP joint that occurred several years after a cheilectomy.

Another example is that of a ruptured EHL tendon at the IP joint of the hallux seen in a professional soccer player with a history of a trauma during a game. The player reported a hyperdorsiflexion injury of the MTP joint in conjunction with severe plantar flexion of the IP joint. The patient reported significant pain, an inability to play and had difficulty walking for several months. On exam, he was noted to have a 1-cm healed scar from the superficial tearing of the skin and weakness of dorsiflexion of the IP joint. A bone contusion was seen on magnetic resonance imaging (MRI) of the proximal phalangeal base and dorsal metatarsal head and a medial plantar plate injury of the MTP joint. At the time of surgery, a

defect was noted in the EHL tendon and dorsal capsule at the IP joint, with discontinuity of the tendon. The EHL was repaired, the MTP joint debrided, and the plantar plate repaired medially. The athlete returned to full function for several succeeding seasons without difficulty.

Sim and Deweerd[27] reported on a spontaneous rupture of the EHL on the anterior aspect of the ankle in a skier. Spontaneous ruptures have also been reported after a hyper–plantar-flexion injury in a taekwondo athlete[15] and from chronic impingement because of a dorsal talar osteophyte.[8] One case of delayed rupture after injury from radiofrequency ablation during arthroscopic surgery has also been reported.[32]

McMaster[17] stated that spontaneous rupture of a tendon rarely occurs without predisposing factors such as chronic disease. Successful surgical treatment centers on early diagnosis and prompt surgical intervention. Sim and Deweerd[27] and Skoff[29] repaired the tendon primarily,

Langenberg[14] used a free tendon graft, and Menz and Nettle[18] transferred the peroneus tertius tendon to reconstruct the EHL. All had excellent results.

With delayed treatment of an old EHL rupture, Berens[5] noted that on initial exploration the proximal portion of the tendon could not be identified. Therefore the extensor hallucis brevis tendon was transferred into the distal stump of the extensor hallucis brevis. Menz and Nettle[18] noted that a primary repair was not possible and used the tendon of the peroneus brevis that was mobilized and sutured it directly to the EHL. Hoelzer and Kalish[11] also reported an EHL tendon disruption and noted at exploration 4 months after injury that the proximal end had retracted. The tendon of the EDL to the second toe was split and anastomosed to the distal stump of the EHL. Allografts and autografts have also been reported as a means to bridge significant defects with delayed treatment of EHL injuries with satisfactory results[8,21,30,32,34]

Postoperative scarring and adhesion formation can lead to diminished postoperative motion[29] and may be a source of pain, but this is uncommon. Floyd et al[9] reported that 38% of those injured had a painful scar.

Conclusion

With only one reported exception, the results of surgical repair of acute disruption of the EHL tendons have been good.

The actual site of injury is an important factor in developing a plan for treatment of a disruption of the EHL. If the injury is distal to the extensor expansion, nonsurgical treatment is considered, as long as the hallux can be maintained in a neutral position with tendon apposition. An injury proximal to the extensor expansion may be treated with a primary repair. Treatment of EHL injuries 6 weeks or later after injury is often associated with an inability to reapproximate the tendon ends. A tendon transfer or tendon graft may be necessary to bridge the interval gap (Fig. 24-11 and Video Clip 114). In these cases, one should assess the amount of tendon loss by placing moderate

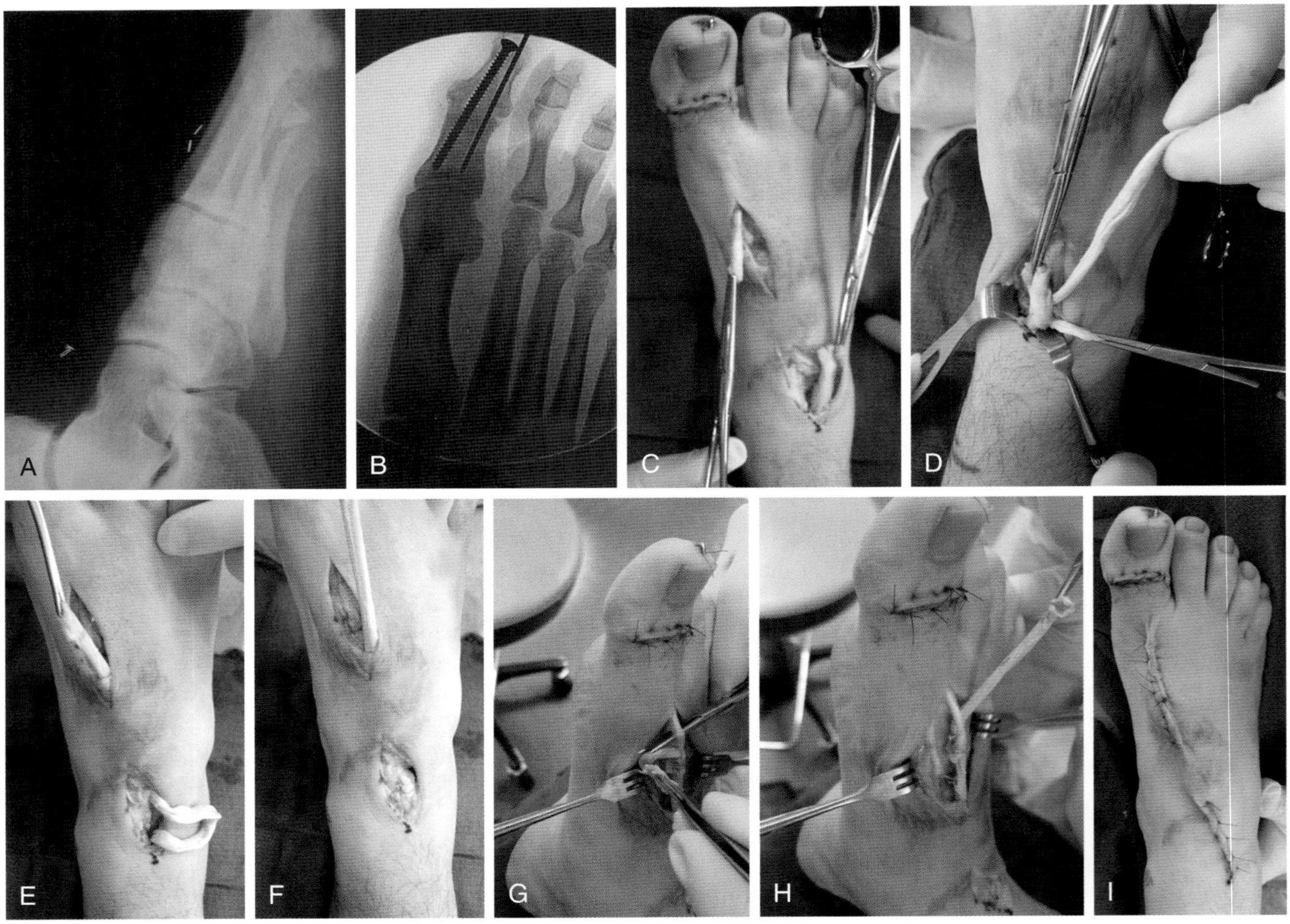

Figure 24-11 Delayed repair of extensor hallucis longus laceration, 1 year after injury (zone 4 injury). **A,** Lateral radiograph shows clips at ends of distal stump and proximal stump with retraction beneath the extensor retinaculum. **B,** Interphalangeal joint fusion completed. **C,** Krakow-type suture placed in proximal end of distal stump. Distal end of proximal stump grasped with clamp (3-4 cm gap in tendon). **D,** Allograft weaved through proximal stump. **E** and **F,** Allograft is pulled distally beneath skin bridge. **G** and **H,** Pulvertaft weave of tendon graft through the distal stump. **I,** Completed delayed extensor hallucis longus reconstruction.

tension on the tendon ends and placing the ankle and hallux in neutral position. When the tendon ends cannot be opposed without excessive tension, a tendon slide, using healthy proximal EHL tendon for defects up to 4 to 5 cm, may be attempted. For anything greater than a 5-cm gap, a tendon transfer may be performed. Although in the past a common reported transfer was the peroneus tertius,[18] a split of the extensor to the second toe for use in lacerations distal to the ankle joint[11] is a good alternative. Allograft and autograph tendon transfers have become more popular to bridge obvious tendon gaps.[8,21,30,32,34]

Aggressive surgical treatment of open lacerations about the foot is most important. Adequate exploration and debridement and anatomic restoration of tendons are usually appropriate. Although Griffiths[10] noted that the EHL tendon might heal spontaneously and that formal repair is not indicated, review of the literature does not support the notion that conservative management is warranted. Surgical repair of the EHL is important when feasible. On the other hand, with significant soft tissue loss, an EHL repair might not be feasible, but secondary tendon grafting can be considered if there is a distal stump, pliable tissues without extensive fibrosis along the tendon path, and no evidence of infection.

ANTERIOR TIBIAL TENDON RUPTURE

Subcutaneous rupture of the anterior tibial tendon has received little attention in the literature, and relatively few ruptures have been reported. Anagnostakos et al[36] reviewed the literature and noted 110 published cases of anterior tibial tendon disruption; in only four series were there more than four cases, the remaining being case reports or very small series.[3,16,68,77] In one of the largest series reported to date, Markarian et al[68] described 16 anterior tibial tendon disruptions, including 10 ruptures and 6 lacerations. At this time, less than 150 cases (case reports or series) of anterior tibial tendon rupture have been reported in the literature.

Anatomy

The anterior tibial tendon functions as the major dorsiflexor of the ankle,[48] primarily during the swing phase, heel strike, and early stance phase of the walking cycle.[41,81] It originates from the proximal half of the anterior tibia, the lower lateral tibial condyle, lateral tibia, and the interosseous membrane and inserts on the plantar medial aspect of the first cuneiform and the plantar base of the first metatarsal (Fig. 24-12). At the level of the lower and middle thirds of the tibia, it becomes tendinous and is surrounded by a synovial sheath. Anagnostakos et al[36] reported on the dissection of 53 cadaveric specimens and reported three different patterns of insertion of the anterior tibial tendon into the medial midfoot. In 36 cases (68%), the tendon inserted into the medial cuneiform and base of the first metatarsal, and in 13 cases (25%), it inserted only into the medial aspect of the first cuneiform.

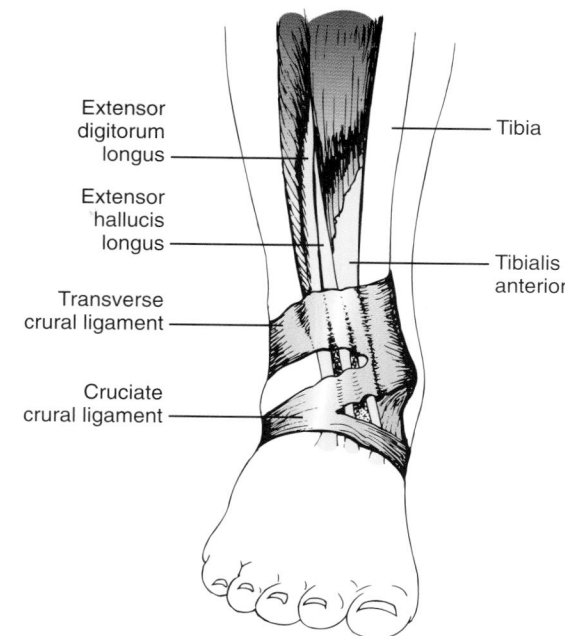

Figure 24-12 The anterior tibial tendon courses beneath the transverse crural ligament and cruciate crural ligament before inserting on the plantar medial aspect of the first cuneiform and plantar base of the first metatarsal.

In four feet (7%), the tendon inserted into both the cuneiform and the metatarsal, but there was an additional accessory tendon that inserted onto the base of the first metatarsal.

Innervated by the deep peroneal nerve, the anterior tibial tendon functions to dorsiflex and invert the foot and provides controlled plantar flexion at heel strike. The tendon is active in heel-strike phase in an *eccentric* mode because it allows the ankle to slowly plantar flex until foot flat. It is active again in the swing phase in a *concentric* mode, dorsiflexing the ankle and keeping the forefoot from dragging. Congenital absence of an anterior tibial muscle and tendon is a rare occurrence[42] and may be associated with clawing of the toes because of recruitment of the EHL and EDL to assist in dorsiflexion of the foot and ankle.

The tendon passes beneath the superior extensor retinaculum and the upper and lower limbs of the inferior extensor retinaculum. Petersen et al[78] investigated the structure and vascular pattern of the tibialis anterior tendon by using injection techniques, light and transmission electron microscopy, and immunohistochemistry. They found a well-vascularized peritenon, with blood vessels penetrating the tendon and anastomosing with a longitudinally oriented intratendinous network. Despite a well-vascularized posterior surface of the tendon, they found an avascular zone where the tendon runs under the superior and inferior retinacula. This results in an area 1 to 2 cm from the insertion that is at risk for rupture.

Not only is the tendon vulnerable to spontaneous rupture here but, as the tendon passes beneath these

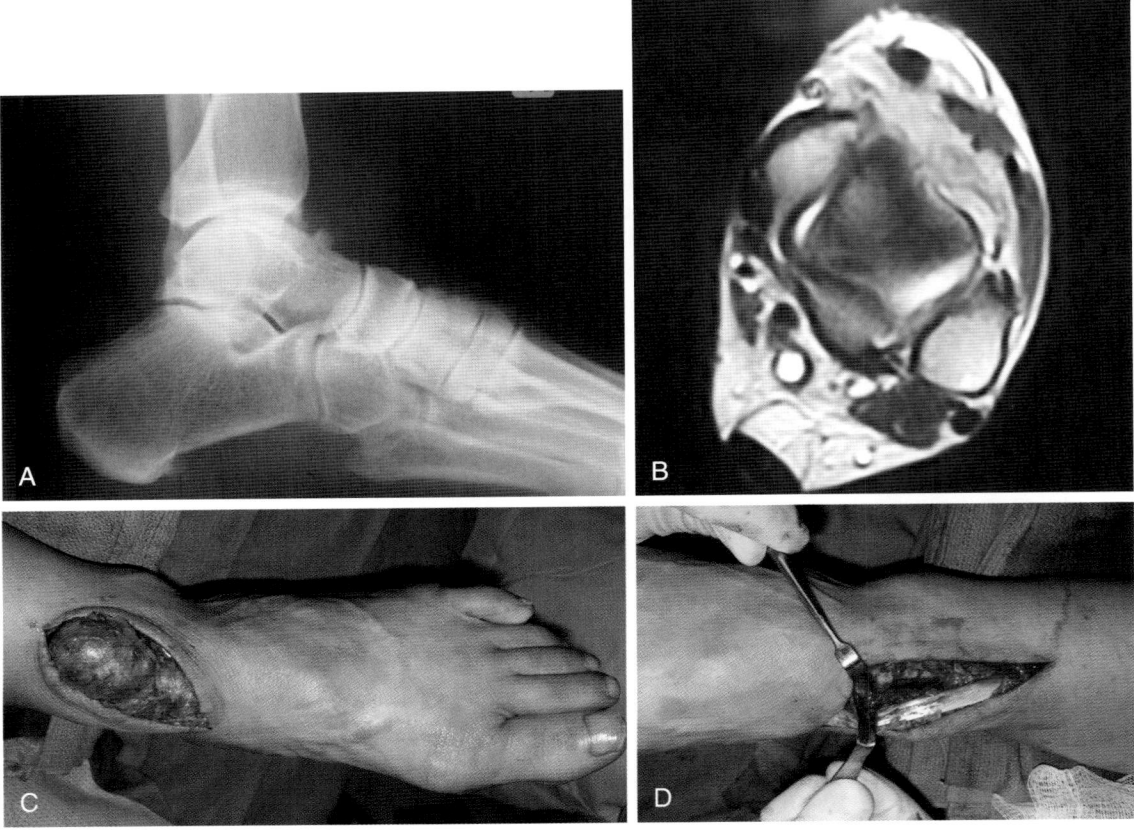

Figure 24-13 Ganglion of the anterior ankle region eroding the anterior tibial tendon, masquerading as a tendon rupture. **A,** Lateral radiograph with dorsal talar spur. **B,** Magnetic resonance image demonstrating a mass anterior to the anterior tibial tendon. **C,** Mass at surgery. **D,** After resection, the anterior tibial tendon is intact. The joint is exposed to remove the osteophytes.

retinacular structures, it also lies on the distal surface of the tibia and is at risk for injury with fracture of the tibia or a laceration.[69] Lipscomb and Kelly[16] stated that the tendon had 6 to 7 cm of excursion at this level.

An acute disruption of the anterior tibial tendon can occur with trauma at any age from fracture of the tibia or laceration.[43,45,65,68,69] Three quarters of these disruptions occur in male patients. A spontaneous rupture can occur from an underlying degenerative process.[50,51,66] Inflammatory arthritis,[49,62] gout,[58] rheumatoid arthritis,[46,68,77] impingement from an underlying exostosis, a local steroid injection,* and diabetes† have all been cited as contributing factors in anterior tibial tendon rupture. A ganglion in the region of the anterior ankle can masquerade as a rupture of the anterior tibial tendon, with the formation of an enlarged mass (Fig. 24-13).[82]

Ruptures occur near the anterior tibial tendon's insertion, most often close to or within 2 to 3 cm of the insertion (Fig. 24-14). They can be caused by chronic wear from an exostosis at the talonavicular, naviculocuneiform, or metatarsocuneiform joints or by attrition from

*References 36, 46, 49, 55, 80, and 81.
†References 38, 46, 49, 62, 64, and 77.

rubbing against the edge of the inferior extensor retinaculum.[54] McMaster[17] noted that ruptures occur in the presence of an abnormal tendon structure. This correlates well with the deficiency in the tendon's vascular supply.

Markarian et al[68] have described "acute on chronic" tears manifesting as a degenerative tear in the anterior tibial tendon. These ruptures usually occur in men between the fifth and seventh decades of life and most often are reported in the seventh decade.[38,44] They appear to develop as an age-related phenomenon. A prodromal phase is unusual, and patients do not routinely complain of pain before tendon rupture. Patients may notice an enlarged nodule on the degenerative tendon before rupture.

Anterior tibial tendon ruptures occur with forced or excessive plantar flexion against a contracted anterior tibial muscle.[38,64,71,81] An acute rupture is usually one of two different clinical presentations. With acute trauma in a younger patient who is involved with a higher functional level of activity, the rupture is associated with the acute onset of pain but infrequently with severe trauma. Walking down a ramp or slope can trigger eccentric contracture of the anterior tibial muscle, which may precipitate a tendon rupture. Decreased dorsiflexion strength is

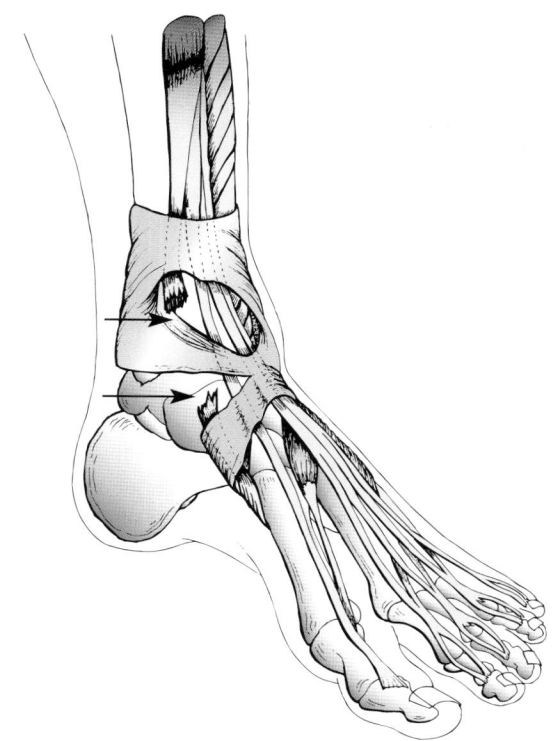

Figure 24-14 Spontaneous rupture of anterior tibial tendon *(arrows)* typically occurs in distal 3 cm of tendon.

noted at the time of injury, which usually prompts the patient to seek medical evaluation and treatment soon after injury. On the other hand, an older patient typically has no history of antecedent trauma and often presents several months after the incident with a complaint of a painless footdrop.[79] Frequently, a patient does not remember a precipitating event,[81] and the older patient often is unaware of the condition.[44] Markarian et al[68] reported an average 10-week delay in diagnosis in their series of 16 anterior tibial tendon disruptions. Late diagnosis is common, and permanent disability is rare.

The patient often experiences a snapping sensation that is associated with a brief episode of sharp pain over the anterior aspect of the ankle and is accompanied by swelling. Ambulation may be difficult in the initial few hours after rupture, but the pain subsides rapidly. A patient might note lack of coordination, a slapping gait, or an inability to clear the toes with ambulation. In time, the anterior tibial muscle atrophies. Both Frigg et al[50] and George et al[51] have reported cases of simultaneous degeneration of the anterior tibial and posterior tibial tendons that required hindfoot arthrodeses and anterior tibial tendon reconstructions.

The anterior tibial tendon, on occasion, may be involved with tendinopathy (tendinitis or tendinosis), as described by Burman,[39] Goldman,[53] and Hamilton.[56] Beischer et al[37] has described a series of 29 cases of tendinosis that were characterized by swelling over the insertion, nocturnal pain, and, on examination, point

tenderness over the insertion of the anterior tibial tendon. Beischer et al observed longitudinal split tears in the distal tendon in 19 of 29 cases and typical tendinosis on those that were explored. They found a much higher incidence of involvement in females in this series and speculated that this may be a different clinical entity than the typical patient (typically elderly males) who sustains a spontaneous rupture of the tendon. Beischer et al suggested a provocative "stretch" test to assess tendinosis, which included forced ankle plantar flexion, midfoot eversion, and abduction with a pronation force applied to the foot in an attempt to acutely passively stretch the anterior tibial tendon. A positive test was characterized by aggravation of the typical pain the patient had previously experienced. In a follow-up study on the operated patients in this series, Grundy et al[54] reviewed the results of 12 cases, mostly women, who were explored for tendinosis and longitudinal tears of the distal anterior tibial tendon. Although there was evidence of macroscopic tendinosis in all cases, those with less than 50% degeneration were treated with a debridement while those with greater than 50% degeneration were treated with debridement and an EHL tendon augmentation. Later rupture in those who only had a debridement, led the authors to recommend more aggressive reconstruction and use of the EHL augmentation on a routine basis.

Insertional tendinopathy can occur after prolonged walking or running. Besides the localized pain, patients may complain of pain in the anterior ankle and lower leg. At times, it will manifest as anterior "shin splints" or even chronic exertional compartment syndrome. The repetitive eccentric load at the bone tendon interface of the contracted anterior tibial tendon musculotendinous unit during impact on heel strike induces microtears that generate a localized inflammatory response. The condition can be exacerbated while descending slopes or inclines, when the sudden jarring at the insertion of the anterior tibial tendon at the cuneiform is maximized. Avoiding these stresses and wearing cushioned heeled shoes can help the tendon to recover. For more intractable cases, patients will benefit from a CAM-boot or an ankle–foot orthosis (AFO). Platelet-rich plasma derived from peripheral blood, or bone marrow injected at the tendon insertion can be helpful in conjunction with immobilization when bracing alone is unsuccessful.[59] Steroid injections at this location should be avoided to minimize the risk of tendon rupture (Fig. 24-15).

History and Physical Examination

A patient with anterior tibial tendon rupture often complains of swelling of the anterior ankle and foot, has weak dorsiflexion, and reports catching the foot on irregular or uneven ground.[79] Footdrop may be significant or minimal. The mild pain associated with a tendon rupture usually subsides quickly.[64,68] Swelling of the anterior ankle can disguise the rupture, although with time a palpable defect becomes apparent.[62,64,71] A fixed lump or mass on the

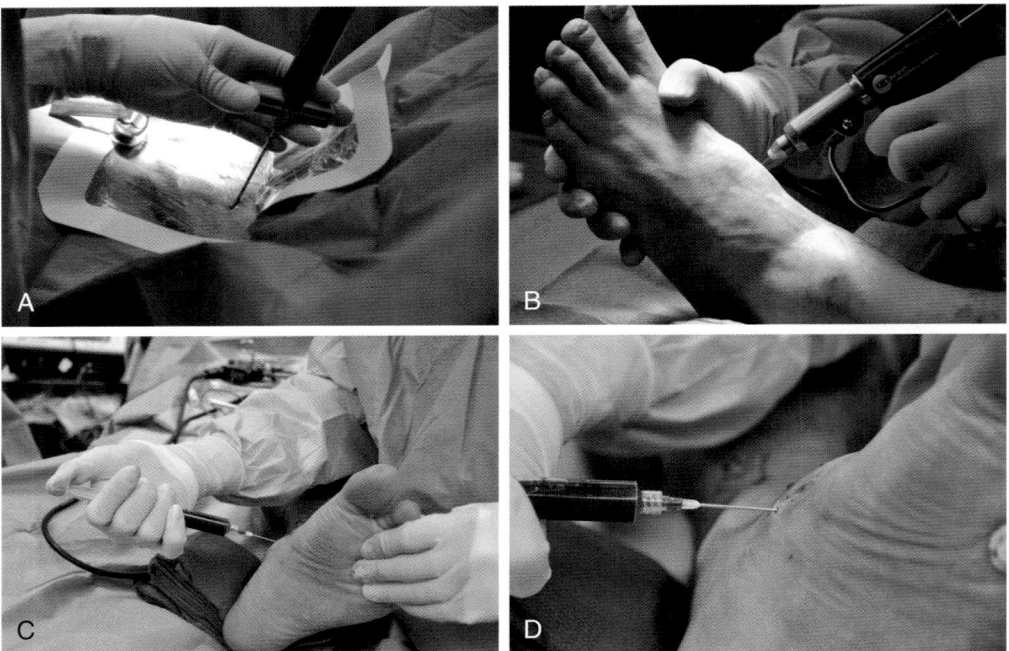

Figure 24-15 Method of plasma-rich protein injection with bone marrow concentrate from the iliac crest. **A,** Aspiration technique using a trocar placed between the tables of the anterior iliac crest 3 cm behind the anterior superior iliac spine (ASIS). Five-mL aliquots are withdrawn, and then the trocar is backed out 1 cm for more aspiration to obtain the maximum cellular content. This is done with several trocar trajectories. Aspirate is then concentrated by a special chamber in a centrifuge. **B,** Midfoot area prepared with 0.045-inch Kirschner wire drilling of the cuneiform, with penetration of the tendon at its insertion. **C,** Injection of concentrate. **D,** Close-up of injection.

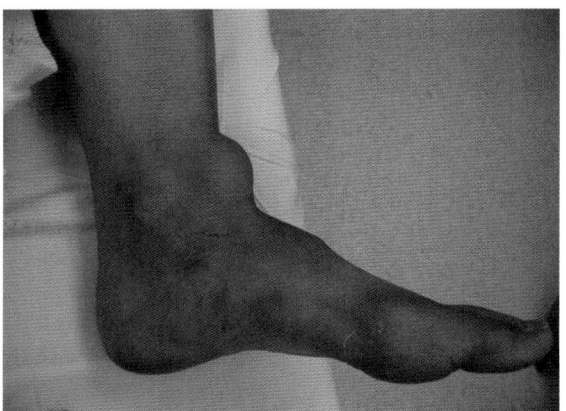

Figure 24-16 Rupture of anterior tibial tendon can manifest with a lump on the anterior aspect of the ankle region.

anterior ankle can develop from the bulbous end of the proximal tendon segment (Fig. 24-16). The proximal tendon often retracts to the level of the ankle joint, and the mass is found deep to the extensor retinaculum and is often adherent to the synovial sheath.[38,64] Typically, the area of the anterior tibial tendon lacks normal contour as it crosses the ankle.

A lack of dorsiflexion power might not be appreciated by the examiner unless muscle strength is compared with the contralateral side (Fig. 24-17). However, weakness in dorsiflexion against resistance can make the diagnosis more apparent.[16,43,62,64] The patient is typically unable to walk on the heel. Many patients are able to dorsiflex the ankle using the remaining dorsiflexors (EHL, EDL),[16] and Moberg[72] has reported that anterior tibial tendon function can be replaced to a large extent by the toe extensors. Patients often do not recognize anterior tibial dysfunction because of the remaining dorsiflexion power of the EHL and EDL and do not seek treatment until many months after injury (Fig. 24-18). Typically, with an attritional rupture, the anterior tibial tendon becomes attenuated. There is a subtle loss of power initially. When examining the patient's dorsiflexion strength, the ankle and foot dorsiflex, but the first metatarsal remains relatively plantar flexed because of an imbalanced peroneus longus. The ankle may achieve a neutral position, but often there is valgus of the forefoot and eversion at the midfoot, with relative weakness of dorsiflexion and inversion (Fig. 24-19).

Without anterior tibial tendon function, a gait disturbance typically occurs.[38,68,81] With a footdrop, footslap, or steppage gait, typically after heel strike, the patient is unable to plantar flex the foot slowly in a controlled manner.[16,38,70,71] The abnormal gait occurs with ambulation as the patient attempts to clear the toes from catching on the ground.

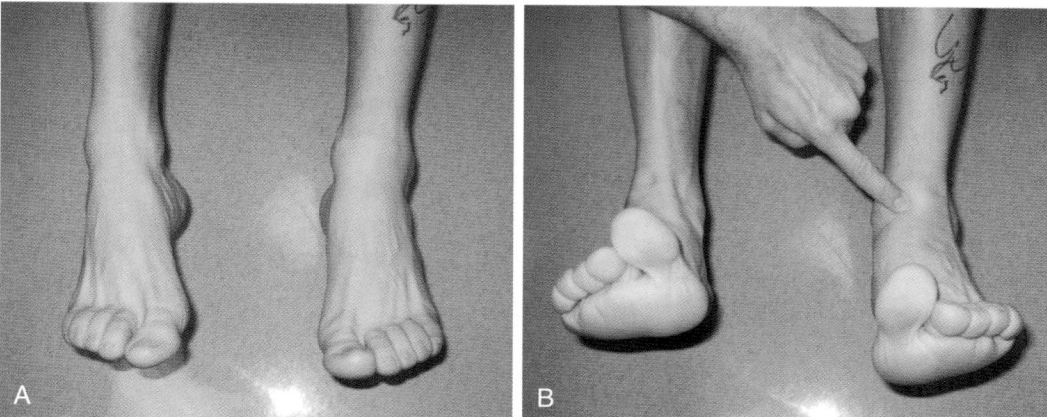

Figure 24-17 Examination after rupture of the anterior tibial tendon. **A,** An absence of dorsiflexion power is not seen with the feet in plantar flexion. **B,** With dorsiflexion, the rupture is obvious with an absence of the anterior tibial tendon on the left.

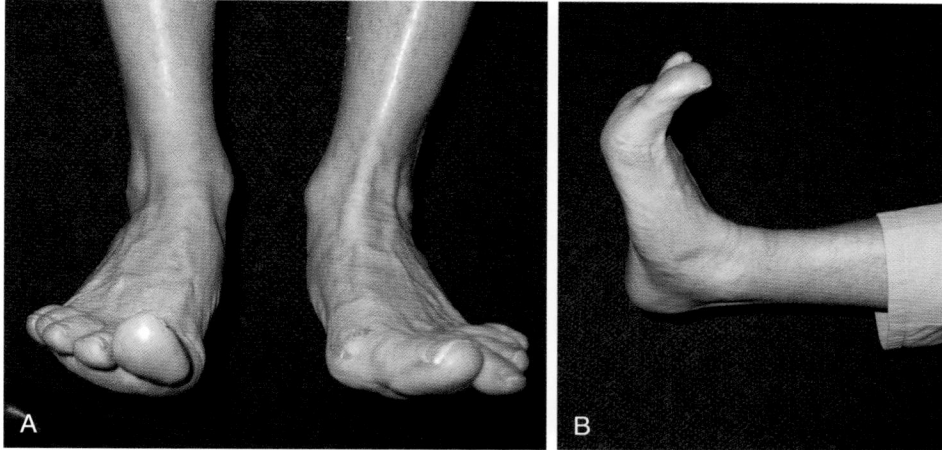

Figure 24-18 **A,** Intact anterior tibial tendon on the left foot, rupture on the right. **B,** The extensor digitorum longus and extensor hallucis longus are recruited to dorsiflex the ankle. Note extension of toes with ankle dorsiflexion. The injured ankle dorsiflexes less and everts more because of the tendon imbalance. The medial ray is still relatively plantar flexed.

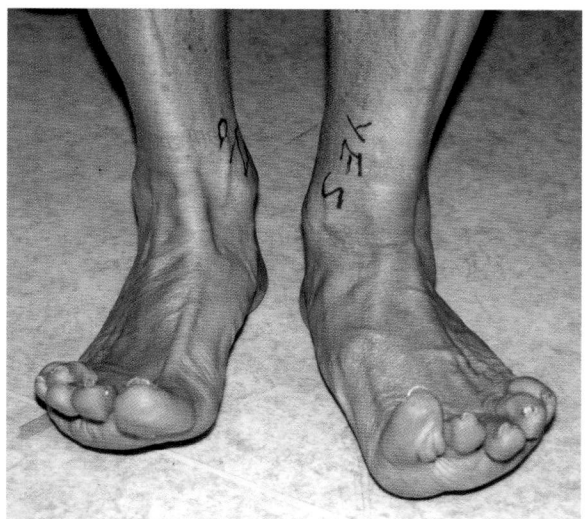

Figure 24-19 The left ankle has neutral dorsiflexion with compensatory over pulling of the EHL and EDL. The forefoot is in valgus and midfoot in eversion relative to the right side.

Mensor and Ordway[70] reported a slight loss (10 to 15 degrees) of dorsiflexion after anterior tibial tendon rupture. Burman[40] and Moberg[72] reported development of a spontaneous flatfoot deformity after anterior tibial tendon rupture.

This condition can be misdiagnosed as a peroneal palsy or confused with an L4-5 radiculopathy.[71,74] Peroneal nerve palsy and lumbar disk syndrome can easily be ruled out on neurologic examination with normal sensation on the dorsum of the foot, normal sensation in the first web space, and normal function of the other extensor tendons with active dorsiflexion of the toes.[62] Heel varus and eversion weakness in conjunction with the loss of dorsiflexion suggests a common peroneal nerve palsy or radiculopathy and makes the diagnosis of tibialis anterior rupture unlikely. In patients with acute anterior tibial disruption, the injury is often associated with laceration or a distal tibial fracture. Open injuries after a fracture or laceration can occur but require assessment of motion and strength of the anterior tibial tendon so that a tendon disruption is not overlooked. Surgical exploration of traumatic wounds should be considered if there is any notion of weakness, a gap, or deformation of the anterior ankle. Mechrefe et al[69] have reported a case of a distal tibial fracture and a simultaneous avulsion of the anterior tibial tendon insertion, with entrapment of the tendon within the fracture site (Fig. 24-20).

Imaging

Magnetic resonance imaging can be helpful in defining an anterior tibial tendon rupture.[60,61,64,76,77] Normal tendons have a low signal intensity and contrast well with surrounding fat, which has a high signal intensity. Both sagittal and axial images are helpful. In patients presenting late, who do not recall a precipitating accident or event, MRI can be helpful in making a diagnosis of rupture or tendon degeneration (Fig. 24-21).[36,54,81]

Treatment

Ruptures of the anterior tibial tendon are uncommon. No consensus in the literature appears to exist regarding recommendations of surgical versus nonsurgical treatment; however, foot and ankle experts generally agree that surgical repair is reasonable to achieve the ultimate goal of improved function without a brace. When an anterior tibial tendon rupture is diagnosed early in a younger active patient, surgical repair is likely to improve ambulation and decrease morbidity. Treatment of an old rupture is more controversial and appears to lead to unpredictable results.[81] Unfortunately, ruptures in older patients are often initially unnoticed.

For the older patient, bracing or a polypropylene AFO or a double upright brace may be prescribed. Ouzounian and Anderson[77] noted that of five patients treated conservatively, three refused a brace or found it too restrictive. Two patients who used a brace found it improved their level of activity. Compliance in the older patient can be difficult. With nonsurgical treatment, the proximal tendon segment usually becomes adherent in the area of the anterior ankle. Some loss of ankle dorsiflexion strength and motion develops. In elderly, sedentary patients with

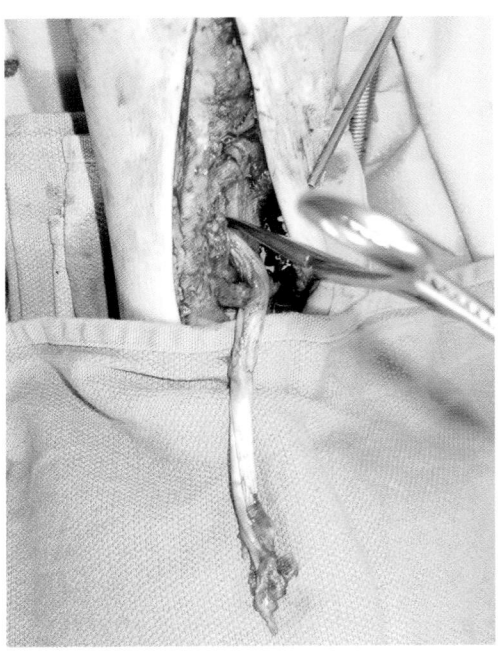

Figure 24-20 Fractured distal tibia with avulsion of anterior tibial tendon. Open exposure of tibial fracture (knee superior, ankle inferior). The anterior tibial tendon was avulsed with a bony fragment from the medial cuneiform and base of the first metatarsal, and interposed in the fracture site, preventing reduction. (From Mechrefe AP, Walsh EF, DiGiovanni CW: Anterior tibial tendon avulsion with distal tibial fracture entrapment: case report, *Foot Ankle Int* 27:645–647, 2006. Used with permission.)

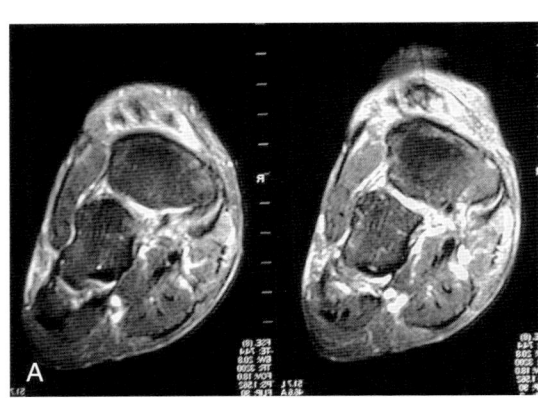 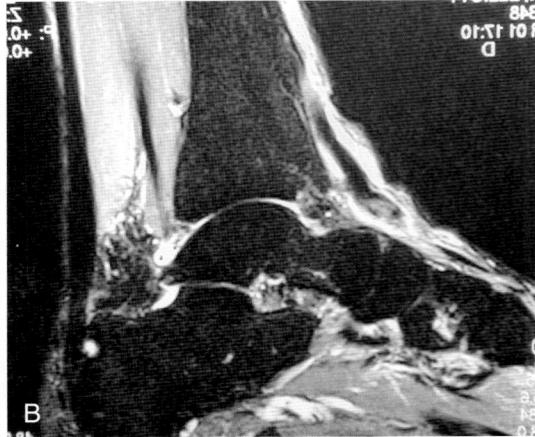

Figure 24-21 Magnetic resonance image demonstrates rupture of the left anterior tibial tendon off its insertion. **A,** At the level of the naviculum, the anterior tibial tendon is indistinct dorsomedially. **B,** Sagittal view demonstrates the anterior tibial tendon, which appears wavy because of loss of tension. It is surrounded by synovial fluid, and distally the tendon cannot be traced, ending abruptly in a widened fibrotic mass just dorsal to the naviculum.

a low level of activity, a normal gait pattern actually may be achieved, justifying conservative treatment.[44,71]

Markarian et al[68] found no significant difference in the conservative and surgical treatment in elderly patients and suggested that nonsurgical treatment was a viable option and "should not adversely affect overall foot and ankle function."

Decreased dorsiflexion strength,[49,71] lack of coordination or a slapping gait,[70] and progressive flatfoot deformity[49] may be associated with nonsurgical treatment. Although full functional recovery might not be obtained, function and gait in the older, less active patient may be acceptable.[44,68,71,72,74]

For patients who want a higher level of function, surgical repair is indicated. Surgical intervention can entail direct repair for the acute rupture or reconstruction of the anterior tibial tendon with either a tendon transfer or an interposition tendon graft for delayed treatment.

Both surgical and conservative treatments have been advocated for anterior tibial tendon ruptures, and treatment should be tailored to the individual patient depending on age, level of activity, time elapsed since the rupture occurred, current level of disability, and local and systemic contraindications to surgery. Nonsurgical treatment is preferred in the older patient with fewer demands, and surgical repair is typically indicated in the younger and middle-aged active athlete. Markarian et al[68] concluded that although primary repair is the optimal treatment for a ruptured anterior tibial tendon, when diagnosis is delayed longer than 4 weeks, the treating physician should "consider the physical demands and goals of the patient" before automatically recommending surgery.

Acute Surgical Treatment

With a laceration of the anterior tibial tendon, the proximal segment may be found anywhere along the course of the tendon. Often it retracts to the level of the ankle joint. With a rupture, the proximal stump is often found deep to the extensor retinaculum and is often adherent to the synovial sheath. The site of the rupture is typically just proximal to the site of the tendon insertion and just distal to the inferior border of the superior extensor retinaculum.

Lipscomb and Kelly[16] and others[36,45,57,75] have recommended a direct repair of the anterior tibial tendon. Its reinsertion into the navicular with a suture anchor or into a bony tunnel are alternatives with an avulsion fracture or distal rupture.[46] The technique of repair and reconstruction depends on the pathologic process present and the time delay in diagnosis. Ouzounian and Anderson[77] recommended a direct repair with reinsertion of the anterior tibial tendon into bone.

With delay in diagnosis and retraction of the proximal tendon stump or with injury to a large segment of tendon, direct repair may be impossible. Tendon reconstruction is then an option. An extensor tendon graft, tendon transfer,[52,77,83-85] or partial tendon advancement[67] are

surgical options for reconstruction. Although the tendon may be advanced through a drill hole,[46] it may be reinforced with bone anchors or a pull-out wire as well.[47]

PRIMARY REPAIR OF RUPTURED ANTERIOR TIBIAL TENDON
Surgical Technique

1. The patient is placed in a supine position with a thigh tourniquet for hemostasis as warranted. An anterior curvilinear incision is made on the inferomedial aspect of the anterior tibial tendon and extended from the level of the first cuneiform proximally to the level of the superior extensor retinaculum.

2. The anteroinferior extensor retinaculum is divided, and the anterior tibial tendon is identified and traced to its insertion in the first cuneiform. A *square wave* cutting of the more proximal retinaculum may be indicated to facilate repair of the retinaculum to prevent bowstringing of the tendon (Fig. 24-22).

3. The dorsalis pedis artery and deep peroneal nerve lie on the lateral aspect of the EHL, and the dissection is deepened on the medial aspect of the EHL to protect the neurovascular bundle.

4. Because the proximal stump of the tendon often retracts to the level of the ankle joint after rupture, exploration should proceed proximally to identify the end of the tendon. With a rupture, the proximal stump is often found deep to the extensor retinaculum and is often adherent to the synovial sheath. The site of rupture is typically just proximal to the site of the tendon insertion and just distal to the inferior border of the superior extensor retinaculum. The tendon sheath is incised longitudinally and the hematoma debrided (Figs. 24-23A and 24-24A and B). After debridement of the tendon ends, a No. 1 nonabsorbable suture is used to approximate the tendons with a Bunnell, Krackow (Fig. 24-23B, see Fig. 24-4), or modified Kessler technique (Fig. 24-24C). The tendon edges are then oversewn with an interrupted absorbable suture. If the tendon has avulsed or is lacerated from its distal attachment, a suture anchor can be inserted into the cuneiform and the tendon secured to the periosteum. The periosteum should be elevated locally and the bone drilled or chiseled to activate a more robust healing response (Figs. 24-23C and 24-24D-F). If adequate length is available, it can be passed through an osseous tunnel and secured with the suture anchor (see Fig. 24-23D and E).

5. The synovial sheath is repaired, but the inferior extensor retinaculum is not repaired to prevent formation of adhesions (Fig. 24-24G).

6. The skin is approximated in a routine manner.

Postoperative Care

A below-knee cast or splint is applied with the foot in maximum dorsiflexion. Weight bearing and walking is permitted in a cast, boot brace, or an AFO 2 to 3 weeks after surgery. Immobilization is continued for 12 weeks

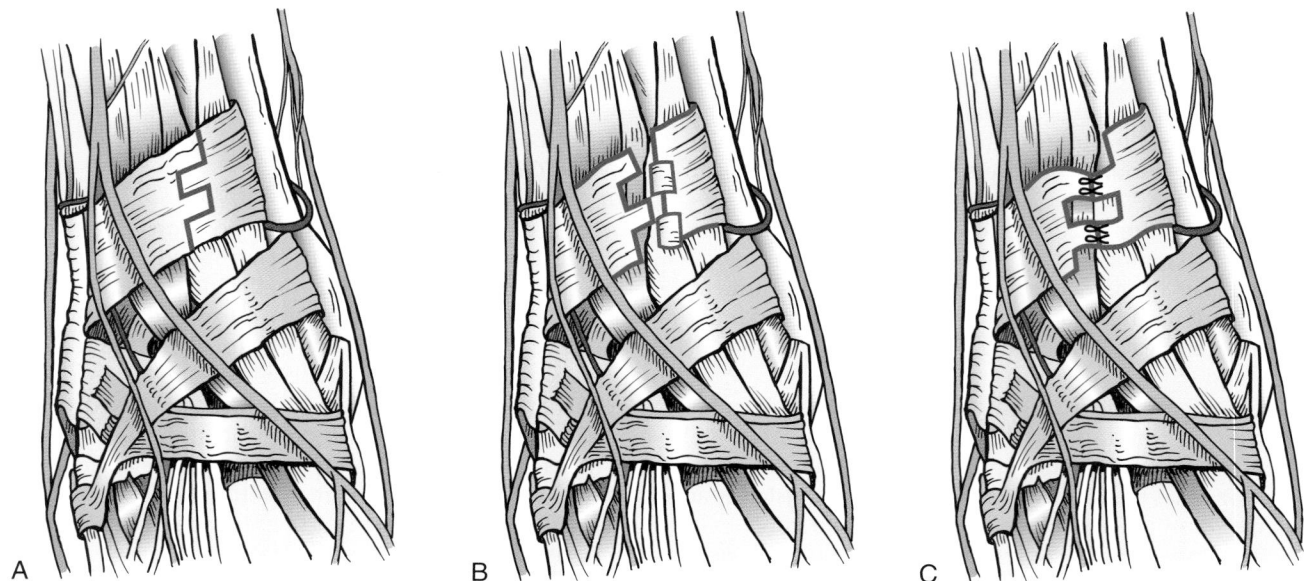

Figure 24-22 **A,** The retinaculum is cut in a step-cut fashion. This allows exposure of the extensor tendons below. **B,** The square wave is then closed with the squares shifted so that the extra capacity is achieved to make room for a tendon reconstruction. **C,** After repair of retinaculum in lengthened fashion.

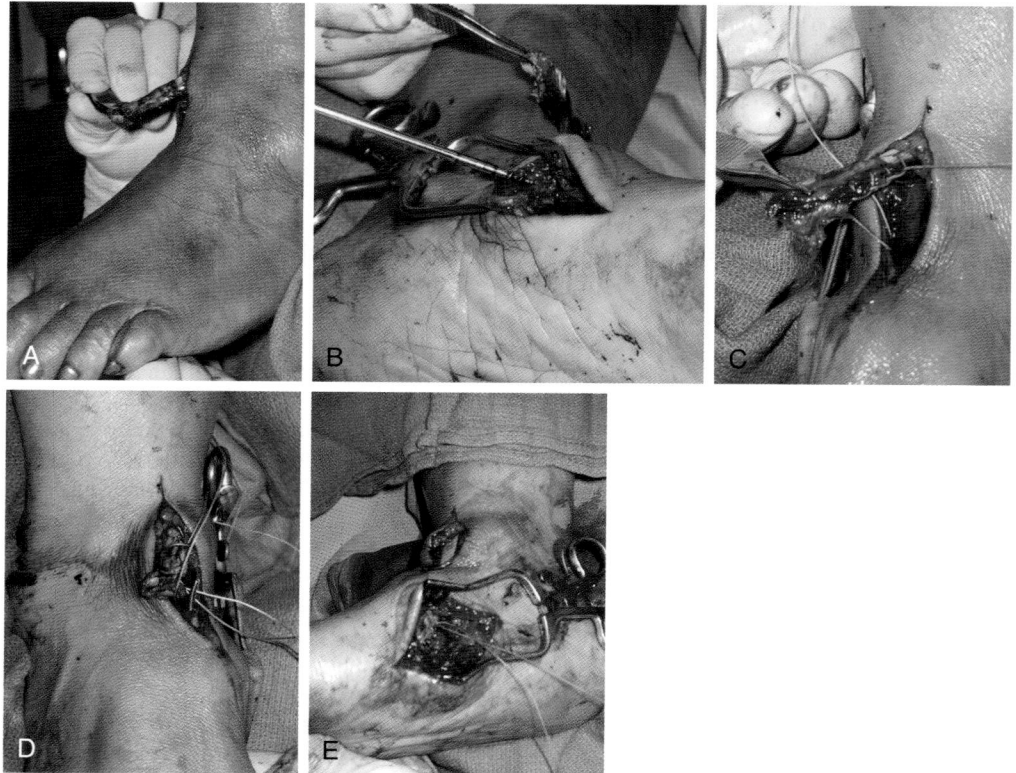

Figure 24-23 **A,** Patient with acute rupture of the anterior tibial tendon. **B,** Krackow suture placed in the distal tendon stump. **C,** A suture anchor is placed at the old insertion site, which is prepared by lifting off local periosteum. **D,** Distal tendon is passed through a tunnel into its position at the plantar medial aspect of the medial cuneiform. **E,** After repair of the anterior tibial tendon to suture anchor.

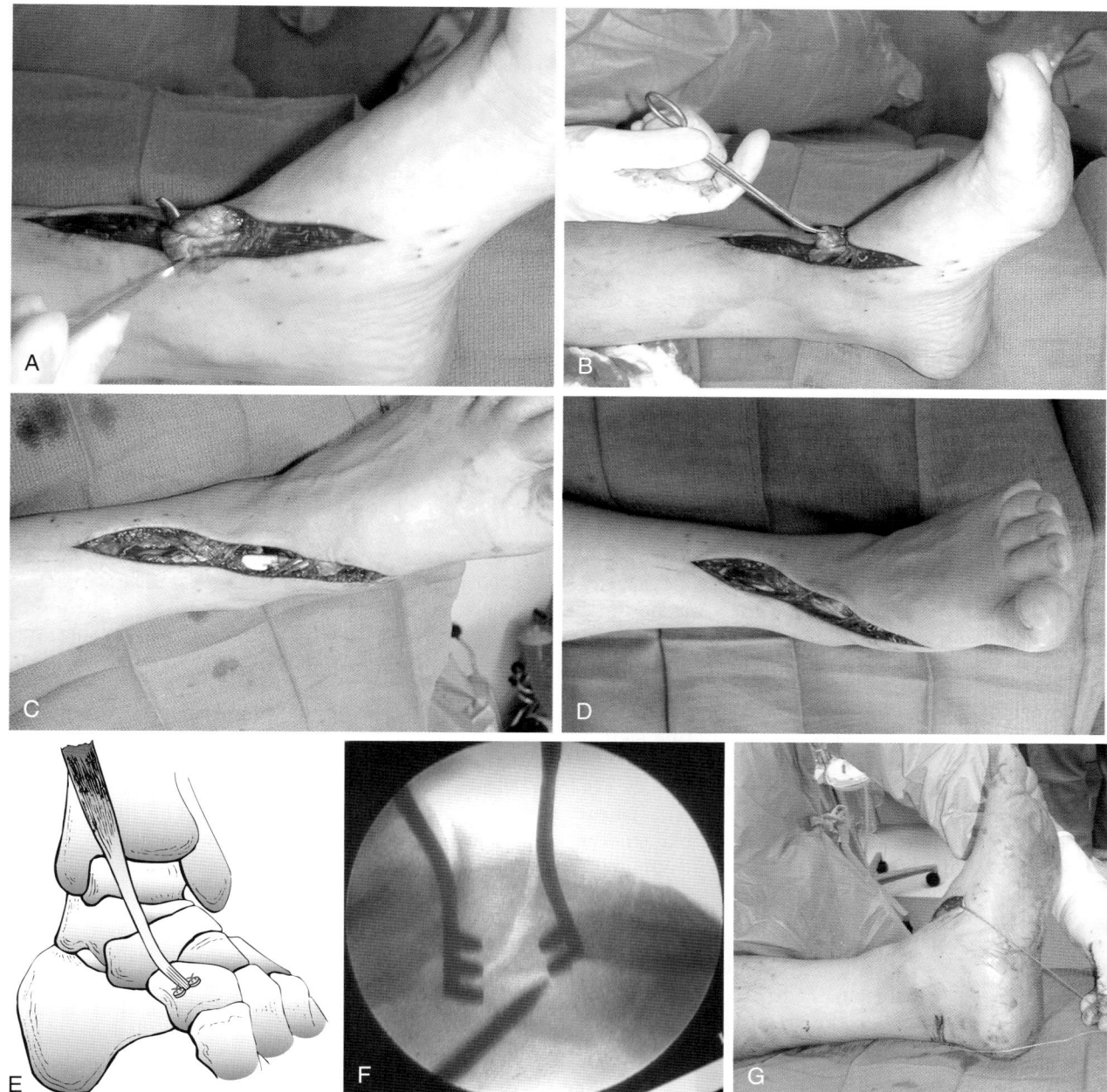

Figure 24-24   A, Intraoperative photograph demonstrates a hematoma at the site of a recent anterior tibial tendon rupture. **B,** Ruptured anterior tibial tendon is pulled into the wound. **C** and **D,** Intraoperative photograph demonstrates primary repair of the tendon, with adequate dorsiflexion of ankle after repair. **E,** Placement of suture anchor into the navicular and placement into the cuneiform **(F). G,** Lateral view of ankle brought into dorsiflexion with securing of the tendon to the suture anchor.

during the day and at night as well. For those who object to wearing their boot at night because of bulkiness or for hygiene reasons, a more open "breathable" lightweight padded or air-cushioned night splint can be worn. Dorsiflexion exercises with deep knee bends, performed five times a day for 20 minutes for each episode, can maintain muscle tone and prevent development of an Achilles contracture. Full range-of-motion exercises are initiated 6 to 8 weeks after surgery. Progressive resumption of walking

without the brace is initiated 8 to 12 weeks after surgery. Jogging, jumping, running, or aggressive athletic activities are initiated as tolerated.

Alternate Techniques
The anterior tibial tendon also may be lengthened using a sliding anterior tibial tendon graft that spans the rupture site, anastomosing the proximal and distal segments of the tendon[62,67] Turn-down tendon grafts have

been advocated, as well, to bridge or span deficient areas.[50,51] Several different tendon transfers have been described to bridge a gap in the anterior tibial tendon. Forst et al[49] accomplished a delayed repair by bridging an extensive defect with a peroneus brevis tendon graft. Smith[83] and others* have used a hamstring autograft or allograft to bridge the defect. Moberg[72] and others[65] recommended an EHL tendon transfer to the distal stump of the anterior tibial tendon. The more proximal EHL tendon is tenodesed to the distal anterior tibial tendon stump, which is secured through a drill hole into the medial cuneiform or into the distal stump of the anterior tibial tendon. Postoperative care is similar to that described for a primary repair. An EDL transfer has been used as well.[65]

Results and Complications

Mankey[67] reported that uniformly good results were achieved with reconstruction of a ruptured anterior tibial tendon. Morris et al[73] reported that patients with repaired anterior tibial tendons had weakness in dorsiflexion relative to the contralateral side. Despite finding a 75% average peak torque strength and 62% of work capacity compared with the contralateral side, there was no functional impairment.[73] Most studies recommend surgical reconstruction for a symptomatic patient with moderate or greater levels of physical activity. Other than failure of reconstruction, no significant complications have been reported in the literature. The patient should be alerted to potential complications, including adhesions, rerupture, neuroma formation, and decreased function not only at the rupture site but also at the donor site, where a tendon is harvested to aid in the anterior tibial tendon reconstruction. Kopp et al[65] reported on the treatment of 10 anterior tibial tendon ruptures. Five were successfully treated with a primary repair, and five required augmentation with either an EHL or EDL tendon transfer. The authors did, however, observe that even with a repair of the ruptured tendon, there remained a decrease in strength on the operative side when the average peak torque in dorsiflexion was measured.

Delayed Surgical Treatment

There are five options in delayed treatment of an anterior tibial rupture: primary repair, reconstruction with a free graft (allograft or autograft), reconstruction with a turn-down procedure, reconstruction with an adjacent tendon transfer, and conservative management. Whichever option is chosen, it is important to recognize that a secondary Achilles tendon contracture may be present. Typically, if a contracture is identified, aggressive stretching preoperatively and postoperatively can minimize its consequences. If the Achilles is determined to be too contracted, with a 10- to 15-degree difference compared with the contralateral side, an Achilles lengthening or Strayer procedure may be beneficial.

---

*References 35, 36, 50, 52, 84, and 85.

A similar surgical approach is used for a delayed repair as for an acute repair. If an end-to-end repair is not possible after the proximal segment is mobilized, the gap may be bridged with a tendon graft. This may be a sliding tendon graft using the anterior tibial tendon, although the sliding graft can leave a scar beneath the more proximal extensor retinaculum.[63,67,68]

ANTERIOR TIBIAL TENDON SLIDING GRAFT OR TURN-DOWN

Surgical Technique

1. The patient is placed in a supine position with a thigh tourniquet for hemostasis.
2. An anterior curvilinear incision is made on the inferomedial aspect of the anterior tibial tendon and extended from the level of the first cuneiform proximally to the level of the superior extensor retinaculum.
3. The anteroinferior extensor retinaculum is divided, and the anterior tibial tendon is identified. The distal stump is traced to its insertion in the first cuneiform. The proximal stump is identified. It may have retracted several centimeters proximally.
4. The proximal tendon end is grasped and pulled. If there is no springiness to the musculotendinous complex, then a tendon transfer may be necessary. With good springiness of at least 1 cm, a sliding graft or a turn-down may be performed (Fig. 24-25).
5. The tendon is mobilized proximally. Distally, the residual tendon should be identified. Occasionally, the tendon is very scarred and cannot be identified, particularly with a very distal rupture. In these situations, the path of the old tendon should be recreated down to the cuneiform.

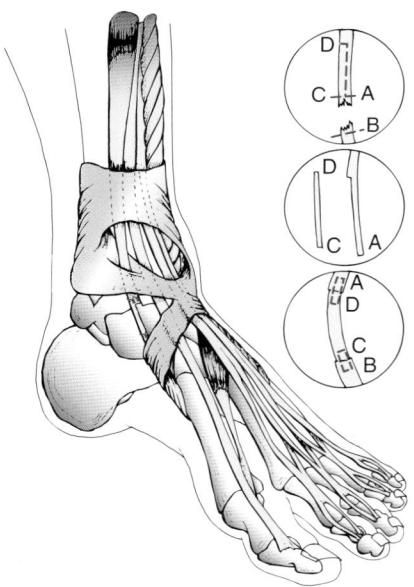

Figure 24-25 Technique of sliding tendon graft as a delayed repair to bridge a defect in the tendon. (*A*, Distal portion of proximal segment. *B*, Transverse cut on proximal aspect of distal segment. *C* and *D*, Ends of free segment to be transferred.)

6. With the ankle held in dorsiflexion and the tendon ends pulled toward each other, the gap is measured. For this procedure, the length of the graft harvested should permit an overlap of 1.5 cm for each anastomosis. Thus for a gap of 4 cm, a 7-cm section of proximal tendon is harvested that includes 3 cm for the overlap (1.5 cm at each anastomosis). Next, half the width of the tendon is harvested from the proximal tendon and transferred distally as a free graft or as a turn-down.

7. A modified Bunnell, Krackow, or Kessler suture is used to anastomose the tendon graft at the proximal and distal ends (see Fig. 24-4A-C). The ankle is held in a neutral position during the repair and until the splint is applied in a neutral position at the conclusion of the reconstruction.

8. The tendon sheath is repaired, but the inferior extensor retinaculum is not repaired in order to prevent formation of adhesions.

9. The skin is approximated in a routine manner, and the postoperative splint is applied.

Postoperative Care

A posterior and/or U splint, or a below-knee cast, is applied with the foot in the maximally dorsiflexed position. Weight bearing is permitted 2 to 3 weeks after surgery using a CAM-boot or AFO. Immobilization is continued for 12 weeks during the day and at night. At night, the patient may wear a lightweight padded or air-cushioned night splint. Dorsiflexion exercises with deep knee bends, performed five times a day for 20 minutes with each exercise episode, can help to maintain muscle tone and prevent an Achilles contracture. Full range-of-motion exercises are initiated 9 to 12 weeks after surgery. The patient is cautioned to avoid jumping, running, or aggressive athletic activity for at least 12 to 16 weeks after surgery.

When the proximal stump of the anterior tibial tendon is of insufficient length for repair, the adjacent EHL or EDL tendon or an allograft can be used as a graft to span the defect.[44,72,76] The authors recommend attempting the tendon slide or turn-down or allograft when the musculoskeletal complex is not fibrotic and tissue is adequate. When these two conditions are not met, the authors would then consider an EHL tendon transfer or tendon graft.

EXTENSOR HALLUCIS LONGUS TRANSFER
Surgical Technique

1. A similar exposure is used as described for the technique of a primary repair or sliding tendon graft.

2. After the fibrous tissue and hematoma are debrided at the rupture site, the EHL tendon is dissected distally at the level of the first MTP joint and is anastomized to the extensor hallucis brevis tendon before transection (Fig. 24-26A and see Fig. 24-27D).

3. The proximal stump of the anterior tibial tendon is sutured to the adjacent EHL tendon, providing that the musculotendinous unit is not fibrotic.

4. The EHL tendon is divided distally and tenodesed to the EHB tendon (Fig. 24-27).

5. The EHL tendon is tunneled into the cuneiform and tensioned with the ankle in dorsiflexion. A horizontal

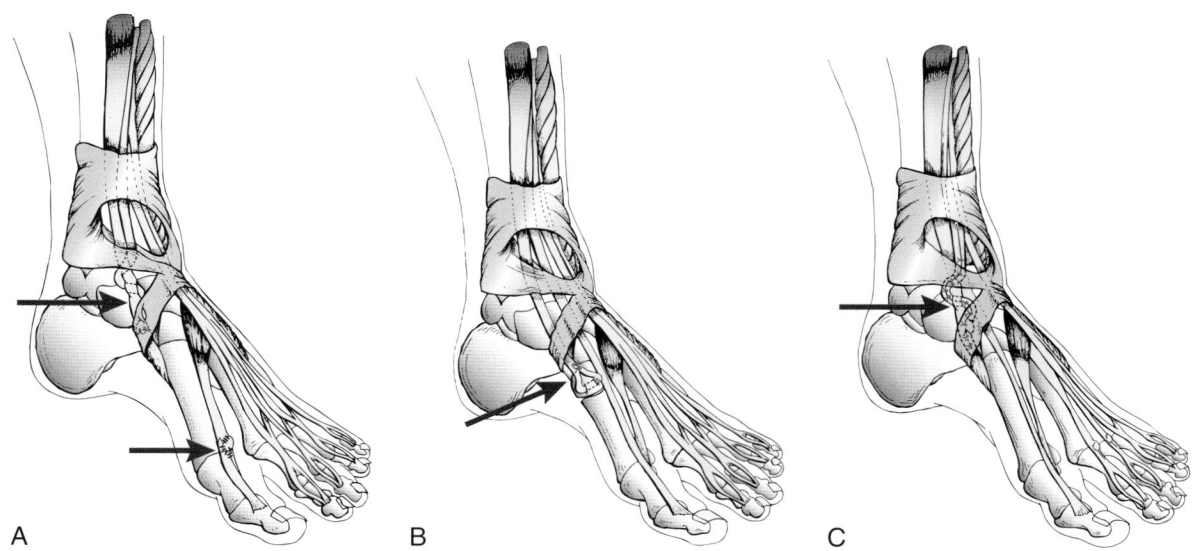

A   B   C

Figure 24-26 **A,** Reconstruction of anterior tibial tendon using Pulvertaft weave of extensor hallucis longus tendon into distal anterior tibial tendon. **B,** Reconstruction of distal rupture of anterior tibial tendon. Tendon is advanced through a horizontal drill hole in the navicular or first cuneiform and sutured to itself. **C,** Reconstruction of ruptured anterior tibial tendon using Kelikian procedure. Extensor digitorum longus (EDL) tendon to second and third toes is woven through anterior tibial tendon. EDL tendon to second and third toes is tenodesed to the extensor digitorum brevis. (**A** and **C,** Modified from Markarian G, Kelikian A, Brage M, et al: Anterior tibialis tendon ruptures: an outcome analysis of operative versus nonoperative treatment, *Foot Ankle Int* 19:792–802, 1998.)

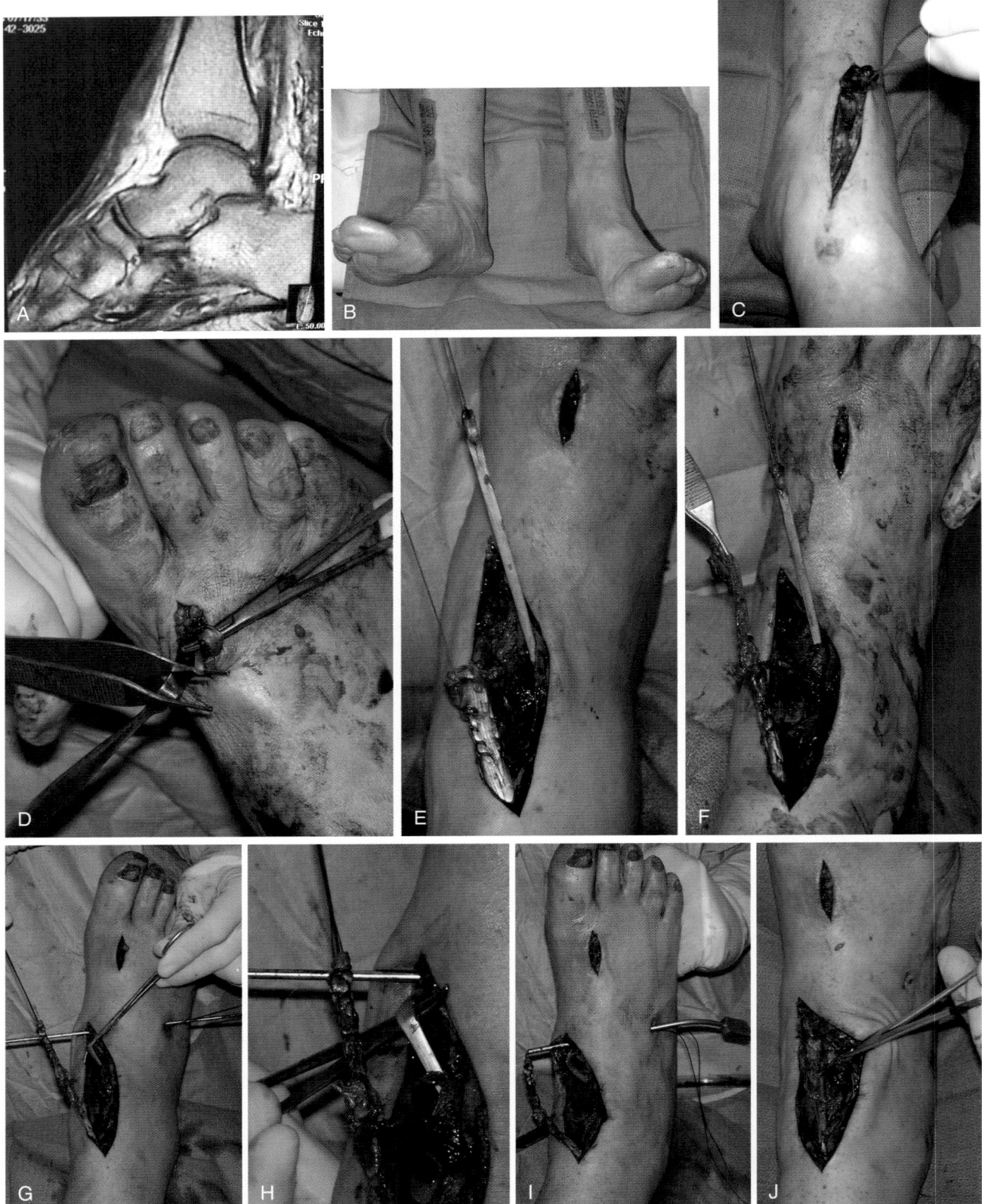

Figure 24-27   Reconstruction of chronic anterior tibial tendon with turn-down and extensor hallucis longus (EHL) tendon graft. **A,** Sagittal magnetic resonance image demonstrating a long zone of fibrotic ruptured anterior tibial tendon. **B,** Clinical appearance of chronic anterior tibial tendon rupture. **C,** End of ruptured tendon. **D,** EHL tendon is identified distally and anastomosed to the extensor hallucis brevis before transection. **E,** The Krackow stitch is placed in the anterior tibial tendon, and the EHL is prepared for transfer. The anterior tibial tendon is too short, so the sutures are removed and a turn-down (**F**) is performed. **G,** The EHL is tunneled through a drill hole through all the cuneiforms from medial to lateral. The tunnel is wide enough to insert the anterior tibial tendon as well. The drill bit demonstrates the pathway. The clamp is under the EHL, whose suture protrudes laterally. **H,** A close-up of the transfers. **I,** A suction tip is placed from lateral to medial to help pass the anterior tibial tendon graft. **J,** The tendons are in the tunnel and fixed with suture anchors medially and laterally under proper tension.

or vertical drill hole is made in the first cuneiform, and the tendon is passed through the bony tunnel and fixed with either a pull-out wire or a bone anchor (Fig. 24-26B and C). Because the EHL graft is long, it is possible to drill from the first cuneiform to the third, exiting just dorsal to the cuboid laterally. This tunnel can be drilled using the guidewire for the cannulated 6.5-, 7.0-, or 7.3-mm screw systems and then over-drilled once a proper position is established with the set's cannulated drill bit. Using a suction tip from the lateral side, the sutures in the EHL tendon can be passed from medial to lateral.

6. The EHL tendon is sewn to itself and/or secured with a tenodesis screw while tension is applied to the graft with the ankle held in dorsiflexion. A soft tissue interference screw can be inserted medially and, if necessary, an additional one can be inserted laterally.
7. The sutures that had been placed in the EHL tendon should be passed through the bone and tied, if the tendon is not secured to itself.

In the presence of a tendon avulsion from the medial cuneiform insertion or with minimal tendon retraction, the tendon can be advanced and reinserted through a drill hole or with a suture anchor in the first cuneiform. Another option is an extensor tendon transfer to augment the anterior tibial tendon reconstruction, performed with direct repair or turn-down/slide reconstruction (Figs. 24-27 and 24-28).[47]

HAMSTRING AUTOGRAFT OR ALLOGRAFT RECONSTRUCTION[83]
Surgical Technique (Video Clip 115)

1. The patient is placed in a supine position on the operating room table. A thigh tourniquet may be used for hemostasis.
2. A longitudinal incision is centered over the dorsal medial aspect of the foot in line with the anterior tibial tendon. The incision is carried from the medial cuneiform proximally to the anterior ankle joint. The proximal stump of the anterior tibial tendon, which often retracts to the level of the ankle joint, is identified.
3. The degenerative area of the tendon stump is debrided along with any scar or hematoma.
4. A gracilis tendon is harvested from the ipsilateral knee (or an allograft is obtained) and then sutured to the proximal anterior tibial tendon stump using a Pulvertaft weave (Fig. 24-29A).
5. The medial cuneiform is identified (fluoroscopy may be used to ensure accuracy).
6. A dorsal to plantar drill hole is placed through the medial cuneiform. It is important to retain a sufficient medial bony bridge to avoid fracture of this bone with the tendon graft transfer.
7. The free end of the tendon graft is then pulled through the drill hole, tensioned adequately with the ankle in

a neutral position, and sutured back onto itself and the proximal anterior tibial tendon (Fig. 24-29B-D).
8. The wound is closed in a routine fashion.
9. Alternatively, the free tendon graft may be passed through the proximal tendon and then secured distally with an interference screw (Fig. 24-30).

Postoperative Care
A posterior splint, combined with a U-splint or a below-knee cast, is applied with the foot in a maximally dorsiflexed position. Weight bearing is permitted 2 to 3 weeks after surgery, using a boot brace or AFO. Immobilization is continued for 12 weeks during the day and at night. At night the patient may wear a lightweight padded or air-cushioned night splint. Dorsiflexion exercises with deep knee bends, performed five times a day for 20 minutes for each episode, can minimize atrophy and prevent equinus contracture. Full range-of-motion exercises are initiated 9 to 12 weeks after surgery. The patient is cautioned to avoid jumping, running, or aggressive athletic activity for at least 12 to 16 weeks after surgery.

Other Techniques
Kelikian and Kelikian[63] suggested transferring the EDL tendon of the second and third toes to the distal stump of the anterior tibial tendon. A tenodesis of the EDB to the distal stumps of the EDL of the second and third toes is then performed (see Fig. 24-26C).

Forst et al[49] used a peroneus brevis tendon transfer, tenodesing the peroneus longus and brevis proximally. Then they resected a 9-cm segment of peroneus brevis, using this as a free graft to bridge the defect at the site of the anterior tibial tendon rupture. If the anterior tibial muscle is no longer viable because of fibrosis, the peroneus longus can be used. It is harvested distally by the cuboid and passed from posterior behind the fibula into the anterior compartment and then inserted into the lateral cuneiform. Yamazaki et al[85] reported the use of an autogenous hamstring graft to bridge a large gap in the lower leg after a traumatic injury that left a defect in the anterior tibial tendon (Fig. 24-31).

Results and Conclusion

There are no long-term prospective studies that assess the value of operative treatment, and thus clinicians are left to examine the results of relatively small series in which often operative and nonoperative treatment has been provided. Although ruptures of the anterior tibial tendon occur infrequently, accurate early diagnosis enables a patient and physician to choose between conservative and surgical treatment. For the older patient with a lower level of activity, bracing or nonsurgical treatment may be sufficient. In those desiring a higher level of function, either acute repair or delayed reconstruction with a tendon transfer may be indicated. Although a direct primary repair is preferable, a tendon transfer or

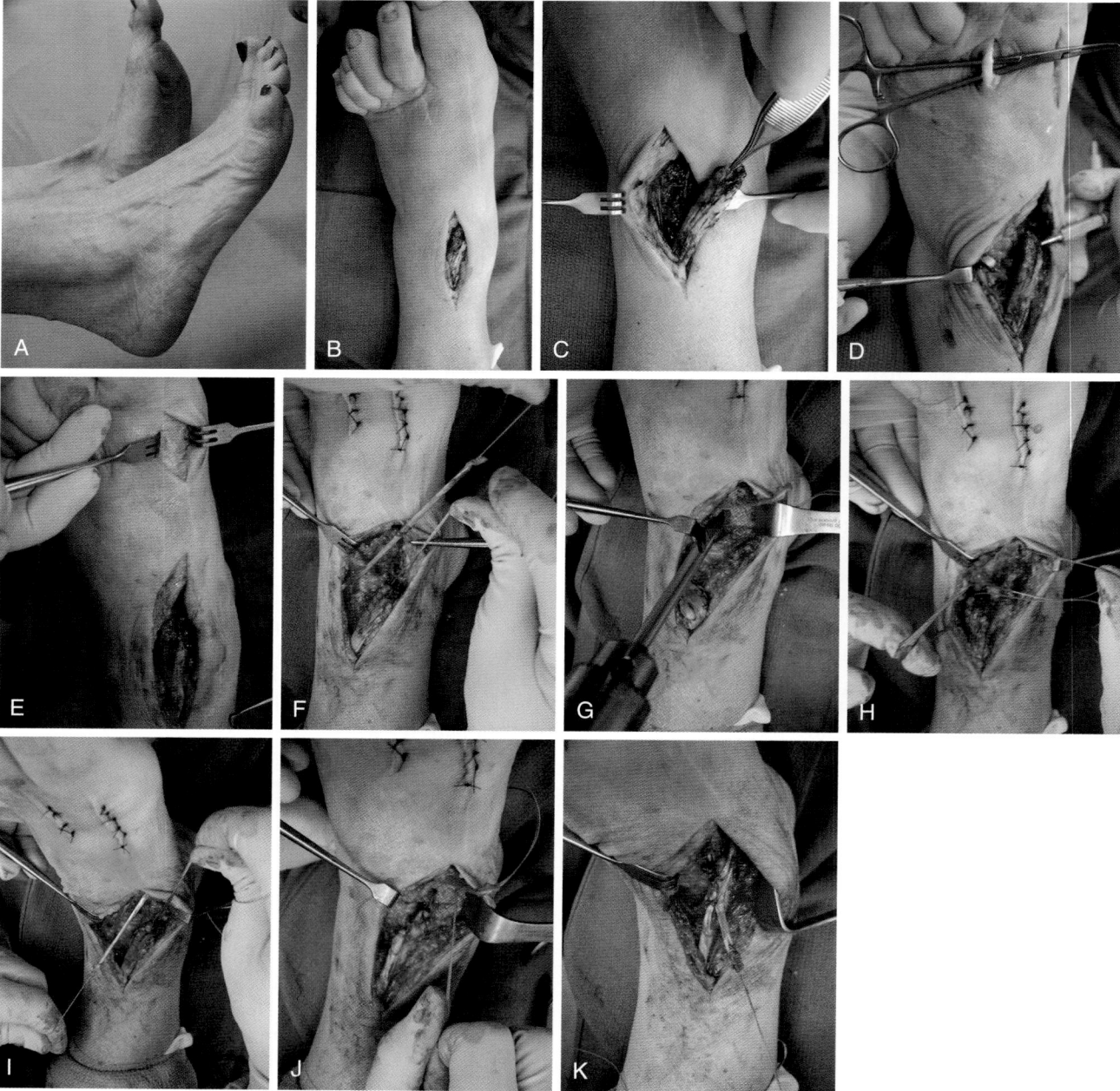

Figure 24-28 Rupture of anterior tibial tendon reconstructed with extensor digitorum longus (EDL) transfer. **A,** Clinical examination demonstrates lack of dorsiflexion of right ankle. **B,** Initial exposure demonstrating rupture of anterior tibial tendon. **C,** After debridement of tendon stump. **D,** Distal exposure of extensor to the second toe and exposure of extensor hallucis longus. **E,** After tenodesis of distal extensor tendon of the second toe to the extensor hallucis longus. **F,** After release of the EDL to second toe, the proximal tendon is pulled into the dorsal wound (there is plenty of EDL tendon length for the reconstruction). **G,** A transverse drill hole is placed in the medial cuneiform. **H,** The EDL tendon is pulled into the drill hole. (Note Krakow suture in the distal anterior tibial tendon stump.) **I** and **J,** The stump of the anterior tibial tendon is sutured to the EDL tendon, which is pulled through the drill hole in the cuneiform and tensioned. **K,** Final sutures in the reconstruction.

graft may be necessary to span a significant gap. The ultimate goal is improved function, and treatment should be adapted to the patient's needs. Nonsurgical treatment is probably sufficient in the older, less active patient, and surgical repair is indicated in the more active, younger patient.

FLEXOR TENDONS

Flexor Digitorum Longus Tenosynovitis

The flexor digitorum longus (FDL) is the primary plantar flexor of the lateral four toes. Innervated by the tibial nerve, the FDL originates on the posterior tibia below the

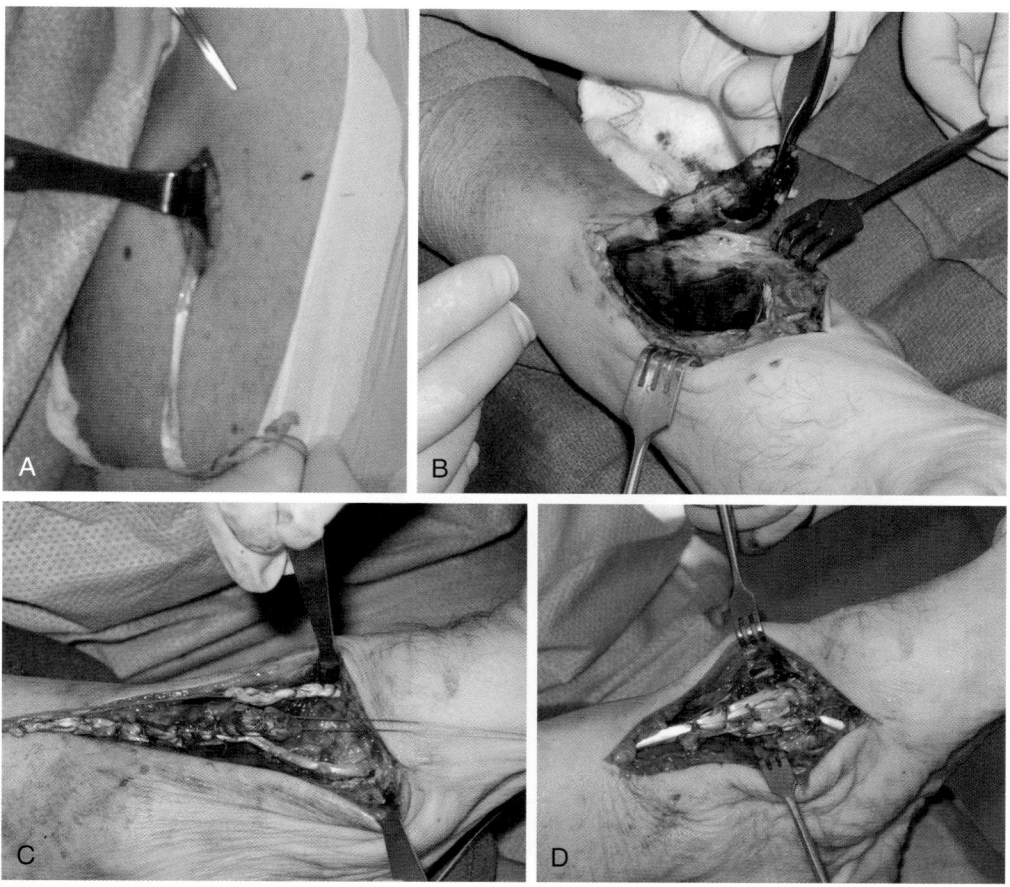

Figure 24-29 Reconstruction of anterior tibial tendon rupture with gracilis tendon autograft. **A,** Harvest of gracilis autograft from ipsilateral knee. **B,** Ruptured anterior tibial tendon stump. **C,** The gracilis tendon autograft is passed through a drill hole in the medial cuneiform from plantar to dorsal. **D,** Completed anterior tibial tendon reconstruction with gracilis tendon autograft sutured in place. (From Smith B, Coughlin M: Technique tip: reconstruction of an acute anterior tibial tendon rupture with a gracilis tendon autograft, *Med Chir Pied* 24:1–3, 2008.)

soleal line and functions to plantar flex the toes and to plantar flex and invert the foot. Lying just posterior to the posterior tibial tendon at the ankle, it courses on the plantar aspect of the tarsus in the deep midfoot before inserting on the distal phalanx of the lateral four toes. It is at risk for laceration in the toes as well as more proximally in the ball of the foot or arch with penetrating injuries.

History and Physical Examination

Although no cases of spontaneous FDL tendon rupture have been reported, flexor tendon ruptures after cortisone injections for interdigital neuromas have been appreciated (Fig. 24-32). FDL tenosynovitis can occur in patients with a posterior tibial tendon disruption caused by the patient overcompensating for the inversion weakness by flexing their toes. Infectious FDL tenosynovitis can occur when a toe or metatarsal ulcer tracks into the FDL sheath. In these cases, a midarch or ankle abscess can develop. There are also reports of tuberculous tenosynovitis requiring multiple surgical procedures.[94] Besides

injection-induced ruptures and overuse, an FDL tendon rupture is almost always associated with a penetrating laceration. A patient often describes a history of stepping on a piece of glass or sharp object, with resultant loss of plantar flexion power to one or more of the lesser toes. Concomitant sensory loss may be noted as well. The penetrating injury may result in wound issues and infection. It is important to note that an FDL tendon deficit is often seen because the FDL tendon is frequently harvested for posterior tibial tendon reconstructions and occasionally for Achilles or peroneal tendon reconstructions. Patients who have had this surgery will report minor dysfunction, such as weakness of lesser toe curling, particularly in the third, fourth, and fifth toes. Occasionally, they will note a lack of stability when rising on their toes or balancing on the forefoot. Patients might complain that the toe gets caught on the inside of a shoe or sock as they dress.

On physical examination, a laceration distal to the knot of Henry is often associated with weakness or absence of plantar flexion of the lesser toes. Most patients have poor individual control of flexion and extension of

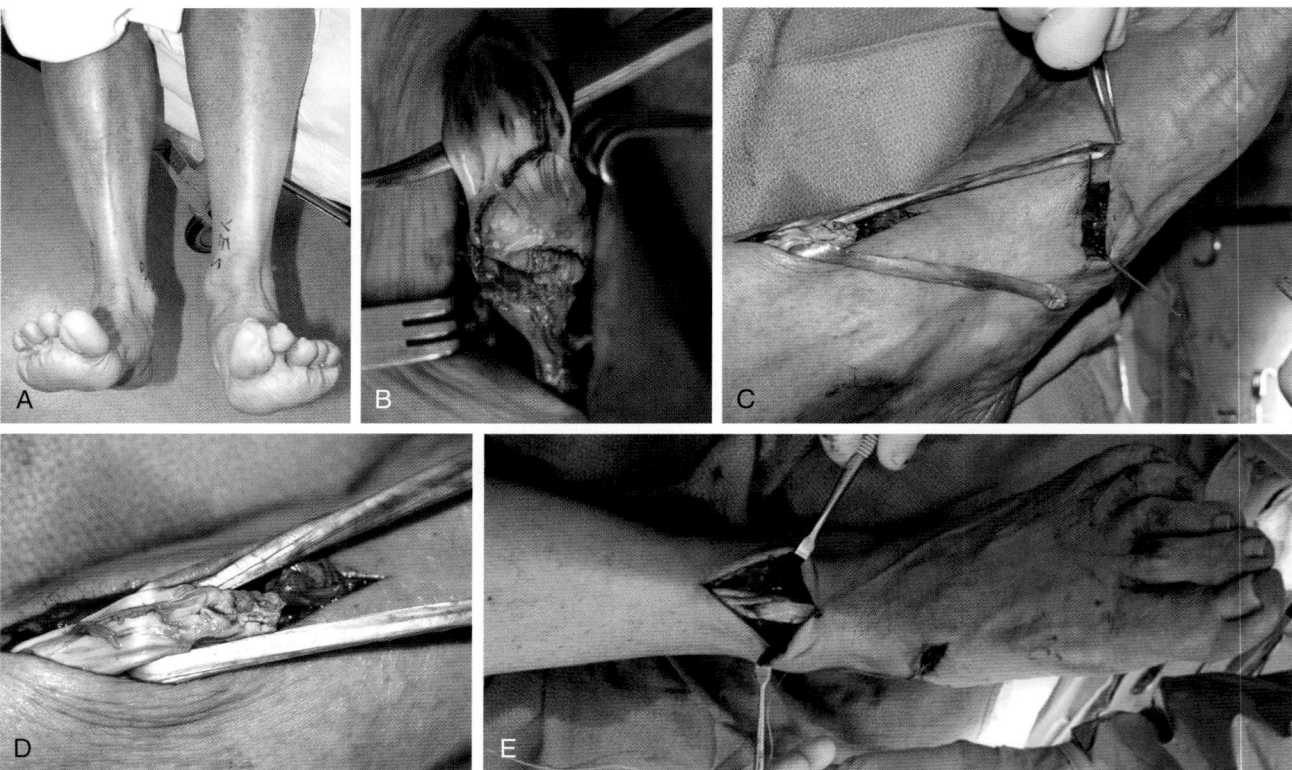

Figure 24-30 A, Delayed diagnosis of rupture of anterior tibial tendon (left ankle). Note that the injured ankle dorsiflexes less and everts more. The medial ray is still relatively plantar flexed. **B,** Intraoperative photograph of rupture. **C,** Free tendon graft is passed through the distal end of the healthier aspect of the tendon, creating two graft ends for attachment. One limb is passed into a tunnel in the dorsal aspect of the cuneiform, and the other is passed into a more plantar medial tunnel as indicated by the protruding wires. The graft is secured using 6- to 7-mm–wide soft tissue interference screws. **D,** Close-up of graft through the anterior tibial tendon. **E,** After completion of repair. Tensioning the graft is critical to achieve dorsiflexion.

the lesser toes, but diagnosis of FDL tendon disruption can be demonstrated by stabilizing the MTP joint and asking the patient to plantar flex the tip of the toe. Weakness or absence of plantar flexion strength to one or more of the lesser toes can demonstrate an isolated disruption of the FDL to an individual toe or a complete disruption of the FDL.[23] Because specific function of the FDL is at the DIP joint, lack of flexion power indicates a rupture (Figs. 24-33 and 24-34).

Proximal to the master knot of Henry, because of a connecting slip from the flexor hallucis longus (FHL), flexion of the DIP joint can remain despite a proximal disruption of the FDL tendon. It is typical that the second toe will maintain flexion based on the FHL tendon attachment, but the third toe can also be connected by a slip. At the ankle level, an FDL injury is often associated with tibial nerve symptoms. In the midtarsus, an FDL tendon laceration is often associated with medial plantar nerve symptoms. Often, at the distal metatarsal level or toe level, injury to an adjacent digital sensory nerve is associated with injuries of the FHL or FDL tendons. Chronic FDL tendon rupture can lead to a hammer toe or swan neck deformity.

Surgical Treatment

While exploring a laceration, the surgeon should keep in mind the principles of trauma care, including adequate irrigation and debridement of the wound. The wound should be explored in a way that does not complicate or exacerbate the injury. Extension of the laceration longitudinally allows an extensile exposure. When possible, a primary repair of the injured tendons is appropriate by using a Bunnell repair, modified Kessler technique, or Krackow tendon repair (see Fig. 24-4A-C).

Postoperative care necessitates immobilization in a below-knee cast for 4 to 6 weeks if the disruption is at or proximal to the master knot. Extension of the cast over the dorsal aspect of the toes prevents excessive dorsiflexion and protects the repair. If the laceration is distal to the master knot, the toe can be held flexed after repair by gluing a metal hook to the toenail and attaching it to a rubber band that is connected proximally and plantarly to a splint or dressing (Fig. 24-35).

In a review of preferences of many orthopaedic surgeons, Yancey[137] found that 80% to 93% thought repair of the FHL was important, but only 53% to 73% thought surgical repair of a lacerated FDL tendon was indicated.

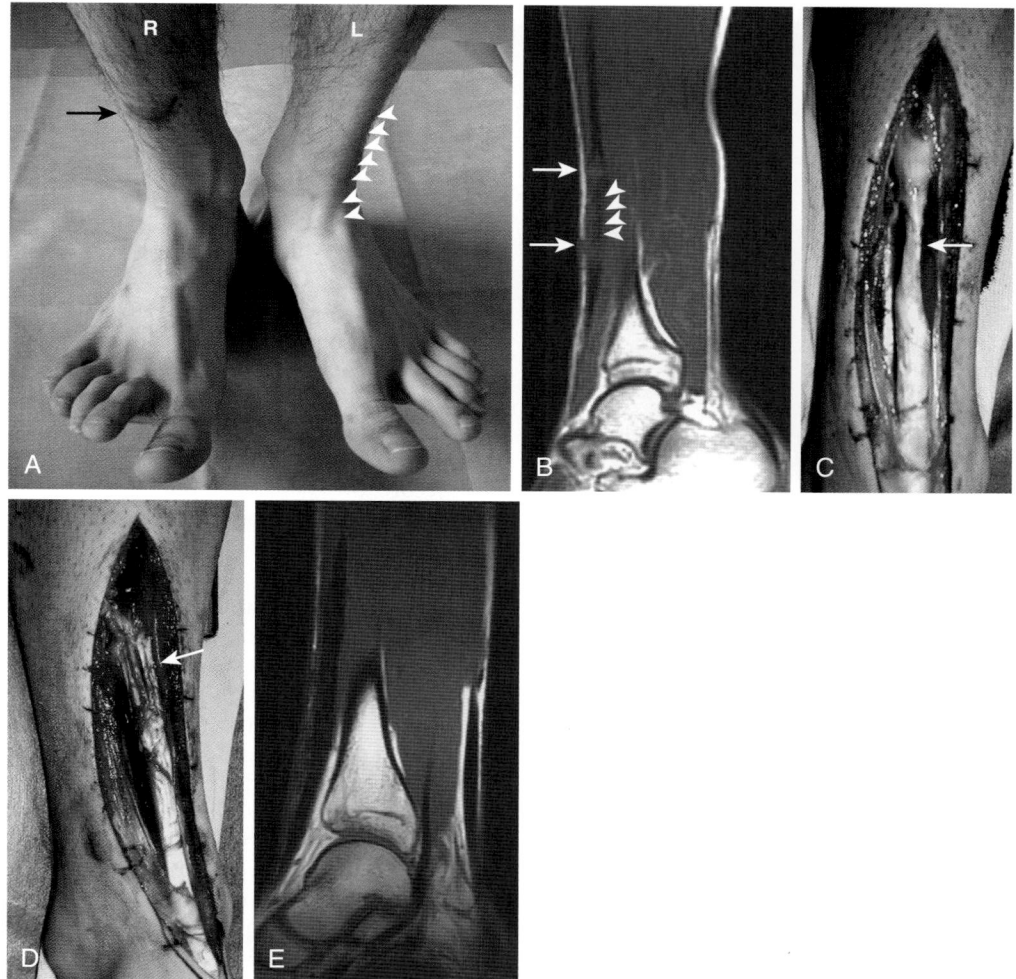

Figure 24-31   Reconstruction of anterior tibial tendon with quadruple gracilis tendon graft. **A,** Six weeks after injury, note scar on right shin, with loss of anterior tibial tendon contour. The *white arrowheads* denote the normal contour of the tendon; the *large black arrow* denotes the transverse scar. **B,** Preoperative T1- weighed sagittal magnetic resonance image (MRI) of the right leg shows a gap between stumps of the tendon (*white arrows and arrowheads*). **C,** Thin cord of fibrous scar tissue (*white arrow*) connects the two tendon stumps of the anterior tibial tendon. **D,** After quadrupled gracilis graft bridges the tendon gap. *White arrow* denotes area of tendon repair. **E,** Postoperative MRI at 1 year shows the reconstructed anterior tibial tendon. (From Yamazaki S, Majima T, Yasui K, et al: Reconstruction of chronic anterior tibial tendon defect using hamstring tendon graft: a case report, *Foot Ankle Int* 28:1190–1193, 2007. Used with permission.)

One FDL tendon laceration was not repaired and had a satisfactory result. Floyd et al[9] reported on lacerated FDL tendon in seven patients: Five underwent a primary repair, one underwent a secondary repair, and one was left unrepaired. The six patients undergoing surgical repair did well. The patient who did not have a repair developed a claw toe deformity. Griffiths[10] reported on one patient who underwent a primary repair with an acceptable result. Wicks et al[33] reported on eight patients who underwent primary repair of a lacerated FDL tendon with six satisfactory results. A hyperextension deformity of the lesser MTP joint developed in the two patients with poor results.

Korovessis et al[106] reported on disruption of the FDL and posterior tibial tendons more proximally at the site of a fractured tibia that was repaired primarily with good result.

The actual site of injury is an important factor in developing a treatment plan for FDL tendon disruption. An injury distal to the knot of Henry leaves the patient without plantar flexion power, whereas an injury proximal to the knot of Henry might leave plantar-flexion power because of the crossover attachment of the FHL tendon.[202] Remaining function can obviate the need for a surgical repair. Treatment of an FDL tendon injury 4 to 6 weeks or longer after injury is likely to be associated with difficulty in reapproximating the tendon.

Aggressive evaluation and repair of open lacerations around the foot are most important. The wound must be explored and debrided, and when possible, an anatomic restoration of the tendons of the FDL tendon is warranted. With significant soft tissue loss, repair of these structures might not be possible. The overall priority is to achieve adequate wound healing and maintain a good plantar weight-bearing surface for ambulation. If a

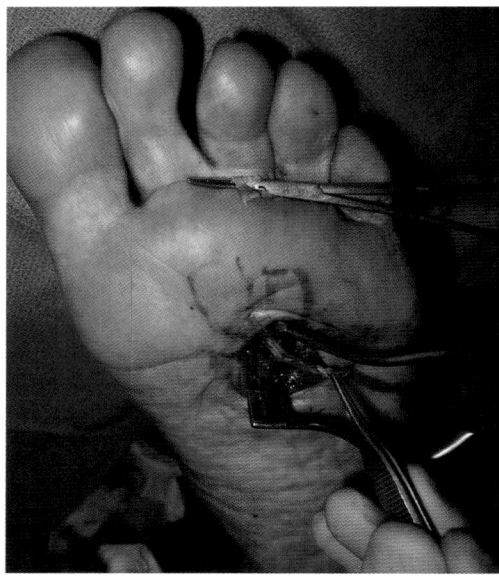

Figure 24-32 Rupture of flexor digitorum longus. The patient had received multiple cortisone injections as treatment for interdigital neuromas. He ultimately developed a bothersome dorsiflexion posture of the toe and an unstable painful metatarsophalangeal joint and an inability to flex the toe. At surgery, the flexor tendon was identified distal and proximal to the weight-bearing plantar fat pad. The tendon ends proximally and distally are sutured with a free graft of extensor digitorum brevis, which was interposed. The tendon is passed through the sheath with a clamp and secured.

hyperextension deformity occurs postoperatively, the surgeon should consider an extensor tenotomy, extensor tendon lengthening, or MTP joint capsulotomy to rebalance clawed toes.

Flexor Hallucis Longus

The FHL tendon is the major plantar flexor of the great toe. It assists with maintaining balance and generating power during walking, running, jumping, climbing, lunging, and squatting. It permits rising up onto the ball of the foot and descending downward in a controlled fashion, as seen in relevé and grand plié in ballet. It is useful during gripping with the toes, particularly with rock climbing, various dance forms, and certain types of kicking sports. Shoes such as sandals or flip flops may not be secure on the foot without the power of the FHL tendon. It works in conjunction with the intricately structured plantar plate and the multiple short flexors to stabilize the MTP joint. Although its action occurs at the MTP, IP, and ankle joints, it assists in stabilizing the subtalar and midfoot joints as well. It is more powerful than the FDL tendon but weaker than the posterior tibial tendons.[131] Its role is important when considering that during normal gait, twice the load of the lesser toes is supported by the great toe,[132] which during jogging and running can approach two to three times body weight. Furthermore, when a running jump is performed, these forces increase to eight times body weight.[117]

The FHL tendon originates from the inferior two thirds of the fibula and the interosseous membrane and courses along the posterior aspect of the tibia and talus. Along the posterior aspect of the talus, there are two tubercles (medial and lateral). The flexor hallucis longus tendon courses between these two tubercles. The os trigonum is the ununited lateral tubercle of the talus (Fig. 24-36). It is

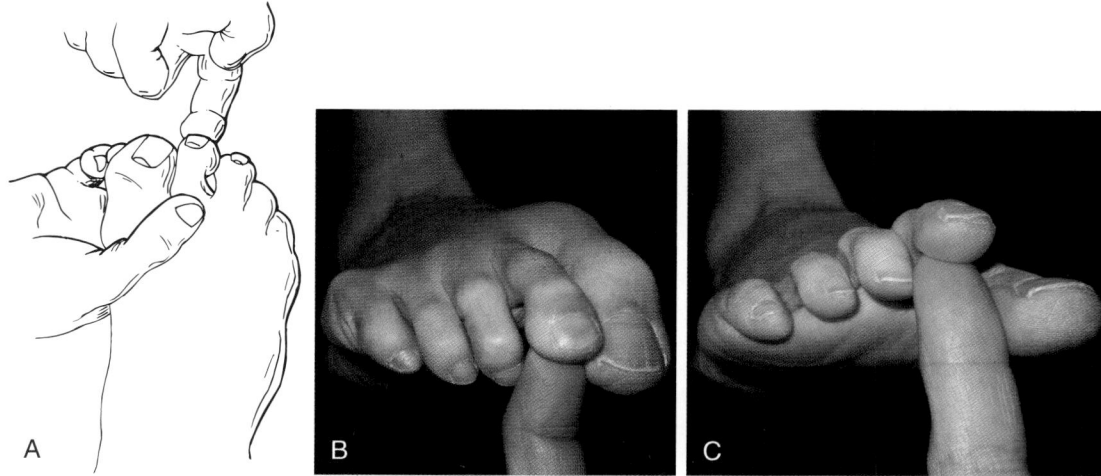

Figure 24-33 **A,** Function of the flexor digitorum longus tendon can be assessed by grasping the forefoot, stabilizing the metatarsophalangeal joint, and requesting the patient to flex the tip of the toe against resistance. **B,** Clinical photograph of intact tendon. **C,** Absence of flexor strength after disruption of the flexor digitorum longus. (**A,** Modified from Rooks M: Tendon, vascular, nerve and skin injuries. In Gould JS, editor: *Operative foot surgery,* Philadelphia, 1994, WB Saunders, p 518.)

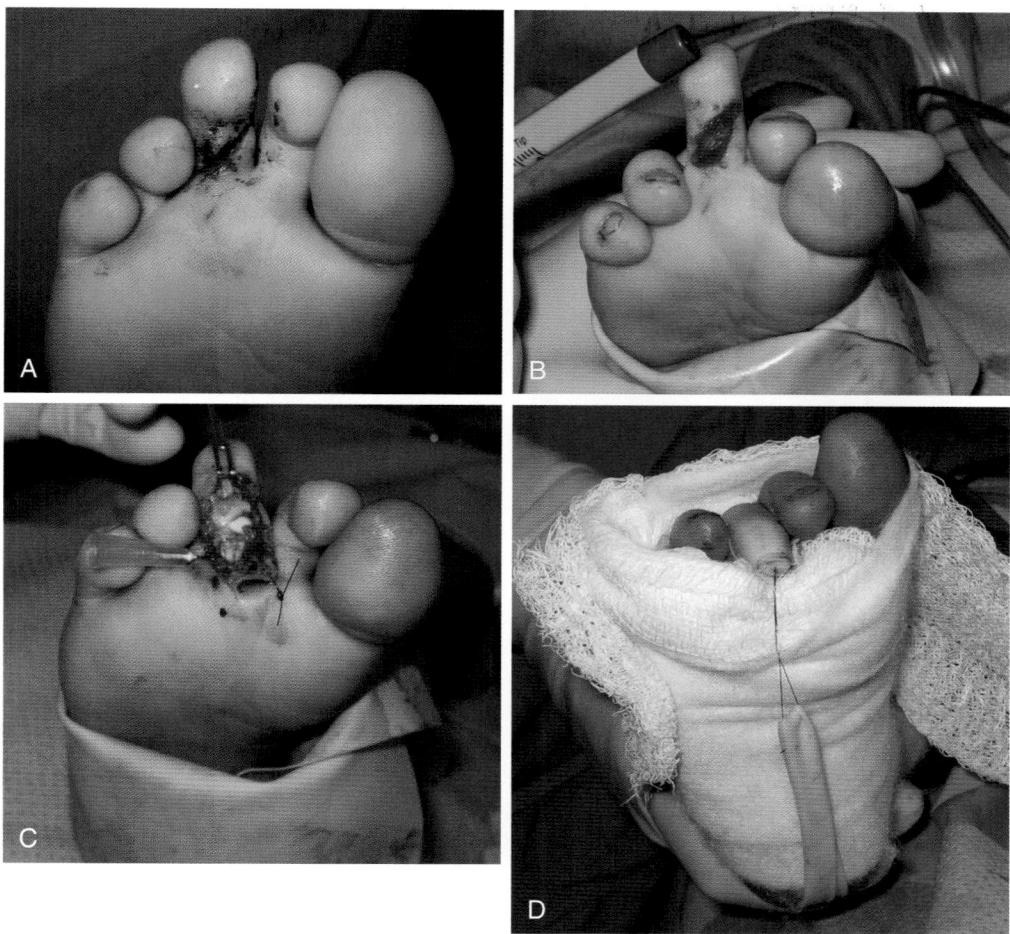

Figure 24-34 **A,** An acute laceration on the underside of the toe penetrated the flexor digitorum longus (FDL), flexor digitorum brevis, and plantar proximal interphalangeal capsule. **B,** There is no resistance to extension of the digit. **C,** The laceration is extended, creating a Z-shaped incision. The flap of skin is sutured to the sole of the foot to permit retraction. A 25-gauge needle is passed through the proximal tendon once the FDL tendon is delivered into the wound to keep it in position during suturing. One limb of the FDL is repaired—not both—to avoid bulk and difficulty reestablishing tendon gliding. The flexor digitorum brevis and capsule are also repaired. The sutures were placed in all the structures, and then the knots were tied with the toe in the flexed position. **D,** 3-0 Nylon is placed through the tip of the nail and then looped around a Penrose drain, which is anchored into the dressing to maintain flexion.

present in 2% to 7% of individuals and is bilateral in 50% of individuals.[87] The tendinous extension of the FHL courses inferior to the sustentaculum tali in a fibroosseous tunnel.[156] Distally, it crosses the flexor digitorum longus at the master knot of Henry, traverses the sole of the foot, and courses between the two heads of the flexor hallucis brevis (FHB) before inserting on the plantar aspect of the distal phalanx. Innervated by the tibial nerve, the FHL tendon flexes the distal phalanx of the hallux and plantar flexes and inverts the foot. The FHL muscle is a strong muscle because the muscle fibers run obliquely to the pull of the tendon (oblique pennation). In muscles with oblique pennation, the cross-sectional diameter of the muscle that is perpendicular to the fibers is greater than the cross-sectional diameter of muscles whose fibers are collinear with the tendon, which are typically better suited to greater excursion than to strength.[89]

Petersen et al[121] studied the blood supply of the FHL tendon by using injections and immunohistochemical studies of cadaver tendons. They found that peritendinous blood vessels penetrated the tendon and anastomosed with a longitudinally oriented intratendinous network. Two avascular zones were demonstrated: one near the posterior talus and the other at the first metatarsal head. The researchers thought that these explained the most typical areas for tendon degeneration and rupture.

Flexor Hallucis Longus Tenosynovitis

Tenosynovitis of the FHL tendon has been described by Lapidus and Seidenstein[108] and others.[110-112] Approximately 50 cases have been described in the literature, mainly as case reports, although series have been reported by Hamilton[100] (17 cases) and others.[101,105,127]

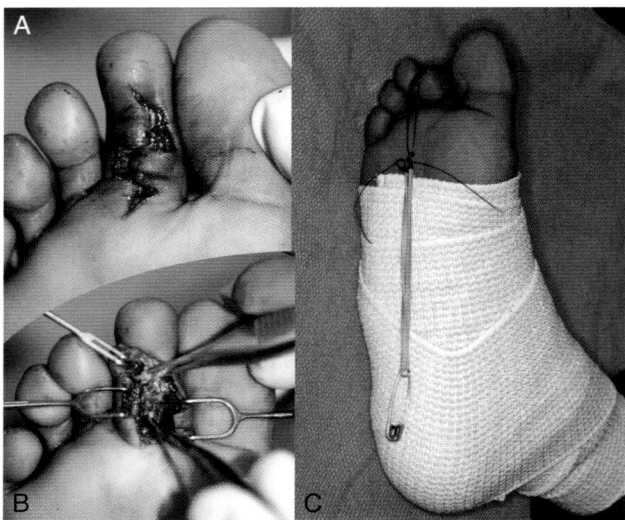

Figure 24-35 Laceration of the flexor digitorum longus in the phalangeal region. **A,** Acute injury. **B,** After repair. **C,** Use of dynamic splint to protect repair.

Most often, tenosynovitis develops proximally at the level of the sustentaculum tali as the tendon enters the fibroosseous tunnel. Often associated with a plantar flexion en pointe position in ballet dancers (Fig. 24-37),[93,98,100,128,136] various pathologic conditions, including hypertrophy of the tendon, synovial adhesions, a more distal insertion of the FHL muscle, longitudinal degenerative tears, and nodularity in the region of the fibroosseous tunnel, have been associated with this condition. McCarroll et al[114] and Kolettis et al[105] have implicated muscle elongation and a distal insertion of the FHL muscle as a cause of this condition.[101]

Gould[99] and Trevino et al[135] have observed that a distal stenosing tenosynovitis could occur at the level where the FHL courses between the sesamoids. Longitudinal tears of the FHL have been reported in association with tenosynovitis.[88,96,128] Hamilton[100] reported FHL tenosynovitis associated with a symptomatic os trigonum, although Kolettis et al[105] noted many cases without an os trigonum.

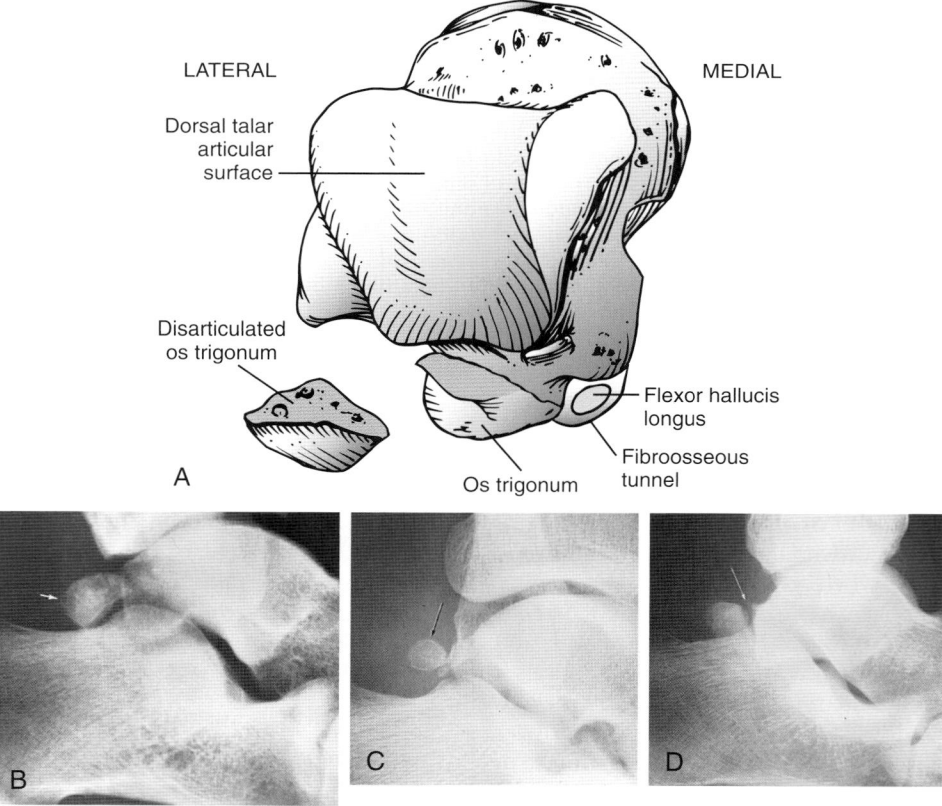

Figure 24-36 **A,** Flexor hallucis longus tenosynovitis may be exacerbated by an adjacent os trigonum. **B** to **D,** Varying sizes and shapes of the os trigonum. (**B, C,** and **D** from Keats TE: *Atlas of Normal Roentgen Variants That Simulate Disease,* ed 4. St. Louis, Mosby, 1987.)

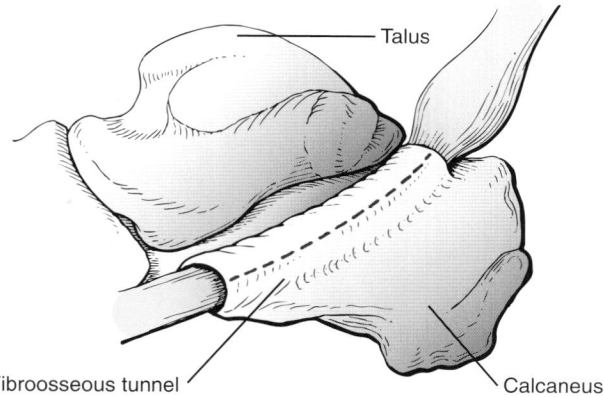

Talus
Fibroosseous tunnel
Calcaneus

Figure 24-39 The flexor hallucis longus can be triggered from nodularity or tendon thickening with restricted motion in the fibroosseous tunnel.

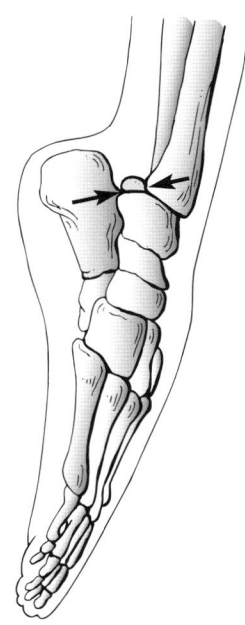

Figure 24-37 Tenosynovitis of the flexor hallucis longus may be associated with an os trigonum and may be exacerbated with forced plantar flexion typical of the en pointe position in ballet dancers.

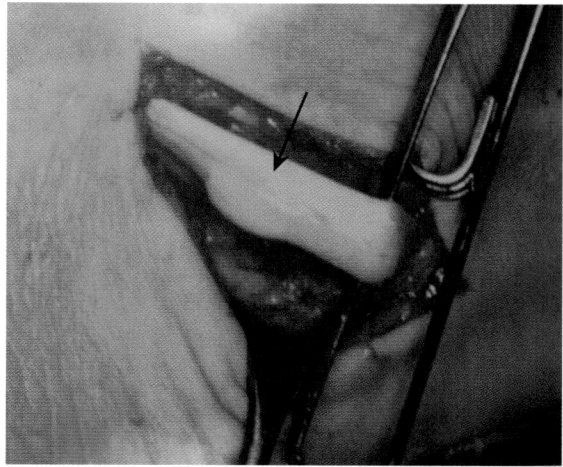

Figure 24-38 Nodule on the flexor hallucis tendon causing triggering of the hallux (arrow). (Courtesy William Hamilton, MD, New York.)

The spectrum of tenosynovitis, FHL triggering, nodularity (Fig. 24-38), and tendon thickening in its natural course can lead to a degenerative tear of the FHL tendon (Fig. 24-39). Frenette and Jackson[97] and others[98,100,128] have described stenosing tenosynovitis. Trepman et al[134] reported a patient who developed posteromedial ankle pain produced with active plantar flexion and passive dorsiflexion of the hallux. The patient had a tearing sensation in the posteromedial ankle with concomitant swelling and ecchymosis. On exploration, a longitudinal tear of the FHL tendon was identified and treated with a primary repair. Fusiform thickening, erosion of the tendon, and eventual triggering can develop from an overuse syndrome.

Another similar case is that of a professional dancer who had a history of triggering of the FHL tendon behind the ankle and suddenly developed a more acute pain associated with a catching or locking of the hallux, which precluded dance. On exploration, a flap tear of the FHL tendon was encountered in addition to the stenosis of the FHL tendon sheath. After release of the sheath and excision of the flap tear, the patient was able to return to Broadway as a principal dancer (Fig. 24-40). Thus the mechanical irritation of the tendon not only may be a source of pain but can also be a risk factor for rupture or tear. This has been observed by several authors, including Sammarco and Miller,[128] who reported fusiform thickening of the FHL tendon with rupture of the central fibers. Kolettis et al[105] reported stenosis of the tendon sheath, synovial hypertrophy, adhesions, mucoid degeneration, tendon nodularity, and several cases of partial FHL tendon tears. Several partial ruptures have also been reported.[107,122,128] These can result from forced extension and against a contracted FHL muscle. Thickening or hypertrophy of the FHL tendon[114] and the presence of a flexor digitorum accessorius longus[116] can lead to constriction in the fibroosseous tunnel with subsequent tenosynovitis.

Entrapment or scarring of the FHL tendon can also occur after distal tibial, ankle, or calcaneus fractures with a different presentation and prognosis that is important to recognize.[91,126,130] Patients complain of inability to roll through the forefoot and often a lack of dorsiflexion flexibility at the ankle as well. In these cases, the deformity increases with dorsiflexion and decreases with plantar flexion of the ankle. This checkrein deformity has treatment implications. If the tendon is adherent to the local bone or soft tissues, it is amenable to release. If the tendon

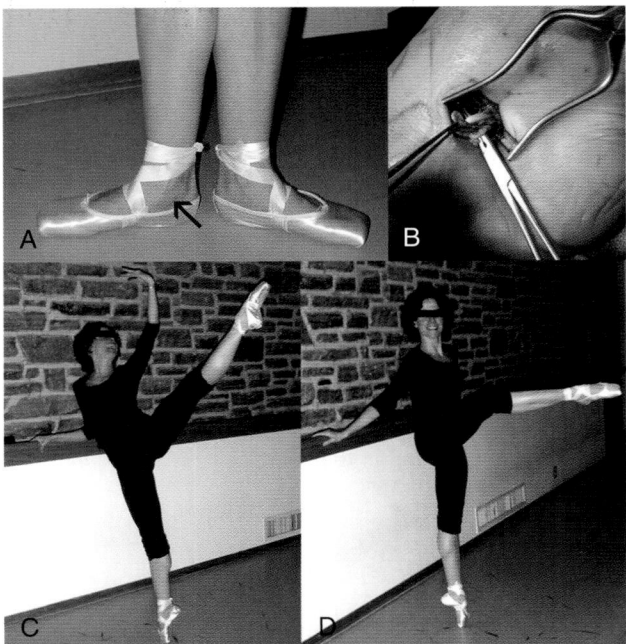

Figure 24-40 Flexor hallucis longus (FHL) tenosynovitis in a professional dancer. **A,** Preoperative swelling of the tendon sheath with a painful limited range of motion of the ankle and great toe. **B,** Intraoperative photograph of tendon sheath release. A flap tear of the tendon is identified and resected. Successful return to dancing with full power in the FHL to permit weight-bearing pointe work **(C)** and ability to perform flexion and extension without triggering, weakness, or pain **(D).**

is adherent and the muscle belly is fibrosed or bound down to the posterior tibia, then release is less productive, and muscle belly excision or tendon transection is necessary. Most of the time with these injuries, there is not enough function of the FHL that lengthening the tendon in the arch of the foot distal to the master knot of Henry is advised. In these cases, the muscle is functional, but the fibrosis that has occurred proximally is thought to be too great to relieve with a release (Fig. 24-41).

In addition to the mechanical factors, the tendon can develop pathologic processes associated with inflammatory arthropathy (rheumatoid arthritis, reactive arthritis, infection, gout, ulcerative colitis).[113] Baan et al[86] reported an 18% incidence of rupture of the flexor hallucis longus tendon in patients (11/60 patients) with long-term rheumatoid arthritis. Reduced first metatarsophalangeal joint motion and pes planus were noted in the study group with a ruptured tendon.

Other reported pathologic conditions include calcific myonecrosis,[120] giant cell tumor of the FHL tendon sheath (Fig. 24-42),[95] osteochondromatosis of the flexor hallucis longus (Fig. 24-43),[118] and degenerative tendinoses of the FHL tendon (Fig. 24-44). Pigmented villonodular synovitis of the anterior ankle may also be associated with an FHL tendon rupture (Fig. 24-45).

History and Physical Examination

Patients often complain of a pain in the area of stenosis, a catching sensation, and some weakness during running,

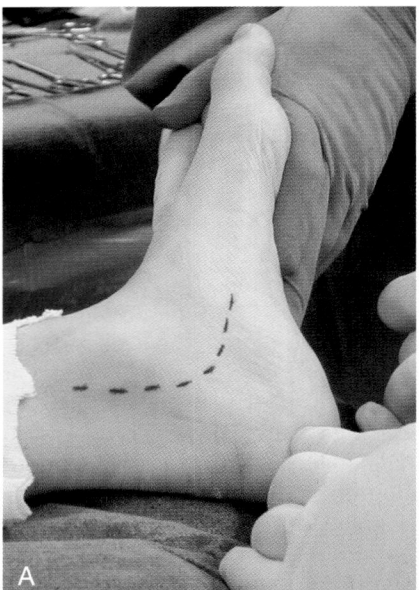
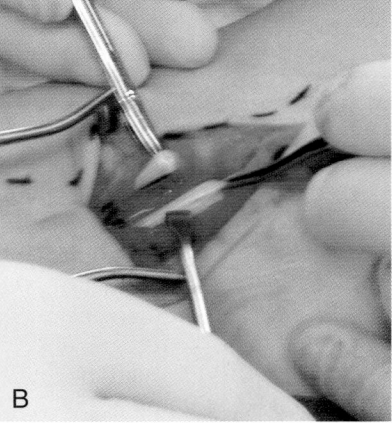
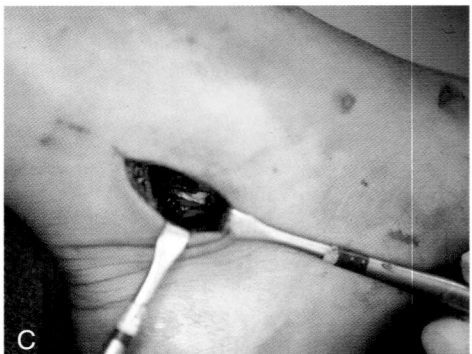

Figure 24-41 Flexor hallucis longus (FHL) tenosynovitis. **A,** Course of the tendon below the sustentaculum tali. **B,** Intraoperative photograph of tendon release. Note the flexor digitorum longus tendon just superior to the FHL. **C,** Small medial incision is used to release the FHL tendon sheath. Note the distal course of the muscle belly leading to stenosis in the tunnel.

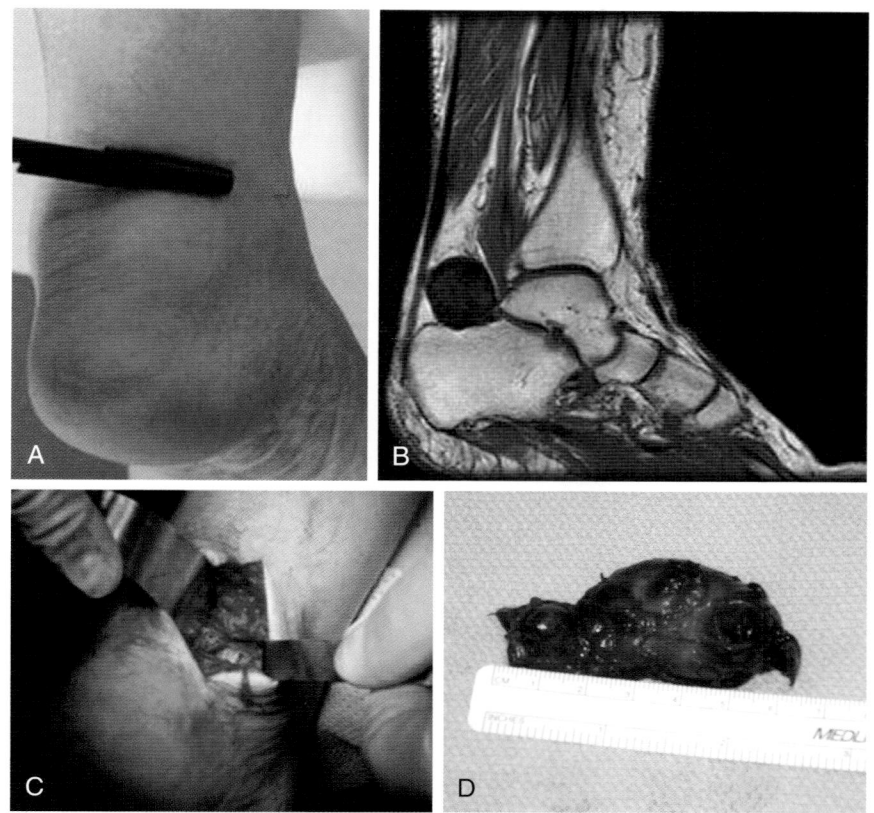

Figure 24-42 Giant cell tumor of flexor hallucis longus tendon sheath. **A,** Clinical presentation of soft tissue mass. **B,** Magnetic resonance image displaying mass on posterior aspect of the medial ankle joint. **C,** Intraoperative photograph of resection of tumor. **D,** Resected specimen demonstrating large giant cell tumor. (From Findling J, Lascola NK, Groner TW: Giant cell tumor of the flexor hallucis longus tendon sheath: a case study, *J Am Podiatr Med Assoc* 101:187–189, 2011. Used with permission.)

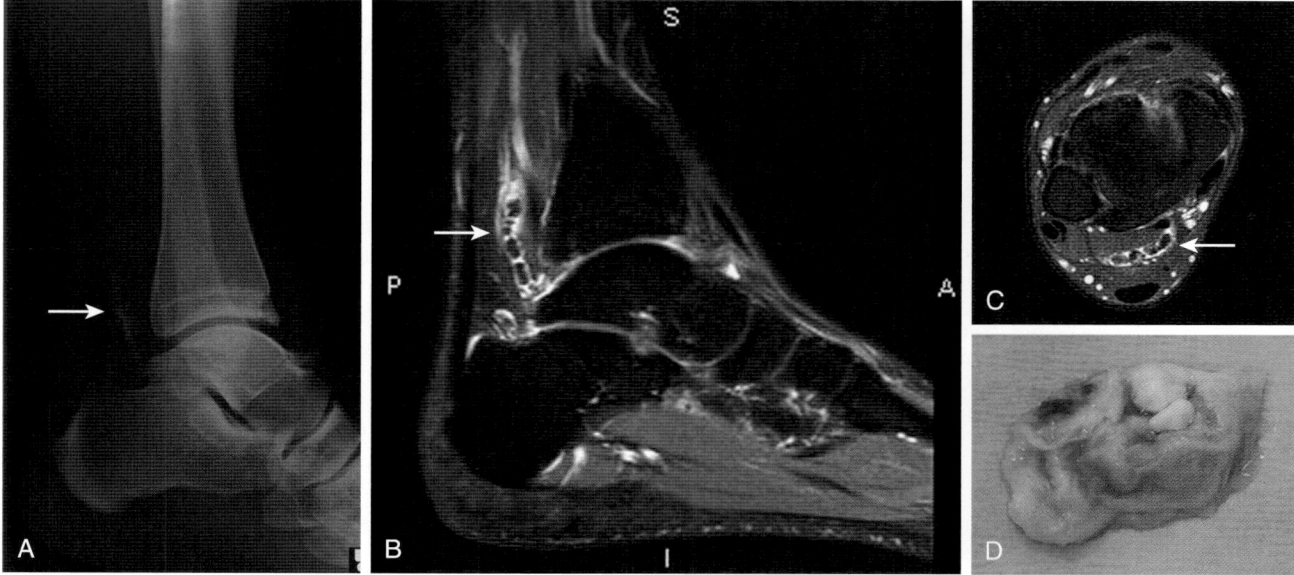

Figure 24-43 Tenosynovial osteochondromatosis of the flexor hallucis longus tendon. **A,** Lateral radiograph of osteochondromal lesions (*arrow*). **B,** Fat-suppressed magnetic resonance image demonstrating multiple calcific nodules (*arrow*). **C,** Axial image showing multiple calcific nodules (*arrow*). **D,** Excised specimen containing multiple osteochondromatous nodules. (A-C, From Oakley J, Yewlett A, Makwana N: Tenosynovial osteochondromatosis of the flexor hallucis longus tendon, *Foot Ankle Surg* 16:148–150, 2010. Used with permission. D, Courtesy J. Oakley, MRCS Ed, MBBCH, Shropshire, United Kingdom.)

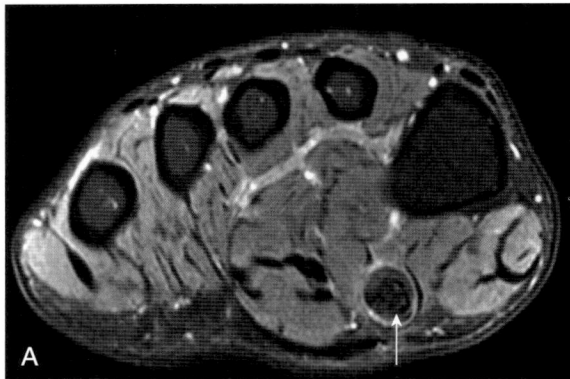

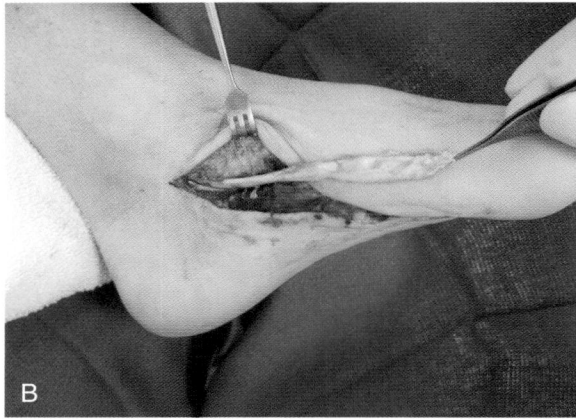

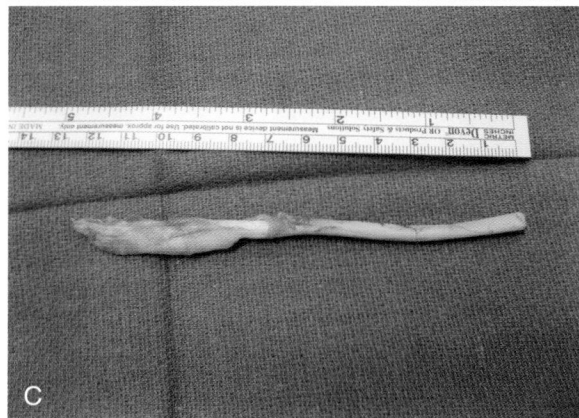

Figure 24-44 Tendinosis of the distal flexor hallucis longus tendon. **A,** Coronal magnetic resonance image demonstrating marked tendinosis of the flexor hallucis longus (FHL) tendon. **B,** Operative exposure demonstrating tendinosis of the distal FHL. **C,** Excised segment distal to the fibroosseous tunnel, with marked tendinosis. (Courtesy Shane Schutt, MD, Omaha, Neb.)

cutting, jumping, squatting, pushing off, or rising on the ball of the foot. Pain along the medial aspect of the ankle or subtalar joint with these mechanical stressors is often noted. Some report an audible pop or a tearing sensation in association with the onset of acute pain. In ballerinas, an en pointe position can exacerbate symptoms. Also, the dancers note that when non–weight bearing and just

repetitively pointing (plantar flexing the ankle and toes) and relaxing the foot and ankle they experience pain, clicking, popping, and a triggering of the hallux. Crepitus is often present on physical examination, but triggering is less common.

Kolettis et al[105] reported this condition in female ballet dancers who had chronic symptoms of FHL tenosynovitis on the medial aspect of the ankle joint. The main symptoms were pain and tenderness over the medial ankle. All patients lost the ability to stand en pointe. An os trigonum was present in only 1 of 13 cases. The differential diagnosis besides tenosynovitis includes a longitudinal tear of the FHL tendon and systemic inflammatory arthropathy.

On examination, the FHL tendon sheath often feels thickened. Examination often reveals no active flexion of the interphalangeal joint with the hallux held in extension. There may be pain on palpation, depending on the area of disease. The pain may be localized to the posteromedial ankle, in the midfoot beneath the knot of Henry, or distally in the area of the FHL tendon insertion. Pain typically occurs with active plantar flexion of the hallux against resistance. With a partial tendon rupture, the patient can have swelling, ecchymosis, and pain with prolonged walking or running. Passive flexion and extension is typically painless. Active flexion may be absent or weak, depending on the degree of stenosis or the presence of a partial rupture. The patient can develop a mild flexion tenodesis of the MTP joint with passive ankle dorsiflexion. When the condition is severe, crepitation and triggering may be noted. If a nodule becomes incarcerated in the fibroosseous tunnel, the toe remains in extension. Passive range of motion of the hallux causes less pain than restricted active range of motion.

When flexor hallucis longus tenosynovitis manifests with pain in the posterior ankle, distinguishing between posterior ankle impingement and FHL tendinitis can be challenging. Because the two structures are close to each other, and these conditions can coexist in dancers, careful attention to diagnostic features is warranted. Both conditions can manifest with pain induced by active plantar flexion of the foot and ankle, but the trigonal or posterior ankle impingement usually occurs with passive full plantar flexion of the ankle, whereas FHL tendinitis does not. Dorsiflexion of the great toe while in the fully plantar-flexed position does not usually induce symptoms in impingement conditions but can in FHL tendinitis. The point of maximum tenderness in posterior impingement is usually posterolateral, whereas it is usually posteromedial with FHL tendinitis.

The Tomassen sign is another helpful diagnostic finding for FHL stenosis. With the ankle in dorsiflexion, MTP joint dorsiflexion is lost because of the tightness of the FHL tendon and a low-lying muscle belly as it courses through the fibroosseous tunnel. Further distinction is possible with lateral radiographs of the ankle taken in neutral and full plantar flexion; these views show abutment of the os trigonum between the tibia and the talus

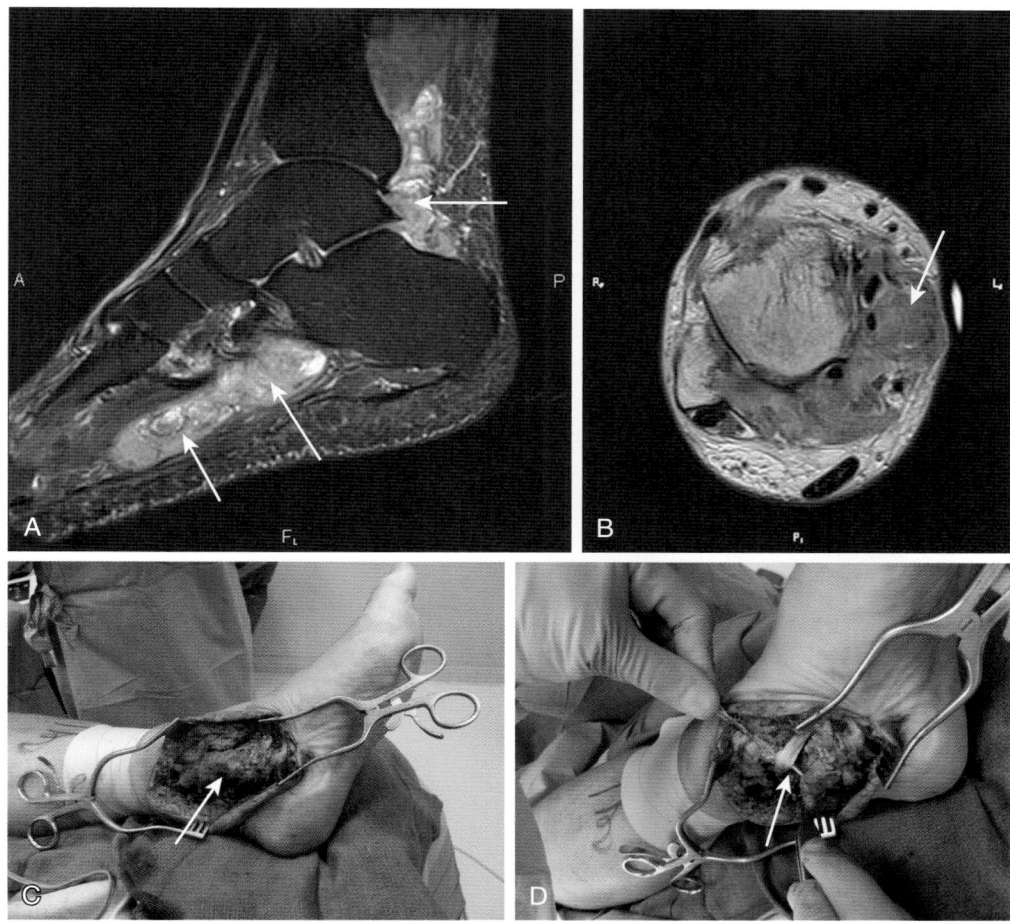

Figure 24-45 Pigmented villinodular synovitis of the flexor hallucis longus tendon. Sagittal **(A)** and axial plane **(B)** magnetic resonance images demonstrating soft tissue mass *(arrows)* encompassing the flexor hallucis longus (FHL) tendon. **C,** Operative exposure of the mass *(arrow).* **D,** After excision of mass *(arrow)* and debridement of the FHL tendon.

and calcaneus or subluxation of the talus and tibiocalcaneal abutment.

Radiographic Examination

Although Trepman et al[134] and others[90,125] have noted the usefulness of MRI in diagnosing FHL tenosynovitis and tears (Fig. 24-46), Beauperthuy[88] observed that an MRI was negative in three patients with longitudinal FHL tears. In Sammarco's series,[127] only eight patients had MRI evaluations before surgery, but clinical correlation was found to be an important factor in interpreting the MRI. Oloff et al[119] reported that some patients with flexor hallucis longus tendinitis also had plantar fasciitis and tarsal tunnel syndrome. In their series, they found that MRI proved valuable in establishing the correct primary diagnosis in their series.

Conservative Treatment

Nonsurgical treatment includes restricted activity, change in dancing and training technique, physical therapy, nonsteroidal anti-inflammatory drugs (NSAIDs), ice and

contrast baths, whirlpool, and orthotics. Immobilization did diminish symptoms.[40] Occasionally, a corticosteroid injection into the tendon sheath is used judiciously. An injection under fluoroscopic or ultrasonic control is often advantageous to ensure the location of the needle and steroid (Fig. 24-47).[115] In cases where conservative treatment has failed or if the symptoms recur, a corticosteroid injection can often give dramatic relief of symptoms. Kolettis et al[105] reported a risk of weakening or rupture of the FHL tendon after a steroid injection. Care must be taken to avoid an intratendinous injection, and Reinhertz[123] stressed that steroid injections are not routinely recommended because they can contribute to spontaneous rupture. Surgery is indicated with the failure of conservative therapy (Fig. 24-48).

Surgical Treatment

Surgical intervention may be considered if conservative care is unsuccessful. During surgery, the sheath can be three to four times thicker than normal according to Lynch and Pupp.[113] Degenerative changes within the

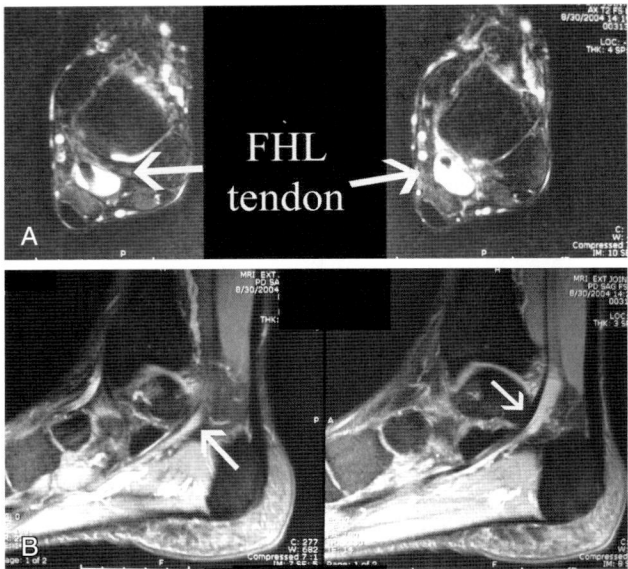

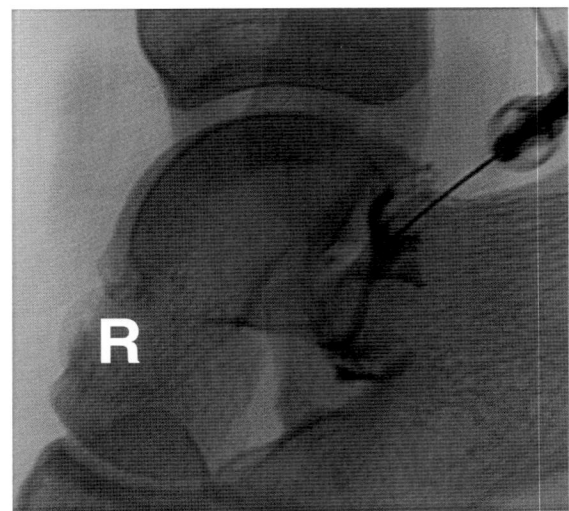

Figure 24-46 T2-weighted magnetic resonance images 5 months after an incomplete tear of the flexor hallucis longus (FHL). **A,** Axial views demonstrate flexor tenosynovitis with increased signal intensity and abnormal but intact FHL tendon. **B,** Sagittal view demonstrates course of tendon with tenosynovitis behind the ankle and under the sustentaculum talus.

Figure 24-47 Technique of injection of flexor hallucis longus tendon sheath under fluoroscopic control.

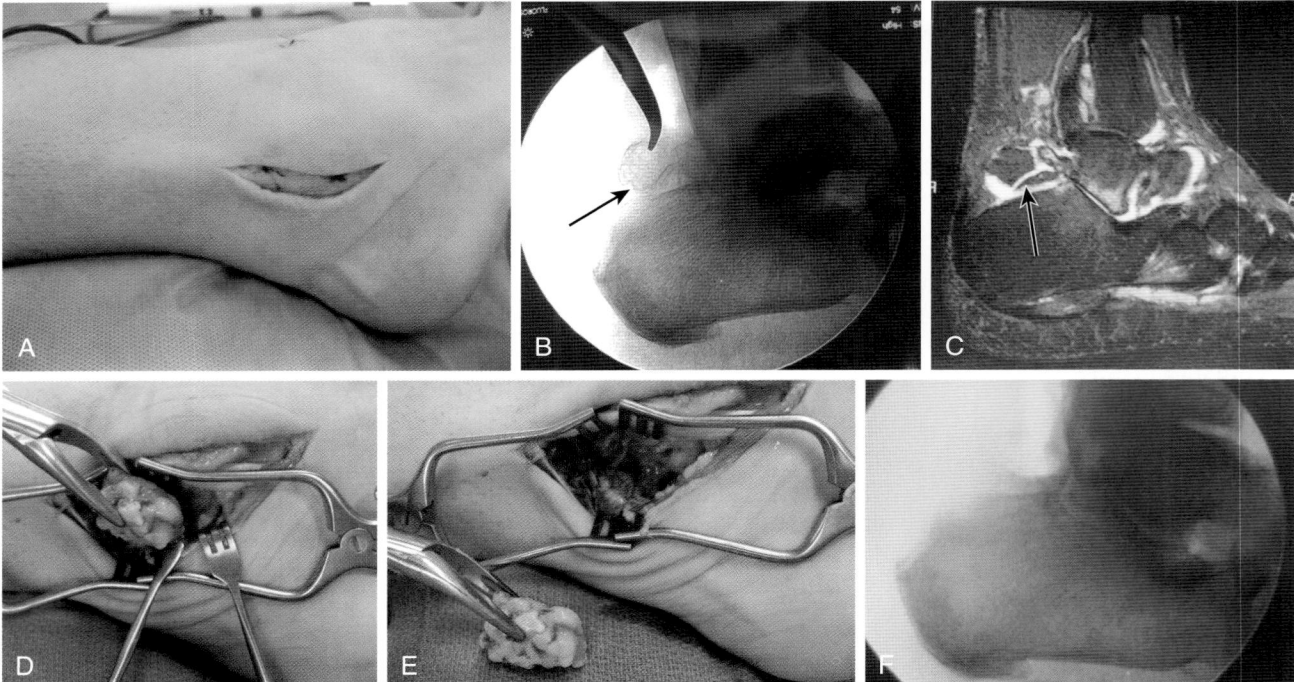

Figure 24-48 Excision of os trigonum from lateral approach. **A,** Lateral incision. Lateral radiograph **(B)** and sagittal **(C)** magnetic resonance images demonstrating large os trigonum *(arrows)*. **D** and **E,** Operative removal of os trigonum. **F,** Final lateral radiograph after removal.

tendon at the time of surgical exploration are typically characterized by yellowing, calcification, or degenerative tears. The pathologic tendon sheath is incised in a step-wise process. If the tendon continues to catch or if the thickness is more than 1 or 2 mm wider, the thickened area of the tendon is resected. Very rarely, new pulleys in the retinacular area are needed to stabilize the tendon. If an os trigonum is present or if there is a large trigonal process, resection is considered if there was preoperative posterior impingement symptoms or if there is persistent catching after releasing. A partial FHL tendon tear is repaired or resected or a nodular area is contoured if necessary. An alternative to open release is posterior ankle arthroscopy in the prone position. In the case of excision of an os trigonum as well, there are alternatives for surgical exposure. A posterior debridement and os trigonum excision can be performed from a medial or lateral approach. The lateral approach is favored in the presence of isolated posterior impingement without a history of FHL tenosynovitis. A medial approach is favored with the combined presence of both FHL tenosyovitis and posterior impingement. Hamilton[101] has favored a medial approach with exposure of the neurovascular bundle, unless there is a clear-cut case of merely a symptomatic os trigonum. Although some have advocated removing the os trigonum arthroscopically, an adequate release of the FHL during this approach is challenging. Keeling and Guyton[104] reported in a cadaveric anatomic study that access to the FHL sheath during posterior arthroscopy is limited.

OPEN RELEASE OF THE FLEXOR HALLUCIS LONGUS
Surgical Technique

1. With the patient in a supine position, a pneumatic tourniquet may or may not be used for hemostasis. A 3- to 5-cm curvilinear incision is made posterior to the medial malleolus and directed toward the navicular.
2. The neurovascular bundle is retracted, revealing the FHL in its fibroosseous sheath. Alternatively, the FDL tendon sheath can be opened and the dissection directed to the bone with retraction of the FDL tendon posteriorly with the neurovascular bundle. The deep aspect of the sheath is then released to gain exposure to the FHL tendon.
3. The retinaculum is released proximally to the level of the sustentaculum tali, and the tendon is inspected.
4. A tenosynovectomy is performed. Any nodules are excised. Longitudinal tears are repaired.
5. With a tear that extends into the midarch, Boruta and Beauperthuy[88] recommend releasing the knot of Henry to debride and repair a longitudinal tear. The interconnecting tendon between the FHL and FDL is excised.
6. Any prominent distal muscle fibers are excised.
7. The hypertrophic tenosynovial tissue is debrided, and if a longitudinal tear is present, it is repaired primarily. The hallux is then flexed and extended to demonstrate

excursion of the tendon. The FHL is released until the retinaculum no longer prohibits its gliding motion. If the surgery is done under local anesthetic with intra-venous sedation, it is useful to have the patient aggressively flex and extend the ankle and toes while the ankle is palpated for persistent crepitance.
8. The tendon sheath is not closed, but the distal soft tissue is approximated. The skin is closed in an interrupted fashion (see Fig. 24-41).

EXCISION OF THE OS TRIGONUM THROUGH A LATERAL APPROACH
Surgical Technique (Video Clip 15)

1. With the patient in a lateral decubitus or prone position, a pneumatic tourniquet may be applied and used to achieve hemostasis.
2. A curvilinear incision is made just posterior to the posterior border of the fibula. The fatty tissue that contains the sural nerve and vascular structures are reflected posteriorly as a unit as the dissection is performed directly over the peroneal retinaculum. The retinaculum is incised just behind the peroneal tendon sheath. Care is taken to identify and protect the sural nerve (Fig. 24-48A-C).
3. The dissection is deepened posteriorly and medially to the peroneal tendons in the interval between the FHL tendon medially and the peroneal tendons laterally.
4. The posterior ankle capsular is incised, and the os trigonum is exposed on the superior aspect of the calcaneus just lateral to the tendon of the flexor hallucis longus (Fig. 24-48D). It is useful to place two small Hohman retractors. One is placed over the dorsal aspect of the os trigonum and the other just posterior. A small-toothed laminar spreader can then be inserted to further facilitate exposure.
5. The os trigonum is excised by a circumferential dissection that releases numerous fibrous attachments to the surrounding tissue. Any dissection medially must be performed judiciously because of the presence of the neurovascular bundle. Using a curet placed deep to the medial aspect of the fragment to lift and elevate the bone away from dense medial soft tissue attachments can minimize inadvertently leaving a small avulsed fragment behind. Attention should also be directed to identify visually, radiographically, and by palpation any loose bodies or sharp bone fragments around the os trigonum or adjacent to the flexor tendon sheath.
6. After removal of the os trigoum, the ankle is maximally dorsiflexed and plantar flexed to ensure there is no residual impingement between the calcaneus and the tibia (Fig. 24-48E). Intraoperative fluoroscopy of the ankle in both plantar flexion and dorsiflexion is helpful. Several oblique angles for fluoroscopy (10-20 degrees internally and externally) can sometimes reveal a small retained fragment or bony prominence.

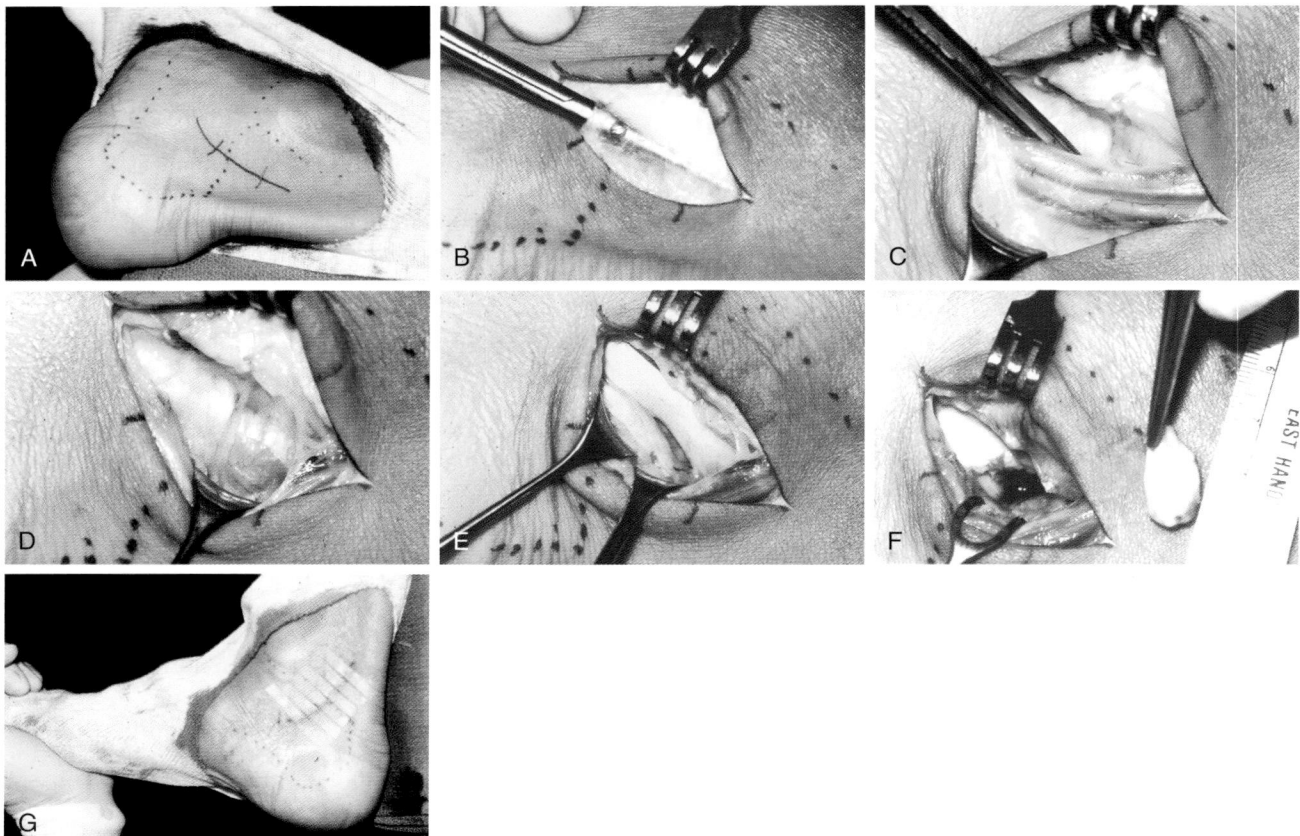

Figure 24-49 **A,** Posteromedial incision. **B,** Division of the laciniate ligament. **C,** Exposing the neurovascular bundle. **D,** The underlying flexor hallucis longus (FHL) tendon. **E,** Tenolysis of the FHL tendon. **F,** Removal of the adjacent trigonal process. **G,** Closure of the wound in neutral dorsiflexion. (Courtesy William Hamilton, MD, New York.)

7. A layered closure is then performed with absorbable sutures. The ankle is splinted for 1 to 2 weeks after surgery to ensure adequate soft tissue healing (Fig. 24-48F).

EXCISION OF THE OS TRIGONUM THROUGH A MEDIAL APPROACH[28,101]

 Surgical Technique (Video Clip 15)

1. With the patient in a supine position, a pneumatic tourniquet may be used to create a bloodless field.
2. A curvilinear incision is centered over the neurovascular bundle just posterior to the medial malleolus, beginning just above the upper border of the os calcis and continuing to a point just inferior to the tip of the medial malleolus. The incision is deepened through the fascia and laciniate ligament, with care taken to protect the neurovascular bundle (Fig. 24-49A).
3. The surgeon then must choose whether to dissect anterior or posterior to the neurovascular bundle. Posteriorly, the sensory branches to the calcaneus are encountered. The anterior exposure, in general, is preferable, taking the entire posterior tibial nerve and

branches posterior. Different branching patterns of the nerve occur in this area, and the nerve should be carefully exposed and protected with blunt retractors or vessel loops (Fig. 24-49B and C). Alternatively, the FDL tendon sheath can be opened and the dissection kept on the tibia and talus with retraction of the FDL tendon posteriorly with the neurovascular bundle. The deep aspect of the sheath is then released to gain exposure to the FHL tendon.

4. The tendon of the flexor hallucis longus is exposed (Fig. 24-49D), and a tenolysis is performed (Fig. 24-49E). The sheath can be quite thickened in this area but thins as it courses beneath the sustentaculum tali.
5. The tendon should be inspected for fibrillation, tears, and loose bodies within the sheath. If present, tears should be carefully excised or repaired.
6. Next, the freed tendon can be retracted posteriorly along with the entire neurovascular bundle. The os trigonum can now be visualized on the lateral aspect of the tunnel of the FHL.
7. Once the os trigonum is identified, it can be resected with a circumferential dissection, staying right on the

bone as it is excised. Once the os trigonum has been removed, the posterior ankle joint is inspected for loose bodies or remaining bone fragments. In some cases, a large prominent articular facet on the superior surface of the os calcis remain, (this previously articulated with the os trigonum). When present, it should be resected using a thin osteotome or chisel (Fig. 24-49F).

8. The wound is closed in layers with absorbable sutures while holding the ankle in the neutral position (Fig. 24-49G). The tunnel of the FHL tendon should not be closed. A well-padded posterior plaster splint or below-knee cast is applied. The patient remains non–weight bearing postoperatively.

Postoperative Care

The foot and ankle are enclosed in a soft dressing and a below-knee splint or cast for 7 to 14 days, and the patient remains non–weight bearing. Then the splint or cast is removed and physical therapy is initiated, including strengthening exercises, range-of-motion activities, and full weight bearing.[113] The use of a protective boot for ambulation for another 6 weeks is helpful to prevent reinjury.

Results

Kolettis et al[105] reported on 13 female ballet dancers who had chronic symptoms of FHL tenosynovitis on the medial aspect of the ankle. The major symptoms were pain and tenderness over the medial aspect of the subtalar joint at an average of 6 months before surgery. All patients had lost the ability to stand en pointe. Hamilton[100] reported on 17 cases of FHL tenosynovitis and combined a soft tissue release with excision of a symptomatic os trigonum. Routinely good and excellent results have been reported after surgical exploration, tenosynovectomy, and repair of the longitudinal degenerative tears of the FHL tendon, when present.[98,100,105,128,136]

Hamilton et al[101] reported their results of surgically treating posterior ankle pain in dancers, with an average follow-up of 7 years. Thirty-seven dancers underwent 41 operations: 26 operations for tendinitis and posterior impingement, 9 for isolated tendinitis, and 6 for isolated posterior impingement syndrome. Thirty ankles had a good or excellent result, 6 had a fair result, and 4 had a poor result. The results were good or excellent for 28 of the 34 ankles in professional dancers, compared with only 2 of the 6 ankles in amateur dancers. This discrepancy can reflect the higher expectations and a poorer ability to compensate in the amateur population.

Sammarco et al[127] reported on FHL tendon injuries in dancers and nondancers. Thirty-one cases of flexor hallucis longus injuries in 26 patients were treated over a 16-year period. The two groups were compared with regard to age, activity, duration of symptoms, operative findings, histopathology, and postoperative time to resumption of full activities. These patients required surgery for unsuccessful nonoperative treatment. In the dancers, 71% of patients had a partial longitudinal tear of the flexor hallucis longus compared with 30% in nondancers. Isolated tenosynovitis occurred in only 21% of the dancers but in 53% of the nondancers. Dancers tended to have symptoms for a longer period before seeking treatment than did nondancers. Surgical intervention for the tenosynovitis and tendon tears yielded good or excellent results in 14 of 15 dancers and 9 of 11 nondancers.

Oloff et al[119] reported on a cohort of patients with FHL tendinitis. In their retrospective series of 19 consecutive cases, they reported that the condition occurred in primarily nonathletic, male, and middle-aged patients. The mean symptom duration was 20 months, with frequent previous misdiagnosis. They found overlapping signs and symptoms of flexor hallucis longus tendinitis, plantar fasciitis, and tarsal tunnel syndrome. MRI and tenography proved valuable in establishing the correct primary diagnosis in their series. Flexor hallucis longus tenolysis was successful in each case, with a mean return to regular activity at 9 weeks.

Gould,[99] who believed that trauma was a causative agent, reported three cases that responded to a lidocaine anesthetic injection that basically lysed adhesions. He also reported six other cases that required an open tenolysis. Sanhudo et al[129] described additional cases of distal stenosis at the sesamoid area.

With cases that have stenosis or synovitis at areas other than the ankle and subtalar joints, after attempted conservative treatment, consideration of a soft tissue release at the site of tendon constriction is warranted.

Flexor Hallucis Longus Rupture

Although isolated spontaneous ruptures have been reported in the literature, the major reason for a loss of continuity is laceration of the tendon.[9,33,97,123,124] Bann et al[86] has reported a high rate of flexor hallucis longus ruptures in patients with long-standing rheumatoid arthritis. Intraoperative transection of the FHL can happen inadvertently during harvest of the FDL tendon for a posterior tibial tendon reconstruction procedure performed through a medial infranavicular approach. The tendon slip that connects the FDL to the FHL tendon tethers the FHL as the FDL is drawn more medially to permit its sectioning. Because the FDL is cut at the depths of the exposure, it is possible to be unaware that the FHL tendon is inadvertently being transected simultaneously. Loss of resting tone of the hallux is noted when this occurs. While flexing the hallux and performing further distal sharp dissection through the fibrous arcade of the FHB, the distal end of the FHL should be identified for repair (Fig. 24-50). An injury to the FHL can occur anywhere along the course of the tendon. The site of disruption can be divided into the following zones:

■ Zone 1: distal to the sesamoids in the area just proximal to the FHL insertion

■ Zone 2: between the sesamoids and the knot of Henry
■ Zone 3: proximal to the knot of Henry

The reason for the designation of different zones of injury is that a disruption in zone 3 leads to proximal retraction of the tendon. Injuries in zones 1 and 2 are not characterized by retraction of the proximal segment because of the fibrous slip connecting the FHL and FDL (Fig. 24-51).[92] With zone 1 injuries, a laceration leaves the

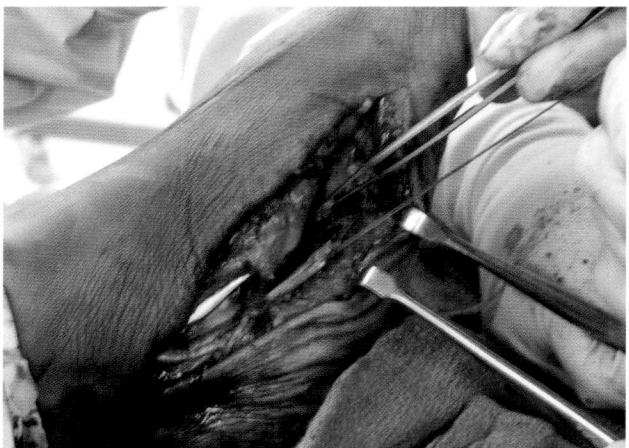

Figure 24-50 Flexor hallucis longus tendon laceration in the sole of the foot.

tendon edges in proximity in a fairly subcutaneous region; however, the tendon is surrounded by a tendon sheath, and fibrous scarring is common. In zone 2, although the FHL is located in the deep arch of the foot, retraction is uncommon. Zone 2 injuries are characterized by a lesser degree of postoperative adhesions.

On the plantar aspect of the foot, the tendons and neurovascular structures are vulnerable to penetrating injuries. Frenette and Jackson[97] reported a high incidence of nerve disruption after lacerations of the FHL. The first common digital nerve and proper digital nerve course along the medial and lateral aspect of the FHL tendon in a superficial area and are vulnerable to injury along with laceration of the FHL. The authors noted that in 75% of injuries in which a laceration was distal to the origin of the FHB, the proper or common digital nerve was lacerated as well. Wicks et al[33] reported that 60% of feet in their series demonstrated nerve injury.

Frenette and Jackson[97] reported that 80% of injuries in their series resulted from stepping on glass while barefoot. They noted 3 of 10 injuries distal to the plantar flexion crease at the MTP joint, 5 in the distal longitudinal arch where the FHL lies between the two bellies of the FHB, and 2 localized to the proximal longitudinal arch.

History and Physical Examination
After injury, a patient might note subjective loss of push-off power and a feeling of giving way. A prodromal period followed by a sudden snap can herald an FHL tendon

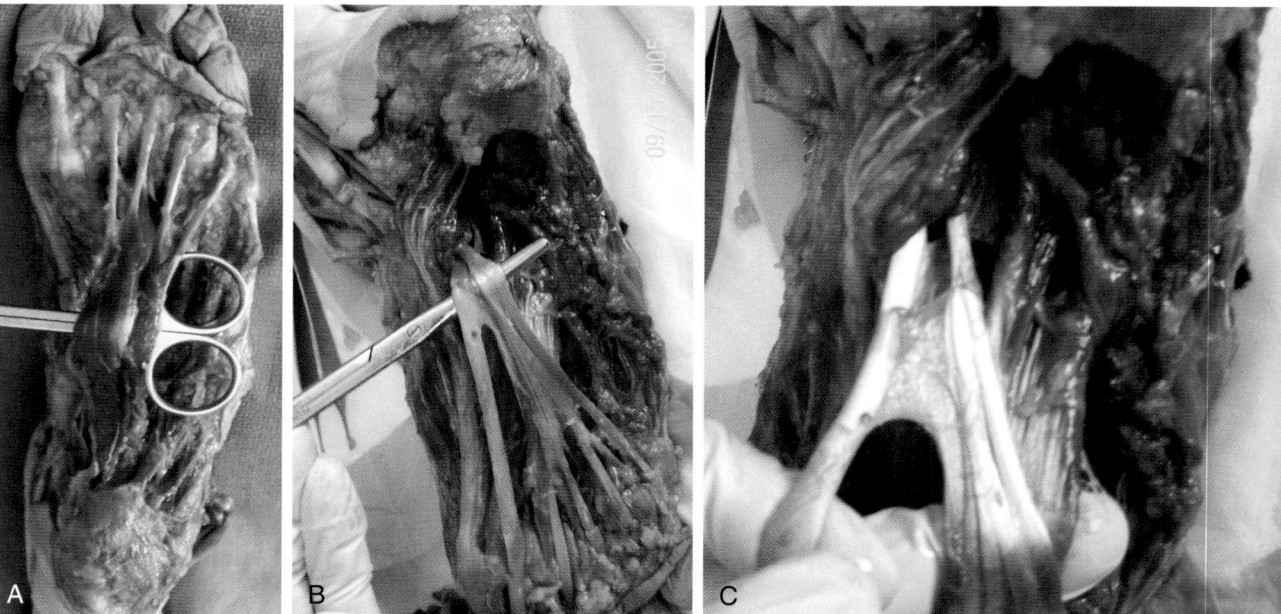

Figure 24-51 Anatomic dissection demonstrates tendon connection between the flexor hallucis longus (FHL) and flexor digitorum longus (FDL). **A,** FDL. **B,** Minor connection between FHL and FDL. **C,** Close-up view. (Courtesy Nick Goucher, MD, Ogden, Utah.)

rupture.[102,125,133] The recognition of spontaneous dorsiflexion of the toe and discomfort with pressure of the hallux against the top of the toe box may be coupled with an inability to flex the tip of the toe. A patient might give a history of forced dorsiflexion against resistance or of being involved in a repetitive activity, such as rising on the ball of the foot or running, cutting, and jumping. Rupture of the FHL tendon can also be associated with systemic disease, trauma, and athletic or dance activity. In patients with a spontaneous rupture, a popping or tearing sensation may be associated with the disruption.

On physical examination, normal active extension of the hallux IP joint is present, but typically, no active plantar flexion is possible. Passive flexion and extension of the hallux is typically painless. Active flexion at the MTP joint denotes function of the FHB. Occasionally, simultaneous rupture of the FHL and FHB tendons can occur. This should be evaluated by examining for flexion of the MTP and IP joints. Further assessment of the plantar plate with attempted dorsal drawer or translation of the proximal phalanx relative to the metatarsal head should be performed. A side-by-side comparison facilitates this evaluation. After rupture, swelling and tenderness on the plantar aspect of the hallux and tenderness at the MTP joint and sesamoid region can denote a distal rupture. Pain and swelling in the posteromedial aspect of the ankle can develop with a proximal FHL tendon rupture. If a rupture occurs distal to the knot of Henry, active flexion of the hallux IP joint is typically absent.

The fibrous slip connecting the FHL and FDL tendons prevents retraction of the proximal tendon into the arch or calf.[109] When the rupture occurs proximal to this fibrous slip attachment, action of the FDL tendon may be transmitted through the fibrous slip to the distal portion of the FHL. Thus there may be weak but apparent active flexion of the hallux. On the other hand, this allows retraction of the proximal segment.

Knowledge of position of the tendon rupture is important in planning a surgical reconstruction either in the medial plantar arch or at the level of the ankle. The location of the rupture can be at the musculotendinous junction, in the tendinous portion, or distally at the level of the insertion.

Radiographic Examination

Routine anteroposterior (AP) and lateral radiographs usually do not aid in the diagnosis of an FHL tendon disruption. MRI has been advocated in the patient with weakness, pain, or dysfunction when a diagnosis is not clear or when the level of retraction of the proximal segment is unknown (Figs. 24-52, 24-53, and 24-54).[125,133,134]

Surgical Treatment

Yancey,[137] in a survey of 88 foot and ankle surgeons, reported that 80% to 93% thought a primary repair of a disrupted FHL tendon was important, whereas only

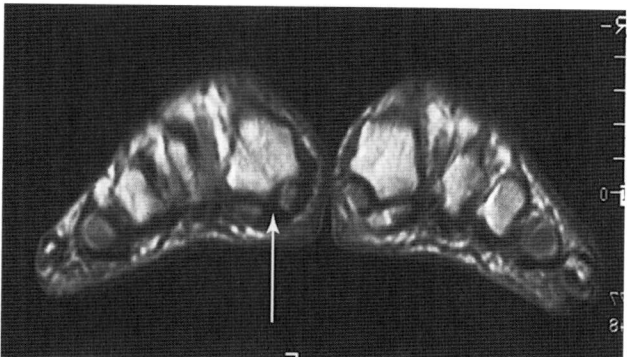

Figure 24-52 A coronal view of a magnetic resonance image demonstrating distal flexor hallucis longus rupture *(arrow)*. (Courtesy M. Romash, MD, Chesapeake, Va.)

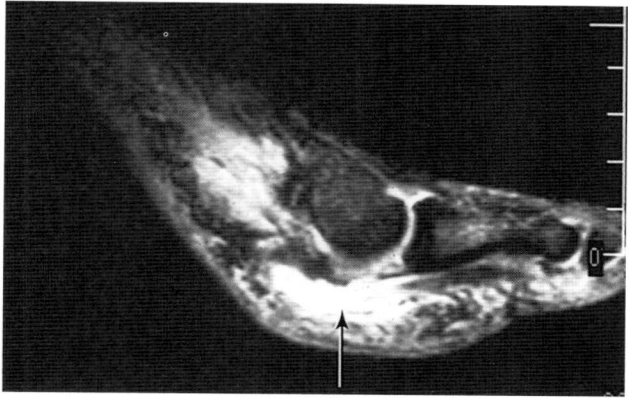

Figure 24-53 A sagittal view of a magnetic resonance image demonstrating distal flexor hallucis longus rupture *(arrow)*. (Courtesy M. Romash, MD, Chesapeake, Va.)

half thought the other lesser-toe flexor tendons were important to repair. Frenette and Jackson[97] recommended repair only if the tendon ends were easily found within the depths of the laceration. They noted that the distal FHL tendon can be tenodesed to the FHB tendon. However, disruption of both the FHL and the FHB tendons has a poor prognosis that can eventually lead to hyperextension of the hallux. Rasmussen and Thyssen[122] repaired the FHL tendon after a distal rupture but observed minimal IP joint motion. They concluded that repair of the FHL tendon did not seem to be "essential in achieving good functional results in cases of rupture or laceration."

An untreated FHL tendon laceration can lead to a cock-up deformity of the hallux. Thompson et al[133] stated that hyperextension of the great toe was an indication for surgical intervention. The options are either primary repair for a distal rupture with acute open or closed trauma or tenodesis of the FHL and FDL tendons

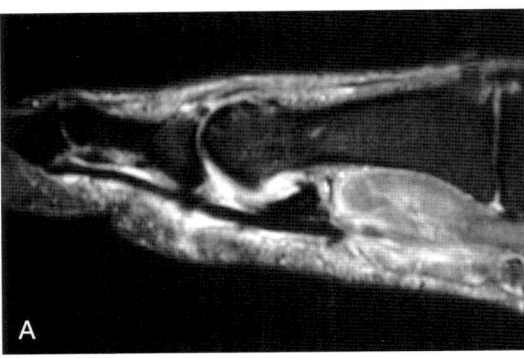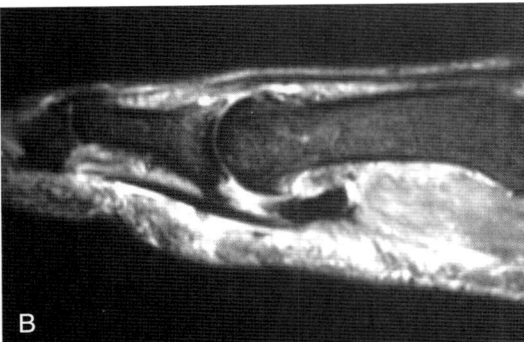

Figure 24-54 **A,** Sagittal view of the first metatarsophalangeal joint on a magnetic resonance image showing flexor hallucis longus (FHL) tenosynovitis. The FHL can be traced from beneath the sesamoid to the base of the proximal phalanx. The sesamoidal phalangeal ligament, which is the continuation of the flexor hallucis brevis tendon, is absent, indicating rupture. **B,** The medial sesamoid shown here has retracted proximally and is no longer under the metatarsal head. The sesamoidal phalangeal ligament and plantar plate has ruptured. The FHL is visualized plantarly, surrounded by edema from the ligament and plantar plate rupture. The extensor hallucis longus can be seen dorsally.

distal and proximal to the sustentaculum tali with a more proximal rupture. They further stated that although a tendon graft might be possible, it seemed "unnecessarily complex." When a rupture is at or adjacent to the fibroosseous tunnel, a primary repair is often unsuccessful. In these cases, a tendon transfer using the FDL tendon to the second toe should be considered, particularly in active or athletic patients.

Krackow[107] observed that the strength of push-off may be improved after repair, and if the patient's physical and athletic activities require high performance, repair should be considered.

PRIMARY REPAIR OF RUPTURED FHL TENDON
Surgical Technique
1. Under tourniquet control, a laceration is explored by extending the incision distally and proximally. The location of the laceration, as previously noted, determines the degree of retraction of the proximal segment. With a closed rupture, the area of maximal tenderness and swelling often determines the location of surgical exploration.
2. The tendon ends are repaired with a modified Bunnell, Krackow, or Kessler suture technique (see Fig. 24-4A-C).

Postoperative Care
The patient is managed in a below-knee cast or splint in plantar flexion at the ankle with an extended toe plate to prevent passive dorsiflexion at the MTP joint. At 2 weeks after surgery, active flexion is permitted. At 4 to 6 weeks after surgery, the ankle is brought to the neutral position. Depending on the tension of the reconstruction, limited dorsiflexion (usually around 20 degrees) and plantar flexion can be initiated at the MTP joint with the ankle in neutral flexion. Active inversion and eversion can be performed with some resistance to maintain muscle function. At 12 weeks, protection is discontinued.[125]

Results and Complications
Primary rupture of the FHL tendon has been described in individual case reports by eight authors (Fig. 24-55). Typically, these injuries occurred in association with athletics after running, dancing, tennis, diving, and soccer, although in one case a rupture occurred after prior first-ray surgery.[90] Locations include distal ruptures[90,107,122,125] and proximal ruptures at the level of the sustentaculum.[102,103,133] A rupture in the midarch just distal to the knot of Henry was reported in a marathon runner.[92]

Trepman et al[134] reported a longitudinal tear of the FHL tendon. They performed a tenolysis, tenosynovectomy, and excision of the prominent distal muscle fibers.

The other major reports of FHL tendon disruption are concerned with traumatic injuries. Floyd et al[9] and others[33,97] reported on a total of 35 disruptions of the FHL tendon at varying locations along the course of the tendon. Iatrogenic injury to the FHL tendon in zone 1 can occur with a phalangeal osteotomy (Akin procedure); careful retraction is necessary to avoid injury to either the FHL or EHL tendons with this procedure (Fig. 24-56).

Primary repair of distal injuries have been reported,[107,122,125] although they are associated with minimal postoperative IP joint motion. Proximal ruptures have been treated with tenodesis of the FDL tendon,[133] fascia lata tendon graft,[103] or primary repair.[102] Proximal repairs tend to be associated with a higher level of active IP joint motion.

Treatment of lacerations of the FHL has been reported in several series. Frenette and Jackson[97] reported on 10 lacerations, of which 6 underwent a primary repair and 4 were left unrepaired. Of those undergoing a primary repair, two thirds had no active IP joint motion. Floyd et al[9] reported on 13 lacerations, 10 of which underwent a primary repair, 2 underwent a delayed repair, and 1 was left unrepaired. Of the 12 repaired, 75% had active IP joint motion. Distal nerve lacerations were reported in 50% of cases, and 70% had acceptable results. In

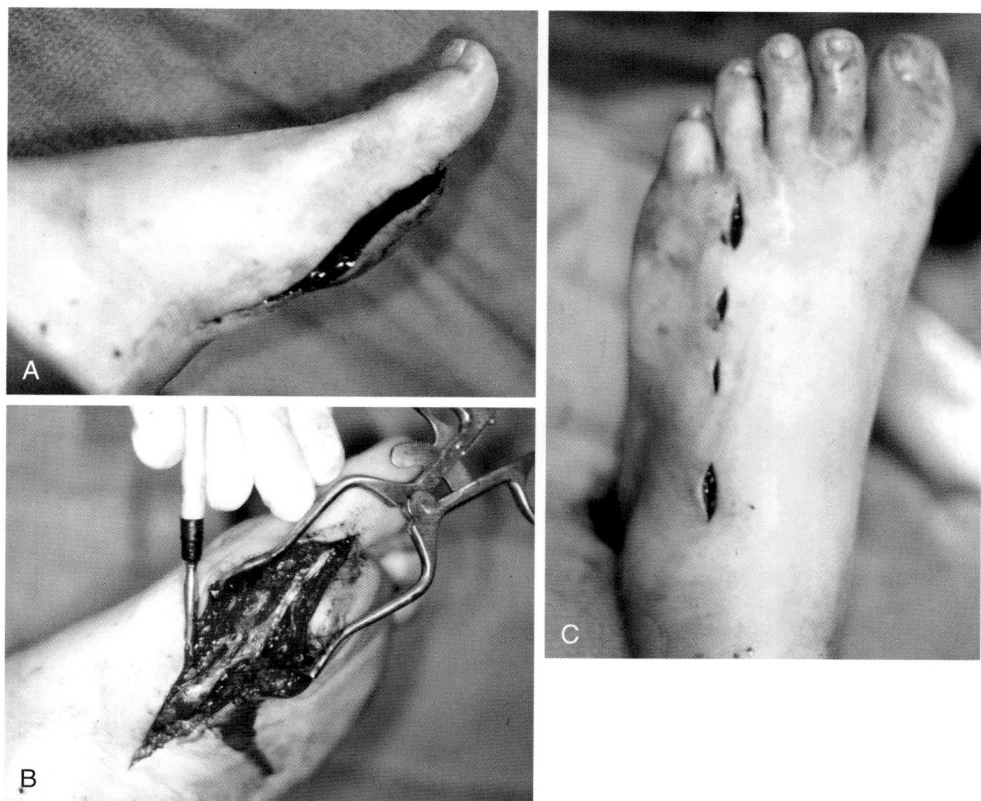

Figure 24-55 Distal rupture of the flexor hallucis longus treated with extensor digitorum brevis (EDB) free graft transfer. **A,** The patient underwent bunion surgery, which resulted in progressive weakness of the flexor hallucis longus (FHL). Once she could no longer flex her great toe, the FHL tendon was approached plantar-medially. **B,** The FHL was found to be attenuated and fibrotic. **C,** The fourth-toe EDB was harvested through multiple small incisions and used as a free tendon graft, successfully bridging the gap.

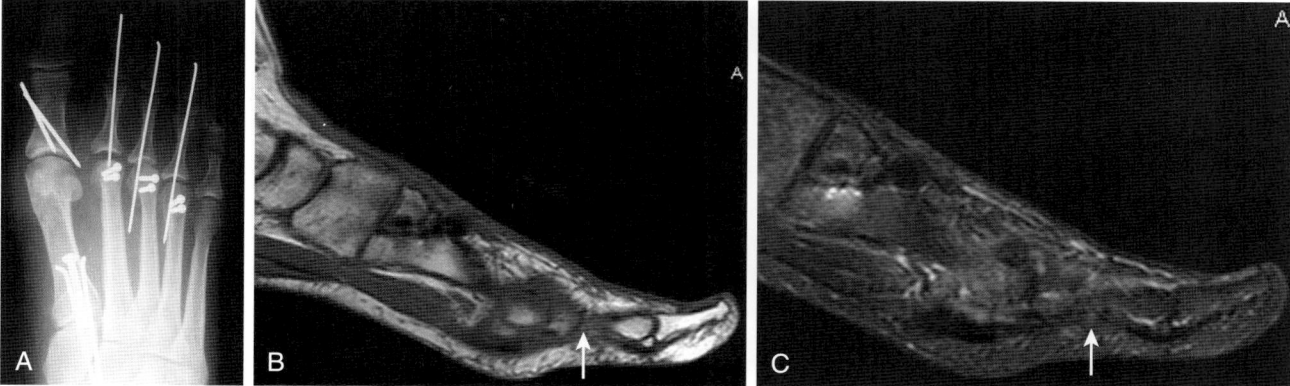

Figure 24-56 Iatrogenic injury to flexor hallucis longus (FHL) with Akin osteotomy. **A,** Postoperative radiograph demonstrating Akin osteotomy and bunion correction. **B** and **C,** Postoperative magnetic resonance images demonstrating discontinuity of distal FHL in zone 1 *(arrows).*

Floyd's series, a more proximal rupture had a greater chance of achieving postoperative IP joint motion than distal ruptures near the IP joint. With closed ruptures of the tendon at the level of the IP joint, return of IP joint motion should not be expected. A closed rupture implies a failure of the tendon under tension. On the other hand, with a laceration, the tendon is cut cleanly and may be more amenable to repair, especially if this occurs in the arch. Wicks et al[33] reported 12 cases of FHL laceration that underwent a primary repair. Sensory nerve injury was noted in 60%, and 55% had acceptable results.

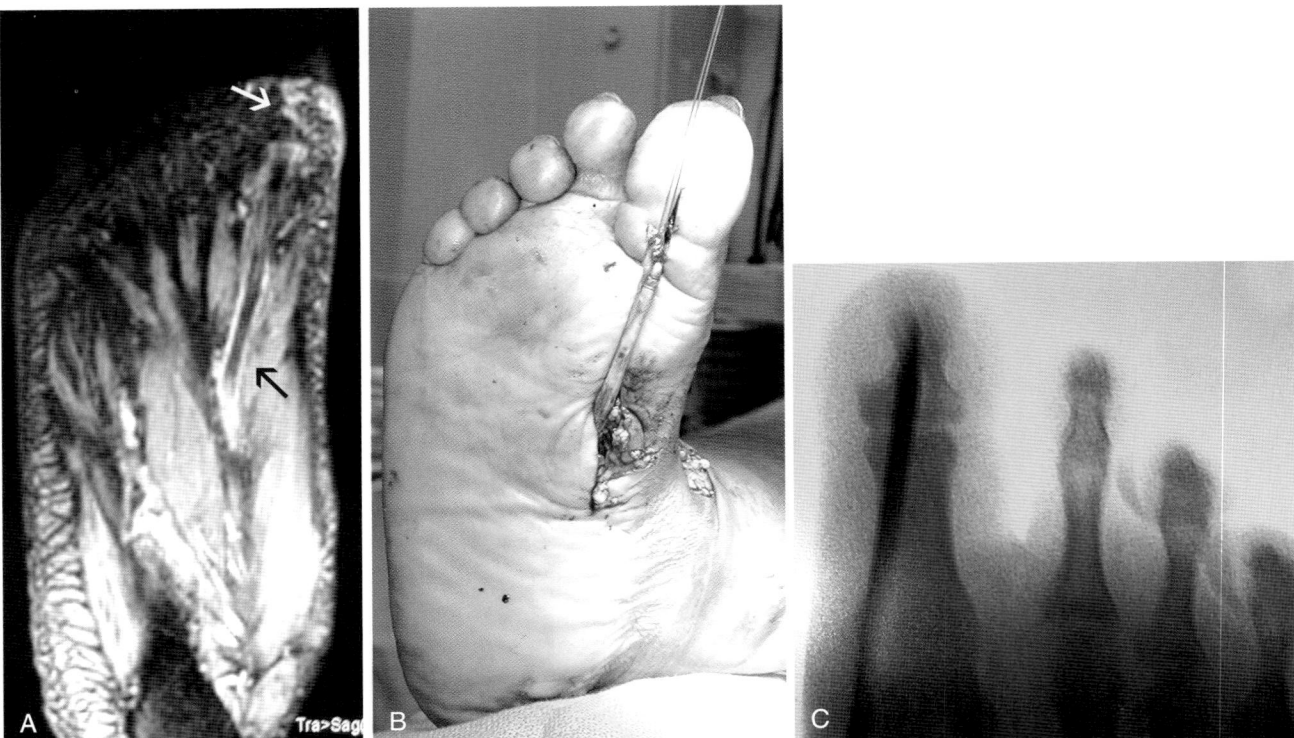

Figure 24-57 The flexor hallucis longus (FHL) tendon had spontaneously ruptured off the distal phalanx. **A,** The magnetic resonance image demonstrates the FHL is intact except for the insertion. **B,** Intraoperative photograph shows ruptured FHL. **C,** The FHL is tunneled between the sesamoids and secured to the suture anchor (3.5 mm) in the distal phalanx.

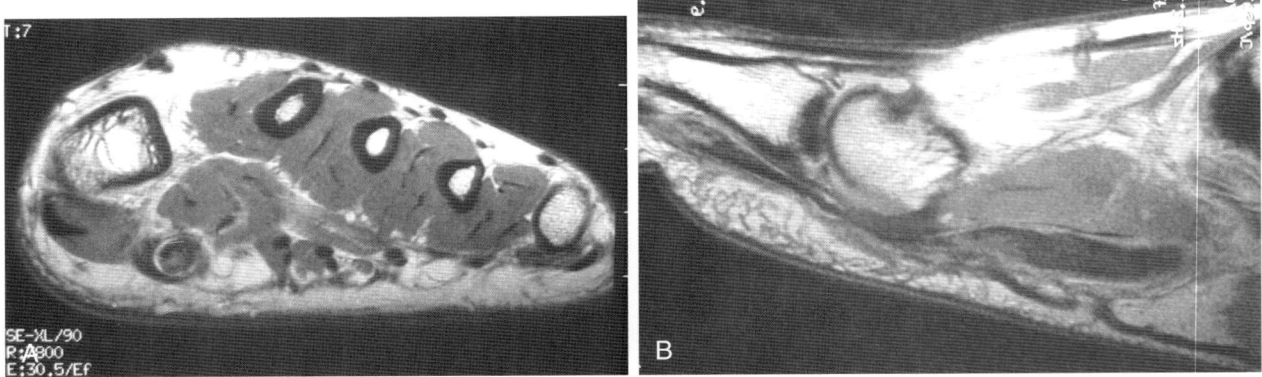

Figure 24-58 This athlete sustained an injury to the metatarsophalangeal joint, which was treated with a steroid injection. Subsequently, the athlete continued to have pain and then felt a giving-way sensation and weakness in the foot. Clinically, there was loss of flexion of the interphalangeal joint of the hallux. A magnetic resonance image (MRI) showed a flexor hallucis longus (FHL) rupture. **A,** A coronal MRI shows the fibrotic ruptured FHL, plantar to the first metatarsal. **B,** The sagittal view demonstrates the FHL rupture proximal to the metatarsal head.

Primary repair has also been reported in several small series and case reports (Fig. 24-57). Boruta and Beauperthuy[88] reported three cases of longitudinal tear of the FHL at the knot of Henry primarily repaired with simultaneous resection of the interconnecting branch. Inokuchi and Usami[103] reported a proximal rupture at the level of the talus treated with a fascia lata interposition graft that

achieved 50% postoperative motion of the IP joint (Figs. 24-58 and 24-59).

Thus the treatment options for disruption of the FHL tendon include nonsurgical treatment, primary repair, tenodesis to the FDL tendon, tenodesis of the distal FHL tendon to the remnant of the FHB, tendon transfer using a slip of the FDL tendon to attach distally to the toe,

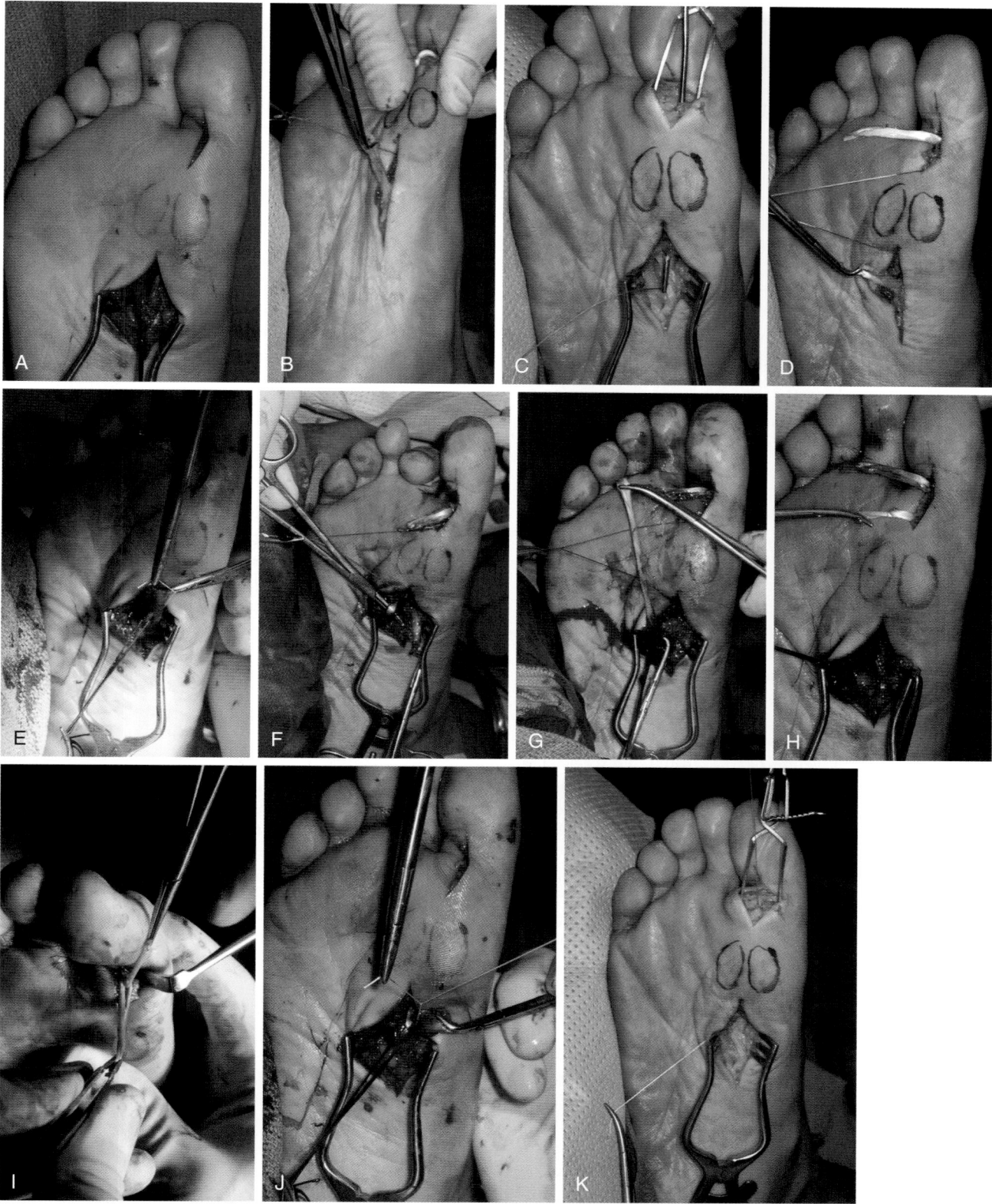

Figure 24-59 The rupture of the flexor hallucis longus (FHL) tendon occurred in the zone just proximal to the sesamoids, making an anastomosis difficult because exposure would violate the weight-bearing fat pad and be vulnerable to stenosis between the sesamoids. **A,** The tendon sheath between the sesamoids is identified and explored. **B,** The FHL is seen in the base of the proximal incision. **C,** A suture is passed through this tunnel for subsequent identification. **D,** Both tendons are brought forth from the incisions; note the length of the distal tendon stump. **E,** The proximal end is pulled distally to display where the anastomosis would have to occur if a direct repair were to be done. **F,** The flexor digitorum longus (FDL) to the second toe will be harvested to add motor strength to the weakened muscle of the FHL and to permit an anastomosis distal to the sesamoids. The FDL slip to the second toe is tensioned by the hemostat, causing flexion of the second toe. **G,** The FDL is cut at the plantar aspect of the second toe just proximal to the distal interphalangeal crease and withdrawn from the incision. **H,** The FDL is passed with the previously placed suture through the sheath of the FHL and into the distal incision, where it lies next to the distal stump of the FHL. **I,** The FDL is secured to the FHL distally. **J,** The proximal end of the FHL is then secured to the FDL. **K,** The repaired FHL and transferred FDL from the second toe have good mechanical integrity.

and anastomosing the FHL to the proximal FDL tendon and tendon graft (probably an unnecessarily complex procedure).

Significant complications after FHL tendon repair or reconstruction include restricted IP joint motion[107,125] and contracture at the IP joint from a tight FHL tendon.[92] Coghlan and Clarke[92] reported that a Z-lengthening of the FHL tendon was necessary to achieve an acceptable result. Romash[125] and others[107,122] did not find that a stiff IP joint led to major disability. Rasmussen and Thyssen[122] observed that FHL tendon function does not seem to be essential in achieving a satisfactory long-term result after rupture or laceration. Floyd et al[9] stated that not repairing the FHL tendon can result in mild deformity with essentially no functional deficit. Patients who remain untreated or who have an unsuccessful repair and develop a hyperextension deformity can ultimately be treated with an IP joint fusion and transfer of the extensor hallucis longus to the first metatarsal head (Jones transfer).

Other potential complications after surgery include postoperative scarring, pain at the surgical site, traumatic neuroma, skin slough, and infection.

Bell and Schon[4] observed that the FHL tendon is especially vulnerable to penetrating injuries to the sole. The depth of the injury in the midfoot makes exposure of the tendon difficult and can require substantial extension of the incision. When possible, an incision should avoid the plantar aspect of the foot. A primary repair can be carried out with either a modified Kessler or Bunnell suture technique. Postoperatively, the foot should be splinted in mild equinus, with weight bearing initiated 4 weeks after surgery. Cast or brace protection with limited extension of the hallux is continued for 8 to 12 weeks after repair.

Romash[125] observed that with a closed rupture, IP joint motion should not be expected postoperatively. With repair of the FHL tendon after laceration, more than 60% of patients noted some active IP joint motion.

The surgical approach to a plantar laceration goes far beyond the question of whether the FHL tendon should be repaired or not repaired. Adequate wound management includes irrigation, debridement, exploration to determine the magnitude of the injury and relation of injury to other structures, including plantar nerves and vessels, and when possible, restoration of normal anatomy. This is best done in the operating room under adequate anesthesia where adequate exploration and wound management can be performed. After either a spontaneous rupture or a laceration with disruption of the FHL tendon, a repair should be performed when feasible. On the other hand, the magnitude of the exploration and the morbidity involved with such surgery should be weighed against the expected end result of surgery. If a patient develops postoperative weakness of the IP joint or a hyperextension deformity, a delayed IP joint fusion of the hallux can treat symptoms after nonsurgical treatment or an unsuccessful repair of an FHL tendon injury.

Although the literature supports primary repair of an FHL laceration, a patient should be informed that after repair, active flexion of the IP joint is uncommon. Still, despite lack of IP flexion, a reasonable goal with repair may be to restore some plantar-flexion power to the MTP joint and to the ankle joint. Perhaps there is also merit in repairing the tendon to regain some proprioceptive input from the FHL. The inconvenience or functional problems after treatment with benign neglect might not be well documented in the literature, but the authors recommend attempts at repair of the FHL tendon in the case of laceration or rupture, especially in young, active patients.

PERONEAL TENDONS

Peroneus Longus

Reports of dysfunction of the peroneus longus tendon are uncommon.[224] Peroneal tendon tenosynovitis, longitudinal ruptures or partial tears of the peroneus longus tendon, and disruption or pathologic changes isolated to the os peroneum constitute the major pathologic conditions associated with the peroneus longus (Fig. 24-60).

Anatomy

The peroneus longus muscle originates on the lateral condyle of the tibia and the head and midlateral aspect of the fibula and inserts onto the inferior aspect of the

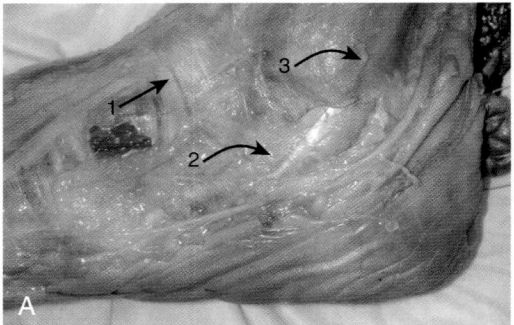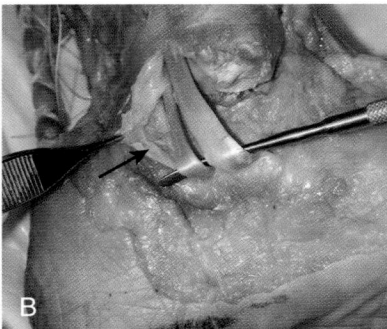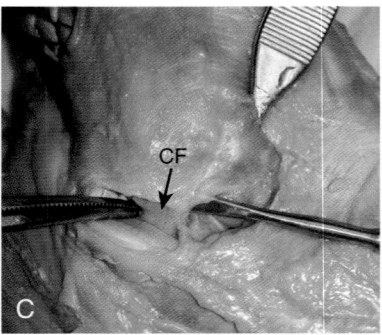

Figure 24-60 Anatomic dissections of the peroneal tendons. **A,** Anatomy of the lateral ankle (*1,* extensor retinaculum; *2,* inferior peroneal retinaculum; *3,* superior peroneal retinaculum). **B,** Turn-down of superior peroneal retinaculum *(arrow)* off of the fibula exposing the peroneal tendons. **C,** Calcaneofibular *(CF)* ligament just superior to the peroneal tendons.

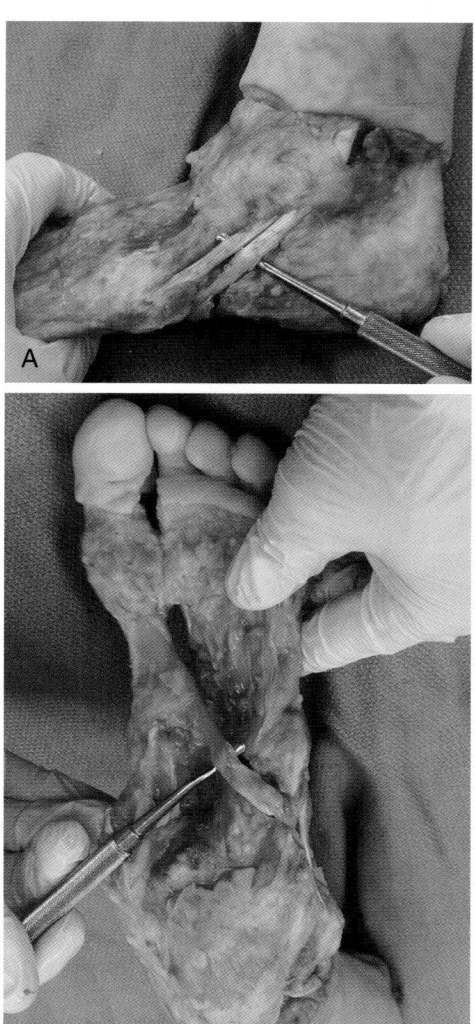

Figure 24-61 **A,** Lateral view demonstrating peroneus longus and brevis. **B,** Plantar view demonstrating the course of the peroneus longus.

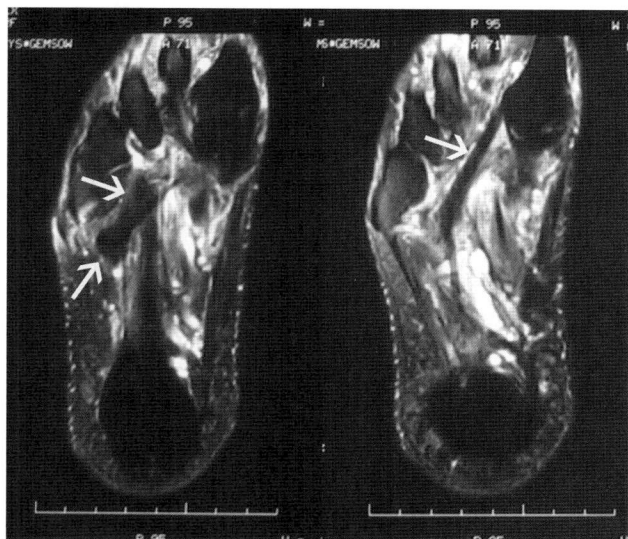

Figure 24-62 Magnetic resonance image of the course of the peroneus longus. Note the thickened tendon *(left),* where the tendon courses around the cuboid. *Right,* the deeper slice of the same foot shows the course of the tendon proximal and plantar to the bases of the second through fourth metatarsals and onto the lateral base of the proximal first metatarsal.

first cuneiform and the inferolateral aspect of the first metatarsal (Fig. 24-61). Innervated by the superficial peroneal nerve, the peroneus longus acts to plantar flex and evert the foot as well as to support the arch. It also plantar flexes the first metatarsal. In its muscular portion, the peroneus longus lies posterior and lateral to the peroneus brevis muscle and becomes tendinous proximal to the ankle joint. It courses posterior to the peroneus brevis at the level of the distal fibula and then runs beneath the trochlear process of the calcaneus in an inferomedial direction. As the tendon crosses over the peroneal tubercle, it turns sharply and obliquely across the plantar aspect of the foot. After traversing the cuboid tunnel, it runs along the metatarsocuneiform (MTC) joints and inserts on the plantar lateral aspect of the first metatarsal (Fig. 24-62).

On the lateral aspect of the calcaneus, the peroneal tubercle can vary in size.[170] Along the course of the tendon,

from a point just proximal to the tip of the fibula and extending to the cuboid tunnel, the peroneus longus is surrounded by a synovial sheath. From a point approximately 4 cm above the lateral malleolus to the peroneal tubercle, the peroneus longus and brevis share a common sheath.[302] Distally, the sheath bifurcates at the level of the peroneal tubercle (Fig. 24-63). At this point, the peroneus brevis extends onward to its insertion into the base of the fifth metatarsal, and the peroneus longus courses toward the plantar surface of the cuboid, finally inserting on the plantar aspect of the first metatarsal.

Within the substance of the peroneus longus, the *os peroneum* may be present.[87] Its frequency has been debated in orthopaedic literature. Sarrafian[255] stated it is always present and may be in either a cartilaginous or a fibrocartilaginous state, whereas Pfitzner[237] noted it to be present in 8.5% of anatomic specimens. The os peroneum may be fully ossified, less than fully ossified, or multipartite. The os peroneum and tendon of the peroneus longus together are closely associated with both the lateral border of the calcaneus and the plantar lateral aspect of the cuboid (Fig. 24-64).

The course of the sural nerve in relation to the peroneal tendons is important. Above the tip of the fibula, the tendons are anterior to the nerve, although there can be a communicating branch from the sural nerve to the superficial peroneal nerve in this location. Distal to the bone, two or more branches may cross the tendons. One branch, usually between 1 and 2 cm, and the other about 4 cm distal to the tip of the fibula are noted. The main trunk of the nerve crosses over the peroneus longus tendon about 2 cm proximal to the calcaneocuboid joint,

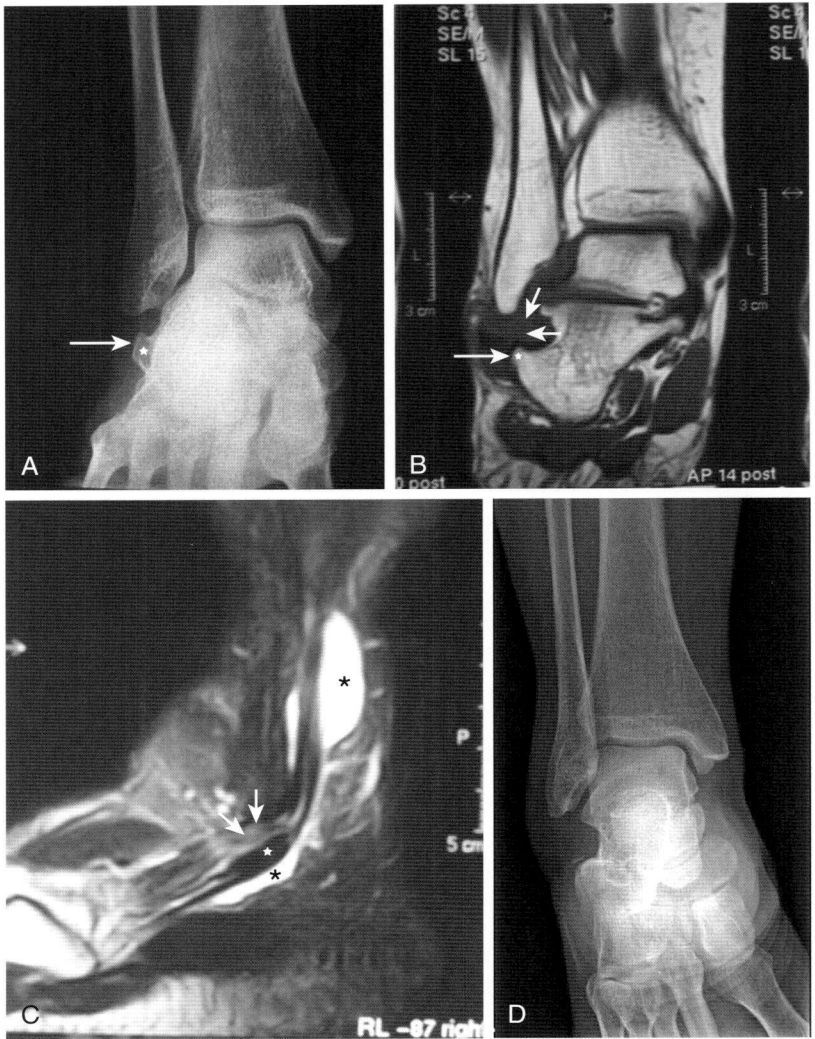

Figure 24-63 Large peroneal tubercle. Anteroposterior (AP) radiograph **(A)** and coronal magnetic resonance image (MRI) **(B)** demonstrating large hypertrophied peroneal tubercle *(arrows)*. **C,** Sagittal MRI demonstrating enlarged tubercle with effusion *(white arrows)* of the peroneal tendon sheath. **D,** AP radiograph after excision of the tubercle. (From Boya H, Pinar H: Stenosing tenosynovitis of the peroneus brevis tendon associated with hypertrophy of the peroneal tubercle, *J Foot Ankle Surg* 49:188–190, 2010. Used with permission.)

and then over the peroneus brevis 1 cm proximal to the calcaneocuboid joint. The blood supply of the peroneus longus has been studied by Petersen et al.[235] They found avascular regions where the peroneus longus tendon courses around the lateral malleolus and the anterior part of the tendon by the peroneal trochlea of the calcaneus. Another avascular zone exists where the tendon runs around the cuboid. These are the regions where the tendon is particularly vulnerable to tears.

Peroneal Tenosynovitis

Etiology
Tenosynovitis of the peroneal tendons was first described by Hildebrand[185] in 1907 and later by Hackenbroch.[181]

Since then, there have been numerous cases of peroneal tendon tenosynovitis reported in the literature.

Tenosynovitis can develop at different levels. It may be associated with hypertrophy of the peroneal tubercle* and can occur along the course of the peroneal tendons,[138,185] at the level of the lateral malleolus,[181] or at the ankle joint.[174,296] Burman[40] reported eight cases at the level of the peroneal tubercle. He hypothesized that this condition developed from a congenitally enlarged peroneal tubercle or after trauma to the peroneal tendons (a direct blow, strain or sprain, fracture, inflammatory arthropathy, overuse, or from an injury to the os peroneum). Burman believed that Hildebrand did not describe

---

*References 40, 152, 184, 229, 238, 278, 285, and 302.

stenosing tenosynovitis but rather subluxation of the peroneal tendons. Aberle-Horstenegg[138] described five cases of localized pain, along the course of the peroneus longus as it passes beneath the cuboid, that were successfully treated with conservative measures.

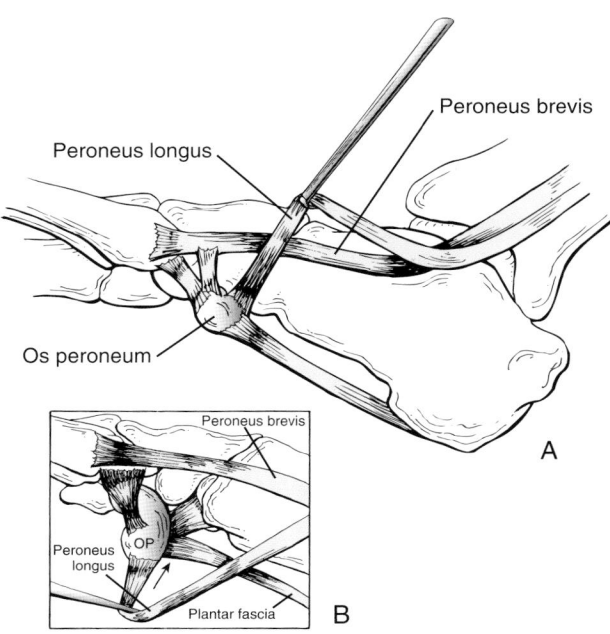

Figure 24-64 The os peroneum (*OP*) has four soft tissue attachments, including plantar fascial band, fifth metatarsal band, band to peroneus brevis **(A),** and the fourth band to cuboid **(B).** (Redrawn from Sobel M, Pavlov H, Geppert M, et al: Painful os peroneum syndrome: a spectrum of conditions responsible for plantar lateral foot pain, *Foot Ankle* 15:112–124, 1994.)

History and Physical Examination

With tenosynovitis of the peroneal tendons, a patient typically complains of vague pain on the posterolateral aspect of the hindfoot that is increased with activity and diminished by rest. Cutting activities or running around curves can induce pain. A traumatic episode, such as an inversion injury to the ankle may be associated with the onset of discomfort. A patient might not recall a specific episode related to the onset of symptoms but instead might cite an increase in athletic training or physical activity associated with discomfort.

Tenosynovitis can develop after a lateral ankle sprain, direct blow to the peroneal tubercle, foreign body penetration,[299] fracture of the calcaneus or fibula, or other episodes of direct or indirect trauma. The patient often notes pain with palpation along the course of the peroneal tendons inferior to the fibula. A palpable thickening may also be noted. Pain may be elicited with passive inversion of the foot or active eversion or pronation of the forefoot against resistance.

Radiographic Examination

Zivot et al[302] and Palmer[233] suggested that peroneal tenography may be helpful in defining the architecture of tendons and determining the presence or distortion of the peroneal tendons from tenosynovitis. Chen et al[158] demonstrated the diminution of the tendon sheath after calcaneal fractures (Fig. 24-65). MRI may be helpful in distinguishing tenosynovitis from either a complete disruption or a partial tear of the peroneus longus (Fig. 24-66).[193,265] However, there is a marked decrease in sensitivity in the detection of peroneal tendon tears with MRI in comparison with other tendons of the foot and ankle because of the *magic angle effect.*[197] The postioning of the

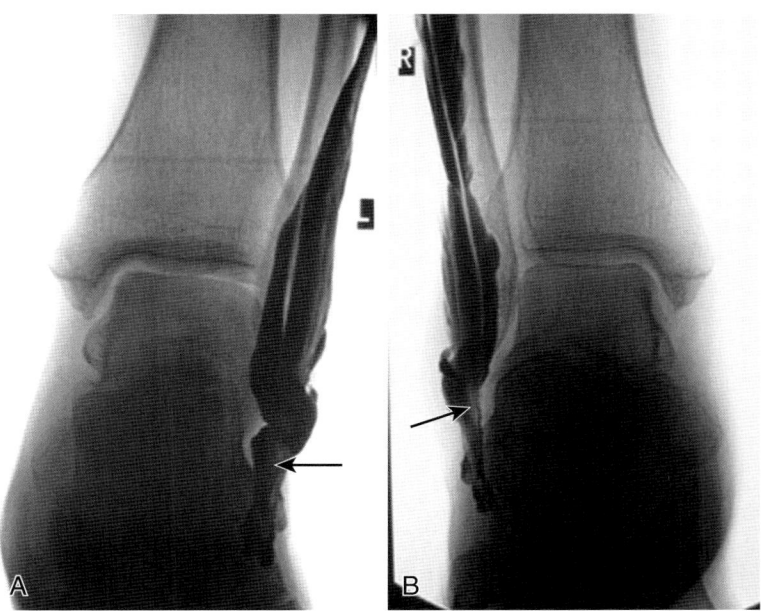

Figure 24-65 Peroneal tenogram to evaluate tendons after calcaneus fracture. **A,** Normal tenogram *(arrow).* **B,** Lateral compression from expanded calcaneal fracture compresses tendon sheath *(arrow).* (From Chen W, Li X, Su Y, et al: Peroneal tenography to evaluate lateral hindfoot pain after calcaneal fracture, *Foot Ankle Int* 32:789–795, 2011. Used with permission.)

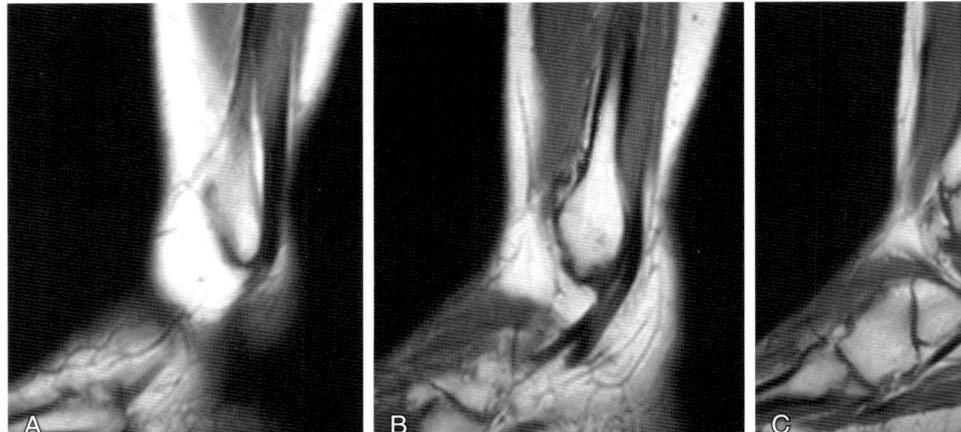

Figure 24-66 Magnetic resonance images of the peroneal tendons. The sequential images demonstrate the peroneal tendon anatomy. **A,** Posterior to the fibula, the peroneus longus is visualized, but on this slice, the peroneus brevis is seen inserting distally onto the fifth metatarsal. **B,** The tendons are seen in the region posterior to the tip of the fibula, where peroneus brevis tears often occur. The brevis is more anterior and medial. **C,** This deeper slice demonstrates the peroneus longus running over the distal calcaneus toward the inferior aspect of the cuboid. This is where peroneus longus tears occur. Note in this slice posterior to the fibula that the tendons are seen within the groove.

extremity may make a dramatic difference in the sensitivity, because Mengiardi et al[214] have demonstrated a higher accuracy when the patient is positioned prone for the study. Ultrasound assessment of the tendon can be useful, particularly in dynamic conditions, such as with tendon subluxation or dislocation.

Conservative Treatment

Nonsurgical treatment for symptomatic peroneal tenosynovitis includes orthotic devices, physical therapy, change in training techniques, and a stirrup or CAM-boot.[173] A below-knee walking cast or brace may be used for 3 to 4 weeks to decrease symptoms. Because sudden changes in training patterns, alterations in surface conditions, and increases in intensity or duration of exercise (or both) can lead to symptoms, eliminating or controlling these factors can allow resolution. With continued symptoms of swelling and thickening consistent with peroneal tenosynovitis, some experts have advocated that a carefully placed corticosteroid injection into the tendon sheath may relieve symptoms. To minimize the risk of rupture, the foot and ankle should be immobilized after the injection. With continued pain and swelling, surgical intervention may be indicated. Platelet-rich plasma derived from bone marrow or peripheral blood may be helpful for treating tendinopathy, provided that the tendon has not lost continuity or stretched beyond function.

Surgical Treatment

Simple division of the tendon sheath was reported as effective in relieving symptoms. Anderson[143] noted that symptoms were poorly defined and that excision of the roof of the tendon sheath is usually successful. Pierson and Inglis[238] released the retinaculum and shaved

a hypertrophied peroneal tubercle with good results. Interposing the retinaculum between the raw osseous surfaces of the calcaneus and the peroneus longus is recommended. It is possible that the benefit seen was due to the instigation of a healing response after a surgical trauma. Perhaps the growth factors and cells released during the resection of bone or the debridement of tissues per se were therapeutic.

PERONEAL TENOSYNOVECTOMY
Surgical Technique

1. With the patient placed in a lateral decubitus position, a thigh tourniquet may be used to facilitate visualization.
2. A curvilinear incision is begun at the base of the fifth metatarsal and extended to the tip of the fibula. With subcutaneous dissection, care is taken to define and protect the sural nerve and its branches.
3. The peroneal tendons are visualized through a longitudinal incision dividing the tendon sheaths (Fig. 24-67).
4. With a stenotic area of the tendon sheath, a longitudinal section is removed from the sheath. Any degenerated areas of tendon or partial ruptures are resected or repaired. The peroneal tubercle is inspected and, if hypertrophied, may be resected or smoothed.
5. The peroneus longus tendon is inspected for the presence of an os peroneum. If the os peroneum is enlarged, irregular, or damaged, it may be resected and the tendon of the peroneus longus primarily repaired. With a tear of the peroneus brevis, a repair or reconstruction is performed (see discussion under "Peroneus Brevis").
6. The tendon sheaths are left unrepaired. If the superior peroneal retinaculum was incised to enable exposure,

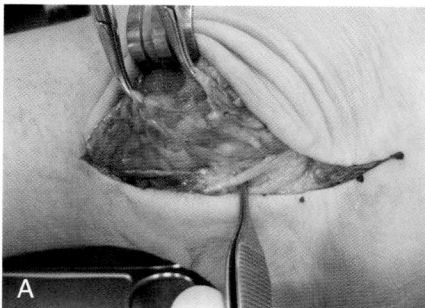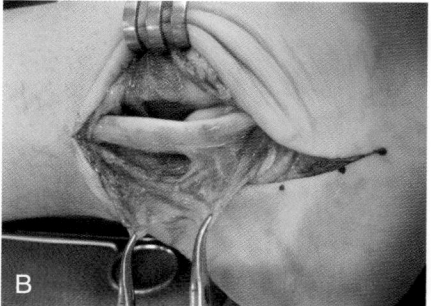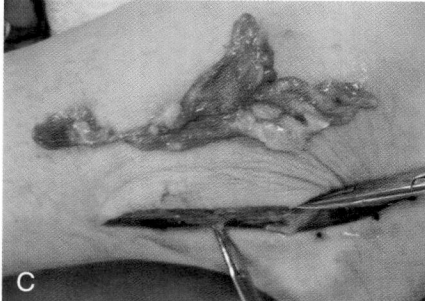

Figure 24-67 Exploration for peroneal tendon tenosynovectomy. **A,** Incision just posterior to the distal fibula. Note sural nerve and expanded peroneal retinaculum from tenosynovitis. **B,** Tenosynovectomy of the peroneus longus. **C,** The entire synovial specimen is removed from both tendons.

it must be repaired meticulously to prevent postoperative subluxation or dislocation.

7. The subcutaneous tissue is closed with absorbable sutures. The skin is approximated with interrupted or running sutures.

Postoperative Care

A below-knee non–weight-bearing cast or splint is placed with the foot and ankle in a neutral position. Two weeks after surgery, a below-knee walking cast or brace is applied. Range-of-motion activities and physical therapy are initiated 2 to 4 weeks after surgery. Strengthening exercises are also begun.

Results

Pierson and Inglis[238] reported a case of stenosing tenosynovitis of the peroneus longus associated with hypertrophy of the peroneal tubercle and os peroneum. They released the retinaculum and excised the hypertrophied tubercle. The retinaculum was interposed between the raw osseous surface of the calcaneus and the peroneus longus.

The differential diagnosis of a symptomatic peroneus longus tendon includes an acute fracture of the os peroneum or diastasis of a partite os peroneum, chronic diastasis of a previously fractured os peroneum, stenosing peroneus longus tenosynovitis, a tear of the peroneus longus distal or proximal to the os peroneum, attrition or complete rupture of the peroneus longus tendon proximal or distal to the os peroneum,[190] and an enlarged peroneal tubercle (see Fig. 24-63). Sobel et al[269] suggested that a painful os peroneum syndrome should be included with other diagnoses in the differential diagnosis, including lateral ankle sprain, peroneus brevis or extensor digitorum brevis avulsion, proximal fifth metatarsal fracture, and fracture of the anterior process of the calcaneus.

Tendon Disruption

Isolated injuries of the peroneus longus tendon are uncommon and typically limited to case reports in the literature (Fig. 24-68).[150,157,190,262] The os peroneum is

often a useful marker in the diagnosis of the rupture. Its position is noted to be slightly proximal to the normal position, providing a clue about the rupture. Thompson and Patterson[282] thought that the presence of an os peroneum predisposed the structure to a degenerative tear in the peroneus longus tendon just distal to the sesamoid. Jahss[186] reported that spontaneous ruptures can occur in the peroneus longus secondary to rheumatoid arthritis and psoriasis. Truong et al[286] stated that concomitant diabetes or hyperparathyroidism can lead to nontraumatic rupture of either the peroneus longus or the os peroneum. A local steroid injection has as well been implicated in peroneus longus tendon rupture.[151,271] Tears of the peroneus longus have been associated with gouty infiltration (Fig. 24-69).[199,243] Pierson and Inglis[238] found that the most common locations for irritation of the peroneus longus are at the level of the peroneal tubercle and the inferior retinaculum. The differential diagnosis of a symptomatic peroneus longus tendon includes an acute fracture of the os peroneum or diastasis of a partite os peroneum, chronic diastasis of a previously fractured os peroneum, stenosing peroneus longus tenosynovitis, a tear of the peroneus longus distal or proximal to the os peroneum, attrition or complete rupture of the peroneus longus tendon proximal or distal to the os peroneum,[190] and an enlarged peroneal tubercle (Fig. 24-70, see Fig. 24-63 and Video Clip 103). Sobel et al[269] suggested that a painful os peroneum syndrome should be included with other diagnoses, including lateral ankle sprain, peroneus brevis or extensor digitorum brevis avulsion, proximal fifth metatarsal fracture, and fracture of the anterior process of the calcaneus.

History and Physical Examination

The onset of acute plantar lateral ankle pain can occur after a traumatic episode (e.g., ankle inversion, supination injury). In chronic cases, symptoms of instability and recurrent episodes of "ankle sprains" or plantar lateral foot pain after athletic activity may be noted.[150] The symptoms can be vague and nonspecific. MacDonald and Wertheimer[205] stressed that diagnosis may be significantly delayed with peroneus longus injuries. Zermatten and

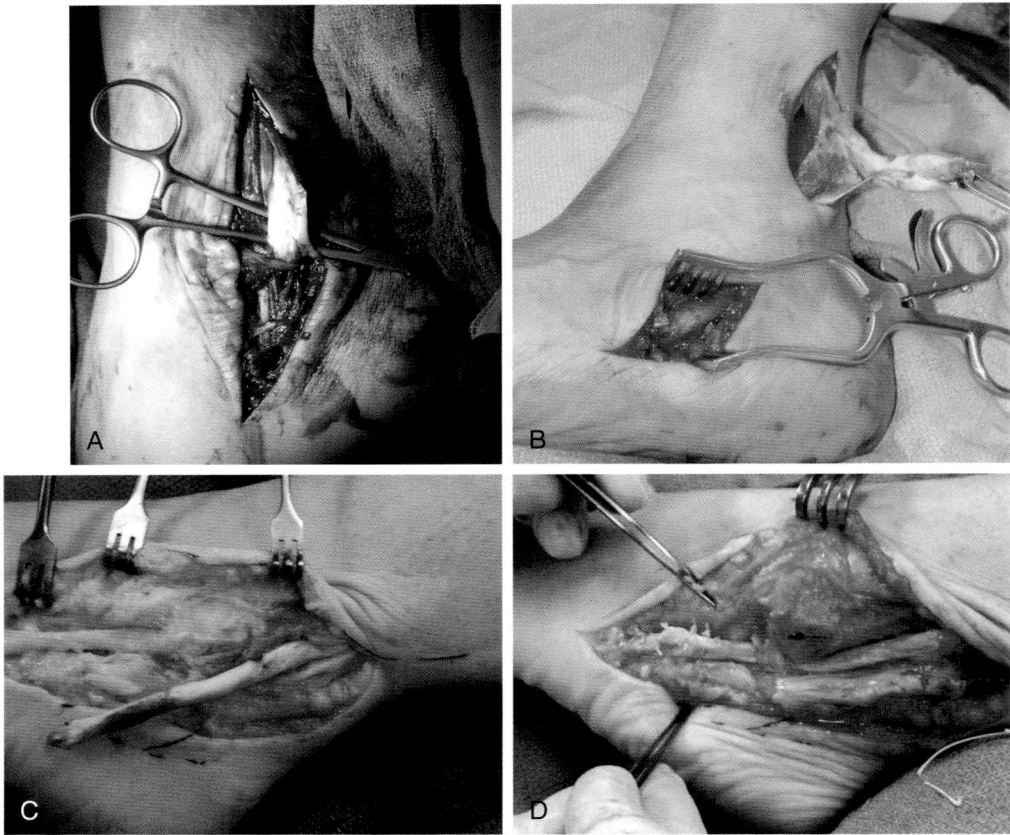

Figure 24-68 Complete rupture of the peroneus longus tendon is demonstrated at surgical exploration. **A,** Flattened tear with multiple perforations of the peroneus longus. **B,** Distal disruption with proximal migration requiring extensive exploration to retrieve the proximal portion. **C,** Rupture of the peroneus longus 10 years after a Watson-Jones repair that sacrificed the peroneus brevis. With rupture, the patient lost the ability to evert her foot. **D,** Salvage with tenodesis of the peroneus longus stump to the brevis, with takedown of the Watson-Jones repair. The patient retained good ankle stability.[190]

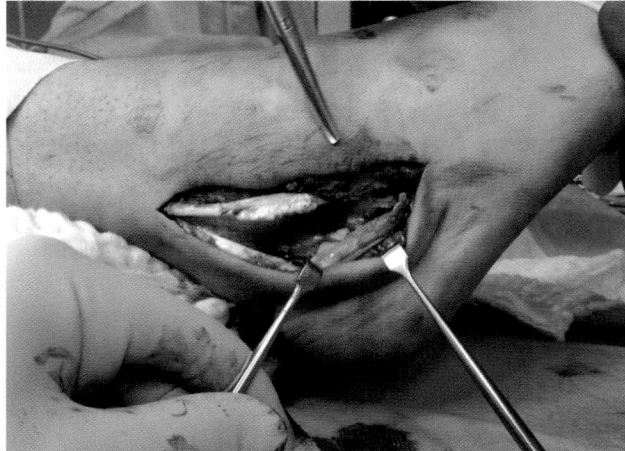

Figure 24-69 Gouty infiltration of peroneal tendons. (From Radice F, Monckeberg JE, Carcuro G: Longitudinal tears of peroneus longus and brevis tendons: a gouty infiltration, *J Foot Ankle Surg* 50:751–753, 2011. Used with permission.)

Crevoisier[301] diagnosed an avulsion fracture of the insertion of the peroneus longus on the base of the first metatarsal with the use of computed tomography (CT) scanning.

Well-localized tenderness, synovitis, or thickening along the course of the distal peroneus longus tendon may be observed. Palpation may demonstrate significant tenderness over the peroneal tubercle, over the os peroneum, or where the peroneus longus enters the cuboid tunnel. Dysesthesia along the distal aspect of the sural nerve can develop. Pain may be increased with resistive plantar flexion of the first ray. Patients can also demonstrate pain or weakness with forced eversion of the foot.

Thompson and Patterson[282] did not find that a loss of function of the peroneus longus led to the formation of a dorsal bunion. They did note, however, the development of a second metatarsal stress fracture in one case.

Radiographic Examination

Initial imaging includes AP, lateral, and oblique radiographs of the foot and ankle. Thompson and Patterson[282] stated that the position of the os peroneum is a useful marker, especially with serial radiographs. Oblique

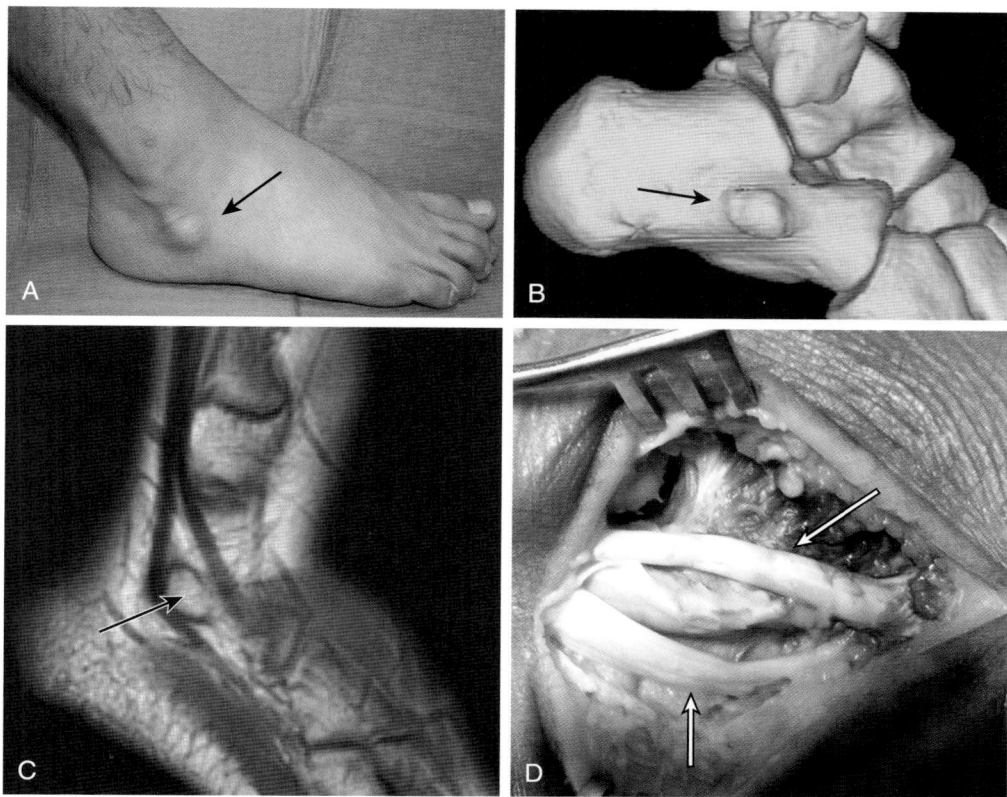

Figure 24-70 Enlarged peroneal tubercle leading to peroneal tendon dysfunction. **A,** Large osseous prominence representing peroneal tubercle *(arrow).* **B,** Three-dimensional computed tomography image of enlarged tubercle *(arrow).* **C,** T1- weighted magnetic resonance image showing peroneus longus pushed inferiorly below enlarged tubercle *(arrow).* **D,** Intraoperative photograph showing enlarged tubercle separating two tendons *(arrows),* leading to tenosynovitis of the peroneus longus. **(A-C,** From Taki K, Yamazaki S, Majima T, et al: Bilateral stenosing tenosynovitis of the peroneus longus tendon associated with hypertrophied peroneal tubercle in a junior soccer: a case report, *Foot Ankle Int* 28:129–132, 2007. Used with permission. **D,** From Heller E, Robinson D: Traumatic pathologies of the calcaneal peroneal tubercle, *Foot (Edinb)* 20:96–98, 2010.)

radiographs can demonstrate proximal retraction of the sesamoid (Figs. 24-71 and 24-72).[218,282] An enlarged peroneal tubercle may be observed as well.[156,193] Truong et al[286] encouraged the use of MRI to diagnose an os peroneum fracture, and Kilkelly and McHale[193] recommended MRI in the diagnosis of a ruptured peroneus longus tendon. A radionucleotide scan can demonstrate increased uptake in the os peroneum after a fracture or disruption (Fig. 24-73). Chadwick et al[157] demonstrated the accuracy of MRI in differentiating a fractured os perineum from edema in the adjacent proximal tendon (Fig. 24-74).

Ultrasound can be useful in experienced hands to diagnose peroneal tendon disease, especially in situations where a dynamic real-time evaluation is warranted.[228]

Conservative Treatment

Treatment depends on the magnitude and duration of a patient's symptoms. Nonsurgical treatment includes immobilization with a below-knee cast, air brace, or splint; taping; a compression dressing; orthotic devices; and physical therapy.[246] Sobel et al[269] reported that in

addition to their one case of successful treatment, seven other patients cited in the literature recovered successfully with nonsurgical treatment. Smith et al[262] found that a minimally displaced os perineum fracture can be successfully treated with immobilization, with the expectation of a return to a high level of activity. Although treatment of acute conditions can be nonoperative, chronic problems are less likely to respond to these measures. Sobel et al[269] found cast immobilization was successful in 20% of patients with chronic peroneus longus symptoms but that 80% eventually required surgery. Although a corticosteroid injection may be considered for chronic cases, more than one corticosteroid injection should be discouraged.

Surgical Treatment

With continued pain, swelling, and dysfunction, surgical intervention may be considered. The location of symptoms generally determines the surgical approach. Pain in the area of a symptomatic os peroneum combined with positive imaging studies can necessitate exploration and

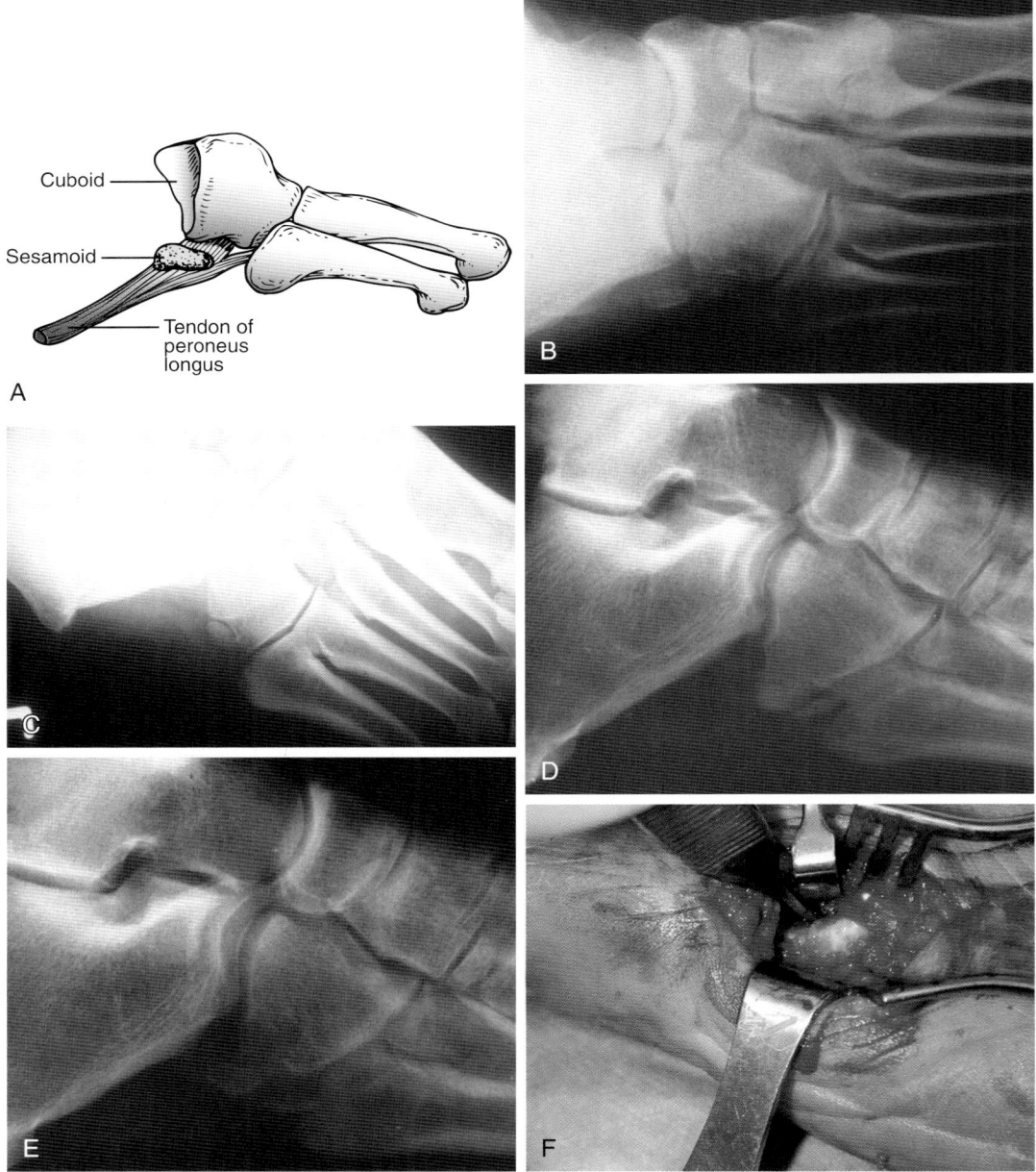

Figure 24-71 A, An os peroneum is contained within the tendon of the peroneus longus and articulates with the lateral border of the cuboid. **B,** More proximal location of the os peroneum can denote distal peroneus longus rupture. **C,** Normal location of os peroneum. **D,** Fragmentation of os peroneum. **E,** Proximal migration of os. Note a fragment of the os perineum is located distally, and the os has migrated proximally. **F,** Surgical excision of painful fragmented os peroneum.

excision of the os peroneum. More proximal symptoms can herald a longitudinal tear or disruption of the peroneus longus tendon.

OS PERONEUM EXCISION
The os peroneum may be excised with or without repair of the tendon. In Sobel's series[269] the os was excised in several cases and the peroneus longus tendon repaired as well. Of nine patients with chronic symptoms, four had a complete rupture of the peroneus longus distal to the os peroneum, and five had a chronic diastasis of a multipartite os peroneum.

Surgical Technique (Fig. 24-75 and Video Clip 106)
1. The patient is placed in a lateral decubitus position, and a thigh tourniquet may be used to facilitate hemostasis.
2. A longitudinal incision is extended from the tip of the fibula approximately 4 cm distally toward the tip of the fifth metatarsal.

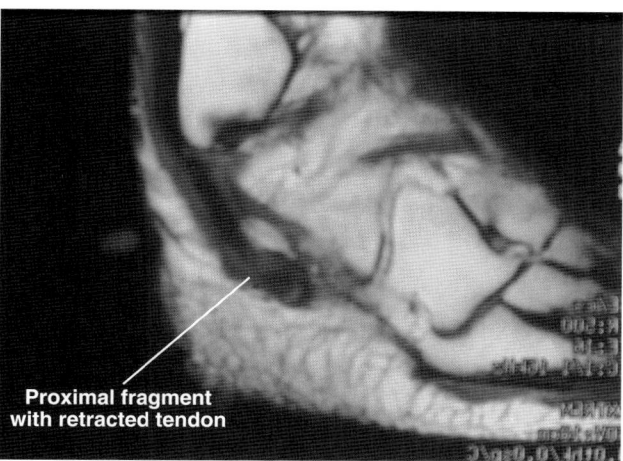

Figure 24-72 Magnetic resonance image demonstrating proximal retraction of fragment of os perineum, entrapped in the inferior peroneal retinaculum. (From Sammarco VJ, Cuttica DJ, Sammarco GJ: Lasso stitch with peroneal retinaculoplasty for player: a case report, *Clin Orthop Relat Res* 468:1012-1017, 2010. Used with permission.)

3. The dissection is carried down to the peroneus longus tendon, and the tendon sheath is incised. Care is taken to protect the adjacent sural nerve and its branches.

4. The os peroneum is carefully identified and, when disrupted or degenerated, is carefully shelled out of the peroneus longus tendon. If the peroneus longus is intact, it may be reinforced with interrupted No. 1 nonabsorbable suture. If the tendon is ruptured, it may be approximated with a modified Bunnell, Kessler, or Krackow suture. It can be difficult to close the void left by the os peroneum, and it is often challenging to get a grip of the distal aspect of the tendon. Thus it is useful to insert the suture distal to the os before excising it to minimize this latter problem. A strip of peroneus longus tendon may be needed to span the resultant gap to address the former situation. One additional option, if the peroneus longus tendon cannot be reconstructed, is attaching to the cuboid with a suture anchor.

5. The tendon sheath is not closed. The overlying soft tissue and skin are approximated in a routine manner.

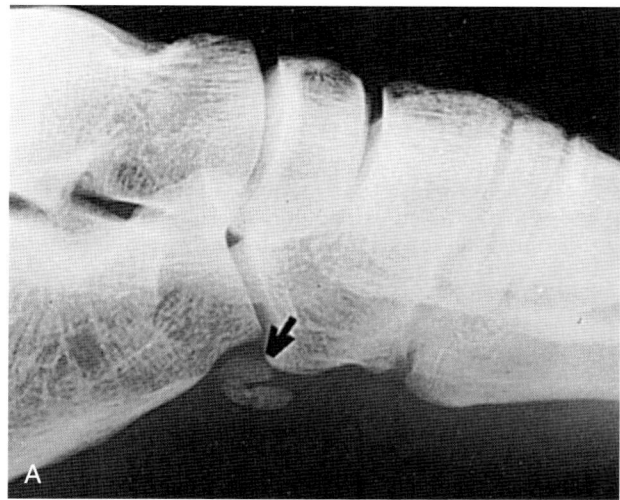

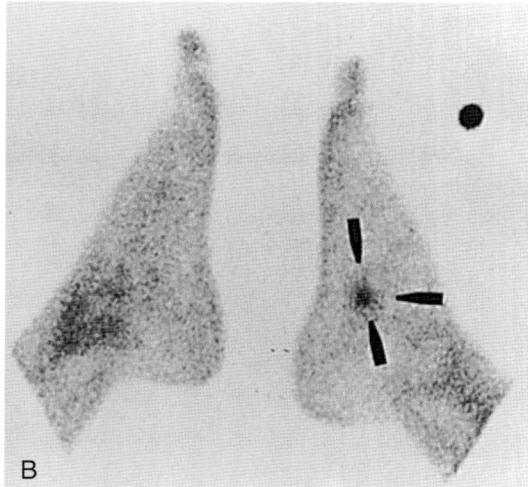

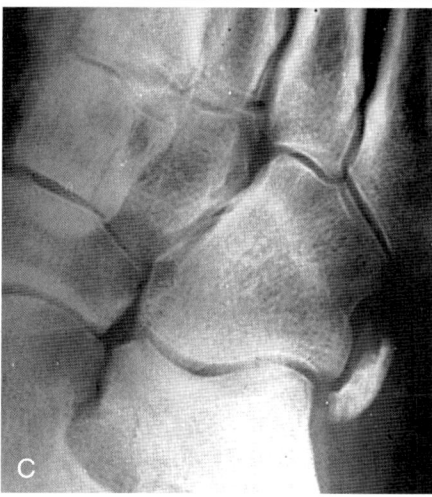

Figure 24-73 **A,** Osteochondritis of the os peroneum is demonstrated by its fragmentation *(arrow).* **B,** Technetium bone scan demonstrates increased uptake in os peroneum *(arrowheads).* **C,** Osteochondritis of os peroneum as demonstrated by sclerotic appearance of sesamoid. The os peroneum is at risk for rupture.

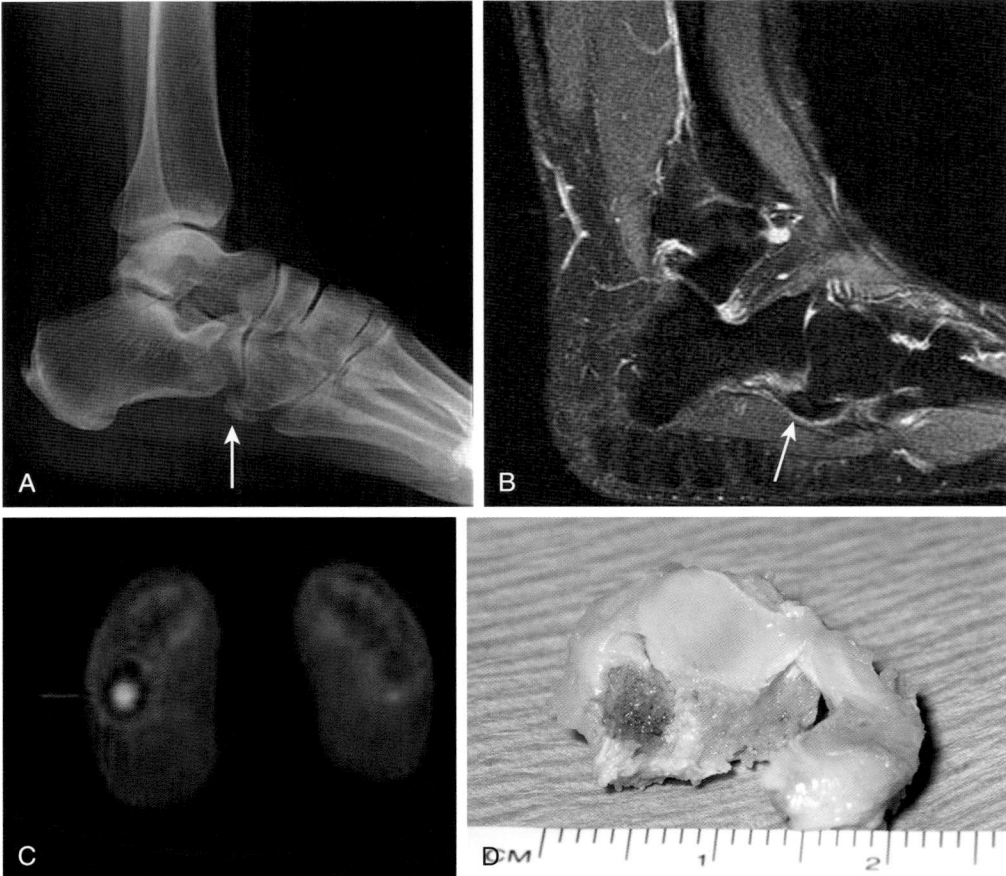

Figure 24-74 Symptomatic os perineum. **A,** Lateral radiograph showing bipartite os perineum *(arrow)*. **B,** Short tau inversion recovery magnetic resonance imaging (STIR MRI) scan showing edema in the tendon of the peroneus longus *(arrow)*. **C,** Single photon emission computed tomography (SPECT) scan showing focal uptake in os peroneum. **D,** Excised fragment after excision and repair of the peroneus longus tendon. (From Chadwick C, Highland AM, Hughes DE, Davies MB: The importance of magnetic resonance imaging in a symptomatic "bipartite" os peroneum: a case report, *J Foot Ankle Surg* 50:82–86, 2011. Used with permission.)

Postoperative Care

A below-knee splint is applied with the foot in a neutral position and the ankle in slight eversion. A below-knee walking cast or CAM-boot is applied 2 to 4 weeks after surgery. Immobilization is continued for 6 more weeks, after which physical therapy and progressive passive and active resistive exercises are initiated. A soft brace or a stirrup brace may be helpful during the subsequent 6 to 16 weeks. Involvement in sports should be curtailed until at least 12 weeks after surgery.

PERONEAL TENDON TENODESIS[282]
Surgical Technique (Video Clips 106 and 107)

1. The patient is positioned in a lateral decubitus position, with a thigh tourniquet used for hemostasis as needed.
2. A longitudinal incision is extended from the base of the fifth metatarsal to the tip of the fibula. Care is

taken to identify and protect the sural nerve and its branches.

3. The dissection is deepened to the peroneus longus and brevis tendons, and the tendon sheath is incised longitudinally.
4. The tendon of the peroneus longus is identified. With a distal rupture, the os peroneum might have migrated proximally toward the tip of the fibula, but it typically does not retract farther proximally. The proximal remnant of the peroneus longus is resected, as is the os peroneum. If it is long enough, the distal aspect of the peroneus longus is then woven through the peroneus brevis distal to the fibula and reinforced with interrupted nonabsorbable sutures. The proximal segment of the peroneus longus may be tenodesed to the peroneus brevis if sufficient tendon is present (Fig. 24-76). It is critical that a bulky anastomosis is not created in the area beginning 1 cm distal to tip of the fibula and 3 cm proximal to this point, to avoid stenosis.

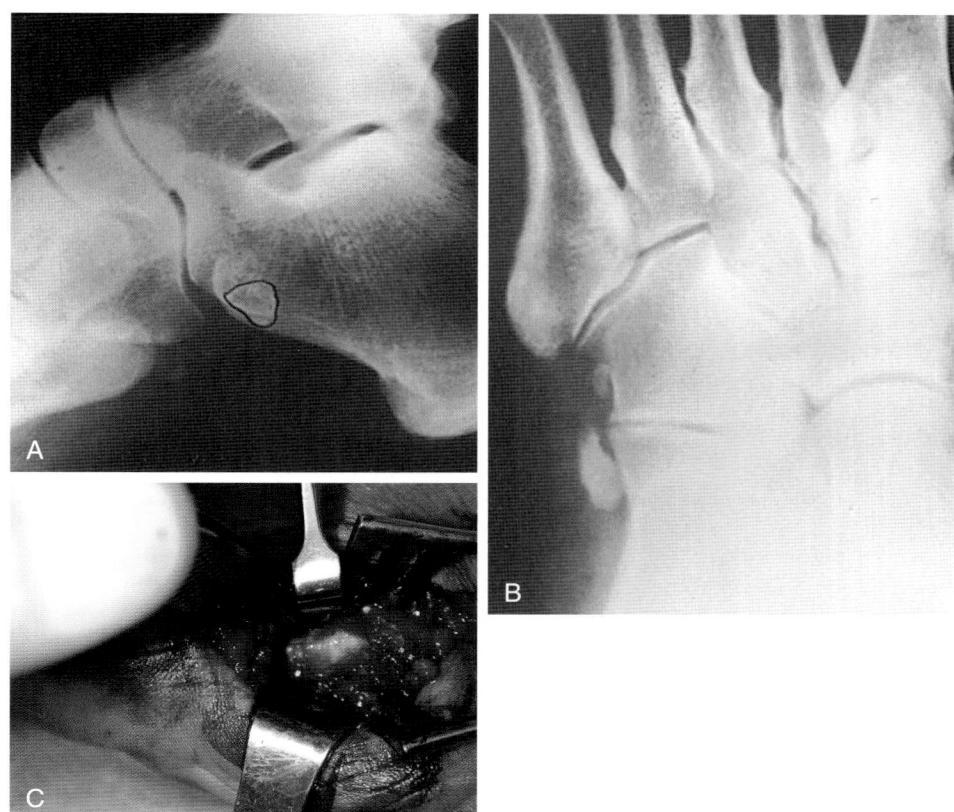

Figure 24-75 **A,** Onset of pain in a 56-year-old man on the lateral aspect of the foot and ankle, with the os peroneum slightly proximal to the normal position. **B,** Oblique radiograph of a 72-year-old man 2 months after onset of lateral foot pain demonstrates proximal migration of os peroneum to the level of the calcaneocuboid joint. **C,** Intraoperative photograph demonstrates rupture of the peroneus longus at the level of the os peroneum with proximal retraction. (**A** and **B,** From Thompson F, Patterson A: Rupture of the peroneus longus tendon. Report of three cases, *J Bone Joint Surg Am* 71:293–295, 1989.)

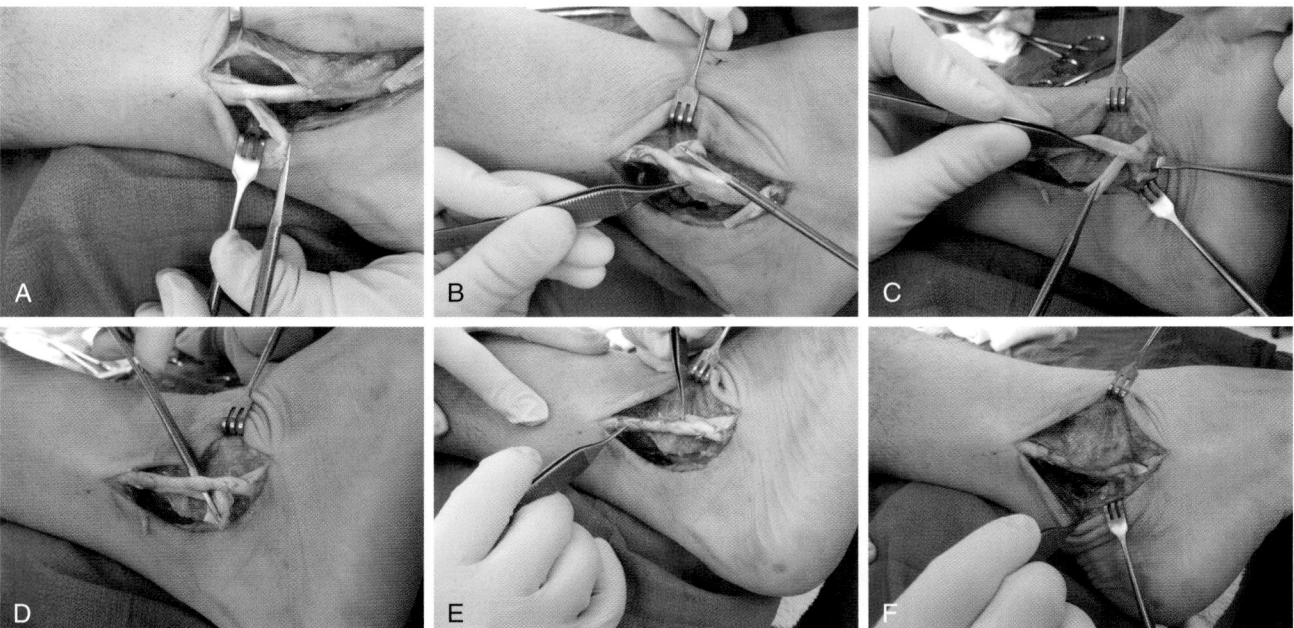

Figure 24-76 Technique of tenodesis (proximal and distal for incompetent peroneus brevis; the proximal tenodesis can be used for peroneus longus disruption as well. **A** and **B,** Peroneus brevis has been resected and proximal segment is woven through the proximal peroneus longus tendon. **C** and **D,** Distal weaving of tendon. **E,** Completion of weaving procedure. **F,** Tendons reduced behind fibula.

5. The tendon sheath is not closed except for the area incised proximal to the tip of the fibula. The overlying soft tissue is closed with interrupted sutures.

6. The skin is approximated in a routine manner (Fig. 24-76).

Postoperative Care

A postoperative splint is applied with the foot and ankle in neutral position. Two to 3 weeks after surgery, sutures are removed, and a below-knee walking cast or CAM-boot is applied. Six weeks later, the full immobilization is discontinued, and a stirrup or cloth brace may be used. Physical therapy commences with range-of-motion and strengthening exercises. Careful avoidance of forceful passive inversion and active eversion against resistance is recommended.

Results

Acute fractures of the os peroneum have been reported infrequently in the literature. A diagnosis may be difficult to make based on the presence of a multipartite or bipartite os peroneum. Sobel et al[269] reported on five patients with chronic diastasis of either a previous os peroneum injury or a multipartite os peroneum. The authors extensively reviewed the literature and identified 17 reports describing 26 patients with os peroneum and peroneus longus injuries. They concluded either that this was an overuse syndrome or that disruption of the os peroneum developed after trauma.

With an acute fracture of the os peroneum, diastasis can result with disruption of the peroneus longus tendon. Chronic diastasis with later development of stenosing peroneus longus tenosynovitis can occur as well. Likewise, attrition of the peroneus longus tendon either proximal or distal to the os peroneum, frank rupture of the peroneus longus either proximal or distal to the os peroneum, and an enlarged peroneal tubercle were all recognized by Sobel et al[269] as leading to chronic plantar lateral foot pain. With a disrupted os peroneum, thickening can develop along the course of the peroneus longus tendon inferior to the fibula or at the level of the peroneal tubercle or cuboid tunnel.

Guineys[180] and others[194,246,262,269] reported on nonsurgical treatment with cast immobilization, orthoses, steroid injection, and taping and noted successful results in 12 cases.

Surgical exploration of the peroneus longus tendon with excision of the os peroneum remains a primary form of treatment. Excision of the os peroneum and tenodesis of the peroneus longus to the peroneus brevis[269] were noted to have theoretic disadvantages, with the possible development of a dorsal bunion, although Thompson and Patterson[282] did not observe this in their experience. Coughlin and Schon have treated a case of peroneus longus rupture that had developed a dorsal bunion. A painful os peroneum may be surgically excised,[179,276,280] excised with primary repair of the peroneus longus tendon,[207,234,236,291] or excised with tenodesis of the

peroneus longus and peroneus brevis.[269,282] In advanced cases, exploration and excision of the peroneus longus may be necessary. Grisolia[179] and others have reported 18 cases treated surgically with excision of a painful os peroneum and primary repair when necessary; 17 (94%) had acceptable results. Sammarco et al[253] reported two cases of a primary repair with suturing for an acute fracture.

Longitudinal Tears

Traumatic rupture or tears of the peroneus longus tendon have been reported in the literature. Twenty-eight tears of the peroneus longus not associated with an os peroneum disruption, one disruption of the peroneus longus at the musculotendinous junction,[163] and 32 ruptures associated with an os peroneum injury have been reported. Thirty-four of these were treated surgically, and 32 had satisfactory results. Twelve ruptures that were treated conservatively had good results. In general, tears of the peroneus longus are decidedly less common that those of the peroneus brevis. In the area of the distal fibula, although occasionally a dual tear is observed,[199,243,247,271] much more commonly only a peroneus brevis tear is noted (Fig. 24-77).

Several cases of calcific tendinitis of the peroneus longus have been reported.[160,194,220,251,297] Sobel et al[269] suggested that these cases actually may be a presentation of chronic degenerative changes in the peroneus longus tendon. The calcification develops in the area of the os peroneum and can follow a chronic disruption of the os peroneum. Williams[297] noted the onset of swelling, warmth, and tenderness in this region, with calcification over the dorsolateral aspect of the cuboid. Klammer et al[194] suggested that rest with short-term immobilization and NSAIDs permitted resolution of the inflammation without surgery.

There have been several reports of ruptures of both the peroneus longus and brevis tendons. Abraham and Stirnaman[139] reported simultaneous ruptures of the peroneus longus and brevis tendons in a 48-year-old diabetic woman. The tendons were repaired primarily. Evans[172] reported on a 20-year-old athlete who developed chronic lateral ankle pain. At exploration, a peroneus longus tear was noted inferior to the lateral malleolus and was treated with a tenodesis of the peroneus longus to the peroneus brevis. Burman[155] also observed a partial tear of the peroneus longus thought to result from an enlarged peroneal tubercle. This was treated with resection of the torn portion, excision of the enlarged tubercle, and tenodesis of the peroneus longus to the peroneus brevis. Kilkelly and McHale[193] reported a traumatic rupture of the peroneus longus at the level of the peroneal tubercle successfully treated with a primary repair. Bassett and Speer[146] and others[151,193,247,259,271] have reported 18 cases of longitudinal tears of the peroneus longus treated with primary repair with routinely good results. Rapley et al[247] augmented his repair with acellular dermal matrix. Thompson and Patterson[282] reported three other cases of peroneus

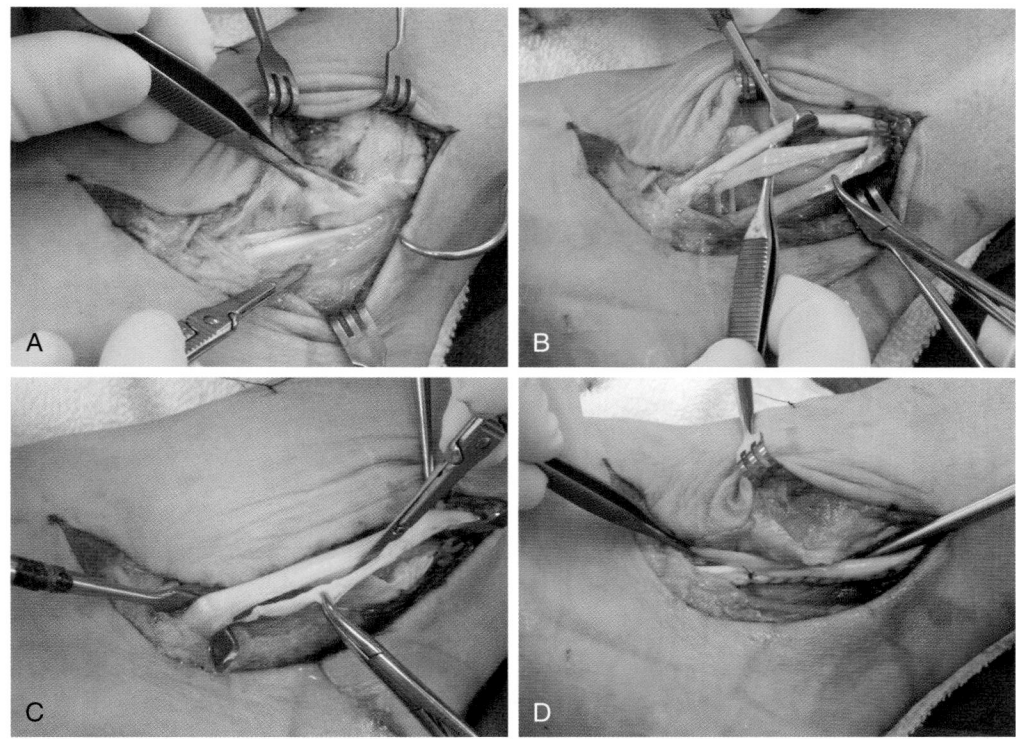

Figure 24-77 Treatment of dual tear of peroneal tendons. **A,** Debridement and synovectomy. **B,** Peroneus longus (at *top*) is retracted showing longitudinal tear of peroneus brevis. **C,** Debridement of small longitudinal tear of peroneus longus. **D,** Tubularization of peroneus brevis and reduction of the two tendons behind the fibula.

longus disruption in older patients (average age 65 years), who were treated with tenodesis of the peroneus longus and brevis with good results.

Several studies have reported on tears of the peroneus longus and noted the presence of lateral ankle ligamentous incompetence, combined peroneus brevis and longus tendon tears, low-lying peroneus brevis muscle belly (see Fig. 24-80A to C), chronic peroneal tendon subluxation or dislocation, and hindfoot varus deformity. With a longitudinal tear, resection of the degenerated portion and primary repair are performed. With complete disruption and proximal migration of the proximal segment, a tenodesis of the peroneus longus and brevis tendons is recommended in less active people. When both tendons are unhealthy or torn, an FDL tendon transfer to bypass the diseased tendon maybe considered.[294] Addressing the primary and associated disease is necessary for successful resolution of symptoms.[166,249,257]

Treatment of peroneus longus tears can be achieved with direct repair, turn-down, free graft (autograft or allograft), or with an FDL or FHL tendon transfer if there is significant muscular atrophy or fibrosis. Typically, as the complexity and chronicity increases, the likelihood of needing a valgus lateral translation calcaneal osteotomy, fibular groove deepening, lateral ligament reconstruction, talar osteochondral defect repair and impinging ankle osteophyte resection also increases

Peroneus Brevis

Approximately 200 cases of longitudinal tears or ruptures of the peroneus brevis tendon have been reported in the literature, although most references cite individual case reports. Approximately 85% of reported cases are contained in seven studies.* With the advent of accessible MRI and a growing awareness among specialists of brevis disorder, more of these acutely and chronically abnormal tendons are being identified.

Although injuries to the lateral ligamentous complex of the ankle typically involve the anterior talofibular ligament and the calcaneofibular ligament, a spectrum from various degrees of rupture, longitudinal tear, or subluxation and dislocation of the peroneal tendons can occur as well. Minor or major foot and ankle trauma could be the one event that triggers the condition, but additionally, overuse can result in tendon disorders. Patients with long-standing lateral ligamentous instability will often develop peroneal tendinopathy resulting from overcompensation. Furthermore, patients with idiopathic or neuromuscular cavovarus feet are vulnerable to pathologic changes in their peroneal tendons. Whatever the cause, acute injuries or chronic insidious degenerative tears are often associated with the signs and symptoms of synovitis of the peroneal tendon sheath.

---

*References 154, 165, 186, 203, 249, 252, and 272.

Anatomy

The peroneus brevis muscle originates from the midportion of the lateral fibula and functions to evert and plantar flex the foot. Innervated by the superficial peroneal nerve, it becomes tendinous on the posterior aspect of the fibula. It courses on the posterior aspect of the fibula and lateral malleolus anterior to the peroneus longus. The peroneus brevis then crosses the peroneal tubercle and inserts onto the base of the fifth metatarsal. The peroneus longus, in contrast, is positioned inferior to the peroneal tubercle and runs beneath the cuboid and across the plantar aspect of the foot, inserting into the plantar base of the first metatarsal and first cuneiform. In the proximal peroneal canal, the peroneus longus tendon actually occupies the major portion of the floor of the canal and only partially overlaps the peroneus brevis tendon. In the lower canal, the peroneus longus tendon overlies the brevis and can compress it.[145] More distally, the peroneus longus tendon is the more posterior of the two tendons and distal to the fibula. Each of the peroneal tendons is maintained within an individual tendon sheath, although they are contained within one common tendon sheath proximal to the tip of the fibula. The posterolateral aspect of the lateral malleolus forms a bony ridge that normally prevents the peroneal tendons from subluxating.

Peroneus longus and brevis injuries can be differentiated by their location. Peroneus longus injuries often are more distal and located in the region of the os peroneum, whereas peroneus brevis injuries are localized to the distal aspect of the fibula.

Etiology

Meyer,[215] in 1924, initially described three anatomic specimens with attritional or longitudinal tears of the peroneus brevis tendon localized to the area of the distal fibula. Later, Sammarco and DiRaimondo,[252] Bassett and Speer,[146] and DiGiovanni et al[165] reported on several patients who underwent surgery for lateral ankle instability and were observed to have longitudinal tears of the peroneus brevis tendon.

Bassett and Speer[146] hypothesized that the cause of a longitudinal peroneus brevis tear is likely an extrinsic phenomenon, with the tendon injured by a portion of the distal fibula or the peroneus longus. In cadaver studies, they observed that with plantar flexion of 15 to 25 degrees, the peroneus brevis impinged on the tip of the fibula with pressure from the peroneus longus. They found that with significant plantar flexion (>25 degrees) the peroneal tendons were well seated in the fibular groove. With lesser amounts of plantar flexion (15-25 degrees) the tendons were "perilously draped across the distal fibula" and at risk for injury. With an inversion injury in plantar flexion, the peroneal retinaculum can be injured, with subsequent injury to the peroneus brevis tendon (Fig. 24-78).

Longitudinal tears of the peroneus brevis probably occur from mechanical irritation or attrition within the fibular groove.

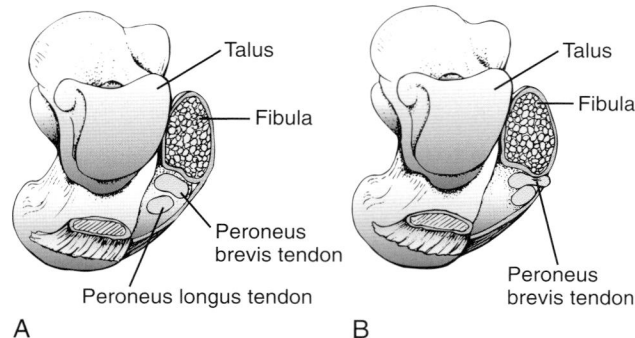

Figure 24-78 Cross section of lower leg at the ankle. **A,** Normal peroneal tendon anatomy. **B,** Compression of the peroneus brevis between the distal fibula and peroneus longus.

Based on a biomechanical study of the peroneal tendon groove, Title et al[283] found that the peroneal tendons sweep distally around the calcaneofibular ligament after riding over the posterior surface of the fibula. Over the distal 2 cm of bone, pressures develop on the tendon. Perhaps over time, especially combined with wear and tear as well as injury, these pressures result in fraying and tearing of the tendon.

Tears can occur with ankle trauma[252,267] and may be associated with lateral ankle instability or an incompetent superior peroneal retinaculum. Distal tears have also been reported associated with a hypertrophic peroneal tubercle.[229] Sobel et al,[266] in an anatomic analysis of cadaveric peroneus brevis tendons with longitudinal tears, demonstrated that the tears were centered over the posterior margin of the distal fibula. These tears demonstrated "an ample source of blood supply to the region of the tear." Vascular proliferation was noted at the site of the rupture. The authors concluded that the primary mechanism of the tendon injury was a mechanical disruption and not hypovascularity. Tears were noted to range in length from 2.5 to 5 cm (average 3.3 cm). The incidence of tears in anatomic cadaver dissections varied from 11% to 37%.[264,266] Of interest, in these same anatomic dissections, no tears of the peroneus longus were noted. In all cases, the central portion of the longitudinal tear was centered over the distal tip of the fibula in the region of the fibular groove.

Later, Sobel et al[267] inspected a large number of peroneal tendons in a laboratory setting. With tension placed on the peroneus longus and with the foot in inversion, compression was placed on the peroneus brevis at the fibular groove. The authors noted that a "flattened peroneus brevis" tendon splayed, with the anterior portion of the peroneus brevis slipping forward out of the fibular groove and over the anterior lip of the fibula. The peroneus brevis was wedged against the sharp posterior edge of the fibula, and the authors found that the peroneus brevis splits all occurred at this level. They then separated peroneus brevis splits into the following four grades:

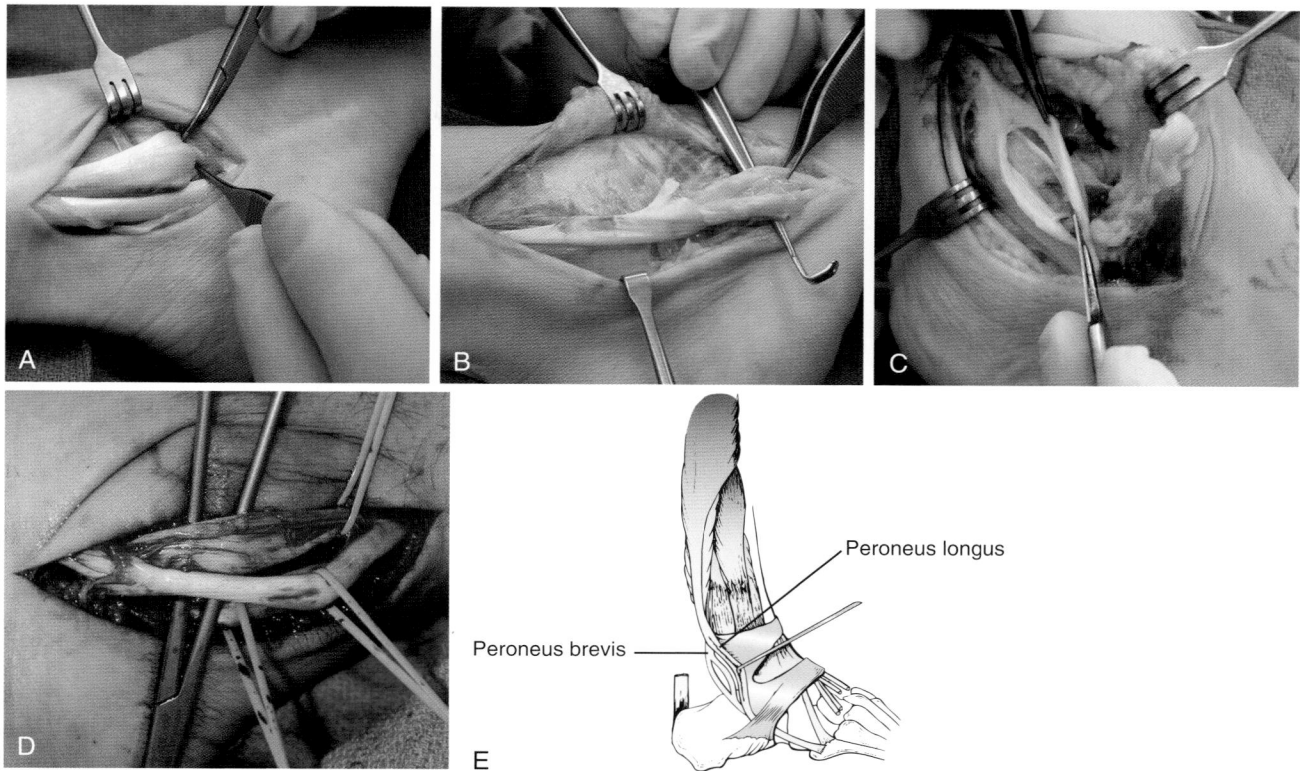

Figure 24-79 Splits (tears) in the peroneus brevis tendon. **A,** Grade 1 tear with splayed or flattened peroneus brevis. **B,** Grade 2 partial-thickness split, 2 cm long. **C,** Grade 3 full-thickness split, 2.5 cm long. **D,** Grade 4 full-thickness split with complete degeneration of this segment of the peroneus brevis. **E,** Diagram of full-thickness split demonstrates three-part tear of peroneus brevis and longitudinal tear of peroneus longus.

Grade 1: splayed or flattened out (Fig. 24-79A)

Grade 2: partial-thickness split, less than 1 cm in length (Fig. 24-79B)

Grade 3: full-thickness split, 1 to 2 cm in length (Fig. 24-79C)

Grade 4: full-thickness split, greater than 2 cm in length (Fig. 24-79D and E)

Sobel et al[267] concluded that longitudinal tears or splits in the peroneus brevis were caused by acute or repetitive mechanical trauma. A sharp posterior edge of the fibula can contribute to tendon stability, but it also may be the site of peroneus brevis injury.

With redundancy or laxity of the superior peroneal retinaculum, the anterior edge of the peroneus brevis can subluxate anteriorly, resulting in attrition and longitudinal tears of the tendon. Other causes include tenosynovitis, hypertrophy of the peroneus longus, anomalous distal insertion of the peroneus brevis muscle, and presence of a peroneus quartus tendon, which can lead to overcrowding within the peroneal tendon sheath[268] (Fig. 24-80).

Munk and Davis[226] suggested that the peroneus longus is pulled tightly against the peroneus brevis, entrapping the peroneus brevis between the peroneus longus and the fibular malleolus and peroneal tubercle. The peroneus longus thus acts as a wedge, pressing on the underlying flattened peroneus brevis and creating a longitudinal cleft in the tendon. Thus the cause of peroneus brevis tears, as Meyer[215] and Sobel et al[264,266,267] have observed, appears to emanate from compression of the peroneus brevis against the ridge on the lateral malleolus (by compression from the peroneus longus). Sobel et al[268] found the peroneus quartus present in 22% of 124 cadaver dissections; more recently, Athavale et al[145] observed an incidence of 28.5% in 60 cadaveric dissections. A large percentage of these cases also showed significant hypertrophy of the peroneal tubercle, which is the insertion site of the peroneus quartus. The authors concluded that the peroneus quartus may be associated with longitudinal attrition of the peroneus brevis.

In a report on 24 patients with longitudinal peroneus brevis tears, Brodsky and Krause[154] observed that all had redundancy of the superior peroneal retinaculum. The level of tears corresponded to the region of the distal 3 cm along the posterolateral edge of the fibula, where the tendon appeared to subluxate over the sharp edge of bone (Fig. 24-81). Sammarco and DiRaimondo[252] noted that all lesions occurred in a segment of tendon that "bends around the lateral malleolus during tendon excursion." They observed one case of bony impingement in the

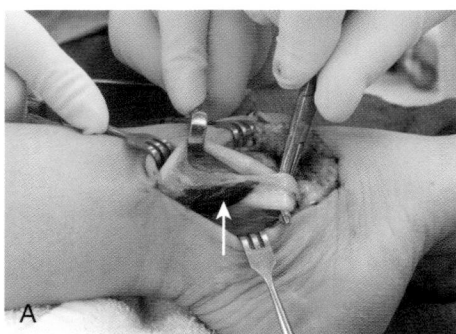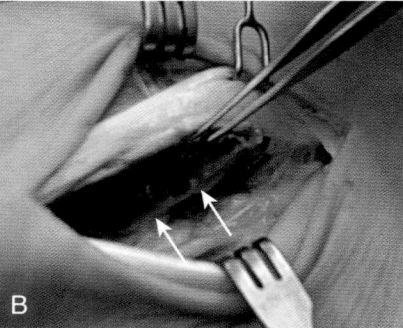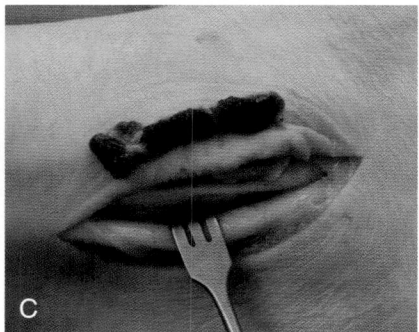

Figure 24-80 Distal muscle of the peroneus brevis is identified. **A,** Low-lying peroneus brevis *(arrow).* **B,** Peroneus longus is retracted superiorly showing the muscle *(arrows)* demonstrating low-lying tendon *(arrows).* **C,** Resected muscle.

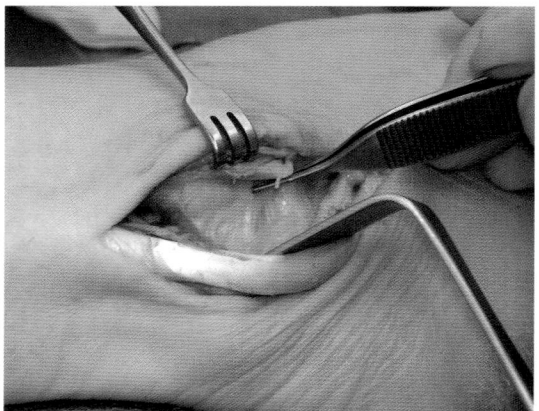

Figure 24-81 The posterior lateral edge of the distal fibula presents a sharp edge that can lead to tendon tears with subluxation.

peroneal groove and suggested that compression of the peroneus brevis occurred from the peroneus longus. Of 13 patients, 12 had a history of ankle trauma.

The blood supply of the peroneus brevis has been studied by Petersen et al[235] with injection techniques and immunohistochemically by using antibodies against laminin. They found avascular regions in both the peroneus longus and brevis tendons in the retromalleolar region. The peroneus longus tendon had an extended zone adjacent to the peroneal trochlea and another area where the peroneus longus curves around the cuboid.[235] These are the areas where the tendon is particularly vulnerable to tears.

The importance of a low-lying muscle belly of the peroneus brevis as a cause of peroneus brevis tendon tears is controversial. Geller et al[178] reported on 30 human cadaveric specimens and the location of the musculotendinous junction (MTJ). The authors found degenerative longitudinal tears in 4 cases. The MTJ was significantly more distal, and the tendon was thicker in the 4 torn specimens versus the untorn specimens, suggesting that a lower peroneus brevis MTJ might influence the development of degenerative tears. Athavale et al[145] found a low-lying muscle belly in 70% of specimens in which only 5 of 60 demonstrated peroneus brevis tendon tears. Freccero et al[175] evaluated MRIs of patients with and without peroneal tears and noted those with tears had a peroneus brevis muscle belly of 8 mm more distal than those with no associated lesion. Also, Unlu et al,[287] in an investigation of 115 cadaveric specimens, found those with peroneus brevis tendon tears had a muscle belly 11 mm higher than those without tears. Although many may associate peroneus brevis tendon tears with a low-lying muscle belly, this conflicting information clouds the issue on the importance of low-lying muscle belly being associated with tendon degeneration.

Weber and Krause[295] reported on 30 of 70 patients who had posterolateral antiglide fibula plates with symptoms of peroneal tendinitis. In their series, of the 30 patients with symptoms, there were nine peroneus brevis lesions and three peroneus longus lesions. The authors recommended that if a low placement of a plate below the distal 2 cm of the fibula (in the osteosynovial canal of the fibula) was needed for fracture fixation, avoiding screw placement in the distal hole would reduce symptoms. If a screw was needed in this distal hole, it should be fully sunk into the plate and not prominent. Thus obliquely placed distal screws in this distal hole are to be avoided.

History and Physical Examination

A patient might note a sudden pop or recall an episode of tearing in the region of the lateral ankle. Although edema may be present, ecchymosis is infrequently noted. A patient might not recall a specific traumatic episode and only seek treatment after a chronic period of discomfort or disability. Pain is typically isolated posterior to the region of the lateral malleolus and is increased with ambulation. Recalcitrant synovitis and swelling over the peroneal tendons in the region of the ankle may be presenting symptom. Weakness, fatigue, and ankle instability can be the first sign of a tendon rupture. Some patients have reported that they experienced the development of a progressive everted gait and that their foot was not "level on the ground" as they ambulated. Surprisingly, sometimes the pain, lateral ankle swelling, and weakness are tolerated, and a stress fracture of the fifth metatarsal eventually develops, necessitating an orthopaedic evaluation.

A history of ankle injury or sprain has been noted in several reports.[200,203,252,274] Sammarco and DiRaimondo,[252] reporting on 13 patients with peroneus brevis tears, noted that two tears were diagnosed preoperatively, four were suspected, and the rest were unsuspected and discovered at surgical exploration. Brodsky and Krause[154] reported that 70% of patients in their series of 24 peroneus brevis tears had a significant delay in diagnosis.

Patients with persistent lateral foot or ankle pain with a history of an ankle sprain or injury should be considered susceptible to a peroneus brevis tendon injury. Although Sammarco and DiRaimondo[252] noted no patients with a history of inflammatory arthropathy or prior steroid injections, these conditions can predispose a patient to peroneal tendon injury.

Symptoms similar to those demonstrated with peroneal tendon tenosynovitis may be observed in a patient with a concomitant peroneus brevis tendon tear. Pain may be elicited with palpation along the course of the peroneus brevis posterior to the distal fibula. Decreased peroneal strength with eversion may be noted, and pain may be elicited with increased active eversion of the foot. Likewise, pain can occur with passive inversion of the foot. Moderate-to-significant soft tissue swelling may be present along the course of the peroneal tendon. Webster[296] noted a large, bulbous pseudotumor in the area of the peroneus brevis.

Testing for peroneus brevis strength can be challenging because the patient may have sufficient power in the peroneus longus to still permit eversion of the foot. Side-to-side comparison examination typically will help distinguish the relative weakness on the affected side. Also, the patient should be instructed to evert against resistance, starting with the foot held in an inverted position and then making an arc of motion to eversion. This helps the examiner to identify eversion weakness. To complete this evaluation, the patient is instructed to hold the foot everted, and the examiner should then attempt to push the patient's foot into inversion while he or she forcefully resists. The amount of resistance and the final position of the foot relative to the axis of the leg should be noted. Also, observing the patient walk will often help to identify the subtle varus of the calcaneus and highlight the lack of functional eversion associated with peroneus brevis weakness or early insufficiency.

The magnitude of warmth and edema is often determined by the magnitude of the degenerative process. Subluxation of the peroneal tendons may be diagnosed by palpating the posterior edge of the fibula as the patient dorsiflexes and everts the foot. On examination, a painful click may be present when a longitudinal peroneus brevis split tear subluxates anteriorly over the anterior edge of the fibula. Circumduction of the foot and ankle should be performed while the examiner palpates the tendons

in the retrofibular groove. The frequency and intensity of tendon popping and the magnitude of the tenderness in this area should be compared with the contralateral side. This maneuver may provoke subluxation, dislocation, or symptomatic gliding of one tendon around the other.

Sobel et al[267] described the "peroneal compression test." With the patient sitting, the knee flexed to 90 degrees, and with the foot and ankle in a relaxed plantar-flexed position, the physician places a thumb over the superior retinaculum just on the posterior edge of the fibula. Slight pressure is applied to the peroneal tendons. The patient then forcibly everts and dorsiflexes the foot and ankle. Pain, crepitation, and popping with palpation over a longitudinal tear may be noted. A triggering or clicking sensation can occur with subluxation of a portion of the peroneus brevis tendon.

Mizel et al[223] used local bupivacaine injections into the peroneal tendon sheath to aid in diagnosis. They injected contrast material as well. This test might not be 100% sensitive because, in approximately 15% of cases, the injection communicated with the ankle or the subtalar joint, or both. The authors observed that the peroneus longus and brevis sheaths filled simultaneously and that the extravasation rate was 10%. Although some false-positive and false-negative results occurred, the authors believed this was a useful test in diagnosing peroneal tendon disorder.

Radiographic Examination

Although standard radiographs are obtained to evaluate the painful ankle, they usually do not demonstrate an abnormality with a peroneus brevis injury.[203] Tenography may be used[252] but largely has been replaced by MRI, which may be helpful in identifying a longitudinal tear, hypertrophy, distal insertion of the peroneal musculature, or a peroneus quartus muscle.[203,259] Sobel et al[265] suggested that MRI can aid in the diagnosis of peroneal tendon disorder and demonstrated its usefulness in evaluating a large number of cadaver specimens. Khoury et al[192] correlated the MRI findings to surgical findings and found the studies useful in establishing the diagnosis of tears. However, there is a marked decrease in sensitivity in the detection of peroneal tendon tears with MRI in comparison with other tendons of the foot and ankle because of the *magic angle effect.*[197] The positioning of the extremity may make a dramatic difference in the sensitivity, because Mengiardi et al[214] have demonstrated a higher accuracy when the patient is positioned prone for the study.

Neustadter et al[228] found sonography useful for diagnosing peroneal tendon tears. These studies are cost-effective; however, the results depend on individual technique.

Included in the differential diagnosis for chronic lateral ankle pain is lateral ankle instability, subtalar instability, peroneal tendon subluxation, tarsal coalition, lumbosacral radiculopathy, peroneal tendon rupture, longitudinal peroneal tendon tear, peroneal tendinitis, or tenosynovitis.

Conservative Treatment

Nonsurgical care for chronic lateral ankle pain includes NSAIDs, reduced activity, shoe modifications, custom insoles, and lateral heel wedges. Immobilization with a below-knee walking cast can diminish symptoms and allow the inflammatory process to subside. An ankle or stirrup brace that diminishes inversion and eversion may be useful to stop the traumatic stresses while permitting full ankle function in the sagittal plane. For resistant cases with partial ruptures, platelet-rich plasma from peripheral blood or bone marrow concentrate may be of help.[59]

With tears of the peroneus brevis, however, symptoms typically do not subside. Brodsky and Krause[154] noted that conservative treatment failed in 20 of 24 patients (83%) with an average of 8 months of nonsurgical care. The failure of conservative care was noted in several other series as well.[166,249,257]

Surgical Treatment

Typically, two types of tears of the peroneus brevis are identified: a single longitudinal tear or multiple longitudinal tears characterized by areas of fibrillation.[203] With degenerative fibrillation, the shredded fibers may be resected and the major divisions repaired primarily. An attempt should be made to tubulize the remaining tendon (Fig. 24-82).[259] Repairs are carried out with absorbable or nonabsorbable sutures on both the anterior and the posterior aspects of the tendon. An advantage of the nonabsorbable sutures is that the suture remains mechanically intact, assisting with load sharing during early stressing of the tendon repair, and should be considered resulting from the potentially slow healing time of the tendon. The disadvantage, however, is that the suture material or knots may cause friction with local symptoms or stenosis. With severe tendon degeneration, Brodsky and Krause[154] advocated a tenodesis proximal and distal to the peroneus longus. Tenodesis was advocated when viable tendon was less than one third the tendon diameter.

Treatment options include repair of the tendon, resection of a major tear or defect, debridement of up to one half the tendon, turn-down of the tendon proximally to bridge a gap or augment a tendon that has less than 50% remaining, free tendon grafting (autograft or allograft), or tenodesis of the peroneus brevis to the peroneus longus.

TENDON DEBRIDEMENT AND REPAIR
Surgical Technique (Video Clips 104 and 105)

1. The patient is placed in a lateral decubitus position. A thigh tourniquet is used as needed for visualization.
2. A longitudinal incision is centered over the course of the peroneal tendons, beginning above the ankle 1 cm posterior and proximal to the tip of the fibula and then extending distally to the base of the fifth metatarsal,

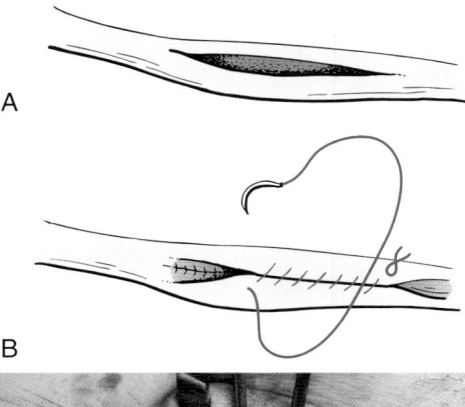

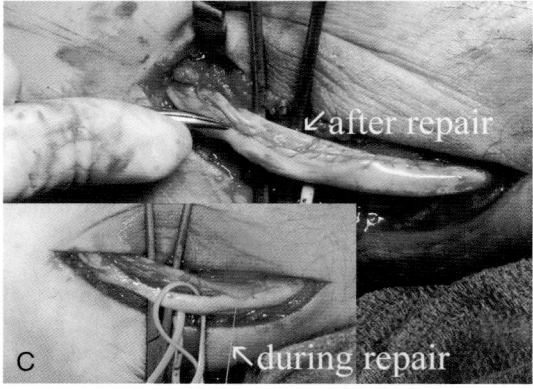

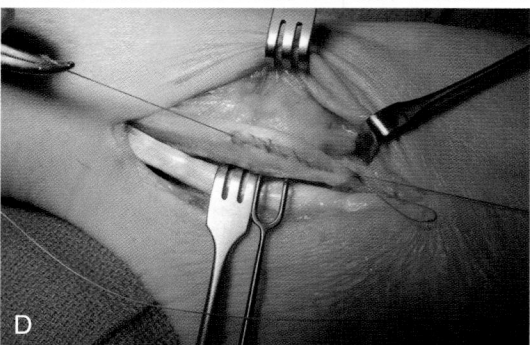

Figure 24-82 Technique of tubulization of a peroneus brevis tear. **A,** Longitudinal tear of peroneus brevis. **B,** Method used to tubulize the peroneus brevis with layered tendon repair. **C,** Tear edges are freshened, and tubulization is performed on superficial and deep areas of the tear. **D,** Another example of tubulization of a peroneus brevis tear.

depending upon location of the tear, based on MRI, ultrasound, or clinical examination. Care is taken to protect the sural nerve, which is posterior to the incision but has branches that cross the incision more distally.
3. The superior peroneal retinaculum is identified and incised 2 to 3 mm posterior to the fibula, providing an anterior soft tissue cuff that can be repaired later.
4. Both tendons are carefully examined, especially the deep side of the peroneus brevis tendon.
5. With a low-lying peroneus muscle belly or a peroneus quartus, the muscle may be debrided or excised. Proliferating synovium is debrided.

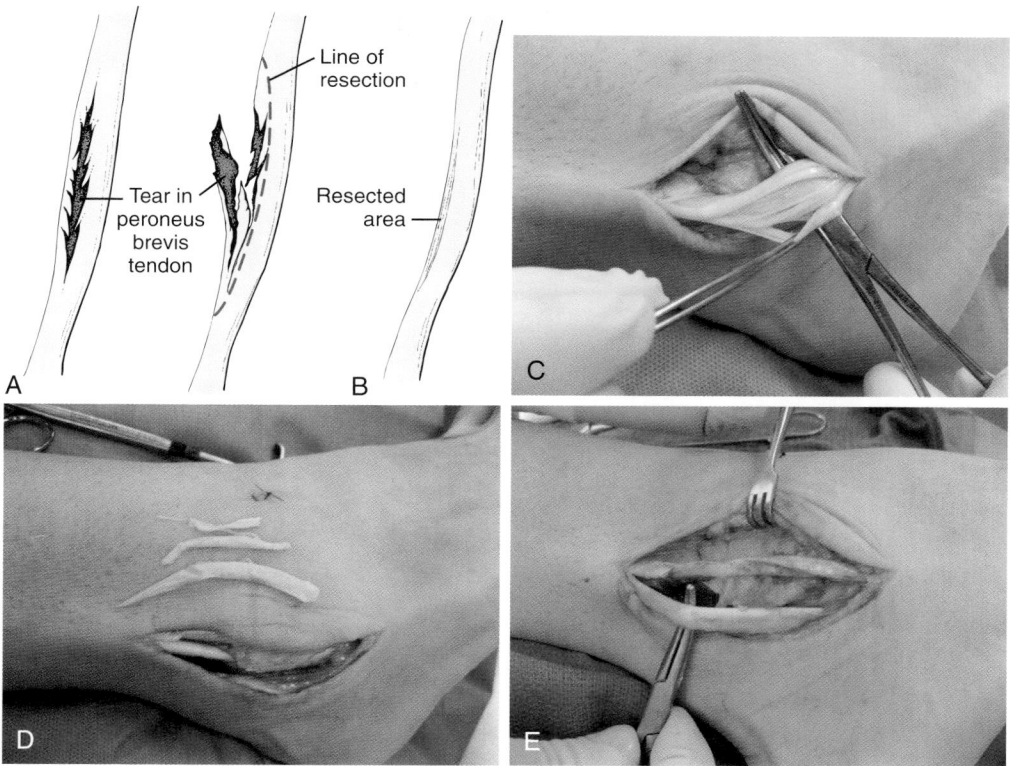

Figure 24-83 Technique of resection of peroneus brevis tear. **A,** Two examples of a peroneus brevis tear. **B,** After resection of the smaller portion. **C,** Triple tear of peroneus brevis tendon. **D,** After debridement. **E,** Remaining tendon after removal of torn segments.

6. A peripheral tear and frayed edges should be resected (Fig. 24-83). If the patient has a shallow retrofibular groove, a groove-deepening procedure may be considered. Also, if the tear is more chronic in onset, and the patient older, the groove deepening may further help unload the repair (see later for groove-deepening technique.)
7. After repair or debridement, the tendons are reduced and the superior peroneal retinaculum repaired.

Postoperative Care
A non–weight-bearing below-knee cast or splint is applied with the foot and ankle in neutral position. After 2 to 4 weeks of non–weight-bearing crutch ambulation, weight-bearing ambulation in a below-knee cast or fixed brace is permitted. Range-of-motion exercises should be initiated 2 weeks after surgery, with progressive strengthening exercises initiated at 8 weeks. In general, a cloth brace or a stirrup brace can be used between 6 to 12 weeks after surgery and then as needed for another 3 months during stressful activities.

TENDON DEBRIDEMENT AND REPAIR WITH TURN-DOWN OF PROXIMAL TENDON
In healthy patients younger than 65 years or in those who are more active, the authors prefer the turn-down repair because there may be some benefit to retaining a two-tendon system for better balance, power, and proprioception. It is indicated when a third or less of the tendon remains. Because the deficit spanned can be as large as 15 cm, the patient should be informed that a long incision is necessary for the tendon harvest.

Surgical Technique
1. The patient is placed in a lateral decubitus position. A thigh tourniquet is used as needed for visualization.
2. A longitudinal incision is centered over the course of the peroneal tendons, beginning above the ankle 1 cm posterior and proximal to the fibula and then extending distally to the posterior distal tip of the fibula and extending to the base of the fifth metatarsal depending upon the location of the tear. Care is taken to protect the sural nerve with its branches that cross distal to the tip of the fibula.
3. The superior peroneal retinaculum is identified and incised 2 to 3 mm posterior to the fibula, providing an anterior soft tissue cuff that can be repaired later.
4. Both tendons are carefully examined, and the exposure is extended to permit final reconstruction.
5. Synovial pathology is addressed. A synovectomy of debridement is performed as warranted.
6. Peripheral tendon tears are debrided, and repairable portions of the tendon are reconstructed with direct suturing.

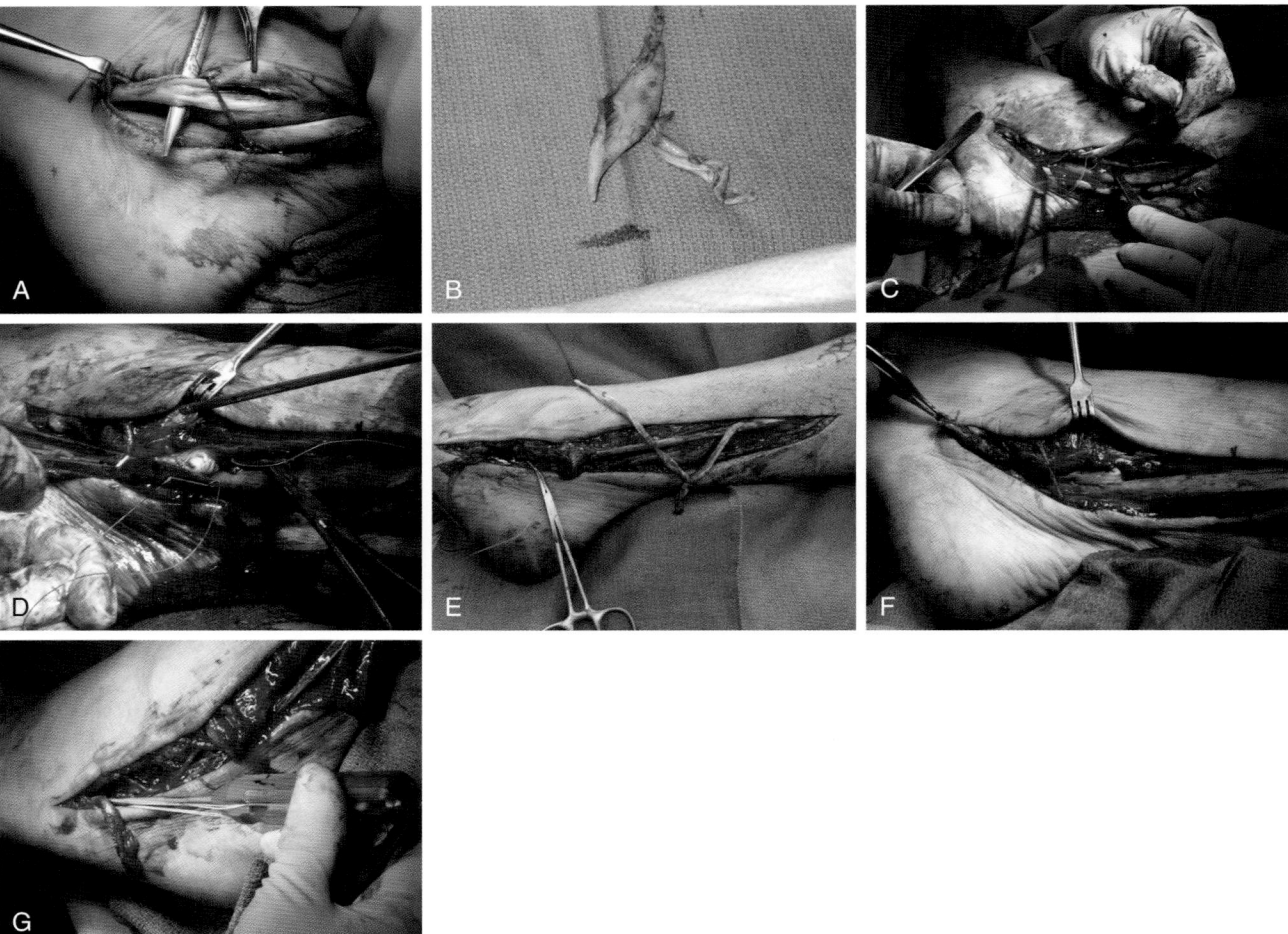

Figure 24-84 Turn-down technique of repair of peroneus brevis rupture. **A,** A patient with large complex longitudinal split tear of the peroneus brevis. The distal aspect of the brevis was frayed and required debridement, leaving a thin section of remaining tendon. The peroneus longus is seen posterior to the brevis. **B,** Resected specimen. **C,** A 6-mm–wide strip of tendon was dissected up to the area of the musculotendinous junction and turned downward. **D,** The area of turn-down was reinforced with interrupted sutures. **E,** The area of the turn-down is chosen above the lower 2 cm of the fibula to avoid a bulky section in the groove. **F,** The distal aspect was prepared and then reattached to the fifth metatarsal by suture anchor **(G).**

7. For more complex tears, the tendon may be adherent to the bone or tendon sheath. Working through this dense scar tissue can be challenging. It is necessary to identify the proximal and distal "normal" sections of the tendon.

8. With a degenerative tear with less than one third of viable peroneus tendon available, a turn-down procedure is performed as follows (Fig. 24-84). The length of the defect or inadequate tendon is measured intraoperatively. In general, if the peroneus brevis is ruptured within 2 cm of the fifth metatarsal insertion, the measurement continues to the base of the fifth metatarsal. If an anastomosis is planned, the overlap between the turn-down and the distal tendon should be at least 1 cm. Also, at the region of the turn-down section, there should be an overlap of at least 1 cm, which means that the surgeon should anticipate doubling this portion. If there is a gap or deficit area of

tendon, it is important to harvest a strip of half of the proximal tendon that will be long enough to turn down, span, and then overlap the area. To be of sufficient length, add to the gap distance the overlap and the turn-down distance, and begin the harvest that far proximally. For example, a 5-cm gap would require a harvest of a 7-cm strip that was obtained 8 cm proximally.

9. At the turn-down portion, the tendon is sutured to itself to reinforce the junction and prevent further propagation of the split in the tendon. This can be achieved with a No. 2 polyester nonabsorbable suture.

10. Distally, the tendon is connected to the fifth metatarsal base with a corkscrew anchor or attached to the distal segment of the tendon with No. 2 or 5 nonabsorbable sutures.

11. Where the tendon turn-down overlaps, the thinned section of remaining tendon, 2-0 nonabsorbable

suture can be used in a modified whip stitch or Krackow-style suture for reinforcement of the repair.

12. Next the surgeon must assess whether a groove deepening is in order.

13. The tendons are reduced, and the superior peroneal retinaculum is repaired.

14. The surgeon may consider injecting bone marrow–derived platelet-rich plasma after a meticulous skin closure.

Postoperative Care

A non–weight-bearing below-knee cast is applied with the foot in neutral position. At 10 to 14 days after surgery, sutures are removed and a CAM-boot in 10 to 20 degrees of equinus is applied to limit any stresses on the tendon reconstruction. After 2 to 6 weeks of non–weight-bearing ambulation with crutches, progressive weight-bearing ambulation in a fixed brace is permitted. Range-of-motion exercises should be initiated 2 weeks after surgery, with progressive strengthening exercises initiated at 8 weeks after surgery.

TENDON DEBRIDEMENT AND REPAIR WITH FREE GRAFT TRANSFER (Video Clip 108)

The free tendon graft is considered as an alternative to a turn-down repair. A semitendinosis autograft or allograft is harvested or procured from the tissue bank. It is necessary to have a healthy muscle proximally for a successful repair. For some, this is a less technically demanding procedure and may remove the variable of the health of a patient's tendon or collagen tissues, in general, from the prognostic uncertainty. For example, patients with Ehlers-Danlos syndrome should generally not have their own tissues used because the collagen deficiency is systemic and makes them vulnerable to postsurgical failure. For healthy patients, however, it may be advantageous to use autograft because the allograft tendon never repopulates with living tenocytes and can lose its elasticity in time. It also does not have self-reparative capabilities and will not eventually hypertrophy as may an autograft or turn-down transfer.

Surgical Technique (Fig. 24-88)

1. The patient is placed in a lateral decubitus position. A thigh tourniquet is used as needed for visualization.

2. A longitudinal incision is centered over the course of the peroneal tendons, beginning above the ankle 1 cm posterior and proximal to the fibula and then extending distally to the posterior distal tip of the fibula and extending to the base of the fifth metatarsal depending on the location of the tear. Care is taken to protect the sural nerve with its branches that cross distal to the tip of the fibula.

3. The superior peroneal retinaculum is identified and incised 2 to 3 mm posterior to the fibula, providing an anterior soft tissue cuff that can be repaired later.

4. Both tendons are carefully examined to permit final reconstruction. Working through dense scar tissue to free tendon from the adjacent bone or tendon sheath can be challenging. All diseased tendon tissue is removed. For the allograft, remaining viable tendon tissue that is thinned is removed.

5. Debridement of synovial tissue is performed as needed.

6. Peripheral tears are debrided and/or are repaired with suture.

7. The free graft procedure is performed as follows. The length of the defect or inadequate tendon is measured. In general, if the brevis is ruptured and a free graft is used, the distal connection is the fifth metatarsal insertion. A corkscrew anchor may be used to attach the distal tendon with a No. 2 or 5 nonabsorbable suture. At the proximal anastomosis, an overlap between the graft and the distal tendon should be at least 1 cm. A Pulvertaft weave technique, using a No. 2 polyester nonabsorbable suture, can be considered and should be performed 4 to 6 cm proximal to the tip of the fibula to avoid a bulky reconstruction. Before using the allograft, the tendon should be stretched with a tensioning device to limit early failure because of creep.

8. It is important to assess whether a groove deepening is necessary.

9. The tendons are reduced after the repair, and the superior peroneal retinaculum is reconstructed.

10. Consider injecting bone marrow–derived platelet-rich plasma after meticulous skin closure.

Postoperative Care

A non–weight-bearing below-knee cast is applied with the foot in a neutral position. At 10 to 14 days, sutures are removed and a CAM-boot in 10 to 20 degrees of equinus is used to limit any stress on the tendon reconstruction. After 2 to 6 weeks of non–weight-bearing ambulation with crutches, progressive weight-bearing ambulation in a fixed brace is permitted. Range-of-motion exercises should be initiated 2 weeks after surgery, with progressive strengthening exercises initiated at 8 weeks.

TENDON DEBRIDEMENT AND REPAIR WITH TENODESIS
Surgical Technique (Video Clip 107)

1. The patient is placed in a lateral decubitus position. A thigh tourniquet is used as needed for visualization.

2. A longitudinal incision is centered over the course of the peroneal tendons, beginning above the ankle 1 cm posterior and proximal to the fibula and then extending distally to the posterior distal tip of the fibula and extending to the base of the fifth metatarsal depending on the location of the tear. Care is taken to protect the sural nerve with its branches that cross distal to the tip of the fibula.

3. The superior peroneal retinaculum is identified and incised 2 to 3 mm posterior to the fibula, providing an anterior soft tissue cuff that can be repaired later.

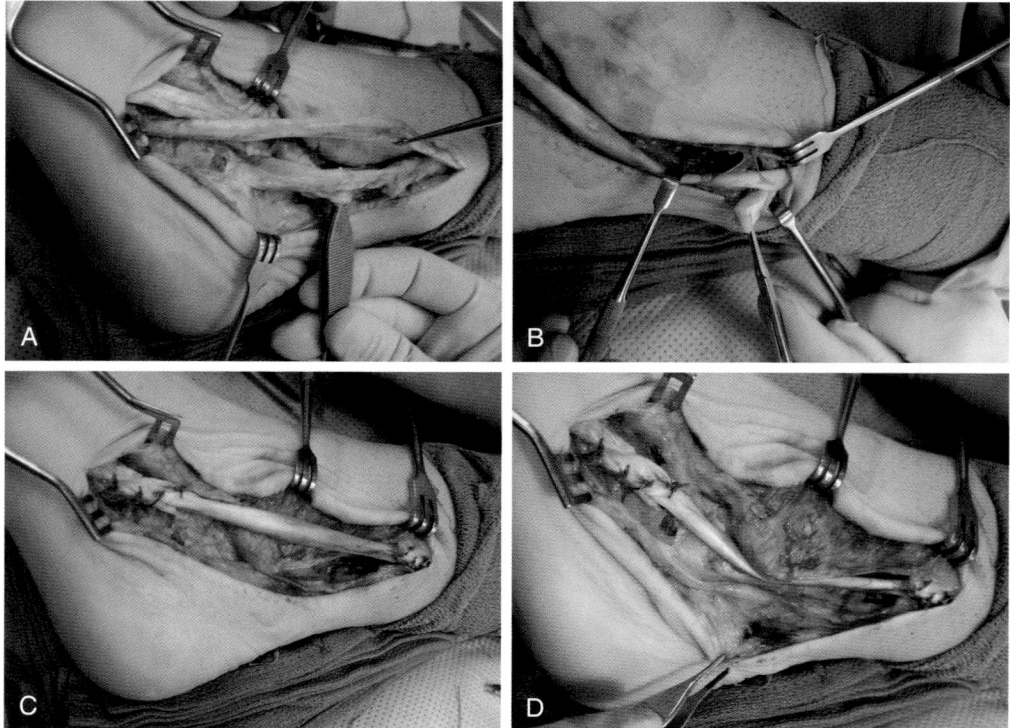

Figure 24-85   Tenodesis of the peroneus brevis and longus. **A,** Complex degenerative tear of the peroneus brevis, requiring tenodesis to the peroneus longus as salvage. **B,** Tendon of peroneus brevis has been excised, and the proximal tendon is woven through the tendon of the peroneus longus. **C,** After Pulvertaft weaving and tenodesis of two tendons proximally and distally. **D,** After reduction of tenodesed tendon behind the fibula and before superior peroneal retinaculum repair.

4. Both tendons are carefully examined.

5. Proliferating synovium is debrided. If a low-lying peroneus muscle belly or a peroneus quartus tendon is present, the muscle may be debrided or excised.

6. A peripheral tear and frayed edges should be resected.

7. The section of tendon that can be repaired is sutured.

8. With a degenerative tear and less than one third of viable peroneus tendon available, a tenodesis is performed between the proximal peroneus brevis and longus at a location 3 cm above the tip of the fibula. The distal peroneus brevis and longus are tenodesed with a Pulvertaft weave or direct anastomosis. The peroneus brevis tendon is woven through in a Pulvertaft repair technique and sutured in place with interrupted nonabsorbable sutures. It is important to appreciate where the anastomosis will move relative to the distal fibula. If at all possible, impingement and stenosis should be avoided. It may be necessary to move the connection higher or lower to avoid vulnerable locations. A direct tendon-to-tendon reconstruction with a core suture technique may be useful to minimize the bulk created by the Pulvertaft weave (Fig. 24-85).

9. After repair or debridement, the tendons are reduced and the superior peroneal retinaculum repaired.

10. In rare cases, with old unrecognized tears of the peroneus brevis and longus tendons that have healed in a lengthened position, a shortening procedure of both tendons may be performed. This reconstruction carries the risk of scarring and the necessity for a repeat tenosynovectomy to reestablish tendon excursion (Fig. 24-86).

Postoperative Care
A non–weight-bearing below-knee cast is applied with the foot in a neutral position. After 2 to 6 weeks of non–weight-bearing using crutches or walker, weight-bearing ambulation in a below-knee cast or fixed brace is permitted. Range-of-motion exercises should be initiated 2 weeks after surgery, with progressive strengthening exercises initiated at 8 weeks.

Results and Complications
Brodsky and Krause[154] noted that with tenodesis, 75% of patients were satisfied postoperatively. Most patients noted gradual resolution of swelling, although a protracted postoperative course was common.

Sammarco and DiRaimondo[252] reported on a series of 14 peroneus brevis tears in 13 patients who complained of ankle instability, with symptoms lasting from 8 months to 20 years. In 11 of 13 patients, lateral ankle instability was treated with a split peroneus brevis tendon graft that incorporated the peroneus brevis tear. Typically, the tendon tear was present at

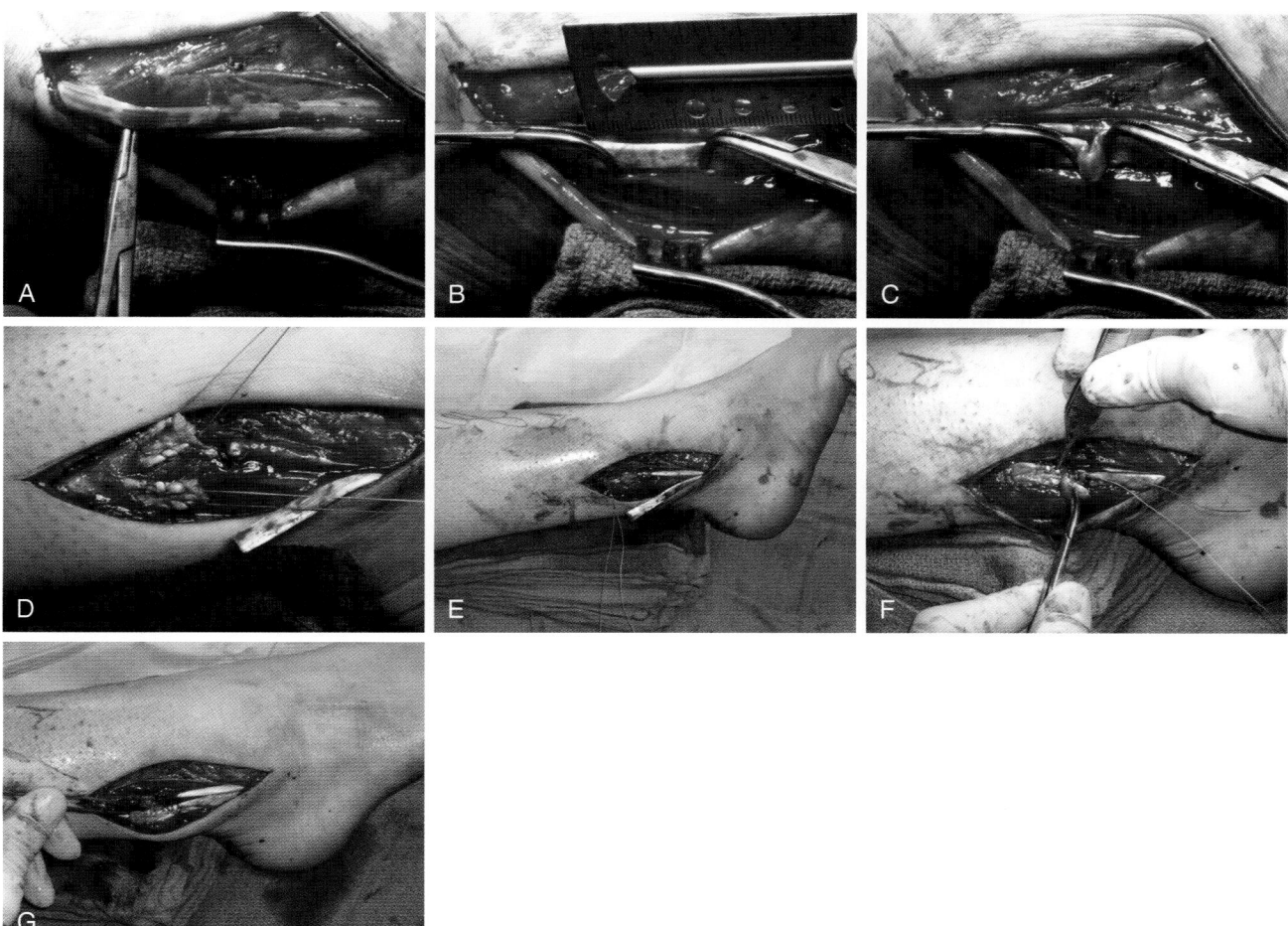

Figure 24-86 Laxity of the peroneals because of prior injury that healed in an elongated manner. A patient with prior injury developed weakness of the peroneals. At the time, no specific tear had been suspected, but later it was determined that she had sustained a peroneus brevis and longus tendon tear that healed. **A,** The tendons had good excursion but marked weakness. **B,** During the surgery with the foot and ankle held in neutral, the tendons had extreme laxity such that the redundant tendons protruded from behind the fibula. The proper tension was determined by bringing the ankle into a neutral position and pulling on the tendon to achieve tension. **C,** It was estimated that a 2-cm shortening was needed to provide the best tension for the tendon. **D,** Next, at the musculotendinous junction, the tendons were cut and final tensioning was performed. The peroneus brevis **(E)** and longus **(F and G)** tendons were then sutured with a modified Krakow suture. The patient ultimately did well and was able to resume athletic activities with excellent power and no instability.

the level of the distal fibula, with the tears 2 to 5 cm in length.

Often, the tendon is somewhat broader or thicker than normal in this region and is dull and yellowed with discoloration. Considerable fibrillation or fraying may be present. With passive dorsiflexion of the ankle, intraoperatively, a longitudinal cleft in the peroneal brevis may be pressed forward onto the anterior aspect of the fibula.

Complications with a peroneal tendon exploration and reconstruction include sural nerve injury and injury to the superficial branch of the peroneal nerve. With an inadequate repair of the superior retinaculum, recurrent subluxation of the peroneal tendons can occur. Recurrent degenerative tears of the remaining tendon can develop, leading to recurrent pain or nonresolution of symptoms.

Saxena[257] reported on 31 peroneus brevis tears; 24 of these were isolated and 7 were combined with peroneus longus tears. The average postoperative American Orthopaedics Foot and Ankle Society (AOFAS) score was 90.8 for isolated tears and 84.3 for combined tears. Most athletes returned to full sporting level. The average return to activity for the peroneus brevis tears group was 3.6 months, and for the group with combined lesions, it was 3.7 months. Dombek[166] reported that 98% of the patients were able to return to full activities after reconstruction, without pain at final follow-up. The minor complication rate was 20%, but clinically significant complications (continued symptoms or revisionary surgery) occurred in an additional 10% of patients.

Steel and DeOrio[271] retrospectively evaluated 30 patients who had peroneal tendon reconstruction (largely for peroneus brevis tendon tears), and although 9 of 10 of those who worked returned to their jobs, 58% complained of scar tenderness, and 54% complained of lateral ankle swelling at an average follow-up of 31 months. Only 46% returned to sporting activities.

In Redfern and Myerson's series,[249] with concomitant tears of the peroneus longus and brevis tendons, the mean postoperative AOFAS score was 82 (range, 20 to 100) points, and 91% of patients achieved normal or moderate peroneal muscle strength. Ankle instability was successfully corrected in all patients, and progressive worsening of varus deformity was prevented.

Options for surgical treatment include resection of bifurcated or trifurcated fragments,[149,200,252,296] resection of degenerated tendon and primary repair,[144,146,161,203,259] reinsertion of the distal attachment (Fig. 24-87),[274] and tenodesis to the peroneus longus.[226,250,296] Mizel et al[224] and others[198,293] suggested using a Hunter tendon rod with a two-stage reconstruction technique for an absent or severely damaged peroneus brevis tendon. After trauma, tumor, or previous surgical intervention, if reconstruction cannot be accomplished with a simple tendon transfer (e.g., FHL), a staged procedure may be performed using a Hunter tendon rod to form a pseudosynovial sheath. Approximately 3 months later, the Hunter tendon rod is removed, and the FHL tendon is transferred into the pseudosynovial sheath and attached to the distal tendon stump or base of the fifth metatarsal. Myerson[249] suggested considering allograft or FDL tendon transfer, or both when both tendons were involved. On occasion a free tendon graft may be used to bridge the gap for a deficient peroneus brevis tendon (Fig. 24-88).

FLEXOR DIGITORUM LONGUS TRANSFER FOR PERONEUS BREVIS LESIONS

Surgery is the procedure of choice for a more active patient who has a chronic degenerative tear of either peroneal tendon that cannot be repaired directly. A long longitudinal attritional rupture in a degenerative tendon or a chronic retracted transverse rupture is an appropriate lesion for this approach. It is an alternative to transection of the diseased tendon and tenodesis to the adjacent healthier tendon. It is particularly appropriate when there has been a prolonged time between tendon rupture and the proposed repair, with the expectation that atrophy or fibrosis of the affected muscle will limit a full reconstruction and recovery. Because this technique adds an additional power source (the FDL muscle), it can be particularly helpful when the involved tendon's muscle is fibrotic and dysfunctional (as seen after multiple recurrent traumas or failed previous surgeries). In the face of a neurologic lesion to the peroneal musculature (common peroneal or high superficial peroneal nerve lesion), or in cases of hereditary sensory motor nerve dysfunction (Charcot-Marie-Tooth disease), this technique may be a consideration. Patients who have neuromuscular conditions and suffer from ruptures of their peroneals are good candidates if their FDL or FHL muscle function is strong. The

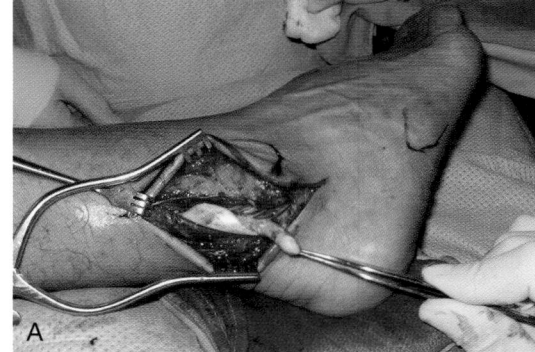
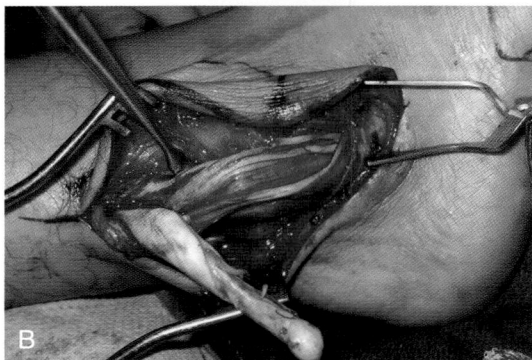
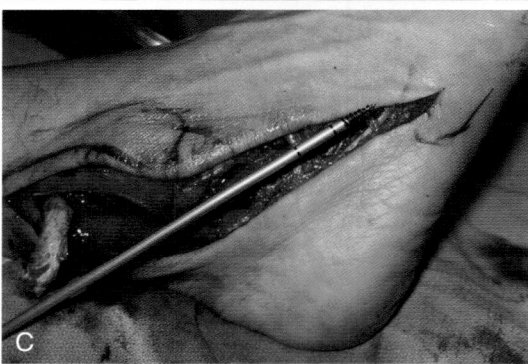

Figure 24-87 Repair of distal rupture of peroneus brevis tendon. **A,** Surgical exposure. **B,** Close-up of ruptured tendon. **C,** Placement of suture anchor for reattachment of tendon into the fifth metatarsal base.

technique has been particularly successful in running athletes who require subtle proprioception and dynamic power needs for cutting and turning, which might not be adequately restored with merely a tenodesis.

More commonly, patients treated with this procedure require adjuvant procedures, such as lateral translational/valgus calcaneal osteotomies, lateral ankle ligament reconstructions, anterior ankle joint osteophyte resections, and possibly a dorsiflexion osteotomy of the first metatarsal.

In the authors' series of 17 FDL tendon transfers for peroneal lesions, 5 were in athletes who had had multiple peroneal surgeries, and 8 were in medium-duty or heavy-duty injured workers with prior failed surgical treatment. Six were in patients with neurologic injury or dysfunction.

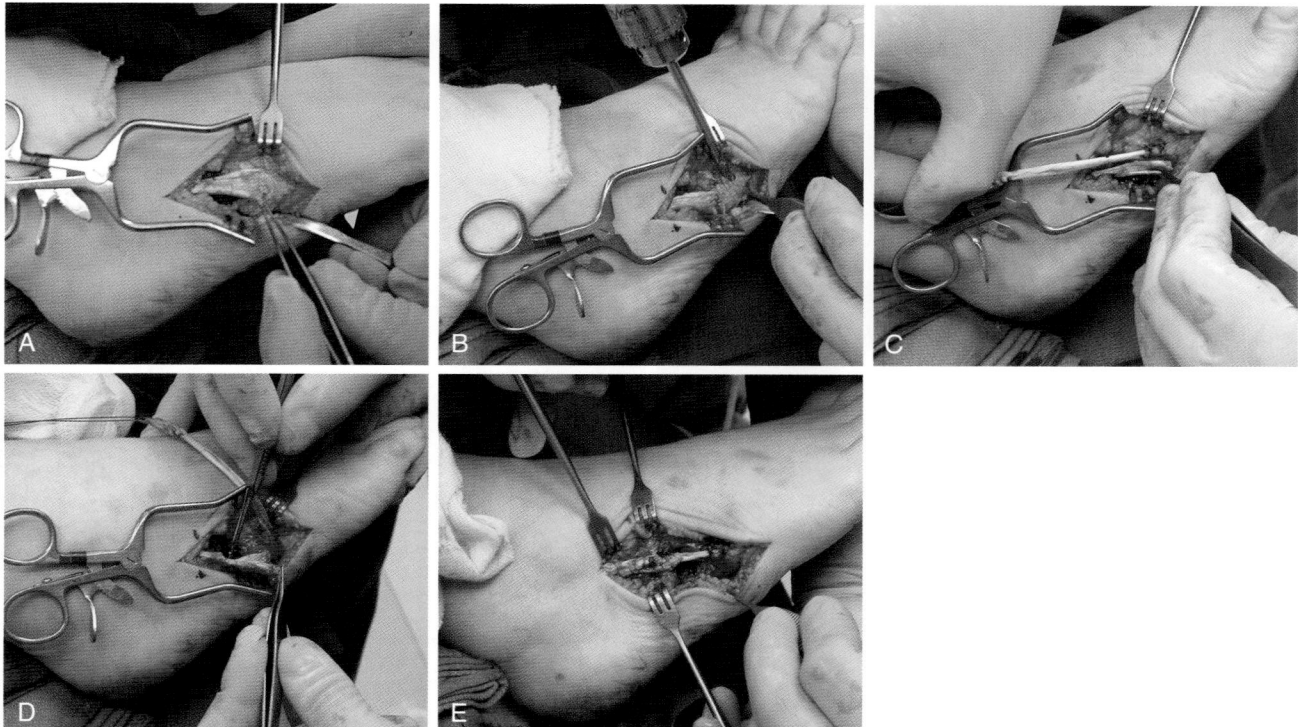

Figure 24-88 Repair of distal peroneus brevis tendinosis with free gracilis tendon autograft. **A,** Degenerated distal peroneus brevis tendon. **B,** Vertical drill hole through the base of the fifth metatarsal. **C,** Attachment of the gracilis tendon autograft through the drill hole. **D,** Resection of the degenerated distal tendon. **E,** Completion of tendon graft repair.

Eleven of the 17 patients had calcaneal varus that required a simultaneous Dwyer osteotomy.

Wapner[294] has also advocated the use of the flexor hallucis longus as a substitution for insufficiency of both peroneal tendons and did delayed repairs with success in a small series.

Surgical Technique

1. The patient is positioned in the lateral decubitus position, with a tilt of approximately 45 degrees.
2. The peroneal tendons are exposed, typically using the previous incisions (Fig. 24-89A-C). Exposure should be sufficient to fully excise or debride the degenerated tendons. The muscle bellies of the involved tendons are assessed by pulling on the musculotendinous unit and feeling the springiness. When there is no springiness, the muscle is useless and should not be anastomosed to the adjacent tendon. If there is minimal muscular fibrosis, the muscle can be salvaged with a proximal tenodesis.
3. The lateral tuberosity of the calcaneus is exposed to address the varus through either prior incisions or a new incision just posterior to the sural nerve (Fig. 24-89D).
4. A laterally based wedge of 5 to 10 mm of bone is removed from the calcaneus. Laminar spreaders are placed to distract the osteotomy site by 10 mm. This permits the osteotomy to be translated laterally for additional correction.
5. The osteotomy is then secured with one or two large-fragment (typically cannulated) screws while the fragments are manually held in reduction (Fig. 24-89E and F).
6. More distally, the fifth metatarsal tuberosity is exposed if the peroneus brevis is the primary pathologic tendon. The zone of exposure should permit insertion of a corkscrew suture anchor deep into the metaphyseal bone. Image intensification should be used to ensure proper placement of the anchor (Fig. 24-89G).
7. A 5- to 10-mm zone of bone should be exposed in anticipation of attachment to the FDL tendon. On the other hand, if the peroneus longus is to be replaced, then exposure is necessary to bypass the degenerated tendon. If there is a chronic dislocation or convex groove in the retrofibular region, a groove-deepening procedure (described later) should be considered.
8. Next, the bean bag is deflated, or the lateral bump is removed to reposition the patients to assist in the exposure of the FDL tendon. When a tendon transfer is needed, the FDL is harvested at or below the master knot of Henry. The exposure can be through an incision on the sole of the foot in the arch or along the medial aspect of the foot just plantar to the cuneiform and first metatarsal. Care is taken to avoid the medial plantar nerve, which is plantar to the FHL and FDL tendons. In an athlete, consideration for tenodesis of

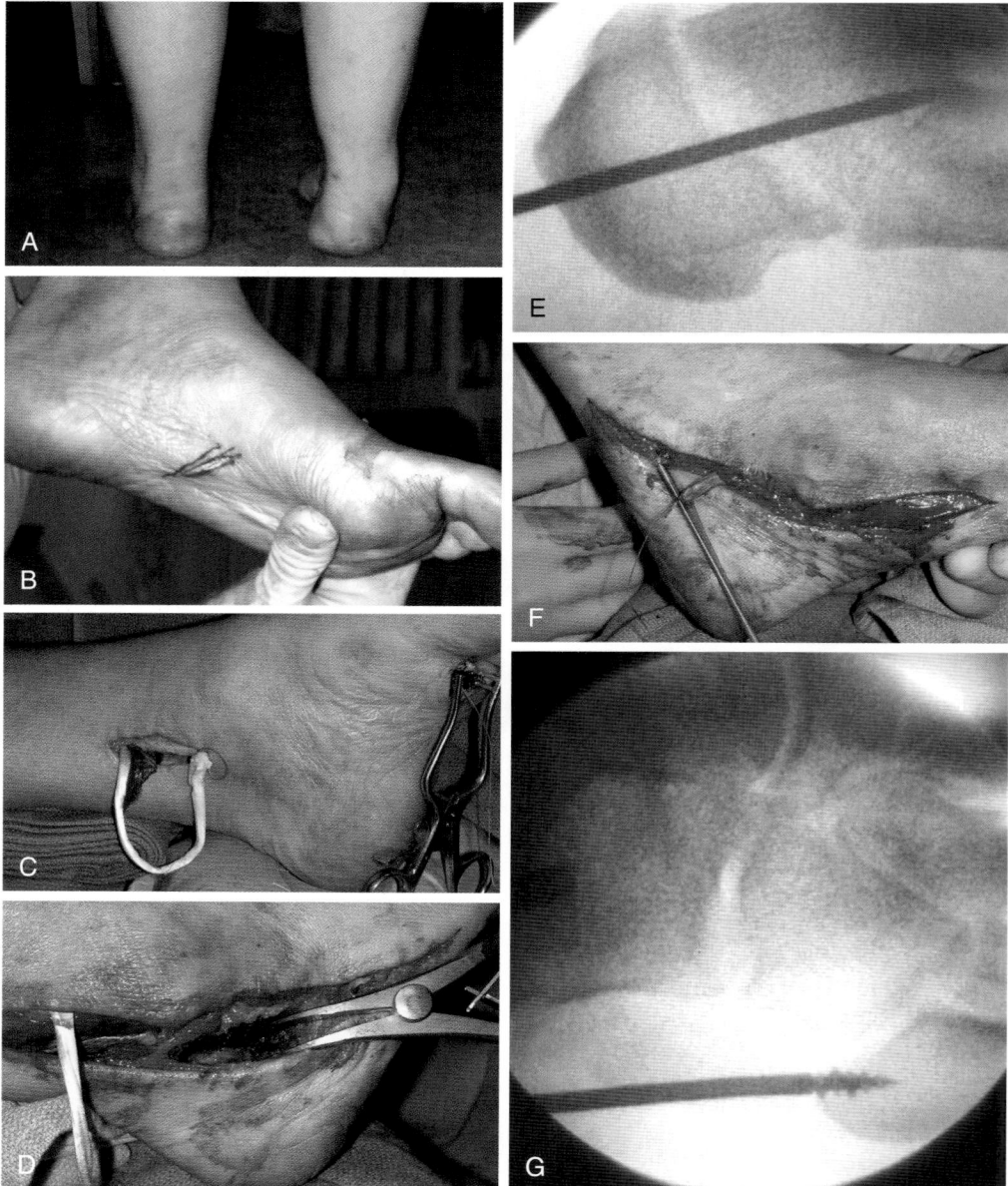

Figure 24-89 Method of reconstruction using flexor digitorum longus (FDL) tendon as free graft for absence of both peroneals. **A,** Marked varus preoperatively with peroneal brevis and longus tendon ruptures. **B,** Incision for harvest of FDL in arch. **C,** After distal detachment of the tendon, the FDL is passed proximally into an incision above the ankle. The FDL tendon is now passed from posterior to the tibia to posterior to the fibula in the peroneal tendon sheath. **D,** A closing-wedge calcaneal osteotomy to correct the varus. The osteotomy is also translated laterally. **E,** Fluoroscopy of osteotomy. **F,** Suture anchor placement into the base of the fifth metatarsal to secure the distal graft. **G,** Fluoroscopy of placement of the suture anchor.

the distal FDL stump to the FHL tendon is appropriate. When less length is needed, the tendon can be sectioned proximal to the knot (see Fig. 24-89B).

9. A second incision is made 7 cm above the medial malleolus and extended for 3 cm proximally. Here the FDL tendon is pulled proximally, with preservation of the distal muscle belly (Fig. 24-89C). A Kelly clamp is passed from the medial incision along the posterior aspect of the tibia until the peroneal sheath is entered.

If the tendon is not already exposed, an incision is made where the clamp penetrates. A second Kelly clamp from the lateral side is then connected to the first, and the tip of the second Kelly clamp is delivered into the medial wound, where it is used to pull the tendon to the lateral side (see Fig. 24-89D).

10. The FDL tendon is then passed through the sheath and distally deep to the sural nerve to the distal anastomosis site or at the fifth metatarsal tuberosity at the

corkscrew anchor site. The length of the transferred tendon is assessed with the tendon taut and the foot and ankle held in eversion. Excess tendon is resected.

11. A modified Krackow technique using one arm of the No. 0 or 2 suture is woven through the FDL up one side and down the other. The other suture strand is then used to advance the tendon to the tuberosity and tied securely. If the attachment is more proximal, the tuberosity site may still be preferred; otherwise, an anastomosis is performed, providing the attachment site is not going to be a bulky impediment to tendon motion. For example, if the anastomosis will occur in the distal retrofibular region, a more proximal or more distal anastomosis is preferable to avoid stenosis.

12. The incisions are then closed with the foot and ankle in a relaxed plantar flexed and everted position. If the surgeon desires, bone marrow–derived platelet concentrate is injected. A U and posterior well-padded splint is applied in this position over a sterile dressing.

Postoperative Care

Postoperatively, the patient is kept non–weight bearing for 6 weeks. Once the sutures are removed at 2 weeks after surgery, gentle range-of-motion activities should be performed to minimize tendon scarring. The patient should avoid dorsiflexion beyond 10 degrees of equinus and 10 degrees of inversion. Passive eversion is encouraged, but active eversion should be limited for 6 weeks. At 6 weeks after surgery, the equinus splinting or bracing is discontinued, and the ankle is held in a neutral position in a brace. Weight bearing can be initiated, followed by active eversion. At 8 to 12 weeks after surgery, the boot brace can be discontinued, and a stirrup brace is worn. During the third through sixth month, the stirrup is worn during walking, running, and stressful activities.

Combined Tears of the Peroneus Brevis and Longus Tendons

It is relatively uncommon to have combined peroneus brevis and longus tears. When this does occur, there will be disruption of the continuity of the tendons or attenuation of one or both tendons (see Fig. 24-86). When present, typically, a varus deformity of the hindfoot occurs that is coupled with a distinct weakness of eversion power in the forefoot. There have been multiple reports of ruptures of both the peroneus longus and brevis tendons.* Steel and DeOrio[271] treated four dual ruptures and successfully repaired both tendons in two cases. Rapley[247] repaired four dual tears with direct tendon repairs augmented with an acellular dermal matrix allograft. Wapner et al[294] reported on seven patients with long-term dual peroneal tendon insufficiency, treated initially with excision of the ruptured tendons and placement of a Hunter tendon rod. On a delayed basis, the rod was removed, and a transfer of the flexor hallucis longus tendon was

---

*References 139, 172, 199, 243, 247, 271, and 294.

performed, attaching the transferred tendon to the base of the fifth metatarsal base. At a follow-up of 4.6 years, six of seven patients had excellent function, relief of pain and good strength. Although this is an uncommon condition, a flexor hallucis longus or flexor digitorum longus transfer can be performed, particularly when there is no peroneal function (Video Clips 112 and 113).

Peroneal Tendon Subluxation–Dislocation

Subluxation–dislocation of the peroneal tendons, although not rare, represents a relatively uncommon condition. Unfortunately, acute peroneal tendon dislocations are often unrecognized or misdiagnosed as "lateral ankle sprains," which often results in chronic instability that requires surgical correction.

Monteggia,[225] (1803) is credited with the first description of peroneal tendon dislocation.[210] Later in the nineteenth century, Blanulet (1875) and Gutierrez (1877)[159] initially proposed surgical treatment.

Most acute peroneal tendon dislocations are associated with a traumatic episode and usually with athletic activities, often including alpine skiing. However, injuries from football, tennis, basketball, soccer, ice skating, and running have been reported as well.[144,211,254] Earle et al[168] estimated that peroneal tendon dislocation accounted for 0.5% of all skiing injuries. In a review of 265 reported cases in the literature, McGarvey and Clanton[211] observed that 71% were related to alpine skiing. Football was the second most common cause of peroneal tendon injury, cited in 7% of reports.

Several more recent reports have highlighted a slightly different perspective on peroneal dislocation and subluxation. Porter's series[241] of 14 cases of subluxation and dislocation included 4 from soccer, 4 from football, 2 from basketball, and 1 each from rugby, dancing, cycling, and baseball. Kollias and Ferkel[196] reported on 13 athletes with subluxation and dislocation. Only one was a skier; the others skated or played softball, basketball, soccer, football, or tennis.

Acute dislocations have been more frequently reported in association with fractures and dislocations of the fibula, talus, and calcaneus. These have occurred in more violent traumatic episodes, such as falls, motor vehicle accidents, and industrial injuries. Because more obvious bone and joint conditions are the focus of the surgeons, the tendon disorder is overlooked. Schon et al[191] reported on 23 chronic intractable peroneal subluxation–dislocations as defined by 12 months of symptoms. In this report, the average time to recognition involved several months of delay. Eight of the 23 patients were athletes, and the other 15 were workers or victims of more serious trauma. Of the seven with calcaneal fractures, six had chronic sural neuritis, one had chronic regional pain syndrome, and five had concomitant peroneal tendon tears. In the athletic subgroup, there were four peroneal tendon tears and two patients with chronic sural neuritis.

Brodsky and Krause[154] reported on 20 patients with peroneal brevis tendon tears. Alanen et al[141] and Tan et al[279] have both reported series of peroneal tendon tears.

Anatomy

At the ankle, the peroneal tendons course through a fibro-osseous tunnel at the level of the distal fibula that is bordered anteriorly by the posterior surface of the lateral malleolus; medially by the posterior talofibular ligament, posterior inferior tibiofibular ligament, and calcaneal fibular ligament[144,254]; and posterolaterally by the superior peroneal retinaculum (SPR). The peroneal tendons are enveloped by a synovial sheath that extends from the inferior border of the peroneal musculature to a point 1 cm below the fibula, where they enter separate and distinct synovial sheaths.[284] Over the course of the distal 2 cm of fibula, the synovial sheath and fascia of the lower calf condense to form the SPR, which is the main primary restraint to subluxation–dislocation of the peroneal tendons as they course around the tip of the fibula. The SPR extends from the posteroinferior edge of the fibula in an inferoposterior direction and inserts on the os calcis.

In an analysis of 30 fibular anatomic specimens, Davis et al[164] determined that the SPR originated from the posterolateral ridge of the fibula in all cases. Although averaging 10 to 20 mm in width, substantial variance was recognized in the width, thickness, and area of insertion. One or two fibrous bands course in a posteroinferior direction, inserting onto the calcaneus in 30%, the Achilles tendon sheath in 60%, and the calcaneus and Achilles tendon in 10% of cases. At least one band typically runs parallel to the calcaneofibular ligament, theoretically placing it at risk for simultaneous injury with a severe ankle sprain.

Edwards[170] examined 178 cadaver fibulas and noted a substantial recess or groove on the posterior aspect of the fibula in 82% and a plantar convex surface in 18% of the specimens. A flat or convex surface on the posterior fibula may be associated with instability of the peroneal tendons. The depth of the groove is variable (2-4 mm), the width is 5 to 10 mm, and the groove is accentuated by an osseous ridge that is covered by a fibrocartilaginous cap, adding another 2 to 4 mm to the overall depth of the sulcus (Fig. 24-90). Edwards[170] speculated that an insufficient lateral ridge predisposed persons to peroneal dislocation. The SPR has no strong attachments to the ridge itself[144] but blends with the periosteum on the lateral surface of the fibula. The inferior peroneal retinaculum attaches superiorly and inferiorly to the lateral wall of the calcaneus just below the sinus tarsi, forming a "pulley" over both peroneal tendons. The inferior retinaculum (IPR) covers both tendons about 2 to 3 cm distal to the tip of the fibula. It is continuous with the inferior extensor retinaculum in the foot and originates near the sinus tarsi. Together they form an arch over the peroneal tendons. The superficial and deep layers of the IPR insert into the calcaneus near the peroneal or posterolateral tubercle. The inferior peroneal retinaculum plays no role in the stability of peroneal tendons at the level of the ankle.

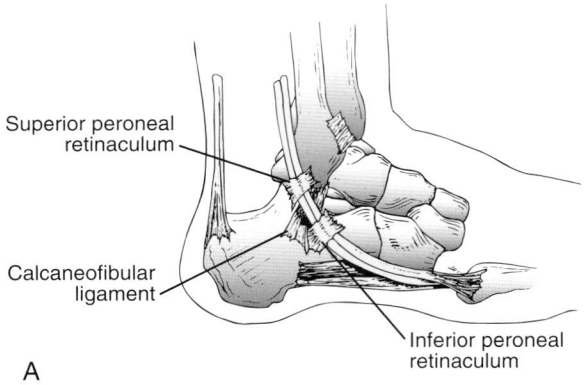

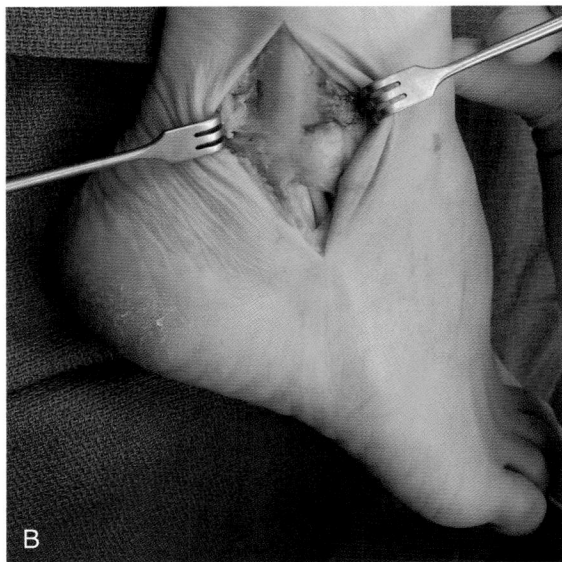

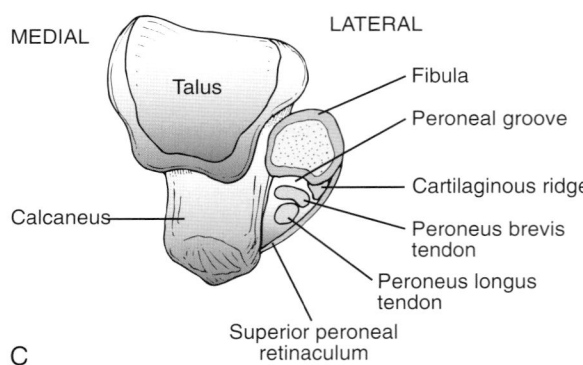

Figure 24-90 **A,** Lateral view of ankle demonstrates peroneal tendons beneath the superior and inferior peroneal retinacula. **B,** Clinical photograph of superior peroneal retinaculum. **C,** Superior view demonstrates position of the peroneus brevis anterior to the peroneus longus tendon.

Mechanism of Injury

Although a disruption or tear of the SPR has been implicated in peroneal tendon dislocation,[187,212,227,240] rupture of the retinaculum rarely occurs.[162,168,169] Typically, the retinaculum is stripped off the fibular insertion[144,162,168] or avulsed with a small fleck of fibular cortex.[248] Das De and

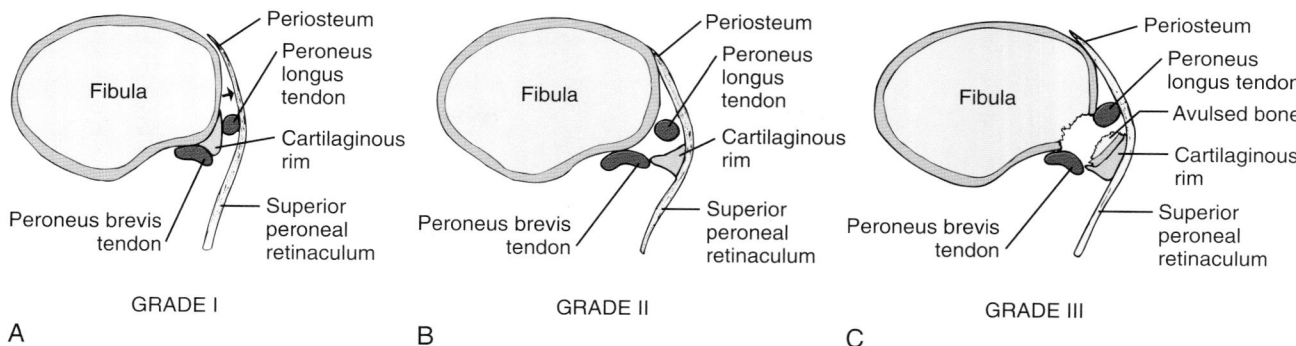

Figure 24-91 Classification of peroneal tendon subluxation–dislocation. **A**, Grade I: superior peroneal retinaculum (SPR) stripped off the fibula; peroneus longus dislocated anteriorly. **B**, Grade II injury: fibrous rim avulsed from posterolateral aspect of the fibula along with the SPR; peroneus longus dislocated anteriorly. **C**, Grade III: bony rim avulsion fracture attached to the SPR, with anterior dislocation of peroneus longus.

Balasubramaniam[162] have likened this to a Bankart lesion of the shoulder, with the creation of a false pouch and laxity of the retinaculum,[275] allowing peroneal tendon dislocation anteriorly.

The mechanism of injury is typically a sudden forceful dorsiflexion and inversion injury of the ankle with a simultaneous violent contraction of the peroneal musculature, leading to a disruption of the SPR. Sobel et al[270] reported a simultaneous rupture of the calcaneofibular ligament with injury to the SPR, and in their report, this isolated case was treated with a Chrisman-Snook ankle reconstruction.

The high incidence of peroneal tendon dislocation associated with skiing injuries supports the premise of both forced dorsiflexion and acute forceful contraction of the peroneal musculature because a ski boot places the ankle in a dorsiflexed position that limits ankle excursion, thus allowing substantial muscle contraction against a fixed ankle. The edging mechanism on the inside edge with alpine skiing places the dorsiflexed ankle in eversion as well, increasing the propensity for an injury with a caught edge.

Chronic subluxation can also occur in patients with recurrent ankle sprains. In the study of associated injuries found in chronic lateral ankle instability by DiGiovanni et al,[165] peroneal tenosynovitis was found in 47 of 61 (77%) cases, attenuated peroneal retinaculum or retinacular avulsion was found in 33 of 61 (54%), and peroneal tendon tears were noted in 15 of 61 (25%). In these cases, the chronic stretching of the SPR can allow expansion of the retrofibular ligamentous structures, thereby predisposing the tendons to roll or jump around each other more without the constraints. With time, the recurrent riding of the peroneal tendons around each other and over the edge can predispose them to longitudinal splits and worsening of the subluxation.

Neuromuscular abnormalities (paralysis, polio) are also associated with peroneal tendon dislocation.[201,275] Kojima et al[195] reported congenital dislocation of the peroneal tendons in 3% of neonates, and this may be a more common entity than appreciated. When untreated,

Table 24-1 Gradations of Peroneal Tendon Dislocations

Grade	Characteristics
I	Superior peroneal retinaculum (SPR) is still attached to the periosteum on the posterior aspect of the fibula. However, the periosteum is elevated from the underlying malleolus by the dissections that are displaced anteriorly.
II	SPR is torn free from its anterior insertion on the malleolus, and the periosteum of the tendons dissects through at this level.
III	SPR is avulsed from the insertion on the malleolus, with avulsion of a small fragment of bone.
IV	SPR is torn from its posterior attachment as tendon dissects through, with the SPR lying deep to the dislocating peroneal tendon.

Modified from Oden R: Tendon injuries about the ankle resulting from skiing, *Clin Orthop Relat Res* 216:63–69, 1987.

almost all cases resolve spontaneously, although one can only speculate whether these patients are at higher risk for peroneal subluxation–dislocation in later life. Some patients recall no specific history of trauma related to peroneal tendon dislocation.

Peroneal tendon subluxation–dislocation is first distinguished as either acute or chronic. Eckert and Davis[169] further differentiated different grades, depending on the type of injury, and documented the incidence of occurrence as follows:

Grade I (51%): The retinaculum is elevated from the lateral malleolus, with the tendons lying between the bone and periosteum (Fig. 24-91A).
Grade II (33%): The fibrocartilaginous ridge is elevated with the retinaculum attached, and the tendons are displaced beneath the ridge (Fig. 24-91B).
Grade III (16%): A thin cortical fragment is avulsed from the fibula with the tendons displaced beneath the fibular fragment (Fig. 24-91C).

Oden[230] added also graded peroneal tendon dislocations and included a rare grade IV, with the retinaculum avulsed or ruptured from the posterior attachment (Table 24-1).

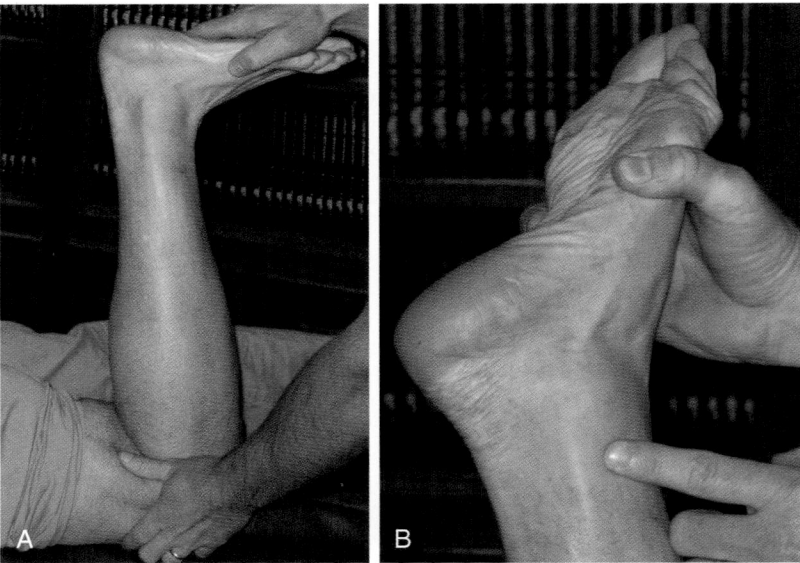

Figure 24-92 Clinical photograph of the technique to examine a patient suspected of having a subluxating peroneal tendon. **A,** Patient in prone position with the knee flexed to 90 degrees. **B,** With the foot and ankle at a comfortable height, the tendon and sheath can be inspected and tested for dynamic instability.

Grade III injuries can often be distinguished on plain radiographic examination, whereas grade I and II can only be differentiated at surgery. Eckert and Davis[169] noted that with reduction of the peroneal tendons, grade III injuries were grossly unstable after reduction. Grade II injuries were also unstable when reduced, but grade I injuries were unstable only in dorsiflexion. This can help to explain the success rate of less than 50% when nonsurgical care is elected after acute rupture. Only with a pure SPR avulsion (with disruption of either a bone or fibrosseous ridge, grades II and III) can success with nonsurgical treatment be reasonably expected.

History and Physical Examination

With an *acute* dislocation, the patient often recalls a significant episode of trauma. A painful snapping sensation may be associated with the actual disruption. Significant pain localized to the retromalleolar area often subsides relatively rapidly.[144] With spontaneous relocation of the peroneal tendons, a patient might relate a history of a "lateral ankle sprain." However, unlike the history of a sprain in which a patient recalls an inversion injury, with peroneal tendon dislocation the mechanism of injury is often vague. With *chronic* instability, a generalized history of "recurrent sprains" is elicited, although occasionally a patient specifically describes peroneal tendon dislocation. The patient might complain of snapping or popping or instability on uneven ground.

On physical examination, subluxation or dislocation is often missed unless it is specifically evaluated (Fig. 24-92). Sarmiento and Wolf[254] and others[142,159,168,227] noted that acute dislocations are rarely diagnosed. Without early diagnosis and prompt appropriate

treatment, dislocation invariably recurs.[144,171] Acutely, a variable amount of swelling and ecchymosis may be present in the retrofibular region, which can obscure the dislocated peroneal tendons. Pain is localized to the posterior aspect of the fibula more proximally and posteriorly than pain associated with an injury to the anterior talofibular ligament. It should not be difficult to differentiate peroneal tendon injury from an acute ankle sprain, but the patient should be evaluated for lateral ankle instability with a drawer and talar tilt examination as well.

With acute peroneal tendon dislocation, palpable crepitus may be noted over the posterior rim of the fibula. The ankle is passively circumducted, and with this maneuver, subluxation may be identified.[182] The patient is then asked to dorsiflex and evert the foot and ankle from a plantar-flexed, inverted position. With tensing of the peroneals, pain may be noted posterior to the fibula. Then, with resisted dorsiflexion and eversion, subluxation or dislocation of the peroneal tendons can occur. With active circumduction of the ankle and foot in clockwise and counterclockwise fashions, the peroneal tendons are palpated in the retrofibular region. Although many normal people have popping of the tendons, there are subtle side-to-side differences that are apparent in most cases. With chronic instability, swelling or ecchymosis is often minimal. An inability to dislocate the peroneal tendons does not necessarily rule out instability.[211]

On occasion, a patient demonstrates anxiety when the foot and ankle are placed in a dorsiflexed and everted position. A high index of suspicion is necessary to make a diagnosis of instability of the peroneal tendons. Examination of the contralateral ankle is important in evaluating the patient for ligamentous laxity. Assessment of the patient while standing and during gait can reveal calcaneal varus. Coexisting ankle ligament instability and peroneal tendon weakness should be identified. Subtalar and ankle disorder may be found in these patients.

Radiographic Examination

Imaging of the injured ankle can occasionally be helpful in ascertaining the diagnosis of peroneal tendon instability. Routine AP, lateral, and mortise radiographs are often normal but can demonstrate a small flake of fibular cortex (0.5 to 1 cm in length), indicating a grade III injury, which is pathognomonic of a tendon dislocation. Ankle stress views for ankle instability may be performed. Computed tomography is infrequently used currently.[231,232] A CT scan may be helpful with an uncertain diagnosis to evaluate the posterior fibular groove.[144,176,277] Ultrasound evaluation is confirmatory in skilled hands (Fig. 24-93).[228] MRI may be helpful in assessing a concomitant peroneal tendon injury (Fig. 24-94).[300]

Acute Dislocation

Treatment of acute peroneal tendon dislocation is controversial.[144]

Conservative Treatment

Nonsurgical treatment is always an option. McGarvey and Clanton[211] considered it a safe treatment, although they recognized the high failure rate. Sarmiento and Wolf[254] stated that an acute dislocation can be casted. Stover and Bryan[275] advocated initial conservative treatment in a well-molded below-knee cast in mild plantar flexion for 5 to 6 weeks. They reported success with casting in 57% and with taping in 40% of cases treated. The purpose of casting is to contain the peroneal tendons while the SPR heals. McLennan[212] noted that although conservative care was satisfactory "in most cases," 44% eventually required surgery. Escalas et al[171] attempted conservative care in 38 patients, 28 of whom (74%) required eventual surgery. Earle et al[168] and others[142,169,227] noted that conservative treatment for acute peroneal tendon dislocation has a success rate of less than 50%.

These injuries tend to occur in young adults and athletes. This population generally wants a speedy return to athletic pursuits, and surgical reconstruction has a much higher rate of success compared with nonsurgical treatment.

When choosing casting, the authors prefer a well-molded below-knee cast in slight plantar flexion and slight inversion. A non–weight-bearing cast for 2 weeks is preferred to allow resolution of swelling.[211] This is followed by a below-knee walking cast or brace for 4 weeks, after which active range-of-motion exercises and physical therapy are initiated.

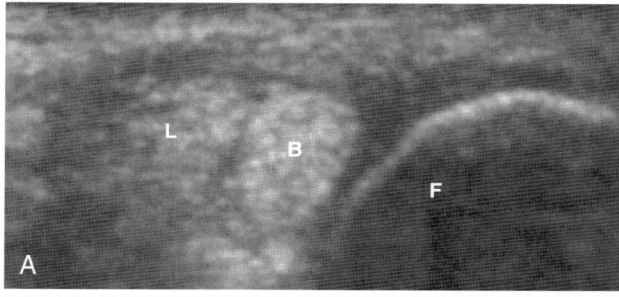

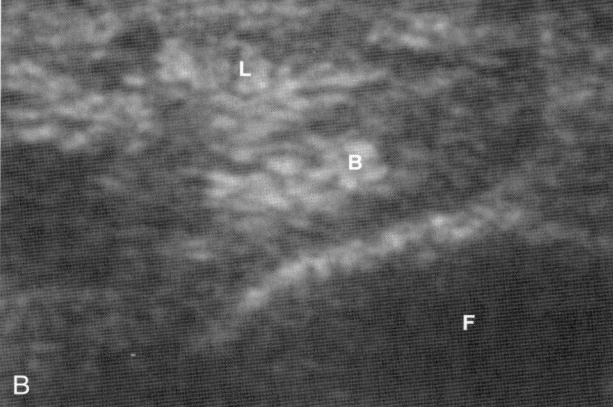

Figure 24-93 A 20-year-old man with typical subluxation of the right peroneal tendon. **A,** Axial sonogram obtained with affected ankle in neutral position shows the peroneus longus *(L)* and peroneus brevis *(B)* tendons in a normal relationship posterior to the distal fibula *(F)*. **B,** Axial sonogram obtained with affected ankle dorsiflexed and everted shows that peroneus longus and peroneus brevis tendons have subluxated anteriorly and now lie superficial relative to the distal fibula.

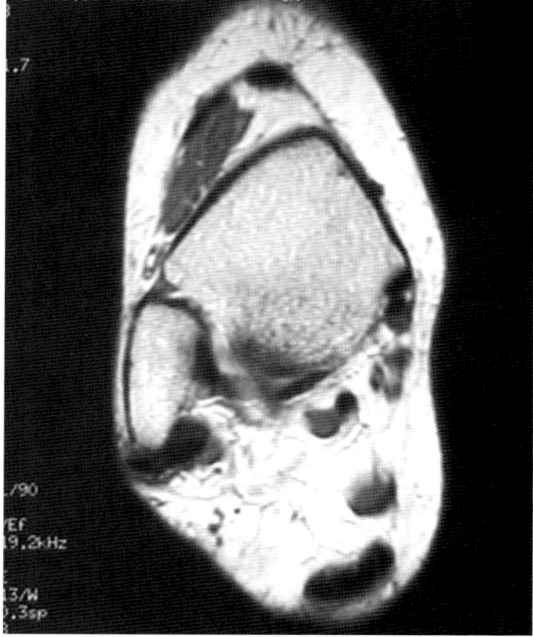

Figure 24–94 Magnetic resonance image demonstrating subluxation of peroneal tendons.

Surgical Treatment

Arrowsmith et al[144] and others have advocated acute repair, citing excellent results and rapid recovery. Arrowsmith et al[144] also have called attention to peroneus brevis tendon tears in patients with chronic peroneal tendon instability, which significantly complicates the recovery process after delayed reconstruction and argues for early repair after peroneal tendon dislocation.

Direct reattachment of the SPR to the posterior periosteum of the fibula through multiple drill holes is the treatment of choice for repair of acute peroneal tendon dislocation. Adachi et al[140] advocated its use for the repair of chronic peroneal tendon dislocation.

DIRECT SUPERIOR PERONEAL RETINACULUM REPAIR
Surgical Technique

1. The patient is placed in a prone position under appropriate anesthesia and with a thigh tourniquet inflated to afford adequate hemostasis. A 6-cm longitudinal incision is centered 1 cm posterior to the fibula and extended from 5 cm proximal to 2 cm distal to the tip of the fibula. Care is taken to protect the sural nerve (Fig. 24-95A).

2. The SPR is identified and incised longitudinally 1 mm to 1 cm from the posterior edge of the fibula (Fig. 24-95B).
3. The fibular ridge can be cross-hatched with an osteotome, and three or four lateral-to-medial drill holes are placed vertically through the cortex and directed slightly posteriorly.
4. The sutures are passed through the drill holes and the SPR, securing the avulsed retinaculum to the fibular ridge.
5. The sutures are tied. The retinaculum is then imbricated along the incision line with absorbable sutures (Fig. 24–95C). The periosteal tissue over the fibula can be elevated off of the bone and advanced to imbricate another layer over the repair.
6. The subcutaneous tissue and skin are approximated in a routine manner (Fig. 24-96).

Postoperative Care

The foot is placed in a non–weight-bearing below-knee cast or splint with the foot in slight equinus and slight eversion. Neutral or slight eversion is acceptable, in contrast to nonsurgical treatment, where slight inversion is advocated to maintain reduction of the peroneal

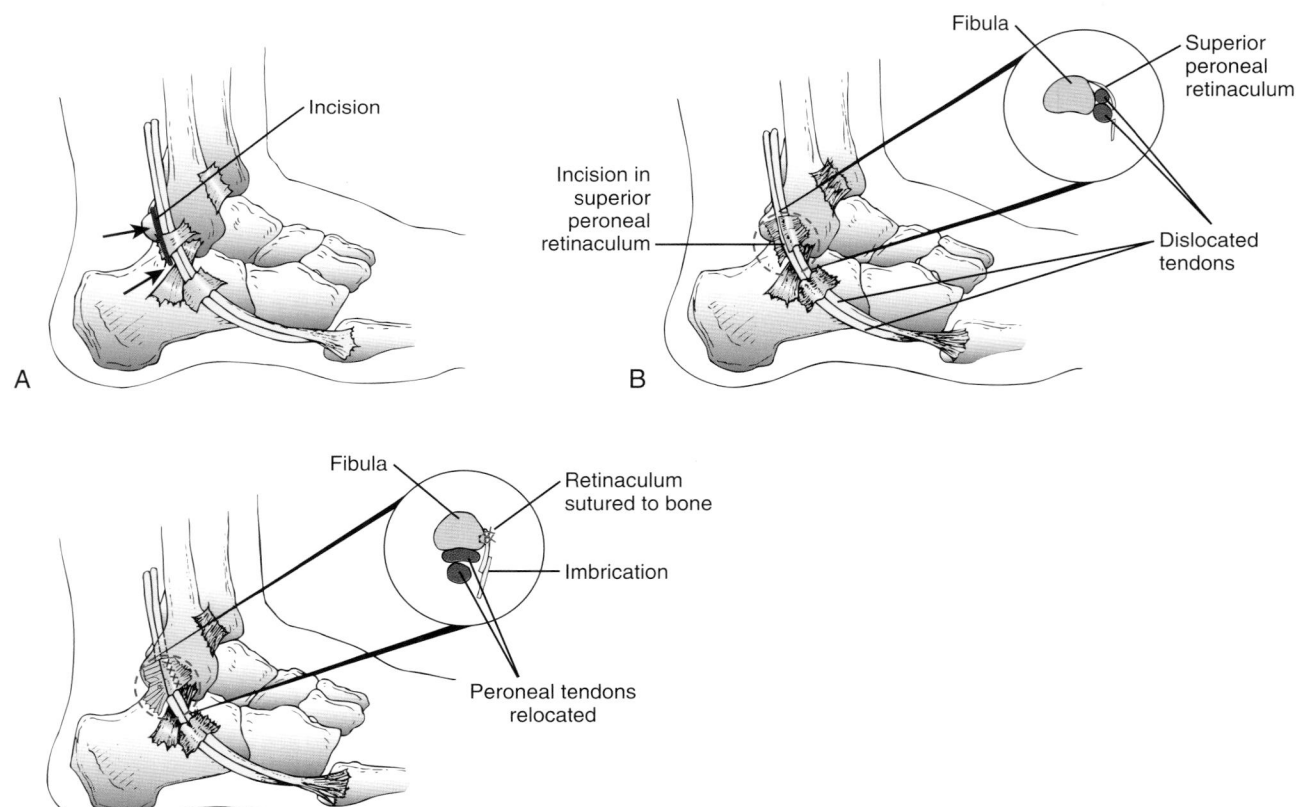

Figure 24-95 Surgical repair of acute peroneal tendon dislocation. **A,** Surgical approach. **B,** Pathologic anatomy demonstrates dislocation of peroneal tendons. **C,** Repair of superior peroneal retinaculum (SPR) with drill holes through the posterolateral portion of fibula and reefing of SPR.

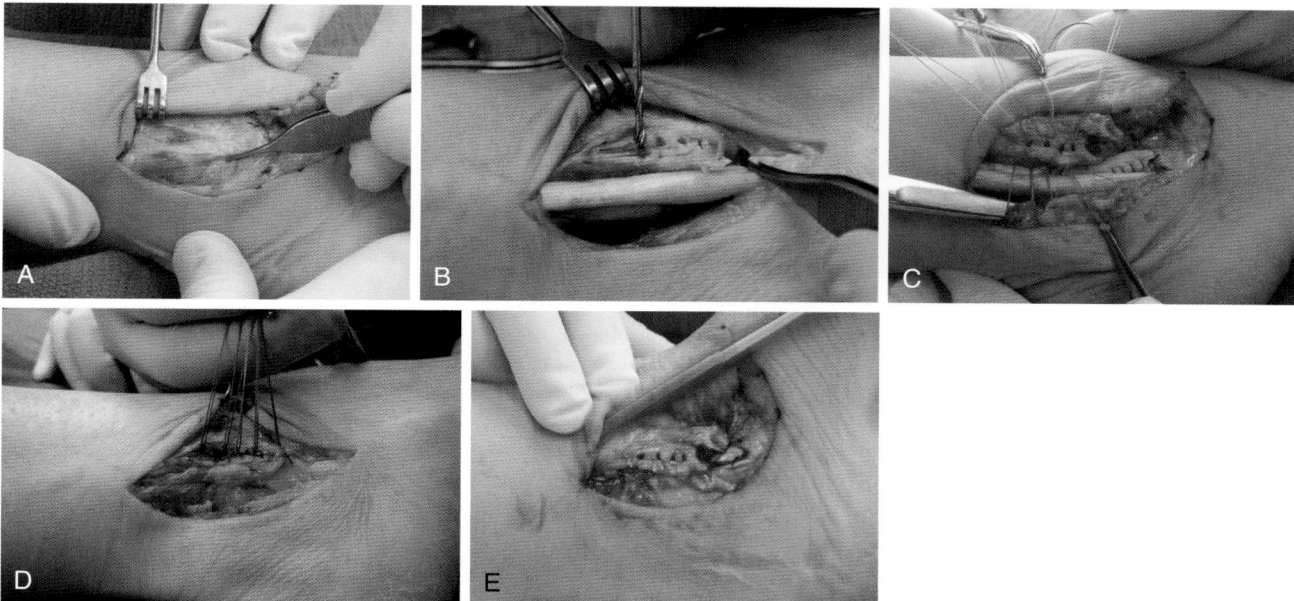

Figure 24-96 Acute repair of peroneal tendon subluxation **A,** Redundant capsule associated with peroneal tendon subluxation. **B,** After repair of small tendon tear, drill holes are placed in posterior fibular ridge. **C,** Sutures have been placed in superior peroneal retinaculum and through the drill holes. The sutures have been tied **(D)** and cut **(E),** completeing the repair.

tendons. After 2 weeks in a non–weight-bearing cast or splint, a plantigrade below-knee cast or CAM-boot is applied, and weight bearing is allowed for 4 weeks. The patient should avoid plantar flexion below 30 degrees and inversion to minimize the risk of disrupting the repair. Boot or cast immobilization is then discontinued and may be replaced by a stirrup brace from which the patient is gradually weaned and physical therapy initiated.

Direct repair of acute peroneal tendon dislocation has been advocated by a number of authors. In 76 reported cases,[142,147,162,168,231] a 96% success rate has been reported.[211]

CHRONIC DISLOCATION

The incidence of missed diagnosis or untreated peroneal tendon dislocation is high, leading often to recurrent dislocation. Casting and other nonsurgical methods can serve to reduce pain or diminish inflammation but have little success in permanent relocation of chronically dislocated peroneal tendons. Numerous surgical procedures have been designed to stabilize chronically dislocating peroneal tendons, attesting to no one technique being uniformly successful, as reported in the literature (Box 24-1). After chronic dislocation of the peroneal tendons, tendon tears may develop, requiring treatment not only for the tendon subluxation but also for tendon pathology as well (Fig. 24-97).

McGarvey and Clanton[211] have grouped the various techniques into the following areas: SPR reinforcement and repair, tissue-transfer techniques, tendon-rerouting techniques, bone-block procedures, and groove-deepening procedures.

Box 24-1 Types of Surgical Reconstruction for Peroneal Tendon Dislocation

Direct repair of peroneal retinaculum[140,162,206,258,263]
Reconstruction of peroneal retinaculum
    Achilles tendon sling[187]
    Plantaris sling[221]
    Peroneus brevis sling[144,272]
    Anomalous muscle[182]
Bone block
    Lateral malleolar osteotomy[188,189]
    Sliding graft (lateral malleolus)[167,216]
Groove deepening with osteoperiosteal flap[144,258,290]
Rerouting procedure beneath calcaneofibular ligament
    Calcaneofibular ligament takedown from fibula with reattachment[153,177,292]
    Calcaneofibular ligament mobilized with bone block from calcaneus[240]
    Calcaneofibular mobilized by osteotomizing the lateral malleolus[242]
    Peroneal tendons divided and rerouted under calcaneofibular ligament[208,254]

SUPERIOR PERONEAL RETINACULUM REINFORCEMENT AND REPAIR

This technique is the same as used for an acute repair with reconstruction of the SPR. When an avulsion of the fibular ridge has occurred, it is reduced and internally fixed. Alm et al[142] and others* reported success with this procedure. Although a simple repair might not adequately stabilize peroneal tendons in the presence of a convex groove or an insufficient SPR, this technique may be combined with other techniques of reconstruction as well.

---

*References 140, 147, 162, 206, 258, and 263.

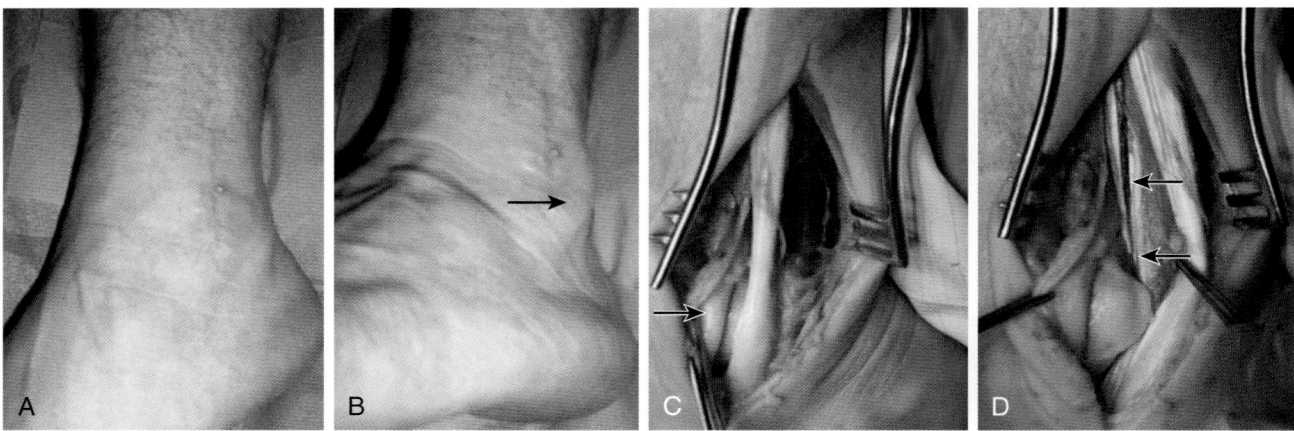

Figure 24-97 Chronic dislocation of the peroneal tendons. Clinical photographs before **(A)** and after **(B)** peroneal tendon subluxation over fibula *(arrow)* (patient had a prior failed ligament repair for subluxation). **C,** Dislocation of peroneus longus *(arrow)* above the fibula. **D,** After retraction, the sharp edge of the fibula is seen, and the peroneus brevis tendon is seen in a reduced position.[219] (From Millar TM, Garg SK: The Singapore operation for chronic recurrent peroneal tendon subluxation— short-term follow-up in four patients, *Foot Ankle Surg* 15:146–148, 2009. Used with permission.)

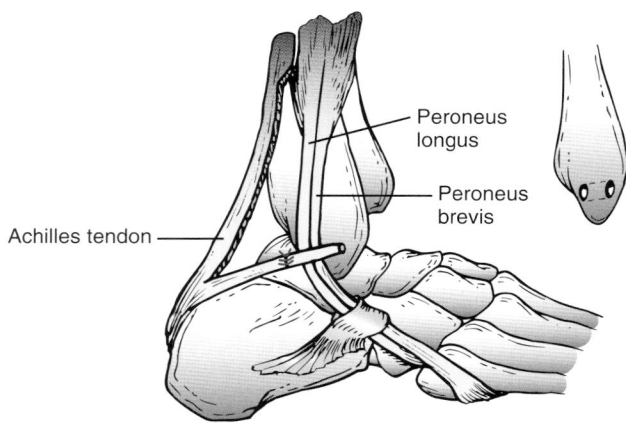

Figure 24-98 Ellis-Jones reconstruction of peroneal retinaculum employing a portion of Achilles tendon.

TISSUE-TRANSFER TECHNIQUES

Jones[187] described the use of a distally attached slip of Achilles tendon routed through the fibula to create a reinforced retinaculum to stabilize the peroneal tendons (Fig. 24-98). Escalas et al[171] and others[169,176] also advocated this technique. The peroneus brevis[217,256,272] and the plantaris[221] tendons have been chosen to reinforce the SPR, but no large series have been reported on these techniques. Miyamoto et al[222] used a gracilis graft to reconstruct insufficient lateral collateral ankle ligaments and simultaneously reconstructed the SPR with the tendon graft for combined lateral ankle and peroneal tendon instability. McGarvey and Clanton[211] noted a 19% complication rate with this technique.

TENDON-REROUTING TECHNIQUES
(Video Clip 109)

Various techniques have been proposed to reroute the peroneal tendons, and most use the calcaneofibular

ligament to stabilize the peroneal tendons. Platzgummer[239] and others[148,273] divided the calcaneofibular ligament near the fibular insertion (Figs. 24-99 and 24-100); Viernstein et al[289] and Poll and Duijfjes[240] performed a distal fibular osteotomy (Fig. 24-101); and Pozo and Jackson[242] transposed the calcaneofibular ligament with a calcaneal bone block (Fig. 24-102). Sarmiento and Wolf[254] and Martens et al[208] divided the peroneal tendons and repaired them after rerouting them beneath the calcaneofibular ligament. No dislocations have been reported, but a high rate of associated sural nerve injury and ankle stiffness has been noted. McGarvey and Clanton[211] noted a complication rate of 61% with this technique.

Coughlin has used the technique described by Sarmiento and Wolf[254] (Fig. 24-103) in skeletally immature patients with good success, and the current authors believe it should be included in the surgeon's armamentarium (Fig. 24-104).

LeNoir[204] described a case of anterior transposition of the peroneal tendons and sheath as an alternative, routing them anterior to the distal fibula. However, no other reports are available on this procedure, and it is not recommended.

Schon has also used a rerouting technique for chronic painful snapping peroneal tendons that did not respond to a groove-deepening procedure. In this procedure, the peroneus longus was placed in a channel that was created obliquely in the distal lateral aspect of the fibula, separating it from the brevis, which was left in the retrofibular groove. A portion of free synovial graft tacked to the bone was used to create a lining for the longus in the new fibula channel. In these two cases, there was an improvement in the painful snapping, better function, and decreased swelling. Both patients continued to have some symptoms, however, despite the benefit.

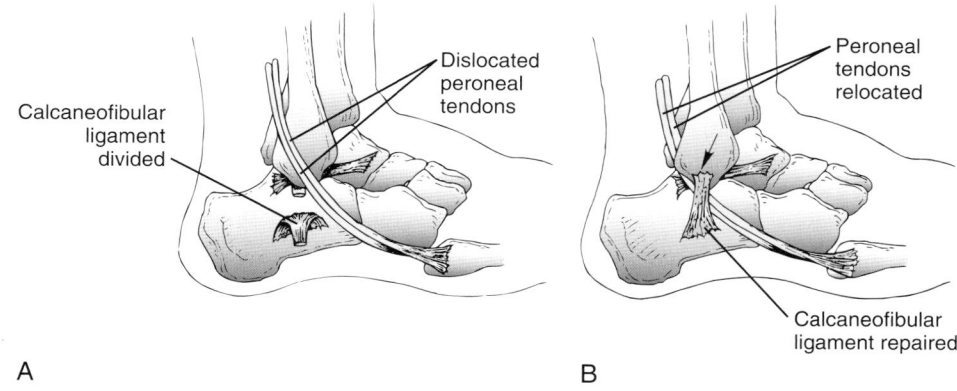

Figure 24-99 Platzgummer method for repair of dislocating peroneal tendons. Peroneal tendons are rerouted beneath the calcaneofibular ligament, which is repaired. **A,** Calcaneofibular ligament has been divided and turned down. **B,** Peroneal tendons have been relocated and calcaneofibular ligament repaired. (Modified from Platzgummer H: [On a simple procedure for the operative therapy of habitual peroneal tendon luxation], *Arch Orthop Unfallchir* 61:144–150, 1967.)

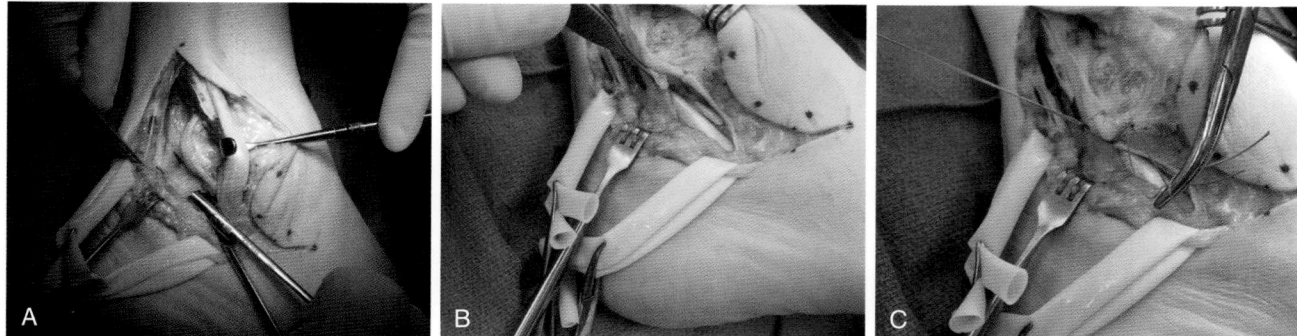

Figure 24-100 Rerouting of peroneal tendons beneath detached calcaneofibular ligament. **A,** With peroneal tendons retracted anteriorly, the calcaneofibular (CF) ligament is clearly seen. **B,** The CF ligament is taken down from its fibular attachment. **C,** The peroneal tendons are reduced, and the calcaneofibular ligament is repaired over them, creating a "new" superior peroneal retinaculum ligament.

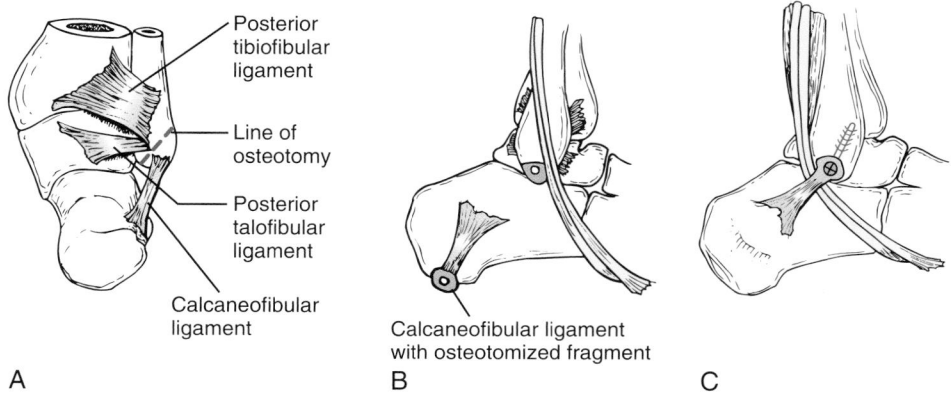

Figure 24-101 Bone block osteotomized from fibula. **A,** Line of osteotomy through fibula. **B,** Osteotomized fibular fragment is attached to the calcaneofibular ligament and turned inferiorly. The hole is predrilled in the fragment before performing the osteotomy. **C,** After peroneal tendons have been reduced, the osteotomized fragment is reattached and stabilized with internal fixation. (Modified from Pozo J, Jackson A: A rerouting operation for dislocation of peroneal tendons: operative technique and case report, *Foot Ankle* 5:42–44, 1984.)

BONE-BLOCK PROCEDURES

Kelly[189] initially described a partial-thickness distal fibular osteotomy that was rotated posteriorly to deepen the fibular groove (Fig. 24-105A and 24-106). DuVries[167] and Micheli et al[216] modified this procedure with variations of the Kelly technique (see Fig. 24-105B). Wirth[298] and others[209,212,216] reported good results after distal fibular osteotomy, although a high rate of complications has been associated with internal fixation, graft fracture, tendon irritation, chronic pain, nonunion, and resubluxation.[201]

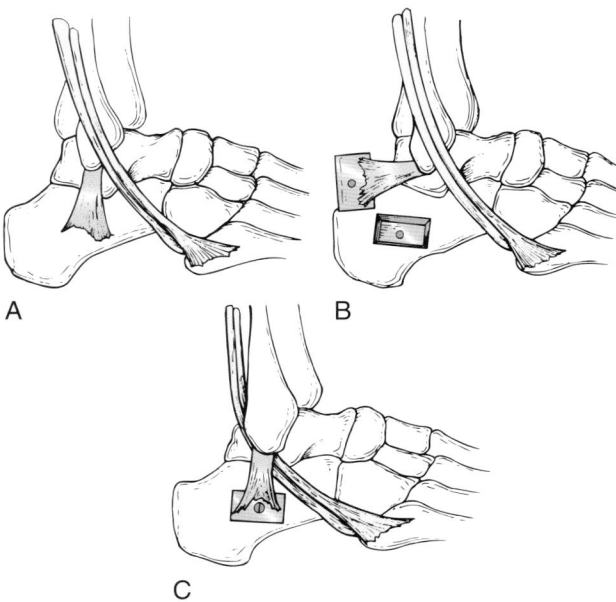

Figure 24-102 Calcaneofibular ligament transferred with bone block from calcaneus. **A,** Tendons are dislocated anteriorly. **B,** Bone block is mobilized from the calcaneus. **C,** After peroneal tendons have been relocated, bone block is internally fixed, stabilizing tendons. (Modified from Poll R, Duijfjes F: The treatment of recurrent dislocation of the peroneal tendons, *J Bone Joint Surg Br* 66:98–100, 1984.)

GROOVE-DEEPENING PROCEDURES

By resecting bone on the posterior aspect of the distal fibula, the peroneal groove is deepened, altering and increasing the stability of the peroneal tendon (Fig. 24-107). These procedures require some technical skill but are useful. Although McGarvey and Clanton[211] reported a 30% complication rate with groove-deepening procedures, Coughlin and Schon have used this technique with very few complications. Tracy[284] stated that peroneal groove deepening was biomechanically an unsound procedure, but Title et al[283] showed biomechanically that pressures within the middle and distal peroneal groove significantly decreased after a groove-deepening procedure when performed in the manner described next. They found it enhanced peroneal stability and decreased pressure on the peroneal tendons, and this can improve peroneal function and decrease retrofibular pain. Zoellner and Clancy[303] and others[144,168,261] have used this technique with good success. Zoellner and Clancy[303] advocated reinforcing the SPR in combination with this procedure.

One other technique for groove deepening, which has been advocated by Mendicino et al[213] and Shawen et al,[260] deserves mention. This method involves deepening the groove by inserting progressively larger drills or burrs through the tip of the distal fibula just anterior to the calcaneofibular ligament (Fig. 24-108). This weakens the posterior cancellous bone that supports the osteocartilaginous posterior aspect of the fibular groove. Next, a bone tamp is inserted, and the posterior fibular surface is impacted into the medullary canal. Although this procedure may be useful, further study is warranted to highlight its benefits over the flap technique as described next.

GROOVE DEEPENING WITH A POSTERIOR OSTEOCARTILAGINOUS FLAP
Surgical Technique (Video Clip 111)

1. After induction of either general anesthesia or a local ankle block with intravenous sedation anesthesia, the patient is placed in a lateral decubitus position.

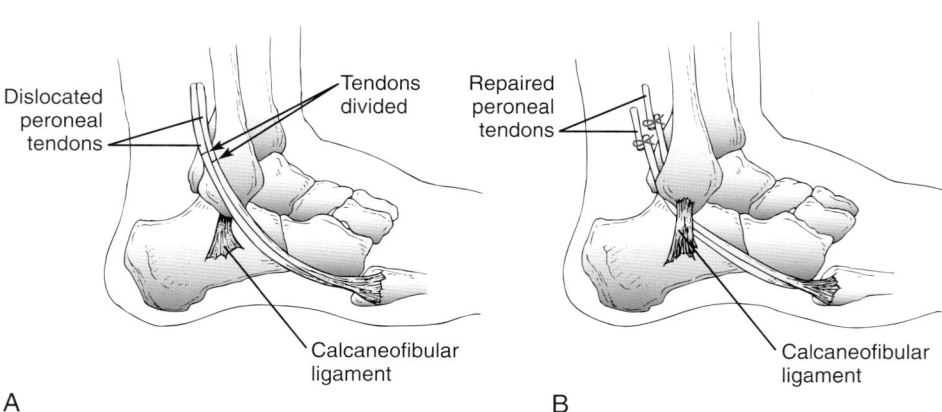

Figure 24-103 Method of rerouting peroneal tendons beneath calcaneofibular ligament by dividing tendons and repairing them. **A,** Pathologic anatomy. **B,** Peroneal tendons are relocated beneath calcaneofibular ligament after division and repair.

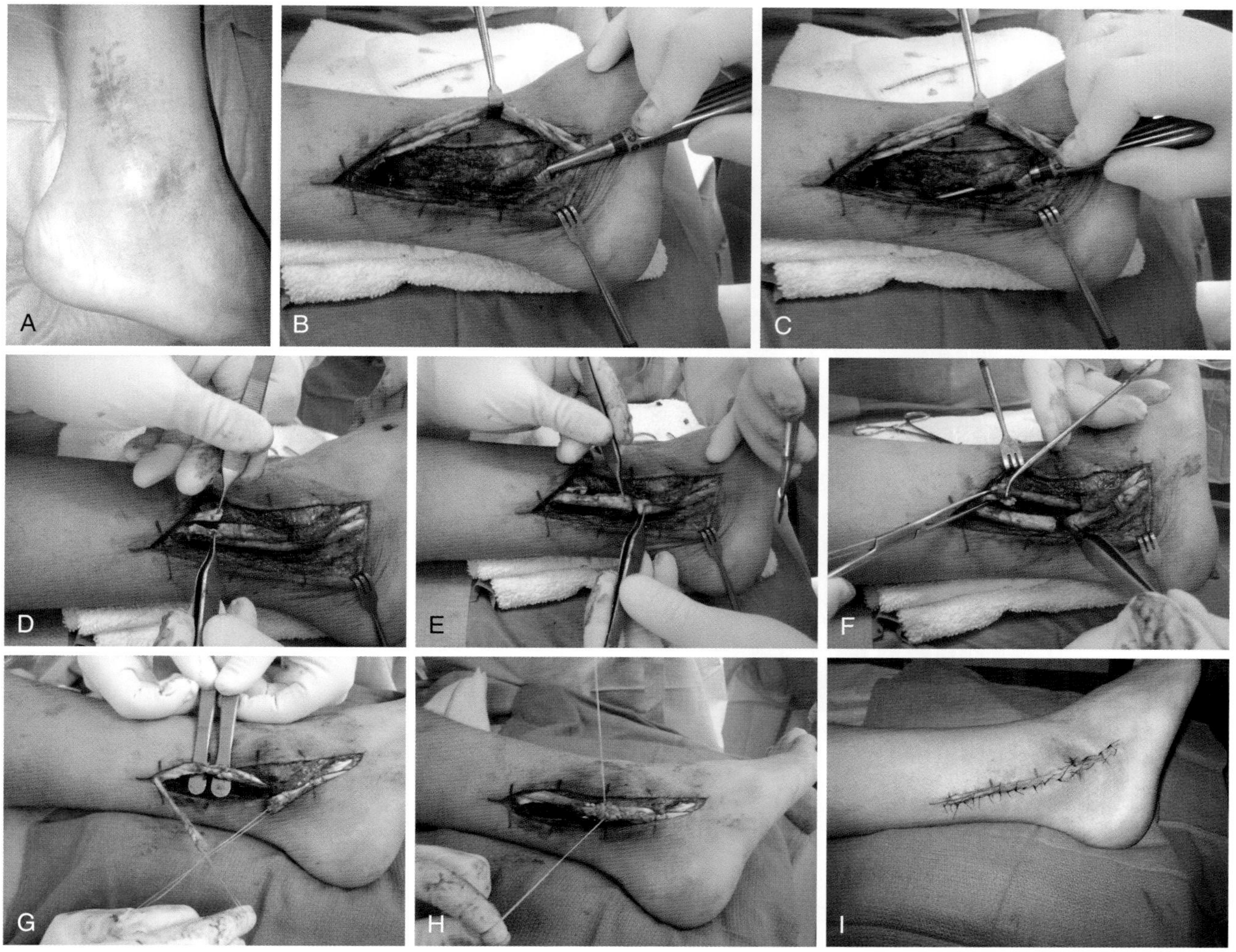

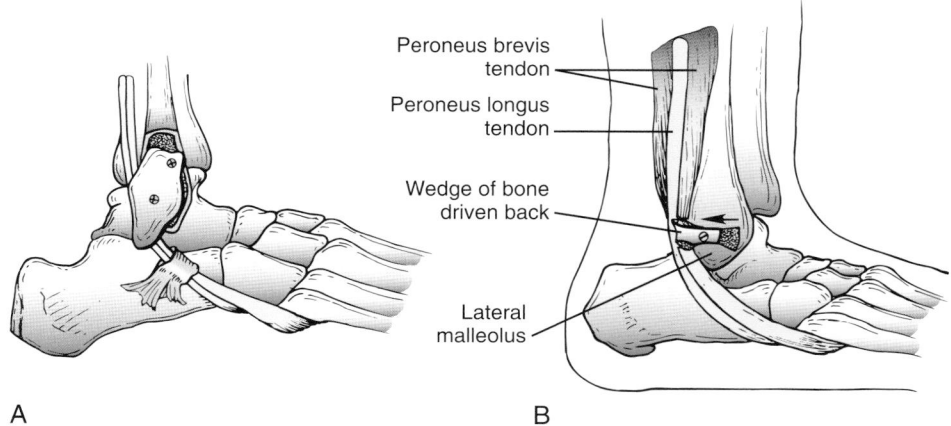

Figure 24-104 Sarmiento procedure for rerouting peroneal tendons beneath the calcaneofibular (CF) ligament. **A,** Clinical photograph of patient with failed superior peroneal retinaculum repair procedure. **B** and **C,** With peroneal tendons retracted, the CF ligament is dilated to ensure easy passage of tendons. **D,** Step-cut of peroneus brevis. **E,** Transverse cut of peroneus longus. **F,** Both tendons have been passed beneath the CF ligament. **G,** Repair of peroneus brevis. **H,** Repair of peroneus longus. **I,** After closure of superior peroneal retinaculum and skin.

Figure 24-105 Bone-block procedures for repair of subluxating peroneal tendons. **A,** Kelly technique for deepening the retromalleolar sulcus by rotating a distal fibular osteotomy. **B,** DuVries modification using distal fibular osteotomy sliding graft. (**A,** Modified from Kelly R: An operation for the chronic dislocation of the peroneal tendons, *Br J Surg* 7:502–504, 1920. **B,** Modified from DuVries H: *Surgery of the foot,* St Louis, 1959, Mosby, pp 253–255.)

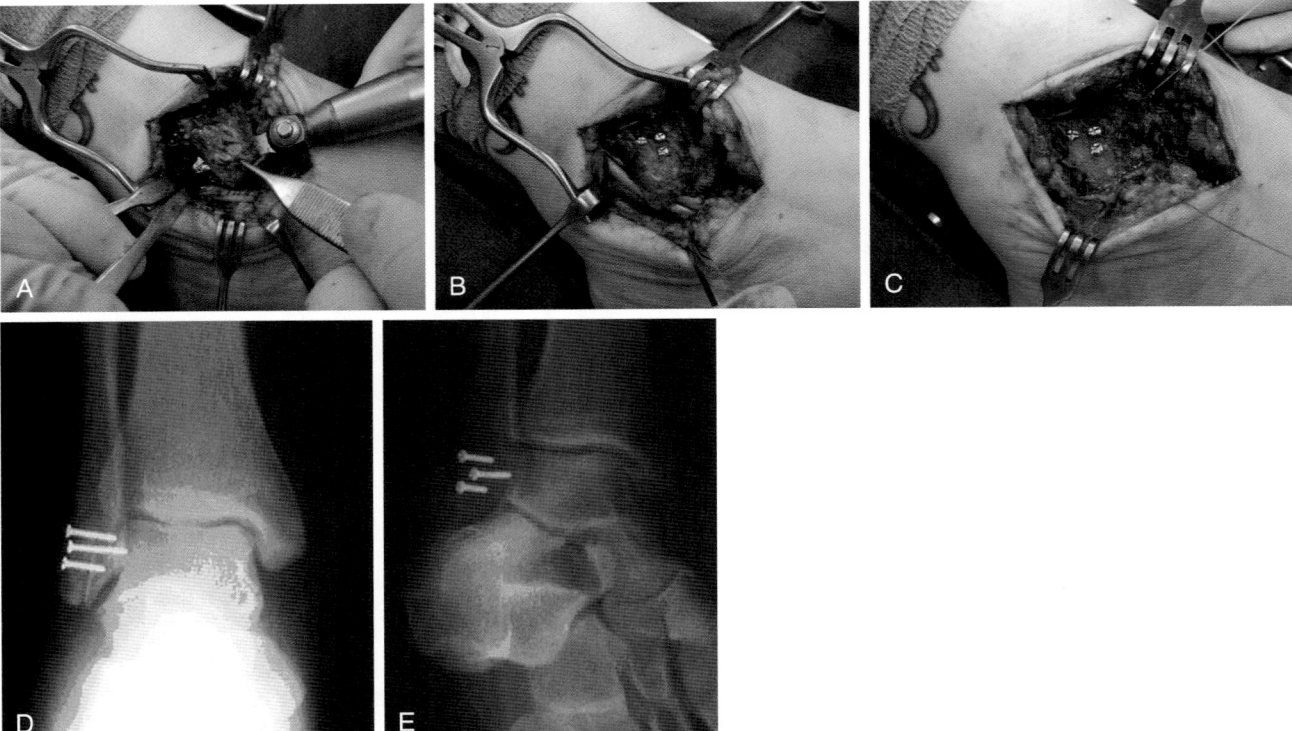

Figure 24-106 Kelly rotational bone-block procedure for dislocating peroneal tendons. **A,** Oblique fibular osteotomy. **B,** Rotation of lateral fragment over peroneal tendons. **C,** After closure of the superior peroneal retinaculum. **D** and **E,** Oblique and anteroposterior radiograph demonstrating position of fibular internal fixation. (From Kaz A, Coughlin M: Technique tip: distal fibula rotational osteotomy for subluxating peroneal tendons, *Med Chir Pied* 23:68–71, 2007. Used with permission.)

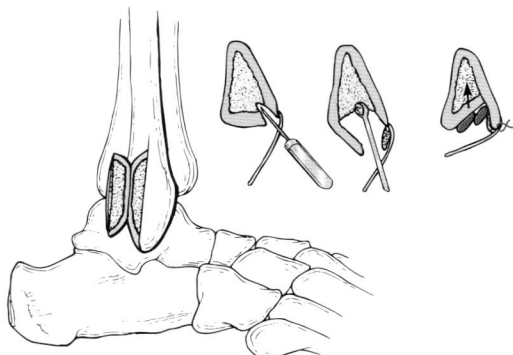

Figure 24-107 Groove-deepening procedure with osteoperiosteal flaps. Decancellation of posterior surface of the lateral malleolus and recessing of cortex to deepen groove. (Modified from Arrowsmith S, Fleming L, Allman F: Traumatic dislocations of the peroneal tendons, *Am J Sports Med* 11:142–146, 1983.)

2. A 4-cm incision is made over the posterior edge of the fibula, curving around the lateral malleolus anteriorly for 5 to 10 mm of the distal incision. Care is taken to avoid the branch of the sural nerve (Fig. 24-109A).

3. The subcutaneous tissues are dissected, and the peroneal tendon sheaths are examined. The ankle is passively manipulated in dorsiflexion, plantar flexion, eversion, and inversion to observe subluxation of the tendons.

4. The tendon sheath is incised 1 mm posterior to the fibula. Peroneal tendons are checked for abnormal pathologic processes (tendinitis or tears), and the shape of retromalleolar groove is examined. Depending upon what is seen intraoperatively, tenosynovectomy or repair of a ruptured retinaculum or peroneal sheath is performed.

5. The anterior sheath of the retinaculum is sharply elevated off the fibula, and the fibula periosteum is raised for an area of 1 to 1.5 cm.

6. With a chisel, a 2- to 3-mm posterior osteocartilaginous flap is detached from the retromalleolar groove with subchondral bone from lateral to medial. The cortex of the medial aspect of the fibula is penetrated to free the flap. The flap is 3 to 4 cm long and includes the distal aspect of the groove, and the flap is 8 to 11 mm wide and includes the entire posterior surface of the fibula groove (Fig. 24-109B and C).

7. Two Homan retractors are placed behind the medial edge of the posterior fibula, reflecting the flap and tendons posteriorly. Using a burr, the groove is deepened by removing 4 to 7 mm of cancellous bone (Fig. 24-109D).

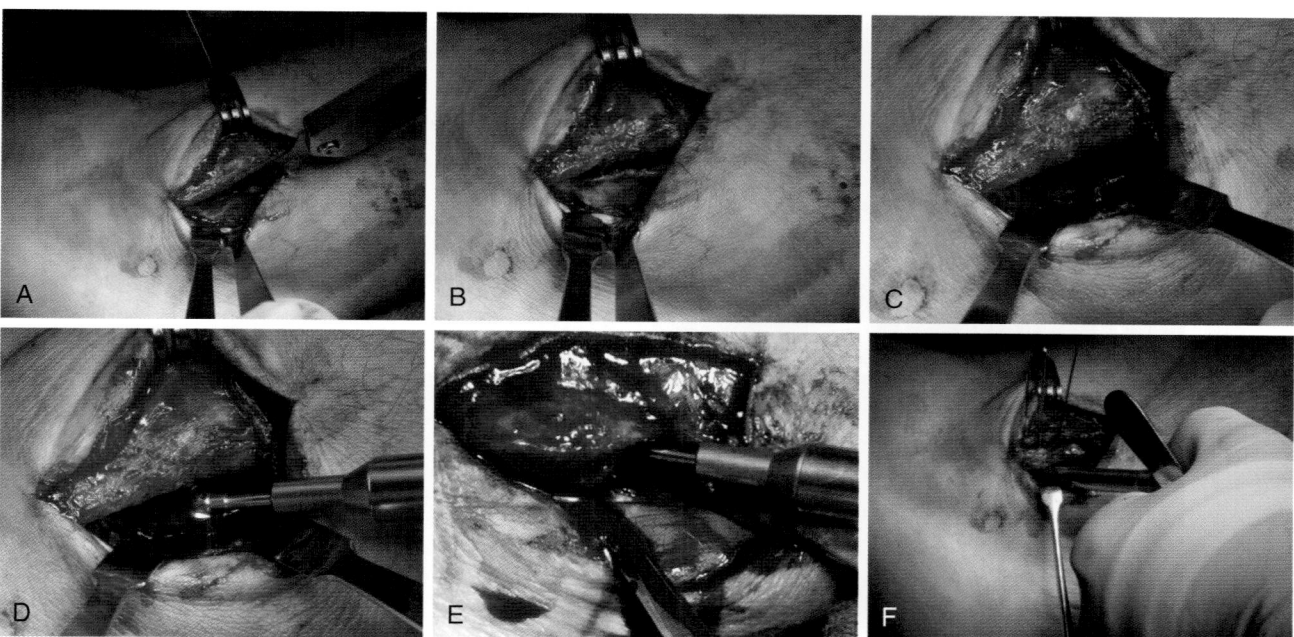

Figure 24-108 Groove deepening. **A,** With an open technique, a chisel is used to create a bony flap, which is osteotomized through the medial cortex (**B**). **C,** The tendons are reflected posteriorly by to Homan refractors. **D,** The burr is used to deepen the groove. **E,** Four to 7 mm of cancellous bone is removed. **F,** The bone flap is tamped back into position.

8. Next, 0.045-inch Kirschner wires are used to create three or four tunnels in the posterior and lateral edge of the fibula. Each wire is left in place and cut immediately before the suture is ready to be passed. The tunnels are started 4 mm anterior to the posterior edge, and they exit in the posterior cancellous bone just inside the remaining lateral wall of the fibula. These wires should not substantially block the flap from being repositioned.

9. The flap is placed onto the cancellous surface, and the tendons are returned to the groove (Fig. 24-109E). If the flap is unstable, the tendons should be positioned in place; if the surgeon is uncomfortable with the motion of the fragment, a 2-mm mini-fragment screw can be inserted from posterior to anterior to stabilize the fragment.

10. Using a 2-0 polyester (Ethibond; Ethicon, Somerville, N.J.) suture, a modified Kessler method is used to hold the most anterior edge (1 to 2 mm) of the posterior aspect of the sheath and retinaculum. The sutures are placed from bone to tissue and then back to bone, but they are not tied until all the throws are placed. These sutures will pull the retinaculum into the posterior lateral aspect of the groove inside the lateral wall the fibula, helping to secure the tendons and the flap and providing a cover for the raw bone surface at the fibula edge. The sutures are tied (Fig. 24-109F-H).

11. The anterior aspect of the periosteum that had been raised is advanced posteriorly and oversewn to the posterior retinaculum and sheath with 2-0 polyglactin (Vicryl; Ethicon, Somerville, N.J.) suture, taking care to avoid the tendons within. The skin is then closed with 4-0 nylon suture. The foot is placed in a bulky Jones dressing in the neutral position.

12. Alternatively, the surgeon may use a burr to decompress the posterior fibula either in a closed technique (see Fig. 24-111 and Video Clip 110) or with open exposure (Fig. 24-108A). With the closed technique, once the tendons have been retracted, a burr can be pushed from the tip of the fibula proximally, and then the lateral wall is impacted with a bone punch to "cave-in" the wall, creating room for the peroneal tendons. The SPR is repaired in a fashion as described above.

13. With an open technique, after exposure of the lateral wall of the fibula, a saw is used to cut along the anterior edge of the peroneal canal (see Fig. 24-108B). The wall is elevated (see Fig. 24-108C). Then wall is removed (see Fig. 24-108D) and a burr used to decompress the canal (see Fig. 24-108E). The wall is compressed with a bone tamp (see Fig. 24-108F), and the tendons are replaced underneath the shelf and the SPR repaired (Fig. 24-110).

Postoperative Care

The splint is removed at 10 days, and a fixed-ankle CAM-boot is applied. The patient is allowed to ambulate with full weight bearing and may do gentle ankle range-of-motion activities, avoiding plantar flexion of greater than 20 degrees and any inversion. At 6 weeks after surgery, a lace-up cloth or Aircast-type stirrup ankle brace is applied.

The patient may use an elliptic trainer or exercise bike with the brace and may begin jogging at 8 to 10 weeks.

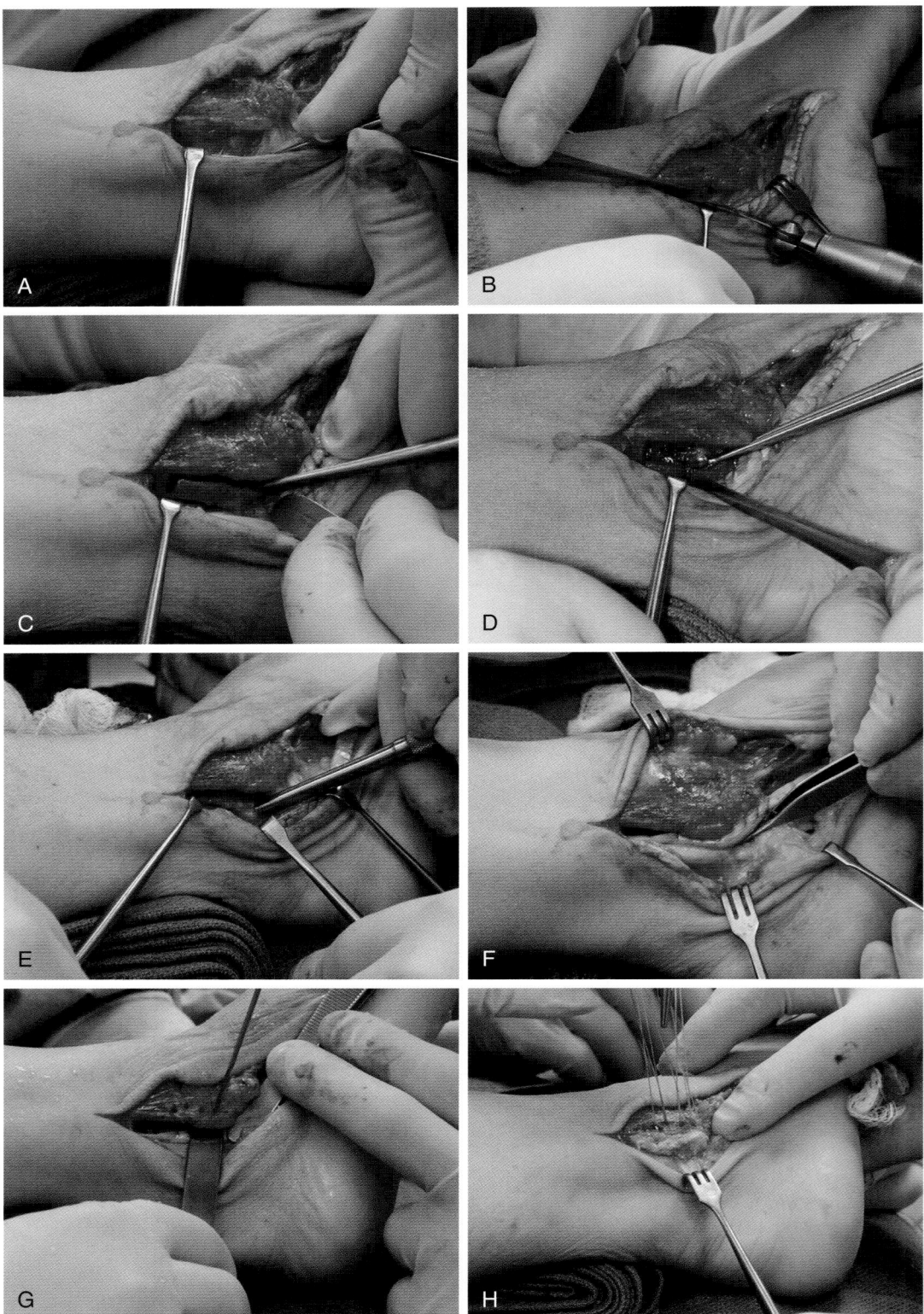

Figure 24-109 **A,** Operative exposure for groove deepening procedure. Parallel saw cuts are used to create a trap door **(B),** which is hinged **(C)** posteriorly, exposing cancellous bone. **D,** Curet or bur is used to decompress this area. **E,** Trap door is impacted into place, creating an offset and deepening the recess posterior to the fibula. **F,** Peroneal tendons are relocated. **G,** Drill holes are placed in the fibular lip. **H,** Sutures are tied securing the superior peroneal retinaculum.

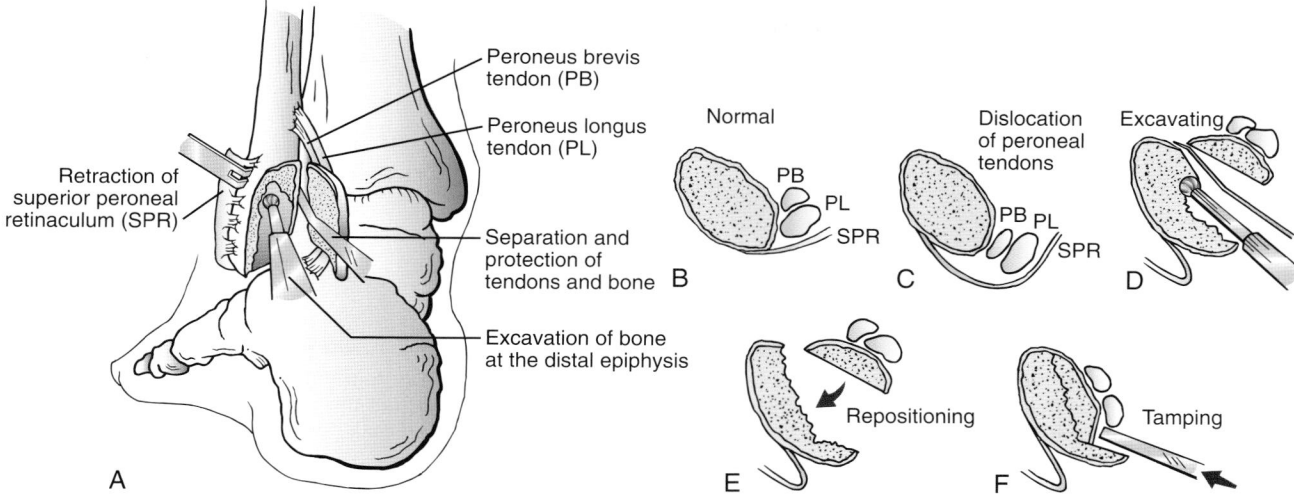

Figure 24-110 **A,** Operative exposure for groove-deepening procedure. Parallel saw cuts are used to create a trap door **(B),** which is hinged **(C)** posteriorly, exposing cancellous bone. **D,** Curet or burr is used to decompress this area. **E,** Trap door is impacted into place, creating an offset and deepening the recess posterior to the fibula. **F,** Peroneal tendons are relocated. **G,** Drill holes are placed in the fibular lip. **H,** Sutures are tied securing the superior peroneal retinaculum.

Cutting activities can begin after the patient has successfully progressed from large figures of eight to small figures of eight, typically at 12 weeks.

Results and Complications
This method does offer treatment to the 18% of patients who have a shallow or convex posterior fibular surface, and it can be helpful even in the presence of a normal groove. Peroneal tendon groove-deepening procedures have become more widely accepted. These procedures are claimed to be less complicated than other bone procedures, while correcting the underlying anatomic deformity, preserving the gliding surface, alleviating pain and subluxation, and preserving essential tendons, ligaments, and range of motion.

Complications associated with peroneal tendon groove deepening include redislocation, decreased range of motion, sural nerve injury, and friction of the tendon after repair. In an unpublished series of 36 groove-deepening procedures performed by Schon, 23 patients had peroneal dislocations, and 13 patients had chronic peroneal tendon pain. In the latter group, 10 of 13 were athletic-induced injuries, and 3 of 13 were trauma-induced injuries. This group was interesting because 5 of the 13 had abnormal grooves, 3 of the 13 had revision surgery for peroneal tendon tears in the face of normal grooves, and 5 of the 13 (all athletes) had normal tendons and grooves but had chronic retromalleolar pain relieved with a local injection. Overall in the 36 patients, there were no redislocations of the peroneal tendons. Two patients had snapping of the tendons, and it was necessary to reroute the tendons, creating a separate channel for the peroneus longus in the lateral aspect of the fibula, which terminated the rolling of the longus and the brevis. In this series, 1 patient had a partial bone flap detachment and

2 patients had lateral distal fibula fragmentation without any consequences to the patient. Transient sural neuritis was seen in 6 patients, but all cases resolved spontaneously between 2 and 3 months after surgery.

Porter et al[241] used a fibular groove-deepening procedure very similar to Coughlin and Schon's technique, performing a complete removal of the bone flap, which allowed a symmetric bone removal and deepening of the groove. Porter et al reported no recurrent dislocations in 14 ankles, all patients returned to sports, and there were no bony complications from detachment of the bone flap. Saxena et al[258] reported on 31 patients who underwent SPR reinforcement and, when needed, a groove-deepening procedure; they reported a return to sporting activity at an average of 3 months after surgery. Walther et al[290] reported on 23 patients, at an average age of 34 years, who had a modified groove-deepening procedure using an intramedullary drill to decompress the fibula beneath the canal and then impact the outer cortex, deepening the groove. The authors reported excellent results with this procedure (Fig. 24-111).

This result might suggest that peroneal groove deepening is not only an excellent procedure to correct peroneal tendon subluxation or dislocation but also a viable option in patients with chronic retrofibular peroneal pain without obvious tendon or groove pathology, as well as in patients with peroneal tendon tears in the presence of an abnormal peroneal groove. This suggestion is borne out by Title et al[283] in a biomechanical cadaveric study that looked at the pressure changes in the peroneal groove before and after a groove-deepening procedure. The pressures over the distal 2 cm of the posterior fibula just proximal to the calcaneofibular ligament decreased significantly after the procedure. This led the authors to suggest that combining the groove deepening with

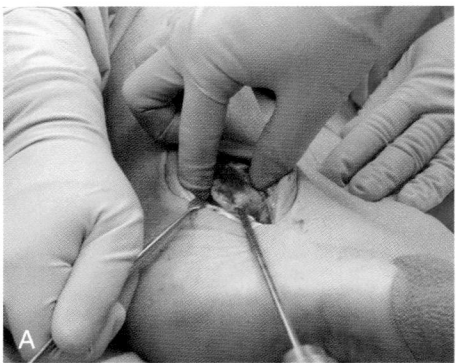 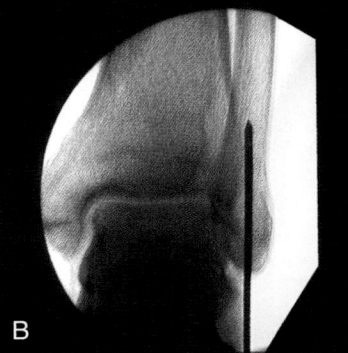 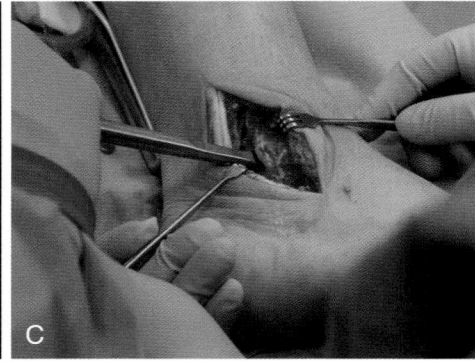

Figure 24-111 Semi-closed technique to drill and "cave-in" fibular cortex. **A,** Clinical photograph demonstrating method of drilling the hole in the fibula. **B,** Radiograph demonstrating guide pin for the reamer within the fibula. **C,** Tamp used to compress the posterior fibular groove in order to deepen it but leave a smooth gliding surface for the tendons.

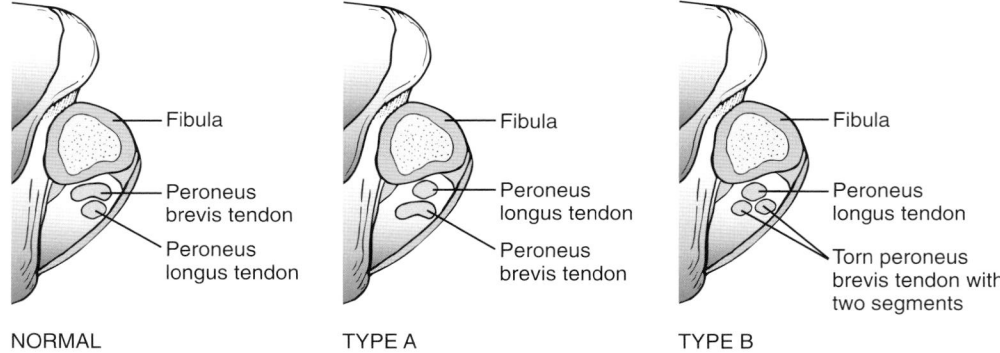

Figure 24-112 Intrasheath subluxation of the peroneal tendons. **A,** Normal position. **B,** Subluxation with peroneus longus deep to brevis. **C,** Peroneus brevis tear with subluxation of longus through the tear. (Modified from Raikin SM, Elias I, Nazarian LN: Intrasheath subluxation of the peroneal tendons, *J Bone Joint Surg Am* 90:992–999, 2008. Used with permission.)

tendon debridement or repair may be advantageous for treatment of peroneal tendon tears or peroneal tendinitis. Although a small number of cases have been reported using this technique, a very high rate of success has been noted.*

The most common complication after nonsurgical or surgical treatment for peroneal dislocation is redislocation, which is decidedly higher in the nonsurgical group. Other reported complications include decreased range of motion, friction on the tendon after repair, and degenerative tendon tears. Skin sensitivity and sural nerve injury have been reported postoperatively but can be avoided with careful surgical technique.

Intrasheath Peroneal Subluxation

McConkey and Favero[210] reported one case and Harper[183] two cases of subluxation of the peroneus brevis on top of the peroneus longus within the tendon sheath. Both groups reported a "rising up" of the peroneus brevis tendon. A thickened peroneus brevis has been observed with 2 of 3 patients with a history of chronic ankle sprains, suggesting a concomitant peroneus brevis tendon

injury. Thomas et al[281] reported on peroneal "intrasheath" subluxation within the canal in 7 patients as confirmed by ultrasound. They noted that this "intrasheath" subluxation was associated with either a "low-lying peroneal muscle belly" or a peroneus quartus tendon. Six of 7 had a tear of one or both of the peroneal tendons (Fig. 24-113). Operative repair of the tendon pathology resulted in elimination of the subluxation symptoms. Raikin and Nazaran[244,245] reported on a large series of 57 patients with peroneal tendon subluxation. Of these, 43 subjects subluxated their tendons out of the canal, while 14 could not. Evaluation of this subset under ultrasound demonstrated that the two tendons were seen to switch their relative positions (the peroneus longus switched deep to the peroneus brevis tendon), and then an audible and painful click occurred. Operative findings included a flat or convex posterior fibular surface in 13 of 14 cases. Five patients had peroneal tendon tears. Treatment consisted of a groove-deepening procedure, repair of peroneal tendon tears, and repair of the superior peroneal retinaculum. Raiken reported that 13 of 14 surgical repairs were successful (Fig. 24-112). Vega et al[288] reported the tendoscopic treatment of 6 patients with intrasheath subluxation of the peroneal tendons. A low-lying peroneus muscle belly or peroneus quartus was resected in 5

---

*References 191, 196, 213, 241, 258, 283, and 290.

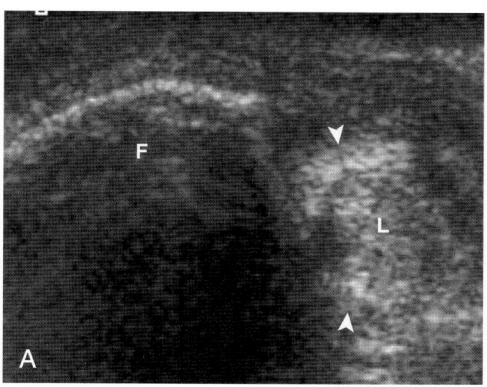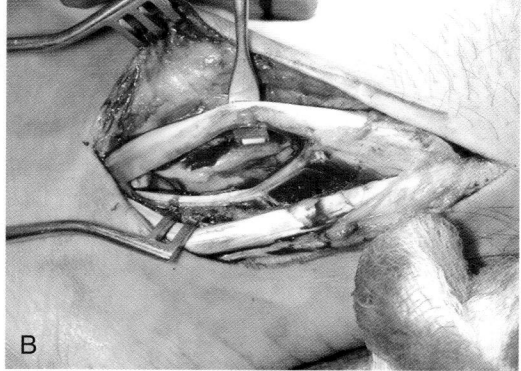

Figure 24-113 **A,** Dynamic ultrasound image demonstrating type B intrasheath subluxation. The peroneus longus tendon has subluxated through the split peroneus brevis tendon. The *white arrowheads* mark the two split portions of the peroneus brevis tendon, *F* marks the fibula, and *L* marks the peroneus longus tendon. **B,** Intraoperative photograph demonstrates a longitudinal split tear of the peroneus brevis through which the peroneus longus can subluxate, causing painful snapping. (*F* is fibula; *B* is peroneus brevis). (From Raikin SM, Elias I, Nazarian LN: Intrasheath subluxation of the peroneal tendons, *J Bone Joint Surg Am* 90:992–999, 2008. Used with permission.)

cases, and a groove-deepening procedure was performed in 2 cases with satisfactory results at 1.5 years.

Patients with dislocation as a result of major trauma are more likely to have sural nerve problems preoperatively.[283] Also, some patients without nerve symptoms postoperatively did have transient neuralgia that may have developed from the exposure, retraction, or the injections from the ankle block.

The reports of both peroneus longus tendon tears[208] and peroneus brevis tears[144] associated with chronic peroneal tendon dislocations make an argument for early definitive repair of peroneal tendon instability.

The peroneal tendons should be carefully inspected at the time of either ankle reconstruction or peroneal tendon stabilization procedures.

Conclusion

Acute subluxation and dislocation of the peroneal tendons may be misdiagnosed or not treated, leading to chronic instability. A high level of suspicion and awareness of the condition leads to early diagnosis and successful treatment. Most often these injuries occur in a young, athletically active population. Anatomically, a deficient SPR or a shallow or absent posterior fibular sulcus is often associated with instability.

Delayed conservative treatment of acute peroneal tendon dislocations is successful in approximately half of cases. Surgical reconstruction is the treatment of choice for young, active patients and those with chronic instability. Although many surgical techniques are available, SPR reconstruction, groove-deepening procedures, and occasionally tendon-rerouting procedures are excellent methods with which to treat acute and chronic peroneal tendon instability successfully. Results are usually excellent after proper diagnosis and appropriate treatment of this condition.

Posterior Tibial Tendon Subluxation–Dislocation

Traumatic dislocation of the posterior tibial tendon occurs rarely, having been reported in less than 50 cases in the English literature. It was first described as a case report by Martius[316] who self-described the injury he sustained when he fell from a balloon in 1874.

Often, these cases have a delay in diagnosis, having been treated for a variety of diagnoses, including ankle sprains,[322-324] tendinitis,[330] subtalar joint injury[315] or some other traumatic event.* Delay in diagnosis and treatment has not appeared to have a deleterious effect on outcomes in reported cases in the literature.

Conservative care has been noted to be uniformly unsuccessful.

The diagnosis is made with a careful history and physical examination, but after acute trauma, the diagnosis may be difficult to make. Most commonly, a traumatic injury is characterized by inversion of the foot with either forced dorsiflexion or plantar flexion associated with a violent contraction of the posterior tibial tendon. At surgical exploration, various findings include elevation of the retinacular-periosteal sleeve,[318,330] a tear or avulsion of the retinaculum,[†] a lax retinaculum,[307,310,320,325,328] or a shallow retromalleolar groove.[311,322,326,330] In these series, the patients often present with a protracted history of symptoms and unsuccessful conservative care. In the authors' experience of four patients, the symptoms of posterior tibial tendon dislocation were severe medial and posteromedial pain with features of tibial neuralgia. Three of the four patients had been erroneously diagnosed with complex regional pain syndrome because of the severity of the dysesthesias, tenderness, and lack of function. Surgical repair is usually successful in returning

---

*References 304, 308, 309, 313, 314, 317, 321, 327, and 329.
†References 305-307, 309, 312, 315, 319, 322, and 326.

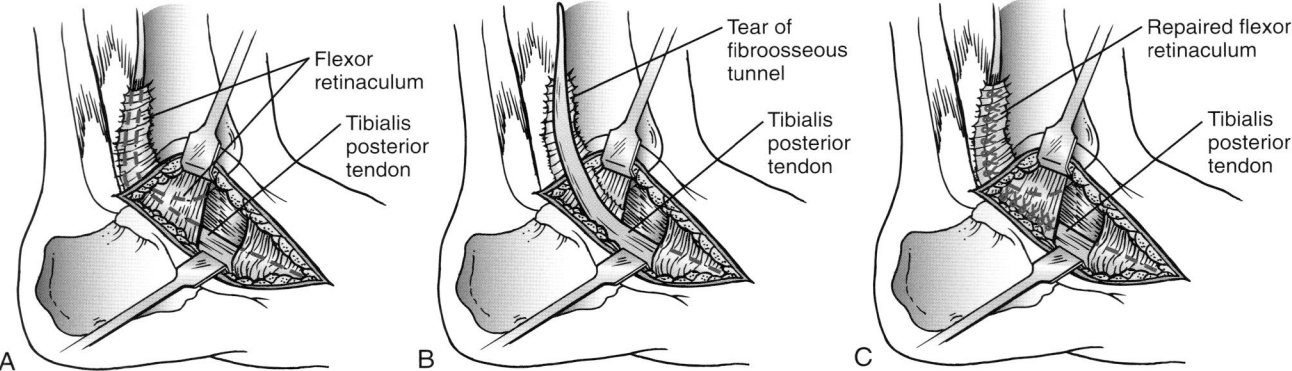

Figure 24-114 **A,** Posterior tibial tendon seen within the flexor retinaculum and fibroosseous tunnel. **B,** Tear of flexor retinaculum and disruption of fibroosseous tunnel allows anterior dislocation of the posterior tibial tendon. **C,** Repair of the flexor retinaculum and fibroosseous tunnel with relocation of the posterior tibial tendon.

patients to full activity. Surgical stabilization is performed by relocating the posterior tibial tendon and repairing or reconstructing the flexor retinaculum with or without a groove-deepening procedure. Most patients were able to return to their preinjury level of function.

Anatomy

The posterior tibial tendon is contained in a strong fibro-osseous tunnel directly posterior to the medial malleolus. The flexor retinaculum, which restrains the posterior tibialis tendon (PTT), originates on the tip of the medial malleolus and inserts on the calcaneus (Fig. 24-114A). The neurovascular bundle and flexor digitorum longus and flexor hallucis longus tendons are less superficial and typically are not involved in the dislocation. Disruption of the fibroosseous tunnel and retinaculum allow the PTT to dislocate anteriorly over the medial malleolus (Fig. 24-114B and C). Soler et al[326] analyzed anatomic variation in the retromalleolar groove in 25 cadaveric specimens. The variations in the width of the groove was quite substantial, ranging from 6 to 15 mm in width, and 1.5 to 4 mm in depth. Often, routine multiplanar radiography is unsuccessful in making the diagnosis of posterior tibial tendon dislocation. The diagnosis has been successfully made by tenography,[323] CT,[324,326] and MRI.[305,315,320,324,330]

Surgical Treatment

There is no consensus regarding the best method of treatment. Simple retinacular repair has been performed[306,312,318,319,326] as well as a complex reconstruction using a periosteal sleeve,[326] Achilles tendon flap,[305,326] and with the use of suture anchors.[320,330] In several cases, the surgeons deepened the retromalleolar groove.*

Surgical Technique to Repair Dislocating Posterior Tibial Tendon (Fig. 24-115)

1. With the patient in a supine position, a pneumatic tourniquet is used for hemostasis.

———————————————————————
*References 310, 311, 323, 325, 326, and 328.

2. A 5-cm curvilinear incision is centered directly posterior to the medial malleolus.
3. The posterior tibial tendon retinaculum is incised and reflected posteriorly, exposing the tendon and any synovial tissue.
4. The tendon is debrided of any small tears, or they are repaired if substantial.
5. The retromalleolar groove is assessed, and if shallow, two parallel cuts are made and a window of bone is elevated. A curet or burr is used to remove cancellous bone beneath the window, and then the bone window is replaced and tamped into place, creating a deepening of the groove.
6. The posterior tibial tendon is relocated.
7. Several drill holes are placed in the anterior edge of the groove, and the retinaculum is secured to the bone with interrupted sutures. A periosteal flap is elevated off the medial malleolus so that it can further secure the reconstruction.
8. After routine soft tissue closure, a posterior splint of boot is applied.

Postoperative Care

The lower extremity is protected in a below-knee cast or boot for 6 weeks. The patient refrains from weight bearing for 3 weeks, and then full weight bearing is allowed. Six weeks after surgery, range-of-motion exercises are commenced. The ankle is protected for another 4 weeks with a CAM-boot, and then aggressive physical therapy is initiated.

Results

Ouzonian and Myerson[322] reported the largest series of posterior tibial tendon dislocations. They reported on seven dislocations (six traumatic and one after several corticosteroid injections). The average time to diagnosis of the dislocation was 9 months. These patients had undergone a variety of treatments without success before the diagnosis. At surgery, the retromalleolar groove was noted to be shallow in four of the cases, and an inflamed tendon was noted in three cases. Ouzonian and Myerson

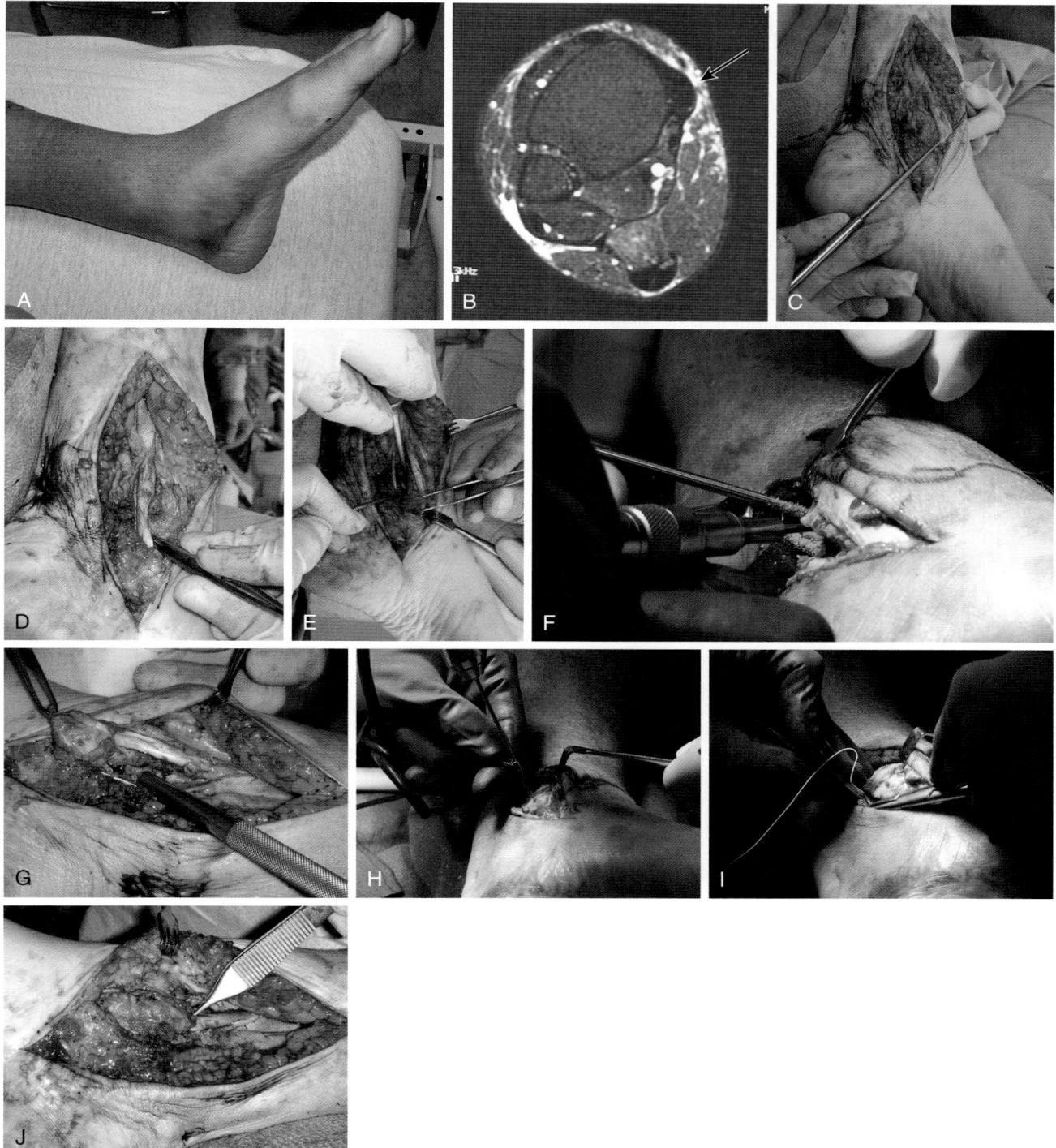

Figure 24-115 **A,** Clinical appearance with dislocation of posterior tibial tendon. **B,** Magnetic resonance image demonstrating dislocation of posterior tibial tendon (PTT). **C,** Surgical exposure demonstrating dislocated PTT anterior to the medial malleolus. **D,** PTT relocated posterior to the medial malleolus. **E,** Osteotomy of medial wall for groove deepening. **F,** Groove deepening with power burr. **G,** Relocation of the anterior wall after groove deepening. **H and I,** Drilling converging holes for repair of the retinaculum and placement of sutures. **J,** After repair of retinaculum.

performed a retinacular repair with reconstruction of the adjacent soft tissue in all these cases, and a groove-deepening procedure in two cases. Six of the seven patients reported satisfactory results.

Bencardino et al[307] reported on MRI findings in seven cases with posterior tibial tendon dislocation. The method of injury was marked dorsiflexion of the ankle in two cases and trauma in five cases. The retinaculum was torn in two and avulsed from the tibia in five cases. Only two patients underwent surgical repair.

Several other publications[304-306,308-321,323-330] list 28 cases that have been reported elsewhere in the literature, almost all of them as a single-case report. A torn flexor retinaculum or an avulsion of the retinaculum from the tibia was noted in seven reports totaling eight cases.* A redundant retinaculum without a disruption of the soft tissue was reported in four cases.[310,320,325,328] In two series, an elevated retinacular attachment was reported.[318,312] A shallow posterior malleolar groove was observed in three reports[310,311,323] and in three series, a normal retromalleolar groove was noted.[306,315,330]

In the 27 cases that have been reported detailing mostly the surgical treatment of a single case, reduction of the posterior tibial tendon, groove deepening (when necessary), and reconstruction of the retinaculum ended with a satisfactory result. The key issue with this condition is making an early diagnosis, especially in the presence of underlying trauma where other more obvious injuries are diagnosed and treated.

TENDON TRANSFERS

A tendon transfer is used to help reestablish balanced muscle function around the foot and ankle to create a plantigrade foot. The plantigrade foot can also enable the patient to obtain a better gait pattern by placing the knee and hip in a more natural orientation for ambulation. Many factors need to be considered with tendon transfers.

Biomechanical Principles

The main biomechanical principle that should be considered in contemplating a tendon transfer involves the axes of the ankle and subtalar joint and the relationship of any tendon to these axes. Other factors are the specific strengths of individual muscles and their phasic activity (stance versus swing phase).

Figure 24-116 illustrates the axes around the foot and ankle. Muscles located anterior to the ankle axis are dorsiflexors, and muscles posterior to the axis are plantar flexors. In relationship to the subtalar joint axis, muscles lying medial to this axis invert the foot, and muscles lying lateral to the axis evert the foot. Because motion can occur about both these axes simultaneously, muscles lying posterior to the ankle axis and medial to the subtalar axis

*References 305, 306, 312, 315, 319, 323, and 326.

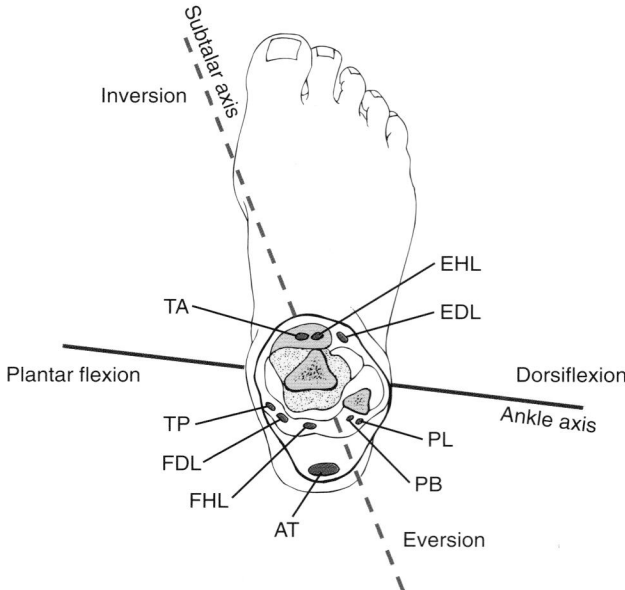

Figure 24-116 Diagram demonstrates rotation that occurs around subtalar and ankle axes. Various muscles around the subtalar and ankle axes are divided into four quadrants, using axes of the ankle and subtalar joint as reference points. *AT,* Achilles tendon; *EDL,* extensor digitorum longus; *EHL,* extensor hallucis longus; *FDL,* flexor digitorum longus; *FHL,* flexor hallucis longus; *PB,* peroneus brevis; *PL,* peroneus longus; *TA,* tibialis anterior.

plantar flex and invert the foot, whereas those posterior to the ankle axis and lateral to the subtalar joint axis plantar flex and evert the foot. Muscles lying anterior to the ankle axis and lateral to the subtalar axis dorsiflex and evert the foot. By visualizing these relationships, the surgeon can then deduce which muscles are deficient and the resultant deformity. This visualization also enables the surgeon to ascertain which muscles are still available for transfer and where they should be placed to correct the deformity.

Principles of Muscle Function

Although clinicians tend to view muscle function around the foot and ankle as a balance of strength between dorsiflexors and plantar flexors and invertors and evertors, Silver et al[131] have demonstrated that this balance is much more complex. In examining the relative strengths of the muscles around the ankle, the authors emphasized that an imbalance exists between the dorsiflexor and plantar flexor musculature. Using a numbering system based on fiber length and muscle mass, the authors stated that the relative strength of the dorsiflexors was 9.4 units and that of the plantar flexors 69 units. The evertors were assigned 11.9 units and the invertors 60.9 units (Table 24-2).

In view of this imbalance, control of muscle balance around the foot and ankle clearly is not based solely on one muscle group balancing another. Rather, the central nervous system (CNS) provides a modulating effect that

Table 24-2 Relative Strengths of Muscles	
Tendon	**Units**
Plantar Flexion	
Soleus	29.9
Gastrocnemius, medial	13.7
Gastrocnemius, lateral	5.5
Flexor hallucis longus	3.6
Flexor digitorum longus	1.8
Posterior tibial	5.5
Peroneus longus	5.5
Peroneus brevis	2.6
Total plantar flexion	69.0
Dorsiflexion	
Anterior tibial	5.6
Extensor digitorum longus	1.7
Extensor hallucis longus	1.2
Peroneus tertius	0.9
Total dorsiflexion	9.4
Inversion	
Posterior tibial	6.4
Flexor hallucis longus	3.6
Flexor digitorum longus	1.8
Gastrocnemius–soleus complex	49.1
Total inversion	60.9
Eversion	
Peroneus longus	5.5
Peroneus brevis	2.6
Extensor digitorum longus	1.7
Extensor hallucis longus	1.2
Peroneus tertius	0.9
Total eversion	11.9

maintains muscle balance around the foot and ankle. When the cerebral balance has been upset as a result of a CNS abnormality (e.g., cerebral palsy, cerebrovascular accident, head injury), the effects of imbalance become quite apparent. Thus, after loss of this central balancing mechanism, clinicians observe, in an equinovarus deformity, the response to the relative strengths of the plantar flexors and invertors in relationship to the dorsiflexors and evertors.

The phasic activity of muscles must be considered as well. Muscle function around the foot and ankle is generally divided into muscles that function during the swing phase and those that function during stance phase. The swing-phase muscles consist of those in the anterior compartment that bring about dorsiflexion of the ankle joint and control initial plantar flexion after heel strike. The stance-phase muscles, which include muscles from both the posterior and the lateral compartments, function during the period of midstance and control the forward movement of the tibia over the fixed foot and then initiate plantar flexion of the ankle joint.

A frequent question regarding muscle transfers is whether a stance-phase muscle can be converted to a swing-phase muscle. Most investigators agree that, on a voluntary basis, a patient with a lower motor neuron (LMN) lesion can usually bring about active dorsiflexion after transfer of a stance-phase posterior tibial muscle or toe flexor muscle. When this patient walks and concentrates on using the transferred muscle, the stance-phase muscle usually functions as a swing-phase muscle. Waters,[342] however, has questioned whether over time true phase conversion persists. In general, a surgeon should attempt to transfer a swing-phase muscle to replace an absent swing-phase muscle and, conversely, transfer a stance-phase muscle to replace an absent stance-phase muscle. Occasionally this is not possible. Nonphasic transfers more likely tend to function as a tenodesis than as an active muscle transfer.

A surgeon also must be aware of the consequences of transferring a muscle from one part of the foot to another. Transferring the peroneus longus in the presence of a normal anterior tibial tendon can result in dorsiflexion of the first metatarsal and a subsequent dorsal bunion. This occurs because the normal agonist–antagonist relationship between these two muscles has been disrupted. As a result, a dorsal bunion can develop. A similar problem has been noted if the anterior tibial tendon is transferred too far laterally or if the posterior tibial tendon is transferred, particularly in a younger patient. A pronation deformity can result.

The particular type of muscle balance present plays a role in the tendon transfer selected. An LMN lesion that produces a flaccid paralysis is easier to evaluate and treat than an upper motor neuron (UMN) lesion that results in spasticity. With flaccid paralysis, it is relatively simple to evaluate which muscles are functioning and the relative strength compared with a UMN lesion in which spasticity is present. When spasticity is present, it is often difficult for a patient to cooperate sufficiently to permit adequate muscle examination because of their lack of selective voluntary control. Under these circumstances, a tendon release or lengthening or a tendon transfer can result in a new deformity because of a change in the balance present in the foot. For this reason, dynamic electromyographic analysis is often helpful in evaluating the patient with spasticity.[338]

The overall posture of the foot must be evaluated to ensure that the foot is plantigrade. If a deformity is present and the foot cannot be placed in a plantigrade position, other surgical procedures must be considered before a tendon transfer. A tendon transfer is unable to function if passive motion is not present in the direction that the transfer is expected to function.

Patient Evaluation

Natural History of Muscle Imbalance

A thorough understanding of the type of muscle imbalance that is present and its natural history is important in determining appropriate treatment. It is important to appreciate whether the muscle balance is progressive or nonprogressive and whether it represents a UMN or an LMN lesion. Both types of motor deficiencies can lead to a progressive deformity, but only the LMN lesion can at times result in a nonprogressive deformity. Typically, the patient who has sustained an LMN lesion has a nonprogressive deformity (e.g., peroneal, sciatic nerve injury). Other types of LMN disease (e.g., peripheral neuropathies, myopathies) can demonstrate a progression of deformity. Although UMN lesions are often considered to result in spasticity (e.g., myelodysplasia), a flaccid paralysis or occasionally a mixed picture may be present.

Age of Patient

When evaluating a child with muscle imbalance, the examiner must carefully consider the effects of later growth on future deformity. In the younger child, the surgeon must be concerned about what can occur after the tendon transfer (e.g., dorsal bunion, flatfoot deformity). In the older child, the surgeon must be concerned that a long-standing muscle imbalance can lead to a distorted postural deformity in which the foot is no longer plantigrade. In general, in the adult patient, no significant bone abnormality is present because often the muscle balance developed after skeletal maturity was reached. Fixed contractures may be present, but in general, the overall bone architecture is normal.

Diagnosis

Diagnostic evaluation of a patient begins with an in-depth history of the problem, the methods of bracing used, and whether the patient's overall gait pattern is stable or deteriorating. Analysis of the range of motion of lower extremity joints and the relative muscle strengths of foot and ankle dorsiflexors and plantar flexors must be determined. When inspecting the posture of the foot, the surgeon must determine whether the foot is plantigrade. If it is not plantigrade, factors to be considered are muscle imbalance, a fixed contracture, and abnormal bone architecture. A determination must be made as to the type of gait evaluation necessary. This may be as simple as observing the patient walking or may be more sophisticated, with the use of motion analysis of the lower extremity and dynamic electromyographic data.[331,338]

Surgical Treatment

Surgical Principles

To achieve a successful tendon transfer, the surgeon should consider the following basic principles.

A plantigrade foot must be present before the tendon transfer. This can be created by performing a tendon lengthening, release of a joint contracture, or, if necessary, joint arthrodesis. The tendon lengthening can involve the Achilles or a posterior tibial or other tendon. The release of a joint contracture can consist of a posterior capsulotomy. A joint arthrodesis can vary from a subtalar or triple arthrodesis to a pantalar arthrodesis.

The muscles to be transferred should be of adequate strength and, if possible, of similar fiber length and of the same phasic activity to provide an optimal tendon transfer. A transferred muscle usually loses one grade of strength (e.g., from normal to good), and therefore, if the muscle strength is only good to fair, the transfer might not be successful.

There are several technical considerations for a tendon transfer. The tendon transfer should be performed in the presence of adequate soft tissue coverage. Dense scar tissue should be resected and, if possible, replaced with soft tissue coverage that provides a gliding surface for the tendon transfer. If the tendon is transferred through the interosseous membrane, a soft tissue window of adequate size should be developed. The line of tendon pull between the muscle and its insertion should be as straight a line as possible to provide maximum efficiency. The transferred tendon should preferably be implanted into bone, and sutures should be placed between the periosteum and the tendon to prevent failure at the insertion site. A bone anchor may be used to reinforce the repair.

Adequate postoperative immobilization and subsequent physical therapy and retraining should be undertaken.

Tendon transfers are generally grouped into anterior, split tendon, posterior, lateral, and distal transfers. A brief discussion of each type is presented here.

ANTERIOR TENDON TRANSFER

Anterior tendon transfers of the posterior tibial tendon or other flexor tendons are performed to reestablish dorsiflexion power. For this type of transfer to succeed, adequate passive dorsiflexion must be present before the procedure. If adequate dorsiflexion is not present, release of a posterior contracture is essential before the tendon transfer (Fig. 24-117).

When the transfer is performed for flaccid paralysis, a posterior tibial transfer through the interosseous membrane is often performed.[337] At times, this transfer may be reinforced by the FHL and FDL tendons. The excursion of the posterior tibial tendon is approximately 2 cm because of the shape of its muscle fibers, whereas the overall excursion of the long flexor tendons is approximately 3 cm, which enables them to move the ankle through a greater range of motion. When several tendons are transferred through the interosseous septum, an adequate soft tissue window must be created to minimize the possibility of adhesions, which can lead to restricted motion postoperatively.

With instability of the subtalar joint from loss of more than just dorsiflexor power, it may be necessary to stabilize the subtalar joint or perform a triple arthrodesis before the tendon transfer (Fig. 24-118).

Occasionally, the EDL tendon may be used to provide increased dorsiflexion power at the ankle joint. This phasic transfer can provide enough extra dorsiflexion power to permit the patient to ambulate without a brace. The EDL is usually transferred into the second or third cuneiform.

After a transfer in a patient with spasticity, even with the addition of the FDL, several problems can result. The

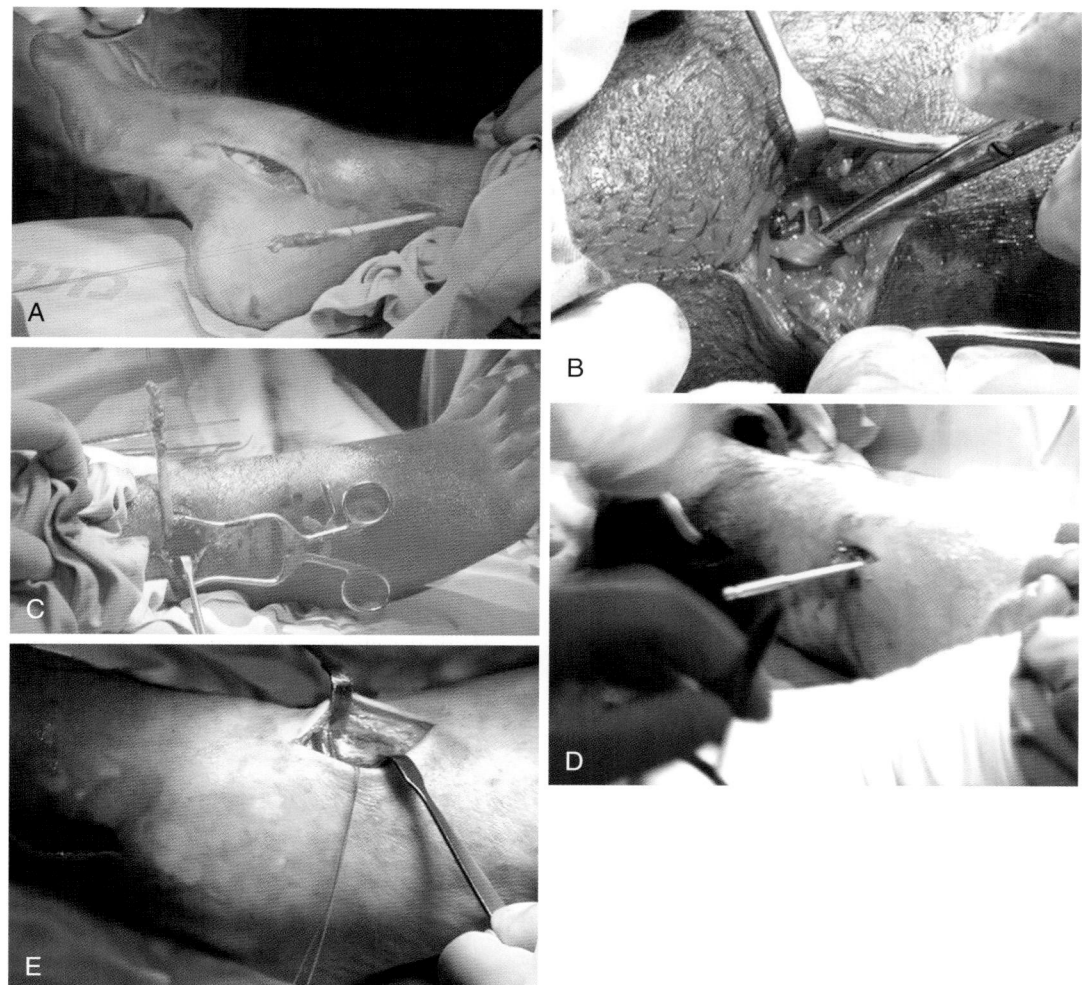

Figure 24-117 Patient with a sciatic nerve injury and footdrop. **A,** The posterior tibial tendon was harvested with additional length by distally including a strip of periosteum from the cuneiform. The hemostat was passed from posterior to anterior through the interosseous membrane. The membrane opening was widened by spreading the clamp and then pushed anteriorly through the anterior compartment. An incision was made at the point where the clamp tented the skin. **B,** It is not uncommon to identify the superficial peroneal nerve here. **C,** With care taken not to damage the nerve, the tendon is passed anteriorly. **D,** The tendon is passed through a tunnel superficially over and distal to the extensor retinaculum, where another incision is placed over the lateral cuneiform. A tunnel is then created from the lateral cuneiform to the medial cuneiform. **E,** The suture will be pulled through the tunnel and the tendon secured laterally. The suture should be tied through the medial cuneiform, creating a second anchor point.

original deformity can persist or recur[340]; the original deformity can be altered, resulting in a calcaneal or calcaneovalgus deformity[340]; and phase conversion can fail to occur during gait, although the patient has the ability of voluntary control.[331,340]

SPLIT TENDON TRANSFER

The split anterior tibial tendon transfer is performed to provide a yoke-type tendon configuration to the dorsum of the foot.[333] This tendon transfer is based on the principle that by tightening the lateral aspect of the yoke, a more plantigrade foot posture is achieved while using a muscle of the same phase. This transfer is most useful in a patient with spasticity with overpull of the invertors of the foot. When this procedure is performed, adequate dorsiflexion must be present. If adequate dorsiflexion is not present, Achilles tendon lengthening and possibly a posterior tibial tendon lengthening should be added to the procedure. The lateral band of the yoke must be tightened sufficiently at the tendon transfer to pull the foot into an everted position, or the procedure will fail (Fig. 24-119).

The posterior tibial split tendon transfer has been used to correct a varus hindfoot deformity. This transfer has the advantage in a younger patient of minimizing the chance of a postoperative flatfoot deformity. With this transfer, an in-phase muscle is used to provide improved muscle function.[332,335,336]

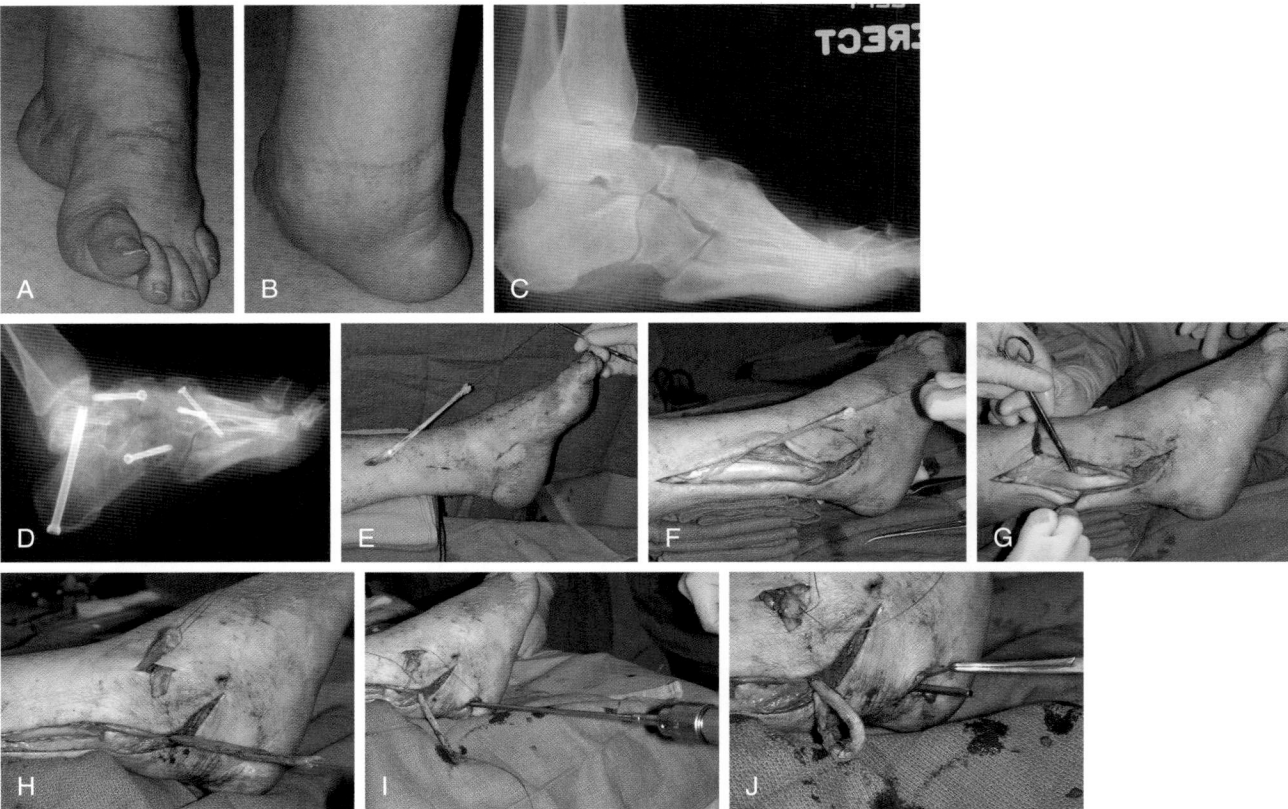

Figure 24-118 Patient had a sensory motor neuropathy with bilateral lower extremity weakness and deformities. **A** and **B,** Clinical photographs of severe cavo varus. **C,** Weight-bearing radiograph demonstrates the cavovarus deformity and plantar flexion of the first metatarsal. **D,** After a triple arthrodesis to align the hind foot, a tendon transfer for a footdrop was performed because of continued dynamic varus position. The posterior tibial tendon was harvested **(E)** and transferred to the lateral side of the foot **(F)** instead of a more central position. **G** and **H,** The nonfunctioning peroneal tendons were used to stabilize the lateral ankle joint through a drill hole **(I)** from lateral to medial. **J,** To pass the peroneal tendon through the calcaneus, a suction tip is used to pull the suture medialward, where it is secured.

A further modification of the split tendon transfer has been used in the treatment of footdrop. Rodriguez[339] described a transfer of the posterior tibial tendon through a hole in the anterior tibial tendon. The tendon transfer was subsequently inserted into the second cuneiform. The peroneus longus tendon was then rerouted anterior to the lateral malleolus and tightened to help provide additional mediolateral balance to the foot. The advantage of this procedure is that by tightening the medial and lateral bands, a plantigrade foot is created along with simultaneous reestablishment of dorsiflexion strength.

POSTERIOR TENDON TRANSFER
Posterior tendon transfers into the Achilles tendon are typically used to prevent or retard the development of a calcaneal deformity and to restore plantar flexion power. Even if only weak plantar flexion is achieved after this type of transfer, it is better and easier to brace a foot in an equinus posture than to manage a calcaneal deformity.

Depending on the muscle function present, posterior transfer of the anterior tibial tendon through the interosseous septum or posterior transfer of the peroneus longus or posterior tibial tendon is done. If possible, a phasic transfer is more desirable, although it appears that the anterior tibial tendon can undergo phase conversion and function as a plantar flexor during gait.[331,341]

LATERAL TENDON TRANSFER
A lateral tendon transfer is used for loss of peroneal muscle function. The peroneus brevis is a powerful evertor of the subtalar joint, whereas the peroneus longus functions mainly to plantar flex the first metatarsal and is a weak evertor. In the patient who has selectively lost peroneus brevis function (e.g., tendon laceration or rupture), the surgeon may consider using the peroneus longus as a transfer to help reestablish eversion function. A split anterior tibial transfer can likewise be used for this condition. Because most of these muscles involve phasic transfers, uniformly good results can be expected.

DISTAL TENDON TRANSFER
The Jones tendon transfer[334] is used to correct a cock-up deformity of the first metatarsophalangeal joint that

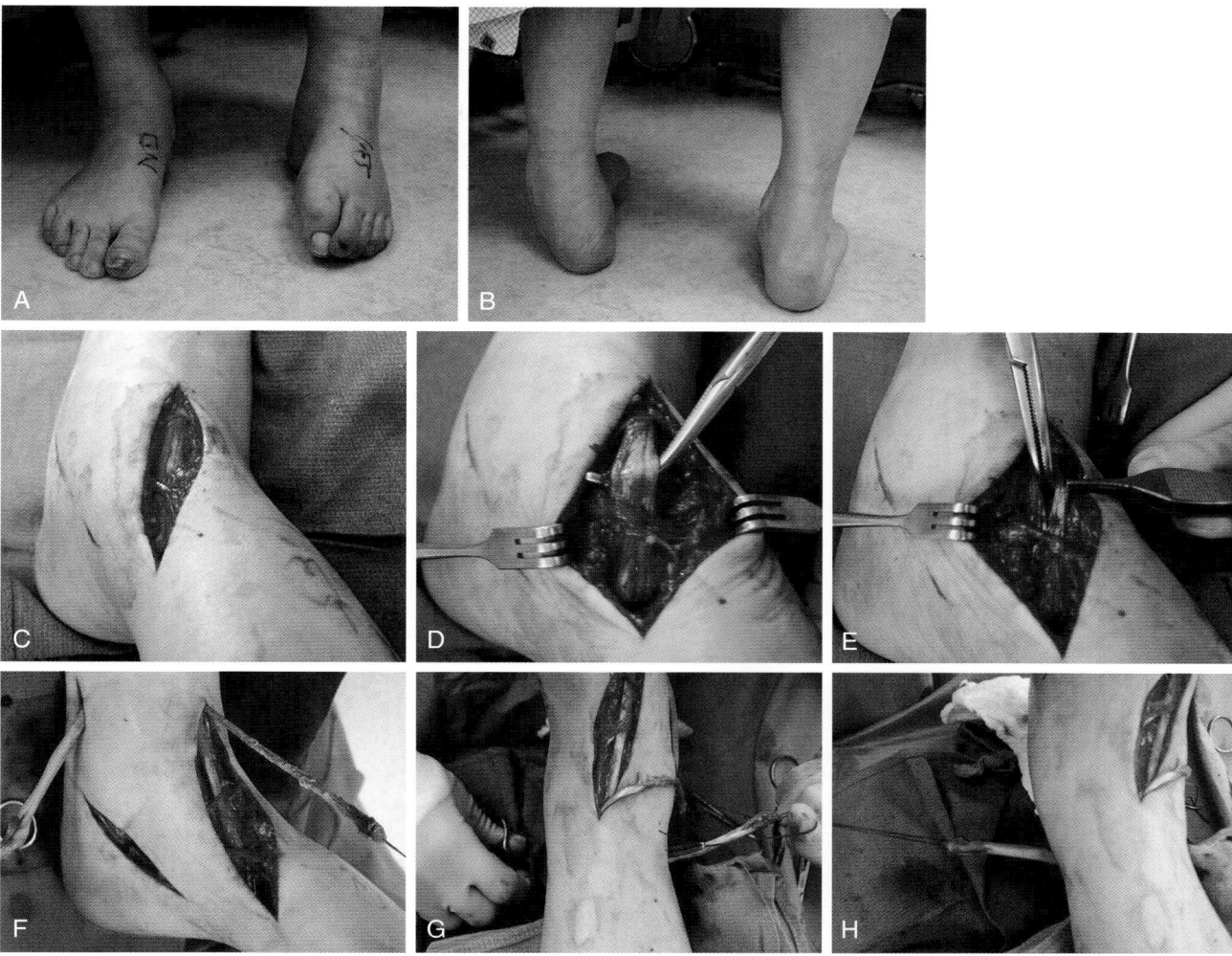

Figure 24-119 This patient had a head injury and a mildly spastic supinated foot with severe varus and no peroneal muscular strength. Anterior clinical **(A)** and posterior clinical **(B)** views. **C,** A split anterior tibial tendon transfer (SPLATT) was performed. The incision is made over the distal aspect of the anterior tibial tendon. **D,** The tendon is split proximally above the ankle joint. **E,** The lateral half is prepared for transfer. **F,** The posterior tibial tendon was harvested from the naviculum. **G,** The posterior tibial tendon was transferred behind the tibia with assistance of Kelly clamps. **H,** The tendon is transferred into the peroneal tendon sheath to be connected to the peroneus brevis. The SPLATT is completed by attaching the lateral aspect of the tendon to the lateral cuneiform.

develops because of weakness of dorsiflexion by the anterior tibial muscle. Subsequently, the EHL is used as a secondary dorsiflexor of the ankle joint. The EHL tendon is transferred into the first metatarsal metaphysis to provide increased dorsiflexion power of the foot. At the same time, this typically corrects the chronic plantar flexion posture of the first metatarsal. A fusion of the interphalangeal joint of the hallux is necessary to offset the unopposed pull of the FHL tendon. Occasionally, an osteotomy of the base of the first metatarsal is performed to dorsiflex the first metatarsal (see Chapter 26).

An FDL tendon transfer is performed when a dynamic deformity of the lesser toes results in flexible hammering of the lesser toes. This tendon transfer involves detachment of the long flexor tendon from its insertion. The tendon is split and transferred on the medial and lateral aspect of the proximal phalanx to the extensor hood mechanism on the dorsum of the proximal phalanx. At the transfer, no fixed contracture of the proximal interphalangeal joint or spasticity must be present. Spasticity can lead to a swan-neck deformity. With a fixed contracture, the flexor tendon transfer may be unsuccessful (see Chapter 7).

REFERENCES
Extensor Tendons

1. Akhtar M, Levine J: Dislocation of extensor digitorum longus tendons after spontaneous rupture of the inferior retinaculum of the ankle. Case report, *J Bone Joint Surg Am* 62:1210–1211, 1980.
2. Al-Qattan MM: Surgical treatment and results in 17 cases of open lacerations of the extensor hallucis longus tendon, *J Plast Reconstruct Aesthet Surg* 60:360–367, 2007.

3. Anzel SH, Covey KW, Weiner AD, Lipscomb PR: Disruption of muscles and tendons; an analysis of 1,014 cases, *Surgery* 45:406–414, 1959.
4. Bell W, Schon L: Tendon lacerations of the toe and foot, *Foot Ankle Clin* 1:355–372, 1996.
5. Berens TA: Autogenous graft repair of an extensor hallucis longus laceration, *J Foot Surg* 29:179–182, 1990.
6. Bronner S, Ojofeitimi S, Rose D: Repair and rehabilitation of extensor hallucis longus and brevis tendon lacerations in a professional dancer, *J Orthop Sports Phys Ther* 38:362–370, 2008.
7. Duke HF, Greenberg PJ: Distal extensor hallucis longus tenotomy, *J Foot Surg* 30:133–136, 1991.
8. Fadel GE, Alipour F: Rupture of the extensor hallucis longus tendon caused by talar neck osteophyte, *Foot Ankle Surg* 14:100–102, 2008.
9. Floyd DW, Heckman JD, Rockwood CA Jr: Tendon lacerations in the foot, *Foot Ankle* 4:8–14, 1983.
10. Griffiths JC: Tendon injuries around the ankle, *J Bone Joint Surg Br* 47:686–689, 1965.
11. Hoelzer W, Kalish S: Traumatic severance of the anterior tibial and extensor hallucis longus tendons, *J Foot Surg* 13:96–97, 1974.
12. Kass JC, Palumbo F, Mehl S, Camarinos N: Extensor hallucis longus tendon injury: an in-depth analysis and treatment protocol, *J Foot Ankle Surg* 36:24–27, discussion 80, 1997.
13. Kriza CG, Mushlin TG: An avulsion fracture at the extensor digitorum brevis muscle origin, *J Foot Surg* 24:82–83, 1985.
14. Langenberg V: Die spontanruptur der Schne des Musculus extensor hallucis longus, *Zentbl Chir* 114:400–403, 1989.
15. Lee KT, Choi YS, Lee YK, et al: Extensor hallucis longus tendon injury in taekwondo athletes, *Phys Ther Sport* 10:101–104, 2009.
16. Lipscomb PR, Kelly PJ: Injuries of the extensor tendons in the distal part of the leg and in the ankle, *J Bone Joint Surg Am* 37:1206–1213, 1955.
17. McMaster P: Tendon and muscle ruptures: clinical and experimental studies on the causes and location of subcutaneous ruptures, *J Bone Joint Surg* 15:705–722, 1933.
18. Menz P, Nettle WJ: Closed rupture of the musculotendinous junction of extensor hallucis longus, *Injury* 20:378–381, 1989.
19. Mulcahy DM, Dolan AM, Stephens MM: Spontaneous rupture of extensor hallucis longus tendon, *Foot Ankle Int* 17:162–163, 1996.
20. Noonan KJ, Saltzman CL, Dietz FR: Open physeal fractures of the distal phalanx of the great toe. A case report, *J Bone Joint Surg Am* 76:122–125, 1994.
21. Park H, Lee B, Sim J: Autogenous graft repair using semitendinoses tendon for a chronic multifocal rupture of the extensor hallucis longus tendon: a case report, *Foot Ankle Int* 24:506–508, 2003.
22. Poggi JJ, Hall RL: Acute rupture of the extensor hallucis longus tendon, *Foot Ankle Int* 16:41–43, 1995.
23. Rooks M: Tendon, vascular, nerve and skin injuries. In Gould J, editor: *Operative foot surgery*, Philadelphia, 1994, WB Saunders, pp 515–566.
24. Sarrafian S: *Anatomy of the foot and ankle*, Philadelphia, 1983, JB Lippincott, pp 199–205.
25. Satku K, Wee JT, Kumar VP, et al: The dropped big toe, *Ann Acad Med Singapore* 21:222–225, 1992.
26. Scaduto AA, Cracchilo A 3rd: Lacerations and rupture of the flexor or extensor hallucis longus tendons, *Foot Ankle Clin* 5:725–736, 2000.
27. Sim FH, Deweerd JH Jr: Rupture of the extensor hallucis longus tendon while skiing, *Minn Med* 60:789–790, 1977.
28. Simonet WT, Sim L: Boot-top tendon lacerations in ice hockey, *J Trauma* 38:30–31, 1995.
29. Skoff H: Dynamic splinting after extensor hallucis longus tendon repair. A case report, *Phys Ther* 68:75–76, 1988.
30. Smith B, Coughlin M: Reconstruction of a chronic extensor hallucis longus tendon laceration with a gracilis tendon autograft, *Orthopedics* 31:1047, 2008.
31. Tomlinson MP, Williams LA: Extensor hallucis longus calcific tendonitis: a case report, *Foot Ankle Int* 27:144–145, 2006.
32. Tuncer S, Aksu N, Isiklar U: Delayed rupture of the extensor hallucis longus and extensor digitorum communis tendons after breaching the anterior capsule with a radiofrequency probe during ankle arthroscopy: a case report, *J Foot Ankle Surg* 49:490 e491–e493, 2010.
33. Wicks MH, Harbison JS, Paterson DC: Tendon injuries about the foot and ankle in children, *Aust N Z J Surg* 50:158–161, 1980.
34. Zielaskowski L, Ponticus J: Extensor hallucis longus tendon rupture repair iusing a fascia lata allograft, *J Am Podiatr Med Assoc* 92:467–470, 2002.

Anterior Tibial Rupture
35. Aderinto J, Gross A: Delayed repair of tibialis anterior tendon rupture with Achilles tendon allograft, *J Foot Ankle Surg* 50:340–342, 2011.
36. Anagnostakos K, Bachelier F, Furst OA, Kelm J: Rupture of the anterior tibial tendon: three clinical cases, anatomical study, and literature review, *Foot Ankle Int* 27:330–339, 2006.
37. Beischer AD, Beamond BM, Jowett AJ, O'Sullivan R: Distal tendinosis of the tibialis anterior tendon, *Foot Ankle Int* 30:1053–1059, 2009.
38. Benzakein R, Wakim WA, DeLauro TM, Marcus R: Neglected rupture of the tibialis anterior tendon, *J Am Podiatr Med Assoc* 78:529–532, 1988.
39. Burman M: Stenosing tendovaginitis of the foot and ankle: studies with special reference to the stenosing tendovaginitis of the peronea tendons of the peroneal tubercle, *AMA Arch Surg* 67:686–698, 1953.
40. Burman M: Subcutaneous rupture of the tendon of the tibialis anticus, *Ann Surg* 100:368–372, 1934.
41. Cornwall MW, McPoil TG: The influence of tibialis anterior muscle activity on rearfoot motion during walking, *Foot Ankle Int* 15:75–79, 1994.
42. Cosculluela PE, Varner KE: Bilateral congenital absence of the anterior tibialis tendon: case report, *Foot Ankle Int* 31:1115–1117, 2010.
43. Crosby LA, Fitzgibbons TC: Unrecognized laceration of tibialis anterior tendon: a case report, *Foot Ankle* 9:143–145, 1988.
44. Dooley BJ, Kudelka P, Menelaus MB: Subcutaneous rupture of the tendon of tibialis anterior, *J Bone Joint Surg Br* 62:471–472, 1980.
45. Ebrahimi FV, Tofighi M, Khatibi H: Closed tibial fracture associated with laceration of tibialis anterior tendon, *J Foot Ankle Surg* 49:86 e19–e22, 2010.
46. ElMaraghy A, Devereaux MW: Bone tunnel fixation for repair of tibialis anterior tendon rupture, *Foot Ankle Surg* 16:e47–e50, 2010.
47. Fennell CW, Ballard JM, Pflaster DS, Adkins RH: Comparative evaluation of bone suture anchor to bone tunnel fixation of tibialis anterior tendon in cadaveric cuboid bone: a biomechanical investigation, *Foot Ankle Int* 16:641–645, 1995.
48. Fennell CW, Phillips P 3rd: Redefining the anatomy of the anterior tibialis tendon, *Foot Ankle Int* 15:396–399, 1994.
49. Forst R, Forst J, Heller KD: Ipsilateral peroneus brevis tendon grafting in a complicated case of traumatic rupture of tibialis anterior tendon, *Foot Ankle Int* 16:440–444, 1995.
50. Frigg AM, Valderrabano V, Kundert HP, Hintermann B: Combined anterior tibial tendon rupture and posterior tibial tendon

dysfunction in advanced flatfoot, *J Foot Ankle Surg* 45:431–435, 2006.

51. George AT, Babu A, Davis J: Traumatic rupture of the tibialis anterior tendon associated with chronic tibialis posterior dysfunction, *Foot Ankle Surg* 15:46–52, 2009.

52. Goehring M, Liakos P: Long-term outcomes following anterior tibialis tendon reconstruction with hamstring autograft in a series of 3 cases, *J Foot Ankle Surg* 48:196–202, 2009.

53. Goldman F: Snapping of the tibialis anterior tendon, *J Am Podiatry Assoc* 73:29–30, 1983.

54. Grundy JR, O'Sullivan RM, Beischer AD: Operative management of distal tibialis anterior tendinopathy, *Foot Ankle Int* 31:212–219, 2010.

55. Gwynne-Jones D, Garneti N, Wyatt M: Closed tibialis anterior tendon rupture: a case series, *Foot Ankle Int* 30:758–762, 2009.

56. Hamilton GA, Ford LA: Longitudinal tear of the tibialis anterior tendon, *J Am Podiatric Med Assoc* 95:390–393, 2005.

57. Imade S, Mori R, Tanaka T, et al: Strong tendon repair using SLLS technique for traumatic disruption of tibialis anterior tendon and extensor hallucis longus tendon to enable early rehabilitation after surgery, *Foot Ankle Int* 32:1012–1015, 2011.

58. Jerome JT, Varghese M, Sankaran B, et al: Tibialis anterior tendon rupture in gout—case report and literature review, *Foot Ankle Surg* 14:166–169, 2008.

59. Jia X, Peters PG, Schon L: The use of platelet-rich plasma in the management of foot and ankle conditions, *Oper Tech Sports Med* 19:177–184, 2011.

60. Kabbani YM, Mayer DP: Magnetic resonance imaging of tendon pathology about the foot and ankle. Part I. Achilles tendon, *J Am Podiatr Med Assoc* 83:418–420, 1993.

61. Kabbani YM, Mayer DP: Magnetic resonance imaging of tendon pathology about the foot and ankle. Part II. Tendon ruptures, *J Am Podiatr Med Assoc* 83:466–468, 1993.

62. Kashyap S, Prince R: Spontaneous rupture of the tibialis anterior tendon. A case report, *Clin Orthop Relat Res* 216:159–161, 1987.

63. Kelikian A, Kelikian H: *Disorders of the foot and ankle*, Philadelphia, 1984, WB Saunders, pp 782–785.

64. Khoury NJ, el-Khoury GY, Saltzman CL, Brandser EA: Rupture of the anterior tibial tendon: diagnosis by MR imaging, *AJR Am J Roentgenol* 167:351–354, 1996.

65. Kopp FJ, Backus S, Deland JT, O'Malley MJ: Anterior tibial tendon rupture: results of operative treatment, *Foot Ankle Int* 28:1045–1047, 2007.

66. Lee WC, Moon JS, Kim JY, Ko HT: Fracture of an ossified tibialis anterior tendon, *Orthopedics* 32:132, 2009.

67. Mankey M: Anterior tibial tendon ruptures, *Foot Ankle Clin* 1:315–324, 1996.

68. Markarian GG, Kelikian AS, Brage M, et al: Anterior tibialis tendon ruptures: an outcome analysis of operative versus nonoperative treatment, *Foot Ankle Int* 19:792–802, 1998.

69. Mechrefe AP, Walsh EF, DiGiovanni CW: Anterior tibial tendon avulsion with distal tibial fracture entrapment: case report, *Foot Ankle Int* 27:645–647, 2006.

70. Mensor MC, Ordway GL: Traumatic subcutaneous rupture of the tibialis anterior tendon, *J Bone Joint Surg Am* 35:675–680, 1953.

71. Meyn MA Jr: Closed rupture of the anterior tibial tendon. A case report and review of the literature, *Clin Orthop Relat Res* 113:154–157, 1975.

72. Moberg E: Subcutaneous rupture of the tendon of the tibialis anterior muscle, *Acta Chir Scand* 95:455–460, 1947.

73. Morris GD, O'Malley M, Deland J, et al: Anterior tibial tendon ruptures: results of surgical treatment. Presented at the 31st Annual Meeting of the American Orthopaedic Foot and Ankle Society, San Francisco, Calif, March 3, 2001.

74. Moskowitz E: Rupture of the tibialis anterior tendon simulating peroneal nerve palsy, *Arch Phys Med Rehabil* 52:431–433, 1971.

75. Neumayer F, Djembi YR, Gerin A, Masquelet AC: Closed rupture of the tibialis anterior tendon: a report of 2 cases, *J Foot Ankle Surg* 48:457–461, 2009.

76. Ouzounian TJ: Combined rupture of the anterior tibial and posterior tibial tendons: a new clinical entity, *Foot Ankle Int* 15:508–511, 1994.

77. Ouzounian TJ, Anderson R: Anterior tibial tendon rupture, *Foot Ankle Int* 16:406–410, 1995.

78. Petersen W, Stein V, Bobka T: Structure of the human tibialis anterior tendon, *J Anat* 197(Pt 4):617–625, 2000.

79. Prieskorn D, Plattner P: Tendons and bursae. In Helal B, Rowley D, Cracchiolo A, et al, editors: *Surgery of disorders of the foot and ankle*, London, 1996, Martin Dunitz, pp 369–398.

80. Richter R, Schlitt R: [Subcutaneous rupture of the tibialis anterior tendon. (Report of 3 cases) (author's transl)], *Z Orthop Ihre Grenzgeb* 113:271–273, 1975.

81. Rimoldi RL, Oberlander MA, Waldrop JI, Hunter SC: Acute rupture of the tibialis anterior tendon: a case report, *Foot Ankle* 12:176–177, 1991.

82. Rodriguez, NN, Blitz, NM: Hemorrhagic ganglion of the tibialis anterior tendon: report of an unusual variant, *J Foot Ankle Surg* 47:571–575, 2008.

83. Smith B, Coughlin M: Technique tip: reconstruction of an acute anterior tibial tendon rupture with a gracilis tendon autograft, *Med Chir Pied* 24:1–3, 2008.

84. Stavrou P, Symeonidis PD: Gracilis tendon graft for tibialis anterior tendon reconstruction: a report of two cases, *Foot Ankle Int* 29:742–745, 2008.

85. Yamazaki S, Majima T, Yasui K, et al: Reconstruction of chronic anterior tibial tendon defect using hamstring tendon graft: a case report, *Foot Ankle Int* 28:1190–1193, 2007.

Flexor Tendons

86. Baan H, Drossaers-Bakkers WK, Dubbeldam R, et al: Flexor Hallucis longus tendon rupture in RA-patients is associated with MTP 1 damage and pes planus, *BMC Musculoskelet Disord* 8:110, 2007.

87. Bizarro AH: On sesamoid and supernumerary bones of the lims, *J Anat* 55:256–268, 1921.

88. Boruta PM, Beauperthuy GD: Partial tear of the flexor hallucis longus at the knot of Henry: presentation of three cases, *Foot Ankle Int* 18:243–246, 1997.

89. Botte M: Personal communication, September 30, 2004.

90. Brand JC Jr, Smith RW: Rupture of the flexor hallucis longus after hallux valgus surgery: case report and comments on technique for adductor release, *Foot Ankle* 11:407–410, 1991.

91. Carr JB: Complications of calcaneus fractures entrapment of the flexor hallucis longus: report of two cases, *J Orthop Trauma* 4:166–168, 1990.

92. Coghlan BA, Clarke NM: Traumatic rupture of the flexor hallucis longus tendon in a marathon runner, *Am J Sports Med* 21:617–618, 1993.

93. Cowell HR, Elener V, Lawhon SM: Bilateral tendinitis of the flexor hallucis longus in a ballet dancer, *J Pediatr Orthop* 2:582–586, 1982.

94. Diwanji SR, Shah ND: Tuberculous tenosynovitis of flexor digitorum longus tendon, *Orthopedics* 31:499, 2008.

95. Findling J, Lascola NK, Groner TW: Giant cell tumor of the flexor hallucis longus tendon sheath: a case study, *J Am Podiatr Med Assoc* 101:187–189, 2011.

96. Fond D: Flexor hallucis longus tendinitis—a case of mistaken identity and posterior impingement syndrome in dancers: evaluation and management, *J Orthop Sports Phys Ther* 5:204–206, 1984.

97. Frenette JP, Jackson DW: Lacerations of the flexor hallucis longus in the young athlete, *J Bone Joint Surg Am* 59:673–676, 1977.

98. Garth WP Jr: Flexor hallucis tendinitis in a ballet dancer. A case report, *J Bone Joint Surg Am* 63:1489, 1981.

99. Gould N: Stenosing tenosynovitis of the flexor hallucis longus tendon at the great toe, *Foot Ankle* 2:46–48, 1981.

100. Hamilton WG: Stenosing tenosynovitis of the flexor hallucis longus tendon and posterior impingement upon the os trigonum in ballet dancers, *Foot Ankle* 3:74–80, 1982.

101. Hamilton WG, Geppert MJ, Thompson FM: Pain in the posterior aspect of the ankle in dancers. Differential diagnosis and operative treatment, *J Bone Joint Surg Am* 78:1491–1500, 1996.

102. Holt KW, Cross M: Isolated rupture of the flexor hallucis longus tendon. A case report, *Am J Sports Med* 18:645–646, 1990.

103. Inokuchi S, Usami N: Closed complete rupture of the flexor hallucis longus tendon at the groove of the talus, *Foot Ankle Int* 18:47–49, 1997.

104. Keeling JJ, Guyton GP: Endoscopic flexor hallucis longus decompression: a cadaver study, *Foot Ankle Int* 2007:28: 810–814.

105. Kolettis GJ, Micheli LJ, Klein JD: Release of the flexor hallucis longus tendon in ballet dancers, *J Bone Joint Surg Am* 78:1386–1390, 1996.

106. Korovessis P, Spastris P, Katsardis T, Sidiropoulos P: Simultaneous rupture of the tibialis posterior and flexor digitorum longus tendons in a closed tibial fracture, *J Orthop Trauma* 5:89–92, 1991.

107. Krackow KA: Acute, traumatic rupture of a flexor hallucis longus tendon: a case report, *Clin Orthop Relat Res* 150:261–262, 1980.

108. Lapidus PW, Seidenstein H: Chronic non-specific tenosynovitis with effusion about the ankle: report of three cases, *J Bone Joint Surg Am* 32:175–179, 1950.

109. LaRue BG, Anctil EP: Distal anatomical relationship of the flexor hallucis longus and flexor digitorum longus tendons, *Foot Ankle Int* 27:528–532, 2006.

110. Lewin P: *The foot and ankle: their injuries, diseases, deformities, and disabilities*, Philadelphia, 1947, Lea & Febiger, pp 207–208.

111. Lipscomb P: Chronic nonspecific tenosynovitis and peritendinitis, *Surg Clin North Am* 24:780–797, 1944.

112. Lipscomb P: Non-suppurative tenosynovitis and paratendinitis, *Instr Course Lect* 7:254–261, 1950.

113. Lynch T, Pupp GR: Stenosing tenosynovitis of the flexor hallucis longus at the ankle joint, *J Foot Surg* 29:345–348, 1990.

114. McCarroll JR, Ritter MA, Becker TE: Triggering of the great toe. A case report, *Clin Orthop Relat Res* 175:184–185, 1983.

115. Mehdizade A, Adler RS: Sonographically guided flexor hallucis longus tendon sheath injection, *J Ultrasound Med* 26:233–237, 2007.

116. Nathan H, Gloobe H, Yosipovitch Z: Flexor digitorum accessorius longus, *Clin Orthop Relat Res* 113:158–161, 1975.

117. Nigg BM: Biomechanical aspects of running. In Nigg BM, editor: *Biomechanics of running shoes*, Champaign, Ill, 1986, Human Kinetics, pp 1–25.

118. Oakley J, Yewlett A, Makwana N: Tenosynovial osteochondromatosis of the flexor hallucis longus tendon, *Foot Ankle Surg* 16:148–150, 2010.

119. Oloff LM, Schulhofer SD: Flexor hallucis longus dysfunction, *J Foot Ankle Surg* 37:101–109, 1998.

120. Papanna MC, Monga P, Wilkes RA: Post-traumatic calcific myonecrosis of flexor hallucis longus. A case report and literature review, *Acta Orthop Belg* 76:137–141, 2010.

121. Petersen W, Pufe T, Zantop T, Paulsen F: Blood supply of the flexor hallucis longus tendon with regard to dancer's tendinitis: injection and immunohistochemical studies of cadaver tendons, *Foot Ankle Int* 24:591–596, 2003.

122. Rasmussen RB, Thyssen EP: Rupture of the flexor hallucis longus tendon: case report, *Foot Ankle* 10:288–289, 1990.

123. Reinherz RP: Management of flexor hallucis longus tendon injuries, *J Foot Surg* 23:366–369, 1984.

124. Reinherz RP, Zawada SJ, Sheldon DP: Recognizing unusual tendon pathology at the ankle, *J Foot Surg* 25:278–283, 1986.

125. Romash MM: Closed rupture of the flexor hallucis longus tendon in a long distance runner: report of a case and review of the literature, *Foot Ankle Int* 15:433–436, 1994.

126. Rosenberg GA, Sferra JJ: Checkrein deformity—an unusual complication associated with a closed Salter–Harris type II ankle fracture: a case report, *Foot Ankle Int* 20:591–594, 1999.

127. Sammarco GJ, Cooper PS: Flexor hallucis longus tendon injury in dancers and nondancers, *Foot Ankle Int* 19:356–362, 1998.

128. Sammarco GJ, Miller EH: Partial rupture of the flexor hallucis longus tendon in classical ballet dancers: two case reports, *J Bone Joint Surg Am* 61:149–150, 1979.

129. Sanhudo JA: Stenosing tenosynovitis of the flexor hallucis longus tendon at the sesamoid area, *Foot Ankle Int* 23:801–803, 2002.

130. Sanhudo JA, Lompa PA: Checkrein deformity—flexor hallucis tethering: two case reports, *Foot Ankle Int* 23:799–800, 2002.

131. Silver RL, de la Garza J, Rang M: The myth of muscle balance. A study of relative strengths and excursions of normal muscles about the foot and ankle, *J Bone Joint Surg Br* 67:432–437, 1985.

132. Stokes IA, Hutton WC, Stott JR, Lowe LW: Forces under the hallux valgus foot before and after surgery, *Clin Orthop Relat Res* 142:64–72, 1979.

133. Thompson FM, Snow SW, Hershon SJ: Spontaneous atraumatic rupture of the flexor hallucis longus tendon under the sustentaculum tali: case report, review of the literature, treatment options, *Foot Ankle* 14:414–417, 1993.

134. Trepman E, Mizel MS, Newberg AH: Partial rupture of the flexor hallucis longus tendon in a tennis player: a case report, *Foot Ankle Int* 16:227–231, 1995.

135. Trevino S, Gould N, Korson R: Surgical treatment of stenosing tenosynovitis at the ankle, *Foot Ankle* 2:37–45, 1981.

136. Tudisco C, Puddu G: Stenosing tenosynovitis of the flexor hallucis longus tendon in a classical ballet dancer. A case report, *Am J Sports Med* 12:403–404, 1984.

137. Yancey HA Jr: Lacerations of the plantar aspect of the foot, *Clin Orthop Relat Res* 122:46–52, 1977.

Peroneal Tendons

138. Aberle-Horstenegg A: Über einen eigenartigen Fußschmerz (tendovaginitis der distalen Schnenscheide des peronaeus longus), *Munchener Med Wochn* 79:946–948, 1932.

139. Abraham E, Stirnaman JE: Neglected rupture of the peroneal tendons causing recurrent sprains of the ankle. Case report, *J Bone Joint Surg Am* 61:1247–1248, 1979.

140. Adachi N, Fukuhara K, Tanaka H, et al: Superior retinaculoplasty for recurrent dislocation of peroneal tendons, *Foot Ankle Int* 27:1074–1078, 2006.

141. Alanen J, Orava S, Heinonen OJ, et al: Peroneal tendon injuries. Report of thirty-eight operated cases, *Ann Chir Gynaecol* 90:43–46, 2001.

142. Alm A, Lamke LO, Liljedahl SO: Surgical treatment of dislocation of the peroneal tendons, *Injury* 7:14–19, 1975.

143. Andersen E: Stenosing peroneal tenosynovitis symptomatically simulating ankle instability, *Am J Sports Med* 15:258–259, 1987.

144. Arrowsmith SR, Fleming LL, Allman FL: Traumatic dislocations of the peroneal tendons, *Am J Sports Med* 11:142–146, 1983.

145. Athavale SA, Swathi V: Anatomy of the superior peroneal tunnel, *J Bone Joint Surg Am* 93:564–571, 2011.

146. Bassett FH 3rd, Speer KP: Longitudinal rupture of the peroneal tendons, *Am J Sports Med* 21:354–357, 1993.

147. Beck E: Operative treatment of recurrent dislocation of the peroneal tendons, *Arch Orthop Trauma Surg* 98:247–250, 1981.

148. Behfar AS: [Dislocation of the peroneal tendons], *Sportverletz Sportschaden* 1:223–228, 1987.

149. Berg EE: Intraoperative peroneus brevis tendon rupture: a technique to salvage the graft during ankle ligament reconstruction, *Foot Ankle Int* 17:349–351, 1996.

150. Blitz NM, Nemes KK: Bilateral peroneus longus tendon rupture through a bipartite os peroneum, *J Foot Ankle Surg* 46:270–277, 2007.

151. Borland S, Jung S, Hugh IA: Complete rupture of the peroneus longus tendon secondary to injection, *Foot (Edinb)* 19:229–231, 2009.

152. Boya H, Pinar H: Stenosing tenosynovitis of the peroneus brevis tendon associated with hypertrophy of the peroneal tubercle, *J Foot Ankle Surg* 49:188–190, 2010.

153. Boykin RE, Ogunseinde B, McFeely ED, et al: Preliminary results of calcaneofibular ligament transfer for recurrent peroneal subluxation in children and adolescents, *J Pediatr Orthop* 30:899–903, 2010.

154. Brodsky J, Krause J: Peroneus brevis tendon tears: pathophysiology, surgical reconstruction, and clinical results, *Foot Ankle Int* 19:271–279, 1998.

155. Burman M: Subcutaneous tear of the tendon of the peroneus longus; its relation to the giant peroneal tubercle, *AMA Arch Surg* 73:216–219, 1956.

156. Burman M, Lapidus P: The functional disturbances caused by the inconstant bones and sesamoids of the foot, *Arch Surg* 22:936–975, 1931.

157. Chadwick C, Highland AM, Hughes DE, Davies MB: The importance of magnetic resonance imaging in a symptomatic "bipartite" os peroneum: a case report, *J Foot Ankle Surg* 50:82–86, 2011.

158. Chen W, Li X, Su Y, et al: Peroneal tenography to evaluate lateral hindfoot pain after calcaneal fracture, *Foot Ankle Int* 32:789–795, 2011.

159. Cohen I, Lane S, Koning W: Peroneal tendon dislocations: a review of the literature, *J Foot Surg* 22:15–20, 1983.

160. Cox D, Paterson FW: Acute calcific tendinitis of peroneus longus, *J Bone Joint Surg Br* 73:342, 1991.

161. Cross MJ, Crichton KJ, Gordon H, Mackie IG: Peroneus brevis rupture in the absence of the peroneus longus muscle and tendon in a classical ballet dancer. A case report, *Am J Sports Med* 16:677–678, 1988.

162. Das De S, Balasubramaniam P: A repair operation for recurrent dislocation of peroneal tendons, *J Bone Joint Surg Br* 67:585–587, 1985.

163. Davies JA: Peroneal compartment syndrome secondary to rupture of the peroneus longus. A case report, *J Bone Joint Surg Am* 61:783–784, 1979.

164. Davis WH, Sobel M, Deland J, et al: The superior peroneal retinaculum: an anatomic study, *Foot Ankle Int* 15:271–275, 1994.

165. DiGiovanni B, Fraga CJ, Cohen BE, Shereff MJ: Associated injuries found in chronic lateral ankle instability, *Foot Ankle Int* 21:809–815, 2000.

166. Dombek MF, Lamm BM, Saltrick K, et al: Peroneal tendon tears: a retrospective review, *J Foot Ankle Surg* 42:250–258, 2003.

167. DuVries H: *Surgery of the foot*, St Louis, 1959, Mosby, pp 253–255.

168. Earle AS, Moritz JR, Tapper EM: Dislocation of the peroneal tendons at the ankle: an analysis of 25 ski injuries, *Northwest Med* 71:108–110, 1972.

169. Eckert WR, Davis EA Jr: Acute rupture of the peroneal retinaculum, *J Bone Joint Surg Am* 58:670–672, 1976.

170. Edwards M: The relations of the peroneal tendons to the fibula, calcaneus, and cuboideum, *Am J Anat* 42:213–253, 1988.

171. Escalas F, Figueras JM, Merino JA: Dislocation of the peroneal tendons. Long-term results of surgical treatment, *J Bone Joint Surg Am* 62:451–453, 1980.

172. Evans JD: Subcutaneous rupture of the tendon of peroneus longus. Report of a case, *J Bone Joint Surg Br* 48:507–509, 1966.

173. Folan JC: Peroneus longus tenosynovitis, *Br J Sports Med* 15:277–279, 1981.

174. Ford LT, Parvin RW: Stenosing tenosynovitis of the common peroneal tendon sheath; report of two cases, *J Bone Joint Surg Am* 38:1352–1357, 1956.

175. Freccero DM, Berkowitz MJ: The relationship between tears of the peroneus brevis tendon and the distal extent of its muscle belly: an MRI study, *Foot Ankle Int* 27:236–239, 2006.

176. Frey CC, Shereff MJ: Tendon injuries about the ankle in athletes, *Clin Sports Med* 7:103–118, 1988.

177. Gaulke R, Hildebrand F, Panzica M, et al: Modified rerouting procedure for failed peroneal tendon dislocation surgery, *Clin Orthop Relat Res* 468:1018–1024, 2010.

178. Geller J, Lin S, Cordas D, Vieira P: Relationship of a low-lying muscle belly to tears of the peroneus brevis tendon, *Am J Orthop* 32:541–544, 2003.

179. Grisolia A: Fracture of the os peroneum: review of the literature and report of one case, *Clin Orthop Relat Res* 28:213–215, 1963.

180. Guineys L: Fracture isolée d'un os sumumeriare du tarse (os peroneum) traitment par l'infiltration novocainique, *Rev Orthop* 26:943–947, 1939.

181. Hackenbroch M: Eine seltene Lokalisation der stenosierenden Tendovaginitis an der Sehnenscheide der peroneen, *Munchener Med Wochn* 74:932, 1927.

182. Hammerschlag WA, Goldner JL: Chronic peroneal tendon subluxation produced by an anomalous peroneus brevis: case report and literature review, *Foot Ankle* 10:45–47, 1989.

183. Harper MC: Subluxation of the peroneal tendons within the peroneal groove: a report of two cases, *Foot Ankle Int* 18:369–370, 1997.

184. Heller E, Robinson D: Traumatic pathologies of the calcaneal peroneal tubercle, *Foot (Edinb)* 20:96–98, 2010.

185. Hildebrand O: Tendovaginitis chronica deformans and Luxation der peronealsehnen, *Deut Z Chir* 86:526–531, 1907.

186. Jahss M: Tendon disorders of the foot and ankle. In Jahss M, editor: *Disorders of the foot and ankle: medical and surgical management*, ed 2, Philadelphia, 1991, WB Saunders, pp 1461–1512.

187. Jones E: Operative treatment of chronic dislocation of the peroneal tendons, *J Bone Joint Surg Am* 14:574–576, 1932.

188. Kaz A, Coughlin M: Technique tip: distal fibula rotational osteotomy for suxluxating peroneal tendons, *Med Chir Pied* 23:68–71, 2007.

189. Kelly R: An operation for the chronic dislocation of the peroneal tendons, *Br J Surg* 7:502–504, 1920.

190. Kennedy MP, Coughlin MJ: Peroneus longus rupture following a modified Evans lateral ankle ligament reconstruction, *Orthopedics* 26:1059–1060, 2003.

191. Khazen GE, Adam N, Wilson MD, Schon LC: Peroneal groove deepening via a posterior osteocartilaginous flap: a retrospective analysis. Presented at the 21st Annual American Orthopaedic Foot and Ankle Society Summer Meeting, Boston, July 15–17, 2005.

192. Khoury NJ, el-Khoury GY, Saltzman CL, Kathol MH: Peroneus longus and brevis tendon tears: MR imaging evaluation, *Radiology* 200:833–841, 1996.

193. Kilkelly FX, McHale KA: Acute rupture of the peroneal longus tendon in a runner: a case report and review of the literature, *Foot Ankle Int* 15:567–569, 1994.

194. Klammer G, Iselin LD, Bonel HM, Weber M: Calcific tendinitis of the peroneus longus: case report, *Foot Ankle Int* 32:638–640, 2011.

195. Kojima Y, Kataoka Y, Suzuki S, Akagi M: Dislocation of the peroneal tendons in neonates and infants, *Clin Orthop Relat Res* 266:180–184, 1991.

196. Kollias SL, Ferkel RD: Fibular grooving for recurrent peroneal tendon subluxation, *Am J Sports Med* 25:329–335, 1997.

197. Kuwada, GT: Surgical correlation of preoperative MRI findings of trauma to tendons and ligaments of the foot and ankle, *J Am Podiatr Med Assoc* 98:370–373, 2008.

198. LaBarbiera AP, Solitto RJ: Silastic tendon graft: Its role in neglected tendon repair, *J Foot Surg* 29:439–443, 1990.

199. Lagoutaris ED, Adams HB, DiDomenico LA, Rothenberg RJ: Longitudinal tears of both peroneal tendons associated with tophaceous gouty infiltration. A case report, *J Foot Ankle Surg* 44:222–224, 2005.

200. Larsen E: Longitudinal rupture of the peroneus brevis tendon, *J Bone Joint Surg Br* 69:340–341, 1987.

201. Larsen E, Flink-Olsen M, Seerup K: Surgery for recurrent dislocation of the peroneal tendons, *Acta Orthop Scand* 55:554–555, 1984.

202. LaRue BG, Anctil EP: Distal anatomical relationship of the flexor hallucis longus and flexor digitorum longus tendons, *Foot Ankle Int* 27:528–532, 2006.

203. LeMelle DP, Janis LR: Longitudinal rupture of the peroneus brevis tendon: a study of eight cases, *J Foot Surg* 28:132–136, 1989.

204. LeNoir JL: A new surgical treatment of peroneal subluxation–dislocation. A case report with a 27-year follow up, *Orthopedics* 9:1689–1691, 1986.

205. MacDonald BD, Wertheimer SJ: Bilateral os peroneum fractures: comparison of conservative and surgical treatment and outcomes, *J Foot Ankle Surg* 36:220–225, 1997.

206. Maffulli N, Ferran NA, Oliva F, Testa V: Recurrent subluxation of the peroneal tendons, *Am J Sports Med* 34:986–992, 2006.

207. Mains DB, Sullivan RC: Fracture of the os peroneum. A case report, *J Bone Joint Surg Am* 55:1529–1530, 1973.

208. Martens MA, Noyez JF, Mulier JC: Recurrent dislocation of the peroneal tendons. Results of rerouting the tendons under the calcaneofibular ligament, *Am J Sports Med* 14:148–150, 1986.

209. Marti R: Dislocation of the peroneal tendons, *Am J Sports Med* 5:19–22, 1977.

210. McConkey JP, Favero K: J: Subluxation of the peroneal tendons within the peroneal tendon sheath. A case report, *Am J Sports Med* 15:511–513, 1987.

211. McGarvey W, Clanton T: Peroneal tendon dislocations, *Foot Ankle Clin* 1:325–342, 1996.

212. McLennan JG: Treatment of acute and chronic luxations of the peroneal tendons, *Am J Sports Med* 8:432–436, 1980.

213. Mendicino RW, Orsini RC, Whitman SE, Catanzariti AR: Fibular groove deepening for recurrent peroneal subluxation, *J Foot Ankle Surg* 40:252–263, 2001.

214. Mengiardi B, Pfirrmann CW, Schottle PB, et al: Magic angle effect in MR imaging of ankle tendons: influence of foot positioning on prevalence and site in asymptomatic subjects and cadaveric tendons, *Eur Radiol* 16:2197–2206, 2006.

215. Meyer A: Further evidences of attrition in the human body, *Am J Anat* 34:241–267, 1924.

216. Micheli LJ, Waters PM, Sanders DP: Sliding fibular graft repair for chronic dislocation of the peroneal tendons, *Am J Sports Med* 17:68–71, 1989.

217. Mick CA, Lynch F: Reconstruction of the peroneal retinaculum using the peroneus quartus. A case report, *J Bone Joint Surg Am* 69:296–297, 1987.

218. Milgram J: Muscle ruptures and avulsions with particular reference to the lower extremities, *Inst Course Lect* 10:233–243, 1953.

219. Millar TM, Garg SK: The Singapore operation for chronic recurrent peroneal tendon subluxation—short-term follow-up in four patients, *Foot Ankle Surg* 15:146–148, 2009.

220. Miller C: Occupational calcaneus peritendinitis of the feet, *AJR Am J Roentgenol* 61:506–510, 1949.

221. Miller JW: Dislocation of peroneal tendons—a new operative procedure. A case report, *Am J Orthop* 9:136–137, 1967.

222. Miyamoto W, Takao M, Komatu F, Uchio Y: Reconstruction of the superior peroneal retinaculum using an autologous gracilis tendon graft for chronic dislocation of the peroneal tendons accompanied by lateral instability of the ankle: technical note, *Knee Surg Sports Traumatol Arthrosc* 15:461–464, 2007.

223. Mizel MS, Michelson JD, Newberg A: Peroneal tendon bupivacaine injection: utility of concomitant injection of contrast material, *Foot Ankle Int* 17:566–568, 1996.

224. Mizel M, Michelson J, Wapner K: Diagnosis and treatment of peroneus brevis injury, *Foot Ankle Clin* 1:343–354, 1996.

225. Monteggia G: *Instiuzini chirurgiche parte secondu*, Milan, Italy, 1803, University of Milan, pp 336–341.

226. Munk RL, Davis PH: Longitudinal rupture of the peroneus brevis tendon, *J Trauma* 16:803–806, 1976.

227. Murr S: Dislocation of the peroneal tendons with marginal fracture of the lateral malleolus, *J Bone Joint Surg Br* 43:563–565, 1961.

228. Neustadter J, Raikin SM, Nazarian LN: Dynamic sonographic evaluation of peroneal tendon subluxation, *AJR Am J Roentgenol* 183:985–988, 2004.

229. Ochoa LM, Banerjee R: Recurrent hypertrophic peroneal tubercle associated with peroneus brevis tendon tear, *J Foot Ankle Surg* 46:403–408, 2007.

230. Oden R: R: Tendon injuries about the ankle resulting from skiing, *Clin Orthop Relat Res* 216:63–69, 1987.

231. Orthner E, Polcik J, Schabus R: [Dislocation of peroneal tendons], *Unfallchirurg* 92:589–594, 1989.

232. Orthner E, Weinstabl R, Schabus R: [Experimental study for clarification of the pathogenic mechanism in traumatic peroneal tendon dislocation], *Unfallchirurg* 92:547–553, 1989.

233. Palmer D: G: Tendon sheaths and bursae involved by rheumatoid disease at the foot and ankle, *Australas Radiol* 14:419–428, 1970.

234. Perlman MD: Os peroneum fracture with sural nerve entrapment neuritis, *J Foot Surg* 29:119–121, 1990.

235. Petersen W, Bobka T, Stein V, Tillmann B: Blood supply of the peroneal tendons: Injection and immunohistochemical studies of cadaver tendons, *Acta Orthop Scand* 71:168–174, 2000.

236. Peterson DA, Stinson W: Excision of the fractured os peroneum: a report on five patients and review of the literature, *Foot Ankle* 13:277–281, 1992.

237. Pfitzner W: Beitrage zur Kenntniss des Menschlichen extremitatenskelets: VII. Die variationen in Aufbau des Fusskelets. In Schwalbe, editor: *Morbologische Arbeiten*, Jena, 1896, Gustav Fischer, pp 245–527.

238. Pierson JL, Inglis AE: Stenosing tenosynovitis of the peroneus longus tendon associated with hypertrophy of the peroneal tubercle and an os peroneum. A case report, *J Bone Joint Surg Am* 74:440–442, 1992.

239. Platzgummer H: [On a simple procedure for the operative therapy of habitual peroneal tendon luxation], *Arch Orthop Unfallchir* 61:144–150, 1967.

240. Poll RG, Duijfjes F: The treatment of recurrent dislocation of the peroneal tendons, *J Bone Joint Surg Br* 66:98–100, 1984.

241. Porter D, McCarroll J, Knapp E, Torma J: Peroneal tendon subluxation in athletes: fibular groove deepening and retinacular reconstruction, *Foot Ankle Int* 26:436–441, 2005.

242. Pozo JL, Jackson AM: A rerouting operation for dislocation of peroneal tendons: operative technique and case report, *Foot Ankle* 5:42–44, 1984.

243. Radice F, Monckeberg JE, Carcuro G: Longitudinal tears of peroneus longus and brevis tendons: a gouty infiltration, *J Foot Ankle Surg* 50:751–753, 2011.

244. Raikin, SM: Intrasheath subluxation of the peroneal tendons. Surgical technique, *J Bone Joint Surg Am* 91(Suppl 2, Pt 1):146–155, 2009.

245. Raikin SM, Elias I, Nazarian LN: Intrasheath subluxation of the peroneal tendons, *J Bone Joint Surg Am* 90:992–999, 2008.

246. Raikin SM, Parks BG, Noll KH, Schon LC: Biomechanical evaluation of the ability of casts and braces to immobilize the ankle and hindfoot, *Foot Ankle Int* 22:214–219, 2001.

247. Rapley JH, Crates J, Barber A: Mid-substance peroneal tendon defects augmented with an acellular dermal matrix allograft, *Foot Ankle Int* 31:136–140, 2010.

248. Rask M, Steinberg L: The pathognostic sign of tendoperoneal subluxation, *Orthop Rev* 8:65–68, 1979.

249. Redfern D, Myerson M: The management of concomitant tears of the peroneus longus and brevis tendons, *Foot Ankle Int* 25:695–707, 2004.

250. Regan TP, Hughston JC: Chronic ankle "sprain" secondary to anomalous peroneal tendon: a case report, *Clin Orthop Relat Res* 123:52–54, 1977.

251. Roggatz J, Urban A: The calcaneous peritendinitis of the long peroneal tendon, *Arch Orthop Trauma Surg* 96:161–164, 1980.

252. Sammarco GJ, DiRaimondo CV: Chronic peroneus brevis tendon lesions, *Foot Ankle* 9:163–170, 1989.

253. Sammarco VJ, Cuttica DJ, Sammarco GJ: Lasso stitch with peroneal retinaculoplasty for repair of fractured os peroneum: a report of two cases, *Clin Orthop Relat Res* 468:1012–1017, 2010.

254. Sarmiento A, Wolf M: Subluxation of peroneal tendons. Case treated by rerouting tendons under calcaneofibular ligament, *J Bone Joint Surg Am* 57:115–116, 1975.

255. Sarrafian SK: Osteology. In Sarrafian SK, editor: *Anatomy of the foot and ankle*, Philadelphia, 1983, JB Lippincott, pp 35–106.

256. Savastano A: Recurrent dislocation of the peroneal tendons. In Bateman J, Trott A, editors: *The foot and ankle: a selection of papers from the American Orthopaedic Foot Society Meeting*, New York, 1980, Decker, pp 110–115.

257. Saxena A, Cassidy A: Peroneal tendon injuries: an evaluation of 49 tears in 41 patients, *J Foot Ankle Surg* 42:215–220, 2003.

258. Saxena A, Ewen B: Peroneal subluxation: surgical results in 31 athletic patients, *J Foot Ankle Surg* 49:238–241, 2010.

259. Saxena A, Pham B: Longitudinal peroneal tendon tears, *J Foot Ankle Surg* 36:173–179, discussion 255, 1997.

260. Shawen SB, Anderson RB: Indirect groove deepening in the management of chronic peroneal tendon dislocation, *Tech Foot Ankle Surg* 3:118–125, 2004.

261. Slatis P, Santavirta S, Sandelin J: Surgical treatment of chronic dislocation of the peroneal tendons, *Br J Sports Med* 22:16–18, 1988.

262. Smith JT, Johnson AH, Heckman JD: Nonoperative treatment of an os peroneum fracture in a high-level athlete: a case report, *Clin Orthop Relat Res* 469:1498–1501, 2011.

263. Smith SE, Camasta CA, Cass AD: A simplified technique for repair of recurrent peroneal tendon subluxation, *J Foot Ankle Surg* 48:277–280, 2009.

264. Sobel M, Bohne WH, Levy ME: Longitudinal attrition of the peroneus brevis tendon in the fibular groove: an anatomic study, *Foot Ankle* 11:124–128, 1990.

265. Sobel M, Bohne WH, Markisz JA: Cadaver correlation of peroneal tendon changes with magnetic resonance imaging, *Foot Ankle* 11:384–388, 1991.

266. Sobel M, DiCarlo EF, Bohne WH, Collins L: Longitudinal splitting of the peroneus brevis tendon: an anatomic and histologic study of cadaveric material, *Foot Ankle* 12:165–170, 1991.

267. Sobel M, Geppert MJ, Olson EJ, et al: The dynamics of peroneus brevis tendon splits: a proposed mechanism, technique of diagnosis, and classification of injury, *Foot Ankle* 13:413–422, 1992.

268. Sobel M, Levy ME, Bohne WH: Congenital variations of the peroneus quartus muscle: an anatomic study, *Foot Ankle* 11:81–89, 1990.

269. Sobel M, Pavlov H, Geppert MJ, et al: Painful os peroneum syndrome: a spectrum of conditions responsible for plantar lateral foot pain, *Foot Ankle Int* 15:112–124, 1994.

270. Sobel M, Warren RF, Brourman S: Lateral ankle instability associated with dislocation of the peroneal tendons treated by the Chrisman–Snook procedure. A case report and literature review, *Am J Sports Med* 18:539–543, 1990.

271. Steel MW, DeOrio JK: Peroneal tendon tears: return to sports after operative treatment, *Foot Ankle Int* 28:49–54, 2007.

272. Stein RE: Reconstruction of the superior peroneal retinaculum using a portion of the peroneus brevis tendon. A case report, *J Bone Joint Surg Am* 69:298–299, 1987.

273. Steinbock G, Pinsger M: Treatment of peroneal tendon dislocation by transposition under the calcaneofibular ligament, *Foot Ankle Int* 15:107–111, 1994.

274. Stiehl JB: Concomitant rupture of the peroneus brevis tendon and bimalleolar fracture. A case report, *J Bone Joint Surg Am* 70:936–937, 1988.

275. Stover CN, Bryan DR: Traumatic dislocation of the peroneal tendons, *Am J Surg* 103:180–186, 1962.

276. Stropeni L: Frattura isolata di un osso soprannumerairo del tarso (os peroneum externo), *Arch Ital Chir* 2:556–564, 1920.

277. Szczukowski M Jr, St Pierre RK, Fleming LL, Somogyi J: Computerized tomography in the evaluation of peroneal tendon dislocation. A report of two cases, *Am J Sports Med* 11:444–447, 1983.

278. Taki K, Yamazaki S, Majima T, et al: Bilateral stenosing tenosynovitis of the peroneus longus tendon associated with hypertrophied peroneal tubercle in a junior soccer player: a case report, *Foot Ankle Int* 28:129–132, 2007.

279. Tan V, Lin SS, Okereke E: Superior peroneal retinaculoplasty: a surgical technique for peroneal subluxation, *Clin Orthop Relat Res* 410:320–325, 2003.

280. Tehranzadeh J, Stoll DA, Gabriele OM: Case report 271. Posterior migration of the os peroneum of the left foot, indicating a tear of the peroneal tendon, *Skeletal Radiol* 12:44–47, 1984.

281. Thomas JL, Lopez-Ben R, Maddox J: A preliminary report on intra-sheath peroneal tendon subluxation: a prospective review of 7 patients with ultrasound verification, *J Foot Ankle Surg* 48:323–329, 2009.

282. Thompson FM, Patterson AH: Rupture of the peroneus longus tendon. Report of three cases, *J Bone Joint Surg Am* 71:293–295, 1989.

283. Title CI, Jung HG, Parks BG, Schon LC: The peroneal groove deepening procedure: a biomechanical study of pressure reduction, *Foot Ankle Int* 26:442–448, 2005.

284. Tracy E: The calcaneo-fibular ligaments and its neighborhood, based on dissections, *Bost Med Surg J* 160:369–371, 1909.

285. Trevino S, Baumhauer JF: Tendon injuries of the foot and ankle, *Clin Sports Med* 11:727–739, 1992.

286. Truong DT, Dussault RG, Kaplan PA: Fracture of the os peroneum and rupture of the peroneus longus tendon as a complication of diabetic neuropathy, *Skeletal Radiol* 24:626–628, 1995.

287. Unlu MC, Bilgili M, Akgun I, et al: Abnormal proximal musculotendinous junction of the peroneus brevis muscle as a cause of peroneus brevis tendon tears: a cadaveric study, *J Foot Ankle Surg.* 49:537–540, 2010.

288. Vega J, Golanö P, Dalmau A, Viladot R: Tendoscopic treatment of intrasheath subluxation of the peroneal tendons, *Foot Ankle Int* 32:1147–1145, 2011.

289. Viernstein K, Rosemeyer B: [A method of operative treatment of recurrent displacement of peroneal tendons], *Arch Orthop Unfallchir* 74:175–181, 1972.

290. Walther M, Morrison R, Mayer B: Retromalleolar groove impaction for the treatment of unstable peroneal tendons, *Am J Sports Med* 37:191–194, 2009.

291. Wander DS, Galli K, Ludden JW, Mayer DP: Surgical management of a ruptured peroneus longus tendon with a fractured multipartite os peroneum, *J Foot Ankle Surg* 33:124–128, 1994.

292. Wang CC, Wang SJ, Lien SB, Lin LC: A new peroneal tendon rerouting method to treat recurrent dislocation of peroneal tendons, *Am J Sports Med* 37:552–557, 2009.

293. Wapner K, Taras J, Lin S, et al: Peroneus brevis reconstruction with passive Hunter rods and secondary flexor hallucis longus transfer as a salvage for chronic peroneus tendon tears: a surgical demonstration. Presented at the 61st Annual Meeting of the American Academy of Orthopaedic Surgeons, New Orleans, February 24-March 1, 1994.

294. Wapner KL, Taras JS, Lin SS, Chao W: Staged reconstruction for chronic rupture of both peroneal tendons using Hunter rod and flexor hallucis longus tendon transfer: a long-term followup study, *Foot Ankle Int* 27:591–597, 2006.

295. Weber M, Krause F: Peroneal tendon lesions caused by antiglide plates used for fixation of lateral malleolar fractures: the effect of plate and screw position, *Foot Ankle Int* 26:281–285, 2005.

296. Webster F: Peroneal tenosynovitis with pseudotumor, *J Bone Joint Surg Am* 50:153–157, 1968.

297. Williams CR: Acute calcification of the peroneal tendons in a sheep shearer, *Foot Ankle Int* 17:49–50, 1996.

298. Wirth CJ: [A modified Viernstein and Kelly surgical technic for correcting chronic recurrent peroneal tendon dislocation], *Z Orthop Ihre Grenzgeb* 128:170–173, 1990.

299. Yewlett A, Oakley J, Makwana N, Patel HJ: Retained blackthorn causing peroneal tendonitis: a case report, *Foot Ankle Surg* 15:205–206, 2009.

300. Zeiss J, Saddemi SR, Ebraheim NA: MR imaging of the peroneal tunnel, *J Comput Assist Tomogr* 13:840–844, 1989.

301. Zermatten P, Crevoisier X: Avulsion fracture of the peroneus longus tendon insertion at the base of the first metatarsal: report of a case, *Foot Ankle Surg* 17:e10–e12, 2011.

302. Zivot ML, Pearl SH, Pupp GR, Pupp JB: Stenosing peroneal tenosynovitis, *J Foot Surg* 28:220–224, 1989.

303. Zoellner G, Clancy W Jr: Recurrent dislocation of the peroneal tendon, *J Bone Joint Surg Am* 61:292–294, 1979.

Posterior Tibial Tendon Subluxation/Dislocation

304. Aguiar RO, Cabral MV, Moura BB, Marchiori E: Dislocation of the flexor digitorum longus and posterior tibial tendons without fracture dislocation of the ankle: a case report, *Foot Ankle Int* 28:1187–1189, 2007.

305. Ballesteros R, Chacon M, Cimarra A, et al: Traumatic dislocation of the tibialis posterior tendon: a new surgical procedure to obtain a strong reconstruction, *J Trauma* 39:1198–1200, 1995.

306. Beidert R: Dislocation of the tibialis posterior tendon, *Am J Sports Med* 20:775–776, 1992.

307. Bencardino J, Rosenberg ZS, Beltran J, et al: MR imaging of dislocation of the posterior tibial tendon, *AJR Am J Roentgenol* 169:1109–1112, 1997.

308. Boss AP, Hintermann B: Tibialis posterior tendon dislocation in combination with achilles tendon rupture: a case report, *Foot Ankle Int* 29:633–636, 2008.

309. Goucher NR, Coughlin MJ, Kristensen RM: Dislocation of the posterior tibial tendon: a literature review and presentation of two cases, *Iowa Orthop J* 26:122–126, 2006.

310. Healy W, Starkweather KD: Chronic dislocation of the posterior tibial tendon: a case report, *Am J Sports Med* 23:776–777, 1992.

311. Langan P, Weiss CA: Subluxation of the tibialis posterior, a complication of tarsal tunnel decompression: a case report, *Clin Orthop Relat Res* 146:226–227, 1980.

312. Larsen E, Lauridsen F: Dislocation of the tibialis posterior tendon in two athletes, *Am J Sports Med* 12:429–430, 1984.

313. Lee K, Byun WJ, Ha JK, Lee WC: Dislocation of the tibialis posterior tendon treated with autogenous bone block: a case report, *Foot Ankle Int* 31:254–257, 2010.

314. Lohrer H, Nauck T: Posterior tibial tendon dislocation: a systematic review of the literature and presentation of a case, *Br J Sports Med* 44:398–406, 2010.

315. Loncarich DP, Clapper M: Dislocation of posterior tibial tendon, *Foot Ankle Int* 19:821–824, 1998.

316. Martius C: Notes sur un cas de luxation du muscle tibial posterieur, etc, *Bull R Med Belg* 4:103, 1874.

317. Mitchell K, Mencia MM, Hoford R: Tibialis posterior tendon dislocation: a case report, *Foot (Edinb)* 21:154–156, 2011.

318. Mittal RL, Jain NC: Traumatic dislocation of the tibialis posterior tendon, *Int Orthop* 12:259–260, 1988.

319. Nava BE: Traumatic dislocation of the tibialis posterior tendon at the ankle. Report of a case, *J Bone Joint Surg Br* 50:150–151, 1968.

320. Nuccion SL, Hunter DM, Difiori J: Dislocation of the posterior tibial tendon without disruption of the flexor retinaculum. A case report and review of the literature, *Am J Sports Med* 29:656–659, 2001.

321. Oakley J, Yewlett A, Makwana N: Avulsion fracture of the medial malleolus following posterior tibialis tendon dislocation: a case report, *Foot Ankle Surg* 17:94–97, 2011.

322. Ouzounian TJ, Myerson MS: Dislocation of the posterior tibial tendon, *Foot Ankle* 13:215–219, 1992.

323. Perlman MD, Wertheimer SJ, Leveille DW: Traumatic dislocations of the tibialis posterior tendon: a review of the literature and two case reports, *J Foot Surg* 29:253–259, 1990.

324. Rolf C, Guntner P, Ekenman I, Turan I: Dislocation of the tibialis posterior tendon: diagnosis and treatment, *J Foot Ankle Surg* 36:63–65, 1997.

325. Sharon S, Knudson H, Gastwirth C: Post-traumatic recurrent dislocation of the tibialis posterior tendon: a case report, *J Am Pod Med* 68:500–502, 1978.

326. Soler R, Gastany F, Ferret J, Ramiro S: Traumatic dislocation of the tibialis posterior tendon at the ankle level, *J Trauma* 26:1049–1052, 1986.

327. Soulier R, Fallat L: Irreducible Salter Harris type II tibial physeal fracture secondary to interposition of the posterior tibial tendon: a case report, *J Foot Ankle Surg* 49:399e5–399e9, 2010.

328. Stanish WD, Vincent N: Recurrent dislocation of the tibialis posterior tendon—a case report with a new surgical approach, *Can J Appl Sport Sci* 9:220–222, 1984.

329. Vialis O, Montojo R, Sorroche P: Traumatic dislocation of the tibialis posterior tendon: a case report in a Tae-Kwon-Do athlete, *Clin J Sport Med* 1:68–69, 2009.

330. Wong YS: Recurrent dislocation of the posterior tibial tendon secondary to detachment of a retinacular-periosteal sleeve: a case report, *Foot Ankle Int* 25:602–604, 2004.

Tendon Transfers

331. Close JR, Todd FN: The phasic activity of the muscles of the lower extremity and the effect of tendon transfer, *J Bone Joint Surg Am* 41:189–208, 1959.

332. Green NE, Griffin PP, Shiavi R: Split posterior tibial-tendon transfer in spastic cerebral palsy, *J Bone Joint Surg Am* 65:748–754, 1983.

333. Hoffer MM, Reiswig JA, Garrett AM, Perry J: The split anterior tibial tendon transfer in the treatment of spastic varus hindfoot of childhood, *Orthop Clin North Am* 5:31–38, 1974.

334. Jones R: An operation for paralytic calcaneocavus, *Am J Orthop Surg* 5:371–383, 1908.

335. Kaufer H: Split tendon transfers, *Orthop Transplant* 1:191, 1977.

336. Kling TF Jr, Kaufer H, Hensinger RN: Split posterior tibial-tendon transfers in children with cerebral spastic paralysis and equinovarus deformity, *J Bone Joint Surg Am* 67:186–194, 1985.

337. Lipscomb P, Sanchez J: Anterior transplantation of the posterior tibial tendon for persistent palsy of the common peroneal nerve, *J Bone Joint Surg Am* 43:60–66, 1961.

338. Perry J, Hoffer MM: Preoperative and postoperative dynamic electromyography as an aid in planning tendon transfers in children with cerebral palsy, *J Bone Joint Surg Am* 59:531–537, 1977.

339. Rodriguez RP: The Bridle procedure in the treatment of paralysis of the foot, *Foot Ankle* 13:63–69, 1992.

340. Schneider M, Balon K: Deformity of the foot following anterior transfer of the posterior tibial tendon and lengthening of the Achilles tendon for spastic equinovarus, *Clin Orthop Relat Res* 125:113–118, 1977.

341. Turner JW, Cooper RR: Anterior transfer of the tibialis posterior through the interosseus membrane, *Clin Orthop Relat Res* 83:241–244, 1972.

342. Waters R: Acquired neurologic disorders of the adult foot. In Mann R, editor: *Surgery of the foot*, ed 5, St Louis, 1986, Mosby, p 339.

Pes Planus

Steven L. Haddad, Jonathan T. Deland

POSTERIOR TIBIAL TENDON DYSFUNCTION

Very few conditions in the realm of foot and ankle surgery incite as much controversy as management of the adult-acquired flatfoot. Perhaps most of this controversy extends from a lack of complete understanding of the condition, despite the passage of more than 50 years since the first published reports recognizing the disorder. Like many aspects of medicine, treatment of the adult-acquired flatfoot has evolved into philosophical ideas based in certain camps of academics, each camp purporting its views as reaching the ultimate solution for explaining and correcting the deformity.

Wisdom gained through experience, however, leads the veteran clinician to assimilate these philosophies into a spectrum of management options, incorporating components of each lesson into a unified whole. With this approach, each patient is respected individually for the specific pathologic components in tibialis posterior tendon dysfunction that cause pain and disability. The clinician can then address these specific components from the proven methodologies created thus far. Thus there is no one "right answer" in managing tibialis posterior tendon dysfunction, but one can gain significant insight by learning from the literature provided to date.

History

The roots of posterior tibial tendon (PTT) insufficiency are found in early writings on tenosynovitis. In 1818, Velpeau described the first case of noninfectious tenosynovitis in the hand. In 1895, de Quervain described stenosis-related tendovaginitis in the first compartment of the dorsal carpal ligament of the wrist in more than 900 patients. Kulowski,[105] in 1936, was the first to publish tenosynovitis of the sheath of the posterior tibial tendon, documenting one case. More than a decade later, the first large series of PTT tenosynovitis was published by Lipscomb at the Mayo clinic.[113] Lapidus and Seidenstein[109] commented on two cases of PTT tenosynovitis in 1950, stating, "nonspecific chronic tenosynovitis must be considered a rarity, particularly at the ankle." These early published reports underestimate its prevalence.

In 1955, A.W. Fowler[107] reported on seven cases of PTT tenosynovitis. He found "the condition was seldom diagnosed early, and it was often mistaken for osteoarthritis of the ankle and treated conservatively without relief. At operation, the tendon sheath was swollen and thickened and the tendon greatly enlarged. The inflamed synovium was excised, with relief in all cases." Although anecdotal, this was the first documented series in which tenosynovectomy was used and found to be successful. This concept was reinforced by Langenskiöld,[107] who, in 1967, documented six cases of PTT tenosynovitis treated surgically after failure of conservative management. These patients experienced great pain relief after debridement of the proliferative granulation tissue.

Key,[98] in 1953, documented the first case of PTT rupture (partial). In the prelude, he states that the case should be of interest, showing great foresight. This worker's compensation case documented the classic signs and symptoms of the condition, including the not-so-unusual missed early diagnosis. This partial rupture was treated with excision of the torn component and debridement of the residual thickened tendon, leaving the patient with 15% disability at the ankle.

Griffiths,[67] in 1965, recognized the difficulty in correcting deformity after late reconstruction of PTT rupture, but all of his "spontaneous" ruptures were in patients with rheumatoid arthritis. Thus confounding factors obviate the direct correlation between PTT rupture and deformity correction. Sixteen years after Key's article, Kettelkamp and Alexander[97] explored spontaneous PTT rupture in four patients without systemic disease. Missed in this article was the prevalence of spontaneous rupture because the authors begin by stating that this mechanism is a rarity. However, the authors pinpoint the challenge of correcting deformity created by delay in treatment. Three of the four patients were treated operatively without correction of tendon length (the retracted tendon was bridged with extensor digitorum longus tendon graft or filled with a Z-plasty lengthening), leaving the patients with residual pain and no correction of deformity. Results at best were rated fair.

In 1974, Goldner[61] revisited the topic of progressive talipes equinovalgus in traumatic and degenerative conditions of the posterior tibial tendon. This article studied nine patients with either of these etiologies, all resulting in the common pathway of an acquired flatfoot deformity. The authors correctly recognized a disorder of the medial plantar calcaneonavicular ligament resulting in limited support through elongation resulting from repetitive stress. Surgical intervention was done for deformity correction as well as pain relief. Transfer of the flexor hallucis longus to substitute for the deficient or absent PTT was done in all cases. The tendon was sutured to the periosteum under the navicular. This tendon was chosen over the flexor digitorum longus (FDL) because of its "more tendinous" structure, larger muscle mass, and the potential ability to elevate the sustentaculum tali to combat hindfoot valgus. In addition, the medial plantar calcaneonavicular ligament was plicated, after experience in not doing so resulted in persistent or progressive deformity. The authors also found failure in simply advancing or plicating the posterior tibial tendon. They also believed that a contracted gastrocnemius–soleus complex contributes to the deformity and must be addressed at the time of surgery.

Eight years later, in 1982, the concept of spontaneous rupture of the PTT resurfaced with a scientific presentation by Mann and Specht.[122] The authors reviewed eight patients undergoing a variation on Goldner's flexor hallucis longus (FHL) tendon transfer by using the FDL tendon as the source replacement tendon. Rationale for avoiding the use of the FHL tendon for transfer centered

on the importance of maintaining full flexion strength in the hallux in compromised patients. This paper will be reviewed more thoroughly in the surgical section of this chapter.

After the preceding article, the history of PTT dysfunction has followed the standard course of newly recognized syndromes in the history of medicine: a search for etiology, pathophysiology, and successful treatment options among multiple investigators. The ideas presented by these investigators will unfold in the following sections.

Anatomy and Function

The substance of a tendon is formed by a group of fasciculi. An epitenon surrounds the tendon and contains an outer synovial layer. Next, a paratenon, made of loose areolar tissue, surrounds the epitenon, carrying the tendinous structures. The next layer comprises the synovial sheath. The synovial sheath is usually continuous with the epitenon, forming a mesotenon that acts as a vascular channel for the tendon.[7] The mesotenon of the PTT sheath is not continuous. This anatomic variant will derive clinical significance as the potential for vascular insult is explored.

The posterior tibialis muscle arises from the interosseous membrane and adjacent surfaces of the tibia and fibula in the proximal one third of the leg. The myotendinous junction appears in the distal one third of the leg. The PTT courses directly behind the medial malleolus at a relatively acute angle. The groove is shallow, and the flexor retinaculum binds the tendon tightly into this groove. Thus the tendon passes posterior to the axis of the tibiotalar joint and medial to the axis of the subtalar joint, plantar flexing and inverting the hindfoot.[174] In fact, the PTT is located farther medially from the axis of the subtalar joint than any other tendon about the ankle, and it therefore has the greatest degree of leverage to bring about inversion of the subtalar joint. It then passes beneath the calcaneonavicular ligament to insert into the tuberosity of the navicular. It is unique in that it has eleven insertion domains: the navicular, the sustentaculum tali, the medial, middle, and lateral cuneiforms, the cuboid, and the bases of the second, third, and fourth metatarsals.[74,174] By its insertion into the midfoot, the tibialis posterior both adducts and supinates the forefoot.

Tendons possessing synovial sheaths have altered directional courses or are bound by tunnels or retinacula. Linear tendons (e.g., the Achilles tendon) often do not have sheaths. Tendons that contain a synovial sheath are generally located at the distal portions of the upper and lower extremities.[186] The sheath consists of three layers: a parietal layer lining the deep fibrous surface or fibroosseous canal, a visceral layer covering the tendon, and a mesotenon connecting the visceral and parietal layers serving as one source of the tendon's blood supply. The PTT is unique in that it does not contain a complete mesotenon and must receive its vascular supply through other channels. Synovial sheaths act to decrease the frictional forces encountered during tendon motion.[186] As gliding occurs, the visceral layer glides against the parietal layer. The mean length of the tendon sheath is 71 mm in men and 66 mm in women. The tendon sheath runs approximately 45 mm proximal to the apex of the medial malleolus and continues approximately 26 mm distal to the peak of the malleolus.[170] The excursion of the PTT is only 2 cm.

The PTT receives its blood supply from four regions: the vessels proximal to the muscle insertion, the connective tissue peritendinous arterial network, the arteries running to the tendon in the triangular vincula, and vessels from the periosteal insertion of the tendon.[170] Frey et al[54] found that the tendon receives its blood supply at the musculotendinous junction via the posterior tibial artery. They noted that a mesotenon was present in the PTT proximally, providing an additional network of vascular channels from the posterior tibial artery. The visceral layer also provides additional proximal blood supply, using this mesotenon as a conduit. This visceral layer remains closely adherent to the epitenon proximally. Distally, at the tendon–bone interface, the periosteal vessels provide the tendon's blood supply. These periosteal vessels are terminal segments for both the medial plantar branch of the posterior tibial artery, supplemented two thirds of the time by the medial tarsal artery, a branch of the dorsalis pedis artery.

The PTT functions to stabilize the hindfoot against valgus forces or eversion. The tibialis posterior is a stance phase muscle, firing from heel strike to shortly after heel lift-off.[89] It decelerates subtalar joint pronation after heel contact through eccentric contraction.[7] At midstance, it stabilizes the midtarsal joints. During the propulsive phase of stance, the tibialis posterior adducts the transverse tarsal joint, initiating inversion of the subtalar joint. This action has two beneficial effects on the gastrocnemius–soleus complex: it locks the transverse tarsal joint, allowing the gastrocnemius–soleus complex to maximize the plantar- flexion force during gait, and it shifts the direction of pull of the Achilles tendon further medially, allowing the gastrocnemius–soleus complex to become the primary invertor of the subtalar joint through increased leverage. In doing so, the foot can become a rigid lever that supports the propulsive phase of gait.

Quantifying this action with respect to gait, during the normal walking cycle, eversion occurs in the subtalar joint at the time of initial ground contact. The tibialis posterior becomes functional at about 7% of the cycle, the soleus muscle at about 10% of the cycle, and the lateral head of the gastrocnemius muscle at about 25% of the gait cycle. Dynamic electromyography suggests that this initial eccentric contraction of the posterior tibial muscle lasts from 7% to 30% of the gait cycle during stance. After this, progressive inversion occurs, starting at approximately 30% of the cycle through concentric contraction of the tibialis posterior.[161,175] The tibialis posterior muscle is silent during swing phase, where its antagonists enjoy maximal benefit. The primary antagonist of the posterior tibial muscle is the peroneus brevis muscle, functioning to abduct the midfoot and evert the hindfoot. Cross-sectional area studies note that the peroneus brevis muscle is 41% as strong as the posterior tibial muscle (relative strength of the PTT is 6.4, and of the peroneus brevis, 2.6).[165] Physiologically, this is manifested through the primary function of the peroneus brevis in unlocking the transverse tarsal joints and everting the hindfoot during the non–weight-bearing swing phase of gait.

Finally, stabilization of the longitudinal arch by the PTT remains a topic of debate. Most authors agree, however, that there are both static and dynamic forces at work. Static support theorists fall into two camps, those believing the foot acts as a truss and those believing the foot acts as a beam. The truss theory is supported by Lapidus.[108] A truss works by creating two struts that meet at an apex, supported at the base by a tie rod, thus forming a triangle. As the apex is loaded, compressive forces are applied to the struts, and tensile forces are applied to the tie rod. As long as the tie rod remains intact, the struts do not collapse, and the truss holds firm. Relating this model to the anatomy of the foot, the tie rod becomes the plantar aponeurosis. Hicks[75] believes that this model becomes critical at toe-off, when the windlass mechanism has maximal effect.

The beam theory, proposed by Sarrafian,[161] supports a less rigid construct. In this model, the foot is a curved beam that sags when it is loaded. Forces generated at the midportion of the beam are compressive on the convex side of the beam and tensile on the concave side. The curved portion of the beam consists of the bones of the midtarsus. Thus tension directly affects the structures on the concave side of these bones, namely, the plantar ligaments. Anatomically, these ligaments consist of the long and short plantar ligaments, the calcaneonavicular (spring) ligament, and the bifurcate ligament. All are attachment sites for the posterior tibial tendon.

The spring ligament consists two distinct bands: a stronger superior medial calcaneonavicular ligament and the inferior calcaneonavicular ligament just lateral to it. The latter structure has a medial plantar oblique and the plantar inferior band.

Dynamic support of the arch revolves around the tibialis posterior muscle and the intrinsic musculature of the foot. Support of the arch by the intrinsics is discussed in the next section. With respect to the posterior tibialis muscle's contribution, Kapandji[92] suggests that contraction of the tibialis posterior adducts and plantar flexes the navicular on the talar head. In doing so, it buttresses the medial longitudinal arch against collapse. In addition, the ligamentous attachments of the PTT have an effect by pulling the cuboid medially along with the navicular through the bifurcate ligament. This cuboid then pulls the calcaneus medially through the strong calcaneocuboid ligament, providing additional support to the talar head through the anterior and middle facets.

Pathophysiology of Posterior Tibial Tendon Rupture

The PTT has a limited excursion of only 2 cm. Thus any insult, no matter how minor, that lengthens this tendon has an adverse effect on its function. This lengthening may be gradual or acute, depending on the underlying pathologic process. The inversion power provided by the PTT has been underestimated by some, the thought process being that all of the posterior compartment muscles act to provide this function. Jahss[85] noted that the normal inversion power of all posterior calf muscles combined is 12 to 15 pounds of torque. Patients with PTT rupture undergo a substantial reduction in this force, lowering the torque to 3 to 6 pounds and emphasizing the importance of this tendon.

In acute situations, the integrity of the longitudinal arch may be initially maintained through static restraints. The valgus deformity of the hindfoot created by unopposed pull of the peroneus brevis through loss of the PTT secondarily causes loss of this integrity. According to Duchene[42] this allows the gastrocnemius–soleus complex to act with a downward force at the talonavicular joint. Downward and medial pressure of the talar head stretches the calcaneonavicular ligaments. The plantar ligaments placed medially that unite the tarsus and metatarsus are comparatively much weaker than those on the lateral side. Eventually, the passive structures of the longitudinal arch give way under continued dynamic insult, and a flatfoot deformity results. In the beam theory, the natural curved beam of the bony architecture of the foot becomes straightened by repetitive tensile forces on its concave surface. In particular, the spring ligament is at risk of failure.

This view is supported by Niki and Sangeorzan[141] who examined the progression to flatfoot deformity in a biomechanical study. The authors evaluated the sequential cause of the acquired flatfoot by creating a custom acrylic foot-loading frame to simulate heel strike, stance, and heel rise by altering tendon tension through regulated pneumatic cylinders. Simultaneously, axial compressive loads were applied to the tibias of these cadaveric specimens. Absence of posterior tibialis function was simulated simply by not activating the pneumatic cylinder attached to this tendon, while continuing normal cylinder load on all other tendons crossing the ankle. Thus, through cyclic evaluation, the authors studied the foot architecture with all tendons loaded in the absence of the posterior tibial tendon and, finally, with activation of the PTT (simulating repair). Small but statistically significant changes in the angular orientation of the bone architecture of the foot were noted after release of the posterior tibial tendon. These changes were not of the magnitude seen in a true flatfoot. This led the authors to surmise that the intact osteoligamentous structure of the foot is at least initially able to maintain normal alignment after acute PTT dysfunction. Of interest, when the PTT was restored in the flatfoot model, it did not restore the angular

changes to anatomic magnitude. Again, these data support the importance of progressive longitudinal arch collapse through attenuation of the spring (and other plantar) ligaments.

The source of the attenuation may be directly related to a disorder within the gastrocnemius–soleus complex and its mechanical orientation. The valgus deformity of the hindfoot created by dysfunction of the PTT substantially alters the mechanical pull of the Achilles tendon. The Achilles tendon is placed lateral to the axis of the subtalar joint, allowing it to become an evertor of the hindfoot, accelerating the valgus deformity. Equally important, the moment arm of the plantar flexion force becomes the talonavicular joint rather than the metatarsal heads.[55] This proximal alteration in force concentration comes directly from the perpetual valgus hindfoot's unlocking the transverse tarsal joint, eliminating the rigid lever of the foot at toe-off. This action accelerates attrition of the spring ligament with each gait cycle.

The intrinsic musculature attempts to compensate for the deficient arch by increased work. According to Mann and Inman,[121] the intrinsics stabilize the transverse tarsal joint and thus create a more efficient lever. As expected, flatfooted persons require increased muscle action to maintain a rigid lever in light of the lack of support at other portions of the arch. Activity of the intrinsics thus begins at an earlier portion of the stance phase of gait, measured at 10% of the cycle rather than the normal 40%.

This cascade of events leads to a common pathway as the PTT fails and a flatfoot develops. Changes in the bone architecture are as those found by Niki,[141] involving plantar flexion of the talus, eversion together with internal rotation of the calcaneus, and eversion of the navicular and the cuboid. Clinically, the hindfoot drifts into valgus and the forefoot into abduction. The posterior tibialis muscle fires earlier and longer to stabilize the hypermobile foot and to control the increased pronation and deviation. This increased demand on the muscle leads to fatigue. The deltoid ligament becomes involved late, as the severe flatfoot deformity places increased demand on the medial soft tissues, creating a valgus deformity and arthritic wear at the tibiotalar joint. Late-term effects occur as the calcaneus falls into further valgus. Abutment against the inferior tip of the fibula creates subfibular impingement. In addition, the relative shortening of the gastrocnemius–soleus complex leads to a permanent contraction, creating a relative equinus deformity of the ankle.

Etiology

Spontaneous rupture of the PTT was first suggested by Kettelkamp and Alexander[97] in 1969. Before that time, the authors were unable to locate a case of spontaneous rupture of the PTT in the literature. Controversy exists as to whether spontaneous rupture is truly spontaneous. McMaster[126] noted that spontaneous rupture did not occur in rabbits. In fact, even with a 75% iatrogenic laceration of the tendon, no ruptures occurred when normal stresses were applied. He stated that some form of disease process must be present to predispose the tendon to rupture.

Trauma of the magnitude to create a complete rupture of the PTT is rare. Funk[55] reported that of 19 patients treated for PTT tenosynovitis, only 4 could recall an inciting event. The authors agreed with McMaster,[126] stating that the lack of proximity of major trauma suggests that rupture of the PTT is more likely related to an intrinsic abnormality or biomechanical failure rather than an extrinsic traumatic factor.

Myerson noted in a group of elderly patients with rupture of the PTT that only 37 (14%) recalled a specific inciting traumatic event.[139] In contrast, Funk and Johnson[55] noted antecedent trauma in one half of the younger population in their study. Thus trauma to the tendon may be age stratified. This becomes evident from the case reports in the literature documenting acute rupture of the PTT resulting from ankle fractures. The first such report, by Giblin,[58] appeared in 1980: An interposed distal stump of a ruptured PTT prevented reduction of an isolated medial malleolus fracture. The patient had no prior symptoms of PTT dysfunction. In 1983, De Zwart[39] noted that two patients sustained rupture of the PTT at the level of a fractured medial malleolus in bimalleolar ankle fractures. A third report[169] suggested a common theme of a small flake of bone avulsed and visualized radiographically at the medial tibial metaphysis, just proximal to the medial malleolus fracture on oblique views.

A second theme[162] suggests that acute rupture of the PTT is more commonly seen in ankle fractures caused by pronation and external rotation. The tight binding of the PTT by the flexor retinaculum contributes to acute rupture through sudden trauma. Fracture of the medial malleolus is not necessary,[131] because the ruptured and interposed PTT may be seen with a deltoid ligament rupture associated with a pronation–external rotation fracture. This can even be seen in children,[1] raising the index of suspicion to prevent delayed flatfoot from developing after fracture of the ankle. Finally, there is some suggestion in the literature that acute injury to the PTT is the mechanism of disruption in dancers, rather than a slower degenerative process.[36] This article reviewed four dancers with either split tearing or more significant destruction of the PTT of acute onset. Often diagnosed initially with flexor hallucis longus tenosynovitis, the authors found this population did not present with a flatfoot, given their preexisting cavus consistent with high-level ballet dancers. Advanced diagnostic imaging was required to hone the diagnosis, and the pathology found at surgery suggested a more proximal location (directly posterior or superior to the medial malleolus) to the lesion than commonly seen in the more distal insidious ruptures.

More likely, repetitive microtrauma can lead to the indolent progression of symptoms through an inflammatory response that ultimately leads to tendon disruption.

A tendon will not tolerate more than 1500 to 2000 cycles per hour. Tendon overloading can cause microtears that trigger an inflammatory response.[7] Such microtears fail to heal, exacerbating the inflammatory response. As persons age, the tendon's elastic compliance decreases through changes in the collagen structure, predisposing the tendon to damage.[124] Myerson's[139] group of older patients reported the onset of symptoms at an average age of 60 years, seeking treatment at an average age of 64 years.

It is possible, however, that inflammation (preexisting tenosynovitis or tendinitis) has no involvement in disruption of the posterior tibial tendon. Mosier et al[133] evaluated gross and histologic specimens of 15 surgically resected posterior tibial tendons excised for rupture. Control tendons were those obtained from cadavers with no known disorder to the posterior tibial tendon, confirmed by gross inspection of the tendons at the time of harvest.

Direct inspection of the diseased tendons revealed a characteristic increased length from the malleolus to the insertion point when referenced with the cadaver tendons. Loss of normal tendon sheen and color was noted, and the tendon had a dull, white appearance. Incomplete longitudinal splitting was present without transverse rupture. Microscopic specimens stained appropriately revealed increased mucin content and myxoid degeneration. Excess mucin was found to alter the normal linear orientation of the tendon collagen bundles. Myxoid degeneration was consistent with a rupture within the substance of the tendon. At the insertion of the posterior tibial tendon, fibroblastic hypercellularity and chondroid metaplasia were present. Again, this had the effect of disrupting the linear collagen orientation. This haphazard or wavy configuration of the collagen leads to decreased tensile strength within the tendon, potentially leading to "spontaneous" rupture. This, of course, would validate McMaster's concept of predisposition.[126] Most important, the authors found no signs of inflammatory infiltrates within either the tendon or the tenosynovium. This suggests that a degenerative condition, rather than an inflammatory one, creates disruption of the posterior tibial tendon.

An evaluation of the biochemical influences upon the PTT with reference to hormonal influence on PTT disease was explored by Bridegman et al.[90] The authors noted the higher propensity of PTT dysfunction in perimenopausal and postmenopausal women, leading to a concern that changes in hormone physiology might be the source of this observation. Evaluating both male and female patients through direct biopsy in those undergoing reconstruction, the authors used the adjacent flexor digitorum longus tendon as a control. Using a centrifuge to isolate tendon ribonucleic acid (RNA), followed by reverse transcription to isolate estrogen receptors in the specimens, the authors noted no difference in receptor expression between male and female patients. In addition, the diseased posterior tibial in female patients expressed a higher estrogen receptor level than the comparative control tendons. However, the sample size was not large enough to draw a statistically significant conclusion. A larger cohort will be required to discern this potential influence upon PTT dysfunction and the relative partiality towards female patients.

Trevino,[180] in 1981, performed the first histopathologic examination of diseased posterior tibial tendons. The authors found a stenosing tenosynovitis characterized by a loose, wavy configuration of the collagen. Other authors[38,135] confirmed this wavy configuration to the collagen, with irregular spaces between bundles. In fact, all of these investigators found little evidence of inflammation in patients with rupture of the posterior tibial tendon. Also, although no complete transverse ruptures were visualized, incompetence of the tendon in combination with elongation of the tendon was clear. Sutherland[175] suggested, through electromyographic studies, that the magnitude of elongation sufficient to reduce the ability of the PTT to act as a dynamic stabilizer of the longitudinal arch was as little as 1 cm. Clearly, degenerative changes manifested as intrasubstance collagen disruption is enough to create this length deficit.

Changes in the composition of the collagen matrix in disrupted posterior tibial tendons was explored by Goncalves-Neto et al.[62] The authors confirmed the alteration in the normal linear orientation of collagen bundles in involved tendons. They noted neovascularization—an increase in size, number, and branching of blood vessels—in conjunction with an increased number of fibroblasts. These findings suggest attempts at repair. More important, they noted a shift in the type of collagen within the diseased tendon. Normal tendons are composed of type I collagen, with minor amounts of type III, IV, and V collagen. Incompetent posterior tibial tendons shifted the makeup of this collagen from 95% to approximately 56% type I. In addition, type III collagen increased 54%, and type V increased 26%. Investigators have found that as the percentages of type III and type V collagen increase within the extracellular matrix, the diameter of the collagen fibrils undergoes a marked reduction. Damaged tendon makes an attempt to heal itself, and it does so with this poorer quality collagen.

Even normal anatomic PTT exhibits alterations in collagen composition at specific locations. Petersen et al[143] found a change in composition of the superficial zone of the PTT directly adjacent to the pulley of the posterior medial malleolus. Using both light and transmission electron microscopy in combination with immunohistochemical methods, the authors noted increased type II collagen as well as acid glycosaminoglycans consistent with fibrocartilage rather than the standard composition of dense connective tissue. The authors believe the physiologic basis of this shift in composition is related to the character of the posterior tibial tendon's changing from a traction tendon to a gliding tendon (subject to intermittent compressive and shear stresses) as it courses behind the medial malleolus.

The only portion of the PTT that exhibited composition consistent with fibrocartilage is the portion directly adjacent to the pulley, which is consistent with the most common site of spontaneous rupture. The fibrocartilage does not penetrate the entire diameter of the tendon at this location; rather, it remains superficial. This finding is physiologic, rather than pathologic, in the posterior tibial tendon. Thus it remains a point of weakness irrespective of the underlying disease process, but it remains vulnerable to any disease process affecting the tendon. From such an insult, a poor repair response occurs from the relatively avascular tissue. Repetitive stress or microtrauma can create such an insult because of the suspected lower resistance to tensile forces.

Despite this information, clinicians cannot eliminate the impact that inflammation has during the early stages of PTT dysfunction. Jahss first suggested a possible link between seronegative spondyloarthropathies and PTT tenosynovitis in 1982.[85] Seronegative disorders are inflammatory conditions generally occurring outside the synovium. They disproportionately involve sites of attachment of the capsule, ligament, and tendon to bone, known as entheses. These arthropathies are generalized and often involve multiple sites in the upper and lower extremities. Common concurrent connective tissue disorders include inflammatory bowel disease, psoriasis, urethritis, uveitis, conjunctivitis, and oral ulcers. Myerson[139] concluded that the majority of younger patients with PTT disorders have signs of systemic enthesopathies. This patient population was predominantly female. Symptoms of systemic disease occur at an average age of 27 years, and patients seek treatment at an average age of 39 years. Two thirds of the patients had, in addition to PTT tenosynovitis, other areas of inflammatory involvement. More than half had a first-degree relative with evidence of a connective tissue disorder.

Myerson[139] determined that two separate patient populations developed PTT tenosynovitis and subsequent dysfunction. Both populations underwent human leukocyte antigen (HLA) typing, supporting the association between age and seronegative spondyloarthropathies. Although only two patients in the older group had positive HLA markers, a majority of the younger population had HLA markers in their blood. Of particular interest is the *Cw6* allele, the primary allele for psoriasis. Nearly half (47%) of the younger patient group had this allele compared with none in the older group. Only 12% in the institutional control group had *Cw6* in their blood. This constellation of symptoms and laboratory results strongly suggests that inflammation plays a role in the inciting event of PTT dysfunction, at least in persons afflicted at a younger age. The younger population had a more rapid progression toward PTT rupture, encouraging prompt recognition of this potential cause and allowing earlier intervention. Stratifying the condition on an age-related basis has value only in patients with associated systemic conditions because degenerative tendinopathy has strong supportive evidence not only in Myerson's older category of patients but also in the literature just noted.

In contrast to seronegative diseases that demonstrate an inflammatory cause inciting PTT dysfunction, rheumatoid arthritis has yet to show that it has a direct role in tendon destruction. Downey[41] thinks that the chronic inflammatory mediators noted in rheumatoid arthritis are the predisposing factor for tenosynovitis. Michelson[128] suggested such a cause exists in as many as 64% of patients afflicted with rheumatoid disease. However, when he narrowed his criteria for diagnosis to include loss of a longitudinal arch, inability to perform a single-limb heel stance, and the inability to palpate the posterior tibial tendon, the incidence dropped to 11%.

The problem with all such studies is the concurrent destruction of the ligament complex at the subtalar and talonavicular joints known to occur in rheumatoid disease. This disorder confuses the specific cause of flatfoot. Any of the signs of PTT rupture noted by Michelson can be seen in patients with joint destruction from the synovitis of rheumatoid disease that creates flatfoot.

Jahss[94] examined the PTT in rheumatoid patients undergoing arthrodesis of the hindfoot for symptomatic flatfoot and found the tendon normal in appearance. Kirkham and Gibson[101] studied 50 patients with rheumatoid arthritis and noted no instance of PTT dysfunction in those with progressive longitudinal arch collapse and hindfoot valgus. Finally, Keenan[95] performed electromyography on five patients with rheumatoid arthritis and hindfoot valgus and observed that muscle activity actually increased in this patient population versus controls. These data suggest that the PTT is actually overpulling in an attempt to correct the hindfoot valgus, rather than undergoing destruction by the underlying disease process. Thus attempts at linking the inflammation of rheumatoid arthritis to destruction of the PTT remain in question.

A vascular cause of PTT dysfunction has been suggested by numerous authors. Holmes and Mann[80] performed a review of 67 patients with a diagnosis of PTT rupture. This epidemiologic study found a statistical correlation between tendon rupture and both obesity ($P = .005$) and hypertension ($P = .025$). This patient population was older, ranging in age from 51 to 87 years, and the correlation remained strong in spite of the general population prevalence of these conditions in this age category. In addition, diabetes and steroid use (both oral and injection) were linked to PTT dysfunction.

All four associated conditions directly or indirectly compromise the blood supply to the posterior tibial tendon. Diabetes promotes vascular hyperplasia and sclerosis, leading to stiffness of the arterioles, luminal narrowing, and blood flow resistance. Steroids lead to local vascular attenuation, creating avascular tissue. Such ischemic insults can compromise an already tenuous blood supply to select portions of the posterior tibial tendon, leading to degenerative tendinopathy. This is supported by Kennedy and Willis,[96] who have shown through

tendon-loading studies that steroid injections into the tendon sheath significantly weaken the tendon for up to 2 weeks. They found that the tendon disruption is related to collagen necrosis at the site of injection. Compromise in a tenuous blood supply can also occur in patients who have undergone previous surgery on the medial portion of the foot and ankle.

The PTT receives its blood supply primarily from the posterior tibial artery (although the insertion of the tendon might receive its blood supply from branches of the dorsalis pedis artery). There has been debate as to the significance of its aberrant blood supply contributing to tendon disorder. Frey and Shereff[54] used a modified Spaltholz technique to study the blood supply of the posterior tibial tendon. In doing so, they injected 28 cadaveric limbs with an India ink–gelatin suspension. This mixture was cleared via the Spaltholz technique, destroying the normal histology of the tendon while allowing visualization of the gross external and internal vasculature. To confirm isolated aberration in the PTT blood supply, they examined the adjacent flexor digitorum longus as a control.

Using this technique, Frey and Shereff[54] discovered that an important hypovascular zone (14 mm long) is present approximately 40 mm proximal to the insertion of the posterior tibial tendon.[80,174] This zone of relative avascularity generally begins at the medial malleolus as the tendon courses out of the groove. Of interest, no mesotenon was present at this level, and the visceral layer of the synovial sheath was hypovascular. In the control flexor digitorum longus tendon, no such zone existed, and consistent vascularity was noted throughout the tendon.

This hypovascular zone has a corollary in the supraspinatus tendon, where Rathbun and Macnab[152] noted that tension in a select portion of the tendon can wring out the blood supply. Without an adequate blood supply, cells require surrounding extracellular fluid to provide nutrition through diffusion. The limits of diffusion are clear, however. Smith[165a] suggests that nutrition will not be adequate when travel distance from source to destination exceeds 1 to 2 cm. Frey et al[54] thus reasoned that the hypovascular zone allows PTT deterioration with age.

There have been critics of this theory, however. In 2002, Petersen et al[144] used a different method to assess blood supply to the posterior tibial tendon. They criticize the Spaltholz technique as providing a large number of false-positive and false-negative results because of its subjective nature. Instead, they used a combination injection of ^{99m}Tc, India ink, and gelatin, specifically studying the laminin. According to the authors, laminin is a basic component of the basement membrane, and staining with ^{99m}Tc reliably and objectively detects blood vessels in the dense connective tissues.

Macroscopic assessment of the tendon at the level of the medial malleolus revealed an avascular, rather than hypovascular, segment. The majority of the avascular tissue was concentrated directly where the tendon is in contact with the malleolus. Confirmation was achieved through the immunohistochemical findings, which revealed an absence of laminin in this same location. Laminin was noted in the posterior quarter (farthest from the contact zone against the malleolus) of the PTT and proximal and distal to the malleolus.

Vascular theories explaining PTT degeneration and rupture have been challenged by Mosier et al.[133] The disorder of the collagen was discussed earlier. In addition to the increased mucin and myxoid degeneration, the authors noted neovascularization in the degenerative zone of the posterior tibial tendon. They surmised that the tendon cannot be avascular or hypovascular in these zones because the new blood vessels had to arise from existing circulation. In addition, they postulated that the fibroblast hypercellularity that they noted on the microscopic sections indicates increased metabolic activity within the presumed hypovascular zone, which is counterintuitive to the absence of vascular flow.

Two anatomic theories exist in the literature as to why the PTT is especially prone to developing long-standing inflammation and degeneration. The first potential agent is the overlying flexor retinaculum, which Jahss[85] suggests can cause compression and constriction of the tendon through synovial enlargement. This can impede circulation, fueling tendon degeneration. Second, the sharp turn or angle behind the malleolus creates excessive frictional forces with physical activity.[174] The excessive friction can contribute to the indolent inflammatory process.

In line with repetitive mechanical torque creating deficiency in the PTT are theories that congenital pes planus contributes to the disorder. Cozen[28] suggested that greater stress is placed on the PTT because of both the increased subtalar motion and medial column sag seen in patients with flexible flatfoot. This is supported by Dyal et al,[45] who reviewed radiographs of patients with PTT insufficiency and compared them with radiographs on the contralateral (asymptomatic) side. Using angular measurements defined by Bordelon[10] and Sangeorzan et al,[160] the authors noted that 84% of asymptomatic feet and 86% of symptomatic feet had flatfoot deformities. These results were stratified to reveal that 23% of asymptomatic feet and 32% of symptomatic feet were moderately or severely flat. Interobserver reliability was highly correlated ($P = .0001$) among three surgeon observers, strengthening their results. Of course, this study does not prove that asymptomatic congenital pes planus is a potential cause of PTT insufficiency, but the suggestion is strong.

Indirectly, the contribution of a congenital flatfoot to PTT dysfunction is supported by Imhauser et al.[84] The authors created an in vitro model evaluating PTT function at heel rise. Unlike previous models, this construction allowed rotation of the tibia to contribute to a more physiologic gait pattern simulation. After creating a flatfoot deformity (through ligament sectioning), the authors noted a medial shift in load acting on the foot, placing undue stress on the PTT (and other medial structures) at

heel lift. Such repetitive stress has already been discussed as a potential cause in PTT dysfunction.

This latter concept is supported by a 2006 paper by Uchiyama et.al.[181] This study compared the gliding resistance of the PTT within its sheath both in simulated flatfoot and without pathology at different ankle positions. Gliding resistance mimics friction applied to the tendon in both static (standing) and dynamic (walking) situations. The authors extrapolated a validated technique developed to measure gliding resistance of tendons in the hand, which they found highly repeatable. Before flatfoot, the gliding resistance with the ankle in neutral averaged 77 N. After flatfoot deformity, this resistance increased to 104 N, on average. The authors postulated that this increased gliding resistance may accelerate tendon degeneration in both preexisting congenital flatfoot deformity and in progressive adult acquired flatfoot disorders.

Finally, the presence of an accessory navicular has a high correlation with developing PTT dysfunction.[12,93]

It is obvious that the cause of PTT insufficiency is most likely multifactorial and patient-specific. It is important for the clinician to assimilate the information discussed here to arrive at the correct underlying mechanism creating the disorder.

Physical Findings

Physical examination of the patient with PTT dysfunction begins with the patient standing barefoot, with the lower extremity exposed proximal to the knee. The examiner must ensure that the patient is standing with both knees facing forward because the patient tends to externally rotate the involved extremity. Depending on the stage of presentation (see Clinical Staging section later in this chapter), the alignment may be anatomic and symmetric, or the flatfoot deformity may be pronounced (Fig. 25-1). In this position, swelling or fullness about the medial ankle may be apparent. In advanced stages, forefoot abduction is obvious, as is impingement of the distal fibula against the calcaneus through hindfoot valgus collapse. The skin may be wrinkled laterally in this subfibular region. Direct palpation to the subfibular region with the ankle and hindfoot loaded elicits pain. In addition, in this position, with the feet symmetrically loaded, the examiner can take one finger and place it underneath the arch until striking soft tissue. By comparison with the opposite extremity in the same location, a rough estimate of arch collapse is noted.

From this position, the patient is asked to externally rotate the involved extremity 90 degrees, maintaining a fully loaded state. Collapse of the talonavicular joint may be appreciated by viewing the foot medially in this position. Calluses plantar to the talar head may be seen, and collapse at the first metatarsal–cuneiform joint may be noted. Rotating the leg 180 degrees to visualize the lateral foot and ankle, the examiner can develop a better appreciation of subfibular impingement. In this position, range of motion of the ankle may be checked and compared

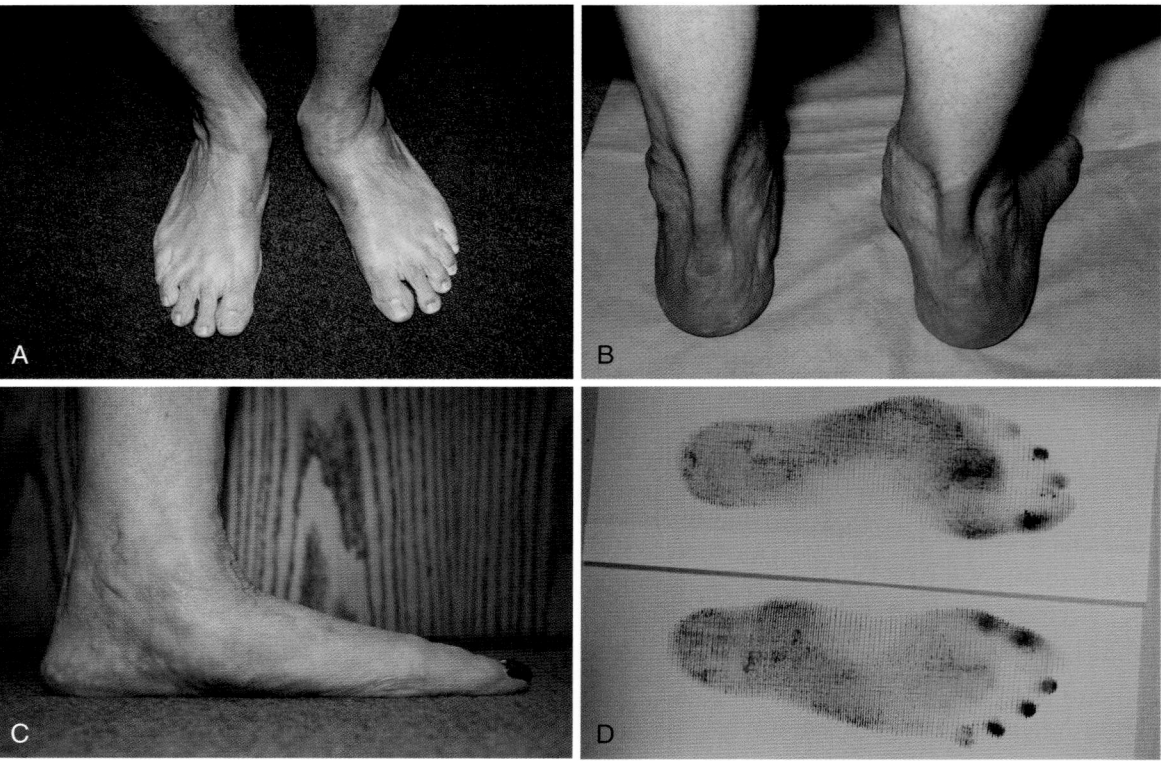

Figure 25-1 Clinical photographs of deformity after rupture of posterior tibial tendon. **A,** Dorsal view demonstrating increased abduction and a prominent talar head secondary to subluxation of the talonavicular joint. **B,** Posterior view demonstrating increased valgus of the calcaneus, increased abduction of the foot, and prominent talar head along the medial border of the foot. **C,** Medial view demonstrating collapse of the longitudinal arch and the prominence of the talar head. **D,** Harris mat demonstrating flattening of the longitudinal arch on the right in a patient with posterior tibial tendon dysfunction.

with the opposite extremity. It is important to examine ankle range of motion in a loaded state to avoid misrepresentation by compensation from the Chopart joint and forefoot joints. In the most advanced cases, this compensation becomes apparent as the patient passively dorsiflexes beyond neutral and the heel rises off the ground while the midfoot joints collapse.

The patient is next asked to face opposite the examiner, again with the knees symmetrically aligned forward. Hindfoot valgus should be noted and can be roughly estimated by visualizing through a goniometer to the patient's hindfoot. The proximal limb of the goniometer is positioned along the axis of the patient's leg, the hinge at the talus, and the inferior limb along the calcaneal axis. With practice, this method gives surprisingly accurate measurements of loaded valgus. Also, in this position, the examiner can note medial ankle fullness or swelling. Even in early stages, before valgus collapse of the hindfoot, this fullness is apparent when compared with the contralateral extremity. In addition, forefoot abduction becomes obvious when viewed from behind. The too-many-toes sign indicates more advanced disease and is sensitive in patients with congenital flatfoot as a comparative test.

One method of testing PTT muscle strength and integrity, the heel-rise test, is performed in this position. First,

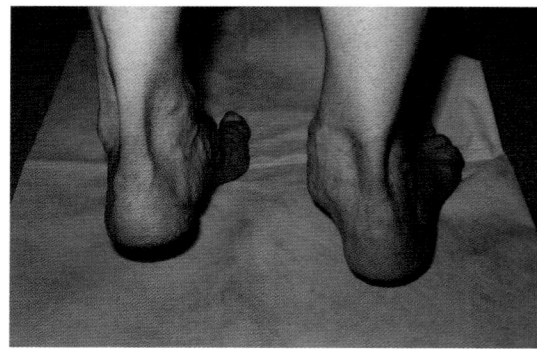

Figure 25-2 Double and single toe rise is an integral part of the physical examination. Note that on the involved (right) side, inversion of the subtalar does not occur.

the examiner asks the patient to rise up onto both tiptoes. While doing so, the examiner looks for symmetric hindfoot inversion. Lack of symmetry indicates that the affected PTT is incompetent to invert the subtalar joint, lock the transverse tarsal joint, and allow heel rise through gastrocnemius–soleus complex power (Fig. 25-2). This is confirmed by asking the patient to perform a single-limb heel rise. The patient may rest a few fingers on an adjacent table or wall for balance, but the examiner must be sure that the patient does not lean forward or bend the knee while attempting to rise on one limb. Altering the body's center of gravity or recruiting adjacent muscle power by cheating in this fashion invalidates the test. In addition, the patient may be able to stand on the tiptoes of the involved extremity after rising up on both legs and lifting the contralateral extremity off the ground.

Returning to the truss theory, if a patient is able to remain standing on the toes without a functioning posterior tibial tendon, it is the plantar aponeurosis that brings about plantar flexion of the metatarsal heads and thus inversion of the calcaneus. In this theory, the longitudinal arch is maintained, and the gastrocnemius–soleus complex maintains the ankle joint in plantar flexion. Thus patients without a functioning PTT may be unable to initiate standing on tiptoes but are able to maintain the position once they have gotten on their toes because the mechanism of action of the PTT is bypassed.

The examination now shifts to a seated patient. Passive range of motion of the ankle, subtalar, and the transverse tarsal joints is assessed. Excess mobility of the first metatarsocuneiform joint is assessed by firmly grasping both the first metatarsal and the midfoot and evaluating for subluxation of this joint surface in the sagittal plane. Simple dorsiflexion and plantar flexion of the first metatarsal while the midfoot is held rigid may be deceptive, and it must be compared with the opposite foot. Still, this maneuver may be useful for assessing midfoot pain and potential arthritis.

Direct palpation along the course of the PTT can elicit pain, although in later-stage disease, where tendinopathy supersedes tenosynovitis, pain might not be present. The examiner feels for increased swelling, fluid within the sheath, and increased warmth. There is some suggestion that palpable pitting edema is a valid clinical finding supplanting the need for advanced diagnostic imaging.[168] Retrospective analysis of this visible depression or deep indentation after direct pressure to the PTT found 86% sensitivity and 100% specificity of fluid within the tendon sheath confirmed via follow-up magnetic resonance imaging (MRI). Although the examiner can certainly make note of this finding on examination, clinical utility of this finding remains suspect because it may be evident only in inflammatory conditions leading to PTT dysfunction and has no predictive outcome on treatment.

Isolating the PTT for strength testing is difficult but possible. The examiner places the patient's ankle into a plantar-flexed position, everting the hindfoot, to negate the effect of the anterior tibial tendon. The patient must relax the toes to prevent overpull by the flexor hallucis longus and flexor digitorum longus.[124] In this position, the patient inverts against resistance applied by the examiner's hand against the medial first metatarsal (Fig. 25-3). Strength and reproduction of pain are noted and compared with the opposite extremity. Comparison is critical because patients can maintain some PTT strength with an incompetent tendon. As noted in the physiology section, the excursion of the PTT is only 1 to 2 cm. Thus a length

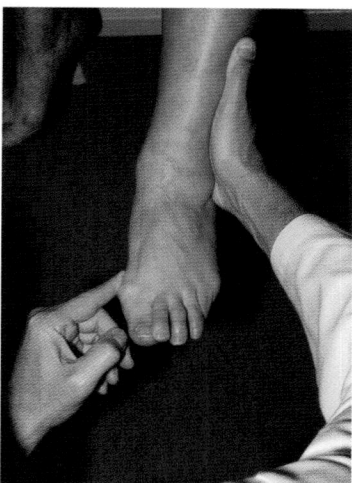

Figure 25-3 Evaluation of posterior tibial tendon function. The foot is placed into full inversion and some plantar flexion, and the patient is asked to resist pressure from the examiner's finger.

deficit of 1 cm because of rupture or tendinopathy can still provide some inversion strength while having no functional value.

Inversion strength has been quantified by Houck et al[81] via a subtalar inversion and forefoot adduction test using a force transducer and oscilloscope. The authors used the premise that muscle force assessment is directly related to the physiologic cross-sectional area of that particular muscle. The authors also sought to suppress the influence of the anterior tibial tendon on this tested plane of motion by plantar flexion of the ankle during testing. Quantification of this influence was determined by electromyographic (EMG) data, confirming suppression of its impact to less than 10% normal inversion strength. The authors noted they were only able to keep only 60% of the control population and 40% to 50% of the diseased subjects from using less than 10% of the anterior tibial tendon in this plane of motion. With this in mind, the authors determined a 20% to 30% deficit in subtalar inversion and forefoot adduction strength, in those with stage 2 PTT dysfunction, versus control subjects. Whether a clinician can manually perceive this discrepancy during examination remains to be determined. However, this protocol can certainly be used to provide objective information during physical therapy, to assess strength recovery of the diseased posterior tibial tendon.

The patient is then asked to lie flat, and the ankle range of motion is assessed with the knee flexed and extended. The Silversköldt test specifically measures gastrocnemius contracture by alternately relaxing and incorporating the muscle because of its origin proximal to the knee joint. This test should be done while holding the subtalar joint in neutral, to avoid subtalar compensation for a tight gastrocnemius muscle. With the legs fully extended and the subtalar joint held in neutral, an assessment for fixed forefoot varus is performed. In the normal foot, a line

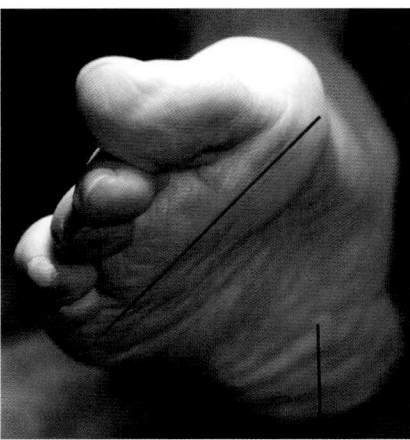

Figure 25-4 Demonstration of forefoot varus. The degree of forefoot varus is determined by placing the heel in neutral position, covering the head of the talus with the navicular, and then observing the relationship of the metatarsal heads to the neutral hindfoot. In fixed forefoot varus, the lateral border of the foot is more plantar flexed than the medial border.

visually drawn across the plantar metatarsal heads is perpendicular to the long axis of the tibia and calcaneus. Patients with long-standing PTT dysfunction can develop fixed varus (Fig. 25-4) of the forefoot as a compensation for increasing hindfoot valgus (they are attempting to maintain a plantigrade foot). The visual metatarsal line is thus inclined medially. The rigidity of this condition may be evaluated by continuing to hold the subtalar joint in neutral while providing a manual dorsiflexion force on the lateral column of the foot through the fourth and fifth metatarsals. Normally, the lateral column of the foot is mobile, and the visual line should return to the anatomic axis. In fixed conditions, the medial inclination remains.

The patient is then placed in a prone position. Here, subtalar joint motion can be measured with the knee flexed 90 degrees and the ankle plantar flexed. Relaxing the gastrocnemius–soleus complex releases outside influence on the subtalar joint and allows accurate measurements to be obtained. This may be done with a goniometer, again placing one limb of the device along the axis of the distal tibia, the hinge at the talus, and the second limb along the axis of the calcaneus. The importance of achieving accuracy in both subtalar motion assessment and fixed forefoot varus deformity will become clear as surgical procedures are discussed.

Finally, gait should be assessed through direct observation and formal analysis. A motion analysis system has been used, revealing prolonged stance phase and diminished stride length, cadence, and walking speed in PTT dysfunction.[140] When segmenting regions of individual pathologic feet, the authors note that gait alteration can be explained through diminished dorsiflexion and increased eversion of the hindfoot, decreased plantar flexion of the forefoot, and diminished dorsiflexion of the hallux. The examiner can use this information in both

surgical planning and in the manufacturing of orthotics or braces to support conservative care. Regardless, this dynamic component of assessment of PTT dysfunction is equally important to standing assessment and should be a part of every evaluation.

Before completing the examination, the patient's shoes are inspected for aberrant wear patterns. This becomes evident as medial heel wear in older shoes because valgus hindfoot asymmetrically erodes the heel through repetitive strike.

Clinical Staging

Posterior tibial tendon dysfunction should be viewed as a syndrome in which there is a spectrum of clinical presentations. This spectrum ranges from patients with recent onset (synovitis can create pain, yet motor function is preserved) to patients with long-standing disease (marked collapse of the hindfoot and midfoot is present and motor function is absent).

The general classification system proposed by Johnson and Strom[89] enables clinicians to organize their thoughts when evaluating this condition. The authors based this classification system on disorder, clinical presentation, and radiographic findings.

Stage 1 patients present with swelling and pain along the medial aspect of the hindfoot, generally at the tip and distal to the medial malleolus along the course of the posterior tibial tendon. In this stage, tenosynovitis is the predominant source of pain. Thus the length of the tendon is preserved and, along with it, motor strength. The patient is usually able to perform a single toe raise, with normal varus tilt to the hindfoot while on the toes. This maneuver might not cause symptoms, but repetitive toe raises reproduce the symptomatic pain. With respect to the above-mentioned parameters in physical examination, hindfoot valgus is absent, too-many-toes sign is absent, and deformity is absent.

Stage 2 patients have undergone elongation and degeneration of the posterior tibial tendon. Deformity of the foot is obvious at this stage. The hindfoot is in valgus, and the forefoot may be in abduction. Collapse at the talonavicular joint is apparent. The patient may be able to perform a single-limb heel rise early in this stage, but as the deformity progresses, the patient is unable to do so. Most important, the deformity remains flexible at this stage. Thus the examiner can passively correct both the hindfoot valgus and forefoot abduction while the patient is seated. Recently, this stage has been subclassified into an "a" stage, where symptoms are primarily medial, the collapse is mild, and the patient can still perform a single-limb heel rise, and a "b" stage, where subfibular impingement develops along with complete incompetence of the posterior tibial tendon.

Stage 3 patients have developed a rigid deformity. Forefoot varus is fixed and usually 10 to 15 degrees at the minimum. The subtalar joint no longer reduces in a seated position, and any attempt to place the calcaneus in the anatomic axis reveals the compensatory supinated forefoot. The gastrocnemius–soleus complex is tight. Often the medial ankle pain is absent in this stage, and patients complain more of pain in the lateral ankle, which, upon examination, is subfibular. Pain at rest might become apparent as arthritis becomes a component of the condition. The patient is unable to perform a single-limb heel rise.

Stage 4 was added by Myerson.[117] Chronic eccentric loading of the ankle joint in valgus creates lateral compartment arthritic wear patterns. The lateral ankle pain with which a patient in stage 3 would present is now only partially subfibular impingement and more directly related to ankle arthritis. This valgus load eventually leads to a valgus deformity of the talus and attenuation of the deltoid ligament.

A more recent classification system, by Raikin et al,[151] attempts to create an algorithmic approach to providing not only static diagnosis but also therapeutic intervention. This Roger A. Mann (RAM) classification system uses the structural outline of the Johnson and Strom system but complements that system by providing specific pathology to the hindfoot, ankle, and midfoot. However, this system is currently descriptive, based on the authors' observations, and it will require validation through clinical testing before widespread use.

Imaging Evaluation

Radiography

Diagnostic modalities for evaluation of the PTT have evolved since Kulowski's report on tenosynovitis in 1936.[105] However, a standard protocol for PTT imaging has yet to be accepted. In 1986, Funk et al[55] noted that four different types of PTT lesions were found during surgical exploration. The authors reported the impossibility of distinguishing the four groups by clinical or radiographic measures before surgery. Funk et al looked at 19 patients who underwent surgical exploration after failed primary conservative treatment for PTT dysfunction. They determined that preoperative radiographs were of little added value in diagnosis, and the various lesions that might be present in the PTT can be suspected clinically, but a precise diagnosis cannot be made until the tendon is exposed surgically. In this study, the preoperative radiograph was the only advanced imaging modality used.

Despite this forewarning, plain radiography is a useful adjunct in evaluating PTT dysfunction. Weight-bearing radiographs are used to appreciate the deformity, and they are useful in proposing management options. The standard series includes three views of the foot and, at the very least, an anteroposterior (AP) view of the ankle (Fig. 25-5). Additional radiographs can include a complete ankle series (Fig. 25-6) and a hindfoot alignment radiograph (Fig. 25-7).[158] Patients who have a congenital flatfoot undergo radiographs of the opposite foot for comparison.

Although the radiographs are normal in stage 1 disease, they are useful to rule out structural diagnoses that could be contributing to the patient's flatfoot and pain. Tarsal coalition, degenerative arthritis, accessory navicular, and old trauma, such as a Lisfranc injury, can be contributing to this constellation of symptoms. As the disorder progresses, characteristic changes are seen. In a general sense, lateral subluxation of the talonavicular joint is evident on the AP radiograph, and talonavicular joint sag is noted on the lateral radiograph. The lateral radiograph also provides useful information about the status of the first metatarsocuneiform joint because subluxation or arthritis of this joint surface can contribute to the flatfoot. Subluxation also occurs at the subtalar joint, manifested as an indistinct joint surface on the lateral film. Ankle radiographs can demonstrate arthritis and subfibular impingement.

To quantify these findings, measurements have been proposed that assist in static assessment of the disorder, while enabling the surgeon to follow progression. Sangeorzan et al[160] suggested that, on the lateral radiograph, the important parameters are the lateral talocalcaneal angle, the lateral talometatarsal angle, and the cuneiform height. The lateral talocalcaneal angle is indicated by a line drawn midway between the superior and inferior portions of the talar body and neck and a second line drawn midway between the superior and inferior portions of both the tuberosity and the sustentaculum tali (see Chapter 3). The lateral talometatarsal angle is measured using the same line through the talus as for the lateral talocalcaneal angle and a second line drawn along a point halfway between the superior and inferior portions of the proximal and distal metaphyseal–diaphyseal junction of the metatarsal (avoiding inconsistencies with the flares distally and proximally) (see Chapter 3). Cuneiform height is measured between the medial cuneiform and the fifth metatarsal base. Cuneiform height can also be measured between the medial cuneiform and the ground, which is less sensitive.

On the AP view, the important parameters are the talocalcaneal angle, the talometatarsal angle, and the articular congruity angle. The talocalcaneal angle uses a point midway between the medial and lateral articular surface and a second point midway between the margins of the talar neck. This line intersects with a line drawn along the lateral border of the calcaneus (see Chapter 3). The talometatarsal angle uses the talus as one axis (with the lines drawn in an identical fashion to that on the sagittal image). The second axis is drawn in the first metatarsal, midway between two points measured along the metaphyseal–diaphyseal junction (proximal and distal) (see Chapter 3).

The articular congruity angle is measured by first drawing a line connecting the articular margins of the talus and navicular. A perpendicular line is drawn at the midpoint of each line. The angle created by the intersection of these two lines represents talonavicular coverage (see Chapter 3). Normal values for these angles include an assessment by Gould,[64] who suggested that the lateral talometatarsal angle should fall between −4 degrees and +4 degrees. Saltzman[157] suggested that 95% of the population has a talocalcaneal angle of less than 12 degrees. The lateral talocalcaneal angle increases in patients with acquired flatfoot, as does the talometatarsal angle. Dyal[45] found the lowest correlation between

symptomatic and asymptomatic flatfeet was at the cuneiform-to-fifth metatarsal measurement, suggesting that this might be the best measurement to determine congenital pes planus versus adult acquired flatfoot. In addition, this measurement has the best interobserver reliability, making its consistency the most accurate measurement of flatfoot.

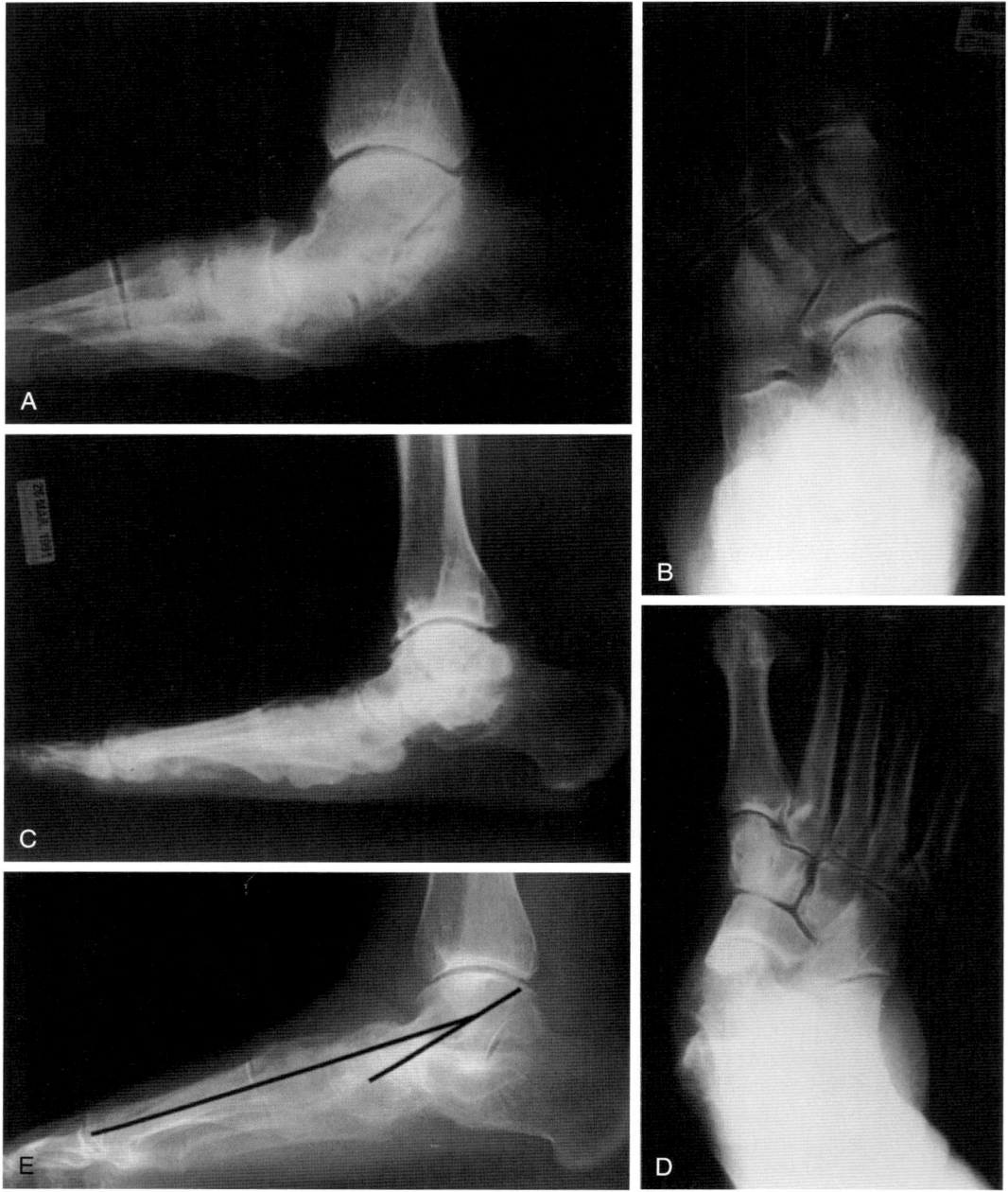

Figure 25-5 Radiographic findings associated with posterior tibial tendon dysfunction. **A** and **B,** Radiographs demonstrate significant talonavicular sag in the lateral radiograph and minimal abduction in the anteroposterior (AP) radiograph. **C** and **D,** Radiographs demonstrate minimal sag at the talonavicular joint on the lateral radiograph yet significant abduction on the AP radiograph. **E** and **F,** Moderate degree of sagging of the talonavicular joint in the lateral radiograph and abduction on the AP radiograph.

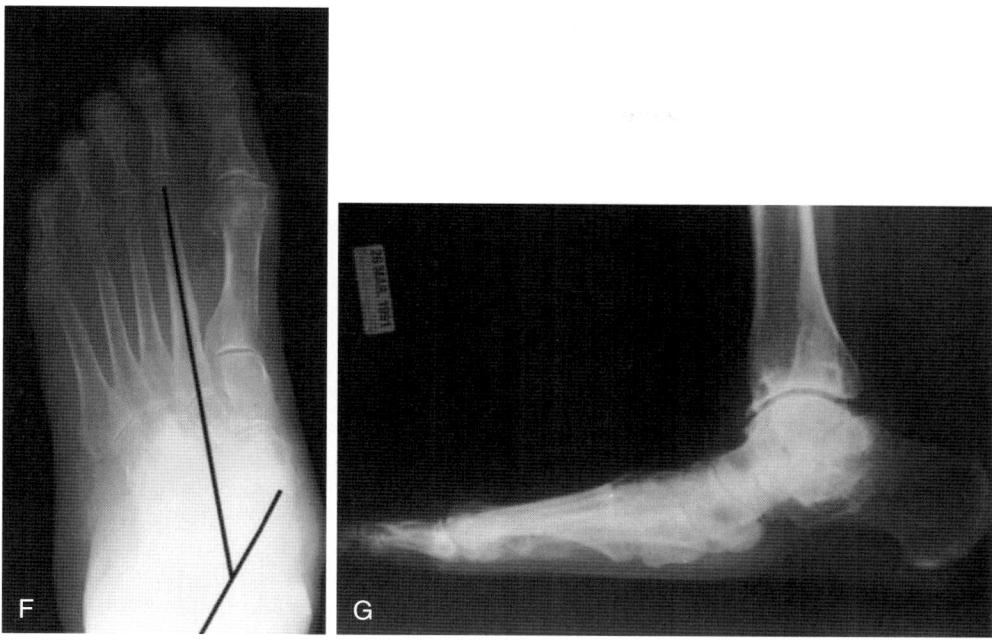

Figure 25-5, cont'd   G, Minimal changes at the talonavicular joint but a moderate sag at the naviculocuneiform joint.

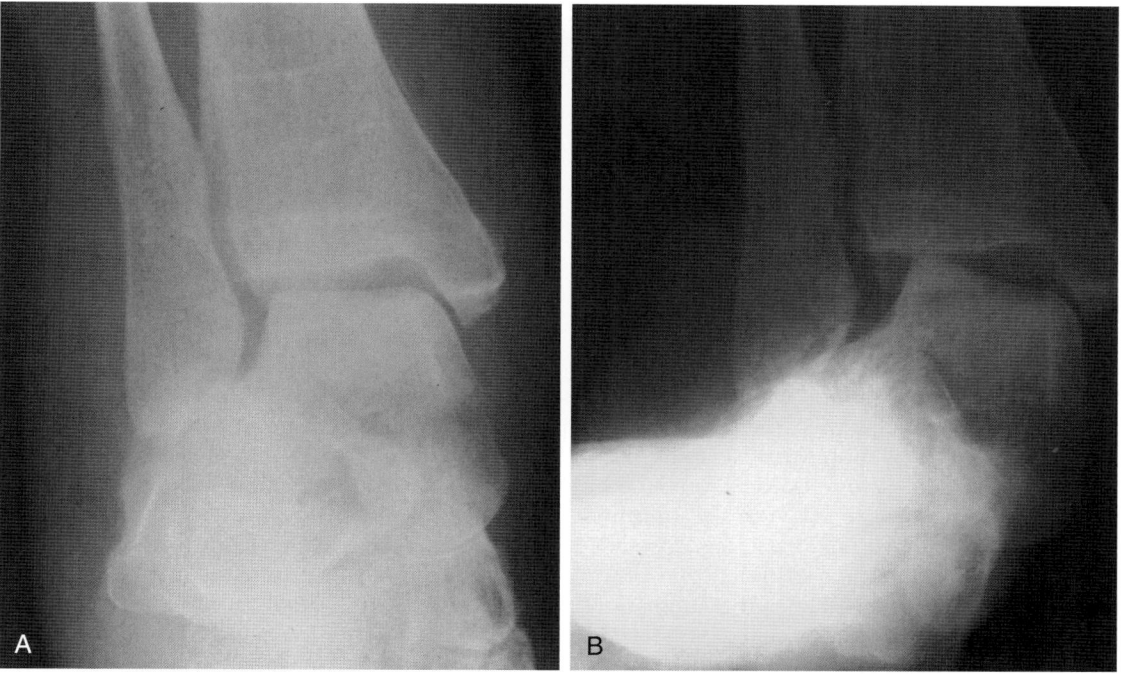

Figure 25-6   Ankle joint changes associated with posterior tibial tendon dysfunction. **A,** Anteroposterior (AP) non–weight-bearing radiograph of the ankle joint demonstrating slight talar tilt. **B,** Weight-bearing radiograph demonstrating significant valgus tilt associated with a marked valgus deformity of the calcaneus.

An alternative to angular measurements, as a radiographic indication to PTT dysfunction, was proposed by Pomeroy et al.[148] Linear measurements are made to quantify uncovering of the talar head upon the navicular. A bilateral standing AP radiograph of the feet is used to evaluate this congruence by choosing an arbitrary fixed point on the medial aspect of the talar head and connecting it to an arbitrary fixed point on the medial edge of the navicular. Using identical points on the opposite foot reveals a discrepancy in length in patients with acquired

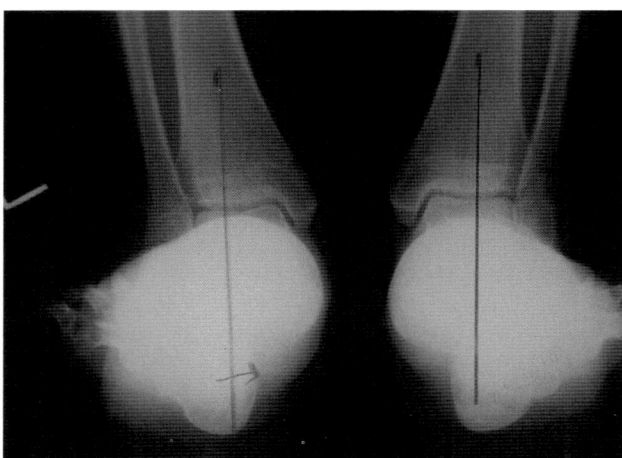

Figure 25-7 Axial radiograph of the hindfoot alignment view. This radiographic view is useful in determining the magnitude of valgus hindfoot deformity and thus planning the appropriate surgical intervention.

flatfoot. Lateral foot radiographs of both feet undergo a similar comparison through lines drawn from the base of the fifth metatarsal to the anterior-inferior corner of the medial cuneiform. This line is drawn perpendicular to the weight-bearing axis of the floor and decreases in patients with flatfoot. The final linear measurement involves use of a bilateral AP ankle radiograph. The total height of the ankle is measured by dropping a perpendicular line from the superior talus (in the ankle mortise) to the floor. Collapse from acquired flatfoot is evident by a decreased ankle height.

Magnetic Resonance Imaging and Computed Tomography

Advanced diagnostic modalities are also available. Before the advent of MRI and computed tomography (CT), tenography was the primary method for assessing ankle tendons.[186] Tenography is rarely used today because the clinician has less invasive and more sensitive and specific techniques for imaging soft tissue disorders. Tenography does show the tendon structure and reveals abnormal villous thickening of the tenosynovium in tenosynovitis. It is also adequate for determining disorders within the sheath, including entrapment and sheath compression. However, it does not allow direct visualization of the posterior tibial tendon; therefore partial ruptures or longitudinal split tears go undetected. Injections into the tendon sheath can be difficult, especially when adhesions obliterate the synovial space. Alexander et al[2] have shown that the results of tenography correlate poorly with the surgical findings. In addition, Hogan[79] explains that the flexor digitorum longus tendon, which lies directly medial to the posterior tibial tendon, can be injected inadvertently. On occasion, the two synovial sheaths communicate, giving false-negative results when true disorder exists.

CT scans show bony anatomy well, but they have limited soft tissue contrast resolution. Rosenberg et al[154] performed CT imaging on 49 patients with a suspected PTT rupture. By correlating surgical findings on these patients, they found CT was accurate 96% of the time in diagnosing and classifying the magnitude of tendon disruption. The authors were able to subclassify tendon damage into partial rupture (with tendon hypertrophy and longitudinal split tears versus tendon attenuation) and full-thickness rupture. They found periostitis of the posterior distal tibia along the course of the PTT in cases with rupture. This secondary phenomenon was noted in 68% of the study group, making it a useful adjunct in diagnosing PTT dysfunction.

Limitations, however, were noted. Longitudinal split tears were underrepresented by CT scanning, with CT missing both the magnitude and volume of such tears. In addition, CT demonstrated less fraying and degeneration of the PTT than was seen during surgical exploration, again underestimating the magnitude of the condition. Synovial inflammation was indistinguishable from damaged tendon, underestimating tenosynovitis. In this 1988 study, the authors predicted the newly developed MRI would supplant CT as a diagnostic modality for PTT dysfunction. Today, CT has value only if MRI is contraindicated.

MRI is an excellent modality for detecting sheath inflammation, soft tissue resolution, and anatomic detail of the tendon.[189] It is superior to CT for tendon definition, resolution of synovial fluid, soft tissue edema, and tissue degeneration.[153] Alexander et al[2] first discussed its usefulness in a 1987 case report on a 44-year-old patient with a complete rupture of her posterior tibial tendon, as diagnosed by MRI and confirmed at surgery. Rosenberg et al[153] found the sensitivity of MRI versus CT is 95% versus 90%, the specificity of MRI versus CT is 100% and 100%, and the accuracy of MRI versus CT is 96% versus 91%. Elusive longitudinal split tears not visualized on CT scanning were easily seen with MRI scanning. Thus the percentage of tears that were diagnosed and classified correctly was greater with MRI (73%) than with CT (59%).

The examination should take place with the patient supine and the ankle in a neutral and slightly plantarflexed position. Axial images are most useful in assessing size, shape, and internal content of the posterior tibial tendon. However, patient position is critical to obtaining good axial images. To negate the magic angle effect of MRI, a true axial plane perpendicular to the tendon at the level of the medial malleolus is required. The magic angle effect is noted on short-TE (T1-weighted) images, where the acute 55-degree angle of the PTT, as it exits the medial malleolus, creates simulated rupture on MRI. This effect is due to the ability of the excitable protons to move in limited planes of the tightly packed collagen of the posterior tibial tendon. This effect is not visualized on long-TE (T2-weighted) images. To negate this effect, an oblique axial image may be obtained by placing the image plane approximately 45 degrees between true axial and coronal image planes.[100] Anatomically, this plane is perpendicular to the posterior facet of the subtalar joint. In addition, the tendon is occasionally lost in the homogenous signal of the medial malleolus. By plantar flexing the ankle slightly, the relaxed tendon moves away from the bone, enhancing its signal. Careful evaluation of sagittal images can reveal the location of the tendon rupture and the length of tendon involved. This ability may be enhanced by rotating the ankle slightly medially during the examination.

Normal tendon substance on MRI appears as a black and homogenous signal with an ovoid shape on all spin-echo images. This appearance is due to the dense collagen within the posterior tibial tendon. The PTT is normally two to three times larger than the flexor digitorum longus tendon. A small amount of fluid within the sheath is normal, although it should not be more than 1 to 2 mm wide, and it should not be circumferential. In tenosynovitis, T2-weighted images show pronounced fluid surrounding the tendon and edema within the tendon sheath. The synovial effusion appears as a bright signal and is best seen on T2 images.[91]

The hallmark of tenosynovitis is a homogenous tendon with fluid in the tendon sheath. T1 images are useful for evaluating the synovial membrane and the substance of the PTT (Fig. 25-8). These structures are hypertrophied, and the PTT occasionally reaches sizes 5 to 10 times that of the adjacent flexor digitorum longus tendon. T1 images also evaluate intratendinous disorders by showing foci of increased signal, revealing longitudinal split tears.[91] The synovial sheath of the PTT ends before its insertion. Thus there is no true tenosynovitis noted distally. Increased signal around the tendon close to its insertion is peritendinitis and is not normal.

The width of the synovial sheath is significantly increased in stage 1 PTT tenosynovitis.[17] In stage 2 or 3 disease, it is less common to find a fluid-filled synovial sheath and tendon hypertrophy. These stages are more likely to reveal tendon disorders such as split tears, ruptures, and tendon elongation.[17] Thus MRI is especially useful for evaluation and diagnosis of stage 1 disease. MRI is more sensitive than surgical exploration in predicting disorders and successful surgical outcome.[91] MRI can detect an intrasubstance tear in the tendon that may be missed intraoperatively, leading to its predictive value.

Elongation of the tendon becomes apparent on MRI as the patient progresses to clinical stage 2 disease. The diameter of the tendon might in fact be less than the adjacent flexor digitorum longus tendon. When stage 3 deformity is reached, complete rupture is often visualized on T1 images. The inflammatory response may be absent in the tendon sheath, and mucinous degeneration may be apparent within the tendon gap. Findings in the lateral ankle may become apparent, recognized as sinus tarsi syndrome and subfibular impingement. MRI detects absence of the normal sinus tarsi fat signal with low signal on T1-weighted images. T1 images reveal fibrosis within the sinus tarsi and absence of the supporting talocalcaneal interosseous ligament and cervical ligament.[4] T2-weighted images can reveal increased signal consistent with edema in the sinus tarsi in less chronic conditions. Balen and Helms[4] found such changes in the sinus tarsi in 72% of patients who have PTT dysfunction (versus 36% of control patients scanned for ankle pain).

Other adjunct MRI findings in the syndrome of PTT dysfunction are valuable in planning surgical reconstruction. Wacker et al[183] studied the physiologic quality of both the posterior tibial and flexor digitorum longus muscle belly in patients with adult acquired flatfoot deformity. The authors found that in patients with a complete rupture of the posterior tibial tendon, the muscle belly underwent significant fatty infiltration. This nonfunctional muscle was noted within 10 months of the injury having created complete rupture. Those patients with posterior tibial tendinosis without complete rupture demonstrated a mean of 10.7% for atrophy of the muscle belly, with compensatory hypertrophy (mean, 17.2%) of the flexor digitorum longus muscle belly. The clinical implications of this study are discussed in the surgery section of this chapter.

The plantar calcaneonavicular ligament (spring ligament) has also been studied with MRI (Fig. 25-9). Yao[190] had independent radiologists evaluate MRI studies done *preoperatively* on patients who had intraoperative findings of spring ligament insufficiency. The MRI evaluations were done retrospectively, after definitive surgical confirmation of disorder. The control population in this series was patients without spring ligament disorder. The radiologists consistently found signal heterogeneity on axial short TE (T1-weighted) within the medial portion (superomedial calcaneonavicular) of the ligament only. Rather than finding an attenuated ligament, the medial ligament

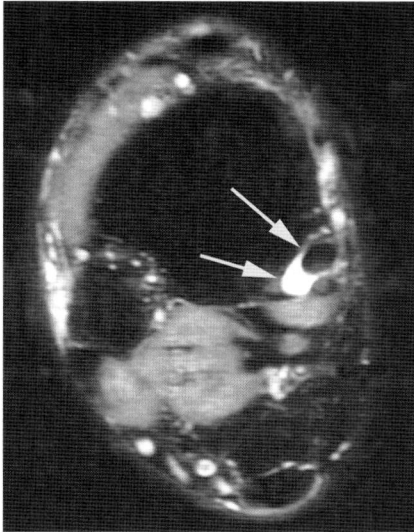

Figure 25-8 Magnetic resonance imaging demonstrates fluid *(arrows)* within the sheath of the posterior tibial tendon.

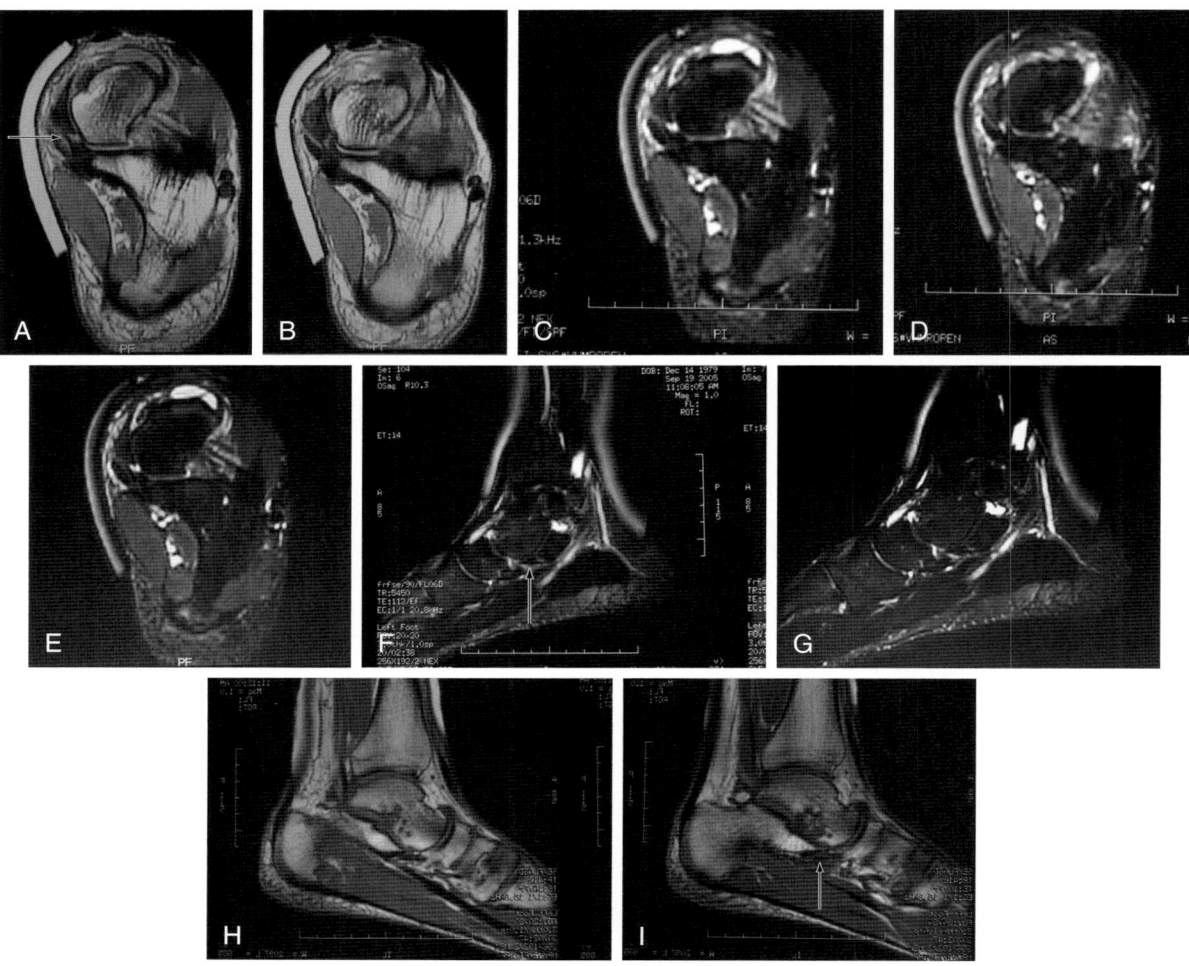

Figure 25-9 Magnetic resonance imaging (MRI) demonstrates a complete rupture of the superior calcaneal navicular portion of the spring ligament. **A** and **B,** T1 images reveal the ruptured ligament *(arrow)*. **C** to **E,** T2 images reveal increased signal at the site of rupture. **F** and **G,** The sagittal T2 images emphasize the lack of support of the talar head created by the rupture of the superior calcaneonavicular ligament. **H** and **I,** The sagittal T1 images show an attenuated and ruptured ligament.

was thickened to more than 5 mm. Poor correlation between radiologists was noted with the plantar (inferior calcaneonavicular) ligament. This ligament is inherently thin, and MRI evaluation was unreliable. Biomechanical studies demonstrate that this component of the ligament plays a minor role in statically stabilizing the longitudinal arch. Overall, the sensitivity for evaluation of the medial ligament was 54% to 77%, and the specificity was 100%. Note that this evaluation was done on chronic ligament disorders, not acute ruptures. In the latter scenario, the MRI diagnosis is more reliable because T2-weighted images demonstrate bright foci consistent with edema and hematoma.

Balen and Helms[4] found 92% of patients with advanced PTT dysfunction (MRI confirmed) had MRI changes consistent with superior calcaneonavicular ligament disorders. Using Yao's[190] criteria, they studied 25 patients with such disease noted in the posterior tibial tendon. Only 28% of the patients in the control group had disorders similar to spring ligament disorders.

Lateral hindfoot impingement (talocalcaneal or sub-fibular) can also be assessed via MRI.[40] Talocalcaneal impingement was seen at the opposing surfaces of the lateral talar process and the lateral wall of the calcaneus, manifesting as marrow edema, cystic change, or sclerosis. Subfibular impingement was evident as soft tissue entrapment or osseous contact between the fibula and calcaneus, or marrow edema of the fibula. MRI findings worsened as the degree of PTT disruption increased, although this was a trend, and not of statistical significance. Despite the non–weight-bearing nature of this form of imaging, the authors were able to detect the magnitude of hindfoot valgus deformity, which was statistically significant in patients with both talocalcaneal and subfibular impingement, rather than each component in isolation. Finally, peroneal tendon subluxation was evident in only advanced hindfoot valgus.

The accuracy of MRI has been supported. Khoury[100] reported that 9 of 11 preoperative MRI diagnoses of various stages of PTT disorder were confirmed through surgical visualization. Such pathologic states included peritendinitis, tendinosis, and partial and complete ruptures. Peritendinitis is found as fluid about the tendon sheath with a normal tendon. Tendinosis is noted with tendon thickening with or without intrasubstance degeneration or deep tears. Partial tears, normally within the portion of the tendon with tendinosis, are distinguished by reaching the surface of the tendon, whereas tears not reaching the surface are classified as tendinosis. Complete rupture reveals a gap filled with fluid or fibrous tissue, as noted above. These four entities were clearly discernible on MRI.

Ultrasonography

Ultrasonography is now recognized as a cost-effective and accurate modality for evaluating tendon disorders in the foot and ankle.[83] A normal tendon appears hyperechoic, and a degenerated tendon is hypoechoic on ultrasound imaging (Fig. 25-10). Normal PTT diameter is 4 to 6 mm.[129] Tenosynovitis manifests with large amounts of fluid surrounding the tendon.[17] A hypoechoic rim visible on the longitudinal sonogram and a target sign on transverse sonogram is pathognomonic for PTT tenosynovitis. The term *target sign* was coined to describe a homogeneous, continuous hyperechoic tendon surrounded by a hypoechoic fluid halo. The halo represents excessive surrounding synovial fluid. Ultrasonography can also reveal a swollen tendon, an irregular tendon contour, longitudinal split tears, heterogeneous echogenicity, and surrounding hypoechoic shadows in patients with tenosynovitis. In contrast, tendon rupture features an empty tibial groove at the level of the medial malleolus.[83]

Chen and Liang[17] have shown that on average the PTT measures 3.30 mm in diameter. A tendon afflicted with tenosynovitis averages 4.61 mm. In addition, an increased synovial sheath diameter is noted in tenosynovitis and is a reliable marker for predicting intraoperative findings. The average diameter of a normal tendon sheath is 3.64 mm. In tenosynovitis, the measurement increases to 7.24 mm ($P < .0001$). Therefore ultrasonography will detect both a mildly enlarged tendon and a significant increase in sheath diameter resulting from fluid accumulation.

Chen and Liang[17] confirmed their ultrasound findings through surgical exploration. All 14 patients with PTT tenosynovitis requiring surgical exploration had an intact PTT and surrounding fluid and hypertrophic tenosynovium. Although this study entertained no false-positive results, the authors caution that misdiagnosis may be common in the hands of an inexperienced examiner reviewing longitudinal scans. The authors suggest that ultrasonography is superior to MRI based on speed, convenience, low cost, and its dynamic nature. This study is limited, however, by lack of double-blinding because the surgeon was given the ultrasound results in advance of the operation, potentially influencing intraoperative findings.

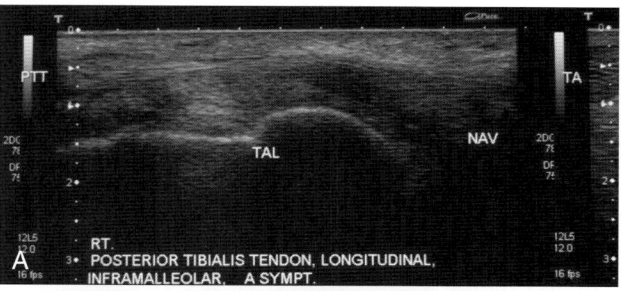
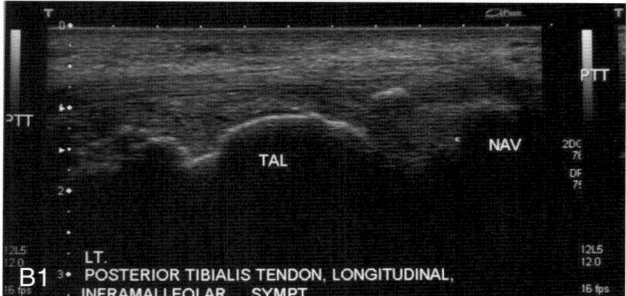
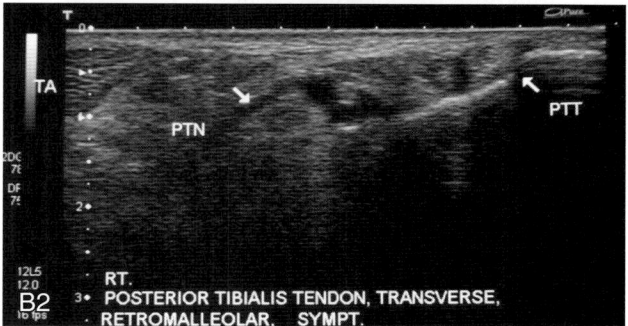
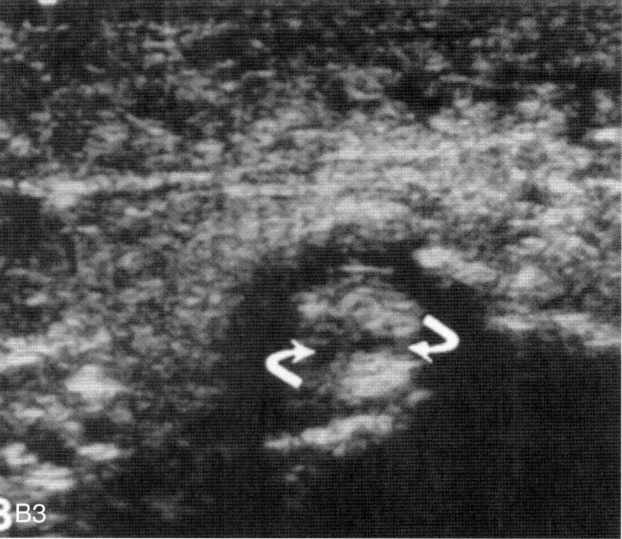

Figure 25-10 Ultrasound examination of posterior tibial tendon. **A,** Normal longitudinal orientation of the posterior tibial tendon, medial to the talus *(TAL)* and navicular *(NAV)*. **B1** to **B3,** Pathologic posterior tibial tendon. The pathologic tendon has a longitudinal split tear within it *(arrows)*. **(B3,** From Miller SD, Van Holsbeeck M, Boruta PM, et al: Ultrasound in the diagnosis of posterior tibial tendon pathology. *Foot Ankle Int* 17:555-558, 1996.)

Studies have suggested that sensitivity and specificity for ultrasonography is similar to those for MRI.[129] Miller et al[129] surgically explored 17 patients with PTT tenosynovitis who had undergone preoperative ultrasound examination. The authors found ultrasonography successful in confirming intraoperative findings in all 17. They concurrently performed preoperative MRI examinations on these 17 patients. Two patients with tendon damage visible on surgical exploration had normal tendon readings on MRI.

Gerling et al[57] performed a double-blinded study on fresh cadaveric feet, creating longitudinal split tears in the posterior tibial tendon. Four separate scans were done on each cadaveric limb, the first with no tear, followed by progressively creating a split tear of 1, 2, and 4 cm in length. Each limb was evaluated with ultrasonography and MRI. The authors found the sensitivity of MRI versus ultrasonography was 73% versus 69%; the specificity of MRI versus ultrasonography was 69% versus 81%; and the accuracy of MRI versus ultrasonography was 72% versus 72%. Interobserver reliability was excellent with MRI (0.86) and only fair with ultrasonography (0.37). It remains difficult to interpret the clinical value of this study because the absence of in vivo perfusion and physiologic tendon function alters the natural environment of these radiographic modalities. The significant deviation from prior studies evaluating MRI sensitivity and specificity echo the questionable validity of this cadaveric study.

Premkumar et al[150] studied 44 tendons in patients with a clinical diagnosis of PTT dysfunction. The authors found the most useful criteria for diagnosing tendinosis and peritendinosis on MRI was enhancement of the tendon. On color-flow Doppler sonography, increased flow was most useful in this regard. Under these criteria, the positive predictive value of MRI was 83%. The positive predictive value of ultrasonography was 90%. When directly compared with MRI, the ability of ultrasonography to diagnose tendinopathy was 80% sensitive and 90% specific. The ability of ultrasonography to diagnose peritendinosis was 90% sensitive and 80% specific. Again, these results are difficult to interpret because no surgical exploration was performed, and thus no pathologic specimens were available to confirm diagnosis.

Additional comparative imaging between MRI and ultrasonography in patients with spring ligament pathology are supplied by Harrish et al.[149] The authors evaluated sixteen patients with tibialis posterior tendon dysfunction, comparing the readings on both MRI and ultrasonography. The studies were symmetric in their interpretation 94% of the time. Within statistical significance, they were equivalent in diagnosing spring ligament disruption in patients with preexisting PTT insufficiency.

These clinical data suggest that ultrasonography is as effective a modality as MRI in the diagnostic algorithm of PTT dysfunction. However, careful analysis of the data finds flaws in the experimental design. Thus readers must interpret this conclusion with caution and use the most effective modality available at their institution. These

thoughts were echoed by Wertheimer,[186] who cautions that interpretation of ultrasonography requires an experienced examiner, which is not always necessary for MRI interpretation.

Magnetic Resonance Imaging Staging

Conti et al[24] have developed a classification system based on MRI observations.

Type 1, consistent with tenosynovitis, is manifested as synovial swelling, occasional fine longitudinal splits, and a homogenous black signal (tendon) on T1 images. This type is divided into two subcategories: type 1A has one or two fine longitudinal splits, and type 1B has increased splits and mild surrounding fibrosis.

Type 2 disease consists of a narrower tendon signal, with evidence of intramural degeneration. This appears as a gray substance within the black tendon signal on T1 images. Wider longitudinal split tears are present. The tendon can taper in the diseased segment and appear bulbous at the extremes of this segment.

Type 3 is manifested as diffuse synovial swelling and prominent, uniform degeneration. This type is also divided into two subcategories: type 3A has uniform degeneration and a few strands of intact tendon, and type 3B has complete rupture and replacement by scar tissue in the gapped segments.

This study compared the above-mentioned magnetic resonance grading with intraoperative surgical grading according to prior clinical classification schemes. Conti et al[24] found that 55% of their patients had less extensive disease within the PTT upon direct visualization than predicted by the MRI classification. The authors found, however, that their MRI classification system did a better job of predicting successful surgical outcome than the surgical classification system. The value of this analysis, however, is clouded because the surgical techniques used (side-to-side flexor digitorum longus tendon anastomosis to the diseased posterior tibial tendon) is no longer performed as an isolated procedure in PTT dysfunction of the magnitude seen in this study. Thus it is impossible, currently, to state that their MRI classification system is a better predictor of surgical outcome than surgical grading because the techniques used at present have a far better clinical outcome. The value of MRI classification remains in question.

Treatment

Conservative Treatment
In most instances, conservative therapy should be instituted before contemplating surgical reconstruction for PTT insufficiency. Although a standard protocol has not been developed and would inherently depend on the stage of the disease when the patient presents at the office, common themes are recognized that involve rest of the tendon, medication, physical therapy, and management of orthotics and braces.

Resting or relieving the tension on the PTT may be done in a graduated fashion. The first level of rest involves a rigid stirrup brace or lace-up sport brace. This type of brace crosses the ankle joint and thus limits excursion of the posterior tibial tendon. However, it offloads only the inversion component to PTT activation, ignoring restriction on sagittal motion.[117] Thus the PTT still glides within the sheath, allowing further aggravation from inflammation and repetitive stress. Still, in more mild conditions, unloading inversion is sufficient for pain relief.

If the first level of rest is ineffective, patients may wear a CAM (controlled ankle movement) walker boot. This device has the added benefit of eliminating motion in the sagittal plane. It retains the advantage over casting by allowing simultaneous functional rehabilitation. A below-knee cast, however, provides ultimate tendon rest and absolute compliance. Calf atrophy can compromise rehabilitation, and risk of deep venous thrombosis is present with the below-knee cast. The weight-bearing status with either device is predicated on pain relief. Patients may bear weight in a CAM boot or cast if they are completely asymptomatic. In fact, Blake and colleagues[7] emphasize that protected weight bearing encourages tendon repair by organizing new collagen along the direction of stress. The time frame of use ranges from 4 to 6 weeks.[23,117,120]

Antiinflammatory medication is used simultaneously with rest of the tendon. With controversy surrounding complications of some nonsteroidal antiinflammatory medications, the orthopedist should determine the appropriate medicine for each patient in conjunction with the patient's primary care physician. It is suggested that the patient take the medicine as prescribed for a complete 2-week course. This will allow appropriate serum concentrations to be established, and continued ingestion will maintain this therapeutic level sufficiently to eliminate the inflammatory component to PTT tenosynovitis.

Oral corticosteroids, and for that matter, injectable corticosteroids, are not used in the author's practice. As suggested in the discussion of etiology, steroids can create local microvascular attenuation, further compromising healing of the insulted posterior tibial tendon. Johnson and Strom[89] felt that steroid injections were contraindicated because of accelerated tendon weakening. In fact, Holmes and Mann[80] reported that in an age-stratified population, 28% of the younger patients and 17% of the older patients with rupture of the PTT had a history of multiple steroid injections or a history of oral corticosteroid use.

Physical therapy can decrease inflammation surrounding the PTT in a nontoxic fashion. Iontophoresis, in which dexamethasone is repelled into the deep soft tissues with electrical current, has an antiinflammatory effect without documented risk of tendon rupture (Fig. 25-11). Cryotherapy, or ice massage, can be done as part of a home program and is especially useful after exercise or activity. Extravasation of humoral mediators is highest after exercise, and icing the tendon sheath slows this

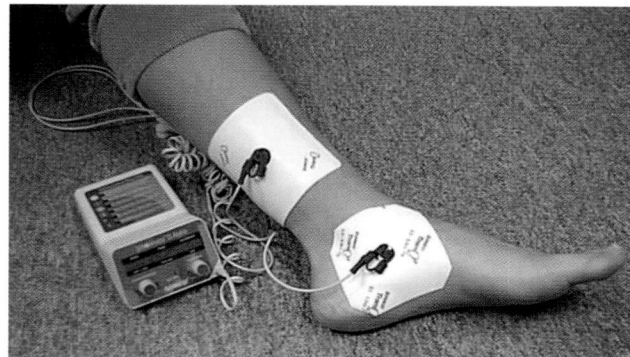

Figure 25-11 Ionotophoresis may decrease inflammation about the tendon through transcutaneous penetration of corticosteroid.

release. Ultrasonography is a heat-applied treatment and can exacerbate inflammatory symptoms, limiting its usefulness. Pulsed ultrasonography can have a role to reduce tendinopathy pain, and it does not have the consequence of increasing inflammation through heat.

Isolated strengthening of the PTT should be avoided until the above-mentioned treatment protocol eliminates the patient's pain. Aggressive strengthening used while the tendon remains painful will only exacerbate the symptoms and lengthen recovery. Selective activation of the PTT was explored by Kulig et al.[103] The authors used MRI to evaluate changes in muscle activation during exercise. They found the greatest increase in posterior tibial muscle activation occurred with resisted foot adduction by using resistance bands (Thera-Band) (activation increased 50%) compared with the surrounding musculature (average increase, 5%). Heel rise and resisted forefoot supination produced less than half of the activation of the posterior tibial muscle when compared with foot adduction. Anatomically, the perpendicular course of the PTT relative to the oblique midtarsal joint axis allows contraction of the muscle belly to adduct at the oblique midtarsal axis. Therapeutic strengthening must be focused on this plane of motion to maximize effectiveness.

Such therapeutic strengthening, along with stretching the gastrocsoleus complex, has shown proven benefit.[5] The authors, Kulig et al,[103] studied patients with PTT pain (both by palpation and ambulation) that lasted at least 3 months, combined with weakened single–toe-rise testing. Using validated tests, such as the Foot Function Index and Visual Analogue Scale (VAS), the authors assessed the ability of both eccentric posterior tibialis exercised and gastrocsoleus stretching (with knee bone extended and flexed) to relieve pain and improve function. It should be noted that an additional variable was introduced by asking the participants to wear orthotics for 90% of their waking hours. The authors added to their evaluation armamentarium by performing gray-scale ultrasonography and Doppler image acquisition to diagnose tendon abnormalities both before and after intervention. Although the studies lasted 6 months, it was noted that by 10 weeks posttreatment a significant improvement in symptoms (pain relief, function, and strength) allowed the patients to return to normal activities. However, this protocol did not change the character of the PTT with respect to neovascularization (a measure of inflammation) or morphology. Thus it remains to be seen whether symptoms recurred after the cessation of this research protocol because the authors did not study the population beyond 6 months.

Orthotic and brace management has been a large focus of attention in conservative management of PTT dysfunction. Simply put, attempts to lessen strain across the PTT may be instituted by elevating the medial arch and eliminating pronation. Before instituting orthotic management, it is important for the clinician to determine if the deformity is fixed or flexible because the orthotist will benefit from specific instructions in fitting this device, and patient satisfaction hinges on appropriate construction.[184] When the patient has a flexible deformity, the heel must be in a subtalar neutral position when the orthotist makes the mold for the orthosis. In this case, the orthosis will have true corrective power, lessening the stress applied to the posterior tibial tendon. If the deformity is rigid, the orthosis is molded in situ, without attempts at correction. In this situation, comfort and pain relief will be enhanced by not attempting to correct an uncorrectable foot.

Patients with milder deformities can achieve success with a semirigid orthosis with a medial heel wedge and a medial column post.[86] This may be particularly effective in stage 1 disease (Fig. 25-12). However, as the patient enters stage 2, with the deformity remaining flexible, a total-contact rigid orthosis or a University of California Biomechanics Laboratory (UCBL) brace may become necessary (Fig. 25-13). The UCBL brace has been shown to significantly affect the orientation and movement of the subtalar joint (and the ankle and knee joints) by reducing the degree and duration of abnormal pronation during the stance phase of gait.[112] The biomechanical principle of the UCBL is to stabilize the heel in neutral and prevent abduction of the forefoot. Abduction is blocked by building up the lateral border of the foot piece. This maneuver helps to reestablish the longitudinal arch.

Chao et al[16] used the UCBL with medial posting in patients with flexible deformities defined as less than 10

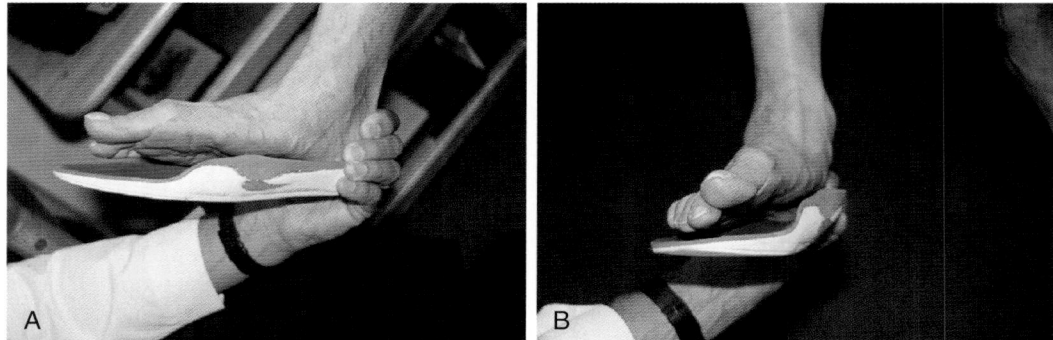

Figure 25-12 Orthotic device used for posterior tibial tendon dysfunction. **A,** Medial view demonstrates a fixed varus deformity of the forefoot, which requires medial posting to provide adequate support. **B,** Frontal view demonstrates the fixed forefoot varus in relation to the orthosis. The medial side of the foot requires adequate support for the orthotic device to be functional.

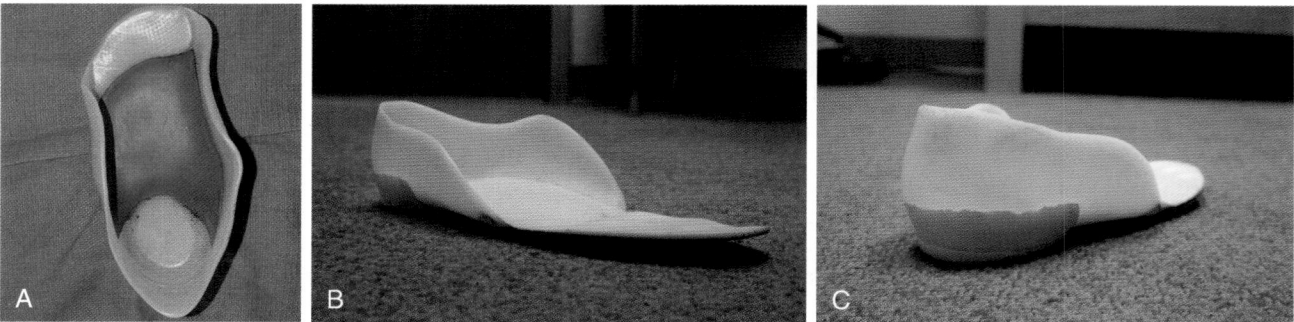

Figure 25-13 **A,** University of California Biomechanics Laboratory (UCBL) orthosis. This orthosis functions by stabilizing the heel in neutral and by building up the lateral wall of the device to prevent abduction of the forefoot, thereby helping to reestablish a longitudinal arch in the flexible foot. **B,** Note higher heel counter allowing better control of heel valgus. **C,** Note posting of posterior orthosis to assist with hindfoot correction.

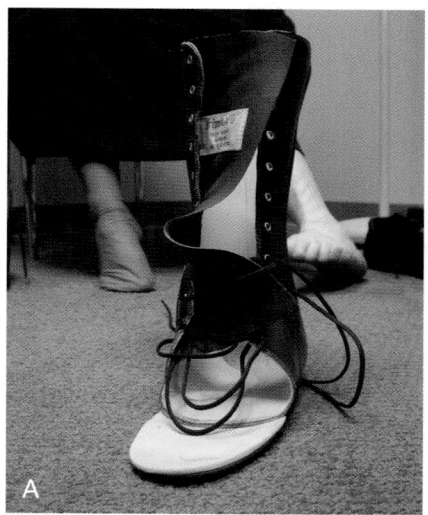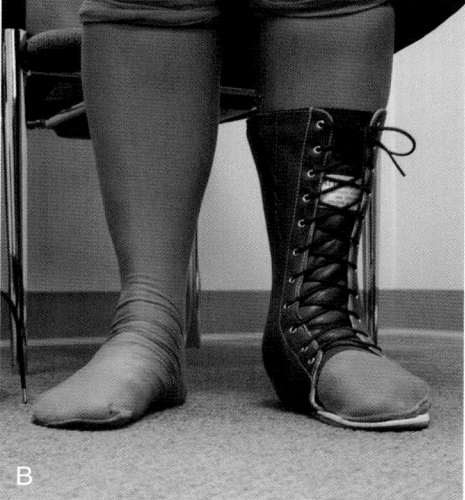

Figure 25-14 A, The Arizona brace is a lace up corset that crosses the ankle joint to provide increased stability preventing collapse of the medial column. **B,** Clinical use of the Arizona brace.

degrees of residual forefoot varus in a subtalar neutral position. Those with rigid deformities were treated with a molded solid-ankle ankle–foot orthosis (AFO). This study did not specifically look at the effectiveness of the UCBL brace; rather, its purpose was to assess the success of brace management for PTT dysfunction. The authors found that 67% of patients achieved a good-to-excellent result with both braces (UCBL or AFO) as a nonoperative adjunct to treating the condition.

Augustin et al[3] evaluated the use of the Arizona brace, first introduced in 1988, in nonoperative management of PTT dysfunction (Fig. 25-14). Unlike the UCBL, this device has no significant impact on stabilizing the hindfoot, but it can restore the arch and midfoot kinematics. Augustin[3] studied 21 patients who had stage 1, 2, and 3 disease and wore the brace an average of 10 hours per day. All patients with stage 1 and 2 disease showed pain relief referable to the brace, and 60% of patients with stage 3 disease showed similar improvement. Overall, 90% demonstrated statistically significant improvement with the Arizona brace. This thorough study evaluated patients with three separate scoring systems: the American Orthopaedic Foot and Ankle Society (AOFAS) Hindfoot Score, the Foot Function Index, and the SF-36 Health Survey. With all three scoring systems, the Arizona brace demonstrated statistically significant improvement in patient outcome.

If patients reach stage 3 disease, where the deformity is rigid and potentially arthritic, accommodation rather than correction becomes the primary function of the brace. The orthosis or brace is not molded in subtalar neutral. A more supportive device for both the ankle and the foot, such as a thermoplastic solid-ankle AFO, may be required for pain relief (Fig. 25-15). A variety of additional braces, such as the Marzano articulated ankle brace, have been attempted with success in cases of more advanced PTT dysfunction. Patients in stage 4, with

arthritic ankle symptoms, require a nonarticulated brace for comfort, such as a solid-ankle AFO. Care must be taken to avoid pressure over bony prominences in patients with more severe valgus deformities. Attempting to correct such a deformity by molding the AFO to negate ankle valgus can place undue pressure across the lateral malleolus, hindfoot, or fifth metatarsal base, causing pain or ulceration.

The effectiveness of an AFO in controlling forefoot abduction has been questioned by Neville and Lemley.[112] These authors studied the ability of a custom AFO (both solid and articulated), an over-the-counter AFO, and a regular shoe (as a control device) to correct a variety of foot postures adopted in stage 2 PTT dysfunction. Throughout the gait cycle, all three devices were found to be no better than the control shoe in correcting forefoot abduction. Hindfoot inversion was only controlled significantly with the articulated AFO. This study led to concern that advanced bracing technologies were not correcting all planes of deformity, and, as such, could lead to failure in treatment or progression of the disorder. This finding is supported by additional data in the literature.[82]

Footwear modifications can enhance conservative treatment by stabilizing the foot, that is, by limiting pronation and strain on the posterior tibial tendon. Measuring the offset heel area can be done with the patient standing in the shoes to be modified, with equal weight placed on both feet.[172] A straight ruler drops from the medial malleolus to the floor (perpendicular to the floor). This line forms a triangle with a second line drawn to the base of the shoe and a third line drawn from the base of the shoe to the malleolus. This triangle is the offset heel area, which is filled in on the shoe to establish stabilization of the longitudinal arch. According to Streb and Marzano,[172] this offset should be approximately two thirds of the height of the medial shoe quarter. In

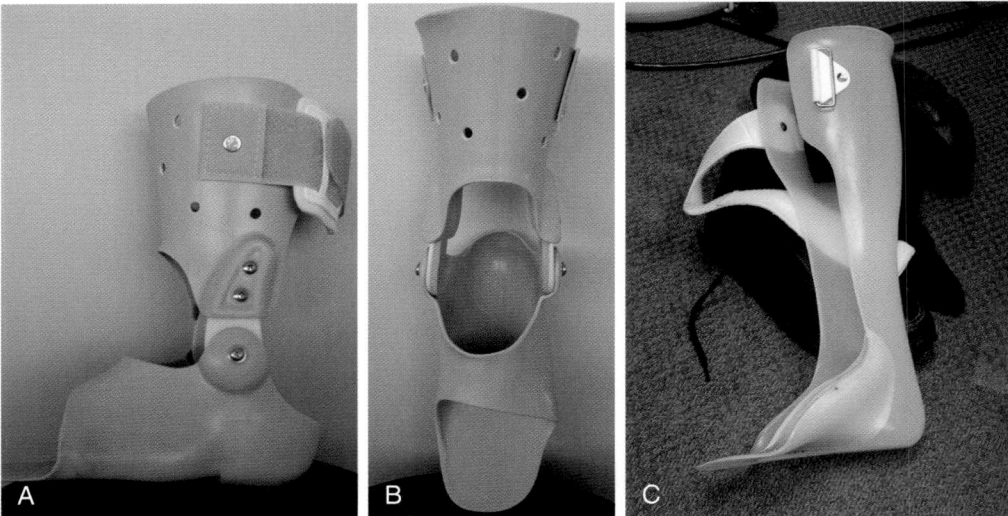

Figure 25-15 An ankle–foot orthosis (AFO). **A,** This device can be used to stabilize both the ankle and the foot in patients with stage 3 disease. **B,** The foot piece can be molded to provide support similar to a University of California Biomechanics Laboratory (UCBL) orthosis. **C,** Alternatively, a solid ankle foot orthosis can be used in more advanced, stage 3 disease to provide absolute stabilization.

addition, the offset can be made more effective by adding $\frac{1}{8}$-inch to $\frac{1}{4}$-inch additional medial post. Other footwear modifications include flanged heels, extended Thomas heels, and posting the medial heel and sole of the shoe from $\frac{1}{4}$ inch to $\frac{1}{2}$ inch to create support from heel to toe.

Often overlooked in the athlete with PTT dysfunction is the ability of appropriate shoe management to limit pain and lessen recurrence of tenosynovitis. According to Conti,[23] athletes should wear a running shoe with a flared heel and not run more than 400 miles on any one pair of shoes. Midfoot cushioning significantly dissipates after 400 miles, resulting in less arch support, less ability to control pronation, and increased tension on the posterior tibial tendon.

Combining orthotic management with a concentrated, aggressive exercise program has support in lessening symptoms of PTT dysfunction, as noted by Alvarez et al.[156] The authors evaluated 47 consecutive patients with stage 1 or 2 PTT dysfunction. No advanced diagnostic imaging was used in this study to quantify tendon disease. An above-ankle articulated device (70%) or orthotic (30%) was used in combination with a high-repetition strengthening and stretching therapy and home program over a 4-month interval (median). The authors considered a successful outcome to be 90% improvement in strength, manifested as the ability to perform 50 single-limb rises without pain and ambulate 100 feet on toes, among other criteria. Their methods demonstrated statistical significance with respect to said strength, and 89% were satisfied after the conclusion of treatment (although only 83% had successful subjective and objective outcomes).

Some authors[85] have suggested that conservative treatment has a limited role in PTT dysfunction because it gives no relief and can allow the condition to worsen.

However, most authors agree that unless a severe structural deformity is present, a 3- to 6-month trial of conservative management is indicated for PTT dysfunction.[7,147,155,174] The treating physician must pay careful attention to the patient, however, to look for signs of progressive deformity. The only circumstance that can cause the clinician to consider operative intervention sooner is in patients afflicted with seronegative spondyloarthropathy and PTT tenosynovitis. Myerson et al[139] suggest that failure of conservative care over a 6-week period should prompt surgical tenosynovectomy to prevent potential tendon rupture.

Surgical Treatment for Stage 1 Dysfunction
TENOSYNOVECTOMY
Indications
Although indications are defined for tenosynovectomy of the posterior tibial tendon, the procedure is often not necessary. Symptoms often resolve with conservative treatment. Still, in refractory cases, tenosynovectomy is indicated as an isolated procedure in patients with persistent inflammatory symptoms without perceptible deformity of the hindfoot. In stage 1 disease, length of the PTT is normal, and thus repair of the tendon is limited to small longitudinal split tears within the tendon. Timing of tenosynovectomy is influenced by the suspected cause of the condition. Patients with florid tenosynovitis resulting from conditions such as the seronegative spondyloarthropathies benefit from tenosynovectomy after a 6-week trial of conservative care.[139] In contrast, patients with more classic stage 1 disease—inflammation resulting from mechanical phenomena or more advanced age—can continue conservative care for up to 3 months before tenosynovectomy is considered. There is some

consideration toward performing tendoscopy to treat stage 1 PTT dysfunction, as noted by Khazen and Khazen.[99] The authors used a 3.5-mm arthroscopic shaver to debride the tendon. Eight of nine patients showed subjective and objective improvement, though no measurement criteria is provided in this study. However, given the limited critical support for this technique in the literature, only the open procedure will be considered below.

Contraindications

The main contraindication to performing an isolated tenosynovectomy is disease within the substance of the posterior tibial tendon. Patients with degenerative changes or intrasubstance rupture of the PTT require more advanced procedures. Static deformity apparent through clinical and radiographic examination also warrants more advanced procedures.

There is recent evidence that repair of the PTT without flexor digitorum longus tendon transfer is valid even under circumstances where the tendon demonstrates more significant splitting or tearing. High-level dancers require strong flexor digitorum longus tendon strength in their lesser toes to achieve demi-point, and thus sacrificing that tendon in transfer may compromise their career.[36] As such, Deland and Hamilton[36] successfully performed repair rather than sacrifice the posterior tibial tendon, allowing the dancer's toe return to 90% function under guarded circumstances. Career choice plays a part in operative decision making under select circumstances.

Preoperative Evaluation

Direct palpation over the PTT medially elicits pain. The medial ankle might feel boggy or fluctuant over the posterior tibial tendon. Strength testing is normal, although repetitive single–heel rises can reproduce the patient's symptoms of pain. Clinical inspection reveals symmetric feet and ankles, without hindfoot valgus or forefoot abduction. When viewed from behind, however, there may be asymmetric posterior swelling of the medial ankle on the affected side. Radiographs are symmetric with the uninvolved side, although MRI reveals fluid within the tendon sheath on T2-weighted images and a possible longitudinal split tear within the tendon on T1-weighted images. No mucinous degeneration is visible within the substance of the tendon.

Preoperative Planning

Extensive preparation is not required for a tenosynovectomy. The surgeon should review the preoperative MRI or ultrasound for a potential longitudinal split tear. This is a soft tissue procedure, and thus requests for hardware or power equipment are not necessary.

Surgical Technique

1. The patient is placed in a supine position. The normal external rotation of the extremity provides adequate exposure of the medial aspect of the foot. If that is not the case, placing a rolled bump under the opposite hip provides excellent external rotation of the involved extremity.

2. A thigh tourniquet is suggested to improve visualization of the inflamed tenosynovium.

3. The incision is centered along the course of the posterior tibial tendon. The length of the incision is from the navicular insertion to approximately 4 cm proximal to the tip of the medial malleolus.

4. The tendon sheath is opened with a knife and incised with scissors. In patients with systemic conditions, there is often an effusion of fluid. Patients with degenerative disease causing PTT insufficiency do not have an effusion of fluid.

5. Synovitis is visible as reddish-brown friable tissue adherent to the lining of the tendon sheath as well as to the tendon itself. All such tissue must be removed (Fig. 25-16).

6. The tendon itself is carefully inspected. The surgeon evaluates the tendon for fusiform thickening and visible fissures. In particular, the surgeon must inspect the undersurface of the tendon because friction in this location often causes one or multiple split tears. If a fissure or split tear is noted, it should be repaired with a tubalization suture technique.

7. The surgeon must check the excursion of the tendon. As noted above, the normal excursion of the PTT is 1 to 2 cm. Excursion is easily detectable by marking the tendon at the apex of the medial malleolus and applying manual traction. A definitive number may be measured. If the tendon does not demonstrate this excursion, it is not a stage 1 deformity and therefore requires more aggressive intervention.

8. With respect to disorders, the PTT should be inspected for avulsion from its insertion on the navicular. Although it may be tempting to simply repair the tendon directly to the navicular, often this is not feasible because of the limited excursion of the tendon and thus the higher failure rate after primary repair. In this instance, a flexor digitorum longus tendon transfer is performed, followed by a side-to-side tenodesis with the nascent posterior tibial tendon. This is the only instance where the native PTT may be preserved because the tendon itself has no intrasubstance disorders.

9. The sheath is then reapproximated in its entirety, preventing dislocation in the postoperative period. If a tourniquet was used, it is important to deflate it before closure to prevent copious scar tissue from compromising the result. The subcutaneous tissue and skin are closed, and the patient is placed in a sugar-tong plaster splint with a posterior mold or in a short-leg cast.

Postoperative Care

The goal of the postoperative period is to rapidly mobilize the patient (relatively) to limit scar tissue accumulation, maximize excursion, and minimize calf atrophy. The splint or cast is removed at 10 days after surgery, and the

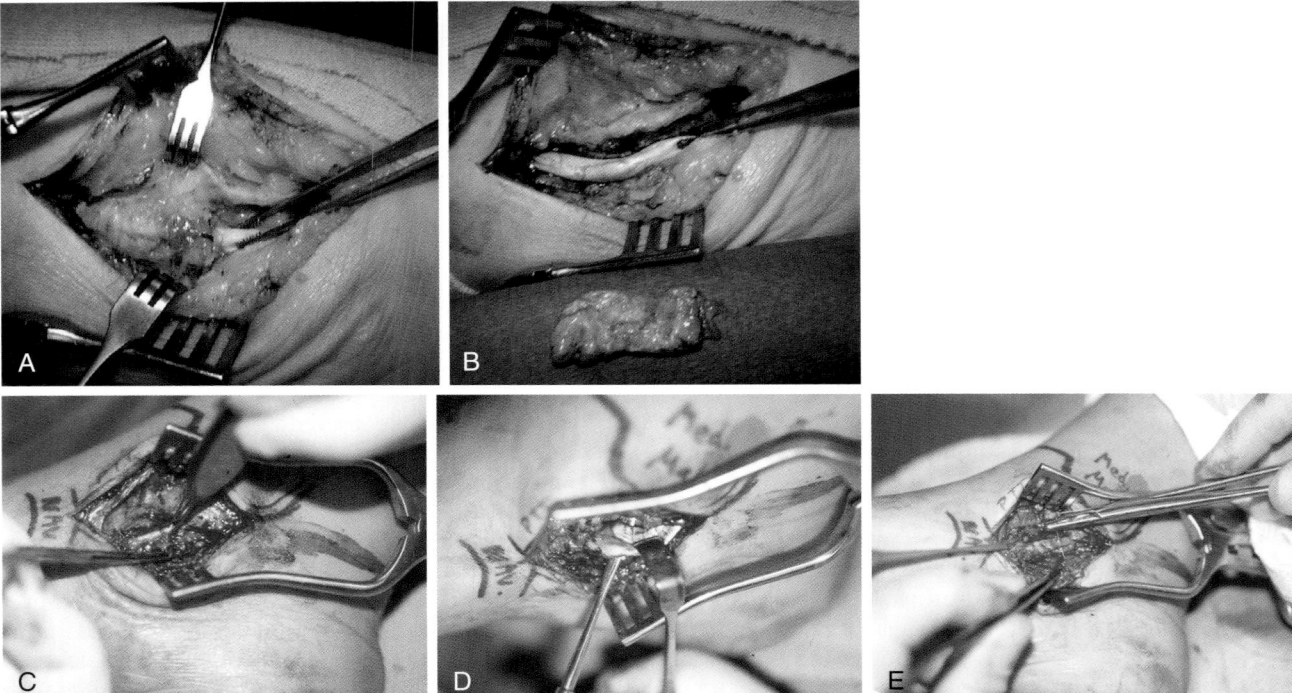

Figure 25-16 Synovitis of the posterior tibial tendon. **A,** Severe synovial proliferation about the posterior tibial tendon. Forceps are on the tendon. **B,** Appearance of the tendon after synovectomy. Synovial tissue that was encircling the tendon is below the wound. **C,** Less significicant synovitis can still reveal disease beneath the inflamed tissue, as this tenosynovectomy illustrates. **D,** The surgeon must inspect the undersurface of the tendon for a longitudinal split tear. **E,** This type of split tear is repaired by tubularizing the tendon at the site of the defect.

sutures are removed. The patient is given a walker boot and begins full weight bearing in this device.

The patient begins physical therapy, with attention directed toward mobilizing the tendon within the sheath. Passive and active range-of-motion therapy begins. Upon complete healing of the surgical incision, deep massage commences to prevent scar accumulation, and iontophoresis may be used to limit inflammation around the tendon sheath. If scar tissue begins to develop, ultrasonography may be used to combat it.

The boot is removed by 6 weeks after surgery to limit calf atrophy and maximize the functional outcome.

Results and Complications

Funk et al[55] performed the above-mentioned procedures on 19 patients with stage 1 disease. In this 1986 paper, the authors found that 12 patients experienced complete pain relief, four had minor pain, and three had persistent moderate or severe pain. Subjectively, 11 felt significant improvement, 5 were somewhat better, and 3 were the same.

Four patients failed the surgery; three of these patients presented with a complete or partial avulsion of the PTT off of the navicular insertion. The authors postulate that preexisting deformity was not recognized at the time of surgery and that although the tendon proximal to the insertional rupture appeared normal, in fact it was not.

Two of these patients later required triple arthrodesis to correct the deformity and eliminate the pain. This honest assessment of their data stresses that the correct surgical procedure must be chosen for this condition. The surgeon must recognize the preoperative deformity and critically assess the quality of the PTT intraoperatively. Failure to do so will result in less-than-adequate surgery and subsequently an unsatisfied patient.

Myerson et al[139] evaluated 76 patients with stage 1 disease caused by seronegative spondyloarthropathies or by degenerative conditions. Fourteen of these patients underwent tenosynovectomy. All reported both subjective and objective improvement after the debridement. Just more than half (57%) were afflicted by seronegative disease. It was clear to the authors that patients with seronegative disorders require earlier surgical debridement if they fail to respond to conservative measures. This type of tenosynovitis was found to be more aggressive intraoperatively and thus had a higher propensity to cause rupture of the PTT if left untreated.

Teasdall and Johnson[177] evaluated 19 patients undergoing tenosynovectomy for stage 1 disease. Fourteen patients experienced complete pain relief, and two complained of moderate-to-severe pain postoperatively. Again, this operation did not bring 100% pain relief to this population because only 84% felt "much better" after the procedure. Two patients required subtalar arthrodesis at a later date for progressive deformity and continued pain. These results mirror Johnson's previous work on stage 1 disease and the need for a careful preoperative and intraoperative assessment of the disorder before performing a simple tenosynovectomy.

Crates and Richardson[29] evaluated seven patients with stage 1 dysfunction who underwent tenosynovectomy. Three patients required simultaneous repair of a split tear or fissure. None had an inflammatory arthropathy. Follow-up averaged 3.5 months, through which six out of seven patients were pain free. The seventh patient had significant intrasubstance degeneration of the PTT at the time of surgery. The authors still proceeded with a tenosynovectomy and repair of a degenerative split tear. This patient developed progressive deformity and pain, necessitating a lateral column lengthening procedure and flexor digitorum tendon transfer at 1 year after the index procedure. Once again, the tendon must be accurately assessed intraoperatively, with advancement to a more aggressive procedure if indicated. Failure to do so will result in a poor outcome and necessitate additional surgery.

McCormack et al[125] reviewed eight competitive athletes with stage 1 disease who underwent tenosynovectomy at an average age of 22 years. Average time from initial evaluation by the authors to surgical intervention was 8 weeks. One patient required simultaneous repair of a longitudinal split tear in the PTT. All were allowed to return to sports at 6 to 8 weeks postoperatively. No patient had tenderness or swelling about the PTT on follow-up examination. Telephone interviews were performed at an average of 22 months after the procedure. Seven athletes (88%) continued to participate at their sport without incident. One cited occasional pain while playing football competitively. The authors recommend early intervention in this subset of patients with stage 1 disease after an aggressive trial of conservative care.

Complications for tenosynovectomy of the PTT (and sheath) include infection, nerve damage causing permanent numbness, incisional wound necrosis, progression of deformity and tendon disease, and deep venous thrombosis.

Surgical Treatment for Stage 2 Dysfunction
The procedures for stage 2 dysfunction will be discussed in tandem. Flexor digitorum longus tendon transfer is rarely done as an isolated procedure. At the very least, it is performed in combination with a calcaneal osteotomy.

FLEXOR DIGITORUM LONGUS TENDON TRANSFER
Indications
Flexor digitorum longus (FDL) tendon transfer is indicated in stage 2 PTT dysfunction (Fig. 25-17 and Video Clip 116). Once incompetence of the PTT is demonstrated, the tendon is nonviable and the diseased segment is unsalvageable. To substitute for this ineffectual tendon, a transfer is required. The FDL tendon has been chosen

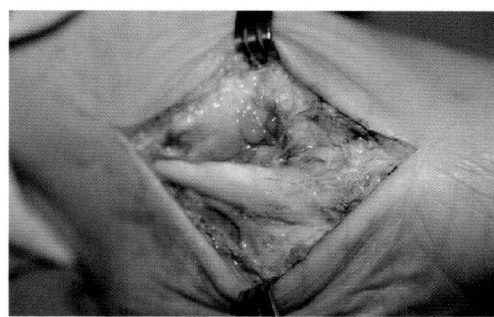

Figure 25-17 Partial avulsion at the insertion of the posterior tibial tendon into the navicular. Note the thickening of the tendon just proximal to the insertion and the way the tendon narrows more proximally.

as the most appropriate tendon to substitute for the PTT, for several reasons. First, the origin of the FDL is the posterior tibia, directly adjacent to the origin of the PTT. These tendons are directly adjacent to each other posterior to the medial malleolus. Thus they have the same line of pull. Second, although it has only 30% of the strength of the PTT, the FDL matches the strength of the peroneus brevis (the PTT antagonist). Thus it is capable of balancing the valgus-deforming pull of the peroneus brevis muscle. Third, the FDL and PTT are in-phase muscles (tendons), both functioning primarily in the midstance phase of gait. They differ in electromyographic activity, with the PTT functioning for a longer duration than the FDL through each stance phase.[115] Finally, the FDL is expendable because of its attachment to the flexor hallucis longus, maintaining lesser toe flexion. In addition, a majority of the push-off force during the terminal stance phase occurs through the flexor hallucis longus and the great toe, rather than through the lesser digits.

For the FDL tendon transfer to be functional, and thus indicated, two criteria must be met. First, there must be adequate subtalar joint motion to allow the FDL tendon to assist in overcoming the hindfoot valgus posture. In general, 15 degrees of subtalar inversion is required. The FDL tendon cannot invert against a fixed deformity at the subtalar joint. Second, transverse tarsal motion must also be supple. In the transverse plane, the patient must demonstrate at least 10 degrees of adduction to permit motion that can lock the transverse tarsal joint, allowing heel rise during gait.

Contraindications
Contraindications for the FDL tendon transfer include rigidity to subtalar and transverse tarsal motion to the degree mentioned above. In addition, a relative contraindication is a fixed forefoot varus deformity greater than 10 to 12 degrees. In the past, this was considered an absolute contraindication because this deformity would cause the subtalar joint to evert during midstance, negating the transfer. However, supplementary procedures, such as an opening-wedge medial cuneiform osteotomy,

a closing-wedge plantar-flexion first metatarsocuneiform arthrodesis, or a naviculocuneiform arthrodesis to correct the fixed forefoot varus, can establish metatarsal balance and negate the impact of fixed forefoot varus. Symptomatic arthritis of the subtalar, talonavicular, or calcaneocuboid joints is a contraindication for this procedure as well. Age is *not* a contraindication in the active patient. Obesity, however, may be a contraindication because of the limited power of the tendon transfer to correct valgus deformity. Obese patients with severe valgus deformity and dysfunction of the PTT might obtain better results through triple arthrodesis.

Preoperative Evaluation

The clinician must carefully examine the hindfoot to ensure the supple nature of the joints mentioned above. In addition to direct manipulation, indirect estimates of a supple hindfoot may be determined through observation of a double heel rise (in patients unable to perform a single heel rise). The hindfoot should demonstrate inversion in a double heel rise. It might not be the same degree as that seen on the contralateral extremity, but it should still be visible.

Hindfoot valgus can be assessed with a goniometer while viewing the patient from behind. Holding one limb of the goniometer along the axis of the tibia, while the second limb is placed along the axis of the calcaneus, gives a relative indication of hindfoot valgus deformity. The contralateral limb must be assessed as well. More objective data can be incorporated through the hindfoot alignment view popularized by Saltzman and El-Khoury[158] (see Fig. 25-7). These authors found that 95% of asymptomatic patients have a point of heel-to-floor contact on the calcaneus within 15 mm of the long axis of the tibia. In theory, without increased hindfoot valgus, the FDL tendon transfer may be considered as an isolated procedure.

Fixed-forefoot varus is assessed by correcting the hindfoot to neutral with the patient in a seated position. The examiner can then assess for elevation of the first metatarsal head relative to the fifth metatarsal head, which is not passively reducible by derotation of the transverse tarsal joints (see Fig. 25-4).

A standard physical examination and radiographic examination should be performed as noted in prior sections.

Preoperative Planning

Planning for an FDL tendon transfer revolves around assessing the need for supplementary procedures. Once the surgeon has determined that the hindfoot joints are supple enough to warrant the tendon transfer, he or she needs to evaluate the foot and ankle carefully to ensure that the appropriate procedures are done in concert with the transfer. These decisions should be made *preoperatively* rather than intraoperatively because the transfer itself will distort the architecture of the talonavicular joint, making assessment difficult. These procedures are discussed later.

Thus, in brief, if hindfoot valgus is significant, the surgeon will add a medial-slide calcaneal osteotomy to the procedure. If fixed forefoot varus is present, the surgeon can add a naviculocuneiform rotational arthrodesis to the procedure, or, if arthritis is present at the first metatarsocuneiform joint, a closing-wedge plantar-flexion arthrodesis of that joint. If the surgeon corrects the hindfoot to neutral and the Silversköldt test reveals an isolated gastrocnemius contracture, a Strayer procedure (or variation thereof) will be performed. Finally, if lateral column pain and subfibular impingement are noted, along with significant abduction of the forefoot, a lateral-column lengthening procedure may be considered. Performing any combination of these procedures should be determined *preoperatively* based on physical examination and radiographic appearance.

If an MRI is available, the surgeon should review it to determine the location of the tendinosis or rupture of the posterior tibial tendon. This will ensure that the entire compromised tendon is excised, minimizing the potential for postoperative pain medially.

Surgical Technique

1. The patient is position supine, with the leg externally rotated. A thigh tourniquet is applied, protected with a 10 × 10–inch adhesive drape to insulate the skin underneath the tourniquet from substances involved in preparing the extremity.
2. The initial incision begins at the tip of the medial malleolus, extending toward the navicular bone. In most circumstances, this incision is extended proximally, just posterior to the medial malleolus and along the posterior border of the tibia. This allows exposure of the PTT proximal to the flexor retinaculum.
3. The PTT sheath is opened with a knife. In cases with aggressive synovitis (seronegative disease), an effusion of fluid accompanies this incision. The remaining sheath is then opened with scissors.
4. The tendon is explored to determine the extent of the tendinosis. This varies from fissuring of the tendon to absence of the tendon within the sheath. In chronic situations, the diseased tendon may become adherent to the sheath, making definition of the tendon difficult. The tendon is often exposed proximal to the flexor retinaculum to allow visualization of proximal disease (Fig. 25-18A-D).
5. After confirming tendon disorder, the incision is extended along the medial aspect of the foot, along the dorsal border of the abductor hallucis to the proximal first metatarsal shaft.
6. The entire diseased segment of the PTT is excised. If possible, a 1-cm stump is preserved distally to facilitate attachment of the FDL tendon transfer. Proximally, the tendon is sectioned proximal to the medial malleolus.
7. The lesser toes are flexed and extended while palpating deep to the former posterior tibial tendon, distal

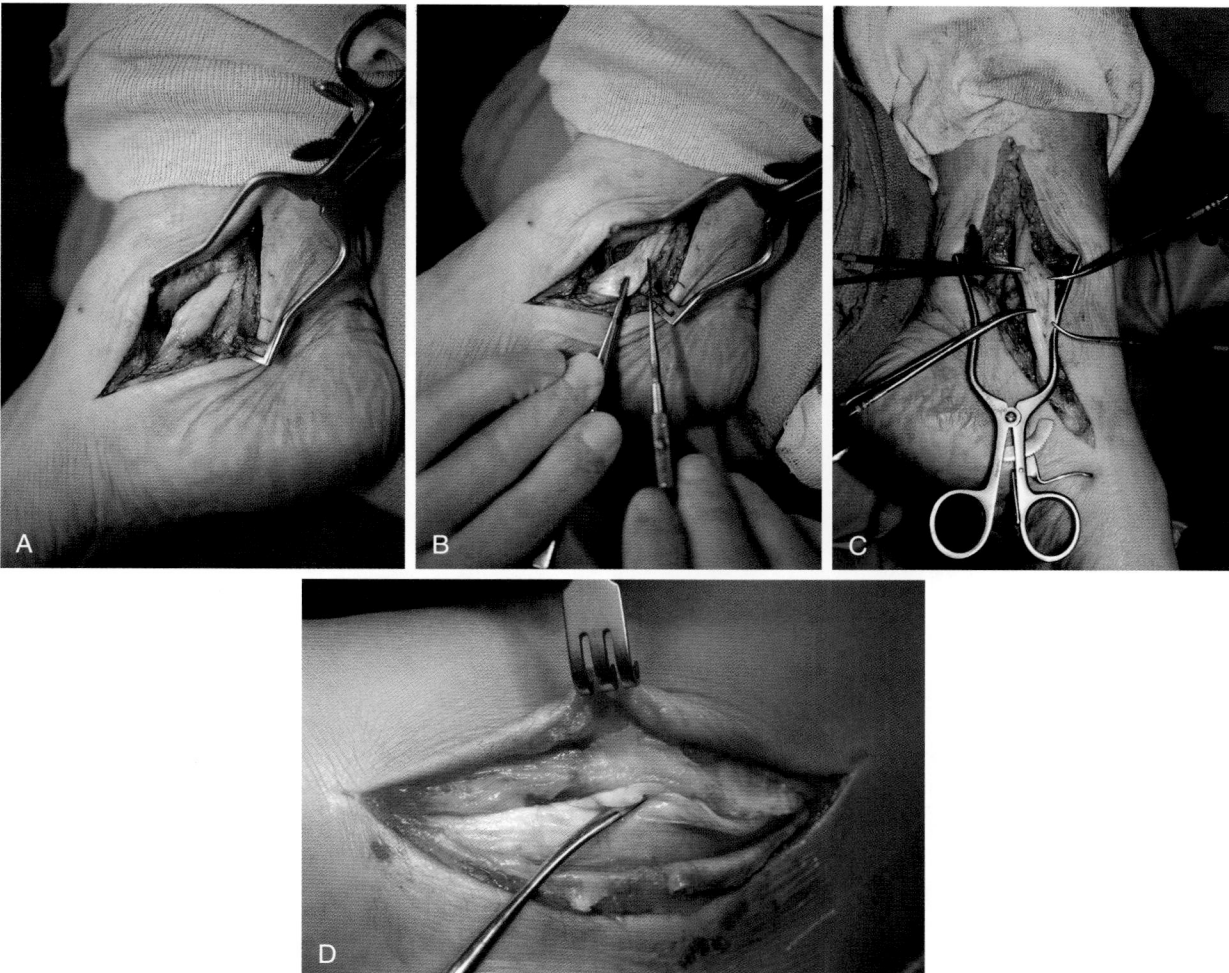

Figure 25-18 Examples of tendon pathology noted in posterior tibial tendon dysfunction. **A,** Grossly thickened tendon. **B,** Underside of tendon demonstrates fissuring. **C,** Marked cavitation of the tendon. **D,** Hypertrophy along the dorsal aspect of the tendon but otherwise minimal pathology observed.

to the medial malleolus. Flexing and extending the toes makes the FDL tendon palpable, and a knife is used to incise the sheath.

8. Scissors are used to complete the opening of the sheath proximally. This dissection is carried proximal to the medial malleolus to allow the FDL tendon to assume the position of the former PTT posterior to the medial malleolus.

9. Distally, the abductor hallucis muscle is visualized. The deep fascia is released, and the muscle belly is reflected plantarward. This brings into view the flexor hallucis brevis muscle. The muscle is traced proximally to its origin and released. This maneuver exposes the FDL and FHL tendons, which lie just laterally (Fig. 25-19A and B).

10. The FDL is now traced into the plantar surface of the foot. This is a meticulous dissection because the plantar veins are always encountered. Bipolar cautery may be used to prevent injury to the branches of the medial plantar nerve. Plantar retraction of the

abductor hallucis muscle belly assists in exposure of the FDL tendon. Emphasis is placed on achieving cauterization of all plantar veins surrounding the FDL distally, which will prevent hematoma after release of the tourniquet.

11. The fibrous connection between the FDL and flexor hallucis longus is reached and traced distally as far as possible. A side-to-side tenodesis of the two tendons is carried out.

12. A Krakow-suture weave is placed through the FDL tendon with nonabsorbable suture.

13. The dorsomedial aspect of the navicular bone is exposed by dissecting deep to the dorsal skin flap for a distance of about 2 to 3 cm. The width of the navicular bone is determined by observing the talonavicular bone and naviculocuneiform joints after this dissection. Alternatively, fluoroscopic imaging may be used to localize the most medial portion of the navicular.

14. The location of the tendon transfer is rationally determined by noting the biomechanical axis of the

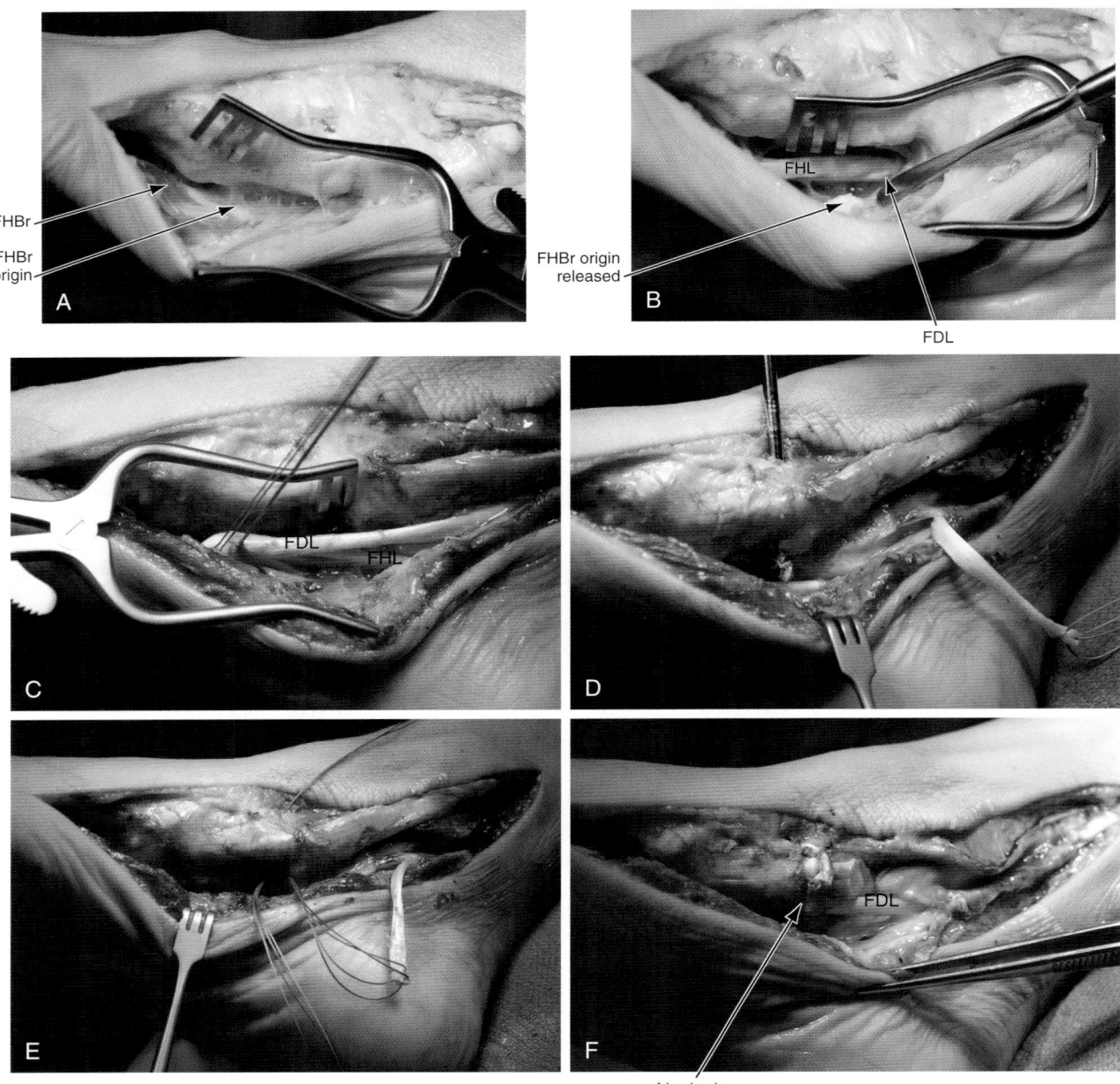

Figure 25-19 Technique of posterior tibial tendon reconstruction using the flexor digitorum longus muscle. **A,** With abductor hallucis muscle retracted plantarward, the flexor hallucis brevis *(FHBr)* can be visualized. The flexor hallucis brevis origin is a tendinous structure as noted in the picture. **B,** Releasing the flexor hallucis brevis origin brings the flexor hallucis longus *(FHL)* and the flexor digitorum longus *(FDL)* tendons into view. **C,** The FDL and FHL tendons are dissected distally and sutured together. The FDL tendon is then released. **D,** A vertical drill hole is made in the tarsal navicular in its medial portion. Bringing the drill through the soft tissues beneath it makes it easier to thread the tendon through the bone. **E,** The suture is passed through the hole in the navicular and the FDL tendon is pulled through the navicular, bringing the foot into some adduction and inversion. **F,** FDL tendon has been passed through the navicular and sutured to the surrounding periosteum.

subtalar joint, which is the fulcrum about which the PTT revolves. Physics defines work as *force × distance;* so, placing the lever arm of the tendon transfer as far as possible from the fulcrum of the subtalar joint will maximize leverage. Anatomically, the bone farthest away from this axis is the navicular bone. Therefore the drill hole placed for the tendon transfer should be

made as far medial on the navicular as possible (Fig. 25-19C and D). If a guidewire is available from screws used to secure supplementary procedures, such as a calcaneal osteotomy, that guidewire may be inserted into the navicular as far medially as possible. Position is then confirmed by fluoroscopic imaging, followed by drilling with a cannulated drill. This method avoids inadvertent fracture of the bone bridge between the drill hole and the medial cortical wall of the navicular.

15. The inferior surface of the navicular is cleared of soft tissue attachments to facilitate the tendon transfer. Using the previously placed suture in the FDL tendon, the tendon is passed from inferior to superior through the navicular (Fig. 25-19E-F).

16. The tendon transfer is tensioned. The FDL tendon is pulled maximally while adducting the transverse tarsal joints and inverting the subtalar joint. The tendon is then marked at its position with respect to the drill hole in the dorsal navicular. All tension is released, and the tendon is marked on the dorsum of the navicular at this most relaxed state. A tendon transfer is appropriately tensioned by suturing the tendon at a point halfway between both marks. If the tendon is tensioned under maximal pull, the surgeon is functionally creating a tenodesis rather than a tendon transfer. Excursion of the FDL tendon must be maintained, while simultaneously allowing the sarcomeres to function under tension, maximizing pull. Thus preference is given to tensioning the tendon halfway between maximal and minimal tension.

17. The tendon may be sutured back upon itself, if possible, under this tension. Alternatively, it is sutured to the PTT tendon stump inferiorly, and the portion placed through the drill hole is kept within the drill hole by using the previously placed Krakow suture, anchoring it to superior soft tissue (see Fig. 25-19F). All sutures should be nonabsorbable. Conversely, a shorter length of FDL tendon can be used, with less dissection, and held in the tunnel with a soft tissue interference screw.

18. The proximally sectioned PTT is now evaluated. This portion is grasped firmly with a clamp, and the excursion is evaluated. If the muscle is noted to be viable proximally through adequate excursion, a side-to-side tenodesis with nonabsorbable suture is performed with the FDL tendon. This is done proximal to the medial malleolus, to avoid impingement within the pulley posterior and inferior to that structure. As a general rule, younger patients with systemic or traumatic conditions causing PTT insufficiency retain viable proximal muscle, warranting tenodesis. Older patients with chronic degenerative ruptures often have poor-quality muscle proximally, which would negate the effect of the FDL tendon transfer by creating a tenodesis effect.

19. The tourniquet is now released to ensure adequate hemostasis and minimize scar tissue. The sheath is closed in its entirety with absorbable suture, the abductor hallucis fascia is reapproximated, and the subcutaneous tissue and skin are closed in a standard manner.

20. The patient is placed into a below knee cast, or sugar-tong splint with a posterior mold, in slight adduction and equinus. Immobilization does not require positioning the foot in the extremes of these planes because the surgeon has ensured strong attachment of the tendon to the bone intraoperatively. Excessive positioning in plantar flexion and inversion can lead to rigidity not recoverable through physical therapy. It is appropriate to have some tension on the sarcomeres of the FDL muscle belly to limit atrophy during immobilization.

Postoperative Care

The patient is kept immobilized for 6 weeks of non–weight bearing on this extremity. This restriction on weight bearing is more often due to the supplementary procedures performed at the time of the FDL tendon transfer than to the transfer itself.

After this immobilization, the patient is placed into walker boot, and physical therapy is instituted. It is important that the surgeon have a working relationship with the physical therapist so that a protocol can be followed. Overly aggressive physical therapy, such as early institution of a heel rise, can damage the tendon transfer and lead to failure of the procedure. The patient may bear full weight in the walking boot and begins inversion strengthening with a resistance band (Thera-Band). In the first few weeks, standing balance exercises (with 25% of the weight borne on the opposite foot) may be instituted, allowing recruitment of the tendon transfer without stressing the repair. Gentle forward lunges may also be incorporated. At 9 weeks after surgery, the patient may begin leg presses on a weight machine (such as a Total Gym), with bilateral squats and double heel rises with the plane of the bench at 30 degrees of elevation from supine. The incline is gradually increased, until 12 to 14 weeks postoperatively, with the patient standing to do these maneuvers. Activation of the tendon transfer early (without stressing the transfer) prevents the patient from delayed progression of rehabilitation upon removal from the CAM-boot. Single heel rise is avoided until 3 to 4 months after surgery.

At 12 weeks after surgery, the patient may progress to a commercially available lace-up sport brace for an additional month.

Results and Complications

Studies on isolated flexor digitorum longus tendon transfer are few. Michelson et al[127] found that 50% of isolated soft-tissue reconstructions failed within 1 year. Other authors have not had such a dismal experience, but they admit that the indications for an isolated FDL tendon transfer are narrow.

Mann and Thompson[123] reviewed 17 patients (14 FDL tendon transfers, 3 PTT advancements) with stage 2 PTT dysfunction. Twelve of their patients had an excellent result (painfree, excellent strength), 1 noted a good result (pain free, some loss of strength), 3 had a fair result (good function with persistent pain), and 1 had a poor result that was revised to fusion. Correction of flatfoot with an isolated transfer was not so successful because only 4 achieved correction, with 7 improved and 4 unchanged. Two patients deteriorated with respect to correction. Average follow-up for this study was 33 months. There was no difference in time of follow-up between all stratifications of results. Finally, there is no mention in the paper of a difference between the FDL tendon transfer and the PTT advancement with respect to clinical outcome.

Mann et al[118] reviewed 73 patients (75 feet) undergoing isolated FDL transfer for stage 2 disease. The average age of these patients was 54 years (range, 20-72 years). The mean follow-up was 73 months. The patient satisfaction review indicated that 64 patients (88%) were satisfied and 11 (15%) were dissatisfied. Of the 11 patients who were dissatisfied, 7 had either a fixed hindfoot valgus deformity or fixed forefoot varus in excess of 15 degrees. The strength of the transfer was always rated as 4 or 5 (good or normal). In the patients with no fixed deformity, the satisfaction index averaged 4.28, in which maximum satisfaction was 5, and the AOFAS score was 87. In patients who had a fixed forefoot varus deformity of greater than 15 degrees or fixed hindfoot valgus, the satisfaction index averaged 1.8, and the AOFAS score was 40.

Factors that negatively affected the results were fixed forefoot varus or fixed hindfoot valgus. Factors that were neutral (did not affect outcome) were greater than 60 months of follow-up; age greater than or equal to 60 years; spring ligament reconstruction, which was carried out in only 26 of the 75 feet in this study; a proximal tenodesis of the remaining PTT into the tendon transfer above the malleolus; and body weight more than 40 pounds over ideal.

Mann[119] reiterated the necessity of appropriate indications of an isolated FDL tendon transfer in a more recent article in 2001. At the conclusion of this article, the author agreed that flatfoot is not corrected by this procedure in isolation. He also noted that in his series of more than 100 isolated tendon transfers, less than 5% have required subsequent fusion at long-term follow-up. When the author did not adhere to the indications mentioned above (i.e., supple subtalar and transverse tarsal joints without fixed forefoot supination), fully 90% of his patients required revision to a fusion at a later date. Mann also stated that a medial slide calcaneal osteotomy is required with the index procedure approximately 80% of the time because of increased hindfoot valgus.

CALCANEAL OSTEOTOMY

As noted earlier, the flexor digitorum longus transfer is rarely done as an isolated procedure. Most studies with follow-up on this procedure incorporate a medial slide calcaneal osteotomy. The idea of shifting the calcaneus or mechanically changing the axis of the calcaneus to restore a more neutral position of the hindfoot was first described by Gleich[59] in 1893. Dwyer[44] added interposition bone graft into the osteotomy to treat flatfoot in cerebral palsy in 1959. It was Koutsogiannis[102] who first suggested that sliding the calcaneus medially will improve outcome in flexible pes planus. This idea was resurrected in the mid-1990s and has now been supported by numerous clinical studies.

Biomechanically, the purpose of the calcaneal osteotomy is twofold: First, it shifts the mechanical pull of the Achilles tendon medially, which both supports the relatively weak FDL tendon transfer and improves inversion power. Second, it shifts the weight-bearing axis of the heel closer to the long axis of the tibia. This theoretically lowers the risk of progressive valgus deformity after tendon transfer.

Cadaveric studies have explored the calcaneal osteotomy and its relationship to correcting PTT insufficiency and hindfoot valgus. Nyska et al[142] used 10 cadaveric limbs with normal longitudinal arches to define the value of the calcaneal osteotomy with respect to the contribution of altering Achilles tendon function. The authors radiographically tested the cadavers in various stages, progressing from an unloaded foot with a normal longitudinal arch through creation of a flatfoot deformity, loading the Achilles tendon, and finally through a medial slide calcaneal osteotomy. The authors found that loading the Achilles tendon in a flatfoot model increased the flatfoot deformity. They found that the addition of a medial slide calcaneal osteotomy improved the flatfoot deformity radiographically. More important, loading the Achilles tendon after the medial slide calcaneal osteotomy did *not* increase the flatfoot deformity. From these results, the authors surmised the calcaneal osteotomy has the added effect of preventing further flatfoot deformity by eliminating the negative effect of Achilles tendon load on progressive flatfoot.

Sung et al[173] evaluated the ability of the medial slide calcaneal osteotomy to decrease the force required for the PTT to achieve early heel rise. The authors used 13 cadaveric limbs mounted on a loading apparatus to measure the force required by the PTT to achieve early heel rise (defined as 7 degrees of calcaneal plantar flexion and 5 degrees of calcaneal inversion) with and without a medial slide calcaneal osteotomy. Before calcaneal osteotomy, the force required for the PTT to achieve these parameters was 399 N. The statistically significant decrease in force required after medial slide calcaneal osteotomy was 329 N. This effect was confirmed by noting that the Achilles tendon force required to achieve heel rise decreased from 1012 N to 981 N after medial slide calcaneal osteotomy. Again, cadaveric results support the calcaneal osteotomy in improving the outcome of FDL tendon transfer.

Finally, Hadfield et al[71] evaluated pressure changes in the forefoot after medial displacement calcaneal osteotomy. Using 14 cadaveric limbs, they used a pressure-sensitive mat to evaluate plantar-foot pressures in loaded specimens both before and after medial displacement calcaneal osteotomy. The authors found a statistically significant decrease in pressure under the first and second metatarsals. The authors postulated that this alteration in load was directly due to increased pull of the Achilles tendon medially. Although not correlated clinically, this study suggests a detrimental effect of calcaneal osteotomy in patients with forefoot varus because the lateral pressure on the metatarsal increases with the procedure.

Indications

The medial slide calcaneal osteotomy is never done as an isolated procedure in PTT dysfunction. It is always done in combination with the FDL tendon transfer, and thus the indications for that technique coincide with the indications for calcaneal osteotomy. However, one additional indication for the calcaneal osteotomy is a flexible hindfoot valgus deformity that is of greater magnitude when compared with the opposite extremity (Fig. 25-20A and Video Clip 117).

Contraindications

Again, contraindications are similar to those for the FDL tendon transfer. Risk of difficulty in healing the lateral incision should be assessed preoperatively with noninvasive arterial Doppler studies if suspicion is present.

Preoperative Evaluation

The patient is evaluated for supple hindfoot valgus by manual examination and the double heel rise. The magnitude of valgus deformity may be measured by the technique described earlier.

Preoperative Planning

The hindfoot alignment view can assist in determining the magnitude of correction required by shift of the posterior tuberosity.

Surgical Technique

1. The patient is placed into a lateral decubitus position. It is helpful to place the patient on a bean bag so the patient can be easily rolled into a supine position intraoperatively. This will facilitate the FDL tendon transfer and any additional medial procedures after the calcaneal osteotomy. A thigh tourniquet is applied, protected with a 10- × 10-inch adhesive drape to insulate the skin underneath the tourniquet from substances involved in preparing the extremity.

2. The incision begins proximally at the superior aspect of the posterior tuberosity of the calcaneus, anterior to the Achilles tendon insertion and posterior to the peroneal tendons (Fig. 25-20B). In practice, this is approximately 1 cm posterior to the fibula and 2 cm proximal to the superior aspect of the calcaneus. This incision extends distally at a 45-degree angle with the plantar surface of the foot. Alternatively, the small fluoroscopy unit that will be used to assess the cut line and position of the calcaneal tuberosity may also be used to confirm the location of the incision.

3. The sural nerve will invariably be encountered, normally anterior to the surgical approach. Thus initial dissection is done with scissors dissection until the nerve is mobilized anteriorly. After retraction of the nerve safely out of the surgical field, dissection may proceed with a scalpel directly to the bone of the calcaneus. While stripping the periosteum off of the lateral wall, care is taken to avoid detachment of the insertion of the calcaneofibular ligament.

4. Again, using a mini-fluoroscopy unit is helpful to confirm location of the osteotomy to ensure that the osteotomy will be anterior enough to create a significant shift of the posterior tuberosity, while allowing adequate bone distally (anteriorly) for screw fixation. In general, the plane of the osteotomy is slightly posterior to the peroneal tendon sheath. The plane is perpendicular to the longitudinal axis of the calcaneus or at an approximate 45-degree angle from the plantar surface of the foot.

5. Before the cut, small Hohman retractors are placed at the superior location of the osteotomy to protect the Achilles tendon and at the inferior aspect of the osteotomy to protect the plantar fascia and lateral plantar nerve branches.

6. The cut is made with a wide and long blade from a macrosagittal oscillating saw. This allows a smooth cut to be made through the soft cancellous bone of the calcaneus. The lateral wall is scored first, followed by penetration to the medial cortex. Upon reaching the medial cortex, the saw blade is gently bounced off the medial wall until it penetrates. Caution while penetrating the medial cortex is critical. The palm of the surgeon's opposite hand may be placed on the medial hindfoot to assist in determining penetration of the saw blade. Greene et al[65] studied the medial neurovascular anatomy in relation to the calcaneal osteotomy. The authors found, on average, that four neurovascular structures crossed the osteotomy site. Most were branches of the lateral plantar nerve and posterior tibial artery. The most common branches of the lateral plantar nerve at risk were the calcaneal sensory branch and the second branch. The medial plantar nerve was not at risk.

7. After completion of the osteotomy, a 25-mm straight osteotome is inserted into the plane of the cut, gently distracting the surfaces (Fig. 25-20C and D). A smooth lamina spreader is also inserted to distract the osteotomy site (Fig. 25-20E). Care must be taken to avoid crushing the soft bone of the calcaneus with this device, especially in older or rheumatoid patients. The medial periosteum is then freed with the use of a Freer elevator.

8. With the posterior tuberosity now mobile, the ankle is placed on an elevated bump, and the knee is flexed to release gastrocnemius tension. This allows medial translation of the posterior tuberosity without superior migration from Achilles tendon pull. In general, the magnitude of the shift is 1 cm (Fig. 25-20F and G).

9. Provisional fixation of the osteotomy is done with a 0.062-inch Kirschner wire (K-wire), followed by placement of the guidewire from the cannulated screw system. The wire is placed laterally in the posterior

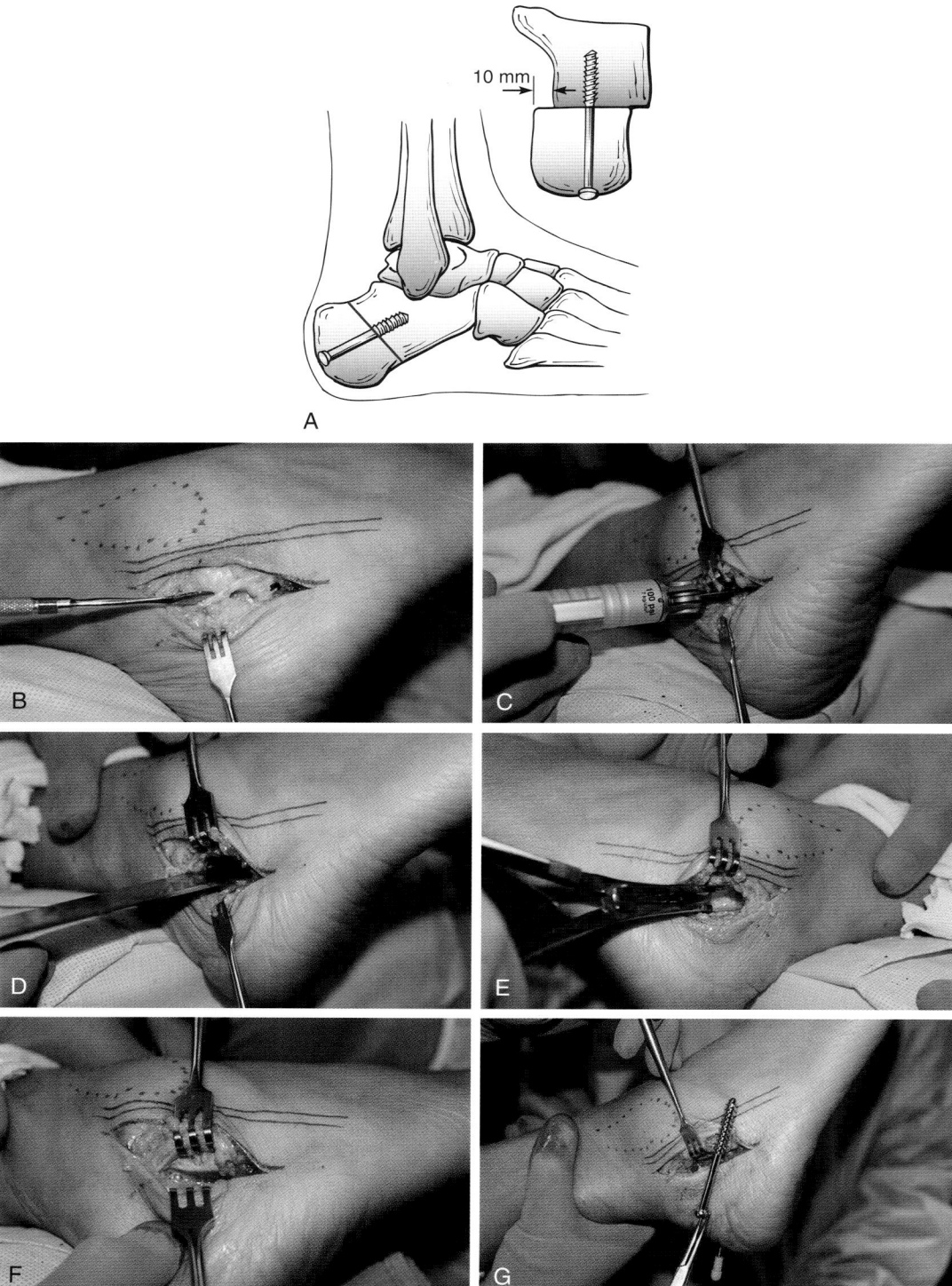

Figure 25-20 Calcaneal osteotomy. **A,** Diagram demonstrates osteotomy and fixation. **B,** Skin incision. The Freer elevator is pointing to the sural nerve. **C,** Osteotomy is cut perpendicular to the long axis of the calcaneus and about 1 cm posterior to the posterior facet of the calcaneus. **D,** Upon completion of the osteotomy, a wide osteotome is used to open the osteotomy site. **E,** A lamina spreader is used to open the osteotomy site so that the periosteum on the medial side can be gently teased off the bone. **F,** Medial displacement of the osteotomy site of about 1 cm. **G,** The partially threaded screw is used to fix the osteotomy site. Preferably, the threads will all be on the distal part of the osteotomy.

tuberosity to accommodate the medial shift and stay within the anterior calcaneus (see Fig. 25-20G). The mini-fluoroscopy unit can be used to ensure the appropriate placement of this guidewire on the sagittal and axial planes. The axial image can be used to determine the appropriate magnitude of tuberosity shift. The lateral image can be used to ensure that the posterior tuberosity is not superiorly or inferiorly translated. One large cannulated screw is acceptable, although some use two smaller screws to (theoretically) control rotation. The contact surface of the osteotomy is large, and the bone is cancellous. Thus the union rate is high.

10. The overhanging edge is beveled with a chisel and rasped smooth. Bone wax may be applied to this exposed surface to minimize adherent scar.

11. The tourniquet is released, and hemostasis is achieved to minimize hematoma formation. During closure, it is important to avoid entrapment of the sural nerve. This will create a painful neuroma or sensory deficit (or both) in the lateral foot.

12. The bean bag is released, allowing the patient to assume a supine position for the additional medial procedures.

Postoperative Care

No additional treatment besides that mentioned for the FDL tendon transfer is required for the calcaneal osteotomy. The postoperative protocol is not altered by addition of this technique.

Results and Complications

Results of the medial slide calcaneal osteotomy are based on its use in conjunction with the flexor digitorum longus tendon transfer (Fig. 25-21).

Myerson and Corrigan[138] reviewed 32 patients treated with a medial slide calcaneal osteotomy and FDL tendon transfer. Mean follow-up was 20 months. Thirty (94%) were satisfied with the outcome of the procedure, exhibiting pain relief, arch improvement, and return to normal footwear without orthotic support. Of this group, 28 (88%) experienced no pain, 3 (9%) had mild pain, and 1 had persistent pain. The last patient eventually underwent triple arthrodesis for progressive deformity and pain. By 6 months, 78% were able to perform a single heel rise, and by 12 months, 88% were able to do so. Radiographic improvements were noted, with the AP talometatarsal angle improving from 26 degrees to 6 degrees and the complementary lateral angle improving from 28 degrees to 13 degrees. The talonavicular coverage angle improved from 37 degrees to 15 degrees.

Guyton et al[68] evaluated 26 patients undergoing a medial slide calcaneal osteotomy in combination with an FDL tendon transfer at an average of 36 months after surgery. Pain relief was rated excellent by 75% and good by 16%. Twenty-three (88%) could perform a single heel rise at the time of follow-up. Of the 3 who could not perform this maneuver, 2 had failures of fixation of the

FDL tendon transfer, necessitating late subtalar arthrodesis. The third patient failed the procedure late, after pregnancy nearly 6 years after the index procedure. Eliminating those requiring subtalar fusion, subtalar motion averaged 81% of the contralateral (normal) extremity. Radiographic assessment showed an improvement in the AP talometatarsal angle from 21 degrees to 7 degrees and the lateral talometatarsal angle from 20 degrees to 13 degrees. Talonavicular coverage improved from 22 degrees to 10 degrees. Similar to Myerson's results, radiographic improvement was present, but complete correction was not provided by these procedures. Only 50% of patients felt the conformation of their foot had noticeably changed, and only 1 (4%) found the improvement significant. Finally, the median length of time to the patient's rating of maximal improvement was 10 months.

Fayazi et al[53] reviewed 23 patients undergoing both calcaneal osteotomy and FDL tendon transfer at an average of 35 months. Twenty-two patients (96%) were subjectively better, 1 (4%) was the same. Objectively, AOFAS scores on 21 patients evaluated in person (the rest were by telephone) improved from 50 to 89. Two (9%) were able to perform a single heel rise before surgery, 18 (78%) were able to perform this postoperatively. Twenty-one (91%) stated they would have the procedure again (1 unsatisfied patient was under workers' compensation, the second sustained a deep venous thrombosis postoperatively).

Wacker et al[184] reviewed 48 patients undergoing the procedures. Twenty-five (52%) were completely satisfied, 19 (40%) were satisfied with minor reservations, 2 (4%) were satisfied with reservations, and 2 (4%) were dissatisfied. The latter 2 had revision to calcaneocuboid arthrodesis. Visual analogue scores for pain noted an improvement from 7.3 to 1.7. Although improvement in visible alignment was noted in 92%, only 25% had fair clinical alignment. Sixteen required orthoses after the operation.

Myerson et al[137] reviewed 129 patients undergoing the procedure at an average of 5.2 years postoperatively. An assessment of strength with a dynamometer designed for torque measurements of concentric and eccentric muscle action revealed 95 patients (74%) experienced inversion and plantar-flexion strength symmetric with the contralateral (normal) extremity. Eighteen patients (14%) were mildly weak (<25% of normal), and 4 (3%) were moderately weak (>50% loss of strength). With respect to the opposite extremity, subtalar motion was normal in 56 (44%), slightly decreased in 66 (51%), and moderately decreased in 7 (5%) patients. Most patients (108, 84%) were able to wear normal shoes without orthotic support. Radiographic assessment noted an improvement in the AP talometatarsal angle from 25 degrees to 6 degrees and the lateral talometatarsal angle from 27 degrees to 12 degrees. Talonavicular coverage improved from 37 degrees to 16 degrees. A positive subjective outcome was directly related to radiographic improvement. The mean time to self-rated maximal improvement was 14 months.

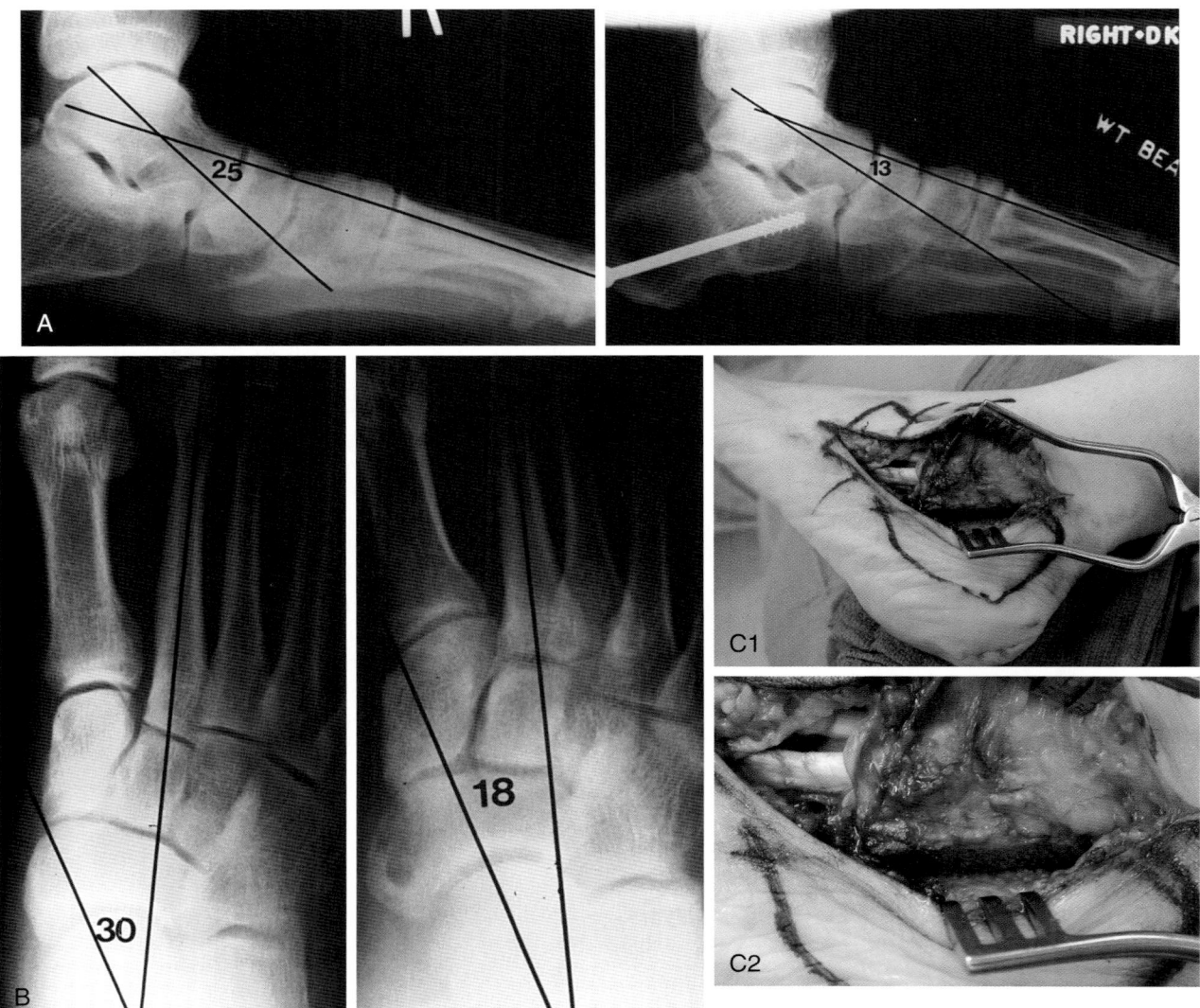

Figure 25-21 A, Preoperative and postoperative lateral radiographs demonstrating correction obtained after a medial displacement calcaneal osteotomy. **B,** Preoperative and postoperative anteroposterior radiographs demonstrate correction of the flatfoot deformity after a calcaneal osteotomy. **C1** and **C2,** Intraoperative photographs demonstrate the 1-cm medial shift normally performed for the procedure.

Complications include sural nerve neuritis or neuroma, infection, incisional wound necrosis, overcorrection (varus hindfoot), nonunion and malunion (rare), injury to medial neurovascular structures, peroneal tendon adhesions, hardware irritation, and deep venous thrombosis.

SPRING LIGAMENT REPAIR AND RECONSTRUCTION

The ligament most commonly involved in posterior tibial tendon dysfunction (PTTD) is the spring ligament, or better termed spring ligament complex.[35] The spring ligament complex is made of three ligaments: the superomedial, the medial plantar oblique, and the plantar inferior, formerly called the plantar spring ligament. The superomedial spring ligament is the largest and is immediately lateral to the posterior tibial tendon. It originates on the sustentaculum tali and inserts onto the medial/dorsal navicular. The superomedial spring ligament blends in with the superficial deltoid ligament superiorly. The plantar inferior spring ligament originates at the junction of the medial and anterior subtalar joint facets and inserts onto the plantar navicular. The medial oblique spring ligament is the thinnest of the three ligaments and is adjacent to the superomedial ligament but immediately plantar and lateral to it, lying in between the two aforementioned ligaments.

How common is involvement of the spring ligament complex in PTTD? In a study of 31 feet with PTTD, 87% of the patients with PTTD showed greater than 50% of the ligament degenerated, attenuated, or with tears in the superomedial spring ligament.[35] The plantar inferior

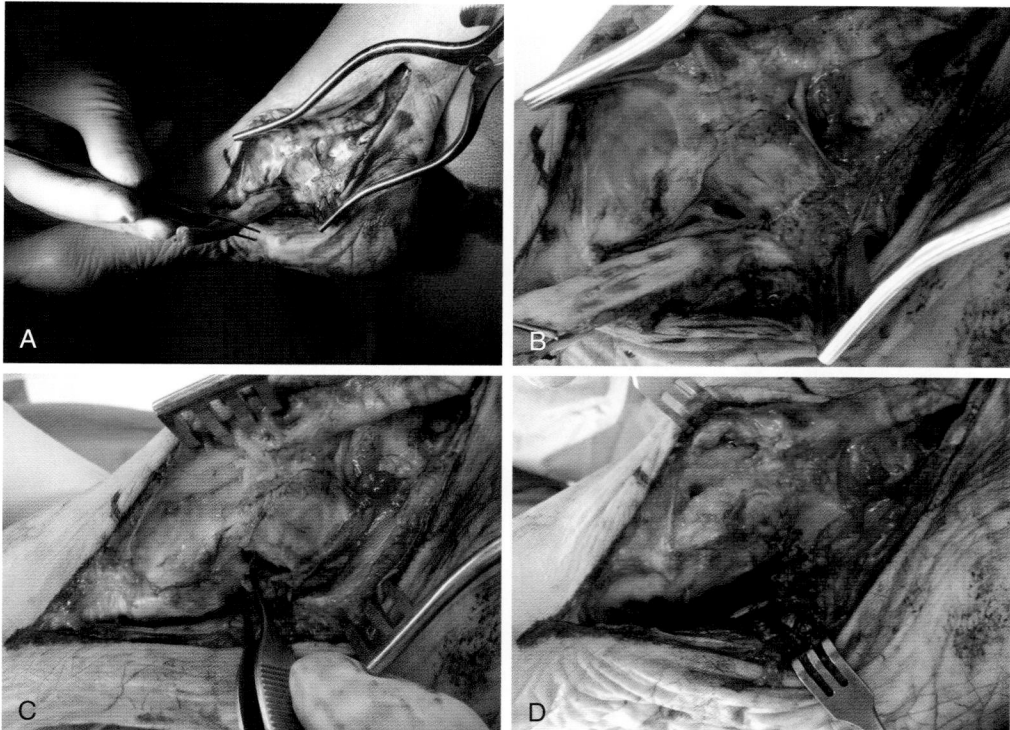

Figure 25-22 **A,** Intraoperative photograph of retracted diseased posterior tibial tendon reveals ruptured spring ligament. **B,** Closer view demonstrates true pathology to spring ligament, with large rent visible as well as multiple small tears. **C,** Poor-quality tissue remains at chronically ruptured site. **D,** Primary end-to-end repair attempted, although better methods are now available.

spring ligament was involved in more than 50% of cases. It should be noted that these ligaments can be "degenerated"—appearing clinically "intact" but actually being stretched out and incompetent.

Indications

Spring ligament repair is indicated for a visible repairable tear or laxity in the ligament when demonstrated in the operating room (Fig. 25-22). Studies that document the efficacy of repair in a series of patients are lacking because the procedure is most often done in combination with a tendon transfer and corrective bony procedures.[56,60,136] It is therefore difficult to separate out the effects of these procedures and document the efficacy of repair. Nevertheless, it is logical with visible tears or gross laxity to repair the ligament and restore it to near its original length. Unfortunately, there is most often degenerated tissue in varying amounts. This needs to be taken into account when doing the repair and when predicting the efficacy of repair. It should not be expected that repair of a spring ligament by itself will not correct the alignment of the flatfoot.

Contraindications

If the tissue available for repair is attenuated or quite degenerated, then the repair is not likely to be efficacious.

Also, if the deformity is fixed or the talonavicular joint is unable to be passively brought into inversion, ligament repair is again not likely to be useful. Spring ligament reconstruction is indicated when in the operating room after lateral column lengthening, there is persistent abduction at this talonavicular joint (>30%), and/or plantar talonavicular sag (>10 degrees).[188] It is contraindicated if the bony procedures have not corrected 50% of the original subluxation at the talonavicular joint (Fig. 25-23). If such failure of bony correction is occurring, a triple arthrodesis is performed. For spring ligament reconstruction, there needs to be flexible deformity as described above and correction of 50% of deformity at the talonavicular joint by the bony procedures, such as lateral column lengthening and medial slide calcaneal osteotomies. If the correction by bony procedures is less than this, there may not be enough secondary ligamentous support to enable the success of a spring ligament reconstruction.

Preoperative Planning

Major planning is not required for spring ligament repair or reconstruction. Reconstruction along with the other procedures makes for a long procedure. There is the option of using allograft tendon or the peroneus longus tendon. A series of reconstructions with the allograft

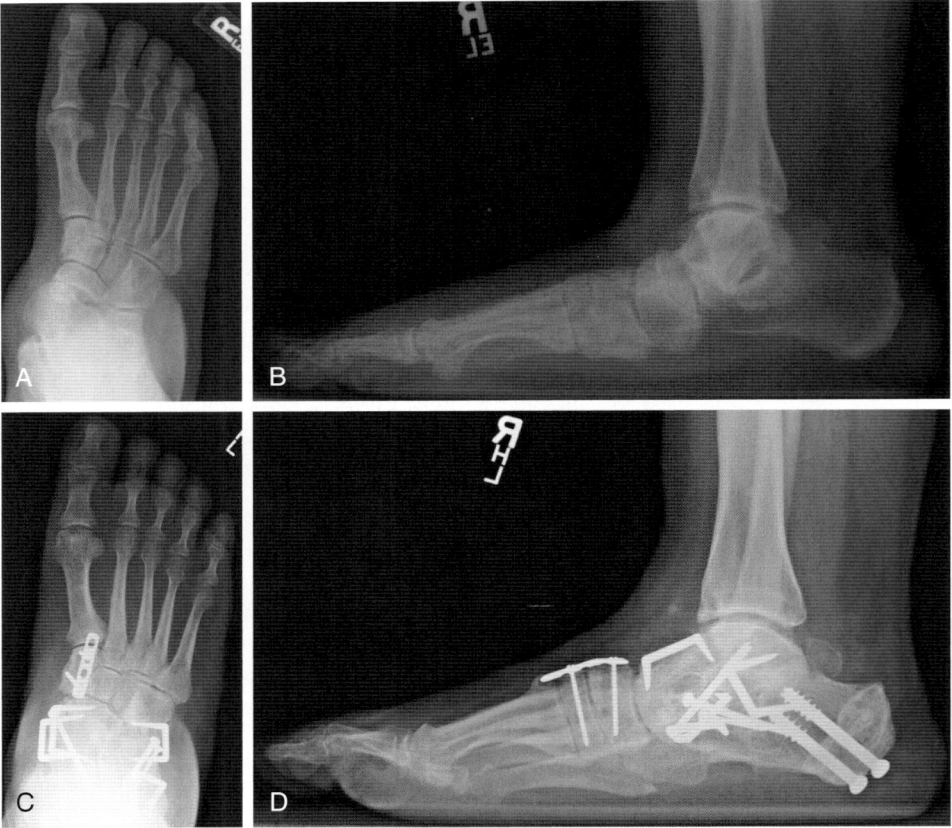

Figure 25-23 Preoperative anteroposterior **(A)** and lateral **(B)** views of a patient with severe fixed deformity. In the operating room, even after lateral capsular release, the patient's talonavicular joint could not be brought into inversion and therefore a triple arthrodesis was performed. **C** and **D,** Postoperative views showing correction. The plate for the Cotton osteotomy is too long but was asymptomatic. Plates for Cotton osteotomies are not recommended as they are far too prominent and not necessary (use simple screw fixation).

tendon has not been published, and therefore confirmation of the efficacy of allograft reconstruction has not been done. However, use of allograft Achilles tendon is currently under trial. A set of cannulated reamers that include sizes from 7 to 9 mm is very helpful when doing this procedure. Preoperative standing AP and lateral radiographs of the foot should be studied to determine if the deformity is a primarily abduction, primarily plantar flexion, or, most commonly, combined.

Surgical Technique for Spring Ligament Repair

1. The medial incision used for FDL tendon transfer is used for plication of the ligament.
2. The easiest and strongest method to repair the spring ligament is through a transverse incision, without excising redundant tissue
3. Closure is done through a pants-over-vest suture. The foot is held in position with the talonavicular joint reduced, and markings are made on the ligament, outlining the overlap of the redundant ligament.
4. Nonabsorbable suture is then placed from the distal segment to the proximal mark. A second set of

nonabsorbable sutures is placed from the proximal segment to the distal mark.
5. These sutures are not tied until after the flexor digitorum longus tendon is brought through the hole drilled into the navicular but before the tendon transfer is tied down. This prevents undue tension on the spring ligament repair. In fact, the appropriate tension to be applied to the FDL tendon transfer should be done before tying the spring ligament sutures (i.e., the FDL tendon must be marked at the appropriate tension as well so that the tendon is under moderate tension with the foot in slight inversion). Once the FDL tendon is brought through the drill hole, the ligament sutures are tied. The FDL tendon is then secured to the stump of the posterior tibial tendon, during which time the assistant continues to hold the talonavicular joint in reduction.
6. This method has value in that it is a reinforced approach to repairing the ligament. Simply excising the redundant segment and repairing the ligament end to end has a potentially higher rate of failure because of the compromised tissue.

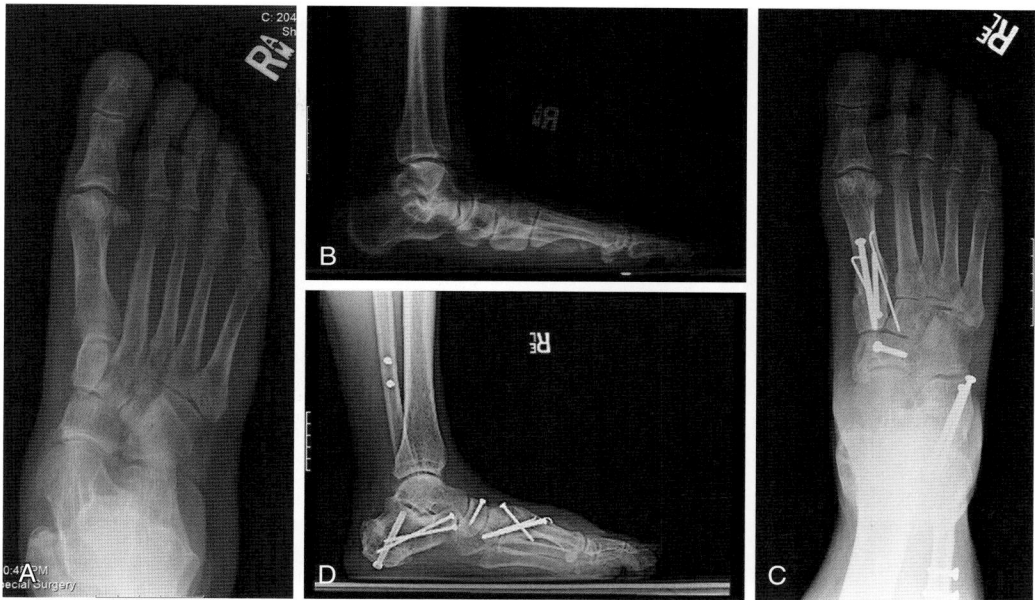

Figure 25-24 Preoperative anteroposterior **(A)** and lateral **(B)** radiographs of a patient with combined abduction and plantar-flexion deformity. **C** and **D,** Patient was treated with an Evans lateral column lengthening, posterior first metatarsal fusion, and spring ligament reconstruction.

Surgical Technique for Spring Ligament Reconstruction (Figs. 25-24 to 25-29)

1. The navicular tunnel for the tendon transfer must be centrally placed in the navicular in the proximal-to-distal plane, with an adequate bone bridge so that widening the tunnel to 7 or 8 mm will not result in navicular fracture when the graft is placed. Place a K-wire in the navicular with a good surrounding bone bridge, and check AP and lateral fluoroscopic views for proper position. Once good position is confirmed, put the guidewire in the K-wire hole and sequentially enlarge the hole to reach 7 or 8 mm, stopping before the bone bridge becomes thin.

2. In the case of a combined or primarily abduction deformity, a tibial bone tunnel is then made (Fig. 25-27). A K-wire is placed in between the colliculi at the medial malleolus and positioned to exit directly dorsally at the medial tibial metaphysis. Using fluoroscopy, check the wire position on AP ankle view to confirm that enlarging the hole will not violate the medial gutter.

3. Pass a suture attached to a snap at the dorsal end of the navicular tunnel through the navicular to the medial malleolus and up through the tibial tunnel. Pull on the free end of the suture to confirm that this path will reduce the deformity. If it does not, consider using the alternative technique described in step 8. If correction is confirmed, measure the length of the suture from the dorsal navicular to the proximal end of the tibial tunnel with the foot in neutral and add 1 cm to avoid too short a graft.

4. If the deformity is primarily the talar head sag type, the same navicular tunnel is used but not the tibial tunnel. A calcaneal tunnel from just underneath the sustentaculum tali to the lateral calcaneus is made; exiting just above the osteotomy site (Fig. 25-28). Expose the sustentaculum tali and retract the FHL medially and plantarly. Place a trial K-wire and then replace with a guide pin from underneath the sustentaculum to the lateral calcaneus. Using the guide pin, drill the calcaneal hole, usually 8 mm in diameter. Place a suture and measure the length of this graft, again adding 1 cm.

5. The tendon graft is then prepared. Use a cylinder sizer to confirm that the tendon graft (allograft or peroneal longus) is not too large to pass through the tunnels. Two No. 2 nonabsorbable sutures are woven at the end of the graft for a strong hold.

6. If a peroneus longus autograft is used, care is taken to confirm by direct inspection that the brevis is of adequate quality because it will be the remaining evertor for the foot. If the brevis is in poor condition, an allograft is definitely used for reconstruction instead of the longus. If used, the peroneus longus is harvested proximally just distal to its musculotendinous junction. The proximal stump is tenodesed to the brevis. The longus is brought through the cubital tunnel, after releasing its attachments to the lateral aspect of the foot. It is then passed through the navicular from dorsal to plantar and into the tibial tunnel. If an Achilles tendon allograft is used, a small bone block with the calcaneal insertion is kept, ending up in the navicular tunnel. Two No. 2 nonabsorbable sutures are woven into each end of the graft. The allograft (nonbone end first) is passed through the navicular from dorsal to plantar, fixed at the navicular tunnel,

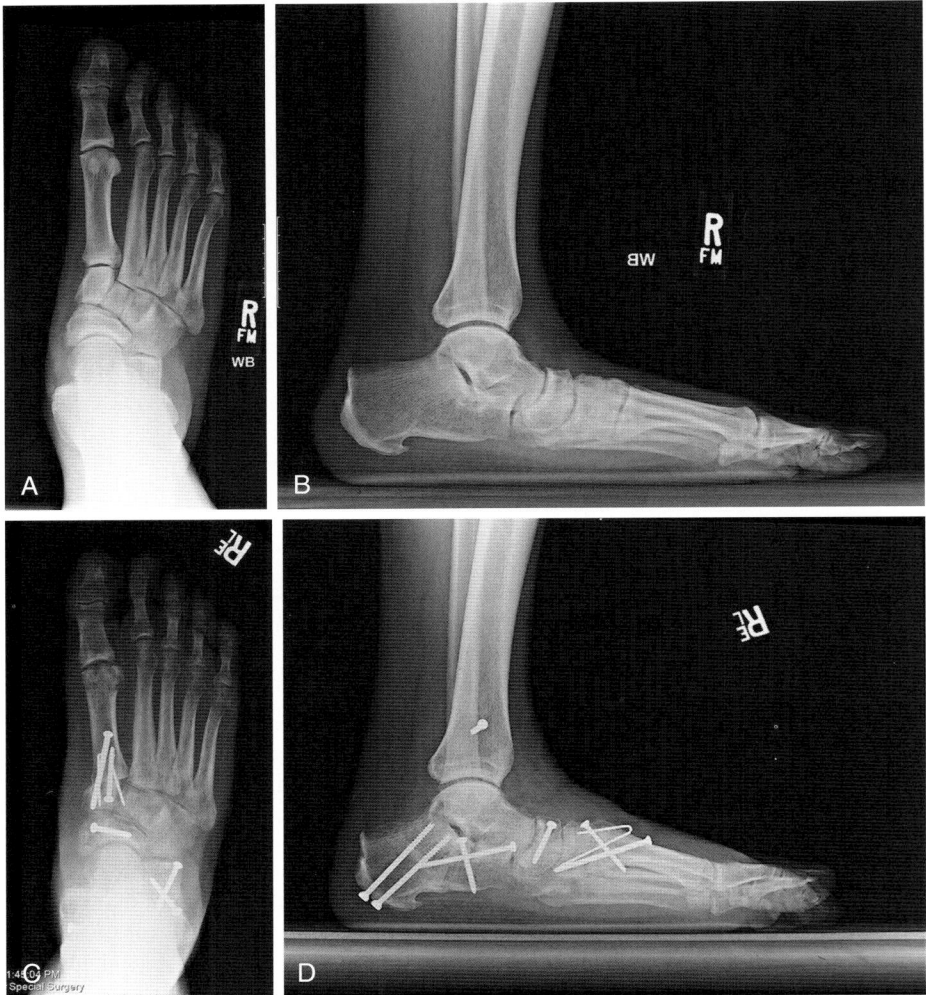

Figure 25-25 **A** and **B**, Patient with a primarily plantar-flexion deformity. **C** and **D**, The patient was treated with a lateral column lengthening, first metatarsal–tarsal fusion, and spring ligament reconstruction. The plantar flexion did not correct with the lateral column lengthening, and therefore a spring ligament reconstruction was done. The patient achieved good radiographic correction. However, correction was not just based on radiographic parameters but leaving near-normal eversion motion.

and finally passed into the tibial tunnel. The bone end of the graft is fixed at the navicular tunnel by sutures from the graft tied to a dorsal screw as a post.

7. Having fixed the graft at the navicular tunnel, pull on graft/sutures at the exit of the tibial tunnel, confirming reduction of the deformity and good tension on the graft. Tie down the No. 2 sutures to screw as a post on the medial tibia and place bone graft in the tunnels.

8. If the abduction or combined deformity does not reduce with the trial suture or tendon graft, an alternative technique can be used which is under clinical trial (Fig. 25-29). A drill hole is made in the navicular and two drill holes are made in the calcaneus at the inferior aspect of the sustentaculum tali. The first calcaneal drill hole is at the distal aspect of the sustentaculum tali, and the second more posteriorly. The calcaneal drill holes exit laterally above the level of a calcaneal

osteotomy. Confirm that the graft is sized to easily slide through the navicular and calcaneal bone tunnels. The graft is first placed through the navicular drill hole and then each limb is placed through the calcaneal drill hole under tension as depicted in Figure 25-29. The graft can be fixed by interference screws in the calcaneal tunnels once the talonavicular joint is reduced and temporarily pinned in the corrected position. The grafts can also be sewn to one another at the lateral calcaneus.

Results and Complications

No study has proven that spring ligament repair (not reconstruction) adds to the correction or the clinical result. Although it is difficult to confirm the efficacy of spring ligament repair when other procedures are done at the same time, the authors of this chapter think it may still be reasonable to repair the spring ligament if there

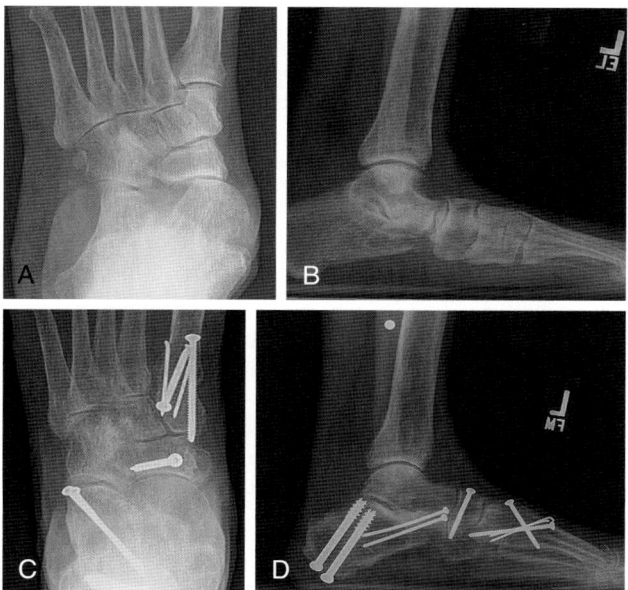

Figure 25-26 **A** and **B,** Preoperative severe deformity at the talonavicular joint, which was reducible into an inverted position of the joint. **C** and **D,** Postoperative radiographs showing good correction from the spring ligament reconstruction, which was added after the bony correction had not adequately reduced the deformity.

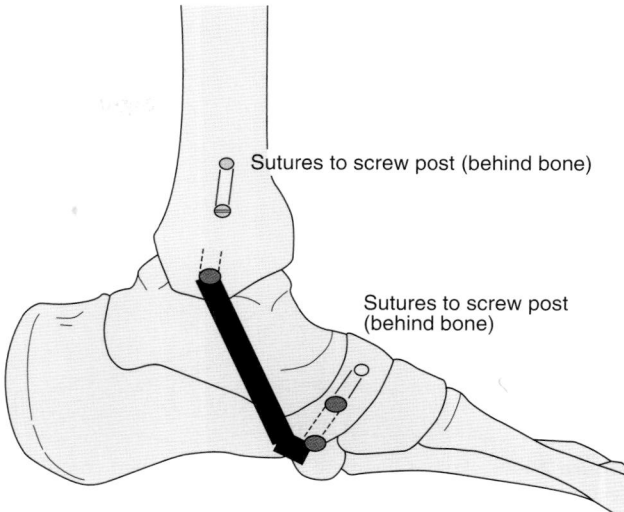

Figure 25-27 Spring ligament reconstruction. Drill holes for combined abduction and plantar-flexion deformity are shown. Also used for primarily abduction deformity. Graft goes from navicular to talus.

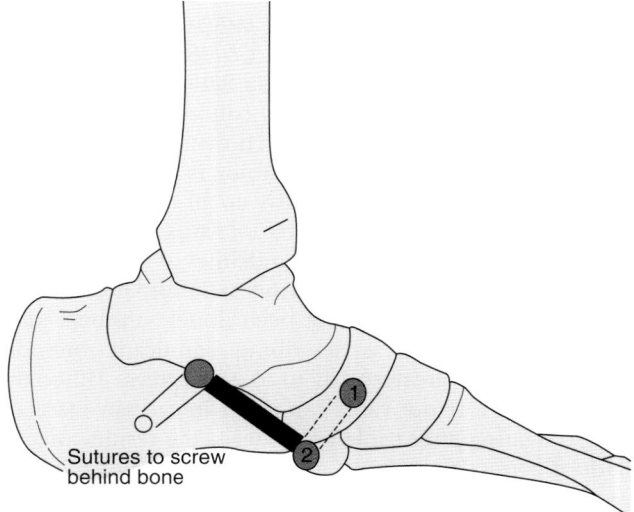

Figure 25-28 Spring ligament reconstruction showing drill holes for a primarily plantar-flexion deformity, where graft goes from navicular to calcaneus.

is adequate tissue and clear laxity present. In a biomechanical study, Choi[18] found that the peroneus longus tendon graft functioned best when the entire reconstruction was performed (i.e., a combined repair with both the superomedial and inferior portions done). A better clinical result from combined repair has not yet been reported in the literature. The spring ligament reconstruction results so far show correction with either a navicular to tibial or navicular to calcaneal technique in properly selected patients.[188] A combined repair using both the navicular to tibial and navicular to calcaneal techniques (or the other combined technique described in step 6, using the talar neck) could result in more supporting tissue. Because of the risk of navicular fracture and the difficulty of a combined procedure, particular care should be taken if two grafts are placed in the navicular tunnel. It is for this reason that the technique in step 8 is under clinical trial.

It should be remembered that the dorsal aspect of the superomedial spring ligament inserts at the dorsal navicular and interlaces with the superficial deltoid. Therefore it is not illogical that a medial attachment point on the tibia (or talus) should be used. Although potentially a stronger repair, the efficacy of the combined techniques awaits clinical follow-up. Also, whether allograft tissue results in a reconstruction more likely to stretch out has not been determined.

Follow-up from the peroneus longus study, good correction was noted in the AP talonavicular coverage angle but was not statistically significant for the other angle measurements.[188] Most patients kept good, but not full,

triple joint motion. For the 14 feet treated, 10 were capable of a single-stance heel rise and inversion of the heel, with 2 being unable invert the heel. However, it should be remembered that spring ligament reconstruction was done in feet that did not get adequate correction with the use of a medial heel slide and lateral column lengthening, and the procedure was performed as an alternative to a triple arthrodesis. No patient had to be converted to a triple arthrodesis. Care was taken that reconstruction was done only when lateral column lengthening and a medial heel slide gave 50% correction or more of the abduction deformity but clearly left too much deformity without

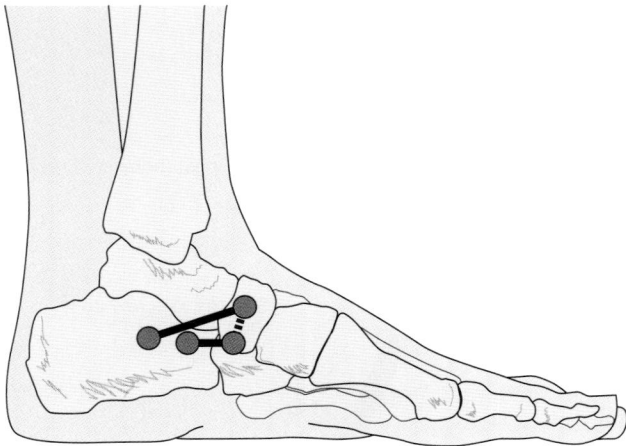

Figure 25-29 Spring ligament reconstruction with combined technique simultaneously replacing superomedial and inferior spring ligament. Technique is presently under clinical trial.

reconstruction. Spring ligament reconstruction is a reasonable alternative to arthrodesis in patients who have partial but incomplete correction with osteotomies.

PLANATAR-FLEXION OPENING-WEDGE (COTTON) OSTEOTOMY OF THE MEDIAL CUNEIFORM

In the patient with a symptomatic flatfoot, elevation of the first ray or forefoot varus is a concern. After flatfoot reconstruction, collapse of the arch distal to the talonavicular joint as well as at that joint is an undesirable outcome. It is therefore attractive to bring the first ray down and correct significant forefoot varus when present. However, there are no precise guidelines as to when this is necessary, and studies proving symptomatic benefit from this procedure have not been done. Numbers that have been suggested as describing significant forefoot varus have been greater than 10 to 15 degrees. Although leaving such forefoot varus can result in excessive lateral weight bearing after triple arthrodesis, the results after a flatfoot correction without a fusion of the talonavicular joint in the setting of forefoot varus have not been studied. It is nevertheless reasonable to maintain the tripod of the foot with good plantar alignment of the first and fifth metatarsal heads in a flatfoot reconstruction. In the setting of moderate deformity at the naviculocuneiform joint, a Cotton osteotomy can be used as an alternative to naviculocuneiform fusion if the first metatarsal–tarsal joint is stable.

A dorsal opening-wedge osteotomy of the medial cuneiform, described by Cotton,[25] can bring the first ray down. The relative efficacy of this procedure versus a first metatarsal–tarsal fusion, to correct elevation of the first ray, has also not been well studied. It is true that both procedures can bring the first ray down. If the Cotton osteotomy does this as well as the first metatarsal–tarsal fusion, the osteotomy has the advantage of being faster and easier to perform and probably has a higher union rate. Because it is being performed adjacent to intact Lisfranc and intercuneiform ligaments, there is likely to be a limitation in the amount of correction possible because of tensioning the ligaments with an opening-wedge osteotomy. Certainly, release of these ligaments is not a good option. In Dr. Jonathan Deland's personal experience there is a limitation to how much a Cotton osteotomy can bring down the first ray. Until data is available, the Cotton osteotomy may therefore be best used to correct moderate elevation of the first ray. In cases of severe elevation or considerable instability at the first metatarsal–tarsal joint, a first metatarsocuneiform fusion may be the more reliable choice because the limitation from ligament tension is less likely to be a factor. The surgeon should be aware that some shortening of the first ray occurs with this fusion, and plantar flexion and shortening of the first metatarsal can dorsiflex the first metatarsophalangeal joint. Excessive shortening or plantar flexion of the first ray should be minimized.

Indications

The osteotomy is indicated with significant forefoot varus (greater than 10 degrees) and a stable first metatarsal–tarsal joint. It can produce a better-appearing arch, but whether it achieves a better outcome is a different question. It is not known whether this procedure clinically decreases excessive lateral weight bearing from a lateral column lengthening because the lateral weight bearing may be at least in part from the postlengthening stiffness along the lateral column as well as elevation of the first ray. It is better to ensure maintenance of both adequate flexibility (eversion) along the lateral column as well as normal eversion of the foot, rather than bring the first ray down. The surgeon should not correct the elevation of the first ray as an antidote for excessive stiffness along the lateral column. Bringing the first ray down and leaving the lateral column stiff still results in symptoms from a stiff lateral column.

Contraindications

This procedure is contraindicated in patients with osteoarthritis of the first metatarsal–cuneiform joint. These patients are better served with an arthrodesis with careful plantar resection to bring the first ray down in good alignment with the second metatarsal head. Patients with gapping at the plantar first metatarsal–tarsal joint, or considerable instability of that joint, are likely to be better served with arthrodesis.

Preoperative Evaluation

Patients are examined in both a seated and standing position to evaluate the forefoot varus. Correction of the subtalar joint to neutral reveals elevation of the first ray in patients with forefoot varus. Palpation of the plantar metatarsal heads while correcting the hindfoot to neutral shows the magnitude of this elevation. Adequate vascularity must be present in the distal foot to support healing of the bone graft. Thus noninvasive Doppler studies with toe pressures are helpful in this evaluation.

Preoperative Planning

Care should be given to incision placement. The incision for this osteotomy is dorsally based. The surgeon should either not carry the medial incision too distally for the FDL transferred, to avoid an insufficient skin bridge, or make the medial incision for the transfer more plantar to the medial cuneiform to maximize the skin bridge. Also, if the alternative of a first metatarsal–tarsal fusion is chosen, the incision for that should be over the lateral edge of the first metatarsal rather than directly over the first metatarsal–tarsal joint, to avoid too small a skin bridge.

There is the choice of allograft or autograft for the bone graft. Both are quite acceptable. There is minimal chance of allograft or autograph collapse as long as there is a good bicortical strut in the graft perpendicular to the osteotomy line.

SURGICAL TECHNIQUE FOR COTTON OSTEOTOMY

1. The patient is in a supine position, with the foot vertical (not internally or externally rotated).
2. A dorsal incision is made overlying the medial cuneiform (Fig. 25-30C).
3. The extensor hallucis longus is retracted medially, and dissection proceeds to the medial cuneiform. Care is taken to avoid the superficial and deep peroneal nerves and the dorsalis pedis artery, which lie just

lateral to the osteotomy. The branch of the superficial peroneal nerve is most at risk.

4. Fluoroscopic imaging is used to locate the middle of the medial cuneiform, the location of the osteotomy.
5. A transverse osteotomy is made with a microsagittal saw from dorsal to plantar, with retractors protecting the lateral structures mentioned above and the extensor hallucis longus (EHL) medially. The osteotomy should not violate the deep plantar cortex but stop about 5 mm short of it. Measuring the depth of the bone with K-wires, on either side of the osteotomy and appropriately marking the depth on the saw blade, is helpful.
6. A straight osteotome placed dorsal to plantar is used to lever the medial cuneiform open at the osteotomy site. The same K-wires used in the last step can be used to open the osteotomy with a laminar spreader–type device.
7. The width of the dorsal base of the graft can be determined by either of two methods. The assistant wedges the dorsal cuneiform open with an osteotome until the surgeon feels a precise balance to the metatarsal heads, and the dorsal gap is measured. It is important to measure the depth of the graft as well, to create an interference fit. The second method involves wedging the medial cuneiform open, while using a lateral

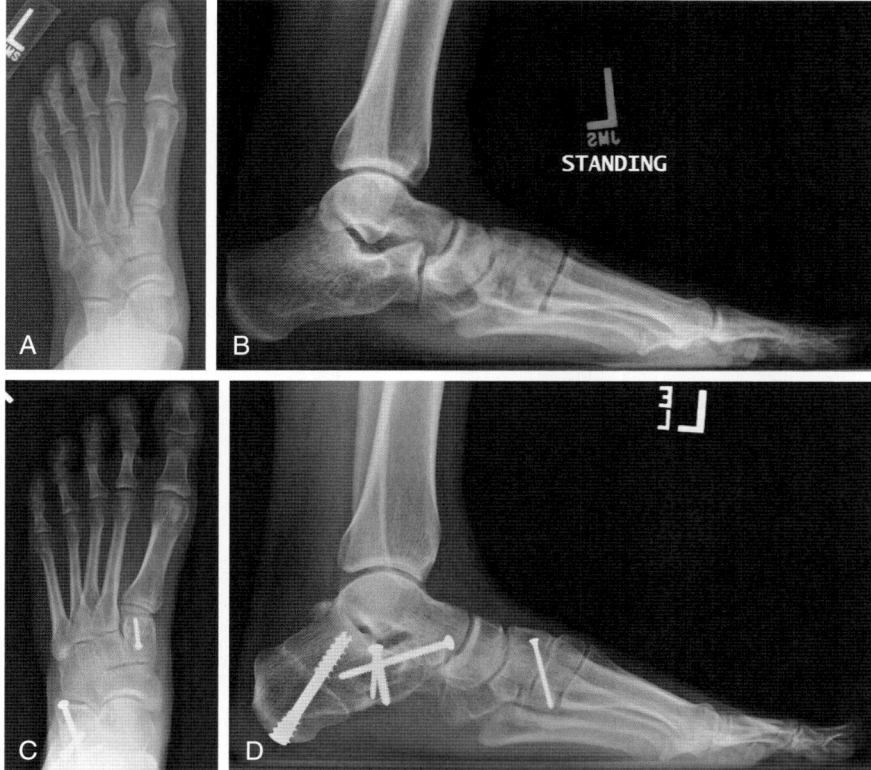

Figure 25-30 **A** and **B,** Preoperative radiographs of a flatfoot patient. **C** and **D,** postoperative radiographs following posterior calcaneal osteotomy, stepcut osteotomy and Cotton osteotomy. Note the single screw fixation of the Cotton osteotomy. This deformity is flexible and remained painful with orthotic management.

fluoroscopic image and looking for appropriate dec-lination of the first metatarsal. This latter method is susceptible to difficulty in judging the position of the first ray because of not obtaining a perfect lateral view. Once a good position is confirmed, the dorsal gap is measured.

8. The bone graft is harvested in a standard fashion, or the allograft is used after soaking in an antibiotic solution.

9. After interposition of the appropriate graft size, lateral fluoroscopic radiographs may be used to ensure excel-lent fit and the appropriate talus–first metatarsal angle. If the fit is not precise, the surgeon can improve the fit by inserting the saw blade from the microsagittal saw into the osteotomy site (proximally and distally), with the graft in place, and creating a perfect fit by dorsal-to-plantar cutting with the blade. This technique is very helpful, but it must be done carefully to prevent shortening the graft or altering the shape of the wedge.

10. This graft is stable and thus does not require fixation. However, the surgeon can use a cannulated screw from dorsal-proximal to plantar-distal.

11. The wound is closed in layers.

Results and Complications

The only study in the literature looking specifically at this osteotomy, used in conjunction with an adult-acquired flatfoot deformity and pediatric congenital flatfoot, comes from Hirose and Johnson.[77] Using the above-mentioned technique, the authors reviewed 16 feet.[77] Two separate populations were studied: adult and pediatric. The average time to union was 7 weeks in the pediatric population and 12 weeks in the adult population. The authors noted a statistically significant improvement in the lateral first talometatarsal angle, the calcaneal pitch, and the plantar medial cuneiform–to-floor height. They also noted the power of this procedure to correct forefoot varus with an adjustment in wedge width and taper.

Complications include painful hardware because of the lack of fat cushioning between the skin and hardware; neuromas of the superficial peroneal nerve, deep peroneal nerve, or saphenous nerve; and also nonunion. A small proximal dorsal-to-plantar distal screw can help avoid prominent hardware, and the neuromas can be avoided by careful dissection and retraction. Nonunion with good apposition and fixation is uncommon (Fig. 25-31). The Cotton osteotomy is useful if the first metatarsal–tarsal joint is stable and the surgeon wishes to bring the first ray down in the setting of the moderate deformity. It is best used to make the plantar first and fifth metatarsal heads approximately equal in alignment in the setting of signifi-cant elevation, but not use it to counteract a lateral column lengthening that has created too much supina-tion or to offset a triple arthrodesis set in supination.

LATERAL COLUMN LENGTHENING

Although originally thought to be a procedure that might not stand the test of time, lateral column lengthening has grown in use in patients with PTTD. It has allowed patients with more severe deformity to gain adequate correction of the triple joint complex (talonavicular,

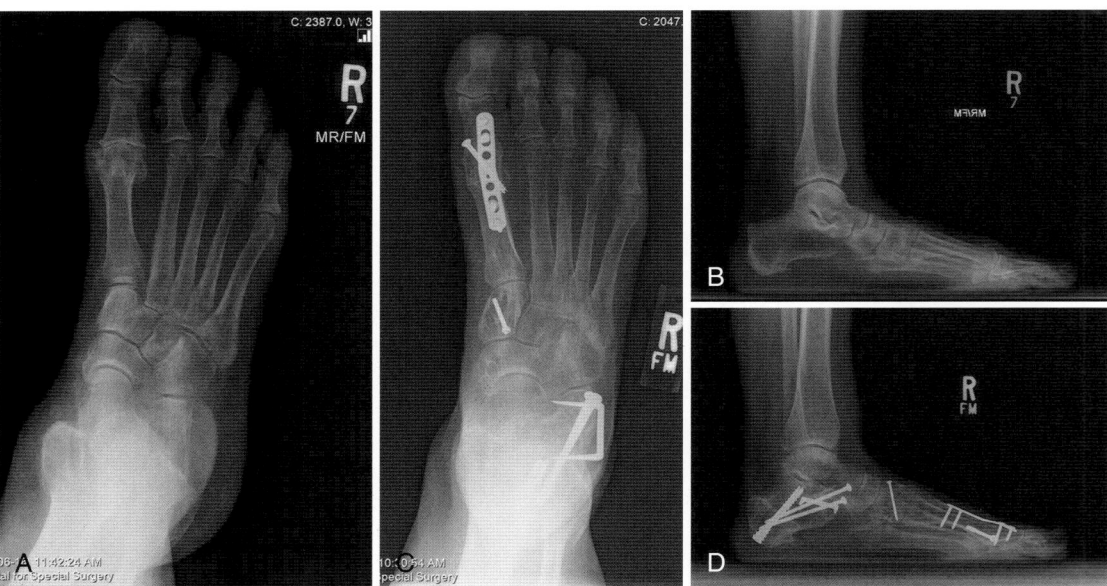

Figure 25-31 Patient with hindfoot **(A)** and midfoot **(B)** deformity as well as elevation of the first ray and first metaphalangeal (MP) arthritis. The preoperative radiographs did not reflect the extent of the deformity at the talonavicular joint (patient did not let arch collapse for the radiograph, deformity was demonstrated fluoroscopically in the operating room). The deformity was corrected with a medial heal side **(C)** and Evans-type lateral **(D)** column lengthening, leaving good eversion motion remaining. The first MP arthritis was treated with a first MP fusion, and the elevation of the first ray was corrected with a Cotton osteotomy fixed with a single screw at the medial cuneiform.

subtalar, and calcaneocuboid joints) but avoid fusion of at least two of those joints: the talonavicular and subtalar joints.* These latter joints are important joints for motion and if fused can eventually promote arthritis of the ankle.

Specifically, lateral column lengthening is for patients with severe flexible deformity whose triple joint complex subluxation cannot be adequately addressed by a medial slide osteotomy and who would otherwise need to be addressed by fusion in the triple joint complex, The deformity includes abduction/plantar sag at the talonavicular joint and subluxation at the subtalar joint resulting in a pronated valgus hindfoot. A severe pronation deformity ultimately results in lateral impingement. The lateral impingement has been found to be at the angle of Gissane in the sinus tarsi and, in the most severe cases, at subfibular area with calcaneal abutment against the fibula.[47,114] One solution for this impingement is to fuse one or more of the joints of the triple joint complex in a corrected position. Another solution is to lengthen the lateral column, as long as it adequately corrects deformity. It most commonly adequately corrects deformity as well as stiffens the hindfoot. If properly used, it should stiffen it to a much lesser degree than an arthrodesis. If done properly, it leaves good motion in the triple joint complex. So far lateral column lengthening, although it may increase pressure in the calcaneocuboid joint, has not led to a high incidence of adjacent joint arthritis.[25,136]

Although it is well-known that lateral column lengthening can lead to lateral discomfort or pain,[47,49] why lateral column lengthening has the potential to cause lateral symptoms is not completely understood. Dumontier et al,[43] in a cadaveric study of lateral column lengthening, showed that the talonavicular joint rotates not as a perfect sphere but takes a path around the ellipsoid talar head. The authors hypothesized that the long plantar ligament and other soft tissue structures may have a role in the correction gained by lengthening the lateral column. The spring ligament complex, whatever part of it is still functioning, probably acts as a ligamentous fulcrum for correction during lateral column lengthening. Therefore correction occurs around the ellipsoid talar head and is dependent on the remaining ligaments mentioned above. Whatever the mechanism, if adequate ligaments remain, the foot becomes increasingly supinated with lateral column lengthening with potential of overstiffening of the lateral hindfoot. In effect, the correction can be so powerful that not only does it eliminate the excessive eversion and abduction motion of the deformity but reduces normal subtalar motion. If too much motion is lost, the foot will become too stiff, with limited eversion resulting in excessive lateral weight bearing. It is a powerful corrector of deformity, with just a 2 to 3 extra millimeters of extra lengthening often having a significant effect on position as well as stiffness. Therefore it has been helpful to gauge correction not just by radiographic correction but by eversion motion intraoperatively. Thus the

goal is to remove the excessive eversion/abduction motion but retain normal or near-normal eversion motion and thereby minimize lateral stiffness and overload. Although both radiographic correction of deformity and motion are important, the primary determinant of correction becomes the elimination of excessive eversion motion but retaining near-normal eversion/abduction motion to achieve the most comfortable foot.

Some surgeons use lateral column lengthening by itself, without a medial slide osteotomy, and others in combination with it.* If used with a medial slide osteotomy, careful attention must be given to the combined effect of the two osteotomies, with each temporarily fixed so that the surgeon can assess the foot for proper position of the heel and midfoot as well as the remaining eversion/adduction motion. The goals are

1. Central position of the heel, no varus
2. Near-normal eversion motion remaining with mild restriction of eversion at the subtalar joint
3. Radiographic correction of the talonavicular joint minimizing remaining abduction or plantar flexion

Varus of the heel or failure to maintain normal eversion/abduction motion will risk stiffness and lateral weight bearing. Slight stiffness is acceptable; considerable stiffness results in unacceptable symptoms. Progressive arthritis of the calcaneocuboid joint, originally thought to be a possible frequent complication of lateral column lengthening, is uncommon, and when it occurs, is usually minimally symptomatic.[134]

Two procedures, the Evans lateral column lengthening and a lateral column lengthening stepcut osteotomy (a modification of the Vander Griend osteotomy), are highlighted below.[66,153] The Evans procedure, developed for the treatment of painful adolescent flatfoot, is the more frequently used at present and has been well studied clinically.[153] However, the stepcut osteotomy, with its longitudinal arm, provides an area of healing that is not dependent upon interpositional bone graft and minimizes the chance of elevation of the distal fragment or graft collapse.[32,66] Although the Vander Griend, or stepcut, osteotomies can potentially still fail to heal, loss of correction is less likely because of the longitudinal arm. Also, the osteotomy has the potential to be displaced in a primarily rotatory fashion, as described by Vander Griend.[66] The modification of the Vander Griend osteotomy uses a stepcut, which is the same type of cut as in the Vander Griend but with a trapezoidal graft, rather than the rotatory correction with some lengthening that Vander Griend described. The term *lateral column lengthening stepcut osteotomy,* or LCL stepcut osteotomy, will be used in the remainder of this chapter because the technique involves trapezoidal wedges. It therefore creates more distraction at the osteotomy site and is likely to gain more correction. The correction of a Vander Griend osteotomy versus an

*References 6, 19, 33, 52, 70, 134, 145, and 179.

*References 9, 32, 38, 68, 76, 178, and 189.

LCL stepcut osteotomy needs to be studied, but it is likely that the probable greater correction of the stepcut can lead to lateral overload. Any lateral column lengthening can be combined or not combined with a medial slide osteotomy, if the medial slide osteotomy is necessary to correct remaining excessive valgus of the heel.

Indications

Indications for lateral column lengthening include (1) lateral impingement or (2) abduction or combined abduction/plantar-flexion deformity at the talonavicular joint that is not likely to be addressed by a medial slide osteotomy. A medial slide osteotomy does not commonly give a large amount of correction to abduction or plantar-flexion deformity. Although this second indication of abduction/eversion deformity is not precise, it can be tested by temporarily fixing the medial slide in the operating room and looking at correction of the talonavicular joint fluoroscopically and assessing eversion motion before a lateral column lengthening is done. Preoperative radiographs are helpful, but surgeons must remember that they are limited by how much the patient lets his or her arch collapse while the radiograph is taken, and the radiograph should be compared with an observation of the patient standing and letting the arch collapse. Uncoverage of the talar head on a standing AP of the foot of more than 30%, and certainly at 40% in a symptomatic flatfoot, suggests the need for lateral column lengthening. Also, because suggestive, excessive passive eversion motion of the hindfoot should be examined.

The talonavicular coverage angle or the incongruency angle may be a more precise measurement than the percentage uncovered, but the former measurements have not been as frequently used in the literature.[50] The AP radiograph must be taken with the patient fully weight bearing on the foot and with the patient letting the arch pronate. The x-ray beam should be centered as much as possible directly dorsal to the talonavicular joint. Confirmation of the uncoverage can be done under fluoroscopy in the operating room.

Contraindications

Patients with stage III disease (fixed hindfoot deformity in the triple joint complex) are not candidates for lateral column lengthening. The deformity must be passively correctible with the talonavicular joint being able to be manipulated past neutral into inversion or adduction. There are cases of severe deformity in which the talonavicular joint cannot be adducted in the office, but after release of the lateral talonavicular joint capsule, the joint can be brought into adduction. Also, patients with symptomatic or severe arthritis in the triple joint complex are not good candidates for lateral column lengthening.

Preoperative Evaluation

Flexibility of the hindfoot joints, allowing good correction of the foot, must be confirmed preoperatively. Specifically, correction of the position of the heel and the to

bring the talonavicular joint into inversion with reduction of the subtalar joint should be confirmed by physical examination. If necessary, a stress AP radiograph of the foot with the foot placed into inversion can be used to demonstrate the ability to bring the talonavicular joint into adduction.

Standing AP and lateral radiographs of the foot and a standing AP radiograph of the ankle should be assessed for the amount of deformity (Fig. 25-32). Care should be taken to check for valgus deformity of the ankle on a standing AP ankle radiograph because that can be missed if the ankle radiograph is not done. Also, a patient can appear clinically to have severe deformity in the foot, yet the radiograph evaluation is not impressive. This most commonly occurs because the patient is not fully weight bearing when the radiographs are taken or the patient is leaning back. If the radiographs are unimpressive compared with the physical examination, they should be repeated with the patient letting the arch completely collapse with full weight bearing. A Saltzman (hindfoot alignment view) is also a very helpful radiograph (Fig. 25-34) and should be considered a routine radiographic view for this condition. It is very helpful in visualizing and measuring the amount of hindfoot valgus. An equation has been developed to predict the amount of correction needed in the operating room.[14] This equation needs to be applied to a large group of patients for confirmation of its usefulness and accuracy. However, there is benefit

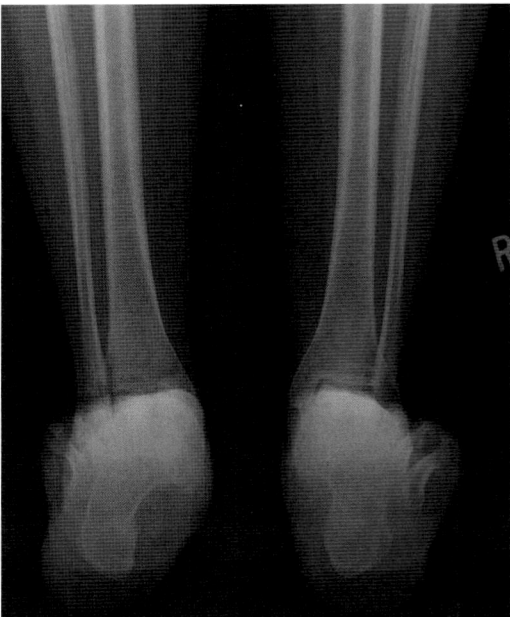

Figure 25-32 This hindfoot alignment view, as described by Saltzman,[158] is used to measure the hindfoot moment arm. This view and measurement accurately depicts the hindfoot deformity and can be used to estimate the amount of correction needed. In this example, this patient with bilateral flat feet needs a large medial slide on the left but not on the right. The hindfoot alignment view is best taken as a single view for each side.

to visualizing the amount of hindfoot valgus and measuring it so the result can be used as an estimate of how much to slide the heel, minimizing the chance of over- or undercorrection. A lateral column lengthening also affects the position of the heel, although it is likely that it will not correct heel valgus to the same degree as a medializing calcaneal osteotomy. When using that osteotomy with a lateral column lengthening, it is important to realize that there will be some correction of the heel from the lengthening procedure. Both osteotomies should be temporarily fixed and the position of the heel assessed in the operating room by looking at the position of the heel from an end-on view (Fig. 25-33), as well as palpating the heel to make sure that the heel is not in varus but centrally placed.

Care should be taken not to perform a lateral column lengthening in the setting of minimal deformity because this can result in an adducted, stiff, uncomfortable foot. It is important to achieve adequate correction of deformity and eliminate excessive eversion while retaining adequate (near-normal) eversion of the hindfoot. Thus performing a lateral column lengthening when there is not excessive eversion will overstiffen the foot.

Surgical Technique for Evans Procedure (Fig. 25-34)
A lateral column lengthening requires good access to the lateral hindfoot with the patient in the lateral decubitus position or in the supine position with the leg internally rotated to gain access to the lateral hindfoot. Fluoroscopic imaging to obtain an AP and lateral view of the foot is essential. The leg should be able to be rotated to a position to allow eversion of the foot and simulate loading of the foot to judge correction and subtalar motion.

1. This procedure can be performed with or without a medial slide osteotomy. By the end of the foot reconstruction, the patient should have central position to a central slight valgus of the heel. The medial calcaneal osteotomy can be performed first in a patient with severe heel valgus but should not be permanently fixed until after the lateral column lengthening has been set. Failure to check the position of the heel and adjust as necessary after the lateral column lengthening can result in improper position of the heel, most commonly varus. The lateral column lengthening does change the position of the posterior heel but does not as much as a medial slide osteotomy.

2. Under thigh tourniquet, an incision is made longitudinally along the sinus tarsi just above its floor, ending at the calcaneocuboid joint. In general, the dissection should remain well above the level of the floor of the sinus tarsi and the peroneal tendons to avoid possible injury to the sural nerve. Once on the floor of the sinus tarsi, dissection is made subperiosteally over the anterolateral calcaneus, mobilizing and retracting the peroneal tendons away from the lateral calcaneus. The very dorsal aspect of the calcaneocuboid joint is also exposed to confirm the calcaneocuboid joint line.

3. A K-wire is placed as a guide for the osteotomy cut. To avoid too small a distal fragment, place the pin 1.5 cm proximal to the calcaneocuboid joint, aiming 10 to 15 degrees posteriorly from a direct perpendicular to the lateral calcaneus. This should place the pin just anterior to the middle facet or at the junction of the anterior and middle facets. A blunt elevator or Freer elevator can be used to locate the middle facet. It is preferable to stay distal to the medial facet with the bone cut.

4. Check pin placement on AP and lateral views of the foot. Note that the saw cut will be made on the distal side of the pin, with retractors in place to protect the peroneal tendons.

5. Make the cut, taking care not to plunge through the medial cortex. The medial cortex can be weakened by

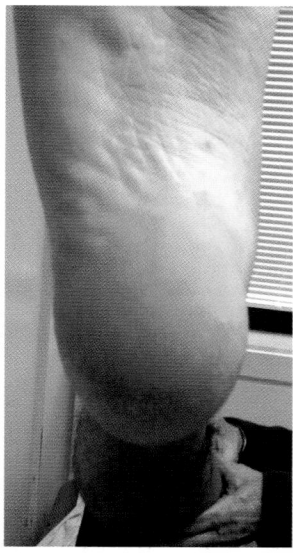

Figure 25-33 Clinical photograph demonstrating a useful position to assess heel alignment in the operating room. Heel should be centrally placed in relation to the ankle and calf, without varus but neutral to slight valgus.

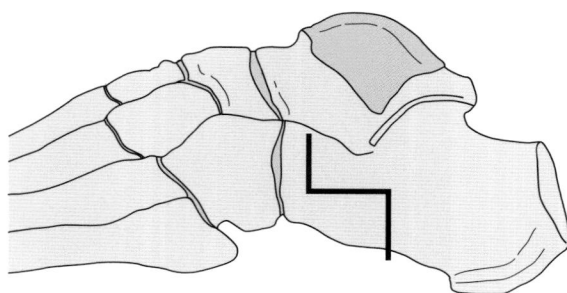

Figure 25-34 Diagram of lateral column lengthening stepcut osteotomy. Note that the longitudinal arm of the osteotomy gives an area of primary bone healing and graft is placed at the vertical arms at either end of the osteotomy. The vertical arms are shorter than those described by Vander Griend, to minimize the chance of fracturing through the intact bone.

small motions of the saw to preserve medial perios-teum and soft tissue. Irrigation is helpful to avoid thermal necrosis.

6. Open the osteotomy site laterally. (Distraction will usually occur on the medial side, but it is best not to overdistract the medial side.)

7. With the use of trial wedges or a laminar spreader, try different amounts of lengthening to gain correction yet not overstiffen the midfoot and hindfoot. The authors prefer using trial wedges because, with wedges in place, easy manipulation of the foot is allowed, to judge both the amount of correction at the talona-vicular joint and the eversion motion of the triple joint complex. Two millimeters of correction can make a very significant difference to the patient in terms of stiffness or over-/undercorrection. Fluoros-copy with the foot everted should be used to check the position of the talonavicular joint on the AP and lateral views. Correction of the joint should occur, but the amount of correction should not be judged purely radiographically. Eversion/abduction motion must also be checked to confirm that normal or near-normal motion remains with manipulation of the calcaneus and hindfoot. This latter motion must remain for the patient to have the least risk of lateral discomfort or pain from stiffness. However, leaving excessive eversion motion (with residual abduction of the talonavicular joint or excessive valgus of the heel) can lead to recurrence of lateral impingement.

8. Once good position and motion is confirmed, the trial wedge or space determined by the laminar spreader is used to fashion the tricortical bone graft.

9. The surgeon has the option of either using allograft or iliac crest autograft. Good results have been reported with both, although there may be less chance of graft collapse with autograft.

10. Using a laminar spreader, the tricortical graft is placed in the osteotomy site. No space should be seen either dorsally or laterally at the interfaces of the graft and host bone. AP and lateral fluoroscopy is also used to confirm good fit of the graft. If space is present, care-fully shave the appropriate location on the graft or host bone so that excellent contact is achieved. If at the correct size, take care not to shorten the graft later-ally because this will change the correction.

11. Pin the osteotomy site with two longitudinal K-wires from the distal fragment to the proximal fragment. Place a long lag screw from the distal fragment across the graft and into the proximal calcaneus. A 3.5-mm lag screw is used; a smaller screw or larger screw is preferred by some surgeons. Most important, good fixation as well as compression and apposition should be achieved. Compression fixation using a thin lateral plate or a compression staple device can be very helpful in addition to the screw.

12. After fixation is placed, check that the graft is stable and good apposition is present.

Surgical Technique for LCL Stepcut Osteotomy (Fig. 25-35A-D)

1. Incision is the same as for the Evans, except that is extended 1 to 2 cm more proximally, to the distal tip of the fibula (Video Clip 119).

2. Similar dissection is made laterally over the anterior calcaneus. However, this dissection is carried proximal

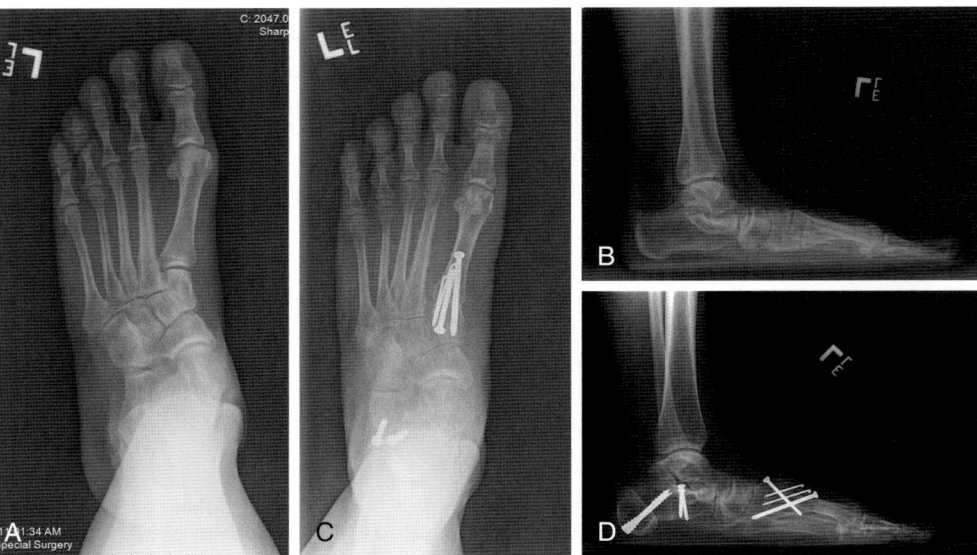

Figure 25-35 **A** and **B**, Patient with advanced abduction and plantar-flexion deformity in the hindfoot and midfoot, showing combined plantar flexion and abduction at the talonavicular joint. **C** and **D**, Correction with lateral column lengthening stepcut osteotomy for lateral column lengthening as well as medial slide calcaneal osteotomy and metatarsal–tarsal fusion.

and plantar to the peroneal tubercle. The peroneus longus is held against the lateral calcaneus by a sheath attached to the peroneal tubercle. Open this sheath and make sure both peroneal tendons are mobilized away from the lateral calcaneus proximally as well as dorsally. A pin is placed, retracting the peroneal tendons inferiorly and proximally, giving maximal exposure of the lateral calcaneus. The proximal bone cut, in particular, risks injuring the peroneal tendons. A pin can be placed proximally and plantarly pushing the peroneal tendons out of the way.

3. Pins are placed to mark the elbows of the stepcut osteotomy. The first pin is placed just over 1 cm proximal to the calcaneocuboid joint at the junction of the dorsal one third and plantar two thirds of the bone. The second pin is placed 2 cm proximal to this at the junction of the dorsal two thirds and plantar one third of the bone. These placements of the pins help minimize the risk of fracturing at the proximal and distal arms of the osteotomy. These vertical arms are shorter than as described by Vander Griend; the shorter arms, which minimize risk of saw cuts straying vertically in the wrong direction, are depicted in Figure 25-35A.

4. Cut the longitudinal 2-cm arm, being careful to retract the peroneal tendons. After cutting the lateral cortex, carefully cut the medial cortex so as not to plunge.

5. Cut the distal dorsal arm, but do not to stray inferiorly and weaken the distal fragment. Be sure to cut the elbow junctures well because this can help avoid difficulty in mobilizing the osteotomy later.

6. Cut the dorsal aspect of the proximal plantar cut, being careful to protect the peroneal tendons. If the plantar portion of the proximal plantar cut is too difficult to make because of the peroneal tendons, dissect around the peroneal tendons and sural nerve and retract them dorsally to gain access to the plantar area for the cut. Protect the tendons and soft tissue with wide retractors when performing these cuts.

7. Mobilize the osteotomy site with an osteotome, but do not hinge aggressively on the dorsal distal or proximal plantar limbs. If the osteotomy does not move easily, check with the saw that the cuts are complete medially, especially at the elbows.

8. Place a pin in the distal more plantar aspect of the calcaneus adjacent the calcaneocuboid joint but away from the elbow of the cut. Place another pin in the more dorsal proximal aspect beyond the osteotomy so that the osteotomy can be distracted with a laminar spreader or pin distractor device. With the device, spread the osteotomy open, making sure that the longitudinal cut remains apposed.

9. Use the laminar spreader to hold the correction, or better, use a trial wedge/spacer of appropriate size in the dorsal arm to judge the amount of correction. The criteria for correction are the same as with the Evans procedure described above.

10. Place tricortical autograft or allograft at the dorsal arm of the osteotomy site keeping the longitudinal arm well opposed. This graft can be gently wedged into the distal arm. The osteotomy should be manually compressed to confirm excellent apposition and a snug stable fit of the graft as described for step 10 of the Evans procedure.

11. Drill a longitudinal K-wire from distal to proximal, from the dorsal aspect of the calcaneus across the graft and into the posterior calcaneus. Start a second K-wire just distal and lateral to the posterior facet and drill it dorsal to plantar for both temporary fixation and the path for a second screw.

12. Replace the proximal-to-distal K-wire with a 3.5-mm lag screw and place a second screw along the path of the dorsal-to-plantar K-wire hole.

13. Wedge a carefully sized tricortical graft into the plantar arm for a snug fit. Trim away any prominent tricortical wedge bone at the distal dorsal arm of the osteotomy to avoid impingement against the talus and smooth any sharp edges along the lateral calcaneus.

14. Check for impingement in the sinus tarsi with eversion range of motion. If necessary, shave away prominent bone on the anterior aspect of the lateral talar process at the posterior facet joint, to avoid bony impingement at the angle of Gissane.

TREATMENT OF DELTOID INSUFFICIENCY

Deltoid ligament insufficiency or disruption occurs late in the course of PTT insufficiency and has been quantified as stage 4 disorder. Although there are components of the deltoid ligament that merge with the spring ligament, for purposes of this discussion, only the failure of the strongest bands will be considered: the tibiocalcaneal (superficial) and posterior (deep) tibiotalar ligaments.[11] The integrity of the deltoid ligament has been shown to be critically important in the maintenance of normal biomechanics of the ankle joint. Sectioning of the deltoid ligament has been shown to decrease the tibiotalar contact area by 43%.[46] Thus, in advanced PTT insufficiency with a valgus deforming force already present, if the disrupted deltoid is left unchecked, the increases in peak pressures leads to the eventual development of osteoarthritic changes within the ankle joint.

Indications

Deltoid ligament reconstruction is indicated if rupture is visible or laxity is noted upon direct inspection intraoperatively. Valgus and/or external rotation stress testing showing increased talar tilt or rotation suggests the necessity of ligament reconstruction. Note that restoration of the medial column of the foot is not sufficient to take the strain and subsequent deforming force upon the ankle.[167] Significant increase in strain upon the deltoid, if present with heel rise even after said reconstructions, allows degenerative wear upon the ankle joint because of improper biomechanics. Finally, similar to other soft tissue procedures mentioned in this chapter, isolated reconstruction of the deltoid ligament is rarely performed and is almost exclusively done in combination with other realignment procedures.

Contraindications

The only relative contraindication to deltoid ligament reconstruction is advanced degenerative disease that may require ankle arthrodesis. With advancement in ankle replacement technology, it is clear that reconstruction under these circumstances remains a relative contraindication. If the patient has potential to undergo total ankle arthroplasty to correct advanced degenerative disease, then reconstruction of the deltoid ligament becomes an indicated component to advanced flatfoot reconstruction.

Preoperative Evaluation

If available, MRI is a useful adjunct to planning deltoid ligament repair because of both its sensitivity and specificity. The location and the poor quality of the tissue can be mapped, allowing the surgeon to decide if any residual deltoid tissue will have value in assisting the reconstruction. Plain radiographs document a tibiotalar tilt, even if subtle, on weight-bearing ankle views. The surgeon must look carefully for this tilt because its presence dictates deltoid instability. Finally, stressing the ankle in both eversion and external rotation tests the rigidity of the deltoid ligament, creating pain that must be discerned from PTT pain based on location. Of note, the deep deltoid component is directly inferior to the posterior tibial tendon, and thus direct palpation of that ligament has less value in confirming ligament disruption because the diseased tendon is generally in this same location.

Preoperative Planning

Planning for deltoid reconstruction primarily involves determination of incision placement commensurate with the additional surgical procedures planned in flatfoot reconstruction. The incision for deltoid reconstruction through tendon transfer requires exposure of the superficial deltoid ligament insertion, which is at the sustentaculum tali of the calcaneus. This incision is virtually vertical, which does not have the same curvilinear slope of the flexor digitorum longus tendon transfer incision directed toward the navicular. As such, the surgeon must plan compromise of both incisions to achieve both goals. Similar to spring ligament reconstruction, patient positioning does matter, as external rotation of the extremity will help to gain access to the medial ankle.

Surgical Technique for Deltoid Reconstruction

There are a variety of procedures in the literature developed to reconstruct the deficient deltoid ligament.[8,34,69] All involve tendon transfers on some level because repair of the chronically insufficient deltoid ligament more often than not results in failure resulting from poor-quality tissue under significant tension. Unlike lateral ligament reconstruction, deltoid reconstruction requires significant tension to prevent recurrent valgus deformity.

HADDAD TECHNIQUE[69]

1. A thigh tourniquet is used for this procedure but must be deflated before closure to ensure adequate hemostasis and prevent postoperative hematoma.
2. A semitendinosus allograft is soaked in antibiotic solution to allow thawing. Graft length should approach 300 mm. The graft is tubularized to facilitate passage. Tension is placed on the graft to minimize late creep of the tendon (Fig. 25-36A).
3. Medial exposure is critical, and thus external rotation of the involved extremity is helped by placing a bump beneath the opposite hip. Note, however, that at certain points in the procedure the surgeon will require access to the lateral hindfoot, and thus the bump is normally removed after deep medial exposure is complete (Fig. 25-36B).
4. As noted above, exposure involves an incision over the intercollicular groove of the medial malleolus, extending distally over the sustentaculum tali. This incision is nearly vertical. Note that to address both the PTT and the deltoid ligament the surgeon may need to alter this incision by beginning just posterior to the medial malleolus and extending toward the navicular. However, this modification should incorporate a larger curvature to incorporate the sustentaculum tali.
5. The PTT is exposed and retracted to expose the deep deltoid insertion, and the flexor hallucis longus is traced to expose the sustentaculum tali. Structures at risk are the tibial nerve, primarily at the inferior portion of the incision near the sustentaculum tali (Fig. 25-36C-E).
6. Drill holes will be placed beginning medially at the insertion of both the superficial and deep deltoid ligaments. These drill holes are through and through the calcaneus and talus, respectively (Fig. 25-36F). To position the drill holes without violation of offending bone structures, the drill holes are placed over guidewires. The guidewires serve a secondary purpose of allowing exact measurement of the length of the drill holes, which is critical in establishing appropriate graft length. The direction of the talus guidewire is from the insertion point of the deep deltoid, 1 cm posterior and inferior to the intercollicular groove, and exiting anterior to the fibula. The central portion of the sustentaculum tali is the starting point for the guidewire, given the small size of this projection and the subsequent potential for the drill to fracture this portion of bone. The wire is directed both inferiorly and anteriorly, exiting 1 cm proximal to the calcaneocuboid joint, and at the inferior margin of the calcaneus (Fig. 25-36G). This direction allows the wire (and drill hole) to avoid the sinus tarsi. Both guidewire lengths within the bone are measured. In general, the talar length is 45 mm, and the calcaneal length is 55 mm.
7. A third guidewire begins at the intercollicular groove of the medial malleolus, directed in the central medial malleolus both anterior and lateral. This wire exits in the central metaphyseal tibia. This length is also mea-

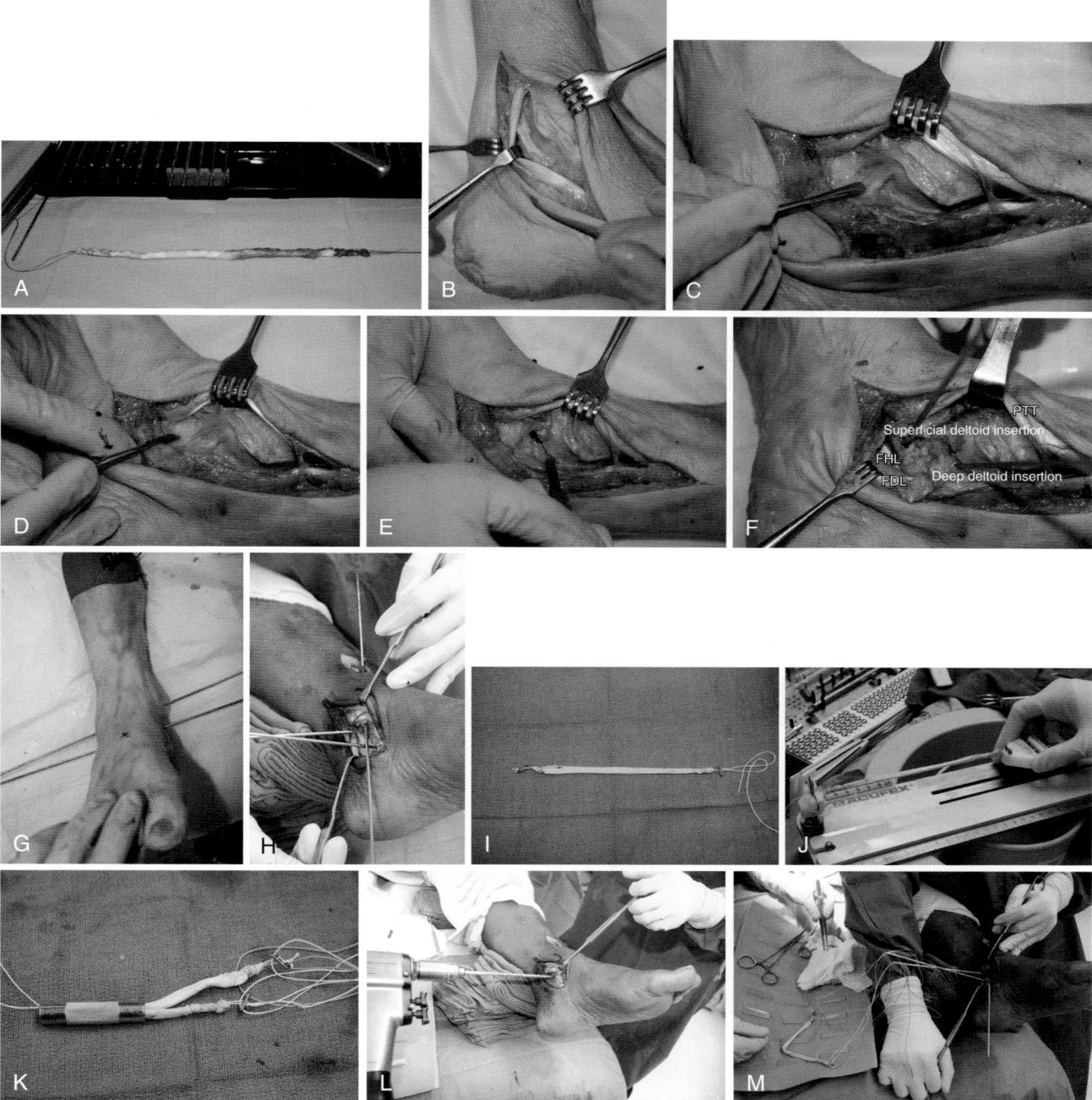

Figure 25-36 **A,** Isolated anterior tibial tendon graft after tubularization and with No. 2 Ethibond suture, undergoing Krakow suture weave on both ends. **B,** Standard medial approach to the ankle, with the posterior tibial tendon retracted posteriorly. This approach allows excellent visualization of the deltoid ligament complex. **C-E,** Visualization of the deltoid ligament complex deep to the posterior tibial tendon. The fibers of the deep deltoid *(a)* and superficial deltoid *(d)* are easily recognizable by their footprint and orientation. After defining both the deep and superficial deltoid ligaments, they are sectioned *(e)*. **F** and **G,** Medial ankle visualization **(F),** with tendons identified (*FDL,* flexor digitorum longus tendon; *FHL,* flexor hallucis longus tendon; *PTT,* posterior tibial tendon). Guidewire insertion points are labeled for both the superficial and deep deltoid ligaments, based on their footprints and anatomic locations. Anterior view of the ankle **(G)** showing orientation of guidewires and exit points inferior and anterior to fibula. **H,** Actual patient with orientation of three guidewires visualized in the operating room. Note the orientation of the tibial guidewire from the intercollicular groove, exiting at the anterior tibia. **I-K,** Graft preparation was performed by first attaching the suture buttons to each end of the sutured tendon graft **(I).** This graft is then pretensioned to minimize creep **(J).** The graft is then sized for absolute width and doubled width **(K)** to determine appropriate tunnel size. **L-O,** Graft passage first required the use of cannulated reamers set to the appropriate tunnel depth, leaving a 1-cm "bone bridge" laterally to maintain the holding power of the suture button **(L).** The sutures that facilitate suture button passage are placed through the respective holes within the medial guidewires **(M),** allowing each end to be passed through a separate cannulated drill hole (one end in the talus and the other in the calcaneus).

Continued

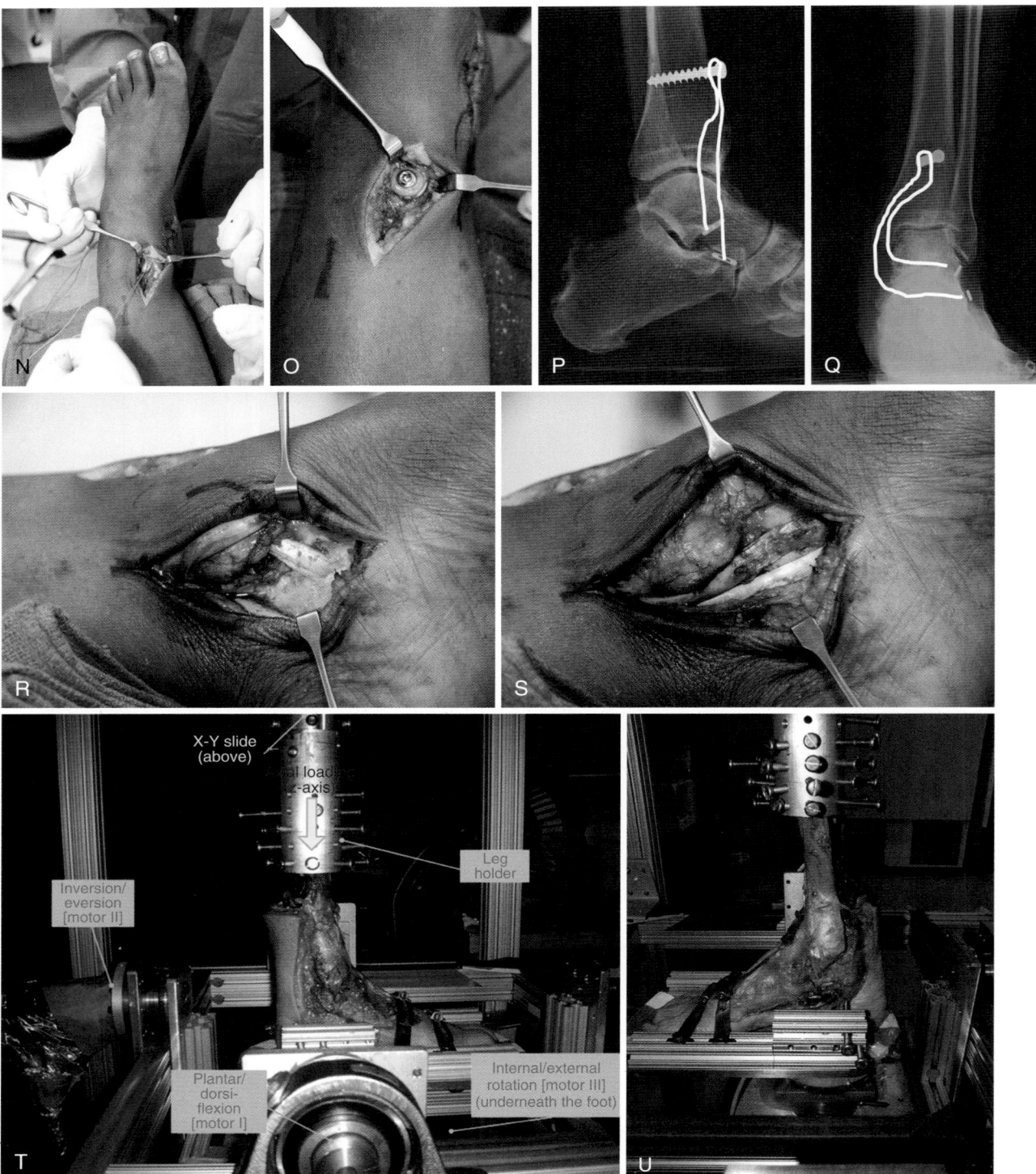

Figure 25-36, cont'd The looped end of the graft is then pulled through the tibial tunnel **(N)** with the assistance of a suture through the loop. Note the power of maximal tension pulling the foot into varus. Fixation is then achieved with a spiked ligament washer over a 6.5-mm cancellous screw post **(O)**. **P** and **Q,** Final radiographs demonstrating graft passage in as a white line. Note that in the lateral radiograph **(P)** the suture buttons are secure against the drill holes, both being placed anterior and inferior to the fibula to facilitate passage. The anteroposterior radiograph **(Q)** again demonstrates the security of the suture button passage, and the lack of violation of the medial articular surface of the ankle joint. **R** and **S,** Final construct demonstrates lack of bulk associated with this tendon transfer medially **(R)**. In fact, the posterior tibial tendon and flexor digitorum longus tendons sit appropriately within the medial malleolar groove **(S)** without the tendency for dislocation. **T** and **U,** The custom multiaxis ankle testing apparatus with active driving in plantar/dorsiflexion, inversion/eversion, and internal/external rotation by motors I, II, and III, respectively **(R** and **S)**. The tibia was loaded axially through the vertical Z slide and was free to move mediolaterally and anteroposteriorly along the X and Y slides.

sured and is doubled to measure the looped component of the tendon transfer (Fig. 25-36H).

8. Summation is now done for graft length—talus length + calcaneal length + (tibial length × 2) + distance between origin and insertion point of deep and superficial deltoid ligaments – distance between suture button and allograft tendon (the latter is usually 1 cm per button).

9. The allograft is then cut to size, with strong Krakow weave stitches placed at either end.

10. A metallic button is secured with a 1-cm distance between the tendon graft and buttons. Multiple ties are placed to secure this button.

11. The talus and calcaneus drill diameters are normally 5 mm, although the graft diameter needs to be sized (Fig. 25-36L).

12. The metallic buttons are passed through the talus and calcaneus, respectively, and flipped to provide secure lateral fixation of each tendon end (Fig. 25-36M). This leaves a loop medially. The graft is pulled upon to ensure the buttons are engaging the lateral cortex.

13. A drill hole is now made in the medial malleolus, following the third guidewire. The diameter of this drill hole is normally 7.5 mm. Again, the graft diameter is sized as a looped construct. An incision is made at the exit point of this guidewire, usually medial to the anterior tibial tendon to avoid the neurovascular complex deep.

14. The graft is now passed through the medial malleolus drill hole by passing a looped suture through the anterior tibial cortex, exiting at the medial malleolus. This suture is used to pull the graft through the tibia, exiting the anterior tibial cortex (Fig. 25-36N).

15. The graft is maximally tensioned, secured over a screw and post construct, with a spiked ligament washer placed over the post (screw) (Fig. 25-36O). Again, this graft is placed at maximal tension (Fig. 25-36P-S).

DELAND TECHNIQUE[34]

1. The technique begins with a 16- to 18-cm incision in the lateral midcalf. Allograft tendon can be used instead of peroneus longus autograft. With allograft tendon the sinus tarsi end of the incision is necessary but not an incision above the tip of the fibula.

2. Peroneus longus tendon is transected proximally at the junction of the proximal two thirds and distal one third of the calf, just distal to where the peroneus longus tendon is well formed. This allows for a long graft that is still attached distally, easily long enough to make it through the described talar and tibial bone tunnels below. Incise the longus tendon proximally enough for adequate length. Bone tunnels can be drilled and measured first so proper length of graft can be checked.

3. Side-to-side tenodesis of the peroneus longus to peroneus brevis tendon is done proximally. Weave two No. 2 permanent sutures into the free end of the graft for a strong hold.

4. Similar to the approach above, the deltoid is exposed through a near-vertical incision along its anterior border. A second surgical approach is through the sinus tarsi.

5. A bone tunnel of sufficient diameter to accommodate the peroneus longus tendon is drilled from the lateral neck of the talus (visualized through the sinus tarsi approach) exiting the medial talar body directly inferior to the medial malleolus. This is the insertion point of the deep deltoid, at the center of rotation of the talus. This tunnel is nearly parallel to the dome of the talus and exits medially inferior to the intercollicular notch of the distal medial malleolus. Confirmation of a good isometric point on the talus during ankle range of motion can be confirmed by placing a small K-wire at the proposed medial talar exit point and dorsiflex and plantar flex the ankle.

6. Once the position for the medial talar exit hole is confirmed, drill a K-wire hole from medial to lateral, exiting in the sinus tarsi dorsally but staying in the middle of the talar neck to minimize chance of subsequent stresss fracture. A lateral fluoroscopic view with the K-wire in place can be taken to confirm position of the pin. The pin is then replaced with the guide pin for use with the cannulated drill.

7. Drill the talar hole of sufficient size for the graft, often an 8- to 9-mm drill hole.

8. The peroneus longus tendon is passed from lateral to medial through this tunnel.

9. A second tunnel is made from the tip of the medial malleolus, exiting at the medial tibial metaphysis as described in step 6 of the Haddad technique.

10. The graft is tensioned at the talar exit point, followed by secondary tensioning at the medial tibial exit point at the medial tibial metaphysis. Simulated weight-bearing intraoperative radiographs confirm the talus is reduced to neutral in the mortise.

11. Under tension, the graft is secured with No. 2 permanent sutures already woven into the end of the graft and tied under tension with the ankle reduced (ankle pinned if desired) to a screw on the medial tibia. Do not drill for this screw until the graft is tensioned, so that good screw placement is confirmed.

Myerson Technique[8,87]

1. This technique uses medial allograft tendon for the reconstruction. To allow appropriate reduction, it is used only in stage IVA PTT insufficiency patients because a flexible deformity is the "A" group.

2. The graft is first passed in the medial distal tibia (straight medial) and approximately 2 cm proximal to the tibial plafond and anchored securely in the tunnel with an interference screw.

3. The graft is then passed through a subcutaneous tunnel overlying the medial malleolus and split for transfer into the talus and calcaneus.

4. Krakow suture weave technique is performed on both limbs of the split graft.

5. The talar tunnel is created first through a drill hole at the medial center or tibiotalar rotation, exiting at the lateral junction of the talar dome and neck.

6. One limb of the split graft is placed through this tunnel and anchored under tension with an interference screw.

7. A calcaneal tunnel is then created from the sustentaculum tali exiting 1 cm superior to the peroneal tubercle laterally. The other graft limb is placed through this tunnel and anchored with an interference screw.

8. The superior limb of the tendon graft is sutured to the patient's natural deltoid ligament at the apex of the medial malleolus, to add additional stability and prevent the graft from shifting too much.

Postoperative Care

Patients are generally in a cast for 6 weeks, with inversion applied to the cast to minimize risk of tendon rupture. In addition, if these techniques involve an osteotomy or arthrodesis, ultimate weight bearing will depend on the strength of the fusion or osteotomy. Progressive weight bearing begins first in a walking boot, followed by a shoe with a stirrup splint. In general, patients are back into a shoe without protective ankle devices by 3 months postsurgery; although, if there is any tendency toward medial column collapse of the foot, a medial posted orthosis is placed in the shoe.

Results and Complications

This Haddad technique has undergone biomechanical testing to ensure anatomic strength (Fig. 25-36T and U). External rotation and eversion laxity, calculated as angular displacement at 2-Nm level torque, was significantly greater in the sectioned group compared with the deltoid reconstruction group, with $P = .006$ and $P = .017$, respectively. There was no statistical difference in laxity in external rotation and eversion (tested at 2 Nm of torque) between the deltoid intact and reconstructed group, with $P = .865$ and $P = .470$, respectively. Loading the specimens at 2 Nm of torque revealed the deltoid ligament reconstruction was 98.1% ± 22.2% and able to withstand angular displacement when compared with the intact ligament in external rotation (Fig. 25-37A). Although, the laxity of the reconstruction was significantly reduced compared with the sectioned state in internal rotation ($P = .034$), the reconstruction was only able to withstand 52.3 ± 7.0% angular displacement in internal rotation compared with the intact ligament (Fig. 25-37B). At 2-Nm torque in eversion, the deltoid ligament reconstruction was able to withstand 92.4 ± 37.4% of the angular displacement compared with the intact ligament (Fig. 25-37C).

Sectioning of the deltoid ligament increased inversion laxity by only 44.1 ± 41.4% compared with the deltoid intact condition. There was no significant difference in inversion laxity between the intact and reconstruction groups ($P = .986$) (Fig. 25-37C). Angular displacement was not statistically significant in plantar flexion between groups. Dorsiflexion laxity did show a statistically significant difference between reconstruction and sectioned groups ($P = .014$), but the magnitude of this difference was small, with only a 25.6 ± 21.3% increase in dorsiflexion laxity in the sectioned state.

Stiffness was statistically significant in eversion but not inversion between the reconstructed and sectioned groups ($P = .022$ and $P = .202$, respectively). The stiffness of the reconstruction was 89.8 ± 54.3% compared with the intact ligament (Fig. 25-37E). Stiffness was statistically significant in external but not internal rotation between the reconstructed and sectioned groups ($P = .001$ and $P = .161$ respectively) (Fig. 25-37F). The stiffness of the reconstruction was 136.4 ± 40.2% compared with the intact ligament. Stiffness data was not statistically insignificant in both plantar flexion and dorsiflexion between the reconstructed and sectioned groups ($P = .050$ and $P = .126$, respectively). Mode of failure was then analyzed for the six specimens in the reconstruction group. Three of the six specimens failed at the knot over the suture button in the tibiocalcaneal bundle, with the tibiotalar bundle intact. In one specimen, the knot over the suture button failed at both tunnels. The medial malleolus fractured, with both bundles intact in one specimen. The final specimen failed by fracture of the roof of the tibiocalcaneal bone tunnel.

The Deland technique has undergone recent clinical follow-up at an average of 8.9 years after the index operation.[48] The authors revisited the five patients on whom they performed this technique in the original 2004 study. Both residual valgus talar tilt (via weight-bearing radiographs) and ankle range of motion (with standing hindfoot alignment) were used in combination with clinical assessment tools.

Valgus tilt improved from 7.7 degrees preoperative to 2.1 degrees postoperative, and ankle range of motion averaged 47 degrees (no preoperative assessment quantified). In addition, clinical hindfoot alignment averaged 4 degrees of valgus. Confounding the quantification of correction was concomitant surgical procedures (bone work) done for realignment. Finally, there is no known "acceptable" level of valgus correction in patients with valgus deformity secondary to deltoid ligament insufficiency. The authors assume angular measurements within 5 degrees are within an acceptable range, but there is no validation of this figure.

The Myerson technique has also undergone clinical follow-up for eight patients at an average of 3 years.[87] Again, concomitant procedures were performed, including triple arthrodesis. Using more stringent criteria—3 degrees or less of valgus at final follow-up being considered successful—the authors found that 5 patients reached radiographic success (this patient population averaged 2 degrees of valgus tilt). Based on these results, the authors felt that the upper limit of corrective power of their technique in valgus talar tilt was 10 degrees.

Complications revolve around violation of the structures near the site of surgery. As noted above, the tibial nerve may sustain injury at the site of the sustentaculum tali. In addition, the sustentaculum tali itself might sustain fracture with drilling, especially if a

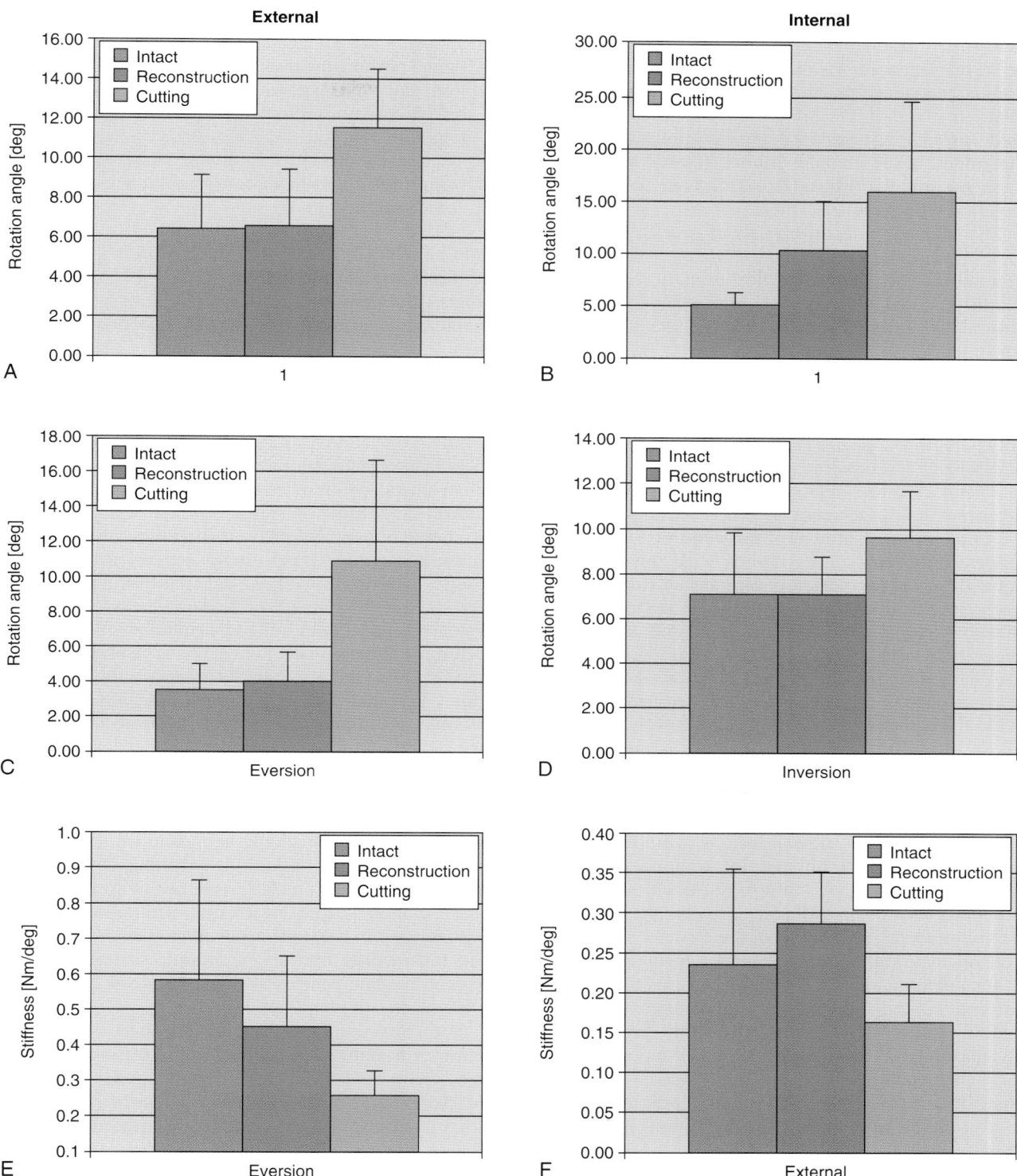

Figure 25-37 **A** and **B,** Average and standard deviation of angular displacements in external **(A)** and internal **(B)** rotation. Note the strength of the repair in external rotation when compared with the intact native ligament. **C,** Average and standard deviation of angular displacements in eversion. Note the strength of the repair in eversion when compared with the intact native ligament. **D,** Average and standard deviation of angular displacements in inversion. Note the strength of the repair in inversion when compared with the intact native ligament. **E,** The stiffness of the reconstruction in eversion was 89.8 ± 54.3% compared with the intact ligament. **F,** The stiffness of the reconstruction in external rotation was 136.4 ± 40.2% compared with the intact ligament.

subtalar fusion is done commensurate with the deltoid reconstruction and the middle facet is prepared for fusion. Screw placement for fusion can shear the graft within the body of the talus if the graft is passed before screw placement. The author, Dr. Steven Haddad, prefers to place guidewires for fixation of the subtalar joint and then place the guidewire for the talus tunnel to avoid screw placement for subtalar arthrodesis. This then prevents graft violation with screw placement.

The allograft and autograft can sustain creep, and thus appropriate tensioning before graft insertion is important. Also, large diameter, nonabsorbable suture should be used to secure the graft ends to the metal buttons to prevent failure at this weakest point in the construct.

SUBTALAR ARTHRODESIS TO TREAT POSTERIOR TIBIAL TENDON DYSFUNCTION

Subtalar arthrodesis has been described for the treatment of deformity for the adult acquired flatfoot.[21] With the use of lateral column lengthening procedures for flexible deformity, it appears to be used less commonly but still has a role in the treatment of this condition.

Deformity correction is noted with this procedure, naturally at the talocalcaneal joint and to some extent at transverse tarsal joint. It is appropriate for fixed or considerable symptomatic deformity at the subtalar joint not corrected by osteotomies or when symptomatic degenerative changes are present. In particular, lateral subluxation at the subtalar joint, if present, is not corrected by a lateral column lengthening. This subluxation can be appreciated on weight-bearing coronal CT imaging or simulated weight-bearing if available. Care should be taken not to put the subtalar joint in varus because this can easily lead to symptomatic lateral weight bearing.

In a large series of subtalar fusions, symptomatic varus deformity did occur (although not commonly) as well as leaving too much valgus at the joint. As with other reconstruction procedures for flatfeet, care should be taken to carefully reduce subluxation of the foot and, if excessive heel valgus is still present, perform a medial slide calcaneal osteotomy as well. For forefoot varus not based in deformity of the talonavicular joint or severe naviculocuneiform joint subluxation, a Cotton procedure or metatarsal–tarsal fusion can achieve better positioning of the first metatarsal head and better appearance of the arch. Do not malposition the subtalar joint into varus or just fuse it "in situ" in an everted position. It should be fused in neutral.

Surgical Technique for Subtalar Arthrodesis (Video Clips 26 and 27)

1. Prepare the joint surface as described in Chapter 20 (Treatment of Hindfoot and Midfoot Arthritis).
2. A laminar spreader can be used to reduce the subtalar joint. A spreader is placed in the sinus tarsi between the lateral talar tuberosity and the anterior calcaneus, to help reduce the deformity. Care is taken to position

the subtalar joint into neutral and to maintain good apposition of the posterior facet for fusion.
3. Before pinning the joint, apply compression across the joint and confirm good bony apposition. Also confirm neutral and not supinated or pronated position of the joint.
4. Fixation is done with 2 cannulated 6.5, 7.0, or 7.3 mm compression screws or a compression screw and lateral compression staple.

SINGLE AND DOUBLE ARTHRODESIS (Video Clips 28 and 29)

Single arthrodesis of the talonavicular joint has been used in the adult acquired flatfoot, although not commonly. Because it is a key joint for alignment of the triple joint complex, it is logical that fusion of this joint can correct deformity. However, in stage III, it is common for significant deformity to be present at the subtalar joint, with the most common operation for stage 3 being a triple arthrodesis.

In late-stage 2b, talonavicular (TN) fusion can be used when lateral column lengthening does not adequately address deformity and spring ligament reconstruction is not being done. Confirmation should be made that significant deformity or pain is not present at the subtalar joint, which would require a subtalar fusion as well.

A calcaneocuboid (CC) fusion can be added to a TN fusion because it does not add significant loss of motion. Deformity at the subtalar joint is not to be likely addressed by a TN/CC double arthrodesis. Therefore, although uncommonly indicated, if the primary deformity is at the TN joint and there is minimal subtalar joint deformity or pain, a TN or a TN and CC fusion is an option. Another double arthrodesis, TN and a subtalar fusion, has been described because patients can have their deformity adequately corrected using this combination.[159] Finally, a CC distraction arthrodesis with a tricortical graft should be mentioned. This is essentially a type of lateral column lengthening. Originally, this was thought to be advantageous because of the potential for lateral column lengthening to cause significant CC arthritis. Symptomatic CC arthritis is uncommon both in the short and intermediate term.[6,134,145] Arthritic changes, although present in some patients at this joint, do not commonly cause significant symptoms.

The distraction CC arthrodesis does have a higher incidence of nonunion than other lateral column lengthenings, (Evans or LCL stepcut techniques). From this perspective and possible additional loss of motion, it is not attractive to use a distraction CC arthrodesis. Nevertheless, a lengthening CC arthrodesis does correct deformity as does a lateral column lengthening.

TRIPLE ARTHRODESIS

Triple arthrodesis is indicated for fixed deformity in the subtalar and talonavicular joints. The joints can neither be passively manipulated into inversion and adduction, nor can they be rendered stable in a good position by procedures other than fusions. The key to this procedure is properly positioning the triple joint complex and obtaining good alignment of the foot. It is important to reduce both the talonavicular and subtalar joints (Fig. 25-38). It is equally important to achieve an even plantar tripod: heel plus first and fifth metatarsal heads. Adjunct procedures to a triple arthrodesis are a posterior medial slide calcaneal osteotomy to correct residual excessive heel valgus and a Cotton osteotomy or first metatarsal–tarsal arthrodesis to correct forefoot varus.

When performing a triple arthrodesis for the adult acquired flatfoot, undercorrection is more common than overcorrection, although both are possible. Within the triple joint complex, the main reduction occurs at the talonavicular joint. Care needs to be taken to reduce the subtalar joint, without placing it in varus. Lateral wound problems are a risk in severe valgus deformities.

A single medial incision technique for severe valgus deformities has been described. One series of 17 patients has been presented.[88] Access to the calcaneocuboid joint is difficult by using one medial incision. Two calcaneal-cuboid nonunions occurred in this series but were well tolerated. Although no other clinical series has been presented, this approach is a consideration in the setting of severe valgus deformity. Below is a technique description using the standard incisions, highlighting how to achieve a plantigrade well-aligned foot.

Technique Triple Arthrodesis

1. Incisions are made along the sinus tarsi and anteromedial talonavicular joint (Video Clip 30).
2. Standard preparation of the joint surfaces to keep the curvilinear shape of the talonavicular and subtalar joints is done with removal of all cartilage, perforating the subchondral bone with multiple K-wire holes, light burring with irrigation, and fish scaling the sclerotic surfaces. The calcaneocuboid joint preparation is performed with minimal lateral bone resection so that the lateral column is not shortened.
3. Position the joints using fluoroscopy to confirm good position and apposition. Commonly, the talonavicular joint will need to be brought out of an abducted and plantar sagged position. Push on the talar head medially to eliminate the abduction, and bring the navicular and medial column down, out of its dorsiflexed and abducted position. If a lateral gap is present at that CC joint, a small amount of additional curvilinear resection can be done at the talonavicular joint to allow good apposition of both joints. Check that there is no prominent bone at the medial CC joint or medial talonavicular joint causing the talonavicular joint to gap laterally. Also, check that the cuboid can be elevated so that, with final positioning of the foot, the cuboid is not prominent plantarly.
4. Once the subtalar and talonavicular joints are in place, they are compressed and temporarily pinned. It is important to place both joints in a good position and compress them for the temporary fixation. An assistant can be useful to pin the joints while the surgeon positions and compresses the joints. Reduction of both

joints must be confirmed clinically and with AP and lateral fluoroscopy.

5. Examine the tripod, if excessive heel valgus remains, through a standard posterior lateral incision. Then perform a medial slide calcaneal osteotomy to correct remaining excessive valgus.
6. If the first ray is elevated in comparison to the second, by assessing the plantar position of the first and second metatarsal heads (residual forefoot varus), bring the first metatarsal down by a Cotton osteotomy or first metatarsal tarsal fusion, the latter being done when there is considerable instability or a plantar gap. The forefoot varus should have been at least partially addressed by setting the position of the talonavicular joint out of dorsiflexion. After these procedures, the plane of the metatarsal heads should not be in forefoot varus or valgus by more than 10 degrees. If elevation of the first ray is primarily from deformity at the naviculocuneiform joint, that may need to be addressed with fusion at that location. This is only done for severe dorsiflexion deformity at the naviculocuneiform joints because these joints have a significant nonunion rate. Some residual dorsiflexion of the naviculocuneiform joints is rarely a problem.
7. A final check of the alignment of the hindfoot, midfoot, and forefoot is then done. With good alignment set, final fixation is placed, usually in the following order: (1) subtalar joint (with medial slide calcaneal osteotomy, if performed); (2) first metatarsal–tarsal fusion or Cotton osteotomy, if performed; (3) talonavicular joint; and finally, (4) the calcaneaocuboid joint. If a gap is present at the CC joint, bone graft is used with tricortical graft being an option but not commonly necessary. The CC joint is fixed with compression screws and/or staples. For the medial calcaneal osteotomy and subtalar fusion, one or two compression screws are used from the heel to the talar body. The talonavicular joint is fixed with compression screws or a compression screw and compression staple. Fluoroscopy is used to confirm good apposition at the joints. If apposition is not good laterally at the TN joint, a separate incision over the lateral talonavicular joint can be made and a screw placed under compression from the navicular into the talus.
8. The foot and ankle is then dorsiflexed to check that it can be brought to neutral. If neutral cannot be achieved with the knee straight but can be with the knee bent, a gastrocnemius lengthening is performed at that time or may have been performed at the beginning of the procedure. The gastrocnemius lengthening (Strayer procedure) can be done at the beginning of the procedure, with the contracture having been demonstrated with the foot manipulated into the corrected position and neutral (not plantar-flexed) position confirmed with the knee bent to 90 degrees. If the hindfoot and ankle remain plantar flexed with the knee flexed, a tricut Achilles lengthening is necessary.

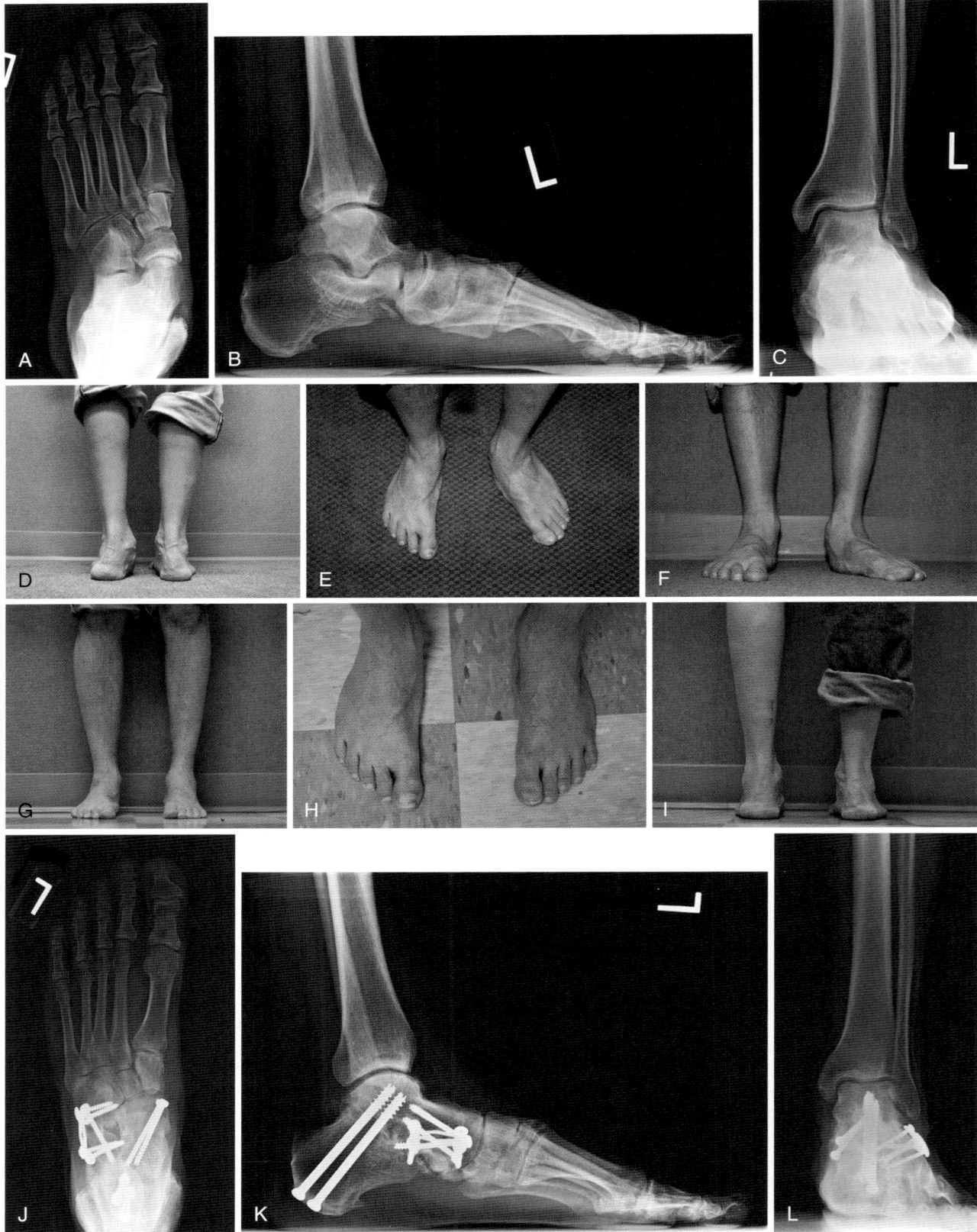

Figure 25-38 **A,** Preoperative radiograph of severe forefoot abduction in rigid stage 3 flatfoot deformity. **B,** Preoperative lateral radiograph in rigid deformity noting plantar flexion of talus and subtalar arthritis. **C,** Preoperative anteroposterior (AP) ankle radiograph demonstrating no valgus tilt or ankle arthritis despite long-standing valgus deformity. **D,** Preoperative clinical photograph of heels showing severe valgus and medial column collapse. **E,** Preoperative clinical AP photograph of feet demonstrating resting forefoot abduction without attempts at correcting foot alignment. **F,** Preoperative clinical photograph of lower limb documenting uncorrected medial column collapse, with rotation evident as callus at medial intraphalangeal joint of great toe. **G,** One and half years postcorrection, with standing lower limb foot position, confirmed with alignment of knees at neutral. **H,** One and a half years postcorrection AP clinical photograph of feet, with knees in neutral. **I,** One and a half years postcorrection with hindfoot alignment restored. Note required Strayer procedure to assist with postoperative motion. **J,** One and a half years postcorrection AP radiograph of foot. Note that a simultaneous lateral column lengthening was performed through the calcaneocuboid joint to achieve forefoot abduction correction. **K,** One and a half years postcorrection lateral radiograph of foot with elevation of the talus. Note autocorrection of sagging medial column through rigid hindfoot correction. This is not possible with joint-preserving operations. **L,** One and a half years postcorrection AP view of ankle without arthritic changes and elimination of subfibular impingement.

RIGID FLATFOOT ASSOCIATED WITH ADULT TARSAL COALITION

Incidence

The majority of the world's literature pertaining to tarsal coalition involves the adolescent patient. Tarsal coalition results from failure of differentiation of the primitive mesenchyme with the resultant lack of joint formation. This concept was first proposed by Leboucq in 1890.[110] The overall incidence is less than 1%.[104] However, a number of studies debate this point, stating that tarsal coalition goes unrecognized in asymptomatic persons and in nonosseous variants. Solomon et al[166] suggest that the incidence of talocalcaneal coalition may be as high as 12.7%. The incidence of bilaterality varies in the literature, ranging from 20% to 60% in talocalcaneal coalitions and 40% to 68% in calcaneonavicular coalitions. A review of the literature by Stormont and Peterson[171] noted that the incidence of talocalcaneal coalitions was 48.1%, calcaneonavicular was 43.6%, talonavicular was 1.3%, and other coalitions were 5.7%.

Although most patients with this entity present between the ages of 8 and 16 years,[72] symptomatic coalitions do occur in the adult population. Presentation is most often associated with a traumatic event, such as a severe ankle sprain sustained through sports activity or an incidental injury during activities of daily living. It is rare for such a patient to have prior problems with the involved foot. According to Varner and Michelson,[182] the lack of prior symptoms may be due to the neutral alignment of most adults with tarsal coalition and lack of spasm about the peroneal tendons. Only 7 of 32 adults (22%) presenting with tarsal coalition had a valgus deformity of their hindfeet. In fact, their cohort included 11 asymptomatic tarsal coalitions, and only one of these patients had a valgus hindfoot.

Physical Examination

Physical examination often reveals a flatfoot deformity of variable rigidity. Patients with a talocalcaneal coalition demonstrate no inversion of the calcaneus upon single-limb heel rise, and those with a calcaneonavicular coalition might demonstrate a percentage of inversion when compared with the unaffected side. Preservation of up to 70% of subtalar motion may be found in patients with a calcaneonavicular coalition. Transverse tarsal motion is preserved in patients with a talocalcaneal coalition, but it is severely restricted in patients with a calcaneonavicular bar.

Pain may be elicited medially directly over the anterior middle facets and inferior to the medial malleolus in patients with a talocalcaneal coalition. Often, the clinical appearance of a medial bony prominence is noted in patients with a talocalcaneal bar. Pain to palpation might also be noted in the anterior portion of the sinus tarsi and around the lateral and dorsolateral portion of the talonavicular joint. Stressing the coalition by manipulating the subtalar and transverse tarsal joints can elicit pain directly at the site of the coalition. Paresthesias or frank numbness may be present in the distribution of the deep or superficial peroneal nerve in patients with significant talar beaking. Tarsal tunnel syndrome has been reported in conjunction with a talocalcaneal coalition[111] because of impingement on the medial plantar nerve from a bony prominence at the sustentaculum tali.

Peroneal spastic flatfoot is a misnomer. Patients might demonstrate periodic spasm of the peroneal tendons because of attempted inversion against relatively shortened peroneal tendons. The shortening occurs from chronic and rigid valgus of the hindfoot. The peroneal tendons elicit a protective mechanism of contracting to minimize pain specifically at the rigid subtalar joint, and thus they might go into spasm because of the length deficit.

Radiographic Studies

Plain radiography has value in the form of weight-bearing AP, oblique, and lateral images. These routine images are inspected for distortion in the normal bone architecture suggesting union (fibrous or bony) between the involved bones. In addition, the lateral radiograph can demonstrate beaking of the talus. This traction spur at the dorsum of the talus is a secondary sign of tarsal coalition and is believed to occur through an aberrant hingelike motion of the navicular upon the talus with dorsiflexion. Subtalar joint rigidity prevents the normal forward subluxation of the calcaneus upon the talus with dorsiflexion, creating a rigid hinge motion of the navicular upon the talus rather than the normal gliding motion. This hinging creates periosteal disturbance upon the head of the talus, which manifests a traction spur at that specific location.

Primary signs may be visualized on the 45-degree lateral oblique radiograph, where the calcaneonavicular coalition becomes evident as either complete osseous union or extension of the anterior neck of the calcaneus to the navicular (the anteater nose sign). The talocalcaneal coalition can also be visualized on plain radiography as narrowing of the posterior subtalar joint, failure to see the middle facet, rounding of the lateral process of the talus (on ankle radiographs), or flattening or concavity of the undersurface of the talar neck. The C sign, described by Brown et al,[13] is a bean-shaped density noted on the lateral radiograph and was initially thought to be diagnostic for talocalcaneal coalition. This sign relies on a prominent inferior outline of the sustentaculum tali to create an overlap or hyperdense region in combination with the medial outline of the talar dome and a bony bridge between the talar dome and sustentaculum tali. Brown found that although the sign is specific (not sensitive) for flatfoot in general, it is neither specific nor sensitive for talocalcaneal coalition. Clearly, the ability of the technologist to obtain a true lateral radiograph of the foot is pivotal in appropriately interpreting that radiograph for tarsal coalition. A true lateral radiograph should allow visualization of the middle and posterior facets, which are parallel. Any rotation of the hindfoot, or nonperpendicular beam positioning, will erroneously lead the interpreter to suggest tarsal coalition because the facets are not visible.

An important primary sign of talocalcaneal coalition may be detected through the Harris axial view[73] and requires the patient to stand on the radiographic cassette while dorsiflexing the ankle 10 degrees. The beam is projected downward from posterior to plantar at 45 degrees from vertical. Additional views are taken at 40 degrees and 50 degrees to capture the parallel nature of the posterior and middle facets. Assistance in determining the appropriate orientation of the beam comes from assessing the angle of the posterior and middle facets with reference to the vertical on the true lateral radiograph. Irregularity of the joint contour suggests a fibrous coalition, and complete obliteration of the joint is pathognomonic for bony coalition.

Despite the advanced diagnostic modalities mentioned below, unenhanced radiography has value in assessment for tarsal coalition. Crim and Kjeldsberg[30] performed a two-phase study in patients with a mean age of 29 years.

The first phase involved retrospectively reviewing radiographs in patients with known tarsal coalitions (confirmed by CT, MRI, or surgery), intermixed with known controls, and assessing diagnostic accuracy. Radiographs provided to the examiners were only AP and lateral foot views, to provide consistency with routine screening radiographs obtained in an office setting. The second phase was prospective—reviewing 150 radiographs in patients with nontraumatic foot and ankle pain and following up suspected coalitions with CT. The authors found that in the first phase, talocalcaneal diagnosis through plain radiographs was sensitive 100% of the time and specific 88% of the time. Calcaneonavicular coalitions ranged from 80% to 100% sensitive and 97% to 98% specific. Observers in this study were a junior musculoskeletal radiologist, a junior radiology resident, and a junior orthopaedics resident, all provided with a 30-minute tutorial before reviewing radiographs. In the second phase of the study, all expected coalitions were confirmed by CT scan, with no false positives noted.

CT has superseded plain radiography in diagnostic accuracy for tarsal coalition. The coronal view may be obtained by having the patient supine with the hips and knees flexed and the feet plantar flexed 20 degrees at the ankle. The image provided is perpendicular to the posterior and middle facets and will confirm an osseous talocalcaneal coalition. In addition, the coronal view will demonstrate the nature and cross-sectional area of the coalition. CT has the added benefit of detecting early degenerative joint disease at adjacent surfaces, which can influence treatment options.

In the past, the ability of CT to evaluate calcaneonavicular coalitions was questioned. Hochman and Reed[78] investigated the ability of CT to make this diagnosis. The authors found that axial CT images provided the best assessment of calcaneonavicular coalition. They also noted, however, that coronal images provide assistance through two features: lateral bridging (an abnormal bone mass lateral to the head of the talus) and abnormal rounding of the head of the talus. In particular, lateral bridging was a definitive finding in all patients studied with a confirmed calcaneonavicular coalition. Thus the authors suggest that while reviewing the coronal CT scan for a potential talocalcaneal coalition, the examiner must focus attention on the additional signs mentioned earlier, to avoid overlooking a calcaneonavicular coalition. If coalition is suspected, the axial images should be reviewed for absence of the normal triangle of soft tissue seen anterolateral to the calcaneus. If a coalition is present, this triangle is replaced by bony protrusions from the calcaneus and the navicular.

The limitations of CT stem from fibrous coalitions, where its accuracy may be compromised.[146,185] Fibrous or cartilaginous coalition is suggested indirectly by an abnormal angulation of the facet, joint space irregularity, subchondral sclerosis, or articular narrowing. However, the actual fibrous tissue is not well visualized. MRI becomes the better modality to assess this particular component.

In particular, the T1-weighted images reveal intermediate-to-low signal bridging the gap in the suspected fibrous coalitions. In addition, osseous coalitions are confirmed by continuity of the bone marrow across the proposed site. More recently, an ill-defined hyperintense pattern was detected on short T1 inversion recovery (STIR) or T2 images in the subchondral bone adjacent to the coalition.[164] It is suspected that this pattern is due to abnormal stresses across the rigid coalition, creating microfractures and edema within the bone.

The value of MRI over CT in fibrous tarsal coalitions remains in question. Emery et al[51] reviewed 40 MRI and CT scans taken on 20 patients with symptoms suggesting tarsal coalition. The authors found 15 feet in 9 patients demonstrated tarsal coalition by both MRI and CT scans. Ten coalitions were confirmed through surgical exploration. In this study, 71% of the subjects were patients with a fibrous coalition. Sensitivity and specificity were compared, revealing that CT scanning was 94% sensitive and 100% specific, whereas MRI was 88% sensitive and 100% specific. The authors found a 97.5% agreement between CT and MRI in rendering diagnosis of tarsal coalition, despite the large percentage of fibrous coalitions. Thus the choice of study depends on the physician's expected findings in a particular case; cost-effectiveness currently favors a CT scan in patients with isolated tarsal coalitions, but if additional soft tissue disorder (PTT disorder) is sought, MRI is the better diagnostic modality.

COMBINED FLATFOOT CORRECTION AND COALITION TREATMENT

It has been noted that failure to correct a moderate-to-severe flatfoot deformity can lead to a poor result in a patient who is having a coalition resection. In fact, the resection of the coalition without surgical treatment of the symptomatic flatfoot deformity has been reported to result in increased deformity and failure of the clinical result.[35] Symptoms from the flatfoot deformity can be present and be misinterpreted as being purely from the coalition on initial evaluation. This misinterpretation leads to just resection of the coalition alone without correction of the symptomatic flatfoot.

There is scant literature on simultaneous surgical correction of a flatfoot and resection of the coalition. The present author has found this combination to be effective and not to the detriment of the coalition resection. Retaining maximum motion from a coalition resection has been a concern in these patients. Mosca[132] in a recent study found simultaneous resection of coalition and correction of the flatfoot gave a good result.

Mosca, in his recent article, documented results of correcting the flatfoot with a calcaneal lengthening osteotomy (not a medial slide osteotomy) in patients with talocalcaneal coalitions.[132] His largest group of patients were treated with correction of the flatfoot alone and not resection of the coalition. These patients did well. The patients with resection of the coalition and correction of the flatfoot deformity also did well, although the numbers in this study are small. The patients who did not do well were those with deformity or arthritis who had resection of coalitions previously without correction of the flatfoot deformity.

Cain[14] reported a series of patients who underwent a medial slide osteotomy for correction of the flatfoot. The medial slide osteotomy was done from a medial approach with resection of bone medially to give more correction. These patients did not get good correction of their pes planus, although good pain relief was reported.

Overall, it is likely that the same rules apply to correction of flatfoot deformity that has been described in this chapter to the patients with symptomatic flatfoot and coalitions, whether they be talocalcaneal or calcaneonavicular. It is important to remember that a mild flatfoot is likely to be an asymptomatic flatfoot and coalition resection alone is reasonable, while a severe flatfoot is commonly symptomatic from the flatfoot itself. In the adult with moderate flatfoot deformity, it is still probably best to correct the flatfoot. If the coalition is asymptomatic and the restriction of motion does not interfere with gaining good alignment, the coalition can be left alone. If the restriction of motion must be taken down to achieve good alignment, then take it down for the correction and leave it resected or fuse the joint, fusion being more likely to be necessary in the case of an extensive talocalcaneal coalition.

Treatment

Most tarsal coalitions are asymptomatic. If a coalition is detected radiographically when evaluating for a separate problem, the patient should be informed about the condition, but no treatment beyond simple observation is necessary.

Pain in conjunction with the adult tarsal coalition is often in associated with a traumatic event, most often an ankle sprain. Thus it is important to maintain clinical suspicion when examining a patient with an ankle sprain, evaluating for rigidity in subtalar motion. Patients who present late after sustaining an ankle sprain must be carefully evaluated for tarsal coalition.

Conservative Treatment

Conservative management for tarsal coalition begins with antiinflammatory medication, icing, and modifying activity. Persistent pain mandates cast immobilization. The clinician must decide the weight-bearing status in the cast based on consultation with the patient. One may certainly use a short-leg walking cast for 6 weeks, but if the patient remains symptomatic after cast removal, a second casting (with a non–weight-bearing cast) will be required. Thus this protocol might extend the casting for a second interval, which can be avoided by making the first cast non–weight bearing. Regardless, it is Dr. Steven Haddad's experience that 60% to 70% of patients respond to immobilization if they have had no prior symptoms from the coalition. This experience is not supported in the literature, where only one third of patients were found to respond to conservative measures.[26,106] Many clinicians recommend that when the patient fails attempts at casting, surgical intervention is appropriate.

Longer-term conservative management can incorporate a medial heel wedge, Thomas heel, or medial longitudinal arch support.[26] In general, in rigid flatfoot, use of a rigid device that attempts to correct the collapsed arch actually increases the patient's symptoms and limits compliance with the device. Thus accommodative orthotics made of Plastizote, or semirigid devices that accommodate rather than correct the arch, have higher satisfaction. A UCBL orthosis or a lace-up ankle brace may be required for continued sports participation to minimize stress across the coalition. In patients who do not participate in sports, a polypropylene AFO may be required. Cowell and Elener[27] found that patients with a fixed hindfoot valgus deformity and a talocalcaneal coalition fared poorly with conservative care when compared with a hindfoot in neutral.

Surgical Treatment
CALCANEONAVICULAR COALITION
Surgical treatment of the calcaneonavicular coalition in an adult with minimal or no secondary changes (arthrosis) consists of resection of the coalition (Fig. 25-39). The goal is to eliminate painful motion at the coalition site while potentially increasing hindfoot motion. The suspected location of pain arising from the coalition appears to be the site around the coalition rather than the actual coalition itself. In particular, the hyperintense ill-defined areas noted on MRI of tarsal coalition[164] can represent bone contusion or edema that creates coalition pain. It is clear that the hyperintensity is present in the subchondral bone and not within the coalition itself. Thus a generous resection of the coalition invariably removes the diseased segment of bone, providing pain relief for the patient.

Indications
Indications for resection of a calcaneonavicular coalition are pain refractory to conservative care, and limited function from extreme rigidity.

Contraindications
Improvement with conservative care is a contraindication to surgery. If the patient is asymptomatic, resection of the coalition is not indicated. In addition, if the adjacent joints are arthritic, resection of the coalition is not sufficient, and a double or triple arthrodesis becomes the best alternative.

Preoperative Evaluation
Patients are evaluated radiographically for coalition. Plain radiographs include the 45-degree oblique view, which demonstrates the coalition. CT scanning reveals the extent of the coalition and whether it is osseous or fibrous. More important, the CT scan assists in evaluating adjacent joint surfaces for arthritic wear. For example, posttraumatic

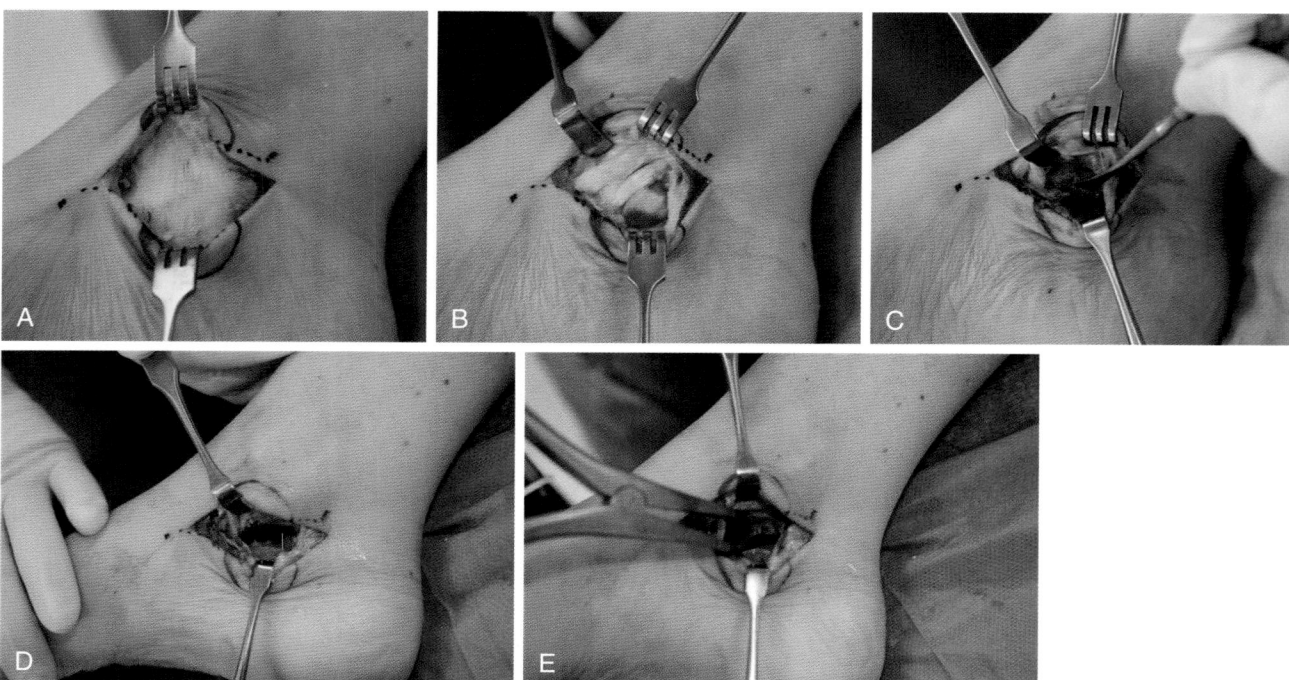

Figure 25-39 **A,** Medial exposure for sustentacular coalition. **B,** The tendons of the flexor hallucis longus and flexor digitorum longus are retracted. **C,** The coalition is seen deep to the tendons. **D,** Resection of the coalition. **E,** The joint is distracted with a lamina spreader to ensure lysis of any remaining fibrous adhesions.

arthritis of the cuboid or subtalar joint can mimic symptoms of a tarsal coalition. Such arthritis warrants fusion rather than resection.

The severity of the planovalgus foot deformity is assessed clinically. The literature does not address correction of the flatfoot deformity in conjunction with coalition resection. However, it must remain a consideration, especially in patients with subfibular impingement (separate from pain at the site of the coalition) or pain medially underlying the talar head. Such patients become candidates for simultaneous medial slide calcaneal osteotomies, lateral column lengthenings, or medial cuneiform opening-wedge osteotomies.

Preoperative Planning

Radiographs and three-dimensional imaging studies are reviewed to determine the extent and location of the coalition.

Surgical Technique

1. Equipment required includes a sharp beveled chisel or a set of sharp straight osteotomes, a rongeur or large pituitary rongeur, and bone wax to cover the exposed bone surfaces (Video Clip 89).
2. The patient is positioned supine with adequate support placed under the ipsilateral hip. Elevation of the lateral hip allows internal rotation of the extremity, facilitating exposure of the coalition.
3. It is helpful to incorporate a popliteal block when considering anesthetic, and if an indwelling popliteal catheter may be used, the patient will experience outstanding pain relief for at least 3 days after the procedure. In fact, the entire procedure can be performed with this block, with the use of a calf tourniquet. If a general anesthetic or spinal anesthetic is chosen, a thigh tourniquet may be used to facilitate hemostasis.
4. The incision begins 1 cm distal to the tip of the fibula and is carried obliquely to the base of the third metatarsal.
5. Two nerves that are subcutaneous at the portion of the foot are at risk. The intermediate dorsal cutaneous branch of the superficial peroneal nerve crosses the surgical path and should be identified and protected with a vessel loop. The anterior branch of the sural nerve can also be found at the proximal portion of the incision.
6. The origin of the extensor digitorum brevis muscle is detached from the lateral surface of the talus and reflected distally.
7. The anterior process of the calcaneus is identified and traced toward the navicular. The coalition is identified as a broad surface of bone (or a surface interrupted by fibrous tissue) connecting the anteromedial aspect of the calcaneus to the plantar-lateral portion of the navicular.
8. The parameters of the coalition are carefully identified. This is critical, to avoid violation of the articular surface of the navicular or the calcaneocuboid joint. For confirmation, the surgeon can use intraoperative fluoroscopy.
9. The ligaments between the talus and navicular and the calcaneus and cuboid are preserved. Damage to the talonavicular ligaments will allow the navicular to sublux upon the talus. Similarly, damage to the calcaneocuboid ligament will allow the cuboid to shift upon the calcaneus.
10. With a straight osteotome or sharp chisel, the navicular portion of the coalition is resected with an oblique angle, ensuring that the plantar-lateral portion is resected. The calcaneal portion is resected with a parallel cut beginning at the superior-medial articular surface of the calcaneocuboid joint.
11. The block of bone and fibrous tissue removed may be as large as 2 cm by using these resection margins. After removing the coalition, the surgeon looks for additional bone fragments impinging upon the talonavicular or calcaneocuboid joint. All such fragments are removed at this time.
12. Manipulation of the transverse tarsal joint assists in evaluating for impingement along the lateral aspect of the calcaneocuboid joint. On occasion, an abnormally shaped calcaneocuboid joint is detected that can block abduction of the foot. This abnormally shaped bone arises from the calcaneus and must be removed to facilitate abduction of the cuboid. Under normal circumstances, the amount of bone removed at this location is small.
13. Bone wax is applied to all cut bone surfaces.
14. The origin of the extensor digitorum brevis may now be interposed into the defect. Keith needles threaded with absorbable suture are placed into the tendinous origin of the muscle. These needles are passed plantarward and may be tied on either side of the plantar fascia through a small separate incision. With this technique, a button may be avoided.
15. The tourniquet is deflated before closure to minimize the risk of hematoma and subsequent scar formation. Hemostasis is very important at this stage, and if drainage is persistent, a suction drain is placed deep in the area of the coalition.
16. The extensor fascia is approximated, as is the subcutaneous tissue and skin.
17. A plaster splint limiting inversion and eversion, or a short-leg fiberglass cast, is applied intraoperatively.

Postoperative Care

If it was not done before the procedure, the popliteal block with an indwelling catheter can be performed in the recovery room to facilitate pain control.

Sutures are removed at 10 days after surgery, unless significant swelling suggests an incisional wound complication. In this instance, sutures are left in place for 3 weeks. The patient is given a walker boot, and ambulation is encouraged. Physical therapy may be instituted simultaneously to encourage aggressive passive range of motion of the transverse tarsal and subtalar joints. Gains achieved intraoperatively will be maintained or enhanced through this activity. A compression stocking, or a more formal lymphedema clinic, should be used to minimize soft tissue edema. Swelling compromises motion at this critical juncture.

The CAM walker boot should be discontinued by 4 weeks postoperatively, which will further encourage range of motion of the hindfoot.

TALOCALCANEAL COALITION

Similar to the calcaneonavicular coalition, surgical treatment of the talocalcaneal coalition in an adult with minimal or no secondary changes (arthrosis) consists of resection of the coalition. Again, the goal is to eliminate painful motion at the coalition site while potentially increasing hindfoot motion.

Indications

Surgical resection of a talocalcaneal coalition is indicated after failure of two trials of conservative care (casting). Pain is the primary indication because recovery of subtalar motion might not be significant enough as an isolated indication.

Contraindications

Previously, it was thought that a coalition that occupied more than 50% of the total articular surface of the subtalar would have a poor result.[163] Scranton[163] chose this value based on CT data, and using this arbitrary figure, the author evaluated his own results, finding good results in 13 of 14 patients. He has been misquoted in many orthopaedic texts over the years, leading to the misconception that he found poor results in patients with coalitions occupying greater than 50% of the *middle* facet as an isolated entity.

It has been shown by Comfort and Johnson[22] that 77% of patients undergoing resection of a talocalcaneal coalition involving less than one third of the *total* joint surface (anterior, middle, and posterior facets) experience good or excellent results. This study evaluated 20 patients by using CT to map the surface area of the posterior, anterior, and middle facets. The authors used these data to determine the location and extent of the talocalcaneal coalition as a percentage of the surface area of the entire joint construct. All patients in the study group had the coalition resected for symptoms. On average, these coalitions involved 66.5% of the anterior and middle facets (these facets are contiguous 67% of the time[161]) and 29.8% of the total joint surface area. With outcome based on level of activity, pain, and subtalar motion, 60% of the results were rated good or excellent. A strong correlation was found between the size of the coalition and the clinical outcome, noting that fair or poor results were found in 75% of the patients sustaining coalitions occupying more than one third of the total joint surface. Age was not correlated with surgical outcome. It has been suggested that increased age correlates with more poor results because

resection allows increased motion across degenerative joint surfaces. This study places that contraindication in question.

Finally, the authors compared their results with Scranton's guidelines and found that if they had followed his initial guidelines for resection, their entire group would be candidates for resection because no coalition involved more than 50% of the total joint surface. In that case, they would have had a much greater percentage of fair or poor results than those illustrated by Scranton. Thus this study, based on Wilde's criteria for measuring surface area of the subtalar joint,[187] suggests that surgery is contraindicated in talocalcaneal coalitions occupying greater than one third of the total articular surface of all three facets of the subtalar joint.

Preoperative Evaluation

Patients are evaluated for coalition radiographically. Plain radiographs include the Harris axial view, which demonstrates the coalition. CT scanning reveals the extent of the coalition and whether it is osseous or fibrous. More important, the CT scan assists in evaluating adjacent joint surfaces for arthritic wear. For example, posttraumatic arthritis of the subtalar joint can mimic symptoms of a tarsal coalition, and if arthritis is present, it warrants fusion over resection.

Clinically, severity of the planovalgus foot deformity is assessed. The literature does not address correction of the flatfoot deformity in conjunction with coalition resection. However, it must remain a consideration, especially in patients with subfibular impingement (separate from pain at the site of the coalition) or pain medially underlying the talar head. Such patients become candidates for simultaneous medial slide calcaneal osteotomies, lateral column lengthenings, and/or medial cuneiform opening-wedge osteotomies. Correction of the symptomatic flatfoot is at least as important as resection of the coalition, as documented by Mosca[139] in a recent study.

Preoperative Planning

Radiographs are reviewed to determine the extent and location of the coalition. Whereas the resection of a calcaneonavicular coalition is relatively simple, the resection of a talocalcaneal coalition is technically demanding and requires adequate exposure, careful orientation, and cautious dissection.

Surgical Technique

1. Equipment required includes a sharp beveled chisel or a set of sharp straight osteotomes, a rongeur or large pituitary rongeur, and bone wax to cover the exposed bone surfaces (Video Clip 90).
2. It is helpful to incorporate a popliteal block when considering anesthetic, and if an indwelling popliteal catheter can be used, the patient will experience outstanding pain relief for at least 3 days after the procedure. In fact, the entire procedure can be performed with this block, with the use of a calf tourniquet. If a

general anesthetic or spinal anesthetic is chosen, a thigh tourniquet may be used to facilitate hemostasis.

3. The patient is positioned supine, with adequate support placed under the contralateral hip to facilitate external rotation of the operative extremity.

4. The incision is made along the inferior aspect of the PTT sheath, beginning 1 cm distal to the tip of the medial malleolus and extending distal to the talonavicular joint.

5. The incision is deepened through the subcutaneous tissue and fat to expose the PTT sheath. The inferior aspect of the sheath is opened and the tendon is retracted superiorly.

6. Deep to this, the sheath for the flexor digitorum longus is encountered. This sheath passes along the medial surface of the talus, superior to the sustentaculum tali and thus the location of the coalition.

7. The flexor digitorum longus is retracted superiorly to expose the inferior edge of its tendon sheath. This inferior edge should be exposed from the medial malleolus to the talonavicular joint. Plantar to the flexor digitorum longus tendon is the neurovascular bundle, which should be identified and protected.

8. The area of the coalition can be identified by locating the posterior facet of the subtalar joint proximally and the inferior aspect of the talonavicular joint distally. The coalition lies between these two landmarks.

9. Using an osteotome or a chisel, a wedge of bone is removed to excise the coalition. The apex of the wedge is lateral. It may be easiest to start at the proximal point of the coalition, at the medial aspect of the posterior facet, and proceed distally. The surgeon must excise sufficient bone to visualize the joint surfaces. Once a sufficient amount of bone has been removed from the middle facet, the tarsal canal is visualized. The sustentaculum tali is not removed in its entirety. In addition, although sufficient bone must be resected to regain a portion of subtalar motion, the surgeon must take care to avoid removing excessive bone because the subtalar joint will become destabilized, accelerating arthritic wear.

10. Subtalar motion is checked and is often less than 50% of that detected on the opposite, normal side.

11. Bone wax is placed over the exposed bone surfaces.

12. The tourniquet is deflated, and meticulous hemostasis is performed. Limiting hematoma will limit subsequent scar tissue and enhance motion.

13. The tendon sheaths are approximated, restoring the tendons to their normal anatomic position.

14. The subcutaneous tissue and skin are sutured.

15. A plaster splint limiting subtalar motion, or a short-leg fiberglass cast, is applied.

Postoperative Care

If not done before the procedure, the popliteal block with an indwelling catheter can be performed in the recovery room to facilitate pain control.

Sutures are removed 10 days postoperatively, unless significant swelling suggests an incisional wound complication. In this instance, sutures are left in place for 3 weeks. The patient is then placed into a walker boot, and ambulation is encouraged. Physical therapy may be instituted simultaneously to encourage aggressive and passive range of motion of the transverse tarsal and subtalar joints. Gains achieved intraoperatively will be maintained or enhanced through this activity. A compressive stocking, or a more formal lymphedema clinic, should be used to minimize soft tissue edema. Swelling compromises motion at this critical juncture.

The walker boot should be discontinued by 4 weeks postoperatively, which will further encourage range of motion of the hindfoot.

Results and Complications

Results of both talocalcaneal and calcaneonavicular coalitions are reviewed.

Swiontkowski et al[176] performed a follow-up study of 40 patients who underwent 57 procedures for tarsal coalition. In total, 44 calcaneonavicular coalitions and 13 talocalcaneal coalitions were reviewed. Thirty-nine of the 44 calcaneonavicular coalitions underwent resection, whereas 5 underwent triple arthrodesis. At an average follow-up of 4.6 years, 29 (66%) were asymptomatic and 7 (16%) had symptoms with strenuous activity. In all, 90% improved considerably through surgical intervention. In the talocalcaneal group, 5 patients underwent resection and 9 had an arthrodesis (both triple and subtalar). At a mean follow-up of 3.1 years, four of five resections were asymptomatic. Of those undergoing arthrodesis, 78% were symptom-free. In both series, talar beaking had no influence on outcome and is not a contraindication. The authors experienced no complications in any of their procedures, other than some coalition resections requiring arthrodesis for persistent pain.

Mann et al[120] evaluated 10 patients with a talocalcaneal coalition undergoing subtalar arthrodesis. This adult population (average age, 26 years) was followed for an average 7.5 years. None were candidates for resection of the coalition. *Preoperative* pain index improved from 3.5 (out of 4) to 1, and postoperative function improved from 3.2 (out of 4) to 0.7. The final modified AOFAS score was 93. Sixty percent (6 out of 10) demonstrated radiographic evidence of mild talonavicular arthrosis, which was not present preoperatively, but none were symptomatic. The authors prefer subtalar arthrodesis for severe flatfoot associated with talocalcaneal coalition over triple arthrodesis, to preserve some of the motion at the Chopart joint. Such limitations clinically amounted to a 40% decrease in transverse tarsal motion, dorsiflexion decrease by 30%, and plantar-flexion decrease of 9%.

Gonzalez and Kumar[63] evaluated 48 patients who underwent resection of a calcaneonavicular coalition in 75 feet. They divided their population into two groups. Group A (32 feet) patients were directly evaluated by the authors in follow-up. Group B (43 feet) patients were evaluated retrospectively. The authors found that 84% of the patients in group A achieved a good or excellent result. Those with a fair result did not warrant conversion to arthrodesis. Group B patients demonstrated 72% good or excellent results, with 7% overall requiring revision to a triple arthrodesis. Combining both groups yielded 77% good or excellent results from resection of a calcaneonavicular coalition. Again, talar beaking did not preclude a good outcome clinically. The result did not deteriorate over time, and some patients followed for more than 20 years maintained a good or excellent result.

Cohen et al[20] evaluated 13 feet undergoing resection for calcaneonavicular coalition. This cohort consisted of adult patients (average age, 33 years), with 77% demonstrating preexisting degenerative arthritis radiographically. With an average 3-year follow-up, 85% (11 of 13) had subjective relief of preoperative symptoms, and 2 of 13 underwent secondary arthrodesis (one subtalar, one triple). Subtalar motion improved an average of 10 degrees. *Preoperative* degenerative arthritic changes were noted in the naviculocuneiform joint (23%), the subtalar joint (23%), and the talonavicular joint (46%). Preexisting arthritis was mild or minimal in 12 of 13 patients, and the one patient with moderate osteoarthritis (multiple peripheral osteophytes in the absence of significant joint space narrowing) later required a subtalar arthrodesis. Complications stemmed from the initial use of the extensor digitorum brevis muscle as an interposition graft with a pull-out suture placed medially. This technique resulted in a 50% lateral wound-dehiscence rate. Using bone wax before restoring the extensor digitorum brevis to its anatomic position eliminated this complication.

REFERENCES

1. Abosala A, Tumia N, Anderson D: Tibialis posterior tendon rupture in children, *Injury* 34:866–867, 2003.
2. Alexander IJ, Johnson KA, Berquist TH: Magnetic resonance imaging in the diagnosis of disruption of the posterior tibial tendon, *Foot Ankle* 8:144–147, 1987.
3. Augustin JF, Lin SS, Berberian WS, Johnson JE: Nonoperative treatment of adult acquired flat foot with the Arizona brace, *Foot Ankle Clin* 8:491–502, 2003.
4. Balen PF, Helms CA: Association of posterior tibial tendon injury with spring ligament injury, sinus tarsi abnormality, and plantar fasciitis on MR imaging, *AJR Am J Roentgenol* 176:1137–1143, 2001.
5. Kulig K, Lederhaus ES, Reischl S, et al: Effect of eccentric exercise program for early tibialis posterior tendinopathy, *Foot Ankle Int* 30:877–885, 2009. doi:10.3113/FAI.2009.0877.
6. Beals TC, Pomeroy GC, Manoli A 2nd: Posterior tibial tendon insufficiency: diagnosis and treatment, *J Am Acad Orthop Surg* 7:112–118, 1999.
7. Blake RL, Anderson K, Ferguson H: Posterior tibial tendinitis. A literature review with case reports, *J Am Podiatr Med Assoc* 84:141–149, 1994.
8. Blumen E, Myerson M: Stage IV posterior tibial tendon rupture, *Foot Ankle Clin* 12:341–362, 2007.
9. Bolt PM, Coy S, Toolan BC: A comparison of lateral column lengthening and medial translational osteotomy of the calcaneus for the reconstruction of adult acquired flatfoot, *Foot Ankle Int* 28:1115–1123, 2007.
10. Bordelon RL: Correction of hypermobile flatfoot in children by molded insert, *Foot Ankle* 1:143–150, 1980
11. Boss PA, Hintermann B: Anatomical study of the medial ankle ligament complex, *Foot Ankle Int* 23:547–553, 2002.
12. Brahms MA: The posterior tibial tendon, *J Am Podiatry Assoc* 56:502–503, 1966.
13. Brown RR, Rosenberg ZS, Thornhill BA: The C sign: more specific for flatfoot deformity than subtalar coalition, *Skeletal Radiol* 30:84–87, 2001.
14. Cain TJ, Hyman S: Peroneal spastic flat foot: its treament by osteotomy of the os calcis, *J Bone Joint Surg Br* 60:527–529, 1978.
15. Chan JY, Williams BR, Nair P, et al: The contribution of medializing calcaneal osteotomy on hindfoot alignment in the reconstruction of the stage II adult acquired flatfoot deformity, *Foot Ankle Int* 34:159–166, 2013. doi:10.1177/1071100712460225.
16. Chao W, Wapner KL, Lee TH, et al: Nonoperative management of posterior tibial tendon dysfunction, *Foot Ankle Int* 17:736–741, 1996.
17. Chen YJ, Liang SC: Diagnostic efficacy of ultrasonography in stage I posterior tibial tendon dysfunction: sonographic-surgical correlation, *J Ultrasound Med* 16:417–423, 1997.
18. Choi K, Lee S, Otis JC, Deland JT: Anatomical reconstruction of the spring ligament using peroneus longus tendon graft, *Foot Ankle Int* 24:430–436, 2003.
19. Coetzee JC, Hansen ST: Surgical management of severe deformity resulting from posterior tibial tendon dysfunction, *Foot Ankle Int* 22:944–949, 2001.
20. Cohen BE, Davis WH, Anderson RB: Success of calcaneonavicular coalition resection in the adult population, *Foot Ankle Int* 17:569–572, 1996.
21. Cohen BE, Johnson JE: Subtalar arthrodesis for treatment of posterior tibial tendon insufficiency, *Foot Ankle Clin* 6:121–128, 2001.
22. Comfort TK, Johnson LO: Resection for symptomatic talocalcaneal coalition, *J Pediatr Orthop* 18:283–288, 1998.
23. Conti SF: Posterior tibial tendon problems in athletes, *Orthop Clin North Am* 25:109–121, 1994.
24. Conti S, Michelson J, Jahss M: Clinical significance of magnetic resonance imaging in preoperative planning for reconstruction of posterior tibial tendon ruptures, *Foot Ankle* 13:208–214, 1992.
25. Cotton FJ: Foot statics and surgery, *N Engl J Med* 214:353–362, 1936.
26. Cowell HR: Talocalcaneal coalition and new causes of peroneal spastic flatfoot, *Clin Orthop Relat Res* 85:16–22, 1972.
27. Cowell HR, Elener V: Rigid painful flatfoot secondary to tarsal coalition, *Clin Orthop Relat Res* 177:54–60, 1983.
28. Cozen L: Posterior tibial tenosynovitis secondary to foot strain, *Clin Orthop Relat Res* 42:101–102, 1965.
29. Crates JM, Richardson EG: Treatment of stage I posterior tibial tendon dysfunction with medial soft tissue procedures, *Clin Orthop Relat Res* 365:46–49, 1999.
30. Crim JR, Kjeldsberg KM: Radiographic diagnosis of tarsal coalition, *AJR Am J Roentgenol* 182:323–328, 2004.
31. Danko AM, Allen B Jr, Pugh L, Stasikelis P: Early graft failure in lateral column lengthening, *J Pediatr Orthop* 24:716–720, 2004.
32. Deland JT: Adult-acquired flatfoot deformity, *J Am Acad Orthop Surg* 16:399–406, 2008.
33. Deland JT, Arnoczky SP, Thompson FM: Adult acquired flatfoot deformity at the talonavicular joint: reconstruction of the spring ligament in an in vitro model, *Foot Ankle* 13:327–332, 1992.
34. Deland JT, de Asla RJ, Segal A: Reconstruction of the chronically failed deltoid ligament: a new technique, *Foot Ankle Int* 25:795–799, 2004.

35. Deland JT, de Asla RJ, Sung IH, et al: Posterior tibial tendon insufficiency: which ligaments are involved? *Foot Ankle Int* 26:427–435, 2005.

36. Deland JT, Hamilton WG: Posterior tibial tendon tears in dancers, *Clin Sports Med* 27:289–294, 2008. doi:10.1016/j.csm.2007.12.001.

37. Deland JT, Otis JC, Lee KT, Kenneally SM: Lateral column lengthening with calcaneocuboid fusion: Range of motion in the triple joint complex, *Foot Ankle Int* 16:729–733, 1995.

38. Deland JT, Page A, Sung IH, et al: Posterior tibial tendon insufficiency results at different stages, *HSS J* 2(2):157–160, 2006. doi: 10.1007/s11420-006-9017-0.

39. De Zwart DF, Davidson JS: Rupture of the posterior tibial tendon associated with fractures of the ankle. A report of two cases, *J Bone Joint Surg Am* 65:260–262, 1983.

40. Donovan A, Rosenberg ZS: Extraarticular lateral hindfoot impingement with posterior tibial tendon tear: MRI correlation, *AJR Am J Roentgenol* 193:672–678, 2009. doi: 10.2214/AJR.08.2215.

41. Downey DJ, Simkin PA, Mack LA, et al: Tibialis posterior tendon rupture: a cause of rheumatoid flat foot, *Arthritis Rheum* 31:441–446, 1988.

42. Duchene GG: *Physiology of motion*, Philadelphia, 1949, JB Lippincott, pp 303–369.

43. Dumontier TA, Falicov A, Mosca V, Sangeorzan B: Calcaneal lengthening: investigation of deformity correction in a cadaver flatfoot model, *Foot Ankle Int* 26:166–170, 2005.

44. Dwyer FC: Osteotomy of the calcaneum for pes cavus, *J Bone Joint Surg Br* 41:80–86, 1959.

45. Dyal CM, Feder J, Deland JT, Thompson FM: Pes planus in patients with posterior tibial tendon insufficiency: asymptomatic versus symptomatic foot, *Foot Ankle Int* 18:85–88, 1997.

46. Earll M, Wayne J, Brodrick C, et al: Contribution of the deltoid ligament to the ankle joint contact characteristics: a cadaver study, *Foot Ankle Int* 17:317–324, 1996.

47. Ellis SJ, Deyer T, Williams BR, et al: Assessment of lateral hindfoot pain in acquired flatfoot deformity using weightbearing multiplanar imaging, *Foot Ankle Int* 31:361–371, 2010.

48. Ellis SJ, Williams BR, Deland JT, et al: Deltoid ligament reconstruction with peroneus longus autograft in flatfoot, *Foot Ankle Int* 31:781–789, 2010. doi:10.3113/FAI.2010.0781.

49. Ellis SJ, Williams BR, Garg R, et al: Incidence of plantar lateral foot pain before and after the use of trial metal wedges in lateral column lengthening, *Foot Ankle Int* 32:665–673, 2011.

50. Ellis SJ, Yu JC, Williams BR, et al: New radiographic parameters assessing forefoot abduction in the adult acquired flatfoot deformity, *Foot Ankle Int* 30:1168–1176, 2009.

51. Emery KH, Bisset GS 3rd, Johnson ND, Nunan PJ: Tarsal coalition: a blinded comparison of MRI and CT, *Pediatr Radiol* 28:612–616, 1998.

52. Evans, D: Calcaneo-valgus deformity, *J Bone Joint Surg Br* 57:270–278, 1975.

53. Fayazi AH, Nguyen HV, Juliano PJ: Intermediate term follow-up of calcaneal osteotomy and flexor digitorum longus transfer for treatment of posterior tibial tendon dysfunction, *Foot Ankle Int* 23:1107–1111, 2002.

54. Frey C, Shereff M, Greenidge N: Vascularity of the posterior tibial tendon, *J Bone Joint Surg Am* 72:884–888, 1990.

55. Funk DA, Cass JR, Johnson KA: Acquired adult flat foot secondary to posterior tibial-tendon pathology, *J Bone Joint Surg Am* 68:95–102, 1986.

56. Gazdag AR, Cracchiolo A 3rd: Rupture of the posterior tibial tendon. Evaluation of injury of the spring ligament and clinical assessment of tendon transfer and ligament repair, *J Bone Joint Surg Am* 79:675–681, 1997.

57. Gerling MC, Pfirrmann CW, Farooki S, et al: Posterior tibialis tendon tears: comparison of the diagnostic efficacy of magnetic resonance imaging and ultrasonography for the detection of surgically created longitudinal tears in cadavers, *Invest Radiol* 38:51–56, 2003.

58. Giblin MM: Ruptured tibialis posterior tendon associated with a closed medial malleolar fracture, *Aust N Z J Surg* 50:59–60, 1980.

59. Gleich A: Beitrag zur operativen *Plattfussbehandlung. Arch Klin Chir* 46:358–362, 1893.

60. Goldner JL: Tendon transfers in rheumatoid arthritis, *Orthop Clin North Am* 5:425–444, 1974.

61. Goldner JL, Keats PK, Bassett FH 3rd, Clippinger FW: Progressive talipes equinovalgus due to trauma or degeneration of the posterior tibial tendon and medial plantar ligaments, *Orthop Clin North Am* 5:39–51, 1974.

62. Goncalves-Neto J, Witzel SS, Teodoro WR, et al: Changes in collagen matrix composition in human posterior tibial tendon dysfunction, *Joint Bone Spine* 69:189–194, 2002.

63. Gonzalez P, Kumar SJ: Calcaneonavicular coalition treated by resection and interposition of the extensor digitorum brevis muscle, *J Bone Joint Surg Am* 72:71–77, 1990.

64. Gould N: Graphing the adult foot and ankle, *Foot Ankle* 2:213–219, 1982.

65. Greene DL, Thompson MC, Gesink DS, Graves SC: Anatomic study of the medial neurovascular structures in relation to calcaneal osteotomy, *Foot Ankle Int* 22:569–571, 2001.

66. Vander Griend RA: "Z" osteotomy of the calcaneus, *Tech Foot Ankle Surg* 7:257–263, 2008.

67. Griffiths JC: Tendon injuries around the ankle, *J Bone Joint Surg Br* 47:686–689, 1965.

68. Guyton GP, Jeng C, Krieger LE, Mann RA: Flexor digitorum longus transfer and medial displacement calcaneal osteotomy for posterior tibial tendon dysfunction: a middle-term clinical follow-up, *Foot Ankle Int* 22:627–632, 2001.

69. Haddad SL, Dedhia S, Ren Y, et al: Deltoid ligament reconstruction: a novel technique with biomechanical analysis, *Foot Ankle Int* 31:639–651, 2010. doi:10.3113/FAI.2010.0639.

70. Haddad SL, Myerson MS, Younger A, et al: Symposium: adult acquired flatfoot deformity, *Foot Ankle Int* 32:95–111, 2011.

71. Hadfield M, Snyder J, Liacouras P, et al: The effects of a medializing calcaneal osteotomy with and without superior translation on Achilles tendon elongation and plantar foot pressures, *Foot Ankle Int* 26:365–370, 2005.

72. Harris RI: Rigid valgus foot due to talocalcaneal bridge, *J Bone Joint Surg Am* 37:169–183, 1955.

73. Harris RJ, Beath T: Etiology of peroneal spastic flatfoot, *J Bone Joint Surg Br* 30:624–634, 1948.

74. Helal B: Tibialis posterior tendon synovitis and rupture, *Acta Orthop Belg* 55:457–460, 1989.

75. Hicks JH: The mechanics of the foot. II. The plantar aponeurosis and the arch, *J Anat* 88:25–30, 1954.

76. Hintermann B, Valderrabano V, Kundert HP: Lengthening of the lateral column and reconstruction of the medial soft tissue for treatment of acquired flatfoot deformity associated with insufficiency of the posterior tibial tendon, *Foot Ankle Int* 20:622–629, 1999.

77. Hirose CB, Johnson JE: Plantar flexion opening wedge medial cuneiform osteotomy for correction of fixed forefoot varus associated with flatfoot deformity, *Foot Ankle Int* 25:568–574, 2004.

78. Hochman M, Reed MH: Features of calcaneonavicular coalition on coronal computed tomography, *Skeletal Radiol* 29:409–412, 2000.

79. Hogan JF: Posterior tibial tendon dysfunction and MRI, *J Foot Ankle Surg* 32:467–472, 1993.

80. Holmes GB Jr, Mann RA: Possible epidemiological factors associated with rupture of the posterior tibial tendon, *Foot Ankle* 13:70–79, 1992.

81. Houck JR, Nomides C, Neville CG, Samuel Flemister A: Effect of Stage II posterior tibial tendon dysfunction on deep compartment muscle strength: a new strength test, *Foot Ankle Int* 29:895–902, 2008. doi:10.3113/FAI.2008.0895.

82. Neville C, Flemister A, Houck JR: Effect of AirLift PTTD brace on foot kinematics with stage II posterior tibial tendon dysfunction. *Orthop Sports Phys Ther* 39:201–209, 2009. doi:10.2519/jospt.2009.2908.

83. Hsu TC, Wang CL, Wang TG, et al: Ultrasonographic examination of the posterior tibial tendon, *Foot Ankle Int* 18:34–38, 1997.

84. Imhauser CW, Siegler S, Abidi NA, Frankel DZ: The effect of posterior tibialis tendon dysfunction on the plantar pressure characteristics and the kinematics of the arch and the hindfoot, *Clin Biomech (Bristol, Avon)* 19:161–169, 2004.

85. Jahss MH: Spontaneous rupture of the tibialis posterior tendon: clinical findings, tenographic studies, and a new technique of repair, *Foot Ankle* 3:158–166, 1982.

86. Janisse DJ, Wertsch JD, Del Toro DR: Foot orthoses and prescription shoes. In Redford JB, Basmajian JV, Trautman P, editors: *Orthotics, clinical practice and rehabilitation Technology*, New York, 1995, Churchill Livingstone, pp 64–65.

87. Jeng CL, Bluman EM, Myerson MS: Minimally invasive deltoid reconstruction for stage IV flatfoot, *Foot Ankle Int* 32:21–30, 2011. doi:10.3113/FAI.2011.0021.

88. Jeng CL, Vora AM, Myerson MS: The medial approach to triple arthrodesis. Indications and technique for management of rigid valgus deformities in high-risk patients, *Foot Ankle Clin* 10:515–521, vi–vii, 2005.

89. Johnson KA, Strom DE: Tibialis posterior tendon dysfunction, *Clin Orthop Relat Res* 239:196–206, 1989.

90. Bridgeman JT, Zhang Y, Donahue H, et al: Estrogen receptor expression in posterior tibial dysfunction: a pilot study, *Foot Ankle Int* 31:1081–1084, 2010. doi:10.3113/FAI.2010.1081.

91. Kadakia AR, Haddad SL: Hindfoot arthrodesis for the adult acquired flat foot, *Foot Ankle Clin* 8:569–594, x, 2003.

92. Kapandji I: *The physiology of the joints*, New York, 1970, Churchill Livingston, pp 170–194.

93. Karasick D, Schweitzer ME: Tear of the posterior tibial tendon causing asymmetric flatfoot: radiologic findings, *AJR Am J Roentgenol* 161:1237–1240, 1993.

94. Kaye RA, Jahss MH: Tibialis posterior: a review of anatomy and biomechanics in relation to support of the medial longitudinal arch, *Foot Ankle* 11:244–247, 1991.

95. Keenan MA, Peabody TD, Gronley JK, Perry J: Valgus deformities of the feet and characteristics of gait in patients who have rheumatoid arthritis, *J Bone Joint Surg Am* 73:237–247, 1991.

96. Kennedy JC, Willis RB: The effects of local steroid injections on tendons: a biomechanical and microscopic correlative study, *Am J Sports Med* 4:11–21, 1976.

97. Kettelkamp DB, Alexander HH: Spontaneous rupture of the posterior tibial tendon, *J Bone Joint Surg Am* 51:759–764, 1969.

98. Key JA: Partial rupture of the tendon of the posterior tibial muscle, *J Bone Joint Surg Am* 35:1006–1008, 1953.

99. Khazen G, Khazen C: Tendoscopy in stage I posterior tibial tendon dysfunction, *Foot Ankle Clin* 17:399–406, 2012. doi:10.1016/j.fcl.2012.06.002.

100. Khoury NJ, el-Khoury GY, Saltzman CL, Brandser EA: MR imaging of posterior tibial tendon dysfunction, *AJR Am J Roentgenol* 167:675–682, 1996.

101. Kirkham BW, Gibson T: Comment on the article by Downey et al, *Arthritis Rheum* 32:359, 1989.

102. Koutsogiannis E: Treatment of mobile flat foot by displacement osteotomy of the calcaneus, *J Bone Joint Surg Br* 53:96–100, 1971.

103. Kulig K, Burnfield JM, Requejo SM, et al: Selective activation of tibialis posterior: evaluation by magnetic resonance imaging, *Med Sci Sports Exerc* 36:862–867, 2004.

104. Kulik SA Jr, Clanton TO: Tarsal coalition, *Foot Ankle Int* 17:286–296, 1996.

105. Kulowski J: Tendovaginitis (tenosynovitis), general discussion and report of one case involving the posterior tibial tendon. *J Missouri State Med Assoc* 33:135–137, 1936.

106. Kumar SJ, Guille JT, Lee MS, Couto JC: Osseous and non-osseous coalition of the middle facet of the talocalcaneal joint, *J Bone Joint Surg Am* 74:529–535, 1992.

107. Langenskiöld A: Chronic non-specific tenosynovitis of the tibialis posterior tendon, *Acta Orthop Scand* 38:301–305, 1967.

108. Lapidus PW: Kinesiology and mechanical anatomy of the tarsal joints, *Clin Orthop Relat Res* 30:20–36, 1963.

109. Lapidus PW, Seidenstein H: Chronic non-specific tenosynovitis with effusion about the ankle; report of three cases, *J Bone Joint Surg Am* 32:175–179, 1950.

110. Leboucq H: De la soudure congenitale de certains os du tarse, *Bull Acad Royale Med Belg* 4:103–112, 1890.

111. Lee MF, Chan PT, Chau LF, Yu KS: Tarsal tunnel syndrome caused by talocalcaneal coalition, *Clin Imaging* 26:140–143, 2002.

112. Lemley FR, Neville C: Effect of ankle foot orthotic devices on foot kinematics in Stage II posterior tibial tendon dysfunction, *Foot Ankle Int* 33:406–414, 2012. doi:10.3113/FAI.2012.0406.

113. Lipscomb P: Non-suppurative tenosynovitis and paratendinitis, *Instr Course Lect* 7:254, 1950.

114. Malicky ES, Crary JL, Houghton MJ, et al: Talocalcaneal and subfibular impingement in symptomatic flatfoot in adults, *J Bone Joint Surg Am* 84:2005–2009, 2002.

115. Mann RA: Tendon transfers and electromyography, *Clin Orthop Relat Res* 85:64–66, 1972.

116. Mann RA: Acquired flatfoot in adults, *Clin Orthop Relat Res* 181:46–51, 1983.

117. Mann RA: Adult acquired flatfoot deformity: treatment of dysfunction of the posterior tibial tendon, *J Bone Joint Surg Am* 78:780–792, 1996.

118. Mann RA: Flatfoot in adults. In Coughlin MJ, Mann RA, editors: *Surgery of the foot and ankle*, St Louis, 1999, Mosby, pp 733–767.

119. Mann RA: Posterior tibial tendon dysfunction. Treatment by flexor digitorum longus transfer, *Foot Ankle Clin* 6:77–87, vi, 2001.

120. Mann RA, Beaman DN, Horton GA: Isolated subtalar arthrodesis, *Foot Ankle Int* 19:511–519, 1998.

121. Mann R, Inman VT: Phasic activity of intrinsic muscles of the foot, *J Bone Joint Surg Am* 46:469–481, 1964.

122. Mann R, Specht T: *Posterior tibial tendon rupture*. Presented at the Annual Winter Meeting of the American Orthopedic Foot and Ankle Society, Las Vegas, Nev, 1982.

123. Mann RA, Thompson FM: Rupture of the posterior tibial tendon causing flat foot. Surgical treatment, *J Bone Joint Surg Am* 67:556–561, 1985.

124. Marcus RE, Pfister ME: The enigmatic diagnosis of posterior tibialis tendon rupture, *Iowa Orthop J* 13:171–177, 1993.

125. McCormack AP, Varner KE, Marymont JV: Surgical treatment for posterior tibial tendonitis in young competitive athletes, *Foot Ankle Int* 24:535–538, 2003.

126. McMaster PE: Tendon and muscle ruptures. Clinical and experimental studies on the causes and location of subcutaneous ruptures, *J Bone Joint Surg* 15:705, 1933.

127. Michelson J, Conti S, Jahss MH: Survivorship analysis of tendon transfer surgery for posterior tibial tendon rupture, *Orthop Trans* 16:30–31, 1992.

128. Michelson J, Easley M, Wigley FM, Hellmann D: Posterior tibial tendon dysfunction in rheumatoid arthritis, *Foot Ankle Int* 16:156–161, 1995.

129. Miller SD, Van Holsbeeck M, Boruta PM, et al: Ultrasound in the diagnosis of posterior tibial tendon pathology, *Foot Ankle Int* 17:555–558, 1996.

130. Momberger N, Morgan JM, Bachus KN, West JR: Calcaneocuboid joint pressure after lateral column lengthening in a cadaveric planovalgus deformity model, *Foot Ankle Int* 21:730–735, 2000.

131. Monto RR, Moorman CT 3rd, Mallon WJ, Nunley JA 3rd: Rupture of the posterior tibial tendon associated with closed ankle fracture, *Foot Ankle* 11:400–403, 1991.

132. Mosca VS, Bevan WP: Talocalcaneal tarsal coalitions and the calcaneal lengthening osteotomy: the role of deformity correction, *J Bone Joint Surg Am* 94:1584–1594, 2012.

133. Mosier SM, Lucas DR, Pomeroy G, Manoli A 2nd: Pathology of the posterior tibial tendon in posterior tibial tendon insufficiency, *Foot Ankle Int* 19:520–524, 1998.

134. Mosier-LaClair S, Pomeroy G, Manoli A 2nd: Operative treatment of the difficult stage 2 adult acquired flatfoot deformity, *Foot Ankle Clin* 6:95–119, 2001.

135. Mueller TJ: Acquired flatfoot secondary to tibialis posterior dysfunction: biomechanical aspects, *J Foot Surg* 30:2–11, 1991.

136. Myerson, MS: Adult acquired flatfoot deformity: treatment of dysfunction of the posterior tibial tendon, *Instr Course Lect* 46:393–405, 1997.

137. Myerson MS, Badekas A, Schon LC: Treatment of stage II posterior tibial tendon deficiency with flexor digitorum longus tendon transfer and calcaneal osteotomy, *Foot Ankle Int* 25: 445–450, 2004.

138. Myerson MS, Corrigan J: Treatment of posterior tibial tendon dysfunction with flexor digitorum longus tendon transfer and calcaneal osteotomy, *Orthopedics* 19:383–388, 1996.

139. Myerson M, Solomon G, Shereff M: Posterior tibial tendon dysfunction: its association with seronegative inflammatory disease, *Foot Ankle* 9:219–225, 1989.

140. Ness ME, Long J, Marks R, Harris G: Foot and ankle kinematics in patients with posterior tibial tendon dysfunction, *Gait Posture* 27:331–339, 2008.

141. Niki H, Ching RP, Kiser P, Sangeorzan BJ: The effect of posterior tibial tendon dysfunction on hindfoot kinematics, *Foot Ankle Int* 22:292–300, 2001.

142. Nyska M, Parks BG, Chu IT, Myerson MS: The contribution of the medial calcaneal osteotomy to the correction of flatfoot deformities, *Foot Ankle Int* 22:278–282, 2001.

143. Petersen W, Hohmann G, Pufe T, et al: Structure of the human tibialis posterior tendon, *Arch Orthop Trauma Surg* 124:237–242, 2004.

144. Petersen W, Hohmann G, Stein V, Tillmann B: The blood supply of the posterior tibial tendon, *J Bone Joint Surg Br* 84:141–144, 2002.

145. Phillips GE: A review of elongation of os calcis for flat feet, *J Bone Joint Surg Br* 65:15–18, 1983.

146. Pineda C, Resnick D, Greenway G: Diagnosis of tarsal coalition with computed tomography, *Clin Orthop Relat Res* 208:282–288, 1986.

147. Plattner PF: Tendon problems of the foot and ankle. The spectrum from peritendinitis to rupture, *Postgrad Med* 86:155–162, 167–170, 1989.

148. Pomeroy GC, Pike RH, Beals TC, Manoli A 2nd: Acquired flatfoot in adults due to dysfunction of the posterior tibial tendon, *J Bone Joint Surg Am* 81:1173–1182, 1999.

149. Harish S, Kumbhare D, O'Neill J, Popowich T: Comparison of sonography and magnetic resonance imaging for spring ligament abnormalities: preliminary study, *J Ultrasound Med* 27: 1145–1152, 2008.

150. Premkumar A, Perry MB, Dwyer AJ, et al: Sonography and MR imaging of posterior tibial tendinopathy, *AJR Am J Roentgenol* 178:223–232, 2002.

151. Raikin SM, Winters BS, Daniel JN: The RAM classification: a novel approach to adult acquired flatfoot, *Foot Ankle Int* 17:169–181, 2012. doi:10.1016/j.fcl.2012.03.002.

152. Rathbun JB, Macnab I: The microvascular pattern of the rotator cuff, *J Bone Joint Surg Br* 52:540–553, 1970.

153. Rosenberg ZS: Chronic rupture of the posterior tibial tendon, *Magn Reson Imaging Clin N Am* 2:79–87, 1994.

154. Rosenberg ZS, Jahss MH, Noto AM, et al: Rupture of the posterior tibial tendon: CT and surgical findings, *Radiology* 167: 489–493, 1988.

155. Ross JA: Posterior tibial tendon dysfunction in the athlete, *Clin Podiatr Med Surg* 14:479–488, 1997.

156. Alvarez RG, Marini A, Schmitt C, Saltzman CL: Stage I and II posterior tibial tendon dysfunction treated by structured non-operative management protocol: an orthosis and exercise program, *Foot Ankle Int* 27:2–8, 2006.

157. Saltzman CL, Brandser EA, Berbaum KS, et al: Reliability of standard foot radiographic measurements, *Foot Ankle Int* 15: 661–665, 1994.

158. Saltzman CL, el-Khoury GY: The hindfoot alignment view, *Foot Ankle Int* 16:572–576, 1995.

159. Sammarco VJ, Magur EG, Sammarco GJ, Bagwe MR: Arthrodesis of the subtalar and talonavicular joints for correction of symptomatic hindfoot malalignment, *Foot Ankle Int* 27:661–666, 2006.

160. Sangeorzan BJ, Mosca V, Hansen ST Jr: Effect of calcaneal lengthening on relationships among the hindfoot, midfoot, and forefoot, *Foot Ankle* 14:136–141, 1993.

161. Sarrafian SK: *Anatomy of the foot and Ankle*, Philadelphia, 1983, JB Lippincott, pp 43–61, 216–219, 375–425.

162. Schaffer JJ, Lock TR, Salciccioli GG: Posterior tibial tendon rupture in pronation–external rotation ankle fractures, *J Trauma* 27:795–796, 1987.

163. Scranton PE Jr: Treatment of symptomatic talocalcaneal coalition, *J Bone Joint Surg Am* 69:533–539, 1987.

164. Sijbrandij ES, van Gils AP, de Lange EE, Sijbrandij S: Bone marrow ill-defined hyperintensities with tarsal coalition: MR imaging findings, *Eur J Radiol* 43:61–65, 2002.

165. Silver RL, de la Garza J, Rang M: The myth of muscle balance. A study of relative strengths and excursions of normal muscles about the foot and ankle, *J Bone Joint Surg Br* 67:432–437, 1985.

165a. Smith JW: Blood supply of tendons, *Am J Surg* 109:272–276, 1965.

166. Solomon LB, Ruhli FJ, Taylor J, et al: A dissection and computer tomograph study of tarsal coalitions in 100 cadaver feet, *J Orthop Res* 21:352–358, 2003.

167. Song SJ, Lee S, O'Malley MJ Deltoid ligament strain after correction of acquired flatfoot deformity by triple arthrodesis, *Foot Ankle Int* 21:573–577, 2000.

168. DeOrio JK, Shapiro SA, McNeil RB, Stansel J: Validity of posterior tibial edema sign in posterior tibial tendon dysfunction, *Foot Ankle Int* 32:189–192, 2011. doi:10.3113/FAI.2011.0189.

169. Stein RE: Rupture of the posterior tibial tendon in closed ankle fractures. Possible prognostic value of a medial bone flake: report of two cases, *J Bone Joint Surg Am* 67:493–494, 1985.

170. Stephien M: The sheath and arterial supply of the tendon of the posterior tibialis muscle in man, *Folia Morph (Warsz)* 32:51–61, 1973.

171. Stormont DM, Peterson HA: The relative incidence of tarsal coalition, *Clin Orthop Relat Res* 181:28–36, 1983.

172. Streb HS, Marzano R: Conservative management of posterior tibial tendon dysfunction, subtalar joint complex, and pes planus deformity, *Clin Podiatr Med Surg* 16:439–451, 1999.

173. Sung IH, Lee S, Otis JC, Deland JT: Posterior tibial tendon force requirement in early heel rise after calcaneal osteotomies, *Foot Ankle Int* 23:842–849, 2002.

174. Supple KM, Hanft JR, Murphy BJ, et al: Posterior tibial tendon dysfunction, *Semin Arthritis Rheum* 22:106–113, 1992.

175. Sutherland DH: An electromyographic study of the plantar flexors of the ankle in normal walking on the level, *J Bone Joint Surg Am* 48:66–71, 1966.

176. Swiontkowski MF, Scranton PE, Hansen S: Tarsal coalitions: long-term results of surgical treatment, *J Pediatr Orthop* 3:287–292, 1983.

177. Teasdall RD, Johnson KA: Surgical treatment of stage I posterior tibial tendon dysfunction, *Foot Ankle Int* 15:646–648, 1994.

178. Tellisi N, Lobo M, O'Malley M, et al: Functional outcome after surgical reconstruction of posterior tibial tendon insufficiency in patients under 50 years, *Foot Ankle Int* 29:1179–1183, 2008.

179. Toolan BC, Sangeorzan BJ, Hansen ST Jr: Complex reconstruction for the treatment of dorsolateral peritalar subluxation of the foot. Early results after distraction arthrodesis of the calcaneocuboid joint in conjunction with stabilization of, and transfer of the flexor digitorum longus tendon to, the midfoot to treat acquired pes planovalgus in adults, *J Bone Joint Surg Am* 81:1545–1560, 1999.

180. Trevino S, Gould N, Korson R: Surgical treatment of stenosing tenosynovitis at the ankle, *Foot Ankle* 2:37–45, 1981.

181. Uchiyama E, Kitaoka HB, Fujii T, et al: Gliding resistance of the posterior tibial tendon: *Foot Ankle Int* 27:723, 2006.

182. Varner KE, Michelson JD: Tarsal coalition in adults, *Foot Ankle Int* 21:669–672, 2000.

183. Wacker JT, Calder JD, Engstrom CM, Saxby TS: MR morphometry of posterior tibialis muscle in adult acquired flat foot, *Foot Ankle Int* 24:354–357, 2003.

184. Wacker JT, Hennessy MS, Saxby TS: Calcaneal osteotomy and transfer of the tendon of flexor digitorum longus for stage-II dysfunction of tibialis posterior. Three- to five-year results, *J Bone Joint Surg Br* 84:54–58, 2002.

185. Wechsler RJ, Schweitzer ME, Deely DM, et al: Tarsal coalition: depiction and characterization with CT and MR imaging, *Radiology* 193:447–452, 1994.

186. Wertheimer SJ, Weber CA, Loder BG, et al: The role of endoscopy in treatment of stenosing posterior tibial tenosynovitis, *J Foot Ankle Surg* 34:15–22, 1995.

187. Wilde PH, Torode IP, Dickens DR, Cole WG: Resection for symptomatic talocalcaneal coalition, *J Bone Joint Surg Br* 76:797–801, 1994.

188. Williams BR, Ellis SJ, Deyer TW, et al: Reconstruction of the spring ligament using a peroneus longus autograft tendon transfer, *Foot Ankle Int* 31:567–577, 2010.

189. Woll TS: Posterior tibial tendon dysfunction, *West J Med* 159:485–486, 1993.

190. Yao L, Gentili A, Cracchiolo A: MR imaging findings in spring ligament insufficiency, *Skeletal Radiol* 28:245–250, 1990.

Pes Cavus

Fabian G. Krause, Gregory P. Guyton

Pes cavus describes a foot with a high arch that maintains its shape and fails to flatten out with weight bearing. By majority, the components of pes cavus are an increased calcaneal pitch and varus of the hindfoot, plantar flexion of the medial forefoot, and adduction of the entire forefoot. The predominant deformity in pes cavus may be in the hindfoot, the forefoot, or a combination of both. A precise radiographic definition of pes cavus is difficult because the deformity is made up of various components in the forefoot and hindfoot.

ETIOLOGY

Although the specific etiology of any cavus foot varies with the disease process, all forms result from muscle *imbalance*. Historical attempts to attribute all forms of cavus foot to a single neurologic lesion have proven overly simplistic. Bentzon[2] and Hallgrimsson[16] in 1939 proposed that extrinsic muscle imbalance underlay all deformities. In 1959, Duchenne[9] subsequently proposed that the deformity results from an imbalance between the extrinsics and the intrinsics. Neither approach is fully satisfactory; a cavus foot is best thought of as an end result that a variety of subtle neurologic lesions can produce.

Brewerton et al[5] specifically looked at the cause of pes cavus in a series of 77 patients and found subtle neurologic defects in 66% of them, leaving a large group of "idiopathic" cases. Of these, 11 of the 26 patients had a family history of pes cavus, and 7 of the 26 had nonspecific abnormalities upon electromyographic and nerve conduction velocity examination. Most cases of idiopathic pes cavus likely represent a very subtle neurologic lesion that is below clinical detection. Roughly half of the detectable lesions are variants of Charcot-Marie-Tooth disease, but a host of other less common conditions can also be discovered (Table 26-1).[19]

Neurologic referral is mandatory in situations that might point toward a correctable lesion of the spinal cord, such as a syrinx or spinal cord tumor. These include rapid progression, hyperreflexia, clonus, or significant asymmetry between sides in motor pattern or deformity. A new diagnosis of central neurologic disease is not uncommon in foot and ankle practice.

CHARCOT-MARIE-TOOTH DISEASE

Charcot-Marie-Tooth disease (CMT) should at least be considered in every patient who presents with pes cavus. CMT is not, in fact, a single disease but rather a heterogeneous group of disorders caused by inheritable defects in any of several constituent proteins of the myelin sheath of peripheral nerve. The disorder was described in general terms by the great French neurologist Jean Martin Charcot and his pupil Marie in 1886 and independently by Tooth in England later that year.[6,44] Originally, Charcot attributed the disorder to a spinal defect, and it was Tooth's subsequent work that correctly classified it as a peripheral nerve disorder. The disease is the most common inheritable defect of peripheral nerves, but approximately half of the time it represents a new sporadic chromosomal recombination error.

Table 26-1 Etiology of Pes Cavus

Classification	Specific Etiology
I. Neuromuscular	
A. Muscle disease	Muscular dystrophy
B. Afflictions of peripheral nerves and lumbosacral spinal nerve roots	Charcot-Marie-Tooth disease
	Spinal dysraphism
	Polyneuritis
	Intraspinal tumor
C. Anterior horn cell disease of spinal cord	Poliomyelitis
	Spinal dysraphism
	Diastematomyelia
	Syringomyelia
	Spinal cord tumors
	Spinal musculature atrophy
D. Long-tract and central disease	Friedreich ataxia
	Roussy–Lévy syndrome
	Primary cerebellar disease
	Cerebral palsy
II. Congenital	Idiopathic cavus foot
	Residual of clubfoot
	Arthrogryposis
III. Traumatic	Residuals of compartment syndrome
	Crush injury to lower extremity
	Severe burn
	Malunion of fractured foot

Modified from Ibrahim K: Pes cavus. In Evarts CM, editor: *Surgery of the musculoskeletal system,* New York, 1990, Churchill Livingstone, pp 4015–4034.

The nomenclature associated with CMT is confusing because of the historical lack of understanding of its cause. The archaic term *peroneal muscular atrophy* (PMA) was supplanted by Dyck and Lambert, who developed an extensive classification of inheritable motor neuropathies based upon their electrodiagnostic patterns in the 1960s and 1970s.[12] Their scheme refers to a series of seven *hereditary motor sensory neuropathies* (HMSN-I through HMSN-VII).

Since 1990 there has been an explosion of understanding of the specific genetic defects underlying the CMT disorders,[4] leading to a new and still evolving reclassification of the disease.

CMT-1 is the most common form and accounts for more than 50% of all cases. It is autosomal dominant and demonstrates slow nerve conduction velocities (NCVs) in the range of 10 to 30 m/sec as a result of demyelination. CMT-1 can be further subdivided.

CMT-1A accounts for 80% of CMT-1 cases and is the single most common form of the disease in general. Curiously, it is usually caused by a segmental trisomy along chromosome 17. The area contains the gene for peripheral myelin protein-22 *(PMP-22),* whose function remains unknown. Although some cases have been linked to alternative point mutations in *PMP-22,* the segmental trisomy responsible for most cases indicates CMT can be produced from a *gene dosage effect.* This chromosomal aberration is inheritable in an autosomal dominant fashion, but many cases seem to represent sporadic chromosomal recombination events.

CMT-1B accounts for 5% to 10% of CMT-1 patients and is associated with a point mutation in the myelin P_0 gene. The phenotype is associated with a particularly aggressive form of the disease.

CMT-1C represents the small remainder of CMT-1 patients in whom the genetic defect is still unknown.

CMT-2 is the second most common general form of the disease and represents 20% of patients. It is autosomal dominant like CMT-1 but has dramatically different electrical findings: NCVs are near normal, and there is no evidence of demyelination. Four separate chromosomal loci have been identified, but the product proteins involved remain unknown. In general, the course of CMT-2 is more indolent than that of CMT-1.

CMT-X shows an X-linked inheritance pattern; male patients are affected and female patients are either unaffected or mildly affected carriers. It is found in 10% to 20% of all CMT cases and is associated with defects in yet another myelin constituent protein, connexin 32.

CMT-4 is an autosomal recessive form of the disease and is quite rare. It in fact encompasses a large number of described genetic defects on different chromosomal loci; no product proteins have yet been described.

The foot deformities in CMT do not result from absolute weakness of the motor units powering the foot but of their relative *imbalance.* Initiation of the deformity likely results from an imbalance of the failing foot intrinsics and the preserved extrinsics.[3] Subsequently, a specific pattern of extrinsic motor weakness is common in CMT in which the anterior and lateral compartment musculature is selectively affected, with certain curious exceptions. The disease almost always affects the peroneus brevis but spares the peroneus longus. This was first observed clinically by Mann and Hsu[33] and subsequently confirmed by Tynan et al,[45] who demonstrated that the cross-sectional area of the peroneus longus was preserved on magnetic resonance imaging (MRI) of patients with the disease. An additional oddity can be observed in the anterior compartment musculature; the extensor hallucis muscle can be spared while the anterior tibialis is affected. This occurs despite the more distal location of the extensor hallucis longus (EHL) and their shared peroneal innervation.

The reasons for the unusual patterns of motor weakness in CMT remain poorly understood. The selective denervation affects certain muscles in the anterior and lateral compartments, and only very late posterior compartment involvement is seen. Denervation in CMT progresses very differently from a classic symmetric polyneuropathy, such as that encountered in diabetes. At least some speculation has been centered upon the possibility that some element of nerve compression can play a role.[14]

Regardless of the cause of the patterns of weakness, each of the deformities of the disease can be explained in

Table 26-2 Foot Deformities in Charcot-Marie-Tooth Disease

Deformity	Weak Agonist Muscle(s)	Intact Antagonist Muscle(s)	Action
Equinus	Tibialis anterior	Gastrocnemius–soleus complex (triceps-surae)	Plantar flexion
Adduction and hindfoot varus	Peroneus brevis	Tibialis posterior	Adducts the foot, inverts the subtalar joint
Plantar flexion of the first ray	Tibialis anterior	Peroneus longus	Plantar flexes the first ray, creates a secondary forefoot cavus
Toe deformities	Foot intrinsics	Long toe flexors	Clawing occurs as the extrinsic forces are unmodified by the intrinsics; also depresses the metatarsal heads and accentuates cavus
Hallux claw toe	Foot intrinsics	EHL and FHL	Severe hallucal clawing occurs when a spared EHL is used to assist a weak tibialis anterior dorsiflex the foot

From Guyton GP, Mann RA: The pathogenesis and surgical management of foot deformity in Charcot-Marie-Tooth disease, *Foot Ankle Clin* 5:317–326, 2000.
EHL, extensor hallucis longus; *FHL,* flexor hallucis longus.

the form of a weak agonist muscle and a *more normally functioning* antagonist (Table 26-2). There is *no* evidence of spasticity in the motor units that remain innervated.

The functional peroneus longus serves to plantar flex the first ray while the denervated anterior tibialis fails to provide any counterbalancing dorsiflexion. The first metatarsal head is depressed and a forefoot cavus results. Next to a relative talus dorsiflexion, an equinus contracture develops as the Achilles tendon (triceps surae) is unopposed by the anterior tibialis. In addition, the toe extrinsics force the toes into a clawed position that is not counterbalanced by the denervated foot intrinsics. This also serves secondarily to depress the metatarsal heads and raise the arch. The supination and adduction of the foot is worsened because the posterior tibialis is unopposed by the weakened peroneus brevis. In cases with sparing of the EHL, the claw toe deformity of the hallux is worsened even more dramatically because the patient uses the EHL to dorsiflex the foot and compensate for the weak anterior tibialis.

It is rare in clinical practice to encounter a patient at such an early stage of disease that the foot is entirely supple with no hindfoot or forefoot contractures. However, rebalancing the foot through tendon transfers can help prevent the development of further deformity if it is done early enough.[38] For instance, the overpull of the peroneus longus that forces the forefoot into cavus can be eliminated by transferring the tendon to the peroneus brevis. This also serves to help oppose the tibialis posterior and prevent adduction. The emphasis in early-stage surgery on CMT should be on tendon transfers rather than lengthening motor units. Because the long-term outcome of CMT is one of progressive, inexorable weakness, strength should be preserved whenever possible.

POLIOMYELITIS

The last great epidemic of polio in the United States occurred in New England in 1955. Although the residual

effects of the disease are now encountered with increasing rarity, it still serves as a useful model of a process that can produce either a forefoot cavus or a hindfoot cavus.[8]

Paralytic polio is the result of a ribonucleic acid (RNA) virus that primarily affects the thalamus, hypothalamus, motor centers of the brain stem and cerebellum, and the anterior tracts of the spinal cord. There is a wide variety of clinical presentations depending upon what portions of the central nervous system (CNS) are affected, but as a practical matter the lower extremity weakness patterns of polio come from a strikingly selective destruction of the anterior motor neurons in the spinal cord itself, preserving function both proximal and distal to the lesion.

After an initial incubation period of 6 to 20 days, the acute phase of the disease is associated with the most dramatic paralysis and lasts approximately 7 to 10 days. Clinically detectable weakness usually occurs when more than 60% of the motor neurons to a muscle group are affected. Muscle function can recover gradually thereafter; the most substantial gains occur in the first 4 months, and some return of function is usually seen up to 2 years after the illness.

Patterns of Foot Deformity in Polio

Hindfoot Cavus

The gastrocnemius–soleus complex is the critical variable in determining what variety of foot deformity will develop. The classic cavus foot deformity resulting from polio is that of a hindfoot cavus associated with a dramatically high calcaneal pitch angle. This is the result of the paralysis of the gastrocnemius–soleus complex with preservation of the remainder of the posterior compartment, the intrinsic foot musculature, and the anterior tibialis. When appropriate tension is missing from the Achilles tendon, the long toe flexors still function to depress the metatarsal heads, raising the arch. The intrinsics foreshorten the distance between the metatarsals and the calcaneus, functioning much like a bowstring to raise the calcaneal pitch. The result is a vertical posture of the calcaneus.

Forefoot Cavus

A lesion slightly higher in the spinal cord can spare the gastrocnemius–soleus complex but affect the tibialis anterior selectively. This situation results in two particular imbalances that drive depression of the first ray and a forefoot cavus. First, just as in CMT, the peroneus longus is unopposed and directly plantar flexes the first ray. Second, the extensor hallucis longus is still functional and serves as an accessory dorsiflexor of the foot. This creates a claw toe as the foot is pulled up through the toe rather than the usual midfoot insertion of the tibialis anterior. The claw toe deformity itself also serves to depress the metatarsal head.

Other Deformities

Because the motor neuron destruction in poliomyelitis is often patchy and recovery is sometimes incomplete, the patterns of motor weakness cannot always be so neatly categorized. When the tibialis posterior is affected, either alone or in combination with the tibialis anterior, the result is a progressive planovalgus foot rather than a cavus foot. Rarer still is isolated involvement of the peroneals, which usually results in a very mild cavus foot dominated more by varus of the hindfoot with attendant instability of the ankle. The critical lesson is that, like all peripheral neural lesions, the motor weakness patterns in polio all must be evaluated and treated individually.

OTHER NEUROLOGIC LESIONS

Although CMT and polio represent the most historically prominent etiologies of the cavus foot, a wide variety of other lesions can lead to the deformity.

Friedreich ataxia is a familial progressive ataxia in which posterior column function is steadily lost.[36] It occurs in an autosomal recessive form with an earlier age of onset (11.75 years) and in a dominant form with a later age of onset (20.4 years). No cases of onset after the age of 25 have been reported. The disease is usually associated with pronounced and progressive symmetric cavus foot deformities with severe claw toe formation. In numerous instances, the foot deformities have been the presenting complaint.

A heterogeneous group of *hereditary cerebellar ataxias* are also associated with cavus foot, but they are less easy to categorize than Friedreich ataxia, which primarily shows spinal cord involvement.

Roussy-Lévy syndrome is a rare syndrome of cavus foot, sensory ataxia without obvious long-tract signs, peripheral motor atrophy, and kyphoscoliosis. Because it shares characteristics of both diseases, it was poorly differentiated from Friedreich ataxia and CMT for many years.[37] The onset occurs very early in childhood and runs a relatively benign course.

Spinal muscular atrophy is a heterogeneous group of disorders that are usually present from birth but have some late-onset forms.[41] They are characterized by an inexorably progressive loss of anterior motor neuron cells. The disorders are characterized by hypotonia and can be associated with the cavus foot deformity, although it is rarely the presenting feature.

Structural spinal cord disease often manifests with cavus foot deformity and requires a high degree of suspicion to detect. In particular, the unexplained onset of a progressive bilateral cavus deformity, or essentially any unilateral deformity, should warrant an imaging workup. *Spinal cord tumors* are notorious for their early absence of symptoms, and foot deformity might be the initial complaint. *Syringomyelia* is a cavitation in the center of the spinal cord that usually occurs in the cervical cord but can also interrupt the neural pathways to the lower extremities and result in spasticity or deformity. *Diastematomyelia* is a rare disorder in which a spicule of bone or fibrous band sagittally divides the spinal canal in the thoracic or high lumbar regions and separates the spinal cord into two pieces, each surrounded by dura. Because the cord and axial skeleton grow at different rates, a traction myelopathy very slowly develops as the child matures. The findings can be subtle, but making the diagnosis is critical.

Spinal dysraphism in all its forms (spina bifida, myelocele, myelomeningocele) is certainly more common and can manifest with a variety of postural foot disorders depending upon the particular patterns of involvement. Fortunately, the diagnosis is almost always well established early in life.

Cerebral palsy is, by definition, a static encephalopathy and can result in a variety of foot deformities, including pes cavus. Although the neurologic lesion is not progressive, the flexibility of the postural disorders deteriorates with time.

POSTTRAUMATIC CAVOVARUS FOOT DEFORMITIES

Any traumatic condition that leads to an imbalance of the intrinsic and extrinsic foot musculature can lead to a cavus deformity. The deep posterior compartment of the leg is most commonly involved in traumatic compartment syndromes, and a Volkmann contracture in that location will lead to a cavus foot with a prominent claw toe component. Crush injuries of the leg and severe burns or soft tissue loss can also have the same result, both from direct injuries to the musculature and indirectly through tibial nerve injury. Compartment syndromes confined to the foot most commonly occur with calcaneus fractures or with crush injuries to the forefoot; they have been associated with the late development of claw toes but not with cavus deformity.

Several forms of fracture malunion can also result in a fixed cavovarus deformity. Most commonly, a talar neck fracture with substantial medial comminution can fall into a varus malunion. This substantially limits subtalar joint eversion and leads secondarily to the calcaneus assuming a varus malalignment. Alternatively, a varus hindfoot can result from residual deformity from an intraarticular calcaneus fracture or even medial impaction of the tibial plafond.

CONGENITAL PES CAVUS

Clubfoot Residuals

The cavus foot deformity is one of four components of the congenital clubfoot, easily remembered by the mnemonic CAVE (cavus, adductus, varus, equinus). Adult clubfoot residuals encountered after childhood casting usually result from a failure of early casting to adequately elevate the first ray before abducting the foot about the fulcrum of the talar head as described by Morcuende et al.[35] The most severe deformities that result from improper casting technique are usually not those of residual cavus but of a rocker-bottom foot that results when the equinus is inappropriately corrected while the calcaneus remains locked under the talus; the foot then dorsiflexes through the midfoot rather than through the ankle.

A wave of enthusiasm for surgical clubfoot correction in the 1970s and 1980s is also now yielding residual effects in the adult foot and ankle population. The results of clubfoot correction surgery have proved to be substantially less reliable than once thought.[30,42] A patient presenting with problems with a postsurgical clubfoot is just as likely to have overcorrection into planovalgus as residual undercorrection in cavovarus. The one constant in the surgically corrected clubfoot is a remarkable amount of stiffness in adults. In a dynamic gait analysis study, Huber and Dutoit[18] specifically identified late subtalar stiffness as the primary feature associated with a poor result after childhood clubfoot surgery. It is rare that anything short of triple arthrodesis can be entertained to address the residual complaints.

The Idiopathic Cavus Foot

Despite the litany of potential known causes of the cavus deformity, the largest single group of cases encountered is symmetric and has no known cause. They can manifest because of stiffness in the hindfoot, stress fractures along the lateral column, recurrent ankle instability, or, commonly, for symptoms totally unrelated to the conformation of the arch.

EVOLUTION OF DEFORMITY

Pes cavus must be viewed as a spectrum of deformities in which the underlying abnormality is that of an elevated longitudinal arch, but after that a variety of bony and soft tissue deformities can be present. The spectrum can range from a mild cavus foot, with flexible claw toes as the only significant clinical problem, to a severe fixed deformity,

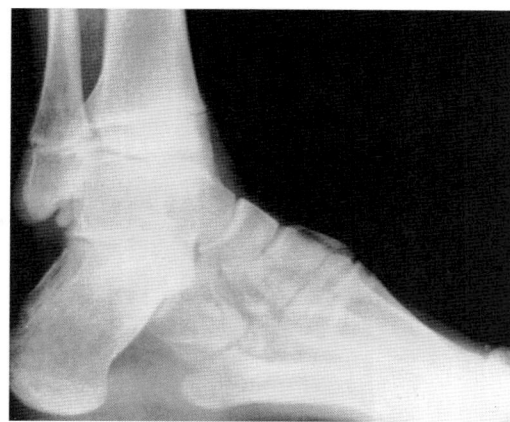

Figure 26-1 Pes cavus with a predominant hindfoot deformity. Note the dramatically high pitch angle of the calcaneus.

with altered weight bearing, callosities, lateral ankle laxity, stress reactions, and pain. The shape of the foot varies with the cause and duration of the motor imbalance that created the deformity. When muscular imbalance in pes cavus begins before maturation of the skeleton, there can be substantial change of healthy osseous morphology. After skeletal maturity, there is usually little or no change in the morphology.[1] The cavus foot is best understood by systematically analyzing the bone deformities, the soft tissue deformities, and the specific muscle functions that are imbalanced.

The bony deformity may be predominantly in the hindfoot, the forefoot, or a combination of both. A *hindfoot cavus* describes an elevated pitch of the long axis of the calcaneus, which is usually greater than 30 degrees in a cavus foot (Fig. 26-1). Hindfoot cavus was a very common deformity in the era of widespread poliomyelitis; the focal nature of the disease in the anterior horn cells of the spinal cord often led to gastrocnemius weakness but sparing of the tibialis anterior and often the foot intrinsics. The resultant imbalance of forces then often led to dramatic calcaneal pitch angles and subsequent soft tissue contractures. Pure hindfoot cavus is now less common, while *hindfoot varus* is a predominant finding in pes cavus with underlying neurologic disease. Elevated calcaneal pitch is still encountered as a component of a combined deformity in the idiopathic cavus foot with no clear neurologic cause.

Most neurologic cavus deformities are thought to occur from a forefoot-driven hindfoot varus resulting from a muscle imbalance as in CMT. The peroneus longus tendon is a direct antagonist to the tibialis anterior tendon. Often spared by the neuropathy, the strong peroneus longus muscle overpowers the affected tibialis anterior and initializes the deformity by plantar flexion of the medial forefoot (Fig. 26-2). The tibialis posterior muscle induces the hindfoot varus, and the Achilles tendon further enhances the varus stress secondary to the plantar-flexed first ray and varus heel alignment, which alters the

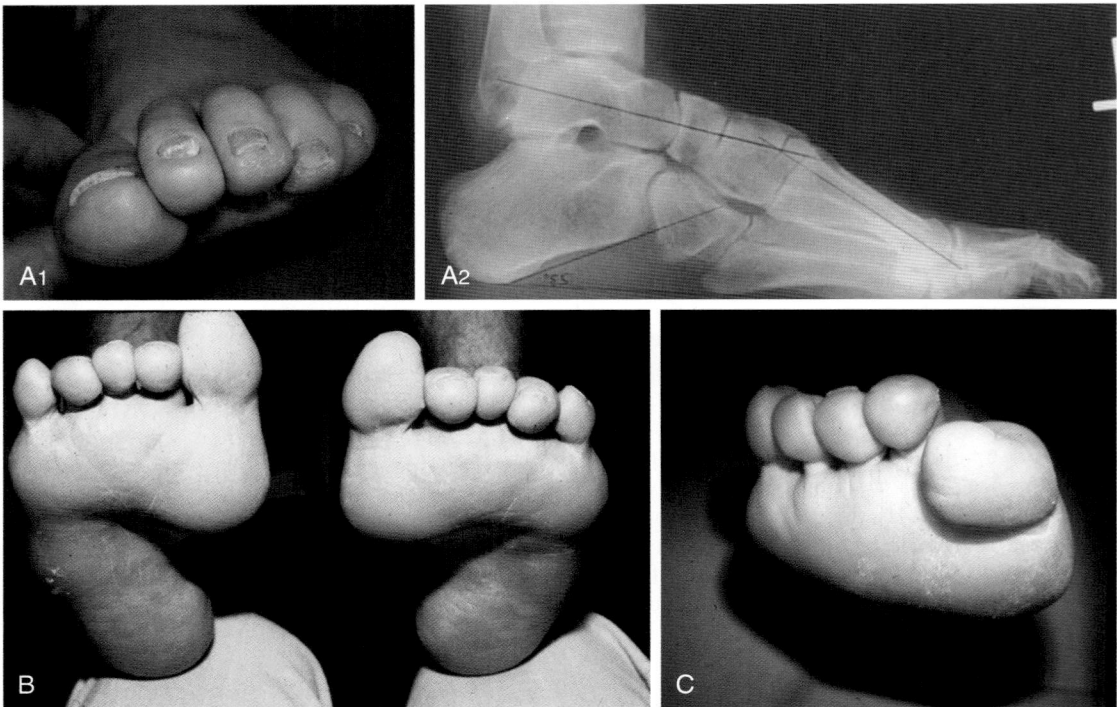

Figure 26-2 Left pes cavus of Charcot-Marie-Tooth patient with a predominant forefoot deformity. **A,** The driving force is the plantar-flexed and adducted forefoot, clinically seen as depression of the first metatarsal head. The radiograph demonstrates plantar flexion and adduction of the first metatarsal relative to the axis of the talus (talo–first metatarsal angle). **B,** Bilateral plantar flexion of the first metatarsal accompanied by a varus heel deformity. **C,** Some cases demonstrate a more generalized forefoot deformity with generalized forefoot equinus.

transmission of axial forces through the ankle joint. With inversion of the hindfoot, the lateral foot supinates and the peroneus longus muscle further plantar flexes the first ray to restore the tripod position and a plantigrade foot.[1] Soft tissue contracture converts a flexible to a fixed cavus deformity over time.

Toe deformities are thought to occur from early degeneration of the intrinsic muscles of the foot. Because the lumbricals are not acting to stabilize the metatarsalphalangeal (MTP) joint (intrinsics effect: MTP flexion, proximal interphalangeal [PIP] and distal interphalangeal [DIP] extension), the unopposed extensor digitorum longus hyperextends the unstable lesser toes at the MTP level while the flexor digitorum longus and brevis flex the phalanges.[1] The plantar-flexed metatarsal heads and plantar fascia shortening amplify forefoot plantar flexion. The deformities might be as mild as flexible clawing of the MTP joints in association with mild flexion of the interphalangeal joints, or they can manifest as fixed claw toe deformities. Once severe fixed claw toe deformities are present, the forces from the extrinsic toe extensors serve to hold the metatarsal heads in a plantar-flexed position (Fig. 26-3). Of importance, the plantar fat pad is displaced distally in severe cases as the toes pull up into extension. Not only are the metatarsal heads driven plantarward by the deformity, but they are also deprived of their normal cushioning layer of fat.

The plantar fascia commonly develops a contracture with time in all forms of cavus foot. It is anatomically much thicker on the medial aspect of the foot, and as the contracture develops, it not only holds the longitudinal arch in an elevated position but also holds the forefoot adducted and keeps the calcaneus inverted (Fig. 26-4). Although some bony procedures can secondarily relax the plantar fascia by altering the shape of the arch, they are not always adequate by themselves.

Early in the development of many cases of forefoot cavus the deformities remain relatively flexible. The arch might not flatten while standing, but muscle forces are holding it in position rather than bone and joint contractures. This is typical, for instance, of a very young patient with Charcot-Marie-Tooth disease. The subtalar joint compensates for the forefoot deformity by falling into a varus alignment (Fig. 26-5). As the disease progresses, the capsule and interosseous ligament of the subtalar joint become contracted, and the once-flexible hindfoot deformity becomes fixed.

BIOMECHANICAL CONSEQUENCES OF PES CAVUS

The mechanics of all variants of the foot are similar. The axes of the talus and the calcaneus are more collinear. The talar head remains over the anterior process of the

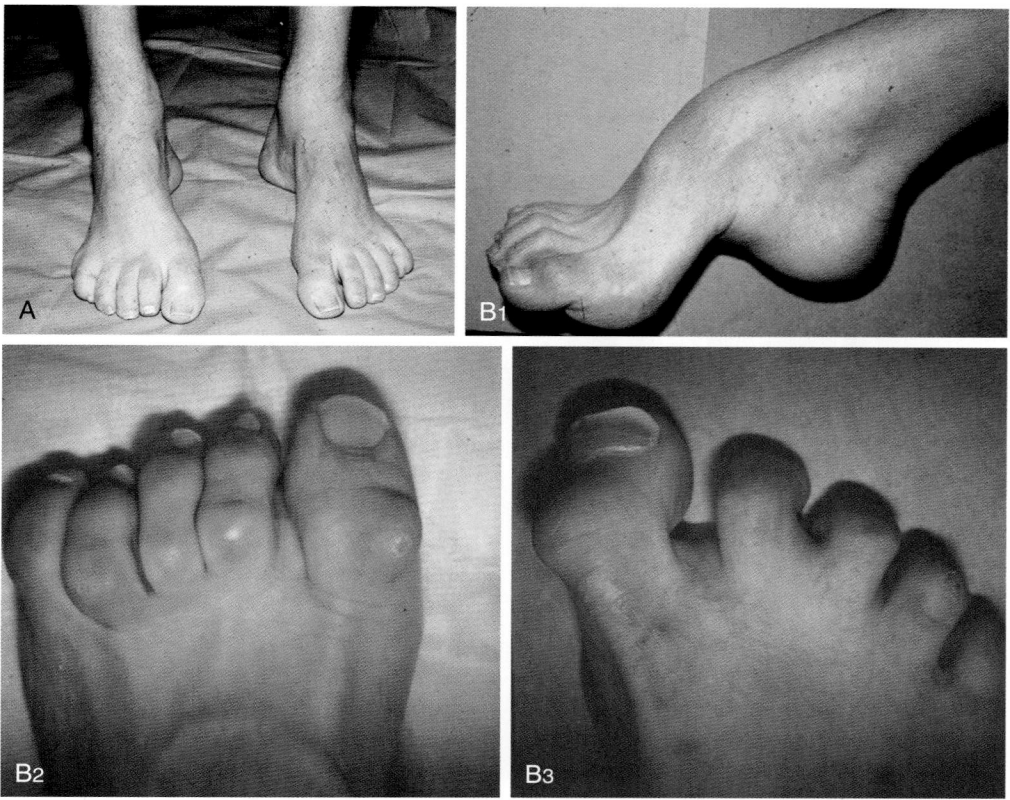

Figure 26-3 Metatarsophalangeal (MTP) joint deformities. **A,** Mild claw toes of the right foot with a near-normal left foot. **B,** Examples of severe clawing of the MTP joints, including clawing of the hallux from the use of the extensor hallucis longus as an accessory dorsiflexor.

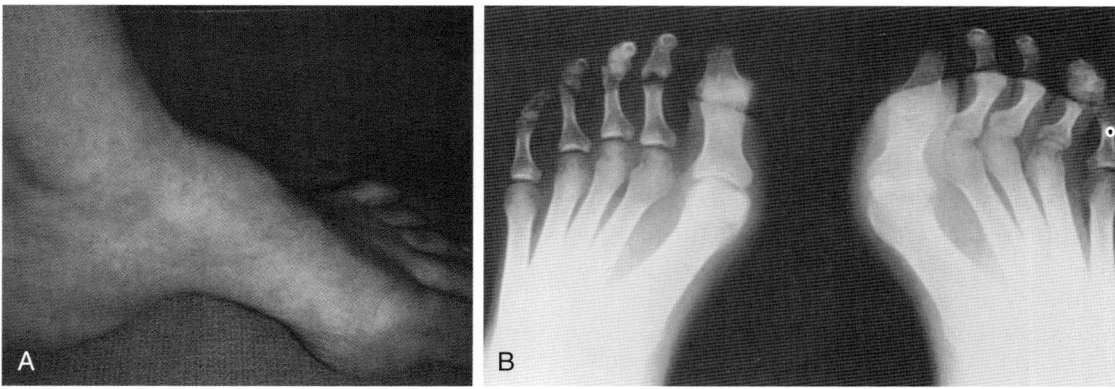

Figure 26-4 Contracture of the plantar fascia contributes to and fixes the deformity. The tight medial band of the plantar fascia holds the forefoot in adduction and the hindfoot in varus. **A,** Cavus foot demonstrates adduction of the forefoot, an elevated longitudinal arch, and varus of the calcaneus. **B,** Radiograph demonstrating severe adduction of the forefoot.

calcaneus, and the navicular moves to a superior instead of a medial position to the cuboid; the subtalar joint axis is more vertical; and the Chopart joint function is impaired.[1] When the hindfoot is locked in inversion, there is less subtalar and transversal tarsal motion during gait than in the normal foot. The ability of the foot to absorb the impact of walking by pronation during the early part of stance phase is diminished, and the first metatarsal head and the lateral border of the foot are overloaded.[1] A cavus foot is always stiffer than one of normal conformation.

The relative dorsiflexion of the talus within the ankle mortise is caused by plantar flexion of the medial forefoot, limits ankle dorsiflexion, and is accompanied by

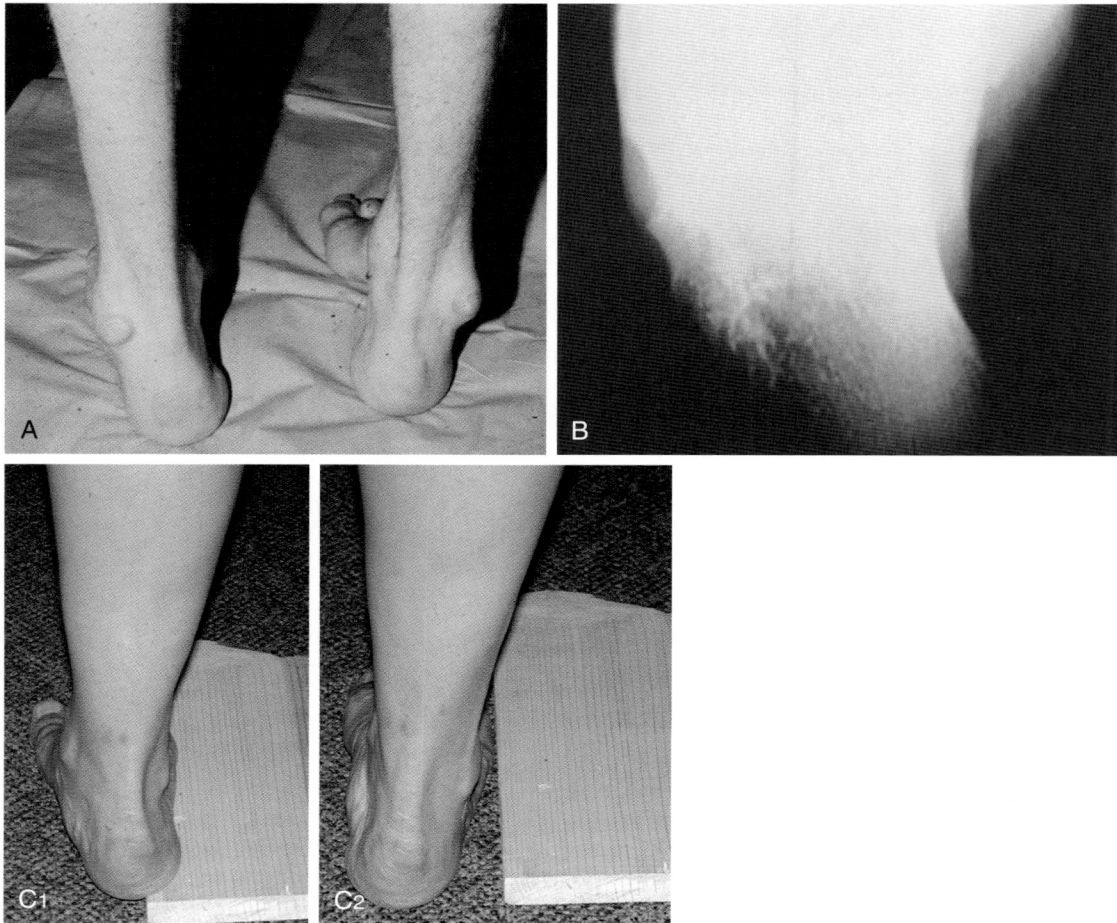

Figure 26-5 Varus heel deformity. **A,** In cases of forefoot-driven cavus, the varus heel is initially present as the natural standing posture of the heel when the first ray is plantar flexed and adducted. With time, the hindfoot deformity can become fixed. The presence of the deformity can be best assessed from behind. **B,** An axial view of the calcaneus demonstrates marked varus deformity. **C,** The Coleman block test can be used to demonstrate persistent flexibility of the hindfoot. If the heel can be forced into valgus by weight bearing on a block supporting only the lateral column of the foot, the subtalar joint remains flexible. In this case, the cavus can be corrected by addressing the forefoot deformity alone.

anterior ankle impingement. Together with the hindfoot varus position, relative talus dorsiflexion is thought to contribute to an increased anteromedial contact stress in the ankle joint. The association between lateral ankle instability, cavovarus deformity, and ankle arthritis has been discussed in the literature.[13,46] A significant pressure increase and reduction of the area loaded in the ankle joint was also demonstrated in simulated pes cavus and is considered to lead to ankle arthritis in long-standing deformities with, but also without, lateral ligament instability.[24]

In the forefoot, the weight-bearing area beneath the metatarsal heads and heel pad is decreased, leading to substantially higher plantar pressures in both locations. In addition, because of the clawing and hyperextension of the MTP joints, the toes do not participate in weight bearing during toe-off, and power is diminished. The plantar fascia normally functions as a passive windlass mechanism to elevate the longitudinal arch, plantar flex

the metatarsals, and invert the calcaneus. In the cavus foot, all three of these conditions are present permanently, and the plantar fascia becomes contracted.

The muscle weakness patterns seen around the foot vary with the cause of the condition, but adduction of the forefoot is commonly seen when the posterior tibialis is active in the presence of a weak peroneus brevis. Metatarsus adductus exacerbates the already considerable tendency for excessive pressure in the lateral column of the foot, and stress reactions of the fifth metatarsal can result.

Physical Examination

The patient encounter begins with a careful history of the condition and a detailed family history. Generalized lateral column pain seems to be the most common presenting symptom associated with the cavus foot. Frequently, patients report ongoing lateral hindfoot instability despite one or more previous lateral hindfoot ligament repairs or reconstructions that failed later because the predisposing hindfoot statics were not corrected.

The patient's gait is carefully observed for the nature of ground contact, the position of the heel, and the position of the toes during stance. Any fall of the heel toward further varus as weight transfers onto the limb should be noted by observing the patient walk from behind. During swing phase, the examiner should check for the possibility of a footdrop and the use of the extensor hallucis longus as an accessory dorsiflexor, leading to a cock-up deformity of the first MTP joint.

The heel pad could be seen easily from the front ("peek a boo") with the patient standing and feet aligned straight ahead. In a normal foot, the heel pad is not visible on the medial side of the foot when viewed from the front because of the slight amount of valgus positioning of the average heel, which places the heel pad behind the normal hindfoot.

The relative position of the hindfoot to the forefoot must be noted along with the rigidity of that relationship. The normal hindfoot will be positioned in slight valgus when standing flat and deviate into varus when rising onto the toes. The patient is asked if he or she experiences a subjective instability in the tiptoe position.

The Coleman block test can be used to determine the ability of the hindfoot to fall back into an appropriate valgus posture. The heel alone or heel and lateral column of the foot are supported on a small flat wooden block while the forefoot or the medial column, respectively, remain unsupported. If the hindfoot is not fixed and the deformity is being driven by a first ray fixed in plantar flexion, the calcaneus will noticeably tilt into valgus when viewed from behind. In theory, a foot that exhibits flexibility on the Coleman block test can be corrected by working on the forefoot deformity alone.

With the patient seated, the examiner observes active and passive range of motion of the ankle, subtalar, transverse tarsal, and MTP joints. The forefoot should also be examined after manual correction of the hindfoot varus deformity to assess the amount of fixed forefoot pronation and to determine the need for medial metatarsals dorsiflexion osteotomies. Limited and painful ankle dorsiflexion may demonstrate anterior or anteromedial ankle impingement because of the relative talar dorsiflexion within the ankle mortise. The hindfoot is assessed for any chronic ligamentous incompetence. Clinical signs of the lateral border overload range from calluses to proximal diaphyseal or metaphyseal fractures of the lateral metatarsals. Peroneal tendon pathology, including tears and subluxation, are commonly present, as is tightness of the gastrocnemius–soleus complex.

Muscle function is very carefully assessed and documented for evaluation disease progression. Special attention should be paid to the ability of the peroneus longus to selectively plantar flex the first ray because this can point to the potential for a tendon transfer to effectively assist in treatment. A patient who does not carry a known neurologic diagnosis should also undergo a neurologic screening, including testing for long-tract signs, reflexes, hamstring tightness, and any asymmetry. Intrinsic wasting is usually easier to pick up in the upper extremity, and in suspected cases of CMT or other systemic peripheral neuropathies, an examination of the intrinsic musculature of the hands is in order. Subtle disease can usually be discerned in the loss of muscle mass and strength of the first dorsal interosseous along the radial border of the second metacarpal. The patient exhibits weakness in abducting the index digit away from the midline with the rest of the hand held in a neutral position to isolate the intrinsics.

Because of the very subtle findings associated with structural disease of the spinal cord, substantial unexplained asymmetry or rapid progression of the deformity warrants a neurologic referral and corresponding imaging.

INVESTIGATIONS

Standing anteroposterior (AP) and lateral radiographs of the foot and ankle are essential. A line drawn down the axis of the talus should pass through the axis of the first metatarsal on both AP and lateral weight-bearing images of the foot in the normal situation. The axes should ordinarily be collinear, 0 degrees ± 5. The lateral talo–first metatarsal angle (the Meary angle) can be used to assess the severity of a forefoot plantar flexion, whereas, as opposed to other measured angles, the extent appears to correlate with the development of anteromedial ankle arthritis.[24] The AP talo–first metatarsal angle defines the amount of forefoot adductus. The calcaneal pitch angle is elevated in cases of hindfoot cavus.

Further findings on the lateral radiographs are an increased navicular height, an increased Hibbs angle (measured by a line through the axis of the calcaneus and the first metatarsal—in normal feet the angle is 45 degrees, and in cavus feet, it is near 90 degrees), and a posterior fibula with a "flat-topped" talus. The latter appearance is an artifact because in pes cavus a standard lateral view is in fact an oblique view.

On the AP radiograph of the foot, the talocalcaneal angle is almost parallel in moderate and severe hindfoot varus. The presence of any associated metatarsus adductus should be noted by drawing of the AP talo–first metatarsal angle because this can require some degree of additional surgical attention or limit the degree of correction that can be achieved.

The extent and progression of any ankle arthritis and talar tilt is recorded on extra AP and lateral standing ankle radiographs. The Saltzman view can be added to assess the angles of the tibiotalar and the subtalar joint.

Computed tomography (CT) examination with the foot supported in the typical 90-degree position, with sagittal and coronal reformats, and three-dimensional modeling rules out occult degenerative joint disease and tarsal coalitions. MRI or ultrasound can occasionally be helpful to reveal any inflammation, splitting, or tears of the tendons. MRI can also detect early cartilage degeneration and osteochondral lesions when arthritis is not yet visible on plain radiographs or CT.

A digital dynamic pedobarography can be helpful to determine a pathologic plantar pressure distribution. Associated changes are the lateralization of the line of center of pressure and increased zone of pressure under the first metatarsophalangeal joint in case of a plantar-flexed first metatarsal.

Conservative Treatment

Many cases of cavus deformity represent stable or slowly progressive deformities that are appropriately managed, at least initially, by nonoperative means. In the case of an adolescent with progressive deformity and a still-supple foot, however, there may be much to be lost by delay. Soft tissue surgery alone might manage the deformity early in the course of the disease, avoid ankle arthritis, and prevent the necessity of osteotomies or fusions.

A stretching program to maintain motion is an important component of conservative management, particularly in cases of neurologic origin. Eversion and dorsiflexion should be emphasized. Metatarsalgia might be an early presenting complaint from uncovering of the metatarsal heads as claw toes develop. Accommodative manufactured shoes with extra-depth toe boxes can be of substantial benefit.

Orthoses are a valuable adjunct to the conservative treatment of cavus feet. The reduced weight-bearing area in cavovarus feet is enlarged with orthotic devices. Typical custom foot orthotics for cavus may include an elevated heel to accommodate a tight gastrocnemius muscle and a recess under the first metatarsal head to accommodate the plantar-flexed first ray and allow some degree of hindfoot eversion.[34] A forefoot wedge, beginning just lateral to the first metatarsal recess, extends to the lateral border of the device to mirror the forefoot pronation.

Basically, the more fixed the cavus deformity is, the less likely is much benefit from orthoses, and discomfort and calluses may develop in supported areas. Once the deformity becomes fixed, patients tolerate corrective orthoses poorly. For lateral ankle instability, a high-top boot or an off-the-shelf ankle brace offer hindfoot stabilization. Lace-up braces are easier to fit inside a shoe or boot and stabilize the ankle comparably to plastic upright braces. Preexisting ankle instability usually worsens by high-arched orthoses amplifying hindfoot varus.

Severe muscle weakness is usually treated with full-length custom ankle–foot orthoses (AFOs) to prevent foot drop. The integration of orthotic modifications into the AFO improves proprioception and ankle stability more than the brace alone. Many patients can be managed by hinged AFOs with dorsiflexion assistance to allow a much more normal gait pattern. In some cases of equinus deformity, full clamshell braces or casts are needed because the strong or unopposed plantar flexors will overcome the correction obtained with a posterior brace or anterior strap.

Surgical Treatment

Decision Making

The goal of surgical management is to produce a plantigrade, stable foot, to alleviate discomfort, and to improve function. Surgical realignment should be recommended when signs of tendon or hindfoot joint degeneration arise, resulting from recurrent hindfoot instability or elevated hindfoot joint contact stresses by varus alignment. Earlier surgery may be appropriate due to lateral column pain or progressive deformity.

Basics of dynamic and static realignment are that tendons contributing to the deformity should be transferred to a more functional location (i.e., peroneus longus to brevis), contracted structures should be released to allow restoration of normal foot shape (i.e., plantar fascia), and osteotomies are preferred over arthrodesis of nonarthritic joints to help realign the foot to a more functional position (calcaneal osteotomy instead of corrective subtalar fusion). If the deformity is fixed, however, an arthrodesis might be necessary to produce a plantigrade foot.

There is no simple boilerplate approach applicable to all cavus feet. A suggested algorithm is provided in Figure 26-6. The key to surgical decision making is to adopt procedures that are necessary to match each specific deformity. It is not uncommon to have a foot with a combination of fixed and supple deformities; a particular case might require a combination of bone and soft tissue procedures.

Soft Tissue Procedures
PLANTAR FASCIA RELEASE (STEINDLER STRIPPING)
The contracted plantar fascia plays a major role in maintaining height of the longitudinal arch and varus positioning of the calcaneus in the patient with pes cavus. Release and stripping of the plantar fascia often help to reduce the height of the longitudinal arch in patients who retain some degree of flexibility (Video Clip 47).[43] At times, the procedure may be carried out in conjunction with a lateralizing calcaneal osteotomy, a triple arthrodesis, or a first metatarsal osteotomy.

Surgical Technique
1. The patient is placed in a supine position. The normal external rotation of the lower extremity provides adequate visualization of the foot. A tourniquet is used around the thigh.
2. An oblique skin incision is made, starting distal to the weight-bearing area of the calcaneal fat pad and passing over the contracted plantar fascia. This incision does not put the medial calcaneal branches to the heel pad at risk of being cut.
3. The incision is deepened through the fat, exposing the plantar fascia on the plantar aspect of the foot as well as medially over the fascia of the abductor hallucis muscle.

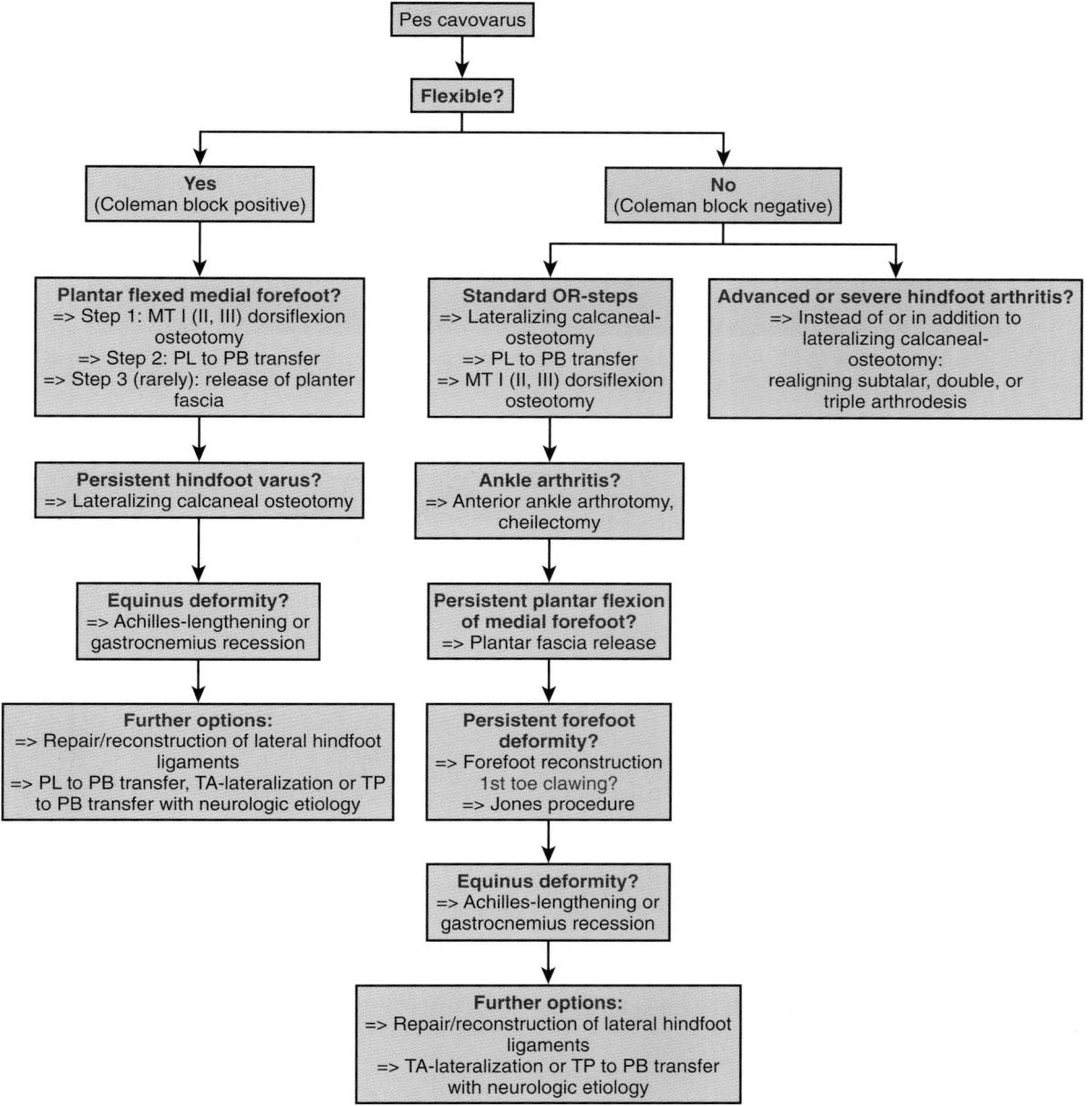

Figure 26-6 Pes cavovarus treatment algorithm. *PB,* Peroneus brevis tendon; *PL,* peroneus longus tendon; *TA,* tibialis anterior tendon; *TP,* tibialis posterior tendon.

4. The origin of the plantar fascia is transected while tension is being applied to it by dorsiflexing the MTP joints. In this way, the plantar fascia will separate as it is cut. Often, some deeper septa must be carefully transected. The lateral plantar nerve passes just distal to the cut, so the surgeon must be cautious when transecting the septa.

5. After releasing the plantar fascia, the surgeon palpates along the medial aspect of the foot, particularly in a severely deformed case, to release the superficial and deep fascia surrounding the abductor hallucis muscle. This is a very important part of the release, particularly

in cases involving significant adduction of the forefoot.

6. Once the cuts have been made by blunt dissection and stretching the fascia, the wound is carefully inspected to ensure that no tight bands of fascia remain, either on the plantar aspect of the foot or along the abductor muscle.

Postoperative Care
The patient is placed into a short-leg compression dressing incorporating plaster splints. The sutures are removed in 12 to 14 days, after which the patient is placed in a

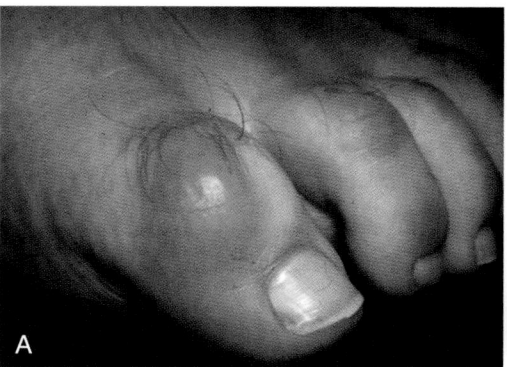
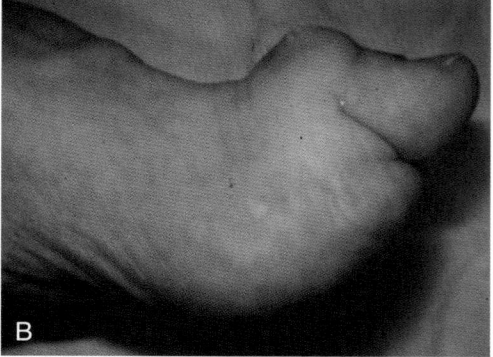

Figure 26-7 Cock-up deformity of the first metatarsophalangeal joint from the use of the extensor hallucis longus as an accessory dorsiflexor with a weak anterior tibialis. **A,** Resting. **B,** With active attempted dorsiflexion of the ankle.

short-leg cast. Weight bearing is begun as tolerated, whereas 4 weeks of immobilization is usually adequate if plantar fascia release is carried out as an isolated procedure.

FIRST-TOE JONES PROCEDURE

The procedure is used to correct a hyperextension deformity of the first MTP joint caused by weakness of the tibialis anterior. Although the EHL is also located in the anterior compartment and is innervated more distally than the tibialis anterior, its function can be spared in a surprising number of conditions. In modern practice, this is usually seen in CMT or variants of cerebral palsy, but it was historically common in polio.[22] In these cases, the EHL is functioning as an accessory dorsiflexor of the ankle joint, which results in hyperextension of the MTP joint and secondary flexion of the interphalangeal joint (Fig. 26-7). Moving the insertion of the EHL tendon into the base of the first metatarsal facilitates dorsiflexion of the ankle and also relieves the cock-up deformity of the MTP. To prevent a floppy first toe, a fusion of the interphalangeal joint is usually performed.

Surgical Technique

1. The procedure is carried out with the patient supine. A tourniquet is used around the thigh (Fig. 26-8 and Video Clip 51).

Interphalangeal Joint Arthrodesis

2. An elliptic skin incision is centered over the dorsal aspect of the interphalangeal joint of the hallux. The collateral ligaments are cut to expose the articular surfaces.
3. The extensor hallucis longus tendon is freed from its retinacular attachments along its mediolateral aspect.
4. The surfaces of the interphalangeal joint are removed with a power saw to create two flat surfaces. The interphalangeal joint is placed in a few degrees of plantar flexion and neutral varus/valgus alignment.
5. A 2.5-mm hole is drilled in an antegrade manner from proximal to distal through the midportion of the

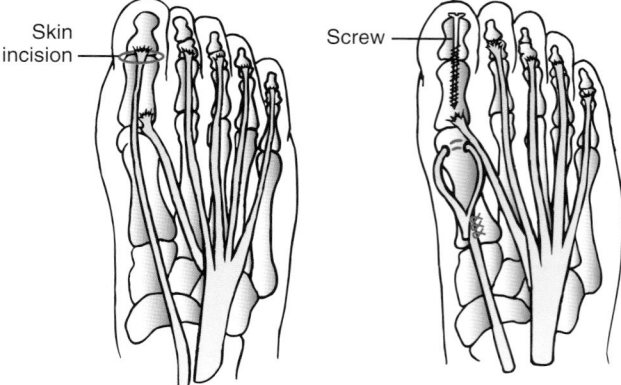

Figure 26-8 The first-toe Jones procedure moves the pull of the extensor hallucis longus (EHL) tendon from the great toe to the neck of the first metatarsal. Interphalangeal joint arthrodesis of the hallux is then performed to prevent a floppy toe. The procedure aids the ability of the EHL to serve as an accessory dorsiflexor and helps eliminate depression of the first metatarsal head. (From Mann RA, Coughlin MJ: *The video textbook of foot and ankle surgery*, St Louis, 1991, Medical Video Productions.)

distal phalanx. Where the drill bit begins to pressure the skin on the tip of the toe, a generous transverse incision is made to prevent maceration of the tissue.
6. The drill bit is removed and brought back through the hole from distal to proximal. Holding the interphalangeal joint in a reduced position, the surgeon extends the drill hole into the proximal phalanx.
7. The hole is measured. A 4.0-mm solid-shaft cancellous lag screw or headless screw is inserted, providing compression to the arthrodesis site.
8. A Kirschner wire (K-wire) may be placed obliquely across the interphalangeal joint to control any rotational forces. This is removed after approximately 4 weeks.

Extensor Hallucis Longus Tendon Transfer

9. A longitudinal incision is made over the dorsal aspect of the first metatarsal.

10. The extensor tendon, which was previously freed distally, is now freed proximally and delivered into the wound.
11. A transverse drill hole is made and cleaned in the distal portion of the first metatarsal. The size is selected to snugly fit the tendon.
12. The extensor hallucis longus tendon is passed through the drill hole and sutured onto itself, holding the ankle in 10 degrees of dorsiflexion and placing a moderate amount of tension on the tendon transfer.

Postoperative Care
The patient is placed into a short-leg compression dressing incorporating plaster splints. A popliteal block can be useful to control postoperative pain. The sutures are removed at 10 to 12 days, and the patient is placed in a short-leg walking cast for 4 weeks. At 6 weeks postoperatively, ambulation as tolerated is allowed. If the interphalangeal joint fusion is not complete at that time, an additional period of ambulation in a postoperative shoe may be necessary.

PERONEUS LONGUS TO BREVIS TRANSFER
Many cases of cavus foot, particularly in CMT, are associated with preserved function of the peroneus longus muscle in the presence of a failing tibialis anterior.[15] This pulls the first ray plantarward and leads to a forefoot cavus deformity as well as a secondary hindfoot varus. A transfer of the peroneus longus to the peroneus brevis can dramatically improve the situation by both weakening the plantar pull on the first metatarsal and augmenting the function of the usually failing peroneus brevis.

Surgical Technique
1. The surgery is carried out with the patient supine. A small bump under the ipsilateral hip can facilitate access to the lateral aspect of the foot. A thigh tourniquet is used (Video Clip 49).
2. A 4-cm incision is made over the anterior margin of the peroneus longus on the lateral aspect of the foot as it courses toward the cuboid to turn underneath the foot. This incision is then deepened through the subcutaneous fat to access the peroneus brevis. Care should be taken to avoid injury to the sural nerve, which usually passes through the proximal aspect of the incision.
3. The peroneus longus and peroneus brevis each lie in separate sheaths in this area, and they must be released to access the tendons. The peroneus longus crosses underneath the brevis and is not always easy to find.
4. The peroneus longus is then cut as far distally as possible as it makes the turn around the cuboid to pass underneath the midfoot. If an os peroneum is present in the tendon, it is excised and the cut is made through this area.
5. The foot is held in maximum eversion, and the peroneus longus is woven two or three times in Pulvertaft fashion through the distal aspect of the peroneus

brevis. A 2-0 coated polyester suture (Ethibond; Ethicon360, Menlo Park, Calif.) is used to join the tendons. If other procedures are to be carried out on the foot, the final tensioning and suture of the tendon is saved until the end of the case.

Postoperative Care
The foot is placed in a short-leg compression dressing reinforced with plaster splints. After 10 to 12 days, the sutures are removed and a short-leg weight-bearing cast is applied. If no other procedures are being performed, a transition to regular footwear is usually made after a total of 4 to 6 weeks of immobilization.

TIBIALIS ANTERIOR LATERALIZATION
The transfer of the insertion of the anterior tibial tendon to the lateral cuneiform is a very powerful step of the dynamic realignment when sufficient strength remains in the tendon. It provides both hindfoot stability and lateral shift of the ankle center of force by changing the strong inversion moment into a light eversion moment while still maintaining dorsiflexion power. Minimal risk of overcorrection is present with transfer of the tendon to the lateral cuneiform, and the procedure is technically simpler than the split anterior tibialis transfer previously advocated.[17] A long history of the procedure exists in the treatment of mild clubfoot residuals after cast correction by the Ponseti method.[35] However, because transferred muscles generally lose one fifth of their strength, tibialis anterior muscle strength of at least 4 of 5 preoperatively is required for a reasonable effect, and the procedure may not be appropriate in cases of CMT.[47]

Surgical Technique
1. The procedure is carried out with the patient supine. A tourniquet is used around the thigh.
2. A medial longitudinal 3- to 4-cm incision is made from the tuberosity of the navicular to the base of the first metatarsal, and the tendon is released at its insertion to bone.
3. A second 3- to 4-cm longitudinal anterior incision is made slightly above the superior extensor retinaculum. The retinaculum is incised as needed to pull out the tendon.
4. The tendon end is grasped with a thick nonabsorbable suture. It is then rerouted subcutaneously to the level of the lateral cuneiform and pulled out through a third 3-cm longitudinal incision centered over the lateral cuneiform.
5. There the fibers of the extensor digitorum brevis muscle are bluntly separated, and the correct entry point of the bone tunnel (dorsolateral edge of the center of the lateral cuneiform) is verified fluoroscopically.
6. A 6-mm hole is drilled from there through all the cuneiforms to the medial cuneiform, and the tendon is drawn into this tunnel until appropriate tension is obtained. It is fixed by transosseous suture at the

medial cuneiform and into the surrounding soft tissues at the lateral entry. Alternatively, a dorsal to plantar tunnel can be created through the lateral cuneiform and fixation achieved with an interference screw.

Postoperative Care
A short-leg compression dressing reinforced with plaster splints is applied. The sutures are removed after 12 to 14 days, and a short-leg weight-bearing cast is applied. If this is the only procedure, a transition to regular footwear is usually made after a total of 4 to 6 weeks of immobilization.

Results and Complications
Patients who undergo tibialis anterior transfer were seen to have a lower mean talo–first metatarsal angle than those who had not, suggesting that, in its native position, the tibialis anterior may contribute to cavus.[47] In general, tendon tranfers result in a decrease in their overall strength. The tibialis anterior also typically loses strength with progression of the Charcot-Marie-Tooth disease, and over time, the transfer may become less effective.

CLAW TOE CORRECTIONS
Associated claw toe deformities are common in pes cavus. Often, dynamic claw toes resolve with realignment of the hindfoot and midfoot deformity. Treatment of the claw toe deformity depends upon whether a fixed or flexible deformity is present. With fixed deformity at the MTP joints, release of the extensor tendons and joint capsules is required. To hold the toes in the neutral position, usually a flexor tendon transfer needs to be done. With fixed deformity of the proximal interphalangeal joint (hammer toe), a proximal interphalangeal joint arthrodesis or a DuVries phalangeal arthroplasty with removal of the distal portion of the proximal phalanx is indicated. Some authors prefer one of the latter two procedures as the standard procedure because they have a similar effect on the long flexor tendons, require less dissection, and are more reliable, particularly in neurologic diseases.[29] However, if the claw toe deformity is passively correctible, a flexor tendon transfer alone usually suffices.

The surgical techniques for flexor tendon transfer (Girdlestone procedure), DuVries phalangeal arthroplasty to correct a hammer toe, and release of the MTP joints in a fixed contracture are described in Chapter 7 (Video Clip 75).

LATERAL LIGAMENT REPAIR/RECONSTRUCTION
Regardless of the repair or reconstruction technique to restore lateral hindfoot stability, the operation will likely fail when hindfoot varus static is not realigned at the same time. The association of lateral ligamentous hindfoot instability, cavus deformity and ankle arthritis has been made by various authors who all advise not only correction of the deformity with osteotomies and tendon transfers but also lateral hindfoot ligament reconstruction to prevent recurrence.[13,40,46]

The surgical techniques for lateral hindfoot ligament repair and reconstruction are described in Chapter 30.

Bony Procedures
OSTEOTOMIES
At times, a specific bony deformity is present in pes cavus that significantly impairs the patient's ability to maintain a plantigrade foot, but the remainder of the foot remains relatively supple. This usually takes the form of a fixed varus deformity of the hindfoot or a fixed plantar flexion of the first ray. If the fixed deformity can be corrected, a plantigrade foot can be achieved without an arthrodesis. In general, an osteotomy that includes the first metatarsal or calcaneus or both is carried out in conjunction with a plantar fascia release and peroneus longus to brevis tendon transfer.

DORSIFLEXION OSTEOTOMY OF THE FIRST RAY
Particularly in cases of CMT, plantar flexion of the first metatarsal can become fixed, with a resultant fixed forefoot valgus deformity. This forefoot equinus deformity can also involve the second and, rarely, the third metatarsal. As a result of this deformity, as the head of the first metatarsal contacts the ground, the forefoot is twisted into an inverted position. If this is associated with a varus deformity of the calcaneus, a weak peroneus brevis muscle, or a contracted plantar fascia, dramatic increases in stress on the lateral ankle ligaments can result. This stress can lead to chronic lateral ankle ligament instability over time.

Dorsiflexion of the first ray is achieved either by a dorsally closing osteotomy of the medial cuneiform (reversed Cotton osteotomy), by a corrective first metatarsocuneiform arthrodesis when the joint is arthritic, or by a dorsally closing osteotomy of the first metatarsal.

DORSIFLEXION OSTEOTOMY OF THE FIRST METATARSAL
In general, a first metatarsal osteotomy is carried out not as an isolated procedure but as part of a more comprehensive cavus foot correction. In the patient with mild and flexible deformity, sometimes only a plantar fascia release and a dorsiflexion osteotomy of the first metatarsal are required. More often, however, a calcaneal osteotomy, plantar fascia release, and first metatarsal osteotomy are done together. The first-toe Jones procedure can also be added without complication. In a similar but more powerful technique, a dorsiflexion of the first ray can also be achieved by removal of a dorsally based wedge of the medial cuneiform (reversed Cotton osteotomy), whereas the osteotomy is sometimes difficult to close because of the Lisfranc ligament.

Surgical Technique
1. The patient is placed in a supine position. If this is an isolated procedure, the first metatarsal osteotomy can be carried out under an ankle block only. If it is part

of a more comprehensive cavus foot correction, general anesthesia is used (Video Clip 50).

2. An incision is made over the dorsal aspect of the first metatarsal, starting over the medial cuneiform and ending over the distal third of the metatarsal.

3. The incision is deepened to the extensor tendon, which is immobilized and retracted medially or laterally.

4. The metatarsocuneiform (MTC) joint is identified, and the proposed osteotomy site is marked on the bone starting about 1.5 cm distal to the joint (Fig. 26-9A and B).

5. A 2.7-mm or 3.5-mm screw is centered in the proximal portion of the metatarsal above the proposed osteotomy.

6. A 0.062-inch K-wire is used to make a transverse drill hole in the dorsal part of the metatarsal 1 cm distal to the osteotomy.

7. The osteotomy is a dorsal closing wedge that usually removes 4 to 6 mm of bone, depending upon the degree of plantar flexion of the first metatarsal that must be corrected.

8. The first cut is made parallel to the MTC joint. A convergent cut is then made distally, aiming for the plantar cortex. Care is taken to leave the plantar cortex intact. A greenstick fracture is made as the osteotomy is closed, resulting in a more stable construct than if the cuts were fully completed. It is better to undercut the osteotomy than to remove too large a segment.

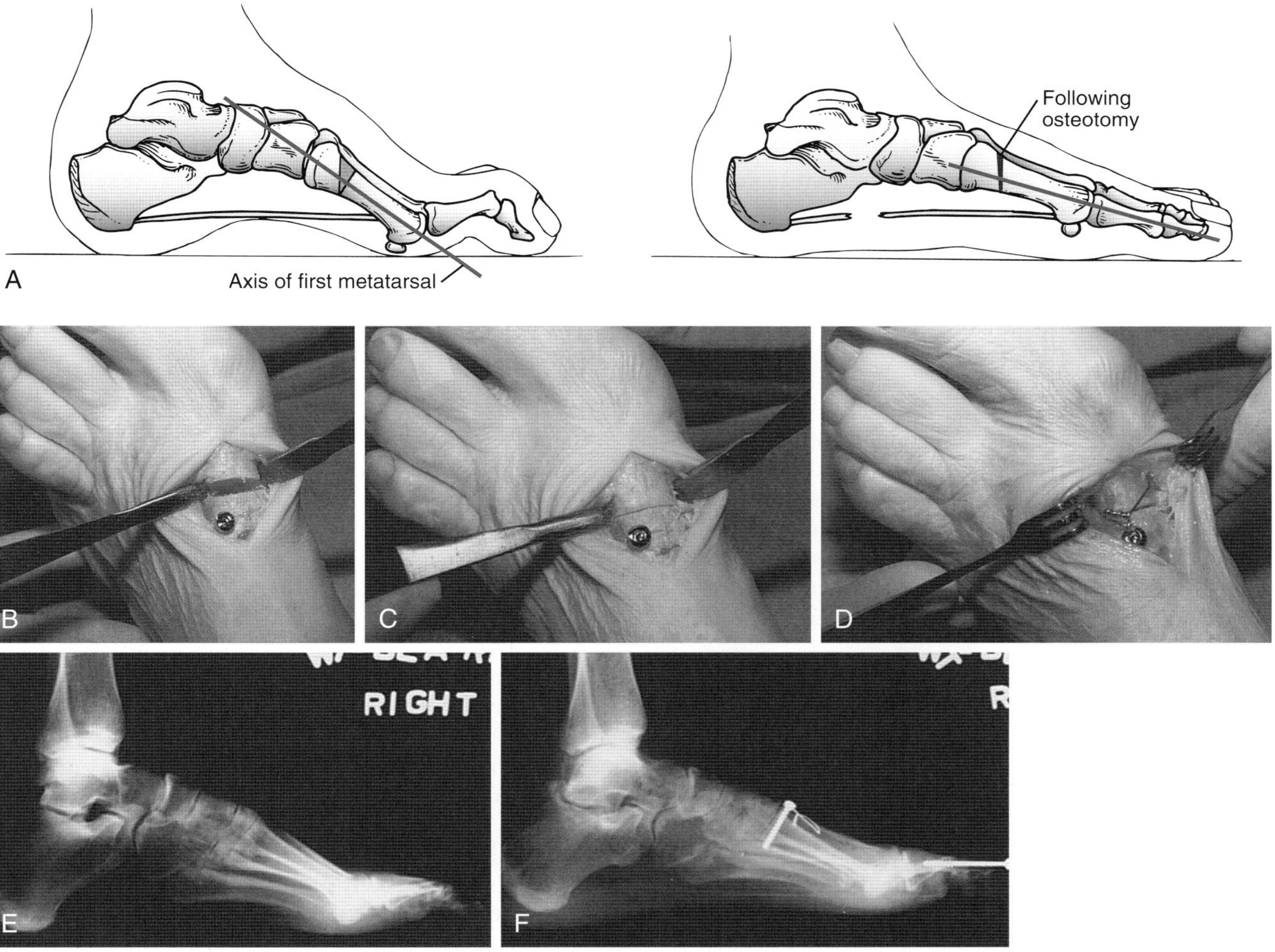

A — Axis of first metatarsal

Following osteotomy

B

C

D

RIGHT

E

F

Figure 26-9 Technique of the dorsiflexion osteotomy of the first metatarsal. **A,** A dorsally based wedge of bone is removed approximately 1 cm distal to the first metatarsocuneiform joint. The plantar fascia is often released when carrying out this procedure for a cavus foot. **B,** A 3.5-mm screw is placed in the proximal fragment to serve as a post. **C,** The osteotomy site is closed down, and the plantar aspect of the foot carefully palpated. If the first metatarsal is still too plantar flexed, a larger wedge is removed. **D,** The osteotomy site is fixed by placing a length of 22-gauge wire through a transverse drill hole in the distal fragment and then fixing it to the screw. **E** and **F,** Preoperative and postoperative radiographs demonstrate dorsiflexion of the first metatarsal after proximal osteotomy. (From Mann RA, Coughlin MJ: *The video textbook of foot and ankle surgery,* St Louis, 1991, Medical Video Productions.)

9. After the osteotomy has been created, the plantar cortex is loosened by rocking the bone back and forth until the dorsal gap can be closed (Fig. 26-9C).

10. To determine whether enough bone has been removed, the ankle is brought up into dorsiflexion and the forefoot is carefully evaluated, comparing the level of the first and fifth metatarsals in relation to the long axis of the leg. The surgeon must imagine that the foot is in a plantigrade position and that the first and fifth metatarsals are on the same plane.

11. If the size of the osteotomy cut is correct, internal fixation is inserted.

12. A piece of 22-gauge wire is passed through the transverse drill hole that was made distal to the osteotomy site in step 6. The wire is then brought up around the screw head in the proximal portion of the metatarsal and tightened with a wire twister while the osteotomy is held closed (Fig. 26-9D).

13. Once the osteotomy site has been completely closed, the bottom of the forefoot is again carefully examined. If the degree of dorsiflexion is adequate, the surgeon may proceed with closure of the wound. If it is not adequate, the wire is removed and more bone is removed from the osteotomy site (Fig. 26-9E). Alternatively, a 3-hole 2.0 DCP is used to compress the osteotomy site by eccentric drilling.

14. Occasionally, the second metatarsal needs to be dorsiflexed, which is done using the same procedure.

15. The foot is placed in a compression dressing. If this is the only procedure being carried out, splints are not required.

Postoperative Care

A popliteal block can be useful to control postoperative pain. If this is the only procedure being carried out, the patient is permitted to ambulate as tolerated in a postoperative shoe. If it is done in conjunction with other procedures, the patient is placed in a short-leg non–weight-bearing cast. In general, the osteotomy heals in approximately 6 weeks, after which ambulation is permitted as tolerated.

CALCANEAL OSTEOTOMIES

Patients with a moderate-to-severe cavus deformity usually have a varus deformity of the hindfoot. A fixed varus deformity is treated with the lateralizing calcaneal osteotomy, that is, as described by Dwyer,[10,11] Malerba and De Marchi,[32] or Knupp.[10,11,23,32] Whenever possible, realigning osteotomies are preferred over arthrodesis. If the patient lacks adequate dorsiflexion and has a high calcaneal pitch angle (a hindfoot cavus), a Samilson[39] osteotomy is carried out to allow the calcaneal tuberosity and the attached Achilles tendon to slide vertically, thereby effectively lengthening the gastrocnemius–soleus complex and correcting the effective pitch angle of the calcaneus. These procedures are usually carried out with a plantar fascia release and a first metatarsal osteotomy.

In the presence of a horizontal ankle joint line and a cavus foot, it appears more reasonable to redistribute the ankle joint contact forces by realigning the foot deformity rather than by creating a new deformity, that is, with a supramalleolar osteotomy. Furthermore, this would create additional problems in the forefoot by accentuating the plantar flexion of the first ray.

Calcaneal osteotomies act by shifting the ground contact point and, consequently, the weight-bearing axis through the ankle joint. They are particularly useful in patients with recurrent hindfoot sprains as a result of heel varus and can be used with either a supple or a stiff subtalar joint.[34] The lateralizing calcaneal osteotomies also lateralize the lever arm of the Achilles tendon during toe-off. The contribution of the Achilles tendon toward the tibialis posterior is thus reduced in favor of the peroneus brevis. From recent static biomechanical studies, there is evidence that in simulated pes cavus common lateralizing calcaneal osteotomies substantially contribute to normalize the elevated contact stress in the anteromedial ankle joint, which is thought to cause ankle arthritis in long-standing pes cavus.[24] Osteotomies that include lateralization of the tuberosity, including a simple slide and the Z-osteotomy with additional lateralization of the tuberosity,[23] reduced contact stresses more effectively than, for instance, the Z-osteotomy without additional lateralization of the tuberosity[32] and are therefore recommended for moderate-to-severe hindfoot varus realignment.

Both the Dwyer osteotomy and its modifications with translation, as well as the Z-osteotomy, can accomplish correction of hindfoot varus and are described below.

DWYER CALCANEAL OSTEOTOMY WITH OPTIONAL LATERAL AND/OR DORSAL TRANSLATION
Surgical Technique

1. The patient is placed in a lateral or in a supine position with a bolster beneath the ipsilateral hip for adequate exposure of the lateral aspect of the calcaneus. A tourniquet is used on the thigh.

2. The skin incision is perpendicular to the axis of the calcaneus, begins about 2 cm posterior to the tip of the fibula, and is carried obliquely past the tip of the fibula toward the plantar aspect of the calcaneocuboid joint (Fig. 26-10A and Video Clip 48).

3. The deep incision is carried just below the peroneal tendon sheath, and the calcaneus is exposed as required. Care is taken not to injure the sural nerve. Dorsally and plantarly, the soft tissues are stripped off to place Hohman retractors.

4. A transverse osteotomy is made in the calcaneus that starts about 2 cm posterior to the posterior facet of the subtalar joint and runs in line with the skin incision, perpendicular to the calcaneus axis. If possible, the medial cortex of the calcaneus is left intact.

5. A second cut is now created, removing a pie-shaped wedge of bone from the lateral aspect of the calcaneus. The size of the wedge depends upon the severity of the

varus deformity. Usually, 5 to 7 mm of calcaneus is removed with the second cut (Fig. 26-10B).

6. Once the second cut is completed, a greenstick fracture is made on the medial side of the calcaneus by manipulating the fragments back and forth. The osteotomy is then closed. Sometimes, temporary insertion of a stout pin into the posterior tuberosity can serve as a joystick to facilitate closing the osteotomy. The

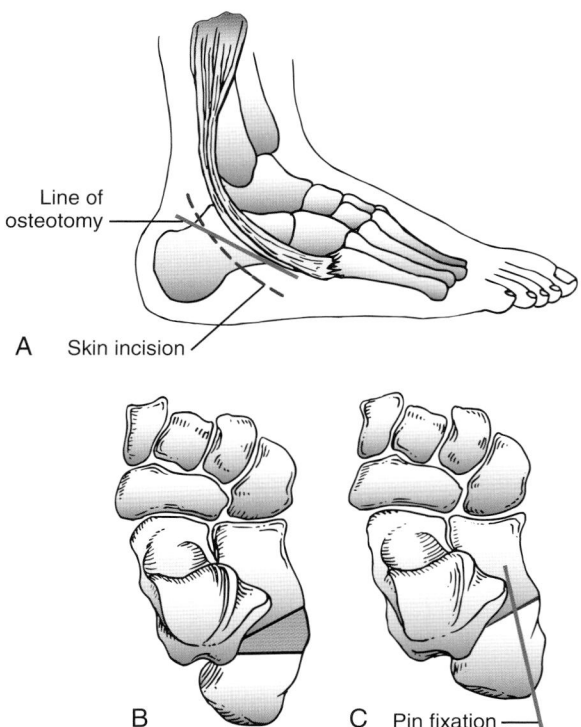

Line of osteotomy —

A   Skin incision

B   C   Pin fixation —

Figure 26-10 The Dwyer calcaneal osteotomy. **A,** Skin incision is made along the inferior margin of the peroneal tendons, with caution taken to avoid injury to the sural nerve. **B,** A lateral closing wedge of bone is taken of sufficient size to correct the deformity. **C,** Fixation is achieved with a longitudinal pin, a longitudinal screw, or a lateral staple. (From Mann RA, Coughlin MJ: *The video textbook of foot and ankle surgery,* St Louis, 1991, Medical Video Productions.)

position of the bone is carefully evaluated. If an inadequate degree of correction has been obtained, more bone needs to be removed. This may result in substantial hindfoot shortening.

Alternatively, the tuberosity is fully osteotomized. This allows further correction in two planes, including further lateralization of up to 7 mm for more severe deformities and vertical translation to reduce the calcaneal pitch. Vertical translation accomplishes the goals of the "Samilson" osteotomy, an operation designed purely to address the excessive calcaneal pitch in poliomyelitis.[22]

7. The osteotomy site is fixed with single or multiple 5.0- to 7.3-mm screws placed down the long axis of the calcaneus through a separate stab incision (Fig. 26-10C). If a screw is used, it should be placed lateral to the midline, and the patient should be warned that it may require later removal if it irritates the back of the foot against the heel counter of a shoe.

Postoperative Care

The patient is placed into a short-leg compression dressing incorporating plaster splints. A popliteal block can be useful in controlling postoperative pain. The sutures are removed 10 to 12 days after the procedure, and a short-leg non–weight-bearing cast is applied. Ambulation is permitted in the cast 4 weeks after the procedure, and casting is discontinued 8 weeks postoperatively if radiographs demonstrate union.

Results and Complications

The postoperative results after a Dwyer calcaneal osteotomy are usually most satisfactory in mild-to-moderate hindfoot varus (Fig. 26-11). Occasionally, the sural nerve becomes entrapped in scar tissue or disrupted, which can create a problem for the patient.

Sometimes it is difficult to judge whether adequate bone has been removed. The surgeon must attempt to line up the calcaneus with the long axis of the leg when trying to decide if a sufficient degree of correction has been achieved.

The only significant error that can be made when performing this procedure is to fail to remove sufficient

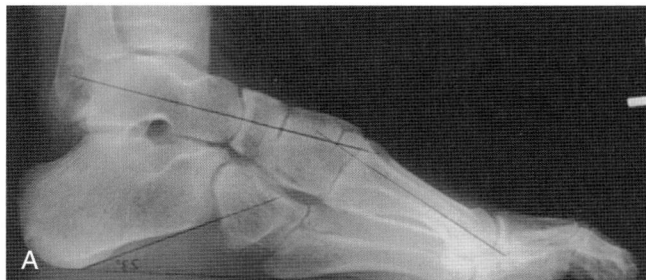
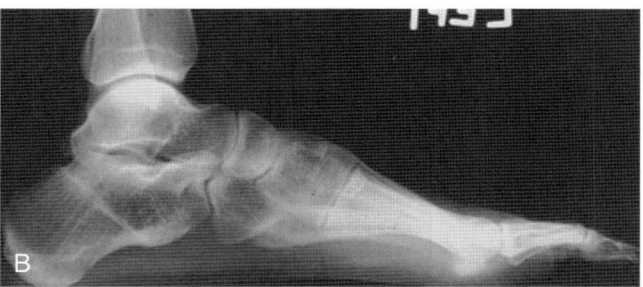

Figure 26-11 Preoperative **(A)** and postoperative **(B)** radiographs demonstrate the results of the Dwyer calcaneal osteotomy. The tarsal canal is visible on end preoperatively, indicating a varus deformity of the heel, whereas the position of the subtalar joint changes once the heel is brought into valgus.

bone, leaving the hindfoot in varus. In cases that require much correction, removal of large wedges may result in substantial hindfoot shortening, whereas the moment arm of the Achilles tendon is decreased, weakening toe-off. Alternatively, the tuberosity may be fully osteotomized and lateralized 6 to 8 mm.

Because translation of the calcaneal ground contact point by lateral sliding is more effective than rotation by lateral closing wedges, translating or combined translating-rotating osteotomies are usually preferable for the realignment of more severe hindfoot varus.[28]

Z-OSTEOTOMY[23,32]
Surgical Technique
1. The patient is placed in a supine position with a bolster beneath the ipsilateral hip or in the lateral position for adequate exposure of the lateral aspect of the calcaneus. A tourniquet is used on the thigh.
2. The skin incision is perpendicular to the axis of the calcaneus, begins about 3 cm posterior to the tip of the fibula, and is carried obliquely past the tip of the fibula toward the plantar aspect of the calcaneocuboid joint (Figs. 26-12 to 26-14 and Video Clip 118).
3. The deep incision is carried just below the peroneal tendon sheath, and the calcaneus is exposed as required. Care is taken not to injure the sural nerve.

Dorsally and plantarly, the soft tissues are stripped off to place Hohman retractors. The exposure of the calcaneus should extend from its dorsal aspect behind the fibula to just proximal to the calcaneocuboid joint.
4. Hohman retractors are used to protect the soft tissues. K-wires should be inserted and checked under fluoroscopy to ensure that the osteotomy is appropriately positioned and perpendicular to the calcaneal axis. The horizontal part of the osteotomy is about 2 cm long and parallel to the plantar fascia. The anterior vertical cut is made 1 to 2 cm posterior and parallel to the calcaneocuboid joint, and the posterior vertical cut is placed in the posterior half of the cavity of the tuberosity. Sparing the Achilles insertion is important.
5. Four K-wires are then used to define the corners of the wedge to be removed. The base of the wedge is 8 to 10 mm in width, depending on the desired amount of correction. The wedge is mobilized with the oscillating saw and osteotomes without harming the soft tissues. A laminar spreader is used to mobilize the osteotomy. The lateral gap is then carefully closed as described by Malerba and De Marchi.[32] An additional lateral displacement of the tuberosity fragment (6-10 mm) is done as described by Knupp et al.[23] An option is that the calcaneus can also be lengthened by displacing the tuberosity posteriorly.

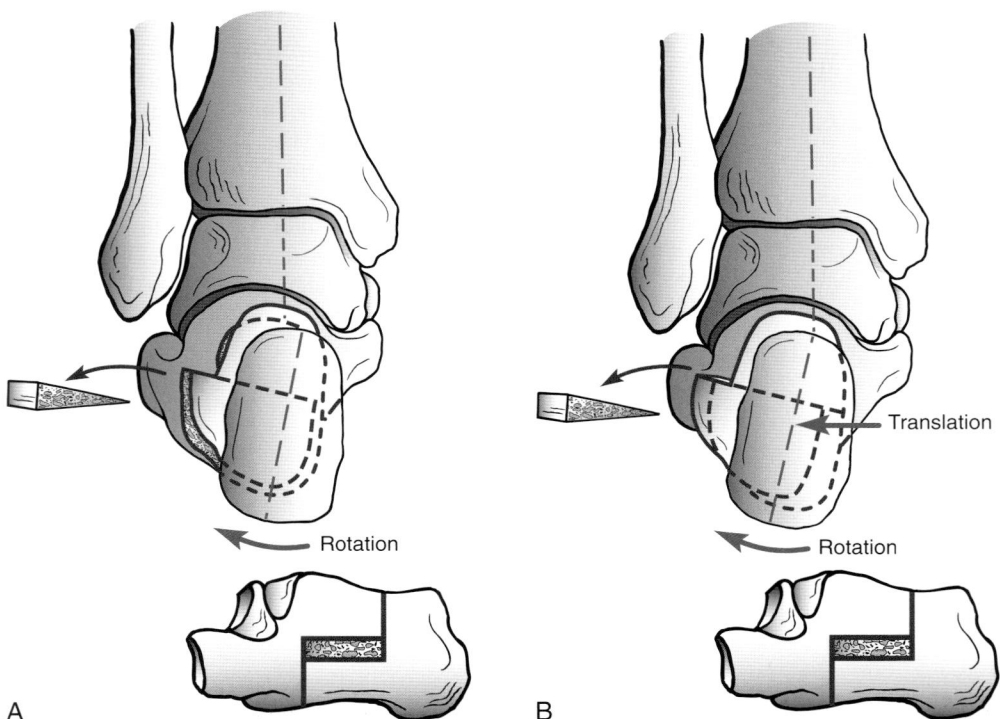

A

B

Figure 26-12   The Z-osteotomy with removal of a laterally based wedge of 8 to 10 mm **(A)**, according to Malerba (rotation of the ground point). A more powerful correction is achieved with additional lateralization of the tuberosity **(B)** according to Knupp and Hintermann (rotation and translation of the ground point). (Modified from Krause FG, Sutter D, Waehnert D, et al: Ankle joint pressure changes in a pes cavovarus model after lateralizing calcaneal osteotomies. *Foot Ankle Int* 31:741-746, 2010. Used with permission.)

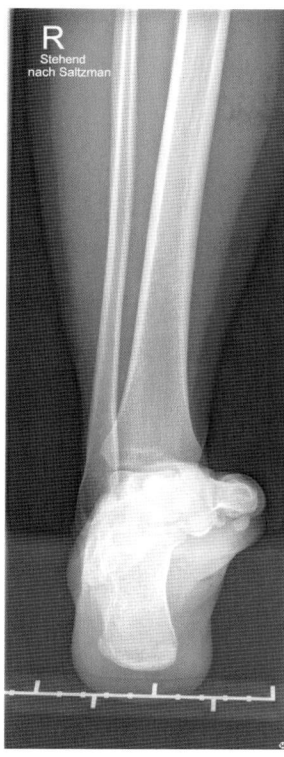

Figure 26-13 Preoperative Saltzman hindfoot view of a hindfoot varus. Intraoperative lateral and axial fluoroscopy, and postoperative Saltzman hindfoot view after a Z-osteotomy of the calcaneus with lateralization of the tuberosity, according to Knupp and Hintermann. A peroneus longus to brevis tendon transfer and a dorsiflexion osteotomy of the first metatarsal were added. (Courtesy M. Knupp, MD, Department of Orthopaedic Surgery, Kantosspital Liesthal, Switzerland. Used with permission.)

6. The osteotomy is secured with one or two K-wires. The desired correction is carefully evaluated clinically and under fluoroscopy. The osteotomy site is fixed by one or two 3.5-mm or larger screws placed down the long axis of the calcaneus through a separate stab incision.

Postoperative Care

The patient is placed into a short-leg compression dressing incorporating plaster splints. A popliteal block can be useful in controlling postoperative pain. The sutures are removed 10 to 12 days after the procedure, and a short-leg non–weight-bearing cast is applied. Partial weight bearing is permitted in the cast 3 to 4 weeks after the procedure, and casting is discontinued 6 to 8 weeks postoperatively if radiographs demonstrate union.

Results and Complications

Transient and irreversible tibial nerve palsy after lateralizing calcaneal osteotomies has been described.[27] Particularly after large corrections in CMT cases and posttraumatic cases, the rate is substantial. Although the

nerves themselves do not appear noticeably enlarged by the eye, CMT nerves may be slightly thicker and more sensitive to compression compared with normal nerves.[14] A routine release of the nerve's compartment (inferior flexor retinaculum) when performing a lateralizing calcaneal osteotomy for hindfoot varus in patients with Charcot-Marie-Tooth disease is therefore recommended.[27]

Consolidation of the osteotomy is reported to be fast and reliable, and most patients show consolidation on the radiographs 6 weeks postoperatively.

MIDTARSAL OSTEOTOMIES

Various types of midfoot osteotomies have been proposed for the patient with a forefoot equinus or anterior cavus deformity with the apex located at the Chopart and midtarsal joints. These include the Cole osteotomy, which consists of removing a dorsal wedge of bone from the navicular, cuneiforms, and cuboid.[7] A similar, more distal osteotomy has been proposed by Japas, in which a V-shaped osteotomy is made within the tarsal bones.[21] The distal portion is then depressed to allow the forefoot to be brought out of its equinus position.

Although, in theory, midfoot osteotomies are preferred because they correct a typical deformity closer to its apex than a basilar osteotomy of the first metatarsal, in practice, this is not the case. Inevitably, all variations of the midfoot osteotomies result in multiple intraarticular cuts that can lead to early arthritis. The residual deformity from the much safer extraarticular osteotomy through the first metatarsal is well tolerated, and this approach should be universally preferred. Midfoot procedures should be reserved for patients who already have arthritis, and the joints should then be arthrodesed in conjunction with the cavus correction.

ARTHRODESIS PROCEDURES

The triple arthrodesis is the requisite operation for more severe, fixed postural deformities of the hindfoot of any kind. In the cavus foot, it is important to remember that other procedures, such as a first metatarsal osteotomy or Jones procedure, can be carried out in addition to a triple arthrodesis if the conditions warrant. Routine joint preparation and cartilage removal often prove adequate for milder degrees of deformity. Because the posterior facet of the subtalar joint is approached from the lateral side, there is a natural tendency to remove more bone laterally and position the calcaneus toward valgus using standard techniques, just as one would perform a triple arthrodesis for hindfoot arthritis.

Long-term follow-up studies of standard triple arthrodesis for patients with Charcot-Marie-Tooth disease and cavus deformity have shown a high incidence of osteoarthritis of the remaining foot joints after this procedure. One study reported degenerative changes of the ankle and midfoot in 77% and the need for subsequent ankle arthrodesis for the treatment of degenerative joint disease in 20% after an average follow-up of 20 years.[48] Also, a literature review reveals poor results in as many as 47%

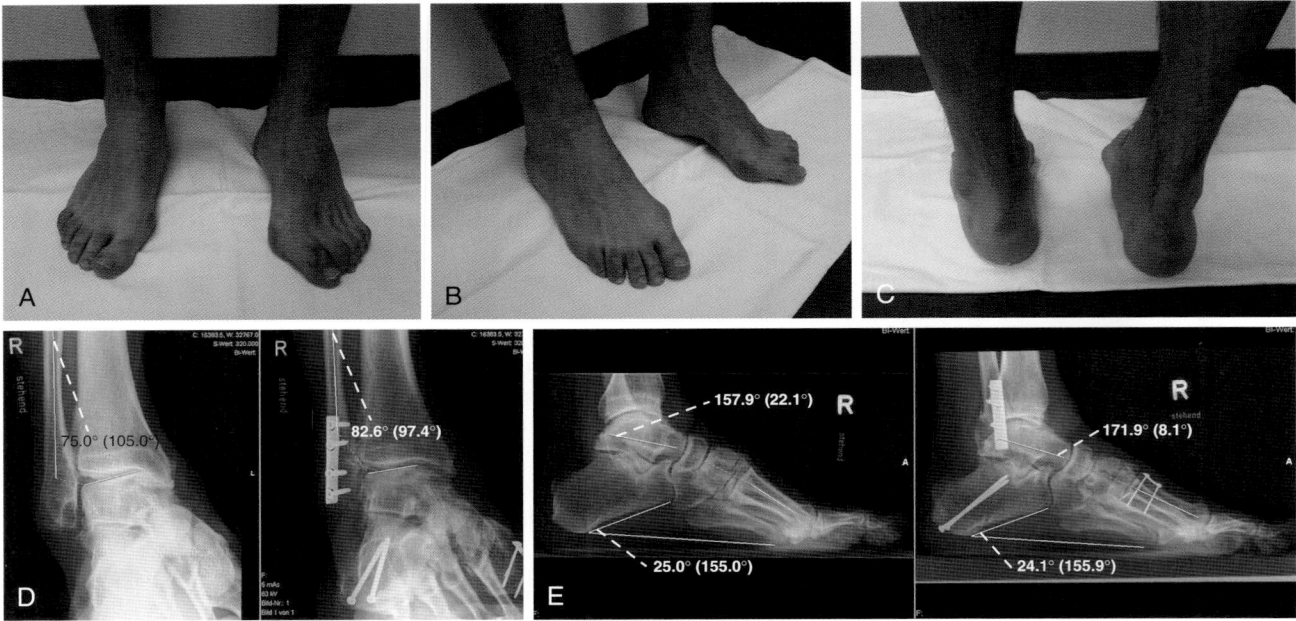

Figure 26-14 Preoperative anterior **(A)**, oblique **(B)**, and posterior **(C)** photographs and postoperative anteroposterior **(D)** and lateral **(E)** weight-bearing radiographs of a 56-year-old male patient with idiopathic pes cavus and grade III anteromedial ankle arthritis. Operative deformity correction included a lateralizing sliding osteotomy of the calcaneal tuberosity, dorsiflexion osteotomy of the first metatarsal, peroneus longus to brevis transfer, and lateral malleolus shortening osteotomy to reduce the varus tilt of the talus. No progression of the ankle arthritis was seen at latest follow-up 4 years postoperatively.

of patients, recurrence rates of 9% to 20%, nonunion in 6% to 33% of patients, and incomplete correction of the deformity in as many as 70% of patients.

Because hindfoot joints usually are already stiff in severe cavus deformities, there is little, if any, motion loss after a triple arthrodesis.[34] Therefore reducing the foot into normal heel valgus with a triple arthrodesis may result in further plantar flexing an already plantar-flexed first ray in long-standing deformities. The ankle will tip into varus postoperatively if this is not corrected with a dorsiflexion osteotomy. A satisfactory plantigrade position is essential for good results.[34]

Outcome

Few level III and IV studies have been published that assess the outcome of operative treatment of mainly fixed neurologic and idiopathic cavus deformities. Because of various etiologies and the limited number of patients treated, the reader is unable to draw definite conclusions. Nevertheless, each study offers some information about successful operative treatment and the pitfalls of certain treatment choices. The natural course of the disease without operative treatment has not yet been described. The surgeon must therefore thoughtfully apply the lessons learned from the available literature.

An overview is given in Table 26-3. The outcome of various procedures reveals significant improvements of function and relief of pain and about two thirds good and excellent results, even in the long term. Worse outcome

after cavus realignment is reported when advanced ankle arthritis stage II and above is present preoperatively, indicating the importance of detecting ankle arthritis early and preventing its progression.[20,26] Another study revealed an association of radiographic evidence of ankle arthritis with a higher Foot Function Index (FFI) pain subscore, which suggests that arthritis prevention may have a greater impact on patient outcome than achievement of radiographic alignment.[47] The unfavorable combination of recurrent lateral ankle sprains or chronic instability and hindfoot varus as commonly seen in pes cavus likely increases the risk for accelerated ankle arthritis, but it is also common in patients without instability because of elevated anteromedial ankle contact stresses in pes cavus.[24,46] To prevent arthritis progression, a more aggressive dynamic and static realignment with slight overcorrection is recommended.

Worse outcomes after surgery have also been reported for patients with neurologic as opposed to idiopathic pes cavus. Despite appropriate pes cavus realignment, neurologic patients appear to suffer more from pain and activity impairments.[31]

After joint-preserving realignment surgery, cavus patients were seen to have a slower gait velocity and lower cadence, but the proportion of time spent in stance and swing phase was near that of normal individuals.[47] Although patients may have some deformity recurrence postoperatively, most are able to wear normal shoes and do not need orthoses.[47]

Table 26-3 Pes Cavus Outcome Studies of the Last Decade

Author	Number	Mean Age at Surgery	Etiology	Flexibility	Ankle Arthritis at Surgery	Procedure	Mean Follow-up (months)	Outcome (Mean)	Radiographic Findings at Follow-up	Evidence
Sammarco et al, 2001	21 ft 15 pts	33	All neurologic	Flexible	None	A, B, H	71	AOFAS: from 46 to 89 Maryland Foot Score: from 72 to 90	Lateral talo–MT I angle decreased 6.5 degrees Arch height decreased 6.8 mm	III
Fortin et al, 2002	13 ft 10 pts	51	All idiopathic	Flexible and rigid	Stage 1-3	A, B, D, F	33	Karlsson score: from 33 to 82	Not reported	III
Vienne et al, 2007	9 ft 8 pts	25	Idiopathic and residual clubfoot	Flexible	Stage 0-2	A, C, D	37	AOFAS: from 57 to 87	Not reported	III
Ward et al, 2008	41 ft 25 pts	16	All neurologic	Flexible	None	B, C, G, H, K	312 (26 years)	SF36 mental: 50 SF36 physical: 38 FFI pain: 35 FFI disability: 41 FFI activity limit: 22	OA most often in TMT 1 joints	IV
Kroon et al, 2009	19 ft 15 pts	40	Idiopathic 11 Neurologic 4	Flexible and rigid	None	2xA, B, C, E, F, G, I	50	AOFAS: 83 FFI pain: 13 FFI activity limit: 13	Talo–first metatarsal angle from 22 to 17 degrees	IV
Irwin et al, 2010	22 ft 22 pts	48	All idiopathic	Rigid	Group 1 stage 0-1 Group 2 stage 2-3	A, B, C, D, G, H	60	AOFAS group 1: 86, group 2: 59 VAS: 21 and 40 resp.	Arthritis progression mainly in group 2	IV
Maskell et al, 2010	29 ft 23 pts	43	All idiopathic	Rigid	None	A, B, C, D, E, J	51	AOFAS: from 45 to 90	Talo–first metatarsal angle from 9.9 to 2.4 degrees	III
Krause et al, 2013	13 ft 13 pts	47	Idiopathic 7 Neuropathic 6	Rigid	Stage 1-3	A, B, C, D, E, J	84	AOFAS: from 45 to 71		III

AOFAS, American Orthopaedic Foot and Ankle Society; *EHL,* extensor hallucis longus; *FFI,* Foot Function Index; *IP,* interphalangeal; *OA,* osteoarthritis; *pts,* patients; *SF36,* 36-item short Form Health Survey; *TMT,* tarsometatarsal; *VAS,* visual analog scale.
Operative procedures: *A,* lateralizing calcaneal osteotomy; *B,* first metatarsal dorsiflexion osteotomy; *C,* peroneus longus to brevis transfer; *D,* lateral ligament reconstruction; *E,* Achilles lengthening tenotomy; *F,* anterior ankle debridement (cheilectomy) for osteophytes; *G,* EHL transfer (Jones procedure) and IP fusion; *H,* plantar fascia release; *I,* tibialis posterior transfer to lateral cuneiform; *J,* gastrocnemius recession; *K,* tibialis anterior transfer to lateral cuneiform; *L,* deltoid ligament release; *M,* fibula osteotomy.

REFERENCES

1. Aminian A, Sangeorzan BJ: The anatomy of cavus foot deformity, *Foot Ankle Clin* 13:191–198, v, 2008.
2. Bentzon PGK: Pes cavus and the m. peroneus longus, *Acta Orthop Scand* 4:50, 1933.
3. Berciano J, Gallardo E, Garcia A, et al: New insights into the pathophysiology of pes cavus in Charcot-Marie-Tooth disease type 1A duplication, *J Neurol* 258:1594–1602, 2011.
4. Bertorini T, Narayanaswami P, Rashed H: Charcot-Marie-Tooth disease (hereditary motor sensory neuropathies) and hereditary sensory and autonomic neuropathies, *Neurologist* 10:327–337, 2004.
5. Brewerton DA, Sandifer PH, Sweetnam DR: "Idiopathic" pes cavus: an investigation into its aetiology, *Br Med J* 2:659–661, 1963.
6. Charcot JM, Marie P: Sur une forme particulaire d'atrophie musculaire progressive souvent familiale débutant par les pieds et les jambes et atteignmant plus tard les mains, *Rev Med* 6:97–138, 1886.
7. Cole WH: The treatment of claw foot, *J Bone Joint Surg Am* 22:895–908, 1940.
8. Dhillon MS, Sandhu HS: Surgical options in the management of residual foot problems in poliomyelitis, *Foot Ankle Clin* 5:327–347, 2000.
9. Duchenne GB: *The physiology of motion (trans EB Kaplan)*, Philadelphia, 1959, WB Saunders.
10. Dwyer FC: Osteotomy of the calcaneum for pes cavus, *J Bone Joint Surg Br* 41:80–86, 1959.
11. Dwyer FC: The present status of the problem of pes cavus, *Clin Orthop* 106:254–275, 1975.
12. Dyck PJ, Lambert EH: Lower motor and primary sensory neuron diseases with peroneal muscular atrophy. I. Neurologic, genetic, and electrophysiologic findings in hereditary polyneuropathies, *Arch Neurol* 18:603–618, 1968.
13. Fortin PT, Guettler J, Manoli A: Idiopathic cavovarus and lateral ankle instability: recognition and treatment implications relating to ankle arthritis, *Foot Ankle Int* 23:1031–1037, 2002.
14. Guyton GP: Peroneal nerve branching suggests compression palsy in the deformities of Charcot-Marie Tooth disease, *Clin Orthop Relat Res* 451:167–170, 2006.
15. Guyton GP, Mann RA: The pathogenesis and surgical management of foot deformity in Charcot-Marie-Tooth disease, *Foot Ankle Clin* 5:317–326, 2000.
16. Halgrimsson S: Pes cavus, seine Behandlung und einige Bemerkungen uber seing Aetiologie, *Acta Orthop Scand* 10:73, 1939.
17. Henderson CP, Parks BG, Guyton GP: Lateral and medial plantar pressures after split versus whole anterior tibialis tendon transfer, *Foot Ankle Int* 29:1038–1041, 2008.
18. Huber H, Dutoit M: Dynamic foot-pressure measurement in the assessment of operatively treated clubfeet, *J Bone Joint Surg Am* 86-A:1203–1210, 2004.
19. Ibrahim K: Pes cavus. In Evarts CM, editor: *Surgery of the musculoskeletal system*, New York, 1990, Churchill Livingstone, pp 4015–4034.
20. Irwin TA, Anderson RB, Davis WH, Cohen BE: Effect of ankle arthritis on clinical outcome of lateral ankle ligament reconstruction in cavovarus feet, *Foot Ankle Int* 31:941–948, 2010.
21. Japas LM: Surgical treatment of pes cavus by tarsal V-osteotomy. Preliminary report, *J Bone Joint Surg Am* 50:927–944, 1968.
22. Jones R: An operation for paralytic calcaneocavus, *Am J Orthop Surg* 5:371, 1908.
23. Knupp M, Horisberger M, Hintermann B: A new Z-shaped calcaneal osteotomy for 3-plane correction of severe deformity of the hindfoot, *Tech Foot Ankle Surg* 7:90–95, 2008.
24. Krause F, Windolf M, Schwieger K, Weber M: Ankle joint pressure in pes cavovarus, *J Bone Joint Surg Br* 89:1660–1665, 2007.
25. Krause FG, Henning J, Pfander G, et al: Cavovarus foot realignment to treat anteromedial ankle arthrosis, *Foot Ankle Int* 34:54–64, 2013.
26. Krause FG, Klammer G, Benneker LM, et al: Biochemical T2* MR quantification of ankle arthrosis in pes cavovarus, *J Orthop Res* 28:1562–1568, 2010.
27. Krause FG, Pohl MJ, Penner MJ, Younger AS: Tibial nerve palsy associated with lateralizing calcaneal osteotomy: case reviews and technical tip, *Foot Ankle Int* 30:258–261, 2009.
28. Krause FG, Sutter D, Waehnert D, et al: Ankle joint pressure changes in a pes cavovarus model after lateralizing calcaneal osteotomies, *Foot Ankle Int* 31:741–746, 2010.
29. Krause FG, Wing KJ, Younger AS: Neuromuscular issues in cavovarus foot, *Foot Ankle Clin* 13:243–258, vi, 2008.
30. Kremli MK: Fixed forefoot adduction after clubfoot surgery, *Saudi Med J* 24:742–744, 2003.
31. Kroon M, Faber FW, van der Linden M: Joint preservation surgery for correction of flexible pes cavovarus in adults, *Foot Ankle Int* 31:24–29, 2010.
32. Malerba F, De Marchi F: Calcaneal osteotomies, *Foot Ankle Clin* 10:523–540, vii, 2005.
33. Mann DC, Hsu JD: Triple arthrodesis in the treatment of fixed cavovarus deformity in adolescent patients with Charcot-Marie-Tooth disease, *Foot Ankle* 13:1–6, 1992.
34. Manoli A, Graham B: The subtle cavus foot, "the underpronator," *Foot Ankle Int* 26:256–263, 2005.
35. Morcuende JA, Dolan LA, Dietz FR, Ponseti IV: Radical reduction in the rate of extensive corrective surgery for clubfoot using the Ponseti method, *Pediatrics* 113:376–380, 2004.
36. Pandolfo M: Friedreich ataxia, *Semin Pediatr Neurol* 10:163–172, 2003.
37. Pareyson D: Differential diagnosis of Charcot-Marie-Tooth disease and related neuropathies, *Neurol Sci* 25:72–82, 2004.
38. Roper BA, Tibrewal SB: Soft tissue surgery in Charcot-Marie-Tooth disease, *J Bone Joint Surg Br* 71:17–20, 1989.
39. Samilson RL: Crescentic osteotomy os calcis for calcaneovarus feet. In Bateman JE, editor: *Foot science*, Philadelphia, 1976, WB Saunders, p 18.
40. Sammarco GJ, Taylor R: Combined calcaneal and metatarsal osteotomies for the treatment of cavus foot, *Foot Ankle Clin* 6:533–543, vii, 2001.
41. Schmalbruch H, Haase G: Spinal muscular atrophy: present state, *Brain Pathol* 11:231–247, 2001.
42. Simbak N, Razak M: Residual deformity following surgical treatment of congenital talipes equinovarus, *Med J Malaysia* 53(Suppl A):115–120, 1998.
43. Steindler A: Operative treatment of pes cavus: stripping of the os calcis, *Surg Gynecol Obstet* 24:612–615, 1917.
44. Tooth HH: *The peroneal type of progressive muscular atrophy*, London, 1886, HK Lewis.
45. Tynan MC, Klenerman L, Helliwell TR, et al: Investigation of muscle imbalance in the leg in symptomatic forefoot pes cavus: a multidisciplinary study, *Foot Ankle* 13:489–501, 1992.
46. Valderrabano V, Hintermann B, Horisberger M, Fung TS: Ligamentous posttraumatic ankle osteoarthritis, *Am J Sports Med* 34:612–620, 2006.
47. Ward CM, Dolan LA, Bennett DL, et al: Long-term results of reconstruction for treatment of a flexible cavovarus foot in Charcot-Marie-Tooth disease, *J Bone Joint Surg Am* 90:2631–2642, 2008.
48. Wetmore RS, Drennan JC: Long-term results of triple arthrodesis in Charcot-Marie-Tooth disease, *J Bone Joint Surg Am* 71:417–422, 1989.

Index

Page numbers followed by "f" indicate figures, "t" indicate tables, and "b" indicate boxes.

Crucial angle of Gissane, of calcaneus, 2044, 2044f
Cryptococcus neoformans infection, 763
Crystal induced arthropathies, 922-929
    calcium pyrophosphate dihydrate deposition disease, 927-929
    gouty arthropathy, 922-927
CUBED mnemonic, for malignant melanoma diagnosis, 843t
Cuboid dislocations, 1927-1928, 1928f
Cuboid fractures, 2164-2166
    avulsed, 2164-2165, 2164f
        conservative treatment, 2164
        operative treatment, 2165
        preferred treatment method, 2165
    compressed, 2165-2166
        nonoperative treatment, 2165
        operative treatment, 2165-2166
    insufficiency/stress, 2166
        nonoperative treatment, 2166
        operative treatment, 2166
        preferred treatment method, 2166
Cuneiform, bipartite first, 555-556
    anatomy and incidence of, 555-556, 555f-556f
    clinical significance of, 556, 557f
Cuneiform/cuboid osteotomies, for metatarsus adductus, 1843-1844, 1843f
    postoperative care, 1843-1844
Cuneiform dislocations, 1926-1927, 1926f-1927f
Cuneiform fractures, 2166-2167
    avulsed, 2166-2167
        mechanism of injury, 2166
        nonoperative treatment, 2166
        operative treatment, 2166-2167
        preferred treatment method, 2167
    crush injury, 2167
        nonoperative treatment, 2167
        operative treatment, 2167
        preferred treatment method, 2167
Cuneocuboid dislocations, 1926-1928
    preferred method of treatment, 1928, 1929f
Curly toe deformity, 325
    association with mallet toe, 356-357
    flexor tenotomy in treatment of, 357, 357f
Custom foot orthoses, 123-124, 123f
Cutaneous larva migrans, 765-766, 766f
Cuticle. *See* Eponychium.
Cystic bone lesions, 850-852

D
Danis-Weber classification, of ankle fractures, 2005, 2006f-2007f
Daptomycin, 772
Darier disease, toenail pathology in, 576, 579f
Decompression/shortening osteotomies, 972, 977f

Deep peroneal nerve, 672-673, 672f, 1932
Deep peroneal nerve block, 145, 146f
Deep peroneal nerve entrapment, 672-675
    etiology of, 673, 673f
    evaluation of, 673-674
        imaging and nerve conduction studies, 674
        physical examination, 673-674
    incidence of, 673
    nonsurgical treatment of, 674
    surgical treatment of, 674-675
Deep peroneal nerve release, 674-675
    postoperative care, 674
    results of, 674-675
    surgical technique, 674
Deep posterior tibiotalar ligament, 1595
Degenerative arthritis, 868-871. *See also* Ankle osteoarthritis.
    arthroscopic treatment of, 1771-1772
    conservative treatment of, 869-871
    diagnosis of
        history and physical examination, 869
        radiographic, 869, 870f
    of hallux, 941-942, 944f. *See also* Hallux rigidus
        conservative treatment, 941, 941f
        surgical treatment, 941, 943f
    of hindfoot, 871-875. *See also under* Hindfoot
    of interphalangeal joints, 941-942, 944f-945f
    of midfoot, 875-879. *See also under* Midfoot
    pathophysiology of, 868
    surgical treatment of, 871
Degenerative bone cyst, 851-852
Deland technique, in deltoid ligament reconstruction, 1343-1346
Delayed onset muscle soreness, and chronic leg pain in athletes, 1555
Deltoid ligament complex, 1595, 1596f, 2003-2004, 2004f. *See also* Medial ankle sprains.
    biomechanics of, 1596-1597
    chronic instability of, 1599-1601
        conservative treatment, 1600
        diagnosis, 1599-1600, 1600f
        reconstructive treatment, 1600-1601, 1601f
        in athletic population, 1600-1601
Deltoid ligament reconstruction, 1339
    contraindications to, 1340
    indications for, 1339-1340
    postoperative care in, 1344
    preoperative evaluation in, 1340
    preoperative planning in, 1340
    results and complications of, 1344-1346

Deltoid ligament reconstruction *(Continued)*
    surgical techniques, 1340
        Deland technique, 1343-1346
        Haddad technique, 1340-1343
        Myerson technique, 1343-1344
DeOrio technique, distal chevron osteotomy, fifth metatarsophalangeal joint, 468-470, 470f
Depth/ischemia classification, of diabetic foot ulceration, 1391-1392, 1391f
Dermabrasion, in scar tissue management, 824
Dermal tumors, 837
Dermatobia hominis infection, 764-765, 766f
Dermatofibroma, 837
Dermatologic conditions, 777
    diagnosis of, importance of, 792
    papules, plaques, nodular, 784-789
        benign, 784-787
        malignant, 787-789
    papulosquamous, 778-783
        infectious, 782-783
        primary, 778-782
    purpuric eruptions, 789-792
Desmoid tumors, 836-837
Diabetes mellitus, 1385-1386
    metabolic control in, 1386
Diabetic foot, 1386, 1386f
    ankle fractures in, 1467-1469
        immobilization duration, 1469-1471
        postoperative complications, 1470-1471
        treatment options, 1468-1469, 2035
    care algorithm for, 1392f
    clinical conditions associated with, 1388-1405
        Charcot neuropathic arthropathy, 1393-1399. *See also* Charcot arthropathy
        ulceration, 1388-1393. *See also* Ulceration
            classification systems, 1390-1393
    infections of, 1400-1405
        abscess, 1444
        cellulitis, 1444
        hyperbaric oxygen treatment, 1450
        osteomyelitis, 1403, 1444-1450
        surgical site, 1403-1405, 1443-1450
    and limb salvage, 1471
    neurologic evaluation of, 1406-1407
    osteomyelitis in, treatment/surgical procedures, 1403, 1444-1450
        ankle, 1450
        first metatarsal, 1446-1447
        hallux sesamoids, 1446
        hindfoot, 1449-1450
        lesser metatarsals, 1447-1448

Klaue device, 171-172, 173f
  modified, 173-174, 173f
Koch-Mason dressing, 750, 752f
Koebner phenomenon, 779, 781f
Koilonychia, 573, 603, 604f
Krackow tendon repair, 1190, 1191f
Kuwada surgical technique, for flexible
    hammer toe deformity, 355, 355f
  results and complications, 355-356

L

Lamotrigine (Lamictal), for complex
    regional pain syndrome, 717
Lange partial foot prosthesis, 1512f-
    1513f, 1513
Lapidus procedure, 407-410
  postoperative care in, 408
  results and complications of, 408-410
  surgical technique, 407-408,
    408f-409f
Lasting, definition of, 130
Lasts, for making shoes, 132, 132f
Lateral ankle instability, 1770
  arthroscopic treatment of, 1770-1771
    indications/contraindications, 1770
    postoperative care, 1771
    preoperative evaluation/planning,
      1770
    surgical technique, 1771
  chronic, conservative treatment, 1570
  tendon transfers in, 1577-1579, 1578f
Lateral ankle sprains, 1555-1579
  acute, 1566-1570
    conservative treatment, 1566-1568
    surgical repair, 1568-1569, 1569f
      complications, 1570
      postoperative care, 1569-1570
  anatomic structures involved in,
    1556-1558, 1557f, 1579f
  chronic injury/instability, 1570-1579,
    1570b
    conservative treatment, 1570
    diagnosis, 1570
    diagnostic arthroscopy, 1570-1571,
      1571f
    secondary repair or reconstruction,
      1571-1579
    surgical treatment, 1570
      complications, 1575-1577
      lateral ligament reconstruction
        with tendon transfer,
        1577-1579, 1578f
      modified Bronström procedure,
        1575-1577, 1575f-1576f
      modified Chrisman-Snook
        procedure, 1577
      postoperative care, 1577-1579,
        1579f
      results, 1572-1575, 1573t-1574t
  classification of, 1565, 1565b
  diagnosis of, 1559-1564
    anterior drawer maneuver,
      1560-1561, 1561f

Lateral ankle sprains (Continued)
    arthrographic examination,
      1562-1564
    inversion stress test of calcaneus,
      1561
    magnetic resonance imaging, 1564,
      1564f
    peroneal or posterior tibial tendon
      involvement, 1561
    peroneal tenography, 1564
    physical examination, 1560
    ultrasonography, 1564
  pathology of ligament injury in,
    1559
  prevention of, 1565-1579
  prognosis in, 1564
  radiologic evaluation of, 1561-1564
    anterior drawer test, 1562, 1563f
    talar tilt, 1562, 1562f
  surgical treatment of, 1568-1570
    acute sprains, 1568-1570
    chronic sprains and instability,
      1570
Lateral body displacement, in gait
    kinematics, 9, 9f
Lateral collateral ligament complex, of
    ankle, 2004-2005, 2005f
Lateral column, 1917
Lateral column lengthening, in posterior
    tibial tendon dysfunction,
    1334-1339
  contraindications to, 1336
  Evans procedure surgical technique,
    1337-1338
  indications for, 1336
  lateral column lengthening (LCL)
    stepcut osteotomy procedure,
    1338-1339
  preoperative evaluation in,
    1336-1337
Lateral condylectomy, fifth metatarsal,
    460-463
  contraindications to, 460
  dislocation after, 489f
  indications for, 460
  postoperative care in, 460
  results and complications of,
    460-463, 462f-463f
  surgical technique, 460, 461f-462f,
    478f
Lateral distal tibial angle (LDTA), 1164,
    1165f
Lateral ligament complex, of ankle,
    2004, 2004f
Lateral ligament repair/reconstruction,
    1374
Lateral malleolar osteotomy, 2128-2129,
    2131f
Lateral malleolus, 2003
Lateral plantar nerve
  calcaneal branches, 665-667,
    666f-667f
  first branch of, 663-665, 664f

Lateral plantar nerve (Continued)
    first branch release procedure, 665
      postoperative care, 665
      results, 665
      surgical technique, 665, 666f
Lateral plantar nerve entrapment, 663-667
  calcaneal branches, 665-667
    evaluation, 667
    management and results, 667, 667f
  first branch, 663-665, 664f
    diagnosis, 665
    etiology, 664
    incidence, 664
    surgical treatment, 665
    symptoms, 665, 665f
Lateral process fractures, of talus,
    2140-2142, 2140f
  classification of, 2141, 2141f
  evaluation of, 2140
    radiographic, 2140-2141, 2141f
  incidence of, 2140
  mechanism of injury in, 2140
  treatment of, 2141
    outcomes, 2141-2142
    preferred method, 2142, 2142f
Lateral talocalcaneal ligament,
    1557-1558
Lateral tendon transfer, 1282
Lateral ulceration, of diabetic foot,
    1440-1441, 1440f
Lateral weight bearing foot
    measurement, 80f
Latissimus dorsi flap, 812-813, 813f
Lauge-Hansen classification, of ankle
    fractures, 2005, 2006f-2007f
LDTA (lateral distal tibial angle), 1164,
    1165f
Leeches, for postsurgical venous
    congestion, 818-819, 819f
Leg pain. See Chronic leg pain.
Length deformity, 1163, 1164f
Lentigo, 573
Lesser metatarsal(s), 46-47, 47f
Lesser metatarsal head(s)
  multiple, ulcerations, surgical
    procedures, 204
  osteomyelitis in, treatment/surgical
    procedures, 1447-1448, 1447f
  ulceration beneath, surgical
    procedures, 186f, 188f, 204
Lesser toe(s)
  amputation of, 1488-1490. See also
    under Lesser toe deformities
    pitfalls and complications,
      1489-1490
    postoperative care, 1489
    in severe rheumatoid arthritis, 904,
      905f
    surgical technique, 1487f, 1489,
      1489f
  anatomy of, 328-332
    extensor digitorum muscle and
      tendon, 328-330, 329f

Night splints, for plantar fascia stretching during inactivity, 691-692, 692f
Nitinol implant, surgical technique, 340-341
Nociceptive pain, 706, 706b
Nodules. *See* Papules, plaques, nodules.
Nonoperative/nonsurgical treatment. *See* Conservative treatment.
Nonsteroidal antiinflammatory drug(s), 136-137, 136t, 870
　for complex regional pain syndrome, 715
　for gouty arthritis, 925
　for neuralgia in tarsal tunnel syndrome, 647
　and paracetamol combination, 137
　for rheumatoid arthritis, 888
Nonweight bearing views, of ankle, 63-66, 64f
Normal alignment, of lower limb, 1163-1167, 1164f
Nuclear medicine imaging, 76-86
　gallium-67 bone and white cell scan, 84-85
　radiopharmaceuticals used in, 76
　science of, 76-85
　single photon emission computed tomography (SPECT), 84
　technetium-99m bone scan, 82-84
　uses of, 76, 85-86
　　fibular stress fracture, 85f
　　occult fractures, 86f
　　os peroneum syndrome, 85f

O

Oblique metatarsal osteotomy, for treatment of plantar keratoses, 438-447
　postoperative care, 440, 441f
　results of, 440
　surgical technique, 438-440, 440f
Obliquity of ankle axis
　estimation of, 19-20, 20f
　in gait biomechanics, 19-20, 20f
Obstructive sleep apnea, anesthesia considerations in patients with, 138-139, 139t
Occlusive hydrocolloid wound dressing, 801
Ofloxacin, 772
Olmstead syndrome, 782f
One-legged hop test, 1584
Onychauxis, 592-593, 603
　treatment of, 594
Onychectomy
　complete, 610
　partial, 581f, 608-610, 609f
Onychia (onychitis), 573, 598
Onychoclasis, 573
Onychocryptosis, 573, 589-592, 590f
　acute symptoms relief, 591, 592f-593f
　causes of, 591, 591f

Onychocryptosis *(Continued)*
　congenital predisposition to, 591
　pathology and stages of, 591-592
　prevention of, 589-590, 590f
　Syme amputation of nail unit in severe, 591, 593f
　treatment of, 590-592, 591f
Onychogryphosis, 573, 593, 594f
　treatment of, 593
Onycholysis, 572-573, 572f, 598
Onychoma, 573
Onychomadesis, 571, 573, 598
Onychomalacia, 573
Onychomycosis, 573, 594-598, 763f, 782-783, 783f
　candidal, 596-598, 596f
　categories of, 594
　chronic, 595
　distal subungual, 595-596, 596f
　examples of, 574f
　organisms causing, 594-595, 595b
　prevalence of, 594-595
　proximal subungual, 596, 596f
　risk factors and conditions associated with, 594, 595b
　treatment of, 762-763
　white superficial, 596, 596f, 596t
Onychophosis, 573, 602
Onychopsittacus, 574, 575f, 598-599
Onychoptosis defluvium, 573
Onychorrhexis, 573
Onychoschizia, 572f, 573, 603, 604f
Onychosis (onychopathy), 574
Onychotrophia, 574
Open fractures, soft tissue reconstruction in, 821
Opioid(s)
　for complex regional pain syndrome, 714-715
　topical, for neuralgia in tarsal tunnel syndrome, 647
Opioid agonist(s), 138
　and monoamine reuptake inhibitor, combined, 136t, 138
Opioid anesthesia, changing role of, 135
Opioid consuming patients, anesthesia considerations, 139, 140t
OpSite wound dressing (3M), 801, 806-807
Oregon ankle prosthesis, 1082
Orthonyx, 574
Orthopedic Trauma Association classification, of pilon fractures, 1974, 1978f
Orthoplastic philosophy, of limb salvage, 796
Orthoses. *See* Ankle-foot orthoses; Foot orthoses.
Os aponeurosis, 543, 547f
Os calcaneus secundarius, 540-542
　anatomy and incidence of, 540-541, 541f-542f

Os calcaneus secundarius *(Continued)*
　clinical significance of, 541-542, 543f-545f
Os cuboides secundarium, 543-544
　anatomy and incidence of, 543-544, 547f-548f
　clinical significance of, 544
Os cuneo-I metararsale-I plantare, 555, 555f
Os cuneo-I metararsale-II dorsale, 555, 555f
Os intercuneiforme, 554-555
　anatomy and incidence of, 554-555, 554f
　clinical significance of, 555
Os intermetatarseum, 189-190, 190f, 556-559, 559f
　clinical significance of, 557-559, 559f
Os peroneum, 530-534, 531f
　abnormalities of, 530-531, 533-534, 533f
　clinical significance of, 531-534, 533f
　excision of, and tenodesis of peroneus longus, 534, 1240-1244
　　postoperative care, 534, 1242-1244
　　results and complications, 1244
　fractures of, 530-531, 532f, 533
　incidence of, 530-531, 533f
　location of, 530, 531f, 1233
　osteochondritis of, 530-531, 532f, 1238-1239, 1241f
　within peroneus longus tendon, 1233, 1240-1242, 1240f
　soft tissue attachments of, 530, 531f, 1235f
　symptomatic, 1242f
Os retinaculi, 537, 537f
Os subcalcis, 543, 547f
Os subfibulare, 535-537
　anatomy and incidence of, 535-537, 536f
　clinical significance of, 537
Os subtibiale, 534-535
　anatomy and incidence of, 534-535, 534f-535f
　clinical significance of, 535
Os sustentaculi, 542-543
　anatomy and incidence of, 542-543, 546f
　clinical significance of, 543, 546f-547f
Os talonaviculare dorsale (os supratalare), 544
　anatomy and incidence of, 544, 549f
　clinical significance of, 544, 549f
Os trigonum, 537-540, 1781f
　anatomy and incidence of, 537-538, 537f-538f
　arthroscopic treatment of, 1781-1782
　　indications/contraindications, 1781
　　preoperative evaluation/planning, 1781-1782